DISEASES/CONDITIONS AND ICD-9-CM CODE

DISEASES/CONDITIONS AND ICD-9-CM CODES *(Continued)*

Intracerebral hemorrhage	.431
Iron deficiency anemia	280.0-280.9
Irritable bowel syndrome	.564.1
Jellyfish sting	.989.5
Juvenile rheumatoid arthritis	.714.3**
Keloids	.701.4
Laryngitis	.464.00
Lead poisoning	.984*
Legionnaires' disease	.482.84
Leishmaniasis	.085*
Leprosy	.030*
Lichen planus	.697.0
Low back pain	.724.2
Lyme disease	.088.81
Lymphogranuloma venereum	.099.1
Malabsorption	.579*
Malaria	.084.6
Measles (rubeola)	.055.9
Meconium aspiration	.770.1
Melanoma, malignant	.172*
Ménière's disease	.386.0**
Meningitis	.320-322
Menopausal	.627.2
Migraine headache	.346**
Mitral valve prolapse	.424.0
Monilial vulvovaginitis	.121.1
Multiple myeloma	.203.0**
Multiple sclerosis	.340
Mumps	.072.9
Myasthenia gravis	.358.0**
Mycoplasmal pneumonias	.483.0
Mycosis fungoides	.202.1**
Nausea and vomiting	.787.01
Neoplasm of the vulva	.239.5
Neutropenia	.288.0
Nevi	.216*
Newborn physiologic jaundice	.774.6
Nongonococcal urethritis	.099.4**
Non-Hodgkin's lymphomas	.202.8**
Non-autoimmune hemolytic anemia	.283.1**
Normal delivery	.650
Obesity	.278.0**
Obsessive-compulsive disorders	.300.3
Onychomycosis	.110.1
Optic neuritis	.377.3**
Osteoarthritis	.715**
Osteomyelitis	.730**
Osteoporosis	.733.00
Otitis externa	.380.10
Paget's disease of bone	.731.0
Panic disorder	.300.01
Pap smear	V72.3
Parkinsonism	.332.0
Paronychia	.681.0**
Partial epilepsy	.345.4**
Patent ductus arteriosus	.747.0
Pediculosis	.132*
Pelvic inflammatory disease	.614*
Peptic ulcer disease	.533*
Pericarditis	.432.9
Peripheral arterial disease	.443.9
Peripheral neuropathies	.356*
Pernicious anemia	.281.0
Personality disorder	.301**
Pheochromocytoma	.227.0
Phobia	.300.2**
Pigmentary disorders—vitiligo	.709.01
Pinworms	.127.4
Pityriasis rosea	.696.3
Placenta previa	.641**
Plague	.020*
Platelet-mediated bleeding disorders	.287.1
Pleural effusion	.511.9
Polycythemia vera	.238.4
Polymyalgia rheumatica	.725
Porphyria	.277.1
Postpartum hemorrhage	.666.1**
Post-traumatic stress disorder	.309.81
Pregnancy	V22.2
Pregnancy-induced hypertension	.642**
Premature beats	.427.6**
Premenstrual tension syndrome (PMS)	.625.4
Prescribed oral contraceptive	V25.01
Pressure ulcers	.707.0
Preterm labor	.644.2**
Primary glomerular disease	.581-583
Primary lung abscess	.513.0
Primary lung cancer	.162.9
Prostate cancer	.185

Prostatitis	.601*
Pruritus	.698.9
Pruritus ani	.698.0
Pruritus vulvae	.698.1
Psittacosis (ornithosis)	.073*
Psoriasis	.696.1
Pulmonary embolism	.415.1
Pyelonephritis	.590**
Q fever	.083.0
Rabies	.071
Rat-bite fever	.026*
Relapsing fever	.087*
Renal calculi	.592
Reye syndrome	.331.81
Rheumatic fever	.390
Rheumatoid arthritis	.714.0
Rib fracture	.807.0**
Rocky Mountain spotted fever	.082.0
Rosacea	.695.3
Roseola	.057.8
Rubella	.056*
Salmonellosis	.003.0
Sarcoidosis	.135
Scabies	.133.0
Schizophrenia	.295**
Seborrheic dermatitis	.690.1**
Septicemia	.038*
Sézary's syndrome	.202.2**
Shoulder dislocation	.831.0**
Sickle cell anemia	.282.6**
Silicosis	.502
Sinusitis, chronic	.473*
Skull fracture	800, 801, 803
Sleep apnea	.780.57
Sleep disorders	.780.50
Snakebite	.989.5
Stasis ulcers	.454.0
Status epilepticus	.345.3
Stomach cancer	.151*
Streptococcal pharyngitis	.034.0
Stroke	.436
Strongyloides infection	.127.2
Subdural or subarachnoid hemorrhage	.852**
Sunburn	.692.71
Syphilis	.090-097
Tachycardias	.785.0
Tapeworm infections	.123*
Telogen effluvium	.704.02
Temporomandibular joint syndrome	.524.6**
Tendonitis	.726.90
Tetanus	.037
Thalassemia	.282.4**
Therapeutic use of blood components	V59.0**
Thrombotic thrombocytopenic purpura	.446.6
Thyroid cancer	.193
Thyroiditis	.245*
Tinea capitis	.110.0
Tinnitus	.388.3**
Toe fracture	.826.0
Toxic shock syndrome	.040.82
Toxoplasmosis	.130*
Transient cerebral ischemia	.435*
Trauma to the genitourinary tract	.958,959
Trichinellosis	.124
Trichomonal vaginitis	.131.01
Trigeminal neuralgia	.350.1
Tuberculosis, pulmonary	.011**
Tularemia	.021*
Typhoid fever	.002.0
Typhus fevers	080, 081
Ulcerative colitis	.556*
Urethral stricture	.598*
Urinary incontinence	.788.30
Urticaria	.708*
Uterine inertia	.661.0**
Uterine leiomyoma	.218*
Varicella	.052*
Venous thrombosis	.453.8
Viral pneumonia	.480.9
Viral respiratory infections	.465.9
Vitamin deficiency	.264-269
Vitamin K deficiency	.269.0
Warts (verrucae)	.078.10
Wegener's granulomatosis	.446.4
Whooping cough (pertussis)	.033*
Wrist fracture	.814.0**

*4th digit needed

**5th (or 4th and 5th) digit needed

CONN'S
Current
Therapy
2010

Edward T. Bope, MD

Director, Riverside Family Practice
    Residency Program
Clinical Professor, Department of Family Medicine
The Ohio State University College of Medicine
Columbus, Ohio

Robert E. Rakel, MD

Professor, Department of Family and
    Community Medicine
Baylor College of Medicine
Houston, Texas

Rick Kellerman, MD

Professor and Chair, Department of Family and
    Community Medicine
University of Kansas School of Medicine—Wichita
Wichita, Kansas

LATEST APPROVED METHODS OF TREATMENT FOR THE PRACTICING PHYSICIAN

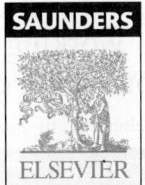

SAUNDERS

ELSEVIER

SAUNDERS
ELSEVIER

1600 John F. Kennedy Blvd.
Ste 1800
Philadelphia, PA 19103-2899

CONN'S CURRENT THERAPY 2010   ISBN: 978-1-4160-6642-2

Notice

Knowledge and best practice in this field are constantly changing. As new research and experience broaden our understanding, changes in research methods, professional practices, or medical treatment may become necessary.

Practitioners and researchers must always rely on their own experience and knowledge in evaluating and using any information, methods, compounds, or experiments described herein. In using such information or methods they should be mindful of their own safety and the safety of others, including parties for whom they have a professional responsibility.

With respect to any drug or pharmaceutical products identified, readers are advised to check the most current information provided (i) on procedures featured or (ii) by the manufacturer of each product to be administered, to verify the recommended dose or formula, the method and duration of administration, and contraindications. It is the responsibility of practitioners, relying on their own experience and knowledge of their patients, to make diagnoses, to determine dosages and the best treatment for each individual patient, and to take all appropriate safety precautions.

To the fullest extent of the law, neither the Publisher nor the authors, contributors, or editors, assume any liability for any injury and/or damage to persons or property as a matter of products liability, negligence or otherwise, or from any use or operation of any methods, products, instructions, or ideas contained in the material herein.

Library of Congress Cataloging-in-Publication Data
Current therapy; latest approved methods of treatment for the practicing physician.
Editors: H. F. Conn and others
  v. 28 cm. annual
   ISBN 978-1-4160-6642-2
  1. Therapeutics. 2. Therapeutics, Surgical. 3. Medicine—Practice.
  I. Conn, Howard Franklin, 1908–1982 ed.

RM101.C87 616.058 49–8328 rev*

Acquisitions Editor: Druanne Martin
Developmental Editor: Joan Ryan
Publishing Services Manager: Frank Polizzano
Project Manager: Jeff Gunning, Lee Ann Draud
Design Direction: Steve Stave

Printed in the United States of America

Last digit is the print number: 9 8 7 6 5 4 3 2 1

Contributors

Charles S. Abrams, MD
Associate Chief, Division of Hematology-Oncology, University of Pennsylvania School of Medicine; Staff Physician, Division of Hematology-Oncology, University of Pennsylvania Medical Center, Philadelphia, Pennsylvania
Platelet-Mediated Bleeding Disorders

Mark J. Abzug, MD
Professor of Pediatrics (Infectious Diseases), University of Colorado Denver School of Medicine; Medical Director, The Children's Hospital Clinical Trials Organization, The Children's Hospital, Aurora, Colorado
Viral Meningitis and Encephalitis

Paul C. Adams, MD
Professor of Medicine, University of Western Ontario Faculty of Medicine; Chief of Gastroenterology, University Hospital, London, Ontario, Canada
Hemochromatosis

Tod C. Aeby, MD
Residency Program Director, Department of Obstetrics, Gynecology, and Women's Health, University of Hawaii John A. Burns School of Medicine, Honolulu, Hawaii
Uterine Leiomyomas

Gorav Ailawadi, MD
Assistant Professor of Surgery, University of Virginia School of Medicine, Charlottesville, Virginia
Acquired Diseases of the Aorta

Lee Akst, MD
Assistant Professor, Department of Otolaryngology, Loyola University Chicago Stritch School of Medicine, Maywood, Illinois
Hoarseness and Laryngitis

Mark R. Albertini, MD
Associate Professor of Medicine, Section of Hematology/Medical Oncology, University of Wisconsin School of Medicine and Public Health; Director, Melanoma Disease Oriented Working Group, University of Wisconsin Carbone Cancer Center, Madison, Wisconsin
Melanoma

Brian K. Albertson, MD
University Physicians Group, Harrisburg, Pennsylvania
Osteomyelitis

Tina S. Alster, MD
Director, Washington Institute of Dermatologic Laser Surgery, Washington, DC
Keloids

Navin M. Amin, MD
Professor of Family Medicine, University of California, Irvine, School of Medicine, Irvine; Associate Professor of Medicine, David Geffen School of Medicine at UCLA, Los Angeles; and Associate Professor of Medicine, Stanford University School of Medicine, Stanford, California
Infective Endocarditis

Girish Anand, MD
Fellow in Gastroenterology, Albert Einstein Medical Center, Philadelphia, Pennsylvania
Dysphagia and Esophageal Obstruction

Deverick J. Anderson, MD
Clinical Associate, Duke University Medical Center, Durham, North Carolina
Rickettsial and Ehrlichial Infections

Kelley P. Anderson, MD
Clinical Associate Professor of Medicine, University of Wisconsin School of Medicine and Public Health–Marshfield Clinic Campus, Marshfield, Wisconsin
Heart Block

Gregory M. Anstead, MD
Associate Professor of Medicine, University of Texas Health Science Center at San Antonio School of Medicine; Director, Immunosuppression and Infectious Diseases Clinics, South Texas Veterans Healthcare System, San Antonio, Texas
Coccidioidomycosis

Paul M. Arguin, MD
Medical Epidemiologist and Chief, Domestic Malaria Unit, Centers for Disease Control and Prevention, Atlanta, Georgia
Malaria

Aydin Arici, MD
Professor, Department of Obstetrics, Gynecology, and Reproductive Sciences, Yale University School of Medicine, New Haven, Connecticut
Abnormal Uterine Bleeding

Ann M. Aring, MD
Assistant Clinical Professor, Department of Family Medicine, The Ohio State University College of Medicine; Assistant Program Director, Family Medicine Residency, Riverside Methodist Hospital, Columbus, Ohio
Fever

Isao Arita, MD
Chairman, Agency for Cooperation in International Health, Kumamoto, Kumamoto City, Japan
Smallpox

v

William Aughenbaugh, MD
Assistant Professor and Vice Chair for Education, Department of Dermatology, University of Wisconsin School of Medicine and Public Health, Madison, Wisconsin
Cutaneous Fungal Infections

Gopal H. Badlani, MD
Vice Chairman, Department of Urology, Long Island Jewish Medical Center, New Hyde Park, New York
Benign Prostatic Hyperplasia

Adrianne Williams Bagley, MD
Pediatrician, Lincoln Community Health Center, Inc., Durham, North Carolina
Pelvic Inflammatory Disease

Arna Banerjee, MD
Assistant Professor of Anesthesiology and Surgery, Department of Anesthesiology and Critical Care and Department of Surgery, Vanderbilt University Medical Center, Nashville, Tennessee
Delirium

J. Ryan Bariola, MD
Assistant Professor of Medicine (Infectious Diseases), University of Arkansas for Medical Sciences College of Medicine, Little Rock, Arkansas
Blastomycosis

James C. Barton, MD
Clinical Professor, Department of Medicine, University of Alabama at Birmingham School of Medicine; Medical Director, Southern Iron Disorders Center, Birmingham, Alabama
Iron Deficiency

Buddha Basnyat, MD
Nepal International Clinic, Kathmandu, Nepal
Typhoid Fever

Minoo Battiwalla, MD
Assistant Professor, State University of New York at Buffalo School of Medicine and Biomedical Sciences; Staff Physician, Department of Medicine, Roswell Park Cancer Institute, Buffalo, New York
Myelodysplastic Syndromes

Nurcan Baykam, MD
Associate Professor of Infectious Diseases, University of Ankara Faculty of Medicine; Staff, Infectious Diseases and Clinical Microbiology Clinic, Ankara Numune Education and Research Hospital, Ankara, Turkey
Brucellosis

Carolyn E. Beck, MD, MSc
Assistant Professor, University of Toronto Faculty of Medicine; Staff Paediatrician, Division of Paediatric Medicine, The Hospital for Sick Children, Toronto, Ontario, Canada
Parenteral Fluid Therapy for Infants and Children

Meg Begany, RD, CSP, LDN
Clinical Neonatal Dietitian, The Children's Hospital of Philadelphia, Philadelphia, Pennsylvania
Normal Infant Feeding

Wilma Bergfeld, MD
Professor of Dermatology and Pathology, Co-Director of Dermatopathology, and Director of Dermatopathology Fellowship, Cleveland Clinic, Cleveland, Ohio
Diseases of the Hair

David I. Bernstein, MD
Professor of Medicine and Environmental Health, University of Cincinnati College of Medicine, Cincinnati, Ohio
Hypersensitivity Pneumonitis

John P. Bilezikian, MD
Professor, Department of Medicine, Columbia University College of Physicians and Surgeons; Attending Physician, NewYork-Presbyterian Hospital, New York, New York
Primary Hyperparathyroidism and Hypoparathyroidism

Brian G. Blackburn, MD
Clinical Assistant Professor and Co-Director, Clinical Services, Division of Infectious Diseases and Geographic Medicine, Stanford University School of Medicine; Clinical Assistant Professor, Stanford Hospital and Clinics, Stanford, California
Travel Medicine

Mary Ann Bonilla, MD
Assistant Clinical Professor, Columbia University College of Physicians and Surgeons, New York, New York; Attending Physician, St. Joseph's Regional Medical Center, Paterson, New Jersey
Neutropenia

Zuleika L. Bonilla-Martinez, MD
Wound Healing Fellow, Department of Dermatology and Cutaneous Surgery, University of Miami Miller School of Medicine, Miami, Florida
Venous Ulcers

Herbert L. Bonkovsky, MD
Professor, University of Connecticut School of Medicine, Farmington, Connecticut; Professor, University of North Carolina College of Medicine; Vice President for Research, Carolinas Health Care System, Charlotte, North Carolina
Porphyria

Patrick Borgen, MD
Chief, Breast Service, Department of Surgery, Memorial Sloan-Kettering Cancer Center, New York, New York
Diseases of the Breast

Krystene I. Boyle, MD
Clinical Instructor, Department of Obstetrics and Gynecology, University of Cincinnati College of Medicine; Clinical Fellow, Department of OB/GYN, Division of Reproductive Endocrinology, University of Cincinnati Medical Center, Cincinnati, Ohio
Menopause

Robert Bradsher, MD
Richard V. Ebert Professor of Medicine, University of Arkansas for Medical Sciences College of Medicine; Program Director, Internal Medicine Residency and Infectious Diseases Fellowship Training Program; Vice-Chairman, Department of Internal Medicine; Director, Division of Infectious Diseases, University of Arkansas for Medical Sciences, Little Rock, Arkansas
Blastomycosis

Mark E. Brecher, MD
Adjunct Professor, Department of Pathology and Laboratory Medicine, University of North Carolina at Chapel Hill School of Medicine, Chapel Hill; Chief Medical Officer/Senior Vice President, Laboratory Corporation of America, Burlington, North Carolina
Therapeutic Use of Blood Components

Patricia D. Brown, MD
Associate Professor of Medicine, Division of Infectious Diseases, Wayne State University School of Medicine; Chief of Medicine, Detroit Receiving Hospital, Detroit, Michigan
Pyelonephritis

Patrick Brown, MD
Assistant Professor of Oncology and Pediatrics, Johns Hopkins
University School of Medicine; Director, Pediatric Leukemia and
Lymphoma Program, Sidney Kimmel Comprehensive Cancer Center
at Johns Hopkins, Baltimore, Maryland
Acute Leukemia in Children

Richard B. Brown, MD
Professor of Medicine, Tufts University School of Medicine,
Boston; Senior Clinician, Baystate Medical Center, Springfield,
Massachusetts
Toxic Shock Syndrome

Peter Buckley, MD
Professor and Chairman, and Associate Dean for Leadership
Development, Medical College of Georgia, Augusta, Georgia
Schizophrenia

Irina Burd, MD, PhD
Instructor, Department of Obstetrics and Gynecology, University of
Pennsylvania School of Medicine; Staff, Hospital of the University of
Pennsylvania, Philadelphia, Pennsylvania
Menopause

Jeffrey Burgess, DDS, MSD
Director, Oral Care Research Associates, Seattle, Washington
Temporomandibular Disorders and Orofacial Pain

Craig N. Burkhart, MD, MS
Assistant Professor (Clinical) of Dermatology, University of North
Carolina at Chapel Hill School of Medicine; Staff, Department of
Dermatology, University of North Carolina Hospitals, Chapel Hill,
North Carolina
Bullous Diseases

Daniel Buroker, MD
Hematology-Oncology Fellow, University of Iowa Hospitals and
Clinics, Iowa City, Iowa
Pernicious Anemia and Other Megaloblastic Anemias

Diego Cadavid, MD
Consultant in Immunology and Inflammatory Diseases,
Massachusetts General Hospital, Charlestown, Massachusetts
Relapsing Fever

Grant R. Caddy, MD
Consultant Physician and Gastroenterologist, Ulster Hospital, Belfast,
Northern Ireland
Cholelithiasis and Cholecystitis

Umberto Capitanio, MD
Resident in Training, Vita-Salute University, Milan, Italy
Prostatitis

Thomas R. Caraccio, PharmD
Associate Professor of Emergency Medicine, Stony Brook University
Medical Center School of Medicine, Stony Brook; Assistant Professor
of Pharmacology and Toxicology, New York College of Osteopathic
Medicine, Old Westbury, New York
*Medical Toxicology: Ingestions, Inhalations, and Dermal and Ocular
Absorptions*

Enrique V. Carbajal, MD
Associate Clinical Professor of Medicine, University of California,
San Francisco School of Medicine, San Francisco; Staff Physician–
Cardiology, Veterans Affairs Central California Health Care System,
Fresno, California
Premature Beats

Steve Carpenter, MD
Associate Professor, Baylor College of Medicine, St. Luke's Episcopal
Hospital, Houston, Texas
Hodgkin's Disease: Radiation Therapy

Petros E. Carvounis, BMBCh
Assistant Professor, Baylor College of Medicine, Houston, Texas
Uveitis

Donald O. Castell, MD
Professor of Medicine, Division of Gastroenterology and Hepatology,
Medical University of South Carolina, Charleston, South Carolina
Gastroesophageal Reflux Disease

Alvaro Cervera, MD
University of Barcelona, Barcelona, Spain; National Stroke Research
Institute, Heidelberg Heights, Victoria, Australia
Ischemic Cerebrovascular Disease

Lawrence Chan, MD
Professor of Medicine, Rutherford Chair, and Division Chief,
Diabetes, Endocrinology, and Metabolism, Baylor College of
Medicine; Chief, Diabetes, Endocrinology, and Metabolism, St. Luke's
Episcopal Hospital, Houston, Texas
Dyslipoproteinemias; Primary Aldosteronism

Miriam M. Chan, BSc, PharmD
Clinical Assistant Professor of Family Medicine, College of Medicine
and Public Health, and Clinical Assistant Professor of Pharmacy,
College of Pharmacy, The Ohio State University, Columbus, Ohio;
Adjunct Assistant Professor of Pharmacy, Ohio Northern University,
Ada, Ohio; Affiliate Faculty of Pharmacy Practice, Idaho State
University, Pocatello, Idaho; Director of Pharmacy Education,
Riverside Family Medicine Residency, Riverside Methodist Hospital,
Columbus, Ohio
*Popular Herbs and Nutritional Supplements; New Drugs in 2008 and
Agents Pending FDA Approval*

Rakesh Chandra, MD
Associate Professor of Otolaryngology—Head and Neck Surgery,
Northwestern University Feinberg School of Medicine, Chicago,
Illinois
Sinusitis; Nonallergic Perennial Rhinitis

Aarthi Chary, MD
Fellow, Division of Infectious Diseases and Geographic Medicine,
Stanford University School of Medicine, Stanford, California
Travel Medicine

Emery Chen, MD
Endocrine Surgeon, Woodland Clinic, Woodland, California
Thyroid Cancer

Venkata Sri Cherukumilli, BS
Medical Student, University of California, San Diego, School of
Medicine, La Jolla, California
Rheumatoid Arthritis

Meera Chitlur, MD
Assistant Professor of Pediatrics, Wayne State University School of
Medicine; Staff Physician, Carman and Ann Adams Department of
Pediatrics, Division of Hematology/Oncology, Children's Hospital of
Michigan, Detroit, Michigan
Hemophilia and Related Bleeding Disorders

Stella T. Chou, MD
Assistant Professor of Pediatrics, University of Pennsylvania School of
Medicine; Attending Physician, The Children's Hospital of
Philadelphia, Philadelphia Pennsylvania
Nonimmune Hemolytic Anemia

Dimitrios Christoforidis, MD
Chief, Clinic, Centre Hospitalier Universitaire Vaudois, Lausanne, Switzerland
Hemorrhoids, Anal Fissure, and Anorectal Abscess and Fistula

Jeffson Chung, MD
Division of Thoracic Surgery, University of Toronto Faculty of Medicine, Toronto, Ontario, Canada
Pleural Effusion and Empyema Thoracis

Maria C. Cid, MD
Associate Professor, University of Barcelona Medical School; Consultant in Systemic Autoimmune Disease, Hospital Clinic, Barcelona, Spain
Polymyalgia Rheumatica and Giant Cell Arteritis

Peter E. Clark, MD
Associate Professor of Urologic Surgery, Vanderbilt University School of Medicine, Nashville, Tennessee
Malignant Tumors of the Urogenital Tract

Claus-Frenz Claussen, MD
Julius-Maximilians-Universität Würzburg, Würzburg; Head, 4-G Research Institute, Neurootologisches Forschungsinstitut, Bad Kissingen, Germany
Tinnitus

Debbie L. Cohen, MD
Assistant Professor of Medicine, University of Pennsylvania School of Medicine, Philadelphia, Pennsylvania
Hypertension

Gary C. Coleman, DDS, MS
Associate Professor, Department of Diagnostic Sciences, Baylor College of Dentistry, Dallas, Texas
Diseases of the Mouth

Robert A. Copeland, Jr., MD
Department of Ophthalmology, Howard University Hospital, Washington, DC
Conjunctivitis

Jorge E. Cortes, MD
Professor of Medicine and Deputy Chair, Department of Leukemia, University of Texas M. D. Anderson Cancer Center, Houston, Texas
Chronic Leukemias

Fiona Costello, MD
Clinical Associate Professor, Departments of Clinical Neurosciences/Surgery, University of Calgary Faculty of Medicine, Calgary, Alberta, Canada
Optic Neuritis

John F. Coyle II, MD
Clinical Professor, Department of Medicine, University of Oklahoma College of Medicine–Tulsa, Tulsa, Oklahoma
Disturbances Caused by Heat

Lester M. Crawford, PhD
Formerly Research Professor, Georgetown University School of Medicine, Washington, DC, and Head, Department of Physiology, University of Georgia College of Medicine, Athens, Georgia
Foodborne Illness

Rosella Creed, MD
Department of Dermatology, University of Texas Medical School at Houston, Houston, Texas
Viral Diseases of the Skin

Daniel A. Culver, DO
Staff Physician, Department of Pulmonary, Allergy, and Critical Care Medicine, Cleveland Clinic, Cleveland, Ohio
Sarcoidosis

Burke A. Cunha, MD
Professor of Medicine, Stony Brook University Medical Center School of Medicine, Stony Brook; Chief, Infectious Disease Division, Winthrop-University Hospital, Mineola, New York
Viral and Mycoplasmal Pneumonias; Urinary Tract Infections in Women

Anne B. Curtis, MD
Division of Cardiovascular Disease, University of South Florida, Tampa, Florida
Atrial Fibrillation

F. William Danby, MD, FRCPC
Adjunct Assistant Professor of Medicine (Dermatology), Dartmouth Medical School, Hanover; Associated Admitting Staff, Elliot Hospital; Consulting Staff, Catholic Medical Center, Manchester, New Hampshire
Anogenital Pruritus

Ralph C. Daniel, MD
Department of Dermatology, St. Dominic-Jackson Memorial Hospital, Jackson, Mississippi
Diseases of the Nails

Athena Daniolos, MD
Associate Professor, Department of Dermatology, University of Wisconsin School of Medicine and Public Health; Attending Physician, University Health Services, University of Wisconsin, Madison, Wisconsin
Condyloma Acuminata (Genital Warts)

Stella Dantas, MD
Physician, Department of Obstetrics and Gynecology, Beaverton Medical Office, Northwest Permanente PC Physicians and Surgeons, Beaverton, Oregon
Uterine Leiomyomas

Andre Dascal, MD, FRCPC
Associate Professor, Departments of Medicine, Microbiology, and Immunology, McGill University Faculty of Medicine; Senior Infectious Disease Physician, Sir Mortimer B. Davis–Jewish General Hospital, Montreal, Quebec, Canada
Acute Infectious Diarrhea

Susan Davids, MD, MPH
Associate Professor of Medicine, Medical College of Wisconsin; Associate Program Director, Internal Medicine Residency, Clement J. Zablocki Veterans Affairs Medical Center, Milwaukee, Wisconsin
Acute Bronchitis

Susan A. Davidson, MD
Associate Professor, University of Colorado Denver School of Medicine; Chief, Gynecologic Oncology, University of Colorado Hospital, Aurora, Colorado
Neoplasms of the Vulva

Terry F. Davies, MD
Baumritter Professor of Medicine, Mount Sinai School of Medicine, New York; Director, Division of Endocrinology and Metabolism, James J. Peters Veterans Affairs Medical Center, Bronx, New York
Hypothyroidism

Prakash C. Deedwania, MD
Professor of Medicine, University of California, San Francisco, School of Medicine, San Francisco; Chief, Cardiology Section, Veterans Affairs Central California Health Care System, Fresno, California
Premature Beats

Richard De La Garza, PhD
Associate Professor, Baylor College of Medicine, Houston, Texas
Treatment for Addiction

Marc de Perrot, MD
Associate Professor, Division of Thoracic Surgery, University of Toronto Faculty of Medicine and Toronto General Hospital, Toronto, Ontario, Canada
Pleural Effusion and Empyema Thoracis

Stephen R. Deputy, MD
Assistant Professor of Neurology, Louisiana State University School of Medicine; Staff Neurologist, Children's Hospital, New Orleans, Louisiana
Traumatic Brain Injury in Children

Richard D. deShazo, MD
Professor of Medicine and Pediatrics and Billy S. Guyton Distinguished Professor, University of Mississippi College of Medicine; Chair, Department of Medicine, University of Mississippi Medical Center, Jackson, Mississippi
Pneumoconiosis

Clio Dessinioti, MD, MSc
Attending Dermatologist, Andreas Sygros Hospital, Athens, Greece
Parasitic Diseases of the Skin

Luis A. Diaz, MD
Professor and Chair of Dermatology, University of North Carolina at Chapel Hill School of Medicine; Staff, Department of Dermatology, University of North Carolina Hospitals, Chapel Hill, North Carolina
Bullous Diseases

Douglas DiOrio, MD
Adjunct Clinical Professor, The Ohio State University College of Medicine; Fellowship Director, Riverside Sports Medicine, Riverside Methodist Hospital, Columbus, Ohio
Common Sports Injuries

Jack A. DiPalma, MD
Professor of Medicine and Director, Division of Gastroenterology, University of South Alabama College of Medicine, Mobile, Alabama
Constipation

Sunil Dogra, MD, DNB, MNAMS
Assistant Professor, Department of Dermatology, Venereology and Leprology, Postgraduate Institute of Medical Education and Research, Chandigarh, India
Leprosy

Basak Dokuzoguz, MD
Chief, Infectious Diseases and Clinical Microbiology Clinic, Ankara Numune Education and Research Hospital, Ankara, Turkey
Brucellosis

Joseph Domachowske, MD
Professor of Pediatrics, Microbiology, and Immunology, State University of New York Upstate Medical University, Syracuse, New York
Infectious Mononucleosis

Geoffrey A. Donnan, MD
Department of Neurology, University of Melbourne Faculty of Medicine, Dentistry, and Health Sciences; Florey Neuroscience Institutes, Carlton South, Victoria, Australia
Ischemic Cerebrovascular Disease

Craig L. Donnelly, MD
Dartmouth Medical School, Hanover; Chief, Child and Adolescent Psychiatry, Dartmouth-Hitchcock Medical Center, Lebanon, New Hampshire
Attention-Deficit/Hyperactivity Disorder

Douglas A. Drevets, MD, DTM&H
Professor and Interim Chief, Section of Infectious Diseases, University of Oklahoma Health Sciences Center School of Medicine; Staff Physician, Veterans Affairs Medical Center, Oklahoma City, Oklahoma
Plague

Jean Dudler, MD
Associate Professor of Medicine, Division of Rheumatology, Centre Hospitalier Universitaire Vaudois and University of Lausanne, Lausanne, Switzerland
Rat-Bite Fever

Peter R. Duggan, MD
Assistant Clinical Professor of Medicine, University of Calgary Faculty of Medicine; Hematologist, Foothills Medical Center, Calgary, Alberta, Canada
Acute Leukemia in Adults

Kim Eagle, MD
Albion Walter Hewlett Professor of Internal Medicine, Chief of Clinical Cardiology, and Director, Cardiovascular Center, University of Michigan Health System, Ann Arbor, Michigan
Angina Pectoris

Julian Elliott, MB, BS, FRACP
Conjoint Senior Lecturer, National Centre in HIV Epidemiology and Clinical Research, University of New South Wales, Sydney; Infectious Diseases Physician, Alfred Hospital, Melbourne; HIV Clinical Advisor, International Health Research Group, Macfarlane Burnet Institute for Medical Research and Public Health, Melbourne, New South Wales, Australia
Psittacosis

Sean P. Elliott, MD
Assistant Professor, University of Minnesota Medical School, Minneapolis, Minnesota
Trauma to the Genitourinary Tract

John M. Embil, MD, FRCP(C), FACP
Associate Professor, Department of Medicine and Medical Microbiology, Section of Infectious Diseases, University of Manitoba Faculty of Medicine; Director, Infection Prevention and Control Unit, Health Science Centre, Winnipeg, Manitoba, Canada
Necrotizing Skin and Soft Tissue Infections

Scott K. Epstein, MD
Dean for Educational Affairs and Professor of Medicine, Tufts University School of Medicine, Boston, Massachusetts
Acute Respiratory Failure

Georgina Espígol-Frigolé, MD
Specialist, Department of Autoimmune and Systemic Diseases, Hospital Clinic, Barcelona, Spain
Polymyalgia Rheumatica and Giant Cell Arteritis

x

Walid Farhat, MD
Associate Professor, Department of Surgery, Pediatric Urologist,
The Hospital for Sick Children, Toronto, Ontario, Canada
Childhood Incontinence

Dorianne Feldman, MD, MSPT
Instructor of Physical Medicine and Rehabilitation, Johns Hopkins
University School of Medicine, Baltimore, Maryland
Rehabilitation of the Stroke Patient

Gregory Feldman, MD
Surgical Resident, Stanford Hospitals and Clinics, Stanford,
California
Peripheral Arterial Disease

Steven R. Feldman, MD, PhD
Professor of Dermatology, Wake Forest University School of
Medicine, Winston-Salem, North Carolina
Acne Vulgaris and Rosacea

Robert S. Fisher, MD
Lorber Professor of Medicine and Chief, Gastroenterology Section
and Digestive Disease Center, Temple University School of Medicine,
Philadelphia, Pennsylvania
Irritable Bowel Syndrome

Alan B. Fleischer, Jr., MD
Professor and Chair, Department of Dermatology, Wake Forest
University School of Medicine, Winston-Salem, North Carolina
Acne Vulgaris and Rosacea

Brian J. Flynn, MD
Associate Professor of Urology, University of Colorado Denver
School of Medicine, Aurora, Colorado
Urethral Strictures

Robert J. Fox, MD
Assistant Professor of Neurology, Cleveland Clinic Lerner College of
Medicine; Staff Neurologist and Medical Director, Mellen Center for
Multiple Sclerosis, Cleveland Clinic Foundation, Cleveland, Ohio
Multiple Sclerosis

Ellen W. Freeman, PhD
Research Professor, Departments of Obstetrics/Gynecology and
Department of Psychiatry, University of Pennsylvania School of
Medicine, Philadelphia, Pennsylvania
Premenstrual Syndrome

Theodore M. Freeman, MD
Jacobs, Ramirez, and Freeman Allergy & Immunology, San Antonio,
Texas
Allergic Reaction to Stinging Insects

Jeremy N. Friedman, MB, ChB
Associate Professor, Department of Paediatrics, University of Toronto
Faculty of Medicine; Head, Division of Paediatric Medicine,
The Hospital for Sick Children, Toronto, Ontario, Canada
Parenteral Fluid Therapy for Infants and Children

R. Michael Gallagher, DO
Director, Headache Center of Central Florida, Melbourne, Florida
Headache

Andrea Gallina, MD
Resident in Training, Vita-Salute University–San Raffaele Hospital,
Milan, Italy
Prostatitis

John Garber, MD
Instructor in Medicine, Harvard Medical School; Fellow in
Gastroenterology, Massachusetts General Hospital, Boston,
Massachusetts
Acute and Chronic Viral Hepatitis

Ana García-Martínez, MD
Specialist, Department of Emergency Medicine, Hospital Clinic,
Barcelona, Spain
Polymyalgia Rheumatica and Giant Cell Arteritis

Shekhar A. Ghamande, MD
West Virginia University, Morgantown, West Virginia
Sleep Apnea

Khalil G. Ghanem, MD, PhD
Assistant Professor of Medicine, Division of Infectious Diseases,
Johns Hopkins University School of Medicine, Baltimore,
Maryland
Gonorrhea

Paul L. F. Giangrande, MD
Senior Lecturer in Haematology, University of Oxford; Consultant
Haematologist, Oxford Haemophilia Centre and Thrombosis Unit,
Churchill Hospital, Oxford, United Kingdom
Venous Thrombosis

Carla M. Giannoni, MD
Assistant Professor, Bobby R. Alford Department of
Otolaryngology–Head and Neck Surgery, Baylor College of Medicine,
Houston, Texas
Streptococcal Pharyngitis

Donald L. Gilbert, MD, MS
Associate Professor of Medicine, University of Cincinnati College of
Medicine; Associate Professor, Cincinnati Children's Hospital
Medical Center, Cincinnati, Ohio
Gilles de la Tourette Syndrome

Robert Giusti, MD
Assistant Professor of Pediatrics, State University of New York
Downstate Medical Center College of Medicine; Director, Cystic
Fibrosis Center; Interim Chairman, Department of Pediatrics,
Long Island College Hospital, Brooklyn, New York
Cystic Fibrosis

Robert C. Goldstein, MD
Fellow, Infectious Diseases, Beth Israel Medical Center, New York,
New York
Toxoplasmosis

Erica V. Gonzalez, MD
Division of Diabetes and Endocrinology, Department of Medicine,
Baylor College of Medicine, Houston, Texas
Hypopituitarism

Marlís González-Fernández, MD, PhD
Assistant Professor of Physical Medicine and Rehabilitation,
Johns Hopkins University School of Medicine; Medical Director,
Outpatient Physical Medicine and Rehabilitation Clinics, Johns
Hopkins Hospital, Baltimore, Maryland
Rehabilitation of the Stroke Patient

E. Ann Gormley, MD
Professor of Surgery (Urology), Dartmouth Medical School,
Hanover; Staff Urologist, Dartmouth-Hitchcock Medical Center,
Lebanon, New Hampshire
Urinary Incontinence

Eduardo Gotuzzo, MD
Principal Professor of Medicine, Universidad Peruana Cayetano Heredia; Chief, Department of Infectious, Tropical, and Dermatologic Diseases, Hospital National Cayetano Heredia, Lima, Peru
Cholera

Mark A. Granner, MD
Associate Professor of Neurology, University of Iowa Carver College of Medicine; Director, Iowa Comprehensive Epilepsy Program, University of Iowa Hospitals and Clinics, Iowa City, Iowa
Seizures and Epilepsy in Adolescents and Adults

Jane M. Grant-Kels, MD
Professor and Chair, Department of Dermatology; Dermatology Residency Director; and Assistant Dean of Clinical Affairs, University of Connecticut School of Medicine; Director of Dermatopathology and Director of Cutaneous Oncology and Melanoma Center, University of Connecticut Health Center, Farmington, Connecticut.
Melanocytic Nevi

Joseph Greensher, MD
Professor of Pediatrics, Stony Brook University Medical Center School of Medicine, Stony Brook; Medical Director and Associate Chair, Department of Pediatrics, Long Island Regional Poison and Drug Information Center, Winthrop-University Hospital, Mineola, New York
Medical Toxicology: Ingestions, Inhalations, and Dermal and Ocular Absorptions

David Gregory, MD
Assistant Clinical Professor of Family Medicine, University of Virginia School of Medicine; Charlottesville; Assistant Clinical Professor of Family Medicine, Virginia Commonwealth University School of Medicine, Richmond; Director of Didactic Curriculum, Lynchburg Family Medicine Residency; Staff Physician in Family Medicine and Obstetrics, Lynchburg General Hospital and Virginia Baptist Hospital, Lynchburg, Virginia
Resuscitation of the Newborn

Priya Grewal, MD
Assistant Professor, Division of Liver Diseases, Mount Sinai School of Medicine, New York, New York
Cirrhosis

Charles Grose, MD
Professor of Pediatrics, University of Iowa Carver College of Medicine; Director of Infectious Diseases Division, Children's Hospital of Iowa, Iowa City, Iowa
Varicella (Chickenpox)

Eva C. Guinan, MD
Associate Professor of Pediatrics and Director, Linkages Program, Harvard Catalyst, Harvard Medical School, Boston, Massachusetts
Aplastic Anemia

Tawanda Gumbo, MD
Associate Professor of Medicine, University of Texas Southwestern Medical School; Attending Physician, Parkland Memorial Hospital and University Hospital–St. Paul, Dallas, Texas
Tuberculosis and Other Mycobacterial Diseases

Juliet Gunkel, MD
Assistant Professor, University of Wisconsin School of Medicine and Public Health; Staff Physician, University of Wisconsin Hospitals and Clinics and Meritor Hospital, Madison, Wisconsin
Premalignant Cutaneous and Mucosal Lesions

Amita Gupta, MD, MHS
Assistant Professor, Division of Infectious Diseases, Johns Hopkins University School of Medicine, Baltimore, Maryland
The Patient with HIV Disease

David Hadley, MD
Urology Resident, University of Utah Health Sciences Center, Salt Lake City, Utah
Urethral Strictures

Thorvardur Halfdanarson, MD
Clinical Assistant Professor, University of Iowa Carver College of Medicine; Clinical Assistant Professor, University of Iowa Hospitals and Clinics; Staff Hematologist/Oncologist, Iowa City Veterans Affairs Medical Center, Iowa City, Iowa
Pernicious Anemia and Other Megaloblastic Anemias; Polycythemia Vera

Ronald Hall II, PharmD
Associate Professor, Texas Tech University Health Sciences Center School of Pharmacy, Dallas, Texas
Tuberculosis and Other Mycobacterial Diseases

Rashidul Haque, MB, PhD
Scientist, Laboratory Sciences Division, International Centre for Diarrhoea Disease Research, Bangladesh (ICDDR, B), Dhaka, Bangladesh
Amebiasis

David R. Harnisch, Sr., MD
Associate Professor, Department of Family Medicine, University of Nebraska Medical Center, Omaha, Nebraska
Dysmenorrhea

Rachel Haroz, MD
Assistant Professor of Emergency Medicine, UMDNJ-Robert Wood Johnson Medical School at Camden; Attending Physician, Department of Emergency Medicine, Cooper University Hospital, Camden, New Jersey
Spider Bites and Scorpion Stings

George D. Harris, MD, MS
Professor and Dean, Year 1 and 2 Medicine, University of Missouri–Kansas City School of Medicine; Faculty, Family Medicine Residency Program at Truman Medical Center–Lakewood, Kansas City, Missouri
Osteomyelitis

Shannon Harrison, MBBS, MMed
Private Practice, Dermatology, Battery Point, Tasmania, Australia
Diseases of the Hair

Weldon W. Haw, MD
Associate Clinical Professor of Cornea, Cataract, and Refractive Surgery, Department of Ophthalmology, University of California, San Diego, School of Medicine, La Jolla, California
Vision Correction Procedures

Peiman Hematti, MD
Assistant Professor of Medicine, University of Wisconsin School of Medicine and Public Health; University of Wisconsin Carbone Cancer Center, Madison, Wisconsin
Myelodysplastic Syndromes

J. Claude Hemphill III, MD, MAS
Associate Professor of Clinical Neurology and Neurological Surgery, University of California, San Francisco, School of Medicine; Director, Neurocritical Care, San Francisco General Hospital, San Francisco, California
Intracerebral Hemorrhage

Shane E. Hendon, DO
Instructor in Medicine and Fellow in Gastroenterology, University of
South Alabama College of Medicine, Mobile, Alabama
Constipation

José Hernández-Rodríguez, MD
Teaching Collaborator, University of Barcelona; Senior Specialist,
Department of Autoimmune and Systemic Diseases, Hospital Clinic,
Barcelona, Spain
Polymyalgia Rheumatica and Giant Cell Arteritis

Emily J. Herndon, MD
Assistant Professor, Department of Family and Preventive Medicine,
Emory University School of Medicine; Staff Physician, Department
of Community Medicine, Grady Health System, Atlanta, Georgia
Contraception

David G. Hill, MD
Yale University School of Medicine, New Haven; Waterbury
Pulmonary Associates, Waterbury, Connecticut
Cough

Micah Hill, MD
Otolaryngologist, Palo Alto, California
Sinusitis; Nonallergic Perennial Rhinitis

Christopher D. Hillyer, MD
Transfusion Medicine Program, Department of Pathology and
Laboratory Medicine, Emory University School of Medicine,
Atlanta, Georgia
Adverse Effects of Blood Transfusion

Stacey Hinderliter, MD
Clinical Assistant Professor of Family Medicine, University of
Virginia School of Medicine, Charlottesville; Clinical Assistant
Professor of Family Medicine, Virginia Commonwealth University
School of Medicine, Richmond; Pediatric Faculty, Lynchburg Family
Medicine Residency; Staff Physician, Lynchburg General Hospital,
Lynchburg, Virginia
Resuscitation of the Newborn

Molly Hinshaw, MD
Assistant Professor of Dermatology, University of Wisconsin School
of Medicine and Public Health, Madison; Dermatopathologist,
Dermpath Diagnostics, Brookfield, Wisconsin
Autoimmune Connective Tissue Disease

David C. Hodgson, MD, MPH
Associate Professor, Department of Radiation Oncology, University
of Toronto Faculty of Medicine; Radiation Oncologist, Princess
Margaret Hospital, Toronto, Ontario, Canada
Hodgkin's Lymphoma

Raymond J. Hohl, MD, PhD
Professor of Internal Medicine and Pharmacology, University of Iowa
Carver College of Medicine, Iowa City, Iowa
Thalassemia

Sarah A. Holstein, MD, PhD
Fellow, Division of Hematology, Oncology, and Blood-Marrow
Transplantation, University of Iowa Carver College of Medicine, Iowa
City, Iowa
Thalassemia

Marisa Holubar, MD
Clinical Teaching Fellow, Warren Alpert Medical School of Brown
University, Providence, Rhode Island
Severe Sepsis and Septic Shock

E. Ekramul Hoque, MBBS, MPH (Hons), PhD
Research Fellow, Centre for Asian Health Research and Evaluation,
School of Population Health, University of Auckland, Auckland,
New Zealand
Giardiasis

Lewis L. Hsu, MD, PhD
Associate Professor and Interim Chief, Pediatric Hematology, Drexel
University College of Medicine; Interim Director, Marian Anderson
Comprehensive Sickle Cell Center, St. Christopher's Hospital for
Children, Philadelphia, Pennsylvania
Sickle Cell Disease

Samuel S. Hsu, MD
Assistant Professor, University of Maryland School of Medicine,
Baltimore, Maryland
Tetanus

Christine Hudak, MD
Summa Health System, Akron, Ohio
Vulvovaginitis

Joseph M. Hughes, MD
Associate Professor of Clinical Medicine, Columbia University
College of Physicians and Surgeons, New York; Attending Physician,
Department of Medicine, Division of Endocrinology, Bassett
Healthcare, Cooperstown, New York
Adrenocortical Insufficiency

Scott A. Hundahl, MD
Professor of Surgery, University of California, Davis, School of
Medicine, Sacramento; Chief of Surgery, Veterans Affairs Northern
California Health Care System, Mather, California
Tumors of the Stomach

Stephen P. Hunger, MD
Professor of Pediatrics, University of Colorado Denver School of
Medicine; Section Chief, Center for Cancer and Blood Disorders, and
Ergen Family Chair in Pediatric Cancer, The Children's Hospital,
Aurora, Colorado
Acute Leukemia in Children

Nader Husseinzadeh, MD
Professor, Department of Obstetrics and Gynecology, Division of
Gynecologic Oncology, University of Cincinnati School of Medicine,
Cincinnati, Ohio
Cancer of the Uterine Cervix

Jimee Hwang, MD, MPH
Medical Epidemiologist, Centers for Disease Control and Prevention,
Atlanta, Georgia
Malaria

Humza Ilyas, MD
Staff Physician, The Dermatology Group and Morristown Hospital,
Morristown, New Jersey
Cancer of the Skin

Robert D. Inman, MD
Professor of Medicine and Immunology, University of Toronto
Faculty of Medicine; Director, Arthritis Center of Excellence,
University Health Network, Toronto, Ontario, Canada
Ankylosing Spondylitis

Gerald A. Isenberg, MD
Associate Professor of Surgery and Director of Surgical
Undergraduate Education, Jefferson Medical College of Thomas
Jefferson University; Program Director, Colorectal Residency,
Thomas Jefferson University Hospital, Philadelphia, Pennsylvania
Tumors of the Colon and Rectum

Sei Iwai, MD
Professor of Clinical Medicine and Director, Cardiac
Electrophysiology Fellowship Program, Stony Brook University
Medical Center School of Medicine; Director, Complex Arrhythmia
Ablation Program, Stony Brook University Medical Center, Stony
Brook, New York
Tachycardias

Alan C. Jackson, MD, FRCPC
Professor of Medicine (Neurology) and Medical Microbiology,
University of Manitoba Faculty of Medicine; Head, Section of
Neurology, Winnipeg Regional Health Authority, Winnipeg,
Manitoba, Canada
Rabies

Danny O. Jacobs, MD, MPH
David C. Sabiston Jr. Professor and Chair, Department of Surgery,
Duke University School of Medicine, Durham, North Carolina
Diverticula of the Alimentary Tract

Kurt M. Jacobson, MD
Cardiovascular Medicine Fellow, University of Wisconsin Hospitals
and Clinics, Madison, Wisconsin
Mitral Valve Prolapse

Robert M. Jacobson, MD
Professor of Pediatrics, Mayo Clinic College of Medicine; Chair,
Department of Pediatric and Adolescent Medicine, and Consultant in
Pediatric and Adolescent Medicine, Mayo Clinic, Rochester,
Minnesota
Office-Based Immunization Practices

James J. James, MD, DrPH, MHA
Director, Center for Public Health Preparedness and Disaster
Response; Editor-in-Chief, *Journal of Disaster Medicine and Public
Health Preparedness*, American Medical Association, Chicago,
Illinois
*Toxic Chemical Agents Reference Chart: Symptoms and Treatment;
Biologic Agents Reference Chart–Symptoms, Tests, and Treatment*

Camila K. Janniger, MD
Clinical Professor and Chief, Pediatric and Geriatric Dermatology,
UMDNJ–New Jersey Medical School, Newark, New Jersey
Pigmentary Disorders

Jeff Jarrett, MD
Nebraska Pulmonary Specialties, Lincoln, Nebraska
Primary Lung Abscess

Nathaniel Jellinek, MD
Department of Dermatology, Warren Alpert Medical School of
Brown University, Providence, Rhode Island
Diseases of the Nails

Roy M. John, MD, PhD
Clinical Assistant Professor, Harvard Medical School; Associate
Director, Cardiac Electrophysiology Laboratory, Brigham and
Women's Hospital, Boston, Massachusetts
Cardiac Arrest: Sudden Cardiac Death

Philip C. Johnson, MD
Professor and Director, Division of General Medicine, and Vice
Chairman, Department of Internal Medicine, University of Texas
Medical School at Houston; Attending Physician, Memorial
Hermann Hospital, Texas Medical Center, and Lyndon Baines
Johnson General Hospital, Houston, Texas
Histoplasmosis

James F. Jones, MD
Research Medical Officer, Chronic Viral Diseases Branch, National
Center for Zoonotic, Vector-Borne, and Enteric Diseases, Centers for
Disease Control and Prevention, Atlanta, Georgia
Chronic Fatigue Syndrome

Joseph L. Jorizzo, MD
Professor, Founder, and formerly Chair, Department of Dermatology,
Wake Forest University School of Medicine, Winston-Salem,
North Carolina
Cutaneous Vasculitis

Ari Kalechstein, PhD
Adjunct Assistant Professor, Baylor College of Medicine, Houston, Texas
Treatment for Addiction

Harmit Kalia, DO
Division of Gastroenterology, UMDNJ-New Jersey Medical School,
Newark, New Jersey
Cirrhosis

Patrick S. Kamath, MD
Professor of Medicine, Mayo Clinic College of Medicine, Rochester,
Minnesota
Bleeding Esophageal Varices

Hagop M. Kantarjian, MD
Professor and Chair, Department of Leukemia, University of Texas
M. D. Anderson Cancer Center, Houston, Texas
Chronic Leukemias

Walter Kao, MD
Associate Professor of Medicine, University of Wisconsin School of
Medicine and Public Health; Attending Cardiologist, Heart Failure
and Transplant Program, University of Wisconsin Hospitals and
Clinics, Madison, Wisconsin
Heart Failure

Pierre I. Karakiewicz, MD
Associate Professor, Department of Urology, University of Montreal
Faculty of Medicine; Urologic Oncologist and Director, Cancer
Prognostics and Health Outcomes Unit, University of Montreal
Health Center, Montreal, Quebec, Canada
Prostatitis

Matthew E. Karlovsky, MD
Staff Urologist (Voiding Dysfunction/Female Urology), Private
Practice, Center for Urological Services, PC, Phoenix, Arizona
Benign Prostatic Hyperplasia

Andreas Katsambas, MD, PhD
Professor of Dermatology, Department of Dermatology, University
of Athens School of Medicine; Andreas Sygzos Hospital, Athens,
Greece
Parasitic Diseases of the Skin

Philip O. Katz, MD
Clinical Professor of Medicine, Jefferson Medical College of Thomas
Jefferson University; Chairman, Division of Gastroenterology, Albert
Einstein Medical Center, Philadelphia, Pennsylvania
Dysphagia and Esophageal Obstruction

Arthur Kavanaugh, MD
Professor of Medicine, University of California, San Diego, School of
Medicine, La Jolla, California
Rheumatoid Arthritis

Clive Kearon, MRCPI, FRCPC, PhD
Professor of Medicine, McMaster University Faculty of Health Sciences; Attending Physician, Henderson General Hospital, Hamilton, Ontario, Canada
Venous Thromboembolism

Jennifer Kelly, DO
Assistant Professor of Medicine, Division of Endocrinology, Diabetes and Metabolism, State University of New York Upstate Medical University College of Medicine, Syracuse, New York
Diabetes Insipidus

Stephen F. Kemp, MD
Professor of Medicine and Associate Professor of Pediatrics, University of Mississippi College of Medicine; Director, Allergy and Immunology Fellowship Program, Departments of Medicine and Pediatrics, University of Mississippi Medical Center, Jackson, Mississippi
Anaphylaxis and Serum Sickness

Kevin A. Kerber, MD
Assistant Professor, Department of Neurology, University of Michigan Health System, Ann Arbor, Michigan
Episodic Vertigo

Sripathi R. Kethu, MD
Digestive Health Associates of Texas, Richardson Regional Medical Center, Richardson, Texas
Gastritis and Peptic Ulcer Disease

Haejin Kim, MD
University of Cincinnati Medical Center, Cincinnati, Ohio
Hypersensitivity Pneumonitis

Robert S. Kirsner, MD, PhD
Vice Chairman and Stiefel Laboratories Professor, Department of Dermatology and Cutaneous Surgery, University of Miami Miller School of Medicine, Miami, Florida
Venous Ulcers

Joseph E. Kiss, MD
Associate Professor of Medicine, Division of Hematology-Oncology, University of Pittsburgh School of Medicine; Medical Director, Hemapheresis and Blood Services, The Institute for Transfusion Medicine, Pittsburgh, Pennsylvania
Thrombotic Thrombocytopenic Purpura

Joel D. Klein, MD, FAAP
Professor of Pediatrics, Jefferson Medical College of Thomas Jefferson University, Philadelphia, Pennsylvania; Division of Pediatric Infectious Diseases, Alfred I. duPont Hospital for Children, Wilmington, Delaware
Mumps

Luciano Kolodny, MD
Adjunct Assistant Professor of Medicine, University of Minnesota Medical School, Minneapolis, Minnesota; Regional Medical Director, External Scientific Medical Affairs, Merck & Company, North Wales, Pennsylvania
Erectile Dysfunction

Gerald B. Kolski, MD, PhD
Clinical Professor of Pediatrics, Temple University School of Medicine; Adjunct Clinical Professor of Pediatrics, Drexel University College of Medicine, Philadelphia; Attending Physician, Crozer Chester Medical Center, Upland, Pennsylvania
Asthma in Children

Frederick K. Korley, MD
Robert E. Meyerhoff Assistant Professor of Emergency Medicine, Johns Hopkins University School of Medicine; Staff, Johns Hopkins Medical Institutions, Baltimore, Maryland
Disturbances Due to Cold

Thomas R. Kosten, MD
J. H. Waggoner Chair and Professor of Psychiatry, Pharmacology, and Neuroscience, Baylor College of Medicine; Director, Veterans Affairs National Substance Use Disorders Quality Enhancement Research Initiative, M. E. DeBakey Veterans Affairs Medical Center, Houston, Texas
Anxiety Disorders

Milind J. Kothari, DO
Professor of Neurology and Vice Chair of Education and Training, Pennsylvania State College of Medicine, University Park, Pennsylvania
Myasthenia Gravis and Related Disorders

Kristin Kozakowski, MD
Pediatric Urology Senior Fellow, The Hospital for Sick Children, Toronto, Ontario, Canada
Childhood Incontinence

Robert Kraft, MD
Clinical Assistant Professor, Department of Family and Community Medicine, University of Kansas School of Medicine, Wichita; Associate Director, Smoky Hill Family Medicine Residency Program, Salina, Kansas
Nausea and Vomiting

Robert A. Kratzke, MD
John Skoglund Chair of Lung Cancer Research, University of Minnesota Medical School; Associate Professor, University of Minnesota Medical Center, Minneapolis, Minnesota
Primary Lung Cancer

Jeffrey A. Kraut, MD
Professor of Medicine, David Geffen School of Medicine at UCLA; Chief of Dialysis, Veterans Affairs Greater Los Angeles Healthcare System, Los Angeles, California
Chronic Renal Failure

Jacques Kremer, PhD
Postdoctoral Program, Institute of Immunology, National Laboratory of Health, Luxembourg, Luxembourg
Measles (Rubeola)

John N. Krieger, MD
Professor of Urology, University of Washington School of Medicine; Chief of Urology, Veterans Affairs Puget Sound Health Care System, Seattle, Washington
Bacterial Infections of the Male Urinary Tract; Epididymitis; Nongonococcal Urethritis

Roshni Kulkarni, MD
Professor, Department of Pediatrics and Human Development, Michigan State University College of Medicine, East Lansing, Michigan
Hemophilia and Related Bleeding Disorders

Bhushan Kumar, MD, MNAMS
Former Professor and Head, Department of Dermatology, Postgraduate Institute of Medical Education and Research, Chandigarh, India
Leprosy

Seema Kumar, MD
Assistant Professor of Pediatrics, Mayo Clinic College of Medicine; Consultant, Division of Pediatrics, Endocrinology, and Metabolism, Department of Pediatrics, Mayo Clinic, Rochester, Minnesota
Obesity

Lori M. B. Laffel, MD, MPH
Associate Professor of Pediatrics, Harvard Medical School; Chief, Pediatric, Adolescent, and Young Adult Section, and Investigator, Section on Genetics and Epidemiology, Joslin Diabetes Center, Boston, Massachusetts
Diabetes Mellitus in Children and Adolescents

Julius Larioza, MD
Attending Physician, Bay State Medical Center, Springfield, Massachusetts
Toxic Shock Syndrome

Jerome Larkin, MD
Assistant Professor of Medicine, Warren Alpert Medical School at Brown University; Attending Physician, Rhode Island Hospital, Providence, Rhode Island
Severe Sepsis and Septic Shock

Andrew B. Lassman, MD
Department of Neurology and Brain Tumor Center, Memorial Sloan-Kettering Cancer Center, New York, New York
Brain Tumors

Barbara A. Latenser, MD
Clara L. Smith Professor of Burn Treatment, Department of Surgery, University of Iowa Carver College of Medicine; Medical Director, Burn Treatment Center, University of Iowa Hospitals and Clinics, Iowa City, Iowa
Burn Treatment Guidelines

Christine L. Lau, MD
Assistant Professor of Surgery, Division of Thoracic and Cardiovascular Surgery, University of Virginia School of Medicine, Charlottesville, Virginia
Atelectasis

Yung R. Lau, MD
Professor of Pediatric Cardiology, University of Alabama at Birmingham School of Medicine, Birmingham, Alabama
Congenital Heart Disease

Susan Lawrence-Hylland, MD
Clinical Assistant Professor, Rheumatology Section, University of Wisconsin Hospital and Clinics, Madison, Wisconsin
Autoimmune Connective Tissue Disease

Miguel A. Leal, MD
Clinical Instructor and Cardiovascular Medicine Fellow, University of Wisconsin Hospital and Clinics, Madison, Wisconsin
Pericarditis and Pericardial Effusions

Jerrold B. Leikin, MD
Professor of Emergency Medicine, Northwestern University Feinberg School of Medicine; Professor of Medicine, Rush Medical College, Chicago; Director of Medical Toxicology, Evanston Northwestern Healthcare–Omega, Glenbrook Hospital, Glenview, Illinois
Disturbance Due to Cold

Bruce B. Lerman, MD
Professor of Medicine and Chief, Division of Cardiology, Weill Cornell Medical College; Director, Cardiac Electrophysiology Laboratory, NewYork-Presbyterian Hospital, New York, New York
Tachycardias

Jeffrey A. Linder, MD, MPH, FACP
Assistant Professor of Medicine, Harvard Medical School; Associate Physician, Division of General Medicine and Primary Care, Brigham and Women's Hospital, Boston, Massachusetts
Influenza

Gary H. Lipscomb, MD
Professor and Director, Division of General Obstetrics and Gynecology, Department of Obstetrics and Gynecology, Northwestern University Feinberg School of Medicine, Chicago, Illinois
Ectopic Pregnancy

James A. Litch, MD, DTMH
Clinical Assistant Professor, University of Washington School of Medicine and School of Public Health and Community Medicine, Seattle, Washington
High-Altitude Illness

Rita Lloyd, MD
Associate Professor of Dermatology, University of Wisconsin School of Medicine and Public Health, Madison, Wisconsin
Contact Dermatitis

James Lock, MD
Professor of Child Psychiatry and Pediatrics, Stanford University School of Medicine; Medical Director, Eating Disorder Program, Lucile Packard Children's Hospital, Stanford, California
Bulimia Nervosa

Frederick L. Locke, MD
Fellow, Hematology/Oncology, Department of Medicine, University of Chicago Medical Center, Chicago, Illinois
Non-Hodgkin's Lymphoma

Benjamin J. Luft, MD
Edmund D. Pellegrino Professor of Medicine, Stony Brook University Medical Center School of Medicine, Stony Brook, New York
Toxoplasmosis

Kelly E. Lyons, PhD
Research Associate Professor, Department of Neurology, University of Kansas School of Medicine, Kansas City, Kansas
Parkinsonism

James M. Lyznicki, MS, MPH
Associate Director, Center for Public Health Preparedness and Disaster Response, American Medical Association, Chicago, Illinois
Toxic Chemical Agents Reference Chart: Symptoms and Treatment; Biologic Agents Reference Chart—Symptoms, Tests, and Treatment

Robert D. Madoff, MD
Professor of Surgery, University of Minnesota Medical School, Minneapolis, Minnesota
Hemorrhoids, Anal Fissure, and Anorectal Abscess and Fistula

Srijoy Mahapatra, MD
Assistant Professor of Medicine and Biomedical Engineering, University of Virginia School of Medicine, Charlottesville, Virginia
Acquired Diseases of the Aorta

Bahaa S. Malaeb, MD
Resident Urologist, University of Minnesota Medical School, Minneapolis, Minnesota
Trauma to the Genitourinary Tract

Edward E. Manche, MD
Professor of Ophthalmology and Director of Cornea and Refractive Surgery, Stanford University School of Medicine, Stanford, California
Vision Correction Procedures

Annette Mankertz, PhD
Assistant Professor, Faculty of Biology, Chemistry, and Pharmacy, Free University of Berlin; Head of Laboratory, Division of Viral Infection, Robert Koch Institute, Berlin, Germany
Rubella and Congenital Rubella Syndrome

Christopher R. Mantyh, MD
Associate Professor and Chief of Gastrointestinal and Colorectal Surgery, Duke University School of Medicine, Durham, North Carolina
Diverticula of the Alimentary Tract

Lynette Margesson, MD, FRCPC
Assistant Professor of Medicine (Dermatology) and Obstetrics and Gynecology, Dartmouth Medical School, Lebanon; Associated Admitting Staff, Elliot Hospital; Consulting Staff, Catholic Medical Center, Manchester, New Hampshire
Anogenital Pruritus

Ali J. Marian, MD
Professor of Medicine (Cardiology) and Molecular Medicine, Brown Foundation Institute of Molecular Medicine, University of Texas Health Science Center; Staff Cardiologist, Texas Heart Institute at St. Luke's Episcopal Hospital, Houston, Texas
Hypertrophic Cardiomyopathy

Thomas J. Marrie, MD
Dean, Dalhousie University Faculty of Medicine, Halifax, Nova Scotia, Canada
Q Fever

Paul Martin, MD
Chief, Division of Hepatology, Schiff Liver Institute/Center for Liver Diseases, University of Miami Miller School of Medicine, Miami, Florida
Cirrhosis

Vickie Martin, MD
Resident, Department of Obstetrics and Gynecology, Kingston General Hospital, Kingston, Ontario, Canada
Amenorrhea

Pierre Marty, MD, PhD
Professor of Parasitology-Mycology, University of Nice; Head, Department of Mycology-Parasitology, Nice Regional Hospital Center, Nice, France
Visceral Leishmaniasis

Maria Mascarenhas, MBBS
Associate Professor of Pediatrics, University of Pennsylvania School of Medicine; Section Chief, Nutrition Division of Gastroenterology and Nutrition; Director, Nutrition Support Service, The Children's Hospital of Philadelphia, Philadelphia, Pennsylvania
Normal Infant Feeding

Pinckney J. Maxwell IV, MD
Assistant Professor of Surgery, Division of Colon and Rectal Surgery, Jefferson Medical College of Thomas Jefferson University, Philadelphia, Pennsylvania
Tumors of the Colon and Rectum

Ali Mazloom, MD
Graduate Student, University of Texas School of Public Health, Houston, Texas
Hodgkin's Disease: Radiation Therapy

Anthony L. McCall, MD, PhD
James M. Moss Professor of Diabetes, University of Virginia School of Medicine; Endocrinologist, University of Virginia Health Care System, Charlottesville, Virginia
Diabetes Mellitus in Adults

Michael T. McCann, MD
Clinical Assistant Professor, Baylor College of Medicine, Houston, Texas
Spine Pain

Laura J. McCloskey, PhD
Assistant Professor of Pathology, Anatomy, and Cell Biology, Jefferson Medical College of Thomas Jefferson University; Associate Director, Clinical Laboratories, Thomas Jefferson University Hospitals, Philadelphia, Pennsylvania
Reference Intervals for the Interpretation of Laboratory Tests

Michael McGuigan, MD
Medical Director, Long Island Regional Poison and Drug Information Center, Winthrop-University Hospital, Mineola, New York
Medical Toxicology: Ingestions, Inhalations, and Dermal and Ocular Absorptions

Dilcia McLenan, MD
Assistant Professor of Pediatrics, Baylor College of Medicine, Pearland, Texas
Care of the High-Risk Neonate

D. Scott McMeekin, MD
Presbyterian Foundation Presidential Professor, University of Oklahoma College of Medicine; Section Chief, Gynecologic Oncology, University of Oklahoma Health Sciences Center, Oklahoma City, Oklahoma
Cancer of the Endometrium

J. Scott McMurray, MD
Associate Professor of Pediatric Otolaryngology, Department of Surgery, University of Wisconsin School of Medicine and Public Health, Madison, Wisconsin
Otitis Media

Donald McNeil, MD
Associate Professor of Clinical Medicine, Department of Immunology, The Ohio State University College of Medicine and Public Health, Columbus, Ohio
Allergic Reactions to Drugs

Mario F. Mendez, MD, PhD
Professor, Department of Neurology and Department of Psychiatry and Biobehavioral Sciences, David Geffen School of Medicine at UCLA; Attending Physician, Neurobehavior Unit, Veterans Affairs Greater Los Angeles Healthcare System, Los Angeles, California
Alzheimer's Disease

Moises Mercado, MD
Professor of Medicine, Faculty of Medicine, Universidad Nacional Autónoma de México; Head, Endocrine Service, and Experimental Endocrinology Unit, Hospital de Especialidades, Centro Médico Nacional Siglo XXI, Instituto Mexicano del Segero Social, Mexico City, Mexico
Acromegaly

Ralph M. Meyer, MD
Edith Eisenhauer Chair in Clinical Oncology and Professor, Departments of Oncology, Medicine, and Community Health and Epidemiology, Queen's University Faculty of Medicine; Director, Institute of Canada Clinical Trials Group at Queen's University, Kingston, Ontario, Canada
Hodgkin's Lymphoma

Brian Miller, MD, MPH
Chief Resident, General Psychiatry, Medical College of Georgia, Augusta, Georgia
Schizophrenia

Peter A. Millward, MD
Medical Director, Transfusion Medicine, William Beaumont
Hospital, Royal Oak, Michigan
Therapeutic Use of Blood Components

Howard C. Mofenson, MD
Professor of Pediatrics and Emergency Medicine, Stony Brook
University Medical Center School of Medicine, Stony Brook;
Professor of Pharmacology and Toxicology, New York College of
Osteopathic Medicine, Old Westbury, New York
*Medical Toxicology: Ingestions, Inhalations, and Dermal and Ocular
Absorptions*

Terry L. Moore, MD
Professor of Internal Medicine, Pediatrics, and Molecular Microbiology
and Immunology, Saint Louis University School of Medicine; Director,
Division of Rheumatology and Pediatric Rheumatology, Saint Louis
University Medical Center, St. Louis, Missouri
Juvenile Idiopathic Arthritis

Enrique Morales, MD
Attending Nephrologist, Hospital 12 de Octubre, Madrid, Spain
Primary Glomerular Diseases

Rita Moretti, MD
Head Researcher, Neurodegenerative Disorders, Department of
Clinical Medicine and Neurology, University of Trieste, Trieste, Italy
Hiccups

Warwick L. Morison, MD
Professor of Dermatology, Johns Hopkins University School of
Medicine, Baltimore, Maryland
Sunburn

Lee E. Morrow, MD, MSc
Associate Professor of Medicine, Department of Internal Medicine,
Division of Pulmonary, Critical Care, and Sleep Medicine, Creighton
University School of Medicine, Omaha, Nebraska
Primary Lung Abscess

Arnold M. Moses, MD, FACP, FACE
SUNY Distinguished Service Professor of Medicine, SUNY Upstate
Medical University College of Medicine; Attending, University
Hospital, Syracuse, New York
Diabetes Insipidus

Scott Moses, MD
Medical Staff, Fairview Lakes Regional Medical Center, Wyoming,
Minnesota
Pruritus

Steven F. Moss, MD
Associate Professor of Medicine, Warren Alpert Medical School of
Brown University; Director, Gastroenterology Fellowship Training
Program, Rhode Island Hospital, Providence, Rhode Island
Gastritis and Peptic Ulcer Disease

Ladan Mostaghimi, MD
Assistant Professor, University of Wisconsin School of Medicine and
Public Health; Clinical Assistant Professor, University of Wisconsin
Hospital and Clinics, Madison, Wisconsin
Psychocutaneous Medicine

Claude P. Muller, MD
Immunology, University of Trier Faculty of Medicine, Trier;
Experimental Medicine, University of Saarland Faculty of Medicine,
Homburg, Germany; HOD Institute of Immunology, National
Laboratory of Health, Luxembourg, Luxembourg
Measles (Rubeola)

Miho Murashima, MD
Staff Physician, Department of Nephrology, Kyoto Katsura Hospital,
Kyoto, Japan
Hypertension

Michael Murphy, MD
Associate Professor, Department of Dermatology, University of
Connecticut School of Medicine; Attending Physician, John Dempsey
Hospital–University of Connecticut Health Center, Farmington,
Connecticut
Melanocytic Nevi

Tashanna K. N. Myers, MD
Fellow in Gynecologic Oncology, University of Oklahoma Health
Sciences Center, Oklahoma City, Oklahoma
Cancer of the Endometrium

Nicole Nader, MD
Instructor, Mayo Clinic College of Medicine; Fellow, Division of
Pediatric Endocrinology and Metabolism, Department of Pediatrics,
Mayo Clinic, Rochester, Minnesota
Obesity

Alykhan S. Nagji, MD
Resident, Department of Surgery, University of Virginia School of
Medicine, Charlottesville, Virginia
Atelectasis

Ramaswami Nalini, MBBS
Assistant Professor of Medicine, Division of Diabetes, Endocrinology,
and Metabolism, Baylor College of Medicine; Endocrine Service, Ben
Taub General Hospital, Houston, Texas
Osteoporosis

David N. Neubauer, MD
Assistant Professor, Johns Hopkins University School of Medicine;
Associate Director, Johns Hopkins Sleep Disorders Center, Baltimore,
Maryland
Sleep Disorders

David H. Neustadt, MD
Clinical Professor of Medicine, University of Louisville School of
Medicine; Senior Attending, University Hospital, Jewish Hospital,
and Norton Hospital, Louisville, Kentucky
Osteoarthritis

Thomas Newton, MC
Professor, Baylor College of Medicine, Houston, Texas
Treatment for Addiction

Douglas E. Ney, MD
Assistant Professor, University of Colorado Denver School of
Medicine; Attending Physician, University of Colorado Hospital,
Aurora, Colorado
Brain Tumors

Richard Ohrbach, DDS, PhD
Department of Oral Diagnostic Sciences, State University of
New York at Buffalo School of Dental Medicine, Buffalo,
New York
Temporomandibular Disorders and Orofacial Pain

David L. Olive, MD
Professor of Obstetrics and Gynecology, University of
Wisconsin School of Medicine and Public Health, Madison,
Wisconsin
Endometriosis

Peck Y. Ong, MD
Assistant Professor of Clinical Pediatrics, Keck School of Medicine of USC; Attending Physician, Children's Hospital Los Angeles, Los Angeles, California
Atopic Dermatitis

Ike Onwere, MD
Hematology/Oncology Fellow, University of Iowa Carver College of Medicine, Iowa City, Iowa
Polycythemia Vera

Finbar D. O'Shea, MB, MRCPI
Spondylitis Fellow, Arthritis Center of Excellence, Toronto Western Hospital, Toronto, Ontario, Canada
Ankylosing Spondylitis

Matthew T. Oughton, MD, FRCPC
Assistant Professor, Department of Medicine, McGill University Faculty of Medicine; Infectious Disease Physician, Sir Mortimer B. Davis–Jewish General Hospital, Montreal, Quebec, Canada
Acute Infectious Diarrhea

Gary D. Overturf, MD
Professor of Pediatrics and Pathology Emeritus, University of New Mexico School of Medicine; Medical Director, Infectious Diseases, TriCore Reference Laboratories, Albuquerque, New Mexico
Bacterial Meningitis

Scott Owings, MD
Clinical Assistant Professor, Department of Family and Community Medicine, University of Kansas School of Medicine, Wichita; Associate Director, Smoky Hill Family Medicine Residency, Salina, Kansas
Gaseousness and Dyspepsia

Kerem Ozer, MD
Instructor, Departments of Medicine and Endocrinology, Baylor College of Medicine, Houston, Texas
Dyslipoproteinemias

Rajesh Pahwa, MD
Professor of Neurology, University of Kansas School of Medicine, Kansas City, Kansas
Parkinsonism

Trish Palmer, MD
Assistant Professor, Departments of Family Medicine and Orthopedic Surgery, Rush Medical College, Chicago, Illinois
Pain

Pratik Pandharipande, MD, MSCI
Associate Professor of Anesthesiology/Critical Care, Vanderbilt University Medical Center, Nashville, Tennessee
Delirium

Sangtae Park, MD, MPH
Clinical Assistant Professor of Urology, University of Chicago Pritzker School of Medicine, Chicago, Illinois
Renal Calculi

Christopher M. Parry, PhD, MRCP, FRCPath
Senior Clinical Research Fellow, Oxford University Clinical Research Unit, Hospital for Tropical Diseases, Ho Chi Minh City, Viet Nam
Typhoid Fever

Jotam Pasipanodya, MD
Research Scientist, University of Texas Southwestern Medical Center at Dallas, Dallas, Texas
Tuberculosis and Other Mycobacterial Diseases

Manish R. Patel, DO
Oncology Fellow, University of Minnesota Medical School, Minneapolis, Minnesota
Primary Lung Cancer

Manisha J. Patel, MD
Assistant Professor of Dermatology, Johns Hopkins University School of Medicine; Medical Director, Johns Hopkins Outpatient Center, Department of Dermatology, Baltimore, Maryland
Cutaneous Vasculitis

Alexander Perez, MD
Assistant Professor of Surgery, Duke University School of Medicine, Durham, North Carolina
Diverticula of the Alimentary Tract

Allen Perkins, MD, MPH
Professor and Chairman, Department of Family Medicine, University of South Alabama College of Medicine, Mobile, Alabama
Marine Poisonings, Envenomations, and Trauma

Jay Peters, MD
Professor of Medicine, University of Texas Health Science Center at San Antonio School of Medicine; Chief, Pulmonary and Critical Care Division, University of Texas Health Science Center at San Antonio, San Antonio, Texas
Management of Chronic Obstructive Pulmonary Disease

William A. Petri, Jr., MD, PhD
Chief, Division of Infectious Disease and International Health, University of Virginia Medical Center, Charlottesville, Virginia
Amebiasis

Michael E. Pichichero, MD
Director of Research, Department of Immunology and Center for Infectious Disease, Rochester General Hospital Research Institute, Rochester, New York
Pertussis

Melissa Piliang, MD
Staff, Departments of Dermatology and Pathology, Cleveland Clinic, Cleveland, Ohio
Diseases of the Hair

Pierre-François Plouin, MD
Professor of Cardiovascular Medicine, Université Paris-Descartes; Head, Hypertension Unit, Hôpital Emopeen G. Pompladh, Paris, France
Pheochromocytomas

Daniel K. Podolsky, MD
Professor of Internal Medicine, University of Texas Southwestern Medical School; Philip O'Bryan Montgomery, Jr., MD, Distinguished Presidential Chair in Academic Administration and Doris and Bryan Wildenthal Distinguished Chair in Medical Science, University of Texas Southwestern Medical Center, Dallas, Texas
Inflammatory Bowel Disease: Crohn's Disease and Ulcerative Colitis

Manuel Praga, MD
Associate Professor of Medicine, Universidad Complutense; Head, Nephrology Department, Hospital 12 de Octubre, Madrid, Spain
Primary Glomerular Diseases

Abhiram Prasad, MD
Associate Professor of Medicine, Mayo Clinic College of Medicine, Rochester, Minnesota
Acute Myocardial Infarction

Daniel Pratt, MD
Assistant Professor of Medicine, Harvard Medical School; Director, Liver-Biliary-Pancreas Center, Massachusetts General Hospital, Boston, Massachusetts
Acute and Chronic Viral Hepatitis

Richard A. Prinz, MD
Helen Shedd Keith Professor and Chairman, Department of General Surgery, Rush Medical College; Chairman, Department of General Surgery, Rush University Medical Center, Chicago, Illinois
Thyroid Cancer

David Puchalsky, MD
Associate Professor of Dermatology, University of Wisconsin School of Medicine and Public Health, Madison, Wisconsin
Papulosquamous Eruptions—Psoriasis

David M. Quillen, MD
Department of Community Health and Family Medicine, University of Florida College of Medicine; Attending Physician, Shands at the University of Florida, Gainesville, Florida
Allergic Rhinitis Caused by Inhalant Factors

Beth W. Rackow, MD
Assistant Professor, Department of Obstetrics, Gynecology and Reproductive Sciences, Yale University School of Medicine, New Haven, Connecticut
Abnormal Uterine Bleeding

Peter S. Rahko, MD
Professor of Medicine, University of Wisconsin School of Medicine and Public Health; Director of Echocardiography, University of Wisconsin Hospitals and Clinics, Madison, Wisconsin
Mitral Valve Prolapse

Kirk D. Ramin, MD
Associate Professor and Director, Maternal-Fetal Medicine Fellowship Program, Department of Obstetrics and Gynecology, University of Minnesota Medical School, Minneapolis, Minnesota
Antepartum Care

Julio A. Ramirez, MD
Professor of Medicine, University of Louisville School of Medicine; Chief, Division of Infectious Diseases, Department of Veterans Affairs Medical Center, Louisville, Kentucky
Legionellosis

Lakshmi N. Ravindran, MD
Assistant Professor, University of Toronto Faculty of Medicine; Staff Psychiatrist, Mood and Anxiety Program, Centre for Addiction and Mental Health, Toronto, Ontario, Canada
Panic Disorder

Elizabeth Reddy, MD
Fellow, Department of Medicine, Division of Infectious Disease, Duke University, Durham, North Carolina
Intestinal Parasites

Guy S. Reeder, MD
Professor of Medicine, Mayo Clinic College of Medicine, Rochester, Minnesota
Acute Myocardial Infarction

Ian R. Reid, MD
Professor of Medicine and Endocrinology, University of Auckland Faculty of Medical and Health Sciences School of Medicine, Auckland, New Zealand
Paget's Disease of Bone

George T. Reizner, MD
Professor of Dermatology, University of Wisconsin School of Medicine and Public Health; Attending Physician, University of Wisconsin Hospital and Clinics, Madison, Wisconsin
Melanoma

Robert L. Reid, MD
Professor, Department of Obstetrics and Gynecology, Queen's University Faculty of Medicine; Chair, Division of Reproductive Endocrinology and Infertility, Kingston General Hospital, Kingston, Ontario, Canada
Amenorrhea

Douglas S. Richards, MD
Professor, Department of Obstetrics and Gynecology, and Director, Obstetric and Gynecologic Ultrasound, University of Florida College of Medicine, Gainesville, Florida
Hemolytic Disease of the Fetus and Newborn

James R. Roberts, MD
Professor of Emergency Medicine and Senior Consultant in Medical Toxicology, Drexel University College of Medicine; Chairman of Emergency Medicine and Director, Division of Toxicology, Mercy Hospital of Philadelphia, Philadelphia, Pennsylvania
Spider Bites and Scorpion Stings

Jason R. Roberts, MD
Gastrointestinal Fellow, Medical University of South Carolina, Charleston, South Carolina
Gastroesophageal Reflux Disease

Jenice Robinson, MD
Assistant Professor of Neurology, Pennsylvania State College of Medicine, Hershey, Pennsylvania
Myasthenia Gravis and Related Disorders

Malcolm K. Robinson, MD
Assistant Professor of Surgery, Harvard Medical School; Metabolic Support Service, Department of Surgery, Brigham and Women's Hospital, Boston, Massachusetts
Parenteral Nutrition in Adults

Griffin P. Rodgers, MD
Director, National Institute of Diabetes, Digestive, and Kidney Disorders; Chief, Molecular and Clinical Hematology Branch, National Institutes of Health, Bethesda, Maryland
Sickle Cell Disease

Nidra Rodriguez, MD
Assistant Professor of Pediatric Hematology, University of Texas Medical School at Houston and University of Texas M. D. Anderson Cancer Center, Houston, Texas
Autoimmune Hemolytic Anemia

Robb L. Romp, MD
Assistant Professor of Pediatric Cardiology, University of Alabama at Birmingham School of Medicine, Birmingham, Alabama
Congenital Heart Disease

Steven P. Roose, MD
Columbia University College of Physicians and Surgeons; New York State Psychiatric Institute, New York, New York
Mood Disorders

Peter G. Rose, MD
Case Western Reserve University School of Medicine; Section Head, Gynecologic Oncology, Cleveland Clinic, Cleveland, Ohio
Ovarian Cancer

Eric Rosenthal, MD, PhD
Professor of Internal Medicine, Nice Sophia Antipolis University Faculty of Medicine; Head, Unit of Internal Medicine, Nice Regional Medical Center, Archet Hospital, Nice, France
Visceral Leishmaniasis

Richard N. Rosenthal, MD
Professor of Clinical Psychiatry, Columbia University College of Physicians and Surgeons; Chairman, Department of Psychiatry, St. Luke's–Roosevelt Hospital Center, New York, New York
Alcoholism

Anne E. Rosin, MD
Associate Professor of Dermatology, University of Wisconsin School of Medicine and Public Health; Attending Physician, University of Wisconsin Hospital and Clinics, Madison, Wisconsin
Warts (Verruca)

David S. Rubenstein, MD, PhD
Professor of Dermatology, University of North Carolina at Chapel Hill School of Medicine; Staff, Department of Dermatology, University of North Carolina Hospitals, Chapel Hill, North Carolina
Bullous Diseases

Beth K. Rubinstein, MD
Assistant Professor of Medicine, Division of Rheumatology, Allergy, and Immunology, Virginia Commonwealth University School of Medicine, Richmond, Virginia
Hyperuricemia and Gout

Bret R. Rutherford, MD
Columbia University College of Physicians and Surgeons; New York State Psychiatric Institute, New York, New York
Mood Disorders

Erik K. St. Louis, MD
Senior Associate Consultant, Departments of Neurology and Medicine, Mayo Clinic and Foundation, Rochester, Minnesota
Seizures and Epilepsy in Adolescents and Adults

Susan L. Samson, MD, PhD
Assistant Professor, Department of Medicine, Baylor College of Medicine; Attending Physician, Ben Taub General Hospital, Houston, Texas
Hyponatremia; Hypopituitarism

Steven R. Sarkisian, Jr., MD
Clinical Assistant Professor, University of Oklahoma Health Sciences Center; Dean, McGee Eye Institute, Oklahoma City, Oklahoma
Glaucoma

J. Terry Saunders, PhD
Assistant Professor of Medical Education in Internal Medicine, University of Virginia School of Medicine, Charlottesville, Virginia
Diabetes Mellitus in Adults

Barry M. Schaitkin, MD
Professor of Otolaryngology, University of Pittsburgh School of Medicine; Residency Program Director, University of Pittsburgh Medical Center, Pittsburgh, Pennsylvania
Acute Peripheral Facial Paralysis (Bell's Palsy)

Ralph M. Schapira, MD
Professor and Vice Chair, Department of Medicine, Medical College of Wisconsin; Staff Physician, Milwaukee Veterans Affairs Medical Center, Milwaukee, Wisconsin
Acute Bronchitis

Michael Schatz, MD, MS
Clinical Professor, Department of Medicine, University of California, San Diego, School of Medicine, La Jolla; Chief, Department of Allergy, Kaiser Permanente, San Diego, California
Asthma in Adolescents and Adults

Stacey A. Scheib, MD
Resident Physician, Department of Obstetrics and Gynecology, Thomas Jefferson University Hospital, Philadelphia, Pennsylvania
Menopause

Lawrence R. Schiller, MD
Clinical Professor of Internal Medicine, University of Texas Southwestern Medical School; Attending Physician, Digestive Health Associates of Texas; Program Director, Gastroenterology Fellowship, Baylor University Medical Center, Dallas, Texas
Malabsorption

Kerrie Schoffer, MD, FRCPC
Assistant Professor in Neurology, Dalhousie University Faculty of Medicine; Neurologist, QEII Health Sciences Centre, Halifax, Nova Scotia, Canada
Peripheral Neuropathies

Kevin Schroeder, MD
Program Director, Transitional Year, and Medical Director of Acute Dialysis, Riverside Methodist Hospital, Columbus, Ohio
Acute Renal Failure

Robert A. Schwartz, MD, MPH
Professor and Head of Dermatology, UMDNJ–New Jersey Medical School, Newark, New Jersey
Pigmentary Disorders

Carlos Seas, MD
Associate Professor of Medicine, Universidad Peruana Cayetano Heredia; Chief, Inservice Department, Hospital National Cayetano Heredia, Lima, Peru
Cholera

Steven A. Seifert, MD, FAACT, FACMT
Professor, University of New Mexico School of Medicine; Medical Director, New Mexico Poison Center, Albuquerque, New Mexico
Venomous Snakebite

Edward Septimus, MD
Affiliated Professor, George Mason University School of Public Policy, Fairfax, Virginia; Medical Director, Infection Prevention, HCA Healthcare System, Nashville, Tennessee
Bacterial Pneumonia

Daniel J. Sexton, MD
Professor of Medicine, Duke University School of Medicine, Durham, North Carolina
Rickettsial and Ehrlichial Infections

Beejal Shah, MD
Assistant Professor, Department of Medicine, Baylor College of Medicine; Attending Physician, Ben Taub General Hospital, Houston, Texas
Hyponatremia; Primary Aldosteronism

Mrunal Shah, MD
Clinical Assistant Professor of Family Medicine, The Ohio State University College of Medicine and Public Health; Assistant Program Director, Riverside Family Practice Residency Program, Riverside Methodist Hospital, Columbus, Ohio
Syphilis

Vijay H. Shah, MD
Professor of Medicine, Mayo Clinic College of Medicine, Rochester, Minnesota
Bleeding Esophageal Varices

Morali Sharma, MD
Associate Professor, Department of Medicine, Division of Endocrinology, Baylor College of Medicine, Houston, Texas
Hyperprolactinemia

Chelsea A. Sheppard, MD
Transfusion Medicine Program, Department of Pathology and Laboratory Medicine, Emory University School of Medicine, Atlanta, Georgia
Adverse Effects of Blood Transfusion

Mona Shimshi, MD
Assistant Professor, Mount Sinai School of Medicine, New York; Staff Physician, James J. Peters Veterans Affairs Medical Center, Bronx, New York
Hypothyroidism

Julie Shott, MD
Sports Medicine Fellow, Riverside Methodist Hospital, Columbus, Ohio
Common Sports Injuries

Tamara Simpson, MD
Assistant Professor of Medicine in Pulmonary/Critical Care, University of Texas Health Science Center at San Antonio School of Medicine; Staff, Pulmonary Division, University of Texas Health Science Center at San Antonio, San Antonio, Texas
Management of Chronic Obstructive Pulmonary Disease

Upinder Singh, MD
Assistant Professor of Medicine (Infectious Diseases), Stanford University School of Medicine, Stanford, California
Travel Medicine

Michael J. Smith, MD, MSCE
Assistant Professor, Department of Pediatrics, University of Louisville School of Medicine; Attending Physician, Division of Pediatric Infectious Diseases, Kosair Children's Hospital, Louisville, Kentucky
Cat-Scratch Disease

Sonali M. Smith, MD
Assistant Professor of Medicine, University of Chicago Pritzker School of Medicine, Chicago, Illinois
Non-Hodgkin's Lymphoma

Stephen N. Snow, MD
Professor of Dermatology, University of Wisconsin School of Medicine and Public Health; Staff Physician, University of Wisconsin Hospital and Clinics, Madison, Wisconsin
Cancer of the Skin

Miguel Angel Solis, Jr., MD
Sports Medicine Physician, Laredo Sports Medicine Clinic, Laredo, Texas
Bursitis, Tendinitis, Myofascial Pain, and Fibromyalgia

Suman L. Sood, MD
Instructor of Medicine, Division of Hematology/Oncology, University of Pennsylvania School of Medicine; Attending Physician, Penn Comprehensive Hemophilia and Thrombosis Program, Hospital of the University of Pennsylvania, Philadelphia, Pennsylvania
Platelet-Mediated Bleeding Disorders

Murray B. Stein, MD
Professor of Psychiatry and Family and Preventive Medicine, University of California, San Diego, School of Medicine, La Jolla; Adjunct Professor of Psychology, San Diego State University, San Diego, California
Panic Disorder

Dennis L. Stevens, MD, PhD
Professor of Medicine, University of Washington School of Medicine, Seattle, Washington; Chief, Infectious Diseases, Veterans Affairs Medical Center, Boise, Idaho
Bacterial Diseases of the Skin

Catherine Stevens-Simon, MD*
Formerly Associate Professor of Pediatrics, Division of Adolescent Medicine, University of Colorado Denver School of Medicine; Staff Physician, The Children's Hospital, Aurora, Colorado
Chlamydia trachomatis

A. Keith Stewart, MB, ChB
Senior Associate Consultant, Mayo Clinic, Scottsdale, Arizona
Multiple Myeloma

Christopher D. Still, DO
Medical Director, Center for Nutrition and Weight Management, Department of Gastroenterology and Nutrition, Geisinger Health Care System, Danville, Pennsylvania
Obesity

Brenda Stokes, MD
Assistant Clinical Professor of Family Medicine, University of Virginia School of Medicine, Charlottesville; Assistant Clinical Professor, Department of Family Medicine, Virginia Commonwealth University School of Medicine, Richmond; Medical Staff, Centra Health–Lynchburg General and Virginia Baptist Hospitals, Lynchburg, Virginia
Hypertensive Disorders of Pregnancy; Postpartum Care

Harris Strokoff, MD
Child and Adolescent Psychiatrist, Northwestern Counseling and Support Services, Saint Albans, Vermont
Attention-Deficit/Hyperactivity Disorder

Shyam Subramanian, MD
Baylor College of Medicine, Houston, Texas
Sleep Apnea

Paniti Sukumvanich, MD
Fellow, Breast Service, Department of Surgery, Memorial Sloan-Kettering Cancer Center, New York, New York
Diseases of the Breast

Prabhakar P. Swaroop, MD
Assistant Professor of Internal Medicine, University of Texas Southwestern Medical Center at Dallas, Dallas, Texas
Inflammatory Bowel Disease: Crohn's Disease and Ulcerative Colitis

Jessica P. Swartout, MD
Fellow in Maternal-Fetal Medicine, Department of Obstetrics and Gynecology, University of Minnesota Medical School, Minneapolis, Minnesota
Antepartum Care

Matthew D. Taylor, MD
Resident, Department of Surgery, University of Virginia Medical Center, Charlottesville, Virginia
Atelectasis

*Deceased

Edmond Teng, MD, PhD
Assistant Professor, Department of Neurology, David Geffen School of Medicine at UCLA; Neurobehavior Unit and Geriatric Research Education and Clinical Center, Veterans Affairs Greater Los Angeles Healthcare System, Los Angeles, California
Alzheimer's Disease

Ellen J. Teng, PhD
Assistant Professor, Department of Psychiatry, Baylor College of Medicine; Clinical Research Psychologist and Director of Psychology Training, Michael E. DeBakey Veterans Affairs Medical Center, Houston Texas
Anxiety Disorders

Joyce M. C. Teng, MD, PhD
Assistant Professor of Dermatology and Pediatrics, University of Wisconsin School of Medicine and Public Health; Attending Physician, University of Wisconsin Hospital and Clinics, Madison, Wisconsin
Urticaria and Angioedema

Manish Thapar, MD
Instructor, University of Missouri College of Medicine; Attending Physician, University Hospital, Columbia, Missouri
Porphyria

Nathan Thielman, MD, MPH
Duke Global Health Institute, Duke University, Durham, North Carolina
Intestinal Parasites

David R. Thomas, MD
Professor of Medicine, Division of Geriatric Medicine, Saint Louis University School of Medicine; Attending Physician, Saint Louis University Hospital, St. Louis, Missouri
Pressure Ulcers

Rodger E. Tiedemann, MB, ChB, PhD
Clinical Senior Lecturer in Medicine, University of Auckland Faculty of Medical and Health Sciences School of Medicine, Auckland, New Zealand; Research Associate, Mayo Clinic, Scottsdale, Arizona
Multiple Myeloma

Kenneth Tobin, DO
Clinical Assistant Professor, Western University of Health Sciences, College of Osteopathic Medicine of the Pacific, Pomona, California
Angina Pectoris

Paola Torre, MD
Head Researcher, Neurodegenerative Disorders, Department of Clinical Medicine and Neurology, University of Trieste, Trieste, Italy
Hiccups

Matthew P. Traynor, MD
Center for Sight, Idaho Falls, Idaho
Glaucoma

Maria Trent, MD, MPH
Assistant Professor of Pediatrics, Johns Hopkins University School of Medicine; Active Staff, Johns Hopkins Hospital Children's Center, Baltimore, Maryland
Pelvic Inflammatory Disease

Elaine B. Trujillo, MS, RD
Nutritionist, National Cancer Institute, National Institutes of Health, Bethesda, Maryland
Parenteral Nutrition in Adults

Papapit Tuchinda, MD
Instructor, Faculty of Medicine, Siriraj Hospital, Mahidol University, Bangkok, Thailand
Keloids

Arvid E. Underman, MD, FACP, DTMH
Clinical Professor of Medicine and Microbiology, Keck School of Medicine of USC, Los Angeles; Director of Graduate Medical Education, Huntington Hospital, Pasadena, California
Salmonellosis

Erin Vanness, MD
Clinical Assistant Professor, University of Wisconsin School of Medicine and Public Health, Madison, Wisconsin
Erythema Multiforme, Stevens-Johnson Syndrome, and Toxic Epidermal Necrolysis

Michele Van Vranken, MD
Staff Physician, Teenage Medical Services, Children's Hospital Minnesota, Minneapolis; Medical Director, West Suburban Teen Clinic, Excelsior; Medical Director, Annex Teen Clinic, Robbinsdale, Minnesota
Chancroid, Granuloma Inguinale (Donovanosis), and Lymphogranuloma Venereum

Vahan Vartanian, BS
Department of Urology, University of Chicago Pritzker School of Medicine, Chicago, Illinois
Renal Calculi

Brenda R. Velasco, MD
Gastroenterology Fellow, Temple University Hospital, Philadelphia, Pennsylvania
Irritable Bowel Syndrome

Donald C. Vinh, MD, FRCP(C), Dip(ABIM)
Division of Infectious Diseases, Department of Medicine, and Department of Medical Microbiology, McGill University Health Center, Montreal General Hospital, Montreal, Quebec, Canada
Necrotizing Skin and Soft Tissue Infections

Todd W. Vitaz, MD
Assistant Professor, Department of Neurological Surgery, University of Louisville School of Medicine; Director of Neurosurgical Oncology; Co-Director, Neurosciences ICU, Norton Hospital, Louisville, Kentucky
Management of Head Injuries

Jeffery T. Vrabec, MD
Associate Professor, Department of Otolaryngology–Head and Neck Surgery, Baylor College of Medicine; Clinical Associate Professor, Department of Head and Neck Surgery, University of Texas M. D. Anderson Cancer Center; Active Staff, Otolaryngology–Head and Neck Surgery, The Methodist Hospital; Courtesy Staff, Otolaryngology Service, Texas Children's Hospital, Houston, Texas
Otitis Externa

Ellen R. Wald, MD
Professor and Chair, Department of Pediatrics, University of Wisconsin School of Medicine and Public Health; Pediatrician-in-Chief, American Family Children's Hospital, Madison, Wisconsin
Urinary Tract Infections in Infants and Children

Shobha Wani, MD
Fellow, Section of Rheumatology, Washington Hospital Center, Washington, DC
Lyme Disease

Rungsima Wanitphakdeedecha, MD, MA, MSc
Instructor, Faculty of Medicine, Siriraj Hospital, Mahidol University, Bangkok, Thailand
Keloids

Bryan K. Ward, MD
Resident Physician, Johns Hopkins University School of Medicine, Baltimore, Maryland
Acute Peripheral Facial Paralysis (Bell's Palsy)

Anthony P. Weetman, MD, DSc
Professor of Medicine, The Medical School, University of Sheffield; Honorary Consultant Endocrinologist, Sheffield Teaching Hospitals, Sheffield, United Kingdom
Thyroiditis

Arthur Weinstein, MD, FACP, FACR
Professor of Medicine, Georgetown University School of Medicine; Associate Chairman, Department of Medicine, and Director, Section of Rheumatology, Washington Hospital Center, Washington, DC
Lyme Disease

Mitchell J. Weiss, MD, PhD
Associate Professor of Pediatrics, University of Pennsylvania School of Medicine; Attending Physician, The Children's Hospital of Philadelphia, Philadelphia, Pennsylvania
Nonimmune Hemolytic Anemia

David N. Weissman, MD
Adjunct Professor of Medicine and Microbiology (Immunology), West Virginia University School of Medicine; Director, Division of Respiratory Disease Studies, National Institute for Occupational Safety and Health, Morgantown, West Virginia
Pneumoconiosis

Robert C. Welliver, Sr., MD
Professor, State University of New York at Buffalo School of Medicine; Co-Director, Division of Infectious Diseases, Women and Children's Hospital of Buffalo, Buffalo, New York
Viral Respiratory Infections

Ryan Westergaard, MD
Postdoctoral Fellow, Division of Infectious Diseases, Johns Hopkins University School of Medicine, Baltimore, Maryland
The Patient with HIV Disease

Isaiah D. Wexler, MD, PhD
Department of Pediatrics and CF Center, Hadassah University Hospital-Mount Scopus Campus, Hadassah Hebrew University Medical Center, Jerusalem, Israel
Diabetic Ketoacidosis

David C. Whitcomb, MD, PhD
Giant Eagle Foundation Professor of Cancer Genetics; Professor of Medicine, Cell Biology, and Physiology; and Professor of Genetics, University of Pittsburgh School of Medicine; Chief of Gastroenterology, Hepatology, and Nutrition, University of Pittsburgh Medical Center, Pittsburgh, Pennsylvania
Acute and Chronic Pancreatitis

Russell D. White, MD
Professor, Department of Community and Family Medicine; Director, Sports Medicine Fellowship Program, University of Missouri-Kansas City School of Medicine, Truman Medical Center Lakewood, Kansas City, Missouri
Bursitis, Tendinitis, Myofascial Pain, and Fibromyalgia

William Wierda, MD, PhD
Associate Professor of Medicine, University of Texas Medical School at Houston/M. D. Anderson Cancer Center, Houston, Texas
Chronic Leukemias

Eliot C. Williams, MD
Professor, University of Wisconsin School of Medicine and Public Health; Attending Physician, University of Wisconsin Hospital and Clinics, Madison, Wisconsin
Disseminated Intravascular Coagulation

Steven R. Williams, MD
Clinical Assistant Professor, Department of Obstetrics and Gynecology, The Ohio State University College of Medicine and Public Health, Columbus, Ohio
Infertility

Robert A. Williamson, MD
Assistant Professor, Otology and Neurotology, Department of Otolaryngology–Head and Neck Surgery, Baylor College of Medicine, Houston, Texas
Meniere's Disease

Elaine Winkel, MD
Associate Professor of Medicine, University of Wisconsin School of Medicine and Public Health; Attending Cardiologist, Heart Failure and Transplant Program, University of Wisconsin Hospital and Clinics, Madison, Wisconsin
Heart Failure

Christopher M. Wise, MD
W. Robert Irby Professor of Medicine, Department of Medicine, Division of Rheumatology, Allergy, and Immunology, Virginia Commonwealth University School of Medicine, Richmond, Virginia
Hyperuricemia and Gout

Gary S. Wood, MD
Professor and Chairman, Department of Dermatology, University of Wisconsin School of Medicine and Public Health; Attending Physician, Veterans Affairs Medical Center, Madison, Wisconsin
Cutaneous T-Cell Lymphomas, Including Mycosis Fungoides and Sézary Syndrome

Jamie R. S. Wood, MD
Instructor in Pediatrics, Harvard Medical School; Research Associate, Sections on Genetics and Epidemiology and Vascular Cell Biology, and Staff Physician, Pediatric, Adolescent, and Young Adult Section, Joslin Diabetes Center, Boston, Massachusetts
Diabetes Mellitus in Children and Adolescents

Jon B. Woods, MD
Associate Professor of Pediatrics, Uniformed Services University of the Health Sciences F. Edward Hébert School of Medicine, Bethesda, Maryland; Pediatric Infectious Diseases, Wilford Hall Medical Center, Lackland Air Force Base, San Antonio, Texas
Anthrax

Steve W. Wu, MD
Assistant Professor, University of Cincinnati College of Medicine; Assistant Professor, Cincinnati Children's Hospital Medical Center, Cincinnati, Ohio
Gilles de la Tourette Syndrome

Yaohui G. Xu, MD, PhD
Assistant Professor, University of Wisconsin School of Medicine; Assistant Professor/Staff Physician, Department of Dermatology, University of Wisconsin Hospital and Clinics, Madison, Wisconsin
Cancer of the Skin

Vijay Yechoor, MD
Assistant Professor of Medicine, Division of Diabetes, Endocrinology, and Metabolism, Baylor College of Medicine, Houston, Texas
Cushing's Syndrome

Ronald F. Young, MD
Director of Neurosurgery, California Neuroscience Institute, St. John's Regional Medical Center, Oxnard, California
Trigeminal Neuralgia

David Zangen, MD
Senior Lecturer, Division of Pediatric Endocrinology, Hadassah Hebrew University Medical Center; Consultant in Pediatrics and Pediatric Endocrinology and Head of the Juvenile Diabetes and Pediatric Endocrinology Service, Hadassah Mt. Scopus and Hadassah Hebrew University Medical Center, Jerusalem, Israel
Diabetic Ketoacidosis

Jami Star Zeltzer, MD
Associate Professor, Department of Obstetrics and Gynecology, Division of Maternal-Fetal Medicine, University of Massachusetts Medical School, Worcester, Massachusetts
Vaginal Bleeding in Late Pregnancy

Wei Zhou, MD
Associate Professor of Surgery, Stanford University School of Medicine, Stanford, California
Peripheral Arterial Disease

Mary Zupanc, MD
Heidi Marie Bauman Chair of Epilepsy and Professor, Departments of Neurology and Pediatrics; Chief, Division of Pediatric Neurology, Medical College of Wisconsin; Director, Pediatric Comprehensive Epilepsy Program, and Director, Pediatric Neurology, Children's Hospital of Wisconsin, Milwaukee, Wisconsin
Epilepsy in Infants and Children

Preface

Conn's Current Therapy has appeared on the bookshelves of physicians and practices since 1949 when Dr. Conn developed and authored the first edition. His concept was to provide in one source the most recent advances in therapy for conditions encountered in practice. Experts were asked to give their "method" of treatment in a format that allowed quick reference for the busy doctor. Some less common diseases have always been included in Current Therapy because, although they may present less often, they can have serious consequences if not recognized, and because they are rarer, the need is even greater for guidance. Robert Rakel, MD, well-known scholar, became the editor in 1984 after Dr. Conn's rather sudden death and has continued the traditions of Current Therapy. Edward Bope, MD, teacher and clinician, joined Dr. Rakel in 2001 and serves today as the chief editor. Rick Kellerman, MD, joins Drs. Rakel and Bope this year.

Each year, new experts are asked to write their method for every topic. They are chosen based on recommendations from other experts and authors or because of their scholarly activity and research. Changing authors each year keeps the book crisp and up to date. Having experts explain their method adds a personal and practical tone to the book. Such practical wisdom is of immense value to today's physician, who typically is inundated with sometimes conflicting information from multiple sources. The authors provide references for their chapters in case the reader needs additional information or wants to see the evidence firsthand. Each year the topics are reviewed and new ones are added to keep the book current.

New features are also added, such as access to previous editions. Using this process, the reader can compare articles from year to year and find favorite topics and authors. It is possible to note variation in the way a disease is managed, which provides options that fit the physician's practice style and population needs.

Current Therapy is indeed an international book. Contributing authors from around the world offer advice about the diagnosis and management of conditions not common in the United States but increasingly seen here because we have a mobile society. The contribution of these international experts adds greatly to the comprehensive nature of the book, making it one of the only sources for treatment of diseases of the world.

Each chapter includes tables for Key Diagnostic and Key Therapeutic lists. These allow quick reference on a busy day or a review of material previously read. As always, tables, graphs, and figures are used when possible to present in-depth data in a convenient format. Authors are asked to present evidence for their treatment choices when possible. Careful attention is given to ensuring that all the information is correct and current. All of the material is reviewed by our pharmacist, Miriam Chan, PharmD, and by Drs. Bope, Rakel, and Kellerman for accuracy and readability. It is our habit to use trade names as well as generic drug names to help the clinician identify the treatment by whatever name is most familiar. The treatment recommendations are those that the author has found work best. When a drug is not approved by the FDA for the use indicated, a footnote is added with this information. Such notations may merely reflect that approval for the indication being discussed was never requested. Dosages outside the usual FDA-approved range are also noted.

We greatly appreciate the assistance of the very capable editorial staff at Elsevier and are always humbled by and grateful for the knowledge and experience of our pharmacist reviewer, Miriam Chan.

Robert E. Rakel, MD

Edward T. Bope, MD

Rick Kellerman, MD

Contents

SECTION 7
The Digestive System

SECTION 8
Metabolic Disorders

Contents

xxx

SECTION **9**
The Endocrine System

SECTION **10**
The Urogenital Tract

SECTION **11**
The Sexually Transmitted Diseases

SECTION 15
The Locomotor System

SECTION 16
Obstetrics and Gynecology

SECTION 17
Psychiatric Disorders

SECTION 18
Physical and Chemical Injuries

SECTION 19
Appendices and Index

Symptomatic Care Pending Diagnosis

Pain

Method of
Trish Palmer, MD

Pain is one of the major determinants of quality of life. To this extent, it is imperative to assess and manage pain, regardless of the diagnosis. The patient experiences pain physically, psychologically, and psychosocially, especially when it is chronic. All of these aspects of pain must be taken into account for effective pain management.

According to the National Center for Health Statistics, one in four adults suffered a day-long bout of pain within the last month, and 1 in 10 adults reports pain lasting longer than 1 year. Low back pain is the most common, followed by headache and joint pain (usually at the knee).

Classification

Definitions of acute and chronic pain vary. Acute pain has a definite start date, is abrupt in onset, and lasts less than 6 weeks, whereas chronic pain is more gradual in onset and lasts for more than 6 weeks. Acute pain in general is expected to resolve; with chronic pain, the expectation is to use long-term tools to manage the pain.

Pain is also commonly classified as nociceptive, neuropathic, or a mixture of both. Nociceptive pain results from irritated musculoskeletal tissue (somatic) or organ tissue (visceral). Neuropathic pain involves irritation of nerves. Some painful problems (cancer, back pain) can have a mixed origin. Although not always possible, it is quite helpful to localize the pain generator or to narrow the diagnosis to the most specific cause possible, because this opens up many disease-specific management options. Migraines can respond to triptans, diabetic peripheral neuropathy can respond to pregabalin (Lyrica), and rheumatoid arthritis can respond to disease-modifying antirheumatic drugs (DMARDs) or biologicals (Box 1).

Pain as a Vital Sign

It is important to assess pain at every medical visit when pain is a complaint. Think of pain as a vital sign. Ask about the level of pain at every visit, and attach a number to it. Use a numerical rating scale, with a rating of 0 to 10, 0 representing the absence of pain and 10 representing the worst pain imaginable. The validity of this approach is well documented. This helps the physician, as well as the patient, to follow the pain level to assess the effectiveness of different interventions. Try to avoid making your own assumptions about the severity of pain, which can lead to undertreatment of pain and underdiagnosis of pain-related urgencies. It is often surprising how well different people deal with pain and a change in their abilities. Ask about current function. This may be the most telling aspect of your conversation and helps to drive disease-specific interventions.

Treatment

Pain is an individual experience. The treatment plan should be tailored to the patient with options for self-management. The objective is to empower the patient as much as possible. What is appealing or acceptable differs from one person to another. Try to understand what your patient is willing to try to decrease the pain, and remember that some of these preferences might stem from their culture or gender. Keep an open mind about how to work within the patient's own framework of dealing with pain. The goal is to decrease pain with methods that the patient understands and accepts, otherwise the pain will not be decreased.

The overriding goals of pain management should be established early on in management. At times it is not realistic to expect to completely alleviate pain, as with some cancers and arthritides. The goal may be to make the pain tolerable enough to permit a desired activity level. This often requires a team approach and creativity. Pain should be treated from a multimodal approach, involving a variety of medications, medication vehicles, nondrug approaches, and complementary methods.

Treatment of acute pain often involves the use of short-acting medications on an as-needed basis. Short-acting medications induce a peak–trough phenomenon: The medication takes a certain amount of time to reach peak effectiveness, and after several hours the effect wears off. This is acceptable for treating short-term or milder pain. There is good patient acceptance of these medications due to experience with these medications, especially because some are available over the counter.

For chronic pain, long-acting preparations are more effective for pain control and less likely to cause problems (e.g., confusion about appropriate use, overdosing). Use of long-acting or extended-release formulations avoids the peak–trough effect of short-acting preparations by providing more constant levels of pain medication and therefore a more constant level of pain control. It is imperative to address patient acceptance and concerns of chronic pain management. Many people are concerned about becoming dependent on medications, especially opioids. Most of these patients are ideal candidates for opioids because they are less likely to misuse these medications.

BOX 1   Disease-Specific Medications

Diabetic Neuropathic Pain
First-Line Medications
Duloxetine (Cymbalta)
Oxycodone (OxyContin)[1]
Pregabalin (Lyrica)
Tricyclic antidepressants[1]

Second-Line Medications
Carbamazepine (Tegretol)[1]
Gabapentin (Neurontin)[1]
Lamotrigine (Lamictal)[1]
Tramadol (Ultram)[1]
Venlafaxine ER (Effexor XR)[1]

Fibromyalgia
Pregabalin (Lyrica)

Gout
Allopurinol (Zyloprim)
Colchicine

Migraine
Triptans

Muscle Spasm
Muscle relaxants

Neuropathic Pain
Anticonvulsants
Gabapentin (Neurontin)[1]
Pregabalin (Lyrica)
Tricyclic antidepressants

Rheumatic Process
Biologicals
Disease-modifying antirheumatic drugs

Joint Swelling
Cyclooxygenase 2 inhibitors
Nonsteroidal antiinflammatory drugs
Steroids

Adapted from Argoff CE, Backonja MM, Belgrade MJ, et al: Consensus guidelines: Treatment planning and options. Diabetic peripheral neuropathic pain. Mayo Clin Proc 2006;81: S12-S25.
[1]Not FDA approved for this indication.

Situations that bode poorly for obtaining good pain relief include older patients, patients receiving worker's compensation, disability, or personal injury claims; and drug abusers or diverters. Depression or other psychopathology can make pain more difficult to manage due to the patient's enhanced perception of pain.

The process of addressing concerns proactively may include a pain contract. A pain contract should define the behavior expected of both the patient and physician and should address all aspects of care, goals of treatment, measures of outcome, and consequences for violating the contract (e.g., lost prescriptions, drug testing, failure to complete recommended testing). The patient should also agree to random drug screens as a part of the monitoring process.

PHARMACOLOGIC TREATMENT

There are three general rules for managing pain: Choose medication to fit the pain; start low and titrate up; and reevaluate the pain at intervals.

Determine whether the pain is likely to be short term or long term, and choose medications specific to the situation. For long-term pain management, I use methods that have the least risk of misuse (side effects, interactions, confusion). In this situation, I use long-acting (twice-daily at maximum) regimens.

Start a single medication at a low dose and titrate up to either side effects or reduction of pain. This helps to determine if a medication is causing a side effect, helps to avoid side effects, and helps to avoid confusion. Add in other medications and nondrug therapies one at a time to be able to assess effectiveness.

Reevaluate the treatment frequently (every 1-2 weeks) until pain is well controlled. Also assess for side effects that can limit use of a medication or modality. The objective is to work with the patient to use methods of pain control that are effective for the individual patient and to introduce them in a stepwise manner.

Medications

Acetaminophen

Acetaminophen (Tylenol, 500-1000 mg PO q6h) is commonly considered to have the least risk, and it is therefore commonly recommended as first-line treatment for many types of pain. It is very effective and often overlooked as a treatment for acute pain and as an adjunct to potentially decrease the dosing of other pain medications.

Many prescription and nonprescription medications contain acetaminophen, and for this reason accidental overdose is a common cause of drug-induced liver failure. Patients at increased risk for liver toxicity include those who fast or have inadequate protein intake (eating disorder) and those who use alcohol on a regular basis.

Nonsteroidal Antiinflammatory Drugs

Nonsteroidal antiinflammatory drugs (NSAIDs) include traditional NSAIDs such as ibuprofen, cyclooxygenase 2 (COX-2) inhibitors, and salicylates (Table 1). These medications are commonly used and are effective for many types of pain. One advantage is that they can decrease joint swelling, which by itself causes pain and needs to be treated directly. These medications are also used as adjuncts to decrease the dosing of other pain medications. They are relatively safe to use in the short term. Long-term use requires periodic monitoring of complete blood count (CBC) and kidney and liver function.

Celecoxib (Celebrex) is safer for those with a history of peptic ulcer, who are older than 65 years, or who use warfarin (Coumadin) or steroids. For protection against drug-induced peptic ulcer, non-acetylated salicylates or NSAIDs (prefereably etodolac [Lodine] or

TABLE 1 Nonopioid Pain Medications

Drug	Dose Range	Frequency
Cyclooxygenase 2 Inhibitor		
Celecoxib (Celebrex)	100-400 mg	Daily
Nonsteroidal Antiinflammatory Drugs		
Diclofenac (Cataflam, Voltaren)	50-100 mg[3]	q8h
Etodolac (Lodine)	200-300 mg	q8h
Mefenamic acid (Ponstel)	250 mg	q6h
Ibuprofen (Motrin)	400-800 mg	q8h
Ketorolac (Toradol)	15-30 mg	xxx
Naproxen (Anaprox, Naprelan, Naprosyn)	250-550 mg	q12h
Salicylates		
Choline magnesium trisalicylate (Trilisate)	500-1000 mg	q8h
Diflunisal (Dolobid)	250-500 mg	q8-12h

Data from Monthly Prescribing Reference. Available at http://www.prescribingreference.com/(accessed April 24, 2008).
[3]Exceeds dosage recommended by the manufacturer.

meloxicam [Mobic]) combined with a proton pump inhibitor or misoprostol (Cytotec) are recommended. Peptic ulcer occurs without warning symptoms, and it is not related to the dyspepsia also potentially caused by these medications. The U.S. Food and Drug Administration (FDA) recommends all NSAIDs and COX-2 medications be given "at the lowest dose and for the shortest time needed."

NSAIDs and COX-2 medications increase the risk of myocardial infarction or cerebral vascular accident in those who take these medications for longer periods and in those who have heart disease. These drugs should never be used just before or after heart surgery, especially coronary artery bypass graft.

Aspirin for cardioprotection should be taken 2 hours before ibuprofen because of the potential for competition for the same binding sites.

Because several NSAIDs are available in a nonprescription strength, it is imperative to know what over-the-counter medications the patient is taking.

Steroids

Steroid (prednisone, Medrol dose pack[1]) medication can be particularly effective for treating pain and swelling. I prescribe prednisone 50 mg PO daily for 5 days, as is commonly done for asthma

---

[1]Not FDA approved for this indication.

exacerbations, for acute treatment of severe inflammatory pain. Long-term use of steroids is associated with avascular necrosis, osteoporosis, and adrenal suppression and therefore is avoided.

Tramadol

Tramadol (Ultram 50-100 mg PO q6h or Ultram ER 100-300 mg PO qd) is considered a non-narcotic opioid. It can potentiate seizures in those who are epileptic or who take selective serotonin reuptake inhibitors (SSRIs), tricyclic antidepressants, or opioids. Tramadol can also potentiate serotonin syndrome if taken concomitantly with SSRIs (documented cases), and caution is also recommended if it is taken with monoamine oxidase inhibitors, other antidepressants, or opioids. Symptoms include nausea, tachycardia, agitation, seizure, coma, and hypertension.

Opioids

Opioid medications may be effective in several ways. Short-acting opioids, especially in combination with adjuvants (acetaminophen or NSAIDs) work well on an as needed or short-term scheduled basis for acute pain and as-needed for breakthroughs of chronic pain or exacerbations of pain. Long-acting preparations on a scheduled basis are especially useful for managing chronic pain. The advantage is that these medications have no maximum dose, and dosing is only limited by side effects (Table 2).

TABLE 2 Opioid-Based Medications

Drug	Availability	Formulation	Frequency
Butorphanol (Stadol)	IR	1 mg nasal spray	q1-4h
Codeine + acetaminophen	IR	30-60/300 mg tab Liquid	q4h
Dihydrocodeine + acetaminophen + caffeine (Panlor DC, Panlor SS)	IR	16/356.4/30 mg tab 32/712.8/60 mg tab	q4h
Dihydrocodeine + aspirin + caffeine (Synalgos-DC)	IR	16/356.4 mg tab	q4h
Fentanyl (Fentora)	IR	100-800 µg buccal tab	q30min Max: 4 doses
Fentanyl (Duragesic)	ER	12-100 µg/h patch	q3d
Hydrocodone + acetaminophen (Lortab, Maxidone, Norco, Vicodin, Xodol, Zydone)	IR	2.5-10/300-750 mg tab Exilir (Lortab)	q6h
Hydrocodone + ibuprofen (Vicoprofen)	IR	7.5/200 mg	q6h
Hydromorphone (Dilaudid)	IR	2-8 mg tab Liquid Rectal suppository Injection	q4h
Meperidine (Demerol)	IR	50-100 mg tab Liquid	q4h
Morphine sulfate (Avinza)	IR and ER	15-200 mg cap, tab	qd
Morphine sulfate (Kadian, MS Contin, Oramorph SR)	ER	15-200 mg cap, tab	qd
Morphine sulfate (MSIR)	IR	15-30 mg tab, cap Oral sol'n	q4h
Nalbuphine (Nubain)	IR	10-20 mg injection (SC, IM, IV)	q3-6h
Oxycodone (OxyIR)	IR	5 mg cap Liquid	q6h
Oxycodone (OxyContin)	ER	10-80 mg tab	q12h
Oxycodone + acetaminophen (Percocet, Tylox)	IR	2.5-10/325-650 mg tab	q6h
Oxycodone + acetaminophen (Roxicet)	IR	Liquid	q6h
Oxycodone + aspirin (Percodan)	IR	4.8/325 mg	q6h
Oxycodone + ibuprofen (Combunox)	IR	5/400 mg tab	q6h
Oxymorphone (Opana)	IR	5-10 mg tab	q4h
Oxymorphone (Opana ER)	ER	20-40 mg tab	q12h
Pentazocine + acetaminophen (Talacen)	IR	25/650 mg tab	q4h
Pentazocine + naloxone (Talwin-NX)	IR	50/0.5 mg tab	q3-4h
Propoxyphene (Darvon, Darvon N)	IR	65-100 mg tab	q4h
Propoxyphene + acetaminophen (Balacet, Darvocet N50, Darvocet N100, Darvocet A500)	IR	50-100/325-650 mg tab	q4h
Propoxyphene + aspirin + caffeine (Darvon Compound 32, Darvon Compound 65)	IR	32-65/389/32.4 mg tab	q4h

Data from Monthly Prescribing Reference. Available at http://www.prescribingreference.com/(accessed April 24, 2008).
cap = capsule; ER = extended release; IR = immediate release; max = maximum; sol'n = solution.

CURRENT DIAGNOSIS

- Associated constitutional symptoms should prompt a timely work-up for infection and malignancy.
- Bowel or bladder changes associated with back or neck pain should prompt an immediate work-up for cauda equina syndrome.
- Pain that does not follow a typical course deserves a further work-up: blood testing to look for metabolic causes, a second type of imaging, and specialist referral.

Dose-limiting side effects include constipation, nausea and vomiting, sedation, cognitive impairment, and pruritus. I specifically ask about each of these side effects at each visit, because they can occur at any time with opioid use and are easier to manage if treated early. Most side effects decrease over 2 to 3 days after starting the medication or changing the dosing, except for constipation. Constipation is almost universal, and I recommend when starting an opioid medication to begin a bowel regimen with stimulant or emollient laxatives. It is reasonable to give 100-200 mg daily of docusate with senna, 2 pills bid.

Opioid intolerance often results from pseudoallergy due to histamine release causing pruritus. This is most likely with use of codeine, morphine, and meperidine (Demerol); using other opioids often avoids this side effect. Combination products (with acetaminophen, NSAIDs) potentially decreases the amount of opioid necessary to decrease pain and are considered opioid sparing. However, there is a ceiling on dosing these products, usually because of the adjunct.

Chronic pain should be treated with long-acting medications on a scheduled basis to avoid the rollercoaster phenomenon. Change in activity amount or type, changes in weather, and progression of disease can worsen chronic pain, causing breakthrough pain. Making a plan for treating breakthrough pain, with a prescription for acetaminophen, an NSAID, or a short-acting opioid is effective and lessens anxiety.

Routes of Administration

Typically, pain medication is given by pill, but other methods exist. Many are available in oral liquid, nasal spray, rectal, injectable, transdermal, epidural, or intrathecal forms. These routes minimize gastrointestinal side effects and drug interactions at times. Direct introduction of pain-decreasing modalities to the pain generator can also be more effective than oral dosing.

Topical agents commonly used include capsaicin (Capsin, Zostrix) and lidocaine (Lidoderm). Capsaicin tends to burn initially and needs to be applied several times per day. Lidocaine 5% patch (Lidoderm) is applied for 12 hours per day. Topical NSAIDs are available as Flector Patch and Voltaren Gel. Intraspinal administration tends to avoid gastrointestinal, skin, and sedation problems. Injectables commonly used for osteoarthritis include cortisone and viscosupplementation into the joint. American patients often prefer pills, but these other routes may be more effective and safer for the patient with multiple medical problems.

NONPHARMACOLOGIC TREATMENT

Pay attention to the whole patient. Depression is a common comorbid condition in patients with chronic pain. Try to elicit their concerns because they may be afraid they have cancer, will be debilitated, or will die as a result of their pain. Allaying fears is a powerful method of decreasing pain.

Formal education and support groups can empower the patient to learn to self-administer methods to decrease the pain. The Arthritis Foundation has a self-help course for managing arthritis pain. Some counselors and psychologists specialize in pain control and can help decrease pain and increase functionality. A pain clinic can combine several drug and nondrug aspects of pain control.

For many types of pain (osteoarthritis, low back pain, any source of lower extremity pain), more weight causes more pain. I initially approach the overweight patient with the idea of weight maintenance. I explain that gaining weight will likely make the problem worse. This is a nice introduction for most patients to the idea of trying to lose weight through dietary modification and daily exercise.

Bracing is effective for many types of musculoskeletal pain. There are braces built to offload the medial or lateral joint compartment of the knee to decrease pain due to osteoarthritis and for the lower back to decrease low back pain. Splints and braces are available for almost every joint in the body, some off the shelf, some custom made. Crutches and walkers can offload a lower extremity joint for pain control.

Physical and occupational therapy might help the patient to regain range of motion, decrease swelling, restore better biomechanics, and learn positioning to protect the body part(s). Modalities such as electrical stimulation, ultrasound, iontophoresis, and phonophoresis can decrease swelling and pain. Assistive devices can help the patient to attend to activities of daily living that have become difficult.

Interruption of neural pathways can decrease pain. This is accomplished by injection of alcohol[1] or phenol[1] or by radiofrequency, cryoanalgesia, or surgery. When specific bone or soft tissue structures are the cause of pain, surgery may be effective.

Osteoarthritis of the knee is managed effectively with several nondrug treatments. Acupuncture has been shown to be effective to decrease pain due to osteoarthritis of the knee. Supplements such as glucosamine,[1,7] methylsulfonylmethane (MSM),[1,7] and S-adenosylmethionine (SAM-e)[1,7] are proven effective to decrease joint pain due to osteoarthritis. Fish oil supplements[1,7] are likely beneficial in decreasing pain because of their omega-3 fatty acid content. Supplements are not regulated by the FDA, and patients should be advised to use those that have the USP label (which decreases product variability). Avocado and soybeans might slow progression of osteoarthritis of the hip. Steroid or hyaluronic acid (Orthovisc, Synvisc, Hyalgan, Euflexxa, Supartz) injection into the joint might decrease pain. Specific braces to offload the medial or lateral joint space can decrease pain. Joint replacement surgery can decrease pain and improve mobility.

Issues in Pain Management

Understanding the issues of addiction, dependence, and tolerance is essential for those who are involved in any type of pain management. There is no validated method to predict patient misuse of opioid medication. Published rates of abuse and addiction in chronic pain populations are approximately 10%. A personal or family history of substance abuse and comorbid psychiatric disorders put a patient at risk for misuse of pain medication.

Addiction is a craving for or excessive or persistent use despite adverse consequences. In patients with pain, addiction is rare, especially with long-term use of the medication. Look for the three Cs of addiction: consequences, control, and craving. Consequences of personal harm resulting from use or misuse include intoxication, somnolence, sedation, declining activity level, labile mood, increasing sleep disturbance, increasing pain complaints, and increasing relationship dysfunction. Impaired control over use can be indicated by reports of lost or stolen prescription or medications, frequent early renewal requests, urgent calls or unscheduled visits, abusing other drugs or alcohol, not being able to produce other medications on request, withdrawal noted on clinic visits, and reports of overuse or sporadic use by observers. Signs of craving include frequently missed appointments unless opioid renewal is expected, avoidance of nonopioid treatments, inability to tolerate multiple medications, and failure to improve.

---

[1]Not FDA approved for this indication.
[7]Available as dietary supplement.

CURRENT THERAPY

- Pain management is individual.
- Use a stepwise approach to pain medications.
- Drug and nondrug therapies are effective and should be used concomitantly.
- Combinations of medications can decrease total dose and side effects.

Undertreatment of pain often leads to patients exhibiting drug-seeking behavior, which for the patient is actually an appropriate response. To prevent this, it is important to educate the patient on realistic expectations (pain might not be eliminated) and to see the patient frequently until pain is well controlled.

Dependence is a normal physiologic response to regular use of opioids for more than a few days. Dependence leads to withdrawal on abrupt cessation of the medication. Fear of dependence often leads both patients and physicians to avoid opioid medication, thereby potentially precluding adequate pain relief.

Tolerance is a condition in which progressively larger doses of opioid are needed to produce the same level of analgesia; it is usually limited to the initial phase of drug titration and rarely seen afterward. What seems to be tolerance after pain control is achieved may be a worsening of the underlying condition causing the pain.

Fear of litigation should not limit use of opioids in appropriate patients. All of the legal cases have been based on inappropriate behavior by physicians, consisting of prescribing for themselves or for those who are not their patients, prescribing without a reasonable indication for opioids, failure to address addictive behavior, and lack of documentation of history or physical examination.

Often, patients taking opioids desire to stop the medication. Although this may be understandable, it is often an unrealistic goal. If the pain is not resolvable, it is more realistic to continue medication to maintain pain control. This should not induce fear or concern on the part of the physician or patient, because some types of pain are not resolvable. Just as diabetic patients need to continue insulin, or they will develop symptoms and complications of diabetes, patients with chronic pain need to continue pain medication. Many medical problems are not curable, yet they can be effectively managed.

Pain Emergencies

Any type of pain that is associated with constitutional symptoms such as fevers, chills, night sweats, or weight loss should prompt an investigation looking for infection and malignancy. Back or neck pain associated with bowel or bladder changes indicates possible cauda equina syndrome, which requires immediate surgical evaluation. Any pain that does not follow a typical course deserves a further work-up, including blood testing to look for metabolic causes, a second type of imaging, or specialist referral. A patient with known cancer and an acute pain increase or a new pain should be urgently evaluated.

REFERENCES

Agency for Healthcare Research and Quality. Assessment and management of chronic pain. Available at http://www.guidelines.gov/summary/summary.aspx?doc_id=10724&nbr=005586&string=chronic+AND+pain (accessed April 24, 2008).

American Society of Addiction Medicine, American Academy of Pain Medicine, American Pain Society. Definitions related to the use of opioids for the treatment of pain. Consensus statement; 2001. Available at http://www.ampainsoc.org/advocacy/opioids2.htm (accessed April 24, 2008).

Bope ET, Douglass AB, Gibovsky A, et al. Pain management by the family physician: The Family Practice Pain Education Project. J Am Board Fam Pract 2004;17:S1–12.

Berman BM, Lao L, Langenberg P, et al. Effectiveness of acupuncture as adjunctive therapy in osteoarthritis of the knee: A randomized controlled trial. Ann Intern Med 2004;141(12):901–10.

Catella-Lawson F, Reilly MP, Kapoor SC, et al. Cyclooxygenase inhibitors and the antiplatelet effects of aspirin. N Engl J Med 2001;345:1809–17.

Federal Drug Administration. Medication guide for non-steroidal anti-inflammatory drugs (NSAIDs). Available at www.fda.gov/cder/drug/infopage/COX2/NSAIDmedguide.htm (accessed April 24, 2008).

Hardy M, Coulter I, Morton SC, et al. S-Adenosyl-L-methionine (SAMe) for depression, osteoarthritis, and liver disease. Evidence Report/Technology Assessment Number 64. Rockville, Md: Agency for Healthcare Research and Quality, US Department of Health and Human Services; 2002. AHRQ publication 02-E033. Available at http://www.ahrq.gov/clinic/tp/sametp.htm (accessed April 24, 2008).

Jensen MP, Karoly P. Self-report scales and procedures for assessing pain in adults. In: Turk DC, Melzack R, editors. Handbook of Pain Assessment. 2nd ed. New York: Guilford Press; 1991. pp 15–35.

Lequesne M, Maheu E, Cadet C, Dreiser RL. Structural effect of avocado/soybean unsaponifiables on joint space loss in osteoarthritis of the hip. Arthritis Rheum 2002;47:50–8.

Richard J, Reidenberg MM. The risk of disciplinary action by state medical boards against physicians prescribing opioids. J Pain Symptom Manage 2005;29(2):206–12.

Spiller H, Gorman S, Villalobos D, et al. Prospective multicenter evaluation of tramadol exposure. J Toxicol Clin Toxicol 1997;35:361–4.

Usha PR, Naidu MUR. Randomised, double-blind, parallel, placebo-controlled study of oral glucosamine, MSM, and their combinations. Clin Drug Invest 2004;24:353–64.

Nausea and Vomiting

Method of
Robert Kraft, MD

Nausea is the sensation of the need to vomit and requires consciousness through the cerebrum. The coordinated and forceful retrograde expulsion of gut contents produces vomiting. The pathophysiology of vomiting is more precisely understood than that of nausea, but it still involves a highly complex interplay of neurotransmitters and receptors (e.g., histaminic, muscarinic, dopaminergic, serotonergic), sites of action (e.g., higher-level central nervous system [CNS], brainstem, labyrinth, gut), and stimuli (e.g., enterotoxins, medications, mechanical stimuli, neurologic stimuli). Nausea and vomiting are extremely common complaints in the primary care setting, yet they can be the presenting symptoms for rare and life-threatening diseases. The causes and the potential outcomes of nausea and vomiting are equally broad. The primary care physician is well served by a thorough understanding of their presentation, work-up, and treatment.

CURRENT DIAGNOSIS

- Nausea and vomiting have a wide variety of causes.
- Assessing for complications (e.g., dehydration) should be a high priority.
- The physical examination should be guided by the history.
- Testing beyond routine laboratory and plain film radiographs is rarely required.

CURRENT THERAPY

- Correcting complications of vomiting is the first priority of treatment.
- Nausea and vomiting can often be treated with dietary changes alone.
- After more life-threatening conditions are ruled out, a trial of an antiemetic chosen based on the etiology is reasonable.
- Nonpharmacologic agents are often tried first during pregnancy.

Differential Diagnosis

Infectious causes of nausea and vomiting are relatively common in young children (<3 years old) and in the third decade of life and are seasonally more common in the autumn and winter. Nausea and vomiting tend to be relatively acute in onset; they may be associated with fever, diarrhea, and abdominal pain and tend to be self-limited in scope. Possible etiologic agents include viruses such as rotaviruses, reoviruses, and adenoviruses. Bacteria such as *Salmonella*, *Shigella*, and *Campylobacter* can produce nausea and vomiting associated with bloody diarrhea. Opportunistic infections such as cytomegalovirus can cause symptoms in the immunocompromised patient.

Gastrointestinal disorders commonly cause nausea and vomiting. Obstruction anywhere along the gut, whether mechanical or functional, elicits nausea and vomiting that can be insidious and intermittent for the gastric outlet or more acute with pain and abdominal distention for the small bowel. Gastroparesis and other disorders of gut motility induce nausea after meals. Dyspepsia may elicit nausea and vomiting through delayed gastric emptying. Intraabdominal inflammatory disorders adjacent to or including the gastrointestinal tract, such as appendicitis, pancreatitis, or cholecystitis, tend to have an acute onset and relatively typical pain presentations along with nausea and vomiting.

Medication reactions and toxic insults commonly produce nausea and vomiting. The best-known and best-studied medication reaction is post-chemotherapy nausea and vomiting (PCNV). Certain types of chemotherapeutic agents are particularly emetogenic: cisplatinum (Cisplatin, Platinol) and nitrogen mustard (Mustargen). PCNV may occur shortly after treatment through direct effects on specific emetogenic receptors in the brain. It can also occur as a delayed effect through less well understood mechanisms and with less satisfactory treatment options. Chemotherapy-associated nausea and vomiting may also be anticipatory, especially in those with underlying anxiety. Radiation treatment, especially that overlapping the upper abdomen, also induces nausea and vomiting.

Because the list of medications with nausea and vomiting as a side effect is almost as long as the list of medications that can be prescribed, pinpointing a causative agent for a patient's symptoms may be challenging. Common offenders include pain medications, such as nonsteroidal antiinflammatory drugs and narcotics, antibiotics, and hormonal medications. Alcohol ingestion, both acute and chronic, should not be forgotten as a potential cause of nausea and vomiting.

Pregnancy leads the endocrinologic causes of nausea and vomiting. It usually peaks at about the ninth week of gestation and may actually be protective, because nausea and vomiting not reaching the severity of hyperemesis gravidarum is associated with positive pregnancy outcomes. Hyperemesis complicates up to 5% of pregnancies and can cause potentially dangerous fluid and electrolyte abnormalities. Other important endocrine disease states produce nausea and vomiting, including uremia, diabetic ketoacidosis, thyroid and parathyroid dysfunction, and Addison's disease.

Nausea and vomiting can also signify CNS problems. Labyrinthine diseases, such as motion sickness, labyrinthitis, and Meniere's disease, often manifest with nausea and vomiting associated with vertigo and nystagmus in a mechanism mediated primarily through histaminic and muscarinic receptors. Increased intracranial pressure resulting from masses, infarctions, or infections typically manifest with additional signs and symptoms, such as headache, meningismus, or focal neurologic signs. Migraines, seizures, and various psychiatric illnesses can also elicit nausea and vomiting.

Postoperative nausea and vomiting (PONV) complicates a significant percentage of surgical procedures—up to 75%, depending on clinical factors. Risk factors include general anesthesia, younger age, female gender, and certain procedure types (gynecologic, middle ear, and intraabdominal procedures). PONV is also one of the most studied forms of nausea and vomiting, and the options for prevention and treatment are better defined than with other causes.

Miscellaneous conditions account for the rest of the differential diagnosis of nausea and vomiting. This grab bag of causes ranges from cyclic vomiting syndrome (also known as abdominal migraine), to cardiac causes (including myocardial infarction and congestive heart failure) and functional nausea and vomiting.

History: Defining the Illness

Evaluation of nausea and vomiting initially requires attention to the ABCs of emergency care. Is the patient's airway, breathing or circulation compromised? Emergency conditions requiring immediate intervention, such as an acute abdomen, significant gastrointestinal bleeding, or CNS signs, must be ruled out.

After immediate, life-threatening conditions are ruled out or treated, the history and physical examination to assess for a cause should commence. The importance of the exactness of the history cannot be overstated. Generalities elicited from the patient or caretaker should prompt directed questioning for specific details. Matters of timing, including duration and frequency, acuteness of onset, and association with other events (e.g., meals) help narrow the range of possible causes. Characteristics of the vomitus, such as bright red blood, undigested food, and bilious or feculent emesis, help pinpoint the location of an obstruction or the possibility of gastrointestinal bleeding. The location, timing, and quality of any associated abdominal pain may identify a specific cause. Fever, headache, vertigo, focal neurologic symptoms, diarrhea, malaise, weight loss, and other associated signs and symptoms should be sought and clearly defined.

Physical Examination

The historical findings should guide the physical examination. The initial evaluation should focus on signs of dehydration—poor skin turgor, delayed capillary refill, hypotension, and orthostasis. The abdominal examination takes high priority. Notation of distention, location, and nature of pain and auscultatory findings is mandatory. Decreased or absent bowel sounds suggest ileus or peritonitis. Early intestinal obstruction may be suspected with increased bowel sounds or late obstruction when high-pitched, rushing bowel sounds coincide with abdominal pain. The rectal examination can reveal rectal bleeding, help pinpoint the nature and location of abdominal pain, or discover and possibly treat rectal impaction. The neurologic examination can be equally important. Cranial nerve testing, ophthalmoscopy, and gait testing are essential aspects of the neurologic examination for patients with nausea and vomiting. The ears, nose, and throat; the lungs; the heart; and the extremities should be examined as thoroughly as the history warrants.

Laboratory and Diagnostic Testing

Blood tests, radiographs, and diagnostic tests are often not required in the evaluation of nausea and vomiting and should be ordered only as the clinical situation warrants. Complete blood counts and chemistries are most often helpful in the evaluation of infectious processes, anemia, and electrolyte abnormalities. Pregnancy testing should not be overlooked in women of childbearing age. A wide variety of other laboratory tests (e.g., thyroid-stimulating hormone, pancreatic enzymes, and drug levels) may be useful but should be ordered for specific clinical scenarios.

Flat and upright abdominal x-rays are usually the initial images of choice and help discriminate obstruction and perforation. Multiple air-fluid levels and distended loops of bowel most likely indicate obstruction. Free air found on an upright plain film points to a perforated viscus. Computed tomography with oral and intravenous contrast is more sensitive and specific for causes of nausea and vomiting and is indicated if a diagnosis is not apparent from the history, physical examination, and plain radiographs. Oral contrast should be used whenever possible but may be omitted if intractable vomiting prohibits its use. Esophagoduodenoscopy and upper gastrointestinal barium study, with or without small bowel follow-through, examine the proximal gastrointestinal tract for obstruction or lesions. Enteroclysis provides more sensitive evaluation of the small bowel but is more invasive than an upper gastrointestinal barium study. Intubation through the esophagus is required for esophagoduodenoscopy and enteroclysis and is often used in upper gastrointestinal barium studies but may not be advisable in patients with significant esophagitis. Barium, which is not water soluble, is contraindicated in intestinal obstruction or perforation. Enteroclysis, even with water-soluble contrast, is relatively contraindicated in patients with suspected complete bowel obstruction or bowel infarction. Diagnostic testing in the setting of an acute abdomen should be performed in conjunction with a surgical consultation. If necessary, gastric emptying scintigraphy evaluates motor functioning of the stomach. Additional testing of dysmotility includes electrogastrography or antroduodenal manometry.

Treatment

The first step in treatment of nausea and vomiting is identifying and correcting complications that have developed. This includes correcting fluid and electrolyte imbalances. Prolonged vomiting and reduced oral intake result in dehydration, hypokalemia, and metabolic alkalosis. Oral fluid with appropriate electrolyte concentrations, such as Pedialyte or other commercially available sports drinks, should be used to replace fluid losses; if necessary, intravenous solutions may be administered. Treatment of the causative agent is the next step, if it is identified and treatable, but often no specific treatment is available or warranted, and supportive measures are all that can be offered. Finally, symptomatic treatment, both pharmacologic and nonpharmacologic, can be offered and is safe and effective.

Diet modification is an important step in the treatment of nausea and vomiting. Frequent offerings of small volumes of clear fluid should be the first attempts at oral intake. This should be followed by small meals of low fat content and low indigestible residue. Diet can then be advanced as tolerated. Some clinical scenarios mandate a nasogastric tube for stomach decompression or long-term use of a modified diet, including liquid formulation of calories.

Medications to treat nausea and vomiting are divided into the antiemetics and the prokinetics. Specific agents are chosen based on clinical circumstances, with the presumed involved receptors dictating which agents should be most effective. However, because multiple receptors are usually involved, treatment outcomes are often incomplete. Medication usage is also often limited by side effects. Effective treatment of PCNV includes the prophylactic use of serotonin receptor (5-HT_3) antagonists in combination with dexamethasone started 30 minutes before the initiation of emetogenic chemotherapy. Table 1 outlines representative agents for the treatment or prevention of various types of nausea and vomiting available in the United States.

Nonpharmacologic interventions are also used for special clinical scenarios. This is most apparent in pregnancy-induced nausea and vomiting, because the treatment must avoid potential side effects on the developing fetus, if possible. Acupuncture (point P6), ginger root[7] (250 mg PO qac and qhs), and pyridoxine[1,7] (vitamin B_6, 25-50 mg PO daily) offer some level of efficacy in pregnancy. Acupuncture has also been tried in chemotherapy-induced nausea and vomiting and PONV.

---

[1]Not FDA approved for this indication.
[7]Available as dietary supplement.

TABLE 1 Common Antiemetic and Prokinetic Pharmacologic Agents Available in the United States with Dosages, Indications, and Side Effects

Medication	Dose	Indications	Side Effects	Pregnancy Safety Category*
Anticholinergic				
Scopolamine (Transderm Scōp)	1.5-mg patch TD q3d	Motion sickness, adjunct for PCNV,[1] PONV prophylaxis	Dry mouth, drowsiness, blurred vision, angle-closure glaucoma	C
Antihistamines				
Meclizine (Antivert)	25-50 mg PO q8-12h	Motion sickness, vertigo, migraine[1]	Drowsiness, dry mouth, thickened bronchial secretion, constipation, urinary retention, confusion, blurred vision	B
Diphenhydramine (Benadryl)	25-50 mg PO/IV/IM q4-6h	Motion sickness	Same as meclizine	B
Dimenhydrinate (Dramamine)	50-100 mg PO/IV/IM q4-6h	Motion sickness	Same as meclizine	B
Hydroxyzine (Atarax, Vistaril)	25-100 mg PO/IM q6h	Nausea and vomiting	Same as meclizine	C

Continued

TABLE 1 Common Antiemetic and Prokinetic Pharmacologic Agents Available in the United States with Dosages, Indications, and Side Effects—Cont'd

Medication	Dose	Indications	Side Effects	Pregnancy Safety Category*
Phenothiazines				
Prochlorperazine (Compazine)	5-10 mg IV/IM q3-4h 5-10 mg PO q6-8h 25 mg PR q12h	Severe nausea and vomiting, vertigo,[1] motion sickness,[1] migraine,[1] PONV prophylaxis,[1] PCNV[1]	Drowsiness, dry mouth, blurred vision, constipation, urinary retention, extrapyramidal effects, cholestatic jaundice, sudden death, prolonged QT interval, seizures, hyperprolactinemia, NMS, blood abnormalities	C
Promethazine (Phenergan)	12.5-25 mg PO/PR/IV/IM q4-6h	Nausea and vomiting, motion sickness	Same as prochlorperazine	C
Chlorpromazine (Thorazine)	10-25 mg PO q4-6h 12.5-50 mg IM q4-6h	Nausea and vomiting	Same as prochlorperazine	C
Benzamides				
Metoclopramide (Reglan)	5-10 mg PO/IV/IM q6-8h	Nausea and vomiting,[1] gastroparesis, adjunct PCNV treatment, PONV	Drowsiness, restlessness, depression, extrapyramidal effects, hypotension, NMS, cardiac rhythm disturbances	B
Trimethobenzamide (Tigan)	300 mg PO q6-8h 200 mg IM q6-8h	Nausea and vomiting associated with gastroenteritis, PONV	Same as metoclopramide	C
5-HT₃ Antagonists				
Ondansetron (Zofran)	4-8 mg PO/IV q8-12h For PCNV prophylaxis: up to 32 mg IV or 24 mg PO × 1 dose For PONV: 16 mg × 1 dose	Severe nausea and vomiting,[1] PCNV, PONV	Headache, constipation, fever, asthenia, diarrhea, dizziness, ataxia, tremor, somnolence, thirst, nervousness, prolonged QT interval	B
Granisetron (Kytril, Granisol)	1-2 mg PO/IV q12-24h	PCNV, PONV	Same as ondansetron	B
Dolasetron (Anzemet)	12.5-100 mg PO/IV q24h	PCNV, PONV	Same as ondansetron	B
Cannabinoids				
Dronabinol (Marinol)	5-15 mg/m² PO q2-4h × 4-6 doses/d	Refractory PCNV, AIDS wasting syndrome	Drowsiness, euphoria, dizziness, somnolence, diarrhea, flushing, hallucinations	C
Benzodiazepines				
Lorazepam (Ativan)	0.5-2.5 mg PO/IV/IM q8-12h	Anticipatory and PCNV[1]	Sedation, amnesia, hypotension, respiratory depression, ataxia, hallucinations	D
Corticosteroids				
Dexamethasone (Decadron)	4 mg PO/IV/IM q6h	Adjunct PCNV treatment[1]	Gastrointestinal upset, anxiety, insomnia, hyperglycemia, facial flushing, euphoria	C
Butyrophenones				
Droperidol (Inapsine)	0.625-1.25 mg IV/IM q3-4h[3]	Anticipatory and PCNV,[1] PONV	Sedation, dizziness, hypotension, tachycardia, extrapyramidal effects, hallucinations, prolonged QT interval, torsades de pointes	C
Other				
Erythromycin	3 mg/kg IV q8h acutely, then 250 mg PO q8h for 5-7 d	Gastroparesis[1]	Abdominal pain, nausea, rash, prolonged QT interval, *C. difficile* diarrhea	B

5-HT₃, serotonin type 3 receptor; IM, intramuscular; IV, intravenous; NMS, neuroleptic malignant syndrome; PCNV, post-chemotherapy nausea and vomiting; PO, per mouth; PONV, postoperative nausea and vomiting; PR, per rectum; TD, transdermal.
[1]Not FDA approved for this indication.
[3]Exceeds dosage recommended by the manufacturer.
*Pregnancy Safety Categories: A = Presumed safe from human studies; B = Presumed safe on the basis of animal studies; C = Uncertain safety—no human studies, and animal studies show a risk; D = Unsafe, but risk may be justified in certain circumstances; X = Highly unsafe—use in pregnancy unjustified.

REFERENCES

American College of Obstetricians and Gynecologists. Nausea and Vomiting of Pregnancy (ACOG Practice Bulletin No. 52). Washington, DC: ACOG; 2004, 1–13.

Hasler WL. Approach to the patient with nausea and vomiting. In: Yamada T, editor. Textbook of Gastroenterology. 4th ed. Philadelphia: Lippincott Williams & Wilkins; 2003, pp 760–80.

Herlinger H, Maglinte DDT, Yao T. Enteroclysis technique and variations. In: Herlinger H, editor. Clinical Imaging of the Small Intestine. 2nd ed. New York: Springer; 2001. p. 95–124.

Mahadevan U, Kane S. American Gastroenterological Association Institute medical position statement on the use of gastrointestinal medications in pregnancy. Gastroenterology 2006;131:278–82.

Parkman HP, Hasler WL, Fisher RS. American Gastroenterological Association Medical Position Statement: Diagnosis and Treatment of Gastroparesis. Gastroenterology 2004;127:1589–91.

Quigley EM, Hasler WL, Parkman HP. AGA technical review on nausea and vomiting. Gastroenterology 2001;120:263–86.

Sadostu AT, Browne BJ. Vomiting, diarrhea, and constipation. In: Tintinalli JE, editor. Emergency Medicine: A Comprehensive Study Guide. New York: McGraw-Hill; 2000. p. 567–74.

Schwartz DT. Abdominal radiology: Patient 1. In: Schwartz DT, editor. Emergency Radiology: Case Studies. New York: McGraw-Hill; 2007. p. 147–65.

Scorza K, Williams A, Phillips D, Shaw J. Evaluation of nausea and vomiting. Am Fam Physician 2007;76:76–84.

Torres LS, Norcutt TLW, Dutton AG. Care of patients during imaging examinations of the gastrointestinal system. In: Torres LS, Norcutt TLW, Dutton AG, editors. Basic Medical Techniques and Patient Care in Imaging Technology. 6th ed. Philadelphia: Lippincott Williams & Wilkins; 2003. p. 220–37.

Gaseousness and Dyspepsia

Method of
Scott Owings, MD

Gaseousness

Gaseousness includes three disorders: belching, flatulence, and bloating. Because patients may interpret symptoms of abdominal pain, early satiety, nausea, and constipation as excess gas, it is important for the physician to elicit a careful description of the patient's complaint. Often, an exact etiology is not found, making treatment difficult. Although the symptoms are usually benign and secondary to diet and eating habits, one must consider etiologies such as gastrointestinal infection, obstruction, malabsorptive processes, dysmotility syndromes, irritable bowel syndrome (IBS), and psychiatric illness.

NORMAL PHYSIOLOGY

The normal volume of gas in the gastrointestinal tract is less than 200 mL, and normal expulsion during a 24-hour period averages 600 to 700 mL. Up to 25 episodes of flatus daily is considered normal, with the average being 14. Ninety-nine percent of intestinal gas consists of nitrogen (N_2), oxygen (O_2), carbon dioxide (CO_2), hydrogen (H_2), and methane (CH_4). The concentration and quantity of gas are determined primarily by three mechanisms: air swallowing, intraluminal production, and diffusion from blood. Air swallowing is responsible for the majority of N_2 and O_2. Intraluminal gas production is responsible for the majority of CO_2, H_2, and CH_4, which are products of bacterial metabolism. Some CO_2 can be produced by the interaction of acid and bicarbonate. The majority of gas in flatus is a product of colonic bacterial metabolism.

PATHOGENESIS

Gaseousness, in particular symptoms of bloating and increased flatus, are most commonly the result of excess gas production, abnormal gas transit, or increased visceral sensitivity to normal amounts of gas. Increased intestinal gas production is commonly caused by carbohydrate maldigestion, such as that seen in patients with lactose intolerance or a diet high in fructose, sorbitol, and starches, which are poorly absorbed. High-fiber diets, celiac disease, and small intestine bacterial overgrowth can increase gas production. Dysmotility is seen with gastroparesis and chronic intestinal pseudo-obstruction, both of which are associated with diabetes mellitus, scleroderma, amyloidosis, and endocrine disease. Patients with previous Nissen fundoplication, fat intolerance, and various familial conditions may have dysmotility. Increased visceral sensitivity is thought to be the pathophysiology in patients with functional bowel disorders such as IBS and functional dyspepsia.

EVALUATION

Typically, a thorough history and physical examination are all that are needed in the evaluation of gaseousness, unless underlying organic disease is suggested. Symptoms such as weight loss, rectal bleeding, fever, vomiting, steatorrhea, nocturnal abdominal pain, and diarrhea indicate structural disease and warrant further evaluation. The dietary history may reveal a close association with specific foods such as certain vegetables and fruits, legumes, or foods containing lactose or fructose. The history may also elicit underlying anxiety or psychiatric illness. The physical examination should include a detailed abdominal inspection and a search for signs of endocrine or neurologic processes as well as nutritional deficiency. Laboratory testing should be aimed at excluding organic disease and may include a complete blood count (CBC), complete metabolic profile (CMP), amylase, erythrocyte sedimentation rate, thyroid-stimulating hormone, and stool studies. Serum testing for antiendomysium (EMA) and tissue transglutaminase (TTG) antibodies is helpful in screening for celiac sprue. Imaging techniques such as plain films, barium studies, ultrasonography, and computed tomography may be helpful, particularly if ileus or obstruction is suspected. Endoscopy may be warranted when biopsies are necessary. Hydrogen breath testing is indicated in the work-up of carbohydrate maldigestion or of small intestinal bacterial overgrowth. Gastric emptying scanning and gastrointestinal manometry are helpful in the evaluation of dysmotility syndromes and chronic intestinal pseudo-obstruction.

Belching

Belching, or eructation, is the retrograde expulsion of esophageal or gastric gas from the mouth. It may result from increased air swallowing with eating meals; drinking carbonated beverages; chewing gum; smoking; anxiety; or aerophagia, which is a functional disorder caused by habitual air swallowing. Patients with gastroesophageal reflux disease (GERD) often increase air swallowing in an attempt to decrease heartburn. It may also be caused by relaxation of the lower esophageal sphincter, which is associated with certain foods such as mints and chocolate. Treatment should be aimed at decreasing air swallowing by eating and drinking slowly, avoiding causative agents, stopping smoking, and treating heartburn.

Flatulence

As mentioned earlier, up to 25 episodes of flatus daily is considered normal. Most patients complaining of increased flatus are not exceeding this level. Because gas volume is difficult to determine, counting episodes of flatus over a 24-hour period is the most reliable measure. Because increased flatus is a common early symptom in patients with maldigestive diseases, the diagnosis should be considered in patients found to have excessive flatus production. A thorough history and physical examination may be all that are necessary for the evaluation of flatulence. If no organic etiology is suspected, treatment should be aimed at dietary modifications. Undergarments and cushions made to reduce malodorous flatus are available.

Bloating

Bloating is perceived by patients to be the sensation of excess abdominal gas. However, studies have failed to confirm a difference in volume or composition of gas between patients complaining of bloating and asymptomatic controls. Although more studies are needed, the symptom of bloating that accompanies functional bowel disorders, such as IBS, is thought to be caused by delayed transit times and visceral hypersensitivity. Functional bloating is a diagnosis of exclusion, and causes such as dysmotility syndromes, malabsorptive processes, infection, and intestinal obstruction should be considered.

TREATMENT

If a cause of gaseousness is not found, treatment may be difficult. Mainstays of management include dietary modification and prescription of nonmedicinal and medicinal therapies. Avoiding foods that

CURRENT DIAGNOSIS

Gaseousness

- Perform a thorough history and physical examination.
- Identify associated triggers such as smoking, medication, diet, and psychosocial factors.
- Identify warning symptoms, such as weight loss, rectal bleeding, fever, vomiting, steatorrhea, and diarrhea, that warrant further work-up.
- Laboratory and imaging studies should be reserved for ruling out organic disease.
- Hydrogen breath testing is done for maldigestion, malabsorption, and bacterial overgrowth.
- Gastric emptying scanning and manometry are done for dysmotility syndromes and pseudo-obstruction.

Dyspepsia

- Rule out common diagnoses (gastroesophageal reflux disease, use of nonsteroidal antiinflammatory drugs, peptic ulcer disease, irritable bowel syndrome).
- If patient is <55 years of age and no alarm features are present, test for *Helicobacter pylori*.
- *H. pylori* testing is done by serology, urea breath test, stool antigen, or biopsy.
- If patient is >55 years of age or alarm features are present, consider esophagogastroduodenoscopy.
- Alarm features include family history of upper gastrointestinal cancer, weight loss, gastrointestinal bleeding, persistent vomiting, dysphagia, and anemia.
- In 60% of cases, the diagnostic evaluation does not identify a cause; this is termed functional dyspepsia.

are contributory, such as those containing lactose, fructose, sorbitol, high fiber, and starches, may be all that is necessary. Various cooking methods have been proposed, as well as a low-gas diet that includes decreased amounts of complex carbohydrates. Hypnotherapy may be helpful in reducing bloating and flatulence in IBS patients and in patients with intractable eructation.

Many medications are available to treat gaseousness and bloating, but there are limited data to support their use. Enzyme preparations such as B-galactosidase (lactase) and encapsulated pancreatic enzymes may be helpful if a deficiency is suspected. Bacterial α-galactosidase (Beano)[7] may be helpful in legume-rich diets. Simethicone (Mylicon) has not been proven to be helpful. Activated charcoal[1] and bismuth compounds such as Pepto-Bismol[1] have some supporting evidence in decreasing the amount of flatus and its odor. Antibiotics are helpful when small intestinal bacterial overgrowth is suspected. Prokinetics such as metoclopramide (Reglan) are helpful in dysmotility syndromes such as diabetic gastroparesis but are not beneficial in the treatment of postoperative ileus. Cisapride (Propulsid) and tegaserod (Zelnorm), both prokinetics pulled from the U.S. market, were beneficial in specific populations. At this point, there are insufficient data to support the use of probiotics such as *Lactobacillus* and *Acidophilus*. In general, narcotics and anticholinergics should be avoided.

Dyspepsia

Dyspepsia has recently been redefined by the so-called Rome III committee, replacing the previous definition of a persistent or recurrent pain or discomfort centered in the upper abdomen. The new definition requires one or more symptoms of postprandial fullness, early satiation, or epigastric pain or burning. Dyspepsia need not be associated with meals, as the term "indigestion" would suggest. Classic heartburn and regurgitation are not included in the definition and are typically more indicative of GERD. The diagnosis is often difficult clinically, because there is significant overlap between symptoms and the pathophysiology is poorly understood.

DIFFERENTIAL DIAGNOSIS

The differential diagnosis can be divided into the categories of functional (nonulcer) dyspepsia and dyspepsia caused by structural or biochemical disease. Functional dyspepsia is defined as symptoms of persistent or recurrent dyspepsia experienced for at least 12 weeks during the preceding 12 months with no evidence of organic disease. Functional dyspepsia accounts for up to 60% of patients with dyspepsia. The pathogenesis is unclear, but current investigation involves the study of gastric motor function, visceral sensitivity, *Helicobacter pylori* infection, and psychosocial factors.

The three most common causes of structural disease are peptic ulcer disease (15%-25%), reflux esophagitis (5%-15%), and gastric or gastroesophageal cancer (1%-2%). Other causes of structural disease include biliary tract disease, gastroparesis, pancreatitis, ischemic bowel disease, and chronic abdominal wall pain. Causes of biochemical disease include drug-induced dyspepsia, carbohydrate malabsorption, and metabolic disturbances.

DIAGNOSIS AND MANAGEMENT

Because functional dyspepsia is a diagnosis of exclusion, a thorough workup is necessary. The medical history may be helpful to identify other common diagnoses, such as GERD, use of nonsteroidal antiinflammatory drugs or cyclooxygenase 2 inhibitors, peptic ulcer disease, and IBS. The physical examination is usually normal in isolated dyspepsia. Signs of anemia or other disease processes should be investigated. Stool should be checked for occult blood. Laboratory studies should include a CBC to check for anemia. Other testing may include pancreatic enzyme levels, liver function tests, and electrolytes if other etiologies are suggested.

The American Gastroenterological Association suggests that patients 55 years of age or younger who have none of the so-called alarm symptoms should be tested for *H. pylori*, using the urea breath test or a stool antigen test, and treated if positive. If *H. pylori* tests are negative or symptoms persist despite eradication, then it is reasonable to try a proton pump inhibitor (PPI) for 4 to 6 weeks. If symptoms continue, the physician should consider doubling the dose of the PPI or assessing the patient with esophagogastroduodenoscopy. Patients older than 55 years of age and younger patients with alarm features should be directly evaluated with endoscopy and *H. pylori* testing. If the work-up is negative and a trial of a PPI has failed, then reevaluation is indicated. If no other source is found and IBS, gastroparesis, and pancreatic, colon, biliary tract, and psychological disorders can be reasonably excluded, then the condition should be treated as for functional dyspepsia.

THERAPY

If a cause of dyspepsia is diagnosed, treatment should be aimed at the underlying diagnosis. The remainder of this section focuses solely on the treatment of functional dyspepsia. It is important to validate the diagnosis, provide education, and reassure the patient of the benign nature of the diagnosis. The physician should set realistic treatment goals while limiting invasive testing and targeting pharmacotherapy toward predominant symptoms. Patients should be advised to quit smoking, discontinue ulcerogenic medications if feasible, and avoid foods or other contributory triggers. Addressing associated psychosocial factors may help alleviate symptoms.

Multiple trials have been performed to evaluate the effectiveness of a wide range of pharmacologic treatments, primarily by comparing them to placebo response (which is 30%-60%). Groups of medications with insufficient evidence of effectiveness or lack of a

---

[1]Not FDA approved for this indication.
[7]Available as dietary supplement.

CURRENT THERAPY

Gaseousness

- Etiology indentified; treat appropriately
- Decrease air swallowing (stop smoking, carbonated beverages, and chewing gum; eat and drink more slowly, treat heartburn)
- Avoid causative agents (lactose, fructose, sorbitol, high fiber, starches, caffeine, mint, chocolate)
- Simethicone (Mylicon) has not proved to be helpful.
- Enzyme preparations such as lactase and pancreatic enzymes if deficiency is suspected
- Bacterial α-galactosidase (Beano)[7] in legume-rich diets
- Antibiotics for small intestinal bacterial overgrowth
- Prokinetics such as metoclopramide (Reglan) for dysmotility syndromes
- Avoid narcotics and anticholinergics.
- Cisapride (Propulsid) and tegaserod (Zelnorm) have been pulled from the U.S. market.

Dyspepsia

- Etiology indentified; treat appropriately
- *Helicobacter pylori* eradication
- Functional dyspepsia
  - Validate diagnosis; provide education and reassurance.
  - Address associated psychosocial factors.
  - Smoking cessation
  - Avoidance of triggers
  - Antidepressants, prokinetics, and H_2 receptor antagonist therapy are beneficial in some groups.
  - Empiric proton pump inhibitor therapy has established efficacy.

---

[7]Available as dietary supplement.

---

statistically significant response include H_2 receptor antagonists, prokinetics, misoprostol (Cytotec),[1] sucralfate (Carafate),[1] anticholinergics and antimuscarinics, antidepressants, psychological therapies, herbal therapies, and antacids, although some treatment trials do support the use of antidepressants, prokinetics, and H_2 receptor antagonist therapy in selected groups. PPI therapy has established efficacy in the treatment of functional dyspepsia. If *H. pylori* is present, eradication may improve symptoms.

---

[1]Not FDA approved for this indication.

REFERENCES

Bazaldua OV, Schneider FD. Evaluation and management of dyspepsia. Am Fam Physician 1999;60(6):1773–84, 1787–8.

Hasler WL. Approach to the patient with gas and bloating. In: Yamada T, editor. Textbook of Gastroenterology. Philadelphia: Lippincott Williams & Wilkins; 2003. p. 802–10.

Longstreth GF. Functional dyspepsia. UpToDate; June 2008. Available at http://www.uptodate.com (accessed May 26, 2009).

Suzuki H, Nishizawa T, Hibi T. Therapeutic strategies for functional dyspepsia and the introduction of the Rome III classification. J Gastroenterol 2006; 41(6):513–23.

Talley NJ. American Gastroenterological Association medical position statement: Evaluation of dyspepsia. Gastroenterology 2005;129(5):1753–5.

Talley NJ, Holtmann G. Approach to the patient with dyspepsia and related functional gastrointestinal complaints. In: Yamada T, editor. Textbook of Gastroenterology. Philadelphia: Lippincott Williams & Wilkins; 2003. p. 655–71.

Talley NJ, Vakil NB, Moayyedi P. American Gastroenterological Association technical review on the evaluation of dyspepsia. Gastroenterology 2005; 129:1756–80.

Hiccups

Method of
Rita Moretti, MD, and Paola Torre, MD

Hiccup is a distinctive sound caused by contractions of the inspiratory muscles and terminated abruptly by the closure of the glottis. The closure occurs almost immediately after the onset of diaphragmatic contraction, minimizing the ventilatory effect. The frequency of hiccupping is modulated by arterial P_{CO_2}. Accordingly, hiccups are most common at maximal inspiration, because the vagal afferents are inhibited by maximal lung inflation.

The real nature of hiccups is not perfectly clear; it has been proposed that hiccups are an abnormal reflex, or myoclonus, generated by repetitive activity of the inspiratory solitary nucleus due to release of higher nervous system inhibitory-regulatory control.

Etiology

Hiccup, therefore, may be due to a persistent disturbance of one of its reflex arc components, which include vagal and phrenic sensory afferents, medullary respiratory center, descending fibers to the C3 to C5 spinal region, and the efferent motor phrenic fibers to the diaphragm. Recent reports hypothesized that a hiccup-like reflex can be elicited by electrical stimulation to a limited area within the medullary reticular formation, the hiccup-evoking site (HES), and hiccups are rapidly suppressed after microinjection of baclofen (Lioresal)[1] into the HES. Following injections of cholera toxin subunit B into the HES, retrograde-labeled cells were found distributed in the lower brainstem and, in particular, in the nucleus raphe magnus, which contains γ-aminobutyric acid (GABA) cells. It is hypothesized that the nucleus raphe magnus is most likely to be the source of the GABAergic inhibitory inputs to the hiccup reflex arc.

Chronic hiccup is defined as persisting symptoms for more than 24 hours or recurring as repetitive attacks.

Hiccup is typically defined as of peripheral or central origin. In the first case, it has been described as due to gastric distension, sudden changes in temperature, and rapid and abundant ingestion of alcohol. Often it has been observed that gastroesophageal reflux, achalasia, and esophageal or small bowel obstruction can cause hiccups. By irritation of the thoracic afferent fibers, mediastinal diseases and thoracic aortic aneurysms can cause hiccups. Many other causes,

---

[1]Not FDA approved for this indication.

CURRENT DIAGNOSIS

- Hiccup is a distinctive sound caused by contractions of the inspiratory muscles terminated abruptly by the closure of the glottis. The closure occurs almost immediately after the onset of diaphragmatic contraction, minimizing the ventilatory effect.
- It has been proposed that hiccups are an abnormal reflex, or myoclonus, generated by repetitive activity of the inspiratory solitary nucleus due to release of higher nervous system inhibitory-regulatory control.
- Chronic hiccup is defined as persisting symptoms for more than 24 hours or recurring as repetitive attacks.
- Hiccup is typically defined as of peripheral or central origin.
- Intractable hiccups can be associated with potentially fatal consequences, and safe management can require inpatient rehabilitation.

such as irritation of the efferent phrenic nerve fibers, subphrenic and hepatic disease, pleural effusion, and lateral myocardial infarction determine hiccups. The involvement of the auricular branch of the vagus nerve might explain the association of hiccups with a foreign body in the external auditory meatus. Systemic disorders such as uremia, diabetes mellitus, hyponatremia or hypocalcaemia, and Addison's disease can cause intractable hiccups. Many drugs, such as doxycycline (Doryx), ceftriaxone (Rocephin), imipenem and cilastatin (Primaxin) dopamine agonists, and chemotherapeutics in general, somehow cause intractable hiccups.

The origin of central hiccups is tightly related to structural or functional pathologies of the medullary region of the vagal nuclei and of the nucleus tractus solitarius. An occlusion in the territory of the posterior inferior cerebellar artery, brainstem tumors, tuberculoma of the brain, sarcoidosis, infections (such as viral encephalitis, HIV encephalopathy), and demyelination of various origins (multiple sclerosis, lupus erythematosus, vasculitis) of the medullary region can produce intractable hiccups.

Treatment

Treatment of hiccups is sometimes unsatisfactory, and it is still debated. Reversing or treating any underlying causative factors may be useful. A beneficial effect can be derived from stimulation of the pharynx opposite C2 and C3, but this is not easy to perform. Some benefits have been reported from different drugs, such as chlorpromazine (Thorazine),[1] haloperidol (Haldol),[1] droperidol (Inapsine),[1] olanzapine (Zyprexa),[1] intravenous midazolam (Versed),[1] baclofen (Lioresal),[1] dexamethasone (Decadron)[1] alone or plus metoclopramide (Reglan)[1] or plus mycophenolate mofetil (Cellcept),[1] amitriptyline (Elavil),[1] intravenous high-dose methylprednisolone (Solu-Medrol),[1] high-dose nifedipine (Procardia)[1] and fludrocortisone (Florinef),[1] amantadine (Symmetrel),[1] and various antiepileptic drugs. Currently, 3 mL of 4% topical lidocaine (Xylocaine)[1] in a small-particle nebulizer seems to be a promising treatment, but the patient must be instructed to avoid eating or drinking 30 minutes before and 2 hours after administration to decrease the risk of aspiration due to a short-term loss of the gag reflex.

Benefits have been reported from these treatments, but because of the low number of treated patients, the short time of follow-up, and mainly the potentially dangerous long-term side effects of the suggested therapies, none has been uniformly recommended to treat hiccups.

---

[1]Not FDA approved for this indication.

 CURRENT THERAPY

- Reversing or treating any underlying causative factors may be useful.
- Some benefits have been reported from drugs such as chlorpromazine,[1] droperidol,[1] olanzapine,[1] intravenous midazolam,[1] baclofen,[1] dexamethasone[1] alone or plus metoclopramide[1] or plus mycophenolate mofetil,[1] amitriptyline,[1] intravenous high-dose methylprednisolone,[1] high-dose nifedipine[1] and fludrocortisone,[1] amantadine,[1] and various antiepileptic drugs.
- One promising treatment is 3 mL of 4% topical lidocaine.[1] The patient must be instructed to avoid eating or drinking 30 minutes before and 2 hours after taking the drug to decrease the risk of aspiration due to a short-term loss of the gag reflex.
- Many reports show good and persistent results using gabapentin[1] for chronic hiccups. An α2δ ligand, pregabalin,[1] has been employed with good results.

---

[1]Not FDA approved for this indication.

Many reports show good results using gabapentin for the persistent treatment of chronic hiccups. Gabapentin (Neurontin)[1] is a novel amino acid derived by the addition of a cyclohexyl group to the chemical backbone of GABA, the major inhibitory neurotransmitter in the mammalian brain. Gabapentin possesses low inherent toxicity; it is not metabolized and does not affect hematologic or biochemical variables to any significant degree. Recent studies with ^{3}H-gabapentin reveal a specific site of binding in brain but not in other organs. Some electrophysiologic studies suggest that gabapentin acts as a partial agonist at the glycine modulatory site of the N-methyl-D-aspartate (NMDA) receptor. More recently, an α2δ ligand, pregabalin (Lyrica),[1] has been employed with good results.

Intractable hiccups' impact on quality of life has been evaluated, and hiccups are related to other significant complications, including aspiration pneumonia, respiratory arrest, and nutritional depletion. Intractable hiccups can have potentially fatal consequences, and safe management can require inpatient rehabilitation.

It is widely demonstrated that there is a direct GABAergic modulation of the hiccup reflex arc. GABA is an inhibitory neurotransmitter that decreases the transmission of monosynaptic extensor and polysynaptic flexor reflexes at the spinal cord level. Gabapentin[1] causes an enhancement of GABA-mediated inhibition or a modulation of voltage-dependent ion channels involved in action potential propagation or burst generation. Pregabalin[1] is a lipophilic analogue of GABA that can diffuse over the blood–brain barrier; however, it is not pharmacologically active at GABA receptors. It exerts its actions at the α2δ binding site that is located on voltage-gated Ca^{2+} channels in the central nervous system. Binding at calcium-ion channels causes a decreased depolarization-induced calcium influx, resulting in a reduction in the release of excitatory neurotransmitters.

It has been reported that gabapentin causes an elevation of central nervous system serotonin, which plays an important role in the inhibition of pain via the raphe–spinal descending control system. This system carries signals from the raphe magnus to inhibit nociception in the substantia gelatinosa of the spinal cord, which contains a high density of projections from the raphe magnus and substance P terminals, opiate receptors, and serotonin terminals. Interestingly, the nucleus raphe magnus is most likely the source of the GABAergic inhibitory inputs to the hiccup reflex arc.

---

[1]Not FDA approved for this indication.

REFERENCES

Brown J, Boden P, Singh L, Gee N. Mechanism of action of gabapentin. Rev Contempo Pharmacother 1996;7:203–14.

Fodstad H, Nilson S. Intractable singultus: A diagnostic and therapeutic challenge. Br J Neurosurg 1993;7(3):255–60.

Howard R. Persistent hiccups. BMJ 1992;305(6864):1237–8.

Jatzko A, Stegmeier-Petroianu A, Petroianu GA. Alpha-2-delta ligands for singultus (hiccup) treatment: Three reports. J Pain Symptom Manage 2007;33(6):756–60.

Kumar A, Droemrick A. Intractable hiccups during stroke rehabilitation. Arch Phys Med Rehabil 1998;79(6):697–9.

Moretti R, Torre P, Antonello RM, et al. Gabapentin as a drug therapy of intractable hiccup because of vascular lesion: A three year follow-up. Neurologist 2004;10(2):102–5.

Oshima T, Sakamoto M, Tatsuta H, Arita H. GABAergic inhibition of hiccup-like reflex induced by electrical stimulation in medulla of cats. Neurosci Res 1998;30(4):287–93.

Rao M, Clarenbach P, Valensieck M, Krätzschmar S. Gabapentin augments whole blood serotonin in healthy young men. J Neural Transm 1988;73:129–34.

Samuels L. Hiccup: A ten years review of anatomy, etiology and treatment. Can Med Assoc J 1952;67:315–22.

Acute Infectious Diarrhea

Method of
Matthew T. Oughton, MD, FRCPC, and
Andre Dascal, MD, FRCPC

Diarrhea is defined as production of at least 200 g of stool per day. However, accurate measurement of stool mass is impractical and is most often used only in clinical trials. A more functional definition of diarrhea is an increase in stool frequency and liquidity compared to the patient's usual bowel habit. Diarrhea is generally classified as acute if it lasts no more than 14 days, persistent if longer than 14 days, and chronic if longer than 30 days.

Clinically, there are two major types of diarrhea. Secretory diarrhea is watery, usually produced in large volumes, and contains little or no blood or leukocytes. Inflammatory diarrhea is bloody, usually has leukocytes, and is produced in smaller volumes. Recognizing the class of diarrhea can be useful in suggesting etiologies and in managing the diarrhea.

The precise cause of a case of diarrhea is usually difficult to ascertain, because diarrhea is a nonspecific reaction by the intestine to numerous insults, including infections, toxins, and autoimmune disorders. Acute infectious diarrhea, by definition, is caused by a microbial pathogen. Although infections are the leading cause of diarrhea, many different pathogens cause acute infectious diarrhea, and the likelihood of any particular agent depends on the patient's age, symptoms, and epidemiologic risk factors.

In immunocompetent adults in the developed world, acute infectious diarrhea is most often a minor and self-resolving ailment. Recent data for the United States estimate an annual burden of between 211 million and 375 million cases, with more than 900,000 hospitalizations and 6000 deaths. However, acute infectious diarrhea can cause severe illness in infants, immunocompromised patients, and malnourished patients; it remains a major cause of global morbidity and mortality. The World Health Organization (WHO) estimates that more than 4 billion cases of acute infectious diarrhea occur each year worldwide and attributes 2 million deaths (5% of all deaths) to diarrheal diseases annually. Most of these deaths are in children who are younger than 5 years and live in developing countries.

Thorough investigation of a patient with acute diarrhea should include a detailed history, physical examination, and laboratory tests (Boxes 1 and 2). In general, clinical investigation of an individual case of acute infectious diarrhea is more useful in identifying sequelae of diarrhea, such as dehydration, than it is in revealing the exact etiologic agent. However, identification of the causative organism can sometimes reveal the existence of a common-source outbreak. One well-known example occurred in 1994, when the state public health laboratory in Minnesota noted an increase in *Salmonella* serotype enteritidis detected in submitted samples; this ultimately led to the recognition of a multistate *Salmonella* outbreak related to improperly cleaned ice cream trucks.

Etiology

It is uncommon to identify the exact etiologic agent in a case of acute infectious diarrhea. However, in some clinical situations, exact identification is important for determining optimal management or possible sequelae. The treatment of inflammatory diarrhea varies depending on the causative organism, and some diseases require alterations in therapy (e.g., suspected *Campylobacter* resistance to fluoroquinolones) or even avoidance of antibiotic therapy (e.g., enterohemorrhagic *Escherichia coli*, in which antibiotic therapy has been associated with more frequent adverse outcomes) (Boxes 3 and 4).

BOX 1 Clinical History for Acute Infectious Diarrhea

- Description of diarrhea
  - Duration
  - Frequency
  - Presence of blood, pus, "grease" in stool
  - Symptoms of fever, tenesmus, dehydration
  - Weight loss
- Other GI symptoms
  - Anorexia
  - Cramping
  - Emesis
  - Nausea
- Previous episodes with similar symptoms
- Ill contacts with similar symptoms
- Recent antibiotic exposure
- Other medication exposure
  - Anticholinergics
  - Antimotility agents
  - Aspirin (ASA)
  - Proton pump inhibitors (PPIs)
- Recent dietary history
  - Shellfish
  - Undercooked meat (chicken)
  - Unsanitary water
- Animal contacts
  - Turtles
  - Other reptiles
- Travel history
  - Travel to endemic or epidemic areas
- Sexual history
- Vaccination history
- Contact with institutions, e.g., hospitals, nursing homes, daycare facilities
- Employment history
- Immune status
  - Presence of HIV
  - Presence of other congenital or acquired immunodeficiencies

---

BOX 2 Physical Examination for Acute Infectious Diarrhea

- Vital signs
  - Blood pressure (look for postural changes)
  - Heart rate (look for postural changes)
  - Respiratory rate
  - Temperature
  - Weight (particularly useful to assess effects of rehydration)
- Cardiovascular examination
  - Volume status (jugular venous pressure)
- Respiratory examination
- Rule out hyperventilation (compensatory respiratory alkalosis for metabolic acidosis due to dehydration and loss of bicarbonate)
- Abdominal examination
  - Focal tenderness
  - Guarding
  - Hepatosplenomegaly
  - Consider rectal examination (look for bloody stool)
- Integument examination
  - Lymphadenopathy
  - Rashes (rose spots)

BOX 3   Etiologic Agents of Predominantly Secretory Diarrhea

Bacterial
- Enteroaggregative *Escherichia coli* (EAEC)
- Enterotoxigenic *E. coli* (ETEC)
- Vibrio cholerae

Viral
- Adenovirus (types 40 and 41)
- Astrovirus
- Caliciviruses (Norwalk, Sapporo)
- Rotavirus

Protozoal
- *Cryptosporidium*
- *Cyclospora*
- *Dientamoeba fragilis*
- *Giardia lamblia*
- *Isospora belli*
- Microspora species (especially *Enterocytozoon bieneusi*)

BOX 4   Etiologic Agents of Predominantly Inflammatory Diarrhea

Bacterial
- *Aeromonas* sp.
- *Bacteroides fragilis* (enterotoxigenic strains)
- *Campylobacter* sp. (particularly FQ-resistant strains)
- *Clostridium difficile* (toxigenic strains)
- *Escherichia coli* (enterohemorrhagic, enteroinvasive)
- *Pleisomonas* sp.
- *Shigella* sp.
- *Salmonella enterica* serotypes *typhi* and *paratyphi*
- Nontyphoid *Salmonella* species
- Noncholera *Vibrio* species
- *Yersinia*

Protozoal
- *Entamoeba histolytica*

BACTERIA

Escherichia coli

E. coli is a versatile pathogen that causes a wide spectrum of disease affecting numerous organ systems. This is illustrated by the wide variety of diarrheagenic *E. coli*, including enterotoxigenic (ETEC), enteroaggregative (EAEC), enterohemorrhagic (EHEC), enteropathogenic (EPEC), and enteroinvasive (EIEC) strains. In general, people are exposed to diarrheagenic *E. coli* by consuming contaminated food and water.

ETEC is a major cause of infantile diarrhea and traveler's diarrhea. Infantile diarrhea affects infants usually in developing countries, particularly during warm and wet conditions, and traveler's diarrhea affects the immunologically naive tourist under similar conditions. In both cases, a large inoculum is required to cause disease. Major virulence factors of ETEC strains include species-specific fimbriae for enterocyte adherence, as well as heat-stable and heat-labile plasmid-encoded enterotoxins. After a relatively brief incubation period of 1 to 2 days, the infected patient develops a secretory diarrhea that lasts up to 5 days. The cornerstones of management are prevention (through dietary hygiene) and adequate rehydration. Antibiotics use is controversial and usually reserved for moderate to severe disease.

EAEC is recognized as a major cause of children's and traveler's diarrhea. Since the initial identification of EAEC in 1985, studies have identified numerous putative virulence factors, including specific aggregative adherence fimbriae. However, no one factor has been identified in all EAEC strains. This suggests that apart from their aggregative adherence to enterocytes, EAEC strains are probably a heterogeneous collection. However, the clinical disease caused by EAEC is relatively consistent and includes persistent secretory diarrhea with low-grade fever. Management of disease from EAEC requires adequate rehydration; the role of antibiotics remains controversial.

The notorious virulence of EHEC (also known as Shiga-like toxin–producing *E. coli*) has led to frequent media reports of "hamburger disease." *E. coli* O157:H7 is the most common strain of EHEC, although several others have been documented. Unlike most other categories of diarrheagenic *E. coli*, EHEC can cause disease with an infectious dose as low as 10 to 100 organisms. Sequelae of EHEC infection include hemorrhagic diarrhea, hemolytic-uremic syndrome, and thrombotic thrombocytopenic purpura. The primary virulence factor is Shiga-like toxin, which damages ribosomes. The gene for Shiga-like toxin is transmitted between EHEC strains by a bacteriophage vector. A separate virulence plasmid has been identified in certain strains of EHEC, but its significance is uncertain. Management of EHEC disease is supportive, because some evidence suggests that antibiotics can enhance the release of Shiga-like toxin and increase the risk of developing hemolytic-uremic syndrome.

EPEC has been associated most strongly with pediatric diarrhea in both epidemic and sporadic forms. EPEC adheres to enterocytes, causing the pathognomic attaching and effacing lesion seen on pathologic section. It then secretes proteins that initiate signal transduction within the enterocyte, ultimately resulting in secretory diarrhea. Because EPEC causes persistent diarrhea that can lead to significant dehydration, rehydration and antibiotic therapy are usually indicated.

As its name implies, EIEC invades enterocytes, where it then replicates and spreads to adjacent cells. The resulting diarrhea may be secretory or inflammatory and lasts up to 7 days. EIEC is closely related to *Shigella* genetically and in the clinical disease that they both cause. As with *Shigella*, antibiotic treatment reduces duration of symptomatic illness.

Shigella Species

The genus *Shigella* consists of four serovars pathogenic to humans: *Shigella sonnei* (Group A), *Shigella flexneri* (Group B), *Shigella boydii* (Group C), and *Shigella dysenteriae* (Group D). *S. sonnei*, the most commonly isolated species, typically causes secretory diarrhea, and the remaining *Shigella* species cause bacillary dysentery with fever, bloody diarrhea, cramping, and tenesmus. As with the typhoid group of *Salmonella*, humans are the sole host for *Shigella* species; however, the low infectious dose required by *Shigella* species to cause disease is more similar to the nontyphoid *Salmonella* species.

Salmonella Species

For clinical purposes, the genus *Salmonella* can be divided into two broad groups: typhoid and nontyphoid.

The typhoid group, consisting of *Salmonella enterica* serotypes *typhi* and *paratyphi*, causes typhoid (enteric) fever. These organisms exclusively infect human hosts and are transmitted via contaminated food or water. A large inoculum of typhoid group bacteria is required to experimentally produce infection. Some infected persons become chronic carriers who can transmit infection to others, such as the infamous Typhoid Mary. Typhoid fever is endemic in the developing world. The classic presentation of typhoid fever evolves over 3 weeks: a stepwise fever with temperature-pulse dissociation in the first week, abdominal pain and rose spots on the trunk in the second week, and hepatosplenomegaly with intestinal bleeding in the third week. Because these species are only transmitted between human hosts, identification of one case of typhoid fever becomes a public health issue that mandates contact tracing. Possible complications include bacteremia, gastrointestinal bleeding or perforation, cholangitis, pneumonia, and osteomyelitis.

The nontyphoid group consists of all *Salmonella* species except *S. enterica* serotypes *typhi* and *paratyphi*. These species generally incubate in animals and are transmitted to humans through consumption of contaminated food or water; direct human-to-human transmission is exceedingly rare. In contrast to the typhoid group, nontyphoid *Salmonella* species can cause disease with inocula as low as 10 to 100 organisms. The disease that results is most often a gastroenteritis with fever, emesis, and diarrhea that can be secretory or inflammatory, lasting up to 7 days. Possible complications include bacteremia, endovascular infection from seeding of atherosclerotic plaques or prosthetic grafts, and Reiter's syndrome.

Campylobacter Species

Campylobacter species are common bacterial causes of acute infectious diarrhea; *Campylobacter jejuni* is the major species that causes human disease. Infection is contracted through consumption of contaminated poultry, milk, or water. After an incubation period of 2 to 7 days, the patient develops bloody diarrhea. *Campylobacter* diarrhea is also notable for its manifold extraintestinal complications, including autoimmune phenomena such as reactive arthritis and Guillain-Barré syndrome. Antibiotic therapy is usually reserved for severe disease or immunocompromised patients, in whom recurrent disease is more frequent.

Vibrio cholerae

Vibrio cholerae is the prototype of an enterotoxic bacterium that causes secretory diarrhea. It is almost exclusively a disease of developing countries with poor sanitation. There have been several pandemics in the last century, with the most recent affecting South America and Central America as well the more typical regions in Africa and Asia. The only two serotypes to cause human disease are O1 and O139; serotype O1 is divided into biotypes *cholerae* and *eltor*. Cholera toxin affects enterocytes to produce a secretory diarrhea described as *rice-water stools*. Disease severity ranges from mild to severe with profound dehydration. Rehydration is the cornerstone of treatment, via oral or intravenous routes as dictated by clinical severity.

Clostridium difficile

Clostridium difficile has been recognized as one cause of antibiotic-associated diarrhea and the leading cause of pseudomembranous colitis since the late 1970s. *C. difficile*–associated diarrhea was conventionally thought to only be a health issue for institutionalized patients who have had recent exposure to antibiotics or chemotherapy. In the last 5 years, however, significant expansions in *C. difficile*–associated diarrhea disease severity and host range have been described by researchers in North America and Europe. Disease severity ranges from asymptomatic colonization to mild diarrhea to fulminant pseudomembranous colitis resulting in colectomy, need for intensive care, and high attributable mortality rate.

Other Bacteria

Several other bacteria are less-common causes of acute infectious diarrhea. They merit some discussion because of their specific clinical presentations or potential for causing severe disease.

Vibrio parahemolyticus

Vibrio parahemolyticus causes gastrointestinal illness associated with consumption of raw or undercooked oysters and other seafood. The spectrum of illness varies widely. Immunocompetent patients usually develop self-limited secretory diarrhea or gastroenteritis with fever lasting from 1 to 3 days, and immunocompromised patients present with severe diarrhea, septicemia, and a profound hemolytic anemia.

Staphylococcus aureus

Staphylococcus aureus causes a variety of gastrointestinal illnesses. It is a common cause of enterotoxin-mediated foodborne illness, manifesting with emesis, watery diarrhea, and cramping after a brief incubation period of 1 to 6 hours. *S. aureus*, particularly methicillin-resistant *S. aureus* (MRSA), is also an uncommon but recognized cause of pseudomembranous colitis.

Bacteroides fragilis

Although *Bacteroides fragilis* is recognized as part of the normal flora of the large intestine, certain strains produce a metalloprotease that has been associated with diarrhea in several studies of human and animal populations. Some studies have suggested that these enterotoxigenic *B. fragilis* strains may be more likely than nontoxigenic strains to cause blood infections.

Clostridium perfringens

Clostridium perfringens is a ubiquitous pathogen that is a common cause of enterotoxin-mediated secretory diarrhea. Its specific enterotoxin (CPE) has been found in all five toxinotypes of *C. perfringens*. Gastrointestinal disease can result from ingestion of preformed toxin, with a short incubation period before clinical disease, or ingestion of a large bacterial inoculum, requiring a longer incubation before disease. Treatment is usually supportive.

PROTOZOA

Giardia lamblia

Giardia lamblia is a protozoan pathogen that causes diarrhea that can be chronic and refractory to treatment. The infectious cyst form is ingested in contaminated food or water, and the trophozoite then attaches to the intestinal wall. *Giardia* has expanded its environmental niche in recent years from the beaver fever endemic to isolated rivers and lakes, becoming a global pathogen.

Entamoeba histolytica

Entamoeba histolytica can cause amoebic dysentery, which can manifest as acute, subacute, or chronic diarrhea. Diagnosis of *E. histolytica* is complicated by the highly similar but nonpathogenic *Entamoeba dispar*. Other than the rare situation where microscopy of stool detects ingested erythrocytes (pathognomic of *E. histolytica*), the two species are morphologically identical and can only be distinguished by methodologies such as serology, antigen detection, or nucleic acid testing.

VIRUSES

Rotavirus

Rotavirus primarily affects infants and children from 3 to 36 months of age, resulting in a spectrum of disease from asymptomatic shedding to severe gastroenteritis with dehydration. Globally, it is the leading viral cause of severe gastroenteritis. Other groups affected include travelers, the immunocompromised, and patients in hospitals or other institutions.

Calicivirus

Norwalk virus is the most well-known member of the calicivirus family. Outbreaks of Norwalk often occur in long-term care facilities, cruise ships, and hospitals. It is highly contagious, with attack rates often greater than 10%. The clinical syndrome of Norwalk infection usually features rapid onset of severe nausea and emesis along with varying degrees of diarrhea.

Differential Diagnosis

OTHER INFECTIONS

Infections that cause diarrhea are not necessarily primarily gastrointestinal (Box 5). Systemic infections that result in diarrhea are probably underrecognized as a distinct etiology; however, the astute clinician should usually be able to recognize a systemic infection after a proper history, physical examination, and appropriate laboratory tests. Bacterial infections such as Group A streptococcosis,

BOX 5 Diseases That Can Mimic Acute Infectious Diarrhea

Infectious Etiologies
- Dengue fever
- *Francisella* sp.
- Hantavirus
- *Legionella* sp.
- Leptospirosis
- Lyme borreliosis
- Malaria
- SARS

Noninfectious Etiologies
- Antibiotic-associated diarrhea
- Bacterial overgrowth
- Brainerd diarrhea (infectious etiology suspected but unproved)
- Endocrinopathies (e.g., VIPoma)
- Inflammatory bowel disease
- Irritable bowel syndrome
- Other medications

Abbreviations: SARS = severe acute respiratory syndrome; VIP = vasoactive intestinal peptide.

legionellosis, leptospirosis, and some tick-borne infections (including borreliosis, ehrlichiosis, tularemia, and Rocky Mountain spotted fever) can manifest with diarrhea as an initial symptom. Septicemia, caused by a variety of pathogens such as gram-negative enteric organisms, can also cause diarrhea and other gastrointestinal symptoms. Viremia is another cause of diarrhea; the most common cause is probably influenza, but other viruses including severe acute respiratory syndrome–associated coronavirus (SARS-CoV), hantaviruses, dengue virus (*Flavivirus* sp.), and hemorrhagic fever viruses should be considered in the presence of correlating exposures. *Plasmodium falciparum* malaria can result in diarrhea severe enough to mimic bacillary dysentery, particularly in children, and severe diarrhea has been associated with poor outcome.

OTHER NONINFECTIOUS ETIOLOGIES

A variety of noninfectious causes can result in acute diarrhea (see Box 5). For instance, diarrhea is a common adverse effect of antimicrobial agents and other medications. The mechanism varies by antibiotic, but common reasons include direct stimulation of gut motility, increased gut osmolality, and disruption of the normal gut flora.

Although not strictly an infection, diarrhea is one of the most common symptoms of bacterial overgrowth. This disease occurs after disruption of host mechanisms that normally regulate bacterial intestinal colonization, such as pancreatitis or intestinal dysmotility. Definitive treatment should address the underlying condition, but broad-spectrum antibiotics can result in a long-lasting cure.

Brainerd diarrhea was initially described after an outbreak in Brainerd, Minnesota, in 1983. It manifests as an acute secretory diarrhea that can last for several months. Its etiology remains unknown, but several outbreaks have demonstrated epidemiologic links to consumption of unpasteurized milk and undertreated water.

Some endocrinopathies, such as VIPoma, can cause profuse diarrhea. Inflammatory bowel diseases (e.g., Crohn's disease, ulcerative colitis) can manifest with an inflammatory diarrhea and constitutional symptoms. Irritable bowel syndrome can result in periods of diarrhea; however, there are alternating periods of constipation and a lack of constitutional symptoms.

Special Cases

TRAVELER'S DIARRHEA

According to the Centers for Disease Control and Prevention (CDC), 20% to 50% of international travelers develop diarrhea related to their travels. The etiologic agents vary by exposure, geographic region, and local outbreaks. Bacteria are the most commonly implicated pathogens, with ETEC being the most commonly identified cause. Other etiologic agents include the other common bacterial, viral, and protozoal enteric pathogens described earlier. Diarrhea is usually mild to moderate and self-limited; 90% of patients report resolution of symptoms after 1 week, and 98% after 4 weeks. Although it is usually a nuisance rather than a severe threat to health, diarrhea can significantly limit the traveler's activities.

Because traveler's diarrhea is self-limited, investigations of the cause are usually reserved for diarrhea that is prolonged or manifests with higher-risk features such as fever or bloody stool. Stool should be examined for ova and parasites (O&P) if the travel history is supportive.

The focus for management should be supportive care. People seen for travel medicine advice should be counseled to avoid consuming water or food not known to be safe. The safest diet for travelers consists of freshly prepared foods served thoroughly heated, fruits and vegetables that are peeled or are washed with safe water, and beverages that are bottled or boiled before consumption. Ice and tap water should be considered contaminated. Patients for whom diarrhea could be catastrophic should be advised to avoid traveling unless it is strictly necessary.

After the traveler has developed diarrhea, a variety of medications are available for treatment (Box 7). One review determined that antibiotics shorten the duration of traveler's diarrhea but had higher rates of adverse effects compared with placebo.

IMMUNOCOMPROMISED STATES

Gastrointestinal illness is a common problem in immunocompromised patients. Apart from the infectious etiologies of diarrhea described earlier, other causes found in immunocompromised patients include the agent causing the immunocompromised state (such as HIV or chemotherapeutic agents), opportunistic organisms, adverse effects of medications, dysfunction of intestinal absorption, and idiopathic enteropathies.

Opportunistic organisms that can cause diarrhea include parasites (e.g., *Cryptosporidium parvum*, *Cyclospora cayetanensis*, *Isospora belli*, microsporidia), fungi (e.g., disseminated fungal infections from *Histoplasma capsulatum* and *Cryptococcus neoformans*), bacteria (e.g., *Mycobacterium avium-intracellulare* complex), and viruses (e.g., cytomegalovirus, herpes simplex virus). In general, treatment requires prolonged courses of antimicrobial agents and can be complicated by concomitant medications or diseases; consultation with an appropriate specialist is suggested.

Prevention

Methods of prevention are listed in Box 6.

BOX 6 Prevention of Acute Infectious Diarrhea

- Avoidance
- Hygiene
- Prophylactic antibiotics
- Probiotics
- Vaccines
  - Cholera/ETEC (Dukoral)[2]
  - Rotavirus (RotaTeq)
  - *Salmonella typhi* (Vivotif Berna, Typhim Vi)

[2]Not available in the United States.
Abbreviation: ETEC = enterotoxigenic *Escherichia coli*.

AVOIDANCE

An effective method for preventing acute infectious diarrhea is to eliminate exposures that put one at risk. This applies particularly to patients who would be at high risk for contracting acute infectious diarrhea or having adverse outcomes, for example, patients who are immunocompromised or physically debilitated. Exposure avoidance is usually situational and patient-specific, such as suggesting that travel be postponed to a region currently undergoing a cholera epidemic or cautioning against consumption of raw seafood.

HYGIENE

Proper handwashing by health care workers caring for patients with acute diarrhea is essential to prevent institutional transmission, and its importance cannot be overstated. Barrier precautions are also commonly implemented, particularly if the patient is incontinent of stool. Other precautions, such as tailoring environmental cleaning practices to specific pathogens during outbreaks, are also proven effective.

PROPHYLACTIC ANTIBIOTICS

There is a limited role for antibiotics in preventing acute infectious diarrhea, particularly traveler's diarrhea. The normally mild severity and self-limited nature of the disease, along with the risk of adverse effects from antibiotics, means that prophylactic antibiotics are most often reserved for brief durations in patients at high risk for contracting acute infectious diarrhea or for experiencing adverse outcomes.

PROBIOTICS

There has been a surge of publications concerning the role of probiotics in preventing diarrhea of varying etiologies. Although individual studies have produced varied results for diarrhea caused by *C. difficile*–associated diarrhea and traveler's diarrhea, one meta-analysis of 34 studies supported a role for probiotics in preventing diarrhea, with an overall risk reduction of at least 21%. Stratification by type of diarrhea found a much larger reduction in antibiotic-associated (52%) than traveler's (8%) diarrhea. However, these findings were challenged due to the variety of organisms and treatment regimens between different studies, and the low proportion of adult patients in those studies reporting reductions in antibiotic-associated diarrhea.

VACCINES

Rotavirus

A live human-bovine reassortant rotavirus oral vaccine (RotaTeq) has been licensed since February 2006 in the United States for infants 6 to 32 weeks of age. The vaccine appears efficacious in preventing rotaviral gastroenteritis, and consequently it reduces the need for outpatient and inpatient assessment. A large phase III trial demonstrated no increased risk over placebo at intussusception, an adverse effect that led to the withdrawal of a previous rotavirus vaccine. An attenuated human rotavirus vaccine (RotaRix) is licensed in countries throughout Europe, Asia, and Africa, but not North America.

Vibrio cholerae and ETEC

An oral inactivated cholera vaccine (Dukoral), available in Canada but not in the United States, has demonstrated some efficacy in preventing traveler's diarrhea. The B subunit of *V. cholerae* toxin used in this vaccine has sufficient structural homology with ETEC heat-labile toxin to provide moderate short-term protection against this common cause of traveler's diarrhea, lasting up to 3 months.

Salmonella typhi

Enteral and parenteral vaccines are available to prevent typhoid. The enteral form (Vivotif Berna) is a live attenuated strain of *S. typhi*, which is taken as four capsules over 7 days and confers immunity

CURRENT DIAGNOSIS

History

- Duration and frequency of diarrhea
- Other gastrointestinal symptoms (emesis, tenesmus, abdominal pain)
- Presence of bloody stool, fever
- Medication use, including recent antibiotic use
- Recent contact with ill persons, travel, and animal contact
- Consumption of raw or undercooked poultry or seafood
- Immunocompromised state (rule out)

Physical Examination

- Hydration status
- Gastrointestinal examination
- Other systems as indicated by symptoms

Laboratory Tests

- For limited secretory diarrhea: usually none
- For bloody diarrhea: complete blood count (CBC), stool for culture (rule out O157:H7); consider ova and parasites test (O&P)
- For chronic diarrhea: consider *C. difficile* assay, O&P
- For traveler's diarrhea: CBC, stool for culture and O&P
- For immunocompromised patients: CBC, stool for culture and O&P

for approximately 5 years. The parenteral form (Typhim Vi) is purified capsular polysaccharide that is given as a single intramuscular injection. This is the preferred route for patients with contraindications to live attenuated vaccines, such as immunocompromised status. Neither vaccine is completely protective, and neither provides protection against *S. paratyphi*.

Treatment

Management of acute infectious diarrhea is listed in Box 7.

BOX 7   Management of Acute Infectious Diarrhea

Rehydration
- Enteral
  - World Health Organization formulation
  - Commercially available rehydration solutions
  - Home remedies
- Parenteral
  - Intravenous
  - Intraosseus
  - Enteroclysis

Medications
- Antidiarrheals
  - Bismuth subsalicylate
  - Morphine derivatives
- Antibiotics
- Probiotics

CURRENT THERAPY

- Supportive care
- Rehydration (always replace previous losses and provide maintenance)
  - Enteral
  - Parenteral (intravenous, intraosseus, enteroclytic)
- Antidiarrheal medications (only if patient is afebrile and stools are not bloody)
  - Morphine derivatives
  - Bismuth subsalicylate (Pepto-Bismol)
- Antibiotics (only if necessary as indicated by symptoms, severity, and risk factors)
  - Empiric therapy
    - Adults
      - Ciprofloxacin (Cipro) 500 mg PO bid for 3-5 d
      - Levofloxacin (Levaquin)[1] 500 mg PO qd for 3-5 d
    - Children
      - Azithromycin (Zithromax)[1] 5-10 mg/kg PO qd for 3-5 d
      - Trimethoprim-sulfamethoxazole (Septra) 5-25 mg/kg/d PO in two equally divided doses for 3-5 d *plus*
      - Erythromycin 10 mg/kg/d PO qid for 5 d
  - Specific therapy as directed by pathogen identification and susceptibilities
- Probiotics

---

[1]Not FDA approved for this indication.

REHYDRATION

Maintaining adequate hydration is usually the cornerstone of management for acute diarrhea. The route of administration depends on the patient's hydration status and disease severity; enteral hydration is preferred to parenteral, if possible.

In 2003 the WHO reformulated their well-known oral rehydration solution (ORS). The new lower-osmolarity formula has been found to reduce stool volume, emesis, and the need for switching to intravenous therapy in children with diarrhea. This new formulation has 75 mmol/L sodium, 75 mmol/L glucose, and a total osmolarity 245 mOsm/L, which can be achieved with a recipe of 2.6 g sodium chloride, 13.5 g anhydrous glucose, 1.5 g potassium chloride, 2.5 g sodium bicarbonate and 1.5 g trisodium citrate dihydrate per liter of water.

A homemade solution can be prepared with 40 mL sugar and 5 mL table salt per liter of clean water; however, this preparation lacks potassium. Furthermore, commercially prepared rehydration solutions should be preferred to homemade in order to minimize the chance of errors in preparing the solution. Most sports drinks are not equivalent to actual rehydration solutions, because sports drinks often have higher carbohydrate and lower electrolyte loads.

Parenteral rehydration is usually intravenous, although intraosseus administration can be used for infants in whom intravenous access cannot be obtained and enteroclysis can be used in adult patients with difficult vascular access who do not require large volumes of replacement fluid. Sufficient volumes of fluid should be given to replace preexisting fluid deficits as well as ongoing losses and maintenance requirements.

ANTIDIARRHEAL MEDICATIONS

Some medications reduce intestinal motility by affecting the myenteric motor plexus to inhibit peristalsis. Opioid derivatives, such as loperamide (Imodium), are the class of medications most commonly used for this purpose. Although licensed for use with acute, chronic, and traveler's diarrhea, loperamide is contraindicated in the presence of fever or bloody stool or in situations where inhibition of peristalsis is otherwise undesirable or potentially harmful.

Other medications are classified as antidiarrheal but have different mechanisms of action. Bismuth subsalicylate (Pepto-Bismol) appears to function by multiple mechanisms including intestinal secretion reduction, intestinal reabsorption of fluids and electrolytes, toxin binding, and direct antimicrobial effects. It has proven efficacy in the management of traveler's diarrhea, although its dosing frequency may be difficult for some patients. Racecadotril (or acetorphan)[2] is a new synthetic enkephalinase inhibitor that acts by the same mechanism as the opioid derivatives and has been studied for its antidiarrheal effect in pediatric patients.

ANTIBIOTICS

Antibiotics should be used cautiously in the treatment of acute infectious diarrhea. Most clinical cases adequately resolve without antibiotic therapy. Furthermore, their use may lead to further diarrhea (including antibiotic-associated diarrhea), contribute to selective pressures favoring development of antibiotic-resistant organisms, and prolong the carriage of certain pathogens. Recommendations in the empiric and pathogen-specific treatment of acute infectious diarrhea are given in Tables 1 and 2.

PROBIOTICS

As with the prevention of diarrhea, a growing body of evidence has yet to provide definite conclusions on the use of probiotics for treating acute infectious diarrhea. One of the major limitations to using probiotics is the variation in species and doses used in different clinical trials. However, there may be a class effect that is most likely a combination of competition for intestinal binding sites or nutritional resources, elaboration of antibacterial compounds, and immune

---

[2]Not available in the United States.

TABLE 1 Empiric Therapy of Diarrheal Disease

Clinical Syndrome	Adult Patients	Pediatric Patients
Febrile dysenteric diarrhea in industrialized regions, or moderate to severe traveler's diarrhea	Ciprofloxacin (Cipro) 500 mg PO bid or levofloxacin (Levaquin)[1] 500 mg PO qd for 3-5 d	Azithromycin (Zithromax)[1] 5-10 mg/kg PO qd for 3-5 d *or* trimethoprim-sulfamethoxazole (Septra) 5-25 mg/kg/d PO in two divided doses for 3-5 d *plus* erythromycin[1] 10 mg/kg PO qid for 5 d
Persistent diarrhea (≥14 d in duration) in industrialized countries	Consider anti-*Giardia* therapy: metronidazole (Flagyl)[1] 250 mg PO tid for 7 d	Consider anti-*Giardia* therapy: metronidazole (Flagyl)[1] 20 mg/kg/d PO in three divided doses for 7 d

Adapted from Montes M, DuPont HL: Enteritis, enterocolitis and infectious diarrhea syndromes. In Cohen J, Powderly WD: Infectious Diseases, 2nd ed. St Louis: Mosby, 2004, pp 477-489.
[1]Not FDA approved for this indication.

TABLE 2 Pathogen-Specific Therapy of Diarrheal Disease

Pathogen	Adult Patients	Pediatric Patients
Campylobacter jejuni	Azithromycin (Zithromax)[1] 500 mg PO qd for 3 d	Erythromycin stearate[1] 40 mg/kg/d in four divided doses for 5 d *or* azithromycin[1] 10 mg/kg/d
Clostridium difficile	Initial disease: metronidazole (Flagyl) 250 mg PO qid for 10-14 d or vancomycin (Vancocin) 125-500 mg PO qid for 10-14 d	Initial disease: metronidazole 20 mg/kg/d in three divided doses for 10-14 d or vancomycin 125-500 mg PO qid for 10-14 d
EAEC, EIEC, EPEC, ETEC	Same as empiric therapy for febrile dysentery and traveler's diarrhea (see Table 1)	Azithromycin[1] 10 mg/kg/d. If resistance is suspected, use ceftriaxone (Rocephin),[1] cefixime (Suprax),[1] or cefotaxime (Claforan)[1]
EHEC*	No antimicrobial therapy (increased risk of increasing toxin release and hemolytic-uremic syndrome)	No antimicrobial therapy (increased risk of increasing toxin release and hemolytic-uremic syndrome)
Entamoeba histolytica	Metronidazole 500 mg PO tid for 10 d or tinidazole (Tindamax) 1 g PO bid for 3 d Follow with paromomycin (Humatin) 500 mg PO tid for 7 d	Metronidazole 50 mg/kg/d IV in three divided doses plus diiodohydroxyquin (Yodoxin) 40 mg/kg/d in three divided doses for 20 d
Giardia lamblia	Metronidazole[1] 250 mg PO tid for 7 d *or* albendazole (Albenza)[1] 400 mg PO qd for 5 d *or* tinidazole 2 g PO in one dose	Metronidazole[1] 20 mg/kg/d in three divided doses for 7 d *or* furazolidone (Furoxone) 6 mg/kg/d divided in four doses for 7 d
Shigella sp.	Ciprofloxacin (Cipro) 500 mg PO bid for 3-5 d *or* levofloxacin (Levaquin)[1] 500 mg PO qd for 3-5 d	Azithromycin[1] 10 mg/kg/d. If resistance is suspected, use ceftriaxone,[1] cefixime,[1] or cefotaxime[1]
Salmonella sp. non-typhoid group	Asymptomatic or mild: no antimicrobial therapy At risk for complications: ciprofloxacin[1] 500 mg PO bid or levofloxacin[1] 500 mg PO qd for 5-7 d Alternatives: azithromycin[1] or erythromycin stearate (Erythrocin stearate)[1] 500 mg PO bid for 5 d	≤6 mo old: ceftriaxone[1] 50 mg/kg IV qd >6 mo old and healthy, and asymptomatic or with mild illness: no antimicrobial therapy At risk for complications: ceftriaxone[1] 50 mg/kg IV qd (not to exceed 2 g/d)
typhoid group	Ciprofloxacin (Cipro) 500 mg PO bid for 7-10 d or levofloxacin (Levaquin)[1] 500 mg PO OD for 7-10 d or ceftriaxone 2 g IV q 24h for 14 d	Ceftriaxone 75-100 mg/kg IVq 24h for 14 d (not to exceed 4 g/d) or azithromycin 20 mg/kg PO OD for 5-7 d (not to exceed 1 g/d)
Vibrio cholerae	Doxycycline 300 mg PO for one dose or ciprofloxacin[1] 1 g PO for one dose Recurrent disease can require prolonged courses of antibiotics or adjunctive therapy (e.g., IVIG,[1] resins[1])	TMP-SMX (Septra)[1] 1 DS tab PO bid for 3 d or azithromycin[1] 20 mg/kg PO for one dose (not to exceed 1 g)

Adapted from Montes M, DuPont HL: Enteritis, enterocolitis and infectious diarrhea syndromes. In Cohen J, Powderly WD: Infectious Diseases, 2nd ed. St Louis: Mosby, 2004, pp 477-489.
[1]Not FDA approved for this indication.
*Shiga toxin and Shiga-like toxin–producing *E. coli.*
Abbreviations: DS = double strength; EAEC = enteroaggregative *E. coli;* EHEC = enterohemorrhagic *E. coli;* EIEC = enteroinvasive *E. coli.*
EPEC = enteropathogenic *E. coli;* ETEC = enterotoxigenic *E. coli;* IVIG = intravenous immunoglobulin; TMP-SMX = trimethoprim-sulfamethoxazole.

stimulation. Another recognized limitation is the rare but serious case of blood infection from the probiotic organism; documented cases have occurred not only in recipients but also in other patients being cared for in close proximity to the recipient.

REFERENCES

Aranda-Michel J, Giannella RA. Acute diarrhea: A practical review. Am J Med 1999;106:670–6.
DuPont HL. What's new in enteric infectious diseases at home and abroad. Curr Opin Infect Dis 2005;18:407–12.
Dupont HL, the Practice Parameters Committee of the American College of Gastroenterology. Guidelines on acute infectious diarrhea in adults. Am J Gastroenterol 1997;92(11):1962–75.
Guerrant RL, Van Gilder T, Stiner TS, et al. Practice guidelines for the management of infectious diarrhea. Clin Infect Dis 2001;32:331–50.
Hahn S, Kim Y, Garner P. Reduced osmolarity oral rehydration solution for treating dehydration due to diarrhea in children: Systematic review. Br Med J 2001;323:81–5.
Helton T, Rolson DD. Which adults with acute diarrhea should be evaluated? What is the best diagnostic approach? Cleve Clin J Med 2004;71(10):778–85.
Musher DM, Musher BL. Contagious acute gastrointestinal infections. N Engl J Med 2004;351(23):2417–27.
Reisinger EC, Fritzsche C, Krause R, Krejs GJ. Diarrhea caused by primarily non-gastrointestinal infections. Nat Clin Practice Gastroenterol Hepatol 2005;2(5):216–22.
Sazawal S, Hiremath G, Dhingra U, et al. Efficacy of probiotics in prevention of acute diarrhoea: A meta-analysis of masked, randomised, placebo-controlled trials. Lancet Infect Dis 2006;6:374–82.
Thielman NM, Guerrant RL. Acute infectious diarrhea. N Engl J Med 2004;350:38–47.
World Health Organization. Oral rehydration salts: Production of the new ORS. 2006. PDF available at http://www.who.int/child-adolescent-health/New_Publications/CHILD_HEALTH/WHO_FCH_CAH_06.1.pdf (accessed April 5, 2007).

Constipation

Method of
Shane E. Hendon, DO, and Jack A. DiPalma, MD

Constipation is a very common condition that affects millions of people in the United States and other developed countries. In the United States, it results in 2.5 million patient visits to physicians and approximately 92,000 hospitalizations each year. Many other people do not seek professional medical care for what they presume to be constipation and treat the condition themselves. The prevalence in North America has ranged from 1.9% to 27.2%, with most estimates falling between 12 and 19%. In the United States, more than $400 million is spent annually on over-the-counter laxatives, and 5 million laxative prescriptions are written each year. The full economic impact of evaluating and treating patients with constipation is unknown.

Definition

There is no single definition of constipation. Patients and physicians seemingly vary in their definitions of constipation. Most patients define constipation by one or more symptoms: hard stools, infrequent stools (typically fewer than three per week), the need for excessive straining, a sense of incomplete bowel evacuation, and excessive time spent on the toilet or in unsuccessful defecation. The Rome criteria for functional gastrointestinal disorders were developed to help standardize the definition of functional bowel disorders, including functional constipation. Currently, the Rome III criteria for functional constipation give physicians and researchers a consensus definition of constipation. Subjective and objective definitions of constipation are listed in Table 1 and include

- Straining, hard stools, infrequent stools, or incomplete evacuation
- Fewer than 3 bowel movements per week, daily stool weight less than 35 g/day, or straining more than 25% of the time
- Prolonged whole gut or colonic transit

Although the term constipation may have different meanings for patients and doctors, it is the doctors' responsibility to make sure that they know what patients mean by constipation, so that any misunderstandings are avoided and unnecessary tests and inappropriate treatments are not undertaken.

Demographics

Constipation is more common in women than in men, with a 2.2:1 ratio; the incidence increases with age, particularly after age 65 years. It is more frequent in non-Caucasians than in Caucasians. An increased prevalence of constipation was found to correlate with low socioeconomic status and lower education levels in several studies, although these differences were more dramatic in studies that used self-report of constipation as the case definition.

Causes and Pathophysiology

Constipation is frequently multifactorial and can be the result of many conditions. Table 2 lists some common medical conditions associated with constipation. Behavioral issues such as diets low in fiber and water, decreased physical activity, inconvenient toilet facilities, voluntary suppression of defecation, and psychiatric disorders can cause constipation. If constipation is caused by another disease, it is referred to as secondary constipation. If there is no known underlying disorder, constipation is referred to as primary. Primary constipation can be classified into three categories based on the underlying pathophysiology: normal-transit constipation, disorders of defecatory or rectal evacuation, and slow-transit constipation. In a study of 1000 patients with chronic constipation, normal-transit constipation was the most prevalent type (59%), with disorders of defecatory or rectal evacuation occurring in 25%, slow-transit in 13%, and a combination of the latter two in 3% of patients.

NORMAL-TRANSIT CONSTIPATION

Normal-transit constipation (functional constipation) is the most common form of chronic constipation that is seen by physicians. As can be inferred by its name, stool traverses through the colon at a normal rate, and stool frequency is normal. Despite the normal rate and frequency of bowel movements, patients believe they are constipated. In this group of patients, constipation is likely to be characterized as a perceived difficulty with evacuation or the presence of hard stools. However, the stool texture is not abnormally hard when tested objectively, so the complaint of hard stool most likely reflects difficulty with evacuation. Patients may complain of abdominal pain or discomfort and bloating, and they may exhibit increased psychosocial distress. With normal-transit constipation, symptoms typically respond to increased dietary fiber, alone or with the addition of an osmotic laxative.

DEFECATORY DISORDERS

Disorders of defecatory or rectal evacuation are most commonly caused by the inability to appropriately coordinate the muscles of the pelvic floor and abdomen that are involved in successful defecation. Normally, continence is maintained by contraction of the puborectalis muscle, which wraps around the anorectum creating an anorectal angle between 80 and 110 degrees, and of the internal anal sphincter. During defecation, the anorectal angle straightens by at least 15 degrees due to relaxation of the pelvic floor muscles; the internal and external anal sphincters relax; and the perineum descends by 1.0 to 3.5 cm. The discoordination most typically seen with defecatory disorders takes the form of paradoxical contraction of the external anal sphincter, which may be accompanied by a failure of the pelvic floor muscles to relax when straining to defecate. This may be the result of prolonged avoidance of pain associated with passage of a large, hard stool; anal fissure; or hemorrhoid. As previously stated, behavioral issues, including voluntary suppression of defecation and psychosexual problems, may contribute to constipation. Less often, structural abnormalities such as rectocele or excessive perineal descent can lead to dyssynergic defecation.

SLOW-TRANSIT CONSTIPATION

Slow-transit constipation is typically seen in young women with one or fewer bowel movements per week; it is associated with an infrequent urge to defecate, bloating, and abdominal pain or discomfort. It may be related to a decreased number of high-amplitude propagated contractions, which leads to prolonged residence time of fecal residue in the proximal colon, or to increased uncoordinated motor activity in the distal colon that offers a functional barrier or resistance to normal transit.

In those patients with minimal delay in colonic transit times, a high-fiber diet may increase stool weight, decrease colon transit time, and relieve constipation. However, patients with more severe slow-transit constipation typically have a poor response to dietary fiber and laxatives. Histopathologic studies in such patients have shown alterations in the number of myenteric plexus neurons expressing the excitatory neurotransmitter substance P, abnormalities in the inhibitory transmitters vasoactive intestinal peptide and nitric oxide, and a reduction in the interstitial cells of Cajal, which regulate gastrointestinal motility.

Hirschsprung's disease is an extreme form of slow-transit constipation in which ganglion cells in the distal bowel are absent due to an arrest in the caudal migration of neural-crest cells through the gut during embryonic development; this allows for bowel narrowing in places that lack ganglion cells. Most patients are diagnosed in infancy or early childhood, but others may present later in life.

SECONDARY CONSTIPATION

Secondary constipation may result from numerous medical conditions (see Table 1), including endocrine and metabolic diseases, neurologic disorders, collagen vascular disorders, and mechanical obstruction. In a study comparing more than 7000 patients with chronic constipation and 7000 normal subjects, the relative risk for chronic constipation in patients with diabetes, thyroid disease, Parkinson's disease, and multiple sclerosis was 1.33, 1.91, 5.04, and 11.02, respectively. Mechanical obstruction from malignancy within the bowel wall or from external compression must be considered.

CURRENT DIAGNOSIS

- Constipation is common, with a prevalence ranging from 2% to 28%.
- There is no single definition of constipation.
- Constipation is frequently multifactorial and can be related to behavioral issues, medical conditions, and use of medications.
- Primary constipation can be classified into three basic categories
    - Normal-transit constipation
    - Slow-transit constipation
    - Disorders of defecatory or rectal evaluation
- A careful history and physical examination can help identify most causes of constipation.

TABLE 3 Drugs That May Cause Constipation

Drug Class	Drugs
Analgesics	Opioids and related narcotics Nonsteroidal antiinflammatory drugs
Anticholinergic drugs	Atropine, dicyclomine (Bentyl), hyoscyamine (Levsin), clidinium (Quarzan)[2] Tricyclic antidepressants Antipsychotic and neuroleptic agents Anti-parkinsonian drugs
Antihypertensive agents	Calcium channel antagonists Central α-adrenergic agonists Monoamine oxidase inhibitors Methyldopa (Aldomet)
Anticonvulsants	Phenobarbital, phenytoin (Dilantin)
Antihistamines	Diphenhydramine (Benadryl), etc.
Metal ions and minerals	Aluminum (antacids, sucralfate [Carafate]) Iron supplements Calcium supplements Barium sulfate Heavy metal intoxication (lead, mercury, arsenic)
Chemotherapeutic agents	Vinca alkaloids
Resins	Cholestyramine (Questran) Sodium polystyrene sulfonate (Kayexalate)

Modified from Rutland TJ, Adeniji OA, DiPalma JA: Prevalence of medication-associated constipation. Am J Gastroenterol 2004;99:S103-S104.
[2]Not available in the United States.

Chronic use of medications, whether over-the-counter or prescribed, can increase the risk of developing chronic constipation (Table 3). The *Physician's Desk Reference* lists more than 900 drugs that are reported to cause constipation. More than 100 entries included constipation as an adverse experience that occurs in more than 3% of patients using the product. In a review of more than 300 patients with self-reported constipation, 59.3% were found to be using constipating medications. Opioids, diuretics, antidepressants, antihistamines, antispasmodics, anticonvulsants, and aluminum acids are some of the medications associated with the highest risk of developing constipation. Medication use is an important factor to consider in the management of this condition.

Evaluation of Chronic Constipation

HISTORY AND PHYSICAL EXAMINATION

As previously stated, there is no clear definition of constipation. The first step in the assessment of chronic constipation is for the physician to clearly understand what the patient means by constipation. Patients should be asked how they define constipation and how the onset, severity, and duration of each symptom relate to their normal bowel habits, and questioned about their description of bowel patterns. Identification of social or environmental factors that may affect bowel habits, evaluation of cognitive and functional abilities, cultural beliefs and expectations regarding bowel patterns, and review of diet and fluid intake are also important. A careful history and complete physical examination help rule out most secondary causes of constipation. One must pay careful attention to relevant associated risk factors, including age, gender, lifestyle, medical conditions, and use of medicines.

A careful rectal examination should be performed in every patient with constipation. The perianal area should be examined for scars, fistulas, fissures, and the presence of external hemorrhoids. A digital examination of the rectum should be performed to determine whether fecal impaction, anal stricture, or rectal masses are present. The perineum should be observed with the patient at rest and bearing down to determine perineal descent, which is normally 1.0 to 3.5 cm. Reduced descent may indicate an inability to relax the pelvic floor muscles during defecation. Excessive perineal descent may indicate laxity of the perineum, which may result from childbirth or excessive straining.

LABORATORY TESTS AND IMAGING

Laboratory tests may be done initially to help exclude potential secondary causes of constipation, including thyroid dysfunction, electrolyte and glucose abnormalities, and other metabolic conditions (see Table 2).

Imaging of the colon is required to exclude the possibility of structural diseases such as colon cancer, but only in patients who exhibit warning symptoms or signs. These alarm symptoms may include new onset or worsening of constipation, onset after age 50 years, rectal bleeding or hematochezia, weight loss, fevers, anorexia, nausea, vomiting, or a family history of inflammatory bowel disease or colon cancer. Patients 50 years of age or older should undergo colon cancer screening regardless of the absence or presence of constipation.

PHYSIOLOGIC TESTING

Physiologic testing may be necessary for patients who have constipation refractory to standard treatment with high-fiber diet and laxatives. Physiologic tests include colonic-transit testing, anorectal manometry, balloon expulsion test, and defecography. In patients with physical findings or symptoms suggestive of a defecatory disorder, the initial physiologic tests to consider are anorectal manometry and balloon expulsion. Defecography may be considered if the results of these tests are equivocal or if there is suspicion of a structural abnormality in the rectum that is impeding defecation. In patients with no clinical features that suggest a defecatory disorder, the initial physiologic test to consider is measurement of the colonic transit time, distinguishing slow-transit from normal-transit constipation.

TREATMENT OF CHRONIC CONSTIPATION

Lifestyle modifications should include encouraging patients to avoid postponing defecation and to monitor bowel habits by means of a daily diary of bowel frequency and characteristics together with any abdominal symptoms. Dietary patterns, a sedentary lifestyle, and inadequate fluid intake may contribute to the risk of constipation, particularly in the elderly. However, increases in fluid intake and physical activity do not appear to relieve constipation, except in patients who are dehydrated. All medications, both over-the-counter and prescribed, should be reviewed. Whenever possible, alternative medications should be substituted for those that are likely to cause constipation.

DIETARY FIBER AND MEDICINAL BULKING AGENTS

Initially, a gradual increase in dietary fiber is recommended for treatment of constipation. Fiber increases the intraluminal volume, stimulates motility, increases stool weight, and reduces colon transit time. Fiber intake should be increased to 20 to 25 g/day by altering the diet or by the addition of a commercial fiber supplement. Patients initiating a course of increased fiber consumption need to be advised that it may take several weeks before any benefits become evident and that they should not discontinue the treatment prematurely. Compliance with the prescription of increased fiber intake is relatively poor, in part because of the associated bloating and gas caused by fermentation of undigested fiber in the colon.

CURRENT THERAPY

Summary

- Lifestyle modifications that promote regular bowel habits should be encouraged.
- Increased dietary fiber may be used initially, followed by an osmotic laxative if there is no response; stimulant laxatives may be used on a short-term basis.
- Polyethylene glycol (PEG-3350 [MiraLax]) is safe for relief of medication-induced and chronic constipation.
- Lubiprostone (Amitiza) activates intraluminal ClC2 channels to promote secretion; it is approved for the treatment of chronic idiopathic constipation and constipation-predominant irritable bowel syndrome.
- Methylnaltrexone (Relistor) may be used to treat opioid-induced constipation.
- Biofeedback, if available, should be considered first-line therapy in patients with pelvic floor dysfunction.
- Surgery should be considered only after all medical therapies have failed.

PHARMACOLOGIC THERAPY

Laxatives

If a patient does not improve with lifestyle and dietary modifications, then a laxative may be used. Most authorities recommend first trying an osmotic laxative before considering use of a stimulant laxative. Osmotic laxatives include sorbitol, lactulose (Cephulac), magnesium hydroxide (Milk of Magnesia), and polyethylene glycol. Osmotic laxatives are poorly absorbed or nonabsorbed substances that result in the secretion of water into the intestinal lumen to maintain isotonicity with plasma. Most osmotic agents take several days to work, but they may be effective in as little as 30 minutes to 3 hours. Dehydration can occur if osmotic laxatives are overused. In patients with cardiac or renal insufficiency, excessive absorption of sodium, magnesium, or phosphate may lead to electrolyte abnormalities and volume overload.

High-molecular-weight polyethylene glycol, or PEG-3350 (MiraLax) is an inert polymer with a high osmotic activity that sequesters water in the intestinal lumen. Polyethylene glycol, dosed at 17 g/day, has been shown to be effective for relief of medication-induced constipation. It has also been shown to be safe and effective for chronic use and relief of chronic constipation. Significant benefit from low doses (17 g/day) may not be seen until the second week of treatment. In contrast, a single high dose of PEG-3350 (68 g)[3] provides overnight improvement in constipation.

Stimulant laxatives exert their primary effects by enhancing motility and altering electrolyte transport across the intestinal mucosa. These medications include surface-acting agents (docusate sodium [Colace], bile salts), diphenylmethane derivatives (bisacodyl [Dulcolax]), ricinoleic acid (castor oil [Neoloid]), and anthraquinones (senna [Senokot], cascara sagrada, aloe,[1,7] rhubarb[1,7]). Stimulant laxatives are discouraged because they have been implicated as promoting a cathartic colon or causing melanosis coli, damage to the myenteric plexus, acid-base and electrolyte disorders, and dependency. Stimulant laxatives are recommended only for short-term use, after organic causes of constipation have been excluded and other interventions have proved unsuccessful.

---

[1]Not FDA approved for this indication.
[3]Exceeds dosage recommended by the manufacturer.
[7]Available as dietary supplement.

Lubiprostone (Amitiza)

Lubiprostone is a member of a new class of prostaglandin E_1 derivatives known as prostones. Lubiprostone is minimally absorbed from the gastrointestinal tract and appears to act intraluminally to activate ClC2 channels located on the apical membrane of intestinal epithelial cells. When it is activated, an efflux of chloride through the ClC2 channels promotes secretion into the lumen of the intestinal tract. Sodium ions follow to maintain electrical neutrality, and water passively follows to maintain isotonicity. Lubiprostone has been shown to be effective for treatment of chronic constipation. Lubiprostone is approved for treatment of chronic idiopathic constipation at a dose of 24 μg PO twice daily and for treatment of constipation-predominant irritable bowel syndrome at a dose of 8 μg PO twice daily.

Methylnaltrexone (Relistor)

Opioid-induced constipation is predominantly mediated by gastrointestinal μ-opioid receptors. Methylnaltrexone is the result of *N*-methylation of the uncharged systemic opioid antagonist naltrexone. Methylnaltrexone has restricted ability to cross the blood-brain barrier in humans because of its polarity and low lipid solubility. In a study investigating the safety and efficacy of subcutaneous methylnaltrexone for treatment of opioid-induced constipation, 48% of treated patients experienced defecation within 4 hours, compared with 15% of patients receiving placebo. Treatment did not appear to affect central analgesia or to precipitate opioid withdrawal. Dosing of methylnaltrexone is weight based. Patients weighing less than 38 kg or more than 114 kg are dosed at 0.15 mg/kg SC every other day. Within that range, patients weighing 38 to 61 kg are given 8 mg SC every other day, and those weighing 62 to 114 kg are given at 12 mg SC every other day.

Miscellaneous Drugs

Colchicine,[1] a drug that is used to treat gout and is known to induce diarrhea as a side effect, increases stool frequency and lessens the need for rescue laxatives in patients with chronic constipation. It provides a clinical benefit in about 10% of patients.

Misoprostol (Cytotec)[1] also has diarrhea as a common side effect. This prostaglandin analogue increases the rate of intestinal transit in healthy volunteers, as well as in patients with constipation, and probably directly stimulates intestinal secretion and contractility. Misoprostol can increase stool frequency in chronic constipation when 200 μg is administered 2 to 4 times per day. This drug may also induce cramping and has the potential to stimulate uterine contractions. Approximately 25% of patients respond to misoprostol at doses titrated below the threshold for severe abdominal cramping.

NONPHARMACOLOGIC TREATMENTS

Biofeedback

For patients with pelvic floor dysfunction, biofeedback should be considered first-line therapy if it is available. During biofeedback for constipation due to defecatory disorders, patients receive visual or auditory feedback, or both, related to the functioning of their anal sphincter and pelvic floor muscles. Biofeedback can be used to train patients to relax their pelvic floor muscles during straining and to coordinate this relaxation with abdominal maneuvers to enhance the entry of stool into the rectum. This technique is not widely available, and there are only limited data from clinical trials to support the feasibility of this approach for long-term management in most patients with chronic constipation.

Surgery

Total colectomy and subtotal colectomy with ileorectal anastomosis should be considered only for patients without defecatory disorders and only after all medical therapies have failed. A majority of patients still experience abdominal pain and continue to use laxatives or enemas. Incontinence as well as small bowel obstruction are not uncommon complications after surgery. Surgery should be performed in units with special expertise in this area.

REFERENCES

American Gastroenterological Association, Clinical Practice and Practice Economic Committee. AGA Technical Review on Constipation. Gastroenterology 2000;119:1766–78.

Cash BD, Chang E, Talley NJ, Wald A. Fresh perspectives in chronic constipation and other functional bowel disorders. Rev Gastroenterol Disord 2007;7:116–33.

DiPalma JA, Cleveland MB, McGowan J, Herrera JL. A comparison of polyethylene glycol laxative and placebo for relief of constipation from constipating medications. South Med J 2007;100:1085–90.

DiPalma JA, Cleveland MV, McGowan J, Herrera JL. An open-label study of chronic polyethylene glycol laxative use in chronic constipation. Aliment Pharmacol Ther 2007;25:703–8.

DiPalma JA, Cleveland MV, McGowan J, Herrera JL. A randomized, multicenter, placebo-controlled trial of polyethylene glycol laxative for chronic treatment of chronic constipation. Am J Gastroenterol 2007;102:1436–41.

DiPalma JA, Schiller LR. Update on chronic constipation. Clinical Symposia 2005;55(2):1–35.

Johanson JF, Morton D, Greenen J, Ueno R. Multicenter, 4-week, double-blind, randomized, placebo-controlled trial of lubiprostone, a locally-acting type-2 chloride channel activator, in patients with chronic constipation. Am J Gastroenterol 2008;103:170–7.

Lembo A, Camilleri M. Chronic constipation. N Engl J Med 2003;349:1360–8.

Longstreth GF, Thompson WG, Chey WD, et al. Functional bowel disorders. Gastroenterology 2006;130:1480–91.

Rutland TJ, Adeniji OA, DiPalma JA. Prevalence of medication-associated constipation. Am J Gastroenterol 2004;99:S103–4.

Talley NJ. Management of chronic constipation. Rev Gastroenterol Disord 2004;4:18–24.

Thomas J, Karver S, Cooney GA, et al. Methylnaltrexone for opioid-induced constipation in advanced illness. N Engl J Med 2008;358:2332–43.

Fever

Method of
Ann M. Aring, MD

Patients often come to the physician's office with a fever. Fever can be present in a wide variety of clinical presentations ranging from self-limited viral illnesses to serious bacterial infections. Most febrile conditions can be easily diagnosed with other presenting symptoms and a problem-focused physical examination. However, fever produces anxiety for patients, parents, and health care providers, which can lead to overtreatment. Typically, fever is transient and only requires treatment to provide patient comfort.

Definitions

The definition of fever is arbitrary, because temperature varies daily within individual persons. The hypothalamic thermostat maintains core body temperature at about 37°C (98.6°F). Normal body temperature varies in a regular pattern each day. This circadian temperature rhythm, or diurnal variation, results in lower body temperatures in the early morning and temperatures approximately 1°C higher in the late afternoon or early evening.

The word *fever* is derived from the Latin *fovere* (to warm). In adults and children older than 12 years, fever is generally accepted as a rectal temperature higher than 38°C (100.4°F), an oral temperature higher than 37.5°C (99.5°F), or an axillary temperature higher than 37°C (98.6°F).

---

[1]Not FDA approved for this indication.

CURRENT DIAGNOSIS

- The definition of fever is arbitrary, because temperature varies within individual persons daily. Oral temperatures of 37.5°C (99.5°F) or rectal temperatures of 100.4°F (38°C) are consistent with fever.
- Temperature accuracy depends on the measurement technique. Oral temperatures are preferred in patients older than 5 years. Rectal temperatures are preferred in infants.
- Fever in infants younger than 3 months or in neutropenic patients is considered a medical emergency that warrants immediate further evaluation.
- Fever is beneficial but is associated with increased cardiac demand and increased metabolic needs. Benign febrile seizures can occur in young children with a fever.
- Fever of unknown origin (FUO) in children merits a thorough evaluation based on the age of the child. FUO in adults is defined as a temperature higher than 101°F that is of at least 3 weeks' duration and whose cause remains undiagnosed after 3 days in the hospital or after three outpatient visits.
- Hyperthermia is characterized by a temperature above the upper limit of the hypothalamic set point of 41.1°C (106°F).

The methods of determining body temperature are oral, rectal, and axillary. The oral route of determining temperature is preferred in children older than 5 years and in adults. Typically, rectal temperatures are obtained in infants by placing a lubricated thermometer in the rectum. In general, axillary temperatures are inaccurate and should not be used. Liquid crystal strips applied to the forehead and temperature-sensitive pacifiers are popular with parents but are inaccurate and miss fevers in many children.

The temperature considered to be the physiologic limit to febrile illness is 41.1°C (106°F). Hyperthermia is characterized by a temperature higher than this hypothalamic set point. Hyperthermia is due to an interference within the normal mechanisms that balance heat production and dissipation or an insult to the hypothalamus.

When the cause of a fever is unknown, two terms may be used: fever of unknown origin (FUO) and fever of unknown source. The definition of FUO in adults includes a temperature higher than 101°F that is of at least 3 weeks' duration and whose source remains undiagnosed after 3 days in the hospital or after three outpatient visits. FUO is also used to define a fever that occurs at different periods over weeks or months. Fever of unknown source is defined as a fever in the first week of an illness.

Pathogenesis and Physiology

Fever is a physiologic mechanism that occurs when an inciting stimulus causes an inflammatory response. Fever may be caused by infections, vaccines, tissue injury, malignancy, drugs, collagen vascular diseases, granulomatous disease, inflammatory bowel disease, endocrine disorders such as thyrotoxicosis and pheochromocytoma, and central nervous system abnormalities. Dehydration, increased physical activity, and heat exposure can all cause an elevation in temperature. Infections cause most fevers in all age groups.

Monocytes or tissue macrophages are activated by the microbial or nonmicrobial stimuli to produce various cytokines with pyrogenic activity. The list of currently recognized pyrogenic cytokines includes interleukin-1 (IL-1), tumor necrosis factor α (TNF-α), IL-6, interferon-β (IFN-β), and interferon-γ (IFN-γ). These cytokines activate the arachadonic acid cascade and increase production of prostaglandin E_2 (PGE$_2$). PGE$_2$ then resets the thermoregulatory set point in the hypothalamus at a higher level.

Thermoregulatory responses include redirecting blood to or from cutaneous vascular beds, increased or decreased sweating, and behavioral responses such as seeking warmer or cooler environmental temperatures. The body dissipates heat via evaporation of water from the body surface and lungs through radiation (60%), convection (12%), and conduction (3%).

Risks and Benefits of Fever

Fever is beneficial and not usually harmful to the host, with a few exceptions. Fever is associated with increased cardiac demand and increased metabolic needs. In pregnancy, fever is associated with harmful clinical effects. Many animal studies have shown that fever enhances the immunologic response to infectious agents. Use of antipyretic medications to lower fever increases both morbidity and mortality in infected laboratory animals and prolongs varicella infections in humans.

Febrile seizures are usually benign but can cause considerable parental anxiety. Febrile seizures are divided into two types: simple (generalized, last <15 minutes, and do not recur within 24 hours) and complex (prolonged, recur more than once in 24 hours, or are focal). Recent studies have shown that in previously normal children, most simple febrile seizures are not associated with recurrent seizures or brain damage.

Fever of Unknown Origin

ADULTS

The evaluation of FUO remains among the most challenging problems facing the clinician. There are four categories. Classic FUO is commonly caused by infections, drug fever, malignancy, and inflammatory diseases. Neutropenic FUO (neutrophils <500/mm³) is seen in periodontal and perianal infections; candidemia and aspergillosis are major causes. Nosocomial FUO is commonly caused by septic thrombophlebitis, drug fever, and *Clostridium difficile* colitis. In HIV-associated FUO, *Mycobacterium avium* complex infections, tuberculosis, non-Hodgkin's lymphoma, cytomegalovirus, and drug fever are important etiologies.

CHILDREN

Febrile illness in infants and young children is common. A complete history and physical examination, including vital signs, skin color and exanthems, behavior state, and hydration status, do not reveal a source of infection in 20% of febrile children. The child's age determines the need for further investigation. Febrile infants younger than 28 days should have a complete blood count (CBC) with differential; electrolytes; serum glucose; cerebrospinal fluid (CSF) Gram stain and cell count; cultures from blood, CSF, and urine; group B streptococcal antigen from urine and CSF; and a chest x-ray. Management requires hospitalization and empiric parenteral antibiotics.

For children 28 to 90 days old, obtain a CBC with differential and urinalysis with culture. A low-risk child is defined as a previously healthy term infant who has no focal bacterial infection on examination. If the white blood cell count (WBC) is greater than 15,000/mm³, blood cultures should be obtained, as well as CSF Gram stain, culture, cell count, glucose, and protein. For a positive CSF Gram stain or abnormal CSF count, the patient should be admitted and parenteral antibiotics should be given. For negative CSF Gram stain, normal CSF cell count, and negative urinalysis, the child should be given ceftriaxone (Rocephin) 50 mg/kg (maximum dose, 1 g) and reevaluated in 24 hours. For a positive urinalysis or urine culture, the patient may be given oral antibiotics as an outpatient and reexamined in 24 hours. If the child cannot take oral antibiotics, he or she must be admitted for parenteral antibiotics. For a WBC less than 15,000 mm³ with a negative urinalysis and CSF Gram stain, the child may be followed closely as an outpatient. The child should be reevaluated in 24 hours. High-risk infants are toxic appearing with lethargy, signs of poor perfusion, hypoventilation, hyperventilation, or cyanosis. High-risk infants need to be admitted to the hospital with parental antibiotics.

CURRENT THERAPY

- Antipyretic therapy for children includes acetaminophen 10 to 15 mg/kg every 4 to 6 hours for children older than 3 months or ibuprofen 10 mg/kg every 6 hours for children older than 6 months.
- Antipyretic therapy for adults and adolescents includes acetaminophen 650 mg to 1000 mg every 6 hours to a maximum of 4000 mg per day, or ibuprofen 200 to 400 mg every 6 hours.
- Aspirin (salicylic acid) should not be used in children due to the risk of Reye's syndrome. In adults, the dose is 325 to 650 mg every 6 hours as needed for fever.
- Combining two antipyretics for fever, such as ibuprofen and acetaminophen, has not been proved to produce quicker or longer-lasting responses.
- Sponge bathing should be done with tepid water and no alcohol.

For children 3 to 36 months old who have a fever without a source, no diagnostic tests or antibiotics are needed if the child appears well and the fever is less than 39°C (102.2°F) (low risk). Acetaminophen (Tylenol) 10 mg/kg may be given with instructions to give every 6 hours as needed. The child's caregiver should also be instructed to return to the clinician if the fever persists longer than 48 hours or if the patient's condition worsens. If the temperature is greater than 39°C, obtain a CBC with differential. In addition, a boy younger than 6 months or a girl younger than 2 years should have a urine culture. Blood cultures are indicated if the WBC is greater than 15,000/mm^3 and the fever is higher than 39°C. CSF cultures are indicated when the diagnosis of sepsis or meningitis is suspected based on history, observation, and physical examination. Empiric antibiotic therapy with ceftriaxone 50 mg/kg (maximum dose, 1 g) should be given if the temperature is higher than 39°C and the WBC is greater than 15,000/mm^3. The child needs to be followed up in 24 to 48 hours. High-risk children in this age group should be admitted to the hospital for broad-spectrum parenteral antibiotics.

Treatment

Antipyretic medications are commonly used for the symptomatic relief of fever. Acetaminophen, ibuprofen (Advil, Motrin), and aspirin are inhibitors of hypothalamic cyclooxygenase, thus inhibiting PGE$_2$ synthesis. These drugs are all equally effective antipyretic agents. Ibuprofen and aspirin are also antiinflammatory agents; acetaminophen does not have any antiinflammatory properties.

Acetaminophen is available in a wide variety of dosage forms including drops, elixir, syrup, capsule, tablet, chewable tablet, and suppository. Dosing is generally 10 to 15 mg/kg every 4 to 6 hours in children older than 3 months. For adults, acetaminophen dosing is 650 to 1000 mg every 6 hours. Maximum daily dose of acetaminophen is 75 mg/kg (or 720 mg) in children and 4000 mg in adolescents and adults.

Ibuprofen is a nonsteroidal antiinflammatory (NSAID) drug that may be given to febrile children 6 months or older. Ibuprofen is quickly absorbed and produces a more rapid temperature fall and longer duration of action than acetaminophen. This advantage might not be maintained after the first dose is given. Dosing in children is 10 mg/kg every 6 to 8 hours. Adults and adolescents may take doses of 200 to 400 mg every 6 hours. Ibuprofen is also available in a wide variety of dosage forms including drops, elixir, syrup, capsule, tablet, and chewable tablet.

Aspirin (salicylic acid) remains an effective treatment for fever in adults. Because aspirin is associated with Reye's syndrome in children, aspirin is not recommended for treating fever in children. Adult dosing is 325 to 650 mg every 4 to 6 hours as needed.

Combining two antipyretics for fever, such as ibuprofen and acetaminophen, is common clinical practice. Combinations have not been proved to produce quicker or longer-lasting responses. The American Academy of Pediatrics (AAP) cautions against using multiple antipyretics because of an increase in the likelihood of dosing errors. Combining drugs is more expensive and could also delay proper diagnosis or therapy.

Nonpharmacologic treatment can also provide relief from the discomfort of fever. Extra oral fluids should be encouraged to prevent dehydration. Sponge bathing with tepid water may be used. Alcohol or ice water should not be used for sponge bathing. Alcohol is absorbed through the skin and can cause hypoglycemia or dehydration. Both alcohol and ice water increase shivering and can cause more discomfort.

REFERENCES

Aronoff DM, Neilson EG. Antipyretics: Mechanisms of action and clinical use in fever suppression. Am J Med 2001;111(4):304–15.

Baraff LJ. Management of fever without source in infants and children. Ann Emerg Med 2000;36:602–14.

Crocetti M, Moghbeli N, Serwint J. Fever phobia revisited: Have parental misconceptions about fever changed in 20 years? Pediatrics 2001;107(6): 1241–6.

Finkelstein JA. Fever in pediatric primary care: Occurrence, management, and outcomes. Pediatrics 2000;105:260–6.

Greisman LA, Mackowiak PA. Fever: Beneficial and detrimental effects of antipyretics. Curr Opin Infect Dis 2002;15(3):241–5.

Kourtis AP, Sullivan DT, Sathian U. Practice guidelines for the management of febrile infants less than 90 days of age at the ambulatory network of a large pediatric health care system in the United States: Summary of new evidence. Clin Pediatr 2004;43(1):11–6.

Knockaert DC, Vanderschueren S, Blockmans D. Fever of unknown origin in adults: 40 years on. J Intern Med 2003;253:263–75.

Mackowiak PA. Temperature regulation and the pathogenesis of fever. In: Mandell GL, Bennett JE, Donlin R, editors. Principles and Practices of Infection Diseases, Vol 1. Philadelphia: Churchill Livingstone; 2000. pp 604–22.

McCarthy PL. Fever without apparent source on clinical examination. Curr Opin Pediatr 2004;16(1):94–106.

Mourad O, Palda V, Detsky A. A comprehensive evidence-based approach to fever of unknown origin. Arch Intern Med 2003;163:545–51.

Roth AR, Basello GM. Approach to the adult patient with fever of unknown origin. Am Fam Phys 2003;68(11):2223–8.

Cough

Method of
David G. Hill, MD

Cough is among the most common presenting complaints of outpatients in the United States. It serves as a protective reflex against foreign material and as a method to clear secretions from the airway. The cough center is located in the medulla, and the cough reflex is mediated by way of multiple nervous system pathways including the trigeminal, glossopharyngeal, vagus, and phrenic nerves. Cough is mediated by separate neural pathways from bronchoconstriction. When cough occurs there is a synchronized activation of muscles, the glottis opens, and the lungs expand. At the peak of inspiration the glottis closes and expiratory muscles contract. This results in increased intrathoracic pressure; when the glottis opens airflow can reach 500 miles per hour. The cough reflex varies in different patient populations. Women have a more sensitive cough reflex than men. Smokers' cough reflexes are depressed despite the increased frequency of cough in this population. Patients who have a decreased cough sensitivity following cerebral vascular accidents have an increased incidence of pneumonia. Angiotensin-converting enzyme (ACE) inhibitors increase cough reflex sensitivity and have been shown to decrease the risk of pneumonia in patients with cerebrovascular accidents. The evaluation of cough as a patient complaint may best be pursued by examining the duration of the symptoms. Cough can be subcategorized into acute and chronic cough. Cough that occurs following an acute respiratory infection may narrow the differential diagnosis and is addressed separately.

Acute Cough

Acute cough may be defined as cough that has been present for less than 8 weeks. Because all causes of chronic coughs initially cause acute symptoms, patients with acute cough may actually have cough caused by one of the etiologies discussed later in this section; however, acute cough more commonly is the result of a less indolent process (Box 1). Infectious etiologies are a frequent cause of acute cough. Most acute cough is the result of viral infections, specifically the common cold. Most cough resulting from the common cold is self-limited and lasts less than 3 weeks. Most episodes of sinusitis are of viral etiology; however, bacterial sinusitis can also result in acute cough. The presence of a significant smoking history raises the possibility of an acute exacerbation of chronic obstructive pulmonary disease (COPD) as the cause of acute cough, especially in patients with previously documented COPD. *Bordetella pertussis* infection may also be the etiology of an acute episode of cough. Noninfectious processes that lead to acute cough include allergic rhinitis, congestive heart failure, asthma, and aspiration. The clinical history, physical examination, and diagnostic testing are of particular importance in differentiating these disease states and often point to the diagnosis.

Postinfectious Cough

Postinfectious cough begins with an acute upper respiratory tract infection but persists following the resolution of the other acute symptoms (Box 2). Postnasal drip syndrome may present following the common cold or sinusitis. Bronchospasm may lead to postinfectious cough either as a result of a single episode of postinfectious wheezing or an exacerbation of underlying asthma. Postinfectious cough may be the initial presentation of asthma. Recurrent episodes of airflow obstruction are required to confirm the diagnosis of this chronic illness. Because *B. pertussis* can present with an indolent course, this infection can be confused with a postinfectious cough. Similarly, bacterial sinusitis can be confused with postinfectious cough. Both of these etiologies of cough are the result of ongoing infection rather than true postinfectious cough. *Mycoplasma pneumoniae* and *Chlamydia pneumoniae* infections may also result in postinfectious cough likely because of persistent airway inflammation and increases in cough reflex sensitivity.

Chronic Cough

Chronic cough presents the most difficult diagnostic dilemma for the health care practitioner. Cough of greater than 8 weeks' duration can be considered chronic. Lesser duration of symptoms may still be indicative of one of the etiologies discussed in this section, but such cough is more likely the result of one of the infectious or postinfectious etiologies described previously. In patients who have never smoked, chronic cough is most likely the result of asthma, postnasal drip syndrome, or gastroesophageal reflux. These three etiologies are the most common cause of chronic cough regardless of patient age. In nonsmokers with a normal chest radiograph who are not taking an ACE inhibitor, these three etiologies alone or in combination are the cause of more than 85% of chronic cough (Box 3). Postnasal drip syndrome is the most common of these etiologies. Cough may be the sole presenting symptom of any of these conditions; they are not mutually exclusive and may coexist, particularly in the patient with troublesome, persistent symptoms. Most patients with problematic, persistent cough have multiple etiologies contributing to their symptoms. COPD must be considered in current smokers and in those patients with a significant smoking history. Smokers can have a cough of any etiology, however, and it should not be assumed that their cough is the result of smoking or COPD. Although smokers frequently admit to cough when a history is taken, they infrequently seek medical attention for this symptom. Cough resulting from the use of ACE inhibitors must be considered in all patients being treated with these medications. Less common, yet frequent causes of cough include chronic bronchitis from irritants other than tobacco smoke and eosinophilic bronchitis. Occasionally, chronic cough may be the result of:

- Bronchogenic carcinoma
- Metastatic carcinoma
- Bronchiectasis
- Sarcoidosis
- Pulmonary fibrosis
- Pneumoconiosis
- Hypersensitivity pneumonitis
- Congestive heart failure
- Chronic infection, such as tuberculosis or *Mycobacterium avium* complex
- Recurrent aspiration because of pharyngeal or esophageal abnormalities

Key Diagnostic Points

The evaluation of acute cough should focus on the history and physical examination. Most acute cough will be the result of self-limited viral upper respiratory infections. More thorough evaluation is necessary in the workup of cough of longer duration particularly if the cough has been present for more than 2 months. The history of onset of the cough and whether it was associated with an acute infectious episode should be elicited. Exposure to sick contacts particularly to a known case of *B. pertussis* are important historic considerations. The timing and nature of the cough and any associated sputum must be described. Factors that mitigate or worsen the cough should be examined, and prior history of episodic cough, allergies, wheezing, asthma, and gastroesophageal reflux should be questioned. A thorough medication history particularly regarding use of ACE inhibitors must be obtained. Environmental factors both at home and in the work place

All Patients Presenting With Cough

- Perform thorough history and physical examination.
- Review timing and nature of cough along with exacerbating or mitigating factors.
- Review prior history of cough, allergies, asthma, or gastroesophageal reflux.
- Take medication history, particularly use of ACE inhibitors.
- Focus physical examination on head, neck, and thorax.

Patients With Postinfectious or Chronic Cough

- Obtain chest radiograph, particularly in patients with an abnormal respiratory examination.
- Evaluate airflow obstruction with spirometry.
- Stop ACE inhibitors and assess for improvement.
- Administer empiric therapy for postnasal drip, asthma, or gastroesophageal reflux.
- Consider methacholine challenge testing to evaluate for airway hyperreactivity.
- Induce sputum for eosinophils or empiric trial of corticosteroids for eosinophilic bronchitis.
- If cough persists, consider esophagoscopy, 24-hour pH probe monitoring, high-resolution chest CT, or bronchoscopy.

Abbreviations: ACE = angiotensin-converting enzyme; CT = computed tomography.

should be reviewed. Although smoking history is important, it is again noted that smoking-related cough is an infrequent reason for a patient to seek medical attention. The physical examination should focus most on the head, neck, and thorax with a thorough examination of the upper respiratory tract including the auditory canal, nose, and oropharynx. The cardiopulmonary examination should also be thorough to elicit signs of less common illnesses.

Acute cough associated with an acute respiratory illness and prominent upper airway symptoms can be assumed to be secondary to the common cold. Diagnostic testing is not indicated in such patients; a chest radiograph would be normal and is thus not recommended. Patients who have abnormal sinus transillumination, purulent nasal secretions, sinus pain or tenderness, or maxillary toothache could possibly have bacterial sinusitis. Again, a viral etiology of sinusitis is more likely than bacterial sinusitis, and antibiotic therapy should be initiated only in patients with persistent symptoms despite symptomatic therapy. Patients with documented COPD who present with acute cough, purulent sputum, dyspnea, and wheezing have an exacerbation of their underlying COPD and should be treated appropriately. Allergic rhinitis usually presents with a clear clinical history of episodic nasal and other allergy symptoms, and allergen avoidance can be initiated. It is important to note that allergic rhinitis can present with perennial symptoms.

Postinfectious cough should be evaluated with thorough history and physical examinations followed by limited diagnostic evaluation and empiric therapies. Patients should be treated for postnasal drip syndrome, particularly in the setting of described rhinitis, postnasal drip, or frequent throat clearing. The presence of nasal inflammation and congestion, cobblestoning of the pharyngeal mucosa, or mucus in the oropharynx should also lead to empiric therapy for postnasal drip syndrome. If cough persists in the patients with suspected postnasal drip syndrome, evaluation of the sinuses with imaging and treatment of those patients with evidence of bacterial sinusitis should be pursued. Computed tomography

(CT) imaging of the sinuses is the gold standard for diagnosing bacterial sinusitis. Patients with postinfectious cough and an abnormal respiratory examination should have a chest radiograph. Patients with a normal radiograph and evidence of bronchospasm can be empirically treated for airway hyperreactivity. Again, the diagnosis of asthma requires recurrent airflow obstruction and cannot be made on the basis of a single episode of postinfectious wheezing or airway hyperreactivity. In subjects with cough and vomiting, known exposure to a case of *B. pertussis*, or in the presence of a *B. pertussis* epidemic in the community, empiric therapy for this illness should be pursued.

Before the vaccine era, *B. pertussis* was an endemic disease, which occurred in cyclic epidemics. It has been documented that *B. pertussis* continues to circulate in the adult population despite control of the disease in the pediatric population by vaccination. Immunity to *B. pertussis*, whether as a result of primary infection or immunization, is shortlived. The longer the elapsed interval since prior infection or immunization and repeat infection, the more likely repeat infection will be symptomatic. Perhaps repeat adolescent and adult booster immunization programs should be implemented to effectively control or eliminate this infection.

History and physical examinations remain paramount in the patient presenting with chronic cough. The majority of patients should have a chest radiograph obtained as part of their evaluation. If the history and physical examination suggest that postnasal drip, asthma, or gastroesophageal reflux is the etiology of a patient's symptoms, empiric therapy for these conditions should be initiated. Cough triggered by environmental factors or changes may be secondary to rhinitis and postnasal drip or airway hyperreactivity and asthma. Substernal burning or a sour taste in the mouth, particularly when triggered by supine positioning or bending, should increase the suspicion of gastroesophageal reflux.

If asthma is suspected, spirometry should be performed to document whether airflow obstruction is present. Response to inhaled bronchodilator with normal spirometry is indicative of airway hyperreactivity. Improvement in symptoms and spirometry with empiric asthma therapy even in the setting of normal baseline flow rates also confirms an asthmatic etiology. A methacholine challenge can be performed to confirm airway hyperreactivity. If cough in the setting of a positive methacholine challenge shows absolutely no response to empiric asthma therapy with inhaled corticosteroids and bronchodilators, consider a trial of systemic steroids. If the cough does not respond to aggressive asthma therapy, the methacholine challenge test results were probably false positive; asthma therapy can be discontinued and diagnostic efforts focused elsewhere.

Cough patients being treated with ACE inhibitors should cease these medications. Up to 30% of patients treated with ACE inhibitors will develop a persistent cough, more commonly in women, nonsmokers, and patients of Chinese ancestry. It may take 4 weeks or more for cough caused by ACE inhibitors to resolve following cessation of these medications. In the presence of ACE inhibitor use, further evaluation of dry cough should not be pursued until the patient has been withdrawn from these medications for 1 month.

An abnormal chest radiograph can direct further diagnostic studies and therapies, whereas a normal chest radiograph makes less common etiologies of chronic cough such as carcinoma, congestive heart failure, sarcoidosis, or interstitial lung disease unlikely. Evidence of basilar infiltrates or fibrosis may suggest interstitial lung disease or chronic aspiration. Severe gastroesophageal reflux must be considered in those patients with radiographic evidence of chronic aspiration.

Chronic cough without a definitive etiology can be troubling to both patient and health care provider. A systematic approach can simplify both diagnosis and treatment (Figure 1). It is again stressed that such a cough may be the result of multiple etiologic factors. In the absence of specific factors that help to point to an etiology of chronic cough, empiric treatment for postnasal drip syndrome should be pursued. Methacholine challenge testing will rule out asthma if it is negative and should also be performed early in the evaluation of chronic cough. Cough may be the sole manifestation

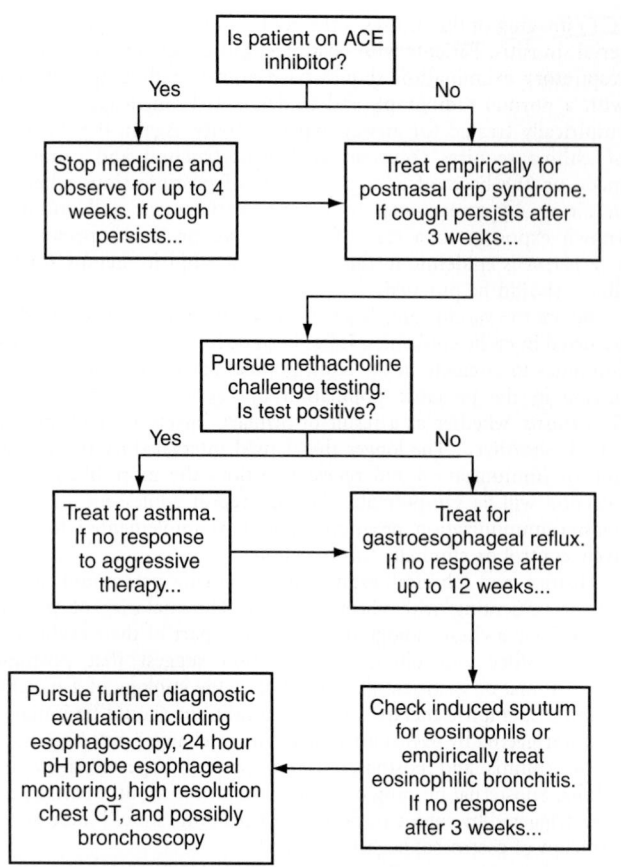

FIGURE 1. Approach to chronic cough of uncertain origin. ACE = angiotensin-converting enzyme; CT = computed tomography

of asthma in nearly 60% of patients presenting with chronic cough. A positive methacholine challenge does not have 100% predictive value but should lead to empiric asthma therapy.

Empiric therapy for silent gastroesophageal reflux should be initiated in those who do not respond to treatment for postnasal drip syndrome and do not have evidence of or respond to treatment for asthma. Cough may be the only manifestation of gastroesophageal reflux up to 30% of the time. Definitive diagnosis of gastroesophageal reflux requires invasive testing and may require more than one testing modality. Therefore it is recommended that empiric therapy for reflux be pursued before diagnostic testing. Reflux therapy should include conservative approaches such as dietary and lifestyle changes, bed positioning, and pharmacologic treatment. Gastroesophageal reflux–related cough can be particularly troublesome and persistent and may take weeks or months to respond to appropriate and intensive antireflux therapy. This may include higher-than-normal doses of proton pump inhibitors and promotility agents. Surgical treatment of reflux may be necessary to effectively treat reflux related cough in some patients. In patients with persistent cough, the common etiologies of cough often coexist and exacerbate one another. Therapy should often be additive, for instance treating both asthma and reflux, rather than mutually exclusive. Persistent cough should result in further diagnostic evaluation including sputum studies, esophagoscopy, 24-hour pH probe esophageal monitoring, high-resolution chest CT, and possibly bronchoscopy. In the presence of normal chest imaging, bronchoscopy is unlikely to yield beneficial diagnostic information in the patient with chronic cough.

Eosinophilic bronchitis in the absence of asthma is also a frequent cause (up to 13% of cases) of chronic cough. Patients with eosinophilic bronchitis will have normal spirometry and a negative methacholine challenge. The disease may be diagnosed by appropriate induced sputum analysis showing at least 3% eosinophils. Alternatively it can be empirically treated with a course of inhaled corticosteroids. Most patients appear to respond to inhaled corticosteroids within 3 weeks. Systemic corticosteroids may be required to improve the symptoms in some cases. There may be an association of gastroesophageal reflux with eosinophilic bronchitis. Patients with gastroesophageal reflux have been found to have increased sputum eosinophilia.

Bronchiectasis may infrequently result in chronic cough. Bronchiectasis is characterized by the abnormal dilatation of one or more branches of the bronchial tree. It can effectively be diagnosed by high resolution CT scan of the thorax. Bronchiectasis may occur following a severe infection, distal to an area of airway obstruction, congenitally, from chronic inflammatory processes, and as a result of chronic parenchymal scarring and traction. Patients with bronchiectasis may present with productive or nonproductive coughs. They may have recurrent episodes of infection resulting from persistent colonization of the abnormal bronchial segment. Infectious agents may include routine bacterial organisms and typical or atypical mycobacterium. Bronchiectasis may be seen in a variety of chronic illnesses. The presence of bronchiectasis in a patient without a known predisposing cause should prompt the clinician to look for appropriate clinical states such as:

- Primary or acquired immunodeficiencies
- Abnormalities of ciliary function, such as ciliary dyskinesia or cystic fibrosis
- Postinfectious inflammatory processes, such as allergic bronchopulmonary aspergillosis
- Collagen vascular diseases
- Inflammatory bowel disease
- Sarcoidosis
- Yellow nail syndrome

The presence of localized bronchiectasis may be an indication to pursue flexible fiberoptic bronchoscopy to rule out an obstructing lesion and to obtain appropriate culture specimens. Treatment of bronchiectasis is aimed at the underlying disease state if one can be identified. Infections should be treated with appropriate antibiotics. Clearance of bronchial secretions can be aided with mucolytics and chest physiotherapy including use of percussive devices. In some cases surgical therapy to remove the bronchiectatic segment can be considered.

Treatment

The key treatments for cough are best described based on the suspected etiology. Acute cough therapy should focus on supportive treatment of the underlying suspected etiology, which will likely be a viral upper respiratory infection. Therapy for exacerbation of chronic obstructive pulmonary disease, allergic rhinitis, bacterial sinusitis, or B. pertussis infection is more specific. Postinfectious cough should focus on therapy for postnasal drip syndrome or airways reactivity if suspected. In chronic cough of uncertain etiology (see Figure 1), cough therapy should begin with empiric treatment of postnasal drip syndrome, evaluation and treatment of asthma, empiric treatment of gastroesophageal reflux syndrome, and finally evaluation or empiric therapy for eosinophilic bronchitis.

Cough is a frequent and troublesome symptom for both patient and health care provider. Acute cough although at times troubling is usually self-limiting. Postinfectious cough and chronic cough are more problematic, but can effectively be evaluated and treated by performing a thorough history and physical examination and pursuing a systematic approach to diagnostic evaluation and both empiric and guided therapies. The resolution of chronic troubling cough is a therapeutic relief for the patient and a gratifying experience for the caregiver.

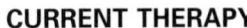

CURRENT THERAPY

Treatment of Acute Cough

- Common cold: Supportive care with dexbrompheniramine, 6 mg, and pseudoephedrine, 120 mg (Drixoral Cold and Allergy Tablets); or ipratropium nasal spray (Atrovent, 0.06%), two 42-mcg sprays in each nostril 3 times daily for 4 to 7 d depending on duration of symptoms.
- Acute sinusitis: Treat as a common cold. Add oxymetazoline (Afrin), two sprays twice daily for three days. If symptoms persist, consider antibiotic therapy directed against *Haemophilus influenzae* and *Streptococcus pneumoniae* such as azithromycin (Zithromax), 500 mg daily for 3 d.
- Exacerbation of chronic obstructive pulmonary disease: Antibiotics directed against *H. influenzae* and *S. pneumoniae* for 3 to 7 d such as clarithromycin (Biaxin), 500 mg twice daily for 7 d; systemic corticosteroids such as prednisone (Deltasone), 40 mg tapered over 10 d; inhaled anticholinergics such as tiotropium (Spiriva), one inhalation daily; and short-acting β-agonists such as albuterol (Proventil), two inhalations every 4 h as needed; smoking cessation.
- Allergic rhinitis: Nasal corticosteroids such as mometasone (Nasonex), two sprays in each nostril daily; nonsedating antihistamines such as fexofenadine (Allegra), 180 mg daily; allergen avoidance if possible.
- *Bordetella pertussis*: Erythromycin 500 mg four times daily for 14 d or trimethoprim 160 mg/sulfamethoxazole (Bactrim DS),[1] 800 mg twice daily for 14 d. Other macrolide antibiotics such as azithromycin (Zithromax)[1] or clarithromycin (Biaxin)[1] are likely effective and may be better tolerated.

Treatment of Postinfectious Cough

- Postnasal drip syndrome: Dexbrompheniramine, 6 mg, and pseudoephedrine (Drixoral Cold and Allergy Tablets), 120 mg for up to 3 wk; ipratropium (Atrovent), 0.06% nasal spray for up to 3 wk; azelastine (Astelin) nasal spray (137 mcg), two sprays each nostril twice daily for up to 3 wk.
- Bronchospasm: Inhaled corticosteroid such as budesonide (Pulmicort),[1] two inhalations daily with or without inhaled long-acting β-agonist such as formoterol (Foradil), two inhalations twice daily; short-acting β-agonist such as albuterol (Ventolin), two puffs every 4 h as needed. Oral steroids such as prednisone (Deltasone), 40 mg tapered over 10 d.

- *Bordetella pertussis*: Erythromycin, 500 mg four times daily for 14 d, or trimethoprim 160 mg/sulfamethoxazole, 800 mg (Bactrim DS)[1] twice daily for 14 d. Other macrolide antibiotics such as azithromycin (Zithromax)[1] or clarithromycin (Biaxin)[1] are likely effective and may be better tolerated.
- Bacterial sinusitis: Dexbrompheniramine, 6 mg, and pseudoephedrine (Drixoral Cold and Allergy Tablets), 120 mg for up to 3 wk; oxymetazoline (Afrin), two sprays twice daily for 3 d; azithromycin (Zithromax), 500 mg daily for 3 d.
- Chlamydia/mycoplasma: Clarithromycin (Biaxin), 500 mg twice daily for 14 d.

Treatment of Chronic Cough

- Postnasal drip syndrome
  Nonallergic: Dexbrompheniramine, 6 mg, and pseudoephedrine (Drixoral Cold and Allergy Tablets), 120 mg for up to 3 wk; ipratropium (Atrovent), 0.06% nasal spray for up to 3 wk; azelastine (Astelin) nasal spray (137 mcg), two sprays each nostril twice daily for up to 3 wk.
  Allergic: Fluticasone (Flonase) (50 mcg), two sprays each nostril daily; fexofenadine (Allegra), 180 mg daily; allergen avoidance.
- Asthma: Albuterol (Proventil), two puffs every 4 hours as needed; inhaled corticosteroid such as budesonide (Pulmicort), two inhalations daily with or without inhaled long-acting β-agonist such as formoterol (Foradil), two inhalations twice daily; combination of long-acting β-agonist and inhaled steroid such as fluticasone/salmeterol (Advair) (100/50 mcg), inhaled twice daily; montelukast (Singulair), 10 mg daily; prednisone (Deltasone), 40 mg daily with tapering dose over 10 d.
- Gastroesophageal reflux: Dietary and lifestyle modifications, lansoprazole (Prevacid), 30 mg daily for up to 3 mo; metoclopramide (Reglan), 10 mg before meals and sleep.
- Eosinophilic bronchitis: Fluticasone (Flovent)[1] (110 mcg), two inhalations twice daily; prednisone (Deltasone), 30 mg daily for 3 wk.
- ACE inhibitor: Discontinue medication.

---

[1]Not FDA approved for this indication.

REFERENCES

Barnes TW, Afessa B, Swanson KL, Lim KG. The clinical utility of flexible bronchoscopy in the evaluation of chronic cough. Chest 2004; 126:268–72.

Breitling CE, Ward R, Goh KL. Eosinophilic bronchitis is an important cause of chronic cough. Am J Respir Crit Care Med 1999;160:406–10.

Cherry JD. Epidemiological, clinical, and laboratory aspects of pertussis in adults. Clin Infect Dis 1999;28(Suppl2):S112–7.

Cohen M, Sahn SA. Bronchiectasis in systemic diseases. Chest 1999; 116:1063–74.

Irwin RS, Madison JM. Symptom research on chronic cough: A historical perspective. Ann Intern Med 2001;134:809–14.

Irwin RS, Madison JM. The diagnosis and treatment of cough. N Engl J Med 2000;343:1715–21.

Irwin RS, Madison JM. The persistently troublesome cough. Am J Respir Crit Care Med 2002;165:1469–74.

Kiljander TO. The role of proton pump inhibitors in the management of gastroesophageal reflux disease-related asthma and chronic cough. Am J Med 2003;115(3A):S65–71.

Pruritus

Method of
Scott Moses, MD

Because pruritus is the most common symptom in dermatology, clinicians are often asked to reduce its distressing effect on comfort and sleep. Left untreated, itch and its associated persistent scratching increases risk of chronic skin changes and secondary infection. Although pruritus is most often caused by a dermatologic condition, it can also be a symptom of underlying systemic disease.

The sensation of itch starts in the skin's free nerve endings, travels via unmyelinated C-fibers to the spine, and finally travels via the spinothalamic tract to the brain. Histamine, commonly associated with allergic rhinitis and urticaria, is only one of several chemical mediators of pruritus. Serotonin is integral to the pruritus of uremia, cholestasis, polycythemia vera, lymphoma, and morphine-associated pruritus. In atopic dermatitis, proinflammatory mediators (e.g., cytokines) are released in an immune-mediated response. Pruritus has been attributed to neuropathy in a wide variety of conditions including herpes zoster, brachioradial pruritus, notalgia paresthetica, spinal tumors, and multiple sclerosis.

Diagnosis

History is the key to identifying the cause of pruritus. Most causes are evident from the associated dermatitis (Box 1), distribution (Figure 1), or exogenous exposure history (Box 2). Clinicians should focus on the timing of pruritus and associated rash development, food and medication exposures, possible allergen and irritant exposures, pet exposure, and travel history.

In children, pruritus rarely has a systemic cause. However, clinicians should be alert for children who demonstrate red flag symptoms such as growth failure, anorexia, fatigue, associated bowel or bladder changes, and nighttime awakenings due to pruritus.

Underlying systemic disease is responsible for up to 50% of pruritus in older adults and should be considered in refractory cases and where skin findings are absent. Reassuring findings that suggest a non-systemic cause include recent onset, localized itch, pruritus

---

BOX 1 Dermatitis-Associated Causes of Pruritus

Allergic Contact Dermatitis
- Sharply demarcated erythematous lesion with overlying vesicles
- Reaction within 2-7 d of exposure (see Box 4)

Atopic Dermatitis
- Atopic patients (allergic rhinitis, asthma) with the itch that rashes
- Affects flexor wrists and ankles, antecubital and popliteal fossa

Bullous Pemphigoid
- Initially pruritic urticarial lesions, often in intertriginous areas
- Tense blisters form after urticaria

Cutaneous T-Cell Lymphoma (Mycosis Fungoides)
- Oval eczematous patch on non–sun-exposed skin (e.g., buttocks)
- Can also manifest as erythroderma (exfoliative dermatitis)
- Can also manifest as a new eczematous disorder in older adults

Dermatitis Herpetiformis
- Rare vesicular dermatitis affects lumbosacral spine, elbows, knees

Folliculitis
- Pruritus out of proportion to appearance of dermatitis
- Papules and pustules at follicular sites on chest, back, or thighs

Lichen Planus
- Lesions often on the flexor wrists
- 6 Ps: pruritus, polygonal, planar, purple papules and plaques

Lichen Simplex Chronicus
- Complication of chronic scratching (e.g., atopic dermatitis)
- Thickened plaques over lower legs, posterior neck, and groin

Parasitic Skin Infections
Insects
- Chigger bites (harvest mite): Southeastern United States
- Cutaneous myiasis (bot fly): Central and South America, Africa
- Leishmaniasis (sand fly): Central and South America, Africa, Asia

Pediculosis (lice)
- Occiput of school-aged child
- Genitalia affected in adults (STD)

Scabies
- Burrows at hand web spaces, axillae, and genitalia
- Hyperkeratotic plaques, pruritic papules or scale present
- Face and scalp affected in children but not adults

Prurigo nodularis
- Complication of chronic scratching (variant of lichen simplex)
- 1-2 cm nodules on extensor arms and legs

Psoriasis
- Plaques on extensor extremities, low back, palms, soles, and scalp

Sunburn
- Consider photosensitizing causes (e.g., NSAIDs, cosmetics)

Xerotic Eczema
- Intense itching during winter in northern climates
- Involves back, flanks, abdomen, waist, and distal extremities

---

Abbreviations: NSAIDs = nonsteroidal anti-inflammatory drugs; STD = sexually transmitted disease.

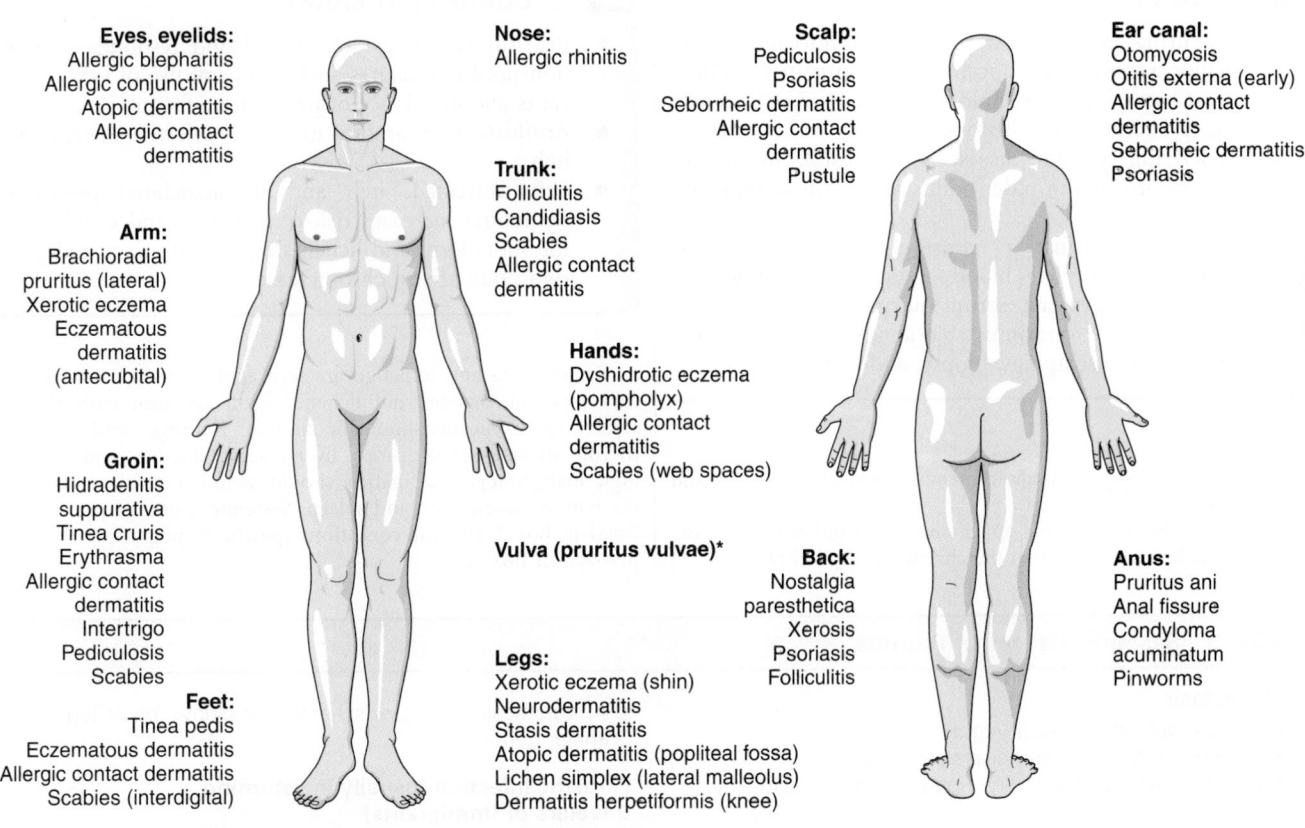

Eyes, eyelids:
Allergic blepharitis
Allergic conjunctivitis
Atopic dermatitis
Allergic contact
dermatitis

Nose:
Allergic rhinitis

Scalp:
Pediculosis
Psoriasis
Seborrheic dermatitis
Allergic contact
dermatitis
Pustule

Ear canal:
Otomycosis
Otitis externa (early)
Allergic contact
dermatitis
Seborrheic dermatitis
Psoriasis

Arm:
Brachioradial
pruritus (lateral)
Xerotic eczema
Eczematous
dermatitis
(antecubital)

Trunk:
Folliculitis
Candidiasis
Scabies
Allergic contact
dermatitis

Hands:
Dyshidrotic eczema
(pompholyx)
Allergic contact
dermatitis
Scabies (web spaces)

Groin:
Hidradenitis
suppurativa
Tinea cruris
Erythrasma
Allergic contact
dermatitis
Intertrigo
Pediculosis
Scabies

Vulva (pruritus vulvae)*

Legs:
Xerotic eczema (shin)
Neurodermatitis
Stasis dermatitis
Atopic dermatitis (popliteal fossa)
Lichen simplex (lateral malleolus)
Dermatitis herpetiformis (knee)

Back:
Nostalgia
paresthetica
Xerosis
Psoriasis
Folliculitis

Anus:
Pruritus ani
Anal fissure
Condyloma
acuminatum
Pinworms

Feet:
Tinea pedis
Eczematous dermatitis
Allergic contact dermatitis
Scabies (interdigital)

*—Causes of pruritus vulvae: prepubertal girls—poor hygiene, streptococcal infection, *Escherichia coli* infection, pinworms, scabies, allergic contact dermatitis; young women—vaginitis, allergic contact dermatitis, hidradenitis suppurativa, lichen simplex chronicus; postmenopausal women—atrophic vaginitus, lichen sclerosus, vulvar cancer, Paget's disease; females with diabetes mellitus—candidiasis, other dermatophyte infections.

FIGURE 1. Causes of pruritus (by distribution). (Adapted from Moses S: Pruritus. Am Fam Physician 2003;68:1135-1146.)

BOX 2 Exposure-Related Pruritus

Allergic Contact Dermatitis
- Topical medications: Neomycin, benzocaine (Americaine)
- Nickel, latex, cosmetics, black hair dye
- Laundry detergents or fabric softeners
- Paint-on tattoos (paraphenylenediamine)
- Tattoo dye: cadmium yellow, mercuric sulfide (red)
- Ointments highly concentrated in inert oil

Heat Exposure
- Miliaria rubra (prickly heat)
- Cholinergic urticaria (response to hot bath, fever, exercise)

Occupational Exposure
- Dyes (e.g., glyceryl monothioglycolate)
- Potassium dichromate in cements and dyes
- Rosins or epoxy resins in adhesives
- Rubber, methyl methacrylate, fiberglass

Systemic Medications
- Drug hypersensitivity (rifampin [Rifadin], vancomycin [Vancocin])
- Itraconazole (Sporanox), fluconazole, ketoconazole (Nizoral)
- Niacinamide (niacin), B vitamins, aspirin, quinidine (Quinidex)
- Nitrates (food preservatives)
- Spinal narcotics (pruritus affects face, neck, and upper chest)

Water Exposure
- Aquagenic pruritus (associated with polycythemia vera)
- Cholinergic urticaria (response to warm water)
- Itching within 15 min of any water contact
- Polycythemia vera
- Swimmer's itch (7-d eruption after freshwater swimming)

CURRENT DIAGNOSIS

- Reassuring findings that suggest a nonorganic cause include recent onset, localized itch, pruritus limited to exposed skin, household members also with pruritus, and recent travel history.
- Underlying systemic disease is responsible for up to 50% of pruritus in older adults and is uncommon in children.
- Laboratory testing to consider in atypical cases includes a complete blood count, ferritin, thyroid-stimulating hormone, serum bilirubin, alkaline phosphatase, serum creatinine, blood urea nitrogen, HIV test, and skin scrapings, biopsy, and culture.

CURRENT THERAPY

- Pruritus is usually self-limited and responds well to nonspecific measures such as liberal use of skin lubricants and avoidance of provocative factors.
- Antihistamines are not uniformly effective in reducing itch.
- Left untreated, itch and its associated persistent scratching increases risk of impetigo and cellulitis in the short term and lichen simplex chronicus and prurigo nodularis in chronic cases.

limited to exposed skin, household members also with pruritus, and recent travel history.

Dermatitis distribution and appearance often indicate the cause. The examination can also reveal the chronicity of pruritus.

Excoriations and impetigo are seen acutely, and postinflammatory pigment changes and lichenification are seen with chronic scratching. Clinicians should be alert for findings consistent with thyroid disease, renal disease, liver disease, anemia, and hematologic malignancy. Examination should include careful palpation of the lymph nodes, liver, and spleen. Systemic causes of pruritus are listed in Box 3. Pruritic conditions specific to pregnancy are summarized in Box 4.

BOX 3   Systemic Causes of Pruritus

Cholestasis
- Intense itching, worse at night
- Affects hands, feet, and pressure sites
- Reactive hyperpigmentation spares midback (butterfly appearance)

Chronic Renal Failure
- Severe paroxysms of generalized itching
- Worse in summer

Delusions of parasitosis
- Focal erosions on exposed areas of arms and legs

Human Immunodeficiency Virus
- Pruritus is a common presenting symptom due to secondary causes
- Causes: Eczema, drug reaction, eosinophilic folliculitis, seborrhea

Hodgkin's Lymphoma
- Prolonged generalized pruritus often precedes diagnosis

Hyperthyroidism
- Skin is warm and moist
- Pretibial edema may be present
- Onycholysis, hyperpigmentation, and vitiligo have been associated

Iron-Deficiency Anemia
- Other dermatologic signs include glossitis and angular cheilitis

Malignant Carcinoid
- Intermittent head and neck flushing
- Explosive diarrhea

Multiple Myeloma
- Affects elderly with bone pain, headache, cachexia, anemia, and renal failure

Neurodermatitis or Neurotic Excoriations
- Bouts of intense itching that can awaken the patient from a sound sleep

- Affects scalp, neck, wrist, extensor elbow, outer leg, ankle, perineum

Parasitic Infection (usually in returning travelers or immigrants)
- Filariasis: Tropical parasite responsible for lymphedema
- Onchocerciasis: Transmitted by black fly in Africa, Latin America
- Schistosomiasis: Fresh water exposure in Africa, Mediterranean, South America
- Trichinosis: Undercooked pork, bear, wild boar, or walrus meat

Parvovirus B19
- Slapped cheek appearance in children
- Arthritis in some adults

Peripheral Neuropathy
- Brachioradial pruritus: Affects lateral arms of white patients in the tropics
- Notalgia paresthetica: Midback pruritus with hyperpigmented patch
- Herpes zoster: Accompanies painful prodrome 2 d before rash

Polycythemia Rubra Vera
- Pricking-type itch persists for hours after hot shower or bath

Scleroderma
- Nonpitting extremity edema, erythema, and intense pruritus
- Edema phase with pruritus precedes fibrosis of the skin

Urticaria
- Response to allergen, cold, heat, exercise, sunlight, or direct pressure

Weight Loss (Rapid) in Eating Disorders
- Other signs include hair loss or fine lanugo hair on back and cheeks
- Also yellow skin discoloration and petechiae

BOX 4 Causes of Pruritus in Pregnancy

Pruritic Urticarial Papules and Plaques of Pregnancy
- Common in the third trimester
- Intense pruritus involves abdomen
- Spreads to thighs, buttocks, breasts, and arms

Prurigo of Pregnancy
- Common in second half of pregnancy
- Extensor arms and abdomen with excoriated papules and nodules
- Associated with atopic dermatitis

Herpes Gestationis or Pemphigoid Gestationis
- Uncommon
- Autoimmune condition associated with Graves' disease
- Vesicles and bullae on abdomen and extremities in second half of pregnancy
- Responds to prednisone[1] 0.5 mg/kg (Level A)

Intrahepatic Cholestasis of Pregnancy
- Uncommon
- Trunk and extremity itching without rash in late pregnancy
- Jaundice not present in the mild form (prurigo gravidarum)
- Responds to cholestyramine (Questran) and Vitamin K_1 (Aquamephyton)[1](Level B)

Pruritic Folliculitis of Pregnancy
- Uncommon, occurs in second half of pregnancy
- Erythematous follicular papules over trunk, with spread to extremities
- May be a variant of prurigo of pregnancy

Other Common Pruritic Conditions Exacerbated in Pregnancy
- Atopic dermatitis
- Contact dermatitis

[1]Not FDA approved for this indication.
Levels of evidence: Level A: Evidence from high-quality randomized controlled clinical trials or meta-analyses; Level B: Evidence from nonrandomized clinical studies or nonquantitative systematic reviews.

In cases refractory to 2 weeks of symptomatic therapy or in which an underlying systemic cause is considered, a limited laboratory evaluation is indicated and is summarized in Table 1. When itch persists or is refractory to general measures, remember that up to one half of older adults have pruritus caused by an underlying systemic problem.

Treatment

Pruritus is usually self-limited and responds well to nonspecific measures such as liberal use of skin lubricants and avoidance of provocative factors (Box 5). Oral antihistamines are not uniformly effective in all causes of pruritus. Specific management of dermatitis, as with atopic dermatitis, scabies, and contact dermatitis, can relieve symptoms.

In the atypical case, where these measures fail, a systemic condition may be uncovered. In these patients, the itch should be alleviated by treating the underlying condition, as with thyroid replacement in hypothyroidism or iron supplementation in iron deficiency anemia. Uremia and cholestasis-related pruritus have established effective therapies beyond treating the causative chronic renal or hepatic insufficiency (Box 6).

Complications

Itch and the scratch it induces are not benign. When scratching is left unchecked, fingernails introduce bacteria into abraded skin, and impetigo or cellulitis can ensue. Lichen simplex chronicus and prurigo nodularis are chronic skin changes seen with long-term scratching and in particular with atopic dermatitis.

Medications to treat pruritus are also not without adverse effects. Antihistamines can affect alertness and learning if used during the day, and with chronic use, the associated dry mouth can predispose to tooth decay.

Follow-Up

General measures to treat pruritus should be reviewed at each visit. Consistent practice of these simple home strategies can prevent sleepless nights, frequent evaluations, unnecessary medications, and the complications of scratching.

TABLE 1 Diagnostic Evaluation of Pruritus for Atypical, Persistent, or Refractory Cases

Tests	Findings
Complete blood count,* serum ferritin*	Iron deficiency anemia, polycythemia rubra vera, Hodgkin's lymphoma, multiple myeloma, parasitic infection
Serum bilirubin, alkaline phosphatase*	Cholestasis (e.g., cirrhosis)
Serum creatinine, blood urea nitrogen*	Uremia (e.g., chronic renal failure)
Thyroid stimulating hormone*	Hyperthyroidism
Microscopy of skin scrapings, skin culture, skin biopsy	Dermatophytes, scabies; skin bacterial, fungal or viral infection; mastocytosis, mycosis fungoides, bullous pemphigoid
HIV test	HIV infection
Chest radiograph	Hodgkin's lymphoma, multiple myeloma
Stool tests	Parasites, *Helicobacter pylori* Children: pinworms, perianal streptococcus

*Denotes a first-line test. Unmarked tests are performed if history indicates.

BOX 5 Nonspecific Management of Pruritus

- Use skin lubricants liberally
  - Petrolatum or skin lubricant cream at bedtime
  - Apply alcohol-free, hypoallergenic lotions frequently during day
- Avoid excessive bathing
  - Briefly pat dry after bath and immediately apply skin lubricants
  - Decrease bathing frequency
  - Limit bathing to brief exposure to tepid water
- Limit soap use
  - Use mild, unscented, hypoallergenic soap 2 or 3 times per wk
  - Daily use of soap only in groin and axillae; spare legs, arms, and torso
- Minimize dryness
  - Humidify dry indoor environment (especially in winter)
- Choose clothing that does not irritate the skin
  - Doubly rinsed cotton clothes and silk are best
  - Add bath oil (e.g., Alpha Keri) to rinse cycle when washing sheets
  - Avoid heat-retaining fabrics (synthetics)
  - Avoid wool and smooth-textured cotton clothes
- Avoid vasodilators
  - Avoid caffeine, alcohol, spices, hot water, and excessive sweating
- Avoid provocative topical medications
  - Avoid prolonged topical corticosteroids (risk of skin atrophy)
- Avoid topical anesthetics and antihistamines
  - May sensitize exposed skin and risk contact dermatitis
- Standard antipruritic topical agents
  - Menthol and camphor (e.g., Sarna Lotion)
  - Oatmeal baths (e.g., Aveeno)
  - Pramoxine[1] (e.g., PrameGel [pramoxine + menthol], Pramosone [pramoxine + hydrocortisone])
  - Calamine lotion (Use on weeping lesions only, not on dry skin)
- Antipruritic topical agents for refractory cases (used in severe atopic dermatitis)
  - Doxepin 5% cream (Zonalon)
  - Burow's solution (wet dressings with aluminum acetate 5% in water)
  - Unna's boot[1] (zinc oxide paste bandages)
  - Coal tar emulsion[1] (Zetar)
- Systemic antipruritic agents (used in allergic and urticarial disease)
  - Doxepin (Sinequan)[1] 1 mg/kg up to 25 mg at bedtime (Level A)
  - Hydroxyzine (Atarax) 0.5 mg/kg up to 25-50 mg at bedtime
  - Nonsedating antihistamines (e.g., Fexofenadine [Allegra], Level A)
- Prevent complications of scratching
  - Keep fingernails short and clean
  - Rub skin with palms if urge to scratch is irresistible

[1]Not FDA approved for this indication.
Level A: Evidence from high-quality randomized controlled clinical trials or meta-analyses.

BOX 6 Specific Management of Pruritic Conditions

Cholestasis
- Cholestyramine (Questran) (Level B)
  - Adult: 4 g 30 min before meals
  - Child: 240 mg/kg/d divided tid (up to 6 g/d)
- Ursodiol (Actigall)[1] 15 mg/kg/d divided before meals
- Ondansetron (Zofran)[1] 4-8 mg IV, then 4 mg PO q8h (Level B)
- Opioid receptor antagonist (Level A)
  - Naloxone (Narcan)[1] 0.002 mcg/kg/h IV, titrate to max 0.25 mcg/kg/h
  - Naltrexone (Revia)[1] 12.5 mg PO qd (advance to 50 mg PO qd)
- Rifampin (Rifadin)[1] 10 mg/kg/d divided bid (max: 300 mg bid) (Level B)
- Bile duct stenting from extrahepatic cholestasis (Level A)
- Lidocaine (Xylocaine)[1] IV has been used
- Bright light therapy (Level B)
- Plasmapheresis

Neurotic Excoriation
- Pimozide (Orap)[1] for delusions of parasitosis
- Selective serotonin reuptake inhibitor (SSRI)

Notalgia Paresthetica
- Topical capsaicin (Zostrix)[1] applied 4-6 times per d for several wk (Level B)

Polycythemia Vera
- Aspirin[1] 500 mg PO q8-24h (Level B)
- Paroxetine (Paxil)[1] 10-20 mg PO qd (Level B)
- Interferon-α (Intron A)[1] 3-35 million IU/wk (Level B)

Spinal Opioid–Induced Pruritus
- Ondansetron (Zofran)[1] 8 mg IV concurrent with opioid (Level A)
- Nalbuphine (Nubain)[1] 5 mg IV concurrent with opioid (Level B)

Uremia
- UV B phototherapy twice weekly for 1 mo (Level A)
- Activated charcoal[1] 6 g/d (Level A)
- Topical capsaicin[1] 0.025% cream to localized areas (Level A)
- Ondansetron and naltrexone are not efficacious in uremia (Level A)

[1]Not FDA approved for this indication.
Level A: Evidence from high-quality randomized controlled clinical trials or meta-analyses; Level B: Evidence from nonrandomized clinical studies or nonquantitative systematic reviews.

REFERENCES

Belsito DV. The diagnostic evaluation, treatment and prevention of allergic contact dermatitis in the new millennium. J Allergy Clin Immunol 2000; 105:409–20.

Bender BG. Sedation and performance impairment of diphenhydramine and second-generation antihistamines: A meta-analysis. J Allergy Clin Immunol 2003;111:770–6.

Bergasa NV. An approach to the management of the pruritus of cholestasis. Clin Liver Dis 2004;8:55–66.

Berger R, Gilchrest BA. Skin disorders. In: Duthie EH, Katz PR, editors. Practice of Geriatrics. 3rd ed. Philadelphia: WB Saunders; 1998. p. 467–72.

Boiko S, Zeiger R. Diagnosis and treatment of atopic dermatitis, urticaria, and angioedema during pregnancy. Immunol Allergy Clin North Am 2000;20:839.

Callen JP, Bernardi DM, Clark RAF, Weber DA. Adult-onset recalcitrant eczema: A marker of noncutaneous lymphoma or leukemia. J Am Acad Dermatol 2000;43:207–10.

Correale CE, Walker C, Lydia M, Craig TJ. Atopic dermatitis: A review of diagnosis and treatment. Am Fam Physician 1999;60:1191–210.

Cyr PR, Dreher GK. Neurotic excoriations. Am Fam Physician 2001;64: 1981–4.

Diehn F, Tefferi A. Pruritus in polycthaemia vera: Prevalence. Laboratory Correlates and Management 2001;115:619–21.

Fagan EA. Intrahepatic cholestasis of pregnancy. Clin Liver Dis 1999;3: 603–32.

Finn AF, Kaplan AP, Fretwell R, et al. A double-blind, placebo-controlled trial of fexofenadine HCl in the treatment of chronic idiopathic urticaria. J Allergy Clin Immunol 1999;103:1071–8.

Fisher AA. Aquagenic pruritus. Cutis 1993;51:146–7.

Gelfand JM, Rudikoff D. Evaluation and treatment of itching in HIV-infected patients. Mt Sinai J Med 2001;68:298–308.

Ghent CN. The pruritus of cholestasis. Hepatology 1999;29:1003–6.

Gupta MA, Gupta AK, Voorhees JJ. Starvation-associated pruritus: A clinical feature of eating disorders. J Am Acad Dermatol 1992;27:118–20.

Habif TP. Clinical Dermatology. 3rd ed. Chicago: Mosby–Year Book; 1996.

Harrigan E, Rabinowitz LG. Atopic dermatitis. Immunol Allergy Clin North Am 1999;19:383–96.

Heymann WR. Chronic urticaria and angioedema associated with thyroid autoimmunity: Review and therapeutic implications. J Am Acad Dermatol 1999;40:229–32.

Koblenzer CS. Itching and atopic skin. J Allergy Clin Immunol 1999;104:S109–13.

Krajnik M, Zylicz Z. Understanding pruritus in systemic disease. J Pain Symptom Manage 2001;21:151–68.

Kroumpouzos G, Cohen LM. Dermatoses of pregnancy. J Am Acad Dermatol 2001;45:1–19.

Leung AKC. Pruritus in children. J Roy Soc Health 1998;118:280–6.

Lidofsky S, Scharschmidt BF. Jaundice. In: Feldman M, Scharschmidt BF, Sleisenger MH, Fordtran JS, editors. Sleisenger and Fordtran's Gastrointestinal and Liver Disease. 6th ed. Philadelphia: WB Saunders; 1998. p. 230–1.

Moses S. Pruritus. Am Fam Physician 2003;68:1135–46.

Parker F. Structure and function of skin. In: Goldman L, Bennett JC, editors. Cecil Textbook of Medicine. 21st ed. Philadelphia: WB Saunders; 2000. p. 2266.

Paus R, Schmeiz M, Biró T, Steinhoff M. Frontiers in pruritus research: Scratching the brain for more effective itch therapy. J Clin Invest 2006;116:1174–85.

Robinson-Bostom L, DiGiovanna JJ. Cutaneous manifestations of end-stage renal disease. J Am Acad Dermatol 2000;43:975–86.

Shellow WVR. Evaluation of pruritus. In: Goroll AH, Mulley AG, editors. Primary Care Medicine. 4th ed. Philadelphia: Lippincott Williams & Wilkins; 2000. p. 1001–4.

Stambuk R, Colvin R. Dermatologic disorders. In: Gabbe SG, Niebyl JR, Simpson JL, editors. Obstetrics: Normal and Problem Pregnancies. 4th ed. New York: Churchill Livingstone; 2002. p. 1283–90.

Tennyson H. Neurotropic and psychotropic drugs in dermatology. Dermatol Clin 2001;19:179–97.

Tormey WP, Chambers JPM. Pruritus as the presenting symptom in hyperthyroidism. Br J Clin Pract 1994;48:224.

Valsecchi R, Cainelli T. Generalized pruritus: A manifestation of iron deficiency. Arch Dermatol 1983;119:630.

Veien NK, Hattel T, Laurberg G, Spaun E. Brachioradial pruritus. J Am Acad Dermatol 2001;44:704–5.

Villamil AG, Bandi JC, Galdame OA, et al. Efficacy of lidocaine in the treatment of pruritus in patients with chronic cholestatic liver disease. Am J Med 2005;118:1160–3.

Waxler B, Dadabhoy Z, Stojiljkovic L, Rabito SF. Primer of postoperative pruritus for anesthesiologists. Anesthesiology 2005;103:168–78.

Zirwas MJ, Seraly MP. Pruritus of unknown origin: A retrospective study. J Am Acad Dermatol 2001;45:892–6.

Tinnitus

Method of
Claus-Frenz Claussen, MD

Tinnitus is noise(s) in the ear, which is usually subjective and can be extremely disturbing and frustrating to those affected. According to studies of the American Tinnitus Association, approximately 36 million Americans older than 40 years suffer from tinnitus.

Tinnitus has been regarded as a disease entity for many centuries. During the second half of the 20th century, physicians were able to discriminate among several different kinds of tinnitus including bruits, maskable tinnitus, and nonmaskable tinnitus. Under the influence of Shulman and his team, the term *tinnitology* was coined.

The present interest of researchers in the field of tinnitology is split into two fields of action: suggestions for improvement of objective and quantitative differential diagnostics in tinnitus and research and development to improve various types of treatment for different kinds of tinnitus.

General Phenomena of Tinnitus

A noise without any human information function, a tinnitus, can be a normal as well as a pathologic function of human hearing. On the one hand, tinnitus can be regarded as a problem of acoustic resolution of the inner ear microphone, that is, the cochlear noise-to-signal ratio. In a well-dampened soundproof chamber, most normal-hearing persons experience a sizzling sound in their ears because of their perception of molecular vibrations from inner ear fluids (as known from thermodynamics). Yet this underlying percept is masked in everyday life by normal environmental noise.

On the other hand, tinnitus patients regularly tell their physicians about subjective ear noises that they describe, for example, as pulsating, humming, roaring, whistling, hissing, fullness of the ear, and pressure and/or pain in the ear.

Table 1 presents the subjective sensational qualities of tinnitus in 823 tinnitus patients (77.52% male and 22.48% female with a mean age of 50.87 years ± 8.68 years) from Bad Kissingen, Germany, who underwent clinical inpatient rehabilitation therapy for several weeks for severe disabling tinnitus.

 CURRENT DIAGNOSIS

Irritating subjective or objective perception of irritating acoustic noise or sound in the ear, head, or body that may be described, for example, as:
- Pulsating
- Humming
- Roaring
- Whistling
- Hissing

TABLE 1 Subjective Classification of Ear Noises in 823 (=100%) Tinnitus Patients

Complaints	Right Ear (%)	Left Ear (%)
Pulsating	1.94	1.94
Humming	7.41	6.93
Roaring	14.10	14.22
Whistling	50.67	51.76
Hissing	9.96	10.81
Pressure in the ear	6.32	5.83
Pain in the ear	14.10	14.22

TABLE 2 Subjective Classification of Different Time/Intensity Patterns of Tinnitus in 823 (=100%) Patients

Time/Intensity Patterns	%
Permanent	59.17
Intermittent	19.97
Swelling up and going down	43.26

In these same patients, we looked for descriptions of different time/intensity patterns of their tinnitus (Table 2), and the subjective background of discomfort was investigated as shown in Table 3. Additionally, the patients named the most irritating factors related to their tinnitus (Table 4).

Sleep disturbance is a common and frequent complaint. Scientific studies report decreased tolerance and increased discomfort when insomnia and depression are associated with tinnitus.

In 1991, a sample of 338 New Zealanders regularly experiencing tinnitus completed and returned questionnaires to associations for people with tinnitus or hearing impairment. Nearly half the sample was sometimes depressed because of tinnitus. Those reporting depression and those reporting more severe problems as a consequence of the tinnitus saw more health care professionals and used more coping strategies. Most respondents did not remember exactly when they first noticed the tinnitus.

A questionnaire investigation comprising 1091 patients from Bispebjerg Hospital, Copenhagen (1993), concerning "tinnitus-incidence and handicap," was conducted at a hearing center. A majority of patients, 59%, claimed that they were troubled by tinnitus. Neither a greater degree of hearing loss nor a longer duration of tinnitus was associated with more severe tinnitus. Among patients with both subjective hearing loss and tinnitus, 23% stated that tinnitus was the greater problem, and 38% said that tinnitus and hearing loss were equally troublesome. The corresponding figures for patients with hearing impairment of such a degree that a hearing aid was deemed necessary were 9% and 41%,

TABLE 3 Subjective Classification of Subjective Background of Discomfort in 823 (=100%) Patients

Subjective Complaints About Factors of Discomfort	%
Headache	69.02
Migraine	4.13
Exhaustion	59.99
Lacking in drive	42.16
Feeling of weakness	55.29
Forgetfulness	68.41
Disorientation	0.49
Daze	44.84
Tiredness	63.91
Insomnia	69.50

TABLE 4 Subjective Classification of Most Irritating Factors Related to Their Tinnitus in 823 (=100%) Patients

Most Irritating Factors Related to Tinnitus	%
All patients with specific additional statements	25.76
Difficulties in going to sleep	10.69
Difficulties in sleeping through the night	11.06
Depression	0.24
Abnormal sounds (also hallucinations)	2.67
Acute hearing loss	8.38

respectively. Stress symptoms such as headache, tension of facial muscles, and sleep disturbances were correlated to tinnitus. Of patients with tinnitus, 83% were interested in obtaining treatment for it.

The so-called Copenhagen Male Study reported on the results from a 10-year follow-up examination concerning hearing and factors known to cause hearing problems. The original sample comprised 5050 subjects, and at the present examination, 3387 (67%) men at a median of 63 years of age (range, 53 to 75 years) participated. An increasing prevalence of 30% to 40% of hearing problems was demonstrated with increasing age. A prevalence of 17% of tinnitus of more than 5 minutes' duration was found; 3% indicated that tinnitus was so annoying that it interfered with sleep, reading, and/or concentration. The prevalence of tinnitus increased up to 70 years of age and seemed to remain constant thereafter.

In Norway, 15% of the adult population has experienced shorter or longer periods of tinnitus. Three percent of these, in total approximately 7000 to 10,000 persons, suffer from continuous tinnitus followed by symptoms that represent a handicap or occupational disability. Similar observations were reported from many other countries.

Clinical Types

Tinnitus is no longer considered to be a syndrome or a single disease. Because of improvements in neuro-otometry, several different types of tinnitus can be differentiated.

By means of modern audiometry, the framework for normal hearing can be described objectively and quantitatively. Therefore, in any tinnitus case, a thorough analysis of the hearing function and pathways needs to be performed including threshold audiometry, audiometric tinnitus masking (if possible), acoustic dynamics between the measurable thresholds of hearing and acoustic discomfort, speech audiometry, otoacoustic emissions, acoustic brainstem-evoked potentials, and acoustic late-evoked potentials. Thereby signs of pathology within the hearing pathways between the ear and the human brain cortex can be measured.

Thus, we know from thorough neuro-otologic studies that approximately 24% of cases of disabling tinnitus have their source within the otoacoustic periphery (i.e., inner ear and the eighth cranial nerve). Approximately 35% originate from the acoustic pathways within the brainstem. Approximately 41% have their cause within supratentorial structures and/or functions. These pathologies also should serve as basic information for planning systematic pharmacotherapy directed to the central nervous system (CNS) focus of dysfunction.

At least four different kinds of tinnitus (Figure 1) can be discriminated, which can be determined by the physician using a simple question-and-answer procedure as follows.

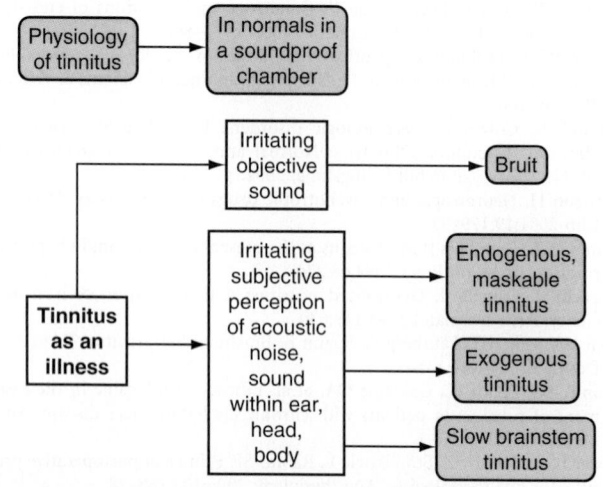

FIGURE 1. Categories of physiologic and clinical types of tinnitus.

BRUITS

Q: Has someone informed you that he or she could hear a noise coming from your head?
A: Yes. Their description of what they heard listening from outside my head is similar to what I perceive.

By means of auscultation through a stethoscope or a microphone, a real sound can be objectively heard emanating from the patient's skull. Patients frequently report, for example, a bubbling, hissing, or pulsating sound.

The cause can be vascular in origin, that is, abnormal curling of blood caused by atheromas, vascular dissections, scars, compressions, or high blood pressure amplitudes, for example.

Bruits also can originate from the middle ear and its connections toward the epipharynx: middle ear inflammations with bubbling sounds of gas from within the effusions, whizzing middle ear muscles, or an open eustachian tube.

Cracking sounds, which are misinterpreted as tinnitus, are reported from arthritic and other mandibular joint disorders. Also, sounds can be transferred from the cervical spine and its joints as well as its vessels into the cranial structures so that they become misinterpreted as tinnitus.

ENDOGENOUS TINNITUS

Q: Where is your feeling of well-being better, in a busy and noisy environment or in cavelike silence?
A: I much prefer a busy and noisy environment.

The patient with a maskable or endogenous tinnitus prefers covering it with external sounds. When using masking procedures, easily three zones of tinnitus can be discriminated within the hearing field:

1. Low-tone tinnitus (at and below 750 Hz)
2. Middle-frequency tinnitus (1 to 2 kHz)
3. High-frequency tinnitus (above 2 kHz until 10 kHz or even 12 kHz)

Low-tone tinnitus is more frequently found in Ménière's disease and some other cochlear-apical disorders, and middle-tone tinnitus is more frequently found in diseases such as otosclerosis. Most frequently tinnitus is matched in the high-tone range and is related, for example, to noise trauma, whiplash, head and skull trauma, cardiovascular failure, stress, acoustic neuromas, and toxic events including those associated with pharmaceutical, nicotine, or drug abuse. Also, several masking points may exist simultaneously.

Dysfunctions of the inner ear contribute to the development of tinnitus. But tinnitus by itself depends on a cortical process of the human brain. A sleeping patient does not suffer from any kind of tinnitus.

Since approximately 1985, the Würzburg neuro-otology group of Claussen et al. has been able to detect by means of vestibular evoked potentials (VestEP) and brain electrical activity mapping (BEAM) groups of patients suffering from a maskable or endogenous tinnitus that respond cortically in a typical, reproducible, and measurable manner:

1. Location of the site of the potentials around the upper gyrus of the temporal lobe (Brodmann's area 41)
2. Typical shortening of the latencies of evoked quantitative electroencephalograms (QEEGs) (i.e., VestEP waves I, II, III)
3. Enlarged DC shift of the evoked QEEGs (i.e., difference between VestEP waves III and IV)
4. Typical cortical electrical burst expansion in three phases on the brain surface

Since approximately 1990, the New York group of Shulman, Strashun, and Goldstein has followed a neuroradiologic path for deciphering the cortical modalities in tinnitus patients by using single-photon emission computer tomography (SPECT). They discovered remarkably elevated metabolic processes in the temporal lobes of patients suffering from a maskable tinnitus.

Thereafter we were able to prove in therapeutic trials with pharmacotherapy (e.g., extractum ginkgo biloba [EGB 761]*), as well as with physiotherapy (competitive kinesthetic interaction therapy [KKIT]), that the subjective reduction or abolition of tinnitus goes together with an electrophysiologic measurable normalization of the VestEP with BEAM or QEEG. So the endogenous tinnitus could be proven to be a CNS network phenomenon.

EXOGENOUS TINNITUS

Q: Where is your feeling of well-being better, in a busy and noisy environment or in cavelike silence?
A: I much prefer a cavelike silence because noise and/or a group of people speaking at the same time are most confusing. It provokes ringing and shrieking sounds within my ears.

Unlike endogenous tinnitus, patients suffering from exogenous tinnitus cannot benefit from masking noises from their surroundings. Some physicians wrongly call this condition *hyperacusis*, but these patients do not hear better as this term suggests. Seemingly better is the named syndrome of the hypersensitive ear.

In exogenous tinnitus, pure-tone audiometry may be normal or exhibit regular deficits of the hearing threshold, but there is no maskable tinnitus. However, when measuring the acoustic dynamics by adding the audiometrically recorded discomfort threshold, the discomfort level, which is usually between 1 and 8 kHz below 95 dB, rises below this level to values of 90 to 60 dB or even 50 dB. The person being exposed to sound exceeding the level of his low discomfort threshold experiences a loss of understanding together with subjective pain and noise in the ears accompanied by possible vegetative reactions.

Hearing aids can adjust the incoming sounds by filtering, peak clipping, and cleaning of the sound signals so they fit optimally into the remaining acoustic dynamics of the individually existing hearing field. Thus, hearing aids are the first choice for treating exogenous tinnitus. Some other methods for treating this type of tinnitus are physiotherapy, psychotherapy, stress reduction, and supportive pharmacotherapy.

TINNITUS IN SLOW BRAINSTEM SYNDROME (CLAUSSEN)

Q: How would you best describe your tinnitus?
A: I am becoming increasingly more in a daze and more disoriented and hear ringing and other sounds, which I cannot really localize in my ears or my head. The noise disturbs me as much as my mental instability.

We regularly see older patients who complain about a hazy tinnitus in combination with vertigo, giddiness, and dizziness and also report a reduced state of alertness. These patients have a connected statoacoustic problem. Objectively, affected patients exhibit an increase in the latencies of the experimentally provoked vestibular nystagmus as well as of the acoustically evoked brainstem potentials.

Especially in this group, we have noted by evaluating our therapeutic responses that a combination of cocculus† (picrotoxin), conium† (coneine), amber and petrol oil (Vertigoheel†) has a so-called tuning-up effect on the brainstem. Then the typical symptoms also disappear.

COMBINED ENDOGENOUS AND EXOGENOUS TINNITUS

A combination of both types of subjective tinnitus, endogenous and exogenous, is also found in tinnitus patients. Affected patients report that the noise they hear is present during both the day and night; however, the noise fluctuates. Especially the intensity of the noise can be very increased, for example when the patient is in a

---

*Available as dietary supplement.
†Available as homeopathic remedy.

noisy environment or busy place or in a conversation with several participants.

Even though patients with combined endogenous and exogenous tinnitus have maskable tinnitus, they report that therapeutic acoustic maskers do not reduce their symptoms. They need a thorough audiometric and neuro-otologic workup.

Contemporary and Practical Treatment

Modern therapy of tinnitus appears to be complex and sometimes incomprehensible. But when talking about therapy of disabling tinnitus, we emphasize a main therapeutic approach in the sense that we have to break and inhibit the psychosomatic cycle of deterioration from tinnitus to stress, to insomnia, to panic. Some aspects of this reactional behavior are similar to pain.

The steps for individual tinnitus therapy must be chosen according to the kind of tinnitus diagnosed. Tinnitus is frequently associated with conditions such as stress, hearing loss, noise trauma, otorhinolaryngologic disorders (e.g., Ménière's disease, otosclerosis, perilymphatic fistula, acoustic neuroma), high blood pressure, metabolic disorders, allergy, intoxications, whiplash and other head and neck traumas, functional disorders of the neck, burnout syndrome, mandibular joint problems, and extracranial and intracranial vascular problems.

The Current Therapy box lists different therapeutic approaches to tinnitus. These ten therapies must be individually interrelated with the different types of tinnitus (see Figure 1). Besides the severe disabling types of tinnitus, minor forms of tinnitus also occasionally occur that may be event related or may be time limited.

CURRENT THERAPY

- Avoidance of noise, ototoxic drugs, allergens
- Treatment of bruits by medical or surgical measures
- Instrumental therapy
- Tinnitus maskers
- Hearing aids
- Electrostimulation
- Specific pharmacotherapy
  - Lidocaine (Xylocaine)[1]
  - Carbamazepine (Tegretol)[1]
- Calming pharmacotherapy
  - Diazepam (Valium)[1]
  - Amitriptyline (Elavil)[1]
- Nontropic pharmacotherapy
  - Gingko*
  - Flunarizine[2]
- Neurotransmitter-directed pharmacotherapy
  - Betahistine*
  - Gabapentin (Neurontin)
- Psychotherapy
  - Retraining therapy (TRT)
- Physiotherapy
  - Competitive kinesthetic interaction therapy (KKIT)
- Other therapies
  - Hypnotherapy
  - Counseling
  - Acupuncture

---

[1]Not FDA approved for this indication.
[2]Not available in the United States.
*Available as dietary supplement.

NOISE AVOIDANCE AND BASICS OF THERAPY

Avoidance can help in noise-related tinnitus by the prevention of noise exposure or at least by wearing ear protection. The use of ototoxic drugs must be controlled and limited. Inflammatory ear disease needs specific treatment of the external and the middle ear with antibiotics and anti-inflammatory drugs. Control and maintenance of a satisfactory degree of aeration of the middle ear is necessary. Acoustic neuroma calls for surgical removal of the tumor. Surgery is also necessary in otosclerosis and perilymphatic fistula. Specific gnatholic therapy by a dentist is recommended in a temporomandibular joint syndrome.

INSTRUMENTATIONS FOR THERAPY

Instrumentations currently available and frequently used according to the type and the chronicity of tinnitus are as follows:

1. Tinnitus maskers/tinnitus instruments, tapes/CDs for masking and relaxation
2. Acoustic ultra-high-frequency stimulation
3. Hearing aids
4. External electrical stimulations
5. External magnetic stimulation

PHARMACOTHERAPY

Pharmacotherapy, that is, treatment with pharmaceutical agents, is important in the management of tinnitus. It may be the main therapy or may play only a supportive, palliative, or intermittent role. The four lines of therapeutic agents used in the treatment of tinnitus may overlap and may be combined.

First-Line Agents

First-line therapeutic agents can relieve tinnitus either slowly or quickly. Lidocaine (Xylocaine),[1] a local anesthetic drug, only has a temporary effect in suppressing tinnitus. It is an aminoethylamide, which is well soluble in water.

A daily intravenous dose of lidocaine of 1 mg per kg of body weight can temporarily alleviate the phenomenon of endogenous tinnitus. The duration, however, depends on the blood level. As soon as the level of lidocaine in the blood is lowered below a threshold, tinnitus returns.

In tinnitus, lidocaine is best applied by iontophoresis through an electrical field with an active electrode in the external ear and a passive electrode at an arm, after instillation of a solution of lidocaine (1:100,000) into the external meatus.

This therapy temporarily relieves the disturbing tinnitus, so that the patients at least get some hours of rest and sleep. However, the untoward side effects of lidocaine also have to be taken into consideration.

Some forms of tinnitus also have an acoustic hallucinatory component, as in epilepsy. Therefore, carbamazepine (Tegretol),[1] which is an important antiepileptic agent used for bipolar affective disorders, is also used in tinnitus with a supratentorial focus. We have seen beneficial effects in very specific cases of endogenous tinnitus. Chemically, carbamazepine belongs to the tricyclic antidepressants. In adults, we give a daily dose of 200 mg. However, renal, hepatic, and hematologic parameters have to be monitored thoroughly.

Second-Line Agents

This group of drugs is especially used to treat the emotional effects seen in endogenous tinnitus, exogenous tinnitus, and combined endogenous and exogenous tinnitus, which can lead via sleeplessness to anxiety and panic. Here we see an indication for alprazolam (Xanax)[1] and similar substances. Alprazolam is administered to tinnitus patients in a daily dosage of 0.75 to 1.5 mg. Also chlordiazepoxide (Librium)[1] can alternatively be applied in a daily dosage of 15 to 30 mg. Even diazepam (Valium)[1] is used in a daily dosage of 4 to 30 mg.

The mood changes associated with tinnitus can lead to psychosis and insomnia. Here a tricyclic antidepressant such as amitriptyline (Elavil)[1] in a daily dosage of 75 to 150 mg can be helpful.

---

[1]Not FDA approved for this indication.

Additionally, this agent has a desired sedative component. Other sedatives and psychotropic drugs are also used to treat the psychologic effects associated with tinnitus, but they must be applied very carefully.

Third-Line Agents

Third-line therapeutic agents comprise the so-called nootropic drugs. These are pharmacologic agents that activate brain function through improved metabolism, leading to a better adaptation and interconnection. They were originally developed to treat senile dementia. Within this group, in Germany, we use piracetam (Nootrop, Normabraïn) in a daily dosage of 800 to 1200 mg.

We have seen very beneficial effects from extract of ginkgo biloba (EGB 761*) (Tebonin, Rökan), which is administered in a daily dosage of 120 mg.

We also use calcium channel antagonists, among which flunarizine (Sibelium),[2] in a daily dosage of 15 to 30 mg, is effective in tinnitus with irritative foci, especially in mesencephalic and diencephalic areas. Cinnarizin[2] was the predecessor. This holds especially for the endogenous tinnitus group.

Fourth-Line Agents

The fourth line of therapy involves neurotransmitter-directed pharmacotherapy. According to the chemical structures of the neurotransmitters, we mainly use one system of the amines (i.e., the histamine mechanism) and one system of amino acids (i.e., γ-aminobutyric acid [GABA]).

Because it is known that inner ear functions are regulated at the neurotransmission level of the histaminergic H_1, H_2, and H_3 receptors, betahistine (Serc)[2] plays an important role in inner ear receptor-targeted therapy. The daily dosage that we administer in peripheral cochlear tinnitus is 16 to 48 mg.

The inhibitory neurotransmitter GABA is extremely potent in its ability to alter neuronal discharges because of failures in the supratentorial CNS neurotransmission. According to recent findings, endogenous tinnitus with a supratentorial dysregulation can be influenced by gabapentin (Neurontin).[1] It is used in dosages starting with 300 mg daily and can be increased to 900 mg daily. Originally gabapentin was used as an additional therapy in partial epilepsia without secondary generalized seizures. Like with other antiepileptic drugs, the parameters from kidney, liver, and blood have to be supervised.

ADAPTED PSYCHOTHERAPY

Nowadays so-called tinnitus retraining therapy (TRT) is widely applied. It includes a therapeutic wide-band low-level noise generator. It is based on habituation, which is defined as a reduced response to a stimulus after repeated exposure. It is a state in which the tinnitus signal no longer elicits any response. Resetting or reprogramming neuronal networks involved in subcortical signal detection brings about habituation.

Also, in cases with a known interrelation of stress and tinnitus, a stress–diathesis model for tinnitus was proposed by Shulman et al. Stress management techniques require a counselor and the close cooperation of the patient, physician, biofeedback therapist, and psychologist.

A cognitive therapy that provides significant support to the patient with severe disabling tinnitus, particularly for control of the effect, is strongly recommended and encouraged.

ADAPTED PHYSIOTHERAPY

A specific program of physiotherapy successfully applied in endogenous tinnitus is KKIT. This therapy uses expressive movements of body language. In a special rehabilitation program, different groups of muscles in the hand, arm, leg, foot, and body, rising from the feet up to the face, are activated, which guides the tinnitus patient into a situation of peaceful resting, reduction of tension, and finally into relaxation. This scheme was adapted from a program of treating pain. KKIT points toward mechanisms of interference of expressive gestural movements with facilitating tinnitus from around the basal ganglia of the brain.

OTHER METHODS OF THERAPY

During the recent years, the external magnetotherapy in tinnitus cases of the type of endogenous tinnitus has been developed. Several authors have proved that pulsating electromagnetic fields applied over the temporal lobe of the brain can reduce the tinnitus complaints or even abolish the complaints during the application. The effect can also be longer lasting after the application. The basis of assessment for the magnetic intensities of the pulsating fields should extend from 2 to 100 mT. The frequency rate should lie between 3 and 12 Hz.

Worldwide, many innovations now take place in this field of a broadened scope of modern tinnitus therapy in special cases. Other methods of tinnitus therapy recommended in the literature include acupuncture, counseling, group therapy, and hypnotherapy.

ACKNOWLEDGMENT

Sponsored by grant Projekt D. 1417, durch die LVA Baden-Württemberg, Stuttgart, Germany.

REFERENCES

Alster J, Shemesh Z, Ornan M, Attias J. Sleep disturbance associated with chronic tinnitus. Biol Psychiatry 1993;34:84–90.

Arnesen AR, Engdahl B. Tinnitus—etiology, diagnosis and treatment. Tidsskr Nor Laegeforen 1996;116:2009–12.

Bergmann JM, Bertora GO. Cortical and brainstem topodiagnostic testing in tinnitus patients—a preliminary report. Int Tinnitus J 1996;2:151–8.

Bertora GO, Bergmann JM. Tinnitus: Supratentorial areas study through brain electric tomography (LORETA), ASN 2004;2:2. ISSN 1612–3352. Available at http://www.neurootology.org.

Claussen CF. Treatment of the slow brainstem syndrome with Vertigoheel. Biol Med 1985;3:447–70, 4:510–4.

Claussen CF. Medical classification of tinnitus between bruits: exogenous and endogenous tinnitus and other types of tinnitus. ASN 2004;2 (ISSN):1612–3352. Available at http://www.neurootology.org.

Claussen CF, Kolchev C, Schneider D, Hahn A. Neurootological brain electrical activity mapping in tinnitus patients. Proceedings of the 4th International Tinnitus Seminar. Bordeaux 1991;1092:351–5.

Claussen CF, Schneider D, Koltchev C. On the functional state of central vestibular structures in monaural symptomatic tinnitus patients. Int Tinnitus J 1995;1:5–12.

George RN, Kemp S. A survey of New Zealanders with tinnitus. Br J Audiol 1991;25:331–6.

Jastreboff PJ, Hazell JWP. A neurophysiological approach to tinnitus: clinical implications. Br J Audiol 1993;27:1–11.

Kersebaum M. Clinical therapy of tinnitus by means of exogenous magnetic stimulation. 19th IFOS-Congress. Sao Paulo, Brasil; 2009.

Kleinjung T, Eichhammer P, Langguth B, et al. Long-term effects of repetitive transcranial magnetic stimulation (rTMS) in patients with chronic tinnitus. Otolaryngol Head Neck Surg 2005;132:566–9.

Parving A, Hein HO, Suadicani P, et al. Epidemiology of hearing disorders. Some factors affecting hearing. The Copenhagen Male Study. Scand Audiol 1993;22:101–7.

Plewnia C, Bartels M, Gerloff C. Transient suppression of tinnitus by transcranial magnetic stimulation. Ann Neurol 2003;53:263–6.

Quaranta A, Assennato G, Sallustio V. Epidemiology of hearing problems among adults in Italy. Scand Audiol Suppl 1996;42:9–13.

Shulman A. A final common pathway for tinnitus—the medial temporal lobe system. Tinnitus J 1996;2:115–26.

Shulman A, Aran JM, Feldmann H, et al. Tinnitus diagnosis/treatment. Philadelphia: Lea & Febiger; 1991.

Shulman A, Strashun AM, Afriyie M, et al. SPECT imaging of brain and tinnitus—neurotologic/neurologic implications. Int Tinnitus J 1995;1:13–29.

---

*Available as dietary supplement.
[1]Not FDA approved for this indication.
[2]Not available in the United States.

Spine Pain

Method of
Michael T. McCann, MD

Back pain is one of the most common musculoskeletal complaints seen in primary care practices; empirical treatment is frequently based on conjecture. Our understanding of the pathophysiology of spine and radicular pain has increased dramatically over the last decade as a result of new technology and more advanced diagnostic testing. Early and accurate diagnosis is imperative if we are to provide specific lesion-based treatment to optimize patient outcomes and health care spending.

Although patients are satisfied with their care for most major illnesses, 20% to 25% of surveyed patients were dissatisfied with their care for back pain. Only headache treatment also received such poor scores. The top reason patients listed for dissatisfaction with their physician's care was inadequate explanation of why they hurt.

Although muscle strain is the most common reason given to patients as the cause of their back pain, it is actually highly unlikely to be the etiology for back pain severe enough for a patient to seek medical care or for pain that lasts more than 2 weeks. An underlying spinal disorder is usually present, leading to overlying myofascial tenderness and tightness. Isolated back pain is not a neurologic problem. Rather, it is an orthopedic problem, as will be evident from the following discussion.

Epidemiology

Eighty percent of the U.S. population develops back pain, limiting day-to-day activities, at some time in their lives. The peak incidence of such pain is between 35 and 65 years of age, declining thereafter. Based on radiographic degeneration alone, we would expect the incidence to increase linearly with age. In 80% of patients, episodes are self-limited, but in 15% to 20%, the pain chronically restricts function. Direct and indirect economical costs are estimated to be between $80 and $100 billion per year in the United States and, from an insurer's standpoint, costs may exceed expenditures on pediatric and obstetrical care combined. The majority of treatment expenditures are on the 20% of patients whose pain does not resolve spontaneously: recurrent or chronic back pain sufferers. To limit expenditures and optimize patient outcomes, it is vital that we prevent progression to a chronic state. Such prevention can best be achieved by early and accurate diagnosis and treatment.

Pathophysiology

Somatic (nociceptive) pain is caused by noxious stimulation of nerve endings in the vertebrae, joints, ligaments and disks, whereas radicular (neuropathic) pain is produced by evoked ectopic impulses in the dorsal root ganglia (Figure 1).

Somatic Pain

In primary somatic back pain, we try diagnostically to separate the pain generators into two anatomic categories based on their relation to the spinal canal. Treatment is significantly different based on the site of the lesions. Note that primary spinal nerve or cord pathology does not in and of itself produce axial back pain.

Pain generators in the anterior column are the disks and vertebral bodies. Only the outer third of a disk's annulus is innervated. Tears of these outer annular fibers produce exquisite pain and back spasm even without complete disruption of the disk. This is a frequent missed cause of nonspecific back pain because these internal disk

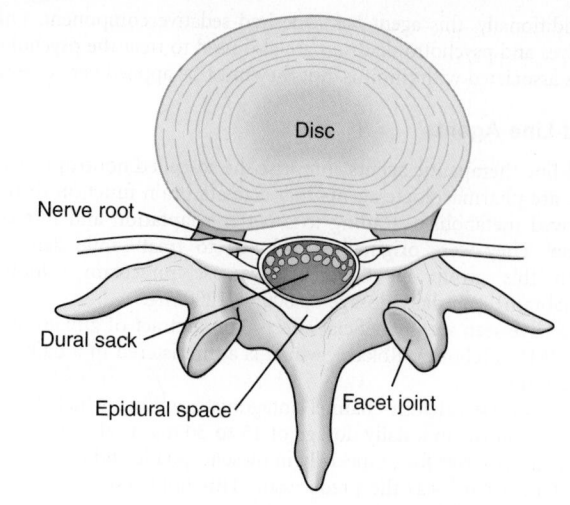

FIGURE 1. Spine cross section.

disruptions are rarely visualized on routine spine magnetic resonance imaging (MRI) or computer tomography (CT) scans. If noted on MRI, a high-intensity zone (HIZ) finding in a disk is highly suggestive of a painful internal annular tear. Definitive diagnosis is established with manometric provocative CT diskography. Diskitis, although rare, is also suggested by MRI findings, although aspiration may be necessary to establish an inflammatory or infectious etiology definitively.

Vertebral compression fractures, whether osteoporotic, traumatic, or pathologic, also contribute to anterior column primary axial pain. CT scanning or plain radiographs generally confirm the diagnosis; however, bone scanning may be necessary to confirm acuteness of a finding and to help rule out metastatic foci. Osteomyelitis should also be considered in any fracture with associated fever or a recent septic source.

The posterior column sources of back pain include the facet joints from the atlanto-occipital articulation caudad to the sacroiliac joints. All are true diarthrodial joints. The surfaces are capped with articular cartilage and lined with a synovial membrane. These paired innervated structures are subject to degeneration and painful traumatic injuries. In double-blind placebo controlled studies, the cervical facets appear to be the source of pain in 59% of patients with post-whiplash cervicalgia. Estimates regarding the lumbar spine place the incidence of facet-based low back pain between 15% and 40%, and the incidence increases significantly after 65 years of age.

Spondylolisthesis refers to a shift in the alignment between two vertebrae. With associated stress fractures of the pars interarticularis (spondylolysis), it is another posterior column source of pain. In chronic cases, instability leads to associated fibrosis under the pars fractures that produce radicular compression and neuropathic extremity pain. The slippage may also lead to central and foraminal stenosis with neurogenic claudication.

Neuropathic Pain

The most common cause of lumbar radicular pain in young patients is disk herniation (98%). Nerve compression alone, however, does not offer a satisfactory explanation for the pain produced. In human studies, root compression alone produces distal extremity paresthesias and numbness but no pain. Isolated lumbar radiculopathy does not cause significant back pain, and disk herniation size does not correlate with severity of pain on straight leg raise testing. Nucleus pulposus placed within the epidural space produces extreme inflammation with a 100,000-fold increase in phospholipase-A_2 immunoreactivity that can be directly correlated with mechanical hyperalgesia. In the complete absence of root compression, nucleus pulposus stimulates sustained discharges of Aδ and Aβ pain fibers in the dorsal root ganglia and causes a conduction delay in the roots. Intravenous methylprednisolone (Solu-Medrol)[1] prevents this conduction delay. Radicular pain appears to be caused by a combination of mechanical irritation in an otherwise chemically sensitized root.

Other sources of radicular pain include central spinal and lateral recess stenosis caused by facet arthropathies, ligamentous hypertrophy, and spondylolisthesis. Even more etiologies include neuromeningeal anomalies, neoplasms, infections, and vascular malformations. Peripheral neuropathies, including thoracic outlet, cubital and carpal tunnel syndromes, piriformis syndrome, tarsal tunnel, and other primary mononeuropathies, may also mimic or exist in conjunction with radiculopathies.

Assessment

The goal of the initial assessment is to screen for emergent causes of back or radicular pain including aneurysms, infections, segmental instability, fractures, tumors, and myelopathy. A careful history and examination should help delineate referred cardiac, pulmonary, gastrointestinal, urologic, gynecologic, and vascular sources.

History

For all patients presenting with back or radicular pain, the screening history should include weight loss, recent fevers or infections, and significant change in bowel or bladder function, including incontinence. For patients with cervicothoracic or upper extremity radicular pain, a cardiac history should be added. Abdominal symptoms, hematuria, dysuria, or vaginal discharge should be included for lumbar pain.

---

[1]Not FDA approved for this indication.

 CURRENT DIAGNOSIS

Emergent or Urgent Conditions Associated with Back Pain (Red Flags)

Associated symptoms	Condition
New onset bowel or bladder incontinence	Myelopathy
Balance difficulties	Myelopathy
Diffuse distal weakness or immobility	Myelopathy
Recent weight loss	Tumor
Severe chest or abdominal pain	Aortic aneurysm

History	Condition
Osteoporosis	Fracture
Recent trauma	Fracture
Intravenous drug use	Infection
Recent infection	Infection
Immunosuppressed state	Infection

Age	Condition
<15 y or >60 y	Tumor suspicion
Male >55 y (M:F 4:1)	Aortic aneurysm

Associated signs	Condition
Tender abdomen	Aortic aneurysm
Saddle sensory loss	Cauda equina syndrome
Hyperreflexia with positive clonus, Babinski's sign, and Hoffmann's sign	Myelopathy

Radicular pain is lancinating with superficial and deep components that extend in distinct, but not necessarily dermatomal, distributions. Pain may extend partially or entirely in the distribution of the affected spinal nerve. Somatic referred pain is deep, aching, and diffuse. It can overlap with radicular symptoms in the proximal extremities. Proximal extremity pain can be radicular, whereas distal extremity pain is not necessarily always radicular.

Diffuse distal symptoms with dysesthesia, complaints of bowel or bladder urgency or incontinence, and a history of balance difficulties are red flags for myelopathy. Most patients also give a history of cervicothoracic or associated radicular pain. If accompanied by severe low back pain and complaints of saddle numbness, consider cauda equina syndrome, a surgical emergency.

Claudication symptoms are suggestive of spinal stenosis and usually there is little pain at rest. Differentiation from vascular claudication is sometimes difficult, but pain with neurogenic claudication is usually not worsened with supine positioning and leg elevation.

Examination

Although clinical exam may establish the presence of a radiculopathy or localize the segmental pain level, etiology must be established by other means. Tumors, cysts, stenosis spondylolisthesis, and disk herniations may all cause very similar clinical signs.

Muscle pain and spasm should not be considered the primary source of the patient's back pain unless all other potential sources are ruled out or an objective rheumatologic etiology is identified pointing to a myositis. An antalgic gait from distal degenerative joint disease may cause lumbar muscular aching, but rarely is the back the site of greatest pain. This is not to say that muscles cannot be painful, but rather that in the majority of primary back pain cases, the muscles are simply reacting to an underlying derangement in the spine itself.

More specifically, examination should note hyperreflexia and clonus and test for Babinski's and Hoffmann's signs to note upper motor neuron irritability. Screening cardiovascular and abdominal examination helps rule out other sources of back pain.

Natural Course of the Disease

For lumbar radicular pain in patients treated conservatively, 50% of patients can expect to have resolution of radicular symptoms after 4 weeks. At 12 months, in 49% of males and 33% of females, radicular pain remains improved. Unfortunately, 60% to 70% of these patients developed back pain by 4 weeks that persisted at 12 months regardless of the radicular pain improvement.

For patients treated surgically versus conservatively, at 10 years there appears to be little statistically significant difference in outcome for radicular pain, with both groups achieving approximately 60% good results and poor results in 7% to 8%. This only holds true if surgery is not applied randomly, but as a last resort for patients who fail to respond to conservative care.

For cervical radiculopathic symptoms, 70% can be expected to improve with time and 20% become asymptomatic. In patients for whom surgery was an option, 90% are improved or only mildly incapacitated at long-term follow-up. Isolated recurrences are seen in 32% of cases, whereas 10% have moderate to severe persistent disability.

Although studies exist detailing favorable outcomes overall for radicular symptoms, the same does not necessarily hold true for mechanical back pain. Although 80% of patients appear to have resolution of initial symptoms independent of their course of care, 20% develop progressive or unrelenting pain. It appears that approximately 35% of persons have intermittent recurrences that limit their activities.

Management

Take an algorithmic approach to the patient presenting with back and/or radicular symptoms of new onset. If initial history and examination suggest an emergent cause for these symptoms, appropriate additional diagnostic testing and referral should be made. Indications for urgent surgical interventions are few but include progressive motor deficit and cauda equina syndrome—progressive neurologic deterioration with loss of bowel and bladder function.

Once an emergent source of pain is ruled out, studies show that primary care physicians who prescribe the least amount of analgesics and place the fewest restrictions on activities have the best patient outcomes. In many cases, a more aggressive approach may reinforce illness behavior and foster a fear of future debilitation.

Radicular Pain Predominating

If radicular pain predominates in a minimally distressed patient, simple reassurance and an explanation of the natural course of recovery may suffice. Avoiding bed rest and activity modification to prevent axial loading should be discussed (no lifting in a forward flexed position and no repetitive flexion activities). A 2-week reassessment allows any insidious red flag conditions to be picked up, provides reassurance, and allows adjustment of treatment.

 CURRENT THERAPY

Acute Presentation without Red Flags: Treatment Ladders (Frequent Reassessment as Indicated)

BACK OR NECK PAIN PREDOMINATING

- Education, activity modification, and reassurance
- Limited course of analgesics dependent on stress
  - NSAIDs
  - Opioids
  - Muscle relaxants
  - Consider steroid taper regimen
- Physical therapy with spinal stabilization regimen
- Screening radiographs with flexion and extension views (rule out gross instability)
- Referral for spinal diagnostic assessment or orthopedic spine evaluation
- Fusion or disk replacement as indicated

RADICULAR PAIN PREDOMINATING

- Education, activity modification, and reassurance
- Early treatment of inflammation with steroid taper regimen
- Limited course of analgesics and muscle relaxants
- Early initiation of neuropathic pain medications
  - Gabapentin (Neurontin)[1]
  - Duloxetine (Cymbalta)[1]
  - Pregabalin (Lyrica)[1]
- Physical therapy guided by McKenzie assessment
- MRI (with gadolinium contrast for cancer, spinal cord pathology, and postoperative spine cases)
- Selective transforaminal steroid injection
- Surgical assessment for decompression

Abbreviations: NSAIDs = nonsteroidal anti-inflammatory drugs.
[1]Not FDA approved for this indication.

For more significantly distressed patients with acute radicular pain, additional analgesics and more frequent follow-up may be required. Although no analgesic regimen alters the natural course of recovery, based on the inflammatory pathogenesis of radicular pain a pulse dose of prednisone or methylprednisolone with a taper can be considered over a week. However, in randomized controlled trials, the nonsteroidal anti-inflammatory drugs (NSAIDs) piroxicam (Feldene) and indomethacin (Indocin) did not offer any greater analgesia or enhance recovery more than placebo. A limited course of muscle relaxants and opioid analgesics may be prescribed but often provide little relief in cases of true neuropathic pain. The limited duration of these prescriptions should be explained to the patient at the outset. Despite ongoing pain, the goal is to avoid dependency and reliance on these medications for activities that may be detrimental to the natural course of the disorder.

Currently, greater success may be found with early initiation and titration of gabapentin (Neurontin)[1] for radicular pain. With low toxicity and few side effects, tolerance is usually good. Initiate dosing at night with 100 to 300 mg (lower dosing in patients <65 years old), escalating every 1 to 3 days as tolerated up to 1200 mg three times daily. If improvement is not obtained by 600 mg three times daily, further escalation is unlikely to be efficacious.

For distressed patients, duloxetine (Cymbalta)[1] may be efficacious while providing additional anxiolysis and antidepressant effects. Because nausea is a frequent side effect for the first few days upon initiation of dosing, we start with 30 mg every morning and advance to 60 mg every morning after 1 week. If sedation occurs, change to every-evening dosing. Symptomatic improvement is often seen by 7 to 10 days.

If at follow-up significant progress is not made and reassessment still lacks red flags, physical therapy with instructions for a McKenzie assessment and therapy over 2 weeks is indicated, with a home program to follow. Again, no scientific studies validate any particular regimen of therapy. However, from a spinal education standpoint, and as an impetus to maintaining function, an empirical recommendation can be made. Follow-up should be scheduled and if progress is partial, another 2 weeks of therapy could be considered.

Failure to improve or deterioration of function at any point would be an indication for additional imaging studies. An MRI provides the most comprehensive survey of causes for radicular symptoms. It does not, however, guarantee that anatomic changes are definitively the source for a patient's symptoms. In asymptomatic patients younger than 40 years, 30% had abnormal spine MRIs, whereas 60% to 70% of patients older than 40 years had abnormal MRIs. The prevalence of asymptomatic disk herniations alone ranged between 20% and 40% in patients between 40 and 60 years of age.

Evidence-based review of the literature currently does not support the use of electromyogram and nerve conduction velocity (EMG/NCV) studies) for diagnosis in cases of radiculopathic pain. Pain is mediated through Aδ and C fibers, and an EMG tests activity in Aα motor fibers. H and F reflexes similarly lack specificity in clinical trials with radiculopathy, despite proposed theoretical foundations. EMG/NCV testing would be indicated in cases where peripheral neuropathy or nerve entrapment is suspected and when objective muscle strength testing is suspect or primary myopathy may be present.

Recent prospective randomized blinded studies support selective nerve root injection (i.e., fluoroscopically guided transforaminal epidural steroid or epiradicular injections) as the next line of treatment. This highly selective procedure may reduce the need for surgical intervention in up to 59% of radicular cases and should be considered in cases where lack of improvement is noted as soon as 2 weeks. Serial MRI studies in humans show statistically significant improvement in the rate of disk reabsorption and symptoms in patients treated with transforaminal injections as compared to controls. The older regimen of translaminar epidural steroid injections is not nearly as efficacious and in some studies appears no more effective than placebo. Partial improvement at 10- to 14-day follow-up would be an indication for repeat injection. An automatic series of three

---

[1]Not FDA approved for this indication.

injections is no longer considered standard of care, and response to a single transforaminal injection should guide additional treatment. Lack of improvement or further functional decline would lead to surgical assessment.

Long-term management of a patient with radicular pain either unrelieved with surgery or in the patient for whom surgical options do not exist falls into the realm of neuropathic pain control. Narcotic regimens should be avoided because long-term efficacy has never been demonstrated. Medication options are limited, but gabapentin (Neurontin)[1] and duloxetine (Cymbalta)[1] are efficacious in reducing pain for a large number of patients with both radicular and other sources of neuropathic pain. The newest drug with indications for neuropathic pain is pregabalin (Lyrica)[1]. Efficacy for radicular pain is as yet undetermined but is expected to approximate gabapentin with fewer dose-related side effects. Other drugs to be considered include mexiletine (Mexitil),[1] tricyclic antidepressants,[1] and some of the newer anticonvulsants including levetiracetam (Keppra),[1] oxcarbazepine (Trileptal),[1] zonisamide (Zonegran),[1] and tiagabine (Gabitril).[1] All modify neuropathic pain in the presence and absence of associated depression.

For patients in whom neuropathic extremity pain far exceeds any mechanical back pain, despite optimization of all conservative treatment and surgical options, spinal cord stimulation may be considered. This modality is efficacious in between 60% and 70% of patients with neuropathic extremity pain predominating. It is not indicated for mechanical back pain. For permanently implanted patients, 70% continue to have approximately 50% improvement in neuropathic pain at 5-year follow-up.

Axial Pain Predominating

For patients with nonurgent acute back or neck pain, again the level of distress helps guide care. Studies regarding early treatment and analgesic regimens for nociceptive back pain lack validity and specificity because early diagnosis is not usually sought because of the high incidence of spontaneous improvement. Early treatment thus remains empirical.

In a minimally distressed patient, supportive education and activity modification support the natural course of recovery. For an initial episode, physical therapy with spinal stabilization exercises, followed by a home program, is recommended to provide back education and to help reduce recurrences.

For the more distressed patient, oral analgesics may be indicated. Because the source of axial pain is nociceptive, NSAIDs should be considered as a first-line analgesic, with opioids reserved for very severe pain and again only for a limited duration. Failure to improve is not an indication for continued daily use of opioids. For moderate to severe pain where a significant inflammatory component is suspected, a bolus/taper dose of steroids over 1 week is often efficacious, and risks are low with this regimen. Muscle spasms are best managed with gradual stretching and paced activities. In severe cases, however, muscle relaxants may be beneficial, and even a limited course of benzodiazepines can be considered.

If at 2-week reassessment progress is not seen, physical therapy over 1 month (usually 3 to 4 times per week) for range of motion and stabilization exercise should be considered. Partial improvement would be an indication for another month of therapy or, in the motivated patient, another month of a home exercise program.

The goal of therapy is to maintain range of motion, strengthen supportive musculature, and maintain activities of daily living without additional injury. To this end, almost all exercise regimens claim efficacy, although no valid studies as yet show that any specific therapy actually alters the natural history.

Should a patient with primary back or neck pain fail to improve with therapy, screening radiographs may be indicated. Plain radiographs for mechanical back pain should always be obtained with flexion and extension views to rule out gross instability as well as other mechanical derangements, including spondylolisthesis, spondylolysis, and compression fractures.

Unfortunately, although all radiographic studies of the spine demonstrate anatomic abnormalities, they cannot show whether these abnormalities are painful. With physical examination also notoriously unreliable for making a definitive diagnosis, referral for more advanced spinal diagnostic assessment may often be indicated in patients who fail to improve or who have frequent recurrences.

For the 20% of patients whose function remains limited by back pain despite maximized conservative care, identification of the exact pain source is imperative to improving outcomes. These patients are prone to seek numerous opinions, undergo fruitless operations, and pay for unproven modality-based treatments. Physicians tend toward making diagnoses based on response to treatment as opposed to the other way around. An early definitive diagnosis allows realistic treatment options and prognosis to be given. Patients can thus adjust their lifestyle to function within the limits imposed by their spinal condition.

Significant advances are being made in the field of diagnosing back pain. Select spinal injection techniques are refined to isolate the exact source of a patient's pain in the majority of cases. Validity testing can also determine if a patient's complaint has an anatomic basis or if symptom magnification is present.

CT-provocative diskography is the only test available to document internal disk anatomy precisely and to determine if a disk is the source of a patient's back pain. Studies show that compared with surgical findings, its anatomic accuracy exceeds MRI and CT myelography. With the use of manometry, intradiskal symptomatic pressures help determine the proper surgical technique to optimize patient outcomes. Diagnostic facet injections can also identify a symptomatic joint precisely, further helping determine options for treatment.

New nonsurgical or minimally invasive treatments are now validated, including radiofrequency thermocoagulation (RFTC) lesioning for desensitization of painful facet joint arthropathies, intradiskal electrothermal therapy (IDET) for treatment of painful disk lesions, and percutaneous disk decompression by both mechanical and laser techniques. For vertebral compression fracture, vertebroplasty and kyphoplasty may offer remarkable and rapid relief of associated fracture pain but do carry a risk of severe neurologic injury and embolism. Treatment outcomes for all of these procedures rely heavily on obtaining an exact diagnosis using the preceding tests.

Surgical assessment for nonemergent back pain should be reserved for those patients who fail conservative management and are not candidates for minimally invasive treatment or who have identifiable gross segmental spinal instability. Unlike radicular pain, decompression alone does not improve primary back pain. For mechanical back pain from segmental instability, the only surgical option is fusion. Poor pain relief is seen most frequently in patients who undergo fusion procedures for back pain based on radiographic findings alone. Provocative testing to isolate the actual pain generators and to determine the integrity of surrounding support structures maximizes the chances for success. For patients with isolated diskogenic pain, validated with manometric CT diskography, newer disk replacement techniques hold promise. Fusions cause a load shift to adjacent spinal motion segments causing degeneration. This leads to a 30% reoperation rate for fusion patients within 10 years. The hope is that disk replacements will prevent this transitional zone degeneration and lower the reoperation rate.

Not all patients are candidates for surgical reconstruction. In many cases, surgical intervention may only serve to worsen a patient's state. Tolerance of symptoms with acceptance of functional limitations is the preferred course.

To conclude, patients presenting with pain of spinal origin should be divided into those with predominantly radicular symptoms and those with primarily mechanical back or neck pain. In the vast majority of cases, back and neck pain originates from derangements of the facets, disks, or vertebrae, not the muscles. Radicular pain is most likely secondary to a compressive lesion with associated underlying inflammation.

Proper diagnosis is paramount to optimizing patient treatment (both conservative and surgical) and to prevention of progress to a chronic

---

[1]Not FDA approved for this indication.

TABLE 1 Clinical Pearls

Muscle strain is a very unusual cause of back pain severe enough to seek medical attention.
For back pain, think facets, disks, and vertebrae.
Referred back and neck pain can extend into the extremities and mimic radicular patterns.
Radicular pain does not always extend into the distal extremities (L5 radiculopathy can mimic hip trochanteric bursitis).
Magnetic resonance imaging (MRI) cannot tell you what hurts, only what might be causing pain.
MRI does not rule out all spinal pathology that can cause pain.
Order MRI with gadolinium contrast only if:
   You suspect cancer.
   You suspect a primary spinal cord lesion.
   Spine surgery was performed in the suspect region.
Laminectomy alone should not be used to treat predominant back pain (only radicular pain).
Fusions and disk replacements are for predominant back pain.
Only spinal diagnostic testing (selective computer tomography [CT] diskography, facet blocks, and transforaminal injections) can isolate the
   source of pain in refractory cases.
Electromyogram and nerve conduction velocity (EMG/NCV) studies should be used only if you:
   Suspect an underlying peripheral neuropathic process (double crush).
   Suspect lack of effort on motor testing.
   Suspect a primary myopathy.
Early referral for accurate diagnostic testing is the key to optimizing care: the more accurate the diagnosis, the more accurate the care.

dysfunctional state. MRIs have limitations in what they are able to visualize and do not guarantee that anatomic derangements are actually the source of the patient's pain. For an accurate diagnosis in a patient who fails to respond to initial conservative care, more specialized interventional spinal diagnostic testing is indicated (Table 1).

Identification and isolation of specific spinal pain generators has allowed for the development of specific lesion-based minimally invasive treatments. These include transforaminal injections for radiculopathy, RFTC desensitization for facet-based pain, and percutaneous decompression for disk displacement pain. Decompressive surgery is very effective at relieving severe radicular pain unresponsive to conservative care and injections, but it is complicated by postlaminectomy spinal instability. Spinal fusion surgery for well-diagnosed painful segmental instability remains the definitive treatment for this disorder; newer disk replacement surgery may offer an alternative to fusion for primary diskogenic back or neck pain.

The Infectious Diseases

The Patient with HIV Disease

Method of
Ryan Westergaard, MD, and
Amita Gupta, MD, MHS

Since its first description in the early 1980s, the acquired immunodeficiency syndrome (AIDS) has become one of the most devastating epidemics in human history. Millions of new infections occur every year, predominantly in resource-poor settings where access to diagnosis and treatment of human immunodeficiency virus (HIV) infection remains inadequate. The natural history of HIV infection remains one of progressive immune system dysfunction with inevitable acute and chronic infectious complications. With few exceptions, the inexorable decline in T-lymphocyte function eventually leads to the death of untreated patients. Remarkable advances in therapeutics, leading to the development of highly-active antiretroviral therapy (HAART), have transformed HIV infection from an almost universally fatal illness to a chronic disease that can be managed over decades with an enlarging repertoire of treatment options. This chapter provides an overview of the current understanding of HIV pathogenesis and epidemiology and reviews guidelines for the initial evaluation and long-term management of HIV infection in adult patients.

Epidemiology

Global statistics continue to paint a discouraging picture of the continued spread of the HIV pandemic. According to the Joint United Nations Programme on HIV/AIDS, an estimated 33 million people were living with HIV at the end of 2007; roughly half of them were women, and more than 2 million were children. Of the estimated 7400 new infections that occur daily, 96% occur in low- and middle-income countries, and approximately 1000 of those infected are children younger than 15 years of age. The prevalence of HIV infection in populations varies widely across the world, with the highest documented rates occurring in southern Africa, where prevalence rates derived from surveillance of asymptomatic pregnant women have exceeded 30% in some settings. AIDS is now the leading cause of death worldwide for persons aged 15 to 59 years, and this trend is associated with particularly dire social and economic consequences in sub-Saharan Africa, where more than half of global AIDS deaths occur. In some sub-Saharan countries such as Swaziland, Botswana, and Lesotho, life expectancy has been reduced by more than 20 years. However, with a rapid and significant increase in funding and commitment from the U.S. government (President's Emergency Plan for AIDS Relief [PEPFAR]) and many multilateral agencies such as the Global Fund, a dramatic increase in prevention, care, and treatment services is now underway. A stabilization and initial trend illustrating a global decrease in AIDS deaths is being observed.

North America has experienced a striking decline in AIDS deaths since the advent of HAART, although a sizeable reduction in the annual number of new HIV infections has not yet been achieved. In the United States, an estimated 1.1 million people are living with HIV. The Centers for Disease Control and Prevention (CDC) estimates that 21% of these individuals are unaware of their HIV status. The CDC estimates that approximately 56,300 people were newly infected with HIV in 2006 (the most recent year for which data are available); a new infection occurs every 9.5 minutes in the United States. Ethnic minorities, particularly African Americans, are disproportionately represented among those with new infections. As is the case worldwide, sexual contact accounts for the majority of HIV transmission for both men and women. In the United States, male-to-male sexual contact represents the mode of acquisition for the majority (61%) of new cases among men, whereas most women are infected via heterosexual contact. Injection drug use accounts for roughly 20% of new HIV infections in both men and women.

The estimated risk of HIV transmission per exposure has been estimated from studies of discordant couples and cohort studies. The average risk of HIV transmission per coital act in serodiscordant heterosexual couples is approximately 0.1%. The presence of other sexually transmitted infections and higher viral load (VL) increase the risk of transmission; condom use and male circumcision considerably reduce the risk. Female-to-male transmission is less effective than male-to-female transmission. Receptive anal intercourse is associated with a higher risk of transmission compared with vaginal intercourse. Even though the risk of transmission by oral sex is very low, it should not be considered completely safe.

Mother-to-child transmission can occur in utero, in the peripartum period, and during breast-feeding. The probability of transmission is most influenced by maternal plasma VL. Other risk factors include maternal $CD4^+$ T-cell count (discussed later), hepatitis C infection, premature rupture of membranes, preterm birth, and duration of breast-feeding. In United States, mother-to-child transmission has been markedly reduced (from 20%-25% to <1%) through routine HIV testing and effective interventions. These interventions include HAART, elective cesarean delivery if the VL is greater than 1000 copies per milliliter at week 38, and recommendation to avoid breast-feeding. The risk of HIV transmission with breast-feeding is 10% to 16% in the absence of intervention and is thought to be highest during the first 2 to 4 months. Factors that increase transmission include inflammatory or ulcerative conditions of the breast, mastitis, and breast abscess. Infants with thrush are more likely to acquire HIV from an infected mother via breast-feeding. In many low-income countries where breast-feeding is critical for infant nutrition and survival, the issue is complex and is the subject of ongoing investigation.

Pathophysiology

HIV is an enveloped, single-stranded RNA virus belonging to the family Retroviridae. It was recognized as the causative agent of AIDS within 3 years after the initial description of the syndrome in 1981, and ongoing characterization of its molecular biology has provided the identification of multiple targets for drug development. Two human immunodeficiency viruses exist: HIV-1 and HIV-2. HIV-1 has worldwide distribution, accounts for most infections outside western Africa, and is the focus of this chapter.

HIV-2 infection causes a similar clinical syndrome but is less efficiently transmitted and results in lower levels of viremia and slower progression to AIDS. A key difference in terms of management between HIV-1 and HIV-2 is that HIV-2 is naturally resistant to non-nucleoside reverse transcriptase inhibitors (see later discussion). For this reason, it is important to assess for HIV-2 by Western blot in persons who are from regions of the world where HIV-2 is present or coexists with HIV-1.

Genetic heterogeneity of HIV-1 is reflected in categorization of the virus into three groups (M, O, and N) and several clades (e.g., B, C, D, AE, CRF01_AE), some of which have overlapping geographic distribution around the world. Subtype C is prevalent in southern and eastern Africa, China, India, South Asia, and Brazil and accounts for 50% of HIV subtypes, whereas subtype B, the most common subtype in the United States, accounts for 12%.

The HIV viral genome is encoded in single-stranded RNA, packaged in core protein structures, and surrounded by a lipid bilayer envelope that is derived from the cell membrane of the host cell as the virus buds from the cell surface after replication. This outer viral membrane contains HIV-specific glycoproteins, including gp120 and gp41, which facilitate attachment and entry into host cells through interaction with the cell surface receptor, CD4, and coreceptors CCR5 and CXCR4. $CD4^+$ helper T lymphocytes are the predominant host cell affected by HIV; this molecular tropism explains the immune system destruction manifested in chronic HIV infection and provides the rationale for clinical staging of HIV infection using $CD4^+$ T-cell counts. The interaction of HIV with the coreceptor CCR5 has been an area of research interest leading to the recent development of coreceptor antagonist drugs.

After host cell entry, the key enzyme responsible for viral replication is reverse transcriptase, an RNA-dependent DNA polymerase that is packaged within the virion core. This enzyme facilitates conversion of the HIV genome into a double-stranded DNA intermediate molecule. The second key enzymatic step is integration of this intermediate nucleic acid product into the host genome, which is facilitated by the viral protein integrase. Protein synthesis with packaging of new viral particles ensues, utilizing an HIV-specific protease. The integrase inhibitor class of drugs acts by blocking this step of integration.

Natural History

The natural history of HIV infection reflects the progressive depletion of circulating $CD4^+$ cells, in addition to diverse effects on other immune cells and tissues that are incompletely understood. Within 1 to 4 weeks after the initial HIV infection, seroconversion may be accompanied by a nonspecific, self-limited illness, often referred to as the acute retroviral syndrome. This illness has variable manifestations but may include fever, malaise, myalgias, arthralgias, generalized lymphadenopathy, pharyngitis, and rash. The associated rash has been described as maculopapular, urticarial, or roseola-like. An illness resembling acute infectious mononucleosis syndrome, similar to that caused by Epstein-Barr virus or cytomegalovirus (CMV), and aseptic meningitis have been described. Very rarely has an acute opportunistic infection (OI) been reported in the setting of acute seroconversion. The proportion of patients experiencing such an illness is not precisely known, because many do not present to medical facilities, and for those who do, HIV infection is commonly not considered. Diagnosis of acute HIV infection requires a high index of suspicion, which does not commonly occur unless the patient reports a recent history of a high-risk exposure.

During the acute phase of infection, high levels of viremia are present (often exceeding 10 million copies per milliliter) as HIV becomes widely disseminated throughout the body and the host defenses are just beginning to counteract circulating virus through cell-mediated and humoral (antibody-mediated) immune mechanisms. Antibodies against HIV usually become detectable between 2 and 4 months after infection. The initial, high-level viremia becomes attenuated as neutralizing antibodies are established and equilibrium is reached whereby ongoing replication is partially controlled by the immune response, resulting in a steady-state level of viremia. This so-called virologic set point differs from patient to patient and is one of the determinants of the rate of disease progression. A small number of HIV-infected persons are able to control viral replication to levels below the limit of detection, and they tend to have a more benign course of disease. In these patients, designated elite suppressors by researchers, HIV replication continues to occur, and HIV RNA can be isolated from latently infected cells by means of specialized laboratory techniques.

After the establishment of HIV infection and seroconversion, a period of asymptomatic infection ensues, during which patients are free of evidence of immune suppression and OIs are uncommon. This phase of clinical latency lasts a median of 8 to 10 years, based on observational studies in the West from the pre-HAART era. Ongoing viral replication leads to gradual decline in the CD4 count.

The symptomatic stage of HIV infection can begin at any time after infection, but clinical manifestations become more likely as the CD4 count falls farther below the normal range of 800 to 1200 cells/mm^3. Both the absolute CD4 count and the percentage of $CD4^+$ T cells correlate with the risk of developing OIs and should be monitored longitudinally to assess patients' candidacy for prophylactic interventions and initiation of HAART. For example, *Pneumocystis jirovecii* (formerly *Pneumocystis carinii*) pneumonia (PCP) usually occurs in patients with a CD4 count of less than 200 cells/mm^3 or a percentage of less than 10%. CMV retinitis occurs almost exclusively in patients with a CD4 count of less than 50 cells/mm^3 or a percentage of less than 5%. Mucocutaneous candidiasis (oral thrush), herpes zoster, HIV-associated nephropathy, peripheral neuropathy, tuberculosis, and community-acquired bacterial pneumonia occur with increased frequency at earlier stages of infection and are less reliably predicted by $CD4^+$ cell measurement.

Diagnosis

Diagnosis of HIV infection during the acute retroviral syndrome requires detection of circulating HIV RNA because of the absence of HIV-specific antibodies at this stage. Other laboratory findings that can raise the suspicion for acute HIV infection include a decreased total lymphocyte count; the T-cell count characteristically decreases during the first several weeks after infection and later often returns to preinfection levels, after the initial spike in viremia is brought under control by immune defenses. The erythrocyte sedimentation rate and hepatic transaminases may also be elevated. Cerebrospinal fluid pleocytosis has been documented in patients undergoing lumbar puncture in the setting of acute HIV infection.

HIV RNA can be detected by reverse transcriptase polymerase chain reaction (RT-PCR) or branched-chain DNA testing. In the acute retroviral syndrome, the VL is usually very high, and ultrasensitive RT-PCR is not generally needed. Although commercially available PCR and branched DNA tests are licensed for disease monitoring and not for diagnosis of HIV infection, their specificity is sufficiently high that finding high levels of HIV RNA in a patient with suspected acute HIV infection provides convincing evidence for infection. In all such cases, close follow-up with repeat HIV antibody testing to confirm seroconversion within 2 to 4 months is essential.

Diagnosis of HIV at all other stages of disease relies on commercially available assays for detecting HIV-specific antibodies. A standard protocol involves screening with the highly sensitive enzyme immunoassay (EIA) that detects antigens of both HIV-1 and HIV-2. Negative EIA is sufficient to rule out HIV infection, except in cases where acute HIV infection is suspected, as just described.

Positive EIA tests require further confirmation with the more specific Western blot test. The CDC has established criteria for Western blot positivity, which include the presence of at least two of the HIV-specific bands p24, gp41, and gp160/120. The Western blot is considered negative if no bands are present and indeterminate if an HIV band is present but the criteria for positivity are not met. Indeterminate Western blot results usually include a single p24 band and can occur during early infection, while seroconversion is in progress, or in advanced AIDS when antibody production is impaired. Causes of indeterminate Western blot results that are unrelated to HIV include pregnancy, autoimmune disease, and cross-reacting antibodies resulting from blood transfusion or organ transplantation.

Other HIV antibody kits have been developed for ease of administration or achievement of rapid results, and they have utility in settings such as community-based screening programs, emergency departments, and even patient-initiated home testing. OraSure, an office-based test that employs a special swab for collecting oral fluid specimens rather than blood, was licensed in 1996. Specimens are collected at the point of care and sent to a central laboratory, where antibodies are detected; the sensitivity and specificity are similar to those of traditional blood-based methods. OraQuick Advance, a rapid HIV test that can utilize whole blood, plasma, or oral fluid, was approved in 2004 and can provide results comparable in accuracy to EIA within about 20 minutes. An advantage of this technique is the ability to provide reliable negative results at the point of care. Positive results still need to be confirmed with standard EIA and Western blot serologic testing.

Screening

The traditional paradigm for screening of asymptomatic patients for HIV has included targeting patients with behavioral risk factors for HIV transmission and patients seeking care for sexually transmitted diseases. Documentation of separate, written consent and administration of formal pretest and posttest counseling has been recommended and is still required by statute in many U.S. states.

In response to the consistent observations that many people are not diagnosed with HIV until late in the course of disease and that transmission rates for infected persons who are unaware of their serostatus are several times higher than for persons who are aware that they are infected, the CDC issued new guidelines for routine HIV testing in September 2006 to make HIV testing a routine part of medical care. Voluntary (opt-out) screening is now recommended in health care settings for all persons aged 13 to 64 years, regardless of risk. Screening should be repeated annually for persons with behavioral risk factors for HIV and should be repeated each time a person seeks treatment for symptoms related to sexually transmitted disease. The CDC advocates that requirements for separate, written consent for HIV testing are no longer needed; instead, general consent to receive medical care can be considered sufficient.

CURRENT DIAGNOSIS

- Revised national guidelines recommend universal screening for HIV infection for patients aged 13 to 64 years in all settings after notification that testing will be done, unless the patient specifically declines (opt-out testing). Patients with behavioral risk factors, sexually transmitted diseases, or tuberculosis should be screened annually.
- Acute HIV infection is recognized as a variable syndrome including fever, pharyngitis, rash, and arthralgias.
- As antiretroviral therapy has prolonged survival for patients living with HIV, non–HIV-related outcomes such as cardiovascular and renal disease have gained importance as preventable causes of morbidity and mortality.

Approach to the Patient with HIV Infection

HIV care is a continuously evolving field, and new drugs and classes of drugs have been introduced in recent years. Professional guidelines for antiretroviral therapy (ART) are updated frequently as data from clinical trials are published and accumulating clinical evidence influences beliefs about best practices in HIV care. For these reasons, the receipt of appropriate care by HIV$^+$ patients is determined in large part by the experience of the care provider. The volume of HIV$^+$ patients seen in one's practice is known to correlate with measures of quality care. A U.S. Department of Health and Human Services panel recommends that HIV patients receive care from a health care provider who routinely cares for at least 20 and preferably 50 HIV-infected patients. Referral to a specialist is warranted in cases of treatment failure due to drug resistance or for management of complications of HIV or antiretroviral drugs. Because of the multifaceted nature of the longitudinal care of HIV-infected patients, an interdisciplinary approach, integrated and coordinated by an experienced primary care provider, is optimal.

The initial history and physical examination of HIV-infected patients should be systematic and comprehensive, owing to the multiorgan system nature of diagnoses associated with HIV infection. A thorough review of current and recent symptoms should assess for presence of OIs and malignant or premalignant conditions. Symptoms such as unexplained weight loss, fever, chronic diarrhea, recurrent oral or genital ulcers, dysphagia, dyspnea, or gastrointestinal bleeding should prompt further investigation for the presence of undiagnosed manifestations of HIV-related complications. Because patients with HIV infection have a higher incidence of cognitive impairment, mental illness, and substance abuse than the general population, symptoms of neurocognitive impairment (e.g., impaired memory), depression, suicidality, and unhealthy alcohol and drug use should also be carefully assessed.

The past medical and surgical history should focus on conditions that may follow a more malignant course in the setting of HIV infection, such as chronic viral hepatitis, and conditions that can be exacerbated by HIV or by ART, such as cardiovascular or renal disease and metabolic abnormalities such as dyslipidemia or impaired glucose tolerance. The circumstances surrounding the patient's HIV acquisition should be formally assessed. The provider should understand previous and current patterns of risk behaviors for the purpose of counseling regarding transmission prevention (positive prevention) and to assess the patient's risk of acquisition of drug-resistant virus and current risk for concomitant sexually transmitted infections.

A complete physical examination should be performed at the time of initial evaluation and at subsequent visits. Signs such as temporal wasting, lymphadenopathy, and hepatomegaly or splenomegaly can provide clues to the stage of disease and alert the provider to the presence of OIs or AIDS-related malignancies. The oral cavity should be examined for the presence of thrush, oral hairy leukoplakia, and mucosal lesions of Kaposi sarcoma. A complete skin examination is important on initial evaluation and longitudinally, because many OIs and medication toxicities have cutaneous manifestations. A funduscopic examination should be done, and, in those patients with a CD4 count of less than 50 to 100 cells/mm^3, referral to an ophthalmologist is necessary to screen for evidence of CMV retinitis. Close examination of the anogenital area may identify treatable sexually transmitted infections and premalignant lesions associated with human papillomavirus infection. Recommended laboratory evaluations are presented in Table 1.

Antiretroviral Therapy

Antiretroviral drugs that are currently approved for the treatment of HIV fall into six classes: nucleoside reverse transcriptase inhibitors (NRTIs), non-nucleoside reverse transcriptase inhibitors (NNRTIs), protease inhibitors (PIs), fusion inhibitors, integrase inhibitors, and chemokine (CC) receptor 5 (CCR5) antagonists (Table 2). The goals of therapy are to increase disease-free survival, achieve maximal and sustained suppression of viral replication to undetectable levels (<50 copies/mL), preserve immunologic function, and improve quality of life.

(Text continued on p. 51)

TABLE 1 Initial Laboratory Evaluation

Test	Frequency	Comments
HIV antibody testing	At initial visit	If prior documentation is not reliable or if HIV RNA is undetectable
CD4$^+$ T-cell count	At initial visit, then every 3–6 mo	Levels may be falsely elevated in splenectomized patients and with concurrent HTLV-1 infection.
Plasma HIV RNA (viral load)	At initial visit, before ART initiation, every 3 mo while on ART	Ultrasensitive viral load assay detects levels as low as 50 copies/mL and should be used to monitor response while on treatment
Resistance testing	At initial visit, and with treatment failure before change in ART regimen	Genotype and phenotype tests are available; genotypes are more commonly used.
HLA-B*5701 testing	Before treatment initiation if considering abacavir (Ziagen)	—
Coreceptor tropism assay	Before treatment initiation if considering CCR5 antagonist (maraviroc [Selzentry])	—
Complete blood count	At initial visit, then every 3–6 mo	AZT can cause bone marrow suppression and macrocytosis.
Serum chemistry panel	At initial visit	Up to 75% of HIV-infected patients have elevated hepatic transaminases at diagnosis.
Fasting lipid profile and blood glucose level	At initial visit	Every 3–6 mo
Hepatitis screen (anti-HCV, anti-HAV, anti-HBsAg, anti-HBcAg)	At initial visit	HAV, HBV vaccinations are indicated for nonimmune patients
Syphilis serology	At initial visit and annually in sexually active patients	Confirm with FTA-ABS test if positive; up to 6% of HIV-infected patients have biologic false-positive RPR result
Urine NAAT for gonorrhea and *Chlamydia*	Consider at initial visit and annually in sexually active patients	Testing every 3–6 mo is recommended for very-high-risk patients.
Toxoplasma gondii serology	At initial visit and if CD4$^+$ count is <100 cells/mm^3	Most cases of toxoplasmosis represent reactivation of latent infection.
Tuberculin skin test (PPD)	At initial visit, then annually in high-risk persons (e.g., homeless, injection drug users) if initial test is negative	Cutoff of >5 mm of induration is indication for treatment of LTBI
PAP smear	At initial visit	Annually
G6PD screen	At initial visit	Identifies patients at risk for hemolysis induced by dapsone or primaquine
Chest radiograph	If patient has pulmonary symptoms or a positive PPD result	Not recommended routinely

Abbreviations: ART = antiretroviral therapy; AZT = azidothymidine (zidovudine); FTA-ABS = fluorescent treponemal antibody, absorbed; G6PD = glucose-6-phosphate dehydrogenase; HAV = hepatitis A virus; HBcAg = hepatitis B core antigen; HBsAg = hepatitis B surface antigen; HCV = hepatitis C virus; HLA = human leukocyte antigen; HTLV-1 = human T-lymphotropic virus 1; LTBI = latent tuberculosis infection; NAAT = nucleic acid amplification test; PAP smear = Papanicolaou test; PPD = purified protein derivative; RPR = rapid plasma reagin test.

TABLE 2 Approved Antiretroviral Medications

Generic Name (Trade Name)	Abbreviation	Formulations and Coformulations	Recommended Adult Dosing	Important Points
Nucleoside Analogue Reverse Transcriptase Inhibitors (NRTIs)				
Abacavir (Ziagen)	ABC	300 mg tablets; 20 mg/mL oral solution *Coformulations:* Trizivir (ABC 300 mg + ZDV 300 mg + 3TC 150 mg) Epzicom (ABC 600 mg + 3TC 300 mg)	300 mg bid or 600 mg qd Trizivir 1 tablet bid Epzicom 1 tablet qd	Hypersensitivity reaction (FDA black box warning); screen patients for the HLA-B*5701 haplotype Possible increase in acute MI No food restrictions
Didanosine (Videx)	ddI	125, 200, 250, 400 mg capsules; 2, 4 g powder for oral solution	Body weight ≥60 kg: 400 mg (with TDF 250 mg) qd Body weight <60 kg: 250 mg (with TDF 200 mg) qd	Pancreatitis, peripheral neuropathy, nausea, lactic acidosis; concurrent use of TDF causes increased ddI levels and higher rate of toxicity Take on an empty stomach Must be swallowed whole
Emtricitabine (Emtriva)	FTC	200 mg capsule; 10 mg/mL oral solution *Coformulations:* Atripla (EFV 600 mg + FTC 200 mg + TDF 300 mg) Truvada (FTC 200 mg + TDF 300 mg)	200 mg capsule qd or 240 mg (24 mL) oral solution qd Atripla 1 tablet qd Truvada 1 tablet qd	Skin discoloration, rare nausea and vomiting No food restrictions

Continued

TABLE 2 Approved Antiretroviral Medications—Cont'd

Generic Name (Trade Name)	Abbreviation	Formulations and Coformulations	Recommended Adult Dosing	Important Points
Lamivudine (Epivir)	3TC	150, 300 mg tablets; 10 mg/mL oral solution *Coformulations:* Combivir (3TC 150 mg + ZDV 300 mg) Epzicom (see ABC) Trizivir (see ABC)	150 mg bid or 300 mg qd Combivir 1 tablet bid	Minimal toxicity Requires dosage adjustment in renal insufficiency. No food restrictions
Stavudine (Zerit)	d4T	15, 20, 30, 40 mg capsules; 1 mg/mL oral solution	30 mg bid (weight-based dosing is no longer recommended)	Peripheral neuropathy, lipodystrophy, pancreatitis, lactic acidosis, dyslipidemia No food restrictions
Tenofovir (Viread)	TDF	300 mg tablet *Coformulations:* Atripla (see FTC) Truvada (see FTC)	1 tablet qd	Renal insufficiency, Fanconi's syndrome, headache, nausea, vomiting, diarrhea No food restrictions
Zidovudine (Retrovir)	AZT, ZDV	100 mg capsules; 300 mg tablets; 10 mg/mL IV solution; 10 mg/mL oral solution *Coformulations:* Combivir (see 3TC) Trizivir (see ABC)	300 mg bid or 200 mg tid	Bone marrow suppression (macrocytic anemia, neutropenia), GI disturbance, lactic acidosis with hepatic steatosis (rare) No food restrictions
Non-nucleoside Analogue Reverse Transcriptase Inhibitors (NNRTIs)				
Delavirdine (Rescriptor)	DLV	100, 200 mg tablets	400 mg tid (four 100-mg tablets may be dispersed in >3 oz water to produce a slurry; 200-mg tablets should be taken as intact tablets)	Rash, elevated hepatic transaminases, headache No food restrictions
Efavirenz (Sustiva)	EFV	50, 200 mg capsules; 600 mg tablets *Coformulation:* Atripla (see FTC)	600 mg qd on an empty stomach at or before bedtime	Rash, CNS symptoms (vivid dreams, impaired concentration, dizziness), hyperlipidemia, false-positive cannabinoid test Take on an empty stomach, preferably at bedtime
Etravirine (Intelence)	ETR	100 mg tablets	200 mg bid after a meal	Rash, nausea Take after a meal Tablets may be dispersed in water
Nevirapine (Viramune)	NVP	200 mg tablets; 50 mg/5 mL oral suspension	200 mg qd for 14 d, then 200 mg PO bid	Hepatotoxicity, rash, lipodystrophy No food restrictions
Protease Inhibitors (PIs)				
Atazanavir (Reyataz)	ATV	100, 150, 200, 300 mg capsules	PI-naive patients only: ATV 400 mg qd PI-experienced patients: 300 mg (with RTV 100 mg) qd (when given with TDF, EFV, NVP)	Indirect hyperbilirubinemia, first-degree atrioventricular block, hyperglycemia, fat maldistribution, nephrolithiasis. Avoid taking simultaneously with antacids. Take with food.
Darunavir (Prezista)	DRV	75, 300, 400, 600 mg tablets	PI-naive patients only: 800 mg (with RTV 100 mg) qd PI-experienced patients: 600 mg (with RTV 100 mg) bid	Rash (contains sulfa moiety), hepatotoxicity, diarrhea, nausea, headache, hyperlipidemia, hyperglycemia, fat maldistribution Take with food.
Fosamprenavir (Lexiva)	FPV	700 mg tablet or 50 mg/mL oral suspension	PI-naive patients only: 1400 mg bid *OR* 1400 mg (with RTV 100-200 mg) qd *OR* 700 mg (with RTV 100 mg) bid PI-experienced patients: 700 mg (with RTV 100 mg) bid (once-daily dosing not recommended)	Rash, GI intolerance, headache, hyperlipidemia, hepatotoxicity, fat maldistribution No food restrictions

Continued

TABLE 2 Approved Antiretroviral Medications—Cont'd

Generic Name (Trade Name)	Abbreviation	Formulations and Coformulations	Recommended Adult Dosing	Important Points
Indinavir (Crixivan)	IDV	100, 200, 333, 400 mg capsules	800 mg q8h *OR* 800 mg (with RTV 100–200 mg) bid	Nephrolithiasis, GI intolerance, indirect hyperbilirubinemia, hyperlipidemia, headache, blurred vision, alopecia Should be administered without food but with water 1 h before or 2 h after a meal for optimal absorption
Lopinavir/ritonavir (Kaletra)	LPV/r	100 mg (+RTV 25 mg), 200 mg (+RTV 50 mg) tablets; 400 mg (+RTV 100 mg)/5 mL oral solution	PI-naive patients only: 4 × 200/50 mg tablets or 10 mL qd PI-experienced patients: 2 × 200/50 mg tablets or 5 mL bid	GI intolerance, diarrhea, hyperlipidemia, elevated hepatic transaminases, hyperlipidemia, fat maldistribution No food restrictions
Nelfinavir (Viracept)	NFV	250, 625 mg tablets; 50 mg/g oral powder	1250 mg bid *OR* 750 mg tid	Diarrhea, hyperlipidemia, hyperglycemia, fat maldistribution, elevated hepatic transaminases Take with food May be dispersed in water
Ritonavir (Norvir)	RTV	100 mg capsules; 80 mg/mL oral solution	Refer to other PIs for dosing recommendations	GI intolerance, headache, hyperlipidemia, hyperglycemia, dysgeusia, paresthesias Take with food
Saquinavir (Invirase)	SQV	200 mg hard gel capsules; 500 mg tablets	1000 mg (with RTV 100 mg) PO bid	GI intolerance, headache, elevated hepatic transaminaes, hyperlipidemia, hyperglycemia, fat maldistribution Take within 2 h after a meal
Tipranavir (Aptivus)	TPV	250 mg capsules	500 mg (with RTV 200 mg) PO bid	Hepatotoxicity, rash (contains sulfa moiety), rare cases of intracranial hemorrhage have been reported Take with food
Fusion Inhibitor Enfuvirtide (Fuzeon)	T20	90 mg/1 mL powder for injection	90 mg SQ bid	Injection site reactions (erythema, pain, induration), increased risk of bacterial pneumonia, hypersensitivity reaction
Coreceptor (CCR5) Antagonist Maraviroc (Selzentry)	MVC	150, 300 mg tablets	150 mg bid when given with strong CYP3A inhibitors (± CYP3A inducers) including PIs (except TPV/RTV) *OR* 300 mg bid when given with NRTIs, T20, TPV/RTV, NVP, and other drugs that are not strong CYP3A inhibitors *OR* 600 mg bid when given with CYP3A inducers (e.g., EFV, ETR, rifampin) without a CYP3A inhibitor	Abdominal pain, cough, dizziness, musculoskeletal symptoms, pyrexia, rash, upper respiratory tract infections, hepatotoxicity, orthostatic hypotension. No food restrictions
Integrase Inhibitor Raltegravir (Isentress)	RAL	400 mg tablets	400 mg bid	Nausea, headache, diarrhea, fever, CPK elevation No food restrictions

Abbreviations: ART = antiretroviral therapy; CNS = central nervous system; CPK = creatine phosphokinase; CYP3A = cytochrome P-450 isoenzyme 3A; GI = gastrointestinal; HLA = human leukocyte antigen; MI = myocardial infarction.

WHEN TO INITIATE ANTIRETROVIRAL THERAPY

In the mid-1990s, when combination HAART became available, the treatment paradigm was to "hit early and hit hard," because it was believed that the virus could be eradicated with treatment and rapid immune restoration could be achieved. However, as more data accumulated, there was recognition that the virus establishes itself within hours after infection and cannot be eradicated with HAART. In addition, during this early HAART era, it was observed that several of the regimens used were complicated, were associated with several toxicities and reduced quality of life, and, importantly, were not associated with marked clinical benefits. Therefore, between 1996 and 2006, the recommended CD4 count threshold for starting therapy steadily declined, with 2006 recommendations of the U.S. Department of Health and Human Services (DHHS), the International AIDS Society–USA, and the British HIV Society all generally indicating a threshold of 200 cells/mm^3 for initiation of treatment in asymptomatic patients.

More recently, however, accumulating evidence of the beneficial effects of earlier versus later treatment has resulted in a shift toward earlier initiation of HAART. There are now several classes of drugs, and many of the newer ART regimens are more potent, better tolerated, and less complex than before (i.e., low pill burden and once-daily dosing). The newer regimens, such as PIs boosted with ritonavir (Norvir) and NNRTIs used in triple-drug combinations, are more effective at achieving and sustaining virologic suppression (HIV-1 RNA <50 copies/mL) than the older regimens that used unboosted PIs and NRTIs. Most cases of virologic failure now occur when patients are lost to follow-up, are nonadherent, or discontinue their treatment. Furthermore, there is mounting evidence from several cohorts with long-term follow-up of HIV-infected patients that demonstrates a benefit of starting ART earlier. Consistently, persons starting treatment at a CD4 count threshold below 200 cells/mm^3 have a two to four times greater risk of AIDS or death than patients who start when their CD4 count is between 201 and 350 cells/mm^3.

There is also increasing recognition of the importance of non–AIDS-defining illnesses, such as cardiovascular, renal, and liver disease, at higher CD4 counts (>350 cells/mm^3). Cohort data (e.g., North American AIDS Cohort Collaboration on Research and Design [NA-ACCORD], ART-Collaborative) and one large trial (Strategies for Management of Anti-Retroviral Therapy [SMART]) reported significant benefits in reducing these complications when ART was initiated at higher CD4 thresholds (>350 or >500 cells/mm^3). Earlier initiation of HAART also appears to be associated with reduced risk of transmission, greater preservation of the R5-tropic virus, improved immune restoration (including CD4 counts); it also may be cost-effective.

CURRENT RECOMMENDATIONS FOR ANTIRETROVIRAL THERAPY

Current guidelines for HIV treatment in the United States are shown in Tables 3 and 4. Current guidelines advocate treating all patients with a CD4 count of less than 350 cells/mm^3 and any patient with

---

TABLE 3 US DHHS Guidelines for HIV Treatment, 2008

Clinical Condition or CD4 Count (cells/mm^3)	Recommendation	Strength and Quality of Evidence*
Patients with a history of AIDS-defining illness		AI
CD4 count <200		AI
CD4 count 200–350		AII
Patients with HIV-associated nephropathy	ART should be initiated.[†]	AI
Patients with HBV infection, when treatment for HBV is indicated		BIII
Pregnant women		AI
CD4 count >350	Optimal time to initiate ART is not well defined; patient scenarios and comorbidities should be taken into account.	

From U.S. DHHS Guidelines for HIV Treatment, 2008. Available at http://www.aidsinfo.nih.gov/Guidelines/ (accessed June 5, 2009).
*Strength of recommendations: A = strong evidence to support the recommendation; B = moderate evidence to support the recommendation. *Quality of evidence:* I = randomized trials with either clinical or validated laboratory outcomes (e.g., viral load); II = nonrandomized trials or well-designed observational cohort studies with long-term clinical outcomes; III = recommendation based on expert opinion.
[†]The necessity for the patient adherence to long-term ART should be discussed in depth (AIII) and barriers to adherence addressed.
Abbreviations: ART = antiretroviral therapy; HBV = hepatitis B virus; US DHHS, U.S. Department of Health and Human Services.

TABLE 4 International AIDS Society–USA Guidelines, 2008

Measure	Recommendation (Rating)	Strength and Quality of Evidence*
Symptomatic HIV disease	ART recommended[†]	AI
CD4 count <350 cells/mm^3	ART recommended[†]	AIIa, AIIb
CD4 count ≥350 cells/mm^3	ART should be individualized[†]	AIIa, AIIb
	Considerations include	
	High viral load (>100,000 copies/mL)	
	Rapid decline in CD4 count (>100 cells/mm^3/y)	
	High risk of cardiovascular disease	
	Active hepatitis B or C co-infection	
	HIV-associated nephropathy	
	Pregnancy with consideration for drug interruption in the postpartum period	

From Hammer SM, Eron JJ Jr, Reiss P, et al: Antiretroviral treatment of adult HIV infection. 2008 Recommendations of the International AIDS Society–USA Panel. JAMA 2008;300(5):555–570.
*Strength of recommendations: A = strong evidence to support the recommendation; B = moderate evidence to support the recommendation. *Quality of evidence:* I = randomized trials with either clinical or validated laboratory outcomes (e.g., viral load); II = nonrandomized trials or well-designed observational cohort studies with long-term clinical outcomes; III = recommendation based on expert opinion.
[†]Perform intensive adherence assessment and counseling to prevent secondary transmission.

an AIDS-defining illness. For patients whose CD4 count is greater than 350 cells/mm³, current guidelines recommend considering individualized treatment for specific scenarios such as active hepatitis B co-infection or pregnancy. Critical to all these recommendations, however, is ensuring that the patient is ready to start therapy and understands the regimen, the importance of adherence to it, and the need to continue therapy for life.

SELECTION OF AN ANTIRETROVIRAL REGIMEN

Table 5 presents the regimens recommended for ART initiation in treatment-naive HIV-1–infected adults residing in the United States and other high-income countries. Current ART strategies that represent the standard of care are based on combining at least three potent antiretroviral agents. Therapy is individualized in high-income settings and takes into account several factors such as comorbidities, concomitant medications, possible drug interactions, pill burden, dosing schedule, adherence issues, risk for side effects, and pregnancy. Triple-NRTI regimens are inferior to PI- and NNRTI-containing regimens and therefore are not recommended.

Efavirenz (Sustiva) is the preferred NNRTI because it has the best long-term treatment response to date, based on clinical trial data. It is available with tenofovir (Viread) and emtricitabine (Emtriva) in a coformulation, called Atripla (efavirenz 600 mg + tenofovir 300 mg + emtricitabine 200 mg), that can be taken once a day. Nevirapine (Viramune) is an alternative NNRTI; it should not be used in women with a CD4 count of less than 250 cells/mm³ or in men with less than 400 cells/mm³, because it is associated with increased risk of severe hepatotoxicity in such patients. Efavirenz-based regimens are equivalent to boosted-PI regimens in terms of efficacy and durability but have the advantages of low pill burden and limited long-term toxicity. The main drawback to NNRTI-containing regimens is their low barrier to resistance; for this reason, NNRTIs are less favored in patients for whom adherence is likely to be a problem.

The preferred PIs are the newer ones: atazanavir (Reyataz) boosted with ritonavir, lopinavir coformulated with ritonavir (Kaletra), and darunavir (Prezista) boosted with ritonavir. They are potent, have a high genetic barrier to resistance, and can be dosed once daily in many treatment-naive patients. The main drawbacks with PIs as a class are their interactions with other drugs, gastrointestinal intolerance, and metabolic complications (for most members of the class). Darunavir, a very potent PI, is generally reserved for second-line therapy but can be used as first-line treatment, especially in patients who have very high VLs (>100,000 copies/mL). The relative advantages and disadvantages of initial ART regimens are shown in Table 6.

TABLE 5 Starting Regimens for Antiretroviral-Naive Patients*

	Column A			Column B
	NNRTI	OR	PI	+ Dual NRTI
Preferred	EFV		ATV/r (qd) LPV/r (bid) FPV/r (bid)	TDF/FTC (qd) ABC/3TC (qd)
Alternative	NVP		LPV/r (qd) FPV/r (qd) SQV/r (bid) ATV (qd) FPV (bid)	ZDV/3TC (bid) ddl + FTC or 3TC

From U.S. DHHS Guidelines for HIV Treatment, 2008. Available at http://www.aidsinfo.nih.gov/Guidelines/ (accessed June 5, 2009).
*Select one component from column A (NNRTI or PI) and one from column B (dual NRTI combination).
Abbreviations:; 3TC = lamivudine (Epivir); ABC = abacavir (Ziagen); ATV = atazanavir (Reyataz); ddl = didanosine (Videx); EFV = efavirenz (Sustiva); FPV = fosamprenavir (Lexiva); FTC = emtricitabine (Emtriva); LPV/r = lopinavir/ritonavir (Kaletra); NRTI = nucleoside reverse transcriptase inhibitor; NNRTI = non-nucleoside reverse transcriptase inhibitor; NVP = nevirapine (Viramune); PI = protease inhibitor; r = ritonavir (Norvir); SQV = saquinavir (Invirase); TDF = tenofovir (Viread); ZDV = zidovudine (Retrovir).

TABLE 6 Advantages and Disadvantages of Initial Antiretroviral Regimens

Drugs	Advantages	Disadvantages
Non-nucleoside Reverse Transcriptase Inhibitors (NNRTIs)		
Entire Class	Extensive experience Saves PI option Fewer drug interactions than PIs Pharmacologic barrier to resistance	Low genetic barrier to resistance Class resistance with single mutation Drug interactions, especially with methadone (Dolophine) ADRs: skin rash (especially NVP)
Efavirenz (Sustiva, EFV)	Potent and never beaten in a clinical trial Low pill burden (coformulated with TDF and FTC as Atripla), once-daily dosing Central nervous system toxicity	Teratogenic (avoid in pregnancy or with pregnancy potential) Compared to LPV/r: lower CD4 response, more resistance mutations, and increased lipoatrophy
Nevirapine (Viramune, NVP)	Single dose to prevent perinatal transmission is safe and effective Low pill burden ART potency comparable to EFV	ADRs: rash and hepatotoxicity including hepatic necrosis Contraindicated with baseline CD4 count >250 cells/mm³ (in women) or >400 cells/mm³ (in men) Single dose may cause class resistance
Protease Inhibitors (PIs)		
Entire Class	Extensive experience Saves NNRTI option Higher genetic barrier to resistance	ADRs: metabolic complications Multiple drug interactions GI intolerance
Atazanavir (Reyataz, ATV)	High genetic barrier to resistance with boosting Potency Once-daily dosing Low pill burden No hyperlipidemia RTV boosting not required (preferred) Less GI intolerance	ADRs: jaundice (harmless) and PR interval prolongation (usually inconsequential) Drug interaction with TDF and EFV (can be overcome by using ATV/r 400/100 mg qd with EFV) Absorption requires food and gastric acid

Continued

Drugs	Advantages	Disadvantages
Lopinavir coformulated with ritonavir (Kaletra, LPV/r)	Potency Coformulated with RTV No food effect Option for once-daily therapy in treatment-naive patients Preferred in pregnancy	ADRs: GI intolerance RTV boosting required (coformulated) Hyperlipidemia
Fosamprenavir (Lexiva) + ritonavir (Norvir) combination (FPV/r)	Potency No food effect Option for once-daily dosing RTV boosting not required in naive patients (preferred) Appears to be equivalent to LPV/r	ADRs: skin rash Cross-resistance with DRV/r
Indinavir (Crixivan) + ritonavir (Norvir) combination (IDV/r)	No food requirement with RTV Twice-daily dosing with RTV boosting	ADRs: nephrolithiasis, sicca syndrome Requirement for >500 mL/d fluid intake
Nelfinavir (Viracept, NFV)	Substantial and favorable experience in pregnancy (1250 mg bid)	ADRs: diarrhea High rate of virologic failure Fatty food requirement No boosting with RTV
Saquinavir (Invirase) + ritonavir (Norvir) combination (SQV/r)	Potency Reduced pill burden with saquinavir 500-mg tablet Once-daily option	ADRs: GI intolerance Boosting with RTV required
NRTI Combinations		
AZT/3TC/ABC	Coformulated (Trizivir) Minimal drug interactions Low pill burden ABC may be associated with risk of cardiovascular disease and higher rate of viral failure in patients with baseline viral load >100,000 copies/mL	ADRs (ABC): hypersensitivity ADRs (AZT): marrow suppression, GI intolerance HBV flare*
AZT/3TC	Extensive experience Coformulated (Combivir) No food effect	ADRs (AZT): GI intolerance, marrow suppression (AZT) HBV flare* Requires twice-daily dosing (AZT)
d4T/3TC or d4T/FTC	No food effect Once-daily dosing	ADRs (d4T): lipoatrophy, hyperlipidemia, lactic acidosis, peripheral neuropathy HBV flare*
TDF/FTC†	Well tolerated Coformulated (Truvada) Long half-life of each drug may provide pharmacologic barrier to resistance No TAMs Extensive experience Once-daily dosing	HBV flare* Rare cases of nephrotoxicity (TDF) HBV flare* Food effect
ABC/3TC†	Coformulated (Epzicom) Once daily No food effect	ADRs (ABC): hypersensitivity HBV flare* Risk of cardiovascular disease
Nucleoside Combinations to Avoid		
d4T/ddl	-	ADRs: peripheral neuropathy, lipoatrophy, pancreatitis, lactic acidosis High rate of virologic failure
TDF/3TC/ABC or TDF/3TC/ddl	-	
Any NNRTI/ddl/TDF	-	High rate of virologic failure
d4T/AZT	-	Antagonistic
TDF/ddl	-	Drug interaction requiring dose adjustment; avoid with NNRTIs

*In hepatitis B virus (HBV) co-infection (HBV surface antigen positive), hepatitis B flare may be caused by discontinuation of agent or by HBV resistance to NRTI (3TC, FTC, TDF).

†FTC and 3TC are similar except for convenience of coformulations; FTC has a longer intracellular half-life and less extensive experience.

Abbreviations: ADRs = adverse drug reactions; ART = antiretroviral therapy; 3TC = lamivudine (Epivir); ABC = abacavir (Ziagen); AZT = zidovudine (Retrovir); d4T, stavudine (Zerit); ddl = didanosine (Videx); DRV = Darunavir (Prezista); FTC = emtricitabine (Emtriva); GI = gastrointestinal; r = RTV as a booster; RTV = ritonavir (Norvir); TAMs = thymidine analogue resistance mutations; TDF = tenofovir (Viread).

MONITORING RESPONSE TO ANTIRETROVIRAL THERAPY

After ART is initiated, the CD4 count usually increases within a few weeks, largely because of redistribution of cells. Subsequently, the CD4 count improves over years of therapy, at an average rate of 100 cells/mm³ per year, and then reaches a plateau. The starting CD4 count appears to influence the plateau reached (i.e. people starting at a lower count also plateau at a lower count than do those whose baseline count was higher). In approximately 5% to 10% of individuals, the CD4 response is less than this or does not increase from baseline. This is not evidence of treatment failure if the VL is undetectable. The plasma HIV VL rapidly decreases after initiation of HAART, and by 4 weeks most patients have at least a 1 $\log_{10}$ drop in VL. In most individuals, it should become undetectable (<50 copies/mL) by 24 weeks.

The CD4 count should be assessed at 3 months after ART initiation and then every 3 to 6 months thereafter. The VL should be measured 2 to 8 weeks after ART initiation, every 1 to 2 months until undetectable, and thereafter every 3 to 4 months. If a patient has been on a long-term stable suppressive regimen, visits can be reduced to every 6 months, with VL and CD4 testing performed at that interval. If a change in ART is motivated by drug toxicity or regimen simplification, it is recommended that VL be measured 2 to 8 weeks afterward, to confirm potency of the new regimen.

Other laboratory tests and their frequency of monitoring are shown in Table 1.

Treatment Failure

Treatment failure can be virologic, immunologic, or clinical. Virologic failure is defined as failure to achieve a VL of less than 400 copies/mL by 24 weeks or less than 50 copies/mL by 48 weeks, or a consistent finding (two consecutive measurements) of more than 50 copies/mL after a fall to less than 50 copies/mL. Most patients should have a decrease of at least 1 $\log_{10}$ in VL within 4 weeks. Immunologic failure is the failure to increase the CD4 count by 25 to 50 cells/mm^3 during the first year. In treatment-naive patients, current regimens are associated with an average increase of 150 cells/mm^3 in the first year. Clinical failure is the occurrence or recurrence of HIV-related events 3 months or longer after HAART initiation; this is not to be confused with immune reconstitution syndromes (discussed later).

Today, with the use of appropriate combinations, newer fixed-dose formulations, and more tolerable regimens, treatment failure in patients on their first-line therapy usually occurs because of inadequate adherence or treatment discontinuation (e.g., loss to follow-up, intolerance) rather than regimen inefficacy. Occasionally, pharmacokinetic issues such as a reduced drug level due to genetic polymorphism or a drug interaction (e.g., omeprazole [Prilosec] with atazanavir [Reyataz]) or transmitted resistance can be causes of treatment failure. In the United States, primary resistance seems to be declining, and in most places it is identified in fewer than 10% of HIV-infected acute seroconverters assessed.

Drug Resistance and Resistance Testing

A patient may be infected with a drug-resistant HIV virus to begin with (primary resistance), or, more commonly, resistance can emerge as a result of treatment (secondary resistance).

Several NNRTI-associated resistance mutations confer resistance to other NNRTIs, including K103N, 106M, and Y181C.

Among NRTIs, the resistance mutation most commonly detected when regimens containing lamivudine (Epivir) or emtricitabine are used is M184V. This mutation also makes the virus hypersusceptible to tenofovir or zidovudine (Retrovir), so in many situations lamivudine or emtricitabine may be kept in the regimen if tenofovir or zidovudine is being used. Other NRTIs can be associated with thymidine analogue mutations, or TAMS (e.g., 41L, 210W, 215Y); accumulation of TAMS or presence of multinucleoside mutations (e.g., Q151M, T69 insertion) confers cross-resistance to other NRTIs.

With PIs, accumulation of mutations generally leads to significant cross-resistance. Ritonavir-boosted PIs, particularly lopinavir (i.e., Kaletra) and darunavir, have high barriers to resistance, so development of resistance does not occur as easily as with the NNRTI class. Indications for resistance testing include the baseline resistance (prior to initial therapy), acute HIV infection, suboptimal viral suppression (VL >1000 copies/mL), and virologic failure with VL greater than 1000 copies/mL. Resistance testing should be performed while the patient is on therapy or within 1 month after discontinuation, because after that point, the wild-type virus may re-emerge and predominate.

Current standard methods of genotyping do not detect minority variants (resistant virus populations accounting for <10% to 20% of plasma virus). Resistance testing is usually a genotypic test and should be performed early in cases of virologic failure. The phenotypic resistance assay is more expensive and is typically used in patients who have multiple resistance mutations after multiple virologic failures. Interpretation of resistance testing should include adherence assessment, prior history of antiretroviral agents, and prior resistance testing results, because a history of resistance mutations remains relevant even if they are not detected on the current resistance test. Because resistance testing interpretation is complex, special expertise should be sought.

Adverse Drug Reactions and Drug-Drug Interactions

Adverse drug reactions (ADRs) are common with ART and are a reason for patient nonadherence or treatment discontinuation. ADRs can be idiosyncratic, dose related, time related (delayed), or dose and time related (cumulative). A particular ADR may be drug specific (e.g., hypersensitivity to abacavir [Ziagen]) or class related (e.g., hyperlipidemia because of PIs). It is important to inform patients of potential common or serious ADRs associated with their therapy. Often, the challenge in managing ADRs is that the patient is taking several concomitant medications that may have overlapping toxicities and ADR profiles. A symptom-based approach is often most practical (Table 7). Although many of the ADRs can be managed conservatively, some, such as symptomatic lactic acidosis, systemic hypersensitivity reactions, Stevens-Johnson syndrome, acute pancreatitis, and severe hepatotoxicity, are potentially life threatening. Serious ADRs necessitate withdrawal of the offending drug, and rechallenge with the drug should not be attempted in these situations.

Numerous important drug-drug interactions exist among antiretroviral agents and other medications of various classes. Familiarity with common interactions and ready access to reliable HIV pharmacology reference materials or a clinical pharmacologist with expertise in ART is essential for the clinician prescribing ART. Table 8, although not exhaustive, lists important drug-drug interactions, including combinations that are contraindicated and those that require adjustments to prescribe dosages. Tables 9 and 10 show dose adjustments that must be made with coadministration of certain antiretroviral drugs.

CURRENT THERAPY

- Multiple studies have demonstrated that superior clinical outcomes are achieved in patients who receive care from clinicians with substantial experience in HIV care.
- Accumulating evidence suggests that earlier initiation of antiretroviral therapy (with CD4$^+$ T-cell counts of 350–500 cells/mm^3) improves outcomes.
- U.S. and European guidelines recommend consideration of individualized antiretroviral therapy for HIV-infected persons with CD4 counts >350 cells/mm^3 for the following: high viral load (>100,000 copies/mL), rapid decline of CD4 count (>100 cells/year), HIV-associated nephropathy, active hepatitis B or C virus co-infection, pregnancy with consideration of drug interruption in postpartum period.
- New classes of antiretroviral medications, including integrase inhibitors and CCR5 coreceptor antagonists, give treatment-experienced patients additional therapeutic options.
- Revised and updated guidelines for prevention and management of opportunistic infections were released in 2009, with emphasis on the importance of antiretroviral therapy for prevention and treatment of opportunistic infections, especially for those for which specific therapy does not exist.

Adverse Effect	Manifestations	Causative Drugs		Stepwise Action
		Antiretrovirals	Other Drugs	
SJS/TEN[†]	Usually in first few weeks, with rash, mucosal ulcerations (± blistering), fever, hepatic dysfunction	NVP (0.5%-1%); less common with EFV (0.1%), ETR (<1%); rare with FPV, DRV, TPV, LPV/r, ATV, IDV, ABC, ZDV, ddI	Cotrimoxazole (Bactrim), sulfadiazine, dapsone, atovaquone (Mepron), voriconazole (Vfend)	Discontinue all antiretroviral agents and any other possible drug; manage like severe burns; do not rechallenge with offending drug
Hypersensitivity reaction[‡]	In rank order: high fever, diffuse rash, nausea, headache, abdominal pain, diarrhea, arthralgias, pharyngitis, dyspnea. Almost all have two or more systems involved. Always progresses with ABC, 90% present within first 6 wk	ABC (6%-7%); very rare if HLA-B*5701 is negative. Less common in African Americans	Cotrimoxazole, sulfadiazine, dapsone	Discontinue ABC and any other possible drug; rule out other causes; do not rechallenge with ABC. Symptoms resolve 48 h after ABC is stopped
Skin rash	Maculopapular rash ± pruritus	NVP, EFV, FPV > TPV >> ABC, DRV/r[§]	Cotrimoxazole, sulfadiazine, dapsone, atovaquone, voriconazole	Rule out SJS/TEN and hypersensitivity Antihistamines; continue offending drug; watch for progression of rash (if so, discontinue)
GI intolerance[¶]	Anorexia, nausea, vomiting, epigastric pain; begins with first dose	PIs, ddI, ZDV; common	Isoniazid (Nydrazid), rifamycins, pyrazinamide	Administer with food (not for ddI or unboosted IDV); antiemetics; switch to less emetogenic antiretroviral agent
	Diarrhea; usually begins with first dose.	PIs, especially NFV, LPV/r, and buffered ddI formulations	Clindamycin (Cleocin), atovaquone	Antimotility agents, calcium salts, bulk-forming agents; rehydration (if needed)
Hepatotoxicity[#]	Abrupt onset of GI symptoms, fever, rash, jaundice, eosinophilia, hepatic necrosis; encephalopathy can occur	NVP (usually ≤6 wk but up to 18 wk reported) Increased risk for baseline CD4 >250 (women) or CD4 >400 (men)	Isoniazid, rifamycins, pyrazinamide	Discontinue all antiretroviral agents and any other possible drug; rule out viral hepatitis; supportive management; do not rechallenge with NVP
	Symptomatic or subclinical hepatic enzyme elevations	NNRTIs, especially d4T, ddI, ZDV PIs, especially TPV, MVC 3TC, FTC, TDF can cause this with HBV co-infection and NRTI withdrawal or HBV resistance	Isoniazid, rifamycins, pyrazinamide, azithromycin (Zithromax), clarithromycin (Biaxin), all azole antifungals	If symptomatic, discontinue all antiretroviral agents and switch to nonhepatotoxic antiretrovirals after normalization; if asymptomatic, monitor closely Many discontinue drugs if ALT >5-10 × upper limit of normal
Lactic acidosis, fatty liver**	Nonspecific GI symptoms, wasting, fatigue, tachypnea, tachycardia, hepatomegaly, pancreatitis, hyperlactatemia, respiratory or multiorgan failure	d4T + ddI > d4T > ddI > ZDV (rare or never with other NRTIs); associated with long duration of use, female gender, obesity	Metformin (Glucophage)	Discontinue all antiretroviral agents; hydration; supportive care; roles of intravenous thiamine[1]/ riboflavin,[1] steroids, carnitine,[7] plasmapheresis are unclear; switch to ABC/3TC/TDF or NRTI-sparing regimen
Pancreatitis**	Epigastric pain (postprandial), vomiting, fever, elevated amylase, lipase	ddI, d4T, high-dose RTV; concurrent d4T, ddI, and TDF without ddI dose adjustment; ddI + ribavirin contraindicated	Alcohol, cotrimoxazole, pentamidine (Pentam)	Discontinue offending drugs; manage like acute pancreatitis related to any other cause; do not rechallenge

Continued

TABLE 7 Approach to Adverse Drug Reactions in the HIV-Infected Patient*—Cont'd

Adverse Effect	Manifestations	Causative Drugs		Stepwise Action
		Antiretrovirals	**Other Drugs**	
Peripheral neuropathy**	Numbness, paresthesia (often painful after weeks to months); depressed ankle jerks; recovery possibly incomplete	ddI, d4T (10%-30% or higher based on duration)	Isoniazid	Switch to ABC/3TC/TDF; gabapentin (Neurontin), tricyclic antidepressants, narcotic analgesics
Myopathy**	Myalgia, muscle tenderness, proximal weakness, elevated creatine kinase	ZDV (uncommon with current doses)	Statins, fibrates, steroids	Switch to another NRTI; improves in 3–4 wk after discontinuation; roles of coenzyme Q10,[7] L-carnitine[7] are unproven
Nephrolithiasis, crystalluria[††]	Flank pain, nondescript abdominal pain, dysuria, hematuria, renal dysfunction	IDV	Cotrimoxazole, sulfadiazine, acyclovir (Zovirax)	Discontinue IDV; hydration and analgesics; IDV can be resumed with plenty of oral fluids; if symptoms recur, consider switching
Nephrotoxicity	Renal dysfunction; nephrogenic diabetes insipidus; Fanconi's syndrome	IDV, TDF Occurs primarily in patients with inadequate dose adjustment, baseline renal dysfunction, or concurrent nephrotoxic drugs Risk for Fanconi's with TDF associated with older age, low BMI, low CD4	Acyclovir, amphotericin B (Fungizone), cotrimoxazole, pentamidine	Discontinue offending drug; hydration; generally reversible
Hematologic	Anemia, neutropenia usually after weeks to months[‡‡]	ZDV	Cotrimoxazole, dapsone, sulfadiazine, pyrimethamine (Daraprim), flucytosine (Ancobon), trimetrexate (Neutrexin), amphotericin B, ganciclovir (Cytovene), valganciclovir (Valcyte), rifabutin (Mycobutin)	Discontinue concomitant marrow suppressant, if any; exclude marrow involvement by opportunistic infections/malignancy; erythropoietin (Procrit) or filgrastim (Neupogen); switch to another NRTI
	Bleeding tendency in hemophiliacs	PIs	—	Factor VIII infusion (Advate); consider NNRTI-based regimens
	Eosinophilia	Enfuvirtide (Fuzeon)	Cotrimoxazole, dapsone, sulfadiazine	Exclude disseminated strongyloidiasis, malignancy; watch for hypersensitivity
Central nervous system symptoms[§§]	Drowsiness, insomnia, vivid dreams, nightmares, hallucination, impaired concentration/attention Usually resolves in 2–3 wk Worsening of psychiatric disorders, suicidal ideation	EFV; effects can begin with first dose	Isoniazid, dapsone, steroids	Usually resolves in 2-4 wk; consider discontinuation, if symptoms are persistent or psychiatric illness is exacerbated
Fat atrophy	Loss of subcutaneous fat (face, buttocks, extremities) Associated with long-term use	d4T > ZDV, ddI; less common with EFV	Steroids	Discontinue d4T, ZDV early if possible; either slow reversal or irreversible changes
Fat accumulation	Increase in abdominal girth, breast size, buffalo hump	PIs, EFV	—	Consider change in regimen for cosmetic reasons; restorative surgery
Hyperlipidemia	Increase in total and low-density lipoproteins, triglycerides; begins within weeks	PIs, except ATV (rank: TPV/r > LPV/r, FPV/r > IDV/r > SQV/r), EFV, d4T	—	Follow NCEP guidelines, statins (preferably pravastatin, atorvastatin, rosuvastatin [Crestor] but may need dose adjustment)[¶¶]

Continued

TABLE 7 Approach to Adverse Drug Reactions in the HIV-Infected Patient*—Cont'd

Adverse Effect	Manifestations	Causative Drugs		Stepwise Action
		Antiretrovirals	Other Drugs	
Insulin resistance	Fasting blood sugar >126 mg/dL, abnormal glucose tolerance test, DM symptoms More likely with family history of DM	PIs, except ATV	—	Diet, exercise, if indicated: metformin, rosiglitazone (Avandia), insulin (no major drug interactions with antiretroviral agents); consider switch to other non-PI regimens

Based on Guidelines for the Use of Antiretroviral Agents in HIV-1-Infected Adults and Adolescents, U.S. Department of Health and Human Services, January 2008.

[1] Not FDA approved for this indication.

[2] Not available in the United States.

[7] Available as dietary supplement.

*Only common and serious side effects are dealt with; side effects such as osteoporosis, avascular osteonecrosis (PIs), unconjugated hyperbilirubinemia, retinoid-like effects (IDV), and cranial malformations (EFV) are also known to occur.

†Approximately 0.3%-1% with NVP; a low dose lead-in period for NVP may decrease the risk; less common (0.1%) with EFV; occurs in the initial weeks after initiation; safety of replacing NVP with another NNRTI is unknown.

‡Approximately 5% with ABC; once-daily dosing possibly increases the risk; if ABC-related, symptoms resolve within 48 h after discontinuation of ABC.

§FPV and TPV are sulfonamide derivatives; potential cross-hypersensitivity with sulfonamides.

¶Symptoms begin with first doses; may abate with time.

#Low-dose lead-in period for NVP may reduce the risk; onset within the first few weeks with NNRTIs, after weeks to months with PIs, and after months to years with NRTIs; discontinuation of 3TC, FTC, or TDF in HBV co-infected patients may cause acute flare-up of hepatitis; safety of replacing NVP with another NNRTI is unknown.

**Class-specific adverse effect of NRTIs, because of mitochondrial toxicity; do not combine ddI/d4T/ddC; ABC, 3TC, and TDF are less prone; all four syndromes can occur in variable combinations; symptomatic lactic acidosis is rare but is associated with high mortality.

††Approximately 10% of patients taking IDV experience at least one episode of colic; occurrence is seen in only 50%, if fluid intake is improved (at least 1.5-2 L of noncaffeinated fluid, preferably water).

‡‡Almost all ZDV-treated patients have isolated macrocytosis; anemia and neutropenia occur in approximately 1%-4% and 2%-8%, respectively.

§§Occurs during initial weeks of treatment; patients are to be warned to restrict risky activities.

¶¶Only atorvastatin (Lipitor) and pravastatin (Pravachol) among statins, and gemfibrozil (Lopid) and fenofibrate (Triglide) among fibrates, can be coadministered with PIs.

Abbreviations: 3TC = lamivudine (Epivir); ABC = abacavir (Ziagen); ALT = alanine aminotransferase; ATV = atazanavir (Reyataz); BMI = body mass index; CD4 = CD4⁺ T-cell count (in cells/mm³); d4T = stavudine (Zerit); ddC = zalcitabine (Hivid)[2]; ddI = didanosine (Videx); DM = diabetes mellitus; DRV = darunavir (Prezista); EFV = efavirenz (Sustiva); ETR = etravirine (Intelence); FPV = fosamprenavir (Lexiva); FTC = emtricitabine (Emtriva); GI = gastrointestinal; HBV = hepatitis B virus; HLA = human leukocyte antigen; IDV = indinavir (Crixivan); LPV/r = lopinavir/ritonavir (Kaletra); MVC = maraviroc (Selzentry); NARTI = nucleoside reverse transcriptase inhibitor; NCEP = National Cholesterol Education Program; NFV = nelfinavir (Viracept); NNRTI = non-nucleoside reverse transcriptase inhibitor; NVP = nevirapine (Viramune); PI = protease inhibitor; r = RTV as a booster; RTV = ritonavir (Norvir); SJS = Stevens-Johnson syndrome; SQV = saquinavir (Invirase); TDF = tenofovir (Viread); TEN = toxic epidermal necrolysis; TPV = tipranavir (Aptivus); ZDV = zidovudine (Retrovir).

TABLE 8 Drug Interactions with Antiretroviral Agents*

Class	Agent	Antiretroviral Agent	Comments
α-Adrenergic blockers	Alfuzosin (Uroxatral)	RTV, All PIs	Consider tamsulosin (Flomax) or doxazosin (Cardura)
Antianginals	Ranolazine (Ranexa)	All PIs	—
Antiarrhythmics	Flecainide (Tambocor), propafenone (Rythmol), amiodarone (Cordarone), quinidine	All PIs	—
Antihistamines	Astemizole (Hismanal)[2], terfenadine (Seldane)[2]	All PIs, EFV	Loratadine (Claritin), fexofenadine (Allegra), cetirizine (Zyrtec), or desloratadine (Clarinex)
Antimycobacterials	Rifampin (Rifadin) Rifapentine (Priftin)	All PIs, NVP All PIs, NNRTIs	Use rifabutin (Mycobutin) with PIs Rifabutin
Antineoplastics	Irinotecan (Camptosar)	ATV, caution with other PIs	—
Calcium channel blockers	Bepridil (Vascor)	All PIs	—
Ergot alkaloids	Ergotamine (Cafergot)	All PIs, EFV	Sumatriptan (Imitrex)
Gastrointestinal agents	Cisapride (Propulsid)[2] Proton pump inhibitors	All PIs, EFV ATV, NFV	Metoclopramide (Reglan)
Herbs	St. John's wort[7]	All PIs, NNRTIs	Other antidepressants
Intranasal steroids	Fluticasone (Flonase)	All PIs	Beclomethasone (Beconase AQ)
Lipid-lowering drugs	Simvastatin (Zocor), lovastatin (Mevacor)	All PIs	Pravastatin (Pravachol), fluvastatin (Lescol), possibly atorvastatin (Lipitor), rosuvastatin (Crestor)
Neurotropics	Pimozide (Orap)	All PIs	—
Psychotropics	Midazolam (Versed), triazolam (Halcion)	All PIs	Temazepam (Restoril), lorazepam (Ativan)

Adapted from John G. Bartlett's Pocket Guide to Adult HIV/AIDS Treatment 2008-2009. Fairfax, VA, Johns Hopkins HIV Care Program, 2008.

[2] Not available in the United States.

[7] Available as dietary supplement.

*Delavirdine (Rescriptor) drug interactions are not shown as this drug is no longer used in clinical practice. Detailed information about drug interactions and searchable drug interaction databases are available at http://www.hopkins-aids.edu/, http://www.hiv-druginteractions.org/, http://hivinsite.ucsf.edu.

Abbreviations: ATV = atazanavir (Reyataz); EFV = efavirenz (Sustiva); NFV = nelfinavir (Viracept); NRTI = nucleoside reverse transcriptase inhibitor; NNRTI = non-nucleoside reverse transcriptase inhibitor; NVP = nevirapine (Viramune); PI, protease inhibitor; RTV = ritonavir (Norvir).

The Patient with HIV Disease

57

TABLE 9 Combinations Requiring Dose Adjustments: NRTIs

Drug	Zidovudine (Retrovir, AZT)	Stavudine (Zerit, d4T)	Didanosine (Videx, ddI)	Tenofovir (Viread, TDF)
Methadone (Dolophine)	AZT AUC increase 40%; no dose change Monitor CBC	d4T decreased 27%; no dose change	ddI EC: no interaction	No change in methadone or TDF levels
Didanosine (Videx, ddI)	—	Increased toxicity: pancreatitis, peripheral neuropathy lactic acidosis Avoid	-	ddI increases 44% >60 kg: 250 mg/d ddI EC <60 kg: 200 mg/d ddI EC
Ribavirin (Rebetol)	Monitor for severe anemia In vitro inhibition of AZT activation; not shown in vivo	No data	Magnifies ddI toxicity; contraindicated	Ribavirin unchanged; no data on TDF level
Atazanavir (Reyataz, ATV)	AZT AUC unchanged but C_{min} decrease 30%; significance unknown	No data	Buffered ddI: take ATV 2 h before or 1 h after ddl or use ddI EC (separate dosing due to food restrictions)	ATV AUC decreases 25%; TDF AUC increases 24% Avoid concomitant use unless ATV is combined with RTV (ATV/r)
Indinavir (Crixivan, IDV)	—	No data	Buffered ddI: take 1 h apart	IDV C_{max} increases 14%; clinical significance unknown
Cidofovir (Vistide), ganciclovir (Cytovene), valganciclovir (Valcyte)	Ganciclovir + AZT increases marrow toxicity Monitor CBC	No data	ddI and oral ganciclovir: ddI AUC increased 111% (PO) and 50%-70% (IV); use with caution or avoid	Combination may increase levels of both drugs; monitor for toxicity
Lopinavir/ritonavir (Kaletra, LPV/r)	No pharmacokinetics data but interaction unlikely due to favorable clinical data	No data	No data	TDF AUC increases 34% Use standard doses and monitor for TDF toxicity
Tipranavir (Aptivus, TPV)	AZT decreased 33%-43%; clinical significance unknown	No interaction	Separate dose of ddI EC by >2 h	TPV AUC decreases 9%-18%; clinical significance unknown

Adapted from John G. Bartlett's Pocket Guide to Adult HIV/AIDS Treatment 2008–2009. Fairfax, VA, Johns Hopkins HIV Care Program, 2008.
Abbreviations: AUC = area under the concentration-versus-time curve; CBC = complete blood count; C_{max} = maximum plasma concentration; C_{min} = minimum plasma concentration; EC = enteric coated; NRTI = nucleoside reverse transcriptase inhibitor.

TABLE 10 Combinations Requiring Dose Adjustments: PIs and NNRTIs

Drug	Efavirenz (Sustiva, EFV)	Nevirapine (Viramune, NVP)	Etravirine (Intelence, ETR)
Atazanavir (Reyataz)/ritonavir (Norvir, RTV) combination (ATV/r)	ATV 400 mg + RTV 100 mg (with food) + EFV SD (avoid coadministration in PI-experienced patients)	Avoid	Avoid
Darunavir (Prezista)/ritonavir combination (DRV/r)	DRV/r SD + EFV SD (dose not established; consider TDM)	DRV/r SD + NVP SD (dose not established; consider TDM)	DRV/r-SD + ETR-SD
Fosamprenavir (Lexiva, FPV)	FPV 1400 mg qd + RTV 300 mg qd + EFV SD FPV 700 mg bid + RTV 100 mg bid + EFV SD	FPV 700 mg + RTV 100 mg bid + NVP SD	Avoid
Indinavir (Crixivan, IDV)	IDV 1000 mg q8h + EFV SD IDV 800 mg q12h + RTV 200 mg bid + EFV SD	IDV 1000 mg q8h + NVP SD IDV 800 mg q12h + RTV 200 mg q12h + NVP SD	Avoid
Lopinavir/ritonavir coformulation (Kaletra, LPV/r)	LPV/r 600/150 mg bid + EFV SD	LPV/r 600/150 mg bid + NVP SD	ETR: SD LPV/r: SD
Nelfinavir (Viracept, NFV)	NFV SD + EFV SD	NVP SD + NFV SD	Avoid
Saquinavir Invirase, SQV)	SQV/r 1000/100 mg bid + EFV SD	SQV 1000 mg bid + RTV 100 mg bid + NVP SD	SQV/r 1000/100 mg bid + ETR SD
Tipranavir (Aptivus)/ritonavir combination (TPV/r)	TPV 500 mg bid + RTV 200 mg bid + EFV SD	Inadequate data; NVP may decrease TPV	Avoid

Adapted from John G. Bartlett's Pocket Guide to Adult HIV/AIDS Treatment 2008-2009. Fairfax, VA, Johns Hopkins HIV Care Program, 2008.
Abbreviations: SD = standard dose; NNRTI = non-nucleoside reverse transcriptase inhibitor; PI = protease inhibitor; TDM = therapeutic drug monitoring.

Complications

DIAGNOSIS AND MANAGEMENT OF OPPORTUNISTIC INFECTIONS

OIs are the most common cause of disability and death in patients who are not receiving ART. Clinical experience from the pre-HAART era demonstrated that the risk of OIs increases proportionately with the severity of immune system dysfunction and can be roughly predicted by the CD4 count in patients receiving and not receiving HAART. Guidelines for initiating and discontinuing antimicrobial prophylaxis against OIs are based on the CD4 count, as summarized in Table 11.

Diagnosis of OIs requires that clinicians recognize that a diverse array of bacterial, fungal, viral, and parasitic pathogens can cause overlapping clinical syndromes. A broad differential diagnosis must be considered when evaluating an HIV-infected patient with specific or generalized symptoms. Aside from infectious complications, symptoms may arise from toxicities inherent to antiretroviral or other medications. Patients infected with HIV have increased rates of cardiovascular, renal, and hematologic abnormalities, which may also cause nonspecific symptoms. A syndromic approach to recognizing complications of HIV infection is described in the following paragraphs. Recommended treatment regimens for the most common OIs are presented in Table 12. Detailed treatment guidelines that are periodically updated are available from the CDC and the HIV Medicine Association of the Infectious Diseases Society of America (http://aidsinfo.nih.gov/contentfiles/Adult_OI.pdf [accessed June 5, 2009]).

Neurologic Complications

Both central nervous system disease and peripheral nerve abnormalities are common in advanced AIDS. Peripheral neuropathy has been associated with some NRTI medications, most commonly stavudine (d4T, Zerit), as a result of the mitochondrial toxicity inherent to these drugs. HIV infection can directly cause distal sensory neuropathy, which may manifest as dysesthesia or hypersensitivity, decreased reflexes, and chronic neuropathic pain. Inflammatory demyelinating polyneuropathy (e.g., Guillain-Barré syndrome), which has known associations with some enteric pathogens, causes ascending motor weakness, typically without sensory involvement. CMV infection may cause polyradiculopathy, transverse myelitis, and encephalitis/ventriculitis in patients with CD4 counts lower than 50 cells/mm^3. CMV end-organ disease, including retinitis (a vision-threatening condition), requires prompt diagnosis and initiation of appropriate anti-CMV therapy.

TABLE 11 Antimicrobial Prophylaxis for Opportunistic Infections

Infection	Indications for Initiating Prophylaxis	Preferred Regimen	Alternative Regimen	Indications for Discontinuing Prophylaxis
Pneumocystis jirovecii pneumonia (PCP)	CD4 <200	TMP-SMX (Bactrim DS) 1 DS tablet PO qd, or TMP-SMX (Bactrim SS) 1 SS tablet PO qd	TMP-SMX (Bactrim DS) 1 DS tablet PO three times weekly[3] Dapsone[1] 100 mg PO qd or 50 mg PO bid Dapsone 50 mg PO qd + pyrimethamine (Daraprim)[1] 50 mg PO weekly + leucovorin[1] 25 mg PO weekly Aerosolized pentamidine (NebuPent) 300 mg via Respirgard II nebulizer monthly Atovaquone (Mepron) 1500 mg/d Atovaquone 1500 mg/d + pyrimethamine 25 mg/d + leucovorin 10 mg/d	CD4 >200 for 3 mo in response to HAART
Toxoplasma gondii encephalitis	CD4 <100 and toxoplasma IgG positive	TMP-SMX[1] 1 DS tablet PO qd	TMP-SMX 1 DS tablet PO three times weekly TMP-SMX 1 SS tablet PO qd Dapsone[1] 50 mg PO qd + pyrimethamine 50 mg PO weekly + leucovorin[1] 25 mg PO weekly Dapsone 200 mg + pyrimethamine 75 mg + leucovorin 25 mg, all PO weekly Atovaquone[1] 1500 mg ± pyrimethamine 25 mg + leucovorin 10 mg, all PO qd	CD4 >200 for 3 mo in response to HAART
Mycobacterium avium-intracellulare (MAI)	CD4 <50	Azithromycin (Zithromax) 1200 mg PO once weekly Clarithromycin (Biaxin) 500 mg PO bid Azithromycin 600 mg PO twice weekly	Rifabutin (Mycobutin) 300 mg PO qd	CD4 >100/mm^3 for 3-6 mo and undetectable viral load in response to HAART
Mycobacterium tuberculosis	Positive diagnostic test for LTBI	Isoniazid (INH) 300 mg PO qd (or 900 mg PO twice weekly for 9 mo) + pyridoxine 50 mg PO qd	Rifampin (Rifadin) 600 mg PO qd × 4 mo	Completion of treatment for LTBI

[1]Not FDA approved for this indication.
Abbreviations: CD4 = CD4$^+$ T-cell count (in cells/mm^3); DS = double-strength; HAART = highly active antiretroviral therapy; IgG = immunoglobulin G; LTBI = latent tuberculosis infection; SS = single-strength; TMP-SMX = trimethoprim-sulfamethoxazole.

TABLE 12 Recommended Treatment for Opportunistic Infections

Infection	Preferred Regimen	Alternative Regimen	Maintenance Therapy	Important Points
Pneumocystis jiroveci pneumonia (PCP)	TMP-SMX (Bactrim) (15–20 mg TMP and 75–100 mg SMX)/kg/day IV divided q6h or q8h May switch to PO after clinical improvement Duration of therapy: 21 d	Pentamidine (Pentam) 4 mg/kg IV q24h infused over ≥60 min, or Primaquine[1] 15–30 mg PO q24h + clindamycin[1] (Cleocin) 600–900 mg IV q6–8h or 300–450 mg PO q6–8h	Drug regimens for secondary prophylaxis same as for primary prophylaxis	Indications for corticosteroids: PaO$_2$ <70 mm Hg on room air, A-a gradient >35 mm Hg Prednisone[1] doses: 40 mg PO bid on days 1–5, 40 mg qd on days 6–10, 20 mg qd on days 11–21
Toxoplasma gondii encephalitis	Pyrimethamine (Daraprim) 200 mg PO × 1, then 50 mg (weight <60 kg) or 75 mg (≥60 kg) PO qd + sulfadiazine 1000 mg (<60 kg) or 1500 mg (≥60 kg) PO q6h + leucovorin[1] 10–25 mg PO qd	Pyrimethamine + leucovorin in same doses as for preferred regimen + clindamycin[1] 600 mg IV or PO q6h, or TMP-SMX[1] (5 mg/kg TMP and 25 mg/kg SMX) IV or PO bid	Pyrimethamine 25–50 mg PO qd + sulfadiazine 2000–4000 mg PO qd (in two to four divided doses) + leucovorin 10–25 mg PO qd	Duration of acute therapy: at least 6 wk; longer if clinical or radiographic response is incomplete at 6 wk
Mycobacterium avium-intracellulare (MAI)	At least two drugs as initial therapy with clarithromycin 500 mg PO bid + ethambutol (Myambutol)[1] 15 mg/kg PO qd Optional third drug in severe disease: rifabutin (Mycobutin)[1] 300 mg PO qd (dosage adjustment may be necessary based on drug-drug interactions)	Azithromycin (Zithromax) 500–600 mg + ethambutol 15 mg/kg PO qd Alternative third drugs include fluoroquinolones: levofloxacin (Levaquin),[1] ciprofloxacin (Cipro),[1] moxifloxacin (Avelox),[1] amikacin (Amikin)[1]	Same as initial treatment	Criteria for discontinuing therapy: CD4 is >100 × 6 mo as a result of ART, symptoms have resolved, and at least 12 mo of therapy has been received
Cryptococcus neoformans meningitis	Induction therapy: amphotericin B deoxycholate 0.7 mg/kg IV qd + flucytosine 100 mg/kg PO qd in 4 divided doses for at least 2 wk	Lipid formulation amphotericin B 4–6 mg/kg IV qd + flucytosine 100 mg/kg PO qd in 4 divided doses for at least 2 wk, or Amphotericin B (without flucytosine) at same dose, or Fluconazole 400–800 mg PO once daily for 10–12 weeks	Consolidation therapy: Fluconazole 400 mg PO qd for 8–10 wk after induction therapy Maintenance therapy: Fluconazole 200 mg PO qd lifelong or until CD4 ≥200 for >6 mo as a result of ART	Managing elevated intracranial pressure is key to preventing morbidity and mortality; serial lumbar puncture and lumbar drainage is indicated in some cases
Cytomegalovirus (CMV) retinitis	Sight-threatening lesions: Ganciclovir intraocular implant + valganciclovir 900 mg PO (bid for 14–21 d, then once daily) Small or peripheral lesions: Valganciclovir 900 mg PO bid for 14–21 d, then 900 mg PO qd	Ganciclovir 5 mg/kg IV q12h for 14–21 d, then valganciclovir 900 mg PO qd, or Foscarnet 60 mg/kg IV q8h or 90 mg/kg IV q12h for 14–21 d, then 90–120 mg/kg IV q24h, or Cidofovir 5 mg/kg/wk IV for 2 wk, then 5 mg/kg every other week	Valganciclovir 900 mg PO qd, or ganciclovir implant (may be replaced q6–8mo) + valganciclovir 900 mg PO qd until immune recovery	Maintenance therapy for CMV retinitis can be safely discontinued in patients with inactive disease and sustained CD4 >100 for ≥3–6 mo; consultation with ophthalmologist is advised
CMV esophagitis or colitis	Ganciclovir 5 mg/kg IV q12h for 21–28 d or until symptoms resolve Oral valganciclovir may be used if symptoms are not severe enough to interfere with oral absorption	Foscarnet 60 mg/kg IV q8h or 90 mg/kg IV q12h for 21–28 d	Maintenance therapy is usually not necessary but should be considered after relapses	Patients with CMV gastrointestinal disease should undergo ophthalmologic screening
Esophageal candidiasis	Fluconazole 100 mg (up to 400 mg) PO or IV qd for 14–21 d	Itraconazole oral solution 200 mg PO qd Voriconazole 200 mg PO or IV bid Posaconazole 400 mg PO bid Caspofungin 50 mg IV qd Micafungin 150 mg IV qd Anidulafungin 100 mg IV × 1, then 50 mg IV qd Amphotericin B deoxycholate 0.6 mg/kg IV qd	Not routinely recommended	Patients with fluconazole-refractory oropharyngeal or esophageal candidiasis with response to echinocandin should be started on voriconazole or posaconazole for secondary prophylaxis until ART produces immune reconstitution

[1]Not FDA approved for this indication.
Abbreviations: A-a gradient = alveolar-arterial difference in partial pressure of oxygen (PaO$_2$ − PaO$_2$); ART = antiretroviral therapy; CD4 = CD4$^+$ T-cell count (in cells/mm^3); PaO$_2$ = arterial-partial pressure of oxygen.

Focal central nervous system lesions may be caused by infectious and malignant conditions. Cerebral toxoplasmosis usually occurs in patients with prior exposure to *Toxoplasma gondii* who develop reactivation disease when the CD4 count is lower than 100 cells/mm^3. The main differential diagnosis for one or several enhancing brain lesions includes toxoplasmosis and primary central nervous system lymphoma (PCNSL). PCNSL is almost always associated with Epstein-Barr virus, and detection of nucleic acid for Epstein-Barr virus in cerebrospinal fluid carries a high specificity for this condition in the proper radiographic context. Progressive multifocal leukoencephalopathy, a rare and potentially devastating demyelinating condition, is caused by reactivation of JC virus and can manifest as focal neurologic deficit, seizures, or cognitive dysfunction. *Cryptococcus neoformans* is a common cause of meningitis in AIDS patients and can also manifest with central nervous system mass lesions, pulmonary disease, or gastrointestinal disease. Worldwide, tuberculosis accounts for a large proportion of HIV-associated meningitis; less commonly, it can manifest as single or multiple focal lesions (tuberculomas). Neurosyphilis should be considered in patients with unexplained neurologic disease and sexual risk factors.

Respiratory Complications

Respiratory illnesses are among the most common causes of morbidity in HIV patients. Community-acquired bacterial pneumonia occurs at a significantly higher rate in HIV-infected compared with HIV-noninfected hosts, regardless of CD4 count, and is one of the most common reasons for hospitalization. *Pneumocystis jirovecii* (formerly *Pneumocystis carinii*) pneumonia (PCP) manifests with fever, cough, and dyspnea. Findings on physical examination and chest radiography can be variable, making the diagnosis difficult in the absence of high clinical suspicion. Elevated lactate dehydrogenase and oxygen desaturation with ambulation can be diagnostic clues. More than 90% of cases occur among patients with CD4 counts lower than 200 cells/mm^3. The diagnosis is established by visualization of organisms in induced sputum (sensitivity, 50%-90%) or in bronchoalveolar lavage specimens (sensitivity, 90%-99%), most commonly with the use of immunofluorescent staining. Slight worsening of clinical symptoms after initiation of treatment for PCP is common, particularly when adjunctive corticosteroids are not administered.

The risk of reactivation of latent TB is increased 100-fold in patients with HIV infection. HIV$^+$ persons who are latently infected have a 10% annual risk of developing symptomatic tuberculosis, compared with a 10% lifetime risk among the general population. The risk of reactivation increases with decreasing CD4 count, and patients with counts lower than 350 cells/mm^3 are more likely to have atypical radiographic presentations, including middle- and lower-lobe infiltrates without cavitation. Patients with very low CD4 counts are more likely to have extrapulmonary tuberculosis. Diagnostic approaches to tuberculosis are similar in HIV$^+$ and HIV$^-$ patients. Tuberculin skin testing can still be used to diagnose latent tuberculosis infection, although the recommended cutoff for a positive test is 5 mm of induration. Treatment of co-infection with *Mycobacterium tuberculosis* and HIV requires consultation with experienced clinicians and pharmacists because of extensive drug-drug interactions among antiretroviral drugs and rifamycins.

Gastrointestinal Complications

Diagnosis of OIs affecting the gastrointestinal tract is made difficult by the numerous infections and complications of therapies that can result in nonspecific syndromes such as nausea, vomiting, abdominal pain, and diarrhea. Oropharyngeal candidiasis (thrush) commonly manifests as white plaques on the tongue, palate, or buccal mucosa that are painless and can easily be scraped off. Although thrush is typically uncomplicated and easily treatable with topical preparations such as nystatin (Mycostatin) and clotrimazole (Mycelex troches), in the proper clinical setting it can alert the clinician to the presence of esophageal candidiasis. Esophageal involvement should be suspected in patients with dysphagia and odynophagia; retrosternal chest pain may also be present. Thrush is usually present but is not required for the diagnosis, which is often made on clinical grounds rather than

being confirmed with endoscopy. Patients with esophageal candidiasis typically respond after several days of treatment, and 7 to 14 days of antifungal therapy is usually sufficient. For cases not responsive to empiric treatment for candidiasis, referral for endoscopy should be considered. Esophagitis caused by CMV or herpes simplex virus requires a histopathologic diagnosis.

Acute diarrhea, defined as three or more loose or watery stools per day for 3 to 10 days, is common among HIV$^+$ patients, and more than 1000 different enteric pathogens have been described. Data from a large cohort indicate that the most common pathogens isolated are *Clostridium difficile*, *Shigella* spp., *Campylobacter jejuni*, *Salmonella* spp., *Staphylococcus aureus*, and *Mycobacterium avium-intracellulare* (MAI). Culture of the stool can yield a microbiologic diagnosis in many cases, particularly for acute diarrheal illnesses caused by *Campylobacter*, *Yersinia*, *Salmonella*, and *Shigella* species. Infection with *C. difficile*, the most common bacterial enteric pathogen in the United States for both HIV-infected and HIV-uninfected persons, is diagnosed in most settings by detection of cytotoxin in the stool, although the more laborious tissue culture is considered the gold standard. Enteric viruses are present in 15% to 30% of HIV-infected persons with acute diarrhea. Definitive diagnosis is not feasible in most clinical laboratories; viral enteritis should be suspected in the setting of community outbreaks, because of the high transmissibility of viral pathogens. Treatment is supportive with fluid resuscitation and antimotility agents.

Chronic diarrhea (duration >30 days) was a common manifestation of advanced-stage AIDS in the pre-HAART era and is still considered an AIDS-defining condition. Most pathogens that cause acute gastroenteritis can also cause chronic symptoms. Pathogens that should be suspected in cases of chronic watery diarrhea include protozoa such as *Cryptosporidium parvum*, *Isospora belli*, and *Microsporidia* spp. These entities are self-limited in the absence of severe immunosuppression. In advanced HIV, pathogen-specific antimicrobial therapy is infrequently effective, and symptoms commonly do not improve without immune reconstitution in response to ART. *Giardia lamblia* causes watery diarrhea, abdominal bloating, and occasionally malabsorption syndrome and can occur at any CD4 count. CMV infection can affect any segment of the gastrointestinal tract and is a common cause of chronic diarrhea. Diagnosis of gastrointestinal CMV disease is difficult without biopsy. Detection of CMV viremia with PCR does not correlate well with presence of CMV disease in HIV-infected patients, and CMV can be undetectable in serum in patients with extensive gastrointestinal disease.

Other Conditions

Mycobacterium avium and *Mycobacterium intracellulare* are closely related mycobacteria that are ubiquitous in the environment. They are discussed as a single pathologic entity and referred to as MAI or *Mycobacterium avium* complex (MAC). MAI is a common cause of chronic pulmonary disease in patients with structurally abnormal airways. In advanced HIV infection, it can cause a multiorgan system disease characterized by fever, night sweats, diarrhea, and abdominal pain. Infiltration of the bone marrow and liver may occur, leading to hematologic abnormalities and abnormal liver function tests, which can be a clue to the diagnosis. Biopsy of a lymph node or of bone marrow is sometimes necessary to diagnose disseminated MAI, but it is most often diagnosed by means of blood culture using specialized culture media.

IMMUNE RECONSTITUTION INFLAMMATORY SYNDROME

Recovery of cellular and humoral immune system function in response to ART is occasionally associated with severe symptoms resulting from inflammatory responses directed against opportunistic pathogens. Risk factors for this immune reconstitution inflammatory syndrome (IRIS) include a low nadir CD4 count, a high baseline VL, and PI-containing HAART regimens. Most cases of IRIS occur within the first 2 months after initiation of HAART, and onset can occur as early as within the first week. Disseminated MAI accounts for up to one third of the cases of IRIS in the United States. Other important causes of IRIS are tuberculosis, CMV infection, viral hepatitis, and candidal infections. It may be possible to decrease the risk of IRIS by delaying initiation of HAART by several weeks, until therapy for OIs has been instituted, but the risks of other complications of untreated AIDS often outweigh any potential benefit of this strategy. When it occurs, IRIS usually can be managed with nonsteroidal anti-inflammatory drugs or corticosteroids. HAART should not be interrupted except in life-threatening illnesses.

Management of HIV in Pregnant Women

Periodically updated guidelines for the treatment of HIV in pregnancy are available on the U.S. Department of Health and Human Services AIDSinfo website (http://www.aidsinfo.nih.gov [accessed June 5, 2009]). Pregnancy is not known to have an effect on HIV progression. HIV progression has been shown to increase rates of preterm delivery and low birth weight in developing countries, but this link has not been established in resource-rich settings. All pregnant women should be offered HAART to reduce perinatal transmission and improve maternal health, regardless of CD4 count or VL. Guidelines for ART are otherwise similar for pregnant and nonpregnant patients, with the important exception that drugs with unacceptable or inadequately studied safety profiles should be avoided. Efavirenz, tenofovir, didanosine (Videx), and stavudine should be avoided. If possible, preferred regimens should include zidovudine and lamivudine with either lopinavir/ritonavir (Kaletra) or nelfinavir (Viracept). Data suggest that nevirapine (Viramune) should be avoided in women who have CD4 counts higher than 250 cells/mm^3 at the time of initiation of therapy. This recommendation does not pertain to the practice of giving a single dose of nevirapine in the intrapartum period in resource-poor settings to prevent perinatal transmission. Elective cesarean should be offered at 38 weeks gestation to women who are likely to have VLs greater than 1000 copies/mL at the time of delivery. After delivery, administration of zidovudine to the infant for 6 weeks is also recommended.

Postexposure Prophylaxis of HIV Infection

The scarcity of data describing occupationally acquired HIV infection makes it difficult to quantify the risk of transmission associated with exposure of health care workers to an HIV-infected source. Pooled data from multiple studies demonstrated HIV transmission in 20 health care workers, out of more than 6000 workers who sustained a needlestick injury from an HIV-infected patient, yielding a transmission rate of 0.33%. HIV transmission due to mucosal exposure was even more uncommon (0.09%), and transmission from exposure of intact skin has not been described.

Despite poorly characterized risks and benefits, postexposure prophylaxis with ART is recommended for health care workers sustaining percutaneous, mucus membrane, or nonintact skin exposure to an HIV-infected source. HIV antibody testing of the worker should be done at the time of exposure and repeated at 6 weeks, 12 weeks, and 6 months after exposure. If given, prophylaxis should be administered as soon as possible, preferably within hours after the exposure. Recommended prophylactic regimens typically contain a two-drug combination of NRTIs; coformulations of zidovudine plus lamivudine (Combivir) and emtricitabine plus tenofovir (Truvada) are used extensively and have good tolerability. Three-drug HAART regimens including a PI are recommended for more severe exposures. The duration of postexposure prophylaxes is typically 4 weeks. The recommendations for prophylaxis have been expanded to include nonoccupational exposures such as unanticipated sexual or needle-sharing behavior. Most recently, strategies for preexposure prophylaxis have been discussed as a strategy for HIV prevention in settings where unsafe sexual practices or injection drug use are likely.

REFERENCES

Adult Prevention and Treatment of Opportunistic Infections Guidelines Working Group. Guidelines for prevention and treatment of opportunistic infections in HIV-infected adults and adolescents [draft]. 2008. Available at: http://aidsinfo.nih.gov/contentfiles/Adult_OI.pdf [accessed June 5, 2009].

Branson B. Current HIV epidemiology and revised recommendations for HIV testing in health care settings. J Med Virol 2007;79(Suppl. 1): S6–10.

Hammer SM, Eron JJ Jr, Reiss P, et al. Antiretroviral treatment of adult HIV infection: 2008 recommendations of the International AIDS Society–USA Panel. JAMA 2008;300(5):555–70.

Hirsch MS. Initiating therapy: What to start, what to use. J Infect Dis 2008;197(Suppl. 3):S252–60.

Joint United Nations Programme on HIV/AIDS. 2008 Report on the Global AIDS Epidemic. Available at: http://www.unaids.org/en/KnowledgeCentre/HIVData/GlobalReport/2008/2008_Global_report.asp [accessed June 5, 2009].

Landon BE, Wilson IB, McInnes K, et al. Physician specialization and the quality of care for human immunodeficiency virus infection. Arch Intern Med 2005;165(10):1133–9.

Panel on Antiretroviral Guidelines for Adults and Adolescents. Guidelines for the use of antiretroviral agents in HIV-1-infected adults and adolescents, Department of Health and Human Services; 2008. Available at: http://www.aidsinfo.nih.gov/ContentFiles/AdultandAdolescentGL.pdf [accessed June 5, 2009].

Amebiasis

Method of
Rashidul Haque, MB, PhD, and
William A. Petri, Jr., MD, PhD

Amebiasis, a disease caused by the protozoan parasite *Entamoeba histolytica*, is estimated to be the third leading parasitic cause of deaths worldwide in humans. There are noninvasive species of ameba including *Entamoeba dispar* and *Entamoeba moshkovskii* that are morphologically indistinguishable from *E. histolytica* by traditional light microscopy. Amebiasis is distributed worldwide, but the majority of cases are found in developing countries. The World Health Organization estimates that approximately 50 million people suffer from invasive amebiasis each year, resulting in 40,000 to 100,000 deaths annually. For example, a prospective study of preschool children in an urban slum of Dhaka, Bangladesh, demonstrated a 39% incidence of *E. histolytica* infection during the first year of observation.

Human beings are the only known host of the parasite *E. histolytica*. Individuals become infected with *E. histolytica* when they ingest cysts in fecally contaminated food or water. When these cysts reach the intestine, they swell and release the motile, symptom-inducing form of *E. histolytica*, called the trophozoite. Trophozoites can remain in the intestine and even form new cysts without causing disease symptoms. They colonize the large intestine by adhering to colonic mucins via a galactose and *N*-acetyl-d-galactosamine (Gal/GalNAc)–specific lectin. Reproduction of trophozoites is without a recognized sexual cycle, and the overall population structure of *E. histolytica* appears to be clonal. Aggregation of amebae in the mucin layer likely signals encystation via the Gal/GalNAc lectin. Cysts excreted in stool perpetuate the life cycle by further fecal–oral spread. Invasive disease results when the trophozoite penetrates the intestinal mucus layer, which acts as barrier to invasion by inhibiting amebic adherence to the underlying epithelium and by slowing trophozoite motility. In addition, trophozoites can be carried through the blood to other organs, most commonly the liver, where they form life-threatening abscesses.

Intestinal Amebiasis

There are several clinical classifications of amebiasis based on the invasiveness and site of infection with different treatments. Intestinal amebiasis is a term that encompasses the entire spectrum of clinical intestinal disease, including amebic colitis. Patients with amebic colitis typically present with a several week history of cramping abdominal pain, weight loss, and watery or, less commonly, bloody diarrhea. The insidious onset and variable signs and symptoms make diagnosis difficult, with fever and grossly bloody stool absent in most cases. Differential diagnosis of a diarrheal illness with occult or grossly bloody stools should include *Shigella*, *Salmonella*, *Campylobacter*, and enteroinvasive and enterohemorrhagic *Escherichia coli*. Noninfectious causes include inflammatory bowel disease, ischemic colitis, diverticulitis, and arteriovenous malformation.

Unusual manifestations of amebic colitis include acute necrotizing colitis, toxic megacolon, ameboma, and perianal ulceration with potential fistula formation. Acute necrotizing colitis is rare (<0.5% of cases) and is associated with a greater than 40% mortality. Patients with acute necrotizing colitis are typically very ill-appearing with fever, bloody mucoid diarrhea, abdominal pain with rebound tenderness, and peritoneal signs of irritation. Surgical intervention is indicated if there is bowel perforation or if the patient fails to improve on antiamebic therapy. Toxic megacolon is rare (approximately 0.5% of cases) and typically is associated with corticosteroid use.

Amebic Liver Abscess

Amebic liver abscess is 10 times more common in men than women and is a rare disease in children. Approximately 80% of patients with amebic liver abscess present with symptoms that develop relatively acutely (typically < 2 to 4 weeks in duration) with fever, cough, and a constant, dull, aching abdominal pain in the right upper quadrant or epigastrium. Involvement of the diaphragmatic surface of the liver may lead to right pleural pain or referred shoulder pain. Associated gastrointestinal symptoms occur in up to 10% to 35% of cases and include nausea, vomiting, abdominal cramping, abdominal distention, diarrhea, or constipation. Hepatomegaly with point tenderness over the liver, below the ribs, or in the intercostal spaces is a typical finding. Complications from amebic liver abscess may arise from rupture of the abscess with extension into the peritoneum, pleural cavity, or pericardium. Extrahepatic amebic abscesses have occasionally been described in the lung, brain, and skin, and presumably reach these sites hematogenously.

Diagnosis

Historically, diagnosis of amebiasis was complicated and often unreliable for various reasons. The signs and symptoms of amebiasis can provide means to obtain clinical diagnosis. However, the confirmation of an amebic infection rests with laboratory identification. Over the last 25 years, various molecular diagnostic tests have been developed to diagnose *E. histolytica*. The diagnosis of intestinal amebiasis must be based on tests that distinguish *E. histolytica* from *E. dispar*. *E. histolytica*-specific antigen detection test and polymerase chain reaction (PCR) tests are now available for specific diagnosis of *E. histolytica* (Table 1). Enzyme-linked immunoabsorbent assay–based antigen detection kits are now commercially available. Field studies that directly compared PCR to stool culture or antigen-detection tests for the diagnosis of *E. histolytica* infection suggest that these three different methods perform equally well. An important aid to antigen detection and PCR-based tests is the detection of serum antibodies to amebae, which are present in 70% to 90% of patients with symptomatic *E. histolytica* infection. A drawback of current serologic tests is that patients remain positive for years after infection, making it difficult to distinguish new from past infection in regions of the world where amebiasis is endemic. Colonic mucosal biopsies and

TABLE 1 Sensitivity of Laboratory Tests for the Diagnosis of Amebiasis

Laboratory Tests	Amebic Colitis	Amebic Liver Abscess
Microscopy (stool)*	25%–60%	8%–44%
Microscopy (abscess fluid)	N/A	<20%
Stool antigen detection†	>90%	40%
Serum antigen detection†	<65%	>90% (before therapy)
PCR/real-time PCR (stool)	>90%	>40%
PCR/real-time PCR (abscess fluid)	N/A	90%–100% (before therapy)
Serology		
Acute	50%–70%	70%–90%
Convalescent	>90%	>90%

*Does not distinguish *Entamoeba histolytica* from the commensal parasites *Entamoeba dispar* and *Entamoeba moshkovskii*.
†TechLab *E. histolytica* II antigen detection test.
Abbreviation: PCR = polymerase chain reaction.

exudates can reveal a range in histopathologic appearance and severity of intestinal lesions associated with amebic colitis.

Amebic liver abscess patients may reveal a mild to moderate leukocytosis and anemia. Patients with an acute presentation of amebic liver abscess tend to have a normal alkaline phosphatase and elevated aspartate transaminase with the opposite true for patients with a chronic presentation. Ultrasound, abdominal computed tomography scan, and magnetic resonance imaging of the liver are all excellent imaging modalities for detecting liver lesions (most commonly single and in the right lobe) but are not specific for amebic liver abscess. The differential diagnosis of a liver mass should include pyogenic liver abscess, necrotic hepatoma, and echinococcal cyst (usually an incidental finding that would not be the cause of fever and abdominal pain). Patients with amebic abscess are more likely than patients with pyogenic liver abscesses to be male and younger than age 50 years; have immigrated from or traveled to an endemic country; and lack jaundice, biliary disease, or diabetes mellitus. Fewer than half of patients with amebic liver abscess have parasites detected in their stool by antigen detection. Helpful clues to the diagnosis include the presence of epidemiologic risk factors for amebiasis and the presence of serum antiamebic antibodies (present in 70% to 80% of patients at the time of presentation; see Table 1). Occasionally, aspiration of the abscess is required to rule out a pyogenic abscess. Amebae are visualized in the abscess pus in a minority of patients with amebic liver abscess. Traditional PCR and real-time PCR tests can be used for the detection of *E. histolytica* DNA in the stool and liver abscess pus samples and have been found to be sensitive and specific (see Table 1).

Therapy

Therapy differs for invasive versus noninvasive infections (Table 2). Noninvasive infections can be treated with lumen active agents such as paromomycin (Humatin) to eradicate cysts and lumen-dwelling trophozoites. Nitroimidazoles, particularly metronidazole (Flagyl), are the mainstay of therapy for invasive amebiasis (see Table 2). Nitroimidazoles with longer half-lives (namely tinidazole [Tindamax], secnidazole,[2] and ornidazole[2]) are better tolerated and allow shorter duration of treatment; they are recently available in the United States. Approximately 90% of patients presenting with mild to moderate amebic colitis or dysentery respond to nitroimidazole treatment. In the rare case of fulminant amebic colitis, it is prudent to add broad-spectrum antibiotics to treat intestinal bacteria that may spill into the peritoneum, with patients occasionally requiring

[2]Not available in the United States.

TABLE 2 Drug Therapy for the Treatment of Amebiasis*

Type of Infection	Drug	Adult Dosage	Pediatric Dosage
Asymptomatic intestinal colonization	Paromomycin (Humatin) or	25–35 mg/kg/d in 3 doses × 7 d	25–35 mg/kg/d in 3 doses × 7 d
	Diloxanide furoate (Furamide)*	500 mg tid × 10 d	20 mg/kg/d in 3 doses × 10 d
Amebic liver abscess[†]	Metronidazole (Flagyl) or	750 mg tid × 7–10 d in 3 doses × 7–10 d	35–50 mg/kg/d
	Tinidazole (Tindamax) *followed by luminal agent*	800 mg tid × 5 d[3] in 3 doses × 5 d	60 mg/kg/d[3]
	Paromomycin (Humatin)	25–35 mg/kg/d in 3 doses × 7 d	25–35 mg/kg/d in 3 doses × 7 d
	Diloxanide furoate (Furamide)[5] or	500 mg tid × 10 d in 3 doses × 10 d	20 mg/kg/d
Amebic colitis[†]	Metronidazole (Flagyl) *followed by luminal agent (similar to amebic liver abscess)*	500–750 mg tid × 7–10 d in 3 doses × 7–10 d	35–50 mg/kg/d

[3]Exceeds dosage recommended by the manufacturer.
[5]Investigational drug in the United States.
*The information is updated annually by the Medical Letter on Drugs and Therapeutics at http://www.medletter.com/htmlprm.htm#Parasitic.
[†]Treatment of amebic liver abscess and amebic colitis should be followed by a treatment with a luminal agent.

surgical intervention for acute abdomen, gastrointestinal bleeding, or toxic megacolon. Parasites persist in the intestine in as many as 40% to 60% of metronidazole (Flagyl)-treated patients. Therefore, metronidazole (Flagyl) treatment should be followed with paromomycin (Humatin) or the second-line agent diloxanide furoate (Furamide) 2 to cure luminal infection (see Table 2). Do not treat with metronidazole (Flagyl) and paromomycin (Humatin) at the same time because the diarrhea, a common side effect of paromomycin (Humatin), may make it difficult to assess response to therapy.

Therapeutic aspiration of an amebic liver abscess is occasionally required as adjunctive treatment to antiparasitic therapy. Abscess drainage should be considered in patients who fail to clinically respond to drug therapy within 5 to 7 days or those with high risk of abscess rupture as defined by cavity size greater than 5 cm or location in the left lobe. Bacterial coinfection of amebic liver abscess has been occasionally observed (both prior to and as a complication of drainage), and it is reasonable to add antibiotics or drainage, or both, to the treatment regimen if a prompt response to nitroimidazole therapy is not observed. Imaging-guided percutaneous treatment (needle aspiration or catheter drainage) has replaced surgical intervention over more recent years as the procedure of choice for therapeutically reducing abscess size.

REFERENCES

Diamond LS, Clark CG. A redescription of *Entamoeba histolytica* Schaudin 1903 (amended Walker 1911) separating it from *Entamoeba dispar* (Brumpt 1925). J Eukaryot Microbiol 1993;40:340–4.

Haque R, Mollah NU, Ali IKM, et al. Diagnosis of amebic liver abscess and intestinal infection with the TechLab *Entamoeba histolytica* II antigen detection and antibody tests. J Clin Microbiol 2000;38:3235–9.

Haque R, Ali IKM, Akther S, Petri Jr WA. Comparison of PCR, isoenzyme analysis, and antigen detection for diagnosis of *Entamoeba histolytica* infection. J Clin Microbio 1998;36:449–52.

Haque R, Ali IKM, Sack RB, et al. Amebiasis and mucosal IgA antibody against the *Entamoeba histolytica* adherence lectin in Bangladeshi children. J Infect Dis 2001;183:1787–93.

Haque R, Huston CD, Hughes M, et al. Current concepts: Amebiasis. N Engl J Med 2003;348:1565–73.

Petri WA Jr, Haque R, Lyerly D, Vine RR. Estimating the impact of amebiasis on health. Parasitol Today 2000;16:320–1.

Petri WA Jr, Singh U. State of the art: Diagnosis and management of amebiasis. Clin Infect Dis 1999;29:1117–25.

Stanley SL Jr. Amoebiasis. Lancet 2003;22(9362):1025–34.

Tanyuksel M, Petri WA Jr. Laboratory diagnosis of amebiasis. Clin Microbiol Rev 2003;16:713–29.

World Health Organization WA. Amoebiasis. Wkly Epidemiol Rec 1997;72:97–100.

Giardiasis

Method of
M. Ekramul Hoque, MBBS, MPH (Hons), PhD

Background

Giardiasis is a parasitic infection of the upper small intestine caused by a flagellated protozoan, *Giardia lamblia* (also called *Giardia intestinalis* and *Giardia duodenalis*). This ubiquitous parasite is a major cause of intestinal infection among adults and children in developing and developed countries. The existence of this parasite was reported in the prehistoric era across the continents. However, pathogenicity of the organism among humans was known only in the latter part of the last century.

Organism

Giardia is a microscopic organism that exists in two life forms. The trophozoite, which is environmentally unstable, causes clinical illness, and the resistant cysts are responsible for the transmission of infection. Trophozoites are binucleated, flagellated, and pear shaped, measuring 12 to 15 µm long and 6 to 8 µm wide. They have a pair of claw-shaped median bodies and a concave ventral disk used for nourishment and attachment on the wall of the small intestine of vertebrate hosts. Cysts are smaller and oval, usually 8 to 12 µm long and 7 to 10 µm wide, and contain four nuclei.

Epidemiology

Giardiasis is one of the most common intestinal infections in the world. More than 200 million people are reported to have symptoms of giardiasis, and some 500,000 new cases are reported annually. Some estimates suggest the worldwide prevalence of giardiasis is 20% to 60%. Others report from 2% to 7% in industrialized countries and 20% to 30% in developing countries. In the United States, giardiasis became nationally notifiable in 2002. In 2005, there were 20,075 giardiasis cases reported from 49 states, with an incidence rate of 6.8 cases per 100,000 population. The incidence varied by state from 1.4 to 30 cases per 100,000 population; rates were higher in the northern states than the southern states. *Giardia* infection is highly underreported, and therefore the true burden of giardiasis in the United States is probably underestimated. An estimate suggests there are 2 million giardiasis cases in the United States annually, and 5000 people are hospitalized due to severe infection. New Zealand reports nearly 30 cases of giardiasis per 100,000 population every year, which is one of the highest among the industrialized countries. *Giardia* infection is reported to be more prevalent in urban areas than in rural populations.

Humans are the primary reservoir of the parasite. Other possible hosts are farm, wild, and domestic animals. Polymerase chain reaction (PCR) testing of samples of human feces from different geographic locations has so far associated *G. intestinalis* genotypes (assemblages) A and B with human infections. The role of animals in transmitting *G. intestinalis* to humans and the most likely routes of infection remain unclear.

Transmission of the *Giardia* infection is through the fecal-oral route following direct or indirect contact with cysts of *Giardia*. Cysts are infectious immediately after being excreted in feces. An infected person can excrete a maximum of 10^9 cysts per day for several months. Cysts may be killed by simple drying and heat, but they can survive for several weeks in cool and wet environments. Infectious dose is low; ingestion of as few as 10 cysts can cause infection. Commonly, the organism spreads by water or food or directly through person-to-person contact. Outbreaks of waterborne giardiasis have been reported year round, suggesting frequent contamination of water sources and longer survival of cysts in water.

Giardiasis shows a bimodal pattern of age distribution, peaking in children younger than 5 years and in adults 25 to 44 years (Figure 1). Incidence of infection varies by season, peaking in late summer and early autumn and dropping in winter. Persons at increased risk for infection include (among others) children of diaper age, children attending daycare centers, daycare workers, immunocompromised persons, pregnant women, institutionalized persons, travelers to endemic regions, people drinking contaminated water during outdoor activities, sewage and irrigation workers, and men who have sex with men.

It is not clear whether giardiasis causes malnutrition or malnutrition predisposes to *Giardia* infection. However, nutritional insufficiency can contribute to chronicity of the disease. Repeated exposure to the parasite can elicit an immune response, which might explain asymptomatic giardiasis cases. Breast-fed infants of immune mothers might acquire temporary protection against giardiasis, but this is not conclusive.

Pathogenesis

Clinical illness results from the interaction of *Giardia* organisms with the human host and the host's subsequent response to the parasite. *Giardia* isolates can vary in virulence, which might further explain the intensity of the symptoms.

After a person ingests *Giarda* cysts, excystation begins in the duodenum in the presence of gastric acid, pancreatic enzymes, and parasite-derived cysteine protease. Two tropozoites are formed from each cyst by binary fission (miotic division). The motility of parasites and the inflammatory cytokine response to parasitic attachment on the mucosal brush borders results in secretion of fluid and electrolytes, hence diarrhea and malabsorption. Trophozoites frequently slough off villi, which are swept into the fecal stream and replaced by new sets. After 4 to 15 days of colonization, some trophozoites encyst in the jejunum under an alkaline environment of bile secretion. Immotile cysts undergo a single cell division to form four nuclei, which are then passed intermittently in the feces.

Giardia trophozoites remain adherent to the intestinal mucosa but are not invasive. This close association might directly affect the brush border and its enzyme system. Hospital-based investigation observed partial villous atrophy in up to 25% of patients. Malabsorption of vitamin B_{12} occurs in 20% to 40% cases. Parasites are also found in extraintestinal sites such as the gallbladder and the urinary tract.

Clinical Features

Clinical manifestations of giardiasis vary from asymptomatic infection to severe diarrhea. The incubation period for *Giardia* infection varies from 1 week to several weeks. However, a period of 5 to 25 days is average.

Freshly exposed persons in an endemic area can present with acute symptoms that usually begin about 15 days (range, 1–46 days) following exposure. The symptoms include nausea, anorexia, upper abdominal discomfort, malaise, low-grade fever, and chills followed by the sudden onset of explosive, watery, foul-smelling diarrhea associated with foul flatulence and abdominal distention. Generally, the acute stage resolves spontaneously within 2 to 4 weeks. Some patients become asymptomatic passers of cysts for a period. Others have periodic brief recurrences of acute symptoms.

About 30% to 50% of infected patients go on to a subacute or chronic stage. Overseas travelers to *Giardia*-endemic areas often do not recognize or remember the infection during their travel and subsequently present periodically with persistent or recurrent mild to moderate symptoms. Features of subacute to chronic *Giardia* infection include flatulence, mushy foul stools, upper abdominal cramps, abdominal distention, steatorrhea, marked weight loss, and fatigue. Uncommon manifestations are cholecystitis, pancreatitis, immunologic reactions (including arthritis, retinal arteritis, and iridocyclitis), and occasionally rash and urticaria, mostly in adults. In rare cases, symptoms persist for years, but most cases resolve spontaneously after a variable period of weeks or months.

Generally, 10% to 30% of infected people remain symptom free, but the true percentage may be as high as 60%. The prevalence of asymptomatic infection is higher among children than among adults, especially among those in daycare. The duration of the asymptomatic cyst-passing state is not determined.

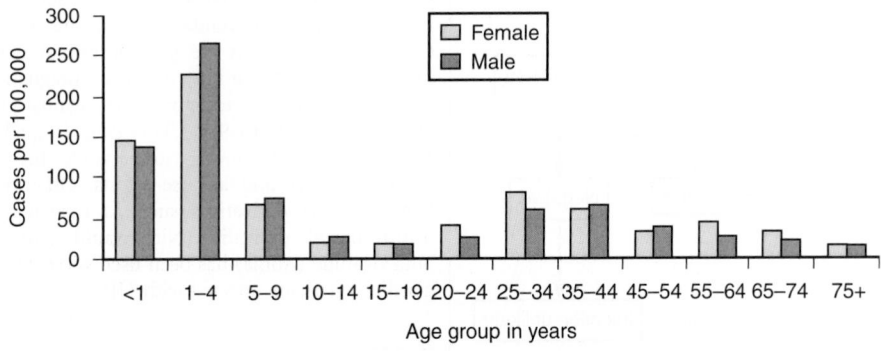

NOTIFICATION RATE OF GIARDIASIS BY AGE AND GENDER IN NZ

FIGURE 1. Notification rate of giardiasis in New Zealand by age and gender.

Diagnosis

Clinical signs and symptoms along with the history of risk behavior and exposure to *Giardia* risk factors can lead to a preliminary diagnosis of the disease. Laboratory diagnostic procedures are then applied to confirm the infection (Figure 2)

Traditionally, diagnosis is based on microscopic detection of *Giardia* cysts or trophozoites in the fecal specimens. At least three specimens of feces collected on consecutive days may be required to recover the parasite. The sensitivity of parasite detection is 50% to 70% in one specimen and 90% in three specimens.

Immunologic methods for detecting *Giardia* have superior sensitivity and specificity compared with other conventional methods of diagnosis. Widely used methods are enzyme immunoassay (EIA) detecting soluble antigens, direct fluorescent antibody (DFA) detecting intact organisms, and immunochromatographic lateral-flow immunoassays or rapid assay. Sensitivity of immunoassay varies between 94% and 97%, and specificity varies between 99% and 100%. EIA and rapid assay can pick up antigens of recently cured cases; DFA detects *Giardia* cysts. Immunoassay tests are quick and costs are reasonable.

Serologic tests do not have great diagnostic value in clinical practice because immunoglobulin G (IgG) persists even after infection; IgM, however, can indicate active infection. Negative serology does not exclude infection.

Duodenal aspirates or string test and duodenal mucosal biopsy are costly and invasive. They should be reserved for situations when giardiasis is strongly suspected despite persistent negative feces tests. PCR is used mostly in epidemiologic studies.

Treatment

Giardiasis, if diagnosed, should be treated. There are unresolved debates on the significance of treatment of asymptomatic cases. However, asymptomatic cases can remain a potential source of infection and can turn symptomatic at any moment.

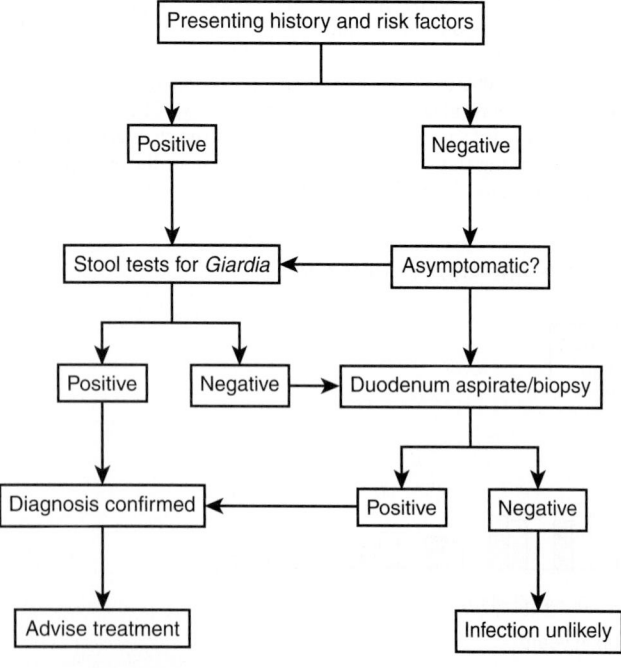

FIGURE 2. Diagnostic algorithm for giardiasis.

 CURRENT DIAGNOSIS

- Giardiasis is a common parasitic infection of the small intestine.
- Children, caregivers, travelers, and persons exposed to contaminated water are at greater risk for infection.
- Clinical manifestations vary widely.
- A large fraction of infected persons remain asymptomatic.
- Infective cysts pass intermittently with patients' feces.
- Diagnosis is by detection of *Giardia* parasites in feces by repeated microscopy or by immunologic assays.
- Assays can give false positives in recently cured persons.
- Infection can resolve spontaneously or can go into a chronic stage lasting for months with marked weight loss.

PHARMACOLOGIC THERAPY

A number of effective antigiardial drugs are available (Table 1).

Metronidazole (Flagyl)[1] is preferred and widely used because of its broad-spectrum coverage. It is not approved by the FDA for routine treatment of giardiasis in the United States. Metronidazole is effective and well tolerated and has a cure rate of 80% to 95%. The common side effects are gastrointestinal upset, headache, nausea, leukopenia, and metallic taste in the mouth. It is contraindicated in the first trimester of pregnancy due to its suspected carcinogenic, teratogenic, and mutagenic effects. Although the drug on therapeutic doses has shown no significant increased risk of cancer in humans. Other minor side effects are peripheral neuropathy, seizures, depression, irritability, restlessness, and insomnia. Drug resistance is not yet widespread.

Furazolidone (Furoxone)[2] is the primary drug of choice in the United States. It is available in liquid form and is widely used to treat children. Cure rates are between 80% and 89%. It is not recommended in pregnancy. Side effects include gastrointestinal disturbances, hemolytic anemia, disulfiram-like reactions with alcohol, hypersensitivity reactions, brown discoloration of the urine, orthostatic hypotension, and hypoglycemia.

Albendazole (Albenza)[1] is an anthelminthic whose efficacy is equal to that of metronidazole and with cure rates of 62% to 95%. Absence of anorexia in using this drug is an advantage for treating children. Notable side effects are gastrointestinal upset, abdominal pain, nausea, vomiting, diarrhea, dizziness, vertigo, fever, increased intracranial pressure, alopecia, and (reversible) increase in serum transaminases after prolonged use. Albendazole is contraindicated in pregnancy due to teratogenicity. Paromomycin (Humatin)[1] is a poorly absorbed aminoglycoside that is excreted in the feces without being metabolized. Its efficacy rate is between 60% and 70%. It is recommended for giardial infection in pregnant patients. Common side effects are nausea, increased gastrointestinal motility, abdominal pain, and diarrhea. 5-Nitroimidazole compounds, tinidazole (Tindamax) ornidazole (Tiberal), and secnidazole (Noameba-DS, Secnil)[1,2] are effective as first-line agents and have a cure rate of 90%. They have longer serum half-lives than metronidazole and are effective in single doses. Common side effects are gastrointestinal upset, vertigo, and bitter taste. They need caution to use in pregnant patients. Quinacrine[2] was one of the most effective drugs against giardial infection, with a cure rate of 92% to 95%. This drug is no longer produced in the United States and elsewhere in the world due to a number of pharmacokinetic issues and adverse effects. Other potential drugs include benzimidazole derivatives such as mebendazole (Vermox)[1] and a 5-nitrothiazole derivative (Nitazoxanide), which are not used widely. Nitazoxanide (Alinia) has been used successfully in France in resistant giardiasis patients infected with HIV.

---

[1]Not FDA approved for this indication.
[2]Not available in the United States.

TABLE 1 Therapeutic Doses of Antigiardial Drugs

Drugs	Adult Dose	Pediatric Dose
Metronidazole (Flagyl)[a]	250 mg tid × 5–7 d	5 mg/kg tid × 5–7 d
Tinidazole (Tindamax)[b]	2 g single dose	50 mg/kg single dose (max, 2 g)
Ornidazole (Tiberal)[c]	2 g single dose	40–50 mg/kg single dose (max, 2 g)
Secnidazole (Noameba-DS, Secnil)[b]	2 g single dose	30 mg/kg single dose
Quinacrine (Atabrine)[c]	100 mg tid × 5–7 d[e]	2 mg/kg tid × 5–7 d (max 300 mg/d)[e]
Furazolidone[d]	100 mg qid × 7–10 d	1.5 mg/kg qid × 10 d
Paromomycin[a]	500 mg tid × 10 d[f]	8–10 mg/kg tid × 5–10 d[f]
Albendazole	400 mg qd × 5 d	15 mg/kg/day × 5–7 d (max 400 mg/d)
Nitrazoxanide	500 mg bid × 3 d	7.5 mg/kg bid × 3 d

[a]Not a U.S. FDA approved indication; [b]Not available in the U.S.; [c]No longer produced in the U.S.; [d]Available in liquid formulation; [e]After meal; [f]With meal
qd, once a day; bid, twice a day; tid, three times a day; qid, four times a day

OTHER MEASURES

Diet modification can reduce acute symptoms, improve host defense mechanisms, and inhibit growth and replication of *Giardia* trophozoites in the lumen of the intestine. General advice is to consume a diet of whole foods that is high in fiber, low in simple carbohydrates, and low in fat.

Follow-up

Follow-up stool tests are advised to ensure resolution of infection. Hygiene practices should be enhanced during outbreaks. Symptomatic persons should be kept away from public contact.

Prognosis

Giardiasis is usually a self-limited intestinal infection. Effective antigiardial agents shorten the infection period. If untreated, giardiasis often resolves spontaneously in a few weeks. Prognosis is, therefore, generally excellent.

 CURRENT THERAPY

- Metronidazole (Flagyl)[1] is widely used because of its broad-spectrum coverage, but it is contraindicated in the first trimester of pregnancy.
- Furazolidone (Furoxone)[2] is available in liquid form to treat children.
- Absence of anorexia with albendazole (Albenza)[1] is an advantage for treating children.
- Paromomycin (Humatin)[1] is recommended in pregnancy due to its poor absorption rate.
- Tinidazole (Tindamax), ornidazole (Tiberal); and secnidazole (Noameba-DS, Secnil)[2] are effective in single doses.
- Nitazoxanide (Alinia) is used in drug-resistant giardiasis.
- Some diet modifications can reduce acute symptoms, improve host defense, and inhibit trophozoite replications.

[1]Not FDA approved for this indication.
[2]Not available in the United States.

Prevention

Eradication of giardiasis is not possible because the disease is endemic in the human population, animal population, and environment. Prevention and control methods are the way forward. Health departments in all countries, including the Centers for Disease Control and Prevention in the United States, publish recommendations for prevention and control of giardiasis. These include decontamination of water supplies and sanitary and hygiene practices. Potentially contaminated water may be treated by boiling for more than 1 minute or filtering through a pore size of 1 μm or smaller. Chlorination and iodination are unreliable. Laws and regulations to protect provisions of safe water should be enforced and monitored. Regular surveillance and reviews of sanitation can ensure quality.

People involved in recreational water activities and persons traveling overseas must be informed about the possibility of exposure to the parasite. Persons with symptomatic infection should not swim in a pool until 2 weeks after the treatment. Other occupational groups (e.g., daycare workers, medical personnel, irrigation and sewage workers) need to be cautioned. In daycare centers, hand washing with soap after changing diapers and a separate diaper-changing area should be implemented. All symptomatic family members, daycare center teachers, and children in daycare should be treated for giardiasis. Treatment of asymptomatic cases should be considered if the infected person is suspected to be a potential source of transmission of the disease.

REFERENCES

Cacciò SM, Thompson RCA, McLauchlin J, Smith HV. Unravelling *Cryptosporidium* and *Giardia* epidemiology. Trends Parasitol 2005;21 (9):430–7.

Centers for Disease Control and Prevention. Parasitic disease information: Giardiasis fact sheet. Available at http://www.cdc.gov/ncidod/dpd/parasites /giardiasis/factsht_giardia.htm [accessed 5.04.07].

Escobedo AA, Cimerman S. Giardiasis: a pharmacotheraphy review. Expert Opin Pharmacother 2007;8(12):1885–902.

Falagas ME, Walker AM, Jick H. Late incidence of cancer after metronidazole use: a matched metronidazole user/nonuser study. Clin Infect Dis 1998;26 (2):384–8.

Gardner TB, Hill DR. Treatment of giardiasis. Clin Microbiol Rev 2001;14 (1):114–28.

Hanson KL, Cartwright CP. Use of an enzyme immunoassay does not eliminate the need to analyze multiple stool specimens for sensitive detection of *Giardia lamblia*. J Clin Microbiol 2001;39(2):474–7.

Hetsko ML, McCaffery JM, Svard SG, et al. Cellular and transcriptional changes during excystation of *Giardia lamblia* in vitro. Exp Parasitol 1998; 88(3):172–83.

Hlavsa MC, Watson JC, Beach MJ. Giardiasis surveillance—United States, 1998–2002. MMWR Surveill Summ 2005;54(SS01):9–16.

Hoque ME, Hope VT, Scragg R. *Giardia* infection in Auckland and New Zealand: Trends and international comparison. The N Z Med J 2002;115(1150):121–3.

Institute of Environmental Science and Research Limited. Notifiable and other diseases in New Zealand: Annual report 2006. Available at http://www.surv.esr.cri.nz/PDFsurveillance/AnnSurvRpt/2006AnnualSurvRpt.pdf [accessed 14.05.08].

Islam A, Stoll BJ, Ljungstrom I, et al. *Giardia lamblia* infections in a cohort of Bangladeshi mothers and infants followed for one year. J Pediatr 1983;103 (6):996–1000.

Kulda J, Nohynkova E. Flagellates of the human intestine and of intestines of other species. In: Kreier JP, editor. Protozoa of Veterinary and Medical Interest, vol. II. New York: Academic Press; 1978. p. 69–104.

Lebwohl B, Deckelbaum RJ, Green PHR. Giardiasis. Gastrointest Endosc 2003;57(7):906–13.

Mineno T, Avery MA. Giardiasis: Recent progress in chemotherapy and drug development. Curr Pharm Des 2003;9:841–55.

New Zealand Ministry of Health. Communicable disease control manual. Wellington: New Zealand Ministry of Health; 1998.

Yoder JS, Beach MJ. Giardiasis surveillance–United States, 2003–2005. MMWR 2007;56(SS07):11–8.

Severe Sepsis and Septic Shock

Method of
Jerome Larkin, MD, and Marisa Holubar, MD

Epidemiology

The true prevalence and incidence of sepsis remain unknown. A study by Martin and colleagues in 2003 analyzed data from the National Hospital Discharge Survey from 1979 to 2000. Although some limitations apply, particularly shifts in the understanding of and use of coding, their findings have the advantage of assessing a large sample size over a prolonged period of observation. The most striking finding was a rise in the incidence of sepsis in the United States over this period, from an annual occurrence of 164,000 cases in 1979 to 660,000 cases in 2000. This reflects an average annual increase on average of 8.7% for more than 20 years. Coincident with this increase was a rise in the percentage of patients with a diagnosis of sepsis due to fungal organisms (4.6% in 2000). Gram-positive organisms supplanted gram-negatives as the largest group of pathogens after 1987 (52% versus 37%).

Mortality was highest among African American men and was associated with failure of three or more organs. Men were more likely to become septic than women (relative risk, 1.90). In-hospital mortality fell from 27.8% to 17.9% between 1995 and 2000. Total mortality increased, most likely as a result of the increase in the total burden of disease. This increase, although perhaps in part attributable to greater use of the diagnostic code for sepsis, is thought to have resulted from a combination of aging of the population, greater numbers of immunosuppressed individuals surviving longer, greater use of prosthetic devices, and greater number and more invasive medical interventions. Diabetes, hypertension, chronic obstructive pulmonary disease, congestive heart failure, and HIV infection all increased as a proportion of medical conditions contributing to sepsis, whereas the proportion of patients with cancer and that of pregnant patients declined. The percentage of patients with one or more organs failing (i.e., severe sepsis) increased from 17% to 35% of all patients with a diagnosis of sepsis.

A study by Dombrovskiy and associates described an even greater increase in the proportion of severe sepsis, from 25.6% in 1993 to 43.8% in 2003. They also found an absolute increase in the number of cases of sepsis, as well as an increase in total mortality, again likely due to increased incidence. Case-fatality rates fell from 45.8% to 37.8%, but mortality was substantially higher at both the beginning and the end of their study period than was described by Martin. These findings suggest acceleration in both severity and incidence of severe sepsis and septic shock.

Sepsis is the 10th most common cause of death in the United States. The incidence is highest during the winter, most likely reflecting increased respiratory viral infections that precede the development of community-acquired pneumonia, which is itself a medical condition with increased risk of developing severe sepsis.

A remarkable aspect of sepsis, severe sepsis, and septic shock is the relatively small number of associated pathogens out of the more than 1000 microorganisms known to cause human disease. *Staphylococcus aureus*, streptococci, enterococci, and gram-negative rods are the most commonly isolated species. *Escherichia coli, Klebsiella, Pseudomonas, Serratia, Acinetobacter, Enterobacter, Citrobacter,* and *Neisseria meningitidis* (a gram-negative coccus) constitute the most common gram-negative pathogens. This relative paucity of etiologic bacterial pathogens has implications for empiric antimicrobial therapy. The emergence of resistant organisms, particularly methicillin-resistant *S. aureus* (MRSA) and gram-negative bacteria harboring extended-spectrum β-lactamases, increases the risk of antibiotic failure and attendant mortality. Fungal pathogens, particularly non-candidal species, continue to increase in incidence. This is most likely the result of better empiric management of gram-negative and candidal sepsis in patients with hematologic malignancies.

Although sepsis is most typically a disease of the elderly, the immune suppressed, and those with chronic medical problems, otherwise young and healthy individuals can also be stricken with no clear cause or known risk factor, such as in meningococcemia, toxic shock syndrome, and necrotizing fasciitis.

Definitions

The term sepsis derives from a Greek word that generally implies putrefaction. It also has a colloquial meaning, understood by most lay people to mean a serious, potentially overwhelming infection. Historically, it has been intuitively understood by physicians to mean an infection, once localized, that has now disseminated and is life threatening. Bacteremia is implied if not always proven. Sepsis was usually fatal in the preantibiotic era, and its morbidity and mortality remain substantial.

In 2001, a consensus conference, sponsored by the American College of Chest Physicians and the Society of Critical Care Medicine and involving the European Society of Intensive Care Medicine, the Surgical Infection Society, and the American Thoracic Society, was convened to arrive at a specific definition of sepsis. Achieving such a definition is critically important to ongoing research on interventions aimed at improving mortality. Their deliberations, building on the work of a previous conference and published in 2003, elaborated several key concepts. They defined systemic inflammatory response syndrome (SIRS) as a state of immune activation characterized by the findings of fever with tachycardia, tachypnea, and/or leukocytosis or leukopenia. Although sensitive, this definition is so overly broad as to be rather unhelpful to an experienced clinician who would not need to resort to such terms to understand that a patient is seriously ill. Nonetheless, it provides a useful construct in beginning to arrive at a specific definition of sepsis. Both infectious and noninfectious processes—severe burn and pancreatitis being the most notable examples of the latter—can cause SIRS.

Sepsis is defined as the finding of SIRS in the presence of known or suspected invasion by a microbe into a normally sterile body site. Severe sepsis is sepsis that has become more generalized. The cardinal finding is organ dysfunction that is unrelated to the primary site of infection. Other typical findings include hyperglycemia, thrombocytopenia, hyperbilirubinemia, acidosis, coagulopathy, edema, oliguria, hypotension, ileus, hypoxia, and poor perfusion. Heart, kidney, and respiratory failure are the most common forms of organ dysfunction. Altered sensorium is also common. Septic shock refers to the presence of hypotension with systolic blood pressure lower than 90 mm Hg or mean arterial pressure lower than 60 mm Hg despite adequate fluid resuscitation. These terms (sepsis, severe sepsis, and septic shock) are all part of a continuum, implying a progressively graver degree of illness with associated increasing mortality. No single symptom, physical finding, organ dysfunction, or laboratory abnormality serves to make or exclude the diagnosis, although isolation of a microorganism in the setting of such findings is highly suggestive. Increasing numbers of physical findings and other abnormalities correlates with an increasing likelihood of the diagnosis of sepsis.

The consensus conference put forward a staging system for sepsis based on host predisposition, nature of infection, host response, and organ dysfunction (mnemonic: PIRO). By this, it is understood that a given patient may be predisposed to infection based on medical conditions such as diabetes, vascular disease, sickle cell anemia, or inherited or acquired immunodeficiencies. Additionally, there are likely to be more subtle genetic predispositions to the development of sepsis, as well as age-related factors. The nature of infection in terms of the site, inoculum, and virulence of the infecting organism clearly plays a role in determining the development of sepsis. The host response—ranging from localization and clearing of the infection without deleterious effect on the host to a state of immunologic dissonance whereby the inflammatory response is itself the driver of pathology—is signaled by the development of organ dysfunction. This staging system allows patients to be stratified at different points and serves as a template for evaluating the efficacy of various interventions as the characterization of sepsis and research into novel therapies progresses.

Pathophysiology

Infection of the immunocompetent host by a microorganism typically leads to immune activation. This serves to isolate the site and source of infection. Local tissue is often damaged, but eventually the infection is cleared, and repair and regeneration occur. This process is highly regulated, with a number of different cell types and mediators involved, all in delicate balance between proinflammatory and antiinflammatory effects. The patient may have few or no symptoms, or there may be systemic evidence of infection (i.e., SIRS). Sepsis is the failure of localization such that the process becomes generalized and leads to tissue destruction remote from the site of infection. Why the immune system enters this state of dysregulation remains unknown, although an enormous amount of research over the last 4 decades has elucidated many of the pathways and mediators involved. Tumor necrosis factor, platelet-activating factor, interleukins, eicosanoids, interferons, and nitric oxide are among the biologically active molecules characterized to date. Particular microbes also contribute to this process through the elaboration of toxins (typically by gram-positive organisms) and endotoxins (gram negative–derived lipopolysaccharide). These events lead to tissue destruction as a result of ischemic insult, direct cytotoxicity, and accelerated apoptosis. The characterization of inflammatory mediators has led to attempts to modify the immune response through the use of novel therapies such as monoclonal antibodies directed against tumor necrosis factor. To date such attempts have not met with success, and investigation continues.

Diagnosis

The diagnosis of sepsis ultimately relies on the clinical suspicion of infection in the setting of SIRS. A constellation of other supportive evidence establishes a greater or lesser likelihood of the presence of sepsis (see the Current Diagnosis box). It is rare that specific microbiologic evidence for infection is available in a manner timely enough to determine that sepsis is present or to help guide the initial, typically urgent, therapy. When it is available, it usually is a Gram stain or other type of specialized microbiology stain that confirms the presence of a potential pathogen in a site where none should be (e.g., gram-positive cocci in cerebrospinal fluid). Early therapy therefore relies on aggressive resuscitative measures and the administration of empiric antibiotics.

 CURRENT DIAGNOSIS

Systemic inflammatory response syndrome (SIRS)

- Diagnosis is based on the presence of two or more of the following:
  - Temperature >38°C or <36°C
  - Pulse >90 beats/min
  - Respirations >20 breaths/min or arterial partial pressure of carbon dioxide ($Paco_2$) <32 mm Hg
  - White blood cell count >12,000 or <4000 cells/mm^3 or >10% bands

Sepsis

- Diagnosis is based on a finding of SIRS plus proven or suspected infection as the cause

Severe Sepsis

- Diagnosis is based on a finding of sepsis plus organ dysfunction of one or more major systems (typically kidney, lung, or heart; less often, central nervous system)

Septic Shock

- Diagnosis is based on a finding of severe sepsis plus persistent hypotension despite aggressive fluid resuscitation (i.e., vasopressors are required to maintain mean arterial pressure >65 mm Hg)

Supportive Laboratory Findings

- Hyperglycemia
- Lactic acidosis
- Hyperbilirubinemia
- Acute renal failure
- Thrombocytopenia
- Coagulopathy
- Leukocytosis or leukopenia
- Elevated erythrocyte sedimentation rate or C-reactive protein

Supportive Physical Findings

- Decreased capillary refill or mottling of skin
- Mental status changes or obtundation
- Tachypnea or respiratory failure
- Tachycardia
- Anuria or oliguria
- Edema

Treatment

EARLY GOAL-DIRECTED RESUSCITATION: THE FIRST SIX HOURS

Initial treatment of sepsis should focus on correction of hemodynamic parameters, early administration of antibiotics, and source control of potential sites of infection. The 2008 guidelines from the Surviving Sepsis Campaign, an international initiative to improve sepsis outcomes, emphasized the importance of aggressive fluid resuscitation. Therapy should be implemented according to a protocol directed at achieving the following specific goals:

- Central venous pressure 8 to 12 mm Hg, or 12 to 15 mm Hg in those who are mechanically ventilated or have decreased left ventricular compliance
- Central venous or mixed venous oxygen saturation 70% or greater
- Mean arterial pressure (MAP) 65 mm Hg or greater
- Urine output 0.5 mL/kg/hour or greater

Administration of fluid boluses of 1000 mL or more of crystalloids or 300 to 500 mL of colloids over 30 minutes should begin as soon as hypoperfusion is recognized. There is no evidence that one type of fluid is superior to the other, although crystalloid is substantially cheaper. In cases of profound intravascular volume depletion, more rapid and more frequent fluid administration may be needed. Hemodynamic improvement (decreased heart rate, increased blood pressure, increased urine output) and the goal central venous pressure should direct the need for continued infusion of fluid while avoiding the development of volume overload and pulmonary edema. Transfusion of packed red blood cells should be considered if anemia is present, with a goal of achieving a hemoglobin level of 7.0 to 9.0 g/dL. If tissue hypoperfusion or hypoxia persists (central mixed venus oxygen saturation <70%) despite achieving a central venous pressure of 12 mm Hg, therapy with dopamine (Intropin) or norepinephrine (Levophed) should be initiated with a goal of achieving a MAP of 65 mm Hg. There is no role for the use of low-dose dopamine for renal protection. An arterial line for more precise and continuous measurement of blood pressure should be inserted as soon as possible after the initiation of vasopressor therapy. Ideally, vasopressors should not be introduced to increase MAP until after the fluid deficit has been corrected. However, in cases of severe shock, vasopressor therapy may be needed early in the resuscitation effort to improve perfusion to the peripheral vascular beds. If there is no response to dopamine and norepinephrine, the patient should be treated with epinephrine (Adrenalin).[1]

Appropriate antibiotics should be administered within 1 hour after diagnosis of severe sepsis or septic shock, because mortality increases in a linear fashion with each hour of delay. All efforts should be made to obtain appropriate cultures, in particular at least two sets of blood cultures. At least one of these should be peripheral, with the second from any long-term (>48 hours) vascular device. Cultures of urine, sputum, wounds, abscesses, and cerebrospinal fluid should also be obtained as appropriate and before the administration of antibiotics, assuming that such specimens can be obtained during the first hour. Specific antibiotic choices are discussed later.

SOURCE CONTROL

A survey for potential sources of infection should be performed, and early resuscitation efforts should occur concomitantly. Elimination of the source of infection is critical to reversing septic shock. Conditions that require emergent intervention, such as necrotizing fasciitis, cholangitis, and intestinal infarction, should be ruled out within the first 6 hours after presentation. Potentially infected indwelling devices should be removed as soon as possible. Necrotic tissue should be débrided and abscesses drained if either condition is detected. Practitioners must consider the risks and benefits of the specific invasive procedures and the timing of such interventions for each patient individually. Every effort should be made to limit the invasiveness of necessary procedures, to avoid further stress in patients with an already hemodynamically fragile state. Imaging studies such as computed tomography of the head, chest, abdomen, and pelvis are necessary to identify or rule out potential sources of infection. An exception to the mandate to drain or débride infected collections is the presence of infected pancreatic necrosis, in which case surgical intervention should be delayed.

OTHER INTERVENTIONS

After hemodynamic parameters have been stabilized with fluid and vasopressors, cultures have been obtained, antibiotics have been administered, and initial source control of infected foci has been achieved, other interventions may be appropriate. Many of these are typical components of good critical care.

---

[1]Not FDA approved for this indication.

CURRENT THERAPY SUMMARY

Initial Six Hours

- Initiate fluid resuscitation with crystalloid or colloid to achieve central venous pressure of 12 mm Hg (or 15 mm Hg if intubated).
- Add dopamine (Intropin) or norepinephrine (Levophed) for persistent hypotension (mean arterial pressure <65 mm Hg).
- Obtain blood, urine, and other appropriate cultures (cerebrospinal fluid, abscess drainage, catheter tip, tissue, sputum).
- Administer empiric antimicrobial therapy.
- Perform appropriate imaging studies with urgent source control as indicated and allowed by clinical status; remove potentially infected foreign bodies.
- All interventions should be undertaken simultaneously and initiated within 1 hour after making a presumptive diagnosis of sepsis.

Subsequent Interventions

- Maintain glycemic control with a target blood glucose level of less than 150 mg/dL.
- Use unfractionated or low-molecular-weight heparin for prophylaxis against deep venous thrombosis.
- Use a histamine 2 (H_2) blocker or proton pump inhibitor for gastric ulcer prophylaxis.
- Initiate therapy with dobutamine (Dobutrex) for low cardiac output in the face of adequate filling pressures.
- Consider therapy with activated protein C (drotrecogin alfa [Xigris]) for patients with an Acute Physiology and Chronic Health Evaluation (APACHE) II score of 25 or greater.
- Consider therapy with hydrocortisone (Solu-Cortef)[1] for patients with continued hypotension despite adequate fluid resuscitation and vasopressors.
- Achieve adequate sedation.

---

[1]Not FDA approved for this indication.

Cardiac Dysfunction

Patients who have adequate left ventricular filling pressures (as determined by a central venous pressure ≥12 mm Hg) but low cardiac output may benefit from therapy with dobutamine (Dobutrex) to increase cardiac output and improve tissue perfusion.

Corticosteroid Therapy

Activation of the hypothalamic-pituitary axis and the consequent increase in serum cortisol levels are vital aspects of the body's acute stress response to shock. Recent data suggest that critical illness–related corticosteroid insufficiency is more prevalent in septic shock than previously thought, with rates as high as 60%. Therapy with corticosteroids is indicated only for those patients who have continued hypotension in the face of adequate fluid resuscitation and vasopressor support. Hydrocortisone (Solu-Cortef)[1] should be administered intravenously 200–300 mg/day for seven days either divided every 6 hours or as a continuous infusion. Dexamethasone (Decadron)[1] should not be used unless hydrocortisone is not available. Because of the unclear long-term benefits and the known immunosuppressive side effects of corticosteroids, patients should

---

[1]Not FDA approved for this indication.

be weaned from hydrocortisone as soon as vasopressors are no longer necessary. If another form of corticosteroid other than hydrocortisone is used, then fludrocortisone (Florinef)[1] at a dose of 50 mcg/day should be added for mineralocorticoid effect.

Activated Protein C

Patients who are at increased risk of death with Acute Physiology and Chronic Health Evaluation (APACHE) II scores of 25 or higher and those with multiple organ dysfunction may benefit from infusion of activated protein C (drotrecogin alfa [Xigris]). This drug has numerous contraindications, including current active bleeding, recent (within 3 months) hemorrhagic stroke, recent (within 2 months) severe head trauma or intracranial or intraspinal surgery, trauma with a risk of life-threatening bleeding, presence of an epidural catheter, and intracranial neoplasm or mass lesion or evidence of herniation. It is not recommended for use in children. It is given as a 96-hour continuous infusion.

Glycemic Control

Maintenance of the blood glucose concentration lower than 150 mg/dL is associated with decreased mortality and length of stay in the intensive care unit. Control should be achieved with intravenous insulin, paying close attention to serum glucose levels every 1 to 2 hours until stable, with adjustments made on the basis of a validated protocol. Patients receiving intravenous insulin should simultaneously receive some form of glucose as a calorie source to minimize the risk of hypoglycemia.

Sedation and Paralytics

Sedation and treatment of pain should be aggressively managed according to validated protocols. Daily interruption of sedation allows for more accurate titration of drug and decreases the total time of mechanical ventilation. Paralytics should be avoided or used only briefly if required.

---

[1]Not FDA approved for this indication.

Anticoagulation

Patients should receive prophylaxis for deep venous thrombosis with either low-molecular-weight heparin or unfractionated heparin unless contraindicated by severe thrombocytopenia, recent intracranial bleeding, or coagulopathy. Those patients who cannot receive heparin should receive prophylaxis with graduated compression stockings or intermittent compression devices. Patients who are at especially high risk for deep venous thrombosis (e.g., prior history of clot, orthopedic surgery, trauma) should receive both pharmacologic and mechanical prophylaxis. Low-molecular-weight heparin is preferred to unfractionated heparin in high-risk patients.

Ulcer Prophylaxis

Patients should receive prophylaxis with a proton pump inhibitor or a histamine 2 (H$_2$) blocker to prevent upper gastrointestinal bleeding.

Bicarbonate Therapy

There is no role for the administration of bicarbonate to correct acidosis or improve hemodynamic status.

ANTIBIOTICS

Antibiotic choices should take into account the most likely pathogens for the suspected site or process. In general, initial empiric therapy (Table 1) should be broad, with an intention to narrow therapy once a microorganism has been isolated or a more precise clinical diagnosis has been made. Such a reevaluation should take place approximately 72 hours after the initiation of therapy. Numerous studies have documented the mortality associated with initial therapy that did not include agents active against the pathogen eventually isolated. In general, drugs from the β-lactam and related classes of antibiotics should be preferred for at least a part of most empiric regimens.

Special considerations include patients with neutropenia and fever, who should always be treated with at least one agent active against *Pseudomonas*. Some debate continues regarding the use of

TABLE 1 Empiric Antibiotic Choices for Severe Sepsis*

Source	Antibiotic and Dose	Comments
Community-acquired pneumonia	Ceftriaxone (Rocephin) 2 g q24h *plus* azithromycin (Zithromax) 500 mg q24h	Should include atypical coverage; alternative is moxifloxacin (Avelox)
Health care–associated pneumonia	Piperacillin/tazobactam (Zosyn) 4.5 g q6h *or* meropenem (Merrem)[1] 2 g q8h[3] *plus* vancomycin (Vancocin)[1] 1 g q12h	Should cover for *Pseudomonas* and other resistant gram-negative rods
Neutropenia/fever	Piperacillin/tazobactam[1] 4.5 g q6h *or* meropenem[1] 2 g q8h[3]	Consider empiric fungal coverage for prolonged neutropenia
Abdominal sepsis	Ampicillin/sulbactam (Unasyn) 3 g q6h *or* piperacillin/tazobactam 4.5 g q6h	Consider coverage for yeast, MRSA
Urosepsis	Ampicillin/sulbactam[1] 3 g q6h *or* piperacillin/tazobactam[1] 4.5 g q6h	Obtain imaging and decompression as appropriate
Foreign body/vascular catheter–related sepsis	Piperacillin/tazobactam[1] 4.5 g q6h *or* meropenem[1] 2 g q8h[3] *plus* vancomycin 1 g q12h	Vascular catheters or other foreign bodies should be removed urgently
Meningitis	Ceftriaxone 2 g q12h *plus* vancomycin[1] 750 mg q8h *plus* rifampin (Rifadin)[1] 600 mg q24h	Consider steroid therapy before or simultaneously with administration of antibiotics
Soft-tissue infection	Cefazolin (Ancef) 2 g q8h *plus* vancomycin 1 g q12h	Image for abscess with débridement as appropriate
Necrotizing fasciitis	Ampicillin/sulbactam 3 g q6h *plus* vancomycin 1 g q12h *plus* clindamycin (Cleocin) 900 mg q8h	Obtain urgent surgical consultation
Unknown	Piperacillin/tazobactam 4.5 g q6h *or* meropenem 2 g q8h[3] *plus* vancomycin 1 g q12h *plus* tobramycin (Tobrex) 7 mg/kg q24h	Obtain appropriate imaging studies, especially of abdomen, pelvis, central nervous system

[1]Not FDA approved for this indication.
[3]Exceeds dosage recommended by the manufacturer.
*In all cases, prior antimicrobial therapy, kidney and liver dysfunction, and the probable source of sepsis should be carefully considered. Always consider coverage for methicillin-resistant *Staphylococcus aureus* (MRSA) in areas where incidence in bloodstream isolates is >10%.

two anti-pseudomonal drugs as part of the initial antibiotic regimen. Given the possibility of resistance on the part of this pathogen, it would seem reasonable to use two drugs initially, until *Pseudomonas* has been isolated (if present) and its susceptibilities are known, allowing coverage to be narrowed. The Surviving Sepsis Campaign guidelines advocate this approach. There is no benefit in treating with two drugs known to be active in an attempt to achieve a supposed synergy.

Patients with hematologic malignancies are at increased risk for sepsis from fungal organisms. Severe sepsis or septic shock in such patients warrants empiric treatment with an echinocandin, a broad-spectrum azole such as voriconazole (Vfend) or posaconazole (Noxafil), or amphotericin (Fungizone).

MRSA continues to increase in incidence nationally and is now common as a community-acquired pathogen. It is also to be suspected as a cause of postinfluenza bacterial pneumonia. Empiric treatment with an antibiotic active against this bacterium, such as vancomycin (Vancocin), linezolid (Zyvox), or daptomycin (Cubicin), should be strongly considered in septic patients in communities where the rate of MRSA in bloodstream infections exceeds 10%. This pathogen should always be considered in a patient with a long-term intravenous catheter, prosthetic device, or other indwelling foreign body. Although vancomycin-resistant *S. aureus* is extremely rare, caution should be taken when using daptomycin and linezolid as empiric therapy, because resistance has been reported.

Prior administration of antibiotics and the attendant risk of infection by a pathogen resistant to the previous therapy should be considered in arriving at a course of empiric therapy. A typical scenario is a patient who presents with a catheter-related bloodstream infection while taking vancomycin. One would expect a gram-negative bacterium, a fungal organism, or, potentially, a vancomycin-resistant enterococcus as the pathogen. Recent hospitalization or residence in a nursing home places patients at risk for colonization and subsequent infection with resistant gram-negative rods.

Prognosis and Limits of Care

Patients who present with severe sepsis or septic shock often have substantial prior medical morbidity, decreasing their chance of survival. The overall mortality rate remains between 20% and 40%. Patients often have expressed wishes regarding limits of care to family members or others close to them before becoming ill. It is always appropriate to discuss goals of therapy, possible and probable outcomes, and plans for further evaluation and treatment with patients (if possible) and their proxies in all instances. Decisions to proceed with or limit care should be made within the context of a patient's expressed or expected wishes and should take into account unfolding clinical data and circumstances. Time spent in this endeavor can substantially decrease the amount of futile care rendered to a patient and lead to care that more truly reflects the patient's wishes regarding life-prolonging measures. The stress and anxiety experienced by family members may also be reduced.

Substantial progress has been made in the last 3 decades in decreasing the mortality associated with severe sepsis and septic shock. Nevertheless, the mortality rate remains unacceptably high, and the overall incidence and severity of disease appear to be increasing, by as much as 1.5% annually by some estimates. The risk of death for an individual patient appears to stabilize approximately 6 months after the original illness. Many patients who do survive remain with the same risk factors (e.g., diabetes, vascular disease, prosthetic devices, immunosuppression) that contributed to their infection and therefore are at risk for recurrence. Moreover, certain organisms, such as MRSA, resistant gram-negative rods, and fungi, remain difficult to treat, and success rates are relatively low despite aggressive, timely, and prolonged therapy.

There is some cause for optimism. The Surviving Sepsis Campaign has now entered phase III. This is a program in which a core set of recommendations, described in the guidelines, are being implemented with opportunities to measure outcomes, assess physician behavior, and provide feedback to improve survival through evidence-based interventions. This effort involves more than 12,000 patients in 239 hospitals in 17 countries and will undoubtedly change the future course of this lethal disease.

REFERENCES

Bone RC. Immunologic dissonance: A continuing evolution in our understanding of the systemic inflammatory response syndrome (SIRS) and the multiple organ dysfunction syndrome (MODS). Ann Intern Med 1996; 125:680–7.

Delinger RP, Levy MM, Carlet JM, et al. Surviving Sepsis Campaign: Intartonal guidelines for management of severe sepsis and septic shock—2008. Crit Care Med 2008;36:296–327.

Dombrovskiy VY, Martin AA, Sunderram J, Paz HL. Rapid increase in hospitalization and mortality rates for severe sepsis in the United States: A trend analysis from 1993 to 2003. Crit Care Med 2007;35:1244–50.

Ibrahim EH, Sherman G, Ward S, et al. The influence of inadequate antimicrobial treatment of bloodstream infections on patient outcomes in the ICU setting. Chest 2000;118:146–55.

Jimenez MF, Marshall JC. Source control in the management of sepsis. Intensive Care Med 2001;27(Suppl. 1):S49–62.

Kumar A, Roberts D, Wood KE, et al. Duration of hypotension before initiation of effective antimicrobial therapy is the critical determinant of survival in human septic shock. Crit Care Med 2006;34:1589–96.

Leibovici L, Shraga I, Drucker M, et al. The benefit of appropriate empirical antibiotic treatment in patients with bloodstream infection. J Intern Med 1998;244:379–86.

Levy MM, Fink MP, Marshall JC, et al. 2001 SCCM/ESICM/ACCP/ATS/SIS International Sepsis Definitions Conference. Intensive Care Med 2003;29:530–8.

Martin GS, Mannino DM, Easton S, et al. The epidemiology of sepsis in the United States from 1979 through 2000. N Engl J Med 2003;348:1546–54.

McDonald JR, Friedman ND, Stout JE, et al. Risk factors for ineffective therapy in patients with bloodstream infection. Arch Intern Med 2005;165:308–13.

Miller PJ, Wenzel RP. Etiologic organisms as independent predictors of death and morbidity associated with bloodstream infection. J Infect Dis 1987;156:471–7.

Sasse KC, Nauenberg E, Long A, et al. Long-term survival after intensive care unit admission with sepsis. Crit Care Med 1995;23:1040–7.

Brucellosis

Method of
Basak Dokuzoguz, MD, and Nurcan Baykam, MD

Brucellosis is a common bacterial zoonotic disease. It has become more significant in recent years as a bioterrorism agent. Brucellosis is known as a historic disease, and the sequencing of the *Brucella melitensis* genome was completed in 2002.

Etiology

The disease is caused by bacteria of the genus *Brucella*, which are nonmotile, gram-negative, aerobic, unencapsulated cocci or short rods. *Brucella* species are divided into six subtypes based on the main host animals (Table 1). Of these, *B. abortus*, *B. melitensis*, *B. suis*, and *B. canis* are known human pathogens. Two new species, provisionally called *B. pinnipediae* and *B. cetaceae*, have been shown to cause human diseases.

Epidemiology

Brucellosis is one of the major zoonotic diseases and occurs all over the world. Some countries in Europe and North America have achieved control and prevention of the disease based on vaccination

TABLE 1 Subtypes and Hosts of *Brucella* Species

Species	Host Animal	Human
B. abortus	Cows, camels, yaks, buffalo	+
B. melitensis	Goats, sheep, camels	+
B. suis	Pigs, wild hares, caribou, reindeer, wild rodents	+
B. canis	Canines	+
B. neotomae	Rodents	−
B. ovis	Sheep	−
B. pinnipediae	Minke whales, dolphins	+
B. cetaceae	Seals	+

programs. However, brucellosis remains endemic in other parts of the world, especially in the Mediterranean, the Middle East, Central Asia, Africa, and Latin America. The real incidence of the disease is not known because underreporting of the disease is believed to be common.

The most common causes of human brucellosis are reported as *B. melitensis* followed by *B. abortus*. The biotypes of *Brucella* species vary by geographic region.

The disease is transmitted to humans by direct contact with infected animals, by ingestion of raw or unpasteurized milk and milk products, through cuts and abrasions, or by inhalation of aerosols. It is an occupational disease of farmers, veterinarians, slaughterhouse workers, and health care workers, especially laboratory staff. Some individual cases occur as a result of ingesting contaminated dairy products, handling infected animal tissue or body fluids, or handling aborted animal fetuses and placentas. However, the transmission route for outbreaks is usually inhalation of aerosols. Human-to-human transmission of brucellosis is very rare, but there are a few case reports of humans infected through sexual contact, transplacental transmission, or transplantation.

Pathogenesis

The *Brucella* species are pathogenic for humans and animals. *Brucella* species prefer to survive and multiply within phagocytic cells of the host. Unlike other pathogenic bacteria, they do not have classic virulence factors such as exotoxins, cytolysins, capsules, fimbria, plasmids, and endotoxic lipopolysaccharides. Instead of these factors, the bacteria have molecular determinants that are necessary for cell invasion and survival in the cellular compartment. The major one of these molecular determinants is S lipopolysaccharide (S LPS).

The bacteria are phagocytosed by M cells, macrophages, and neutrophils after invasion of mucosa. Fc receptors, complement, lectin, and fibronectin receptors mediate the bacteria for internalization. Most intracellular *Brucella* species are eliminated in phagolysosomes, but some of them reproduce in the acidic compartment. The intracellular mechanism of the organism is not completely described, but intracellular replication of bacteria does not destroy the cell or the cell's function. Replication of *Brucella* spp. within human osteoblastic cell lines can directly mount a proinflammatory response which may have a role in the chronic inflammation and bone/joint destruction in osteoarticular brucellosis.

After they are taken up by local tissue lymphocytes, the bacteria disseminate into the circulation, and with tropism to the reticuloendothelial system, they become localized within bone marrow, liver, spleen, and lymph nodes. The characteristic feature of the disease is the formation of granulomas in these tissues.

As a host humoral immune response to the disease, the titers of IgM antibodies increase within the first week of infection, and IgG synthesis follows after the second week. Cell-mediated immunity is probably the main mechanism for recovery from the infection.

Clinical Features

Human brucellosis is a multisystem disease that can manifest with a broad spectrum of clinical features. The musculoskeletal, genital, cardiac, respiratory, and nervous systems are involved. The definition and the classification of cases recommended by the World Health Organization (WHO) is presented in Box 1. Some authors classify the disease course as acute, subacute, or chronic, but such a classification has no clinical significance.

The onset of symptoms can be insidious or acute after the incubation period, which is 2 to 8 weeks. A broad spectrum of symptoms such as fever, headache, back pain, weakness, profuse sweating, chills, depression, and joint pain can be observed. These symptoms can also mimic various infectious and noninfectious diseases. Usually an undulant fever pattern is accompanied by so much sweating that the patient needs to change clothes frequently. On the other hand, the physical examination might not reveal any specific finding (Table 2). In children, the range of clinical signs and symptoms may be different than in adults, because children have fewer constitutional symptoms but more hepatic and splenic involvement.

Hepatomegaly, elevated transaminase levels, and granulomatous lesions are the presentations of hepatic involvement in brucellosis. The most common complication of brucellosis is osteoarticular disease, which occurs as peripheral arthritis, sacroiliitis, and spondylitis. This complication is reported in 10% to 80% of cases, and this range may be related to the age and genetic predisposition (HLA-B39) of patients and the infecting *Brucella* species. Genitourinary system involvements exist in 2% to 20% of patients with brucellosis.

BOX 1 Recommended Case Definitions and Classifications by the World Health Organization

Clinical Description

An illness characterized by acute or insidious onset, with continued, intermittent, or irregular fever of variable duration; profuse sweating, particularly at night; fatigue; anorexia; weight loss; headache; arthralgia and generalized aching. Local infection of various organs can occur.

Laboratory Criteria for Diagnosis

- Isolation of *Brucella* spp. from clinical specimen *or*
- Brucella agglutination titer (e.g., standard tube agglutination tests: STA>160) in one or more serum specimens obtained after onset of symptoms *or*
- ELISA (IgA, IgG, IgM), 2-mercaptoethanol test, complement fixation test, Coombs' test, fluorescent antibody test (FAB), radioimmunoassay for detecting antilipopolysaccharide antibodies, counterimmunoelectrophoresis (CIE)

Case Classification

Suspected

A case that is compatible with the clinical description and is epidemiologically linked to suspected or confirmed animal cases or contaminated animal products.

Probable

A suspected case that has a positive rose bengal test.

Confirmed

A suspected or probable case that is laboratory confirmed.

Abbreviations: ELISA = enzyme-linked immunosorbent assay; Ig = immunoglobulin.

TABLE 2 Clinical Presentation and Laboratory Findings of Human Brucellosis

Feature	Percentage
Signs and Symptoms	
Fever	72–91
Constitutive symptoms (e.g., malaise, arthralgias)	26–90
Hepatic involvement	17–31
Splenomegaly	14–16
Osteoarticular involvement	9–22
CNS disorder	3–13
Lymphadenopathy	2–7
Genitourinary involvement	1–5.7
Respiratory disorders	0.2–6
Cardiovascular disorders	0.4–1.8
Skin rashes	0.4–3
Laboratory Findings	
Hematologic	
Relative lymphocytosis	40
Anemia	31
Leukopenia	2–27
Thrombocytopenia	5–15
Pancytopenia	2
Biochemistry	
Elevated transaminase	24–31

Data derived from Aygen B, Doganay M, Sümerkan B, et al: Clinical manifestations, complications and treatment of brucellosis: An evaluation of 480 patients. Med Mal Infect 2002;32:485–493; Dokuzoguz B, Ergonul O, Baykam N, et al: Characteristics of *B. melitensis* versus *B. abortus* bacteremias. J Infect 2005;50(1):1–5; Pappas G, Akritidis N, Bosikovski M, Tsianos E: Brucellosis. N Engl J Med 2005;352:2325–2336.
Abbreviation: CNS = central nervous system.

Prostatitis, epididymo-orchitis, cystitis, pyelonephritis, interstitial nephritis, exudative glomerulonephritis, and renal abscess are the clinical manifestations of this complication. Neurobrucellosis can develop at any stage of disease and can have widely variable manifestations, including encephalitis, meningoencephalitis, radiculitis, myelitis, peripheral and cranial neuropathies, subarachnoid hemorrhage, and psychiatric manifestations. Brucellosis can cause a variety of ocular lesions and different types of skin rash that are nonspecific and reported rarely. Another rare (<2%) but severe complication of brucellosis is endocarditis, which most often involves the aortic valve and requires surgery. Mortality from brucellosis is rare and is usually related to endocarditis.

Diagnosis

The absolute diagnosis of brucellosis is based on identification of bacteria from blood, bone marrow, and materials from affected organs such as cerebrospinal fluid, liver, lymph nodes, synovial fluid, or prostatic fluid by culture. The rate of bacteria isolation from the blood is between 15% and 70%. Lysis centrifugation technique and automated systems improve the range of culture positivity. Lysis centrifugation technique is inexpensive and easier method which can be used in laboratories with limited expertise or equipment if all safety precautions are taken.

Compatible clinical findings with a serum agglutinin titer of at least 1/160 in the standard tube agglutination test (STA) have diagnostic value. In endemic areas, the titer of at least 1/320 is recommended in the diagnosis. False-negative results of STA may be attributed to blocking antibodies; results can be improved by testing with 2-mercaptoethanol or antihuman immunoglobulin. Negative results in the early phase of the disease can be overcome by repeating the test after 2 weeks. Diagnosis of *B. canis* infection is unavailable with routine STA. False-positive results may be related to cross-reactions of some gram-negative bacterial infections.

CURRENT DIAGNOSIS

- The common symptoms of brucellosis, which can also mimic various infectious and noninfectious diseases, are fever, headache, back pain, weakness, profuse sweating, chills, depression, and joint pain.
- The absolute diagnosis of brucellosis is based on identification of bacteria from blood, bone marrow, and materials of affected organs such as cerebrospinal fluid, liver, lymph nodes, synovial fluid, and prostatic fluid by culture.
- Compatible clinical findings with a serum agglutinin titer of $\geq 1/160$ in the standard tube agglutination test (STA) have diagnostic value.

CURRENT THERAPY

- The treatment requires combined regimens for their synergistic effect plus agents with good penetration capacity into the macrophages.
- At least 6 weeks of therapy may be extended to 6 months, according to the complications of the disease.
- Rifampin (Rifadin)[1] plus doxycycline (Vibramycin) treatment is a favorable regimen and the most synergistic one.
- Rifampin may be replaced by streptomycin or gentamycin (Garamycin)[1] as the first-line therapy choice.
- Combinations with trimethoprim-sulfamethoxazole (TMP-SMX; Bactrim)[1] is usually recommended in the second-line treatment regimens.
- Quinolones[1] are alternative drugs in cases with side effects due to first-line drugs and relapses.
- Rifampin in a combination with TMP-SMX[1] or an aminoglycoside are the main regimens for children younger than 8 years.
- Rifampin and TMP-SMX[1] combination is preferred in pregnancy
- Although the use of ceftriaxone (Rocephin)[1] is controversial in brucellosis, it could be preferred in the treatment of central nervous system involvement.
- Rifampin[1] (600–900 mg qd) plus doxycycline (100 mg bid) regimen for 2–3 weeks is recommended as postexposure prophylaxis.

[1]Not FDA approved for this indication.

Enzyme-linked immunosorbent assay (ELISA) is another serologic test that has higher specificity and sensitivity compared with STA. Although it is not used in current clinical practice because of standardization problems, polymerase chain reaction (PCR) is a promising diagnostic tool in brucellosis. Duration of diagnosis can be shortened by automated culture systems and PCR techniques. Rose bengal and a new dipstick test are also rapid tests useful for early diagnosis, but positive results should be confirmed by STA.

Treatment

Because the *Brucella* species are intracellular pathogens, treatment requires not only combined regimens for their synergistic effect but also agents with good penetration into the macrophages. For success

TABLE 3 Drug Combinations Used to Treat Brucellosis

Generic Name (Trade Name)	Adult Dose	Pediatric Dose	Dose Adjustment		Adverse Effects
			Renal Failure	Hepatic Insuffiency	
Ciprofloxacin[1] (Cipro)	500–750 mg PO q12h *or* 400 mg IV q8–12h	Not suggested	Necessary	No change	Drug fever, rash, seizures, Achilles tendon rupture or tendinitis
Doxycycline (Vibramycin, Vibra-tabs)	100 mg PO q12h	2.2–4.4 mg/kg[3] PO div q12h (≥ 8 y)	No change	No change	Nausea, vomiting, eosinophilia, photosensitivity
Gentamicin[1] (Garamycin)	2 mg/kg IM/IV q8h *or* 5 mg/kg IM/IV q24h[1] *or* 240 mg q24h	2.5 mg/kg q8–12h IM/IV	Necessary	No change blockade (rapid infusion)	Ototoxicity, nephrotoxicity, neuromuscular
Ofloxacin[1] (Floxin, Oflox)	400 mg PO bid	Not suggested	Necessary	Moderate: no change Severe: necessary	Drug fever, rash, mild neuroexcitatory symptoms
Rifampin[1] (Rifadin, Rimactane)	600–900 mg PO qd	20 mg/kg PO qd Do not exceed 600 mg qd	No change	Moderate: caution Severe: avoid	Red/orange discoloration of body secretions, flu-like symptoms, elevated AST/ALT, drug fever, rash, thrombocytopenia
Streptomycin	15 mg/kg IM q24h *or* 1 g IM qd for 2–3 wk	20–40 mg/kg IM qd	Necessary	No change	Ototoxic, nephrotoxic
TMP-SMX[1] (Bactrim, Septra)	1 DS tab PO q12h (160 mg TMP/800 mg SMX)	Do not exceed 1 g qd 8–12 mg/kg TMP PO q12h	Necessary; avoid use	No change	Folate deficiency, hyperkalemia, leukopenia, thrombocytopenia, hemolytic anemia ± G6PD, aplastic anemia, elevated AST/ALT, hypersensitivity reactions (Stevens-Johnson syndrome, erythema multiforme)

[1]Not FDA approved for this indication.
[3]Exceeds dosage recommended by the manufacturer.
Abbreviations: ALT = alanine aminotransferase; AST = aspartate aminotransferase; DS = double strength; G6PD = glucose-6-phosphate dehydrogenase; TMP-SMX = trimethoprim-sulfamethoxazole.

of the therapy, adequate duration of drug therapy is another important factor. At least 6 weeks of drug therapy is recommended by the WHO. This duration may be extended to 6 months, depending on such complications of the disease as neurobrucellosis, spondylodiskitis, and abscessers.

The drug combinations listed in Table 3 are widely used in brucellosis. Rifampin (Rifadin)[1] plus doxycycline (Vibramycin) treatment for human brucellosis was recommended by WHO two decades ago; it is still a favorable regimen and was found to be the most synergistic one. Rifampin may be replaced by streptomycin or gentamycin (Garamycin)[1] as first-line therapy choices. According to a recently reported meta-analysis, doxycycline-streptomycin resulted in a significantly higher rate of failure than doxycycline-rifampicin-aminoglycoside regimen. Combinations with trimethoprim-sulfamethoxazole (TMP-SMX, Bactrim)[1] is usually recommended in second-line treatment regimens. Combination rifampin plus a quinolone[1] is not preferred in the initial therapeutic regimen because of the reported decreased activity in pH 5 and lack of synergism between quinolones and other antibiotics that are used in brucellosis. Quinolones are alternative drugs for patients who have relapses or who have side effects from first-line drugs.

Rifampin[1] in combination with TMP-SMX[1] or an aminoglycoside are the main regimens for children younger than 8 years. The rifampin and TMP-SMX combination may be prescribed for pregnant patients.

Although the use of ceftriaxone (Rocephin)[1] is controversial in brucellosis, it may be preferred for treating central nervous system involvement. Because their activity is decreased in an acidic environment, macrolides are not used in brucellosis treatment.

Because there are no significantly important resistance problems for antibiotics targeted to *Brucella* species, susceptibility tests are not recommended routinely except in epidemiologic studies and for some rare recurrent cases. Most of the recurrences are related to non-compliance or to short duration of therapy. In tuberculosis-endemic populations, community-acquired rifampin resistance should be taken into consideration in treating brucellosis.

Supportive therapy might be useful depending on the clinical situation. The cognitive and emotional disturbances in neurobrucellosis can be improved by antibiotics without any antidepressant or antipsychotic therapy.

In the management of *Brucella* endocarditis, medical treatment alone is often effective in patients with early diagnosis and no cardiac failure. However, in most cases, surgery is required in addition to medical treatment.

Prevention

Various vaccines have been applied to humans in some countries in the 20th century, but an acceptable vaccine has not yet been developed for humans. Although investigations of the *B. melitensis* outer membrane protein 25 and cytoplasmic protein BP26 are promising for future vaccine development, prevention of the disease in humans is related to controlling and eliminating animal brucellosis. In this respect, vaccination and slaughter programs of animals, pasteurization of milk and milk products, and education programs about contact precautions for persons at risk must be emphasized.

Because *Brucella* bacteria can be transmitted via the inhalational route, laboratory workers should be warned about the risk, and biosafety level 2 prevention measures should be applied.

---

[1]Not FDA approved for this indication.

Because of laboratory accidents and biological warfare, rifampin[1] (600–900 mg qd) plus doxycycline (100 mg bid) for 2 to 3 weeks is recommended as postexposure prophylaxis.

REFERENCES

Aygen B, Doganay M, Sümerkan B, et al. Clinical manifestations, complications and treatment of brucellosis: An evaluation of 480 patients. Med Mal Infect 2002;32:485–93.

Baykam N, Esener H, Ergonul O, et al. In vitro antimicrobial susceptibility of *Brucella* species. Int J Antimicrob Agents 2004;23(4):405–7.

Bossi P, Tegnell A, Baka A, et al. Bichat guidelines for the clinical management of brucellosis and bioterrorism-related brucellosis. Euro Surveill 2004;9(12):E15–6.

Dokuzoguz B, Ergonul O, Baykam N, et al. Characteristics of B. melitensis versus B. abortus bacteremias. J Infect 2005;50(1):1–5.

Delpino MV, Fossati CA, Baldi PC. Proinflammatory response of human osteoblastic cell lines and osteoblast-monocyte interaction upon infection with Brucella spp. Infect Immun. 2009;77(3):984–95.

Eren S, Bayam G, Ergonul O, et al. Cognitive and emotional changes in neurobrucellosis. J Infect 2006;53:184–9.

Ergonul O, Celikbas A, Tezeren D, et al. Analysis of risk factors for laboratory-acquired *Brucella* infections. J Hosp Infect 2004;56:223–7.

Espinosa BJ, Chacaltana J, Mulder M, et al. Comparison of culture techniques at different stages of brucellosis. Am J Trop Med Hyg 2009;80(4):625–7.

Falagas ME, Bliziotis IA. Quinolones for treatment of human brucellosis: Critical review of the evidence from microbiological and clinical studies. Antimicrob Agents Chemother 2006;50(1):22–33.

Giannacopoulos I, Nikolakopoulou NM, Eliopoulou M, et al. Presentation of childhood brucellosis in Western Greece. Jpn J Infect Dis 2006;59:160–3.

Joint Food and Agriculture Organization/World Health Organization, FAO-WHO Expert Committee on Brucellosis (sixth report). In: WHO Technical Report Series No. 740. Geneva: World Health Organization, 1986. p. 56–7.

Pan American Health Organization. Case definition: Brucellosis, Epidemiol Bull 2000;21(3):13. PDF available at http://www.paho.org/english/dd/ais/EB_v21n3.pdf [accessed 27.04.07].

Pappas G, Akritidis N, Bosilkovski M, Tsianos E. Brucellosis. N Engl J Med 2005;352:2325–36.

Skalsky K, Yahav D, Bishara J, et al. Treatment of human brucellosis: systematic review and meta-analysis of randomised controlled trials. BMJ 2008;336(7676):701–4.

Young EJ. *Brucella* species. In: Mandel GL, Bennett JE, Dolin R, editors. Mandell, Douglas and Bennett's Principles and Practice of Infectious Diseases, 6th ed. Philadelphia: Churchill Livingstone; 2005. p. 2669–72.

---

[1]Not FDA approved for this indication.

Varicella (Chickenpox)

Method of
Charles Grose, MD

Chickenpox is caused by varicella zoster virus (VZV). After chickenpox occurs, VZV enters the sensory nerve and establishes latency in the dorsal root ganglia along the spinal cord. When VZV reactivates in late adulthood, the virus causes the disease known as shingles (herpes zoster).

Pathogenesis of Chickenpox

Chickenpox is an airborne infection. The virus first infects the mucosa tissues of the nose and subsequently establishes an infection in the tonsils or lymph nodes around the neck. After 4 to 6 cycles of replication, the primary viremia occurs (Figure 1). The virus then disperses to multiple organs in the body. After a second period of replication, the second viremia occurs. The virus is carried within lymphocytes in the bloodstream. The vesicular lesions occur after the virus exits the capillaries and enters the epidermis.

Epidemiology after Approval of the Vaccine

The varicella vaccine was approved for administration to children in the United States in 1995, and the vast majority of states have approved the administration of varicella vaccine to all young children. Approximately 4 million cases of chickenpox occurred annually in the United States prior to 1995. There were also approximately 100 deaths annually, the vast majority in otherwise healthy children, and more than 14,000 hospitalizations per year.

More than 10 years later, the effect of universal varicella immunization in the United States is dramatic. The number of hospitalizations and deaths was reduced by 75%. Similarly, the total number of cases of chickenpox in the United States has also decreased dramatically. Nevertheless, more than one half million cases of chickenpox will probably continue to occur annually. These cases will include many immunocompromised children who remain unimmunized.

ADMINISTRATION OF VARICELLA VACCINE

Varicella vaccine is a live attenuated virus. Each dose of vaccine (0.5 mL) is administered subcutaneously. The virus must replicate in the infected child for an immune response to occur (Figure 2). The initial virus replication can cause a few vesicles near the site of infection. The replication can also lead to a viremia with a short-lived rash anywhere on the body. The vaccine virus can, in very few cases, replicate to a sufficient extent that the infection transfers to another person who will subsequently develop a mild case of vaccine-related chickenpox. In 1995, a single dose of varicella vaccine was originally recommended. As of 2007, two doses of varicella vaccine are recommended for every child. The first dose is given between 12 and 15 months. The second dose is routinely recommended between 4 and 6 years. Instead of single-dose vials of vaccine (Varivax), the vaccine can also be administered as a component of the 4-in-1 vials of measles-mumps-rubella-varicella vaccine (Pro Quad). This approach reduces the number of injections given to a child. Children 13 years and above, who have never received varicella vaccine, should be given 2 doses of vaccine (Varivax), separated by a 4-week interval.

RISK FACTORS FOR BREAKTHROUGH CHICKENPOX

Breakthrough chickenpox refers to a wild-type chickenpox that is usually a mild illness with less than 50 vesicles that occurs in children given varicella vaccine at least 42 days previously. Thus, breakthrough chickenpox is a form of vaccine failure. Breakthrough chickenpox was believed to be relatively uncommon during the prelicensure clinical studies. However, by 2000 it was apparent that breakthrough chickenpox was not a rare event. Several reports documented large outbreaks of wild-type chickenpox in immunized children who were attending large daycare facilities or grade schools.

A major risk factor is believed to be immunization with one dose of vaccine. The 2-dose regimen of varicella vaccine should eliminate most cases of breakthrough chickenpox.

 CURRENT DIAGNOSIS

- Diagnosis of chickenpox is usually made by observation or rash.
- Diagnosis is confirmed by a rapid viral diagnosis kit performed on a vesicle smear.
- Diagnosis of past varicella infection is made by serology.
- Commercial antibody kits may not be sensitive enough to detect serum antibody after varicella vaccination.

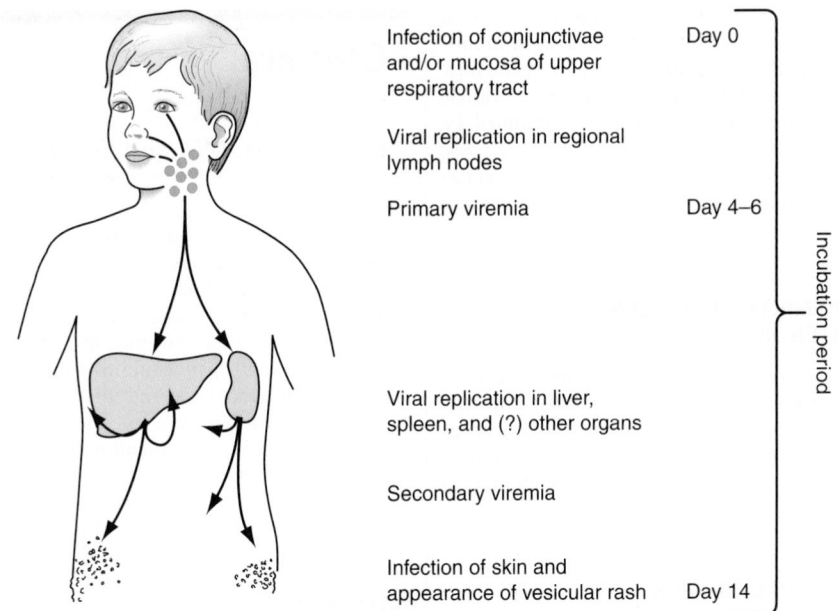

FIGURE 1. Diagrammatic representation of the pathogenesis of acute varicella infection. There are two viremias during the 14-day incubation period. The first viremia occurs after local replication at the site of infection. The typical chickenpox rash appears at the end of the second viremia. See Grose (2005) for a more detailed description.

Infection of conjunctivae and/or mucosa of upper respiratory tract — Day 0

Viral replication in regional lymph nodes

Primary viremia — Day 4–6

Viral replication in liver, spleen, and (?) other organs

Secondary viremia

Infection of skin and appearance of vesicular rash — Day 14

Incubation period

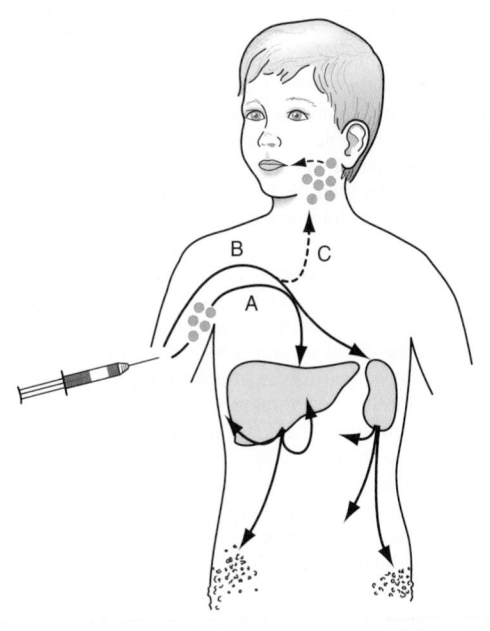

FIGURE 2. Pathways of infection following administration of varicella vaccine. Pathway A shows a rash that sometimes appears at the site of injection after local replication of the virus. Pathway B shows a viremia with appearance of a few small papulovesicular lesions on the skin distant from the site of injection. Pathway C shows the virus as it travels to the respiratory tract where infection can be spread on rare occasions to other individuals. See Grose (2005) for a more detailed description.

Treatment

TREATMENT OF SEVERE CHICKENPOX IN HEALTHY CHILDREN

Chickenpox is considered a more severe disease in children younger than 1 year and in postpubertal adolescents. VZV is highly susceptible to acyclovir and two second-generation antiviral agents: famciclovir (Famvir) and valacyclovir (Valtrex). Acyclovir is now a generic drug and very economic. Every case of chickenpox in a child younger than 1 year should be treated with acyclovir. The oral dosage is 20 mg/kg four times a day for 5 to 7 days. Chickenpox in children older than 1 year can also be treated with acyclovir to reduce the severity and duration of disease. The maximum dosage is 800 mg four times a day. Acyclovir is available in a liquid suspension and tablets containing 200, 400, or 800 mg. The 800-mg tablet is very large and may be difficult for some children to swallow.

Famciclovir (Famvir) or valacyclovir (Valtrex) are the preferred antiviral agents for adolescents because these are better adsorbed than acyclovir. However, they are much more expensive. The dosage of famciclovir (Famvir) is 500 mg orally three times a day. The dosage of valacyclovir (Valtrex) is 1 g three times a day. For most adolescents, a 5-day regimen should be sufficient treatment.

TREATMENT OF CHICKENPOX IN CHILDREN WITH AN UNDERLYING IMMUNODEFICIENCY

Children with HIV infection who contract chickenpox can usually be managed with oral acyclovir treatment as long as their HIV is under control. The majority of children diagnosed with acute chickenpox who have cancer or have undergone organ transplantation should be considered for admission to the hospital and begin immediate treatment with intravenous (IV) acyclovir. The dosage of IV acyclovir is 10 mg/kg every 8 hours. The dosage can be raised to 15 mg/kg every 8 hours in patients presenting varicella pneumonia or varicella encephalitis. The serum creatinine level should be monitored daily and the acyclovir dosage adjusted downward if the serum creatinine reaches 1 mg/dL.

CURRENT THERAPY

- Severe chickenpox in infants and immunosuppressed children is treated with intravenous acyclovir (30 mg/kg/d).
- Severe chickenpox in healthy children is treated with oral acyclovir (80 mg/kg/d).
- Severe chickenpox in adolescents is treated with either famciclovir (Famvir) (500 mg tid) or valacyclovir (Valtrex) (1 g tid).
- Prophylaxis following exposure to chickenpox can be managed with a course of oral acyclovir (40 mg/kg/d).

The efficacy of oral famciclovir or valacyclovir is better than oral acyclovir, allowing older children with chickenpox and an immuno-suppressive condition to be discharged more quickly from the hospital. Discharge is generally considered after no new vesicle formation is noted for 24 hours. Antiviral therapy (combined IV and oral) for 10 to 14 days is usually suggested, although each case must be assessed individually. Children who have varicella encephalitis or varicella pneumonia may require more than 2 weeks of antiviral therapy.

TREATMENT OF CHICKENPOX IN CHILDREN RECEIVING CORTICOSTEROIDS

Children receiving high-dose oral corticosteroid treatment for conditions such as acute asthma are also at high risk of severe chickenpox. These children should be treated with antivirals just as aggressively as those with cancer. Children receiving only intermittent inhaled corticosteroids do not appear to be at high risk of severe chickenpox.

TREATMENT OF ZOSTER IN CHILDREN

Zoster in otherwise healthy children is usually a benign illness. The disease is normally improving by the time the diagnosis is made. However, zoster in immunocompromised children may persist for 2 weeks or longer, requiring immediate treatment with one of the oral antiviral drugs recommended. The dosage is the same as for severe chickenpox.

ALTERNATIVES TO VARICELLA-ZOSTER IMMUNE GLOBULIN

Varicella-zoster immune globulin (VZIG) has been given in the past to infants and children with cancer who were exposed to chickenpox. VZIG has been discontinued after 2005. Physicians can consider the administration of IV gammaglobulin as a single infusion of 500 mg/kg for infants who are exposed to varicella shortly after birth. An alternative regimen is oral acyclovir suspension at 40 mg/kg per day divided every 6 hours. Acyclovir should be initiated on the day of exposure and continued for 10 days.

Prophylaxis with oral acyclovir also can be considered for VZV-nonimmune children with cancer after an exposure to chickenpox. The recommended dosage is one half of the therapeutic dosage, meaning oral acyclovir can be given at 40 mg/kg per day. The daily dosage for children who can swallow tablets can be divided three times a day rather than four times a day during the 10-day therapy period. Children who develop chickenpox despite oral acyclovir treatment should be admitted to the hospital for treatment with IV acyclovir at 10 mg/kg every 8 hours. There are extremely few examples of true acyclovir-resistant VZV; most failures are caused by inadequate absorption of the oral formulation.

REFERENCES

Davis MM, Patel MS, Gebremariam A. Decline in varicella-related hospitalizations and expenditures for children and adults after introduction of varicella vaccine in the United States. Pediatrics 2004;114:786–92.

Grose C. Varicella vaccination of children in the United States: Assessment after the first decade, 1995–2005. J Clin Virol 2005;33:89–95.

Grose C, Widerman J. Generic acyclovir vs. famciclovir and valacyclovir. Pediatr Infect Dis J 1997;16:838–41.

Hay M, Kimura H, Oshiro M, et al. Varicella exposure in a neonatal medical center: Successful prophylaxis with oral acyclovir. J Hosp Infect 2003;54:212–5.

Nguyen HQ, Jumaan AO, Seward JF. Decline in mortality due to varicella after implementation of varicella vaccination in the United States. N Engl J Med 2005;352:450–8.

Takahashi M. Effectiveness of live varicella vaccine. Expert Opin Biol Ther 2004;4:199–216.

Cholera

Method of
Carlos Seas, MD, and Eduardo Gotuzzo, MD

Cholera is an ancient scourge recognized since the time of Hippocrates. More accurate descriptions of the disease began approximately in 1817. Since then, cholera has caused seven pandemics, affecting all continents, and it remains endemic in almost all affected areas. Recent examples of severe epidemics are the Latin American extension of the seventh pandemic in Peru in 1991, explosive epidemics among refugees in Africa, and unexpected epidemics of cholera due to a new serogroup in Asia since 1992. We can conclude from these epidemics that it is very difficult to predict when a new epidemic will start, that appropriate treatment reduces the mortality to values less than 1%, and that the pathogen continues to evolve in the environment despite interventions to control its spread.

Etiology

Cholera is caused by a curved gram-negative bacillus that belongs to the family Vibrionaceae. Two serogroups, O1 and O139, are associated with clinical cholera, and both cause the same clinical entity. These serogroups have shown both regional and pandemic potential. *Vibrio cholerae* is a natural inhabitant of certain aquatic environments, where it lives attached to copepods, algae, and crustacean shells in a symbiotic association. If conditions are not favorable for growth, *V. cholerae* adopts a dormant state. In this state it remains metabolically inactive for long periods. The switch to a metabolically active state occurs when conditions become suitable for division. Humans get the infection by consuming contaminated water, beverages, or food. During epidemics, a single source can be identified, but usually multiple routes of transmission play a role simultaneously. Epidemics tend to occur during the warmest months of the year, and association with climate variability and El Niño southern oscillation has been recently documented.

V. cholerae O1 and O139 secrete a number of potent exotoxins that induce the characteristic isotonic dehydration of cholera. The better studied toxin is the cholera toxin, which has two subunits, A and B. The B subunit allows the toxin to attach to a specific receptor present along the small intestine of humans, and the A subunit activates the adenylate cyclase enzyme. The chain of events that follows this enzymatic activation is mediated by cyclic adenosine monophosphate (cAMP) and includes blockage of the absorption of sodium and chloride by the microvillus and promotion of secretion of chloride and water by crypt cells. The result of these events is the massive liberation of water and electrolytes into the intestinal lumen, as shown in Table 1.

CURRENT DIAGNOSIS

- History of travel to an endemic area.
- Acute voluminous watery diarrhea with rice-water appearance, leading to severe dehydration in a matter of hours.
- Muscle cramps, vomiting, and signs of severe dehydration such as loss of skin elasticity (slow skin-pinch retraction), hoarse voice, sunken eyes, and wrinkled hands and feet (washerwoman hands).
- Fever is absent in most patients.
- Milder forms of dehydration cannot be distinguished from other common causes of acute diarrhea.
- Stool culture using proper media is positive for *V. cholerae* O1 or O139. Dark field microscopy of a fresh stool sample can detect the presence of vibrio; specific antisera confirm the serogroup.

TABLE 1 Electrolyte Concentrations (mmol/L)

Substance	Sodium	Chloride	Potassium	Bicarbonate	Osmolality
Cholera Stool					
Adults		130	100	20	44
Children		100	90	33	30
Rehydration Solution					
Ringer's lactate*	130	109	4	28*	271
Normal saline	154	154	0	0	308
Rice-based ORS	75	65	20	10	180
WHO ORS‡	75	65	20	10†	245

*Ringer's lactate contains lactate instead of bicarbonate.
†Bicarbonate is replaced with trisodium citrate, which stays fresh longer than bicarbonate in sachets.
‡Reduced osmolality formula.
Abbreviations: ORS = oral rehydration solution; WHO = World Health Organization.

Treatment

The objectives of therapy are to replace the fluid and electrolyte losses caused by diarrhea and vomiting, to maintain hydration, and to reduce the volume of diarrhea and excretion of vibrios to the environment. The treatment is divided into two phases: the rehydration phase and the maintenance phase.

REHYDRATION PHASE

The objective of the rehydration phase is to replace the losses that occurred before the patient was admitted. This phase begins with a thorough evaluation of the degree of dehydration. Table 2 shows the clinical signs according to the degree of dehydration.

Patients with severe dehydration present with a constellation of signs that reflect a deficit of at least 10% of body weight. The pulse is feeble and very rapid, the blood pressure is not measurable, the skin elasticity is lost, the eyes are sunken, and the voice is inaudible or hoarse. The intravenous route is recommended for rehydrating all patients with severe dehydration. The rate and speed of the infusion is recommended at 50 to 100 mL/kg/hour for the first 2 to 4 hours. After this time, the patient must be fully rehydrated to begin the maintenance phase. The preferred intravenous solution is Ringer's lactate solution. If this solution is not available, normal saline may be used, but the recovery from metabolic acidosis is less efficient. Oral rehydration solutions (ORS) should be started as soon as possible in these patients.

Milder forms of dehydration due to cholera cannot be clinically distinguished from other common causes of acute diarrhea. Symptoms due to some degree of dehydration are seen when water deficit is greater than 5% of body weight. The intravenous route may be used in these patients if the stool output is high (<10–20 mL/kg/hour) or if the patient does not tolerate the oral route. The great majority of patients with milder forms of dehydration can be rehydrated by the oral route.

Laboratory abnormalities in patients with severe cholera reflect hemoconcentration and include a high hematocrit, increase in white blood cell count, azotemia, and elevation of specific gravity and total proteins. These laboratory parameters are good indicators of the degree of dehydration on admission, but they are not useful for following the rehydration status. Metabolic acidosis with a high anion gap is typically seen in patients with severe cholera. Hypokalemia or normal values (due to acidosis) and normal or low serum sodium and chloride are also observed in these patients. Hyperglycemia results from high levels of epinephrine, glucagon, and cortisol stimulated by hypovolemia. Hypoglycemia is rare but carries a poor prognosis, particularly in children.

MAINTENANCE PHASE

The maintenance phase begins when the patient has been fully rehydrated. A good indicator of the recovery of the normal hydration status is not only the absence of clinical signs of dehydration but also the volume of urine output. Urine outputs greater than 0.5 mL/kg/hour are expected in fully hydrated patients. The maintenance phase has the objective of preserving the normal hydration status, and it lasts until the diarrhea abates.

The oral route is advised for the maintenance phase, and the ORS recommended by the World Health Organization (WHO) is the preferred oral solution. Recently, WHO has promoted the use of ORS with lower osmolality (75 mmol/L of sodium and total osmolality of 245 mOsm/L vs. the former solution containing 90 mmol/L of sodium and total osmolality of 311 mOsm/L) to treat all kinds of acute diarrheal diseases. Adults should be observed for hyponatremia when using this reduced-osmolality ORS. ORS uses the principle of common transportation of solutes, electrolytes, and water not affected by cholera in the intestine. ORS containing rice instead of glucose is also preferred, because the purging rate is lower with solutions containing rice than with glucose-based solutions. If ORS in packets is not available, a solution can be made with 2.6 g sodium chloride, 2.9 g sodium citrate, 1.5 g potassium chloride, and 13.5 g glucose or 50 g rice powder to 1 L of boiled water.

The amount of oral fluids should match the ongoing losses to prevent dehydration during this phase. Periodic review of the patient's chart is advised for this purpose. Predesigned forms to register intake and output and vital signs should be available to monitor the hydration status regularly. Cholera cots or cholera chairs facilitate the collection and measurement of stools and urine during treatment.

TABLE 2 Clinical Findings by Degree of Dehydration

Clinical Finding	Degree of Dehydration	
	Some	**Severe**
Loss of fluid (% of body weight)	5%–10%	>10%
Mentation	Restless	Drowsy or comatose
Radial pulse rate	Rapid	Very rapid
Radial pulse intensity	Weak	Feeble or impalpable
Respiration	Normal or deep	Deep and rapid
Systolic blood pressure	Low	Very low or undetectable
Skin elasticity	Retracts slowly	Retracts very slowly
Eyes	Sunken	Very sunken
Voice	Hoarse	Not audible
Urine production	Scant	Oliguria

CURRENT THERAPY

- Identify the degree of dehydration on admission.
- Register the intake and output regularly in predesigned charts.
- Rehydrate the patient in two phases. The rehydration phase lasts 2–4 hours. The maintenance phase lasts until diarrhea abates.
- Use the intravenous route for patients who have severe dehydration during the rehydration phase, those who purge more than 10–20 mL/kg/h, and those who do not tolerate the oral route during the maintenance phase. The amount and speed of the intravenous infusion vary between 50 and 100 mL/kg/h.
- The preferred intravenous solution is Ringer's lactate solution. Normal saline may be used, but the acidosis resolves less efficiently.
- Use the oral rehydration solution advised by the World Health Organization during the maintenance phase for severely dehydrated patients and for milder forms of dehydration in the rehydration phase. The amount of oral fluids advised is 500–1000 mL/h.
- Start antibiotics once the patient can tolerate the oral route. Doxycycline (Vibramycin) in a single dose of 300 mg, is the preferred regimen, given with a light meal.
- Start a normal diet as soon as the patient tolerates anything by mouth.
- Discharge patients when all the following criteria are fulfilled: oral tolerance <600–800 mL/h, stool output >400 mL/h, urine output <30–40 mL/h.

Discharging patients from the hospital is a critical issue, particularly when health centers are overloaded with patients with varying degrees of dehydration. Patients can be safely discharged if all the following criteria are met: oral intake between 600 and 800 mL/hour, urine output between 30 and 40 mL/hour, and stool output lower than 400 mL/hour. Case fatality rates in centers with experience in the treatment of cholera are extremely low, about 0.14%.

PHARMACOLOGIC THERAPY

An oral antibiotic is advised to reduce the volume of diarrhea, the requirement for intravenous fluids, and the hospital stay. Antibiotics are not lifesaving and should not be offered if the patient cannot tolerate the oral route. A reduction in almost 50% of the volume and duration of diarrhea and a reduction in the excretion of vibrios to 1 to 2 days have been documented with the use of effective antimicrobials. Single-dose regimens are preferred over multiple-dose regimens. A single dose of doxycycline (Vibramycin) 300 mg, given with a light meal, is the preferred regimen. Alternative regimens are listed in Table 3.

The quinolones are the group of antimicrobials more extensively studied to date, and excellent results in both clinical and bacteriologic parameters have been reported in clinical trials. Quinolones should not be used in children or pregnant women. Resistance to the quinolones has emerged in endemic areas of India and Bangladesh. Oral azithromycin (Zithromax)[1] (1 g in a single dose) is an alternative to treat infections by quinolone-resistant strains in both children and adults. Chemoprophylaxis with antimicrobials to prevent transmission of cholera is not recommended.

Complications and Prognosis

The most severe complication of cholera is acute renal failure. A careful evaluation of the medical charts of these patients disclosed improper replacement of fluids during the rehydration or maintenance phases. The nonoliguric form predominates. All age groups are affected, and the mortality rate is very high.

The presentation of cholera in children is similar to that in adults. Certain features are distinctive in children, however, such as fever, seizures, mental alteration, and hypoglycemia.

Cholera in the elderly carries a bad prognosis. The common presence of comorbidities, the difficulties in properly evaluating the hydration status, and the higher incidences of acute renal failure and pulmonary edema account for the higher mortality observed in this population.

Cholera in pregnant women is associated with more severe illness and with fetal losses.

---

[1]Not FDA approved for this indication.

TABLE 3 Antimicrobial Regimens for the Treatment of Cholera

| Drug | Antimicrobial Regimen | |
	Adult	Children
Preferred Regimen		
Doxycycline (Vibramycin)	300 mg with food	
Alternative Regimens		
Azithromycin (Zithromax)[1]	1 g as a single dose	20 mg/kg as a single dose
Ciprofloxacin (Cipro)[1]	1 g single-dose or 250 mg qd for 3 d or 500 mg bid for 3 d	Not recommended
Cotrimoxazole (Bactrim)[1]	TMP 160 mg and SMX 800 mg bid for 3 d	TMP 8 mg/kg and SMX 40 mg/kg divided in 2 doses for 3 d
Doxycycline (Vibramycin)	300 mg as a single dose	Not evaluated
Erythromycin[1]	250 mg qid for 3 d	12.5 mg/kg q6h for 3 d
Furazolidone (Furoxone)	100 mg qid for 3 d	5 mg/kg qid for 3 d or 7 mg/kg as a single dose
Norfloxacin (Noroxin)[1]	400 mg bid for 3 d	Not recommended
Tetracycline	500 mg qid for 3 d	50 mg/kg body weight qid for 3 d*

[1]Not FDA approved for this indication.
*Only for children older than 8 years.
Abbreviations: SMX = sulfamethoxazole; TMP = trimethoprim.

REFERENCES

Griffith DC, Kelly-Hope LA, Miller MA. Review of reported cholera outbreaks worldwide, 1995–2005. Am J Trop Med Hyg 2006;75:973–7.

Khan WA, Bennish ML, Seas C, et al. Randomized controlled comparison of single-dose ciprofloxacin and doxycycline for cholera caused by *Vibrio cholerae* O1 or O139. Lancet 1996;348:296–300.

Khan WA, Saha D, Rahman A, et al. Comparison of single-dose azithromycin and 12-dose, 3-day erythromycin for childhood cholera: A randomized, double-blind trial. Lancet 2002;360(9347):1722–7.

Nalin DR, Hirschhorn N, Greenough III W, et al. Clinical concerns about reduced-osmolarity oral rehydration solution. JAMA 2004;291:2632–5.

Sack DAW, Sack RB, Nair GB, Siddique AK. Cholera. Lancet 2004;363:223–33.

Saha D, Karim MM, Khan WA, et al. Single-dose azithromycin for the treatment of cholera in adults. N Engl J Med 2006;354:2452–62.

Seas C, Gotuzzo E. Cholera. In: Mandell GL, Bennett JE, Dolin R, editors. Principles and Practice of Infectious Diseases. Philadelphia: Churchill-Livingstone; 2005. p. 2536–44.

Foodborne Illness

Method of
Lester M. Crawford, PhD

History

In the 1920 edition of *Principles and Practice of Medicine*, Sir William Osler devoted three of the 1168 pages to food poisoning. He got virtually everything right, even by today's standards. He just had very little to report on a disease complex that was vitally important in his time. Today, the Centers for Disease Control and Prevention (CDC) estimates approximately 76 million illnesses, 325,000 hospitalizations, and 5000 deaths from foodborne disease each year in the United States. Viruses account for 67% of these infections, bacteria for 30%, and parasites for 2%.

Therapy of foodborne disease has passed through a variety of stages. In Osler's time, treatment primarily consisted of stomach lavage and enemas. After World War II, antibiotics were freely used. By the 1980s, competitive exclusion by antibiotic-resistant bacteria had dictated a more conservative approach that relied on supportive therapy including fluids. In severe cases, selective use of specific targeted antibacterials remained necessary. The remarkable success rate of oral rehydration therapy under primitive conditions in developing countries underscored the critical importance of maintaining fluid balance. Today, fluid therapy has become the cornerstone of the treatment of foodborne disease.

Etiology, Diagnosis, and Treatment

There are 30 principal foodborne diseases. Waterborne diseases are classified as foodborne diseases. Six of the 30 diseases are dealt with in other chapters. These are hepatitis, salmonellosis, typhoid, cholera, giardiasis, and toxoplasmosis. This chapter deals with the remaining major causes of this group of diseases.

AEROMONAS SPECIES

Although the role of *Aeromonas* in foodborne disease was elucidated in the 1890s, it has only recently been appreciated as the ubiquitous pathogenic organism that it is. These are, in fact, aquatic organisms, but *Aeromonas* has been isolated from a variety of plants, animals, and foodstuffs. *Aeromonas* has also been found in stool cultures, skin, and sputum samples from healthy persons. Gastrointestinal infections caused by this organism are characterized by mucoid, bloody stools, watery diarrhea typical of dysentery, and low-grade fever. This syndrome can progress to pneumonia, arthritis, osteomyelitis, endocarditis, and urinary tract infections, particularly in children, the elderly, and immunocompromised patients. *Aeromonas* can affect virtually any organ system and can cause hemolytic uremic syndrome.

The organism is amenable to antibiotic therapy and may be successfully treated with trimethoprim-sulfamethoxazole (Bactrim),[1] aminoglycosides, tetracyclines, cephalosporins, and the quinolones. Antibiotic resistance has now become a problem; it has been demonstrated that *Aeromonas* spp. can produce β-lactamases and transferable tetracycline R-plasmids. Therefore, it may be preferable to initiate therapy with trimethoprim-sulfamethoxazole or one of the fluoroquinolones when *Aeromonas* is isolated.

BACILLUS CEREUS

Bacillus cereus was not recognized as a significant foodborne pathogen until the 1950s, and the first major outbreak was not until 1971 in England. This organism is ubiquitous in the environment but is not pathogenic until conditions favor its growth. Pathogenesis is accomplished through a wide variety of extracellular toxins and enzymes. There is a diarrheagenic toxin and an emetic toxin.

Foods become toxic when the levels of *B. cereus* approach millions of organisms per gram. The usual syndrome involves nausea (but not vomiting), watery diarrhea, rectal straining, and abdominal pain. There is an incubation period of 8 to 19 hours; the duration of illness is usually 12 to 24 hours. In some cases, an emetic syndrome occurs that is more severe and acute than the diarrheal syndrome. The emetic syndrome is characterized by an incubation period of approximately 3 hours and is typified by severe vomiting. Diarrhea is generally not present in the emetic syndrome. The emetic syndrome closely mirrors staphylococcal food poisoning.

The diarrheal syndrome generally requires minimal therapeutic intervention other than monitoring of fluid and food intake. The emetic syndrome, although brief, can require intravenous fluids and medication such as phenobarbital[1] to moderate the frequency of vomiting.

CALICIVIRUSES

Caliciviruses cause the majority of foodborne illness in the United States and, most likely, the rest of the world. Indeed, without the cases caused by norovirus, cases of foodborne disease would be reduced by approximately two thirds according to some estimates, and there would likely be little need for or interest in this chapter.

Norwalk, Ohio, was the site of the first reported outbreak (1968) of this disease complex. The virus was therefore named *Norwalk virus*. The name was later changed to *Norwalk-like virus* (NLV), and the current name is *norovirus*.

There are three genotypes of enteric caliciviruses. In addition to norovirus, the calicivirus family includes Desert Shield virus, Hawaii virus, Mexico virus, Snow Mountain virus, and others.

Etiology

Fecal-oral transmission is the most common route of infection, but vomitus can also transmit infectious doses of the agent. Although swimming pools and uncooked or partially cooked food can transmit the infection, the primary source is drinking water. The recent spate of cruise ship infections has generally been traced to drinking water. Properly chlorinated water is generally safe, but nonchlorinated water is problematic. Inadequately chlorinated or brominated water can transmit norovirus, as can chlorinated water that comes from an overwhelmingly contaminated source. Leakage of sewage into treated water can result in individual cases or outbreaks.

Diagnosis

The disease entity is characterized by epidemic diarrhea. Symptoms include gastroenteritis, vomiting, diarrhea, headache, and 2 to 3 days

---

[1]Not FDA approved for this indication.

of low-grade fever. People of all ages are affected. In the United States, older children and adults are more likely to be infected, and in the Third World, young children are more often involved. Diagnosis may be by isolation of the virus from feces and confirmation by radioimmunoassay (RIA) or enzyme-linked immunosorbent assay (ELISA), or both.

Treatment

There is no specific treatment for norovirus infection. Supportive therapy, especially including fluids, is generally adequate for most patients. For patients in developing countries, oral rehydration therapy is generally the treatment of choice.

A specific vaccine for norovirus is being developed. The virus has been isolated, cloned, and sequenced, and an experimental vaccine is in clinical trials.

CAMPYLOBACTER SPECIES

Campylobacter has gone from not being recognized as a human pathogen to being the leading cause of bacterial diarrhea in just over 25 years. The agent is estimated to cause about 2.5 million illnesses, which is 12% of all foodborne disease in the United States. Moreover, serious sequelae such as Guillain-Barré syndrome (1:1000 cases) and Reiter's syndrome (1:100 cases) infrequently supervene.

Diagnosis

Difficulty in culturing *Campylobacter* prevented isolation and characterization of the organism until the early 1970s. *Campylobacter jejuni* is the species most associated with foodborne illness. Campylobacteriosis is characterized by abdominal pain, diarrhea, and fever lasting 2 to 5 days. Longer durations of illness and relapses are not uncommon. Diagnosis is confirmed by direct microscopic examination of the stool or through the use of selective media.

Treatment

Seriously ill patients should be treated with antibiotics, as should infants, older people, and the immunosuppressed. Seriously ill patients are defined as those with persistent high fever or refractory or bloody diarrhea. Clarithromycin (Biaxin)[1] is generally accepted as the antibiotic of choice, and fluoroquinolones such as ciprofloxacin (Cipro)[1] are the first alternative. The tetracyclines are also useful. Campylobacteriosis is resistant to the cephalosporins, vancomycin (Vancocin), and rifampin (Rifadin). Supportive therapy aimed at electrolyte replacement and hydration is also important.

CLOSTRIDIUM BOTULINUM

Clostridium botulinum elaborates one of the most potent substances in nature. One nanogram per kilogram of body weight is sufficient to paralyze an otherwise healthy person. When the toxin is ingested in food in sufficient quantities to cause illness, near total paralysis occurs in humans, often requiring artificial ventilation for extended periods. Mild botulism can consist of nothing more than double vision or a few days of dysphagia.

The mechanism of action of botulism is to block release of acetylcholine at the neuromuscular junction by attaching to specific receptors on the nerve terminal side of the junction. Nerve conduction restores activity at the neuromuscular junction.

Any food can contain botulinum toxin, but the most common vehicles in the United States are fruits and vegetables. Infant botulism is usually associated with consumption of honey.

Diagnosis

Diagnosis is confirmed by isolation of botulinum toxin either from the suspect food or from the patient's blood serum or feces. Resorting to symptomatic diagnosis can lead to confusing botulism with Guillain-Barré syndrome or even stroke.

Treatment

Therapy must center around the management of respiratory impairment. This requires accessibility to an intensive care unit. The Centers for Disease Control and Prevention (CDC) can provide polyvalent vaccines[5,10] that are effective against the six botulism toxins (A, B, C, D, E, F). The toxin can persist in the patient's serum for as much as a month after ingestion, and relapses and exacerbations are possible. The toxicity to the neuromuscular junctions can continue for months and, in rare cases, for as long as a year. Careful management and diagnostic advances have reduced mortality to well under 10%.

CLOSTRIDIUM PERFRINGENS

McClane has written, "*Clostridium perfringens* is ideally suited for its role as a major foodborne pathogen." He was referring to its ubiquity in soil and in human and animal feces; moreover, the organism has a doubling time of less than 10 minutes once established in foods. Finally, *C. perfringens* is heat resistant and it elaborates two toxins that can induce specific pathology in the human intestinal tract. Indeed, *C. perfringens* is the third leading cause of foodborne illness in the United States, after norovirus and *B. cereus*.

Diagnosis

The two forms of human disease caused by this organism are *C. perfringens* type A food poisoning and *C. perfringens* type C food poisoning, better known as necrotic enteritis. The type A syndrome is much more common but type C is a more serious disease.

Abdominal cramps and diarrhea typify the type A disease. These symptoms develop 8 to 16 hours after ingestion of contaminated food and persist for 12 to 24 hours, with a complete recovery in most patients. However, severe illness and even death can supervene in older or debilitated patients.

The necrotic enteritis form of the disease is characterized by vomiting, intense abdominal pain, bloody diarrhea, and severe gastroenteritis. The incubation period is 1 to 5 days after exposure. The more advanced cases can progress to jejunal necrosis and death if not managed well.

Treatment

Treatment for the type A disease is supportive therapy. Necrotic enteritis can require surgical repair of the small intestine, including removal of the affected area. *C. perfringens* is quite susceptible to penicillin, and some authorities report that the antibiotic may be useful in the management of severe cases of type C.

ENTEROBACTER SAKAZAKII

Enterobacter sakazakii causes meningitis or necrotizing enterocolitis in neonates, which results in a mortality rate of 40% to 80%. Surviving patients sometimes develop hydrocephalus, paralysis, or neurologic deficits. *E. sakazakii* has been isolated from dry infant formulas. The natural source of the organism is not well known.

Enterobacters are generally resistant to the cephalosporins but are responsive to medium-spectrum penicillins, such as carbenicillin (Geocillin),[1] piperacillin (Pipracil),[1] and ticarcillin (Ticar).[1] The aminoglycosides and the fluoroquinolones are also indicated.

ESCHERICHIA COLI O157:H7

This variant of *Escherichia coli* burst on the scene in North America in the late 1970s, and now it can be found in practically every country in the world. The reservoir for the disease is believed to be cattle, but wildlife of various kinds can likewise harbor the organism. In cattle, the disease is silent, causing no overt signs.

In humans, the verocytotoxin, a Shiga-like toxin that has been genetically incorporated into the organism, can cause hemorrhagic

---

[1]Not FDA approved for this indication.

---

[1]Not FDA approved for this indication.
[5]Investigational drug in the United States.
[10]Available in the United States from the Centers for Disease Control.

colitis and hemolytic-uremic syndrome, which leads, in some cases, to disseminated intravascular coagulation (DIC). DIC can result in a layer of fibrin forming in the glomerular capillary bed and acute renal failure. These sequelae are most likely to occur in children and older persons and in pregnant women. The young patients generally fully recover but sometimes require dialysis.

The number of cases is low and the fatality rate is small, but the severity and permanence of some of the sequelae have given great prominence to the disease. Major outbreaks such as the Jack-in-the-Box event of 1993 and the 2006 spinach outbreak have focused public attention on *E. coli* O157:H7. Control of this organism depends on proper cooking and handling of food, assiduous hand washing, and effective water-treatment programs. There is much interest in a vaccine for cattle or humans for *E. coli* O157:H7.

Diagnosis

Diagnosis is made by serotyping for specific antibodies to *E. coli* O157:H7. Transmission of the organism generally occurs from ingesting contaminated food but can occur from direct contact. The incubation period is 12 to 60 hours.

Treatment

Therapy consists of fluid replacement. Antibiotics are of no use because the lesional insult is caused by a combination of toxins that continue to be pathogenic for a period of time after the elaborating organism is no longer active. In fact, the U.S. Food and Drug Administration (FDA) has issued (January 2007) a warning against the use of antibiotics in enterohemorrhagic *E. coli* cases because such therapy could adversely affect the outcome. Dialysis is indicated in cases that progress to kidney failure. In the more severe cases of intestinal hemorrhage, blood transfusion may be necessary.

LISTERIA MONOCYTOGENES

Although *Listeria monocytogenes* infects a relatively small number of patients, listeriosis results in a 25% to 40% fatality rate, and severe aftereffects are relatively common in affected patients. It is extremely difficult to identify the specific food responsible because of the highly variable incubation period, which ranges from 3 to 70 days.

There are three modes of transmission: contaminated food, direct contact with the organism or with contaminated soil, and inhalation of the organism. Initial symptoms include fever, headache, and vomiting, but these may be followed by endocarditis, meningoencephalitis, and septicemia. These later symptoms can lead to hemorrhagic shock, disorientation, and coma. Listeriosis is a leading cause of stillbirth and miscarriage and must be handled aggressively in pregnant women. Neonatal cases likewise must be managed with care. Almost one half of all listeriosis cases are in neonates.

Confirmation of the diagnosis is accomplished by isolation of the organism from blood or cerebrospinal fluid. Virtually all β-lactam antibiotics are effective against *L. monocytogenes* including potassium penicillin G (Pfizerpen). Erythromycin (Ery-Tab),[1] tobramycin (Nebcin),[1] and other antibiotics in the macrolide and aminoglycoside families also are effective against *L. monocytogenes*.

STAPHYLOCOCCUS AUREUS

Whereas most food borne illnesses have incubation periods of days and even weeks, *Staphylococcus aureus* infections usually trigger symptoms in 2 to 6 hours. The organism elaborates a complex system of toxins in food under certain conditions that results in nausea, vomiting, retching, and abdominal cramping. Severe cases result in muscle cramping, vacillations in blood pressure and heart rate, and severe headaches. The disease usually runs its course in 2 days, but some cases last longer. Death can occur in the young, the elderly, and the debilitated.

Incriminated foods in *Staphylococcal* outbreaks are generally those that require a great deal of human handling such as salads and various meats, although canned foods have caused clusters of infection.

The usual inciting factor is not keeping the prepared foods hot enough or cold enough to prevent the proliferation of organisms and the formation of the causative toxins. Stored foods should be maintained at temperatures of 45°F (7.2°C) or kept warm at 140°F (60°C). Foods should be brought to these temperatures as rapidly as technologically possible.

Supportive therapy is indicated. Antibiotic therapy is not useful because the causative agent, the toxin, is not affected by antibiotics. Persistent vomiting or dehydration can indicate fluid therapy, such as 5% dextrose, together with electrolyte replacement, particularly potassium.

REFERENCES

Allos BM, Blaster MJ. *Campylobacter jejuni* and the expanding spectrum of related infections. Clin Infect Dis 1995;20:1092–101.

Ball JM, Graham DY, Opekum AR, et al. Recombinant Norwalk-like particles given orally to volunteers: Phase I study. Gastroenterology 1999;117:40–8.

Bennett RW. *Bacillus cereus*. In: Labbé RG, García S, editors. Guide to Foodborne Pathogens. New York: John Wiley and Sons; 2001. p. 51–60.

Gill DM. Bacterial toxins: A table of lethal amounts. Microbiol Rev 1982;46:86–94.

Greatorex JS, Thorne GM. Humoral immune response to Shiga-like toxins and *Escherichia coli* O157:H7 lipopolysaccharide in hemolytic-uremic syndrome patients and healthy subjects. J Clin Microbiol 1994;32:1172–8.

Lawrence GW. The pathogenesis of enteritis necroticans. In: Rood JA, McClane, Songer JG, et al (editors). The Clostridia: Molecular Genetics and Pathogenesis. London: Academic Press; 1997. p. 198–207.

Lederberg J, Shope RE, Oaks SC, editors. Emerging Infections: Microbial Threats to Health in the United States. Washington, DC: National Academies Press; 1992.

Miliotis MD, Bier JW, editors. International Handbook of Foodborne Pathogens. New York: Marcel Dekker; 2003.

Olsen SJ, MacKinnon LC, Goulding JS, et al. Surveillance for foodborne-disease outbreaks—United States, 1993–1997. MMWR CDC Surveill Summ 2000;49(1):1–62.

Schlech WF. Foodborne listeriosis. Clin Infec Dis 2000;31:770–5.

Necrotizing Skin and Soft Tissue Infections

Method of
*John M. Embil, MD, FRCP(C), FACP, and
Donald C. Vinh, MD, FRCP(C), Dip(ABIM)*

Necrotizing skin and soft tissue infections (SSTIs) are a heterogeneous group of infections that progress unimpeded across anatomic boundaries, producing destruction of the subcutaneous, fascial, or muscle layers of the integument, resulting in gangrenous cellulitis, necrotizing fasciitis, or myonecrosis, respectively. These infections have an acute onset, usually the patient appears toxic, and the infection is potentially limb- or life-threatening. Although necrotizing SSTIs are relatively uncommon, early recognition and appropriate interventions are crucial for optimal outcome. Thus, clinicians assessing a patient presenting with an SSTI should always consider the possibility of an underlying necrotizing process that would require consultation with a surgeon and infectious disease specialist.

Etiology

Necrotizing SSTIs are most often bacterial in origin and can be either monomicrobial (type II) or polymicrobial (type I). Much less often, fungal pathogens cause such infections.

Polymicrobial necrotizing SSTIs are, by far, most common. These infections are caused by the synergistic interaction between mixed

---

[1]Not FDA approved for this indication.

TABLE 1 Causes and Risk Factors for Monomicrobial Acute Necrotizing Skin and Soft Tissue Infections

Pathogen	Risk Factors
Aeromonas hydrophila	Wounds contaminated by freshwater (e.g., lakes, rivers, streams)
Clostridium perfringens (gas gangrene)	Contamination of traumatic wounds (e.g., by soil)
	Deterioration in a postsurgical wound (e.g., dehiscence, duskiness, bullae)
Clostridium septicum	Malignancy (e.g., colon cancer, hematologic malignancy)
Community-acquired methicillin-resistant *Staphylococcus aureus*	No established regular risk factors
	Close contacts who have a recent history of furuncles or difficult-to-treat skin abscesses may be suggestive
Group A streptococci (*S. pyogenes*)	Breaks in integrity of skin
	Impaired lymphatic or venous circulation
	Diabetes mellitus
	Superinfection of chickenpox
Pseudomonas aeruginosa	Ecthyma gangrenosum:
	Immunocompromise (hematologic malignancy, neutropenia)
	Malignant otitis externa: Diabetes mellitus
Vibrio vulnificus	Wounds contaminated by saltwater (e.g., Atlantic Gulf Coast)
	Wounds exposed to saltwater crustaceans and other seafood
	Chronic liver disease or cirrhosis
	Chronic renal failure or dialysis

facultative anaerobic and obligate anaerobic gram-positive and gram-negative bacteria, such as *Escherichia coli*, *Klebsiella spp*, *Proteus spp*, the staphylococci, the streptococci, and *Bacteroides spp*. On average, 4 or 5 different organisms are involved. The polymicrobial nature can be suggested by the location of the infected site; most commonly, they occur in the head and neck area (especially if odontogenic), the abdominal area (e.g., postsurgical sites), the pelvic, genital, and perineal areas (e.g., Fournier's gangrene, infections following gynecologic procedures, and infections originating from sacral decubitus ulcers), and extremities with neglected care (especially diabetic foot infections). Culture and susceptibility testing (C&S) should be performed on any discharge or deep tissue to guide therapy.

Monomicrobial necrotizing SSTIs occur less often (Table 1). These pathogens should be especially considered among patients with certain risk factors (see Table 1) who present with community-acquired infections. By far the most common isolate responsible for this condition is group A streptococcus (*Streptococcus pyogenes*), which might or might not cause concomitant streptococcal toxic shock syndrome and which can have devastating consequences. Because no clinical features are absolutely diagnostic for a specific pathogen, cultures should be obtained.

Fungal pathogens are emerging as an important cause of acute necrotizing SSTIs. Most commonly, these are due to saprophytic septated molds (e.g., *Aspergillus spp*, *Fusarium spp*, *Paecilomyces spp*) and to the aseptated zygomycetes producing mucormycosis. Major risk factors include diabetic ketoacidosis, iron overload states and deferoxamine (Desferal) therapy, immunocompromised states (prolonged neutropenia, hematologic malignancy, corticosteroid therapy, solid organ or stem cell transplant), and soft tissue trauma (e.g., burns, contaminated wounds).

Clinical Features

The distinction between necrotizing SSTIs and uncomplicated SSTIs (e.g., cellulitis) may be difficult. Both usually manifest with erythema, edema, and tenderness of a localized area of skin. A systematic approach for clinical features favoring the presence of a necrotizing SSTI should be undertaken, including a systemic evaluation of the patient, a focused assessment of the involved region, and laboratory investigations (Table 2).

TABLE 2 Clinical Clues to the Presence of Acute Necrotizing Skin and Soft Tissue Infections

Systemic Features	Local Features	Laboratory Investigations
Altered mental status (e.g., delirious, stuporous, obtunded)	Anesthesia of the affected area	Myonecrosis (e.g., increased creatine kinase, increased myoglobin)
	Crepitus	Radiography: Gas in the soft tissues
Hypotension (systolic BP <90 mm Hg or <5th percentile by age for children <16 years)	Rapidly progressive spread of erythema or pain	WBC $\geq$ 12,000 cells/μL or $\leq$4000 cells/μL or >10% immature granulocytes
	Focal areas of dermal necrosis	
Hypothermia or fever (temperature $\leq$36°C or $\geq$38°C)	Foul smell	Acidosis
Hypoxia	Purulent discharge, particularly if grayish or blackish or with gas bubbles	Electrolyte derangements (e.g., hyponatremia, hypocalcemia)
Tachycardia (heart rate $\geq$ 90 bpm)	Dusky, violaceous, or brownish discoloration	Anemia
	Bullae (serum filled or blood filled)	
Tachypnea (respiratory rate $\geq$ 20 breaths/min)	Generalized erythematous macular rash with or without desquamation	Thrombocytopenia with or without DIC
Toxic appearance	Exquisite tenderness out of proportion to the appearance of the affected area	Organ dysfunction (e.g., increased serum creatinine, increased hepatic transaminase)

Note: A patient who has a necrotizing soft tissue infection might also have limited clinical findings, and thus the history and clinical acumen will be of great value in helping to guide therapeutic interventions.
Abbreviations: DIC = disseminated intravascular coagulation; WBC = white blood cell count.

Diagnosis

A key component in diagnosing a necrotizing SSTI is to clinically suspect it. Imaging modalities (e.g., plain radiographs, computed tomographic [CT] scans, magnetic resonance image [MRI] scans) may be useful to delineate the depth and extent of infection. However, the time required to obtain such investigations can lead to inappropriate delays in diagnostic and life-saving interventions. The most important diagnostic procedure in suspected cases is surgical exploration to determine the gross and microscopic appearance of the subcutaneous, fascial, and muscle layers. Hence, early surgical consultation is necessary. Specimens of the tissue itself (rather than a swab) should be sent for Gram stain and microbiological culture and susceptibility testing; these results will help in guiding management.

Treatment

Effective management of all forms of necrotizing SSTIs requires a combined surgical and medical approach. Early and aggressive débridement of gangrenous tissue is crucial. Repeated exploration and débridements are commonly necessary. Amputation is required in some cases.

Medical therapy consists of early initiation of appropriate antimicrobial therapy and supportive care (usually in an intensive care unit) (Table 3). In the case of STSIs, adjunctive therapy with intravenous immunoglobulin (IVIG, Baygam)[1] may be used. Because these infections may be difficult to treat, consultation with an infectious disease specialist is encouraged.

[1]Not FDA approved for this indication.

TABLE 3 Empiric Antimicrobial Therapy for Necrotizing Skin and Soft Tissue Infections

Pathogen(s)	Empiric Antimicrobial Therapy*	
	First Line	**Alternative**[†]
Polymicrobial		
Aerobic or anaerobic gram-negative or gram-positive bacteria	Ticarcillin-clavulanate (Timentin) 3.1 g IV q6h *or* Piperacillin/tazobactam (Tazocin, Zosyn) 3.375 g IV q6h *or* Meropenem (Merrem) 1 g IV q8h *or* Imipenem-cilastatin (Primaxin) 500 mg IV q6h	Vancomycin (Vancocin) 1 g IV q12h *plus* a fluoroquinolone *plus* metronidazole (Flagyl) 500 mg IV q8h *or* Vancomycin 1 g IV q12h *plus* aztreonam (Azactam) 1 g IV q8h *plus* metronidazole 500 mg IV q8h *or* Ceftriaxone (Rocephin) 1 g IV q24h *plus* clindamycin (Dalacin, Cleocin) 600 mg q8h
Monomicrobial		
Group A streptococcus (*S. pyogenes*)	Penicillin G 4 million units IV q4h *plus* clindamycin 600–900 q4h *plus* mg IV q8h	Clindamycin 600–900 mg IV q8h
Clostridium perfringens, Clostridium septicum	Penicillin G 4 million units IV q4h *plus* clindamycin 600–900 mg IV q8h	Clindamycin 600–900 mg IV q8h or Metronidazole 500 mg PO or IV q8h
Aeromonas hydrophila	Ciprofloxacin (Cipro) 400 mg IV q12h or levofloxacin (Levaquin) 750 mg IV q24h	Trimethoprim-sulfamethoxazole (TMP/SMX, Septra, Bactrim)[1] 10 mg/kg/d (based on TMP) IV divided q6h or Ceftriaxone[1] 1 g IV q12h or Cefotaxime (Claforan)[1] 1 g IV q8h
Vibrio vulnificus	Minocycline (Minocin, Dynacin)[1] 100 mg IV q12h plus either ceftriaxone[1] 1 g IV q12h or cefotaxime[1] 1 g IV q8h	Ciprofloxacin (Cipro)[1] 400 mg IV q12h
Pseudomonas aeruginosa	Ciprofloxacin 400 mg IV q12h or Ceftazidime (Fortaz, Tazicef) 1 g IV q8h or Piperacillin-tazobactam 4.5 g IV q8h or Meropenem 1 g IV q8h	
Community-acquired methicillin-resistant *Staphylococcus aureus*	Vancomycin 1 g IV q12h	TMP/SMX[1] 10 mg/kg/d (based on TMP) IV divided q6h or Linezolid (Zyvox) 600 mg PO/IV q12h *or* Daptomycin (Cubicin) 4 mg/kg IV qd[‡]
Fungal		
Septated molds (e.g., *Aspergillus spp, Fusarium spp, Scedosporium spp*)	Amphotericin B deoxycholate (Fungizone) 1–1.5 mg/kg/d *or* Amphotericin B lipid-based formulations: Amphotericin B lipid complex (ABLC, Abelcet)[1] 5 mg/kg IV qd or Liposomal amphotericin B (L-AmB, AmBisome)[1] 5 mg/kg IV qd	Voriconazole (Vfend) 6 mg/kg IV q12h × 1 d, then 4 mg/kg IV q12h[‡]
Zygomycetes or mucormycosis	Amphotericin B deoxycholate 1–1.5 mg/kg/d *or* Amphotericin B lipid-based formulations: Amphotericin B lipid complex[1] 5 mg/kg IV qd *or* Liposomal amphotericin B[1] 5 mg/kg IV qd	Posaconazole (Noxafil) 200 mg PO qid[1,‡,§]

[1]Not FDA approved for this indication.

*The dosages of antimicrobial agents provided are based on normal renal function in adults weighing ≥70 kg and may need to be modified in patients with renal insufficiency. Drug serum levels should be monitored where appropriate.

[†]Alternative recommended regimens may be used in patients with a history of type 1 hypersensitivity reaction (anaphylaxis) to penicillin or other β-lactams. Other regimens with equivalent coverage are also appropriate.

[‡]Currently, there is a paucity of published clinical experience with these agents for necrotizing SSTIs.

[§]Posaconazole is available only orally.

CURRENT DIAGNOSIS

- Appropriate diagnosis and management of a necrotizing skin and soft tissue infection (SSTI) require early clinical suspicion and a prompt comprehensive examination. Focus on the following:
    - Systemic evaluation: Presence of certain risk factors, hemodynamic instability, respiratory distress, toxic appearance, delirium
    - Local features: Rapidly progressive erythema or pain, pain out of proportion to appearance of infection, dermal necrosis, bullae, crepitus, undermining of the skin, and tissue planes that separate when a blunt probe is passed through openings in the skin
    - Key laboratory investigations: Hematologic derangement, organ failure, gas in the soft tissues
- Diagnosis is best established by prompt surgical assessment of the involved soft tissue for gross and microscopic evaluation. Tissue specimens should be sent for immediate Gram stain, culture, and susceptibility testing.

CURRENT THERAPY

- Expeditious and aggressive surgical débridement is mandatory; second look surgeries with repeated débridements are usually required.
- Broad-spectrum antimicrobial therapy covering aerobic and anaerobic gram-positive and gram-negative organisms should be initiated empirically. Once culture results are available, the antimicrobial regimen can be tailored.

Because most necrotizing SSTIs are polymicrobial, it is usually most prudent to initiate broad-spectrum empiric antimicrobial therapy that covers the typical mixed aerobic and anaerobic flora of such infections. No single regimen is superior to others. Given the usual toxicity of such patients, intravenous therapy should be used, at least initially. In patients with a history of penicillin allergy, alternative regimens must be created that cover the same spectrum of pathogens (gram-positive, gram-negative, and anaerobic bacteria). Examples of recommended regimens are provided in the Current Therapy box.

Monomicrobial necrotizing SSTIs do not, in theory, require empiric broad-spectrum therapy. However, because it may be difficult to confidently predict either the monomicrobial nature of the infection on initial presentation or the specific single pathogen involved, it may be most prudent to administer broad-spectrum antibiotic coverage empirically. Once results of cultures and susceptibilities become available, the regimen can be focused on the isolated pathogen.

Fungal necrotizing SSTIs should be empirically treated with amphotericin B (either deoxycholate [Fungizone] or lipid-based formulation [Abelcet, AmBisome]), because this is currently the only antifungal agent with generally reliable coverage against septated molds and zygomycetes (although exceptions do occur). In addition, the underlying immunocompromised state, if possible, should be reversed (e.g., discontinue or decrease steroids and other immunosuppressive therapies).

Once the results of cultures and susceptibilities are available, the antimicrobial regimen can be tailored. The duration of antimicrobial therapy should be individualized.

REFERENCES

Bisno AL, Stevens DL. Streptococcal infections of skin and soft tissues. N Engl J Med 1996;334:240–5.
DiNubile MJ, Lipsky BA. Complicated infections of skin and skin structures: When the infection is more than skin deep. J Antimicrob Chemother 2004;53:37–50.
Ellis MW, Lewis 2nd JS. Treatment approaches for community-acquired methicillin-resistant *Staphylococcus aureus* infections. Curr Opin Infect Dis 2005;18:496–501.
Eron LJ, Lipsky BA, Low DE, et al. Managing skin and soft tissue infections: Expert panel recommendations on key decision points. J Antimicrob Chemother 2003;52:3–17.
Nichols RL, Florman S. Clinical presentations of soft-tissue infections and surgical site infections. Clin Infect Dis 2001;33(Suppl. 2):S84–93.
Lipsky BA, Berendt AR, Deery HG, et al. For the Infectious Disease Society of America: Diagnosis and treatment of diabetic foot infections. Clin Infect Dis 2004;39:885–910.
Stevens DL, Bisno AL, Chambers HF, et al. For the Infectious Disease Society of America: Practice guidelines for the diagnosis and management of skin and soft-tissue infections. Clin Infect Dis 2005;41:1373–406.
Vinh DC, Embil JM. Rapidly progressive soft tissue infections. Lancet Infect Dis 2005;5:501–13.
Vinh DC, Embil JM. Rapidly progressive soft tissue infections—Authors' reply. Lancet Infect Dis 2006;6:66–7.

Toxic Shock Syndrome

Method of
Julius Larioza, MD, and Richard B. Brown, MD

Toxic shock syndrome (TSS) is an acute illness caused by the production of local exotoxins capable of diffusing into the mucosa and exerting an exaggerated immunologic response resulting in the development of multisystem disease. These substances are superantigens belonging to a family of pyrogenic toxins produced by bacteria that include *Staphylococcus aureus* and *Streptococcus pyogenes*. The former produces classic TSS, whereas the latter causes a modified form of TSS known as toxic shock-like syndrome (TSLS). A high burden (colonization or infection) with these organisms in the setting of certain parameters allows for the production of superantigens and the subsequent development of the syndrome.

CURRENT DIAGNOSIS

- Toxic shock syndrome (TSS) and toxic shock-like syndrome (TSLS) are rapid-onset illnesses causing fever, hypotension, rash, vomiting, diarrhea, and the potential for multiorgan failure.
- TSS and TSLS are associated with elaboration of bacterial toxins, which results in a vigorous cytokine cascade, rather than direct bacterial invasion.
- Diagnosis of TSS and TSLS is based on fulfillment of criteria that involve identification of a constellation of clinical and laboratory data.

CURRENT TREATMENT

- Bacteremia is present more commonly in TSLS and may contribute to higher mortality.
- Treatment consists of strategies to decrease bioburden and toxin production, directed antibiotic therapy at maximal parenteral doses, and clinical support with close monitoring of end-organ function.

Epidemiology

TSS was first described in 1978 and is now recognized in both menstrual and nonmenstrual forms. The former, as initially described, was typically noted after several days of menstruation and was commonly related to use of high-absorbency tampons, such as the Rely brand, which have since been taken off the market. Currently, nonmenstrual TSS has become almost as common as menstrual TSS, with most cases reported after surgical procedures (e.g. sinonasal manipulation with packing). It has also been linked with use of contraceptive diaphragms, chronic peritoneal dialysis catheters, viral influenza, sinusitis, intravenous drug use, and burn wounds.

TSLS was first described in 1987. Similar in clinical appearance to TSS, it was associated with *S. pyogenes* and was initially labeled as streptococcal toxic shock syndrome. Most commonly, organisms produce streptococcal pyrogenic exotoxin type A. However, other toxins and other streptococci have been occasionally implicated. Although those at the extremes of life and persons with underlying comorbidities appear to be at risk, most cases of TSLS occur in otherwise healthy persons between the ages of 20 and 50 years. It may be a result of the absence of protective immunity.

Clinical Manifestations

TSS is a rapid-onset illness that causes fever, hypotension, rash, vomiting, diarrhea, and, eventually, multiple organ failure. If not treated promptly, it can be lethal. TSLS displays many of the typical TSS symptoms with the addition of severe soft tissue necrosis. Menstrual and nonmenstrual TSS share similar features. The rash is most commonly a diffuse erythema that may resemble severe sunburn. However, a rash mimicking that of scarlet fever may also be seen. Hyperemia of conjunctiva and mucous membranes and strawberry tongue may also be present. Desquamation of the palms and soles, as noted in many bacterial toxin-mediated disorders, often appears during convalescence. When it occurs after surgery, the classic signs of localized infection, such as erythema, tenderness, and purulence, may be absent, making diagnosis more difficult. Multiple organ involvement may include the gastrointestinal, hepatic, renal, musculoskeletal, hematologic, or central nervous systems.

There are several notable differences between TSS and TSLS. The skin is often the portal of entry in TSLS, with soft tissue infections developing in 80% of patients. Cutaneous signs may include localized erythema and edema, a bullous or hemorrhagic cellulitis, necrotizing fasciitis, myositis, or gangrene. Soft tissue involvement of this nature is uncommonly encountered in TSS. Bacteremia is present in more than 50% of patients with TSLS, compared to 15% of those with TSS. Perhaps as a result of this fact, the mortality rate is as much as five times greater with TSLS, reaching 25%.

Pathogenesis

Production of toxic shock syndrome toxin type 1 (TSST-1) has been associated with the majority of menstrual TSS cases (90%); nonmenstrual cases are mediated by TSST-1 or by staphylococcal enterotoxins B and C. The dependence of menstrual TSS on TSST-1 may be related to the ability of this protein, but not other pyrogenic toxins, to cross vaginal mucosa. Toxin production is regulated by the *agr* gene, which is expressed under conditions that include high protein levels, relatively neutral pH, and high partial pressures of CO_2 and O_2. All of these conditions are met when menstruation occurs in the setting of high-absorbency tampon use.

Most TSS-susceptible patients lack specific antibodies capable of blocking the responsible superantigens. Nonmenstrual onset of TSS is most likely related to clinically trivial *S. aureus* infections in the vagina and elsewhere (e.g., sinonasal passages). A major subclass of nonmenstrual TSS is viral influenza–associated. *S. aureus,* which can infect nasopharyngeal tissues damaged by influenza infection and cause TSS by secreting TSST-1 or staphylococcal enterotoxins.

S. pyogenes causes TSLS by secreting streptococcal pyrogenic exotoxins of three serotypes: A, B, and C. Infection usually occurs after minor injury or surgery, although a portal of entry may never be identified.

Diagnosis

The diagnosis of TSS or TSLS is based on identification of a constellation of clinical and laboratory data proposed by the Centers for Disease Control and Prevention (Table 1).

Differential diagnosis for patients presenting with components of this syndrome includes sepsis caused by other bacteria, staphylococcal scalded skin syndrome, Rocky Mountain spotted fever, meningococcemia, exanthematous viral syndromes, and leptospirosis. Noninfectious causes include severe hyperthermia, drug reactions, and insect-related allergic reactions.

Additional laboratory data that are helpful in diagnosis include complete blood count (CBC) with differential, serum electrolytes, assessment of muscle enzymes, and renal and liver function studies. Urinalysis, chest radiography, and electrocardiography may also help in identification of end-organ complications. Blood, wound, urine, and respiratory cultures should always be performed before initiation of antibiotic therapy. If menstrual TSS is suspected, vaginal cultures for *S. aureus* should be obtained. Testing for TSST-1 should be undertaken if the test is available.

TABLE 1 Diagnostic Criteria for Toxic Shock Syndrome (Staphylococcal) and Toxic Shock-Like Syndrome (Streptococcal)

TSS*	TSLS
Fever	Isolation of group A streptococci from a sterile site (definite case) or from a nonsterile site (probable case)
Hypotension	Hypotension
Diffuse macular rash with subsequent desquamation	Plus two of the following: Renal dysfunction Liver dysfunction Erythematous macular rash Coagulopathy Soft tissue necrosis Adult respiratory distress syndrome
Plus involvement of three of the following organ systems: Liver Blood Renal Mucous membrane Gastrointestinal Muscular Central nervous system Negative serologic tests for measles, leptospirosis, Rocky Mountain spotted fever Negative cultures from blood or cerebrospinal fluid for organisms other than *Staphylococcus aureus*	

Adapted from McCormick JK, Yarwood JM, Schlievert PM. Toxic Shock syndrome and bacterial superantigens: An update. Annu Rev Microbiol 2001; 55:77–104.

*Proposed revision of diagnostic criteria for TSS secondary to *Staphylococcus aureus* includes isolation of *S. aureus* from a mucosal or normally sterile site, production of TSS-associated superantigen by the isolate, lack of antibody to the implicated toxin at the time of acute illness, and development of antibody to the toxin during convalescence.

TSLS = toxic shock-like syndrome; TSS = toxic shock syndrome.

TABLE 2 Recommended Doses of Selected Antibiotics Useful in the Management of Toxic Shock Syndrome and Toxic Shock-Like Syndrome

Agent	Dose
Vancomycin* (Vancocin)	15 mg/kg q12h
Daptomycin* (Cubicin)	6 mg/kg q24h
Clindamycin (Cleocin)	900 mg q8h

*Adjust for renal dysfunction.

Treatment

Treatment strategies for TSS and TSLS are similar. Initial management should include cleaning of any obvious wounds, removal of foreign bodies (e.g. tampons, nasal packing), and drainage or débridement of affected tissues. Such strategies result in decreased bioburden and toxin production.

Antibiotics active against offending pathogens should be employed parenterally and in the highest dose appropriate for the patient's circumstances. With the emergence of methicillin-resistant *Staphylococcus aureus* (MRSA), vancomycin (Vancocin) and daptomycin (Cubicin) are agents likely to be effective against typical pathogens, even if associated with bacteremia. The former is often monitored by measuring trough levels and maintaining them at 15 to 20 μg/mL. The latter has the additional potential advantage of killing organisms without major cell lysis, which may spare cytokine release and elaboration of sepsis cascades. Clindamycin (Cleocin) should be employed as a second agent, because of its activity against likely pathogens and because it may terminate toxin production at a cellular level. Table 2 depicts usual doses. Because of their potential for affecting renal function, agents such as vancomycin and daptomycin need to be assessed carefully for optimal dosing during the period of illness. Duration of therapy is typically 7 days, although bacteremic patients may be treated for more extended periods.

As appropriate, local wound management may include use of topical agents. In vitro studies of silver sulfadiazine (Silvadene)[1] cream suggest that sublethal concentrations may actually increase toxin production by *S. aureus*. For that reason, mupirocin (Bactroban) or povidine iodine (Betadine) may be a better choice. Management and monitoring of end organs and treatment of shock are mandatory, and severely ill patients are best managed in the critical care unit. Corticosteroids and specialized forms of intravenous gamma globulin[1] have been employed but are not considered standard care.

Prevention

Awareness of these syndromes may help with prevention. Patients who have developed menstrual TSS should be encouraged to avoid tampon use for at least three cycles, and to then employ the lowest-absorbency tampon feasible. Careful cleansing of skin wounds, drainage of abscesses, and judicious use of topical antimicrobials for injuries may help to prevent colonization and subsequent toxin production.

REFERENCES

Davies HD, McGeer A, Schwartz B, et al. Invasive group A streptococcal infections in Ontario, Canada. Ontario Group A Streptococcal Study Group [see comment and author reply]. N Engl J Med 1996;335:547–54.

Edwards-Jones V, Foster HA. The effect of topical antimicrobial agents on the production of toxic shock syndrome toxin-1. J Med Microbiol 1994;41:408–13.

Jamart S, Denis O, Deplano A, et al. Methicillin-resistant *Staphylococcus aureus* toxic shock syndrome. Emerg Infect Dis 2005;11(4):636–7.

Manders SM. Toxin-mediated streptococcal and staphylococcal disease. J Am Acad Dermatol 1998;39:383–98.

McCormick J, Yarwood JM, Schlievert PM, et al. Toxic shock syndrome and bacterial superantigens: An update. Ann Rev Microbiol 2001;55:77–104.

Parsonnet J, Hansmann MA, Delaney ML, et al. Prevalence of toxic shock syndrome toxin 1-producing *Staphylococcus aureus* and the presence of antibodies to this superantigen in menstruating women. J Clin Microbiol 2005;43(9):4628–34.

Schlievert PM. Staphylococcal toxic shock syndrome: Still a problem. Med J Aust 2005;182(12):651–2.

Stevens DL. The toxic shock syndromes. Infect Dis Clin North Am 1996;10 (4):727–46.

Tierno PM Jr. Reemergence of staphylococcal toxic shock syndrome in the United States since 2000. J Clin Microbiol 2005;43(4):2032; author reply 2032–3.

Wood TF, Potter MA, Jonasson O. Streptococcal toxic shock-like syndrome: The importance of surgical intervention. Ann Surg 1993;217:109–14.

Influenza

Method of
Jeffrey A. Linder, MD, MPH, FACP

Influenza is a highly contagious viral infection that should be considered in any patient with respiratory symptoms between October and May in North America. Influenza infects 5% to 20% of the population of the United States in a typical year and is responsible for up to 226,000 hospitalizations and 36,000 deaths per year. Influenza can range in severity from mild illness to life-threatening disease. Those at highest risk of hospitalization, death, or complications from influenza are children younger than 5 years, adults older than 65 years, adults older than 50 years who have underlying medical conditions, those infected with HIV, and pregnant women.

Information about influenza changes rapidly. To optimally care for patients with influenza-like illness during the influenza season, clinicians need to keep abreast of updated recommendations and the current prevalence of influenza in their community. The influenza vaccine remains the best means of reducing the incidence, severity, and complications from influenza, but antiviral medications and symptomatic treatments have an important role in the prevention and treatment of influenza as well (Box 1).

Microbiology

There are two types of influenza viruses, A and B. Influenza A is separated into subtypes based on two surface antigens: hemagglutinin (H) and neuraminidase (N). The predominant circulating strains of influenza in recent decades have been influenza A (H1N1), influenza A (H3N2), and influenza B. Influenza A (H3N2) subtypes generally cause more severe influenza and are associated with higher mortality than other types. Influenza viruses undergo slight genetic changes from year to year, termed *antigenic drift*. Major changes in surface glycoproteins are termed *antigenic shift* and can result in severe pandemic influenza in a nonimmune population. Because of antigenic drift and because immunity to a given type or subtype of influenza provides limited cross-immunity to other types and subtypes, the influenza vaccine needs to be reformulated and administered each year.

Patients contract influenza by being exposed to large-sized respiratory droplets from an infected person or contact with surfaces harboring influenza virus. Influenza has a latency of 1 to 4 days before the onset of symptoms. Adults are infectious from the day before symptom onset through about day 5 of illness, but immunosuppressed adults and children shed virus for longer periods. Symptoms generally last from 7 to 14 days.

Highly pathogenic influenza A (H5N1), also called *avian influenza*, spreads rapidly among birds and has very high mortality. To date, there have been several hundred cases of influenza A (H5N1) among humans, with about 60% mortality. Influenza A (H5N1), if it acquires the ability to be highly transmissible among humans, is a threat to cause pandemic influenza. To date, there have also been several hundred cause of a novel swine-origin influenza A (H1N1) virus, which also has the potential to cause pandemic influenza.

Prevention

Influenza vaccination is between 30% and 90% effective in preventing influenza or complications of influenza. Influenza vaccination is highly cost-effective and can even be cost-saving in high-risk groups. Influenza vaccination is less effective in younger children, in adults older than 65 years, in adults with comorbid conditions, and if there is a poor match between the influenza vaccine and circulating influenza. The Centers for Disease Control and Prevention's (CDC) Advisory Committee on Immunization Practices puts out annual recommendations and supplementary updates on the prevention and treatment of influenza (www.cdc.gov/flu). At present, there are two types of influenza vaccine: the trivalent inactivated vaccine (TIV) and the live, attenuated influenza vaccine (LAIV).

The TIV (Fluzone, Fluvirin, Fluarix, FluLaval, Afluria) is administered as an intramuscular injection. The main adverse effect of the TIV is soreness at the injection site. Patients often report a mild immune response of fever, malaise, myalgia, and headache that can last for 1 to 2 days, but rates of most of these symptoms are no different from those who receive placebo injection. The TIV should not be administered to patients with egg allergies. Allergic reactions to egg proteins or other vaccine components (e.g., antibiotics and inactivating compounds) include angioedema, hives, asthma, and anaphylaxis. Vaccination should be deferred in patients with acute febrile illness, but patients with more moderate illness can be vaccinated. Guillain–Barré syndrome was associated with the 1976 swine flu vaccine, but there is no consistent evidence that modern influenza vaccines are associated with Guillain–Barré syndrome.

The LAIV (FluMist) is administered as a nasal spray and is approved for patients ages 2 to 49 years. The LAIV is contraindicated in children with recurrent wheezing, in patients with comorbid conditions, in pregnant women, and in family members or close contacts of severely immunosuppressed patients who require a protected environment (e.g., hematopoetic stem cell transplant recipients). The LAIV should not be administered to those with severe nasal congestion. Adverse effects of the LAIV include runny nose, nasal congestion, headache, sore throat, chills, and tiredness, although these are only slightly more common than in patients receiving placebo. Those receiving the LAIV should avoid contact with severely immunosuppressed persons for 7 days.

Patients should begin to be vaccinated in the fall when the seasonal vaccine becomes available, generally starting in October. In the event of vaccine shortages, higher-risk patients should receive priority. Patients should continue to be vaccinated until February and beyond because in the majority of recent influenza seasons, the peak has been February or later. Children 6 months to 8 years of age who have not been previously immunized against influenza should be given two doses separated by at least 4 weeks for both vaccines.

Evaluation

COMMUNITY PREVALENCE OF INFLUENZA

In caring for a patient with suspected influenza, the single most important piece of data is the community prevalence of influenza among patients with influenza-like illness. This ranges from near 0% during summer months to about 30% during a typical influenza seasonal peak. The prevalence may be higher during a particularly severe outbreak. Clinicians can check the local prevalence of influenza among patients with influenza-like illness through the CDC (www.cdc.gov/flu) and their state department of public health.

HISTORY AND PHYSICAL EXAMINATION

Beyond the local prevalence of influenza, the diagnosis of influenza rests on the patient's history. All methods of diagnosing influenza—symptom complexes, clinician judgment, and testing—generally are highly specific but have poor sensitivity. Thus, it is important to consider a diagnosis of influenza in any patient with respiratory symptoms during influenza season. Influenza is classically described as the very sudden onset of fever, headache, sore throat, myalgias, cough, and nasal symptoms. Children can also have otitis media, nausea, and vomiting. In differentiating influenza from nonspecific upper respiratory tract infections, it is most useful to consider the circulating prevalence of influenza, the abruptness of onset, and the severity of symptoms.

Certain symptom complexes have been shown in trials of antiviral treatment to strongly suggest influenza. For example, in an area with circulating influenza, the acute onset of cough and fever can have a positive predictive value as high as 85%. Similarly, several clinical trials found patients likely to have influenza while influenza was circulating if patients had symptoms for 48 hours or less, subjective fevers, or a measured temperature of at least 100.5°F, and any two symptoms of headache, cough, sore throat, or myalgias. Other studies, outside of clinical trials, have shown that clinician judgment performed as well as or better than hard-and-fast symptom complexes or rapid testing.

The physical examination in influenza primarily serves to identify the severity of influenza, complications, and worsening of underlying medical conditions. Clinicians should record vital signs and perform examinations of the ears, nose, sinuses, throat, neck, lungs, and heart for all patients suspected to have influenza.

TESTING

Rapid influenza test kits, some of which can distinguish influenza A from influenza B, can provide a point-of-care result in about 30 minutes and are available as nasopharyngeal swabs, nasal washes, and nasal aspirates. All forms of rapid testing have a sensitivity of about 70% and are more than 90% specific. Testing is likely most useful when there is an intermediate probability of influenza (e.g., a community prevalence of influenza among patients with influenza-like illness of 10%-30%), and patients have an intermediate probability of complications from influenza. If circulating prevalence of influenza is low (e.g., <10%), testing is unlikely to be positive and is not necessary. If the circulating prevalence of influenza is high (e.g., >30%), the relatively low sensitivity of rapid tests makes the risk of a false-negative test unacceptably high. In the event of a high prevalence of influenza or a high risk of complications from influenza, empiric antiviral treatment is indicated. Testing may be particularly helpful for hospitalized patients to rule out a need for antibiotics. Chest radiography, cultures, and blood tests are not routinely indicated, but they should be obtained for patients with suspected pneumonia or to identify other suspected complications.

Complications

Complications of influenza include primary complications, suppurative complications, and worsening of comorbid conditions. Primary complications of influenza include viral pneumonia, which is a feared complication and is likely a main cause of mortality in pandemic influenza. Other, less common primary complications of influenza include myositis and rhabdomyolysis, Reye's syndrome, myocarditis, pericarditis, toxic shock syndrome, and central nervous system disease (e.g., encephalitis, transverse myelitis, and aseptic meningitis). Children can have a severe course with influenza, including signs and symptoms of sepsis along with febrile seizures. Suppurative complications of influenza include bacterial pneumonia, otitis media, and sinusitis. Influenza can cause worsening of comorbid conditions like asthma, chronic obstructive pulmonary disease, congestive heart failure, and chronic kidney disease.

Chemoprophylaxis

Antiviral medications can be used to prevent influenza in patients who did not receive the influenza vaccine, cannot receive the influenza vaccine, received the vaccine in the prior 2 weeks (before reliable immunity develops) or in the event of poor matching between vaccine and circulating influenza strains (Table 1). Chemoprophylaxis should also be considered for close contacts of patients with confirmed influenza or for patients with immune deficiency who are unlikely to respond to the influenza vaccine but who are at high risk for having complications from influenza.

Amantadine (Symmetrel) and rimantadine (Flumadine) are no longer recommended for chemoprophylaxis or treatment because of a high prevalence of resistant influenza A strains. The neuraminidase inhibitors oseltamivir (Tamiflu) and zanamivir (Relenza) had been shown to be about 80% effective in preventing influenza in household contacts of persons with influenza and more than 90% effective in preventing influenza in institutional settings. However, most influenza A (H1N1) strains circulating early in the 2008–2009 influenza season were resistant to oseltamivir. Chemoprophylaxis should be taken for a minimum of 2 weeks or until 1 week after the end of an outbreak. For patients allergic to or unable to respond to the vaccine, chemoprophylaxis should be used for the duration of circulating influenza. The TIV can be given to patients receiving chemoprophylaxis. The LAIV should not be given from 2 days before to 14 days after taking an antiviral medication. Patients who receive the LAIV in this window should be revaccinated at a later date.

CURRENT DIAGNOSIS

- Influenza should be considered in any patient with respiratory symptoms between October and May in North America.
- The single most important piece of information when considering a diagnosis of influenza is the community prevalence of influenza.
- During outbreaks, sudden onset of fever and cough has a positive predictive value of about 85%.
- Rapid testing should be used when the community prevalence of influenza among patients with influenza-like illness is between 10% and 30%.

TABLE 1 Antiviral Agents for the Treatment and Prophylaxis of Influenza

Antiviral Agent	Treatment* Children	Treatment* Adults	Prophylaxis† Children	Prophylaxis† Adults	Comments
Oseltamivir (Tamiflu)	Approved for children ≥ 1 y Dose for 5 d bid: ≤15 kg: 30 mg 16–23 kg: 45 mg 24–40 kg: 60 mg >40: 75 mg	75 mg bid for 5 d	Approved for children ≥1 y Dose qd: ≤15 kg: 30 mg 16–23 kg: 45 mg 24–40 kg: 60 mg >40: 75 mg	75 mg qd	Oseltamivir should only be used if predominant circulating strains are influenza A (H3N2) or influenza B or testing is positive for influenza B. For patients with creatinine clearance <30 mL/min, oseltamivir dosing should be reduced to qd for treatment and to qod for prophylaxis.
Zanamivir (Relenza)	Approved for children ≥7 y 10 mg (2 inhalations) bid for 5 d	10 mg (2 inhalations) bid for 5 d	Approved for children ≥ 5 y 10 mg (2 inhalations) qd	10 mg (2 inhalations) qd	

Adapted from Centers for Disease Control and Prevention: Prevention and control of influenza: Recommendations of the Advisory Committee on Immunization Practices (ACIP), 2008. MMWR 2008:57(RR-7); 1–60 and interim recommendations from the Centers for Disease Control and Prevention.
*Treatment must be started within the first 48 hours of symptoms.
†Prophylaxis should be given for at least 2 weeks or until 1 week after the end of an outbreak.

CURRENT THERAPY

- The influenza vaccine is the best means of preventing influenza. The trivalent inactivated influenza vaccine is recommended for health care workers, children aged 6 months to 4 years, all persons 50 years old and older, and patients with chronic conditions.
- The antivirals zanamivir (Relenza; for all influenza types) and oseltamivir (Tamiflu; for influenza A [H3N2] and influenza B) can be used for prophylaxis of influenza in unimmunized patients, in close contacts of infected patients, and during institutional outbreaks of influenza.
- Zanamivir (for all influenza types) and oseltamivir (for influenza A [H3N2] and influenza B) can be used to treat influenza, but they must be started within 48 hours of symptom onset.

Treatment

The influenza vaccine is the best means of reducing influenza-related morbidity and mortality, but its limitations include production problems, low vaccination rates, and the variable effectiveness of the vaccine itself. Given these limitations, there is an important role in management for influenza-specific antiviral medications (see Table 1). Antiviral medications reduce the duration of influenza symptoms by 1 to 2 days, reduce complications requiring antibiotics by 30% to 40%, might decrease hospitalizations and mortality, and are cost-effective.

Again, amantadine and rimantadine are no longer recommended for the treatment of influenza because of a high prevalence of resistant influenza A strains, and oseltamivir should not be used if the influenza strain is likely to be influenza A (H1N1). To date, swine-origin influenza A (H1N1) has been sensitive to both oseltamivir and zanamivir. Zanamivir is taken as an oral inhaled powder and is not recommended for patients with underlying lung or heart disease. Adverse effects of zanamivir include worsening of underlying lung disease and allergic reactions. Oseltamivir is taken as a capsule or oral suspension. The dose of oseltamivir should be reduced in patients with renal disease. Adverse effects of oseltamivir include nausea, vomiting, and, extremely rarely, behavioral changes.

Antibiotics are generally not necessary, but they should be prescribed to treat suppurative complications of influenza. Antitussives such as guaifenesin with codeine (Robitussin AC) help coughing patients sleep at night. β-Agonists, such as albuterol (Proventil),[1] can help patients with cough, especially if there is wheezing on examination. Analgesics and antipyretics like acetaminophen (Tylenol) and ibuprofen (Motrin) reduce fever and generally help patients feel better. Patients should be encouraged to rest and drink plenty of fluids. Patients with suspected influenza should minimize contact with others to avoid spreading the infection.

REFERENCES

Centers for Disease Control and Prevention. Prevention and control of influenza: Recommendations of the Advisory Committee on Immunization Practices (ACIP), 2008. MMWR 2008;57(RR-7):1–60.

Cooper NJ, Sutton AJ, Abrams KR, et al. Effectiveness of neuraminidase inhibitors in treatment and prevention of influenza A and B: Systematic review and meta-analyses of randomised controlled trials. BMJ 2003;326 (7401):1235.

Falsey AR, Murata Y, Walsh EE. Impact of rapid diagnosis on management of adults hospitalized with influenza. Arch Intern Med 2007;167 (4):354–60.

Rothberg MB, Bellantonio S, Rose DN. Management of influenza in adults older than 65 years of age: Cost-effectiveness of rapid testing and antiviral therapy. Ann Intern Med 2003;139:321–9.

Stein J, Louie J, Flanders S, et al. Performance characteristics of clinical diagnosis, a clinical decision rule, and a rapid influenza test in the detection of influenza infection in a community sample of adults. Ann Emerg Med 2005;46(5):412–9.

Visceral Leishmaniasis

Method of
Pierre Marty, MD, PhD, and
Eric Rosenthal, MD, PhD

Leishmanias are vector-borne diseases transmitted by sandfly bite; they are characterized by diversity and complexity. Depending on virulence factors of the parasite and on the immune response established by the host, a spectrum of diseases can appear: visceral, cutaneous, and mucosal leishmaniasis, all resulting from obligated replication of the protozoa in macrophages in the mononuclear system. Visceral leishmaniasis (VL) is a disseminated infection in which macrophages of the liver, spleen, and bone marrow are preferentially invaded by the parasite and support intracellular replication. Diagnosis of VL is based on clinical suspicion. According to sanitary conditions, the diagnosis is confirmed with the use of serologic tests, parasite demonstration, or molecular tests. Most often, the criteria for response to treatment are clinical, without parasitologic confirmation. Once established, the clinical course of untreated VL exhibits high mortality.

CURRENT DIAGNOSIS

Suspicion

- Clinical: irregular fever, pallor, splenomegaly, with or without hepatomegaly
- Living or past travel in endemic area: Mediterranean basin, Latin America (northeast Brazil), China (Xia Jiang, Sichian, Gansu provinces)
- Biology: anemia, leukoneutropenia, thrombopenia, hyperproteinemia, hypergammaglobulinemia
- Immunosuppression: HIV infection, corticotherapy, transplantation, very young age, malnutrition

Confirmation

- Serology
- Leukoconcentration and microscopic examination
- Culture on special medium
- Polymerase chain reaction (PCR)
- Confirmation bone marrow aspirate* (PCR, microscopic examination, culture on special medium)

*If serology and PCR results are positive and the results of leukoconcentration and microscopic examination and of cultured special medium are negative, confirmation using bone marrow aspirate is necessary.

---

[1]Not FDA approved for this indication.

CURRENT THERAPY

- Two major pentavalent antimonials are currently used: sodium stibogluconate (Pentostam)[10] and meglumine antimoniate (Glucantime).[2] The drugs are given intravenously or intramuscularly and are equal in efficacy when used in equivalent doses. Disadvantages of antimonials include the parenteral mode of administration, the long duration of therapy, and adverse reactions.

- Lipid derivatives of amphotericin B have been developed to increase the therapeutic index. AmBisome is a lipid formulation of amphotericin B in which the drug is packaged along with cholesterol and other phospholipids within a small unilamellar liposome. The highly specialized liposomal formulation of AmBisome has several characteristics that increase its efficacy against visceral leishmaniasis (VL) while minimizing toxicity.

- Miltefosine (Impavido)[5] is the first orally administered treatment effective for VL; however, it has toxic effects on reproductive capacity in female animals (pregnancy should be avoided for 2 months after completion of therapy).

- Injectable paromomycin[5] has been tested by OneWorld Health as a treatment for VL.

- In antimonial-resistant VL, pentamidine isethionate (Pentam)[1] may be used.

- Recommendations in the treatment of VL may be differentiated according to the setting.

---

[1]Not FDA approved for this indication.
[2]Not available in the United States.
[5]Investigational drug in the United States.
[10]Available in the United States from the Centers for Disease Control and Prevention.

Epidemiology

VL is present in 61 countries on four continents, where approximately 200 million people are exposed. The incidence is 500,000 cases per year, with 90% occurring in only five countries: India, Nepal, Bangladesh, Sudan, and Brazil. Severe epidemics have occurred in India (300,000 cases between 1977 and 1980 in the Bihar state, with 2% mortality) and in Sudan (100,000 deaths between 1989 and 1994). In the Mediterranean basin, three countries of North Africa (Morocco, Algeria, and Tunisia) are particularly concerned, because 95% of cases are observed in the children younger than 5 years of age. In the north part of the Mediterranean area, sporadic cases of VL are observed in children but also in adults with or without permanent immunosuppression.

Since the 1980s, VL has been an emerging opportunistic disease in southwestern Europe (Portugal, Spain, France, and Italy), where more than 2500 cases of HIV-*Leishmania* co-infection have been reported. Although not recognized as an AIDS-defining criterion, VL constitutes an opportunistic disease in HIV-infected patients. Several studies have demonstrated that patients with HIV/AIDS living in *Leishmania*-endemic areas are at greater risk for development of VL and that dual infection accelerates the clinical course of HIV disease. Clinical presentations are often atypical, with unusual parasite localizations and frequent relapses. The introduction of highly active antiretroviral therapy as a standard treatment for HIV patients in southern Europe has resulted in a significant decrease in the incidence of VL in this population. Finally, the number of asymptomatic carriers demonstrated by transitory parasitemia in the human population and the role of humans as a reservoir of *Leishmania infantum* related to sharing of syringes by intravenous drug users raise new questions.

Two epidemiologic types of VL must be considered:

- Zoonotic VL is caused by *L. infantum* (syn. *Leishmania chagasi* in Latin America) with the dog as reservoir. This animal is frequently killed by the disease, but asymptomatic forms are not rare. Zoonotic VL is observed in China, Pakistan, Latin America, and the Mediterranean basin.
- Anthroponotic VL, with humans serving as a unique reservoir, is caused by *Leishmania donovani* and is an epidemic disease in Sudan, Ethiopia, India, Nepal, and Bangladesh.

After contamination by the parasitic sandfly bite, the evolution from an asymptomatic carrier state to the stage of patent VL may occur based on the following risk factors: genetic susceptibility, acquired or iatrogenic immunosuppression, dose of inoculated parasites, and virulence of the strain.

Diagnosis

The clinical signs of the classic Mediterranean zoonotic VL in young children are constant, irregular fever persistent over several weeks and splenomegaly associated with hepatomegaly in 50% to 70% of cases. Pallor is almost always present, and lymphadenopathies are rare. Adult cases of zoonotic VL are increasingly frequent in southwestern Europe (two thirds of total cases), and the characteristic clinical signs are less constant in this population than in children. In half of adult cases, a permanent immunosuppression is present (e.g., HIV infection, immunosuppressive treatment for neoplastic disease or transplantation).

Anthroponotic VL is diagnosed in adults or children; pallor; high, irregular fever; and splenomegaly are quasi-constant. Lymphadenopathy and cutaneous manifestations such as darkening or even blackening of the skin, affecting especially the face, hands, and upper torso, are frequently associated in India, where the disease is called *kala azar* ("black sickness" in Sanskrit).

Pancytopenia is present with anemia, leukoneutropenia, and thrombocytopenia, and there is an associated inflammatory syndrome (hyperproteinemia or polyclonal hypergammaglobulinemia).

Serologic tests allow diagnosis in almost all cases. The gold standard is the indirect immunofluorescence antibody test (IFAT), but enzyme-linked immunosorbent assay (ELISA) is becoming more frequently used. The specificity and sensitivity of ELISA tests depend on the antigens used. ELISA is especially useful for field work, because samples may be collected on filter papers and eluted directly into microtiter wells. The direct agglutination test (DAT) of fixed parasites is inexpensive and useful in field conditions. The new generation of this test is very sensitive (97% to 100%), as are the rapid immunochromatographic tests (dipstick with a band impregnated with recombinant protein antigen, especially rK 39). Western blotting is very specific and very sensitive but also extremely expensive. This test is able to discriminate between people with patent VL and asymptomatic carriers. It is appealing for epidemiologic studies.

The parasitologic diagnosis is based on visualization of the amastigote form of the parasite in bone marrow aspirate (Latin tradition) or spleen aspirate (British tradition, particularly in India). Parasites can be detected in peripheral blood after concentration, particularly in severely immunosuppressed patients. The culture of blood or bone marrow on special medium (NNN/Schneider's medium) is useful, especially for characterization of the strain. Fortuitous diagnosis of atypical localizations is possible with digestive or cutaneous biopsies or with bronchoalveolar lavages in at least one third of patients with HIV co-infection. The molecular diagnosis is very sensitive but again expensive. Polymerase chain reaction (PCR) is used to decrease the number of false-negative results obtained with parasitologic methods. PCR is particularly useful for follow-up after therapy and to diagnose relapses.

Available Drugs

Pentavalent Antimony

Organic salts of pentavalent antimony (Sb^V) have been the cornerstone of the treatment for all the leishmanias for more than 60 years. Two major pentavalent antimonials are currently used: sodium stibogluconate (Pentostam),[10] containing antimony 100 mg/mL and meglumine antimoniate (Glucantime),[2] containing antimony 85 mg/mL. The drugs are given intravenously or intramusculary and are equal in efficacy when used in equivalent doses. The recommended regimen consists of once-daily injections of full-dose drug (20 mg/kg) for 30 days (Table 1). Disadvantages of antimonials include the parenteral mode of administration, the long duration of therapy, and adverse reactions. Systemic toxicity normally relates to total dose administered. Secondary effects are frequent, albeit usually reversible, and include fatigue, body aches, electrocardiographic abnormalities, raised aminotransferase levels, and chemical pancreatitis. Severe adverse events remain rare; sudden death due to arrhythmia and acute pancreatitis with a fatal evolution have been reported.

Lipid-Associated Formulations of Amphotericin B

The antifungal agent amphotericin B (Fungizone, AmBisome, Abelcet, Amphotec[1]) has long been recognized as a powerful leishmanicidal drug. Largely because of the decline of antimonials in some areas and the failure of pentamidine[1] as a satisfactory substitute, amphotericin B has been rediscovered as an effective treatment for VL. Infusion-related side effects and renal toxicity of conventional amphotericin B are major problems. Lipid derivatives of amphotericin B have been developed to increase the therapeutic index. AmBisome is a lipid formulation of amphotericin B in which the drug is packaged along with cholesterol and other phospholipids within a small unilamellar liposome. The highly specialized liposomal formulation of AmBisome has several characteristics that increase its efficacy against VL while minimizing toxicity. The small size of the liposome (<100 nm) promotes wide distribution and penetration into tissues. The high transition temperature (55°C, compared with 25°C for an amphotericin B lipid complex formulation [Abelcet]) ensures liposome stability, which minimizes the release of the drug until contact is made with the pathogen. Tissue penetration is highest in the liver and spleen, and therapeutic levels persist in these organs for several weeks or longer after doses of AmBisome. Pharmacokinetic studies demonstrate that high initial doses (at least 5 mg/kg,[3] with doses up to 50 mg/kg[3] tested in animals) give better tissue penetration and longer persistence in viscera than frequent low doses, suggesting that initial loading doses may increase efficacy. In humans, the terminal elimination half-life after repeated administration of AmBisome is approximately 7 hours, with a trough level in blood by 24 hours. Although transient rises in creatinine can occur, acute and chronic toxicity from AmBisome is low even with doses of up to 15 mg/kg.[3]

First used to treat antimonial-resistant VL in 1991, lipid formulations of amphotericin B (AmBisome) have been proven to increase the efficacy and limit the toxicity of conventional amphotericin B (Fungizone). Thirteen clinical trials of AmBisome for treatment of VL have been published. One objective was to find the lowest total dose with acceptable efficacy due to affordability concerns. A single dose of 7.5 mg/kg[3] resulted in a 90% cure rate at 6 months in a fairly

---

[1]Not FDA approved for this indication.
[2]Not available in the United States.
[10]Available in the United States from the Centers for Disease Control and Prevention.

[3]Exceeds dosage recommended by the manufacturer.

TABLE 1 Key Treatment for Visceral Leishmaniasis

Type of VL	First-Line Drug	Total Dose (mg/kg)	Regimen	Primary or Secondary Unresponsiveness	Total Dose (mg/kg)	Regimen
Zoonotic VL	Liposomal amphotericin B (AmBisome)	20	*10 mg/kg on days 1 and 2[3] or in smaller divided doses, but initial dose of at least 5 mg/kg is recommended[3]	Not documented		
Anthroponotic VL	Pentavalent antimony (Pentostam,[10] Glucantime[2])	600	20 mg/kg qd for ≥30 d	Liposomal amphotericin B or combination regimen without antimonial drugs	10 to 20	Various short schedules, such as liposomal amphotericin B plus miltefosine or liposomal amphotericin B plus paromomycin (Humatin)[1]
HIV co-infection	Liposomal amphotericin B	20–40	†100 mg/d × 21 days[3] or †4 mg/kg/d on days 1–5, 10, 17, 31, and 38	Cross-over with first-line regimen		
	Pentavalent antimony	600	20 mg/kg qd for ≥30 d	Or miltefosine (Impavido)[5]		In adults: 100 mg/d for 28 d or longer

[1]Not FDA approved for this indication.
[2]Not available in the United States.
[3]Exceeds dosage recommended by the manufacturer.
[5]Investigational drug in the United States.
[10]Available in the United States from the Centers for Disease Control and Prevention.
*This schedule needs to be validated in adults.
†Use of higher daily doses with shorter schedule needs to be evaluated.

large Indian trial. In Europe, clinical trials demonstrated 90% to 98% efficacy with a total AmBisome dose of 18 to 21 mg/kg in immunocompetent patients. A variety of regimens are currently in use:

- In Italy, 3 mg/kg on days 1 through 5 and on day 10, for a total dose of 18 mg/kg
- For imported cases in the United States, 3 mg/kg on days 1 through 5 and on days 14 and 21, for a total dose of 21 mg/kg
- In New Zealand, 1 to 1.5 mg/kg for 21 days or 3 mg/kg for 10 days
- In southern Europe, published case series and current pediatric practice suggest good efficacy for a total dose of 20 mg/kg, with many pediatricians currently using a regimen of 10 mg/kg/day[3] for 2 consecutive days.

In HIV co-infected patients, there have been no formal randomized clinical trials of AmBisome treatment and secondary prophylaxis regimens and only two open label dose-finding studies. The efficacy of antimonials and AmBisome were comparable in most case series, but the lower rate of toxicity for AmBisome has caused most clinicians to consider it the antileishmanial drug of choice in HIV co-infected patients. Secondary prophylaxis with doses of AmBisome or other antileishmanials every 2 to 4 weeks after initial clinical cure of VL is now the standard of care in Europe.

Other Drugs

Miltefosine

Hexadecylphosphocholine (miltefosine [Impavido][5]) is one of a series of alkylphosphocholines. It was developed as an antineoplastic agent. The mechanisms of action of miltefosine against *Leishmania* have not been well determined, although miltefosine has been shown to block the proliferation of *Leishmania* and to alter phospholipid and sterol composition. The activity of miltefosine on *Leishmania* is caused by a direct cytotoxicity and the activation of cellular immunity. Miltefosine is the first orally administered treatment that has proved effective for VL, including antimony-resistant infections. The treatment is 100 mg/day for 28 days in adults and children older than 10 years of age. Vomiting and diarrhea are the most common side effects. Miltefosine has toxic effects on reproductive capacity in female animals, and pregnancy should be strictly avoided while on the drug and for 2 months after completion of therapy. Because of the long half-life, subtherapeutic levels of miltefosine may remain for some weeks after a 4-week course, and it is feared that this characteristic might encourage the emergence of resistance in the future.

Paromomycin

Paromomycin (Humatin)[1] is an aminoglycoside antibiotic with antiparasitic activity. Injectable paromomycin[5] has been tested in Indian VL in Bihar: 667 patients were randomly assigned in a 3:1 ratio to receive paromomycin (11 mg/kg body weight IM daily for 21 days) or amphotericin B (Fungizone; 1 mg/kg IV every other day for 30 days). Paromomycin was shown to be noninferior to amphotericin B, with final cure rates of 94.6% and 98.8%, respectively. Adverse effects were significantly more common among patients receiving paromomycin (6% versus 2%) and consisted mostly of injection-site pain (55%).

Diamidine

In antimonial-resistant VL, pentamidine isethionate (Pentam)[1] 4 mg/kg IM was administered 3 times weekly for 6 weeks. However, side effects (myalgia, nausea, headache, and hypoglycemia) were common at this dose and included exceptional risks of irreversible diabetes. At present, in antimonial-resistant areas, second-line treatment with pentamidine alone achieves poor response rates, which limits interest in pentamidine use.

Therapeutic Strategies

The declining activity and the toxicity of traditional leishmanicidal drugs stress the need for alternative compounds and for optimization of therapeutic protocols. Recommendations in the treatment of VL may be differentiated according to the setting.

ZOONOTIC VISCERAL LEISHMANIASIS

Over the past decade, AmBisome has been used with increasing frequency to treat VL. In some European countries (Cyprus, France, and Italy), AmBisome is used as a first-line drug. In others (Greece, Israel, Portugal, and Spain), both AmBisome and pentavalent antimony are employed. Compared with existing antileishmanial drugs, AmBisome has the highest therapeutic index, supporting its use as first-line therapy. A total AmBisome dose of 20 mg/kg is adequate to treat immunocompetent children and adults. According to the recommendations of the World Health Organization, the exact dosing schedule can be flexible (divided into doses of 10 mg/kg[3] on 2 consecutive days or in smaller divided doses), but AmBisome pharmacokinetics suggest that the initial dose provides better tissue levels if at least 5 mg/kg[3] is given. The schedule of 10 mg/kg[3] on 2 consecutive days needs to be validated in adults with zoonotic visceral leishmaniasis. In contrast, in countries with less gross domestic product per capita (Northern African and Middle Eastern countries), pentavalent antimony is still used exclusively.

ANTHROPONOTIC VISCERAL LEISHMANIASIS

The first-line treatment remains antimonial pentavalent compounds, with a minimal dose of 20 mg/kg/day for 28 days. Suboptimal doses, incomplete treatment, and substandard drugs may lead to clinical resistance. When unresponsiveness (primary and secondary) to antimonial drugs exceeds 10% in an area, policy makers should strongly consider a shift to an alternative first-line regimen. According to recent World Health Organization recommendations, two possible alternatives are an amphotericin B formulation (AmBisome, at a total dose of 20 mg/kg) and a combination regimen that does not include antimonial drugs. Use of combination antileishmanial drug regimens should be promoted to prevent the development of resistance to existing drugs. With respect to AmBisome, combinations of AmBisome with miltefosine, with paromomycin, and with pentavalent antimonials (in areas with <10% primary unresponsiveness to pentavalent antimonials) should be evaluated. Another approach should be combined sequential treatment, as was recently evaluated in India with single-dose AmBisome followed by short-course oral miltefosine.

HIV CO-INFECTION

Access to highly active antiretroviral therapy is high priority for patients co-infected with HIV and *Leishmania*. For HIV patients whose immune reconstitution is incomplete, data are insufficient to make firm recommendations regarding the best regimens for primary treatment and secondary prophylaxis of VL. Multicentered trials of first-line treatment and secondary prophylaxis of VL in HIV-infected patients are needed, and AmBisome regimens should be included in these trials.

REFERENCES

Adler-Moore J, Proffitt RT. AmBisome: Liposomal formulation, structure, mechanism of action and preclinical experience. J Antimicrob Chemother 2002;49(Suppl. 1):21–30.

Alvar J, Canavate C, Guttierez-Solar B, et al. *Leishmania* and human immunodeficiency virus coinfection: The first ten years. Clin Microbiol Rev 1997;10:298–319.

Bern C, Adler-Moore J, Berenguer J, et al. Liposomal amphotericin B for the treatment of visceral leishmaniasis. Clin Infect Dis 2006;43:917–24.

---

[1]Not FDA approved for this indication.
[3]Exceeds dosage recommended by the manufacturer.
[5]Investigational drug in the United States.

---

[3]Exceeds dosage recommended by the manufacturer.

Bryceson A. A policy for leishmaniasis with respect to the prevention and control of drug resistance. Trop Med Int Health 2001;6:928–34.

Deniau M, Canavate C, Faraut-Gambarelli F, Marty P. The biological diagnosis of leishmaniasis in HIV-infected patients. Ann Trop Med Parasitol 2003; 97:S115–33.

Desjeux P. Leishmaniasis: Current situation and new perspectives. Comp Immunol Microbiol Infect Dis 2004;27:305–18.

Gradoni L, Soteriadou K, Hecmi L, et al. Drug regimens for visceral leishmaniasis in Mediterranean countries. Trop Med Int Health 2008;13:1–5.

Kafetzis DA, Velissariou IM, Stabouli S, et al. Treatment of paediatric visceral leishmaniasis: Amphotericin B or pentavalent antimony compounds? Int J Antimicrob Agents 2004;25:26–30.

Le Fichoux Y, Quaranta JF, Aufeuvre JP, et al. Occurrence of *Leishmania infantum* parasitemia in asymptomatic blood donors living in an area of endemicity in southern France. J Clin Microbiol 1999;37:1953–7.

Rosenthal E, Marty P, Del Giudice P, et al. HIV and *Leishmania* coinfection: A review of 91 cases with focus on atypical locations of *Leishmania*. Clin Infect Dis 2000;31:1093–5.

Singh S, Dey A, Sivakumar R. Applications of molecular methods for *Leishmania* control. Expert Rev Mol Diagn 2005;5:251–65.

Sundar S, Jha TK, Chandreshwar P, et al. Injectable paromomycin for visceral leishmaniasis in India. N Engl J Med 2008;356:2571–81.

Sundar S, Jha TK, Thakur CP, et al. Oral miltefosine for Indian visceral leishmaniasis. N Engl J Med 2002;347:1739–46.

Sundar S, Jha TK, Thakur CP, et al. Single-dose liposomal amphotericin B in the treatment of visceral leishmaniasis in India: A multicenter study. Clin Infect Dis 2003;37:800–4.

Leprosy

Method of
Bhushan Kumar, MD, MNAMS, and
Sunil Dogra, MD, DNB, MNAMS

Leprosy is a chronic, very mildly infectious disease of the skin and peripheral nerves caused by *Mycobacterium leprae*. The first historical descriptions of leprosy came from India in about 600 BC when it was called *kushta*. Leprosy is also known as *Hansen's disease* after the demonstration of *M. leprae* by Gerhard Armauer Hansen in 1873. The damage to peripheral nerves results in sensory and motor impairment with the characteristic hideous deformities and disabilities so deeply associated with the disease. Leprosy was once widely distributed in Europe and Asia but now occurs mainly in resource-poor countries in tropical and warm temperate regions. Stigma remains a major obstacle to leprosy control, despite advances in bacteriology, chemotherapy, and epidemiology.

Epidemiology

At the beginning of 2008, only 3 countries (Brazil, Nepal, and Timor-Leste) were yet to achieve the leprosy elimination goal. The registered prevalence of leprosy globally was 212,802; the number of new cases detected during 2007 was 254,525. The global detection of new cases declined by 11,100 cases (4%) during 2007 compared with 2006. India, which has the highest number of leprosy cases in the world, achieved national-level elimination of leprosy in December 2005. *Elimination* is defined as less than one case per 10,000 population, and the prevalence in India was 0.84 per 10,000 population as of the end of March 2006.

After the successful implementation of and subsequently very encouraging results reported with multidrug therapy (MDT), a highly effective treatment regimen, in 1991 the World Health Assembly developed the global strategy for eliminating leprosy as a public health problem by 2000. The goal to reduce the prevalence of leprosy to less than one case per 10,000 population at the global level by 2000 was achieved; however, several countries had not done so at the national level. Therefore, the deadline for achieving the goal for these countries was extended to the end of 2005.

Major achievements of the leprosy elimination strategy have included achieving elimination in more than 120 countries (including cure of more than 18 million patients), free supply of MDT drugs, increased coverage of leprosy services, and integration of the leprosy elimination strategy within general health services.

However, reaching a prevalence level of less than one per 10,000 population is not the end of leprosy or leprosy work. The new challenge is to build on the success of the leprosy campaign and deliver sustainable care for leprosy patients who have been treated successfully or who are likely to trickle in because of the long incubation of the disease.

Etiopathogenesis

Modern-day leprosy dates from 1873 following the discovery of *M. leprae* (the first bacillus to be associated with a human disease). *M. leprae* is an acid- and alcohol-fast, gram-positive, obligate intracellular, noncultivable bacterium, which has been successfully inoculated and has multiplied in the nine-banded armadillo and nude mouse.

The principal means of transmission of *M. leprae* is probably through nasal or respiratory mucosa and skin-to-skin transmission in contacts of heavily infected multibacillary (MB) patients. The incubation period varies widely from months to 30 years, and the average time is usually 5 to 7 years. Apart from humans, nine-banded armadillos and, very rarely, sooty mangabey monkeys are the only known reservoir of infection.

More than 95% of adults are resistant to the infection. Subclinical infections occur more commonly in endemic areas, but clinical disease manifests in only a small fraction having specific impairment of cell-mediated immunity (CMI) to *M. leprae*.

The disease presents a broad spectrum of clinical and histopathologic manifestations ranging from bacteriologically scanty tuberculoid to highly bacilliferous lepromatous leprosy. The clinicopathologic bipolarity stems from the immunologic status, which guides the dual response of monocytes and macrophages to *M. leprae*. In cases located at the tuberculoid pole, these cells can destroy and eliminate all the bacilli; in cases near the lepromatous pole, the bacilli proliferate and persist in these cells and can be also partially killed simultaneously.

Clinical Features

The clinical features of leprosy reflect the pathology, which in turn depends on the balance between bacillary multiplication and the host cell–mediated immune response (Table 1). Leprosy affects skin and nerves and produces systemic involvement in lepromatous disease. Patients commonly present with skin lesions, weakness or numbness caused by involvement of a peripheral nerve trunk, deformities, resorption of fingers and toes, or a burn or ulcer in an anesthetic hand or foot. Sometimes patients present with nerve pain, sudden palsy, new skin lesions, painful red eye, or a systemic febrile illness.

Inspection of the whole body in good light is important because otherwise lesions with faint erythema or slight hypopigmentation (more often on covered areas in borderline disease) might be missed. Skin lesions should be examined for hypoesthesia to light touch and temperature and for anhidrosis.

TYPES OF LEPROSY

Indeterminate Leprosy

The classic skin lesion of indeterminate leprosy is most commonly found on the face, the extensors of the limbs, the buttocks, or the trunk. There may be one or more slightly hypopigmented or erythematous macules, a few centimeters in diameter, with poorly defined margins (Figure 1). Hair growth and nerve function are usually not affected. A biopsy might show perineurovascular infiltrate;

TABLE 1   Characteristics of the Ridley-Jopling Classification*

Observation	TT	BT	BB	BL	LL
Number of lesions	Usually 1 (up to 3)	Single, few (up to 10)	Several (10–30)	Many, asymmetric (>30)	Multiple, symmetric
Size of lesions	Variable, usually large	Variable, some are large	Variable	Variable, not very large†	Small
Surface	Very dry, scaly, lesions look turgid	Dry	Dull, slightly shiny	Shiny	Shiny
Sensations in lesions	Absent	Markedly diminished	Moderately diminished	Slightly diminished	Minimally diminished or not affected
Hair growth in lesions	Absent	Markedly diminished	Moderately diminished	Slightly diminished	Not affected
AFB in lesions	Nil	Nil or scanty	Moderate number	Many	Very many (globi)
Lepromin	Strongly positive (++++)	Weakly positive (+ or ++)	Negative	Negative	Negative

*Compartmentalization of the features is not very stringent. All these features occur in various combinations as the disease progresses.
†Presence of large lesions indicates downgrading of the disease from a higher spectrum.
Abbreviations: AFB = acid fast bacilli; BB = borderline borderline leprosy; BL = borderline lepromatous leprosy; BT = borderline tuberculoid leprosy; LL = lepromatous leprosy; TT = tuberculoid leprosy.

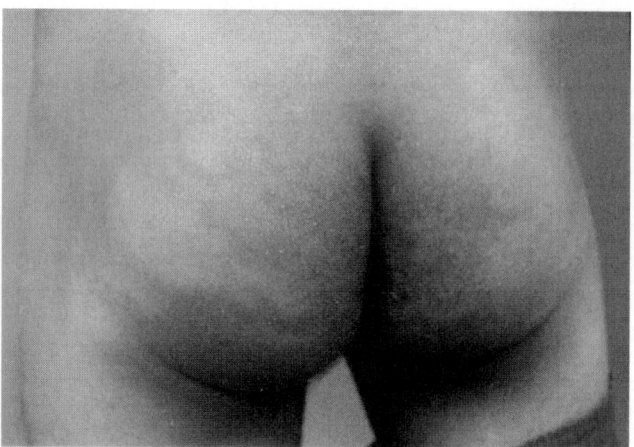

FIGURE 1. Indeterminate leprosy.

however, acid-fast bacilli (AFB) are mostly not demonstrable. Many patients do not notice such lesions and present only with characteristic determinant lesions at some point. Perhaps three out of four indeterminate lesions heal spontaneously and the rest become determinate and enter the clinical spectrum.

Tuberculoid Leprosy

Tuberculoid leprosy (TT) often has one or few skin lesions, and lesions seldom measure more than 10 cm in diameter. The typical lesion is a well-defined erythematous plaque with a raised and clear-cut edge sloping toward a rather flattened and usually hypopigmented center, acquiring an annular configuration. Erythema might not be apparent on dark skin. The surface is dry, hairless, anesthetic, and sometimes scaly. Sensory impairment may be difficult to demonstrate on the face because of the generous supply of sensory nerve endings. Less commonly, the lesion is a dry, anesthetic macule with sparse hair; the lesion appears erythematous on light skin and hypopigmented (never depigmented) on dark skin. Usually, a solitary peripheral nerve trunk is thickened in the vicinity of a TT lesion—for example, a thickened ulnar nerve if the lesion is on the arm.

Borderline Tuberculoid Leprosy

The skin lesions of borderline tuberculoid (BT) leprosy resemble those of tuberculoid leprosy, but there is evidence that the disease is not contained. Individual lesions do not show the well-defined margins, and the edge in part might fade imperceptibly into normal skin (Figure 2). There may be satellite lesions. The number of lesions can vary from three to ten and show variation in size and contour. Loss of sensation is less intense than in the lesions of tuberculoid leprosy. Xerosis, scaling, and erythema or hypopigmentation are also less conspicuous than in the TL form.

Several of the peripheral nerves are likely to be enlarged irregularly and in an asymmetric pattern. Nerve damage is an important characteristic of BT leprosy, and anesthesia or motor deficit is often found at the time of presentation.

Borderline Borderline Leprosy

Borderline borderline (BB) disease is unstable and mostly downgrades toward the lepromatous pole, especially when it is untreated. There are many skin lesions of all shapes and sizes including papules, nodules, plaques, and circinate lesions. Characteristic skin lesions are annular or dimorphic. In annular lesions, the inner edge is abrupt, and the outer edge slopes toward normal skin and has islands of clinically normal-looking skin within the plaque, giving a Swiss cheese appearance. The classic dimorphic lesion is shown in Figure 3.

The face might show infiltration, with occasional nodules over the ears and chin. Because of immunologic instability, the BB state is

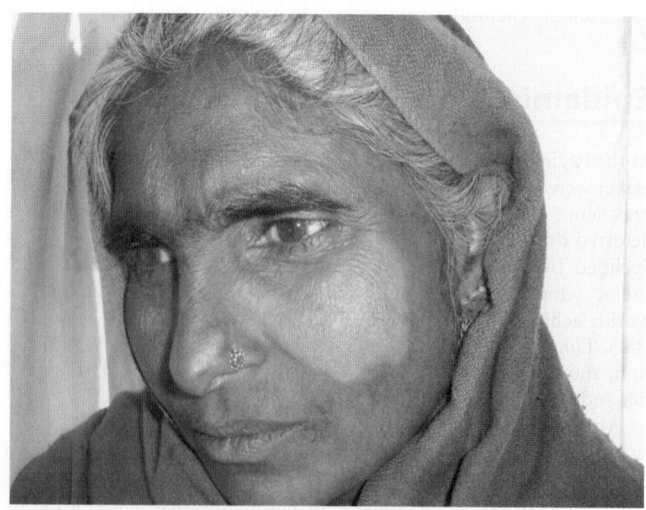

FIGURE 2. Borderline tuberculoid leprosy.

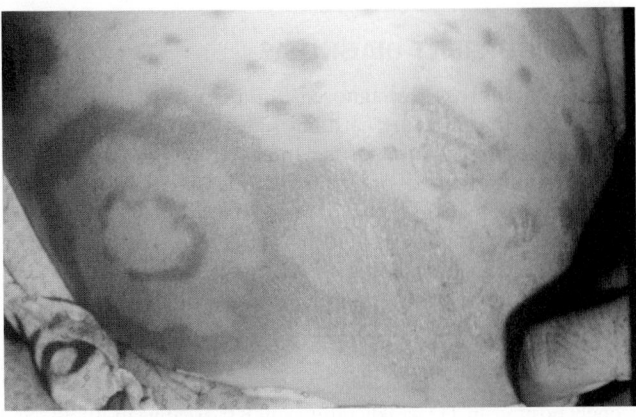

FIGURE 3. Borderline borderline leprosy.

short-lived, and such patients are evidently rarely seen; the disease usually changes rapidly to borderline lepromatous (BL) or BT leprosy. Many nerves are involved, although not symmetrically as in lepromatous leprosy.

Borderline Lepromatous Leprosy

There are numerous skin lesions in BL, and they are classically distinct but not so well defined. There occur slightly infiltrated macules variable in shapes in not so symmetric distribution, with areas of apparently normal skin in between. With disease progression, papules, nodules, and plaques can develop, although they usually have sloping margins that merge imperceptibly into normal skin (Figure 4). Associated large lesions and of variable morphology indicate downgrading of disease from a higher spectrum. Eyebrows are not completely lost. Peripheral nerve trunks become thickened and develop corresponding anesthesia and paresis but lack symmetry. Nerves are, however, unlikely to be damaged as quickly as in BB and BT leprosy.

Lepromatous Leprosy

The early lesions of lepromatous leprosy (LL) are minimally infiltrated macules that are innumerable, widely disseminated, and symmetrically distributed. The edges are indistinct, and their surface is shiny and erythematous rather than hypopigmented. In rapidly progressive cases, they coalesce so that the skin is diffusely involved. The early macules of LL are not anesthetic.

If the disease is untreated and allowed to progress, the affected skin takes on a waxy appearance and feels full. Thickness of skin is most marked over the face, especially the forehead, earlobes, eyebrows, nose, and malar surfaces (Figure 5). The eyebrows and,

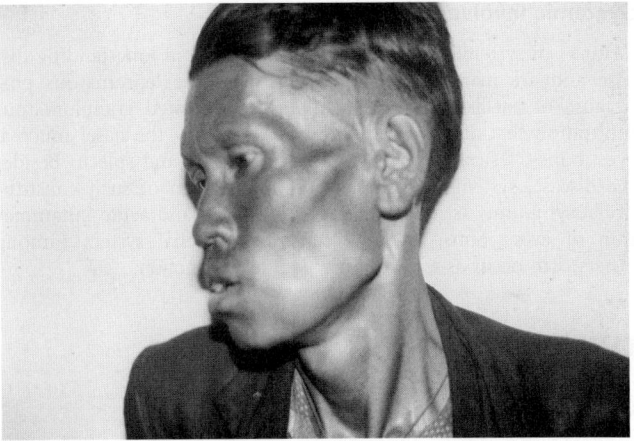

FIGURE 5. Lepromatous leprosy (diffuse infiltration).

ultimately, the eyelashes are lost. The thickened skin accentuates into folds, producing the classic leonine facies. Nodules and even plaques on the face and other areas of the body can follow. By this time, peripheral anesthesia is extensive and is accompanied by anhidrosis, with compensatory hyperhidrosis of the trunk and axillae.

The sensory loss is symmetric and is first detected over the extensors of forearms, legs, hands, and feet, which gradually results in the typical glove-and-stocking distribution. Weakness usually starts in the intrinsic muscles of the hands and feet.

EXTENT OF INVOLVEMENT

Nerve Involvement

Nerve damage occurs in two settings: peripheral nerve trunks and small dermal nerves. Small dermal sensory and autonomic nerves are affected in the early part of disease establishment, producing hypoesthesia and anhidrosis within skin lesions. The posterior tibial is the most commonly affected nerve trunk, followed by the ulnar, median, lateral popliteal, and facial nerves. Involvement of these nerves produces enlargement, with or without tenderness, and regional sensory and motor loss. Thickening of the greater auricular nerve is better seen than felt (Figure 6). Rarely, nerve abscess is encountered in peripheral nerve trunks, mostly in the ulnar and lateral popliteal nerves.

The morbidity and disability associated with leprosy are secondary to nerve damage. About 25% of leprosy patients have some degree of disability, which is greatest in patients with BL and LL disease. Early recognition and treatment are crucial to prevention of deformities.

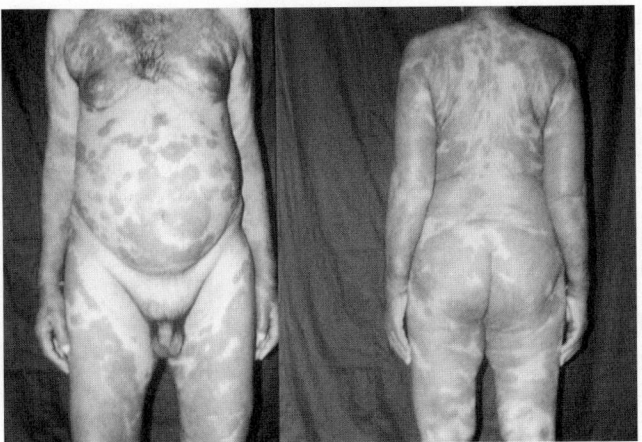

FIGURE 4. Borderline lepromatous leprosy.

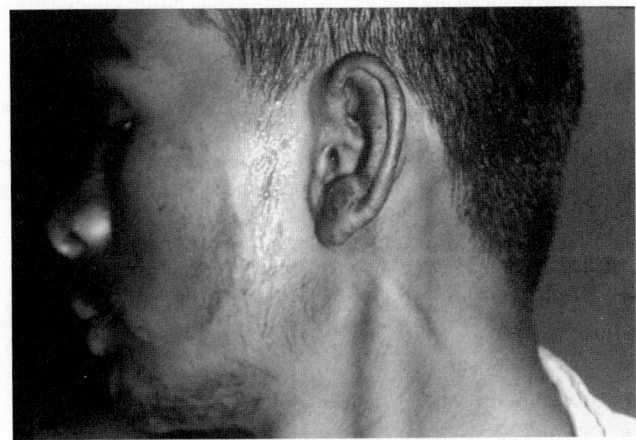

FIGURE 6. Nerve involvement (greater auricular nerve thickening).

Systemic Involvement

Features of systemic involvement occur usually in longstanding disease and are mainly seen in patients near the lepromatous pole because of bacillary infiltration and the associated granulomatous infiltration that affects various organs, especially the nasal mucosa, eyes, bones, testes, kidneys, lymph nodes, liver, and spleen. Besides the disease, systemic manifestations in the form of such constitutional symptoms as fever, malaise, joint pains, and acute inflammation of eyes, joints, and the reticuloendothelial system (among others) can occur as a part of a type 2 lepra reaction.

Diagnosis

CLINICAL DIAGNOSIS

The diagnosis and classification of leprosy have been based on clinical features and skin smears when facilities are available. Clinical diagnosis of leprosy is based on patients having one or more of the three cardinal signs. The cardinal signs are hypopigmented or erythematous skin lesion(s), with definite loss of or impairment of sensations; involvement of the peripheral nerves, as demonstrated by definite thickening, with sensory impairment; and skin smear positive for AFB.

LABORATORY DIAGNOSIS

Laboratory diagnostic tests such as slit skin smears, histologic examination of involved tissues, serology, and polymerase chain reaction (PCR) studies have been confined to areas where such facilities are available and in academic and research centers.

Slit Skin Smears

The diagnostic specificity of skin smears is almost 100%; however, the sensitivity is rarely more than 50% because smear-positive patients represent only 10% to 50% of cases. The inherent problems of skin smears are the logistics and the reliability of the technique of taking, staining, and interpreting the smears. Skin smears help identify patients with MB disease and patients who are experiencing clinical relapse.

Skin Biopsies

The biopsy helps to confirm the clinical diagnosis and classification of disease, but it cannot be regarded as the diagnostic gold standard because a number of the histologic features can be nondiagnostic or doubtful. In practice, a clinical and histopathologic correlation may be necessary for resolving a diagnostic difficulty.

Serology and Polymerase Chain Reaction

Serology and PCR are rarely used in endemic countries because of their limited availability and lack of uniform diagnostic values across the disease spectrum. The basis of serologic tests is to determine the presence of anti-phenolic glycolipid-1 (PGL-1) antibodies by the *M. leprae* particle agglutination assay (MLPA) and the enzyme-linked immunosorbent assay (ELISA) techniques. The PGL-1 antibody test is specific and more sensitive in patients with MB disease, but unfortunately it is not very helpful in the diagnosis of paucibacillary (PB) disease, and it has low predictive value for diagnosis of early disease. Antibodies to the 35-kD protein of *M. leprae* have been studied for their role in diagnosis of disease with comparable results. PCR for detection of *M. leprae* DNA encoding specific genes is highly sensitive and specific, because it detects *M. leprae* DNA in 95% of MB and 55% of PB patients. Currently, PCR is not used in routine clinical practice.

Lepromin Test

The lepromin test is not a diagnostic test, but it is helpful for identifying the level of CMI against *M. leprae* in a given patient. It is a nonspecific test of some value in classifying a case of leprosy. It is

CURRENT DIAGNOSIS

A case of leprosy is diagnosed in a person who has one or more of the following cardinal signs and who has yet to complete a full course of treatment:

- Hypopigmented or erythematous skin lesion(s) with definite loss or impairment of sensations
- Involvement of the peripheral nerves, as demonstrated by definite thickening with sensory impairment
- Skin smear positive for acid-fast bacilli

strongly positive in TL; weakly positive in BT; negative in BB, BL, and LL; and unpredictable in indeterminate leprosy. Lepromin (lepromin A, 160 million bacilli/mL) 0.1 mL is injected intradermally, and the reaction is read at 48 hours (Fernandez reaction) and at 3 to 4 weeks (Mitsuda reaction). Neither test is diagnostic, because both may be positive in persons with no evidence of leprosy. However, close contacts of an MB patient who have negative lepromin tests have a greater risk of developing disease.

Classification Of Disease

Ridley and Jopling (1966) defined five groups on the basis of clinical, bacteriologic, histologic, and immunologic features. These groups are tuberculoid, borderline tuberculoid, midborderline (borderline borderline), borderline lepromatous, and lepromatous leprosy. This is a very useful classification for research purposes, but it is often not feasible in field conditions and primary health centers. This classification does not include the indeterminate and pure neuritic type of leprosy. In general, PB disease is equivalent to indeterminate, tuberculoid, and BT leprosy, and MB disease is equated with BB, BL, and LL disease.

In 1998, the WHO Expert Committee on Leprosy declared skin-slit smears as not essential for institution of MDT. This was necessitated by the unavailability or unreliability of technical expertise for the skin smear in many leprosy-control programs and the potential for transmitting HIV and hepatitis by nonsterile techniques.

Recently, for field workers, WHO has classified leprosy based on the number of skin lesions for treatment purposes. PB leprosy is leprosy with one to five skin lesions. MB leprosy includes more than five skin lesions. If facilities are available, any patient with a positive slit-skin smear should be considered to have MB leprosy.

Rare Variants

Lucio Leprosy

Lucio leprosy (LuLp) is a diffuse form of LL. It is common in Mexico and Costa Rica and less common in the Gulf Coast, but it is quite rare in the rest of the world. It manifests as slowly progressive, diffuse, shiny infiltration of skin of the face and most of the body (*lepra bonita*, "beautiful leprosy"). There is loss of eyebrows, hoarseness of voice, and numbness and edema of hands and feet that mimic myxedema. This form of the disease is liable to the most severe of all reactional states, the Lucio phenomenon, in which destructive vasculitis leads to skin necrosis and ulcers.

Pure Neuritic Leprosy

Pure neuritic leprosy is characterized in the absence of any skin patch by an area of sensory loss along the distribution of a thickened nerve trunk with or without motor deficit. This form is seen most often, but not exclusively, in India and Nepal, where it accounts for 5% to 10% of leprosy cases. Histology of a cutaneous nerve might reveal an infiltrate that is characteristic of any type of leprosy.

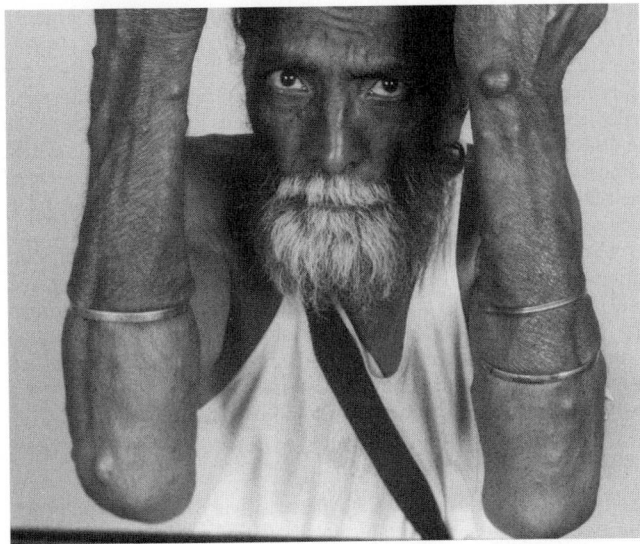

FIGURE 7. Histoid leprosy.

Histoid Leprosy

Histoid leprosy, first described in 1960, is now a well-recognized but rarely reported entity. Controversy still remains whether to consider histoid leprosy as a separate entity. It usually occurs in patients who had received irregular or inadequate treatment or dapsone monotherapy or as a spectrum under lepromatous leprosy. It manifests as superficially or deeply fixed cutaneous nodules, plaques, or pads (Figure 7). In a given patient, the number of lesions can vary from a few to a hundred. Histopathologically, the striking feature is predominance of spindle-shaped cells and unusually large numbers of AFB.

Treatment

The concept of chemotherapy for leprosy has undergone a phenomenal change over the last two decades. The WHO MDT has been successful in eliminating leprosy in many countries. However, the search for new drugs and new drug regimens continues. The goals of advanced therapy include improved patient compliance, alternative agents against clofazimine- and rifampin-resistant bacilli, more efficient killing of persistent bacteria, uniform MDT for all types of leprosy, and supervised short regimens for preventing drug resistance.

WHO MULTIDRUG THERAPY

The MDT introduced in 1982 has proved to be the most effective tool in controlling leprosy. More than 18 million patients have been cured of the disease, with acceptable cumulative relapse rates of 0.77% for MB and 1.07% for PB disease. MDT as recommended by WHO remains the current and most accepted treatment by all countries with endemic leprosy. A single dose of rifampin (Rifadin)[1] 600 mg plus ofloxacin (Floxin)[1] 400 mg and minocycline (Minocin)[1] 100 mg (ROM therapy) is an acceptable and cost-effective alternative regimen for PB leprosy with one skin lesion, although most still favor the conventional WHO MDT PB regimen.

OTHER REGIMENS FOR SPECIAL SITUATIONS

Drug Substitutions

For adult MB patients who cannot take rifampin, the Seventh WHO Expert Committee on Leprosy recommended daily administration of 50 mg of clofazimine (Lamprene), together with two of the following

---

[1]Not FDA approved for this indication.

Multidrug Therapy Regimen for Paucibacillary Leprosy (6 months)

ADULT (50–70 KG)

- Dapsone: 100 mg daily
- Rifampin (Rifadin)[1]: 600 mg once a mo under supervision

CHILD (10–14 Y)

- Dapsone: 50 mg daily
- Rifampin: 450 mg once a mo under supervision

Adjust dose appropriately for a child younger than 10 y. For example, dapsone 25 mg daily and rifampicin 300 mg given once a mo under supervision.

Multidrug Therapy Regimen for Multibacillary Leprosy (12 months)

ADULT (50–70 KG)

- Dapsone: 100 mg daily
- Rifampin:[1] 600 mg once a mo under supervision
- Clofazimine (Lamprene): 50 mg daily and 300 mg once a mo under supervision

CHILD (10–14 Y)

- Dapsone: 50 mg daily
- Rifampin[1]: 450 mg once a mo under supervision
- Clofazimine: 50 mg daily and 150 mg once a mo under supervision

Adjust dose appropriately for a child less than 10 y. For example, dapsone 25 mg daily and rifampin 300 mg given once a mo under supervision, clofazimine 50 mg given twice a wk, and clofazimine 100 mg given once a mo under supervision.

---

[1]Not FDA approved for this indication.

---

three drugs: 400 mg ofloxacin,[1] 100 mg minocycline,[1] or 500 mg clarithromycin (Biaxin)[1] once daily for 6 months, followed by daily administration of 50 mg clofazimine plus 100 mg minocycline or 400 mg ofloxacin for at least an additional 18 months. For MB patients who cannot take clofazimine, clofazimine should be replaced with ofloxacin 400 mg daily or minocycline 100 mg daily. Alternatively, the patient may be treated with a monthly administration of a combination consisting of rifampin[1] 600 mg, ofloxacin 400 mg, and minocycline 100 mg (ROM therapy) for 24 months. MB patients who cannot tolerate dapsone should receive only daily clofazimine with no substitution; in PB cases dapsone should be replaced with clofazimine.

Accompanied Multidrug Therapy

Accompanied MDT (A-MDT) recommended by WHO is an essential element of the "flexible and patient friendly MDT delivery system" suitable to migrant populations, patients living in remote areas, and patients living in areas of civil war. In this policy, the patient is provided the entire supply of MDT drugs at the time of diagnosis: 6 months of medication for a PB patient and 12 months for an MB patient, while asking "someone close or important to the patient" to assume the responsibility of helping the patient complete the full course of treatment. However, poor adherence to self-administration of treatment, a common phenomenon in tuberculosis and leprosy patients, and the associated risk of drug resistance and relapses are to be expected.

---

[1]Not FDA approved for this indication.

BOX 1   Newer Drugs and Alternate Drugs

Quinolones
- Clinafloxacin[5]
- Moxifloxacin (Avelox)[1]
- Ofloxacin (Floxin)[1]
- Pefloxacin (Pefocin)[2]
- Sparfloxacin (Zagam)[2]
- Temafloxacin (Omniflox)[2]

Macrolides
- Clarithromycin (Biaxin)[1]

Tetracyclines
- Minocycline (Minocin)[1]

Ansamycins
- KRM-1648[5]
- KRM-1657[5]
- KRM-1668[5]
- Rifabutin (Mycobutin)[1]
- Rifapentine (Priftin)[1]

[1]Not FDA approved for this indication.
[2]Not available in the United States.
[5]Investigational drug in the United States.

Pregnancy and Lactation

Leprosy is exacerbated during pregnancy, so it is important that the standard multidrug therapy be continued during pregnancy. The standard MDT regimens are safe, both for the mother and the child, and therefore should be continued unchanged during pregnancy and lactation.

Concomitant Active Tuberculosis

If the patient has both leprosy and active tuberculosis, it is necessary to treat both infections at the same time. Give appropriate antituberculosis therapy in addition to the MDT appropriate to the type of leprosy. Rifampin is common to both regimens, and it must be given in the doses required for tuberculosis.

Concomitant HIV Infection

The management of a leprosy patient infected with HIV is the same as that of any other leprosy patient without infection with HIV.

NEWER DRUGS

A few new drugs are available to complement or replace the currently used MDT (Box 1). The objective of the new drugs is not to induce quick clinical regression but to minimize relapses or to address special situations like drug resistance or drug intolerance. Promising bactericidal activity of ofloxacin,[1] clarithromycin,[1] and minocycline[1] against *M. leprae* has been demonstrated in the mouse foot-pad system and then confirmed in clinical trials. Strong bactericidal effects against *M. leprae* of moxifloxacin (Avelox),[1] rifapentine (Priftin),[1] and other derivatives have been identified in in vitro studies. However, no precise recommendation of their use is available yet.

Reactions

During the course of leprosy, immunologically mediated episodes of acute or subacute inflammation known as *reactions* can occur. Most reactions belong to one of the two major types; reversal reaction

[1]Not FDA approved for this indication.

(RR or type 1) or erythema nodosum leprosum (ENL or type 2). Reversal reactions can occur throughout the spectrum of leprosy but are more common in patients with borderline leprosy. On the other hand, ENL occurs exclusively in patients with MB disease, especially lepromatous and borderline lepromatous leprosy. Reactions can be disastrous; they cause acute nerve damage resulting in deformities. Almost 30% of MB patients develop reactions during the course of their disease. Reactions may be seen at presentation, during treatment, and even after treatment.

The principles of treatment of reactions are to control the acute inflammation in skin and nerves, ease the pain, halt eye damage, and prevent spread of the disease. Standard antileprosy chemotherapy should be started or continued along with antireaction treatment. Clinical evidence of ongoing neuritis (nerve tenderness, new anesthesia, motor loss) should be carefully sought and, if neuritis is present, corticosteroid treatment should be started immediately.

TYPE 1 REACTIONS

The type 1 reaction is a type IV hypersensitivity (delayed-type hypersensitivity) reaction, and it typically occurs in borderline disease. It is characterized by acutely inflamed skin lesions or acute neuritis, or both. Existing skin lesions become erythematous or edematous and can desquamate or, rarely, ulcerate. Often, new small lesions also appear at distant sites (Figure 8). Occasionally, edema of face, hands, or feet is the presenting symptom; however, constitutional symptoms are unusual. Although type 1 reactions can occur spontaneously and at any time during the course of the disease, the usual times are after starting treatment and during the puerperium.

Because of the high risk of permanent damage to peripheral nerve trunks, RR needs to be diagnosed as soon as possible and managed adequately. The drug of choice is prednisolone (Delta-Cortef). The usual course begins with 40 to 60 mg daily (up to a maximum of 1 mg/kg), gradually reducing the dose weekly or biweekly and eventually stopping in about 12 weeks. Neural impairment of up to 6 months' duration may be helped by systemic corticosteroid therapy tapered over a period of 4 to 6 months. Adverse effects associated with long-term corticosteroid therapy must be kept in mind.

TYPE 2 REACTIONS

The type 2 reaction, a type III hypersensitivity reaction (immune-complex mediated) occurs in patients with LL and BL disease. Attacks are often acute in onset but can become chronic or recur over several years. ENL typically manifests as painful, red evanescent nodules on the face and extensor surfaces of the limbs. Rarely, they appear as bullous, pustular, necrotic forms. ENL is often accompanied by systemic symptoms producing fever and malaise, and in severe form it may be complicated by uveitis, dactylitis, arthritis, neuritis, lymphadenitis, myositis, and orchitis.

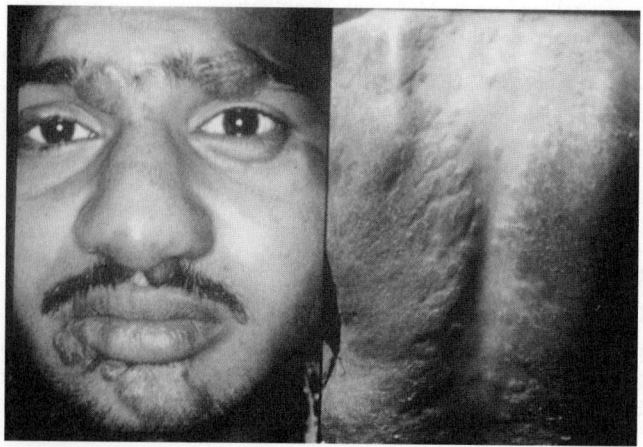

FIGURE 8. Borderline tuberculoid leprosy with type 1 reaction.

Acute or subacute neuritis with or without nerve function impairment is one of the major criteria for distinguishing mild and severe ENL. The treatment of ENL should start with general measures as in type 1 reaction. Mild ENL can be treated with analgesics like aspirin. In moderate and severe ENL, corticosteroids or thalidomide (Thalomid) are more useful and may be life saving. Thalidomide (100 mg q8h) has a dramatic effect in controlling ENL, and it may be useful in preventing recurrent ENL, but its teratogenic effects preclude its use in women of childbearing age. Clofazimine (Lamprene) has a useful anti-inflammatory effect in ENL and can be used at 300 mg daily in divided doses as an adjuvant to prednisolone and tapered over several months. Injectable antimonials are often used by Indian leprologists.

LUCIO'S PHENOMENON

The Lucio phenomenon occurs only in patients with Lucio leprosy. It results from infarction consequent on deep cutaneous vasculitis, causing the appearance of irregularly shaped erythematous patches. The patches sometimes darken and heal, but sometimes they form bullae that necrose, leaving deep, painful ulcers that are slow to heal. The systemic features are severe and can be fatal. Treatment with glucocorticoids (prednisolone) should be instituted at doses of 60 to 80 mg in two equal daily doses supplemented preferably with an augmented daily dose (200–300 mg) of clofazimine.

Prevention of Disabilities and Rehabilitation

The socioeconomic impact resulting from the physical and psychological disabilities of leprosy continues to be a burden in endemic countries. Approximately 25% of leprosy patients have some degree of disability, which is greatest in patients with long-standing BL and LL disease.

Preventing patients with nerve damage from progressing to disability and deformity is a challenge that will last for the patient's lifetime. Among the important efforts for prevention are periodic measurement of neural impairment, early and adequate management of reactions, and advice for care of eyes, hands, and feet. Special footwear needs to be provided for patients with foot deformities to prevent ulceration. Early detection and treatment of reactions significantly reduce and prevent such complications as nerve damage with its resultant impairment, eye involvement, and loss of vision. Socioeconomic rehabilitation is another important component of caring for patients.

Prevention

Large population-based trials in different countries suggest that bacille Calmette-Guérin (BCG) vaccine[1] gives variable protection against leprosy, ranging from 34% to 80%. Therefore, BCG immunization of children for tuberculosis can contribute to leprosy control.

In a recently published large study from India, vaccine containing cultivable mycobacterium, ICRC,[5] provided a protective efficacy of 65% (heat-killed *M. leprae* BCG provided 64% protective efficacy). The role of chemoprophylaxis with bactericidal drugs in contacts of leprosy patients is still debated.

WHO Strategy for 2006 Through 2010

The WHO Technical Advisory Group (TAG) recognizes that new cases will continue to appear in most of the currently endemic countries, and therefore, expertise will have to be maintained at the appropriate level even within an integrated system. The main aim of the strategy is to sustain antileprosy services and the gains made so far. It is expected that by 2010 the disease burden will be further reduced to very low levels through services that would ensure enhancing community awareness, quality diagnosis, adequate management of patients including referral facilities, reduction of stigma, prevention of disabilities, rehabilitation, long-term care of the disabled, and effective partnerships among all stake holders.

REFERENCES

Abulafia J, Vignale RIA. Leprosy: Pathogenesis updated. Int J Dermatol 1999;38:321–34.
Bhattacharya SN, Sehgal VN. Reappraisal of the drifting scenario of leprosy multi-drug therapy: New approach proposed for the new millennium. Int J Dermatol 2002;41:321–6.
Britton WJ, Lockwood DN. Leprosy. Lancet 2004;363:1209–19.
Grosset JH. Newer drugs in leprosy. Int J Lepr Other Mycobact Dis 2001;69 (2 Suppl.):S14–8.
Gupte MD. South India immunoprophylaxis trial against leprosy: Relevance of the findings in the context of trends in leprosy. Lepr Rev 2000;71 (Suppl.):S43–7; discussion S47–9.
Kumar B, Dogra S, Kaur I. Epidemiological characteristics of leprosy reactions: 15 years experience from North India. Int J Lepr Other Mycobact Dis 2004;72:125–33.
Kumar B, Kaur I, Dogra S, Kumaran MS. Pure neuritic leprosy in India: An appraisal. Int J Lepr Other Mycobact Dis 2004;72:284–90.
Lockwood DN, Kumar B. Treatment of leprosy. BMJ 2004;328:1447–8.
Naafs B. Current views on reactions in leprosy. Indian J Lepr 2000;72:97–122.
Noordeen SK. Vision beyond 2005. Indian J Lepr 2004;76:171–2.
Pfaltzgraff RE, Bryceson A. Clinical leprosy. In: Hastings RC, editor. Leprosy. New York: Churchill Livingstone; 1989. p. 134–76.
WHO Expert Committee on Leprosy. Seventh Report. WHO Technical Report Series No. 874. Geneva: World Health Organization, 1998.
World Health Organization. The Weekly Epidemiological Record 2008;83 (33):293–300. PDF available for download at http://www.who.int/wer/2008/wer8333/en/index.html [accessed May 14, 2009].

Malaria

Method of
Jimee Hwang, MD, MPH, and
Paul M. Arguin, MD

Malaria is an intraerythrocytic infection caused by protozoa of the genus *Plasmodium*. It is transmitted by the bite of an infective female *Anopheles* mosquito, which serves as the vector and definitive host.

Malaria is one of the most important parasitic diseases in the world, with an unacceptably high global burden. There were an estimated 247 million clinical cases and 881,000 deaths in 2006, mostly among children younger than 5 years of age living in sub-Saharan Africa, making it one of the world's leading killers. World Malaria Report 2008 stated that 109 countries and territories had areas at risk of malaria transmission, placing some 3.3 billion people at risk for malaria infection. Although malaria has been eliminated from the United States, approximately 1500 cases of malaria are reported annually. Most cases occur among travelers to malaria-endemic areas, but occasional instances of local transmission occur.

Malaria should be considered in the differential diagnosis of fever in a returning traveler from a malarious area and in a patient with fever of unknown origin regardless of travel history. Prompt diagnosis and treatment are imperative, because untreated *Plasmodium falciparum* and occasionally *Plasmodium vivax* infections can progress to coma, renal failure, pulmonary edema, and death. Appropriate chemoprophylaxis and the use of personal protective measures are important in preventing malaria infection.

---

[1]Not FDA approved for this indication.
[5]Investigational drug in the United States.

CURRENT DIAGNOSIS

- Fever or influenza-like symptoms in a person who has been to a malarious area, especially within the past 2 months
- Laboratory abnormalities including anemia, thrombocytopenia, and elevated liver function tests, especially hyperbilirubinemia
- Severe malaria can manifest as prostration, impaired consciousness, convulsions, pulmonary edema, circulatory collapse, abnormal bleeding, jaundice, and hemoglobinuria. Laboratory findings of severe malaria include severe anemia, acidosis, hypoglycemia, and hyperparasitemia.
- Blood smears demonstrating intraerythrocytic protozoa are the gold standard for diagnosis.

CURRENT THERAPY

- Prompt diagnosis and treatment are essential and potentially life-saving.
- Determine where the patient acquired the infection to assess local drug resistance patterns.
- Distinguish between uncomplicated and severe malaria.
- Severe malaria should be treated with parenteral therapy (i.e., quinidine or artesunate[5]) and in an intensive care setting, if possible.
- In uncomplicated malaria, distinguish between falciparum and non-falciparum types; if falciparum malaria is diagnosed, strongly consider admitting the patient to hospital.

[5]Investigational drug in the United States.

Transmission

Malaria is most commonly transmitted through the bite of an infective female *Anopheles* mosquito. Rarely, it can be transmitted through exposure to infected blood and blood products, organ transplantation, or contaminated needles (induced malaria) or by vertical transmission (congenital malaria). In nonendemic countries, most cases of malaria are acquired during traveling in an endemic area (imported malaria), posing a potential for reintroduction. In the United States from 1957 to 2003, 63 outbreaks of locally acquired mosquito-borne malaria transmission (introduced malaria) occurred. Such outbreaks result when a local mosquito acquires the parasite by biting an infected individual and then transmits the infection to another individual.

Etiology and Life Cycle

Infection with protozoa of the genus *Plasmodium* causes malaria. Typically, four species of *Plasmodium* cause clinical disease in humans: *P. falciparum, P. vivax, Plasmodium ovale,* and *Plasmodium malariae;* however, recent data from Southeast Asia describe an increasing number of human infections caused by *Plasmodium knowlesi,* a simian strain. The life cycle of malaria starts with inoculation of sporozoites into the human bloodstream from the bite of a female *Anopheles* mosquito; the organisms travel rapidly to the liver, where asexual replication occurs (exoerythrocytic cycle, or

tissue schizogony). Numerous merozoites are released from the infected liver cells to invade red blood cells, where they multiply every 24 to 72 hours, depending on the species (erythrocytic cycle, or blood schizogony). Some parasites differentiate into gametocytes (sexual erythrocytic stage), which can be ingested by subsequent female *Anopheles* mosquitoes, develop in the midgut, and migrate into the salivary glands, continuing the transmission of malaria (Fig. 1).

In *P. vivax* and *P. ovale* infections, some sporozoites do not enter the exoerythrocytic cycle but instead develop into latent hepatic forms, or hypnozoites. These forms may reactivate later and cause acute illness. The resulting infection, a relapse, can occur months to years after the initial infection and can occur repeatedly. However, if *P. vivax* or *P. ovale* infection is acquired congenitally or through exposure to blood or blood products, no liver phase occurs, and therefore relapses cannot occur. Neither *P. falciparum* nor *P. malariae* has a latent hepatic form, but recurrence of parasitemia, called recrudescence, can occur in all species after suboptimal therapy. For example, if *P. malariae* infection is not treated, symptomatic recrudescences, often associated with immunosuppression, can occur decades after the primary infection.

The incubation period, or the period from infection to the appearance of symptoms, is species dependent. It is usually 9 to 14 days for *P falciparum,* 12 to 17 days for *P. vivax,* 16 to 18 days for *P. ovale,* and 18 to 40 days (or longer) for *P. malariae.* Individuals taking chemoprophylaxis and those who have acquired partial immunity from repeated exposure to malaria infection may experience a prolonged incubation period.

Epidemiology

Malaria is endemic to much of Africa, Asia, and parts of Central Asia, Oceania, Central America, South America, the Caribbean, and the Middle East. *P. falciparum* is the most common species in the tropics and subtropics. *P. malariae* follows a similar geographic distribution but is less common. *P. vivax* is prevalent in many temperate zones as well as in the tropics and subtropics and has the widest geographic distribution. *P. ovale* is most common in West Africa. *P. knowlesi,* a simian strain, has been reported to infect humans in Southeast Asia. Together, *P. falciparum* and *P. vivax* account for more than 90% of clinical malaria illnesses worldwide.

The development of resistance to antimalarial drugs has complicated malaria prophylaxis and treatment. Notably, chloroquine-resistant *P. falciparum* is widespread with few exceptions, and chloroquine-resistant *P. vivax* is an issue in Papua New Guinea, Indonesia, and East Timor. *P. falciparum* resistance to sulfadoxine-pyrimethamine (Fansidar) is widespread in the Amazon River basin, much of Southeast Asia, and Africa, whereas mefloquine (Lariam) resistance is limited to Southeast Asia. Knowledge of species-specific resistance patterns is essential to making appropriate decisions about chemoprophylaxis and treatment. The most up-to-date information regarding geographic-specific risk and rapidly evolving resistance information can be found on websites of the Centers for Disease Control and Prevention (CDC), http://www.cdc.gov/malaria/risk_map/ or http://wwwn.cdc.gov/travel/default.aspx (both accessed May 5, 2009).

Clinical Manifestations

The clinical presentation of malaria is nonspecific; therefore, clinicians must maintain a high index of suspicion for malaria and routinely obtain a travel history from febrile patients. The clinical presentation of malaria can vary substantially, depending on the infecting species, the level of parasitemia, and the immune status of the patient. The initial clinical symptoms usually include a flu-like prodrome, with headache, malaise, and myalgias, that is followed by fever.

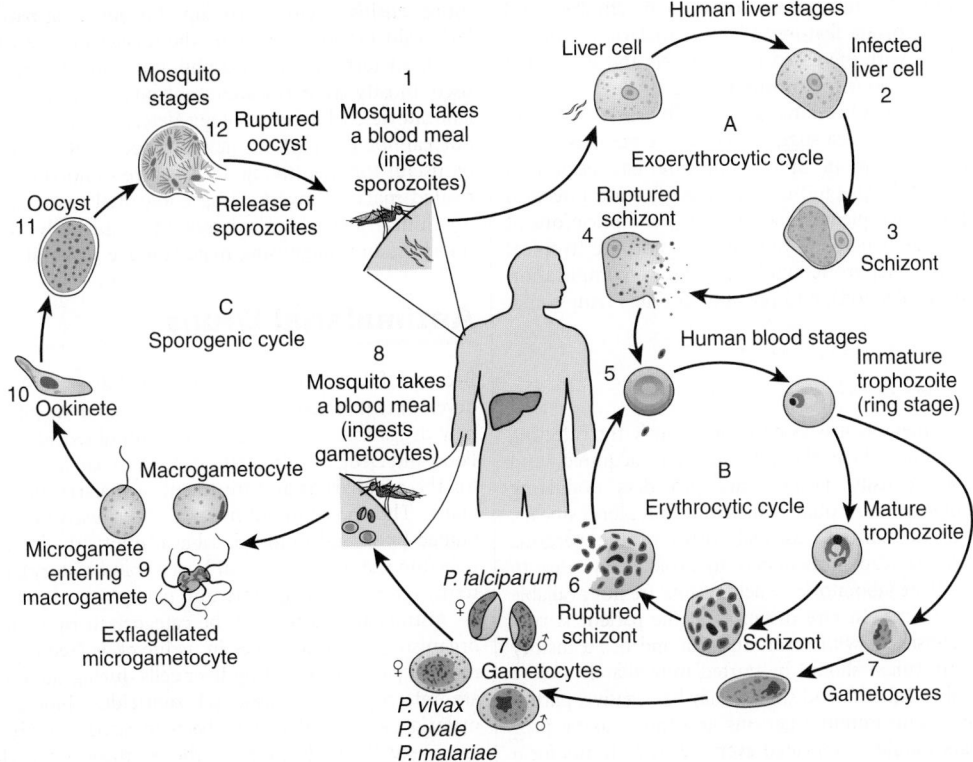

FIGURE 1. The malaria parasite life cycle involves two hosts and three cycles of development. During a blood meal, a malaria-infected female *Anopheles* mosquito inoculates sporozoites into the human host (1). Sporozoites infect liver cells (2) and mature into schizonts (3), which rupture and release merozoites (4). (In *P. vivax* and *P. ovale,* a dormant stage [hypnozoites] can persist in the liver and cause relapses by invading the bloodstream weeks or years later.) After this initial replication in the liver, known as the exoerythrocytic cycle (A), the parasites undergo an asexual multiplication cycle in the erythrocytes (B). Merozoites released from the schizont infect red blood cells (5). The ring-stage trophozoites mature into schizonts, which rupture, releasing more merozoites (6). Blood-stage parasites are responsible for the clinical manifestations of the disease. Some parasites differentiate into sexual erythrocytic stages, called gametocytes (7), which are ingested by an *Anopheles* mosquito during a blood meal (8). The parasites' multiplication in the mosquito is known as the sporogenic cycle (C). While in the mosquito's stomach, the microgametes (male) penetrate the macrogametes (female), generating zygotes (9). The zygotes develop into motile and elongated ookinetes (10), which invade the midgut wall of the mosquito, where they develop into oocysts (11). The oocysts grow, rupture, and release sporozoites (12), which make their way to the mosquito's salivary glands. Inoculation of the sporozoites into a new human host perpetuates the malaria life cycle.

Malaria paroxysms of chills, high fevers, and then sweats are produced when infected red blood cells rupture and release merozoites. After a number of cycles of erythrocytic schizogony, the release of merozoites may become synchronized, resulting in classic cyclic fevers. With *P. falciparum, P. vivax,* and *P. ovale* infections (tertian malaria), the paroxysms may occur in 48-hour cycles, whereas with *P. malariae* infections (quartan malaria), the cycles last 72 hours. However, patients, particularly those with *P. falciparum,* may not develop cyclic paroxysms at all, so a lack of cyclic fevers should not rule out a diagnosis of malaria. Other symptoms include headache, febrile seizures, rigors, cough, chest pain, diarrhea, nausea, vomiting, myalgias, and abdominal pain. On physical examination, a patient may appear well without physical findings or may have signs of jaundice, tachycardia, hypotension (usually secondary to dehydration), mild hepatomegaly, and splenomegaly. Laboratory abnormalities in cases of uncomplicated malaria may include anemia, an elevated reticulocyte count, thrombocytopenia, lymphopenia, hyperbilirubinemia, and mildly elevated transaminases. Appropriately treated, uncomplicated malaria has good outcomes, with a mortality rate of approximately 0.1%.

An uncomplicated malaria infection can progress to severe disease or death within hours. Risk factors for severe malaria include age older than 50 years, delays in treatment, inadequate or inappropriate treatment, a high parasite burden, and lack of acquired immunity. *P. falciparum,* more than any other species of *Plasmodium,* is responsible for the severe disease and death associated with malaria. This severity is attributed to several factors unique to this species. The tissue and blood schizonts release a larger number of merozoites

when they rupture, resulting in a rapid rise in parasitemia, and they can invade red blood cells of all ages, producing worse anemia. In addition, the processes of cytoadherence of *P. falciparum*–infected erythrocytes to the vascular endothelium, rosetting of infected erythrocytes with uninfected erythrocytes, and agglutination of infected erythrocytes with other infected erythrocytes contribute to tissue hypoxia and end-organ dysfunction. Even the immune response itself contributes to many of the cellular and humoral processes that manifest in severe malaria illness.

Severe malaria due to *P. falciparum* is associated with a 15% to 20% mortality rate. Signs and symptoms of severe malaria include impaired consciousness, coma (cerebral malaria), generalized seizures, severe anemia, acute renal failure, acute respiratory distress syndrome (ARDS), circulatory collapse, disseminated intravascular coagulation, abnormal bleeding, metabolic (lactic) acidosis, hypoglycemia, hemoglobinuria, jaundice, and a parasitemia greater than 5%.

Cerebral malaria, an ominous complication with an estimated 10% to 40% mortality rate, is characterized by diffuse symmetric encephalopathy. Coma or impaired mental status caused by malaria must be distinguished from other causes of altered mental status, including hyperpyrexia, hypoglycemia, and concurrent infections such as meningitis. Signs of cerebral malaria may range from odd behavior to delirium to coma with extensor posturing or opisthotonos. Children are more likely than adults to suffer from cerebral malaria and its residual neurologic sequelae. On the other hand, ARDS, jaundice, and renal impairment occur more frequently in adults. ARDS can occur even after signs of initial improvement.

Severe anemia and hypoglycemia, more common in children and pregnant women, are important features of severe malaria predicting poor prognosis. Acidosis with increased lactate levels and associated acidotic breathing are also poor prognostic factors.

With other species, complications are usually rare, although recent studies from Southeast Asia suggest that severe manifestations of *P. vivax* are not uncommon. Splenic rupture has been also described in patients with long-standing untreated *P. vivax* infection who have developed massive splenomegaly. Chronic complications of malarial infections include hyperreactive malarial syndrome (tropical splenomegaly syndrome), nephrotic syndrome (a rare complication of persistent *P. malariae* infection), and possibly Burkitt's lymphoma.

Diagnosis

To provide appropriate therapy, it is essential to identify the infecting malaria species, determine where the infection was acquired, and determine the parasite density. Health care providers evaluating patients for possible malaria must obtain thick and thin blood smears, the gold standard, to demonstrate asexual forms of the parasite. Malaria smears should be read immediately to avoid delays due to sending these tests to offsite laboratories where results are not available for extended periods of time. In rare instances, if the patient is very sick with symptoms consistent with severe malaria and has a history of malaria exposure, treatment should be started immediately, before results might be available. Initial blood smears may be negative, particularly in symptomatic, semi-immune persons and those taking prophylaxis. Blood smears should be repeated every 12 to 24 hours for a total of 48 to 72 hours (3 sets) before the diagnosis of malaria can be excluded. Initial laboratory evaluation of individuals with suspected malaria should include a complete blood count (CBC), electrolytes, creatinine, urea, glucose, and liver function tests. In patients with severe disease or respiratory symptoms, lactate level, arterial blood gases, and additional coagulation studies should also be obtained.

Blood smears should be prepared with Giemsa stain (pH 7.2) and examined under light microscopy. Both thick and thin smears should be scanned at low magnification and then examined under oil immersion (1000× magnification). The thick smear concentrates the parasites, resulting in a higher diagnostic sensitivity than the thin smear. The easiest way to determine the percentage of parasitemia using the thin smear is to count the parasitized erythrocytes among 500 to 2000 erythrocytes, divide that number by the total number of erythrocytes counted, and multiply by 100. To avoid missing low-density infections, at least 200 high-power fields should be examined before a slide is considered negative. Further details about preparation and interpretation of smears can be found at the CDC's Division of Parasitic Diseases diagnostic Internet site, http://www.dpd.cdc.gov/dpdx (accessed May 5, 2009).

The relationship between parasitemia and clinical severity is complex. Although severe malaria can occur even with apparently low parasitemia, persons with greater than 5% parasitemia are at higher risk of dying. Therefore, it is essential to determine the parasite burden at the time of diagnosis, as an assessment of disease severity. Sequential smears every 12 to 24 hours are useful for monitoring the response to treatment and detecting potential drug failure. Gametocytes may persist much longer and are not a sign of treatment failure.

Malaria should be considered in any febrile patient who has a history of travel to an area of malaria transmission, even if the patient was taking prophylaxis. Information on the location and duration of the trip, the date of return, the history of prophylaxis choice and adherence, and the date of symptom onset enables the physician to assess the risk of malaria and, if necessary, choose an appropriate course of treatment.

Alternative methods for diagnosis are available. Rapid diagnostic tests detect the presence of falciparum antigens by measuring histidine-rich protein-2 (HRP-2) or plasmodial enzymes such as aldolase and lactate dehydrogenase (pLDH). Determination of parasite density is not possible with these methods, but they can be useful if microscopy is unavailable. One assay, BinaxNOW, which detects two different malaria antigens (HRP-2 and aldolase), is available in the United States. The polymerase chain reaction method may be more sensitive than microscopy for detecting parasites. It is particularly valuable for identifying the species of a parasite when that cannot be determined by morphology alone. Currently, this method is used mostly as a research tool and is available only in reference laboratories. Malaria serology detects antibodies to all four species but cannot be used to diagnose acute infections. However, it may be useful for identifying an infective donor in cases of transfusion-related malaria, investigating congenital cases, assessing the validity of clinical malaria diagnoses in empirically treated nonimmune travelers, and diagnosing hyperreactive malarial syndrome.

Antimalarial Drugs

Because of the emergence and spread of drug resistance, the slow rate of development of new antimalarial drugs, and the infrequency with which new drugs that are developed are submitted for approval to the U.S. Food and Drug Administration (FDA), relatively few drugs are available for the prophylaxis and treatment of malaria infections in the United States. The choice of antimalarial drugs used for treatment should be guided by several factors: local availability, the infecting species, where infection was acquired (or at least a travel history), drug resistance patterns, severity of symptoms, and percentage of parasitemia.

Antimalarial drugs can be categorized by their ability to kill the organism at various stages in its life cycle (see Fig. 1). Drugs that kill malaria parasites infecting liver cells during the exoerythrocytic cycle are referred to as tissue schizonticides; blood schizonticides kill malaria parasites that have been released into the bloodstream and are asexually replicating in the erythrocytic cycle. Rapidly acting blood schizonticides are the essential components of acute malaria treatment regimens. Some drugs also have activity against the gametocytes. This activity does not affect a patient's clinical response but can decrease transmission. There are currently no medications available that have activity against malaria sporozoites.

Quinine sulfate (Qualaquin, an oral formulation), and its dextro-isomer, quinidine gluconate (a parenteral drug), are used for the treatment of malaria in the United States. They are blood schizonticides that are effective against the erythrocytic stages of all four species of plasmodia and are also active against the gametocytes of *P. vivax, P. ovale,* and *P. malariae.* Parenteral quinidine is currently the only FDA-approved treatment for severe malaria in the United States, but intravenous or intramuscular formulations of quinine[2] are used in other countries. Both intravenous quinine and quinidine should be administered with telemetry monitoring because of potential cardiac toxicity. Common side effects include cinchonism (a syndrome of tinnitus, deafness, headache, nausea, and visual disturbance) and hyperinsulinemic hypoglycemia. The longer the duration of therapy, the higher the risk of adverse events. To shorten the course of therapy, quinine and intravenous quinidine often can be combined with doxycycline (Vibramycin),* tetracycline,* or clindamycin (Cleocin),* except in cases acquired in Southeast Asia. Artesunate,[5] described in detail later in this section, is an alternate parenteral option available in the United States through the CDC. These drugs are described later and in Table 1.

Chloroquine phosphate (Aralen) and hydroxychloroquine sulfate (Plaquenil) are used for prevention and treatment of malaria. They are blood schizonticides that are active against the erythrocytic stages of all four *Plasmodium* species and have gametocytocidal activity against *P. vivax, P. ovale,* and *P. malariae.* Chloroquine is the treatment of choice for susceptible strains of all *Plasmodium* species, although chloroquine-resistant forms of *P. falciparum* and *P. vivax* have become major public health concerns. Chloroquine can be taken safely by pregnant women and children. Side effects include gastrointestinal disturbance, dizziness, blurred vision, insomnia, headache, and pruritus. In extremely rare cases, long-term administration over

---

*Although not FDA approved for this indication, it is an official CDC approved treatment.

[5]Investigational drug in the United States.

TABLE 1 Recommended Drugs for Treatment of Specific Types of Malaria

Diagnosis	Recommended Drug
Uncomplicated chloroquine-sensitive *P. falciparum*	Chloroquine phosphate (Aralen)
Uncomplicated chloroquine-resistant *P. falciparum* OR Resistance unknown OR Species unknown	Quinine sulfate* (Qualaquin) **plus one of the following**: Doxycycline[†,‡] or Tetracycline[†,‡] or Clindamycin (Cleocin)[‡] **OR** Artemether-lumefantrine (Coartem) **OR** Atovaquone/proguanil (Malarone) **OR** Mefloquine[§] (Lariam)
Uncomplicated *P. malariae* or *P. knowlesi*	Chloroquine phosphate (Aralen)
Uncomplicated *P. vivax* or *P. ovale* (except chloroquine-resistant *P. vivax*)	Chloroquine phosphate (Aralen) **plus** primaquine phosphate[¶]
Uncomplicated chloroquine-resistant *P. vivax*	Quinine sulfate* (Qualaquin) **plus** primaquine phosphate[¶] **plus one of the following**: Doxycycline[†,‡] **OR** Tetracycline[†,‡] **OR** Mefloquine[§] (Lariam) **plus** primaquine phosphate[¶] **OR** Atovaquone-proguanil (Malarone) **plus** primaquine phosphate[¶]
Chloroquine-sensitive malaria during pregnancy	Chloroquine phosphate (Aralen)
Chloroquine-resistant *P. falciparum* during pregnancy	Quinine sulfate* (Qualaquin) **plus** clindamycin (Cleocin)[‡]
Chloroquine-resistant *P. vivax* during pregnancy	Quinine sulfate* (Qualaquin)
Severe malaria	Parenteral quinidine gluconate **plus one of the following**: Doxycycline[†,‡] or Tetracycline[†,‡] or Clindamycin (Cleocin)[‡] **OR** Parenteral artesunate** followed by another oral treatment (investigational new drug; contact CDC for information)

*Quinidine/quinine course = 7 days if infection was acquired in Southeast Asia; = 3 days if infection was acquired in Africa or South America.
[†]Doxycycline and tetracycline are not indicated for use in children younger than 8 years.
[‡]Although not FDA approved for this indication, it is an official CDC approved treatment.
[§]Because of resistant strains, treatment with Mefloquine is not recommended in persons who have acquired infections in parts of Thailand, Burma, Cambodia, Laos, China, and Vietnam.
[¶]All persons who take primaquine should have a documented normal G6PD level prior to starting the medication.
**Available in the United States through the CDC as an investigational new drug.

many years of chloroquine for malaria prevention can lead to retinopathy, ototoxicity, and peripheral neuropathy.

Mefloquine (Lariam) is a long-acting blood schizonticide that is used for prevention and treatment of malaria. It is effective against the erythrocytic stages of all four species. Side effects include nausea, vomiting, diarrhea, abdominal pain, myalgia, a mild skin rash, fatigue, and mild neuropsychiatric complaints (dizziness, headache, somnolence, sleep disorders). Mefloquine has also been associated with rare serious adverse reactions, such as seizures and psychoses, at prophylactic doses. Although mefloquine can be used to treat chloroquine-resistant *P. falciparum*, adverse reactions are more common at the higher doses used for treatment. Because other options that have fewer adverse events are available for treatment, mefloquine is usually not recommended. Mefloquine is contraindicated for use in patients with known hypersensitivity to the drug and persons with a history of psychiatric disease. Mefloquine also is contraindicated in persons with a history of seizures (not including febrile seizures in childhood). It should be avoided in patients with cardiac conduction disorders, because it prolongs the QTc interval, and should be used with caution in persons taking β-blockers. Concomitant administration of mefloquine and quinine or quinidine should be avoided, because it may produce arrhythmias and increase the risk of seizures. Mefloquine prophylaxis in the second and third trimesters is not associated with an adverse fetal or pregnancy outcome. More limited data suggest that it is probably safe in the first trimester. Any traveler receiving a prescription for mefloquine must receive a copy of the FDA Medication Guide found at http://www.fda.gov/cder/foi/label/2003/19591s19lbl_Lariam.pdf (accessed May 5, 2009).

Atovaquone-proguanil (Malarone), a fixed-combination antimalarial drug that is both a blood and tissue schizonticide, can be used for chemoprophylaxis and for treatment of chloroquine-resistant *P. falciparum*. It does not prevent relapses of *P. vivax* and *P. ovale*. Side effects are rare, but abdominal pain, nausea, vomiting, and headache have been reported. Treatment efficacy, safety, and pharmacokinetic data in children weighing 5 to 11 kg have been extrapolated, allowing for prophylactic doses in these children; this constitutes an off-label use in the United States. Atovaquone-proguanil is contraindicated in children who weigh less than 5 kg, pregnant women, women who are breast-feeding infants who weigh less than 5 kg, and persons with severe renal impairment.

Tetracyclines* are blood schizonticides that are effective against the erythrocytic stages of all four species of *Plasmodium*. Because of their relatively slow onset of action, tetracyclines should never be used alone for treatment. Combined with quinine or quinidine, they are effective against chloroquine-resistant *P. falciparum* and *P. vivax*. Doxycycline (Vibramycin) alone is effective as prophylaxis against chloroquine-resistant and mefloquine-resistant *P. falciparum*. Side effects include

---

*Although not FDA approved for this indication, it is an official CDC approved treatment.

gastrointestinal symptoms, *Candida* vaginitis or stomatitis, and idio-syncratic photosensitivity reactions. Tetracyclines should not be used in pregnant women or in children younger than 8 years old.

Clindamycin (Cleocin)* is active against blood schizonts of all four species of *Plasmodium*. Like the tetracyclines, it has a slow onset and should never be used alone for treatment of malaria. Clindamy-cin can be used in combination with quinine to treat chloroquine-resistant *P. falciparum* infections in people who are not able to take tetracyclines. Side effects include diarrhea, nausea, and skin rashes.

Derivatives of artemisinin (e.g., artesunate,[5] artemether,[2] dihy-droartemisinin[2]) are compounds derived from the Chinese medicinal plant quinghaosu (*Artemisia annua*) that are active against blood schizonts and gametocytes. Artemisinin and its derivatives are short-acting, highly effective antimalarial drugs for the treatment of uncomplicated multidrug-resistant *P. falciparum* and severe *P. falci-parum* infection. These drugs are available in oral, rectal, and intrave-nous formulations. Although they can be used alone for at least 7 days, combining them with other antimalarial drugs treats malaria infections effectively, decreases the length of treatment, and safe-guards against selection for drug-resistant parasites. Commonly used artemisinin-based combination therapies include artesunate copack-aged with mefloquine (Artequin)[2] and artemether coformulated with lumefantrine[2] (Coartem or Riamet). Artemether-lumefantrine (Coar-tem) has been recently approved by the FDA and is available in the United States. Parenteral artesunate is available through the CDC as an investigational drug for treating severe malaria.

Primaquine phosphate, a tissue schizonticide with gametocytocidal activity, is the only drug available to prevent relapse of *P. vivax* and *P. ovale* infections. Primaquine (up to 30 mg/day)[3] has the following uses: primary prophylaxis, especially for travelers to destinations where *P. vivax* is the main species*; presumptive anti-relapse therapy (PART), to treat the liver stages (hypnozoites) of *P. vivax* and *P. ovale*, generally indicated for persons who have had prolonged exposure in malaria-endemic areas (e.g., missionaries, Peace Corps volunteers, military per-sonnel)*; and radical cure to prevent relapses of *P. vivax* and *P. ovale* infection. Primary prophylaxis with primaquine obviates the need for PART. The duration of therapy for PART and radical cure is 14 days after the patient has left the malarious area, and the drug is best given in conjunction with a blood schizonticide. Primaquine can cause hemolysis and methemoglobinemia in persons with glucose-6-phos-phate dehydrogenase (G6PD) deficiency, which must be ruled out by appropriate laboratory testing before it is used. The most common side effects are abdominal pain and headache. Primaquine is contrain-dicated in pregnant and breast-feeding women.

Other antimalarials often encountered in malaria-endemic countries include sulfadoxine-pyrimethamine (Fansidar), amodiaquine (Camoquin),[2] proguanil (Paludrine),[2] and halofantrine (Halfan).[2] These agents are not recommended for use in the United States because of limited efficacy or their side effect profile.

Treatment

GENERAL INFORMATION

Ideally, treatment for malaria should not be initiated until the diagno-sis has been confirmed by laboratory investigations. However, health care providers should not delay treatment if malaria is strongly sus-pected and smear results are not available in a timely manner. Once the diagnosis is confirmed, appropriate antimalarial therapy must be initiated immediately. The choice of treatment should be guided by the species of *Plasmodium* found, the level of parasitemia, the clinical status of the patient, and the likely drug susceptibility of the infecting species (as determined by where the infection was acquired). Although all four species require treatment with a rapidly acting blood

schizonticide, patients with *P. vivax* or *P. ovale* also require treatment with primaquine phosphate to decrease the likelihood of a relapse.

Species identification is necessary to distinguish falciparum malaria from non-falciparum malaria. *P. falciparum* can cause rapid progres-sion of disease and death; therefore, patients with *P. falciparum*, mixed infections with *P. falciparum*, or infections in which the species cannot be identified immediately should be hospitalized and monitored closely to assess for the development of severe malaria and subsequent complications. If the infecting species or probable origin of infection cannot be determined, patients should be treated for multidrug-resistant *P. falciparum* until the organism is otherwise identified. All patients should have repeat blood smears 12 to 24 hours after initia-tion of treatment to assess for appropriate response.

Using available clinical and laboratory data, physicians must determine whether a patient has uncomplicated or severe malaria. Individuals with uncomplicated malaria typically can be treated with oral therapy but may need parenteral therapy if they are unable to tolerate oral medications. Individuals with severe malaria should be immediately started on parenteral therapy and monitored in an intensive care setting, if available.

For detailed treatment information, including doses and frequency of therapy, refer to Tables 1 and 2.

DRUG-RESISTANT *P. FALCIPARUM*

For *P. falciparum* infections acquired in chloroquine-resistant areas, there are four treatment options: quinine sulfate (Qualaquin) plus doxycycline,* tetracycline,* or clindamycin (Cleocin)*; artemether-lumefantrine (Coartem) alone; atovaquone-proguanil (Malarone) alone; and mefloquine (Lariam) alone. Because mefloquine has a higher rate of severe neuropsychiatric reactions at treatment doses, it is recommended only if the other two options are not available. Also, mefloquine is not recommended for the treatment of falci-parum malaria in persons who acquired the infection in Southeast Asia, especially Thailand, Cambodia, Burma (Myanmar), Laos, or Vietnam, because of the potential for mefloquine-resistant strains.

CHLOROQUINE-SENSITIVE *P. FALCIPARUM*, *P. VIVAX*, *P. OVALE*, AND *P. MALARIAE*

For *P. malariae*, *P. ovale*, *P. knowlesi*, chloroquine-sensitive *P. vivax*, and chloroquine-sensitive *P. falciparum* infection, prompt treatment with oral chloroquine phosphate (Aralen) is recommended. In addition, infections with *P. vivax* and *P. ovale* require primaquine to reduce the likelihood of a relapse. Before starting primaquine treatment, patients must have a documented normal level of G6PD activity.

DRUG-RESISTANT *P. VIVAX*

Chloroquine-resistant *P. vivax* should be treated with quinine sulfate plus doxycycline* or tetracycline* or with mefloquine alone. In addi-tion to either of those regimens, persons with a normal level of G6PD activity infected with *P. vivax* should be treated with primaquine phosphate to prevent relapse.

SEVERE MALARIA

Patients diagnosed with severe malaria, regardless of species, and those who are unable to take oral medications should be treated with parenteral antimalarial therapy. Severe malaria is a medical emergency, and treatment with intravenous medication should be initiated imme-diately (see Tables 1 and 2). In the United States, quinidine gluconate is the only parenteral rapidly acting blood schizonticide approved by the FDA. Under an investigational new drug protocol, artesunate, a parenteral drug for the treatment of severe malaria, is available through the CDC. Health care providers caring for patients with severe malaria should contact the CDC to assess the need for artesunate (CDC Malaria Hotline: 770-488-7788, M-F 8 AM-4:30 PM Eastern time; emergency consultation after hours: 770-488-7100).

---

*Although not FDA approved for this indication, it is an official CDC approved treatment.

[2]Not available in the United States.

[3]Exceeds dosage recommended by the manufacturer.

[5]Investigational drug in the United States.

---

*Although not FDA approved for this indication, it is an official CDC approved treatment.

TABLE 2 Treatment Dosages of Antimalarial Drugs

Drug	Adult Dose	Pediatric Dose*
Artemether-lumefantrine (Coartem)	1 tablet = 20 mg artemether and 120 mg lumefantrine. 3 day treatment schedule of 6 total doses. The patient should receive the initial dose, followed by the second dose 8 hours later, then 1 dose PO bid for the following 2 days 4 tablets per dose.	1 tablet = 20 mg artemether and 120 mg lumefantrine 3 day treatment schedule of 6 total doses. The patient should receive the initial dose, followed by the second dose 8 hours later, then 1 dose PO bid for the following 2 days. 5–<15 kg: 1 tablet per dose 15–<25 kg: 2 tablets per dose 25–<35 kg: 3 tablets per dose ≥35 kg: 4 tablets per dose
Artesunate[†] (available only through the CDC in the United States)	2.4 mg/kg IV push at 0, 12, 24, and 48 h	2.4 mg/kg IV push at 0, 12, 24, and 48 h
Atovaquone-proguanil (Malarone)	4 Adult tablets (each adult tablet contains 250 mg atovaquone and 100 mg proguanil) PO as a single daily dose for 3 consecutive days	Dosage based on weight (each pediatric tablet contains 62.5 mg atovaquone and 25 mg proguanil); daily dose to be taken for 3 consecutive days: 5–8 kg: 2 pediatric tablets 9–10 kg: 3 pediatric tablets 11–20 kg: 1 adult tablet 21–30 kg: 2 adult tablets 31–40 kg: 3 adult tablets ≥41 kg: 4 adult tablets
Chloroquine phosphate (Aralen)	600 mg base (= 1 g salt) PO, then 300 mg base (= 500 mg salt) at 6, 24, and 48 h	10 mg base/kg PO, then 5 mg base/kg at 6, 24, and 48 h
Clindamycin—oral (Cleocin)[‡]	20 mg base/kg/day PO divided tid for 7 d	20 mg base/kg/d PO divided tid for 7 d
Clindamycin—parenteral (Cleocin)[‡]	10 mg base/kg IV followed by 5 mg base/kg IV q8h; switch to oral clindamycin as soon as patient is able to complete 7-d course	10 mg base/kg IV followed by 5 mg base/kg IV q8h; switch to oral clindamycin as soon as patient is able to complete 7-d course
Doxycycline[‡,§]	100 mg PO or IV bid for 7 d	2.2 mg/kg PO or IV bid for 7 d[§]
Mefloquine (Lariam)	750 mg salt (= 684 mg base) PO followed by 500 mg salt (= 456 mg base) PO 6–12 h after the initial dose	15 mg salt/kg (= 13.7 mg base/kg) PO followed by 10 mg salt/kg (= 9.1 mg base/kg) PO 6–12 h after the initial dose
Primaquine phosphate[¶]	30 mg base* PO qd for 14 d**	0.5 mg base/kg[3] PO qd for 14 d**
Quinidine gluconate	6.25 mg base/kg (= 10 mg salt/kg) loading dose[††] IV over 1–2 h, then 0.0125 mg base/kg/min (= 0.02 mg salt/kg/min) continuous infusion for at least 24 h. An alternative regimen is 15 mg base/kg (= 24 mg salt/kg) loading dose IV infused over 4 h, followed by 7.5 mg base/kg (= 12 mg salt/kg) infused over 4 h q8h, starting 8 h after the loading dose. Once parasite density is <1% and patient can take oral medication, complete treatment with oral quinine.	6.25 mg base/kg (= 10 mg salt/kg) loading dose[††] IV over 1–2 h, then 0.0125 mg base/kg/min (= 0.02 mg salt/kg/min) continuous infusion for at least 24 h. An alternative regimen is 15 mg base/kg (= 24 mg salt/kg) loading dose IV infused over 4 h, followed by 7.5 mg base/kg (= 12 mg salt/kg) infused over 4 h q8h, starting 8 h after the loading dose. Once parasite density is <1% and patient can take oral medication, complete treatment with oral quinine.
Quinine sulfate (Qualaquin)	650 mg salt (= 542 mg base) PO tid for 3 d (7 d if acquired in Southeast Asia)	10 mg salt/kg (= 8.3 mg base/kg) PO tid for 3 d (7 days if acquired in Southeast Asia)
Tetracycline[‡,§]	250 mg PO qid for 7 d	25 mg/kg/d PO divided qid for 7 d[§]

*Pediatric dose should never exceed adult dose.
[†]Investigational drug in the United States.
[‡]Although not FDA approved for this indication, it is an official CDC approved treatment.
[§]Doxycycline and tetracycline are not indicated for use in children younger than 8 years.
[¶]All persons who take primaquine should have a documented normal glucose-6-phosphate dehydrogenase level prior to starting the medication.
**Exceeds dosage recommended by the manufacturer.
[††]Patients should be given a loading dose of quinidine unless they have received more than 40 mg/kg of quinidine in the preceding 48 hours or if they received mefloquine treatment within the preceding 12 hours.

In addition to antimalarial therapy, patients should receive the necessary supportive care. The patient should be admitted to an intensive care unit with continuous blood pressure and cardiac monitoring (to assess the QTc interval) and regular measurements of blood glucose. Fluid status, level of consciousness, and vital signs should be monitored closely. Because these patients are at risk for hypoglycemia, severe anemia, renal failure, and acidosis, regular assessment of blood glucose, hemoglobin/hematocrit, creatinine, urea, electrolytes, and acid-base status also is required. Severe anemia requires blood transfusion with packed red blood cells. Hemodialysis or hemofiltration is usually needed in patients with acute renal failure. Oxygen and other respiratory support may be required in individuals with ARDS. One should consider exchange transfusion if parasitemia is greater than 10% or if the patient has altered mental status, ARDS, or renal complications. Blood smears should be repeated every 12 hours to monitor response. Once parasite density is lower than 1% and the patient is able to eat and drink, the treatment course should be completed with oral medications.

Various adjunctive therapies have been shown to be not effective and some even harmful, including corticosteroids[1] for the treatment of cerebral malaria, phenobarbital for seizure prophylaxis, heparin for coagulation abnormalities, iron chelators[1] to reduce parasite clearance time, pentoxifylline (Trental)[1] to inhibit tumor necrosis factor, and dichloroacetate[1] for treatment of metabolic acidosis.

CONGENITAL AND PREGNANCY-ASSOCIATED MALARIA

Malaria in pregnancy affects both the mother and her fetus. Infection with *P. falciparum* during pregnancy can increase the mother's risk of developing severe disease and anemia as well as increasing the risk of stillbirth, prematurity, and low birth weight, especially for women in

[1]Not FDA approved for this indication.

their first or second pregnancies and those who are immunocompromised. Babies born to mothers with acute malaria are at risk for congenital malaria, but empiric treatment is not recommended. Treating physicians should judge each case individually, considering such factors as reliability of follow-up and access to medical care. Simply educating the mother about the risk of congenital malaria and instructing her to seek medical care if the infant develops symptoms of malaria may be appropriate in most cases, whereas presumptive treatment of the newborn may be warranted in others. Primaquine treatment of infants is unnecessary, because there is no liver phase with congenital infections. If the infant's blood smear is negative at the time of delivery, health care providers should remain alert for the development of signs and symptoms consistent with malaria and should initiate a prompt diagnostic evaluation. Congenital malaria often manifests as fever, anemia, or failure to thrive at 1 to 2 months of age and can be difficult for an unsuspecting clinician to detect.

For pregnant women diagnosed with uncomplicated malaria caused by *P. malariae, P. ovale,* chloroquine-sensitive *P. vivax,* or chloroquine-sensitive *P. falciparum,* prompt treatment with chloroquine (Aralen) is recommended. For pregnant women diagnosed with chloroquine-resistant *P. vivax,* treatment with quinine (Qualaquin) for 7 days is recommended. After treatment, all pregnant women with *P. vivax* and *P. ovale* should be given chloroquine prophylaxis for the duration of the pregnancy to avoid relapses; women can be treated with primaquine after delivery if they have a normal G6PD screening test. For pregnant women diagnosed with uncomplicated chloroquine-resistant *P. falciparum* malaria, prompt treatment with quinine and clindamycin (Cleocin)* is recommended. Primaquine should never be given during pregnancy because of the risk of G6PD-mediated hemolysis in the fetus.

MALARIA IN CHILDREN

For pediatric patients, treatment options are the same as for adults except that the drug dose is adjusted for patient weight. The pediatric dose should never exceed the recommended adult dose. For treatment of chloroquine-resistant *P. falciparum* in children younger than 8 years of age, doxycycline and tetracycline should not be used;

---

*Although not FDA approved for this indication, it is an official CDC approved treatment.

atovaquone-proguanil alone (if weight is >5 kg) or quinine sulfate given in combination with clindamycin* is the recommended treatment option. Mefloquine (Lariam) may be considered if these options are not available. In rare instances, doxycycline* or tetracycline* can be used in combination with quinine in children younger than 8 years old if other treatment options are not available or are not tolerated and the benefit of adding doxycycline or tetracycline is judged to outweigh the risk.

Prevention

A combination of personal protective measures and chemoprophylaxis can be highly effective in preventing malaria in travelers and in those living in malaria-endemic areas. Malaria-endemic countries have focused on delivering personal and household protection through use of insecticide-treated nets and indoor residual spraying with insecticides. Chemoprophylaxis in the form of intermittent preventive treatment of high-risk groups, pregnant women, and infants has been adopted by several malaria-endemic countries.

Other protective measures include avoiding being outdoors during the peak *Anopheles* biting period between dusk and dawn, wearing clothing that minimizes the amount of exposed skin, and applying insect repellents that contain diethylmethyl-toluamide (DEET). DEET may be used on adults and children including infants older than 2 months of age. Higher concentrations of DEET may have a longer repellent effect; however, concentrations greater than 50% provide no added protection. Travelers who are not staying in well-screened or air-conditioned rooms should sleep under insecticide-treated bed nets.

For travelers, the choice of prophylactic medication should be made with consideration of destination, length of stay, presence of resistant strains, and patient age, drug allergies, other medications, and medical history. Often, potential side effects, convenience of the dosing regimen, and cost affect patients' choices of medications. Detailed prophylaxis recommendations are presented in Table 3.

---

*Although not FDA approved for this indication, it is an official CDC approved treatment.

TABLE 3 Malaria Chemoprophylaxis Recommendations

Drug	Usage	Adult Dose	Pediatric Dose	Comments
Atovaquone-proguanil (Malarone)	Prophylaxis in all malaria risk areas	1 Adult tablet PO qd (each adult tablet contains 250 mg atovaquone and 100 mg proguanil hydrochloride)	Pediatric tablets contain 62.5 mg atovaquone and 25 mg proguanil hydrochloride; daily dose: 5–8 kg[1]: $\frac{1}{2}$ pediatric tablet 9–10 kg[1]: $\frac{3}{4}$ pediatric tablet 11–20 kg: 1 pediatric tablet 21–30 kg: 2 pediatric tablets 31–40 kg: 3 pediatric tablets ≥41 kg: 1 adult tablet	Begin 1–2 d before travel to malarious areas. Take daily at the same time each day while in the malarious area and for 7 d after leaving such areas. Contraindicated in persons with severe renal impairment (creatinine clearance <30 mL/min). Atovaquone-proguanil should be taken with food. Not recommended for prophylaxis for children <5 kg and pregnant women. Partial tablet dosages may need to be prepared by a pharmacist and dispensed in individual capsules.
Chloroquine phosphate* (Aralen and generic)	Prophylaxis only in areas with chloroquine-sensitive *P. falciparum*	300 mg base (= 500 mg salt) PO q wk	5 mg/kg base (= 8.3 mg/kg salt) PO q wk, up to maximum adult dose of 300 mg base	Begin 1–2 wk before travel to malarious areas. Take weekly on the same day of the week while in the malarious area and for 4 wk after leaving such areas. May exacerbate psoriasis.

Continued

TABLE 3 Malaria Chemoprophylaxis Recommendations—Cont'd

Drug	Usage	Adult Dose	Pediatric Dose	Comments
Doxycycline[†]	Prophylaxis in all malaria risk areas	100 mg PO qd	≥8 y of age: 2 mg/kg up to adult dose of 100 mg/d[†]	Begin 1–2 d before travel to malarious areas. Take daily at the same time each day while in the malarious area and for 4 wk after leaving such areas. Contraindicated in children <8 y and pregnant women.
Hydroxychloroquine sulfate (Plaquenil)	An alternative to chloroquine for prophylaxis only in areas with chloroquine-sensitive *P. falciparum*	310 mg base (= 400 mg salt) PO q wk	5 mg/kg base (= 6.5 mg/kg salt) PO q wk, up to maximum adult dose of 310 mg base	Begin 1–2 wk before travel to malarious areas. Take weekly on the same day of the week while in the malarious area and for 4 wk after leaving such areas.
Mefloquine (Lariam and generic)	Prophylaxis in areas with mefloquine-sensitive *P. falciparum*	228 mg base (= 250 mg salt) PO q wk	≤9 kg: 4.6 mg/kg base (= 5 mg/kg salt) PO q wk 10–19 kg: $\frac{1}{4}$ tablet q wk 20–30 kg: $\frac{1}{2}$ tablet q wk 31–45 kg: $\frac{3}{4}$ tablet q wk ≥46 kg: 1 tablet q wk	Begin 1–2 wk before travel to malarious areas. Take weekly on the same day of the week while in the malarious area and for 4 wk after leaving such areas. Contraindicated in persons allergic to mefloquine or related compounds (e.g., quinine, quinidine) and in persons with active depression, a recent history of depression, generalized anxiety disorder, psychosis, schizophrenia, other major psychiatric disorders, or seizures. Use with caution in persons with psychiatric disturbances or a previous history of depression. Not recommended for persons with cardiac conduction abnormalities.
Primaquine phosphate[‡]	Prophylaxis in areas with mainly *P. vivax*	30 mg base (= 52.6 mg salt)[§] PO qd	0.5 mg/kg base (= 0.8 mg/kg salt)[§] up to adult dose PO qd	Begin 1–2 d before travel to malarious areas. Take daily at the same time each day while in the malarious area and for 7 d after leaving such areas. Contraindicated in persons with G6PD deficiency.[‡] Also contraindicated during pregnancy and lactation unless the infant being breast-fed has a documented normal G6PD level.
Primaquine phosphate[‡]	Used for presumptive anti-relapse therapy (terminal prophylaxis) to decrease the risk of relapses of *P. vivax* and *P. ovale*	30 mg base (= 52.6 mg salt)[§] PO qd for 14 d after departure from the malarious area	0.5 mg/kg base (= 0.8 mg/kg salt)[§] up to adult dose PO qd for 14 d after departure from the malarious area	Indicated for persons who have had prolonged exposure to *P. vivax* or *P. ovale* or both. Contraindicated in persons with G6PD deficiency.[‡] Also contraindicated during pregnancy and lactation unless the infant being breast-fed has a documented normal G6PD level.

*All pregnant women with *P. vivax* and *P. ovale* should be given chloroquine prophylaxis for the duration of pregnancy to avoid relapses and can be treated with primaquine after delivery.
[†]Doxycycline is not indicated for use in children younger than 8 years.
[‡]All persons who take primaquine should have a documented normal glucose-6-phosphate dehydrogenase level prior to starting the medication.
[§]Exceeds dosage recommended by the manufacturer.

Malaria infection in pregnant women can be more severe than in nonpregnant women. Women who are pregnant or are likely to become pregnant should be advised to avoid travel to high-risk areas. However, pregnant women who choose to travel to these areas should take appropriate antimalarial prophylaxis and use personal protective measures.

Travelers should be advised that they can contract malaria despite the use of prophylaxis and personal protective measures. Travelers should be aware of the signs and symptoms of malaria and should urgently seek medical care if they develop fever or experience flu-like symptoms. Because many health care providers do not always ask about travel, travelers should be advised to specifically inform providers of their recent travel to a malaria-endemic area so that the appropriate diagnostic evaluation and treatment can be initiated.

REFERENCES

Baird JK. Effectiveness of antimalarial drugs. N Engl J Med 2005;352 (15):1565–77.

Centers for Disease Control and Prevention. Guidelines for Treatment of Malaria in the United States. Available at: http://www.cdc.gov/malaria/pdf/treatmenttable.pdf [accessed May 5, 2009].

Cox-Singh J, Davis TM, Lee KS, et al. *Plasmodium knowlesi* malaria in humans is widely distributed and potentially life threatening. Clin Infect Dis 2008;46(2):165–71.

Genton B, D'Acremont V, Rare L, et al. *Plasmodium vivax* and mixed infections are associated with severe malaria in children: A prospective cohort study from Papua New Guinea. PLoS Med 2008;5(6):e127.

Griffith KS, Lewis LS, Mali S, et al. Treatment of malaria in the United States: A systematic review. JAMA 2007;297(20):2264–77.

Lalloo DG, Hill DR. Preventing malaria in travellers. BMJ 2008;336(7657): 1362–6.

Mali S, Steele S, Slutsker L, et al. Malaria surveillance—United States, 2006. MMWR Surveill Summ 2008;57(5):24–39.

Phu NH, Hien TT, Mai NT, et al. Hemofiltration and peritoneal dialysis in infection-associated acute renal failure in Vietnam. N Engl J Med 2002; 347(12):895–902.

Riddle MS, Jackson JL, Sanders JW, et al. Exchange transfusion as an adjunct therapy in severe *Plasmodium falciparum* malaria: A meta-analysis. Clin Infect Dis 2002;34(9):1192–8.

Rosenthal PJ. Artesunate for the treatment of severe falciparum malaria. N Engl J Med 2008;358(17):1829–36.

World Health Organization. Severe falciparum malaria: World Health Organization, Communicable Diseases Cluster. Trans R Soc Trop Med Hyg 2000; 94(Suppl. 1):S1–90.

World Health Organization. World Malaria Report 2008. WHO: Geneva; 2008.

Bacterial Meningitis

Method of
Gary D. Overturf, MD

Acute bacterial meningitis occurs in all age groups, but predominantly in children younger than 2 years and the elderly (older than 60 years). With the introduction of effective protein conjugate vaccines for *Haemophilus* and pneumococcal infection, the incidence of bacterial meningitis is rapidly declining in children, and adults are now the major population affected. Bacterial meningitis is a medical emergency requiring rapid and decisive action to prevent death or neurologic sequelae. Since the introduction of chloramphenicol (Chloromycetin) in the early 1950s, the mortality has remained between 5% and 40% depending on the age of the patient and the etiology. Of the survivors, 10% to 30% suffer permanent neurologic deficits. Prognosis is affected by the timeliness of therapy, the age of the patient, and the etiology. Presumptive diagnosis and administration of therapy are critical.

Diagnosis

Acute bacterial meningitis must be considered in the differential diagnosis of persons of any age presenting with fever and headache or signs of meningeal irritation or acute central nervous system dysfunction. Presentations can be subtle at the extremes of age or in patients who have received partially effective antibiotic therapy. The diagnosis of bacterial meningitis requires the examination of the cerebrospinal fluid (CSF), which must be performed as expeditiously as possible. Studies indicate that lumbar puncture may be safely performed on patients who have normal mental status or are without focal neurologic signs or papilledema; clinical impression are predictive of the computed tomography (CT) findings. If there are signs or symptoms suggesting the presence of an intracranial mass

CURRENT DIAGNOSIS

- Patient age and epidemiology:
  - Clinical symptoms: Fever, headache, meningeal signs
  - CSF examination: High opening pressure >300 mm Hg
  - Elevated white blood cell count (>10–>5000)
  - >60% polymorphonuclear cells
- Low CSF glucose (<40 mg/dL or <50% serum glucose)
- High CSF protein (>50–>1.0 g/dL)
- Bacteria present on Gram stain of CSF

Abbreviation: CSF = cerebrospinal fluid.

(e.g., tumor, cerebral hematoma, or brain abscess), blood cultures should be obtained and empirical antibiotics should be administered prior to the performance of a CT scan.

The CSF findings in bacterial meningitis include a cell count of greater than 500 to 5000 white blood cells (WBC) per mm^3 with a predominance of neutrophils, a protein concentration of greater than 150 mg/mL, and a low glucose (e.g., less than 35 to 40 mg/dL). No single value is absolute, and a single value may be normal in up to a third of the cases. The Gram-stained sediment of centrifuged CSF is the critical examination leading to a specific diagnosis. In patients who have not received antibiotics capable of reaching the CSF, the Gram stain is positive in 80% to 90% of culture-confirmed cases. In persons previously treated with antibiotics (e.g., beta-lactam antibiotics, tetracycline, fluoroquinolones), the frequency of positive Gram stains is much reduced (e.g., 60% to 70%), but the cells, cell type, protein, and glucose concentrations are not significantly affected. CSF antigen tests are not reliable, and high false-positive and false-negative rates direct against relying on the use of such tests. Clinical judgment is paramount, and antibiotics should be given in situations of ambiguous results of the CSF examination.

Antibiotic Selection

The outcome of bacterial meningitis is closely related to the timely use of antibiotics. Hypotension, seizures, an altered mental status, and hypoglycorrhachia at the time of initial antibiotic administration are predictive of higher case fatality and neurologic sequelae. Because prompt administration of antibiotics is critical, the choice of antibiotics usually is made before results of the CSF cultures are known. If organisms are seen on Gram stain, therapy may be directed by the probable bacterial etiology (Table 1). In the event the CSF Gram stain fails to reveal a possible pathogen, empirical antibiotic therapy should be begun based on the age of the patient for those persons who have acquired their infection in the community (Table 2). For those persons who are members of special risk groups, empirical therapy should be based on the likely etiology (Table 3). Once the CSF cultures are completed, therapy can be modified according to results of the culture and sensitivity data.

Antibiotics used in bacterial meningitis should be rapidly bactericidal and achieve high concentrations in the CSF. Antibiotics should be given in maximal doses (Table 4). Because the bactericidal activity of antibiotics in CSF is dose dependent, the fractional CSF-to-serum ratio is very small. Finally, the use of combinations of antibiotics should be minimized to avoid antagonizing the bactericidal activity.

Special Considerations for Antibiotic Therapy

During the past two decades, resistance to penicillin and some third-generation cephalosporins (e.g., ceftriaxone [Rocephin], cefotaxime [Claforan]) has steadily increased among strains of *Streptococcus*

TABLE 1 Cerebrospinal Fluid Gram Stain Morphology and Antibiotic Recommendations

Morphology	Possible or Probable Pathogens	Treatment Options	Alternative Therapies
Gram-positive cocci, short chains or pairs	Streptococcus pneumoniae, Streptococcus agalactiae (group B streptococci)	Ceftriaxone (Rocephin) or cefotaxime (Claforan) plus vancomycin (Vancocin)	Chloramphenicol (Chloromycetin)
Gram-positive cocci, clusters; or gram-positive bacilli	Staphylococcus aureus, Listeria monocytogenes	Vancomycin, ampicillin plus gentamicin (Garamycin)	Nafcillin (Unipen) or Oxacillin, trimethoprim-sulfamethoxazole (Bactrim)
Gram-negative diplococci	Neisseria meningitidis	Ceftriaxone or cefotaxime	Ampicillin, Penicillin G, or chloramphenicol
Gram-negative coccobacilli	Haemophilus influenzae	Ceftriaxone or cefotaxime	Chloramphenicol
Gram-negative bacilli	Escherichia coli, Klebsiella species, Pseudomonas aeruginosa	Cefepime (Maxipime) or ceftazidime (Fortaz)	Imipenem (Primaxin) or meropenem (Merrem)

TABLE 2 Antibiotic Recommendations for Bacterial Meningitis Acquired in the Community, by Age Group and Probable Pathogen

Age Group	Probable Pathogens	Empirical Therapy
Neonate < 1 mo	Group B streptococcus; Escherichia coli, or other gram-negative enteric rod; occasionally Listeria monocytogenes	Ampicillin plus cefotaxime (Claforan)
Infants 1–3 mo	H. influenzae, N. meningitidis, S. pneumoniae, Group B streptococci	Ceftriaxone (Rocephin) or cefotaxime (Claforan)
Children 3 mo–7 y and older children and adults 7–50 y	H. influenzae, S. pneumoniae, N. meningitidis	Ceftriaxone or cefotaxime plus vancomycin (Vancocin)
Older adults > 50 y	S. pneumoniae, N. meningitidis, and L. monocytogenes	Ceftriaxone plus ampicillin

TABLE 3 Antibiotic Recommendations for Presumed Bacterial Meningitis in Persons with Special Risks

Condition or Risk Factor	Common Pathogens	Antibiotic Recommendations
Impaired immunity (e.g., HIV, early complement deficiency, agammaglobulinemia)	Listeria monocytogenes, Streptococcus pneumoniae, Haemophilus influenzae	Ampicillin plus ceftriaxone (Rocephin) or cefotaxime (Claforan)
Closed head trauma with CSF leak	S. pneumoniae, H. influenzae	Ceftriaxone or cefotaxime plus vancomycin (Vancocin)
Asplenia	S. pneumoniae, H. influenzae	Ceftriaxone or cefotaxime plus vancomycin
Terminal complement deficiency	Neisseria meningitidis	Ceftriaxone or cefotaxime
Neurosurgical procedures	Staphylococcus aureus	Vancomycin plus ceftriaxone or cefotaxime
CSF shunt infections	Coagulase-negative staphylococci, gram-negative bacilli	
Elderly patients (> 65 y)	S. pneumoniae, Listeria monocytogenes	Ceftriaxone or cefotaxime plus vancomycin
Recurrent bacterial meningitis (see CSF leak)	Streptococcus pneumoniae	Ceftriaxone or cefotaxime plus vancomycin
Alcoholic patients	Streptococcus pneumoniae and gram-negative bacilli	Ceftriaxone or cefotaxime plus vancomycin

Abbreviation: CSF = cerebrospinal fluid.

pneumoniae. Currently, approximately 30% to 50% of isolates are either intermediately (inhibitory concentration, 0.1 to 1.0 µg/mL) or fully (inhibitory concentration more than 2.0 µg/mL) resistant to Penicillin G and ampicillin. Resistance to ceftriaxone (Rocephin) and cefotaxime (Claforan) may occur as well in 10% to 15% of strains. Vancomycin (Vancocin) is recommended in those regimens for meningitis when pneumococci are considered. However, higher maximal doses are required for vancomycin because of its relatively poor penetration into the CSF. In general, lumbar puncture with CSF culture should be repeated in 48 hours in those cases where

vancomycin therapy is the primary drug because of demonstrated penicillin or cephalosporin resistance.

Meningitis caused by gram-negative bacilli such as Pseudomonas aeruginosa, Escherichia coli, or Enterobacter cloacae should be treated with a cephalosporin with an extended spectrum of gram-negative activity, such as ceftazidime (Fortaz) or cefepime (Maxipime). A carbapenem, such as imipenem (Primaxin) or meropenem (Merrem), can also be used for antibiotic-resistant gram-negative enteric and pseudomonas meningitis. Meropenem is associated with less risk of drug-induced seizures and may be a better choice for bacterial meningitis.

TABLE 4 Antibiotic Doses for Adults and Children for Treatment of Bacterial Meningitis

Antibiotic	Daily Adult Dose	Daily Pediatric Dose	Dose Interval
Amikacin (Amikin)	15 mg/kg	15–20 mg/kg	8 h
Ampicillin	12 g	200–400 mg/kg	4–6 h
Cefotaxime (Claforan)	12 g	200–300 mg/kg	4–6 h
Ceftriaxone (Rocephin)	4 g	100 mg/kg	12 h
Ceftazidime (Fortaz)	6 g	150–200 mg/kg	8 h
Cefepime (Maxipime)	6 g	100–150 mg/kg	8 h
Gentamicin (Garamycin)	5 mg/kg	7.5 mg/kg	8 h
Meropenem (Merrem)	6 g	120 mg/kg	8 h
Nafcillin (Unipen)	12 g	200 mg/kg	4–6 h
Penicillin G	24 million U	250,000 units/kg	4 h
Tobramycin (Nebcin)	5 mg/kg	6–7.5 mg/kg	8 h
Trimethoprim-sulfamethoxazole (Bactrim)	10–15 mg/kg	10–20 mg/kg	8 h
Vancomycin (Vancocin)	2 g	60 mg/kg	12 h

Adapted from Bradley JS, Nelson JD: 2002–2003 Nelson's Pocket Book of Pediatric Antimicrobial Therapy, 15th ed. Philadelphia and New York, Lippincott Williams & Wilkins, 2002.
Gilbert DN, Moellering RC, Sande MA. The Sanford Guide to Antimicrobial Therapy 2005. Hyde Park, Antimicrobial Therapy Inc., 2005.

Patients with ventriculoatrial and ventriculoperitoneal shunt–associated meningitis and ventriculitis usually require removal of the shunt for cure, as well as the administration of antibiotics to clear the infection. Certain patients with infections caused by organisms of reduced virulence, such as coagulase-negative staphylococci, or those with exquisitely antibiotic-susceptible infections, can be treated with a trial of antibiotics alone.

Because of the extreme sensitivity of *Neisseria meningitidis* to antibiotics, uncomplicated meningitis may be treated with as little as 5 to 7 days of antibiotics. Pneumococcal meningitis may be treated with 10 to 14 days of antibiotics and haemophilus infections are treated successfully with 7 to 10 days of antibiotics. Gram-negative meningitis was treated in the past with 3 weeks of aminoglycosides, but current experience with newer extended-spectrum cephalosporins (ceftriaxone, cefotaxime, carbapenems) suggests that 2 weeks of therapy is often sufficient in neonates as well as in some elderly patients and postoperative infections.

All patients with bacterial meningitis should be monitored carefully throughout the treatment period. Infectious disease consultation is recommended for most infections of the central nervous system.

CURRENT THERAPY

- Neonates < 2 mo
  - Group B streptococcal infection: cefotaxime (Claforan) or ampicillin
  - Gram-negative rods, other than *Pseudomonas:* cefotaxime
  - *Pseudomonas:* cefepime (Maxipime), ceftazidime (Fortaz), or meropenem (Merrem)
  - *Listeria:* Ampicillin + gentamicin (Garamycin)
- Children > 2 mo
  - Empirical for unknown etiology: cefotaxime or ceftriaxone (Rocephin)
  - *Streptococcus pneumoniae:* cefotaxime or ceftriaxone
  - *Haemophilus influenzae:* cefotaxime or ceftriaxone
  - *Neisseria meningitidis:* ampicillin or cefotaxime
- Older children and adults
  - Empirical for unknown etiology: cefotaxime or ceftriaxone
  - *S. pneumoniae:* cefotaxime or ceftriaxone
  - *N. meningitidis:* ampicillin or cefotaxime
  - Gram negative, postoperative, or *Staphylococcus aureus* (see Tables 1–4)
  - Add vancomycin if at risk for infection with resistant pneumococcus

Repeated lumbar punctures are not routinely recommended for patients with fully susceptible bacterial isolates or in those who show good response to therapy. Repeated sampling of the CSF with lumbar puncture or, when appropriate, shunt or ventricular reservoir puncture should be performed in those with known resistant bacterial isolates, in patients who have an inadequate response, in those patients who deteriorate on therapy, or in those for whom clinical response may correlate poorly with the microbiologic response (shunt infections, neonates, and elderly patients).

Adjunctive Therapy

Corticosteroids reduce the incidence of permanent neurologic sequelae in children with bacterial meningitis, particularly when caused by *Haemophilus influenza* type b. Data in support of steroids in either pneumococcal or meningococcal infections are less robust. Dexamethasone (Decadron[1]), 0.15 mg/kg every 6 hours for the first 2 to 4 days of treatment, was evaluated in children older than 2 months with bacterial meningitis. The first dose of dexamethasone should be given before, at the start, or within no later than 12 hours after beginning antibiotics.

Use of corticosteroids in adults is more controversial. Although doses of dexamethasone are recommended by some experts for adults with bacterial meningitis, its efficacy in adult meningitis has not been evaluated in a well-designed prospective trial. A recent study in adults found that corticosteroids significantly reduced the risk for unfavorable outcomes, particularly in patients with pneumococcal meningitis. There has been concern that the anti-inflammatory properties of dexamethasone may decrease the penetration of antibiotics, especially vancomycin, into the CSF. One study in children did not show this to be the case. Dexamethasone[1] should be administered in adults with proven or suspected pneumococcal meningitis, only if it can be given prior to the first dose of antibiotics in a dose of 10 mg every 6 hours for 4 days. In patients with meningitis caused by *Streptococcus pneumoniae* highly resistant to penicillin (minimum inhibitory concentration [MIC] >2.0 µg/mL) or cephalosporins (MIC >4.0 µg/mL), vancomycin should not be used as a single agent if corticosteroids are used. The addition of rifampin (Rifadin[1]) is often recommended in these situations.

Chemoprophylaxis for Bacterial Meningitis

Prophylactic antibiotics are recommended in case of meningitis caused by *Neisseria meningitidis* and *Haemophilus influenzae* type b. Prophylaxis is provided to eliminate the carriage of organisms among

---

[1]Not FDA approved for this indication.

contacts and prevent spread to hosts susceptible to invasive disease. In cases of meningococcal meningitis, prophylaxis is indicated only for those with household or close intimate contact with the index case. Administration of prophylaxis to large groups (e.g., college students, schoolchildren, or preschool classes) requires a special assessment and a recommendation of local or regional health departments. Chemoprophylaxis is not necessary for casual contacts or medical personnel unless there is a direct exposure to respiratory secretions. The recommended dose of rifampin (Rifadin) is 10 mg/kg (600 maximal, adults) twice a day for 2 days; ciprofloxacin (Cipro[1]), 500 mg as single dose, is also effective for adults. Third-generation cephalosporins used in treatment of the index case of meningitis are sufficient to eliminate carriage of the organism.

Chemoprophylaxis for *H. influenzae* type b is recommended for all household contacts of an index case if one of the contacts is an unvaccinated child younger than 4 years. If the index case is treated with ceftriaxone (Rocephin) or cefotaxime (Claforan), prophylaxis is not required, but if treated with ampicillin or chloramphenicol (Chloromycetin), prophylaxis is recommended to eliminate carriage. The recommended regimen for prophylaxis is rifampin,[1] 20 mg/kg (or 600 mg in adults) once a day for 4 days. With the near elimination of invasive infections caused by *Haemophilus influenzae* type b, with the use of routine immunization of children with conjugate haemophilus vaccines, *Haemophilus influenzae* types A, F, and rarely other serotypes have emerged, and the use of prophylaxis is not recommended in these situations because sufficient data are not available to support its efficacy, nor has spread within contacts been documented.

Vaccines for Bacterial Meningitis

The universal recommendation for the use of protein-polysaccharide conjugate *Haemophilus influenzae* type b (HIB) vaccines in 1987 reduced the incidence of bacterial meningitis by this organism by greater than 97%. Three HIB vaccines (PedvaxHIB, ActHIB, HibTITER), licensed in the United States, are routinely given to children in dosage schedules employing three to four doses by 12 to 18 months of age (see www.cdc.gov).

A pneumococcal protein-polysaccharide conjugate vaccine (Prevnar) licensed in 2000 is routinely recommended for children and has markedly reduced the incidence of invasive infections with seven serotypes of pneumococci in children. This vaccine is also recommended for children at high risk of pneumococcal infections (e.g., HIV infection, asplenia, sickle cell disease, and others). A pneumococcal polysaccharide vaccine (Pneumovax 23) is recommended for adults older than 65 years or for those over 50 years with risk factors (e.g., alcoholism, diabetes or other metabolic or renal disease, chronic pulmonary or cardiac disease). Although clear evidence for prevention of bacterial meningitis is lacking, evidence supports its efficacy against invasive pneumococcal diseases, many of which are the preceding infections leading to bacteremia and meningitis.

Currently two vaccines remain available for prevention of meningococcal disease caused by four serotypes, A, C, Y, and W-135. The meningococcal polysaccharide vaccine (Menomune) was recommended for persons older than 2 years at high risk for severe meningococcal infections including adolescents and college students (particularly those residing in dormitories), military recruits, and those with complement deficiencies and asplenia. A quadrivalent protein-polysaccharide conjugate vaccines (Menactra) was licensed in 2005. This vaccine is now recommended for routine immunization of all children 11 to 12 years of age and adolescents and college students at high risk as well as those more than 2 to 55 years of age with high-risk factors for meningococcal infection, including all those for whom the polysacharide vaccine was previously recommended.

---

[1]Not FDA approved for this indication.

REFERENCES

Anderson EJ, Yogev LR. A rational approach to the management of ventricular shunt infections. Pediatric Infect Dis J 2005;24:557–8.

Andes DR, Craig WA. Pharmacokinetics and pharmacodynamics of antibiotics in meningitis. Infect Dis Clin North Am 1999;13(2):595–618.

De Gans J, van de Beek. Dexamethasone in adults with bacterial meningitis. N Engl J Med 2002;347:1549–64.

Gray LD, Fedorko DP. Laboratory diagnosis of bacterial meningitis. Clin Microbiol Rev 1992;5:130–45.

Hussein AS, Shafran SD. Acute bacterial meningitis in adults: A 12-year review. Medicine (Baltimore) 2000;79:360–8.

Klinger G, Chin C-Y, Beyene J, et al. Predicting the outcome of neonatal bacterial meningitis. Pediatrics 2000;106:477–82.

Klein JO. Bacterial sepsis and meningitis. In: Remington JS, Klein JO, editors. Infectious Diseases of the Fetus and Newborn Infant. 5th ed. New York and Saint Louis: WB Saunders; 2002. p. 943–98.

Odio CM, Faingezicht I, Paris M, et al. The beneficial effects of early dexamethasone administration in infants and children with bacterial meningitis. N Engl J Med 1991;324:1525–31.

Ronan A, Hogg GG, Klug CL. Cerebrospinal fluid shunt infections in children. Pediatr Infect Dis J 1995;14:782–6.

Schuchat A, Robinson K, Wenger JD, et al. Bacterial meningitis in the United States in 1995. N Engl J Med 1997;337:970–6.

Unhanand M, Mustapha MM, McCracken GH, et al. Gram-negative enteric bacillary meningitis: A twenty-one year experience. J Pediatr 1993;122:15–7.

Van de Beek D, de Gans J, Spanjaard L, et al. Clinical features and prognostic factors in adults with bacterial meningitis. N Engl J Med 2004;351:1849–58.

Infectious Mononucleosis

Method of
Joseph Domachowske, MD

Infectious mononucleosis (IM) is a clinical syndrome consisting of fever, lymphadenopathy, exudative tonsillopharyngitis, splenomegaly, and atypical lymphocytosis. Because most cases are caused by Epstein-Barr virus (EBV), many clinicians use the term IM synonymously with acute EBV infection. Less common causes of IM include primary cytomegalovirus infection, hepatitis A, hepatitis B, toxoplasmosis, HIV, adenovirus, and rubella.

CURRENT DIAGNOSIS

- Fever
- Lymphadenopathy
- Exudative pharyngitis
- Splenomegaly
- Atypical lymphocytosis

CURRENT THERAPY

- Supportive therapy including hydration and analgesics
- Antiviral medications are not effective.
- Glucocorticoids are reserved for patients with airway obstruction.

Classic Syndrome and Disease Course

Humans are the only known reservoir for EBV. Transmission occurs efficiently, usually through direct contact with oral secretions. The incubation period of EBV in IM is between 30 and 50 days. This is followed by a prodrome characterized by malaise, headache, and fatigue, after which fever, sore throat, and cervical lymphadenopathy occur. The adenopathy is symmetrical and involves the posterior and anterior cervical lymph node chains. More generalized adenopathy is not uncommon. The pharynx is erythematous with an associated white or green-gray exudate. Severe fatigue can be predominant. Less common signs include palatal or pharyngeal petechiae; periorbital, palpebral, or forehead edema; and a maculopapular or morbilliform rash, particularly if the patient takes penicillin or amoxicillin (Amoxil). Gastrointestinal complaints are also relatively common. The nausea and anorexia may be secondary to mild hepatitis, which is present in almost all infected individuals. Splenomegaly is also common, whereas jaundice and hepatomegaly are uncharacteristic.

Although most patients with IM develop pharyngitis, adenopathy predominates in the so-called glandular form of IM, and there are minimal or no pharyngeal symptoms. Patients may also present with a more systemic illness characterized by prolonged fever and fatigue. The vast majority of individuals who develop IM recover uneventfully. Acute symptoms resolve in 1 to 2 weeks, although fatigue often persists for months. The frequency with which clinical signs and symptoms occur in children and in adults are summarized in Table 1.

Complications of Infectious Mononucleosis

SPLENIC RUPTURE

As many as 2 patients per 1000 develop splenic rupture as a direct complication of IM. Approximately half of these events are spontaneous, and, for reasons that are poorly understood, almost all are reported in males. Rupture has occurred between days 4 and 24 of symptomatic infection and was not able to be predicted based on symptom severity, laboratory findings, or even physician-documented palpable splenomegaly. Despite the life-threatening potential of splenic rupture, fatalities are rare. Nonoperative treatment with intensive supportive care is successful for some patients, whereas others require splenectomy. Specific guidelines have not been established

regarding the timing of safe return to athletic participation after IM without risk of splenic rupture. Because rupture can occur even in the absence of trauma, precluding strenuous activity, including weight lifting and contact sports, for the first 3 to 4 weeks after the onset of illness is usually recommended. For patients who compete in higher-risk contact sports, radiologic evaluation of spleen size may be reasonable before clearance, although this approach remains a debated issue.

AIRWAY OBSTRUCTION

Obstruction of the upper airway is another known complication of IM. Patients with massive lymphadenopathy, mucosal edema, and severe tonsillopharyngitis need to be carefully evaluated and monitored. The administration of glucocorticoids is advocated for individuals with incipient obstruction. Some patients require endotracheal intubation or tracheostomy placement.

Unusual Manifestations of Infectious Mononucleosis

A full spectrum of illness and laboratory abnormalities have been described for primary EBV- associated IM. Mild hematologic abnormalities (anemia, mild thrombocytopenia, atypical lymphocytosis) are common (Table 2), and more severe changes can also occur. Hemolytic anemia, aplastic anemia, thrombocytopenic purpura, hemolytic uremic syndrome, and disseminated intravascular coagulation are among the most serious hematologic perturbations described. EBV infection is also the most commonly recognized infectious trigger for the development of hemophagocytic lymphohistiocytosis (sometimes called macrophage activation syndrome). Patients with this syndrome develop fever, generalized lymphadenopathy, hepatosplenomegaly with hepatitis, pancytopenia, and coagulopathy. A detailed discussion of the important association of EBV infection with the development of lymphoproliferative disorders (including those seen in transplant patients), Burkitt's lymphoma, T-cell lymphoma, smooth muscle tumors, Hodgkin's disease, and nasopharyngeal carcinoma are beyond the scope of this chapter.

Neurologic manifestations of primary EBV infection may include meningoencephalitis, "Alice in Wonderland" syndrome with associated metamorphopsia (visual-spatial hallucinations), Guillain-Barré syndrome, facial nerve palsy, optic neuritis, and peripheral neuritis. Patients with neurologic manifestations of EBV infection may not have other evidence of IM.

TABLE 1 Clinical Signs and Symptoms of Primary Epstein-Barr Virus Infection in Children and Adults

Sign or Symptom	Frequency (%) Children <16 y	Adults
Lymphadenopathy	94–100	93–100
Malaise/fatigue	85–100	90–100
Fever	92–100	63–100
Tonsillopharyngitis	67–75	70–91
Pharyngeal exudate	45–59	40–74
Splenomegaly	53–82	32–51
Hepatomegaly	30–63	6–24
Cough	15–51	5–31
Rash	17–34	3–15
Nausea, abdominal pain	0–17	2–14
Eyelid or forehead edema	10–14	5–34
Genital ulcers	1–2	Uncommon, perhaps underreported
Meningoencephalitis and other neurologic findings	Uncommon	Uncommon

TABLE 2 Laboratory Abnormalities in Acute Epstein-Barr Virus Infectious Mononucleosis

Findings	% Positive
EBV-specific antibody	100
Lymphocytosis	95–100
Elevated liver transaminases	80–100
Atypical lymphocytosis	90–99
Heterophile antibody	80–90 in adults*
Leukocytosis	60–80
Neutropenia	60–80
Anemia (mild-moderate)	40–60
Thrombocytopenia (usually mild)	25–45
Increased cold agglutinins	10–45
Leukopenia	10–20
Positive direct Coombs' test	Rare
Significant anemia	Rare
Anti-platelet antibodies	Rare
False-positive HIV ELISA	Rare

*Age dependent (see text).
EBV, Epstein-Barr virus; ELISA, enzyme-linked immunosorbent assay.

Lymphoproliferative disorders and malignancies associated with EBV persistence and reactivation are recognized complications in immunocompromised individuals; however, persistent, recurrent, or reactivated EBV infection is extremely rare in immunocompetent individuals. Care must be taken to carefully interpret laboratory results of EBV antibody titers (see later discussion). If IM does recur in an otherwise healthy individual, it is likely that the separate episodes of IM were each caused by a different etiologic agent (e.g., EBV and then cytomegalovirus), rather than true recurrence of the EBV infection.

Diagnosis

The clinical diagnosis of IM is not always straightforward, so confirmatory testing is usually performed. In addition, hematologic and liver enzyme perturbations are common, so complete blood counts with evaluation of the peripheral smear and detection of serum liver transaminases are prudent. By the second week of infection, it is not uncommon to see 20% or more atypical lymphocytes on the peripheral blood smear. These atypical cells, sometimes referred to as Downey cells, have a higher cytoplasm-to-nucleus ratio than normal lymphocytes, and prominent nucleoli are occasionally seen. The cytoplasm is more basophilic and vacuolated than usual, so an untrained eye might suspect the presence of peripheral blasts. These lymphocytes represent activated T lymphocytes that are directed against the EBV-infected B lymphocytes.

Most cases of IM are caused by EBV, so confirming the etiologic agent of IM starts with EBV testing. Primary EBV infection stimulates the production of serum antibodies directed against viral antigens, as well as unrelated antigens found on sheep and horse erythrocytes. The latter antibodies, referred to as heterophile antibodies, are a group of proteins (mostly immunoglobulin M [IgM]) that do not recognize EBV antigens. Although it is not specific for a diagnosis of EBV infection (i.e., other conditions can lead to the production of heterophile antibodies), a positive heterophile antibody test result obtained from an adolescent or adult patient with symptoms consistent with IM is presumptive evidence for EBV infection. Although the heterophile antibody tests have a sensitivity of up to 90% in patients older than 12 years of age, these types of tests are not recommended for use in young children, because children do not reliably generate these nonspecific antibody responses. Approximately 50% of children between 2 and 4 years of age, and fewer than 10% of children younger than 2 years with primary EBV infection are heterophile antibody positive.

A number of rapid spot tests are commercially available for the detection of heterophile antibodies. The assay itself is simple and inexpensive to perform and requires minimal training. The results can be available within minutes, making this an attractive, popular diagnostic tool that is available in many office and urgent care settings.

The specific diagnosis of acute EBV infection is based on the appearance of IgM antibody directed against the EBV viral capsid antigen (anti-EBV-VCA-IgM). This is the first EBV-specific antibody produced, and it is usually detectable by the time the patient is symptomatic. The detection of anti-EBV-VCA-IgM establishes that the patient has a current (or has had a very recent) primary EBV infection and is the single most useful EBV specific antibody titer used to diagnose the etiologic agent of IM. Further on during the course of the illness, the patient also develops additional antibodies directed against the VCA (anti-EBV-VCA-IgG), early antigen (anti-EBV-EA), and nuclear antigen (anti-EBNA). Many clinical laboratories perform these antibody tests as an EBV antibody panel, requiring interpretation of each of the results. Table 3 provides details regarding the appearance and persistence of each of these antibodies. Because IgG titers to VCA and EBNA can persist for life, their presence alone simply confirms a past infection.

The most common cause of EBV-negative IM is cytomegalovirus infection, but toxoplasmosis, hepatitis A, hepatitis B, HIV, adenovirus, and rubella are recognized to cause fever, adenopathy, and fatigue with atypical lymphocytosis. The diagnosis of IM caused by these other agents can be established by standard serologic testing. IgM testing is available to establish toxoplasmosis, hepatitis A, hepatitis B, and rubella. Alternatively, IgG antibody titers can be collected from the patient's serum during the acute phase of infection and compared with titers obtained during convalescence (usually 4–6 weeks apart). A fourfold rise in IgG antibody titer establishes the etiologic agent. HIV testing is performed as a two-step process consisting of a screening enzyme linked immunoassay for anti-HIV IgG antibodies, followed by confirmatory Western blotting. Adenovirus infection can be confirmed by viral culture or nucleic acid–based amplification tests, if available.

Treatment

The mainstay of treatment for individuals with IM is supportive care. Acetaminophen (Tylenol) or nonsteroidal antiinflammatory medications are recommended for the treatment of fever and throat pain. Maintaining adequate hydration in the face of fevers and severe pharyngitis can be challenging. Intravenous hydration is necessary in a minority of cases. No specific treatment has been identified to relieve the prolonged fatigue that many adolescents and young adults experience after the acute infection.

The use of corticosteroids for uncomplicated IM remains controversial. Studies evaluating steroids for use in IM suggest that they do reduce lymphoid and mucosal swelling, and clinicians should consider administering steroids to patients with impending airway obstruction. However, routine use of glucocorticoids is probably best avoided. The clinical manifestations of IM represent the immune response to infection with EBV, a herpes-group virus that establishes lifelong latency and has oncogenic potential. For this reason, therapy with immunomodulatory agents (e.g., glucocorticoids) could alter the immune response potentially predisposing the patient to a lifelong lymphoproliferative complication.

Specific antiviral therapy of acute EBV infection with oral and intravenous acyclovir (Zovirax)[1] has been tested. Although short-term

---

[1]Not FDA approved for this indication.

TABLE 3 Serologic Testing for Epstein-Barr Virus Infection

Antibody	Time of Appearance from Onset of Symptoms	Patients with Positive Test (%)	Antibody Persistence
Heterophile	End of 1st wk	See text	Up to 1 y
VCA-IgM	1–3 wk	100	2–3 mo
VCA-IgG	<3 wk	100	Lifelong
Early antigen	After the 1st wk	70–80	3–6 mo
EBNA	3–4 wk	100	Lifelong

EBNA, Epstein-Barr nuclear antigen; Ig, immunoglobulin; VCA, viral capsid antigen.

suppression of virus shedding can be demonstrated, measurable clinical benefits are lacking. These results are not unexpected, because there is little evidence that ongoing viral replication contributes to disease pathogenesis. Available data support the hypothesis that the symptoms of IM are secondary to the immunopathology generated in response to EBV-transformed lymphocytes during the acute phase of the disease.

REFERENCES

Barnes CJ, Alió AB, Cunningham BB, et al. Epstein-Barr virus-associated genital ulcers: An under-recognized disorder. Pediatr Dermatol 2007;24:130–4.

Cameron B, Bharadwaj M, Burrows J, et al. Prolonged illness after infectious mononucleosis is associated with altered immunity but not with increased viral load. J Infect Dis 2006;193:664–71.

Candy B, Hotopf M. Steroids for symptom control in infectious mononucleosis. Cochrane Database Syst Rev 2006;(3):CD004402.

Domachowske JB, Cunningham CK, Cummings DL, et al. Acute manifestations and neurologic sequelae of Epstein Barr virus encephalitis in children. Pediatr Infect Dis J 1996;15:871–5.

Gershburg E, Pagano JS. Epstein-Barr virus infections: Prospects for treatment. J Antimicrob Chemother 2005;56:277–81.

Gulley ML, Tang W. Laboratory assays for Epstein-Barr virus-related disease. J Mol Diagn 2008;10:279–92.

Klein E, Kis LL, Klein G. Epstein-Barr virus infection in humans: From harmless to life endangering virus-lymphocyte interactions. Oncogene 2007;26:1297–305.

Kutok JT, Wang F. Spectrum of Epstein-Barr virus-associated diseases. Annu Rev Pathol 2006;1:375–404.

Stephenson JT, Dubois JJ. Nonoperative management of spontaneous splenic rupture in infectious mononucleosis: A case report and review of the literature. Pediatrics 2007;120:e432–5.

Thompson SK, Doerr TD, Hengerer AS. Infectious mononucleosis and corticosteroids: Management practices and outcomes. Arch Otolaryngol Head Neck Surg 2005;131:900–4.

Waninger KN, Harcke HT. Determination of safe return to play for athletes recovering from infectious mononucleosis: A review of the literature. Clin J Sport Med 2005;15:410–6.

Chronic Fatigue Syndrome

Method of
James F. Jones, MD

Definition

Chronic fatigue syndrome (CFS) is the name applied to an illness of unknown origin that at face value resembles unresolved infections, depression, endocrinologic and metabolic disorders, sleep disorders, and many other conditions that include fatigue in their diagnostic criteria.

In the modern era, interest in this illness began with the question of a relationship with a chronic active Epstein-Barr virus infection. Subsequent studies did not support Epstein-Barr virus as the only cause of this syndrome, but several recent studies have found 10% of patients with acute infectious mononucleosis and other infectious diseases might have a similar illness or postinfection fatigue syndrome.

The lack of association with a specific infectious agent led to the generation in 1988 of a definition based on the presence of incapacitating fatigue and varying combinations of signs and symptoms. Any preexisting medical or psychiatric condition was exclusionary. Evaluation of this definition at a number of centers in the United States, Great Britain, and Australia led to the current definition published in 1994 (Box 1). The definition was altered so that preexisting medical conditions that were treated satisfactorily were allowed, as well as

---

BOX 1 International Consensus Definition of Chronic Fatigue Syndrome

- Clinically evaluated, unexplained, persistent or relapsing chronic fatigue (lasting more than 6 months) that is of new or definite onset (has not been lifelong); is not the result of ongoing exertion; is not substantially alleviated by rest; and results in substantial reduction in previous levels of occupational, educational, social, or personal activities.
- Four or more of the following symptoms are concurrently present for more than 6 months:
  - Impaired memory or concentration
  - Multijoint pain
  - Muscle pain
  - New headaches
  - Postexertional malaise
  - Sore throat
  - Tender cervical or axillary lymph nodes
  - Unrefreshing sleep
- Exclusionary clinical diagnoses:
  - Any active medical condition that could explain the chronic fatigue
  - Any previously diagnosed medical condition whose resolution has not been documented beyond reasonable clinical doubt and whose continued activity can explain the chronic fatiguing illness
  - Psychotic major depression, bipolar affective disorder, schizophrenia, delusional disorders, dementias, anorexia nervosa, bulimia nervosa
  - Alcohol or other substance abuse within 2 years prior to the onset of the chronic fatigue and at any time afterward

Adapted from Fukuda K. Straus SE, Hickie I, et al: The chronic fatigue syndrome: A comprehensive approach to its definition and study. Ann Intern Med 1994;121:953–959.

---

certain psychiatric and syndromic diagnoses. Additional changes in the definition included a decrease in the number of symptoms and removal of the signs; signs had been shown to be somewhat arbitrary, and patients could be identified in their absence. The greater number of symptoms in the 1988 version did not allow identification of a specific illness, and they increased the possibility that patients who had primary psychiatric illnesses (e.g., somatiform disorders) would be mislabeled with CFS. The 1994 definition still requires more than 6 months of fatigue, but it dropped the 50% level of activity present in the 1988 definition because the requirement was impossible to apply evenly across all patients.

The diagnostic criteria, including exclusion of other illnesses, are described in the Current Diagnosis box. The definition was originally designed as a research tool and included suggestions for unifying the measurement of fatigue and evaluation of the mental status of patients.

Epidemiology

The prevalence of the syndrome using the 1988 definition is approximately 13 per 100,000, whereas the 1994 definition identified approximately 300 per 100,000. Application of an empiric definition (see later) in a population recruited with unwellness, rather than fatigue, identified a higher prevalence of CFS (Reeves et al, 2007). An increase in CFS cases in an unwell population highlights the need to address illness in general and not just fatigue when considering this diagnosis. One demographic variable that has remained stable is the 3:1 ratio of women to men.

BOX 2   Screening Laboratory Tests

- Alanine aminotransferase
- Albumin
- Alkaline phosphatase
- C-reactive protein
- Complete blood count
- Creatinine
- Electrolytes
- Globulin
- Glucose
- Thyroid-stimulating hormone and free T_4
- Total protein
- Urinalysis

Abbreviation: T_4 = thyroxine.

Diagnosis

Diagnosis of CFS begins with exclusion of other illness processes associated with fatigue and unwellness and subsequent suspicion of the syndrome after taking a history and performing a physical examination and screening laboratory tests (Box 2). It should not be assumed that a patient with fatigue as a presenting complaint has CFS. The history shows whether the illness began acutely or more gradually and whether there are preexisting symptoms. History often provides insight into previously identified factors that influence patient perception of illness. Questioning about typical episodes provides information about cyclic events, possible triggers of symptoms, and possible exposures.

The interviewer gives the patients the opportunity to describe the history of the illness. The interviewer simply guides the patient and tries not to ask leading questions. This process not only gathers information but also serves as an ice breaker between the interviewer and the patient. It allows the interviewer to determine the mental status of the patient, the patient's concentration and memory capabilities, and what may be on the patient's agenda. It usually allows the examiner to determine the kind and scope of prior medical and alternative care evaluations the patients has received.

The diagnosis of CFS should not be made on the first visit. Attempts should be made to determine the duration, the mode of onset, the magnitude, and the consequences of each complaint, although these are not included in the working definition. Only with such thorough questioning will an underlying process responsible for the illness be identified or suspected.

A more recent application of the definition uses three validated questionnaires: the Medical Outcomes Survey Short Form-36 (SF-36), the Multidimensional Fatigue Inventory (MFI), and the CDC Symptom Inventory. These questionnaires provide numeric scores that identify persons with CFS and provide a record of their level of impairment. The Symptom Inventory collects information about the presence, frequency, and intensity of 19 fatigue- and illness-related symptoms during the month preceding the interview; these include all eight CFS-defining symptoms (postexertional fatigue, unrefreshing sleep, problems remembering or concentrating, muscle aches and pains, joint pain, sore throat, tender lymph nodes and swollen glands, and headaches). Perceived frequency of each symptom is rated on a four-point scale (1 = a little of the time, 2 = some

of the time, 3 = most of time, 4 = all of the time), and severity or intensity of symptoms is measured on a three-point scale (1 = mild, 2 = moderate, 3 = severe).

The case definition specifies that CFS causes substantial reduction in occupational, educational, social, or recreational activities. *Substantial reduction* is defined as scores lower than the 25th percentile on the SF-36 using the following four factors: physical function (≤ 70), or role physical (≤ 50), or social function (≤ 75), or role emotional (≤ 66.67) subscales of the SF-36, related to published norms of the U.S. population according to Ware and Sherbourne. We defined severe fatigue using the Multidimensional Fatigue Inventory as a score of 13 or higher on the general fatigue scale or 10 or higher on the reduced activity scales of the MFI (their respective medians). Finally, because the case definition specifies that characteristic symptoms accompany fatigue, subjects reporting at least 4 symptoms and scoring at least 25 on the Symptom Inventory Case Definition Subscale were considered to have substantial accompanying symptoms.

Routine laboratory evaluations are recommended to address contributory illnesses (see Box 2). Routine testing does not include specific antibody testing, tests of immune function per se, or single-photon emission computed tomography (SPECT) or magnetic resonance imaging (MRI) of the brain. Negative screening test results do not automatically exclude an alternative diagnosis. Specific testing, for example, for a sleep disorder or chronic sinusitis may be necessary. A mental status examination, either informally or by using a standard instrument when indicated, is equally important.

A working diagnosis of CFS may then be made if the evaluation fails to identify an underlying illness. This approach is warranted because the patient's underlying disease might declare itself in the future. Continued adherence to a diagnosis of CFS in the face of an evolving or readily identifiable medical or psychiatric illness is the single most detrimental outcome of a premature or prolonged diagnosis of CFS.

Additional laboratory or other diagnostic testing is based on the individual patient's complaints. The interview techniques listed earlier assist in this process. An additional valuable tool that will lead the interviewer to identify a specific illness or symptoms requiring intervention is simply to ask the patient to list the problems described in decreasing order of magnitude. Which problem causes the most difficulty? Or which problems interfere with the ability to carry out daily functions? Patients often use this exercise to list the consequences of their illness.

Therapy

Treatment regimens vary with the needs of the individual patient and how he or she perceives the illness. The goals of treatment depend on the person's specific symptoms and eventually the patient's identified needs within a framework of providing reentry into their premorbid condition. Complete return to normal might not be possible immediately, however, nor is this goal appropriate if it is too lofty. In fact, the desire for total immediate recovery can hamper clinical improvement. The patient's adaptation to this new, albeit temporary, state is often a more realistic short-term goal. Therapeutic modalities include education regarding the boundaries and limitations of the diagnosis, development of coping skills, institution of a graduated exercise program when possible, and use of medications to treat symptoms. If the patient is being seen in a multidisciplinary setting, these approaches may be combined into a specific program. If CFS is an infrequent diagnosis in a practice, identifying the problems that cause loss of function becomes critical.

EDUCATION

All physicians who make the diagnosis must provide information regarding the illness in general and the specific criteria that allowed recognition of the problem. Just as education regarding asthma and diabetes mellitus is a critical component of therapy for those diseases, education regarding the origin, specific components, and outcome of the syndrome is more critical in this situation.

CURRENT DIAGNOSIS

- Identify duration of fatigue and its consequences.
- Identify primary symptoms.
- Exclude other illnesses/diseases.
- Reconsider the diagnosis on an ongoing basis.
- Chronic fatigue syndrome is a working diagnosis.

CURRENT THERAPY

- Education regarding the advantages and disadvantages of CFS as a diagnosis
- Development of coping skills
- Cognitive behavior therapy
- Initiation of a graded exercise program
- Symptomatic medication

The literature supports CFS as a condition that is not life threatening or progressive. Lay representations, which are readily available, are often incorrect in painting a uniformly dismal outcome. Physicians should counsel their patients that all illness symptoms should not be attributed to CFS, and patients should seek medical advice when new problems arise or old problems become more prominent. Patients should also be taught that persistent efforts to find a cure via experiences of their acquaintances or the newest information in magazines or on the Internet are not as productive as their participation in a specifically designed program as outlined here. Paramount in this process is their consideration of acceptance of their current, albeit temporary, status. Wanting their lives back and attempting to regain them with a pill are not effective approaches.

A major part of the education and treatment process is the interview process. Giving the patient the opportunity to describe the illness and its consequences in a nonjudgmental situation is critical to gaining the patient's confidence. A physician who makes the diagnosis of CFS literally establishes a contract for long-term care with the patient, and it must be based on mutual trust.

DEVELOPMENT OF COPING SKILLS

To recommend coping strategies, the provider must know the needs of the patient, another rationale for the patient-generated problem list. If the patient complains of problems with memory and concentration, simple advice regarding using lists and audiotaping activities or needs is logical. If they cannot perform on the job or their behavioral responses to these complaints aggravate the consequences, formal neuropsychological testing or therapy, or both, is required. Assistance with understanding losses is also very important. Depending on the magnitude of the consequences of their illness, patients can lose self-respect and the appreciation of their families, employees, and coworkers. They need to learn that as individuals they are not responsible for these losses but that they are responsible, at least in part, for their recovery. They need to go through a grieving process and then learn how to adapt to their current state. They need to learn to accept and desire incremental levels of progress. Formal psychological therapy may be required to achieve these goals.

The origin of the illness and the character of the fatigue dictate the approach in many cases. If the origin is with an apparent, usually unidentified, flu-like illness that does not resolve, or if the character of the fatigue simulates the malaise of such an illness, the patient needs to know that the symptoms are normal responses. The duration and consequences in the eyes of society and the individual patient are the factors that differentiate a normal resolution of an illness from a prolonged or chronic condition.

The patient also needs to know that resumption of normal activity is not the correct approach. Most patients have symptoms on a daily basis, but they also have days when the symptoms are more or less pronounced (bad and good days). A typical patient performs on the good days as if there were no illness. This action is then followed in 1 or 2 days by an exacerbation of symptoms. Learning to compartmentalize activities and to never exceed their personal limits are critical steps in coping with CFS.

On the other hand, total acceptance of such a program is not appropriate either. Usually, acute-onset patients notice that they can be more active without exacerbation of symptoms regardless of their therapeutic program. This observation usually heralds resolution of the illness. In some instances, the illness is resolving, but the patient perceives the outcome of increased physical activity (e.g., muscle aches and tiredness) as illness symptoms rather than simply the expected consequences of increased activity. The recurrence of the patient's whole syndrome following activity, however, suggests that resolution has not taken place.

EXERCISE

It seems contradictory to follow the discussion about listening to one's body and avoiding excessive activity with a section that recommends regular exercise. The studies on muscle function show that patients are tired after performing repetitive acts and that there appears to be no primary problem in muscle function. There may a problem in fitness or conditioning, however. Whether this result is a consequence of the illness or the inactivity that accompanies the syndrome is not known.

Lessons from the rehabilitation of patients with cardiac and pulmonary diseases teach us that anaerobic exercise to regain strength should precede exercises to improve aerobic fitness and overall conditioning. A program that includes active stretching followed by range-of-motion contractions and extensions that eventually includes resistance is usually an effective start. Five minutes per day is a typical starting point for a patient who has been totally inactive. The endpoint of each session should be preset by the clock or number of repetitions and should be reached before the patient becomes tired. This endpoint is based on the fact that either tiredness is a trigger for the production of biological changes that are a part of the host's attempt to limit activity or the perception that tiredness triggers illness behavior. At this stage in the understanding of the illness, prevention of activation of either of these pathways and an increase in overall fitness are appropriate goals. This section may be summarized by the adage that no exercise is bad, some is good, and too much exercise is not helpful.

The previous sections on education, coping skills, and exercise provide the kinds of therapy that are offered in cognitive behavior therapy programs.

SYMPTOMATIC THERAPY

One usually associates symptomatic therapy with medication. Some interventions require alterations in patient habits or changes in biological processes that do not require medication per se.

Sleep Therapy

The primary example is treatment of sleep problems. A very large percentage of patients presenting for evaluation of fatigue, many of whom carry the diagnosis of CFS, have sleep disorders or disturbances. Some have problems with sleep hygiene. They may read or watch television for prolonged periods (longer than 15 minutes) before trying to go to sleep. This habit can actually allow arousal of the brain within several hours following sleep onset, thus leading to interrupted sleep. Caffeine ingestion after 6 PM and exercise within 4 hours of bedtime can impede getting to sleep.

Patients are often given medication for insomnia that is manifested by going to bed at 11 PM but not being able to get to sleep until 1 or 2 AM, with a waking time of 10 AM. A hypnotic might be prescribed that allows induction of sleep at an earlier time, but the patient might still not experience restorative sleep. One explanation for this series of events is that the patient has a phase-delay syndrome and needs to alter the sleep cycle with prescribed light therapy before improvement is expected. Appropriate use of hypnotics may be important in allowing initial normalization of sleep cycling, but these agents are not sufficient as the sole mode of therapy, nor should they be used for prolonged periods.

Daytime sleepiness is another common problem with multiple origins. Ill-advised symptomatic therapy includes self- or physician-generated use of stimulants. These drugs include caffeine, herbs that contain ephedrine such as Ma huang (Ephedra sinica), and antidepressants that actually serve as stimulants (serotonin and norepinephrine reuptake inhibitors [SNRIs]). These substances might allow short-term improvement in daytime function, but they block identification of the underlying nighttime or daytime origin of the sleep problem.

Pharmacologic Therapy

Premature treatment can prevent adequate diagnosis and treatment of readily remediated problems. However, symptomatic medications have a definite place in the therapy of CFS. Many CFS patients do not tolerate standard doses of any of the medications used for symptomatic relief.

Classes of drugs that might have beneficial effects for symptom relief include hypnotics of various types, antidepressants of several types if depression is evident, and non-narcotic analgesics. As used in the treatment of fibromyalgia, tricyclic antidepressants and SNRIs are used for symptomatic therapy in the absence of formal depression. Because these classes of medications are being used as adjuncts to the other modes of therapy, they are not always successful. They might need to be changed during the course of the illness.

Often patients come to the physician using a large number of medications. It might not be possible to determine by the history alone whether the patient's symptoms are not at least in part due to the medication regimen. Often the medications need to be tapered and stopped to sort out their influence on the manifesting complaints.

Popular remedies for CFS are discussed primarily to familiarize the practitioner with them and to support previous warnings regarding lack of efficacy. The primary problem with their use is that proof is lacking that such intervention has been uniformly beneficial. This statement is particularly true in cases of parenteral (injectable) repetitious therapy with any substance.

Alternative Therapies

The effectiveness of diet manipulations and ingestion of herbs, enzymes, amino acids, vitamins, minerals, or hormones, although usually safe, is equally unproven. These agents constitute a large component of the therapeutic armamentarium in use by patients with CFS. Herbs are particularly in vogue. Many of them have medicinal qualities and if taken in excessive amounts may be injurious. Because many of these substances are readily available, they are used by patients who are anxious for improvement in their illness. If the reader has such patients or is such a patient, one must make sure that the remedy in question is safe and that its use is affordable and does not hide illness parameters that require specific identification.

If patients are intent on taking these types of remedies, they should be advised to at least seek the advice of a responsible care provider who is knowledgeable in their use and adverse consequences. Alternative care in many forms is also in vogue and may be helpful if provided in a responsible fashion. Some patients with myalgias and other pain complaints find particular benefit from acupuncture and therapeutic massage.

Therapeutic Plan

Therapy for CFS patients continues to be directed at relieving symptoms and consequences of the syndrome. It is clear, however, that one approach or one medication is not satisfactory for all patients. Identifying the patient's most problematic symptoms and using a variety of modalities that address those problems in the treatment plan are the most effective ways of assisting the patient. Patients should be reminded not to expect total return to their premorbid state to occur immediately.

Because the use of medications remains arbitrary, failure of one regimen may be followed by successful relief using the more effective modes of therapy, such as cognitive behavior therapy and graduated exercise. Eventually the origins of symptom production will be understood and therapy can be directed with some authority. As it stands now, one must always be careful that whatever the treatment, it must not aggravate the illness.

REFERENCES

Bazelmans E, Prins JB, Lulofs R, et al. The Netherlands Fatigue Research Group Nijmegen. Cognitive behaviour group therapy for chronic fatigue syndrome: A non-randomised waiting list controlled study. Psychother Psychosom 2005;74(4):218–24.

Jones JF, Maloney EM, Boneva RS, et al. Complementary and alternative medical therapy utilization by people with chronic fatiguing illnesses in the United States. BMC Complement Altern Med 2007;7:12.

Jones JF, Nisenbaum R, Reeves WC. Medication use by persons with chronic fatigue syndrome: Results of a randomized telephone survey in Wichita, Kansas. Health Qual Life Outcomes 2003;I(1):74.

Moss-Morris R, Sharon C, Tobin R, Baldi JC. A randomized controlled graded exercise trial for chronic fatigue syndrome: Outcomes and mechanisms of change. J Health Psychol 2005;10(2):245–59.

Nater UM, Wagner D, Solomon L, et al. Coping styles in people with chronic fatigue syndrome identified from the general population of Wichita, KS. J Psychosom Res 2006;60(6):567–73.

Reeves WC, Jones JF, Maloney E, et al. Prevalence of chronic fatigue syndrome in metropolitan, urban, and rural Georgia. Popul Health Metr 2007;5:5.

Reeves WC, Wagner D, Nisenbaum R, et al. Chronic fatigue syndrome: A clinically empirical approach to its definition and study. BMC Med 2005;3(1):19.

Wagner D, Nisenbaum R, Heim C, et al. Psychometric properties of the CDC Symptom Inventory for assessment of chronic fatigue syndrome. BioMed Central Popul Health Metr 2005;3:8.

Ware JE, Sherbourne CD. The MOS 36-item short form health survey (SF-36): Conceptual framework and item selection. Med Care 1992;30:473–83.

Whiting P, Bagnall AM, Sowden AJ, et al. Interventions for the treatment and management of chronic fatigue syndrome: A systematic review. JAMA 2001;286:1360–8.

Mumps

Method of
Joel D. Klein, MD, FAAP

Mumps is a respiratory viral infection caused by mumps virus, an RNA virus in the family Paramyxoviridae. The virus is spread from human to human through direct contact with airborne droplets.

Epidemiology

Before the introduction of mumps vaccine, there were large yearly epidemics, usually occurring in the winter and early spring. Infection generally occurred among young children (younger than 15 years), with rare cases in young adults. With the introduction of the mumps vaccine in 1967, there was a dramatic decrease in the number of cases. However, in 1986 and 1987, there was a resurgence of mumps among teenagers and young adults, most of whom were born before routine immunization with the mumps vaccine.

Outbreaks were also seen among some children who had received mumps vaccine, because a single dose of the vaccine did not always confer immunity. In 1989, a second dose of mumps vaccine was recommended to address this issue. Mumps vaccine currently is usually administered as part of a combined vaccine such as measles-mumps-rubella (MMR) or most recently measles-mumps-rubella-varicella (MMRV) (Proquad).

Despite these changes, outbreaks of mumps occasionally occur, usually among college-aged persons. Recent examples include an epidemic in the United Kingdom in the winter of 2004 to 2005 and in the United States in 2006.

Clinical Manifestations

The incubation period of mumps is 14 to 25 days and involves nonspecific complaints of malaise, low-grade fever, and anorexia. The single most diagnostic physical finding in mumps is unilateral or bilateral parotitis, which occurs in up to 40% of cases. Mumps

CURRENT DIAGNOSIS

- Painful parotid swelling
- Edema of the face in the area of the parotid
- Elevation of serum amylase
- Headache and occasional meningismus
- Viral isolation or serology can confirm diagnosis

parotitis can occur early in the disease and may be associated with swelling and pain in other salivary glands. There often is erythema of the area and tenderness with palpation of the affected parotid. Patients at times also complain of earache and headache. Swelling over the parotid and related glands can occur rapidly and can result in distortion of the contours of the face, pushing the earlobe upward and outward. Edema can extend to the anterior chest wall as well. Examination of the oral cavity can reveal erythema of the orifice of Stensen's duct without purulent discharge. Parotitis generally resolves within 1 week.

The most commonly reported complications of mumps are aseptic meningitis and encephalitis, which can occur individually or together. Meningitis occurs in 10% to 15% of cases but probably is underreported. There is a typical viral-like pleocytosis in the cerebrospinal fluid (CSF), but the CSF glucose may be low. Encephalitis is rare and is seen in 1 or 2 per 100,000 cases.

Orchitis, either unilateral or bilateral, may be seen in as many as 50% of infected men. This complication can have a rapid onset and can be associated with increased fever, abdominal pain, nausea, and testicular swelling. This complication generally resolves within 1 week and can result in testicular atrophy but rarely infertility. Pancreatitis is sometimes seen, is usually mild, and may be associated with transient hyperglycemia. Table 1 lists the incidence of complications of mumps.

Diagnosis

Diagnosis of mumps is usually made by clinical examination and history. It should be considered in any patient with sudden onset of parotid swelling and fever. Mumps virus isolation may be attempted on fluids obtained by nasopharyngeal swab and urine. Virus may be excreted for 1 week before and 1 week after the onset of parotitis. When available, PCR may also be used to detect mumps virus in secretions.

Serum amylase determinations, although not specific, may be helpful in situations where mumps is suspected. Serology, which is readily available, may be diagnostic as well. Mumps IgM obtained during the acute infection is usually elevated and diagnostic. Acute and convalescent-paired sera can also be used to retrospectively confirm the diagnosis. Other commonly ordered laboratory tests, including complete blood count (CBC) are not particularly helpful. The CBC might show mild leukopenia with lymphocytosis.

Differential diagnosis of mumps parotitis includes many infections that are listed in Box 1.

TABLE 1   Complications of Mumps Infection

Mumps Complications	Incidence of Complications
Central nervous system	40%–50%
Orchitis and epididymitis	15%–30%
Oophoritis	7%
Pancreatitis	2%–5%
Deafness	1 in 20,000 reported cases
Myocarditis	Rare
Arthritis	Rare
Thyroiditis	Rare

BOX 1   Differential Diagnosis of Mumps Parotitis

- Parainfluenza virus infection
- Enterovirus infection
- Epstein-Barr virus
- Cytomegalovirus infection
- HIV
- Suppurative bacterial infection *(Staphylococcus aureus, Streptococcus pneumoniae)*
- Nontuberculous mycobacterial infection

Treatment

There is no specific therapy for mumps. Adequate analgesia is important, because many patients are quite uncomfortable. Because most patients are febrile, hydration also plays an important role. This is particularly critical because there may be difficulty swallowing and pain with mastication.

Children with mumps should be excluded from school for 9 days from onset of parotid swelling. Droplet precautions are recommended for patients with mumps admitted to the hospital for a period of 9 days from onset of parotid swelling.

Prevention

Mumps vaccine should be administered to children at age 12 to 15 months. A second dose should be given at age 4 to 6 years. Patients with HIV who are not severely immunocompromised may receive a combination mumps vaccine. Adults born in 1957 or later, in whom immunity is not known, should receive one dose of a mumps combination vaccine (MMR). Persons born before 1957 are usually considered immune, but they might benefit from immunization during a mumps community outbreak.

CURRENT THERAPY

- Analgesia for pain
- Warm or cold compresses
- Droplet isolation in the hospital
- Patient may return to school 5 days after the onset of parotid swelling

REFERENCES

American Academy of Pediatrics Committee on Infectious Diseases. Mumps. In: Pickering LK, editor. Red Book: 2006 Report of the Committee on Infectious Diseases. 27th ed. Elk Grove Village, Ill: American Academy of Pediatrics; 2006. p. 464–8.

Cherry JD. Mumps Virus. In: Feigin RD, Cherry JD, Demmler GJ, Kaplan SL, editors. Textbook of Pediatric Infectious Diseases. 5th ed. Philadelphia: WB Saunders; 2004. p. 2305–14.

Gupta RK, Best J, MacMahon E. Mumps and the UK epidemic 2005. BMJ 2005;330:1132–5.

Litman N, Baum SG. Mumps virus. In: Mandell GL, Bennett JE, Dolin R, editors. Principles and Practice of Infectious Diseases. 6th ed. Philadelphia: Churchill Livingstone; 2005. p. 2003–8.

Maldonado Y. Mumps. In: Behrman RE, editor. Nelson Textbook of Pediatrics. 17th ed. Philadelphia: WB Saunders; 2004. p. 1035–6.

McQuone SJ. Acute viral and bacterial infections of the salivary glands. Otolaryngol Clin North Am 1999;32(5):793–811.

Plague

Method of
Douglas A. Drevets, MD, DTM&H

Plague caused by *Yersinia pestis* is an ancient disease, and historical descriptions indicate that it probably caused Justinian's Plague (AD 541) that led into the first plague pandemic. The second plague pandemic, also known as the Black Death, began in Central Asia in 1347 and then spread to Europe, Asia, and Africa. It killed an estimated 50 million persons. The third and current plague pandemic began in China and then disseminated throughout the world by shipping routes in 1899–1900. *Y. pestis* is a gram-negative, nonmotile, facultatively anaerobic, non-spore-forming coccobacillus that is approximately 0.5 to 0.8 μm in diameter and 1 to 3 μm in length. Genomic sequencing shows that *Y. pestis* is a recently emerged clone of *Y. pseudotuberculosis*.

Epidemiology

Plague is a zoonosis that is usually spread between mammalian hosts by the bite of infected fleas. The most important enzootic reservoirs are urban and sylvatic rodents; however, domestic cats and dogs also are linked to human disease. Human plague occurs in North and South America, Asia, and Africa. An average of 2547 cases of human plague were reported yearly to the World Health Organization between 1988 and 1997, 76% of which were from Africa, with an overall case fatality rate of 7.1%. In North America, 82% of 295 indigenous cases were from Arizona, Colorado, and New Mexico. Bubonic plague is the most common form in humans, accounting for 97% of cases in a recent outbreak in Madagascar. Similarly, 84% of U.S. cases reported between 1947 and 1996 were the bubonic form, with septicemic and pneumonic plague accounting for 13% and 2%, respectively.

Modes of Transmission

Most human infections are transmitted from rodent to humans via the bite of an infected flea. Infection also can be acquired by contact with body fluids from infected animals, such as during field dressing of game or by inhalation of respiratory droplets from animals, particularly cats, or humans with pneumonic plague.

Bioterrorism Threat

Plague was used as an agent of biowarfare by the Japanese in World War II and was a focus of intensive research and development in the former Soviet Union during the Cold War. Primary pneumonic plague is the most likely form of exposure because of biowarfare or bioterrorism.

Pathogenesis and Clinical Syndromes

Transdermal inoculation of bacilli from the bite of an infected flea ultimately leads to infection of the regional lymph nodes in which massive replication of bacteria creates the bubo (derived from the Greek "bubon" or "groin"), a swollen, erythematous, and painful lymph node in the groin, axilla, or cervical region. Bacteremia and septicemia frequently develop and lead to secondary infection of other organs including lungs, spleen, and the central nervous system. Primary pneumonic plague is a rare natural occurrence and results

from the inhalation of respiratory droplets containing *Y. pestis* bacilli from another case of pneumonic plague, usually in humans or in cats. Secondary pneumonic plague results from seeding of the lungs by blood-borne bacteria in the setting of either bubonic or septicemic plague. Septicemic plague also begins with a transdermal exposure but manifests as primary bacteremia/septicemia without the bubo. Less common manifestations include meningitis, pharyngitis, and gastroenteritis.

Bubonic plague is an acute febrile lymphadenitis that develops 2 to 8 days after inoculation. Inflamed lymph nodes are usually 1 to 6 cm and painful. Abrupt onset of fever is an almost universal finding and occurs simultaneously with, or up to 24 hours before, the appearance of the bubo. Headache, malaise, and chills are frequent, along with nausea, vomiting, and diarrhea. Most patients are tachycardic, hypotensive, and appear prostrate and lethargic with episodic restlessness. Leukocytosis with a left shift is typical. Complications include pneumonia, shock, disseminated intravascular coagulation, purpuric skin lesions, acral cyanosis, and gangrene. The differential diagnosis of bubonic plague includes tularemia and Group A β-hemolytic streptococcal adenitis with bacteremia.

The symptoms of septicemic plague are not distinct from those caused by other gram-negative bacteria, and they are very similar to those of bubonic plague except that abdominal pain is more common in septicemic plague. Septicemic plague must be differentiated from fulminate septicemia caused by other gram-negative bacteria. Primary pneumonic plague has an abrupt onset of fever and influenza-like symptoms 1 to 5 days after inhalation exposure. Symptoms include shortness of breath, cough, chest pain, and bloody sputum with rapid progression to fulminate pneumonia and respiratory failure. Patients with secondary pneumonic infection show respiratory symptoms in addition to those attributed to the bubo or sepsis. Radiographic findings include patchy bronchopneumonia, multilobar consolidations, cavitations, and alveolar hemorrhage and are not pathognomonic of *Y. pestis*. Plague pneumonia must be differentiated from severe influenza, inhalation anthrax, and overwhelming community-acquired pneumonia.

Diagnosis

Plague is diagnosed by demonstrating *Y. pestis* in blood or body fluids such as a lymph node aspirate, sputum, or cerebrospinal fluid. A tentative diagnosis of bubonic plague can be made rapidly with fluid aspirated from a bubo showing gram-negative coccobacilli with bipolar staining. Serology showing a fourfold rise in antibody titers to F1 antigen or a single titer of more than 1:128 is also diagnostic.

Treatment

The aminoglycosides gentamicin (Garamycin) and streptomycin, the fluoroquinolones ciprofloxacin (Cipro), levofloxacin (Levaquin), and ofloxacin (Floxin), and tetracyclines (i.e., doxycycline [Vibramycin]) are the first-, second-, and third-line classes of antibiotics, respectively. Typical minimal inhibitory concentrations for 90% (MIC_{90}) of tested strains for the fluoroquinolones are less than 0.03 to 0.25 μg/mL compared with less than 1.0 μg/mL and less than 1.0 μg/mL to

CURRENT THERAPY

- Prompt administration of gentamicin or ciprofloxacin.
- Aggressive supportive care.
- Respiratory isolation of hospitalized cases.
- Postexposure prophylaxis to close contacts.

4.0 µg/mL for gentamicin and streptomycin, respectively, and less than 1.0 µg/mL for doxycycline. Streptomycin (15 mg/kg up to 1 g intermuscularly [IM] every 12 hours) and gentamicin (5 to 7 mg/kg/day intravenously [IV]/IM in one or two doses daily) are the drugs of choice for severe infection. Standard doses for the fluoroquinolones include ciprofloxacin, 400 mg IV/500 mg orally every 12 hours; levofloxacin, 500 mg IV/orally daily; and ofloxacin, 400 mg IV/orally every 12 hours. Doxycycline is administered at 100 mg IV/orally every 12 hours. Chloramphenicol (25 mg/kg IV/orally every 6 hours) can be used in select circumstances. Antibiotic therapy should be continued for a total of 10 days.

Prevention and Control

Standard infection control procedures that should be used when caring for patients with suspected plague include a disposable surgical mask, latex gloves, devices to protect mucous membranes, and good hand washing. Hospitalized patients with known or suspected pneumonic plague should be placed in strict isolation for at least 48 hours after appropriate antibiotics are initiated. Postexposure prophylaxis should be given to individuals with close contact (defined as less than 2 meters) with an infectious case or who have had a potential respiratory exposure. The recommended adult antibiotics for prophylaxis are doxycycline or ciprofloxacin in the same doses used for treatment. Postexposure prophylaxis can be given orally and should be continued for 7 days following exposure. Currently, there is no licensed plague vaccine.

REFERENCES

Butler T. A clinical study of bubonic plague. Observations of the 1970 Vietnam epidemic with emphasis on coagulation studies, skin histology and electrocardiograms. Am J Med 1972;53:268–76.

Boulanger LL, Ettestad P, Fogarty JD, et al. Gentamicin and tetracyclines for the treatment of human plague: Review of 75 cases in New Mexico, 1985–1999. Clin Infect Dis 2004;38:663–9.

Cler DJ, Vernaleo JR, Lombardi LJ, et al. Plague pneumonia disease caused by *Yersinia pestis.* Semin Respir Infect 1997;12:12–23.

Gage KL, Dennis DT, Orloski KA, et al. Cases of cat-associated human plague in the Western US, 1977–1998. Clin Infect Dis 2000;30:893–900.

Hull HF, Montes JM, Mann JM. Septicemic plague in New Mexico. J Infect Dis 1987;155:113–8.

Inglesby TV, Dennis DT, Henderson DA, et al. Plague as a biological weapon: Medical and public health management. Working Group on Civilian Biodefense. JAMA 2000;283:2281–90.

Perry RD, Fetherston JD. *Yersinia pestis*—etiologic agent of plague. Clin Microbiol Rev 1997;10:35–66.

Prentice MB, Rahalison L. Plague. Lancet 2007;369:1196–1207.

Ratsitorahina M, Chanteau S, Rahalison L, et al. Epidemiological and diagnostic aspects of the outbreak of pneumonic plague in Madagascar. Lancet 2000;355:111–3.

Wong JD, Barash JR, Sandfort RF, Janda JM. Susceptibilities of *Yersinia pestis* strains to 12 antimicrobial agents. Antimicrob Agents Chemother 2000;44:1995–6.

Anthrax

Method of
Jon B. Woods, MD

Anthrax has been a significant disease for both humans and their livestock for millennia. It was the first disease to fulfill Koch's postulates in 1876, as well as the first bacterial disease for which an effective vaccine was developed, for livestock, in 1880. This gram-positive rod-shaped bacillus species differs from the more benign members of its genera in containing two additional plasmids, one encoding for an antiphagocytic poly-D-glutamic acid capsule and the other encoding for two toxins. Three distinct toxin components combine to form two toxins, edema toxin and lethal toxin; the common component, protective antigen (PA), forms a pore through eukaryotic cell walls that allows the other two toxin components, edema factor (EF) and lethal factor (LF), to enter affected host cells. EF is an adenylate cyclase affecting many cell types and is responsible for the edema associated with anthrax infections. LF is a zinc metalloprotease that seems to have its greatest affect on macrophages; within the cells it cleaves mitogen-activated protein kinase and disrupts the cellular response to infection.

Background

Anthrax is an enzootic, and occasionally epizootic, disease of grazing animals worldwide. The incredibly durable spores of this bacillus can persist in soil for decades. These spores, when inadvertently ingested by herbivores while grazing, can germinate and then replicate in a rapid progression to bacteremia and subsequent death of the animal. At the time of death these animals can have as many as 10^8 vegetative bacilli per milliliter of blood. Those bacilli, which are exposed to oxygen upon the animal's death, can sporulate and then reenter the soil to begin the cycle anew.

Human anthrax can take several forms, most commonly cutaneous, but also intestinal, oropharyngeal, and inhalational disease. Naturally occurring human anthrax disease has typically been the result of exposure to infected animals or contaminated animal products such as hair or wool, bone meal, hides, or meat. Less commonly, human cutaneous anthrax has resulted from the bites of flies that have recently fed on infected animals. Gastrointestinal and oropharyngeal anthrax can result from ingestion of the raw or inadequately cooked flesh of an animal infected with anthrax. Endemic inhalational anthrax, or woolsorter's disease, results from inhalation of anthrax spores aerosolized during the manipulation of contaminated animal products, especially hair or wool; this was an exceedingly rare form of disease even prior to the institution of more stringent control measures and closure of most of the U.S. textile mills processing foreign-acquired goat hair by the 1970s. More recently, inhalational anthrax and cutaneous cases have resulted from exposure to spores intentionally processed and disseminated as biologic weapons. The extreme environmental stability of the spores, their ease of production, and their infectivity via the aerosol route are some features that have made *Bacillus anthracis* a top candidate for both nations and terrorists seeking biologic weapons. An apparently accidental aerosol release of dried anthrax spores from a biologic weapons facility in the Soviet city of Sverdlovsk in 1979 resulted in as many as 68 deaths because of inhalational anthrax. More recently, anthrax spores intentionally sent through the U.S. postal system resulted in 11 cases of inhalational anthrax and perhaps as many as 11 cases of cutaneous anthrax.

Clinical Features

Cutaneous anthrax represents approximately 95% of naturally occurring human anthrax cases. It typically occurs 1 to 7 days after exposure to infected livestock or contaminated livestock products, but rarely it is transmitted to humans by the bites of flies that have recently fed on infected animals. The lesion begins as a painless or mildly pruritic papule at the site of spore inoculation, progressing into an expanding round ulcer by the following day. Over the following several days the ulcer dries to a dark, almost black eschar, which resolves over the ensuing 1 to 2 weeks. The lesion can be surrounded by significant local edema and may be accompanied by regional lymphadenopathy. Treated, cutaneous anthrax is rarely fatal, although without antibiotics, progression to bacteremia and ultimately death can occur in up to 10% to 20% of cases.

Both forms of gastrointestinal anthrax are acquired via ingestion of insufficiently cooked meat from infected animals. The infectious dose is unknown. Intestinal anthrax may be initially misdiagnosed as either gastroenteritis or acute abdomen, typically presenting 1 to 6 days following contaminated meat consumption with fever, nausea, vomiting, and focal abdominal pain. Without prompt initiation of antibiotic therapy, disease can progress to hematemesis, hematochezia or melena, massive serosanguineous or hemorrhagic ascites, and sepsis, with mortality rates greater than 50%. Oropharyngeal anthrax typically presents after a 1- to 6-day incubation period with severe pharyngitis and fever, followed by appearance of pharyngeal or tonsillar ulcers. Gray or tan pseudomembranes can form over the ulcers, which are often accompanied by significant cervical lymphadenopathy and unilateral neck edema. Mortality of oropharyngeal anthrax varies from 10% to 50%.

Inhalation of aerosolized anthrax spores into the pulmonary alveoli can result in inhalational anthrax. The lethal dose via inhalation for 50% of humans (LD_{50}) is thought to be between 8000 and 55,000 spores. The alveolar spores are ingested by macrophages and carried to regional lymphatics, where they can germinate and replicate, eventually leading to hemorrhagic mediastinitis. The incubation period is presumably dose dependent, and although typically 1 to 6 days was suspected in at least one human case to be 43 days. Early inhalational anthrax presents suddenly as a nonspecific syndrome consisting of fever, malaise, headache, fatigue, and drenching sweats. Other common symptoms include nausea, vomiting, confusion, a nonproductive cough, and mild chest discomfort. Upper respiratory symptoms are notably absent. Physical findings are nonspecific in the early phase of the disease, but tachycardia is common. Auscultatory lung exam is typically normal at this stage, but dullness to percussion can develop over time in the lower lung fields as hemorrhagic pleural effusions accumulate. These early findings generally persist for 2 to 5 days before progressing fulminantly to tachypnea, cyanosis, shock, and multiorgan system failure. These late findings typically herald impending death within 24 to 36 hours. Gastrointestinal hemorrhage and hemorrhagic meningitis are common at autopsy. Prognosis is poor in the absence of intensive supportive care and early initiation of appropriate antibiotic combinations. Mortality ranges from 45% to more than 85% historically.

Diagnosis

None of the forms of human anthrax disease can be diagnosed on the basis of clinical findings alone (Table 1). For example, diagnosis of cutaneous anthrax requires the presence of a compatible skin lesion accompanied by confirmatory laboratory studies; an exposure history, or a known risk may also be present. Both forms of gastrointestinal anthrax are typically accompanied by a history of ingestion of the meat of anthrax-infected animals. Early intestinal anthrax can be difficult to differentiate clinically from other causes of gastrointestinal illness to include acute gastroenteritis, dysentery, or even peritonitis. Later in the course of intestinal disease, surgical or autopsy findings may include ileal or cecal ulceration, and bowel edema and necrosis is

TABLE 1 Empirical Antibiotic Therapy for Anthrax*

Cutaneous Anthrax (without Systemic Symptoms)	Inhalational, Gastrointestinal, or Cutaneous Disease with Systemic Symptoms
Ciprofloxacin (Cipro[1]) • 500 mg PO twice daily (adults) • 15 mg/kg (up to 500 mg/dose) PO twice daily (children) *or* Doxycycline (Vibramycin) • 100 mg PO twice daily (adults) • 2.2 mg/kg (up to 100 mg/dose) PO bid (children < 45 kg) *or (if strain susceptible):* Penicillin G procaine (Bicillin C-R) • 1,200,000 U IM q12h (adults) • 25,000 U/kg (maximum 1,200,000 U) q12h (children) *or* Penicillin V Potassium (Veetids) • 500 mg PO q6h (adults) *or* Amoxicillin (Amoxil[1]) • 500 mg PO q8h (adults and children > 40 kg) • 15 mg/kg q8h (children <40 kg) According to CDC recommendations, amoxicillin prophylaxis is appropriate only after 14–21 d of fluoroquinolone or doxycycline and only for populations with relative contraindications to the other drugs (children pregnancy)	Ciprofloxacin (Cipro IV[1]) • 400 mg IV q12h (adult) • 15 mg/kg/dose (up to 400 mg/dose) q12h (children) *or* Doxycycline (Vibramycin IV) • 200 mg IV, then 100 mg IV q12h (adults) • 2.2 mg/kg (100 mg/dose maximum) q12h (children < 45 kg) *or (if strain susceptible):* Penicillin G (Pfizerpen) • 4 million U IV q4h (adults) • 50,000 U/kg (up to 4M U) IV q6h (children) *plus* One or two additional antibiotics with activity against anthrax. Clindamycin (Cleocin[1]) plus rifampin (Rifadin[1]) may be a good empiric choice, pending susceptibilities. Potential additional antibiotics include one or more of the following clindamycin (Cleocin[1]), rifampin (Rifadin[1]), gentamicin[1] (generic), macrolides (erythromycin [generic], vancomycin (Vancocin[1]), imipenem (Pimaxin[1]), and chloramphenicol[1] (generic). Convert from IV to oral therapy when patient is stable, to complete at least 60 d of antibiotics. **Meningitis** Add Rifampin (Rifadin[1]) 20 mg/kg IV once daily or vancomycin (Vancocin[1]) 1 g IV q12h Oral dosing may be necessary for treatment of systemic disease in a mass casualty situation.

Adapted from Woods JB (ed): USAMRIID's Medical Management of Biological Warfare Casualties Handbook, 6th ed. 2005.
[1]Not FDA approved for this indication.
*Should be adjusted for susceptibilities.
Abbreviations: CDC = Centers for Disease Control and Prevention; IV = intravenous; PO = orally.

CURRENT DIAGNOSIS

Cutaneous/Oropharyngeal

- Painless or pruritic lesion beginning 1–7 d after exposure
  - Typical lesion progression from papule to ulcer to dark eschar (see text), often with significant edema

Plus

- Lesion gram stain, culture usually positive if patient has not received antibiotics
  - If negative, punch biopsy of lesion margin for IHC may still be positive
- Blood culture rarely positive in absence of systemic symptoms

Acute and convalescent serology or may give evidence of infection.

Gastrointestinal

- Gastrointestinal symptoms (variable) beginning 1–6 d after ingestion exposure.
  - Focal abdominal pain with hematochezia or melena common.
  - Nonspecific bowel wall edema, air–fluid levels, and ascites on radiographs.

Plus

- Stool culture (variably +).
- Blood culture (variably +).
- Acute and convalescent serology or blood sample for PCR may give evidence of infection.
- Ascites: often hemorrhagic.
  - Gram stain and culture, and IHC or PCR, if available, may be positive.

Surgical findings: hemorrhagic mesenteric adenitis, bowel edema, ileal and/or cecal ulcerations.

Inhalational

- Nonspecific febrile syndrome beginning abruptly 1–6 (but up to 43) d after aerosol exposure (see text).
  - Absence of upper respiratory findings, no pneumonia.
  - Widened mediastinum ± effusions on CXR or chest CT in *all* cases.

Plus

- Blood culture often positive if patient has not received antibiotics.
- Acute and convalescent serology or blood sample for PCR may give evidence of infection.
- Laboratory studies show hemoconcentration, mildly increased WBC with left shift, mildly increased AST and ALT, hypoalbuminemia.
- CSF (if meningitis) and pleural effusions are hemorrhagic.
- Gram stain and culture often positive.

If negative, IHC or PCR may be positive.

Abbreviations: AST = serum aspartate aminotransferase (level); ALT = serum alanine aminotransferase (level); CSF = cerebrospinal fluid; CXR = chest radiograph; CT = computed tomography study; IHC = immunohistochemical staining; PCR = polymerase chain reaction (study); WBC = white blood count.

associated with hemorrhagic mesenteric adenitis and serosanguineous to hemorrhagic ascites. Oropharyngeal anthrax can clinically resemble diphtheria, with pharyngeal lesions and an edematous so-called bull neck. Early inhalational anthrax is a nonspecific febrile syndrome that may be difficult to distinguish clinically from many other infectious diseases. However, the presence of mental status changes, profuse sweating, and absence of upper respiratory symptoms or pneumonia in inhalational anthrax may aid in differentiating it from influenza-like respiratory illnesses.

Gram stain and culture of skin lesions are ideally performed on the fluid of an unopened vesicle and are often positive in the cutaneous anthrax patient who has not received antibiotics. Tissue biopsy can be performed on lesions for immunohistochemical staining in culture-negative patients. Blood culture should be collected in any systemically ill patient suspected of having any form of anthrax disease. *B. anthracis* grows quickly in standard laboratory culture media. Paired acute and convalescent serologic studies may suggest infection in patents that have negative cultures, albeit these studies are not well validated. Stool culture can be positive in intestinal anthrax, although it is only variably so. Peritoneal fluid, pleural effusions, or cerebrospinal fluid (CSF) (when meningitis is present) can potentially demonstrate organisms on Gram stain and culture or may be positive via immunostaining or polymerase chain reaction (PCR) studies.

For patients with inhalation anthrax during the attacks of 2001, the complete blood count (CBC) revealed a mean white blood cell count of 9800/µL, with a predominance of neutrophils and a mildly elevated hematocrit. Mildly elevated serum sodium, aspartate transaminase (AST), and alanine aminotransferase (ALT) were common, as was hypoalbuminemia.

A widened mediastinum caused by adenitis, as well as pleural effusions, may be visible on chest radiograph in patients with inhalational anthrax. Negative chest radiograph in a patient suspected of inhalational

anthrax should prompt a chest computerized tomography (CT) scan. In the 2001 attacks, either the chest radiograph or CT was abnormal in all cases of inhalational disease. Abdominal radiographs in intestinal anthrax may demonstrate any number of nonspecific findings, to include ascites, diffuse air–fluid levels, and bowel edema.

Treatment

Patient survival for all forms of severe anthrax disease hinges on prompt initiation of appropriate antibiotics. Initial empirical therapy for patients with inhalational anthrax, gastrointestinal anthrax, or cutaneous anthrax with systemic symptoms should include intravenous (IV) ciprofloxacin (Cipro IV) or doxycycline (Vibramycin IV) combined with one or two additional antibiotics effective against anthrax (Table 2). One suggested combination includes a quinolone (ciprofloxacin [Cipro IV]), clindamycin (Cleocin[1]), and rifampin (Rifadin[1]). Antibiotic choices should be adjusted to reflect the specific susceptibilities of the infecting strain. Rifampin (Rifadin[1]), vancomycin (Vancocin[1]), or chloramphenicol[1] (generic) should be added if meningitis is suspected. IV antibiotics can be switched to oral treatment as the patent's clinical condition improves, to complete at least 60 days of total antibiotic therapy. Specific antidotes for anthrax toxins are in development, including human anthrax immune globulin, which may be available as an investigational therapy for severe anthrax disease through the Centers for Disease Control and Prevention (CDC).

---

[1]Not FDA approved for this indication.

CURRENT THERAPY

<table>
<tr><td>

Cutaneous Anthrax (without Systemic Symptoms)

- Oral antibiotics (see Table 2 for details)
  - Doxycycline (Vibramycin), or
  - Ciprofloxacin (Cipro[1])
- Consider nonsteroidal anti-inflammatory agents (NSAIDs) or corticosteroids for severe edema
- Infection control:
  - Contact precautions

Do not debride lesions

</td><td>

Inhalational, Gastrointestinal, or Cutaneous Disease with Systemic Symptoms

- Supportive care
  - May need assisted ventilation and/or vasopressors
  - Drain pleural effusions and large peritoneal fluid collections
- Combination IV antibiotics (see Table 2 for details)
  - Doxycycline (Vibramycin IV), or
  - Ciprofloxacin (Cipro IV[1])

Plus

  - One or two additional antibiotics
- Consider corticosteroids for severe edema or meningitis
- Consider human anthrax immune globulin (investigational), if available
- Infection control:
  - Contact precautions (not transmitted by droplet or aerosol)

Avoid autopsy or invasive procedures prior to receipt of antibiotics.

</td></tr>
</table>

[1]Not FDA approved for this indication.

Patients with systemic anthrax disease often require aggressive supportive therapy, including fluid resuscitation, blood products, vasopressor agents, and airway management. Patients may also benefit from drainage of large hemorrhagic pleural or peritoneal fluid accumulations. Although clinical data are lacking, severe edema or meningitis in anthrax disease may benefit from administration of corticosteroids.

Uncomplicated naturally acquired cutaneous anthrax should be treated empirically with 7 to 10 days of either oral ciprofloxacin (Cipro[1]) or doxycycline (Vibramycin). For cutaneous disease thought to have been acquired via exposure to an anthrax aerosol, at least 60 days of antibiotics is recommended.

A licensed anthrax vaccine (BioThrax) has been available in the United States to the armed forces, veterinarians, and textile and laboratory workers since 1970. It is derived from the sterile supernatant of a liquid culture of an attenuated (nonencapsulated) strain of *B. anthracis* and is administered subcutaneously in a six-shot primary series over 18

months followed by annual boosters. The vaccine is licensed only for preexposure prophylaxis of persons 18 to 65 years of age but is available investigationally for postexposure and pediatric use.

Individuals exposed to aerosolized anthrax spores should immediately receive postexposure prophylaxis consisting of both oral antibiotics and anthrax vaccine. Oral doxycycline (Vibramycin) or ciprofloxacin (Cipro) are the preferred empiric antibiotics for postexposure prophylaxis. Antibiotics should be continued for variable lengths of time depending on the patient's anthrax immune status and the suspected inhaled dose of anthrax (Table 2). Exposed individuals should also receive the anthrax vaccine[1] (BioThrax) to counter delayed incubation of residual alveolar anthrax after discontinuation of antibiotics.

[1]Not FDA approved for this indication.

TABLE 2 Anthrax Aerosol Postexposure Prophylaxis*

Immunized[†]	Not Immunized and Vaccine Available	Not Immunized and Vaccine Not Available
Ciprofloxacin (Cipro) • 500 mg PO bid for adults • 10–15 mg/kg PO twice daily (up to 1 g/d) for children *or* Doxycycline (Vibramycin) • 100 mg PO bid for adults or children > 8 y and > 45 kg • 2.2 mg/kg PO bid (up to 200 mg/d) for children < 8 y		
If antibiotic susceptibilities allow, patients who cannot tolerate tetracyclines or quinolone antibiotics can be switched to amoxicillin (Amoxil[1]), 500 mg PO tid for adults and 80 mg/kg divided tid (≥ 1.5 g/d) in children.		
Continue antibiotics for *at least* 30 d	Receive at least 3 doses of anthrax vaccine[1] (BioThrax) at 2-wk intervals, and then continue antibiotics for *at least* 1–2 wk after receipt of 3rd dose of vaccine.	Continue antibiotics for *at least* 60 d.
Patients should be closely observed after discontinuation of antibiotics.		
If suspected clinical signs of anthrax disease occur, then resume empirical antibiotics.		

Adapted from Woods JB (ed): USAMRID's Medical Management of Biological Warfare Casualties Handbook, 6th ed. 2005.
[1]Not FDA approved for this indication.
*Unknown antibiotic susceptibilities.
[†]Immunized = completed 6 doses of anthrax vaccine and up to date on boosters, or minimum of 3 doses within past 6 mo. Those who have already received 3 doses within 6 mo of exposure should continue with their routine vaccine schedule.
Abbreviation: PO = orally.

REFERENCES

Beatty ME, Ashford DA, Griffin PM, et al. Gastrointestinal anthrax, a review of the literature. Arch Intern Med 2003;163:2527–31.

Centers for Disease Control and Prevention. Notice to readers: Use of anthrax vaccine in response to terrorism: Supplemental recommendations of the Advisory Committee on Immunization Practices. MMWR 2002;51(45):1024–26.

Inglesby TV, O'Toole T, Henderson DA, et al. Anthrax as a biological weapon 2002: Updated Recommendations for Management. JAMA 2002;287 (17):2236–52.

Jernigan JA, Stephens DS, Ashford DA, et al. Bioterrorism-related inhalational anthrax: The first 10 cases reported in the United States. Emerg Infect Dis 2001;7:933–44.

Kuehnert MJ, Doyle TJ, Hill HA, et al. Clinical features that discriminate inhalational anthrax from other acute respiratory illnesses. Clin Infect Dis 2003;36:328–36.

Turnbull PCB. Guidelines for the Surveillance and Control of Anthrax in Humans and Animals. 3rd ed. World Health Organization Report WHO/EMC/ZDI/98.6; 1998.

Woods JB editor. USAMRIID's Medical Management of Biological Warfare Casualties Handbook; 2005. 6th ed.

Psittacosis

Method of
Julian Elliott, MB, BS, FRACP

Epidemiology

Psittacosis is the disease caused by infection with the bacterium *Chlamydophila psittaci*, formerly known as *Chlamydia psittaci*. It affects men more than women, and the main age group affected is adults older than 40 years. The main reservoir for psittacosis is birds, particularly psittacine birds (parrots, parakeets, budgerigars, and cockatoos), but other bird species and mammals can be infected. The most common form of acquisition is exposure to infected birds, by breathing in an aerosol of dried feces or from nose or eye secretions.

Risk factors for disease include contact with pet birds—especially a new, sick, or dead bird—and occupational exposure, for example work as a veterinarian, as a zoo keeper, or in a poultry-processing plant. Most cases are sporadic, but outbreaks have occurred associated with pet shops, aviaries, and poultry-processing plants and with mowing lawns in areas with large numbers of psittacine birds. Person-to-person transmission is rare. There is no evidence of infection acquired through ingestion of poultry products.

Clinical Features

The incubation period varies from 4 to 14 days or longer. The typical presentation of psittacosis is of an influenza-like illness with sudden onset of fever, chills, and prominent headache, but a more gradual onset is also seen. Rigors may be present. Cough is usually later in onset, dry, and not very marked. There may also be diarrhea, pharyngitis, altered mental state, or shortness of breath. Chest examination is usually abnormal, but the findings are often minimal and less prominent than symptoms or x-ray findings would suggest. Pleural effusions are rare.

Patients might present with a fever of unknown origin without obvious respiratory involvement, or the disease can be misdiagnosed as meningitis due to prominent headache, sometimes with photophobia. The degree of illness varies from asymptomatic to life threatening. Elderly persons and pregnant women are susceptible to more severe illness.

Other, less common findings include hemoptysis, proteinuria, hepatosplenomegaly, and encephalitis. Cardiac manifestations include relative bradycardia and rarely myocarditis, culture-negative endocarditis, and pericarditis. Erythema nodosum and other skin manifestations have also been described. *C. psittaci* has also been demonstrated by PCR to be present in a variable proportion of ocular adnexal MALT lymphomas with up to one half of cases responding to antibiotic treatment.

Diagnosis

Diagnosis depends on eliciting a history of recent bird contact from a patient with a compatible clinical syndrome, most commonly an influenza-like presentation, community-acquired pneumonia (CAP), or fever of unknown origin. The diagnosis should also be considered in a patient with CAP and prominent headache, splenomegaly, or failure to respond to β-lactam antibiotics. If the presentation is of an atypical CAP, the differential diagnosis includes infection with *Legionella* species, *Mycoplasma pneumoniae*, or *Chlamydophila pneumoniae*.

The white cell count is usually normal or slightly elevated, but there is often a left shift or toxic changes. Increases in the C-reactive protein (CRP) and erythrocyte sedimentation rate (ESR) are common. Mildly abnormal liver function tests, hyponatremia, and mild renal impairment are also common. The cerebrospinal fluid sometimes contains a few mononuclear cells but is otherwise normal. The chest x-ray usually shows more than predicted by the examination findings, but is nonspecific. The most common finding is lobar consolidation, but bilateral consolidation or interstitial opacities are also commonly seen.

Culture of *C. psittaci* is difficult and hazardous, so confirmation of diagnosis is more commonly performed using serology. The complement fixation (CF) test is widely used, but it cannot differentiate between *Chlamydophila* species. A fourfold rise in titer, using samples collected at least 14 days apart, or a single titer of 1:128 or higher, is interpreted as a positive result. The antibody rise may be delayed or diminished by antibiotic treatment. A microimmunofluorescent (MIF) test is more specific for each *Chlamydophila* species, with a fourfold rise in titer or an IgM antibody titer of 1:16 interpreted as positive, but this test is not widely available. Polymerase chain reaction (PCR) assays have been developed, but they are not yet available for routine clinical use.

CURRENT DIAGNOSIS

- The key to successful management of psittacosis is considering it as a possible diagnosis and asking about bird contact.
- The commonest clinical scenarios are influenza-like illness, community-acquired pneumonia, or fever of unknown origin. The typical presentation is sudden onset of fever and chills, with prominent headache. The diagnosis should also be considered in a patient with community-acquired pneumonia and failure to respond to β-lactam antibiotics.
- Nonspecific findings on investigation include a normal or slightly elevated white blood cell count with a left shift or toxic changes, increase in C-reactive protein (CRP) or erythrocyte sedimentation rate (ESR), mildly abnormal liver function tests, hyponatremia, mild renal impairment, and a chest x-ray with more abnormalities than predicted by the examination findings.
- Diagnosis can be confirmed with serology using either the complement fixation test, which is widely used but unable to differentiate between *Chlamydia* species, or the microimmunofluorescent test, which is specific for individual *Chlamydia* species. Either a single high titer or a fourfold rise in titer using samples collected at least 14 days apart are interpreted as positive.

CURRENT THERAPY

- Empiric therapy should be commenced when the diagnosis is suspected on clinical presentation and initial investigations.
- Tetracyclines are the drugs of choice; for example, doxycycline (Vibramycin) 100 mg bid for 10 to 14 days.
- Macrolides are usually recommended for pregnant women, children, and people with intolerance of tetracyclines, but they are probably less effective.
- Defervescence and improvement in symptoms usually occur within 24 to 48 hours of initiating a tetracycline; subsequent mortality is less than 1%.
- Notification to health authorities facilitates public health investigation and interventions to reduce transmission and control outbreaks.

Management

When the diagnosis is suspected on clinical presentation and initial investigations, empiric therapy should be commenced. Tetracyclines are the drugs of choice, for example, doxycycline (Vibramycin) 100 mg bid for 10 to 14 days. This class usually leads to defervescence and improvement in symptoms within 24 to 48 hours, and subsequent mortality is less than 1%. Macrolides are usually recommended for pregnant women, children, and patients with intolerance of tetracyclines, but erythromycin (Erythrocin)[1] has been shown to fail in situations where a tetracycline was effective, and there are few clinical data on the efficacy of the other agents in this class. Some data suggest that quinolones may be effective, but further evidence is needed. Tetracycline hydrochloride[2] or doxycycline (4.4 mg/kg/d divided into two infusions) is given intravenously for critically ill patients.

Notification of health authorities is important for initiating public health investigations and interventions to reduce transmission and control of outbreaks.

REFERENCES

Centers for Disease Control and Prevention. Compendium of measures to control *Chlamydia psittaci* infection in humans (psittacosis) and pet birds (avian chlamydiosis), 2000. MMWR Morb Mortal Wkly Rep 2000;49 (RR08):1–17.
Crosse BA. Psittacosis: A clinical review. J Infect 1990;21:251–9.
Grayston JT, Thom DH. The chlamydial pneumonias. Curr Clin Top Infect Dis 1991;11:1–18.
Gregory DW, Schaffner W. Psittacosis. Semin Resp Infect 1997;12:7–11.
Hughes P, Chidley K, Cowie J. Neurological complications in psittacosis: A case report and literature review. Respir Med 1995;89:637–8.
Husain A, Roberts D, Pro B, et al. Meta-Analyses of the association between Chlamydia psittaci and ocular adnexal lymphoma and the response of ocular adnexal lymphoma and the response of ocular adnexal lymphoma to antibiotics. Cancer 2007;110:809–15.
Richards M. Psittacosis, UpToDate 2006; Available at http://www.uptodate.com/physicians/pulmonology_toclist.asp [accessed August 18, 2007; subscription required].
Williams J, Tallis G, Dalton C, et al. Community outbreak of psittacosis in a rural Australian town. Lancet 1998;351:1697–9.
Yung AP, Grayson ML. Psittacosis: A review of 135 cases. Med J Aust 1988;148:228–33.

---

[1]Not FDA approved for this indication.
[2]Not available in the United States.

Q Fever

Method of
Thomas J. Marrie, MD

CURRENT DIAGNOSIS

- Q fever should be considered in patients who have a prolonged febrile illness, pneumonia, or hepatitis after contact with cattle, sheep, goats, or parturient cats in areas endemic for this illness.
- Diagnosis of sporadic cases in nonendemic areas is more difficult and requires a high index of suspicion.

CURRENT THERAPY

- Acute Q fever can be treated with a 10-day course of doxycycline (Vibramycin) or a fluoroquinolone.[1]
- Q fever during pregnancy should be treated with trimethoprim-sulfamethoxazole (Bactrim)[1] for the duration of the pregnancy and doxycycline and hydroxychloroquine (Plaquenil)[1] for 1 year after delivery.
- Chronic Q fever requires prolonged therapy with doxycycline and hydroxychloroquine or a fluoroquinolone plus rifampin (Rifadin).[1]

---

[1]Not FDA approved for this indication.

Q fever is an zoonosis. The most common reservoirs of this organism are infected goats, sheep, and cattle. In some areas such as the Maritime Provinces of Canada, infected parturient cats have been a reservoir. The organism, *Coxiella burnetii*, which is an intracellular pathogen, is trophic for the placenta and mammary glands. It reaches high concentrations in the placenta, and during parturition the environment is contaminated. The organism, which forms spores, can survive for long periods and germinate under favorable conditions. Winds can spread the organism from the contaminated environment up to 10 km from the source. Inhalation of just one microorganism can result in illness.

The epidemiology of the disease is dictated by its reservoirs and contaminated fomites. Typically, outbreaks (in humans) occur during the birthing season in areas in which this infection is endemic in the animal reservoir. However, because of spore formation and contamination of fomites (dust, straw, and cosmetics made with the use of animal placental material), the epidemiology of infection due to this microorganism is protean. *C. burnetii* is a potential bioterrorism agent.

Diagnosis

Serologic testing is the mainstay of diagnosis, although the organism can be cultured in special laboratories or its DNA can be amplified using polymerase chain reaction techniques. A four fold rise between acute and convalescent samples is diagnostic. In acute Q fever, the antibody titer to phase I antigen is always higher than that to phase II, whereas in chronic Q fever, the phase I titer is very high, often greater than 1:8192.

Disease States

Q fever is typically divided into acute and chronic varieties.

TABLE 1 Treatment of Acute and Chronic Q Fever

Syndrome	Treatment
Acute Q Fever	
Inapparent infection	None, unless patient has valvular heart disease, in which case careful follow-up is necessary regarding endocarditis
Pneumonia	Doxycycline (Vibramycin) 200 mg PO followed by 100 mg bid for 10 to 14 d; or a fluoroquinolone, preferably levofloxacin (Levaquin)[1] or moxifloxacin (Avelox)[1]
Hepatitis (can also be chronic)	As for pneumonia; prednisone[1] 0.5 mg/kg/d can be used for those who remain febrile for ≥5 d after onset of antibiotic therapy
Chronic Q Fever	
Endocarditis or endovascular infection	Doxycycline 100 mg PO bid plus hydroxychloroquine (Plaquenil)[1] 200 mg PO tid to achieve a chloroquine level of 1 mg/L OR Doxycycline 100 mg PO bid plus a quinolone[1] or quinolones—ciprofloxacin (Cipro),[1] levofloxacin (Levaquin),[1] or moxifloxacin (Avelox)[1] OR Rifampin (Rifadin)[1] 600 mg qd plus a quinolone *In pregnancy:* trimethoprim-sulfamethoxazole (Bactrim)[1] 1 double-strength tablet bid for the duration of the pregnancy, followed by doxycycline and hydroxychloroquine[1] for 18 mo as for endocarditis treatment

[1]Not FDA approved for this indication.

Acute Q Fever

Most infections are inapparent and manifest as a nonspecific febrile illness of short duration. Prolonged fever, pneumonia, and hepatitis are the most common clinical manifestations. Radiographically, pneumonia may manifest as multiple rounded opacities or may be indistinguishable from any other cause of pneumonia. Patients with hepatitis typically have doughnut granulomas on liver biopsy, and some patients remain febrile despite antibiotic therapy. Meningitis, encephalitis, pericarditis, myocarditis, pancreatitis, acute cholecystitis, splenic rupture, orchitis, and priapism are other manifestations of acute Q fever.

Chronic Q Fever

Most commonly, chronic Q fever manifests as endocarditis. Both native and prosthetic valves can be affected. The vegetations can be visualized by transesophageal echocardiography. Infection of aortic aneurysms, osteomyelitis, and occasionally hepatitis are other manifestations of chronic Q fever. Q fever during pregnancy should also be considered as a manifestation of chronic Q fever.

Post-Q Fever Fatigue Syndrome

In some areas, a prolonged fatigue state follows acute Q fever in up to 20% of cases.

Treatment

Treatment options are outlined in Table 1. Patients with acute Q fever and valvular heart disease should be treated preemptively with 1 year of treatment, because they are at high risk for chronic Q fever. Patients with chronic Q fever should have antibody titers performed every 3 months. Once the immunoglobulin G phase I titer has fallen to 1:256 or less, antibiotic therapy can be discontinued.

Patients who are receiving hydroxychloroquine (Plaquenil)[1] therapy should be monitored for retinal toxicity, and the risks of phototoxicity should be emphasized when doxycycline (Vibramycin) and/or quinolone therapy is instituted.

REFERENCES

Ayres JG, Flint N, Smith EG, et al. Post infection fatigue syndrome following Q fever. Q J Med 1998;91:105–23.
Hawker JI, Ayres JG, Blair MR, et al. A large outbreak of Q fever in the West Midlands: Windborne spread into a metropolitan area. Commun Dis Public Health 1998;1:180–7.
Marrie TJ. Epidemiology of Q fever. In: Marrie TJ, editor. Q Fever: The Disease, vol. 1. Boca Raton, FL: CRC Press; 1990. p. 49–70.
Marrie TJ, Durant H, Williams JC, et al. Exposure to parturient cats: A risk factor for acquisition of Q fever in Maritime Canada. J Infect Dis 1988;158:101–8.
Raoult D, Fenollar R, Stein A. Q fever during pregnancy: Diagnosis, treatment and followup. Arch Intern Med 2002;162:701–4.
Raoult D, Houpikian P, Tissot Dupont H, et al. Treatment of Q fever endocarditis: Comparison of 2 regimens containing doxycycline and ofloxacin or hydroxychloroquine. Arch Intern Med 1999;159:167–73.
Raoult D, Tissot-Dupont H, Foucault C, et al. Q fever, 1985–1998: Clinical and epidemiologic features of 1,383 infections. Medicine (Baltimore) 2000;79:109–23.

[1]Not FDA approved for this indication.

Rabies

Method of
Alan C. Jackson, MD, FRCPC

Rabies is an acute infection of the nervous system caused by rabies virus, which is a member of the family Rhabdoviridae in the genus *Lyssavirus*. Other lyssaviruses have only very rarely caused rabies in Europe, Africa, and Australia.

Pathogenesis

Rabies virus is usually transmitted by bites from rabid animals. Transmission has rarely occurred through an aerosol route (in a laboratory accident or bat cave containing millions of bats) or by transplantation of infected organs and tissues. The virus is in the saliva of the rabid animal and inoculated into subcutaneous tissues or muscles. During most of the long incubation period (lasting 20 to 90 days or longer), the virus is close to the site of inoculation.

The virus binds to the nicotinic acetylcholine receptor at the post-synaptic neuromuscular junction and travels toward the central nervous system (CNS) in peripheral nerves by retrograde fast axonal transport. There is rapid dissemination throughout the CNS by fast axonal transport. Under natural conditions, degenerative neuronal changes are not prominent, and it is thought that the rabies virus induces neuronal dysfunction by mechanisms that are not well understood. In rabies vectors, the encephalitis is associated with behavioral changes that lead to transmission by biting. After the CNS infection is established, the virus spreads by autonomic and sensory nerves to multiple organs, including the salivary glands in which the virus is secreted in high titer.

Clinical Features

In North America, where the bat is the most common rabies vector, a history of an animal bite is usually absent, and there may be no known contact with animals. The incubation period is usually between 20 and 90 days, but it may occasionally last 1 or more years. Prodromal features are nonspecific and include malaise, headache, and fever, and patients may also have anxiety or agitation. Approximately half of patients may experience pain, paresthesias, or pruritus at the site of the wound, which has often healed; this may reflect involvement of local sensory ganglia. Approximately 80% of patients with rabies have encephalitic rabies; approximately 20% have paralytic rabies. In encephalitic rabies, there are characteristic periods of generalized arousal or hyperexcitability separated by lucid periods. Autonomic dysfunction occurs frequently and includes hypersalivation, gooseflesh, cardiac arrhythmias, and priapism. Hydrophobia is the most characteristic feature of rabies and occurs in 50% to 80% of patients; contractions of the diaphragm and other inspiratory muscles occur on swallowing. This may become a conditioned reflex, and even the sight or thought of water can precipitate the muscle contractions. Hydrophobia is thought to be caused by inhibition of inspiratory neurons near the nucleus ambiguus.

In paralytic rabies, prominent muscle weakness usually begins in the bitten extremity and progresses to quadriparesis; typically there is sphincter involvement. Patients have a longer clinical course than in encephalitic rabies. Paralytic rabies is frequently misdiagnosed as the Guillain-Barré syndrome. Coma subsequently develops in both clinical forms. With aggressive medical therapy, a variety of medical complications develop, and multiple organ failure is a frequent occurrence. Survival is very rare and has usually occurred in the context of incomplete postexposure rabies prophylaxis that included administration of some rabies vaccine.

Epidemiology

Worldwide more than 55,000 human deaths per year are attributed to rabies. The impact is particularly significant in terms of years of life lost because children are frequently the victims. Most human rabies cases occur through transmission from dogs in developing countries with endemic dog rabies, particularly in Asia and Africa. In the United States and Canada, the most common human cases are from insect-eating bats, and often, there is no known history of a bat bite or exposure to bats. A bat bite may not be recognized. The rabies virus variant responsible for most human cases is found in silver-haired bats and eastern pipistrelle bats. These are small bats not frequently in contact with humans. There are a variety of other rabies vectors in North American wildlife, including skunks, raccoons, and foxes, but these species are rarely responsible for transmission to humans. This is likely because of effective postexposure rabies prophylaxis.

Diagnosis

Most cases of rabies can be diagnosed clinically or the diagnosis strongly suspected, which is particularly important to initiate appropriate barrier nursing techniques and prevent exposures of many health care workers. Some cases may be candidates for an aggressive therapeutic approach. A serum neutralizing titer can be useful in a previously unimmunized individual, but a positive titer may not develop until the second week of clinical illness, and the result of the test may not be readily available. Detection of rabies virus antigen on a skin biopsy obtained from the nape of the neck using a fluorescent antibody technique is a useful diagnostic test. Detection of rabies virus ribonucleic acid (RNA) in saliva using reverse transcription polymerase chain reaction (RT-PCR) amplification is an important recent advance in rapid rabies diagnosis. Rabies virus antigen can be detected in brain tissue obtained by brain biopsy or postmortem.

Prevention

After recognition of a rabies exposure, rabies can be prevented with initiation of appropriate steps, including wound cleansing and active and passive immunization. After a human is bitten by a dog, cat, or ferret, the animal should be captured, confined, and observed for a period of at least 10 days. The animal should also be examined by a veterinarian prior to its release. If the animal is a stray, unwanted, shows signs, or develops signs of rabies during the observation period, the animal should be killed immediately, and its head should be transported under refrigeration for a laboratory examination. The brain should be examined via an antigen-detection method using the fluorescent antibody technique and viral isolation using cell culture or mouse inoculation.

The incubation period for animals other than dogs, cats, and ferrets is uncertain; these animals should be killed immediately after an exposure, and the head submitted for examination. If the result is negative, one may safely conclude that the animal's saliva did not contain rabies virus and, if immunization has been initiated, it should be discontinued. If an animal escapes after an exposure, it should be considered rabid unless information from public health officials indicates this is unlikely, and rabies prophylaxis should be initiated. The physical presence of a bat may warrant postexposure prophylaxis when a person (such as a small child or sleeping adult) is unable to reliably report contact that could have resulted in a bite.

Local wound care should be given as soon as possible after all exposures, even if immunization is delayed, pending the results of an observation period. All bite wounds and scratches should be washed thoroughly with soap and water. Devitalized tissues should be debrided.

CURRENT THERAPY

- Details of an exposure determine whether postexposure rabies prophylaxis should be initiated.
- Wound cleansing is very important after a potential rabies exposure.
- Active immunization with a schedule of 5 doses of rabies vaccine at intervals is recommended.
- Passive immunization (if previously unimmunized) consists of human rabies immune globulin infiltrated into the wound and the remainder of the 20 IU/kg dosage given intramuscularly.

Purified chick embryo cell culture vaccine (RabAvert) and human diploid cell vaccine (Imovax) are licensed rabies vaccines in the United States and Canada. Other vaccines grown in either primary cell lines (hamster or dog kidney) or continuous cell lines (Vero cells) are also satisfactory and available in other countries. A regimen of five 1-mL doses of rabies vaccine should be given intramuscularly (IM) in the deltoid area (anterolateral aspect of the thigh is also acceptable in children). Ideally, the first dose should be given as soon as possible after exposure, but failing that, it should be given regardless of the length of a delay. Four additional doses should be given on days 3, 7, 14, and 28. Pregnancy is not a contraindication for immunization. Live vaccines should not be given for 1 month after rabies immunization. Local and mild systemic reactions are common. Systemic allergic reactions are uncommon, and anaphylactic reactions may be treated with epinephrine and antihistamines. Corticosteroids may interfere with the development of active immunity. Immunosuppressive medications should not be administered during postexposure therapy unless they are essential. The risk of developing rabies should be carefully considered before deciding to discontinue vaccination because of an adverse reaction. A serum neutralizing antibody determination is necessary only after immunization of immunocompromised patients. Less expensive vaccines, derived from neural tissues, are still used in some developing countries; these vaccines are associated with serious neuroparalytic complications.

Human rabies immune globulin (Imogam or BayRab) should also be administered as passive immunization for protection before the development of immunity from the vaccine. It should be given at the same time as the first dose of vaccine and no later than 7 days after the first dose. Rabies vaccine and human rabies immune globulin should never be administered at the same site or in the same syringe. The recommended dose of human rabies immune globulin is 20 international units (IU)/kg; larger doses should not be given because they may suppress active immunity from the vaccine. After wounds are washed, they should be infiltrated with human rabies immune globulin (if anatomically feasible), and the remainder of the dose should be given IM in the gluteal area. If the exposure involves a mucous membrane, the entire dose should be administered IM. With multiple or large wounds, the human rabies immune globulin may need to be diluted for adequate infiltration of all of the wounds. Adverse effects of human rabies immune globulin include local pain and low-grade fever.

After an exposure, a previously immunized patient should receive two 1-mL doses of rabies vaccine on days 0 and 3, but the patient should not receive human rabies immune globulin.

Management of Human Rabies

Only seven people have survived rabies, and six received rabies vaccine prior to the onset of their disease. The possibilities for an aggressive approach were recently reviewed (see Jackson et al., 2003). There was one survivor in Wisconsin in 2004 who did not receive rabies vaccine. It is now doubtful whether the therapy she received played a significant role in her favorable outcome because a similar approach has failed in many cases (Wilde et al. 2008). Palliation is an alternative approach and may be appropriate for many patients who develop rabies.

REFERENCES

Centers for Disease Control and Prevention. Human rabies prevention—United States, 1999: Recommendations of the Advisory Committee on Immunization Practices (ACIP). MMWR 1999;48(RR-1):1–21.
Jackson AC. Human disease. In: Jackson AC, Wunner WH, editors. Rabies. 2nd ed. London: Elsevier, Academic Press; 2007. p. 309–40.
Jackson AC. Rabies. Curr Treat Options Infect Dis 2003;5:35–40.
Jackson AC. Rabies: New insights into pathogenesis and treatment. Curr Opin Neurol 2006;19(3):267–70.
Jackson AC, Warrell MJ, Rupprecht CE, et al. Management of rabies in humans. Clin Infect Dis 2003;36:60–3.
Jackson AC, Wunner WH. Rabies. 2nd ed. London: Elsevier, Academic Press; 2007.
Wilde H, Hemachudha T, Jackson AC. Viewpoint: management of human rabies. Trans R Soc Trop Med Hyg 2008;102:979–82.
World Health Organization. WHO expert consultation on rabies. First report (First Report Edition). Geneva: WHO; 2005.

Rat-Bite Fever

Method of
Jean Dudler, MD

Rat-bite fever (RBF) is a systemic febrile disease caused by infection with *Streptobacillus moniliformis*. As its name implies, it is transmitted by rat bite. However, it can also be transmitted by simple contact with infected rats or even through ingestion of food contaminated with rat excreta. Diagnosis can be difficult, and a high degree of awareness is necessary to make a correct diagnosis. Recognition and early treatment are crucial, because case fatality can be higher than 10% in untreated cases.

Epidemiology

S. moniliformis is part of the normal respiratory flora of the rat. From 50% to 100% of healthy wild, laboratory, and pet rats harbor *S. moniliformis* in the nasopharynx. *S. moniliformis* is also excreted in the urine, and *Spirillum minus* has been demonstrated in conjunctival secretions and blood. Thus, rat-bite fever can be transmitted not only from a bite but also through scratches, handling of dead rats, and even handling of litter material.

Although the rat is the natural reservoir and major vector of the disease, *S. moniliformis* has also been found in other rodents such as mice, squirrels, and gerbils, as well as in other mammals such as weasels and in pets that prey on rodents, such as cats and dogs, which can also act as vectors of the disease.

The major risk factor is exposure to rats, either as an occupational hazard for persons such as laboratory workers, veterinarians, or pet shop employees, or for persons who have rats for pets or feed rats to snakes, especially children. Classically, homelessness and lower socioeconomic status were described as major factors, but most cases reported in the last few years have involved pet rats.

No precise data are available on the true incidence of rat-bite fever because it is not a reportable disease. It appears to be unusual in Western countries, a rarity that could reflect failed diagnosis or a spontaneous recovery in most cases, considering the high percentage of *S. moniliformis* carriage, the frequency of contacts between humans and rats in modern society, and the fairly high risk—estimated around 10%—of developing rat-bite fever after being bitten or scratched.

Clinical Presentation

Rat-bite fever is a systemic febrile disease. Classically, following a rat bite and a short incubation of 1 to 3 days (but up to 3 weeks), systemic dissemination of the organism is associated with an abrupt onset with intermittent relapsing fever, rigors, myalgias, arthralgias, headache, sore throat, malaise, and vomiting. These symptoms are followed within the first week by the development of a maculopapular rash in 75% of patients. The rash can be pustular, purpuric, or petechial, and it typically involves the extremities, in particular the palms and soles. The bite site typically heals promptly, with minimal inflammation and absent or minimal regional adenopathy.

Up to 50% of infected patients develop an asymmetric migrating polyarthritis, which appears to be exceedingly painful and affects large and middle-sized joints. Joint effusion appears more common in adults. Infection can occur in any tissues. Anemia, meningitis, bronchitis, pneumonia, endocarditis, myocarditis, pericarditis, brain abscess, and infarcts of the spleen and kidneys have been reported as complications of rat-bite fever.

Although most cases seem to resolve spontaneously within 2 weeks, persistence up to 2 years has been reported. The mortality rate in untreated cases is around 10% to 15%, and it rises to more than 50% in the rare cases with cardiac involvement.

Two closely related variants have been described. In Havervill fever, the organism is transmitted by ingestion of contaminated food. It tends to occur in epidemics and also causes rashes and arthritis, but upper respiratory tract symptoms and vomiting appear more prominent. Sodoku is a rat-bite fever caused by *Spirillum minus*; it is common in Japan. The course is more subacute, arthritic symptoms are rare, and if the bite initially heals, it then ulcerates and is associated with regional lymphadenopathy and a distinctive rash.

Diagnosis

Diagnosis is difficult, with nonspecific clinical findings, broad differential diagnosis, and difficulties in identifying the responsible organism. Rat-bite fever should not be dismissed in the absence of bite history, because transmission can occur without a bite, and pet lovers or laboratory workers can minimize or forget the bite, especially in the absence of a local reaction.

No reliable serologic test is available, and the definitive diagnosis requires isolation of *S. moniliformis* from the wound, the blood, or the synovial fluid. The microbiology laboratory should be specifically notified of any clinical suspicion because of the hurdles in identification.

CURRENT DIAGNOSIS

- The examiner must maintain a high index of suspicion.
- Nonspecific initial symptoms are followed by a maculopapular rash and septic arthritis.
- Exposure to rats is the major risk factor. Transmission can occur with simple contact with infected animals or excreta.
- Notify microbiology laboratory of suspicion (slow growth, 5%–10% CO_2 microaerophilic conditions, 20% normal rabbit serum media supplementation, and avoidance of sodium polyanethol sulfonate).

S. moniliformis is a highly pleomorphic, nonencapsulated, nonmotile gram-negative rod, which may stain positively on Gram stain. It is often dismissed as proteinaceous debris because of its numerous bulbous swellings with occasional clumping (*moniliformis* = "necklace-like"). It grows slowly and requires a microaerophilic environment with 5% to 10% CO_2 or anaerobic conditions and media supplementation with 20% normal rabbit serum. Cultures should be held for more than 5 days and should not be dismissed as contamination. *S. moniliformis* is also inhibited by sodium polyanethol sulfonate, a common adjunct in most commercial blood culture media. Identification using polymerase chain reaction amplification and gene sequencing has been used. It can be performed on samples from the patient or animal in question if available.

Differential Diagnosis

Differential diagnosis is broad and depends on the clinical presentation. Malaria, typhoid fever, and neoplastic disease can cause relapsing fevers, and the presence of a rash and polyarthritis might suggest viral and rickettsial diseases. An asymmetric oligoarthritis points more toward a bacterial etiology, in particular disseminated gonococcal and meningococcal diseases in the context of cutaneous lesions. Lyme disease or secondary syphilis occasionally have such a clinical presentation, but 25% to 50% of patients infected with *S. moniliformis* or *S. minus* have a false-positive VDRL (Venereal Disease Research Laboratory) test. Finally, when classic infectious symptoms such as fever or rash are missing, any causes of polyarthritis, from crystal-related arthropathies to rheumatoid arthritis, can be entertained.

Treatment

All established cases of rat-bite fever should be treated with antibiotics. Despite being potentially lethal, rat-bite fever is easily treatable by a simple course of penicillin. The Centers for Disease Control and Prevention recommends intravenous penicillin G 1.2 million units per day for 5 to 7 days followed by oral penicillin V (Pen Vee K)[1] or

---

[1]Not FDA approved for this indication.

CURRENT THERAPY

Bite Site

- Clean and disinfect bite site.
- Local treatment does not prevent further dissemination.
- Administer tetanus toxoid (Td), if indicated.
- Do not give antirabies prophylaxis.

Established Cases

- Intravenous penicillin G (Bicillin) 1.2 million U/d for 5 to 7 d, followed by oral penicillin V[1] or ampicillin (Omnipen)[1] 500 mg qid for an additional wk (CDC recommendations).
- Oral tetracycline[1] 500 mg qid or streptomycin[1] 7.5 mg/kg bid IM are alternatives.
- Numerous other antibiotics are reported useful (macrolides, cephalosporins, quinolones).

Prophylaxis

- The role of prophylactic antibiotic is unknown. Some authors recommend oral penicillin V.[1]
- Encourage patients with an occupational risk to use protective gloves to handle animals or cages.

---

[1]Not FDA approved for this indication.

ampicillin (Omnipen)[1] 500 mg qid for an additional week. For allergic patients, or if an intravenous line cannot be established, oral tetracycline (Achromycin)[1] 500 mg qid or streptomycin[1] 7.5 mg/kg bid intramuscularly are alternatives. Numerous other antibiotics have been reported to be potentially useful, including clarithromycin (Biaxin),[1] cephalosporins, and quinolones, but none has been subjected to any clinical trial.

Typically the bite site heals promptly. It should be cleaned and disinfected, even if local treatment does not appear to prevent further dissemination. Tetanus prophylaxis (Td) administration is indicated as required by the patient's immunization record, but antirabies prophylaxis is usually not required for rodent bite.

The role of prophylactic antibiotics is unknown, but some authors recommend the use of oral penicillin V.[1] Primary prevention by using protective gloves to handle animals or cages should be encouraged for patients with occupational risk.

REFERENCES

Abdulaziz H, Touchie C, Toye B, Karsh J. Haverhill fever with spine involvement. J Rheumatol 2006;33:1409–10.

Albedwawi S, LeBlanc C, Show A, Slinger RW. A teenager with fever, rash and arthritis. CMAJ 2006;175:354.

Berger C, Altwegg M, Meyer A, Nadal D. Broad range polymerase chain reaction for diagnosis of rat-bite fever caused by Streptobacillus moniliformis. Pediatr Infect Dis J 2001;20:1181–2.

Centers for Disease Control and Prevention. Fatal rat-bite fever—Florida and Washington, 2003. MMWR Morb Mortal Wkly Rep. 2005;53:1198–202.

Holroyd KJ, Reiner AP, Dick JD. Streptobacillus moniliformis polyarthritis mimicking rheumatoid arthritis: An urban case of rat bite fever. Am J Med 1988;85:711–4.

Rupp ME. Streptobacillus moniliformis endocarditis: Case report and review. Clin Infect Dis 1992;14:769–72.

Schachter ME, Wilcox L, Rau N, et al. Rat-bite fever. Canada Emerg Infect Dis 2006;12:1301–2.

Stehle P, Dubuis O, So A, Dudler J. Rat bite fever without fever. Ann Rheum Dis 2003;62:894–6.

van Nood E, Peters SH. Rat-bite fever. Neth J Med 2005;63:319–21.

Washburn RG. Streptobacillus moniliformis (rat-bite fever). In: Mandell GL, Bennett R, Dolin R, editors. Mandell, Douglas, and Bennett's Principles and Practice of Infectious Diseases. 4th ed. Philadelphia: Churchill-Livingstone; 2000. p. 2422–4.

[1]Not FDA approved for this indication.

Relapsing Fever

Method of
Diego Cadavid, MD

Relapsing fever is one of several diseases caused by spirochetes. Other human spirochetal diseases are syphilis, Lyme disease, and leptospirosis. Notable features of spirochetes are wavy and helical shapes, length-to-diameter ratios of as much as 100 to 1, and flagella that lie between the inner and outer cell membranes. The spirochetes that cause relapsing fever are in the genus *Borrelia*. Other *Borrelia* species cause Lyme disease, avian spirochetosis, and epidemic bovine abortion. Table 1 shows the main *Borrelia* species of relapsing fever, their vectors, and an estimate of their geographic ranges. In the United States relapsing fever was considered a disease endemic only in the West. However, the recent finding of relapsing fever–like *Borrelia* in ticks and dogs in the eastern United States suggests that the risk of relapsing fever may extend into the East.

Epidemiology

There are two forms of relapsing fever: epidemic transmitted to humans by the body louse *Pediculus humanus* (louse-borne relapsing fever, LBRF) and endemic transmitted to humans by soft-bodied ticks of the genus *Ornithodoros* (tick-borne relapsing fever, TBRF). In LBRF itching caused by skin infestation with lice leads to scratching, which may result in crushing of lice and release of infected hemolymph into areas of skin abrasion. Louse infestation is associated with cold weather and a lack of hygiene. Migrant workers and soldiers at war are particularly susceptible to this infection. Historically, massive outbreaks of LBRF occurred in Eurasia, Africa, and Latin America, but currently the disease is found only in Ethiopia and neighboring countries. However, immigrants can spread LBRF to other parts of the world.

The main risk factor for TBRF is exposure to endemic areas (Table 1). The risk of infection increases with outdoor activities in areas where rodents nest, like entering caves or sleeping in rustic cabins. *Ornithodoros* ticks are soft-bodied and feed for short periods of time (minutes), usually at night. They can live many years between blood meals and may transmit spirochetes to their offspring transovarially. Infection is produced by regurgitation of infected tick saliva into the skin wound during tick feeding. There are several natural vertebrate reservoirs for TBRF, but most common are rodents (deer mice, chipmunks, squirrels, and rats). In contrast, the body louse *Pediculus humanus* is a strict human parasite, living and multiplying in clothing.

Clinical Diagnosis

Relapsing fever should be suspected in any patient presenting with two or more episodes of high fever and constitutional symptoms spaced by periods of relative well-being. The index of suspicion increases if the patient has been exposed to endemic areas for TBRF or to countries where LBRF still occurs (Table 1). Whereas LBRF is usually associated with a single febrile relapse, TBRF usually has multiple relapses (up to 13). In LBRF the second episode of fever is typically milder than the first; in TBRF the multiple febrile periods are usually of equal severity. The febrile periods last from 1 to 3 days, and the intervals between fevers last from 3 to 10 days. During the febrile periods, numerous spirochetes are circulating in the blood. This is called spirochetemia and is sometimes unexpectedly detected during routine blood smear examinations. Between fevers, spirochetemia is not observed because the numbers are low. The fever pattern and recurrent spirochetemia are the consequences of antigenic variation of abundant outer membrane lipoproteins of relapsing fever *Borrelia* species that are the target for serotype-specific antibodies.

CURRENT DIAGNOSIS

- There are two forms of relapsing fever: epidemic and endemic.
- Epidemic relapsing fever is transmitted from person to person by the body louse *Pediculus humanus*.
- Endemic relapsing fever is transmitted from rodent reservoirs to humans exposed to endemic areas by soft-bodied ticks of the genus *Ornithodoros*.
- The hallmark of relapsing fever is two or more febrile episodes separated by periods of relative well-being.
- The diagnosis is confirmed by visualization of the etiologic spirochetes in thin peripheral blood smears prepared at times of febrile peaks by phase-contrast or darkfield microscopy or light microscopy after Wright or Giemsa staining.

TABLE 1 Relapsing Fever *Borrelia* Species Pathogenic to Humans

Relapsing Fever	*Borrelia* Species	Arthropod Vector	Distribution of Disease
Endemic	B. hermsii	Ornithodoros hermsi	Western North America
	B. turicatae	O. turicata	Southwestern North America and northern Mexico
	B. venezuelensis	O. rudis	Central America and northern South America
	B. hispanica	O. marocanus	Iberian peninsula and northwestern Africa
	B. crocidurae	O. erraticus	North and East Africa, Middle East, southern Europe
	B. duttoni	O. moubata	Sub-Saharan Africa
	B. persica	O. tholozani	Middle East, Greece, Central Asia
	B. uzbekistan	O. pappilipes	Tajikistan, Uzbekistan
Epidemic	B. recurrentis	Pediculus humanus	Worldwide (recently only in East Africa including immigrants to Europe)

The mean latency between exposure to ticks in the endemic form or to lice in the epidemic form and onset of symptoms is 6 days (range, 3 to 18 days). Because *Ornithodoros* ticks feed briefly and painlessly at night, patients with TBRF may not be able to recall having been bitten by a tick. The clinical manifestations of TBRF and LBRF are similar, although some differences do exist. Table 2 lists the frequency of the most common manifestations of TBRF. The usual initial presentation is sudden onset of chills followed by high fever, tachycardia, severe headache, vomiting, myalgia and arthralgia, and often delirium. In the early stages, a reddish rash may be seen over the trunk, arms, or legs. The fever remains high for 3 to 5 days, and then it clears abruptly. After an asymptomatic period of 7 to 10 days, the fever and other constitutional symptoms can reappear suddenly. The febrile episodes gradually become less severe, and the person eventually recovers completely. As the disease progresses, fever, jaundice, hepatosplenomegaly, cardiac arrhythmias, and cardiac failure may occur, especially with LBRF. Jaundice is more common at times of relapses. Patients with LBRF are more likely to develop petechiae on the trunk, extremities, and mucous membranes; epistaxis; and blood-tinged sputum. Rupture of the spleen may rarely occur. Multiple neurologic complications can occur as a result of disseminated intravascular coagulation in LBRF and as a result of infection of the meninges and cranial and spinal nerve roots by spirochetes in TBRF. The most common neurologic complications of TBRF are aseptic meningitis and facial palsy. Relapsing fever in pregnant women can cause abortion, premature birth, and neonatal death. Sometimes patients can have nonfebrile relapses, consisting of periods of severe headache, backache, weakness, and other constitutional symptoms without fever that occur at the time of expected relapses. Delirium may persist for weeks after the fever resolves, and rarely symptoms may be protracted.

Relapsing fever may be confused with many diseases that are relapsing or cause high fevers. These include typhoid fever, yellow fever, dengue, African hemorrhagic fevers, African trypanosomiasis, brucellosis, malaria, leptospirosis, rat-bite fever, intermittent cholangitis, cat-scratch disease, echovirus 9 infection, among others. Relapsing fever *Borrelias* have antigens that are cross reactive with Lyme disease *Borrelias* and inasmuch as the endemic areas of relapsing fever and Lyme disease overlap to some extent, confusion between the two infections can be expected.

Laboratory Diagnosis

Although the pattern of recurring fever is the clue to diagnosing relapsing fever, confirmation of the diagnosis requires demonstration of spirochetes in peripheral blood taken during an episode of fever. The comparatively large number of spirochetes in the blood during relapsing fever provides the opportunity for the simplest method for laboratory diagnosis of the infection, light microscopy of Wright or Giemsa stained thin blood smears or darkfield or phase-contrast microscopy of a wet mount of plasma. The blood should be obtained during or just before peaks of body temperature. Between fever peaks, spirochetes often can be demonstrated by inoculation of blood or cerebrospinal fluid (CSF) into special culture medium (BSK-H with 6% rabbit serum available from Sigma) or experimental animals. Enrichment for spirochetes is achieved by using the platelet-rich fraction of plasma or the buffy coat of sedimented blood. In the United States the most common causes of relapsing fever are *Borrelia hermsii* and *Borrelia turicatae*; both grow in BSK-H medium and in young mice or rats. Whereas direct visual detection of organisms in the blood is the most common method for laboratory confirmation of relapsing fever, immunoassays for antibodies are the most common means of laboratory confirmation for Lyme disease. Although serologic assays have been developed for the agents of relapsing fever, these are not widely available and of dubious utility. The antigenic variation displayed by the relapsing fever species means there are hundreds of different "serotypes." If a different serotype or species is used for preparing the antigen, only antibodies to conserved antigens may be detected. For this reason, a standardized enzyme-linked immunosorbent assay (ELISA) with Lyme disease *Borrelia* as antigen may be the best available serologic assay for relapsing fever. ELISA for *Borrelia burgdorferi* antibodies is routinely done across the United States and Europe. If a positive result for IgM or IgG antibodies is obtained, the Western blot for antibodies to *B. burgdorferi* antigens would be expected to discriminate current or past Lyme disease from relapsing fever, as well as from syphilis, another cause of false-positive Lyme disease ELISA results. Other frequent laboratory abnormalities can occur in relapsing fever but are not diagnostic. These include elevated white blood cell count with increased neutrophils, thrombocytopenia, increased serum bilirubin, proteinuria, microhematuria, prolongation of the prothrombin time (PT) and partial thromboplastin time (PTT), and elevation of fibrin degradation products.

TABLE 2 Frequent Clinical Manifestations of Tick-Borne Relapsing Fever

Sign or Symptom	Frequency (%)
Headache	94
Myalgia	92
Chills	88
Nausea	76
Arthralgia	73
Vomiting	71
Abdominal pain	44
Confusion	38
Dry cough	27
Ocular pain	26
Diarrhea	25
Dizziness	25
Photophobia	25
Neck pain	24
Rash	18
Dysuria	13
Jaundice	10
Hepatomegaly	10
Splenomegaly	6

Treatment

Relapsing fever *Borrelias* are very sensitive to several antibiotics, and antimicrobial resistance is rare. Table 3 summarizes the treatment options for adults and children younger than 8 years. Children older than 8 years can be treated with the same antibiotics as adults, but the doses should be adjusted by weight. Before antibiotics are given, the possibility of causing the Jarisch-Herxheimer reaction should be considered (see later). The tetracycline antibiotics are most commonly used for treatment of LBRF and TBRF. The first antibiotic of choice in adults and children older than 8 years is doxycycline (Doryx). In general, shorter treatments are needed for LBRF than for TBRF. Single-dose therapy is usually recommended for LBRF. In contrast, in TBRF even multiple doses of tetracyclines for up to 10 days may fail to prevent relapses, and retreatment can be required.

Alternative oral antibiotics to the tetracyclines are erythromycin (E-Mycin),[1] azithromycin (Zithromax),[1] amoxicillin (Amoxil),[1] penicillin,[1] and chloramphenicol (Chloromycetin).[1] However, oral chloramphenicol is no longer available in the United States. Erythromycin, azithromycin, and penicillin do not appear as effective as the tetracyclines; however, they are recommended for children younger than 8 years and for pregnant women. Amoxicillin is another alternative for young children with early Lyme disease; however, it is ineffective for human granulocytic ehrlichiosis, which sometimes occurs as a co-infection with Lyme disease.

Although treatment with antibiotics is usually given orally, they may need to be given intravenously if severe vomiting makes swallowing impractical. If there are symptoms and signs of meningitis or encephalitis without clinical and/or radiologic signs of increased intracranial pressure, the CSF should be examined to rule out central nervous system (CNS) infection. The finding of elevation of CSF cells and protein demands the use of parenteral antibiotics, such as penicillin G or ceftriaxone (Rocephin). Optimally, antibiotic treatment

[1]Not FDA approved for this indication.

TABLE 3 Treatment Options for Tick-Borne Relapsing Fever*

Adults
Nonsevere forms

1. Doxycycline (Doryx oral), 100 mg PO bid for 1–2 wk[†]
2. Tetracycline (Sumycin), 500 mg PO qid for 1–2 wk
3. Erythromycin (Erythrocin),[1] 500 mg PO tid for 1–2 wk

Severe forms

1. Ceftriaxone (Rocephin),[1] 2 g IV qd for 1–2 wk
2. Penicillin G parenteral aqueous (Pfizerpen),[1] 4 million U IV q4h for 1–2 wk

Children (≤8 y)
Nonsevere forms

1. Erythromycin suspension oral (EryPed),[1] 30–50 mg/kg/d divided tid for 1–2 wk
2. Azithromycin oral suspension (Zithromax),[1] 20 mg/kg on the first day followed by 10 mg/kg/d for 4 more days
3. Penicillin V (Pen-Vee K),[1] 25–50 mg/kg/d divided qid for 1–2 wk
4. Amoxicillin (Amoxil),[1] 50 mg/kg/d divided tid for 1–2 wk

Severe forms

1. Ceftriaxone (Rocephin),[1] 75–100 mg/kg/d IV for 1–2 wk
2. Penicillin G parenteral aqueous (Pfizerpen),[1] 300,000 U/kg/d given IV in divided doses q4h for 1–2 wk

[1]Not FDA approved for this indication.
*The same oral agents are used for treatment of louse-borne (epidemic) relapsing fever but given as a single dose.
[†]In general, treatment for 1 wk is recommended in early/milder cases and for up to 2 wk for more severe cases.
Abbreviations: IV = intravenous; PO = orally.

CURRENT THERAPY

- The antibiotic of choice for treatment of relapsing fever is doxycycline (Doryx) except in children or pregnant women. In children < 8 y, erythromycin (E-Mycin)[1] or oral penicillin[1] is used instead of tetracycline (Table 3).
- Relapsing fever if severe or complicated with neuroborreliosis requires treatment with the intravenous antibiotics ceftriaxone (Rocephin) or penicillin G (Table 3).
- The louse-borne epidemic form is treated with a single dose, whereas the endemic tick-borne form is treated with multiple doses for at least 1 week (Table 3).
- Antibiotic treatment of relapsing fever results in the Jarisch-Herxheimer reaction in as many as 60% of cases, more often in the epidemic than in the endemic form. It is characterized by the sudden onset of tachycardia, hypotension, chills, rigors, diaphoresis, and high fever. To reduce the risk of the JHR, antibiotics should be started between but not at times of febrile peaks.

[1]Not FDA approved for this indication.

should be started during afebrile periods when the spirochetemia is low. Starting therapy near the peak of a febrile period may induce the Jarisch-Herxheimer reaction, in which high fever and a rise and subsequent fall in blood pressure, sometimes to dangerously low levels, may occur. Dehydration should be treated with fluids given intravenously. Severe headache can be treated with pain relievers such as codeine, and nausea or vomiting can be treated with prochlorperazine.

Jarisch-Herxheimer Reaction

Antibiotic treatment of relapsing fever causes the Jarisch-Herxheimer reaction (JHR) in as many as 60% of cases. The JHR is more common in LBRF than in TBRF. It is characterized by the sudden onset of tachycardia, hypotension, chills, rigors, diaphoresis, and high fever. Patients with the JHR have said that they felt as if they were going to die. The JHR is caused by the rapid killing of circulating spirochetes 1 to 4 hours after the first dose of antibiotic, which results in the release of large amounts of *Borrelia* lipoproteins in the circulation followed by massive release of tumor necrosis factor and other cytokines. If possible, patients with the JHR should be transferred to an intensive care unit for close monitoring and treatment. During several hours, the temperature declines and the patient feels better. Large amounts of intravenous fluids (0.9% sodium chloride solution) may be required to treat hypotension. Steroids and nonsteroidal antiinflammatory agents have no effect on the frequency or severity of the JHR. One study found that pretreatment with anti-TNF-alpha monoclonal antibody (Humira)[1] suppressed the JHR after penicillin treatment for LBRF and reduced the associated increases in plasma cytokines. Death can occur as a result of the JHR secondary to cardiovascular collapse in up to 5% of patients with treated LBRF and much less frequently in TBRF.

Outcome

Complete recovery occurs in 95% or more of adequately treated patients. The prognosis for untreated cases or if treatment is delayed varies. Mortality as high as 40% is reported in untreated epidemics of LBRF. Relapsing fever also has a high mortality in neonates. Some neurologic sequelae can occur in patients with TBRF complicated with neuroborreliosis.

[1]Not FDA approved for this indication.

Prevention

Prevention of TBRF involves avoidance of rodent- and tick-infested dwellings such as animal burrows, caves, and abandoned cabins. Wearing clothing that protects skin from tick access (e.g., long pants and long-sleeved shirts) is also helpful. Repellents and acaricides provide additional protection. Diethyltoluamide (DEET) repels ticks when applied to clothing or skin, but it must be used with caution. It loses its effectiveness within 1 to several hours when applied to skin and must be reapplied; it is absorbed through the skin and may cause CNS toxicity if used excessively. Picaridin (KBR 3023), which has been used as an insect repellent for years in Europe and Australia, is now available in the United States in 7% solution as Cutter Advanced Repellent (Spectrum Brands). The U.S. Centers for Disease Control and Prevention (CDC) is recommending it as an alternative to DEET. Permethrin Insect Repellent, an acaricide, is more effective than DEET but should not be applied directly to skin. When applied to clothing, it provides good protection for 1 day or more. In LBRF, prevention can be achieved by promoting personal hygiene and by dusting undergarments and the inside of clothing with malathion[1,2] or lindane powder[2] when available. Widespread antibiotic use may be necessary to control epidemics of LBRF, using one or two doses of 100 mg doxycycline given within 1 week of exposure.

REFERENCES

Barbour AG, Hayes SF. Biology of *Borrelia* species. Microbiol Rev 1986;50:381–400.

Bryceson AD, Parry EH, Perine PL, et al. Louse-borne relapsing fever. Q J Med 1970;39:129–70.

Cadavid D, Barbour AG. Neuroborreliosis during relapsing fever: Review of the clinical manifestations, pathology, and treatment of infections in humans and experimental animals. Clin Infect Dis 1998;26:151–64.

Fekade D, Knox K, Hussein K, et al. Prevention of Jarisch-Herxheimer reactions by treatment with antibodies against tumor necrosis factor alpha. N Engl J Med 1996;335:311–5.

Kazragis RJ, Dever LL, Jorgensen JH, Barbour AG. In vivo activities of ceftriaxone and vancomycin against *Borrelia* spp. in the mouse brain and other sites. Antimicrob Agents Chemother 1996;40:2632–6.

Melkert PW. Fatal Jarisch-Herxheimer reaction in a case of relapsing fever misdiagnosed as lobar pneumonia. Trop Geogr Med 1987;39:92–3.

Southern P, Sanford J. Relapsing fever. Medicine 1969;48:129–49.

Taft W, Pike J. Relapsing fever. Report of a sporadic outbreak including treatment with penicillin. JAMA 1945;129:1002–5.

---

[1]Not FDA approved for this indication.
[2]Not available in the United States.

Lyme Disease

Method of
*Arthur Weinstein, MD, FACP, FACR, and
Shobha Wani, MD*

Epidemiology

Lyme disease, or borreliosis, is a tick-transmitted infection caused by *Borrelia burgdorferi*. It is the most common insect-borne illness in the United States with more than 20,000 new cases reported annually. It occurs worldwide with hyperendemicity in temperate regions. In the United States, most cases originate from states in the Northeast, mid-Atlantic, upper Midwest, and Pacific coast regions. The life cycle of the Ixodes tick ensures that most cases of human borrelial infection occur from spring to fall. Three genospecies of *B. burgdorferi* account

for human disease: *B. burgdorferi sensu stricto*, *B. garinii*, and *B. afzelii*. Although all three are found in Europe and the latter two in Asia, *B. burgdorferi sensu stricto* is the only cause of Lyme disease in the United States. Lyme disease occurs in all age groups with highest frequencies in young children and adults older than 30 years and is equally common in men and women. It often manifests clinically in stages, with exacerbations and remissions in each stage.

Clinical Features

EARLY LYME DISEASE

Localized skin infection and early disseminated infection occur within days to weeks after the bite of an infected tick. Erythema migrans (EM) rash, the hallmark of early Lyme disease, occurs in up to 70% to 80% of patients at the site of the tick bite. It usually is macular and asymptomatic but may burn or itch, and it is commonly found at the belt line, inguinal area, or in and around the axilla. It expands over days, often to a very large circumference and with central clearing, giving a bull's-eye appearance. Approximately 10% of patients have multiple skin lesions (disseminated EM), a sign of hematogenous spread of the borrelia. At this early stage, patients may have nonspecific flulike complaints, namely fever, fatigue, myalgia, arthralgia, and headache, resembling a viral syndrome. These symptoms occasionally occur without the rash. In untreated patients, EM resolves spontaneously within days to several weeks after onset, but treatment often accelerates its resolution.

Early disseminated disease occurs days to weeks after the tick bite and may occur without preceding localized EM. Certain subtypes of *B. burgdorferi* are associated with higher frequency of spirochetemia and dissemination to other organs. For instance, in Europe, EM is often an indolent, localized infection, whereas in the United States, it is associated with more intense inflammation and signs that suggest dissemination of the spirochete. The clinical manifestations of dissemination can be highly variable and may include disseminated EM rash and neurologic, cardiac, and musculoskeletal features either alone or in combination. Neurologic features (neuroborreliosis) are seen in approximately 10% of patients and include acute lymphocytic meningitis, cranial neuropathy, especially facial paresis, which may be bilateral, and radiculoneuritis. Neuroborreliosis is more common in Europe where neurotropic subspecies of borrelia (*B. garinii, B. afzelii*) are found. Meningitis usually resolves spontaneously, whereas treatment of other neurologic features can hasten recovery and prevent progression to the later stages of Lyme disease. Carditis, which includes varying degrees of atrioventricular block or mild myopericarditis, may develop in approximately 8% of untreated patients, but early treatment can prevent its occurrence. In more recent series, the incidence of Lyme carditis was reported as less than 1% in the United States. Rheumatic features at this stage consist of migratory, episodic joint, tendon, or bursal pains with or without objective signs of inflammation. Typically there is acute localized pain that lasts days to weeks, remits spontaneously, and then recurs in another region. Inflammatory polyarthritis is not a feature of early or late Lyme disease.

The diagnosis of early Lyme disease relies to a great degree on the clinical presentation. In an endemic area, with a history of possible tick exposure, the presence of a classical EM lesion is sufficient for the diagnosis. With very early infection and isolated EM, laboratory tests for antibodies to *B. burgdorferi* may be negative. Conversely, with disseminated early Lyme disease, antibody testing is frequently positive.

LATE LYME DISEASE

Late Lyme disease occurs months to years after initial infection (mean, 6 months) and may present de novo without prior features of early Lyme disease. Systemic symptoms are generally minimal or absent. Musculoskeletal complaints, the most common manifestation, are seen in 80% of untreated patients and include intermittent oligoarthritis (50%) and acute or subacute inflammatory arthritis that most often affects one or both knees. This arthritis may begin abruptly with knee pain and a large joint effusion. Synovial fluid is inflammatory with white counts ranging in the thousands or tens of thousands. Radiographs may be normal except for soft-tissue swelling and joint effusion but may also demonstrate osteopenia, bone cysts, and even mild cartilage loss with small erosions. Untreated, these attacks of arthritis generally last many months, recur for several years but eventually may remit. *B. burgdorferi* is not culturable from the synovial fluid of patients with Lyme arthritis, but borrelial DNA can be detected by polymerase chain reaction (PCR) in over 80% of untreated patients. The PCR test is generally negative after appropriate antibiotic therapy.

Neurologic features of late Lyme disease are seen more frequently in Europe because *B. garinii* is the most neurotropic subspecies. There are a wide range of neurologic abnormalities, especially encephalomyelitis and peripheral neuropathy. In the United States, Lyme encephalopathy or polyneuropathy is described with subtle disturbances of memory and concentration, spinal radicular pain, or distal paresthesias. Nerve conduction studies reveal axonal polyneuropathy. Pleocytosis of the cerebrospinal fluid (CSF) is unusual in late neurologic Lyme disease. High CSF protein may be seen, but borrelial organisms by culture or PCR are not commonly found. Important to the diagnosis of neuroborreliosis is the demonstration of increased intrathecal synthesis of borrelia-specific antibodies.

A chronic skin lesion, acrodermatitis chronica atrophicans, caused by *B. afzelii*, is seen most commonly in Europe.

Laboratory Testing in Lyme Disease

Lyme disease should not be diagnosed purely on serologic tests because false-positive tests are common. Instead, serologic tests should be used to confirm the diagnosis in the appropriate clinical setting. Even a true positive test only confirms recent or past exposure to *B. burgdorferi*, but this must be evaluated in the context of the patient's past and current symptoms.

Despite these methodologic and diagnostic issues, measurement of antibodies to *B. burgdorferi* by enzyme-linked immunoassay (ELISA) is a useful screening test for early and late Lyme disease. This so-called Lyme test is positive in most cases of late Lyme disease and virtually always positive in late Lyme arthritis. It may be negative very early after infection or in those individuals who receive early antibiotic therapy. However, the high rate of false positivity has led to a two-test strategy whereby all sera that show positive or equivocal ELISA tests for borrelial antibodies are tested again by more specific Western (immuno) blotting. In patients with CNS disease, demonstration of intrathecal antibodies by ELISA in relatively higher concentration than serum antibodies is suggestive of neuroborreliosis.

CURRENT DIAGNOSIS

- Erythema migrans is usually asymptomatic and expansile.
- Lyme disease can present with only flulike symptoms: fever, arthralgia, myalgia.
- Antibody testing for borrelial infection is often negative during early infection.
- A two-test strategy (serum ELISA, immunoblot) is recommended for diagnosis.
- IgM antibodies are commonly seen in early infection (4–8 wk) but may persist for many months.
- IgG antibodies are characteristic of late Lyme disease, especially Lyme arthritis.
- Intrathecal antibody synthesis is an important diagnostic marker for neuroborreliosis.
- Clinical symptoms combined with antibody status are of diagnostic importance.

Abbreviation: ELISA = enzyme-linked immunosorbent assay.

Immunoblotting is usually performed for both IgM and IgG antibodies to borrelial proteins. Although this technique is not as automated or quantitative as ELISA, it is more specific because it identifies the borrelial antigens to which the antibodies are directed. There are recommendations for standardized testing and interpretation of Western blot results. IgM antibodies usually appear 2 to 4 weeks after EM, peak at 6 to 8 weeks, and decline thereafter, although IgM reactivity may occasionally persist for many years. An IgM blot is considered to be positive if two of three specified bands (23, 39, 41 kd) are present. The results of an IgM blot are best interpreted in the first weeks after symptom onset when the true positive rate exceeds the false-positive rate. A positive IgM blot found in a patient with long-standing symptoms should be interpreted with caution because it likely represents a false-positive result. IgG antibodies appear after 4 to 6 weeks, peak at 4 to 6 months, and then remain positive for many years, even decades. An IgG immunoblot is considered to be positive if 5 of 10 specified bands (18, 23, 28, 30, 39, 41, 45, 58, 66, 93 kd) are present. IgG seroconversion, with or without IgM seroconversion, can be taken as presumptive evidence of exposure to *B. burgdorferi* and in the proper clinical context supports the diagnosis of Lyme disease. However, a positive IgG immunoblot does not necessarily mean current or ongoing borreliosis. Conversely, a negative IgG immunoblot is presumptive evidence against the diagnosis of late Lyme disease. An ELISA assay for antibodies to a borrelial-specific surface protein (C6 peptide of VlsE) was demonstrated to be a sensitive and specific single test for the diagnosis of Lyme disease and is commercially available.

Culture of *B. burgdorferi* requires special medium and conditions and takes many weeks. Even so, in expert laboratories the organism can be recovered from the EM lesion in a high percentage of patients and from the blood in patients with disseminated early Lyme disease. Risk for spirochetemia starts the day the patient notices the rash and continues for 2 weeks.

B. burgdorferi is cultured only rarely from the CSF of patients with neuroborreliosis.

PCR to detect borrelial DNA is also positive with the same or higher frequency as culture from the skin, blood, and CSF. However, it is most useful in the synovial fluid of patients with suspected and untreated Lyme arthritis where it can be positive in more than 80% of patients despite universally negative cultures. PCR analysis of synovial tissue may be more likely to yield positive results than synovial fluid because *B. burgdorferi* associates with connective tissue. However, because virtually all cases of Lyme arthritis are strongly positive by ELISA and immunoblotting for IgG antibodies to *B. burgdorferi*, the diagnosis can usually be made with reasonable certainty using these tests alone.

Treatment

The goals of treatment of Lyme disease are to resolve the clinical symptoms by eradication of the organism and to prevent late stage disease with early therapy. Although most manifestations resolve spontaneously without treatment, clinical trials demonstrated that treatment with antibiotics hastens resolution and prevents late manifestations of Lyme borreliosis. In most of the trials, treatment of 3 weeks' duration was effective. Revised evidence-based guidelines for treatment have recently been published by the Infectious Diseases Society of America. Generally, early Lyme disease is treated with antimicrobials for 2 to 3 weeks, although studies showed that EM treatment with oral doxycycline for 10 days is as effective as treatment for 20 days. Effective oral medications include doxycycline (Vibramycin),[1] tetracycline, second-generation cephalosporins such as cefuroxime axetil (Ceftin), and amoxicillin (Amoxil).[1] Erythromycin (E-Mycin)[1] and azithromycin (Zithromax)[1] are somewhat less effective. Doxycycline and tetracycline should not be used in children younger than 8 years or in pregnant women. Oral therapy is sufficient for certain clinical features: EM, facial palsy without signs of meningitis, and first-degree heart block. Oral therapy with doxycycline (Vibramycin) is associated with

[1]Not FDA approved for this indication.

CURRENT THERAPY

- Early antibiotic therapy hastens resolution of symptoms and prevents late complications.
- In adults, oral therapy with doxycycline (Vibramycin)[1] is preferred for most features of Lyme disease.
- Neuroborreliosis is usually treated with IV ceftriaxone.
- Duration of therapy is generally 2–4 wk.
- Lyme disease is cured after antibiotic treatment (one or two courses) in most patients.
- Some patients with Lyme arthritis develop persistent antibiotic-resistant synovitis, which may be autoimmune and is treated with antirheumatic drugs.
- Patients with chronic fatigue, arthralgia, and myalgia that begins, persists, or recurs after antibiotic treatment for Lyme disease generally have a post–Lyme disease syndrome and not ongoing infection.
- There is no scientific support for prolonged courses of oral or IV antibiotics for Lyme disease.

---

[1]Not FDA approved for this indication.
Abbreviation: IV = intravenous.

---

fewer side effects and is much less expensive than the also employed intravenous (IV) therapy with ceftriaxone (Rocephin).[1] Although amoxicillin and doxycycline appear to be equally efficacious, doxycycline has the distinct advantage of also being effective in treating *Anaplasma phagocytophila* infection, which causes human granulocytic ehrlichiosis (HGE) and is also transmitted by the Ixodes tick. In general, patients with neurologic manifestations, either early or late, other than

isolated facial palsy, are treated de novo with IV ceftriaxone (Rocephin)[1] for 3 to 4 weeks, although aqueous penicillin (Penicillin G)[1] is also effective. Carditis with heart block may resolve spontaneously, but patients with higher grades of heart block and with cardiomyopathy are generally treated with IV antibiotics. If the oral regimen fails, as may occur with 20% of patients, parenteral therapy with ceftriaxone or cefotaxime (Claforan)[1] is warranted. In patients with persistent symptoms, a second parenteral regimen is usually administered. There is no need to change the medication because *B. burgdorferi* does not show resistance to any of the antimicrobials recommended.

Oral and parenteral therapies are both used with success in treating Lyme arthritis with treatment duration of 3 to 4 weeks. Occasionally a second month of treatment is needed to eradicate the organism from the joint. Even with successful treatment, the arthritis may resolve quite slowly with synovitis persisting over several months (Table 1).

PERSISTENT (TREATMENT-RESISTANT) LYME ARTHRITIS

Approximately 10% of patients with Lyme arthritis in the United States are treatment resistant, with recurrent inflammatory effusions, usually in one knee, for months to several years despite appropriate antibiotic therapy. This antibiotic-resistant Lyme arthritis is thought to be related to an intra-articular autoimmune response in predisposed individuals. There is no evidence for persistent infection because borrelial DNA by PCR in synovial fluid or synovial tissue is not found in these individuals. A genetic predisposition is suggested by the increased frequency of HLA-DR4 and HLA-DRB1*0401, 0101, and related alleles, similar to that seen in rheumatoid arthritis. In this situation, treatment consists of nonsteroidal anti-inflammatory drugs, intraarticular steroid injections, and antirheumatic agents such as hydroxychloroquine (Plaquenil),[1] sulfasalazine (Azulfidine),[1] and even methotrexate (Rheumatrex).[1] In some cases, arthroscopic synovectomy proves effective. This arthritis usually remits after several years.

---

[1]Not FDA approved for this indication.

TABLE 1 Suggested Treatment of Lyme Disease

Clinical Features/Indication	Antibiotic regimen	Regimen		Duration of Therapy
		Adults	**Children**	
Early Infection (Local and Disseminated Disease)	Doxycycline (Vibramycin)[1]	100 mg bid	<8 y: not recommended >8 y: 1–2 mg/kg bid; maximum 100 mg	2–3 wk
	Tetracycline[1]	500 mg qid	Not for pregnant women	2–3 wk
	Amoxicillin[1]	500 mg tid	As above	2–3 wk
	Cefuroxime axetil (Ceftin)	500 mg bid	50 mg/kg/d in 3 divided doses	2–3 wk
	Azithromycin (Zithromax)[1]	500 mg daily	30 mg/kg/d in 2 divided doses	7–10 d
	Erythromycin[1]	500 mg qid	50 mg/kg/d	2–3 wk
Neuroborreliosis Failure to Respond to Oral Therapy	Ceftriaxone (Rocephin)[1]	2 g IV daily	75–100 mg/kg/d	2–4 wk
	Cefotaxime (Claforan)[1]			
	Penicillin G[1]	2 g IV tid	90–180 mg/kg/d in 3–4 divided doses	2–4 wk
		4–5 million U IV q4h	2–4 million U IV q4 h	2–4 wk
Carditis	Oral or IV regimen			2–3 wk
Late Lyme Arthritis	Oral or IV regimen			4 wk*
Pregnancy	Amoxicillin Penicillin G Ceftriaxone Cefotaxime			2–4 wk

*May give another course if poor response.
[1]Not FDA approved for this indication.
Abbreviation: IV = intravenous.

POST–LYME DISEASE SYNDROME

Although the long-term prognosis of treated Lyme disease is excellent, some patients develop arthralgia, myalgia, and fatigue, during or soon after infection, which persists despite adequate courses of antibiotics. Other features of this symptom complex include memory and concentration difficulties, neuropathic pains, headache, and unrefreshed sleep. This condition is often called post–Lyme disease syndrome, post-treatment chronic Lyme disease, or chronic Lyme disease. The actual frequency of this condition after Lyme disease is unclear but is likely no more than 5%. Some studies suggested that delay in initiating antibiotic treatment for borrelial infection is more likely to result in post–Lyme disease syndrome. In none of these studies did current serologic status correlate with persistent symptoms. Although these patients have significant somatic complaints and functional disability, they lack objective findings of an inflammatory condition. Although virtually all patients with this syndrome complain of problems with memory and concentration, demonstrable abnormalities on neurocognitive testing are not universally present. The pathogenesis of this chronic post-treatment symptomatic state and its relationship to Lyme disease are unclear. Patients may feel better during antibiotic therapy, but the effect is not durable and relapse is common when antibiotics are discontinued. The symptoms wax and wane, but the overall course is chronic. Controversy has raged as to whether chronic, relatively resistant borrelial infection plays a role and hence whether chronic antibiotic therapy is warranted. However, an important study on post–Lyme syndrome patients failed to document the presence of *b. burgdorferi* in the plasma or spinal fluid of these patients by culture or PCR. In addition, a controlled trial failed to show a response to a 3-month course of antibiotics (1 month of IV ceftriaxone [Rocephin][1] followed by 2 months of oral doxycycline[1]). This suggests that chronic infection is not the cause of post–Lyme disease syndrome, that the condition spontaneously waxes and wanes, and that prolonged antibiotic treatment does not result in long-term symptom remission.

Prevention

The best currently available method for preventing infection with *B. burgdorferi* and other tick-transmitted infections is to avoid tick infested areas through the summer. If exposure is unavoidable, use of protective clothing (shirt tucked into pants and pants tucked under socks) may interfere with attachment by ticks. Wearing light-colored clothing makes it easier to identify ticks. Daily inspection of the entire body to locate and remove ticks also decreases the transmission of infection. Attached ticks should promptly be removed with fine-toothed forceps, if possible. Tick and insect repellent applied to the skin and clothing provides additional protection. The most effective repellent is DEET (diethyltoluamide). Permethrin, a pesticide that kills ticks and mites when applied to clothing, decreases the risk of tick bite. Strategies to reduce the number of ticks may be somewhat effective in decreasing tick-borne illnesses, including the application of acaricides and landscaping to provide desiccating barriers. Although vaccination is available for dogs and a recombinant outer surface protein A (OspA)-based vaccine (LYMErix) is effective and relatively safe in humans, currently no marketed vaccine is available to prevent Lyme disease in humans.

AFTER TICK BITE

It is not recommended to treat all patients after a tick bite because several prospective studies demonstrated that the risk of drug-associated rash is as great as the risk of developing Lyme disease. Conversely, it may be reasonable to treat persons believed to be at higher risk for the development of borrelial infection prophylactically. Studies showed that transmission of *B. burgdorferi* from tick to host occurs with greater frequency when there has been tick attachment for more than 48 hours resulting in a blood-engorged tick. Because a controlled study demonstrated that a single 200-mg dose of doxycycline[1] effectively prevents

Lyme disease when given within 72 hours of a tick bite, the threshold for treating patients after tick bites with this benign regimen is lower than in the past.

REFERENCES

Klempner MS, Hu LT, Evans J, et al. Two controlled trials of antibiotic treatment in patients with persistent symptoms and a history of Lyme disease. N Engl J Med 2001;345:85–92.

Nadelman RB, Nowakowski J, Fish D, et al. Prophylaxis with single dose doxycycline for the prevention of Lyme disease after an Ixodes scapularis tick bite. N Engl J Med 2001;345:79–84.

Recommendations for test performance and interpretation from the Second National Conference on Serologic Diagnosis of Lyme Disease. MMWR 1995;44:590–1.

Steere AC. Lyme disease. N Engl J Med 2001;345:115–25.

Steere AC, Dhar A, Hernandez J, et al. Systemic symptoms without erythema migrans as the presenting picture of early Lyme disease. Am J Med 2003;114:58–62.

Steere AC, Sikand VK, et al. The presenting manifestations of Lyme disease and the outcomes of treatment. N Engl J Med 2003;348:2472–4.

Treatment of Lyme disease. The Medical Letter 2005;47:41–3.

Tugwell P, Dennis DT, Weinstein A, et al. Clinical guideline 2: Laboratory evaluation in the diagnosis of Lyme disease. Ann Intern Med 1997;127:1109–23.

Weinstein A, Britchkov M. Lyme arthritis and post-Lyme disease syndrome. Curr Opin Rheum 2002;14:383–7.

Wormser GP, Dattwyler RJ, Shapiro ED, et al. The clinical assessment, treatment, and prevention of Lyme disease, human granulocytic anaplasmosis, and babesiosis: Clinical practice guidelines by the Infectious Diseases Society of America. Clin Infect Dis 2006;43:1089–134.

Wormser GP, Ramanathan R, Nowakowski J, et al. Duration of antibiotic therapy for early Lyme disease. A randomized, double-blind, placebo-controlled trial. Ann Intern Med 2003;138:697–704.

Rubella and Congenital Rubella Syndrome

Method of
Annette Mankertz, PhD

Postnatal rubella is a benign illness associated with rash and fever. Rubella virus (RUBV) is a teratogenic agent, and infection in early pregnancy may result in spontaneous abortion, stillbirth, or congenital defects known as congenital rubella syndrome (CRS). Because RUBV is limited to humans, CRS can be eliminated by vaccination. Accordingly, the World Health Organization has proclaimed an elimination goal, which has been achieved in the Americas but not yet worldwide.

CURRENT DIAGNOSIS

- Although rubella virus (RUBV) no longer circulates endemically in the Americas, rubella and congenital rubella syndrome cases continue to occur due to importations.
- Because of the nonspecific symptoms of rash and fever, rubella is easily misdiagnosed. Therefore, clinical diagnosis should be confirmed by laboratory testing.
- Serologic testing for immunoglobulin M is the most common method for diagnosis; virus isolation and reverse transcriptase polymerase chain reaction are also available.

---

[1]Not FDA approved for this indication.

CURRENT THERAPY

- Postnatal rubella infections are normally mild and self-limited, and there is no specific therapy.
- Two doses of measles, mumps, rubella vaccine (MMR) are recommended by the World Health Organization and the Centers for Disease Control and Prevention and induce effective protection against rubella.
- Pregnant women with a laboratory-confirmed acute RUBV infection up to gestational week 20 should be counseled about the risk of congenital defects.
- Infants with congenital rubella syndrome should be evaluated and treated under the care of appropriate specialists.

Background and Epidemiology

RUBV (family Togaviridae, genus *Rubivirus*) particles have a diameter of 60 to 70 nm and consist of a nucleocapsid wrapped in a lipid envelope. The genome is a linear, single-stranded RNA of 9757 nucleotides. There is no animal reservoir for RUBV. RUBV is moderately contagious and is transmitted through aerosol inhalation, person-to-person contact, and contact with freshly infected articles. The average incubation period is 14 days, with a range of 12 to 23 days. Persons with RUBV infection shed virus from 7 days before rash onset to 5 to 7 days afterward.

Before the implementation of the rubella vaccination program, rubella epidemics occurred worldwide every 4 to 9 years. The World Health Organization proclaimed a goal of eliminating rubella and CRS in the Americas and Europe by the year 2010. By the end of 2008, all countries and territories of the Americas had implemented the recommended vaccination strategies, but the risk for rubella importations from other continents is still prevailing.

Clinical Features and Diagnosis

A characteristic, nonconfluent, maculopapular rash usually appears 14 days after infection, starting on the face and neck and progressing downward to the trunk and limbs. It occurs in 50% to 80% of RUBV-infected persons and lasts for up to 3 days. Prepubertal children usually do not develop constitutional features, but adults can experience a 1- to 5-day prodrome with malaise and low-grade fever. Headache, sore throat, mild coryza, cough, and conjunctivitis may also occur. Postauricular, occipital, and posterior cervical lymphadenopathy typically precedes the rash by 5 to 10 days. Moreover, arthralgia and arthritis are seen in up to 70% of adult females with RUBV infection. Between 20% and 50% of RUBV infections occur subclinically and escape the notice of patients and practitioners. Because other illnesses associated with rash and fever may be misdiagnosed as rubella, clinical diagnosis of suspected rubella cases is not reliable, and confirmation by a laboratory test is indispensable.

Acute primary RUBV infection can be confirmed directly through detection of the virus by reverse transcriptase polymerase chain reaction (RT-PCR) or virus isolation from blood or serum, nasal and throat swabs, urine, or cerebrospinal fluid specimens. Detection of RUBV-specific immunoglobulin M (IgM) in serum samples by capture or indirect enzyme-linked immunosorbent assay (ELISA) is the method of choice for diagnosis of postnatally and congenitally acquired infections, but IgM antibodies might not be present before day 5 after rash onset. False-positive serum RUBV IgM tests have occurred in patients with cross-reacting IgM antibodies against measles, parvovirus B19, Epstein-Barr virus, or cytomegalovirus and in those with a positive rheumatoid factor.

Differential diagnosis should cover human herpesviruses 6 and 7 as well as enterovirus and group A streptococcus infections.

Depending on the epidemiologic situation in the respective country, dengue, West Nile fever, chikungunya, Sindbis fever, and Ross River virus infection may also be considered.

In addition to IgM, an increase in RUBV IgG antibody titer in two consecutive samples indicates an infection with RUBV. For this application, two serum samples should be collected, the first (acute) sample during the first 10 days after rash onset and the second 10 to 30 days later during convalescence. If the samples are tested in parallel, a fourfold increase in IgG titer indicates an acute RUBV infection.

Complications

Rubella disease is usually mild and results in very few complications. Transient arthralgia or arthritis occurs in up to 70% of RUBV-infected women. Other complications include thrombocytopenic purpura (1 in 3000 cases) and encephalitis (1 in 6000 cases). The most serious complication is associated with intrauterine RUBV infection acquired during the first trimester of pregnancy. It can result in miscarriage, stillbirth, or the constellation of severe birth defects known as CRS.

CONGENITAL RUBELLA SYNDROME

CRS is the most serious consequence of rubella. The World Health Organization estimates the incidence of CRS as 1 of every 100,000 births. If a pregnant woman develops a primary RUBV infection during the first 12 weeks of gestation, 80% of the infants will be infected, and 85% of those infected infants will develop CRS. Because reinfection has a less pathogenic potential, it is important to differentiate between primary and secondary RUBV infection. After the first trimester of pregnancy, the risk of CRS declines rapidly, and RUBV infection after week 20 is not considered harmful to the child.

The most common congenital defects of CRS are eye defects (e.g., cataracts, microphthalmos), cardiac defects (e.g., patent ductus arteriosus, pulmonary artery stenosis), and deafness or hearing impairment. Other clinical manifestations may include microcephaly, mental and motor retardation, purpura, meningoencephalitis, hepatosplenomegaly, and low birth weight. Prenatal confirmation of CRS can be obtained only by specialized invasive diagnostic testing. Usually, this involves a test for RUBV-specific IgM antibodies in the infant's cord blood and virus detection by RT-PCR using fetal blood or amniotic fluid.

A pregnant patient with clinically confirmed rubella should be counseled about the risk of congenital defects in her child and her options. Newborn babies of mothers who had rubella during pregnancy should be tested for RUBV-specific IgM and persisting IgG. Infants with CRS can shed virus from body secretions for up to 1 year and are considered infectious.

MANAGEMENT OF RUBELLA VIRUS EXPOSURE DURING PREGNANCY

As part of routine prenatal care, all women of child-bearing age should be vaccinated twice with MMR/V prior to pregnancy. Pregnant women without written proof of twofold RUBV vaccination should be tested for rubella immunity. IgG positive women with a titer of more than 10–15 IU/mL and without a recent history of exposure to rubella are considered immune. Seronegative women can be retested for IgM and IgG at week 16 to exclude a fresh RUBV infection. In addition, unprotected family members should be vaccinated.

If a pregnant woman develops a rash or has been exposed to RUBV, a blood specimen should be taken and tested for RUBV IgG and IgM antibody. The sample should be stored for possible retesting. Collection of urine and throat swabs for virus detection is also advisable. RUBV IgM is a marker for an acute RUBV infection and can be detected usually 5 days after rash onset. However, the presence of rheumatoid factor, RUBV-specific IgG, or cross-reacting nonspecific IgM can produce a false-positive result, and RUBV-specific IgM may persist, so a positive IgM test does not suffice to recommend termination of the pregnancy. Moreover, it is highly important to discriminate between a recent and an acute infection.

The latter is highly likely if two distinct IgM tests (indirect and μ-capture) are positive, RUBV-specific IgG of low avidity has been detected, and RUBV late protein E2 IgG is not yet seen in a Western blot reaction.

In addition, a positive result on RT-PCR and virus cultivation indicates an acute RUBV infection or reinfection. Reinfection is more likely in vaccinees and normally does not endanger the unborn child.

Treatment and Vaccination

There is no effective therapy for RUBV infection. RUBV-specific IgG[2] may be administered 3 to 5 days after RUBV exposure in pregnant women. There is no specific therapy for CRS; however, infants should be evaluated and provided early intervention by specialists who treat the identified CRS defects.

Rubella vaccine is available in most countries as a monovalent formulation (Meruvax II); in a combination measles, mumps, and rubella vaccine (MMR), or as a measles, mumps, rubella, and varicella vaccine (MMRV; Proquad). Live attenuated rubella vaccine RA 27/3 (Meruvax II) produces immunity in 95% of vaccinees after one dose and in 97% after a second dose. Immunity is considered to last for a lifetime, but the effect of decreased RUBV circulation on immunity has not been evaluated. In some individuals, seroconversion is not observed despite repeated vaccination. Nevertheless, they are thought to be protected from RUBV infection, because most of them show a secondary immune response after revaccination, indicative of immunity.

A personal history of rubella or clinical diagnosis of rubella is highly unreliable and not acceptable as proof of immunity. Evidence of RUBV immunity includes a positive serologic test for RUBV-specific IgG in absence of IgM, birth before 1957, or written documentation of vaccination with at least one dose of RUBV-containing vaccine shortly before or after the first birthday. Earlier vaccination may interfere with maternally derived immunity and is not recommended.

Vaccination is contraindicated during pregnancy, but inadvertent rubella vaccination is no indication for abortion. Women found to be susceptible during pregnancy should be vaccinated immediately after delivery. In the United States, the period of time after rubella vaccination during which a woman should avoid getting pregnant has been shortened from 3 months to 28 days.

REFERENCES

Centers for Disease Control and Prevention. Revised ACIP recommendation for avoiding pregnancy after receiving a rubella-containing vaccine. MMWR Morb Mortal Wkly Rep 2001;50:1117.

Centers for Disease Control and Prevention. Elimination of rubella and congenital rubella syndrome—United States, 1969–2004. MMWR Morb Mortal Wkly Rep 2005;54:279–82.

Centers for Disease Control and Prevention. Progress toward elimination of measles and prevention of congenital rubella infection—European region, 1990–2004. MMWR Morb Mortal Wkly Rep 2005;54:175–8.

Best JM. Rubella. Semin Fetal Neonatal Med 2007;12:182–92.

Best JM, Enders G. Laboratory diagnosis of rubella and congenital rubella. In: Banatvala C, Peckham C, editors. Rubella Viruses. Philadelphia: Elsevier; 2007. p. 39–77.

Hofmann J, Liebert UG. Significance of avidity and immunoblot analysis for rubella IgM-positive serum samples in pregnant women. J Virol Methods 2005;130:66–71.

Matter L, Kogelschatz K, Germann D. Serum levels of rubella virus antibodies indicating immunity: Response to vaccination of subjects with low or undetectable antibody concentrations. J Infect Dis 1997;175:749–55.

Plotkin SA, Reef S. Rubella vaccine. In: Plotkin SA, Orenstein WA, editors. Vaccines. 4th ed. Philadelphia: WB Saunders; 2004. p. 707–43.

Robinson JL, Lee BE, Preiksaitis JK, et al. Prevention of congenital rubella syndrome: What makes sense in 2006? Epidemiol Rev 2006;28:81–7.

---

[2]Not available in the United States.

Measles (Rubeola)

Method of
Claude P. Muller, MD, and Jacques Kremer, PhD

Measles is an acute systemic disease associated with a maculopapular rash, fever, and respiratory symptoms caused by a single-stranded RNA virus of the family of Paramyxoviridae and the genus *Morbillivirus*.

Epidemiology

With a basic reproduction number of 15, measles virus is the most infectious pathogen. It is transmitted via aerosol to susceptibles (e.g., in kindergarten classes or doctors' offices), and humans are the only natural host. At least 95% of a population must be immune in order to prevent the virus from circulating.

Before the introduction of vaccination, epidemics occurred at regular intervals, and virtually all children had measles during early childhood. Measles induces high levels of antibodies and lifelong protection against the disease. Although vaccine-induced immunity is probably somewhat less robust than immunity after natural infection because of lower and waning antibodies, measles morbidity and mortality have dramatically declined since the introduction of a live-attenuated vaccine in 1963.

As of 2004, endemic circulation of the virus had been interrupted in the Western Hemisphere, as well as in several countries in Europe and the Western Pacific. The success in measles control has encouraged the World Health Organization (WHO) to introduce a timetable for measles elimination in most regions of the world.

In many developing countries, where 98% of global measles deaths occur, measles continues to be a serious condition. Although the 197,000 deaths estimated in 2007 represent a 74% reduction in global measles mortality compared with 1999, measles vaccines are still underused in many developing countries.

Clinical Features

Eight to 14 days after infection, the patient develops characteristic prodromal symptoms including fever and cough, coryza, or conjunctivitis. A maculopapular rash appears 2 to 4 days later (typically on day 12 after exposure) behind the ears and the hairline, spreading from the head to the trunk and the extremities. One or 2 days before the onset of rash, Koplik's spots, the pathognomonic enanthema, appear on the buccal mucosa and fade again as the skin rash evolves.

Uneventful measles lasts about 7 to 10 days, and cough is usually the last symptom to disappear. Patients are infectious from 4 to 5 days before until 4 days after the onset of rash. The course of disease can be complicated by otitis media (3%–9%), bronchitis or bronchopneumonia (1%–6%), and gastrointestinal and neurologic involvement. Postinfectious encephalitis complicates about 1 in 1000 infections, and subacute sclerosing panencephalitis (SSPE) affects approximately 1 in 1,000,000 cases, usually 7 to 10 years after acute measles. Measles also causes immunosuppression, facilitating secondary bacterial infections, which are responsible for most measles deaths, especially in developing countries.

Measles outbreaks have sometimes been observed in highly vaccinated populations. A mild, vaccine-modified form of measles, not necessarily covered by the clinical case definition, can occur in vaccinated persons with low-level immunity. In contrast, patients who contracted measles after vaccination with a formalin-inactivated measles vaccine, licensed in 1961 and withdrawn from the market in 1966, suffered from a severe illness referred to as *atypical measles*.

CURRENT DIAGNOSIS

- Fever (>38.3°C) and maculopapular rash (≥3 d) in association with cough, conjunctivitis, or coryza or some combination of these (CDC clinical case definition)
- Pathognomonic Koplik's spots on the buccal mucosa
- Detection of measles-specific IgM or increase in measles-specific IgG in paired sera
- Detection of viral RNA by reverse transcriptase polymerase chain reaction (RT-PCR) in nasopharyngeal swabs, oral fluid, urine, peripheral blood mononuclear cells (PBMCs), (or dried blood spots) with or without virus isolation

Diagnosis

The clinical case definition includes any person with fever (>38.3°C), maculopapular rash (≥3 d), and at least one of the symptoms of cough, coryza, or conjunctivitis. Laboratory confirmation is based on measles-specific IgM by enzyme-linked immunosorbent assay (ELISA), detected from onset of rash until weeks later. When IgM and IgG are negative early after onset of rash, repeat testing is warranted. The diagnosis can also be confirmed by an increase in measles-specific IgG between paired sera, detection of viral RNA by reverse-transcriptase polymerase chain reaction (RT-PCR), or virus isolation. Nasopharyngeal swabs, oral fluid, peripheral blood mononuclear cells (PBMCs), and the cellular fraction of urine are appropriate specimens for measles RT-PCR and virus isolation, as well as for genotyping of the virus in specialized laboratories. In most countries, confirmed or even suspected cases must be reported to the national health authorities.

Treatment

There is no specific treatment for acute measles. Supportive therapy includes hydration, antipyretics, bedrest, and protection from light for patients with photophobia. Secondary bacterial infections are treated with antibiotics. Vitamin A supplementation[1] has been shown to improve the clinical outcome in malnourished patients and patients with vitamin A deficiency. Ribavirin (Virazole)[1] and isoprinosin,[2] combined with interferon-α (IFN-α), have been used with limited success in experimental treatments of SSPE.

Prevention

Measles virus has only one serotype, and current live-attenuated vaccines are effective against all of the 23 known genotypes. Vaccination induces long-lasting protection against the disease even after a single dose. Transplacentally acquired maternal antibodies and immaturity of the infant immune system interfere with seroconversion rates, which, after the first dose, range between 80% and 95% depending on the age of the vaccinee. Improper handling of the vaccine can be another reason for primary vaccine failures. Therefore, two-dose vaccination programs are necessary to achieve a population immunity greater than 95%, which is necessary to interrupt virus circulation.

[1]Not FDA approved for this indication.
[2]Not available in the United States.

CURRENT THERAPY

Treatment

- There is no specific therapy for treating acute measles.
- Patient care is limited to supportive therapy.
- Secondary bacterial infections are treated with antibiotics.
- Vitamin A supplementation[1] might improve the clinical outcome.

Supportive Therapy

- Hydration
- Antipyretics
- Rest
- Protection from light
- Vitamin A[1]
- Treatment for secondary bacterial infections

[1]Not FDA approved for this indication.

Measles vaccination is recommended in virtually all countries, but immunization schedules depend on the specific epidemiologic situation of each country. Many industrialized countries use measles-mumps-rubella (MMR) combined vaccines, with a first dose given at 12 to 15 months of age and a second dose at 3 to 6 years of age to catch up children with primary or secondary vaccine failure after the first dose. In many developing countries with large birth cohorts and a higher measles incidence, monovalent measles vaccines (Attenuvax) are administered at 6 to 9 months of age to offset the higher risk of early exposure to wild-type virus and the earlier loss of maternal antibodies. A second dose should be provided as a routine revaccination during early childhood or in follow-up campaigns including broader age groups. Transient fever and rash are observed in 5% to 10% of patients vaccinated with live attenuated strains. Much publicized links to autism or other chronic diseases have never been confirmed by national or international scientific panels.

The vaccine is not recommended for children with primary or acquired severe immunodeficiency, except for children with asymptomatic HIV infection. The disease may be prevented in susceptible persons by hypergammaglobulin given within 6 days or by active immunization within 3 days after exposure. Passive immunization is also recommended in persons with some malignant diseases or deficits in cellular immunity.

REFERENCES

Bannister BA, Begg NT, Gillespie SH. Childhood Infections: Measles. Infectious Disease. Oxford: Blackwell Science; 1996. p. 256–60.

Campbell C, Levin S, Humphreys P, et al. Subacute sclerosing panencephalitis: Results of the Canadian Paediatric Surveillance Program and review of the literature. BMC Pediatr 2005;5:47.

Gershon AA. Measles virus. In: Mandell GL, Bennett JE, Dolin R, editors. Principles and Practice of Infectious Diseases. New York: Churchill Livingstone; 1995. p. 1519–25.

Griffin DE. Measles virus. In: Knipe DM, Howley PM, editors. Fields Virology. Philadelphia: Lippincott Williams & Wilkins; 2001. p. 1401–24.

World Health Organization. Progress in reducing global measles deaths: 1999–2004. Wkly Epidemiol Rec 2006;81(10):90–4.

Tetanus

Method of
Samuel S. Hsu, MD

Tetanus is a toxin-mediated infectious disease that is acquired from wounds and that results in muscular hyperexcitability and autonomic instability. It has a high mortality rate despite optimal treatment. It is best managed by prevention, which is accomplished with a highly effective low-cost vaccine. Victims are typically inadequately immunized.

Etiology

The causative agent of tetanus is *Clostridium tetani*, a spore-forming, gram-positive bacillus. The vegetative form is an obligate anaerobe, but the spores remain viable at ambient oxygen concentrations. The spores are ubiquitous in soil, are highly resistant to extremes in temperature and humidity, and can survive indefinitely. When spores enter wounds, they might not germinate immediately if tissue conditions are unfavorable. They can activate well after the wound has healed, which might account for cases of tetanus that have no identifiable source. When conditions are favorable, the spores germinate into mature bacilli, which release the toxin tetanospasmin.

Tetanospasmin is responsible for the clinical manifestations of tetanus. It enters peripheral nerves and travels via retrograde axonal transport to the central nervous system. Tetanospasmin then enters presynaptic neurons and disrupts the release of γ-amino butyric acid (GABA) and glycine, which are inhibitory neurotransmitters. This results in a disinhibition of end-organ neurons, such as motor neurons and those of the autonomic nervous system. Recovery depends on synthesis of new presynaptic components, a process that occurs over 2 to 3 weeks.

Epidemiology

Most cases occur in developing countries. In 2005, the World Health Organization (WHO) received reports of more than 15,000 cases, two thirds of which occurred in neonates. In contrast, tetanus is a disease of older adults in developed countries. According to the latest data from the Centers for Disease Control and Prevention (CDC), there are an average of 43 cases of tetanus per year in the United States, and the incidence is 0.16 per million population.

Even with optimal treatment, the mortality of tetanus is very high. The global fatality rate is estimated to be 30% to 50%. In the United States, the fatality rate ranges from 11% to 25%. Older adults have a higher mortality, 40% in those older than 60 years compared with 8% in those ages 20 to 59 years.

Lack of immunization is the greatest risk factor for contracting tetanus. The largest groups with the lowest rates of immunization in the United States are older adults and immigrants from Latin America. Serologic surveys show that although 95% of those 6 to 39 years old are adequately immunized, only 74% of those older than 60 years and 59% of those older than 70 years are adequately immunized. Only 75% of Latin American immigrants are adequately immunized. The result is a higher incidence of tetanus in these groups: 0.35 per million adults older than 60 years and 0.38 per million Latin Americans.

Clinical Features

An acute injury precedes most cases of tetanus, the most common being puncture wounds and lacerations. Nonacute etiologies include chronic wounds, IV drug use, and complications of diabetes. Cases have occurred without a clear etiology. The median time between an injury and onset of symptoms is 7 days, but there have been delayed presentations of up to 3 months. A more rapid onset correlates to a more severe clinical presentation.

CURRENT DIAGNOSIS

- Tetanus is diagnosed on clinical grounds alone.
- Involuntary muscle spasms are the hallmark of tetanus.
- Generalized tetanus is the most common form. Characteristic features include trismus (lockjaw), risus sardonicus, and opisthotonos.
- Sensory function and mental status are preserved.
- Mimics of tetanus can be excluded by physical findings and select laboratory tests.

There are four clinical forms of tetanus representing the extent and location of neurons involved: generalized, local, cephalic, and neonatal.

In the United States and other developed countries, generalized tetanus is the most common form. The initial symptom in 50% to 75% of cases is trismus ("lockjaw") secondary to masseter muscle spasm. Risus sardonicus, the "ironical smile of tetanus," can occur due to facial muscle contraction. Nuchal rigidity and dysphagia can also be initial complaints. As the disease spreads, generalized muscle spasms occur, either spontaneously or to minor stimuli such as touch or noise. Opisthotonos, a tonic contraction very similar to decorticate posturing, is classically described with tetanus. Severe spasms can result in bone fractures, tendon detachments, and rhabdomyolysis. Mental status is not affected, and spasms are experienced with severe pain.

In the acute phase, death results from acute respiratory failure due to diaphragmatic paralysis or laryngeal spasms. In severe cases, autonomic instability can occur, resulting most importantly in labile hypertension, tachycardia, and pyrexia. Hypotension and bradycardia can also occur. Arrhythmias and myocardial infarction are the most common fatal events. The exact mechanism of this syndrome is unclear but likely involves disinhibition of the sympathetic nervous system.

Local tetanus manifests as persistent muscle rigidity close to a site of injury. The rigidity can linger for weeks to months and often resolves without sequelae. Localized tetanus rarely progresses to generalized tetanus.

Cephalic tetanus is an uncommon variant of localized tetanus that involves the cranial nerves. Cephalic tetanus uniquely results in nerve palsies and muscle spasms. The seventh cranial nerve is most often involved, followed by the sixth, third, fourth, and 12th in decreasing order of frequency. With its predilection for the seventh cranial nerve, it commonly mimics Bell's palsy. Cephalic tetanus also manifests with trismus, but cranial nerve deficits precede the onset of trismus about 40% of the time. Head trauma and otitis media are commonly cited etiologies. About two thirds of cases progress to generalized tetanus.

Neonatal tetanus is generalized tetanus that occurs in newborns around the first week of life. Symptoms begin with nonspecific irritability and poor feeding, and they rapidly progress to generalized spasms. The portal of entry is the freshly cut umbilical cord. The risk of contracting neonatal tetanus is directly related to maternal immunization status, because passive transfer of maternal immunoglobulins is protective. Mortality is very high, 50% to 100%, due to the high load of toxin per body weight in neonates. In the United States, there were three reports of neonatal tetanus in the 1990s, all involving inadequately immunized mothers.

Diagnosis

The diagnosis of tetanus must be made on clinical grounds alone. There are no laboratory tests that can diagnose or exclude tetanus. Wound cultures rarely yield *C. tetani* and are not available quickly enough to aid diagnosis. Fortunately, the presentation of tetanus is so characteristic that a presumptive diagnosis can be made in most cases. When faced with a potential case of tetanus, it is useful to recall that sensory function and mental status remain normal.

The differential diagnosis is minimal. Most possibilities can be excluded by history, examination, and select laboratory tests. Exact mimics of tetanus occur with strychnine poisoning, which disables glycine release as tetanospasmin does, and hypocalcemia. These are easily excluded by laboratory tests. The differential for trismus includes peritonsillar/odontogenic abscesses and dystonic reactions. Cephalic tetanus without trismus can be easily mistaken for Bell's palsy, central nervous system tumor, or stroke. Neonatal tetanus initially manifests much like a host of other disorders. Once generalized spasms begin, the diagnosis is obvious.

Apte and Karnad describe a bedside test for tetanus in which a spatula is inserted into the pharynx. If the patient gags and tries to expel the spatula, the test is negative for tetanus; if the patient bites the spatula due to reflex masseter spasm, the test is positive for tetanus. The researchers reported 94% sensitivity and 100% specificity.

Treatment

Treatment involves neutralizing tetanospasmin, removing the source of the toxin, and providing supportive care for muscle spasms, respiration, and autonomic instability. Human tetanus immunoglobulin (hTIG, BayTet) 500 IU IM neutralizes circulating tetanospasmin. It cannot inactivate toxin already within neurons. Its half-life is 25 days; only a single dose is necessary. Doses of hTIG up to 10,000 IU have been used, but the lower dose is effective and has the advantage of requiring fewer injections to deliver. This feature is not insignificant, because hTIG is supplied in 250-IU doses, and injections are powerful stimuli for spasms. The adult and pediatric doses are the same. The burden of tetanospasmin, not the patient's size, determines the amount of hTIG needed.

To prevent ongoing production of toxin, antibiotics are needed to eliminate reservoirs of *C. tetani*. Metronidazole (Flagyl) in standard dose is the drug of choice. Penicillin, the historic drug of choice, does not penetrate devascularized wounds and abscesses well. Penicillin also has GABA-antagonist activity, which can potentiate the effects of tetanospasmin. In addition to antibiotics, obviously dirty wounds, abscesses, or devitalized tissue must be cleaned, drained, or excised to decrease the bacterial load.

 CURRENT THERAPY

ACUTE TETANUS

- Human tetanus immune globulin (hTIG, BayTet) 500 IU IM neutralizes tetanus toxin.
- Metronidazole (Flagyl) eliminates reservoirs of *Clostridium tetani*.
- Wounds and abscess must be débrided and drained.
- Benzodiazepines are the drugs of choice to control muscle spasms. In severe cases, paralytics and mechanical ventilation may be required.
- Tetanus immunization must be initiated because surviving tetanus does not confer immunity.

PROPHYLAXIS IN ACUTE WOUNDS

- Administer tetanus toxoid (Td) if the last booster was more than 10 y ago in non–tetanus-prone or more than 5 y ago in tetanus-prone wounds.
- Administer hTIG 250 IU IM if the patient never completed a primary immunization series and has a tetanus-prone wound.
- Pregnancy is not a contraindication to appropriate use of Td or hTIG.

Benzodiazepines are the drug of choice for muscle spasms because of their GABA-agonist and sedative properties. Daily doses of hundreds or thousands of milligrams have been used to control spasms. For severe cases, paralytics and mechanical ventilation may be needed. Vecuronium (Norcuron)[1] is an ideal agent for immediate and long-term control due to its minimal cardiovascular effects.

Treatment of autonomic instability has been problematic and is the subject of ongoing research. No therapeutic regimen has proved to be universally effective. α-Blockers,[1] β-blockers,[1] clonidine (Catapres),[1] and magnesium[1] have yielded variable success. Fentanyl (Sublimaze)[1] centrally decreases sympathetic outflow and has produced more consistent control of hypertension and tachycardia.

Supportive care includes placing the patient in a quiet, dark environment, minimizing patient manipulation, and treating for complications, most significantly rhabdomyolysis. Importantly, survivors must also receive a tetanus immunization series. The amount of tetanospasmin produced in clinical tetanus is small and partially sequestered in neurons; consequently, an immune response does not occur. Unimmunized survivors of tetanus have become victims a second time.

Prevention

Tetanus is preventable with proper use of tetanus toxoid and hTIG. Tetanus toxoid is an inactivated form of tetanospasmin. It is available as a single-antigen tetanus toxoid (TT) and combined with diphtheria and pertussis vaccine. The combination vaccines (e.g., Td for adults) are preferable because concurrent immunization is appropriate. The recommended primary immunization schedule is shown in Table 1. Adults should receive boosters every 10 years to maintain immunity.

Common adverse reactions to tetanus toxoid include erythema, swelling, and tenderness at the injection site. Nonspecific systemic effects such as fever, malaise, and anorexia can also occur. Reactions tend to occur more often and more severely if boosters are given more frequently than the recommended schedule. Patients who give a history of "allergy" to tetanus vaccine are most likely referring to a local or nonspecific systemic reaction. These are not contraindications to receiving tetanus toxoid. Other false contraindications include mild, acute illness; fever; and family history of an adverse reaction to vaccination. Anaphylactic reactions, neuropathies, and encephalopathies are rare and constitute the only true contraindications for giving toxoid. Patients who give a history of anaphylaxis should be referred for skin testing because they might no longer be reactive and can receive future vaccinations.

hTIG is derived from human plasma. It is available as 250-IU doses and is approved only for intramuscular use. Intradermal injection causes local irritation due to the concentration of the product and does

---

[1]Not FDA approved for this indication.

TABLE 1 Tetanus Primary Immunization

Age	Vaccine	No. of Doses	Schedule
<7 y	DTaP or DT	5	Doses 1–4 at 2, 4, 6, 15 mo Dose 5 between 4 and 6 y
>7 y	Td	3	First 2 doses more than 4 wk apart Dose 3 at 6 mo after dose 2

From Immunization Practices Advisory Committee: Diphtheria, tetanus, and pertussis: Recommendations for vaccine use and other preventive measures: Recommendations of the Immunization Practices Advisory Committee (ACIP). MMWR 1991;40(RR-10):1–28.
Abbreviations: DT = diphtheria and tetanus (adult); DTaP = diphtheria and tetanus toxoids and acellular pertussis; Td = diphtheria and tetanus (pediatric).

TABLE 2 Tetanus Prophylaxis in the Acute Wound

Wound Status	Primary Immunization			
	Completed or Last Booster			Not Completed
	<5 y	>5 y	>10 y	
Clean				
Td*	Yes	No	No	Yes
Tetanus-prone				
Td	Yes	No	Yes	Yes
TIG	Yes	No	No	No

Adapted from Immunization Practices Advisory Committee: Diphtheria, tetanus, and pertussis: Recommendations for vaccine use and other preventive measures: Recommendations of the Immunization Practices Advisory Committee (ACIP). MMWR 1991;40(RR-10):1–28.
*DTaP or DT for children younger than 7 years.
Abbreviations: DT = diphtheria and tetanus (adult); DTaP = diphtheria and tetanus toxoids and acellular pertussis; Td = diphtheria and tetanus (pediatric); TIG = tetanus immune globulin.

not represent an allergy to hTIG. Because of this reaction, hTIG should not be infiltrated into the wound. Intravenous injection can cause hypotension. Adverse reactions to properly administered hTIG are rare and consist largely of discomfort at the injection site and slight temperature elevation.

In the setting of an acute injury, the CDC recommendations for tetanus prophylaxis depend on the wound characteristics and the patient's immunization history (Table 2). Many acute wounds can be considered not tetanus prone: recent wounds, linear wounds with sharp edges, well-vascularized wounds, and wounds not obviously contaminated or infected. All other wounds are considered tetanus prone, particularly those resulting from blunt trauma and bites and those that are grossly contaminated or infected.

If the patient has completed primary immunization, a booster is given if the last dose was longer than 5 years ago in a tetanus-prone wound or more than 10 years ago in a non–tetanus-prone wound. Patients with a contraindication to tetanus toxoid must be treated with hTIG alone.

If the patient has not completed primary immunization and the wound is tetanus prone, hTIG 250 IU IM is indicated. hTIG should be given at a site contralateral to the tetanus toxoid to prevent interaction between the two. A tetanus booster is also required, and the patient will need follow-up to complete primary immunization.

Due to an aging immune system, in elderly patients tetanus antibodies after vaccination do not form as quickly, do not have as high a peak, and do not persist as long as in younger persons. With low rates of baseline immunity, elderly patients who receive only a tetanus booster can not develop protective levels of antibodies quickly enough in the setting of an acute injury. More liberal use of hTIG in these patients, regardless of primary immunization, may be warranted to ensure protection against tetanus if the last booster was significantly longer than 10 years ago.

Td is safe in pregnancy. Generally, routine immunizations are avoided in the first trimester; however there is considerable evidence that Td is not teratogenic. In the setting of acute wounds, Td should not be withheld if indicated. hTIG is also safe in pregnancy. The main risk with donated biological products is infection, not teratogenesis. Other immune globulin products, such as Rh immune globulin (Rho-Gam), are commonly used during pregnancy without adverse effects.

REFERENCES

Ahmadsyah I, Salim A. Treatment of tetanus: An open study to compare the efficacy of procaine penicillin and metronidazole. Br J Med (Clin Res Ed) 1985;291:648–50.
American College of Obstetrics and Gynecology. Immunization during pregnancy. ACOG Committee Opinion No. 282. Obstet Gynecol 2003;101:207–12.
Apte NM, Karnad DR. Short report: The spatula test: A simple bedside test to diagnose tetanus. Am J Trop Med Hyg 1995;53(4):386–7.

Bleck TP, Brauner JS. Tetanus. In: Scheld JWM, Whitely RJ, Durack DT, editors. Infections of the Central Nervous System. 2nd ed. Philadelphia: Lippincott-Raven; 1997. p. 629–53.
Centers for Disease Control: Prevention. Diphtheria, tetanus, and pertussis: Recommendations for vaccine use and other preventive measures: Recommendations of the Immunization Practices Advisory Committee (ACIP). MMWR 1991;40(RR-10):1–28.
Centers for Disease Control and Prevention. Tetanus surveillance—United States, 1998–2000. MMWR Surveill Summ 2003;52(SS-3):1–8.
Dietz V, Galazka A, Loon F, et al. Factors affecting the immunogenicity and potency of tetanus toxoid: Implications for the elimination of neonatal and non-neonatal tetanus as public health problems. Bull World Health Org 1997;75(1):81–93.
Sanford JP. Tetanus—forgotten but not gone. N Engl J Med 1995;332(12):812–3.
Silveira CM, Caceres VM, Dutra MG, et al. Safety of tetanus toxoid in pregnant women: A hospital-based case-control study of congenital anomalies. Bull World Health Org 1995;73:605–8.
Talan D, Abrahamian F, Moran G, et al. Tetanus immunity and physician compliance with tetanus prophylaxis practices among emergency department patients presenting with wounds. Ann Emerg Med 2004;43(3):305–14.

Pertussis

Method of
Michael E. Pichichero, MD

Pertussis, or whooping cough, is a highly contagious acute respiratory tract infection caused by *Bordetella pertussis*. It causes prolonged cough illness, without associated fever, characterized by paroxysms of coughing, inspiratory "whoops," and post-tussive vomiting in severe cases and persistent intermittent staccato cough episodes in teenagers and adults. The incidence of pertussis is rising in the United States despite record-high vaccination coverage. In 2004, more cases occurred in adolescents and in adults than children.

Microbiology and Pathophysiology

B. pertussis is a gram-negative coccobacillus that is difficult to grow with standard media. *B. pertussis* does not invade the human host; bacteremia does not occur. The systemic effects of illness are produced by the organism's toxins, especially pertussis toxin. *B. pertussis* attaches to the nasopharynx and tracheobronchial tree with adhesins such as fimbriae, filamentous hemagglutinin, and pertactin where it produces toxins such as pertussis toxin, adenylate cyclase toxin, and tracheal cytotoxin that paralyze the respiratory cilia, resulting in inflammation of the respiratory tract.

Epidemiology

B. pertussis is a human pathogen transmitted from person to person via aerosolized droplets. Pertussis is highly contagious, similar to varicella, infecting 80% to 90% of susceptible contacts. Persons with pertussis are most contagious in the 2 weeks before cough onset and during the first 2 weeks of cough, typically a time frame before medical care is sought or clinicians consider the possibility of the diagnosis.

In 2004, approximately 20,000 cases of pertussis were reported to the Centers for Disease Control and Prevention (CDC); because substantial underreporting is a recognized problem, current estimates of true pertussis incidence per year in the United States probably is in the range of 1 to 3 million cases. A new development is the recognition that pertussis is a disease of adolescents and adults as well as children. Several studies showed that among teenagers and adults who seek care for cough illness of more than 1 week duration, approximately 20% have pertussis.

Immunity

It has been known for decades that immunity to tetanus wanes over time and boosters are needed approximately every 10 years to sustain protective antibody levels. The phenomenon of waning immunity to pertussis is a newer observation and one of the explanations of the rising incidence of pertussis in the United States. Apparently boosters of pertussis vaccines are also needed, perhaps, like tetanus, approximately every 10 years. Two new adolescent/adult pertussis vaccine formulations that are combined with tetanus and diphtheria vaccines (Boostrix, Adacel) were licensed and recommended for universal use in 2005 to address this problem.

Clinical Symptoms

Classic pertussis is a 30- to 90-day illness that presents in three stages: catarrhal, paroxysmal, and convalescent. The stages may be shorter in immunized children, adolescents, and adults. Pertussis is most severe when it occurs during the first 6 months of life.

In the catarrhal stage, nonspecific symptoms similar to the common cold predominate. The paroxysmal stage is characterized by a persistent cough, sometimes with bursts of numerous rapid coughs. A long inspiratory effort sometimes causes a high-pitched whoop. Typically, the patient is afebrile and, between coughing attacks, usually appears normal. The paroxysmal stage usually lasts 6 weeks. The cough gradually lessens over 2 to 3 weeks during the convalescent period. Milder paroxysms may recur with subsequent respiratory infections for many months following a pertussis infection. Infants may appear very ill and distressed during the paroxysmal stage and require close observation and supportive care. Older children, adolescents, and adults have a prolonged cough with paroxysms but no whoop.

Complications

Complications occur most commonly among young infants with pertussis. The most common complication is secondary bacterial pneumonia. Hypoxia or effects of pertussis toxin may contribute to neurologic complications including seizures and encephalopathy. In the United States, 90% of deaths occur in children younger than 6 months. Complications from pertussis in adolescents and adults are not uncommon (Table 1).

TABLE 1 Complications From Pertussis in Adolescents and Adults

Symptoms/Signs	Minnesota	Massachusetts Adolescents	Adults
Paroxysmal cough	100%	85%	87%
Whooping	26%	30%	35%
Post-tussive emesis	56%	45%	41%
Apnea	–	19%	37%
Cyanosis	–	6%	9%
Hospitalization	0%	1.4%	3.5%

Diagnosis

A clinical diagnosis of pertussis is typically made based on the characteristic cough, although patients are often seen several times before the correct diagnosis is considered absolute lymphocytosis (>10,000 lymphcytes/mm^3) may be seen during the late catarrhal and paroxysmal stages but is less common among adults and immunized children. Chest radiographs may show peribronchial consolidation, interstitial edema, or variable atelectasis. The presence of fever and consolidation with pertussis suggests a secondary bacterial pneumonia.

Isolation of *B. pertussis* from a culture of nasal secretions remains the gold standard for laboratory diagnosis. A nasopharyngeal specimen is obtained by inserting a small flexible Dacron or calcium alginate swab through the nose to the posterior nasopharynx (attempting to touch the adenoids) where it is held for a few seconds, perhaps inducing a cough. The specimen is transferred to *Bordetella*-specific transport media and subsequently plated on Regan-Lowe charcoal agar or Stainer-Scholte agar. Cultures are usually positive if obtained in the catarrhal or early paroxysmal stage of disease. Success in isolating *B. pertussis* diminishes if patients have received pertussis vaccine or recent antimicrobials or if specimens are obtained beyond the first 2 weeks of cough.

Polymerase chain reaction (PCR) is more sensitive among persons with mild or atypical symptoms and those who have received prior antimicrobial therapy. The CDC recommends using PCR as a presumptive assay in conjunction with culture. Direct fluorescent antibody (DFA) testing has a low sensitivity and variable specificity, requiring experienced laboratory personnel for consistent results. DFA testing should only be performed as a adjunct to culture or PCR. Serologic testing methods have recently emerged as a very valuable diagnostic tool. Single samples of 100 μL of blood can be used to measure pertussis antibodies that are compared to age-specific standards to confirm a clinical diagnosis. These methods are not widely available in hospitals or private laboratories, but state laboratories often can provide this testing.

Treatment

Infants and children with severe cough paroxysms associated with cyanosis or apnea require hospitalization and intensive care. Infants younger than 3 months should be admitted routinely for observation of their paroxysmal episodes, their need for supportive interventions, and their ability to feed appropriately. Continuous monitoring of heart rate, respiratory rate, and oxygen saturation is indicated.

All patients should receive antibiotics. Macrolides are the treatment of choice: erythromycin, clarithromycin (Biaxin),[1] azithromycin (Zithromax),[1] or telithromycin (Ketek).[1] Fluoroquinolones are also effective therapy for pertussis. Trimethoprim-sulfamethoxazole (Bactrim)[1] is an alternative choice although less effective.

Prevention

Pertussis is a preventable disease by vaccination. Vaccines are available and recommended for universal use in infants, children, adolescents, and selected adult populations (health care workers, adults

---

[1]Not FDA approved for this indication.

TABLE 2 Licensed Vaccines for the Prevention of Pertussis in Infants, Children, Adolescents, and Adults

Indicated Age Group	Sanofi Pasteur Tripedia infants/ children[†]	GlaxoSmithKline Infanrix* Infants/ children[†]	Sanofi Pasteur Daptacel infants/ children[†]	GlaxoSmithKline Boostrix adults/ adolescents	Sanofi Pasteur Adacel adults/ adolescents
Antigens					
PT (µg)	23.4	25	10	8	2.5
FHA (µg)	23.4	25	5	8	5
PRN (µg)	–	8	3	2.5	3
FIM 2 + 3 (µg)	–	–	5	–	5
D (Lf)	6.7	25	15	2.5	2
T (Lf)	5	10	5	5	5

*PEDIARIX also contains these DTaP components
[†]6 wk to < 7 y
Abbreviations: D = diphtheria toxoid; FHA = filamentous hemagglutinin; FIM 2 + 3 = fimbrial agglutinogen 2 and 3; PRN = pertactin; PT = pertussis toxoid; T = tetanus toxoid.

caring for infants younger than 6 months, and those with chronic respiratory conditions, e.g., chronic obstructive pulmonary disease). Table 2 lists the vaccines licensed in the United States.

REFERENCES

Farizo KM, Cochi SL, Zell ER, et al. Epidemiological features of pertussis in the United States, 1980–1989. Clin Infect Dis 1992;14(3):708–19.

Lee LH, Pichichero ME. Costs of illness due to *Bordetella pertussis* in families. Arch Fam Med 2000;9(10):989–96.

Pichichero ME, Rennels MB, Edwards KM, et al. Combined tetanus, diphtheria, and 5-component pertussis vaccine for use in adolescents and adults. JAMA 2005;293(24):3003–11.

Purdy KW, Hay JW, Botteman MF, et al. Evaluation of strategies for use of acellular pertussis vaccine in adolescents and adults: A cost-benefit analysis. Clin Infect Dis 2004;39:20–8.

Skowronski DM, De Serres G, MacDonald D, et al. The changing age and seasonal profile of pertussis in Canada. J Infect Dis 2002;185(10):1448–53 [Epub 2002 Apr 22].

Strebel P, Nordin J, Edwards K, et al. Population-based incidence of pertussis among adolescents and adults, Minnesota, 1995–1996. J Infect Dis 2001;183(9):1353–9 [Epub 2001 Mar 30].

Yih WK, Lett SM, des Vignes FN, et al. The increasing incidence of pertussis in Massachusetts adolescents and adults, 1989–1998. J Infect Dis 2000;182(5):1409–16 [Epub 2000 Oct 09].

Office-Based Immunization Practices

Method of
Robert M. Jacobson, MD

Routine immunizations represent the cutting edge for consensus-driven, evidence-based practice guidelines in the care of children and adults. Perhaps no other office-based task is as universally accepted and evidenced as immunizations. We should model the rest of our practices on the success that we have enjoyed with immunizations.

That is not to say that we are providing immunizations as well as we should; the practice of immunization is difficult, complex, and evolving. Other chapters deal with the specific diseases to which we direct our vaccines, but office practitioners must consider a variety of aspects that go beyond the understanding of the individual vaccine-preventable diseases. These include the adoption of a comprehensive immunization schedule, using a number of immunization-specific practices, and the understanding of common problems associated with immunization in the office.

The Adoption of a Comprehensive Immunization Schedule

In recent years, we have benefited from efforts made at the national level to harmonize and systematically update recommended schedules for routine immunizations (Tables 1 and 2). The Advisory Committee on Immunization Practices (ACIP), sponsored by the Centers for Disease Control and Prevention (CDC), works closely with the American Academy of Pediatrics (AAP) and the American Academy of Family Physicians (AAFP) to publish a single set of recommendations for routine immunizations for infants, children, and adolescents up to 18 years of age. The Adult Immunization Schedule is similarly approved by the ACIP, the American College of Obstetricians and Gynecologists, the AAFP, and the American College of Physicians (Table 3). These are published widely in a number of journals as well as on the internet. The harmonized schedules address the use of both individual vaccine components as well as all licensed combination vaccines. The vaccine schedules give ranges of target age ranges for immunization rather than prescribe individual ages. For example, the measles-mumps-rubella combination is to be given from 12 to 15 months of life rather than either 12 months or 15 months. Furthermore, the pediatric schedule includes catch-up schedules for children who did not receive immunizations at the recommended ages. The adult schedule includes common conditions with vaccine-specific recommendations (such as for pregnancy).

Each of the 50 states in the United States has specific immunization requirements for day care, school, and even college attendance. These vary state by state and in some states affect not only initial enrollment but also continued participation in schools. The Immunization Action Coalition collates and publishes online (www.immunize.org/laws/) an up-to-date listing of the state-specific state mandates on immunization and vaccine-preventable diseases as well as links to the individual state health departments.

(Text continued on p. 152)

TABLE 1 Recommended Childhood and Adolescent Immunization Schedule

Recommended Immunization Schedule for Persons Aged 0 Through 6 Years—United States • 2009
For those who fall behind or start late, see the catch-up schedule

Vaccine ▼ Age ►	Birth	1 month	2 months	4 months	6 months	12 months	15 months	18 months	19–23 months	2–3 years	4–6 years
Hepatitis B[1]	HepB	HepB		see footnote 1	HepB						
Rotavirus[2]			RV	RV	RV[2]						
Diphtheria, Tetanus, Pertussis[3]			DTaP	DTaP	DTaP	see footnote 3	DTaP				DTaP
Haemophilus influenzae type b[4]			Hib	Hib	Hib[4]	Hib					
Pneumococcal[5]			PCV	PCV	PCV	PCV				PPSV	
Inactivated Poliovirus			IPV	IPV		IPV					IPV
Influenza[6]						Influenza (Yearly)					
Measles, Mumps, Rubella[7]						MMR		see footnote 7			MMR
Varicella[8]						Varicella		see footnote 8			Varicella
Hepatitis A[9]						HepA (2 doses)				HepA Series	
Meningococcal[10]										MCV	

Range of recommended ages

Certain high-risk groups

This schedule indicates the recommended ages for routine administration of currently licensed vaccines, as of December 1, 2008, for children aged 0 through 6 years. Any dose not administered at the recommended age should be administered at a subsequent visit, when indicated and feasible. Licensed combination vaccines may be used whenever any component of the combination is indicated and other components are not contraindicated and if approved by the Food and Drug Administration for that dose of the series. Providers should consult the relevant Advisory Committee on Immunization Practices statement for detailed recommendations, including high-risk conditions: http://www.cdc.gov/vaccines/pubs/acip-list.htm. Clinically significant adverse events that follow immunization should be reported to the Vaccine Adverse Event Reporting System (VAERS). Guidance about how to obtain and complete a VAERS form is available at http://www.vaers.hhs.gov or by telephone, 800-822-7967. http://www.cdc.gov/vaccines/recs/schedules/downloads/child/2009/09_0-6yrs_schedule_bw.pdf

1. **Hepatitis B vaccine (HepB).** *(Minimum age: birth)*
   At birth:
   - Administer monovalent HepB to all newborns before hospital discharge.
   - If mother is hepatitis B surface antigen (HBsAg)-positive, administer HepB and 0.5 mL of hepatitis B immune globulin (HBIG) within 12 hours of birth.
   - If mother's HBsAg status is unknown, administer HepB within 12 hours of birth. Determine mother's HBsAg status as soon as possible and, if HBsAg-positive, administer HBIG (no later than age 1 week).
   After the birth dose:
   - The HepB series should be completed with either monovalent HepB or a combination vaccine containing HepB. The second dose should be administered at age 1 or 2 months. The final dose should be administered no earlier than age 24 weeks.
   - Infants born to HBsAg-positive mothers should be tested for HBsAg and antibody to HBsAg (anti-HBs) after completion of at least 3 doses of the HepB series, at age 9 through 18 months (generally at the next well-child visit).
   4-month dose:
   - Administration of 4 doses of HepB to infants is permissible when combination vaccines containing HepB are administered after the birth dose.

2. **Rotavirus vaccine (RV).** *(Minimum age: 6 weeks)*
   - Administer the first dose at age 6 through 14 weeks (maximum age: 14 weeks 6 days). Vaccination should not be initiated for infants aged 15 weeks or older (i.e., 15 weeks 0 days or older).
   - Administer the final dose in the series by age 8 months 0 days.
   - If Rotarix® is administered at ages 2 and 4 months, a dose at 6 months is not indicated.

3. **Diphtheria and tetanus toxoids and acellular pertussis vaccine (DTaP).** *(Minimum age: 6 weeks)*
   - The fourth dose may be administered as early as age 12 months, provided at least 6 months have elapsed since the third dose.
   - Administer the final dose in the series at age 4 through 6 years.

4. ***Haemophilus influenzae* type b conjugate vaccine (Hib).** *(Minimum age: 6 weeks)*
   - If PRP-OMP (PedvaxHIB® or Comvax® [HepB-Hib]) is administered at ages 2 and 4 months, a dose at age 6 months is not indicated.
   - TriHiBit® (DTaP/Hib) should not be used for doses at ages 2, 4, or 6 months but can be used as the final dose in children aged 12 months or older.

5. **Pneumococcal vaccine.** *(Minimum age: 6 weeks for pneumococcal conjugate vaccine [PCV]; 2 years for pneumococcal polysaccharide vaccine [PPSV])*
   - PCV is recommended for all children aged younger than 5 years. Administer 1 dose of PCV to all healthy children aged 24 through 59 months who are not completely vaccinated for their age.

   - Administer PPSV to children aged 2 years or older with certain underlying medical conditions (see *MMWR* 2000;49[No. RR-9]), including a cochlear implant.

6. **Influenza vaccine.** *(Minimum age: 6 months for trivalent inactivated influenza vaccine [TIV]; 2 years for live, attenuated influenza vaccine [LAIV])*
   - Administer annually to children aged 6 months through 18 years.
   - For healthy nonpregnant persons (i.e., those who do not have underlying medical conditions that predispose them to influenza complications) aged 2 through 49 years, either LAIV or TIV may be used.
   - Children receiving TIV should receive 0.25 mL if aged 6 through 35 months or 0.5 mL if aged 3 years or older.
   - Administer 2 doses (separated by at least 4 weeks) to children aged younger than 9 years who are receiving influenza vaccine for the first time or who were vaccinated for the first time during the previous influenza season but only received 1 dose.

7. **Measles, mumps, and rubella vaccine (MMR).** *(Minimum age: 12 months)*
   - Administer the second dose at age 4 through 6 years. However, the second dose may be administered before age 4, provided at least 28 days have elapsed since the first dose.

8. **Varicella vaccine.** *(Minimum age: 12 months)*
   - Administer the second dose at age 4 through 6 years. However, the second dose may be administered before age 4, provided at least 3 months have elapsed since the first dose.
   - For children aged 12 months through 12 years the minimum interval between doses is 3 months. However, if the second dose was administered at least 28 days after the first dose, it can be accepted as valid.

9. **Hepatitis A vaccine (HepA).** *(Minimum age: 12 months)*
   - Administer to all children aged 1 year (i.e., aged 12 through 23 months). Administer 2 doses at least 6 months apart.
   - Children not fully vaccinated by age 2 years can be vaccinated at subsequent visits.
   - HepA also is recommended for children older than 1 year who live in areas where vaccination programs target older children or who are at increased risk of infection. See *MMWR* 2006;55(No. RR-7).

10. **Meningococcal vaccine.** *(Minimum age: 2 years for meningococcal conjugate vaccine [MCV] and for meningococcal polysaccharide vaccine [MPSV])*
    - Administer MCV to children aged 2 through 10 years with terminal complement component deficiency, anatomic or functional asplenia, and certain other high-risk groups. See *MMWR* 2005;54(No. RR-7).
    - Persons who received MPSV 3 or more years previously and who remain at increased risk for meningococcal disease should be revaccinated with MCV.

The Recommended Immunization Schedules for Persons Aged 0 Through 18 Years are approved by the Advisory Committee on Immunization Practices (www.cdc.gov/vaccines/recs/acip), the American Academy of Pediatrics (http://www.aap.org), and the American Academy of Family Physicians (http://www.aafp.org).
DEPARTMENT OF HEALTH AND HUMAN SERVICES • CENTERS FOR DISEASE CONTROL AND PREVENTION

Continued

TABLE 1 Recommended Childhood and Adolescent Immunization Schedule—Cont'd

Recommended Immunization Schedule for Persons Aged 7 Through 18 Years—United States • 2009
For those who fall behind or start late, see the schedule below and the catch-up schedule

Vaccine ▼ Age ►	7–10 years	11–12 years	13–18 years	
Tetanus, Diphtheria, Pertussis[1]	see footnote 1	Tdap	Tdap	Range of recommended ages
Human Papillomavirus[2]	see footnote 2	HPV (3 doses)	HPV Series	
Meningococcal[3]	MCV	MCV	MCV	
Influenza[4]		Influenza (Yearly)		
Pneumococcal[5]		PPSV		Catch-up immunization
Hepatitis A[6]		HepA Series		
Hepatitis B[7]		HepB Series		
Inactivated Poliovirus[8]		IPV Series		Certain high-risk groups
Measles, Mumps, Rubella[9]		MMR Series		
Varicella[10]		Varicella Series		

This schedule indicates the recommended ages for routine administration of currently licensed vaccines, as of December 1, 2008, for children aged 7 through 18 years. Any dose not administered at the recommended age should be administered at a subsequent visit, when indicated and feasible. Licensed combination vaccines may be used whenever any component of the combination is indicated and other components are not contraindicated and if approved by the Food and Drug Administration for that dose of the series. Providers should consult the relevant Advisory Committee on Immunization Practices statement for detailed recommendations, including high-risk conditions: http://www.cdc.gov/vaccines/pubs/acip-list.htm. Clinically significant adverse events that follow immunization should be reported to the Vaccine Adverse Event Reporting System (VAERS). Guidance about how to obtain and complete a VAERS form is available at http://www.vaers.hhs.gov or by telephone, 800-822-7967. http://www.cdc.gov/vaccines/recs/schedules/downloads/child/2009/09_7-18yrs_schedule_bw.pdf

1. **Tetanus and diphtheria toxoids and acellular pertussis vaccine (Tdap).** *(Minimum age: 10 years for BOOSTRIX® and 11 years for ADACEL®)*
   - Administer at age 11 or 12 years for those who have completed the recommended childhood DTP/DTaP vaccination series and have not received a tetanus and diphtheria toxoid (Td) booster dose.
   - Persons aged 13 through 18 years who have not received Tdap should receive a dose.
   - A 5-year interval from the last Td dose is encouraged when Tdap is used as a booster dose; however, a shorter interval may be used if pertussis immunity is needed.
2. **Human papillomavirus vaccine (HPV).** *(Minimum age: 9 years)*
   - Administer the first dose to females at age 11 or 12 years.
   - Administer the second dose 2 months after the first dose and the third dose 6 months after the first dose (at least 24 weeks after the first dose).
   - Administer the series to females at age 13 through 18 years if not previously vaccinated.
3. **Meningococcal conjugate vaccine (MCV).**
   - Administer at age 11 or 12 years, or at age 13 through 18 years if not previously vaccinated.
   - Administer to previously unvaccinated college freshmen living in a dormitory.
   - MCV is recommended for children aged 2 through 10 years with terminal complement component deficiency, anatomic or functional asplenia, and certain other groups at high risk. See *MMWR* 2005;54(No. RR-7).
   - Persons who received MPSV 5 or more years previously and remain at increased risk for meningococcal disease should be revaccinated with MCV.
4. **Influenza vaccine.**
   - Administer annually to children aged 6 months through 18 years.
   - For healthy nonpregnant persons (i.e., those who do not have underlying medical conditions that predispose them to influenza complications) aged 2 through 49 years, either LAIV or TIV may be used.
   - Administer 2 doses (separated by at least 4 weeks) to children aged younger than 9 years who are receiving influenza vaccine for the first time or who were vaccinated for the first time during the previous influenza season but only received 1 dose.

5. **Pneumococcal polysaccharide vaccine (PPSV).**
   - Administer to children with certain underlying medical conditions (see *MMWR* 1997;46[No. RR-8]), including a cochlear implant. A single revaccination should be administered to children with functional or anatomic asplenia or other immunocompromising condition after 5 years.
6. **Hepatitis A vaccine (HepA).**
   - Administer 2 doses at least 6 months apart.
   - HepA is recommended for children older than 1 year who live in areas where vaccination programs target older children or who are at increased risk of infection. See *MMWR* 2006;55(No. RR-7).
7. **Hepatitis B vaccine (HepB).**
   - Administer the 3-dose series to those not previously vaccinated.
   - A 2-dose series (separated by at least 4 months) of adult formulation Recombivax HB® is licensed for children aged 11 through 15 years.
8. **Inactivated poliovirus vaccine (IPV).**
   - For children who received an all-IPV or all-oral poliovirus (OPV) series, a fourth dose is not necessary if the third dose was administered at age 4 years or older.
   - If both OPV and IPV were administered as part of a series, a total of 4 doses should be administered, regardless of the child's current age.
9. **Measles, mumps, and rubella vaccine (MMR).**
   - If not previously vaccinated, administer 2 doses or the second dose for those who have received only 1 dose, with at least 28 days between doses.
10. **Varicella vaccine.**
   - For persons aged 7 through 18 years without evidence of immunity (see *MMWR* 2007;56[No. RR-4]), administer 2 doses if not previously vaccinated or the second dose if they have received only 1 dose.
   - For persons aged 7 through 12 years, the minimum interval between doses is 3 months. However, if the second dose was administered at least 28 days after the first dose, it can be accepted as valid.
   - For persons aged 13 years and older, the minimum interval between doses is 28 days.

The Recommended Immunization Schedules for Persons Aged 0 Through 18 Years are approved by the Advisory Committee on Immunization Practices (www.cdc.gov/vaccines/recs/acip), the American Academy of Pediatrics (http://www.aap.org), and the American Academy of Family Physicians (http://www.aafp.org).
DEPARTMENT OF HEALTH AND HUMAN SERVICES · CENTERS FOR DISEASE CONTROL AND PREVENTION

TABLE 2 Recommended Catch-Up Immunization Schedule

Catch-up Immunization Schedule for Persons Aged 4 Months Through 18 Years Who Start Late or Who Are More Than 1 Month Behind—United States • 2009

The table below provides catch-up schedules and minimum intervals between doses for children whose vaccinations have been delayed. A vaccine series does not need to be restarted, regardless of the time that has elapsed between doses. Use the section appropriate for the child's age.

CATCH-UP SCHEDULE FOR PERSONS AGED 4 MONTHS THROUGH 6 YEARS

Vaccine	Minimum Age for Dose 1	Minimum Interval Between Doses			
		Dose 1 to Dose 2	Dose 2 to Dose 3	Dose 3 to Dose 4	Dose 4 to Dose 5
Hepatitis B[1]	Birth	4 weeks	**8 weeks** (and at least 16 weeks after first dose)		
Rotavirus[2]	6 wks	4 weeks	**4 weeks**[2]		
Diphtheria, Tetanus, Pertussis[3]	6 wks	4 weeks	4 weeks	6 months	6 months[3]
Haemophilus influenzae type b[4]	6 wks	**4 weeks** if first dose administered at younger than age 12 months **8 weeks (as final dose)** if first dose administered at age 12-14 months **No further doses needed** if first dose administered at age 15 months or older	**4 weeks**[4] if current age is younger than 12 months **8 weeks** (as final dose)[4] if current age is 12 months or older and second dose administered at younger than age 15 months **No further doses needed** if previous dose administered at age 15 months or older	**8 weeks** (as final dose) This dose only necessary for children aged 12 months through 59 months who received 3 doses before age 12 months	
Pneumococcal[5]	6 wks	**4 weeks** if first dose administered at younger than age 12 months **8 weeks (as final dose for healthy children)** if first dose administered at age 12 months or older or current age 24 through 59 months **No further doses needed** for healthy children if first dose administered at age 24 months or older	**4 weeks** if current age is younger than 12 months **8 weeks** (as final dose for healthy children) if current age is 12 months or older **No further doses needed** for healthy children if previous dose administered at age 24 months or older	**8 weeks** (as final dose) This dose only necessary for children aged 12 months through 59 months who received 3 doses before age 12 months or for high-risk children who received 3 doses at any age	
Inactivated Poliovirus[6]	6 wks	4 weeks	4 weeks	4 weeks[6]	
Measles, Mumps, Rubella[7]	12 mos	4 weeks			
Varicella[8]	12 mos	3 months			
Hepatitis A[9]	12 mos	6 months			

CATCH-UP SCHEDULE FOR PERSONS AGED 7 THROUGH 18 YEARS

Vaccine	Minimum Age for Dose 1	Dose 1 to Dose 2	Dose 2 to Dose 3	Dose 3 to Dose 4	
Tetanus, Diphtheria/ Tetanus, Diphtheria, Pertussis[10]	7 yrs[10]	4 weeks	**4 weeks** if first dose administered at younger than age 12 months **6 months** if first dose administered at age 12 months or older	**6 months** if first dose administered at younger than age 12 months	
Human Papillomavirus[11]	9 yrs	Routine dosing intervals are recommended[11]			
Hepatitis A[9]	12 mos	6 months			
Hepatitis B[1]	Birth	4 weeks	**8 weeks** (and at least 16 weeks after first dose)		
Inactivated Poliovirus[6]	6 wks	4 weeks	4 weeks	4 weeks[6]	
Measles, Mumps, Rubella[7]	12 mos	4 weeks			
Varicella[8]	12 mos	**3 months** if the person is younger than age 13 years **4 weeks** if the person is aged 13 years or older			

1. **Hepatitis B vaccine (HepB).**
   - Administer the 3-dose series to those not previously vaccinated.
   - A 2-dose series (separated by at least 4 months) of adult formulation Recombivax HB® is licensed for children aged 11 through 15 years.
2. **Rotavirus vaccine (RV).**
   - The maximum age for the first dose is 14 weeks 6 days. Vaccination should not be initiated for infants aged 15 weeks or older (i.e., 15 weeks 0 days or older).
   - Administer the final dose in the series by age 8 months 0 days.
   - If Rotarix® was administered for the first and second doses, a third dose is not indicated.
3. **Diphtheria and tetanus toxoids and acellular pertussis vaccine (DTaP).**
   - The fifth dose is not necessary if the fourth dose was administered at age 4 years or older.
4. ***Haemophilus influenzae* type b conjugate vaccine (Hib).**
   - Hib vaccine is not generally recommended for persons aged 5 years or older. No efficacy data are available on which to base a recommendation concerning use of Hib vaccine for older children and adults. However, studies suggest good immunogenicity in persons who have sickle cell disease, leukemia, or HIV infection, or who have had a splenectomy; administering 1 dose of Hib vaccine to these persons is not contraindicated.
   - If the first 2 doses were PRP-OMP (PedvaxHIB® or Cornvax®), and administered at age 11 months or younger, the third (and final) dose should be administered at age 12 through 15 months and at least 8 weeks after the second dose.
   - If the first dose was administered at age 7 through 11 months, administer 2 doses separated by 4 weeks and a final dose at age 12 through 15 months.
5. **Pneumococcal vaccine.**
   - Administer 1 dose of pneumococcal conjugate vaccine (PCV) to all healthy children aged 24 through 59 months who have not received at least 1 dose of PCV on or after age 12 months.
   - For children aged 24 through 59 months with underlying medical conditions, administer 1 dose of PCV if 3 doses were received previously or administer 2 doses of PCV at least 8 weeks apart if fewer than 3 doses were received previously.
   - Administer pneumococcal polysaccharide vaccine (PPSV) to children aged 2 years or older with certain underlying medical conditions (see *MMWR* 2000;49[No. RR-9]), including a cochlear implant, at least 8 weeks after the last dose of PCV.

6. **Inactivated poliovirus vaccine (IPV).**
   - For children who received an all-IPV or all-oral poliovirus (OPV) series, a fourth dose is not necessary if the third dose was administered at age 4 years or older.
   - If both OPV and IPV were administered as part of a series, a total of 4 doses should be administered, regardless of the child's current age.
7. **Measles, mumps, and rubella vaccine (MMR).**
   - Administer the second dose at age 4 through 6 years. However, the second dose may be administered before age 4, provided at least 28 days have elapsed since the first dose.
   - If not previously vaccinated, administer 2 doses with at least 28 days between doses.
8. **Varicella vaccine.**
   - Administer the second dose at age 4 through 6 years. However, the second dose may be administered before age 4, provided at least 3 months have elapsed since the first dose.
   - For persons aged 12 months through 12 years, the minimum interval between doses is 3 months. However, if the second dose was administered at least 28 days after the first dose, it can be accepted as valid.
   - For persons aged 13 years and older, the minimum interval between doses is 28 days.
9. **Hepatitis A vaccine (HepA).**
   - HepA is recommended for children older than 1 year who live in areas where vaccination programs target older children or who are at increased risk of infection. See *MMWR* 2006;55(No. RR-7).
10. **Tetanus and diphtheria toxoids vaccine (Td) and tetanus and diphtheria toxoids and acellular pertussis vaccine (Tdap).**
    - Doses of DTaP are counted as part of the Td/Tdap series
    - Tdap should be substituted for a single dose of Td in the catch-up series or as a booster for children aged 10 through 18 years; use Td for other doses.
11. **Human papillomavirus vaccine (HPV).**
    - Administer the series to females at age 13 through 18 years if not previously vaccinated.
    - Use recommended routine dosing intervals for series catch-up (i.e., the second and third doses should be administered at 2 and 6 months after the first dose). However, the minimum interval between the first and second doses is 4 weeks. The minimum interval between the second and third doses is 12 weeks, and the third dose should be given at least 24 weeks after the first dose.

Information about reporting reactions after immunization is available online at http://www.vaers.hhs.gov or by telephone, 800–822–7967.
Suspected cases of vaccine-preventable diseases should be reported to the state or local health department. Additional information, including precautions and contraindications for immunization, is available from the National Center for Immunization and Respiratory Diseases at http://www.cdc.gov/vaccines or telephone, 800-CDC-INFO (800–232–4636).
DEPARTMENT OF HEALTH AND HUMAN SERVICES · CENTERS FOR DISEASE CONTROL AND PREVENTION

TABLE 3 Recommended Adult Immunization Schedule

Recommended Adult Immunization Schedule UNITED STATES • 2009

Note: These recommendations must be read with the footnotes that follow containing number of doses, intervals between doses, and other important information.

Recommended adult immunization schedule, by vaccine and age group

VACCINE ▼ AGE GROUP ►	19–26 years	27–49 years	50–59 years	60–64 years	≥65 years
Tetanus, diphtheria, pertussis (Td/Tdap)[1,*]	Substitute 1-time dose of Tdap for Td booster; then boost with Td every 10 yrs				Td booster every 10 yrs
Human papillomavirus (HPV)[2,*]	3 doses (females)				
Varicella[3,*]	2 doses				
Zoster[4]				1 dose	
Measles, mumps, rubella (MMR)[5,*]	1 or 2 doses		1 dose		
Influenza[6,*]	1 dose annually				
Pneumococcal (polysaccharide)[7,8]	1 or 2 doses				1 dose
Hepatitis A[9,*]	2 doses				
Hepatitis B[10,*]	3 doses				
Meningococcal[11,*]	1 or more doses				

*Covered by the Vaccine Injury Compensation Program.

▨ For all persons in this category who meet the age requirements and who lack evidence of immunity (e.g., lack documentation of vaccination or have no evidence of prior infection)	▨ Recommended if some other risk factor is present (e.g., on the basis of medical, occupational, lifestyle, or other indications)	☐ No recommendation

Report all clinically significant postvaccination reactions to the Vaccine Adverse Event Reporting System (VAERS). Reporting forms and Instructions on filing a VAERS report are available at www.vaers.hhs.gov or by telephone, 800-822-7967.

Information on how to file a Vaccine Injury Compensation Program claim is available at www.hrsa.gov/vaccinecompensation or by telephone, 800-338-2382. To file a claim for vaccine Injury, contact the U.S. Court of Federal Claims, 717 Madison Place, N.W., Washington, D.C. 20005; telephone, 202-357-6400.

Additional information about the vaccines in this schedule, extent of available data, and contraindications for vaccination is also available at www.cdc.gov/vaccines or from the CDC-INFO Contact Center at 800-CDC-INFO (800-232-4636) in English and Spanish, 24 hours a day, 7 days a week.

Use of trade names and commercial sources is for identification only and does not imply endorsement by the U.S. Department of Health and Human Services.

Vaccines that might be indicated for adults based on medical and other indications

INDICATION ► VACCINE ▼	Pregnancy	Immuno-compromising conditions (excluding human immunodeficiency virus [HIV])[12]	HIV infection[3,12,13] CD4+ T lympho-cyte count		Diabetes, heart disease, chronic lung disease, chronic alcoholism	Asplenia[12] (including elective splenectomy and terminal complement component deficiencies)	Chronic liver disease	Kidney failure, end-stage renal disease, receipt of hemodialysis	Health-care personnel
			<200 cells/μL	≥200 cells/μL					
Tetanus, diphtheria, pertussis (Td/Tdap)[1,*]	Td	Substitute 1-time dose of Tdap for Td booster; then boost with Td every 10 yrs							
Human papillomavirus (HPV)[2,*]		3 doses for females through age 26 yrs							
Varicella[3,*]	Contraindicated				2 doses				
Zoster[4]	Contraindicated				1 dose				
Measles, mumps, rubella (MMR)[5,*]	Contraindicated				1 or 2 doses				
Influenza[6,*]	1 dose TIV annually								1 dose TIV or LAIV annually
Pneumococcal (polysaccharide)[7,8]	1 or 2 doses								
Hepatitis A[9,*]	2 doses								
Hepatitis B[10,*]	3 doses								
Meningococcal[11,*]	1 or more doses								

*Covered by the Vaccine Injury Compensation Program.

▨ For all persons in this category who meet the age requirements and who lack evidence of immunity (e.g., lack documentation of vaccination or have no evidence of prior infection)	▨ Recommended if some other risk factor is present (e.g., on the basis of medical, occupational, lifestyle, or other indications)	☐ No recommendation

These schedules indicate the recommended age groups and medical indications for which administration of currently licensed vaccines is commonly indicated for adults ages 19 years and older, as of January 1, 2009. Licensed combination vaccines may be used whenever any components of the combination are indicated and when the vaccine's other components are not contraindicated. For detailed recommendations on all vaccines, including those used primarily for travelers or that are issued during the year, consult the manufacturers' package inserts and the complete statements from the Advisory Committee on Immunization Practices (www.cdc.gov/vaccines/pubs/acip-list.htm).

The recommendations in this schedule were approved by the Centers for Disease Control and Prevention's (CDC) Advisory Committee on Immunization Practices (ACIP), the American Academy of Family Physicians (AAFP), the American College of Obstetricians and Gynecologists (ACOG), and the American College of Physicians (ACP).

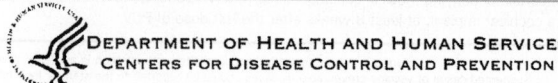

DEPARTMENT OF HEALTH AND HUMAN SERVICES
CENTERS FOR DISEASE CONTROL AND PREVENTION

CDC

Recommended Adult Immunization Schedule—United States • 2009

For complete statements by the Advisory Committee on Immunization Practices (ACIP), visit www.cdc.gov/vaccines/pubs/ACIP-list.htm.

1. Tetanus, diphtheria, and acellular pertussis (Td/Tdap) vaccination

Tdap should replace a single dose of Td for adults aged 19 through 64 years who have not received a dose of Tdap previously.

Adults with uncertain or incomplete history of primary vaccination series with tetanus and diphtheria toxoid-containing vaccines should begin or complete a primary vaccination series. A primary series for adults is 3 doses of tetanus and diphtheria toxoid-containing vaccines; administer the first 2 doses at least 4 weeks apart and the third dose 6–12 months after the second. However, Tdap can substitute for any one of the doses of Td in the 3-dose primary series. The booster dose of tetanus and diphtheria toxoid-containing vaccine should be administered to adults who have completed a primary series and if the last vaccination was received 10 or more years previously. Tdap or Td vaccine may be used, as indicated.

If a woman is pregnant and received the last Td vaccination 10 or more years previously, administer Td during the second or third trimester. If the woman received the last Td vaccination less than 10 years previously, administer Tdap during the immediate postpartum period. A dose of Tdap is recommended for postpartum women, close contacts of infants aged less than 12 months, and all health-care personnel with direct patient contact if they have not previously received Tdap. An interval as short as 2 years from the last Td is suggested; shorter intervals can be used. Td may be deferred during pregnancy and Tdap substituted in the immediate postpartum period, or Tdap may be administered instead of Td to a pregnant woman after an informed discussion with the woman.

Consult the ACIP statement for recommendations for administering Td as prophylaxis in wound management.

2. Human papillomavirus (HPV) vaccination

HPV vaccination is recommended for all females aged 11 through 26 years (and may begin at 9 years) who have not completed the vaccine series. History of genital warts, abnormal Papanicolaou test, or positive HPV DNA test is not evidence of prior infection with all vaccine HPV types; HPV vaccination is recommended for persons with such histories.

Ideally, vaccine should be administered before potential exposure to HPV through sexual activity; however, females who are sexually active should still be vaccinated consistent with age-based recommendations. Sexually active females who have not been infected with any of the four HPV vaccine types receive the full benefit of the vaccination. Vaccination is less beneficial for females who have already been infected with one or more of the HPV vaccine types.

A complete series consists of 3 doses. The second dose should be administered 2 months after the first dose; the third dose should be administered 6 months after the first dose.

HPV vaccination is not specifically recommended for females with the medical indications described in Figure 2, "Vaccines that might be indicated for adults based on medical and other indications." Because HPV vaccine is not a live-virus vaccine, it may be administered to persons with the medical indications described in Figure 2. However, the immune response and vaccine efficacy might be less for persons with the medical indications described in Figure 2 than in persons who do not have the medical indications described or who are immunocompetent. Health-care personnel are not at increased risk because of occupational exposure, and should be vaccinated consistent with age-based recommendations.

3. Varicella vaccination

All adults without evidence of immunity to varicella should receive 2 doses of single-antigen varicella vaccine if not previously vaccinated or the second dose if they have received only one dose unless they have a medical contraindication. Special consideration should be given to those who 1) have close contact with persons at high risk for severe disease (e.g., health-care personnel and family contacts of persons with immunocompromising conditions) or 2) are at high risk for exposure or transmission (e.g., teachers; child care employees; residents and staff members of institutional settings, including correctional institutions; college students; military personnel; adolescents and adults living in households with children; nonpregnant women of childbearing age; and international travelers).

Evidence of immunity to varicella in adults includes any of the following: 1) documentation of 2 doses of varicella vaccine at least 4 weeks apart; 2) U.S.-born before 1980 (although for health-care personnel and pregnant women, birth before 1980 should not be considered evidence of immunity); 3) history of varicella based on diagnosis or verification of varicella by a health-care provider (for a patient reporting a history of or presenting with an atypical case, a mild case, or both, health-care providers should seek either an epidemiologic link with a typical varicella case or to a laboratory-confirmed case or evidence of laboratory confirmation, if it was performed at the time of acute disease); 4) history of herpes zoster based on health-care provider diagnosis or verification of herpes zoster by a health-care provider; or 5) laboratory evidence of immunity or laboratory confirmation of disease.

Pregnant women should be assessed for evidence of varicella immunity. Women who do not have evidence of immunity should receive the first dose of varicella vaccine upon completion or termination of pregnancy and before discharge from the health-care facility. The second dose should be administered 4–8 weeks after the first dose.

4. Herpes zoster vaccination

A single dose of zoster vaccine is recommended for adults aged 60 years and older regardless of whether they report a prior episode of herpes zoster. Persons with chronic medical conditions may be vaccinated unless their condition constitutes a contraindication.

5. Measles, mumps, rubella (MMR) vaccination

Measles component: Adults born before 1957 generally are considered immune to measles. Adults born during or after 1957 should receive 1 or more doses of MMR unless they have a medical contraindication, documentation of 1 or more doses, history of measles based on health-care provider diagnosis, or laboratory evidence of immunity.

A second dose of MMR is recommended for adults who 1) have been recently exposed to measles or are in an outbreak setting; 2) have been vaccinated previously with killed measles vaccine; 3) have been vaccinated with an unknown type of measles vaccine during 1963–1967; 4) are students in postsecondary educational institutions; 5) work in a health-care facility; or 6) plan to travel internationally.

Mumps component: Adults born before 1957 generally are considered immune to mumps. Adults born during or after 1957 should receive 1 dose of MMR unless they have a medical contraindication, history of mumps based on health-care provider diagnosis, or laboratory evidence of immunity.

A second dose of MMR is recommended for adults who 1) live in a community experiencing a mumps outbreak and are in an affected age group; 2) are students in postsecondary educational institutions; 3) work in a health-care facility; or 4) plan to travel internationally. For unvaccinated health-care personnel born before 1957 who do not have other evidence of mumps immunity, administering 1 dose on a routine basis should be considered and administering a second dose during an outbreak should be strongly considered.

Rubella component: 1 dose of MMR vaccine is recommended for women whose rubella vaccination history is unreliable or who lack laboratory evidence of immunity. For women of childbearing age, regardless of birth year, rubella immunity should be determined and women should be counseled regarding congenital rubella syndrome. Women who do not have evidence of immunity should receive MMR upon completion or termination of pregnancy and before discharge from the health-care facility.

6. Influenza vaccination

Medical indications: Chronic disorders of the cardiovascular or pulmonary systems, including asthma; chronic metabolic diseases, including diabetes mellitus, renal or hepatic dysfunction, hemoglobinopathies, or immunocompromising conditions (including immunocompromising conditions caused by medications or human immunodeficiency virus [HIV]); any condition that compromises respiratory function or the handling of respiratory secretions or that can increase the risk of aspiration (e.g., cognitive dysfunction, spinal cord injury, or seizure disorder or other neuromuscular disorder); and pregnancy during the influenza season. No data exist on the risk for severe or complicated influenza disease among persons with asplenia; however, influenza is a risk factor for secondary bacterial infections that can cause severe disease among persons with asplenia.

Occupational indications: All health-care personnel, including those employed by long-term care and assisted-living facilities, and caregivers of children less than 5 years old.

Other indications: Residents of nursing homes and other long-term care and assisted-living facilities; persons likely to transmit influenza to persons at high risk (e.g., in-home household contacts and caregivers of children aged less than 5 years old, persons 65 years old and older and persons of all ages with high-risk condition[s]); and anyone who would like to decrease their risk of getting influenza. Healthy, nonpregnant adults aged less than 50 years without high-risk medical conditions who are not contacts of severely immunocompromised persons in special care units can receive either intranasally administered live, attenuated influenza vaccine (FluMist®) or inactivated vaccine. Other persons should receive the inactivated vaccine.

7. Pneumococcal polysaccharide (PPSV) vaccination

Medical indications: Chronic lung disease (including asthma); chronic cardiovascular diseases; diabetes mellitus; chronic liver diseases, cirrhosis; chronic alcoholism, chronic renal failure or nephrotic syndrome; functional or anatomic asplenia (e.g., sickle cell disease or splenectomy [if elective splenectomy is planned, vaccinate at least 2 weeks before surgery]); immunocompromising conditions; and cochlear implants and cerebrospinal fluid leaks. Vaccinate as close to HIV diagnosis as possible.

Other indications: Residents of nursing homes or long-term care facilities and persons who smoke cigarettes. Routine use of PPSV is not recommended for Alaska Native or American Indian persons younger than 65 years unless they have underlying medical conditions that are PPSV indications. However, public health authorities may consider recommending PPSV for Alaska Natives and American Indians aged 50 through 64 years who are living in areas in which the risk of invasive pneumococcal disease is increased.

8. Revaccination with PPSV

One-time revaccination after 5 years for persons with chronic renal failure or nephrotic syndrome; functional or anatomic asplenia (e.g., sickle cell disease or splenectomy); and for persons with immunocompromising conditions. For persons aged 65 years and older, one-time revaccination if they were vaccinated 5 or more years previously and were aged less than 65 years at the time of primary vaccination.

9. Hepatitis A vaccination

Medical indications: Persons with chronic liver disease and persons who receive clotting factor concentrates.

Behavioral indications: Men who have sex with men and persons who use illegal drugs.

Occupational indications: Persons working with hepatitis A virus (HAV)-infected primates or with HAV in a research laboratory setting.

Other indications: Persons traveling to or working in countries that have high or intermediate endemicity of hepatitis A (a list of countries is available at wwwn.cdc.gov/travel/contentdiseases.aspx) and any person seeking protection from HAV infection.

Single-antigen vaccine formulations should be administered in a 2-dose schedule at either 0 and 6–12 months (Havrix®), or 0 and 6–18 months (Vaqta®). If the combined hepatitis A and hepatitis B vaccine (Twinrix®) is used, administer 3 doses at 0, 1, and 6 months; alternatively, a 4-dose schedule, administered on days 0, 7 and 21 to 30 followed by a booster dose at month 12 may be used.

10. Hepatitis B vaccination

Medical indications: Persons with end-stage renal disease, including patients receiving hemodialysis; persons with HIV infection; and persons with chronic liver disease.

Occupational indications: Health-care personnel and public-safety workers who are exposed to blood or other potentially infectious body fluids.

Behavioral indications: Sexually active persons who are not in a long-term, mutually monogamous relationship (e.g., persons with more than 1 sex partner during the previous 6 months); persons seeking evaluation or treatment for a sexually transmitted disease (STD); current or recent injection-drug users; and men who have sex with men.

Other indications: Household contacts and sex partners of persons with chronic hepatitis B virus (HBV) infection; clients and staff members of institutions for persons with developmental disabilities; international travelers to countries with high or intermediate prevalence of chronic HBV infection (a list of countries is available at wwwn.cdc.gov/travel/contentdiseases.aspx); and any adult seeking protection from HBV infection.

Hepatitis B vaccination is recommended for all adults in the following settings: STD treatment facilities; HIV testing and treatment facilities; facilities providing drug-abuse treatment and prevention services; health-care settings targeting services to injection-drug users or men who have sex with men; correctional facilities; end-stage renal disease programs and facilities for chronic hemodialysis patients; and institutions and nonresidential daycare facilities for persons with developmental disabilities.

If the combined hepatitis A and hepatitis B vaccine (Twinrix®) is used, administer 3 doses at 0, 1, and 6 months; alternatively, a 4-dose schedule, administered on days 0, 7 and 21 to 30 followed by a booster dose at month 12 may be used.

Special formulation indications: For adult patients receiving hemodialysis or with other immunocompromising conditions, 1 dose of 40 µg/mL (Recombivax HB®) administered on a 3-dose schedule or 2 doses of 20 µg/mL (Engerix-B®) administered simultaneously on a 4-dose schedule at 0, 1, 2 and 6 months.

11. Meningococcal vaccination

Medical indications: Adults with anatomic or functional asplenia, or terminal complement component deficiencies.

Other indications: First-year college students living in dormitories; microbiologists who are routinely exposed to isolates of *Neisseria meningitidis*; military recruits; and persons who travel to or live in countries in which meningococcal disease is hyperendemic or epidemic (e.g., the "meningitis belt" of sub-Saharan Africa during the dry season [December-June]), particularly if their contact with local populations will be prolonged. Vaccination is required by the government of Saudi Arabia for all travelers to Mecca during the annual Hajj.

Meningococcal conjugate (MCV) vaccine is preferred for adults with any of the preceding indications who are aged 55 years or younger, although meningococcal polysaccharide vaccine (MPSV) is an acceptable alternative. Revaccination with MCV after 5 years might be indicated for adults previously vaccinated with MPSV who remain at increased risk for infection (e.g., persons residing in areas in which disease is epidemic).

12. Selected conditions for which *Haemophilus influenzae* type b (Hib) vaccine may be used

Hib vaccine generally is not recommended for persons aged 5 years and older. No efficacy data are available on which to base a recommendation concerning use of Hib vaccine for older children and adults. However, studies suggest good immunogenicity in persons who have sickle cell disease, leukemia, or HIV infection or who have had a splenectomy; administering 1 dose of vaccine to these persons is not contraindicated.

13. Immunocompromising conditions

Inactivated vaccines generally are acceptable (e.g., pneumococcal, meningococcal, and influenza [trivalent inactivated influenza vaccine]), and live vaccines generally are avoided in persons with immune deficiencies or immunocompromising conditions. Information on specific conditions is available at www.cdc.gov/vaccines/pubs/acip-list.htm.

For your office practice, you are encouraged to adopt a more specific schedule. For example, where the harmonized schedule might give you some latitude with what age to give the dose for the measles-mumps-rubella vaccine, it would be more appropriate for you and your colleagues to pick either 12 or 15 months. When all practitioners sharing an office adopt a uniform practice, they prevent parental and staff confusion and misunderstanding as well as mistakes in vaccine administration and patient scheduling.

Adoption of Immunization-Specific Practices

EDUCATION OF SELF AND STAFF

Immunization practices certainly have evolved over the last century, and much of the development has accelerated since the enactment of the National Childhood Vaccine Injury Act of 1986 (PL 99-660), which established the national Vaccine Injury Compensation Program (VICP), a no-fault alternative to the tort system for resolving vaccine injury claims. This legislation protects vaccine providers and manufacturers from frivolous lawsuits directed against routine childhood immunization.

Although in the 1980s it was routine for a child in the first year of life to receive three injections and three oral doses of polio, now the typical infant by 12 months of age may receive 24 separate injections against vaccine-preventable disease. Almost each year the routine childhood vaccine schedule is altered in a substantive way. Most recently, the newest routine vaccination schedule includes annual influenza vaccinations for children and adolescents through 18 years of age. Such changes require a practitioner's continuing education and practice advancement.

A number of electronic web sites provide announcements and updates of vaccines in form delivered for health care practitioners; the CDC provides a web site (www.cdc.gov/vaccines) with information resources for both parents and health care practitioners including sections on updates. In addition, the Immunization Action Coalition, a not-for-profit group dedicated to the dissemination of scientifically correct immunization information, also has a very useful web site (www.immunize.org). The latter invites practitioners to sign up for routine mailings of updates on immunization practices. Similarly, providers can access the CDC's Morbidity and Mortality Weekly Report (MMWR) online. These provide updates and statements from ACIP. Furthermore, the AAP publishes on its web site (www.aap.org) its policy statements and recommendation online for members and nonmembers alike.

Paper-based resources are more difficult to keep up to date, but important ones include the paper-based publication *MMWR* published by the CDC and the *Red Book* published by the AAP. The *Red Book* not only does an outstanding job with vaccine-related issues but also includes a host of information for a general practitioner on pediatric and adolescent infectious diseases. The CDC publishes the "Pink Book" both in paper and online too. It is formally entitled *Epidemiology and Prevention of Vaccine Preventable Diseases.*

The CDC and the Medical University of South Carolina have sponsored the development of an electronic-based educational program called Teaching Immunization Delivery and Evaluation (TIDE). Its web site is http://www2.edserv.musc.edu/tide, and the program is endorsed by the Ambulatory Pediatric Association and the Society of Adolescent Medicine. It is a flexible tool to teach immunization delivery, and it uses clinical scenarios that inspire problem solving. Self-contained modules are available that provide continued education credit.

ASSESSMENT OF INDIVIDUAL NEEDS

Each patient is unique, but the success of the routine immunization schedule depends on its universality. Precautions and contraindications exist, and the children and adults who most frequently attend health care providers' offices have relatively higher rates of chronic conditions than the general population. These conditions raise questions of contraindications and precautions. Therefore, individuals must be assessed for their individual needs. Even misperceptions of contraindications can lead to delays and require catch-up. Practitioners should be familiar with the routine schedules (Tables 1 and 2) as well as the general precautions of contraindications associated with each vaccine.

One of the most important resources available for the busy practitioner is a chart developed by the CDC organized by condition that specifies which vaccines are contraindicated by that condition. This chart is on the CDC web site under the tab of Healthcare Professionals. It is entitled "Guide to Contraindications" (www.cdc.gov/vaccines/recs/vac-admin/contraindications.htm).

The CDC has developed survey tools that are available freely to download from its web site (www.cdc.gov/vaccines). The practitioner can use this with the individual patient to assess vaccine needs. Assessment tools are available online for both adults and children.

PATIENT EDUCATION

Patient and parent education is incredibly important in applying immunizations. After all, we are giving a form of a biologic with known rates and associations with adverse events to large numbers of persons who are often well and without a medical need or condition. We should inform the patient, and, in the case of a child or adolescent not yet at the age of majority, the parent as best we can about the immunizations, the diseases for which we are vaccinating, the nature of the benefits from the vaccines, as well as the common adverse reactions and possible severe adverse reactions that might occur. The patients and parents should learn who should receive the vaccines and who should not and what they should do in case of an adverse event. This information is complex in depth and breadth, but the National Childhood Vaccine Injury Act of 1986 that created protection for vaccine providers and manufacturers at the same time created regulations with a uniform system of vaccine information statements to be provided. The National Immunization Program publishes brief vaccine-specific statements for all of the routine vaccines given to children and adults. These Vaccine Information Statements (VISs) are published in a highly readable format (www.cdc.gov/vaccines/pubs/vis) and are required by U.S. law to be provided to the parent and recipient before each dose of certain vaccines including those on a routine childhood vaccine schedule. VISs also exist for some of the more exotic vaccines, such as the Japanese encephalitis vaccine, the smallpox vaccine, the typhoid vaccines, the yellow fever vaccine, as well as for the rabies vaccines. The Immunization Action Coalition (www.immunize.org) has partnered with the CDC and has translated the VISs for each vaccine into more than 20 different languages. More detailed information for the vaccines can be obtained from the statements from the ACIP (www.cdc.gov/vaccines/recs/acip), the Food and Drug Administration-approved package inserts, and the AAP's *Red Book.*

PREVACCINATION PREPARATION

Not only should the parent and recipient of the vaccine be provided the VIS, but efforts should be taken to minimize the discomfort of the recipient. Information plays a large role. A study done at the Mayo Clinic demonstrated that informing the child prior to the visit actually decreased the amount of distress observed at the time of the visit. Furthermore, efforts at the time of the visit including distraction or relaxation techniques can prevent or reduce distress associated with the vaccine. Office staff should learn methods of successful communication, distraction, and relaxation techniques to facilitate routine immunizations.

CURRENT DIAGNOSIS

- At each patient contact, practitioners should review the patient's immunization record for vaccines due and overdue.

For some of the vaccines, antipyretics such as acetaminophen (Tylenol) or ibuprofen (Advil) might be administered at the time of immunization and then at regular intervals specific to that drug for the following 24 hours to reduce the occurrence and the severity of fever as well as the local injection pain that might occur with immunization.

The *Red Book* Committee, the Committee on Infectious Diseases of the AAP, recommends that practitioners consider a variety of efforts to minimize the discomfort of immunization including specific injection techniques, the use of multiple vaccinators to immunize simultaneously rather than serially, as well as possibly local anesthetics and nonpharmacologic agents.

VACCINE DELIVERY

Some vaccines are given intramuscularly (IM) or subcutaneously (SC); still others, via the mouth or nose. IM vaccines should be given deep into a muscle mass. Practitioners should use the anterolateral thigh muscle injections for children younger than 18 months and then move to the deltoid muscle in children older than 18 months when the muscle mass of the deltoid is large enough. SC injections should be given in subcutaneous fat of the anterolateral thigh or triceps with a shorter needle inserted at an angle.

PREVENTION OF NEEDLE INJURY

For the safety of the patient, parent, and provider, efforts should be made to minimize the exposure to an accidental needle stick. Although the risk of accidental inoculation with the patient's blood is minimal in immunization, as with the use of sharps in any office, employees should examine the safety needles available and choose a safety needle appropriate for minimizing accidental needle sticks. The office should provide a child-proof sharps container that allows for rapid disposal of the needle with a minimal amount of effort. The container should be checked regularly for function and emptied frequently to avoid overfilling during the workday.

DOCUMENTATION AND RECORDS

All offices should adopt a standard of documentation of immunizations. The physician's or nurse's order for a vaccine should not be used in place of documentation that the vaccine was given. Documentation of the vaccine administered should include the species and the brand name given as well as the lot number. The patient record should also include the location, date, and time. Such a record would be made more useful if all the vaccine-antigens could be viewed at once with regard to series and dates. To best manage combinations currently available as well as future possibilities, the record should be organized by vaccine-antigen and not common vaccine combinations. This requires that a combination vaccine then appear in several antigen categories. Furthermore, the record would be enhanced by clarification when vaccines were not given because of precaution or contraindication as the basis. We have an ongoing problem with the adoption of chickenpox vaccine (Varivax). Those children who previously acquired chickenpox do not need the chickenpox vaccine, but we need to document the occurrence of that disease and its date to prevent overvaccination.

CURRENT THERAPY

- Providing routine immunizations requires an office to organize its educational activities, practice standards, communication methods, and documentation strategies.

RECORD SHARING AND REGISTRIES

Vaccine registries at the community level or regional level dramatically reduce the miscommunication and the need for occurrence of both overimmunization as well as empowering physicians and nurses to feel better about taking advantage of missed opportunities in vaccinating children. Most parents whose children are undervaccinated report that their children are "up to date." Records that accurately reflect the child's full vaccine record would better equip the practitioner in best managing those patients.

VACCINE STORAGE

Storage requirements are much more complex than traditionally practiced. Offices must provide proper refrigeration as well as freezers for vaccines. Certain vaccines require refrigeration, other vaccines require freezing, and some vaccines are more heat labile or cold labile than others. Proper care and maintenance of refrigerator includes the purchase of appropriate dedicated equipment, the monitoring of the temperatures, the purchase of proper containers to be used on the shelves, and adequate space to allow for prevention of errors with storage. Furthermore, the staff must be trained and scheduled to provide oversight in the case of a power or equipment failure.

ASSESSMENT OF THE OVERALL PROCESS AND ITS OUTCOMES

Assessing an individual's immunization needs, providing the vaccines, and recording them properly in the individual's record is no longer adequate for the assessment of the overall process. Each office should make efforts to assess its overall practice. Each office must monitor the rates of on-time immunizations as well as up-to-date immunization and look for opportunities to improve these metrics. The effort of collecting this information has led to improvements in rates of on-time vaccination. Immunization practices are evolving and the maintenance of quality as well as the rapid adoption and improvement of practices require regular office meetings of staff. Physicians, nurses, and receptionists must be aware of new changes. Receptionists' misunderstanding of the vaccine needs frequently leads to missed opportunities to vaccinate. Misunderstanding between physicians and other clinicians can also lead to failed attempts. Regular office meetings should occur throughout the year to evaluate the vaccine schedule, the success of vaccinating the panel of patients, and considerations for practice improvements.

STANDING ORDERS

One of the most successful approaches in the office to make real efforts to improve immunization rates above and beyond that driven by the well child care schedule is to create standing orders that permit nursing staff to provide vaccines to patients without a doctor visit. This is particularly helpful with flu season and for acute care contacts with the patient. Such standing orders need to be written in such a way that they meet state law, facilitate nurse assessment of the patient's vaccine needs, as well as rule out any precautions or contraindications for the child's immunization. Materials exist online at the Immunization Action Coalition (www.immunize.org) that can help in writing such standing orders.

RECALL REMINDERS AND TRACKING

A second method for improving office vaccination rates are recall reminders and tracking. Providers should develop proactive approaches toward their patient panels to ensure compliance with the routine childhood schedule. Offices should contact patients when vaccines are due. Additional efforts should be made for those subjects who are behind in immunizations. Finally, offices should have systems to identify those children in families for whom the flu vaccine is indicated and make efforts every autumn to contact the families proactively and schedule immunization visits. The broadening of the flu vaccine indications has made this a major issue for office practices who care for either children or adults or both.

REPORTING ADVERSE EVENTS

The same laws that created the vaccine information statements and the protection for vaccine providers from frivolous lawsuits have also created the Vaccine Adverse Events Reporting System (VAERS). This system, set up by the federal government, collects information on adverse events believed to be related to immunization. These include certain ones required by regulation as well as those temporally associated with the immunizations that strike the provider or family as potentially significant. Vaccine manufacturers and providers are in fact required to report certain adverse events occurring after immunization whether or not they were caused by the immunization.

VAERS has actually led to the discontinuation of certain office-based immunization practices including the use of the tetravalent oral rhesus rotavirus vaccine (RotaShield). It has also helped to protect vaccines from unwarranted claims of harm. Although it has its weaknesses, statistical approaches have made it a powerful tool. Participation for providers of vaccines is required. All office staff, including receptionists, must understand the legal requirements of reporting.

VACCINES FOR CHILDREN

The U.S. government set up a program entitled Vaccines for Children (VFC) that enables providers to receive free-of-charge vaccines that can be given to patients with certain conditions including those who are younger than 18 years and are Medicaid eligible, uninsured, American Indian or Alaska Native, or whose health insurance benefit plan does not include vaccinations. Some recipients may be charged a vaccine provider fee, which is a limited amount. The federal government purchases vaccine for the VFC program and then distributes it to the state's health departments, which redistributes to the qualified providers. To learn how an office can participate, the VFC program can be contacted at the CDC through its web pages.

Common Problems

Offices that provide vaccines to their patients struggle with common problems in immunization practice. These include missed or delayed vaccinations, vaccine shortages, catch-up, change-ups, decisions not to vaccinate, true and false contraindications, multiple providers, and incomplete records. One cannot make these problems disappear, but one can prepare for them, prevent them from happening in many cases, and minimize the harm when they do occur.

MISSED OR DELAYED VACCINATIONS

Although daycare and school-based requirements have resulted in very high vaccine rates by school entry, on-time immunization is tragically low. Many children do not get their vaccines when due and are left at risk. Although this occurs more frequently among those with multiple providers and those who do not have health insurance, practitioners can change their office practices to reduce the problems in delayed immunizations. First of all, do not relegate routine immunization to the well child visit. Second, be assertive in obtaining the complete vaccine records from your patient's previous providers of health care. Third, create standing order policies to facilitate your office staff providing vaccines without a physician visit.

Furthermore, the practitioner should have charts available in the office explaining how to proceed with a child who has not received vaccines on time. Practitioners cannot be expected to memorize this information. It is complex, age dependent, and vaccine specific. The information must be available for ready reference. With the American Academies of Pediatrics and Family Practitioners, the ACIP has created catch-up schedules (www.cdc.gov/vaccines/recs/schedules).

There are two catch-up schedules: one for children 4 months to 6 years of age and one for 7 to 18 years of age (Table 2).

LOCUS OF RESPONSIBILITY

Providers cannot expect their patients or their patients' parents to take responsibility for timely vaccination. Patient-held immunization records have failed to improve vaccination rates. Office practitioners must also consider that even in a specialty practice their patients may be expecting them to monitor their immunization needs along with providing them the vaccines that they need. Providers, whether of specialty or primary care, must assess their individual patients and determine who is monitoring the patients' vaccination status and needs. Specialists must never assume that the patient is cognizant of the need or that a primary care provider is actively playing that role. All too often, patients relinquish their relationships with primary care providers once they begin an ongoing relationship with a specialist.

VACCINE SHORTAGES

Ongoing shortages do occur with vaccine supplies. Most famously are the shortages with the influenza vaccine, but we also have shortages with vaccines when there have been changes in use or recommendations such as the adoption of the adolescent diphtheria/tetanus (Td) at 11 years of age and the rapid acceptance of the pneumococcal conjugate vaccine (Prevnar). Manufacturers struggle to produce adequate supplies knowing the expense of creating inadequate supplies actually leads to distrust and anger directed toward the manufacturer as well as difficulties in completing on-time immunizations. Manufacturing too much vaccine can lead to unusable stockpiles of expired vaccine product. Therefore manufacturers seek to reach a balance. Shortages are communicated best to office practices in the United States through the online web site (http://www.cdc.gov/vaccines/vac-gen/shortages/) at the CDC where information is provided for the basis of shortages as well as explanations for what the practitioners should do during this time. In most situations the vaccine providers are expected to record those people who have not received the vaccine on time because of the shortage and are to be called back in a timely manner when vaccine supplies are available.

CATCH-UP

Catching children up on missed or delayed vaccinations is a major problem. This activity results not just because of shortages but because of parents' delays in immunization. The third and fourth children in a family often suffer delays in immunizations because of parents' issues with the organization and scheduling of appropriate on-time well child visits. Offices that rely on the well child visit schedules as the only basis for immunization have higher rates of vaccine delays and more problems with catch-up than those who use every opportunity of every visit to assess vaccine status of the child and to vaccinate on time. To make matters worse, the current schedule when on time can call for five injections at once. Imagine the child who has accumulated significant delays and now needs to be caught up. One of the major difficulties of catch-up is the problem of information. I previously mentioned the chart that all vaccine providers should have available to facilitate catching up immunizations (see Table 2).

CHANGE-UPS

Change-ups are also difficult because the new adoption of a vaccine can lead to some confusion for those who previously received an older moiety. For example, the recipients of the meningococcal polysaccharide vaccine (Menomune) are not due for the meningococcal conjugate vaccine (Menacta), but those who previously received the adolescent tetanus-diphtheria (Td) vaccine may certainly benefit from the new adolescent tetanus-diphtheria-reduced-dose-acellular pertussis vaccine (Adacel, Boostrix).

DECISIONS NOT TO VACCINATE

There are many reasons why patients may fail to be vaccinated. Common reasons include misunderstandings by the practitioner or parent of contraindications regarding vaccines. These are vaccine specific and complex in language in application. Many more people fail to get vaccines because of contraindications than those who truly have them. Other common reasons include parents' failure to attend to the well-visit schedule and the practitioners' failures to use other visits as the basis for immunization.

Some parents, however, actually consider immunization and choose to refuse. They are suspicious that the vaccines do not work, are not necessary or at least no longer necessary, are not safe, weaken the immune system, provide a poorer immunity than the actual diseases they target, that children receive too many vaccines, and that some vaccine lots are contaminated. Practitioners should be familiar with these concerns and their rebuttals. Two good sources for information on these include CDC (www.cdc.gov/vaccines) and the Immunization Action Coalition (www.immunize.org). The latter organization has actually collected stories of parents who chose not to vaccinate their children and then suffered the consequences of vaccine-preventable disease.

TRUE AND FALSE CONTRAINDICATIONS

Perhaps one of the most common problems with immunization delivery in the United States with regard to the failure of the provider stems from common misconceptions regarding the presence or absence of contraindication to immunization. Although some contraindications are vaccine specific, certain principles apply. First, family histories of adverse events are never contraindications to immunization. Second, household pregnancy or breast-feeding is never a contraindication to immunization. Third, the presence of an illness or injury by itself is not a contraindication. If the illness is moderate or severe, with or without a fever, then a vaccine's administration may be contraindicated. Although local and systemic adverse reactions do occur with vaccines, these are in general not contraindications to further doses.

It would be impossible for a practitioner to memorize contraindications. The CDC (www.cdc.gov/vaccines) has prepared a user-friendly online table that is indexed by disease and condition to guide the practitioner. This table should be available for ready use throughout the day.

MULTIPLE PROVIDERS AND INCOMPLETE RECORDS

Both under- and overimmunization occur much more frequently among patients who use more than one provider. Regional registries that allow practitioners to share their vaccine records greatly reduce both missed opportunities to vaccinate as well as the inadvertent administration of unnecessary doses. Practitioners should work with their local and state health departments to develop regional vaccine registries.

For all of the problems we face, for all of the intricacies of practices we must adopt, there is perhaps no one practice more important to the health of the community than the delivery of routine immunizations. Although it is worth the effort, it requires an ongoing commitment to continuing education, practice assessment, and evidence-based improvement of the office practice.

REFERENCES

American Academy of Family Physicians. AAFP Immunization Resources, http://www.aafp.org/online/en/home/clinical/immunizationres.html; 2009 [Accessed May 8, 2009]. This web site provides links to specific AAFP recommendations for immunizations.

American Academy of Pediatrics. AAP Policy. http://aappolicy.aappublications.org/ [Accessed May 8, 2009]. This web site provides links to the AAP policies including its online Red Book with its recommendations regarding vaccines and immunization.

Centers for Disease Control and Prevention. ACIP Recommendations. http://www.cdc.gov/vaccines/pubs/ACIP-list.htm. This page last modified on February 5, 2009 [Accessed May 8, 2009]. This web site provides links to the ACIP recommendations, which are updated annually as new data dictate. All of the documents listed on this page are current, regardless of their publication dates.

Centers for Disease Control and Prevention. 2009 Child & Adolescent Immunization Schedules, http://www.cdc.gov/vaccines/recs/schedules/child-schedule.htm. This page last modified on February 26, 2009 [Accessed May 8, 2009]. This web site provides the harmonized schedule for children and adolescents with informative footnotes and additional charts for catch-up for children between the ages of 4 months and 18 years.

Centers for Disease Control and Prevention. Adult Immunization Schedule. http://www.cdc.gov/vaccines/recs/schedules/adult-schedule.htm. This page last modified on April 7, 2009 [Accessed May 8, 2009]. This web site provides a harmonized schedule for anyone over 18 years old with informative footnotes.

Centers for Disease Control and Prevention. Vaccine Information Statements. http://www.cdc.gov/vaccines/pubs/vis/default.htm. This page last modified on May 6, 2009 [Accessed May 8, 2009]. This web page lists links to all of the federally mandated Vaccine Information Statements that vaccine providers must use when informing parents of the recommended vaccines to be given to children.

Centers for Disease Control and Prevention. Vaccine Management: Recommendations for Storage and Handling Selected Biologicals. November 15, 2007. http://www.cdc.gov/vaccines/pubs/vac-mgt-book.htm; 2007. This page last modified on July 21, 2008 [Accessed May 8, 2009]. This document provides vaccine-specific instructions on storage of vaccines.

Immunization Action Coalition. State Mandates on Immunization and Vaccine-Preventable Diseases. http://www.immunize.org/laws/. Last updated December 18, 2008 [Accessed May 8, 2009]. This web site provides specific state-by-state rules for school and day-care attendance.

Pickering LK, Baker CJ, Long SS, McMillan JA, editors. Red Book: 2006 Report of the Committee on Infectious Diseases. 27th ed. Elk Grove Village, IL: American Academy of Pediatrics; 2006.

Shefer A, Briss P, Rodewald L, et al. Improving immunization coverage rates: an evidence-based review of the literature. Epidemiologic Rev 1999;21 (1):96–142. A systematic review of the published studies of interventions to improve vaccine uptake.

Travel Medicine

Method of
Aarthi Chary, MD, Upinder Singh, MD, and Brian G. Blackburn, MD

Every year, more than 700 million travelers cross international borders, and more than 50 million people from industrialized countries travel to the developing world. It is estimated that 20% to 70% of these travelers develop illness associated with their travel, and up to 8% seek medical care. Given the magnitude of global travel, emerging infections, and increasing knowledge about travel-related illnesses, the field of travel medicine has grown rapidly.

Travel medicine is devoted to the overall safety of the traveler, including environmental risks, infectious diseases, and other health concerns. Primary care physicians are the first point of contact for many patients planning travel and should be able to advise the subset of travelers who are in good health, have simple itineraries, and are visiting low-risk destinations. Providers must have an understanding of travel-related infectious diseases, noninfectious health concerns, indications for vaccination and chemoprophylaxis, and recognition and management of major syndromes in the ill returned traveler. They should be well versed in the resources available to providers and patients, including organizations, websites, textbooks, and journals. As suggested by the Infectious Diseases Society of America, travelers with special needs, preexisting medical issues, or complex itineraries should seek care in a specialized travel clinic.

Pretravel Counseling

GENERAL CONSIDERATIONS

History taking during the pretravel visit should include preexisting medical conditions, allergies and current medications, vaccination and prior travel history, and previous travel-related illnesses. In addition, pregnancy and other immunocompromised states can significantly alter advice on risk and management of disease. Itinerary information that should be considered includes specific destinations, duration and nature of travel, potential food and water sources, anticipated climate and altitude, medical care accessibility, and planned modes of travel. Questions regarding specific activities—such as work in refugee camps or hospitals, adventure travel, or exposure to domestic animals or wildlife—are also helpful in assessing the risk of certain infectious diseases.

Individuals who are returning to their country of origin to visit friends or relatives (called VFR travelers) are a distinct population. These persons comprise 25% to 40% of travelers from industrialized countries to developing nations. As a group, they (and their children) are less likely to seek pretravel health advice, be adequately vaccinated, or adhere to recommendations regarding arthropod avoidance or chemoprophylaxis. This behavior is often related to incorrect perceptions of immunity and risk of transmissible diseases. Furthermore, VFR travelers are more likely than others to have increased contact with local residents, to stay in less developed conditions, to travel for longer durations, and to observe fewer food restrictions. Several lines of evidence show that they are more likely than other travelers to acquire serious infectious diseases while traveling. Because VFR travelers are less likely to seek pretravel care, primary care physicians should ask immigrant patients about potential or impending travel plans so that appropriate pretravel counseling can be pursued.

ARTHROPOD AVOIDANCE

One of the most important measures in preventing several travel-related infections is avoiding insect bites. Travelers should wear clothing that reduces the amount of exposed skin, sleep under insecticide-impregnated bed nets, stay in well-screened or air-conditioned rooms, and use insect repellant. The most effective topical insect repellant is diethyl-m-toluamide (DEET). Higher concentrations provide longer duration of protection; recommended concentrations of 20% to 50% provide coverage for at least 4 hours, and longer-acting formulations exist. DEET is safe for infants and children older than 2 months of age and during the second and third trimesters of pregnancy. DEET should be applied before sunscreen; otherwise, it can decrease the efficacy of the sunscreen. The insecticide permethrin (Permanone) can be used to treat clothing, bedding, and mosquito nets for long-lasting protection against insects.

ENVIRONMENTAL PRECAUTIONS

Sunscreen application (sun protection factor ≥15) and safe practices regarding water and food should be emphasized. Pretravel counseling should address avoidance of swimming in fresh water in areas endemic for schistosomiasis or leptospirosis, such as sub-Saharan Africa, Southeast Asia, the Middle East, north/northeastern South America, and the Caribbean.

For travelers to high altitudes, acute mountain sickness and high-altitude pulmonary edema (HAPE) or cerebral edema (HACE) are important considerations. Manifestations range from headache, nausea, and dizziness to coma and death over hours to days. Factors that contribute to acute mountain sickness include rate of ascent, altitude reached, and altitude at which the traveler sleeps. Approximately 25% of those who rapidly ascend to 2500 m, 50% of those who ascend to 4000 m within a week, and up to 80% of those who fly directly to 3800 m develop acute mountain sickness. Therefore, gradual ascent with acclimatization periods is recommended. Sleeping altitudes should not increase by more than 300 to 500 m per night, and each 1000 m ascended necessitates an extra day of acclimatization. Acetazolamide (Diamox) 125 to 250 mg twice daily, beginning 1 to 2 days before ascent and continuing for at least 48 hours after reaching maximum altitude, may prevent or mitigate acute mountain sickness. Mild symptoms may resolve if further ascent is not attempted, but for more severe or persistent symptoms or symptoms of HACE or HAPE, descent is paramount. In such cases, acetazolamide 250 to 500 mg twice daily should be administered. Dexamethasone (Decadron)[1] may be used in severe cases, and nifedipine (Adalat)[1] is sometimes used for severe HAPE, but only by experienced practitioners. Oxygen and hyperbaric therapy can serve as temporizing measures while emergency descent is achieved.

DEEP VENOUS THROMBOSIS AND JET LAG

Prolonged immobilization during air travel can increase the risk of deep venous thrombosis, especially in patients with additional risk factors (e.g., smoking, pregnancy, prior thrombosis, malignancy, obesity, recent surgery, use of oral contraceptives). Travelers should exercise their calf muscles, limit alcohol ingestion, maintain hydration, and avoid restrictive clothing, particularly on flights lasting 6 hours or longer. Below-the-knee compression stockings are also beneficial.

Jet lag may be an issue, particularly with travel across five or more time zones; eastward travel is associated with more symptoms than westward travel. Although no interventions are proven effective, the use of melatonin[1,7] 2 to 5 mg at bedtime beginning on the first night of travel and continuing for several nights thereafter may decrease symptoms. Changing activities and lighting patterns to correspond with the destination time zone before travel and use of short-acting hypnotics such as benzodiazepines or zolpidem (Ambien)[1] have also been advocated.

PERSONAL SAFETY

Injuries, primarily caused by road traffic accidents, are the leading cause of preventable death in travelers, and appropriate preventive precautions should be undertaken. Travelers should also remain abreast of political and civil conflicts in their planned destination. Up-to-date safety information for travelers to particular destinations can be obtained from the U.S. Department of State website (http://travel.state.gov/ [accessed May 8, 2009]). Sexually transmitted diseases are another concern in travelers.

MEDICAL KITS

Patients should prepare a personal medical kit, including analgesics, topical care for rashes and insect bites, basic first aid supplies, and destination-specific supplies (e.g., sunscreen, altitude-sickness medications), as well as antihistamines, antidiarrheals, antiemetics, antimalarials, or prophylactic antibiotics as appropriate. Patients with preexisting medical conditions should take adequate supplies of their own medications, and travelers should consider supplemental travel, health, and evacuation insurance, especially on prolonged trips. Excellent resources include the U.S. Department of State (http://travel.state.gov/ [accessed May 8, 2009]) for information regarding travel insurance and listings of health care professionals and hospitals abroad. The websites of the Centers for Disease Control and Prevention (CDC) (http://www.cdc.gov/travel [accessed May 8, 2009]) and the World Health Organization (http://www.who.int/ith [accessed May 8, 2009]) offer outbreak and travel notices for destination countries.

Immunizations

Vaccine-preventable infections are a major cause of morbidity among international travelers. The risk is dependent on the traveler's itinerary, nature of travel, and personal medical history. Vaccines considered at the pretravel visit should include both routine and destination-specific immunizations. In addition, each patient must be assessed for contraindications for each vaccination. Table 1 summarizes vaccines commonly used for travelers.

---

[1]Not FDA approved for this indication.
[7]Available as dietary supplement.

TABLE 1 Recommended and Required Travel-Related Immunizations*

Vaccine Name	Type (Route)	Schedule	Dosage	Indication	Comments, Adverse Effects, and Precautions[†]
Hepatitis A Havrix, Vaqta	Inactivated virus (IM)	Adults and children ≥1 y: 2 doses at 0 mo and 6–18 mo	Age 1–18 y: 720 EU Havrix or 25 U Vaqta (0.5 mL) Age ≥19 y: 1440 EU Havrix or 50 U Vaqta (1.0 mL)	Now a universally recommended childhood vaccine in US For unvaccinated travelers: travel to most developing countries	Two doses appear to provide lifelong immunity (no booster recommended); use either vaccine interchangeably for 1st and 2nd dose; 2nd dose is still effective if given late. Protective antibody may appear as early as 2 wk after vaccination; immune globulin still is sometimes given instead to travelers with imminent departure. May cause LR, occasional fever, headache. Pregnancy: safety unknown
Hepatitis B Engerix-B	Recombinant hepatitis B surface antigen (IM)	Age 0–19 y: 3 doses at 0, 1, and 6 mo Age ≥20 y: 3 doses as above or 4 doses at 0, 1, 2, and 12 mo	Age 0–19 y: 10 μg (0.5 mL) Age ≥20 y: 20 μg (1.0 mL)	Now a universally recommended childhood vaccine in US For unvaccinated travelers: persons likely to be in contact with blood or body fluids; persons residing in areas of intermediate to high endemicity	Use interchangeably with Recombivax-HB in 3rd dose only. No need to restart if schedule is interrupted. May cause LR (uncommon), fever (rare). Pregnancy: not contraindicated
Recombivax-HB	Recombinant hepatitis B surface antigen (IM)	Age 0–19 y: 3 doses at 0, 1, and 6 mo, OR for age 11–15 y only, 2 doses at 0 and 4–6 mo Age ≥20 y: 3 doses at 0, 1, and 6 mo	Age 0–19 y: 5 μg (0.5 mL) if 3 doses are given, or 10 μg if 2 doses are given Age ≥20 y: 10 μg (1.0 mL)	Same indication as for Engerix-B	Use interchangeably with Engerix-B in 3rd dose only. No need to restart if schedule interrupted. May cause LR (uncommon), fever (rare). Pregnancy: not contraindicated
Hepatitis A and B (Combined) Twinrix	Inactivated hepatitis A plus recombinant hepatitis B surface antigen (IM)	Age ≥18 y: 3 doses at 0, 1, and 6 mo, OR 4 doses at 0 d, 7 d, 21–31 d, and 12 mo (accelerated schedule)	Age ≥18 y: 720 EU (hepatitis A) and 20 μg (1.0) (hepatitis B)	See individual vaccines above.	See individual vaccines above. Pregnancy: safety unknown
Immune Globulin Immune globulin, GamaSTAN	Human immune globulin (IM)	Travel <3 mo: single dose given before travel Travel >3 mo: give 1 dose before travel, then for travel >5 mo repeat dose every 4–5 mo	Travel duration <2–3 mo: 0.02 mL/kg body weight Travel duration >2–3 mo: 0.06 mL/kg body weight	For prevention of hepatitis A in travelers to areas of intermediate to high endemicity Indicated for unvaccinated older adults, immunocompromised persons, and patients with liver disease or other chronic medical conditions who have <2 wk before departure (give in combination with initial dose of vaccine); persons who cannot receive or decline hepatitis A vaccination (including persons <1 y of age and those allergic to vaccine component); nonimmune persons based on pretravel hepatitis A antibody testing	Should not be given <2 wk after or <3 mo before measles, mumps, rubella, or varicella vaccine; give at a separate anatomic site from any simultaneous dose of hepatitis A vaccine. Single dose provides approximately 3 mo of effective protection.

Continued

Travel Medicine

157

TABLE 1 Recommended and Required Travel-Related Immunizations*—Cont'd

Vaccine Name	Type (Route)	Schedule	Dosage	Indication	Comments, Adverse Effects, and Precautions†
Meningococcal Infection					
Menomune (MPSV4)	Inactivated bacterial polysaccharide (SC) Quadrivalent (serotypes A, C, Y, and W-135)	Age >2 y (vaccine of choice for age >55 y): single dose. *Booster:* at 5 y in adults and children ≥4 y, or at 2–3 y in children 2–4 y	50 µg (0.5 mL)	Travelers to areas with epidemic meningococcal disease (e.g., African "meningitis belt" in dry season); religious pilgrims to Saudi Arabia; persons with asplenia or certain complement-deficiency conditions	May cause mild LR, low-grade fever, headache. Pregnancy: can be considered
Menactra (MCV4)	Inactivated bacterial conjugate vaccine (IM) Quadrivalent (serotypes A, C, Y, and W-135)	Age >2 y (vaccine of choice for age 2–55 y): single dose	4 µg of each antigen (0.5 mL total)	Now a universally recommended childhood vaccine in US Unvaccinated travelers: same indication as for MPSV4	As for MPSV4 PLUS Recommended to those who received MPSV4 ≥3 y earlier and are still at increased risk of meningococcal disease. May cause LR more frequently than MPSV4
Yellow Fever					
YF-VAX	Live, attenuated virus (SC)	Age ≥9 mo: single dose 10 d–10 y before travel‡ *Booster:* every 10 y	0.5 mL	Travel to endemic area (tropical South America and equatorial Africa)	Documentation required for entrance to some countries in Africa and Asia. Commonly causes fever, myalgia, headache; rarely causes hypersensitivity, viscerotropic or neurologic disease. Contraindicated in children <6 mo and persons with hypersensitivity to eggs; avoid in persons with thymus disorders or immune deficiencies; caution in persons age 6–9 mo or ≥60 y. Pregnancy: if high-risk travel, discuss the risks and benefits with an expert before considering vaccination.
Typhoid					
Typhim Vi (injectable, ViCPS)	Vi capsular polysaccharide antigen (IM)	Age ≥2 y: single dose *Booster:* every 2 y if ongoing risk	25 µg (0.5 mL)	Travel to most developing countries	Avoid in setting of acute febrile illness. May cause LR, headache, fever (rare). Pregnancy: safety unknown; avoid if possible.
Vivotif Berna (oral, Ty21a)	Live, attenuated Ty21a strain of *S. typhi* (PO)	Age ≥6 y: 4 doses of 1 capsule every other day *Booster:* every 5 y if ongoing risk	1 capsule	Same indication as for Typhim Vi	Must be refrigerated, taken with cool liquid 1 h before a meal; should not be taken with other antibiotics; if taken with mefloquine, separate doses by 24 h. Avoid in setting of acute febrile or GI illness; avoid in immunocompromised persons. May cause GI disturbance or rash (rare). Pregnancy: safety unknown, avoid if possible.

Poliomyelitis§

Vaccine	Type	Schedule	Dose	Indications	Comments
IPOL, Poliovax (injectable)	Enhanced potency inactivated virus (IM)	*Primary series:* Age >6 wk: 3 doses at 0, 1–2, and 6–18 mo (preferred interval: 2–8 mo between 2nd and 3rd doses) 4th dose: at age 4–6 y if primary series was completed before age 4 y. Booster: single dose	0.5 mL	A universally recommended childhood vaccine in US. For travelers to Asia or Africa: one lifetime booster dose at age ≥18 y if primary series was completed	Contraindicated in persons with severe allergy to streptomycin, polymyxin B, or neomycin. May cause mild LR. Pregnancy: relatively contraindicated; avoid if possible.

Rabies

Vaccine	Type	Schedule	Dose	Indications	Comments
Imovax (HDCV)	Inactivated virus in human diploid cell vaccine (IM)	*All ages:* Before exposure: 3 doses at 0, 7, and 21–28 d. After exposure if not previously immunized: 5 doses at 0, 3, 7, 14, and 28 d PLUS 1 dose RIG¶. After exposure if previously immunized: 2 doses at 0 and 3 d	1.0 mL (2.5 IU)	Travelers with high-risk exposures (e.g., spelunkers, veterinarians, medical and laboratory workers, animal-control and wildlife workers in rabies-epizootic areas); other travelers with itineraries and activities with high risk for rabies (dogs are a primary threat in developing regions)	Full course should be given with same vaccine; boosters are based on risk and antibody response. Immunosuppressed persons may not mount protective antibody response: check titers if high-risk travel cannot be avoided. May cause mild LR; mild headache, myalgia, nausea; occasional (6%) immune complex–like reaction with malaise, urticaria, pruritus after booster. Pregnancy: not contraindicated
RabAvert (PCEC)	Inactivated virus in purified chick embryo cell (IM)				

Japanese Encephalitis

Vaccine	Type	Schedule	Dose	Indications	Comments
JE Vax	Inactivated virus (SC)	Age ≥1 y: 3 doses at 0, 7, and 30 d. *Booster:* single dose at 24-mo interval (duration of protection unknown) Complete series ≥10 d before departure	Age 1–2 y: 0.5 mL; Age ≥3 y: 1.0 mL	Travelers with high-risk exposures (e.g., >1 mo in endemic rural areas during transmission season); other travelers with itineraries and activities with high risk	Monitor patient for 30 min after each dose and advise avoiding travel for ≥10 d after last dose of vaccine. Avoid if history of multiple allergies or anaphylaxis; avoid if history of allergy to mouse-derived vaccines or thimerosal. May cause LR lasting 1–3 d; mild systemic symptoms such as fever, myalgia, headache, GI disturbance (10%); allergic reactions such as urticaria, angioedema, rash, respiratory distress (0.6%); encephalitis or death (rare). Pregnancy: safety unknown; avoid if possible.

Data from the following CDC Web pages (accessed May 9, 2009): Travelers' Health, available at http://wwwn.cdc.gov/travel/contentVaccinations.aspx; CDC Health Information for International Travel 2008 (The Yellow Book), available at http://wwwn.cdc.gov/travel/content/yellowbook/home-2008.aspx; Immunization Schedules (ACIP guidelines), available at http://www.cdc.gov/vaccines/recs/schedules/default.htm.

*Routine immunizations are not listed; ACIP routine immunization schedules are available at http://www.immunize.org/acip/ (accessed May 8, 2009).

†Avoid any vaccine if a serious allergic reaction to previous dose of vaccine or vaccine component has occurred.

‡Live, attenuated virus vaccines should generally be given simultaneously or separated by at least 4 wk.

§Oral polio virus, OPV, is no longer available in US.

¶RIG, rabies immune globulin: 20 IU/kg administered at bite site as possible, with remainder given IM in area away from vaccine site.

ACIP, Advisory Committee on Immunization Practices (Centers for Disease Control and Prevention [CDC]); CNS, central nervous system; EU, ELISA units; GI, gastrointestinal; LR, local reaction; *S. typhi, Salmonella enterica* serovar Typhi; US, United States.

ROUTINE IMMUNIZATIONS

The pretravel visit is an excellent opportunity to ensure that travelers are up-to-date on routine, age-appropriate vaccinations (http://www.cdc.gov/vaccines/ [accessed May 8, 2009]). These include diphtheria, tetanus, pertussis, *Haemophilus influenzae* type B, pneumococcus, poliovirus, measles, mumps, rubella, varicella, and hepatitis B. Although consideration should be given to vaccination of all North American adults against hepatitis B, particular emphasis should be given to nonimmune travelers to areas of intermediate or high endemicity (hepatitis B surface antigen prevalence >2%).

Additional booster doses of vaccines may also be indicated. For example, adults who have completed the primary polio vaccination series should receive one lifetime booster dose of inactivated polio vaccine if they will be traveling to regions (primarily in countries in Asia and Africa) in which polio transmission is occurring (see http://www.polioeradication.org [accessed May 8, 2009]).

Although measles is no longer endemic in the United States, imported infections have been reported, with documented transmission to nonimmune adults and children. All travelers should therefore be appropriately vaccinated. Children older than 12 months of age should receive two doses of the measles, mumps, and rubella vaccine (MMR), at least 28 days apart, before travel, and infants 6 to 11 months of age who are believed to be at risk should be given a single dose before travel. Adults born after 1956 who had only a single childhood dose should receive a second, booster dose.

Influenza is the most common vaccine-preventable illness in travelers. Influenza vaccination should be a particular priority in children younger than 5 years and adults older than 50 years of age, based on seasonal influenza activity both in the region of origin and at the destination. For example, travel to the temperate Northern or Southern Hemisphere during the local winter season, or travel to the tropics year-round, confers risk of influenza; cruise ships are another situation where year-round transmission is possible. Immunization with vaccines available in the United States may not confer immunity to strains of influenza present in other regions of the world, and vaccines are often difficult to obtain except during the U.S. influenza transmission season.

A special consideration for some travelers is avian (H5N1) influenza. Most cases are thought to result from direct contact with infected poultry, but rare cases of human-to-human transmission have occurred. Symptoms range from mild, influenza-like symptoms to severe respiratory illness, gastrointestinal effects, and neurologic changes. Routine chemoprophylaxis is not recommended, and the influenza vaccine is not protective against avian influenza. Travelers to areas where outbreaks have been reported should avoid direct contact with birds and their feces or secretions, cook poultry and eggs thoroughly, practice careful hand-washing hygiene, and monitor closely for influenza-like illness.

RECOMMENDED IMMUNIZATIONS

Additional vaccinations are recommended based on planned travel-related exposures.

Hepatitis A is the second most common vaccine-preventable illness in travelers, and it is now a routine childhood immunization in the United States. It is indicated for all nonimmune travelers to regions where hygiene may be poor. In general, it is recommended for persons traveling anywhere except the United States, Canada, Australia, New Zealand, Japan, or Western Europe. Antibodies to hepatitis A develop within 2 weeks after the first vaccine dose in most people. Therefore, although vaccination is recommended 1 month before departure, late vaccination may still confer significant protection. The vaccine (Havrix, Vaqta) is approved for children 1 year of age or older; at-risk infants and other persons who cannot receive the vaccine, as well as those who receive it less than 2 to 4 weeks before departure, may be given immune globulin before travel. A combination vaccine for hepatitis A and hepatitis B (Twinrix) is available for adults in a three-dose schedule.

Enteric fever is a term that encompasses both typhoid fever (caused by *Salmonella enterica* serovar Typhi) and paratyphoid fever (caused by *S. enterica* Paratyphi types A, B, and C). Enteric fever is common in travelers, particularly immigrant VFR travelers. Although it is 10-fold less common in travelers than hepatitis A, considerable geographic variability exists; for example, the incidence of enteric fever on the Indian subcontinent is extremely high. Protective acquired immunity does not persist after typhoid infection, with relapse (and reinfection) occurring in 5% to 10% of individuals who have had enteric fever. Given this risk and the growing antibiotic resistance of these organisms in many countries, appropriate vaccination for typhoid has become increasingly important. Typhoid vaccine is recommended for travelers to most of the developing world, in particular Central and South America, Africa, and Asia, especially the Indian subcontinent. Travelers 6 years old and older can be given an oral live, attenuated typhoid vaccine (Ty21a; Vivotif Berna), which is protective for 5 years. These capsules need to be refrigerated and taken every other day for a total of 4 doses. Importantly, no other antibiotics should be given from 1 day before until 7 days after the course. An intramuscular Vi capsular polysaccharide vaccine (ViCPS; Typhim Vi) is available for adults and children 2 years of age and older and should be given at least 2 weeks before travel; the redosing interval for the injectable vaccine is 2 to 3 years. Both of these vaccines offer 50% to 80% protection against typhoid fever, and Ty21a may also have some effect against *S. enterica* Paratyphi, but they are not a substitute for careful selection of food and drink.

Meningococcal vaccine is recommended for adults and children 2 years of age and older who are traveling to endemic areas, particularly to the so-called "meningitis belt" in sub-Saharan Africa during the dry season (December through June). Travelers to other areas who will have extensive, close contact with local populations (especially in dormitories, refugee camps, or health care settings) also should consider vaccination. Vaccination is required by Saudi Arabia for pilgrims traveling to Mecca during the Hajj and Umrah. Two quadrivalent vaccines against *Neisseria meningitidis* serotypes A, C, Y, and W-135 are available. The meningococcal polysaccharide-protein conjugate vaccine (MCV4; Menactra) is the recommended vaccine for persons 2 to 55 years of age; tetravalent meningococcal polysaccharide vaccine (MPSV4; Menomune) is recommended for those older than 55 years of age but is approved for all persons 2 years of age and older. The vaccine should be administered at least 7 to 10 days before departure.

Yellow fever is a disease transmitted by *Aedes* mosquitoes in equatorial Africa and South America that carries a 20% mortality rate. Although yellow fever vaccine is one of the few remaining vaccines required by international health regulations, it is estimated that only 10% to 30% of Americans traveling to endemic regions have been immunized. In the United States, administration of the vaccine is regulated by public health authorities. Documentation of appropriate vaccination is required on arrival to many countries in yellow fever–endemic zones, and on return from such regions to nonendemic countries; however, these regulations are not always strictly enforced. The vaccine (YF-Vax) is a live, attenuated vaccine prepared in eggs, so it generally should not be given to pregnant or immunocompromised patients, to those allergic to eggs, or to infants younger than 9 months of age. If travel to an endemic region is unavoidable, patients in these groups should be counseled about the relative risks of the vaccine compared with the risks of acquiring yellow fever when traveling to an endemic area without vaccination. During the high-transmission seasons, the risk of infection may approach 1 in 1000 travelers per month in West Africa and 1 in 10,000 travelers per month in South America, although great individual variation exists depending on the region traveled and mosquito exposure. Patients with a history of a thymus disorder or thymectomy and individuals 60 years of age and older have a higher risk for vaccine-associated viscerotropic and neurologic disease; for these patients, the risks and benefits should be discussed before vaccination is considered. The vaccine should be given at least 10 days before departure, and the revaccination interval is 10 years. Only vaccination clinics certified by the World Health Organization—a list of which may be found on the CDC Travelers' Health website (see Table 4)—may administer the yellow fever vaccine and issue the validation stamp.

Rabies is present on all continents except Antarctica and is highly endemic in parts of Africa, Asia, and Central and South America. Because there is no treatment for rabies, preexposure and postexposure prophylaxis is critical. Travelers to high-risk areas who are planning extensive outdoor activities, spelunking, or other occupational or recreational activities with exposure to animals, especially those in locations where rabies postexposure prophylaxis may not be available, should be counseled on animal-bite prevention and may be candidates for the rabies vaccine (Imovax, RabAvert). Three preexposure vaccine doses should be given before travel.

Japanese encephalitis is an arboviral infection present in most Asian and some Western Pacific countries. The disease is uncommon in travelers, and the vaccine (JE-Vax) carries a relatively high risk of hypersensitivity reactions; therefore, it need be considered only for travelers who plan a prolonged (≥4 weeks) stay in an endemic country during the transmission season and those who will be in rural areas or have heavy mosquito exposure. Risk is highest in areas where flood irrigation is practiced (e.g., rice paddies) and with nighttime outdoor exposure, given the feeding habits of the *Culex* vector. Regional and seasonal transmission risks for endemic countries are published in the CDC's Health Information for International Travel, known as The Yellow Book (see Table 4).

Tick-borne encephalitis virus is endemic primarily in Eastern and Central Europe, Scandinavia, and Siberia during warmer months. Travelers at risk are primarily those who spend extended time in forested, nonurban areas and those who consume unpasteurized dairy products. Because the vaccine is not available in the United States and must be given over the course of 9 to 12 months, prevention depends primarily on avoidance of tick bites (especially during the late spring to early fall months) and avoidance of unpasteurized dairy products. Travelers who plan to spend extensive time outdoors in rural, endemic areas may consider being vaccinated in Canada or Europe.

Cholera vaccine[2] is not currently recommended for routine use in travelers but may be considered for some who plan to work in refugee camps or as health care providers in endemic regions. Anthrax and smallpox vaccines are also not recommended and are unavailable for the general public.

CONTRAINDICATIONS AND PRECAUTIONS

It is important to review the vaccination and allergy histories of each patient to ensure that the patient is not allergic to eggs or other vaccine components. Immunizations generally should not be given in the setting of an active, moderate to severe illness. If multiple live virus vaccines (e.g., varicella vaccine [Varivax], MMR, and YF-Vax) are to be given, immune interference should be avoided. The vaccines should be given simultaneously or separated by 4 weeks, and they should not be given in the period from 2 weeks before to 3 months after any administration of immune globulin.

In most circumstances, live virus vaccines should not be given to pregnant or immunocompromised patients, although the risks must be weighed against potential benefit. Information on immunizations and other health-related travel issues for immunocompromised travelers, pregnant women, and other travelers with specific needs is detailed in the CDC's Yellow Book.

Those traveling with infants should also be informed of any recommended or required immunizations that are not generally given before a certain age. For example, YF-Vax should not be administered to infants younger than 9 months of age, and the meningococcal vaccines (Menomune, Menactra) are approved only for children 2 years old or older.

Protection against Malaria

Malaria, an illness transmitted by *Anopheles* mosquitoes and caused by one of the five human parasites of the genus *Plasmodium*, is a major global health problem. It is one of the most frequent causes of fever and the leading preventable infectious cause of death in travelers. Among the five species—*Plasmodium falciparum, Plasmodium vivax, Plasmodium ovale, Plasmodium malariae,* and

---

[2]Not available in the United States.

Plasmodium knowlesi—*P. falciparum* has by far the greatest potential to cause severe disease and death. There were 1564 reported cases of malaria in the United States in 2006, and all were imported. The highest case rate was seen among travelers returning from Western Africa (the vast majority of whom had *P. falciparum* infection), but an increased number of cases were from Asia. Six deaths were reported, five due to *P. falciparum* and one to *P. malariae*.

Because there is no malaria vaccine, adequate protection, including chemoprophylaxis and prevention of *Anopheles* mosquito bites, is paramount. Among the U.S. travelers with malaria in 2006 for whom such information was available, only one third reported adherence to an appropriate chemoprophylactic drug regimen. In addition, given the potential risk and severity of malaria, travelers should be instructed to urgently seek care if they develop a fever while abroad or within 1 year after return from travel.

PREVENTION

The necessity and choice of malaria prophylaxis depend on the specific planned travel destination. Risk of malaria transmission also depends on the types of accommodations and activities planned, duration of stay, seasonal factors, elevation, and adherence to preventive measures. In the United States, malaria prophylaxis is generally recommended if any part of a traveler's itinerary includes a malaria-endemic area. Specific information on the distribution of malaria is available in the Yellow Book (http://wwwn.cdc.gov/travel/yellowBookCh4-Malaria.aspx [accessed May 8, 2009]). In general, malaria risk exists in both cities and rural areas in the most heavily endemic countries (e.g., most of sub-Saharan Africa, Oceania, India), but in less malaria-endemic countries (e.g., most of Latin America, Southeast Asia, the Middle East), it is concentrated more in rural, lowland areas and is less likely to be present in larger cities. Areas endemic for malaria and antimicrobial resistance patterns are shown in Figure 1.

CHEMOPROPHYLAXIS

Chloroquine (Aralen) is the drug of choice for areas that still have chloroquine-sensitive malaria (e.g., Central America west of the Panama Canal, the Dominican Republic and Haiti, parts of the Middle East). Chloroquine is generally well tolerated but can cause gastrointestinal disturbances, headache, blurred vision, and, if overdosed, arrhythmias. It is safe for use in children and in pregnant women. Chloroquine is a once-weekly drug that should be taken for 1 week before exposure to the malarious area, during exposure, and for 1 month after exposure concludes. Table 2 lists dosages for chloroquine and other chemoprophylactic medications.

Chloroquine-resistant *P. falciparum* is now prevalent in most other regions of the world, and chloroquine-resistant *P. vivax* is common in Indonesia and Papua New Guinea. In areas with chloroquine-resistant malaria, there are three primary choices for chemoprophylaxis, which all have similar efficacies but differing side effect profiles. In general, malaria chemoprophylaxis is extremely effective if taken appropriately.

Atovaquone-proguanil (Malarone) is a fixed-dose, once-daily combination drug that is usually the best tolerated but most expensive option. It can cause headaches, gastrointestinal disturbances, liver enzyme elevations, and mouth ulcers. It should be avoided in pregnant and breast-feeding mothers and in patients with a creatinine clearance rate of less than 30 mL/min. It is probably safe in children between 5 and 11 kg, but in the United States it is approved only for those weighing more than 11 kg. Atovaquone-proguanil should be taken for 1 or 2 days before exposure to the malarious area, during exposure, and for 1 week after exposure concludes. Like other antimalarials, it acts on blood-stage parasites, but, because it also acts on actively replicating parasites (schizonts) in the liver, the duration for which it must be continued after travel is shorter.

Mefloquine (Lariam) is a once-weekly medication that has many adverse effects, including dizziness, headache, insomnia, and disturbing dreams. More severe neuropsychiatric effects that require drug discontinuation occur in approximately 5% of users. Most adverse effects occur early in use; if a patient tolerates the first three doses, severe adverse effects are less likely to develop later. Mefloquine

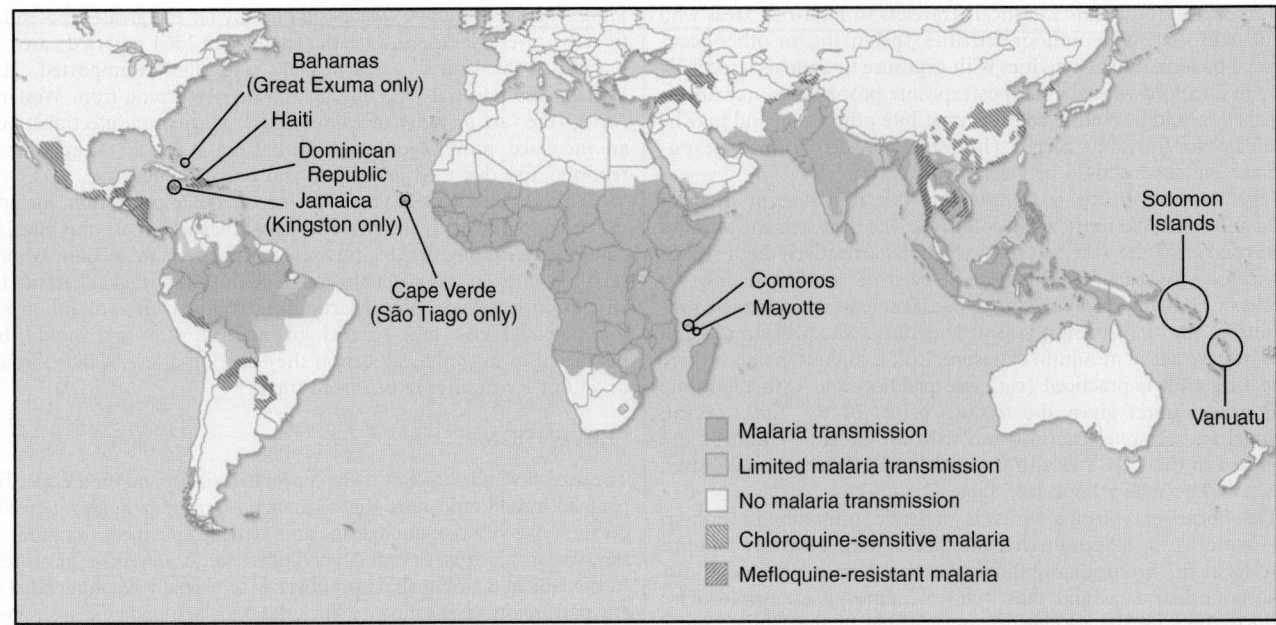

FIGURE 1. Areas endemic for malaria and antimicrobial resistance patterns. Reprinted with permission from Freedman DO: Clinical practice: Malaria prevention in short-term travelers. N Engl J Med 2008;359:603–12.

should be avoided in travelers with a preexisting psychiatric disorder, seizure disorder, or cardiac arrhythmia. It is a category C drug for pregnant women, but is probably safe in the second and third trimesters if necessary. It is safe for use in children. Mefloquine should be taken for 1 to 3 weeks before exposure to the malarious area, during exposure, and for 1 month after exposure concludes. Mefloquine should not be used if the travel itinerary includes the regions in Southeast Asia with mefloquine-resistant *P. falciparum* (e.g., the Burmese borders with Thailand, China, and Laos; Thai-Cambodian border areas; parts of eastern Burma, western Cambodia, and southern Vietnam).

Doxycycline (Vibramycin) is the least expensive alternative for malaria prophylaxis. Like atovaquone-proguanil, it is taken once daily and can prevent infection by multidrug-resistant *P. falciparum*. The drug may be associated with gastrointestinal side effects and photosensitivity, and it can cause vaginal candidiasis in women. Patients should be advised to use sunscreen. Doxycycline may interact with other prescription drugs; it decreases the efficacy of oral contraceptive pills, and concurrent use of bismuth subsalicylate decreases absorption of doxycycline. It is contraindicated in children younger than 8 years of age and in pregnant women. Doxycycline should be taken for 1 to 2 days before exposure to the malarious area, during exposure, and for 1 month after exposure concludes.

Primaquine is an alternative agent for patients who are unable to take any other antimalarial drug. Taken once daily, it is effective against chloroquine-resistant malaria. It also prevents relapses of *P. vivax* and *P. ovale*, which can persist in the liver (as dormant hypnozoites) and cause clinical malaria months to years after travel. Other antimalarials do not eradicate the hypnozoite forms of the parasite. Primaquine is therefore the drug of choice for so-called terminal prophylaxis in travelers who are returning from prolonged stays in areas highly endemic for *P. vivax* or *P. ovale*; it is taken for 14 days after departure from the malarious area. Primaquine can cause severe hemolytic anemia in persons with glucose-6-phosphate dehydrogenase (G6PD) deficiency, and all persons should have a G6PD level determined before initiation of therapy. Primaquine should not be given to pregnant women nor to lactating women unless the breast-feeding infant has been documented to have normal G6PD levels. In rare situations when primaquine is used for primary prophylaxis, it should be taken for 1 to 2 days before exposure to the malarious area, during exposure, and for 1 week after exposure concludes. The use of primaquine for malaria chemoprophylaxis should be reviewed by an infectious disease specialist or a physician certified in travel medicine.

Travelers to chloroquine-sensitive areas who are unable to tolerate chloroquine or the related drug hydroxychloroquine (Plaquenil) may take any of the other four agents for prophylaxis.

TREATMENT

Some authorities recommend that travelers bring a malaria self-treatment course with them, for use under certain predefined circumstances. The specific management of malaria is briefly addressed later in this chapter (see "Illness in the Returned Traveler") and is covered in more detail in the chapter on Malaria.

Protection against Traveler's Diarrhea

Traveler's diarrhea (TD) is a very common travel-related illness. Classic TD is defined as three or more unformed stools in a 24-hour period, in addition to at least one associated symptom (cramps, tenesmus, fecal urgency, nausea, vomiting, fever, or blood in the stools); dysentery is defined as diarrhea with fever, bloody stools or both. The incidence of TD is highly variable depending on the individual traveler's exposures and activities. In general, risk is related to local hygienic conditions, duration of travel, type of travel, and host immunity. Low-risk countries for TD include the United States, Canada, Australia, New Zealand, Japan, and Northern and Western Europe. Intermediate-risk countries include those in Eastern Europe, South Africa, and some of the Caribbean islands. High-risk areas include most of Asia, the Middle East, Africa, and Central and South America. In high-risk areas, 30% to 50% of travelers will develop TD during a stay of 1 to 2 weeks.

The most common etiologic organisms include enterotoxigenic (ETEC) or enteroaggregative (EAEC) strains of *Escherichia coli*, *Campylobacter*, *Shigella*, *Salmonella*, *Vibrio* spp., *Yersinia enterocolitica*, and *Aeromonas*. Less common agents include viruses (although norovirus outbreaks commonly occur on cruise ships) and parasites such as *Giardia intestinalis*, *Cryptosporidium* spp., *Entamoeba histolytica*, and *Cyclospora cayetanensis*. Symptoms usually occur during the first week of travel, and more than 90% within the first 2 weeks. TD is typically self-limited; although the illness usually is not severe, significant discomfort and inconvenience often result. Infants, children, and young adults are at highest risk for TD and dehydration. Hospitalizations and fatalities have been occasionally reported, and chronic complications (e.g., development of irritable bowel syndrome) may be associated with TD.

TABLE 2 Malaria Chemoprophylaxis

Medication	Adult Dosage	Pediatric Dosage	Comments and Precautions
Areas of Chloroquine-Sensitive Malaria*			
Chloroquine phosphate (Aralen)	300 mg base (= 500 mg salt) q wk	5 mg/kg base (= 8.3 mg/kg salt), up to adult dose, q wk	Begin 1 wk before entering risk area, take while in risk area, and continue for 4 wk after leaving. May cause bitter taste, GI disturbance, headache, pruritus, QT prolongation; may exacerbate psoriasis. Use in pregnancy: appears safe
Hydroxychloroquine sulfate (Plaquenil)	310 mg base (= 400 mg salt) q wk	5 mg/kg base (= 6.5 mg/kg salt), up to adult dose, q wk	As for chloroquine. Use in pregnancy: appears safe
Areas of Chloroquine-Resistant Malaria†			
Atovaquone-proguanil (Malarone)	Adult tablets contain 250 mg atovaquone combined with 100 mg proguanil; take 1 tablet qd	Pediatric tablets contain 62.5 mg atovaquone with 25 mg proguanil 5–8 kg: $\frac{1}{2}$ pediatric tablet qd‡ ≥8–10 kg: $\frac{3}{4}$ pediatric tablet qd‡ 11–20 kg: 1 pediatric tablet qd 21–30 kg: 2 pediatric tablets qd 31–40 kg: 3 pediatric tablets qd >40 kg: 1 adult tablet qd	Begin 1–2 d before entering risk area, take while in risk area, and continue for 1 wk after leaving. Also recommended for primary prophylaxis in areas with mefloquine-resistant *P. falciparum* (see below); avoid in patients with creatinine clearance <30 mL/min. Should be taken with food or milky drink. May cause GI disturbance, headache (common); increased transaminases (occasional); rash (rare); generally well-tolerated. Use in pregnancy: no (insufficient data to recommend use in pregnant women)
Mefloquine HCl (Lariam)	228 mg base (= 250 mg salt) 1 tablet q wk	<5 kg: 4.6 mg/kg base (= 5 mg/kg salt)‡ q wk <10 kg: 4.6 mg/kg base (= 5 mg/kg salt) q wk 10–19 kg: $\frac{1}{4}$ tablet q wk 20–30 kg: $\frac{1}{2}$ tablet q wk 31–45 kg: $\frac{3}{4}$ tablet q wk >45 kg: 1 tablet q wk Pharmacy can compound ingredients into 1 tablet if splitting medication is too difficult for the patient.	Begin 1 wk before entering risk area, take while in risk area, and continue for 4 wk after leaving; consider starting several weeks before travel to assess tolerability. Contraindicated in patients with active or recent depression, major psychiatric disorder, seizures, cardiac conduction abnormalities, or quinine allergy. May cause CNS effects (somnolence, psychiatric effects, mood alteration, vivid dreams), bradycardia, GI disturbance; rare adverse events include seizures and psychosis. Use in pregnancy: likely safe, especially in 2nd and 3rd trimesters, if necessary
Doxycycline (Vibramycin)	100 mg PO qd	≥8 y: 2 mg/kg/d, up to maximum dose of 100 mg/d	Begin 1 wk before entering risk area, take while in risk area, and continue for 4 wk after leaving. Also recommended for primary prophylaxis in areas with mefloquine-resistant *P. falciparum* (see below). Contraindicated in children <8 y of age. Caution for drug interactions: bismuth subsalicylate, oral contraceptives, other antimicrobials. May cause photosensitivity, GI disturbance, *Candida* vaginitis. Use in pregnancy: no
Rare Circumstances: Alternative if other Prophylactic Agents are Contraindicated or Unavailable			
Primaquine	30 mg base (= two 26.3-mg tablets) qd	0.6 mg/kg base (= 1 mg/kg salt) qd, up to adult dose	Consult with a travel or infectious diseases specialist before use—second line for primary prophylaxis. Begin 1–2 d before entering risk area, take while in risk area, and continue until 7 d after leaving. Must check G6PD level first: contraindicated in patients with G6PD deficiency because of potential hemolytic anemia. May cause GI disturbance, leukopenia (uncommon). Use in pregnancy: no

Continued

TABLE 2 Malaria Chemoprophylaxis—Cont'd

Medication	Adult Dosage	Pediatric Dosage	Comments and Precautions
Areas of Mefloquine-Resistant Malaria[§]			
Atovaquone-proguanil	See above.		
Doxycycline	See above.		
Primaquine	See above; should be used only in consultation with a travel or infectious diseases specialist.		
Terminal Prophylaxis to Prevent Relapse of *P. vivax* and *P. ovale*			
Primaquine	30 mg base (two 26.3-mg tablets) qd for 14 d at completion of travel	0.6 mg/kg base (= 1 mg/kg salt) qd, up to adult dose, for 14 d at completion of travel	As above.

Data, including off-label pediatric dosing, based on CDC Health Information for International Travel 2008 (The Yellow Book), available at http://wwwn.cdc.gov/travel/content/yellowbook/home-2008.aspx (accessed May 8, 2009).

*Areas of chloroquine-sensitive malaria are Haiti, the Dominican Republic, Central America west of the former Panama Canal Zone, much of the Middle East (except Iran, Oman, Saudi Arabia, and Yemen), Argentina, Paraguay, and parts of China and northern Africa.

[†]Areas of chloroquine-resistant malaria are Central America east of the former Panama Canal Zone, South America (except Paraguay and Argentina), parts of the Middle East, most of Africa, and Asia and Oceania.

[‡]Off-label use; dose recommended by CDC.

[§]Areas of mefloquine-resistant malaria are parts of Southeast Asia, specifically Burmese borders with Thailand, China, and Laos; Thai-Cambodian border areas; and parts of eastern Burma, western Cambodia, and southern Vietnam.

CDC, Centers for Disease Control and Prevention; CNS, central nervous system; G6PD, glucose-6-phosphate dehydrogenase; GI, gastrointestinal.

PREVENTION

There is no vaccine against TD available in the United States, although vaccines against ETEC are currently being studied. The oral cholera vaccine (Dukoral)[1] also confers some protection against ETEC but is not available in the United States, and there are few data regarding its efficacy in protecting Western travelers against TD. Prevention through safe food and water consumption is therefore paramount. When traveling to areas where hygiene is poor, travelers should avoid consumption of untreated tap water and items prepared with untreated water (e.g., ice cubes, prepared fruit juices, salads, raw vegetables, unpeeled fruit), unpasteurized dairy products, undercooked or underheated foods, and open buffets.

CHEMOPROPHYLAXIS

Routine antimicrobial chemoprophylaxis is not recommended for the general population, given concerns for adverse effects, tolerability, and emergence of resistant organisms. A prophylactic antibiotic course of no longer than 2 to 3 weeks' duration may be considered for travelers to high-risk regions who fall into one of the following groups:

- Travelers for whom remaining well during the trip is critical
- Travelers who are at risk for severe or complicated diarrhea, such as immunocompromised persons and those with achlorhydria, inflammatory bowel disease, or chronic diarrhea
- Travelers who ae more susceptible to dehydration (e.g., those taking diuretics)
- Travelers who would have difficulty coping with diarrhea, such as those with colostomies

When used in these circumstances, prophylaxis typically consists of a fluoroquinolone, such as ciprofloxacin (Cipro)[1] 500 mg, levofloxacin (Levaquin)[1] 500 mg, norfloxacin (Noroxin)[1] 400 mg, or ofloxacin (Floxin)[1] 300 mg; these are given once daily during travel and for 2 days after return. Data suggest that such regimens have an 80% protective efficacy. Rifaximin (Xifaxan),[1] a poorly absorbed oral rifamycin with activity against a wide range of enteric organisms, appears to have a protective efficacy of 70% to 80% for TD in Latin America (where ETEC is most common etiologic agent and invasive pathogens are less common). Given its excellent side effect profile and minimal alterations of bowel flora, rifaximin may be safe to use more liberally as chemoprophylaxis, but currently it is not FDA approved for this indication. It is less clear what the role of these regimens should be in Asia, where the rates of fluoroquinolone-resistant *Campylobacter* are very high and where rifaximin has been less well studied against the prevalent invasive pathogens. Azithromycin (Zithromax)[1] has not been well studied for use as prophylaxis but may be an alternative to consider.

A non-antibiotic agent, bismuth subsalicylate (Pepto-Bismol),[1] also decreases the incidence of TD, with a protective efficacy of 60% to 65%. Drawbacks include dosing inconvenience and a black discoloration of the tongue and of the stool, which can be mistaken for melena. Bismuth subsalicylate should be avoided by children younger than 3 years of age, persons allergic to salicylates, patients taking anticoagulants or doxycycline, and patients with gout or renal insufficiency.

TREATMENT

If diarrhea does occur during travel, aggressive fluid and electrolyte replacement should be advised, particularly in children, the elderly, and individuals with severe diarrhea. Oral rehydration salts (Cera-Lyte) are available in the United States and throughout the world. In adults and children older than 2 years, mild diarrhea without fever or bloody stools can be treated initially with loperamide (Imodium).

Antibiotics decrease the duration of symptoms of TD, and travelers are often given a small supply of appropriate antibiotics for self-treatment if indicated. A short antibiotic treatment course is warranted for travelers who have moderate to severe diarrhea, diarrhea that is not improving after 24 hours, or dysentery. Trimethoprim-sulfamethoxazole (Bactrim)[1] is no longer recommended because of increasing resistance; ciprofloxacin or levofloxacin[1] is usually the drug of choice (Table 3). A single dose of a fluoroquinolone

---

[1]Not FDA approved for this indication.

TABLE 3 Self-Treatment for Traveler's Diarrhea

Drug	Dosage*	Comments and Precautions
Antimotility Medications		
Bismuth subsalicylate (active ingredient in Pepto-Bismol)	1 oz liquid or 2 tablets q30min until symptomatic relief is obtained, up to 8 doses Not to be used longer than 3 weeks	May cause tinnitus and blackening of tongue and stool. Avoid in patients <3 y; those with renal insufficiency, gout, or aspirin allergy; those taking anticoagulation therapy or doxycycline; and children with possible influenza or varicella (increased risk of Reye's syndrome)
Loperamide (Imodium)	Do not use longer than 48 hours Adults and children >12 y: 4 mg LD, then 2 mg after each loose stool until symptomatic relief, to maximum of 16 mg/d Children 2–5 y: 1 mg LD, then 1 mg prn, to maximum of 3 mg/d Children 6–11 y: 2 mg LD, then 1 mg prn to maximum of 4–6 mg/d	Avoid in children <2 y. Not for use in dysentery. Discontinue promptly if abdominal distention, ileus, or constipation develops.
Antibiotics		
Azithromycin[1] (Zithromax)	Adults: 1000 mg once, OR 500 mg qd × 3 d Children: 10 mg/kg/d	Preferred in children and in women who might be pregnant.
Fluoroquinolones[1]:		Not FDA-approved for use in children <18 y.
Ciprofloxacin (Cipro)	500 mg bid × 1–3 d	Adjust dose for renal insufficiency; can interact with anticoagulation therapy.
Levofloxacin (Levaquin)	500 mg bid × 1–3 d	Resistance is increasing, particularly among *Campylobacter*, especially in Southeast Asia
Norfloxacin (Noroxin)	400 mg bid × 1–3 d	May cause GI disturbance, CNS effects.
Ofloxacin (Floxin)	300 mg bid × 1–3 d	Not FDA-approved for use in children <12 y.
Rifaximin (Xifaxan)	200 mg tid × 3 d	May cause GI disturbance, headache.

[1]Not FDA approved for this indication.
*All doses are oral.
CNS, central nervous system; GI, gastrointestinal; LD, loading dose.

is often adequate for treatment of mild to moderate TD, but if evidence of invasive disease is present (e.g., fever, chills, bloody stools), a 3-day course should be completed. Loperamide in conjunction with effective antibiotics has been shown to offer an advantage over antibiotics alone in achieving early clinical cure of TD, and its early use may decrease the symptoms and duration of illness in mild to moderate diarrhea. More severe diarrhea can also be treated with an antibiotic and loperamide, but the latter should not be used in cases of dysentery. Medical care should be sought if self-treatment does not result in symptom improvement within 48 hours or if symptoms worsen despite empiric therapy.

In areas with a high prevalence of fluoroquinolone-resistant *Campylobacter*, such as Southeast Asia and the Indian subcontinent, azithromycin[1] is a more suitable empiric therapy. Single-dose azithromycin was as effective and as well tolerated as single-dose ciprofloxacin or levofloxacin in a study involving travelers to Mexico. Azithromycin is safe to use in children 2 years of age and older and in pregnant women (although there are no well-controlled studies of azithromycin in pregnant women), so it may be a reasonable choice for empiric treatment of TD in all destinations.

Rifaximin has also been approved for treatment of TD in individuals 12 years of age and older who have TD with no fever, chills, or bloody stools. In several multicenter, randomized, double-blind, placebo-controlled studies, it was safe and as effective in treating TD as ciprofloxacin. Dosing for non-invasive strains of *E. coli* is 200 mg three times a day. However, rifaximin has not been approved for use in persons with dysentery or with suspected *Shigella*, *Salmonella*, or *Campylobacter jejuni* infection, nor in children younger than 12 years of age. There may also be some risk of emergence of resistance in ETEC isolates after rifaximin use.

[1]Not FDA approved for this indication.

Travelers should carry a supply of loperamide and an antibiotic, and detailed advice should be given on when and how to self-treat TD, as well as when to seek medical care if symptoms worsen or fail to improve after self-treatment.

Illness in the Returned Traveler

Up to 8% of travelers to the developing world (4 million persons annually) seek medical care during or just after travel. Febrile illness, diarrhea, and dermatologic conditions are the three most common clinical syndromes in returning travelers. Given the broad differential diagnosis, a careful work-up is necessary, with attention given to clinical signs and symptoms, epidemiologic factors, detailed travel history, and vaccination and chemoprophylactic measures taken.

FEVER

Approximately 3% of short-term international travelers develop a febrile illness related to their trip. Most patients present within 1 month, but some present more than 6 months after return from travel. Fever in the returned traveler requires immediate evaluation, because potentially life-threatening infections are often considerations. Evaluation should include, at minimum, a complete blood count (CBC) with differential, renal and hepatic panels, blood cultures, and thick and thin blood smears. Other tests, such as urinalysis, stool culture or ova and parasite examination, chest radiography, or specific serologic testing, may be performed based on clinical suspicion.

The travel itinerary is an important consideration when attempting to stratify the likelihood of potential diagnoses. Among travelers to sub-Saharan Africa, malaria is overwhelmingly the most common cause of febrile syndromes. For travelers to Southeast Asia and the Caribbean, dengue fever is most common, whereas enteric fever is an important consideration for travelers returning from South Asia. Other common causes of fever in returned travelers include mononucleosis, rickettsial infection (particularly in those returning from southern Africa, because of African tick bite fever), and leptospirosis. Other viral illnesses, such as acute HIV infection, hepatitis A, influenza, and chikungunya, may also be considerations based on exposure history.

An estimation of the possible range of the incubation period, based on symptom onset in relationship to the travel dates, is helpful. Dengue has a short incubation period (4–8 days), whereas for typhoid fever it is usually 1 to 3 weeks. For malaria, the minimum incubation period is about 1 week but can be as long as months or years. Hepatitis A (median incubation period, 4 weeks) and schistosomiasis (typical incubation period, 4–8 weeks) may manifest well after return from travel.

Helminthic infections (acute hookworm, ascariasis, trichuriasis, strongyloidiasis, toxocariasis, and trichinosis) should be considered in travelers with eosinophilia, fever, and gastrointestinal symptoms. Acute schistosomiasis (Katayama fever) is caused by a blood fluke acquired by contact with infested fresh water through bathing or swimming. Symptoms include fever, eosinophilia, rash, respiratory symptoms, and hepatosplenomegaly. Schistosomiasis occurs in returned travelers predominantly from Africa but also from the Middle East, north/northeastern South America, the Caribbean, and Southeast Asia.

Malaria

Malaria causes 350 to 500 million infections annually, resulting in 1 million deaths worldwide. Malaria is endemic in more than 100 countries and remains a major cause of febrile illness among travelers to the developing world. Almost all reported U.S. cases are imported, although autochthonous transmission is possible because of the endemic anophelines in the southern states. The highest rates of malaria are in sub-Saharan Africa, and VFR travelers are at particularly high risk for acquiring malaria. Illness severity depends on the *Plasmodium* species, the degree of parasitemia, and the host response. Because no chemoprophylactic antimalarial agent is 100% effective, both patient and provider should be aware of the clinical signs and symptoms of malaria.

Most patients with malaria present with fever. Classic cyclic fever patterns are described—48-hour intervals for *P. falciparum*, *P. vivax*, and *P. ovale*, and 72-hour intervals for *P. malariae*—but, in practice, these distinct patterns are rarely seen. Other common symptoms include sweats, vomiting, diarrhea, and cough. Thrombocytopenia and anemia are common. More serious complications include disseminated intravascular coagulation, jaundice, shock, renal failure, respiratory distress, hypoglycemia, and altered mental status (usually related to *P. falciparum* hyperparasitemia). Malaria does not usually cause rash or lymphadenopathy.

Almost all malaria fatalities are caused by *P. falciparum*, so differentiating it from the other species that cause malaria is essential. *P. falciparum* is responsible for 62% of the annual cases of malaria in the United States for which species identification is made. Among U.S. travelers with malaria, those exposed in sub-Saharan Africa have *P. falciparum* approximately five times more commonly than the other malaria species. For individuals exposed in Asia and Latin America (except Haiti), other species are six to seven times more common than *P. falciparum*. Persons infected with *P. falciparum* usually begin to exhibit symptoms of malaria within 1 month after returning from travel. In contrast, more than 40% of those infected with *P. vivax* or *P. ovale* have onset of disease 1 month or longer after returning. Some patients with *P. vivax* or *P. ovale* infection present months or even years after travel; however, these late relapses are rarely fatal. Therefore, the travel destination and incubation period are critical considerations when evaluating travelers with possible malaria.

Diagnosis is made by the Giemsa-stained thick and thin blood smears, which can reveal the presence and magnitude of parasitemia and often identify the infecting *Plasmodium* species. If the first evaluation is negative and suspicion for malaria is high, two or three additional smears should be obtained, preferably collected 12 to 24 hours apart, during fever paroxysms. The first antigen-based malaria rapid diagnostic test was licensed in the United States in 2007 for use by laboratories to facilitate diagnosis. These tests may provide a rapid alternative to microscopy in some situations, but issues of cost and accuracy currently limit widespread use, and it is currently recommended that positive results be confirmed and quantified by microscopy. Malaria polymerase chain reaction (PCR) tests are another emerging diagnostic tool. They can establish species identification and seem to be as sensitive and specific as blood smears, although they are not yet widely available.

Once a diagnosis of malaria is established, treatment with antimalarials should begin immediately, with the assistance of an infectious disease specialist. Based on susceptibility patterns in the region of travel, the species of *Plasmodium* identified, and the status of the patient, treatment may consist of either oral therapy (if the patient has low levels of parasitemia and no serious clinical signs or symptoms) or parenteral therapy. Most patients with malaria caused by *P. vivax*, *P. ovale*, or *P. malariae* recover without major sequelae. *P. knowlesi* may be misidentified as *P. malariae* but appears to have the potential to cause a more severe and sometimes fatal form of disease. *P. falciparum* infections can be fatal, and outcome is often related to parasite burden. Because falciparum malaria can progress quickly to death, U.S. patients should generally be admitted for treatment and monitoring. Malaria patients with greater than 5% parasitemia or the serious complications noted earlier are at higher risk for death and should be admitted to an intensive care setting for monitoring and supportive care in addition to antimalarial therapy.

Dengue

Dengue fever, caused by an arthropod-borne flavivirus, is endemic to the tropics and subtropics, and more than 2.5 billion persons worldwide live in at-risk areas. Annually, there are 100 million infections, 250,000 cases of dengue hemorrhagic fever, and 25,000 deaths. With the notable exception of sub-Saharan Africa, where malaria predominates, dengue is among the most common causes of fever in travelers to most regions. In Southeast Asia, it occurs more frequently than all other causes of travel-related fever combined. Dengue is transmitted by *Aedes* mosquitoes, which, unlike the anopheline vectors of malaria, feed during the day, particularly in the morning and late afternoon. Furthermore, *Aedes* predominate in urban environments, in contrast to the rural anophelines. Almost all U.S. cases are imported, although *Aedes* vectors are endemic to the southeastern United States, where they create the potential for autochthonous transmission. The incubation period is usually 4 to 8 days and is rarely longer than 2 weeks.

Most commonly, dengue infection is subclinical or presents as a mild, self-limited, febrile illness. Classic dengue is associated with sudden-onset fevers, headaches, retro-orbital pain, and arthralgias and myalgias, the severity of which have earned dengue the moniker "break-bone fever." Nausea, vomiting, lymphadenopathy, and a maculopapular or petechial rash may also be observed. Leukopenia, thrombocytopenia, and elevated transaminases are very common. The rash is classically biphasic, transiently appearing during the first few days and then reappearing near the time of defervescence as erythema surrounding islands of normal-appearing skin.

Dengue hemorrhagic fever and dengue shock syndrome are complications that occur primarily at the time of defervescence and are responsible for most of the morbidity and mortality associated with dengue. Although the mechanisms that lead to these complications are complex, infection with a second dengue serotype seems to be involved, particularly in children. Therefore, these syndromes are rare in tourist travelers and are more common in VFR travelers, who may have had previous dengue infections. Hemorrhagic symptoms, severe thrombocytopenia, and manifestations of capillary plasma leakage, including ascites and pleural effusions, are hallmarks of dengue hemorrhagic fever. An acute drop in platelet count at about the time of defervescence, followed by an increase in hematocrit, can be a sign of impending dengue hemorrhagic fever. Bone marrow suppression and renal failure may also be seen. Dengue shock syndrome is characterized by circulatory collapse.

Diagnosis can be made in the first days of illness by PCR tests or culture of the virus, and later by serologic assays. However, these tests are not usually rapidly available at the time of presentation, so the diagnosis should be made primarily on clinical criteria. Treatment is supportive, but frequent monitoring for hematologic and circulatory abnormalities should be performed to assess for dengue hemorrhagic fever or shock syndrome. Admission should be considered for patients with a platelet count lower than $100,000/mm^3$, especially around the time of defervescence or if there is a concurrent rise in hematocrit.

Enteric Fever

Enteric fever, caused by *S. enterica* Typhi and *S. enterica* Paratyphi, is another major cause of febrile illness among travelers. Enteric fever is endemic to most of the developing world, with highest incidence in South Asia. Transmission is through ingestion of contaminated water or food. VFR travelers are at particularly high risk for typhoid.

Classic enteric fever is characterized by abdominal discomfort, fever, constipation (usually in adults) or diarrhea (usually in children or in HIV-positive adults). On examination, hepatomegaly, splenomegaly, and lymphadenopathy may be noted. A small proportion of patients demonstrate so-called rose spots, a blanching, erythematous, maculopapular rash on the trunk. Relative bradycardia is considered a classic finding but is not consistently seen in clinical practice. Laboratory examination may reveal mild pancytopenia and elevation of transaminases. Diagnosis is made by blood or stool culture; bone marrow cultures are even more sensitive.

Enteric fever is usually mild, and fatality rates are low. Most patients do not seek care or have their infection treated on an outpatient basis. However, cardiovascular, neurologic, and gastrointestinal complications occur in 10% to 15% of patients. Relapses, seen in 5% to 10% of patients, usually occur within 1 month and may be treated with a longer course of antimicrobials. In addition, up to 4% of patients become chronic carriers and may excrete the organism in their stool or urine for up to 1 year. This may pose a public health risk, particularly if the patient is in the food service industry.

Treatment of enteric fever in the developed world is usually with ciprofloxacin or ceftriaxone (Rocephin),[1] although there is increasing resistance to fluoroquinolones, particularly in South Asia. Azithromycin[1] appears to be another good option. The initial choice of antimicrobial can be based on the regional prevalence of drug resistance, with further therapy guided by antibiotic susceptibility testing. In addition to routine susceptibility testing, patients should be screened for nalidixic acid (NegGram) resistance, because resistance to this parent quinolone compound is associated with fluoroquinolone treatment failure even if the isolate appears susceptible by routine testing.

Other Destination-Specific Febrile Illnesses

Chikungunya, an alphavirus and a re-emerging infection, is transmitted predominantly by *Aedes* mosquitoes. Chikungunya is endemic to the Indian Ocean basin and sub-Saharan Africa, and an outbreak has also been reported in Italy. Patients usually experience fevers, headaches, nausea and vomiting, abdominal pain, and severe muscle and joint pains similar to those associated with dengue. Patients often have persistent arthralgias, predominantly in the small joints of the hands, wrists, feet, and ankles, which may last for longer than 1 year. During the first week of illness, diagnosis is by reverse transcriptase-PCR; thereafter, virus-specific antibodies can be detected. Treatment is supportive, but nonsteroidal antiinflammatory agents

may be useful in treating arthralgias. Although chikungunya is clinically similar to dengue, no hemorrhagic or shock syndrome has been associated with this viral disease.

DIARRHEA

Diarrhea occurring during travel is most commonly caused by ETEC, *Campylobacter jejuni*, *Salmonella*, *Shigella* spp., norovirus, rotavirus, and enteric adenoviruses. In most cases of TD caused by bacterial or viral pathogens, the disease is self-limited or can be managed by self-treatment during travel. However, bacterial diarrhea may manifest after return from travel, especially from Southeast Asia, where *Campylobacter* or *Shigella* is often the cause. This may be due in part to the increasing prevalence of antibiotic-resistant bacteria; fluoroquinolone-resistant *C. jejuni* is particularly common in Southeast Asia.

The likelihood of identifying a causal pathogen decreases as the duration of the diarrhea episode increases. Between 5% and 10% of returned travelers report diarrhea lasting at least 2 weeks, and 1% to 3% report diarrhea lasting 4 weeks or longer. Chronic diarrhea (defined as diarrhea lasting ≥4 weeks) is more likely to be caused by a parasitic infection (e.g., *G. intestinalis*, *Cryptosporidium* spp., *E. histolytica*, *C. cayetanensis*, *Strongyloides stercoralis*). Chronic diarrhea after travel with malabsorption and weight loss should prompt evaluation for giardiasis or tropical sprue. TD, especially when caused by enteroinvasive bacteria, may exacerbate inflammatory bowel disease. Development of irritable bowel syndrome after an episode of TD has also been reported in returned travelers, both in retrospective studies of North American travelers to Mexico and in a prospective study of Israeli travelers, primarily to Asia. Compared with tourist travelers, VFR travelers seem to have lower rates of acute and chronic diarrhea but higher rates of intestinal parasite infection.

Patients with acute or chronic diarrhea should have a CBC with differential; stool culture; stool acid-fast stain; stool assays for *Cryptosporidium*, *Giardia*, and *E. histolytica*; three stool ova and parasite examinations; and other stool or serologic studies performed based on clinical suspicion.

DERMATOLOGIC CONDITIONS

Dermatologic problems are common in returned travelers and are usually caused by insect bites, allergic or contact dermatitides, photosensitivity, scabies, or skin abscesses. The work-up comprises exposure history, physical examination, and basic laboratory tests including CBC and differential, specific serologic tests, and skin biopsy. The differential diagnosis is often determined by the type of lesion.

Serpiginous Lesions

Cutaneous larva migrans manifests with a track-like, migratory, pruritic rash, often occurring on the feet. Disease is caused by direct skin contact with contaminated soil or sand, followed by migration and death of animal hookworms in the superficial tissue. Strongyloidiasis may also be associated with a migratory rash or with a serpiginous rash called larva currens.

Nodular Lesions

Nodules or discrete swellings may be caused by tissue infestation with fly larvae (myiasis). Disease is caused by invading larvae (commonly tumbu fly in Africa, botfly in Latin America) and results in painful papules or furuncles. Occasionally, the posterior end of the larva can be seen through a small, central punctum. Burrowing sand fleas (tungiasis) may cause similar painful or pruritic lesions, usually on the soles and interdigital webs of the foot. Other causes of nodular skin eruptions include bacterial furuncles, Calabar swellings (from the nematode, *Loa loa*), trypanosomiasis, and gnathostomiasis. Human schistosomes found in fresh water produce a pruritic papular rash, which occurs as the larval forms of the parasite (cercariae) penetrate exposed skin.

---

[1]Not FDA approved for this indication.

TABLE 4 Travel Medicine Websites for Travelers and Providers*

Organization	Web Page Title and Content	Address
Centers for Diseases Control and Prevention (CDC)	Travelers' Health: international travel and health	http://www.cdc.gov/travel/index.htm
	Health Information for International Travel (The Yellow Book): destination-specific and disease-specific information for travelers	http://wwwn.cdc.gov/travel/contentYellowBook.aspx
	Malaria: Topic Home	http://www.cdc.gov/malaria/
World Health Organization (WHO)	International Travel and Health	http://www.who.int/ith/en/
	Epidemic and Pandemic Alert and Response (EPR): disease outbreak news	http://www.who.int/csr/don/en/
U.S. Advisory Committee on Immunization Practices (ACIP)	Recommendations and Guidelines: vaccine schedules and guidelines	http://www.cdc.gov/vaccines/recs/acip/
	Vaccine Information Statements: information sheets for patients	http://www.cdc.gov/vaccines/pubs/vis/
Immunization Action Coalition	Vaccination Information for Healthcare Professionals, including link to ACIP guidelines	http://www.immunize.org/
U.S. Department of State Bureau of Consular Affairs	International Travel: travel warnings and consular information	http://www.travel.state.gov/travel
Public Health Agency of Canada	Travel Health: travel health and current travel advisories	http://www.phac-aspc.gc.ca/tmp-pmv/index-eng.php
U.S. Occupational Safety and Health Administration (OSHA)	Safety and Health During International Travel: technical information bulletin for international business travelers	http://www.osha.gov/dts/tib/tib_data/tib20020412.pdf
Central Intelligence Agency	The World Factbook: country profiles including major infectious diseases	https://www.cia.gov/library/publications/the-world-factbook/index.html
International Association for Medical Assistance to Travelers (IAMAT)	Home page: health advice for travelers	http://www.iamat.org/
International Society of Travel Medicine	Home page	http://www.istm.org/
American Society of Tropical Medicine and Hygiene	Home page	http://www.astmh.org/
Global Infectious Diseases Epidemiology Online Network (GIDEON)	Home page: reference database in tropical and infectious diseases diagnosis, epidemiology, microbiology and antimicrobials (requires subscription)	http://www.gideononline.com/
Travel Medicine	Home page: products and information for safe travel	http://www.travmed.com/
Travax and Travax Encompass	Shoreland home page: travel medicine resource for providers (requires subscription)	http://www.shoreland.com/
Travel Health Online (derived from U.S. Travax)	Home page: free travel health information for travelers (no subscription, for personal use only)	http://www.tripprep.com/

*All websites were accessed May 8, 2009.

Ulcerative Lesions

Infection with *Leishmania* spp. can have variable clinical syndromes based on the infecting species, which differ geographically. Cutaneous disease is especially common among travelers to South and Central America and usually manifests as granulomatous or crusted ulcerations or, occasionally, as lymphocutaneous lesions.

Post-travel Counseling

Providers who care for travelers should be vigilant for travel-related health issues. Travelers should be advised to seek care immediately if they develop fever or other concerning symptoms for up to 1 year after travel. They should inform the physician about their travels, and a thorough evaluation and work-up should be initiated. Providers should be able to recognize, diagnose, and treat or refer major infectious and noninfectious conditions that may occur in travelers during or after travel. A detailed travel history should always be obtained and may be relevant to active medical issues for months to years after travel. Given the complexity of evaluating for exposure risks, itinerary-specific recommendations, and the potential for unusual travel-related illnesses, providers should be cognizant of the resources available through subspecialists and travel clinics, the CDC, the World Health Organization, and many other electronic and organizational sources (Table 4).

REFERENCES

Abramowicz M, Zuccotti G. Advice for travelers. Treatment guidelines from the Medical Letter 2006;4:25–34.

Centers for Disease Control and Prevention. ACIP Recommendations. Available at http://www.cdc.gov/vaccines/pubs/ACIP-list.htm. Accessed September 8, 2009. This page last modified on September 1, 2009.

Centers for Disease Control and Prevention. Travelers' Health—Yellow Book Available at http://wwwn.cdc.gov/travel/content/yellowbook/home-2010.aspx. Accessed September 8, 2009. This page last modified on July 27, 2009.

DuPont AW, DuPont HL. Travelers' diarrhea: modern concepts and new developments. Curr Treat Options Gastroenterol 2006;9:13–21.

Freedman DO. Clinical practice. Malaria prevention in short-term travelers. N Engl J Med 2008;359:603–12.

Freedman DO, Weld LH, Kozarsky PE, et al. Spectrum of disease and relation to place of exposure among ill returned travelers. N Engl J Med 2006;354:119–30.

Leder K, Tong S, Weld L, et al. Illness in travelers visiting friends and relatives: a review of the GeoSentinel Surveillance Network. Clin Infect Dis 2006;43:1185–93.

Lederman ER, Weld LH, Elyazar IR, et al. Dermatologic conditions of the ill returned traveler: an analysis from the GeoSentinel Surveillance Network. Int J Infect Dis 2008;12:593–602.

Ryan ET, Wilson ME, Kain KC. Illness after international travel. N Engl J Med 2002;347:505–16.

Steffen R, Tornieporth N, Clemens SA, et al. Epidemiology of travelers' diarrhea: details of a global survey. J Travel Med 2004;11:231–7.

Toxoplasmosis

Method of
Robert C. Goldstein, MD, and
Benjamin J. Luft, MD

Toxoplasmosis is the disease caused by the ubiquitous, obligate intracellular protozoan *Toxoplasma gondii*. Samuel T. Darling first described toxoplasmosis in the adult human in 1908. B. H. Kean and R. G. Grocott suggested *Toxoplasma* as the identity of the organism in 1945. In the immunocompetent host, toxoplasmosis is usually self-limited and may cause asymptomatic lymphadenopathy or, rarely, acute chorioretinitis. If *Toxoplasma* is acquired within 3 months of conception or during the first or second trimester of pregnancy, potentially grave congenital infection may result. If it is acquired during the third trimester, transmission occurs with greater frequency but the infant tends to be asymptomatic at birth, only to have manifestations of the disease later in life. The immunocompromised host is especially at risk for newly acquired infection (e.g., through solid organ transplantation) and for reactivation of latent organisms (e.g., AIDS, bone marrow transplantation, severe immunosuppression secondary to chemotherapy) with infection involving all tissues but manifesting most prominently within the central nervous system.

Pathophysiology and Epidemiology

The protozoan exists in three main forms: sporozoite, tachyzoite, and bradyzoite. Although *T. gondii* may infect humans, other mammals, and birds (intermediate hosts), its definitive host is the cat family, Felidae. It is only in the cat that the organism can undergo its entire life cycle. Asexual and then sexual replication of the organism occurs in the epithelium of cat small intestine, producing environmentally hardy oocysts. Oocysts are shed in cat feces for 3 to 14 days after the primary infection. In favorable environmental conditions (i.e., soil of high humidity and moderate temperatures [4°C-37°C]), sporulation occurs in 2 to 5 days, creating a sporozoite within the oocyst. This infectious state may remain for up to a year, or possibly longer.

The sporozoites are ingested by hosts in contaminated meat, water, and soil to initiate the tachyzoite form. In the intermediate host, this is produced by an extraintestinal asexual cycle. In this rapidly multiplying stage, tachyzoites disseminate in the bloodstream and infect many tissues, including central nervous system, heart muscle, skeletal muscle, liver, spleen, and placenta. Clinical manifestations are caused by the inflammatory response to tachyzoite infestation. This includes helper T-cell (Th1) production and production of cytokines interleukin-12, tumor necrosis factor-α, and interferon-γ. In turn, this response leads to the formation of bradyzoites within cysts, which can persist in tissues, causing latent infection.

Transmission to humans occurs by oral ingestion of infected undercooked meat containing cysts, eating of undercooked food that has come into contact with infected meat, ingestion of contaminated water or soil containing sporulated oocysts, organ transplantation from an infected donor, blood transfusion, laboratory accidents, and vertically by congenital transmission.

Seroprevalence of infection increases with age; is roughly equal in males and females; is lower in regions that are cold, hot, arid, or of high elevation (possibly because *T. gondii* oocysts do not survive well in the soil of these areas); and varies according to health and hygiene practices. Prevalence is higher in Western Europe (e.g., 65%-85% in France) than in the United States (20%-40%). This may be related to higher consumption of raw or undercooked meat in Europe. This also holds true for tropical parts of South America and sub-Saharan Africa, where the humid climate favors survival of oocysts and there is an abundance of cats.

CURRENT DIAGNOSIS

- *Toxoplasma*-specific immunoglobulin G can be used as an initial screening test for all patients.
- *Toxoplasma*-specific immunoglobulin M can be used to help differentiate between acutely acquired and latent infection, but results may not be fully reliable, and samples should be sent to a *Toxoplasma* reference laboratory for confirmation.
- Treat all immunocompromised patients who have multiple ring-enhancing brain lesions for presumed toxoplasmosis and monitor for response.

Each year in the United States, there are between 400 and 4000 congenital infections, 1.26 million cases of ocular infection, and many cases of systemic or neurologic infection among immunocompromised persons. Approximately 23% of U.S. adolescents and adults have been exposed to *T. gondii*. There are approximately 750 deaths per year, with 50% to 60% of these infections probably acquired through food. Overall, *Toxoplasma* complications account for 21% of food-related deaths, third after *Salmonella* and *Listeria*.

In a recent study conducted by the Centers for Disease Control and Prevention (CDC), the overall age-adjusted seroprevalence of persons aged 6 to 49 years in the United States was 10.8%. Seroprevalence is lower among U.S.-born individuals than among immigrants. For example, the seroprevalence was 7.7% among U.S-born women and 28.1% among foreign-born women. There was also a higher prevalence among people living below the poverty index level. When looking at ethnic groups of U.S.-born persons between 1999 and 2004, the immunoglobulin G (IgG) seroprevalence was highest in non-Hispanic blacks and lowest in Mexican Americans, with non-Hispanic whites being in between. Among U.S. and foreign-born members of different ethnic groups between 6 and 49 years of age, Mexican Americans had the highest prevalence (13.7%) and non-Hispanic whites the lowest (8.7%). Overall, there was a significant drop in seroprevalence among U.S.-born persons between 12 and 49 years of age between 1988–1994 (14.1%) and 1999–2004 (9.0%). This may be due to improved food, livestock, and pet hygiene.

Diagnosis and Testing

Detection is available via indirect methods (serology) and directly (polymerase chain reaction [PCR] of DNA, hybridization, culture, and pathology). Serology is often used for diagnosis in immunocompetent patients (Fig. 1). Immunocompromised patients often require direct evidence to definitively establish the diagnosis; biopsy with evidence of tachyzoites is diagnostic of acute infection.

IgG is used as a screening test in all categories of patients, including immunocompromised patients, pregnant patients, newborns, and those with eye infection. The Sabin-Feldman dye test, the IgG avidity test, the immunofluorescent antibody test, the enzyme-linked immunosorbent assay (ELISA), or the agglutination and differential agglutination (AC/HS) test can be used for IgG detection. Antibody develops within 1 to 8 weeks after infection and persists for life. In newborns, maternal IgG may persist for up to 1 year, so differentiation is needed by a Western blot or enzyme-linked immune filtration assay (ELIFA).

A positive IgG high avidity test, which measures the strength with which IgG binds to *Toxoplasma*, can be used to rule out infection within the past 3 to 5 months in pregnant patients and in those with ocular infection. High-avidity antibodies develop 12 to 16 weeks after infection, depending on the testing kit used. A positive result in a pregnant woman during the first 3 months of pregnancy indicates that the woman most likely was infected before she became pregnant,

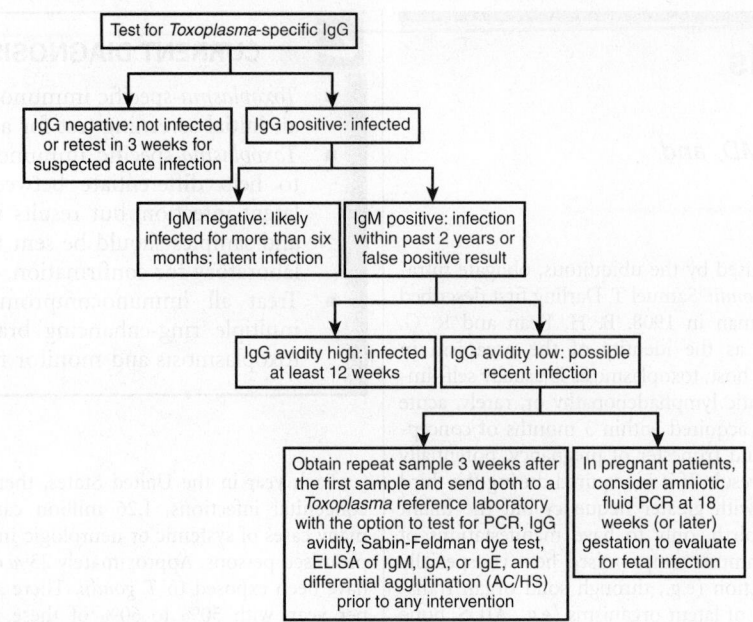

FIGURE 1. Suggested algorithm for serologic testing of *Toxoplasma gondii* in people older than 1 year of age. Equivocal results should be repeated and sent for confirmatory testing at a reference laboratory. *Abbreviations:* AC/HS = agglutination and differential agglutination test; ELISA = enzyme-linked immunosorbent assay; Ig = immunoglobulin; PCR = polymerase chain reaction. (Adapted with permission from Wilson M, Jones JL, McAuley JB: Toxoplasma. In Murray PR, Baron EJ, Landry ML, et al [eds]: Manual of Clinical Microbiology, 9th ed. Washington, DC, ASM Press, 2007, pp 2070–2081.)

so the fetus is not at high risk for having acquired *Toxoplasma*. The absence of IgG antibodies in early pregnancy identifies mothers who are at risk for acquiring acute infection.

IgM, detectable within 2 weeks, is generally used to rule out recently acquired infection. A negative IgM test during the first two trimesters of pregnancy rules out infection. In early pregnancy, more power can be attained by testing for both IgM and IgG. Negative results with ocular disease may indicate reactivation of congenital infection, whereas high titers may signify an acutely acquired infection. IgM can also be used for neonatal screening of toxoplasmosis. The particularly sensitive and specific IgM immunosorbent agglutination assay (ISAGA) can be used for this purpose. IgM has low sensitivity in immunocompromised patients. Confirmation of positive results should be attained from a *Toxoplasma* reference laboratory, because many commercially available IgM testing kits have had problems with specificity (ranging from 77.5% to 99.1%), leading to high rates of false-positive results. In a recent examination of 100 consecutive serum samples of IgM-positive results received for confirmatory testing by the Palo Alto Medical Foundation Toxoplasma Serology Laboratory, 62% were found to be negative. Therefore, the greatest benefit of a positive IgM antibody test is that it demonstrates the possibility of a recently acquired infection, making it necessary to send the sample for confirmatory testing at a reference laboratory.

IgA, peaking in 2 months, can persist for prolonged periods (usually 1 to 5 years) and can be used in newborn testing. Combining IgA and IgM tests greatly increases sensitivity in neonates. Up to 75% of affected infants can be identified.

IgE is highly specific in pregnant patients but has low sensitivity. It can be used in combination with other serologic tests.

In addition to tissue diagnosis by immunohistochemistry, cell culture, and mouse inoculation, PCR amplification of specific genes can be used for direct detection. Amniotic fluid, blood, urine, vitreous or aqueous fluid, cerebrospinal fluid, peritoneal fluid, pleural fluid, bone marrow aspirate, and organ tissue can all be tested using PCR. With appropriate precautions to minimize contamination, PCR specificity and positive predictive value approach 100%. Mixed

results are obtained with sensitivity and negative predictive value when dealing with amniotic fluid, although PCR is useful in prenatal testing for *T. gondii* by allowing for early diagnosis. PCR testing of amniotic fluid after 18 weeks of gestation caries a sensitivity of approximately 60% and a specificity of 100%. Amniotic fluid PCR should be considered in pregnant women with serology results suggestive of recently acquired infection, in those with ultrasound findings of possible toxoplasmosis, and in patients who are immunocompromised. Caution is advised, however, for pregnant women with HIV infection who may be coinfected with *T. gondii,* because of the risk of infecting the fetus with HIV during the amniocentesis. PCR is of great utility in immunocompromised patients, but it may not distinguish between acute (e.g., tachyzoites) and chronic (e.g., tissue cysts) infection. In immunocompromised patients, PCR amplification can be combined with parasite isolation from body fluids to demonstrate tachyzoites and tissue histologic findings.

Histologic findings in lymph nodes infected with *T. gondii* include reactive follicular hyperplasia, irregular clusters of epithelial-like histiocytes encroaching on germinal centers, and monocyte-like cells causing distention of sinuses. Neural tissue findings consist of multiple foci of necrosis and microglia nodules. Presence of tissue cysts indicates past infection but does not, on its own, indicate active infection. Wright-Giemsa stain may be used to visualize the cysts, but immunoperoxidase staining is more sensitive.

Neuroimaging should be done for any focal or nonfocal clinical neurologic findings in immunocompromised patients. In cases of *Toxoplasma* encephalitis, they may guide therapy and aid in diagnosis. Clinical and radiologic response to therapy, usually seen within 10 to 14 days, supports a diagnosis of toxoplasmosis without the need of invasive brain biopsy. Computed tomography or magnetic resonance imaging (MRI) may be used, although the latter is more sensitive. A noncontrast computed tomogram of the brain may show hypodense lesions with surrounding vasogenic edema in acute or subacute cases. Chronic lesions, especially after treatment, may appear calcified. MRI, preferably with gadolinium contrast, may show multiple ring-enhancing lesions that can occupy the basal ganglia, lobar gray-white junction, periventricular white matter, cerebral cortex, or posterior fossa. Surrounding edema is often disproportionately large compared with the lesion size. It is difficult to differentiate between toxoplasmosis brain lesions and lymphoma (an important differential in immunosuppressed patients). Positron emission tomography and single-photon emission tomography may have a role in making this distinction in the near future.

Infection in Immunocompetent Patients

Infection in immunocompetent hosts, including pregnant women, is usually asymptomatic. Between 10% and 20% of patients develop a nonspecific flu-like or mononucleosis-like illness with low-grade fever, malaise, or predominantly isolated cervical or occipital lymphadenopathy that is nontender. Nodes may stay enlarged for up to 6 weeks, but a fluctuating, chronic form has also been described. Myocarditis, polymyositis, encephalitis, pneumonitis, and hepatitis are possible but rare. In general, if signs and symptoms develop, they are self-limited and resolve within weeks to months.

Important and more common differential diagnoses that can cause similar symptoms are cytomegalovirus and Epstein-Barr virus infection. The differential diagnosis also includes cat scratch disease, lymphoma, tuberculosis, sarcoidosis, and metastatic cancer. To help establish a diagnosis, serology and lymph node biopsy should be performed.

Infection in Immunocompromised and AIDS Patients

Infection in immunocompromised patients usually occurs as a result of reactivation of chronic infection and may be life threatening. Multiorgan involvement is possible, including *Toxoplasma* pneumonia and septic shock, but the most typical findings involve the central nervous system. Meningeal signs rarely occur, but there may be altered mental status, seizures, cerebellar signs, focal neurologic deficits (i.e., speech abnormalities and hemiparesis), and neuropsychiatric findings.

The finding of multiple brain abscesses in an immunocompromised patient is highly suggestive of *Toxoplasma* encephalitis. There is usually bilateral hemisphere involvement, especially in the basal ganglia. Pulmonary toxoplasmosis is another possibility; it may manifest as a pneumonia, pneumonitis, or effusion.

Ocular Toxoplasmosis

Ocular infection may produce acute chorioretinitis, which can lead to necrotizing retinitis. The vitreous humor may become exudative, with tachyzoites and cysts possibly visible within the retina. The typical finding is areas of white focal lesions with a surrounding vitreal inflammatory reaction, the classic "headlight in the fog."

Ocular disease may result from congenital or acutely acquired infection. Acute infection is thought to be more common. Patients with congenitally acquired infection typically have bilateral eye disease, whereas those with acutely acquired infection usually have unilateral signs.

Congenital Toxoplasmosis and Toxoplasmosis in Pregnancy

In the United States, approximately 85% of women of child-bearing age are at risk for acquiring *T. gondii*. Mother-to-fetus vertical transmission can occur through an infected placenta. If a mother obtains a primary infection more than 3 months before conception (i.e., only

CURRENT THERAPY

- Pyrimethamine (Daraprim) plus sulfadiazine[1] plus folinic acid (Leucovorin)[1] is the mainstay of therapy for toxoplasmosis.
- Spiramycin (Rovamycine)[2] should be used for therapy in pregnancy if treatment is needed before 18 weeks of gestation, because of the possible teratogenic effects of pyrimethamine.
- Prophylactic treatment should be initiated for immunocompromised patients who have a CD4[+] count of less than 100 cells/mm^3 and should be continued for the life of the patient or until immunosuppression has ended.

[1]Not FDA approved for this indication.
[2]Not available in the United States.

positive IgG is present), there is little risk to the fetus. There is a small but discernible increased risk if the infection is obtained within 3 months of conception, and this risk progressively increases throughout gestation. The frequency of transmission is inversely related to the severity of disease. Although the rate of toxoplasmosis transmission between mother and fetus is low (10%-20%), maternal infection in the first two trimesters can result in severe congenital toxoplasmosis and possibly fetal death. Maternal third-trimester infection leads most often to fetal toxoplasmosis (80%-90%) but also often results in subclinical infection in newborns. If this is left untreated, chorioretinitis and growth retardation may develop in the second or third decade of life. Immunocompromised patients with chronic infection can rarely transmit infection via the placenta.

There are no specific diagnostic ultrasound findings of fetal toxoplasmosis. Findings include increased placental thickness, intracranial calcifications, ventricular dilatation, liver enlargement, and ascites. Hydrocephalus demonstrated by ultrasonography has been used as an indication to terminate pregnancy.

In infected infants, pathologic examination of brain tissue typically reveals periaqueductal and periventricular vasculitis and necrosis. Calcification of necrotic areas may be revealed on imaging. Hydrocephalus can develop secondary to obstruction. However, the classic triad of hydrocephalus, chorioretinitis, and cerebral calcifications is a rare occurrence. Instead, several nonspecific signs are microcephaly, blindness, strabismus, epilepsy, mental retardation, anemia, thrombocytopenia, hepatosplenomegaly, jaundice, and rash. These signs are included in the TORCH (toxoplasmosis, other infections, rubella, cytomegalovirus, and herpes simplex) syndrome.

Treatment

Suggested toxoplasmosis treatment regimens are summarized in Table 1.

IMMUNOCOMPETENT HOSTS

Lymphadenitis usually is not treated unless symptoms persist or are severe. Combination therapy with pyrimethamine (Daraprim), sulfadiazine,[1] and folinic acid (leucovorin)[1] for 2 to 6 weeks is the typical regimen. Infection acquired through blood products or laboratory accidents is usually more serious and requires treatment.

[1]Not FDA approved for this indication.

TABLE 1 Suggested Toxoplasmosis Treatment Regimens

Population	Drug	Dosage	Duration
Acute infection in an immunocompetent patient or in a pregnant patient infected ≥6 mo before conception	Treatment not recommended *or,* if acutely ill, Pyrimethamine (Daraprim) *plus*	200 mg PO loading dose, then 50–75 mg PO daily 1–1.5 g PO q6h	4–6 wk, or 1–2 wk after symptoms resolve
	Sulfadiazine[1] *plus* Leucovorin (folinic acid)[1]	5–20 mg PO TIW	During and 1 week after pyrimethamine use
Acute infection in a pregnant patient acquired <18 wk gestation ≥18 wk gestation	Spiramycin (Rovamycine)[2] See fetal infection (or, if amniotic PCR test is negative, consider switch to spiramycin)	1g PO q8h without food	Throughout pregnancy or until fetal infection is documented
Fetal infection (after 16–18 wk gestation)	Pyrimethamine *plus*	Loading dose 50 mg PO q12h × 2 d, then 50 mg PO daily	Throughout pregnancy
	Sulfadiazine[1] *plus*	Loading dose 75 mg/kg PO, then 50 mg/kg q12h (maximum, 4 g daily)	Throughout pregnancy
	Leucovorin	10–20 mg PO daily	During and for 1 wk after pyrimethamine use
Congenital infection in the infant	Pyrimethamine *plus*	Loading dose 2 mg/kg PO daily × 2 d, then 1 mg/kg PO daily × 2–6 mo, then 1 mg/kg TIW	1 y
	Sulfadiazine *plus*	50 mg/kg PO q12h	1 y
	Leucovorin *and possibly*	10 mg PO TIW	During and for 1 wk after pyrimethamine use
	Prednisone (if CSF protein is ≥1 g/dL and if chorioretinitis threatens vision)	1 mg/kg daily in two divided doses	Until signs resolve
Adult chorioretinitis	Pyrimethamine[1] *plus*	200 mg PO loading dose, then 50–75 mg PO daily	1–2 wk after symptoms resolve
	Sulfadiazine *plus*	1–1.5 g PO q6h	1–2 wk after symptoms resolve
	Leucovorin *and possibly*	5–20 mg PO TIW	During and 1 wk after pyrimethamine use
	Prednisone	1 mg/kg daily in two divided doses	Until signs and symptoms resolve
Immunocompromised patients and patients with encephalitis*	Pyrimethamine *plus*	Loading dose 200 mg PO, then 50–75 mg PO daily	At least 4–6 wk after signs and symptoms resolve
	Leucovorin *plus either*	10–20 mg PO or IV or IM daily (maximum, 50 mg daily)	During and for 1 wk after pyrimethamine use
	Sulfadiazine *or*	1–1.5 g PO q6h	At least 4–6 wk after signs and symptoms resolve
	Clindamycin (Cleocin)[1] *Alternatives:*	600 mg PO or IV q6h (maximum, 1200 mg q6h)	Same as above
	Trimethoprim-sulfamethoxazole (Bactrim)[1] alone, or	5 mg/kg trimethoprim PO or IV q12h (maximum, 15–20 mg/kg/day)	Same as above
	Pyrimethamine *plus* leucovorin *plus one of the following:*	Same as above pyrimethamine/leucovorin doses	
	Clarithromycin (Biaxin)[1]	1 g PO q12h[†]	
	Atovaquone (Mepron)[1]	750 mg PO q6h	
	Azithromycin (Zithromax)[1]	1200–1500 mg PO daily	
	Dapsone[1]	100 mg PO daily	
Primary prophylaxis for immunocompromised patients (i.e., CD4$^+$ count ≤100 cells/mm^3)	Trimethoprim-sulfamethoxazole (Bactrim DS)[1] *Alternatives:*	1 double-strength tablet (160/800 mg) PO daily	For life or until immunosuppression has abated (see text)
	Pyrimethamine[1] *plus* dapsone[1] *plus* leucovorin	50–75 mg/wk pyrimethamine *plus* 50 mg/day dapsone *plus* 25 mg/wk leucovorin	
	Pyrimethamine-sulfadoxine (Fansidar)[1] *plus* leucovorin	1 tablet twice weekly Fansidar *plus* 25 mg/wk leucovorin	Same as above

Adapted with permission from Montoya JG, Liesenfeld O: Toxoplasmosis. Lancet 2004;363(9425):1965–1976.
[1]Not FDA approved for this indication.
[2]Not available in the United States.
*After the initial phase of therapy, maintenance therapy must be continued as long as the patient remains immunocompromised. See text for details.
[†]In a recent CDC report, doses of clarithromycin above 500 mg twice daily may be associated with increased mortality in patients treated for disseminated *Mycobacterium avium* complex.
Abbreviations: CSF = cerebrospinal fluid; IM = intramuscular; PCR = polymerase chain reaction; PO = orally; TID = three times daily; TIW = three times per week.

PREGNANCY

Although not universally utilized, spiramycin (Rovamycine),[2] available through the CDC, is recommended for suspected or confirmed acute maternal infection acquired during gestation in the first and early second trimester or pyrimethamine plus sulfadiazine[1] in the late second and third trimesters. Definitive diagnosis of acute infection requires conversion of a negative titer to a positive one or a significant rise in titers. In addition, infection of the mother does not necessarily indicate infection of the fetus. Therefore, it is necessary to have prenatal diagnostic testing by amniotic fluid PCR (sensitivity ranges from 68% to 98.8%).

If the PCR result is negative, spiramycin prophylaxis should be given until at least the 17th week of pregnancy. In Austria and Germany, this is followed by 4 weeks of pyrimethamine plus sulfadiazine[1] plus leucovorin.[1] In the United States and France, spiramycin[2] is continued throughout pregnancy, in addition to monthly ultrasound examinations.

If the PCR result is positive and the possibility of fetal infection is high (e.g., by ultrasound findings) or the infection was acquired after 18 weeks of gestation, it is recommended to use the pyrimethamine and sulfadiazine regimen after 18 weeks of gestation (although in some countries this may start as early as 16 weeks). In some countries, this regimen is alternated with spiramycin, but it does not reliably cross the placenta to treat fetal infection. Treatment is continued throughout pregnancy, along with monthly ultrasound examinations and folinic acid to reduce bone marrow toxicity. Pyrimethamine is potentially teratogenic and should not be given during the first 16 to 18 weeks of pregnancy. In most countries, treatment is continued for the newborn through the first year of life.

Treatment of acute infection during pregnancy has been associated with a reduction in the rate of fetal infection of about 50%. The European Research Network on Congenital Toxoplasmosis sponsored studies of the effects of treatment in pregnant mothers. One of the studies confirmed prenatal infection with amniocentesis or cordocentesis. These women were treated with pyrimethamine plus sulfadiazine or pyrimethamine plus sulfadoxine (Fansidar).[1] The congenital transmission rate was 39% in women who received therapy and 72% in those who did not; this difference was not statistically significant when time of gestation was taken into account. The percentage of infants born with severe congenital signs of toxoplasmosis in mothers who received prenatal treatment was 3.5%, compared with 20% in those who did not receive treatment. The earlier antibiotics were given, the greater their efficacy in preventing severe infection. Additionally, The National Collaborative Chicago-Based Congenital Toxoplasmosis Study prospectively studied 120 infected infants who were treated between 1981 and 2004 with pyrimethamine, sulfadiazine, and leucovorin for 1 year; there were significantly fewer occurrences of cognitive, motor, vision, and hearing abnormalities. Patients with congenital toxoplasmosis who are not treated or are treated for only 1 month have been shown to have poor outcomes.

Caution must be taken in the use of antibiotics to treat congenital infection. Sulfonamides given late in pregnancy have been associated with kernicterus in the newborn. Pyrimethamine is a folic acid antagonist (dihydrofolate reductase inhibitor) that can cause neural tube defects, because folic acid serves as a coenzyme in the formation of DNA, RNA, myelin, and lipids. Folinic acid (leucovorin)[1] should be given with pyrimethamine to compensate for the reduction of folic acid. Pyrimethamine has also been associated with kidney and heart malformations in newborns and with increased risk of central nervous system cancers in children. There is also danger of bone marrow suppression in mother and fetus from treatment with pyrimethamine and sulfadiazine (a dihydrofolate synthetase inhibitor), requiring weekly blood count monitoring. Risks and benefits must be weighed before treatment for toxoplasmosis is implemented in the pregnant patient.

CHORIORETINITIS

Treatment is recommended for severe inflammatory reaction and for close proximity of retinal lesions to the fovea or optic disk. Small peripheral retinal lesions in immunocompetent patients may not need treatment, because the disease may be self-limited. If treatment is warranted, a common regimen consists of pyrimethamine (with leucovorin), sulfadiazine, and prednisone continued for at least 1 week after the resolution of symptoms. Alternatively, clindamycin (Cleocin)[1] and trimethoprim-sulfamethoxazole (TMP/SMX [Bactrim])[1] may be used. In cases of recurrent chorioretinitis, a long-term intermittent regimen of TMP-SMX may be of benefit. A short course of steroids may be given to patients with ocular or neural toxoplasmosis if there is suspicion of a significant inflammatory component of pathology.

IMMUNOCOMPROMISED HOSTS

In patients who have undergone organ transplantation, particularly those who are donor positive and recipient negative for *T. gondii*, prophylactic treatment with TMP-SMX[1] is recommended.

Immunocompromised patients are particularly susceptible to toxoplasma encephalitis. Neuroimaging by computed tomography or MRI should be done for any suspicion of neurologic infection. It is standard practice to initiate anti-*Toxoplasma* therapy in the setting of multiple ring-enhancing lesions found on imaging with positive IgG titers in an immunocompromised patient. The most common regimen consists of pyrimethamine (with leucovorin) plus sulfadiazine[1] (or clindamycin[1] in sulfa-allergic patients) continued for at least 4 to 6 weeks after resolution of signs and symptoms. TMP-SMX[1] may be an acceptable alternative to pyrimethamine plus sulfadiazine, especially in developing countries where there is a limited supply of medications. Other alternatives, in combination with pyrimethamine and leucovorin, include atovaquone (Mepron)[1] (750 mg PO every 6 hours), dapsone[1] (100 mg PO daily), clarithromycin (Biaxin)[1] (1 g PO every 12 hours),* azithromycin (Zithromax)[1] (1200–1500 mg PO daily), and clindamycin[1] (600–1200 mg IV or PO every 6 hours).

After the initial phase of therapy has ended, maintenance therapy should be continued. This usually consists of the same regimen of medications, but at half the doses, for the life of the patient or until immunosuppression has concluded. In AIDS patients whose symptoms of toxoplasmosis have resolved, this usually coincides with a $CD4^+$ count greater than 200 cells/mm^3 that has been sustained for at least 6 months and an HIV PCR viral load that has been controlled for at least 6 months.

Prevention

The best treatment is prevention. HIV-positive patients and pregnant women should avoid extensive contact with cats whenever possible. If cats are present, they should not be fed undercooked meat, and they should be kept indoors to avoid contact with potentially infected soil. Litter boxes should be cleaned daily (and gloves should be worn) and disinfected with near-boiling water for 5 minutes before refilling. Petting of cats probably poses little risk of transmission of *Toxoplasma*. This may be due to generally frequent self-grooming by housecats and the fact that not much, if any, fecal material adheres to cat fur. Serologic testing of cats has not been shown to be of clinical utility. Cats may not develop antibodies during the oocyst-shedding period; they may test positive after already having shed the oocysts; and they may shed oocysts more than once. In addition, cats shed oocysts for only 1 to 2 weeks, making stool testing unhelpful.

Gloves should be worn when handling soil or gardening. It is also important to thoroughly wash the hands after contact with animals, soil, and raw meat and to appropriately cook meat. Beef, lamb, and veal roasts and steaks should be cooked to at least 145°F. Pork, ground meat, and wild game should be cooked to at least 160°F. Poultry should be

---

[1]Not FDA approved for this indication.
[2]Not available in the United States.

---

[1]Not FDA approved for this indication.
*In a recent CDC report, doses of clarithromycin above 500 mg twice daily may be associated with increased mortality in patients treated for disseminated *Mycobacterium avian* complex.

cooked to 180°F in the thigh. Fruits and vegetables need to be thoroughly washed or peeled before eating. Freezing food to −12°C can kill tissue cysts, and appropriate levels of irradiation may kill oocysts. Microwave ovens are not reliable because of uneven heating. Cooking utensils and appliances should be cleaned if they are contacted by undercooked or raw foods. To prevent contamination of food and water, felines should be kept away from farms and water sources.

Although there is no currently available human vaccine, prophylactic treatment should be offered to immunocompromised patients who are IgG positive. AIDS patients who have a CD4$^+$ count of less than 100 cells/mm^3 and are seropositive for *T. gondii* can receive primary prophylaxis with one double-strength tablet of TMP-SMX (160/800 mg [Bactrim DS])[1] daily. Alternative regimens although less effective, include pyrimethamine 50 to 75 mg/week plus dapsone[1] 50 mg/day or, as another option, pyrimethamine/sulfadoxine (Fansidar)[1] one tablet twice weekly. It has been suggested that primary prophylaxis should be discontinued in those patients who have responded to an effective HIV regimen and maintain a CD4 count >200 cells/mm^3 for more than 3 months.

Other options in preventing the spread of toxoplasmosis include health care provider and patient education about treatment and the interpretation of tests. Universal prenatal screening is used in some European nations (e.g., Austria, France). Cost-benefit analysis is still underway to determine whether the United States may adopt these methods, but there is the overlying risk of equivocal and false-positive results that may lead to further testing, stress, and unnecessary treatment.

REFERENCES

Bakshi R. Neuroimaging of HIV and AIDS related illnesses: A review. Front Biosci 2004;9:632–46.

Chirgwin K, Hafner R, Leport C, et al. Randomized phase II trial of atovaquone with pyrimethamine or sulfadiazine for treatment of toxoplasmic encephalitis in patients with acquired immunodeficiency syndrome: ACTG 237/ANRS 039 Study. Clin Infect Dis 2002;34:1243–50.

Fisher MA, Levy J, Helfrich M, et al. Detection of *Toxoplasma gondii* in the spinal fluid of a bone marrow transplant recipient. Pediatr Infect Dis 1987;6:81–3.

Foulon W, Villena I, Stray-Pedersen B, et al. Treatment of toxoplasmosis during pregnancy: A multicenter study of impact on fetal transmission and children's sequelae at age 1 year. Am J Obstet Gynecol 1999;180:410–5.

Hughes JM, Colley DG, Lopez A, et al. Preventing congenital toxoplasmosis. Morb Mortal Wkly Rep MMWR 2000;49(RR02):57–75.

Jones JL, Kruszon-Moran D, Sanders-Lewis K, et al. *Toxoplasma gondii* infection in the United States, 1999–2004: Decline from the prior decade. Am J Trop Med Hyg 2007;77(3):405–10.

Jones JL, Lopez A, Wilson M. Congenital toxoplasmosis. Am Fam Physician 2003;67(10):2131–8.

Jones JL, Lopez A, Wilson M, et al. Congenital toxoplasmosis: A review. Obstet Gynecol Surv 2001;56(5):296–305.

Kaplan JE, Benson C, Holmes KH, et al. Guidelines for prevention and treatment of opportunistic infections in HIV-infected adults and adolescents: Recommendations from CDC, the National Institutes of Health, and the HIV Medicine Association of the Infectious Diseases Society of America. MMWR Recomm Rep 2009;58:1–207.

Luft BJ, Conley F, Remington JS, et al. Outbreak of central-nervous system toxoplasmosis in Western Europe and North America. Lancet 1983;1:781–3.

Luft BJ, Hafner R, Korzun AH, et al. Toxoplasmic encephalitis in patients with acquired immunodeficiency syndrome: Development of objective criteria for early diagnosis and treatment. N Engl J Med 1993;329(14): 995–1000.

Luft BJ, Remington JS. Acquired toxoplasmic encephalitis. In: Remington JS, Swartz M, editors. Current Clinical Topics in Infectious Diseases, vol. 6. New York: McGraw-Hill; 1985.

McAuley JB. Toxoplasmosis in children. Pediatr Infect Dis J 2008;27:161–2.

McLeod R, Boyer K, Karrison T, et al. Outcome of treatment for congenital toxoplasmosis, 1981–2004: The National Collaborative Chicago-Based, Congenital Toxoplasmosis Study. Clin Infect Dis 2006;42(10):1383–94.

Montoya JG, Liesenfeld O. Toxoplasmosis. Lancet 2004;363:1965–76.

Montoya JG, Remington JS. Management of *Toxoplasma gondii* infection during pregnancy. Clin Infect Dis 2008;47(4):554–66.

Remington JS. Toxoplasmosis in the adult. Bull N Y Acad Med 1974;50(2):211–26.

Wilson M, Jones JL, McAuley JB. Toxoplasma. In: Murray PR, Baron EJ, Landry M, et al., Manual of Clinical Microbiology. 9th ed. Washington, DC: ASM Press; 2007. p. 2070–81.

---

[1]Not FDA approved for this indication.

Cat-Scratch Disease

Method of
Michael J. Smith, MD, MSCE

Cat-scratch disease (CSD), regional lymphadenopathy following a cat scratch or bite, has been described since the 1950s. *Bartonella henselae*, a pleomorphic, facultative intracellular gram-negative bacillus, was not identified as the etiologic agent until 40 years later. As the laboratory detection of *B. henselae* has improved, it has become associated with an increasing number of clinical entities. These have traditionally been divided into typical CSD, the classic finding of unilateral regional lymphadenopathy following a cat scratch or bite, and atypical CSD, which includes all other presentations.

Epidemiology

As CSD is not a reportable disease, the true incidence remains unknown. However, there are an estimated 24,000 cases in the United States each year. Predominantly a disease of childhood and adolescence, CSD has the highest age-specific incidence rate occurring in children younger than 10 years of age. Although less frequent, CSD does occur in older individuals as well. A recent study found that 6% of patients with confirmed CSD were older than the age of 60 years.

Nearly 90% of patients with CSD have exposure to cats and approximately half recall a definitive scratch or bite. Early epidemiologic evidence suggested an increased risk of CSD in patients with kittens as compared to patients with adult cats. It was subsequently shown that kittens have a higher rate of *B. henselae* bacteremia than adult cats. In contrast, adult cats are more likely to have antibodies indicative of past infection. Most bacteremic cats are asymptomatic, so even a healthy-appearing animal can transmit disease.

The cat flea, *Ctenocephalides felis*, has been implicated in the transmission between cats. Consequently, CSD is more prevalent in warm and humid environments that support the growth of fleas with infection occurring primarily in the fall and winter months. To date, no evidence exists for human to human transmission.

Clinical Manifestations

Typical CSD is the most common form of CSD in immunocompetent patients. Initially, papules develop at the site of inoculation within the first week after a cat scratch or bite. This is followed by the gradual onset of unilateral regional lymphadenopathy over the next several weeks. Occasionally these lymph nodes may suppurate. The location of lymphadenopathy depends on the site of inoculation but most commonly occurs in the axillary, inguinal or cervical chains. In contrast to bacterial lymphadenitis, the lymph nodes are not inflamed. Patients are usually well-appearing and afebrile. Lymphadenopathy gradually resolves over several months without specific therapy.

The most common form of atypical CSD is Parinaud's oculoglandular syndrome (POGS), which occurs when bacteria are inoculated directly into the eye or eyelid. Small papules develop, almost always in the palpebral conjunctiva, in association with ipsilateral preauricular lymphadenopathy. There is also a painless, nonpurulent conjunctivitis. Similar to typical CSD, these symptoms resolve without antimicrobial therapy over several weeks.

Typical CSD and POGS share a similar pathophysiology; direct inoculation followed by a local immune response. In contrast, the other types of atypical CSD are due to systemic infection with *B. henselae*. These include hepatosplenic CSD, osteomyelitis, endocarditis, encephalitis, and neuroretinitis. *Bartonella* has also been implicated in the etiology of fever of unknown origin (FUO). One recent study revealed that 5% of all children with FUO of infectious etiology had antibodies against *B. henselae* indicative of current or recent infection.

In immunocompromised individuals, *B. henselae* can cause life-threatening invasive disease. Bacillary angiomatosis (BA), which is also caused by other *Bartonella* species, is caused by the angioproliferative effects of *Bartonella* and results in multiple vascular tumors in the skin and subcutaneous tissues. Bacillary peliosis (BP) is another form of vasoproliferative disease that leads to the development of blood-filled cysts in the reticuloendothelial element of the liver, spleen, and bone marrow of severely immunocompromised patients.

Diagnosis

A detailed history and physical examination are essential for the diagnosis of CSD. Any contact with cats or kittens, especially if bites or scratches occurred, should raise suspicion for CSD, regardless of the patient's age and clinical presentation.

Bartonella is a fastidious organism that takes several weeks to grow, making culture impractical. Therefore, serologic testing has become the mainstay of diagnosis. Indirect fluorescent antibody testing for IgM and IgG against *B. henselae* is performed by most commercial laboratories as well as the Centers for Disease Control. A single elevated titer or a fourfold or greater increase between acute and convalescent titers is diagnostic of CSD.

CURRENT DIAGNOSIS

- Suspect CSD in any patient with lymphadenopathy and a history of cat exposure, regardless of age.
- Serologic testing can confirm the diagnosis.
- If biopsy is performed, specimens should be sent for pathology as well as fungal, mycobacterial, and routine bacterial cultures.
- Granulomas with central necrosis are characteristic of CSD but are not specific. When available, PCR is highly specific for CSD.

Abbreviations: CSD = cat-scratch disease; PCR = polymerase chain reaction.

CURRENT THERAPY

Immunocompetent Patients

- Typical CSD only requires supportive treatment.
- No antibiotics are indicated.
- For atypical CSD there are no definitive treatment recommendations.
- Endocarditis requires surgery and antibiotic therapy, which should include at least 14 days of an aminoglycoside.

Immunocompromised Patients

- BA or BP treatment for at least 3 months with either
  - Erythromycin (E.E.S.)[1] 500 mg PO qid or
  - Doxycycline (Vibramycin) 100 mg PO bid.

---

[1]Not FDA approved for this indication.
Abbreviations: BA = bacillary angiomatosis; BP = bacillary peliosis; CSD = cat-scratch disease.

The combination of history, physical examination, and serologic testing may obviate the need for biopsy in cases of typical CSD. If a node is removed, the characteristic histopathologic finding is the formation of granulomas with microabscesses and central necrosis. Rarely, gram-negative bacilli may be identified using the Warthin-Starry silver stain. These are both nonspecific findings, and any patient undergoing biopsy should have samples sent for cytology as well as fungal, mycobacterial, and standard bacterial culture and sensitivity to rule out other etiologies of lymphadenopathy. Polymerase chain reaction (PCR) testing of tissue is emerging as a highly specific diagnostic tool. Sensitivity of PCR testing varies with the specific DNA target used but is usually quite high. It is becoming increasingly available in commercial laboratories.

Treatment

Treatment of typical CSD is supportive and mainly consists of needle aspiration of suppurative lymph nodes when required. There is no evidence to suggest that treatment with antibiotics significantly alters the course of disease. In the only prospective, randomized, double blinded study of typical CSD, a 5-day course of azithromycin (Zithromax) or placebo was given to 29 patients with clinical CSD. Although the subjects who received azithromycin had a more rapid reduction in lymphadenopathy as measured by ultrasound at 30 days, the long-term outcomes were identical for both groups.

Evidence for the treatment of atypical CSD in immunocompetent patients is limited to case reports and retrospective reviews. Success has been reported using a range of oral antibiotics including trimethoprim-sulfamethoxazole (Bactrim, Septra),[1] rifampin (Rifadin),[1] azithromycin (Zithromax),[1] doxycycline (Vibramycin), and ciprofloxacin (Cipro),[1] as well as intravenous gentamicin (Garamycin).[1] Nevertheless, most cases of atypical CSD are thought to resolve without antibiotic therapy. A notable exception is endocarditis, which requires surgical replacement of the damaged valve in addition to antibiotic therapy. One retrospective review found that treatment of endocarditis with a regimen that included an aminoglycoside for at least 14 days was significantly associated with a higher rate of survival.

Immunocompromised patients with BA or BP warrant antimicrobial treatment. There have been no controlled studies to determine optimal therapy, but either erythromycin (E.E.S.)[1] or doxycycline (Vibramycin) is effective. Most experts recommend a treatment course of at least 3 months to prevent relapse.

Prevention

Cat owners should avoid activities that may result in a cat scratch or bite, and should promptly wash any cat-inflicted wounds. Appropriate flea control will also reduce the likelihood of CSD. Because of the risk for invasive disease caused by *B. henselae*, immunocompromised individuals should be specifically warned of the risks of cat exposure. If possible, they should avoid purchasing or adopting kittens.

REFERENCES

American Academy of Pediatrics. Cat-scratch disease. In: Pickering LK, editor. Red Book: 2003 Report of the Committee on Infectious Diseases. 26th ed. Elk Grove Village, IL: American Academy of Pediatrics; 2006. p. 232–4.

Bass JW, Freitas BC, Freitas AD, et al. Prospective randomized double blind placebo-controlled evaluation of azithromycin for treatment of cat-scratch disease. Pediatr Infect Dis J 1998;17:447–52.

Batts S, Demers DM. Spectrum and treatment of cat-scratch disease. Pediatr Infect Dis J 2004;23:1161–2.

Ben-Ami R, Ephros M, Avidor B, et al. Cat-scratch disease in elderly patients. Clin Infect Dis 2005;41:969–74.

Hansmann Y, DeMartino S, Piemont Y, et al. Diagnosis of cat scratch disease with detection of *Bartonella henselae* PCR: A study of patients with lymph node enlargement. J Clin Microbiol 2005;43:3800–06.

Jacobs RF, Schutze GE. *Bartonella henselae* as a cause of prolonged fever and fever of unknown origin in children. Clin Infect Dis 1998;26:80–4.

---

[1]Not FDA approved for this indication.

Massei F, Gori L, Machhia P, Maggiore G, et al. The extended spectrum of bartonellosis in children. Infect Dis Clin North Am 2005;19:691–711.

Raoult D, Fournier PE, Vandenesch F, et al. Outcome and treatment of *Bartonella* endocarditis. Arch of Int Med 2003;163:226–30.

Rolain JM, Brouqui P, Koehler JE, et al. Recommendations for treatment of human infection caused by *Bartonella* species. Antimicrob Agents Chemother 2004;48:1921–33.

Zangwill KM, Hamilton DH, Perkins BA, et al. Cat scratch disease in Connecticut: Epidemiology, risk factors, and evaluation of a new diagnostic test. N Engl J Med 1993;329:8–13.

Salmonellosis

Method of

Arvid E. Underman, MD, FACP, DTMH

Salmonellosis refers to a group of infections caused by members of the genus *Salmonella*. This genus is named after Salmon, a pathologist who first isolated the organism, later designated as *Salmonella choleraesuis*, from the intestine of pigs with diarrhea. *Salmonellae* are widely distributed throughout nature and are adapted to a myriad of warm and cold-blooded hosts. In humans there are four main clinical presentations:

1. Acute gastroenteritis
2. Bacteremia
3. Focal extraintestinal infection
4. Chronic carriage (Table 1)

Microbiology

Salmonellae are motile, Gram-stain negative, nonspore-forming bacilli that are differentiated from other *Enterobacteriaceae* by inability to ferment lactose and sucrose while producing acid, hydrogen sulfide, and gas (except *Salmonella typhi*). Members of the genus were more accurately classified into serotypes using the Kauffman-White schema that differentiated and grouped them serologically dependent on their lipopolysaccharide somatic (O) and flagellar (H) antigens.

TABLE 1 Clinical Presentations of Salmonellosis

Acute gastroenteritis (90%–95% of cases)
Bacteremia (< 5% of cases)
- Transient during acute gastroenteritis
- Enteric fever (nontyphoid)
- Persistent or recurrent (especially HIV)
Focal complications following bacteremia
- Bronchopneumonia, empyema, chest wall abscess
- Aortitis with mycotic aneurysm
- Prosthetic graft or valve infection
- Endocarditis, endarteritis
- Osteomyelitis (especially with sickle cell anemia)
- Septic arthritis
- Soft tissue abscess
- Hepatic or splenic abscess
- Meningitis or brain abscess
- Suppurative urogenital disease
Carriage (asymptomatic)
- Convalescent excretors (<2 mo)
- Convalescent carriers (2–12 mo)
- Chronic carriers (> 12 mo)

More recently, DNA analysis has divided the genus into two species. Initially the first of the two species was named *Salmonella choleraesuis* and was divided into six subspecies, each of which was then divided into more than 2400 serotypes (serovars) by Kauffman-White methodology. The second species, *Salmonella Bongori*, is inconsequential. Serotypes were named historically from the host or the geographic locale of the first isolate, such as *Salmonella typhimurium* or *Salmonella dublin*. However, under the new DNA division, *choleraesuis* was both a species and a serotype. To avoid confusion the name *Salmonella enterica* has been widely adopted. The first of the six subspecies (Group I) is also named *enterica*. It contains the more than 1400 serotypes that occur in warm-blooded animals. Using nomenclature employed by the United States Centers for Disease Control and the World Health Organization (WHO), the species and subspecies name is understood; and the serotype is capitalized. Thus, the formal *S. enterica* subspecies *enterica* serotype *typhimurium* becomes simply *S. Typhimurium*, which except for the capital T is where we started!

Epidemiology

In the last 25 years, the incidence of nontyphoid salmonellosis has increased two- to threefold with approximately 1.5 million cases occurring annually in the United States. This is an underestimate because most cases are sporadic (endemic) and go unreported. Children younger than 5 years of age have the highest incidence of gastroenteritis and constitute the greatest number of cases.

Animals are the source of nontyphoid salmonella infection in humans. Infection occurs from food of animal origin such as meat, poultry, eggs, and dairy products. Contamination may occur during the production, slaughter, processing, or distribution of these products. Outbreaks have been associated with eggs, ice cream, and processed meats. Increasingly there have been outbreaks associated with raw vegetables (e.g., scallions) that are crosscontaminated during growth and distribution. Restaurant or home outbreaks occur in the context of improper preparation, cooking, and refrigeration. Most of the outbreaks can be attributed to centralized mass production and preparation of food along with globalization of the food trade. Novel sources of human salmonella include pet turtles, lizards, iguanas, African hedgehogs, rattlesnakes, and even marijuana contaminated by manure.

Emergence of antibiotic resistant species is a formidable problem. It is believed that resistance is driven worldwide by improper antibiotics use. However, in developed countries it is attributable to widespread use in animal feeds. Large numbers of transferable resistance plasmids have been described. Resistance rates of more than 50% to ampicillin, chloramphenicol (Chloromycetin), and trimethoprim-sulfamethoxazole (TMP-SMZ) (Bactrim) occur in parts of Asia, Africa, and Latin America. One strain of *S. Typhimurium* (DT104) is resistant to five antimicrobials; the three mentioned previously plus tetracycline and streptomycin. This organism has spread widely in livestock throughout the United States, Canada, United Kingdom, Europe, and the Middle East. Likewise, resistance to third-generation cephalosporins is increasing and is mediated by plasmids producing both regular and extended-spectrum beta-lactamases (ESBLs). Even more disturbing is fluoroquinolone resistance caused by mutated DNA gyrase, topoisomerase IV, or efflux pumps. The latter literally expel the quinolone from the bacterium before it can act on its target. Fluoroquinolone resistance is most pronounced in Southeast Asia, Europe, and the Middle East.

Pathogenesis

Human infection usually requires 10^6 organisms. Fewer organisms may cause disease in patients who have hypochlorhydria or achlorhydria, have impaired cellular immunity, are at the extremes of age, or are taking certain drugs (Table 2). *Salmonellae* predominately infect the terminal ileum and proximal colon through

TABLE 2 Predisposing Factors for Salmonellosis

Gastrointestinal
- Achlorhydria
- Gastric surgery
- Inflammatory bowel disease

Immune or structural compromise
- Age (<6 mo, >60 y)
- Lymphoma
- Splenectomy
- Cirrhosis with portal hypertension
- Diabetes mellitus
- Chronic uremia
- Hemolytic anemia (iron overload)
- Sickle cell (bone infarct, autosplenectomy)
- Systemic lupus
- Atheromata, aortic aneurysm

Infections
- HIV/AIDS (decreased T-cells)
- Malaria
- Bartonellosis
- Schistosomiasis

Drugs
- H_2-blockers, $H+^+$ proton pump inhibitors
- Antibiotic administration
- Antimotility agents
- Chemotherapy
- Corticosteroids
- Transplant antirejection agents

attachment. Initially host response is by neutrophils followed by lymphocytes and macrophages. Strains vary genetically in their virulence and invasiveness. The organisms can survive intracellularly, thus avoiding antibiotic agents that lack intracellular penetration. Bacteria that are not contained regionally in the gut or lymph nodes may enter the blood. There are many predisposing factors associated with this and subsequent focal complications (see Table 2).

Clinical Presentation

GASTOENTERITIS

Acute gastroenteritis is by far the most common clinical presentation of salmonellosis. It should be emphasized that there is considerable overlap in its presentation with other infectious intestinal pathogens such as *Campylobacter* species. Given this, the incubation ranges from 6 to 96 hours but most commonly occurs between 12 and 48 hours. Initial symptoms include nausea and vomiting, followed by headaches, myalgias, malaise, chills, low-grade fever, abdominal cramps, and diarrhea. High temperatures (40°C [104°F]) should alert the clinician to invasive disease. Stools may be merely loose or profuse and watery. On direct examination, they may or may not contain

CURRENT DIAGNOSIS

- More than 95% of nontyphoid Salmonellosis presents as uncomplicated acute gastroenteritis.
- The clinical presentation of different causes of gastroenteritis and diarrhea overlaps significantly.
- The physician should be familiar with groups of patients at risk for complicated Salmonellosis.
- Specific diagnosis requires culture of the stool or blood.
- Focal complications are always suspect in high-risk patients who are blood culture positive for nontyphoid *Salmonellae* (e.g., aortitis or mycotic aneurysm in patients older than age 60 years with atherosclerosis).

polymorphonuclear leukocytes or occult blood. The presence of mucus or gross blood in the absence of hemorrhoids or fissures should alert the clinician to organisms causing dysentery such as *Shigella* species. The white count is most often normal or slightly elevated, with a left shift containing 10 to 15 bands. Low white counts with greater numbers of bands should alert the clinician to possible bacteremia or enteric fever. The diagnosis can be confirmed only by stool or blood culture. Serum serology examinations are not helpful. Most healthy adults have a self-limited, uncomplicated course, with resolution of symptoms without treatment within 48 to 72 hours.

Treatment

FLUID AND ELECTROLYTE REPLACEMENT

The sine qua non in the treatment of diarrhea is fluid and electrolyte replacement. In most cases increased oral intake of bland juices coupled with clear broth and temporary elimination of lactose-containing foods will suffice. Commercial electrolyte solutions (Pedialyte) may be useful. Although not readily available in the United States, rehydration salts are widely employed in many developing countries. WHO distributes packets containing its recommended formula of 90 mmol of sodium, 20 of potassium, 80 of chloride, 30 of bicarbonate, along with 111 mmol of glucose to dissolve in 1 L of sterile or boiled water. This mixture should be consumed at a rate sufficient to compensate for diarrheal losses while maintaining an adequate output of dilute appearing urine. Within 24 to 48 hours, the diet can be supplemented with bland, soft foods given in small, frequent feedings. If the patient has profuse vomiting or severe dehydration as determined by orthostatic changes in blood pressure, parenteral rehydration should be used. Frequently, this can be accomplished as an outpatient in an infusion room or with a home agency rather than through admission to hospital. When there is persistent emesis, profuse diarrhea, systemic toxicity, or abnormalities in serum electrolytes, parenteral rehydration in hospital is prudent.

ANTIMOTILITY AND ANTINAUSEA AGENTS

The use of agents such as atropine-diphenoxylate (Lomotil) or loperamide (Imodium) should be discouraged. Although they may result in symptomatic improvement in cramps and diarrhea, they can increase complications and even predispose to bacteremia. In general, if the patient has a fever and the diarrhea contains blood or mucus, their use should be eschewed. Most pediatricians feel they should never be used in children younger than 5 years of age. An alternative is bismuth subsalicylate (Pepto-Bismol). The adult dose is 1 ounce (2 tablespoons) or 2 tablets (262.5 mg) every 30 minutes for 8 hours. The pediatric dose is 1.1 mL/kg at 4-hour intervals for up to 5 days. Although nausea and vomiting are occasional presenting symptoms with enterocolitis, they rarely persist. Prochlorperazine (Compazine) or trimethobenzamide (Tigan) may be helpful. Both are available in oral, suppository, or parenteral form, even though injectable prochlorperazine (Compazine) has been in short supply. Suppositories usually stimulate further diarrhea. Vomiting may preclude oral administration. A singular muscular injection of prochlorperazine (Compazine) 5 to 10 mg, is often all that is needed. This may be repeated every 4 to 6 hours as needed. Promethazine hydrochloride (Phenergan) is more frequently used in children and may be used orally (0.5 mg/pound or 1 mg/kg every 6 hours) or intramuscularly in the same doses. A 5-HT$_3$ receptor antagonist such as ondansetron (Zofran)[1] is expensive and inefficacious.

ANTIBIOTICS

The routine empiric use of antibiotics, especially fluoroquinolones, for any and all cases of diarrhea is not only unjustifiable but should

---

[1]Not FDA approved for this indication.

CURRENT THERAPY

- Fluid and electrolyte replacement is of paramount importance.
- The physician should avoid routine empiric antibiotic in acute uncomplicated patients.
- The physician should avoid antimotility agents for diarrhea presenting with fever or with mucus and blood present.
- More than 95% of patients with nontyphoid salmonellosis *will get better* on their own.
- Fluoroquinolone antibiotics should be reserved for when they are truly indicated clinically.
- Increasing resistance mandates sensitivity testing (including tests for ESBL) to guide therapy of bacteremia and its complications.
- Do not prescribe *prophylactic* antibiotics to prevent diarrhea in travellers.
- Stress personal hygiene and prudent food choice with proper preparation.

Abbreviation: ESBL = extended spectrum beta lactamases.

be decried. Certainly antibiotics are not needed in the treatment of uncomplicated *Salmonella* gastroenteritis in otherwise healthy children or adults. Studies have shown that they neither shorten the course nor improve symptoms. No doubt some of this usage is patient driven. However, overuse is contributing to the emergence of resistance, and may increase risk of symptomatic and bacteriologic relapse. Indeed antibiotic use may actually prolong the convalescent excretion or contribute to chronic carriage of the organism. Postponing antibiotic therapy until the return of a stool culture often provides the physician with a way to avert the frequent demand for antibiotic therapy. Often patients are better by the time results become available. Nevertheless, high-risk patients, as previously identified (see Table 2), should receive treatment to prevent potential complications from bacteremia. Additionally, if patients are sick enough to require hospitalization, antibiotic therapy should be considered.

Appropriate antibiotic therapy should be guided by susceptibility testing. Initially, TMP-SMZ (cotrimoxazole, Bactrim, or Septra)[1] may be administered to the nonsulfonamide-sensitive patient. The dose is 5 to 8 mg/kg trimethoprim every 12 hours for children or 1 double-strength tablet (160 mg trimethoprim/800 mg sulfamethoxazole) every 12 hours for adults. Although widely used, trimethoprim-sulfamethoxazole has not yet received FDA approval. If the organism is susceptible, ampicillin, 50 mg/kg orally to 100 mg/kg/day intravenously, each in four divided doses for children, or 2 to 4 g/day in four divided doses for adults, may be administered. Amoxicillin (Amoxil)[1] in equivalent oral dosage may be substituted. The duration of therapy is generally 5 days.

Newer fluoroquinolone antibiotics, such as ciprofloxacin,[1] ofloxacin,[1] and norfloxacin,[1] are among the most effective agents with excellent oral bioavailability and intracellular concentration. They are contraindicated in prepubertal children and pregnant women. Adult doses are ciprofloxacin (Cipro), 500 mg twice daily; ofloxacin (Floxin), 400 mg twice daily; or norfloxacin (Noroxin), 400 mg twice daily. It must be emphasized that the trend in the United States to use these agents empirically for all suspected bacterial diarrhea should be vigorously resisted by the thoughtful clinician.

---

[1]Not FDA approved for this indication.

Bacteremia and Focal Infection

Bacteremia in acute uncomplicated *Salmonella* gastroenteritis is infrequent. Therefore, blood cultures are not routinely necessary except for patients who are in high-risk categories. Shaking chills or high fever (40°C [104°F]) should alert the clinician to possible bacteremia. Focal suppurative infection following bacteremia is also infrequent but may occur at any site. Thus, *Salmonella* has been associated with bronchopneumonia, soft tissue infection, aortic mycotic aneurysms, endocarditis, septic arthritis, splenic or hepatic abscesses, meningitis, and osteomyelitis. The clinician should suspect an endovascular mycotic aneurysm in all blood culture positive patients older than 50 years of age. *Salmonella* should always be suspected in individuals with sickle cell disease in whom bone and joint infection is the most frequent cause of extraintestinal infection. Meningitis occurs primarily in infants younger than 5 months of age. The diagnosis of a *Salmonella* bacteremia in HIV patients will almost always be accompanied by recurrent episodes.

Treatment

ANTIBIOTICS

Bacteremia and localized suppurative infection require antibiotic therapy. The choice of effective treatment is less predictable with the emergence of resistance. Therapy must be altered according to the results of susceptibility testing. Therefore the recovery of the organism is extremely important, and adequate cultures of blood or infected material must be obtained before initiation of therapy.

Parenteral ampicillin, 100 to 200 mg/kg/day divided into four doses, or TMP/SMZ,[1] 8 to 10 mg/kg of trimethoprim per day in three divided doses, may be used. In the case of resistance or allergy to the foregoing, third-generation cephalosporins such as cefotaxime (Claforan) or ceftriaxone (Rocephin) have reasonable activity, but intracellular concentrations are not optimal. Cefotaxime, 1 to 2 grams every 6 to 8 hours for adults, or 100 to 200 mg/kg/day in three or four divided doses for children, has been found effective in bacteremia, osteomyelitis, septic arthritis, and a variety of other focal *Salmonella* infections. The use of chloramphenicol (Chloromycetin) is not recommended but a preparation of it in oil (Typhomycine)[2] is in use in developing countries. Ciprofloxacin (Cipro)[1] 7.5 mg/kg intravenously twice daily is becoming a favored agent; not only is it effective but oral bioequivalence facilitates the change to 500 to 750 mg by mouth twice daily. If fluoroquinolone resistance is encountered, imipenem (Primaxin)[1] may be tried. Efficacy data for it or other agents such as azithromycin (Zithromax)[1] are scant.

SURGERY

Focal infection often requires surgery. Often this is as simple as the drainage of localized suppuration or lavage of a septic joint. However, in the case of infected aortic aneurysms, extensive resection and vascular reconstruction are required. Infected prosthetic grafts must be removed in nearly all cases with courses of antibiotics before and after surgery.

The duration of therapy for simple bacteremia is 10 to 14 days. Septic arthritis is usually treated 4 weeks whereas osteomyelitis and endovascular infections require 6 weeks. Oral fluoroquinolones such as ciprofloxacin (Cipro), 500 mg twice daily, may be helpful in treating osteomyelitis. TMP-SMZ (Bactrim)[1] can also be used in this manner. Both have adequate blood levels after oral administration. I have had to use continuous prophylaxis of either TMP-SMZ or ciprofloxacin in several HIV patients to prevent recurrent bacteremia. Because prophylactic TMP-SMZ is used chronically for *Pneumocystis*, it may be preferred.

---

[1]Not FDA approved for this indication.
[2]Not available in the United States.

Enteric Fever

The clinical picture of nontyphoid *Salmonella* enteric fever is indistinguishable from that of typhoid fever, which is discussed elsewhere in this publication. However, the following discussion also applies to enteric fever caused by nontyphoid *Salmonellae*.

TREATMENT

The adjunct and antibiotic therapy of nontyphoid enteric fever parallels that of the treatment of typhoid. Antibiotics should be adjusted and altered once the results of susceptibility testing are available. Acceptable regimens include ampicillin, amoxicillin,[1] and TMP-SMZ (Bactrim),[1] along with third-generation cephalosporins and fluoroquinolone antibiotics. My preference was cefotaxime (Claforan)[1] in the same doses as for bacteremic salmonellosis. The duration is 10 to 14 days. Relapse rates are low and is seen within 2 to 6 weeks. Relapse requires an equivalent course of therapy in both dose and duration. Currently, I prefer ciprofloxacin (Cipro)[1] intravenously 7.5 mg/kg every 12 hours continued until the patient is afebrile and clinically able to start it orally. Comparative studies are ongoing using both third-generation cephalosporins, such as ceftriaxone (Rocephin)[1] or cefixime (Suprax),[1] and oral fluoroquinolones in short-course therapy of typhoid as well as nontyphoid enteric fever. Although these show some promise, they are currently not the standard of practice in the United States. Nevertheless, a strong case can be made for oral fluoroquinolones use, with obvious cost saving. Otherwise healthy young adults may be treated orally as outpatients. This advantage, if for no other reason, should *prevent* the physician from prescribing quinolones for uncomplicated gastroenteritis or other self-limited diarrheas of bacterial origin.

Adjunctive measures are of importance, including attention to fluid and electrolyte balance and nutrition. As in typhoid the routine use of corticosteroids is controversial. Use in patients who are steroid dependent or believed to be hypoadrenal is indicated. In those who are delirious, obtunded, comatose, or in shock it may be warranted; but there are little supportive data. It has been my overall impression that nontyphoid enteric fever is somewhat milder than typhoid itself, and complications such as gastrointestinal bleeding or ileal perforation are exceedingly rare.

Carrier State

Asymptomatic excretion of organisms invariably occurs following clinical *Salmonella* gastroenteritis. It exceeds 8 weeks in 5% to 10% of patients. Chronic carriage, either in the stool or urine, is defined as excretion of the organism for more than 1 year. Its incidence is stated to be 1% in adults and 5% in children younger than 5 years of age. This is somewhat less than that seen with *S. typhi*. Convalescent excreters need only maintain strict personal hygiene to prevent transmission of the organism. Those involved in food preparation or in child and health care should be kept off work until three successive cultures are negative at intervals required by the public health department. It goes without saying that all positive cases of salmonellosis are reportable by law to local public health authorities.

Recently, oral quinolones have been used (ciprofloxacin [Cipro],[1] 500 to 750 mg twice daily for 5 to 14 days), to curtail institutional outbreaks, as in nursing homes or psychiatric facilities. Although this may be expeditious, eliminating or preventing the source of the outbreak in a prospective fashion is preferable. In the case of food handlers and health or child care workers, some feel that quinolone therapy eliminates the problem of convalescent excretion, hence individuals may return to work without delay. The data are debatable and the successive negative stool requirement will not be obviated.

---

[1]Not FDA approved for this indication.

The management of the chronic carriage of nontyphoidal salmonellosis is the same as that of *S. typhi*, which is discussed in detail elsewhere. A 4- to 6-week course of oral antibiotics may be tried when no evidence of gallbladder disease exists. However, if chronic cholecystitis and/or cholelithiasis are present, cholecystectomy is almost always necessary. Despite cholecystectomy, a certain number of individuals will continue to excrete organisms thought to be of hepatobiliary origin. Chronic carriage is seen, albeit rarely, in the United States with either *Schistosoma mansoni* or *Schistosoma haematobium*. When these parasites are treated, subsequent therapy of the *Salmonella* results in termination of the stool or urinary carrier state.

Prevention

Prevention of salmonellosis has both personal and public health dimensions. Food and leftovers should be rapidly refrigerated. I recommend separate plastic (not wood) cutting boards for meats and vegetables that are washed after each use. Spillage of raw animal juices should be immediately cleaned. All preparation surfaces should be washed and dried after each meal. Detergent rather than antibacterial cleaners should be used; bleach is beautiful.

Public health surveillance is essential with regular inspection of restaurants, food retailers, and industrial food processors. National efforts to coordinate and computerize surveillance systems such as FoodNet should be expanded and fully funded so as to guarantee our food supply. Preservation technologies including irradiation need study.

Finally, the practicing physician should take the time to reiterate to patients with HIV, malignancies or other immune compromised patients (see Table 2) how they can avoid food-borne pathogens.

REFERENCES

Brenner FW, Villar RG, Angulo FJ, et al. Salmonella nomenclature. J Clin Microbiol 2000;38:2465.

Fierer J, Swancutt M. Non-typhoid *Salmonella*: A review. In: Remington JS, Swartz MN, editors. Current Clinical Topics in Infectious Diseases 20. Boston: Blackwell Science; 2000. p. 134–57.

Herikstad H, Hayes P, Mokhtar M, et al. Emerging quinolone-resistant Salmonella in the United States. Emerg Infect Dis 1997;3:371–2.

Molbak K. Human health consequences of antimicrobial drug resistant *Salmonella* and other foodborne pathogens. Clin Infect Dis 2005;41:1613–20.

Sirinivan S, Garner P. Antibiotics for treating Salmonella gut infections. Cochrane Database Sys Rev 2000;93:CD001167.

Su LH, Chiu CH, Chu CS, et al. Antimicrobial resistance in nontyphoid *Salmonella*: A global challenge. Clin Infect Dis 2004;39:546–51.

Voetsch AC, Van Gilder TJ, Angulo FJ, et al. FoodNet estimate of the burden of illness caused by nontyphoidal Salmonella infections in the United States. Clin Infect Dis 2004;38(Suppl. 3):S127–34.

Typhoid Fever

Method of
Christopher M. Parry, PhD, MRCP, FRCPath, and Buddha Basnyat, MD

Typhoid fever is an acute systemic illness caused by *Salmonella enterica* serovar Typhi. Paratyphoid fever, caused by *S. enterica* ser. Paratyphi A (or occasionally by Paratyphi B or C), causes an indistinguishable clinical syndrome that can be as severe as typhoid fever. Collectively, these infections are known as enteric fever, and their management is identical.

Epidemiology

An estimated 27 million cases of enteric fever occur worldwide each year, with about 200,000 deaths. In the Indian subcontinent, Central and Southeast Asia, Indonesia, and sub-Saharan Africa, rates of transmission are high, and annual incidence rates exceeding 100 cases per 100,000 population have been recorded. Most cases of enteric fever are caused by ser. Typhi, although in some areas of south Asia the proportion of cases due to Paratyphi A has been increasing. Sources of typhoid transmission are excretions from chronic or convalescent carriers and the acutely infected. Transmission occurs through contamination by carriers of food or water through effluents containing infected urine or feces. In affluent countries, enteric fever is seen in travelers returning from vacation or from visiting friends and relatives abroad in areas of endemicity. It may occasionally occur when food or water safety measures fail.

Clinical Features

Typhoid and paratyphoid fever commonly occur in infants, children, and young adults. The infection is characterized by prolonged fever and is associated with vague abdominal discomfort, alteration in bowel habit (constipation or diarrhea or both), headache, dry cough, malaise, and anorexia. The incubation period ranges from 3 to 60 days, but most infections occur 7 to 14 days after exposure. Physical findings are usually sparse but may include hepatomegaly or splenomegaly and, variably, an exanthema (rose spots) on the trunk. The clinical picture can range from a mild febrile illness to life-threatening complications. Patients with advanced illness may display the so-called typhoid facies—a thin, flushed face with a staring, apathetic expression.

Complications

Severe and complicated disease develops in up to 5% to 10% of patients and is usually encountered in patients with untreated disease lasting 2 or more weeks. Occasionally, a complication dominates the clinical picture and deflects attention from the underlying diagnosis of typhoid. Many complications are described, but the most common ones are gastrointestinal bleeding, perforation, and encephalopathy. Gastrointestinal bleeding from ileal ulcers occurs in up to 30% of patients but is usually self-limited. Intestinal perforation of the ileal ulcers causing peritonitis occurs in 1% to 3% of hospitalized patients. An encephalopathic presentation with altered mental state, frequently with hemodynamic shock, is associated with a high fatality rate. Patients may progress from obtundation to delirium and terminal coma. Other severe complications include hepatitis, cholecystitis, myocarditis, pneumonia, nerve lesions, psychotic symptoms, disseminated intravascular coagulation, and renal failure.

CURRENT DIAGNOSIS

- Typhoid and paratyphoid fever (the enteric fevers) should be considered in the differential diagnosis of febrile patients in endemic areas and in travelers returning from these areas.
- The principal method for confirming the diagnosis is by isolation of *Salmonella enterica* serovar Typhi or Paratyphi from blood or another sterile site.
- Gastrointestinal bleeding, intestinal perforation, and a syndrome of mental confusion and shock are the principal life-threatening complications of typhoid fever.

The disease may be complicated by relapse, usually with the development of the same symptoms 2 to 3 weeks after initial recovery. Transient convalescent and chronic (>1 year) fecal excretion due to gallbladder carriage can occur after the end of treatment in typhoid and paratyphoid fever. Urinary carriage is rare and may be associated with schistosomiasis.

Diagnosis

Many viral, bacterial, and protozoal infections, as well as noninfectious conditions characterized by fever, including lymphoproliferative disorders and vasculitides, can resemble enteric fever. Patients usually have a total white cell count within the normal range. A mild normochromic anemia, mild thrombocytopenia, and an increased erythrocyte sedimentation rate are commonly observed.

The definitive diagnosis of enteric fever requires the isolation of *S. enterica* ser. Typhi or Paratyphi from blood, bone marrow, cerebrospinal fluid, or rose spots. Successful culture from blood can be achieved in up to 80% of patients but depends on culturing adequate volumes of blood. Blood cultures are most likely to be positive in the first 7 to 10 days of illness. Culture of a bone marrow aspirate can be positive in up to 90% of cases, even after treatment has begun, but is difficult to employ routinely. Isolation of the organism allows antimicrobial susceptibility testing to be performed. Isolation of the organism from feces and urine may indicate chronic carriage rather than acute infection.

Serologic methods are also used for diagnosis. The low-cost Widal test is widely available in developing countries and measures agglutinating antibodies against the O lipopolysaccharide somatic antigen and the H protein flagella antigen. The interpretation of the test is complicated by false-positive and false-negative results. A serologic test using an immunoblot of serum has been shown to have good performance characteristics but is not easy to perform. A number of new, rapid kit-based serologic tests have been developed to measure immunoglobulin G (IgG) and IgM, or just IgM antibodies, against various typhoid antigens. Although these tests have a better performance than the Widal test, none is sufficiently robust to be widely recommended.

Treatment

Treatment of typhoid fever requires supportive measures, such as good hydration and adequate nutrition, in addition to an appropriate antimicrobial therapy. Many patients in endemic areas are managed as outpatients. Patients who are vomiting or have developed severe or complicated disease require treatment in hospital. The choice of antimicrobial agent in enteric fever has become increasingly complicated with changing patterns of resistance in different areas. Local guidelines should be considered.

Variable levels of multidrug resistance (MDR) to the older antimicrobials chloramphenicol (Chloromycetin), amoxicillin (Amoxil),[1] and trimethoprim-sulfamethoxazole (TMP-SMX [Bactrim])[1] occur in Asia and Africa. In areas with MDR infections, fluoroquinolones, such as ciprofloxacin (Cipro), have been widely used, but resistance has also appeared against them. Isolates with decreased susceptibility to ciprofloxacin (DCS) are particularly common in Asia and are sporadically reported from Africa. These isolates have a decreased ciprofloxacin minimum inhibitory concentration (0.1–1.0 µg/mL) but are reported as susceptible using current disc susceptibility breakpoints. Infections with these isolates are associated with prolonged recovery times and increased failure rates. Most are resistant to nalidixic acid (NegGram), and this has proved to be a useful, albeit not 100% sensitive, surrogate marker of DCS status.

Ceftriaxone (Rocephin),[1] azithromycin (Zithromax),[1] or later-generation fluoroquinolones such as gatifloxacin (Tequin)[2] can be

---

[1]Not FDA approved for this indication.
[2]Not available in the United States.

used for infections with MDR or MDR/DCS isolates. Ceftriaxone requires parenteral administration, and the response to treatment is often slow. Oral azithromycin is effective in uncomplicated typhoid fever and appears to produce low levels of relapse. Gatifloxacin should not be used in diabetics or in the elderly, but current evidence suggests that it has an acceptable safety profile in the younger age group. Resistance to ceftriaxone and azithromycin is currently rarely reported, but full resistance to ciprofloxacin is reported in India, and it is unclear whether gatifloxacin will work against such infections. Currently recommended regimens are presented in Table 1. Syndromic therapy of undifferentiated fever may be required in areas where microbiology facilities are unavailable. Once malaria has been excluded, azithromycin may be a good choice to cover enteric fever, leptospirosis, and most types of typhus.

In severe typhoid fever, ceftriaxone or a fluoroquinolone is probably the optimal therapy and should be used for a minimum of 10 days. In patients with an altered level of consciousness associated with typhoid encephalopathy, high-dose intravenous dexamethasone (Decadron)[1] (an initial dose of 3 mg/kg,[3] by slow intravenous infusion over 30 minutes, followed by eight doses of 1 mg/kg[3] every succeeding 6 hours) should be given in addition to the antimicrobial and can be lifesaving. Intestinal perforation requires prompt surgical intervention, and the antimicrobial coverage should be broadened to cover the gastrointestinal flora contaminating the peritoneum. Relapse occurs in 5% to 20% of apparently successfully treated acute cases; it may be as severe as the initial illness but can usually be treated with the same antimicrobial as in the initial episode.

Eradication of carriage is advised in those still excreting at 3 months, particularly if they are at risk for communicating infection to others. Eradication of carriage requires a prolonged, high-dose antimicrobial regimen. Choice of antimicrobial should depend on the susceptibility profile of the isolated organism; some suggested regimens are presented in Table 2. Cholecystectomy may be considered if antimicrobial therapy fails and there are additional indications for the operation.

---

[1]Not FDA approved for this indication.
[3]Exceeds dosage recommended by the manufacturer.

CURRENT THERAPY

- Antimicrobial therapy reduces mortality and complications and shortens the illness.
- Resistance to first-line antimicrobials (chloramphenicol [Chloromycetin], amoxicillin [Amoxil],[1] trimethoprim-sulfamethoxazole [Bactrim][1]) is common in many areas of Asia and Africa.
- Fluoroquinolones (ciprofloxacin [Cipro], ofloxacin [Floxin][1]), extended-spectrum cephalosporins (ceftriaxone [Rocephin][1]), and azithromycin (Zithromax)[1] are available alternatives for multidrug-resistant infections.
- Decreased susceptibility to ciprofloxacin (DCS, nalidixic acid resistance) is widespread in Asia and occurs sporadically in Africa.
- Older fluoroquinolones, such as ciprofloxacin and ofloxacin, should not be used in infections caused by isolates with DCS, but the newer fluoroquinolone, such as gatifloxacin (Tequin),[2] extended-spectrum cephalosporins (ceftriaxone), and azithromycin are appropriate alternatives.

---

[1]Not FDA approved for this indication.
[2]Not available in the United States.

Prevention

The elimination of typhoid requires provision of safe drinking water; safe disposal of sewage; legal enforcement of high standards of food hygiene; programs to detect, monitor, and treat chronic carriers; and prompt investigation and intervention when these safeguards are breached. Many endemic areas currently struggle to fulfill these requirements.

TABLE 1 Antimicrobial Treatment of Typhoid Fever

Antimicrobial	Total Daily Dose (mg/kg)	Route*	Doses per Day	Duration (d)	
				Nonsevere	Severe[†]
Chloramphenicol (Chloromycetin)[‡]	50–100[3]	PO/IM/IV[§]	4	14	14–21
Trimethoprim-sulfamethoxazole (Bactrim)[1,¶]	6.5–10 trimethoprim; 40 sulfamethoxazole	PO/IM/IV	2–3	14	14
Amoxicillin (Amoxil)[1]	75–100[3]	PO/IM/IV	3	14	14
Ceftriaxone (Rocephin)[1]	50–75[3]	IM/IV	2	10–14	14
Cefixime (Suprax)[1]	20[3]	PO	2	14	—
Ciprofloxacin (Cipro)[¶]	20–25[3]	PO/IV	2	7–10	14
Ofloxacin (Floxin)[1,¶]	20[3]	PO/IV	2	7–10	14
Gatifloxacin (Tequin)[2,**]	10[3]	PO	1	7	14
Azithromycin (Zithromax)[1]	10–20[3]	PO	1	7	—

[1]Not FDA approved for this indication.
[2]Not available in the United States.
[3]Exceeds dosage recommended by the manufacturer.
*Oral therapy is satisfactory for most patients. Parenteral therapy is generally reserved for severely ill patients.
[†]In intestinal perforation, the antibiotic therapy should also cover other aerobic and anaerobic gastrointestinal bacteria contaminating the peritoneum. In severe typhoid (characterized by delirium, obtundation, coma, or shock), dexamethasone (Decadron)[1] is beneficial (see text).
[‡]May cause bone marrow suppression.
[§]The oral route is preferred; there are reports of lower blood levels of chloramphenicol in patients given parenteral therapy.
[¶]May cause allergic reactions and nephrotoxicity. Not suitable for children younger than 2 years of age or for pregnant women.
[¶]Infection with isolates that have low-level fluoroquinolone resistance (nalidixic acid resistance) may not respond.
**Has been associated with hyperglycemia and hypoglycemia in some patients. Avoid in the elderly and in patients with diabetes.

TABLE 2 Treatment of Carriers

Antimicrobial	Total Daily Dose (mg/kg)	Route	Doses per Day	Duration
Amoxicillin [Amoxil][1] with probenecid	100[3]	PO	3–4	3 mo*
Trimethoprim-sulfamethoxazole [Bactrim][1,†]	6.5–10 trimethoprim	PO	2	3 mo
Ciprofloxacin [Cipro][1]	20–25[3]	PO	2	28 d

[1]Not FDA approved for this indication.
[3]Exceeds dosage recommended by the manufacturer.
*The duration of treatment can be shortened if parenteral therapy is given (e.g., amoxicillin IV q8h for 2 weeks).
[†]May cause allergic reactions and nephrotoxicity. Not suitable for children younger than 2 years or pregnant.

Two vaccines are available. The parenteral Vi polysaccharide vaccine (Typhim Vi) is given as a single intramuscular injection repeated every 3 years and is approximately 70% effective. The oral live attenuated vaccine (Ty21a, Vivotif Berna) is available in a liquid formulation[2] or in enteric-coated capsules and is given in three to four oral doses, each 2 days apart. The Ty21a vaccine has a protective efficacy of 60% to 70% but should not be given to immunosuppressed persons or to those taking mefloquine (Lariam) or antimicrobials. Vaccination is recommended by the World Health Organisation for children living in highly endemic areas, particularly where there are high levels of drug resistance; in the management of outbreaks; and for travelers. The current vaccines do not protect against paratyphoid infection, and the protection afforded by vaccination can be overcome by large inocula of bacteria. The current vaccines are unsuitable for children younger than 2 years of age. A number of new vaccines are being developed or evaluated, notably a Vi conjugate vaccine,[5] single-dose oral vaccines, and vaccines to protect against paratyphoid fever. The intention is to develop vaccines suitable for use in infants that can be incorporated into the Expanded Programme of Immunisation.

REFERENCES

Basnyat B, Maskey AP, Zimmerman MD, et al. Enteric fever (typhoid) fever in travellers. Clin Infect Dis 2005;41:1467–72.

Bhan MK, Bahl R, Bhatnager S. Typhoid and paratyphoid fever. Lancet 2005;366:749–62.

Bhutta ZA. Current concepts in the diagnosis and treatment of typhoid fever. BMJ 2006;333:78–82.

Chart H, Cheasty T, de Pinna E, et al. Serodiagnosis of *Salmonella enterica* serovar Typhi and *Salmonella enterica* serovars Paratyphi A, B and C human infections. J Med Microbiol 2007;56:1161–6.

Dolecek C, Tran TP, Nguyen NR, et al. A multi-center randomised controlled trial of gatifloxacin versus azithromycin for the treatment of uncomplicated typhoid fever in children and adults in Vietnam. PLoS One 2008;3:e2188.

Effa EE, Bukirwa H. Azithromycin for treating uncomplicated typhoid and paratyphoid (enteric fever). Cochrane Database Syst Rev 2008;(4): CD006083.

Pandit A, Arjal A, Day JN, et al. An open randomised comparison of gatifloxacin versus cefixime for the treatment of uncomplicated enteric fever. PLoS One 2007;2:e542.

Parry CM, Ho VA, Phuong LT, et al. Randomized controlled comparison of ofloxacin, azithromycin, and an ofloxacin-azithromycin combination for treatment of multidrug-resistant and nalidixic acid-resistant typhoid fever. Antimicrob Agents Chemother 2007;51:819–25.

Parry CM, Threlfall EJ. Antimicrobial resistance in typhoidal and nontyphoidal salmonellae. Curr Opin Infect Dis 2008;21:531–8.

Thaver D, Zaidi AKM, Critchley J, et al. Fluoroquinolones for treating typhoid and paratyphoid fever (enteric fever). Cochrane Database Syst Rev 2008; (4):CD004530.

[1]Not FDA approved for this indication.
[2]Not available in the United States.
[5]Investigational drug in the United States.

Rickettsial and Ehrlichial Infections

Method of
Deverick J. Anderson, MD, and
Daniel J. Sexton, MD

Rickettsial Infections

ROCKY MOUNTAIN SPOTTED FEVER

Rocky Mountain spotted fever (RMSF) is the most lethal of several tickborne illnesses that occur in the United States. Between 20% and 25% of infections are fatal if not treated appropriately. *Rickettsia rickettsii*, the obligate intracellular bacterium that causes RMSF, circulates in nature in a complex cycle between ticks and small rodents. Humans are only occasional and accidental hosts for this organism.

Epidemiology

RMSF is a highly seasonal disease that predominantly occurs in the spring and early summer months; cases occasionally occur in the autumn and even the winter in warmer climates. RMSF occurs with varying frequency in western Canada, much of the continental United States, Mexico, Central America, Brazil, and Colombia. The incidence of RMSF varies by geographic area and, although reporting of cases of RMSF is primarily through passive surveillance, the average reported annual incidence of RMSF is approximately 2.2 cases per 1 million persons.

Pathogenesis

In the United States, *R. rickettsii* is primarily transmitted by *Dermacentor variabilis* (the American dog tick) in the eastern United States and *Dermacentor andersoni* (the wood tick) in the western United States. Recently, *Rhipicephalus sanguineus* (the common brown dog tick) was recognized as the vector for RMSF in an outbreak in eastern Arizona; this finding is not surprising because this vector also transmits RMSF in Mexico and Central America. Although most infections occur after a tick bite, transmission rarely occurs from crushing or removing infected ticks from humans or animals. Indeed, infection can be experimentally induced with aerosols of infected tick tissues or by mucosal contact. Tick bites are painless and often go unnoticed. Thus, many patients with RMSF have no knowledge of a tick bite prior to the onset of their illness.

Clinical Features and Diagnosis

After inoculation from a tick bite, *R. rickettsii* proliferates and spreads throughout the body via the bloodstream and lymphatics, as well as by contiguous spread from cell to cell. *R. rickettsii* has a specific tropism for endothelial cells, resulting in widespread vasculitis, increased vascular permeability, edema, and activation of the humoral inflammatory and coagulation mechanisms. Organ dysfunction, hypovolemia, and shock can result from microvascular thrombosis and hemorrhage. Risk factors associated with increased severity and fatal outcomes include increasing age, male gender, diabetes mellitus, glucose-6-phosphate dehydrogenase (G6PD) deficiency, alcohol use, and delay in effective therapy for longer than 6 days after onset of symptoms.

The incubation period for RMSF ranges from 2 to 14 days. Most patients with RMSF develop a rash between the third and fifth days of illness. The typical rash of RMSF begins on the ankles and wrists and spreads both centrally and to the palms and soles. The skin rash often begins as a macular or maculopapular eruption and then usually becomes petechial. As many as 10% of patients do not, however, develop a rash (*spotless RMSF*). Additionally, the rash can be difficult to recognize in patients with dark skin.

Other symptoms of RMSF are nonspecific and include fever, headache, myalgias, malaise, and anorexia. As the disease progresses and becomes more severe, symptoms such as cough, bleeding, nausea, vomiting, abdominal pain, edema (especially in children), delirium, and focal neurologic symptoms (including seizures) can occur. In the absence of the classic triad of tick bite, fever, and rash, patients with RMSF may be erroneously believed to have an array of other infections such as ehrlichiosis, infectious mononucleosis, viral hepatitis, viral meningitis, measles, influenza, toxic shock syndrome, meningococcemia, leptospirosis, or typhoid fever. Because of shared residence and shared risks for tick exposure, family clusters of infection occasionally occur. When such clusters do occur, assumed person-to-person transmission of a viral or bacterial pathogen may lead to misdiagnosis and delay in treatment. If ineffective antibiotics are prescribed empirically before a typical rash appears, patients with RMSF may be erroneously assumed to have a drug eruption. Such cases can end tragically if the rash is presumed to occur because of (ineffective) drug therapy rather than in spite of it.

Most patients with RMSF have normal white blood cell (WBC) counts. As the severity of illness progresses, thrombocytopenia almost always develops, and WBC counts can become quite low. Although fibrinogen concentrations may be low and fibrin split products can become elevated in patients with RMSF, disseminated intravascular coagulation is uncommon. Other common laboratory abnormalities in patients with RMSF include hyponatremia, elevated serum transaminases, hyperbilirubinemia, and elevated creatinine.

There is no timely diagnostic test for RMSF in the early phase of illness. Thus, it is imperative that therapy be based on individual clinical features and the epidemiologic setting. Patients who have symptoms suggesting RMSF and who present in the spring or summer in an endemic area usually require empiric therapy.

Treatment

The preferred therapy is doxycycline (Vibramycin) 100 mg orally or intravenously every 12 hours for adults and children who weigh more than 45 kg. For children younger than 8 years or for children older than 8 years but weighing less than 45 kg, the dose is 2.2 mg/kg divided into two doses (maximum dose 200 mg/day).[1] In severe cases, adjunctive therapy such as mechanical ventilation, oxygen therapy, or hemodialysis may be necessary and useful.

---

[1]Not FDA approved for this indication.

CURRENT DIAGNOSIS

- There are no widely available tests to rapidly and accurately diagnose Rocky Mountain spotted fever (RMSF) in its early phases.
- If morulae are not found in patients with HME or HGA, the diagnosis cannot be established with certainty in the acute phases of these illnesses.

The optimal duration of therapy is unknown. Doxycycline can usually be discontinued 2 or 3 days after the patient becomes afebrile. Most clinicians treat patients with RMSF for 7 to 10 days, but this is probably longer than is necessary for cure in all but the most severe cases. Therapy can and should be discontinued within 4 or 5 days in children with RMSF who respond promptly to treatment because the risk of dental staining is minimal when short courses of doxycycline are given. In general, doxycycline use should be avoided in pregnant women. Instead, pregnant women should be given chloramphenicol (Chloromycetin) 500 mg intravenously or orally every 6 hours. Doxycycline may, however, be the preferred agent for treatment of RMSF in pregnant women at the end of pregnancy because chloramphenicol use in such situations can result in the gray baby syndrome, a potentially fatal drug reaction due to chloramphenicol's effect on bilirubin conjugation in term infants.

Although the diagnosis of RMSF can rarely be made in its acute phase by immunohistochemical staining of skin biopsy samples or by polymerase chain reaction, these diagnostic techniques are available only in a few large referral centers. In routine practice, the diagnosis of RMSF is usually proved long after symptoms and treatment have ceased. The mainstay of diagnosis is indirect fluorescent antibody testing, which is available through all state health laboratories. Antibodies typically appear 10 to 12 days after the onset of illness. The optimal time to obtain a convalescent antibody titer is 14 to 21 days after the onset of symptoms. The minimum diagnostic titer in most laboratories is 1:64.

Prevention

Prevention of many cases of RMSF is impossible because ticks are ubiquitous and many patients with RMSF are unaware of having had a tick bite. Persons with frequent exposure to tick-infested environments should frequently inspect their bodies and clothes for ticks. Early detection and removal of attached ticks can prevent disease transmission. Several hours of feeding are usually required for an infected tick to transmit *R. rickettsii*; thus, RMSF might not occur if infected ticks are removed during this preactivation period. Embedded ticks should be carefully removed by tweezers or by fingers shielded by a cloth, tissues, paper towels, or gloves. Prophylactic antimicrobial therapy is *not* recommended following tick exposure, because only a minuscule percentage of ticks in endemic areas are infected with *R. rickettsii.*

OTHER RICKETTSIAL INFECTIONS

Rickettsiae other than *R. rickettsii* can also cause human infection. For example, a single case of *Rickettsia parkeri* infection was reported in an otherwise healthy 40-year-old man from coastal Virginia in 2002. *R. parkeri* was first isolated from Gulf Coast ticks in the southern United States more than 60 years ago, but until this Virginia case was recognized, *R. parkeri* was not known to cause infections in humans. The patient presented with symptoms similar to those of RMSF and multiple eschars on his lower extremities. Erythematous papules, which then developed into eschars, preceded the other symptoms by 4 days. The patient failed to respond to other antibiotics but improved with doxycycline therapy. Subsequently, the authors of a serologic study of 15 patients with presumed RMSF reported that four of these 15 patients had higher titers for *R. parkeri* than for *R. rickettsii*, suggesting that infection with *R. parkeri* may be more common than previously realized and that some patients with presumed RMSF actually have *R. parkeri* infection.

Ehrlichial Infections

Ehrlichia and *Anaplasma* are obligate intracellular bacteria that grow within membrane-bound vacuoles in human and animal leukocytes. As yet, there is no clear understanding of the mechanism by which *Ehrlichia* produces disease in humans. Humans infected with *Ehrlichia* do not show tissue necrosis, abscess formation, or a severe inflammatory response. Ehrlichial and anaplasmal infections do not lead to vasculitis, thrombosis, or acute endothelial injury as seen in rickettsial infections. *Ehrlichia* replicates within phagosomes in infected leukocytes and produces intracellular colonies called *morulae*.

Ehrlichiosis typically leads to one of two types of illness in humans: human monocytotropic ehrlichiosis (HME) caused by *Ehrlichia chaffeensis* or human granulocytic anaplasmosis (HGA) caused by *Anaplasma phagocytophilum*.

EPIDEMIOLOGY

Like other tickborne diseases, the actual incidence of ehrlichiosis is difficult to ascertain because reporting is based on a passive surveillance system that undoubtedly fails to detect or report many cases.

The best available evidence suggests that HME has an annual incidence of approximately 0.7 cases per 1 million persons and primarily occurs in the southeastern, south-central, and mid-Atlantic regions of the United States. *E. chaffeensis* was first isolated from a soldier in Fort Chaffee, Arkansas, in 1990. Since then, cases of HME have been recognized in New England and the Pacific Northwest as well. First described in 1994, HGA has an annual incidence of approximately 1.6 cases per 1 million persons and has been described in the upper Midwest, California, and almost the entire Atlantic seaboard.

PATHOGENESIS

The principal vector of *E. chaffeensis* is *Amblyomma americanum* (the Lone Star tick); the principal vector of *A. phagocytophilum* is *Ixodes scapularis* (the black-legged tick) in the eastern United States and *I. pacificus* (the western black-legged tick) in the western United States. As opposed to rickettsia, survival of ehrlichia requires horizontal transmission by ticks to and persistent infection in a wild vertebrate host (typically the white-tailed deer or white-footed mouse).

At least two other ehrlichial genogroups cause human disease. Infection of the neutrophils by *E. ewingii* causes mild disease that has mainly been diagnosed in immunocompromised patients in the Midwest. The ehrlichial-like *Neorickettsia sennetsu* group causes a mild mononucleosis-like illness that has never been reported outside East and Southeast Asia.

CLINICAL FEATURES AND DIAGNOSIS

Both HGE and HMA typically occur from May to September and have similar symptoms. After an incubation period of 7 to 14 days, patients most often present with fever, malaise, myalgias, headaches, and chills. An important minority of patients have nausea, vomiting, arthralgias, cough, or neurologic symptoms including altered mental status or stiff neck. Rash is uncommon in ehrlichiosis, though a faint rash occurs more commonly in patients with HGE than in those with HMA. When a rash is present as a prominent sign, coinfection with another rickettsial or other tickborne pathogen should be suspected. Rarely, patients with severe illness develop meningoencephalitis, septic shock, respiratory insufficiency, congestive heart failure, and acute renal failure.

Mortality rates of 3% for patients with HGE and 1% for patients with HMA have been reported, but these numbers may be inaccurate because many mild cases or cases that are empirically treated with doxycycline escape detection or definitive diagnosis. Immunocompromised patients may have severe illnesses and higher mortality rates.

The most common laboratory abnormalities seen in patients with ehrlichiosis are leukopenia and thrombocytopenia, but elevated serum transaminases, lactate dehydrogenase, and alkaline phosphatase levels also occur commonly. Cerebrospinal fluid abnormalities including pleocytosis are common and can mimic the changes seen in patients with viral or other forms of aseptic meningitis.

Distinguishing between RMSF and ehrlichiosis on the basis of clinical features may be impossible, although the presence of leukopenia and the absence of rash are more typical of ehrlichiosis. There are five methods to diagnose ehrlichiosis:

- Examination of peripheral blood or buffy coat for the presence of characteristic morulae in leukocytes

- Indirect fluorescent antibody (IFA) testing
- Polymerase chain reaction testing of tissues
- Immunochemical staining of erhlichial or anaplasmal antigens in tissue
- Synthesis of the history, clinical, laboratory, and epidemiologic features of individual cases

Culture of *Ehrlichia* is extremely difficult, and laboratories able to perform such cultures are few and often inaccessible to clinicians in daily practice. Although only a minority of patients with ehrlichiosis have morulae detectable in blood smears, a blood film should be examined in all patients with suspected infection; morulae are more commonly seen in patients with HGA than in those with HME.

Convalescent serologic antibody testing should be performed 2 to 3 weeks after onset of symptoms. The minimum diagnostic IFA titer is 1:64, and a fourfold-antibody rise is considered confirmatory of recent infection.

TREATMENT

As with rickettsial infection, doxycycline[1] is the treatment of choice for ehrlichiosis. Doxycycline can be administered either orally or intravenously at a dose of 100 mg twice per day. For children who weigh less than 45 kg or are younger than 8 years old, the recommended dose is 2.2 mg/kg each day in two divided doses.[1]

There have been no randomized trials of optimal therapy for either HME or HGA, but the consensus of most experienced clinicians is that therapy should be continued for approximately 7 days or for 3 days after defervescence. Defervescence typically occurs within 48 hours of initiation of therapy.

---

[1]Not FDA approved for this indication.

 CURRENT THERAPY

- In most patients with Rocky Mountain spotted fever (RMSF), human monocytotropic ehrlichiosis (HME), or human granulocytic anaplasmosis (HGA), the cornerstone of management is empiric therapy based on clinical judgment and the epidemiologic setting.

- Doxycycline 100 mg PO or IV bid is the treatment of choice for patients with RMSF, HME, and HGA.

- For children who weigh <45 kg or who are younger than 8 y, the recommended dose of doxycycline is 2.2 mg/kg/d in two divided doses.[1]

- Most clinicians treat patients with RMSF for 7 to 10 d; treatment can usually be discontinued 2 to 3 d after the patient becomes afebrile.

- Treat ehrlichiosis for approximately 7 d or for 3 d after defervescence.

- Chloramphenicol (Chloromycetin) 500 mg IV every 6 h should be used to treat pregnant patients with RMSF and patients with adverse reactions to tetracyclines.

- Alternative therapies for HGE and HMA include chloramphenicol and rifampin (Rifadin),[1] although these should only be used to treat HGE or HMA in pregnant patients or in patients with adverse reaction to doxycycline. Doxycycline, however, may be necessary when life-threatening illness occurs in a pregnant patient.

---

[1]Not FDA approved for this indication.

All tetracyclines can cause dental staining, but this risk remains low if a short course is administered. Chloramphenicol[1] has also been used effectively, but, given the higher risk of hematologic toxicity, this medication should be reserved for pregnant patients or patients with adverse reaction to doxycycline. Additionally, some ehrlichia have been shown to be resistant to chloramphenicol in vitro. Thus, doxycycline may be necessary when life-threatening illness occurs in a pregnant patient. Rifampin (Rifadin)[1] has been used to successfully treat a few pregnant patients with HGA, but at present the efficacy of such therapy can only be considered an anecdotal observation; rifampin does not have an FDA approval for this indication.

REFERENCES

Bakken JS, Dumler JS. Human granulocytic ehrlichiosis. Clin Infect Dis 2000;31:554–60.

Chapman AS, Bakken JS, Folk SM, et al. Diagnosis and management of tick-borne rickettsial diseases: Rocky Mountain spotted fever, ehrlichioses, and anaplasmosis—United States: A practical guide for physicians and other health-care and public health professionals. MMWR Recomm Rep 2006;55(RR-4):1–27.

Holman RC, Paddock CD, Curns AT, et al. Analysis of risk factors for fatal Rocky Mountain spotted fever: Evidence for superiority of tetracyclines for therapy. J Infect Dis. 2001;184:1437–44.

Kaplan JE, Schonberger LB. The sensitivity of various serologic tests in the diagnosis of Rocky Mountain spotted fever. Am J Trop Med Hyg 1986;35:840–4.

Kirk JL, Sexton DJ, Fine DP, Muchmore HG. Rocky Mountain spotted fever: A clinical review based on 48 confirmed cases. Medicine (Baltimore) 1990;69:35–45.

Paddock CD, Holman RC, Krebs JW, Childs JE. Assessing the magnitude of fatal Rocky Mountain spotted fever in the United States: Comparison of two national data sources. Am J Trop Med Hyg 2002;67:349–54.

Parola P, Raoult D. Ticks and tickborne bacterial diseases in humans: An emerging infectious threat. Clin Infect Dis 2001;32:897–928.

Pretzman C, Daugherty N, Poetter K, Ralph D. The distribution and dynamics of *Rickettsia* in the tick population of Ohio. Ann N Y Acad Sci 1990;590:227–36.

Stone JH, Dierberg K, Aram G, Dumler JS. Human monocytic ehrlichiosis. JAMA 2004;292:2263–70.

[1]Not FDA approved for this indication.

Smallpox

Method of
Isao Arita, MD

This chapter discusses the diagnosis and treatment of smallpox. However, in the unlikely event that a patient appears to have smallpox, it is essential to contact your local public health service office to obtain any updates, including vaccination, other methods of preventing further transmission, and protection for yourself and your personnel from the infection.

In 1980, the World Health Organization (WHO) declared that smallpox was eradiated throughout the world and would not return to the human community, and they recommended that smallpox vaccination be discontinued based on their assessment that risk of return of the disease is unlikely. Thus, all the nations in the world discontinued smallpox vaccination, and smallpox virus stocks in laboratories were destroyed except for those in two WHO collaborating centers in the United States and the Soviet Union. These stocks have been maintained to complete necessary research under strict biocontainment measures.

Since then, there has been no smallpox despite continuing global surveillance of the disease. Although the world has been apparently enjoying the benefit of successful smallpox eradication, the terrorist suicide attacks in New York City and Washington D.C. on September 11, 2001 completely altered the situation: Subsequent deliberate delivery of *Bacillus anthracis* from an unknown source alerted the U.S. and global community to the potential threat of bioterrorism, including smallpox as the bioweapon.

These circumstances urgently revived the necessity to remember the experience in smallpox eradication, which was once thought to be the technology of the past and which did not progress much in terms of prevention and treatment. Fortunately, such experience was described in detail and comprehensively by the experts who actually worked in the eradication program in WHO's 1988 publication "Smallpox and Its Eradication." In this section, special efforts are made to describe salient features of such experiences and knowledge for medical professionals at medical facilities, who may employ them in their emergency work for minimizing possible hazard, if smallpox infection occurs.

As in the past, there is no specific treatment for smallpox. In fact, this was one of the reasons international efforts were made to eradicate smallpox. Smallpox was greatly feared because of its 30% case-fatality rate and its ability to spread in any country and in any season. The second reason was that vaccination had been a very effective tool for prevention, but the complications, such as postvaccinal encephalitis, eczema vaccinatum, and progressive vaccinia, were relatively frequent and severe. For example, 10 to 50 persons per 1 million primary vaccinees suffered adverse effects in the United States. These complications prompted a strong consensus that the only way to eliminate such vaccine complications was to eradicate the disease, thereby making vaccination unnecessary.

Clinical Features

The clinical pictures of smallpox is distinct for diagnosis and surveillance. There is no subclinical infection of epidemiologic significance. If the national security office warns of a possible return of smallpox, the disease ought to be, without much difficulty, suspected by medical personnel, who are concerned about the risk.

Surveillance of deliberate release of smallpox virus will be done by the appropriate national security offices, which require full cooperation by medical professionals. In fact, such cooperation is indispensable. Experience has shown that medical facilities are a common contact point, where persons infected with such severe disease as smallpox will visit, seeking consultation and medical treatment.

Clinical Course

After the incubation period (usually 10–14 days, ranging rarely 7–19 days), prodromal symptoms begin with fever and malaise. The exanthem develops in a very regular stepwise fashion of macules, papules, vesicles, and pustules (Figure 1). The exanthem is quite characteristic, with uniform features at each step and typical distribution on the body. The lesions are distributed more on the face and extremities, the extensor side is more affected than the flexor side, and there are fewer lesions on the trunk. The appearance is so classic that medical personnel can suspect smallpox once they have seen the good pictures of smallpox exanthems.

Within one week, the skin lesions become pustules, which, in a few days, become confluent and reach maximum size. By the end of the second week, scabbing starts. The scabs fall from the skin, leaving depigmented spots in the affected skin (see Figure 1H). The scabs can persist for as long as 1 month. Within a few months, the depigmented areas become blackish pigmented spots. These are signs with which surveillance identified the presence of transmission retrospectively in the affected community in the recent past, if the surveillance missed the actual presence of smallpox. Finally, the pustules on the face become pockmark scars.

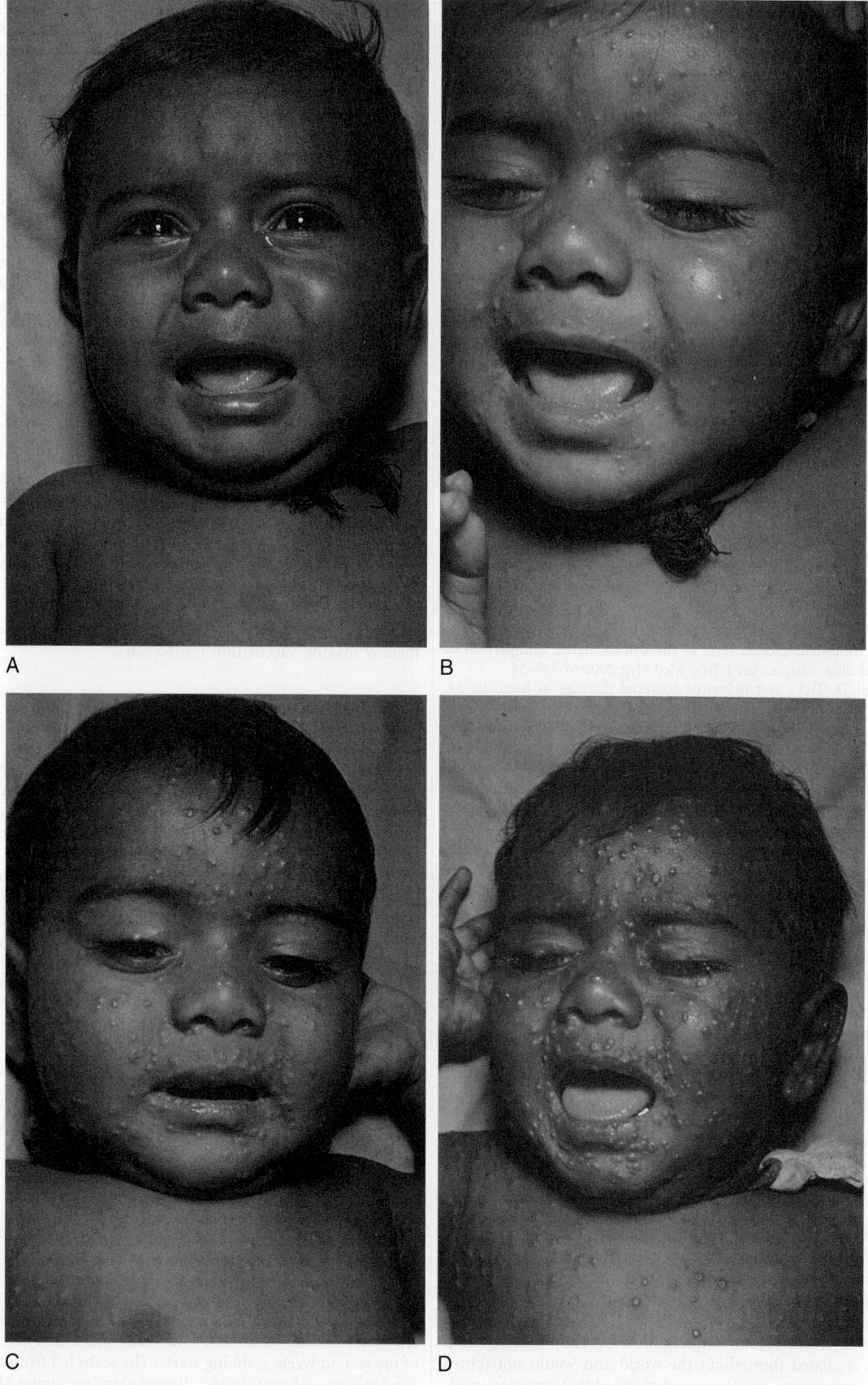

FIGURE 1. Lesions of smallpox. **A,** Day 1: The rash appears 1 day after the onset of fever. A few small papules are visible on the face and upper arms. An enanthem is usually present in the oropharynx at this time, but it cannot be seen in this photograph. **B,** Day 3: Additional lesions continue to appear, and some of the papules are becoming obviously vesicular. **C,** Day 4: All lesions have usually appeared by this time. Those that appeared earliest on the face and upper extremities are somewhat more mature than those that appeared later on other parts of the body, but on any specific area of the body all lesions are at approximately the same stage of development. Lesions are present on the palms. **D,** Day 5: Almost all the papules have now become vesicular or pustular, the true vesicular stage usually being very brief. Some of the lesions on the upper arms show early umbilication.

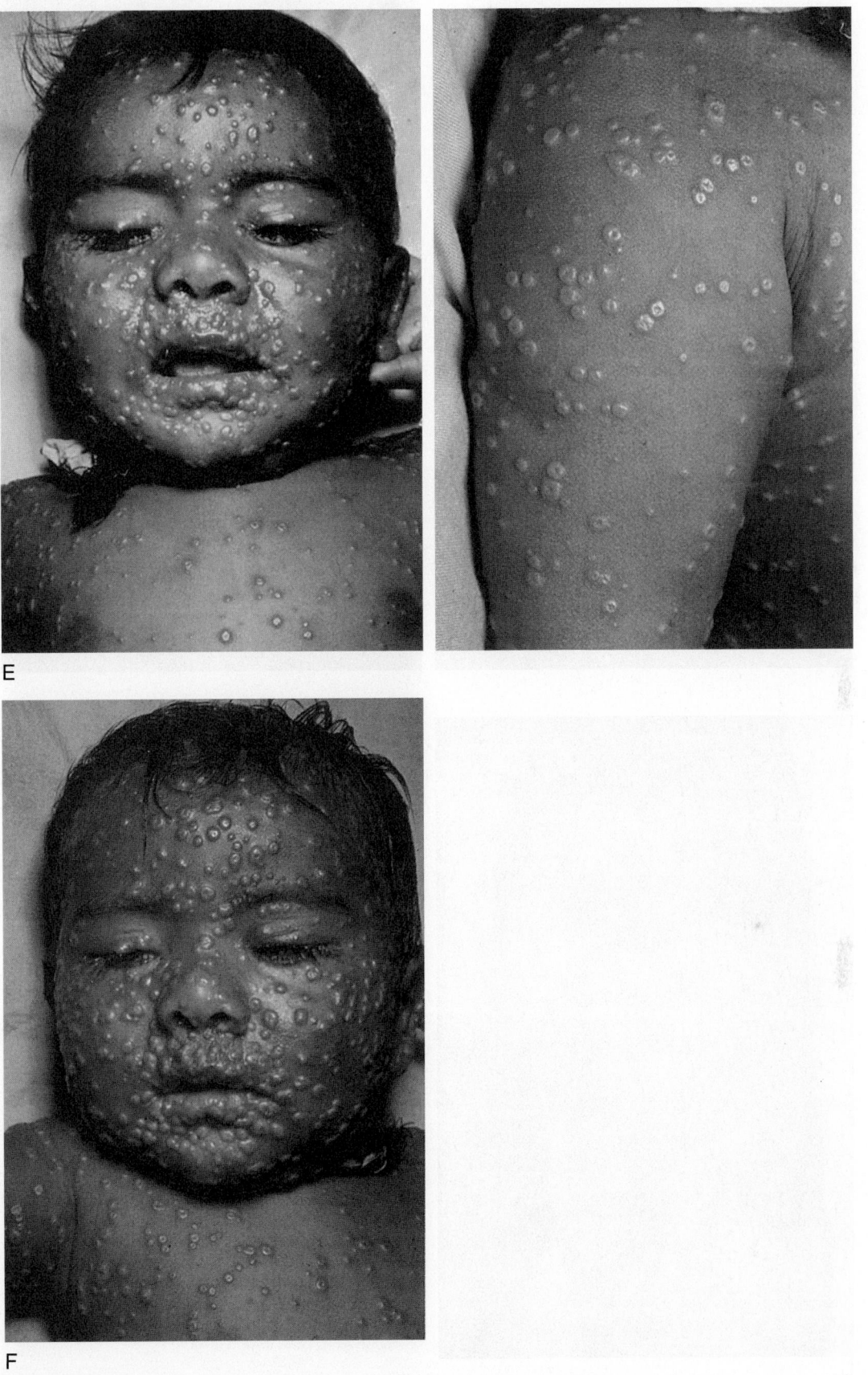

FIGURE 1. (Cont'd) E, Day 6: All the vesicles have now become pustules, which feel round and hard to the touch ("shotty"), like a foreign body. **F,** Day 7: Many of the pustules are now umbilicated and all lesions now appear to be at the same stage of development.

(Continued)

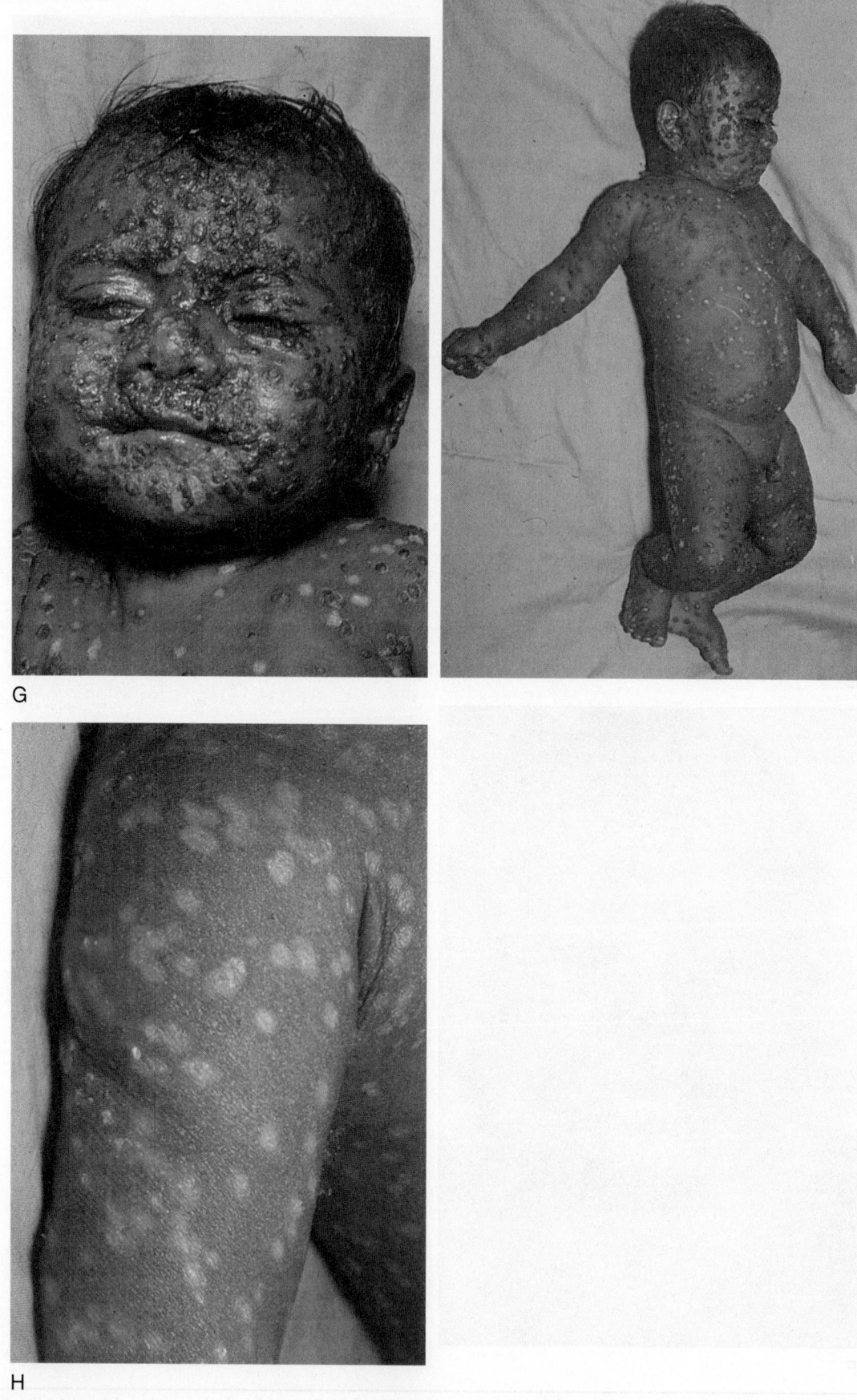

FIGURE 1. (Cont'd) G, Day 13: The lesions are now scabbing, but the eyelids are more swollen than at earlier times. There is no evidence of secondary bacterial infection of the skin lesions. **H,** Day 20: The scabs have separated except on the palms and the soles, leaving depigmented areas.

As for the severity of the disease, *Variola major* is the severest type, with a fatality rate of 30%. For smallpox terrorism, *V. major* is the likely strain. *V. minor* causes mild disease, with a fatality rate of a few percent. Intermediate-type disease has been found in some areas, including Africa. The clinical pictures of mild and intermediate smallpox are similar to those caused by *V. major*. Hence, *V. minor* disease should be treated just as *V. major* disease is in practice, when surveillance and control measures are to take place. Only laboratory study can verify the type of *V.* virus. Pregnancy appears to augment the severity of the disease.

History of smallpox vaccination modifies the course of the disease. Vaccinated patients who have smallpox have an accelerated clinical course and fewer skin lesions. This applies to persons vaccinated either before immunization programs ended, when smallpox had not yet been eradicated, or during special containment vaccination programs against the risk of infection. However, the percentage of unvaccinated persons among the global population is rapidly increasing. For clinical diagnosis, it is important to refer to the clinical characteristics, as described earlier.

Meanwhile, in emergency or unexpected circumstances, where the public health service has not yet been ready to organize personnel, persons who were vaccinated in the past may be requested (subject to their agreement to help), after a fresh vaccination, to participate in some emergency activities for surveillance or related activities.

Differential Diagnosis and Laboratory Studies

During the program of smallpox eradication (1967–1980), surveillance was based on the clinical diagnosis in endemic nations, and only during the last 3 years of the program was laboratory diagnosis practiced by WHO reference laboratories in the United States and the Soviet Union. However, in today's world, it is important to pay special attention to the differential diagnosis, both clinical and laboratory, because a diagnosis of smallpox will necessarily result in a national health emergency including control of traffic, social events, and economic affairs and psychological calamity.

CURRENT DIAGNOSIS

- Smallpox was declared eradicated in 1980.
- Smallpox is one of the priority diseases requiring biodefense preparedness.
- Preliminary diagnosis of smallpox should be regarded as a national emergency.
- Smallpox has a characteristic progression of exanthems after prodromal symptoms: macules, papules, vesicles, and pustules. The entire rash is uniform at each stage. The rash lasts about 1 wk after the onset of fever. Check the type of rash on the patient against photos of the exanthems.
- If you suspect smallpox, report it to the local public health service office immediately to get instructions for further emergency action.
- Be prepared to collect specimens from the rash, based on established procedures, and to dispatch them to the designated laboratory.

The clinical differential diagnosis includes varicella and other diseases of rash and fever (Table 1). In varicella, the features of the exanthem are different from those of smallpox. The varicella exanthem is a mixture of different types of rash, and the lesions are more abundant on the trunk (Figure 2). For clinicians, it may be difficult to suspect smallpox for the first 2 to 3 days of smallpox rash, because the rash may be mistaken for varicella or some other skin eruption. However, by day 3 to 4, it should be apparent that the rash is smallpox. Human monkeypox is another possible diagnosis, because the type of rash and distribution on the skin are very similar to those of smallpox, but the lymphadenopathy (maxillar, inguinal, etc.) is distinctive in monkeypox (Figure 3).

In the differential diagnosis of smallpox, it is important to pay attention to the case history of the patient regarding whether the patient has had contact with a smallpox-like disease. In the case of

TABLE 1 Alternative Diagnoses in Suspected but Unconfirmed Cases of Smallpox

Final Diagnosis	Case Series		
	England and Wales, 1946–1948* *(Variola major)*	India, 1976[†] *(Variola major)*	Somalia, 1977–1979[‡] *(Variola minor)*
Chickenpox	41	53	20
Erythema multiforme	7	1	0
Allergic dermatitis	7	1	1
Drug rash	6	2	1
Syphilis	3	4	4
Impetigo	3	2	0
Scabies	1	1	0
Psoriasis	1	1	0
Vaccinia	5	0	1
Herpes	2	0	0
Measles	2	0	0
Rubella	1	0	0
Molluscum contagiosum	0	0	1
Septicemia	4	0	0
Skin diseases (various)	14	5	0
Other (including no diagnosis made)	0	30	1
Total	97	100	29

Source: World Health Organization.
*Data from Conybeare ET: Cases in which smallpox was suspected but unconfirmed. Mon Bull Min Health Public Health Lab Serv 1950:9:56–61.
[†]During posteradication surveillance in India. Data from Basu RN, Jezek Z, Ward NA: The eradication of smallpox from India. New Delhi: World Health Organization, 1979.
[‡]During posteradication surveillance in Somalia. Data from Jezek Z, Kriz B, Masar I, et al: [Liquidation of the last foci of variola in the world—Somalia (author's transl)] Cesk Epidemiol Mikrobiol Imunol 1981;30(12):113–124, Czech.

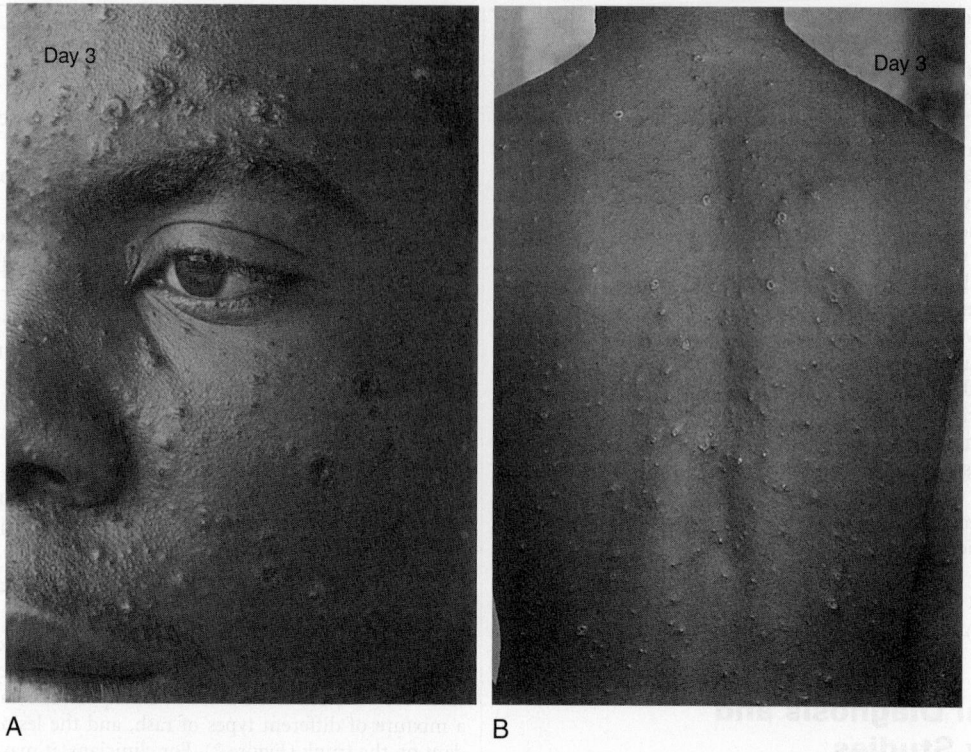

FIGURE 2. Chickenpox. **A** and **B**, On the third day of rash, pocks are at different stages of development (papules and vesicles). There are many lesions on the trunk (**B**) and few on the limbs. (Photographs from the World Health Organization.)

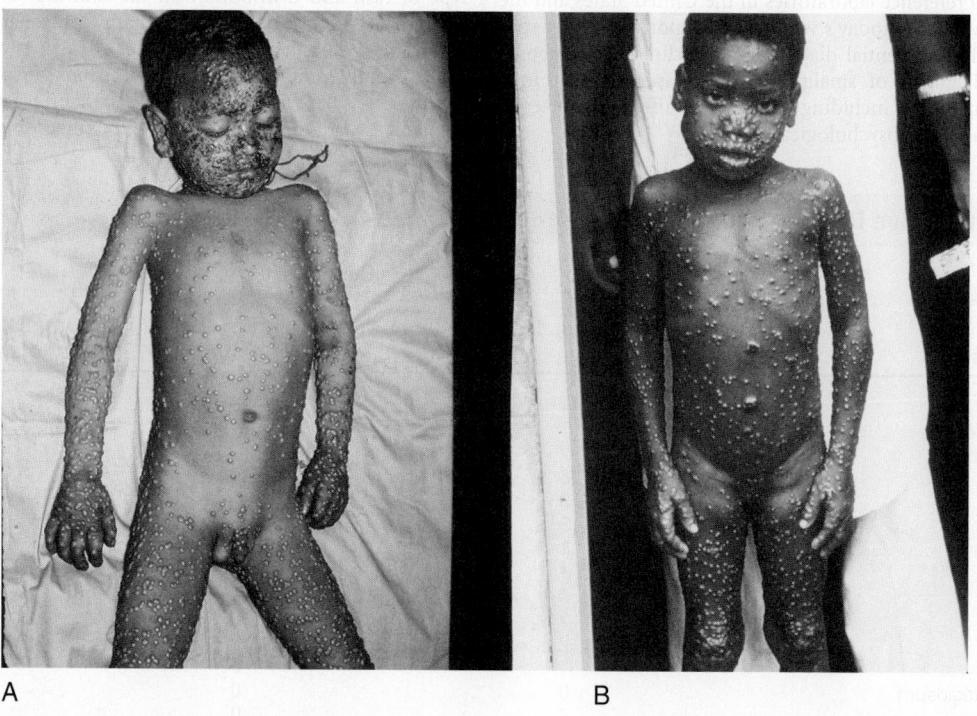

FIGURE 3. Similar exanthem in patients infected with smallpox virus (**A**) and monkeypox virus (**B**) on day 7 of exanthem. (Photographs from the World Health Organization.)

a smallpox attack, there are two possible scenarios. In the first one, a case of deliberate release of smallpox virus through aerosol or contaminated materials, the case history does not arouse suspicion. The second scenario is a patient with secondary transmission from a primary smallpox patient. In this situation, the case history might show the contact with a smallpox-like disease within 17 days before the onset of rash.

The methods of laboratory diagnosis include electron microscopic test, rapid DNA test, virus isolation, and genetic sequence study. These should be operative services of a laboratory network of either

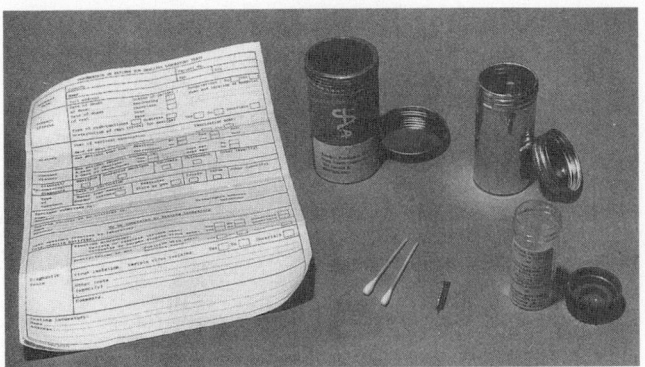

FIGURE 4. Container for smallpox specimen collection. Transportation of dangerous pathogens or specimens requires a special double container to ensure safety. (Photograph from the World Health Organization.)

a national reference laboratory or a contracted reference laboratory from another country. WHO should be in a position to assist in these laboratory networks.

The electron microscopic or rapid DNA test can be completed within a day, and virus isolation and genetic sequence tests can be completed in a few days in a designated laboratory in the network. Collection and dispatch of specimens (usually from skin lesions) should be according to the accepted protocol, namely, specimen placed in a leak-proof double container and packed according to the rules of the International Association of Transportation Regulators (IATR) (Figure 4).

The preparedness of the laboratory network is the first priority in any nation that wishes to handle smallpox bioterrorism surveillance properly.

Treatment

The patient with diagnosed smallpox must be safely transported and admitted to an isolated station or ward for treatment by trained hospital personnel. Patients with suspected smallpox should be also isolated and vaccinated. Patients with suspected smallpox *must not* be treated in the same isolation facilities with smallpox patients.

Currently, there is no effective therapeutic substance licensed for treating smallpox in humans. Before and after the smallpox eradication period (1967–1980), strenuous efforts were made to develop treatment for smallpox, but they have failed. As recently experienced in the United States, immunization of the population as preparedness for biodefense has also failed due to vaccine complications. Most nations, to date, are not in favor of conducting mass vaccination campaigns as preemptive measures. Thus, the research to produce a safer vaccine and the research on an antiviral drug are warranted and continued.

 CURRENT THERAPY

- We have no specific antiviral drug or treatment of smallpox.
- Provide supportive care as symptoms suggest.
- Consult the local health service office for all the necessary pubic health measures, such as protection for yourself and your staff from infection, disinfection, isolation, vaccination, transport, and other relevant containment methods as required.

If smallpox reemerges, all patients should receive supportive care. Supportive care can include infection control, such as antibiotics to prevent secondary infection, and intensive rehydration therapy. Ventilator assistance may be needed. In special cases, such as the severe type of hemorrhagic smallpox, patients must also be treated for shock. Attention should be paid to likely renal failure and malnutrition. These medical practices are complicated by the precautions for protection and disinfection that are necessary to prevent smallpox virus contamination of the environment and population.

Experience has shown that smallpox vaccination during the incubation period, within 4 to 5 days after the exposure to the infection, can prevent the infection. However, in practice, any person in contact with a smallpox patient or suspected smallpox patient should be vaccinated as soon as possible. Vaccinia immune globulin intravenous (VIGIV) can reduce some complications of vaccination, but there has been no evidence that it is effective for treating smallpox.

Smallpox was once eradicated by the unified efforts of humankind. The strategy was through immunization as a preventive measure, not through curative treatment, which is not available even today, when bioterrorism by smallpox is threatening us. Research is needed to develop a further attenuated vaccine and antiviral drug as well, but use of the vaccine should still play a greater role, as was done in the eradication efforts a quarter century ago.

This article was written in 2006, and because the technical progress will be very rapid, readers are requested to seek updated information that will be available from the World Health Organization (http://www.who.int/csr/disease/smallpox/en/) and the U.S. Centers for Disease Control and Prevention (http://www.bt.cdc.gov/agent/smallpox/index.asp) in 2008.

Acknowledgments

I am grateful to Dr. D. A. Henderson of Johns Hopkins University, who advised on the preparation of this article and to Ms. M. Nakane of the Agency for Cooperation in International Health (in Japan), who sorted out all important references during the preparation of this article.

REFERENCES

Arita I. Smallpox vaccine and its stockpile in 2005. Lancet Infect Dis 2005;5 (10):647–52.

Breman JG, Henderson DA. Diagnosis and management of smallpox, N Engl J Med 2002;346(17):1300–8. Available from http://content.nejm.org/cgi/content/full/346/17/1300 [accessed May 30, 2007].

Centers for Disease Control and Prevention. Smallpox response plan and guidelines: Annex 1: Overview of smallpox, clinical presentations, and medical care of smallpox patients, Available from http://www.bt.cdc.gov/agent/smallpox/response-plan/files/annex-1-part1of3.pdf [accessed May 30, 2007].

Centers for Disease Control and Prevention. Smallpox response plan and guidelines: Annex 2: General Guidelines for Smallpox Vaccination Clinics. Available from http://www.bt.cdc.gov/agent/smallpox/response-plan/files/annex-2.pdf [accessed May 30, 2007].

Centers for Disease Control and Prevention. Smallpox response plan and guidelines: Annex 3: Guidelines for Large Scale Smallpox Vaccination Clinics: Logistical Considerations and Guidance for State and Local Planning for Emergency, Large-Scale, Voluntary Administration of Smallpox Vaccine in Response to a Smallpox Outbreak. Available from http://www.bt.cdc.gov/agent/smallpox/response-plan/files/annex-3.pdf [accessed May 30, 2007].

Centers for Disease Control and Prevention. Slides and notes: Smallpox disease and its clinical management. Available from http://www.bt.cdc.gov/agent/smallpox/training/overview/pdf/diseasemgmt.pdf [accessed May 30, 2007].

Centers for Disease Control and Prevention. Smallpox fact sheet: Reaction after smallpox vaccination. Available from http://www.bt.cdc.gov/agent/smallpox/vaccination/pdf/reactions-vacc-public.pdf [accessed May 30, 2007].

Fenner F, Henderson DA, Arita I, Jezek Z, Ladnyi ID. Smallpox and Its Eradication. Geneva, Switzerland: World Health Organization, 1988. PDF available at http://whqlibdoc.who.int/smallpox/9241561106.pdf [accessed May 15, 2007].

Institute of Medicine. Assessment of Future Scientific Needs for Live Variola Virus. Washington, DC: National Academies Press; 1999.

University of Pittsburgh Medical Center Center for Biosecurity. Smallpox FAQ, 2005 [on the Internet, cited October 2, 2006], Available from http://www.upmc-biosecurity.org/website/bioagents/smallpox/smallpox_faq_2005.html.

Diseases of the Head and Neck

Vision Correction Procedures

Method of
Weldon W. Haw, MD, and
Edward E. Manche, MD

Background and Definitions

Refractive surgery is the art of surgically correcting refractive error. Refractive error occurs when parallel rays of light entering the nonaccommodating eye (i.e., one in which the focusing muscle or ciliary body is relaxed) are not focused on the retina. This results in blurry vision. The refractive state of a patient's eye can be described according to the following classification.

CURRENT DIAGNOSIS

- Refractive error (nearsightedness, farsightedness, astigmatism) and presbyopia are prevalent in the U.S. population and result in blurry vision.
- Elective surgical therapeutic options exist and usually include reshaping of the corneal surface or intraocular surgical procedures.

CURRENT THERAPY

- Spectacles
- Contact lenses
- Refractive surgery
- Corneal refractive surgery: photorefractive keratectomy, laser in situ keratomileusis (LASIK), epithelial LASIK
- Intraocular refractive surgery: phakic intraocular lenses, clear lens extraction
- Surgical correction of presbyopia

Emmetropia

In emmetropia (no refractive error), parallel light rays entering an nonaccommodating eye are focused exactly on the retina (Fig. 1). Distance vision is intact without any corrective lenses. Near vision is also intact until the natural onset of presbyopia near the age of 40 years.

Ametropia

In ametropia, refractive error is present. There are three types:

Myopia (Nearsightedness)

In myopia, the focusing power of the eye is too strong. This usually occurs because the length of the eye is longer than normal or the cornea is steeper than normal. The resulting focus point is anterior to the retina. This condition is corrected by diverging the light rays entering into the eye, such as by use of a concave lens (spectacle or contact lens) (Fig. 2). Patients usually have blurry distance vision but relatively intact near vision.

Hyperopia (Farsightedness)

In hyperopia, the focusing power of the eye is too weak. This usually occurs because the length of the eye is shorter than normal or the cornea is flatter than normal. This results in a focus point posterior to the retinal surface. This condition is corrected by converging the light rays entering into the eye, such as by use of a convex lens (spectacle or contact lens). Young patients with mild levels of hyperopia may not be symptomatic because the ciliary body can accommodate and self-correct for this condition. Eventually, as the patient ages, the near vision becomes blurrier, followed by the distance vision, as age-related decline in the ability to accommodate occurs.

Astigmatism

Myopia and hyperopia can occur with or without astigmatism. Significant astigmatism results in blurry vision at all distances. It occurs because light rays in one plane are at a different focus point than light rays in the corresponding plane 90 degrees away (Fig. 3).

Presbyopia

Although it is not truly a refractive error, presbyopia is considered here because its correction has similarities to the correction of refractive errors. Presbyopia is the gradual and progressive decline of accommodation by the ciliary body that manifests as a progressive deterioration in a patient's near vision. This is a natural process that occurs in all individuals regardless of their refractive error. In a patient without refractive error (emmetropia), there is a gradual decline in near vision, which results in the need for reading glasses. Patients with myopia may not be symptomatic because their natural

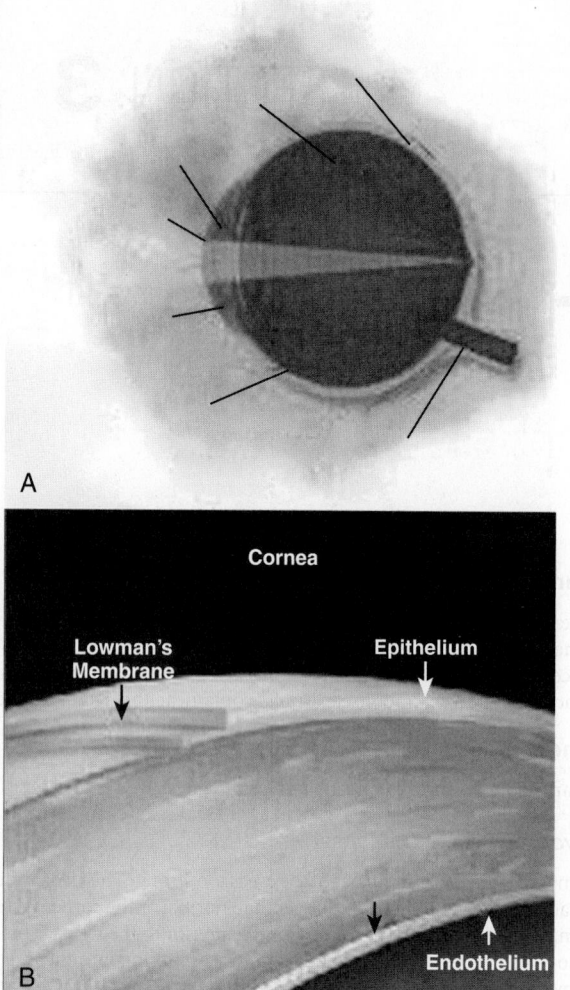

FIGURE 1. A, Basic anatomy of the eye and emmetropia. In eyes without refractive error (emmetropia), parallel light rays entering the eye are focused on the retina. Most refractive surgery procedures involve reshaping of the corneal surface. **B,** Basic anatomy of the cornea. The surface of the cornea, the epithelium, regenerates spontaneously. This layer is therefore expendable, unlike the underlying layers of the cornea (i.e., stroma).

focus point is already set for near vision; they may be able to remove their distance spectacles and still read without readers. However, patients whose myopia is corrected with spectacles or contact lenses may have difficulty reading by their forties due to presbyopia. In a patient with hyperopia, presbyopia and the need for reading spectacles manifests itself at a much earlier age (late thirties to forties).

Epidemiology

Approximately three quarters of the American population older than 40 years of age have refractive errors greater than 0.5 diopter (D). About 150 million Americans currently use some form of eyewear to correct refractive errors, including 36 million who use contact lenses. Population-based studies indicate that approximately 40% of people in their forties have myopia, and 20% have hyperopia. Astigmatism of more than 0.5 D is common in adults and the prevalence increases to approximately 28% in persons in their forties.

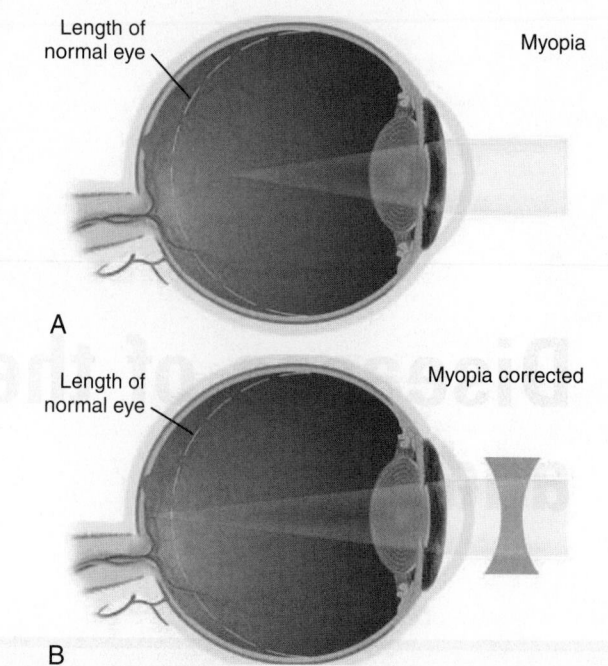

FIGURE 2. Myopia or nearsightedness. **A,** Myopia results when the focusing power of the eye is too strong. **B,** Myopia can be corrected by flattening the central cornea or placing a concave spectacle lens in front of the eye.

Surgical Management of Refractive Error

The need to correct refractive error depends on the patient's visual demands and symptoms. Many patients with small levels of refractive error or with minimal visual demands do not require any correction. Symptomatic refractive error can be managed with nonsurgical techniques such as spectacles or contact lenses. However, these aids have limitations that include suboptimal optical quality, discomfort with use, inconvenience, and poor peripheral vision. In some cases, patients simply become intolerant of contact lens use, necessitating a review of alternative optical correction methods. Also, use of contact lenses may result in permanent vision-threatening consequences (e.g., corneal infections).

For whatever reason, many motivated patients elect to proceed with surgical correction of their refractive error. In the last decade, there have been a multitude of technologic advancements that allow for more reliable and reproducible reduction of refractive error. Despite these

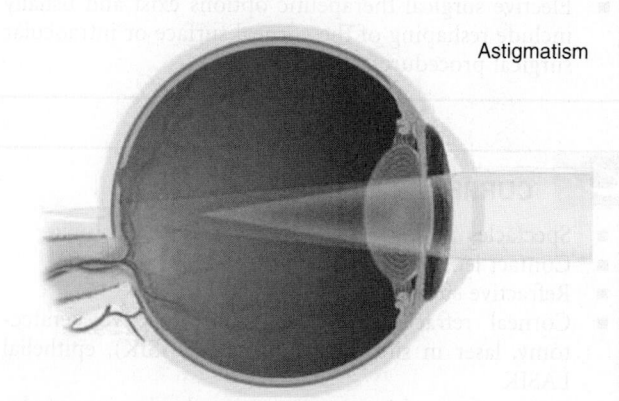

FIGURE 3. Astigmatism occurs when the refractive power of the eye is not symmetrical. One axis has a stronger refractive power than another axis.

TABLE 1 Summary of the More Common Refractive Surgery Procedures

Surgical Procedure	Advantages	Disadvantages
Photorefractive keratectomy (PRK)	Avoids flap complications; more untouched normal corneal tissue (less risk for ectasia)	Discomfort; slower visual recovery; corneal scarring
Laser in situ keratomileusis (LASIK)	No discomfort; rapid vision recovery; rapid healing; minimal corneal scarring	Potential for severe flap complications; results in less normal corneal tissue (potential for ectasia)
Epithelial-LASIK or LASEK	Similar to PRK	Similar to PRK
Conductive keratoplasty (CK)	Spares central visual axis	Initial overcorrection; regression of refractive effect; induction of astigmatism
Intracorneal ring segments (ICRS or Intacs)	Spares central visual axis; segments can be removed	Can only correct low levels of myopia or ectasia
Phakic intraocular lenses	Retains accommodation in pre-presbyopic patient; can correct high levels of myopia or hyperopia; good quality of vision	Intraocular surgery, so more potential for severe vision-threatening complications
Clear lens extraction	Same as phakic intraocular lenses, except may sacrifice accommodation	Intraocular surgery, so more potential for severe vision-threatening complications

advancements, refractive surgery is not always predictable, nor does it always result in satisfied patients. For these reasons, and because these procedures are elective, a thorough informed consent of the risks, benefits, alternatives, and limitations must be obtained. The informed consent process typically includes a discussion of the expected refractive outcome, the possibility of undercorrection or overcorrection (especially in eyes requiring large-level corrections), the need for reading spectacles for presbyopic patients corrected for distance vision, the risk of loss of visual acuity despite glasses, the risk of poor quality of vision (particularly in low-ambient-light conditions) and glare and halos at night (especially in eyes with large pupils), the risk of infection, and other potential vision-threatening complications.

Surgical correction of refractive error includes procedures that are performed on the ocular surface (i.e., cornea) and those that are performed within the eye (i.e., intraocular surgeries) (Table 1).

CORNEAL REFRACTIVE SURGERY

Most of the bending of light rays occurs along the air-tear interface. The shape of this interface can be directly affected by shaping the corneal surface, because changes in the corneal surface are translated to the tear surface. These changes often are induced by a nonthermal excimer laser, which can be used to reliably ablate corneal tissue. By changing the ablation pattern, a variety of refractive errors can be corrected. If more corneal tissue is ablated centrally than peripherally, the central corneal surface is flattened, weakening the refractive power of the eye and correcting myopia. Conversely, ablation of more corneal tissue in the midperiphery steepens the central cornea, increasing the refractive power of the eye and correcting hyperopia. By preferential ablation along a particular axis, astigmatism can be corrected. These corneal refractive surgeries are office-based procedures (i.e., they do not require an operating room); they can often be completed in minutes with the patient under topical anesthesia, and they have a very low risk of severe vision-threatening complications.

Photorefractive Keratectomy

Photorefractive keratectomy (PRK) was the first excimer laser procedure approved by the FDA in 1995. In this procedure, the corneal epithelium is removed mechanically, chemically, or with the excimer laser. The excimer laser is subsequently used to directly ablate the corneal surface (Bowman's membrane and corneal stroma) in a preset pattern according to the patient's refractive error. The higher the refractive error, the more tissue is ablated. Because the ablation occurs directly on the corneal surface, a corneal abrasion is created, and the patient may experience mild to moderate discomfort during the postoperative period. The surface heals within 3 to 5 days. The vision is functional but continues to improve over the next few months. Disadvantages of this procedure include mild discomfort for 3 to 5 days, slower visual rehabilitation, and potential for corneal scarring resulting in suboptimal vision.

Laser In Situ Keratomileusis (LASIK)

In LASIK, a partial-thickness corneal flap is created by a mechanical blade (microkeratome) or by a laser (femtosecond laser) (Fig. 4). The flap is lifted, and the excimer laser is used to apply the ablation profile to the underlying corneal stroma. The flap is then repositioned. Because the corneal flap is left attached by a hinge, it can be lifted and repositioned easily. The performance of the laser ablation under the flap results in several benefits. Unlike PRK, LASIK does not create a corneal abrasion; therefore, it is much more comfortable, results in

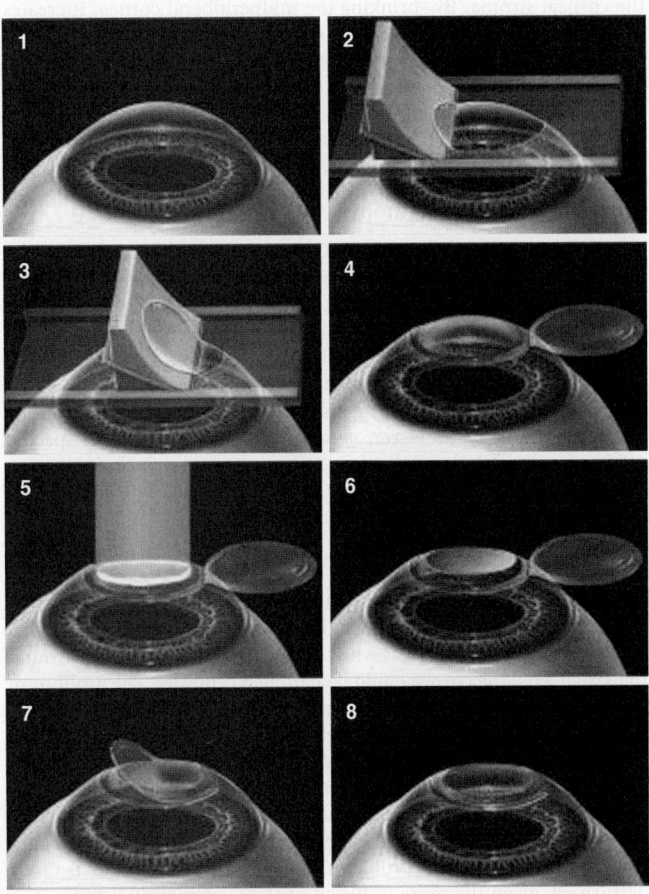

FIGURE 4. LASIK procedure. Image 1 shows the normal cornea. A microkeratome (or laser) is used (2 and 3) to create a partial-thickness corneal flap attached at a hinge. The corneal flap is lifted (4), and the excimer laser ablates the corneal stroma (5). The corneal stroma is then reshaped (6), and the corneal flap is repositioned (7 and 8).

more rapid vision recovery (1 day), and is not subject to as many problems of corneal surface healing (i.e., there is less corneal scarring). However, the creation of the flap in LASIK exposes the patient to potential complications such as flap dislocation, wrinkles or striae in the flap, and epithelial in-growth under the flap. In addition, cutting a flap into the cornea has several potential negative implications: first, the corneal nerves are also cut, which predisposes to a neurotrophic cornea and risk of dry eye; second, cutting a cornea flap weakens the cornea, resulting in a higher risk of corneal bulging (ectasia) than with PRK. Many of these flap-induced complications result in permanent and significant loss of spectacle-corrected vision.

Epithelial LASIK

Epithelial LASIK (LASEK or Epi-LASIK) is a newer development that seeks to merge the advantages of PRK and LASIK. In this procedure, a corneal flap is created with a chemical (i.e., dilute alcohol) or with a mechanical blunt separator or blade, followed by application of the excimer laser directly under this superficial flap. In contrast to LASIK, the flap is a superficial flap that removes only corneal epithelium (i.e., corneal stroma is not traumatized). Because the corneal epithelial layer is naturally regenerated over the course of 3 to 5 days, it is potentially expendable. This hybrid procedure aims to retain the comfort and more rapid visual recovery while avoiding the potentially severe flap complications that can result from LASIK. In reality, the postoperative outcomes are similar to those of PRK, and the healing, return to comfort, and vision recovery are significantly slower than in LASIK.

Conductive Keratoplasty

In conductive keratoplasty, a probe is inserted into the cornea to focally deliver radiofrequency energy, which shrinks collagen within the corneal stroma. By shrinking the midperipheral cornea, it creates a belt-like tightening effect that steepens the central cornea. This technology spares the central visual axis and can be used to reduce hyperopia and to temporarily reduce presbyopia. Disadvantages include the induction of astigmatism and early postoperative overcorrection. Additionally, there are questions regarding long-term stability and regression of the refractive effect over time.

Intracorneal Ring Segments

The intracorneal ring segments (ICRS or Intacs) procedure involves placement of arcuate-shaped plastic segments into channels created in the midperiphery of the cornea. The central corneal shape is altered by the configuration and location of these segments. Intracorneal ring segment technology was initially approved in 1999 for low-level correction of myopia. The narrow range of correction and lack of ability to reliably correct astigmatism have limited the applications for this technology. However, it can also be used to correct specific types of corneal bulging (ectasia). The advantages include sparing of the visual axis and reversibility (segments can be removed without long-term consequences).

Corneal Incisions (Radial Keratotomy)

Radial keratotomy was the first-generation attempt at correcting myopia and gained favor in the 1980s. By placement of four or eight radial incisions (like the spokes of a wheel) at 90% depth in a pattern around the visual axis, the cornea could be flattened centrally. The amount of correction can be tailored by placing additional incisions, placing the incisions deeper, or extending them more centrally. However, these deep incisions inherently destabilize the cornea, resulting in significant diurnal variation of vision and progression of farsightedness over many years. In addition, irregular astigmatism; propensity to rupture with minimal eye trauma; and glare, halos, and starbursts around light sources are all significant problems. Currently, this technique is rarely performed, given the more viable alternatives previously listed.

Contraindications

Contraindications to corneal refractive surgery procedures include an unstable refractive measurement, abnormalities of the cornea (thinning as in keratoconus, edema, loss of sensation or neurotrophic cornea, extensive vascularization), irregular astigmatism (e.g., corneal

warpage from contact lens use), other ocular morbidities (e.g., visually significant cataract, uncontrolled glaucoma, uncontrolled external disease such as dry eye), uncontrolled connective tissue or autoimmune disease, and unrealistic patient expectations. In addition, because corneal laser procedures remove corneal tissue, a calculation should be performed before every corneal surgery to ensure adequate corneal thickness for the proposed ablation. The postoperative central corneal thickness should be a minimum of 250 to 300 μm, to prevent postoperative corneal bulging (ectasia).

Caution should be exercised in patients who are monocular (i.e., have only one eye); in those who have other ocular conditions that limit visual function, a history of ocular involvement by herpes simplex or herpes zoster, dry eye disease, large pupils, prior corneal surgeries, or systemic immunosuppression; in those who are taking certain systemic medications, including isotretinoin (Accutane), amiodarone (Cordarone), sumatriptan (Imitrex), levonorgestrel implants (Jadelle),[2] and colchicine; and patients younger than 18 years of age.

Outcomes

Most patients do well after corneal refractive surgery. However, even despite a well-performed surgery in an excellent surgical candidate, patients may notice a subtle loss in contrast or glare and halos during low ambient lighting (e.g., at night). Also, subjective visual function and patient satisfaction do not always correlate with objective measurements. The advancement of excimer laser software and technology has incrementally improved on these results. The ability to measure subtle optical aberrations in a patient's eye with so-called wavefront technology has allowed surgeons to customize a patient's preoperative profile. Custom laser ablation profiles are now possible that can treat these subtleties on an individual basis. Eye-tracking software that allows the excimer laser to follow small patient eye movements that occur during laser surgery has maximized the benefit of the custom laser treatments.

INTRAOCULAR REFRACTIVE SURGERY

Unlike corneal refractive surgical procedures, intraocular surgeries are typically performed in the well-controlled sterile environment of a hospital or ambulatory surgery center operating room. These procedures are typically quite costly, because an anesthesiologist and operating room staff are usually present. The potential for infection and severe vision-threatening consequences does exist with intraocular surgery. These complications include endophthalmitis (infection within the eye), retinal detachment, rapidly progressing glaucoma (angle-closure glaucoma), irreversible corneal edema or decompensation, and cataract formation (in patients receiving phakic intraocular lenses [IOLs]). Because the potential complications are more severe, intraocular surgeries are usually reserved for patients who are not candidates for the previously mentioned corneal refractive surgery procedures. Potential candidates include patients who have higher levels of myopia or hyperopia, previous corneal refractive surgery, abnormal corneal shape or thickness (e.g., bulging of the cornea or ectasia), or insufficient residual corneal thickness that prohibits the use of the excimer laser. These procedures often result in a better quality of vision, compared with corneal refractive procedures, in these subgroups.

Phakic Intraocular Lenses

Specially designed phakic IOLs (also called implantable contact lenses) can be surgically placed within the eye with retention of the natural crystalline lens. Accommodation and the ability to focus remain uncompromised in patients who are not affected by presbyopia. Advantages include rapid visual recovery, stability of achieved correction, and ability to perform high-level corrections. Currently, only two phakic IOLs have been approved by the FDA: the Verisyse Phakic IOL (Advanced Medical Optics) and the Visian Implantable Contact Lens (STAAR Surgical).

---

[2]Not available in the United States.

Clear Lens Extraction

Removal of the clear crystalline lens before development of a cataract is known as clear lens extraction. A new artificial lens, specifically calculated for the patient's eye, is placed within the eye to correct the refractive error. Advantages include rapid rehabilitation and predictability of refractive outcome. Disadvantages include loss of accommodation and the previously listed complications of intraocular surgery. Newer lens implants are available that allow for the partial recovery of near vision without sacrificing distance vision. These lenses currently have limitations and do not restore accommodation to normal levels. There are three FDA-approved premium IOLs that have the capability of enhancing near vision: ReSTOR (Alcon), ReZOOM (Advanced Medical Optics), and Crystalens (Bausch and Lomb).

Treatment of Presbyopia

Nonsurgical approaches to correction of presbyopia include use of reading spectacles, bifocal or progressive spectacles, or monovision with contact lenses. The surgical correction of presbyopia is challenging, because many of the previously mentioned procedures involve changing the focus point of a patient's eye, which sacrifices distance vision to achieve reading vision.

Currently, the most common surgical method of managing presbyopia involves monovision. In monovision, the patient's dominant eye is treated for distance vision, and the nondominant eye is set for near vision. Although monovision patients have an excellent range of vision (distance and near), depth perception and binocular vision are sacrificed, because the two eyes will never be focused together at a single focal point. The repercussions include loss of the ability to perceive depth, which can be difficult in most daily tasks such as reaching for a cup, judging distance when driving, or hitting a tennis ball. Many patients cannot adjust, and the most successful candidates for surgical correction of presbyopia with monovision are those who have already experienced it through the use of contact lenses. Patients who have undergone a successful trial with contact lenses are potential candidates for monovision, which can be achieved with excimer laser ablation or conductive keratoplasty. For patients undergoing clear lens extraction or cataract surgery, the presbyopia-correcting premium IOLs (e.g., ReSTOR, ReZOOM, Crystalens) can be used.

Future Outlook

Refractive surgery technology continues to evolve. More advanced methods of measuring subtle aberrations in the eye and the ability to refine the treatment of these aberrations with the excimer laser on an individualized basis will continue to be important components of successful corneal refractive surgery. Expanded indications for phakic IOLs to correct hyperopia are now being used in Europe and may soon be applied in the United States.

The correction of presbyopia through creation of a multifocal cornea (PresbyLASIK) is currently being evaluated by a number of excimer laser companies. However, although a multifocal optical system may improve the range of vision, previous experience with multifocal systems (IOLs) has demonstrated difficulties including poor quality of vision and the presence of glare and halos. These problems will need to be evaluated before widespread application. Reversible corneal implants on top of (onlays) and within (inlays) the cornea are being evaluated to treat presbyopia. These corneal implants can be removed, and they have the potential ability to recover near vision without sacrificing distance vision.

Improvements in IOL technology, such as true accommodating lenses, are on the horizon. These implantable lenses have the potential to restore the more natural physiologic process of near vision recovery without the obvious disadvantages of multifocal optical systems.

Summary

Refractive errors are extremely prevalent in the United States and result in blurry vision. Correction can be performed with the use of spectacles, contact lenses, or refractive surgery. Most surgical techniques involve reshaping of the corneal surface and can be performed as an outpatient procedure with the patient under topical anesthesia. Results are excellent for most refractive errors. In eyes that are not candidates for corneal refractive surgery, intraocular refractive surgery can be considered. The future continues to be bright for the continual advancement of refractive surgery technology, with expansion of indications and more refined results.

REFERENCES

Haw WW, Manche EE. Conductive keratoplasty and laser thermal keratoplasty. Int Ophthalmol Clin 2002;42(4):99–106.
Katz J, Tielsch JM, Sommer A. Prevalence and risk factors for refractive errors in an adult inner city population. Invest Ophthalmol Vis Sci 1997;38:334–40.
Manche EE, Carr JD, Haw WW, Hersh PS. Excimer laser refractive surgery. West J Med 1998;169(1):30–8.
Wang Q, Klein BE, Klein R, Moss SE. Refractive status in the Beaver Dam Eye Study. Invest Ophthalmol Vis Sci 1994;35:4344–7.

Conjunctivitis

Method of
Robert A. Copeland, Jr., MD

The conjunctiva is a unique mucous membrane that covers the inner surface of the eyelids and extends to the limbus on the surface of the globe. The major functions of the conjunctiva are to produce mucus for the tear film layer and to provide immune cells and antimicrobial agents to protect the ocular surface. The conjunctiva is divided into three anatomic areas: palpebral, forniceal (cul-de-sac), and bulbar. The conjunctiva is loosely attached to the eye and allows free movement. Similar to most mucous membranes, the conjunctiva has an epithelial layer and a deeper substantia propria.

Conjunctivitis is an inflammation of the conjunctiva that may have an infectious or noninfectious cause (Table 1). Noninfectious entities include allergic, immunologic, and toxic causes. Infectious agents include bacteria, viruses, and chlamydia.

Allergic Conjunctivitis

Ocular allergies encompass a variety of entities and are classically divided into five categories: seasonal allergic conjunctivitis, vernal keratoconjunctivitis, giant papillary conjunctivitis, atopic keratoconjunctivitis, and contact conjunctivitis. These varied diseases of the conjunctiva correlate with one or more of the four types of hypersensitive reactions described by Gell and Coomb. Allergic diseases affect approximately 10% of the general population, and most allergy sufferers have a family history. These patients develop symptoms and signs in childhood.

Seasonal allergic conjunctivitis is an acute process that is IgE mediated and triggered by airborne pollen, dander, mold, and house dust. This IgE mediation results in degranulation of conjunctiva, edema, erythema, and itching. Other, more severe forms of allergic conjunctivitis include vernal keratoconjunctivitis, which occurs in people with atopic dermatitis. Giant papillary conjunctivitis occurs in contact lens wearers who in most cases have lens surface deposits.

TABLE 1 Differential Diagnosis of Conjunctivitis

Cause	Signs and Symptoms	Diagnostic Tests	Treatment	Differential Diagnosis
Bacterial	Lids stuck together in morning, visible discharge in tear film and/or caruncle, conjunctival injection, membrane or pseudomembranes	Gram stain, blood agar, chocolate agar, thioglycolate broth	Erythromycin, polymyxin B plus trimethoprim, bacitracin, aminoglycosides, fluoroquinolones	Allergic conjunctivitis, dry eye syndrome, viral conjunctivitis, chlamydial conjunctivitis, Parinaud's oculoglandular syndrome, sebaceous gland carcinoma, drug-induced allergic conjunctivitis, floppy lid syndrome
Chlamydial	Chronic unilateral or bilateral mucopurulent conjunctivitis	McCoy cell culture, ELISA, direct immunofluorescent monoclonal antibody stain	Tetracycline 250 mg PO qid for 3 wk; Doxycycline 100 mg bid PO for 3 wk; Erythromycin 500 mg PO qid[3]* for 3 wk	Bacterial conjunctivitis, viral conjunctivitis
Drug-induced allergic conjunctivitis	Ocular itching (moderate-severe), inferior conjunctiva vasodilation, lid edema (lower more than upper), ±dermatitis of the lower lid, relentless progression	Conjunctival scraping, acute eosinophils, chronic lymphocytes and mononuclear cells	Avoiding the offending agents, nonpreserved artificial tears and ointments, antihistamine and vasoconstrictor, cold compresses	Seasonal allergic conjunctivitis, bacterial conjunctivitis, superior limbic keratoconjunctivitis
Dry eye syndrome	Ocular burning, foreign body sensation, photophobia, blurred vision	Tear breakup test, fluorescein and rose Bengal stains, Schirmer's test, conjunctival impression cytology	Artificial tears, lubricants, ointments, restasis, punctal occlusion	Seasonal allergic conjunctivitis, drug-induced conjunctivitis, superior limbic keratoconjunctivitis
Gonococcal	Hyperpurulent conjunctivitis, beefy-red conjunctival injection	Gram stain, chocolate agar, Thayer-Martin media	Topical bacitracin or erythromycin; systemic antibiotics	Chlamydial conjunctivitis, viral conjunctivitis
Seasonal allergic conjunctivitis	Bilateral itching, conjunctival edema, injection, lid edema, tearing	Conjunctival scraping, eosinophils 20%-80%	Artificial tears, antihistamines, mast cell stabilizers, NSAIDs	Vernal keratoconjunctivitis, atopic keratoconjunctivitis, giant papillary conjunctivitis, contact conjunctivitis
Viral	Serous discharge starting unilaterally and then spreading bilaterally, itching, photophobia, conjunctival injection, membranes or pseudomembranes, preauricular and submandibular adenopathy	Viral cultures, immunofluorescent techniques	Cold compresses, dark glasses, vasoconstrictors, cycloplegia, antivirals	Allergic conjunctivitis, drug-induced allergic conjunctivitis, bacterial conjunctivitis

[3]Exceeds dosage recommended by the manufacturer
*Usually erythromycin is 250 mg qid or 500 mg bid.
ELISA = enzyme-linked immunosorbent assay; NSAID = nonsteroidal antinflammatory drug.

Seasonal allergic conjunctivitis is controlled by avoiding the offending allergen if possible. Initially, artificial tear supplements and a topical antihistamine and decongestant can be used to treat acute symptoms. The nonsteroidal antiinflammatory drug ketorolac (Acular) is effective in relieving itching. Cromolyn sodium 4% (Crolom) and lodoxamide (Alomide) are mast cell stabilizers and can be used prophylactically before exposure to offending allergens. A new classification of antihistamines and mast cell stabilizers, including ketotifen fumarate (Zaditor), levocabastine (Livostin),[8] olopatadine (Patanol), emedastine difumarate (Emadine), nedocromil sodium (Alocril), and azelastine (Optivar), is expected to play an increasing role in treating seasonal allergic conjunctivitis. The low-dose corticosteroid

[8]Orphan drug in the United States.

loteprednol etabonate (Alrex) has been used to relieve signs and symptoms of allergic conjunctivitis and in refractory cases. Because of the side effects of cataract formation and secondary glaucoma, however, this drug should be used with the supervision of an ophthalmologist.

Patients with vernal keratoconjunctivitis, atopic keratoconjunctivitis, and giant papillary conjunctivitis should usually be referred to an ophthalmologist for management.

Viral Conjunctivitis

Viral conjunctivitis can be caused by coxsackievirus, enterovirus, Epstein–Barr virus, herpes simplex virus (HSV), and herpes zoster virus (HZV). Most cases of conjunctivitis (pink eye) are caused by adenovirus. Two syndromes of external ocular adenovirus infection—epidemic keratoconjunctivitis and pharyngoconjunctival fever—have been described.

Epidemic keratoconjunctivitis has been reported to occur worldwide from 11 virus serotypes; 8, 11, and 19 are the most common causative strains. Patients present with watery discharge, redness, photophobia, mild foreign body sensation, and preauricular nodes. The peak intensity of the follicular conjunctivitis occurs 5 to 7 days after the onset of symptoms. The fellow eye is involved in at least 50% of cases. Adenovirus keratitis progresses through six stages characterized by an orderly sequence of superficial epithelial infiltrates. Often pharyngoconjunctival fever is indistinguishable from epidemic keratoconjunctivitis.

Diagnosis is usually based on clinical features, and only select cases are confirmed by rapid immunodetection of adenovirus antigens or viral cultures.

The treatment for adenovirus keratoconjunctivitis is mainly supportive. Cold compresses, artificial tears, topical decongestants, and prophylactic topical antibiotics may be given. The use of topical corticosteroids is controversial; corticosteroids should not be used without consultation with an ophthalmologist.

A primary ocular HSV infection typically manifests as a unilateral blepharokeratoconjunctivitis. If external vesicles of the skin are not present, this often is indistinguishable from epidemic keratoconjunctivitis. Primary ocular HSV is a self-limited condition, but topical and oral antiviral agents may be used for 1 week.

Bacterial Conjunctivitis

Bacterial conjunctivitis, which is uncommon, can be categorized into three subsets: acute, hyperacute, and chronic (Box 1). Bacterial conjunctivitis is the result of bacterial overgrowth with a secondary infiltrate of the conjunctival epithelium and sometimes the substantia propria as well. It is usually self-limited, but the severity depends on the inoculum size and the bacterial virulence factors.

ACUTE BACTERIAL CONJUNCTIVITIS

The most common form of bacterial conjunctivitis is the acute mucopurulent form. Cases can occur spontaneously or in epidemics. Common manifestations are modest mucopurulent discharge, diffuse conjunctival hyperemia, and, sometimes, preauricular nodes. In adults, acute mucopurulent conjunctivitis is usually caused by *Staphylococcus aureus*, *Streptococcus pneumoniae*, or *Streptococcus viridans*. In children, *Haemophilus influenzae*, *S. aureus*, and *S. pneumoniae* are the usual causes of acute mucopurulent conjunctivitis.

BOX 1   Causes of Bacterial Conjunctivitis

Acute (hours to days)
Haemophilus influenzae biotype III
H. influenzae
Staphylococcus aureus
Streptococcus pneumoniae

Hyperacute (6 to 24 hours)
Neisseria gonorrhoeae
Neisseria meningitidis

Chronic (days to weeks)
S. aureus
Moraxella lacunata
Enterobacteriaceae
Pseudomonas species

Topical antibiotic therapy should be based on Gram-stained morphology of conjunctivitis caused by gram-positive organisms. This condition can be treated with erythromycin or polymyxin B–bacitracin (Polysporin) ointment or polymyxin B–trimethoprim (Polytrim) solution. Cases caused by gram-negative coccobacilli should be treated with polymyxin B–trimethoprim. Topical aminoglycosides and fluoroquinolones should be reserved for cases refractory to initial therapy.

HYPERACUTE BACTERIAL CONJUNCTIVITIS

Hyperacute bacterial conjunctivitis manifests itself with an explosive onset of severe purulent conjunctivitis, severe chemosis, and massive exudation. If left untreated, it can progress to corneal infiltrates, melting, and perforation. The organism most commonly responsible is *Neisseria gonorrhoeae*. Cases of infection with *Neisseria meningitidis* have been reported, however. Gram stain and cultures on Thayer-Martin medium should be performed. The treatment is with systemic and topical antibiotics.

CHRONIC BACTERIAL CONJUNCTIVITIS

A unilateral or bilateral conjunctivitis that lasts more than 3 to 4 weeks is considered chronic. *S. aureus* is the most common causative organism. A vigorous lid hygiene regimen and topical antibiotics are used initially. In refractory cases, conjunctival swabs for culture and sensitivity should be performed and the patient treated accordingly.

Adult Inclusion Conjunctivis

Adult inclusion conjunctivitis is a chronic follicular conjunctivitis associated with mucopurulent discharge and palpable preauricular adenopathy and is caused by *Chlamydia trachomatis* (serotypes D through K). The diagnosis is made by a direct fluorescent antibody assay, enzyme immunoassay, or a Giemsa stain of the conjunctiva. Treatment is with systemic tetracycline or erythromycin. Topical therapy is optional. The patient's sexual contacts should also be treated with systemic therapy.

Neonatal Conjunctivitis

Neonatal conjunctivitis, or ophthalmia neonatorum, is a distinct entity that occurs in the first 4 weeks of life. Because some of the infectious agents can lead to severe localized eye infection and possible serious systemic infection, precise identification and treatment are essential. Neonatal conjunctivitis is caused by a myriad of entities (Table 2).

Chemical conjunctivitis classically occurs in 90% of neonates from the instillation of silver nitrate drops used first by Crede in 1881 to protect against gonococcal infection. Although this form of conjunctivitis is 2.5 to 12 times more common when 1% silver nitrate is used, it has also been reported with topical erythromycin and tetracycline agents. The symptoms of a mild conjunctivitis and erythema and lid edema occur in the first 24 hours of life. Gram stain shows neutrophils with no organisms. This is a self-limited condition that resolves in 48 hours in most cases. In many countries, silver nitrate has been replaced by topical erythromycin or tetracycline ointment, both of which are effective against *Neisseria* and *Chlamydia* species.

Conjunctival cultures of vaginally delivered neonates reflect the flora of the vaginal canal, whereas the conjunctivae of neonates delivered by cesarean section within 3 hours of membrane rupture are culture negative. The conjunctival flora of the neonate is correlated with the method of delivery. The most common causes of neonatal bacterial conjunctivitis are *S. aureus*, *S. viridans*, *H. influenzae*, *S. pneumoniae*, *Branhamella catarrhalis*, *Enterococcus* species, *Escherichia coli*, and *Klebsiella* species. These bacterial species generally cause

TABLE 2 Neonatal Conjunctivitis

Cause	Time of Onset	Microscopic Features of Conjunctival Smear	Culture	Treatment
Chemical (silver nitrate)	1–36 h	Neutrophils (Gram)	None	None
Neisseria gonorrhoeae	24–48 h	Bacteria, intracellular diplococci, neutrophils (Gram)	Chocolate agar, Thayer-Martin media	IM ceftriaxone (Rocephin) or IV/IM cefotaxime (Claforan) plus topical erythromycin
Bacteria Staphylococcus Streptococcus Haemophilus	3–5 d	Bacteria, neutrophils (Gram)	Blood agar, thioglycolate broth	Gram positive erythromycin ointment Gram-negative tobramycin/ gentamicin
Viruses	3–15 d	Lymphocytes, plasma cells, multinucleated giant cells (Gram); eosinophilic intranuclear inclusions in epithelial cells (Papanicolaou)	Viral culture	Topical trifluridine (Viroptic), systemic acyclovir (Zovirax)[1]
Chlamydial	5–14 d	Neutrophils, lymphocytes, plasma cells (Gram)	McCoy cell culture	Topical erythromycin and tetracycline ointment, systemic erythromycin

[1]Not FDA approved for this indication.

a mild, acute, mucopurulent conjunctivitis 3 to 5 days after birth. Serious complications are few except in the case of nosocomial infections caused by Pseudomonas aeruginosa, which can cause corneal complications and endophthalmitis. Systemically, there may be sepsis, which can lead to death. Gram stain and cultures are needed to make the diagnosis. Topical aminoglycosides are indicated for gram-negative organisms, and erythromycin or bacitracin ointment is recommended for gram-positive organisms and fortified antibiotics for Pseudomonas aeruginosa.

Neonatal conjunctivitis caused by N. gonorrhoeae has decreased significantly since the advent of prophylaxis. Gonococcal conjunctivitis in the neonate consists of excessive mucopurulent discharge, eyelid edema, and profound chemosis 24 to 48 hours after birth. This condition is a medical emergency. Therapy must be started immediately based on presumptive diagnosis from the Gram stain, which typically shows gram-negative intracellular diplococci. The neonate is hospitalized and the ophthalmologist is consulted. Recommended treatment consists of a single intramuscular dose of ceftriaxone (Rocephin) 25–50 mg/kg or IM or IV cefotaxime (Claforan) 100 mg/kg, (50 mg/kg in newborns) every 24 hours for 7 days. Either of these regimens should be combined with saline irrigation of the conjunctiva and application of topical erythromycin ointment.

The most common cause of neonatal conjunctivitis in the United States is C. trachomatis serotypes D through K. Infants whose mothers have untreated chlamydia infections have a 30% to 40% chance of developing conjunctivitis and a 10% to 20% chance of developing pneumonia. Neonatal chlamydial conjunctivitis differs clinically from the adult form of the infection: There is no follicular response in the newborn, newborns have greater amounts of mucopurulent discharge, and newborns have a greater percentage of Giemsa-stained intracytoplasmic inclusions. There is better response to topical medications in newborns. Gram and Giemsa stains of conjunctival scrapings are recommended with conjunctivitis to identify C. trachomatis and N. gonorrhoeae as well as other possible causative agents. Systemic erythromycin (Ery-Tab) 50 mg/kg orally divided into four doses a day for 14 days is recommended, even though inclusion conjunctivitis in the newborn usually responds to topical erythromycin.

Viral conjunctivitis is rare in neonates and is predominantly herpetic and seen in 40% to 50% of infants born to mothers with active genital infections. These infections are usually herpes type 2, but type 1 has been isolated. The onset of herpes keratoconjunctivitis is usually between 1 and 2 weeks postpartum, manifesting as serous discharge with moderate conjunctival infection. Herpes almost always manifests as a unilateral infection. This entity can be associated with central nervous system herpes or disseminated systemic disease. The diagnosis is confirmed by the characteristic vesicular skin lesions or a corneal dendrite, if present; otherwise a maternal history is helpful. To aid in the diagnosis, conjunctival smears and viral cultures can be implemented. The treatment for topical disease is trifluridine (Viroptic) 1 drop every 2 hours or vidarabine (Vira-A) ointment five times a day for 7 days. For systemic disease, treatment is oral acyclovir (Zovirax)[1] 30 mg/kg divided every 8 to 10 hours for 10 days.

[1]Not FDA approved for this indication.

Optic Neuritis

Method of
Fiona Costello, MD

Idiopathic optic neuritis (ON) is an acquired, inflammatory, demyelinating optic nerve injury that commonly affects young adults. ON can occur as a clinically isolated syndrome (CIS) or in association with multiple sclerosis (MS). In 20% of cases, patients present with ON as their first manifestation of MS; and a significant proportion of MS patients develop ON during the course of their disease.

Clinical Presentation

Patients with ON often describe acute to subacute onset of vision loss, with associated pain on eye movement. Women make up the majority of cases, and approximately one third of patients experience positive visual phenomena, such as sparkles, flashes of light, or other photopsias. Loss of color vision, or dyschromatopsia, is also common. A variety of visual field loss patterns occur, including cecocentral, arcuate, and altitudinal defects. Patients with unilateral ON have a relative afferent pupil defect in the affected eye, but this clinical

CURRENT DIAGNOSIS

- Age greater than 45 years
- Optic disc pallor at "acute" presentation
- Bilateral simultaneous vision loss
- Absence of pain, or pain that progresses over weeks
- Atypical fundus features (abundant vitreous cells, florid optic disc edema, hemorrhages, and exudates)
- Poor or no visual recovery
- History of myelitis with poor clinical recovery
- Associated systemic signs and symptoms (rash, joint swelling, fever, or lymphadenopathy)

finding may be absent in cases of bilateral ocular involvement. The fundus examination is normal in most adult patients at presentation, but mild hyperemia of the optic disc occurs in approximately one third of cases. Visual recovery typically occurs 4 to 6 weeks after symptom onset, at which time optic disc pallor often becomes evident in the affected eye.

Atypical clinical features such as hemorrhages and exudates should serve as "red flags" and prompt the clinician to consider possible ON mimics. Failure of clinical improvement, for example, may indicate an underlying compressive lesion, such as an optic nerve sheath tumor or a suprasellar mass. Bilateral simultaneous vision loss may lead to a diagnosis of Leber's hereditary optic neuropathy. Abundant vitreous cells or florid optic disc edema at the time of presentation suggests the diagnosis of neuroretinitis, and careful clinical follow-up of these patients often reveals the development of a "macular star." Patients with vascular risk factors may present with abrupt-onset vision loss and optic disc swelling due to anterior ischemic optic neuropathy. In such cases, the patients have a specific morphologic appearance of the optic disc, with a small or absent physiologic cup to suggest the diagnosis. Posterior ischemic optic neuropathy may be more challenging to distinguish from ON, because optic disc swelling is not apparent at initial presentation. Again, a compatible clinical history and clinical course should suggest this diagnosis, which is considered one of exclusion. Systemic clinical manifestations including fever, rash, joint pain, alopecia, and lymphadenopathy are not typical for ON, and patients with these signs and symptoms should be investigated for underlying disorders including lymphoma, sarcoidosis, or systemic lupus erythematosus.

Neuromyelitis optica is a severe inflammatory process of the optic nerves and spinal cord that is associated with poor clinical recovery. In addition to optic nerve involvement, patients with neuromyelitis optica typically develop clinical and magnetic resonance imaging (MRI) evidence of myelitis, with absent lesions on brain imaging. The recently described neuromyelitis optica immunoglobulin G autoantibody can be used to expedite diagnosis and treatment of this distinct clinical syndrome.

Investigations

ON remains a clinical diagnosis, yet its association with MS serves as an impetus for additional investigations, including cranial MRI. Many ON patients demonstrate clinically silent lesions on their baseline MRI study (50%-70%) and harbor abnormal cerebrospinal fluid constituents (60%-70%), increasing their future risk of MS. The Optic Neuritis Treatment Trial (ONTT) experience has shown that the presence or absence of white matter lesions on the baseline cranial MRI scan can predict the future risk of clinically definite MS (CDMS) after ON. Twenty-five percent of ON patients with no brain lesions on their baseline cranial MRI scan developed CDMS after 15-years of follow-up, compared with 72% of patients with one or more lesions. Furthermore, among ON patients with no MRI lesions, male gender, optic disc swelling, and atypical clinical features

(e.g., no light perception vision, lack of pain, severe optic disc edema, peripapillary hemorrhages, retinal exudates) were associated with a reduced future risk of CDMS.

Current Approach to Therapy: Acute and Long-term Management

Much of our understanding regarding the clinical presentation and acute management of ON has come from the ONTT, which was designed to compare the speed and level of visual recovery after treatment with oral prednisone, intravenous methylprednisolone (IVMP; Solu-Medrol), or placebo. Patients were randomized into three groups within 8 days after symptom onset. Those treated with oral prednisone (1 mg/kg/day for 14 days) demonstrated an increased incidence of recurrent ON, compared to those treated with IVMP (250 mg every 6 hours for 3 days in hospital, followed by an oral taper for 11 days), or those given oral placebo (for 14 days). IVMP therapy decreased the likelihood of developing CDMS after 2 years, although this effect was not sustained after 3 years. According to the American Academy of Neurology practice parameter for the role of corticosteroids in the management of acute monosymptomatic ON, oral prednisone in doses of 1 mg/kg/day has not demonstrated efficacy in promoting visual recovery and therefore has no proven value in treating ON. Higher-dose oral corticosteroids or IVMP may hasten the speed of visual recovery, but there is no evidence of long-term benefit for visual function. Hence, the decision to use these medications should be made with the intention to increase the speed of recovery but not to improve eventual visual outcome.

In light of the future risk of MS after ON, efforts have become more proactive to initiate disease-modifying drug therapies as early as the first demyelinating event so as to delay or possibly prevent this diagnosis. Three studies have addressed the role of interferon therapy in patients with ON and other CIS. The first of these was the Controlled High-Risk Subjects Avonex Multiple Sclerosis Prevention Study (CHAMPS), which included 383 CIS patients who were enrolled into a randomized, placebo-controlled trial if they had two or more clinically silent lesions on their baseline cranial MRI scan. Fifty percent (192 patients) of the CIS patients included in this study had ON. After initial treatment with high-dose IVMP, half of the patients received weekly interferon beta-1a (Avonex)[1] 30 μg once weekly, and half received placebo. There was a significantly lower rate (44%) of MS and a relative reduction of new MRI lesions in patients treated with interferon versus placebo. A second study, the Early Treatment of Multiple Sclerosis (ETOMS) study, enrolled 308 CIS patients with four asymptomatic white matter lesions (or three

---

[1]Not FDA approved for this indication.

CURRENT THERAPY

- Investigate for clinical mimics in patients with atypical signs or symptoms.
- Request cranial magnetic resonance imaging to predict future risk of multiple sclerosis.
- Avoid standard dose of oral prednisone (1 mg/kg/day).
- Consider treatment with high-dose corticosteroids (equivalent to intravenous methylprednisolone 1000 mg/day) to enhance the rate of visual recovery in appropriate patients.
- Consider initiating a disease-modifying therapy in optic neuritis patients deemed to be at high risk for multiple sclerosis in the future.

lesions if one of them enhanced with gadolinium) on the baseline cranial MRI scan. Half of the patients received subcutaneous interferon beta-1a (Rebif)[1] 22 μg once weekly, and half received placebo. After 2 years, 45% and 34% of treated patients had developed MS. More recently, the Betaferon in Newly Emerging Multiple Sclerosis for Initial Treatment (BENEFIT) trial included CIS patients with at least two brain MRI lesions, who were randomized to receive interferon beta-1b (Betaseron)[1] 250 μg subcutaneously on alternate days or placebo until the diagnosis of CDMS or a 24-month follow-up point was reached. Treatment with interferon beta-1b delayed the time to diagnosis of MS.

Prognosis and Future Considerations

Most patients with ON have an excellent visual prognosis, with 95% of patients achieving visual acuity of 20/40 or better after 12 months of follow-up. Nevertheless, many patients report subtle and persistent visual problems after ON, including loss of stereovision, loss of depth perception, and altered motion perception. Patients with prior ON may also describe Uhthoff's phenomenon, which refers to recurrent symptoms of visual disturbance induced by exercise or increased body temperature.

The prognosis for ON patients depends in large part on their risk of recurrent MS-related relapses, and long-term management must be tailored to meet the needs of the individual. Patients with MRI abnormalities who are deemed to be at future risk of MS can benefit from early treatment, and initiation of disease-modifying drug therapy should be considered in these individuals.

REFERENCES

Beck RW, Cleary PA, Anderson MM. A randomized controlled trial of corticosteroids in the treatment of acute optic neuritis. N Engl J Med 1992; 326:581–8.

Comi G, Filippi M, Barkof F. Effect of early interferon treatment on conversion to definite multiple sclerosis: A randomized study. Lancet 2001;357: 1576–82.

Hickman SJ, Dalton CM, Miller DH. Management of acute optic neuritis. Lancet 2002;360:1953–62.

Jacobs LD, Beck RW, Simon JH. Intramuscular interferon beta-1a therapy initiated during a first demyelinating event in multiple sclerosis. N Engl J Med 2000;343:898–904.

Kappos L, Polman CH, Freedman MS, et al. Treatment with interferon beta-1b delays conversion to clinically definite and McDonald MS in patients with clinically isolated syndromes. Neurology 2006;67:1242–9.

Kaufman DI, Trobe JD, Eggenberger ER, et al. Practice parameter: The role of corticosteroids in the management of acute mononysymptomatic optic neuritis. Neurology 2000;54:2039–44.

Lennon VA, Wingerchuk DM, Kryzer TJ, et al. A serum autoantibody marker of neuromyelitis optica: Distinction from multiple sclerosis. Lancet 2004;354:2106–12.

Miller D, Barkhof F, Montalban X, et al. Clinically isolated syndromes suggestive of multiple sclerosis. Part 1: Natural history, pathogenesis, diagnosis and prognosis. Lancet Neurol 2005;4:281–8.

Optic Neuritis Study Group. The clinical profile of optic neuritis: Experience of the Optic Neuritis Treatment Trial. Arch Ophthalmol 1991;109: 1673–8.

Optic Neuritis Study Group. High and low risk profiles for the development of mutiple sclerosis within 10 years after optic neuritis. Arch Ophthalmol 2003;121:944–9.

Optic Neuritis Study Group. Multiple sclerosis risk after optic neuritis: Final optic neuritis treatment trial follow-up. Arch Neurol 2008;65: 727–32.

Soderstrom M, Ya-Ping J, Hillert J. Optic neuritis prognosis for multiple sclerosis from MRI, CSF, and HLA findings. Neurology 1998;50:708–14.

[1]Not FDA approved for this indication.

Uveitis

Method of
Petros E. Carvounis, BMBCh

Uveitis refers to intraocular inflammation: it comprises multiple disease entities, some of which are caused by infectious agents and some of which are immune mediated. Uveitis can be classified by the predominant anatomic location of the inflammation: if it is in the anterior chamber, it is an anterior uveitis (previously known as iritis or iridocyclitis); if it is in the vitreous, it is an intermediate uveitis; and if it is in the retina or choroid, it is a posterior uveitis. In panuveitis, inflammation involves all of these sites. Uveitis is said to be limited if it lasts less than 3 months or persistent if it lasts longer than 3 months.

Clinical Features and Diagnosis

ANTERIOR UVEITIS

Anterior uveitis is the most commonly encountered type. It typically manifests with sudden-onset severe photosensitivity, pain, blurred vision, and red eye. Clinical examination documents decreased vision, limbal injection, keratic precipitates (cells and protein on the corneal endothelium), and an anterior chamber reaction (white cells and flare-increased light scatter in the anterior chamber caused by the increased protein concentration resulting from inflammation-induced vascular permeability). The anterior uveitis associated with juvenile idiopathic arthritis in children may be asymptomatic.

Anterior uveitis is commonly idiopathic but may be associated with human leukocyte antigen (HLA) B27; other HLA-B27 conditions, such as ankylosing spondylitis, Achilles' tendonitis, plantar fasciitis, and dactylitis, should be sought. It may also be associated with psoriatic arthropathy, Reiter's syndrome (although conjunctivitis is its most common feature), inflammatory bowel disease (which is also associated with intermediate uveitis), or sarcoidosis. Rheumatoid arthritis does not cause uveitis, although it may cause scleritis. In a patient with prior intraocular surgery or recent trauma, postoperative infectious endophthalmitis is a possibility. Infectious causes such as tuberculosis, syphilis, and Lyme disease need to be excluded, because they are curable. Viral infections (e.g., herpes simplex virus, varicella-zoster virus) can lead to an anterior uveitis, but they more frequently cause keratitis. Other rare associations are possible.

A good history, including a very thorough systems review combined with a good clinical examination including dilated funduscopy (to rule out retina or choroid involvement) by an ophthalmologist with expertise and interest in uveitis is mandatory for appropriate diagnosis and management.

A first occurrence of anterior uveitis that readily responds to topical corticosteroids (see later discussion) does not require further investigation unless there is strong suggestion of an associated systemic disorder based on the history and general physical examination. Investigation for anterior uveitis that is recurrent or is unresponsive to topical corticosteroids should be tailored based on the clinical examination findings but should not neglect to rule out syphilis, tuberculosis, Lyme disease, and HIV.

INTERMEDIATE UVEITIS

Intermediate uveitis typically manifests in a young or middle-aged adult with pain, photosensitivity, blurred vision, and floaters. The most important finding on clinical examination is a vitreitis (white cells in the vitreous and vitreous haze).

Intermediate uveitis is commonly idiopathic (pars planitis) or may be associated with tuberculosis, sarcoidosis, Lyme disease, syphilis, inflammatory bowel disease, or, rarely, multiple sclerosis. Intraocular lymphoma should be considered in patients older than 50 years of age who have vitreitis. Investigation of intermediate uveitis is mandatory, because it is usually unresponsive to topical corticosteroid drops.

CURRENT DIAGNOSIS

- The most common form of uveitis is anterior uveitis.
- Anterior uveitis is commonly idiopathic.
- Posterior uveitis is most likely infectious.
- In any form of uveitis, syphilis, tuberculosis, and Lyme disease need to be ruled out.
- In immunosuppressed individuals, the uveitis is most likely infectious: the patient's HIV status needs to be determined, because a positive status completely changes the diagnostic approach.
- The key to correct diagnosis is a good history, including a thorough review of systems and a careful ophthalmologic examination as well as dilated funduscopy; laboratory and radiographic investigations, sometimes including aqueous or vitreous polymerase chain reaction or cytologic studies, are frequently necessary.
- Involvement of an ophthalmologist with expertise in the diagnosis and treatment of uveitis is mandatory.

POSTERIOR UVEITIS

Posterior uveitis is commonly infectious. Patients complain of visual loss and floaters. Clinical signs include decreased visual acuity, vitreous cells and haze, and some of the following: retinal infiltrates, serous retinal detachment, retinal hemorrhage, chorioretinal scars, choroidal granulomas, venular sheathing, or arteriolar sheathing.

The most common cause of posterior uveitis is *Toxoplasma* retinochoroiditis. Viral infections such as varicella-zoster or herpes simplex can uncommonly cause acute retinal necrosis, and cytomegalovirus retinitis can be devastating in immunocompromised individuals. Tuberculosis, Lyme disease, and syphilis are bacterial causes of posterior uveitis. *Pneumocystis jiroveci* (formerly called *Pneumocystis carinii*) and *Cryptococcus* can cause a choroiditis in the immunocompromised individual. Sarcoidosis can also cause posterior uveitis. There is a plethora of well-defined posterior uveitides without associated systemic findings (e.g., serpiginous chorioretinitis). Intraocular lymphoma can masquerade as posterior uveitis and needs be considered in older patients.

Unless a clinical diagnosis is possible (e.g., in *Toxoplasma* chorioretinitis), further investigations are required. If a rapid plasma reagin test is negative, a diagnostic vitrectomy should be considered in all patients and is mandatory in immunocompromised patients; otherwise, tailored laboratory and radiographic investigations need be performed.

PANUVEITIS

Panuveitis combines the signs and symptoms of anterior and posterior uveitis, although early in the course one location may predominate. Bacterial or fungal endophthalmitis needs be considered. Vogt-Koyanagi-Harada syndrome is a common cause in the Far East and in patients of Native American ancestry. Adamantiades-Behçet syndrome, sympathetic ophthalmia, tuberculosis, syphilis, and, rarely, Lyme disease need be considered, among others.

Sequelae and Complications of Uveitis

Uncontrolled uveitis can be a blinding condition. Visual loss results commonly from cystoid macular edema or from cataracts, glaucoma, band keratopathy, hypotony maculopathy, macular scar, macular necrosis, or retinal detachment.

Current Treatment

Almost all of the medications employed in the treatment of uveitis are used off-label (FDA approved for an indication other than the treatment of uveitis).

ANTERIOR UVEITIS

If photosensitivity is a prominent complaint, topical cycloplegia affords considerable relief. Homatropine (Isopto Homatropine) 2% or 5%, scopolamine (Isopto Hyoscine) 0.25%, or tropicamide (Mydriacyl) 1% may be used. Cyclopentolate (Cyclogyl) should be avoided, because it has chemoattractant properties in vitro. Topical cycloplegia is also necessary with severe anterior uveitis to prevent posterior synechiae.

Topical corticosteroid drops are the first line of treatment for anterior uveitis (e.g., prednisolone acetate [Pred Forte] 1% 1 drop every 2 hours while awake).[3] Patient education to ensure compliance is of paramount importance. Rimexolone (Vexol) 1% is considered an alternative by some authorities.

After 1 to 2 weeks, a slow taper of the drops is commenced (administer four times daily for 7–10 days, then taper by 1 drop every 7–10 days), provided that the anterior chamber cells have resolved. If there is an increase in activity during the taper, an increase in the dosing frequency to re-achieve a complete response, followed by a slower taper, is performed. Occasionally, patients have to be maintained for the long term on topical prednisolone; this is acceptable, provided that no adverse side effects occur.

---

[3]Exceeds dosage recommended by the manufacturer.

CURRENT THERAPY

- Uveitis resulting from a systemic infection (e.g. syphilis, Lyme disease, tuberculosis) needs to be treated as a central nervous system infection.
- Idiopathic anterior uveitis or anterior uveitis related to an autoimmune disease responds to topical corticosteroids (e.g., prednisolone acetate [Pred Forte] 1% 1 drop every 2 hours while awake[3]) and cycloplegia (e.g., homatropine [Isopto Homatropine][1] 2% 1 drop three times daily).
- Periocular steroids (posterior or anterior sub-Tenon's steroid injection) is useful in the management of severe anterior uveitis and in intermediate uveitis.
- Intraocular triamcinolone acetonide injection (Kenalog)[1] or implantation of a sustained-release fluocinolone implant (Retisert) is reserved for cases of severe uveitis.
- Oral steroids (prednisone 1–2 mg/kg PO) can be effective in cases of severe uveitis that is unresponsive to topical, periocular, and intraocular steroids.
- Systemic immunosuppressants can control uveitis unresponsive to steroids or be used as steroid-sparing agents. Some specific uveitides mandate systemic immunosuppression as first-line treatment.
- Commonly used immunosuppressants are azathioprine (Imuran),[1] methotrexate (Trexall),[1] cyclosporine (Neoral),[1] and mycophenolate mofetil (CellCept).[1]
- Anti-tumor necrosis factor-α agents are promising immunomodulators.

---

[1]Not FDA approved for this indication.
[3]Exceeds dosage recommended by the manufacturer.

If there is incomplete response prednisolone acetate 1% given every 2 hours or if the drops cannot be tapered without recurrence and investigations are negative, the next step to be considered could be a sub-Tenon's (under the conjunctiva) injection of 0.5 to 1.0 mL triamcinolone acetonide 40 mg/mL (Kenalog),[1,6,*] which forms a depot providing continuous steroid release for up to 6 months; alternatively, oral corticosteroids (usually prednisone) may be used in patients with especially severe bilateral uveitis, although this is uncommon. For the rare severe anterior uveitis that is unresponsive to these treatments or to decreases in the steroid dose, immunosuppressant medications such as methotrexate,[1] cyclosporine,[1] or mycophenolate mofetil[1] or an anti-tumor necrosis factor-α (anti-TNF-α) agent such as infliximab)[1] may be given (see later discussion for recommended doses).

It cannot be overemphasized that a severe "anterior uveitis," especially with a hypopyon, occurring after recent intraocular surgery or trauma should alert the physician to the possibility of endophthalmitis. Emergent anterior chamber and vitreous cultures need be obtained, and intravitreous nonpreserved vancomycin (Vancocin) 1.0 mg/0.1 mL[6] and ceftazidime (Fortaz) 2.25 mg/0.1 mL[6] must be injected.

The main side effects of topical steroid use are cataract formation and ocular hypertension, which can lead to glaucoma. Untreated uveitis can cause the same side effects; therefore, inflammation needs be controlled promptly, and then the corticosteroids need to be tapered off as soon as possible without precipitating a recurrence. Topical steroid use also predisposes to cornea infection, including reactivation of herpes simplex or varicella-zoster keratitis.

INTERMEDIATE UVEITIS, POSTERIOR UVEITIS, AND PANUVEITIS

Uveitis associated with systemic infection (e.g. syphilis, Lyme disease) is treated in consultation with an infectious disease specialist, because intraocular involvement is considered central nervous system involvement. Adjuvant topical corticosteroids and mydriatics can afford relief without jeopardizing cure in most cases (as for anterior uveitis).

Ocular toxoplasmosis, the most common posterior uveitis, is self-limited. Treatment is required in cases in which the optic nerve or macula is threatened or the vitreitis is particularly severe. Treatment consists of pyrimethamine (Daraprim) (loading dose 50 mg, then 25 mg twice daily), sulfadiazine (1 g four times daily), and folinic acid (Leucovorin)[1] 5 mg three times weekly. More recently, clindamycin (Cleocin)[1] 150 to 300 mg PO four times daily or trimethoprim-sulfamethoxazole[1] (Bactrim DS 800 mg sulfamethoxazole/160 mg trimethoprim twice daily) have been found to be equally efficacious and are more widely used. Prednisone 40 mg/day is added 24 to 48 hours later. Treatment duration is usually 30 to 40 days, with a prednisone taper guided by the clinical response.

For intermediate uveitis, posterior uveitis, or panuveitis not associated with systemic infection, treatment options are to be considered in the following order:

1. Periocular steroids (posterior sub-Tenon's injection of triamcinolone acetonide)[1] are commonly efficacious for intermediate uveitis.
2. Oral corticosteroids are very efficacious but have ocular as well as systemic side effects. If the uveitis cannot be controlled with less than prednisone 10 mg after 6 months of treatment, one of the other options needs to be considered.
3. In very severe cases of intermediate uveitis and in cases of severe posterior uveitis or panuveitis, intravitreous triamcinolone acetonide (Kenalog 4 mg[1,*] or a fluocinolone implant (Retisert) inserted with a pars plana vitrectomy can be used; whether the latter is superior to systemic immunosuppression is the subject of an

ongoing clinical trial (the Multicenter Uveitis Steroid Treatment [MUST] trial).

4. Systemic immunosuppression with azathioprine (Imuran)[1] up to 2.5 to 4 mg/kg/day, cyclosporine (Neoral)[1] 2.5 to 5.0 mg/kg/day in 2 divided doses, tacrolimus (Prograf)[1] 0.15 to 0.30 mg/kg/day, mycophenolate mofetil (CellCept)[1] 500 to 1000 mg twice daily, methotrexate (Trexall)[1] (12.5 to 25 mg weekly, or an anti-TNF-α agent (e.g., infliximab [Remicade])[1] have all been used with success as steroid-sparing agents or to control uveitis poorly responsive to corticosteroids alone.

There are specific uveitis entities that mandate the use of immunosuppression as first-line treatment (together with steroids initially). These include Wegener's retinal vasculitis, Adamantiades-Behçet's syndrome, sympathetic ophthalmia, and possibly birdshot choroidopathy, uveitis related to Vogt-Koyanagi-Harada syndrome, and serpiginous chorioretinitis.

REFERENCES

Harper SL, Chorich LJ, Foster CS. Diagnosis of uveitis. In: Foster CS, Vitale A, editors. Diagnosis and Treatment of Uveitis. Philadelphia: WB Saunders; 2002. p. 79–97.

Jabs DA, Rosenbaum JT, Foster CS, et al. Guidelines for the use of immunosuppressive drugs in patients with ocular inflammatory disorders: Recommendations of an expert panel. Am J Ophthalmol 2000;130:492–513.

Nussenblatt RB. Philosophy, goals and approaches to medical therapy. In: Nussenblatt SM, Whitcup SM, editors. Uveitis, Fundamentals and Clinical Practice. 3rd ed. Philadelphia: Mosby; 2004. p. 95–136.

The Standardization of Uveitis Nomenclature (SUN) working group. Standardization of uveitis nomenclature for reporting clinical data: Results of the first international workshop. Am J Ophthalmol 2005;140:509–16.

[1]Not FDA approved for this indication.

Glaucoma

Method of
*Matthew P. Traynor, MD, and
Steven R. Sarkisian, Jr., MD*

Glaucoma can be classified by the anatomy of the anterior chamber angle, which may be open or closed. Gonioscopy, a detailed evaluation of the angle using a mirrored lens, is required to differentiate types of glaucoma. Elevated intraocular pressure (IOP) has long been synonymous with glaucoma but is now recognized as only one of many risk factors for the development of glaucoma. Elevated IOP contributes to retinal ganglion cell death and changes to the structure and appearance of the optic nerve head. Visual field defects emerge in the areas subtended by the damaged retinal ganglion cells. Central vision loss is typically a late finding in glaucoma.

Glaucoma is seen predominantly in older individuals. Nevertheless, glaucoma does affect children and young adults. Glaucoma in young children includes both primary glaucoma (caused by abnormal development of the anterior chamber angle), and secondary glaucoma (associated with systemic abnormalities or other ocular disease).

[1]Not FDA approved for this indication.
[6]May be compounded by pharmacists.
*Kenalog is commercially available as 40 mg/mL. Special compounding is needed for the concentration of 4 mg/mL.

Types of Glaucoma

PRIMARY OPEN-ANGLE GLAUCOMA

The most common form of glaucoma is primary open-angle glaucoma (POAG). Increased resistance to outflow of the aqueous humor through the trabecular meshwork leads to gradual and painless elevation of IOP; hence, it is typically asymptomatic. POAG is bilateral but can be asymmetrical. The existence of a subgroup of POAG patients without elevated IOP (normal-pressure glaucoma) suggests that other factors may be significant, such as insufficient vascular flow to the optic nerve head, accelerated programmed cell death (apoptosis), diurnal fluctuations of IOP, and autoimmunity.

Diseases such as diabetes mellitus, systemic hypertension, and vasospastic disorders have been associated with glaucoma but are not clearly linked to the disease. Increasing age is a risk factor: 8% of the population older than 70 years but only 0.1% of those younger than 40 years of age are affected by glaucoma. African American patients have a 5 to 15 times greater risk than white patients. Immediate family members of glaucoma patients have a 10- to 15-fold increased risk for developing glaucoma.

The prolonged asymptomatic phase of POAG can be discovered only by ocular evaluation. Complete eye examination is recommended every 2 to 4 years for patients older than 40 years of age and every 1 to 2 years for those older than 65 years. Patients with risk factors (age, race, family history) should be evaluated earlier and more frequently.

Screening in the primary care setting can include a family and medical history, vision (and possibly IOP) screening, and examination of the optic nerve head by direct ophthalmoscopy. Early clinical findings of glaucoma may be subtle and difficult to detect. Visual acuity is often normal until late in the course of glaucoma. Decreased central vision secondary to glaucoma suggests advanced disease. Normal confrontation visual fields cannot exclude glaucoma because of this technique's low sensitivity in identifying glaucomatous visual field loss. Formal visual field testing is the preferred method for evaluating and monitoring visual field damage. Elevated IOP is a risk factor for glaucoma and should lead to more thorough evaluation. Optic nerve examination of patients with glaucoma shows enlarged cupping of the optic nerve head or asymmetry between the optic nerves or both. Focal loss of neural rim tissue (notching) may occur, and flame hemorrhages may be seen at the disc margin, especially in actively progressing disease. If glaucoma is suspected, a patient should be referred for further ophthalmologic evaluation.

CURRENT DIAGNOSIS

- The most common form of glaucoma in the United States is primary open-angle glaucoma (POAG).
- Risk factors for POAG include elevated intraocular pressure (IOP), advanced age, African American race, decreased corneal thickness, and a positive family history.
- Screening for POAG is recommended every 2 to 4 years after age 40 years and every 1 to 2 years after age 65 years.
- If risk factors for POAG are present, screening is recommended every 2 to 4 years after age 30 years and every 1 to 2 years after age 65 years.
- Ninety-five percent of patients with POAG and 5% of normal patients may experience IOP elevation of greater than 15 mm Hg while taking steroids; therefore, patients with known glaucoma who are taking long-term steroids (>1 month) need close follow-up with an ophthalmologist.
- Primary angle-closure glaucoma has an acute onset with pain, haloes, red eye, decreased vision, and nausea and vomiting. Emergent ophthalmologic referral is required.

Patients with suggestive findings but no definitive glaucomatous damage are classified as glaucoma suspects. The Ocular Hypertension Treatment Study, a recent multicenter randomized, controlled clinical trial, conducted a long-term follow-up of glaucoma suspects with elevated IOP, normal optic nerve appearance, and no visual field defects. This study found that, over 5 years, maintaining IOP at 20% below baseline reduced the rate of progression to POAG from 9.5% to 4.4%.

SECONDARY OPEN-ANGLE GLAUCOMA

Secondary open-angle glaucomas result from ocular or systemic disorders that lead to decreased outflow through the trabecular meshwork. Examples of secondary open-angle glaucoma include pigmentary glaucoma, pseudoexfoliation glaucoma, traumatic glaucoma, and steroid-induced glaucoma.

Pigment dispersion syndrome and pseudoexfoliation syndrome demonstrate deposition of iris pigment and fibrillar protein, respectively, in the trabecular meshwork. Almost 50% of patients with these disorders develop glaucoma due to aqueous outflow obstruction and secondarily elevated IOP. Blunt ocular trauma (often remote) is a common cause of unilateral glaucoma because of structural changes in the trabecular meshwork.

Chronic use of glucocorticosteroids can create resistance to trabecular outflow and subsequent IOP elevation, resulting in a glaucoma resembling POAG. Steroid-induced pressure elevation generally correlates with the dose and length of administration. Although it is most often seen with topical and periocular use, it can also result from systemic or inhaled administration. Steroid responses of greater than 15 mm Hg IOP elevation develop in 95% of patients with POAG and in only 5% of patients without glaucoma. All patients with a known diagnosis of glaucoma should be evaluated by an ophthalmologist within 1 month after initiating a long-term steroid regimen for systemic diseases.

PRIMARY ANGLE-CLOSURE GLAUCOMA

Primary angle-closure glaucoma can have an acute, subacute, intermittent, or chronic presentation. Attacks of acute angle closure are ocular emergencies that can lead to irreversible vision loss within hours. Anatomic narrow anterior chamber angles are a major risk factor for the development of primary angle closure. If the pupillary margin of the iris contacts the lens for 360 degrees, flow of the aqueous humor from the posterior to the anterior chamber may be blocked. With the aqueous humor trapped behind the iris due to pupillary block, the peripheral iris may be pushed anteriorly into apposition with the trabecular meshwork, obstructing outflow. The IOP may rise rapidly to greater than 60 mm Hg. Pupillary block can frequently occur in anatomically susceptible eyes when the iris is mid-dilated.

In Asian populations, primary angle-closure glaucoma is more common than open-angle glaucoma. The risk increases with age, with most cases occurring during the sixth or seventh decade. Women have primary angle-closure glaucoma attacks 2 to 4 times more often than men. Environmental circumstances may trigger an acute attack of angle closure in predisposed eyes; such factors include movie theaters or dark rooms (physiologic mydriasis), sudden anxiety or pain (sympathetic stimulation causing pupil dilation), or medications causing mild mydriasis (anticholinergics and adrenergic stimulants such as sleep and cold medications).

The diagnosis of an acute angle-closure glaucoma attack requires gonioscopic evidence of a closed anterior chamber angle preventing aqueous flow into the trabecular meshwork. Patients may complain of ocular pain, brow ache, rainbow-colored halos around lights, or blurred vision. They may experience intense nausea and vomiting, bradycardia, and sweating. Ocular examination reveals elevated IOP, conjunctival vascular injection, a cloudy cornea (if the IOP rose acutely and recently), a shallow anterior chamber, a closed angle by gonioscopy, and a globe that is firm to palpation.

SECONDARY ANGLE-CLOSURE GLAUCOMA

Scarring and adhesions between the peripheral iris and the anterior chamber angle may block outflow of aqueous. Diabetes mellitus may result in neovascularization of the retina, which can progress to neovascularization of the anterior segment including the iris and angle, blocking aqueous outflow or closing the angle or both. The resultant neovascular glaucoma can be devastating and refractory to treatment. Central retinal vein occlusion, a vascular accident closely linked to uncontrolled hypertension and diabetes, can also lead to retinal neovascularization and a similar process. Uveitis from systemic diseases such as sarcoidosis or autoimmune arthropathies can produce intraocular scarring and secondary angle closure if not controlled.

Sulfonamide-based systemic medications can rarely cause swelling of the ciliary body, which anteriorly displaces the lens and iris. This can produce a secondary acute angle-closure glaucoma, which requires discontinuation of the medication and urgent lowering of the IOP. This phenomenon has also been reported with topiramate (Topamax).

CHILDHOOD GLAUCOMA

Congenital or childhood glaucoma develops from aqueous outflow obstruction caused by abnormal anatomic development of the angle, ocular inflammation, or trauma. Primary congenital glaucoma often manifests in infancy with the classic triad of photophobia, epiphora (tearing), and blepharospasm, but these signs are unnecessary for diagnosis. Buphthalmos (enlarged eye) may occur secondary to increased IOP if the glaucoma develops during the first 3 years of life. Juvenile glaucoma is similar in etiology to POAG and has been linked to several specific genetic loci. Enlargement of the cornea and sclera is not seen in this subtype.

CURRENT THERAPY

- Although primary open-angle glaucoma (POAG) is typically treated first medically, in selected circumstances laser and incisional surgery may be appropriate first-line interventions.
- Glaucoma medications lower intraocular pressure by decreasing production of aqueous humor or increasing its outflow.
- Whereas topical β-blockers have been the traditional primary medical therapy for POAG, prostaglandin analogues have now emerged as the first-line choice.
- Laser trabeculoplasty increases aqueous outflow through the trabecular meshwork.
- Incisional filtering surgery creates a new outflow drain that bypasses the dysfunctional trabecular meshwork.
- Primary angle-closure attacks require emergent treatment both medically and with laser iridotomy to prevent further attacks.
- Secondary angle-closure glaucoma can be difficult to manage medically and often requires surgery.

Treatment

The Glaucoma Preferred Practice Pattern Committee of the American Academy of Ophthalmology suggests a target of 20% to 30% reduction of IOP from the untreated levels. Traditionally, medical treatment has been attempted first. However, recent studies such as the Glaucoma Laser Trial and Collaborative Initial Glaucoma Treatment Study have demonstrated a role for laser and incisional surgery as first-line therapy. Parameters that factor into selection of medications include efficacy in lowering IOP, systemic and localized side effect profiles, ease of compliance, and cost (Table 1).

Noncompliance with treatment regimens may be responsible for 10% of visual loss in glaucoma; in one study, approximately 60% of patients failed to use eyedrops as prescribed. If medications fail to control IOP, changes in optic nerve structure and visual field function may occur. Surgical treatment may become necessary to slow the progression of glaucomatous damage.

PROSTAGLANDIN ANALOGUES

This newest class of antiglaucoma agents has become the most commonly prescribed initial medical treatment because of efficacy and lack of major systemic side effects. These medications reduce IOP by increasing aqueous humor outflow. Latanoprost (Xalatan), bimatoprost (Lumigan), and travoprost (Travatan) require only once-daily dosing. Side effects include conjunctival hyperemia during the first several weeks of therapy, eyelash lengthening and thickening, occasional iris and periocular skin hyperpigmentation, and, rarely, exacerbation of ocular inflammation. Capitalizing on the eyelash-lengthening side effect of prostaglandin analogues, bimatoprost has recently been approved by the FDA for hypotrichosis under the trade name Latisse.

β-ADRENERGIC ANTAGONISTS

β-Adrenergic antagonists very effectively lower IOP by decreasing the production of aqueous humor. They include timolol (Timoptic, Betimol, Istalol), carteolol (Ocupress), metipranolol (OptiPranolol), and levobunolol (Betagan). Topical formulations may be absorbed into the bloodstream, and potential side effects are similar to those of systemic β-blockers, including exacerbation of chronic obstructive or reactive pulmonary disease, worsening of heart block or heart failure, bradycardia, systemic hypotension, mood effects or altered mental status, decreased libido, and masking of hypoglycemic symptoms in diabetic patients. Care should be taken in patients who are already taking systemic β-blockers, because additive side effects may develop. Use of Betaxolol (Betoptic), a selective β1-antagonist, may minimize the pulmonary side effects, but it still must be used cautiously in patients with asthma or chronic obstructive pulmonary disease.

Topical β-blockers are dosed once or twice daily, depending on the formulation of the eyedrop. Multiple fixed-combination drops that include timolol are available. Combigan is a fixed combination of 0.5% timolol and 0.2% brimonidine approved for twice-daily dosing. Cosopt, a fixed combination of 0.5% timolol and 2% dorzolamide, has recently gone off patent and is now available in generic form. Xalcom is a fixed combination of 0.5% timolol and latanoprost but is not available in the United States.

TABLE 1 Medications Used to Treat Glaucoma

Topical Medications	Efficacy	Local Side Effects	Systemic Side Effects	Dosing	Cost
Prostaglandin analogues	+++	++	none to +	Once daily	+++
β-Blockers	++	+	+++	bid	++*
α2-Agonists	++	++	++	bid-tid	+++*
Carbonic anhydrase inhibitors	++	++	+ to ++	bid-tid	+++*†

*= generic form is available;
† = systemic form is less costly; +++ = high; ++ = moderate; + = low.

α₂-ADRENERGIC AGONISTS

α_2-Agonists such as apraclonidine (Lopidine) and brimonidine (Alphagan) lower IOP by decreasing aqueous humor production. They are dosed two or three times daily. Major systemic side effects include somnolence and dry mouth. These medications are contraindicated in infants and young children because of the risk of respiratory depression. α_2-Agonists are also contraindicated in patients who are taking monoamine oxidase (MAO) inhibitors because of potential systemic hypertension. The most frequent ocular side effect is allergic follicular conjunctivitis, which may necessitate discontinuation.

CARBONIC ANHYDRASE INHIBITORS

Carbonic anhydrase inhibitors decrease the production of aqueous humor. Systemic carbonic anhydrase inhibitors such as acetazolamide (Diamox) and methazolamide (Neptazane) have been used to treat glaucoma for decades, but up to 60% of patients are intolerant of the side effects. These include metallic taste alteration, loss of appetite, fatigue, confusion, nausea and vomiting, paresthesias, polyuria, urolithiasis, and hearing dysfunction or tinnitus. Rare side effects include Stevens-Johnson syndrome (in patients with sulfonamide allergies) and idiosyncratic aplastic anemia. Oral agents may also lower serum potassium levels, and patients who are taking diuretics or digoxin (Lanoxin) should be monitored closely.

Dorzolamide (Trusopt) and brinzolamide (Azopt) are topical preparations of carbonic anhydrase inhibitors that are administered two or three times daily. Systemic side effects are minimized, but ocular stinging, localized allergic responses, and metallic taste alteration may occur. Systemic carbonic anhydrase inhibitors are somewhat more efficacious, but the improved tolerability of the topical agents has made them the standard for this class of medication. Moreover, the combination of systemic and multiple topical antiglaucoma agents usually necessitates a discussion or referral for incisional glaucoma surgery.

NONSPECIFIC SYMPATHOMIMETICS AND PARASYMPATHOMIMETICS

Nonspecific sympathomimetic and parasympathomimetic drugs have historically been used for the treatment of glaucoma, but, with the newer agents available, these are rarely prescribed. The mechanism for both classes involves increasing aqueous humor outflow. The sympathomimetic agents include epinephrine (Epifrin) and dipivefrin (Propine). Potential adverse effects are systemic hypertension, headache, cardiac arrhythmias including premature ventricular contractions and tachycardia, and anorexia. Parasympathomimetic medications such as pilocarpine (Pilocar) can cause gastrointestinal cramping, diarrhea, vomiting, syncope, hypotension, increased sweating, and pupillary constriction.

TREATMENT FOR ACUTE ANGLE CLOSURE

Patients with acute angle closure require emergent ophthalmologic referral and treatment to prevent severe permanent sequelae. If this is not immediately possible, treatment should be initiated promptly with a topical β-blocker and a topical α_2-agonist every 30 minutes and a single dose of oral acetazolamide (Diamox) 250 mg × 2 tablets. Oral glycerin (Osmoglyn) or intravenous mannitol (Osmitrol) 1.0 to 1.5 g/kg may be used if necessary. Pilocarpine should be used cautiously because it may worsen underlying inflammation and even the extent of angle closure if given in too high a concentration. Once the attack has been broken medically, the corneal edema will clear and a laser peripheral iridotomy can be made to prevent future attacks. This opening in the peripheral iris allows aqueous flow to bypass any obstruction caused by pupillary block. Prophylactic iridotomy of the other eye is recommended if the eye is anatomically at risk.

The management of chronic angle-closure glaucoma is similar to that for POAG. Chronic angle-closure glaucoma occurs when a patient has received a laser peripheral iridotomy and the IOP is still elevated due to permanent damage to the trabecular meshwork. This damage is caused by the presence of scar tissue over and in the outflow pathway due to inflammation and trauma caused by the previous attack of angle closure. It should be noted that, once a patient with primary angle-closure glaucoma has undergone laser peripheral iridotomy, that patient is no longer at risk for an attack of angle closure secondary to ingestion of the medications mentioned earlier (i.e., anticholinergics and adrenergic stimulants such as sleep and cold medications).

LASER

Laser may also be used to treat open-angle glaucomas. Argon laser trabeculoplasty or the newer selective laser trabeculoplasty lowers IOP by facilitating aqueous outflow. For patients with pigmentary glaucoma, pseudoexfoliative glaucoma, or POAG, laser trabeculoplasty has been shown to be an effective method to lower IOP.

SURGERY

Surgical measures to control glaucoma include filtering procedures such as trabeculectomy or aqueous shunt placement, which increase aqueous outflow by creating alternative filtration pathways. Patients are warned of an increased lifetime risk for serious ocular infection after trabeculectomy and are advised to report to an ophthalmologist immediately if any changes such as redness, pain, or decrease in vision occur.

Recent surgical advances include the Ex-Press mini glaucoma shunt, a metal shunt that is magnetic resonance imaging compatible; it used as an adjunct to trabeculectomy to reduce the risk of hypotony while achieving pressure reduction similar to that seen with traditional trabeculectomy. Canaloplasty is a new approach to glaucoma surgery that focuses on improving the aqueous drainage distal to the trabecular meshwork and avoids creation of a filtering bleb. In endoscopic cyclophotocoagulation, a small, intraocular endoscope provides direct visualization while photocoagulation is applied to the ciliary body. This can be performed in patients who have had previous cataract surgery or in conjunction with cataract surgery.

For poor surgical candidates with severely advanced disease, more powerful cyclodestructive procedures can be performed in the office, ambulatory surgery center, or hospital as needed to decrease aqueous production by ablating the ciliary body. If glaucomatous damage has left an eye with no vision, the only reason to treat IOP is to control pain. In most cases, topical agents are sufficient. If pain becomes frequent and severe, injections of retrobulbar absolute alcohol or even enucleation of the blind, painful eye may be offered.

REFERENCES

Allingham RR. Shields' Textbook of Glaucoma. 5th ed. Philadelphia: Lippincott Williams & Wilkins; 2005.

American Academy of Ophthalmology. Glaucoma: Basic and Clinical Science Course, 2008–2009. San Francisco: American Academy of Ophthalmology; 2008 [Section 10].

American Academy of Ophthalmology Online. Preferred practice patterns: Primary angle closure glaucoma, primary open angle glaucoma, primary open angle glaucoma suspect 2005, Available at: http://www.aao.org/ [accessed May 20, 2009].

Glaucoma Laser Trial Research Group. The Glaucoma Laser Trial (GLT): 2. Results of argon laser trabeculoplasty versus topical medicines. Ophthalmology 1990;97:1403–13.

Kass MA, Heuer DK, Higginbotham EJ, et al. The ocular hypertension treatment study: A randomized trial determines that topical ocular hypotensive medication delays or prevents the onset of primary open-angle glaucoma. Arch Ophthalmol 2002;120:701–13.

Lichter PR, Musch DC, Gillespie BW, et al. Interim clinical outcomes in the Collaborative Initial Glaucoma Treatment Study comparing initial treatment randomized to medications or surgery. Ophthalmology 2001;108:1943–53.

Maris PJ Jr, Ishida K, Netland PA. Comparison of trabeculectomy with Ex-PRESS miniature glaucoma device implanted under scleral flap. J Glaucoma 2007;16:14–9.

Morrison JC, Pollack IP. Glaucoma: Science and Practice. New York: Thieme; 2003.

Netland PA. Glaucoma Medical Therapy. New York: Oxford University Press; 2008.

Tsai JC, Forbes M. Medical Management of Glaucoma. 2nd ed. West Islip, NY: Professional Communications; 2004.

Otitis Externa

Method of
Jeffrey T. Vrabec, MD

Otitis externa is defined as an acute infection originating in or limited to the external auditory canal. This common affliction may occur in any age group and may be caused by a variety of infectious agents.

Anatomy and Physiology

Functionally, the ear canal serves two purposes. It is important for sound localization and because of resonance effects it improves sound perception in the frequency range from 2500 to 4000 hertz (Hz). The ear canal is approximately 25 mm in length and has a diameter of approximately 7.5 mm. The medial half is an osseous channel formed by the merger of the tympanic bone with the mastoid posteriorly and the squamous portion of the temporal bone superiorly. The lateral half of the canal wall is cartilaginous with a thick squamous epithelium that contains sebaceous glands, sweat glands, and hair follicles. The medial skin covering the bony canal is quite thin, measuring only 0.2 mm in thickness. The medial skin lacks a subcutaneous layer and is in continuity with the outermost layer of the tympanic membrane.

The external canal receives its blood supply from the superficial temporal and posterior auricular branches of the external carotid artery. Venous drainage is to the external jugular vein. The external canal receives sensory innervation via multiple cranial nerves. The trigeminal nerve supplies sensation to the superior and anterior aspect of the canal, the facial nerve supplies the anterior inferior area, and the glossopharyngeal and vagus nerves innervate the inferior and posterior regions. Because of the diverse nerve supply, otalgia may often reflect referred pain from oral cavity, nasal, or pharyngeal sources.

Several anatomic features serve to protect the external canal and tympanic membrane (TM) from injury or infection. The gentle curvature of the canal and the narrowing at the bone–cartilage junction (the isthmus) reduce the probability of large objects penetrating the TM. The hair and cerumen also protect the canal, trapping airborne particles that enter the external meatus. Cerumen has the additional benefit of repelling water. The acidic composition of cerumen lowers the ambient pH of the external canal, making it less hospitable to infectious organisms. The phenomenon of epithelial migration is documented in the ear canal. Surface epithelium moves laterally from the umbo to the annulus of the TM and then laterally to the external meatus. Epithelial movement on the TM proceeds at a rate of 0.05 mm per day and is typically slower in the external canal. Lateral migration helps clear the medial canal of surface epithelium and attached debris. This migratory pattern is arrested in chronic infection of the external canal.

Diagnosis

Infections develop in the external canal when organisms breach the anatomic barriers. Trauma to the canal skin, excessive removal of the cerumen, and excessive moisture in the canal may all facilitate otitis externa. Presenting symptoms of an external ear infection include pain, itching, and hearing loss. Pain develops rapidly, is typically constant, and may be quite severe. Manipulation of the ear or jaw movement exacerbates the pain. Conductive hearing loss occurs because of accumulation of debris in the external canal and is exacerbated by concurrent edema. Persistent symptoms despite treatment are a matter of great concern and may indicate a developing osteitis. Cranial nerve deficits are ominous symptoms and indicate an advanced osteitis of the temporal bone.

Physical examination findings typically include erythema, edema, and drainage. Differences in examination findings can help distinguish

bacterial from fungal infections. Bacterial infections usually produce marked edema of the canal skin, especially in the lateral cartilaginous canal. Drainage is usually scant and may have a mucoid or mucopurulent consistency and often has a foul odor. In contrast, fungal infections typically involve the medial canal skin and produce little edema. Drainage is thick and surface spore formation is evident. Focal granulation tissue develops in areas with invasive disease and TM perforations are occasionally present. Bloody drainage can be seen with either bacterial or fungal infections because of maceration of the canal skin or from granulation tissue formation.

Regional or systemic symptoms are uncommon in otitis externa. Periaural erythema, mild lymphadenopathy, and low-grade fever are possible. The presence of regional symptoms indicates a more virulent infection.

Treatment

The initial approach to outer ear infections involves aural toilet and avoidance of further trauma or moisture. Topical antibiotics are prescribed in accordance with the likely infectious organism. Many preparations have a rather broad spectrum of efficacy so routine culture of aural discharge is not performed. It is prudent to obtain culture and sensitivity data in recalcitrant cases. Analgesics are prescribed as necessary to control pain. Narcotics are occasionally required. Patients are instructed to avoid or minimize water exposure. With appropriate treatment, symptoms improve rapidly, and complete healing is seen in 2 weeks or less.

The most common organism identified in routine cases of external otitis is *Pseudomonas aeruginosa*. Staphylococcal species are the next most common. Topical fluoroquinolone or aminoglycoside antibiotics are the most appropriate choice for treatment. Preparations that include a steroid are recommended. Drops are instilled three times daily until resolution of the infection, usually 7 to 10 days. When severe edema of the canal skin is present, a wick is inserted into the canal to facilitate drug delivery. Persistent symptoms indicate inadequate treatment, although this may also be because of inappropriate antibiotic, inefficient drug delivery, noncompliance, or progressive infection.

Differential Diagnosis and Treatment

There are many other infectious disorders of the external canal, although each can usually be distinguished by characteristic clinical findings. Malignancy may also mimic chronic infection. Biopsy is recommended for abnormal tissue that does not quickly resolve with treatment.

 CURRENT DIAGNOSIS

Presenting symptoms include:

- Pain: develops rapidly, typically constant; exacerbated by movement of ear or jaw
- Itching
- Hearing loss: exacerbated by concurrent edema

Exam findings include:

- Erythema
- Edema
- Drainage: sometimes bloody
- Bacterial infections: often have edema of the canal skin with minimal drainage that has foul odor
- Fungal infections: involve the medial canal skin with slight edema, thick drainage, evident surface spore formation

ACUTE INFECTIONS

Furuncles occur at the external meatus in the hair-bearing skin. Erythema and edema are localized, and skin a few millimeters away from the infection has a healthy appearance. Pain can be severe and is exacerbated by pressure or manipulation of the auricle. Furuncles are caused by staphylococcal infection. Spontaneous rupture of the lesion leads to resolution of the infection and pain. If fluctuance is present at presentation, the lesion is drained under local anesthesia. Topical antibiotics (bacitracin, neomycin, or mupirocin [Bactroban] ointment or solution) are a useful adjunct.

The physical findings in otomycosis were outlined earlier. The predominant organisms are *Aspergillus* and *Candida* with considerable variation in prevalence according to geographic region. Fungal infections produce more destruction of the canal skin but less edema. Granulation tissue and TM perforations are not uncommon, although most perforations heal spontaneously after eradication of the infection. Treatment requires meticulous cleaning of debris and topical antifungals. Clotrimazole (Lotrimin) solution is effective for *Candida* species, but eradication of *Aspergillus* species is most efficient with ketoconazole (Nizoral) cream applied directly to the affected skin.

Bullous external otitis is diagnosed based on the characteristic finding of hemorrhagic vesicles in the external canal. Spontaneous rupture of the lesions produces bloody otorrhea. The lesions are quite painful, and lancing the bullae to drain the fluid does not provide relief as is seen in bullous myringitis. Involvement of the medial canal skin is typical. The etiology of this infectious process is unclear. However, the disease responds to a broad spectrum of topical antibiotics. Topical or oral analgesics are a useful adjunctive treatment.

Herpes zoster oticus, or Ramsay Hunt syndrome, occurs because of reactivation of latent varicella zoster virus in the geniculate ganglion. Vesicles may develop in the sensory distribution of the facial nerve. The appearance of skin lesions is characteristic of zoster eruptions. Initially, the vesicles are erythematous with a straw-colored fluid. Spontaneous rupture results in a crusted ulcer that may take several weeks to heal. Facial paralysis, dysgeusia, dizziness, and sensorineural hearing loss are typical in herpes zoster oticus but extremely rare in other infectious diseases of the external ear canal. Treatment of the facial paralysis is the primary objective, necessitating systemic steroids and antivirals. The skin lesions of the ear canal usually heal without incident, but secondary bacterial otitis externa is possible.

CHRONIC INFECTIOUS DISORDERS

Skull base osteitis occurs when disease extends from soft tissues of the canal into the temporal bone. Elderly patients, diabetics, and immunocompromised individuals are at increased risk of developing osteitis. The diagnosis is suspected when pain, discharge, fever, and/or granulation tissue persist despite treatment. Progressive involvement of the skull base may lead to cranial nerve palsies, vascular thrombosis, and intracranial infection. Laboratory testing reveals a markedly increased sedimentation rate. Technetium-99m bone scan displays increased uptake throughout the course of the disease and is useful for initial diagnosis. Computed tomography (CT) of the temporal bone displays bone erosion in advanced cases. Magnetic resonance imaging (MRI) is useful to detect soft-tissue and dural involvement. Biopsy of infected tissue or bone may be necessary to identify the responsible organism. Systemic antibiotics are selected according to culture and sensitivity data and should be continued until the sedimentation rate returns to normal. This may require months of treatment.

CURRENT THERAPY

- Provide aural toilet and encourage avoidance of further trauma and water exposure.
- Obtain culture and sensitivity data in recalcitrant cases.
- Prescribe topical antibiotics that include a steroid and analgesics (for pain) as needed.

Osteoradionecrosis is a late complication of temporal bone irradiation. Contemporary stereotactic techniques should significantly reduce the incidence of this problem. The process is typically limited, and symptoms are much less severe than in skull base osteitis. Exposed necrotic bone with slight granulation and purulent drainage is seen on examination. Local débridement and topical antibiotics are usually sufficient to control the infection. Recurrence is common because the irradiated ear canal is highly susceptible to infection after exposure to water or minor trauma.

MISCELLANEOUS

With the exception of herpes zoster oticus, none of the entities just described typically involves the pinna. Inflammation of the external canal in conjunction with pinna involvement may signify dermatologic disease. Some common entities include eczema, neomycin allergy, relapsing polychondritis, and erysipelas.

REFERENCES

Clark WB, Brook I, Bianki D, Thompson DH. Microbiology of otitis externa. Otolaryngol Head Neck Surg 1997;116:23–5.

Hawke M, Wong J, Krajden S. Clinical and microbiological features of otitis externa. J Otolaryngol 1984;13:289–95.

Hurst WB. Outcome of 22 cases of perforated tympanic membrane caused by otomycosis. J Laryngol Otol 2001;115:879–80.

Litton WB. Epithelial migration over tympanic membrane and external canal. Arch Otolaryngol 1963;77:254–7.

Lucente FE. Fungal infections of the external ear. Otolaryngol Clin North Am 1993;26:995–1006.

Sreepada GS, Kwartler JA. Skull base osteomyelitis secondary to malignant otitis externa. Curr Opin Otolaryngol Head Neck Surg 2003;11:316–23.

Sweeney CJ, Gilden DH. Ramsay Hunt syndrome. J Neurol Neurosurg Psychiatry 2001;71:149–54.

Otitis Media

Method of
J. Scott McMurray, MD

Ear infections, their complications and sequelae, comprise most patient-clinician interactions. Estimates suggest nearly $3 billion in direct and indirect cost for acute otitis media (AOM) and otitis media with effusion were spent in 1995 alone. In 2000 more than 16 million office visits were made for otitis media and 802 prescriptions per 1000 visits were written for a total of more than 13 million prescriptions. As common as the problem may be, it continues to be a source of confusion and controversy in terms of its diagnosis, treatment, and expectation for outcomes. Recently, there has been a renewed interest in determining the appropriate evaluation and management of these afflicted children, based on evidence-based medicine.

Along with new diagnostic protocols and realigned treatment strategies, there is a realization that children may fall into different at-risk groups and will therefore benefit from different treatment options. In his recent editorial in the International Journal of Pediatric Otolaryngology on a practical classification of otitis media subgroups, Richard Rosenfeld quoted Stanley Hoerr saying, "It is difficult to make the asymptomatic patient feel better." Yet, he added, much of the research on which we base our decisions to treat or not to treat children with otitis media has been formulated on those who would otherwise do well without treatment, the so-called innocent bystander. Children in the at-risk or suffering groups have been excluded from research trials for ethical reasons against withholding treatment. It is possible to group children into four subgroups with otitis media:

1. Innocent bystander
2. Susceptible child

3. At-risk child
4. Suffering child

These different subgroups imply different treatment limbs. The innocent bystander may do well without any therapy and may tolerate careful observation, whereas the suffering child with a similar disease process deserves rapid and intensive medical or surgical treatment or both.

The stratification of children into different subgroups may appear daunting at first glance but after closer reflection answers the problem of conflicting research data and perhaps uses more common sense (confirmed by clinical trials) in determining treatment. Otherwise developmentally and physically healthy children may be closely observed rather than treated medically or surgically for their acute ear infection or middle ear effusion (MEE). Other children who are at risk for developmental delays, physically challenged, or suffering from the effects or side effects of AOM or otitis media with effusion should be treated more aggressively with either the appropriate medical or surgical plan of care. Unfortunately, this increases the number of possible permutations when determining the appropriate treatment for the afflicted child. Fortunately, however, this new paradigm allows more freedom in determining the appropriate treatment option to be followed. Our challenge lies in honing our abilities to make a correct diagnosis and an accurate assessment of risk so that an appropriate treatment protocol with adequate follow-up can be implemented.

In 2004, the American Academy of Pediatrics, the American Academy of Family Practice, and the American Academy of Otolaryngology Head and Neck Surgery combined forces to create two separate clinical guidelines for AOM and otitis media with effusion. These guidelines serve as an excellent frame on which to build a knowledge base and understanding for the treatment of all children with AOM or otitis media with effusion. These references are invaluable and are recommended reading for all who treat children with ear pathology.

Definitions

Acute otitis media is defined as an abrupt onset of inflammation of the middle ear space. This contrasts with otitis media with effusion, which is fluid in the middle ear without signs and symptoms of inflammation. Otitis media with effusion is much more common than AOM but may be seen as a residual finding of a recently resolved infection. The distinction between the two and the ability of the clinician to distinguish between these disease entities is paramount to decision making and appropriate treatment.

The signs and symptoms of AOM are found in an abrupt onset of fluid in the middle ear with redness or distinct pain. Children suffering with AOM may or may not also exhibit systemic signs of infection, such as fever. Fever, pain, and irritability are seen in 90% of children with AOM, but it is also seen in 76% of children with upper aerodigestive tract viral illnesses as well. History alone may lead to an erroneous conclusions and unnecessary treatment. The distinction lies in the physical findings of MEE with inflammation. Fullness or bulging of the tympanic membrane, air fluid levels, opacification of the tympanic membrane, or bullous vesicles on the tympanic membrane are signs suggesting AOM when associated with acute inflammation. Visualization of the tympanic membrane and the use of pneumatic otoscopy should confirm the presence of a MEE and inflammation. Tympanometry can confirm suspicion of a MEE, but the clinician should work to be proficient with pneumatic otoscopy.

Otitis media with effusion alone may result from a resolved infection or from eustachian tube dysfunction alone. The physical findings are similar to those described but without the signs of acute inflammation. Although the tympanic membrane may be red in the otherwise healthy child crying at the displeasure of being examined, pain and an effusion are not generally associated with normal health.

Treatment Recommendations

Children with AOM should have adequate pain management. Acetaminophen, ibuprofen, and occasionally narcotics are useful in treating the pain of AOM. Rarely, myringotomy is required to relieve the discomfort of an acute ear infection.

If an acute bacterial infection in the middle ear is recognized, antibacterial therapy may be used in all age groups. If the diagnosis is uncertain, antibacterial therapy is recommended in the very young, younger than age 6 months. Antimicrobials may also be administered if one is uncertain of the diagnosis, if the illness is severe in those from 6 months to 2 years of age. If the child is older than age 2 years and the diagnosis is uncertain, observation and close follow-up is recommended.

If antibacterial treatment is instituted, amoxicillin at 80 to 90 mg/kg/day is used as a first line of therapy. If severe illness is encountered or if coverage for beta-lactamase–positive organisms such as *Haemophilus influenzae* or *Moraxella catarrhalis* is required, amoxicillin-clavulanate (Augmentin) is suggested (90 mg/kg/day of the amoxicillin component).

Children who are allergic to amoxicillin, but not with urticaria or anaphylaxis, may be given cefdinir (Omnicef), cefpodoxime (Vantin), or cefuroxime (Ceftin). Children with type-1 hypersensitivity to amoxicillin may be given azithromycin (Zithromax), clarithromycin (Biaxin), erythromycin-sulfisoxazole (Pediazole), or sulfamethoxazole-trimethoprim (Bactrim). In AOM where the organism is thought to be penicillin resistant *Streptococcus pneumoniae*, clindamycin is a reasonable choice.

Patients who fail to respond within 48 to 72 hours, whether in the observation or antibacterial therapy group, should be reassessed and treatment changed depending on the findings. Reduction of risk factors for AOM is encouraged for everyone. No recommendations were made regarding the efficacy of complementary and alternative medicine for the treatment of AOM.

 CURRENT DIAGNOSIS

- The diagnosis of AOM requires acute signs of illness such as fever and pain along with signs of middle ear inflammation such as fluid and erythema.
- Associated symptoms of AOM include fever, pain, and irritability.
- Visualization of the tympanic membrane and pneumatic otoscopy are required to confirm the diagnosis of AOM.
- Fluid behind the tympanic membrane does not necessarily indicate an infection in the middle ear space.

Abbreviation: AOM = acute otitis media.

 CURRENT THERAPY

- Adequate pain management is key in treating AOM.
- If a child has an acute bacterial otitis media, antibiotics are indicated.
- Amoxicillin at 80 to 90 mg/kg/day is the first therapy of choice in nonallergic children.
- Children older than age 2 years may be observed without antibiotic therapy if the diagnosis is uncertain.
- Children younger than age 2 years may be treated with antibiotics if the diagnosis is uncertain.

Abbreviation: AOM = acute otitis media.

Otitis media with effusion is common after resolution of acute otitis. Some children also present with asymptomatic otitis media with effusion as well. Treatment of children with persistent middle effusion depends on their at-risk grouping. Children at risk for speech, language, or other learning problems should be treated more promptly than other children not at risk. The at-risk groups include children with a permanent hearing loss independent of the otitis media, suspected or known speech and language delays, autism-spectrum disorder or other pervasive developmental disorder, syndromes or craniofacial disorders, blindness or uncorrectable visual impairment, cleft palate with or without associated syndrome, or developmental delay. The management of the child with otitis media with effusion in these at-risk groups should include hearing tests, speech and language assessment and therapy, hearing aids or other amplification devices for hearing loss independent of the otitis media, tympanostomy tube placement, and assessment of hearing after resolution of the otitis media with effusion to detect underlying hearing loss independent of the middle ear fluid.

Children who do not fall in the at-risk group may be watched for 3 months before intervention. If the MEE persists for longer than 3 months, audiometric assessment of hearing should be obtained. Intervention is then based on the presence of a hearing loss of generally greater than 20 decibels, suspicion of language development delay, or other impending complications related to the MEE. If the hearing loss is mild (21 to 39 decibels), strategies to optimize the listening and learning environment and/or surgical intervention should be suggested. If the hearing loss is greater than 40 decibels, surgical intervention to correct the MEE is indicated and most efficacious.

Initial surgical treatment of a problematic persistent MEE as described earlier is tympanostomy tube placement. Adenoidectomy is reserved for children who have other distinct indications, such as nasal airway obstruction or chronic adenitis, or in whom another set of pressure equalization tubes are necessary. Approximately 20% to 50% of children relapse after their tympanostomy tubes extrude and will require additional tubes. When adenoidectomy is performed with the second set of tubes, the rate of recidivism is decreased by 50%. This advantage is seen in children as young as age 2 years, with the greatest effect seen in children aged 3 years and older, regardless of adenoidal size. Children older than age 4 years may also benefit from adenoidectomy and myringotomy without tube placement. Myringotomy alone without tympanostomy tube insertion and/or tonsillectomy alone solely for the treatment of otitis media with effusion has not been found to be efficacious.

Conclusion

The key to successful management of a child with AOM or otitis media with effusion, as it is with any medical problem, is based on the clinician's ability to correctly diagnose and stratify at-risk groups. The new recommended clinical pathways developed by the AAP, AAFP, and AAO-HNS for AOM and otitis media with effusion may at first seem to increase complexity of treatment because it increases the number of pathways possible. Closer reflection, however, will reveal an easier paradigm. It is the clinician's responsibility to attain the skills and knowledge set to make the correct initial diagnosis and assessment of risk for the patient. The support from the evidence-based-medicine clinical pathways will then help in the decision making and treatment formulation.

REFERENCES

American Academy of Family Physicians, American Academy of Otolaryngology Head and Neck Surgery, American Academy of Pediatrics Subcommittee on Otitis Media with Effusion. Otitis media with effusion. Pediatrics 2004;113(5):1412–29.
American Academy of Pediatrics Subcommittee on Acute Otitis Media. Diagnosis and management of acute otitis media. Pediatrics 2004;113(5):1451–65.
Bell LM. The new clinical practice guidelines for acute otitis media: An editorial. Ann Emerg Med 2005;45(5):514–6.
Bluestone CD. Epidemiology and pathogenesis of chronic suppurative otitis media: Implications for prevention and treatment. Int J Pediatr Otorhinolaryngol 1998;42(3):207–23.
Ohlms LA, Chen AY, Stewart MG, Franklin DJ. Establishing the etiology of childhood hearing loss. Otolaryngol Head Neck Surg 1999;120(2):159–63.
Paradise JL, Campbell TF, Dollaghan CA, et al. Developmental outcomes after early or delayed insertion of tympanostomy tubes. N Engl J Med 2005;353(6):576–86.
Rosenfeld RM. A practical classification of otitis media subgoups. Int J Pediatr Otorhinolaryngol 2005;69(8):1027–9.
Rosenfeld RM, Culpepper L, Doyle KJ, et al. Clinical practice guideline: Otitis media with effusion. Otolaryngol Head Neck Surg 2004;130(5 Suppl.):S95–118.
Rosenfeld RM, Lous J, Bluestone CD, et al. Recent advances in otitis media. 8. Treatment. Ann Otol Rhinol Laryngol Suppl 2005;194:114–39.

Episodic Vertigo

Method of
Kevin A. Kerber, MD

Vertigo is a type of dizziness symptom. Dizziness is a nonspecific term that refers to any sensation of spatial disorientation; vertigo means an illusion of movement—typically, true visualized spinning of the environment. Vertigo can also mean a sense of linear displacement or tilt, although it is best to report these symptoms using the patient's own words. Other common types of dizziness include lightheadedness, presyncope, and unsteadiness while walking. True vertigo is highly suggestive of vestibular system involvement, although by itself it cannot differentiate a peripheral localization (i.e., inner ear or vestibular nerve) from a central localization (i.e., brainstem or cerebellum). Because vertigo does not discriminate peripheral from central pathology, localization of the lesion and subsequent diagnosis depend on the features of the vertigo and the presence or absence of other signs or symptoms.

To effectively evaluate patients who present with vertigo, an understanding of the key aspects of the vestibular system is of central importance, because the dilemma is often discriminating a benign peripheral vestibular disorder from a small focal brain lesion. Many clinicians make a diagnosis of peripheral disease if other neurologic features (e.g., motor, sensory, or language deficits) are not present, but this approach is flawed. A more effective approach is to aim to diagnose one of the specific peripheral vestibular disorders. If a specific peripheral vestibular disorder does not fit, then a work-up for a central nervous system lesion may be warranted. The three common peripheral vestibular disorders all have highly characteristic history and examination features.

The Vestibular System

The peripheral vestibular system maintains a balanced tonic input to the brain. The input represents the circuitry linking the inner ear to brain structures that control eye movements. This circuitry is called the vestibulo-ocular reflex. A normal functioning vestibulo-ocular reflex is important for balance and for maintaining clear vision when moving. When an imbalance is caused by a lesion or aberrant stimulation, then vertigo ensues. A hallmark sign of vestibular system imbalance is nystagmus.

Nystagmus is a term used to describe rhythmic slow and fast movements of the eyes in opposite directions. The slow phase is caused by the imbalance in the vestibular system, whereas the fast phase represents the brain's attempt to correct for the slow drift. The pattern of nystagmus is determined by the location of pathology and whether the pathology is inhibitory or stimulatory. Pathology at the level of the semicircular canal causes nystagmus in the plane of the affected canal. In other words, vertical canals (i.e., posterior and anterior canals) lead to vertical and torsional nystagmus, whereas the horizontal canal leads to nystagmus in the horizontal plane. At the vestibular nerve level (i.e., cranial nerve 8), a mixed horizontal-torsional pattern of nystagmus is generated, because inputs from all of the semicircular canals converge at this level, and the signals from the vertical canals mostly cancel each other out. Patterns of nystagmus become less predictable with central lesions, although some general rules apply. Patterns of central dysfunction include the following: pure vertical (downbeat or upbeat) spontaneous nystagmus, bidirectional gaze-evoked nystagmus (look left, beats left; look right, beats right), gaze-evoked down-beating nystagmus, and persistent down-beating positional nystagmus.

Another hallmark sign of vestibular disturbance is a positive head-thrust test. A subject with an intact vestibulo-ocular reflex will maintain gaze on a stationary, straight-ahead target after a brief, small amplitude, high acceleration movement of the head to one side. A subject with vestibular impairment on one side loses this reflex on the ipsilateral side and therefore, after the quick head movement, needs to make a refixation voluntary eye movement (i.e, a "saccade") back to the target because the eyes moved with the head. This so-called catch-up or corrective saccade is easily appreciated at the bedside and indicates vestibular de-afferentation.

THREE COMMON PERIPHERAL VESTIBULAR DISORDERS

The three common peripheral vestibular disorders are vestibular neuritis, Meniere's disease, and benign paroxysmal positional vertigo (BPPV). Each has characteristic bedside features.

A patient with vestibular neuritis presents with the abrupt onset of severe vertigo, nausea, and imbalance. No other neurologic symptoms are present. The disorder is presumed to be caused by a viral disturbance of the vestibular nerve, although no viral tests are reliable for confirming this cause in individual patients. This situation is analogous to that of Bell's palsy. On examination, the acute peripheral vestibular pattern of nystagmus is seen. This pattern consists of unidirectional spontaneous nystagmus with a horizontal greater than torsional component. "Uni-directional" means that the nystagmus beats toward only one side. Looking in the direction of the fast phase increases the velocity of the nystagmus, whereas looking in the opposite direction decreases the velocity—but the direction of the fast phase never changes. If the nystagmus does change direction, then the pathology localizes to the brain. The affected ear is on the side opposite the fast phase of nystagmus. The other characteristic finding is a corrective saccade after the head-thrust test toward the affected side. Treatment with a short course of an oral corticosteroid within 3 days of symptom onset may result in a more complete recovery of vestibular function than if this therapy is not used. In addition, a program of vestibular rehabilitation can improve the outcome. It is important to note that small strokes of the cerebellum or brainstem can closely mimic vestibular neuritis.

Meniere's disease is characterized by recurrent episodes of vertigo, nausea, and imbalance typically lasting hours. Unilateral auditory features (i.e., hearing loss, roaring tinnitus, or fullness) must be present and prominent to make the diagnosis. Early in the course, auditory symptoms fluctuate along with vertigo attacks, but later the auditory symptoms become fixed and progressive. Some patients develop bilateral Meniere's disease. The initial treatment of Meniere's disease is a low-salt diet (<1500–2000 mg/day) or a diuretic. However, neither of these treatments is of established efficacy. Ablative surgical procedures are appropriate in cases of refractory vertigo. Transient ischemic attacks should be considered in the differential diagnosis whenever the vertigo attacks are brief (minutes) and new in onset. The dizziness of migraine can also closely mimic Meniere's disease.

Patients with BPPV report very brief episodes (<1 minute) of vertigo triggered by certain head movements. The most common positional triggers are tilting the head back to look up, getting in or out of bed, or rolling over in bed. It is important to note that dizziness of any cause may worsen after certain movements, but the dizziness of

CURRENT DIAGNOSIS

Vestibular Neuritis

- A single, severe and prolonged (days) episode of vertigo, nausea, and imbalance
- Nystagmus: spontaneous, unidirectional, horizontal more than torsional; fast phase beats away from affected side
- Head-thrust test: positive toward affected side (e.g. opposite to the direction of fast phase of nystagmus)
- Red flags for stroke: any other pattern of nystagmus, negative head-thrust test, and stroke risk factors

Meniere's Disease

- Recurrent episodes of vertigo (typically lasting hours) with unilateral and prominent auditory features (hearing loss, roaring tinnitus, or fullness)
- Unilateral hearing loss eventually becomes permanent and progressive
- Red flags for transient ischemic attacks: new onset, brief episodes (i.e., minutes), stroke risk factors

Benign Paroxysmal Positional Vertigo (BPPV)

- Recurrent, brief (<1 minute), positionally triggered vertigo attacks
- A burst of upbeat-torsional nystagmus triggered by the Dix-Hallpike test occurs with the most common variant, posterior canal BPPV
- Resolution of positional nystagmus with the Epley maneuver
- Red flags for central structural pathology: persistent down-beating nystagmus, other neurologic signs or symptoms

BPPV is *triggered* by certain movements. The most common form of BPPV occurs when particles that stem from the otolith organ break free and enter the posterior canal. Posterior canal BPPV is identified at the bedside with the use of the Dix-Hallpike test (Fig. 1). In response to the Dix-Hallpike test, the particles move in the canal and, by doing so, trigger a burst of upbeat-torsional nystagmus lasting 20 to 30 seconds. This disorder is cured in minutes by the particle repositioning maneuver described by Fife and others. BPPV is less commonly caused by particles in the horizontal canal or, very rarely, in the anterior canal. If the particles are in one of these other canals, both the pattern of nystagmus and repositioning maneuvers are different. Positional vertigo and nystagmus are common in patients with migraine. If a persistent down-beating nystagmus is seen during the Dix-Hallpike test, a central nervous system cause (e.g., Chiari malformation, cerebellar tumor, cerebellar degeneration) should be considered.

OTHER PERIPHERAL VESTIBULAR DISORDERS

Many other disorders can involve the peripheral vestibular system, but an understanding of the three most common peripheral vestibular disorders allows one to recognize features of pathology that stems from the peripheral structures. Many physicians order magnetic resonance imaging to exclude an acoustic neuroma in patients with vertigo; however, recurrent vertigo is an atypical presentation of this very rare disorder. Although case reports suggest that acoustic neuroma can manifest with isolated recurrent dizziness, epidemiologic research shows that up to one third of the general population report a history of bothersome dizziness, including vertigo. The more typical presentation of acoustic neuroma is gradually progressive unilateral hearing loss.

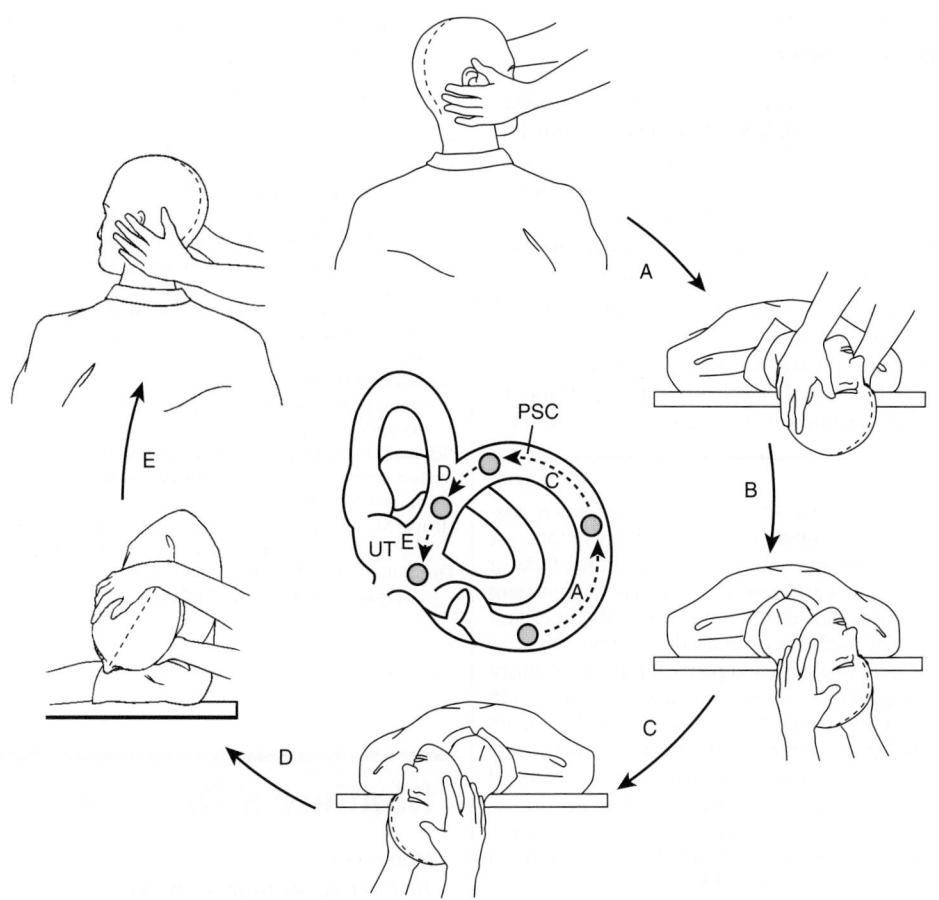

FIGURE 1. Treatment maneuver for benign paroxysmal positional vertigo affecting the right ear. To treat the left ear, the procedure is reversed. The drawing of the labyrinth in the center shows the position of the particle as it moves around the posterior semicircular canal (PSC) and into the utricle (UT). The patient is seated upright, with head facing the examiner, who is standing on the right. **A,** The patient is rapidly moved to head-hanging right position (Dix-Hallpike test). This position is maintained until the nystagmus ceases. **B,** The examiner moves to the head of the table, repositioning hands as shown. **C,** The head is rotated quickly to the left with right ear upward. This position is maintained for 30 seconds. **D,** The patient rolls onto the left side while the examiner rapidly rotates the head leftward until the nose is directed toward the floor. This position is then held for 30 seconds. **E,** The patient is rapidly lifted into the sitting position, now facing left. The entire sequence should be repeated until no nystagmus can be elicited. After the maneuver, the patient is instructed to avoid head-hanging positions to prevent the particles from reentering the posterior canal. (Reprinted with permission from Rakel RE: Conn's Current Therapy 1995. Philadelphia, WB Saunders, 1995, p 839.)

Vestibular paroxysmia is a label for very brief (seconds) spontaneous recurrent vertigo attacks, often preceded by auditory symptoms. The mechanism causing vestibular paroxysmia is believed to be analogous to that of trigeminal neuralgia and hemifacial spasm: aberrant stimulation within the system leads to transient symptoms.

Superior canal dehiscence syndrome is characterized by brief vertigo (seconds) triggered by sound or pressure changes.

CENTRAL VESTIBULAR DISORDERS

The central vestibular system involves many pathways within the brainstem and the cerebellum. Any pathology that affects the central vestibular pathways can cause an imbalance within the system. Acute or recurrent transient pathology causes vertigo; gradually progressive pathology causes abnormal eye movements and unsteadiness.

Stroke should be on the differential diagnosis of any acute vertigo presentation. Although the true probability of stroke as a cause of acute-onset severe vertigo is unknown, the best estimates suggest that between 3% and 20% of patients with acute vertigo harbor a stroke etiology. This probability drops substantially if there are no other neurologic features, the peripheral vestibular pattern of nystagmus is identified, and a corresponding head-thrust test is positive.

Other central structural lesions can cause acute vertigo, but again the likelihood of these causes is extremely low in the absence of central neurologic signs and symptoms. The characteristic finding in a Chiari malformation is down-beating nystagmus triggered by positional testing. Episodic vertigo is a common feature in some types of the genetic disorder known as episodic ataxia.

Approach to the Patient

If the symptom is true vertigo (i.e., visualized spinning of the environment), then the vestibular system is involved. A mild internal spinning sensation is probably less specific for a vestibular system localization. The next step is to define the characteristics of the symptom. Is this a new symptom or recurrent? If it is recurrent, what is the duration and frequency of the episodes, and are there any triggers? Next, ask about aggravating or alleviating factors and about accompanying symptoms. The patient's past medical history may predict a risk for certain disorders. The family history may reveal a familial pattern of similar symptoms (e.g., benign recurrent vertigo often has a familial pattern).

CURRENT THERAPY

- Vestibular neuritis: Both oral corticosteroids and vestibular rehabilitation have a high level of evidence supporting efficacy. Consider a burst and taper of oral corticosteroids if the diagnosis is made within 3 days after onset. Consider referral for vestibular rehabilitation.
- Meniere's disease: Consider a trial of a low-salt diet or a diuretic as initial therapy, although both lack evidence to support efficacy. Consider an ablative surgical procedure in refractory cases.
- Benign paroxysmal positional vertigo (BPPV): The Epley maneuver has a high level of evidence supporting efficacy in the treatment of posterior canal BPPV.

The examination is critical for localizing the lesion. Whenever possible, it is always preferable to examine the patient while symptoms are active. Hearing should be tested one ear at a time with tuning forks or finger rub. If the general medical and general neurologic examinations are unrevealing, then the focus should shift to the ocular motor examination to search for signs of vestibular or brain dysfunction. Does the patient have nystagmus? If so, what type and pattern? Is the head-thrust test positive? Instruct the patient to follow your finger back and forth and assess whether the eyes move smoothly. This is a test of the smooth pursuit system, and pathologically impaired smooth pursuit is a central nervous system sign. If the patient reports that symptoms are triggered by head or body turns, then positional testing should be performed. Start with the Dix-Hallpike test. If this test does not trigger nystagmus, then have the patient lie supine and turn the head to each side; this can trigger the nystagmus of horizontal canal BPPV.

If the patient's features do not fit with a common peripheral vestibular disorder, central nervous system causes should be considered. There are two main questions to ask when trying to decide whether the vertigo localizes to the brain: Are there other symptoms that must stem from the brainstem or cerebellum? and Are there examination findings (e.g., central pattern of eye movements) that localize to the brainstem or cerebellum rather than the peripheral vestibular system?

If the symptom has been present for longer than several months, the features do not fit with a peripheral vestibular disorder, and the neurologic examination is normal, then chronic dizziness or benign recurrent vertigo is the appropriate label. This diagnosis is inclusive of migraine-related dizziness, dizziness with panic disorder, and psychophysiologic dizziness. These causes may represent focal chemical or signaling changes within the brain or a hypersensitivity disorder. Although much remains to be known about the underlying mechanisms of chronic dizziness symptoms, genetics does seem to play a role.

Management

First, attempt to identify a specific disorder and focus on the treatment of that disorder. Patients with prolonged symptoms usually require symptomatic treatment with standard doses of an antihistamine, an antiemetic, or a benzodiazepine. However, these symptomatic medications are not appropriate as long-term therapy. Patients with chronic dizziness may benefit from lifestyle modifications, such as cardiovascular exercise, optimizing sleep and stress management, and eliminating any food triggers. Migraine prophylactic agents are reasonable to try, but their effectiveness for dizziness has not been established.

REFERENCES

Baloh RW, Honrubia V. Clinical Neurophysiology of the Vestibular System. 3rd ed. New York: Oxford University Press; 2001.

Fife TD, Iverson DJ, Lempert T, et al. Practice parameter: Therapies for benign paroxysmal positional vertigo (an evidence-based review). Report of the Quality Standards Subcommittee of the American Academy of Neurology. Neurology 2008;70:2067–74.

Hillier SL, Hollohan V. Vestibular rehabilitation for unilateral peripheral vestibular dysfunction. Cochrane Database Syst Rev 2007;(4):CD005397.

Hilton M, Pinder D. The Epley (canalith repositioning) manoeuvre for benign paroxysmal positional vertigo. Cochrane Database Syst Rev 2004;(2): CD003162.

James AL, Thorp M. Meniere's disease. BMJ Clin Evid 2006;15:797–803.

Kerber KA, Brown DL, Lisabeth LD, et al. Stroke among patients with dizziness, vertigo, and imbalance in the emergency department: A population-based study. Stroke 2006;37:2484–7.

Lee H, Sohn SI, Cho YW, et al. Cerebellar infarction presenting isolated vertigo: Frequency and vascular topographical patterns. Neurology 2006;67: 1178–83.

Lewis RF, Carey JP. Images in clinical medicine: Abnormal eye movements associated with unilateral loss of vestibular function. N Engl J Med 2006; 355:e26.

Neuhauser HK, von Brevern M, Radtke A, et al. Epidemiology of vestibular vertigo: A neurotologic survey of the general population. Neurology 2005;65:898–904.

Newman-Toker DE, Kattah JC, Alvernia JE, Wang DZ. Normal head impulse test differentiates acute cerebellar strokes from vestibular neuritis. Neurology 2008;70:2378–85.

Strupp M, Zingler VC, Arbusow V, et al. Methylprednisolone, valacyclovir, or the combination for vestibular neuritis. N Engl J Med 2004;351:354–61.

Thirlwall AS, Kundu S. Diuretics for Meniere's disease or syndrome. Cochrane Database Syst Rev 2006;(3):CD003599.

Meniere's Disease

Method of
Robert A. Williamson, MD

Background and Epidemiology

Prosper Meniere, in 1861, first described the constellation of episodic vertigo, tinnitus, and fluctuating hearing loss as a disease of the inner ear and not a cerebral disorder, as was commonly thought at the time. Specifically, Meniere's disease (MD) involves a disruption of the fluid and electrolyte homeostasis within the compartments of the inner ear, typically affecting both cochlear and vestibular function. The symptomatology in classic cases reflects involvement of both aspects of inner ear function, and involvement of only one ear is the most common situation.

Epidemiologic studies published over the last 35 years indicate that the prevalence of MD is between 15 and 45 per 100,000, and there is a slightly higher prevalence in females than in males (1.3:1). Onset is most common in the fourth and fifth decades, and the disease is rare overall in the pediatric population. MD occurs in people of northern European descent most commonly, followed by those of Asian descent, and it is much less common in populations of African descent. Finally, there is a strong genetic component in up to 20% of patients. Inheritance is thought to be autosomal dominant with reduced penetrance.

Pathophysiology

To this day, the pathophysiology of MD remains poorly understood and is a focus of active research. The common histopathologic feature in temporal bone studies is dilatation or excess fluid within the endolymphatic compartments of the inner ear, especially visible in the cochlea; for this reason, MD can be characterized by the term endolymphatic hydrops, although not all forms of endolymphatic hydrops lead to clinical symptoms of MD. Perilymphatic compartments of the inner ear are typically unaffected. Postmortem histologic evaluation is the diagnostic gold standard and is the final

CURRENT DIAGNOSIS

- Episodic vertigo lasting 20 minutes or longer, usually associated with nausea
- Hearing loss (usually fluctuating) in the affected ear
- Tinnitus and fullness in the affected ear

criterion for MD according to published diagnostic guidelines (Fig. 1). Most clinical cases do not achieve that level of diagnostic accuracy, so clinical judgment and the natural history of the patient's symptoms become extremely important, and uncertainty can be a source of frustration for the patient and the physician.

There are several factors that can lead to MD (or symptoms that mimic MD), and each should be considered in the history. Acoustic (noise-induced) or mechanical trauma, autoimmune and inflammatory conditions, syphilis and other atypical infectious (viral) processes, metabolic and hormonal derangements, and neoplastic lesions should all be considered. There is a relationship between MD and allergy in approximately 25% of patients, and inheritance should also be reviewed.

Evaluation

An accurate and thorough history is crucial in evaluating MD, because the diagnosis is clinical. All four symptoms should be inquired about: episodes of vertigo and their frequency, fullness or stuffiness in the affected ear, tinnitus (often described as roaring), and hearing loss in the affected ear that waxes and wanes in severity. Many patients also complain that the ear is sensitive to loud or unexpected noises, which can be irritating.

---

1. Recurrent spontaneous and episodic vertigo. A definitive spell of vertigo lasting at least 20 minutes, often prostrating, accompanied by disequilibrium that can last several days; usually nausea or vomiting, or both; no loss of consciousness. Horizontal rotatory nystagmus is always present.

2. Hearing loss (not necessarily fluctuating)

3. Either aural fullness or tinnitus, or both

Certain Meniere's disease

    Definite disease with histopathological confirmation

Definite Meniere's disease

    Two or more definitive episodes of vertigo with hearing loss, plus tinnitus, aural fullness, or both

Probable Meniere's disease

    Only one definitive episode of vertigo with hearing loss, plus tinnitus, aural fullness or both

Possible Meniere's disease

    Definitive vertigo with no associated hearing loss or hearing loss with non-definitive disequilibrium

---

FIGURE 1. Criteria for diagnosis of Meniere's disease according to the Committee on Hearing and Equilibrium of the American Academy of Otolaryngology–Head and Neck Surgery, 1995. (Modified from Committee on Hearing and Equilibrium: Guidelines for the diagnosis and evaluation of therapy in Meniere's disease. American Academy of Otolaryngology–Head and Neck Surgery Foundation Inc. Otolaryngol Head Neck Surg 1995;113:176–178.)

In classic MD, the episodes of vertigo typically last 20 minutes or longer, and they can be preceded by increasing tinnitus and fullness in the ear, a sudden drop in hearing, or both. There are variants of MD that seem to involve mostly cochlear symptoms (hearing loss, tinnitus, and fullness in the ear without vertigo) or vestibular symptoms (episodic vertigo alone with little or no hearing loss, fullness, or tinnitus). The vertigo is typically severe (described as a whirling or spinning sensation), is associated with nausea and vomiting, and can last from 20 minutes to several hours. Most patients are very ill or prostrate and remain in bed or can only crawl to a nearby bathroom. Between episodes, however, most patients feel their balance is normal or only mildly affected and do not complain of disequilibrium. The frequency of vertigo attacks is highly variable among patients; often, there is no warning, and anxiety regarding when the next attack will occur is common. A detailed history of headaches, including family history, should be sought, because migraine-associated dizziness and vertigo can often mimic MD; in this situation, migraine-prevention medications are the mainstays of treatment and are more useful for dizziness than abortive agents.

The physical examination in most patients is normal with regard to the head and neck region. The ears should be inspected carefully, looking for cerumen impaction, middle ear effusion, drainage, or other signs of infection. A full neurologic and cardiovascular examination is also important to rule out common causes of dizziness. Findings in patients with MD are usually normal, and the neurologic examination is nonfocal. During an acute MD attack, physical findings can be dramatic. Patients have a spontaneous horizontal nystagmus and can be nauseated and vomit repeatedly. Most are unable to ambulate, prefer to sit or lie, and appear ill.

Additional work-up should include formal audiometry with both pure-tone testing and an evaluation of speech discrimination. The audiogram most commonly shows an upsloping, low-frequency sensorineural hearing loss (indicating a cochlear process, and not a middle ear, tympanic membrane, or ossicular/conductive process). Over time, the loss tends to worsen in severity and to involve other frequencies, so serial audiometric testing is important in diagnosing and managing MD. Serologic markers for infection, inflammation, and autoimmune abnormalities should be ordered, including erythrocyte sedimentation rate, antinuclear antibodies, rheumatoid factor, and screening tests for syphilis. Complete blood count, fasting glucose level, glycosylated hemoglobin (HbA1c), and thyroid function tests should also be ordered, and indicated conditions should be corrected or treated if abnormal. Finally, if a sensorineural hearing loss is detected on the audiogram, particularly if it is unilateral, consideration should be given to magnetic resonance imaging of the brain and internal auditory canals with contrast enhancement to rule out neoplasms of the eighth cranial nerve and cerebellopontine angle. Additional ancillary tests, such as electronystagmography (ENG) and vestibular testing with calorics, electrocochleography, and glycerol challenge have been used when the etiology of symptoms has been in question, but they are not necessary for the diagnosis of MD.

Management

Once the diagnosis of MD has been made, the mainstays of treatment are reduction of sodium intake to less than 2000 mg/day, diuretic therapy, and lifestyle modification. Because there is no cure for MD, the goals of therapy should be outlined clearly with the patient; reduction in frequency and severity of vertigo attacks is the primary objective, and is achievable in over 90% of patients with conservative medical management alone. Potassium-sparing or combination diuretics such as hydrochlorothiazide/triamterene (Dyazide)[1] are usually first-line options. Patients who have ongoing vertigo attacks can be converted to loop diuretics such as furosemide (Lasix)[1] but may require potassium monitoring or supplementation. Lifestyle modification to reduce or eliminate caffeine and alcohol consumption, reduce stress, and include exercise and adequate rest are also

---

[1]Not FDA approved for this indication.

helpful, as are counseling and reassurance that the disease process can be brought under control. The hearing loss in MD can often be rehabilitated with use of amplification (depending on the severity of the loss, speech discrimination scores, and the amount of fluctuation that occurs), and referral to an audiologist licensed to dispense hearing aids can be useful. The fullness and tinnitus are less responsive to treatment overall but are frequently rendered less bothersome by treatment and by hearing aid use.

Acute attacks and the accompanying vertigo can be managed with vestibular suppressants such as meclizine (Antivert) or promethazine (Phenergan)[1] and antiemetics, and severe episodes respond well to low-dose benzodiazepines (e.g., diazepam [Valium][1]). Prescriptions should be given for patients to have these medications on hand, because attacks are often unpredictable, and access to a physician or emergency department can be difficult. If attacks are frequent and severe, oral steroids such as prednisone[1] are useful; dosing should start at 1 mg/kg for 7 days, followed by gradual tapering over an additional 3 to 7 days. Adjustment of the medical regimen to a stronger diuretic (e.g., furosemide [Lasix]) should also be considered in this situation. In those patients with bilateral MD, aggressive medical management is especially important to help preserve useful hearing as long as possible.

In those 5% to 10% of patients with MD that fails to respond well to the regimen just described, additional treatment options are available and are typically rendered by an otolaryngologist or otologist. Each involves some additional level of risk and should be considered only after the medical regimen has been maximized and has failed. Steroids or gentamicin (Garamycin)[1] can be injected into the middle ear (intratympanic therapy) to allow diffusion into the cochlea and inner ear as a means of modulating or reducing the vestibular dysfunction in MD. Single or multiple injections may be required, depending on the agent used and the patient's response. These procedures are office-based, intermediate steps between medication and surgery and do involve some risk of causing additional hearing loss or imbalance (particularly with the ototoxic effects of gentamicin), tympanic membrane perforation, and otitis media. A low-pressure pulse-generator device has been developed (Meniett device, Medtronic, Jacksonville, Fla.) but requires placement of a pressure-equalization tube.

For those patients who have ongoing or disabling vertigo despite these therapies, surgery can be considered to remove or ablate the offending vestibular input. For patients with poor or nonuseful hearing in the affected ear, labyrinthectomy is offered; those who have useful hearing can undergo vestibular nerve section or neurectomy. Both options are highly successful in controlling vertigo in refractory cases of MD, with success rates of approximately 95%. Endolymphatic sac surgery (via mastoidectomy) has also been used as a nonablative form of surgery to treat MD, but some controversy exists regarding its efficacy.

Vestibular therapy (under the supervision of a well-trained physical or occupational therapist) to address issues of disequilibrium and imbalance, as well as safety and fall-precaution counseling and training, can be useful in MD once the acute vertigo episodes have been brought under reasonable control. It should also be noted that the natural history of the MD typically leads to hearing loss (often severe or profound) in the affected ear, but vertigo attacks also decrease over time (usually several years) and eventually disappear completely in 65% to 70% of patients; therefore, reassurance and frequent monitoring and counseling are important in long-term management.

---

[1]Not FDA approved for this indication.

CURRENT THERAPY

- Low-sodium diet and diuretic therapy are the mainstays of treatment.
- Lifestyle modification to avoid triggers
- Intratympanic injection therapy, surgery, or both in refractory cases

REFERENCES

Committee on Hearing and Equilibrium. Guidelines for the diagnosis and evaluation of therapy in Meniere's disease. American Academy of Otolaryngology–Head and Neck Surgery Foundation Inc. Otolaryngol Head Neck Surg 1995;113:176–8.

da Costa SS, de Sousa LCA, Piza M. Meniere's disease: Overview, epidemiology, and natural history. Otolaryngol Clin North Am 2002;35:455–95.

Merchant SN, Adams JC, Nadol JB. Pathophysiology of Meniere's syndrome: Are symptoms caused by endolymphatic hydrops? Otol Neurotol 2005; 26:74–81.

Sajjadi H. Medical management of Meniere's disease. Otolaryngol Clin North Am 2002;35:581–9.

Sajjadi H, Paparella MM. Meniere's disease. Lancet 2008;372:406–14.

Sinusitis

Method of
Micah Hill, MD, and Rakesh Chandra, MD

Sinusitis is a disease with significant impact on the health care system and on the individuals it affects. Approximately 32 million Americans are diagnosed with chronic sinusitis each year, and the number of acute sinusitis cases is thought to be even greater. Health care expenditures for sinusitis are $5.8 billion annually and include 13.8 million outpatient visits. Patients experience 73 million days of restricted activity per year in relation to the diagnosis. Recent classifications and recommendations from task force groups have aimed to streamline and improve diagnosis and management. This chapter highlights current diagnostic and therapeutic considerations.

Sinusitis refers to inflammation of the paranasal sinuses. The term *rhinosinusitis* is more recently the preferred term, because sinus inflammation is almost always associated with inflammation of the adjacent nasal mucosa. The paranasal sinuses are five sets of pneumatized, paired bony structures lined with ciliated respiratory mucosa. They are contiguous with the nasal cavity through small openings that measure millimeters in diameter. The nose and paranasal sinuses constitute the first line of defense to protect the lower airways against pathogens by "filtering" inspired air. The mucosal epithelium captures particulate matter and sweeps it in a continuously moving mucus layer every 10 to 15 minutes. Both innate and acquired immunity mechanisms respond to the constant exposure to bacteria, viruses, and fungi at this interface. Air is also conditioned and humidified by passage through these sinuses.

Definitions

The most common cause of rhinosinusitis is viral infection, which, strictly speaking, does cause inflammation of the sinonasal membranes. Rhinosinusitis may also be a manifestation of infection with bacteria or fungi, allergic reactions, and other chronic inflammatory processes that affect the respiratory membranes. A careful and systematic approach to diagnosis and treatment was developed by the American Academy of Otolaryngology-Head and Neck Surgery (AAO-HNS) Task Force on Rhinosinusitis to standardize diagnosis based on symptoms and time course.

Rhinosinusitis can be classified into acute, subacute, acute recurrent, and chronic types based on duration of illness. The term acute rhinosinusitis (ARS) typically implies acute *bacterial* rhinosinusitis (ABRS), and, by definition, has a symptom duration of less than 4 weeks. Subacute rhinosinusitis is a more recently described entity that has a duration of 4 to 12 weeks, and chronic rhinosinusitis (CRS) has a duration of greater than 12 weeks. True ABRS must be clinically distinguished from viral rhinosinusitis (VRS) based on presumed etiology (e.g. sick contacts), duration, and symptom

CURRENT DIAGNOSIS

- The clinical diagnosis of acute rhinosinusitis (ARS) consists of three cardinal symptoms: purulent nasal discharge, nasal obstruction, and facial pain, pressure, or fullness with a duration of less than 4 weeks.
- Viral rhinosinusitis should be diagnosed if the ARS symptoms have been present for less than 10 days and the symptoms are not worsening.
- Acute bacterial rhinosinusitis (ABRS) should be diagnosed if the ARS symptoms have been present for 10 or more days since the onset of upper respiratory symptoms or if the symptoms worsen within 10 days after an initial improvement.
- Chronic rhinosinusitis may be diagnosed if symptoms of purulent nasal discharge, hyposmia, nasal obstruction, and facial pain, pressure, or fullness are present for longer than 12 weeks; there is corroborating evidence of inflammation on nasal endoscopy, computed tomography, or allergy and immune testing; and there is no evidence of other sinonasal disorders.
- Recurrent acute rhinosinusitis may be diagnosed if at least four bouts of ABRS occur annually and intervening episodes are free of signs and symptoms.

pattern. Most cases of viral infection are improved by 7 to 10 days, during which time an ABRS would continue to progress. Recurrent ABRS is defined as four or more discreet episodes of ABRS per year separated by symptom-free intervals.

Acute Rhinosinusitis

The diagnosis of ARS is based on identification of three cardinal symptoms: purulent nasal discharge, nasal obstruction, and facial pain, pressure, or fullness. If these three symptoms occur together, the clinician must distinguish between VRS and presumed ABRS based on illness pattern and duration. This differentiation can be difficult, especially in the initial days of the ARS episode, in part because of the overlapping incidences of these disorders. Moreover, a small (0.5% to 2.0%) but significant number of upper respiratory tract infections with associated VRS episodes progress into ABRS. In the early phases, it is important to counsel the patient regarding prolongation of acute symptoms, because ABRS may become further complicated by the clinical extension of inflammation outside the paranasal sinuses and into the adjacent orbital, neurologic, or soft tissues of the head.

When a patient with a suspected diagnosis of ARS is evaluated in the office, particular aspects of the history and physical examination should be emphasized. The history is critical to elicit the three cardinal symptoms, associated symptoms, and duration of illness. There should be no evidence for extension beyond the paranasal sinuses, and patients at high risk for complicated disease courses need to be identified. Pain assessment and vital signs should be included. The physical examination of the head and neck directs particular attention to any swelling, erythema, or edema of the face or orbital area or tenderness of the upper teeth. The posterior oropharynx and nasal cavity should be inspected for purulent postnasal discharge. Proptosis, chemosis, vision loss, and meningeal signs are ominous findings that suggest extension beyond the confines of the sinuses. Culturing of visualized secretions is not recommended, although endoscopically directed cultures from the middle meatus (near the maxillary sinus ostium) may be required in selected cases.

Recommendations for therapy are based on the diagnostic differentiation of VRS and ABRS. VRS treatment includes the option of symptomatic relief with analgesic or antipyretic medication and limited use of a topical or oral decongestant. There is weak evidence for symptomatic improvement with topical nasal steroid sprays in the acute setting.

The treatment for ABRS should be formulated with consideration of the pain assessment (using a visual analog scale), followed by appropriate analgesic therapy. Medications for mild to moderate pain such as acetaminophen (Tylenol) or nonsteroidal antiinflammatory medications given alone or in combination with opioids may be necessary. Symptomatic relief with decongestants, corticosteroids, saline irrigation, and mucolytics may be considered on an individualized basis.

ABRS therapy recommendations include the options of treatment with antibiotics and observation without antibiotics in selected patients. Antibiotic therapy targets the most common pathogens, including *Streptococcus pneumoniae*, *Haemophilus influenzae*, and *Moraxella catarrhalis*. *Staphylococcus aureus* and anaerobes may also be isolated in ARBS. Amoxicillin (Amoxil) is recommended as a first-line agent if antibiotics are prescribed. Trimethoprim-sulfamethoxazole (Bactrim)[1] or macrolides may be considered as first-line therapy for penicillin-sensitive patients. Local area resistance patterns may further influence the choice and strength of antibiotic. *S. pneumoniae* rates of penicillin resistance can be as high as 15% to 25%. High-dose amoxicillin may be considered for areas with high resistance and for contacts of children in daycare. However, amoxicillin is not effective against isolates of *M. catarrhalis* and *H. influenzae* that produce β-lactamase. Patients who have taken antibiotics within the last 4 to 6 weeks have an increased risk of infection with antibiotic-resistant bacteria; for such patients, high-dose amoxicillin-clavulanate potassium (Augmentin XR) 4 g/250 mg daily or fluoroquinolones may be used. The duration of treatment is typically 7 to 10 days.

The option of observation without antibiotics may be considered in some adults who have uncomplicated ABRS with mild pain and a temperature lower than 38.3 °C who will follow up reliably if symptoms worsen. This recommendation is based on data demonstrating that spontaneous improvement occurs in the majority of patients with or without antibiotics after 7 to 14 days. Severe illness, complicated sinus disease, immune deficiency, other comorbid conditions, and poor general health should be taken into consideration as exemptions from the option of observation. Furthermore, if the patient's condition worsens or fails to improve within 7 days after diagnosis, an antibiotic should be initiated or the initial antibiotic switched. Patients should also be examined for signs of possible complicated ABRS.

Chronic Rhinosinusitis

The diagnosis of CRS depends on the persistence of symptoms for longer than 12 weeks in addition to evidence of inflammation. Symptoms include purulent nasal drainage; nasal obstruction; facial pain, pressure, or fullness; and hyposmia. Noncontrast computed tomographic (CT) imaging is the current radiologic gold standard for diagnostic testing, but imaging findings must be corroborated with an endoscopic evaluation, because a subset of CRS patients have nasal polyps (Fig. 1) or comorbid anatomic defects, such as deviated septum. Hyposmia is a frequent complaint in patients with polyps. Those with nonpolypoid CRS are more likely to manifest pain and pressure symptoms, but it is important to correlate the sites of pain or pressure with CT findings. If there is a lack of correlation, nonsinogenic causes of pain (i.e. neurologic causes) must be considered.

CRS is a syndrome (rather than having a single etiology) in which allergic, anatomic, environmental, genetic, and unidentified immunologic factors likely play variable roles, depending on the individual patient. Distinguishing routine CRS from other specific pathologies is critical for appropriate management and to prevent a missed diagnosis, including but not limited to allergic fungal rhinosinusitis, invasive fungal rhinosinusitis, neoplasms of the paranasal sinuses, and Wegener's granulomatosis. Therapy for CRS should include saline nasal irrigation, cessation of tobacco exposure, and control of concomitant sinonasal disorders, including allergic rhinitis. Topical nasal corticosteroids should be considered for patients with comorbid allergic rhinitis and may also be useful empirically for patients with significant obstructive symptoms, even if allergy tests are negative. Some patients

---

[1]Not FDA approved for this indication.

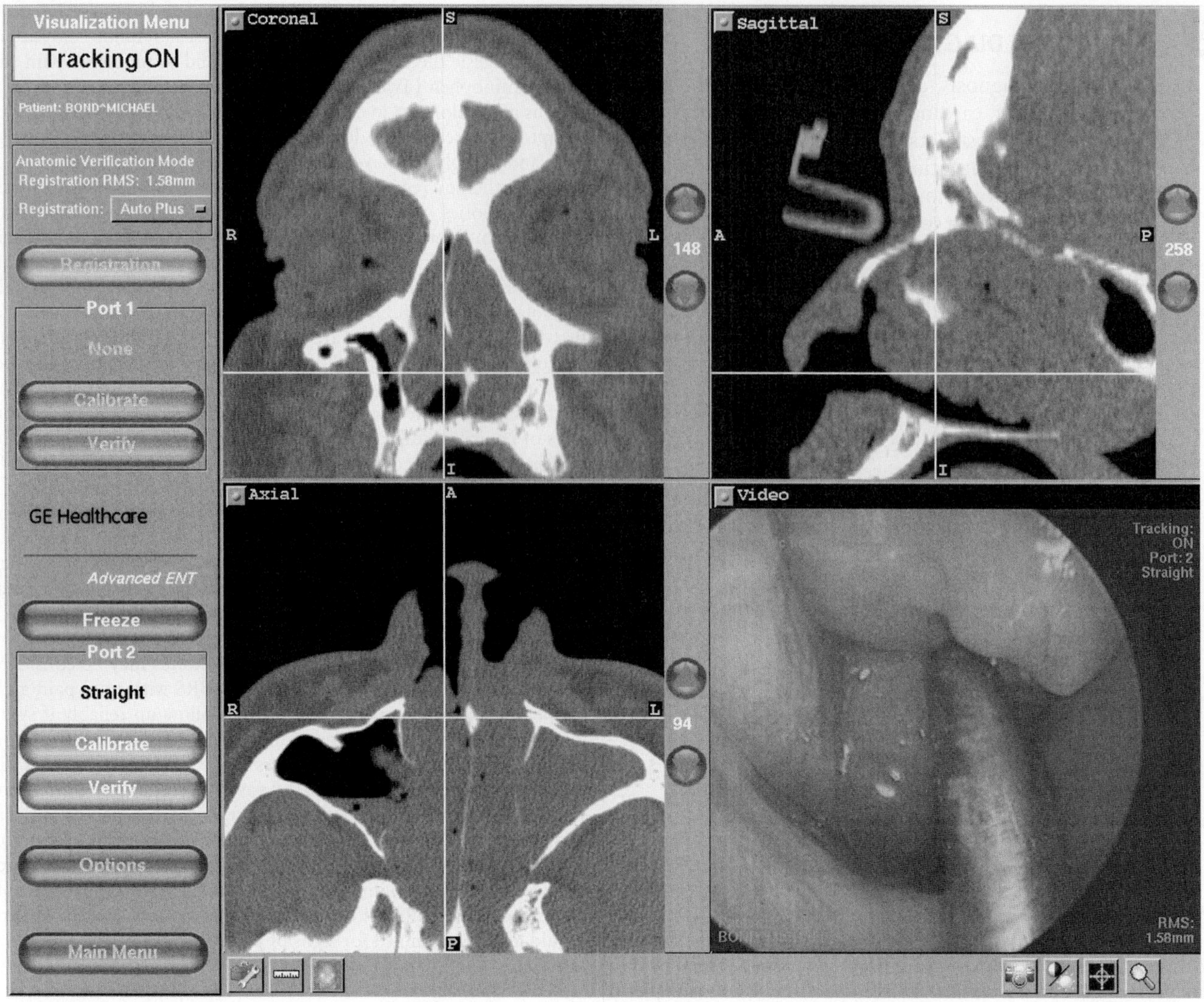

FIGURE 1. Triplanar computed tomographic reconstruction reveals pansinus opacification. The accompanying endoscopic image (*lower right*) demonstrates diffuse sinonasal polyposis.

require chronic topical therapy. Acute exacerbations of CRS can be treated with broad-spectrum antibiotics to cover the pathogens of ABRS plus *S. aureus* and *Pseudomonas aeruginosa*. The prevalence of community-acquired methicillin-resistant *S. aureus* is increasing.

For troubling baseline symptoms or frequent exacerbations, surgery is a consideration. The current consensus is that patients should be treated with 3 to 6 weeks of broad-spectrum antibiotic therapy before consideration of surgery, although the evidence basis for this approach is lacking. Oral corticosteroid bursts may be useful to treat exacerbations, especially in those with polyps, asthma, or allergic disease, and to aid healing in the perioperative period. Surgery for CRS is almost always performed endoscopically; the goals are to resect foci of chronically inflamed (or polypoid) tissue, widen the natural sinus ostia, and drain inspissated fluid, mucin, or purulent secretions (Fig. 2).

Recurrent Acute Bacterial Rhinosinusitis

Recurrent ARS is diagnosed when four or more episodes of ABRS occur per year, separated by periods without symptoms. Although this is a distinct form of rhinosinusitis, only a few studies have examined how this entity may differ from recurrent VRS or CRS. CT imaging during periods without symptoms may help to identify anatomic abnormalities contributing to recurrent disease. Allergy and

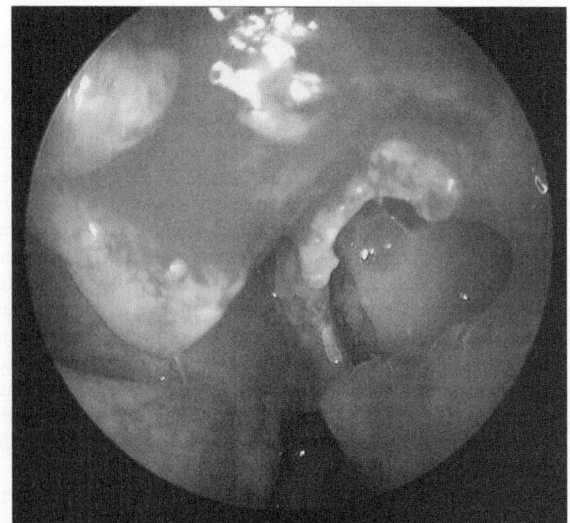

FIGURE 2. Endoscopic view into a surgically enlarged left maxillary sinus, revealing inspissated mucopurulent fluid.

immunology evaluation is recommended. Therapy for recurrent ABRS episodes is similar to that for isolated ABRS. However, patients may also befit from chronic treatment (e.g. topical steroids, antihistamines, saline washes, mucolytics) during the interval times, to reduce coexisting allergic rhinitis or immunologic abnormalities. Selected patients with recurrent ABRS may be surgical candidates, particularly if there are anatomic abnormalities such as deviated septum or variant air cells that are deemed to limit drainage patterns.

Radiographic Imaging

Radiographic evaluation is recommended for rhinosinusitis if there is concern for complications with paranasal extension, CRS, or recurrent ARS. Imaging options for the paranasal sinuses historically have included plain film X-rays, CT scans with and without contrast, and magnetic resonance imaging (MRI). Plain radiographs are now considered obsolete because of lack of sensitivity and the wide availability of CT, which can be performed rapidly and with lower radiation dosages. Noncontrast CT imaging is the current radiologic gold standard for diagnostic testing. However, any radiologic study represents a single snapshot in time and may not reflect the degree of disease during more exacerbated or more quiescent periods. Routine diagnostic sinus CT scans are obtained in the coronal plane with 3-mm sections, although current protocols permit triplanar reconstruction (see Fig. 1). Scans are typically interpreted in bone windows, and it is not necessary to use a contrast agent.

Radiographic imaging is unnecessary in cases of VRS or ABRS without suspected complication. VRS and ABRS appear similarly on imaging, rendering the study unhelpful in diagnosis. A lack of correlation between the anatomic location of symptoms and sites of radiologic disease further decreases the usefulness of imaging in the setting of ARS. If complications of ABRS, invasive fungal disease, or neoplastic disease is suspected, CT scanning with contrast or MRI is recommended to evaluate extension from the sinuses into surrounding tissue and to further characterize the soft tissue.

Complications of ABRS and Differential Diagnosis

Rare but serious complications of ABRS may occur. These result from direct extension of disease into the neurologic, ocular, or soft tissues of the head. Warning signs of intracranial extension include severe headache, cranial nerve palsy, meningismus, and altered mental status. Intracranial complications include abscess, cerebritis, cavernous sinus thrombosis, and meningitis. Deep facial extension manifests with facial swelling and cellulitis. Ophthalmologic extension should be suspected if visual complaints, proptosis, or periorbital inflammation is present, suggesting orbital cellulitis or abscess. Patients with immunocompromised states, recent antibiotic treatment, known nasal polyps or underlying CRS, prior sinus surgery, or other coexisting bacterial illnesses such as otitis media or pneumonia require special attention. These patients are at risk for more severe disease courses or unusual disease presentations and warrant more aggressive evaluation and treatment.

Other disease processes may manifest in a manner similar to rhinosinusitis and should be included in the differential diagnosis. A detailed discussion of these entities is beyond the scope of this chapter. Many of these disorders may be comorbidly present, including allergic rhinitis, eosinophilic nonallergic rhinitis, vasomotor rhinitis, allergic fungal rhinosinusitis, vascular headaches, and migraines. Less common but more serious disease processes are also included in the differential. These include invasive fungal rhinosinusitis, an aggressive and often lethal fungal infection that occurs in immunocompromised patients, and neoplastic disease such as sinonasal carcinoma or natural killer/T-cell lymphoma. Patients with severe or chronic symptoms of rhinosinusitis, especially those with unilateral symptoms, epistaxis, cranial nerve or ocular symptoms, or a personal history of malignancy, should be thoroughly evaluated for underlying neoplasm.

CURRENT THERAPY

- Viral rhinosinusitis: observe; option of symptomatic management
- Acute bacterial rhinosinusitis (ABRS) with antibiotic treatment: amoxicillin (Amoxil) as first-line treatment or a folate inhibitor or macrolide for penicillin-allergic patients
- ABRS with observation option used in selected cases: pain control with reevaluation at 7 days, or sooner if symptoms worsen.
- ABRS pain management: acetaminophen or nonsteroidal antiinflammatory medications alone or in combination with opioids.
- Chronic rhinosinusitis: saline nasal irrigation, cessation of tobacco exposure, control of concomitant sinonasal disorders, antibiotics, nasal and/or oral steroids.
- Surgical management may have a role in chronic rhinosinusitis, recurrent acute rhinosinusitis, and complications of ABRS.

Conclusions

Sinusitis, or more appropriately rhinosinusitis, must be further classified according to the duration and pattern of symptoms. Patients with recurrent ABRS, CRS, or suspected complications should be evaluated by CT and endoscopically. Comorbid conditions, such as allergy or migraines, should be evaluated and managed. The practitioner must bear in mind that other conditions may mimic rhinosinusitis, including neurologic and neoplastic diseases, further underscoring the need for detailed work-up in patients with recurrent, chronic, or severe symptomatology.

REFERENCES

Anand VK. Epidemiology and economic impact of rhinosinusitis. Ann Otol Rhinol Laryngol Suppl 2004;193:3–5.

Benninger MS, Appelbaum PC, Denneny JC, et al. Maxillary sinus puncture and culture in the diagnosis of acute rhinosinusitis: The case for pursuing alternative culture methods. Otolaryngol Head Neck Surg 2002;127(1): 7–12.

Gwaltney JM Jr. Acute community-acquired sinusitis. Clin Infect Dis 1996;23 (6):1209–23; quiz 1224–1225.

Hadley JA, Pfaller MA. Oral beta-lactams in the treatment of acute bacterial rhinosinusitis. Diagn Microbiol Infect Dis 2007;57(3 Suppl.):47S–54S.

Ip S, Fu L, Balk E, et al. Update on acute bacterial rhinosinusitis. Evid Rep Technol Assess (Summ) 2005;124:1–3.

Lethbridge-Cejku M, Schiller JS, Bernadel L. Summary health statistics for U.S. adults: National Health Interview Survey, 2002. Vital Health Stat 2004; 10 (222):1–151.

Malm L. Pharmacological background to decongesting and anti-inflammatory treatment of rhinitis and sinusitis. Acta Otolaryngol Suppl 1994;515:53–5; discussion 55–56.

National Center for Health Statistics. Health, United States, 2005 with Chartbook on Trends in the Health of Americans. Hyattsville, MD: National Center for Health Statistics; 2005.

Pearlman AN, Conley DB. Review of current guidelines related to the diagnosis and treatment of rhinosinusitis. Curr Opin Otolaryngol Head Neck Surg 2008;16(3):226–30.

Rosenfeld RM, Andes D, Bhattacharyya N, et al. Clinical practice guideline: Adult sinusitis. Otolaryngol Head Neck Surg 2007;137(3 Suppl.):S1–S31.

Sharp HJ, Denman D, Puumala S, Leopold DA. Treatment of acute and chronic rhinosinusitis in the United States, 1999–2002. Arch Otolaryngol Head Neck Surg 2007;133(3):260–5.

Williams Jr JW, Aguilar C, Cornell J, et al. Antibiotics for acute maxillary sinusitis. Cochrane Database Syst Rev 2003;(2) CD000243.

Nonallergic Perennial Rhinitis

Method of
Micah Hill, MD, and Rakesh Chandra, MD

Although rhinitis, defined strictly, means "inflammation of the nasal mucosa," it can be generally defined as a disorder of the nasal mucosa characterized by one or more of the common symptoms of sneezing, rhinorrhea, nasal congestion, and nasal pruritus. It is thought to affect as many as 30% of the world population, and it is a significant detriment to quality of life. Rhinitis therefore represents an important disease entity worthy of specific attention by physicians in primary care clinics. For allergic rhinitis alone, the direct costs of medical care and the indirect costs, including loss of productivity and missed days of school or work, are estimated to be greater than $11 billion annually in the United States. It may be assumed that this dollar amount would be much higher if all forms of rhinitis were included. A better understanding of the pathophysiology, diagnosis, and treatment of the various forms of rhinitis can decrease these costs through the employment of more effective therapeutic strategies.

Classification

Rhinitis is a family of disorders with multiple causes (Fig. 1). It can be divided into two categories by making the distinction between infectious (bacterial or viral) and noninfectious etiologies. The non-infectious group can be further divided into allergic and nonallergic forms. Allergic rhinitis is characterized by mucosal inflammation produced by immunoglobulin E–mediated responses to a variety of aeroallergens. Nonallergic rhinitis can produce periodic or perennial nasal symptoms that are not the result of these IgE-dependent mechanisms. Perennial nonallergic rhinitis is loosely defined as the presence of two or more symptoms—such as hypersecretion, sneezing, nasal congestion, and postnasal drip—for more than 3 months per year. It is estimated that up to 25% of rhinitis patients fit into this purely nonallergic category; however, other studies have found that between 44% and 87% of rhinitis patients have mixed disease. As discussed later in this chapter, diagnosis is made on the basis of exclusion of an identifiable allergy, structural abnormality, sinus disease, or cerebrospinal fluid rhinorrhea.

Nasal Physiology

The nose is the gatekeeper between the outside environment and the more fragile lower airways. It performs critical functions, including warming and humidifying inhaled air and filtering out harmful airborne particles before they reach the lungs.

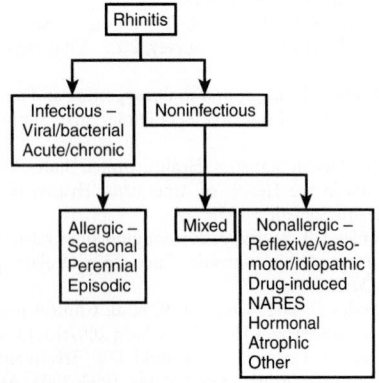

FIGURE 1. Classification of rhinitis. NARES = nonallergic rhinitis with eosinophilia syndrome.

The nasal vasculature consists of an intricate network of resistance vessels (small arteries, arterioles, and arteriovenous anastomoses) and capacitance vessels (valveless veins and venous sinusoids). The sinusoids are particularly numerous in the lamina propria (erectile tissue) of the nasal turbinates. They are fed by inflow from the resistance vessels, which are primarily under sympathetic control. Increased sympathetic stimulation results in α-adrenergically mediated vasoconstriction. This leads to a decrease in blood pooling in the venous sinusoids, turbinate shrinkage, and increased nasal airflow.

Sensory nerve endings are distributed throughout the nasal mucosa from the ophthalmic and maxillary branches of the trigeminal nerve. They are able to detect touch, temperature, pain, itch, and airflow. The small, unmyelinated, nociceptive C-fibers are responsible for the detection of pain and noxious chemical stimuli. Excitation of these fibers induces reflexive parasympathetic responses. The parasympathetic nervous system's primary postganglionic neurotransmitter, acetylcholine, acts on muscarinic (M) receptors concentrated in the glands, blood vessels, and epithelium of the nasal mucosa, leading to an increase in glandular secretion and vasodilation.

Pathophysiology

REFLEXIVE AND IDIOPATHIC (VASOMOTOR) RHINITIDES

Many noninfectious, nonallergic rhinitis syndromes are caused by the reflexive parasympathetic production of nasal congestion or increased nasal secretions in response to C-fiber activation by a known stimulus. Included in this group is gustatory rhinitis, in which patients develop rhinitis after the ingestion of food, especially spicy foods that contain capsaicin. This compound directly activates C-fibers. Cold/dry air and environmental or occupational irritants such as tobacco smoke, perfume, or chemical fumes may also initiate rhinitis symptoms. On the other hand, many patients have no identifiable cause for their rhinitis. The terminology for this condition is in constant flux in the medical literature, but the most commonly used names are idiopathic rhinitis or vasomotor rhinitis.

Although many of these nonallergy stimuli are able to produce mild symptoms in normal subjects, they tend to create far more persistent and intense nasal pathology in rhinitic patients. Some have proposed that the central nervous system is incorrectly interpreting signals from the sensory fibers of the nasal mucosa—a so-called central hyperresponsiveness. Another theory posits that nasal hyperresponsiveness is caused by an imbalance between parasympathetic and sympathetic effects on the nasal mucosa as it reacts to stimuli. Finally, some believe that the underlying mechanism is a phenomenon called neurogenic edema. Nociceptive C-fibers are known to release multiple inflammatory neuropeptides. These neurons can be antidromically stimulated, meaning that their dendrites can be triggered to release neuropeptides by action potentials generated at axon terminals on the same nerve (the so-called axon reflex). Repeated stimuli may lead to high neuropeptide levels in the mucosa. The neuropeptides, in turn, cause increased vascular permeability, vasodilation, and a cascade of inflammatory cell responses leading to edema, nasal congestion, and rhinorrhea.

DRUG-INDUCED RHINITIS

Aspirin-sensitive patients often develop rhinitis symptoms in addition to nasal polyposis and intrinsic asthma. In sensitive patients, aspirin's effects on arachidonic acid metabolism may lead to abnormally high levels of leukotrienes and subsequent inflammation of the nasal mucosa. There may also be some inhibition of eosinophil apoptosis related to the increased levels of leukotrienes.

Rhinitis medicamentosa is a separate type of drug-induced rhinitis caused by excessive use of topical α-adrenergic agonists. These drugs produce vasoconstriction of nasal blood vessels. With long-term use, the α-adrenergic receptors are downregulated, and the patient is forced to use higher and higher doses to achieve adequate symptom relief. Sudden discontinuation of the product leads to an intense rebound nasal congestion. Many other drugs, including such as angiotensin-converting enzyme inhibitors, β-blockers, chlorpromazine (Thorazine), methyldopa (Aldomet), nonsteroidal antiinflammatory drugs, immunosuppressive drugs, and oral contraceptives, can also cause nasal congestion.

NONALLERGIC RHINITIS WITH EOSINOPHILIA SYNDROME (NARES)

Patients with nonallergic rhinitis with eosinophilia syndrome (NARES) have perennial rhinitis symptoms with paroxysmal exacerbations of sneezing, profuse watery rhinorrhea, nasal pruritus, and, occasionally, loss of the sense of smell. They have greatly increased levels (5%-20%) of eosinophils in their nasal secretions. NARES may be an early stage of aspirin sensitivity or nasal polyposis. Nasal biopsies from patients with NARES show mast cells with bound IgE despite no evidence of allergy on skin testing. This may point to a local allergic reaction as the main culprit in symptom production. These patients respond well to nasal corticosteroids.

HORMONAL RHINITIS

Rhinitis symptoms are common during pregnancy but can also occur in conjunction with the menstrual cycle. It is presumed that increased levels of estrogen lead to vascular smooth muscle relaxation, pooling of blood in the venous sinusoids, and increased plasma leakage. Not all pregnant women with rhinitic symptoms have hormonally induced rhinitis, because allergic rhinitis, infectious rhinosinusitis, and rhinitis medicamentosa are also very common in this patient group. A previous history of rhinitis or asthma is not a risk factor for pregnancy-induced rhinitis. Hypothyroidism is believed to cause rhinitis in up to 2% of patients, but a strong link has never been established.

ATROPHIC RHINITIS

Primary atrophic rhinitis is a progressive, chronic nasal disease characterized by atrophy of the nasal mucosa and glands with subsequent resorption of the bone of the nasal turbinates. There is extensive nasal crusting, dryness, and a fetid odor in addition to the sensation of nasal congestion despite widely patent nasal cavities. Infection with the bacteria *Klebsiella ozaenae* is the most commonly implicated cause of primary atrophic rhinitis, although hereditary and vascular anomalies may also play a role.

Secondary atrophic rhinitis can be caused by overly aggressive turbinate surgery, chronic sinus infections, granulomatous disease, trauma, or irradiation.

OTHER CAUSES

Emotional stress (e.g., crying) and sexual arousal can also produce nasal congestion and rhinitic symptoms, presumably through autonomic mechanisms. Gastroesophageal reflux also has been linked to nasal inflammation and subsequent rhinitis.

Diagnosis

As with any medical condition, the proper diagnosis of perennial nonallergic rhinitis begins with a careful history and differential diagnosis (Box 1). Important elements include the age at symptom onset, time course, perennial versus seasonal symptoms, possible inciting factors, detailed questions about occupational exposures, the character of the mucus, pertinent related symptoms such as itching eyes, past medical history, family history, and previous medical evaluation or therapy for the problem. Features of the patient's story that would suggest a nonallergic cause include onset after age 20 years and isolated postnasal drainage. Features that might suggest an allergic cause include seasonal exacerbations, concomitant eye symptoms, and frequent sneezing or nasal pruritus. Rhinitis syndromes with specific inciting factors, such as gustatory rhinitis, cold/dry air rhinitis, or rhinitis medicamentosa, can often be diagnosed from the history alone.

BOX 1 Differential Diagnosis

- Allergic rhinitis
- Nasal obstruction
- Nasal tumors
- Foreign body
- Choanal stenosis
- Septal deviation
- Enlarged turbinates
- Adenoid hypertrophy
- Nasal polyps
- Sinusitis
- Ciliary defects
- Cerebrospinal fluid rhinorrhea

GRANULOMATOUS AND AUTOIMMUNE DISEASES

Another important element of the history is an assessment of how the symptoms affect the patient's quality of life. This is important in establishing a baseline against which symptomatic improvement can be compared.

Next, a thorough head and neck examination is necessary. The careful physician will examine the ears for effusions or other middle ear pathology, palpate the neck for evidence of lymphadenopathy suggestive of an infectious etiology, and inspect the face for classic allergic signs such as periorbital venous congestion (allergic shiners) and the so-called allergic salute—a transverse nasal crease created by frequent wiping of a chronically dripping nose with the back of the hand. The latter two signs are more often found in patients with allergic disease but can be identified in patients with nonallergic rhinitis as well.

A comprehensive nasal examination requires proper lighting with a headlight or indirect light reflected from a head mirror (the use of which has unfortunately been lost in most primary care clinics despite its ubiquity in images of physicians from decades past). A nasal speculum is used to examine the nasal cavity. Septal perforations can cause crusting, nasal irritation, and epistaxis due to the increased air turbulence in the nasal vault caused by air criss-crossing across the hole. Deviations of the nasal septum should be noted, as well as any turbinate hypertrophy, because obstruction can block the flow of nasal secretions and lead to rhinorrhea, postnasal drip, and nasal congestion. The turbinate and nasal mucosa may have a pale appearance or a bluish hue in both allergic and nonallergic rhinitis. It tends to be hyperemic in patients with infections and in those with rhinitis medicamentosa. Quantity and quality of secretions should be noted, with profuse, watery rhinorrhea possible in both allergic and vasomotor rhinitis.

Physicians with expertise in the use of rigid or flexible nasopharyngoscopes may choose to use these instruments when assessing the posterior septum, choanae, nasopharynx, and middle meatus. Adenoidal hypertrophy is a common cause of nasal obstruction and mouth breathing, especially in children. Unilateral choanal atresia is occasionally diagnosed in adults. Patients with unilateral nasal obstruction, discharge, and possibly pain should be assessed for a nasal neoplasm or foreign body. Purulent secretions emanating from the middle meatus may indicate infectious rhinosinusitis. Finally, a scope examination can easily identify nasal polyps, which are distinguished from mucosal hypertrophy because they are freely mobile and insensate and fail to shrink with application of α-adrenergic vasoconstrictors.

In daily clinical practice, the diagnosis of nonallergic rhinitis and its subgroups is based primarily on a thorough history and physical examination. If this evaluation suggests clinically relevant noninfectious rhinitis, other possible diagnoses are excluded in a stepwise fashion (see Current Diagnosis box). Perform nasal cytology (looking for eosinophilia); if the result is positive, consider an oral aspirin challenge.

CURRENT DIAGNOSIS

- Check for possible stimuli and severity and duration of disease.
- Check drug use, exposure at the workplace, hormonal status, and history of asthma.
- Exclude other nasal diseases with an endoscopy.
- Exclude allergy.
- Exclude chronic rhinosinusitis with a computed tomographic scan.
- Exclude cerebrospinal fluid rhinorrhea (if suggested by the history) with a β_2-transferrin test of the nasal fluid.

CURRENT THERAPY

- Make the correct diagnosis of nonallergic perennial rhinitis (diagnosis of exclusion).
- Classify it correctly as to the type of nonallergic perennial rhinitis; effective therapy depends on correct classification of the disorder.
- Evaluate the severity of the disease to confirm need for therapy.
- Lifestyle changes may be sufficient for therapy.
- If medical therapy fails, a vidian neurectomy is an option for treatment.

Although a detailed history and physical examination are often sufficient to establish a diagnosis of allergic versus nonallergic rhinitis and initiate treatment, it is helpful to obtain further testing to clearly delineate the two. The preferred method for doing so is intradermal skin testing. This method is fast, sensitive, and easily performed in the office setting. Serum immunoassays for specific IgE are also available but are, on average, not as sensitive as skin testing.

Treatment

There are many modalities in the clinician's armamentarium against perennial nonallergic rhinitis. An evaluation of the severity of the disease should be performed to confirm the need for therapy.

INTRANASAL CORTICOSTEROIDS

Intranasal corticosteroids have been shown to effectively relieve symptoms in a number of nonallergic rhinitides, especially NARES and idiopathic rhinitis. Because their therapeutic action is predominantly through their antiinflammatory effects, they are much less likely to be effective in noninflammatory conditions such as hormonally induced rhinitis. There are a large number of drugs available in this category, with varying dosage amounts and schedules (Table 1).

No single corticosteroid has been proven to be more effective than any of the others. Local side effects can include a burning or stinging sensation and minor epistaxis, typically manifested as blood-streaked mucus. Septal perforation is rare but can occur if the patient consistently directs the spray at the septum. Proper instruction on delivering the spray in a slightly lateral direction helps avoid this complication. Systemic side effects are rare when these compounds are used at recommended doses.

ORAL ANTIHISTAMINES

Oral antihistamines have been shown to be generally ineffective in relieving symptoms of nonallergic rhinitis. In addition, the first-generation antihistamines, such as diphenhydramine (Benadryl) and hydroxyzine (Vistaril),[1] commonly induce drowsiness and impairment.

INTRANASAL ANTIHISTAMINES

Two intranasal antihistamines are available in the United States, azelastine (Astelin) and olopatadine (Patanase).[1] Both have been shown to be effective compared with placebo for control of rhinorrhea, postnasal drip, and sneezing and reducing nasal congestion. Intranasal azelastine has been shown to be effective in reducing symptoms caused specifically by nonallergic rhinitis. Azelastine comes in a 0.1% aqueous solution, whereas olopatadine is available as a 0.6% aqueous solution. Both are delivered by means of a metered-dose spray device, placing 2 sprays in each nostril twice daily. This should be considered as primary therapy for patients with allergic or nonallergic rhinitis. Systemic absorption does exist and can cause some sedation; patients should be warned of this side effect before initiation of therapy.

TOPICAL DECONGESTANTS

The topical decongestants, all α-adrenergic agonists, include phenylephrine (Neo-Synephrine) and oxymetazoline (Afrin). Both are effective in reducing nasal congestion by decreasing blood flow to the nasal mucosa, but they have no effect on the other symptoms of rhinitis. In addition, both carry the risk of inducing rhinitis medicamentosa, as discussed earlier. Therefore, they are recommended only as short-term therapies (i.e., <4–5 days) for acute exacerbations of rhinitis syndromes.

If rhinitis medicamentosa develops, therapy consists of discontinuation of the offending topical decongestant and initiation of an intranasal corticosteroid to help mitigate rebound nasal congestion. In some cases, surgical reduction of the size of the inferior turbinates may be required.

ORAL DECONGESTANTS

In nonallergic rhinitis patients with nasal congestion, an oral decongestant, such as pseudoephedrine (Sudafed), may be of some benefit. They should be used with caution in patients with medical comorbidities. There is a risk of adverse outcomes in patients with hypertension, vascular disease, hyperthyroidism, closed-angle glaucoma, or bladder obstruction. Even in healthy individuals, these agents can cause unpleasant side effects such as insomnia, palpitations, irritability, and loss of appetite.

TABLE 1 Intranasal Corticosteroids Used to Treat Nonallergic Rhinitis

Generic Drug Name	Trade Name	Adult Dosage (sprays per nostril)
Beclomethasone dipropionate monohydrate	Beconase AQ	1–2 bid
Budesonide	Rhinocort Aqua[1]	1–4 qd
Ciclesonide	Omnaris[1]	2 qd
Flunisolide	Nasarel[1]	2 bid-qd
Fluticasone furoate	Veramyst[1]	2 qd
Fluticasone propionate	Flonase	2 qd
Mometasone	Nasonex[1]	2 qd
Triamcinolone	Nasacort AQ[1]	1–2 qd

[1]Not FDA approved for this indication.

[1]Not FDA approved for this indication.

INTRANASAL ANTICHOLINERGICS

Because the reflexive production of increased nasal secretions is mediated by the parasympathetic nervous system, application of an anticholinergic to the nasal mucosa might be expected to decrease this response. Intranasal ipratropium bromide (Atrovent) has been shown to be effective at decreasing rhinorrhea in nonallergic rhinitis without impairment of normal nasal functions such as olfaction or mucociliary clearance. It comes in 0.3% and 0.6%[1] preparations, with the lower concentration being more commonly used for rhinorrhea associated with perennial nonallergic rhinitis. Ipratropium can also be used safely and effectively in conjunction with an antihistamine or an intranasal corticosteroid. In addition, patients with reflexive rhinitis caused by specific stimuli (e.g., gustatory rhinitis, cold/dry air rhinitis) may benefit from the application of an intranasal anticholinergic agent shortly before exposure to the stimulus.

OTHER PHARMACEUTICAL AGENTS

Several other medications used for the treatment of allergic rhinitis have unclear utility in patients with nonallergic rhinitis. Cromolyn sodium (Nasalcrom)[1] inhibits the degranulation of sensitized mast cells, but the importance of histamine release in the pathogenesis of nonallergic rhinitis is uncertain. Therefore, only a modest benefit may be expected with use of this medication, and studies thus far have shown mixed results.

Despite the possible role of leukotrienes in the development of drug-induced rhinitis, there are no studies that demonstrate a place for leukotriene receptor antagonists, such as montelukast (Singulair),[1] in the treatment of this syndrome.

SALINE RINSES

A favorite of otolaryngologists, saline rinses in either isotonic or hypertonic concentrations may have modest benefits in reducing nasal congestion and sneezing. This is perhaps a result of improved mucociliary clearance, removal of mucosal irritants, and reduction of nasal bacteria and secretions. Delivery method and preparation are not standardized and depend mostly on patient and physician preference. Common delivery methods include squeeze bottles, neti pots, and water picks with irrigating adaptors.

BEHAVIOR MODIFICATION AND AVOIDANCE MEASURES

Patients with known triggers of hyperreactive rhinitis symptoms should be encouraged to avoid them if possible. Also, some rhinitides may respond to simple behavioral modifications. For example, rhinitis of pregnancy may improve with elevation of the head of the bed, gentle exercise, use of nasal valve dilators, and saline rinses. Cautious use of topical decongestants and intranasal corticosteroids may be of benefit if these measures fail.

INTRANASAL CAPSAICIN

A short course of topical applications of capsaicin[1,6] to the nasal mucosal has been shown to control symptoms of nonallergic rhinitis for up to 1 year. Capsaicin therapy is thought to work by repeatedly stimulating nociceptive C-fibers, causing depletion of their inflammatory neuropeptides and eventual nerve degeneration. Capsaicin is not available in any standardized form in the United States, and this therapeutic strategy remains in its experimental phase.

SURGERY

Surgical intervention can often help decrease the sensation of nasal congestion, drainage, and decreased airflow through correction of anatomic abnormalities. Septoplasty, inferior turbinate reduction,

endoscopic nasal polypectomy, adenoidectomy, and nasal valve reconstruction all seek to relieve obstructions to nasal airflow. Multiple methods exist for the performance of each of these procedures, and the particular strategy used depends on the surgeon's expertise and the patient's specific anatomy.

Since the 1960s, when Golding-Wood first described the procedure, vidian neurectomy has been used to treat idiopathic or vasomotor rhinitis that is recalcitrant to medical therapy. The procedure is aimed at eliminating the proposed autonomic imbalance caused by a dominant parasympathetic system. Postganglionic sympathetic neurons from the deep petrosal nerve and preganglionic parasympathetic neurons from the greater superficial petrosal nerve combine to form the vidian nerve as it courses through the vidian canal. Destruction of the vidian nerve as it exits the canal interrupts the parasympathetic input, but most of the sympathetic tone remains, because fibers traveling in the carotid plexus continue to reach the nasal mucosa. Many surgeons have shied away from this procedure over the last several decades because of the difficulties associated with accessing the vidian nerve. Long-term relief of symptoms was rarely achieved, but this may have been related to incorrect identification of the vidian nerve. Newer endoscopic techniques, which allow for direct visualization of the nerve, have led to renewed interest by increasing the safety and effectiveness of the procedure.

Conclusion

The perennial nonallergic, noninfectious rhinitides make up a diverse group of disease entities producing derangements in nasal physiology and aggravating nasal symptoms such as congestion and rhinorrhea. A careful history and physical examination are crucial to proper diagnosis, and treatment options are as varied as the disease entities themselves. It is incumbent on primary care providers to understand the syndromes of rhinitis in order to reduce the burden of rhinitis symptoms in their patients.

REFERENCES

Bachert C, van Cauwenberge P, Khaltaev N, et al. Allergic rhinitis and its impact on asthma. In collaboration with the World Health Organization. Executive summary of the workshop report. Geneva, Switzerland, December 7–10, 1999. Allergy 2002;57(9):841–55.

Dykewicz MS, Fineman S, Skoner DP, et al. Diagnosis and management of rhinitis: Complete guidelines of the Joint Task Force on Practice Parameters in Allergy, Asthma and Immunology. Ann Allergy Asthma Immunol 1998;81(2):478–518.

Greiner AN, Meltzer EO. Pharmacologic rationale for treating allergic and nonallergic rhinitis. J Allergy Clin Immunol 2006;118(5):985–96.

Jaradeh SS, Smith TL, Torrico L, et al. Autonomic nervous system evaluation of patients with vasomotor rhinitis. Laryngoscope 2000;110:1828–31.

Robinson SR, Wormald PJ. Endoscopic vidian neurectomy. Am J Rhinology 2006;20(2):197–202.

Sapci T, Yazici S, Evcimik MF, et al. Investigation of the effects of intranasal botulinum toxin type a and ipratropium bromide nasal spray on nasal hypersecretion in idiopathic rhinitis with eosinophilia. Rhinology 2008;46:45–51.

Sarin S, Undem B, Sanico A, et al. The role of the nervous system in rhinitis. J Allergy Clin Immunol 2006;118(5):999–1014.

van Rijswijk JB, Boeke EL, Keizer JM, et al. Intranasal capsaicin reduces nasal hyperreactivity in idiopathic rhinitis: A double blind randomized application regimen study. Allergy 2003;58:754–61.

Wallace DV, Dykewicz MS, Bernstein DI, et al. The diagnosis and management of rhinitis: An updated practice parameter. J Allergy Clin Immunol 2008;122(2 Suppl):S1–S84.

---

[1]Not FDA approved for this indication.
[6]May be compounded by pharmacists.

Hoarseness and Laryngitis

Method of
Lee Akst, MD

Voice is an essential component of communication. Vocal difficulty is very distressing to patients and can have a negative impact on physical, social, and emotional qualities of life. To understand the pathophysiology, evaluation, and treatment of voice complaints, it is important to understand the anatomy and physiology of normal voice production. Looking first at how good voice quality is achieved makes it readily apparent how alterations in vocal fold vibration, symmetry, or closure can lead to various vocal difficulties.

To aid discussion of voice complaints, clarification of terminology is necessary. Although "hoarseness" is a term that most patients use to describe any type of voice complaint and "laryngitis" is the presumptive explanation that many patients provide for their symptoms, each of these terms has a more precise meaning. Dysphonia is the general term for vocal difficulty. Hoarseness implies a rough or raspy change in voice quality and is one type of dysphonia. Other categories include limited vocal projection, strained vocal effort, and change in pitch—each of which may occur with or without vocal roughness. The term laryngitis specifically describes inflammation of the larynx. This inflammation may be acute or chronic, and again it describes some but certainly not all cases of dysphonia. This distinction will be made clear as the evaluation and management of dysphonia are described.

Normal Laryngeal Function

The larynx plays a central role in voice production by serving as a vibrating instrument that turns airflow from the lungs into sound. The sound is shaped into intelligible speech through the resonating and articulating functions of the pharynx and oral cavity. The ability of the larynx to create vibration and serve as a sound source is a function of its complex layered microanatomy. The deeper layers of the vocal fold include the thyroarytenoid muscle and the vocal ligament, which position the more superficial layers of the superficial lamina propria and epithelium during phonation. Compared with the fibrous nature of the vocal ligament, the superficial lamina propria is a loose gelatinous layer whose pliability allows for voice production.

During inspiration (Fig. 1A), the vocal folds are abducted so that air can move past the larynx without resistance. During phonation (see Fig. 1B), the vocal folds are held in an adducted position while the lungs drive air toward the larynx. Air pressure builds in the subglottis, beneath the vocal folds, until it overcomes the forces of vocal fold closure, pushes past the vocal folds, and generates negative pressure in its wake as it moves past the larynx. A combination of the vocal folds' intrinsic viscoelasticity and the negative pressure created through Bernoulli's effect draws the vocal fold edges back together, allowing subglottic pressure to rebuild and the cycle to repeat. Repeated cycles of opening and closing at the level of the vocal fold edges generate a so-called mucosal wave, which travels from the inferior edge of each vocal fold up across the medial and superior edges (see Fig. 1C). These waves may repeat hundreds of times each second, depending on pitch. This cycled opening and closing of the vocal folds during phonation imparts pressure waves to the air column that moves the vocal folds, generating sound. The ability of vocal folds to vibrate easily and symmetrically in this very rapid fashion allows for clear, smooth voicing.

Evaluation of Dysphonia

Central to the evaluation of dysphonia is the understanding that any disruption of vocal fold closure, symmetry, or vibration impairs the ability of the vocal folds to generate a clear sound source. Most voice complaints arise from anatomic or functional limitations in glottal closure or mucosal wave formation, although other parts of the respiratory tree are also responsible for components of the voice. General points concerning evaluation of dysphonia are discussed in this section, with specific causes discussed afterward.

HISTORY

A careful history can provide many clues that point toward the proper diagnosis in patients with dysphonia. Although many patients offer the complaint of "hoarseness" as a general term, a careful historian distinguishes between complaints related to voice quality, vocal projection, vocal effort or strain, vocal fatigue, and so on. Two questions that can help a patient organize his or her own thoughts related to poor voice are, "What abnormal things does your voice do now that it did not do before?" and "What normal things did your voice do before that it now no longer can do?" The acuteness of onset, duration, severity, and progression of any complaint should be determined.

The history should also determine what other factors or events might have caused or exacerbated the dysphonia. Recent sources of laryngeal inflammation might include intubation, excessive voice use, or upper respiratory tract infection. Baseline conditions that foster chronic laryngeal inflammation include environmental allergies, rhinitis, and laryngopharyngeal reflux. Laryngopharyngeal reflux can exist in the absence of heartburn, with reflux-associated inflammation of the larynx and pharynx providing symptoms of globus pharyngeus, throat clearing, nonproductive cough, effortful swallowing, and even mild dysphagia in association with dysphonia.

Concerning the possibility of laryngeal malignancy, any patient with dysphonia should be asked about smoking and alcohol use, because these are risk factors for squamous cell carcinoma. Another important question in distinguishing inflammatory dysphonia from a mass lesion of the vocal fold concerns whether there are any periods

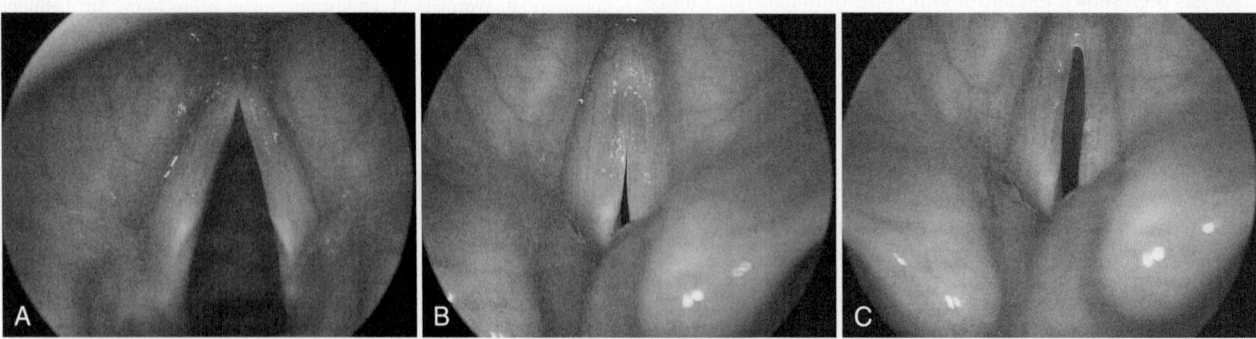

FIGURE 1. A, Normal vocal folds in abducted position for inspiration. **B,** Normal vocal folds in adducted position for phonation. **C,** Displacement of the vocal fold medial edges creates mucosal wave propagation during phonation and produces voice.

of normal voice or the dysphonia is constant—inflammation may wax and wane, but dysphonia associated with mass lesions is usually progressive and unremitting. Finally, the history should elicit other possible head and neck complaints, including dyspnea, stridor, dysphagia, odynophagia, otalgia, sore throat, and pain with speaking (odynophonia). If hoarseness is associated with some of these symptoms for longer than 2 weeks, the suspicion of malignancy is increased.

PHYSICAL EXAMINATION

The physical examination for patients with dysphonia includes a complete head and neck evaluation with focus on the larynx and laryngeal function. Although much of the head and neck examination can be performed in a general setting, some portions of the laryngeal examination require specialized equipment found only in some otolaryngology offices that specialize in voice care. Routine head and neck evaluation should include systematic examination of the ears, nose, oral cavity, oropharynx, and neck.

Complaint of otalgia in the setting of an unremarkable ear examination suggests a possibility of referred pain from a lesion of the larynx or pharynx, and is concerning for possible malignancy. Edematous and erythematous nasal mucosa suggests rhinitis, with the possibility of postnasal drip contributing to laryngeal inflammation. Tremor of the tongue or palate might suggest neurologic disorder, whereas pharyngeal erythema and exudate suggest possible acute infection. Pachydermia (cobblestoning) of the posterior pharyngeal wall suggests the possibility of laryngopharyngeal reflux. Tenderness with manipulation of the hyoid bone suggests tension of the strap muscles and correlates closely with complaint of odynophonia and the possibility of muscle tension dysphonia. A neck mass might represent either metastatic lymphadenopathy from a laryngeal malignancy or a primary lesion which itself compresses the recurrent laryngeal nerve and causes paralytic dysphonia. Surgical scarring along the neck suggests the possibility that prior thyroid surgery, carotid endarterectomy, or anterior approach to the cervical spine might have led to vocal fold paralysis.

LARYNGEAL EXAMINATION

Beyond a general examination of the head and neck, there should be directed evaluation of the larynx and laryngeal function. The examiner should listen to the voice carefully, because vocal characteristics such as roughness, breathiness, strain, vocal breaks, and diplophonia (pitch instability, with two different pitches present simultaneously) can help guide the differential diagnosis of dysphonia. Visual examination of the larynx has many forms, ranging from mirror examination to flexible fiberoptic laryngoscopy to videostrobolaryngoscopy.

Mirror examination offers an adequate view of the vocal folds in many patients but may be limited by patient tolerance, physician inexperience, and inherent limitations of this technique to brightly illuminate the larynx or record the examination for later review. Flexible laryngoscopy is routinely available in almost all otolaryngology offices, is well tolerated by patients, and offers good views of the larynx that can be recorded with appropriate equipment. Mirror examination and flexible laryngoscopy are limited to observation of vocal fold motion and anatomy but cannot observe laryngeal function because they do not visualize vibration of the vocal folds. To examine vocal fold vibration, videostroboscopy uses a strobe light to create the impression of slow motion analysis of mucosal waves. Stroboscopy is typically available only in selected otolaryngology practices in which laryngologists specialize in the treatment of voice disorders.

OTHER TESTING

Videostroboscopic evaluation, combined with a thorough history and routine physical examination, can establish the diagnosis for almost all patients with voice complaints, but further testing is sometimes indicated. For instance, electromyography is used by some laryngologists for further evaluation of vocal fold paralysis or paresis. More commonly, radiographic studies are used for further evaluation of some voice complaints. Computed tomography (CT) scans are ordered most often in the evaluation of suspected laryngeal neoplasms and for patients with vocal fold paralysis.

CURRENT DIAGNOSIS

- The general term to describe vocal difficulty is dysphonia. Hoarseness is a specific term for rough voice quality, which is one type of dysphonia. Laryngitis signifies laryngeal inflammation, which is one possible cause of dysphonia.
- An accurate history and physical examination guide the diagnosis of voice complaints. Although many portions of the examination for dysphonia can be done in a general setting, videostroboscopy is often necessary for diagnosis and may be available only in specialized laryngology offices.
- The most common cause of acute hoarseness is viral laryngitis. Symptoms are self-limited and usually resolve within 2 weeks.
- Dysphonia persisting for longer than 2 weeks suggests the possibility of another diagnosis, such as vocal cord paralysis, neoplasm, phonotraumatic lesion, or chronic laryngitis.
- Indications for referral of a patient with voice complaints to an otolaryngologist include dysphonia that persists for longer than 2 weeks, that is of acute onset during voicing, or that is accompanied by other symptoms such as otalgia, dysphagia, or difficulty breathing.

In the case of neoplasm, CT scanning is useful to assess the extent of the primary lesion and to evaluate possible metastatic cervical lymphadenopathy. In patients with laryngeal malignancy, chest radiography is also important to assess for pulmonary metastases. For patients with vocal fold paralysis who do not have a clear history of surgical injury of the recurrent laryngeal nerve, a CT scan from skull base to thoracic inlet identifies possible lesions along the course of the recurrent laryngeal nerve. Central problems are less likely, but if they are suspected as a cause of vocal fold paralysis, then magnetic resonance imaging of the brain may be indicated as well.

Types of Dysphonia

Although not comprehensive, the conditions discussed here account for the vast majority of voice complaints. Some patients with voice complaints have more than one condition, and not every patient will fit neatly into a single category. Nevertheless, understanding how each of these conditions creates dysphonia, and knowing which particular history and physical examination findings might be associated with each cause, can help a physician to appropriately diagnose and manage voice complaints.

ACUTE LARYNGITIS

Acute laryngitis is the most common cause of hoarseness and dysphonia. It is most often viral in nature, and onset of laryngeal symptoms may be associated with other symptoms of upper respiratory tract infection, including fever, myalgia, sore throat, and rhinorrhea. Viral inflammation of the vocal folds leads to diminished and more effortful vocal fold vibration, yielding a voice characterized by increased effort and a harsh, strained quality with decreased projection. Characteristic findings on laryngoscopy include vocal fold edema and erythema with decreased amplitude of the mucosal wave. Treatment of acute viral laryngitis is supportive, with counseling for hydration, humidification, and mucolytics. Symptoms generally are self-limited and resolve within 2 weeks. During this time, patients should be instructed to use the voice in a comfortable fashion, rather than straining or pushing to get loudness, because pushing behaviors may lead to the development of persistent muscle tension dysphonia.

Bacterial or fungal infections also cause acute laryngitis in rare cases. With appropriate physical findings and in the right clinical setting, antibiotic or antifungal therapy may be used to treat these conditions.

Amoxicillin-clavulanate (Augmentin) is often the antibiotic of choice, and fluconazole (Diflucan) is a commonly used antifungal agent.

CHRONIC LARYNGITIS

Chronic laryngitis is the nonspecific condition of prolonged laryngeal inflammation; the term itself does not indicate an etiology for the inflammation. Among the many possible sources for this inflammation are mechanical irritation from traumatic coughing or prolonged speaking, chemical irritation from environmental irritants (e.g., smoking, inhaled medications), and irritation from postnasal drip or laryngopharyngeal reflux. More than one cause may exist simultaneously. Issues related to cigarette use, excessive voice use, medication effect, and rhinitis can identified with careful history taking. Laryngopharyngeal reflux is a very common source of chronic laryngitis. It may manifest with several nonspecific symptoms, such as throat irritation, globus pharyngeus, frequent throat clearing, and nonproductive cough, with or with accompanying heartburn. Because vocal fold inflammation increases with continued mechanical trauma, the hoarseness of chronic laryngitis typically gets worse with prolonged voice use and improves with voice rest. Examination findings in chronic laryngitis include generalized laryngeal edema and erythema, and careful inspection may also reveal interarytenoid hyperplasia, subglottic edema, laryngeal ventricular obliteration, and an increase in thick glottic secretions.

Treatment of chronic laryngitis is tailored to the cause of the inflammation. Vocal hygiene with moderate voice use and instructions to reduce throat clearing and coughing may diminish mechanical irritation, and smoking cessation is recommended to any smoker with laryngeal complaints. Several studies have suggested that an appropriate trial of proton pump inhibitors for treatment of laryngopharyngeal reflux includes twice-daily therapy for at least 2 months, in contrast to the once-daily dosing often used for typical heartburn complaints. Lifestyle counseling to limit consumption of caffeine, carbonation, alcohol, and acidic foods can improve reflux, and attention to hydration and humidification decreases the viscosity of glottic secretions. For patients who are troubled by vocal difficulties associated with chronic laryngitis, referral to a speech language pathologist for voice therapy can improve compliance with suggested lifestyle changes and help foster vocal improvement.

VOCAL FOLD PARALYSIS

The dysphonia in cases of vocal fold paralysis usually relates to poor vocal fold closure (Fig. 2). The result is a breathy voice with limited projection and increased vocal effort. The farther from midline the immobile vocal fold, the more air leaks through the incompetent glottal valve without being turned into sound. Patients whose immobile vocal fold sits in a lateral position may have severely weak and breathy voices, whereas patients whose immobile vocal fold sits near midline may have a perceptually near-normal conversational voice and complain only of

mild increase in effort, vocal fatigue, or problems with loud projection. Because of their glottal insufficiency, patients may complain of "running out of air" with prolonged speech. Impaired glottal closure may also decrease airway protection during swallowing, so patients with vocal fold paralysis need to be questioned about aspiration as well. Whereas rehabilitation of poor voice may be elective, patients with increased aspiration risk need prompt therapy.

Evaluation of vocal fold paralysis includes identification of the cause of paralysis. Surgical injury to the recurrent laryngeal nerve accounts for almost half of all cases of unilateral vocal fold paralysis, and cervical or thoracic neoplasm and idiopathic paralysis account for most of the remaining cases. In a patient without a clear surgical history explaining the paralysis, CT scanning from skull base to mediastinum can identify any possible lesions along the course of the recurrent laryngeal nerve. In those patients whose histories suggest other possible causes (e.g., central neurologic injury, Lyme disease), further investigations, such as magnetic resonance imaging of the brain or blood work may be indicated as well. Some physicians perform laryngeal electromyography to help with the prognosis of paralysis or to differentiate neurologic injury from cricoarytenoid joint fixation; however, this study is neither standardized nor routine in many practices. Although flexible laryngoscopy alone may be satisfactory to document vocal fold immobility, stroboscopy can be added to investigate the impact of glottal insufficiency on vocal cord vibration and possible vocal fold flutter.

Treatment of vocal fold paralysis might include any combination of voice therapy, injection laryngoplasty, transcervical medialization laryngoplasty, and laryngeal reinnervation. Depending on the cause of the paralysis, some patients experience gradual recovery with synkinetic reinnervation or recovery of purposeful vocal fold motion over a period of several months. Based on the degree of voice and swallowing handicap, treatment of patients with vocal fold paralysis may be optional rather than necessary. Voice therapy can help teach patients to produce a stronger voice despite the paralysis, but by itself will not help a paralyzed vocal cord to recover motion. Various medialization techniques have been developed to help reposition an immobile vocal fold in the midline, where the contralateral mobile vocal fold can provide for complete glottal closure and lead to improved voice and swallowing. Injection medialization can be performed in the office or in the operating room, with temporary or permanent materials; if recovery of vocal fold motion is thought possible, then temporary injection is preferred. Transcervical medialization is a permanent but reversible surgical technique performed by otolaryngologists that repositions an immobile vocal fold in the midline. Laryngeal reinnervation offers the possibility of midline positioning of the immobile vocal fold with restored tone and bulk of the vocal fold musculature; however, because results may not mature for several months, this technique is less commonly performed than either injection or transcervical medialization.

PHONOTRAUMATIC LESIONS: NODULES, POLYPS, AND CYSTS

During vibration, vocal folds are subject to the shearing stresses of vibration. Although vocal fold structure is designed to accommodate these stresses in most circumstances, patients with vocal abuse or excessive voice use are at risk for development of lesions as the result of cumulative phonotrauma. Depending on the location and nature of these lesions, they are categorized as nodules, polyps, or cysts.

Vocal fold nodules are areas of fibrovascular scarring that are located just beneath the epithelium, at the level of basement membrane and superficial lamina propria. They are typically bilateral and symmetrical, sitting at the junction of the anterior one third and the posterior two thirds of each vocal fold. Polyps are typically unilateral lesions that may be edematous or fibrous in nature and may contain hemorrhage (Fig. 3). They usually are exophytic and extend outward from the vocal fold epithelium, although the fibrous base of a polyp may extend into the superficial lamina propria of a vocal fold. In contrast to an epithelial-based lesion such as a polyp, a vocal fold cyst is a subepithelial encapsulated lesion that sits entirely within the vocal fold; its size may exert a mass effect that deforms the medial edge of the involved vocal fold. These cysts are occasionally

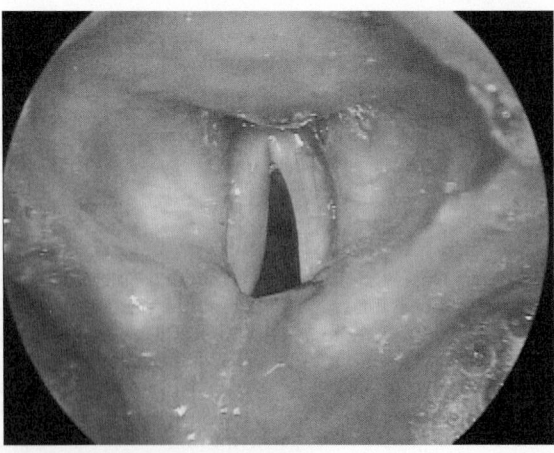

FIGURE 2. Vocal fold paralysis prevents the right vocal fold from closing to midline and creates dysphonia.

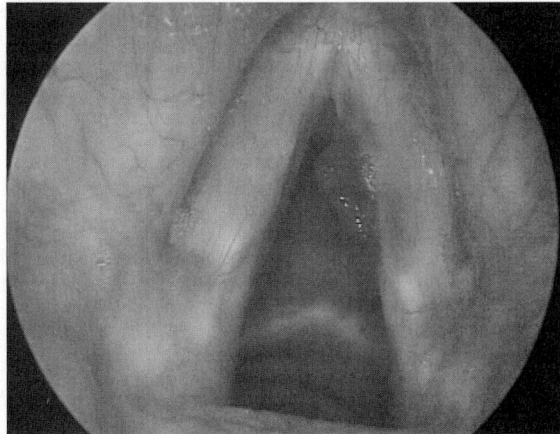

FIGURE 3. A large right hemorrhagic polyp, which can impair vocal fold vibration.

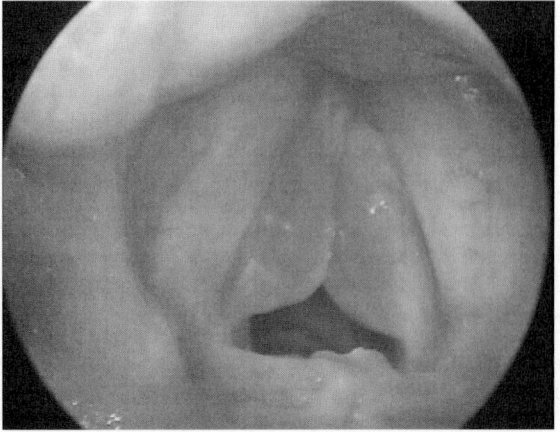

FIGURE 4. Symmetrical polypoid degeneration of the bilateral vocal folds, characteristic of Reinke's edema.

noted as congenital lesions in children, but in adults they are more often caused by traumatic occlusion of the ducts of the seromucinous glands within the larynx.

Nodules, polyps, and cysts cause dysphonia by disturbing vocal fold vibration, leading to rough voice quality. These lesions get larger as traumatic voice use accumulates, and vocal roughness usually becomes more severe and more constant as the lesions progress. Because vibration is more easily disturbed at high pitch, performers with these lesions may notice that high pitch is affected first. Effort of phonation often increases, but projection remains intact. Lesions large enough to limit vocal fold closure may also cause a slightly breathy voice quality. Because patients with excessive voice use are at risk for these lesions, a history of social and occupational voice demands is valuable in cases of suspected phonotrauma.

Treatment for these lesions always begins with voice therapy designed to modify the patient's voice use so as to diminish trauma. Voice therapy may be all that is necessary to allow resolution of some early traumatic changes, particularly in the case of edematous nodules. If dysphonia persists despite voice therapy and other conservative measures, surgery may be considered. Surgery with the goal of voice preservation and restoration (phonosurgery) is typically performed by otolaryngologists who specialize in the care of persons with vocal difficulties. The goal of phonosurgery for these lesions is to remove the lesion that impairs vibration while preserving as much of the remaining, pliable superficial lamina propria as possible, so that vocal fold vibration can be restored.

REINKE'S EDEMA

Reinke's edema, also known as polypoid corditis, is a benign swelling of the vocal folds that is most commonly seen in patients with a long-term smoking history. The edema, a reaction to long-term irritation, accumulates within the superficial lamina propria. The edema is most often bilateral and occurs diffusely along the entire length of the vocal fold, rather than being limited to a more discrete area, as is seen with phonotraumatic polyps (Fig. 4). As vocal fold mass increases with disease progression, the pitch of the voice decreases, and this is the change in voice most associated with Reinke's edema. A classic presentation of this condition is a female in her fifth or sixth decade of life who provides a long history of smoking and progressive deepening of her voice. In rare circumstances, the vocal folds gradually accumulate enough edema to compromise the airway, so breathing complaints should be evaluated as well.

Because a significant smoking history is also a risk factor for vocal fold leukoplakia and malignancy, good visualization of the vocal folds is necessary to evaluate for other lesions in these patients. If benign edema of the vocal folds is truly the only lesion noted, management depends on the degree to which voice quality is disturbing to the patient or the degree to which the airway is narrowed. Smoking cessation can lead to stabilization of pitch at its current level, and

phonosurgery to remove excess vocal fold mass can help lead to normalization of pitch and improve the airway. Phonosurgery may be performed with cold instruments or with the pulsed photoangiolytic lasers, an emerging therapy; in either case, there is a risk of creating a vocal fold scar that might limit vocal fold vibration even as vocal fold contours are improved.

RECURRENT RESPIRATORY PAPILLOMATOSIS

Recurrent respiratory papillomatosis (Fig. 5) is a benign laryngeal neoplasm that is caused by the human papilloma virus. It is the most common source of hoarseness in children, although adults also may be affected. As the lesions grow on the laryngeal epithelium, they create hoarseness and sometimes effortful voice by disrupting vocal fold vibration, particularly if the lesions are located along the medial edge of either vocal fold. Large and bulky lesions may lead to airway compromise, and advanced disease may spread throughout the mucosa of the upper aerodigestive tract rather than being limited to the larynx. Although accurate diagnosis depends on histopathologic analysis, a diagnosis of benign papilloma can be suspected from the characteristic appearance of the vascular fronds, which can be seen under magnified visualization in the office or in the operating room.

Treatment of recurrent respiratory papillomatosis is surgery, which is performed with a carbon dioxide laser, microdebrider, cold instruments, or the emerging technology of pulsed potassium titanyl phosphate (KTP) laser. As its name implies, the condition is recurrent: Even though surgery may reduce or remove the papilloma temporarily, the tissue continues to harbor the papilloma virus, and the disease usually grows back. Because repeated surgeries are expected,

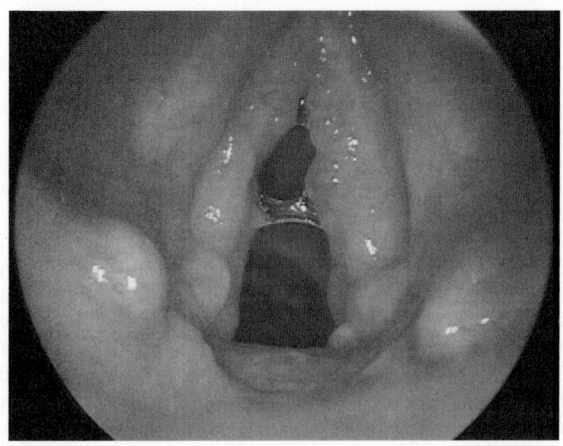

FIGURE 5. Recurrent respiratory papillomatosis, whose presence along each vocal fold medial edge disrupts sound production.

the goal of any single procedure is to remove as much disease as possible while limiting surgical scarring of the vocal folds. Scarring created as a result of surgery is cumulative, and over time patients develop persistent dysphonia caused as much from repeated surgeries as from recurrence of the disease. An ability to treat epithelial lesions while limiting scarring at the level of the superficial lamina propria is one main advantage of pulsed laser photoangiolysis; that these pulsed laser procedures can be performed in the office as well as the operating room is another. To help limit the need for repeated surgical procedures, adjunct medical therapies such as interferon and cidofovir are sometimes used for treatment of advanced disease.

VOCAL CORD CANCER

In 2008, an estimated 12,250 new cases of laryngeal cancer and 3,670 deaths attributable to laryngeal cancer occurred in the United States. The annual incidence of laryngeal cancer is 6.4 cases per 100,000 for men and 1.3 cases per 100,000 for women. Smoking is the single largest risk factor for laryngeal cancer, and excessive alcohol use has a synergistic effect as a risk factor as well. Survival rates for laryngeal cancer depend on the stage of the tumor at the time of diagnosis, which is a function of tumor size and possible tumor spread to the cervical lymph nodes or distant metastatic sites. Cancers that occur on the medial edge of the vocal fold produce dysphonia while still small, and many laryngeal cancers are diagnosed early.

The dysphonia associated with laryngeal cancer is constant, progressive, and unremitting, without the intermittent vocal improvement that may occur in inflammatory conditions. The presence of dysphagia, odynophagia, otalgia, hemoptysis, or unexplained weight loss further increases the index of suspicion for malignancy. Cervical lymphadenopathy is associated with advanced tumors. Diagnosis may be suspected on the basis of laryngeal examination and is confirmed with biopsy. The presence or absence of mucosal waves on the involved vocal fold on videostroboscopic examination can help predict the depth of the lesion. Both a CT scan of the neck and chest radiographs are indicated to assess for tumor size and spread. Early cancers are treated with surgery or radiation therapy, with similar cure rates. Emerging technologies such as pulsed photoangiolytic lasers may allow for surgical treatment of early disease with better preservation of surrounding normal tissue. More advanced tumors are usually treated with a combination of radiation therapy and surgery or chemotherapy.

Leukoplakia, or a raised white plaque on the epithelial surface, is a visual marker for the likely presence of dysplasia or carcinoma in situ. As a very early lesion, vocal fold leukoplakia may manifest with mild dysphonia or may be found incidentally on head and neck examination performed for other reasons. This early disease may take many years before progressing to invasive carcinoma, and recognition of leukoplakia presents an opportunity for early treatment to prevent progression of disease. Pulsed laser photoangiolysis has emerged as a state-of-the-art therapy for treatment of this epithelial lesion with preservation of the underlying vocal fold pliability.

Neurologic Disorders and the Voice

Neurologic conditions that affect the voice usually do so by causing poor coordination of vocal fold motion. Spasmodic dysphonia, for instance, leads to involuntary spasms that either bring the vocal folds tightly together (adductor spasmodic dysphonia) or apart (abductor spasmodic dysphonia) during phonation. These spasms lead to vocal breaks that are strained or breathy, respectively. Although the cause of spasmodic dysphonia is thought to lie within the central nervous system, the gold standard treatment of botulinum toxin is targeted at the end organ. Injection of botulinum toxin (Botox)[1] into appropriate laryngeal muscles can weaken these muscles and diminish the spasm.

Vocal fold tremor is a neurologic disorder that is distinct from spasmodic dysphonia. Its hallmark is tremulous voice quality caused by tremor of the larynx, which may occur both during phonation and at rest. Vocal fold tremor may exist alone or as part of systemic

[1]Not FDA approved for this indication.

tremor. Botulinum toxin[1] can decrease the amplitude of the tremor but may exacerbate the loss of projection that many tremor patients also have as a complaint. Medications such as anxiolytics or β-blockers that are used to treat systemic tremor may also improve the voice in patients with vocal fold tremor without worsening hypophonia.

Functional Voice Disorders

Functional dysphonia may exist by itself or in combination with an anatomic or neurologic source of dysphonia. The most common form of functional voice disorder is muscle tension dysphonia, which describes inappropriate hyperfunction of the supraglottic muscles. This hyperfunction often occurs in response to another source of hoarseness, as the patient tries to force out a strained voice with improved projection rather than accept the limited voice quality that may accompany the other disorder. The hyperfunction may then become an entrenched habit separate from the original pathology. In this sense, a classic scenario for muscle tension dysphonia is a patient who strains to speak more loudly during an acute laryngitis and whose strained, squeezed voice pattern persists even after the acute laryngitis has resolved. Patients with muscle tension dysphonia may complain of odynophonia as tension in the involved supraglottic muscles leads to muscular pain with prolonged speaking. Once other lesions have been evaluated, the treatment of muscle tension dysphonia is expert voice therapy with an emphasis on decreased hyperfunction.

Presbylaryngis

Presbylaryngis is the term that is used to describe the aging voice. It typically manifests in the seventh or eighth decade but can develop earlier. Acoustically, presbylaryngis results in a characteristic thinned voice, often with decreased projection and increased vocal strain. The condition occurs as cumulative voice use leads to traumatic thinning of the superficial lamina propria, particularly at the mid-cord level. This loss of superficial lamina propria leads to deficiency at the medial edge of each vocal fold, and a spindle-shaped defect in glottal closure may be noticed with close evaluation. Many patients with a complaint of presbylaryngis find that appropriate voice therapy to address breath support and vocal projection leads to satisfactory improvement in the voice without altering the vocal fold anatomy. For those patients who remain unsatisfied with their voice after therapy, vocal fold medialization procedures can restore straight vocal cord edges and may lead to improved projection; however, currently available injectables and implants that address contour defects cannot restore pliability.

[1]Not FDA approved for this indication.

 CURRENT THERAPY

- Appropriate treatment of voice complaints depends on accurate diagnosis.
- Supportive therapy is all that is necessary for most cases of acute laryngitis associated with viral upper respiratory tract infections.
- Laryngopharyngeal reflux is a common cause of chronic laryngitis, and appropriate therapy often requires twice-daily administration of proton pump inhibitors for at least 2 months.
- Microlaryngeal phonosurgery may be indicated for some patients with benign phonotraumatic lesions.
- Vocal cord medialization can rehabilitate the voice in a patient with unilateral vocal cord paralysis.
- Many patients with dysphonia benefit from voice therapy, alone or in combination with other treatment strategies.

Conclusion

Understanding the anatomy and physiology of normal voice production provides a framework through which dysphonia can be evaluated. Application of this knowledge during the history and physical examination guides the diagnosis of hoarseness and allows clinicians to distinguish among conditions as varied as acute laryngitis, benign phonotraumatic lesions, vocal fold paralysis, and laryngeal cancer as part of a differential diagnosis. Videostrobolaryngoscopy allows evaluation of vocal fold function as well as structure and can confirm diagnosis. As with any condition, accurate diagnosis directs appropriate therapy. Because no further evaluation or management is necessary for acute viral laryngitis, many patients with hoarseness require no more than a careful history and physical examination. However, if dysphonia persists for longer than 2 weeks or is accompanied by other laryngopharyngeal symptoms that are not thought to be related to an upper respiratory tract infection, referral should be made to an otolaryngologist for further evaluation.

REFERENCES

Koufman JA, Aviv JE, Casiano RR, et al. Laryngopharyngeal reflux: Position statement of the committee on speech, voice, and swallowing disorders of the American Academy of Otolaryngology-Head and Neck Surgery. Otolaryngol Head Neck Surg 2002;127:32–5.

Merati AL, Heman-Ackah YD, Abaza M, et al. Common movement disorders affecting the larynx: A report from the neurolaryngology committee of the AAO-HNS. Otolaryngol Head Neck Surg 2005;133:654–65.

Swibel Rosenthal LH, Benninger MS, Deeb RH. Vocal fold immobility: A longitudinal analysis of etiology over 20 years. Laryngoscope 2007;117:1864–70.

Wilson JA, Deary IJ, Millar A, et al. The quality of life impact of dysphonia. Clin Otolaryngol 2002;27:179–82.

Zeitels SM, Casiano RR, Gardner GM, et al. Management of common voice problems: Committee report. Otolaryngol Head Neck Surg 2002;126:333–48.

Zeitels SM, Healy GB. Laryngology and phonosurgery. N Engl J Med 2003;349:882–92.

Streptococcal Pharyngitis

Method of
Carla M. Giannoni, MD

Acute sore throat, or pharyngitis, accounts for 1.1% of visits to primary care offices (11 million office visits in 2000 in the United States). Overall, the most common cause of acute infectious pharyngitis is viral infection (Table 1). Group A β-hemolytic streptococcus (GABHS) accounts for approximately 30% of cases of acute pharyngitis in school-age children. In young adults and young children, adenovirus is the most common agent causing acute pharyngitis.

Epidemiology

Strep throat is the common term for an acute pharyngitis caused by *Streptococcus pyogenes*, also known as GABHS. Patients with this disease usually present with an acutely sore throat and fever. Patients may also have headache, nausea and vomiting, or abdominal pain. Common physical findings are inflammation of the tonsils, often with tonsillar exudate, and tender anterior lymphadenopathy. Patients may also have palatal petechiae, uvular edema, and a history of recent known contact with an infected patient. Scarlet fever is a manifestation of GABHS pharyngitis with a bacterial strain that produces an erythrogenic toxin. Patients develop a sunburn-like rash, which may later peel, in addition to the other symptoms of GABHS tonsillitis.

TABLE 1 Distribution of Common Causes of Pharyngitis in Children and Adults

Bacterial	
GABHS	*Children:* 15%-30% of acute pharyngitis cases (especially age 5–15 y)
	Adults: 5%-15% of acute pharyngitis cases
Mycoplasma pneumoniae	*Children:* 5%-16% (>6 y)
Viral	
Epstein-Barr virus	Adolescents and young adults (15–30 y)
Adenoviruses	*Children:* most common cause in children <3 y; 4%-10% of pharyngitis cases in school-age children
	Adults: 37%-75% of non-GABHS pharyngitis cases in military recruits
Enteroviruses	*Children:* 8% (1 study); summer and early fall; children are most sensitive cohort
Unknown	30%-35% of pharyngitis cases are of unknown etiology

Abbreviation: GABHS = group A β-hemolytic streptococcus.

Transmission of GABHS and viruses that cause pharyngitis is by hand contact with nasal discharge. The incubation period is 1 to 3 days. The transmission rate with close contact is approximately 35%. The course of GABHS pharyngitis is usually about 5 days (range, 3–10 days). Patients with GABHS pharyngitis are contagious during the acute phase of the illness and for one additional week. Treatment with penicillin renders a patient effectively noncontagious in 24 hours.

Reasons to Treat

Prevention of complications, such as acute rheumatic fever (ARF), has traditionally driven physician treatment of acute pharyngitis with antimicrobials. Patients, on the other hand, generally seek symptom relief, especially pain reduction. In patients with known GABHS pharyngitis, the use of penicillin has been shown to reduce severity and duration of symptoms by 1 to 2 days if started within 48 hours after symptom onset. Appropriate antibiotic use can also reduce transmission of GABHS within 24 hours after antibiotic initiation, and complications such as ARF are significantly reduced when GABHS is treated.

CURRENT DIAGNOSIS

- Acute infectious pharyngitis is caused by a wide variety of infectious agents.
- Viruses are the most common cause of acute pharyngitis.
- Group A β-hemolytic streptococcus (GABHS) accounts for 15% to 30% of pediatric cases of acute pharyngitis.
- GABHS accounts for only 5% to 10% of adult cases of acute pharyngitis.
- Centor criteria (tonsil exudates, fever, tender anterior cervical lymphadenopathy, and no viral symptoms such as cough or conjunctivitis) are often used to predict likelihood of GABHS.
- The rapid antigen detection test (RADT) is a useful diagnostic tool in patients with two or more Centor criteria and suspected GABHS pharyngitis.
- Empiric treatment with antibiotics is considered only for adults who have all four Centor criteria.
- Because of the low incidence of GABHS in adults, throat culture is not recommended if the RADT is negative.
- Because of the higher incidence of GABHS in children, throat culture is recommended if the RADT is negative.

It is important to balance achieving these positive goals with the need to reduce the risks of antibiotic use to the patient and the community. Many antibiotics are provided for viral infections and do not change the disease course. In 2000, there were approximately 6.7 million health care visits by adults for sore throat. Although 70% of adult patients were given an antibiotic prescription for their sore throat, only about 10% are estimated to have actually have had GABHS infection. Use of antibiotics also carries the risks of antibiotic-associated side effects and complications. Because patients are primarily concerned about symptom relief, it is important to provide symptomatic therapy and to remember that effective communication is more important than an antibiotic for patient satisfaction.

Clinical Diagnosis

Classically, the so-called Centor criteria—fever ($>38°C$), acute pharyngitis with or without tonsillar exudates, absence of cough, and tender anterior cervical lymphadenopathy—have been used to assess the likelihood that GABHS is the cause of an infection in a patient with acute pharyngitis. Symptoms of cough, conjunctivitis, rhinorrhea, and diarrhea are associated with viral infections.

In adult patients, the presence of all four positive indicators gives a 56% probability that GABHS is the cause. The incidence decreases if only three, two, one, or zero indicators are present, to 32%, 15%, 6%, and 2.5%, respectively.

GABHS pharyngitis is more common in children, particularly between the ages of 5 and 15 years of age, and occurs more commonly in the late fall, winter, or early spring. Among school-age children during the peak season, the incidence of GABHS pharyngitis in those with three of the four Centor criteria is 59%; in those with all four criteria, it is 75%.

Testing

Throat culture is the gold standard for the diagnosis of GABHS disease (Table 2). In a controlled setting, the specificity of the test is 95% to 99%, and the sensitivity is 88% to 91%, although the sensitivity can be much lower in a physician's office. It is important that the culture collection be thorough, with swabbing of both tonsillar fossae and the posterior pharynx under direct visualization. There is a 24- to 48-hour delay in obtaining a culture result. This delay may be inconvenient and may reduce the benefit of early antibiotic use for symptom reduction, but it does not negatively affect the complication rate or the risk of rheumatic fever. If other bacterial agents are suspected because of an atypical presentation or the presence of epidemiologic features that indicate a risk for gonorrhea, diphtheria, tularemia, or infection with *Arcanobacterium* or *Mycoplasma*, the laboratory should be notified, because the usual culture for GABHS may miss other organisms.

Rapid antigen detection tests (RADTs) have been designed to provide a more immediate diagnosis. An RADT is an enzyme-linked radioimmunoassay that detects the A carbohydrate of the streptococcus organism and is read by a color change on the swab. These tests are almost as accurate as throat culture (85% to 95% sensitivity) and are very specific for GABHS disease (Table 3). The Infectious Diseases Society of American (IDSA) has set forth some recommended guidelines for diagnosis and treatment of acute pharyngitis. They recommend RADT testing for all children with two or more Centor criteria and treatment for those who are RADT positive. RADT is 90% sensitive for pediatric patients with three and four criteria, but only 82% sensitive with two, 65% with one, and 47% zero criteria. Because of the higher incidence of disease and the lower sensitivity of testing in some pediatric groups, patients who are RADT negative should have throat culture performed.

There are many strategies for RADT testing and treatment in adults. The IDSA recommendations for diagnosis and treatment are the same in adults as in children except that, because of the low incidence of GABHS in adult patients, routine culture for RADT-negative patients is not recommended. The Centers for Disease Control and Prevention (CDC), in conjunction with the American College of Physicians–American Society of Internal Medicine/American Academy of Family Physicians (ASIM), has supported the IDSA strategy as an option for diagnosis and treatment but also provides two additional modifications of this strategy as options for adult patients. Evaluation of these different strategies suggests that the IDSA guidelines result in the highest specificity and sensitivity of all the available options, short of obtaining throat cultures from all patients; however, the ASIM option 2 does not sacrifice much specificity and results in fewer RADT tests (Table 4). The ASIM, option 3 results in a significant increase in the unnecessary use of antibiotics and for this reason cannot be recommended (see Table 3).

TABLE 2 Diagnostic Testing in Suspected GABHS Pharyngitis

Test	Key Points
Throat culture	Gold standard test
	Culture medium: 5% sheep blood agar plate with a bacitracin disk
	Sensitivities to common antibiotics are not usually done (penicillin resistance is very rare).
RADT	There are several different test kits available.
	The more popular kits use an ELISA to test for the A carbohydrate of the streptococcus organism.
	Sensitivity varies by test but is usually good to excellent in all age groups; specificity varies in relation to disease incidence.
ASO titer	Detects recent infection by quantitating the antibody response to streptolysin-O
	Most useful in evaluating patients with nonsuppurative sequelae of GABHS
Monospot test	Slide agglutination (heterophil antibody) test for mononucleosis
	Sensitivity in the first week is only 69%; overall sensitivity is 86%, and specificity is 99%.

Abbreviations: ASO = anti-streptolysin O; ELISA = enzyme-linked immunosorbent assay; GABHS = group A β-hemolytic streptococcus; RADT = rapid antigen detection testing.

TABLE 3 Recommended Testing and Treatment Strategy for Adults and Children with Acute Pharyngitis

No. of Centor Criteria Met	Testing Recommendation	Antibiotic Treatment Recommendation
0 or 1	Do not test	Do not treat; provide symptomatic treatment for viral pharyngitis
2 or 3	RADT and throat culture (except RADT(−) adults)*	Treat if RADT or culture is positive
4		
Option 1[†]	RADT and throat culture (except RADT(−) adults)*	Treat if RADT or culture is positive
Option 2[‡]	Do not test	Treat empirically

*Culture is not recommended for RADT(−) adults except to evaluate for other organisms; routine throat culture for RADT(−) children is recommended.
[†]Proposed by ASIM (see Table 4).
[‡]Proposed by ASIM for adults (see Table 4); proposed by various authors for children.
Abbreviation: RADT = rapid antigen detection testing.

TABLE 4 Testing and Treatment of Adults* with Acute Pharyngitis: Characteristics and Implications for Antibiotic Use of Various Strategies

Proposed Strategy	No. of Centor Criteria Met and Antiobiotic Treatment Recommendation	Sensitivity (%)	Specificity (%)	Excess Antibiotic Use (% of Patients)
IDSA/ASIM option 1	2, 3, or 4: treat if RADT+	77	99	0.6
ASIM option 2	2 or 3: treat if RADT+ 4: treat empirically	78	96	3.3
ASIM option 3	2: treat if RADT+ 3 or 4: treat empirically	77	44	44

*For children, both IDSA and ASIM recommend RADT testing of those meeting 2, 3, or 4 Centor criteria and treatment of RADT+ patients only.
Abbreviations: ASIM = Centers for Disease Control and Prevention in conjunction with the American College of Physicians—American Society of Internal Medicine/American Academy of Family Physicians; IDSA = Infectious Diseases Society of America; RADT = rapid antigen detection testing.

Anti-streptolysin-O antibodies (ASO) are produced in response to exposure to the streptococcal extracellular protein, streptolysin-O (see Table 2). An elevated ASO titer is a good indication of recent infection and is most helpful in the diagnosis of nonsuppurative sequelae such as rheumatic fever and glomerulonephritis. A series of titers is usually taken to determine whether infection has occurred, but a single, highly elevated value is adequate to diagnose GABHS infection.

Differential Diagnosis

In contemplating the differential diagnosis for acute pharyngitis, one should consider the likelihood that GABHS is responsible by performing adequate evaluation and testing as described earlier. For those patients who have a low probability of having GABHS or who test negative, one should consider the demographics and the patient's risk factors for contracting one of the more common viral infections or a less common bacterial or viral infection (Table 5; see Table 1). In the absence of fever, noninfectious causes of sore throat, such as silent gastroesophageal reflux or postnasal drainage caused by rhinitis (allergies or sinusitis), should be considered. Chronic cough, a foreign body, and smoking can also cause sore throat. Sometimes, there are distinguishing features that point to the cause. For instance, a prolonged course suggests Epstein-Barr virus infection, and concurrent gingivostomatitis is more commonly seen with herpes simplex . Acute HIV infection is an unusual cause of pharyngitis, but its diagnosis is important for initiating appropriate therapy and should be considered in young, sexually active adolescents. The cause of Kawasaki disease is unknown but is probably an infectious agent; it manifests with fever, conjunctivitis, erythematous oral mucosa, inflamed pharynx, and strawberry tongue. Later, a rash and erythema of hands and feet with peeling of the hands occurs. The most important concern is the potential involvement of coronary arteries.

 CURRENT THERAPY

- The recommended treatment for streptococcal pharyngitis is penicillin or amoxicillin.
- Cephalosporins have a success rate in treating GABHS infections similar to that of the penicillins, but their use is not justified in primary cases because of cost and the risk of development of antibiotic resistance in a community.
- Erythromycin is recommended for penicillin-allergic patients.
- Treatment failures are most commonly caused by an incorrect diagnosis, infection with a copathogen, or antibiotic resistance.

Treatment

Penicillin is the treatment of choice for GABHS pharyngitis (Table 6). Even after more than 50 years of use, GABHS remains almost universally susceptible to penicillin and other β-lactam antimicrobial agents; susceptibility need not be routinely determined. Treatment within 9 days after symptom development provides protection from nonsuppurative complications such as rheumatic fever. A full 10 days of penicillin treatment is necessary for bacteriologic cure and for the prevention of complications.

Alternative drugs are considered mainly for patients who are allergic to penicillin. Erythromycin is the drug of choice in such cases. Cephalosporins are highly effective and may be substituted in some cases of penicillin allergy but should be avoided if there is a history of anaphylaxis with penicillin. Although erythromycin is an alternative choice for patients with penicillin allergy, broader-spectrum macrolides, such as clarithromycin (Biaxin), are not necessary. The use of azithromycin (Zithromax) in lieu of erythromycin is common because of its better tolerance and better compliance, but inadequate dosing can lead to a high failure rate. Tetracyclines and sulfonamides are likely to be ineffective and should not be used. Similarly, fluoroquinolones are not indicated for uncomplicated GABHS pharyngitis.

TREATMENT FAILURE

There are many reasons for treatment failure. Antibiotics do not eliminate GABHS from the pharynx in every patient. Common causes of treatment failure include noncompliance with antibiotic use, repeated exposure to GABHS, presence of copathogens, early treatment suppressing the immune response, and the carrier state. Failure to respond to treatment should raise suspicion that the diagnosis was incorrect. Between 10% and 20% of school-age children are GABHS carriers, and most of them are asymptomatic. If GABHS testing was done and the patient has persistent pharyngitis, then he or she may be a GABHS carrier and may have a different etiology for the acute pharyngitis. Tables 1 and 5 outline a fairly extensive differential diagnosis for acute pharyngitis, of which GABHS is only one common cause. In particular, the diagnosis of mononucleosis syndrome should be considered in children and adolescents who have prolonged symptoms.

Patients with recurrent infections may harbor co-infection with another bacterial pathogen, and treatment with amoxicillin-clavulanate (Augmentin)[1] may be more effective than amoxicillin alone (Table 7). Patients with recurrent GABHS pharyngitis who have mild to moderate symptoms may benefit from delaying treatment for 48 hours, to allow the immune response to develop. Resistance to erythromycin is increasing in the United States, and resistance rates of 25% have been reported in some nonepidemic areas. Cross-resistance among macrolides is universal, so azithromycin and clarithromycin are not appropriate choices in the case of an erythromycin failure. Alternative choices to treat known GABHS infection after failed erythromycin therapy are a cephalosporin or clindamycin (Cleocin).

---

[1]Not FDA approved for this indication.

TABLE 5 Differential Diagnosis of Pharyngitis with Distinguishing Characteristics

Infectious Cause	Comments
GABHS	Children <3 y: atypical presentation with protracted nasal congestion, low-grade fever, tender cervical lymphadenopathy
	Children >3 y and adults: typical presentation with abrupt onset, fever, headache, abdominal pain, nausea and vomiting, exudative pharyngitis, enlarged tender cervical lymphadenopathy, palatal petechiae, and/or inflamed uvula
	Peak incidence in winter and early spring
Non-group A streptococci	Symptoms similar to GABHS
	Can cause poststreptococcal glomerulonephritis but not rheumatic fever
Mycoplasma pneumoniae	Often associated with pneumonia or bronchitis
Neisseria gonorrhoeae	Variable presentation: pharyngeal erythema, edema, exudates, or normal
	Oral-genital transmission
Arcanobacterium spp.	Similar to GABHS in presentation
	Scarlatiniform rash on arms (extensor surfaces) in 50%
	Does not respond to penicillin; erythromycin is drug of choice
Corynebacterium diphtheriae	Consider in patients from endemic regions
	Onset: gradual with rhinitis and/or pharyngitis, malaise, low-grade fever
	Later: at least 1/3 of patients develop a gray adherent membrane in nasopharynx and oropharynx that bleeds if removed
	Can be fatal
Tularemia	Oropharyngeal tularemia: fever, painful ulcerative exudative pharyngitis
	Transmission from poorly cooked wild animal meat or contaminated water
	Unresponsive to penicillin
Viruses (all)	May have concurrent conjunctivitis, coryza, cough, hoarseness, stomatitis, viral exanthems, ulcerative lesions, and/or diarrhea
EBV	Most common cause of mononucleosis syndrome (prodrome of malaise and fever, followed by severe pharyngitis with tonsillar exudates)
	Posterior cervical lymphadenopathy distinguishes it from GABHS
	Prolonged course
	Splenomegaly is seen in 50%, and splenic rupture is possible
	May develop fifth-day rash after treatment with ampicillin or amoxicillin
	Can be concurrent with GABHS
Cytomegalovirus	Similar to EBV (usually with more hepatitis and less severe pharyngitis)
Adenoviruses	Wide range of signs and symptoms; may not have distinguishing findings
	Can cause pharyngitis, croup, bronchitis, and pneumonia
	Usually lasts 5–7 d
	Can present as pharyngoconjunctival fever
HSV	Adolescents: exudative pharyngitis (50%)
	Adolescents: vesicular lip lesion (10%)
	Younger children: gingivostomatitis with ulcerative vesicular lesions
	Culture can confirm; antiviral treatment is given
	Type: most are HSV-1; 15% are HSV-2
Influenza	Usually high fever, cough, headache, and myalgias
	Often associated with community epidemics; treatable
Enteroviruses	Fever, headache, pharyngitis, and myalgias; aseptic meningitis is possible
	Hand-foot-mouth disease: ulcerative lesions of mouth and tongue; vesicular lesions of hands and feet; red rash on buttocks
	Herpangina: caused by Coxsackie A; manifested by small ulcerative vesicles in palate with or without posterior pharynx and fever
Primary HIV	Manifests similarly to EBV; lymphopenia may be present
	HIV risk factors usually within 2–5 wk of presentation
	Consider in sexually active adolescents

Abbreviations: EBV = Epstein-Barr virus; GABHS = group A β-hemolytic streptococcus; HIV = human immunodeficiency virus; HSV = herpes simplex virus.

CARRIER STATE

As noted previously, 10% to 20% of school-age children are carriers of GABHS. In the early stages of the carrier state, the patient is contagious, but after 1 to 2 months, there are diminished numbers of bacteria, reduced bacterial virulence due to loss of M antigens, and reduced transmissibility. Carriers do not appear to have an increased risk of rheumatic fever or suppurative complications. The carrier state does not require treatment unless the person appears to be the source of recurrent household outbreaks of GABHS, works in a hospital or patient care facility, has a history of rheumatic fever, or lives in a community with an outbreak of rheumatic fever. Treatment is usually that recommended for recurrent GABHS pharyngitis (see Table 7).

Complications

SUPPURATIVE COMPLICATIONS

Suppurative complications of GABHS pharyngitis range from the more common ones, peritonsillar cellulitis and abscess, to the much more rare and severe complications of bacteremia, toxic shock syndrome, and necrotizing fasciitis. Peritonsillar cellulitis and abscess are local phenomena that require systemic treatment and, in the case of abscess, usually require drainage of the abscess fluid collection. Peritonsillar abscess is diagnosed by unilateral edema of the palate and medial bulging of the tonsil with a convex medial displacement of the palate on the side of the abscess.

TABLE 6 Treatment for Primary Group A β-Hemolytic Streptococcus Infection

Antimicrobial Agent	Daily Dosing (Maximum Adult Daily Dose; Maximum Duration)	Notes
Penicillin V/Pen VK (Veetids)	<27 kg (60 lb): 250 mg PO bid or tid ≥27 kg (60 lb): 500 mg PO bid or tid	10-Day course is required for eradication Use bid dosing if good compliance is expected
Benzathine Penicillin G (Bicillin LA)	25,000-50, 000 U/kg IM in 1–2 doses (max: 1.2 million U)	IM mode is recommended if compliance is unlikely
Other penicillins	Individualize dosing to the drug	Nafcillin is not effective
Amoxicillin	50 mg/kg in 2–3 doses (max: 750–1500 mg; 6–10 d) (90 mg/kg in 2 doses if concurrent otitis media)	6-Day course is probably sufficient Once-daily dosing may be adequate Better gastrointestinal absorption than penicillin Compliance often better because of better taste
Cephalexin (Keflex)	25–50 mg/kg in 2–4 doses (max: 1000 mg in 2 doses; 10 d)	Very effective, bid dosing approved Much more expensive than penicillins
Other first-generation cephalosporins	Individualize dosing to the drug; 5-d course adequate for some	Concern about development of resistance if wider use of these drugs occurs
Erythromycins (numerous types)	40–50 mg/kg in 3–4 doses (max: 1 g/d)	Penicillin-allergic patients Some increasing resistance is being seen
Azithromycin (Zithromax)	60 mg/kg per course, given as 10–12 mg/kg/d × 5 d (e.g., 750 mg/d for a 70-kg patient)	5-Day course is sufficient Prepackaged course may provide inadequate dose (higher failure rates)

Severe GABHS disease occurs rarely; 4587 cases of bacteremia, toxic shock syndrome, or necrotizing fasciitis were reported to the CDC in 2006. The portal of the infection entry in these severe infections is often through the skin after varicella infection or trauma. Those at the greatest risk for a severe GABHS infection are children with chickenpox; immunosuppressed patients, including patients undergoing steroid treatments or chemotherapy; burn victims; elderly people with cellulitis, diabetes, blood vessel disease, or cancer; and intravenous drug users. However severe GABHS disease may also occur in healthy people who have no known risk factors.

NONSUPPURATIVE COMPLICATIONS

ARF is one of the most feared complications of GABHS pharyngitis and often drives the treatment of acute pharyngitis but is actually an uncommon disease in the United States, with an annual incidence of less than 1 case per 100,000 population. However focal outbreaks of rheumatic fever in school-age children occurred throughout the 1990s in the United States, and ARF is an important health concern worldwide. It occurs almost exclusively in children younger than 15 years of age unless there is a prior history of the disorder. The illness develops a few weeks to 1 month after GABHS infection and is caused by an autoimmune response to infection with a rheumatogenic strain of GABHS. Patients may develop a rash (erythema marginatum), subcutaneous nodules, joint swelling or pain, and heart murmur due to carditis. The heart valves may be permanently scarred and damaged. There appears to be a genetic risk for developing the most serious manifestation of ARF. Although most attention is focused on disease

prevention, treatment is available and should be implemented when ARF is diagnosed. Secondary prophylaxis for all patients who have had rheumatic fever should be continued for at least 5 years or until the person is 21 years of age, whichever is longer. Secondary prophylaxis should be long-term, perhaps for life, in patients with rheumatic heart disease.

Acute glomerulonephritis is similar to ARF. This illness is an autoimmune-mediated complication of GABHS infection, either pharyngitis or impetigo. Patients are usually 7 years of age or younger and most commonly present with hematuria. Renal failure may develop, although the prognosis is usually good.

Sydenham's chorea is a manifestation of ARF. It is the most common cause of chorea in children. The neurologic features include chorea, the most common motor sign, and nonmotor manifestations such as obsessive-compulsive behavior and attention-deficit/hyperactivity disorder. Its morbidity relates to the cardiac lesions of ARF, which are present in 30% to 64% of patients with Sydenham's chorea.

Pediatric autoimmune neuropsychiatric disorders associated with streptococcus infections (PANDAS) is a relatively new diagnosis. The predominant symptoms are obsessive-compulsive behavior or tic disorder or both, with a worsening of symptoms after GABHS infection. The patients most commonly affected are prepubertal children. Behaviorally, there is overlap between Sydenham's chorea and PANDAS; however, there is no cardiac involvement in PANDAS. Some researchers believe that the basal ganglia dysfunction is autoimmune, as in ARF, and is caused by anti-brain antibodies.

TABLE 7 Treatment of Recurrent GABHS Infection

Antimicrobial Agent	Daily Dosing (Maximum Adult Daily Dose; Maximum Duration)	Notes
Amoxicillin/clavulanate (Augmentin)[1]	45 mg/kg in 2 doses (max: 500 mg in 3 doses; 10 d)	Treatment of copathogens may account for better success rates
Amoxicillin (see Table 6) with rifampin	Rifampin (Rifadin)[1]: 15 mg/kg in 2 doses (max: 600 mg; 4 d)	Rifampin is given on the last 4 d of therapy Especially for carriers needing treatment
Cephalosporins	See Table 6	Slightly more effective than the penicillins
Clindamycin (Cleocin)	20 mg/kg in 3 doses (max: 600–1800 mg; 10 d)	Oral suspension has unpleasant taste Some risk of pseudomembranous colitis

[1]Not FDA approved for this indication.

Vaccine Development

There has long been interest in development of a GABHS vaccine that could potentially reduce the infections that trigger ARF and other severe complications of GABHS. This interest has been tempered by concerns that a vaccine might induce antibody production that itself triggers ARF. There are several molecular targets for vaccine development. A 26-valent vaccine that uses the bacterial surface M protein as an antigen target was reported to be well tolerated and immunogenic in adult subjects. Research is ongoing in this area.

REFERENCES

American Academy of Pediatrics. Group A streptococcal infections, In: Pickering L, editor. Red Book: 2006 Report of the Committee on Infectious Diseases. 26th ed. Elk Grove Village, IL: American Academy of Pediatrics; 2006. p. 610–20. Available at:http://aapredbook.aappublications.org/cgi/content/full/2006/1/3.122 [accessed May 20, 2008].

Bisno AL, Gerber MA, Gwaltney JM, et al. Practice guidelines for the diagnosis and management of group A streptococcus pharyngitis. Clin Infect Dis 2002;35:113–25.

Bisno AL, Rubin FA, Cleary PP, Dale JB. Prospects for a group A streptococcal vaccine: Rationale, feasibility, and obstacles. Report of a National Institute of Allergy and Infectious Diseases Workshop. Clin Infect Dis 2005;41:1150–6.

Cooper RJ, Hoffman JR, Bartlett JG, et al. Centers for Disease Control and Prevention: Principles of appropriate antibiotic use for acute pharyngitis in adults: Background. Ann Emerg Med 2001;37(6):711–9.

Gaebler JW. Pharyngitis and tonsillitis. In: Finberg L, Kleinman RE, (editors):. Saunders Manual of Pediatric Practice. 2nd ed. Philadelphia: WB Saunders; p. 710–4.

Gibofsky A, Zabriskie JB. Treatment and prevention of acute rheumatic fever. UpToDate Online 16.2 [online text]. Available at http://www.UpToDate.com/patients/content/topic.do?topicKey=~bzzs5y48epRIMb&selectedTitle=1~81&source=search_result (accessed May 20, 2009).

McIsaac WJ, Kellner JD, Aufricht P, et al. Empirical validation of guidelines for the management of pharyngitis in children and adults. JAMA 2004;291(13):1587–95 [Erratum in JAMA 2005;294(21):2700].

National Institute of Allergy and Infectious Diseases. Severe Strep Infections [online health information]. Available at: http://www3.niaid.nih.gov/topics/strep [accessed May 20, 2009].

Pavone P, Parano E, Rizzo R, Trifiletti RR. Autoimmune neuropsychiatric disorders associated with streptococcal infection: Sydenham chorea, PANDAS, and PANDAS variants. J Child Neurol 2006;21(9):727–36.

Vincent MT, Celestin N, Hussain AN. Pharyngitis. Am Fam Physician 2004;69(6):1465–70.

Wald ER. Approach to diagnosis of acute infectious pharyngitis in children and adolescents. UpToDate Online 16.2 [online text]. Available at:http://www.UpToDate.com/patients/content/topic.do?topicKey=~TNhvxk/E3E/bOv&selectedTitle=4~150&source=search_result [accessed May 20, 2009].

Wald ER, Green MD, Schwartz B, Barbadora K. A streptococcal score card revisited. Pediatr Emerg Care 1998;14(2):109–11.

The Respiratory System

Acute Respiratory Failure

Method of
Scott K. Epstein, MD

The respiratory system serves many complex physiologic functions, the most important of which is gas exchange. Using the interface between the alveolar space and capillaries, O_2 is taken up and CO_2 is eliminated. Acute respiratory failure, a life-threatening entity, is present when this system fails, over the course of minutes to hours, resulting in hypoxemia (type I) or hypercapnia (type II), or both. Most patients with acute respiratory failure present with dyspnea, although the correlation with disease severity is poor. Indeed, dyspnea might seem mild in those with baseline chronic respiratory failure, and it might be absent in those with an underlying neurologic process (e.g., drug overdose). Other symptoms and signs such as cough, chest pain, orthopnea, fever, tachypnea, rales, and wheezing are insensitive and nonspecific.

This chapter outlines the general pathophysiology and therapeutic approach to acute respiratory failure by using the examples of three common entities: acute lung injury (ALI), cardiogenic pulmonary edema (congestive heart failure [CHF]), and acute exacerbation of chronic obstructive pulmonary disease (COPD).

Definitions and Pathophysiology

ACUTE HYPOXIC RESPIRATORY FAILURE

Hypoxic respiratory failure is conventionally defined as an arterial oxygen tension (Pao_2) of less than 60 mm Hg. Because this definition ignores the inspired fraction of oxygen (Fio_2), some favor a Pao_2/Fio_2 ratio of less than 300. To account for the arterial CO_2 tension ($Paco_2$), others favor an alveolar–arterial (A–a) O_2 gradient greater than 250 mm Hg, using the equation

$$A - a \ O_2 \ gradient = PAo_2 - Pao_2$$
$$= (713 \times Fio_2) - (PAo_2 + Paco_2/0.8)$$

where 713 is the barometric pressure (760) minus the water vapor pressure. A normal A–a O_2 is less than 10 mm Hg, but this threshold value increases with age. The determination of Pao_2 requires an invasive test, an arterial blood gas. Oxygenation can be continuously monitored noninvasively by pulse oximetry, which provides an estimate of arterial oxygen saturation (Sao_2). In general, an Sao_2 of 0.90 corresponds to a Pao_2 of 60 mm Hg, but the relation depends on temperature, pH, $Paco_2$, and 2,3-diphosphoglycerate (2,3-DPG).

Accuracy is adversely affected by low perfusion states, dark skin pigmentation, nail polish, dyshemoglobins (e.g., carboxyhemoglobin, methemoglobin), intravascular dyes, motion, and ambient light.

Clinicians tend to focus on Pao_2 and Sao_2, but the real parameter of interest is O_2 delivery (Do_2) to organs and tissues. Do_2 depends on cardiac output and O_2 carrying capacity of arterialized blood (Cao_2):

$$Do_2 = CO \times Cao_2$$

where

$$Cao_2 = k(Hb \times Sao_2) + 0.003 \ Pao_2$$

where k is a constant. Do_2 decreases when cardiac output or hemoglobin is reduced despite a normal Pao_2 and Sao_2. The peripheral response to reduced Do_2 is an increased O_2 extraction ratio (O_2ER), allowing oxygen uptake ($\dot{V}o_2$), an indicator of metabolic demand, to remain constant. Cellular and organ dysfunction occurs when Do_2 and O_2ER are outstripped by metabolic demand. The balance between Do_2 and demand can be estimated by examining the mixed venous O_2 saturation (Mvo_2) using the rearranged Fick equation:

$$Mvo_2 = Sao_2 - (\dot{V}o_2/CO \times Hb)$$

When Mvo_2 falls below 65% to 75%, imbalance is present.

When cellular injury is present, extraction capabilities are limited and cellular hypoxia occurs despite "adequate" Do_2. Under these circumstances, the Mvo_2 can be paradoxically normal. These parameters can be determined using a pulmonary artery catheter. The data obtained may be useful in individual patients, but randomized, controlled trials show no benefit when the pulmonary artery catheter is used routinely to guide therapy.

The pathophysiologic mechanisms of type I respiratory failure are listed in Table 1. The most common mechanism is ventilation–perfusion ($\dot{V}/\dot{Q}$) mismatch, characterized by a widened A–ao$_2$ gradient, a dramatic increase in Pao_2 in response to supplemental O_2, and a variable $Paco_2$. When areas of low $\dot{V}/\dot{Q}$ predominate (e.g., reduced ventilation with normal perfusion), the $Paco_2$ may be low as the patient hyperventilates in an effort (only partially effective) to increase the Pao_2. When areas of high $\dot{V}/\dot{Q}$ predominate, much ventilation is wasted, and hypercapnia is also present. Areas of lung that are perfused but not ventilated characterize shunt. The resulting fall in Pao_2 depends on the percentage of cardiac output circulating through the shunt and the O_2 content of that blood. Supplemental O_2 has minimal or small effect on Pao_2 because the shunted blood is not exposed to the increased Fio_2. Therefore, treatment is aimed at decreasing shunt by improving ventilation to the affected area or reducing perfusion to that area. When shunt results from a unilateral process (e.g., pneumonia, atelectasis), placing the good lung down decreases shunt perfusion, and oxygenation improves.

TABLE 1 Pathophysiologic Mechanisms of Acute Hypoxic Respiratory Failure

Mechanism	A–ao$_2$ Gradient	Paco$_2$	Response to 100% O$_2$	Cause
Diffusion abnormality	↑	↑ normal	↑↑	Severe interstitial lung disease
Hypoventilation	Normal	↑	↑↑↑	Narcotic overdose, obesity hypoventilation syndrome, respiratory muscle weakness
↓ Fio$_2$	Normal	Usually ↓	↑↑↑	High altitude, smoke inhalation
↓ Mvo$_2$	↑	Usually ↓	↑	ALI, shock, CHF, PE
Shunt	↑	Usually ↓	None or ↑	ALI, CHF, atelectasis, PE
V̇/Q̇ mismatch	↑	↑, normal, ↓	↑↑↑	Acute exacerbation of COPD, asthma, PE

↑ = increased; ↓ = decreased; A–ao$_2$ = alveolar–arterial O$_2$; ALI = acute lung injury; CHF = cardiogenic pulmonary edema; COPD = chronic obstructive pulmonary disease; Fio$_2$ = fraction of inspired oxygen; Mvo$_2$ = mixed venous oxygen saturation; Paco$_2$ = partial pressure of arterial CO$_2$; PE = pulmonary embolism: V̇/Q̇ = ventilation–perfusion ratio.

ACUTE HYPERCAPNEIC RESPIRATORY FAILURE

Hypercapneic respiratory failure is defined as a Paco$_2$ greater than 45 mm Hg. The equation used to determine Paco$_2$ provides insight into the three basic mechanisms underlying hypercapnia:

$$\text{Paco}_2 = k(\dot{V}\text{Co}_2)/V_E(1 - V_D/V_T)$$

where k is a constant, V_E is total minute ventilation (respiratory rate times tidal volume) and V_D/V_T is the dead space. Therefore, hypercapnia can result from increased CO$_2$ production ($V\text{co}_2$), increased physiologic dead space (V_D/V_T), and decreased minute ventilation (Box 1). Increased $\dot{V}\text{Co}_2$ alone is usually insufficient to cause hypercapnia because the respiratory system responds by increasing minute ventilation to keep Paco$_2$ normal (37–43 mm Hg). Conversely, with abnormalities of respiratory muscle function or respiratory drive or with increased dead space (and diminished reserve), the respiratory response to increased $\dot{V}\text{Co}_2$ may be insufficient, and hypercapnia results.

Treatment

Treatment of acute hypoxemic and hypercapneic respiratory failure combines nonspecific (e.g., supplemental O$_2$, mechanical ventilation) and specific therapy (Boxes 2 and 3).

BOX 1   Pathophysiologic Mechanisms of Hypercapnia

Increased Carbon Dioxide Production ($\dot{V}\text{co}_2$)
Fever
Overfeeding
Seizure
Sepsis
Thyrotoxicosis

Decreased Ventilation (V_E)
Depressed respiratory drive
Phrenic nerve injury
Respiratory muscle weakness

Increased Dead Space (V_D/V_T)
Acute exacerbation of chronic obstructive pulmonary disease
Interstitial lung disease
Pulmonary vascular disease

OXYGEN THERAPY

In the hospital, 100% O$_2$ is supplied from a wall source with a regulator determining flow rate in liters per minute. The final delivered oxygen concentration (Fio$_2$) depends on this flow rate and the amount of room air breathed by the patient. The O$_2$ flow rate is almost never sufficient to meet all of the patient's ventilatory demands, so varying amounts of room air are entrained to meet these needs. The final inspired oxygen concentration depends on

BOX 2   Causes of and Treatments for Acute Hypoxemic Respiratory Failure

Acute Exacerbation of Chronic Obstructive Pulmonary Disease
Antibiotics
Bronchodilators
Systemic steroids

Acute Lung Injury or Acute Respiratory Distress Syndomre
Efforts to decrease lung water
Lung-protective mechanical ventilation

Congestive Heart Failure
Afterload reduction
Diuretics
Inotropes

Lobar Collapse or Atelectasis
Bronchoscopy
Pulmonary toilet (airway suctioning to improve clearance of secretions)

Pneumonia
Antibiotics
Chest physiotherapy

Pneumothorax
Tube thoracostomy to drain pleural air and facilitate lung re-expansion

Pulmonary Embolism
Anticoagulation
Thrombolytic therapy

Status Asthmaticus
Bronchodilators
Systemic steroids

BOX 3 Causes of and Treatments for Acute Hypercapneic Respiratory Failure

Acute Exacerbation of Chronic Obstructive Pulmonary Disease
Antibiotics
Bronchodilators
Systemic steroids

Acute Respiratory Muscle Weakness (e.g., myasthenic crisis)
Acetylcholinesterase therapy

Drug Overdose
Flumazenil (Romazicon)
Naloxone (Narcan)
Other antidotes

Guillain-Barré Syndrome
Immunoglobulin
Plasmapheresis

Spinal Cord Injury
Intravenous methylprednisolone

Status Asthmaticus
Bronchodilators
Systemic steroids

Toxin (e.g., botulinum toxin)
Antitoxin

binding of CO_2, and minute ventilation inadequate for the amount of CO_2 produced. Therefore, the goal in these patients is to achieve a Pao_2 of 55 to 60 mm Hg (Sao_2 88%–90%) with low-flow oxygen (~24%–28% O_2). If this (often delicate) balance between maintaining tissue oxygenation and avoiding significant respiratory acidosis cannot be achieved, short-term mechanical ventilation may be required. In most nonhypercapneic patients, high flow of oxygen (50%–100%) can be administered safely for 24 hours with a goal Pao_2 of between 65 and 80 mm Hg.

MECHANICAL VENTILATION

Mechanical ventilation can be delivered noninvasively through a tight-fitting face mask or invasively via an endotracheal tube. The goals of mechanical ventilation are to correct severe arterial blood gas abnormalities, provide respiratory support while specific therapy is used, and unload and rest the respiratory muscles. The ventilator should be set to optimize patient–ventilator interaction and avoid dynamic hyperinflation and intrinsic positive end-expiratory pressure (PEEPi). PEEPi can worsen gas exchange, predispose to barotrauma, and cause hypotension.

Noninvasive Ventilation

Noninvasive ventilation is most commonly applied as continuous positive airway pressure (CPAP), when airway pressure is kept constant throughout the respiratory cycle, or by bilevel positive airway pressure (BiPAP), when inspiratory pressure support actively assists each inspiration. Noninvasive ventilation offers numerous advantages over invasive ventilation, including increased comfort; maintenance of normal swallowing, speech, and cough; less need for sedation; and avoiding the trauma of intubation.

The effective application of noninvasive ventilation starts with carefully explaining the procedure to the patient, followed by selection of a proper-fitting face mask. The mask is placed close to the face to acclimate the patient to high inspiratory flow. The mask is then secured using straps (but not too tightly), and ventilator settings are adjusted to minimize leak and ensure comfort. The patient is reassessed frequently. Failure to improve within 2 to 4 hours (e.g., reduction in dyspnea, respiratory rate, accessory muscle use, and hypercapnia) signals noninvasive ventilation failure and need for intubation.

Noninvasive ventilation improves outcome (avoids intubation, decreases length of stay, improves survival) in a number of conditions (Table 3). Although randomized, controlled trials show dramatic benefit in AECOPD, other studies show no or uncertain benefit in

the relative fraction of each gas, total minute ventilation, and the pattern of breathing (including the inspiratory to expiratory ratio). O_2 may be administered using nasal prongs, a facial mask, or high-flow devices designed to deliver higher Fio_2 (Table 2).

In hypercapneic patients (e.g., with acute exacerbation of COPD), high-flow O_2 can lead to worsening hypercapnia and acute respiratory acidosis. The mechanisms are multifactorial: worsening $\dot{V}/\dot{Q}$ matching (increased dead space), decreased intracellular

TABLE 2 Short-Term Oxygen Delivery Systems

Delivery System	O₂ Flow Rate (L/min)	Fio₂ Range	Comments
Basic Systems			
Nasal cannula (prongs)	1–6	0.22–0.40	Comfortable Facilitates communication and oral intake Humidification required at high flow rates
Simple masks	5–6	0.30–0.50	Mask acts as reservoir to increase Fio₂ High flow combats CO₂ rebreathing Less comfortable Must be removed to facilitate communication and oral intake Easily displaced with movement
Reservoir Masks			
Nonrebreathing	4–10	0.60–1.00	One-way valve between the mask and the reservoir bag Inspired O₂ from wall source and reservoir bag
Partial rebreathing	5–10	0.35–0.90	Lacks one-way valve
Venturi masks	4–10	0.24–0.40	Uses Bernoulli principle (fixed amount of entrained room air added to O₂) Maximum delivered Fio₂ can be controlled Often used in COPD to avoid excessive Fio₂ and risk for hypercapnia

COPD = chronic obstructive pulmonary disease; Fio₂ = fraction of inspired oxygen.

TABLE 3 Efficacy of Noninvasive Ventilation in Various Conditions

Condition	Quality of Evidence	Comment
AECOPD	Strong	↓ Need for intubation ↑ Survival
Acute cardiogenic pulmonary edema	Strong	↓ Need for intubation ↑ Survival
Hypoxemic respiratory in ICH with diffuse pulmonary infiltrates	Strong	↓ Need for intubation ↑ Survival
Facilitating weaning in select patients	Strong	↓ Duration of intubation Most effective in AECOPD
High risk for extubation failure	Strong	↓ Need for reintubation
Extubation failure in heterogeneous patient population	Moderate	Not effective, two RCTs
Routinely after extubation	Moderate	Not effective, single RCT
Extubation failure in acute exacerbation of COPD	Moderate	Single case-control study
Type I RF, diffuse infiltrates, not ICH	Moderate	↓ Need for intubation
Asthma	No RCTs	Probably effective in ↓ need for intubation
Obesity hypoventilation	No RCTs	Probably effective in ↓ need for intubation
Postoperative respiratory failure	Small RCTs	Probably effective in ↓ need for reintubation
Do not intubate patients	Observational studies	Most effective with CHF, COPD
Pulmonary fibrosis	Observational studies	Not effective

AECOPD = acute exacerbation of chronic obstructive pulmonary disease; CHF = cardiogenic pulmonary edema; COPD = chronic obstructive pulmonary disease; Fio_2 = fraction of inspired oxygen; ICH = immunocompromised host; RCT = randomized, controlled trial; RF = respiratory failure.

BOX 4   Screening Criteria to Assess Readiness to Undergo a Trial of Spontaneous Breathing

Required Criteria
$Pao_2/Fio_2 \geq 150$ or $Sao_2 \geq 90\%$ or $Fio_2 \leq 40\%$ and (PEEP) ≤ 5 cm H_2O
Absence of hypotension

Additional Criteria (optional criteria)
Weaning parameters*
- Negative inspiratory force < −20- to −25 cm H_2O
- Respiratory rate (f) $\leq$35 breaths/min
- Spontaneous tidal volume (V_T) > 5mL/kg
- $f/V_T < 105$ breaths/L/min

Absence of significant anemia (e.g., Hb $\geq$ 8–10 mg/dL)
Absence of fever (e.g., core temperature $\leq$38.5°C)
Adequate mental status: patient awake and alert or easily aroused

---

*Recent studies indicate that these parameters are often unnecessary in deciding whether to initiate trials of spontaneous breathing.
Hb = hemoglobin; PEEP = positive end-expiratory pressure

dysfunction can result. Most patients require sedation, but excessive sedation levels are associated with worse outcomes. Therefore, strategies to minimize continuous intravenous sedation using a sedation protocol or once-daily interruption of sedation are recommended.

Invasive mechanical ventilation, especially when prolonged, is associated with numerous complications including ventilator-associated pneumonia, sinusitis, airway injury, thromboembolism, and gastrointestinal bleeding. Therefore, once significant clinical improvement occurs efforts should focus on rapidly removing the patient from the ventilator. This is achieved by daily screening for readiness (Box 4) followed by a 30- to 120-minute spontaneous breathing trial on minimal or no ventilator support. Patients tolerating the spontaneous breathing trial are extubated if they have a good cough, manageable respiratory secretions, and an adequate mental status to protect the airway. Approximately 25% of patients do not tolerate the spontaneous breathing trial; they should be returned to full ventilator support for 24 hours and undergo careful evaluation for reversible causes. The clinician should consider a more gradual approach to weaning these patients.

Specific Causes of Acute Respiratory Failure

ACUTE EXACERBATION OF CHRONIC OBSTRUCTIVE PULMONARY DISEASE

Patients with COPD can experience two or three exacerbations per year, especially if they are actively smoking, resulting in 500,000 hospitalizations every year in the United States. Hospital mortality ranges from 2% to 11%, rising to 25% for those requiring critical care.

Acute exacerbation of COPD is defined by increased sputum volume, purulence, and dyspnea. Physical examination is notable for tachypnea, use of accessory respiratory muscles, diminished breath sounds, prolonged expiratory phase with wheezing, thoraco-abdominal paradox (inward inspiratory abdominal motion), and Hoover's sign (inward inspiratory motion of the lower rib cage). The latter two physical signs indicate the presence of dynamic hyperinflation and diaphragmatic dysfunction. Acute exacerbation of COPD is further characterized by hypoxemia (resulting from $\dot{V}/\dot{Q}$ mismatch) and hypercapnia. Patients with more severe underlying disease might demonstrate evidence of acute and chronic respiratory acidosis.

community acquired pneumonia, acute respiratory distress syndrome (ARDS), pulmonary fibrosis, and routinely after planned extubation. One mechanism for improved outcome is the reduction in infection (pneumonia, sepsis) seen with noninvasive ventilation compared with intubated patients. Noninvasive ventilation should not be used in the presence of respiratory arrest, shock, excessive secretions, inability to protect the airway, an agitated or uncooperative patient, and facial abnormalities that preclude proper application of the mask.

Invasive Ventilation

Invasive mechanical ventilation is delivered via an endotracheal tube. The set parameters include Fio_2 and positive end-expiratory pressure (PEEP). For volume-assist control, the clinician chooses respiratory rate and tidal volume. For pressure support, the clinician chooses the inspiratory pressure level above PEEP, and the patient determines respiratory rate. The resulting tidal volume depends on inspiratory pressure level and patient factors including respiratory muscle strength and respiratory system mechanics. Initially the ventilator is set to meet most of the patient's minute ventilation, allowing respiratory muscle rest. Such full support should not be prolonged because diaphragmatic

CURRENT DIAGNOSIS

- History and physical examination can give insight into the etiology of hypoxic and hypercapneic respiratory failure but may be insufficient to make a definitive diagnosis and guide therapy.
- An arterial blood gas is mandatory to define severity and whether hypoxic or hypercapneic (or both) respiratory failure is present.
- Additional diagnostic modalities, including chest radiograph, electrocardiogram, cardiac laboratory tests (troponin, brain natriuretic peptide), echocardiography, and selected use of a pulmonary artery catheter, can help identify a specific etiology.

Etiology and Diagnosis

Approximately 50% of acute exacerbations of COPD result from bacterial infection (e.g., *Pneumococcus* species, *Haemophilus influenzae*, *Moraxella catarrhalis*, and *Pseudomonas* species). The remainder result from viral infection and air pollution. In many cases a cause cannot be identified, although there is increasing appreciation that acute myocardial infarction and pulmonary embolism may be present in up to 25%. Pulmonary embolism may be suggested by a $Paco_2$ lower than baseline and the need for a higher than expected Fio_2 to maintain the Sao_2 at greater than 90%. Computed tomographic pulmonary arteriogram is recommended to make the diagnosis, because $\dot{V}/\dot{Q}$ scanning is nondiagnostic in nearly one half of COPD patients, and false-positive high-probability scans occur.

Treatment

Treatment for acute exacerbation of COPD is based on high-quality evidence consisting of numerous randomized, controlled trials and well-performed meta-analyses. Bronchodilator therapy is essential. Nebulized combination therapy (albuterol and ipratropium [Duo-Neb]) is effective, but it is not demonstrably superior to single-agent therapy delivered via a metered-dose inhaler. Theophylline should generally be avoided because toxicity outweighs benefits.

Antibiotics improve outcome, especially in the presence of fever and increased sputum purulence and volume. Older agents, such as amoxicillin and tetracycline, appear to be less effective than newer macrolides and fluoroquinalones.

Corticosteroids enhance β-agonist activity and counteract the inflammatory state seen in acute exacerbations of COPD. Oral prednisone at a dose of 30 to 40 mg is recommended. Intravenous therapy (methylprednisolone [SoluMedrol] 125 mg every 6 hours for 72 hours followed by oral prednisone) should be used in the critically ill patient or when response to oral therapy is suboptimal.

There is no role for mucolytic agents or chest physiotherapy.

Admission to the intensive care unit (ICU) is indicated for patients with hemodynamic instability, confusion, lethargy and coma, severe dyspnea unresponsive to emergency management, or severely abnormal gas exchange despite initial therapy (Pao_2 <40 mm Hg, $Paco_2$ >60 mm Hg, pH <7.25).

Randomized, controlled trials demonstrate that noninvasive ventilation decreases the risk for intubation and improves survival in acute exacerbations of COPD when there are severe dyspnea, hypoxemia, tachypnea, and significant respiratory acidosis ($Paco_2$ >45 mm Hg and pH <7.35). Patients who fail noninvasive ventilation or who are not candidates require intubation and mechanical ventilation.

A major risk is the development of dynamic hyperinflation (PEEPi), which can worsen gas exchange, predispose to barotrauma (e.g., pneumothorax), and cause hypotension. PEEPi is minimized by keeping delivered minute ventilation at 5 L/min or less; this is achieved by lowering tidal volume (e.g., 6 mL/kg ideal body weight) or respiratory rate (8–10 breaths/min), or by increasing inspiratory flow rate, allowing more time for expiration. PEEPi is suggested by an elevated plateau pressure or persistent expiratory flow at the

CURRENT THERAPY

- Treatment of acute respiratory failure often begins with nonspecific approaches such as oxygen and mechanical ventilation (noninvasive or invasive).
- The goal of mechanical ventilation is to improve gas exchange and rest the respiratory muscles while waiting for the beneficial effects of specific therapy aimed at the underlying cause (e.g., bronchodilators, antibiotics, and corticosteroids in acute exacerbations of chronic obstructive pulmonary disease [COPD]).
- Noninvasive ventilation avoids many complications associated with invasive ventilation and improves outcomes for patients with acute cardiogenic pulmonary edema and acute exacerbations of COPD.
- Invasive mechanical ventilation can be lifesaving but can cause clinical deterioration if not properly administered.
- Using low tidal volumes (6 mL/kg ideal body weight) can help avoid dangerous dynamic hyperinflation in acute exacerbations of COPD and further lung injury in acute lung injury (e.g., volutrauma, barotrauma).
- Once signs of improvement are evident, focus rapidly shifts to liberating the patient from the ventilator using spontaneous breathing trials to assess the need for ventilatory support followed by airway assessment to determine readiness for extubation.

time of the next ventilator breath. PEEPi can also increase work of breathing by increasing the patient's inspiratory effort to trigger the ventilator. When extrinsic PEEP is at or just below the PEEPi level, the patient triggers more easily and work of breathing is reduced.

The approach to weaning and extubation in acute exacerbations of COPD is similar to that for other conditions, although the risk of failing a spontaneous breathing trial is increased.

ACUTE LUNG INJURY AND ACUTE RESPIRATORY DISTRESS SYNDROME

ALI is the result of an acute process and is characterized by hypoxemia (Pao_2/Fio_2 < 300), bilateral diffuse alveolar infiltrates, and no evidence of cardiac etiology. When the Pao_2/Fio_2 is less than 200, the patient is said to have ARDS. ALI results from pulmonary and extrapulmonary etiologies. Pulmonary causes include pneumonia, gastric aspiration, near drowning, toxic gas inhalation, and lung contusion. Extrapulmonary causes include sepsis, pancreatitis, fat embolism, drug overdose, nonthoracic trauma, and massive transfusion. Conditions that can mimic the clinical findings of ALI include CHF, diffuse alveolar hemorrhage (DAH), acute cryptogenic organizing pneumonia (COP), and acute eosinophilic pneumonia (AEP). These latter three entities can be diagnosed by bronchoscopy (DAH, AEP) or by open lung biopsy (COP), all are treated with high doses of corticosteroids. Studies indicate that corticosteroids do not improve the outcome of ALI/ARDS.

Differentiating cardiogenic pulmonary edema from ALI can be challenging, especially because these conditions can coexist. Physical findings of jugular venous distention and a positive third heart sound, abnormal electrocardiogram (ECG), elevated brain natruretic peptide (BNP), and positive cardiac enzymes (troponin) point to a cardiac etiology. A chest radiograph showing cardiomegaly, vascular redistribution, widened vascular pedicle, perihilar alveolar infiltrates and pleural effusions also suggest a cardiac cause. Bedside echocardiography can demonstrate reduced left ventricular function. A pulmonary artery catheter provides definitive evidence of an elevated pulmonary capillary wedge pressure and reduced cardiac output. That said, recent randomized, controlled trials demonstrate no improvement in survival with routine use of the pulmonary artery catheter in ALI.

ALI causes heterogeneous effects in the lung, resulting in poorly ventilated, atelectatic, dependent regions of lung. Traditional tidal volumes of 10 to 15 mL/kg can cause lung injury by creating significant shear stress by repeatedly opening these atelectatic areas (atelectrauma) and overdistending less affected areas (volutrauma, barotrauma). Indeed, experimental and clinical studies demonstrate that a lung-protective strategy, using a tidal volume of 6 mL/kg ideal body weight, improves survival in ALI. Using small tidal volumes often results in significant hypercapnia, which can have an independent protective effect (permissive hypercapnia). The application of PEEP recruits and opens atelectatic lung, thereby reducing harmful shear forces. The optimal level of PEEP remains uncertain: A recent multicenter study found no difference in mortality in patients randomized to high (~14 cm H_2O) or low (~8 cm H_2O) PEEP when all patients received a tidal volume of 6 mL/kg ideal body weight.

CARDIOGENIC PULMONARY EDEMA

CHF occurs in patients with cardiomyopathy or acutely when ischemia is present. Diagnosis is suggested by jugular venous distension, a third heart sound, diffuse rales, abnormal ECG, and a chest radiograph showing cardiomegaly, diffuse alveolar infiltrates, and bilateral pleural effusion. A markedly elevated BNP or pro-BNP further suggests a cardiac etiology.

Therapy consists of oxygen, nitrates, diuretics, afterload reduction, and anti-ischemic therapy if the history or ECG is suggestive. Mechanical ventilation produces positive intrathoracic pressure, which improves cardiac function by decreasing both left ventricular preload and afterload, reversing hypoxemia, and decreasing work of breathing. In hemodynamically stable patients without active ischemia, CPAP at levels of 8 to 12 cm H_2O should be used. A meta-analysis of 15 randomized, controlled trials showed that noninvasive ventilation decreased the need for intubation and improved survival. CPAP and BiPAP appear to be equivalent, although many prefer BiPAP when hypercapnia is present.

Because cardiogenic pulmonary edema is rapidly reversible, intubated patients can often be extubated within 24 hours. That said, the transition from positive pressure ventilation to negative ventilation (e.g., T-piece or extubation) can precipitate pulmonary edema.

REFERENCES

Acute Respiratory Distress Syndrome Network. Ventilation with lower tidal volumes as compared with traditional tidal volumes for acute lung injury and the acute respiratory distress syndrome. N Engl J Med 2000;342:1301–8.

Bach PB, Brown C, Gelfand SE, et al. Management of acute exacerbations of chronic obstructive pulmonary disease: A summary and appraisal of published evidence. Ann Intern Med 2001;134:600–20.

Brower RG, Lanken PN, MacIntyre N, et al. Higher versus lower positive end-expiratory pressures in patients with the acute respiratory distress syndrome. N Engl J Med 2004;51:327–36.

Ely EW, Baker AM, Dunagan DP, et al. Effect on the duration of mechanical ventilation of identifying patients capable of breathing spontaneously. N Engl J Med 1996;335:1864–9.

Epstein SK. Complications in ventilator supported patients. In: Tobin M, editor. Principles and Practice of Mechanical Ventilation. New York: McGraw Hill; 2006. p. 877–902.

Kress JP, Pohlman AS, O'Connor MF, et al. Daily interruption of sedative infusions in critically ill patients undergoing mechanical ventilation. N Engl J Med 2000;342:1471–7.

MacIntyre NR, Cook DJ, Ely EW Jr, et al. Evidence-based guidelines for weaning and discontinuing ventilatory support: A collective task force facilitated by the American College of Chest Physicians, the American Association for Respiratory Care, and the American College of Critical Care Medicine. Chest 2001;120:375S–95S.

Majid A, Hill NS. Noninvasive ventilation for acute respiratory failure. Curr Opin Crit Care 2005;11:77–81.

Masip J, Orque M, Sanchez B, et al. Noninvasive ventilation in acute cardiogenic pulmonary edema: Systematic review and meta-analysis. JAMA 2005;294:3124–30.

Schumaker G, Epstein SK. Management of acute respiratory failure in acute exacerbations of COPD. Resp Care 2004;49:766–82.

Atelectasis

Method of
Christine L. Lau, MD, Alykhan S. Nagji, MD, and Matthew D. Taylor, MD

Atelectasis refers to the collapse of alveoli that affects segmental or lobar regions of the lung or the entire lung and results in hypoventilation. However, recent studies have suggested that the alveoli are not collapsed but are filled with fluid and foam. These hypotheses are not mutually exclusive; collapsed alveoli and fluid- and foam-filled alveoli may be present concurrently in an atelectatic lung. Although atelectasis is considered a benign condition, early treatment, reversal, and prevention are essential to an overall improved outcome.

Etiology

COMPRESSION ATELECTASIS

Compression atelectasis occurs when the transmural pressure distending the alveolus is reduced to a level that allows the alveolus to collapse. To best illustrate this mechanism, consider the patient who has undergone induction of anesthesia. The diaphragm is relaxed and is displaced cephalad. In the supine position, the pleural pressures increase to the greatest extent in the dependent lung regions and can compress the adjacent lung tissue.

SURFACTANT IMPAIRMENT

Surfactant serves to reduce the alveolar surface tension, thereby stabilizing the alveoli and preventing collapse. Reduction in surfactant occurs with certain types of anesthesia. Studies have shown that hyperinflation by means of increased tidal volume, sequential air inflations to the total lung capacity, or even a single cycle of increased tidal volume can increase the release of surfactant, aiding in recruitment and stabilization of alveoli.

GAS RESORPTION

One mechanism by which gas resorption results in atelectasis involves the patent airway. In regions of the lung with increased ventilation compared to perfusion, which produces a ventilation/perfusion ($\dot{V}/\dot{Q}$) mismatch, there is low alveolar oxygen tension. Increasing the fraction of inspired oxygen (F_{IO_2}) initiates a cascade of events that increases alveolar oxygen tension (P_{AO_2}) and decreases alveolar nitrogen tension (P_{AN_2}), which results in loss of alveolar volume secondary to increased absorption of oxygen.

Another mechanism by which gas resorption leads to atelectasis occurs after complete airway occlusion. In such cases, gas is trapped distal to the obstruction. Gas uptake by the proximal blood flow continues without additional gas inflow. This causes the alveoli to collapse.

Pathophysiology

The trapping of air and hyperinflation of the alveoli are produced from the aforementioned mechanisms. The gases that are trapped are absorbed by the blood perfusing through that region of the lung, which eventually causes collapse of the alveoli. The atelectasis produces alveolar hypoxia and pulmonary vasoconstriction to prevent $\dot{V}/\dot{Q}$ mismatching and to minimize arterial hypoxia. This vascular response is effective only if a large part of the lung is not collapsed; otherwise, intrapulmonary shunting occurs.

CURRENT DIAGNOSIS

- Hypoxia
- Tachypnea
- Diminished breath sounds
- Wheezing
- Radiologic signs of atelectasis

Clinical Presentation

The signs and symptoms of atelectasis are often nonspecific. The natural course of atelectasis may lead to fever, cough, tachypnea, wheezing, rhonchi, and chest pain. On physical examination, atelectasis may manifest as an area of localized reduced breath sounds with constant wheeze or reduced chest wall expansion or both.

Diagnosis

Chest radiographs aid in the diagnosis of atelectasis. They provide both direct and indirect signs that may indicate an atelectatic etiology for the patient's symptoms.

Direct signs include:

- Displaced pulmonary vessels
- Air bronchograms
- Displacement of intralobar fissures (most reliable sign)

Indirect signs include:

- Pulmonary opacification
- Diaphragmatic elevation
- Hyperexpansion of unaffected lung
- Tracheal, heart, and mediastinal shift toward atelectic side
- Shift of the hilum toward the collapsed lobe
- Segmental ipsilateral rib approximation

Treatment

Treatment of atelectasis is geared toward the underlying cause. It is important to recognize respiratory distress and to intubate the patient if appropriate.

If the etiology is that of an obstructive atelectasis, chest percussion or vibration and nasotracheal or bronchoscopic suctioning may help in the clearing of secretions. With regard to lung re-expansion, incentive spirometry, continuous or intermittent positive-pressure ventilation, and early ambulation may be used.

Those patients who have a nonobstructive atelectasis caused by a pneumothorax or pleural effusion benefit from tube thoracostomy or thoracentesis. Additionally, appropriate pain management in the postoperative setting allows for proper ventilation.

CURRENT THERAPY

- Chest percussion or vibration
- Nasotracheal or bronchoscopic suctioning
- Incentive spirometry
- Positive-pressure ventilation
- Ambulation
- Postoperative pain control

REFERENCES

Duggan M, Kavanagh BP. Pulmonary atelectasis: A pathogenic perioperative entity. Anesthesiology 2005;102:838–54.

Duggan M, Kavanagh BP. Atelectasis in the perioperative patient. Curr Opin Anaesthesiol 2007;20:37–42.

Hubmayr RD. Perspective on lung injury and recruitment: A skeptical look at the opening and collapse story. Am J Respir Crit Care Med 2002;165:1647–53.

Peroni DG, Boner AL. Atelectasis: Mechanisms, diagnosis and management. Paediatr Respir Rev 2000;1:274–8.

Wagner PD, Laravuso RB, Uhl RR, West JB. Continuous distributions of ventilation-perfusion ratios in normal subjects breathing air and 100 per cent O2. J Clin Invest 1974;54:54–68.

Management of Chronic Obstructive Pulmonary Disease

Method of
Tamara Simpson, MD, and Jay Peters, MD

Chronic obstructive pulmonary disease (COPD) is characterized by airflow limitation that is not fully reversible. The airflow limitation is usually both progressive and associated with an abnormal inflammatory response of the lungs to noxious particles of gases. Under the direction of the National Heart, Lung, and Blood Institute (NHLBI) and the World Health Organization (WHO), collaborative guidelines on the diagnosis and management of chronic obstructive pulmonary disease (COPD) have been assembled by an expert panel: the Global Initiative for Chronic Obstructive Lung Disease (GOLD). These guidelines define the classifications of COPD on the basis of both severity and type of symptoms and explore all new information on the diagnosis and treatment of COPD. The GOLD initiative aims to improve prevention and management of COPD through a concerted worldwide effort of people involved in all facets of health care policy and to encourage a renewed research interest in this extremely prevalent disease.

To assure that recommendations for management of COPD are based on current scientific literature, the GOLD program established a science committee to update the sections of the report on recommendations for management of COPD each year. Although the update of these sections will occur each year and will be posted on the Web site (http://www.goldcopd.com), the full report will be updated and printed every 5 years. The latest update, including new modifications of management, was published in 2007.

Pathophysiology

The pathophysiology of COPD is somewhat different in various patients, and the terms *emphysema* or *chronic bronchitis* were used in the past. Both of these disorders cause airway obstruction. Emphysema is defined pathologically as abnormal permanent enlargement of airspaces distal to the terminal bronchioles, accompanied by destruction of their walls and without obvious fibrosis. This tissue destruction results in enlargement of proximal and distal airspaces and can ultimately form bullae in the lung parenchyma. These bullae result in loss of surface area for gas exchange in the involved lungs. There is also a genetically inherited form of emphysema which is caused by the α_1-antitrypsin (AAT) deficiency. This disorder accounts for less than 1% of COPD cases in the United States. AAT is a protease inhibitor produced by the liver that circulates into tissues. Active proteases are released into the lung by lung macrophages, which can contribute to the development of emphysema. When patients smoke cigarettes, they also recruit a neutrophil population into their lungs. These neutrophils release neutrophil elastase (another type of protease) and other toxic molecules, which can destroy alveolar walls and may also contribute to the production of emphysema. AAT offers protection from these effects, but the protection found in normal people is inadequate in patients with AAT deficiency. Patients who develop emphysema despite normal levels of AAT usually develop emphysema in the fifth or sixth decades of life, whereas patients with AAT deficiency can develop emphysema as early as the third or fourth decades of life, depending on the extent of their deficiency and smoking history.

All patients developing emphysema should be evaluated for AAT deficiency at least once, especially if they present with COPD before the age of 45–50. A normal serum level of AAT is greater than 11 mmol/L (>80 mg/dL). Patients with low levels of AAT should be evaluated by a pulmonologist and may be candidates for AAT replacement therapy.

Chronic bronchitis is defined clinically as the presence of chronic, productive cough for 3 months during each of 2 consecutive years, and for which other causes of chronic cough are excluded. The other most common causes of chronic cough include asthma, gastric reflux, or postnasal drip secondary to sinus disease. The pathologic findings of chronic bronchitis are enlargement of tracheobronchial mucus glands, variable amounts of airway smooth-muscle hyperplasia, inflammation, and bronchial wall thickening. Abnormalities of small airways may be present as well and are accompanied by fibrosis and the presence of a mononuclear inflammatory process. The forced expiratory volume at 1 second (FEV_1) of a COPD patient is inversely proportional to the number of inflammatory cells in the airways. Patients with chronic bronchitis also have increased mucus hypersecretion, goblet cell metaplasia, increased submucosal gland formation, and abnormal matrix deposition.

The use of the terms *emphysema* or *chronic bronchitis* is no longer specified in the GOLD definition of COPD. The inflammation seen in COPD is different from that seen in asthma, but some obstructive lung disease patients do have pathologic changes that can be seen in both diseases, so some overlap does occur.

Epidemiology and Risk Factors

In the United States COPD is presently the fourth leading cause of death and affects more than 21 million people. Death rates have risen more than 22% in the last decade and the disease is responsible for approximately 700,000 hospital stays each year. The disease is now more common in women than men because of increasing amounts of cigarette smoking in women and increased susceptibility. The primary risk factor associated with the development of COPD, cigarette smoking, increases the death rate and disability caused by COPD and causes lung function to deteriorate over time much more rapidly than in a nonsmoker. Cigar and pipe smokers have greater COPD incidence than nonsmokers. Approximately 20% of smokers will develop COPD. The risk of development of COPD is increased in first-degree relatives of patients with COPD, which suggests the importance of genetic factors, but AAT deficiency is the only proved genetic risk factor in COPD. Exposures other than smoking that have been associated with COPD development include passive smoking, ambient air pollution, occupational dust and chemical exposure, and severe respiratory childhood infections.

Diagnosis

The diagnosis of COPD is suggested on the basis of symptoms, which may include those caused by the airway irritation (cough and sputum production) and those reflecting altered lung mechanics (dyspnea, wheezing, and occasionally chest pain). Individuals usually experience cough and sputum production years before the development of airflow limitation, while not all individuals with cough and sputum production go on to develop COPD.

Physical examination of individuals with COPD can reveal hyperinflation, wheezing, diminished breath sounds, hyperresonance, or prolonged expiration. Visual inspection during an examination can reveal signs of increased respiratory rate, increased anteroposterior (AP) chest diameter, hyperresonance to chest percussion, and

impaired respiratory muscle function. Patients with COPD commonly have a respiration rate greater than 16 breaths per minute, and often this is proportional to disease severity; patients with COPD severe enough to exhibit hypercapnia (partial pressure of arterial carbon dioxide [$PaCO_2$] greater than 45 mm Hg) may have breathing rates of greater than 25 breaths per minute. Absence of wheezing does not exclude COPD. Patients with end-stage COPD may adopt body positions that help relieve dyspnea, such as leaning forward or expiring through pursed lips. Use of accessory muscles for respiration, such as the use of the abdominal rectus muscle on expiration, is a sign of advanced disease. Other signs of hyperinflation may include decreased diaphragm movement, tracheal tug, or pulsus paradoxus greater than 20 mm Hg.

Patients with advanced COPD may also have central cyanosis, peripheral edema, and signs of cor pulmonale associated with right heart failure. Other objective findings often include arterial blood gas changes demonstrating hypercapnia, severe hypoxemia, compensated respiratory acidosis with elevated carbon dioxide (CO_2), tension and a normal pH, and elevated serum bicarbonate level. Morning headaches in COPD patients may be indicative of hypercapnia.

The diagnosis of COPD is confirmed by spirometry. The standard pulmonary function test used to measure airway obstruction is the forced expiratory spirogram. This test assesses the rate of change in volume that occurs as a function of time. Pulmonary functions useful in the evaluation of patients presenting with symptoms of COPD include FEV_1, the forced vital capacity (FVC), and the ratio of FEV_1/FVC. The FVC provides a measure of lung volume and the FEV_1 and FEV_1/FVC both provide a measure of obstruction. In most of these patients, other abnormal lung volumes that may exist include increases in both the total lung capacity (TLC) and the residual volume (RV). These increases in lung volumes are caused by hyperinflation and air trapping of the lungs.

An FEV_1/FVC less than 70% of predicted confirms the presence of airflow obstruction. The FEV_1 serves as a marker of severity of the airflow obstruction. Other pulmonary function tests such as the flow volume loop or diffusing capacity for carbon monoxide (DL_{CO}) can help rule out other types of airway obstruction or help quantitate a patient's risk for surgery. Chest radiographs are only helpful for diagnosis in COPD if there are signs of bullous disease or severe hyperinflation or loss of vascular markings. These findings may overlap with other forms of obstructive lung disease. Computed tomography (CT) scanning can show the location of bullous disease which can be helpful in narrowing the differential diagnosis of a patient with airway obstruction and also may be used to help determine if a patient is a candidate for lung reduction surgery.

COPD Classification

The GOLD committee presented a new classification of COPD. The management of COPD is largely symptom driven, and there is only an imperfect relationship between the degree of airflow limitation and the presence of symptoms. The staging therefore is aimed at practical implementation and should be only regarded as an educational tool, and a general indication of the approach to management. All FEV_1 values refer to postbronchodilator FEV_1.

This classification includes stages I to IV (Figure 1).

Stage I: Mild COPD—Characterized by mild airflow limitation (FEV_1/FVC <70% but FEV_1 >80% predicted) and usually, but not always, chronic cough and sputum production. At this stage, the individual may be unaware of abnormal lung function.

Stage II: Moderate COPD—Characterized by worsening airflow limitation (<50% FEV_1 <80% predicted) and usually the progression of symptoms, with shortness of breath typically developing on exertion. This is the stage at which most patients typically first seek medical attention because of dyspnea or an exacerbation of their disease.

Stage III: Severe COPD—Characterized by further worsening of airflow limitation (<30% FEV_1 <50% predicted), increased

Characteristics		I: Mild	II: Moderate	III: Severe	IV: Very severe
Characteristics		• $FEV_1/FVC < 70\%$ • $FEV_1 \geq 80\%$ • With or without symptoms	• $FEV_1/FVC < 70\%$ • $50\% \leq FEV_1 < 80\%$ • With or without symptoms	• $FEV_1/FVC < 70\%$ • $30\% \leq FEV_1 < 50\%$ • With or without symptoms	• $FEV_1/FVC < 70\%$ • $FEV_1 < 30\%$ or $FEV_1 < 50\%$ predicted plus chronic respiratory failure
		Avoidance of risk factor(s); influenza vaccination			
		Add short-acting bronchodilator when needed			
			Add regular treatment with one or more long-acting bronchodilators *Add* rehabilitation		
				Add inhaled glucocorticosteroid if repeated exacerbations	
					Add long-term oxygen if chronic respiratory failure. Consider surgical treatments

FIGURE 1. Therapy for different stages of COPD

shortness of breath, and repeated exacerbations which have an impact on the patient's quality of life.

Stage IV: Very Severe COPD—Characterized by severe air-flow limitation (FEV_1 <30% predicted) or the presence of chronic respiratory failure. Patients may have very severe (Stage IV) COPD even if the FEV_1 is greater than 30% predicted, if respiratory failure is present. At this stage, quality of life is appreciably impaired and exacerbations may be life-threatening.

Management of Stable COPD

The general guidelines to management of COPD include the avoidance of risk factors to prevent disease progression and pharmacotherapy as needed to control symptoms. In addition, patient education including counseling about smoking cessation, instruction in physical exercise, and nutritional advice are necessary components of a comprehensive COPD management plan. The goals of management are to relieve symptoms, increase exercise tolerance, improve quality of life, prevent and treat complications, and decrease disease progression.

Smoking cessation is the single most effective (and cost-effective) intervention to reduce the risk of developing COPD and stop its progression. Comprehensive tobacco elimination policies and programs with clear and repeated nonsmoking messages should be delivered through every feasible system possible. Legislation to establish smoke-free schools, public facilities, and work environments should be encouraged by working with government officials, public health workers, and the public. Guidelines for smoking cessation were published by the U.S. Agency for Health Care Policy and Research (AHCPR) in 2000.

There are numerous effective pharmacotherapies for smoking cessation. Except in the presence of special circumstances, pharmacotherapy is recommended when counseling is insufficient. Nicotine replacement therapy in any form (nicotine gum, inhaler, nasal spray [Nicotrol NS], transdermal patch [Nicoderm], sublingual tablet [Nicorette Microtab],[2] or lozenge [Commit]) reliably increases long-term smoking abstinence rates. The antidepressants bupropion (Zyban) and the nicotinic receptor antagonist varenicline (Chantix), have been shown to significantly increase long-term quit rates. The antihypertensive drug clonidine (Catapres)[1] can also be used to help a patient quit smoking, but side effects should be carefully reviewed

with each patient. Special consideration should be given before using pharmacotherapy in selected populations including patients smoking fewer than 10 cigarettes per day, pregnant patients, and adolescent smokers.

The overall approach to managing stable COPD should be characterized by a stepwise increase in treatment, depending on the severity of the disease. The management strategy is based on an individualized assessment of disease severity and response to various therapies. Disease severity is determined by the severity of symptoms and airflow limitation (using pulmonary function measurements) and other factors such as the frequency and severity of exacerbations, complications, respiratory failure, co-morbidities (cardiovascular disease and sleep-related disorders), and the general health status of the patient. Different types of pharmacologic agents treat patients with COPD (Box 1). Pharmacologic therapy is used to prevent and control symptoms, reduce the frequency and severity of exacerbations, improve health status, and improve exercise tolerance. Initial use should decrease airway obstruction and decrease dyspnea. None of the existing medications for COPD had been shown to alter the inevitable long-term decline in lung function that occurs with COPD; however, they can decrease morbidity and may also delay disability and mortality in some patients. Medications may also decrease the number of exacerbations of COPD occurring per year.

Bronchodilators are primary medications for symptomatic management of COPD. Bronchodilator drugs commonly used include anticholinergics (short and long acting), β_1 agonists (short and long acting), and long-acting methylxanthines. All of these medications have been shown to improve exercise capacity in COPD patients even if the FEV_1 is insignificantly changed. Inhaled drugs tend to have fewer side effects than oral drugs. Short-acting bronchodilators on an as-needed basis are recommended for mild (Stage I) COPD. The GOLD guidelines recommend the use of regular daily treatment with long-acting bronchodilators for moderate (Stage II) or severe (Stages III and IV) COPD and long-acting bronchodilators are preferred to short-acting drugs because of better compliance because of longer duration of action (Box 1). Regular use of a long-acting anticholinergic (tiotropium [Spiriva]) or a long acting β_1-agonist (salmeterol [Serevent] or formoterol [Foradil]) improves health status. Theophylline (Theophylline SR; Theo-Dur) is effective in COPD, but because of its potential toxicity, inhaled bronchodilators are preferred when available. All studies that have shown efficacy of theophylline (Theo-Dur) in COPD were done with slow-release preparations (theophylline [Theo-Dur]). Each of the inhaled bronchodilators requires a delivery device which must be used correctly. Each type of device

[1]Not FDA approved for this indication.
[2]Not available in the United States.

BOX 1   Current Drugs Used to Manage Chronic Obstructive Pulmonary Disease

SABAs
- Albuterol (multiple formulations)

LABAs
- Formoterol (Foradil)
- Salmeterol (Serevent)

Short-acting anticholinergics
- Ipratropium (Atrovent)

Combination SABA + anticholinergic in 1 inhaler
- Albuterol/ipratropium (Combivent)

Long-acting anticholinergics
- Tiotropium (Spiriva)

Methylxanthines
- Theophylline (Theo-Dur)

Inhaled corticosteroids
- Beclomethasone (QVAR)
- Budesonide (Pulmicort)
- Fluticasone (Flovent)
- Mometasone (Asmanex)
- Triamcinolone (Azmacort) and mometasone (Asmanex)

Combination LABA + ICS in 1 inhaler
- Formoterol/budesonide (Symbicort)
- Salmeterol/fluticasone (Advair)

Systemic corticosteroids
- Prednisone
- Methylprednisolone (Medrol)

Abbreviations: LABAs = long-acting β_2 agonists; SABAs = short-acting β_2 agonists.

---

caution in giving these medications to patients receiving monoamine oxidase inhibitors or tricyclic antidepressants. The short-acting anticholinergic agent, ipratropium bromide (Atrovent), causes bronchodilation by competitive inhibition of muscarinic receptors. This agent reverses cholinergically mediated bronchospasm and may decrease mucus-gland secretions. It is effective for 4 to 6 hours after use.

The most recent addition to the long-acting bronchodilators is tiotropium (Spiriva), a long-acting anticholinergic agent that lasts 24 hours, allowing for once-daily administration. Tiotropium (Spiriva) has shown in several recent studies with COPD patients to result in improvement in lung function, improvement in quality of life, and lower rates of respiratory failure. Inhaled LABAs are highly preferred than the extended-release oral formulation because of longer action and fewer side effects. Salmeterol (Serevent) and formoterol (Foradil) are both long-acting, inhaled β_2 agonists, and extended-release albuterol (Proventil Repetabs) are long-acting, β_2 agonists available as oral agents. The long-acting inhaled agents have a slower onset of action and longer duration of action, remaining active for more than 12 hours. The onset of action of formoterol (Foradil) is more rapid than salmeterol (Serevent), but it should not be used for rescue during episodes of acute shortness of breath. It remains a chronic bronchodilator therapy. Like the short-acting inhaled β_2 agonists, the long-acting agents produce bronchodilation by smooth muscle relaxation as a result of adenylate cyclase activation and increasing cyclic AMP in smooth muscle cells. Combining β_2 agonists and anticholinergics may increase the effects of these agents. Several studies have shown superior efficacy for either a SABA or LABA in combination with an anticholinergic.

Theophylline inhibits phosphodiesterase action, which causes smooth muscle relaxation and leads to bronchodilation. It also increases central respiratory drive, diaphragm strength, promotes venous pooling in the legs, and may have some mild anti-inflammatory activity. Therapy with theophylline should be individualized, taking into account such factors as drug interactions, current smoking, the patient's age, and the presence of congestive heart failure or liver disease. Serum theophylline (Theo-Dur) concentrations should be maintained at levels between 5 and 15 µg/mL. Dosage adjustment is based on the patient's clinical response, tolerance to the agent, and serum theophylline levels. Some patients metabolize theophylline very rapidly. Although theophylline (Theo-Dur) is not a preferred first line agent in the management of COPD, it may be a second-line agent in patients with severe COPD.

Inhaled corticosteroids (ICSs) are not recommended as single agents for chronic use in COPD management, which is quite different from the recommendations in asthma. They are recommended in combination therapy with other bronchodilators in severe COPD, and the only Food and Drug Administration (FDA)-approved combinations of ICS and a LABA are fluticasone plus salmeterol (Advair) or formoterol (Foradil) plus budesonide (Symbicort)[4] (see Box 1). In a recent trial combination ICS and a LABA was shown to slow decline in lung function, decrease the number of exacerbations, and improve quality of life. Systemic steroids are clinically beneficial to patients hospitalized with COPD exacerbations and maximum effects of oral steroids after 3 days of intravenous (IV) steroids are achieved by 2 weeks of therapy. Longer use of oral steroids increases side effects without increasing pulmonary functions. Long-term treatment with oral glucocorticosteroids is not recommended in COPD. There is no evidence of a long-term benefit from this treatment. Moreover, a side effect of long-term treatment with systemic glucocorticosteroid is steroid myopathy, which contributes to muscle weakness, decreased functionality, and respiratory failure in patients with advanced COPD. Oral glucocorticosteroid use for long periods of time can also complicate control of diabetes and hypertension as well as causing bone demineralization.

Other pharmacologic treatments have been evaluated by the GOLD committee with some being beneficial. Use of influenza vaccines can reduce serious illness and death in COPD patients by approximately 50%. Use of the influenza vaccine has also been shown to reduce outpatient visits for influenza and reduces both hospital

---

requires patient education and monitoring, and the GOLD guidelines recommend consideration of the delivery device as part of the selection process for drug treatment in a single patient. As symptoms of COPD worsen, several different types of COPD therapy are given simultaneously, and deletion of drug therapy is usually not possible. In general nebulized therapy for a stable patient is unnecessary unless it has been demonstrated to be more effective than conventional metered dose or dry powder inhaler dose therapy in that patient.

Combinations of bronchodilators with different mechanisms and durations of action tend to increase the degree of bronchodilation in COPD patients with increases in FEV_1, FEV_1/FVC, and peak expiratory flow (PEF). Changes in pulmonary function are indirectly additive with increasing the number of bronchodilators being administered, but combinations usually increase pulmonary function more than each agent alone. Short-acting β_2 agonists (SABAs) are quick-relief medications for use only when necessary rather than on a daily, regular schedule. The regular use of a SABA results in twice as much β_2 agonist use without any noted clinical benefits. Increasing use or daily use of a SABA for rescue indicates the need for additional therapy to achieve long-term control. Inhaled SABAs include albuterol (Proventil, Ventolin), bitoterol (Tornalate), pirbuterol (Maxair), terbutaline (Brethaire), and levalbuterol (Xopenex). These medications are effective for 4 to 6 hours after use. Adverse effects of SABAs include palpitations, chest pain, tachycardia, tremor, unstable coronary artery disease or nervousness. Patients with coronary artery disease or cardiac dysrhythmias should also be monitored closely. Use

---

[4]Not yet approved for use in the United States.

costs and death. Vaccines containing killed (Fluzone) or live, inactive viruses (FluMist)[1] are recommended and should be given once (in autumn) or twice[3] (in autumn and winter) each year. A pneumococcal vaccine containing 23 virulent serotypes (Pneumovax-23) has been used in an effort to decrease the number of cases of pneumococcal pneumonia in COPD patients but evidence supporting its effectiveness in COPD patients but evidence supporting its effectiveness in COPD patients is lacking. An oral vaccine* using a strain of nontypeable *Haemophilus influenzae* has been shown to produce short-lived reduction in the number of exacerbations in some groups of COPD patients. The use of antibiotics, other than in treating infectious exacerbations of COPD or other bacterial infections such as pneumonia, is not recommended. Although a few patients with viscous sputum may benefit from mucolytics, the overall benefit is small. Therefore, the widespread use of these agents cannot be recommended.

Cough, although sometimes a troublesome symptom in COPD, has a significant protective role and the regular use of antitussives is contraindicated in stable COPD. The use of doxapram (Dopram), a nonspecific respiratory stimulant available as an intravenous formulation, is not recommended in stable COPD. Almitrine bismesylate (Duxil) also is not recommended for regular use in stable COPD patients. Narcotics are contraindicated in COPD because of their respiratory depressant effects and potential to worsen hypercapnia. Clinical studies suggest that morphine use to control dyspnea may have serious adverse effects, but it may provide benefits to a few select limited patients. Codeine and other narcotic analgesics should be avoided. Nonsteroidal anti-inflammatory agents (Nedocromil [Tilade]) and leukotriene modifiers have not been adequately tested in COPD patients and are not recommended for use. Alternative healing methods including herbal medicine, acupuncture, and homeopathy are not recommended for treatment in COPD.

Nonpharmacologic management of COPD patients includes pulmonary rehabilitation and long-term oxygen therapy. The principal goals of pulmonary rehabilitation are to improve quality of life, decrease symptoms, and increase physical participation in everyday activities. To accomplish these goals, pulmonary rehabilitation addresses a range of nonpulmonary problems, including exercise deconditioning, relative social isolation, altered mood states (especially depression), muscle wasting, and weight loss. COPD patients at all stages of disease benefit from exercise training programs and improve with respect to both exercise tolerance and symptoms of dyspnea and fatigue. These benefits can be sustained even after a single pulmonary rehabilitation program. Benefits have been reported from rehabilitation programs conducted in inpatient, outpatient, and home settings. Ideally, a comprehensive pulmonary rehabilitation program includes exercise training, nutrition counseling, and education. Baseline and outcome assessments of each participant in a pulmonary rehabilitation program should be made to quantify individual gains and target areas for improvement and include a detailed medical history and physical exam; measurement of spirometry before and after a bronchodilator drug; assessment of exercise capacity; measurement of the impact of breathlessness and/or health status; and assessment of inspiratory and expiratory muscle strength and lower limb strength (e.g., quadriceps) in patients who suffer from muscle wasting.

The long-term administration of oxygen (more than 15 hours per day) to COPD patients with chronic respiratory failure has been shown to increase survival. In studies done in Britain by the Medical Research Council Trial and in the United States in the Nocturnal Oxygen Therapy Trial, patients receiving continuous oxygen therapy had increased survival as compared with patients that did not receive oxygen or received oxygen only at night. Oxygen also has a beneficial impact on hemodynamics, hematologic characteristics, exercise capacity, lung mechanics, and mental state. Oxygen therapy also should be used if the patient has evidence of pulmonary hypertension, peripheral edema suggesting either right- or left-sided heart failure, or evidence of polycythemia (hematocrit greater than 55%). Therapy can be given continuously, acutely to combat acute dyspnea, or intermittently during exercise. It is recommended to perform arterial blood gas measurement in patients with FEV_1 less than 40% predicted or with clinical findings suggestive of respiratory failure or cor pulmonale.

Management of Exacerbations

Patients with COPD will have usually two to three exacerbations of symptoms of their disease each year with some requiring hospitalization. The economic and social burden of COPD exacerbations is extremely high. The most common causes of an exacerbation are pulmonary infections (acute bacterial bronchitis) and air pollution. The exact cause of approximately one-third of severe exacerbations cannot be identified and may be related to reactive airway disease. Other conditions that may produce the symptoms of an acute exacerbation of COPD include pneumonia, myocardial ischemia, congestive heart failure, pneumothorax, formation of a pleural effusion, pulmonary embolism, cardiac arrhythmias, esophageal reflux, or noncompliance with medications. The clinical diagnosis of a COPD exacerbation is an increase in amount of sputum production, change in color of sputum, or increase in dyspnea. Exacerbations may also be accompanied by a number of nonspecific complaints such as malaise, insomnia, sleepiness, fatigue, anxiety, depression, confusion, or panic attacks. Patients with exacerbations of COPD may require hospital admission, and some patients will require ICU admission. There is a high incidence of *H. influenzae* infections in patients with a COPD exacerbation caused by infection. Other important bacterial causes include *Streptococcus pneumoniae*, *Moraxella catarrhalis*, and *Pseudomonas aeruginosum*. Hospital admission must be considered in COPD with an exacerbation if they have marked increase in symptoms, failure to respond to outpatient treatment, confusion, lethargy and coma, worsening oxygenation, or development of respiratory acidosis. Oxygen therapy is usually required in a hospitalized patient with an acute exacerbation of COPD; but this may lead to CO_2 retention and acidosis, which in turn could lead to either noninvasive mechanical ventilation, or mechanical ventilation depending on the cause of the exacerbation and the patient's wishes. Hospital mortality for patients with COPD admitted for an acute exacerbation is approximately 10%. Antibiotics, oral prednisone (40–60 mg/day for 5–10 days), and noninvasive positive pressure ventilation have been shown to reduce treatment failure, relapse, and length of hospital stay in patients hospitalized with acute exacerbation of COPD. Ventilator associated pneumonia is also an important risk in a COPD patient treated with invasive mechanical ventilation.

The primary objectives of mechanical ventilatory support in patients with acute exacerbations of severe COPD are to decrease mortality and morbidity and relieve symptoms. Ventilatory support can be given through an orotracheal or nasotracheal tube or tracheostomy connection, which is referred to as invasive (conventional) mechanical ventilation and is particularly suitable in severe acute exacerbations occurring in patients with end-stage disease. Ventilatory support can also be given through a noninvasive means using either negative or positive pressure devices. Fewer complications occur with noninvasive ventilation, but many patients presenting with severe exacerbations of COPD, including respiratory acidosis, may not be candidates for noninvasive ventilation. Noninvasive positive-pressure ventilation (NPPV) involves using a mechanical ventilator connected by tubing to an interface that allows airflow into the nose or the nose and mouth by using a mask or a mouthpiece. Head straps are used to secure the mask tightly to the patient. NPPV allows ventilation without the use of an endotracheal tube. Use of NPPV in acute respiratory failure has been studied in both uncontrolled and randomized controlled trials. The studies show consistently positive results with success rates of 80% to 85%. Taken together they provide evidence that NPPV increases pH, reduces $PaCO_2$, reduces the severity of breathlessness in the first 4 hours of treatment, and decreases the length of hospital stay. More importantly, mortality

245

---

[1]Not FDA approved for this indication.
[3]Exceeds dosage recommended by the manufacturer.
*Investigational[1] drug in the United States.

and intubation rates are reduced by this intervention. However, NPPV is not appropriate for all patients and invasive mechanical ventilation may still be needed to maximize arterial blood gases values. NPPV can be delivered by different types of ventilators: volume-controlled, pressure-controlled, bilevel positive airway pressure, or continuous positive airway pressure. The use of NPPV together with long-term oxygen therapy has been shown to result in a significant improvement in daytime arterial blood gases, total sleep time, sleep efficiency, quality of life, and overnight $PaCO_2$.

Other treatments that can be useful in COPD patients who must be hospitalized include fluid administration as needed to keep the patient normovolemic; nutrition supplementation as needed with careful attention to the amount of carbohydrates given because excessive amounts can increase CO_2 production; and the use of low molecular weight heparin in immobilized patients with or without a history of thromboembolic disease. Manual or mechanical chest percussion and postural drainage may also be beneficial in patients producing greater than 25 mL sputum per day or those with lobar atelectasis.

Surgical Options

Surgical treatments of COPD include bullectomy, lung volume reduction surgery, and lung transplantation. In carefully selected patients, bullectomy can be effective in reducing dyspnea and improving lung function. A thoracic CT scan, arterial blood gases measurement and comprehensive respiratory function tests are essential before making a decision regarding a patient's suitability for resection of a bulla. Specific large bullae may be removed if they are compressing significant amounts of normal lung tissue.

Lung volume reduction surgery (LVRS) is another option for COPD patients and involves removing 20% to 30% of the upper lobes to improve airway mechanics and increase FEV_1. The National Emphysema Treatment Trial (NETT) study was a randomized controlled trial in 1218 patients with severe emphysema who received either LVRS or medical therapy. The results showed no overall survival benefit with LVRS compared with medical therapy, but improved exercise capacity and quality of life. The best outcome of this surgery was in patients with predominantly upper lobe emphysema and initial low exercise capacity. The surgery was prohibitive in patients with an FEV_1 of up to 20% and either a homogeneous distribution of emphysema or a concomitant diffusing capacity of lung for carbon monoxide (DL_{CO}) of up to 20%.

In appropriately selected patients with very advanced COPD, lung transplantation has been shown to improve quality of life and functional capacity. The average 5-year survival rate is approximately 50% when performed by highly skilled medical or surgical teams that specialize in lung transplantation. Appropriate criteria for lung transplantation referral include FEV_1 of up to 25% of predicted, $PaCO_2$ greater than 55 mm Hg, PaO_2 less than 50–60 mm Hg on room air, or the presence of secondary pulmonary hypertension.

Cystic Fibrosis

Method of
Robert Giusti, MD

Cystic fibrosis (CF), an autosomal recessive disease, is the most common lethal inherited disease in the white population. In this population the carrier rate is approximately 1 in 30, with an incidence of 1 in 3200 births. CF also occurs in African Americans (1 in 15,000), Hispanic Americans (1 in 8000) and Asian Americans (1 in 31,000),

but diagnosis may be delayed because of a low index of suspicion in these ethnic groups. Lung disease is the primary cause of morbidity and mortality in CF. Progressive fibrosis and destruction of lung tissue from chronic cycles of infection and inflammation lead to respiratory failure. The median survival for CF patients is 37.4 years.

Pathophysiology

The defect that results in CF is an abnormal gene located on the long arm of chromosome 7 that codes for a protein known as the cystic fibrosis transmembrane regulator (CFTR). This protein becomes incorporated into the lipid bilayer of the epithelial surface of the cell and functions as a chloride channel. Defective cyclic adenosine monophosphate (cAMP)-regulated chloride secretion through a mutated CFTR protein results in dehydrated airway surface fluid, which impedes the normal ciliary function, resulting in chronic infection and atelectasis. In addition, CFTR also down-regulates an epithelial sodium channel (ENaC). When CFTR is defective, this down-regulation is diminished, resulting in increased sodium reabsorption and a further reduction in airway surface fluid. The *CFTR* gene is expressed in the biliary ducts, vas deferens, pancreatic ducts, sweat glands, and the mucous glands of the lung.

More than 1500 specific mutations have been discovered in the CF gene, and the functional consequences of these mutations at the cellular level have been classified into five types. Clinical features correlate with the amount of CFTR activity at the epithelial surface. As the amount of residual CFTR declines, more organ systems are involved. Classes I, II, and III mutations result from abnormal protein production, trafficking through the cell, and regulation at the apical cell surface. These mutations result in 1% CFTR activity and are associated with more severe disease, worse pulmonary function, and pancreatic insufficient (PI) phenotype. The ΔF508 mutation, the most common mutation affecting 70% of CF mutations in the U.S. population, results from the deletion of a phenylalanine at amino acid position 508. In the presence of two copies of this mutation, a patient manifests a PI phenotype.

In Classes IV and V mutations, CFTR is present on the apical surface but chloride channel conduction is defective, resulting in 5% residual CFTR activity and the pancreatic sufficient (PS) phenotype. In the PS phenotype, respiratory symptoms might not present until adulthood, and sufficient pancreatic function is maintained to prevent malabsorption. Because PS patients have residual pancreatic function, there is adequate pancreatic tissue to become inflamed, and these patients might present with recurrent pancreatitis. Residual CFTR function is also manifested in the sweat gland, with sweat tests in the borderline range (40–60 mEq/L). The presence of a class IV or V mutation with a Δ508 mutation results in a PS phenotype.

At the end of intron 8, a noncoding region of the *CFTR* gene, a stretch of 5, 7, or 9 thymidine residues is found, designated the 5T, 7T, or 9T allele. A lower number of thymidines results in less efficient splicing of CFTR transcripts and therefore a lower amount of functional CFTR protein. The 5T allele has been classified as a mutation causing mild disease with partial penetrance. The 5T polymorphism is found on about 21% of the *CFTR* genes derived from patients with congenital bilateral absence of the vas deferens (CBAVD). In CBAVD there is 10% CFTR activity, which is sufficient to have obstructive azoospermia as the only clinical manifestation (Box 1).

Clinical Presentation

GASTROINTESTINAL

About 15% of infants present with meconium ileus, obstruction of the distal ileum with thickened viscid meconium. Prenatal ultrasound might detect echogenic bowel, which suggests CF. Infants present shortly after birth with feeding intolerance and a distended abdomen that requires surgical intervention. Colostomies are placed

BOX 1 Differentiating Between Criteria of CFTR Genotypes

Pancreatic Insufficient

Class I, II, or III mutation
1% CFTR activity
Absent or minimal chloride channel function
Elevated sweat chloride > 60 mmol/L
Classic early presentation (50% diagnosed by 6 months of age)
Median survival is 37.4 years
Patients require pancreatic enzymes
Fecal pancreatic elastase-1 <100 µg/g
Atrophic scarred pancreas
Risk of diabetes mellitus increases with age

Pancreatic Sufficient

Class IV or V mutation
5% CFTR activity
Some chloride channel function
Borderline or mildly elevated sweat chloride (40–60 mmol/L)
Atypical late presentation (sometimes in adulthood)
Survival to 50 years is not uncommon
No pancreatic enzyme supplement required
No enzyme requirement
Fecal pancreatic elastase-1 >250 µg/g
Adequate functional pancreatic tissue to develop recurrent pancreatitis
Lower risk of diabetes mellitus

CFTR = cystic fibrosis transmembrane regulator (protein).

pancreatic lipase and amylase results in fat and protein malabsorption, steatorrhea, failure to thrive, hypoalbuminemia, and edema. The buffering capacity of pancreatic chyle is diminished, resulting in decreased effectiveness of pancreatic enzyme replacement therapy, which is optimally effective at a neutral pH.

The 72-hour recording of dietary intake and stool collection for quantitative determination of fecal fat content is inconvenient and prone to collection errors in the nonresearch setting. The pancreatic enzyme elastase-1 is stable during intestinal transit and is not affected by porcine pancreatic replacement therapy. The measurement of fecal elastase-1 in stool has been found to be a less cumbersome and a sensitive assay to assess pancreatic function. This can be performed on a small specimen and does not require a timed collection.

Treatment with pancreatic enzyme replacement (pancrelipase [Creon, Pancrease]) improves linear growth and weight gain. The recommended dose per meal is 1000 to 2500 U/kg/dose. A high-fat diet is recommended to increase caloric intake to 150 kcal/kg of body weight, which is necessary to ensure optimal growth. The report of the Cystic Fibrosis Foundation Patient Registry indicates that 14% of CF patients are below the 5th percentile for height and 22% are below the 10th percentile for weight. Because nutritional failure as measured by body mass index (BMI) has been shown to be a predictor of progressive pulmonary deterioration, aggressive use of nutritional supplementation and nighttime gastrostomy feeds are advocated to improve the quality of life and lung function. Supplementation of fat-soluble vitamins is necessary to prevent nutritional deficiency.

Because CF patients are living longer, progressive fibrosis of the pancreas results in an increased incidence of diabetes, which is seen in 15% of CF patients. Annual glucose tolerance testing has become the standard of care in adolescents and adults to diagnose glucose intolerance before the onset of diabetes, which has been found to result in deterioration of lung function. Respiratory infection and steroid therapy can result in hyperglycemia, leading to a need for insulin before the patient develops frank diabetes. Because there are reductions of both insulin and glucagon, ketoacidosis is rare.

Infants with CF lose a great deal of salt in their sweat and can develop hyponatremic dehydration, heat prostration, and hypochloremic alkalosis. Salt supplementation is the norm, especially during warm summer months.

PULMONARY

The lungs in CF are normal at birth. In young CF patients *Staphylococcus aureus* and *Haemophilus influenzae* are common early colonizers, but as patients age, *Pseudomonas aeruginosa* becomes the predominant organism and is present in the sputum of 80% of adults. *P. aeruginosa* undergoes a mucoid transformation, which interferes with the effectiveness of antibiotic therapy. Because the acquisition of *P. aeruginosa* has been correlated with a more rapid deterioration of lung function and decreased survival, aggressive antibiotic therapy is initiated when this organism is isolated to prevent chronic colonization of the airway.

Burkholderia cepacia, an organism that is intrinsically resistant to a broad range of antibiotics, has been associated with poorer lung function. Nine genetically distinct species, known as genomovars, make up the *B. cepacia* complex. *Burkholderia cenocepacia* and *Burkholderia multivorans* are most commonly isolated from CF patients. The transmission of these organisms and other multiply resistant gram-negative bacteria from person to person in CF clinics and summer camps has resulted in strict infection-control guidelines.

A chronic cough, recurrent chest infections, purulent sputum, digital clubbing, chronic sinusitis, and nasal polyps are common presenting symptoms in CF. The incidence of recurrent pneumothorax is increased in CF, and chemical pleurodesis or pleurectomy are often required. Massive hemoptysis and recurrent episodes of hemoptysis are often a result of collateral bronchial arteries that can require embolization. CF patients often have opacification of the sinuses and nasal polyposis (Box 2).

to permit irrigation to dilate the underdeveloped microcolon, and resection of the terminal ileum is sometimes required. In utero perforation of the bowel can occur, manifesting with calcifications on abdominal x-ray.

The distal intestinal obstruction syndrome (DIOS) is an intestinal obstruction seen in older CF patients. It manifests with abdominal pain, constipation, and a palpable mass in the right lower quadrant consisting of viscous mucus and undigested fecal material that causes obstruction at the ileocecal valve. This can predispose to intussusception. The obstruction is treated by oral or nasogastric administration of polyethylene glycol and electrolytes (GoLYTELY),[1] an osmotic agent, which causes water to be retained in the intestine, inducing diarrhea. Rectal prolapse and the meconium plug syndrome, in which there is delayed passage of meconium in the newborn period, are additional reasons for referring a child for a sweat test.

Infants might also present with prolonged obstructive jaundice, which can progress to hepatic steatosis, complete biliary obstruction, and acholic stools. In the biliary tree, sludging of bile due to inadequate chloride and fluid transfer into the bile canaliculus can result in focal biliary cirrhosis and cholethiasis. Approximately 2% of patients progress to multilobular cirrhosis with portal hypertension, hypersplenism, and esophageal varices. Progression to liver failure and the need for transplantation is a possibility. Ursodeoxycholic acid (Actigall),[1] a cholorectic bile acid that increases the flow of bile, has been shown to lower hepatic enzymes and delay the progression of liver disease.

Chloride channel dysfunction in the pancreas results in thickened secretions within the pancreatic ducts and obstruction to the flow of pancreatic chyle. Approximately 85% of patients with CF develop exocrine pancreatic insufficiency. The inadequate production of

---

[1]Not FDA approved for this indication.

BOX 2   Clinical Presentation of Cystic Fibrosis

Gastrointesinal

Failure to thrive
Malabsorption
Meconium ileus
Meconium plug syndrome
Rectal prolapse
Recurrent pancreatitis
Steatorrhea

Pulmonary

Bronchiectasis
Chronic cough
Chronic sinusitis
Digital clubbing
Nasal polyps
Purulent bronchitis
Recurrent and persistent pneumonia

Other

Growth failure
Hyponatremia and dehydration
Male infertility

Diagnosis

Sweat testing remains the standard for making the diagnosis of CF. The elevation of the chloride results from CFTR chloride channel dysfunction in the sweat ducts, where reabsorption of chloride occurs. Pilocarpine is iontophoresized into the skin to stimulate sweating. A chloride level greater than 60 mEq/L is consistent with the diagnosis of CF, but the result must be interpreted in the context of the clinical picture. The borderline range for sweat chloride is 40 to 60 mEq/L. Additional testing is necessary to confirm the diagnosis when the sweat test is in the borderline range. False-positive sweat test results can occur with malnutrition, Addison's disease, and ectodermal dysplasia, so it is essential to confirm the diagnosis with a confirmatory sweat test or a genetic analysis, or both. Sweat tests can be performed after 2 weeks of age or when an infant weighs about 8 lbs (3.6 kg), at which time a sufficient quantity of sweat can be collected to ensure a proper analysis.

Genetic analysis for mutations known to cause CF symptoms is an alternative diagnostic approach. The presence of two abnormal CFTR mutations known to cause CF disease predicts with a high degree of certainty that a patient has CF. Prenatal screening is recommended by the American College of Obstetrics and Gynecology for pregnant white women. When both parents are found to be carriers, amniocentesis and chorionic villous sampling can be used to assess the 25% chance of having an infant affected by CE.

The active transport of ions generates a transepithelial electrical potential difference (PD). Abnormalities of chloride ion transport in patients with CF are associated with a different pattern of PD compared with normal epithelium. This assay thus provides a direct view of the physiology at the ion channel level. Nasal PD measurements help to resolve diagnostic dilemmas in atypical patients and a change of PD measurement toward normal is an outcome measure of therapeutic interventions that correct the chloride channel dysfunction.

Three features distinguish the nasal PD in a patient with CF. A high basal PD reflects enhanced sodium transport across a relatively chloride impermeable membrane. A larger inhibition of PD after nasal perfusion with the sodium channel inhibitor amilorlide reflects inhibition of accelerated sodium transport. Little or no change in PD in response to perfusion of the nasal epithelial surface with a chloride-free solution in conjunction with isoproterenol reflects an absence of CFTR-mediated chloride secretion.

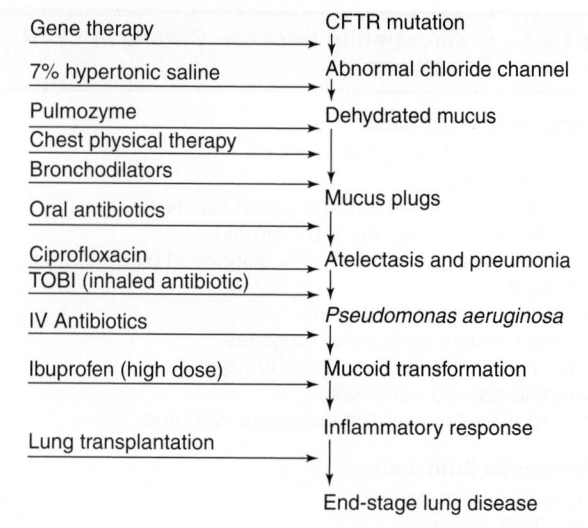

FIGURE 1. Therapeutic interventions for cystic fibrosis lung disease.

Newborn screening for CF has been shown to improve nutritional and neurodevelopmental outcomes. Trypsinogen, a precursor of trypsin, is commonly elevated in the serum of newborns with CF because of in utero obstruction of pancreatic ducts. Infants with CF have elevated immunoreactive trypsinogen (IRT) levels for 2 to 3 weeks after birth. When the IRT is elevated in a blood specimen collected shortly after birth, then an analysis for the presence of CF mutations on the same blood specimen or a persistent elevation of IRT at 2 to 3 weeks of age in a repeat blood specimen are two different methods to determine which infants should be referred for sweat testing. Mutation analysis performed during newborn screening detects carriers of CF mutations, and genetic counseling for these families is warranted to permit informed decisions concerning future pregnancies.

Treatment

Therapeutic interventions are shown in Figure 1.

GENE THERAPY

The goal of gene therapy is to correct the basic defect by inserting a normal functioning gene into the ciliated cells in the submucous glands that express abnormal CFTR function. Initial attempts using the adenovirus as the vehicle for transporting the gene into the cells lining the airway appeared promising; however, the host immune response to the virus has limited the effectiveness of this approach. The ideal vector would efficiently deliver the gene to the appropriate target cell without causing toxicity or an inflammatory response. Although gene therapy offers the potential to correct the basic defect of CF, many technical barriers to effective gene therapy need to be addressed to permit this form of therapy to become an effective treatment. Liposomes are being evaluated as an alternate delivery system for administering the normal gene into epithelial cells.

HYDRATION OF AIRWAY SURFACE FLUID

Hypertonic saline (Hyper-sal), at a 7% concentration,[6] has been shown to increase the hydration of the airway surface fluid and reduce the frequency of pulmonary exacerbations. This recent addition to the therapeutic treatment regimen has been shown to facilitate the clearance of airway mucus, resulting in improved pulmonary function, and to decrease the frequency of pulmonary exacerbations. Hypertonic saline induces coughing and bronchospasm and is administered following bronchodilator therapy.

---

[6]May be compounded by pharmacists.

PHYSICAL THERAPY

Airway clearance can be performed using various techniques, including conventional percussion therapy, pneumatically inflated chest vest percussion device, oscillating positive pressure devices such as the Flutter or Acapella, autogenic drainage, and exercise. These techniques are recommended on a daily basis to help mobilize secretions and prevent the complications related to persistent accumulation of airway mucus.

BRONCHODILATORS

Airway hyperreactivity is present in 50% to 60% of CF patients. β-Agonists keep airways open and facilitate airway clearance by increasing ciliary beat frequency and smooth muscle relaxation. The spirometric response to β-agonists should be monitored because with worsening bronchiectasis and the development of floppy airways, airflow may be impaired. Because anticholinergics alter viscosity of mucus and can have an adverse effect on gastrointestinal motility, this class of bronchodilator has not been recommended for routine use in CF by a consensus conference of the Cystic Fibrosis Foundation.

ANTIBIOTICS

Aggressive use of antibiotics for the chronic bacterial colonization of the airways in CF has resulted in improving longevity and quality of life. Prophylactic inhaled antibiotics have been effective in CF patients to decrease the bacterial burden in the CF airway. Alternate-month therapy with a 300-mg aerosol preparation of tobramycin (TOBI) improves lung function, delays the time to the onset of pulmonary exacerbation, and decreases the need for hospitalization. A preparation of aztreonam (Azactam) for inhalation,[1] which is administered by a very efficient portable nebulizer (eFlow), appears to be promising but has not yet been approved by the FDA.

Pulmonary exacerbations are characterized by an increased cough, copious purulent sputum, decreased appetite, weight loss, and decreased exercise tolerance. Quinolone antibiotics are effective for treating *P. aeruginosa* in an oral preparation, but the development of resistance to this class of drug is a limiting factor. Ciprofloxacin (Cipro) is not approved by the FDA for use in children, but there is considerable experience with this drug in children with CF. When oral and inhaled antibiotics are not effective, hospitalization for aggressive airway clearance and a 10- to 14-day course of IV antibiotics is indicated. A combination of two drugs (usually an aminoglycoside and a β-lactam semisynthetic penicillin or a cephalosporin) is selected based on susceptibility of the organism recovered by culture of sputum or a deep throat swab. In young children who are not able to produce sputum, bronchoscopy is employed to obtain a specimen for culture.

MUCOLYTIC THERAPY

DNase (Pulmozyme) is a nebulized mucolytic agent that cleaves neutrophil-derived DNA that contributes to the thick airway secretions that clog the CF airways. Daily inhalation therapy (2.5 mg) reduces sputum viscosity, facilitating airway clearance and resulting in a 5% improvement in lung function. This therapy has largely replaced treatment with *N*-acetylcysteine (Mucomyst),[1] which causes bronchial irritation.

ANTIINFLAMMATORY THERAPY

There has been growing awareness of the role of the host inflammatory responses in the progression of CF lung disease. Chronic endobronchial colonization with bacteria results in the release of proinflammatory mediators interleukin (IL)-8 and nuclear factor (NF)-κB. These mediators recruit neutrophils into the airway; the neutrophils release elastase, protease, superoxide ions, and hydroxyl radicals, which damage lung tissue and contribute to the development of bronchiectasis.

Corticosteroids

Alternate day-systemic steroids were studied in a multicenter placebo-controlled study as a therapeutic intervention to decrease the inflammatory response in the CF airway. Significant risks of growth impairment, diabetes, and cataracts were found. Although inhaled steroids are commonly prescribed for CF patients, there is no double-blind study to demonstrate benefit of long-term therapy in CF patients who do not have a component of asthma.

Nonsteroidal Antiinflammatory Drugs

Oral administration of twice-daily high-dose ibuprofen[1] (20–30 mg/kg)[3] to achieve peak plasma concentration of 50 to 100 μg/mL interferes with neutrophil migration and inhibits the activation of NF-κB. Konstan studied 85 CF patients and found that ibuprofen therapy results in less decline in lung function, fewer hospitalizations, and improved weight gain. This effect is most pronounced in patients who are younger than 13 years and have minimal lung disease. Although prolonged use of this therapy has been shown to have ongoing benefit, the risk of GI side effects has limited the implementation of this therapy by most CF patients.

Macrolide antibiotics (azithromycin [Zithromax])[1] are not considered effective in the treatment of infection with *P. aeruginosa*, but a number of clinical trials have demonstrated a modest improvement in lung function and a decrease in the frequency of infectious exacerbations and need for antibiotic therapy in CF patients chronically colonized with *P. aeruginosa*. The mechanisms of action are not well understood but are believed to be related to a number of antiinflammatory and immunomodulatory effects of this class of antibiotic. The expression of *P. aeruginosa* pathogenicity factors and neutrophil recruitment appear to be altered by chronic macrolide therapy.

Oxygen therapy to correct alveolar hypoxia is effective to prevent pulmonary hypertension in CF patients with severe lung disease. Pulmonary hypertension results from pulmonary vascular remodeling, which results in increased pulmonary vascular resistance. Cor pulmonale contributes to the morbidity of CF with right heart failure, progressive exercise intolerance, and risk of syncope.

LUNG TRANSPLANTATION

Approximately 150 patients receive bilateral cadaveric lung transplants per year. Evaluation at a lung transplant center is considered when progressive deterioration in lung function results in a forced expiratory volume in one second (FEV_1) less than 30% predicted. Survival rates in CF lung-transplant recipients are comparable with other groups of patients. The availability of donor organs continues to be a limiting factor, and the disparity between donor availability and a growing recipient pool has progressively lengthened the waiting time for organs and has increased the mortality for patients awaiting lung transplantation. Living-donor lobar transplantation, which involves removal of both diseased lungs from the recipient and the implantation of two lower lobes donated by two donors, is an alternative for CF patients awaiting lung transplantation.

REFERENCES

http://www.genet.sickkids.or.ca/cftr/app

Cystic Fibrosis Foundation. Cystic Fibrosis Foundation Patient Registry, 2005 Annual Data Report to the Center Directors. Bethesda Md: Cystic Fibrosis Foundation; 2006.

Solomon MP, Wilson DC, Corey M, et al. Glucose intolerance in children with cystic fibrosis. J Pediatr 2003;142:128–32.

Konstan MW, Byard PJ, Hoppel CL, Davis PB. Effect of high-dose ibuprofen in patients with cystic fibrosis. N Engl J Med 1995;332(13):848–54.

---

[1]Not FDA approved for this indication.

---

[1]Not FDA approved for this indication.
[3]Exceeds dosage recommended by the manufacturer.

Sleep Apnea

Method of
Shekhar A. Ghamande, MD, and Shyam Subramanian, MD

Sleep apnea refers to intermittent cessation of respiration during sleep. There are two main types: obstructive sleep apnea (OSA), which is characterized by intermittent upper airway collapse during sleep, and central sleep apnea (CSA), which is characterized by central cessation of respiration during sleep.

Obstructive Sleep Apnea

OSA is common and can affect children as well as adults. Prevalence is estimated at 2% of women and 4% of men aged 30 to 60 years. This increases among older adults (mean age, 76 years), with an estimated prevalence of 24% to 26%. Among older adults, OSA with daytime sleepiness can cause significant cognitive difficulties, particularly in tests of attention. Risk factors include increased age, male gender, obesity, and high serum cholesterol levels.

There are a number of phenotypic traits that predispose an individual to the development of sleep apnea, and individual variability may ultimately determine who develops apnea and how severe the apnea will be. These traits include upper airway anatomy, the ability of upper airway dilator muscles to respond to rising intrapharyngeal negative pressure and increasing CO_2 levels during sleep, the arousal threshold in response to respiratory stimulation, and loop gain (ventilatory control instability).

During wakefulness, neuromuscular compensatory systems function to increase the activity of the pharyngeal dilator muscles, thus preserving airway patency. This reflex-driven augmented muscle activity is lost at sleep onset, and collapse of the pharyngeal airway occurs. The associated hypoxemia and hypercapnia drive increase respiratory effort, which ultimately leads to arousal from sleep and reestablishment of airway patency and ventilation. Once the patient returns to sleep, the cycle begins again (Box 1). The patient thus suffers the consequences of repeated sleep disruption as well as recurrent hypoxemia and hypercapnia.

CLINICAL PRESENTATION

OSA symptoms develop insidiously and progress with age and increasing weight. Sleep at night is disturbed by loud snoring; sensations of choking, gasping, or snorting; apneas witnessed by bed partners; frequent awakenings; nocturia; and even difficulty staying asleep. Mornings are difficult because of persistent sleepiness and, sometimes, headache or dry mouth. Daytime hypersomnolence, fatigue, difficulties with concentration and short-term memory, and depression can occur as a result of OSA.

BOX 1   Cycle of Sleep Disruption in Obstructive Sleep Apnea

Sleep
Loss of upper airway patency
Airway collapse
Hypoxemia
Increased respiratory effort
Arousal
Reopening of the upper airway
Periodic breathing

Snoring

Snoring is the most frequent symptom of OSA, occurring in up to 95% of patients. However, it has poor predictive value because of the high prevalence of snoring in the general population. Population surveys indicate that 25% of men and 15% of women are habitual snorers. The absence of snoring, on the other hand, makes OSA unlikely.

Excessive Daytime Sleepiness

As many as 30% of the general population report significant sleepiness, so this is not useful as a clinical feature to discriminate between patients with and without OSA. Severity of daytime sleepiness and sleep apnea do not correlate well. Moreover, it may be hard to distinguish EDS from other symptoms such as fatigue. Patients with OSA frequently underestimate the severity of sleepiness or are reluctant to admit the symptom for social or work-related reasons. Tools for measuring excessive daytime sleepiness include the Epworth Sleepiness Score and the Stanford Sleepiness Score.

Witnessed Apneas

Concern by the bed partner about witnessed breathing pauses during sleep is a common reason for referral to a sleep clinic, especially in men. Witnessed apneas are reported in up to 6% of the normal population. These events are a good diagnostic predictor of OSA syndrome but do not predict severity.

Nocturnal Choking

Many patients with OSA report waking at night with a choking sensation. It is quite frightening but almost invariably passes within a few seconds of wakening.

Insomnia

Many patients develop sleep maintenance insomnia and have disturbed sleep with frequent nocturnal awakenings.

Nocturia

More than 70% of patients with sleep apnea have at least two episodes of urination at night time. Clinical signs that suggest OSA are obesity (body mass index >30), especially with a upper body or male pattern of fat distribution, a crowded pharyngeal space, and retrognathia. A neck circumference of greater than 43 cm in men or 41 cm in women increases the risk of OSA. Other craniofacial features that suggest OSA include reduced cricomental space, macroglossia, lateral peritonsillar narrowing, and tonsillar hyperplasia. Use of a score such as the Mallampati classification or the Modified Friedman Score is helpful to quantify these abnormalities.

DIAGNOSIS

Typically, sleep-related questionnaires are used to increase clinical prediction of OSA. The most commonly used instrument is the Epworth Sleepiness Score, which assigns points to the degree of sleepiness in various situations, such as reading, watching TV, sitting as a passenger, and driving. The Berlin questionnaire derives a composite score based on three domains and has been shown to have a high sensitivity and specificity; it is especially useful in a primary care population. Although more complex clinical prediction models using several phenotypic elements may improve diagnostic accuracy, their widespread clinical application is limited.

Overnight polysomnography is the standard for diagnosis of OSA. Full polysomnography involves an overnight stay in a designated sleep laboratory with multichannel monitoring to measure chin and leg electromyography, electro-oculography, chest and abdominal respiratory effort, nasal airflow via a thermistor or nasal cannula, oxygen saturation, and heart rate, in addition to several sleep architecture measures. Polysomnography is the gold standard for the diagnosis of sleep apnea. An obstructive apnea is defined as a 10-second pause in respiration associated with ongoing ventilatory effort.

An obstructive hypopnea is defined as a 50% decrease in flow associated with a 3% drop in oxygen saturation. A diagnosis of OSA syndrome is accepted when a patient has an apnea-hypopnea index (AHI; number of apneas and hypopneas per hour of sleep) of 5 or greater and symptoms of excessive daytime sleepiness. Another index used to quantify OSA severity is the Respiratory Disturbance Index (RDI), which includes respiratory effort–related arousals.

The most widely accepted diagnostic threshold for OSA is an AHI value of 5 or more per hour in association with symptoms or significant comorbidity. This is further stratified as mild OSA (AHI 5–15), moderate OSA (16–30), and severe OSA (AHI >30). Portable home sleep studies using a level 3 portable monitor have been shown to be accurate in the diagnosis of OSA. Their predictive values are best when the AHI is greater than 30 or less than 5.

CLINICAL CONSEQUENCES

The clinical consequences of OSA stem from sleep fragmentation as a result of repeated arousals as well as from the neurohumoral and proinflammatory effects of intermittent hypoxia.

Sleep fragmentation causes excessive daytime sleepiness, which can result in significant social and occupational impairment. Untreated OSA results in a twofold to sevenfold increased risk of being involved in a motor vehicle crash. There is an increased prevalence of OSA among commercial vehicle operators, a situation that calls for aggressive screening strategies. Similarly, there is a higher risk of occupational accidents among people with OSA. In children, poor scholastic performance is seen, and there is a higher likelihood of attention deficit disorder.

CARDIOVASCULAR CONSEQUENCES

Five longitudinal studies performed since 1995 have indicated an increased cardiovascular mortality rate among patients with OSA. Similarly, an increased risk for death or stroke has been reported, with a dose-response relationship between OSA severity and risk.

Hypertension

OSA confers an odds ratio of 2 to 3, depending on its severity, for development of systemic hypertension. An estimated 30% of hypertensive patients have OSA. In drug-resistant hypertension, OSA prevalence has been to shown to be as high as 83%. Treatment of OSA with continuous positive airway pressure (CPAP) has been shown to reduce blood pressure.

Stroke

Presence of moderate OSA confers an adjusted odds ratio for stroke of almost 4. Approximately 70% of stroke victims have OSA, and treatment of OSA with CPAP tends to have a positive impact on neurologic recovery and rehabilitation outcomes.

Heart Disease

Untreated OSA carries an odds ratio of 4.5 for coronary artery disease. Prevalence of OSA in patients with coronary artery disease may be as high as 60%, and OSA has been shown to be an independent predictor of mortality in this disease. Nocturnal desaturation correlates with severity of coronary atherosclerosis. Severe OSA increased the risk of arrhythmias twofold to fourfold, including atrial fibrillation, nonsustained ventricular tachycardia, and complex ventricular ectopy. Treatment of OSA has been shown to improve the mortality rate among patients with coronary artery disease.

Heart Failure

The prevalence of sleep-disordered breathing is 55% to 60% among patients with congestive heart failure. Treatment with CPAP has been shown to improve ejection fraction in patients with systolic congestive heart failure, and CPAP compliance has been shown to improve survival.

Diabetes Mellitus and Metabolic Syndrome

Prevalence of OSA is 50% among patients with diabetes mellitus and correlates with insulin resistance. CPAP therapy may have beneficial effects on glycemic control. OSA is believed to result in leptin resistance, and CPAP therapy has been shown to reverse this effect. There is a high prevalence (up to 67%) of OSA in patients with polycystic ovarian syndrome.

Erectile Dysfunction

Prevalence of OSA among patients with erectile dysfunction is high. The etiology is believed to be multifactorial, with effects that include endothelial dysfunction as well as low serum testosterone levels secondary to OSA. Patients being treated with testosterone replacement need to be screened for OSA. Treatment with CPAP has been shown to be beneficial in patients with erectile dysfunction.

TREATMENT

Weight loss in obese patients with OSA leads to a measurable improvement in AHI, snoring, and sleep efficiency. The most dramatic results are observed in patients with morbid obesity after successful bariatric surgery. A small subset of patents with positional sleep apnea (primarily in the supine position) may be helped with mechanical measures that prevent them from lying on the back.

The mainstay of treatment is CPAP therapy, which consists of a blower connected to the nose or face via a mask. Preset pressurized air maintains a positive airway pressure, which splints the airway open throughout the usage period. The optimal CPAP pressure, determined during polysomnography, is the pressure at which apneas, hypopneas, hypoxia, and snoring are eliminated in all positions and stages of sleep. The commonly reported 50% nonadherence rate to CPAP is a barrier to effective management. Predictors of continued CPAP use include severity of sleepiness, severity of AHI, adequate usage during the first 3 months, and a perceived improvement in symptoms. Adequate education about the CPAP device, mask interface, humidification, and close follow-up improve compliance. Newer, auto-adjusting CPAP units have not consistently been shown to result in greater adherence or effectiveness.

Oral appliances should be considered for mild to moderate OSA as well as for positional OSA if CPAP is not accepted. These devices are custom fitted by a dentist. They lead to pharyngeal dilatation as a result of anterior mandibular advancement, and they also serve the purpose of tongue retention. Although less efficacious than CPAP, oral appliances are often preferred by patients, leading to better patient adherence.

Surgery may be a viable option in carefully selected patients with a favorable pharyngeal anatomy. The most common surgery for sleep apnea is uvulopalatopharyngoplasty, which is intended to enlarge the airway by removing or shortening the uvula and removing the tonsils and adenoids, if present, as well as part of the soft palate or roof of the mouth. Overall, a meta-analysis concluded that both laser-assisted uvulopalatoplasty and radiofrequency ablation did not provide any significant benefits. Other surgical procedures include laser midline glossectomy and linguoplasty, in which part of the tongue is removed. Two others that try to enlarge the airway by moving the jaw forward are maxillomandibular osteotomy or advancement and the two-part inferior sagittal mandibular osteotomy and genioglossal advancement with hyoid myotomy and suspension.

Central Sleep Apnea

There are several forms of CSA. Periodic breathing develops in most individuals ascending to high altitude, if the altitude is high enough, and represents a form of ventilatory instability produced by ambient hypoxia. A form of CSA called Cheyne-Stokes respiration is seen in patients with congestive heart failure and, to a lesser extent, in those with stroke. The prevalence of CSA in patients with heart failure has been found to be as high as 40%; patients with CSA are more likely to be male, to be older, and to have a lower body mass index and a higher pulmonary capillary wedge pressure.

CLINICAL PRESENTATION

Clinical presentation of patients with CSA is predominantly disturbed sleep, frequent awakenings, paroxysmal nocturnal dyspnea, and daytime fatigue. Excessive daytime sleepiness, obesity, and snoring are not observed, in contrast to OSA. Pulmonary congestion, increased cardiac filling pressures, and a prolonged circulation time lead to oscillations of tidal volume, with hyperventilation alternating with apnea (as the arterial partial pressure of CO_2 drops below the apneic threshold), which is called Cheyne-Stokes respiration. Increased AHI from CSA and increased left atrial size are potent predictors of mortality in patients with congestive heart failure.

TREATMENT

Intensified heart failure therapy improves CSA, particularly with diuresis and angiotensin-converting enzyme inhibition. Nocturnal oxygen and theophylline (Uniphyl)[1] improve CSA without changing cardiac outcomes. Theophylline can induce arrhythmias and should be used with caution. Acetazolamide (Diamox)[1] reduced CSA as a single dose at night, but there have been no long-term trials with it. CPAP should be offered selectively to those patients with heart failure and sleep apnea. Newer modalities of positive pressure therapy such as servo ventilation may prove useful in this scenario. Cardiac resynchronization therapy was beneficial in a small study.

REFERENCES

Chowdhuri S. Continuous positive airway pressure for the treatment of sleep apnea. Otolaryngol Clin North Am 2007;40(4):807–27.

Franklin KA, Anttila H, Axelsson S, et al. Effects and side-effects of surgery for snoring and obstructive sleep apnea: A systematic review. Sleep 2009;32(1):27–36.

Hartenbaum N, Collop N, Rosen IN, et al. Sleep apnea and commercial motor vehicle operators: Statement from the Joint Task Force of the American College of Chest Physicians, American College of Occupational and Environmental Medicine, and the National Sleep Foundation. J Occup Environ Med 2006;48(9 Suppl.):S4–37.

Marin JM, Carrizo SJ. Mortality in obstructive sleep apnea. Sleep Med Clin 2007;2(4):593–601.

Patil SP, Schnieder H, Schwartz AR, et al. Adult obstructive sleep apnea: Pathophysiology and diagnosis. Chest 2007;132(1):325–37.

Ramchandran SK, Josephs LA. A meta-analysis of clinical screening tests for obstructive sleep apnea. Anesthesiology 2009;110(4):928–39.

Somers VK, White DP, Raouf A, et al. Sleep apnea and cardiovascular disease: An American Heart Association/American College of Cardiology Foundation scientific statement. Circulation 2008;118:1080–111 [Erratum in Circulation 2009;119:e380.].

Tonelli de Oleveira AC, Martinez D, Vasconcelos LFT, et al. Diagnosis of obstructive sleep apnea syndrome and its outcomes with home portable monitoring. Chest 2009;135(2):330–6.

[1]Not FDA approved for this indication.

Primary Lung Cancer

Method of
Robert A. Kratzke, MD, and Manish R. Patel, DO

Lung cancer is the leading cause of cancer-related death in North America for both men and women. It is not the most common cancer, but most patients with lung cancer are diagnosed at a late stage, accounting for the excess mortality. In the United States, lung cancer accounts for only 13% of new cancer cases but almost one third of cancer-related deaths. Although approximately one third of patients are diagnosed at an early stage, the 5-year survival rate for all patients with lung cancer is less than 20%.

Lung cancer is broadly divided into two groups, small cell lung cancer (SCLC) and non–small cell lung cancer (NSCLC). Approximately 80% of lung cancers are NSCLC, and most of those are squamous carcinomas, adenocarcinomas, or bronchoalveolar carcinomas. Carcinoid tumors and other neuroendocrine tumors are less common, and adenoid cystic carcinomas are rare. Although there is increasing awareness of the importance of histologic subtype in determining responses to newer therapies, the concept of histology-targeted therapy is still evolving, and the standard treatments for NSCLC are generally the same regardless of the histologic subtype.

Epidemiology

Lung cancer occurs most commonly in middle-aged and elderly people. The peak incidence occurs in those aged 65 to 85 years. It is extremely rare in people younger than 30 years of age, and the incidence decreases after 85 years. Before the 1960s, lung cancer was rare among women. However, in North America, the current incidence of lung cancer is almost equal between men and women.

The incidence is decreasing among men and has leveled off in women over the past decade. Lung cancer occurs at a higher frequency in African Americans. This most likely reflects socioeconomic status more than genetic risk, because cigarette smoking remains more common among African Americans. However, there is some evidence that African Americans are more vulnerable to the effects of tobacco-related carcinogens.

Etiology

Cigarette smoking is the established cause of the lung cancer in general. In particular, there is a positive smoking history in 95% of all cases of SCLC. Eighty percent of newly diagnosed lung cancers are in patients who are current or former smokers. Current smokers with a greater than 20-pack-year smoking history have a 2000-fold greater risk of developing lung cancer compared with nonsmokers. Smoking cessation decreases the risk but does not eliminate it. The risk of developing lung cancer in former smokers remains increased by 2-to 10-fold over that in nonsmokers even decades after smoking cessation. There is also clearly a dose-response relationship in tobacco smoke–induced lung cancer in that the risk is highest among those with the greatest prior cigarette exposure. Pipe and cigar smoke also increase the risk of lung cancer. Among nonsmokers, there is a twofold increased risk of developing lung cancer that is clearly associated with inhalation of second-hand smoke.

 CURRENT DIAGNOSIS

- A history of cigarette smoking is the greatest risk factor.
- Cough, dyspnea, and chest pain are the most common presenting symptoms.
- Diagnosis is made by needle biopsy or pleural fluid cytology.
- The initial staging evaluation should include
  - Positron-emission tomography/computed tomography to evaluate for distant metastasis
  - Magnetic resonance imaging of the brain for small cell lung cancer
- Patients with resectable cancers should have an additional evaluation of mediastinum before resection (i.e., mediastinoscopy or endoscopic ultrasonography)

Other environmental factors have been associated with the development of lung cancer. Up to 20% of lung cancer cases occur among nonsmokers, and this population of patients appears to be rising. Certainly, some of this increase is a result of second-hand exposure to cigarette smoke, but this is difficult to quantify. Asbestos exposure has been associated with the development of lung cancer, and the risk is particularly accentuated by combination with cigarette smoke. Radon exposure has also been associated with the development of lung cancer, particularly in uranium mine workers, in whom the risk approaches 10 times that of the general population. Several other environmental exposures, including chromium, arsenic, and polyvinyl chloride, have been implicated in the development of lung cancers; however, a clear causal link is less well established. Although a patient with a family history of lung cancer has an approximately twofold higher risk, the genetic basis of this finding is not well understood.

Clinical Presentation

The location of tumors and the appearance of paraneoplastic syndromes often determine the clinical presentation of patients with lung cancer (Table 1). Many patients with early-stage disease are asymptomatic and have a mass discovered incidentally on chest radiography or computed tomography (CT) scanning done for some other reason. Centrally located tumors often cause symptoms associated with local effects of the tumor, such as cough, hemoptysis, wheezing, or stridor. Obstruction of the bronchi can lead to postobstructive pneumonia (i.e., pneumonia distal to the obstruction) as the presenting sign, and obstruction of the superior vena cava can lead to the superior vena cava syndrome, with facial edema, bluish discoloration of the upper chest, and shortness of breath. Mediastinal lymph node involvement can cause disruption of the recurrent laryngeal nerve, leading to hoarseness. Tumors arising in the superior sulcus (Pancoast tumors) can lead to a lower brachial plexopathy and Horner's syndrome. Peripheral tumors tend to manifest later as pain when they involve the chest wall or pleura. Pleural effusion may also be the presenting sign for lung cancer.

Lung cancer frequently metastasizes early, and symptoms caused by metastatic lesions may be the first sign of malignancy. Brain metastases are a common presentation, particularly in patients with SCLC, but also in NSCLC. Symptoms such as seizures, nausea and vomiting, headache, and focal neurologic signs may be the initial presentation in such patients. Bony metastases are common in all types of lung cancer and can manifest with pain, pathologic fracture, or spinal cord compression. Liver metastases can cause biliary obstruction and jaundice, but this is not particularly common.

Lung cancers are notable for ectopic production of hormones leading to several paraneoplastic syndromes. These are most commonly described in SCLC but also occur in NSCLC. Probably the most common paraneoplastic syndromes in NSCLC are tumor cachexia and hypercalcemia. Although the causes of tumor cachexia are not well characterized, hyperkalemia is mediated by the production of parathyroid hormone–related peptide. This leads to release of calcium from bones and elevation of calcium in the blood. This syndrome is effectively treated with bisphosphonate therapy. Hypertrophic pulmonary arthropathy can occur with NSCLC or SCLC and is characterized by digital clubbing and periostitis of the long bones demonstrable on plain radiographs. SCLC frequently manifests with paraneoplastic syndromes, the most common being the Lambert-Eaton myasthenic syndrome. Approximately 50% of patients who present with this syndrome have an underlying malignancy, and 95% of those are SCLCs. Other paraneoplastic syndromes related to SCLC are the syndrome of inappropriate antidiuretic hormone, Cushing's syndrome caused by ectopic production of corticotropin, and cerebellar degeneration associated with the elaboration of anti-Yo autoantibodies.

Diagnosis and Evaluation

Once lung cancer is suspected, tissue biopsy is required to make a definitive diagnosis. Several methods can be used to obtain tissue, depending on the location of the tumor. Mediastinal involvement can be assessed by mediastinoscopy; endoscopic ultrasonography is also being increasingly used. Transbronchial biopsy can be performed for centrally located tumors, and the yield may be increased by using endobronchial ultrasonography techniques. For peripheral lesions, CT-guided needle biopsy is usually recommended. If equivocal results are obtained, open procedures using video-assisted thoracoscopic surgery (VATS) are occasionally required. For patients presenting with pleural effusion, cytologic examination of pleural fluid can establish the diagnosis.

Once the diagnosis is confirmed, accurate staging of disease is important to determine the prognosis and appropriate therapy. The first step is to rule out metastatic disease. For NSCLC, fusion positron-emission tomography (PET)-CT scanning is often the best test. Although SCLC tumors are PET-avid tumors, the added benefit of PET-CT over the CT scan is not clear for this disease. For NSCLC, additional imaging of the brain or the bones is not necessary unless symptoms warrant additional evaluation. In SCLC, the frequency of metastasis to these sites warrants a baseline evaluation with bone scanning and magnetic resonance imaging of the brain at the time of diagnosis.

In patients that are potentially resectable, accurate staging of the mediastinum becomes paramount. Abnormal lymphadenopathy on CT is not adequate to determine lymph node involvement for NSCLC. PET-CT scans have higher sensitivity and specificity, but these tests do not replace direct sampling of the lymph nodes by mediastinoscopy. Endoscopic and endobronchial ultrasonography techniques are less invasive, can be combined with lymph node sampling, and are emerging as an appropriate method of staging the mediastinum in experienced hands.

All patients should be evaluated with baseline blood work including a complete blood count, liver function tests, and assessment of renal function. Assessment of the patient's performance status has important prognostic and therapeutic implications and should be

TABLE 1 Clinical Manifestations of Lung Cancer

Tumor Local Effects	Distant Metastases	Paraneoplastic Syndromes
Cough	Bone pain	Hypercalcemia
Dyspnea	Neurologic symptoms	SIADH
Hemoptysis	Headache	Lambert-Eaton syndrome
Chest pain	Nausea and vomiting	Cerebellar ataxia
Hoarseness	Weight loss	Encephalitis
Horner's syndrome	Fatigue	Cachexia/anorexia
SVC syndrome	Abdominal pain	Cushing's syndrome
Postobstructive pneumonia	Spinal cord compression	
Pericardial effusion	Pathologic fracture	

Abbreviations: SIADH = syndrome of inappropriate antidiuretic hormone; SVC = superior vena cava.

CURRENT THERAPY

Non–small cell lung cancer

- Stage I: Surgical resection
- Stage II: Surgery + adjuvant chemotherapy
- Stage IIIA: Induction chemotherapy
    - Responders: Surgery with or without XRT
    - Nonresponders: Concurrent chemotherapy + XRT
- Stage IIIB: Concurrent chemotherapy and XRT
- Stage IV: Chemotherapy and drugs targeting the epidermal growth factor receptor
    - 1st line: Platinum doublet chemotherapy with bevacizumab (Avastin) or cetuximab (Erbitux)
    - 2nd line: Pemetrexed (Alimta), docetaxel (Taxotere), or erlotinib (Tarceva) as a single agent

Small cell lung cancer

- Limited stage: Concurrent chemotherapy + XRT; PCI for responders
- Extensive stage:
    - 1st line: Carboplatin (Paraplatin)/etoposide (VePesid) or cisplatinum (Platinol)/irinotecan (Camptosar) for four cycles; PCI for responders; supportive care
    - 2nd line: Topotecan (Hycamtin)

Abbreviations: PCI = prophylactic cranial irradiation; XRT = radiation therapy.

documented for all patients. Furthermore, for patients who are considered surgically resectable, it is important to assess the tolerability of lobectomy or pneumonectomy. A forced expiratory volume in 1 second (FEV_1) greater than 2 L generally predicts the ability to tolerate pneumonectomy, whereas an FEV_1 of less than 1 L predicts worse outcome with lobectomy. The diffusion capacity of carbon monoxide (DL_{CO}) can also be a useful measurement in borderline cases.

Treatment

NON-SMALL CELL LUNG CANCER

For NSCLC, the stage at diagnosis is the best predictor of overall survival and the most appropriate therapy (Tables 2 and 3).

Stage I

In the tumor-node-metastasis (TNM) staging system, stage I comprises T1 (stage IA) and T2 (stage IB) tumors that do not have any nodal involvement (N0) and no evidence of distant metastasis (M0). The primary mode of therapy for these patients is surgical resection, which results in 5-year survival rates of approximately 70%. Whenever possible, lobectomy with complete mediastinal lymph node dissection is recommended for accurate pathologic staging. Occasionally, pneumonectomy is required based on the location of the primary tumor; however, the morbidity and mortality of this procedure are much higher than with lobectomy. Video-assisted thoracoscopy approaches, if possible, are often desirable and may result in lower surgical morbidity. Surgical resection may not be feasible for all patients, particularly those with poor pulmonary function or poor performance status. For such patients, primary radiotherapy

TABLE 3 Staging Groups*

Stage	T	N	M
IA	T1	N0	M0
IB	T2	N0	M0
IIA	T1–2a	N0	M0
	T2b	N0	M0
IIB	T2b	N1	M0
	T3	N0	M0
IIIA	T1–2	N2	M0
	T3	N1	M0
	T4	N0–1	M0
IIIB	T4	N2	M0
	Tx	N3	M0
IV	Tx	NX	M1

*For staging of tumors (T), nodes (N), and metastases (M), see Table 2.

TABLE 2 Tumor-Node-Metastasis (TNM) Staging*

Primary Tumor (T)	
T0	No demonstrable tumor
T_{is}	Carcinoma in situ
T1	Tumor <3 cm
T1a	Tumor <2 cm
T1b	Tumor >2 cm and <3 cm
T2	Tumor >3 cm but <7 cm
T2a	Tumor >3 cm but <5 cm
T2b	Tumor >5 cm but <7 cm
T3	Tumor >7 cm or any of the following: • Directly invades the chest wall, diaphragm, phrenic nerve, mediastinal pleura, pericardium, or main bronchus <2 cm from carina • Atelectasis or obstructive pneumonitis of the entire lung • Separate tumor nodules within the same lobe
T4	Tumor of any size that invades the mediastinum, heart, great vessels, esophagus, trachea, recurrent laryngeal nerve, vertebral body, or carina or separate tumor nodule in a different ipsilateral lobe

Regional Lymph Nodes (N)	
N0	No regional lymph node disease
N1	Ipsilateral involvement of hilar, peribronchial, or interlobar nodes including by direct extension of the primary tumor
N2	Involvement of ipsilateral mediastinal nodes
N3	Involvement of contralateral mediastinal or hilar nodes or involvement of ipsilateral or contralateral scalene or supraclavicular nodes

Distant Metastasis (M)	
M0	No metastasis identified
M1	Distant metastasis
M1a	Separate tumor nodule in contralateral lobe, tumor with pleural nodules, or malignant pleural or pericardial effusion
M1b	Distant metastasis

*For staging groups, see Table 3.

may be considered. Traditional external-beam radiation therapy results in much poorer outcomes than surgery, although newer techniques are emerging; for example, stereotactic radiosurgery is becoming an effective method of providing local control for stage I tumors.

Several studies have evaluated the role of adjuvant chemotherapy in this group of patients, but no clear survival benefit has emerged. The Cancer and Leukemia Group B (CALGB) 9633 study randomized 344 patients with stage IB tumors to receive either surgery alone or surgery followed by carboplatin (Paraplatin)[1] and paclitaxel (Taxol). A survival benefit was demonstrated only for patients with tumors larger than 4 cm. The JBR.10 study, conducted by the National Cancer Institute of Canada, showed a survival benefit for carboplatin and vinorelbine (Navelbine) adjuvant therapy; however, this study included patients with stage IB, II, and III disease. Additional studies from Europe and Asia have also demonstrated advantages to adjuvant chemotherapy in resected NSCLC, but typically not in tumors smaller than 4 cm. The LACE (Lung Adjuvant Cisplatin Evaluation) meta-analysis incorporated data from five large, randomized trials and also found no significant benefit for adjuvant chemotherapy in stage I patients. In light of these findings, adjuvant therapy in NSCLC is not routinely recommended for small stage I tumors (<4 cm) except as part of a clinical trial. Larger stage I tumors may benefit from adjuvant chemotherapy, and this decision is largely left to the practicing oncologist and patient.

There does not appear to be any added benefit for the use of radiation therapy after surgical resection of stage I tumors. If the surgical margins are positive, adjuvant radiation therapy is routinely recommended, but this occurs infrequently. As discussed later, some patients with a clinical stage I NSCLC are upstaged by the finding of malignant disease in the mediastinum, and in this group postoperative radiation therapy improves local control and, potentially, survival when combined with adjuvant chemotherapy.

Stage II

The approach to treating stage II NSCLC is largely the same as for stage I, with surgical resection as the primary modality of treatment. Again, lobectomy using a minimally invasive video-assisted thoracoscopic approach is preferred whenever possible. Adjuvant chemotherapy offers a more clear survival advantage in patients with stage II disease. All of the aforementioned studies and the meta-analysis showed a benefit for adjuvant chemotherapy in stage II patients.

Stage III

Stage III NSCLC denotes metastasis to mediastinal lymph nodes. The hallmark of treatment in stage III patients is a multimodal approach in which surgery, radiation, and chemotherapy all may play a significant role. The division of this stage into IIIA and IIIB denotes ipsilateral and contralateral nodal involvement, respectively. Whereas the overall prognosis in this group of patients is poor, treatment with curative intent results in long-term survival in 10% to 30% of cases. This also represents the stage with the most heterogeneity, so the approach should be individualized, taking into consideration the patient's performance status, resectability, and extent of disease.

Whether patients with stage III disease should undergo resection of the tumor is still open to some debate. The Intergroup 0139 trial randomized stage IIIA and selected stage IIIB patients to receive concurrent chemoradiation with cisplatin (Platinol)[1] and etoposide (VePesid)[1] plus 45 Gy of radiation followed by surgical resection, or the same chemoradiation with 61 Gy of radiation therapy. Patients in the surgical arm who experienced progression while receiving the chemotherapy were given additional radiation therapy to 61 Gy. There was no difference in overall survival between the two groups (23.6 versus 22.2 months for trimodality and chemoradiation therapy, respectively). Recurrence rates and progression-free

survival were much more favorable for the surgery arm. Much of the excess mortality in the surgery arm occurred among those patients who required a pneumonectomy for complete resection. Forty-six percent of patients were downstaged by induction chemotherapy to N0 disease at the time of resection. Among those patients, the 5-year survival rate was 40%, suggesting that good response to induction chemoradiotherapy may predict a benefit for surgical resection. Therefore, for patients with stage IIIA, two cycles of induction chemotherapy with or without irradiation should be offered, followed by restaging. Those with a good response to chemotherapy could be considered for complete resection followed by consolidation chemotherapy. Radiation therapy to the mediastinum should be offered to patients who have residual mediastinal disease at the time of resection. Pneumonectomy for complete resection should be undertaken only in patients who have an excellent performance status and after careful discussion of the risks of this procedure.

In general, stage IIIB disease is inoperable. Patients who have satellite tumors within the same lobe may be considered for resection provided that they do not have disease in the mediastinum and that resection can be accomplished with no more than a lobectomy. For patients with inoperable stage III disease, chemotherapy with irradiation is clearly superior to irradiation alone and can lead to long-term survival, with a 3-year survival rate as high as 30%. The optimal strategy is not known, but a commonly used regimen is the combination of cisplatin[1] and etoposide[1] given concurrently with radiation therapy to 66 Gy for 6 weeks. The use of induction chemotherapy followed by chemoradiation has been evaluated, as has the use of consolidation chemotherapy, but neither regimen has clearly been proven to be superior. For patients with poor performance status, a sequential chemotherapy followed by irradiation might be preferred; for those deemed unfit for chemotherapy, palliative irradiation might be the most appropriate therapy.

Stage IV

For patients with metastatic NSCLC, the treatment is mainly palliative; however, prolongation of survival is a reasonable goal. Despite best therapy, however, median survival time remains less than a year. Several platinum combinations have efficacy in NSCLC. Schiller and colleagues randomized 1207 patients to receive either cisplatin[1] in combination with paclitaxel, docetaxel (Taxotere), or gemcitabine (Gemzar), or a combination of carboplatin[1] and paclitaxel, with survival as the primary endpoint. Response rates were highest with the cisplatin/gemcitabine combination; however, overall survival was not significantly different for any of the groups. Based on tolerability, carboplatin-containing regimens have largely replaced cisplatin doublets for patients with metastatic disease. Carboplatin can be combined with one of the previously mentioned drugs or with newer agents such as pemetrexed (Alimta) and irinotecan (Camptosar).[1] All have demonstrated efficacy, but no single regimen has emerged with clear superiority. Recently, the addition of bevacizumab (Avastin), a monoclonal antibody against vascular endothelial growth factor, to carboplatin and paclitaxel was shown to prolong median survival to 12.3 months, compared with 10.3 months for chemotherapy alone. This study excluded patients with squamous histology and brain metastasis because of the risk of bleeding complications in those subgroups. Therefore, in patients with nonsquamous NSCLC, this regimen is standard of care. It remains to be seen whether the addition of bevacizumab to other platinum doublets results in similar improvements in survival. In one trial, the combination of cisplatin, gemcitabine, and bevacizumab did not provide any additional benefit to cisplatin and gemcitabine alone.

There has also been interest in the use of drugs targeting the epidermal growth factor receptor (EGFR). Data presented at the 2008 American Society of Clinical Oncology annual meeting demonstrated a modest benefit for the addition of cetuximab (Erbitux),[1] a monoclonal antibody against EGFR, to a regimen of cisplatin[1] and

---

[1]Not FDA approved for this indication.

[1]Not FDA approved for this indication.

vinorelbine, compared with the chemotherapy regimen alone, in patients whose tumors expressed EGFR. Targeting of EGFR in combination with chemotherapy has not extended to the oral EGFR tyrosine kinase inhibitors, erlotinib (Tarceva) and gefitinib (Iressa). Four phase III randomized trials, two with gefitinib and two with erlotinib, failed to show a survival benefit for EGFR tyrosine kinase inhibitors in combination with platinum doublet chemotherapy in unselected NSCLC patients, although subgroup analysis did demonstrate a benefit for never-smokers, patients with bronchioalveolar histology, and patients with somatic mutations in EGFR. Therefore, cetuximab with cisplatin and vinorelbine can be considered for first-line therapy, but this should be limited to patients with squamous histology and those who have brain metastases, because such patients are not eligible for bevacizumab therapy.

Patients are commonly evaluated for response after two cycles of treatment and continued for four cycles if they have responsive or stable disease. There has been controversy as to whether additional chemotherapy after four cycles of treatment offers any benefit, and the general trend among North American oncologists is to limit the first-line chemotherapy to four cycles. Thus far, no clear benefit to maintenance chemotherapy or extended chemotherapy beyond six cycles has been demonstrated. It should be noted that in the bevacizumab trial and the cetuximab trial, these agents were maintained after completion of four cycles of chemotherapy, until progression or unacceptable toxicity developed. Maintenance pemetrexed resulted in an improvement in progression-free survival, without a clear improvement in overall survival; but it was not clear whether this strategy was better than simply using second-line pemetrexed at the time of progression.

When relapse occurs, there continues to be a survival and quality-of-life benefit associated with salvage therapy. Single-agent regimens should be used to avoid excess toxicity in this poor-prognosis population. Approved second-line treatments include docetaxel and erlotinib, based on improved survival compared with best supportive care. Pemetrexed has also been approved based on non-inferiority to docetaxel in the second-line setting and is better tolerated than docetaxel. If these therapies fail, salvage therapy can be attempted with several active chemotherapy agents, although none of these has demonstrated a clear survival benefit in this population. Chemotherapy should be considered only for patients who have good performance status, and careful emphasis should be placed on palliation of symptoms.

Supportive care is an important adjunct to chemotherapy in the treatment of stage IV lung cancer. Palliative irradiation can be applied to tumors that are causing significant pain or symptoms. Palliative response is seen in more than 50% of patients. Patients with superior vena cava syndrome benefit from the addition of palliative irradiation, as do patients with obstructive pneumonia. One or a few metastases to the brain should be treated with surgical resection followed by whole-brain radiotherapy whenever possible. Stereotactic radiosurgery is an alternative if surgery is not feasible.

SMALL CELL LUNG CANCER

SCLC is hallmarked by aggressive growth and early metastasis. If it is left untreated, median survival time is only 2 to 4 months. However, these tumors are highly sensitive to chemotherapy, and response rates of 60% to 80% are expected. These tumors are also highly radiosensitive, but radiation therapy is limited by the extent of metastatic disease. Although the TNM staging system for NSCLC is applicable, in practical terms SCLC is usually referred to being of limited stage (if the disease is limited to one radiation field) or extensive stage (if not so limited). Surgery is not usually a viable treatment option except in those with very small tumors and no evidence of metastasis to the mediastinum or distant sites.

Patients with limited-stage disease should be treated with four cycles of cisplatin[1] and etoposide with concurrent radiotherapy to the involved field. With this approach approximately 20% of patients are disease free at 3 years. Extensive-stage SCLC is incurable, and median survival is in the range of 8 to 12 months. Chemotherapy can result in dramatic improvements in performance status, and this is one of the few situations in which chemotherapy should be offered even to very moribund patients. The standard of care is carboplatin[1] plus etoposide. Despite numerous trials of multiagent chemotherapy and novel targeted agents, no other regimen has surpassed the results of the standard of care. The combination of carboplatin and irinotecan[1] was shown to be superior to the standard of care in a large, randomized, phase III trial in Japan, but an American trial showed no benefit for this approach. Therefore, cisplatin and irinotecan could be considered an acceptable alternative to the standard of care. The toxicity profile is similar, with the irinotecan regimen causing significant gastrointestinal toxicity and the etoposide regimen having mainly hematologic toxicity. If first-line therapy fails, topotecan (Hycamtin) has been shown to improve quality of life and overall survival when used as second-line therapy. There are no other second- or third-line agents with proven survival or palliative benefit, and, given the dismal prognosis, patients should be considered for a clinical trial whenever possible.

For both limited- and extensive-stage disease, relapse in the brain is a significant cause of morbidity and mortality and has prompted the use of prophylactic cranial irradiation. This approach has consistently proved to be of benefit for patients who have a good response to primary therapy. The benefit has been seen to prevent symptomatic brain metastasis and also to improve overall survival. Cognitive dysfunction after prophylactic cranial irradiation can occur, particularly if it is given concurrently with chemotherapy. Therefore, whenever possible, it should be given only after chemotherapy is completed.

REFERENCES

Arriagada R, Bergman B, Dunant A, et al. Cisplatin-based adjuvant chemotherapy in patients with completely resected non-small-cell lung cancer. N Engl J Med 2004;350:351–60.

DeVita VT, Hellman S, Rosenberg SA. Cancer: Principles and practice of oncology. 4th ed. Philadelphia: Lippincott; 1993.

Noda K, Nishiwaki Y, Kawahara M, et al. Irinotecan plus cisplatin compared with etoposide plus cisplatin for extensive small-cell lung cancer. N Engl J Med 2002;346:85–91.

Pignon JP, Tribodet H, Scagliotti GV, et al. Lung adjuvant cisplatin evaluation: A pooled analysis by the LACE Collaborative Group. J Clin Oncol 2008;26:3552–9.

Sandler A, Gray R, Perry MC, et al. Paclitaxel-carboplatin alone or with bevacizumab for non-small-cell lung cancer. N Engl J Med 2006;355:2542–50.

Schiller JH, Harrington D, Belani CP, et al. Comparison of four chemotherapy regimens for advanced non-small-cell lung cancer. N Engl J Med 2002;346:92–8.

Shepherd FA, Rodrigues Pereira J, Ciuleanu T, et al. Erlotinib in previously treated non-small-cell lung cancer. N Engl J Med 2005;353:123–32.

Slotman B, Faivre-Finn C, Kramer G, et al. Prophylactic cranial irradiation in extensive small-cell lung cancer. N Engl J Med 2007;357:664–72.

Strauss GM, Herndon JE 2nd, Maddaus MA, et al. Adjuvant paclitaxel plus carboplatin compared with observation in stage IB non-small-cell lung cancer: CALGB 9633 with the Cancer and Leukemia Group B, Radiation Therapy Oncology Group, and North Central Cancer Treatment Group Study Groups. J Clin Oncol 2008;26:5043–51.

van Meerbeeck JP, Kramer GW, Van Schil PE, et al. Randomized controlled trial of resection versus radiotherapy after induction chemotherapy in stage IIIA-N2 non-small-cell lung cancer. J Natl Cancer Inst 2007;99:442–50.

Winton T, Livingston R, Johnson D, et al. Vinorelbine plus cisplatin vs. observation in resected non-small-cell lung cancer. N Engl J Med 2005;352:2589–97.

---

[1]Not FDA approved for this indication.

---

[1]Not FDA approved for this indication.

Coccidioidomycosis

Method of
Gregory M. Anstead, MD

Coccidioidomycosis is caused by soil fungi of the genus *Coccidioides*, divided genetically into *Coccidioides immitis* (California isolates) and *Coccidioides posadasii* (isolates outside California). There are no distinct clinical differences between the two species. *Coccidioides* occurs only in the Western hemisphere, primarily in the southwestern United States (Arizona and parts of California, New Mexico, Utah, Nevada, and Texas) and in northern Mexico, areas characterized by arid to semiarid climates, hot summers, low altitude, alkaline soil, and sparse vegetation. Hyperendemic areas include the San Joaquin Valley of California and Pima, Pinal, and Maricopa Counties in Arizona. *Coccidioides* is also found in parts of Latin America (Guatemala, Honduras, Nicaragua, Argentina, Paraguay, Venezuela, and Colombia). Cases may be observed in nonendemic areas because of travel or reactivation of prior infection. In the United States, an estimated 150,000 cases of coccidioidomycosis occur annually, with the clinical presentation ranging from a self-limited respiratory infection to devastating disseminated disease. Persons with occupations involving exposure to soil are at risk for coccidioidomycosis. Immunocompromised persons are also at high risk, including patients with AIDS, transplant recipients (especially those who received *Coccidioides*-infected organs), patients receiving tumor necrosis factor-α antagonists, pregnant women, and cancer patients. Filipinos, African Americans, and persons with blood group B are also at increased risk for disseminated disease. Outbreaks may occur after dust storms, earthquakes, droughts, and activities causing soil disruption, such as construction and archeological digs.

Coccidioides is dimorphic; in the soil, the organism exists in its mycelial form, which produces barrel-shaped arthroconidia. The usual means of infection is the inhalation of arthroconidia; uncommon routes include direct cutaneous inoculation and organ transplantation. Arthroconidia germinate to produce spherules filled with endospores, the characteristic tissue phase. Spherules rupture to release endospores, which form additional spherules. The spherules become surrounded by neutrophils and macrophages, which leads to granuloma formation. Both B and T lymphocytes are essential for host defense against this pathogen.

Clinical Manifestations

Coccidioidomycosis is asymptomatic in 60% of infected individuals. In the remaining 40% a self-limited, flu-like illness, with dry cough, pleuritic chest pain, myalgias, arthralgia, fever, sweats, anorexia, and weakness, develops 1 to 3 weeks after exposure. Primary infection may be accompanied by immune complex–mediated complications, including an erythematous macular rash, erythema multiforme, and erythema nodosum. Acute infection usually resolves without therapy, although symptoms may persist for weeks. In 5% of these patients, asymptomatic pulmonary residua persist, including pulmonary nodules and cavitation. Immunocompromised patients may develop chronic progressive pulmonary infection, with the evolution of thin-walled cavities that may rupture, leading to bronchopleural fistula and empyema formation.

Extrapulmonary disease develops in 1 of every 200 patients and can involve the skin, soft tissues, bones, joints, and meninges. The most common cutaneous lesions are verrucous papules, ulcers, or plaques. The spine is the most frequent site of osseous dissemination, although the typical lytic lesions may also occur in the skull, hands, feet, and tibia. Joint involvement is usually monoarticular and most commonly involves the ankle and knee. Fungemia may occur in immunocompromised patients and carries a poor prognosis.

In coccidioidal meningitis, the basilar meninges are usually affected. Cerebrospinal fluid findings include lymphocytic pleocytosis (often with eosinophilia), hypoglycorrhachia, and elevated protein levels. The mortality rate is greater than 90% at 1 year without therapy, and chronic infection is the rule. Hydrocephalus or hydrocephalus coexisting with brain infarction is associated with a higher mortality rate.

CURRENT DIAGNOSIS

- Maintain a high index of suspicion in patients from endemic areas and travelers.
- Diagnostic tests include
  - Serologic detection of immunoglobulin M and immunoglobulin G antibodies by immunodiffusion, complement fixation, and enzyme immunoassay
  - Culture of sputum, exudates, cerebrospinal fluid, and tissue
  - Direct observation of *Coccidioides* spherules in histopathologic and cytologic specimens
  - Urine antigen enzyme immunoassay

Coccidioidomycosis is a great imitator and has many diverse clinical presentations, including immune thrombocytopenia, ocular involvement, massive cervical lymphadenopathy, laryngeal and retropharyngeal abscesses, endocarditis, pericarditis, peritonitis, hepatitis, and lesions of the male and female genitals and urogenital tracts.

Diagnosis

Coccidioidomycosis may be diagnosed by direct observation of spherules in tissues or in wet mounts of sputa or exudates. The growth of *Coccidioides* in culture usually occurs in 3 to 5 days, with sporulation after 5 to 10 days. Definitive identification is made by DNA probe or exoantigen testing. Laboratory personnel should exercise extreme caution when handling cultures of *Coccidioides*.

CURRENT THERAPY

Pulmonary Infection

- No risk factors for dissemination; not severe disease—Observe
- Risk factors; prolonged symptoms—Fluconazole (Diflucan)[1] 400 mg/day or itraconazole (Sporanox)[1] 200 mg twice a day for 3 to 6 months
- Diffuse or severe pneumonia—Amphotericin B (Fungizone) 1 mg/kg/day or lipid formulation of Amphotericin (Abelcet, AmBisome)[1] 5 mg/kg/day; after improvement, switch to azole; treat for 1 year
- Chronic fibrocavitary disease—Azole therapy for at least 1 year; resection in selected cases

Disseminated Disease

- Nonmeningeal, severe disease—Amphotericin B 1 mg/kg/day or lipid formulation of Amphotericin[1] 5 mg/kg/day; after improvement, switch to azole for 1 to 2 years; consider posaconazole (Noxafil)[1] 200 mg four times daily in refractory cases
- Nonmeningeal, slowly progressive—Azole therapy for 1 to 2 years; itraconazole[1] preferred for bony involvement; consider posaconazole[1] 200 mg four times daily in refractory cases
- Meningeal, central nervous system involvement—Fluconazole 800 to 2000 mg/day[3]; intrathecal amphotericin B[1] or voriconazole (Vfend)[1] 200 mg twice daily in refractory cases; shunting for hydrocephalus; consider corticosteroids if vasculitis is present

---

[1]Not FDA approved for this indication.
[3]Exceeds dosage recommended by the manufacturer.

Serologic methods are quite useful in establishing the diagnosis and for monitoring the course of the infection. Immunoglobulin M (IgM) antibodies are present soon after infection or relapse but then wane; quantification does not correlate with disease severity. The IgG antibody appears later and remains positive for months. Rising titers of IgG are associated with progressive disease, and declining titers are associated with resolution. The IgG antibodies are able to fix complement when combined with coccidioidal antigen, and can be detected by immunodiffusion for complement fixation (IDCF); titers of 1:16 or greater suggest disseminated disease. In the cerebrospinal fluid, a positive IDCF of any titer is considered diagnostic of meningitis and is much more sensitive than culture in making the diagnosis. An enzyme immunoassay is also available, but it is less specific. Recently, a specific urinary antigen test became available for the diagnosis of coccidioidomycosis; this assay has a sensitivity of 71% in moderate-to-severe disease, compared with 84% for culture, 29% for histopathologic examination, and 75% for serologic testing.

Treatment

In most patients, primary pulmonary infection resolves spontaneously without treatment. However, all patients require observation for at least 2 years to document resolution of infection and to identify any complications as soon as possible. For patients who have risk factors for disseminated disease (listed earlier), treatment is necessary. Other indications for treatment are severe disease (infiltrates involving both lungs or more than half of one lung; significant hilar or mediastinal lymphadenopathy; complement fixation titers >1:16) and highly symptomatic disease (weight loss >10%; night sweats present for >3 weeks; symptoms present for >2 months).

For diffuse or severe pneumonia, therapy with amphotericin B deoxycholate (Fungizone) 0.5 to 1.5 mg/kg/day, or a lipid formulation of amphotericin B (Abelcet or AmBisome)[1] 2 to 5 mg/kg/day should be given for several weeks, followed by an oral azole, such as itraconazole (Sporanox)[1] 200 mg twice daily or fluconazole (Diflucan)[1] 400 to 800 mg/day). The total duration of therapy should be at least 1 year; for immunosuppressed patients, oral azole therapy should be maintained as secondary prophylaxis. In HIV patients with CD4-positive T-cell counts greater than 250 cells/mm^3 who had focal pneumonias that responded to azoles, antifungals may be discontinued. Azole therapy may be used initially for less severe disease. During pregnancy, amphotericin B is the preferred drug, because of the teratogenicity of azoles.

An asymptomatic patient with a solitary nodule or pulmonary cavitation due to C. immitis does not require specific antifungal therapy or resection. However, the development of complications from the cavitation, such as hemoptysis or bacterial or fungal superinfection, necessitates initiation of azole therapy. Resection of the cavities is an alternative to antifungal therapy. Rupture of a cavity into the pleural space requires surgical intervention with closure by lobectomy with decortication, in addition to antifungal therapy. For chronic pneumonia, the initial treatment should be an oral azole for at least 1 year. If the disease persists, one may switch to another oral azole, increase the dose if fluconazole was initially selected, or switch to amphotericin B. Resection should be performed for patients with refractory focal lesions or severe hemoptysis.

The treatment of disseminated infection without central nervous system involvement is based on oral azole therapy, such as itraconazole or fluconazole (400 mg/day, or higher in case of fluconazole). If there is little or no improvement or if there is vertebral involvement, treatment with amphotericin B is recommended (dosage as for diffuse pneumonia). Concomitant surgical débridement or stabilization is also recommended. In patients with refractory coccidioidomycosis that has failed to respond to fluconazole, itraconazole, and

amphotericin B and its lipid formulations, treatment with posaconazole (Noxafil)[1] 200 mg four times daily has been successful.

For coccidioidal meningitis, lifetime treatment with azoles is indicated. Fluconazole, at doses of 800 mg/day or higher,[3] is recommended. There have been a few reports of successful treatment of coccidioidal meningitis with voriconazole (Vfend)[1] 200 mg orally twice daily after a loading dose. Itraconazole is not recommended because of its irregular oral absorption. Obstructive hydrocephalus requires shunting. Intrathecal amphotericin B[1] was previously used for meningeal coccidioidomycosis, but it is now strictly reserved for infections that are refractory to high-dose azoles.

REFERENCES

Anstead GM, Graybill JR. Coccidioidomycosis. Infect Dis Clin North Am 2006;20:621–43.

Blair JE. State-of-the art treatment of coccidioidomycosis skeletal infections. Ann N Y Acad Sci 2007;1111:422–33.

Blair JE. State-of-the-art treatment of coccidiodomycosis skin and soft tissue infections. Ann N Y Acad Sci 2007;1111:411–21.

Crum NF, Lederman ER, Stafford CM, et al. Coccidioidomycosis: A descriptive survey of a reemerging disease—Clinical characteristics and emerging controversies. Medicine (Baltimore) 2004;83:149–75.

Crum-Cianflone NF, Truett AA, Teneza-Mora N, et al. Unusual presentations of coccidioidomycosis: A case series and review of the literature. Medicine (Baltimore) 2006;85:263–77.

Galgiani J, Ampel N, Blair J, et al. Coccidioidomycosis. Clin Infect Dis 2005;41:1217–23.

Parish JM, Blair JE. Coccidioidomycosis. Mayo Clin Proc 2008;83:343–8; quiz 348–349.

Saubolle MA, McKellar PP, Sussland D. Epidemiologic, clinical, and diagnostic aspects of coccidioidomycosis. J Clin Microbiol 2007;45:26–30.

Williams PL. Coccidioidal meningitis. Ann N Y Acad Sci 2007;1111:377–84.

---

[1]Not FDA approved for this indication.
[3]Exceeds dosage recommended by the manufacturer.

Histoplasmosis

Method of
Philip C. Johnson, MD

Histoplasma capsulatum causes a variety of disease states in areas of the world endemic for the organism. Therapeutic modalities have been studied over the last 20 years in response to new presentations of histoplasmosis in a variety of patient groups. Guidelines have been published by the Infectious Diseases Society of America that take into account the changing epidemiology, pathogenesis, and diagnosis of these conditions. New therapeutic options, including lipid preparations of amphotericin B and new triazole antifungals, have improved responses to therapy. This chapter outlines these developments and summarizes the current treatment recommendations for histoplasmosis.

Etiology and Epidemiology

H. capsulatum is a fungus that grows as a mold at ambient temperature and as a yeast at mammalian body temperatures. Similar to *Blastomyces dermatitidis, Paracoccidioides brasiliensis, Sporothrix schenckii,* and *Coccidioides immitis,* it is a dimorphic fungus. It is the mycelia growth phase that produces the small microconidia (spores) that are inhaled as droplet nuclei and carried to the distal alveolar septa of the lung. Once at body temperature, the microconidia germinate and convert to the yeast phase of the organism; the yeast phase is pathogenic.

---

[1]Not FDA approved for this indication.

Skin test surveys performed 40 years ago defined the endemic area for *H. capsulatum* in the United States, which borders the Ohio and Mississippi River valleys. In the Western Hemisphere, the endemic area includes the islands in the Caribbean and Mexico, as well as Central and South America. Cases have been also reported in Asia, Africa, and Europe. Growth of the fungus occurs in soil enriched by nitrogen-containing wastes of bird and bat droppings, which in the midwestern United States usually occurs under tree-lined areas bordering rivers, in caves, and under chicken coops or bird roosts. Microfoci of contaminated soil exist throughout the endemic area. When these are disturbed by the wind or by human activity through walking, spelunking, or using earth moving equipment, aerosolization of microconidia ensues and previously unexposed people are at risk for histoplasmosis. Although the infectious dose is unknown, outbreak studies have found that those with the most serious pulmonary disease have usually been exposed to the highest numbers of organisms concentrated in a small space.

Pathogenesis

Microconidia of *H. capsulatum* are inhaled and carried to the alveoli, where an inflammatory process unfolds. The initial inflammatory process consists of neutrophil infiltration. Within days, macrocytes phagocytize the spores. It is suspected that conversion from mold to yeast occurs intracellularly at that time. Yeast are carried by these cells through lymphatics to regional lymph nodes and the other organs of the reticuloendothelial system, the liver, spleen, and bone marrow. Cell-mediated immunity is the primary immune response to the yeast. Granulomas develop in the lung and other organs where the yeast lodge. These granulomas contain the organisms and eventually heal by fibrosis and calcification. Chest radiographs of people residing in endemic areas typically reveal the presence of small granulomas, representing previous acute pulmonary histoplasmosis. Calcified granulomas can also be found in the spleen and liver.

Several presentations of histoplasmosis result from an exuberant host immune response. These include mediastinal lymphadenitis, mediastinal granuloma, mediastinal fibrosis, pericarditis, and histoplasmoma. If the reaction is primarily one of fibrosis in the mediastinal region, patients will present with symptoms of constriction of vascular structures and airways. If the reaction is peripheral in the lung, an asymptomatic lesion resembling a malignancy will be found on chest radiography.

Patients with centrilobular emphysema or preexisting cavitary lung disease can develop a chronic histoplasmosis infection in the pulmonary cavities. The pathophysiology of this disease is the growth of organisms in pulmonary cavities, where they elude control by cellular immunity. Collections of organisms in the abnormal pulmonary tissue can spill over to other areas of less-diseased lung tissue. Treatment is centered on decreasing the amount of the organisms present in the cavities.

In patients with a deficiency of cell-mediated immunity a variety of disease presentations can occur. These relate in part to the degree of immunodeficiency present. Infants, patients infected with HIV, and patients undergoing cancer chemotherapy or treatment for organ transplantation can present with progressive disseminated histoplasmosis (PDH), which can occur after primary exposure or reactivation. These patients may have pulmonary presentations as well as disease resulting from the involvement of the reticuloendothelial system, with enlargement of lymph nodes, liver, and spleen and bone marrow involvement. Other presentations include involvement of the trachea and vocal cords, skin, brain, and intestines. Rarely, central nervous system histoplasmosis is observed with cerebral lesions.

Diagnosis

The gold standard for diagnosis of *H. capsulatum* infection is culture of the organism from pulmonary secretions, blood, bone marrow, or tissue. This takes time. In acute pulmonary histoplasmosis, the yeast can rarely be identified in pulmonary secretions digested with 10% potassium hydroxide. Culturing of the organism can be cultured in 10% to 15% of cases, but it takes 2 to 6 weeks for presumptive diagnosis. Therefore, for acute pulmonary histoplasmosis, the value of a culture is minimal, because the patient invariably improves before the organism is isolated. Cultures can be of value in chronic pulmonary histoplasmosis, where up to 60% of cultures of respiratory secretions are positive and the diagnosis is usually in doubt because of its resemblance to tuberculosis. Cultures are usually positive in PDH, but the diagnosis can be established more quickly with antigen detection.

Antibody detection by the complement fixation test is useful for outbreak situations but has limited utility in the care of individual patients. A single titer of 1:32 or greater is significant, as is seroconversion. In patients with chronic pulmonary histoplasmosis, a negative result favors another diagnosis.

In PDH, examination of clinical specimens for the yeast form of *H. capsulatum* is difficult but can provide a timely answer. The 2- to 4-μm yeast form can be seen with Gomori methenamine silver or periodic acid–Schiff staining of tissue. Occasionally, organisms can be seen in macrophages with Wright staining of peripheral blood.

The detection of polysaccharide antigen by a test developed by Dr. Joseph Wheat has revolutionized the diagnosis of PDH in patients with AIDS. The urine is the easiest and best specimen to send, but the antigen may also be detected in blood and cerebrospinal fluid. An improved test has been released that is more specific. Monitoring of antigen levels is a useful tool for determining when to alter antifungal therapy in PDH.

Clinical Manifestations

ACUTE PULMONARY HISTOPLASMOSIS

Acute pulmonary histoplasmosis manifests as a flu-like respiratory illness within 7 to 21 days after inhalation in persons not previously exposed to the organism. It is suspected that the majority of those infected do not seek medical attention for this illness. In outbreak situations, only 1% to 4% of patients are hospitalized, and 95% of patients have a resolution of symptoms within 3 weeks. Those who have prolonged symptoms are believed to have been exposed to a larger dose of organisms. Their symptoms consist of prolonged fever, weight loss, and cough. These patients with moderate to severe disease have respiratory insufficiency and hypoxia.

In highly endemic areas patients may develop secondary cases of acute pulmonary histoplasmosis. In these cases, the incubation period is shorter, the symptoms are less, and hilar lymphadenopathy is absent, signaling development of a rapid cell-mediated immune response.

CHRONIC CAVITARY PULMONARY HISTOPLASMOSIS

Patients with chronic cavitary pulmonary histoplasmosis present with a chronic cough, malaise, weight loss, and low-grade fever. Treatment is complicated by the difficulty of getting the antifungal agent to the disease process, because of the altered architecture of the preexisting cavitary lung disease.

PERICARDITIS

Once the immune response to acute pulmonary histoplasmosis has developed and hilar lymph nodes are involved, some of these nodes adjacent to the pericardium can induce a pericarditis. Direct extension of the infection to the covering of the heart is not involved. This disease mimics a viral pericarditis with the additional finding of enlarged hilar lymph nodes. Pericarditis is rare in PDH, because the altered host immunity fails to develop.

RHEUMATOLOGIC SYNDROMES

In outbreaks of histoplasmosis, arthritis, arthralgias, and erythema nodosum occur in 5% to 10% of patients. These represent immune sequelae rather than direct infection. Even in PDH, fungal arthritis is exceedingly rare, and the dermatologic involvement is localized rather than inflammatory.

MEDIASTINAL LYMPHADENITIS

Enlargement of infected mediastinal lymph nodes, where histoplasmosis is contained, leads, particularly in children, to a variety of symptoms resulting from bronchial and esophageal compression by the engorged lymph nodes. Chest pain, cough, atelectasis, and dysphagia are the common symptoms. All are inflammatory in nature and do not represent direct organ involvement with *H. capsulatum*.

MEDIASTINAL GRANULOMA

Mediastinal granuloma is the coalescence of enlarged, infected lymph nodes. These masses may be up to 10 cm in diameter. They are located primarily in the subcarinal and right paratracheal areas. They can obstruct local structures, and their caseous centers can drain to the skin.

MEDIASTINAL FIBROSIS

In mediastinal fibrosis, the inflammatory process results in scarring and fibrosis, rather than lymph node enlargement and compression. The fibrosis can cause obstruction of the superior vena cava, lymphatics, and other structures. The symptoms can include those of superior vena cava syndrome or swelling in the arms, the neck, and, sometimes, the head.

BRONCHOLITHIASIS

Inflammatory lymph nodes may erode into a bronchus, resulting in cough, hemoptysis, and, occasionally, coughing up broncholiths of calcified particles extruded from eroded nodes. This condition is called broncholithiasis; although rare, it can cause a concerning array of symptoms that prompts medical evaluation.

HISTOPLASMOMA

Histoplasmomas are calcified granulomas, created by an exuberant immune response that can yield masses that can reach up to 1 to 2 cm. These lesions are found incidentally on chest radiographs and computed tomographic scans, and they can be differentiated by their calcified concentric rings, which are laid down similar to the peels of an onion. These lesions can be mistaken for coin lesions and are suspicious for lung cancer. They do not produce symptoms and therefore need no treatment. If they are resected because of the suspicion of malignancy, the question then becomes what is the appropriate treatment. None is necessary. The calcified granuloma is an example of the immune system's ability to wall off the organism and effectively contain it.

PROGRESSIVE DISSEMINATED HISTOPASMOSIS

Originally, PDH was reported primarily in infants. Because infants are not able to contain the disease, the organisms disseminate from regional lymph nodes to other area of the reticuloendothelial system. With the advent of chemotherapy for malignancy and organ transplantation, these patient groups were also found to develop this wasting disease. The AIDS epidemic produced another group of patients lacking cellular immunity who developed PDH, and now the majority of patients with PDH have AIDS.

In patients with AIDS, PDH manifests as a febrile illness involving the lymph nodes, spleen, liver, and bone marrow. Patients present with pancytopenia, disseminated pulmonary disease, hepatomegaly, splenomegaly, and sometimes rash. The lung is involved in half of the cases. As with *Pneumocystis jirovecii* pneumonia (PCP), levels of lactate dehydrogenase are elevated. Serum ferritin levels are also elevated. The CD4-positive T-cell count of patients with PDH is usually less than 50 cells/mm^3. The organism can be seen on peripheral blood smears or in tissues, and antigen detection in urine and blood is positive in more than 95% of cases. Tissue biopsy and cultures are invariably positive. Serologic tests are not helpful in the diagnosis.

Prophylaxis in Patients with AIDS

Primary prophylaxis was studied for 1 year in patients with AIDS and a CD4 count of less than 150 cells/mm^3 in a highly endemic area of the United States. Prophylaxis was successful but did not affect survival. A secondary effect on preventing oral candidiasis was demonstrated.

Secondary prophylaxis is better termed suppression therapy in patients with AIDS who have been successfully treated with induction therapy. The practice initially was to continue itraconazole (Sporanox) lifelong, for fear that patients with AIDS would relapse. With the advent of highly active antiviral therapy (HAART), patients with AIDS can recover their immune function to a level at which they are not at risk for opportunistic infections, including a relapse of histoplasmosis. So the question becomes when itraconazole suppression can be stopped. In an observational study, itraconazole was stopped after the CD4 count had increased to 150 cells/mm^3 and the patients had been on antifungal therapy for 12 months and on HAART for at least 6 months. No relapses of PDH were noted in 32 patients who had a median follow-up of 24 months. The use of urine histoplasma antigen has assisted in this question. Antigen levels should be less than 4.1 units.

Treatment

In 2007, the Infectious Diseases Society of America revised their guidelines for the treatment of histoplasmosis (Table 1). They took into consideration new studies with lipid formulations of amphotericin and tackled unresolved issues regarding treatment of histoplasmosis involving the central nervous system, in pregnant women and in children.

Lipid preparations of amphotericin B have become an acceptable alternative to the time-honored treatment with deoxycholate amphotericin B (Fungizone) for certain forms of histoplasmosis. There are several lipid-containing preparations. The most studied form is liposomal amphotericin (AmBisome),[1] which is given in a dose of 3 to 5 mg/kg/day. This compares to an amphotericin B dose of 0.7 to 1.0 mg/kg/day. If amphotericin lipid complex (Abelcet)[1] is used instead of AmBisome, the dose is 5.0 mg/kg/day.

Itraconazole (Sporanox) is given to adults in a regimen of 200 mg three times daily for 3 days, followed by 200 mg twice daily. Absorption of itraconazole can be a problem in certain patients, especially those taking histamine 2 blockers or proton pump inhibitors. It also may be problematic when used with inducers of the cytochrome P-450 system, such as phenytoin (Dilantin), rifampin (Rifadin), and the rifamycins—rifabutin (Mycobutin) and rifapentine (Priftin). In these situations, the guidelines suggest monitoring itraconazole levels. In general, itraconazole 200 mg/day is sufficient for those with mild disease and those who are receiving primary prophylaxis.

For pericarditis, rheumatologic syndromes, and mediastinal lymphadenitis, which are basically immunologic conditions resulting from histoplasma antigen, nonsteroidal antiinflammatory agents are often sufficient to relieve the symptoms. Prednisone is an alternative, but it is given together with itraconazole to cover the possibility of development of PDH. The dose used of prednisone is 0.5 to 1.0 mg/kg/day, which is tapered over 2 to 3 weeks.

Treatment of histoplasmosis in children relies on amphotericin B deoxycholate, which causes less renal insufficiency in children than in adults.

Histoplasmosis in pregnant women has resulted in transplacental passage of the organism to the fetus. Case reports are rare, and treatment guidelines are conjectural.

Despite new presentations of histoplasmosis in different populations, the development of improved understanding of the epidemiology, pathogenesis, diagnosis, and therapy of histoplasmosis has resulted in progress to better manage this unusual fungus infection.

---

[1]Not FDA approved for this indication.

TABLE 1 Treatment Recommendations for Histoplasmosis*

Histoplasmosis	Primary Therapy	Alternative Therapy	Notes
Acute pulmonary disease			
Mild to moderate	Observe if symptoms last <4 wk	Symptoms >4 wk: itraconazole (Sporanox) for 6–12 wk	
Severe	L Ampho B¹ or Ampho B for 2 wk	Follow with itraconazole for 12 wk Add methylprednisolone (SoluMedrol) 0.5–1.0 mg/kg for 1–2 wk	
Chronic cavitary pulmonary disease	Itraconazole for at least 1 yr		Monitor itraconazole levels at 2 wk
Pericarditis	NSAIDs	Oral prednisone 0.5–1.0 mg/kg for 1–2 wk plus itraconazole for 6–12 wk	Pericardiocentesis if patient is hemodynamically compromised
Rheumatologic syndromes	NSAIDs	Oral prednisone as above, if necessary	Steroids are rarely needed
Mediastinal lymphadenitis	NSAIDs	Steroids and oral prednisone for 1–2 wk plus itraconazole for 6–12 wk	Itraconazole if symptoms last >4 wk
Mediastinal granuloma	Observe	Itraconazole 6–12 wk	
Mediastinal fibrosis	Observe	Itraconazole 6–12 wk	Use itraconazole if mediastinal granuloma is present
Broncholithiasis	Observe		
Histoplasmoma	Observe		Differentiate from malignancy
PDH			
Mild to moderate	Itraconazole for 1 yr		Monitor histoplasmosis antigen
Severe	L Ampho B¹ for 2 wk	Ampho B for 2 wk	Itraconazole suppression after 2 wk
Prophylaxis in AIDS	Itraconazole 200 mg/day		If CD4 <150 in highly endemic area
Discontinuation of itraconazole in PDH in AIDS			After 1 yr of treatment if CD4 <150 and antigen level <4.1 units
Pregnancy	L Ampho B¹ for 4–6 wk	Ampho B for 4–6 wk	
CNS disease	L Ampho B¹ for 4–6 wk		Follow with itraconazole for 1 yr
Acute disease in children	Ampho B for 4–6 wk		
PDH in children	Ampho B for 4–6 wk	Itraconazole	

Adapted from Wheat LJ, Freifeld AG, Kleiman MB, et al; Infectious Diseases Society of America: Clinical practice guidelines for the management of patients with histoplasmosis: 2007 Update by the Infectious Diseases Society of America. Clin Infect Dis 2007;45(7):807–825.
¹Not FDA approved for this indication.
*See text for dosages.
Abbreviations: Ampho B = amphotericin B (Fungizone); L Ampho B = liposomal preparation of amphotericin B (AmBisome); CD4 = CD4⁺ T-cell count (in cells/mm³); CNS = central nervous system; NSAIDs = nonsteroidal antiinflammatory drugs; PDH, progressive disseminated histoplasmosis.

REFERENCES

Bamberger DM. Successful treatment of multiple cerebral histoplasmomas with itraconazole. Clin Infect Dis 1999;28(4):915–6.

Goldman M, Zackin R, Fichtenbaum CJ, et al. and the AIDS Clinical Trials Group A5038 Study Group. Safety of discontinuation of maintenance therapy for disseminated histoplasmosis after immunologic response to antiretroviral therapy. Clin Infect Dis 2004;38(10):1485–9.

Johnson PC, Wheat LJ, Cloud GA, et al. Safety and efficacy of liposomal amphotericin B compared with conventional amphotericin B for induction therapy of histoplasmosis in patients with AIDS. Ann Intern Med 2002;137:105–9.

McKinsey DS, Wheat LJ, Cloud GA, et al. Itraconazole prophylaxis for fungal infections in patients with advanced human immunodeficiency virus infection: Randomized, placebo-controlled, double-blind study. National Institute of Allergy and Infectious Diseases Mycoses Study Group. Clin Infect Dis 1999;28:1049–56.

Saccente M, McDonnell RW, Baddour LM, et al. Cerebral histoplasmosis in the azole era: Report of four cases and review. South Med J 2003;96(4):410–6.

Wheat LJ, Freifeld AG, Kleiman MB, et al. Infectious diseases society of America: Clinical practice guidelines for the management of patients with histoplasmosis: 2007 Update by the Infectious Diseases Society of America. Clin Infect Dis 2007;45(7):807–925.

Wheat LJ, Witt J 3rd, Durkin M, Connolly P. Reduction in false antigenemia in the second generation *Histoplasma* antigen assay. Med Mycol 2007;45:169–71.

Whitt SP, Koch GA, Fender B, et al. Histoplasmosis in pregnancy: Case series and report of transplacental transmission. Arch Intern Med 2004;164:454–8.

Blastomycosis

Method of
Robert Bradsher, MD, and J. Ryan Bariola, MD

Epidemiology

Blastomycosis is caused by infection with the thermally dimorphic fungus *Blastomyces dermatitidis*. The organism grows as a yeast form at 98.6°F (37°C) and as a mycelial form at room temperature. In the environment, the fungus is thought to exist in warm, moist soil associated with decomposing vegetation and decaying wood. In North America, *B. dermatitidis* is endemic along the Mississippi and Ohio River basins, in the regions that surround the Great Lakes, and in a small area of New York and Canada along the St. Lawrence River. Hyperendemic areas with very high rates of blastomycosis have been reported within these endemic regions. Cases outside North America have been described most commonly in Africa, but there have been reports of blastomycosis on several continents.

Infection with *B. dermatitidis* usually occurs via inhalation of aerosolized conidia. Cutaneous inoculation has been reported after inadvertent exposure in the laboratory, at autopsy, and after dog bites. Person-to-person transmission has been described in rare cases of sexual and perinatal transmission. The median incubation period is approximately 30 to 45 days.

CURRENT DIAGNOSIS

- Because colonization with *B. dermatitidis* does not occur, identification by culture or histology confirms infection.
- The gold standard for diagnosis is culture of the organism from clinical specimens, which may take up to 4 weeks.
- A presumptive diagnosis may be made by visualization of the typical yeast from clinical specimens in the appropriate setting

Clinical Manifestations

Approximately 50% of infected individuals may be asymptomatic. Pulmonary disease may be acute or chronic. Acute pulmonary blastomycosis presents similarly to bacterial pneumonia with abrupt onset of fever, chills, pleuritic chest pain, myalgias, arthralgias, and cough that is initially nonproductive but later becomes productive of purulent sputum. Chest radiography demonstrates lobar or segmental consolidation; pleural effusion and hilar adenopathy are unusual. Patients diagnosed with blastomycosis may develop progressive, chronic disease that may involve pulmonary and numerous extrapulmonary sites. Patients with chronic pulmonary blastomycosis present with productive cough, hemoptysis, weight loss, pleuritic chest pain, and low-grade fever. Alveolar or fibronodular infiltrates, mass lesions, nodular lesions, and cavitation are seen on chest radiography. Findings may mimic tuberculosis, other endemic mycoses, or bronchogenic carcinoma. Acute respiratory failure may be seen with miliary disease or diffuse pneumonitis and is associated with a very high mortality.

Hematogenous dissemination to almost any other organ may occur. Manifestations in the skin, bone, or genitourinary tract are the most common and may be seen after clearance of pulmonary manifestations. The skin is the most frequently encountered extrapulmonary site of infection. Lesions are usually characterized as verrucous or ulcerative; they may be mistaken for squamous cell carcinoma, atypical mycobacterial infection, pyoderma gangrenosum, or keratoacanthoma. After the skin, bone is the most frequent site of dissemination. Manifestations include osteolytic lesions with associated soft-tissue abscesses or chronic draining sinuses. Genitourinary disease occurs in some male cases, affecting the prostate and epididymis. Although central nervous system (CNS) infection is reported in only a small number of normal hosts, it is a relatively common complication in immunocompromised patients, in whom it may present as an abscess or meningitis. In a review of AIDS patients with blastomycosis, 40% had CNS involvement. Indeed, blastomycosis is more often disseminated and fulminant in patients with AIDS and other types of chronic immunosuppression; mortality rates of 30% to 40% have been reported in these groups.

Diagnosis

The definitive diagnosis of blastomycosis is based on isolation of the organism from cultures of clinical specimens. Mycologic media usually demonstrate growth after an incubation period of 2 to 4 weeks. Conversion from the mycelial form to the yeast phase is required for confirmation.

Because isolation of the organism may take weeks, presumptive diagnosis of blastomycosis is established by identification of the characteristic yeast form in clinical specimens. With a compatible clinical picture, treatment should be initiated if round, broad-based budding yeasts with thick, doubly refractile cell walls are seen on a wet mount preparation with addition of 10% potassium hydroxide to digest mammalian cells. In histopathologic specimens, acute suppurative and granulomatous inflammation are found. Visualization in tissue is improved by the use of special stains, such as the Gomori methenamine silver and periodic acid-Schiff stains. Nucleic acid hybridization tests

are now commercially available and significantly shorten identification time. Most serologic tests are neither adequately sensitive nor specific to be useful in diagnosing blastomycosis, although newer antigen assays may be more reliable. A recently developed assay detects *Blastomyces* antigen in urine, serum, and other body fluids, including cerebrospinal fluid. The test is most sensitive in urine samples, in which 70% to 80% are positive in disseminated blastomycosis, and almost 100% are positive in pulmonary disease. Antigen is detected in serum in approximately 50% of cases. Cross-reactivity can occur in patients with other endemic mycoses. The assay may be used to monitor response to therapy and to detect recurrence.

Treatment

Although spontaneous resolution of acute blastomycotic pneumonia has been reported in immunocompetent hosts, most patients with blastomycosis require treatment. Treatment is indicated in all immunocompromised individuals and in all patients with progressive pulmonary disease or extrapulmonary disease. Factors to consider when initiating therapy include the severity and extent of disease, the immune status of the patient, and the toxicities of the antifungal agents.

PULMONARY DISEASE

For mild to moderate lung disease, itraconazole (Sporanox) is the preferred oral agent because it is efficacious and well tolerated. The initial dose should be 200 to 400 mg daily. Treatment should continue for at least 6 months. Bioavailability of itraconazole capsules is enhanced with food, whereas the oral suspension should be taken while fasting. Attention should be given to the patient's concurrent medications because of the potential for drug–drug interactions. Clinical experience with fluconazole (Diflucan)[1] indicates that this agent is not as efficacious as itraconazole but may be effective at doses of 400 to 800 mg daily. In patients with life-threatening pulmonary disease, progression of disease while on an azole or inability to tolerate an azole, amphotericin B (Fungizone) remains the agent of choice. A dose of 0.7 to 1.0 mg/kg daily should be administered until a cumulative dose of 1.5 to 2.5 g is completed. Some patients may be switched to oral itraconazole at 200 to 400 mg daily after clinical stabilization with amphotericin B. Lipid formulations of amphotericin B have not been adequately studied, but have been used in patients unable to tolerate conventional amphotericin B.

---

[1]Not FDA approved for this indication.

CURRENT THERAPY

- Itraconazole (Sporanox) is the agent used most commonly to treat blastomycosis. It is administered in an oral dose of 200 to 400 mg daily for 6–12 months, depending on the site of infection.
- For life-threatening pulmonary disease (acute respiratory distress syndrome [ARDS]) or severe disseminated disease, amphotericin B (Fungizone) is the drug of choice. After initial improvement, itraconazole may be substituted.
- For CNS blastomycosis, amphotericin is used because itraconazole does not adequately penetrate the CNS. Liposomal amphotericin is used when high doses are needed or adverse effects from amphotericin B are encountered.
- Fluconazole (Diflucan),[1] ketoconazole (Nizoral), and IV itraconazole have lesser roles in the treatment of blastomycosis. Voriconazole (Vfend)[1] has not been studied adequately, but it may hold promise for CNS disease.

---

[1]Not FDA approved for this indication.

NERVOUS SYSTEM DISEASE

CNS infection should be treated with amphotericin B at a dose of 0.7 to 1.0 mg/kg daily to complete a total dose of 2.0 to 2.5 g. Itraconazole and ketoconazole are not recommended because of inadequate CNS penetration; fluconazole at 800 mg daily may be considered if amphotericin B is not tolerated.

EXTRAPULMONARY DISEASE (WITHOUT CNS INVOLVEMENT)

For mild to moderate disease, itraconazole at 200 to 400 mg daily is recommended for a minimum of 6 months. Patients whose disease progresses on this agent should be switched to amphotericin B to complete at least 1.5 g. Bone disease should be treated for at least 1 year. For life-threatening disease, amphotericin B at 0.7 to 1.0 mg/kg daily should be administered for a total dose of 2.0 to 2.5 g. In immunocompromised individuals, many authorities recommend long-term suppressive therapy with itraconazole after a treatment course of amphotericin B. Pregnant women should be treated with amphotericin B because the azoles are teratogenic. Data on blastomycosis in children are sparse, but some authorities suggest initial amphotericin B because of a potential unfavorable response to azoles.

NEW ANTIFUNGAL AGENTS

Voriconazole (Vfend)[1] is active in vitro and in animal models of pulmonary blastomycosis; the in vitro activity against *B. dermatitidis* is similar to itraconazole. Although clinical data in treating blastomycosis in humans are inadequate, voriconazole has good CNS penetration based on reports of successful treatment of CNS aspergillosis. Posaconazole (Noxafil),[1] which has recently been licensed in the United States, is also active in vitro and in animal models. Further data are needed before these agents may be recommended for use in blastomycosis. The echinocandin class of antifungal agents shows variable activity against *B. dermatitidis* and there are no clinical data to support their use.

REFERENCES

Bradsher RW. Clinical features of blastomycosis. Semin Respir Infect 1997;12:229–34.

Bradsher RW, Chapman SW, Pappas PG. Blastomycosis. Infect Dis Clin North Am 2003;17:21–40.

Chapman SW. Blastomyces dermatitidis. In: Mandell GL, Bennett JE, Dolin R, editors. Principles and Practice of Infectious Disease. New York: Churchill Livingstone; 2005. p. 3026–40.

Chapman SW, Dismukes WE, Proia LA, et al. Clinical practice guidelines for the management of blastomycosis: 2008 update by the IDSA. Clin Infect Dis 2008;46:1801–12.

Chapman SW, Lin AC, Hendricks KA, et al. Endemic blastomycosis in Mississippi: Epidemiological and clinical studies. Semin Respir Infect 1997;12:219–28.

Lemos LB, Guo M, Baliga M. Blastomycosis: organ involvement and etiologic diagnosis. A review of 123 patients from Mississippi. Ann Diagn Pathol 2000;4:391–406.

Pappas PG. Blastomycosis in the immunocompromised patient. Semin Respir Infect 1997;12:243–51.

Schutze GE, Hickerson SL, Fortin EM, et al. Blastomycosis in children. Clin Infect Dis 1996;22:496–502.

Sugar AM, Liu X-P. Efficacy of voriconazole in treatment of murine pulmonary blastomycosis. Antimicrob Agents Chemother 2001;45:601–4.

---

[1]Not FDA approved for this indication.

Pleural Effusion and Empyema Thoracis

Method of
Jeffson Chung, MD, and Marc de Perrot, MD

Physiology of Pleural Disease

The pleural space is lined by the parietal and visceral pleurae, which secrete a serous fluid that provides lubrication for movement of the lung against the chest wall during respiration. The rate of secretion is 0.01 mL/kg/hour, and the fluid comes mainly from the parietal pleura. Absorption is up to 0.2 mL/kg/hour and is primarily through the parietal lymphatics. In a healthy adult, secretion and absorption are balanced, and there should be only 5 to 10 mL of fluid in the pleural space. Systemic conditions and local lesions can upset this balance and cause fluid accumulation. Several disease processes and their mechanisms are listed in Table 1. The most common causes of pleural fluid accumulation in adults are congestive heart failure, pneumonia, cancer, and pulmonary embolus. In the pediatric population, the most common causes are pneumonia, congenital heart disease, and malignancy.

Clinical Features of Pleural Effusions and Empyema

The signs and symptoms of pleural effusion and empyema tend to be subtle and nonspecific and may be confounded by those of the underlying illness. Physical examination findings tend to be insensitive but can be fairly specific, with good negative predictive value. Table 2 lists the signs and symptoms. Effusions of less than 300 mL usually produce a normal physical examination, whereas larger volumes produce abnormal findings. Additional symptoms such as sputum or hemoptysis may point toward the etiology.

Etiology

There are many diverse causes of fluid accumulation in the pleural space, each resulting in a fluid that can be characterized as either transudative or exudative. Box 1 lists Light's criteria for an exudate based on laboratory findings.

TRANSUDATIVE PLEURAL EFFUSION

Of the transudative processes, congestive heart failure is by far the most common cause, accounting for 90% of transudative effusions. Often the effusion manifests bilaterally. Other causes of transudates include nephrotic syndrome, uremia, pulmonary embolus, superior vena cava obstruction, and cirrhosis.

Pulmonary embolus is commonly associated with pleural effusions, with one third to one half of patients developing an effusion. The effusions are typically unilateral and small, occupying less than one third of the hemithorax, and they can be either transudative or exudative. Because the effusions tend to be small, treatment is not usually required, although delayed diagnosis can be associated with loculated collections that are more difficult to resolve. Patients with pulmonary embolus are typically treated with anticoagulation, but thoracentesis can still be safe and may be indicated in cases of large effusions or to rule out other etiologies.

Superior vena cava obstruction usually is caused by malignancies but can also be also be associated with benign processes such as central lines, pacemaker wires, dialysis catheters, aortic aneurysms, or primary thromboses. Although the conventional belief is that the fluid is transudative, recent evidence suggests that it can be exudative

TABLE 1 Mechanisms of Pleural Fluid Accumulation

Mechanism	Example of Disease Process
Increased pressure gradient	Heart failure, atelectasis
Decreased serum oncotic pressure	Nephrotic syndrome
Increased capillary permeability	Inflammation, infection, malignancy
Impaired clearance	Lymphatic obstruction
Movement across diaphragm	Ascites

TABLE 2 Symptoms and Signs of Pleural Effusions

Symptoms	Signs
Dyspnea	Decreased vesicular or bronchial breath sounds
Pleuritic chest pain (increases with deep inspiration or lying down; may refer to shoulder)	Dullness to percussion
Cough	Egophony
	Asymmetry of chest expansion and tactile fremitus
Constitutional—fatigue, fever, chills, weight loss	Pleural rub on auscultation

---

BOX 1 Light's Criteria for a Pleural Exudate

The presence of any of these three criteria suggests an exudate:
- Ratio of pleural fluid protein to serum protein >0.5
- Ratio of pleural fluid LDH to serum LDH >0.6
- Pleural fluid LDH >2/3 of normal upper limit for serum LDH

Abbreviation: LDH = lactate dehydrogenase.

---

and chylous, possibly because of impaired lymphatic drainage of the pleural space. Effusions occur in up to 60% of superior vena cava obstructions and can be either unilateral or bilateral. The volume is typically small, but it can be larger if caused by a malignancy.

Hepatic hydrothorax is defined by pleural effusion, usually greater than 500 mL, in the setting of cirrhosis without cardiopulmonary disease. It is an uncommon complication of cirrhosis, occurring in only 4% to 10% of patients. Positive intraabdominal and negative intrathoracic pressures create blebs in the peritoneum that rupture and allow ascites fluid to cross defects in the tendinous portion of the diaphragm and enter the pleural space. Similar to ascites, this fluid collection predisposes to spontaneous bacterial empyema.

EXUDATIVE PLEURAL EFFUSION

The most common causes of exudative pleural effusions are hemothorax, infection (e.g., pneumonia, tuberculosis), and malignancy, followed by postinfarction syndrome, gastrointestinal disease states (e.g., pancreatitis, esophageal rupture, liver abscess), connective tissue diseases (e.g., rheumatoid arthritis, lupus), pulmonary embolus, postsurgical states, and chylothorax. In the case of malignancy, the underlying mechanism is a change in the pleura permeability and lymphatic drainage.

CURRENT DIAGNOSIS

- Clinical suspicion along with a thorough history and physical examination
- Imaging by radiography, ultrasonography, or computed tomography
- Thoracentesis and appropriate laboratory investigations

Chylothorax typically occurs after injury or obstruction of the thoracic duct, with trauma being the most common cause, followed by malignancy. Pleuritic chest pain is rare in this situation, because chyle is a noninflammatory substance. Aspiration of the pleural space will reveal a turbid fluid with increased triglyceride and chylomicron levels.

EMPYEMA

Empyema is defined by purulent fluid in the pleural space. The most common cause is pneumonia. Other causes include lung abscess, trauma, bronchopleural fistula, esophageal perforation, and complications of thoracic surgery.

Laboratory Investigations

The most important investigation is thoracentesis, which can be both diagnostic and therapeutic. Complications of the procedure include pneumothorax, infection, and bleeding. Care must be taken to avoid draining large volumes (>1500 mL) acutely, because this can cause re-expansion pulmonary edema, a potentially life-threatening condition. For large volumes, drainage may have to be done progressively over 24 hours.

The fluid removed can be submitted for studies listed in Box 2. With regard to cytology, predominant neutrophils suggest a parapneumonic effusion or an effusion secondary to pulmonary embolus or pancreatitis, the latter of which may also be accompanied by elevated amylase. Predominant mononuclear cells suggest a chronic process, including malignancy or tuberculosis, which can be confirmed with an acid-fast stain. Eosinophilia (>10%) is often caused by blood or air in the pleural space. Presence of lupus erythematosus cells suggests systemic lupus erythematosus. In the case of bacterial infection, the glucose level may be decreased, and Gram stain, culture, and sensitivity can help guide treatment. Lactate dehydrogenase and protein levels are used for identifying exudates, and chylomicron and triglyceride levels for chylothorax.

BOX 2 Laboratory Studies for Pleural Fluid

Routine Studies
- Cell count
- Culture and sensitivity
- Cytology
- Glucose
- Gram stain

Additional Studies
- Lactate dehydrogenase
- pH
- Protein
- Acid-fast stain
- Amylase
- Bilirubin
- Chylomicrons
- Triglycerides
- Fatty acids
- Creatinine

CURRENT THERAPY

- Systemic antibiotics if there is an infective etiology
- Thorough removal of fluid by drainage
- Débridement and decortication may be necessary for empyema
- Pleurodesis for relapsing malignant effusions

Imaging

Large effusions appear as a whited-out area over the affected region on the radiograph. The diaphragm may be obscured and the meniscus curved. Very large effusions can result in a deviation of mediastinal structures appreciable on radiographic images. Small effusions (20–150 mL) can cause blunting of the costophrenic angle. Layering of the fluid can be detected at even smaller volumes (5–15 mL) on lateral decubitus radiography.

Ultrasound and computed tomographic modalities are useful for identifying loculations and air and for differentiating between effusion and consolidation. Ultrasound can also be used to guide thoracocentesis.

Treatment of Pleural Effusion

The exact management strategy for a pleural effusion depends on whether the effusion is transudative or exudative and on the underlying etiology. In all cases, the goal is to evacuate the pleural space for symptomatic relief and to treat the underlying cause.

Removal of pleural fluid by thoracentesis can be both diagnostic and therapeutic. This procedure is performed with the patient sitting and leaning forward, with the ipsilateral arm raised, or in a lateral decubitus position in the case of an infant. The preferred location for insertion of the catheter is the seventh intercostal space, below the tip of the scapula. This area is cleaned, and a local anesthetic is applied. The catheter is introduced with a syringe attached so that constant suction can be maintained. The first sign of fluid entry into the syringe indicates entry into the pleural space. After aspiration of the fluid, the catheter is removed, and pressure is applied over the area. A chest radiograph should be obtained to rule out pneumothorax.

Chest tube insertion is indicated in situations of respiratory and hemodynamic compromise, hemothorax, infection, or malignant effusion. The preferred location for chest tube insertion is between the anterior and midaxillary lines at the fifth intercostal space. After localized cleaning with povidone-iodine, the skin, subcutaneous tissue, and periosteum are infiltrated with 1% lidocaine (Xylocaine), and an incision made one intercostal space below the rib over which the catheter will pass. After blunt dissection to the upper surface of the rib with a curved hemostat or Kelly clamp, the intercostal muscles and pleura are carefully punctured. The hemostat or clamp is then used to introduce the tip of the chest tube through the tract into the pleural space. Next, the instrument is opened to splint the tract open, while the chest tube is advanced until resistance is met. Finally, the incision is closed with sutures, taking care to encircle the tube to fix it in place, and the area is covered with sterile dressing. A chest radiograph should be obtained to evaluate the position of the chest tube and to rule out pneumothorax. Table 3 lists the appropriate sizes of chest tubes to use in patients of various ages.

TRANSUDATE

In the case of pleural effusion due to congestive heart failure, diuresis may be sufficient if the patient is known to have a background of congestive heart failure and is asymptomatic. Similarly, in a cirrhotic patient, salt restriction to 90 mEq/day and diuresis may be sufficient management of the pleural effusion. However, like peritoneal ascites,

TABLE 3 Sizing of Chest Tube Based on Age of Patient

Age	Chest Tube Size (F)
Newborn-6 mo	10–12
1 yr	16–20
4 yr	20
>10 yr	20–28

pleural effusions may evolve to spontaneous bacterial empyemas, which require antibiotic treatment. If thoracentesis is required every 2 or 3 weeks in spite of salt restriction and diuresis, a transjugular intrahepatic portosystemic shunt may be indicated. Pleurodesis may also be pursued as management of relapsing pleural effusion.

EXUDATE

Exudative pleural fluid can be a sign of early infection that should be approached aggressively by drainage and systemic antibiotics. Small, uncomplicated effusions, however, may be sufficiently treated by antibiotics alone. Complicated effusions are defined in Box 3. Between 5% and 20% of those patients whose effusions are due to infection go on to develop empyemas, in which case surgical intervention may be indicated.

Effusions associated with malignancy are approached with palliative intent, because malignant effusion is typically a sign of late-stage disease. The goal here is simply relief of dyspnea. This can be achieved by obliterating the pleural space through thoracoscopic pleurodesis (instillation of talc or a sclerosant into the cavity). The resulting inflammation causes adhesion of the pleural surfaces, leaving no room for fluid collection. Pleurodesis works only if the lung is able to expand and fill the entire chest cavity; if the lung is trapped, indwelling tunneled Silastic catheters may be used instead.

Treatment of Empyema

Empyema is classically divided into three phases: early/acute exudative, transitional fibrinopurulent, and late/organized. The treatment strategy varies depending on the phase, but the goal is inevitably to thoroughly drain the pleural space and allow re-expansion of the lung. In the early/acute exudative stage of empyema, drainage of the pleural space by thoracentesis or thoracostomy along with systemic antibiotics may be sufficient, because the lung is not trapped and will re-expand once the fluid has been evacuated.

The transitional fibrinopurulent phase typically occurs 1 to 6 weeks after diagnosis of pleural effusion. It is marked by the formation of loculated fluid collections as a result of pleural adhesions. Because of the noncommunicating nature of these collections, simple drainage may not be adequate. Instead, thoracoscopic drainage and débridement under direct visualization is preferred.

The late/organized phase appears at least 5 weeks after the initial diagnosis of pleural effusion. It is characterized by the formation of a thick visceral pleura that prevents the lung from filling the pleural

---

BOX 3 Definition of a Complicated Effusion

The presence of any one of these criteria suggests a complicated effusion:
- pH < 7.2
- Glucose <40 mg/dL
- Lactate dehydrogenase >1000 IU/L
- Positive stain and culture
- Loculations

space. As a result, this space recurrently fills with fluid despite drainage. Management should involve decortication via thoracoscopy or, more commonly, thoracotomy, to allow the lung to re-expand. In the rare cases in which the lung is unable to fully re-expand because of the underlying disease or prior resections, an open pleural window may be necessary to adequately treat the empyema.

Fibrinolytics have been used for years in the treatment of empyema. The belief is that the enzyme instilled into the pleural space can digest fibrous septa and cellular debris that hinder drainage. The formulation is typically 250,000 IU/day of streptokinase (Streptase)[1] or 100,000 IU/day of urokinase (Abbokinase)[1] in 30 to 100 mL of saline, injected through the chest tube 2 to 4 hours before drainage. Efficacy may be improved by splitting the dose to several times per day. Absolute contraindications to this procedure are previous allergic reactions (particularly to streptokinase), bronchopleural fistula, and trauma or surgery within 48 hours. Relative contraindications include major surgery within 2 weeks, history of hemorrhagic stroke, and coagulation defects. Although evidence has shown that fibrinolytic therapy can reduce the need for surgery, surgery remains the standard of care. There is still much controversy regarding the efficacy and the safety profile of fibrinolytic therapy, but it may provide an alternative for poor surgical candidates. Trials are underway for the use of DNAase[2] and tissue plasminogen activator (tPA; Alteplase)[1] in the treatment of empyema.

Postpneumonectomy empyema deserves special mention, because it usually is caused by a bronchopleural fistula. The goal of management here is not only to drain the affected space but also to prevent soiling of the remaining lung.

Outcome

Most pleural effusions respond very well to therapy but may contribute significantly to morbidity and mortality. Those caused by malignancy, however, carry a poor prognosis because of the advanced stage of the underlying disease.

REFERENCES

Agrawal V, Sahn SA. Lipid peural effusions. Am J Med Sci 2008;335 (1):16–20.
Beers SL, Abramo TJ. Pleural effusions. Pediatr Emerg Care 2007;23 (5):330–4.
Cameron RJ, Davies HRHR. Intra-pleural fibrinolytic therapy versus conservative management in the treatment of adult parapneumonic effusions and empyema. Cochrane Database Syst Rev 2008;(2) CD002312. DOI: 10.1002/14651858.CD002312.pub3.
Diaz-Guzman E, Budev MM. Accuracy of the physical examination in evaluating pleural effusion. Cleve J Med 2008;75(4):297–303.
Kashani A, Landaverde C, Medici V, Rossaro L. Fluid retention in cirrhosis: Pathophysiology and management. Q J Med 2008;101:71–85.
Molnar T. Current surgical treatment of thoracic empyema in adults. Eur J Cardiothoracic Surg 2007;32:422–30.
Mulroy JF. Differential diagnosis of pleural effusions: A case study. Dimens Crit Care Nurs 2008;27(3):110–3.
Porcel JM, Light RW. Pleural effusions due to pulmonary embolism. Curr Opin Pulm Med 2008;14:337–42.
Rice T. Pleural effusions in superior vena cava syndrome: Prevalence, characteristics, and proposed pathophysiology. Curr Opin Pulm Med 2007;13:324–7.

---

[1]Not FDA approved for this indication.
[2]Not available in the United States.

Primary Lung Abscess

Method of
Lee E. Morrow, MD, MSc, and Jeff Jarrett, MD

A lung abscess is defined as parenchymal necrosis with confined cavitation that results from pulmonary infection. Abscesses in patients who aspirate or who are otherwise healthy are considered primary. The term secondary lung abscess implies an associated condition (e.g., obstructing neoplasm, foreign body, bronchiectasis) that predisposes to pulmonary infection with cavitation or pulmonary extension of another localized infection.

A primary lung abscess consists of one or two cavities, often with air-fluid levels, in the lung of a patient with signs and symptoms of a respiratory infection. Multiple small (<2 cm) cavities spread throughout the lungs are referred to as necrotizing pneumonia and represent a continuum of the process leading to abscess formation. For anatomic reasons, primary lung abscesses are more common in the right lung. Similarly, abscess formation is more frequent in the superior segments of the lower lobes and the posterior segments of the upper lobes, because these segments are dependent in a supine (unconscious) patient.

Primary lung abscesses are also classified as acute or chronic; if symptoms are present for longer than 1 month before presentation, the condition is considered chronic.

Cause

Aspiration of pathogen-laden secretions is the most common cause of a primary lung abscess and is typically seen in patients with impaired levels of consciousness. Other risk factors for primary lung abscess formation are shown in Box 1. Poor oral hygiene predisposes to colonization of the oropharynx with the anaerobic bacteria (*Bacteroides, Fusobacterium, Peptostreptococcus, Prevotella*) that frequently lead to

---

BOX 1   Risk Factors for Primary Lung Abscess Formation

Anemia
Diabetes mellitus
Impaired consciousness
• Alcohol abuse
• Drug overdose
• Seizure
• Stroke
Impaired swallowing
• Achalasia
• Esophageal obstruction (cancer, stricture)
• Esophageal dysfunction
• Gastroesophgeal reflux disease
• Zenker's diverticulum
Malnutrition
Pneumonia with "necrotizing" pathogens
• Anaerobes
• *Klebsiella* species
• *Nocardia*
• *Staphylococcus aureus*
• *Streptococcus pyogenes*
Poor dentition and oral hygiene

CURRENT DIAGNOSIS

- Clinical findings are suggestive of pulmonary infection
  - Fevers and night sweats
  - Cough, particularly if productive of putrid sputum or blood
  - Pleuritic chest pain
  - Fatigue
- Assess for risk factors predisposing to aspiration
  - Intoxication: alcohol or illicit drugs
  - Sedative-hypnotic use
  - Neurologic disorders: seizures or stroke
  - Swallowing impairment
- Diagnosis is confirmed by radiographic findings of a cavity with an air-fluid level
  - Posteroanterior and lateral chest radiographs should be the initial tests ordered
  - Computed tomographic imaging is used if routine studies are nondiagnostic
- Invasive diagnostic testing has a limited role
- Exclude abscess mimics if there is no clinical response to empiric antibiotics
  - Infected bulla
  - Malignancy
  - Mycobacterial infection
  - Pulmonary infarction
  - Pulmonary sequestration
  - Vasculitis

CURRENT THERAPY

- Therapy is usually empiric, given the limited yield of anaerobic cultures
  - Clindamycin (Cleocin) is first-line therapy.
  - β-Lactam/β-lactamase inhibitors or carbapenems are alternative agents.
  - The metronidazole (Flagyl) failure rate is approximately 50%
- Duration of therapy is unclear and should be determined by the initial severity of illness and the response to therapy: 1 to 3 months of therapy is common
- Risk factors for failure of medical therapy include
  - Large abscess size (>6 cm)
  - Advanced age
  - Immune compromise
  - Infection with aerobic "problem" pathogens
- Refractory abscesses can be effectively treated with computed tomography–guided drain placement
- Surgical resection is possible but rarely indicated

abscess formation. Recent data suggest that *Klebsiella*, staphylococci, and other aerobic organisms are increasingly frequent causes of pulmonary abscesses, most likely a reflection of the increased frequency of patients with more complex medical conditions. *Nocardia*, *Actinomyces*, fungi, and parasites are other rare causes of lung abscesses.

Signs and Symptoms

Patients typically present with vague symptoms such as fevers, night sweats, cough, putrid sputum, hemoptysis, pleuritic chest pain, and fatigue. The physical examination is equally nonspecific early in the disease course, often demonstrating only the findings of risk factors for aspiration: altered mental status, neurologic deficits, an impaired gag reflex, and poor dentition. Progression of clinical symptoms is variable: anaerobic infections may evolve over an extended period, whereas aerobic bacteria manifest more acutely. With advanced disease states, patients may demonstrate tachypnea, hypoxemia, weight loss, and the foul-smelling sputum characteristic of an anaerobic infection. Clubbing of the digits may be seen in chronic cases.

Diagnosis

The diagnosis of an abscess is established by a clinical history of predisposing conditions and confirmatory radiographic studies. Consistent laboratory studies include leukocytosis with a left shift, anemia, and an elevated erythrocyte sedimentation rate. Routine chest radiographs typically demonstrate a thick-walled cavity with an air-fluid level. Alternative explanations for these radiographic findings include an infected bulla, malignancy, mycobacterial infection, pulmonary infarction, pulmonary sequestration, and vasculitis. Computed tomography of the chest may be needed to clearly demonstrate cavitation or to exclude a pleural process.

Whereas culture data from sputum, blood, and pleural effusions may help direct therapy, the diagnostic yield of anaerobic cultures is notoriously low. Positive blood cultures in the presence of multiple abscesses mandates echocardiography to look for a cardiac source of septic emboli. If acceptable sputum cultures cannot be collected and the patient is stable, bronchoscopy may safely be performed. Other reasons for bronchoscopy include assessment of hemoptysis, pulmonary toilet, and exclusion of a secondary abscess (evaluation for an endobronchial malignancy or foreign body). Bronchoscopy is also useful in patients for whom empiric antimicrobial therapy has failed.

Treatment

The most commonly accepted therapy for primary lung abscess is prolonged antimicrobial courses using agents directed against anaerobes and microaerophilic streptococci. Although lung abscesses are usually polymicrobial infections, it is unclear whether all isolated organisms merit specific therapy. Standard treatment at present is clindamycin (Cleocin) 600 mg IV every 8 hours followed by 150 to 300 mg orally four times daily after the patient improves. β-Lactam/β-lactamase inhibitors such as ampicillin-sulbactam (Unasyn),[1] piperacillin-tazobactam (Zosyn),[1] and carbapenems (imipenem [Primaxin],[1] meropenem [Merrem][1]) are acceptable alternatives. Metronidazole (Flagyl) monotherapy is not appropriate, given failure rates of approximately 50%. The optimal duration of therapy is controversial and probably should be individualized, but 1 to 3 months of therapy is typically prescribed.

Risk factors for failure of medical therapy include abscess size greater than 6 cm, old age, immune compromise, and infection with certain aerobic pathogens (*Klebsiella pneumoniae*, *Pseudomonas aeruginosa*, *Staphylococcus aureus*). If signs of sepsis persist after initiation of antibiotic therapy, more than 90% of abscesses can be successfully treated with computed tomography–guided drainage. Failure to respond may indicate a noninfectious etiology (e.g., pulmonary infarct, vasculitis), empyema formation, or development of antimicrobial resistance. Surgical excision of the affected segments is possible, but, given the considerable risk of morbidity and mortality, this approach is reserved for patients with clinical failure persisting beyond 6 weeks or massive hemoptysis.

---

[1]Not FDA approved for this indication.

Prevention

The most effective preventive measures are minimizing aspiration and attention to oral hygiene. Other precautionary measures include adequate nutrition, elevation of the head of the bed, pulmonary toilet, and judicious use of sedative-hypnotics.

REFERENCES

Bartlett JG. The role of anaerobic bacteria in lung abscess. Clin Infect Dis 2005;40:923–5.

Bowling MR, Chin R, Haponik E, et al. Bronchoscopic myths and legends: Bronchoscopy in the treatment of pulmonary abscess. Clin Pulm Med 2007;14:45–8.

Mansharamani NG, Balachandran D, Delaney D, et al. Lung abscess in adults: Clinical comparison of immunocompromised to non-immunocompromised patients. Respir Med 2002;96:178–85.

Wang JL, Chen KY, Fang CT, et al. Changing bacteriology of adult community-acquired lung abscess in Taiwan: *Klebsiella pneumoniae* versus anaerobes. Clin Infect Dis 2005;40:915–22.

Acute Bronchitis

Method of
Susan Davids, MD, MPH, and Ralph M. Schapira, MD

Acute bronchitis is one of the most common diagnoses made by primary care physicians in the United States and accounts for nearly 10 million office visits per year. Acute bronchitis is a transient, self-limited inflammatory process of the upper respiratory tract, specifically the trachea and bronchi. Antibiotics are overprescribed to patients with acute bronchitis; this practice has raised significant concern related to the worldwide rise of antibiotic resistance, which is viewed as one of the world's most pressing public health problems.

Acute bronchitis manifests as an acute respiratory illness of less than 3 weeks' duration, with or without sputum production. Acute bronchitis is a clinical diagnosis and must be distinguished from other respiratory diseases, such as pneumonia, acute exacerbation of chronic bronchitis (episode of worsening of symptoms and expiratory airflow obstruction in patients with chronic obstructive pulmonary disease), and the onset of asthma. Most cases of acute bronchitis occur in the fall and winter. The etiology of acute bronchitis is infectious, and viruses appear to be the cause of most cases. Influenzas A and B are the most common viruses isolated, although a wide variety of infectious agents have been identified, such as adenovirus, coronavirus, parainfluenza virus, respiratory syncytial virus, coxsackievirus, *Mycoplasma pneumoniae, Bordetella pertussis*, and *Chlamydia pneumoniae.*

Diagnosis of acute bronchitis is based on findings of a prominent cough that may be accompanied by wheezing and sputum production. Most patients are otherwise healthy and without preexisting respiratory disease. Nonspecific constitutional symptoms may also be part of acute bronchitis. Appropriate management of acute bronchitis is essential because it is one of the most common illnesses that present to physicians in the outpatient setting. Antibiotics are often prescribed unnecessarily for acute bronchitis and other respiratory tract illnesses; these prescriptions may potentially lead to adverse events (i.e., allergic reactions and gastrointestinal side effects) and bacterial resistance. Other medications, such as inhaled bronchodilators and antitussives, are often prescribed for acute bronchitis despite questionable evidence to support their routine use.

CURRENT DIAGNOSIS

- Normal healthy adult with cough
- Predominance of cough
- Lasts 1 to 3 weeks
- With or without sputum
- Can be accompanied by other respiratory and constitutional symptoms
- Absence of abnormal vital signs and physical exam suggesting pneumonia, particularly
  - Heart rate > 100 beats per minute
  - Respiratory rate >24 breaths per minute
  - Temperature > 100.4°F (38°C)
  - Lung findings suggest a consolidation process

Pathophysiology of acute bronchitis involves an acute inflammatory response involving the mucosa of the trachea and bronchi, resulting in injury to the respiratory tract epithelium. Sputum production is increased and bronchoconstriction (potentially resulting in airflow obstruction and wheezing) can occur. Positron emission tomography (PET) of a patient with acute bronchitis confirms that the primary inflammatory changes occur in the trachea and bronchi and not the remainder of the lower respiratory track.

Diagnosis

Cough, phlegm (which may be purulent as both bacteria and viruses can cause purulent sputum), and wheezing help differentiate acute bronchitis from upper respiratory infections such as pharyngitis and sinusitis. Acute bronchitis must be differentiated from acute bacterial pneumonia. The absence of abnormalities in vital signs (heart rate >100 bpm, respiratory rate >24 breath/min, oral temperature >100.4°F [38°C] and physical examination of the chest) supports the diagnosis of acute bronchitis and makes the need for chest radiography unnecessary in most cases. The treatment and outcome of acute bronchitis and pneumonia are very different; a chest radiograph should always be obtained if there is uncertainty about the diagnosis. Chest radiography will demonstrate no lung infiltrates in a patient with acute bronchitis. In contrast, lung infiltrates are present in pneumonia. Pertussis or whooping cough should be considered in adults with cough in the setting of what appears to be an upper respiratory infection, even in those previously immunized. Typically, the cough of pertussis, unlike acute bronchitis, lasts for longer than 3 weeks. Other respiratory diseases, such as previously undiagnosed asthma, can also mimic acute bronchitis, although several features differentiate asthma from acute bronchitis (see Section 12). Rapid testing to diagnose influenza viruses A and B (the most common causes of acute bronchitis) as a cause of acute bronchitis should be considered given the availability of effective treatment if initiated in the first 48 hours.

Treatment

ANTIBIOTICS, INHALED BRONCHODILATORS, AND ANTITUSSIVES

Existing evidence does not support the routine use of antibiotics for uncomplicated cases of acute bronchitis. Although most cases of acute bronchitis are caused by viral infections, upwards of 60% of patients are prescribed antibiotic therapy, which is contributing to the rise of bacterial resistance to commonly used antibiotics. Meta-analyses examining the effectiveness of antibiotic therapy in patients without underlying lung disease suggest no consistent effect of

CURRENT THERAPY

- Antibiotics not routinely recommended
- If influenza is highly probable and patient is presenting within the first 48 hours, consider treatment with
  - Oseltamivir (Tamiflu) 75 mg PO bid with food for 5 days (influenza A/B)
  - Zanamivir (Relenza) 10 mg bid by inhalation for 5 days (influenza A/B)
  - *Amantadine (Symmetrel) 100 mg bid or 200 mg once daily for 5 days (influenza A)
  - *Rimantadine (Flumadine) 100 mg bid for 5 days (influenza A)
- In patients with evidence of bronchial hyperresponsiveness, consider treatment with
  - β₂-agonists for 1 to 2 weeks
  - Antitussives in those with cough for 2 to 3 weeks
  - Antipyretics and analgesics as needed
  - Smoking cessation
- Education: cough likely to last 3 weeks or more

---

*Due to antiviral medication resistance, the choice of agent to treat influenza should be based on recommendations from the CDC and local health departments.

antibiotics on the severity or duration of acute bronchitis. A recent study evaluated children and patients with colored sputum and found that they also did not benefit from antibiotics. This study also found that compared to other populations, the elderly were less likely to benefit from antibiotics. Smokers with acute bronchitis are even more likely to be prescribed antibiotics. Their response to antibiotics was either equal to or worse than that of nonsmokers.

One possible reason for overuse of antibiotics is the concern by physicians about patient satisfaction. Studies show that patients presenting to the doctor expecting antibiotics were more likely to be prescribed antibiotics; studies also suggest that satisfaction is more related to appropriate patient education than to receiving antibiotics. Patient education should include information regarding the duration of symptoms associated with acute bronchitis. It was found that patients presented on average after 9 days of cough and that the cough persisted for an additional 12 days after the physician visit. This information can impart a realistic expectation of illness duration to the patient.

If influenza is highly suspected and the patient presents within 48 hours of the onset of symptoms, rapid diagnostic testing and treatment should be considered. Both amantadine (Symmetrel) and rimantadine (Flumadine) are effective for influenza A, and neuraminidase inhibitors, inhaled zanamivir (Relenza), and oral oseltamivir (Tamiflu) are effective for influenzas A and B. If these medications are initiated within the first 48 hours of symptoms (and ideally within 30 hours), the duration of illness can be shortened.

The evidence supporting the use of inhaled bronchodilators for the treatment of the symptoms has been variable. Two small trials reported a shorter duration of cough with the use of inhaled β-agonists; another study reported benefit in those with evidence of bronchial hyperresponsiveness. Current recommendations support the use of β-agonists only in patients with evidence of bronchial hyperresponsiveness (wheezing or spirometry demonstrating a forced expiration volume in 1 second [FEV₁] <80% of predicted).

Antitussive agents have not been shown to improve the acute or early cough but did show some improvements in cough lasting longer than 3 weeks. The current recommendations are to use antitussives, namely dextromethorphan (Benylin) or codeine, in patients with cough of 2 to 3 weeks' duration.

Acute uncomplicated bronchitis is most often a viral illness in which antibiotics are not routinely indicated. Patients presenting with an acute respiratory illness, who are younger than 65 years old without existing pulmonary disease or other significant comorbid illness, should have a thorough physical examination, including vital signs. If the vital signs are normal and physical examination of the chest is clear, pneumonia can most likely be ruled out. In patients who present within 48 hours of onset of symptoms, influenza should be considered as effective therapy is available for acute bronchitis caused by influenzas A or B. Otherwise, the evidence for treatment with antibiotics does not support their routine use. Bronchodilators should be considered in those with evidence of bronchial hyperresponsiveness; cough suppressants should be considered in those with 2 to 3 weeks of cough. Patient education is an integral part of the treatment, and patients should receive information that provides realistic expectations regarding the duration of cough.

REFERENCES

Aagaard E, Gonzales R. Management of acute bronchitis in healthy adults. Infect Dis Clin North Am 2004;18:919–37.
Ebell MH. Antibiotic prescribing for cough and symptoms of respiratory tract infection. JAMA 2005;294(3):3062–4.
Fahey T, Smucny J, Becker L, Glazier R. Antibiotics for acute bronchitis. Cochrane Database Syst Rev 2004;(4) CD000245.
Gonzales R, Sande M. Uncomplicated acute bronchitis. Ann Intern Med 2000;133:981–91.
Kicska G, Zhuang H, Alavi A. Acute bronchitis imaged with F-18 FDG positron emission tomography. Clin Nucl Med 2003;28(6):511–2.
Little R, Rumsby K, Kelly J, et al. Information leaflet and antibiotic prescribing strategies for acute lower respiratory tract infection. JAMA 2005;293(24):3029–35.
Linder JA, Sim I. Antibiotic treatment of acute bronchitis in smokers. J Gen Intern Med 2002;17:230–4.
Martinez FJ. Acute bronchitis: State of the art diagnosis and therapy. Compr Ther 2004;30(1):55–9.
Smucny J, Flynn C, Becker L, Glazier R. Beta₂-agonists for acute bronchitis. Cochrane Database Syst Rev 2004;(1) CD001726.

Bacterial Pneumonia

Method of
Edward Septimus, MD

Pneumonia occurs in about 3 to 4 million patients per year in the United States with approximately 1 million patients requiring hospitalization. The symptoms of pneumonia include cough, shortness of breath, sputum production, and chest pain. Physical examination includes fever in most, with crackles and bronchial breath sounds on auscultation in about 80% of cases. Pneumonia is classified by where it was acquired: community-acquired pneumonia (CAP) and health care–acquired pneumonia (HAP, sometimes called *hospital-acquired pneumonia*). This chapter focuses on adult patients with CAP or HAP.

Community-Acquired Pneumonia

CAP remains a leading cause of death in the United States. One study estimated that more than 900,000 cases of CAP occur in persons older than 65 years each year. The emergence of drug-resistant

Streptococcus pneumoniae (DRSP) and less common pathogens including methicillin-resistant *Staphylococcus aureus* (MRSA) is well documented. Pneumonia in long-term care institutions usually resembles HAP and is discussed later.

DIAGNOSTIC TESTING

Symptoms plus an infiltrate by chest radiograph or other imaging studies are required for the diagnosis. Clinical features and physical findings may be absent in the elderly. All patients should be screened by pulse oximetry. Arterial blood gases should be reserved for patients with suspected CO_2 retention. Routine diagnostic studies to determine the etiology for outpatients with CAP are optional. For patients requiring admission, diagnostic studies to determine the etiology of CAP should be attempted. Increased mortality is more common with inappropriate initial empiric therapy. De-escalation of antimicrobial therapy based on pathogen-specific treatment has been shown to decrease adverse drug effects and selection of antimicrobial resistance.

Blood cultures and sputum for Gram stain and culture (in patients with a productive cough) should be obtained in most patients who are admitted to the hospital. Pretreatment blood cultures have a 5% to 14% yield in patients hospitalized with CAP. The most common positive blood culture to be considered a pathogen is *S. pneumoniae*. In some series, false-positive blood cultures (contaminants) exceed positive blood culture with true pathogens. A false-positive blood culture can lead to extra days in the hospital and unnecessary use of antibiotics, especially vancomycin (Vancocin). The highest yield has been demonstrated with severe CAP (Box 1). Pretreatment Gram stain and culture should be performed only if a good quality specimen can be obtained. A Gram stain can direct initial empiric therapy, especially with less common pathogens such as *S. aureus* or gram-negative bacteria.

Patients with pleural effusions greater than 5 cm on a lateral upright chest radiograph or greater than 1 cm on a lateral decubitus film should undergo a thoracentesis for Gram stain and culture. Urinary antigen tests are available for *S. pneumoniae* and *Legionella pneumophila*. These tests are rapid and specific in adults. For pneumococcal pneumonia, studies in adults show a sensitivity of 50% to 80% and a specificity of greater than 90%. False-positives are seen in children colonized with *S. pneumoniae*; therefore, this test is not recommended in children. For *L. pneumophila*, the urinary antigen can only detect *L. pneumophila* serogroup 1, which accounts for 80% to 90% of legionnaires' disease cases in the United States. The urinary antigen has a sensitivity of 70% to 90% and a specificity of greater than 95%. A new polymerase chain reaction (PCR) test can detect all serotypes of *L. pneumophila* in sputum; however, clinical experience is currently limited.

The diagnosis of atypical pneumonia such as *Chlamydophila pneumoniae*, *Mycoplasma pneumoniae*, and *Legionella* species other than *L. pneumophila* rely on acute and convalescent serologies. In general, management on a single acute serology is unreliable; therefore, serologies are often retrospective and usually do not affect initial antimicrobial therapy.

ADMISSION CRITERIA

The initial decision of the treatment of CAP often revolves around severity of illness and if the patient requires hospitalization. Two severity-of-illness scores are commonly used, CURB-65 and the pneumonia severity index (PSI). CURB-65 stands for confusion, uremia (blood urea nitrogen > 20 mg/dL), respiratory rate greater than 30 breaths/minute, systolic blood pressure less than 90 mm Hg, and age older than 64 years. The PSI score is based primarily on history of underlying diseases and age that increase the risk of mortality, whereas CURB-65 does not rely on underlying diseases.

With CURB-65, mortality was higher when three (14.5%), four (40%), or five (57%) factors were present. Patients with a score of 0 or 1 can be treated on an outpatient basis, patients with a score of 2 can be admitted to the floor, and patients with scores higher than 3 often require admission to the intensive care unit (ICU). PSI uses 20 different variables and places patients into five risk groups (Table 1). Risk classes I and II patients can be treated as

---

BOX 1 Criteria for Severe Community-Acquired Pneumonia

Minor Criteria

Confusion or disorientation
Hypotension requiring fluid resuscitation
Hypothermia (<36°C)
Leukopenia (WBC <4000 cell/mm³)
Multilobar infiltrates
$Pao_2/Fio_2 \leq 250$
Respiratory rate ≥ 30
Thrombocytopenia (platelet count <100,000 cells/mm³)
Uremia (BUN ≥ 20 mg/dL)

Major Criteria

Invasive mechanical ventilation
Septic shock requiring vasopressors

Adapted from Mandell LA, Wunderink RG, Anzueto A, et al: Infectious Diseases Society of America/American Thoracic Society Consensus Guidelines on the Management of Community-Acquired Pneumonia in Adults. Clin Infect Dis 2007;44:S27–S72.
BUN = blood urea nitrogen; Fio_2 = fraction of inspired oxygen; Pao_2 = partial pressure of arterial oxygen; WBC = white blood cell count.

TABLE 1 Pneumonia Severity Index

Risk Factors	Points
Demographic factors	
Age for men	Age (yr)
Age for women	Age (yr) −10
Nursing home resident	+10
Coexisting illnesses	
Active neoplastic disease	+30
Chronic liver disease	+20
CHF	+10
Cerebrovascular disease	+10
Chronic renal disease	+10
Physical examination	
Altered mental status	+20
Respiratory rate >30	+20
Blood pressure <90 mm Hg	+20
Temperature <35°C or ≥40°C	+15
Pulse ≥125	+10
Laboratory and radiographic findings	
Arterial pH <7.35	+30
BUN ≥30 mg/dL	+20
Sodium <130 mmo/L	+20
Glucose ≥250 mg/dL	+10
Hematocrit <30%	+10
Pao_2 <60 mm Hg	+10
Pleural effusion	+10

Adapted from Fine MJ, Auble TE, Yealy DM, et al. A predictive rule to identify low-risk patients with community-acquired pneumonia. N Engl J Med 1997;336:243–250.
Risk classes: I = 0; II = 70 (low risk); III = 71–90 (low risk); IV = 91–130 (moderate risk); V >130 (high risk).
BUN = blood urea nitrogen; CHF = congestive heart failure; Pao_2 = partial pressure of arterial oxygen.

outpatients, risk class III patients can be treated on a short hospitalization or observational unit, and risk classes IV and V patients should be treated as inpatients.

ETIOLOGY

CAP may be caused by a number of pathogens, but only a few account for the majority of cases. Box 2 lists the more common pathogens divided by site of care and severity. According to most studies, an etiology is established in only about 40% of patients with CAP. In confirmed cases, *S. pneumoniae* is the most common bacterial pathogen identified. Atypical pathogens are the most common in mild to moderate CAP; *S. aureus*, gram-negative bacilli, and *L. pneumophila* are more common in severe CAP. Nontypable *Haemophilus influenzae* can be seen in patients with underlying chronic lung disease. *S. aureus* is often associated with preceding influenza. Gram-negative bacilli, including *Pseudomonas aeruginosa*, can be seen in patients who are taking steroids or chemotherapy, who have previously used antibiotics, are alcoholics, or who have underlying pulmonary disease.

TREATMENT

Antimicrobial therapy remains the mainstay of treatment. Until better diagnostic tests are available, initial treatment remains largely empiric. Box 3 reviews the most recent recommended empiric antibiotics. Anaerobic coverage should be considered with a history of loss of consciousness in patients with gingival or esophageal disease. Antibiotics should be modified based on local epidemiology and susceptibilities.

Current levels of penicillin and cephalosporin resistance to *S. pneumoniae* do not usually result in failure when appropriate doses are administered. However, recent studies indicate that resistance to macrolides and older fluoroquinolones (levofloxacin [Levaquin] and ciprofloxacin [Cipro]) have resulted in clinical failures in

---

BOX 2 Community-Acquired Pneumonia Pathogens by Site

Outpatient Setting
Chlamydophlia pneumoniae
Haemophilus influenzae
Mycoplasma pneumoniae
Respiratory viruses: adenovirus, influenza, parainfluenza, respiratory syncytial virus
Streptococcus pneumoniae

Inpatient outside Intensive Care Unit
Aspiration
Chlamydophlia pneumoniae
Haemophilus influenzae
Legionella species
Mycoplasma pneumoniae
Respiratory viruses
Streptococcus pneumoniae

Inpatient in Intensive Care Unit
Gram-negative bacilli
Haemophilus influenzae
Legionella species
Staphylococcus aureus
Streptococcus pneumoniae

Adapted from File TM: Community-acquired pneumonia. Lancet 2003;362:1991–2001.

BOX 3 Empiric Antimicrobial Choice for Community-Acquired Pneumonia

Outpatient Treatment
Healthy patient, no prior antibiotics within the previous 3 months
- Macrolide (azithromycin [Zithromax], clarithromycin [Biaxin], or erythromycin) *or*
- Doxycycline (Vibramycin) (weak recommendation)

Patient with comorbidity (e.g., chronic heart, lung, liver, or renal disease; malignancies; alcoholism; asplenia; diabetes mellitus; immunosuppression) or use of antibiotics in previous 3 months
- Respiratory fluoroquinolone (moxifloxacin [Avelox], gemifloxacin [Factive], or levofloxacin [Levaquin] (750 mg) *or*
- β-Lactam (high-dose amoxicillin or amoxicillin-clavulanate [Augmentin]); alternatives are ceftriaxone (Rocephin), cefpodoxime (Vantin), or cefuroxime (Ceftin) plus a macrolide

In regions with a high rate (> 25%) of infection with high-level (MIC ≥ 16 μg/mL) macrolide-resistant *Streptococcus pneumoniae*
- Use a fluoroquinolone or a β-lactam plus either a macrolide or doxycycline

Inpatients Not in Intensive Care
- Fluroquinolone alone *or*
- β-Lactam (e.g., ceftriaxone, cefotaxime [Claforan], ampicillin, ertapenem [Invanz]) plus a macrolide

Intensive Care Unit Patients
- β-Lactam (e.g., ceftriaxone, cefotaxime, or ampicillin-sulbactam [Unasyn]) *plus* either azithromycin or a fluoroquinolone

For *Pseudomonas* infection
- Antipneumococcal, antipseudomonal β-lactam (piperacillin-tazobactam [Zosyn], cefepime [Maxipime], imipenem [Primaxin], or meropenem [Merrem]) plus either ciprofloxacin (Cipro) or levofloxacin (750 mg) *or*
- Antipneumococcal, antipseudomonal β-lactam *plus* an aminoglycoside and azithromycin

Community-Acquired MRSA
- Add vancomycin (Vancocin) or linezolid (Zyvox)

Adapted from Mandell LA, Wunderink RG, Anzueto A, et al: Infectious Diseases Society of America/American Thoracic Society Consensus Guidelines on the Management of Community-Acquired Pneumonia in Adults. Clin Infect Dis 2007;44:S27–S72.
MIC = minimum inhibitory concentration;
MRSA = methicillin-resistant *Streptococcus aureus*.

---

patients with CAP caused by *S. pneumoniae*. Pneumonia caused by community-acquired MRSA may be increasing, especially associated with influenza. Many of these cases are genotypically and phenotypically different from hospital-acquired MRSA. Community-acquired MRSA isolates are less antibiotic resistant and often contain the gene for Panton-Valentine leukocidin (PVL), a toxin associated with necrotizing pneumonia. Anecdotal and in vitro studies suggest clindamycin (Cleocin) (if susceptible) or linezolid (Zyvox) can affect toxin production and improve outcome. More studies are needed to determine the most effective treatment for CAP caused by community-acquired MRSA. Several studies have reported that combination therapy with the combination of a macrolide and a β-lactam for bacteremic pneumococcal pneumonia is associated with lower mortality compared with a single effective drug. A possible explanation might relate to the fact that macrolides have immunomodulatory effects, including cytokine production.

Time to first antibiotic dose for CAP has been studied in two retrospective studies in Medicare patients. These studies demonstrated lower mortality in patients who received timely antimicrobial treatment. The first study showed that if the first dose was given within 8 hours of arrival, mortality was reduced. The second study demonstrated that a 4-hour interval was associated with better outcomes. Treatment should be given for a minimum of 5 days; the patient should be afebrile for 48 to 72 hours and clinically stable. Longer treatment may be needed for CAP caused by *S. aureus*, *L. pneumophila*, or *P. aeruginosa* and in patients with evidence of associated endocarditis, septic arthritis, or meningitis.

PREVENTION

Patients older than 50 years, others at risk for influenza complications, household contacts of high-risk patients, and health care workers with direct patient contact should receive a yearly influenza vaccine. Several reviews have demonstrated that influenza vaccination not only prevents pneumonia but also decreases hospitalizations, decreases cerebrovascular events, and decreases deaths from all causes.

Pneumococcal polysaccharide vaccine (Pneumovax 23) is recommended for all persons older than 65 years and persons with certain underlying illnesses (e.g., functional and anatomic asplenia, cardiopulmonary disease, diabetes). Studies have documented moderate effectiveness for preventing invasive pneumococcal disease (bacteremia and meningitis). The overall efficacy in patients older than 65 years is reported to be between 44% and 75%.

Vaccination status should be determined in all patients admitted to the hospital. Vaccination should be offered year-round for pneumococcal vaccine and during the fall and winter months for influenza vaccine.

Health Care–Acquired Pneumonia

HAP is defined as a pneumonia that occurred more than 48 hours after admission and that was not incubating at the time of admission. Ventilator-associated pneumonia (VAP) is defined as pneumonia that develops 48 to 72 hours after intubation. Health care–associated pneumonia (HCAP) is a new category; HCAP occurs in a patient who attended a hospital or hemodialysis clinic, who was hospitalized in an acute-care hospital for more than 2 days within the prior 90 days, or who resided in a long-term care facility or nursing home. The remaining comments are directed at HAP and VAP.

HAP is the second or third most common health care–associated infection in the United States and is associated with significant morbidity and mortality, resulting in increased length of stay and costs. HAP accounts for about 25% of all ICU infections. VAP occurs in 9% to 27% of intubated patients, and the mortality is double that of similar patients without VAP. The risk of VAP is highest in the first 1 to 2 weeks. Some investigators consider time of onset an important factor in terms of outcomes and pathogens. Early-onset HAP and VAP are pneumonia occurring within 4 to 7 days of hospitalization. Early-onset HAP and VAP usually carry a better prognosis and are more likely to be caused by more sensitive pathogens. Late-onset HAP and VAP are more likely to be caused by multidrug-resistant organisms (MDRO) with a higher mortality.

Aspiration of oropharyngeal secretions or leakage of bacteria around the endotracheal tube is the primary source of bacteria causing HAP or VAP. The stomach and sinuses, blood, and contaminated aerosols are much less common sources. Contaminated biofilm in the endotracheal tube, with subsequent embolization into the lower airway, may be an important factor in the pathogenesis of VAP.

DIAGNOSIS

Unfortunately, there is no universally accepted gold standard for the diagnosis of HAP or VAP. The diagnosis is suspected if a patient has a new or progressive infiltrate along with new-onset fever, purulent sputum (>25 neutrophils per low-power field), leukocytosis, and decreased oxygenation.

Unfortunately, the clinical parameters are overly sensitive; therefore, other diagnostic tests are desirable. For a start, blood and lower respiratory secretions should be collected for culture in all patients with suspected HAP or VAP. A thoracentesis should be performed if a large pleural effusion is present. The microbiological approach favors quantitation or semiquantitation of lower respiratory secretions. The diagnostic threshold used to differentiate colonization versus true infection varies by specimen collection. The proposed diagnostic threshold for endotracheal aspirate is greater than 10^5 colony-forming units (CFU)/mL; for bronchoalveolar lavage, greater than 10^4 CFU/mL; and for protected-specimen brush, greater than 10^3 CFU/mL. A major reservation to this approach is the possibility of false-negative results, which can result if a patient has been started on an antimicrobial agent before the specimens are collected.

TREATMENT

For patients with suspected HAP or VAP, appropriate broad-spectrum antimicrobial therapy should be ordered to cover anticipated pathogens. Consider a Gram stain to guide initial therapy. Whenever possible, select antimicrobial therapy based on local microbiology and epidemiology. Use combination therapy in patients whenever an MDRO is suspected until culture results are available. Risk factors include prolonged hospitalization (>5–7 days), admission from another health care facility, and recent antibiotic therapy. Table 2 summarizes suggested empiric therapy. De-escalation of therapy is strongly recommended when culture results become available. Discontinue antimicrobial therapy if results of cultures and other clinical parameters do not confirm pneumonia. Based on recent studies, a shorter duration of therapy (7–8 days) is now recommended in patients with uncomplicated HAP or VAP who received initial appropriate therapy and have had a good clinical response. *P. aeruginosa*, *Acinetobacter* species, and MRSA can require longer durations of therapy.

PREVENTION

The incidence of HAP and VAP can be reduced by following certain proved measures. An effective infection control program, which includes education, hand-washing compliance, surveillance of ICU infections, and isolation of patients with MDRO to reduce cross-infection should be followed. Noninvasive ventilation should be used whenever possible. If intubation is required, the orotracheal route is preferred to reduce health care–associated infections due to sinusitis and VAP. Consider continuous aspiration of subglottic secretions, if available. Follow a protocol for using sedation with daily interruptions. Perform daily assessment for extubation. For patients on a ventilator, keep the head of the bed at 30 to 45 degrees to prevent aspiration (except when contraindicated). Use agents such as oral chlorhexidine (Peridex) to reduce oropharyngeal colonization. Glucose control to maintain level between 140–180 mg/dL results in lower mortality without increasing the risk of severe hypoglycemia.

TABLE 2 Initial Empiric Therapy for Suspected Health Care–Acquired Pneumonia or Ventilator-Associated Pneumonia

Suspected Pathogen	Recommended Therapy
Patients with No Known Risk Factors for MDRO and Early Onset	

Streptococcus pneumoniae
Haemophilus influenzae
Methicillin-sensitive
  Streptococcus aureus
Antibiotic-sensitive enteric
  gram-negative
  Escherichia coli
Klebsiella pneumoniae
Enterobacter species
Proteus species
Serratia marcescens
	One of the following:
	Ceftriaxone (Rocephin) or
	Fluoroquinolone (levofloxacin
	  [Levaquin], moxifloxacin
	  [Avelox], or ciprofloxacin [Cipro])
	or
	Ertapenem (Invanz)
	or
	Piperacillin-tazobactam (Zosyn)

Patients with Risk Factors for MDRO or Late Onset	

Pathogens listed above and
  MDRO
Pseudomonas aeruginosa
K. pneumoniae (ESBL)*
Acinetobacter species
MRSA
Legionella species†
	Antipseudomonal cephalosporin
	  (e.g., cefepime [Maxipime] or
	  ceftazidime [Fortaz])
	or
	Antipseudomonal carbepenem
	  (e.g., imipenem [Primaxin] or
	  meropenem [Merrem])
	or
	Piperacillin-tazobactam (Zosyn)
	plus
	Aminoglycoside
	or
	Antipseudomonal fluoroquinolone
	  (e.g., ciprofloxacin [Cipro] or
	  levofloxacin [Levaquin])
	plus
	Vancomycin (Vancocin) or linezolid
	  (Zyvox)

Modified from American Thoracic Society; Infectious Diseases Society of America: Guidelines for the management of adults with hospital-acquired, ventilator-associated, and healthcare-associated pneumonia. Am J Respir Crit Care Med 171:388–416, 2005.

*If an ESBL strain, a carbepenem is preferred.

†If *Legionella* suspected, the combination regimen should include either a macrolide (e.g., azithromycin) or a fluoroquinolone.

ESBL = extended-spectrum β-lactamase; MDRO = multidrug-resistant organisms; MRSA = methicillin-resistant *Staphylococcus aureus*.

REFERENCES

American Thoracic Society; Infectious Diseases Society of America. Guidelines for the management of adults with hospital-acquired, ventilator-associated, and healthcare-associated pneumonia. Am J Respir Crit Care Med 2005;171:388–416.

Chastre J, Wolff M, Fagon JY, et al. Comparison of 8 vs 15 days of antibiotic therapy for ventilator-associated pneumonia in adults: A randomized trial. JAMA 2003;290:2588–98.

Fagon JY, Chastre J, Wolff M, et al. Invasive and noninvasive strategies for management of suspected ventilator-associated pneumonia: A randomized trial. Ann Intern Med 2000;132:621–30.

File TM. Community-acquired pneumonia. Lancet 2003;362:1991–2001.

Fine MJ, Auble TE, Yealy DM, et al. A predictive rule to identify low-risk patients with community-acquired pneumonia. N Engl J Med 1997;336:243–50.

Houck PM, Bratzler DW, Nsa W, et al. Timing of antibiotic administration and outcomes for Medicare patients hospitalized with community-acquired pneumonia. Arch Intern Med 2004;164:637–44.

Lim WS, van der Eerden MM, Laing R, et al. Defining community acquired pneumonia severity on presentation to hospital: An international derivation and validation study. Thorax 2003;58:377–82.

Mandell LA, Wunderink RG, Anzueto A, et al. Infectious Diseases Society of America/American Thoracic Society Consensus Guidelines on the Management of Community-Acquired Pneumonia in Adults. Clin Infect Dis 2007;44:S27–72.

Metersky ML, Ma A, Houck PM, Bratzler DW. Antibiotics for bacteremic pneumonia: Improved outcomes with macrolides but not fluoroquinolones. Chest 2007;131:466–73.

NICE-SUGAR Study Investigators. Intensive versus conventional glucose control in critically ill patients. N Engl J Med 2009;360:1283–97.

Richards MJ, Edwards JR, Culver DH, Gaynes RP. Nosocomial infections in medical ICUs in the United States: National Nosocomial Infections Surveillance System. Crit Care Med 1999;27:887–92.

van den Berghe G, Wilmer A, Hermans G, et al. Intensive insulin therapy in the medical ICU. N Engl J Med 2006;354:449–61.

Viral Respiratory Infections

Method of
Robert C. Welliver, Sr., MD

Viral infections of the respiratory tract are among the most common infections in humans, and they account for significant morbidity at all ages. Infants and young children can sustain six to eight such infections annually, and adults have an average of nearly two such infections per year.

Rhinoviruses are the most commonly identified etiologic agents and cause illness year-round. Other common causative agents during winter months include influenza viruses and respiratory syncytial virus, and enteroviruses predominate in summer months. The parainfluenza viruses also commonly cause respiratory infection, particularly in autumn (type 1) and late spring or summer (type 3). Coronaviruses, metapneumoviruses, adenoviruses, and other agents are identified less often.

Although each of these agents can cause a common cold, some viral infections are associated with characteristic patterns of respiratory disease. Most of these viruses can also exacerbate asthma, cystic fibrosis, and chronic obstructive pulmonary disease (COPD).

Common Colds

Colds are the most common of the viral respiratory illnesses. Pharyngitis is usually the earliest sign of a cold, beginning a few days after infection has taken place. Nasal congestion and clear or slightly cloudy rhinorrhea usually follow within 24 to 48 hours. Cough occurs in approximately 30% to 40% of those infected, and fluid can accumulate in middle ear or sinus cavities that have become blocked as a result of mucosal swelling. Ear and sinus cavity infections occur when this fluid is trapped for a week or more. Treatment with antibiotics is ineffective before this time, and they are ineffective especially in the absence of other clinical signs of ear and sinus infections.

Colds are a frequent cause of missed school and work, and even of mild morbidity, but they are rarely serious in otherwise healthy persons. The most appropriate approach to treatment therefore entails rest, with adequate nutrition and hydration. Agents that inhibit the activity of cyclooxygenase probably represent the most effective form of pharmacologic intervention. These compounds include acetaminophen (Tylenol) and the nonsteroidal anti-inflammatory agents (NSAIDs) such as ibuprofen (Motrin). They are effective in reducing fever and, perhaps more importantly in most colds, reducing malaise, headache, and pharyngitis.

Nasal congestion and some rhinorrhea during colds are related to dilation of blood vessels in the nose and sinuses. Vasoconstrictors have therefore been used extensively to attempt to reverse these symptoms. Oral decongestants such as pseudoephedrine (Sudafed) have minimal effect on nasal congestion, and can result in systemic hypertension, anxiety, and difficulty sleeping. The propensity for these compounds to cause cardiac arrhythmias in the very young child has led to recommendations against their use in the first year or two of life. Nasal sprays containing vasoconstricting agents such as oxymetazoline (Afrin) can result in mild temporary relief of nasal obstruction. However, the use of these compounds for more than 3 or 4 days can result in rebound vasodilation and paradoxically increased rhinorrhea.

Numerous investigations have evaluated the role of antihistamines in colds. The release of histamine itself is not associated with fever, cough, or malaise, so effects on these symptoms would not be expected. Furthermore, nasal congestion and discharge may be more related to the release of kinins, and not histamine. Indeed, the administration of antihistamines in adults and, particularly, in children has not demonstrated strikingly positive results. As many as 40% of subjects treated with placebo report beneficial effects. Side effects of histamine use, primarily sedation and dry mouth, are commonly encountered.

Cough can be one of the most irritating symptoms during colds. Cough during colds is principally caused by secretions entering the airway (postnasal drip) and not by inflammation of the airway itself. Therefore, it is not surprising that cough suppressants, especially codeine, have little effect on cough induced by colds. Antihistamines have also been found to be ineffective in relief of cough during colds.

Influenza-Like Illness

The influenza syndrome is defined as the abrupt onset of fever, headache, and striking degrees of malaise and prostration, often with intense myalgia. Respiratory symptoms can occur concurrently, but they might not be prominent features. The principal cause is, of course, influenza virus, although infection with many other viruses can cause similar (although not as intense) symptoms. The illness is generally self-limited, and most symptoms resolve over 4 or 5 days. Lassitude can persist for up to 2 weeks.

Influenza virus infection and influenza-like illness are best treated symptomatically, relying on rest, adequate intake of fluids and calories, and appropriate analgesic therapy. Compounds referred to as *M2 inhibitors* such as amantadine (Symmetrel) and rimantadine (Flumadine) have been approved for therapy. Positive outcomes from therapy with these agents are observed only when therapy is instituted within 48 hours after the onset of symptoms, and benefits are not striking. In recent years, resistance to M2 inhibitors has been commonly observed among circulating epidemic strains of influenza virus.

More recently, inhibitors of the activity of influenza viral neuraminidase have been used in treatment and prevention of influenza virus infection in adults and children. The first such compound released, zanamivir (Relenza), was administered by inhalation but was unpopular because of its irritating effects on the airway.

An oral compound, oseltamivir (TamiFlu), has been used to prevent and to treat influenza virus infection. As with M2 inhibitors, it is believed that treatment should be started within the first 48 hours of symptoms and that prophylaxis should be instituted within 48 hours of exposure. Treatment with oseltamivir shortens the duration of subsequent illness by only about 24 hours. Treatment can prevent some of the complications of influenza infection, including pneumonia. The drug may be more effective as a therapeutic agent, because it may be up to 90% effective in preventing culture-positive symptomatic influenza illness. The recommended dose for adults is 75 mg orally every 12 hours for 5 days. In children, the appropriate dose based on body weight is 30 mg twice daily for children weighing less than 15 kg, 45 mg twice daily for children weighing 15 to 23 kg, 60 mg twice daily for children weighing 23 to 40 kg, and 75 mg twice daily for children weighing more than 40 kg. The principal side effect is nausea, which can be reduced by taking the drug with food.

Croup

Croup is defined by the occurrence of hoarseness or laryngitis, a deep, brassy or barking cough, and inspiratory stridor. Airway obstruction in croup is caused by constriction in the subglottic area, often noted on radiographs by a steeple-shaped narrowing of the air column in this region. Affected children are usually afebrile and nontoxic in appearance.

Parainfluenza virus type 1 is the primary cause of croup, although infection with many different viruses can produce this illness, and influenza virus can cause a particularly severe form of croup. Bacterial secondary infection occurs uncommonly, but it can result in fever and severe obstruction of the airway. Administration of dexamethasone (Decadron)[1] at 0.6 mg/kg either orally or intramuscularly markedly reduces the rate of hospitalization, admission to the intensive care unit, and intubation for croup.

Bronchiolitis

Bronchiolitis represents the most common cause for hospitalization of infants in developed countries. Infants present with a history of several days of upper respiratory symptoms, followed by the rapid onset of wheezing and labored breathing. Respiratory syncytial virus (RSV) is the most common cause and is the agent found in the most severe cases that result in respiratory failure. Contrasting with asthma, obstruction of the airway in bronchiolitis is a result of plugging of bronchioles with detached epithelium and inflammatory cells. Mucus plugging and constriction of smooth muscle are not prominent. Also in contrast with asthma is the absence of a sustained response to bronchodilators and corticosteroids among infants with bronchiolitis.

Therapy of bronchiolitis primarily consists of administration of supplemental oxygen and replacement of fluid deficits as needed. Ribavirin (Virazole)[1] is a compound with antiviral activity against RSV, but controlled studies have not demonstrated meaningful differences

---

[1]Not FDA approved for this indication.

CURRENT DIAGNOSIS

- Rapid diagnostic kits are available for many common respiratory viruses. These tests are used increasingly to establish that antibiotic therapy is not necessary in many patients with febrile respiratory illnesses or with lower respiratory tract infections.
- The presence of wheezing on physical examination virtually excludes bacterial infection from consideration in subjects with lower respiratory disease.

CURRENT THERAPY

- The management of most viral respiratory infections consists of rest, adequate caloric and fluid intake, and management of fever and malaise.
- Corticosteroids are essential in the management of croup.
- Specific antiviral therapy is available only for influenza virus infection, and beneficial effects have been more readily achieved in prevention rather than treatment.

in outcomes between treated and untreated subjects. The compound is quite expensive and must be delivered via a special aerosol generator.

Palivizumab (Synagis), a preparation consisting of a monoclonal antibody against the fusion protein of RSV, has proved to be effective in reducing the rate of hospitalization for RSV infection by approximately 50% when given to high-risk infants. Infants who may be considered candidates for therapy include those with chronic lung disease, those born prematurely, and those with hemodynamically significant congenital heart disease. Doses of palivizumab (15 mg/kg) are given on a monthly basis throughout the local RSV season, usually November through March.

REFERENCES

Akerlund A, Klint T, Olen L, Runderantz H. Nasal decongestant effect of oxymetazoline in the common cold: An objective dose-response study in 106 patients. J Laryngol Otol 1989;103:743–6.

Buckingham SC, Jafri HS, Bush AN, et al. A randomized, double-blind, placebo-controlled trial of dexamethasone in severe respiratory syncytial virus (RSV) infection: Effects on RSV quantity and clinical outcome. J Infect Dis 2002;185:1222–8.

Curley FJ, Irwin RS, Pratter MR, et al. Cough and the common cold. Am J Respir Crit Care Med 1988;138:305–11.

Flores G, Horwitz RI. Efficacy of β_2-agonists in bronchiolitis: A reappraisal and meta-analysis. Pediatrics 1997;100:233–9.

Johnson DW, Jacobson S, Edney PC, et al. A comparison of nebulized budesonide, intramuscular dexamethasone, and placebo for moderately severe croup. N Engl J Med 1998;339:498–503.

Muether PS, Gwaltney JM Jr. Variant effect of first- and second-generation antihistamines as clues to their mechanism of action on the sneeze reflex in the common cold. Clin Infect Dis 2001;33:1483–8.

Randolph AG, Wang EL. Ribavirin for respiratory syncytial virus lower respiratory tract infection. Arch Pediatr Adolesc Med 1996;150:942–7.

Tavorner D, Danz C, Economos D. The effects of oral pseudoephedrine on nasal patency in the common cold: A double-blind single-dose placebo-controlled trial. Clin Otolaryngol 1999;24:47–51.

Treanor JJ, Hayden FG, Vrooman PS, et al. Efficacy and safety of the oral neuraminidase inhibitor oseltamivir in treating acute influenza: A randomized controlled trial. US Oral Neuraminnidase Study Group. JAMA 2000;283:1016–24.

Van Voris LP, Betts RF, Hayden FG, et al. Successful treatment of naturally occurring influenza A/USSR/77 H1N1. JAMA 1981;245:1128–31.

Viral and Mycoplasmal Pneumonias

Method of
Burke A. Cunha, MD

Influenza pneumonia is the most important cause of viral pneumonia in adults. Influenza A is the predominant type of influenza found in adults, and influenza B is more common in children. Influenza A has the potential for severe disease, occurs seasonally, and is the predominant type involved in influenza pandemics. *Mycoplasma pneumoniae* community-acquired pneumonia (CAP) was first recognized decades ago as distinctive from bacterial and viral pneumonias. It was originally described by Eaton as "Eaton agent" pneumonia caused by a pleuropneumonia-like organism (PPLO), later shown to be caused by *M. pneumoniae*. *M. pneumoniae* is a common cause of pneumonia in all age groups, but the peak incidence of *M. pneumoniae* CAP is in young adults. *M. pneumoniae* CAP is a common cause of ambulatory CAP.

The term *atypical pneumonia* was first applied to viral pneumonias because the clinical laboratory and radiologic findings were different from those caused by typical bacterial pulmonary pathogens. In influenza pneumonia, the clinical findings are confined to the trachea, bronchi, lung parenchyma, and central nervous system.

M. pneumoniae CAP is a systemic infection with a pulmonary component. Over the years, atypical pneumonia has come to refer to pneumonia caused by systemic nonviral/nonbacterial pathogen agents that have a pulmonary component. Viral pneumonias are no longer considered atypical pneumonias. Atypical pneumonias may be divided into nonzoonotic and zoonotic atypical CAPs. Nonzoonotic CAPs are most commonly caused by *M. pneumoniae*, *Chlamydia pneumoniae*, or *Legionella* species; whereas the three most common zoonotic atypical pneumonias are caused by *Chlamydia psittaci* (psittacosis), *Francisella tularensis* (tularemia), or *Coxiella burnetii* (Q fever). All of the atypical pneumonias are distinct clinical entities that may be differentiated on the basis of their characteristic pattern of extrapulmonary organ involvement. Although some viruses may occasionally have extrapulmonary manifestations (i.e., influenza, adenovirus with viral pneumonias), the primary clinical features are confined to the lungs. *M. pneumoniae* is a critical cause of nonzoonotic atypical CAP, particularly in the ambulatory setting. *M. pneumoniae* CAP may be severe in patients with impaired host defenses or those with severe, preexisting cardiopulmonary disease.

Influenza (Human, Avian, and Swine)

Viral influenza pneumonia affects children and adults. Influenza B is the primary type causing mild influenza in children and adults. Influenza A is primarily an infection of adults that may be mild to severe. Influenza A has the potential for pandemic spread (e.g., swine influenza [H_1N_1]).

Influenza occurs during the winter months, usually peaking in February. Influenza is spread by aerosolized droplet infection from person to person and via fomites. Influenza A is classified into subtypes based on hemagglutinin (H) and neuramidase (N) surface proteins. An important characteristic of influenza A virus is antigenic drift, which refers to minor changes in surface protein shift in the neuramidase or hemagglutinin receptors. With influenza A, these surface receptor proteins are important in cellular adherence of the influenza virus and spread of influenza from respiratory epithelial cells. The vaccine for the flu season most often includes the influenza hemagglutinin and neuramidase types seen at the end of the preceding year's season. Prevention of attachment and spread of the virus is helpful to controlling the spread of influenza; vaccine protection conferred by specific antibody response to influenza A is highly protective (approximately 80% in noncompromised hosts).

During the years when influenza B has been prevalent, vaccines for the subsequent year contain an influenza B component.

Clinical manifestations of influenza A in adults varies considerably from mild to fatal infection. Mild infection is usually manifested as an acute febrile illness characterized by headache and myalgias with dry unproductive cough and rhinorrhea. Mild influenza may be due to influenza A or B and usually resolves in a few days without complications in normal hosts who have good cardiopulmonary function.

Severe influenza A (human, avian, swine) occurs in normal healthy adults and may be fatal. The onset of severe influenza A (human, avian, swine) is sudden, and the patient often recalls the exact hour of onset. The patient is febrile with early/extreme prostration rendering the patient bedridden. Fever rapidly rises and may be accompanied by chills. Neck soreness, severe headache, and myalgias are typical. Sore throat, eye pain, conjunctival injection, and hemoptysis are frequently present. Chest pain worsened by deep inspiration is not truly pleuritic but rather reflects influenza A myositis of the intracostal muscles. Shortness of breath is related to the degree of hypoxemia. Severe influenza A causes an oxygen diffusion defect as manifested by an increased A-a gradient (>35). Profound hypoxemia may be accompanied by cyanosis. Hypotension caused by hypoxemia and vascular collapse may follow. The course of fulminant viral influenza A is of short duration.

Physical findings are few in viral influenza (i.e., conjunctival suffusion). Auscultation reveals absolutely quiet lungs because the infectious process is interstitial and not alveolar. Routine blood tests are usually unremarkable except for leukopenia, relative lymphopenia, and thrombocytopenia. Atypical lymphocytes are not present, but low titers of cold agglutinins may be present. Cold agglutinins (if present) have low titers less than or equal to 1:18. In fatal cases, a pale bluelike hue of the skin may be noted, and there may be bleeding from multiple orifices preterminally. The chest radiograph in uncomplicated influenza A is unremarkable or may have minimal perihilar bilateral increased prominence of interstitial markings. In severe influenza A pneumonia, the chest radiograph shows bilateral symmetrical perihilar infiltrates without pleural effusions in <48 hours.

Patients may die from severe influenza A without superimposed bacterial pneumonia. Most deaths during the 1918–1919 pandemic were young military recruits who died early of influenza A pneumonia without bacterial pneumonia. Influenza may be complicated by bacterial pneumonia. Bacterial pneumonias complicating influenza may occur concurrently at presentation or may occur 1 to 2 weeks after an interval of improvement after the presentation of influenza. Influenza A presenting concurrently with bacterial pneumonia is caused by Staphylococcus aureus. In contrast to influenza alone, MSSA/CA-MRSA is manifested by an increase in fever, shaking chills, leukocytosis, purulent sputum, localized rales on auscultation, bacteremia, and focal/segmental infiltrates on chest radiograph that rapidly cavitate in less than 72 hours. Alternately, patients with influenza A may develop a secondary bacterial infection 1 to 2 weeks later. Secondary bacterial pneumonia is less severe and is usually caused by Streptococcus pneumoniae or Haemophilus influenzae.

ANTI-INFLUENZA THERAPY

Therapy of viral influenza is directed at inhibiting viral replication and preventing further infection of respiratory epithelial cells. The neuramidase inhibitors zanamivir (Relenza) and oseltamivir (Tamiflu) have anti-influenza A and B activity. Neuramidase inhibitors decrease the severity and duration of influenza symptoms by 1 to 2 days. Current flu strains are resistant to amantadine and rimantadine, but these drugs may still be useful to increase peripheral airway dilatation and oxygenation, which may be of critical importance in severe influenza A with severe hypoxemia. Mild influenza A/B may be treated with neuramidase inhibitors. Mild cases of influenza A should be treated at the onset of the illness. For severe influenza A, neuramidase inhibitors provide optimal anti-influenza therapy (Table 1). For human and avian influenza (H_5N_1), these antiviral drugs may be ineffective, but are effective against swine influenza.

Mycoplasma pneumoniae Pneumonia

M. pneumoniae is a common cause of ambulatory CAP. It affects all age groups, and in normal hosts with intact cardiopulmonary function, Mycoplasma CAP is usually a mild, self-limiting infection.

However, M. pneumoniae derives its importance from difficulty in diagnosis, the necessity for non–β-lactam therapy, and because of its effect on peripheral airways.

Mycoplasma CAP is one of the nonzoonotic causes of CAP (the others being Legionella and Chlamydia pneumoniae). M. pneumoniae is an atypical pneumonia that is a systemic infectious disease with a pulmonary component. It may be distinguished from other atypical pneumonias by its characteristic pattern of extrapulmonary organ involvement. M. pneumoniae CAP most closely resembles C. pneumoniae CAP clinically, but is very different from Legionnaires' disease in terms of its epidemiology, age distribution, pattern of extrapulmonary organ involvement, and severity.

Clinically, M. pneumoniae presents as a subacute febrile illness. Temperatures rarely exceed 102°F (38.9°C). Rigors are not a feature of M. pneumoniae CAP, but patients may complain of chilly sensations. Mild headache and/or myalgias are not uncommon. The most common presenting symptom in Mycoplasma CAP is the prolonged, nonproductive dry cough. Patients with Mycoplasma CAP often complain of or have mild nonexudative pharyngitis. Rhinorrhea and conjunctivitis are not features of M. pneumoniae CAP. Watery diarrhea is commonly present in Mycoplasma CAP, but abdominal pain is not a clinical finding. Other extrapulmonary manifestations are uncommon or rare (e.g., meningoencephalitis, pericarditis, hemolytic anemia, glomerular nephritis, Guillain-Barré syndrome, erythema multiforme). M. pneumoniae has a distinctive pattern of extrapulmonary organ involvement that does not include cardiac involvement (relative bradycardia) or hepatic involvement, including normal serum glutamate-oxaloacetate transaminase (SGOT) or serum glutamate-pyruvate transaminase (SGPT). The distinguishing laboratory feature of M. pneumoniae CAP is elevated cold agglutinin titers. Although a variety of infectious and noninfectious diseases are associated with cold agglutinin elevations, they are usually of low titer (i.e., <1:16). There are no pulmonary infections presenting as CAP that are associated with high elevations of cold agglutinin titers (i.e., ≥1:64). Although elevated cold agglutinins occur early in up to 75% of patients with M. pneumoniae CAP, they are still diagnostically important when present. In a patient with CAP and a cold agglutinin titer greater than or equal to 1:64, the diagnosis of M. pneumoniae CAP is very likely.

M. pneumoniae may be differentiated from the typical bacterial pneumonias because of the presence of extrapulmonary findings, including nonexudative pharyngitis, loose stools or watery diarrhea, erythema multiforme, and high cold agglutinin. Patients with typical bacterial CAP usually have a more acute onset of presentation, a productive cough, and temperatures that may exceed 102°F (38.9°C), often accompanied by chills. Patients with typical pneumonia often have pleuritic chest pain, which is not a feature of M. pneumoniae CAP. Among the atypical pneumonias, the zoonotic pneumonias (i.e., tularemia, psittacosis, Q fever) may be eliminated from consideration if there is a recent zoonotic contact history with the appropriate vector.

C. pneumoniae resembles closely M. pneumoniae CAP. C. pneumoniae may be distinguished by the absence of cold agglutinins and the presence of hoarseness, which is a feature of C. pneumoniae but not M. pneumoniae CAP. Loose stools or watery diarrhea are not usual features of C. pneumoniae CAP. The most common clinical problem is differentiating Legionella from Mycoplasma CAP; this may be done by appreciating the differences in the pattern of extrapulmonary organ involvement with each of these pathogens. Legionella may be clinically differentiated from Mycoplasma by acuteness of onset or severity, the presence of relative bradycardia, temperatures greater than 102°F (38.9°C), and the presence of abdominal pain. From a laboratory standpoint, highly elevated cold agglutinin titers argue strongly against the diagnosis of Legionella and point to M. pneumoniae. Nonspecific laboratory tests in a patient with CAP that suggest Legionella and argue against M. pneumoniae include otherwise unexplained hypophosphatemia, hyponatremia, microscopic hematuria, and increased creatinine. Legionella does not affect the upper respiratory tract as does Mycoplasma (e.g., nonexudative pharyngitis). Ear findings are not a feature of Legionnaires' disease but are common in M. pneumoniae CAP. The finding most likely to cause confusion between M. pneumoniae and Legionella pneumophila is the presence of loose stools or watery diarrhea, which is found in both.

TABLE 1 Adult Anti-Influenza Antivirals

Antiviral	Treatment Dose	Prophylactic Dose
Mild Influenza A/B		
Zanamivir (Relenza)[†]	2 inhalations (5 mg per inhalation) q12h × 5d	2 inhalations (5 mg per inhalation) q24h × 5d
Influenza A		
Oseltamivir (Tamiflu)[†]	75 mg (PO) q12h × 5d*	75 mg (PO) q24h × 7d

*For avian (H5N1) influenza, 150 mg (PO) q12h may be effective.
[†]Currently most human and avian influenza strains are resistant.

CURRENT DIAGNOSIS

Influenza (human, avian, swine)
- Mild influenza A or B presents acutely with headache, fever, sore throat, plus/minus rhinorrhea.
- Severe influenza A presents with an acute onset (patients often able to name the hour the influenza began) and rapidly become bed bound.
- Headache, myalgias, and prostration are severe.
- With swine influenza, gastrointestinal symptoms (e.g., nausea/vomiting or diarrhea) may be prominent.
- Auscultation of the lungs is quiet, disproportionate to the degree of respiratory distress. Influenza is an interstitial process and not alveolar, which explains the absence of rales.
- With severe influenza, patients rapidly become hypoxemic. Hypoxemia is accompanied by an A-a gradient >35, which indicates a interstitial oxygen diffusing defect.
- Severe tracheobronchitis is common and manifested by hemoptysis.
- Relative lymphopenia occurs early followed by thrombocytopenia and later leukopenia. Low titer elevations of cold agglutinins are not infrequent (≥1:18).
- Patients may have chest pain exacerbated by breathing mimicking pleuritic chest pain. This is the result of direct intracostal muscle involvement with the influenza virus, which results in myositis and pain on inspiration.
- The chest radiograph in early influenza, in mild to moderate cases, is normal or near normal, with minimal, if any, increase in perihilar interstitial markings. The chest radiograph in fulminant cases shows symmetrical bilateral patchy infiltrates without pleural effusion in 48 hours.
- Severe influenza A is accompanied by severe hypoxemia cyanosis, and may be followed by an early fatal outcome.
- Influenza pneumonia most often presents alone without bacterial superinfection, but bacterial infection may accompany (MSSA/CA-MRSA) or follow influenza (*S. pneumoniae* or *H. influenzae*).

- Purulent sputum with influenza indicates concurrent bacterial pneumonia usually caused by *S. aureus* (MSSA/MRSA). Bacterial pneumonia following influenza (after 1 to 2 weeks), is suggested by leukocytosis, focal or segmental pulmonary infiltrates, and purulent sputum; the pathogens are not *S. aureus*, but most commonly are *S. pneumoniae* or *H. influenzae*.
- A laboratory diagnosis may be made by DFA staining of respiratory secretions or viral cultures.

Mycoplasma pneumoniae
- In a patient with CAP and a dry nonproductive cough, without severe headache or myalgias, the most likely diagnosis is *M. pneumoniae*. *M. pneumoniae* CAP is commonly accompanied by nonexudative pharyngitis and/or loose stools or watery diarrhea.
- The temperature is usually less than 102°F (38.9°C) and is not accompanied by frank rigors or pleuritic chest pain.
- Relative bradycardia and elevations in the serum transaminases are not features of *M. pneumoniae* CAP.
- Respiratory viruses are often associated with mild elevations of cold agglutinins (≤1:16) but *M. pneumoniae* is the only pathogen causing CAP associated with highly elevated cold agglutinin titers (≥1:64). Elevated cold agglutinin titers occur in up to 75% of patients with *M. pneumoniae*, and occur early and transiently.
- In a patient with CAP, elevated cold agglutinin titers (>1:8) effectively rule out the typical pathogens, as well as *Legionella* species and *C. pneumoniae*.
- Elevated *M. pneumoniae* ELISA IgG titers indicate past exposure/infection and not current infection or co-infection with another pathogen.
- In the absence of an antecedent respiratory tract infection (e.g., nonexudative pharyngitis, otitis, etc., in the preceding 3 months), the presence of an increased *M. pneumoniae* ELISA IgM titer is diagnostic of acute infection.

 CURRENT THERAPY

Viral Influenza
- The aim of therapy is to inhibit the influenza virus and prevent its attachment/spread to uninfected respiratory epithelial cells.
- The neuramidase inhibitors shorten the course of influenza by 1 to 2 days and have antiviral activity. These agents are active against both influenza A and B.
- Most strains of human and avian, but not swine flu strains, are resistant to amantadine (Symmetrel) or rimantadine (Flumadine).
- Amantadine and rimantadine may have an important therapeutic effect in severe influenza A by increasing distal airway dilation and increasing oxygen action.

Mycoplasma pneumoniae
- The agents active against *M. pneumoniae* are macrolides, tetracyclines, quinolones, and ketolides. β-Lactam

antibiotics are not active against *M. pneumoniae* because the organisms do not contain a bacterial cell wall.
- Goals of therapy of *M. pneumoniae* CAP are to eradicate the infection, decrease the shedding of *Mycoplasma* in respiratory secretions posttherapy, and to prevent posttreatment asthma.
- Therapy is equally efficacious with macrolides, doxycycline (Vibramycin), or a respiratory quinolone intravenously, orally, or in combination for 1 to 2 weeks.
- The mode of administration is determined by the severity of the CAP and the setting. Outpatients are usually treated orally. Patients hospitalized with severe CAP are initially treated intravenously and then changed to an oral agent.
- Resistance to *M. pneumoniae* with antimicrobials has not been described and is not a clinical consideration.

M. pneumoniae may be cultured from the throat in viral culture media, but the diagnosis is usually made serologically. An elevated enzyme-linked immunosorbent assay (ELISA) or enzyme immuno-assay (EIA) IgM titer suggests acute or recent infection, but an elevated IgG titer indicates past exposure but not acute infection. Elevated IgG titers regardless of degree of elevation are not diagnostic of current infection with *M. pneumoniae* and only indicate previous antigenic exposure. *M. pneumoniae* ELISA IgM levels may take up to 3 months to decrease. Therefore, clinicians should take into account recent antecedent respiratory illness in order to properly interpret elevated IgM titers, including patients with nonexudative pharyngitis within 3 months prior to the presentation of CAP. The combination of an increased *M. pneumoniae* IgM titer and highly elevated cold agglutinin titers is virtually diagnostic of acute infection. Cold agglutinin titers are elevated transiently early and rapidly fall; the simultaneously elevated cold agglutinins and IgM titers of *M. pneumoniae* indicate active or current infection. In patients with CAP caused by another organism (e.g., *S. pneumoniae*), the presence of elevated *Mycoplasma* IgG titers does not indicate co-infection but only preexisting serologic exposure to *M. pneumoniae*.

THERAPY

M. pneumoniae has a predilection for the respiratory epithelial cells and resides literally on their surface. Mycoplasmas have no definite cell wall like the typical pathogens causing CAP. Their position on the surface of the respiratory epithelium and their absence of a cell wall necessitates the therapeutic approach, which includes non–β-lactam antibiotics with the capacity to penetrate into the *Mycoplasma* organisms. Traditionally, macrolides and tetracyclines have been used successfully to treat *M. pneumoniae*. Both CAP tetracyclines and macrolides are effective against *Mycoplasma* because they interfere with intracellular protein synthesis at the ribosomal level. Tetracyclines penetrate intracellularly better than macrolides, with the exception of penetration into the alveolar macrophage, which is relevant in *Legionella*, but not *M. pneumoniae*, infections. Macrolides and tetracyclines are both active against *Mycoplasma*; the relative lack of penetration by macrolides into respiratory epithelial cells accounts for differences in therapeutic response. Patients treated with macrolides or tetracyclines defervesce rapidly over 24 to 48 hours. Clinical defervescence manifests by an increased feeling of well-being and a decrease in fever. The dry cough persists during and after therapy regardless of the anti-*Mycoplasma* antimicrobial used.

There are important differences in the shedding rates of *Mycoplasma* from respiratory epithelial cells posttherapy when using tetracyclines instead of macrolides. Tetracycline therapy is associated with a more rapid decrease in shedding. Tetracyclines with better ability to penetrate intracellularly, such as doxycycline (Vibramycin), are the most rapid at decreasing *Mycoplasma* shedding, which is an important public health consideration. Mycoplasmas are transmitted by aerosolized droplet infection. Because patients with *Mycoplasma* have a prolonged cough, organisms not eliminated from respiratory epithelial cells may be aerosolized during coughing for weeks following the acute infection, spreading the infection to susceptible individuals via aerosolized droplets. The aim of therapy is to rapidly treat the patient's pneumonia and extrapulmonary sites of involvement. The secondary goal is to rapidly decrease shedding and aerosolization to prevent the spread of *Mycoplasma* to other individuals. An additional therapeutic goal is to decrease the incidence of post-*Mycoplasma* asthma seen in some patients. *M. pneumoniae* CAP may exacerbate preexisting asthma, but may also cause permanent post-CAP asthma in some individuals.

Until recently, doxycycline was the most active antimicrobial to use against *M. pneumoniae*. Currently, the "respiratory quinolones," levofloxacin (Levaquin), or moxifloxacin (Avelox), are highly active anti-*M. pneumoniae* antimicrobials. The respiratory quinolones and doxycycline penetrate cells efficiently and interfere with intracellular enzymes or protein synthesis of intracellular organisms. Respiratory quinolones and doxycycline are highly effective anti-*Mycoplasma* agents and rapidly decrease shedding of *M. pneumoniae* in respiratory secretions.

Therapy for *M. pneumoniae* is ordinarily 1 to 2 weeks. Patients who have impaired cardiopulmonary disease or compromised host

TABLE 2 Antibiotics Effective Against *M. pneumoniae*

Antibiotic	Dose (Adult)
Mild/Moderate CAP	
Doxycycline	100 mg (IV/PO) q12h
Erythromycin	500 mg (base, estolate, stearate) (PO) q6h
Erythromycin lactobionate	1 g (IV) q6h
Clarithromycin (Biaxin)	500 mg (PO) q12h
Azithromycin (Zithromax)	500 mg (IV) q24h × 2 doses, followed by 500 mg (PO) q24h
Severe CAP	
Levofloxacin (Levaquin)	500 mg (IV/PO) q24h, or 750 mg IV/PO q24h (may allow for shorter duration of therapy)
Moxifloxacin (Avelox)	400 mg (IV/PO) q24h

may require 2 full weeks of therapy. In patients with borderline cardiopulmonary function, *M. pneumoniae* as with other relatively low virulence pathogens may present as severe CAP. Antimicrobial therapy for typical or atypical CAP should be directed against the presumed pathogen and not based on co-morbidities. Normal healthy hosts are treated with the same antimicrobial as patients hospitalized with severe CAP. Patients hospitalized with compromised cardiopulmonary function severe *Mycoplasma* CAP are most often initially treated intravenously with doxycycline (Vibramycin), a macrolide, or a respiratory quinolone. Most patients with *M. pneumoniae* CAP present in the ambulatory setting, which permits therapy with oral doxycycline, macrolide, or a respiratory quinolone (Table 2).

REFERENCES

Ali NJ, Sillis M, Andrews BE, et al. The clinical spectrum and diagnosis of *Mycoplasma pneumoniae* infection. Q J Med 1986;58:241–51.

Cunha BA. Hepatic involvement in *Mycoplasma pneumoniae* community-acquired pneumonia. J Clin Microbiol 2003;3:385–6.

Cunha BA. Influenza: Historical aspects of epidemics and pandemics. Infect Dis Clin North Am 2004;18:141–55.

Cunha BA. The atypical pneumonia: Clinical diagnosis and importance. Clin Microbiol Infect 2006;12:12–24.

Cunha BA. Pneumonia Essentials. 3rd ed. Jones & Bartlett, Sudbury, MA, 2010.

Cunha BA. Urosepsis in the Critical Care Unit. In: Cunha BA, editor. Infectious Diseases in Critical Care Medicine. 3rd ed. New York, NY: Informa Healthcare USA, Inc.; 2009.

Cunha BA. Antibiotic Essentials. 8th ed. Sudbury, MA: Jones and Bartlett; 2009.

Debré R, Couvreur J. Influenza: Clinical features. In: Debré R, Celers J, editors. Clinical Virology: The Evaluation and Management of Human Viral Infections. Philadelphia: WB Saunders; 1970. p. 507–15.

File TM. Tan JS: *Mycoplasma pneumoniae* pneumonia. In: Marrié TJ, editor. Community-Acquired Pneumonia. New York: Kluwer Academic/Plenum Publishers; 2001. p. 487–500.

Hammerschlag MR. *Mycoplasma pneumoniae* infections. Curr Opin Infect Dis 2001;14:181–6.

Hurt AC, Selleck P, Komadina N, et al. Susceptibility of highly pathogenic A(H5N1) avian influenza viruses to the neuraminidase inhibitors and adamantanes. Antiviral Res 2007;73:228–31.

Louria DB, Blumenfield HL, Ellis JT. Studies on influenza in the pandemic of 1957–1958. II. Pulmonary complications of influenza. J Clin Invest 1959;38:213–65.

Marrie TJ. Empiric treatment of ambulatory community-acquired pneumonia: Always include treatment for atypical agents. Infect Dis Clin North Am 2004;18:829–41.

Murray HW, Masur H, Senterfit LS, Roberts RB. The protean manifestations of *Mycoplasma pneumoniae* infection in adults. Am J Med 1975;58:229–42.

Nisar N, Guleria R, Kumar S, et al. Mycoplasma pneumoniae and its role in asthma. Postgrad Med J 2007;83:100–4.

Schmidt AC. Antiviral therapy for influenza: A clinical and economic comparative review. Drugs 2004;6:2031–46.

Waites KB, Talkington DF. *Mycoplasma pneumoniae* and its role as a human pathogen. Clin Microbiol Rev 2004;17:697–728.

Legionellosis

Method of
Julio A. Ramirez, MD

In the summer of 1976, an outbreak of approximately 182 cases of pneumonia occurred in persons attending the American Legion convention in Philadelphia. One year later, Dr. McDade reported the identification of *Legionella pneumophila*, the bacterium responsible for the infection. Today, the family of Legionellaceae is composed of more than 40 species, with some species having different serogroups. *L pneumophila* causes approximately 85% of all *Legionella* infections. *L. pneumophila* serogroup 1 is the single most common member of the family causing clinical infections.

Epidemiology

Legionella is an intracellular organism that lives in natural water. In the aquatic environment, the bacteria live and multiply within freshwater amebae. The number of *Legionella* organisms in the water can increase significantly with appropriate local conditions such as warm temperature, lack of biocides, stagnant water, and presence of amebae and other nutrients. These special conditions can be present in artificial water systems such as cooling towers, whirlpools, decorative fountains, and respiratory therapy devices.

The susceptible host acquires the bacteria from water containing the organism. Infection can be acquired by inhaling aerosols containing *Legionella* organisms or by microaspiration of water contaminated with *Legionella*. The hospitalized patient with *Legionella* pneumonia does not require respiratory isolation because legionellosis is not transmitted from person to person.

Clinical Features

Once *Legionella* organisms reach the respiratory tract, based on the interactions of the organism with the host immune system, the patient can have four possible clinical outcomes: asymptomatic infection, Pontiac fever, legionnaires' disease, or extrapulmonary disease involving the liver, heart brain, or other organs. Pontiac fever is a nonpneumonic form of disease characterized by fever, headaches, myalgias, and malaise. The patient has an influenza-like illness, with resolution of disease in a few days without specific antimicrobial therapy. Patients with legionnaires' disease present with community-acquired pneumonia associated with high fever, gastrointestinal complaints such as diarrhea and central nervous system complaints such as headaches or mental status changes. Hospital-acquired pneumonia can occur if *Legionella* is present in the hospital water supply.

Diagnosis

The currently available laboratory tests for diagnosis of *Legionella* infections include the direct fluorescent antibody stain (DFA), culture, antigen detection in the urine, antibody detection in serum by indirect fluorescent antibody testing (IFA), and DNA amplification using the polymerase chain reaction (PCR). The DFA stain can detect all *L. pneumophila* serogroups, but a large number of bacteria need to be present in sputum for a positive result. *Legionella* can be cultured from respiratory specimens on selective media composed of buffered charcoal–yeast extract agar. The urinary antigen detection has a specificity greater than 95%; the disadvantage is that the test detects only the antigen of *L. pneumophila* serogroup 1. Clinical specimens that

have been used to detect *Legionella* by PCR include throat swabs, sputum, tracheal suction, bronchoalveolar lavage fluid, pleural fluid, and lung tissue.

Treatment

In the pulmonary parenchyma, *Legionella* can infect and multiply inside alveolar macrophages, alveolar epithelial cells, and capillary endothelial cells. The poor clinical outcome with β-lactam antibiotics is due to their lack of penetration into cells. Antibiotics with good intracellular penetration that can be used as monotherapy for *Legionella* infections include macrolides, ketolides, tetracyclines, and quinolones (Table 1). Rifampin (Rifadin)[1] is not used as monotherapy because resistance can rapidly emerge when it is used alone.

Therapy of the patient with severe disease is initiated with intravenous antibiotics. Once the patient reaches clinical stability, the intravenous therapy can be switched to oral therapy. Doses for the most common antibiotics for intravenous and oral therapy are depicted in Table 1. In the nonimmunocompromised patient, the recommended duration of therapy is 7 to 10 days. In immunocompromised patients, because they are at risk for relapsing infection, the recommended duration of therapy is 14 to 21 days.

Several antibiotics have demonstrated clinical efficacy in legionnaires' disease. Data with several in vitro and animal studies comparing different anti-*Legionella* antibiotics indicate that erythromycin (Ery-Tab) is a weak anti-*Legionella* agent. If erythromycin is selected for therapy, it is important to add rifampin to the regimen to increase intracellular killing. From the family of macrolides, azithromycin (Zithromax)[1] is the most active. The best bactericidal activity in the laboratory is achieved with quinolones. Retrospective observational studies indicate that patients treated with levofloxacin (Levaquin) have a shorter time to reach clinical stability and shorter duration of hospital stay. These antibiotics are considered primary anti-*Legionella* agents.

In clinical practice, I treat immunocompromised patients who have severe legionnaires' disease with a combination of an intravenous quinolone plus an intravenous macrolide (e.g., levofloxacin plus azithromycin). This regimen is based only on the theoretical consideration that synergistic killing may be obtained using a quinolone to alter DNA synthesis and a macrolide to alter protein synthesis.

---

[1]Not FDA approved for this indication.

TABLE 1 Antibiotic Therapy for *Legionella* Infections

Antibiotic	Oral Dose	Intravenous Dose
Ketolides		
Telithromycin (Ketek)[1]	800 mg qd	—
Macrolides		
Azithromycin (Zithromax)[1]	500 mg qd	500 mg qd
Clarithromycin (Biaxin)[1]	500 mg bid	—
Erythromycin (Ery-Tab)	500 mg q6h	1 g q6h
Quinolones		
Ciprofloxacin (Cipro)[1]	750 mg bid	400 mg bid
Levofloxacin (Levaquin)	750 mg qd	750 mg qd
Moxifloxacin (Avelox)[1]	400 mg qd	400 mg qd
Rifamycins		
Rifampin (Rifadin)[1]	300 mg bid	300 mg bid
Tetracyclines		
Doxycycline (Vibramycin)[1]	100 mg bid	100 mg bid

[1]Not FDA approved for this indication.

Venous Thromboembolism

Method of
Clive Kearon, MRCPI, FRCPC, PhD

Venous thromboembolism (VTE), which includes deep venous thrombosis (DVT) and pulmonary embolism (PE), is the third most common cause of vascular death (after myocardial infarction and stroke) and the leading cause of preventable death among hospitalized patients. Thrombosis starts in the deep veins, and PE occurs when such thrombi break free and lodge in the pulmonary arteries, where they obstruct blood flow and can cause lung damage (i.e., pulmonary infarction). About 90% of the instances of DVT involve the legs, about 5% involve the upper extremities (axillary, subclavian, or jugular veins), and the remaining 5% involve other veins of the body (e.g., internal iliac, renal, ovarian). DVT that is confined to the deep veins of the calf, without involvement of the popliteal vein, is termed isolated distal DVT, whereas that involving the popliteal or a more proximal vein is termed proximal DVT (most proximal DVT also involves the distal veins). Thrombosis of the subcutaneous veins is referred to as superficial vein thrombosis or superficial thrombophlebitis. Superficial vein thrombosis mostly occurs in the legs (e.g., long or short saphenous veins, often in association with varicosities), and its main importance is that it causes pain and swelling and may extend to cause DVT. This chapter focuses on DVT of the legs and PE.

Pathogenesis and Risk Factors

Virchow is credited with identifying stasis, vessel wall injury, and hypercoagulability as the pathogenic triad responsible for thrombosis. This classification of risk factors for VTE remains valuable. Most patients who develop VTE have more than one, and often multiple, risk factors.

VENOUS STASIS

The importance of venous stasis as a risk factor for VTE is demonstrated by the fact that most DVT associated with stroke affects the paralyzed leg, and most DVT associated with pregnancy affects the left leg, due to extrinsic compression of the left common iliac vein by the pregnant uterus and the right common iliac artery. General immobilization, such as in hospitalized patients and in patients with leg injuries or other chronic illness, is also an important risk factor. Venous stasis is thought to predispose to thrombosis by causing local hypoxia (e.g., in venous valve cusps), which attracts inflammatory cells and causes endothelial dysfunction, leading to an increase in the local concentration of clotting factors and tissue factor and an increase in interactions between circulating cells and the venous endothelium.

VESSEL DAMAGE

Venous endothelial damage, usually as a consequence of accidental injury, manipulation during surgery, or iatrogenic injury, is an important risk factor for VTE. Three quarters of proximal DVT that complicates hip surgery occurs in the operated leg, and thrombosis is common with indwelling venous catheters. Venous injury is thought to predispose to thrombosis by exposing blood to subendothelial tissue factor and to collagen, which binds von Willebrand's factor.

HYPERCOAGULABILITY

A complex balance between naturally occurring coagulation and fibrinolytic factors and their inhibitors serves to maintain blood fluidity and hemostasis. Inherited or acquired changes in this balance can predispose to thrombosis. The most important inherited biochemical disorders associated with VTE are defects of the naturally occurring inhibitors of coagulation (i.e., deficiencies of antithrombin, protein C, or protein S and resistance to activated protein C caused by factor V Leiden) and the G20210A prothrombin gene mutation, which is associated with elevated levels of prothrombin. The first three coagulation deficiencies listed are rare in the normal population (combined prevalence, <1%), have a combined prevalence of approximately 5% in patients with a first episode of VTE, and are associated with a 10- to 40-fold increase in the risk of VTE. The factor V Leiden mutation is common, occurring in approximately 5% of Caucasians and 20% of patients with a first episode of VTE (i.e., a fourfold increase in VTE risk). The G20210A prothrombin gene occurs in approximately 2% of Caucasians and 5% of patients with a first episode of VTE (i.e., a 2.5-fold increase in VTE risk).

Elevated levels of a number of coagulation factors (I, II, VIII, IX, XI) are also associated with thrombosis in a dose-dependent manner. It is probable that such elevations are often inherited, and there is strong evidence for this supposition for factor VIII and factor II; for example, the G20210A prothrombin gene is associated with an increase of approximately 25% in factor II (prothrombin). Abnormalities of the fibrinolytic system have a questionable association with VTE.

Acquired hypercoagulable states include estrogen therapy (threefold increase in VTE, highest during the first 6 months), antiphospholipid antibodies (anticardiolipin antibodies or lupus anticoagulants or both), systemic lupus erythematosus, malignancy, chemotherapy for cancer, and surgery. Patients who develop immunologically related heparin-induced thrombocytopenia also have a very high risk for arterial and venous thromboembolism. Unlike the congenital abnormalities, acquired risk factors are often transient, and this fact has important implications for the duration of anticoagulant prophylaxis and treatment.

COMBINATIONS OF RISK FACTORS AND RISK STRATIFICATION

The risk of developing VTE depends on the prevalence and severity of risk factors (Box 1). By assessment of these factors, hospitalized patients can be categorized as having a low, moderate, or high risk

---

BOX 1   Risk Factors for Venous Thromboembolism (VTE)*

Patient Factors
- Previous VTE[†]
- Age older than 40 years, and particularly older than 70 years[†]
- Pregnancy, puerperium
- Marked obesity
- Inherited hypercoagulable state

Underlying Condition and Acquired Factors
- Malignancy[†]
- Estrogen therapy
- Cancer chemotherapy
- Paralysis[†]
- Prolonged immobility
- Major trauma[†]
- Lower limb injuries[†]
- Heparin-induced thrombocytopenia
- Antiphospholipid antibodies

Type of Surgery
- Lower limb orthopedic surgery[†]
- General anesthesia >30 min

---
*Combinations of factors have an at least an additive effect on the risk of VTE.
[†]Common major risk factors for VTE.

TABLE 1 Risk Stratification for VTE in Hospitalized and Postoperative Patients, Frequency of VTE without Prophylaxis, and Recommended Methods of Prophylaxis*

| Risk Factor | Venographic DVT[†] (%) | | Pulmonary Embolism (%) | | Recommended Prophylaxis |
	Calf	Proximal	Symptomatic	Fatal	
Low Risk: Minor (usually same-day) surgery in a mobile patient Medical patients, fully mobile No additional risk factors	2	0.4	0.2	<0.01	Early mobilization
Moderate Risk: Most general surgery patients Most medical patients	20	5	2	0.5	Low-dose UFH (5000 U SQ preoperatively and bid or tid postoperatively) LMWH (~3000 U/d SQ with a preoperative start)[‡] Fondaparinux (Arixtra)[1] GC stockings, alone or with pharmacologic methods
High Risk: Most general surgery patients with previous VTE Major knee or hip surgery Major trauma, spinal cord injury (Heparin-induced thrombocytopenia)	50	15	5	2	LMWH (>3000 U/d) Fondaparinux Warfarin (Coumadin)[§] IPC devices, alone or with GC stockings or pharmacologic methods or both (Specific nonheparin therapy)

[1]Not FDA approved for this indication.
*New anticoagulants (e.g., oral direct thrombin, anti-factor Xa inhibitors) are becoming available for moderate- and high-risk patients.
[†]Asymptomatic DVT detected by screening bilateral venography.
[‡]Higher doses are used in high-risk patients (e.g., ~ 4,000 U once daily with a preoperative start in Europe; ~3,000 U twice daily with a postoperative start in North America).
[§]Usually started postoperatively and adjusted to achieve an international normalized ratio of 2.0-3.0.
Abbreviations: DVT = deep venous thrombosis; GC = graduated compression; IPC = intermittent pneumatic compression; LMWH = low-molecular-weight heparin; UFH = unfractionated heparin; VTE = venous thromboembolism

of VTE (Table 1). Patients with active cancer are among those with the highest risk of thrombosis, because they often have a large number of major risk factors, such as the hypercoagulable state associated with cancer, recent surgery, chemotherapy, generalized immobility from weakness, localized stasis associated with venous obstruction by tumor, and the presence of indwelling venous catheters.

Epidemiology and Natural History of Venous Thromboembolism

The overall incidence of VTE is about 1.5 per 1000 persons per year in adults, with about two thirds of these episodes being symptomatic DVT and about one third being symptomatic PE (with or without symptoms of DVT). However, the incidence of VTE is highly influenced by age. Before the age of 16 years, most likely because the immature coagulation system is resistant to thrombosis, VTE is very rare and is largely confined to children with major provoking factors such as indwelling venous lines. The risk of VTE increases exponentially with advancing age, with an almost twofold increase every decade, from an annual incidence of 0.3 per 1000 at 40 years to 1 per 1000 at 60 years and 4 per 1000 at 80 years of age.

VTE occurs slightly more frequently in men than in women, although this pattern is reversed before 40 years of age because the association of VTE with estrogen-containing contraceptives and pregnancy. The relative frequency of PE to DVT is somewhat higher in the elderly.

About 50% of the cases of VTE are associated with hospitalization (about half before and half after discharge), which emphasizes the

importance of using appropriate prophylaxis to prevent VTE in high-risk patients. Among hospital-associated VTE cases, about half occur in surgical and half in medical patients. About one quarter of VTE cases are associated with cancer; one quarter are associated with minor illnesses, injuries, or estrogen therapy; and one quarter are not associated with any apparent clinical risk factor (referred to as unprovoked or idiopathic VTE). There is overlap among these categories; for example, there is a particularly high risk of VTE among patients with cancer who are hospitalized.

Of all episodes of VTE, about three quarters are first episodes and one quarter are recurrent episodes. Clinically important components of the natural history of VTE are summarized in Box 2.

Diagnosis of Deep Venous Thrombosis

CLINICAL FEATURES

The clinical features of DVT, such as localized swelling, redness, tenderness, and distal edema, are nonspecific, and the diagnosis should always be confirmed by objective tests. About 85% of ambulatory patients with clinically suspected DVT have another cause for their symptoms. The conditions that are most likely to simulate DVT are a ruptured Baker's cyst, cellulitis, muscle tears, muscle cramp, muscle hematoma, external venous compression, superficial thrombophlebitis, and the postthrombotic syndrome. Of patients with symptomatic DVT, about 75% have proximal vein thrombosis; in the rest, thrombosis is confined to the calf. Although clinical features cannot unequivocally confirm or exclude a diagnosis of DVT, clinical assessment can stratify the probability of DVT as high (prevalence of

BOX 2   Natural History of Venous Thromboembolism: Key Points

- Clinical factors can identify high-risk patients.
- VTE starts in the calf veins in >75% of patients.
- Three quarters of asymptomatic DVT detected postoperatively by screening venography are confined to the distal (calf) veins.
- About 20% of symptomatic isolated calf DVT subsequently extends to the proximal veins, usually within 1 week after presentation.
- More than 90% of asymptomatic postoperative DVT resolves without causing symptoms.
- More than 80% of symptomatic DVT involves the popliteal or more proximal veins.
- Symptomatic PE usually arises from proximal DVT.
- Most (70%) patients with symptomatic proximal DVT have asymptomatic PE (high-probability lung scans in 40%), and most patients with symptomatic PE (80%) have DVT.
- Only one quarter of patients with symptomatic PE have symptoms or signs of DVT.
- About 50% of untreated symptomatic proximal DVT is expected to cause symptomatic PE.
- About 10% of symptomatic PE is rapidly fatal.
- Most fatal PE is not diagnosed.
- About 30% of patients with untreated symptomatic nonfatal PE have a fatal recurrence.
- The risk of recurrent VTE after stopping anticoagulant therapy is much lower if VTE was provoked by a reversible risk factor (particularly recent surgery) than if it was unprovoked or provoked by a persistent risk factor.

Abbreviations: DVT = deep venous thrombosis; PE = pulmonary embolism; VTE = venous thromboembolism.

thrombosis, ∼60%), intermediate (∼25%), or low (∼5%) based on: the presence or absence of risk factors (e.g., recent immobilization, hospitalization within the past month, malignancy); whether the clinical manifestations at presentation are typical or atypical and their severity; and whether there is an alternative explanation for the symptoms that is at least as likely as DVT (Table 2).

TABLE 2 Wells Model for Determining Clinical Suspicion of Deep Venous Thrombosis (DVT)*

Variable	Points
Active cancer (treatment ongoing or within previous 6 mo or palliative)	1
Paralysis, paresis, or recent plaster immobilization of the lower extremities	1
Recently bedridden >3 d or major surgery within 4 wk	1
Localized tenderness along the distribution of the deep venous system	1
Entire leg swollen	1
Calf swelling 3 cm greater than on asymptomatic side (measured 10 cm below tibial tuberosity)	1
Pitting edema confined to the symptomatic leg	1
Dilated superficial veins (non-varicose)	1
Alternative diagnosis as likely or greater than that of DVT	−2

*Pretest probability of DVT is calculated from the total points: >2 points, high; 1 or 2, moderate; <1, low.

VENOGRAPHY

Venography, which involves the injection of a radiocontrast agent into a distal vein, is the reference standard for the diagnosis of DVT. Venography detects both proximal and isolated distal DVT. However, it is expensive and technically difficult to perform, can be painful, and requires injection of radiographic contrast, which can cause allergic reactions or renal impairment. For these reasons, venography is now rarely performed.

VENOUS ULTRASONOGRAPHY

Venous ultrasonography is the noninvasive imaging method of choice for diagnosing DVT. It is not painful and is easy to perform. The common femoral vein, the femoral vein (previously called the superficial femoral vein), the popliteal vein, and the calf vein trifurcation (i.e., proximal junction of deep calf veins) are imaged in real time and compressed with the transducer probe (compression ultrasound). Inability to fully compress (i.e., obliterate) the vein lumen with pressure from the ultrasound probe is diagnostic for DVT. Duplex ultrasonography, which combines compression ultrasound with pulsed Doppler or color-coded Doppler technology, facilitates identification of the deep veins (particularly in the calf; see later discussion) and may enable thrombus to be detected if it is not feasible to assess vein compressibility (e.g., iliac or subclavian veins).

Venous ultrasonography is highly accurate for diagnosis of proximal vein thrombosis, with a sensitivity and specificity approaching 95%. The sensitivity for symptomatic calf vein thrombosis is considerably lower and appears to be highly operator dependent. For this reason, many centers do not examine the deep veins of the calf with ultrasonography. Instead, if examination of the proximal veins excludes proximal DVT in a patient with a moderate or high clinical assessment for DVT, the test is repeated in 7 days to detect the small number of calf vein thrombi (∼3%) that subsequently extend into the proximal veins. If the test remains negative after 7 days, the risk that thrombus is present and will extend to the proximal veins is negligible, and it is safe to withhold treatment (Box 3).

If the clinical assessment for DVT is low and the result of an initial proximal venous ultrasound scan is normal, it is not necessary to repeat ultrasonography after 7 days, because the prevalence of DVT is only about 2% (mostly distal). If the calf veins below the level of the calf vein trifurcation are also examined and there is no isolated distal DVT as well as no proximal DVT, then DVT is excluded without the need for repeat ultrasonography after 7 days. However, examination of the calf veins has the disadvantage of resulting in diagnosis and treatment of DVT in substantially more patients than does serial examination of the proximal veins, without further reducing the risk of VTE during follow-up (approximately 1% over 3 months in both groups) in those who are not initially diagnosed with DVT.

Ultrasonography is less accurate when its results are discordant with clinical assessment. Therefore, if the clinical suspicion for DVT is low and the ultrasound study shows a localized abnormality (i.e., less convincing findings), or if clinical suspicion is high and the ultrasound is normal, further diagnostic testing (e.g., venography) should be considered.

D-DIMER BLOOD TESTING

D-dimer is formed when cross-linked fibrin in thrombi is broken down by plasmin. Because it is usually increased in patients with acute VTE, low levels of D-dimer can be used to exclude DVT and PE. A variety of D-dimer assays are available, and they vary markedly in their accuracy as diagnostic tests for VTE. All D-dimer assays have a low specificity for DVT; consequently, an abnormal result is associated with a low positive predictive value and cannot be used to diagnose DVT.

D-dimer assays that are used for diagnosis of VTE can be divided into two groups based on their sensitivity and specificity. Very highly sensitive D-dimer assays (e.g., sensitivity >98%; specificity ∼40%) have a sufficiently high negative predictive value (>98%) that a normal result can be used to exclude VTE without the need to perform additional diagnostic testing. With moderate to highly sensitive D-dimer assays (sensitivity 85%-97%; specificity 50%–70%), a negative result needs

---

BOX 3 Test Results That Confirm or Exclude Deep Venous Thrombosis (DVT)

Diagnostic for First DVT

Venography: Intraluminal filling defect in proximal or distal deep veins

Venous ultrasound: Noncompressible popliteal or common femoral vein

Excludes First DVT

Venography: All deep veins seen, and no intraluminal filling defects

D-dimer:
- Normal result on a D-dimer test with a very high sensitivity (i.e., ≥98%) and at least a moderate specificity (i.e., ≥40%)
- Normal result on a D-dimer test with a moderately high sensitivity (i.e., ≥85%) and specificity (i.e., ≥70%), plus low clinical suspicion for DVT at presentation

Venous ultrasound: Fully compressible proximal veins and one or more of the following:
- Low clinical suspicion for DVT
- Normal result on a D-dimer test with a moderately high sensitivity (i.e., ≥85%) and specificity (i.e., ≥70%) at presentation
- Fully compressible distal deep veins (whole leg ultrasound)
- Normal repeat ultrasound of the proximal veins after 7 days

Diagnostic for Recurrent DVT

Venography: Intraluminal filling defect

Venous ultrasound:
- A new, noncompressible common femoral or popliteal vein segment
- A 4.0-mm increase in diameter of the common femoral or popliteal vein compared with a previous test

Excludes Recurrent DVT

Venogram: All deep veins seen, and no intraluminal filling defects

Venous ultrasound: Normal, or ≤1 mm increase in diameter of the common femoral or popliteal veins compared with a previous test, which remains unchanged on repeat testing after 2 and 7 days

D-dimer:
- Normal result on a D-dimer test with a very high sensitivity (i.e., ≥98%) and at least a moderate specificity (i.e., ≥40%)
- Normal result on a D-dimer test with a moderately high sensitivity (i.e., ≥85%) and specificity (i.e., ≥70%), plus low clinical suspicion for DVT

---

to be combined with another assessment that identifies patients as having a lower prevalence of VTE in order to exclude DVT. Management studies have shown that it is safe to consider DVT excluded in patients who have a normal result on a moderately sensitive D-dimer test in combination with either a low clinical suspicion for DVT or no proximal DVT on venous ultrasonography (see Box 3).

D-dimer testing is much less specific (i.e., fewer negative tests among those without venous thrombosis), and therefore has less clinical utility in postoperative and hospitalized patients and in the elderly (>75 years). Also, D-dimer testing has less clinical utility in patients with a high clinical suspicion of VTE because negative results are rarely obtained, and if a negative test is obtained, its predictive value is lower because of the high prevalence of disease.

COMPUTED TOMOGRAPHIC AND MAGNETIC RESONANCE IMAGING VENOGRAPHY

Computed tomography (CT) and magnetic resonance imaging (MRI) have been reported to have high accuracy (sensitivity and specificity >90%) for the diagnosis of DVT but are rarely used for this purpose, because CT requires the use of radiographic contrast and is associated with high radiation exposure, and both CT and MRI are costly. CT and MRI are expected to be more accurate than ultrasound for DVT that does not involve the limbs, such as that confined to the pelvic veins or the inferior vena cava. Diagnosis of DVT on CT (or, less commonly, on MRI) is most commonly an incidental finding in patients who undergo CT to stage a known malignancy. In this situation, because the clinical suspicion for DVT is low and the examination will not have been designed to diagnose DVT, patients need to be carefully reviewed, often including further testing, before a diagnosis of DVT is accepted.

Diagnosis of Recurrent Deep Venous Thrombosis

The diagnosis of recurrent DVT can be difficult. A negative D-dimer test can exclude recurrent DVT, although the safety of this approach has been less well evaluated than for first episodes of DVT. If D-dimer testing is positive or has not been done, venous ultrasonography is

performed. If the result is normal (i.e., full compressibility of the veins), treatment is withheld, and the test should be repeated twice over the next 7 to 10 days. If the result is positive in the popliteal or common femoral vein segments and the result of a previous test was negative at the same site, a recurrence is diagnosed. Recurrence can also be diagnosed if venous ultrasonography shows other convincing evidence of more extensive thrombosis than was seen on a previous examination (e.g., an increase in compressed thrombus diameter of >4 mm in the common femoral or the popliteal segments; unequivocal extension within the femoral vein of the thigh).

If a comparison between current and previous venous ultrasound findings is equivocal, or if no previous ultrasound is available for comparison, venography should be performed; however, many hospitals no longer perform venography. If the venogram shows an intraluminal filling defect, which is seen with acute rather than remote thrombosis, recurrent DVT is diagnosed. If the venogram outlines all of the deep veins and does not show an intraluminal filling defect, recurrent DVT is excluded. If the venogram is nondiagnostic (i.e., nonfilling of segments of the deep veins) or if venography is not performed in a patient with equivocal findings on ultrasound, the patient can be observed with repeat venous ultrasonography to detect extending DVT or, less satisfactorily, recurrent DVT can be diagnosed based on the results of all assessments, including clinical features. Clinical assessment of the probability of recurrent DVT is less well standardized than for a first episode of DVT; however, many of the factors that are predictive of a first episode are also expected to be predictive of recurrent DVT (Box 3).

Diagnosis of Pulmonary Embolism

CLINICAL FEATURES

Dyspnea is the most common symptom of PE. Chest pain is also common and is usually pleuritic but can be substernal and compressive. Hemoptysis is less frequently present. Tachycardia and tachypnea are common signs. Evidence of right heart failure is less common but of prognostic importance, and a pleural rub may be heard in association

TABLE 3 Wells Model for Determining Clinical Suspicion of Pulmonary Embolism*

Variable	Points
Clinical signs and symptoms of DVT (minimum leg swelling and pain with palpation of the deep veins)	3.0
An alternative diagnosis is less likely than PE	3.0
Heart rate >100 beats/min	1.5
Immobilization or surgery in the previous 4 wk	1.5
Previous DVT/PE	1.5
Hemoptysis	1.0
Malignancy (treatment ongoing or within previous 6 months or palliative)	1.0

*Pretest probability of PE is calculated from the total points: >6 points, high; 4 to 6, moderate; <4, low.
Abbreviations: DVT = deep venous thrombosis; PE = pulmonary embolism.

with pulmonary infarction. Although most patients with PE also have DVT, fewer than 25% have symptoms or signs. The clinical features of PE, like those of DVT, are nonspecific, and PE is diagnosed in only about 20% of those in whom it is suspected.

Two groups have published explicit criteria for determining the clinical probability of PE. The model by Wells and colleagues incorporates an assessment of symptoms and signs, the presence of an alternative diagnosis that could account for the patient's condition, and the presence of risk factors for VTE. With this model, a patient's clinical probability of PE can be categorized as low or unlikely (prevalence of PE <10%), moderate (~25%), or high (~ 60%) (Table 3).

CHEST RADIOGRAPHY AND ELECTROCARDIOGRAPHY

In patients with PE, chest radiographs show either normal or nonspecific findings. However, a chest radiograph is useful for exclusion of pneumothorax and other conditions that can simulate PE (e.g., left ventricular failure). The electrocardiogram also frequently shows normal or nonspecific findings but is valuable for excluding acute myocardial infarction. In the appropriate clinical setting, right ventricular strain can suggest PE and a poorer short-term outcome among those with PE.

VENTILATION/PERFUSION LUNG SCANNING

Ventilation/perfusion lung scanning was the most important test for diagnosing PE in the past. Computed tomographic pulmonary angiography (CTPA) has now supplanted lung scanning, although the latter is still used, particularly if CTPA is contraindicated because of renal failure or associated radiation exposure to the chest (e.g., in young women). A normal perfusion scan excludes PE but is obtained in only about 25% of patients; a higher proportion of normal scans is obtained in patients who are young, who do not have chronic lung disease, or who have a normal chest radiograph. An abnormal perfusion scan is nonspecific. Ventilation imaging improves the specificity of perfusion scanning. If the ventilation scan is normal at the site of two or more large (>75% of a segment) perfusion defects, the lung scan is associated with a greater than 85% prevalence of PE and is termed a high-probability scan. About half of patients with PE have a high-probability lung scan. Therefore, among consecutive patients who are investigated for PE, about 25% have a normal perfusion scan and can have the diagnosis excluded; about 15% have a high-probability scan and can have PE diagnosed (provided that the clinical probability is moderate or high) (Box 4); and about 60% have a nondiagnostic lung scan that requires further diagnostic testing.

COMPUTED TOMOGRAPHIC PULMONARY ANGIOGRAPHY

CTPA, performed using helical CT (also known as spiral or continuous-volume CT), is able to directly visualize the pulmonary arteries. CTPA has rapidly advanced from use of single detector scanners to

BOX 4 Test Results That Confirm or Exclude Pulmonary Embolism (PE)

Diagnostic for PE
Pulmonary angiography: Intraluminal filling defect
Computed tomographic pulmonary angiography (CTPA):
- Intraluminal filling defect in a lobar or main pulmonary artery
- Intraluminal filling defect in a segmental pulmonary artery, plus moderate or high clinical suspicion
Ventilation/perfusion scan: High-probability scan, plus moderate to high clinical suspicion
Diagnostic test for deep venous thrombosis: With a nondiagnostic ventilation/perfusion scan or CTPA

Excludes PE
Pulmonary angiogram: Normal
Perfusion scan: Normal
D-dimer:
- Normal result on a D-dimer test with a very high sensitivity (i.e., ≥98%) and at least a moderate specificity (i.e., ≥40%)
- Normal result on a D-dimer test with a moderately high sensitivity (i.e., ≥85%) and specificity (i.e., ≥70%), plus low clinical suspicion for PE
Nondiagnostic ventilation/perfusion scan or suboptimal CTPA, plus normal venous ultrasound of the proximal veins and one or more of the following:
- Low clinical suspicion for PE
- Normal result on a D-dimer test with at least a moderately high sensitivity (i.e., ≥85%) and specificity (i.e., ≥70%)
- Normal repeat venous ultrasound of the proximal veins after 7 and 14 days

use of progressively larger numbers of detectors (multidetector CT) that enable more rapid and detailed examination of the pulmonary arteries.

Results of the Prospective Investigation of Pulmonary Embolism Diagnosis (PIOPED II) study suggested that CTPA is nondiagnostic in 6% of patients and that, among adequate examinations, sensitivity for PE is 83%, specificity is 96%, positive predictive value is 86% and negative predictive value is 95%. Accuracy varies according to the size of the largest pulmonary artery involved: the positive predictive value was 97% for defects in the main or lobar artery, 68% in segmental arteries, and 25% in subsegmental arteries (4% of PE in this study). Predictive values were also influenced by the clinical assessment of PE probability: the positive predictive value of CTPA was 96% in combination with high, 92% with intermediate, and 58% with low clinical probability (8% of patients); likewise, the negative predictive value was 96% with low, 89% with intermediate, and 60% with high clinical probability (3% of patients). Management studies, in which anticoagulant therapy was withheld in patients with a negative CTPA result suggested that fewer than 2% of patients with a negative CTPA for PE will return with symptomatic VTE during 3 months of follow-up. Taken together, these observations suggest the following conclusions (see Box 4).

- An intraluminal filling defect in a segmental or larger pulmonary artery is generally diagnostic for PE. However, if the clinical probability is low and if there are additional findings that undermine a diagnosis of PE (e.g., technically suboptimal study, negative D-dimer test), further diagnostic testing should be considered (e.g., venous ultrasonography, ventilation/perfusion scanning, repeat CTPA), particularly if the most proximal pulmonary artery involved is at the segmental level.

- A good-quality negative CTPA finding excludes PE. If the CTPA does not show PE but is suboptimal, ultrasonography of the proximal deep veins of the legs should be performed to supplement the findings of the CTPA and exclude DVT.
- Abnormalities suggestive of intraluminal defects that are confined to subsegmental pulmonary arteries are generally nondiagnostic and require further investigation.

MRI is less well evaluated than CTPA for the diagnosis of PE and appears to be less accurate. Both CTPA and MRI have the advantage of identifying alternative pulmonary diagnoses. MRI does not expose the patient to radiation or radiographic contrast media.

D-DIMER BLOOD TESTING

D-dimer testing is a valuable test for the exclusion of PE, either alone (very sensitive D-dimer assay) or in combination with other assessments that are associated with a reduced prevalence of PE (see Box 4 and earlier discussion of D-dimer testing for suspected DVT).

COMPRESSION ULTRASONOGRAPHY

Compression ultrasonography, usually evaluating the proximal deep veins of the legs, can aid in the diagnosis of PE. Demonstration of DVT, which occurs in about 5% of patients with nondiagnostic ventilation/perfusion lung scans, serves as indirect evidence of PE. Exclusion of proximal DVT does not rule out PE in a patient with a nondiagnostic ventilation/perfusion scan, although it does reduce that probability somewhat. However, if there is no proximal DVT on the day of presentation and proximal DVT is not detected on two subsequent examinations performed 1 and 2 weeks later (DVT is diagnosed during serial testing in approximately 2% of patients), anticoagulant therapy can be withheld with a very low risk that the patient will return with VTE (<2% during 3 months of follow-up).

As previously noted for patients with a nondiagnostic ventilation/perfusion lung scan, withholding of anticoagulant therapy and performance of serial ultrasonography is a reasonable approach to management in patients who have a CTPA result that is nondiagnostic, including patients with isolated subsegmental abnormalities.

PULMONARY ANGIOGRAPHY

Although pulmonary angiography was considered to be the reference standard for PE in the past, it is now very rarely performed, because it is invasive and can usually be replaced by CTPA. Combinations of test results that confirm and exclude PE are shown in Box 4.

Prevention of Venous Thromboembolism

The most effective way to reduce mortality from PE and morbidity from the postthrombotic syndrome is to use primary prophylaxis in patients at risk for VTE, particularly during hospitalization. On the basis of well-defined clinical criteria, patients can be classified as being at low, moderate, or high risk for VTE, and use of prophylaxis can then be tailored to the patient's risk (see Table 1). By reducing the need to diagnose and treat VTE, prophylaxis is cost-saving in many situations, rather than just being cost-effective.

Prophylaxis is achieved by reducing blood coagulability or by preventing venous stasis. Anticoagulants, including subcutaneous heparin, low-molecular-weight-heparin (LMWH), and fondaparinux (Arixtra), as well as oral vitamin K antagonists, oral direct thrombin, and factor Xa inhibitors, reduce coagulability. Mechanical methods, including graduated compression stockings and intermittent pneumatic compression (IPC) devices, prevent venous stasis. Antiplatelet agents, such as aspirin,[1] also prevent VTE, but less effectively than the previously stated methods, and they are not usually recommended for this purpose.

Heparin is given subcutaneously at a dose of 5000 U 2 hours before surgery and 5000 U every 8 or 12 hours after surgery. In patients undergoing major orthopedic surgical procedures, low-dose heparin is less effective than LMWH, vitamin K antagonist therapy, or fondaparinux and is not recommended.

LMWH is also given subcutaneously, once or twice a day. It is effective in high-risk patients undergoing elective hip surgery, major general surgery, or major knee surgery and in patients with hip fracture, spinal injury, or acute medical illness. LMWH is more effective than vitamin K antagonist therapy at preventing VTE after major orthopedic surgery while patients are in hospital, but it is also associated with more frequent early postoperative bleeding; both of these differences may be related to the more rapid onset of anticoagulation with LMWH than with vitamin K antagonist therapy.

Graduated compression stockings reduce the risk of venous thrombosis without increasing the risk of bleeding. On their own or in conjunction with IPC, they are indicated in patients who are at high risk for bleeding and in those who are unable to tolerate any bleeding (e.g., neurosurgical patients). In surgical patients, the combined use of graduated compression stockings and pharmacological agents (e.g., low-dose heparin) is more effective than use of either alone. In the absence of a contraindication, pharmacologic prophylaxis is preferred to graduated compression stockings alone, because the evidence of efficacy at preventing PE is greater with the former.

IPC of the legs enhances blood flow in the deep veins and may increase blood fibrinolytic activity. IPC is more effective than graduated stockings alone, particularly after major orthopedic surgery and especially after knee replacement.

Vitamin K antagonist therapy (international normalized ratio [INR], 2.0 to 3.0) is effective for preventing postoperative VTE, including after major orthopedic surgery, but it is difficult to use because of the need for laboratory monitoring.

Fondaparinux, the synthetic pentasaccharide that corresponds to the active component of heparin that binds antithrombin and inhibits factor Xa, has been shown to reduce the frequency of venographically detected DVT by 50%, compared with LMWH, but is associated with an additional risk of bleeding.

GENERAL SURGERY AND MEDICINE

Low-dose heparin or LMWH prophylaxis is the method of choice for moderate-risk general surgical and medical patients. It reduces the risk of VTE by 50% to 70% and is simple, inexpensive, convenient, and safe. If anticoagulants are contraindicated because of an unusually high risk of bleeding, graduated compression stockings, IPC of the legs, or both, should be used. Fondaparinux[1] has also been shown to be effective in these patients.

MAJOR ORTHOPEDIC SURGERY

LMWH, fondaparinux, or vitamin K antagonists provide effective prophylaxis after major orthopedic surgery. If pharmacologic agents are contraindicated because of the risk of bleeding, IPC (with or without graduated compression stockings) is recommended until it becomes safe to use an anticoagulant therapy. Aspirin[1] has also been shown to reduce the frequency of symptomatic VTE and fatal PE after hip fracture; however, because aspirin is expected to be much less effective than anticoagulant therapies, aspirin is not recommended as the sole agent for postoperative prophylaxis. A number of new antithrombotic agents, including oral direct antithrombins (e.g., dabigatran [Pradaxa][2]) and factor Xa inhibitors (e.g., rivaroxaban [Xarelto],[2] apixaban[5]), have been shown to provide effective prophylaxis after major orthopaedic surgery and are being introduced into clinical practice.

A minimum of 10 days of prophylaxis is recommended after major orthopedic surgery, which usually includes treatment after

[1]Not FDA approved for this indication.

[1]Not FDA approved for this indication.
[2]Not available in the United States.
[5]Investigational drug in the United States.

discharge from hospital. In addition, extended prophylaxis for another 10 to 30 days is generally recommended, particularly in patients who have had hip surgery or have other risk factors for thrombosis, such as previous VTE or active cancer.

ENDOSCOPIC GENITOURINARY SURGERY, NEUROSURGERY, AND OCULAR SURGERY

Anticoagulant therapies are avoided in patients undergoing endoscopic genitourinary surgery, neurosurgery, or ocular surgery because of the associated risk of bleeding, particularly close to the time of surgery. Graduated stockings may be used, or IPC in patients with additional risk factors for VTE. If hospitalization is prolonged and the risk of bleeding recedes, patients can subsequently be started on an anticoagulant.

Treatment of Venous Thromboembolism

Anticoagulation is the mainstay of therapy for acute DVT of the leg and PE. The main objectives of anticoagulant therapy are to prevent extension of DVT, early PE, and later recurrences of VTE.

ACUTE ANTICOAGULANT THERAPY

In 1960, it was first established in a randomized trial that heparin (1.5 days) and oral anticoagulants (2 weeks) reduced the risk of recurrent PE and associated death. Based on expert opinion, a regimen of 10 to 14 days of heparin therapy and 3 months of oral anticoagulation became widely adopted in clinical practice. Subsequently, it was shown that 4 or 5 days of intravenous heparin is as effective as 10 days of therapy for the initial treatment of VTE.

In the past 20 years, many trials have established that weight-adjusted LMWH (without laboratory monitoring), given once or twice daily by subcutaneous injection (daily dose of 150–200 IU/kg), is as least as safe and effective as adjusted-dose intravenous unfractionated heparin for the treatment of acute DVT and PE. This enabled treatment of DVT on an outpatient basis, which is now recommended in the absence of very severe symptoms and signs (e.g., impending venous gangrene), severe comorbidity, or marked renal failure that precludes the use of LMWH (which is predominantly renally excreted). Selected patients with PE—those who are without severe symptoms or cardiorespiratory compromise and have good social supports—can also be treated as outpatients, although this approach to treatment has not been evaluated in a randomized trial. In addition to acute anticoagulant therapy, patients with PE should be assessed for possible treatment with thrombolytic therapy (see later discussion).

More recently, once-daily fixed-dose subcutaneous fondaparinux (7.5 mg for body weight 50–100 kg; 5 mg for <50 kg; 10 mg for >100 kg) and twice-daily subcutaneous unfractionated heparin (with or without laboratory monitoring) have also been shown to be as safe and as effective as treatment with LMWH. In the one study that evaluated unmonitored subcutaneous unfractionated heparin, heparin was administered at an initial dose of 333 units/kg followed by 250 units/kg every 12 hours. Danaparoid (Orgaran),[2] argatroban, or lepirudin (Refludan) should be used to treat heparin-induced thrombocytopenia with or without associated thrombosis.

Vitamin K antagonist therapy is usually started on the same day as parenteral anticoagulant therapy. If warfarin (e.g., Coumadin) is used, the initial dose is usually 2.5 to 10 mg, with a lower dose being appropriate in older patients, women, and those with impaired nutrition, and a higher dose being appropriate in younger (<60 years) otherwise healthy outpatients. Subsequent doses should be adjusted to maintain the INR at a target of 2.5 (range, 2.0–3.0). Parenteral anticoagulant therapy is continued until it has been given for 5 days and until the INR is at least 2.0 on two consecutive days.

---

[2]Not available in the United States.

LONG-TERM ANTICOAGULANT THERAPY

The initial demonstration that 3 months of warfarin markedly reduced the frequency of recurrent DVT, compared with 3 months of low-dose subcutaneous heparin, established the need for a prolonged phase of treatment for VTE after initial treatment with intravenous heparin. Subsequently, high-dose subcutaneous heparin and LMWH (50%–75% of the acute treatment dose) was shown to be as effective as warfarin for long-term treatment. Early studies did not monitor patients after anticoagulant therapy was withdrawn to determine whether the risk of recurrent VTE remained acceptable, and they did not compare the risk of recurrence after completion of various durations of therapy to identify the optimal duration. However, during the last 2 decades, a series of well-designed studies have helped to define the optimal duration of anticoagulation for VTE. The findings of these studies can be summarized as follows:

- Shortening the duration of anticoagulation from 3 or 6 months to 4 or 6 weeks results in a doubling of the frequency of recurrent VTE during 1 to 2 years of follow-up.
- Patients with VTE provoked by a transient risk factor have a lower (about one third) risk of recurrence, compared to those with an unprovoked VTE or a persistent risk factor. The greater the provoking transient risk factor (e.g., recent major surgery), the lower the expected risk of recurrence after stopping anticoagulant therapy.
- Three months of anticoagulation is adequate treatment for VTE provoked by a transient risk factor; in the first year after stopping therapy, the risk of recurrence is about 3% if VTE was provoked by a major transient risk factor (e.g., recent surgery) and about 5% if there was a minor risk factor.
- The risk of recurrent VTE is similar if anticoagulant therapy is stopped after 3 months of treatment compared to after 6 or 12 months of treatment; this suggests that 3 months of treatment is sufficient to treat the acute episode of VTE.
- The risk of recurrence is about 10% in the first year, 30% in the first 5 years, and 50% in the first 10 years after stopping anticoagulant therapy in patients with a first unprovoked episode of proximal DVT or PE.
- After 3 months of initial treatment of unprovoked VTE with oral anticoagulants targeted at an INR of 2.5 (range, 2.0–3.0), treatment should be continued as follows:
  - Oral anticoagulation targeted at an INR of approximately 2.5 reduces the risk of recurrent VTE by more than 90%.
  - Oral anticoagulation targeted at an INR of approximately 1.75 reduces the risk of recurrent VTE by about 75%.
  - Oral anticoagulation with a target INR of approximately 2.5 is more effective than with a target of 1.75, without further increasing the risk of bleeding.
- A second episode of VTE suggests a higher risk of recurrence (increased by about 50%). If both episodes of VTE were provoked by a transient risk factor, 3 months of anticoagulant therapy is expected to be adequate, with subsequent aggressive prophylaxis during transient periods of high risk. A second episode of unprovoked proximal DVT or PE is a strong argument for indefinite anticoagulant therapy.
- The risk of recurrence is lower (about one half) after an isolated calf (distal) DVT than after proximal DVT or PE. This argues against treating unprovoked isolated calf DVT for longer than 3 months.
- The risk of recurrence is similar after an episode of proximal DVT or PE. However, recurrent VTE is about three times as likely to be a PE after an initial PE (about 60% of episodes) than after an initial DVT (about 20% of episodes). This effect is expected to increase mortality from recurrent VTE about twofold after a PE compared with a DVT.
- The risk of recurrence is about threefold higher in patients with active cancer. The risk is higher in patients with metastatic rather than localized disease, and it is expected to be lower if VTE occurred while the patient was receiving chemotherapy and the chemotherapy was subsequently stopped.
- Long-term treatment with LMWH, particularly for the first 3 or 6 months, is more effective than warfarin in patients with VTE associated with cancer and is the preferred treatment for such patients.

- Estrogen therapy is a risk factor for first and recurrent episodes of VTE; consequently, the risk of recurrent VTE after stopping anticoagulants is expected to be lower in women who had VTE while on estrogen therapy, provided that they have stopped taking estrogens, and estrogen therapy should be avoided in patients with a previous VTE who are not on anticoagulant therapy.
- The presence of a hereditary predisposition to VTE does not appear to be a clinically important risk factor for recurrence during or after anticoagulant therapy. Consequently, testing for hereditary thrombophilias is not required in selecting the duration of therapy.
- The presence of an antiphospholipid antibody has uncertain significance as a predictor of recurrence independently of clinical presentation (e.g., provoked versus unprovoked). Absence of an antiphospholipid antibody on routine testing is not a good reason to stop anticoagulant therapy at 3 months in a patient with unprovoked proximal DVT or PE, and presence of an antiphospholipid antibody is not a good reason to treat patients with VTE provoked by a transient risk factor for longer than 3 months.
- Elevated D-dimer levels, measured 1 month after stopping anticoagulant therapy, predict a higher risk of recurrence in patients with a first episode of unprovoked VTE. However, further studies are needed to determine whether negative D-dimer results justify stopping anticoagulant therapy at 3 months in all or selected subgroups of patients with unprovoked proximal DVT or PE.
- Women appear to have a lower risk of recurrence than men. However, further studies are needed to determine whether this risk is low enough to justify stopping anticoagulant therapy in women with unprovoked proximal DVT or PE who have completed 3 months of treatment.
- The presence of residual DVT on ultrasound may be a marker of a heightened risk of recurrence in patients with unprovoked VTE. However, the strength of this relationship is uncertain, and further studies are needed to determine whether absence of residual DVT on ultrasound justifies stopping anticoagulant therapy in patients who have had an unprovoked proximal DVT.
- The presence of an inferior vena caval filter increases the long-term risk of DVT, decreases the risk of PE, and has no net effect on the risk of recurrent VTE. Consequently, the presence of an inferior vena caval filter need not influence the duration of anticoagulant therapy.
- The risk of anticoagulant-induced bleeding is highest during the first 3 months of treatment and stabilizes after the first year.
- The risk of bleeding differs markedly among patients depending on the prevalence of risk factors such as advanced age (particularly >75 years), previous bleeding or stroke, renal failure, anemia, antiplatelet therapy, malignancy, and poor anticoagulant control.
- The risk of major bleeding in younger patients (<60 years) without risk factors for bleeding who have good anticoagulant control (target INR, 2.0–3.0) is about 1% per year, and in those aged 60–75 years it is about 2% per year.

Whether anticoagulant therapy (INR, 2.0 to 3.0) is recommended for 3 months or for an indefinite period (with annual review) depends primarily on the presence of a provoking risk factor for VTE (i.e., major or minor transient risk factor, no risk factor, or cancer), risk factors for bleeding, and patient preference (i.e., burden associated with treatment) (Table 4).

THROMBOLYTIC THERAPY

Systemic thrombolytic therapy (e.g., with tissue plasminogen activator) accelerates the rate of resolution of DVT and PE at the cost of an approximately fourfold increase in frequency of major bleeding, and a 10-fold increase in intracranial bleeding. Such therapy can be lifesaving for those who have PE with hemodynamic compromise, and regimens that are administered over 2 hours or less are recommended in this situation. Systemic thrombolytics may reduce the risk of prothrombotic syndrome after DVT, but this does not appear to justify its associated risks.

Catheter-directed therapy, which uses lower doses of thrombolytic agents and is often combined with mechanical disruption of thrombus and stent insertion if there is residual thrombosis, is expected to

TABLE 4 Duration of Anticoagulant Therapy for Venous Thromboembolism

Categories of VTE	Durations of Treatment (Target INR 2.5, Range 2.0–3.0)
Provoked by a transient risk factor*	3 mo
Unprovoked VTE[†]	Minimum 3 mo, then reassess
First unprovoked proximal DVT or PE; no risk factors for bleeding; good anticoagulant control is achievable; and anticoagulation is not a major burden for the patient	Indefinite therapy with annual review
Isolated distal DVT as a first event	3 mo
Second unprovoked VTE	Indefinite therapy with annual review
Cancer-associated VTE	Indefinite treatment[‡]

*Transient risk factors include surgery, hospitalization, or plaster cast immobilization within 3 mo; estrogen therapy; pregnancy; prolonged travel (>8 hr); and lesser leg injuries or immobilizations occurring more recently (≤6 wk). The greater the provoking reversible risk factor (e.g., recent major surgery), the lower the expected risk of recurrence after stopping anticoagulant therapy.
[†]Absence of a transient risk factor or active cancer.
[‡]Initial treatment with LMWH for at least 3 mo is recommended, followed by long-term treatment with either LMWH or warfarin while cancer is active.
Abbreviations: DVT = deep venous thrombosis; INR = international normalized ratio; LMWH = low-molecular-weight heparin; VTE = venous thromboembolism.

be associated with a lower risk of bleeding but requires further evaluation before it can be widely recommended in patients with extensive proximal DVT.

INFERIOR VENA CAVAL FILTERS

Inferior vena caval filters reduce the risk of PE at the expense of increasing the risk of DVT. Their use is usually confined to patients with acute DVT or PE, or both, who cannot be anticoagulated because of a high risk of bleeding. Removable filters can be used for patients with acute VTE who have a temporary contraindication to anticoagulation. Patients who have an inferior vena caval filter inserted should receive anticoagulant therapy if it becomes safe to do so.

GRADUATED COMPRESSION STOCKINGS

Routine early use of graduated compression stockings for 2 years has been shown to reduce the incidence of the postthrombotic syndrome by about 50% after DVT. The efficacy of routinely wearing graduated stockings compared with selectively using stockings in patients who have persistent leg symptoms or new symptoms during follow-up has not been assessed.

Acknowledgment

Dr. Kearon is supported by the Heart and Stroke Foundation of Ontario.

REFERENCES

Anderson FA Jr, Spencer FA. Risk factors for venous thromboembolism. Circulation 2003;107:I-9–I-16.

Bernardi E, Camporese G, Buller HR, et al. Serial 2-point ultrasonography plus D-dimer vs whole-leg color-coded Doppler ultrasonography for diagnosing suspected symptomatic deep vein thrombosis: A randomized controlled trial. JAMA 2008;300:1653–9.

Geerts WH, Bergqvist D, Pineo GF, et al. Prevention of venous thromboembolism: American College of Chest Physicians evidence-based clinical practice guidelines (8th edition). Chest 2008;133:381S–453S.

Kearon C. Natural history of venous thromboembolism. Circulation 2003;107: I-22–I-30.

Kearon C, Kahn SR, Agnelli G, et al. Antithrombotic therapy for venous thromboembolic disease: ACCP evidence-based clinical practice guidelines (8th edition). Chest 2008;133:454S–545S.

Stein PD, Fowler SE, Goodman LR, et al. Multidetector computed tomography for acute pulmonary embolism. N Engl J Med 2006;354:2317–27.

Torbicki A, Perrier A, Konstantinides S, et al. Guidelines on the diagnosis and management of acute pulmonary embolism: The Task Force for the Diagnosis and Management of Acute Pulmonary Embolism of the European Society of Cardiology (ESC). Eur Heart J 2008;29:2276–315.

Wells PS, Owen C, Doucette S, et al. Does this patient have deep vein thrombosis? JAMA 2006;295:199–207.

Sarcoidosis

Method of
Daniel A. Culver, DO

Sarcoidosis is a systemic disease of unknown origin that is characterized by the presence of non-necrotizing granulomatous inflammation in affected organs. Since the first description of sarcoidosis by the British dermatologist Jonathon Hutchinson, in 1869, it has both perplexed and fascinated physicians of all medical specialties. It occurs worldwide, but the incidence, severity, and clinical phenotypes are influenced by race, ethnicity, gender, and age. Although the lungs are affected in most of the cases, the clinical manifestations are protean, and diagnosis is often delayed.

Epidemiology

Sarcoidosis occurs worldwide, but the highest incidence rates are reported in Scandinavia and among African Americans in the United States. In the Detroit, Michigan, area, the age-adjusted incidence rates for disease that is ascertained by discovery during routine health care are 10.9 per 100,000 among whites and 35.5 per 100,000 among blacks. Based on these data, it has been estimated that the lifetime risk for developing sarcoidosis is 0.85% in whites and 2.4% in blacks. Sarcoidosis has a predilection for individuals younger than 40 years of age, although there is also a second peak for older females. In most series, there is a slightly higher risk for females overall. In addition to susceptibility, race also influences disease phenotype, with blacks being far more likely to exhibit chronic disease, multiple organ involvement, and morbidity.

Etiology and Pathophysiology

The exact cause of sarcoidosis remains unknown. Based on epidemiologic evidence, it is believed that development of sarcoidosis requires exposure to an environmental antigen or antigens. This hypothesis is supported by several observations, including epidemiologic studies of disease incidence, reports of clusters of cases in small populations, transmission by organ transplantation, and the worldwide reproducibility of intradermal granulomatous reactions only in sarcoidosis subjects after injection of sarcoidosis lymph node homogenate (the Kveim-Siltzbach test). Molecular analyses, prolonged culture for organisms, and antimicrobial trials have failed to reveal definite evidence for a microbial etiology, but emerging data suggest that mycobacterial proteins could be a contributor in some patients.

Numerous investigators have sought genetic predispositions for sarcoidosis, based on the observations that ethnicity is a risk factor and that there is familial aggregation of disease risk. Much of the data

CURRENT DIAGNOSIS

- Sarcoidosis is a diagnosis of exclusion.
- Sarcoidosis occurs worldwide; in the United States, it more commonly affects African Americans, females, and individuals younger than 40 years of age.
- Diagnosis of sarcoidosis usually requires biopsy demonstration of non-necrotizing granulomas with no evidence of infectious organisms on staining or culture and no exposure to other agents known to induce granulomatous inflammation.
- Asymptomatic organ involvement that is not readily apparent by routine blood tests, electrocardiography, or ophthalmologic examination is unlikely to be clinically important, and extensive screening tests to stage sarcoidosis are not usually necessary.

suggest that the genetic effect on disease risk or severity depends on human leukocyte antigen genes that govern the expression of the type II major histocompatibility complex (MHC) on antigen-presenting cells. These observations fit well with the current concepts of disease pathogenesis, reserving a central role for activation of antigen-specific oligoclonal CD4$^+$ T cells by MHC class II–restricted antigen-presenting cells, which then amplify immune mechanisms that lead to granuloma formation. A number of other genes, most commonly encoding cytokines or chemokines, have been associated with sarcoidosis susceptibility or phenotype. However, lack of validation studies and difficulties with interpopulation genetic variability have limited progress in elucidating the genetic profiles in sarcoidosis. It is most likely that multiple genes in combination inform susceptibility and phenotype. The responsible genes probably differ among populations, possibly depending on the responsible antigens as well.

Sarcoid inflammation is characterized by non-necrotizing granulomas. The granuloma is a compact mass of cells that walls off foreign antigens, typically microbes. Epithelioid histiocytes, together with a few multinucleated giant cells, comprise the core, which is surrounded by an outer rim of T lymphocytes. The lymphocyte population is oligoclonal, with restricted T-cell receptor repertoires, consistent with an antigen-driven process. Inflammation in sarcoidosis is dependent on persistent stimulation by CD4$^+$ T cells.

Most of the pathophysiologic research has focused on the inflammatory, or early, stages of sarcoidosis. Characterization of sarcoidosis inflammation in humans has consistently demonstrated a Th1-predominant cytokine profile, with important roles for interferon-γ, interleukin-12, interleukin-18, and tumor necrosis factor (TNF). The first three are likely to be important in directing the development of the Th1 phenotype and may account for failure of feedback mechanisms to downregulate immune activation. In accordance with this hypothesis, interleukin-12 and interferon-γ knockout mice fail to develop granulomatous inflammation after challenge with granuloma-inducing agents. Additionally, TNF is an essential mediator, directing monocyte proliferation and differentiation of macrophages into the epithelioid cells of granulomas.

Clinical Presentation

The clinical presentation of sarcoidosis is protean. At least one third of patients diagnosed with sarcoidosis are asymptomatic. Constitutional symptoms may occur, especially with acute presentations. Common manifestations include fever (typically low-grade), weight loss, diaphoresis, arthralgias, and fatigue. The fatigue, which can be disabling, is often especially prominent, and it usually resolves more slowly than other symptoms. At the time of diagnosis, a detailed history and physical examination, along with focused testing, are indicated to identify organs with potentially important involvement (Table 1).

TABLE 1 Suggested Initial Evaluation of Sarcoidosis Patients

Complete history with emphasis on occupational and
  environmental exposure
Physical examination
Complete blood count, comprehensive metabolic panel
Posteroanterior chest radiograph
Spirometry, carbon monoxide diffusing capacity
Electrocardiogram
Ophthalmologic examination (with slit lamp)
Purified protein derivative (PPD) test
Urinalysis (if clinically indicated)

Two distinctive clinical syndromes are typically caused by sarcoidosis. The most renowned of these is Löfgren's syndrome, manifested as bilateral hilar lymphadenopathy, erythema nodosum, periarticular ankle arthralgias (usually), and fever (often). Löfgren's syndrome has a predilection to occur in the springtime and is more common in whites, especially Scandinavians. The prognosis is excellent in most cases. Heerfordt's syndrome, or uveoparotid fever, is characterized by fever, facial nerve palsy, parotid gland enlargement, and anterior uveitis.

PULMONARY EFFECTS

Sarcoidosis affects the lungs in approximately 95% of patients. The most common presenting symptoms are nonproductive cough, dyspnea, and substernal chest discomfort. Symptoms of airway hyperreactivity, including wheezing, occur frequently, and many patients are initially misdiagnosed with asthma. The cough in sarcoidosis is also commonly exacerbated by exposure to dusts, cold air, or other irritants. Even with prominent pulmonary symptoms or radiologic findings, the chest examination in sarcoidosis is usually normal, except in patients with narrowing of the airways caused by severe parenchymal disease. Clubbing and rales are rare and may indicate a complication, such as bronchiectasis; if either is found, an alternative diagnosis should also be considered carefully.

The chest radiograph is abnormal in more than 90% of patients at the time of diagnosis. A popular classification system, the Scadding scale, confers a loose sense of the overall prognosis for resolution of sarcoidosis within 5 years after diagnosis (Fig. 1). However, the Scadding scale has not been validated for chest computed tomography (CT), does not describe sequential steps in the natural history of sarcoidosis, has not been validated in all populations, and is not directly correlated with the response to treatment.

Chest CT scanning is more sensitive than radiography for the diagnosis and evaluation of fibrosis. The characteristic finding on high-resolution chest CT is the presence of nodular infiltrates centered along the bronchovascular bundles (Fig. 2). Chest CT is used routinely to plan bronchoscopic diagnosis, especially if transbronchial needle aspiration is entertained. It may also be useful to obtain a chest CT scan if there is a high index of suspicion for sarcoidosis despite a normal chest radiograph, a suspicion of sarcoidosis-induced pulmonary complications (e.g. bronchiectasis, mycetoma, bullae), an atypical radiographic pattern such as unilateral adenopathy, or a suggestion of infection. Some patterns on the initial chest CT, such as consolidation, ground glass opacities, and conglomerate central opacification, suggest a higher likelihood of developing pulmonary fibrosis or respiratory limitations.

Baseline pulmonary function studies are recommended at the time of diagnosis (see Table 1). The most reliable single test is the forced vital capacity (FVC), but the single-breath diffusing capacity

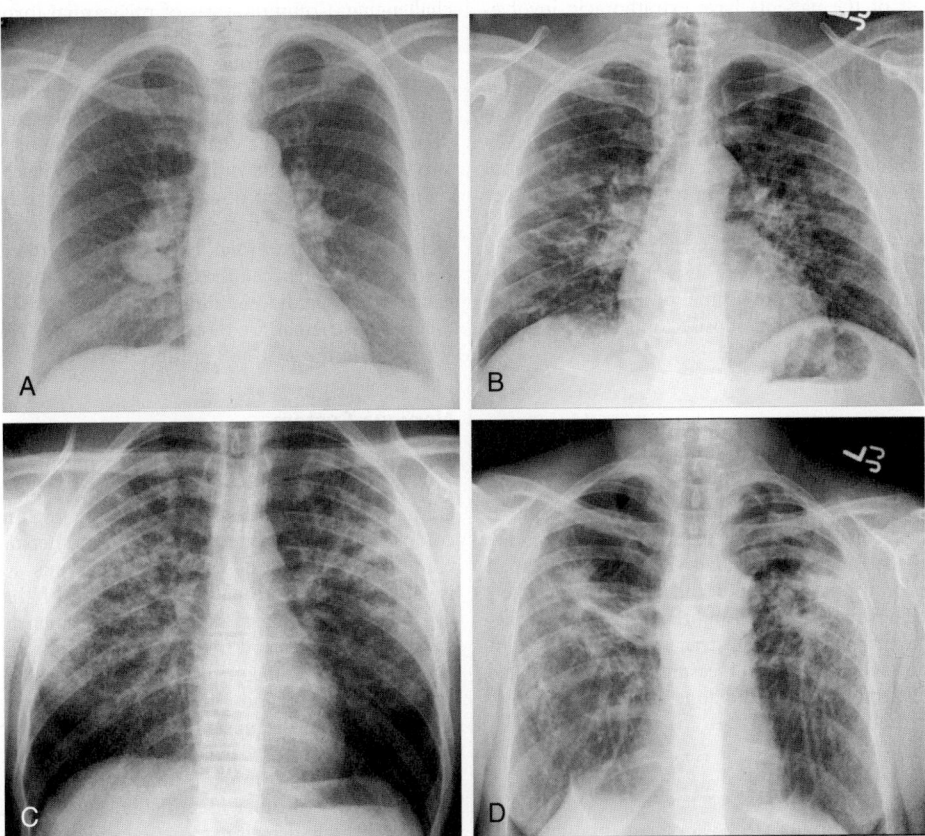

FIGURE 1. Chest radiographic stages of sarcoidosis as described by Scadding. The stages can be loosely correlated with prognosis for spontaneous disease resolution at 5 years. **A,** Stage 1 (bilateral hilar adenopathy), 85%-90% chance of resolution. **B,** Stage 2 (bilateral hilar adenopathy + infiltrates), 50%-60% chance. **C,** Stage 3 (infiltrates alone), 20%-30% chance. **D,** Stage 4 (irreversible scarring), 0% chance. The presence of radiographic changes should not be equated with disease activity.

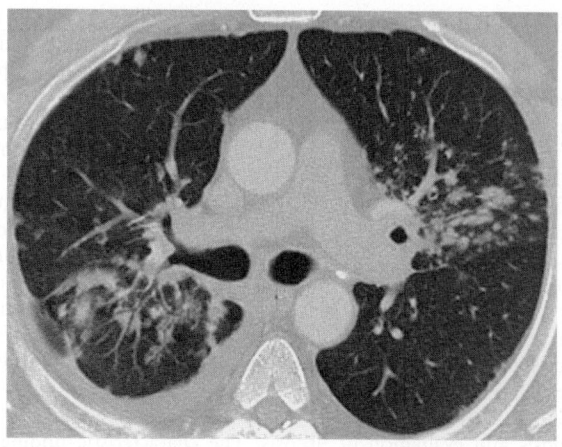

FIGURE 2. Typical parenchymal window computed tomographic findings in sarcoidosis, demonstrating nodular infiltrates centered along the bronchovascular bundles.

of the lung for carbon monoxide (DLCO) independently provides additional useful clinical information. Although restrictive physiology is widely assumed to be typical for sarcoidosis, obstructive lung disease is seen in up to 57% of patients. Similarly, bronchial hyperresponsiveness documented by bronchoprovocation testing is present in 21% to 50% of subjects. The presence of bronchial hyperreactivity is correlated with a higher likelihood of endobronchial sarcoidosis.

EXTRAPULMONARY SARCOIDOSIS

Slightly more than half of the patients have extrathoracic involvement as ascertained by a conventional screen for involvement (see Table 1) at the time of diagnosis. If more aggressive testing is performed, such as routine biopsies of the liver or muscles, the prevalence of involvement is found to be markedly higher for almost all organ systems. However, a general rule of thumb is that clinically occult sarcoidosis is unlikely to be important, so routine use of aggressive diagnostic modalities for the sole purpose of seeking other organ involvement is probably not warranted. Table 2 lists proposed criteria for determining organ involvement in a patient who already has an established diagnosis of sarcoidosis, as well as the reported incidence of organ involvement at the time of diagnosis in the ACCESS (A Case Control Study of Sarcoidosis) cohort.

Eyes

Ocular sarcoidosis may involve any structure in the eye. The most common manifestation is anterior uveitis, but patients may also exhibit lacrimal gland involvement, dacryocystitis, conjunctivitis, scleritis, glaucoma, cataracts, retinal vasculitis, and optic neuritis. If anterior structures (e.g., ciliary body) are involved, symptoms are common and the prognosis is generally good. The development of intermediate or posterior uveitis may be occult and is more likely to lead to vision loss. Therefore, a formal ophthalmologic examination including visual acuity assessment, external examination, slit-lamp examination, intraocular pressure measurement, and dilated vitreous and fundus inspections should be done at least once for all patients diagnosed with sarcoidosis.

Skin

Cutaneous sarcoidosis occurs in 20% to 35% of patients with sarcoidosis. The most common granulomatous manifestations are maculopapular nodules. A wide variety of other forms may be seen, including plaques, hypopigmented or hyperpigmented patches, subcutaneous nodules, alopecia, and mucosal disease. Cutaneous sarcoidosis has a predilection for sites of prior injury and should be sought in scars and tattoos (Fig. 3). It is important to distinguish

localized, sarcoid-like reactions in areas of prior injury from systemic sarcoidosis by searching for extracutaneous disease.

Erythema nodosum, manifested as reddish or violet, tender, indurated lesions typically on the shins, is more common in acute presentations of sarcoidosis. The presence of erythema nodosum in sarcoidosis confers an excellent prognosis. The differential diagnosis of erythema nodosum includes infections, malignancies, inflammatory bowel disease, and medication reactions. Biopsy of the lesions will reveal only a nonspecific panniculitis.

Lupus pernio, depicted in Figure 4, is characterized by disfiguring violaceous plaques and induration around the nose, cheeks, and, occasionally, other facial areas. It is associated with chronic, often refractory disease and frequently with concomitant sinonasal sarcoidosis.

Liver

Hepatic sarcoidosis, as ascertained by liver biopsy or autopsy, is frequent (50%-75%). Elevations of liver enzymes occur in approximately one third of patients, with increased alkaline phosphatase being the most common single abnormality. Hepatomegaly is evident on examination in fewer than 25% of patients. Liver involvement is twice as common in blacks as in whites. Most patients with hepatic involvement are asymptomatic. Abdominal pain or pruritus are the most common symptoms; signs of portal hypertension or synthetic insufficiency are rare. There are no compelling data to suggest that treatment of hepatic sarcoidosis alters the natural course of liver disease, which is generally benign.

Heart

Clinically evident cardiac sarcoidosis occurs in 2% to 7% of patients. The location and extent of granulomas dictates the clinical phenotype, but differentiation of active disease from fibrosis is extremely challenging. Common areas of myocardial involvement, in descending order of frequency, are the septum, the left ventricular free wall, and the right ventricular free wall. Involvement of the atria or the pericardium is rare. The most common manifestations are conduction delays, dysrhythmias (mainly ventricular), and cardiomyopathies. Sudden cardiac death, previously reported to occur in up to two thirds of patients with cardiac disease, has become more uncommon with the advent of advanced imaging techniques, more aggressive treatment, and frequent use of implanted devices. Because the yield of endomyocardial biopsy is low, the diagnosis of cardiac involvement is reached most often when patients with biopsy-proven extracardiac sarcoidosis fulfill specified criteria. Two commonly used diagnostic schemas are those of the Japanese Ministry of Health and Welfare and the ACCESS group criteria (see Table 2).

Nervous System

Either the central nervous system or the peripheral nervous system may be affected by sarcoidosis. Except for the situations of isolated cranial nerve VII palsies or acute aseptic meningitis, neurologic sarcoidosis usually portends chronic and bothersome disease. The most common manifestations of central nervous system sarcoidosis are isolated cranial neuropathies, especially of the optic nerve or the facial nerve; meningeal inflammation, which has a predilection for the basal meninges and frequently leads to headaches; hydrocephalus, which may occur in up to 10% of the cases; pituitary or hypothalamic dysfunction; and intramedullary or extramedullary spinal cord sarcoidosis. The diagnosis of neurosarcoidosis can be difficult. It is most typically reached when findings on neuroimaging or analysis of the cerebrospinal fluid are consistent with the disease (see Table 2), in the absence of other identifiable causes for the abnormality, in a patient with confirmed extraneural sarcoidosis.

Upper Respiratory Tract

Sarcoidosis of the upper respiratory tract is underrecognized and difficult to treat. It can be challenging to diagnose because of the frequency of nasal symptoms in the general population. In addition

TABLE 2 Criteria for Organ Involvement in Patients with Preexisting Sarcoidosis*

Organ	Definite	Probable	Frequency[†] (%)

Lungs	Chest radiography with one of the following:
	  Bilateral hilar lymphadenopathy
	  Diffuse infiltrates
	  Upper lobe fibrosis
	  Restrictive pulmonary function tests
	  Biopsy
		Lymphocytic alveolitis by bronchoalveolar lavage
		Any infiltrates
		Isolated reduction of D$_{LCO}$
			95

Skin	Lupus pernio Annular lesion Erythema nodosum Biopsy	Maculopapular lesion New nodules	16[‡]
Eyes	Lacrimal gland swelling Uveitis Optic neuritis Biopsy	Blindness	12
Liver	Liver function test values >3 times normal Biopsy	Compatible computed tomographic or ultrasound study Elevated alkaline phosphatase	12

Heart	Treatment-responsive cardiomyopathy
	Intraventricular conduction defect or nodal block
	Positive gallium scan of the heart
	Biopsy
		Any of the following (in the absence of other cardiac disease):
		  Ventricular dysrhythmias
		  Cardiomyopathy
		  Positive MRI
		  Positive thallium scan
			2

Nervous system	Enhancement in meninges or brainstem on MRI Increased lymphocytes or protein in cerebrospinal fluid Diabetes insipidus Bell's palsy Cranial neuropathy Biopsy	Other MRI abnormalities Unexplained neuropathy Positive electromyographic findings	5[§]
Bone marrow	Granulomas in bone marrow Unexplained anemia Marked leukopenia Thrombocytopenia Biopsy	—	4
Spleen	Biopsy	Enlargement by examination or imaging	7
Bone and joints	Granulomas on biopsy Cystic changes in phalanges	Asymmetrical, painful clubbing	<1
Lymph node	Biopsy	New palpable node above the waist Lymph node >2 cm by imaging	15
Ear, nose, and throat	Biopsy	Endoscopic examination consistent with granulomatous involvement	4
Parotid and salivary glands	Biopsy Symmetrical parotitis without mumps Gallium scan (Panda sign)		4
Muscles	Biopsy Treatment-responsive elevation of creatine kinase/aldolase	Increased creatine kinase/aldolase	<1
Calcium	Hypercalcemia without other cause	Hypercalciuria Presence of calcium-based renal stone	4
Kidney	Treatment responsive renal insufficiency Biopsy	Treatment-responsive renal insufficiency in patients with diabetes mellitus and/or hypertension	<1

*In the absence of other causes for the abnormality.
[†]Incidence data at the time of diagnosis in A Case Control Study of Sarcoidosis (ACCESS).
[‡]Excluding erythema nodosum.
[§]Excluding small-fiber neuropathy.
Abbreviations: D$_{LCO}$, diffusing capacity of the lung for carbon dioxide; MRI, magnetic resonance imaging.

to the typical manifestations of chronic rhinitis, the nasal mucosa may be very friable with crusting or bleeding, and there may be nodularity or marked thickening (Fig. 5). Other manifestations of sarcoidosis of the upper respiratory tract include otitis media, vestibular symptoms, hearing loss, exocrine gland swelling, xerostomia, chronic sinusitis, oral ulcerations, laryngeal involvement, and oral-nasal fistulas. Adjunctive management may include the use of nasal saline spray and saline irrigation. Topical corticosteroids are sometimes helpful, but systemic therapies are often required.

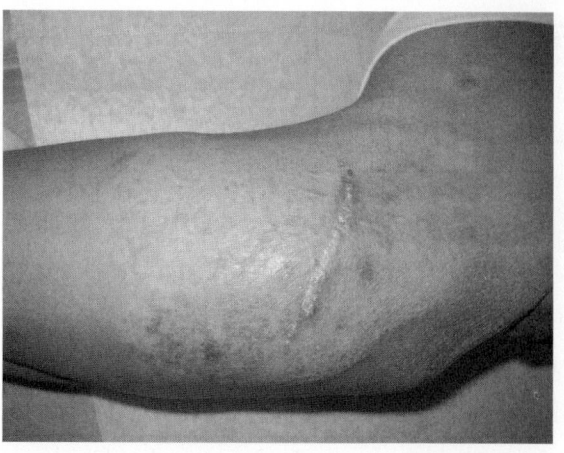

FIGURE 3. Scar sarcoidosis involving the site of a prior motorcycle injury. Note the local diffusion of cutaneous infiltration with hypopigmentation.

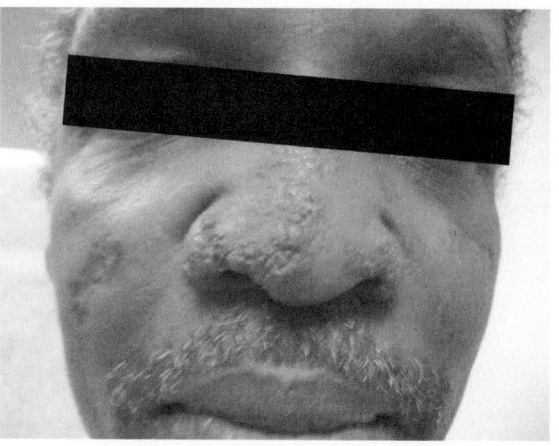

FIGURE 4. Long-standing lupus pernio lesions involving the nose and right cheek.

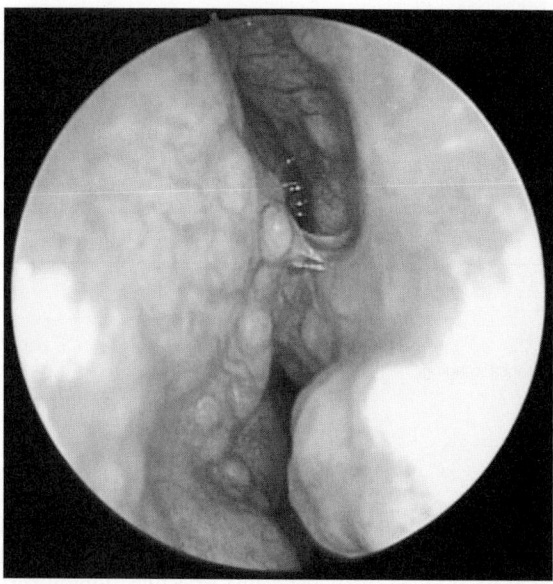

FIGURE 5. Nodular mucosal inflammation caused by sarcoidosis. Similar mucosal findings may be seen throughout the airways.

Calcium Homeostasis

Autonomous, uncontrolled conversion of 25-hydroxy-vitamin D to 1,25-dihydroxy-vitamin D by activated sarcoid macrophages accounts for the presence of hypercalcemia in up to 11% of patients and hypercalciuria in up to 20%. Ectopic vitamin D production usually responds easily to moderate doses of oral corticosteroids or antimalarial agents. Patients with deranged calcium metabolism should be instructed to avoid excessive sunlight and high-calcium diets, including calcium supplements. Decreased bone density is common in sarcoidosis, even in the absence of treatment with corticosteroids. Supplementation with calcium and vitamin D is indicated in these patients unless there is uncontrolled hypercalcemia or problematic hypercalciuria.

Musculoskeletal System

Muscle involvement occurs in up to 80% of random biopsies in some reports, but it is difficult to diagnose in patients. It can cause weakness and sometimes elevated muscle enzymes or pain; the diagnosis is supported by electromyographic abnormalities and enhancement on gadolinium-enhanced magnetic resonance imaging or gallium scanning. Usually, the proximal muscles are most affected, and involvement of the bulbar muscles is very rare. Unrecognized myositis may be an important contributor to fatigue and exercise limitation. Steroid myopathy is an important differential consideration for many patients; the presence of myalgias favors the diagnosis of sarcoidosis myopathy but is not sensitive for it.

Acute arthritis with overt synovitis tends to occur early in the course of the disease and may be the presenting feature. It is usually symmetrical, most commonly with involvement of the ankles, and often involving the knees, hands, wrists, and elbows as well. Chronic arthritis is uncommon (1%-4%) and is almost always associated with multiorgan disease. In the chronic form, the shoulders, knees, wrists, ankles, and hands are affected most frequently, and response to treatment is poor.

Osseous sarcoidosis is often clinically occult; pain and swelling may occur, but symptomatic bony disease is uncommon overall (<5%). Any bony structure may be involved, but the middle and distal phalanges of the hands and feet are the most frequent sites (Fig. 6). Significant symptomatic osseous involvement is associated with multisystem disease and portends a poor prognosis.

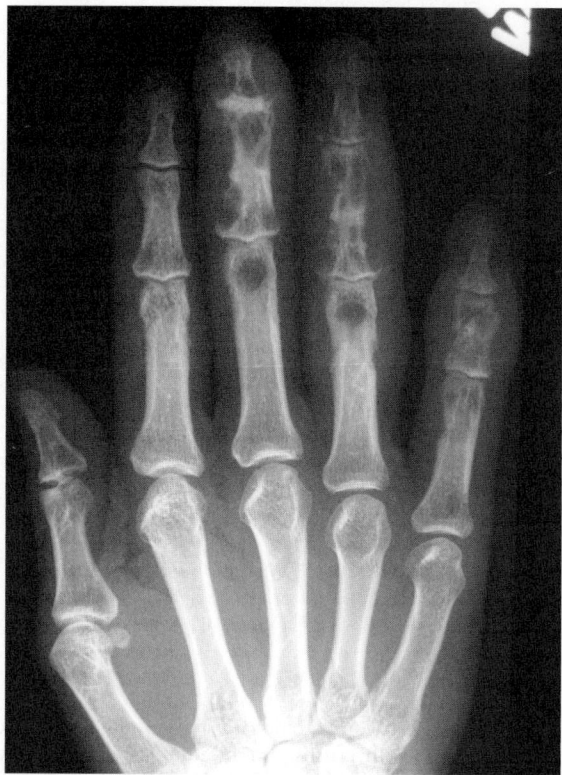

FIGURE 6. Bony involvement in sarcoidosis, with extensive cortical bone loss most dramatic in the third and fourth digits.

SARCOIDOSIS PENUMBRA

When sarcoidosis patients are interviewed about their symptoms and the issues most relevant to them, those symptoms that affect their quality of life most are often nonspecific, difficult to measure, and frustrating to clinicians. These symptoms do not correlate well with parameters such as FVC or chest radiographic stage.

Common complaints include profound fatigue, personality changes, cognitive impairment, and pain syndromes. Many of these can be attributed to the presence of depression, which occurs in 60% to 66% of sarcoidosis patients in the United States. Risk factors for depression include female gender, dyspnea, and perceived lack of access to health care. Fatigue in sarcoidosis may be multifactorial, but a significant proportion of patients develop disabling fatigue; the overall prevalence of fatigue in this population is between 50% and 80%. Sleep apnea syndrome, which occurs in 17% of sarcoidosis patients, is one possible cause and should be actively sought. If no other risk factor is identified, the fatigue is severe, and there is no indication for use of systemic immunosuppressive agents, nonspecific treatment with modafinil (Provigil)[1] or dex-methylphenidate (Focalin)[1] may be useful.

Small nerve fiber dropout (small-fiber neuropathy) may be caused by inflammatory mediators or by a number of diseases. In sarcoidosis, it is frequent and may be the cause for nonspecific pain syndromes or neuropathic symptoms. Treatment of small-fiber neuropathy is difficult.

Diagnosis

Sarcoidosis is a multisystem disease, and the diagnosis is most secure when manifestations of the disease are documented in at least two organs. From a practical standpoint, there are two main pathways to diagnosis: biopsy confirmation in a patient with a clinically compatible presentation, and, less commonly, the presence of an overwhelmingly typical clinical syndrome. The clinical diagnoses that do not mandate a tissue biopsy are primarily ones that portend a benign course, including Löfgren's syndrome, Heerfordt's syndrome, and asymptomatic bilateral hilar lymphadenopathy on chest imaging. However, the more common way to reach the diagnosis is by tissue biopsy. In general, the organ with the most accessible lesion should be targeted for biopsy. Because clinically overt involvement in the lungs (95%) and skin (16% to 25% excluding erythema nodosum) is common, these are the most frequent sites for initial diagnosis. As mentioned earlier, the diagnosis is most secure when involvement of at least two organs can be documented. Table 2 provides a guide for confirmation of involvement of a second organ.

Important aspects of establishing the diagnosis include the presence of negative microbial stains and cultures, absence of relevant exposures or diseases that could cause similar granulomas, and ongoing circumspection regarding the provisional diagnosis if only a single target organ can be identified. Table 3 provides an abbreviated list of the most relevant causes for granulomatous inflammation in the differential diagnosis.

Because the lungs are involved in almost 100% of cases, bronchoscopy with tissue sampling is the best way to make the diagnosis for many patients. Even in the absence of parenchymal infiltrates, random transbronchial biopsies may be diagnostic; at our institution, these are routinely performed in patients with suspected ocular, neurologic, or cardiac sarcoidosis if the diagnosis cannot otherwise be made more easily. The combination of transbronchial biopsies with endobronchial forceps biopsy or transbronchial needle aspiration of enlarged lymph nodes, or both, increases the overall sensitivity. Recently, several groups have reported excellent experiences with ultrasound-guided transbronchial needle aspiration, with sensitivity approaching that of mediastinoscopy.

---

[1]Not FDA approved for this indication.

TABLE 3 Most Frequent Differential Diagnoses for Granulomas in Target Organs

Lung
Mycobacteria, especially nontuberculous species
Fungi, especially endemic species
Pneumocystis jiroveci
Hypersensitivity pneumonitis
Metal exposure (beryllium, aluminum, titanium)
Foreign material aspiration
Granulomatous lesions due to immune deficiency syndromes (e.g., CVID)

Liver
Mycobacteria, especially *M. tuberculosis*
Schistosomiasis
Brucellosis
Primary biliary cirrhosis
Crohn's disease
Lymphoma
Idiopathic granulomatous hepatitis
GLUS syndrome*

Skin
Mycobacteria
Fungi
Foreign body reaction (tattoos, retained debris)

Bone Marrow
Tuberculosis
Histoplasmosis
Lymphoma
Viruses (cytomegalovirus, mononucleosis)
GLUS syndrome*

Lymph Node
Mycobacteria
Fungi
Rare infections (brucellosis, cat-scratch disease, toxoplasmosis)
Lymphoma
Granulomatous histiocytic necrotizing lymphadenitis (Kikuchi disease)
Sarcoid-like reaction in regional lymph nodes from carcinoma
GLUS syndrome*

Adapted from Hunninghake GW, Costabel U, Ando M, et al: ATS/ERS/WASOG statement on sarcoidosis. American Thoracic Society/European Respiratory Society/World Association of Sarcoidosis and Other Granulomatous Disorders. Sarcoidosis Vasc Diffuse Lung Dis 1999;16(2):149-173.
*Granulomatous lesions of undetermined significance (GLUS) is a disorder, thought to be distinct from sarcoidosis, with a generally benign course.
Abbreviation: CVID = common variable immune deficiency.

Natural History

The natural history of sarcoidosis is quite variable, and no single study has comprehensively ascertained which clinical features independently are the best prognostic indicators. Overall, approximately two thirds of patients experience resolution of their disease within 5 years of onset, and the 5-year time point has increasingly been accepted as the differentiating point for labeling sarcoidosis as acute or chronic. Overall, in the United States, the mortality rate is between 1% and 5%, with the actual value likely closer to 1%. As mentioned previously, black race confers a worse prognosis. Other poor prognostic indicators include age older than 40 years at diagnosis, multisystem disease, cardiac sarcoidosis, symptomatic bony sarcoidosis, organomegaly, sarcoidosis of the upper respiratory tract, nephrocalcinosis, advanced Scadding stage, worse lung function, poor socioeconomic status, and the presence of sarcoidosis-related pulmonary hypertension. Good prognostic indicators include white race, Löfgren's syndrome, Scadding stage 0 or 1 on chest radiography, and acute onset. However, recent data from the ACCESS study

- Approximately two thirds of patients experience spontaneous resolution within 5 years of onset. There are insufficient data supporting the hypothesis that early treatment increases the prospects for resolution to warrant routine empiric therapy in all patients.

- Treatment is generally considered to be a strategy to prevent or reverse deterioration of organ function; therefore, treatment regimens lasting at least several months are typically used.

- Treatment is almost always indicated for active neurologic or cardiac involvement of any degree (except isolated cranial nerve VII palsy), severe hypercalcemia, ocular disease refractory to topical therapy, lupus pernio, significant hepatic involvement, symptomatic splenic disease, and bulky lymphadenopathy resulting in symptomatic compression of surrounding structures.

- Treatment for other manifestations requires careful consideration of the expected course of disease, pattern of organ involvement, goals of therapy, and toxicities of the proposed treatment.

- Corticosteroids have traditionally been used to treat acute, severe manifestations of sarcoidosis; for chronic or refractory disease, steroid-sparing alternatives may be considered.

- Comorbidities, including depression, sleep apnea, fibromyalgia, small-fiber neuropathy, and sarcoidosis-related fatigue, often confer the greatest impact on patients' quality of life. Treatment strategies should identify and address these issues if possible.

suggest that need for treatment in the first 6 months after diagnosis may be the single best indicator of future need for systemic treatment.

The British Thoracic Society study of patients with stable but persistent pulmonary sarcoidosis lasting longer than 6 months suggested that routine treatment of stable sarcoidosis has little influence on the natural course of the disease.

Treatment

The decision to treat sarcoidosis with systemic medications can be difficult. Factors to consider include the following:

- Expected natural course of untreated disease in the involved organ
- Presence of definitive treatment indications, such as active neurologic or cardiac involvement of any degree (except isolated cranial nerve VII palsy), severe hypercalcemia, ocular disease refractory to topical therapy, lupus pernio, significant hepatic involvement, symptomatic splenic disease, and bulky lymphadenopathy resulting in symptomatic compression of surrounding structures
- Evidence of disease progression during a period of observation
- Presence of favorable or poor prognostic factors
- Duration of disease, with chronic disease unlikely to remit spontaneously
- Risk for development of and significance of potential medication toxicities in the patient
- Definition of physician and patient expectations of the goals of treatment, with some reconciliation of patient-defined therapeutic goals with those of the physician

Because sarcoidosis is likely to evolve slowly, therapeutic regimens are typically maintained over a period of months to years. The decision to treat pulmonary sarcoidosis is most commonly made when there is clear evidence of deterioration (e.g., 10% decline in pulmonary function test values) or when there are significant symptoms attributable to pulmonary involvement. Neither the presence of infiltrates alone nor fluctuations in asymptomatic intrathoracic lymph node size alone are sufficient to initiate systemic treatment. Other factors that may influence a decision to treat include persistence of infiltrates for longer than 2 to 5 years and the presence of poor CT-defined prognostic features (see "Pulmonary Effects"). If the predominant manifestations are airway-based, such as cough or mild wheezing, a trial of inhaled corticosteroids may be useful. However, the published data on this treatment in symptomatic sarcoidosis suggest mixed results. For extrapulmonary disease, in addition to the definitive treatment indications outlined earlier, the decision to treat must be individualized. In these cases, it is extremely important to define clear therapeutic goals and to consider that asymptomatic manifestations (e.g., incidental finding of bony sarcoidosis or stable persistent elevations in liver function tests) usually do not require treatment.

Corticosteroids have been the mainstay of treatment for more than 50 years, but there is a gradual movement in many centers to use more steroid-sparing regimens if possible. The toxicities of prolonged steroid use are substantial, and it not infrequently causes more morbidity than the underlying disease. For acute sarcoidosis (i.e., <5 years since diagnosis), requiring treatment, a dose of 20 to 40 mg of prednisone daily is usually sufficient. The initial duration of therapy before tapering has not been well studied, but most experts reassess response and consider tapering the dose at 6 to 8 weeks. In a single trial, alternate-day regimens appeared to be as effective as daily dosing, and they may decrease toxicity. For severe, extrapulmonary disease, higher doses of corticosteroids have been advocated by some authors, but it is unclear whether higher doses are actually beneficial, and the rationale for using them may simply reflect the relatively slower therapeutic response in some organs, such as the heart and central nervous system.

For chronic (>5 years since diagnosis) or relapsing acute disease, the role of corticosteroids is more circumscribed. These patients are less likely to successfully taper steroids, and in these settings alternative agents are frequently required. In our practice, corticosteroids are most useful in patients with chronic sarcoidosis when used at higher doses for a short trial to assess reversibility or as part of a maintenance regimen using doses no higher than 10 mg/d.

The choice of steroid-sparing agent is limited by the lack of comparative data. The most widely used ones are hydroxychloroquine (Plaquenil)[1] and methotrexate (Trexall).[1] Hydroxychloroquine monotherapy (200–400 mg daily) is most useful for mild to moderate cutaneous or mucosal disease and for hypercalcemia. It may also be useful in combination with other agents. Methotrexate, administered orally or by injection, has been shown to be useful as a steroid-sparing agent in pulmonary, cutaneous, ocular, and neurologic sarcoidosis. It also appears to have utility in steroid-refractory disease. Typical doses range from 10 mg to 0.3 mg/kg weekly; the full response may require 6 to 9 months to manifest. The presence of hepatic enzyme abnormalities and pulmonary infiltrates in sarcoidosis complicates the use of methotrexate, although both usually improve with therapy.

Azathioprine (Imuran)[1] is also used frequently but has relatively less published data to support it. Like methotrexate, azathioprine requires periodic monitoring of liver function, but it also is probably safe in hepatic sarcoidosis. Typical doses range from 2 to 2.5 mg/kg/day.

---

[1]Not FDA approved for this indication.

Leflunomide (Arava),[1] which antagonizes lymphocyte proliferation, was reported in a single-center observational study to induce partial or complete responses in 25 (78%) of 32 patients with chronic sarcoidosis unresponsive to or intolerant of methotrexate. It may have synergistic effects when used in combination with methotrexate.

It appears that more clinicians have begun using mycophenolate mofetil (Cellcept)[1] and mycophenolate sodium (Myfortic).[1] The published evidence for these medications is limited to scattered case reports. Theoretically, the risk of developing neutropenia may be lower than with traditional agents.

Cyclophosphamide (Cytoxan),[1] an alkylating agent, can be used in oral or intravenous formulations. In at least one report on neurosarcoidosis, it appeared to be more efficacious than methotrexate. The side-effect profile and burdensome monitoring requirements have dampened enthusiasm for its use except in the most severe cases.

Thalidomide (Thalomid)[1] and pentoxifylline (Trental),[1] which inhibit TNF, are used sporadically as third- or fourth-line alternatives in patients who have refractory disease or are intolerant of other agents. Thalidomide also has useful anti-angiogenic properties that may account for some of its effects.

The most recent therapeutic options for treatment of sarcoidosis are the biologic TNF antagonists. The bulk of the evidence to date is for infusion therapy with the monoclonal antibody, infliximab (Remicade);[1] the subcutaneous monoclonal agent, adalimumab (Humira),[1] has also been successful in a handful of cases. A randomized, double-blind, placebo-controlled trial of 138 subjects demonstrated effectiveness of infliximab in chronic pulmonary disease. Others have reported that infliximab is useful for refractory neurologic, ocular, and cutaneous sarcoidosis. Potential toxicities of this approach include infection, especially atypical reactivation syndromes from granulomatous organisms; possible risks of malignancy; and worsening of cardiomyopathy. In a subset of patients with refractory sarcoidosis, infliximab may be dramatically more effective than other therapies.

REFERENCES

Baughman RP, Drent M, Kavuru M, et al. Infliximab therapy in patients with chronic sarcoidosis and pulmonary involvement. Am J Respir Crit Care Med 2006;174(7):795–802.

Baughman RP, Judson MA, Teirstein A, et al. Presenting characteristics as predictors of duration of treatment in sarcoidosis. QJM 2006;99(5): 307–15.

Baughman RP, Teirstein AS, Judson MA, et al. Clinical characteristics of patients in a case control study of sarcoidosis. Am J Respir Crit Care Med 2001;164:1885–9.

Drake WP, Newman LS. Mycobacterial antigens may be important in sarcoidosis pathogenesis. Curr Opin Pulm Med 2006;12(5):359–63.

Gibson GJ, Prescott RJ, Muers MF, et al. British Thoracic Society Sarcoidosis Study: Effects of long term corticosteroid treatment. Thorax 1996; 51:238–47.

Hunninghake GW, Costabel U, Ando M, et al. ATS/ERS/WASOG statement on sarcoidosis. American Thoracic Society/European Respiratory Society/World Association of Sarcoidosis and other Granulomatous Disorders. Sarcoidosis Vasc Diffuse Lung Dis 1999;16(2):149–73.

Iannuzzi MC, Rybicki BA, Teirstein AS. Sarcoidosis. N Engl J Med 2007;357 (21):2153–65.

Judson MA. An approach to the treatment of pulmonary sarcoidosis with corticosteroids. Chest 1999;115:1158–65.

Judson MA. The diagnosis of sarcoidosis. Clin Chest Med 2008;29(3): 415–28.

Rybicki BA, Major M, Popovich J, et al. Racial differences in sarcoidosis incidence: A 5-year study in a health maintenance organization. Am J Epidemiol 1997;145:234–41.

[1]Not FDA approved for this indication.

Pneumoconiosis

Method of
Richard D. deShazo, MD, and
David N. Weissman, MD

Pneumoconiosis

The pneumoconioses are a group of interstitial fibrotic lung diseases predominantly associated with occupational exposures. They are caused by inhalation of particulate matter in the respirable size range (0.3–5 µm mean aerodynamic diameter), especially mineral or metallic dusts (Table 1). These agents interact with pulmonary target cells, including alveolar macrophages and alveolar epithelial cells, to activate a cascade of inflammatory mediators including growth factors. Although exposure to these dusts can induce other types of respiratory disease as well, the final common pathway is alveolar epithelial cell damage and interstitial fibrosis. This chapter focuses on silicosis and asbestosis, two common forms of pneumoconiosis.

Asbestosis

Asbestos is composed of strong, heat-resistant fibers of hydrated magnesium silicate classified morphologically as serpentine (chrysotile) or amphibole (crocidolite [riebeckite asbestos]), amosite [cummingtonite-grunerite asbestos], anthophyllite asbestos, actinolite asbestos, and tremolite asbestos. In addition, certain asbestiform fibers (winchite, richterite, erionite) can cause adverse health effects identical to those of asbestos. Fiber dimensions and persistence in tissues are key determinants of toxicity. There is a dose–response effect between the quantity of asbestos inhaled and the severity of fibrotic lung disease. Asbestos is also a carcinogen, and increasing exposure is associated with increased risk, particularly for lung cancer and mesothelioma.

Although asbestos is no longer mined in the United States, importation of asbestos-containing products continues. Exposures also continue to occur, especially in construction and renovation (due to reservoirs of asbestos that are still present in many older buildings), the heating trades (where asbestos is often encountered), and with exposure to older or imported asbestos-containing automotive friction products such as brake linings and clutch facings. Workers exposed to asbestos can carry it home on their clothing, resulting in exposure of family members. Living near natural amphibole deposits in California has been implicated as a risk factor for mesothelioma.

The Occupational Safety and Health Administration (OSHA) permissible exposure limit (PEL) for asbestos is 0.1 fiber per cc air. This limit was affected in part by the limits of the analytical methodology used in exposure assessment. Exposure to the PEL every day over a 45-year working lifetime has been estimated to be associated with an increased risk of cancer (lung, mesothelioma, and gastrointestinal) of 336 cases per 100,000 exposed persons and an increased risk of asbestosis of 250 cases per 100,000 exposed persons.

Asbestosis causes symptoms of dyspnea and cough. Latency between initial exposure and disease onset is related to exposure intensity. In the United States, this period is generally about two decades. The disease can lead to chronic respiratory failure. Effects of smoking add to the severity of the disease and can cause obstructive findings in addition to the expected decreased lung volume and diffusion capacity associated with fibrotic lung diseases. Bibasilar rubs and inspiratory crackles on auscultation, finger clubbing, and diffuse, bilateral, small, irregular parenchymal opacities and linear streaking at the lung bases on chest x-ray are characteristic.

The International Labour Organization (ILO) has established a system for classification (grading) of radiographs for the presence

TABLE 1 Representative Pneumoconioses

Source	Clinical Features	Occupation	Dust
Crystalline silica	Silicosis, increased susceptibility to TB, airways obstruction, lung cancer	Mining, stone cutting, pottery, foundry work	Free crystalline silica (SiO_2)
Asbestiform fibers	Asbestosis, bronchogenic carcinoma, mesothelioma, various forms of benign pleural disease	Insulation, shipbuilding, construction, some mining (e.g., vermiculite mining in Libby, Mont)	Various asbestiform fibers
Coal	Coal workers' pneumoconiosis, COPD	Coal mining	Coal mine dust
Hard metal	Hard metal lung disease (cobalt lung), asthma	Machinists, metal workers	Hard metal, composed primarily of tungsten carbide and cobalt

COPD = chronic obstructive pulmonary disease; TB = tuberculosis.

of radiographic abnormalities in lung parenchyma and pleura that are associated with pneumoconiosis, as well as their severity. The ILO classification system is widely used in epidemiology, surveillance, administrative, and legal settings. The small opacity profusion grades of 0/1 and 1/0 are often considered as defining the boundary between normal and abnormal lung parenchyma.

High-resolution computed tomography (CT) is the most sensitive imaging method for suspected asbestosis. It detects a range of parenchymal abnormalities related to the fibrotic process, such as ground glass and honeycombing, and pleural abnormalities, such as pleural plaques and diffuse pleural thickening. The presence of pleural plaques on radiography (particularly bilateral calcified pleural plaques); uncoated asbestos fibers or fibers coated with an iron-rich proteinaceous material (asbestos bodies) in sputum, bronchoalveolar lavage, or lung biopsy; and the slower progression of symptoms help differentiate asbestosis from idiopathic pulmonary fibrosis.

CRITERIA FOR DIAGNOSIS

Diagnosis is supported by radiographic chest imaging or lung biopsy findings of interstitial lung disease compatible with asbestos; documentation of exposure to asbestos by history, the presence of pleural plaques (bilateral pleural plaques are essentially pathognomonic for asbestos exposure), or the presence of asbestos bodies or an excessive burden of uncoated asbestos fibers in lung biopsy tissue or possibly via bronchoalveolar lavage or sputum; and no other likely explanation for the diffuse fibrotic lung disease.

ASBESTOS-RELATED BENIGN PLEURAL DISEASE

Pleural plaques are characteristic forms of localized parietal pleural thickening that are usually bilateral and asymmetrical, involve the lower lung fields or the diaphragm, and spare the costophrenic angles and apices. Pleural plaques are a marker for exposure to asbestos and are often associated with other asbestos-related conditions. Pleural plaques result in minimal reductions in forced vital capacity and do not degenerate into malignant lesions.

In contrast, *diffuse visceral pleural thickening* can result in adhesions between the visceral and parietal pleura with major decreases in forced vital capacity, respiratory insufficiency, and the requirement for decortication.

CURRENT DIAGNOSIS

- History of inhalation of mineral or metal dust
- Respiratory symptoms such as cough and dyspnea
- Spirometry and lung volumes show restriction in advanced disease
- Interstitial lung disease can usually be demonstrated by chest imaging. Biopsy is usually unnecessary
- No other likely cause of interstitial lung disease is present

Benign pleural effusions can occur in the first decade after asbestos exposure and contain erythrocytes and a mixed inflammatory cell infiltrate of lymphocytes, neutrophils, and eosinophils. The thickened visceral pleura and adjacent atelectatic lung tissue can result in a pleural-based area of *rounded atelectasis,* simulating a lung mass on chest radiography. CT can reveal the comet sign, a pleural band connecting the apparent mass to an area of thickened pleura.

LUNG CANCER AND MALIGNANT MESOTHELIOMA

Exposure to all forms of asbestos increases the risk of lung cancer. The peak risk occurs at about 30 to 35 years after the onset of exposure. Tobacco smoking increases this risk in a multiplicative fashion, increasing the sixfold risk associated with asbestos exposure alone to a relative risk of about 60-fold. In contrast, smoking does not further increase the asbestos-associated risk for *malignant mesothelioma*. Asbestos-associated malignant mesothelioma can also affect the peritoneum (and sometimes the pericardium), but when it affects the pleura, this disease manifests with dyspnea, chest pain, and bloody pleural effusion (most often unilateral). A latency period of 30 years or longer after initial exposure is common. Special immunochemical stains and electron microscopy of pleural fluid or pleural biopsies may be necessary to differentiate mesothelioma from adenocarcinoma. There is no evidence of benefit from surveillance for lung cancer in asbestos-exposed populations.

TREATMENT

Treatment of asbestosis is symptomatic and similar to that for other patients with chronic lung disease (Box 1). Lung transplantation should be considered in the setting of end-stage lung disease. Treatment of benign pleural disease is also symptomatic; as already noted, decortication is sometimes required for managing diffuse visceral pleural thickening. Depending on extent of disease, mesothelioma may be treated with surgery, radiation, chemotherapy, or some combination of these. In general, prognosis is poor. Mesothelioma-associated malignant pleural effusion can require palliation through procedures such as pleurodesis, pleurectomy, and decortication. Asbestos-associated lung cancer is managed in the same fashion as lung cancer occurring without a history of exposure to asbestos.

Silicosis

Silicosis is a fibrosing interstitial lung disease resulting from the inhalation of crystalline silicon dioxide (silica) in dust of respirable size. The commonest form of crystalline silica is quartz, which is the main component of sand and is present in most rocks. Noncrystalline (amorphous) silica, like that in diatomaceous earth or glass, does not cause silicosis. However, heating amorphous silica, as occurs in foundries when molten metal is poured into clay castings, can convert amorphous silica into cristobalite, a hazardous form of crystalline silica. Mining, stone cutting, sandblasting, and foundry work are all

BOX 1 Recommendations for Managing Patients with Silicosis or Asbestos-Related Lung Disease

Patients

Stop further exposure to silica or asbestos.
Stop smoking, avoid exposure to tobacco products.

Physicians

Provide early treatment of respiratory infections with antibiotics.
Give pneumococcal and influenza vaccinations.
Maintain a high index of suspicion and provide early evaluation of symptoms for lung, laryngeal, and gastrointestinal cancers and mesothelioma in asbestos-exposed patients.
Maintain a high index of suspicion for pulmonary infection with *Mycobacterium tuberculosis*, nontuberculous mycobacteria, and fungi in silica-exposed patients.
Screen silica-exposed patients for latent tuberculosis infection with tuberculin skin test. Treat latent infections with isoniazid (9 mo) or rifampin (4 mo).
Provide empiric treatment with short- and long-acting inhaled bronchodilators and inhaled corticosteroids when they are found to provide symptomatic relief.
Give supplemental oxygen therapy if pulmonary hypertension is present or to prevent pulmonary hypertension if O_2 saturation is less than 85% at rest, with exercise, or with sleep.
Consider lung transplantation in the setting of end-stage lung disease.

---

examples of trades associated with exposure to respirable dust containing crystalline silica. The International Agency for Research on Cancer (IARC) has designated crystalline silica from occupational sources as a Group 1 human lung carcinogen.

The current OSHA PEL for respirable dusts containing crystalline silica is defined according to specified formulas, including one that is most commonly used:

$$(10 \text{ mg/m}^3)/(\% \text{ SiO}_2 \text{ content} + 2)$$

According to this formula, if a respirable dust contains 100% crystalline silica, the PEL for that dust approximates 0.1 mg/m^3.

A number of studies have suggested that this PEL is not fully protective for exposures over an entire working lifetime. The National Institute for Occupational Safety and Health (NIOSH) recommended exposure limit (REL) for respirable crystalline silica should be lower than the PEL, at 0.05 mg/m^3. Reporting of silicosis cases to public health authorities is required in some states.

RADIOGRAPHIC PATTERNS OF SILICOSIS

Three main radiographic patterns of silicosis have been described. Two are nodular interstitial patterns and one is an alveolar-filling pattern. The *simple* pattern is associated with nodules that are smaller than 10 mm and that are predominantly rounded and in the upper lung zones. *Progressive massive fibrosis* (PMF) is found in more advanced interstitial disease. It is associated with multiple coalescent larger nodules, upper lobe fibrosis, upward retraction of the hila, and compensatory hyperinflation of the lower lobes. The large upper-zone opacities can cavitate, sometimes in the setting of superimposed mycobacterial infection. Hilar adenopathy can occur, sometimes with an egg-shell pattern of hilar node calcification. A third radiographic pattern is an alveolar-filling process. Overwhelming silica exposure over a short period can cause a pathologic response called

silicoproteinosis, in which alveoli become flooded with proteinaceous fluid. The condition resembles idiopathic pulmonary alveolar proteinosis. The radiographic alveolar filling pattern favors the lower lung zones and is not associated with the changes of simple silicosis or PMF.

SILICOSIS SYNDROMES

Three syndromes of silicosis can be defined based on clinical course and radiographic pattern. *Chronic silicosis* develops slowly, usually 10 to 30 years after first exposure. It most often has the simple radiographic pattern, but it can be associated with PMF.

Accelerated silicosis develops more rapidly, within 10 years after first exposure. It is associated with higher intensity exposures and can be associated with either the simple or PMF radiographic patterns. Accelerated silicosis is differentiated from chronic silicosis by its more rapid course. Patients with accelerated courses are at greater risk for developing PMF. The clinical presentations of chronic and accelerated silicosis are variable but include cough, dyspnea, and a variety of chest findings ranging from a normal chest examination to crackles, rhonchi, or wheezing. PMF is associated with more severe symptoms and respiratory impairment. Findings compatible with both restrictive and obstructive lung disease (decreased forced vital capacity [FVC], forced expiratory volume at 1 sec [FEV_1], FEV_1/FVC, diffusion capacity) can occur, potentially leading to cor pulmonale and respiratory failure.

Acute silicosis is associated with very intense exposures to silica, leading to symptoms within a few weeks to a few years after exposure. Intense exposure results in lung injury caused by flooding of alveoli with proteinaceous material, or silicoproteinosis. As already noted, the radiographic appearance is that of an alveolar-filling pattern favoring the lower lung zones. Patients present weeks to a few years after exposure with cough, weight loss, fatigue, and occasional pleuritic chest pain, crackles on auscultation, and progression to respiratory failure often complicated by mycobacterial infection.

CRITERIA FOR DIAGNOSIS

The diagnosis of silicosis is predicated on a history of exposure to respirable crystalline silica, typical chest x-ray findings, and the lack of a more likely diagnosis. There is no consensus on the use of high-resolution CT, and lung biopsy is seldom required for diagnosis.

TREATMENT

Treatment is symptomatic and similar to that for other patients with chronic lung disease (see Box 1). Experimental therapies such as oral corticosteroid therapy and whole-lung lavage have been reported, but clinical benefit is unclear. Lung transplantation should be considered for patients with end-stage lung disease.

All forms of silicosis, as well as substantial exposure to crystalline silica in the absence of silicosis, are associated with an increased risk of pulmonary tuberculosis and fungal infections. Patients should be evaluated for latent tuberculosis infection by skin testing with tuberculin purified protein derivative. A positive tuberculin skin test in a patient with a history of substantial silica exposure of at least 10 mm of induration should be considered evidence of tuberculosis infection, regardless of previous immunization with bacille Calmette-Guérin. If the tuberculin skin test is positive, an evaluation for active tuberculosis should be performed and active disease treated. If active tuberculosis is not present, treat for latent infection. For adults, isoniazid (Nydrazid) 5 mg/kg (300 mg maximum) daily or 15 mg/kg (900 mg maximum) twice weekly for 9 months; or rifampin (Rifadin) 10 mg/kg (600 mg maximum) daily for 4 months are effective regimens. Pediatric doses are isoniazid (Nydrazid) 10–20 mg/kg (300 mg maximum) daily or 20–40 mg/kg (900 mg maximum) twice weekly for 9 months; or rifampin (Rifadin) 10–20 mg/kg (600 mg maximum) daily for 4 months. Directly observed therapy must be used with twice-weekly dosing. Pneumococcal vaccine polyvalent (Pneumovax 23, 0.5 mL intramuscularly every 10 years[3]) and yearly influenza immunization should be provided.

---

[3]Exceeds dosage recommended by the manufacturer.

Disclaimer

The findings and conclusions in this report are those of the authors and do not necessarily represent the views of the National Institute for Occupational Safety and Health or the Centers for Disease Control and Prevention.

REFERENCES

American Thoracic Society. Targeted tuberculin testing and treatment of latent tuberculosis infection. MMWR Recomm Rep 2000;49(RR-6):1–54.
Department of Labor. Mine Safety and Health Administration: 30 CFR Parts 56, 57, and 71. Asbestos exposure limit; proposed rule. Fed Reg 2005;70:43950–89.
Miller A. Radiographic readings for asbestosis: Misuse of science—validation of the ILO classification. Am J Ind Med 2007;50:63–7.
Rimal B, Greenberg AK, Rom WN. Basic pathogenic mechanisms of silicosis: Current understanding. Curr Opin Pulm Med 2005;11:169–73.
Ross MH, Murray J. Occupational respiratory disease in mining. Occup Med 2004;54:304–10.
Weissman DN, Banks DE. Silicosis. In: King TE, Schwarz MI, editors. Interstitial Lung Disease. 4th ed. Hamilton, Ontario: B.C. Decker; 2003. p. 387–402.
World Health Organization. Concise international chemical assessment document 24. Crystalline silica quartz. Stuttgart: Wissenschaftliche Verlags GmbH; 2000.

Hypersensitivity Pneumonitis

Method of
David I. Bernstein, MD, and Haejin Kim, MD

Hypersensitivity pneumonitis, also known as extrinsic allergic alveolitis, is an inflammatory disorder of the lungs that is mediated by immunologic hypersensitivity to a specific antigen, usually organic in nature. Table 1 lists causative agents in hypersensitivity pneumonitis.

Pathophysiology

Hypersensitivity pneumonitis is thought to involve primarily type IV (cell-mediated) hypersensitivity. Bronchoalveolar fluid obtained from patients with hypersensitivity pneumonitis shows a predominant CD8+ lymphocytosis supporting T cell–mediated disease. Viruses are thought to play a role in the development of hypersensitivity pneumonitis through upregulation of costimulatory molecules on alveolar macrophages and dendritic cells, leading to increased activation of type 1 helper T cells. Adoptive transfer models in animals have shown that CD4+ T cells and cytotoxic T cells are the most important effector cells in experimental hypersensitivity pneumonitis, rather than cytokines, antibodies, or complement alone.

CURRENT DIAGNOSIS

- Objective evidence of interstitial lung disease by physical exam, spirometry, and radiography associated with exposure to a causative agent
- Improvement in symptoms, lung function, and radiographic abnormalities with avoidance of the causative agent

TABLE 1 Hypersensitivity Pneumonitis: Representative Sources and Causative Agents

Condition or Persons at Risk	Source	Causative Antigens
Dairy farmers	Hay, grains, silage	Thermophilic actinomycetes
Bird fancier's or pigeon breeder's disease	Avian droppings or feathers	Avian proteins
Humidifier lung	Contaminated water	*Aureobasidium pullulans* or other microorganisms
Chemical workers	Polyurethane foam, varnishes, lacquers	Isocyanates
Machine workers	Metalworking fluid	*Pseudomonas fluorescens, Aspergillus niger, Staphylococcus capitis, Rhodococcus* spp., *Bacillus pumilus*
Familial hypersensitivity pneumonitis	Contaminated wood dust in walls	*Bacillus subtilis*
Hot tub lung	Mold on ceiling	*Cladosporium* spp.

From Richerson HB, Bernstein IL, Fink JN, et al: Guidelines for the clinical evaluation of hypersensitivity pneumonitis: Report of the subcommittee on hypersensitivity pneumonitis. J Allergy Clin Immunol 1989;84:839–844; and Hanak V, Golbin JM, Hartman TE, et al: High-resolution CT findings of parenchymal fibrosis correlate with prognosis in hypersensitivity pneumonitis, Chest 2008;134:133–138.

Clinical Presentation and Diagnosis

The main clinical features for hypersensitivity pneumonitis are listed in Table 2. Hypersensitivity pneumonitis is most likely to be diagnosed if the history, physical findings, and pulmonary function tests indicate interstitial lung disease; the chest film is consistent; exposure is documented to a recognized or new causative agent; and there is significant improvement in symptoms, lung function, and radiographic findings with avoidance of the offending cause. Antibody to the offending antigen may be demonstrated but is not required for diagnosis. These are the most widely accepted criteria, but evidence-based diagnostic guidelines have not been established. A careful home, environmental, and occupational history is essential to identify one or more causative antigens.

Treatment

The primary treatment is cessation of exposure to the sources of offending antigens at home or in the workplace. Effective environmental control measures may include modification of work habits, improvement in ventilation, or change in manufacturing procedures. Systemic corticosteroids are often required and aid in recovery during the acute or subacute phases, but there are no long-term studies of their impact on disease progression or survival rates. Referral to a specialist in occupational lung diseases is recommended for proper diagnosis and identification of the sources of causative antigens.

CURRENT THERAPY

- Avoidance of contact with the offending antigen is essential and is often curative if performed early in the course of the disease.
- Systemic corticosteroids are often required during the acute phase of hypersensitivity pneumonitis.

TABLE 2 Clinical Features of Hypersensitivity Pneumonitis

Feature	Acute	Subacute	Chronic
Exposure to antigen	Hours to days	Days to weeks	Months
Symptoms	Influenza-like illness ± cough/dyspnea	Cough and dyspnea with severe cyanosis	Increasing cough and exertional dyspnea; fatigue, weight loss
Physical findings	Fever; lungs normal or bibasilar crackles	Cyanosis; lungs normal or bibasilar crackles	Cyanosis; right-sided heart failure; lungs normal or bibasilar crackles
High-resolution computed tomography	Diffuse ground-glass infiltrates	Reticulation; small centrilobular nodules; air trapping on expiration	Honeycombing, traction bronchiectasis
Pulmonary function testing	↓ FEV_1 and FVC (restrictive pattern); ↓ TLC; ↓ PaO_2 on exercise challenge; ↓ D_{LCO}		
Other findings supportive of a diagnosis of HP	• Positive natural challenge or increase in signs and symptoms on reexposure • Positive precipitating antibodies to HP antigens or antigens cultured directly from the causative environment • Improvement with avoidance • Surgical lung biopsy: interstitial lymphocytic or plasma cell infiltrates and/or noncaseating granulomas; pulmonary fibrosis in advanced cases • BAL lymphocytosis with reduced CD4/CD8 ratio		

From Richerson HB, Bernstein IL, Fink JN, et al: Guidelines for the clinical evaluation of hypersensitivity pneumonitis: Report of the subcommittee on hypersensitivity pneumonitis. J Allergy Clin Immunol 1989;84:839–844; and Bernstein D, Lummus Z, Santilli G, et al: Machine operator's lung: A hypersensitivity pneumonitis disorder associated with exposure to metalworking fluid aerosols. Chest 2006;108:636–641.

Abbreviations: BAL = bronchoalveolar lavage; D_{LCO} = carbon monoxide diffusion in the lungs; FEV_1 = forced expiratory volume in 1 second; FVC = forced vital capacity; HP = hypersensitivity pneumonitis; PaO_2 = arterial partial pressure of oxygen; TLC = total lung capacity.

REFERENCES

Bernstein D, Lummus Z, Santilli G, et al. Machine operator's lung: A hypersensitivity pneumonitis disorder associated with exposure to metalworking fluid aerosols. Chest 2006;108:636–41.

Girard M, Lacasse Y, Cormier Y. Hypersensitivity pneumonitis. Allergy 2009;65:322–34.

Hanak V, Golbin JM, Hartman TE, et al. High-resolution CT findings of parenchymal fibrosis correlate with prognosis in hypersensitivity pneumonitis. Chest 2008;134:133–8.

Jacobs RL, Andrews CP, Coalson JJ. Hypersensitivity pneumonitis: Beyond classic occupation disease: Changing concepts of diagnosis and management. Ann Allergy Asthma Immunol 2005;95:115–28.

Lacasse Y, Assayag E, Cormier Y. Myths and controversies in hypersensitivity pneumonitis. Semin Respir Crit Care Med 2008;29:631–42.

Richerson HB, Bernstein IL, Fink JN, et al. Guidelines for the clinical evaluation of hypersensitivity pneumonitis: Report of the subcommittee on hypersensitivity pneumonitis. J Allergy Clin Immunol 1989;84:839–44.

Schuyler M, Gott K, French V. The role of MIP-1alpha in experimental hypersensitivity pneumonitis. Lung 2004;182:135–49.

Tuberculosis and Other Mycobacterial Diseases

Method of
Jotam Pasipanodya, MD, Ronald Hall II, PharmD, and Tawanda Gumbo, MD

Mycobacterial diseases are some of the oldest documented infectious diseases in humans, and they still cause significant morbidity and mortality. *Mycobacterium tuberculosis* complex, *Mycobacterium avium* complex (MAC), and *Mycobacterium leprae* are slow-growing, acid-fast bacilli that belong to the family Mycobacteriaceae of the order Actinomycetales. This chapter deals with management of diseases caused by *M. tuberculosis*, MAC, and *M. leprae*. A summary of diseases caused by other, less common mycobacteria is presented in Table 1.

Recent evidence suggests that the mycobacteria causing tuberculosis (TB) might have co-evolved with humans. Clues attesting to the success of mycobacteria as human pathogens include the prolonged period of latency and the ability to cause extensive disease in only a narrow host range. DNA evidence suggests that the *M. tuberculosis* strains causing the current waves of TB epidemics most likely evolved from a common ancestor. *Mycobacterium canetti* and the other strains that form the *M. tuberculosis* complex (i.e., *Mycobacterium africanum, Mycobacterium microti*, and *Mycobacterium bovis* strains) also evolved from the ancestral strain through successive loss of DNA. This is contrary to the belief that the *M. tuberculosis* complex evolved from *M. bovis*.

Tuberculosis

EPIDEMIOLOGY

TB remains a global pandemic, with 9.3 million new cases and 1.4 million deaths reported worldwide in 2007. Approximately 1 of every 7 patients who has TB is co-infected with the human immunodeficiency virus (HIV). Whereas global TB incidence trends are stabilizing after reaching a peak in 2004, rates in countries with a low TB burden have been declining gradually. An explanation could be the similar plateau and declines in HIV prevalence observed in the year 2000. On the other hand, this could merely reflect the natural ebbs and increases inherent to epidemic cycles.

Global estimates show that one third of humankind has been infected with *M. tuberculosis*, the TB disease-causing bacillus. About 80% of global TB is accounted for by the 22 high-burden countries. The top five countries in rank order are India, China, Indonesia, Nigeria, and South Africa. TB program priorities and approaches to combating the disease differ among and within countries. These differences are based on the availability of resources and the prevalence of HIV within communities. For example, program goals in areas of low TB incidence, such as the United States, are aimed at TB elimination. Therefore, in the United States, treatment of latent TB is a priority. Reducing TB transmission through increased diagnosis of patients with active TB disease is the primary goal in high-incidence areas.

In 2007, a total of 13,299 TB cases (case rate, 4.4 per 100,000 population) were reported to the Centers for Disease Control and Prevention (CDC) from the 50 U.S. states and the District of

TABLE 1 Species of Mycobacteria

Microbe	Reservoir	Clinical Manifestation
Always Pathogenic in Humans		
M. tuberculosis	Humans	Pulmonary and disseminated tuberculosis
M. bovis	Cattle, humans	TB-like disease
M. africanum	Humans, monkeys	Rarely, TB-like pulmonary disease
M. leprae	Humans	Leprosy
M. canetti	Humans, possibly others	Rarely, TB-like pulmonary disease
Potentially Pathogenic in Humans		
M. avium complex	Soil, water, birds, swine, cattle, environment	Disseminated and pulmonary TB-like disease
M. microti	Rodents, llamas, cats, ferrets, and possibly humans	Rarely, TB-like pulmonary disease
M. kansasii	Water, cattle	TB-like disease
Uncommon or Rarely Pathogenic in Humans		
M. flavescens	Humans, environment	TB-like disease
M. genavense	Humans, birds	Blood-borne disease with AIDS
M. haemophilum	Unknown	Skin, joint, bone, and pulmonary infections in immunocompromised individuals; lymphadenitis in children
M. malmoense	Environment, possibly others	TB-like pulmonary disease in adults; lymphadenitis in children
M. marinum	Fish, water	Skin infections
M. scrofulaceum	Soil, water	Cervical lymphadenitis
M. simiae	Monkeys, water	TB-like pulmonary disease and disseminated disease with AIDS
M. szulgai	Water, environment	TB-like pulmonary disease
M. ulcerans	Humans, environment	Skin infections (Buruli ulcer)
M. xenopi	Water, birds	TB-like pulmonary disease

Adapted from Coberly JS, Chaisson RE: Tuberculosis. In Nelson KE, Williams CM (eds): Infectious Disease Epidemiology: Theory and Practice, 2nd ed. Boston, Jones and Bartlett, 2007.
Abbreviations: M. = genus Mycobacterium; TB = tuberculosis.

Columbia. Foreign-born persons accounted for 58% of the national case total. This means that a high degree of suspicion is needed for the diagnosis of TB when recent immigrants are seen in the clinic. The top five countries of origin for foreign-born persons with TB in the United States were Mexico, the Philippines, India, Vietnam, and China. Since the 1992 TB resurgence peak, the number of cases reported annually in the United States has decreased by 50%.

NATURAL HISTORY

Susceptibility to M. tuberculosis infection and the subsequent progression of that infection to active TB disease is influenced by the complex interaction of host, pathogen, and environmental factors. Between 20% and 30% of people exposed to a person with active TB become infected. Animal models, twin studies, segregation studies, and candidate gene analysis studies provide insight into the role of host genetic factors in susceptibility to TB.

The immune system contains the infection in more than 90% to 95% of persons infected. Protective immunity mediated by subsets of T lymphocytes produces soluble lymphokines that enable macrophages to kill intracellular bacilli. The bacilli are often not completely eradicated and remain dormant in macrophages or other cells, with the potential to reactivate to active disease when the immune system wanes. This is termed latent TB infection (LTBI). The lifetime risk of reactivation to active TB disease is 5% to 10%. This risk of reactivation increases with several factors, including development of the acquired immunodeficiency syndrome (AIDS), renal failure, immunomodulatory therapy, and poorly controlled diabetes mellitus.

In a small subgroup of patients, M. tuberculosis infection is not brought under control during primary infection and quickly progresses to disseminated disease. TB that follows such a course is called progressive primary TB. Primary TB is associated with a higher mortality rate, and death typically occurs within 2 years after infection. The risk of developing TB disease after being infected is higher in males from infancy to 6 years of age. Males older than 45 years of age are also at an increased risk compared to females of the same age.

Diagnosis of Active Tuberculosis

In immunocompetent persons, pulmonary involvement is the most common presentation, followed by isolated extrapulmonary disease. Involvement of only extrapulmonary sites is rare, and most immunocompromised patients present with both pulmonary and extrapulmonary involvement. The presenting signs and symptoms of active TB disease are site specific. However, constitutional symptoms such as fever, night sweats, and fatigue are common and gradually evolve over many weeks. Patients should be specifically asked about constitutional symptoms, because these symptoms raise the index of suspicion. Atypical presentations are common in patients who are immunosuppressed and can delay diagnosis.

Definitive diagnosis is made on the basis of a positive culture. Therefore, all patients with suspected TB must have the appropriate specimens collected for microscopic and, if appropriate, histologic examination. Mycobacterial culture and sensitivity testing should also be performed, if available. Acid-fast bacillus (AFB) staining and microscopy is limited by poor sensitivity (45%-80% with culture-confirmed TB cases) and poor positive predictive value (50%-80%) for TB in settings where nontuberculous mycobacteria are commonly isolated. TB culture results are available only after 2 to 6 weeks. Nucleic acid amplification (NAA) testing can also be used to confirm a TB diagnosis in 24 to 48 hours, even when the specimen sample is limited. NAA tests can detect the presence of M. tuberculosis in 50% to 80% of AFB-negative and culture-positive specimens. The CDC now recommends that evaluation of at least the first diagnostic specimen include NAA testing.

Serial radiologic images can be used to exclude active TB and assess clinical improvement.

Principles of Treatment

The goal of anti-TB therapy is cure. A secondary objective is minimizing the transmission of M. tuberculosis to others by curing the patient. Treatment outcomes are best when patient-centered treatments and care are offered, regardless of whether the treatment facility is private or public. Patient management and supervision plans should be tailored to the patient's clinical and social circumstances. Directly observed therapy (DOT) is recommended by regulatory bodies to help ensure adherence to treatment and is regarded as central to current case management. However, the efficacy of DOT compared with self-administration has been questioned in recent studies. There are three types of anti-TB therapy: prophylaxis, definitive TB therapy for drug-susceptible infection, and therapy for drug-resistant TB.

CHEMOPROPHYLAXIS

The confusing terms preventive therapy and chemoprophylaxis are sometimes used to describe treatment of LTBI. Preventive therapy, in this context, does not actually prevent infection; rather, it prevents development of active TB in those already infected. Therefore, the better descriptive term, treatment of LTBI, is preferred. Treatment of minimal or latent TB infection prevents subsequent evolution to active disease. A series of double-blind, placebo-controlled clinical trials done in the 1950s and 1960s provided evidence demonstrating the effectiveness of treatment of LTBI. Priority is usually given to those patients with the highest risk for reactivation.

Treatment of LTBI, particularly when it is targeted toward persons with higher risks of reactivation, is one of the major strategies for elimination of TB in the United States. Targets include people who have been recently infected and those who were remotely infected but have concurrent disease that puts them at higher risk for developing reactivation disease. There are more than 11 million people with LTBI in the United States, each with a 5% to 10% lifetime risk of developing TB disease.

The Mantoux method of tuberculin skin testing is commonly used to diagnose LTBI as well as active disease. Use of tuberculin skin testing is hampered by low sensitivity in immunocompromised patients, low specificity in persons who have received the bacille Calmette-Guérin (BCG) vaccine, and the requirement to return to a trained person to have the test read after 48 to 72 hours. Results are interpreted based on the patient scenario (Box 1).

Recently, various blood-testing methods that are based on detection of the interferon-γ (IFN-γ) released by T lymphocytes in response to *M. tuberculosis*–specific antigens have become available as an alternative to skin testing. These tests may be more specific than the tuberculin skin test in BCG-vaccinated and immunocompromised populations. However, IFN-γ release assays do not differentiate LTBI from active TB disease. Currently available IFN-γ release assays are QuantiFERON, QuantiFERON-Gold, and ELISPOT. The CDC recommends these tests for LTBI screening of health care workers, recent immigrants, injection drug users, prison and jail inmates and workers, and contacts of TB cases within schools, workplaces, and the military. Prohibitive costs limit the use of these assays in resource-limited places.

Table 2 summarizes the regimens currently recommended by the American Thoracic Society (ATS), CDC, and Infectious Diseases Society of America (IDSA) for treatment of LTBI. Because of high rates of hospitalization and death from liver injury, the ATS and the CDC no longer recommend the 2-month regimen of daily or twice-weekly rifampin (Rifadin) plus pyrazinamide for LTBI. Rifampin or rifabutin (Mycobutin)[1] may be used to treat LTBI in HIV-infected persons exposed to TB that is resistant to isoniazid (INH; Nydrazid) and susceptible to rifampin, with dose adjustments and diligence taken to prevent cytochrome P-450–derived drug interactions with antiretroviral agents.

DEFINITIVE THERAPY

The decision to initiate therapy is made based on local epidemiologic information; the patient's clinical, pathologic, and radiologic data; and the results of microscopic and culture examination. Therapy may be started immediately if the index of suspicion is high or if the patient is gravely ill. However, in general, clinicians should still collect initial specimens for microscopic evaluation and culture before starting treatment. HIV testing and baseline liver function testing, serum creatinine levels, and platelet counts should be conducted as part of standard medical care for patients with suspected or documented TB disease.

---

[1]Not FDA approved for this indication.

BOX 1 Interpretation of a Tuberculin Skin Test

Reaction ≥5 mm of Induration

HIV-positive persons
Recent contacts of TB case patients
Fibrotic changes on chest radiography consistent with prior TB
Organ transplant recipients and other immunosuppressed patients (receiving the equivalent of ≥15 mg/d of prednisone for 1 mo or longer)*

Reaction >10 mm of Induration

Recent immigrants (i.e., ≤5 y) from high-prevalence countries
Injection drug users
Residents and employees[†] of the following high-risk congregate settings:
- Prisons and jails
- Nursing homes and other long-term facilities for the elderly
- Hospitals and other health care facilities
- Residential facilities for patients with AIDS
- Homeless shelters
- Mycobacteriology laboratory personnel

Persons with the following clinical conditions that place them at high risk:
- Silicosis
- Diabetes mellitus
- Chronic renal failure
- Certain hematologic disorders (e.g., leukemias, lymphomas)
- Other specific malignancies (e.g., carcinoma of the head, neck, or lung)
- Weight loss (>10% of ideal body weight)
- Gastrectomy and jejunoileal bypass

Children <4 yr of age; infants, children, and adolescents exposed to adults at high risk

Reaction >15 mm of Induration

Persons with no risk factors for TB

Adapted from Centers for Disease Control and Prevention: Screening for tuberculosis and tuberculosis infection in high-risk populations: Recommendations of the Advisory Council for the Elimination of Tuberculosis. Morb Mortal Wkly Rep MMWR 1995;44(No. RR-11):19–34.
*Risk of TB in patients treated with corticosteroids increases with higher dose and longer duration.
[†]For persons who are otherwise at low risk and are tested at the start of employment, a reaction of >15 mm induration is considered positive.
Abbreviations: AIDS = acquired immunodeficiency syndrome; HIV = human immunodeficiency syndrome; TB = tuberculosis.

Achieving microbiologic cure by killing all bacilli and preventing emergence of clinically significant drug-resistant mutants are the primary goals of definitive TB therapy. Therapy is prolonged despite sputum conversion and resolution of symptoms, because some organisms persist in some tissues. DOT is generally recommended to ensure compliance with prescribed medications.

The four ATS/CDC/IDSA-recommended regimens used for treating TB caused by drug-susceptible organisms are shown in Table 3. Each regimen has an initial phase of 2 months followed

TABLE 2 CDC-Recommended Treatment for Latent Tuberculosis Infection

Drug	Interval*	Oral Dose (mg/kg) Children	Adults	Monitoring
Isoniazid (INH, Nydrazid)	Daily	10–20[3]	5	Monthly, LFTs[†] at baseline, repeat in selected patients if initial results are abnormal; hepatitis risk increases with age and alcohol consumption; pyridoxine[1] 10–25 mg/d may prevent peripheral neuropathy and CNS effects
	Twice weekly	20–40[3]	15	
Rifampin (Rifadin)	Daily	10–20	10	Weeks 2, 4, and 8 with pyrazinamide; contraindicated in patients receiving antiretroviral drugs; baseline
	Twice weekly	—	10	LFTs[†] and CBC and platelets
Rifabutin (Mycobutin)[1]	Daily	—	5	Weeks 2, 4, and 8; baseline LFTs[†] and CBC and platelets; use adjusted daily doses of rifabutin and monitor for decreased antiretroviral activity and rifabutin toxicity if PIs or NNRTIs are taken concurrently; contraindicated with saquinavir (Invirase) or delavirdine (Rescriptor)
	Twice weekly	—	5	
Pyrazinamide[‡]	Daily	—	15-20	Weeks 2, 4, and 8; LFTs[†] at baseline; avoid in first trimester of pregnancy
	Twice weekly	—	50	

Adapted from American Thoracic Society: Treatment of tuberculosis. Am J Respir Crit Care Med 2003;167:603–662.
[1]Not FDA approved for this indication.
[3]Exceeds dosage recommended by the manufacturer.
*All intermittent dosing should be given by directly observed therapy (DOT).
[†]LFTs include aspartate aminotransferase (AST), alanine aminotransferase (ALT), and serum albumin.
[‡]Used with either rifampin or rifabutin in combination therapy for 2–4 mo.
Abbreviations: CBC = complete blood count; CDC = Centers for Disease Control and Prevention; CNS = central nervous system; LFT = liver function test; NNRTI = non-nucleoside reverse transcriptase inhibitor; PI protease inhibitor.

by a choice of several options for the continuation phase of 4 or 7 months. Treatment of previously untreated TB consists of 2 months of an initial phase of four drugs: isoniazid, rifampin, pyrazinamide, and ethambutol (Myambutol) or streptomycin (generally not used in the United States). The newer rifamycins are also first-line drugs used under certain circumstances. Rifabutin[1] is used if rifampin is contraindicated, as in patients taking certain antiretroviral drugs; rifapentine (Priftin) is used in the once-weekly continuation phase with isoniazid in selected patients (see Table 3). If the organisms are later demonstrated to be susceptible to isoniazid and rifampin, ethambutol is discontinued. The continuation phase is usually 4 months of daily or intermittent isoniazid and rifampin or rifapentine. The 7-month continuation phase is recommended only for those patients with cavitary TB caused by susceptible organisms that remains sputum positive after 2 months of DOT, patients whose initial treatment phase did not include pyrazinamide, and patients on weekly isoniazid and rifapentine whose sputum smear was still positive at the end of the intensive phase. There is evidence from many clinical trials done worldwide that demonstrates the efficacy of supervised intermittent therapy is similar to daily dosing in terms of various clinical outcomes. Routine follow-up to monitor adverse events and adherence to the treatment regimen should occur at least monthly.

Approximately 80% of patients who take the four-drug therapy for susceptible organisms are expected to convert from culture positive to negative after 2 months, and 90% to 95% after 3 months. Failure of treatment is defined by positive culture or, at times, positive smears after 4 months of supervised therapy. Relapse is defined by recurrent TB at any time after completion of treatment or apparent cure. Relapses most commonly occur during the first 6 to 12 months after the end of therapy. Treatment of initially susceptible disease can fail for many reasons, including extensive cavitary disease, drug resistance, malabsorption of drugs, laboratory error, and biologic variation in response. In any case, positive smears or cultures after 2 months of supervised therapy should be carefully evaluated to determine the cause. In addition, a full course of therapy is determined by the number of doses completed. Hence, a 6-month daily regimen (including both initiation and continuation phases) consists of at least 182 doses of isoniazid and rifampin and 56 doses of pyrazinamide (see Table 3). All missed doses should be taken. Patients interrupting therapy by more than 14 days during the initial phase or more than 3 months during continuation phase should be restarted on therapy from the beginning.

TREATMENT OF TUBERCULOSIS IN RESOURCE-POOR SETTINGS

Direct observation of patients taking therapy is just one of five elements of DOTS recommended by the World Health Organization and the International Union Against Tuberculosis and Lung Disease for TB treatment programs in resource-poor settings. The five elements of DOTS are:

- Government commitment to sustained TB control activities
- Case detection by sputum microscopy in symptomatic patients self-reporting to health centers
- Standardized treatment regimen of 6 to 9 months for at least all confirmed sputum smear-positive cases, with DOT for at least the intensive phase
- Regular, uninterrupted supply of essential anti-TB drugs
- Standardized recording and reporting system that allows for patient and program assessments

Smear microscopy for AFB is emphasized because of cost concerns and because access to culture facilities is limited in most countries. Three AFB stains that include early-morning sputum smears are recommended for a diagnosis. However, some recent data refute the need for three sputum samples by suggesting that no significant benefit is derived from the third smear when performed in high-burden countries.

Susceptibility testing is strongly recommended for patients who fail to convert to smear-negative status after 2 months of treatment. The prevalence of drug resistance in areas of high TB burden is unknown because of limited laboratory capacity.

Individualized TB care in resource-limited areas is difficult to implement because most decisions are made based solely on clinical judgment or limited radiologic findings. These challenges result in the use of standardized treatments that emphasize cost-effectiveness for utilitarian returns. This "one size fits all" approach is likely to worsen the financial and clinical outcomes of some patients.

[1]Not FDA approved for this indication.

TABLE 3 Drug Regimen for Culture-Positive Pulmonary Tuberculosis Caused by Drug-Susceptible Organisms

Regimen	Drugs	Interval and Minimum Duration*	Dose (Maximum Dose in 24 h or Maximum Duration) Children	Adults
Initial Phase				
1	Isoniazid (INH, Nydrazid)	Once daily on 7 d/wk for 56 doses (8 wk), or	10–20 mg/kg/d[3] (300 mg)	5 mg/kg/d (300 mg)
	Rifampin (Rifadin)	Once daily on 5 d/wk for 40 doses (8 wk)	10–20 mg/kg/d (600 mg)	10 mg/kg/d (600 mg)
	Pyrazinamide		15–30 mg/kg/d (2000 mg)	15–30 mg/kg/d (2000 mg)
	Ethambutol (Myambutol)		15–25 mg/kg/d	15–25 mg/kg/d
2	Isoniazid	Once daily on 7 d/wk for 14 doses (2 wk), then twice weekly for 12 doses (6 wk), or	20–40 mg/kg/d (900 mg)	15 mg/kg/d (900 mg)
	Rifampin		10–20 mg/kg/d (600 mg)	10 mg/kg/d (900 mg)[3]
	Pyrazinamide		50–70 mg/kg/d (4000 mg)	50–70 mg/kg/d (4000 mg)
	Ethambutol	Once daily on 5 d/wk for 10 doses (2 wk), then twice weekly for 12 doses (6 wk)	50 mg/kg/d[3]	50 mg/kg/d[3]
3	Isoniazid	Three times weekly for 24 doses (8 wk)	20–40 mg/kg/d (900 mg)	15 mg/kg/d (900 mg)
	Rifampin		10–20 mg/kg/d (600 mg)	10 mg/kg/d (900 mg)[3]
	Pyrazinamide		50–70 mg/kg/d (3000 mg)	50–70 mg/kg/d (3000 mg)
	Ethambutol		50 mg/kg/d[3]	50 mg/kg/d[3]
4	Isoniazid	Once daily on 7 d/wk for 56 doses (8 wk), or		
	Rifampin			
	Ethambutol	Once daily on 5 d/wk for 40 doses (8 wk)		
Continuation Phase†				
1a	Isoniazid	Once daily on 7 d/wk for 126 doses (18 wk), or	182–130 doses (max. 26 wk)	
	Rifampin	Once daily on 5 d/wk for 90 doses (18 wk)		
1b‡	Isoniazid	Twice weekly for 36 doses (18 wk)	92–76 doses (max. 26 wk)	
	Rifampin			
1c§	Isoniazid	Once weekly for 18 doses (18 wk)	74–58 doses (max. 26 wk)	
	Rifapentine			
2a†	Isoniazid	Twice weekly for 36 doses (18 wk)	62–58 doses (max. 26 wk)	
	Rifampin			
2b§	Isoniazid	Once weekly for 18 doses (18 wk)	44–40 doses (max. 26 wk)	
	Rifapentine (Priftin)			
3a	Isoniazid	Three times weekly for 54 doses (18 wk)	78 doses (max. 26 wk)	
	Rifampin			
4a	Isoniazid	Once daily on 7 d/wk for 217 doses (31 wk), or	273–195 doses (max. 39 wk)	
	Rifampin	Once daily on 5 d/wk for 155 doses (31 wk)		
4b	Isoniazid	Twice weekly for 62 doses (31 wk)	118–102 doses (max. 39 wk)	
	Rifampin			

Adapted from the American Thoracic Society: Treatment of tuberculosis. Am J Respir Crit Care Med 2003;167:603–662.

[3]Exceeds dosage recommended by the manufacturer.

*When directly observed therapy (DOT) is used, drugs may be given on 5 d/wk, with the necessary number of doses adjusted accordingly; therapy administered on 5 d/wk should always be given by DOT.

†Patients with cavitation on initial chest radiography and positive cultures at 2 mo should receive a 7-mo (31-wk) regimen of either 217 (daily) or 62 (twice weekly) doses in the continuation phase

‡Not recommended for HIV-infected patients with CD4+ T-cell count <100 cells/mm³.

§Use only in HIV-negative patients who have negative smears at 2 mo and no cavitation on chest radiography.

TREATMENT OF TUBERCULOSIS IN SPECIAL CIRCUMSTANCES

Multidrug-Resistant Tuberculosis

In resource-poor settings, where susceptibility testing facilities usually are not available, the surrogate terms "retreatment" and "chronic" are used to define various forms of drug-resistant strains. In the United States, about 1.1% of TB cases reported in 2007 had primary multidrug resistance, which is defined as resistance to at least isoniazid and rifampin in a patient with no previous history of TB treatment. Combination therapy including first- and second-line drugs is used to treat multidrug-resistant TB, and at least one of the drugs must be an injectable agent. Some of the second-line TB drugs are levofloxacin (Levaquin),[1] cycloserine (Seromycin), ethionamide (Trecator), p-aminosalicylic-acid (Paser), capreomycin (Capastat), kanamycin (Kantrex),[1] and amikacin (Amikin).[1]

Therapy takes several years to complete. Treatment failure, costs, and drug-related side-effects are higher with the second-line drugs. Patients with suspected treatment failure should be managed at specialized facilities with necessary expertise where the full range of drug susceptibilities can be performed. As a general rule, single drugs should never be added to failing regimens because this leads to acquired resistance to each new drug. Drug resistance in

---

[1]Not FDA approved for this indication.

mycobacteria occurs through random genetic mutations, with minimal lateral transfer of genetic material. Chances of detecting primary resistance are greater when the bacillary load is high, for example in patients with multiple cavitary disease. In addition, selective pressure can induce the emergence of drug-resistant mutants.

Extrapulmonary and Sputum-Negative Tuberculosis

TB can involve any organ or tissue in the body. Therefore, histologic examination or smear microscopy with AFB staining of specimens from appropriate sites is necessary to confirm extrapulmonary TB. The specimens may include cerebrospinal, pleural, pericardial, or ascitic fluids and lymph node tissue, bone, bone marrow, or brain biopsy specimens. The yield of bacilli in staining or culture from body fluids is usually very low (<50% for pericardial fluid). A diagnosis of extrapulmonary TB can also be made based on clinical and radiologic improvement on empiric therapy if it is not possible to obtain a specimen.

The same four drugs and dosing regimens used to treat pulmonary TB are also used for extrapulmonary disease. Use of adjunct corticosteroids in patients with pericardial or meningeal TB was associated with lower mortality in some prospective and retrospective studies. Bone and joint TB is treated for 6 to 9 months, and central nervous system TB (including meningitis) for 9 to 12 months. Duration of treatment for TB in all other sites is 6 months if pyrazinamide is given during the first 2 months; otherwise, the continuation phase is prolonged to 7 months. The ATS/CDC/IDSA guidelines also recommend intermittent therapy. Once-weekly administration of isoniazid and rifapentine should be avoided in the continuation phase, because data to support the efficacy of this regimen in patients with extrapulmonary TB is lacking. However, recent data report poor long-term outcomes despite adequate therapy in patients successfully treated for pericardial and meningeal TB. These and other studies question the wisdom of using the same drug exposures to target organisms in different physiologic spaces, given that drug penetration, and therefore drug concentrations, in these spaces differs.

A diagnosis of sputum-negative TB is made in patients for whom the clinical and radiologic findings strongly suggest TB but the culture and AFB smears are negative. In addition, there is clinical and/or radiologic improvements at the end of 2 months of therapy. A 2-month continuation phase of isoniazid and rifampin is used for these patients, rather than the 4 months used for sputum-positive patients.

Mycobacterium avium Complex Infection

In patients with advanced AIDS and other causes of severe cell-mediated immune deficiency, MAC cause disseminated infections. In others with ill-defined immunologic disorders, and in those who are immunocompetent, MAC causes chronic pulmonary disease. Therapy for these patients is long and complicated, with many adverse effects. The same regimens are used for all patients regardless of their HIV/AIDS status. Drug resistance is frequent.

Culture from blood or other sites (e.g., lymph node, bone marrow) is required to demonstrate invasive or disseminated disease. Bacteriologic diagnosis should be based on positive cultures or smears (or both) from sputum or bronchial wash specimens. If sputum specimens are used to diagnose pulmonary disease, at least three positive sputum smears are needed for diagnosis. Clinical and radiologic findings must also be consistent with MAC.

Combination therapy is used to prevent selection of drug-resistant mutants and to capitalize on the additive and synergistic effects of antimycobacterial drugs. Clarithromycin (Biaxin) or azithromycin (Zithromax) together with ethambutol is now the cornerstone of MAC therapy. Three- or four-drug combinations that included ethambutol, a rifamycin (rifampin[1] or rifabutin), clofazimine (Lamprene),[1] isoniazid,[1] or ciprofloxacin (Cipro)[1] were shown to clear bacteremia better in some AIDS patients, especially those with a

bacillary burden of greater than $2 \log_{10}$ colony-forming units per milliliter. However, adherence to therapy was poor because of toxicity. Two-way interactions between antiretroviral medications (e.g. protease inhibitors, non-nucleoside reverse transcriptase inhibitors) and the rifamycins as well as clarithromycin and rifabutin can make patient management complicated. AIDS patients with CD4-positive T-cell counts lower than 50 cells/mm^3 should be offered prophylactic therapy to protect against disseminated MAC. Azithromycin has greater efficacy, has fewer drug interactions, and can be given once weekly. Resistance has been observed in 16% of patients treated with azithromycin and in 29% to 58% of those treated with clarithromycin. Resistance of MAC to rifamycin is rare.

Mycobacterium leprae

Leprosy is a legendary disease that has been stigmatized throughout many societies and eras of human history. The causative organism is *M. leprae*. The global incidence of this disease has been on the decline. Fewer than 200 cases are diagnosed each year in the United States, almost exclusively in immigrants. Most practitioners in the United States will not encounter patients with this disease.

The important clinical features of leprosy are skin lesions, nerve involvement, disfigurement of the face, and reversal reactions. Skin lesions are hypopigmented anesthetic macules and papules. Peripheral nerve enlargement can also occur, as can disfigurement of parts of the face (e.g., leonine faces). Leprosy has a spectrum of manifestations. Some patients have multibacillary leprosy associated with poor cell-mediated immunity. Others have paucibacillary leprosy resulting in a few skin patches with a robust cell-mediated immunity. Skin reactions encountered in paucibacillary leprosy due to delayed hypersensitivity to *M. leprae* antigens are called reversal reactions. These may also occur when massive numbers of bacilli are killed by chemotherapy.

Diagnosis is established on the basis of a compatible clinical picture and demonstration of *M. leprae* in smears or on histologic analysis of skin and nerve biopsy specimens. The lepromin skin test is nonreactive in multibacillary disease but reactive in paucibacillary disease. Unlike other mycobacteria, *M. leprae* has stringent growth requirements; it can only grow when injected into foot pads of some animals and does not grow on artificial laboratory media.

The aim of leprosy treatment is total cure. As with other slow-growing mycobacteria, multidrug therapy is administered. Therapy consists of rifampin,[1] clofazimine (Lamprene), and dapsone. Recently, fluoroquinolones have been investigated for a role in the treatment of leprosy. In the United States, the therapy for paucibacillary leprosy is oral rifampin 600 mg/day and dapsone 100 mg/day for 6 months, followed by dapsone monotherapy for at least 3 years. The treatment of multibacillary leprosy is similar to that of paucibacillary leprosy, with dual therapy being continued for 3 years. Clofazimine is added for reverse reactions and if there is dapsone resistance. After 3 years of dual or even triple therapy, dapsone monotherapy is continued for 10 years. These regimens differ from those recommended by the World Health Organisation, which are utilized elsewhere.

Mycobacteria Other Than Tuberculosis

Mycobacteria other than tuberculosis (MOTT) are mycobacterial species that may cause human disease but do not cause TB (see Table 1). The incidence of infection is reported to be about 2 in 100,000, but this may be an underestimate. The common mycobacteria identified in the United States are *M. avium, Mycobacterium gordonae, Mycobacterium fortuitum, Mycobacterium kansasii,* and *Mycobacterium chelonae.* MOTT infections are not contagious, but some produce signs and symptoms similar to those of TB, whereas others cause suppurative-like disease. MOTT primarily affect the lungs, and disease progression is slow. MOTT cause reportable disease.

---

[1]Not FDA approved for this indication.

[1]Not FDA approved for this indication.

Diagnosis is based on clinical presentation, radiologic findings, examination of histologic specimens, culture, and smear staining for microscopy of sputa or bronchial washings. The diagnostic criteria for MOTT in AIDS and non-AIDS patients are

- Chest radiographs showing infiltrates or nodular or cavitary disease or computed tomographic scans consistent with bronchiectasis or small nodules
- Three positive cultures with negative AFB smears or two positive cultures and one positive AFB smear from three sputum or bronchial washing specimens obtained within the previous 12 months
- Positive culture from bronchial wash with AFB smear or growth on solid media greater than 2+
- Transbronchial or lung biopsy consistent with mycobacterium histologic features and sputum or bronchial washings that are non-diagnostic of another disease.
- For mycobacteria other than tuberculosis such as *M. abscessus/chelonae* therapy is more with standard antibiotics like ceftriaxone. However, all these patients should be reported to specialist centers.

REFERENCES

Agins BD, Berman DS, Spicehandler D, et al. Effect of combined therapy with ansamycin, clofazimine, ethambutol, and isoniazid for *Mycobacterium avium* infection in patients with AIDS. J Infect Dis 1989;159:784–7.

American Thoracic Society, Centers for Disease Control and Prevention, Council of the Infectious Diseases Society of America. Diagnostic standards and classification of tuberculosis in adults and children. Am J Respir Crit Care Med 2000;161:1376–95.

Bach MC. Treating disseminated *Mycobacterium avium-intracellulare* infection. Ann Intern Med 1989;110:169–70.

Bellamy R, Beyers N, McAdam KP, et al. Genetic susceptibility to tuberculosis in Africans: A genome-wide scan. Proc Natl Acad Sci U S A 2000;97:8005–9.

Blumberg HM, Burman WJ, Chaisson RE, et al. American Thoracic Society/Centers for Disease Control and Prevention/Infectious Diseases Society of America: Treatment of tuberculosis. Am J Respir Crit Care Med 2003;167:603–62.

Brosch R, Gordon SV, Marmiesse M, et al. A new evolutionary scenario for the *Mycobacterium tuberculosis* complex. Proc Natl Acad Sci U S A 2002;99:3684–9.

Cegielski JP, Devlin BH, Morris AJ, et al. Comparison of PCR, culture, and histopathology for diagnosis of tuberculous pericarditis. J Clin Microbiol 1997;35:3254–7.

Centers for Disease Control and Prevention. Reported Tuberculosis in the United States, 2007. Atlanta: U.S. Department of Health and Human Services, CDC; 2007.

Comstock GW. Frost revisited: The modern epidemiology of tuberculosis. Am J Epidemiol 1975;101:363–82.

Comstock GW. Tuberculosis in twins: A re-analysis of the Prophit survey. Am Rev Respir Dis 1978;117:621–4.

Comstock GW, Livesay VT, Woolpert SF. Evaluation of BCG vaccination among Puerto Rican children. Am J Public Health 1974;64:283–91.

Dannenberg AM Jr. Delayed-type hypersensitivity and cell-mediated immunity in the pathogenesis of tuberculosis. Immunol Today 1991;12:228–33.

Engel ME, Matchaba PT, Volmink J. Corticosteroids for tuberculous pleurisy. Cochrane Database Syst Rev 2007;(4) CD001876.

Guerra RL, Hooper NM, Baker JF, et al. Use of the amplified *Mycobacterium tuberculosis* direct test in a public health laboratory: Test performance and impact on clinical care. Chest 2007;132:946–51.

Guerra RL, Hooper NM, Baker JF, et al. Cost-effectiveness of different strategies for amplified *Mycobacterium tuberculosis* direct testing for cases of pulmonary tuberculosis. J Clin Microbiol 2008;46:3811–2.

Gumbo T, Louie A, Deziel MR, et al. Concentration-dependent *Mycobacterium tuberculosis* killing and prevention of resistance by rifampin. Antimicrob Agents Chemother 2007;51:3781–8.

Gumbo T, Louie A, Liu W, et al. Isoniazid bactericidal activity and resistance emergence: Integrating pharmacodynamics and pharmacogenomics to predict efficacy in different ethnic populations. Antimicrob Agents Chemother 2007;51:2329–36.

Haas CJ, Zink A, Palfi G, et al. Detection of leprosy in ancient human skeletal remains by molecular identification of *Mycobacterium leprae*. Am J Clin Pathol 2000;114:428–36.

Iseman MD. A Clinician's Guide to Tuberculosis. Philadelphia: Lippincott Williams & Wilkins; 2000.

Kallmann FJ, Reisner D. Twin studies on the significance of genetic factors in tuberculosis. Am Rev Tuberculosis 1943;47:549–74.

Kramnik I, Demant P, Bloom BB. Susceptibility to tuberculosis as a complex genetic trait: Analysis using recombinant congenic strains of mice. Novartis Found Symp 1998;217:120–31.

Kramnik I, Dietrich WF, Demant P, Bloom BR. Genetic control of resistance to experimental infection with virulent *Mycobacterium tuberculosis*. Proc Natl Acad Sci U S A 2000;97:8560–5.

Mabaera B, Lauritsen JM, Katamba A, et al. Sputum smear-positive tuberculosis: Empiric evidence challenges the need for confirmatory smears. Int J Tuberc Lung Dis 2007;11:959–64.

Mabaera B, Lauritsen JM, Katamba A, et al. Making pragmatic sense of data in the tuberculosis laboratory register. Int J Tuberc Lung Dis 2008;12:294–300.

Mayosi BM, Wiysonge CS, Ntsekhe M, et al. Clinical characteristics and initial management of patients with tuberculous pericarditis in the HIV era: The Investigation of the Management of Pericarditis in Africa (IMPI Africa) registry. BMC Infect Dis 2006;6:2.

Mayosi BM, Wiysonge CS, Ntsekhe M, et al. Mortality in patients treated for tuberculous pericarditis in sub-Saharan Africa. S Afr Med J 2008;98:36–40.

Moonan PK, Weis SE. Assessing the impact of targeted tuberculosis interventions. Am J Respir Crit Care Med 2008;177:557–8.

Moore DF, Guzman JA, Mikhail LT. Reduction in turnaround time for laboratory diagnosis of pulmonary tuberculosis by routine use of a nucleic acid amplification test. Diagn Microbiol Infect Dis 2005;52:247–54.

Nerlich AG, Haas CJ, Zink A, et al. Molecular evidence for tuberculosis in an ancient Egyptian mummy. Lancet 1997;350:1404.

Nuermberger E, Grosset J. Pharmacokinetic and pharmacodynamic issues in the treatment of mycobacterial infections. Eur J Clin Microbiol Infect Dis 2004;23:243–55.

Prasad K, Singh MB. Corticosteroids for managing tuberculous meningitis. Cochrane Database Syst Rev 2000;(1) CD002244.

Stein CM, Nshuti L, Chiunda AB, et al. Evidence for a major gene influence on tumor necrosis factor-alpha expression in tuberculosis: Path and segregation analysis. Hum Hered 2005;60:109–18.

Stein CM, Zalwango S, Malone LL, et al. Genome scan of *M. tuberculosis* infection and disease in Ugandans. PLoS ONE 2008;3:e4094.

Volmink J, Garner P. Directly observed therapy for treating tuberculosis. Cochrane Database Syst Rev 2007;(4) CD003343.

Weis SE, Miller TL, Hilsenrath PE, Moonan PK. Comprehensive cost description of tuberculosis care. Int J Tuberc Lung Dis 2005;9:467–8.

World Health Organisation. Global leprosy situation. Wkly Epidemiol Rec 2005;80:289–95.

World Health Organisation. Global Tuberculosis Control: Epidemiology, Strategy, Financing: WHO Report 2009. Geneva: WHO; 2009.

Zink A, Haas CJ, Reischl U, et al. Molecular analysis of skeletal tuberculosis in an ancient Egyptian population. J Med Microbiol 2001;50:355–66.

The Cardiovascular System

Acquired Diseases of the Aorta

Method of
Srijoy Mahapatra, MD, and Gorav Ailawadi, MD

Aortic disease can occur anywhere along the length of the aorta. The most common conditions are aneurysms, dissections, and traumatic injury. Traditional open surgical treatment is being replaced by less invasive endovascular therapy. Medical therapy may be helpful in slowing progression and can mitigate the risk factors for aortic disease.

Aortic Aneurysms

An aortic aneurysm is a dilation of the vessel beyond at least 50% of the expected baseline. Although the baseline varies among individuals, the mean diameters of the ascending, descending, and abdominal aorta are 2.8, 2.5, and 2 cm, respectively. Aneurysms most commonly affect the infrarenal abdominal aorta (AAA). The most cited risk factors for aneurysms include smoking (fivefold increased risk), age greater than 60 years, male gender, hypertension, family history of aneurysm, and hyperlipidemia. Notably, black race, female gender, and diabetes are negatively associated with AAA.

Although many of the risk factors are associated with occlusive vascular and coronary disease, the pathophysiology of aortic aneurysm appears to be different. At a molecular level, aneurysms are characterized by inflammatory cell infiltration, release of matrix-degrading enzymes, and destruction of the aortic wall media. Specifically, matrix metalloproteinases 1, 2, 3, 9, 12, and 13 are known to be upregulated in aortic aneurysm walls. The inciting event for this process is unclear, although an immune-regulated phenomenon has been suggested. The destruction of extracellular matrix proteins, collagen and elastin, in combination with smooth muscle cell apoptosis weakens the wall and leads to aortic wall dilation.

Thoracic aortic aneurysms include both ascending aortic aneurysms and descending thoracic aortic aneurysms (DTAA). The causes of thoracic aneurysms include cystic medial necrosis, familial diseases (see below), Takayasu's arteritis, and previous aortic dissection. Historically, syphilis was an important cause of thoracic aneurysms, but in current practice this is rare.

Inflammatory aneurysms are nonbacterial, sterile aneurysms with an intense periaortic inflammatory infiltrate; they are associated with retroperitoneal fibrosis. Despite the misnomer, mycotic aneurysms involve bacterial (not fungal) infiltration of the vessel wall, most commonly by *Staphylococcus aureus, Salmonella,* and *Streptococcus* species, resulting in subacute aneurysmal dilation.

INCIDENCE AND NATURAL HISTORY

The incidence of aortic aneurysms is estimated to be as high as 100 per 100,000 person-years. About 9% of men older than 65 years of age have an AAA, as do 15% of men older than age 75. Aneurysms typically grow at a rate of approximately 10% (2–4 mm) per year.

The aorta resists rupture by means of its strong extracellular matrix. As this weakens, the wall expands. The Law of LaPlace predicts that the larger the diameter, the more wall tension is placed on the already weakened wall. This leads to more dilation and sets up a positive feedback loop. Thus, the risk of rupture is proportional to aneurysm size. For example, estimates for annual AAA rupture risk increase by diameter: 5 to 6 cm, 6% rupture risk per year; 6 to 7 cm, 20% risk; 7 to 8 cm, 30% risk; and more than 8 cm, more than 40% risk. Because women have a higher risk of rupture at each diameter, earlier repair may be warranted.

Whereas AAAs tend to rupture, ascending aortic aneurysms tend to dissect. DTAA can either rupture or dissect. Ascending aortic aneurysms larger than 5.5 cm have a 5% annual risk of dissection. DTAAs larger than 6 cm have an 8% annual risk of rupture or dissection.

FAMILIAL DISEASES

Marfan's syndrome is an autosomal dominant defect of the fibrillin gene that results in abnormal elastic fibers with a predisposition toward aneurysmal dilation and dissection. Ehlers-Danlos type IV is an autosomal dominant disorder of type III collagen synthesis that can lead to aneurysmal dilation and rupture.

DIAGNOSIS

Most aneurysms are asymptomatic and are found incidentally on physical examination or on imaging tests ordered for other reasons. Symptoms are related to the location of the aneurysm. Among symptomatic patients with nonruptured AAA, a steady, gnawing pain in hypogastric region or lower back pain is the most common presenting symptom. Movement does not affect the pain. Ascending aneurysms can manifest with chest pain, aortic regurgitation causing heart failure symptoms, or mass effect (compression of the superior vena cava or hoarseness). DTAAs can manifest with chest or back pain, hemoptysis, or hoarseness or dyspnea due to mass effect on the lung or airway. Ruptured aneurysms manifest with acute onset of pain and hypotension.

Physical examination may detect AAA in thin people. Abdominal ultrasound screening for AAA is inexpensive and reproducible, and echocardiography can identify thoracic aortic aneurysms. Computed tomography (CT) is the gold standard test to diagnose and monitor aortic aneurysms. Magnetic resonance angiography may be used for patients who are unable to tolerate intravenous dye. In patients with ascending aortic aneurysms, echocardiography should be performed to evaluate for aortic valve pathology.

TREATMENT

Medical Therapy

No large clinical trial has proved the efficacy of medical therapy, although there are several ongoing trials. Control of blood pressure through the use of β-blockers is commonly accepted therapy but was not found to slow aneurysm progression in one randomized trial. This intent-to-treat analysis was limited by a 40% dropout rate due to side effects of the medication. Nonrandomized data suggest that statins reduce AAA growth rates by 50%. Recent small trials have demonstrated that both losartan (Cozaar)[1] and perindopril (Aceon)[1] slowed the rate of dilation in patients with Marfan's syndrome, perhaps by inhibiting transforming growth factor-β. A larger trial with losartan in a broader population is ongoing.

Surgical Therapy

Surgical treatment is warranted if the risk of rupture is greater than the morbidity and mortality of repair. Randomized trials focusing on small aneurysms (defined as <5.0 cm) have demonstrated no advantage for early surgical repair, with a low 1% yearly rate of rupture. On the other hand, patients with larger aneurysms clearly benefit from repair. The surgical approach is determined by the location and extent of the aneurysm.

Ascending Aorta and Arch

Mortality rates for elective surgical treatment of an ascending aortic aneurysm or AAA are 2% to 5%, increasing to 6% to 15% with the repair of aortic arch aneurysms because the necessity of circulatory arrest and reimplantation of arch vessels. The approach for repair of these aneurysms is through a sternotomy, and cardiopulmonary bypass is used. Typically, ascending aortic aneurysms of 5.5 cm or larger are referred for repair in low- to moderate-risk patients. In the setting of concomitant cardiac surgery or bicuspid aortic valve, the ascending aorta is replaced when it is 5.0 cm or larger. Marfan's patients, because of the high risk of dissection, should have their ascending aorta and root replaced when it is 4.5 cm or larger. Repair or replacement of the aortic valve is dependent on the presence and severity of aortic valve pathology.

Descending and Thoracoabdominal Aorta

Repair of DTAAs and thoracoabdominal aneurysms carries a risk of mortality of 5% to 15% and a risk of paraplegia of 3% to 20%, depending on the anatomy. In adequate-risk patients, repair is recommended when the aneurysm is 6 cm or larger. DTAA repair can often be performed with an endovascular approach, but this is difficult with thoracoabdominal aneurysms because of the involvement of visceral vessels. Open repair is performed through a left thoracotomy, often with the assistance of partial bypass and lumbar cerebrospinal fluid drainage to decrease the risk of paraplegia and renal failure. Whether reimplantation of intercostal vessels minimizes the risk of paraplegia is controversial.

Abdominal Aorta

Mortality for open repair of an AAA is 2% to 5%. Open repair is most commonly performed through a vertical or transverse laparotomy, although retroperitoneal approaches have excellent results as well.

Endovascular Repair

Endovascular repair is gradually becoming more common than open repair of AAAs and DTAAs. At our institution, more than 60% of AAAs are repaired endovascularly. Endovascular repair is more likely to be successful with landing zones of at least 2 cm of normal aorta

---

[1]Not FDA approved for this indication.

---

proximal and distal to the aneurysm, little tortuosity, smaller size, and good renal function. Lifetime follow-up is necessary, because up to 20% of patients develop an endoleak (i.e., a leak around or through the graft into the aneurysm sac). Mid-term results for endovascular repair demonstrated less morbidity and mortality in AAA and DTAA, compared with open repair. Long-term results are currently being evaluated.

SCREENING

Clinical examination alone can miss the diagnosis of AAA. Ultrasound screening programs have not been performed routinely in the United States. Studies indicate that ultrasound screening in men older than 50 years of age can reduce the AAA rupture rate by 50%. Cost analyses support ultrasound screening in men older than age 50 with a history of smoking. Medicare covers a single screening abdominal ultrasound study in white men after the age of 65.

Aortic Occlusive Disease

Atherosclerosis can affect the thoracic or the abdominal aorta. Abdominal disease often occurs with iliac disease. The spectrum can span from mild atheromatous disease to complete occlusion of these large vessels. Symptoms include embolic disease from mobile

 CURRENT DIAGNOSIS

Abdominal and Descending Thoracic Aortic Aneurysms

- Men older than 60 years of age who have a smoking history are at greatest risk.
- Usually asymptomatic and found incidentally
- Ultrasound can be used to screen and should be used in smokers.
- The gold standard diagnostic test is computed tomographic (CT) angiography.

Ascending Aortic Aneurysm

- Men and women are affected equally.
- Associated with aortic insufficiency and familial disorders such as Marfan's syndrome
- Conventional or CT aortography is diagnostic.
- Echocardiography should be performed to evaluate for aortic valve pathology

Aortoiliac Occlusive Disease

- Diagnosis is made by history and examination.
- Measurements of the ankle-brachial index or pulse volume recordings confirm the diagnosis.
- Conventional or CT arteriography or magnetic resonance angiography identify the location and extent of disease.

Acute Aortic Dissection

- Diagnosis is often delayed because this is the great imitator.
- Manifests with chest or back pain
- CT angiography is the gold standard and identifies malperfused branches.
- Transesophageal echocardiography is diagnostic and is preferred in an unstable patient.

Traumatic Aortic Injury

- High index of suspicion based on chest injury
- Chest radiography may be suggestive.
- CT angiography is the gold standard.

plaques, limb or thigh claudication, rest pain, or tissue loss of the lower extremities. Occasionally, symptoms include impotence, diminished femoral pulses, and buttock claudication (Leriche syndrome).

INCIDENCE AND NATURAL HISTORY

Peripheral vascular disease affects 8 million Americans and is associated with a shorter span of life. Risk factors include smoking, diabetes, hypertension, atherosclerosis, coronary artery disease, hyperhomocysteinemia, and African American race. The natural history is not determined by the severity and length of the stenosis but by patient factors, including continued tobacco use, diabetes, and renal failure.

DIAGNOSIS

A history and physical examination are often sufficient to make the diagnosis. Claudication is reproducible exertional pain relieved by rest. It typically occurs in the calf, thigh, or buttock. Embolic disease manifests as infarcts affecting toes bilaterally, termed blue-toe syndrome. Examination demonstrates diminished femoral pulses. Measurements of ankle-brachial index and pulse volume recordings can confirm clinical suspicion. Once the diagnosis is suggested, characterization of disease extent can be determined by CT angiography, magnetic resonance angiography, or conventional angiography.

Thoracic aortic plaques may be identified in a patient with embolic disease or as an incidental finding. They are at risk for embolization during cardiac and aortic surgery and are best diagnosed by transesophageal echocardiography or CT angiography.

TREATMENT

Treatment choice is determined by the severity of symptoms. Treatment of mild to moderate claudication should begin with medical therapy. Smoking cessation should be reinforced regardless of the severity of the disease. Severe claudication, rest pain, and tissue loss warrant intervention.

Medical Therapy

Control of risk factors (including smoking cessation) is critical and may slow the progression of disease. Exercise programs can help recruit collateral vessels and improve symptoms but do not change objective ankle-brachial index measurements. However, exercise programs in randomized studies have documented significant improvements in symptoms. All patients should be prescribed aspirin if tolerated. Cilostazol (Pletal)[1] has been documented to provide symptomatic benefit in patients with claudication in some studies.

Endovascular Therapy

Minimally invasive techniques, including balloon angioplasty and stenting, have become the preferred treatments for isolated or bilateral iliac occlusive disease. However, extensive aortic or aortoiliac disease is treated surgically.

Surgical Therapy

Approaches to improve blood flow to the lower extremities include aortobifemoral bypass, thoracobifemoral bypass, or axillobifemoral bypass. The mortality rate with aortobifemoral bypass is 5%. At 10 years, the patency of an aortobifemoral or thoracobifemoral bypass approaches 85% to 90%, whereas that of an axillofemoral bypass is 60% because of the longer length and smaller caliber of the conduit. As a consequence, axillofemoral bypass is reserved for high-risk patients who are unable to tolerate the other approaches.

Aortic Dissections

An aortic dissection occurs when an intimal tear results in blood propagating into the media of the aortic wall. They are classified by

---

[1]Not FDA approved for this indication.

location. *Stanford A dissections* (62.5%) always involve the ascending aorta and may involve the descending aorta. *Stanford B dissections* (37.5%) involve the descending aorta and may include the aortic arch but not the ascending aorta. An alternative classification is the DeBakey classification: type I, ascending and descending aorta; type II, ascending aorta only; and type III, descending aorta only.

Subacute dissections are those present for longer than 2 weeks, and chronic dissections are those that have been present for longer than 2 months. These less acute dissections do not have the same risk of early mortality as acute dissections. Intramural hematoma is a focal intimal tear that can lead to aortic dissection in 15% to 50% of cases and should be treated as a dissection.

INCIDENCE AND NATURAL HISTORY

The incidence of aortic dissection is estimated to be 3 per 100,000 patient-years. Aortic dissection develops in 30% of patients with Marfan's syndrome. The most important risk factor is hypertension and aortic diameter. However, dissections can occur in normal-diameter aortas. The natural history of dissections varies based on location. The mortality for Stanford A dissections is estimated to be 25% at 24 hours, 50% at 48 hours, and 90% at 1 month.

DIAGNOSIS

Sudden onset of severe, tearing chest or back pain is classic for an aortic dissection and is present in up to 80% of patients. The physical examination should seek aortic insufficiency murmurs, asymmetrical pulses, and neurologic deficits indicating propagation of the dissection into the cerebrovascular system.

Chest radiography may show a widened mediastinum in 50% of the cases, but the definitive diagnostic test is a CT scan, which has a sensitivity and specificity of greater than 99%. If CT is unavailable or the patient is unstable, a transesophageal echocardiogram provides greater than 97% specificity and sensitivity when performed by an experienced operator.

TREATMENT

Stanford Type A Dissection

Initial management includes blood pressure control, but urgent surgical intervention is warranted, because these aortic catastrophes can lead to acute aortic insufficiency, propagation of the dissection into the coronary arteries, pericardial tamponade, or frank rupture. Operative intervention requires cardiopulmonary bypass and replacement of the ascending aorta. Occasionally, coronary artery bypass grafting or aortic valve replacement is necessary. The remaining descending aorta, if involved, should be monitored long term, as for type B dissections.

Stanford Type B Dissection

The initial management involves control of blood pressure with a systolic goal of less than 100 mm Hg. β-Blockers are the preferred agent, because they decrease the pulsatility (dp/dt) of the blood the aorta receives. Placement of an arterial line for continuous blood pressure monitoring and serial examination is recommended. Visceral or extremity ischemia (20% of type B dissection) warrants urgent intervention. Endovascular stenting of the aortic dissection is becoming the preferred approach. The goal with this technique is to cover the entry tear (or tears) with a covered stent, eliminating flow into the false lumen and reestablishing flow in the visceral vessels and lower extremities. Alternatively, angiographically guided fenestration of the dissection flap can be performed. The least desirable alternative, operative intervention, may be necessary in centers where the aforementioned approaches are not available. The 30-day mortality rate for medically managed type B dissection is 10%, whereas that for surgically treated type B dissection is greater than 30%. Patients must be monitored for life, because up to 30% require surgical intervention for recurrent pain, visceral ischemia, or aneurysmal dilation of the dissected aorta.

Traumatic Aortic Injury

Traumatic aortic injury occurs as a result of sheer stress on the mobile aorta, distal to the fixed ligamentum arteriosum, which is sustained with rapid deceleration, most commonly during motor vehicle crashes. The mortality rate is high, and early surgery should be considered.

INCIDENCE AND NATURAL HISTORY

Traumatic aortic injury occurs most often in young men, and 80% of patients die before reaching the hospital. Of the remainder, 50% will die within the first 24 hours, and 25% over the subsequent 2 weeks, without any treatment. In these patients, the transected aorta is kept intact by the overlying adventitia and mediastinal pleura.

CURRENT THERAPY

Abdominal Aortic Aneurysm (AAA)

- There are no proven medical treatments to prevent AAA growth.
- Smoking cessation and blood pressure control are generally accepted.
- Repair is considered when the AAA is larger than 5.0 to 5.5 cm.
- Endovascular repair is being performed more commonly with good results.

Thoracic Aortic Aneurysms

- Repair of an ascending aortic aneurysm is considered if it is larger than 5.5 cm, or larger than 5.0 cm with concomitant cardiac disease or a bicuspid aortic valve.
- Losartan (Cozaar)[1] or perindopril (Aceon)[1] may be helpful in patients with Marfan's syndrome.
- Repair of the ascending aorta is performed in Marfan's patients when the aneurysm is larger than 4.5 cm.
- Repair of a descending thoracic aortic aneurysm is considered when it is larger than 6 cm.
- Selected descending thoracic aortic aneurysms have been repaired endovascularly with good results.

Aortoiliac Occlusive Disease

- Medical treatment includes smoking cessation, glycemic control, statin therapy, and an exercise program.
- Severely symptomatic patients can undergo stenting for isolated lesions.
- Low-risk patients can undergo aortobifemoral bypass, whereas axillofemoral bypass is reserved for high-risk patients.

Acute Aortic Dissection

- Stanford type A dissections are treated with emergent intervention, usually sparing the aortic valve.
- Stanford type B dissections are treated medically, but 30% of patients develop aneurysms later.

Traumatic Aortic Injury

- The physician must have a high index of suspicion based on the mechanism of injury.
- Careful medical observation can be performed in the presence of severe concomitant injuries.
- Endovascular repair is being performed more commonly, with good results.

---

[1]Not FDA approved for this indication.

DIAGNOSIS

A conscious patient may present with chest or back pain, hoarseness, dyspnea, dysphagia, or paralysis and signs of trauma to the chest. Usually, however, these patients are unconscious and the diagnosis is based on imaging. Chest radiography can demonstrate a widened mediastinum or a left pleural effusion. CT angiography is the gold standard at many institutions. Transesophageal echocardiography, although operator dependent, can be useful in the unstable patient.

TREATMENT

Medical Therapy

Initial treatment includes blood pressure control, primarily with β-blockers and afterload reduction if necessary. This is important to allow treatment of other life-threatening traumatic injuries. Many centers are reporting experience with delayed repair after treatment of other injuries and careful hemodynamic monitoring.

Surgical Therapy

Surgical therapy for traumatic aortic injury is evolving. Traditional open repair involves a left thoracotomy in the fourth interspace, clamping of the aorta proximally and distally to the injury, and aortic replacement. Use of left heart bypass and spinal cord drainage may decrease the risk of paraplegia and renal failure. The mortality rate of 30% often depends on concomitant injuries.

Endovascular repair is becoming more common for treatment of traumatic aortic injury. Current limitations include endograft sizes designed for aneurysmal aortas; small-caliber iliac vessels in these previously healthy, young patients; less than ideal proximal landing zone; and poor long-term follow-up. Nonetheless, endovascular repair may be the preferred treatment in patients with significant traumatic injuries. The long-term sequelae of endografts in young patients is unknown.

REFERENCES

Baxter BT, Pearce WH, Waltke EA, et al. Prolonged administration of doxycycline in patients with small asymptomatic abdominal aortic aneurysms: Report of a prospective (phase II) multicenter study. J Vasc Surg 2002;36:1–12.

Birkmeyer JD, Upchurch GR Jr. Evidence-based screening and management of abdominal aortic aneurysm. Ann Intern Med 2007;146:749–50.

Brooke BS, Habashi JP, Judge DP, et al. Angiotensin II blockade and aortic-root dilation in Marfan's syndrome. N Engl J Med 2008;358:2787–95.

Brown SL, Busuttil RW, Baker JD, et al. Bacteriologic and surgical determinants of survival in patients with mycotic aneurysms. J Vasc Surg 1984;1:541–7.

Cao P, Verzini F, Parlani G, et al. Clinical effect of abdominal aortic aneurysm endografting: 7-Year concurrent comparison with open repair. J Vasc Surg 2004;40:841–8.

Etz CD, Halstead JC, Spielvogel D, et al. Thoracic and thoracoabdominal aneurysm repair: Is reimplantation of spinal cord arteries a waste of time? Ann Thorac Surg 2006;82:1670–7.

Golledge J, Muller J, Daugherty A, Norman P. Abdominal aortic aneurysm: Pathogenesis and implications for management. Arterioscler Thromb Vasc Biol 2006;26:2605–13.

Hagan PG, Nienaber CA, Isselbacher EM, et al. The International Registry of Acute Aortic Dissection (IRAD): New insights into an old disease. JAMA 2000;283:897–903.

Powell JT, Brown LC, Forbes JF, et al. Final 12-year follow-up of surgery versus surveillance in the UK Small Aneurysm Trial. Br J Surg 2007;94:702–8.

Propanolol Aneurysm Trial Investigators. Propranolol for small abdominal aortic aneurysms: Results of a randomized trial. J Vasc Surg 2002;35:72–9.

Sukhija R, Aronow WS, Sandhu R, et al. Mortality and size of abdominal aortic aneurysm at long-term follow-up of patients not treated surgically and treated with and without statins. Am J Cardiol 2006;97:279–80.

Thomas SM, Beard JD, Ireland M, et al. Results from the prospective registry of endovascular treatment of abdominal aortic aneurysms (RETA): Mid term results to five years. Eur J Vasc Endovasc Surg 2005;29:563–70.

Tsai TT, Evangelista A, Nienaber CA, et al. Long-term survival in patients presenting with type A acute aortic dissection: Insights from the International Registry of Acute Aortic Dissection (IRAD). Circulation 2006;114:I350–6.

Tsai TT, Fattori R, Trimarchi S, et al. International Registry of Acute Aortic Dissection: Long-term survival in patients presenting with type B acute aortic dissection: Insights from the International Registry of Acute Aortic Dissection. Circulation 2006;114:2226–31.

Wilmink AB, Hubbard CS, Day NE, et al. The incidence of small abdominal aortic aneurysms and the change in normal infrarenal aortic diameter: Implications for screening. Eur J Vasc Endovasc Surg 2001;21:165–70.

Angina Pectoris

Method of
Kenneth Tobin, DO, and Kim Eagle, MD

Angina pectoris is defined as cardiac-induced pain that is a direct result of a mismatch between myocardial oxygen supply and demand. The initial presentation of ischemic heart disease is chronic stable angina in approximately 50% of patients, and it is estimated that 16.5 million Americans have this diagnosis. Ischemic heart disease is the leading cause of death in the United States.

Stable angina refers to predictable chest discomfort during various levels of exertional activity that is predictably resolved with rest or administration of sublingual nitroglycerin (Nitrostat). Unstable angina is an acute ischemic event; this diagnosis includes patients with new-onset cardiac chest pain, angina at rest, postmyocardial infarction angina, or an accelerating pattern of previously stable angina. The terms unstable angina and non–Q wave myocardial infarction are often used interchangeably and should be further defined on the basis of myocardial necrosis as measured by serum biomarkers.

The clinical sensation of angina pectoris is caused by stimulation of chemosensitive and mechanosensitive receptors of unmyelinated nerve cells found within cardiac muscle fibers and around the coronary vessels. This stimulation cascade is thought to occur when lactate, serotonin, bradykinin, histamine, reactive oxygen species, and adenosine are released into the coronary circulation during periods of lactic acidosis. Nerve stimulation via the sympathetic ganglia occurs most commonly between the seventh cervical and fourth thoracic portions of the spinal cord. This explains from an anatomic standpoint why the most commonly recognized pain patterns for angina pectoris involve discomfort in the chest, neck, jaw, and left arm.

The most common cause of angina pectoris is coronary atherosclerosis. As plaque is initially deposited within a coronary vessel, there may be no significant internal luminal compromise during the early positive remodeling phase. However, at the point at which this compensatory mechanism fails, internal luminal compromise ensues. As long as the coronary artery segment distal to the stenosis retains the ability to vasodilate in response to increasing blood flow demands, coronary homeostasis is maintained. Once the critical threshold is passed, the blood supply cannot accommodate this demand, and angina may occur. The four major factors that determine myocardial oxygen demand are heart rate, systolic blood pressure, myocardial wall tension, and myocardial contractility.

Clinical Features

For patients with documented coronary artery disease (CAD) who have predictable episodes of classic symptoms, the diagnosis of angina pectoris is straightforward. Most patients are aware of the levels of exertion that typically induce angina symptoms. Most describe a pain or heaviness across their middle chest that may or may not radiate to the jaw or left arm. Some patients deny chest pain symptoms altogether and instead complain of exertional dyspnea or diaphoresis. Environmental situations such as cold exposure, emotional stress, or heavy meals can induce angina. The Canadian

TABLE 1 Differential Diagnosis of Chest Pain

Cardiac ischemia
Angina
Myocardial infarction
Vasospastic angina
Pericarditis
Aortic dissection (new-onset chest pain and new aortic insufficiency noted on auscultation is an aortic dissection until proven otherwise)
Pulmonary embolism
Esophageal spasm
Gastroesophageal reflux disease
Musculoskeletal pain
Biliary colic
Acute pneumonia

Cardiovascular Society and the New York Heart Association classification systems are used to define angina severity. Both systems use a I through IV scale, with mild angina (class I) referring to episodes that occur with extreme exertion and severe angina (class IV) to episodes that occur with minimal or no exertion. These classification systems are useful for risk stratification and for assessing medical therapy efficacy.

There are clear gender differences in the clinical presentations of angina. Pleuritic, musculoskeletal-type pain, nonexertional pain, and nocturnal pains have been reported as anginal equivalents in women. Fatigue is one of the most common presenting symptoms for CAD in women. The key to the diagnosis in men and women lies in a thorough history, which should always include the quality, location, provoking activities, and duration of pain and factors that relieve the pain. Based on a detailed clinical history, the many diagnoses that can masquerade as angina may be eliminated (Table 1).

Diagnostic Testing

A baseline electrocardiogram (ECG) is often one of the initial tests obtained in a patient with the complaint of chest pain. A normal tracing does not exclude the diagnosis of ischemic heart disease. More than 50% of patients with diagnosed angina have a normal ECG at rest. The baseline ECG may, however, show evidence of pathologic Q waves or left ventricular hypertrophy, either of which increases the statistical probability of significant CAD. Baseline laboratory data should include a fasting lipid panel to help define the patient's risk factor profile.

Stress testing is an appropriate screening tool for the initial diagnosis of CAD, risk stratification after acute ischemic syndrome, and assessment of treatment efficacy. Whenever feasible, it is more advantageous to obtain an exercise stress test rather than a pharmacologically based study. The additional prognostic data obtained through exercise include blood pressure response, heart rate response, heart rate recovery, metabolic equivalent level attained, and ECG assessment of the ST segment. There are several validated exercise protocols that add additional risk stratification measures to the test results.

The predictive value of exercise treadmill stress testing ranges from 40% for single-vessel disease to 90% for three-vessel disease. A baseline left bundle branch block, paced rhythm, poorly controlled atrial arrhythmia, or left ventricular hypertrophy with secondary ischemic changes often renders the test inconclusive when assessing for ischemic changes. However, if stress testing is being performed for attainment of hemodynamic responses and achievable metabolic equivalent levels, these baseline ECG abnormalities may be overlooked.

Stress test accuracy is markedly improved by the addition of an imaging modality such as echocardiography or nuclear perfusion scanning. The sensitivity and specificity of stress echocardiography and stress nuclear imaging are 85% to 90%. Stress echocardiography is believed to be somewhat more specific, and stress nuclear imaging

CURRENT DIAGNOSIS

- The clinical diagnosis of angina depends largely on accurate assessment of a patient's risk factor profile for coronary artery disease and the typicality of the symptom complex.
- The most common symptom of angina pectoris is left-sided chest pain or pressure, with or without associated radiation of pain or pressure to the jaw or left arm, occurring with exertion and relieved with rest or sublingual nitroglycerin.
- Women may present with atypical symptoms such as sharp, nonexertional chest pain; generalized fatigue; or right-sided chest pain.
- Basic screening tests (e.g., 12-lead electrocardiogram, laboratory data, chest radiograph) are normal in most cases.
- For an initial diagnosis, appropriate noninvasive testing or coronary angiography, or both, is important to define the amount of ischemic myocardium and an overall treatment plan.
- Even when invasive procedures are clinically indicated, aggressive medical therapy with high-dose statins, attainment of appropriate blood pressure levels, smoking cessation, and use of antiplatelet therapy is of paramount importance.
- Patients who have clinical evidence of unstable angina and laboratory evidence of myocardial ischemia most often benefit from early invasive treatment strategies.

is thought to be more sensitive. A stress echocardiogram also allows assessment of left ventricular systolic function and valvular function and prediction of right ventricular pressure. In deciding on which stress test to perform, one should rely on the expertise of the testing facility and the individual patient's circumstance.

Risk Factor Management

HYPERTENSION

Hypertension is a commonly occurring, well-established, major cardiovascular risk factor. Although the current guidelines (from the seventh report of Joint National Committee on Prevention, Detection, Evaluation and Treatment of High Blood Pressure, known as JNC 7) define hypertension as pressures greater than 140/90 mm Hg, it has been shown that cardiovascular risk progressively increases at blood pressures greater than 115/75 mm Hg.

A meta-analysis of 61 prospective observational trials of hypertension involving 1 million adults with no known vascular disease at baseline revealed several interesting findings. Patient outcomes were related per decade of age to the usual blood pressure at the start of that decade. For example, from ages 40 to 69, for each increase in 20 mm Hg systolic blood pressure, a twofold increase in cardiovascular death rate occurred. These findings were much more pronounced in patients who were between 80 to 89 years old than in the youngest cohort, 40 to 49 years old. Although the relative risk was much higher in the younger group, the absolute risk was greatest among the octogenarians. These increased cardiovascular risks were not confined to subjects with blood pressures greater than 140/90 mm Hg; rather, there was a threshold of risk shown all the way down to 115/75 mm Hg. Even small reductions in blood pressure can have a significant positive impact on cardiovascular disease. Blood pressure reductions of 4 mm Hg systolic and 3 mm Hg diastolic were shown to reduce cardiovascular events by 15% in a cohort of 20,888 patients.

The Heart Outcomes Prevention Evaluation (HOPE) study asked the question whether all patients with atherosclerosis, regardless of blood pressure, should be treated with an angiotensin-converting enzyme inhibitor. Although many subsequent editorials implied that all patients with CAD could benefit from this therapy, a closer look at the data suggests a different interpretation. The mean blood pressure was 139/79 mm Hg, suggesting that a significant portion of the 9297 participants had a baseline blood pressure higher than this value. Compared with placebo, the treatment group had a 22% reduction in the primary outcome composite of myocardial infarction, stroke, or cardiovascular death. A small substudy using 24-hour ambulatory blood pressure monitoring showed blood pressure differences of 11 mm Hg systolic and 4 mm Hg diastolic in the treatment group compared with the placebo group, which may explain the cardiovascular event reductions reported.

HYPERLIPIDEMIA

Dyslipidemia is an important risk factor for atherosclerotic cardiovascular disease. Increased levels of low-density lipoproteins (LDL) and reduced levels of high-density lipoproteins are the main therapeutic targets. Lowering of LDL-cholesterol has been shown to intimately correlate with reductions in cardiovascular disease event rates.

The medical approach to patients with angina should always include aggressive lipid management. Recent guidelines recommend that LDL levels in patients with known CAD should be less than 70 mg/dL. In most patients, it is difficult to achieve these levels without pharmacologic intervention. It has been shown that, regardless of how cholesterol is lowered, there is a concomitant reduction in atherosclerotic cardiovascular disease. However, statins are the first choice for lowering LDL-cholesterol levels among the available pharmacologic agents because of their tolerability profile, positive non-lipid pleiotropic effects, and ability to dramatically lower LDL levels.

The Cholesterol Treatment Trialists' meta-analysis including 90,056 subjects from 14 trials showed a 12% reduction in all-cause mortality per 38.6 mg/dL (1 mmol/L) reduction in LDL-cholesterol, with a 19% reduction in coronary mortality, a 24% reduction in need for revascularization, a 17% reduction in stroke incidence, and a 21% reduction in any major vascular event during a mean follow-up period of 5 years. These benefits were observed in different age groups, across genders, at different baseline cholesterol levels, and equally among those with and without prior CAD and cardiovascular risk factors.

The Heart Protection Study showed that, in patients with established CAD, other atherosclerotic vascular disease, or diabetes, statin therapy reduced cardiovascular events regardless of the baseline LDL-cholesterol level. The trial, which enrolled 20,536 patients aged 40 to 80 years, showed a 24% reduction in major cardiovascular events, a 25% reduction in stroke, and a 13% reduction in overall mortality with statin therapy.

Patients with a recent acute ischemic syndrome were enrolled in the Pravastatin or Atorvastatin Evaluation and Infection Therapy (PROVE IT) trial, known as Thrombolysis in Myocardial Infarction (TIMI) 22, which compared 80 mg atorvastatin (Lipitor) with 40 mg of pravastatin (Pravachol). The atorvastatin group achieved a median LDL level of 62 mg/dL, compared with 96 mg/dL in the pravastatin group. The relative risk reduction for this reduced LDL level was 16%. A substudy looking at the LDL-cholesterol levels achieved with atorvastatin showed that those subjects achieving a level of 40 to 60 mg/dL had a 22% reduction in events, compared with those achieving a level of 80 to 100 mg/dL. Therefore, it appears that high-dose statin therapy and aggressive LDL lowering in this patient population leads to reduced cardiovascular events.

The Treating to New Targets (TNT) trial was the first to compare a more intensely treated group with a less intensely treated group using the same agent. The design of this 10,000-patient study eliminated concerns that outcome differences were induced from dissimilar statin preparations. The mean LDL level achieved was 101 mg/dL with 10 mg atorvastatin (Lipitor), and 77 mg/dL with the 80 mg dose. This LDL reduction was associated with a relative risk reduction of 27% for the primary endpoint of first major cardiovascular event.

It is apparent from both primary and secondary prevention lipid trials that achieving a lower LDL reduces cardiovascular event rates. Following evidence-based data, patients with established CAD benefit from achieving an LDL-cholesterol level of less than 70 mg/dL.

METABOLIC SYNDROME

The combined presence of insulin resistance, hypertension, dyslipidemia, and abdominal obesity define the metabolic syndrome. There is debate about whether this is a true syndrome or simply a clustering of cardiovascular risk factors in a particular individual. The key concept is that the concomitant presence of these particular cardiovascular risk factors markedly increases a patient's chances of developing diabetes mellitus and coronary atherosclerosis. The approach to treatment for this syndrome is no different from that for the individual components. Recognition of the components is key to the treatment of this disorder.

SMOKING

Cigarette smoking is probably the most important of the identified modifiable cardiovascular risk factors. The incidence of CAD is two to four times higher in smokers than in nonsmokers. The pathophysiologic process that leads to atherosclerosis from smoking stems from induced platelet dysfunction, endothelial dysfunction, smooth muscle cell proliferation, and attenuated high-density lipoprotein–cholesterol levels. Smoking cessation must be sought for every CAD patient.

OTHER LIFESTYLE CHANGES

Exercise should be encouraged in patients with stable angina once all appropriate invasive and noninvasive tests have been completed and a stable medical regimen has been established.

Increasing a patient's aerobic capacity can lower the body's oxygen requirement for a given workload, which can lead to increased exercise tolerance and reduced anginal symptoms. Aerobic exercise can improve endothelial function and positively affect baroreflex sensitivity and heart rate variability in patients with CAD.

Endorphins released during exercise are thought to be mood-enhancers as well as effective muscle relaxants. Exercise itself improves sleep patterns. Cortisol levels are reduced with regular exercise, which may attenuate the body's sensation of stress and anxiety. For these reasons, appropriate exercise programs for patients with stable angina have far-reaching positive benefits. Exercise guidelines for CAD patients have been published and should be reviewed before patients begin aggressive secondary prevention efforts.

Major depression affects approximately 25% of people recovering from a myocardial infarction, and another 40% suffer from mild depression. In any given year, one of every three long-term acute ischemic syndrome survivors will develop depression. The Heart and Soul Study examined 1017 patients with stable CAD over a period of 4.8 years. Patients identified with depression were twice as likely to experience recurrent cardiovascular events. Physical inactivity was associated with a 44% greater rate of cardiovascular events. Patients with symptoms of depression were less likely to follow dietary, exercise, and medication recommendations.

Approach to Treatment

MEDICAL THERAPY

Medications used to treat angina pectoris and typical dosages are listed in Table 2.

Nitrates

Nitrates provide an exogenous source of nitric oxide which serves to relax smooth muscle and inhibit platelet aggregation. Nitrates exert their antianginal effect by reducing myocardial oxygen demand

---

CURRENT THERAPY

Stable Angina Pectoris

- Treatment with β-blockers, nitrates, calcium channel blockers for symptom control
- Consider addition of ranolazine (Ranexa) if symptoms not adequately controlled
- Aggressive cholesterol treatment based on the National Cholesterol Education Program (NCEP-III) updated guidelines
- Blood pressure management
- Antiplatelet therapy
- Lifestyle modifications:
  - Smoking cessation
  - Exercise prescription
  - Dietary guidelines
- Depression assessment

Unstable Angina

- Positive biomarkers for myocardial ischemia: consider coronary angiography
- Negative biomarkers for myocardial ischemia:
  - Consider noninvasive assessment once symptoms are controlled
  - Substantial ischemic burden identified: consider coronary angiography
  - No or minimal ischemia identified: consider increasing medical therapy
- Persistent symptoms: consider other treatment modalities

TABLE 2 Medications Used for the Treatment of Angina Pectoris

Name	Dosage
β-Blockers	
Atenolol (Tenormin)	25–200 mg PO qd
Metoprolol tartrate (Lopressor)	25–200 mg bid
Metoprolol succinate (Toprol XL)	25–200 mg qd
Carvedilol (Coreg)[1]	6.25–25 mg PO bid
Carvedilol phosphate (Coreg CR)[1]	20–80 mg PO qd
Propranolol (Inderal)	80–320 mg/day, divided bid or tid
Propranolol (Inderal LA)	80–160 mg PO qd
Labetalol (Trandate, Normodyne)[1]	200–800 mg bid
Nitrates	
Isosorbide dinitrate (Isordil)	10–40 mg PO bid or tid
Isosorbide mononitrate (Imdur)	30–240 mg PO qd
Nitroglycerin (Nitrostat)	0.4 mg SL q5min
Nitroglycerin transdermal (Nitro-Dur)	0.2–0.8 mg/h 12–14 h patch
Calcium Channel Blockers	
Dihydropyridines	
Amlodipine (Norvasc)	2.5–10 mg PO qd
Felodipine (Plendil)[1]	2.5–10 mg PO qd
Nifedipine (Procardia XL)	30–90 mg PO qd
Nondihydropyridines	
Verapamil (Calan)	80–120 mg PO tid
Verapamil (Calan SR)	120–480 mg PO qd
Diltiazem (Cardizem)	360 mg/day PO, divided tid or qid
Diltiazem (Cardizem LA)	180–360 mg PO qd

[1]Not FDA approved for this indication.

through coronary and systemic vasodilatation. Nitrates are strong venodilators, and in higher doses they can also induce arterial dilatation. Reducing the preload through venodilitation reduces myocardial oxygen demand. Coronary artery dilatation of stenotic vessels and intracoronary collaterals directly increases myocardial oxygen delivery. Through these mechanisms, nitrates have been shown to prevent recurrent episodes of angina and to increase exercise tolerance.

There are several nitrate preparations, which differ mainly in route of administration, onset of action, and effective half-life. Nitrate tolerance can occur with long-term use of any nitrate preparation and can be avoided by providing a 10- to 12-hour nitrate-free interval.

β-Blockers

β-Blockers are considered first-line therapy for patients with chronic stable angina pectoris. They competitively inhibit catecholamines from binding to β-receptors. Over time, β-blocker therapy leads to an increase in β-receptor density. Because of receptor upregulation, acute β-blocker withdrawal may lead to a transient supersensitivity to catecholamines and subsequent angina or even myocardial infarction. There are three classes of β-receptors. Some β-blockers are receptor specific, and some exert an effect over all three receptors. However, at higher doses, even β-selective agents have cross-reactivity for all β-receptors. β-Blockers reduce myocardial oxygen demand through a negative inotropic effect, a chronotropic effect, and a reduction in left ventricular wall stress.

Several cardioselective β-blockers, including atenolol (Tenormin) and metoprolol (Lopressor), have been shown to be effective antianginals that are fairly well tolerated in patients with underlying bronchospastic disease. Dosing is important for β-blocker efficacy. A study comparing atenolol with placebo showed that all doses from 25 through 200 mg/day were effective in reducing angina, but only the two highest doses led to an increase in exercise tolerance. Certain β-blockers have intrinsic sympathomimetic activity, including pindolol (Visken)[1] and acebutolol (Sectral).[1] Although they may be effective in reducing angina, they should be used with caution in patients with a prior history of myocardial infarction and in those with left ventricular dysfunction, because they may not reduce heart rate or blood pressure at rest.

When β-blockers are used to treat angina, a goal resting heart rate should be between 55 and 60 beats/min. Caution should be used in patients with resting bradycardia and in those with known reactive airway disease. Atenolol is renally excreted and should be used with caution in the elderly and in those with known renal dysfunction.

Calcium Channel Blockers

Calcium channel blockers are classified as either dihydropyridines or nondihydropyridines. The former group includes amlodipine (Norvasc), felodipine (Plendil),[1] nifedipine (Procardia), and nicardipine (Cardene); the latter includes diltiazem (Cardizem) and verapamil (Calan). There are differences among the two subclasses in regard to chronotropic, dromotropic, and inotropic effects.

Calcium channel blockers positively alter myocardial oxygen supply and demand, mainly through direct arterial vasodilatation. The nondihydropyridines also exhibit negative chronotropic and inotropic effects, thus further lowering myocardial oxygen demands.

One of the early quick-release preparations of a dihydropyridine calcium channel blocker, nifedipine, was reported to potentially induce myocardial infarction when used to treat angina. This was most likely due to a rapid drop in afterload leading to reflex adrenergic activation. Sustained-release preparations of nifedipine (Procardia XL), as well as the other dihyropyridines, have been proven safe and effective in patients with cardiovascular disease. Although amlodipine and felodipine are tolerated in patients with left ventricular systolic dysfunction, other calcium channel blockers should be avoided in this patient subset.

---

[1]Not FDA approved for this indication.

Ranolazine (Ranexa)

Ranolazine (Ranexa) is a new and unique antianginal drug approved for the treatment of stable angina. It is a sustained-release preparation that has been approved for patients who remain symptomatic while on standard angina pharmacotherapy. Its mechanism of action may be through reduction of fatty acid oxidation or effects on sodium shifts and intracellular calcium levels. QT prolongation has been reported, but a significant increase in arrhythmias has not been seen. Side effects include dizziness, constipation, and nausea. Dosing is 500 or 1000 mg twice daily, and the major route of metabolism is the cytochrome P-450 system. Ranolazine should be used cautiously in patients who are taking other pharmacologic agents that have the potential to prolong the QT interval.

Medication Combinations

Many patients with chronic stable angina require more than one antianginal medication to control their symptoms. There are no published data available to guide firm treatment recommendations. However, it is important to recognize medication side effects when deciding which agents to combine. β-Blockers block the atrioventricular (AV) node and exert a portion of their effectiveness through this mechanism. The nondihydropyridine calcium channel blockers also have AV-nodal blocking properties, and therefore should be used cautiously with β-blockers, especially in patients with preexisting conduction system disease. The dihydropyridine agents do not have AV-nodal blocking effects and may be a safer choice when used in combination with β-blockers. Nitrates do not have a side effect profile that raises concerns when they are used with β-blockers or with calcium channel blockers.

Antiplatelet Therapy

The common etiology leading to an acute ischemic syndrome is a platelet-rich clot occurring at the site of a significant coronary artery stenosis, often after a plaque rupture. Antiplatelet medications have been shown to consistently decrease morbidity and mortality in a wide array of cardiovascular disease patients. A meta-analysis suggested that, for patients with stable cardiovascular disease, low-dose aspirin therapy (50–100 mg daily) is as effective as higher doses (>300 mg). In this patient population, aspirin therapy resulted in a 26% reduction in myocardial infarction; the number of patients needed to treat to prevent a myocardial infarction was 83.

The Antiplatelet Trialists' Collaboration study demonstrated a reduction in myocardial infarction, stroke, and death in high-risk cardiovascular patients treated with antiplatelet therapy. Consensus guidelines recommend indefinite oral aspirin for the secondary prevention of cardiovascular events in all angina patients.

Clopidogrel (Plavix) is an effective alternative to aspirin for the treatment of stable cardiovascular disease in those patients with a true aspirin allergy. However, there are no data to indicate that clopidogrel is superior to aspirin in this particular patient population. In patients with unstable angina, dual antiplatelet therapy with aspirin and clopidogrel is recommended.

INVASIVE ASSESSMENT

The decision to pursue an invasive treatment approach differs significantly in patients with chronic stable angina and in those with acute coronary syndromes. Within both groups, accurate risk stratification is the key consideration in choosing who will benefit from coronary angiography and subsequent percutaneous coronary intervention. An invasive strategy in unstable angina patients has been shown to reduce recurrent acute coronary syndrome events consistently in many trials. A routine invasive strategy is recommended for patients with non-ST segment acute ischemic syndromes who have refractory ischemia, elevated cardiac biomarkers suggesting myocardial necrosis, or new ST-segment depression on ECG monitoring.

In patients with unstable angina, there are significant gender differences in outcomes related to the use of invasive therapy. Both men and women with elevated biomarkers from myocardial necrosis have comparable reductions in rates of death, myocardial infarction, and rehospitalization with invasive treatment strategies. However, in the absence of positive biomarkers, women appear to have potentially negative outcomes with an invasive approach. The current American College of Cardiology and American Heart Association guidelines recommend a conservative approach in such women.

Patients diagnosed with stable angina comprise a vast array of clinical presentations. The two most fueled debates in this arena concern the initial choice of medical therapy versus an invasive approach, and when to cross over from a medical treatment plan to an invasive one. The Atorvastatin Versus Revascularization Treatment (AVERT) trial studied the effects of intensive lipid-lowering therapy on ischemic events in a relatively low-risk population of patients with single- or two-vessel disease compared with percutaneous transluminal coronary angioplasty. AVERT randomized 341 patients to medical therapy plus atorvastatin (Lipitor) 80 mg or to angioplasty followed by usual medical care (which included the option of statin therapy at the choice of the treating physician). The medical treatment group experienced a 36% reduction in the composite endpoint of ischemic events compared with the angioplasty group. This difference was due primarily to repeated angioplasty, coronary artery bypass grafting, or hospitalization for worsening angina. The primary outcome of this trial from a practical standpoint was that high-dose statin therapy was safe in this patient population and did not increase cardiovascular events, compared with an angioplasty-based treatment plan.

One of the keys in interpreting the available data is recognizing that, by the time many of these trials are published, the percutaneous treatment choices are often outdated. Early trials used mainly balloon angioplasty, and later trials used early-generation bare metal stents. Equally as important is to determine what the background medical treatment plans were for any particular trial on this subject. Often, lipid therapy was not aggressive, hypertension management was not confirmed to be adequate, and intravenous glycoprotein IIb/IIIa antagonists were either not available or not used as a standard protocol when indicated.

The Clinical Outcomes Utilizing Revascularization and Aggressive Drug Evaluation (COURAGE) trial was designed to address the potential advantages of current medical therapy over a percutaneous approach in patients with demonstrable ischemia but stable CAD. Of the 35,000 patients screened, only 2287 met the study inclusion criteria. All participants of the COURAGE trial underwent a coronary angiography, and patients with high-risk anatomic findings such as severe left main coronary artery stenosis were excluded. The biggest difference in this trial compared with previous studies was that strict guideline-based medical therapy was followed in both groups. In the entire cohort, 85% of subjects were taking a β-blocker, 93% were taking a statin, and 85% were taking aspirin. The final interpretation of the COURAGE trial results was not that medical therapy is superior for all patients with CAD but that, in selected cohorts, aggressive medical therapy is an appropriate first step in the treatment of ischemic heart disease.

NOVEL THERAPIES

Transmyocardial Laser Revascularization

Transmyocardial laser revascularization is an invasive treatment that can be performed as an open heart procedure or percutaneously. The mechanism was originally thought to be the creation of myocardial channels leading to collateral circulation to ischemic zones, but this concept has been called into question. Current theories suggest cardiac denervation, laser-induced angiogenesis, or placebo effect. Likely selection bias within trials has also limited published outcomes data. In a randomized trial involving patients with class III or IV angina and percutaneously untreatable CAD, there was no reduction in angina, no improvement in exercise tolerance, and no decrease in adverse cardiac events after percutaneous transmyocardial laser revascularization, compared with maximal medical therapy. In this trial, the placebo effect was dramatically reduced through extensive blinding protocols for patients and treating physicians.

Angiogenesis leading to the induction of newly formed coronary vessels has been an active area of research for many years. Three main angiogenic growth factors that have been studied: fibroblastic growth factors, vascular endothelial growth factor, and platelet-derived growth factor. Major research limitations for these agents are that they do not act independently, and their biologic properties are poorly understood. Potential complications such as aberrant vascular proliferation, tumor development or proliferation, and proatherogenic effects have made patient enrollment difficult. Although there are some trial results suggesting that the ischemic burden shown on perfusion imaging may be reduced, no firm positive outcome data have yet been published.

External Counterpulsation

External counterpulsation is a noninvasive method of increasing coronary blood flow through diastolic augmentation. Large blood pressure cuffs are placed on both legs and thighs and are inflated to a pressure of 300 mm Hg in early diastole (triggered by the patient's ECG), promoting venous return to the heart. The mechanism is unclear but may be related to enhanced endothelial function, improved myocardial perfusion, and possibly placebo effect. Several small studies have suggested a clinical reduction in angina episodes, but no positive mortality benefit has yet been published. Contraindications to this treatment include certain aortic valvular diseases, aortic aneurysm, and peripheral vascular disease.

Spinal Cord Stimulation

For patients whose angina is refractory to medical therapy and who are not candidates for revascularization, spinal cord stimulation may be considered. Few intermediate or long-term data are available, but many short-term studies suggest reduced angina episodes. Placement of the device and subsequent stimulation at the C7-T1 level suggests that the mechanism of action is reduced pain sensation.

Other Causes of Angina

SYNDROME X

The cardiac syndrome X refers to patients who have normal or near-normal epicardial coronary arteries and episodic chest pain. This disorder is much more common in women and is often seen in patients younger than 50 years of age. The chest pain episodes may last longer than 30 minutes and may have a variable response to sublingual nitrates. Patients with syndrome X often describe typical stress-induced angina. Risk factors include hypertension, diabetes, and hyperlipidemia. Female patients are typically postmenopausal and frequently have stress-induced symptoms and ischemia on stress imaging. They often respond to standard angina medications and typically have a better prognosis than patients with significant epicardial plaque.

VASOSPASTIC OR PRINZMETAL'S ANGINA

The classic definition of Prinzmetal's angina is chest pain with documented ST-segment elevation during symptoms or during exercise in the face of angiographically normal or near-normal coronary arteries. Over the years, the definition has expanded to include patients who have classic angina symptoms commonly relieved with nitrates or calcium channel blockers and minimal or no CAD. It has been shown that patients with nonobstructive CAD may be prone to focal artery spasm at the stenosis site; therefore, the previous requirement of normal coronary arteries is not an absolute necessity. Other disease states (e.g., Raynaud's phenomenon) can increase a patient's development of coronary artery spasm, as can illicit drug usage (e.g., cocaine). Vasospasm is more common in active smokers. β-Blockers should be used cautiously in these patients, because they may exacerbate coronary spasm. Patients with angiographically documented intramyocardial bridging may be prone to focal coronary spasm and subsequent angina pectoris.

Newer Imaging Techniques

CALCIUM SCORING

Coronary artery calcium scoring is a well-studied imaging modality used to assess a patient's pretest probability of CAD. With respect to evaluation for angina, one must remember that electron-beam computed tomographic (CT) scanning does not offer physiologic data and therefore does not allow determination of myocardial ischemia. This study is most useful in the work-up of a low-risk patient with an atypical chest pain syndrome. If such a patient has an elevated calcium score, other studies may be reasonable.

COMPUTED TOMOGRAPHIC CORONARY ANGIOGRAPHY

CT coronary angiography is a noninvasive way to image the coronary arteries. Like electron-beam CT, it does not provide physiologic data regarding coronary artery perfusion, but it does provide anatomic information such as the presence and percentage of coronary artery stenosis. Although selected patients with stable or unstable angina may be considered candidates for CT angiography, its main utility is in patients being evaluated for chest pain who are otherwise at low risk and have a low pretest probability. Because of the volume of intravenous contrast required by CT angiography, the risk of contrast nephropathy must be considered when contemplating this study.

Summary

The approach to the patient with angina should be based on a global assessment and intensive treatment of all identified cardiovascular risk factors. Noninvasive testing is helpful for an initial diagnosis and to guide the decision for a more invasive approach. Familiarity and adherence to current treatment guidelines is of paramount importance. There are important gender differences that should not be overlooked in the clinical presentation of angina and in the approach to optimal therapy.

REFERENCES

Anderson JL, Adams CD, Antman EM, et al. ACC/AHA 2007 guidelines for the management of patients with unstable angina/non-ST-elevation myocardial infarction: A report of the American College of Cardiology/American Heart Association Task Force on Practice Guidelines. J Am Coll Cardiol 2007;5067:e1–157.

Antithrombotic Trialists C. Collaborative meta-analysis of randomized trials of antiplatelet therapy for prevention of death, myocardial infarction, and stroke in high risk patients. BMJ 2002;423:71–86.

Berger J, Brown D, Becker R, et al. Low-dose aspirin in patients with stable cardiovascular disease: A meta-analysis. Am J Med 2008;121(1):43–9.

Blood Pressure Lowering Treatment Trialists Collaboration. Effects of different blood pressure lowering regimens on major cardiovascular events: Results of prospectively-designed overviews of randomized trials. Lancet 2003;362:1527–45.

Boden WE, O'Rourke RA, Teo KK, et al. Optimal medical therapy with or without PCI for stable coronary disease. N Engl J Med 2007;35:1503–16.

Cholesterol Treatment Trialists' Collaborators. Efficacy and safety of cholesterol-lowering treatment: Prospective meta-analysis of data from 90056 participants in 14 trials of statins. Lancet 2005;366:1267–78.

Gibbons RJ, Abrams J, Chatterjee K, et al. ACC/AHA 2002 guideline update for the management of patients with chronic stable angina: A report of the American College of Cardiology/American Heart Association Task Force on Practice Guidelines (Committee to Update the 1999 Guidelines for the Management of Patients with Chronic Stable Angina), Available at www.acc.org/qualityandscience/clinical/guidelines/stable/stable_clean.pdf (accessed October 2009).

Grundy SM, Cleeman JI, Merz NB, et al. Implications of recent clinical trials for the National Cholesterol Education Program Adult Treatment Panel III guidelines. Circulation 2004;110:227–39.

Heart Outcomes Prevention Evaluation Study Investigators. Effects of an angiotensin-converting-enzyme inhibitor, ramipril, on cardiovascular events in high-risk patients. N Engl J Med 2000;342:145–53.

Mehta SR, Cannon CP, Fox KA, et al. Routine vs selective invasive strategies in patients with acute coronary syndromes: A collaborative meta-analysis of randomized trials. JAMA 2005;293(23):2908–17.

Ray K, Cannon C. Optimal goal for statin therapy use in coronary artery disease. Curr Opin Cardiol 2005;20:525–9.

Stone G, Teirstein P, Rubenstein R, et al. A prospective, multicenter, randomized trial of percutaneous transmyocardial laser revascularization in patients with nonrecanalizable chronic total occlusions. J Am Coll Cardiol 2002;39:1581–7.

Wenger NK. Cardiac rehabilitation: A guide to practice in the 21st century. New York: Marcel Dekker; 1999.

Whooley MA, Jonge P, Vittinghoff E, et al. Depressive symptoms, health behaviors, and risk of cardiovascular events in patients with coronary heart disease. JAMA 2008;300:2379–88.

Cardiac Arrest: Sudden Cardiac Death

Method of
Roy M. John, MD, PhD

Cardiac arrest, or sudden cardiac death, accounts for 60% of deaths from cardiac disease. It may be the initial manifestation or a complication of preexisting heart disease. Most cases are the result of potentially correctable arrhythmias, but the rate of successful resuscitation from an out-of-hospital cardiac arrest to neurologically intact survival remains dismally low. Recognition of patients who are at high risk for sudden cardiac arrhythmic death is critical for prevention. The ability to recognize those at risk for sudden death has increased appreciably, such that prophylactic measures can be implemented in a number of cardiac conditions to minimize risk.

Whereas specific antiarrhythmic drugs have proved disappointing in the prevention of sudden death, drugs that block the effects of β-adrenergic stimulation, angiotensin, and aldosterone have consistently led to reduced mortality among patients with cardiac disease and left ventricular (LV) dysfunction, partly through their salutary effects on sudden death. The implantable cardioverter-defibrillator (ICD) has emerged as a dominant therapeutic strategy based on clinical trials of its efficacy. This review addresses the clinical conditions associated with a high risk for sudden death and the current therapeutic options.

Definition and Causes

Sudden cardiac death is defined as abrupt, unexpected natural death occurring within a short time period (generally <1 hour) after onset of acute symptoms. Primary cardiac arrhythmia is responsible for most of the cases, but acute severe myocardial dysfunction, intracardiac obstruction, and acute aortic dissection are other important causes (Table 1). Structural abnormalities of the myocardium resulting from hypertrophy, scarring, and fibrosis serve as substrates for malignant arrhythmias. The majority of patients who die suddenly have atherosclerotic coronary artery disease (CAD). However, only about 20% of those who survive a cardiac arrest demonstrate evidence of an acute myocardial infarction. Instead, a large number have evidence of prior myocardial infarction and LV dysfunction. It is now recognized that chronic LV dysfunction is the most important predictor of sudden death in ischemic and nonischemic cardiomyopathy.

TABLE 1 Causes of Sudden Cardiac Death

Electrophysiologic abnormalities
  Conduction system disease involving the His-Purkinje
    conduction system
  Primary ventricular arrhythmia associated with cardiac
    conditions listed here
Abnormalities of the QT interval
  Brugada syndrome
  Wolff-Parkinson-White syndrome
  Catecholaminergic ventricular tachycardia
  Idiopathic ventricular fibrillation
  Malignant ventricular arrhythmia resulting from metabolic
    abnormalities
  Commotio cordis
Coronary artery disease
  Atherosclerotic disease
  Congenital anomalies
  Spasm
  Arteritis
  Dissection
  Embolism
Primary cardiomyopathies
  Nonischemic dilated cardiomyopathy
  Hypertrophic cardiomyopathy
Myocarditis
Valvular heart disease
Arrhythmogenic right ventricular dysplasia
Pulmonary hypertension
Hypertensive heart disease
Congenital heart disease
Noncompaction of the left ventricle
Inflammatory and infiltrative diseases of the myocardium
  Sarcoidosis
  Chagas' disease
  Hemochromatosis
  Amyloidosis
  Hydatid cyst
Neuromuscular diseases
  Muscular dystrophy
  Myotonic dystrophy
  Kearns-Sayre syndrome
  Friedreich's ataxia
Intracardiac obstruction
  Primary cardiac tumors (e.g., myxoma)
  Intracardiac thrombus
  Massive pulmonary embolism
Acute aortic dissection

A significant number (10%) of sudden deaths occur in the absence of obvious structural heart disease. Young, active, and otherwise healthy individuals are often the victims. Inherited or spontaneous mutations in genes coding for ion channels are responsible for most of these cases. A number of specific syndromes have been recognized, allowing for screening of relatives.

Tests to Identify Risk for Sudden Death

Electrocardiography (ECG) and echocardiography can provide several clues. Assessment of ventricular function provides the most information in determining the risk for sudden death.

Several noninvasive tests, including detection of microvolt T-wave alternans, signal-averaged ECG, and heart rate variability, have been developed to predict the future risk of sudden death. These tests have poor generalized applicability because of their low positive predictive value. In addition, most have not been coupled with a therapeutic intervention to show that therapy based on them can reduce the risk of dying.

Intracardiac electrophysiologic testing has retained some value, especially in patients with CAD. Inducibility of a sustained arrhythmia can be a marker for arrhythmic events, and therapy based on results of electrophysiologic testing has been shown to reduce mortality.

Treatment

This article summarizes the treatment modalities that have been shown to be effective in the various conditions leading to sudden cardiac death. Data based on randomized clinical trials are limited to common conditions such as CAD and the cardiomyopathies. The rarer diseases lack large clinical experience, and recommendations are based on the current consensus.

ACUTE MANAGEMENT OF SURVIVORS OF CARDIAC ARREST

Once stabilized with the use of standard advanced cardiac life support guidelines, patients should undergo cardiac evaluation by echocardiography and cardiac catheterization. Electrolyte abnormalities should be sought and corrected. Mild hypokalemia (3.0–3.5 mmol/L) is common after a cardiac arrest and resuscitation and is related to hypotension and transient acidosis. Hence, it is often the result and not the cause of the cardiac arrest. Similarly, in the acute phase after resuscitation, it is not uncommon to find global LV hypokinesis, but this should not be taken as a marker for preexisting heart disease. LV function tends to improve over the next 24 to 48 hours and should then be reassessed.

Ventricular fibrillation that occurs during the acute phase of a myocardial infarction (within the first 24–48 hours) is presumed to be secondary to electrical instability resulting from myocardial ischemia and reperfusion. If treated promptly by defibrillation, this arrhythmia has little prognostic value so long as overall myocardial function is preserved.

If acute ischemia or infarction is the documented cause of a cardiac arrest, revascularization by percutaneous angioplasty or coronary bypass surgery is the best treatment. The risk of recurrence is determined by the residual LV ejection fraction. In the Antiarrhythmic Versus Implantable Defibrillator (AVID) trial and Canadian trial of Implantable Defibrillators (CIDS), ICDs did not offer any survival benefit for patients with preserved LV function (>35%). Therefore, postrevascularization electrophysiologic evaluation is recommended only for patients with impaired ejection fraction or significant LV scarring.

Survivors of a malignant arrhythmia other than that due to a reversible cause such as severe metabolic disturbance, toxic drug effect, or acute myocardial infarction are best treated with an ICD. In the largest prospective, randomized trial of drugs versus an ICD (the AVID trial), the ICD reduced mortality by 39% at 1 year and by 31% at 3 years, compared with amiodarone (Cordarone) or sotalol (Betapace). In the absence of specific contraindication, ICD therapy is currently the standard of care for secondary prevention of life-threatening arrhythmic events.

Primary Prevention of Ventricular Arrhythmias and Sudden Cardiac Death

CORONARY ARTERY DISEASE

There are considerable data to guide efforts at primary prevention of sudden death in patients with CAD. β-Adrenergic blockers and angiotensin-converting enzyme inhibitors reduce mortality after myocardial infarction and should be routinely prescribed in the absence of major contraindications (Table 2). Part of the benefit

TABLE 2 Drugs That Have Been Shown to Reduce Sudden Cardiac Death

β-Adrenergic blockers: metoprolol (Lopressor), carvedilol (Coreg)
Angiotensin-converting enzyme inhibitors
Angiotensin receptor blockers
Aldosterone antagonists
Antiplatelet drugs
Lipid-lowering agents
Fish oil[1]

[1]Not FDA approved for this indication.

TABLE 3 Indication for ICD Therapy Based on the ACC/AHA 2008 Guidelines

Class I Indication*
1. Cardiac arrest due to VF or VT not due to a transient or reversible cause
2. Spontaneous sustained VT in association with heart disease
3. Recurrent syncope of undetermined origin in the presence of ventricular dysfunction and inducible ventricular arrhythmias on electrophysiologic study
4. NYHA class II or III heart failure and persistent systolic left ventricular dysfunction with LVEF ≤35%
5. Coronary artery disease and systolic left ventricular dysfunction (LVEF ≤30%) persisting >40 days after myocardial infarction or revascularization
6. Nonsustained VT with coronary disease, prior myocardial infarction, left ventricular dysfunction, and inducible VF or sustained VT on electrophysiologic study

Class II Indication†
1. Familial or inherited conditions with a high risk for life-threatening ventricular tachyarrhythmia
2. Unexplained syncope in the presence of left ventricular dysfunction and nonischemic cardiomyopathy
3. Patients with cardiac sarcoid, Chagas' disease, or giant cell myocarditis
4. Adult congenital heart disease with high risk for sudden cardiac death

*There is good clinical evidence and general agreement that ICD is beneficial.
†There is inadequate data or some divergence of opinion regarding ICD benefit.
ACC/AHA, American College of Cardiology/American Heart Association Task Force; ICD, implantable cardioverter-defibrillator; LVEF, left ventricular ejection fraction; NYHA, New York Heart Association; VF, ventricular fibrillation; VT, ventricular tachycardia.

on mortality offered by these drugs is achieved through reduction of the incidence of sudden death. There is no role for the use of antiarrhythmic drugs in primary prevention. Amiodarone, sotalol, and dofetilide (Tikosyn) have largely neutral effects, but class 1 antiarrhythmic drugs such flecainide (Tambocor) and propafenone (Rythmol) are clearly harmful and increase mortality in patients with ventricular dysfunction.

Ventricular arrhythmias occurring late (>24 hours) after a myocardial infarction usually indicate a persisting propensity for recurrent arrhythmia and risk of death. Commonly, these patients have impaired LV function and benefit from treatment with an ICD; an intracardiac electrophysiologic study is helpful in determining the risk of recurrence. Inducibility of ventricular tachycardia (VT) on electrophysiologic study is considered a predictor of sudden death, and treatment of such patients with an ICD lowers mortality.

For the stable patient with CAD, depressed ejection fraction and nonsustained VT are recognized risk factors for sudden death. If severe LV dysfunction is present (ejection fraction <30%), implantation of an ICD will significantly reduce sudden death mortality. In the presence of moderate LV dysfunction (ejection fraction 30%-40%), a defibrillator is indicated if patients have New York Heart Association class II or III heart failure symptoms. Nonsustained VT occurring in the context of moderate LV dysfunction warrants an intracardiac electrophysiologic study. In 40% and 60% of patients, sustained ventricular arrhythmia is inducible; these patients will benefit from ICD therapy (Table 3).

IDIOPATHIC DILATED CARDIOMYOPATHY

Unlike CAD, nonischemic dilated cardiomyopathy is more variable in its course. This is partly because the etiology is often unclear; the disease process may be progressive in some and self-limited with spontaneous improvement in others. Consequently, benefit from ICD therapy is not as convincing as in patients with CAD. Nonsustained VT, syncope, and heart failure symptoms are predictors of high risk of sudden death in this population. In the Defibrillators in Nonischemic Cardiomyopathy Treatment Evaluation trial (DEFINITE), implantation of an ICD based on the presence of LV dysfunction, symptomatic heart failure, and nonsustained VT resulted in a reduction in arrhythmic mortality. The Sudden Death in Heart Failure trial (SCD Heft) showed that ICDs reduce mortality in the presence of heart failure symptoms and an LV ejection fraction of 35% or less.

Syncope in the presence of cardiomyopathy can be a harbinger of sudden death and merits the use of ICD therapy if another cause of syncope cannot be identified.

HYPERTROPHIC CARDIOMYOPATHY

Hypertrophic cardiomyopathy is a genetically heterogenous disease with an autosomal dominant mode of inheritance caused by mutations in genes coding for sarcomeric proteins. Unrecognized hypertrophic cardiomyopathy is a frequent cause of sudden death in young athletes.

Sudden death in hypertrophic cardiomyopathy is caused by ventricular arrhythmias and can be prevented by implantation of an ICD. A number of risk factors for sudden death have been identified in retrospective studies and are outlined in Table 4. The presence of any one of the major risk factors is an indication for ICD implantation. Electrophysiologic testing has no major value in risk stratification.

There are some families with mutations in the cardiac troponin T gene in whom the phenotypic features may not be diagnostic of hypertrophic cardiomyopathy but who nevertheless have a higher risk of sudden death. Currently, however, the value of genetic screening for risk stratification is unknown and is not considered standard of care.

TABLE 4 Clinical Risk Factors for Sudden Death in Hypertrophic Cardiomyopathy

Major Risk Factors
Cardiac arrest
Spontaneous sustained or nonsustained ventricular tachycardia
History of sudden cardiac death in first-degree relatives
Syncope
Left ventricular thickness ≥30 mm
Abnormal blood pressure response to exercise

Possible Risk Factors
Atrial fibrillation
Myocardial ischemia
Left ventricular outflow obstruction
High-risk mutations
Intense (competitive) physical exertion

ARRHYTHMOGENIC RIGHT VENTRICULAR DYSPLASIA

Arrhythmogenic right ventricular dysplasia is characterized by progressive replacement of myocytes with fibrofatty tissue due to an inherited autosomal dominant abnormality in the genes coding for cell-to-cell junction proteins. Typically, the right ventricle is involved, but progressive involvement of the LV has been described. Right bundle branch blockade with late potentials (epsilon wave) and T-wave inversion in the precordial lead may be present on ECG. Ventricular arrhythmia and sudden death are common modes of presentation between the ages of 20 and 40 years, although occasionally heart failure is the presenting symptom.

Patients presenting with stable VT may respond to radiofrequency ablation and antiarrhythmic therapy, but the recurrence rates are high. Consequently, most patients will require ICD therapy. ICD is the first line of treatment for patients with prior cardiac arrest, inducible ventricular arrhythmias on electrophysiologic study, and unexplained syncope.

Sudden Death Associated with Abnormalities of the QT Interval

Congenital long QT (LQT) syndrome is caused by inherited abnormalities of the potassium channel (LQT1 and LQT2) or of the sodium channel (LQT3) that result in abnormal cardiac repolarization. These patients carry a risk of developing torsades de pointes VT. Torsades de pointes can lead to syncope but is frequently self-limited. However, the arrhythmia can degenerate to ventricular fibrillation, and sudden death may be the initial manifestation.

The mortality rate is high in untreated patients (approximately 1% per year). Once syncopal episodes begin, the risk of death increases; in one study, 20% of patients had died within 1 year after a syncopal spell. However, ideal management of the congenital LQT syndrome remains controversial. β-Adrenergic blockers and left stellate ganglionectomy, at times in conjunction with cardiac pacing, have been shown to reduce symptoms and mortality. However, β-blockers provide incomplete protection for patients with LQT2 or LQT3. Because most patients are children or teenagers at the time of diagnosis, there is concern about long-term therapy with implantable devices because of the need for generator changes, potential lead malfunction, and risk of infection. ICD therapy is currently reserved for high-risk patients identified by prior cardiac arrest, recurrent syncope, or VT while on β-blockers, QTc exceeding 500 msec, siblings with sudden death, and symptoms in the patient with LQT3 and possibly LQT2.

One of the major precipitants of torsades in the asymptomatic patient is iatrogenic effects. Numerous drugs have the potential to prolong the QT interval (Table 5). In addition, hypokalemia

TABLE 5 Drugs Known to Cause QT Prolongation and Torsades de Pointes

Common
Quinidine
Sotalol (Betapace)
Dofetilide (Tikosyn)
Ibutilide (Corvert)
Disopyramide (Norpace)
Procainamide (Pronestyl)

Less Common
Amiodarone (Cordarone)
Antibiotics: clarithromycin (Biaxin), erythromycin, pentamidine (Pentam), sparfloxacin (Zagam)[2]
Antiemetic agents: domperidone (Motilium),[2] droperidol (Inapsine)
Antipsychotic agents: chlorpromazine (Thorazine), haloperidol (Haldol), mesoridazine (Serentil),[2] thioridazine (Mellaril)

[2]Not available in the United States.

and hypomagnesemia can induce QT prolongation and torsades de pointes.

In patients without a recognized QT abnormality, drug-induced torsades is treated by discontinuation and avoidance of the offending drug. A number of risk factors have been recognized for drug-induced torsades. They include female gender, hypokalemia and hypomagnesemia, bradycardia, congestive heart failure, baseline QT prolongation, and high drug concentrations (with the exception of quinidine). Conversion of atrial fibrillation with rapid heart rates to sinus rhythm in the presence of a QT-prolonging drug is a known risk for torsades because of the relative bradycardia interacting with QT prolongation. Administration of class III antiarrhythmic drugs such as sotalol, ibutilide (Corvert), and dofetilide used for conversion and prevention of atrial fibrillation should be commenced under telemetric monitoring. The potential for accumulation of antiarrhythmic drugs in the face of renal dysfunction (e.g., sotalol, dofetilide) should be recognized and dosing adjusted.

A familial form of the short QT syndrome associated with sudden death has been described. A family history of sudden death appears to confer a high risk of sudden arrhythmic death in these patients, warranting ICD therapy.

BRUGADA SYNDROME

Brugada syndrome is characterized by ECG features of incomplete right bundle branch block, J-point elevation with ST-segment elevation in the right precordial leads, normal QT interval, and risk of ventricular fibrillation. The condition has been shown to be caused by an inherited abnormality of the sodium channel involving the same gene (SCN5A) that is responsible for LQT3. The clinical features share similarities with those of LQT3: relative inefficacy of β-blockade, high mortality in symptomatic patients, and sudden death occurring during rest or sleep. Diagnostic criteria are equivocal. ST-segment abnormalities may be transient and dynamic and tend to be augmented by administration of sodium channel blockers.

The general consensus is that symptomatic patients should be treated with an ICD. Asymptomatic patients with a malignant family history should also be considered for ICD therapy. As with the LQT syndromes, drugs have a potential for provoking arrhythmias; sodium channel blockers, including tricyclic antidepressants, have the potential for inducing ventricular arrhythmias and are best avoided in these patients.

CATECHOLAMINERGIC VENTRICULAR TACHYCARDIA

Inherited defects in genes coding for handling of calcium by the sarcoplasmic reticulum result in ventricular arrhythmia triggered by exercise or emotional stress. The resting ECG is normal. Children are usually affected, but late onset of this condition has been recognized. An autosomal dominant form is caused by mutations in the gene coding for the cardiac ryanodine receptor. The autosomal recessive form is caused by mutation in the gene encoding for calsequestrin, a calcium-buffering protein in the sarcoplasmic reticulum. β-Blockers are the primary form of treatment. However, those patients who have had ventricular fibrillation or continue to have VT or syncope despite β-blocker therapy are considered to be at high risk and should receive ICD therapy.

WOLFF-PARKINSON-WHITE SYNDROME

In the Wolff-Parkinson-White (WPW) syndrome, atrial fibrillation can be conducted rapidly via an accessory pathway with a short refractory period, resulting in ventricular fibrillation and death. The risk of sudden death in patients with WPW syndrome is estimated to be less than 1 in every 1000 patient-years of follow-up. Although the risk is reportedly very low among asymptomatic patients, a potentially lethal arrhythmia can be the initial manifestation in a small number of patients (up to 10%).

The treatment of choice for WPW syndrome is catheter ablation of the accessory pathway; this is successful in 95% of patients.

If ablation is ineffective or preferentially avoided because of a high risk of heart block, use of antiarrhythmic drugs such as flecainide or propafenone is an alternative. Rarely, amiodarone may be required to suppress arrhythmias including atrial fibrillation.

Management in the asymptomatic individual who exhibits the WPW pattern on ECG is controversial. Until recently, the consensus was that asymptomatic patients did not require invasive evaluation. Patients with intermittent ventricular preexcitation and those in whom the refractory period of the accessory pathway can be determined to be long are at low risk for sudden death. If a benign nature of the accessory pathway cannot be confirmed by noninvasive evaluation, intracardiac electrophysiologic testing should be considered, with radiofrequency ablation if appropriate. A recent study showed that prophylactic ablation in asymptomatic patients younger than 35 years of age significantly reduced subsequent arrhythmias. Prophylactic ablation should also be considered for individuals in situations in which there is minimal tolerance of a potential for arrhythmias, such as in airline pilots.

Idiopathic Ventricular Fibrillation

A small number of patients who are resuscitated from sudden death episodes have no identifiable structural, electrical, or genetic abnormalities. The term idiopathic ventricular fibrillation is applied to these patients. Clinically silent focal myocarditis, cardiomyopathy, or unrecognized ionic channel abnormalities may be responsible and may become apparent during subsequent follow-up. The current consensus is that drug therapy is ineffective, and ICD therapy is the safest and most effective secondary prevention strategy.

Adult Congenital Heart Disease

A number of congenital heart diseases can be corrected or palliated by surgery, and survival into adulthood is common. However, sudden arrhythmic cardiac death is a leading cause for late mortality. Unexplained syncope in such patients warrants evaluation by electrophysiologic testing. Intracardiac repair of tetralogy of Fallot has been accomplished since the mid-1950s, with favorable long-term outcome. Risk of late arrhythmic death increases with wide QRS duration, right ventricular dilatation from pulmonary regurgitation, and LV dysfunction. Ventricular arrhythmias or complete heart block may lead to sudden death. Syncope in such patients is an ominous symptom and should be investigated by electrophysiologic evaluation. Pulmonary valve replacement is known to reduce subsequent arrhythmia risk. Inducible VT and evidence for spontaneous ventricular arrhythmias should prompt the consideration of ICD therapy.

A rare condition called noncompaction, caused by an arrest in development of the LV, is known to be associated with sudden death. Prophylactic ICD implantation is recommended.

Neuromuscular Diseases

Some neuromuscular diseases are associated with conduction system disease and ventricular arrhythmias leading to sudden death. Myotonic dystrophy and Kearns-Sayre syndrome are situations in which prophylactic cardiac pacing at the first sign of conduction system disease can be life-saving. If evidence of cardiac disease precedes the onset of respiratory muscle disease, the risk of cardiac arrhythmia is high, and ICD implantation is often necessary.

Bradyarrhythmia

Bradyarrhythmias resulting from atrioventricular blockade below the atrioventricular node is a cause for sudden death. Most cases of Mobitz type II block or complete heart block below the His bundle

are caused by sclerodegenerative changes in the specialized conduction system. Occasionally, cardiac sarcoid or other infiltrative diseases may be responsible. Chagas' disease is a common cause in endemic areas in South America. A familial form of progressive heart block caused by a defect in the SCN5A gene has been identified in some families.

Symptomatic bradyarrhythmias and heart block due to disease in the His-Purkinje system are indications for permanent cardiac pacing. In the absence of the other structural heart disease, permanent cardiac pacing can restore longevity to match that of age-matched controls.

REFERENCES

Antiarrhythmics Versus Implantable Defibrillators (AVID) Investigators. A comparison of antiarrhythmic drug therapy with implantable defibrillators in patients resuscitated from near fatal ventricular arrhythmias. N Engl J Med 1997;337:1576–83.

Ezekowitz JA, Armstrong PW, McAlister FA. Implantable cardioverter defibrillators in primary and secondary prevention: A systematic review of randomized, controlled trials [see comments]. Ann Intern Med 2003;138:445–52.

Goldberg I, Moss AJ, Peterson DR, et al. Risk factors for aborted cardiac arrest and sudden cardiac death in children with the congenital long QT syndrome. Circulation 2008;117:2184–91.

Pappone C, Santinelli V, Manguso F, et al. A randomized study of prophylactic catheter ablation in asymptomatic patients with the Wolff-Parkinson-White syndrome. N Engl J Med 2003;349:1803–11.

Priori SG, Schwartz PJ, Napolitano C, et al. Risk stratification in the long-QT syndrome. N Engl J Med 2003;348:1866–74.

Santinelli V, Radinovic A, Manguso F, et al. The natural history of asymptomatic ventricular pre-excitation: A long-term prospective follow-up study of 184 asymptomatic children. J Am Coll Cardiol 2009;53:275–80.

Zipes DP, Camm AJ, Borggrefe M, et al. ACC/AHA/ESC 2006 Guidelines for management of patients with ventricular arrhythmias and the prevention of sudden cardiac death. Circulation 2006;114(10):e385–484.

Atrial Fibrillation

Method of
Anne B. Curtis, MD

Atrial fibrillation (AF) is the most common arrhythmia seen in clinical practice, and it accounts for about one third of hospitalizations for cardiac arrhythmias. The prevalence of AF is 0.4% to 1.0% in the general population, but it increases to about 8% in those older than 80 years. More than 2.3 million people in the United States are estimated to have AF.

Classification

Paroxysmal AF is AF that begins and terminates spontaneously. *Persistent* AF is AF that lasts longer than 7 days or requires intervention, either pharmacologic treatment or electrical cardioversion, to restore sinus rhythm. AF is *permanent* when the arrhythmia has failed to respond to cardioversion or when attempts to restore sinus rhythm have been abandoned.

Presentation

Patients may or may not have symptoms with AF. If they do, they may complain of palpitations, shortness of breath, exercise intolerance, chest discomfort, or fatigue. Many patients have symptomatic

CURRENT DIAGNOSIS

Minimum Evaluation

- Detailed history and physical examination
- 12-lead electrocardiogram
- Transthoracic echocardiogram
- Laboratory tests including thyroid function tests

Additional Tests

- 24-hour Holter monitor or event monitor (to establish diagnosis or to assess rate or rhythm control)
- Exercise testing (to assess adequacy of rate control, reproduce exercise-induced atrial fibrillation, or exclude ischemia)
- Transesophageal echocardiogram (to evaluate for thrombus in the left atrial appendage before cardioversion)

as well as asymptomatic episodes of AF, as demonstrated from arrhythmia logs in permanent pacemakers.

AF increases the risk of stroke and impairs quality of life. It is often found in patients with valvular heart disease, particularly mitral valve disease, and is found in many patients with heart failure from any etiology.

Clinical Evaluation

The most common finding on physical examination in a patient with AF is an irregular pulse. The S1 can vary in intensity, an S3 may be present if there is coexisting heart failure, and an S4 is absent. The A wave is absent in the jugular venous pulse.

When a patient presents with AF, initial evaluation beyond a history and physical examination should include an electrocardiogram and a transthoracic echocardiogram and routine blood chemistries including thyroid function tests. The electrocardiogram (ECG) shows an absence of P waves and irregular R-R intervals. An echocardiogram is useful to evaluate the patient for valvular heart disease, assess left ventricular function, and measure left atrial size. Event monitors may be used to confirm the diagnosis of AF in patients with unexplained palpitations. Holter monitors and exercise stress tests may be useful in assessing the adequacy of rate control in patients with persistent or permanent AF. For a first episode of AF, reversible causes such as pericarditis, pulmonary embolism, or hyperthyroidism, among others, should be considered.

Treatment

When the diagnosis of AF has been established, several decisions must be made regarding patient management. First, the patient should be evaluated for the risk of thromboembolism, and anticoagulation should be initiated as appropriate. Second, a decision must be made about the need for treatment. If treatment is needed, a decision is needed as to whether rate control or rhythm control should be the initial management strategy.

ANTICOAGULATION

The most useful scheme for stratification of patients for risk of thromboembolism is the CHADS$_2$ score (Table 1). In this approach, one point each is assigned for the presence of congestive heart failure, hypertension, age (>75 years), and diabetes mellitus, and two points are assigned for a history of stroke or transient ischemic attack. Patients with no risk factors for thromboembolism do not need anticoagulation with warfarin (Coumadin). They may be managed with aspirin 81 to 325 mg daily. Patients with a CHADS score greater

TABLE 1 The CHADS$_2$ Score for Assessing Risk of Thromboembolism in Patients with Nonvalvular Atrial Fibrillation

Risk Criterion	Score
Cardiac failure	1
Hypertension	1
Age > 75 years	1
Diabetes mellitus	1
Stroke or prior transient ischemic attack	2

than or equal to 2 and patients with rheumatic mitral stenosis should be managed with adjusted-dose warfarin to achieve an international normalized ratio (INR) of 2 to 3. For patients with a CHADS score of 1, anticoagulation with either aspirin or warfarin is reasonable. Patients with AF and no risk factors do not need anticoagulation.

The decision whether and how to anticoagulate should be made on the basis of an assessment of risk factors and not on the type of AF, because there is no evidence that the risk of thromboembolism is different in patients with paroxysmal versus permanent AF. Patients with atrial flutter, although they appear to have a somewhat lower risk of thromboembolism compared with patients with AF, should still receive anticoagulation based on the considerations outlined earlier.

A recent study showed that bleeding risks in elderly patients given warfarin may be higher than previously appreciated, creating some challenges in managing these patients. Elderly patients who are given warfarin should be followed very closely after the drug is initiated because the risk of hemorrhage is highest in the initial months of treatment.

RATE VERSUS RHYTHM CONTROL

When AF is diagnosed, a decision must be made about the management approach. A patient with a first episode of AF that terminates spontaneously or after cardioversion might need no specific therapy aside from consideration of anticoagulation. For patients with recurrent AF, the management approach should be determined based on the patient's symptoms and underlying heart disease. There have been several randomized trials of rate versus rhythm-control strategies for the management of AF. The two largest, the Atrial Fibrillation Follow-up Investigation of Rhythm Management (AFFIRM) and the Rate Control vs. Electrical Cardioversion (RACE) trials, found no significant difference in morbidity or mortality with either strategy. Generally speaking, patients with minimal symptoms or long-standing AF are best managed with a rate-control strategy, and highly symptomatic patients benefit most from a rhythm-control approach.

CURRENT THERAPY

Stroke Prevention

- Aspirin
- Warfarin (Coumadin)

Rate Control

- β-Blockers
- Non-dihydropyridine calcium channel blockers: Diltiazem, verapamil
- Digoxin (Lanoxin)
- AV junction ablation and permanent pacemaker

Rhythm Control

- Cardioversion: Electrical and pharmacologic
- Antiarrhythmic drugs
- Atrial fibrillation ablation
- Surgical maze procedure

Rate Control

Rate control often must be initiated first in any patient presenting with AF, regardless of whether the ultimate goal is rhythm control or rate control, in order to control symptoms from an elevated heart rate. Particularly in elderly patients with minimal to no symptoms from AF, rate control may be the preferred long-term strategy. The goal for heart rate control should be 60 to 80 bpm at rest and 90 to 115 bpm with moderate exercise.

For acute management of the ventricular response in AF, either intravenous β-blockers or non–dihydropyridine calcium channel blockers (diltiazem [Cardizem] or verapamil) may be used. The same drugs may be used orally for long-term control of heart rate in patients with persistent or permanent AF (Box 1). Digoxin (Lanoxin) is not the best choice as a sole agent for controlling the ventricular response in patients with paroxysmal AF. However, it is useful for controlling resting heart rate in sedentary patients or patients with heart failure. In addition, digoxin may be added to other atrioventricular (AV) nodal blockers if heart rate control is not adequate with single agents. Although amiodarone can slow the heart rate in patients with AF, it is not advisable to use this drug for the long term solely for the purpose of rate control because of the side effects potentially associated with its use.

Rhythm Control

The approach to rhythm control in AF depends heavily on the patient's symptoms, the frequency of recurrences, and any underlying structural heart disease (Table 2). For patients with an initial episode of AF or rare

---

BOX 1   Long-term Treatment Options

Stroke Prevention
Aspirin 325 mg/d
Warfarin (Coumadin) (dosed for target INR of 2–3)

Rate Control
Pharmacologic
β-Blockers
• Atenolol (Tenormin) (PO)
• Esmolol (Brevibloc) (IV)
• Metoprolol (Lopressor) (PO or IV; IV drip available)
Calcium channel blockers
• Diltiazem (Cardizem) (PO or IV; IV drip available)
• Digoxin (Lanoxin) (PO or IV)
• Verapamil (Calan) (PO or IV)

Nonpharmacologic
AV junction ablation and pacemaker

Rhythm Control
Antiarrhythmic Drugs*
Amiodarone (Cordarone) 100–400 mg/d
Propafenone (Rythmol) 150–300 mg tid (450–900 mg daily)
Propafenone (Rythmol SR) 225–425 mg bid (450–850 mg daily)
Flecainide (Tambocor) 50–150 mg bid (100–300 mg daily)
Sotalol (Betapace) 80–160 mg bid (160–320 mg daily)
Dofetilide (Tikosyn) 125–500 μg bid (250–1000 μg daily)

Nonpharmacologic Treatment
Catheter ablation
Surgical maze procedure

---

* Quinidine, procainamide, and disopyramide (Norpace) are rarely used anymore for long-term treatment unless patients are intolerant of amiodarone.
AV = atrioventricular; INR = international normalized ratio.

TABLE 2 Guidelines for Choosing Antiarrhythmic Drugs

Underlying Disorder	First Line	Second Line
No structural heart disease	Flecainide (Tambocor) Propafenone (Rythmol) Sotalol (Betapace)	Amiodarone (Cordarone) Dofetilide (Tikosyn)
Left ventricular dysfunction	Amiodarone Dofetilide	
Coronary artery disease	Sotalol	Amiodarone Dofetilide
Hypertension with left ventricular hypertrophy <1.4 cm	Flecainide Propafenone	Amiodarone Dofetilide Sotalol
Hypertension with left ventricular hypertrophy >1.4 cm	Amiodarone	

---

recurrences of AF, particularly those that terminate spontaneously, no specific therapy to control rhythm may be indicated. For patients who have occasional episodes of symptomatic AF in the setting of a structurally normal heart or only mild left ventricular hypertrophy, an excellent option is the pill-in-the-pocket approach. A patient may take either flecainide (Tambocor) 300 mg or propafenone (Rythmol) 600 mg[3] orally as a single dose. It may be best to give either of these drugs in a monitored setting the first time they are administered, in case there are side effects such as marked sinus arrest on termination of AF.

For management of recurrent AF, the presence of underlying heart disease dictates to a large extent the choice of antiarrhythmic drug therapy. Patients with normal hearts or at most mild left ventricular hypertrophy may be treated with flecainide or propafenone orally. Propafenone has β-blocking properties, so it may be used as a sole agent. It is particularly attractive in its sustained-release preparation, in which it is dosed twice daily. Because flecainide has no AV nodal blocking properties, it is usually given in conjunction with either a β-blocker or a calcium channel blocker. Both drugs are usually well tolerated, with minimal extracardiac side effects, and neither prolongs the QT interval. An alternative antiarrhythmic drug in this setting is sotalol (Betapace), which has β-blocking properties as well and can prolong the QT interval. Sotalol is particularly attractive as an initial choice of antiarrhythmic drug therapy in patients with coronary artery disease and preserved ventricular function, both because of its β-blocking properties and because flecainide and propafenone are not recommended in patients with established ischemic heart disease.

When these drugs are ineffective or not tolerated, either amiodarone (Cordarone) or dofetilide (Tikosyn) can be used. However, catheter ablation is now considered an acceptable alternative management approach in such patients when initial antiarrhythmic drug therapy fails to control symptoms.

For patients with heart failure, amiodarone and dofetilide are the drugs of choice for rhythm control. The latter requires in-hospital initiation because of the slight risk of QT prolongation and torsades de pointes. Patients with significant left ventricular hypertrophy should also be treated with amiodarone for rhythm control.

CATHETER ABLATION

One of the most important changes in the 2006 Guidelines for the Management of Patients with Atrial Fibrillation was the elevation of catheter ablation from its status as a last-resort therapeutic approach after failure of all antiarrhythmic drugs (including amiodarone) to a coequal option with amiodarone. The reasons for the change include

---

[3] Exceeds dosage recommended by the manufacturer.

the increasing success rate with catheter ablation and the better understanding and standardization of the procedure itself.

In the course of management of a patient with AF, when one would recommend catheter ablation depends on the type of AF, the presence and severity of underlying heart disease, and the comorbidities of the patient. An ideal candidate is a patient younger than 60 years with paroxysmal AF and a structurally normal heart. In such cases, pulmonary vein isolation alone is often sufficient to cure AF, with success rates approaching 85% to 90% if one includes patients who require second procedures.

Patients with persistent or permanent AF usually require more than just pulmonary vein isolation, with additional ablation lines in both atria and ablation of complex fractionated electrograms as well, depending on the approach in the particular electrophysiology laboratory. Success rates for these patients for an initial procedure are much lower than for patients with paroxysmal AF, often around 33% in patients with permanent AF even in experienced laboratories.

At present, catheter ablation for AF is not recommended solely for the purpose of allowing discontinuation of anticoagulation with warfarin. Long-term studies have not yet been done to show that this approach is safe, and the procedure itself has a number of potentially serious complications associated with it.

Surgical maze procedures have success rates similar to those for catheter-based procedures for AF. Because surgery is more invasive, surgical procedures for management of AF are most often performed in conjunction with cardiac surgery for another reason, such as mitral valve repair for mitral regurgitation.

PACING

In patients who have the tachy–brady syndrome manifested as sinus bradycardia alternating with AF, permanent pacemakers are often considered for managing the bradycardia, and antiarrhythmic drugs and AV nodal blockers are used to manage the tachycardia. Given the success of radiofrequency ablation for cure of paroxysmal AF in patients without significant structural heart disease, ablation should be considered as an initial approach instead of a pacemaker if medical therapy fails, particularly in younger patients.

A number of pacing algorithms have been investigated for preventing AF in order to suppress bradycardia or pauses that can promote the development of AF. None of these approaches has been demonstrated to have a significant impact on AF burden, and so pacemaker therapy cannot be recommended solely for that purpose.

Ablation of the AV node with permanent pacing has fallen out of favor to a large extent, particularly for paroxysmal AF, where curative ablation is preferred. AV node ablation might still be a viable option in patients with existing pacemakers and uncontrollable heart rates from AF, especially when there are significant comorbidities that make a prolonged catheter ablation procedure unattractive.

CARDIOVERSION

Patients who present with AF that does not convert spontaneously may be candidates for cardioversion. If the onset of AF can confidently be determined to have been within 48 hours of presentation, and if anticoagulation with heparin is instituted promptly, one may proceed with cardioversion immediately. If patients are hemodynamically unstable or experiencing acute ischemia from elevated rates in AF, cardioversion should also be performed without delay.

There are several options for cardioversion (Table 3). Electrical cardioversion requires general anesthesia. It should be performed with patches placed in an anterior–posterior configuration, and 200-J biphasic shocks are recommended initially to maximize the chances of conversion to sinus rhythm with a minimal number of shocks. Ibutilide (Corvert) can be used intravenously if the patient has a normal QT interval. Monitoring of the patient must be continued for at least 4 hours after conversion to sinus rhythm, because there is a risk of torsades de pointes if significant QT prolongation occurs. Oral flecainide or propafenone can be administered if the patient has minimal heart disease. These drugs do not prolong the QT interval, so they pose no risk of torsades de pointes. An additional advantage of these drugs is that the patient can be observed in a monitored situation as sinus rhythm is restored. If there are no untoward side effects, such as marked sinus arrest on termination of AF, patients can be given a prescription for either drug to use in the future for recurrent AF according to the pill-in-the-pocket approach. Finally, intravenous amiodarone is another option for chemical cardioversion. Conversion to sinus rhythm may be delayed, but this is a good option for patients in intensive care settings who need ongoing suppression of AF after cardioversion.

If the duration of AF cannot be determined, or if it is known to be longer than 48 hours without adequate anticoagulation, there are two options. A transesophageal echocardiogram can be performed to rule out the presence of thrombus in the left atrium. A transthoracic echocardiogram is inadequate for this purpose. If no clot is seen, cardioversion may be performed, with the patient subsequently anticoagulated with warfarin for a minimum of 4 weeks afterward. Alternatively, the patient may be anticoagulated with warfarin for at least 3 weeks with documented therapeutic INRs before cardioversion, without a transesophageal echocardiogram, followed again by a minimum of 4 weeks of anticoagulation.

POSTOPERATIVE ATRIAL FIBRILLATION

AF commonly occurs postoperatively, especially after cardiothoracic surgery. Both sotalol and amiodarone have been shown to reduce the incidence of AF when used prophylactically. β-Blockers have also been shown to be effective in preventing AF in the postoperative setting. Amiodarone is usually used when AF occurs postoperatively and requires treatment, because it can be given intravenously and has a high efficacy rate.

TABLE 3 Advantages and Disadvantages of Different Approaches to Cardioversion

Method	Advantages	Disadvantages
Electrical (direct current; 200-J biphasic shocks)	Rapid conversion to sinus rhythm	Need for general anesthesia Early recurrence
Ibutilide, 1 mg IV; may repeat one time	No need for general anesthesia	Requires ECG monitoring for at least 4 hours after administration
Flecainide 300 mg PO or propafenone 600 mg PO[3]	No need for general anesthesia Outpatient use (consider observation of response in-hospital for first use)	Effect may be delayed for several hours
Amiodarone IV	No need for general anesthesia Prevention of early recurrence Ideal in postoperative setting	Delayed onset of action

[3]Exceeds dosage recommended by the manufacturer.
ECG = electrocardiogram.

REFERENCES

Alboni P, Botto GL, Baldi N, et al. Outpatient treatment of recent-onset atrial fibrillation with the "pill-in-the-pocket" approach. N Engl J Med 2004;351:2384–91.

Atrial Fibrillation Follow-up Investigation of Rhythm Management (AFFIRM) Investigators. A comparison of rate control and rhythm control in patients with atrial fibrillation. N Engl J Med 2002;347:1825–33.

Calkins H, Brugada J, Packer DL, et al. HRS/EHRA/ECAS Expert Consensus Statement on catheter and surgical ablation of atrial fibrillation: recommendations for personnel, policy, procedures and follow-up. A report of the Heart Rhythm Society (HRS) Task Force on catheter and surgical ablation of atrial fibrillation. Heart Rhythm 2007;4:816–61.

Fuster V, Ryden LE, Cannom DS, et al. ACC/AHA/ESC 2006 Guidelines for the Management of Patients with Atrial Fibrillation—Executive Summary. Circulation 2006;114:700–52.

Hylek EM, Evans-Molina C, Shea C, et al. Major hemorrhage and tolerability of warfarin in the first year of therapy among elderly patients with atrial fibrillation. Circulation 2007;115:2689–96.

Van Gelder IC, Hagens VE, Bosker HA, et al. A comparison of rate control and rhythm control in patients with recurrent persistent atrial fibrillation. N Engl J Med 2002;347:1834–40.

Van Walraven WC, Hart RG, Wells GA, et al. A clinical prediction rule to identify patients with atrial fibrillation and a low risk for stroke while taking aspirin. Arch Intern Med 2003;163:936–43.

Premature Beats

Method of
Prakash C. Deedwania, MD, and
Enrique V. Carbajal, MD

Premature beats are the most common form of cardiac arrhythmia encountered in clinical practice. Premature beats are one of the most common causes of irregular pulse and palpitations. In many instances, premature beats are not associated with any symptoms. They result from electrical depolarization of myocardium that occurs earlier than the sinus impulse. Premature beats have been referred to by a variety of names, including premature contractions, premature complexes, ectopic beats, and early depolarizations. Although no single term is ideal, most electrophysiologists refer to them as premature complexes because although the term *ectopic beat* denotes the abnormal site of origin of the depolarization, it does not necessarily require the beat to be premature, and, in some cases, ectopic rhythm indeed occurs as an escape phenomenon.

Although premature beats generally occur in patients with organic heart disease, they frequently can be seen in the absence of any structural heart disease, especially in elderly patients. Premature beats can be triggered by, or increase in frequency with, myocardial ischemia and heart failure. Premature beats can be provoked by, or occur in association with, a variety of systemic abnormalities, including electrolyte disturbances, acid-base imbalance, toxins from recreational drug and/or alcohol abuse, metabolic perturbations, systemic illnesses such as thyroid disorders, pulmonary disease, infections, and febrile illnesses, and any condition associated with increased catecholamine levels.

Most premature beats occur as a result of enhanced automaticity, but other electrophysiologic mechanisms, including reentry and triggered activity, might play a role. Based on the corresponding site of origin, premature electrical depolarizations are called *premature atrial complexes* (PACs), *premature junctional complexes* (PJCs), and *premature ventricular complexes* (PVCs). Morphologic features and timing of the premature beat on electrocardiographic (ECG) recording(s) help determine the site of origin and the nature of premature complexes. Premature beats can occur in a repetitive fashion as *bigeminy* (after every other normal beat), *trigeminy* (after each sequence of two normal beats), or *quadrigeminy* (after each sequence

of three normal beats). They also can occur as two or three successive premature beats, defined as *couplets* and *triplets*, respectively. In this article, the primary focus is on single premature beats.

Premature Atrial Complexes

PACs are the most common form of atrial arrhythmias that can originate at any site in the atria. The exact morphology of the atrial activation (P wave) varies depending on the site of origin of the PAC. Careful and systematic examination of the ECG features of PACs usually can distinguish them from PVCs.

ELECTROCARDIOGRAPHIC FEATURES

The cardinal features of PACs include their prematurity with reference to sinus beats, abnormal P wave morphology, and, in most cases, QRS morphology that is similar to that of sinus beats. The P wave morphology of the PAC generally differs from the sinus P wave unless the premature complex originates in the high right atrial area adjacent to the sinus node, in which case distinguishing PACs from sinus arrhythmia may be difficult. Although sinus arrhythmias are generally phasic in nature, being influenced by the respiratory cycle, this feature would be helpful in differentiating from high right atrial PACs only when the PACs are frequent and repetitive. When the PAC occurs quite early in the diastolic phase, the P wave may not be obvious on surface ECG because it is often hidden in the preceding T wave and would be evident only by watching carefully for the notched or peaked T wave.

If the PAC is too premature, it might fail to conduct to the ventricles if the atrioventricular (AV) node is refractory owing to conduction of the preceding sinus impulse. Such nonconducted PACs are called *blocked PACs*, and they are important because they can be confused with instances of AV block. Such erroneous interpretation can be avoided by simply remembering a common rule of thumb that requires normal successive P-P intervals for all sinus beats, including the interval for a blocked P wave, before considering the diagnosis of AV block. Although most PACs have a normal or prolonged PR interval, the relationship of the PAC to the subsequent QRS complex depends on the site of origin of the PAC and the prematurity index. For example, a PAC originating in the lower atrial area near the AV node generally has a shorter PR interval, whereas a PAC that is quite premature and originates in the upper left atrial area might have a longer than usual PR interval. In general, the PR interval of a PAC is inversely related to its prematurity.

Because most PACs are able to depolarize the sinus node, they usually can reset the sinus automaticity; therefore, the subsequent pause following most PACs is generally less than compensatory because the sinus node fires earlier than expected. In this case, measurement of the P-P interval between the sinus P wave preceding the PAC and the P wave following the PAC is generally less than twice the basic sinus cycle length. This is in contrast to the full compensatory pause often observed in conjunction with PVCs. In some cases,

---

   CURRENT DIAGNOSIS

- Premature beats are identified by their occurrence at times considerably shorter than the regular sinus rhythm cycles.
- The origin of the premature beats is determined by the presence or absence of P waves, morphology of the P wave (when present), QRS configuration, and the presence or absence of a compensatory period.
- The presence of frequent PVCs (≥10 per hour) during the postdischarge evaluation of survivors of acute MI predicts increased risk of arrhythmic death and overall cardiac mortality.

the PAC collides with the sinus impulse in the perinodal tissue and thus fails to reset the sinus node, thereby resulting in a full compensatory pause.

In general, electrical depolarization below the AV node is normal with PAC and results in an unchanged (baseline) QRS complex. Aberrant conduction, however, may be encountered when the PAC reaches the infranodal tissue during the period when it is still partially refractory. Most frequently, the aberrant conduction usually occurs when a short coupled PAC follows a long pause in patients with sinus bradycardia (long-short cycle). This usually results in a right bundle-branch block pattern and is commonly referred to as the *Ashman phenomenon.*

CLINICAL FEATURES

Although PACs can occur in normal individuals of all ages, they are quite infrequent except in the elderly. Their frequency increases with age; as many as 50% to 70% of the elderly may have occasional PACs. Some elderly individuals without organic heart disease have frequent PACs and occasionally atrial bigeminy or two to three PACs in a row. Whether the increased frequency of PACs in these individuals is secondary to senile amyloidosis, myocardial fibrosis, or diastolic dysfunction secondary to aging-related changes in the heart is not known. PACs are extremely common in patients with heart disease and in patients with acute as well as chronic respiratory failure. The frequency of PACs can increase markedly during periods of acute febrile illness, shock states, and metabolic disorders, especially in patients with hyperthyroidism and conditions associated with increased catecholamine levels. Use of excessive caffeine, alcohol, tobacco, and recreational drugs can increase the frequency of PACs. In patients with acute myocardial infarction (MI), frequent PACs usually are precursors of atrial fibrillation and occur in association with ventricular failure. In general, the presence of frequent PACs in the setting of acute MI is an indicator of poor prognosis.

In general, PACs are benign except when they are a marker of an underlying cardiopulmonary disorder(s). The major clinical importance of PACs is related to the increased risk of atrial tachyarrhythmias in patients with an established history of such arrhythmias as well as in the elderly who are generally at high risk for atrial fibrillation. As indicated earlier, in rare instances the blocked PACs may be confused with episodes of AV nodal block; however, careful examination of the ECG features described previously easily establishes the correct diagnosis and avoids unnecessary pacemaker implantation.

TREATMENT

The correction of an underlying structural cardiopulmonary disorder and other precipitating factors (e.g., electrolyte or metabolic abnormalities) usually is all the treatment that is needed. No specific treatment is generally required in most patients because PACs usually are benign except in patients with a history of recurrent atrial tachyarrhythmias, for example, atrial flutter/fibrillation. In such patients, specific treatment may be indicated and could include a β-blocker or a heart rate-modulating calcium channel blocking agent such as verapamil (Calan) or diltiazem (Cardizem). Recent studies have shown that verapamil is quite effective in patients with frequent PACs and multifocal atrial tachycardia in the setting of acute or chronic ventilatory insufficiency. In patients who are at risk for recurrent atrial fibrillation, treatment with a specific antiarrhythmic agent, such as propafenone (Rythmol) or flecainide (Tambocor), may be beneficial; however, these drugs should be used only when the patient has a history of recurrent atrial flutter/fibrillation because of the increased risk of proarrhythmia, especially in the presence of organic heart disease such as recurrent ischemia or heart failure.

Premature Junctional Complexes

PJCs are rarely seen in normal individuals and are infrequently encountered even in patients with organic heart disease. When present, PJCs can occur due to abnormal automaticity or reentry

CURRENT THERAPY

- In general, premature beats in patients without evidence of organic heart disease do not require any specific antiarrhythmic therapy because generally there is no significant increased risk of life-threatening arrhythmia.
- Correction of any underlying structural cardiopulmonary disorder and other precipitating factors (e.g., electrolyte or metabolic abnormalities).
- Suppression of PVCs using currently available antiarrhythmic drugs (except for amiodarone) is not advisable for most patients primarily because of the increased risk of proarrhythmic effects of these drugs.
- In the occasional patient who is disabled by annoying symptoms due to PVCs, a trial of β-blocker therapy should be considered and often is effective in many patients.

phenomenon. Although digitalis toxicity is cited as a common etiologic factor, PJCs also can occur in the setting of MI, myocarditis, and electrolyte/metabolic disturbances.

ELECTROCARDIOGRAPHIC FEATURES

The ECG characteristics of PJCs are distinct from those of PACs in that the P wave usually is inverted in the inferior leads (II, III, and aVF) because of retrograde conduction to the atria from the ectopic foci in the junctional area. The second feature of PJCs is that the PR interval almost always is shorter than the normal PR interval because of the proximity of ectopic foci to the AV node and bundle of His. In most cases, the P wave might not even be visible on surface ECGs because it lies hidden within the QRS complex. Rarely, the P wave precedes the QRS complex when the ectopic impulse traverses to the atria before traveling down to depolarize the ventricle. In general, the infranodal conduction of PJCs is normal, and thus the QRS morphology of the conducted PJCs is similar to that noted during sinus rhythm. When the PJC is closely coupled to the preceding sinus beat, aberrant conduction might occur if the impulse traverses down the bundle branch during the relative refractory period (most frequently manifesting as a right bundle-branch block pattern). Because in many instances no obvious P wave accompanies a PJC, aberrantly conducted PJCs may be hard to differentiate from PVCs.

In some instances when PJCs occur during the period when the AV node as well as the infranodal conduction systems both are refractory, the PJC may encounter both retrograde and antegrade blocks for impulse propagation. In such situations, no P wave or QRS complex is related to the PJC. Although the ectopic impulse would be invisible on a surface ECG, it would penetrate a portion of the conduction system and thus make it partially or completely refractory to conduction of the subsequent sinus impulse. This would be manifested as a sudden prolongation of subsequent PR interval in case of partial refractoriness or as an episode of "pseudo AV nodal block" due to the blocked sinus beat if the infranodal tissue were unable to conduct the sinus impulse. Thus, even though some PJCs might not have any surface ECG complexes, their presence can be suspected based on their influence on the conduction of the following sinus beat owing to the electrophysiologic phenomenon described as "concealed conduction."

CLINICAL FEATURES

PJCs usually are not seen in normal persons and are rarely encountered in cardiac patients except in the setting of digitalis intoxication and infrequently in the setting of MI or myocarditis. In patients with digitalis toxicity, PJCs may lead to junctional tachycardia, occasionally resulting in palpitation, but are rarely associated with hemodynamic compromise. Because in some cases concealed conduction of PJCs might result in periods of varying degrees of pseudo AV blocks, it is clinically important to recognize their presence in order to prevent undue concern and avoid inappropriate pacemaker implantation.

Premature Ventricular Complexes

PVCs are the most common form of arrhythmia and can be encountered frequently in both healthy individuals as well as in patients with a variety of cardiac disorders. PVCs are often triggered by electrolyte abnormalities, acid-base imbalance, metabolic perturbations, hypoxia, and ischemia.

ELECTROCARDIOGRAPHIC FEATURES

PVCs occur as a result of premature depolarization of the ventricles due to ectopic foci in the ventricular myocardium or Purkinje fibers. In general, PVCs result in wide QRS complexes with the T wave axis usually opposite to that of the QRS. In the vast majority of cases, PVCs do not conduct retrogradely and thus do not result in a distinct P wave. The sinus beats may, however, continue uninterrupted and thus manifest as an instance of AV dissociation in conjunction with PVCs. For the same reason, because PVCs usually do not conduct retrogradely and depolarize the atrium and the sinus node, there usually is a full compensatory pause in contrast to the partial compensatory pause generally seen with PACs. In patients with slow sinus rates, however, interpolated PVCs might occur. If the ectopic foci for PVCs are located high in the His-Purkinje system, the resulting premature complexes may have a narrow QRS morphology quite similar to that seen during sinus rhythm. Additionally, if the PVCs occur rather late, in close proximity to the sinus impulse, there may also be a narrow complex QRS because of fusion between the normal depolarization due to sinus impulse and the abnormal activation sequence from the ectopic foci. In the instance of fusion beats, a normal P wave precedes the QRS. The PR interval is shorter, and the QRS morphology may be only partially altered. In some cases, this might give the appearance of an intermittent bundle-branch block or preexcitation (Wolff-Parkinson-White syndrome) pattern.

Based on the morphologic features of PVCs, they have been classified as *uniform* or *multiform;* they also have been referred to as *unifocal* or *multifocal.* Also recommended is classification of PVCs based on their coupling interval with the preceding sinus beat. PVCs with a short coupling interval near or on the previous T wave have been described as showing R-on-T phenomenon; alternatively PVCs may have long coupling intervals. Based on the underlying electrophysiologic mechanism responsible for PVCs, the coupling interval may be *fixed,* as in reentrant beats, or *variable,* as seen with ventricular parasystole. PVCs may have a repetitive pattern, for example, bigeminy or trigeminy, or they may occur in pairs. It is now believed that repetitive PVCs, such as couplets and triplets, are prognostically more important than just the frequency of isolated PVCs.

CLINICAL FEATURES

PVCs can be recorded frequently in normal individuals, and, similar to PACs, their frequency increases with age. In patients without organic heart disease or without prior evidence of sustained ventricular tachyarrhythmias, the mere presence of frequent PVCs is not considered prognostically important. However, individual exceptions do exist, and the clinician is advised to evaluate each given patient accordingly. In patients with organic heart disease, PVCs are the most common form of arrhythmia and carry significant prognostic importance, especially in survivors of acute MI and patients with recurrent ischemia and advanced heart failure. It has been well established during the past 2 decades that frequent PVCs occurring during the acute phase of MI are associated with an increased risk of sustained ventricular arrhythmias in the initial 48 hours, but they do not predict long-term outcome or risk of arrhythmic events. More recently, it has been shown in patients receiving thrombolytic therapy that PVCs, particularly episodes of nonsustained ventricular tachycardia, increase in frequency but are generally short-lived and represent a sign of myocardial reperfusion. However, the presence of frequent PVCs during the postdischarge evaluation of survivors of MI is indicative of a poor prognosis.

Although as many as 80% to 90% of patients with chronic heart failure have frequent PVCs, the results of several recent studies have shown that only the presence of nonsustained ventricular tachycardia (defined as three or more PVCs in a row) at a rate greater than 100 bpm is strongly predictive of an increased risk of sudden cardiac death in these patients. This is in clear contrast to the findings of several large clinical trials, which showed that more than 10 PVCs per hour in post-MI patients are predictive of a poor prognosis and an increased risk of arrhythmic death.

Overall, the association between PVCs and an increased risk of ventricular tachyarrhythmias and sudden cardiac death appears to be related not only to the frequency and complexity of PVCs but also to the severity of underlying structural heart disease. For example, a patient with mitral valve prolapse and frequent PVCs would be at relatively lower risk for arrhythmic events compared to a patient with advanced heart failure who has repetitive PVCs and episodes of nonsustained ventricular tachycardia. Proper evaluation of the risk of PVCs has become more crucial than ever because most currently available antiarrhythmic drugs have the potential for causing serious adverse reactions, including proarrhythmias, in patients with advanced cardiac disorders.

TREATMENT

In general, PVCs in patients without evidence of organic heart disease do not require any specific antiarrhythmic therapy because generally there is no significantly increased risk of life-threatening arrhythmia. However, when PVCs are associated with disabling palpitations, reassurance and treatment with β-blockers (atenolol [Tenormin], metoprolol [Toprol-XL]) may help in relieving symptoms. In patients with systemic illness or other provoking factors (e.g., electrolyte abnormalities or acid-base imbalance), immediate correction of the underlying abnormality usually is associated with beneficial effects.

Because of the associated poor prognosis with PVCs in the setting of acute MI, common practice in the past consisted of routine administration of intravenous lidocaine (Xylocaine) in an effort to suppress PVCs during the initial phase of acute MI. However, because recent data suggest that the routine use of lidocaine is not necessary and often can be harmful, lidocaine should be avoided because of the risk of serious adverse reactions, especially central nervous system side effects such as seizures in the elderly. With the ready availability of cardiac monitoring, it now is possible to accurately identify a harbinger of ventricular tachyarrhythmias early in the coronary care unit, so prophylactic use of lidocaine is generally not recommended. Furthermore, results from several studies and their meta-analyses have demonstrated that routine use of prophylactic lidocaine during the acute or healing phase of MI does not alter the overall mortality in patients with acute MI.

In contrast, it is well established that the presence of frequent PVCs (≥10 per hour) during the postdischarge evaluation of survivors of acute MI predicts an increased risk of arrhythmic death and overall cardiac mortality. Numerous trials have been conducted with a variety of different antiarrhythmic drugs. Many of the studies demonstrated that suppression of PVCs with most currently available antiarrhythmic drugs is not beneficial in reducing the increased risk associated with PVCs. The Cardiac Arrhythmia Suppression Trials (CAST I and II) clearly demonstrated that, compared to placebo, treatment with class Ic antiarrhythmic drugs (which primarily work by slowing conduction) was associated with an increased risk of arrhythmic death despite adequate suppression of PVCs. The findings from CAST I and II, as well as several other clinical trials, indicate that although frequent PVCs may be a marker for an adverse event, suppression of PVCs with type I antiarrhythmic agents does not favorably influence the associated increased risk of death. Results from the Canadian Amiodarone Myocardial Infarction Arrhythmia Trial (CAMIAT) and the European Myocardial Infarct Amiodarone Trial (EMIAT) suggest that in patients with frequent PVCs in the post-MI setting, use of amiodarone (Cordarone), a complex drug with predominantly class III antiarrhythmic properties, in combination with β-blockers is associated with improved outcome. However, because of the associated drug toxicity with long-term amiodarone use, it is generally considered suitable only for the high-risk cohort (although many patients with low left ventricular ejection fraction now undergo implantation of an automatic internal cardiac defibrillator).

In general, suppression of PVCs using currently available antiarrhythmic drugs (except for amiodarone) is not advisable for most patients, primarily because of the increased risk of proarrhythmic effects of these drugs. In the occasional patient who is disabled by annoying symptoms due to PVCs, an initial trial of β-blocker therapy should be considered and is effective in many patients. Correction of the provoking factors and appropriate management of any underlying heart disease often are beneficial in managing patients with frequent PVCs.

REFERENCES

Barrett PA, Peter CT, Swan HJ, et al. The frequency and prognostic significance of electrocardiographic abnormalities in clinically normal individuals. Prog Cardiovasc Dis 1981;23:299.

Boutitie F, Boissel J-P, Connolly SJ, et al. EMIAT and CAMIAT Investigators: Amiodarone interaction with β-blockers: Analysis of the merged EMIAT (European Myocardial Infarct Amiodarone Trial) and CAMIAT (Canadian Amiodarone Myocardial Infarction Trial) databases. Circulation 1999;99:2268.

Brodsky M, Wu D, Denes P, et al. Arrhythmias documented by 24 hour continuous electrocardiographic monitoring in 50 male medical students without apparent heart disease. Am J Cardiol 1977;39:390.

Cairns JA, Connolly SJ, Roberts R, et al. Randomised trial of outcome after myocardial infarction in patients with frequent or repetitive ventricular premature depolarisations: CAMIAT. Lancet 1997;349:675.

Echt DS, Liebson PR, Mitchell B, et al. Mortality and morbidity in patients receiving encainide, flecainide, or placebo. N Engl J Med 1991;324:781.

Fleg J, Kennedy H. Cardiac arrhythmias in a healthy elderly population. Chest 1982;81:302.

Julian DG, Camm AJ, Frangin G, et al. Randomised trial of effect of amiodarone on mortality in patients with left-ventricular dysfunction after recent myocardial infarction: EMIAT. Lancet 1997;349:667.

Morganroth J. Premature ventricular complexes. Diagnosis and indications for therapy. JAMA 1984;252:673.

Romhilt D, Chaffin C, Choi S, et al. Arrhythmias on ambulatory electrocardiographic monitoring in women without apparent heart disease. Am J Cardiol 1984;54:582.

Rosen KM, Rahimtoola SH, Gunnar RM. Pseudo A-V block secondary to premature nonpropagated His bundle depolarizations: Documentation by His bundle electrocardiography. Circulation 1970;42:367.

Ruskin JN. Ventricular extrasystoles in healthy subjects. N Engl J Med 1985;312:238.

Simpson RJ Jr, Cascio WE, Schreiner PJ, et al. Prevalence of premature ventricular contractions in a population of African American and white men and women: The Atherosclerosis Risk in Communities (ARIC) study. Am Heart J 2002;143:535.

Heart Block

Method of
Kelley P. Anderson, MD

Heart block is at once a syndrome, a set of electrocardiographic (ECG) patterns, and a mechanism of serious signs and symptoms including sudden death and syncope. Interest has accelerated since conventional pacemaker therapy, once considered to be a straightforward, definitive treatment, has been associated with serious consequences in many patients. The development of new forms of pacing has magnified the complexity of pacemaker therapy selection and many aspects remain controversial. This has underscored the importance of recognizing preventable and reversible causes of heart block to reduce the need for permanent pacing and to eliminate unnecessary implantation.

The details of risk stratification of heart block, assessment of the benefits and risks of the therapeutic options, and patient education and guidance are largely in the domain of heart rhythm specialists. However, heart block may be encountered unexpectedly in any patient during any clinical encounter. Furthermore, some patients can require evaluation in the absence of known cardiac disease because of increased risk of conduction disorders in themselves, family members, or future children. A basic understanding of heart block may be useful in order to initiate emergency treatment when necessary and to recognize patients who might benefit from further evaluation or specialist referral.

Mechanisms

The function of the cardiac conduction system is to initiate and coordinate cardiac contractions in order to circulate blood according to physiologic needs. Electrical activation is initiated by pacemaker cells of the sinus node regulated by the autonomic nervous system. Unlike conduction in common electrical circuits in which electrons flow along a conductor according to the voltage gradient, electrical activity in cardiac cells propagates from segment to segment of the cell membrane in cardiac myocytes (myocardial cells) and in specialized cardiac conduction cells. Energy-requiring ion pumps maintain an electrochemical gradient across the insulating cell membrane. Electrical activity opens voltage-sensitive ion channels, causing regenerative electrical activity as ions shift along their electrochemical gradient.

Electrical activity in a single cell excites several adjacent cells via gap junctions. This cascade effect makes it possible for a single cell impulse to spread rapidly throughout the myocardium so that myocytes are excited in the shortest possible time to enhance contraction synchrony, and it provides a vital safety mechanism in that each myocardial cell can be activated by many electrical paths. In addition, specialized conduction cells exhibit automaticity. Although normally latent, because normal activation inhibits spontaneous discharge, when the normal impulse is blocked, discharges from these subsidiary pacemakers provide vital heart rate support.

Block of electrical activation can occur due to failure of any step in the process, such as lack of energy, electrolyte imbalance, inflammatory disruption of the membrane, block of ion channels by drugs, or loss of gap junctions with infiltration of fibrous tissue (Box 1). Because of the

---

BOX 1   Some Mechanisms of Conduction Disturbances

Calcium channel blockade
- Diltiazem
- Verapamil

Cell death
- Ablation
- Apoptosis
- Inflammatory necrosis
- Ischemic necrosis
- Surgical trauma

Cell dysfunction
- Barotrauma
- Inflammation
- Thermal injury

Congenital structural defects
- Endocardial cushion defects

Energy depletion
- Cyanide
- Ischemia

Gap junction disturbances
- Edema
- Fibrosis
- Genetic defects
- Inflammation

Genetic defects
- *NKX2.5* mutation
- *SCN5A* mutation

Prolonged refractory period
- Drugs
- Ischemia
- Vagal activity

Sarcolemmal ion gradient disturbances
- Hyperkalemia
- Hypokalemia

Sodium channel dysfunction
- *SCN5A* mutations
- Sodium channel blocking drugs such as lidocaine, procainamide, flecainide, amiodarone, and imipramine

extensive redundancy and interconnectedness of system elements and because of the capacity to compensate for injury by electrical and anatomic remodeling, extensive damage can occur before signs or symptoms of heart block. Regions of the heart where there are fewer alternative paths for electrical activation, such as proximal portions of the His–Purkinje system, where all conducting fibers are confined to a relatively small area, are more vulnerable to complete block. Subclinical preexisting injury might explain why subsidiary pacemakers often fail to provide adequate rate support when heart block occurs.

If the patient survives the initial insult, there is a possibility for recovery due to remodeling. However, remodeling can be maladaptive and result in an adverse long-term outcome by further conduction system damage, by left ventricular dysfunction, and perhaps by increasing the propensity for bradycardia-induced ventricular tachyarrhythmias (VTAs). The mechanisms of bradycardia-induced VTA are not known, but bradyarrhythmias precipitate torsades de pointes, a specific form of VTA, in the presence of drugs that block potassium channels, electrolyte disturbances, certain genetic abnormalities of ion channel function, heart failure, and myocardial hypertrophy. A comprehensive list of drugs that can account for bradyarrhythmia-related ventricular arrhythmias is available at www.torsades.org.

Etiology

Although there are many potential causes of heart block, the pathophysiology is not known for the vast majority of cases because there are no tests that allow detailed structural or functional examination in patients. By the time of death, morphologic examination can reveal only nonspecific changes such as fibrosis. Instead, most etiologies are inferred by history of recent or past exposures (e.g., trauma or radiation), concomitant disorders (e.g., muscular dystrophy, amyloidosis), abnormal test results (Lyme disease), or family history (Lenègre's disease) (Box 2). Because most etiologies cannot be verified, the clinician must remain open to alternative explanations and accept the likelihood of multiple contributors.

Some patients, usually young, otherwise healthy persons, present with prolonged asystole due to heart block but have no other detectable abnormalities and have excellent outcomes in the absence of intervention beyond counseling. This suggests that autonomic influences alone can cause severe heart block and suppression of subsidiary pacemakers. It is not known if such responses result from an abnormality or an exaggerated normal reflex. However, the identification of such patients is important because most can be managed without pacemakers.

Other patients who should be identified are those with conditions that place them, their relatives, or their unborn children at risk for heart block. This includes patients and family members with genetic disorders associated with heart block. It also includes women with anti-Ro/SSA and/or anti-La/SSB antibodies whose children are at increased risk for congenital heart block, a rare, but devastating disorder. Members of this group can benefit from counseling and anticipatory evaluation and treatment of offspring.

Signs and Symptoms

Most of the symptoms experienced by patients with heart block are common and nonspecific, such as syncope, lightheadedness, fatigue, and dyspnea. Because other arrhythmias and other cardiac and noncardiac disturbances may be responsible for the same symptoms, it is important to document the cause. Proof, which requires documentation of rhythm and the abnormal hemodynamics responsible for the symptoms, is almost never accomplished. Sometimes a cardiac rhythm disturbance can be related to a clinical event, such as several seconds of asystole due to atrioventricular (AV) block and syncope. More commonly, a patient complaining of fatigue or lightheadedness is bradycardic due to high-grade AV block. Asymptomatic complete AV block is also not uncommon. A favorable response to pacemaker implantation is inconclusive due to a powerful placebo effect. Rarely, first-degree AV block results in significant symptoms (e.g., fatigue, palpitations, chest fullness) due to atrial contraction against a partially closed mitral valve. In such cases it is often possible to identify a recent change in PR interval.

BOX 2   Etiologies of Heart Block

Often Permanent or Progressive

Alcohol septal ablation (acute, delayed)
Cardiomyopathies (hypertrophic, idiopathic, mitochondrial)
Catheter ablation (atrioventricular nodal reentry, accessory atrioventricular connections)
Congenital heart block (neonatal lupus)
Congenital heart disease (endocardial cushion defects)
Genetic disorders (sodium channel mutations, Lenègre's disease)
Hypertension
Idiopathic fibrosis and calcification (previously Lev's disease, Lenègre's disease)
Infectious disorders (destructive, e.g., endocarditis)
Infiltrative disorders (amyloidosis)
Myocardial infarction
Neuromyopathic disorders (myotonic dystrophy, Erb's dystrophy, peroneal muscular atrophy)
Noninfectious inflammatory disorders (HLA-B27–associated disorder, sarcoidosis)
Tumors (mesothelioma)
Valvular heart disease

Often Transient or Reversible

Blunt trauma (baseball)
Cardiac surgery (valve replacement)
Cardiac transplant rejection
Central nervous system
Drugs (antiarrhythmics, digoxin, edrophonium [Tensilon])
Electrolyte disturbances (hyperkalemia)
Increased vagal activity
Infectious disorders—nondestructive (Eyme disease)
Metabolic disturbances (hypothermia, hypothyroidism)
Myocardial ischemia
Myocarditis (Chagas' disease, giant cell myocarditis)
Rheumatic fever

ELECTROCARDIOGRAPHIC PATTERNS

Cardiac conduction disturbances are classified by the pattern of ECG complexes. A normal 12-lead ECG lessens the probability of significant fixed conduction disturbances, but it does not eliminate the possibility of transient third-degree block due to reversible functional effects such as intense vagal activity or ischemia. A normal ECG rhythm during symptoms is very helpful for excluding heart block as the mechanism.

PR prolongation and intraatrial delay rarely require immediate action but can have adverse hemodynamic consequences and occasionally cause symptoms due to suboptimal coordination between atrial and ventricular contraction. Significant disease of the His bundle may be electrocardiographically silent, but more often, concomitant distal disease is evident in the form of fascicular or bundle branch block or a nonspecific intraventricular conduction delay. In a patient with syncope, the presence of bifascicular block raises the possibility of transient third-degree block as the mechanism and of progression to permanent complete block.

Most patients with conduction disorders are not symptomatic and do not progress to complete block. However, the combination of right bundle branch block (RBBB) and left posterior fascicle block has a greater tendency to progress to complete block than the more common RBBB and left anterior fascicle block. Nevertheless, conduction disturbances of the His-Purkinje system should not be assumed to be responsible for syncope or cardiac arrest because they are relatively common in patients with cardiovascular disorders that cause syncope or cardiac arrest due to other mechanisms. Conduction disturbances can cause dyssynchronous contraction and result in adverse remodeling. In addition, they can mask or mimic the ECG signs of myocardial infarction.

Alternating bundle branch block is a changing ECG pattern in which both RBBB and left bundle branch block are observed or when the bifascicular block pattern switches between the anterior and posterior fascicle involvement. This pattern is considered a harbinger of complete block with or without symptoms and warrants continuous monitoring and evaluation for permanent pacemaker implantation.

The challenge in second-degree and transient third-degree AV block is distinguishing between block in the AV node, which is rarely permanent, and infranodal block, which often progresses to permanent third-degree block. ECG clues that block is in the AV node include normal QRS duration (<100 ms), type I (Wenckebach) pattern, PR prolongation before blocked impulses and PR shortening after pauses, occurrence during enhanced vagal activity (e.g., sleep), narrow QRS escape complexes, and no factors favoring infranodal block. ECG clues for infranodal block include prolonged QRS duration (120 ms), type II pattern, and escape QRS complexes broader than intrinsic complexes. Whereas type II second-degree AV block is almost always due to block in the His-Purkinje system, other second-degree AV block ECG patterns have poor sensitivity and specificity for the site of the block.

Unsustained polymorphic ventricular tachycardia is an ominous sign in any context and can result from a variety of cardiac, metabolic, and autonomic abnormalities. However, in the presence of heart block it suggests that heart rate support may be necessary to prevent sustained VTA. QT prolongation and post-pause U-wave accentuation should be sought as other harbingers of bradycardia-related VTA.

The importance and value of ECG documentation of heart block to the patient's management and well-being cannot be overemphasized. ECGs are subject to artifact and may be misleading when standards for acquisition and analysis are not followed. Multiple tracings of suspicious events should be obtained in multiple leads when possible. A 12-lead simultaneous rhythm recording mode is available on most modern ECG machines and should be used when continuous recordings are obtained to document arrhythmias.

METHODS USED IN THE ASSESSMENT OF HEART BLOCK

Clinicians encounter heart block in three general contexts. For the patient with documented heart block, the clinician selects therapy based, in part, on whether or not the arrhythmia is permanent or likely to recur. There are no tests that provide information about the pathologic state of the AV conduction system; therefore, these outcomes must be inferred from the ECG and past experience. Additional testing including invasive tests such as electrophysiologic studies, coronary angiography, and myocardial biopsy, as well as a large number of specific laboratory tests are occasionally helpful but usually do not provide information about the choice of therapy for heart block.

Another common context is the patient with symptoms for whom the objective is to verify or exclude heart block as the mechanism by

CURRENT DIAGNOSIS

- Assess risk for heart block in the absence of symptoms or evidence of asystole
- Review ECG pattern, family history, maternal antibodies, cardiac interventions, and surgery
- Evaluate documented heart block with asystole or bradycardia
- Classify bradyarrhythmia: Transient, recurrent, progressive, permanent
- Grade signs and symptoms: none, mild, severe
- Evaluate signs or symptoms of possible transient heart block with no documentation
- Establish temporal pattern: Single, recurrent, rare, often, recent onset, long-standing
- Grade signs and symptoms: none, mild, severe
- Document rhythm during symptoms: Telemetry monitoring, Holter monitor, external loop recorder, implantable recorder

correlating the cardiac rhythm with symptoms. Real-time monitoring, such as inpatient telemetry, is used for patients who might require immediate access to drugs or pacing devices to prevent or terminate asystole or bradycardia-dependent VTA. Holter monitoring is useful for patients who have more than one event in a 24-hour window and for capturing asymptomatic rhythm events. External loop recorders are carried for a month or longer and are very helpful to associate rhythm abnormalities with symptoms and to rule out a rhythm disorder as the cause of symptoms. Patients with infrequent events may be candidates for implantable loop recorders that monitor for longer than 1 year.

Electrophysiologic studies allow precise measurements of AV node and His-Purkinje system function and can provide definitive information regarding the site of block if the conduction disturbance occurs during the study. Additional tests have been developed that stress the AV conduction system, including rapid atrial and ventricular pacing, administration of antiarrhythmic drugs such as procainamide and disopyramide, combinations of drugs, and pacing maneuvers. The provocation of heart block is assumed to indicate a propensity for spontaneous AV block. Unfortunately, the sensitivity is low and a negative test does not imply a low risk of future episodes. Electrophysiologic studies have the additional advantage of providing immediate test results, as well as providing the results of programmed stimulation for provocation of supraventricular and ventricular tachyarrhythmias.

The third important context for clinicians is patients who might be at high risk for adverse consequences of heart block but are asymptomatic. Addressing this is a challenge for the future because few methods are currently available. Possible applications include screening for mutations and polymorphisms that predispose to heart block, measurements of mechanical dyssynchrony to identify patients prone to develop adverse cardiac remodeling due to conduction disorders or right ventricular pacing, and methods capable of assessing electrophysiologic and metabolic function of conducting tissue in vivo.

Treatment

Selecting the correct therapeutic approach balances the risks and benefits of therapy against the risks of heart block for both immediate and long-term management. Pharmacologic agents are useful for emergency, temporary, and standby heart support in select circumstances. The standby mode is accomplished by a prepared infusion at the bedside. To avoid excessive doses at the time of sudden heart block, the optimal dose can be established in advance by test doses starting at low infusion rates.

PHARMACOLOGIC TREATMENT

Atropine 0.5 to 3.0 mg[3] or 0.04 mg/kg IV is useful for treatment or pretreatment of patients who develop heart block at the level of the AV node in the context of elevated vagal tone, such as in association with nausea or endotracheal tube suction. Atropine should be avoided in patients with infranodal AV block because prolonged asystole sometimes occurs due to more frequent His-Purkinje system depolarization from increased sinus rate. Vagal activity inhibits sympathetic activity, and therefore reduction of vagal tone by atropine disinhibits sympathetic activity and can account for the unpredictable effects of atropine on heart rate. Elevations in heart rate after atropine can persist for hours and cannot be readily reversed.

Aminophylline 2.5 to 6.3 mg/kg IV is reported to reverse heart block resistant to atropine and epinephrine by antagonizing adenosine. Stimulation of β-adrenergic receptors increases sinus and subsidiary pacemaker rates, AV node and His-Purkinje system conduction velocities, and myocardial contractility. The effective refractory period shortens in most tissue, but this effect varies with dose and specific tissue type.

Dobutamine 2.5 to 40 μg/kg/minute is a useful β-receptor agonist because it increases cardiac output and lowers filling pressures without excessive rise or fall of blood pressure. Isoproterenol (Isuprel) in a 0.02 to 0.06 mg IV bolus or 0.5 to 10.0[3] μg/min IV infusion, stimulates β1- and β2-adrenergic receptors and enhances vasodilation more than the other catecholamines.

CURRENT THERAPY

Methods of Heart Rate Support

- Immediate: Intravenous catecholamines, transcutaneous pacing
- Short-term: Transvenous temporary pacing
- Long-term: Permanent pacemakers

Pacemaker Configuration

- Number of leads: 1,2,3,4
- Lead locations: Right atrial appendage, Bachmann's bundle, right ventricular apex, outflow tract, left ventricle, coronary sinus
- Programming to minimize ventricular pacing (manufacturer dependent)

This can result in unwanted hypotension in some circumstances, but it is also less likely to cause a reflex increase in vagal tone than other drugs.

Epinephrine in 1 mg IV boluses for cardiac arrest, 0.2 to 1 mg subcutaneously, or 0.5 to 5 μg/min IV stimulates both α- and β-adrenergic receptors. It is recommended for asystolic cardiac arrest in part because it increases myocardial and cerebral flow. However, the increase of systemic vascular resistance may be detrimental by augmenting metabolic acidosis and decreasing cardiac performance in patients with poor left ventricular function. The suggested dose ranges are broad because the response, such as improved AV conduction, to β-adrenergic stimulants varies widely and may be affected by β-adrenergic receptor downregulation in patients with chronic elevations in sympathetic activity, such as patients with long-standing heart failure.

Any of these agents can precipitate tachyarrhythmias by direct electrophysiologic effects mediated by adrenergic receptors and indirect effects such as myocardial ischemia, and they can worsen hemodynamic status. The adverse effects of catecholamines are time dependent and cumulative. Ischemia and receptor-mediated electrophysiologic effects occur immediately after administration, and changes in gene expression of ion channels begin as early as several hours. Long-term changes such as myocardial hypertrophy, apoptosis, and fibrosis usually begin to occur within 24 hours but can progress over much longer periods. This suggests that the duration and dose of catecholamine infusions should be minimized.

PACING

Temporary pacing includes transcutaneous, transvenous, transthoracic, transesophageal, and transgastric approaches. Transcutaneous pacing provides noninvasive heart rate support as well as immediate access to countershock, but it is often painful, so most patients require sedation, and capture is not achieved in some patients. For these reasons, its principal uses are for short-term pacing during cardiopulmonary resuscitation and for standby pacing in patients at risk for bradyarrhythmias. If the risk of bradycardia is high, ventricular capture should be verified in advance. Capture is often difficult to ascertain because transcutaneous stimuli cause large deflections on the ECG, and pectoral muscle stimulation can be confused with a pulse. Capture should be verified by careful ECG analysis at sub- and suprathreshold stimulus amplitudes and confirmed by appropriately timed femoral artery pulses, Korotkoff sounds, or arterial pressure waveforms.

Transvenous insertion of an electrode catheter is the method of choice for most patients who require temporary pacing. This approach is reliable and safe when performed by competent staff with strict aseptic technique, fluoroscopic guidance, and appropriate catheters. Complications include inadequate pacing or sensing thresholds, vascular complications, pneumothorax, myocardial perforation, infection, and dislodgment. Small studies suggest that long-term (>5 days) temporary pacing can be accomplished with active-fixation permanent pacemaker leads attached to an external pulse generator.[1] Tunneling the lead can enhance stability and reduce the risk of infection.

---

[1]Not FDA approved for this indication.

Permanent pacemakers are highly effective, safe, and cost-effective and have few contraindications. Although the complications are rarely life threatening, they should be carefully considered and acknowledged. Septicemia or endocarditis has been reported in 0.5% of patients. In patients with pacemaker-related endocarditis, the in-hospital mortality rate is reported to be greater than 7%, with a 20-month mortality greater than 25%. The rate of significant complications has been reported to be 3.5%. About 10% of pacemakers become infected or develop some other type of failure that can require extraction. In one series, the rate of major complications associated with extraction was 1.4%. There is a long-term continuous risk of infection, thrombosis, and erosion. Conventional pacing, that is, from the right ventricular apex, is now known to be detrimental and can cause adverse ventricular remodeling, atrial fibrillation, heart failure, and premature death.

In young persons there is a periodic need to replace generators and leads, which limits venous access sites, and unused leads accumulate or must be extracted. Perhaps of greater consequence is the constant inconvenience of lifelong follow-up, electromagnetic interference, and false alarms from electronic surveillance devices as well as exclusion from important procedures, such as magnetic resonance imaging of the thorax.

Although it has been shown that patients with reduced left ventricular function are at greater risk for adverse effects, it is not known how to identify other patients at risk. Many strategies for reducing the adverse effects of conventional pacing have been proposed and many have been studied, but there is no consensus about which method should be used in the many settings that are encountered. Therefore, the decision for pacemaker implantation also includes selection of lead configuration, lead locations, and pacing mode. Because some configurations change the short- and long-term risks of implantation, patient guidance and education are more complex as well.

Approach to the Patient

The object of the evaluation and management for heart block is to prevent adverse effects by heart rate support in patients with poorly tolerated bradycardia; monitoring and standby heart rate support in stable patients at high risk for asystole or severe bradycardia; identifying and treating reversible causes of heart block; identifying patients at high risk for sudden death, syncope, or recurrent symptoms; and selecting and implanting the appropriate rate support device as soon as safety permits.

Advanced cardiac life-support guidelines apply to the patient who is unresponsive or severely compromised by heart block. However, heart block is rarely the primary problem. Therefore, evaluation and treatment of other disorders should continue while efforts to increase heart rate are under way.

The initial evaluation should include a thorough history and physical examination, review of current and previous ECGs and rhythm strips, and laboratory tests to determine if heart block is present or if there is a significant risk of heart block occurring in the future and, if so, a differential diagnosis of possible etiologies. The patient should then be stratified for the appropriate level of care: the unstable patient who requires ongoing evaluation and treatment in an intensive care setting, the stable patient at high risk for asystole or complications who needs temporary transvenous pacing or other invasive procedures, the patient at moderate risk who requires continuous monitoring and standby noninvasive heart rate support measures, the patient at low risk who requires rapid but not immediate access to heart rate support measures that hospital monitoring provides, and the patient at low risk who can be evaluated and managed as an outpatient.

Patients who present after resuscitated cardiac arrest or syncope or with ECG abnormalities that indicate conduction system abnormalities usually belong in one of the first four categories. The fifth category usually includes patients with mild symptoms and no suggestive ECG abnormalities and patients whose risk is estimated to be low after inpatient monitoring or previous evaluation. The most common presentation is the patient who has symptoms that could be due to heart block as well as other arrhythmic or nonarrhythmic causes. In such patients, ECG confirmation of the relationship between heart block and symptoms should be obtained.

Determining the need for long-term heart rate support, as well as other issues that can affect selection of implantable devices (e.g., risk for VTAs), should be accomplished as soon as possible because the risks of complications and anxiety associated with temporary heart rate support measures increase over time. Medical societies have developed guidelines for implantable rhythm management devices (http://www.cardiosource/guidelines/index.asp). The reasons for the selected therapy, including the rationale for any deviation from established guidelines, should be documented and provided to the patient. This will reduce future confusion or misunderstanding about the original rationale for implantation that can affect management of patients with device complications and those with a compelling need for device upgrade or explanation.

Patients with acute coronary syndromes require special consideration. The incidence of heart block in patients with myocardial infarction based on creatine phosphokinase as the marker of necrosis is approximately 10%. Although the incidence is probably lower using more sensitive markers such as troponin, heart block is still likely to be associated with increased in-hospital mortality due to larger infarct size. Bradycardia reduces myocardial oxygen consumption. Therefore, overcorrection of heart rate must be avoided, and ischemia should be relieved by increasing perfusion as soon as possible.

Studies in the prethrombolytic era did not demonstrate a benefit in mortality with prophylactic temporary transvenous pacing, and complications were common. The risks of transvenous insertion may be higher in patients requiring administration of thrombolytics and other anticoagulants. Catheter-based revascularization methods should be given strong consideration because of established effectiveness, because thrombolytic drugs might be avoided, and because transvenous temporary pacing, if needed, is readily and safely accomplished during the procedure. Suggestions for standby temporary pacing (Box 3) should take into consideration the risks of transvenous pacing based on local circumstances (e.g., experience, fluoroscopic guidance, insertion site, use of anticoagulants).

Most conduction disturbances associated with myocardial ischemia or infarction resolve quickly but can persist for days or weeks. The need for permanent pacemaker implantation as a consequence of myocardial infarction is rare, and prophylactic pacemaker implantation in high-risk subsets has not been shown to reduce mortality. Guidelines for temporary and permanent pacing in acute myocardial infarction have been published (http://www.escardio.org/guidelines-surveys/esc-guidelines/pages/cardiac-pacing-and-cardiac-resynchronisation-therapy.aspx).

BOX 3   Suggestions for Temporary Pacing in Acute Myocardial Infarction

Transvenous Pacing

Asystole or poorly tolerated bradycardia unresponsive to atropine or aminophylline
Persistent third-degree AV block
Alternating RBBB and LBBB, or RBBB and alternating LAFB and LPFB
Bifascicular block (new)
Second-degree AV block (any type) and QRS ≥110 ms
Any indication listed for standby transcutaneous pacing at time of cardiac catheterization if performed

Standby Transcutaneous Pacing

Any indication listed for transvenous pacing until the transvenous pacing system is inserted
Transient asystole or poorly tolerated bradycardia
Bifascicular block (uncertain time of onset or old)
Second-degree AV block (any type) and QRS <110 ms
New first-degree AV block

AV = atrioventricular; LAFB = left anterior fascicle block; LPFB = left posterior fascicle block; LBBB = left bundle branch block; RBBB = right bundle branch block.

Conclusions

Heart block remains a challenge because the cellular mechanisms responsible are poorly understood, prediction of symptomatic heart block (who and when) is unreliable, treatments that restore normal conduction do not exist for most conditions, and pacemaker therapy can have significant long-term adverse consequences. Fortunately, ongoing clinical trials will provide guidance in pacemaker configurations and programming that will minimize adverse effects. Recent achievements in molecular biology suggest we are on the threshold of advances that will elucidate mechanisms and produce treatments that will relegate artificial pacemakers to museum pieces.

Acknowledgments

The author thanks the Marshfield Clinic Research Foundation for its support through the assistance of Linda Weis and Alice Stargardt in the preparation of this chapter.

REFERENCES

Barold SS, Hayes DL. Second-degree atrioventricular block: A reappraisal. Mayo Clin Proc 2001;76:44–57.
Carlson MD, Wilkoff BL, Maisel WH, et al. Recommendations from the Heart Rhythm Society Task Force on Device Performance Policies and Guidelines Endorsed by the American College of Cardiology Foundation (ACCF) and the American Heart Association (AHA) and the International Coalition of Pacing and Electrophysiology Organizations (COPE). Heart Rhythm 2006;3:1250–73.
Elizari MV, Acunzo RS, Ferreiro M. Hemiblocks revisited. Circulation 2007;115:1154–63.
Pierpont ME, Basson CT, Benson DW Jr, et al. Genetic basis for congenital heart defects: Current knowledge: A scientific statement from the American Heart Association Congenital Cardiac Defects Committee, Council on Cardiovascular Disease in the Young: Endorsed by the American Academy of Pediatrics. Circulation 2007;115:3015–38.
Zipes DP, Camm AJ, Borggrefe M, et al. ACC/AHA/ESC 2006 guidelines for management of patients with ventricular arrhythmias and the prevention of sudden cardiac death: A report of the American College of Cardiology/American Heart Association Task Force and the European Society of Cardiology Committee for Practice Guidelines (writing committee to develop Guidelines for Management of Patients with Ventricular Arrhythmias and the Prevention of Sudden Cardiac Death): Developed in collaboration with the European Heart Rhythm Association and the Heart Rhythm Society. Circulation 2006;114:e385–484.

Tachycardias

Method of
Sei Iwai, MD, and Bruce B. Lerman, MD

The term *tachycardia* translates literally into "fast" (tachy-) "heart" (cardia). Cardiac arrhythmias that result in electrical activation more than 100 times per minute fall under the category of tachycardia.

Mechanisms of Tachyarrhythmias

Tachycardias are initiated or sustained by one of three general mechanisms: reentry, abnormal automaticity, or triggered activity.

Reentry is the most common mechanism of arrhythmogenesis. Reentry typically requires a region of relatively slow conduction in order to become sustained. This creates an excitable gap, preventing the leading edge of a wavefront from colliding with its back end (Fig. 1). Reentry can occur in the setting of an abnormal electrical

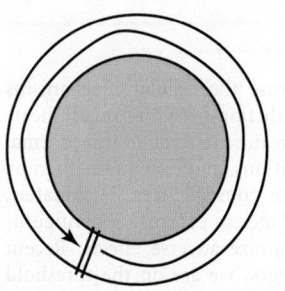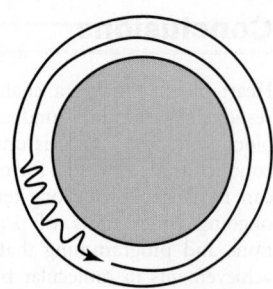

FIGURE 1. Diagrams demonstrate the effect of slow conduction in promoting reentrant circuits. *Gray area* represents an obstacle (e.g., scar). *Left,* In this example, normal conduction velocity around the scar results in termination of the wavefront *(circular line with arrow)*, as the head *(arrow)* of the wavefront meets the tail during refractoriness *(double line)*. *Right,* Due to an area of slow conduction, the head of the wavefront meets the tail after it has recovered *(circular line with arrow)* and can perpetuate reentry.

pathway or connection (e.g., accessory atrioventricular [AV] pathway or dual AV nodal pathway physiology). Alternatively, a barrier to conduction, either anatomic (e.g., tricuspid or mitral valve, venae cavae), or functional (e.g., crista terminalis—due to anisotropic conduction), can provide a setting favorable for reentry. Finally, abnormal impulse propagation, such as through diseased cardiac tissue, can cause sufficient slowing of conduction, allowing recovery of neighboring cells, initiating reentry.

Rhythmic pacemaker activity can occur in various types of cardiac cells. However, there is a normal hierarchy in the frequency of the initiated action potentials from these sites; the sinoatrial node is the dominant pacemaker. Automaticity in the distal conduction system (or myocardium) can compete with that in the sinoatrial node on the basis of enhanced normal or *abnormal automaticity.*

Under certain pathologic conditions, a decrease in the resting membrane potential can occur, resulting in spontaneous phase-4 depolarization in cardiac cells. Abnormal automaticity is defined as spontaneous impulse initiation in cells that are not fully polarized. Perturbations in the ionic balance (state of depolarization), which result in abnormal automaticity, may be due to disturbances in various ion channel currents. For example, during the subacute phase of a myocardial infarction, automatic arrhythmias can arise from the infarct border zones.

Triggered activity has become an increasingly appreciated cause of cardiac arrhythmias. In cardiac cells, oscillations of membrane potential that occur during repolarization or after the action potential are referred to as *afterdepolarizations.* They are divided into two subtypes: early and delayed afterdepolarizations, depending on when they occur relative to the cardiac action potential. When an afterdepolarization achieves sufficient amplitude to reach a threshold potential, a new action potential, or triggered response, is evoked. If this process repeats itself, sustained triggered arrhythmias can develop.

An early afterdepolarization can appear during the plateau (phase 2) or repolarization phase (phase 3) of the action potential (Fig. 2). A prolongation of repolarization by a reduction in outward currents, an increase in inward currents, or a combination of the two is required for the manifestation of early afterdepolarization–induced ectopic activity. Bradycardia or pauses, which prolong repolarization, can potentiate early afterdepolarizations.

Delayed afterdepolarizations are oscillations in membrane potential that occur after repolarization, during phase 4 of the action potential (see Fig. 2). In contrast to automatic rhythms that originate *de novo* during spontaneous diastolic depolarization, delayed afterdepolarizations depend on the preceding action potential and do not occur in the absence of a previous action potential.

During the plateau phase of the normal action potential, calcium enters the cell. The increase in intracellular calcium triggers release of calcium from the sarcoplasmic reticulum. This further elevates intracellular calcium and initiates contraction. Relaxation occurs through sequestration of calcium by the sarcoplasmic reticulum. Delayed afterdepolarizations arise when the cytosol becomes overloaded with

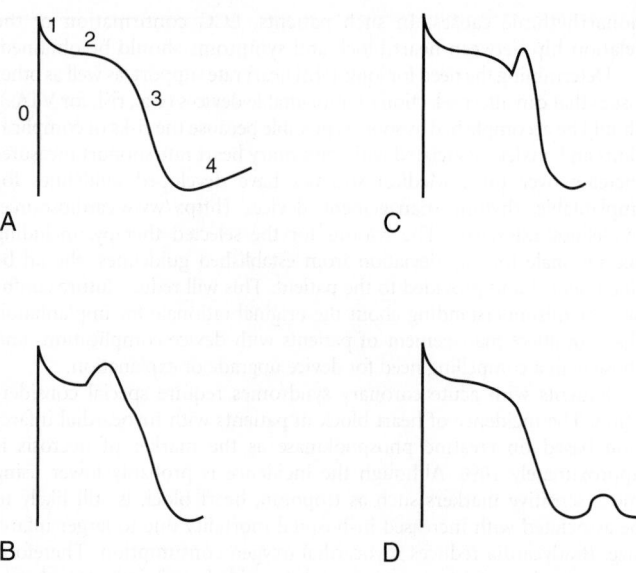

FIGURE 2. **A,** Normal action potential of myocardial tissue and the corresponding phases (0–4). **B,** Early afterdepolarization during phase 2. **C,** Early afterdepolarization during phase 3. **D,** Delayed afterdepolarization occurring during phase 4.

calcium and triggers a transient inward current, I_{Ti}. I_{Ti} is generated by the sodium–calcium exchanger (I_{NaCa}). Delayed afterdepolarizations can originate from myocardial cells, Purkinje fibers, and even mitral valve and coronary sinus tissue.

Tachyarrhythmias can be broadly classified as either supraventricular, which arise from the atria or AV junction, or ventricular, which arise from the ventricles.

Supraventricular Tachyarrhythmias

ATRIOVENTRICULAR NODAL REENTRY

Excluding atrial fibrillation (discussed in the chapter on atrial fibrillation), the most common supraventricular arrhythmia is AV node reentrant tachycardia (AVNRT). AVNRT accounts for more than 50% of the supraventricular tachycardias (SVTs) with a 1:1 atrial-to-ventricular activation pattern. The initiation of AVNRT depends on the presence of dual AV nodal pathway physiology. A fast pathway, located in the anterior portion of the septum, typically has a relatively longer refractory period. A slow AV nodal pathway, usually located in the posterior aspect of the septum, has a shorter refractory period.

The anatomy of the AV node is quite complex and incompletely understood. It appears that the reentry circuit of AVNRT also contains transitional cells in between the atrial portions of the fast and slow pathways. During the typical form of AVNRT, anterograde conduction occurs over the slow pathway, and retrograde conduction is via the fast pathway. Therefore, activation of the atria and ventricles occurs almost simultaneously. As a result, this tachycardia can be described as a short RP′ tachycardia, based on the relation between the R and P waves; that is, the R-P interval is less than the P-R interval (Fig. 3). Thus, in typical AVNRT, the P wave occurs during the QRS complex, or it occurs shortly afterward, in which case it can appear as a pseudo-R′ (Fig. 4). Less common forms of AVNRT include fast–slow (i.e., anterograde conduction down the fast pathway and retrograde conduction via the slow pathway) and slow–slow variants (in which there are two different slow pathways). The former results in a long RP′ tachycardia, and the latter results in an RP′ interval approximately equal to the PR interval. The relation between P wave and QRS complex on an electrocardiogram (ECG) can help in forming a differential diagnosis for the SVT (Box 1).

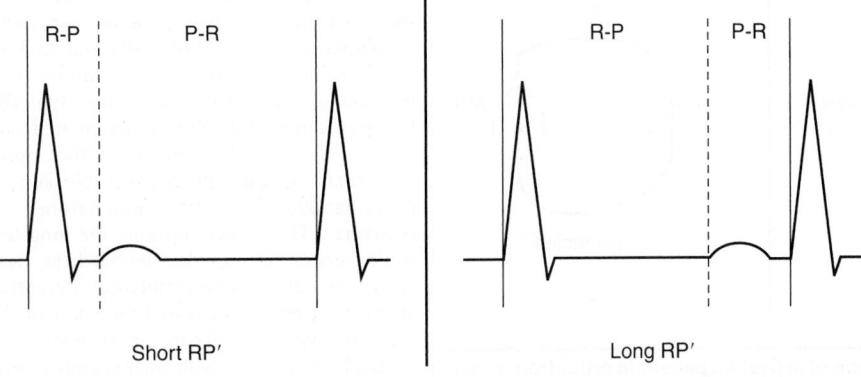

FIGURE 3. Schematic demonstrating the relation of the P wave with respect to the R-R interval. *Left*, Short RP′ tachycardia, with P wave occurring shortly after the preceding QRS complex; thus the R-P interval is short (compared with the P-R interval). *Right*, The P wave occurs just before the following QRS complex (long RP′ tachycardia).

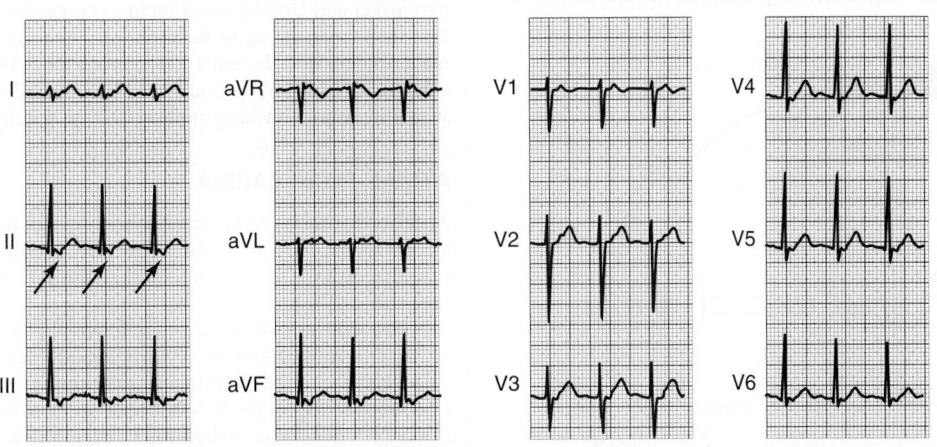

FIGURE 4. A 12-lead electrocardiogram of a short RP′ tachycardia, consistent with typical atrioventricular nodal reentrant tachycardia. *Arrows* identify the retrograde P waves.

BOX 1	Differential Diagnosis of Narrow Complex Supraventricular Tachycardia with 1:1 Atrioventricular Conduction

Short RP′ Tachycardias

Typical atrioventricular (AV) nodal reentry
Orthodromic reciprocating tachycardia
Atrial tachycardia with first-degree AV delay
Junctional tachycardia

Long RP′ Tachycardias

Atypical AV node reentry
Atrial tachycardia
Sinus tachycardia
Permanent form of junctional reciprocating tachycardia

Initiation of AVNRT is usually due to an atrial or ventricular premature complex that blocks in one pathway but conducts via the other with enough delay to allow recovery and activation of the initially refractory pathway in the retrograde direction. First-line therapy for acute termination of AVNRT is adenosine (Adenocard) (typically 6 or 12 mg IV). Other options include intravenous β-blockers or calcium channel blockers such as metoprolol (Lopressor)[1] 5 mg IV or diltiazem (Cardizem) 20 mg IV. Therapeutic options for long-term

---

[1]Not FDA approved for this indication.

therapy include oral β-blockers or calcium channel blockers and radiofrequency catheter ablation.

ATRIOVENTRICULAR RECIPROCATING TACHYCARDIA

The presence of an accessory pathway between the atria and ventricles can result in a reentrant tachycardia called *atrioventricular reciprocating tachycardia* (AVRT). The most common location (>50%) for an accessory pathway is the left free wall. Orthodromic reciprocating tachycardia (ORT) results when anterograde conduction occurs over the AV node, with retrograde conduction occurring over the accessory pathway. Conversely, antidromic reciprocating tachycardia (ART) describes reentry in the opposite direction (Fig. 5). Anterograde conduction evident on ECG during sinus rhythm is a Wolff-Parkinson-White (WPW) pattern.

The combination of a WPW pattern and a history of tachycardia is WPW syndrome. Ventricular preexcitation is present, as manifested by a delta wave on the ECG. A delta wave is formed by AV conduction via the accessory pathway, which occurs without the delay seen during conduction via the AV node and His-Purkinje system (Fig. 6). Thus, the PR interval is shortened. The magnitude of PR interval shortening is related to the proximity of the accessory pathway to the sinus node. Right-sided accessory pathways therefore usually result in shorter PR intervals than left-sided accessory pathways. The accessory pathway can often be concealed; that is, the pathway is capable of retrograde conduction only. In this case, no delta wave is present.

ORT results in a short RP′ tachycardia, owing to relatively rapid conduction over the accessory pathway. However, the RP′ interval is typically longer than that seen in typical AVNRT. This is because

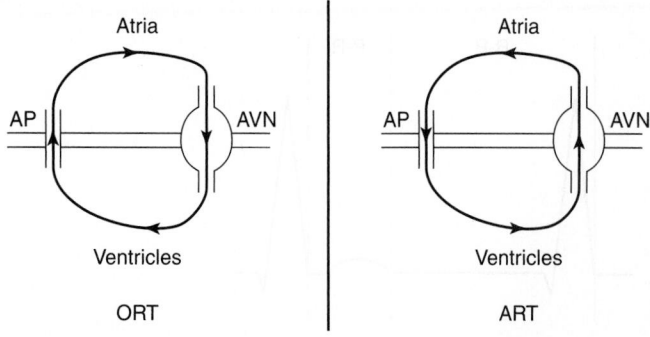

FIGURE 5. Demonstration of activation pattern in orthodromic reciprocating tachycardia (ORT) and antidromic reciprocating tachycardia (ART). ORT involves anterograde conduction down the atrioventricular node (AVN), with retrograde conduction back to the atria via the accessory pathway (AP). ART is due to conduction in the opposite direction and results in a wide (preexcited) QRS complex due to ventricular activation originating at the site of the AP.

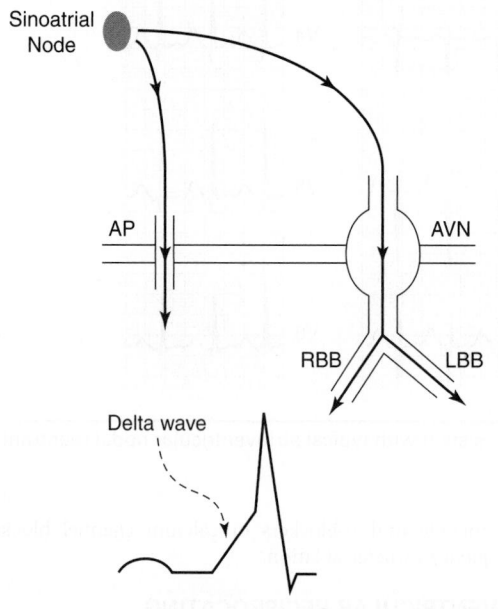

FIGURE 6. The delta wave is a result of fusion of ventricular activation via the atrioventricular node (AVN) and conduction via the accessory pathway (AP). Due to the normal slowing of conduction down the AVN (to the right and left bundle branches [RBB and LBB, respectively], and subsequently the ventricles), a portion of the ventricles is preexcited via the AP, manifesting as a slurred upstroke (curved dashed arrow) of the initial portion of the QRS complex (the delta wave).

the reentry circuit in ORT results in serial, or sequential, activation of the ventricles and the atria, whereas it occurs in parallel in AVNRT. RP′ intervals in AVNRT are rarely greater than 70 ms, and they are rarely less than this in ORT.

ART manifests as a wide complex tachycardia rhythm, with QRS morphology dependent on the location of the accessory pathway. ART is an uncommon arrhythmia. In fact, in patients with WPW syndrome, atrial fibrillation is more common, occurring in up to 40% of patients. The combination of an accessory pathway and atrial fibrillation can result in very rapid activation of the ventricles (via the accessory pathway), with bizarre QRS complexes. Atrial fibrillation with WPW syndrome can lead to syncope or even ventricular fibrillation due to the rapid ventricular stimulation.

Rarely, ORT can result due to reentry using a long, slowly conducting serpentine pathway, with decremental (similar to the AV node) conduction. These tachycardias can be incessant and are termed *permanent form of junctional reciprocating tachycardia*. Permanent form

of junctional reciprocating tachycardia often results in a tachycardia-mediated cardiomyopathy, due to its incessant nature.

Similar to AVNRT, both ORT and ART are usually initiated by an atrial or ventricular premature complex. First-line therapy for acute termination of AVRT is adenosine (typically 6 or 12 mg IV). ART, however, can be difficult to differentiate from ventricular tachycardia, due to its wide QRS complex. Other options include intravenous β-blockers or calcium channel blockers, as well as intravenous procainamide (Pronestyl), amiodarone (Cordarone), or ibutilide (Corvert). Therapeutic options for long-term therapy include oral β-blockers or calcium channel blockers, class I or III antiarrhythmic agents, as well as catheter ablation. Recently, the availability of cryo-ablation energy has increased the safety of ablation of accessory pathways in close proximity to the AV node.

Lastly, in patients with dual-chamber permanent pacemakers only, a specific form of iatrogenic AV reciprocating tachycardia can occur, called *pacemaker-mediated tachycardia*. Typically in this case, a ventricular premature complex conducts retrogradely up to the atria, with enough delay to result in atrial activation after the end of the postventricular atrial refractory period. This atrial activation is sensed by the pacemaker and tracked, resulting in a ventricular paced beat. The paced beat then conducts up to the atria, perpetuating the tachycardia. Pacemaker-mediated tachycardia can be avoided by extending the postventricular atrial refractory period, or, if intrinsic AV conduction is present, switching from a tracking mode (DDD) to a nontracking mode (DDI).

ATRIAL TACHYCARDIA

Atrial tachycardias (ATs) can be broadly subdivided into those that are focal (i.e., arising from a discrete region) and those that are macroreentrant (i.e., reentry occurs around obstacles, either anatomic or functional).

Focal ATs appear to arise preferentially from certain anatomic areas. The most common regions include the tricuspid and mitral valve annuli, crista terminalis, pulmonary vein ostia, and atrial appendages. Although it is difficult to conclusively determine the mechanism of these arrhythmias, triggered activity appears to be the underlying mechanism for most ATs, with microreentry and abnormal automaticity responsible for a smaller fraction.

Macroreentrant AT, as the term implies, involves a reentry circuit that revolves around a relatively large area. As stated above, boundaries that stabilize this form of AT can include anatomic structures (valves, venae cavae, pulmonary veins) as well as functional obstacles (crista terminalis, diseased atrial myocardium). The classic example of macroreentrant AT is typical atrial flutter. The reentry circuit for this arrhythmia revolves around the tricuspid valve (outer, or anterior boundary) with the venae cavae, coronary sinus, fossa ovalis, and crista terminalis helping to form the inner (or posterior) boundary. Macroreentrant ATs can also occur due to the presence of surgical scars (e.g., from prior valve surgery). These are often termed *lesional tachycardias*. In addition, incomplete ablation lesion sets, with gaps within linear lesion sets, can result in an area of slow conduction. This can lead to a larger excitable gap, a favorable condition for the occurrence of macroreentry.

Management of ATs can involve either (ventricular) rate control or attempt at conversion of the arrhythmia to sinus rhythm. Rate control can be attempted with β-blockers or calcium channel blockers, either intravenously (acute management) or orally (chronic). Conversion of a focal AT to sinus rhythm can often be achieved with adenosine (6–12 mg IV), which can terminate ATs resulting from cyclic AMP–mediated triggered activity. In addition, adenosine can transiently suppress (typically for <20 sec) focal ATs that result from abnormal automaticity. Other therapeutic options for these ATs include β-blockers or calcium channel blockers. For ATs that are insensitive to adenosine, class I or III antiarrhythmic agents can be considered. Long-term therapy includes oral forms of the effective agents used in acute management (except for adenosine). In addition, catheter ablation is effective, especially when used in conjunction with a three-dimensional mapping system to help localize the arrhythmia focus or circuit.

Sinus tachycardia has not been included in this discussion, because this arrhythmia is usually secondary to another condition, such as fever, pain, hypotension, hyperthyroidism, or anemia.

Ventricular Tachyarrhythmias

In this section, we highlight the more common and the more important forms of ventricular tachycardia (VT). VTs can be either monomorphic or polymorphic. The term monomorphic signifies that the QRS complex has a consistent morphology from beat to beat. This implies that either the site of origin of each ventricular depolarization is the same, or that the reentrant circuit is uniform for each beat of the tachycardia. Ventricular fibrillation (VF), characterized by chaotic electrical ventricular activity, is discussed in the chapter on cardiac arrest.

OUTFLOW TRACT VENTRICULAR TACHYCARDIA

The most common form of idiopathic VT in North America is outflow tract tachycardia. Although this form of VT was first appreciated in the right ventricular (RV) outflow tract and occurs more commonly (~80% of the time) from this region, origin from the left ventricular outflow tract region is also possible. Less commonly, these arrhythmias can arise from other sites, including the mitral annulus and the RV inflow tract, as well as epicardial sites. These tachycardias are focal in origin, are monomorphic, and most commonly have a left bundle branch block (LBBB) and inferior axis morphology (due to its RV outflow tract origin). Patients with this form of arrhythmia can present with frequent premature ventricular complexes (at rest), with salvos of nonsustained VT, or with sustained VT (usually exertional). This arrhythmia appears to be highly dependent on autonomic tone.

The underlying mechanism of outflow tract VT is delayed afterdepolarizations due to cyclic AMP-mediated triggered activity. β-Adrenergic receptor stimulation increases cyclic AMP, ultimately increasing intracellular calcium via stimulation of L-type calcium current (I_{CaL}) and subsequent calcium-induced calcium release and activation of a transient inward current (I_{ti}). This form of VT is uniquely sensitive to adenosine. Adenosine binds to a G-protein–coupled (A_1-adenosine) receptor and exerts its antiarrhythmic effect on ventricular myocytes via antagonism of β-adrenergic receptor activity. Other pharmacologic options for acute termination of outflow tract VT include intravenous β-blockers and intravenous verapamil (Calan). Long-term therapy includes administration of oral β-blockers or verapamil. Catheter ablation is extremely effective in curing outflow tract tachycardia.

INTRAFASCICULAR VENTRICULAR TACHYCARDIA

After outflow tract tachycardias, intrafascicular VT is the next most common form of monomorphic VT arising in the absence of structural heart disease. This form of VT is usually diagnosed in the second through fourth decades of life and has a male predominance. The distinguishing characteristics of intrafascicular VT include inducibility with rapid atrial pacing, right bundle branch block (RBBB) morphology with relatively narrow QRS complex (≤ 140 ms), and sensitivity to verapamil. Although there has been some debate regarding the exact mechanism of intrafascicular VT, it appears that it is due to a small reentrant circuit involving a portion of one of the fascicles of the left bundle branch (more commonly the posterior fascicle), as well as peri-Purkinje fibers. As a result, this tachycardia most commonly manifests with a RBBB and left superior axis morphology on ECG. However, RBBB and right inferior axis VT can also be observed when the circuit involves the left anterior fascicle. This form of VT is initiated due to conduction block down the fascicle, with conduction down the peri-Purkinje circuit. Retrograde conduction occurs up the adjacent fascicle.

Regarding acute management of intrafascicular VT, intravenous verapamil is effective in terminating the arrhythmia. The efficacy of oral verapamil in chronic therapy for intrafascicular VT is less clear, however. Catheter ablation has emerged as a viable alternative. Current strategies include targeting the earliest retrograde Purkinje potentials in the region of the reentrant circuit.

ARRHYTHMOGENIC RIGHT VENTRICULAR DYSPLASIA OR CARDIOMYOPATHY

It is extremely important to differentiate RV outflow tract VT from VT due to arrhythmogenic right ventricular dysplasia/cardiomyopathy (ARVD/C). Similar to RV outflow tract VT, ARVD/C can manifest with monomorphic VT of LBBB, inferior axis morphology.

ARVD/C is a condition involving progressive infiltration of the right ventricle with fibrosis and fat. The entity appears to have a male predominance, and diagnosis is usually made in the second through fourth decades of life, although this can be quite variable. Because there is no gold standard to diagnose ARVD/C, identifying patients can sometimes be difficult. Currently, diagnosis is made using Task Force criteria, published in 1994, which includes morphologic, functional, ECG, and histologic characteristics of the right ventricle, along with family history. Cardiac magnetic resonance imaging of the RV can demonstrate thinning of the walls and fibrofatty replacement, although this might not be evident early on in the disease. Modified, less stringent, criteria have been proposed for use in screening relatives of patients with ARVD/C to improve sensitivity.

Classically, the fibrofatty infiltration in ARVD/C has been described to involve predominantly the RV apex, diaphragmatic, and infundibular regions, the *triangle of dysplasia*. However, this can progress to involve other parts of the RV as well as the left ventricle. This fibrofatty infiltration predisposes the patient to VT due to reentry.

Several theories have been hypothesized regarding the etiology of ARVD/C. However, recent reports of mutations in plakoglobin, plakophilin, desmoplakin, and desmocollin genes have been reported in families with ARVD/C, pointing to a disorder of the desmosome as the underlying etiology of the disease process.

ARVD patients can present with ventricular arrhythmias as well as progressive RV failure. Due to the catecholamine dependence of VT in patients with ARVD/C, management includes avoidance of extreme physical activity and administration of β-blockers for low-risk patients. Those with a history of ventricular arrhythmias, unexplained syncope, sudden death, or family history of sudden death should consider receiving an implantable cardioverter-defibrillator (ICD) and possibly arrhythmia suppression with antiarrhythmic agents. ICD implantation can be technically difficult because of the thinning of the RV commonly seen in these patients. In some cases, palliative catheter ablation of VT can be performed. If either intractable ventricular tachycardia or end-stage right (or, less commonly, left) ventricular failure occurs, cardiac transplantation may be the only viable option.

LONG QT SYNDROME AND TORSADE DE POINTES

The clinical entity of long QT syndrome (LQTS) is heterogeneous with respect to phenotype and genotype. However, as the name suggests, there is a common ECG manifestation, a prolonged corrected QT interval (>440 ms in men, >460 ms in women), which is associated with an increased risk of syncope and sudden death. The estimated prevalence of LQTS is approximately 1:5000.

LQTS is considered a channelopathy. Hundreds of mutations have been reported in eight distinct ion channel genes, as well as in four channel-related proteins (Table 1). LQTS demonstrates both autosomal dominant (more common) and recessive patterns of inheritance. In addition to the congenital form of LQTS, an acquired form can also occur. In this form, after administration of certain medications, QT

TABLE 1 Long QT Syndrome: Mutations

Gene	Locus	Ion Channel or Protein
LQT1	11p15	I_{Ks}
LQT2	7q35	I_{Kr}
LQT3	3p21	I_{Na}
LQT4	4q25	Ankyrin B
LQT5	21q22	I_{Ks}
LQT6	21q22	I_{Kr}
LQT7	17q23	I_{Kl}
LQT8	9q8A	I_{Ca-L}
LQT9	3p25	I_{Na} or caveolin-3
LQT10	11q23.3	I_{Na}
LQT11	7q21–q22	I_{Ks}
LQT12	20q11.2	I_{Na}

prolongation occurs due to electrolyte abnormalities or due to marked bradycardia. Most patients with acquired LQTS also have an underlying genetic predisposition to QT prolongation.

The most commonly affected gene, *KCNQ1* (LQT1) on chromosome 11, encodes the α-subunit of the slowly activating delayed rectifier potassium channel (I_{Ks}), leading to a loss of function. The next most commonly affected gene, *KCNH2* (or *HERG*; [LQT2]) is located on chromosome 7, resulting in loss of function of the rapidly activating delayed rectifier potassium channel, I_{Kr}. These two gene loci account for approximately 95% of cases of LQTS. LQT3 is due to mutations in a sodium channel (*SCN5A;* chromosome 3), leading to a gain of function of the channel. Abnormalities in this gene account for 3% to 5% of cases of LQTS.

Increased dispersion of repolarization within the ventricular myocardium serves as the substrate for torsade de pointes (TdP), a form of polymorphic VT that has a characteristic appearance of twisting around an isoelectric point. TdP is initiated by an early afterdepolarization (enabled by the prolonged QT interval). The maintenance of TdP is due to reentry facilitated by the dispersion of repolarization between the different layers and regions of the ventricular myocardium. TdP can either terminate spontaneously or can degenerate into VF, causing sudden death.

The circumstances in which TdP is initiated can provide clues regarding the underlying gene involved. Emotional or physical stress or exertion is a common trigger of TdP in LQT1 patients. LQT2 patients can also experience arrhythmias during stress, but sudden auditory stimuli (e.g., alarm clock) are often the culprits. In contrast, LQT3 patients often have TdP during rest or sleep. The ECG can also help differentiate between the genotypes. LQT1 patients often have a prominent, broad-based T wave, and LQT2 manifests with low-amplitude notched T waves. LQT3 patients typically have a long ST segment with a fairly normal T wave. Recently, clinical screening for many of the LQTS mutations has become available.

All patients with suspected LQT1, as well as those with LQT2, should be treated with β-adrenergic antagonists. In addition, these patients should refrain from competitive sports. Higher-risk patients (those with syncope, aborted sudden death, or marked QT prolongation) should consider implantation of an ICD. Family members of those with LQTS should also be screened by careful history an a 12-lead ECG.

CATECHOLAMINERGIC POLYMORPHIC VENTRICULAR TACHYCARDIA

Catecholaminergic polymorphic VT (CPVT) was first described by Reid in 1975 and by Coumel in 1978. Three distinct features were noted: a structurally normal heart, onset of arrhythmia during adrenergic activation, and a typical pattern of bidirectional VT with normal resting ECG. These patients have been found to have polymorphic VT as well. The degree and complexity of ectopy are correlated with increase in physical or emotional stress, and ectopy occurs with heart rates greater than 110 to 120 bpm. Patients usually present early in childhood (mean age 7–9 years; although CPVT is diagnosed in some during their adult years) with syncope or sudden death.

CPVT has a familial distribution, with both autosomal dominant and recessive patterns. Mutations in the gene encoding the cardiac ryanodine receptor (*RyR2*) have been reported, and they occur in an autosomal dominant fashion. *RyR2* mutations account for approximately 50% of patients with CPVT. The autosomal recessive form of CPVT results from mutations in the calsequestrin gene (*CASQ2*), which encodes a protein involved in controlling calcium release from the sarcoplasmic reticulum. CPVT occurs because of uncontrolled calcium release from the sarcoplasmic reticulum, leading to VT due to delayed afterdepolarization–dependent triggered activity. CPVT typically arises from the left and right ventricular outflow tracts or the RV apex. Interestingly, CPVT patients often have supraventricular arrhythmias, including isolated atrial ectopy, and nonsustained atrial fibrillation.

β-Blocker therapy should be administered to all patients with CPVT, including silent carriers of *RyR2* mutations. ICD implantation should be considered for all CPVT patients with aborted sudden death and for those with syncope or VT despite therapy with β-blockers.

Brugada Syndrome

In 1992, the Brugadas described eight patients with aborted sudden death and a distinct ECG pattern. This ECG pattern included RBBB and coved ST segment elevation in leads VI through V3 (with inverted T wave) in the absence of structural heart disease (Fig. 7). This ECG pattern can be intermittent; the findings can be unmasked by the administration of sodium channel blockers such as procainamide (Pronestyl), flecainide (Tambocor), or ajmaline.[2]

Although mutations in *SCN5A*, the gene encoding the α-subunit of the sodium channel, have been reported in patients with Brugada syndrome, the majority of patients do not have a mutation in this gene. In contrast to mutations causing LQTS, SCN5A mutations causing Brugada syndrome lead to a *loss* of function. Other mutations reported to cause Brugada syndrome include those involving the glycerol-3-phosphate dehydrogenase 1-like gene (*GPD1L*) on chromosome 3, which leads to a reduction in sodium current, as well as two other genes encoding the α1-(CACNA1C) and β-(CACNB2b) subunits of the L-type calcium channel.

The underlying abnormality, loss of function of the sodium channel, leaves the transient outward potassium current (I_{to}) unopposed during phase 1 of the action potential. This results in a loss of the normal spike and dome and truncation of the action potential (Fig. 8). The RV subepicardial region is most severely affected, likely

---

[2]Not available in the United States.

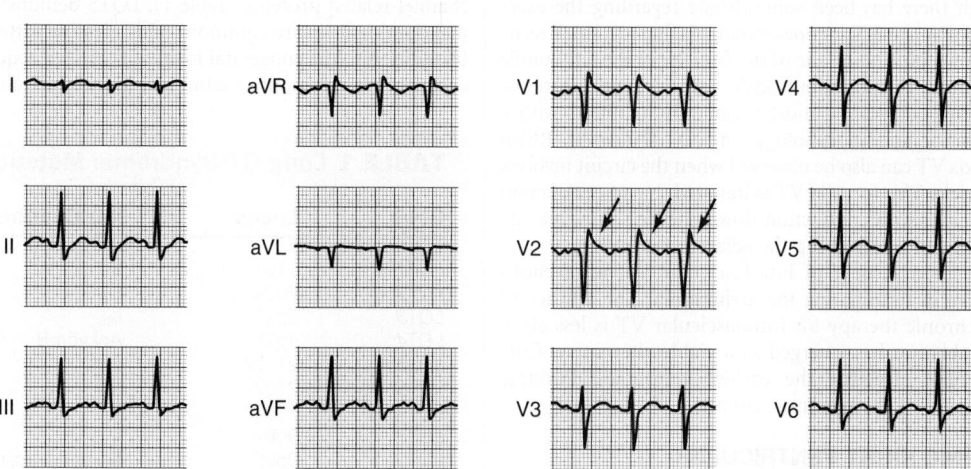

FIGURE 7. 12-lead electrocardiogram in a patient with Brugada syndrome. Note the J-point elevation and coved ST segments in the right precordial leads, most prominent in lead V_2 *(arrows).*

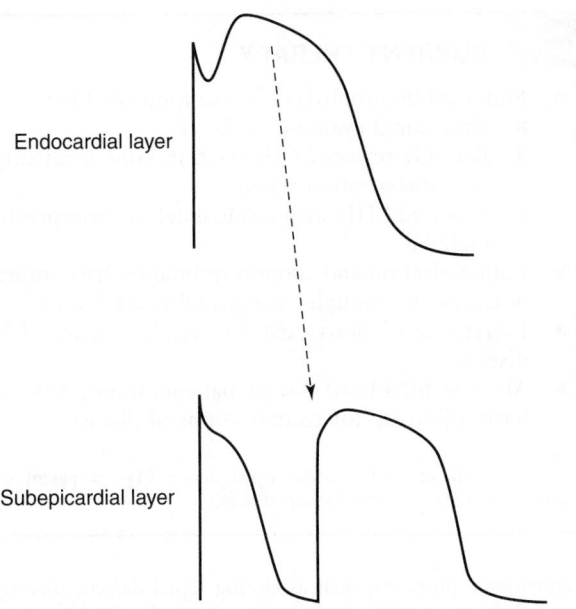

Endocardial layer

Subepicardial layer

FIGURE 8. Typical action potentials in the endocardial *(top)* and subepicardial *(bottom)* layers of the right ventricle in a patient with Brugada syndrome. Note the loss of the spike-and-dome appearance (all-or-none phenomenon) in the subepicardial layer from loss of sodium channel function. This results in heterogeneity of repolarization (i.e., epicardium is fully repolarized when the endocardium is depolarized), which can lead to phase 2 reentry. In this example, propagation proceeds from phase 2 of the endocardial layer to the epicardial layer *(dashed arrow)*, which has already fully repolarized.

due to a higher concentration of I_{to} in this region. As a result, this leads to heterogeneity of repolarization between the epi- and endocardial layers and polymorphic VT/VF due to phase 2 reentry.

There have been isolated case reports of the use of intravenous isoproterenol (Isuprel)[1] in improving the ST segment elevation as well as in preventing VF episodes in patients with Brugada syndrome. The data are limited, however. Recently, oral quinidine has been reported to be efficacious in reducing VT and VF in these patients. Quinidine, although a sodium channel blocker, also blocks I_{to}, which reduces the effect on the action potential of the loss of sodium channel function. Symptomatic patients should be treated with implantation of an ICD.

Much more controversial is the management of the asymptomatic patient with Brugada pattern. The inducibility of ventricular arrhythmias during electrophysiologic testing has met with conflicting results regarding its prognostic usefulness. A spontaneous Brugada pattern on ECG and family history of sudden death from VF, have also been proposed as adverse prognostic risk factors. ICD implantation can be considered on an individual basis in those thought to be at high risk for sudden death.

VENTRICULAR ARRHYTHMIAS IN ISCHEMIC HEART DISEASE

Patients who have had a prior myocardial infarction (MI) are at increased risk for sudden cardiac death due to ventricular arrhythmias. Approximately 2% to 5% of patients develop sustained monomorphic VT during the chronic (healed) phase of an MI. Areas of infarction (scar) provide anatomic obstacles for perpetuation of reentry. Also, the peri-infarct border zone, as well as surviving myocardial cells within the scar, provides the substrate for slow conduction. These areas of slow conduction provide the optimal milieu for sustaining reentrant circuits.

Patients with sustained, hemodynamically significant VT and coronary artery disease should be managed with ICD implantation. ICDs have been shown, in numerous randomized multicenter studies, to reduce overall mortality in patients undergoing implantation for both primary and secondary prevention of sudden death. In those

with frequent episodes of VT, suppressive therapy with antiarrhythmic agents can be considered. However, antiarrhythmic therapy is often ineffective, and it has not been shown to reduce overall mortality. Use of class IC antiarrhythmic agents (e.g., flecainide) is contraindicated in MI patients due to increased mortality. Alternatively, catheter ablation can be effective in decreasing the frequency of VT by disruption of the reentrant circuits.

REFERENCES

Ackerman MJ, Clapham DE. Normal cardiac electrophysiology. In: Chien K, editor. Molecular Basis of Cardiovascular Disease. Philadelphia: WB Saunders; 1999. p. 281–301.

Antzelevitch CA. Brugada syndrome. PACE 2006;29:1130–59.

Brugada P, Brugada J. Right bundle branch block, persistent ST segment elevation and sudden cardiac death: A distinct clinical and electrocardiographic syndrome. J Am Cofl Cardiol 1992;20:1391–6.

Hulot J-S, Jouven X, Empana J-P, et al. Natural history and risk stratification of arrhythmogenic right ventricular dysplasia/cardiomyopathy. Circulation 2004;110:1879–84.

Iwai S, Markowitz SM, Stein KM, et al. Response to adenosine differentiates focal from macroreentrant atrial tachycardia: Validation using three-dimensional electroanatomic mapping. Circulation 2002;106:2793–9.

Jalife J, Delmar M, Davidenko J, et al. Basic Cardiac Electrophysiology For The Clinician. Armonk, NY: Futura; 1999.

Kim RJ, Iwai S, Markowitz SM, et al. Clinical and electrophysiologic spectrum of idiopathic ventricular outflow tract arrhythmias. J Am Coll Cardiol 2007;49:2035–43.

Lerman BB, Stein KM, Markowitz SM. Adenosine-sensitive ventricular tachycardia: A conceptual approach. J Cardiovasc Electrophysiol 1996;7:559–69.

Markowitz SM, Nemirovsky D, Stein KM, et al. Adenosine-insensitive focal atrial tachycardia: Evidence for de novo microreentry in the human atrium. J Am Coll Cardiol 2007;49:1324–33.

McKenna WJ, Thiene G, Nava A, et al. Diagnosis of arrhythmogenic right ventricular dysplasia/cardiomyopathy. Br Heart J 1994;71:215–8.

Napolitano C, Priori SG. Diagnosis and treatment of catecholaminergic polymorphic ventricular tachycardia. Heart Rhythm 2007;4:675–8.

Zipes DP, Camm AJ, Borggrefe M, et al. ACC/AHA/ESC 2006 guidelines for management of patients with ventricular arrhythmias and the prevention of sudden cardiac death. Circulation 2006;114:e385–484.

Congenital Heart Disease

Method of
Robb L. Romp, MD, and Yung R. Lau, MD

Congenital heart disease is the most common type of severe congenital malformation, with a prevalence of approximately 8 per 1000 live births. Proper evaluation of patients for congenital heart disease includes reviewing the past medical history, performing a systematic physical examination, and using selective ancillary testing.

The etiology of most congenital heart disease is unknown, but numerous high-risk populations have been identified. Fetal exposure to maternal diabetes, rubella, or teratogens such as ethanol and retinoic acid leads to an increased incidence of cardiac malformation. Certain chromosomal abnormalities, including Down syndrome (trisomy 21), DiGeorge's syndrome (22q11 deletion), and Turner's syndrome (XO) are associated with specific cardiac lesions. Some forms of congenital heart disease carry increased risk for familial transmission.

Cardiac Evaluation

The physical examination begins with gross inspection for dysmorphic features suggesting syndromes related to congenital heart disease. Next, a thorough review of vital signs including growth parameters, four extremity blood pressures, and oxygen saturation

---

[1]Not FDA approved for this indication.

CURRENT DIAGNOSIS

- History and physical examination, including growth parameters, blood pressures, respiratory rate, pulse oximetry, work of breathing, hepatomegaly, and peripheral pulses
- Cardiac examination, including description of murmur and heart sounds
- Ancillary testing, including chest radiograph and electrocardiogram
- Consultation with pediatric cardiologist for:
- Abnormal examination suggesting congenital heart disease
- High-risk populations (trisomy 21)

CURRENT THERAPY

- Endocarditis prophylaxis is recommended for:
  - Unrepaired cyanotic CHD
  - Recently repaired CHD (<6 months from surgical or catheterization repair)
  - Repaired CHD with residual defects near prosthetic material
- Catheterization and surgical techniques have improved outcomes for complex congenital heart disease
- Exercise restrictions exist for certain congenital heart disease
- All congenital heart disease patients should have long-term follow-up for complications of disease

Abbreviations: ASD = atrial septal defect; PDA = patent ductus arteriosus; VSD = ventricular septal defect.

should be conducted. Normal arterial saturations should be greater than 93% in newborns. In the presence of desaturation, a hyperoxia challenge (measuring partial oxygen pressure of blood while breathing 100% oxygen) can be helpful. Infants with pulmonary disease can typically achieve a partial oxygen pressure in excess of 150 mm Hg, whereas infants with intracardiac right-to-left shunting cannot. Respiratory symptoms, including tachypnea and hyperpnea, are frequent findings in cardiac malformations that cause increased pulmonary blood flow. Hepatomegaly is also common in cardiac malformations with important pulmonary overcirculation. The extremities should be evaluated for evidence of impaired perfusion, clubbing, or edema. Abnormal pulses and brachiofemoral pulse delay are markers for certain types of congenital heart disease.

Evaluation of the heart itself includes observing and palpating the location and size of the cardiac impulse on the precordium. Auscultation of cardiac sounds should focus sequentially on the first and second heart sounds and then on murmurs. The first heart sound is typically single in pediatric patients. The second heart sound varies with respiration, with splitting that widens during inspiration and narrows to a single sound during expiration.

Murmurs are described based on intensity from I (quietest) to VI (loudest), and a palpable thrill is present in murmurs of grades IV to VI. The timing and amplitude of murmurs help to identify the cause of the sound. Systolic ejection murmurs have an onset after the first heart sound and a crescendo-decrescendo quality that terminates before the second heart sound. When such murmurs are soft and vibratory and vary with patient position, they are generally benign or innocent. Harsher and louder ejection murmurs are more likely to represent obstructed blood flow, such as valve stenosis.

Holosystolic murmurs have an onset coincident with the first heart sound. These murmurs are caused most commonly by ventricular septal defects but are also associated with mitral or tricuspid valve insufficiency. Continuous murmurs extend from systole through the second heart sound into diastole and represent flow from the systemic arterial circulation into the pulmonary or venous circulation. Diastolic murmurs are isolated in diastole and can be caused by aortic or pulmonary valve insufficiency. Diastolic rumbles can also be caused by excess flow across the tricuspid or mitral valve due to intracardiac left-to-right shunting. The location of the murmur and direction of radiation are helpful in determining the cause of the sound.

Ancillary testing plays an important role in diagnosing congenital heart disease. Chest radiography can help identify the presence of cardiac enlargement and the prominence of the pulmonary vasculature. These findings help determine whether a heart defect is causing increased, normal, or decreased pulmonary blood flow. The electrocardiogram (ECG) can identify conduction abnormalities that are associated with certain congenital malformations. In experienced hands, echocardiography is the primary tool for diagnosis of congenital heart disease. Most malformations of the heart can be delineated completely by transthoracic echocardiography, and fetal echocardiography can be used to diagnose many cardiac abnormalities prenatally. Although cardiac catheterization has, in the past, played a role in defining congenital heart disease, most catheterizations are now performed for interventional purposes, such as closing septal defects, dilating stenotic valves, or stenting open narrowed vessels. Cardiac computed tomography (CT) and magnetic resonance imaging (MRI) are becoming increasingly important noninvasive diagnostic tools for extracardiac vascular abnormalities and patients in whom only limited transthoracic echocardiographic images can be obtained.

Using an evaluation including only the physical examination, oxygen saturation, and chest x-ray, it should be possible to identify patients with significant congenital heart disease and in turn the urgency of an evaluation by a pediatric cardiologist. This same basic evaluation permits patients to be readily categorized based on the presence or absence of cyanosis and the amount of pulmonary blood flow. Acyanotic lesions include those with increased pulmonary blood flow and those with normal pulmonary blood flow but obstruction of flow from the heart. Cyanotic lesions include those with increased or decreased pulmonary blood flow.

Acyanotic Lesions with Increased Pulmonary Blood Flow

Acyanotic cardiac defects with increased pulmonary blood flow make up the largest category of congenital heart disease and include ventricular septal defect, atrial septal defect, atrioventricular canal defect, and patent ductus arteriosus. Such defects permit left-to-right shunting, the magnitude of which depends on the size of the defect and the relative resistances of the pulmonary and systemic vascular beds. As the pulmonary vascular resistance falls within the first weeks of life, the quantity of shunting increases substantially. This leads to the typical findings of cardiomegaly and increased pulmonary vascularity on the chest radiograph. Symptoms are related to the magnitude of additional pulmonary flow.

VENTRICULAR SEPTAL DEFECT

A ventricular septal defect (VSD), an opening in the ventricular septum, is the most common cardiac malformation. It is present as an isolated lesion in one quarter and as a component of a cardiac malformation in one half of all patients with congenital heart disease. The hemodynamic importance and natural history of a VSD are related to its location and size. A VSD located in the muscular septum, remote from the valves, is the most common type and fortunately the most likely to undergo spontaneous closure. Defects of the perimembranous septum can also decrease in size over time, but perimembranous defects are more likely to be associated with other abnormalities and to require surgical closure. Defects of the inlet and outlet portions of the ventricular septum are relatively rare. Large defects (approaching the size of the aortic annulus) are almost certain to cause symptoms from pulmonary overcirculation and to require surgical closure. Moderate-sized defects (about one half the size of the aortic annulus) can cause sufficient symptoms to require medical management but often spontaneously decrease in size to the point where they no longer require surgical or medical intervention. Small defects (less than one half the aortic annulus) are unlikely to cause symptoms or require intervention.

Most often, a newborn with a VSD has no murmur immediately after birth, due to the relatively high pulmonary vascular resistance, which prevents significant left-to-right shunting. As the pulmonary resistance falls in the first few weeks of life, shunting increases. In small and moderate VSDs, a concomitant decrease in right ventricular pressure occurs and a characteristic harsh holosystolic murmur is heard. In a large VSD, there is little restriction of flow, and no holosystolic murmur is present. Patients with pulmonary overcirculation caused by important left-to-right shunts typically develop symptoms in the first weeks to months of life. Tachypnea is often the first sign, followed by poor feeding, diaphoresis, and eventual failure to thrive. The chest x-ray shows increased cardiac size and pulmonary vascular markings in proportion to the size of the shunt. In rare circumstances, a large VSD can lead to persistent elevation of the pulmonary resistance. Though such patients have no murmur and few symptoms, they are at risk for developing pulmonary vascular obstructive disease.

Management of ventricular septal defects depends on the patient's symptoms and the magnitude of shunting permitted by the defect. Symptomatic patients are usually treated with a combination of diuretics, digoxin (Lanoxin), and afterload reduction. Patients who are refractory to medical management and those with large nonrestrictive defects should undergo surgical closure during infancy to prevent the development of irreversible pulmonary vascular obstructive disease. Surgical closure might also be indicated in asymptomatic children with significant shunting that persists, due to long-term risk of pulmonary vascular obstructive disease. Surgical closure is currently the standard of care for defects requiring closure, but trials are under way for catheter-delivered devices that will play an increasingly important role in VSD closure in the future.

ATRIAL SEPTAL DEFECT

An atrial septal defect (ASD) is an opening in the atrial septum that permits important left-to-right shunting. The magnitude of the shunt depends on the size of the defect and the relative compliance of the ventricles. Despite the increased pulmonary blood flow permitted by a large ASD, such a defect generally does not cause pulmonary hypertension or symptoms during childhood. The increased right ventricular output and flow across the pulmonary valve cause the systolic ejection murmur and widely split second heart sound, which does not narrow during expiration.

If the magnitude of the shunt is substantial, ASD closure should be performed during childhood to avoid the long-term risks of pulmonary vascular disease and atrial arrhythmias. With the exception of large ASDs and some defects located eccentrically within the atrial septum that require surgical closure, most ASDs are now closed using a catheter-delivery system in which a device is positioned within the defect to prevent shunting. Medical therapy is rarely necessary.

ATRIOVENTRICULAR CANAL DEFECT

Atrioventricular (AV) canal defects are malformations caused by incomplete fusion of the endocardial cushions during embryonic development. These cushions normally fuse to form the tricuspid and mitral valves as well as the adjacent portions of the atrial and ventricular septum. Endocardial cushion defects include a spectrum of abnormalities ranging from an isolated defect in the atrial septum, known as a primum ASD, to a common AV canal defect in which there is a single AV valve in association with a large ASD and VSD. A common AV canal defect permits substantial left-to-right shunting at both the atrial and ventricular levels, which leads to early symptoms from both excess pulmonary blood flow and pulmonary hypertension. Patients typically develop early symptoms of congestive heart failure in the first months of life.

Physical findings include tachypnea and hepatomegaly. The cardiac examination reveals a hyperdynamic precordium and a systolic ejection murmur from increased flow across the pulmonary valve. A holosystolic murmur is likely caused by AV valve insufficiency,

which is commonly present, rather than VSD shunting. The chest x-ray shows cardiomegaly and increased pulmonary vascularity. The EGC characteristically reveals left axis deviation.

AV canal defects require surgical repair. Although such patients can benefit from medical treatment with diuretics, digoxin, and afterload reduction, the onset of heart failure symptoms is generally the point at which surgery is considered. Surgical techniques vary and include use of one or two patches (depending on the size of the septal defects) and division of the common AV valve into two separate components.

PATENT DUCTUS ARTERIOSUS

The patent ductus arteriosus (PDA) is a normal prenatal vessel connecting the pulmonary artery and the aorta that permits the output of the right ventricle to bypass the fetal lungs. The PDA typically constricts and closes within the first days of postnatal life. Persistent PDA is present in one in 1250 live births, with an increasing prevalence in premature infants (as common as 80% for infants with a birth weight of less than 750 g). The presence of a PDA permits left-to-right shunting that is related to the size of the PDA and the relative resistance of the pulmonary and systemic vascular beds. Significant shunting leads to volume overload of the left heart and pulmonary vascular bed that manifest clinically as tachycardia, tachypnea, and widened pulse pressures. A large ductus in a patient with low pulmonary vascular resistance causes a continuous murmur. Often the diastolic component of the murmur is diminished in newborns who might have elevated pulmonary resistance, making clinical diagnosis more challenging.

In the infant, the need for closure of a PDA depends on the clinical significance of the shunt. As a general rule, a PDA that causes symptoms or results in dilation of the left heart should be closed. In an older child, closure of a PDA is advisable if a classic murmur is present in order to eliminate the lifetime risk of endocarditis.

Several options are available to close a PDA. Preterm infants often respond to medical management with prostaglandin inhibitors such as indomethacin (Indocin) or ibuprofen (Motrin). If medical therapy is unsuccessful or contraindicated, surgical ligation of the ductus is performed. In older children, interventional catheterization techniques using several available devices are widely used to occlude the ductus.

Acyanotic Lesions with Obstruction

Obstruction of blood flow from the heart can be caused by aortic stenosis, pulmonary stenosis, or coarctation of the aorta. These lesions are not associated with cyanosis, except in cases of critically severe obstruction in neonates.

COARCTATION OF THE AORTA

Coarctation, which has a prevalence of 1 in 3000 live births, is a narrowing of the aortic arch between the origin of the left subclavian artery and the insertion of the ductus arteriosus–ligamentum. Coarctation can manifest in two ways: neonatal critical coarctation and nonneonatal coarctation. Critical coarctation manifests as shock caused by impaired systemic cardiac output when the ductus arteriosus closes spontaneously in the neonatal period. Less severe forms of coarctation cause hypertension in the proximal aorta (best measured in the right arm) and both delayed and diminished pulses in the femoral arteries.

Coarctation should be excluded as the etiology of hypertension in any pediatric patient. The heart sounds are normal unless there is an associated anomaly, such as a bicuspid aortic valve. A continuous murmur may be heard over the back. Chest x-ray findings can include the "3 sign" caused by indentation of the aorta at the point of coarctation and rib notching due to engorged intercostal arteries carrying collateral flow.

Treatment of coarctation depends on the age at presentation. Critical coarctation is initially treated medically with prostaglandin E_1 (Alprostadil) to maintain ductal patency. Surgical repair, involving resection of the coarctation site and elongated anastomosis of the proximal and descending ends of the aorta, is the most widely used therapy in infants. After repair, infants can develop re-coarctation from

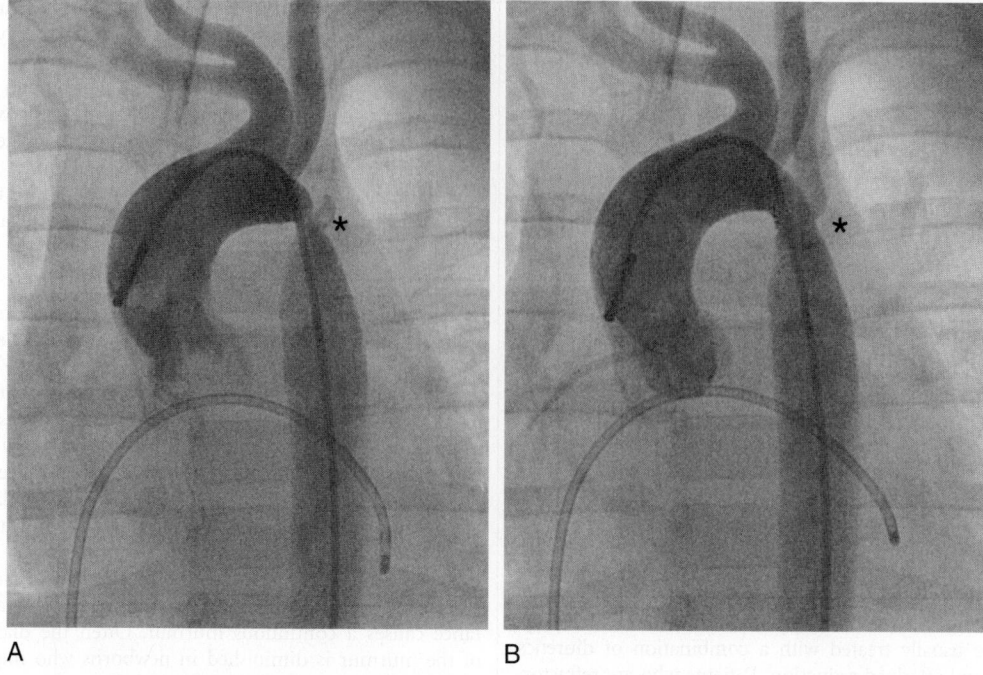

FIGURE 1. Angiography demonstrating aortic coarctation. **A,** There is moderate to severe coarctation with reduced blood flow into the left subclavian artery (*). **B,** Following balloon angioplasty, the obstruction is reduced and filling of the sub-clavian artery is normalized.

anastomotic scarring, which responds well to balloon angioplasty in the catheterization laboratory. Older children and adults may be candidates for catheterization interventions including balloon angioplasty or stenting of native coarctation as an initial intervention (Figure 1).

AORTIC STENOSIS

The incidence of aortic stenosis is as great as 1 in 2600 live births. Obstruction most commonly occurs at the level of the valve itself, due to dysplasia or fusion of the valve leaflets, but it can also involve the region below or above the valve. Critical aortic stenosis manifests as shock in the neonatal period, when systemic cardiac output is compromised. Severe aortic stenosis can manifest with exertional chest pain, syncope, or even sudden death. Mild to moderate aortic stenosis is generally asymptomatic.

Cardiac examination reveals an ejection click and a systolic ejection murmur that radiates to the carotids and increases in intensity in relation to severity of stenosis. With moderate to severe stenosis, a thrill may also be palpated in the suprasternal notch. The ECG is normal with mild stenosis but shows evidence of left ventricular hypertrophy and strain with increasingly severe aortic stenosis. Dilation of the ascending aorta may be apparent on chest x-ray.

Aortic stenosis has a tendency to progress over time and therefore requires close follow-up. With higher degrees of severity, exercise restrictions are recommended. For moderate and severe aortic stenosis, balloon valvuloplasty performed in the catheterization laboratory is recommended to reduce the obstruction. Though generally effective in reducing the stenosis, valvuloplasty can cause aortic insufficiency. Surgery is reserved for patients who have aortic stenosis associated with important insufficiency or stenosis caused by a severely dysplastic valve not responsive to balloon dilation.

PULMONARY STENOSIS

Pulmonary stenosis is a common form of congenital heart disease, with an incidence of 1 in 1250 live births. As in aortic stenosis, the valve leaflets are thickened and they separate incompletely from one another. Critical pulmonary stenosis can result in impaired pulmonary blood flow and cyanosis in newborns (due to right-to-left shunting through the patent foramen ovale), but less severe forms of pulmonary stenosis are generally asymptomatic. An ejection click and systolic ejection murmur are present, with the intensity and duration of the murmur proportional to the severity of stenosis. ECG findings may include right ventricular hypertrophy or strain. Echocardiography can accurately grade the severity of stenosis. Balloon valvuloplasty is the treatment of choice for moderate and severe valvular pulmonary stenosis and provides excellent long-term relief of obstruction.

Cyanotic Lesions with Decreased Pulmonary Blood Flow

Cyanotic lesions with decreased pulmonary vascularity are caused by obstructed pulmonary blood flow and right-to-left shunting within the heart. The most common lesions are tetralogy of Fallot and tricuspid atresia. Affected patients have varying degrees of cyanosis. The absence of pulmonary overcirculation prevents the development of tachypnea seen in patients with congestive heart failure.

TETRALOGY OF FALLOT

Tetralogy of Fallot is the most common form of cyanotic congenital heart disease, with an incidence of about 1 in 3000 live births. Malalignment of the perimembranous ventricular septum leads to the tetralogy, which consists of pulmonary outflow tract obstruction, large ventricular septal defect with aortic override, and right ventricular hypertrophy. The severity of pulmonary outflow tract obstruction dictates the degree of cyanosis, ranging from pulmonary atresia with severe cyanosis to more mild pulmonary stenosis with normal saturations. Hypercyanotic spells are precipitated by spasm of the subpulmonary infundibular muscle, which causes acute worsening of pulmonary outflow tract obstruction and potentially life-threatening cyanosis. Squatting is a maneuver used by older unrepaired patients to increase the systemic vascular resistance and overcome the pulmonary obstruction causing a hypercyanotic spell.

The examination is notable for cyanosis in the case of more severe obstruction of the pulmonary outflow tract. A harsh systolic ejection murmur is present in the pulmonary region. The chest x-ray shows decreased pulmonary vascularity with an absent pulmonary segment and upturned apex of the cardiac silhouette, which gives the classic boot-shaped heart.

Noninvasive Treatments

Patient in calm environment (mother's lap)

Supplemental oxygen

Swaddled knee-chest position to increase systemic afterload

Invasive Treatments

• Morphine or ketamine (Ketalar)

• Volume expansion (packed red blood cells if anemic)

• Phenylephrine (Neo-Synephrine) to increase systemic afterload

• Esmolol (Brevibloc) to relax the infundibular spasm

• Anesthetize and paralyze

• Surgical repair or palliation

Tetralogy does not typically require medical management, and in fact, diuretics and positive inotropes can increase the likelihood of hypercyanotic spells. Hypercyanotic spells are a medical emergency and must be treated aggressively (Box 1). Patients with pulmonary atresia are ductal dependent and require prostaglandin therapy to maintain ductal patency. These patients commonly undergo surgical placement of a modified Blalock-Taussig shunt between the subclavian artery and the pulmonary artery to secure pulmonary blood flow during infancy. Repair of the intracardiac abnormalities can be undertaken as early as the neonatal period, but it is often delayed until later in infancy in the patient with only mild cyanosis.

Surgical repair involves patch closure of the VSD with enlargement of the pulmonary outflow tract by resection of subpulmonary muscle

bundles and enlargement of the pulmonary valve with a transannular patch. Lifelong endocarditis prophylaxis is recommended, but most patients require no other long-term medical management. Although the functional outcomes are excellent during childhood, right ventricular dilation and dysfunction are common long-term complications that can require surgical placement of a competent pulmonary valve.

TRICUSPID ATRESIA

Tricuspid atresia is a rare cardiac malformation with an incidence of 1 in 17,500 live births. In this condition, the tricuspid valve is platelike and does not permit flow from the right atrium to the right ventricle. Instead, the systemic venous return shunts right to left across an atrial septal defect, mixing with the pulmonary venous return in the left atrium. Blood flow to the lungs is either through a VSD to a hypoplastic right ventricle and thereby to the pulmonary artery or is ductal dependent from the aorta to the pulmonary arteries by way of a PDA.

Patients are severely cyanotic from the time of birth but can have relatively quiet hearts without pathologic murmurs. The ECG is helpful in making the diagnosis due to the presence of left axis deviation. The chest x-ray shows diminished pulmonary vascularity and relatively small heart size, similar to tetralogy of Fallot.

Treatment of tricuspid atresia depends on the degree of flow through the hypoplastic right ventricle. Ductal-dependent patients require prostaglandin to maintain ductal patency until placement of a modified Blalock-Taussig shunt in the neonatal period. All patients eventually undergo cavopulmonary anastomosis by means of a modified Glenn operation (superior vena caval anastomosis to pulmonary artery) during infancy and a modified Fontan operation (inferior vena caval anastomosis to pulmonary artery) during early childhood (Figure 2). The cavopulmonary anastomoses permit the systemic venous return to bypass the heart and flow passively through the lungs, allowing the functional single ventricle to be used as the systemic ventricle. The modified Glenn and modified Fontan operations

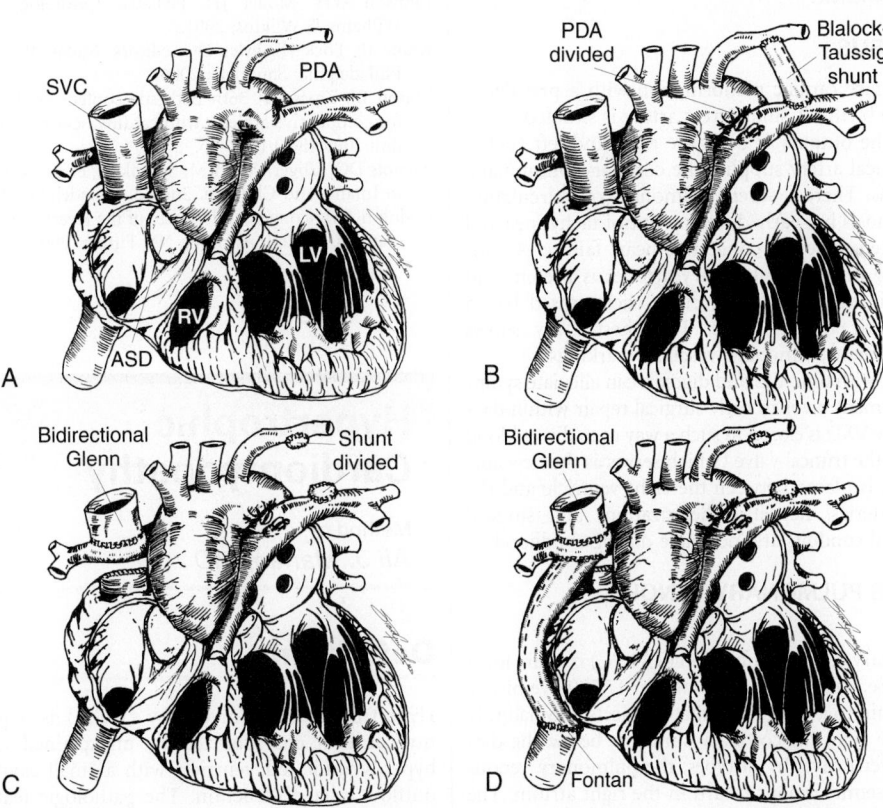

FIGURE 2. Illustrations of tricuspid atresia and surgical palliations. **A,** Pulmonary blood flow originates from the patent ductus arteriosus (PDA), **B,** A modified Blalock-Taussig shunt replaces the PDA as the source of pulmonary blood flow. **C,** Pulmonary blood flow is through the bidirectional Glenn connection of the superior vena cava (SVC) to the right pulmonary artery. **D,** Following the modified Fontan connection of the inferior vena cava to the right pulmonary artery, the systemic venous return bypasses the heart, entirely separating the deoxygenated blood from the oxygenated blood. *Abbreviation:* ASD = atrial septal defect.

are used as a common final pathway in most cardiac malformations resulting in a functional single ventricle.

Cyanotic Lesions with Increased Pulmonary Blood Flow

Cyanosis with increased pulmonary blood flow suggests the presence of an admixture lesion that has both right-to-left and left-to-right shunting. Patients in this category have both cyanosis and early development of tachypnea due to pulmonary overcirculation. The most common lesions include transposition of the great arteries, truncus arteriosus, total anomalous pulmonary venous connection, and hypoplastic left heart syndrome.

TRANSPOSITION OF THE GREAT ARTERIES

Transposition of the great arteries (TGA) has a prevalence of 1 in 4000 live births. In TGA, the aorta arises from the right ventricle and the pulmonary artery arises from the left ventricle. This arrangement of parallel systemic and pulmonary circulations causes severe cyanosis. Mixing between the systemic and pulmonary circulations depends on the presence of an ASD, which permits shunting of the oxygenated pulmonary venous return to the right heart, where it is pumped to the systemic circulation. Cardiac examination reveals a single second heart sound without pathologic murmurs. The chest x-ray shows cardiomegaly with a narrow superior mediastinum related to the parallel orientation of the great arteries.

Treatment of TGA involves prompt recognition and institution of prostaglandin infusion to maintain ductal patency. If an adequate ASD is not present, a balloon atrial septostomy is performed urgently to enhance mixing of systemic and pulmonary circulations. Repair is done in the first week of life by means of an arterial switch operation, which involves transection and relocation of the great arteries so they arise from the correct ventricle.

TRUNCUS ARTERIOSUS

Truncus arteriosus is a rare cardiac malformation with a prevalence of about 1 in 25,000 live births. A single great artery is situated above a large VSD, receiving the outputs of both the right and left ventricles. This ascending truncal artery supplies the coronary, pulmonary, and systemic circulations. There is severe pulmonary overcirculation with relatively mild cyanosis but early development of tachypnea and respiratory distress related to severe congestive heart failure. A continuous murmur of flow into the pulmonary arteries is present and there is often a diastolic murmur and ejection click caused by an insufficient and dysplastic truncal valve. The chest x-ray shows cardiomegaly and prominent pulmonary vascular markings.

Medical management with diuretics and digoxin can alleviate symptoms, but definitive treatment involves early surgical repair within days to weeks of diagnosis. The VSD is closed in such a way as to direct blood from the left ventricle to the truncal valve (which serves as the new aortic valve), and a conduit is placed between the right ventricle and the detached pulmonary arteries. Repeat catheterizations and surgical replacement of obstructed conduits are inevitable during childhood.

TOTAL ANOMALOUS PULMONARY VENOUS CONNECTION

Total anomalous pulmonary venous connection (TAPVC) is a rare form of congenital heart disease, with a prevalence of 1 in 17,500 live births. The pulmonary veins drain to a confluence that connects anomalously to either the innominate vein, the coronary sinus, or below the diaphragm to the inferior vena cava. In all types, the pulmonary venous return mixes with the systemic venous return in the right atrium. The systemic cardiac output is dependent on right-to-left shunting through an ASD. Pulmonary blood flow is increased and the level of cyanosis is generally mild. A systolic ejection murmur is present over the pulmonary valve. The chest x-ray shows cardiomegaly and vascular engorgement. Subdiaphragmatic forms of TAPVC can have obstruction of the anomalous pulmonary venous connection, which can cause respiratory distress and severe cyanosis within hours of birth. Surgical

repair is performed in the neonatal period and involves ASD closure and anastomosis of the pulmonary venous confluence to the left atrium.

HYPOPLASTIC LEFT HEART

Hypoplastic left heart (HLH) is relatively rare, with a prevalence of 1 in 3500 live births. There is hypoplasia of the mitral valve, left ventricle, aortic valve, and ascending aorta to a degree that the left heart is not able to support the systemic circulation. The pulmonary venous return shunts left to right across an ASD to mix with the systemic venous return in the right atrium, and the systemic circulation is dependent on right-to-left shunting across the PDA.

Patients are cyanotic and develop severe pulmonary overcirculation as newborns. Presentation often involves circulatory collapse when the PDA closes, causing impaired systemic perfusion. The examination is notable for cyanosis and a single second heart sound but no important murmurs. The chest x-ray shows cardiomegaly and increased pulmonary vascularity.

Treatment involves early recognition and institution of prostaglandin infusion to maintain ductal patency. Surgical palliation in the first week of life involves the Norwood stage 1 procedure, which has mortality rates approaching 10% at many larger medical centers. Patients require future surgeries during infancy and childhood, including the Glenn and Fontan cavopulmonary anastomoses, which permit passive systemic venous return to the lungs and establish the single right ventricle as the systemic pump. Although such patients have a diminished exercise tolerance and risk of right ventricular failure long term, they can have a reasonable quality of life through childhood.

REFERENCES

Allen HD, Gutgesell HP, Clark EB, Driscoll DK, editors. Moss and Adams' Heart Disease in Infants, Children, and Adolescents. 6th ed. Philadelphia: Lippincott Williams & Wilkins; 2001.
Garson A, Bricker JT, Fisher DJ, Neish SR, editors. The Science and Practice of Pediatric Cardiology. 2nd ed. Baltimore: Williams & Wilkins; 1998.
Johnson WH, Moller JH. Pediatric Cardiology. Philadelphia: Lippincott Williams & Wilkins; 2001.
Keane JF, Lock JE, Fyler DC, editors. Nadas' Pediatric Cardiology. 2nd ed. Philadelphia: Saunders; 2006.
Maron BJ, Zipes DP. 36th Bethesda conference: Eligibility recommendations for competitive athletes with cardiovascular abnormalities. J Am Coll Cardiol 2005;45(8):1312–75.
Nichols DG, Ungerleider RM, Spevak PJ, et al., editors. Critical Heart Disease in Infants and Children. 2nd ed. Philadelphia: Mosby; 2006.
Rudolph AM. Congenital Diseases of the Heart: Clinical Physiological Considerations. 2nd ed. Armonk, NY: Futura; 2001.

Hypertrophic Cardiomyopathy

Method of
Ali J. Marian, MD

Definition

Hypertrophic cardiomyopathy (HCM) is a primary disease of the myocardium characterized by unexplained cardiac hypertrophy, a hyperdynamic left ventricle with a small cavity, and often dynamic outflow tract obstruction. The pathologic features of HCM include myocyte hypertrophy, disarray, and interstitial fibrosis. Myocyte disarray is considered the pathologic hallmark of HCM.

The current clinical diagnosis of HCM is neither specific nor highly sensitive. For example, the presence of systemic hypertension, per convention, excludes the diagnosis of HCM, despite the possibility of concomitant HCM in hypertensive individuals. "Unexplained cardiac hypertrophy" also can occur in storage diseases, mitochondrial disorders, and triplet repeat syndromes. The presence of a hyperdynamic left ventricle, outflow tract obstruction, and asymmetric hypertrophy favors the diagnosis of true HCM. In contrast, depressed global cardiac systolic function, conduction defects, neurologic abnormalities, and skeletal myopathy favor the possibility of a phenocopy.

Prevalence

The prevalence of HCM, defined as a wall thickness of 15 mm or greater on echocardiogram in the absence of a secondary cause, is estimated to be 1:500 in individuals 23 to 35 years old. However, the disease probably is more common, as expression of cardiac hypertrophy is age dependent. Many young individuals with the disease-causing mutation may exhibit mild hypertrophy or express cardiac hypertrophy late in life.

Clinical Manifestations

Clinical manifestations of HCM are variable, ranging from an asymptomatic course to that of severe heart failure and sudden cardiac death (SCD). The majority of patients with HCM are asymptomatic or minimally symptomatic. The most common symptoms are dyspnea, chest pain, palpitations, and lightheadedness. Syncope is an infrequent symptom that often indicates serious cardiac arrhythmias. Atrial fibrillation and nonsustained ventricular tachycardia are the most common cardiac arrhythmias in patients with HCM.

HCM is the most common cause of SCD and often is the first manifestation of the disease in young competitive athletes, accounting for almost half of cases. A history of SCD, syncope, a strong family history of SCD, serious ventricular arrhythmias including frequent episodes of nonsustained ventricular tachycardia, severe cardiac hypertrophy, exertional hypotension, and genetic factors are considered risk factors for SCD. None of the risk factors alone is a reliable predictor; hence, the global risk, which is derived from a combination of multiple risk factors, should be assessed. The overall estimated annual mortality rate of patients with HCM is about 1% in the adult population.

Molecular Genetics

HCM is a genetic disease with an autosomal dominant mode of inheritance. A family history of HCM can be elicited in approximately half to two thirds of cases. The seminal report by Seidman and colleagues in 1999 of the R403Q mutation in the β-myosin heavy chain (β-MyHC) led to elucidation of the molecular genetic basis of HCM. To date, more than 400 causal mutations in more than a dozen different genes, all encoding the sarcomeric proteins, have been identified. Accordingly, HCM is considered a disease of mutant sarcomeric proteins (excluding HCM phenocopy). Mutations in *MYH7* and *MYBPC3*, which encode β-MyHC and myosin-binding protein-C (MyBP-C), respectively, are the most common, each accounting for approximately 30% of HCM cases. Mutations in *TNNT2* and *TNNI3*, which encode cardiac troponin T and cardiac troponin I, respectively, each account for 3% to 5% of HCM cases. The vast majority of causal mutations are missense and private mutations; hence, the frequency of each specific mutation is low.

There is considerable variability in the phenotypic expression of HCM, even among patients with similar or identical causal mutations.

 CURRENT DIAGNOSIS

- Cardiac hypertrophy in the absence of known etiology, usually asymmetric with predominant involvement of the interventricular septum.
- Hyperdynamic left ventricle with a small cavity size
- Outflow tract obstruction

 CURRENT THERAPY

Asymptomatic

- Periodic follow-up for symptoms and risk factors assessment for SCD
- ICD implantation in patients at high risk for SCD

Symptomatic

- ICD implantation in patients at high risk for SCD
- Medical therapy with β-blockers and calcium channel blockers
- Surgical myectomy, transcoronary septal ablation, and dual-chamber pacing in patients refractory to medical therapy, septal thickness >15 mm, and outflow tract obstruction >50 mm Hg
- Atrial fibrillation
  1. Acute: Cardioversion
  2. Chronic: β-Blockers and amiodarone (Cordarone), anticoagulation, and radiofrequency ablation if refractory to medical therapy
- Syncope
  1. β-Blockers and clonidine in patients with inappropriate vasodilatory response
  2. ICD and antiarrhythmic drugs in patients with ventricular arrhythmias
  3. Antiarrhythmic drugs in patients with supraventricular arrhythmias and radiofrequency ablation for refractory cases
  4. Myectomy or transcoronary septal ablation in patients with severe outflow tract obstruction

Abbreviations: ICD = internal cardioverter-defibrillator; SCD = sudden cardiac death.

Multiple mutations are often associated with more severe phenotypes but are present in only a small fraction of cases. The genetic background of individuals, defined by the presence of single nucleotide polymorphisms, is considered an important determinant of phenotypic variability of HCM. In addition, environmental factors, such as isometric exercises, are expected to affect phenotypic expression of HCM.

GENETIC SCREENING

There is considerable interest in genetic testing for the diagnosis and prognostication of HCM patients. Currently, the primary utility of genetic testing is in families in which the causal mutation is already known, which makes possible the accurate diagnosis of mutation carriers from noncarriers. In families in which the causal mutation is unknown, initial genetic linkage mapping could help to identify the putative candidate gene, followed by mutation screening. Genetic testing in isolated cases of HCM is complicated by the need for extensive genetic screening of a large number of genes and a 30% to 40% chance of not finding the causal mutation. However, advances in rapid and high-throughput screening techniques are expected to change the current approach. The significance of genetic testing in clinical prognostication and identification of individuals at risk for SCD remains to be established. In general, information on the causal genes as well as the modifier genes and the environmental factors will be necessary for accurate prognostication and genetic counseling of HCM patients.

Pathogenesis

Elucidation of the molecular genetic basis of HCM has provided significant clues to its pathogenesis. The evolution of phenotype can be categorized into three sets: the initial functional phenotype, the intermediary molecular phenotype, and the final morphologic phenotype.

The collective results of a large number of in vitro and in vivo mechanistic studies indicate that the initial defects are diverse and encompass reduced ATPase activity of the myofibrils, impaired actomyosin cross-bridging, and enhanced Ca^{2+} sensitivity of myofibrils. The intermediary molecular phenotype occurs in response to the functional phenotype and is largely unknown but is expected to include expression and activation of intracellular signaling molecules. The morphologic and histologic phenotypes are the consequence of the intermediary molecular phenotype and, hence, are considered secondary and potentially reversible.

Treatment

The goals in the management of patients with HCM are fourfold: to determine the risk of SCD, to reduce the risk of SCD, to alleviate symptoms, and to provide genetic counseling to patients and family members.

MANAGEMENT ACCORDING TO THE RISK OF SUDDEN CARDIAC DEATH

There is no close correlation between the risk of SCD and the presence of symptoms. Overall, the majority of patients with HCM are at low risk for SCD and are asymptomatic or minimally symptomatic. These individuals require periodic evaluation to determine risk of SCD and to assess symptoms. Accordingly, history, physical examination, electrocardiography, Holter monitoring, and two-dimensional and Doppler echocardiography are performed at least annually. Asymptomatic individuals at high risk for SCD should undergo internal cardioverter-defibrillator (ICD) implantation. Otherwise, no pharmacologic or nonpharmacologic intervention is necessary in asymptomatic patients who are at low risk for SCD.

MANAGEMENT OF SYMPTOMATIC PATIENTS

Therapeutic options in symptomatic patients include pharmacologic therapy, surgical myectomy, and transcatheter septal ablation; the latter two are options for those with significant outflow tract obstruction. Symptomatic patients at high risk for SCD should undergo ICD implantation in addition to medical therapy. Medical treatment of symptomatic patients is largely empiric and limited to β-blockers, verapamil hydrochloride[1] (Calan and Verelan), disopyramide[1] (Norpace), low-dose diuretics, and amiodarone[1] (Cordarone and Pacerone[1]). The goals are to improve diastolic function, reduce outflow tract obstruction, and prevent cardiac arrhythmias. β-Blockers such as atenolol (Tenormin[1]) and metoprolol (Lopressor and Toprol XL[1]) are the first line of therapy and are generally well tolerated. β-Blockers with intrinsic sympathetic activity are avoided. β-Blockers are also the preferred choice in patients with sympathetic-driven symptoms, such as exercise-induced dyspnea, outflow tract obstruction, and chest pain. The most common side effect of β-blocker therapy is easy fatigability. Other side effects include excess bradycardia, hypotension, and bronchospasm.

Verapamil and, to lesser extent, diltiazem (Cardizem, Cartia XT, Dilacor, Tiazac[1]) are the most commonly used calcium channel blockers in patients with HCM. They are commonly used in conjunction with β-blockers. Symptomatic relief with calcium channel blockers presumably is achieved through improving left ventricular relaxation and reducing left ventricular filling pressure. Calcium channel blockers impart a negative inotropic effect, which could contribute to reduction of outflow tract obstruction. Nonetheless, the use of verapamil is primarily restricted to patients without an outflow tract obstruction because of concern about the vasodilatory effect inducing hypotension, syncope, and rarely death. The most common side effect of verapamil is constipation. Nifedipine (Adalat and Procardia) is avoided because of its potent vasodilatory effect.

Disopyramide is commonly reserved for patients who do not respond to β-blockers and/or calcium channel blockers, because of the relatively higher rate of anticholinergic side effects with disopyramide.

The beneficial effect of disopyramide is mediated through its negative inotropic effect, which results in a significant reduction in left ventricular outflow tract gradient and symptomatic improvement. Diuretics are used judiciously to relieve dyspnea while avoiding intravascular volume depletion. Rapid changes in intravascular volume should be avoided because of enhanced susceptibility to hypotension. Mineralocorticoid receptor blockers may be preferable because of their antihypertrophic and antifibrotic effects in addition to their diuretic effects. Angiotensin-converting enzyme inhibitors and angiotensin-II receptor blockers are not conventionally used. However, experimental data favor their use because of their antihypertrophic and antifibrotic effects.

In a small fraction of patients, HCM evolves into advanced heart failure with systolic dysfunction and a congestive state. These patients are treated, as are those with other forms of systolic heart failure, with β-blockers, angiotensin-converting enzyme inhibitors, angiotensin-II receptor blockers, digoxin, and diuretics.

MANAGEMENT OF CARDIAC ARRHYTHMIAS

Patients with palpitations should undergo 12-lead electrocardiography, Holter monitoring, and electrophysiologic studies, if needed, to delineate the etiology and to provide appropriate therapy. Chronic or intermittent atrial fibrillation occurs in approximately 20% of patients. Atrial fibrillation with a fast ventricular rate is not well tolerated and often results in severe dyspnea and hypotension, particularly in those with severe cardiac hypertrophy or left ventricular outflow tract obstruction. Electrical cardioversion is indicated in such patients. Electrical or chemical cardioversion is also warranted in patients with new-onset atrial fibrillation (<48 hours in duration) if they are at low risk for intracardiac thrombus. Otherwise, transesophageal echocardiography should be performed to exclude intracardiac thrombi prior to cardioversion. Patients with chronic or intermittent atrial fibrillation require chronic anticoagulation. Medical treatment of atrial fibrillation includes use of β-blockers, verapamil, diltiazem, and amiodarone. Amiodarone is the most effective, but its long-term use is associated with considerable toxicity; therefore, only low-dose amiodarone (up to 200 mg daily) is recommended. Experience with other antiarrhythmic agents, such as flecainide (Tambocor), for treatment of arrhythmias in patients with HCM is limited. Radiofrequency ablation is reserved for patients refractory to medical therapy.

Patients with frequent nonsustained ventricular tachycardia or sustained ventricular tachycardia should undergo ICD implantation because they are considered at high risk for SCD. In addition, medical treatment with antiarrhythmic drugs such as amiodarone or β-blockers is recommended. Patients with rare episodes of nonsustained ventricular tachycardia should undergo further evaluation to assess the risk of SCD and then treated according to the risk of SCD.

MANAGEMENT OF SYNCOPE

Recurrent syncope is a serious event in patients with HCM because it often heralds SCD. The most common causes of syncope are malignant ventricular or supraventricular arrhythmias, exercise-induced hypotension, severe outflow tract obstruction, and neurally mediated syncope (vasodepressor syncope). Evaluation of patients with syncope includes Holter monitoring, exercise test, tilt-table testing, and, if needed, electrophysiologic studies. Patients with repetitive bursts of nonsustained ventricular tachycardia and those with sustained ventricular tachycardia are candidates for ICD implantation. Ventricular arrhythmia is the main cause of SCD in individuals with HCM. Implantation of an ICD as a preventive measure reduces the risk of SCD.

Patients with syncope due to supraventricular arrhythmias are treated with antiarrhythmic drugs, and those refractory to medical therapy are treated with radiofrequency ablation. Surgical myectomy and transcoronary septal ablation are considered in patients with syncope due to severe outflow tract obstruction. Treatment of patients with syncope due to an inappropriate peripheral vascular response to exercise includes propranolol (Inderal[1]), clonidine (Catapres[1]), and sometimes paroxetine (Paxil[1]).

---

[1]Not FDA approved for this indication.

[1]Not FDA approved for this indication.

MANAGEMENT OF OUTFLOW TRACT OBSTRUCTION

Left ventricular outflow tract obstruction is a dynamic phenotype that is associated with symptoms of heart failure, but its contribution to the risk of SCD is not well established. Most patients with outflow tract obstruction respond well to medical therapy and remain asymptomatic or mildly symptomatic. Treatment with β-blockers alone may suffice. A subset of patients who exhibit significant resting or exercise-induced outflow tract obstruction (>50 mm Hg) remain in New York Heart Association functional class III and IV despite optimal medical therapy. These patients are candidates for percutaneous transcoronary septal ablation or surgical myectomy. The prerequisite for invasive interventions is an interventricular septal thickness of 15 mm and greater. Otherwise, invasive procedures are not warranted because of a potentially excessive risk-to-benefit ratio. Instead, treatment should focus on diastolic dysfunction.

No prospective randomized studies have compared clinical outcomes after surgical myectomy and percutaneous transcoronary septal ablation. Several observational studies suggest the two interventions are equally effective in reducing the left ventricular outflow tract gradient and alleviating symptoms. However, neither is a curative intervention, and additional treatment usually is necessary.

A. **Surgical Myectomy (Myomectomy):** Surgical myectomy involves resection of a small portion of the interventricular septum, commonly at the base, through a transaortic approach (Morrow procedure). It reduces outflow tract obstruction and results in significant improvement of heart failure symptoms. It is best reserved for symptomatic patients with significant outflow tract obstruction at rest who are refractory to pharmacologic therapy. It is the procedure of choice in patients with concomitant valvular disease and/or coronary artery disease. The recurrence rate of outflow tract obstruction is low, and a second intervention is seldom required. The overall mortality rate of surgical myectomy in experienced centers is 1% to 5%, but the rate is higher among the elderly and those with concomitant cardiac surgeries. Surgical myectomy is associated with excellent short-term and long-term symptomatic relief and survival, and it has a favorable impact on the risk of SCD.

B. **Transcoronary Septal Ablation:** The procedure is performed through percutaneous coronary catheterization and injection of 1 to 3 mL of pure ethanol into the main septal perforators of the left anterior descending artery. Accordingly, focal myocardial necrosis, emulating surgical myectomy, is induced. It reduces the outflow tract gradient significantly and improves symptoms. It is indicated in symptomatic patients who are refractory to medical therapy, have an interventricular septal thickness of 15 mm and greater, and have a significant resting left ventricular outflow tract gradient. In those with significant exertional dyspnea, a provoked exercise-induced gradient can be used as a surrogate phenotype for septal ablation.

Overall, the procedure is well tolerated and has relatively low perioperative morbidity and mortality. The most common complication is the development of advanced atrioventricular (AV) conduction defect requiring permanent pacemaker placement in 15% to 20% of patients. There is a small risk of ventricular arrhythmias arising from the localized myocardial necrosis. Progressive left ventricular remodeling occurs predominantly within the first 6 months. Short-term and intermediary follow-up data show favorable outcome that is largely comparable, but probably not equal, to that of surgical myectomy.

C. **Dual-Chamber Pacing:** Dual-chamber pacing is designed to reduce outflow tract obstruction by inducing dyssynchronized left ventricular contraction. Thus, optimal timing of the AV interval is considered essential. Randomized clinical studies show no significant direct benefit to pacing strategy but rather a considerable placebo effect and no discernible improvement in exercise tolerance. Accordingly, dual-chamber pacing is reserved for occasional symptomatic patients who are refractory to medical therapy and are not candidates for either surgical or transcatheter septal ablation.

Experimental Pharmacologic Agents

Recent experimental studies have suggested the potential utility of β-hydroxy-β-methylglutaryl-coenzyme A (HMG-CoA) reductase inhibitors (statins), angiotensin-II receptor blockers, aldosterone blockers, and antioxidants in the prevention, attenuation, and reversal of cardiac phenotype in patients with HCM. Clinical studies testing the potential utility of these agents for treatment of patients with HCM are ongoing.

REFERENCES

Cannan CR, Reeder GS, Bailey KR, et al. Natural history of hypertrophic cardiomyopathy. A population-based study, 1976 through 1990. Circulation 1995;92:2488–95.

Geisterfer-Lowrance AA, Kass S, Tanigawa G, et al. A molecular basis for familial hypertrophic cardiomyopathy: a beta cardiac myosin heavy chain gene missense mutation. Cell 1990;62:999–1006.

Hess OM, Sigwart U. New treatment strategies for hypertrophic obstructive cardiomyopathy: Alcohol ablation of the septum: the new gold standard? J Am Coll Cardiol 2004;44:2054–5.

Marian AJ. Pathogenesis of diverse clinical and pathological phenotypes in hypertrophic cardiomyopathy. Lancet 2000;355:58–60.

Marian AJ. Recent advances in genetics and treatment of hypertrophic cardiomyopathy. Future Cardiol 2005;1:341–53.

Maron BJ, Gardin JM, Flack JM, et al. Prevalence of hypertrophic cardiomyopathy in a general population of young adults. Echocardiographic analysis of 4111 subjects in the CARDIA Study. Coronary Artery Risk Development in (Young) Adults. Circulation 1995;92:785–9.

Maron BJ, Shen WK, Link MS, et al. Efficacy of implantable cardioverter-defibrillators for the prevention of sudden death in patients with hypertrophic cardiomyopathy. N Engl J Med 2000;342:365–73.

Maron BJ, Shirani J, Poliac LC, et al. Sudden death in young competitive athletes. Clinical, demographic, and pathological profiles. JAMA 1996;276:199–204.

Ommen SR, Maron BJ, Olivotto I, et al. Long-term effects of surgical septal myectomy on survival in patients with obstructive hypertrophic cardiomyopathy. J Am Coll Cardiol 2005;46:470–6.

Woo A, Williams WG, Choi R, et al. Clinical and echocardiographic determinants of long-term survival after surgical myectomy in obstructive hypertrophic cardiomyopathy. Circulation 2005;111:2033–41.

Mitral Valve Prolapse

Method of
Kurt M. Jacobson, MD, and Peter S. Rahko, MD

Mitral valve prolapse (MVP) has been known by many names, including floppy valve syndrome, Barlow's syndrome, click/murmur syndrome, myxomatous mitral valve disease, and billowing mitral cusp syndrome. MVP is a common cardiac valvular abnormality characterized by redundant, floppy mitral valve leaflets; it is often detected initially by characteristic nonejection clicks or a middle- to late-peaking crescendo systolic murmur on physical examination.

Prevalence

MVP is the most common congenital cause of mitral regurgitation (MR) in adults and the most common indication for mitral valve surgery in the United States today. Previously, it was one of the most overdiagnosed conditions within cardiology, with suggested prevalence rates ranging from 5% to 15%. With the use of current diagnostic standards, rates are much lower; the overestimation was a consequence of diverse and nonuniformly accepted two-dimensional echocardiographic diagnostic criteria. Freed and colleagues, using the Framingham study population and applying consistent and more stringent echocardiographic diagnostic criteria, demonstrated a much lower prevalence of MVP (approximately 2.4%). The incidence appeared to be similar among men and women. Gender differences do exist, however. Women tend to have a more benign course, whereas men tend to have more advanced myxomatous disease resulting in a greater chance of more severe MR.

Classification

Primary MVP is characterized by idiopathic myxomatous change of the mitral valve leaflets or the chordal structures or both. Secondary MVP is present when underlying conditions such as Marfan's syndrome, Ehlers-Danlos syndrome, osteogenesis imperfecta, or other collagen vascular disorders are evident. Certain congenital cardiac abnormalities, including Ebstein anomaly, aortic coarctation, hypertrophic cardiomyopathy, and ostium secundum atrial septal defects, are also associated with MVP. Familial variants with an autosomal dominant pattern of inheritance have been identified, and work to identify the genes involved is underway. The reported prevalence of MVP in first-degree relatives is between 30% and 50%.

Pathology

Macroscopic and microscopic changes can involve both the anterior and posterior leaflets as well as the chordal structures of the leaflet apparatus. Macroscopically, the surface area of the leaflet is increased, providing the accentuated, billowing appearance of the valve leaflets. Additional notable changes are thickening of the individual leaflets, increased leaflet length, thinning and stretching of the chordae, and increased circumference of the mitral valve annulus. At the microscopic level (Fig. 1), normal mitral valves have three well-defined layers, each containing cells and a characteristic composition and configuration of the extracellular matrix: the fibrosa, composed predominantly of collagen fibers densely packed and arranged parallel to the free edge of the leaflet; the centrally located spongiosa, composed of loosely arranged collagen and proteoglycans; and the atrialis, composed of elastic fibers. In myxomatous mitral valves, the spongiosa layer is expanded by loose, amorphous extracellular matrix that has more proteoglycans but less collagen and more fragmented

elastic fibers. What collagen is present appears to be disorganized and fragmented, giving the appearance of a haphazard layering of the spongiosa. It is this thickening that produces the classic macroscopic appearance of the myxomatous valve on two-dimensional echocardiography.

Clinical Presentation

Most patients with MVP are asymptomatic and will remain so, testifying to the often benign nature of this disease. Previously, various nonspecific symptoms, including fatigue, dyspnea, palpitations, postural orthostasis, anxiety, and panic attacks, were described as an MVP syndrome when present in association with the characteristic nonejection systolic click or middle- to late-peaking crescendo systolic murmur. Other symptoms, including chest discomfort, near-syncope, and syncope, have also been described by patients with MVP. However, in a community-based study, the prevalence of various clinical complaints including chest pain, dyspnea, and syncope was no higher in patients with MVP than in those without evidence of MVP, making such findings nonspecific. In a controlled study that compared symptomatic MVP patients with first-degree relatives with and without echocardiographic evidence of MVP, there also was no association of MVP with atypical chest pain, dyspnea, panic attacks, or anxiety. There was, however, a significant association of MVP with

CURRENT DIAGNOSIS

- A midsystolic click with or without a middle- to late-peaking crescendo systolic murmur is the classic auscultatory finding of mitral valve prolapse (MVP).
- Key examination maneuvers can help differentiate MVP from other valvular heart diseases.
- Diagnostic echocardiographic findings of MVP are systolic billowing of the mitral valve leaflets 2 mm above the annulus into the left atrium.
- The presence of significant myxomatous thickening of the valve leaflets (>5 mm) is significant for prognosis.

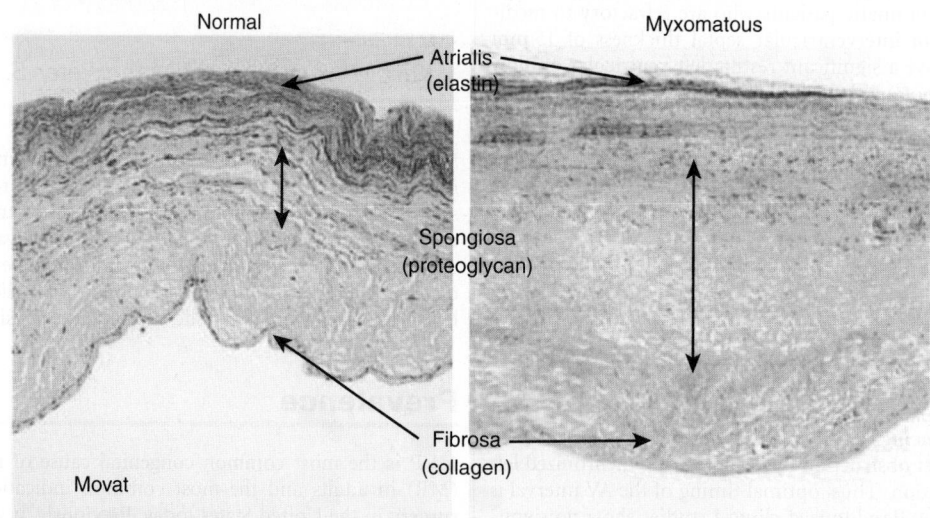

FIGURE 1. Morphologic features of normal mitral valves *(left)* and valves with myxomatous degeneration *(right)*. Myxomatous valves have an abnormal layered architecture: loose collagen in fibrosa, expanded spongiosa strongly positive for proteoglycans, and disrupted elastin in atrialis *(top)*. Movat pentachrome stain (collagen stains yellow, proteoglycans blue-green, and elastin black). (Modified from Rabkin E, Aikawa M, Stone JR, et al: Activated interstitial myofibroblasts express catabolic enzymes and mediate matrix remodeling in myxomatous heart valves. Circulation 2001;104:2525.)

physical findings of systolic clicks, systolic murmurs, thoracic bony abnormalities, low body weight, and low blood pressure. Congestive heart failure, atrial fibrillation, stroke or transient ischemic attack, hypertension, diabetes, and hypercholesterolemia are no more likely in patients with MVP than in those without MVP. However, previous retrospective studies suggested a higher incidence of cerebral embolic events, infectious endocarditis, severe MR, and need for mitral valve replacement in patients with classic (complicated) versus nonclassic MVP. Symptoms of poor cardiac reserve, such as reduced exercise tolerance, dyspnea on exertion, and fatigue, may reflect the presence of significant MR and warrant clinical concern.

Diagnosis

Symptoms are not predictive of the presence or absence of MVP. Certain physical and auscultatory characteristics on examination do support the diagnosis of MVP. Patients with MVP more often have a lower body mass index, have a lower waist-to-hip ratio, and are taller. Findings of scoliosis, pectus excavatum, and hyperextensibility are also prevalent among patients with MVP. The classic auscultatory findings include a midsystolic click and a middle- to late-peaking crescendo systolic murmur heard best at the apex. The auscultatory findings are best elicited with the diaphragm of the stethoscope, and they change in relation to the first and second heart sounds (S_1 and S_2) in response to changes in left ventricular (LV) volume. Therefore, the patient should be examined in several positions: supine (including lateral decubitus), sitting, standing, and, if possible, squatting. Changes in LV filling and volume affect the degree of prolapse.

The most important and most specific finding on auscultation is the presence of a nonejection midsystolic click or clicks caused by snapping of the valve apparatus as parts of the valve leaflets billow into the atrium during systole. Although these clicks can be heard over the entire precordium, they are best heard at the apex. The click can be misinterpreted as a split S_1, a true S_1 with an S_4, or a true S_1 with an early ejection click from a bicuspid valve. It can be differentiated from an ejection click heard in bicuspid aortic valves by its timing relative to the beginning of the carotid upstroke. Ejection clicks occur as the aortic valve opens and therefore precede the carotid upstroke, whereas the nonejection clicks of MVP occur afterward. Clicks from atrial septal aneurysms are uncommon but can be difficult to distinguish from those of MVP. Ejection clicks and clicks from atrial septal aneurysms are not altered by changes in loading characteristics, allowing them to be differentiated from clicks of MVP. Often, but not always, a middle- to late-peaking crescendo systolic murmur can be appreciated by itself or after a click. The murmur terminates with closure of the aortic valve (A2). This represents MR, and, in general, the duration of the murmur correlates with the severity of the MR. The earlier in systole the murmur is detected, the more severe the MR. Eventually, with more severe MR, the murmur becomes holosystolic. MVP manifestations on examination vary, and they may not always be reproducible, even in the same patient.

Certain maneuvers can aid in more accurately diagnosing MVP on examination (Fig. 2). MVP is very sensitive to LV filling, and subtle changes in auscultatory findings elicited by careful examination maneuvers can be instrumental in separating MVP from other valvular abnormalities. Generally, measures that decrease LV volume or increase contractility produce earlier and more prominent systolic prolapse of the mitral leaflets, causing the systolic click and murmur to move closer to S_1. For example, in the transition from squatting to standing, LV volume is reduced, and the onset of the click and murmur is moved closer to S_1. Conversely, anything that increases LV volume, such as leg-raising, squatting, or slowing the heart rate (increased diastolic filling), delays the onset of the click or murmur and usually diminishes its duration and intensity.

Use of Echocardiography

Two-dimensional echocardiography has proved to be the most accurate noninvasive tool for the diagnosis, assessment, and follow-up of clinically suspected MVP. In fact, physical signs of MVP in an asymptomatic patient are an American College of Cardiology/American Heart Association (ACC/AHA) class I indication for use of echocardiography to make the diagnosis of MVP and assess the severity of MR, leaflet morphology, and ventricular size and function. Once the diagnosis is made, follow-up is determined by the severity of MVP. Routine echocardiographic follow-up of asymptomatic patients with MVP is not recommended unless there are significant findings of MR or LV structural changes. Frequency of follow-up in patients with prolapse and MR is determined by the severity of MR and should be at least annual in patients with severe MR.

Diagnostic criteria for MVP on two-dimensional echocardiography are

- Billowing of one or both mitral valve leaflets or their prolapse superiorly across the mitral annular plane in the parasternal long-axis view by greater than 2 mm during systole
- The degree of thickening of the leaflets

Combined leaflet prolapse of greater than 2 mm and leaflet thickness greater than 5 mm are supportive of classic MVP, whereas prolapse in the absence of increased thickness is considered nonclassic MVP. In addition to more often being associated with the auscultative findings of the click and murmur, the classic form is more commonly associated with increased risk of endocarditis, stroke, progressive MR, and need for mitral valve repair or replacement.

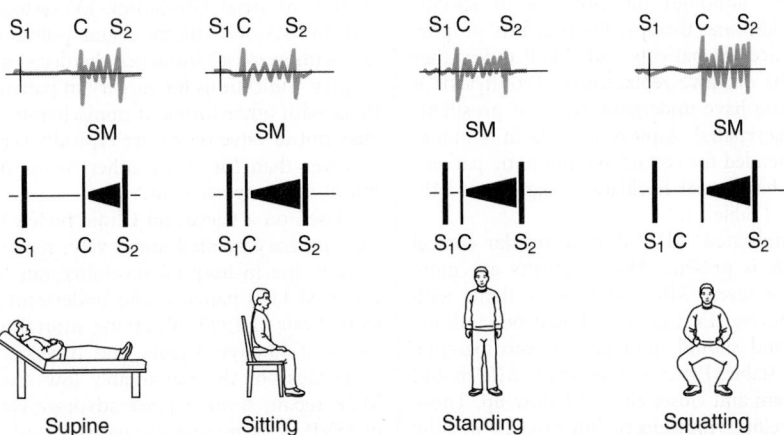

FIGURE 2. Auscultative findings with changes in position in patients with mitral valve prolapse (MVP). *Abbreviations:* C, click of MVP; S_1, mitral valve closure; S_2, aortic valve closure. (Modified from Devereux RB, Perloff JK, Reichek N, et al: Mitral valve prolapse. Circulation 1976;54[1]:3–14.)

CURRENT THERAPY

- Patients with physical findings of mitral valve prolapse (MVP) should have an echocardiogram to confirm the diagnosis, determine the severity of prolapse, determine the amount of myxomatous thickening, document the severity (if present) of mitral regurgitation, and determine left ventricular size and function.
- Uncomplicated MVP without significant mitral regurgitation can be evaluated clinically every 3 to 5 years.
- Complicated MVP (associated with significant mitral regurgitation, left ventricular structural changes, pulmonary hypertension, atrial fibrillation, or stroke) should be observed closely with serial clinical evaluation and echocardiography.
- Surgery may be required for complicated MVP associated with severe mitral regurgitation. Repair rather than replacement is the procedure of choice and should be performed at surgical centers experienced with mitral valve repair.
- Recommendations for surgery are the same for MVP as for other forms of chronic severe mitral regurgitation.

Because the mitral apparatus is saddle-shaped, certain echocardiographic views are more specific than others for determining leaflet prolapse. Most practitioners agree that the parasternal long-axis and apical two-chamber or apical long-axis views are the most accurate for determining prolapse. A finding of prolapse as determined on other views, particularly the apical four-chamber view, is much less specific and frequently leads to a false-positive diagnosis.

Medical Management

Most patients with MVP remain asymptomatic and require no additional management aside from careful observation over time. It is appropriate to provide reassurance that uncomplicated (nonclassic) MVP is a non–life-threatening condition and is unlikely to affect longevity. Periodic clinical evaluation every 3 to 5 years is reasonable. Patients who develop palpitations, lightheadedness, dizziness, or syncope should undergo Holter or event monitoring for detection of arrhythmias. Palpitations are frequently controlled with β-blockers or calcium channel blockers, although the presence of specific arrhythmias may mandate additional therapy. Endocarditis prophylaxis is no longer recommended for patients with MVP unless they have a history of endocarditis or valve replacement. Prophylaxis is recommended for patients who have undergone repair if prosthetic material was used (e.g., in ring repairs). Aspirin or warfarin (Coumadin) therapy may be recommended for certain symptomatic patients with neurologic events who have atrial fibrillation, significant MR, hypertension, or heart failure (Table 1).

Patients with classic (complicated) MVP deserve regular clinical follow-up, particularly if MR is present. These patients are more likely to develop moderate or severe MR over time. Patients with mild to moderate MR and normal LV function should be clinically evaluated at least annually and should undergo echocardiography every second or third year if stable. Patients with severe MR should have an annual echocardiogram and closer clinical follow-up. Those who have severe MR and develop symptoms or impaired LV systolic function require cardiac catheterization and evaluation for mitral valve surgery. Often the valve can be repaired rather than replaced, with a low operative mortality rate and excellent short- and long-

TABLE 1 ACC/AHA Recommendations for Oral Anticoagulation in Patients with Mitral Valve Prolapse

Class	Recommendation
I	ASA therapy (75–325 mg/d) for cerebral TIAs
	Warfarin (Coumadin) therapy for patients ≥65 y in atrial fibrillation with hypertension, MR, or history of congestive heart failure
	ASA therapy (75–325 mg/d) for patients <65 years in atrial fibrillation with no history of MR, hypertension, or congestive heart failure
	Warfarin therapy after stroke for patients with MR, atrial fibrillation, or left atrial thrombus
IIa	ASA therapy is reasonable in patients after stroke who do not have MR, atrial fibrillation, left atrial thrombus, or echocardiographic evidence of thickening >5 mm or redundancy of leaflets
	Warfarin therapy is reasonable after stroke for patients without MR, atrial fibrillation, or left atrial thrombus who have echocardiographic evidence of thickening >5 mm or redundancy of leaflets
	Warfarin therapy is reasonable for TIAs that occur despite ASA therapy
	ASA therapy (75–325 mg/d) can be beneficial for patients with a history of stroke who have contraindications to anticoagulants
IIb	ASA therapy (75–325 mg/d) may be considered for patients in sinus rhythm with echocardiographic evidence of complicated mitral valve prolapse

Adapted from Bonow RO, Carabello BA, Chatterjee K, et al: ACC/AHA 2006 guidelines for the management of patients with valvular heart disease. [Erratum in J Am Coll Cardiol 2007;49(9):1014.] J Am Coll Cardiol 2006;48(3):e1–e148.
Abbreviations: ACC/AHA = American College of Cardiology/American Heart Association; ASA = aspirin; MR = mitral regurgitation; TIA = transient ischemic attack.

term results when performed at experienced centers. Preservation of the native valve allows for lower risks of thrombosis and endocarditis than does prosthetic valve replacement.

Surgical Management

MVP is the most common cause of adult MR requiring mitral valve surgery. Symptoms of heart failure, severity of MR, presence or absence of atrial fibrillation, LV systolic function, LV end-diastolic and end-systolic volumes, and pulmonary artery pressure (at rest and with exercise) influence the decision to recommend mitral valve surgery. Indications for surgery in patients with MVP and MR mirror those with other forms of nonischemic severe MR. Patient outcomes after mitral valve repair are typically very good, and the surgical risk is lower than for many other forms of cardiac surgery, including mitral valve replacement.

Based on a Cleveland Clinic review of 1072 patients who underwent primary isolated mitral valve repair for MR due to myxomatous disease, the in-hospital mortality rate was 0.3%. The Mayo Clinic reviewed 1173 patients who underwent mitral valve repair for MVP from 1980 to 1999, observing mortality rates of 0.7%, 11.3%, and 29.4% at 30 days, 5 years, and 10 years, respectively.

Because of the remarkably low mortality rates associated with MVP repair, some experts advocate earlier rather than later repair of MVP in asymptomatic patients with severe MR and no evidence of LV dysfunction, pulmonary hypertension, or atrial fibrillation. Class I ACC/AHA recommendations for surgery are shown in Table 2.

TABLE 2 ACC/AHA Recommendations for Mitral Valve Surgery in Patients with Chronic Severe Mitral Regurgitation

Class	Recommendation
I	MV surgery is beneficial for patients in NYHA functional class II, III, or IV symptoms in the absence of severe LV dysfunction.*
	MV surgery is beneficial for asymptomatic patients with mild to moderate LV dysfunction.*
	MV repair is recommended over MV replacement in most patients who require surgery, and patients should be referred to experienced surgical centers.
IIa	MV repair is reasonable in experienced surgical centers for asymptomatic patients with normal LV function* if the likelihood of successful repair without residual mitral regurgitation is >90%.
	MV surgery is reasonable for asymptomatic patients with preserved LV function and new onset of atrial fibrillation.
	MV surgery is reasonable for asymptomatic patients with preserved LV function and pulmonary hypertension.†
	MV surgery is reasonable for patients who have a primary abnormality of the mitral apparatus and NYHA class III-IV symptoms and severe LV dysfunction* in whom MV repair is highly likely.
III	MV surgery is not indicated for asymptomatic patients with mitral regurgitation and preserved LV function* if repair seems unlikely.
	Isolated MV surgery is not indicated for patients with mild or moderate mitral regurgitation.

Adapted from Bonow RO, Carabello BA, Chatterjee K, et al: ACC/AHA 2006 guidelines for the management of patients with valvular heart disease. [Erratum in J Am Coll Cardiol 2007;49(9):1014.] J Am Coll Cardiol 2006;48(3):e1-e148.
*Normal (or preserved) LV function is defined as EF >60% and ESD <40 mm; mild to moderate LV dysfunction is defined as EF 30%-60% and/or ESD between 40 and 55 mm; severe LV dysfunction is defined as EF <30% and/or ESD >55 mm.
†Pulmonary hypertension is defined as a pulmonary artery systolic pressure >50 mm Hg at rest or >60 mm Hg with exercise.
Abbreviations: ACC/AHA = American College of Cardiology/American Heart Association; EF = ejection fraction; ESD, end-systolic dimension; LV = left ventricular; MV = mitral valve; NYHA, New York Heart Association.

REFERENCES

Bonow RO, Carabello BA, Chatterjee K, et al. ACC/AHA 2006 guidelines for the management of patients with valvular heart disease: A report of the American College of Cardiology/American Heart Association Task Force on Practice Guidelines (Writing Committee to Revise the 1998 guidelines for the management of patients with valvular heart disease) developed in collaboration with the Society of Cardiovascular Anesthesiologists endorsed by the Society for Cardiovascular Angiography and Interventions and the Society of Thoracic Surgeons. J Am Coll Cardiol 2006;48(3): e1-148 [Erratium in J Am Coll Cardiol 2007;49(9):1014].

Devereux RB, Kramer-Fox R, Brown WT, et al. Relation between clinical features of the mitral prolapse syndrome and echocardiographically documented mitral valve prolapse. J Am Coll Cardiol 1986;8:763–72.

Flack JM, Kvasnicka JH, Gardin JM, et al. Anthropometric and physiologic correlates of mitral valve prolapse in a biethnic cohort of young adults: The CARDIA study. Am Heart J 1999;138:486.

Freed LA, Benjamin EJ, Levy D, et al. Mitral valve prolapse in the general population: The benign nature of echocardiographic features in the Framingham Heart Study. J Am Coll Cardiol 2002;40:1298–304.

Freed LA, Levy D, Levine RA, et al. Prevalence and clinical outcome of mitral-valve prolapse. N Engl J Med 1999;341:1–7.

Gillinov AM, Cosgrove DM, Blackstone EH, et al. Durability of mitral valve repair for degenerative disease. J Thorac Cardiovasc Surg 1998;116(5):734–43.

Levy D, Savage D. Prevalence and clinical features of mitral valve prolapse. Am Heart J 1987;113:1281–90.

Marks AR, Choong CY, Sanfilippo AJ, et al. Identification of high-risk and low-risk subgroups of patients with mitral-valve prolapse. N Engl J Med 1989;320:1031–6.

Rabkin E, Aikawa M, Stone JR, et al. Activated interstitial myofibroblasts express catabolic enzymes and mediate matrix remodeling in myxomatous heart valves. Circulation 2001;104:2525–32.

Savage DD, Devereux RB, Garrison RJ, et al. Mitral valve prolapse in the general population: 2. Clinical features: The Framingham Study. Am Heart J 1983;106:577–81.

Savage DD, Garrison RJ, Devereux RB, et al. Mitral valve prolapse in the general population: 1. Epidemiologic features: The Framingham Study. Am Heart J 1983;106:571–6.

Suri RM, Schaff HV, Dearani JA, et al. Survival advantage and improved durability of mitral repair for leaflet prolapse subsets in the current era. Ann Thorac Surg 2006;82(3):819–26.

Heart Failure

Method of
Elaine Winkel, MD, and Walter Kao, MD

Despite the decrease in the incidence of other circulatory conditions, or perhaps rather because of improvements in the management of related circulatory conditions, heart failure represents the major clinical challenge facing all clinicians who manage patients with cardiac disease today. It continues to be the most common cause of hospitalization for patients older than 65 years of age and results in the expenditure of almost 40 billion dollars annually in the United States. Heart failure is a chronic degenerative disease; if left untreated, it will result in progressively deteriorating functional capacity and premature death. For optimal patient outcome, it must be managed aggressively and proactively.

This discussion focuses exclusively on heart failure resulting from systolic dysfunction, the management of which has been most extensively studied. However, it is now recognized that diastolic dysfunction, particularly of the left ventricle (LV), is an increasingly common condition, particularly in the elderly, and can result in similar symptoms. The optimal management of this vexing condition has yet to be determined with certainty, although there are ongoing efforts to establish evidence-based approaches to this disease as well.

Definition

Although heart failure is defined traditionally as a condition in which the heart is unable to pump enough blood to satisfy the metabolic demands of the body, this expression has little direct clinical relevance. On a practical level, heart failure is perhaps better thought of as a condition involving abnormality of cardiac emptying or filling associated with increased intracardiac filling pressures or decreased cardiac output, exercise intolerance, frequent arrhythmias, and early death. The abnormalities in cardiac structure and function typically precede, often by many years, the onset of symptoms. Therefore, to most effectively treat this disease, it is critically important to affirmatively seek out and diagnose cardiac dysfunction before overt symptoms develop.

History and Physical Examination

In the United States, the most common cause of cardiac dysfunction is coronary artery disease due to atherosclerotic cardiovascular disease (ASCVD). Because ASCVD is typically a systemic rather than a localized phenomenon, any suggestion of atherosclerotic disease in any vascular bed should prompt a thorough cardiac evaluation as well.

Exercise intolerance due to dyspnea or fatigue is the most common presenting symptom in patients with heart failure, although other symptoms may also be present, such as orthopnea, paroxysmal nocturnal dyspnea, dependent edema, or palpitations. Many of these symptoms are nonspecific, and a high index of suspicion is necessary to diagnose underlying heart failure. Other historical findings that should heighten the suspicion for underlying heart failure include the presence of predisposing conditions such as hypertension, diabetes mellitus or metabolic syndrome, obesity, prior exposure to known cardiotoxic agents, ASCVD, and a family history of premature ASCVD, documented cardiomyopathy, or unexplained premature death. When such characteristics are present, particularly in concert with other suggestive findings from the history or physical examination, they should prompt a more directed evaluation, including strong consideration of imaging studies to measure cardiac function.

Physical examination findings are often subtle, especially if the underlying disease has been progressing insidiously for an extended period before presentation, as is often the case. The vital signs may be normal, although the heart rate is frequently elevated due to the compensatory hyperadrenergic state associated with untreated cardiac dysfunction. Tachycardia, especially sinus tachycardia, should always be considered a symptom of underlying systemic disease and should spur further investigation. Chronic arterial hypertension is a frequent cause of heart failure, particularly in non-Caucasian populations; it often persists despite substantial degrees of cardiac dysfunction and should prompt additional cardiac evaluation. Increased central venous pressure may manifest as an elevation in measured jugular venous pressure or as systemic edema; however, the latter symptom is frequently nonspecific, being often seen in older individuals with venous insufficiency, obesity, or sedentary lifestyles. In contrast, visceral edema, when detected, is more specifically associated with increased central venous pressure. The carotid impulse is typically normal, although in patients with severe degrees of LV systolic dysfunction the impulse may be less dynamic than normal. Asymmetrical arterial pulses or bruits suggest systemic atherosclerotic disease, including likely coronary artery disease.

The presence of pulmonary rales, although classically described in patients with cardiogenic or noncardiogenic intraalveolar pulmonary edema, is typically seen only with new and rapid onset of cardiac dysfunction, the prototype of which is acute myocardial infarction with associated LV dysfunction. The compensatory potential of pulmonary venous and lymphatic drainage is such that more insidious, slowly developing cardiac dysfunction is most often not associated with intraalveolar fluid; for this reason, the lung fields may be clear on auscultation or even on radiographic examination. In patients with disease of longer standing, in whom one or both ventricular chambers has had a chance to dilate, the apical (LV) impulse may be laterally displaced; in more severe degrees of LV dysfunction, it may not be palpable at all.

The heart sounds are often subtly decreased in intensity due to decreased LV contractile power, but they remain physiologic in the absence of conduction disease. With an acute onset, gallops may be present, particularly an early diastolic sound (S_3); however, a slowly dilating dysfunctional heart may retain a substantial degree of compliance, lessening the chance of an audible filling sound even if LV filling pressures are elevated. In more advanced stages of disease, evidence of impaired peripheral or end-organ perfusion may be present, such as jaundice, cool extremities, delayed capillary refill, or decreased intensity of peripheral pulses. These symptoms are typically accompanied by unequivocal symptoms or other suggestive cardiopulmonary signs of cardiac disease.

Laboratory and Diagnostic Procedures

The chest radiography and 12-lead electrocardiography are simple, rapid, and low-risk procedures that can frequently add to the initial diagnostic impression. Depending on the degree of cardiac chamber dilation, the radiographic cardiac silhouette may be variably affected. The LV silhouette is most often enlarged in patients with slowly progressive disease, because the LV chamber has had a opportunity to dilate significantly, whereas in instances of acute onset (e.g., acute myocardial infarction without antecedent disease), the LV may appear normal sized. Patients with chronic valvular or coronary atherosclerotic disease may also demonstrate calcification that can be detected on plain chest films. The presence of intraalveolar pulmonary edema typically is easily detected on standard chest radiographs, although pulmonary interstitial edema can be much more subtle and difficult to detect. More commonly, in patients with chronic LV dysfunction and resultant secondary postcapillary pulmonary hypertension, the central pulmonary arteries are dilated and more prominent than normal.

Many electrocardiographic abnormalities associated with heart failure are nonspecific. Because the most common cause of heart failure is coronary artery disease, any indication of ongoing myocardial ischemia or pattern of prior infarction or injury should prompt further intensive evaluation. The presence of arrhythmias, especially those of ventricular origin, also suggests underlying organic cardiac disease.

Standard laboratory results are typically nonspecific but in more advanced cases can yield findings of impaired end-organ perfusion, such as elevations in serum urea nitrogen, creatinine, or liver transaminases. Patients with chronic heart failure may also be anemic and may manifest other chemical evidence of malnutrition or chronic disease. However, patients who have progressed to this degree of impairment typically have a host of other symptoms and signs that point unequivocally to a severe heart failure syndrome. More recently, the presence of elevated levels of plasma brain natriuretic peptide has been associated with cardiac disease in patients with dyspnea. This test has gained increasing popularity as an initial diagnostic tool, although its utility in the diagnosis of nondecompensated heart failure remains to be fully elucidated.

Transthoracic echocardiography has emerged as the most common method of definitively diagnosing LV systolic dysfunction. It is typically available at short notice in most clinical settings and can provide a wealth of structural and functional data in a noninvasive fashion. After the history, physical examination, and standard laboratory studies discussed earlier, echocardiography should be the next diagnostic study performed if cardiac dysfunction is suspected. Although a complete review of the echocardiographic findings typically seen in heart failure is beyond the scope of this discussion, standard studies can establish the diagnosis, provide clues to the underlying etiology, and help guide initial therapy. Moreover, an echocardiographic study obtained at initial diagnosis establishes an important baseline data set to which subsequent studies can be compared to gauge the efficacy of therapy and assist in determining prognosis.

Once the diagnosis of LV systolic dysfunction has been established, an effort should be made to determine the underlying etiology, because it may dictate therapy. Cardiac catheterization, including coronary angiography and right heart catheterization for hemodynamic assessment, should be strongly considered in all patients with newly diagnosed LV systolic dysfunction, because noncontracting or poorly contracting myocardium, if ischemic or hibernating (viable but hypoperfused), may regain contractile strength after proper revascularization. In addition, hemodynamic data obtained during catheterization can assist in guiding medical and surgical therapy for heart failure; moreover, like other initial imaging studies, it can provide valuable baseline information for future comparison. The use of supplemental catheter-based procedures such as endomyocardial biopsy remains controversial, predominantly because of the risk associated with these procedures and the variable sensitivity of routine endomyocardial biopsy in the diagnosis of infiltrative myocardial processes such as myocarditis. In specific cases in which the index of suspicion for certain infiltrative diseases is particularly high, biopsy may be used to confirm the diagnosis. If this procedure is employed, it is important that a sufficient volume and distribution of specimens be collected, to optimize diagnostic yield, and that the procedure be performed by an experienced operator, to minimize the risk of complications.

Provocative testing (e.g., treadmill exercise testing), with or without supplemental imaging modalities such as radionuclide perfusion imaging, is less useful in patients with already established cardiac dysfunction, although the response to exercise testing in a patient with previously undiagnosed heart failure can be revealing. In addition to the likely finding of decreased exercise performance, the blood pressure and heart rate response to increasing exercise demand may be impaired. Further scrutiny (e.g., cardiac catheterization) should follow the demonstration of inducible or fixed myocardial perfusion defects with exercise or of a decreased left ventricular ejection fraction (LVEF). Resting radionuclide ventriculography can also be employed to determine global LV systolic function (LVEF) in patients in whom effective imaging cannot be achieved with echocardiography. Exercise testing with expired gas analysis may be used to determined peak exercise oxygen consumption and has been demonstrated to correlate with prognosis in patients with chronic heart failure. However, its value when measured before optimization of therapy in patients with newly diagnosed heart failure is uncertain.

Classification

Patients with heart failure are classified according to their self-described degree of functional impairment and assigned a New York Heart Association (NYHA) functional class (Table 1). Although it is subjective on the part of both the patient and the interviewer, this classification has long been used for gross estimation of functional status. The NYHA class has been reported to correlate with mortality risk, but its ability to discriminate among patients and its relevance in an individual patient over time remains questionable.

Heart failure can also be classified by evolutionary stage (Table 2), based predominantly on management strategy (pharmacologic, non-pharmacologic, or surgical).

Management of Heart Failure

NONPHARMACOLOGIC THERAPY

Nonpharmacologic heart failure therapy reduces symptoms and improves functional capacity and quality of life. It is vital to provide on-going patient and family education about dietary restrictions, avoidance of unhealthy behaviors, stress reduction, and energy conservation. Participation in an exercise program to combat deconditioning and promote weight loss improves functional capacity. Close outpatient monitoring, including a heart failure disease management program, improves compliance and reduces hospitalization. Identification and treatment of sleep-disordered breathing, present in as many as 40% of patients with heart failure, can dramatically improve symptoms.

PHARMACOLOGIC THERAPY

Angiotensin-converting enzyme (ACE) inhibitors and selected β-blockers have been shown in randomized clinical trials to improve symptoms and survival in patients with LV systolic dysfunction and are the cornerstones of medical therapy for heart failure. Angiotensin receptor

CURRENT DIAGNOSIS

- Identify the presence of characteristics associated with left ventricular systolic dysfunction.
- Document the degree of left ventricular dysfunction by imaging.
- Ascertain clinical volume and perfusion status.
- Determine the cause of cardiac dysfunction, if possible, with special attention to coronary artery disease.

blocking agents, or the combination of hydralazine (Apresoline)[1] and a nitrate, provide similar (but not superior) benefit in patients with contraindications to use of ACE inhibitors. Digoxin (Lanoxin) provides no survival benefit but improves symptoms in patients with atrial fibrillation and in those patients who remain symptomatic on optimal doses of vasodilators. Diuretics provide symptomatic relief if volume overload is present. Antialdosterone agents should be prescribed for all patients with LV dysfunction after acute myocardial infarction and for all other heart failure patients who remain symptomatic despite optimal doses of vasodilator and β-blocker therapy. Antiarrhythmics should be used only for symptomatic atrial or ventricular arrhythmias, because they may be proarrhythmic. Table 3 describes the use of various medications in patients with heart failure.

Parenteral agents for heart failure, including dobutamine (Dobutrex), milrinone (Primacor), and nesiritide (Natrecor), are used primarily in the inpatient setting to treat acutely decompensated heart failure and are beyond the scope of this discussion. However, it should be noted that intravenous inotropic agents (dobutamine, milrinone) have been shown in uncontrolled trials to improve symptoms and quality of life but to increase mortality. Therefore, they should be used only for short periods, at the lowest possible doses, and in a monitored setting. Short-term inpatient use of nesiritide also improves symptoms.

DEVICE THERAPY

Implantable cardioverter-defibrillators (ICDs) have been shown in randomized clinical trials to improve survival in heart failure patients with ischemic or nonischemic cardiomyopathy. Indications for implantation are an LVEF of less than 30% and mild-to-moderate symptoms of heart failure in a patient whose anticipated survival exceeds 1 year or ischemic cardiomyopathy and an LVEF of less than 35% regardless of symptoms.

TABLE 2 New York Heart Association Functional Classification of Chronic Heart Failure

Class*	Symptoms
I	No perceived limitation of physical activity
II A/B	Symptoms with moderate physical exertion
III A/B	Symptoms with low levels of physical exertion (i.e., activities of daily living)
IV	Resting symptoms

*A = early stage; B = late stage.

TABLE 1 Stages of Heart Failure

Stage	Description	Examples
A	High risk for development of HF due to presence of conditions strongly associated with HF development No identified structural or functional abnormalities of the pericardium, myocardium, or cardiac valves No history of signs or symptoms of HF	Systemic hypertension Coronary artery disease Diabetes mellitus Prior cardiac drug therapy Prior alcohol abuse Family history of cardiomyopathy
B	Presence of structural heart disease strongly associated with HF development No history of signs or symptoms of HF	LV hypertrophy or fibrosis LV dilation or dysfunction Asymptomatic valvular heart disease Previous myocardial infarction
C	Current or prior symptoms of HF with underlying structural heart disease	Dyspnea or fatigue from LV systolic dysfunction Asymptomatic patient undergoing treatment for prior symptoms of HF
D	Advanced structural heart disease and marked symptoms of HF at rest despite maximal medical therapy Requirement for specialized interventions	Frequent HF hospitalizations and cannot be discharged In hospital awaiting heart transplantation Home continuous inotropic or mechanical support In hospice setting for HF management

HF, heart failure; LV, left ventricular.

TABLE 3 Heart Failure Medications

Drug Class	Name/Dose	Comments
ACEIs (in enalapril [Vasotec] equivalents)	10–20 mg bid	Likely a class effect, so agent choice depends on duration of action and tolerability. Higher doses decrease hospitalization rates. Hyperkalemia limits use. Reduced doses may be necessary to allow adequate β-blocker dose titration.
Angiotensin receptor blockers	Valsartan (Diovan) 40–160 mg bid Candesartan (Atacand) 4–32 mg/d	The only two agents in this class to show benefit in randomized clinical trials. Good for patients intolerant of ACEIs. Noninferior but not superior to ACEIs, so use second line. Hyperkalemia limits use.
Hydralazine and nitrates	Hydralazine (Apresoline)[1] 25–100 mg qid with isosorbide dinitrate (Isordil Titradose)[1] 20–40 mg qid	Agents of choice in patients with significant renal insufficiency or other contraindications to ACEIs or aldosterone receptor antagonists.
β-Blockers	Metoprolol succinate (Toprol XL) 100–200 mg/d Carvedilol (Coreg) 25–50 mg bid Bisoprolol (Zebeta)[1] 2.5–10 mg/d	The only three agents in this class to show benefit in randomized clinical trials. Dose is based on body size. Some clinical and survival improvement with lower doses, but target dose is recommended.
Loop diuretics (expressed as furosemide [Lasix] equivalents)	40–100 mg qd or bid	Dietary compliance, fluid restriction, and titration of other heart failure drugs affect dose required.
Aldosterone receptor antagonists	Spironolactone (Aldactone) 12.5–25 mg/d	For patients who remain NYHA functional class III despite adequate doses of vasodilators and β-blockers. Hyperkalemia limits use.
	Eplerenone (Inspra) 25–50 mg/d	For patients with left ventricular dysfunction after acute myocardial infarction. Fewer side effects than spironolactone. Hyperkalemia limits use.
Digoxin (Lanoxin)	0.125–0.25 mg/d	Adjust for renal insufficiency. Women need lower doses. Serum level measurement not routinely necessary; only to confirm toxicity.

[1]Not FDA approved for this indication.
Abbreviations: ACEI = angiotensin-converting enzyme inhibitor; NYHA, New York Heart Association.

Cardiac resynchronization therapy, with or without implantation of a cardioverter-defibrillator, has been shown in randomized clinical trials to improve symptoms and survival in selected heart failure patients when added to optimal medical heart failure therapy. One third of heart failure patients with low LVEF and moderate to severe symptoms have ventricular dyssynchronous contraction, which is associated with increased mortality. Indications for cardiac resynchronization therapy include an LVEF lower than 35%, NYHA functional class III-IV symptoms, and a QRS duration of greater than 120 msec, which is a marker for ventricular dyssynchrony.

THERAPY FOR ADVANCED HEART FAILURE

Patients with heart failure that has become refractory to medical and resynchronization therapy should be referred to an advanced heart failure center experienced in the surgical treatment of heart failure. Surgical therapies improve symptoms and survival and are now considered the standard of care for heart failure patients in whom standard medical therapy has failed.

Heart transplantation is the only definitive surgical therapy for advanced heart failure, but alternative surgical approaches include coronary revascularization, valve surgery, LV reconstruction, and the use of ventricular assist devices. In patients with ischemic cardiomyopathy and hibernating myocardium, coronary revascularization improves LV function, functional capacity, and survival, compared with medical therapy. Mitral valve repair or replacement can improve symptoms in selected patients. Ventricular reconstruction may benefit patients with LV aneurysms or recurrent ventricular arrhythmias.

Left ventricular assist devices are implantable pumps that work in parallel with the native heart to provide short-term mechanical circulatory support in patients who are expected to recover heart function (e.g., patients with myocarditis, after acute myocardial infarction, after coronary artery bypass grafting) and in patients awaiting heart transplantation. In addition, these devices are approved as a permanent alternative to transplantation (destination therapy) in patients for whom heart transplantation is not an option. Early identification and referral of patients who might benefit from these therapies is essential for the best surgical outcomes.

Common Management Errors

Heart failure management errors result in increased hospitalizations and mortality. ACE inhibitors remain underused, despite evidence from clinical trials in more than 10,000 patients. Although Losartan (Cozaar)[1] is commonly used for the patient who cannot tolerate ACE inhibitors, only two members of the angiotensin receptor blocker class, valsartan (Diovan) and candesartan (Atacand), have been shown in clinical trials to provide benefit. The combination of hydralazine (Apresoline)[1] and isosorbide dinitrate (Isordil Titradose)[1] is also underused, despite evidence that these drugs improve exercise tolerance and survival.

Only three β-blockers, metoprolol succinate (Toprol XL), carvedilol (Coreg), and bisoprolol (Zebeta),[1] have been shown in trials to improve symptoms and survival in heart failure patients. Metoprolol tartrate (Lopressor)[1] and atenolol (Tenormin)[1] are commonly used as substitutes, even though there are no data supporting their use. β-Blockers are commonly started too early in the course of heart failure, when the patient is experiencing decompensation and fluid overload, and leads to further decompensation.

Patients may receive drugs that worsen the heart failure state, such as first-generation calcium channel blockers, nonsteroidal antiinflammatory drugs, cyclooxygenase 2 inhibitors, and antiarrhythmic drugs. Intravenous inotropic therapy or nesiritide (Natrecor) may be used when the patient would be better served by optimization of his or her oral heart failure regimen. Patients are commonly overdiuresed, which results in symptomatic hypotension and makes initiation and titration of vasodilators and β-blockers difficult.

Many physicians fail to utilize nonpharmacologic therapies as an adjunct to drug therapy. In addition, lack of education and close follow-up can undermine the best medical regimen. Physicians also commonly fail to refer patients who need advanced heart failure therapy, or refer them too late, when end-organ damage is irreversible.

---

[1]Not FDA approved for this indication.

CURRENT THERAPY

- Angiotensin-converting enzyme (ACE) inhibitors, angiotensin receptor blocking agents, β-blockers, and aldosterone receptor antagonists improve survival and are integral to the treatment plan.
- Use nonpharmacologic therapy along with medical therapy. Sodium and fluid restriction, smoking and alcohol cessation, stress reduction and treatment of depression, and exercise and weight loss, all improve symptoms and reduce hospitalization.
- Treat comorbidities that exacerbate the heart failure state (e.g., hypertension, arrhythmias, sleep disordered breathing).
- Consider interventions to treat concomitant structural heart disease, such as coronary revascularization, mitral valve surgery, arrhythmia treatment, and cardiac resynchronization therapy.
- Refer patients with refractory disease early to an advanced heart failure center for implantation of a ventricular assist device or cardiac transplantation.
- Provide palliative care for patients who are not candidates for advanced heart failure therapy.

REFERENCES

Bardy GH, Lee KL, Mark DB, et al. Amiodarone or an implantable cardioverter defibrillator for congestive heart failure. N Engl J Med 2005;352:225–37.

Cleland JG, Daubert JC, Erdmann E, et al. The effect of cardiac resynchronization on morbidity and mortality in heart failure. N Engl J Med 2005;352:1539–49.

Cohn JN, Archibald DG, Ziesche S, et al. Effect of vasodilator therapy on mortality in chronic congestive heart failure: Results of a Veterans Administration Cooperative Study. N Engl J Med 1986;314:1547–52.

Cohn JN, Johnson G, Ziesche S, et al. A comparison of enalapril with hydralazine-isosorbide dinitrate in the treatment of chronic congestive heart failure. N Engl J Med 1991;325:303–10.

The Digitalis Investigation Group. Effect of digoxin on mortality and morbidity in patients with heart failure. N Engl J Med 1997;336:525–33.

The SOLVD Investigators. Effect of enalapril on mortality and the development of heart failure in asymptomatic patients with reduced left ventricular ejection fractions. N Engl J Med 1992;327:685–91.

Metoprolol CR/XL Randomized Intervention Trial in Congestive Heart Failure (MERIT-HF). Effect of metoprolol CR/XL in chronic heart failure. Lancet 1999;353:2001–7.

Hunt SA, Abraham WT, Chin MH, et al. ACC/AHA 2005 Guideline Update for the Diagnosis and Management of Chronic Heart Failure in the Adult: A report of the American College of Cardiology/American Heart Association Task Force on Practice Guidelines (Writing Committee to Update the 2001 Guidelines for the Evaluation and Management of Heart Failure). Developed in collaboration with the American College of Chest Physicians and the International Society for Heart and Lung Transplantation; endorsed by the Heart Rhythm Society. Circulation 2005;112:e154–235.

International Registry for Heart and Lung Transplantation (ISHLT Registry). Available at: http://www.ishlt.org/registries/heartLungRegistry.asp; (accessed May 29, 2009).

Packer M, Bristow MR, Cohn JN, et al. The effect of carvedilol on morbidity and mortality in patients with chronic heart failure. U.S. Carvedilol Heart Failure Study Group. N Engl J Med 1996;334:1349–55.

Pitt B, Zannad F, Remme WJ, et al. The effect of spironolactone on morbidity and mortality in patients with severe heart failure. Randomized Aldactone Evaluation Study Investigators. N Engl J Med 1999;341:709–17.

Rose EA, Gelijns AC, Moskowitz AJ, et al. Long-term mechanical left ventricular assistance for end-stage heart failure. N Engl J Med 2001;345:1435–43.

Infective Endocarditis

Method of
Navin M. Amin, MD

Epidemiologic Changes

Infective endocarditis denotes microbial infection of the cardiac valves and, less frequently, infection of the mural endocardium or of septal defects. At present, infective endocarditis accounts for 1 case per 1000 hospital admissions. The age of patients with endocarditis has increased. In the preantibiotic era, the average age of patients with endocarditis was 32 to 39 years old; currently more than half the cases occur in patients older than 60 years of age. Men are affected twice as often as women; the ratio increases to 5:1 in men older than 60 years of age.

Three major epidemiologic changes are observed in endocarditis:

1. The pattern of infective organisms has changed. Early in the antibiotic era group A *Streptococci* (β hemolyticus), *Pneumococci*, *Gonococci*, and *Meningococci* were the predominant pathogens. *Streptococcus viridans*, *Staphylococcus aureus* (methicillin-sensitive [MSSA] or methicillin resistant [MRSA]), coagulase—negative *Staphylococcus epidermidis* or *lugdunensis*—and gram-negative organisms are more common today.
2. Certain signs and symptoms, once characteristic of endocarditis, are seen in less than 5% of cases today: peripheral lesions involving skin, nails, and eyes—petechiae, subungual hemorrhage, Janeway lesions, Osler nodes, or Roth's spots.
3. Surgical procedures can be both a cause and a cure of endocarditis. Prosthetic valves inserted to improve mechanically malfunctioning valves can predispose recipients to endocarditis. But surgery can be lifesaving in patients with refractory congestive heart failure (CHF) or resistant infections.

Forms of Endocarditis

Endocarditis is classified as acute or subacute on the basis of its clinical course. The acute form, which evolves over days to weeks, is diagnosed within 2 weeks. Invasive organisms such as *Staphylococcus aureus*, *Staphylococcus epidermidis*, *Streptococcus pneumoniae*, group A streptococci, *Neisseria gonorrhoeae*, *Haemophilus influenzae*, *Salmonella*, other Enterobacteriaceae, Serratia, and *Pseudomonas aeruginosa* are usually the cause. Clinically acute endocarditis is associated with high fever, systemic toxicity, and leukocytosis with rapid destruction of the valves. It carries high morbidity and mortality.

Subacute endocarditis has a duration of more than 6 weeks and an indolent course. The most common agents are streptococcal species, with *Streptococcus viridans* the most predominant: *Enterococcus*, HACEK (*Haemophilus*, *Actinobacillus*, *Cardiobacterium*, *Eikenella*, *Kingella*) organisms, fungi, and *Coxiella burnetii*. Clinically subacute endocarditis is associated with prolonged low-grade fever (fever of unknown origin [FUO]), night sweats, weight loss, and vague symptoms such as generalized weakness, lethargy, and myalgia.

Infective endocarditis can also be grouped into three categories:

1. *Native valve endocarditis* usually develops when there is structural damage to the heart valve. Rheumatic/syphilitic valvular disease is responsible in 20% to 40% of the cases. The mitral valve is involved in 85%, and the aortic valve is affected in 50% of the cases. In patients older than age 60 years, 30% of cases occur with degenerative cardiac lesions such as calcified mitral valve annulus and calcified nodular lesions secondary to atherosclerosis or postmyocardial infarction thrombus. Twenty percent of cases with mitral valve prolapse (with thickened leaflets or significant mitral regurgitation) and obstructive cardiomyopathy can predispose to endocarditis. In 6% to 25% of cases, congenital heart disease is a risk factor as is evident in ventricular septal defect (VSD), patent

ductus arteriosus (PDA), tetralogy of Fallot, or coarctation of the aorta. It can also occur with a stenotic or regurgitant valve such as bicuspid aortic valve and pulmonary stenosis. Endocarditis is rare in patients with atrial septal defect (secundum type) because of the low-pressure gradient between the atria. Finally is a group of patients without any structural defect who are susceptible to endocarditis. Tricuspid valve endocarditis can develop in intravenous drug abusers and immunocompromised patients (with chronic renal failure, severe burns, chronic active hepatitis, collagen vascular disease, or neoplasm involving the pancreas, lung, or stomach).

2. *Prosthetic valve endocarditis* (PVE) at present constitutes 20% of all cases of endocarditis. It occurs in 2% to 4% of patients with a prosthetic valve. It can be early or late. Early PVE occurs within 60 days of the valve replacement, and predominant organisms are *Staphylococcus epidermidis* and *S. aureus* (MSSA or MRSA). In the case of late-onset endocarditis, which occurs after 2 months, *Streptococcus viridans* is the main offending pathogen.

3. *Nosocomial endocarditis* commonly affects patients older than age 60 years and seriously ill hospitalized patients. These individuals are subjected to invasive procedures such as insertion of central venous pressure, monitoring lines, hyperalimentation catheters, or intracardiac pacemaker wires that represent nidus of infection. Box 1 summarizes the factors predisposing to endocarditis.

Microbiology

Any microorganism can cause endocarditis (Table 1). Certain pathogens have increased ability to adhere to valvular leaflets, thereby establishing infection. Approximately 70% of the cases are caused by streptococci and staphylococci.

BOX 1   Factors Predisposing to Endocarditis

Native Valve Endocarditis
- Structural Damage
  Rheumatic valvular disease
  Syphilitic valvular disease
  Degenerative
    Calcified mitral/aortic valve
    Calcified post-MI thrombus
  Mitral valve prolapse
  IHSS
  Congenital heart disease
    Regurgitant or stenotic valve, bicuspid aortic valve, PS, Ebstein's anomaly, Marfan's syndrome
    High-pressure shunt, VSD, PDA, coarctation of the aorta, tetralogy of Fallot
- No Structural Damage
  Catheter Induced
  IVDA
  Immunocompromised

Prosthetic Valve Endocarditis
- Early (<2 mo)
  Staphylococcus epidermidis
  Staphylococcus aureus
- Late (>2 mo)
  Staphylococcus viridans

Nosocomial Endocarditis
- Invasive procedures

Abbreviations: IHSS = idiopathic hypertrophic subaortic stenosis; IVDA = intravenous drug abuse; MI = myocardial infarction; PDA = patent ductus arteriosus; PS = pulmonary stenosis; VSD = ventricular septal defect.
Adapted with permission from Amin NM: Infective endocarditis. Consultant 1994;34(3):319–343.

Staphylococci (MSSA or MRSA) are encountered predominantly in intravenous drug abuse (IVDA), in early PVE, in an immunocompromised host, and in nosocomial endocarditis. *S. viridans* is more commonly seen in native valve endocarditis and in late PVE. Gram-negative bacilli commonly cause right-sided endocarditis as in IVDA and in patients with intravascular catheters.

Approximately 10% of patients with endocarditis have a negative blood culture after 48 to 72 hours of incubation. Factors that produce culture-negative endocarditis are (1) antibiotic therapy before cultures are obtained; (2) a low level of bacteremia (common with right-sided and mural endocarditis); (3) infection with fastidious or nutritionally deficient bacteria that require prolonged cultures (2 to 3 weeks) or additional supplements (e.g., pyridoxine) for growth; this group includes HACEK organisms, *Brucella*, and nutritionally deficient streptococci; (4) nonbacterial infectious agents such as fungi, viruses, spirochetes, *Rickettsia, Chlamydia,* or parasites; and (5) noninfectious causes: left atrial myxoma, Libman-Sacks endocarditis, systemic lupus erythematosus, Löffler's hypereosinophilic endocarditis, carcinoid syndromes, and marantic endocarditis associated with malignancies of the pancreas, stomach, or lung.

Clinical Manifestations

The clinical manifestations of infective endocarditis are extremely diverse and can mimic pulmonary, neurologic, renal, or bone and joint disease. The classic manifestations of fever, heart murmur, splenomegaly, and petechiae of the skin and the mucous membranes help establish the diagnosis.

The onset may be abrupt or insidious. The early manifestations may be vague flulike symptoms that occur within 3 weeks after an invasive procedure. The patient may complain of malaise, fatigue, weakness, myalgia, arthralgia, low-grade fever, night sweats, or weight loss. Anorexia is almost universal. When the onset is acute, as in intravenous (IV) drug abuse, PVE, or nosocomial endocarditis, there may be evidence of severe infection heralded by high fever (90% to 95%), shaking chills and rigors, or, more ominous, symptoms of frank heart failure or embolic phenomena.

In patients older than age 60 years, diagnosis is often delayed because 5% may not have fever or are admitted with diagnosis of cerebral vascular accident (CVA), pneumonia, occult neoplasm, degenerative joint disease, or osteomyelitis. Infective endocarditis should always be considered in patients older than age 60 years who have fever and associated unexplained CHF, CVA, renal failure, weight loss, anemia, new-onset murmur, or confusional state.

In 85% of the cases, cardiac manifestations include a heart murmur. In right-sided endocarditis and mural infection, murmur is absent. A new or changing murmur (usually of aortic regurgitation) occurs in 5% to 10% of patients and is a very helpful diagnostic sign. Persistent or progressive CHF is indicative of a serious complication that carries a high mortality rate.

Peripheral cutaneous manifestations take a variety of forms: skin pallor caused by secondary anemia; petechiae found in 20% to 40% of cases concentrated on the conjunctiva, palate, buccal mucosa, and distal extremities; clubbing of nails in 10% to 20% if infection is long-standing; splinter hemorrhages as linear red-to-brown streaks in the middle of the nail bed of fingers and toes; Osler nodes (5% to 20% cases), which are small painful, tender, purplish subcutaneous nodules in the pads of fingers and toes; and Janeway lesions, which are small macular, painless, erythematous or hemorrhagic plaques on the palms or soles.

Ocular manifestations include Roth's spots, which occur in 5% of the patients and appear as oval or boat-shaped white or pale retinal lesions surrounded by hemorrhage and located near the optic disk. In a few cases there may be presence of cotton-wool exudates, petechiae, or flame-shaped hemorrhages.

Embolization can occur in 15% to 35% of cases. A cerebral emboli may produce hemiplegia, monoplegia, aphasia, or unilateral blindness. Mesenteric emboli can result in acute abdominal pain, ileus, or melena. Splenic emboli may cause left upper quadrant pain that radiates to the left shoulder of the chest with a small pleural effusion or splenic frictional rub. Flank pain with hematuria indicates a renal infarction. Peripheral arterial emboli may produce pain or gangrene. Large arterial occlusions are frequently seen with fungal endocarditis.

TABLE 1 Microbiology of Infective Endocarditis

Type of Infection	Specific Associated Risk Factors
Bacterial	
Gram Positive	
Streptococci (40%–60%)	
S. viridans, S. pneumoniae, S. bovis, S. pyogenes, S. sanguis	NVE, late-onset PVE
Enterococci (Group D) (5%–20%)	
S. faecalis, S. faecium, S. durans	Gastrointestinal malignancies
Staphylococci (17%–40%)	IVDA, early PVE
S. aureus (MRSA), *S. epidermidis* (MRSE), *S. lugdunensis*	
Diphtheroids	
Listeria	IVDA, early PVE
Gram Negative	
Cultured easily	
Pseudomonas aeruginosa, Serratia marcescens, Salmonella,	IVDA, immunocompromised, nosocomial endocarditis
Proteus mirabilis, Shigella, Providencia,	
Enterobacter, Neisseria gonorrhoeae, Escherichia coli	
Difficult to culture	
(HACEK) (1%–10%)	
Haemophilus, Actinobacillus, Cardiobacterium, Eikenella, Kingella	
(not HACEK)	
Brucella, Legionella	
Nonbacterial	
Fungi (2%–4%)	
Candida, Aspergillus, Histoplasma, Coccidioides, Blastomyces	IVDA, PVE, cardiac surgery, IV catheters, immunosuppressed
Viruses	
Coxsackie B, adenovirus	
Spirochetes	
Borrelia burgdorferi	Tick bite
Spirillum minus	Rat bite
Rickettsiae	
Coxiella burnetii	Infected livestock or unpasteurized milk
Chlamydia	
C. psittaci	Infected birds
Parasites	
Trypanosoma cruzi (Chagas' disease)	Kissing bug bite

Modified from Amin NM: Infective endocarditis. Consultant 1994;34(3):319–343.
Abbreviations: IVDA, intravenous drug abuse; MRSA, methicillin-resistant *Staphylococcus aureus*; MRSE, methicillin-resistant *Staphylococcus epidermidis*; NVE, native valve endocarditis; PVE, prosthetic valve endocarditis.

Very rarely, emboli to coronary arteries cause acute myocardial infarction, myocardial abscess, or mycotic aneurysm.

Neurologic complications (30% to 40%) include CVA from embolization, mycotic aneurysm causing cerebral of subdural hemorrhage and seizure, and brain abscess or toxic encephalopathy with confusion and nonspecific obtundation.

Renal manifestations are accompanied by microscopic or frank hematuria secondary to renal infarct, diffuse membranoproliferative glomerulonephritis, focal embolic glomerulonephritis, or renal abscess.

Splenomegaly occurs in 25% to 45% of the patients and is more common in subacute than in acute endocarditis.

Diagnosis

Infective endocarditis may mimic any systemic disorder. For this reason and because of its high morbidity and mortality, the diagnosis should be kept in mind whenever a high-risk patient has an unexplained fever, constitutional symptoms, or multiple systemic involvement with a changing or new heart murmur. A high index of suspicion for endocarditis in certain clinical situations is very helpful:

- Intravenous drug abusers with high fever
- Patients older than age 60 years with nonspecific vague symptoms with a calcified mitral valve annulus
- Unknown source of embolization
- Certain virulent infections caused by organisms such as *Staphylococcus* or *Enterococcus*

A thorough history, complete examination, and laboratory tests should establish the correct diagnosis. Box 2 outlines the various laboratory abnormalities in infective endocarditis.

BOX 2 Laboratory Abnormalities in Endocarditis

Hematologic
  Leukocytosis
  Anemia of chronic disorder
  Thrombocytopenia (10% SBE)
  Elevated ESR
  Urine analysis
  Hematuria, microscopic
  Proteinuria
Cardiac abnormality
  ECG: chamber enlargement, conduction defect
Chest x-ray
  Cardiomegaly
  Evidence of congestive heart failure
  Nodular infiltrate (staphylococcal endocarditis)
Diagnostic gold standards
  Echocardiography (transesophageal preferred)
  Three sets of blood (embolus) cultures
Immunologic abnormalities
  Rheumatoid factor (disappears after treatment)
  Hypergammaglobulinemia
  Cryoglobulinemia
  Circulating immune complexes
  Low complement levels

Abbreviations: ECG = electrocardiogram; ESR = erythrocyte sedimentation rate; SBE = subacute bacterial endocarditis.

A baseline electrocardiogram (ECG) is helpful to detect chamber enlargement or possible conduction defect that may indicate underlying valvular or congenital anomalies. Later development of first-degree atrioventricular (AV) block, new bundle branch block, or new ectopic beats may indicate a myocardial abscess, especially in aortic valve endocarditis.

Echocardiography (transesophageal [TEE], M mode, two-dimensional, or Doppler) can confirm the diagnosis, detect complications, and help assess the prognosis. The echocardiogram can detect vegetations larger than 2 to 3 mm on mitral or aortic valves. Sensitivity in detecting vegetations is approximately 87% to 90% with TEE, 30% to 75% with M-mode, 40% to 50% with two-dimensional, and 50% with Doppler echocardiography. False-positive results are seen with old healed vegetations, myxomatous valvular degeneration, arterial myxoma, or a thrombus.

Echocardiogram can detect complications such as torn or perforated valves, ruptured chordae tendineae, myocardial abscess, or pericardiac effusion that may require surgical intervention. Large-sized vegetations in the left side of the heart or in the aortic valve, or myocardial abscess, suggest a relatively poor prognosis, and surgery may be indicated.

Serial blood cultures are required to establish the diagnosis by isolating the offending bacterium or fungus. A minimum of three blood samples should be drawn 30 to 60 minutes apart before initiating empiric antibiotic therapy. If the patient has taken antibiotics in the preceding 2 weeks, two or three additional sets of blood cultures should be taken. Cultures of arterial blood offer no additional advantage over venous blood. Ninety percent of the blood cultures become positive within 7 days of incubation. Negative blood cultures are likely seen in patients who have received prior antibiotics or who have endocarditis caused by fastidious gram-negative (HACEK) bacilli, fungi, or nutritionally deficient streptococci. The microbiology laboratory should be alerted to the suspected endocarditis, and a report for prolonged incubation for 2 weeks included.

In fungal endocarditis, in which there is embolization of large arteries, a culture of the removed embolus can establish the diagnosis. Serologic studies can be helpful in fungal infection (histoplasmosis or coccidioidomycosis) or when rickettsial (Q fever) Legionella or Chlamydia infections are suspected.

Treatment of Infective Endocarditis

The main goal is eradicating the infecting pathogens as quickly as possible to reduce the risks of morbidity and mortality. This can be achieved with antibiotic therapy, surgical intervention, or both.

ANTIBIOTIC THERAPY

In using antibiotics to treat infective endocarditis, the following guidelines are helpful:

- Parental antibiotics are used to sustain bactericidal activity.
- Bactericidal antimicrobials are used for complete eradication of the pathogens. Synergistic bactericidal activity is achieved with combination therapy such as ampicillin and aminoglycosides in treatment of enterococcal endocarditis.
- The drug regimen and appropriate duration of course, 2 to 6 weeks, must be tailored to prevent relapse.
- The bactericidal activity of the antibiotic is monitored by determining the minimum inhibitory concentration (MIC) and the minimum bactericidal concentration (MBC) against the infecting organisms.
- Antibiotic therapy is initiated as quickly as possible. When endocarditis is severe and/or complicated, empiric treatment should be instituted immediately with antibiotics effective against S. aureus and enterococci. A combination of vancomycin (Vancocin) and gentamicin (Garamycin) is recommended. Once a specific organism is identified, appropriate bactericidal antibiotics should be used.

Most streptococci other than enterococci are exquisitely sensitive to penicillin. If MIC is less than 0.2 μg per mL, high-dose penicillin alone or in combination with either gentamicin (Garamycin) or

streptomycin or ceftriaxone (Rocephin) can be used for 4 weeks. If the MIC is below 0.1 μg per mL, treatment should be for 2 weeks. If MIC is greater than 0.2 μg per mL or the MBC to MIC ratio exceeds 10:1, as it occurs in 15% to 20% of cases with S. viridans infection, higher dose of penicillin with aminoglycoside should be used. In penicillin-allergic patients, vancomycin is the best alternative with or without aminoglycoside (Table 2).

In enterococcal endocarditis, ampicillin is recommended in combination with an aminoglycoside. Gentamicin is preferred because 40% of the isolates are resistant to streptomycin. In penicillin-allergic patients, vancomycin with an aminoglycoside is the best choice.

In S. aureus infection, semisynthetic penicillin or first-generation cephalosporins are the agents of first choice. Addition of gentamicin or rifampin (Rifadin)[1] during the first few days rapidly reduces bacteremia. Vancomycin is recommended for patients allergic to penicillin or if the organism is methicillin resistant (MRSA). Addition of rifampin, although controversial, is recommended in patients demonstrating poor bactericidal activity during therapy with beta-lactams or vancomycin and for patients with suppurative complication, such as a valve ring abscess.

Endocarditis with S. epidermidis, which commonly develops on prosthetic valves, is ideally treated with vancomycin and rifampin.[1] An aminoglycoside may be added for 2 weeks.

Gram-negative infections causing high mortality are best treated with broad-spectrum penicillin or, preferably, a third-generation cephalosporin with an aminoglycoside. In most of these patients, valve replacement is necessary.

SURGICAL INTERVENTIONS

Approximately 25% of patients with severe or complicated endocarditis undergo surgery. The chief indications for surgery are refractory moderate or severe CHF; perivalvular invasion or myocardial abscess as evident by persistent fever despite antibiotics or electrocardiographic changes of conduction defects; systemic or arterial embolization; fungal endocarditis; PVE of early onset; large bulky vegetations that increase risk of CHF; persistent infection (particularly with gram-negative bacilli) that does not respond to 7 to 10 days of antibiotic therapy; and staphylococcal endocarditis in IV drug abusers that does not respond to antimicrobials.

PREVENTION OF BACTERIAL ENDOCARDITIS

Transient bacteremia that develops after a variety of manipulations or surgical procedures in patients with structural heart defects causes endocarditis. Prophylactic antibiotics in this situation can be highly effective when given before the procedure. Administration of these agents only once is required 30 minutes to 2 hours before the procedure (Table 3).

In choosing prophylactic therapy, the following questions (Table 4) are useful:

- Is the patient at increased risk for endocarditis with underlying structural defect?
- Is there a high risk the procedure will produce bacteremia with organisms that cause endocarditis, such as S. viridans infection with oral cavity procedures or enterococcal with gastrointestinal or genitourinary procedures?

Antibiotic prophylaxis is recommended for patients with VSD, PDA, pulmonary or aortic stenosis, tetralogy of Fallot, or coarctation of the aorta. Such therapy is needed for patients with rheumatic or syphilitic valvular defects, prosthetic valves, calcified valves, obstructive cardiomyopathy, or mitral valve prolapse with either regurgitant murmur or with thickened mitral valve leaflets.

Endocarditis prophylaxis is not advised for patients with isolated secundum atrial septal defect or those who have undergone surgical repair for VSD or PDA and have no residual defect beyond 6 months. The same is true for those who have coronary artery bypass graft, previous rheumatic fever, or Kawasaki disease without any valve dysfunction. Prophylaxis is not recommended for those who have mitral valve prolapse (MVP) without mitral regurgitation (MR) and for persons with a cardiac pacemaker or implanted defibrillator (Table 5).

---

[1]Not FDA approved for this indication.

TABLE 2 Antibiotic Regimens for Bacterial Endocarditis

Infecting Organism	Antibiotic	Dosage, Route, and Frequency	Duration in Weeks
Penicillin susceptible *Streptococcus viridans*, and *S. bovis* (MIC <0.2 µg/dL)	*Preferred Regimen* Penicillin G	12–16 million U/d IV in 6 divided doses	4
	or		
	Penicillin G PLUS	12–16 million U/d IV in 6 divided doses	4
	Gentamicin	1 mg/kg IM or IV q8h	2
	or		
	Penicillin G PLUS Gentamicin	Dosages same as above regimen	2
	or		
	Ceftriaxone	2 g IV or IM q24h	4
	Alternative Regimen Vancomycin	0.5 g IV q6h	4
Relative penicillin-resistant streptococci (MIC >0.2 µg/dL)	*Preferred Regimen* Penicillin G PLUS	20–30 million U/d IV in 6 divided doses	4
	Gentamicin	1 mg/kg IV or IM q8h	4
	Alternative Regimen Vancomycin	0.5 g IV q6h	4
Staphylococcus epidermidis (MRSE)	*Native Valve* Vancomycin	0.5 g IV q6h	4
	Prosthetic Valve Vancomycin PLUS	0.5 g IV q6h	4–6
	Gentamicin	1 mg/kg IV or IM q8h	2
	or		
	Rifampin	300 mg PO/IV q12h	2
Enterococcus (*S. faecalis*, *S. faecium*, *S. durans*)	*Preferred Regimen* Penicillin G PLUS	20–30 million U/d IV in 6 divided doses	4–6
	Gentamicin	1 mg/kg IM or IV q8h	4–6
	or		
	Ampicillin PLUS	2 g IV q4h	4–6
	Gentamicin	1 mg/kg IM or IV q8h	4–6
	Alternative Regimen Vancomycin PLUS	0.5 g IV q6h	4–6
	Gentamicin	1 mg/kg IM or IV q8h	4–6
Staphylococcus aureus (methicillin sensitive)	*Preferred Regimen* Nafcillin or Oxacillin	2 g IV q4h	4–6
	or		
	Oxacillin PLUS	2 g IV q4h	4–6
	Gentamicin OR/PLUS	1 mg/kg IM or IV q8h	2
	Rifampin	300 mg PO/IV q12h	2
	Alternative Regimen Cefazolin	2 g IV q6h	4–6
	or		
	Vancomycin	0.5 g IV q6h	4–6
S. aureus (methicillin resistant [MRSA])	Daptomycin	6 mg/kg IV once a day	6
	Vancomycin PLUS	0.5 g IV q6h	4–6
	Gentamicin OR/PLUS	1 mg/kg IM or IV q8h	2
	Rifampin[1]	300 mg PO/IV q12h	2
HACEK group (*Haemophilus, Actinobacillus, Cardiobacterium, Eikenella, Kingella*)	Ampicillin	2 g IV q6h	4
	or		
	Ampicillin PLUS	2 g IV q6h	4
	Gentamicin	1 mg/kg IM or IV q8h	4
	or		
	Ceftriaxone	2 g IV q24h	4
Culture negative	Vancomycin PLUS	0.5 g IV q8h	6
	Gentamicin	1 mg/kg IM or IV q8h	6

Modified from Amin NM: Infective Endocarditis. Consultant 1994;34(3):319–343.
[1]Not FDA approved for this indication.
Abbreviation: MIC = minimum inhibitory concentration.

Procedures for which antibiotic prophylaxis is needed are those in which transient bacteremia develops when mucosal surfaces colonized with microorganisms are traumatized. For example, bacteremia may occur following dental manipulation in 80% of cases or in 20% of patients after urethral instrumentation. Prophylactic antimicrobials are recommended for high-risk patients who are scheduled to have certain dental, oropharyngeal, gastrointestinal, or genitourinary manipulations.

Standard antibiotic prophylaxis for patients undergoing oral, dental, or upper respiratory tract manipulations include oral amoxicillin. Clindamycin (Cleocin),[1] cefadroxil (Duricef),[1] cephalexin (Keflex),[1] or azithromycin (Zithromax)[1] or clarithromycin (Biaxin)[1] should be given to those who cannot tolerate or are allergic to penicillin.

Parenteral ampicillin is recommended for patients who cannot take oral antibiotics and for those at high risk for infective endocarditis, such as patients with a prosthetic valve, previous endocarditis, or surgical systemic pulmonary shunts. Clindamycin[1] or cefazolin (Ancef) can be used as an alternative. Patients undergoing gastrointestinal or genitourinary instrumentation should be given vancomycin.

---

[1]Not FDA approved for this indication.

TABLE 3 Preprocedural Antibiotic Prophylaxis for At-Risk Patients

Type of Procedure and Situation	Antibiotic	Dosage, Route, and Frequency
Dental, oral respiratory tract, and esophageal procedures		
Standard prophylaxis	Amoxicillin	2 g PO 1 h before procedure
Patient unable to take oral medication	Ampicillin	2 g IM/IV within 30 min before procedure
Patient allergic to penicillin	Clindamycin (Cleocin*) or	600 mg PO 1 h before procedure
	cefadroxil (Duricef*) or	2 g PO 1 h before procedure
	cephalexin (Keflex*) or	2 g PO 1 h before procedure
	azithromycin (Zithromax*) or	500 mg PO 1 h before procedure
	clarithromycin (Biaxin*)	500 mg PO 1 h before procedure
Patient allergic to penicillin and unable to take oral medication	Clindamycin (Cleocin*) or	600 mg IV within 30 min of starting procedure
	cefazolin (Ancef) or	1 g IV within 30 min of starting procedure
	vancomycin (Vancocin)	1 g IV over 1–2 h within 60 min of starting procedure
Genitourinary/gastrointestinal procedures		
Moderate-risk patient	Amoxicillin or	2 g PO 1 h before procedure
	ampicillin	2 g IM/IV within 30 min of starting procedure
Moderate-risk penicillin-allergic patient	Vancomycin	1 g IV over 1–2 h infusion completed within 30–60 min of starting procedure
High-risk patient	Ampicillin PLUS	2 g IM/IV given within 30 min of starting procedure
	gentamicin 6 h later	1.5 mg/kg IV given within 30 min of starting procedure
	Ampicillin or	1 g IM or IV
	amoxicillin	1 g PO
High-risk penicillin-allergic patient	Vancomycin PLUS	1 g IV over 1–2 h
	gentamicin	1.5 mg/kg IV given within 30 min of starting procedure

Modified from Dajani AS, Taubert KA, Wilson W, et al: Prevention of bacterial endocarditis: Recommendation by the American Heart Association. JAMA 1997;277(22):1794–1801.
*Not FDA approved for this indication.

TABLE 4 Indications for Endocardial Prophylaxis

Cardiac Conditions	Procedures
High-risk category	**Dental**
Prosthetic valve	Dental extraction
Previous endocarditis	Periodontal procedures: surgery, scaling, root planing
Complex cyanotic disease Tetralogy of Fallot, single ventricle	Dental implant replacement
Surgically conducted systemic-pulmonary shunt	Subgingival placement of antibiotic fibers
Moderate-risk category	Intraligamentary local anesthetic injection
Congenital heart disease: VSD, PDA, AS, PS	Cleaning of teeth or implants
Acquired valvular dysfunction Rheumatic/syphilitic	**Respiratory**
Hypertrophic cardiomyopathy	Tonsillectomy/adenoidectomy
MVP with MR or thickened leaflets	Rigid bronchoscopy
	Gastrointestinal
	Sclerotherapy
	Esophageal stricture dilation
	ERCP with biliary obstruction
	Biliary tract surgery
	Surgery involving intestinal mucosa
	Genitourinary
	Prostatic surgery
	Cystoscopy
	Urethral dilation
	Septic abortion

Modified from Dajani AS, Taubert KA, Wilson W, et al: Prevention of bacterial endocarditis: Recommendations by the American Heart Association. JAMA 1997;277(22):1794–1801.
Abbreviations: AS = aortic stenosis; ERCP = endoscopic retrograde cholangiopancreatography; MVP = mitral valve prolapse; MR = mitral regurgitation; PDA = patent ductus arteriosus; PS = pulmonary stenosis; VSD = ventricular septal defect.

TABLE 5 Endocardial Prophylaxis Not Recommended

Cardiac Conditions	Procedures
Isolated secundum ASD	**Dental**
Surgical repair of ASD, VSD, PDA (without residue >6 mo)	Restorative dentistry
	Local anesthetic injections
Previous CABG surgery	Intracanal treatment
MVP without valvular dysfunction	Postoperative suture removal
	Oral impression/radiograph
Functional murmur	Fluoride treatment
Kawasaki disease without valvular dysfunction	Shedding of primary teeth
Previous rheumatic fever without valve dysfunction	**Respiratory**
	Endotracheal intubation
Cardiac pacemaker and implanted defibrillators	Fiberoptic bronchoscopy
Cardiac catheterization, balloon angioplasty	Tympanostomy tube insertion
Coronary stent placement	**Gastrointestinal**
	TEE*
	Endoscopy with/without biopsy*
	Genitourinary
	Vaginal delivery/hysterectomy*
	Cesarean section
	Urethral catheterization
	Uterine dilation and curettage
	Insertion/removal of IUD
	Circumcision

Modified from Dajani AS, Taubert KA, Wilson W, et al: Prevention of bacterial endocarditis: Recommendations by the American Heart Association. JAMA 1997;277(22):1794–1801.
*Prophylaxis optional for high-risk category.
Abbreviations: ASD = atrial septal defect; CABG = coronary artery bypass graft; IUD = intrauterine device; MVP = mitral valve prolapse; PDA = patent ductus arteriosus; TEE = transesophageal echocardiogram; VSD = ventricular septal defect.

CURRENT DIAGNOSIS

- High index of suspicion
- Febrile patient (temperature >38°C [100.4°F]) with
  Valvular or congenital heart defects
  Intravenous drug abuse
  Prosthetic or vascular access
  New onset or changing cardiac murmur
  Unknown source of embolization
- Positive blood cultures on at least two different specimens.
- Presence of vegetation detected on echocardiography (transesophageal [TEE] preferred)

CURRENT THERAPY

- Empiric antibiotics should be started immediately with vancomycin and gentamicin.
- Specific therapy should be started once the pathogen is identified:
  Use combination therapy for synergetic activity.
  Monitor MIC/MBC level whenever possible.
  Administer therapy for 2 to 6 weeks.
- Surgical interventions should be undertaken for severe, refractory, and complicated endocarditis.
- Prophylactic antibiotics are recommended in patients with structural heart defects undergoing surgical procedures or manipulations that can cause transient bacteremia, as recommended by the American Heart Association.
- Administration of antibiotic is usually once and 30 minutes to 1 to 2 hours before the procedure.

Abbreviations: MBC = minimum bactericidal concentration; MIC = minimum inhibitory concentration.

As recommended by the American Heart Association, all prophylactic antibiotics should be used only once before the procedure. There is no need for additional antibiotic administration except in high-risk patients who are undergoing gastrointestinal or genitourinary manipulation and who are given an ampicillin and gentamicin combination.

REFERENCES

Amin NM. Infective endocarditis. Consultant 1994;34(3):319–43.
Bansal RC. Infective endocarditis. Med Clin North Am 1995;79:1205–20.
Bayer AS, Bolger AF, Taubert KA, et al. Diagnosis and management of infective endocarditis and its complications. Circulation 1998;98:2936–48.
Bayer AS, Ward JI, Ginzton LE, Shapiro SM. Evaluation of new clinical criteria for diagnosis of infective endocarditis. Am J Med 1994;96:211–9.
Cunha BA, Gill MV, Lazar JM. Acute infective endocarditis. Infect Dis Clin North Am 1996;10(4):811–34.
Dajanai AS, Taubert KA, Wilson W, et al. Prevention of bacterial endocarditis. Recommendations by American Heart Association. JAMA 1997;277:1794–801.
Giessel BE, Koenig CJ, Blake RL. Management of bacterial endocarditis. Am Fam Physician 2000;61:1725–32.
Karchner AW. Infections on prosthetic valves and intravascular infections. In: Mandell JE, Bennett JE, Dolin R, editors. Mandell, Douglas and Bennett's Principles and Practice of Infectious Diseases. 5th ed. Philadelphia: Churchill Livingstone; 2000. p. 903–17.
Li JS, Sexton DJ, Mick N, et al. Proposed modification to Duke criteria for diagnosis of infective endocarditis. Clin Infect Dis 2000;30:633–8.
Mylonakis E, Calderwood SB. Infective endocarditis in adults. N Engl J Med 2001;345(18):1318–30.

Hypertension

Method of
Miho Murashima, MD, and Debbie L. Cohen, MD

Definition

The current classification of blood pressure (BP) is shown in Table 1. A diagnosis of hypertension (HTN) is based on the average of two or more properly measured BP readings on each of two or more office visits. The highest systolic (SBP) or diastolic (DBP) measurement from the four or more measurements determines the classification. The stage of HTN at the initial visit determines how frequently the patient should be seen and the magnitude of therapy required.

MEASUREMENT OF BLOOD PRESSURE

A mercury manometer should be used to measure BP, because it is the most accurate method. The patient should be seated in a quiet room in a chair with the back supported and the legs uncrossed. The cuff should be applied to an uncovered arm that is supported at the level of the heart. The length of the cuff bladder should encircle 80% of the arm circumference, and the width of the cuff bladder should be 40% of the arm circumference. The bell of the stethoscope is used to auscultate low-intensity Korotkoff sounds over the brachial artery, and then the cuff is slowly deflated by 2 to 3 mm Hg per second. SBP is represented by the first faint tapping sound after cuff deflation, and DBP is the point at which Korotkoff sounds completely cease. At least two or three measurements at 1-minute intervals should be obtained at every visit. Initial BP measurements should include measurement in the contralateral arm. If an electronic sphygmomanometer is used, it must be calibrated against a mercury manometer every 3 to 6 months.

Home BP monitoring can be a useful tool for patient care. Many home devices are not accurate. An objective source of information is available online (http://www.dableeducational.com/sphygmomanometers.html [accessed May 29, 2009]) to help guide physicians' recommendations. The patient should be told to take two seated measurements twice daily after resting for 5 minutes. Values consistently lower than 130/80 mm Hg are normal. Home monitoring is more accurate than office BP measurements and can be useful when making medication adjustments and assessing overall BP control.

Epidemiology

PREVALENCE OF HYPERTENSION

According to the National Health and Nutrition Examination Survey, approximately 65 million adults in the United States have HTN, and about one third of them are unaware that they have it. Approximately 67% of patients receive treatment for HTN, but control is achieved in only 64% of those who receive treatment. There has been an improvement in the control of BP in patients receiving antihypertensive medication, with an increase from 36% in 1988–1994 to 43% in 1999–2004. BP still remains poorly controlled among African Americans, Mexican Americans, and Hispanics.

ASSOCIATION WITH CARDIOVASCULAR RISKS

HTN is one of the modifiable risk factors for cardiovascular disease. At any age, higher BP is associated in a linear manner with increase in death due to coronary heart disease or stroke (Fig. 1). With treatment of HTN, the risks of congestive heart failure, stroke, and cardiovascular disease decrease substantially (Fig. 2). Data from a meta-analysis of individual data for 1 million adults participating in 61 prospective observational studies of BP and mortality demonstrated that even a small, 2 mm Hg fall in mean SBP was associated with a 7% lower risk of coronary heart disease death and a 10% lower

TABLE 1 Classification of Blood Pressure

| Classification | Blood Pressure (mm Hg) | | | Follow-up Recommended |
	Systolic		Diastolic	
Normal	<120	AND	<80	Recheck within 2 y
Prehypertension	120–139	OR	80–89	Recheck within 1 y
Stage 1 hypertension	140–159	OR	90–99	Recheck within 2 mo
Stage 2 hypertension	≥160	OR	≥100	Evaluate or refer to source of care within 1 mo

Modified from Chobanian AV, Bakris GL, Black HR, et al: Seventh report of Joint National Committee on Prevention, Detection, Evaluation and Treatment of High Blood Pressure. Hypertension 2003;42:1206–1252.

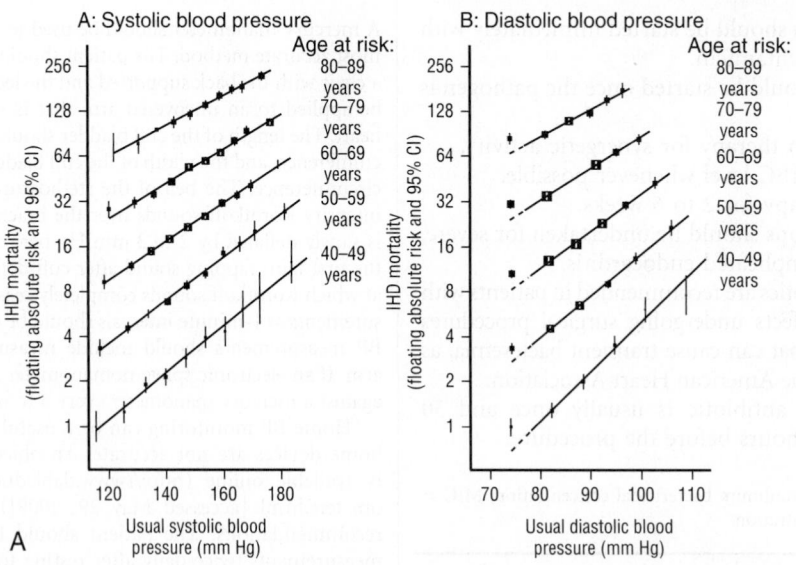

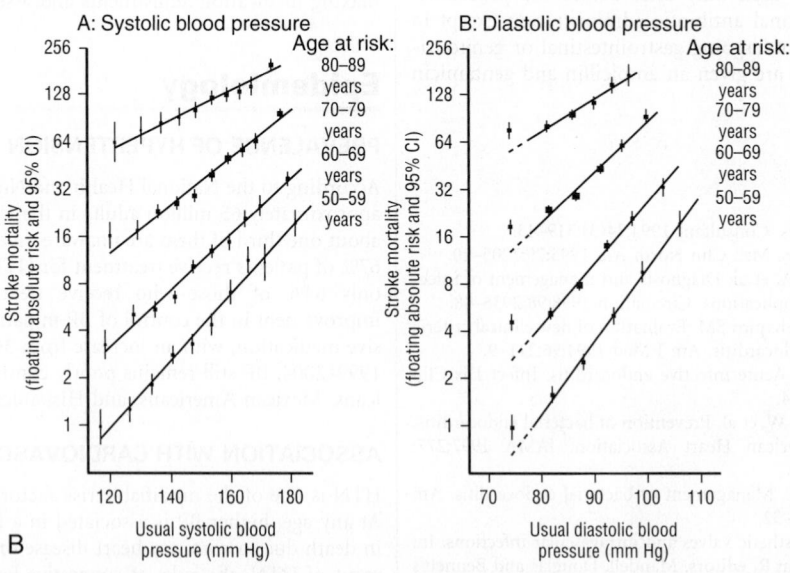

FIGURE 1. **A**, Relationship between ischemic heart disease (IHD) mortality in each decade of age and usual blood pressure at the start of the decade. **B**, Relationship between stroke mortality in each decade of age and usual blood pressure at the start of the decade (Reprinted with permission from Lewington S, Clarke R, Qizilbash N, et al; Prospective Studies Collaboration: Age-specific relevance of usual blood pressure to vascular mortality: A meta-analysis of individual data for one million adults in 61 prospective studies. Lancet 2002;360:1903–1913.)

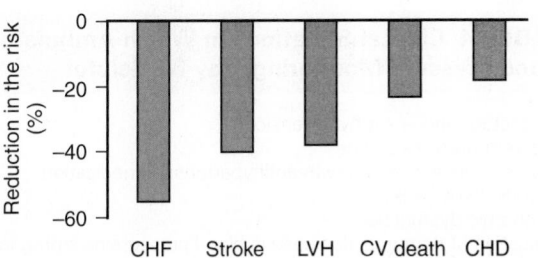

FIGURE 2. The benefit of antihypertensive drug treatment. Abbreviations: CHD = coronary heart disease; CHF = congestive heart failure; LVH = left ventricular hypertrophy. (Modified from Moser M, Hebert PR: Prevention of disease progression, left ventricular hypertrophy and congestive heart failure in hypertension treatment trials. J Am Coll Cardiol 1996;27:1214–1218.)

risk of stroke death, emphasizing that even small reductions in SBP in large populations can have important cardiovascular morbidity and mortality benefits. The impact of treatment of HTN is especially prominent in terms of reduction of CHF and stroke (see Fig. 2).

Prehypertension

The Seventh Report of the Joint National Committee on Prevention and Detection, Evaluation and Treatment of High Blood Pressure (JNC 7) added the new classification of prehypertension (see Table 1). This derives from the notion that there is a linear increase in cardiovascular diseases with BP levels greater than 120/80 mm Hg (see Fig. 1). The Trial of Preventing Hypertension (TROPHY) study randomized subjects with prehypertension to treatment with candesartan (Atacand), an angiotensin receptor blocker, or with placebo for 2 years. Patients were monitored for a 4-year period. Almost two thirds of people with untreated prehypertension developed stage 1 HTN, whereas subjects in the treatment group had a lower incidence. It has not been proven whether treating prehypertension ultimately decreases the risk of cardiovascular morbidity and mortality, and active treatment of patients with prehypertension is not recommended at this time. However, it is critically important to encourage lifestyle modification in this group of patients.

Systolic and Diastolic Blood Pressure

JNC 7 emphasized that systolic HTN is a major risk factor for cardiovascular disease because of the finding that treatment of isolated systolic HTN reduces cardiovascular morbidity and mortality. On the other hand, for the same SBP, a lower DBP is associated with an increase in coronary heart disease (Fig. 3). Coronary blood flow depends on DBP, and the lower DBP is associated with decreased coronary perfusion. Also, lower DBP with the same SBP represents higher pulse pressure, which indicates vascular stiffness. A recent American Heart Association Scientific Statement cautioned against lowering DBP to less than 60 mm Hg in patients with coronary heart disease.

Pathogenesis

There is no single mechanism that explains the etiology of essential HTN, unlike the mechanisms for secondary HTN. Essential HTN is viewed as a polygenic trait with various subsets of genes that are additive. In contrast to first-degree relatives of normotensive patients, first-degree relatives of hypertensive patients are more likely to develop HTN. African Americans tend to have an earlier onset of HTN and to develop more severe HTN than Caucasians do. Excess body weight, sodium and potassium ingestion, alcohol consumption, and physical activity modify the level of BP in an individual patient.

Four major factors are involved in the pathogenesis of HTN: sodium retention, overactivation of the sympathetic nervous system, overactivation of the renin-angiotension-aldosterone system, and dysfunction of the vascular smooth muscle (Fig. 4). In some forms

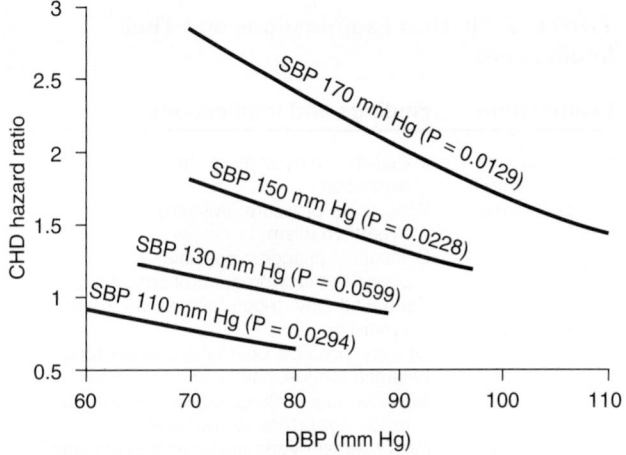

FIGURE 3. Risk of coronary heart disease (CHD) by systolic (SBP) and diastolic (DBP) blood pressure levels. (Reprinted with permission from Franklin SS, Khan SA, Wong ND, et al: Is pulse pressure useful in predicting risk for coronary heart disease? The Framingham Heart Study. Circulation 1999;100:354–360.)

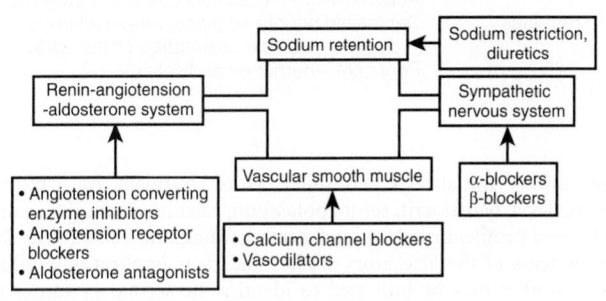

FIGURE 4. Major factors in hypertension and their modulators.

of HTN, the contribution of one factor is dominant. For example, HTN due to pheochromocytoma is caused by the release of catecholamines from the tumor. However, in most cases of HTN, these four factors are present in various degrees. African Americans, diabetics, and elderly patients tend to be more salt sensitive and respond well to diuretics. The major component of HTN in dialysis patients tends to be volume overload. When treating HTN, the contributions of all these factors should be considered in each individual patient. Most patients require a combination of drugs, often three or four drugs, to control BP to goal.

Evaluation

The goals for the initial evaluation are to document that the patient has a sustained elevation in BP, to identify the presence of target organ involvement, to screen for other cardiovascular risk factors (e.g., diabetes mellitus, tobacco use, physical inactivity, obesity, family history), to identify factors that might modify treatment (e.g., asthma), and to diagnose correctable causes of secondary HTN. Table 2 lists the components of the physical examination and their

---

 CURRENT DIAGNOSIS

- Hypertension is defined as a resting blood pressure >140/90 mm Hg on two different occasions.
- A focused history, physical examination, and selected laboratory tests should be performed to identify target organ damage or secondary causes of hypertension.

TABLE 2 Physical Examinations and Their Implications

Examination	Findings and Implications
Blood pressure measurement in both arms	Inequality: coarctation of the aorta, aortic dissection
	Wide pulse pressure: possible hyperthyroidism
	Orthostatic changes: possible pheochromocytoma, autonomic failure
General appearance	Central obesity, moon face, striae: Cushing's syndrome
	Obesity: possible obstructive sleep apnea
	Enlarged tongue, hands, and feet: acromegaly
Fundus	Arteriovenous nicking, copper or silver wire reflex: hypertensive retinopathy
	Papilledema: hypertensive encephalopathy, intracranial hypertension
Neck	Carotid bruits: atherosclerotic disease
	Thyroid enlargement: possible hyperthyroidism
Lungs	Rales: congestive heart failure
Heart	S_4: stiff left ventricle
Abdomen	Palpable kidneys: polycystic kidney disease
	Pulsatile mass: abdominal aneurysm
	Abdominal bruit: possible renal artery stenosis
Extremities	Decreased peripheral pulse: atherosclerotic disease, possible coarctation of the aorta
	Peripheral edema: renal diseases

implications. Initial tests performed before treatment are a fasting glucose level, hematocrit, serum potassium, calcium, creatinine, complete lipid profile, urinalysis, and electrocardiogram. Table 3 lists the components of the laboratory studies and their implications. Additional studies may be indicated to identify the secondary causes of HTN if age (onset before age 30 or after age 55 years), history, physical examination (see Table 2), severity of HTN, or initial laboratory studies (see Table 3) suggest such causes; if BP responds poorly to therapy; if BP begins to increase for unknown reasons after being well controlled, or if the onset of HTN is sudden.

INDICATIONS FOR AMBULATORY BLOOD PRESSURE MONITORING

Ambulatory BP monitoring provides information about BP during daily activities and during sleep. It is the most effective technique for identifying so-called white-coat hypertension (elevated BP at office measurement but normal BP on other occasions), which may be present in as many as 20% of people who are considered to have hypertension by office BP readings. Recent studies suggest that patients with white-coat hypertension likely have a higher risk of developing HTN. Although pharmacologic treatment is not currently indicated for white-coat hypertension, close follow-up is necessary,

TABLE 3 Laboratory Assessment of Hypertension

Findings	Implication
Hypokalemia	Cushing's syndrome, diuretic use, primary hyperaldosteronism
Hyperglycemia	Acromegaly, corticosteroid use, Cushing's syndrome, diabetes mellitus, pheochromocytoma
Hypercholesterolemia	Cushing's syndrome, nephrotic syndrome, hypothyroidism
Increased serum creatinine	Renovascular hypertension, primary renal diseases
Hematuria and proteinuria	Primary renal diseases

TABLE 4 Clinical Situations in Which Ambulatory Blood Pressure Monitoring May Be Helpful

Suspected white-coat hypertension
Apparent drug resistance
Hypotensive symptoms with antihypertensive medication
Episodic hypertension
Autonomic dysfunction
Evaluation of nocturnal decrease in blood pressure as a prognostic factor for target organ disease

Modified from Chobanian AV, Bakris GL, Black HR, et al: Seventh report of Joint National Committee on prevention, detection, evaluation and treatment of high blood pressure. Hypertension 2003;42:1206–1252.

and lifestyle modification should be strongly encouraged. The cardiovascular risk in these patients is considered to be intermediate between normotension and hypertension.

Nighttime BP measured by an ambulatory BP monitor is superior to office BP measurement in predicting cardiovascular events. BP has a reproducible circadian profile, with higher values while awake and active, lower values during rest and sleep, and an early-morning increase for 3 or more hours during the transition from sleep to wakefulness. In most people, BP drops by 10% to 20% during the night (nighttime dipping). Those without nighttime dipping appear to be at higher risk for cardiovascular disease. Recent studies have drawn attention to the importance of controlling not only daytime but also nighttime BP. In this regard, control of the early-morning surge may prove to be particularly important in preventing stroke. The indications for ambulatory BP monitoring are listed in Table 4.

Treatment

TARGET BLOOD PRESSURE

The goal of treating HTN is to reduce morbid events such as renal failure, stroke, and cardiovascular mortality. The target level of BP control differs depending on the presence of comorbid diseases. The recommendations by several organizations are summarized in Table 5.

LIFESTYLE MODIFICATION

Adoption of a healthy lifestyle is a critical part of the treatment of all patients with HTN and prehypertension (Table 6). For overall cardiovascular risk reduction, all patients should be counseled for smoking cessation.

PHARMACOLOGIC THERAPY

There are many classes of antihypertensive medications; they are summarized in Table 7. The algorithm for treatment of HTN recommended by JNC 7 is shown in Figure 5. JNC 7 recommended thiazide diuretics as first-line therapy for most patients with stage 1 disease or as a part of combination therapy for uncomplicated stage 2 HTN. They recommended the adjunctive use of angiotensin receptor blocker, angiotensin-converting enzyme inhibitor (ACEI), β-blocker, or calcium channel blocker (CCB), or some combination of these, as second-line therapy. The basis for this recommendation was that, in trials comparing thiazides with other agents, thiazides were virtually unsurpassed in preventing cardiovascular complications of HTN. However, this recommendation has been challenged by accumulating evidence from more recent studies (Table 8). Increasing evidence indicates that ACEIs and angiotensin receptor blockers may have additional benefits in reducing cardiovascular morbidity and mortality, independent of their BP-lowering effect.

On the other hand, the benefit of β-blockers on reduction of cardiovascular morbidity in uncomplicated HTN has been questioned. Earlier clinical trials on the treatment of HTN used the combination

TABLE 5 Target Goals for Blood Pressure Control

Patient's Condition	JNC 7	NKF	ADA	AHA
No target organ damage and no clinical CV disease	<140/90			
Target organ damage or clinical CV disease	<130/80			<130/80
Diabetes mellitus	<130/80	<130/80	<130/80	
Nondiabetic renal disease	<130/80	<130/80		
Coronary heart disease with left ventricular dysfunction				<120/80

Abbreviations: ADA = American Diabetes Association; AHA = American Heart Association; CV = cardiovascular; JNC 7 = Seventh Report of the Joint National Committee; NKF = National Kidney Foundation.

TABLE 6 Lifestyle Modifications for the Management of Hypertension

Modification	Recommendation	Approximate SBP Reduction (mm Hg)
Weight reduction	Maintain body mass index of 18.5–24.9 kg/m^2	5–20 (10 kg)
DASH diet	Consume a diet rich in fruits, vegetables, and low-fat dairy products with a reduced content of saturated fats and total fat.	8–14
Dietary sodium reduction	Reduce dietary sodium intake to no more than 100 mmol/d (2.4 g sodium or 6 g sodium chloride).	2–8
Physical activity	Engage in regular aerobic exercise, such as brisk walking, at least 30 min/d on most days of the week.	4–9
Moderation of alcohol consumption	Limit consumption to no more than 2 drinks per day for men or 1 drink per day for women.	2–4

Modified from Chobanian AV, Bakris GL, Black HR, et al: Seventh report of Joint National Committee on Prevention, Detection, Evaluation and Treatment of High Blood Pressure. Hypertension 2003;42:1206–1252.
Abbreviations: DASH = Dietary Approaches to Stop Hypertension; SBP = systolic blood pressure.

TABLE 7 Antihypertensive Medications

Drug	Comments
Diuretics (thiazide, loop, and potassium-sparing)	
Hydrochlorothiazide (Oretic)	• Proven to reduce strokes, CHF, and total CV mortality in clinical trials
Chlorthalidone (Hygroton)	• Especially effective for African Americans, the elderly, diabetic patients, patients with systolic heart failure, and patients with excess sodium intake
Chlorothiazide (Diuril)	• Enhance the efficacy of other drug classes and are recommended as a component of combination therapy
Indapamide (Lozol)	
Metolazone (Zaroxolyn)	
Methyclothiazide (Enduron)	• Side effects include hyponatremia, hypokalemia, hyperuricemia
Furosemide (Lasix)	• Essential part of the management of HTN in patients with CKD
Bumetanide (Bumex)[1]	• Torsemide has longer half-life and better bioavailability than furosemide
Torsemide (Demadex)	• All but ethacrynic acid contain a sulfa moiety; use ethacrynic acid in patients with severe sulfa allergy
Ethacrynic acid (Edecrin)[1]	
Amiloride (Midamor)	• Effective adjunctive therapy in resistant HTN
Triamterene (Dyrenium)[1]	
Angiotensin-Converting Enzyme Inhibitors	
Benazepril (Lotensin)	• Reduce mortality in patients with CHF or left ventricular dysfunction and after MI
Lisinopril (Prinivil, Zestril)	• Decrease proteinuria and the rate of progression of CKD
Captopril (Capoten)	• May increase creatinine after initiation of therapy; up to 30% of increase should be accepted
Enalapril (Vasotec)	• Angioedema and chronic dry cough are major side effects
Fosinopril (Monopril)	• May increase serum potassium in patients with CKD
Moexipril (Univasc)	• Contraindicated in pregnancy
Perindopril (Aceon)	
Quinapril (Accupril)	
Ramipril (Altace)	
Trandolapril (Mavik)	
Angiotensin Receptor Blockers	
Candesartan (Atacand)	• Reduce stroke, as well as mortality in CHF and after MI, and rate of progression of diabetic nephropathy in type II diabetes mellitus
Irbesartan (Avapro)	
Olmesartan (Benicar)	• Reduces the development of new-onset diabetes mellitus
Losartan (Cozaar)	• Telmisartan has longest half-life
Valsartan (Diovan)	• Losartan is uricosuric
Telmisartan (Micardis)	• May increase creatinine after initiation of therapy; up to 30% of increase should be accepted
Eprosartan (Teveten)	• Less increase in serum potassium compared with angiotensin-converting enzyme inhibitors
	• Contraindicated in pregnancy

Continued

TABLE 7 Antihypertensive Medications—Cont'd

Drug	Comments
Direct Renin Inhibitor	
Aliskiren (Tekturna)	• BP reduction of about 15 mmHg with maximum daily dose of 300 mg • Reduces proteinuria
Aldosterone Receptor Blockers	
Spironolactone (Aldactone) Eplerenone (Inspra)	• Spironolactone reduces mortality in NYHA class III-IV CHF • Eplerenone reduces mortality after MI
Calcium Channel Blockers (dihydropyridine and nondihydropyridine)	
Amlodipine (Norvasc) Felodipine (Plendil) Nicardipine (Cardene) Nifedipine (Procardia) Nisoldipine (Sular) Isradipine (DynaCirc) Diltiazem (Cardizem) Verapamil (Calan)	• A potent antihypertensive • May cause peripheral edema • Can cause severe bradycardia in combination with a β-blocker • Contraindicated in systolic heart failure
β-Blocker (without or with sympathomimetic activity)	
Atenolol (Tenormin) Betaxolol (Kerlone) Bisoprolol (Zebeta) Metoprolol (Lopressor) Nadolol (Corgard) Nebivolol (Bystolic) Propranolol (Inderal) Acebutolol (Sectral) Penbutolol (Levatol) Pindolol (Visken)	• Reduce mortality in patients with CHF or after MI • Unfavorable metabolic effect (increased blood sugar or cholesterol) • Sudden withdrawal can cause rebound tachycardia or HTN • May cause fatigue, weight gain, depression, claudication, or erectile dysfunction • Nebivolol increases intrinsic nitric oxide and causes vasodilatation
Combined α- and β-Blockers	
• Carvedilol (Coreg) • Labetalol (Trandate)	• Less metabolic adverse effect compared with selective β-blockers
α-Blocker	
Doxazosin (Cardura) Prazosin (Minipress) Terazosin (Hytrin)	• May cause more CHF and stroke compared with thiazide • Not first-line therapy for HTN
Central α2-Agonists and Other Centrally Acting Agents	
Clonidine (Catapres) α-Methyldopa (Aldomet) Reserpine Guanfacine (Tenex)	• Side effects include sedation, dry mouth, and erectile dysfunction • Sudden withdrawal causes rebound HTN and tachycardia • Concomitant use with β-blocker can cause bradycardia • α-Methyldopa can be safely used in pregnancy • Not first-line therapy for HTN
Direct Vasodilators	
Hydralazine (Apresoline) Minoxidil	• Hydralazine can be safely used in pregnancy • Combination of hydralazine and a nitrate reduced mortality in African American with systolic heart failure • Hydralazine can cause lupus-like syndrome • Minoxidil must be used with diuretics and β-blockers • Minoxidil can cause fluid retention, hypertrichosis, and pericardial effusion • Usually used as a last resort for refractory HTN

[1]Not FDA approved for this indication.
Abbreviations: CHF = congestive heart failure, CKD = chronic kidney disease, CV = cardiovascular; HTN = hypertension; MI = myocardial infarction; NYHA = New York Heart Association.

of diuretics and β-blockers, because they were the most commonly used antihypertensive agents at that time. However, more recent studies comparing the effects of various classes of antihypertensive agents have suggested that β-blockers, especially atenolol (Tenormin), may not reduce cardiovascular morbidity and mortality as much as other agents do. The British Society of Hypertension has recommended against use of a β-blocker as first-line treatment for HTN.

The Avoiding Cardiovascular Events Through Combination Therapy in Patients Living with Systolic Hypertension (ACCOMPLISH) trial is a randomized, controlled trial comparing combination therapy for HTN (ACEI + CCB versus ACEI + thiazide). The study showed a relative risk reduction of 19.6% with ACEI + CCB

treatment compared with ACEI + thiazide. This study may influence the recommendation for use of diuretics as the first-line therapy and raises the question of whether diuretics are an essential part of combination therapy.

JNC 8 is currently being drafted and is scheduled for release in 2010. There may be a change in the recommendations for choice of first-line therapy for HTN. The landmark clinical trials on the treatment of HTN and cardiovascular outcomes are summarized in Table 8. For those with comorbidities such as diabetes mellitus, congestive heart failure, or chronic kidney disease, there are compelling indications for the use of certain classes of antihypertensive agents, as shown in Table 9.

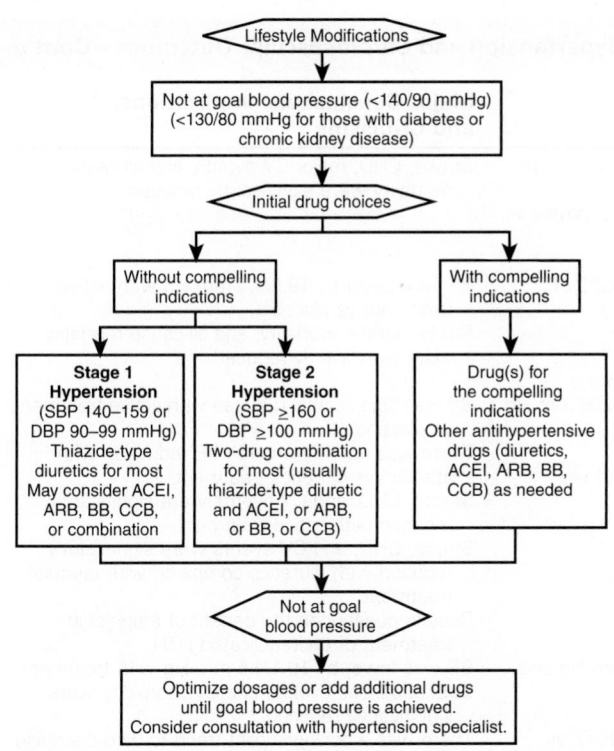

FIGURE 5. Algorithm for treatment of hypertension. (Modified from Chobanian AV, Bakris GL, Black HR, et al: Seventh report of Joint National Committee on prevention, detection, evaluation and treatment of high blood pressure. Hypertension 2003;42:1206–1252.)

Resistant Hypertension

Resistant HTN is defined as BP that cannot be reduced to less than 140/90 mm Hg despite compliance with a regimen of three or more antihypertensive medications in adequate dosage. Although the exact prevalence of resistant HTN is unknown, clinical trials suggest that it involves 20% to 30% of study participants. Before diagnosing resistant HTN, it is important to rule out inaccurate BP measurement (especially use of inappropriately small cuffs for obese patients), white-coat hypertension (by ambulatory BP monitoring or self-monitoring of BP at home), and noncompliance with nonpharmacologic or pharmacologic therapy. Excessive salt intake may contribute to difficulty in controlling BP. Measurement of the 24-hour urine sodium level is useful in estimating the sodium intake. To improve compliance with pharmacologic therapy, once-daily regimens and combination therapies may be useful.

EVALUATION

Patients may be taking prescription and nonprescription drugs or other supplements that can elevate BP (Box 1). Physical examination should be focused on the evaluation of target organ damage and signs of secondary HTN (see Table 2). Laboratory evaluation of resistant HTN should include electrolytes, blood urea nitrogen, creatinine, glucose, urinalysis, and paired plasma renin activity and plasma aldosterone concentration to screen for primary aldosteronism. Even in the setting of ongoing antihypertensive treatment (excluding aldosterone antagonists), the aldosterone-to-renin ratio is an effective screening test for primary hyperaldosteronism, having high negative predictive values. After exclusion of pseudoresistance and offending agents, it is reasonable to consider evaluation for the more common causes of secondary HTN. These include renovascular HTN, renal parenchymal HTN, and obstructive sleep apnea. If a patient has labile HTN or any symptoms suspicious for pheochromocytoma, the best screening test is a plasma metanephrine level. Patients should be cautioned not to ingest acetaminophen for 5 days before having this test.

TABLE 8 The Landmark Clinical Trials* on Treatment of Hypertension and Cardiovascular Outcomes

Trials	Study Design	Major Conclusions, Implications, and Criticisms
VACS on DBP 115–129 mm Hg (JAMA 1967;202:116–122)	143 men with average DBP 115–129 mm Hg Placebo vs HCTZ + reserpine + hydralazine (Apresoline) Follow-up 1.5 y	BP was lower by 43/30 mm Hg with active treatment vs placebo. Mortality, stroke, CHF, and MI were significantly reduced in active treatment group.
VACS on DBP 90–114 mm Hg (JAMA 1970;213:1143–1152)	380 men with average DBP 90–114 mm Hg Placebo vs HCTZ + reserpine + hydralazine Follow-up 5 y	BP was lower by 31.4/18.6 mm Hg with treatment vs placebo. Treatment decreases CV morbidity or mortality from 55% to 18%.
HDFP (JAMA 1979;242:2562–2571)	10,940 participants with HTN Systematic antihypertensive program (stepped care vs referral to community medical therapy) Followup 5 y	BP control was better with stepped care vs referral. Mortality was significantly lower in stepped care group. Mortality was significantly reduced in group with DBP 90–104 mm Hg.
MRC-I (BMJ 1985;291:97–104)	17,354 participants with DBP 90–109 mm Hg Age 35–64 y Bendrofluazide[2] vs propranolol (Inderal) vs placebo Average follow-up 5 y	BP was significantly lower with active treatment. BP control was better with bendrofluazide than with propranolol. Stroke and all CV events were significantly reduced (but not CHD or all-cause mortality) with active treatment vs placebo. Stroke incidence was significantly less with bendrofluazide vs propranolol.
EWPHE (Lancet 1985;1:1349–1354)	840 participants with DBP 90–119 mm Hg and SBP 160–239 mm Hg Age >60 y HCTZ + triamterene (Dyrenium)[1] vs placebo	CV mortality, morbid CV events, and death from MI were significantly reduced with active treatment. There was a nonsignificant decrease in cerebrovascular mortality with active treatment. There was no difference in all-cause mortality.

Continued

TABLE 8 The Landmark Clinical Trials* on Treatment of Hypertension and Cardiovascular Outcomes—Cont'd

Trials	Study Design	Major Conclusions, Implications, and Criticisms
SHEP (JAMA 1991;265:3255–3264)	4736 participants with isolated systolic HTN Age >60 y Chlorthalidone (Hygroton) + atenolol (Tenormin) vs placebo Average follow-up 4.5 y	Stroke, CHD, major CV events, and all-cause mortality were significantly reduced.
STOP (Lancet 1991;338:1281–1285)	1627 participants with SBP 180–230 and DBP >90 mm Hg or DBP 105–120 mm Hg Age 70–84 y β-Blocker + diuretic vs placebo Intervention for 25 mo, follow-up for 65 mo	BP was lower by 19.5/8.1 mm Hg with active treatment vs placebo. Stroke, stroke mortality, and all-cause mortality were significantly reduced.
MRC-II (BMJ 1992;304:405–411)	4396 participants with mean SBP 160–209 mm Hg and mean DBP <115 mm Hg Age 65–74 y Atenolol vs HCTZ + amiloride (Midamor) vs placebo Follow-up for 5 y	BP was significantly reduced with active treatment vs placebo There was no difference in BP reduction with atenolol vs diuretics treatment. Stroke, CHD, and CV events were significantly reduced with active treatment. Stroke, CHD, and CV events were significantly reduced with diuretics compared with atenolol treatment. Results questioned the benefit of atenolol in treatment of uncomplicated HTN.
Syst-EURO (Lancet 1997;350:757–764)	4695 participants with SBP 160–219 mm Hg and DBP <95 mm Hg Age >60 y Nitrendipine[2] ± enalapril (Vasotec) ± HCTZ vs placebo Median follow-up 2 y	BP was lower by 10.1/4.5 mm Hg with treatment. Stroke, cardiac events, and CV morbidity were significantly reduced. There was a nonsignificant trend toward decrease in CV mortality with treatment. There was no difference in all-cause mortality.
HOPE (NEJM 2000;342:145–153)	9297 participants with vascular disease or DM + one other CV risk factor Ramipril (Altace) vs placebo Follow-up 5 y	There no significant difference in BP with treatment vs placebo. There were significant reductions in composite endpoint (MI, stroke, and CV death), CV death, MI, stroke, all-cause mortality, and CHF with treatment.
LIFE (Lancet 2002;359:1004–1010)	1195 participants with HTN, DM, and LVH Losartan (Cozaar) vs atenolol (Tenormin) (thiazide as second-line therapy)	BP was reduced to the same degree in both groups. There were significant reductions in composite CV endpoint (CV death, stroke, and MI), CV death, new-onset DM, and all-cause mortality with losartan vs atenolol.
ALLHAT (JAMA 2002;288:2981–2997)	33,357 participants age ≥55 y with HTN and at least one more CHD risk factor Chlorthalidone vs amlodipine (Norvasc) vs lisinopril (Prinivil) (reserpine or clonidine [Catapres] or atenolol as second step, and hydralazine [Apresoline] as third step) Mean follow-up 4.9 y	There were no differences in rates of CHD, all-cause mortality, or combined CV outcomes. BP was reduced more with chlorthalidone treatment than in the other two groups. This study became the basis for recommending thiazide diuretics as first-line therapy for HTN. Study design was biased against ACEI because a diuretic could not be added.
INVEST (JAMA 2003;290:2805–2816)	22,756 participants with HTN and CHD Age >50 y Atenolol vs verapamil (Calan)	There were no significant differences in BP reduction, composite CV endpoint, MI, stroke, CV mortality, or all-cause mortality. There was significantly less new-onset DM in the verapamil group.
VALUE (Lancet 2004;363:2022–2031)	15,313 participants of age >50 y with HTN and high risk for CV disease Valsartan (Diovan) vs amlodipine (diuretic as second-line agent) Mean follow-up 4.2 y	There was more BP reduction in the amlodipine group. There were no differences in composite CV endpoint or stroke. There was significantly more reduction in MI in the amlodipine group. There was significantly less new-onset DM in the valsartan group. Dose of valsartan was not optimal and should have been higher.
ASCOT-BPLA (Lancet 2005;366:895–906)	19,257 participants with HTN and three or more CV risk factors Atenolol ± bendroflumethiazide[2] vs amlodipine ± perindopril (Aceon)	BP was lower by 2.7/1.9 mm Hg in the amlodipine ± perindopril group. Stroke, CV events, CV mortality, and new-onset DM were significantly less in the amlodipine ± perindopril group.
ON TARGET (NEJM 2008;358:1547–1559)	25,620 participants with CV disease or DM with end-organ damage Ramipril vs telmisartan (Micardis) vs ramipril + telmisartan Median follow-up 56 mo	BP reduction was significantly greater in the telmisartan and combination groups compared with the ramipril group. There were no differences in composite CV endpoints, stroke, MI, CV mortality, or all-cause mortality. There was significantly more renal impairment in the combination group.

Continued

TABLE 8 The Landmark Clinical Trials* on Treatment of Hypertension and Cardiovascular Outcomes—Cont'd

Trials	Study Design	Major Conclusions, Implications, and Criticisms
HYVET (NEJM 2008;358:1887–1898)	3845 participants age >80 y and SBP >160 mm Hg Indapamide (Lozol) ± perindopril vs placebo Follow-up 2 y	BP was lower by 15.0/6.1 mm Hg with active treatment. Deaths from stroke, CV mortality, CHF, and all causes were significantly less with active treatment.
ACCOMPLISH (NEJM 2008;359:2417–2428)	11,506 participants at high risk for CV events Benazepril (Lotensin) + amlodipine vs benazepril + HCTZ Follow-up 3 y	BP was lower by only 0.9/1.1 mm Hg in the benazepril + amlodipine group. There were significantly greater reductions in composite CV endpoints in the benazepril + amlodipine group Results challenge the current guideline of diuretics-based regimen as the first line.

[1]Not FDA approved for this indication.
[2]Not available in the United States.
*Randomized, controlled trials: ACCOMPLISH = Avoiding Cardiovascular Events Through Combination Therapy in Patients Living with Systolic Hypertension; ALLHAT = Antihypertensive and Lipid-Lowering Treatment to Prevent Heart Attack Trial; ASCOT-BPLA = Anglo-Scandinavian Cardiac Outcomes Trial–Blood Pressure Lowering Arm; EWPHE = European Working Party on High Blood Pressure in the Elderly; HDFP = Hypertension Detection and Follow-up Program; HOPE = The Heart Outcomes Prevention Evaluation Study; HYVET = Hypertension in the Very Elderly Trial; INVEST = International Verapamil-Trandolapril Study; LIFE = Losartan Intervention for Endpoint Reduction in Hypertension Study; MRC = Medical Research Council; ON TARGET = Ongoing Telmisartan Alone and in Combination with Ramipril Global End Point Trial; SHEP = Systolic Hypertension in the Elderly Program; STOP = Swedish Trial in Old Patients with Hypertension; Syst-EURO = Systolic Hypertension in Europe Trial; VACS = Veterans Administration Cooperative Study; VALUE: Valsaltan Antihypertensive Long-Term Use Evaluation Trial.
Abbreviations: ACEI = angiotensin-converting enzyme inhibitor; BP = blood pressure; CHD = coronary heart disease; CHF = congestive heart failure; CV = cardiovascular; DBP = diastolic blood pressure; DM = diabetes mellitus; HCTZ = hydrochlorothiazide; HTN = hypertension; LVH: left ventricular hypertrophy; MI = myocardial infarction; SBP = systolic blood pressure.

TABLE 9 Compelling Indications for Individual Drug Classes Based on Clinical Trials and Guidelines

Compelling Indication	Recommended Drugs						Clinical Trial Basis*
	Diuretic	β-Blocker	Angiotensin-Converting Enzyme Inhibitor	Angiotensin Receptor Blocker	Calcium Channel Blocker	Aldosterone Antagonist	
Congestive heart failure	•	•	•	•		•	ACC/AHA Heart Failure Guideline, MERIT-HF, COPERNICUS, CIBIS, SOLVD, AIRE, TRACE, VaHEFT, RALES, CHARM
After myocardial infarction		•	•			•	ACC/AHA Post-Myocardial Infarction Guideline, BHAT, SAVE, CAPRICORN, EPHESUS
High risk for coronary heart disease	•	•	•		•		ALLHAT, HOPE, ANBP2, LIFE, CONVINCE, EUROPA, INVEST
Diabetes mellitus	•	•	•	•	•		NKF-ADA Guideline, UKPDS, ALLHAT
Chronic kidney disease			•	•			NKF Guideline, Captopril Trial, RENAAL, IDNT, REIN, AASK
Stroke prevention	•		•				PROGRESS

Modified from Chobanian AV, Bakris GL, Black HR, et al: Seventh report of the Joint National Committee on Prevention, Detection, Evaluation, and Treatment of High Blood Pressure. Hypertension 2003;42:1206–1252.
*AASK = African American Study of Kidney Disease and Hypertension (Arch Intern Med 2002;162:1636–1643); ACC/AHA = American College of Cardiology/American Heart Association; ADA = American Diabetes Association; AIRE = Acute Infarction Ramipril Efficacy Study (Lancet 1993;342:821–828); ALLHAT = Antihypertensive and Lipid-Lowering Treatment to Prevent Heart Attack Trial; ANBP2 = Australian National Blood Pressure Study 2 (NEJM 2003;348:583–592); BHAT = β-Blocker Heart Attack Trial Research (JAMA 1982;247:1707–1714); CAPRICORN = Carvedilol Post-infarct Survival Controlled Evaluation (Lancet 2001;357:1385–1390); Captopril Trial (NEJM 1993;329:1456–1462); CHARM = Candesartan in Heart Failure–Assessment of Reduction in Morbidity and Mortality Programme (Circulation 2004;110:2618–2626); CIBIS = Cardiac Insufficiency Bisoprolol Study (Circulation 1994;90:1765–1773); CONVINCE = Controlled Onset Verapamil Investigation of Cardiovascular End Points (JAMA 2003;289:2083–2093); COPERNICUS = Carvedilol Prospective Randomized Cumulative Survival Trial (Circulation 2002;106:2194–2199); EPHESUS = Eplerenone Post-AMI Heart Failure Efficacy and Survival Study (NEJM 2003;348;1309–1321); EUROPA = European Trial on Reduction of Cardiac Events with Perindopril in Stable Coronary Artery Disease (Lancet 2003;362:782–788); HOPE = The Heart Outcomes Prevention Evaluation Study; IDNT = Irbesartan Diabetic Nephropathy Trial (NEJM 2001;345:851–860); INVEST = International Verapamil-Trandolapril Study; LIFE = Losartan Intervention for Endpoint Reduction in Hypertension Study; MERIT-HF = Metoprolol CR/XL Randomized Intervention Trial in Congestive Heart Failure (Lancet 1999;353:2001–2007); NKF = National Kidney Foundation; PROGRESS = Perindopril Protection Against Recurrent Stroke Study (Lancet 2001;358:1033–1041); RALES = Randomized Aldactone Evaluation Study (NEJM 1999;341:709–717); REIN = Ramipril Efficacy in Nephropathy Study (Lancet 1997;349:1857–1863); RENAAL = Reduction of End Points in NIDDM with Angiotensin II Antagonist Losartan Study (NEJM 2001;345:861–869); SAVE = Survival and Ventricular Enlargement Trial (NEJM 1992;327:669–677); SOLVD = Studies of Left Ventricular Dysfunction (NEJM 1991;325:293–302); TRACE = Torandolapril Cardiac Evaluation Study (NEJM 1995;333:1670–1676); UKPDS = United Kingdom Prospective Diabetes Study (BMJ 1998;317:713–720); VaHEFT = Valsartan Heart Failure Trial (NEJM 2001;345:1667–1675).

BOX 1 Drugs That Elevate Blood Pressure

- Anabolic steroids
- Nonsteroidal antiinflammatory drugs
- Alcohol
- Amphetamines
- Caffeine
- Tobacco
- Cocaine
- Calcineurin inhibitors: cyclosporine (Sandimmune), tacrolimus (Prograf)
- Disulfiram (Antabuse)
- Erythropoietin (Procrit, Epogen), when hemoglobin is rapidly increasing
- Licorice
- Monoamine oxidase inhibitors, when combined with foods containing tyramine or with amphetamine
- Sympathomimetic drugs such as nasal decongestants or bronchodilators
- Oral contraceptives
- Withdrawal from alcohol, β-blockers, or clonidine

Modified from O'Rorke JE, Richardson WS: Evidence based management of hypertension: What to do when blood pressure is difficult to control. BMJ 2001;322:1229–1232.

TREATMENT OPTIONS

Resistant HTN is almost always multifactorial in etiology. Lifestyle modification is still important and should be strongly encouraged. If a secondary cause is identified, it should be managed appropriately. In most cases of resistant HTN, treatment resistance was in part related to lack of or underuse of diuretic therapy. Addition of or increase in dosage of thiazide diuretics is often effective in controlling BP, and potassium-sparing diuretics (amiloride [Midamor], triamterene [Dyrenium],[1] spironolactone [Aldactone], or eplerenone [Inspra]) can be useful additions to therapy. In patients with a glomerular filtration rate of less than 30 mL/min, a loop diuretic may be necessary. Ultimately, the combination of three or more antihypertensive medications from different classes is usually necessary. Combination of an ACEI or angiotensin receptor blocker with diuretics and a CCB is the most commonly used triple regimen. Addition of a β-blocker, α-blocker, centrally acting agent, or direct vasodilator should be considered on an individual basis.

[1]Not FDA approved for this indication.

CURRENT THERAPY

- Target blood pressure levels are less than 140/90 mm Hg for uncomplicated hypertension; less than 130/80 mm Hg in patients with clinical cardiovascular disease, diabetes mellitus, or chronic kidney disease; and less than 120/80 mm Hg in patients with coronary heart disease or left ventricular dysfunction.
- Lowering blood pressure to the target level is the most important treatment goal to prevent target organ damage. Therapy should be individualized according to underlying comorbidities.
- Certain drug classes have been shown to have potential advantages in decreasing the risks of cardiovascular disease, stroke, and diabetes, and this should be considered when selecting antihypertensive drug therapy.
- Potassium-sparing diuretics are often a useful adjunct to therapy in salt-sensitive patients.
- Consider screening for primary hyperaldosteronism in a patient with resistant hypertension, because this condition is underdiagnosed and accounts for up to 30% of patients with severe hypertension.
- β-Blockers should not be used as initial therapy in patients with uncomplicated hypertension.

Secondary Hypertension

Secondary causes of HTN are summarized in Table 10, along with screening, confirmatory tests, and main treatment options.

Hypertensive Emergencies

Hypertensive emergencies are characterized by severe elevation in BP (>180/120 mm Hg) complicated by evidence of impending or progressive target organ damage. Examples include hypertensive encephalopathy, intracerebral hemorrhage, acute myocardial infarction, acute left ventricular failure with pulmonary edema, unstable angina pectoris, aortic dissection, and eclampsia.

TABLE 10 Secondary Causes of Hypertension

Cause	Screening	Confirmatory Tests	Treatment Options
Obstructive sleep apnea	Continuous pulse oxymetry during sleep	Polysomnography	Continuous positive airway pressure
Renal parenchymal disease	Urinalysis, serum creatinine	Renal ultrasonography, renal biopsy	Depends on the condition
Primary aldosteronism	Aldosterone-to-renin ratio	Salt-loading test, CT or MR imaging of the adrenal glands	Aldosterone antagonists, adrenalectomy for aldosterone-producing adenoma
Renal artery stenosis	CT angiography or MR angiography	Renal angiography	Benefit of angioplasty remains controversial
Pheochromocytoma	Free plasma metanephrine	CT or MR imaging of the adrenal glands	Surgical resection
Cushing's disease	Dexamethasone suppression test	Imaging study and localization test	Surgical resection
Hyperthyroidism	Thyroid function test	—	Depends on the cause
Coarctation of aorta	Blood pressure lower in lower extremities compared with upper extremities	CT angiography	Surgical correction

Abbreviations: CT = computed tomography; MR = magnetic resonance.

TABLE 11 Parenteral Drugs for Treatment of Hypertensive Emergencies

Drug	Dose	Onset of Action	Duration of Action	Adverse Effects	Special Indications
Sodium nitroprusside (Nitropress)	0.25-10 µg/kg/min	Immediate	1–2 min	Cyanide intoxication	Most hypertensive emergencies; caution with high intracranial pressure or azotemia
Nicardipine (Cardene)	5–15 mg/h	5–10 min	15–30 min	Tachycardia, headache	Most hypertensive emergencies except acute heart failure; caution with coronary ischemia
Fenoldopam (Corlopam)	0.1–0.3 µg/kg/min	<5 min	30 min	Tachycardia, headache	Caution with glaucoma
Nitroglycerin	5–100 µg/kg/min	2–5 min	5–10 min	Headache, tolerance with prolonged use	Coronary ischemia
Enalaprilat (Vasotec IV)	1.25-5 mg IV q6h	15–30 min	6–12 h	Precipitous fall in blood pressure in high renin status	Acute left ventricular failure
Hydralazine (Apresoline)	10–20 mg IV	10–20 min	1–4 h	Tachycardia, headache	Eclampsia
Labetalol (Trandate)	20–80 mg IV	5–10 min	3–6 h	Bronchospasm, bradycardia	Most hypertensive emergencies except acute heart failure
Esmolol (Brevibloc)[1]	0.5-2 mg/min	1–2 min	10–30 min	Bradycardia, heart block	Aortic dissection
Phentolamine	5–15 mg IV	1–2 min	10–30 min	Tachycardia, flushing	Catecholamine excess
Clevidipine butyrate (Cleviprex)	1–2 mg/h IV	Immediate	<1 min	Tachycardia	Acute reduction of BP in emergency room and perioperatively in cardiac surgery

Modified from Chobanian AV, Bakris GL, Black HR, et al: Seventh report of Joint National Committee on prevention, detection, evaluation and treatment of high blood pressure. Hypertension 2003;42:1206–1252.
[1]Not FDA approved for this indication.

Patients with hypertensive emergency should be admitted to an intensive care unit and be treated with appropriate parenteral agents (Table 11). Mean arterial BP should be reduced by more than 25% within minutes to 1 hour and then, if the patient is stable, to 160/100 mm Hg within the next 2 to 6 hours. Choice of parenteral agents usually depends on availability and physician comfort with the various agents. Nitroprusside (Nitropress) should be avoided in patients with abnormal renal function.

Hypertensive urgency is defined as BP greater than 180/110 mm Hg without target organ damage. Hypertensive urgency may be treated with short-acting oral medications such as captopril (Capoten), labetalol (Trandate), or clonidine (Catapres). Patients do not always need to be admitted to a hospital, although follow-up is needed within a few days.

Excessive fall in BP may precipitate cerebral, renal, and coronary ischemia. Sublingual nifedipine (Procardia) is no longer recommended for the treatment of hypertensive emergency or urgency.

REFERENCES

Chobanian AV, Bakris GL, Black HR, et al. Seventh report of Joint National Committee on Prevention, Detection, Evaluation and Treatment of High Blood Pressure. Hypertension 2003;42:1206–52.
Rosendorff C, Black HR, Cannon CP, et al. Treatment of hypertension in the prevention and management of ischemic heart disease: A scientific statement from the American Heart Association Council for High Blood Pressure Research and the Councils on Clinical Cardiology and Epidemiology and Prevention. Circulation 2007;115:2761–88.
Calhoun DA, Jones D, Textor S, et al. Resistant hypertension: Diagnosis, evaluation and treatment. A scientific statement from the American Heart Association Professional Education Committee of the Council for High Blood Pressure Research. Hypertension 2008;51:1403–19.
Lewington S, Clarke R, Qizilbash N, et al. Prospective Studies Collaboration: Age-specific relevance of usual blood pressure to vascular mortality: A meta-analysis of individual data for one million adults in 61 prospective studies. Lancet 2002;360:1903–13.

Acute Myocardial Infarction

Method of
Guy S. Reeder, MD, and Abhiram Prasad, MD

The diagnosis of myocardial infarction (MI) is confirmed by a typical rise and fall in biochemical markers of myocardial necrosis with at least one of the following: ischemic symptoms, changes on the electrocardiogram (ECG) of ischemia (ST elevation or depression), development of pathologic Q waves, or percutaneous coronary intervention (PCI).

Incidence

More than 1 million patients suffer an MI every year in the United States. Despite a 50% decline in cardiovascular death due to advances in diagnosis and management related to MI since the 1970s, MI remains a fatal event in one out of three patients.

Pathophysiology

MI results from reduction in myocardial perfusion sufficient to cause cell necrosis. Atherosclerotic plaque rupture or erosion allows the thrombogenic lipid core to be exposed with complete or partial thrombotic occlusion. Epicardial occlusion may also be accompanied by downstream microvascular constriction. Coronary spasm is an uncommon cause of MI, and spontaneous coronary artery dissection, coronary embolus, and hypercoagulable states are among the rare causes.

Clinical Presentation

Patients with MI usually present with central pressure-like chest discomfort that can radiate to the arms, neck, or back. This is often associated with nausea, diaphoresis, and dyspnea. At least 20% of MIs are

TABLE 1 Killip Class and Hospital Mortality

Killip Class	Clinical Classification	Mortality (%)
I	No heart failure	6
II	Mild heart failure, rales, S_3, congestion on chest radiograph	17
III	Pulmonary edema	38
IV	Cardiogenic shock	81

Data from Killip T 3rd, Kimball JT: Treatment of myocardial infarction in a coronary care unit. A two year experience with 250 patients. Am J Cardiol 1967;20(4):457–464.

clinically unrecognized due to atypical presentation without chest pain, especially in elderly, diabetic, or postoperative patients. Symptoms include back pain, epigastric pain, syncope, dyspnea, or confusion. The differential diagnosis of acute MI includes aortic dissection, acute pulmonary embolus, perimyocarditis, musculoskeletal pain, esophagitis, peptic ulcer disease, cholecystitis, biliary colic, and pancreatitis.

Physical examination is often normal. Some patients have signs of left ventricular (LV) dysfunction including tachycardia, pulmonary rales, and third heart sound. Infarction or ischemia leading to papillary muscle dysfunction or rupture can lead to a murmur of mitral regurgitation. Patients with right ventricular (RV) infarction might have an elevated jugular venous pressure and a positive Kussmaul sign, and those with severe LV dysfunction present with cardiogenic shock. An estimation of prognosis at presentation is possible using the Killip classification or the TIMI (Thombolysis in Myocardial Infarction [trial] risk scores (Table 1).

Evaluation of Suspected Acute Myocardial Infarction

The initial evaluation of a patient with suspected MI should include a focused history, physical examination, ECG, blood sample for cardiac biomarkers, and chest radiograph. The patient's rhythm should be continuously monitored and intravenous access should be established.

ELECTROCARDIOGRAM

A 12-lead ECG should be performed within 10 minutes of arrival into an emergency department. In addition, posterior leads (V7-V9) and leads V3R and V4R should be used in patients with suspected posterior and RV infarctions, respectively. The ECG findings differentiate patients with ST elevation MI (STEMI) and ST depression MI (NSTEMI) (Fig. 1). Patients with STEMI require immediate reperfusion therapy, but those with NSTEMI do not unless there is ongoing ischemic pain or hemodynamic instability.

The ECG diagnosis of MI is difficult in the presence of left bundle branch block (LBBB). However, the presence of ST segment elevation of greater than 1 mm concordant with a QRS complex, ST segment depression greater than 1 mm in leads V1 to V3, or ST segment elevation greater than 5 mm discordant with a QRS complex supports the diagnosis.

SERUM MARKERS

Serum biomarkers of myocardial necrosis include troponins, MB isoforms of creatine kinase (CK-MB), creatine kinase (CK), and myoglobin. Measurement of troponin has replaced other biomarkers due to higher sensitivity, specificity, and prognostic value. Measurements of troponin I or T should be performed at presentation and 6 to 9 hours after the onset of symptoms. If troponin levels are elevated, confirmation with CK-MB may be performed to determine acuteness, because troponin can remain elevated for 10 to 15 days after MI. Likewise, CK-MB is useful for detecting reinfarction during a period of persistent troponin elevations from the initial event. Troponin and CK-MB may be elevated following cardiac surgery, myopericarditis, PCI,

tachyarrhythmias, and cardioversion. Troponins may be elevated following pulmonary embolus and decompensated congestive heart failure. All cardiac markers may be initially negative early in acute MI; treatment must never be withheld based on negative initial biomarkers.

Treatment

ST ELEVATION MYOCARDIAL INFARCTION

Initial Approach

These goals should be achieved expeditiously and simultaneously (see Fig. 1): relief of pain, initiation of reperfusion and ancillary therapy, and assessment and treatment of hemodynamic abnormalities. Pain relief is best achieved with oxygen (2 L nasal cannula), nitroglycerin, and morphine sulfate. Patients with ST segment elevation or new LBBB with symptoms for 12 hours or less are candidates for reperfusion therapy.

Reperfusion Therapy

The diagnosis of STEMI mandates immediate reperfusion. PCI is preferred, but it is not promptly available in many areas. Fibrinolytic therapy is widely available, but it is slightly less effective in randomized trials and carries a higher risk of hemorrhagic stroke. The decision regarding which therapy to employ should be made on the basis of a written institution-specific protocol that considers symptom duration, availability of PCI locally, time to transfer to a PCI facility, and fibrinolytic contraindications (Fig. 2). In general, patients presenting within 3 hours of symptom onset derive a large benefit from fibrinolytics; if transfer time to a PCI facility results in a door-to-balloon time of longer than 90 minutes, fibrinolysis is preferred. Guidelines for door-to-needle (30 min) and door-to-balloon (90 min) times recommended by the American College of Cardiology and American Heart Association (ACC/AHA) are one of a number of quality indicators for acute MI care.

Fibrinolytic Therapy

Fibrinolytic therapy should be administered within 30 minutes of arrival to the emergency department. The greatest benefit is seen when this is performed within the first 4 hours of onset of pain resulting in an absolute 3% reduction in mortality, but it is associated with a small (0.4%) increase in stroke rate. There is a 2% absolute reduction in mortality rate for every hour saved in administration of therapy, and no benefit is seen after 12 hours of symptom duration. A benefit is observed in all age groups, including those with prior MI and diabetes, as well as in patients presenting with hypotension and tachycardia. Age older than 75 years, Killip class higher than II, resting tachycardia, hypotension, anterior MI location, and time to reperfusion longer than 4 hours are useful predictors of early mortality, ranging from 0.8% with none of these factors to more than 36% for all (Table 2). Box 1 lists indications and contraindications for fibrinolysis.

Table 3 lists the currently available fibrinolytic agents. These differ primarily with respect to plasma half-life; the longest-acting agent, tenecteplase, requires a single bolus injection. Intravenous heparin must be administered concurrently to reduce the risk of late reocclusion of infarct-related artery.

Primary Percutaneous Coronary Intervention

Although fibrinolytic therapy is easy to administer and widely available, it provides early reperfusion in only 80% of patients and is often not administered due to perceived or actual contraindications in a significant number of patients. In contrast, primary PCI has only rare contraindications and leads to higher reperfusion (approximately 90%). Randomized trials performed in high-volume academic centers comparing fibrinolytic therapy with PCI for acute MI have demonstrated approximately 30% reduction in mortality and reinfarction rates and a significant reduction in cerebrovascular accidents with PCI. Stent deployment during acute MI leads to similar early outcome compared with balloon angioplasty, but it reduces restenosis rates and target vessel revascularization.

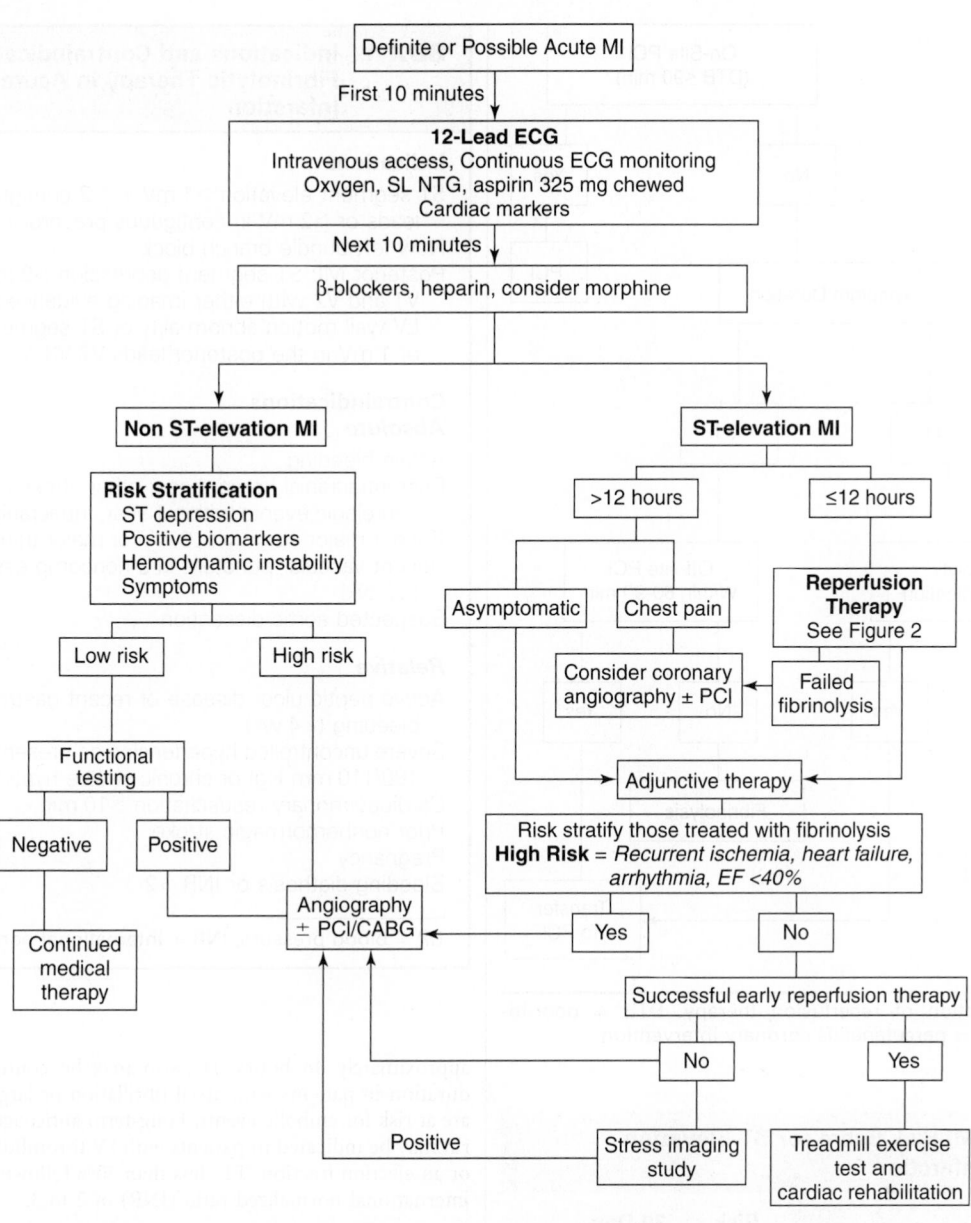

FIGURE 1. Definite or possible acute myocardial infarction (MI). CABG = coronary artery bypass graft; ECG = electrocardiogram; EF = ejection fraction; PCI = percutaneous coronary intervention; SL NTG = sublingual nitroglycerin.

Primary PCI should be performed within 60 to 90 minutes of arrival to the hospital by an interventional cardiologist who performs at least 75 procedures a year in a center that has a volume of at least 200 procedures a year and has cardiac surgery capabilities. PCI should also be considered in specific patient populations listed in Box 2. Transfer from one hospital to another for primary PCI should only be considered if it can be achieved within 60 to 90 minutes (total door-to-balloon time); otherwise, fibrinolytic therapy should be administered without delay.

Adjunct Therapy for STEMI

Agents proved to reduce mortality in patients with STEMI include aspirin, β-blockers, statins, and angiotensin-converting enzyme (ACE) inhibitors (Table 4).

Aspirin

Unless there is history of allergic reaction, aspirin 325 mg should be administered immediately on the patient's arrival to the emergency room and continued indefinitely at a dose of at least 81 mg/day. Chewed aspirin has the most rapid onset of action due to absorption

from the buccal mucosa, with inhibition of platelets within minutes. Clopidogrel (Plavix) may be administered to patients with an aspirin allergy.

Clopidogrel

is a thienopyridine that blocks the platelet ADP receptor, resulting in reduced platelet aggregation. A loading dose of 300 to 600[3] mg is typically administered at the time of PCI. Some data suggest a benefit of 75 to 300 mg administered with thrombolytic therapy; the lower dose might reduce the bleeding risk in patients older than 75 years. Maintenance dose is 75 mg/day; duration of therapy in PCI with stenting is defined by type of stent. Duration of therapy when administered with fibrinolytics is not well established.

Unfractionated Heparin

Unfractionated heparin has been shown to decrease reocclusion following fibrinolytic therapy, and it should be administered at the time of fibrinolytic infusion. A bolus of 60 U/kg (maximum 4000 units) of

---

[3]Exceeds dosage recommended by the manufacturer.

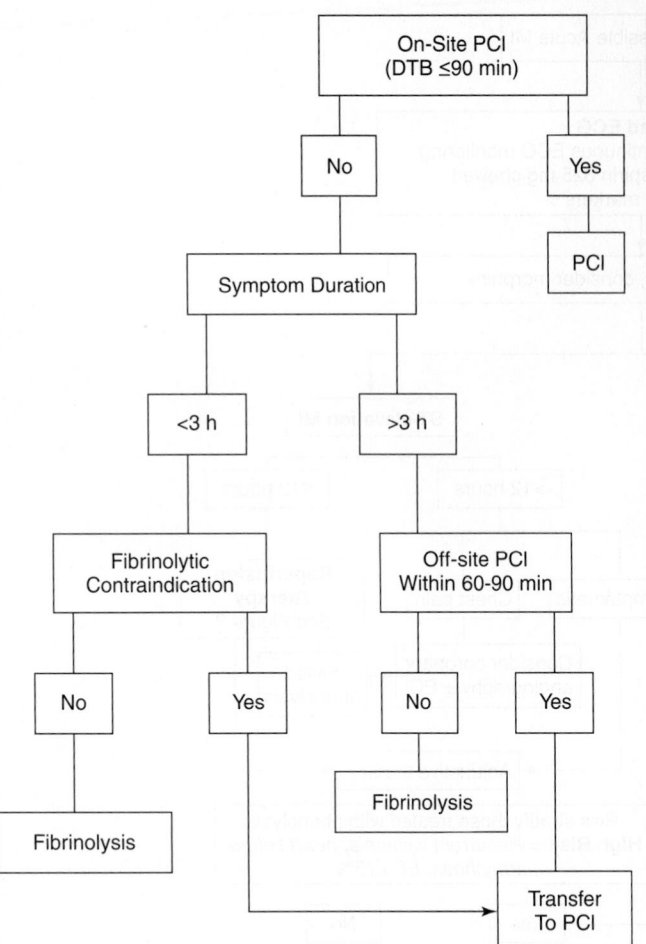

FIGURE 2. Selection of reperfusion therapy. DTB = door-to-balloon time; PCI = percutaneous coronary intervention.

BOX 1   Indications and Contraindications for Fibrinolytic Therapy in Acute Myocardial Infarction

Indications

ST segment elevation ≥1 mV in ≥2 contiguous limb leads or ≥2 mV in contiguous precordial leads

New left bundle branch block

Posterior MI: ST segment depression >2 mV in leads V1 and V2 with either imaging evidence of posterior LV wall motion abnormality or ST segment elevation of 1 mV in the posterior leads V7-V9

Contraindications
Absolute

Active bleeding

Prior intracranial hemorrhage; other strokes or neurologic events within 1 year; intracranial neoplasm

Recent major surgery (<6 wk) or major trauma (<2 wk)

Recent vascular puncture in a noncompressible site (<2 wk)

Suspected aortic dissection

Relative

Active peptic ulcer disease or recent gastrointestinal bleeding (<4 wk)

Severe uncontrolled hypertension on presentation (BP > 180/110 mm Hg) or chronic severe hypertension

Cardiopulmonary resuscitation >10 min

Prior nonhemorrhagic stroke

Pregnancy

Bleeding diathesis or INR >2

BP = blood pressure; INR = international normalized ratio.

TABLE 2   TIMI Risk Score for ST-Elevation Myocardial Infarction

Risk Factor	Points	Risk Score	30-Day Mortality (%)
Age ≥ 75 y	3	0	0.8
Age 65–74 y	2	1	1.6
Diabetes or hypertension	1	2	2.2
Systolic BP <100 mm Hg	3	3	4.4
Heart rate >100/min	2	4	7.3
Killip class II-IV	2	5	12.4
Anterior MI or LBBB	1	6	16.1
Weight <67 kg	1	7	23.4
Time to treatment >4 h	1	8	26.8
		>8	35.9

Data from Morrow DA, Antman EM, Charlesworth A, et al: TIMI risk score for ST-elevation myocardial infarction: A convenient, bedside, clinical score for risk assessment at presentation: An intravenous nPA for treatment of infarcting myocardium early II trial substudy. Circulation 2000;102:2031–2037.

BP = blood pressure; TIMI = Thombolysis in Myocardial Infarction (trial).

---

unfractionated heparin followed by an infusion of 7–12 U/kg/h may be used to initiate therapy. The activated partial thromboplastin time (aPTT) should be checked at 4 to 6 hours after initiation of heparin and then every 6 to 8 hours. The aPTT should be maintained between 50 and 70 seconds, and therapy should be continued for approximately 48 hours. Heparin may be continued for a longer duration in patients with atrial fibrillation or large anterior MI who are at risk for embolic events. Long-term anticoagulation with warfarin may be indicated in patients with LV thrombus, atrial fibrillation, or an ejection fraction (EF) less than 30% following MI with a target international normalized ratio (INR) of 2 to 3.

Low-Molecular-Weight Heparin

Low-molecular-weight heparins (LMWHs) are produced by fragmentation of unfractionated heparin. These agents have advantages over unfractionated heparin, including a more predictable dose response, greater bioavailability, no need for laboratory monitoring, and a lower rate of thrombocytopenia. LMWHs possess greater anti-Xa activity relative to anti-IIa (antithrombin) activity. This may be of potential benefit, because factor Xa generation occurs several steps earlier in the coagulation cascade.

Enoxaparin (Lovenox) is the most widely studied LMWH in STEMI and acute coronary syndromes. Trials of enoxaparin in conjunction with fibrinolysis have shown benefit in terms of preventing reinfarction, no significant mortality advantage, and somewhat increased risk of bleeding. LMWH should be avoided in men with creatinine higher than 2.5 or women with creatinine higher than 2.0.

Glycoprotein IIb/IIIa Antagonists

Platelet glycoprotein IIb/IIIa receptor inhibitors block the final common pathway in platelet aggregation. Currently available drugs include the chimeric monoclonal antibody abciximab (Reopro) and the nonantibody agents tirofiban (Aggrastat) and eptifibatide (Integrilin). Several studies have investigated the role of glycoprotein IIb/IIIa antagonists in STEMI and demonstrated a reduction in the composite endpoints of death, MI, and target vessel revascularization in

TABLE 3 Comparison of Fibrinolytics

Characteristic	Alteplase (Activase) (tPA)	Reteplase (Retavase) (rPA)	Tenecteplase (TNKase)
Dose	15-mg bolus, then 0.75 mg/kg over 30 min (max 50 mg), then 0.5 mg/kg over 60 min (max 35 mg)	10 + 10 MU double bolus 30 min apart	0.5 mg/kg single bolus (max 50 mg)
Plasma half-life	4–6 min	18 min	20 min
Fibrin specificity	++	+	+++
Plasminogen activation	Direct	Direct	Direct
Antigenicity	No	No	No

max = maximum; MU = megaunit; rPA = recombinant plasminogen activator; tPA = tissue plasminogen activator.

BOX 2 Indications for Percutaneous Coronary Intervention in Acute Myocardial Infarction

Failed fibrinolysis (rescue PCI)
Contraindication to fibrinolytics
Shock or markers of increased mortality such as TIMI risk score ≥5 or Killips classes III-IV
Nondiagnostic ECG changes with ongoing pain or hemodynamic instability
As a preferred strategy when available promptly

ECG = electrocardiogram; PCI = percutaneous coronary intervention; TIMI = Thrombolysis in Myocardial Infarction (trial).

---

patients treated with primary PCI. This benefit is due to higher TIMI-3 flow rate in the infarct-related artery, both before and after the coronary intervention procedure. Initial studies investigating the use of glycoprotein IIb/IIIa receptor antagonists with fibrinolytic agents suggested higher TIMI-3 flow rates, but phase III trials have failed to show a superiority of combined therapy over fibrinolytic therapy alone. Thus, intravenous glycoprotein IIb/IIIa inhibitors are indicated in patients being reperfused with PCI, but no indication exists for their combination with fibrinolytic therapy.

β-Adrenergic Antagonist Drugs

Early intravenous β-blocker therapy—metoprolol (Lopressor) 5 mg IV × 3 q5 min, followed by oral administration—is indicated in all patients without contraindications. In patients with borderline LV function, a test dose of intravenous esmolol can be given to assess tolerance to β-blockade. Patients with relative contraindications, such as chronic obstructive pulmonary disease or insulin-dependent diabetes, appear to derive benefit from treatment. Major contraindications to β-blockade include moderate to severe asthma, second- or third-degree atrioventricular block, severe bradycardia, hypotension, and pulmonary edema. β-Blockade should be withheld in these settings.

Angiotensin-Converting Enzyme Inhibitors

ACE activity is markedly increased at the edge of the infarct, and clinical trials have confirmed that ACE inhibitors reduce deleterious LV remodeling. The optimal selection of patients for ACE-inhibitor therapy remains controversial, but the most cost-effective approach is to selectively treat high-risk patients (those with impaired LV function or an anterior MI). However, demonstration of asymptomatic LV dysfunction requires bedside imaging studies, and selection of patients by infarct location alone might not result in early identification of all patients with significant LV dysfunction. Thus, unless the infarct is known to be small, it may be most reasonable to consider initial administration of ACE inhibitors in a nonselective fashion (i.e., in all patients with an acute MI) and then withdraw therapy later based on the absence of high-risk features. Exclusion criteria include allergy to ACE inhibitors, hypotension (systolic blood pressure [BP] <90 mm Hg), shock, history of bilateral renal artery stenosis, and prior worsening of renal function with ACE inhibitors.

ACE inhibitors have a class effect and should be administered orally, initially at low doses, with careful monitoring of the BP. Treatment should be continued indefinitely in patients with symptomatic heart failure or asymptomatic LV dysfunction (LVEF <45%), hemodynamically significant mitral regurgitation, or hypertension. Angiotensin receptor blockers (ARBs) may be used in patients intolerant of ACE inhibitors.

HMG CoA Reductase Inhibitors

Low-density lipoprotein (LDL) cholesterol plays a critical role in the pathogenesis of atherosclerosis. Lipid lowering with HMG CoA (3-hydroxy-3-methyl-glutaryl coenzyme A) reductase inhibitors

---

TABLE 4 Adjunctive Therapies That Reduce Mortality in Patients with Myocardial Infarction

Drug	Indication	Suggested Drugs and Initial Dose	NNT
Aspirin	All	160–325 mg/day	42 patients for 1 mo
β-Blocker	All except patients with moderate or severe asthma, cardiogenic shock, pulmonary edema or ≥second-degree AV block	Metoprolol (Lopressor) 5 mg IV × 3 (at 5-min intervals), and then 50 mg PO bid or Esmolol (Brevibloc) bolus 500 μg/kg and infuse at 50 μg/kg/min	38 patients for 2 y
HMG CoA reductase inhibitors	All	Simvastatin (Zocor) or atorvastatin (Lipitor) 40–80 mg/day	30 patients for 5 y
ACE Inhibitors	Anterior MI, EF <40%, diabetes May consider using in all CAD patients	Captopril (Capoten) 6.25 mg PO tid, increasing at 6h-8h intervals to a maximum of 50 mg tid or Lisinopril (Prinivil, Zestril) 2.5-10 mg PO qd Maintain systolic BP >90 mm Hg	20 patients for 3.5 y

ACE, angiotensin-converting enzyme; AV = atrioventricular; BP = blood pressure; CAD = coronary artery disease; EF = ejection fraction; HMG CoA = 3-hydroxy-3-methyl-glutaryl coenzyme A; MI = myocardial infarction; NNT = number needed to treat to save one life.

(statins) are effective in secondary prevention by reducing mortality, recurrent infarction, ischemia, and heart failure. Preliminary studies indicate that treatment with statins can also lead to modest reductions in recurrent ischemia and infarction during acute coronary syndromes. Thus, a lipid profile should be assessed within 24 hours of the MI (before the inflammatory response from the MI leads to a temporary reduction in lipids) or 6 to 8 weeks later. Either way, improved outcomes have been demonstrated by early intensive statin therapy started in the hospital, with a target LDL cholesterol of 60 to 85 mg/dL.

Nitrates

Potential benefits of nitrate therapy include increased perfusion of ischemic zones, decrease in oxygen consumption, improved diastolic function, and enhanced collateral flow. The infusion of intravenous nitroglycerin should be initiated at 5 to 10 µg/min and gradually increased. The goal should be a 10% reduction in systolic BP in normotensive patients and approximately a 30% reduction in systolic pressure in hypertensive patients. Nitrates should be used with caution in patients with RV infarction or dehydration (who are preload dependent) to avoid excessive hypotension. Long-acting oral nitrates may be indicated with significant residual ischemia or heart failure. A nitrate-free interval of 8 to 12 hours must be provided to prevent nitrate tolerance.

Calcium Channel Blockers

Calcium channel blockers have vasodilative, antianginal, and antihypertensive actions. Calcium channel blockers do not reduce mortality in patients with MI and are not recommended for routine therapy or secondary prevention. In patients in whom β-adrenergic antagonists are contraindicated, verapamil or diltiazem may be appropriate as an alternative.

Antiarrhythmic Therapy

Potentially fatal ventricular arrhythmia occurs most commonly in the first 48 hours after an MI, and numerous trials have investigated the effects of antiarrhythmic agents on mortality and the incidence of ventricular fibrillation. Prophylactic therapy with antiarrhythmic drugs has been shown to be ineffective. Lidocaine may be used for 24 to 48 hours to treat ventricular tachycardia and following resuscitation for ventricular fibrillation. Amiodarone (Cordarone) is safe to use in the setting of MI and is the drug of choice for treating symptomatic ventricular arrhythmia.

Implantable Cardioverter-Defibrillator

ICD implantation reduces the occurrence of sudden death in certain high-risk patients such as those with late (>24 hours after the onset of symptoms) sustained ventricular tachycardia and ventricular fibrillation and in patients with EF persistently less than 30% to 35%. An ICD may also be beneficial in patients with late nonsustained ventricular tachycardia who have an EF of less than 40% and ventricular tachycardia induced during an electrophysiology study. ICD implantation should be considered if the patient is judged to be at continuous high risk for ventricular arrhythmia after revascularization for significant spontaneous or inducible ischemia.

NON–ST-ELEVATION MYOCARDIAL INFARCTION

Incompletely occluding coronary thrombus, or extensive collateral arterial supply (or both) is the underlying pathology of NSTEMI. More common than STEMI, especially in the elderly, the presentation is identical except for the absence of ST elevation.

Initial Therapy

Management differs from STEMI in that urgent reperfusion therapy is not indicated; the administration of fibrinolytics may be harmful. Instead, the focus of initial therapy is intensive medical stabilization with antiplatelet and antithrombotic agents to prevent clot propagation, nitrates and β-blockers for anti-ischemic effects, statins for cholesterol lowering, and other agents to control pain and hemodynamic

TABLE 5　TIMI Risk Score for Unstable Angina and Non–ST-Elevation Myocardial Infarction

Risk Factor	Points	Risk Score	14-Day D, MI, Revascularization
Age ≥65	1	1	4.7
Three risk factors	1	2	8.3
Stenosis ≥50%	1	3	13.2
ST deviation	1	4	19.9
Angina × 2/24 h	1	5	26.2
ASA use	1	6	
Elevated biomarkers	1	7	40.9

ASA = aspirin; MI = myocardial infarction.

compromise. For patients with continued pain or hemodynamic deterioration, immediate angiography and PCI are indicated. All other patients should undergo risk stratification (see Fig. 1). The TIMI risk score for unstable angina and NSTEMI (Table 5) allows separation of low risk from intermediate and high risks. Low-risk patients are suitable for functional testing, whereas all others undergo elective catheterization plus PCI in 4 to 48 hours.

Adjunct Therapy

In addition to aspirin, clopidogrel is beneficial in NSTEMI. The benefit must be weighed against the bleeding risk if coronary bypass surgery is performed within 5 days of drug administration. We elect to not administer clopidogrel until establishment of coronary anatomy and decision regarding need for bypass surgery. Once started, the drug has shown benefit for 9 to 12 months.

Several large studies have investigated the role of glycoprotein IIb/IIIa antagonists in patients with unstable angina or NSTEMI. Overall, the studies using tirofiban and eptifibatide have demonstrated a small but significant risk reduction in composite endpoints, with the greatest benefit in patients with diabetes, patients with troponin elevations, and patients undergoing PCI. In contrast, the GUSTO-IV ACS (Global Utilization of Strategies To open Occluded coronary arteries trial IV in Acute Coronary Syndromes) trial did not demonstrate any benefit of abciximab in the treatment of NSTEMI. Thus, these studies lead us to recommend that glycoprotein IIb/IIIa receptor antagonists should not be routinely used in all patients with NSTEMI, but they should be considered for high-risk patients requiring PCI, especially those with diabetes, resting ST depression, or elevated troponin.

Enoxaparin has shown modest outcome benefits over unfractionated heparin in patients with NSTEMI. This benefit may be counterbalanced by the inability to measure drug effect if PCI is performed. In our center, where PCI is readily available, we prefer unfractionated heparin.

Bivalirudin (Angiomax) is a direct thrombin inhibitor that compares favorably with unfractionated heparin plus glycoprotein IIb/IIIa inhibition in patients with acute coronary syndromes undergoing PCI. It is also commonly used in the catheterization laboratory for patients with a history of heparin-induced thrombocytopenia. We reserve its use for the latter case.

Fondaparinux (Arixtra) is a synthetic pentasaccharide that binds to antithrombin and compares favorably with enoxaparin in patients with NSTEMI.

The use of β-blockers and statins is similar to that in STEMI. The role of ACE inhibitors is less well defined for all patients, but they are selectively useful for treatment of hypertension and in those with LVEF less than 45%.

Meta-analyses of trials of early elective catheterization and PCI versus initial medical therapy have shown lower rates of mortality, recurrent MI, and rehospitalization for recurrent unstable angina after an early invasive approach. Benefits are predominantly limited to higher-risk patients, especially those older than 65 years and those who have resting ST depression or elevated biomarkers.

SPECIAL SITUATIONS

Cardiogenic Shock

Cardiogenic shock occurs in approximately 7% of patients with MI and has a mortality rate of approximately 80%. It is characterized by systemic hypotension (systolic BP <80 mm Hg), reduced cardiac index (<2.2 L/min/m^2), and elevated pulmonary artery wedge pressure (> 16 mm Hg). Initial stabilization should be attempted with inotropes such as dopamine, dobutamine, or epinephrine together with intraaortic balloon counterpulsation. Intraaortic balloon counterpulsation reduces cardiac afterload, improves coronary artery perfusion, and increases systolic BP. However, these interventions do not reduce mortality. Early angiography and revascularization with either PCI or surgery have a significant effect in reducing mortality and should be considered in patients with cardiogenic shock.

Right Ventricular Infarction

RV infarction occurs in approximately 40% of patients with acute inferior MI; however, hemodynamically significant RV dysfunction is less common. Patients usually present with an elevated jugular venous pressure without hemodynamic compromise. Some patients present with hypotension, particularly after the administration of vasodilators such as nitrates. On physical examination, patients might have an elevated jugular venous pressure, Kussmaul sign, clear lungs, and a right-sided gallop. The diagnosis is strengthened by demonstrating the presence of at least 1 mm of ST segment elevation in leads V1, V3R, or V4R or RV dysfunction by echocardiography. The treatment is supportive, with intravenous fluids and inotropic support with dopamine or dobutamine if needed. These interventions may be tailored using guidance from hemodynamic data obtained from a pulmonary artery catheter. Patients with RV infarction are more likely to have complications with bradycardia or atrioventricular block that can require temporary atrial and ventricular pacing. Most patients improve spontaneously after 48 to 72 hours. Patients with shock might benefit from early revascularization with PCI to the right coronary artery.

Mechanical Complications of Acute Myocardial Infarction

Successful reperfusion therapy leads to lower complication rates. Table 6 lists the major ischemic, mechanical, and electrical complications of acute MI and their management.

TABLE 6 Complications Associated with Acute Myocardial Infarction

Complications	Clinical Features	Treatment
Ischemic		
Postinfarction angina	Recurrent chest pain after resolution of symptoms	Medical therapy or revascularization
Infarct extension	Recurrent chest pain and biomarker elevation	Urgent angiography and revascularization
Mitral regurgitation	Murmur, heart failure	Treat ischemia, ACE inhibitors Consider revascularization with or without mitral valve repair
Mechanical		
LV dysfunction (see Killip classification)	Dyspnea, hypoxia, elevated jugular venous pressure, third heart sound, rales	Diuretics, vasodilators Consider revascularization Treat associated mechanical complications
Cardiogenic shock	See text	Inotropes and IABP Urgent revascularization
Papillary muscle rupture	New mitral regurgitation, pulmonary edema, or shock 2–7 days after MI	IABP Emergency mitral valve replacement or repair
Myocardial rupture (lateral wall most often involved)	More common in women, elderly, non-reperfused patients, and inferior MI 3–5 days post MI Recurrent chest pain, pericarditis, vomiting, agitation, bradycardia	Emergency surgery
Ventricular septal defect	Equally prevalent with anterior or inferior MI New pansystolic mumur, heart failure, shock	IABP Urgent surgery
Electrical		
Second-degree AV block Mobitz type I	Asymptomatic, syncope More common after inferior MI	Observe Avoid AV node–blocking drugs
Second-degree AV block Mobitz type II	Asymptomatic presyncope/syncope Presyncope/syncope	Observe if asymptomatic and temporary pacing with symptoms after inferior MI
Third-degree AV block		Temporary ± permanent pacing after anterior MI
Atrial fibrillation/flutter	Asymptomatic, palpitations, heart failure	IV heparin for thromboembolic risk DC cardioversion for ischemia or hemodynamic compromise β-Blockers and digoxin for rate control in asymptomatic patients Sotalol or amiodarone for recurrent episodes
Ventricular premature complexes	Asymptomatic, palpitations	No antiarrhythmics indicated β-Blockers Correct electrolytes
Ventricular tachycardia	Hemodynamic collapse, syncope, palpitations, sudden cardiac death	CPR and DC cardioversion for hemodynamic collapse; otherwise, IV lidocaine or amiodarone
Ventricular fibrillation	Sudden cardiac death	Treat associated ischemia and heart failure Correct electrolytes Consider revascularization If >24 hours after MI, consider EPS and ICD
Torsades de pointes	Hemodynamic collapse, sudden cardiac death	CPR and DC cardioversion Correct hypokalemia or hypomagnesemia Consider temporary pacing for bradycardia or IV phenytoin

ACE = angiotensin-converting enzyme; AV = strioventricular; CPR = cardiopulmonary resuscitation; DC = direct current; EPS = electrophysiologic study; IABP = intraaortic balloon counterpulsation; ICD = implantable cardioverter-defibrillator; LV = left ventricular; MI = myocardial infarction.

Cardiac Rehabilitation and Secondary Prevention

Cardiac rehabilitation should be initiated before discharge from the hospital, with the goals of improving quality of life, facilitating return to normal activities, encouraging regular exercise, and promoting secondary prevention. Secondary prevention is aimed at smoking cessation and at aggressive dietary and pharmacologic treatment for hyperlipidemia, hypertension, and diabetes mellitus. Patients with uncomplicated MI may drive a car after 1 to 2 weeks and return to work at 2 to 4 weeks, whereas those with complicated MI require longer cardiac rehabilitation.

Summary

Early recognition and prompt treatment are essential for management of MI. Atypical and painless presentation must always be considered. Urgent reperfusion with fibrinolytic or primary PCI is lifesaving in STEMI, and in-hospital revascularization is beneficial in high-risk NSTEMI and unstable coronary syndromes. Agents that reduce mortality, including aspirin, β-blockers, ACE inhibitors, and lipid-lowering drugs, should always be employed in the absence of contraindications. Most patients benefit from lifestyle changes and risk factor modification in a continuing outpatient setting.

REFERENCES

Alpert JS, Thygesen K, Antman E, et al. Myocardial infarction redefined—a consensus document of the Joint European Society of Cardiology/American College of Cardiology Committee for the redefinition of myocardial infarction. J Am Coll Cardiol 2000;36:959–69.

Anderson JL, Adams CD, Antman EM, et al. ACC/AHA 2007 guidelines for the management of patients with unstable angina/non-ST-elevation myocardial infarction. I Am Coll Cardiol 2007;50:e1–157.

Antman EM, Anbe DT, Armstrong PW, et al. ACC/AHA guidelines for the management of patients with ST-elevation myocardial infarction: A report of the American College of Cardiology/American Heart Association Task Force on Practice Guidelines (Committee to Revise the 1999 Guidelines for the Management of Patients With Acute Myocardial Infarction). J Am Coll Cardiol. 2004;44(3):E1–211.

Antman EM, Cohen M, Bernink PJ, et al. The TIMI risk score for unstable angina/non-ST elevation MI: A method for prognostication and therapeutic decision making. JAMA 2000;284:835–42.

Cannon CP, Hand MH, Bahr R, et al. Critical pathways for management of patients with acute coronary syndromes: An assessment by the National Heart Attack Alert Program. Am Heart J 2002;143:777–89.

Krumholz HM, Anderson JL, Brooks NH, et al. ACC/AHA clinical performance measures for adults with ST-elevation and non—ST-elevation myocardial infarction: A report of the ACC/AHA task force on performance measures (ST-Elevation and Non-ST-Elevation Myocardial Infarction Performance Measures Writing Committee). J Am Coll Cardiol 2006;47:236–65.

Mehta SR, Cannon CP, Fox KA, et al. Routine vs selective invasive strategies in patients with acute coronary syndromes: A collaborative meta-analysis of randomized trials. JAMA 2005;293:2908–17.

Smith Jr SC, Allen J, Blair SN, et al. AHA/ACC guidelines for secondary prevention for patients with coronary and other atherosclerotic vascular disease: 2006 update endorsed by the National Heart, Lung, and Blood Institute. J Am Coll Cardiol 2006;47:2130–9.

Smith Jr SC, Feldman TE, Hirshfeld Jr JW, et al. ACC/AHA/SCA1 2005 guideline update for percutaneous coronary intervention: A report of the American College of Cardiology/American Heart Association Task Force on Practice Guidelines (ACC/AHA/SCAI Writing Committee to Update the 2001 Guidelines for Percutaneous Coronary Intervention). Circulation 2006;113(7):e166–286.

Weaver WD, Cerqueira M, Hallstrom AP, et al. Prehospital-initiated vs hospital-initiated thrombolytic therapy. The Myocardial Infarction Triage and Intervention Trial. JAMA 1993;270:1211–6.

Pericarditis and Pericardial Effusions

Method of
Miguel A. Leal, MD

Embryologic Origin of the Pericardium

During the fifth week of embryonic development, lateral structures called the pleuropericardial folds begin to grow toward the midline. As the folds move medially, they bring along the phrenic nerves, and the root of each fold migrates ventrally. At the end of the fifth week, the pleuropericardial folds fuse, partitioning the thoracic cavity into a pericardial cavity and two partially formed pleural cavities.

The pericardium comprises two juxtaposed layers of connective tissue, which form the parietal and the visceral pericardium. The virtual space between the two layers is called the pericardial space. It normally contains a very small amount of transudative fluid (approximately 5 mL). Its function is not well established, but it could conceptually minimize friction and trauma to the epicardium during the cardiac cycle.

Pathologic Processes Involving the Pericardium

The pericardium can be secondarily involved in a large number of systemic disorders, and it can be primarily affected in an isolated disease process. Clinically, most disease processes involving the pericardium manifest with varying degrees of inflammation, constituting the clinical syndrome of pericarditis. In addition, the amount of pericardial fluid may be increased and may result in a pericardial effusion, which can be transudative or exudative and is sometimes hemodynamically significant.

Although pericarditis and pericardial effusions are distinct phenomena, both manifestations are present in a large group of patients. In some cases, the clinical presentation of acute pericardial inflammation predominates, and the presence of excess pericardial fluid has no clinical significance. In other cases, the effusion and its clinical consequences, such as hemodynamic instability, are the main pathologic mechanism.

Classification

Classically, pericardial disease has been categorized as inflammatory, neoplastic, degenerative, vascular, or idiopathic. Some of the major causes of inflammatory disease are infections (viral infections, including HIV, Coxsackie A and B viruses, echoviruses, influenza and adenoviruses; purulent pericarditis; tuberculosis), myocardial infarction (Dressler's syndrome), and collagen vascular diseases. Neoplastic disease may be related to breast, lung, esophagus, lymphoma, melanoma, or renal cell carcinoma. Degenerative disease is related to mediastinal radiation, whether recent or remote.

Miscellaneous causes of pericardial disease include cardiac surgery, aortic dissection, cardiac contusion (with recent or remote sharp or blunt chest trauma), iatrogenic causes (usually after cardiac diagnostic or interventional procedures, such as coronary angiography or placement of a pacemaker or defibrillator), metabolic causes (uremia, myxedematous state), and idiopathic causes.

Most of these causes of pericardial disease can produce both dry pericarditis (i.e., pericarditis with minimal or no effusion) and pericardial effusive disease. Some causes (e.g., HIV infection, hypothyroidism) are primarily associated with effusion without a significant amount of pericardial inflammation.

The frequencies reported for specific causes of pericardial disease vary significantly in the medical literature, depending on the epidemiology, the population at risk, and how the diagnosis was established. The diagnostic yield of pericardiocentesis or pericardial biopsy is typically higher in patients who are found to have a pericardial effusion than in those who present with apparent acute pericarditis without concomitant effusion.

Clinical Manifestations

ACUTE PERICARDITIS

The typical clinical manifestations of acute pericarditis are chest pain, which is usually pleuritic in nature (i.e., associated with inspiration and positional changes); a pericardial friction rub; and widespread ST-segment elevation on the 12-lead surface electrocardiogram (ECG). Usually, at least two of these features, with or without an accompanying pericardial effusion, should be present for the clinical diagnosis.

The yield of a full diagnostic evaluation is much lower in patients who present with acute pericarditis than in those presenting with pericardial effusion. In two series with a total of 331 patients, a specific diagnosis was established in only 54 (16%). The most common causes of pericarditis were neoplasia (20 patients), tuberculosis (13 patients), nontuberculous infection (7 patients), and collagen vascular disease (7 patients).

In patients with acute pericarditis for which no cause is identified (idiopathic pericarditis), the etiology is frequently presumed to be viral, but evidence for this is often not pursued, given the expense involved and the time required for the results of viral titers to become available. It is likely that some cases for which an identifiable cause exists are labeled idiopathic as the result of an insufficient diagnostic evaluation. However, complex and exhaustive testing strategies are typically not justified by the limited implications for clinical management. An exception to this recommendation is the absence of a prompt and adequate response to standard treatment.

PERICARDIAL EFFUSION

Pericardial effusions are typically diagnosed by chest radiography (Fig. 1) or transthoracic echocardiography (Fig. 2). The latter may reveal a layer of echo-free space between the epicardium and the pericardial sac, sometimes associated with fibrin strands, hematoma, or amorphous material deposited around the heart. The distribution of causes varies with demographics and diagnostic strategies.

In a review of 322 patients with a moderate to large pericardial effusion on echocardiography, the most common causes were idiopathic (20%), iatrogenic (16%), malignancy (13%), chronic

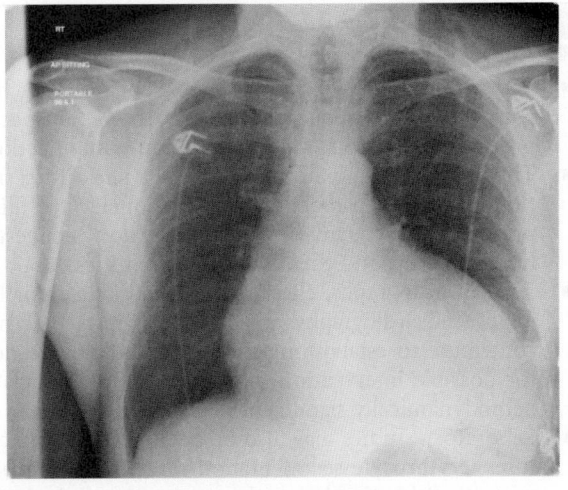

FIGURE 1. Cardiomegaly is demonstrated on a chest radiograph; the double-shadow pattern suggests a large pericardial effusion.

idiopathic effusion (9%), acute myocardial infarction (8%), uremia or end-stage renal disease (6%), and collagen vascular disease (5%).

In a different series, including 75 patients presenting to a tertiary care medical center in the United States with a new, unexplained, large pericardial effusion, a diagnosis was made in 53 patients. The most common causes were malignancy (23%), infection (27%), irradiation (14%), collagen vascular disease (12%), uremia or dialysis (12%), and idiopathic (7%). Examination of pericardial fluid yielded a diagnosis in 26%, mostly of malignancy, whereas examination of pericardial tissue was useful for diagnosis in 23%, mostly with infection.

A higher rate of idiopathic disease was found in a review of 204 patients from France; a specific cause was identified in 107 patients (52%). The following distribution was noted: idiopathic (48%), infection (16%), malignancy (15%), collagen vascular disease (10%), hypothyroidism (10%), and renal failure (2%).

Diagnostic Work-up

A careful history and physical examination may reveal a pericardial friction rub, which is usually triphasic (with early diastolic, late diastolic, and systolic components), and the presence of pulsus paradoxus (a drop of 10–12 mm Hg in the systolic blood pressure with inspiration, reflecting enhanced interventricular dependence in the setting of limited pericardial compliance). In addition, laboratory and imaging studies may contribute to establishing the diagnosis.

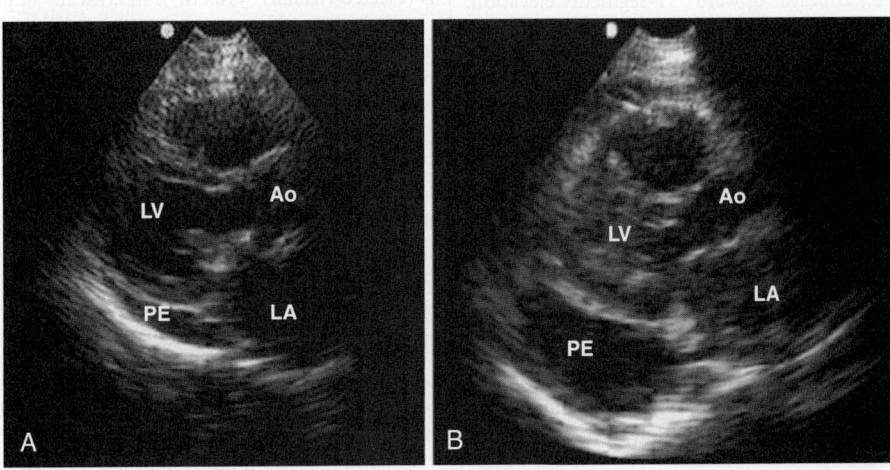

FIGURE 2. Parasternal long-axis views on transthoracic echocardiography demonstrate a large pericardial effusion (PE), lying predominantly posterior to the heart. *Abbreviations*: Ao = aorta; LA = left atrium; LV = left ventricle.

CURRENT DIAGNOSIS

- Pericarditis usually manifests as a pleuritic-type chest pain syndrome, frequently preceded by a nonspecific prodrome (e.g., malaise, fatigue, recent viral infection).
- The physical examination may reveal a pericardial friction rub, pulsus paradoxus, and signs of elevated filling pressures (e.g., jugular venous distention, congestive hepatomegaly, and edema of the extremities).
- Electrocardiography, chest radiography, and transthoracic echocardiography are diagnostic tests that may contribute to establishing the diagnosis and the need for possible intervention, in the case of an associated hemodynamically significant pericardial effusion.
- Laboratory studies may also be helpful, including cultures, erythrocyte sedimentation rate, C-reactive protein, thyroid-stimulating hormone, creatinine, and markers of autoimmune disease.
- Prognosis is usually favorable, except in specific causes such as malignancy, trauma, or aortic dissection.

LABORATORY STUDIES

A complete blood count with differential may show leukocytosis. The erythrocyte sedimentation rate and C-reactive protein level are usually elevated, especially if active inflammation is present. Blood urea nitrogen and creatinine levels should also be checked if uremia is suspected.

Cardiac biomarkers are part of the diagnostic work-up and are abnormal in cases of associated myocarditis or myocardial infarction. In a recent study, an elevated troponin I level was found in 32% of patients with viral or idiopathic pericarditis. This was related to the extent of myocardial inflammation but was not a negative prognostic marker.

Further laboratory work may include blood or viral cultures, tuberculin testing with sputum for acid-fast bacilli, rheumatoid factor, antinuclear antibody, and thyroid function tests.

OTHER STUDIES AND PROCEDURES

Chest Radiography

Chest radiography may demonstrate an enlarged cardiac silhouette, which is sometimes the first indication of a large pericardial effusion.

Electrocardiography

Acute pericarditis classically evolves through stages. Initial ECG changes include diffuse, concave upward ST-segment elevation, except in leads aVR and V_1 (where it is usually depressed). T waves are upright in the leads with ST elevation, and the PR segment deviates opposite to P-wave polarity. Several days later, the ST segments return to baseline, followed by flattening of the T waves. The T waves then become inverted, and the ECG eventually returns to baseline weeks to months after the acute episode. The T-wave inversion may persist indefinitely in the chronic inflammation observed with tuberculosis, uremia, or neoplastic processes.

Electrical alternans, the beat-to-beat variability in QRS voltage caused by excessive cardiac mobility, may be seen with a large-size pericardial effusion.

Echocardiography

Universally recommended, echocardiography should be performed urgently if cardiac tamponade is suspected. Cardiac tamponade occurs when the extracardiac pressure from a large effusion causes collapse of the cardiac chambers during diastole. The collapse occurs in a progressive fashion, with right atrial collapse initially, followed by right ventricular collapse and eventual decrement in the cardiac output once the left-sided chambers are affected.

Echocardiograms are particularly helpful if pericardial effusion is suspected on clinical or radiographic grounds, if the illness lasts longer than 1 week, or if myocarditis or purulent pericarditis is suspected. Other causes of pericardial echo-free spaces that must be considered include pleural effusion, pericardial masses, and epicardial fat. Echocardiography can also be used to evaluate for chamber size, tamponade, and ventricular dysfunction.

Computed Tomography

Effusions are easily detected on computed tomography by virtue of the different X-ray coefficients of fluid and pericardium. The nature of the effusion also may be anticipated, given the different attenuation coefficients for blood, exudates, lipid-rich fluids, and serous fluids. Hemopericardium can be difficult to assess without intravenous contrast, because blood has the same radiodensity as myocardium.

Magnetic Resonance Imaging

Magnetic resonance imaging is a sensitive technique for detecting pericardial effusion and loculated pericardial effusion and thickening.

Cardiac Catheterization

Cardiac catheterization can assist in the differentiation between constrictive and restrictive cardiomyopathy.

Pericardiocentesis

Pericardiocentesis is relatively safe when it is guided by angiography or echocardiography, especially with a large, free anterior effusion. One study reported only 3 minor complications in 117 procedures with ultrasound guidance. Heterogeneous exudates may indicate a potentially difficult pericardiocentesis, especially if the fluid is loculated in pockets—a common finding in autoimmune pericarditis, postsurgical cases, and recurrent disease.

In a large study, diagnostic pericardiocentesis led to a diagnosis in only 6% of cases, compared with 29% diagnosed by therapeutic pericardiocentesis. As such, pericardiocentesis should not be performed unless tamponade or suspected purulent pericarditis is present.

If a pericardiocentesis is performed for drainage, an indwelling catheter should be placed in the pericardial space for continued drainage over several days. If the catheter continues to drain a large amount, a more definitive procedure should be performed.

The pericardial fluid should be analyzed for red cells, total protein level, lactic acid dehydrogenase level, adenosine deaminase activity, and cultures. Cytologic studies are also indicated if malignancy is suspected.

Pericardial Window

In the pericardial window procedure, a small area of the pericardium is resected (usually ≤ 10 cm^2). In critically ill patients, a balloon catheter may be used to create a pericardial window. In some studies almost 25% of patients who underwent the procedure required repeat operation within 2 years. Constrictive pericarditis may be a long-term complication if pathologic healing affects the pericardium and leads to thickening of the pericardial sac, usually beyond 1.5 cm.

Pericardiectomy

Pericardiectomy is used for constrictive pericarditis, effusive pericarditis, or recurrent pericarditis with multiple attacks; steroid dependence; or intolerance to other medical management. Studies demonstrate that failure rates are proportional to the amount of pericardium removed (i.e., the more pericardium removed, the less likely it is that the procedure will fail). In effusive pericarditis, the higher failure rate associated with a pericardial window or partial pericardiectomy is probably secondary to continued fluid production from the remaining pericardium, with sealing of the remaining pericardium to the heart.

The operative mortality rate was 14% in one series, with a range of 1% for New York Heart Association class I-II, 10% for class III, and 46% for class IV. The 5-year survival rate was 80% for class III-IV and approximately 95% for class I-II.

CURRENT THERAPY

- Nonsteroidal antiinflammatory drugs such as ibuprofen (Advil), indomethacin (Indocin),[1] and ketorolac (Toradol) are the usual treatment modality of choice.
- Colchicine[1] may also be used for prevention of disease recurrence.
- Pericardiocentesis and surgical pericardial windows are needed if there is hemodynamic instability (cardiac tamponade).
- Steroids may be used in refractory cases or if autoimmune causes are involved.

[1]Not FDA approved for this indication.

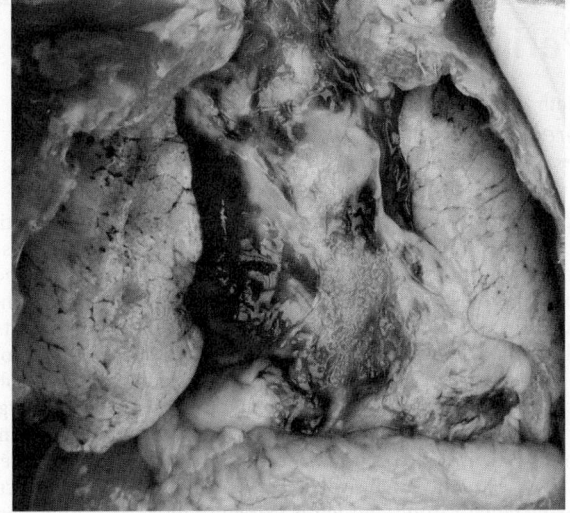

FIGURE 3. Autopsy findings of a large hemorrhagic pericardial effusion.

Treatment

All patients admitted with suspected or established pericarditis, with or without an effusion, should be monitored by telemetry. Other life-threatening causes of chest pain (e.g., myocardial infarction, aortic dissection) should be considered in the differential diagnosis.

In selected cases (young patients with no hemodynamic instability and minor clinical symptoms), pericarditis may be managed on an outpatient basis. In a recent study, fever greater than 38°C, subacute onset, immunosuppression, trauma, oral anticoagulation therapy, failure of therapy with aspirin or nonsteroidal antiinflammatory drugs (NSAIDs), myopericarditis, severe pericardial effusion, and cardiac tamponade were poor prognostic predictors. Patients without these factors were treated on an outpatient basis, without serious complications after a mean follow-up of 38 months.

In another study, the presence of cardiac tamponade and an unfavorable clinical outcome, with persistence of fever, significant pericardial effusion, or general illness lasting longer than 1 week, were highly associated with finding a specific etiology.

If significant clinical activity persists for 3 weeks after admission without an etiologic diagnosis, some authors recommend pericardial biopsy. Complicated cases, such as tuberculous, purulent, or uremic causes, require multidisciplinary involvement, including consultations with a cardiologist, cardiac surgeon, and medical subspecialists (e.g., infectious diseases specialist, nephrologist).

Treatment for specific causes of pericarditis is directed according to the underlying cause. For patients with idiopathic or viral pericarditis, therapy is directed at symptom relief. NSAIDs such as indomethacin[1] (Indocin, 50 mg PO every 8 hours), ibuprofen (Motrin or Advil, 400–800 mg PO every 6–8 hours), or ketorolac (Toradol, 30–90 mg IV/IM every 4 hours[3]) are the mainstay of therapy. These agents have similar efficacies, with relief of chest pain in 85% to 90% of patients within days of treatment. Ibuprofen has the advantage of fewer adverse effects and fewer negative effects on coronary flow. Indomethacin has a poor adverse effect profile and has been shown to reduce coronary flow. Ketorolac is used if the oral route of treatment is not an option. The duration of treatment depends on the clinical course, but common therapeutic courses rarely extend beyond 7 to 10 days.

Aspirin (325 mg PO daily) is recommended for treatment of pericarditis after an ST-elevation myocardial infarction, as part of a secondary prevention regimen against recurrent coronary events. Colchicine[1] (1 mg PO daily), in combination with an NSAID, can be considered in the initial treatment to prevent recurrent pericarditis. Colchicine, alone or in combination with an NSAID, can be considered for patients with recurrent or continued symptoms beyond 14 days.

Corticosteroids (prednisone tapering regimens, starting usually at 40–60 mg PO daily and tapered over the course of 10–14 days) should not be used for initial treatment of pericarditis unless indicated for the underlying disease. Corticosteroids also may be used if the patient has had no response to NSAIDs or colchicine, or if these drugs are contraindicated.

Prognosis

The prognosis depends on the etiology. Pericarditis from idiopathic and viral causes usually has a self-limited course. Purulent, tuberculous, hemorrhagic (Fig. 3) and neoplastic causes of pericarditis and pericardial effusions result in more complicated courses with worse outcomes.

REFERENCES

Atar S, Chiu J, Forrester JS, Siegel RJ. Bloody pericardial effusion in patients with cardiac tamponade: Is the cause cancerous, tuberculous, or iatrogenic? Chest 1999;116:1564–9.

Corey GR, Campbell PT, van Trigt P, et al. Etiology of large pericardial effusions. Am J Med 1993;95:209–13.

Galve E, Garcia-del-Castillo H, Evangelista A, et al. Pericardial effusion in the course of myocardial infarction: Incidence, natural history, and clinical relevance. Circulation 1986;73:294–9.

Permanyer-Miralda G, Sagrista-Sauleda J, Soler-Soler J. Primary acute pericardial disease: A prospective series of 231 consecutive patients. Am J Cardiol 1985;56:623–30.

Sagrista-Sauleda J, Merce J, Permanyer-Miralda G, Soler-Soler J. Clinical clues to the causes of large pericardial effusions. Am J Med 2000;109:95–101.

Spodick DH. Pericardial disease. In: Braunwald E, Zipes DP, Libby P, editors. Heart Disease: A Textbook of Cardiovascular Medicine. New York: WB Saunders; 2001. p. 183–202.

Troughton RW, Asher CR, Klein AL. Pericarditis. Lancet 2004;363:717–27.

Zayas R, Anguita M, Torres F, et al. Incidence of specific etiology and role of methods for specific etiologic diagnosis of primary acute pericarditis. Am J Cardiol 1995;75:378–82.

[1]Not FDA approved for this indication.
[3]Exceeds dosage recommended by the manufacturer.

Peripheral Arterial Disease

Method of
Gregory Feldman, MD, and Wei Zhou, MD

Peripheral vascular disease comprises a diverse group of conditions that result in significant morbidity and mortality and offers an opportunity for the astute clinician to recognize common but under-diagnosed problems for which effective interventions exist. Peripheral vascular disease is defined as pathology of the blood vessels outside the brain and heart, and peripheral arterial disease (PAD) involves that subset that affects arteries. Most manifestations of PAD follow logically from the consequences of reduced perfusion of end organs and tissues downstream from sites of flow obstruction. Common forms of PAD include extracranial carotid stenosis, aortoiliac disease, and lower extremity occlusive disease (LEOD). This chapter focuses on extracranial carotid and lower extremity diseases; venous conditions are described in the next chapter.

Epidemiologic data suggest that the prevalence of PAD is 12.2% for American adults older than 60 years of age, increasing to 23.2% for those older than 80 years. Risk factors include increased age, diabetes, past or current tobacco use, renal insufficiency, hypertension, dyslipidemia, and African American or Hispanic ethnicity. More than 95% of patients with PAD have one or more risk factors for cardiovascular disease, and the diagnosis of either condition should raise suspicion for the other. The 10-year risk of death after a diagnosis of PAD is 40%. Alarmingly, an estimated 68% of patients with PAD are undiagnosed by their primary care physicians, although as a group these patients have mainly less advanced cases of atherosclerosis.

The history and physical examination are of paramount importance in detecting peripheral vascular disease and prompting further evaluation. Risk factors for peripheral vascular disease should merit elicitation of common presenting symptoms, including claudication, limb pain at rest, and nonhealing extremity ulcers for LEOD; and amaurosis fugax, transient ischemic attack (TIA), and stroke for carotid occlusive diseases. An appropriate physical examination includes palpation of radial, aortic, femoral, popliteal, and pedal pulses; careful examination of distal extremities for stigmata of arterial insufficiency; cervical and abdominal auscultation for carotid and renal bruits; and a thorough neurologic evaluation.

CURRENT DIAGNOSIS

Carotid Artery Diseases

- Presentation: transient ischemic attack and stroke
- Physical examination: bruit and lateralized neurologic deficit
- Diagnostic modalities: carotid ultrasonography, magnetic resonance angiography (MRA), computed tomographic angiography (CTA), and carotid angiography

Lower Extremity Occlusive Diseases

- Presentation: claudication, rest pain, tissue loss, and numbness
- Physical examination: diminished pulse, hair loss, pallor, cool extremities, tissue wasting, ulcerations, and delayed capillary refill (>3 sec).
- Imaging modalities: ankle-brachial index, segmental pressures with waveforms, CTA, MRA, and lower extremity angiography

Carotid Artery Disease

Stroke is the most common cause of permanent disability in the United States, and it remains the third leading cause of death in industrialized countries. Atherosclerotic disease involving the extracranial carotid artery is one of the major causes of all strokes and TIAs. Management of stroke consumes $45 billion annually and is responsible for more than 1 million hospital admissions each year in this country. Neurologic sequelae related to cerebrovascular accidents severely limit a patient's ability to carry out activities of daily living and invariably create an enormous burden on health care costs. As a result, the prevention of cerebrovascular accidents through safe treatment of extracranial carotid occlusive disease remains an important health care goal.

PATHOPHYSIOLOGY

The underlying pathophysiology of atherosclerotic plaque formation continues to be an area of active investigation, with explanatory models incorporating elements of flow dynamics, endothelial damage, lipid deposition, and inflammatory mediators. Plaque deposition frequently occurs at sites of bifurcation, and the carotid bifurcation is a common location for plaque formation. The neurologic sequelae from carotid disease mostly result from movement of microemboli or macroemboli of disrupted plaque into the cerebral circulation, with symptoms determined by the vascular territory disrupted and the availability of collateral circulation. Rarely, symptoms can also result from critical flow limitation secondary to severe carotid stenosis, although typically the collateral circulation through the vertebral arteries and the contralateral carotid is adequate to compensate. It is not uncommon to find complete occlusion of a single carotid artery without any perceptible neurologic dysfunction.

Carotid stenosis is categorized as symptomatic or asymptomatic, with divergent therapeutic strategies based on this determination. Most patients are asymptomatic. Symptomatic patients can present with TIA or stroke. Although the classification for neurologic insults is constantly evolving, TIA is defined as a focal neurologic deficit that resolves completely within 24 hours. Symptoms of TIA can include generalized confusion, loss of strength or sensation at contralateral upper or lower extremities, and difficulty with speech, vision, or memory. One example of a TIA is amaurosis fugax, in which painless monocular loss of vision results from temporary occlusion of a retinal artery. Patients often describe this as having the appearance of a curtain being drawn down over the eye. Stroke, in contrast, is defined as a neurologic deficit with acute onset that resolves incompletely or not at all after a thromboembolic or hemorrhagic event.

EVALUATION

Asymptomatic carotid stenosis is detected on auscultation of a cervical bruit (although most stenoses are not accompanied by bruits) or on imaging, which includes screening duplex ultrasonography based on risk factors or, increasingly, incidental findings on computed tomography or magnetic resonance scans performed for other indications. The physical examination for a patient with suspected or confirmed carotid stenosis includes a comprehensive neurologic evaluation, auscultation for cervical bruits, and the palpation of peripheral pulses. Vigorous palpation of carotid pulses is discouraged. Important components of the neurologic examination include a thorough evaluation of cranial nerves, strength, sensation, gait, memory, speech, and comprehension. One needs to pay particular attention to lateralized symptoms.

Imaging modalities are important in diagnosing carotid artery stenosis. The most useful screening imaging modality is a carotid duplex examination, which provides information regarding the estimated degree of stenosis, plaque location and characteristics, and flow dynamics (Fig. 1). Confirmatory imaging includes computed tomographic or magnetic resonance angiography, which can also be used to evaluate intracerebral circulation and to confirm or detect acute or chronic stroke. Of note, magnetic resonance angiography often overestimates the degree of carotid stenosis, particularly for calcified lesions, and should be interpreted in conjunction with duplex results. Carotid and cerebral angiography, historically considered

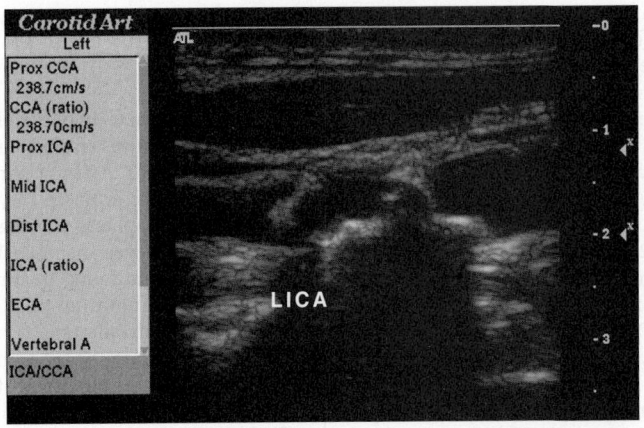

FIGURE 1. Ultrasound scan of left internal carotid artery (LICA) shows severe carotid stenosis and echogenic calcification at the carotid bulb.

the gold standard, is increasingly being supplanted by these noninvasive imaging modalities. Carotid angiography is now generally reserved for patients who had conflicting findings on two noninvasive diagnostic tests and patients for whom percutaneous interventions are contemplated.

MANAGEMENT

Management options for carotid stenosis include medical optimization, carotid endarterectomy (CEA), and carotid angioplasty and stenting (CAS) (Fig. 2). Medical optimization involves strategies for diet and lifestyle modification, blood pressure control, lipid-lowering agents, and antiplatelet therapy.

Surgical intervention most commonly involves CEA, in which the carotid artery is exposed, controlled, and opened, and atherosclerotic plaque is removed. A patch angioplasty is performed during closure

of the artery to avoid luminal narrowing. An estimated 98,000 CEAs were performed in the United States in 2004. Potential perioperative complications include stroke, cranial nerve injury, hematoma, myocardial infarction, and death. Recommendations for surgical intervention are based on balancing the demonstrated benefits of stroke reduction with the incidence of periprocedural complications; such decisions have been shaped by the results of four large, multicenter trials of carotid endarterectomy published during the 1990s. The North American Symptomatic Carotid Endarterectomy Trial (NASCET) randomly assigned 651 patients with severe (70%–99%) symptomatic carotid stenosis to receive either medical therapy alone or CEA in addition to medical therapy. At 2 years, the rate of ipsilateral stroke was 26% in the medical therapy group and 9% in the CEA group, demonstrating a relative risk reduction of 65%. The European Carotid Surgery Trial (ECST) randomized 3024 patients with symptomatic carotid stenosis to CEA versus initial nonoperative

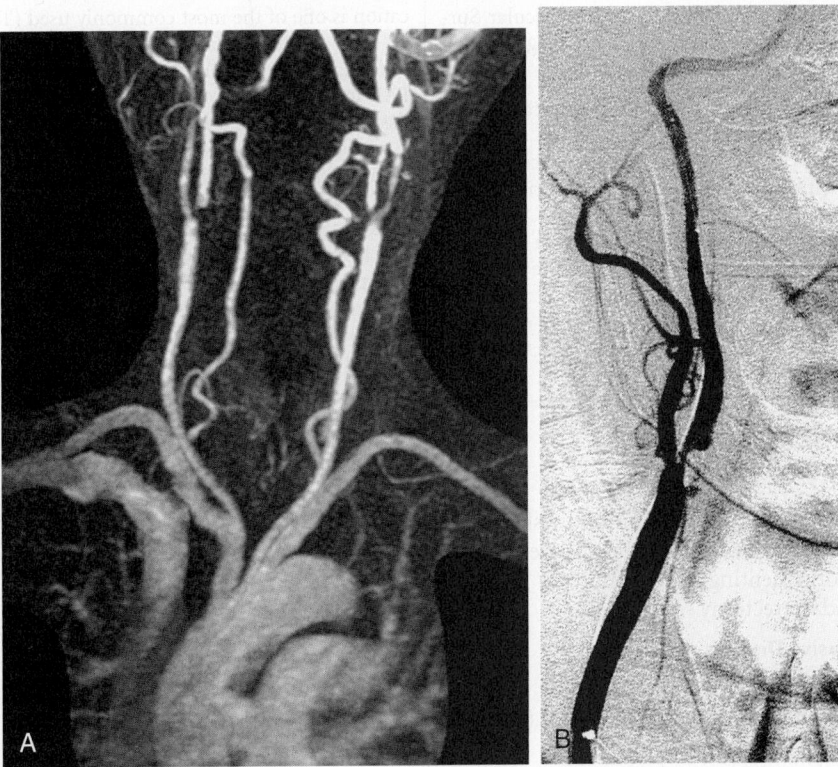

FIGURE 2. A, Time-of-flight magnetic resonance angiogram of the aortic arch and carotid artery demonstrates a severe right carotid artery stenosis. **B**, Carotid angiography confirms a severe stenosis before carotid stenting procedure. A distal protection device is positioned at middle of the internal carotid artery.

management. Rates of stroke, death, and other adverse events were monitored for 3 years and stratified by degree of stenosis. For patients with stenosis equal to or greater than 80%, the risk of major stroke or death at 3 years was 26.5% in the nonoperative group, compared with 14.9% in the CEA group, for a relative risk reduction of 44%. A large Veterans Affairs trial for symptomatic patients with greater than 70% stenosis demonstrated similar results.

The Asymptomatic Carotid Atherosclerosis Study (ACAS) attempted to evaluate the utility of CEA in patients with asymptomatic carotid stenosis. A total of 1662 patients with asymptomatic stenosis of 60% or greater were randomized to CEA or medical treatment. The aggregate risk of ipsilateral stroke and perioperative stroke or death at 5 years was 11.0% for patients treated medically and 5.1% for those treated surgically, with an aggregate risk reduction of 53%. Because this represents an absolute risk reduction of only about 1% per year, considerable controversy still exists as to the degree of asymptomatic stenosis that should prompt surgical intervention.

Endovascular techniques represent a recent addition to the arsenal of available treatments for carotid stenosis. CAS, typically with deployment of a distal protection device to minimize the risk of embolization, has emerged as a promising therapeutic option, and the FDA has approved several devices for this purpose. Long-term data are not yet available, but several recent studies suggest that CAS may be comparable in outcome to CEA in selected populations. Indications for the appropriate use of CAS are still being developed, but it is generally agreed that CAS should be considered for symptomatic patients with significant medical comorbidities or high surgical risks, such as recurrent stenosis after CEA, prior neck irradiation or dissection, and inaccessible lesions above the C2 level. After CAS, a second antiplatelet agent, such as clopidogrel (Plavix),[1] is recommended for at least 6 weeks in addition to lifelong aspirin.

Postprocedure restenosis is an uncommon but well-recognized long-term complication after CEA or CAS. A severe restenosis can lead to neurologic symptoms and warrants reintervention. For this reason, routine ultrasound surveillance of the carotid arteries is necessary after CEA or CAS. Higher rates of restenosis have been reported after CAS, compared with CEA, particularly for patients with prior surgeries.

A recent consensus statement from the Society for Vascular Surgery issued the following recommendations for the management of carotid stenosis:

- Symptomatic patients with <50% stenosis: optimal medical therapy
- Symptomatic patients with >50% stenosis: CEA
- Asymptomatic patients with <60% stenosis: optimal medical therapy
- Asymptomatic patients with >60% stenosis and low perioperative risk: CEA
- Carotid stenting was described as a potential alternative in symptomatic patients with >50% stenosis and high operative risk.

---

[1]Not FDA approved for this indication.

 CURRENT THERAPY

Carotid Artery Diseases

- Medical therapy: lifestyle modification and risk factor reduction, lipid-lowering agents, and antiplatelet agents
- Percutaneous carotid stenting procedures
- Carotid artery endarterectomy

Lower Extremity Occlusive Diseases

- Medical management: lifestyle and risk factor modification, pentoxifylline (Trental), and cilostazol (Pletal)
- Exercise regimen
- Percutaneous interventions: angioplasty, stent, and atherectomy
- Surgery: bypass and endarterectomy

Lower Extremity Occlusive Disease

LEOD is a common form of peripheral vascular disease in which arterial obstruction or stenosis results in inadequate blood flow to meet peripheral tissue demands. Areas of partial or complete occlusion can occur anywhere from the aorta to the pedal vessels, frequently in the iliofemoral, femoropopliteal, or tibial arterial systems. LEOD can best be understood as the peripheral analog to the imbalance between oxygen supply and demand found in coronary artery disease, and it similarly represents a spectrum from mild disease symptomatic only at exertion to severe disease manifesting at rest. The distribution and intensity of symptoms depend on the location and severity of occlusion, the acuteness of onset, and the efficiency of tissue oxygen extraction and utilization. Mild disease can manifest with symptoms of claudication, defined as limb discomfort in specific muscle groups at a reproducible level of exertion. Severe disease can manifest with pain at rest in the affected extremity, tissue loss, or chronic nonhealing wounds.

A distinction should be made between acute and chronic LEOD. Acute LEOD may result from a thrombotic or embolic event and is characterized by an abrupt onset of symptoms. Chronic LEOD is typically less dramatic in presentation and slowly progressive in nature. However, many patients present with acute LEOD. Acute LEOD is a surgical emergency and merits urgent evaluation by a vascular surgeon or specialist.

EVALUATION

The presenting symptoms of PAD are myriad and include cramping or pain in the legs or hips, cool extremities, and diminished extremity sensation. Approximately 50% of patients have atypical symptoms, and the classic symptom of claudication has been observed in only 10% of affected patients in some series. It is worth noting that the term intermittent claudication is frequently misapplied; this term correctly refers to the reproducible nature of the symptoms after a given level of exertion, not to a sporadic manifestation of discomfort. Several classification systems have been established to create uniform standards for evaluation and reporting of PAD. Among them, the Rutherford classification is one of the most commonly used (Table 1).

After careful elicitation of presenting symptoms, a focused physical examination is critical in the diagnosis of LEOD. Physical findings of PAD include reduced or absent pulses, hair loss, pallor, cool extremities, tissue wasting, ulcerations, and delayed capillary refill (>3 seconds).

A useful and inexpensive test for diagnosing and monitoring LOED is the ankle-brachial index (ABI), which can be readily performed in a clinic. Doppler ultrasonography is used to measure systolic blood pressures in bilateral dorsalis pedis, posterior tibial, and brachial arteries. The highest pedal systolic value in each leg is then divided by the highest arm pressure to calculate the ABI. An ABI of greater than 0.9 is considered normal. Claudicants typically have ABIs between 0.5 and 0.9. A value lower than 0.5 is concern for critical limb ischemia, and a value lower than 0.3 is often associated with tissue loss. Diabetic patients and patients with noncompressible tibial vessels secondary to calcification often have falsely elevated ABIs that are not dependable predictors of arterial disease. The numeric value of an ABI might not correlate

TABLE 1 Rutherford Classification for Peripheral Arterial Occlusive Disease

Symptoms	Grade	Category
Asymptomatic	0	0
Claudication		
Mild	I	1
Moderate	I	2
Severe	I	3
Ischemic rest pain	II	4
Tissue loss		
Minor	III	5
Major	III	6

precisely with symptoms or with vascular imaging findings, but it can be used to monitor progression of disease and should be interpreted in the clinical context.

A more sophisticated diagnostic screening test includes segmental pressures with evaluation of arterial waveforms. This test is routinely performed in noninvasive vascular laboratories and can provide both anatomic and functional information regarding blood flow without exposing the patient to radiation or nephrotoxic contrast agents. In segmental pressure measurement, systolic blood pressures are recorded at multiple levels, including the upper thigh, lower thigh, upper calf, ankle, and toes. A decrease of 20 mm Hg pressure between segments indicates significant arterial disease within that segment. For example, a pressure difference of 30 mm Hg between the upper and lower thigh suggests severe superficial femoral artery occlusive disease.

After a careful history and physical examination and noninvasive ultrasound evaluations have been performed, other diagnostic modalities may be required to further delineate anatomy, particularly if interventions are intended. Computed tomographic angiography produces a more detailed anatomic description and is useful for both diagnosis and preoperative planning but requires the use of radiation and intravenous contrast. Magnetic resonance angiography is emerging as a complementary modality, but is typically more expensive than computed tomographic angiography and has limited availability outside academic centers. Traditional angiography is performed if noninvasive modalities are unobtainable. Angiography affords the additional advantage of enabling endovascular intervention at the time of evaluation (Fig. 3).

TREATMENT

Treatment options for PAD include medical optimization, exercise training, and surgical or percutaneous interventions. Patients with mild claudication can benefit from risk factor modification, including smoking cessation and medical optimization for hypertension, diabetes, and dyslipidemia. The role of antiplatelet therapy in mild claudication is controversial, with mixed results from studies on the

FDA-approved agents pentoxifylline (Trental) and cilostazol (Pletal). Most claudicants should be prescribed aspirin (ASA) on the basis of cardiovascular risk factors. Medical management alone can lead to improvement in symptoms in a significant proportion of claudicants (as high as 75% in some series), and there is evidence that multimodality therapy is more effective than any single intervention. It is reasonable to perform a trial of medical optimization before more invasive therapeutic modalities are considered, particularly in patients with mild and moderate symptoms.

Supervised exercise regimens have also demonstrated efficacy for some patients with mild and moderate symptoms and should be considered before surgical or percutaneous interventions.

For patients who have not responded to medical optimization, multiple revascularization options exist. As with any surgical intervention, the risks and benefits of the proposed procedure must be carefully weighed against potential improvements in quality of life. Indications for revascularization include critical limb ischemia with rest pain, tissue loss, or nonhealing lesions. Lifestyle-limiting claudication is a relative indication for revascularization. Surgical revascularization options include bypassing the occluded arterial segment with a venous or synthetic graft and removing plaque from an arterial segment (endarterectomy) with local reconstruction. In the acute setting, removal of thromboembolus can be performed by direct exposure, balloon thrombectomy, or purely endovascular techniques. Commonly performed bypass operations that have achieved durable long-term results include aortofemoral bypass for aortoiliac occlusive disease and femoropopliteal and femorotibial bypass for more distal disease. Perioperative morbidity is not insignificant (2%–6%). In this patient population with substantial comorbidity, complications can include myocardial infarction, wound infection, graft infection, graft thrombosis, limb loss, and death. Long-term surveillance of bypass grafts with regular duplex ultrasonographic evaluations is necessary.

Driven by developments in technology and efforts to decrease periprocedural morbidity and mortality, endovascular interventions are increasingly being performed for the treatment of LEOD.

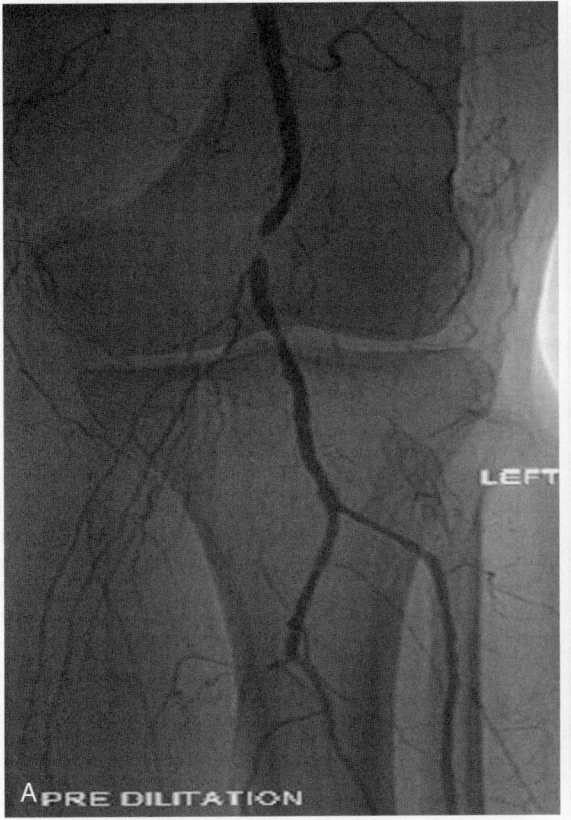
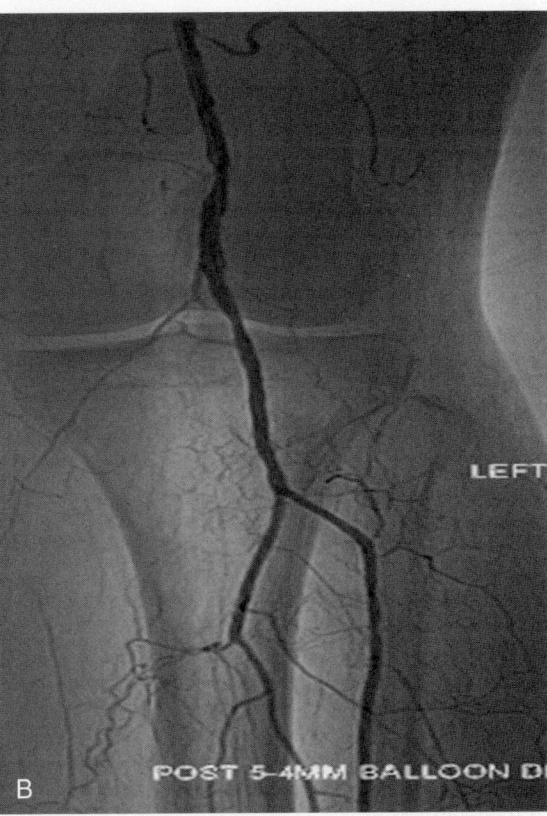

FIGURE 3. A, Lower extremity angiogram shows a focal occlusive lesion of the popliteal artery. **B,** Postprocedure angiogram shows complete resolution of the stenosis after balloon angioplasty.

Endovascular options include angioplasty alone, angioplasty with stenting, and atherectomy (a percutaneous analog of endarterectomy). In general, endovascular treatment is effective and durable for treatment of focal lesions with good distal run-off vessels. Patients with distal three-vessel run-off have better long-term outcome than those with one-vessel run-off or no run-off vessel. Lesion characteristics are also important. Long segments of occlusion, diffuse lesions, and calcified lesions are associated with poor long-term outcomes. The decreased invasiveness and shorter convalescence achieved with percutaneous approaches are appealing, but fewer long-term data are available than for traditional surgical approaches, and complications can be equally devastating. Endovascular technology is an area of active research and development, and improvements may expand the use of endovascular approaches to LEOD in the future. As with open approaches, routine postintervention surveillance is essential to identify severe restenoses that require secondary intervention. Given that percutaneous interventions can limit options for future reconstruction, patients with LEOD are best managed by vascular specialists familiar with the full range of therapeutic techniques as well as the natural history of disease progression.

REFERENCES

Arain F, Cooper L. Peripheral arterial disease: Diagnosis and management. Mayo Clin Proc 2008;83(8):944–50.

Donnan G, Fisher M, Macleod M, Davis SM. Stroke. Lancet 2008;371:1612–23.

European Carotid Surgery Trialists Collaborative Group. Randomised trial of endarterectomy for recently symptomatic carotid stenosis: Final results of the MRC European Carotid Surgery Trial (ECST). Lancet 1998;351:1379–87.

Ferguson G, Eliasziw M, Barr HW, et al. The North American Symptomatic Carotid Endarterectomy Trial: Surgical results in 1415 patients. Stroke 1999;30:1751–8.

Hobson RW 2nd, Mackey WC, Ascher E, et al. Management of atherosclerotic carotid artery disease: Clinical practice guidelines of the Society for Vascular Surgery. J Vasc Surg 2008;48:480–6.

Ostchega Y, Paulose-Ram R, Dillon CF, et al. Prevalence of peripheral arterial disease and risk factors in persons aged 60 and older: Data from the National Health and Nutrition Examination Survey 1999–2004. J Am Geriatr Soc 2007;55(4):583–9.

Rosamond W, Flegal K, Friday G, et al. Heart Disease and Stroke Statistics—2007 Update: A Report from the American Heart Association Statistics Committee and Stroke Statistics Subcommittee. Circulation 2007;115:e69–171.

Selvin E, Erlinger T. Prevalence of and risk factors for peripheral arterial disease in the United States: Results from the National Health and Nutrition Examination Survey, 1999–2000. Circulation 2004;110:738–43.

TASC Working Group. Management of peripheral arterial disease. J Vasc Surg 2000;31(1):S1–296.

White C. Intermittent claudication. N Engl J Med 2007;356:1241–50.

Venous Thrombosis

Method of
Paul L. F. Giangrande, MD

Air Travel and Thrombosis

The subject of air travel and thrombosis has been the subject of much debate in both the lay and medical press in recent years, although a possible link has been recognized for many years, and the very first report concerned a physician who traveled from Boston to Venezuela in 1946. However, venous thromboembolism is not exclusively associated with air travel, and it has also been documented following long car, bus, and train journeys.

A case-control study of 160 consecutive patients with deep venous thrombosis (DVT) showed that 39 of 160 (24.5%) had recently completed a journey by car, train, or plane of longer than 4 hours; nine of these patients had traveled by air. When the patients with DVT were compared with the control group, a history of recent travel was reported four times more often in the subjects with venous thromboembolism (odds ratio [OR] = 4). This correlation has been confirmed by a recent and much larger case-control study, the Multiple Environment and Genetic Assessment (MEGA) study, from the Netherlands, which confirmed that travel by car, bus, train, or plane is associated with an increased risk of venous thrombosis. Thrombosis associated with flight is also by no means restricted to those in the relatively confined conditions of economy class, and thus the alternative term of "travelers' thrombosis" has been suggested.

It is possible to derive some general conclusions from published cases of venous thromboembolism associated with travel. Thromboembolism is rarely observed after flights of less than 5 hours, and typically, the flights are 12 hours or longer. The risk rises with age, and persons older than 50 years are more at risk, whereas those younger than 40 years are less vulnerable. Symptoms of thromboembolism do not usually develop during or immediately after the flight but tend to appear within 3 days of arrival, when the patient may present far away from the airport, and thus the causal link might not be immediately apparent. Symptoms of thrombosis or pulmonary embolism have been reported up to 2 weeks after a long flight. Pulmonary embolism may also be the first manifestation, without any symptoms in the lower limbs. Although most case reports and studies involve DVT in the lower limbs, there are also reports of cerebral venous thrombosis and arterial thrombosis associated with long flights.

The consequences of venous thromboembolism are not insignificant. Quite apart from the pain and discomfort, which can ruin a holiday or business trip, pulmonary embolism is estimated to develop in approximately 10% of cases. The mortality associated with pulmonary embolism rises with increasing age, but it is in the range of 2% to 15% of cases. The inconvenience and side effects of warfarin treatment should also not be overlooked.

Approximately 60% of patients develop postphlebitis syndrome (persistent swelling and discomfort of the leg, often associated with ulceration) within 2 years despite appropriate anticoagulant therapy. A history of thrombosis precludes future prescription of hormone replacement therapy (HRT) or oral contraceptive pills (OCPs) for women, and it can make it difficult to secure travel insurance in the future because of the increased risk of recurrence.

Epidemiology

The precise incidence of thromboembolism in relation to air travel is uncertain, though it has been estimated that at least 5% of all cases of DVT may be linked to air travel. A study based on 56 confirmed cases of pulmonary embolism among 135.3 million passengers passing through one airport in the period between 1993 and 2000 clearly demonstrated an association between duration of travel and risk of pulmonary embolism was significantly higher (1.5 cases per million) for passengers traveling more than 5000 km when compared with a risk of only 0.01 cases per million among passengers traveling less than 5000 km.

Cases of pulmonary embolism clearly only represent the tip of the iceberg of cases of DVT. A recent observational study from New Zealand, based on the study of 878 passengers who traveled extensively (at least 10 hours; mean, 39 hours) reported an incidence of venous thromboembolism of 1%, including four cases of pulmonary embolism and five of DVT. However, the incidence of latent, asymptomatic thrombosis is likely to be even higher. A prospective study of long-haul air passengers older than 50 years reported that 12 of 116 passengers (10%) were found by duplex scanning to have asymptomatic DVT confined to the calf.

Etiology

The etiology of venous thrombosis is usually multifactorial, with a combination of both constitutional and environmental factors responsible for causing a thrombosis in a patient at a given time.

The three underlying causes of thrombosis are classically defined as Virchow's triad: stasis, hypercoagulability of the blood, and vessel wall disease.

Stasis in the venous circulation of the lower limbs is undoubtedly the major factor in promoting the development of venous thromboembolism associated with travel. The potential danger of confinement in cramped conditions has been recognized for some years. An increase in the incidence of fatal pulmonary embolism was reported during the Blitz in London during the Second World War. Simpson recognized that the primary cause was mechanical impairment of venous circulation due to squatting for a prolonged period in air raid shelters, and he recommended that bunks should be installed. The term *economy class syndrome* was coined to describe the phenomenon, and this also emphasizes the role of impaired venous circulation due to prolonged immobility in a cramped position. Ingestion of alcohol also encourages immobility during a flight, and the use of strong sedative medication may also be associated with an increased risk of venous thrombosis.

A number of other risk factors are now also recognized, primarily through clinical experience in the setting of surgery, which predispose to venous thromboembolism. These are listed in Box 1.

The effect of age was highlighted in a recent study from Australia, which concluded that the annual risk of venous thromboembolism is increased by 12% if one long-haul flight is undertaken annually. However, the incidence of thromboembolism was less than 1 per 100,000 arriving passengers younger than 40 years, but it rose steadily to exceed 14 per 100,000 in those aged 75 years or older.

A hematologic abnormality might predispose a person to development of venous thromboembolism. Such disorders include the relatively rare congenital (inherited) deficiencies of natural anticoagulants, such as antithrombin, protein C, or protein S. A recent study demonstrated that an inherited thrombophilic defect or use of an OCP increased the risk of thrombosis associated with air travel 16-fold and 14-fold, respectively. The MEGA study has also demonstrated that positivity for the factor V Leiden thrombophilic mutation, body mass index greater than 30, height greater than 1.9 or less than 1.6 meters, and use of OCPs are strong susceptibility factors. In one small uncontrolled, retrospective study of patients with flight-related DVT, 6 of 20 (30%) subjects had a thrombophilic defect (factor V Leiden in 5). Four subjects had a history of a previous episode of thrombosis, and other potential risk factors were identified in 10 subjects (including malignancy, leg in plaster cast, use of OCP or HRT). Five of the 20 patients had a negative thrombophilia screen and no other identifiable risk factor.

The value of screening passengers for thrombophilic defects before long-haul flights has been raised. It is generally accepted that routine screening of passengers or screening of pilots as part of their medical screening is not justified or cost-effective. Such screening is not, of course, routinely offered in other circumstances associated with an increased risk of thrombosis (e.g., before starting an OCP, pregnancy, before orthopedic surgery), and no case has yet been established for air travel to be treated differently from current practice for thrombophilia screening in other fields.

Some evidence now suggests that exposure to the mild hypobaric hypoxia encountered in pressurized aircraft might also result in activation of the coagulation and thus encourage thrombosis. Aircraft typically fly at altitudes of between 35,000 and 40,000 feet to avoid turbulence and drag, thus benefiting fuel consumption. The cabin air is derived from the outside atmospheric air, which is drawn in and compressed. The maximum pressure in the cabin at cruising altitude is influenced by the allowable differential pressure across the wall of the cabin. This varies with aircraft design, but the lowest pressure permitted by the regulatory authorities for civil aircraft is equivalent to atmospheric pressure at an altitude of 8000 feet. Although the percentage of oxygen in the cabin remains unchanged at around 21%, the partial pressure of oxygen is reduced to around 74% of the sea level value. The very cold air at this altitude (typically around $-50°C$) contains only negligible water vapor, and the humidity in the cabin is thus typically very low.

Markers of activation of coagulation were transiently elevated in an uncontrolled study of 20 healthy male volunteers who were exposed to a hypobaric environment designed to simulate the conditions of an airplane cabin. The plasma levels of prothrombin fragments 1 and 2, thrombin-antithrombin (TAT) complex, and activated coagulation factor VII increased significantly, although the D-dimer level remained unchanged. Treatment with heparin inhibited the development of this apparent activation of the coagulation cascade. Another study of eight subjects who ascended rapidly to high altitudes by helicopter in Nepal documented increases in the levels of prothrombin fragments 1 and 2 and PAI-1 (plasminogen activator inhibitor, a key inhibitor of fibrinolysis). Activation of coagulation associated with flight, reflected by an increase in plasma levels of TAT complex, was also demonstrated in a crossover study in which 71 healthy volunteers were studied in the setting of an 8-hour flight, with the same volunteers monitored in two controlled-exposure situations.

Contrary to the widespread belief that passengers on long-haul flights can develop dehydration through increased insensible loss of water across the skin and mucous surfaces, it has been calculated that the maximum possible increase in insensible loss of water over an 8-hour period in such conditions is only around 100 mL. Although systemic dehydration is not a significant factor in healthy persons, the low humidity in an aircraft cabin can certainly lead to dryness of the mucous membranes and a sensation of thirst. Excessive consumption of alcohol or gastrointestinal infections associated with vomiting and diarrhea can also exacerbate dehydration.

BOX 1 Risk Factors for Venous Thromboembolism

- Age greater than 40 years (but especially the elderly)
- Previous thrombotic episode (especially pulmonary embolism)
- Documented thrombophilic abnormality (e.g., antithrombin deficiency)
- Other hematologic disorders (polycythemia and thrombocythemia)
- Pregnancy and puerperium
- Malignancy
- Congestive heart failure or recent myocardial infarction
- Recent surgery (especially lower limb)
- Chronic venous insufficiency
- Estrogen therapy (e.g., OCP, HRT)
- Obesity
- Prolonged recent immobility (e.g., after recent stroke)
- Dehydration (diarrhea)

Abbreviations: HRT = hormone-replacement therapy; OCP = oral contraceptive pill.

Prevention

A number of general measures may be taken to minimize the risk of thrombosis associated with long flights. Perhaps the most important step is to consider at the outset whether the passenger is actually fit to fly in the first place. For example, it is probably wise to defer long-haul travel after recent major orthopedic surgery. Passengers should be encouraged to carry out leg exercises from time to time while seated (e.g., flexion, extension, and rotation of the ankles help to promote circulation in the lower limbs). However, many airlines discourage unnecessary walking about in the cabin because there is always the possibility of encountering unexpected air turbulence. Hand luggage stowed under seats also restricts movement. Passengers should take advantage of refueling stops on long-haul flights to get off the plane and walk around for awhile. Adequate hydration should be ensured during the flight. It is not necessary to abstain from alcohol, but excessive consumption should be avoided because it promotes diuresis and discourages mobility. Similarly, sedatives are best avoided. Although estrogen-containing OCPs and HRT are recognized risk factors for venous thrombosis,

I do not advocate interrupting such hormonal medication for the period of travel.

A recent review of 10 randomized studies for the Cochrane database has confirmed the value of compression hosiery (flight socks). In the very first study performed, 231 passengers were recruited before long-haul flights and randomized into two groups. Of those who did not wear compression hosiery, 12 of 116 (10%) were found after the flight to have asymptomatic calf DVT with duplex ultrasonography, but none of the 115 who wore compression hosiery was affected. In the LONFLIT-4 study of 372 passengers considered to be at medium to high risk of thromboembolism, none of the 179 subjects wearing compression hosiery developed DVT, but six of 179 (3.35%) controls developed asymptomatic DVT (four DVT, two superficial) ($P <0.002$). In the subsequent LONFLIT-5 study of 224 high-risk passengers who went on an even longer flight, DVT was observed in six of 102 (5.8%) control subjects and only one of 103 (0.97%) subjects wearing compression hosiery ($P <0.0025$). Quite apart from reducing the risk of thrombosis, compression hosiery helps to prevent edema of the legs and feet, which can itself cause discomfort after a long flight.

Flight socks have the advantage of being readily available without prescription and are washable and thus reusable. They apply graduated pressure to the leg that is maximal at the ankle, thus encouraging venous return. The usual full-length stockings used in hospitals for prophylaxis of thromboembolism in patients undergoing surgery are not suitable for use in flight because they provide a lower pressure at the ankle (UK Class I standard: 14–17 mm Hg) because they are designed for recumbent patients. It is also important that the patient is provided with the correct type and size of compression stocking; unfortunately, there is no internationally agreed standard with regard to the degree of compression. The stockings also need to be worn correctly, taking care to ensure that there is no constriction in the popliteal area. Stockings are contraindicated in cases of peripheral vascular disease because the additional compression could provoke ischemia.

Aspirin[1] has been advocated by some in the general prophylaxis of thrombosis associated with travel, but any beneficial effect is weak in absolute terms. Aspirin is certainly very effective in preventing arterial thrombosis, because platelets play a major role in thrombosis in the arterial circulation. Arterial thrombi are rich in platelets on histologic examination, whereas thrombi in the venous circulation consist primarily of red cells enmeshed in fibrin strands but contain few platelets. It has been estimated that if the rate of travel-related DVT is 20 per 100,000 travelers, then 17,000 people would need to be treated with aspirin to prevent just one episode of DVT. Furthermore, there is a significant potential for adverse reactions: 13% of subjects taking aspirin in a study to evaluate its potential in preventing venous thrombosis associated with air travel reported gastrointestinal symptoms such as dyspepsia. Heparin may be considered in the relatively few passengers considered to be at particularly high risk for thrombosis (e.g., history of more than one thrombotic episode and an identified thrombophilic abnormality), although many such subjects are already likely to be on long-term oral anticoagulation anyway.

Unfortunately, there are no consensus guidelines yet and it is clear that there is still a wide difference in practice. This was emphasized by the results of a survey of more than 2000 delegates attending an international conference on thrombosis in Australia, which noted that 80% had taken precautions to prevent travel-related thrombosis. Just 17% wore compression hosiery and 21% relied on aspirin either alone or in combination with other measures.

Summary

It is now generally accepted that there is an association between long-distance air travel as well as other forms of long-distance travel and venous thromboembolism. The risk is largely confined to those with recognized additional risk factors for venous thromboembolism. Leg exercises while seated help to reduce the risk of DVT. There is also clear evidence from prospective and randomized clinical trials to support the use of compression hosiery as a preventive measure. By contrast, there is no firm evidence to support the indiscriminate use of aspirin as a routine prophylactic measure.

---

[1]Not FDA approved for this indication.

REFERENCES

Ashkan K, Nasim A, Dennis MI, Sayers RD. Acute arterial thrombosis after a long-haul flight. J R Soc Med 1998;91:324.

Belcaro G, Cesarone MR, Shah SS, et al. Prevention of edema, flight micro-angiopathy and venous thrombosis in long flights with elastic stockings. A randomized trial: The LONFLIT 4 Concorde Edema-SSL Study. Angiology 2002;53:635–45.

Belcaro G, Cesarone MR, Nicolaides AN, et al. Prevention of venous thrombosis with elastic stockings during long-haul flights: The LONFLIT 5 JAP study. Clin Appl Thromb Hemost 2003;9:197–201.

Bendz B, Rostrup M, Sevre K, et al. Association between hypobaric hypoxia and activation of coagulation in human beings. Lancet 2000;356:1657–8.

Bendz B, Sevre K, Andersen TO, Sandset PM. Low molecular weight heparin prevents activation of coagulation in a hypobaric environment. Blood Coagul Fibrinolysis 2001;12:371–4.

Cannegieter SC, Doggen CJ, van Houwelingen HC, Rosendaal FR. Travel-related venous thrombosis: Results from a large population-based case control study (MEGA study). PLoS Med 2006;3:e307.

Cesarone MR, Belcaro G, Nicolaides AN, et al. Venous thrombosis from air travel: The LONFLIT 3 study—prevention with aspirin vs. low molecular weight heparin (LMWH) in high risk subjects: A randomized trial. Angiology 2002;53:1–6.

Clarke M, Hopewell S, Juszczak E, et al. Compression stockings for preventing deep vein thrombosis in airline passengers. Cochrane Database Syst Rev 2006;(2) CD004002.

Collins REC, Field S, Castleden WM. Thrombosis of leg arteries after prolonged travel. BMJ 1979;2:1478.

Cruickshank JM, Gorlin R, Jennett B. Air travel and thrombotic episodes: The economy class syndrome. Lancet 1988;2:497–8.

Giangrande PLF. Air travel and thrombosis. Br J Haematol 2002;117:509–12.

Hagg S, Spigset O. Antipsychotic-induced venous thromboembolism: A review of the evidence. CNS Drugs 2002;16:765–76.

Homans J. Thrombosis of the deep leg veins due to prolonged sitting. N Engl J Med 1954;250:148–9.

Hughes RJ, Hopkins RJ, Hill S, et al. Frequency of venous thromboembolism in low to moderate risk long distance air travellers: The New Zealand Air Traveller's Thrombosis (NZATT) Study. Lancet 2003;362:2039–44.

Kelman CW, Kortt MA, Becker NG, et al. Deep vein thrombosis and air travel: Record linkage study. BMJ 2003;327:1072–5.

Kuipers S, Cannegieter SC, Middeldorp S, et al. Use of preventive measures for air travel–related venous thrombosis in professionals who attend medical conferences. J Thromb Haemost 2006;4:2373–6.

Lapostolle F, Surget V, Borron SW, et al. Severe pulmonary embolism associated with air travel. N Engl J Med 2001;345:779–83.

Loke YK, Derry S. Air travel and venous thrombosis: How much help might aspirin be? Med Gen Med 2002;4:4. Available at http://www.medscape.com/viewarticle/441153 (accessed June 1, 2007).

Martinelli I, Taioli E, Battaglioli T, et al. Risk of venous thromboembolism after air travel: Interaction with thrombophilia and oral contraceptives. Arch Intern Med 2006;163:2674–6.

Mannucci PM, Gringeri A, Peyvandi F, et al. Short-term exposure to high altitude causes coagulation activation and inhibits fibrinolysis. Thromb Haemost 2002;87:342–3.

Nicholson AN. Dehydration and long haul flights. Travel Med Int 1998;16:177–81.

Pfausler B, Vollert H, Bosch S, Schmutzhard E. Cerebral venous thrombosis: A new diagnosis in travel medicine. J Travel Med 1996;3:165–7.

Rege KP, Bevan DH, Chitolie A, Shannon MS. Risk factors and thrombosis after airline flight. Thromb Haemost 1999;81:995–6.

Rosendaal FR. Venous thrombosis: A multicausal disease. Lancet 1999;353:1167–73.

Schreijer AJM, Cannegieter SC, Meijers JCM, et al. Activation of coagulation system during air travel: A crossover study. Lancet 2006;367:832–8.

Scurr JH, Machin SJ, Bailey-King S, et al. Frequency and prevention of symptomless deep-vein thrombosis in long-haul flights: A randomized trial. Lancet 2001;357:1485–9.

Simpson K. Shelter deaths from pulmonary embolism. Lancet 1940;11:744.

Teenen RP, MacKay AJ. Peripheral arterial thrombosis related to commercial airline flights: Another manifestation of the economy class syndrome. Br J Clin Pract 1992;46:165–6.

Thomassen R, Vandenbroucke JP, Rosendaal FR. Antipsychotic drugs and venous thrombosis. Br J Psychiatry 2001;179:63–6.

Zornberg GL, Jick H. Antipsychotic drug use and risk of first-time idiopathic venous thromboembolism: A case-control study. Lancet 2000;356:1219–23.

The Blood and Spleen

Aplastic Anemia

Method of
Eva C. Guinan, MD

The survival of patients with aplastic anemia has improved dramatically in the past several decades. Improved testing for underlying acquired and congenital genetic defects has served to better segregate patients with idiopathic aplastic anemia from those with the very different prognoses associated with an inherited bone marrow failure syndrome (IBMFS) and myelodysplasia (MDS). For patients in the idiopathic (or acquired) aplastic anemia group, advances in transfusion medicine and other supportive care have also certainly contributed. Refinements in both major arms of treatment, immunosuppressive therapy (IST), and allogeneic hematopoietic stem cell transplantation (HSCT), have also contributed to current outcomes (Fig. 1). Although IST survival curves have been stable in the last decade, survival after HSCT regardless of donor source has continued to improve. Greater understanding of pathophysiology and long-term treatment outcomes are having the largest impact on triage of therapy and standards of practice.

Definition

There is no pathognomonic diagnostic test for aplastic anemia. Accordingly, aplastic anemia continues to be diagnosed by a combination of inclusion and exclusion criteria. The definition established by the International Agranulocytosis and Aplastic Anaemia Study states that patients must have bone marrow hypocellularity with two or more of the following: hemoglobin of less than 10 g/dL, platelet count of less than 50×10^9/L, and neutrophil count of less than 1.5×10^9/L. Most commonly, patients said to have aplastic anemia in fact have severe aplastic anemia, which is defined by the absolute neutrophil count (ANC) as shown in Box 1. Severity grading has become part of the diagnostic algorithm and is increasingly used as a predictor of outcome.

Differential Diagnosis

Because many conditions can fulfill these inclusion criteria, care must be taken to consider infectious, metabolic, and toxic exposures that could result in transient pancytopenia. Specific considerations are listed in many current reviews. These diagnoses are wide ranging and include hypoplastic presentations of lymphoma, leukemia, and MDS; anorexia; and transient severe bone marrow suppression due to drug exposure or, albeit rarely, a spectrum of acute viral illnesses.

Patients should be carefully evaluated for other conditions that can require an alternative management approach. A small fraction of pancytopenic and hypocellular patients have clonal cytogenetic abnormalities despite well-reviewed histology that appears to be free of any evidence of dysplasia or infiltrative disease. Accordingly, best practice should include both fluorescent in situ hybridization (FISH) and routine cytogenetics, because the yield for the latter analysis may be inadequate given the hypocellularity of the bone marrow compartment.

Although the prognostic relevance of clonal cytogenetics remains somewhat debatable, evidence of clonality at diagnosis should certainly provoke consideration of MDS as an alternative diagnosis and mandate an aggressive plan of follow-up and determination of HSCT donor status. Clonality also potentially alters immediate treatment depending on the clinical setting and most current literature. Among infectious problems, perhaps the most important consideration from a diagnostic and management perspective is HIV. However, viruses rarely cause a true aplastic picture, and their diagnosis, at present, does not have much therapeutic importance. Aplastic anemia can occur or recur during pregnancy and can resolve with either delivery or termination.

The most important alternative diagnoses are the IBMFSs (Table 1), which should be considered in virtually all patients and certainly in all pediatric patients. Such a diagnosis has important implications for medical management of the extended family, for genetic counseling, for the choice of therapy, for prognosis of the patient, and, in the setting of HSCT, for donor evaluation. A meticulous patient and family history and physical examination should be performed, although uninformative results do not eliminate the possibility of an IBMFS. Genetic testing is now widely available for some IBMFSs; however, it is clear that these syndromes are polygenic, and the relevant genetic defects have not all been defined. Therefore, testing might not be diagnostic. As additional mutations are described and as the natural history and phenotype of various mutations and polymorphisms become better elucidated, this information should be of increasing value.

In addition to IBMFS, an evaluation for paroxysmal nocturnal hemoglobinuria (PNH) should be undertaken. A clonal population of cells deficient in glycosylphosphatidylinositol (GPI)-linked proteins that characterize PNH can be found in 20% to 40% of adults with aplastic anemia without a concurrent history of clotting or hemolysis. A similar percentage of children has been found to have such cells in their bone marrow. The presence of such cells does not imply a diagnosis of classic PNH, although some patients with apparent aplastic anemia do develop classic PNH. Ongoing clinical investigation into the relation of aplastic anemia and PNH might yield further information that will assist in therapeutic decision making.

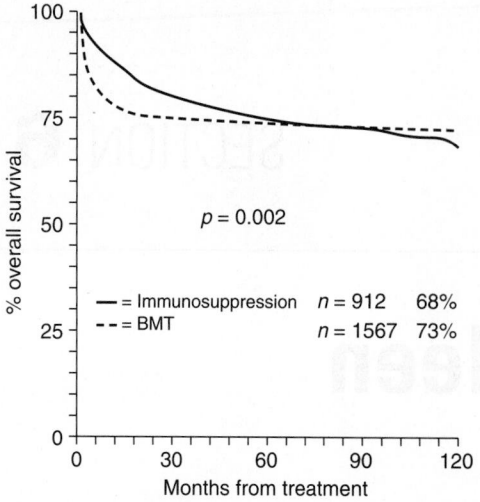

FIGURE 1. The actuarial survival of 2479 patients with acquired severe aplastic anemia. Group A received immunosuppressive therapy (IST) *(solid line)* as first-line therapy and Group B underwent hematopoietic stem cell transplant (BMT) *(dashed line)*. Ten-year survival was 73% with BMT and 68% with IST (*P* < 0.002). Data from Locasciulli A, Oneto R, Bacigalupo A, et al: Outcome of patients with acquired aplastic anemia given first-line bone marrow transplantation or immunosuppressive treatment in the last decade: A report from the European Group for Blood and Marrow Transplantation (EBMT). Haematologica 2007;92:11–18.

Supportive Care

The goals of supportive care in aplastic anemia are alleviating symptoms of anemia and addressing the risks of hemorrhage and infection that result from pancytopenia. Appropriate precautions for minimizing alloimmunization should be taken, such as use of leukodepletion techniques and conservative transfusion goals.

Preemptive counseling can play as important a role as symptom management. There are few evidence-based guidelines for activities of daily living, such as the quality of diet, extent of exercise, and travel restrictions. The best standard is frequent, open communication between physician and patient. Some practical issues, however, are common. For example, the menstrual status of female patients should be ascertained immediately on diagnosis. Because severe menorrhagia

---

BOX 1 Severity Classification of Aplastic Anemia

Severe

Bone marrow cellularity <25%
and
Two peripheral blood findings:
- Absolute neutrophil count <0.5 × 10⁹/L
- Platelet count <20 × 10⁹/L
- Reticulocyte count <20 × 10⁹/L

Very Severe

Same criteria as for severe
and
Peripheral blood absolute neutrophil count <0.2 × 10⁹/L

Nonsevere (Moderate)

Hypocellullar bone marrow
and
Peripheral blood cytopenias not meeting criteria for
    severe aplastic anemia

CURRENT DIAGNOSIS

- Patient must all meet hematologic criteria.
- Assess severity.
- Adequate cytogenetic analysis is essential.
- Consider diagnoses with treatment implications:
  - Causes of transient pancytopenia.
  - Evaluate for inherited bone marrow failure syndromes, paroxysmal nocturnal hemoglobinuria, myelodysplasia syndrome.
  - Evaluate for malignancy (leukemia, lymphoma), HIV.

can occur in the setting of protracted thrombocytopenia, use of hormonal therapy to suppress menstruation should be addressed with patients and with families of younger patients. Particular regard should be paid to anticipation of menarche in pubertal girls.

With regard to infectious risks, standards widely vary by practitioner and institution. Although the largest single cause of death in patients undergoing either HSCT or IST is infection, there is no current standard for infection prophylaxis in aplastic anemia. Clinical trials to define the best possible approaches to this issue, including the role of novel broad-spectrum anti-infectives and their schedule of use, would be very important. At the least, a detailed history taken in the context of exposure and lifestyle issues should be used to develop a plan for fever and infection prophylaxis with which the patient can be compliant.

Benefit from the use of hematopoietic growth factors to support the ANC, or indeed any lineage, has been unclear in patients with idiopathic aplastic anemia. Some concern has been raised about the association of long-term use of granulocyte colony-stimulating factor (G-CSF) (Neupogen)[1] by patients, particularly children, with aplastic anemia and subsequent development of MDS and acute myelogenous leukemia (AML), although this remains uncertain.

Monitoring of iron status should be routine for patients with ongoing red cell transfusion needs. Chelation should be initiated according to accepted guidelines to minimize complications of iron overload.

Treatment

Observation is not a successful treatment option for patients with severe aplastic anemia; older, retrospective data demonstrate a 1-year mortality with supportive care alone of more than 80%, although clearly more effective current transfusion and support strategies would improve on this outcome. Nonetheless, a recent large report from the European Group for Blood and Marrow Transplantation demonstrates that decreased time from diagnosis to treatment, whether IST or HSCT, is a highly significant predictor of survival. A triage of therapy is shown in Figure 2.

IMMUNOSUPPRESSIVE THERAPY

It is generally held that a significant percentage of aplastic anemia has an immune pathogenesis. A variety of data on immune effector cell function and repertoire, cell surface phenotype, and cytokine production support this belief. In practice, this hypothesis is also supported by the observation that IST with cyclosporine (Neoral)[1] (CSA), antithymocyte globulin (Atgam) (ATG), and corticosteroids results in response in roughly 75% of patients.

Age and response are related, and younger patients generally have a higher likelihood of response. It has also been reported that children with IST and very severe aplastic anemia do better than their age peers with severe aplastic anemia and that children (<16 years)

---

[1]Not FDA approved for this indication.

TABLE 1 Inherited Bone Marrow Failure Syndromes Commonly Associated with Pancytopenia*

Syndrome	Common Hematologic Findings	Diagnostic Tests Available[†]
Amegakaryocytic thrombocytopenia	Thrombocytopenia with absent or hypolobulated megakaryocytes Macrocytosis Progressive pancytopenia with marrow hypoplasia	Gene mutation analysis
Dyskeratosis congenita	Macrocytosis Thrombocytopenia Progressive pancytopenia with marrow hypoplasia	Gene mutation analysis Telomere length (may be shortened)
Fanconi's anemia	Macrocytosis Single, bilineage, or trilineage cytopenia Progressive pancytopenia with marrow hypoplasia	Abnormal chromosomal breakage or sister-chromatid exchange in the presence of DNA cross-linkers Cell cycle progression in the presence of DNA cross-linkers Gene mutation analysis
Shwachman-Diamond syndrome	Neutropenia Progressive pancytopenia with marrow hypoplasia	Radiologic bony abnormalities Serum trypsinogen and isoamylase levels (may be decreased) Gene mutation analysis

*Diamond-Blackfan anemia, as well as less common disorders such as Pearson's, Seckel's, and Noonan's syndromes; cartilage–hair hypoplasia; and reticular dysgenesis, can progress to marrow failure meeting the definition of aplastic anemia.
[†]Clinically approved mutation testing is becoming increasingly available, but not all genetic defects have been defined for any of these disorders.

with very severe aplastic anemia have better survival rates than similarly affected adults. Age does not affect the relative survival rate of patients with less severe aplastic anemia.

Randomized studies have demonstrated better response when IST agents are used in combination. In addition to their general immunomodulatory capacity, the immunologic effects of IST may be specific, because direct lympholytic and bone marrow stimulatory activities have been described. The addition of further immunosuppressive medications, such as mycophenolate, to this regimen has thus far not improved outcomes.

IST responses can be of varying degree and duration and can take 3 to 6 months to become evident. Often, responding patients continue to manifest some evidence of bone marrow failure, with mild degrees of cytopenia or residual macrocytosis commonly observed. Slow taper of CSA in IST responders is advisable, generally over longer than 6 months, and a significant fraction of patients demonstrate prolonged dependence on CSA for persistent hematologic improvement. A second course of IST in patients who failed a first course can produce response in 35% to 50% of patients. Complete or partial loss of response occurs in an appreciable number of patients,

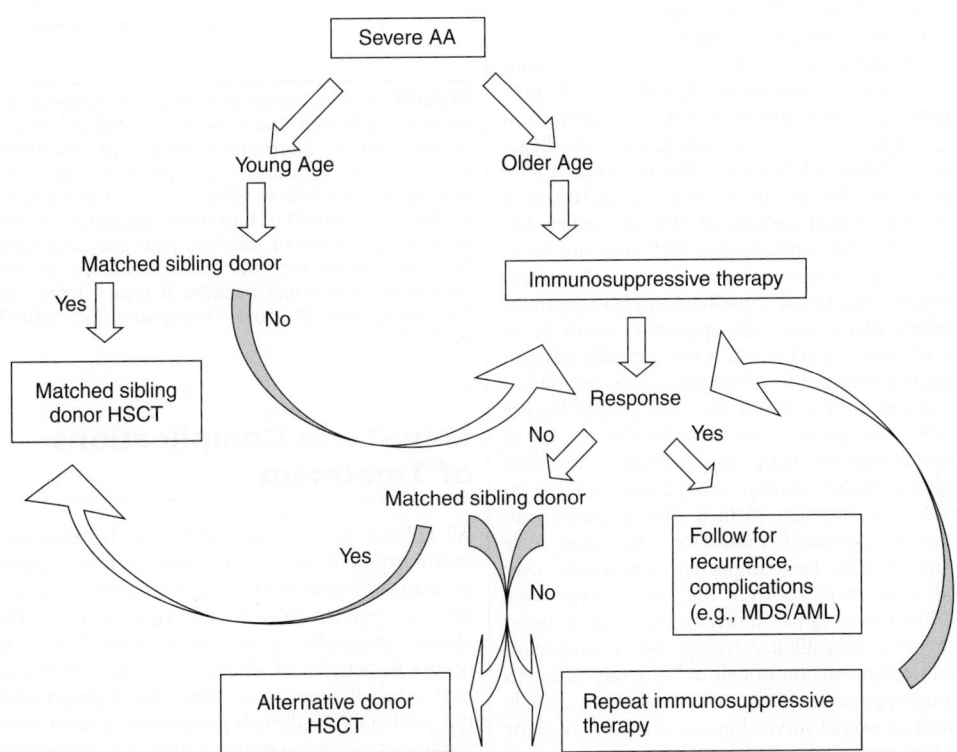

FIGURE 2. Triage of aplastic anemia (AA) therapies. The age limit suggested by young/old is variable from report to report, but generally sits in the 30- to 40-year-old range. AML = acute myelogenous leukemia; HSCT = hematopoietic stem cell transplant; MDS = myelodysplasia.

CURRENT THERAPY

- Minimize interval between diagnosis and initiation of treatment.
- Determine if an MSD is available.
- If the patient is young and has an MSD, proceed to HSCT with non-TBI regimen.
- If has no MSD or is older, proceed to IST with CSA/ATG/steroid.
- For treatment failure, reconsider IST versus HSCT options.

ATG = antithymocyte globulin; CSA = cyclosporine; HSCT = hematopoietic stem cell transplantation; IST = immunosuppressive therapy; MSD = matched sibling donor; TBI = total body irradiation.

approximately one third, and can become manifest years after cessation of IST or immediately on CSA taper. Re-treatment with the same or a similar regimen is often successful.

HEMATOPOIETIC STEM CELL TRANSPLANTATION

HSCT is the only truly curative therapy for aplastic anemia and produces stable survival rates in the range of 60% to 80%, depending on donor type and other HSCT variables (Fig. 3). In young patients with matched sibling donors (MSDs), a short interval from diagnosis to HSCT, and little prior therapy, survival rates up to 97% have been recently reported. Conversely, prior IST or excessive transfusion (or both) are associated with worse outcome. Thus, the general recommendation is for young patients with MSDs to proceed to HSCT as soon as the diagnosis is confirmed. The age cutoff for this decision varies somewhat, but the recommendation certainly holds for patients younger than 30 years and is often implemented for those younger than 40 years.

HSCT for aplastic anemia from MSD can be successfully achieved with radiation-free preparative regimens, of which the most standard and widely used is cyclophosphamide (Cytoxan)[1] (CY) and ATG conditioning. CSA and short-course methotrexate (Trexall)[1] (MTX) provide highly effective graft-versus-host disease (GVHD) prophylaxis in this setting. In a group of adults and children undergoing MSD allogeneic HSCT, this classic CY/ATG/CSA/MTX regimen produced a 96% rate of sustained engraftment, 3% rate of severe acute GVHD, 26% rate of chronic GVHD, and overall survival of 88% at median follow-up of 9 years. A recent study suggests that ATG may not be as essential to this outcome as previously thought. All stem cell sources, including sibling umbilical cord blood, have been used successfully, although use of peripheral blood stem cells appears to result in an unacceptably high rate of chronic GHVD and is not currently advised.

The dearth of alternative therapies for those who fail to respond to IST, coupled with the success of MSD HSCT, have encouraged the use of alternative-donor HSCT for aplastic anemia. Originally, the use of somewhat more aggressive regimens than those necessary with MSD engendered more regimen-related toxicity, and patients coming to alternative-donor HSCT were often late in their clinical course with significant aplastic anemia–associated morbidity. Outcomes were somewhat disappointing. Results have improved significantly over the past decade, and even more so over the past 5 years (see Fig. 3B). Moving HSCT treatment earlier in therapeutic triage, coupled with improvements in histocompatibility typing, better supportive care, and the successful implementation of reduced-intensity regimens and alternative immunosuppressive strategies have produced highly encouraging results, with an overall survival in excess of 70% in some reports. However, the best results are seen when patients are younger, and outcomes in those older than 40 years remain less satisfactory.

[1]Not FDA approved for this indication.

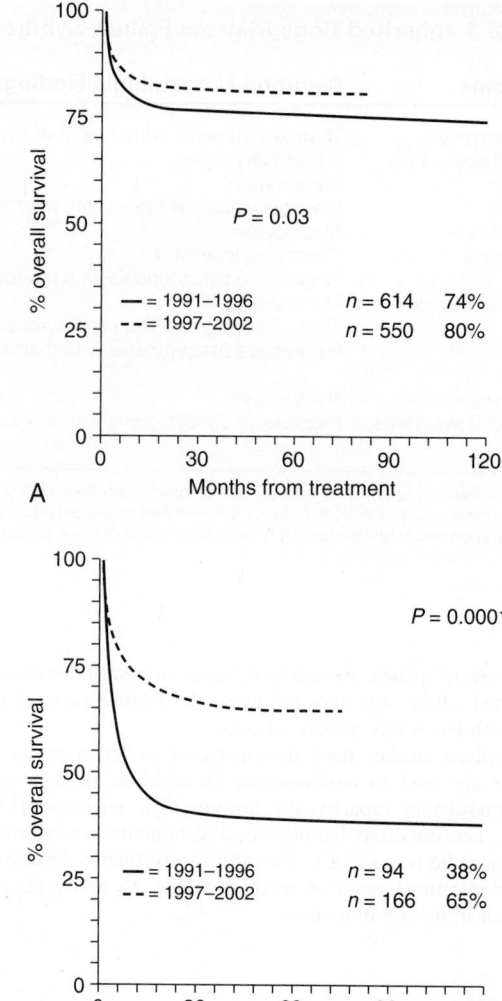

FIGURE 3. The actuarial survival of patients undergoing hematopoietic stem cell transplantation (HSCT) from matched sibling donors **(A)** or alternative donors **(B)** by time periods. Results improved for both donor groups in the later time period (matched sibling donors 74% vs 80%, $P = 0.03$) and alternative donors (38% vs 65%, $P = 0.0001$). Data from Locasciulli A, Oneto R, Bacigalupo A, et al: Outcome of patients with acquired aplastic anemia given first line bone marrow transplantation or immunosuppressive treatment in the last decade: A report from the European Group for Blood and Marrow Transplantation (EBMT). Haematologica 2007;92:11–18.

Long-Term Complications of Treatment

All aplastic anemia treatments can be associated with significant morbidity, be it the iron-overload of chronic transfusion or the more protean problems of IST or HSCT. These include, in both cases, significant regimen-related end-organ toxicity. The development of clonal cytogenetic abnormalities after IST is well described and occurs in patients of all ages, regardless of treatment response, and over a broad time frame. The rate of progression to frank AML is not predictable, although progression is most common in those with monosomy 7 or complex cytogenetic abnormalities. Patients with aplastic anemia who undergo HSCT generally experience fewer toxicities than does the overall HSCT population, in part due to the reduced intensity of aplastic anemia regimens. Growth and fertility may be well preserved, but persistent infectious complications, pulmonary insufficiency, dermatologic pathology, avascular necrosis, and other bone and joint issues, as well as hypothyroidism or other endocrine disturbances, can occur, as can secondary malignancies. Some of these conditions reflect the sequelae of chronic GVHD itself, and others reflect the toxicity of drugs used to manage GVHD. The toll of GVHD is real; decreased quality of life and overall survival are observed in the nearly one half of aplastic anemia patients experiencing chronic GVHD.

Conclusions

Improvements in diagnosis, supportive care, IST, and HSCT have led to significant improvements in survival for patients with severe aplastic anemia. However, there are still controversies over the optimal choice of therapy for individual patients, and any given choice can lead to a number of serious regimen-related toxicities. Further insights into the pathophysiology of bone marrow failure, increased diagnostic accuracy for IBMFS, greater appreciation of the risk and epidemiology of late complications, and steady progress in therapeutics will hopefully combine to yield increasingly well-targeted and more-successful treatment.

Acknowledgments

Eva C. Guinan is a recipient of a Specified Established Researcher Award from the Aplastic Anemia & MDS International Foundation.

REFERENCES

Ades L, Mary JY, Robin M, et al. Long-term outcome after bone marrow transplantation for severe aplastic anemia. Blood 2004;103:2490–7.
Alter BP. Bone marrow failure: A child is not just a small adult (but an adult can have a childhood disease). Hematology (Am Soc Hematol Educ Program) 2005;96–103.
Frickhofen N, Heimpel H, Kaltwasser JP, Schrezenmeier H. Antithymocyte globulin with or without cyclosporin A: 11-year follow-up of a randomized trial comparing treatments of aplastic anemia. Blood 2003;101:1236–42.
Fuhrer M, Burdach S, Ebell W, et al. Relapse and clonal disease in children with aplastic anemia (AA) after immunosuppressive therapy (IST): The SAA 94 experience. German/Austrian Pediatric Aplastic Anemia Working Group. Klin Padiatr 1998;210:173–9.
Kojima S, Horibe K, Inaba J, et al. Long-term outcome of acquired aplastic anaemia in children: Comparison between immunosuppressive therapy and bone marrow transplantation. Br J Haematol 2000;111:321–8.
Kurre P, Johnson FL, Deeg HJ. Diagnosis and treatment of children with aplastic anemia. Pediatr Blood Cancer 2005;45:770–80.
Locasciulli A, Oneto R, Bacigalupo A, et al. Outcome of patients with acquired aplastic anemia given first line bone marrow transplantation or immuno-suppressive treatment in the last decade: A report from the European Group for Blood and Marrow Transplantation (EBMT). Haematologica 2007;92:11–8.
Maciejewski JP, Risitano A, Sloand EM, et al. Distinct clinical outcomes for cytogenetic abnormalities evolving from aplastic anemia. Blood 2002;99:3129–35.
Marsh JCW, Ball SE, Darbyshire P, et al. Guidelines for the diagnosis and management of acquired aplastic anaemia. Br J Haematol 2003;123:782–801.
Parker C, Omine M, Richards S, et al. Diagnosis and management of paroxysmal nocturnal hemoglobinuria. Blood 2005;106:3699–709.
Schrezenmeier H, Passweg JR, Marsh JC, et al. Worse outcome and more chronic GVHD with peripheral blood progenitor cells than bone marrow in HLA-matched sibling donor transplants for young patients with severe acquired aplastic anemia: A report from the European Group for Blood and Marrow Transplantation and the Center for International Blood and Marrow Transplant Research. Blood 2007;110(4):1397–400.
Socie G, Gluckman E. Cure from severe aplastic anemia in vivo and late effects. Acta Haematol 2000;103:49–54.
Socie G, Mary JY, Schrezenmeier H, et al. Granulocyte-stimulating factor and severe aplastic anemia: a survey by the European Group for Blood and Marrow Transplantation (EBMT). Blood 2007;109:2794–6.
Young NS. Paroxysmal nocturnal hemoglobinuria: Current issues in pathophysiology and treatment. Curr Hematol Rep 2005;4:103–9.
Young NS, Calado RT, Scheinberg P. Current concepts in the pathophysiology and treatment of aplastic anemia. Blood 2006;108:2509–19.

Iron Deficiency

Method of
James C. Barton, MD

Iron deficiency is common worldwide. In developed countries, iron requirements of reproductive-age women (menstruation, pregnancy, lactation) and the increased iron requirements for growth in infants and children often exceed dietary iron availability and absorption. Pathologic blood loss in men and postmenopausal women, especially that from the gastrointestinal tract, is also a common cause of iron deficiency. In less well-developed areas, diets poor in absorbable iron, vegetarianism, intestinal parasitism, chronic diarrhea, and multiparity are common causes of iron deficiency.

Successful treatment of iron deficiency depends on identification and management of its cause(s) and administration of a regimen that takes into account the cause and severity of iron deficiency, comorbid disorders, and concomitant medications.

Normal Iron Metabolism

Body iron quantities are regulated by controlled absorption that responds to the rate of erythropoiesis and other body demands. Quantities of total body iron in healthy adults are approximately 4.0 g in men and 3.5 g in women. Hemoglobin in men contains about 2.0 g Fe and in women about 1.5 g Fe. Storage sites in men contain about 1.0 g and in women about 0.3 g. The remaining iron, approximately 6% of total body quantities, is incorporated in myoglobin, heme-containing enzymes, transferrin, and other compounds.

Dietary iron typically consists of heme derived from animal products, nonheme ionic iron in vegetable foods, and inorganic iron added to fortify certain foodstuffs. Iron compounds must be soluble for absorption to occur. Heme iron is readily soluble. Absorption of nonheme iron is facilitated by gastric acid, ascorbic acid (vitamin C), and certain amino acids and sugars that maintain iron solubility at acid values of pH. Other substances commonly present in food, such as tannate in tea and phytates in vegetables, inhibit iron absorption.

Iron is absorbed only from the small intestine, especially the duodenum. Transport of nonheme iron across the microvilli of absorptive enterocytes requires its reduction to a soluble ferrous form and binding to DCT1 (divalent cation transporter), quantities of which are increased in iron deficiency. Heme enters enterocytes via a surface receptor and is cleaved thereafter to release iron. Other iron uptake mechanisms also exist in enterocytes. Transport of iron to transferrin in the blood is modulated by ferroportin (an iron export protein), HFE (hemochromatosis) protein, and transferrin receptor at the basolateral surfaces of enterocytes. On average, 5% to 10% of food iron is absorbed daily.

Iron is highly conserved due to phagocytosis and digestion of senescent erythrocytes by macrophages in the spleen, marrow, and liver and by iron storage in ferritin molecules (or degraded ferritin aggregates known as *hemosiderin*). Hepcidin, a liver-derived polypeptide that is a potent regulator of iron absorption and transport, controls the release of conserved iron into the circulation from macrophages via ferroportin. Iron delivered by transferrin to erythrocytes and other cells via their surface transferrin receptors. Unavoidable iron losses of about 1.0 mg daily occur due to exfoliation of skin and gastrointestinal tract cells, perspiration, and minor trauma. In menstruating women, additional average daily iron losses average 0.5 to 1.0 mg. Average net iron losses with normal term pregnancies are 700 mg. If insufficient quantities of iron are presented to the gastrointestinal tract in a form acceptable for absorption, or if iron absorptive mechanisms are not intact, iron depletion, iron-deficient erythropoiesis, and iron-deficiency anemia develop sequentially in accordance with the rate of net iron loss.

Causes of Iron Deficiency

Some infants and adolescents ingest insufficient dietary iron to meet physiologic demands of rapid growth. Many women of childbearing age develop iron deficiency due to the high iron requirements of menstruation, pregnancy, and lactation. Many otherwise healthy regular blood donors and highly trained athletes develop iron deficiency.

Pathologic blood loss from gastrointestinal tract lesions of diverse etiologies is a common cause. These include erosion or ulceration of the esophagus, stomach, or duodenum, malignant neoplasms (particularly those of the colon, esophagus, or stomach), microangiopathy (inherited or acquired), inflammatory disorders (especially Crohn's disease), diverticula, and polyps. Chronic intestinal blood loss due to hookworms is common in tropical regions. Some patients who receive warfarin (Coumadin) or aspirin therapy have chronic gastrointestinal blood loss without demonstrable anatomic lesions. Nonbleeding gastrointestinal causes in patients with few or no gastrointestinal symptoms include atrophic gastritis, celiac disease, and *Helicobacter pylori* gastritis.

Less commonly, there is urinary tract blood loss from lesions within the kidneys, ureters, or bladder or due to conditions that cause hemoglobinuria (e.g., defective heart valve prostheses, paroxysmal nocturnal hemoglobinuria). Chronic blood loss from the respiratory tract is sometimes caused by recurrent epistaxis or hemoptysis (e.g., idiopathic pulmonary hemosiderosis, lung fluke infestation).

Blood loss during major chest operations or with hip or knee replacement can induce iron deficiency that is unapparent until weeks or months later. Patients on chronic hemodialysis develop iron deficiency due to blood retained in dialysis apparatus, hemolysis, and laboratory testing. Antitransferrin antibodies or mutations of the ceruloplasmin gene have been reported as rare causes.

Signs and Symptoms of Iron Deficiency

Many persons develop weakness, ease of fatigue, or dyspnea with exertion, often before anemia develops. Infants or children can present with retarded motor and intellectual skills.

Pica, the compulsive ingestion of (often) non-nutritive substances, is a distinctive consequence that occurs in approximately one half of persons with iron deficiency, especially women. Ice eating (pagophagia) is the most common form of pica; some patients prefer dirt or clay, salt, sand, paper, cold fruit or lettuce, laundry starch, or other substances.

Some patients report evidence of bleeding. In adults with severe, chronic iron deficiency, sore mouth or tongue, nail and hair changes, dysphagia, paresthesias, and loss of memory and normal affect sometimes occur. Others present with restless legs.

Iron deficiency is diagnosed in a high percentage of children and adults coincidentally when routine physical and laboratory evaluations are performed. The most common physical sign of iron deficiency is pallor, although some patients have angular stomatitis, glossitis, koilonychia, or cricoid or esophageal web.

Laboratory Abnormalities

Laboratory abnormalities associated with iron deficiency and other forms of anemia in the differential diagnosis are displayed in Table 1. Because iron deficiency is more common in women, many laboratories report lower reference limits for iron measures in women than men. Nonetheless, astute clinicians recognize that serum iron measures characteristic of iron deficiency are equally applicable to men and women. Persons with serum ferritin less than 50 ng/mL often have iron depletion or deficiency by bone marrow examination criteria, regardless of the laboratory's lower reference limit for serum ferritin. Other causes of abnormal serum iron measures or anemia occur in some patients with iron deficiency (see Table 1).

TABLE 1 Laboratory Assessment of Iron Deficiency*

Laboratory Measurement	Diagnostic Result
Depletion of Iron Stores	
Serum ferritin concentration	<50 ng/mL
Serum total iron-binding capacity	Increased
Stainable marrow iron	Absent
Iron-Deficient Erythropoiesis	
Serum transferrin saturation	<15%
Mean corpuscular volume	<80 fL
RDW	Increased
Free erythrocyte protoporphyrin concentration	Increased
Reticulocyte index	Low
Serum transferrin receptor concentration	Increased
Iron-Deficiency Anemia	
Hemoglobin concentration	Men: <13.0 g/dL
	Women: <12.0 g/dL

*Consult laboratory-specific reference ranges. The differential diagnosis often includes anemia of chronic disease or inflammation, renal insufficiency, or malignancy, in which total iron-binding capacity is usually decreased, serum ferritin concentration is normal or increased, and RDW is normal. These forms of anemia can also occur concomitantly with iron deficiency. In some patients, the differential diagnosis also includes thalassemia minor, hemoglobinopathy E or Lepore hemoglobinopathy, various forms of sideroblastic anemia, anemia of chronic liver disease, anemia of chronic hemolysis, hypoplastic and aplastic anemias, myeloproliferative and myelodysplastic disorders, congenital dyserythropoietic anemias, anemia of myxedema, and megaloblastic anemia.
Abbreviation: RDW = red blood cell distribution width.

Principles of Iron Replacement Therapy

Treatment should be undertaken after the diagnosis is established and potential benefits and adverse effects of therapy options have been considered (Table 2). Therapy must be individualized and monitored regularly. Many patients can be treated with oral iron preparations. Hematinic combinations should not be used in lieu of an adequate pretreatment evaluation. There is no indication for administering iron therapy except to treat iron deficiency.

Intravenous iron therapy should be reserved for noncompliant patients, those unable to take oral iron, patients who absorb iron poorly, patients who have not had a satisfactory therapeutic response to oral iron replacement, and patients in whom recurrent bleeding causes iron loss in excess of what can be replaced at an acceptable rate with oral therapy. For chronic hemodialysis patients, intravenous iron administration is the only suitable route of replacement. However, intravenous therapy does not induce a more rapid erythropoietic response than is possible with oral replacement. Intravenous iron therapy should be given only by physicians experienced in such treatment who are prepared to treat hypotension or other hypersensitivity symptoms that sometimes occur. I do not recommend single intravenous iron doses greater than 500 mg (see Table 2).

Increasing the quantity of food iron is important in children with iron deficiency, many of whom have other nutritional deficits. Infants and some children need iron supplements; these should be prescribed by experienced pediatricians. In adults, dietary maneuvers as treatment are often ineffective. Multivitamins that contain "daily" amounts of iron (usually 10–20 mg Fe as inorganic iron salts) are usually inadequate for replacement therapy, and there is no basis for advising patients to take these preparations routinely unless they are premenopausal women, vigorous athletes, chronic blood donors, or vegetarians with uncomplicated iron depletion. Erythrocyte transfusion is indicated to elevate the circulating red blood cell mass in persons with iron-deficiency anemia who have vigorous bleeding or cardiac or respiratory compromise.

TABLE 2 Adverse Effects of Iron Replacement Therapy*

Adverse Effect	Form of Iron Therapy	Relative Frequency	Susceptible Patients
Black discoloration of stools	Iron salts,† carbonyl iron†	Very common	Children, adults
Epigastric pain, nausea, constipation, abdominal cramps, metallic taste	Iron salts† (more likely, especially with ascorbic acid), carbonyl iron† (less likely), intravenous iron‡ (unlikely)	Common	Children, adults
Acute iron poisoning	Iron salts†	Common in children; rare in adults	Children: accidental ingestion Adults: accidental ingestion, suicide attempt
Arthralgias, myalgias, bone aches, low-grade fever	Intravenous iron‡ (likely with doses >500 mg Fe), oral iron (less likely)†	Uncommon	Children, adults
Decreased absorption of other medications	Iron salts, carbonyl iron†	Uncommon	Children, adults
Flushing, hypotension	Intravenous iron‡	Uncommon with proper administration	Children, adults
Skin discoloration due to extravasation	Intravenous iron‡	Very uncommon with proper administration	Children, adults
Tooth discoloration (temporary)	Liquid oral iron elixir§	Very uncommon with proper administration	Children
Severe hypersensitivity, anaphylaxis	Intravenous iron‡	Very uncommon with proper administration	Children, adults
Increased susceptibility to infections with *Vibrio vulnificus* and other *Vibrio* species	Intravenous iron (dose-related)‡	Probably uncommon	Hemodialysis patients who consume raw shellfish or are exposed to water from warm seas
Iron overload	Intravenous iron (more likely),‡ oral iron (less likely)†	Rare	Adults

*I do not recommend single intravenous iron doses >500 mg due to risk of post-treatment myalgias, arthralgias, and low-grade fever. I do not recommend intramuscular iron therapy due to risk of severe allergy or anaphylaxis; pain, discoloration, and atrophy of subcutaneous tissues at injection sites; therapy failure due to limitations of iron doses; and rare occurrence of sarcomas at injection sites. Avoid intravenous iron therapy in pregnant women unless the benefit outweighs the potential risk to the fetus. Intravenous iron therapy for children should be undertaken only by pediatricians experienced in such management.
†Feosol Ferrous Sulfate Tablets, 65 mg Fe/tablet; Niferex Film Coated Tablets, 50 mg Fe/tablet; Feosol Carbonyl Iron Tablets, 45 mg Fe; ICAR Pediatric Chewables, 15 mg Fe/tablet; ICAR Pediatric Suspension, 15 mg Fe/1.25 mL.
‡InFeD, 50 mg Fe/mL; Dexferrum, 50 mg Fe/mL; Venofer, 20 mg Fe/mL; Ferrlecit, 12.5 mg Fe/mL.
§Niferex Elixir, 100 mg Fe/5 mL.

ORAL IRON THERAPY

Carbonyl Iron

Carbonyl iron consists of microspheres of pure iron precipitated from the gas iron pentacarbonyl; it is widely used for food iron fortification. This is the oral therapy of choice for most persons, because it causes less gastrointestinal toxicity than iron salts and is equally effective in correcting iron deficiency. Increasing the dosage gradually over a few weeks until the target dose is reached can improve tolerance in some patients.

The usual adult dosage is 45 mg three times daily (Feosol Carbonyl Iron tablets, 45 mg Fe/tablet), preferably taken on an empty stomach. Doses for adolescents (to be divided into three or four equal portions) are higher: For adolescent boys younger than 18 years, the dose is 90 to 135 mg daily, and for menstruating adolescent girls 12 to 18 years, the dose is 45 to 135 mg daily. In preadolescent school-age children, administer up to 6 mg/kg/day (ICAR Pediatric Chewables, 15 mg Fe/tablet); in infants and young children, administer 3 mg/kg/day (ICAR Pediatric Suspension, 15 mg Fe/1.25 mL).

In patients with anemia, the hemoglobin concentration usually increases about 1.0 g/dL weekly. Continue treatment until anemia is corrected and serum ferritin concentration is higher than 50 ng/mL; microcytosis, if present, typically resolves several months after iron stores are replete. In patients who have gastrointestinal symptoms, administer iron with meals or reduce dosing frequency, but expect delayed correction of iron deficiency. Completion of therapy in patients without continuing blood loss typically requires several months.

Iron Salts

Iron salts are suitable for many children and adults. The most commonly used preparation is ferrous sulfate (Feosol Ferrous Sulfate Tablets, 65 mg Fe/tablet; many generic brands); a polysaccharide-iron complex is also popular (Niferex Film Coated Tablets, 50 mg Fe/tablet).

In adults, the dose is one tablet three times daily, preferably on an empty stomach. In older children, the dose is 5 mg/kg of iron daily as tablets or elixir (administered by an adult).

Rate of response of anemia, monitoring of hemoglobin and ferritin concentrations, and dose adjustments for adverse gastrointestinal symptoms attributed to treatment are similar to those for carbonyl iron therapy. Ferrous gluconate, ferrous fumarate, polysaccharide-iron complex, and enteric-coated iron preparations can be used similarly. However, they might contain less iron per tablet than ferrous sulfate or be less absorbable, and thus induce therapeutic responses less rapidly. Most are more expensive.

CURRENT DIAGNOSIS

- Weakness, fatigue, pica, and pallor are common.
- Transferrin saturation is usually <15% (decreased serum iron level, normal or elevated total iron-binding capacity).
- Serum transferrin receptor concentration is elevated in most cases.
- Serum ferritin level is typically <20 ng/mL.
- Serum ferritin level is normal or elevated in patients who also have anemia of chronic disease, active liver disease, renal insufficiency, or malignancy.
- Reticulocytopenia and normal or low erythrocyte count are typical.
- Anemia with or without microcytosis is a late development.

CURRENT THERAPY

- Identify and correct causes of inadequate nutrition and blood loss.
- Individualize therapy and monitor outcomes regularly.
- Many patients can be treated with oral preparations; noncompliance is the most common cause of treatment failure.
- Oral therapy often fails in patients who take antacids, H₂ blockers, proton pump antagonists, or calcium supplements.
- Use intravenous therapy for noncompliance or inadequate response to oral iron, severe iron deficiency, recurrent blood loss, malabsorption, or hemodialysis.
- Many patients with nondialysis chronic renal disease, chronic inflammation, or malignancy and all hemodialysis patients require erythropoietin (Epogen, Procrit, Aranesp) therapy to maximize response to iron replacement.

INTRAVENOUS IRON THERAPY

Iron Dextran

Iron dextran preparations (InFeD or Dexferrum, 50 mg Fe/mL) are indicated for treatment of iron deficiency in persons with normal renal function who fail to respond to or do not tolerate oral iron supplementation. Iron dextran is safe and effective when administered properly (see Table 2). Each infusion in adults should consist of 500 mg Fe in 250 to 500 mL of normal saline. I recommend premedication with intravenous dexamethasone (Deltasone) (10 mg) plus either diphenhydramine (Benadryl) (25 mg), cimetidine (Tagamet) (400 mg), or famotidine (Pepcid) (20 mg) and giving a test dose of 25 mg Fe or approximately 5 mL over 10 to 15 minutes in a freely flowing intravenous line. If there is no immediate adverse effect, the remaining dose should be infused over 2 to 3 hours. Infusions are repeated every 2 to 3 weeks until anemia is corrected and iron stores are replete, as described for oral iron preparations. Many patients who require intravenous iron dextran for initial management have recurrent bleeding and thus require periodic maintenance infusions.

Iron Sucrose

Iron sucrose (Venofer, 20 mg Fe/mL) is indicated for treatment of iron deficiency in patients undergoing chronic hemodialysis who also receive erythropoietin therapy (epoetin alfa, epoetin beta, or darbepoetin). In previously untreated patients, a test dose should be administered before the first infusion as described for iron dextran. Doses of 200 to 300 mg[1] Fe administered intravenously over 2 hours during hemodialysis are safe and effective. In anemic patients with nondialysis-dependent chronic kidney disease, oral and intravenous iron therapies yield similar hemoglobin responses, but intravenous iron is more effective in increasing iron stores. Goals of therapy include maintenance of serum transferrin saturation at least 30%, serum ferritin concentration at least 300 ng/mL, and hemoglobin greater than 11.0 g/dL. Most hemodialysis patients require ongoing or recurrent therapy.

Iron Gluconate

This product (Ferrlecit, 12.5 mg Fe/mL) is also indicated for treating iron deficiency in patients undergoing chronic hemodialysis who are receiving erythropoietin therapy. A test dose should be administered before the first infusion, as described for iron dextran. Typical treatments consist of 125 mg of Fe administered intravenously at each hemodialysis treatment. Adequacy of therapy is monitored in the same manner as for iron sucrose therapy.

---

[1]Not FDA approved for this indication.

FAILURE OF IRON REPLACEMENT THERAPY

The most common cause of unsuccessful therapy with oral iron supplements is poor compliance due to adverse gastrointestinal effects. Another common cause is unrecognized or uncorrectable chronic or recurrent blood loss associated with angiodysplasia of the gastrointestinal tract or chronic anticoagulant therapy. Some commonly prescribed drugs markedly decrease iron absorption, including antacids, H₂ blockers, proton pump antagonists, calcium supplements, and tetracycline. Gastrectomy, duodenectomy, achlorhydria, celiac disease, and gastric or intestinal bypass are often associated with iron malabsorption. Patients suspected to have suboptimal iron absorption unrelated to medications should be evaluated for additional causes of anemia. Many patients who have inadequate responses to oral iron therapy require intravenous iron replacement. In persons with chronic disease or renal insufficiency and in those receiving anticancer chemotherapy, erythropoietin therapy is often necessary to induce a satisfactory erythropoietic response.

REFERENCES

Annibale B, Capurso G, Chistolini A, et al. Gastrointestinal causes of refractory iron deficiency anemia in patients without gastrointestinal symptoms. Am J Med 2001;111:439–45.

Barton JC, Barton EH, Bertoli LF, et al. Intravenous iron dextran therapy in patients with iron deficiency and normal renal function who failed to respond to or did not tolerate oral iron supplementation. Am J Med 2000;109:27–32.

Cook JD, Flowers CH, Skikne BS. The quantitative assessment of body iron. Blood 2003;101:3359–64.

Ferguson BJ, Skikne BS, Simpson KM, et al. Serum transferrin receptor distinguishes the anemia of chronic disease from iron deficiency anemia. J Lab Clin Med 1992;119:385–90.

Hershko C, Bar-Or D, Gaziel Y, et al. Diagnosis of iron deficiency anemia in a rural population of children: Relative usefulness of serum ferritin, red cell protoporphyrin, red cell indices, and transferrin saturation determinations. Am J Clin Nutr 1981;34:1600–10.

Hershko C, Hoffbrand AV, Keret D, et al. Role of autoimmune gastritis, *Helicobacter pylori* and celiac disease in refractory or unexplained iron deficiency anemia. Haematologica 2005;90:585–95.

Ioannou GN, Rockey DC, Bryson CL, et al. Iron deficiency and gastrointestinal malignancy: A population-based cohort study. Am J Med 2002; 113:276–80.

Lozoff B, Beard J, Connor J, et al. Long-lasting neural and behavioral effects of iron deficiency in infancy. Nutr Rev 2006;64:S34–43.

Van Wyck DB, Roppolo M, Martinez CO, et al. A randomized, controlled trial comparing IV iron sucrose to oral iron in anemic patients with nondialysis-dependent CKD. Kidney Int 2005;68:2846–56.

Yates JM, Logan EC, Stewart RM. Iron deficiency anaemia in general practice: Clinical outcomes over three years and factors influencing diagnostic investigations. Postgrad Med J 2004;80:405–10.

Autoimmune Hemolytic Anemia

Method of
Nidra Rodriguez, MD

Hemolysis, the premature destruction of red blood cells (RBCs), leads to hemolytic anemia when the bone marrow cannot compensate for RBC loss. Autoimmune hemolytic anemia (AIHA) occurs as a result of antibody production against self-RBC antigens. Suggested causes for the occurrence of AIHA include alteration in immunoregulatory mechanisms leading to loss of immune tolerance and activation of B cells, T cells, or both. AIHA can be idiopathic, or it can occur secondary to infections, malignancies, or autoimmune disorders. Types of AIHA include warm-antibody AIHA, cold-antibody

BOX 1 Classification of Hemolytic Anemia Mediated by Antibodies

I. Warm-autoantibody type
   A. Primary or idiopathic warm-antibody AIHA
   B. Secondary warm-antibody AIHA associated with
      1. Lymphoproliferative disorders (e.g., Hodgkin's disease, lymphoma)
      2. Rheumatic/autoimmune disorders (e.g., SLE, ulcerative colitis)
      3. Certain nonlymphoid neoplasms (e.g., ovarian tumors)
      4. Ingestion of certain drugs (e.g., α-methyldopa [Aldomet])
II. Cold-autoantibody type
   A. Mediated by cold agglutinins
      1. Idiopathic (primary) chronic cold-agglutinin disease (most exhibit evidence of monoclonal B-lymphoproliferation)
      2. Secondary cold-agglutinin hemolytic anemia associated with
         a. Infections (e.g., *Mycoplasma pneumoniae*, infectious mononucleosis)
         b. Clinically evident malignant B-cell lymphoproliferative disorders
   B. Mediated by cold hemolysins
      1. Idiopathic (primary) paroxysmal cold hemoglobinuria
      2. Secondary
         a. Donath-Landsteiner hemolytic anemia, usually associated with an acute viral syndrome in children
         b. Associated with congenital or tertiary syphilis in adults
III. Mixed cold and warm autoantibodies
   A. Primary or idiopathic mixed AIHA
   B. Secondary mixed AIHA
      1. Associated with the rheumatic disorders, especially SLE
IV. Drug-immune hemolytic anemia
   A. Hapten or drug-adsorption mechanism
   B. Ternary (immune) complex mechanism
   C. True autoantibody mechanism

Adapted from Packman CH: Hemolytic anemia due to warm autoantibodies. Blood Rev 2008;22[1]:17–31.
Abbreviations: AIHA = autoimmune hemolytic anemia; SLE = systemic lupus erythematosus.

BOX 2 Laboratory Values That Suggest Hemolysis

Reticulocytosis >125,000/L of blood
- If automated determination of reticulocyte concentration is unavailable, the value can be derived by multiplying the reticulocyte count (reported as a percentage) by the RBC concentration (RBC/μL) and dividing the total by 100. For example, if the reticulocyte count is 1 and the RBC concentration is 5×10^6/L, the number of reticulocytes per microliter of blood is 50,000.

Indirect bilirubin concentration between 1 and 5 mg/dL
- Patients with Gilbert's disease have an increased indirect bilirubin level in the absence of hemolysis. Unless the patient has underlying liver disease, the direct bilirubin level is rarely elevated in association with hemolysis.

Haptoglobin concentration <50 mg/dL
- Haptoglobin is an acute-phase reactant. When hemolysis occurs in association with inflammatory processes or steroid administration, haptoglobin levels may be within the normal range.

Elevated LDH concentration
- The normal range for LDH depends on the assay and the units of measurement; it therefore varies among laboratories. LDH is mildly to moderately elevated in cases of extravascular hemolysis. Values are much higher in cases of intravascular hemolysis.

Adapted from Rakel RE, Bope ET: Conn's Current Therapy 2008, 60th ed. Philadelphia, Elsevier Saunders, 2008.
Abbreviations: LDH = lactic dehydrogenase; RBC = red blood cells.

AIHA, paroxysmal cold hemoglobinuria (PCH), Evans syndrome, and medication-induced AIHA (Box 1).

General Clinical and Laboratory Findings of AIHA

Patients with AIHA typically present with signs and symptoms of anemia, jaundice, and splenomegaly. Anemia may range from mild to severe, and its symptoms may be of acute or insidious onset.

Laboratory findings include anemia, reticulocytosis, increased mean corpuscular volume due to the presence of reticulocytes, indirect hyperbilirubinemia, increased lactate dehydrogenase (LDH), and decreased haptoglobin (Box 2). A positive direct antiglobulin test or Coombs is seen in more than 95% of patients with AIHA. It may be positive for immunoglobulin G (IgG) only, both IgG and complement, or complement alone. The peripheral smear shows polychromasia, spherocytes, and RBC fragments.

Warm-Antibody AIHA

Warm-antibody AIHA is the most common form of AIHA, with an estimated annual incidence of 1 in 80,000. Approximately half of the cases are classified as idiopathic, whereas the remaining cases are often secondary to a predisposing condition. It is mainly identified in the elderly population. However, it is often described in children in association with viral illnesses.

PATHOGENESIS

The antibodies most commonly involved in warm-antibody AIHA are of the IgG type. These IgG antibodies are typically directed against antigens on the Rh system. They bind RBCs at 37°C, allowing their Fc region to remain exposed. This region is recognized by Fc receptors on the macrophages of the spleen, resulting in

CURRENT DIAGNOSIS

- Confirm presence of immune-mediated hemolysis by performing direct antiglobulin test (DAT).
- Determine type of autoimmune hemolytic anemia (AIHA) based on DAT and clinical findings.
- Consider medications in the differential diagnosis of AIHA.
- Consider other tests, such as Donath-Landsteiner antibody testing and cold agglutinin titers, to establish cause of AIHA.

fragmentation and ingestion of the antibody-coated RBCs. This results in partial or complete phagocytosis. If partial phagocytosis occurs, spherocytes are formed. Splenomegaly results from entrapment of RBCs in the spleen.

EVALUATION

A positive direct antiglobulin test is seen in more than 95% of patients with warm-antibody AIHA. It may be positive for IgG only or for both IgG and complement C3. Most IgG antibodies are of the IgG1 subtype. Fewer than 5% of patients with warm-antibody AIHA have a negative direct antiglobulin test. In these cases, hemolysis is evident by laboratory results and peripheral smear, but more sensitive assays are needed to confirm the diagnosis. A clinical response to corticosteroids is useful to support the diagnosis.

CLINICAL MANAGEMENT

The goal of treatment is to minimize or eliminate hemolysis. Some mild cases may not require medical intervention. For those patients with moderate to severe AIHA, corticosteroids are the treatment of choice. Approximately 80% of patients have a rapid respond to corticosteroids, typically within 1 week after starting therapy. However, most responses are not sustained. The majority of adult patients receive high-dose oral prednisone (60–100 mg)[3] daily during the initial phase of treatment. Intravenous methylprednisolone (Solu-Medrol) may also be used at daily doses of 100 to 200 mg.[3] In the pediatric population, prednisone is given at doses ranging from 2 to 6 mg/kg/day.[3] These high doses in adults and children are commonly maintained for approximately 2 weeks.

Once the hematocrit has increased and remains stable, the dose may be decreased and subsequently tapered at a slow rate over several months. Patients who require more than 10 to 15 mg of prednisone daily to keep an adequate hematocrit may benefit from splenectomy. More than 50% of splenectomized patients have a partial or complete response. Nevertheless, the rate of relapse is high. Corticosteroids are continued when relapse occurs, but usually at lower doses. Patients who are candidates for splenectomy should receive immunizations against encapsulated organisms at least 2 weeks before the procedure.

Rituximab (Rituxan),[1] a monoclonal antibody directed against CD20 antigen on the surface of B lymphocytes, has produced response in patients with warm-antibody AIHA. In a study published by Zecca and colleagues, 13 of 15 pediatric patients with warm-antibody AIHA were successfully treated with rituximab at a dose of 375 mg/m^2 weekly for 2 to 4 weeks. Other studies performed in adults have also demonstrated response to this approach. However, the long-term side effects of rituximab are not entirely clear. Therefore, it should be used with caution, and patients should be monitored for side effects. Immunosuppressive drugs such as cyclophosphamide (Cytoxan),[1] azathioprine (Imuran),[1] and cyclosporine (Neoral)[1] have been used primarily in cases refractory to corticosteroids and splenectomy.

The best-described regimen has been cyclophosphamide 50 mg/kg/day for 4 days. Other treatment options that have been used with some success include danazol (Danocrine)[1] and plasmapheresis. High-dose intravenous immune globulin (IVIG, Gammagard)[1] may be effective in some cases, but the response is short lived (1–4 weeks).

Supportive care includes RBC transfusions for life-threatening situations and folic acid[1] supplementation to compensate for the increased RBC turnover. If RBC transfusions are needed, the least incompatible unit should be transfused slowly over 3 to 4 hours with careful monitoring for signs of an acute hemolytic reaction. The smallest volume of blood should be transfused to keep the patient hemodynamically stable, to avoid volume overload and an increase in the rate of hemolysis. In cases of secondary warm-antibody AIHA, it is recommended that the underlying condition be treated.

---

[1]Not FDA approved for this indication.
[3]Exceeds dosage recommended by the manufacturer.

Cold-Antibody AIHA

Primary cold-agglutinin disease is primarily seen in individuals older than 50 years of age, whereas secondary cold-agglutinin disease is most commonly seen in children and young adults. The primary form is idiopathic. The secondary form is caused by infections, autoimmune diseases, or malignancies. Monoclonal autoantibody formation is seen in the primary form, whereas the secondary form is associated with monoclonal or polyclonal autoantibodies.

PATHOGENESIS

Cold agglutinins are typically IgM autoantibodies that cause RBC agglutination at temperatures lower than 37°C, with maximal RBC agglutination at temperatures lower than 4°C. Cold agglutinins may occur in response to infection, as is commonly seen with *Mycoplasma* pneumonia and infectious mononucleosis. The IgM antibody usually reacts with I/i RBC antigen, resulting in complement activation by fixation of antibody to the antigen at low temperatures. Anti-I is characteristic of *Mycoplasma* pneumonia–induced hemolysis, whereas anti-i is characteristic of infectious mononucleosis. However, cold agglutinins have also been reported with other viral or bacterial illnesses, as well as lymphoproliferative disorders.

EVALUATION

Symptoms of anemia are variable and depend on the severity and rapidity of onset. Symptoms, such as acrocyanosis may also occur as a result of RBC agglutination. However, these usually disappear with warming. Other findings include scleral icterus, splenomegaly, and hemoglobinuria. If lymphadenopathy is present, a lymphoproliferative disorder should be suspected.

The Coombs test is typically positive for complement (C3) and negative for IgG. However, if an IgG antibody is present, the Coombs test may also be positive for IgG. Cold agglutinin titers are considered positive if the titer is greater than 1 in 40. These positive titers are variable, typically greater than 1 in 10,000. Signs of hemolysis are usually not evident until the titer is greater than 1 in 1000. Other blood tests that confirm the presence of cold-antibody AIHA include *Mycoplasma* and Epstein-Barr virus titers.

CLINICAL MANAGEMENT

In children, symptoms are usually mild and self-limited. A general approach is to avoid cold exposure. Supportive care to control the underlying disorder is recommended. RBC transfusions warmed to 37°C may be given for life-threatening situations, and the least incompatible unit should be used. For severe anemia, a trial of cytotoxic drugs such as cyclophosphamide (Cytoxan)[1] or chlorambucil (Leukeran)[1] may be used to decrease the cold agglutinin titer and the rate of hemolysis. Other alternatives that have been used with some success include rituximab[1] and interferon alfa-2b (Intron-A).[1] Plasmapheresis may be used to reduce or eliminate IgM antibodies. However, because its effect is not long-standing, it is used only in the acute setting. Treatment with corticosteroids alone or in combination is generally not effective. In addition, splenectomy is not effective, because the liver is the predominant site of hemolysis.

Paroxysmal Cold Hemoglobinuria

The Donath-Landsteiner autoantibody is responsible for PCH, which is typically characterized by a sudden onset of hemolysis and hemoglobinuria, usually after cold exposure that results in mild to severe anemia. PCH can result from infection, autoimmune disease, syphilis, or it can be idiopathic.

---

[1]Not FDA approved for this indication.

PATHOGENESIS

The Donath-Landsteiner autoantibody is a biphasic, polyclonal IgG that binds RBCs at cooler temperatures (4°C), activates complement, and results in intravascular hemolysis at warmer temperatures (37°C) due to complement fixation. This autoantibody is able to bind several RBC antigens, although its main target is the P antigen.

EVALUATION

The Coombs test is positive for C3 but negative for IgG, because of its dissociation from the RBC surface at warmer temperature. However, the Coombs test may be positive for IgG if it is performed at 4°C. PCH is confirmed by Donath-Landsteiner antibody testing. Plasma is incubated with normal RBCs and cooled to 4°C. If Donath-Landsteiner antibody is present, the cold hemolysin in the plasma binds RBCs. On rewarming to 37°C, the sensitized RBCs are hemolyzed by the complement present in plasma. The presence of hemolysis constitutes a positive antibody test result.

CLINICAL MANAGEMENT

The mainstay of treatment is supportive care and avoidance of cold exposure. Warmed RBCs may be administered in cases of life-threatening hemolysis or symptomatic anemia.

Evans Syndrome

Evans syndrome is the coexistence of Coombs-positive AIHA with immune-mediated thrombocytopenia. The exact pathophysiology is unknown, although defects in immune regulation have been proposed. The typical clinical course is chronic and relapsing, and some patients may also develop neutropenia.

EVALUATION

The Coombs test is positive (often weakly positive) for IgG, C3, or both. Anemia and thrombocytopenia are present with occasional neutropenia or combined cytopenias. Other features of hemolysis are present.

CLINICAL MANAGEMENT

The treatment of choice is corticosteroids, although relapses are frequent during tapering. Other alternatives that have shown some success include intravenous immune globulin (IVIg),[1] immunosuppressive agents, danazol,[1] and splenectomy. Rituximab[1] has been used with varied clinical responses. Supportive care with blood products should be given as needed, although their use should be minimized as possible.

Medication-Induced AIHA

It is well known that medications can cause AIHA. In the past, most cases were secondary to the use of methyldopa (Aldomet) and high-dose penicillin. More recently, the majority of the cases are secondary to the use of cephalosporins.

PATHOGENESIS

Medication-induced AIHA results from three proposed mechanisms based on the interactions among medications, RBC membrane antigens, and antibodies. These mechanisms are induced by drug or hapten adsorption, neoantigen formation, and autoantibody binding (Table 1).

---

[1]Not FDA approved for this indication.

TABLE 1 Major Mechanisms of Drug-Related Hemolytic Anemia and Positive Direct Antiglobulin Tests

	Hapten/Drug Adsorption	Ternary Complex Formation	Autoantibody Binding	Nonimmunologic Protein Adsorption
Prototype drug	Penicillin	Quinidine	α-Methyldopa (Aldomet)	Cephalothin[2]
Role of drug	Binds to RBC membrane	Forms ternary complex with antibody and RBC membrane component	Induces formation of antibody to native RBC antigen	Possibly alters RBC membrane
Drug affinity to cell	Strong	Weak	None demonstrated to intact RBC, but binding to membranes is reported	Strong
Antibody to drug	Present	Present	Absent	Absent
Antibody class predominating	IgG	IgM or IgG	IgG	None
Proteins detected by DAT	IgG, rarely complement	Complement	IgG, rarely complement	Multiple plasma proteins
Dose of drug associated with positive antiglobulin test	High	Low	High	High
Presence of drug required for indirect antiglobulin test	Yes (coating test RBCs)	Yes (added to test medium)	No	Yes (added to test medium)
Mechanism of RBC destruction	Splenic sequestration of IgG-coated RBCs	Direct lysis by complement plus splenic–hepatic clearance of C3b-coated RBCs	Splenic sequestration	None

Adapted from Packman CH: Hemolytic anemia resulting from immune injury. In Lichtman MA, Beutler E, Kipps TJ, et al (eds): Williams Hematology, 7th ed. New York, McGraw-Hill, 2006, Chapter 52.
[2]Not available in the United States.
Abbreviations: DAT = direct antiglobulin test; Ig = immunoglobulin; RBC = red blood cell.

CURRENT THERAPY

Summary

- Corticosteroids are the mainstay of treatment. However, patients unable to be weaned off may require splenectomy.
- Immunosuppressive therapy, primarily cyclophosphamide (Cytoxan),[1] has been used with some success, as has rituximab (Rituxan).[1]
- Red blood cell transfusion may be used for life-threatening situations, and the least incompatible unit should be used.
- Avoid cold exposure if cold-antibody autoimmune hemolytic anemia (AIHA) or paroxysmal cold hemoglobinuria (PCH) is present.
- Discontinue medications if medication-induced AIHA is suspected.

[1]Not FDA approved for this indication.

REFERENCES

Dacie SJ. The immune hemolytic anemias: A century of exciting progress in understanding. Br J Haematol 2001;114:770–85.

D'Arena G, Califano C, Annunziate M, et al. Rituximab for warm-type idiopathic autoimmune hemolytic anemia: A retrospective study of 11 adult patients. Eur J Haematol 2007;79:53–8.

Garratty G. Drug-induced immune hemolytic anemia: The last decade [Review]. Immunohematology 2004;20:138–46.

Glader B. Immune hemolytic anemias. In: Arceci RJ, Hann IM, Smith OP, Hoffbrand A, editors. Pediatric Hematology. 3rd ed. Hoboken, NJ: Wiley-Blackwell; 2006.

Nydegger UE, Kazatchkine MD, Miescher PA. Immunopathologic and clinical features of hemolytic anemia due to cold agglutinins. Semin Hematol 1991;28:66–77.

Packman CH. Hemolytic anemia resulting from immune injury. In: Lichtman E, Beutler E, Kipps TJ, et al, editors. Williams Hematology. 7th ed. New York, McGraw-Hill; 2006 [Chapter 52].

Packman CH. Hemolytic anemia due to warm autoantibodies. Blood Rev 2008;22(1):17–31.

Parker CJ. Autoimmune hemolytic anemia. In: Rakel RE, Bope ET, editors. Conn's Current Therapy. 60th ed. Philadelphia: WB Saunders; 2008.

Zecca M, Nobili B, Ramenghi U, et al. Rituximab for the treatment of refractory autoimmune hemolytic anemia in children. Blood 2003;101:3857–61.

Nonimmune Hemolytic Anemia

Method of
Stella T. Chou, MD, and Mitchell J. Weiss, MD, PhD

The hemolytic anemias (HAs) are a heterogeneous group of disorders characterized by accelerated erythrocyte destruction. Intrinsic causes of hemolysis are usually inherited and include abnormalities in the erythrocyte membrane, metabolic defects, and altered hemoglobin structure. Extrinsic causes include erythrocyte-directed antibodies, trauma, infections, and toxins. Within these categories, there are virtually hundreds of specific etiologies. Here we address the most common and clinically significant disorders, focusing mainly on the congenital HAs.

Diagnosis

Anemia with reticulocytosis, hyperbilirubinemia, and an elevated lactate dehydrogenase (LDH) level strongly suggests hemolysis. The family history is often helpful for diagnosis. In particular, the clinician should inquire about ethnic background and family members with anemia, splenectomy, early gallstones/cholecystectomy, or significant neonatal jaundice. Several forms of HA confer protection against *Plasmodium falciparum* malaria. Accordingly, these disorders are relatively common in malaria endemic regions such as Africa, the Mediterranean basin, and Asia because of positive selective genetic pressure. Assessment of erythrocyte indexes and morphology are critical and frequently reveal distinct diagnostic clues (Table 1). Together, these initial data usually point to a specific diagnosis that can be confirmed by directed specialized testing that includes more detailed examination of erythrocytes and DNA analysis.

In addition, patients with primary hemolytic disorders may present during an aplastic episode, most typically from Parvovirus B19 infection. In this case, erythrocyte production stops temporarily resulting in reticulocytopenia and declining hemoglobin.

Management

Folate replacement is recommended for most patients with moderate to severe congenital hemolytic anemia. Iron from hemolyzed erythrocytes is usually reabsorbed, and supplementation is not necessary. Formation of gallstones is a common complication of HA, and therefore periodic screening abdominal ultrasounds are warranted. Concomitant Gilbert's syndrome, caused by a variant in the uridine diphosphoglucuronate glucuronosyltransferase 1A (UGT1A) gene promoter, increases the propensity for gallstones. Neonatal jaundice is common in many of the inherited disorders and may necessitate exchange transfusion for severe hyperbilirubinemia. Parvovirus BI9–induced aplastic crisis is a life-threatening complication of congenital HA that frequently requires blood transfusion. Therefore, it is essential that patients with known hemolytic disorders be counseled to seek medical attention if they experience symptoms of viral illness, increased pallor, and lethargy.

Splenectomy is an effective treatment for many forms of severe congenital HA. The most significant problem from splenectomy is increased risk of life-threatening infections from encapsulated organisms. Prior to splenectomy, patients should be vaccinated

CURRENT DIAGNOSIS

- Anemia, reticulocytosis and hyperbilirubinemia suggest hemolytic anemia (HA).
- Congenital HA can present with severe neonatal jaundice.
- History, physical examination, and examination of erythrocyte morphology combined with more specialized testing usually provide a specific diagnosis.
- Erythrocyte-intrinsic etiologies for HA are usually inherited abnormalities affecting the erythrocyte membrane, enzymes, or hemoglobin structure.
- Extrinsic causes for HA include antierythrocyte antibodies, trauma, infection, and toxins.
- Reticulocytopenia in the context of chronic HA suggests a Parvovirus-induced aplastic crisis.
- Paroxysmal nocturnal hemoglobinuria is a clonal somatically acquired hematopoietic disorder characterized by intravascular hemolysis, thromboses, and sometimes cytopenias. Diagnosis is made by flow cytometry demonstrating a population of cells that lack glycosyl phosphatidylinositol (GPI)-anchored membrane proteins.

TABLE 1 Causes of Nonimmune Hemolytic Anemia

Type of Defect	Disease Mechanism	Example	Erythrocyte Morphology
Intrinsic erythrocyte defect	Membranopathy	Hereditary spherocytosis	Spherocytes
		Hereditary elliptocytosis	Elliptocytes
		Hereditary stomatocytosis	Stomatocytes
		Hereditary xerocytosis	Target cells, echinocytes
		Hereditary pyropoikilocytosis	Micropoikilocytes, microspherocytes, fragmented erythrocytes
		Paroxysmal nocturnal hemoglobinuria	Macrocytosis
	Enzymopathy	G6PD deficiency	Heinz bodies, bite cells, blister cells, anisocytosis, poikilocytosis
		Pyruvate kinase deficiency	Echinocytes
	Hemoglobinopathy	Sickle cell disease	Sickle cells
		Thalassemia	Microcytosis, target cells
		Unstable hemoglobinopathies	Heinz bodies
Extrinsic erythrocyte defect	Trauma	Heart valve hemolysis (macrovascular)	Schistocytes
		DIC/TTP/HUS (microvascular)	Schistocytes
	Thermal injury	Severe burns	Schistocytes
	Chemicals	Arsenic, lead, copper, and chlorates	Varied
	Toxins	Bee and wasp stings, spider bites, and snake venom	Schistocytes
	Infections	Malaria, *Babesia*, *Bartonella*, clostridia, streptococci, staphylococci, enterococcus, salmonella, mycoplasma, EBV, CMV, HSV, rubeola, influenza A	Intraerythrocytic parasites Schistocytes with bacterial infections

Abbreviations: CMV = cytomegalovirus; DIC = disseminated intravascular coagulation; EBV = Epstein-Barr virus; HSV = herpes simplex virus; HUS = hemolytic uremic syndrome; TTP = thrombotic thrombocytopenic purpura.

CURRENT THERAPY

- Many forms of congenital severe HA are ameliorated by splenectomy.
- Long-term risks of splenectomy include susceptibility to sepsis from encapsulated organisms and possibly increased risk of thrombosis.
- Splenectomized patients should be immunized against *Streptococcus pneumoniae*, *Haemophilus influenzae* type B, and *Neisseria meningitidis*. Daily penicillin prophylaxis is recommended for children.
- Splenectomized patients presenting with fever should receive appropriate parenteral antibiotics until a negative blood culture is documented.
- Aplastic crisis and hyperhemolytic episodes associated with HA are managed with erythrocyte transfusion.
- Folate (folic acid) replacement, 1 mg/d, is recommended for moderate to severe HA.

against *Streptococcus pneumoniae*, *Haemophilus influenzae type B*, and *Neisseria meningitidis*. Daily penicillin prophylaxis is recommended postsplenectomy, particularly for children. Splenectomized patients presenting with fever should be managed promptly with physical examination, blood culture, and appropriate parenteral antibiotics.

Congenital Hemolytic Anemias

ERYTHROCYTE MEMBRANE ABNORMALITIES

The erythrocyte membrane must be flexible and strong enough to withstand multiple passages through small capillary beds. A specialized membrane composed of a lipid bilayer, integral membrane proteins, and an underlying skeletal network formed by numerous proteins supports these requirements. Erythrocyte membrane proteins include alpha and beta spectrin, ankyrin, protein 4.1, and actin. Inherited mutations in these proteins disrupts the integrity of the membrane to cause HA.

Hereditary Spherocytosis

Hereditary spherocytosis is the most common cause of nonimmune HA in populations from Northern Europe and North America, with a prevalence of approximately 1 in 2000.

Pathophysiology

Hereditary spherocytosis is caused by varying degrees of spectrin loss, usually from deficient or dysfunctional ankyrin, band 3 and/or protein 4.2, or, less frequently, a primary spectrin defect. Disruption of the membrane skeleton destabilizes the lipid bilayer causing splenic removal of microvesicles and subsequent spherocyte formation. The molecular basis of hereditary spherocytosis is heterogeneous. Approximately two thirds of cases are autosomal dominant, with the remaining one third being autosomal recessive or arising from new mutations.

Clinical Manifestations and Diagnosis

The severity of hereditary spherocytosis varies from asymptomatic to severe and typically correlates with the degree of spectrin deficiency. Most diagnoses of hereditary spherocytosis are made in childhood, from a positive family history or a clinical presentation of anemia, jaundice, and splenomegaly. New patients occasionally present with a Parvovirus-induced aplastic crisis. In these clinical contexts, an elevated mean corpuscular hemoglobin concentration (MCHC) strongly indicates hereditary spherocytosis. This value reflects a decreased surface-to-volume ratio caused by splenic removal of the erythrocyte membrane. In addition, the red cell distribution width (RDW) reflecting size variation, is elevated. The blood smear demonstrates spherocytes (erythrocytes lacking central pallor). A positive incubated osmotic fragility test, which demonstrates increased susceptibility to hypotonic lysis, supports the diagnosis. However, it is important to note that osmotic fragility is normal in 10% to 20% of hereditary spherocytosis cases. Moreover, other disorders, most notably immune HAs, are also characterized by spherocytes with increased osmotic fragility. A positive direct antiglobulin test (Coombs test) usually distinguishes immune HA from hereditary spherocytosis.

Patients with mild hereditary spherocytosis may have normal or near normal hemoglobin levels, mild reticulocytosis and hyperbilirubinemia, and typically have an uncomplicated course. More severely affected patients experience additional complications including severe neonatal hyperbilirubinemia and hyperhemolytic episodes later in life. The latter are frequently precipitated by viral illness and are characterized by worsening anemia, signs of accelerated hemolysis, and, often, splenic enlargement. Rare complications of severe hereditary spherocytosis include leg ulcers, gout, and extramedullary hematopoiesis.

Management

Aplastic and hyperhemolytic episodes are supported with erythrocyte transfusions. Although splenectomy improves the anemia and reduces the risk of gallstones by removing the site of erythrocyte destruction, splenectomy should be reserved for patients with severe hemolysis, recurrent life-threatening hyperhemolytic episodes, or growth failure. Most clinicians prefer to treat as needed with transfusions until after 5 years of age when the postsplenectomy infection risk declines. In less severely affected patients, the threshold for recommending splenectomy varies among clinicians. In most centers, splenectomy is performed laparoscopically with very low morbidity and rapid recovery times. Moreover, improved vaccines, particularly pneumococcal, reduce the risk for postsplenectomy sepsis. However, some data indicate that splenectomy increases the long-term risk for venous and arterial thromboses, cardiovascular disease, and pulmonary hypertension. Accessory spleens are relatively common and should be searched for at the time of surgery.

Hereditary Elliptocytosis and Pyropoikilocytosis

The hereditary elliptocytoses are a heterogeneous group of inherited HAs with oval-shaped erythrocytes. Hereditary elliptocytosis is relatively common in African, Mediterranean, and Asian populations. Hereditary pyropoikilocytosis is a more rare and severe form of HA with erythrocyte fragmentation in which one parent usually has hereditary elliptocytosis.

Pathophysiology

Most forms of hereditary elliptocytoses are inherited in an autosomal dominant fashion and are relatively mild. The underlying molecular defects are usually mutations in genes encoding alpha or beta spectrin, band 3, or protein 4.1. These mutations all destabilize the latticework of spectrin organization underlying the plasma membrane to induce an oval or elliptical shape. Assorted hereditary elliptocytoses mutations that qualitatively alter membrane proteins produce subtle variations in cell shape that distinguish different clinical subtypes, which are categorized according to erythrocyte morphology. In hereditary pyropoikilocytosis, the patient usually inherits a common hereditary elliptocytosis mutation from one parent and a milder subclinical defect in spectrin synthesis from the other parent.

Clinical Manifestations and Diagnosis

Hereditary elliptocytosis is classified into three subtypes according to morphology: common hereditary elliptocytosis, the most prevalent form, which is characterized by biconcave elliptocytes; spherocytic hereditary elliptocytosis, a phenotype between hereditary spherocytosis and hereditary elliptocytosis; and Southeast Asian ovalocytosis, characterized by oval erythrocytes. Most patients are asymptomatic and diagnosed incidentally with minimal or mild compensated hemolysis. The peripheral smear demonstrates more than 30% elliptocytes. Patients who are homozygous or compound heterozygous have more severe HA. The peripheral blood smear also has budding erythrocytes, fragments, and other poikilocytes. Hereditary pyropoikilocytosis, at the extreme end of this spectrum, causes bizarre fragmented erythrocytes with microspherocytosis and micropoikilocytosis. The mean

corpuscular volume is very low (25 to 75 fL), the osmotic fragility is abnormal, and erythrocytes characteristically demonstrate thermal instability. Hereditary pyropoikilocytosis typically presents in newborns or infants with jaundice and anemia.

Management

Most hereditary elliptocytoses patients have a mild course and do not require treatment. In cases of severe hemolysis because of homozygous or compound heterozygous hereditary elliptocytosis or hereditary pyropoikilocytosis, splenectomy is indicated.

Hereditary Stomatocytosis and Xerocytosis

Hereditary stomatocytosis and xerocytosis are rare inherited causes of hemolytic anemia associated with abnormal erythrocyte cation permeability and volume (increased in stomatocytosis and decreased in xerocytosis). Both disorders are autosomal dominant. Hereditary stomatocytosis patients have erythrocytes with a mouth-shaped (stoma) area of central pallor, whereas hereditary xerocytosis patients demonstrate target cells and echinocytes. The clinical courses of these diseases are highly variable, ranging from asymptomatic to moderate hemolysis and subsequent anemia. Most patients do not require treatment. Importantly, splenectomy is contraindicated in hereditary stomatocytosis because of an increased incidence of life-threatening thrombosis.

ERYTHROCYTE METABOLISM ABNORMALITIES

Erythrocytes rely on two major biochemical pathways: glycolysis for energy to maintain metabolic needs and the hexose-monophosphate shunt for antioxidant pathways. More than 20 enzymes are involved in these two pathways, and defects in each one are associated with various forms of HA. The two most common enzymopathies are deficiencies in glucose-6-phosphate dehydrogenase (G6PD) and pyruvate kinase (PK).

Glucose-6-Phosphate Dehydrogenase Deficiency

G6PD deficiency is the most common erythrocyte metabolism disorder, affecting as much as 3% of the world's population.

Pathophysiology

G6PD is the first enzyme in the hexose-monophosphate pathway, which is required to maintain a high level of reduced glutathione, an important antioxidant. G6PD-deficient erythrocytes undergo increased hemoglobin oxidation leading to hemolysis. G6PD deficiency is an X-linked recessive disorder. More than 300 G6PD genetic variants affect enzyme activity to different extents that determine the severity of HA. Type A⁻ is a genetic variant seen in 10% to 15% of African American males and is associated with mild to moderate G6PD deficiency. Variants causing more severe HA are more prevalent in Mediterranean and Asian populations.

Clinical Manifestations and Diagnosis

G6PD deficiency is an X-linked disorder; therefore, hemizygous males and homozygous females are typically affected. Many G6PD variants are associated with neonatal jaundice. Severe forms of G6PD deficiency can cause chronic ongoing HA, but most commonly, affected individuals are asymptomatic in between hemolytic episodes. However, anemia develops rapidly following a precipitating event related to oxidative stress that induces acute intravascular hemolysis with the severity determined by the G6PD variant and the offending agent. Drugs are the most common inciting event in Africans with the A⁻ variant (Table 2). Other precipitating events include mothball (naphthalene) exposure and infections. In some Mediterranean and Asian variants, ingestion of fava beans can cause acute life-threatening hemolysis. Symptoms can include fever, abdominal pain, nausea, diarrhea, and impressive hemoglobinuria, frequently described as Coca-Cola colored. The spleen is often enlarged and tender. Anemia ranges from mild to life-threatening and is normocytic and normochromic. Morphologic abnormalities include anisocytosis, poikilocytosis, "bite cells" (erythrocytes that

TABLE 2 Drugs Capable of Precipitating Hemolysis in G6PD Deficiency

Analgesics and Antipyretics	Acetanilid*
	Acetylsalicylic acid (aspirin)
Antibacterials	Chloramphenicol
	Furazolidone (Furoxone)*
	Nalidixic acid (NeGram)*
	Nitrofurantoin (Furadantin)*
	Sulfonamides*
	Trimethoprim-sulfamethoxazole (Bactrim)
Antimalarials	Pamaquine*
	Pentaquine*
	Primaquine*
	Quinacrine
Miscellaneous	Dimercaptosuccinic acid (Succimer)
	Methylene blue*
	Phenazopyridine (Pyridium)*
	Urate oxidase*
	Vitamin K

*These drugs have an increased tendency to cause clinically significant hemolysis. Most patients with mild G6PD deficiency alleles tolerate drugs that are not marked by the asterisk. For a more comprehensive list of drug–G6PD interactions, see reading by Beutler.
Abbreviation: G6PD = glucose-6-phosphate dehydrogenase.

are partially destroyed in the spleen), and "blister cells" (a thin strip of membrane overlying a bleb of clear cytoplasm). A methyl violet stain to detect Heinz bodies, indicative of denatured hemoglobin, is typically positive. Immediately after an acute hemolytic event, G6PD levels can be deceptively normal because of an elevated reticulocyte count, which can express significant enzymatic activity in some variants. Therefore, G6PD levels should be tested weeks to months later to obtain a true baseline level.

Management

Treatment of the A⁻ variant of G6PD deficiency is mostly preventive by avoiding oxidant stresses. When acute hemolytic episodes result in symptomatic anemia, erythrocyte transfusions are indicated. Rarely, acute renal failure develops secondary to severe intravascular hemolysis. This is managed by vigorous hydration, alkalinization, electrolyte monitoring, and occasionally hemodialysis.

Pyruvate Kinase Deficiency

Pyruvate kinase (PK) deficiency, which is most commonly seen in Northern European populations, accounts for more than 80% of the HAs due to glycolytic disorders.

Pathophysiology

PK deficiency is genetically heterogeneous, with many different mutations impairing enzyme activity to different extents. Pyruvate kinase deficiency causes decreased production of ATP, impairing erythrocyte survival. Inheritance is usually autosomal recessive; simple heterozygotes with 50% enzyme activity are unaffected.

Clinical Manifestations and Diagnosis

PK deficiency is extremely heterogeneous, ranging from life-threatening HA to asymptomatic compensated hemolysis. Erythrocyte morphology may be normal or show echinocytes (small dense crenated erythrocytes). Quantitation of erythrocyte enzyme activity is usually diagnostic.

Management

General supportive care for chronic hemolysis and supportive erythrocyte transfusions when needed are the mainstays of therapy. Patients with severe hemolysis may benefit from splenectomy, although the response is variable and unpredictable.

HEMOGLOBINOPATHIES

HA can be caused by mutations that alter the α- or β-like globin proteins that contribute to hemoglobin structure. Quantitative defects that impair globin gene expression comprise the thalassemia syndromes, discussed in the article on thalassemia. Qualitative defects are usually caused by missense mutations that alter hemoglobin structure and stability. The most important examples are the sickle syndromes, discussed in the article on sickle cell disease. Numerous other missense mutations that destabilize hemoglobin also cause HA. In these cases, hemoglobin precipitates may be detected by a Heinz body stain. Unstable hemoglobins can also be detected by hemoglobin electrophoresis or increased precipitation upon exposure to heat or isopropanol. If any of these tests are positive in the context of hemolysis, direct globin gene sequencing can provide a definitive diagnosis.

Acquired Nonimmune Hemolytic Anemias

PAROXYSMAL NOCTURNAL HEMOGLOBINURIA

Paroxysmal nocturnal hemoglobinuria (PNH) is a rare acquired disease with chronic HA, thrombosis, and often pancytopenia. The hemolytic anemia results from increased erythrocyte sensitivity to complement-mediated hemolysis.

Pathophysiology

PNH is an acquired clonal disorder caused by a somatically acquired inactivating mutation in the X-linked phosphatidylinositol glycan, class A (PIGA) gene, which encodes an enzyme involved in the synthesis of glycosyl phosphatidylinositol (GPI) anchor proteins. All blood cells derived from the abnormal clone lack surface proteins that require the GPI anchor. Hemolysis occurs from the deficiency of specific GPI-linked surface proteins that inhibit complement activation. The hypercoagulable state seen in PNH is most likely related to complement-mediated platelet activation and elevated levels of ADP from lysed erythrocytes, leading to platelet aggregation. For unknown reasons, PNH commonly progresses to aplastic anemia.

Clinical Manifestations and Diagnosis

PNH can present as a primary hemolytic syndrome with chronic intravascular HA, a thrombotic event, or with pancytopenia. Few patients exhibit the classic nocturnal hemoglobinuria, reporting red or brownish urine in the morning. In most patients hemoglobinuria occurs irregularly and is often precipitated by infection or stress. Iron deficiency can occur from urinary loss. Associated thromboses may be venous or arterial and can involve extremities, the hepatic vein (Budd-Chiari syndrome), other intraabdominal veins, and cerebral veins. Hence, PNH can present as severe abdominal pain or headaches. The majority of patients have defective hematopoiesis, ranging from a macrocytic anemia to severe aplastic anemia and pancytopenia. Rarely, PNH can also evolve into a myelodysplastic syndrome or acute leukemia. The median survival for patients diagnosed with PNH is 10 to 15 years.

Laboratory findings include anemia, variable reticulocytosis, leukopenia, and thrombocytopenia. The bone marrow examination typically reveals erythroid hyperplasia or, in the case of associated aplastic anemia, hypocellularity. Urine hemosiderin is typical. Laboratory diagnosis of PNH previously relied on assays that demonstrated abnormal erythrocyte sensitivity to complement (Ham test, sucrose hemolysis test). The current standard is flow cytometry demonstrating the absence of hematopoietic GPI-linked proteins, typically CD55 and CD59, on some or all circulating cells.

Management

Oral iron supplementation is recommended to replace the urinary losses associated with intravascular hemolysis. Corticosteroids can sometimes improve the hemolysis in the first 24 to 72 hours of a hemolytic episode. A recent phase 3 trial showed that eculizumab, a monoclonal antibody that inhibits activation of the terminal complement complex, is effective for the hemolytic anemia of PNH. Eculizumab was recently FDA-approved and is entering clinical practice. Anticoagulation is indicated for documented thromboses, and thrombolytic therapy can be effective for patients with hepatic vein thrombosis or massive thrombotic events. Short-term prophylactic therapy should be used in the setting of surgery or prolonged immobilization, even if there is no history of thrombosis. HLA-identical bone marrow transplantation is indicated for bone marrow failure associated with PNH. Alternatively, immunosuppressive therapy with antithymocyte globulin and cyclosporine is used for patients without a suitable bone marrow donor.

Hemolytic Anemia Caused by Erythrocyte Fragmentation

Erythrocyte fragmentation can occur in the macrovascular or microvascular circulations. Shear stress produces fragmented erythrocytes (schistocytes). Macroangiopathic hemolysis can occur with prosthetic surfaces, large thromboses, and aged or damaged heart valves, but it is usually mild. Microangiopathic causes of hemolysis include disseminated intravascular coagulation, thrombotic thrombocytopenic purpura, and hemolytic uremic syndrome, which are discussed in their respective articles.

Hemolytic Anemia Caused by Chemical and Physical Agents

Arsenic, lead, copper, and chlorates can cause hemolysis through numerous mechanisms. Most notably, hemolytic anemia may be the presenting feature of the copper toxicity of Wilson's disease. Animal toxins associated with intravascular hemolysis include bee and wasp stings, brown recluse spider bites, and snake venom. Severe burns can also cause fragmentation hemolysis from the thermal injury.

Hemolytic Anemia Caused by Infection

Infections cause hemolysis by direct invasion of the erythrocyte, toxin production, or by immune-mediated mechanisms. Malaria is the most common infectious cause of hemolytic anemia worldwide. *Plasmodium falciparum* invades erythrocytes and is associated with severe hemolysis and hemoglobinuria (blackwater fever). Other parasitic infections associated with hemolysis are *Babesia microti* and *Bartonella bacilliformis*. Bacterial organisms that cause hemolysis via erythrocyte membrane injury and toxins include clostridia, streptococci, staphylococci, enterococcus, and salmonella. Immune hemolysis is associated with *Mycoplasma pneumoniae*, Epstein-Barr virus, cytomegalovirus, herpes simplex, rubeola, and influenza A (see topic in Section 2). Hemolysis improves once the underlying infection resolves.

REFERENCES

Beutler E. Glucose-6-phosphate dehydrogenase deficiency and other red cell enzyme abnormalities. In: Beutler E, et al., editors. Williams Hematology. New York: McGraw-Hill; 2001. p. 527–45.

Bolton-Maggs PH, Stevens RF, Dodd NJ, et al. Guidelines for the diagnosis and management of hereditary spherocytosis. Br J Haematol 2004;126 (4):455–74.

Gallagher P, Lux S. Disorders of the erythrocyte membrane. In: Nathan D, et al., editors. Nathan and Oski's Hematology of Infancy and Childhood. Philadelphia: WB Saunders; 2003. p. 560–684.

Hillmen P, Young NS, Schubert J, et al. The complement inhibitor eculizumab in paroxysmal nocturnal hemoglobinuria. N Engl J Med 2006;355 (12):1233–43.

Parker C, Omine M, Richards S, et al. Diagnosis and management of paroxysmal nocturnal hemoglobinuria. Blood 2005;106(12):3699–709.

Tse WT, Lux SE. Red blood cell membrane disorders. Br J Haematol 1999;104 (1):2–13.

Zanella A, Fermo E, Bianchi P, Valentini G. Red cell pyruvate kinase deficiency; Molecular and clinical aspects. Br J Haematol 2005;130(1):11–25.

Pernicious Anemia and Other Megaloblastic Anemias

Method of
Daniel Buroker, MD, and Thorvardur Halfdanarson, MD

The term pernicious anemia refers to the autoimmune-mediated loss of gastric intrinsic factor (IF) which results in anemia and sometimes pancytopenia that is frequently associated with neuropsychiatric complications. Absence of IF causes failure of the terminal ileum to absorb cobalamin (vitamin B_{12}). Pernicious anemia is one type of megaloblastic anemia. The term megaloblastic anemia identifies disorders of impaired hematopoiesis caused by cobalamin deficiency or folate deficiency. Impaired erythropoiesis is a signature defect of a megaloblastic anemia, but global hematopoiesis can be affected as well. The hallmark defects of erythroid production, red blood cell macrocytosis with macro-ovalocytes, can be seen in the peripheral blood. These vitamin deficiencies impair DNA synthesis in other cell lines as well. Hypersegmented neutrophils and large metamyelocytes may be seen, and macro-megakaryocytes are also observed. Nonhematopoietic cells that also proliferate, such as gastrointestinal cells, may likewise demonstrate megaloblastic features.

Pernicious Anemia

Parietal cells are stomach epithelial cells that secrete both hydrochloric acid and IF. IF binds to dietary cobalamin in the gut and then binds to a receptor in the terminal ileum; the IF-cobalamin complex enters the portal circulation, where the cobalamin binds transport proteins. In pernicious anemia, autoantibodies target both IF and parietal cells of the stomach. There are two types of anti-IF antibodies. One prevents cobalamin binding to IF, and the other prevents binding of the cobalamin-IF complex to receptors in the terminal ileum. Other autoimmune disorders are commonly associated with pernicious anemia, and patients with pernicious anemia are at risk for gastric carcinoma and gastric carcinoid tumors. The term pernicious anemia is used to describe the anemia resulting from this autoimmune mechanism for cobalamin deficiency, but the clinical manifestations of pernicious anemia are the same as in other patients with cobalamin deficiency from nonautoimmune causes (Box 1).

Other Causes of Megaloblastic Anemia

COBALAMIN DEFICIENCY

Dietary cobalamin is found in meat and dairy products. A Western diet may contain 5 to 20 μ/day of cobalamin (vitamin B_{12}). Daily requirements for cobalamin are between 0.5 to 1.0 μg, and total body stores are approximately 2 to 5 mg. Therefore, cobalamin deficiency takes years to develop after dietary absorption of cobalamin is interrupted.

Gastrectomy and gastritis, or any condition that impairs secretion of gastric acid and pepsin, can inhibit cobalamin binding to IF. An

BOX 1   Common Causes of Megaloblastic and Nonmegaloblastic Macrocytosis

Megaloblastic is not synonymous with macrocytic. The following nonexhaustive list contains common causes of megaloblastic and nonmegaloblastic anemia with macrocytosis.

Causes of Nonmegaloblastic Macrocytic Anemia

- Primary bone marrow disorders: aplastic anemia, myelodysplastic disorders, acute leukemia
- Reticulocytosis secondary to acute bleeding or hemolysis
- Chronic ethanol abuse
- Chronic liver disease
- Splenectomy or functional asplenism
- Hypothyroidism

Causes of Megaloblastic Anemia
Cobalamin (Vitamin B₁₂) Deficiency

- Stomach abnormalities including pernicious anemia, gastrectomy, bariatric surgery, and chronic gastritis
- Food-cobalamin malabsorption
- Small-bowel disorders including malabsorption, ileal resection, Crohn's disease, and bacterial overgrowth (blind loops)
- Strict vegan diet
- Medications that inhibit absorption, including neomycin, metformin (Glucophage), proton pump inhibitors, and nitrous oxide blockade of methionine synthase

Folate Deficiency

- Poor oral intake (depression, anorexia, alcoholism, unusual diet preference)
- Malabsorption (sprue, inflammatory bowel disease, surgical resection)
- Increased requirements (pregnancy, chronic hemolysis, dialysis removal)
- Medications, including methotrexate, acyclovir (Zovirax), 6-mercaptopurine (Purinethol), 5-fluorouracil (Adrucil), hydroxyurea (Hydrea), anticonvulsants (particularly phenytoin [Dilantin]), oral contraceptives, metformin (Glucophage), colchicines, and neomycin

CURRENT DIAGNOSIS

- Megaloblastic anemia is almost always caused by the deficiency or impaired absorption of either folate or cobalamin (vitamin B₁₂).
- Pernicious anemia is caused by the autoantibody-mediated impairment of intrinsic factor, which produces reduced absorption of cobalamin in the terminal ileum.
- Serum measurements of cobalamin and red blood cell folate concentrations are reasonable initial screening tests for causes of megaloblastic anemia but suffer from limited sensitivity and specificity.
- Measurements of serum methylmalonic acid and homocysteine are more sensitive indicators for deficiency than measurements of cobalamin and folic acid.
- Measurement of methylmalonic acid is both sensitive and specific for cobalamin deficiency.

Unlike cobalamin, folate does not depend on a specific protein mediator for intestinal absorption. However, as in cobalamin deficiency, disorders that disrupt absorption across the intestinal epithelium also affect folate deficiency. Celiac disease, tropical sprue, inflammatory bowel disease, and bacterial overgrowth may decrease intestinal absorption of folate. Folate absorption is optimal in an acidic gastric environment, and prolonged use of acid-reducing medications such as proton pump inhibitors and histamine 2 antagonists can cause folate deficiency. Anticonvulsants, and in particular phenytoin (Dilantin), can impair folate absorption. Methotrexate and trimethoprim (Proloprim) are medications that inhibit the enzyme dihydrofolate reductase, which is necessary to convert folate into its biologically active form.

Clinical Manifestations

NEUROLOGIC

Cobalamin deficiency and folate deficiency both may produce megaloblastic anemia, but the former produces neurologic deficits, and the latter does not. Cobalamin deficiency impairs myelin formation and produces a symmetrical axonal myeloneuropathy involving both peripheral and central neurons caused by degeneration of dorsal and lateral spinal columns. Paraesthesias, proprioception loss, diminished deep tendon reflexes, loss of sensation, and ataxia are early symptoms. These symptoms can progress to profound weakness, paraplegia, spasticity, and bowel and bladder incontinence. Cognitive impairments may be found as well, including dementia and memory loss. Neurologic deficits may be present before hematologic abnormalities manifest, and there seems to be an inverse relationship between the hematologic manifestations and the neurologic deficits. The hematologic and neurologic manifestations of copper deficiency may mimic those of cobalamin deficiency.

HEMATOLOGIC

Macrocytic anemia with macro-ovalocytes is the hallmark finding in megaloblastic anemia on the peripheral blood smear. Up to 40% of patients with cobalamin deficiency are not anemic, and some have both normal hemoglobin and normal mean corpuscular volume. Coexisting iron deficiency may mask the macrocytosis and should be excluded. Hypersegmented neutrophils, giant metamyelocytes, and macro-megakaryocytes are characteristic of megaloblastic anemia but are not always seen. Serum bilirubin and lactate dehydrogenase can be elevated secondary to ineffective erythropoiesis. Reticulocyte counts are normal or decreased. Neutropenia and thrombocytopenia may be present, and the blood smear may have a leukoerythroblastic appearance, with circulating nucleated red blood cells and immature myeloid forms. Some patients have splenomegaly at the time of diagnosis. Bone marrow examination

acidic environment in the stomach favors cobalamin release from ingested food, and medications that inhibit acid production may lead to cobalamin deficiency. Proton pump inhibitors and histamine 2 blockers may cause cobalamin malabsorption. The inability to release cobalamin from food or intestinal transport proteins is termed food-cobalamin malabsorption syndrome (FCMS). FCMS is characterized by cobalamin deficiency despite sufficient intake of food-cobalamin and no evidence of malabsorption of other nutrients or pernicious anemia.

Surgical resection that includes the terminal ileum also leads to cobalamin deficiency. Diseases affecting the terminal ileum may cause cobalamin deficiency and include disorders such as celiac disease, inflammatory bowel disease, enteritis, tropical sprue, bacterial overgrowth, intestinal tapeworm infestation, and small-intestinal lymphoma.

FOLATE DEFICIENCY

Dietary folate is found in meat and dairy products as well as leafy green vegetables. A Western diet may contain 200 to 400 µg of dietary folate, which is the approximate value range of the daily folate requirement. Compared to cobalamin, tissue stores of folate are more limited. Folate levels decrease within 2 to 4 weeks after folate deprivation, and manifestations of a deficiency may develop a few months thereafter. In most clinical situations, folate deficiency is caused by reduced dietary intake. Patients with alcoholism, dementia, eating disorders, or chronic psychiatric illness are commonly found to have inadequate folate intake.

demonstrates hypercellularity. The erythroid cell line reveals megaloblastic features, with a high ratio of cytoplasmic to nuclear material and hyperplasia. Giant metamyelocytes may be found as well.

Laboratory Diagnosis

Commercial laboratories are available to measure a serum cobalamin level (Box 2). There is some overlap in the normal ranges of these tests, but a definitive cutoff point does not exist. Nevertheless, some rules of thumb for interpreting cobalamin levels are usually safely applied. A serum cobalamin level greater than 300 pg/mL is usually a normal result, and the diagnosis of cobalamin deficiency is unlikely. A cobalamin level lower than 200 pg/mL is often an abnormally low result indicating cobalamin deficiency, but many patients have low cobalamin levels without evidence of clinical deficiency. Results in the intermediate range, from 200 to 300 pg/mL, fall into a borderline category, and cobalamin deficiency is possible. Additional laboratory testing may be helpful in those patients whose serum cobalamin values fall into this intermediate category or as an additional confirmatory step.

Cobalamin has two known roles in humans. It binds to methionine synthase and transfers a methyl group from methyltetrahydrofolate to homocysteine in the formation of methionine. It also binds methylmalonyl-coenzyme A mutase, which is necessary for the formation of succinyl-coenzyme A. Homocysteine and methylmalonic acid are precursor molecules in these reactions. When cobalamin deficiency exists the rate of these synthetic reactions is diminished, and the concentration of precursor molecules increases. Elevated methylmalonic acid is very sensitive and specific for cobalamin deficiency, and it is more specific than homocysteine, because the latter is also elevated in folate deficiency. Serum measurements of homocysteine and methylmalonic acid will demonstrate abnormally high levels if cobalamin deficiency is present, but methylmalonic acid is not elevated in folate deficiency.

The red blood cell folate concentration is, in principle, a better measurement for evaluating folate stores than the serum folate concentration. Red cell folate may be low in cobalamin-deficient patients, limiting the usefulness of the test. Serum folate as a diagnostic test suffers from lack of sensitivity and specificity. Serum folate concentrations should be low in patients with folate deficiency, but folate deficiency can be masked by a recent meal, because serum folate concentrations reflect the last 24 to 48 hours of folate ingestion. A serum folate concentration lower than 4 ng/mL is strong evidence that folate deficiency is present, and a concentration lower than 2 ng/mL is virtually diagnostic.

Folate deficiency also produces an increase in homocysteine concentrations, and it may be reasonable to measure this as a confirmatory step or in those patients with borderline folate concentrations but high suspicion for folate deficiency. It is important to note that serum homocysteine concentrations should not be used as a screening test for folic acid deficiency, because other conditions can elevate homocysteine, including renal insufficiency and hypothyroidism.

BOX 2	Indications for Laboratory Testing to Evaluate for Folate or Cobalamin Deficiency

- Macrocytosis, with or without the presence of anemia or other cytopenias
- Peripheral blood smear demonstrating macro-ovalocytic red cells or hypersegmented neutrophils or both
- Pancytopenia of unexplained etiology
- Neurologic findings, particularly dementia, of uncertain etiology
- Patient from a high-risk population (elderly, alcoholics, drug abusers, patients with eating disorders) who has malnutrition
- Unexplained anemia, even if not macrocytic

CURRENT THERAPY

- Folate supplementation should continue until the underlying cause of the deficiency is corrected.
- Oral cyanocobalamin (B_{12}) replacement is a reasonable alternative to monthly intramuscular injections in appropriate patients.
- Patients' hematologic and clinical responses should be monitored after therapy starts, especially when oral cyanocobalamin is used.

Diagnosing Pernicious Anemia

Commercial laboratory tests are available to determine the presence of anti-IF antibodies in the peripheral blood. Sensitivity ranges up to 80%, and the specificity is almost 100%. In cases of low to borderline cobalamin levels but negative anti-IF antibodies, elevated gastrin levels (>200 ng/L) are strongly suggestive of pernicious anemia. The availability of these tests has largely replaced the need for the Schilling test, which was the historical gold standard for detection of pernicious anemia. The Schilling test involved the use of radiolabeled cobalamin given both orally and intramuscularly, followed by a 24-hour urine collection. Because of the expense and inconvenience of the Schilling test, it is available only at a few institutions and should be reserved for patients with negative anti-IF antibodies and high clinical suspicion for the disorder.

Treatment

Depending on the severity of the hematologic abnormalities, treatment of cobalamin or folate deficiency may require only replacement of those particular nutritional elements. However, replacement of cobalamin or folate produces hematologic improvements slowly, over weeks to months. Some patients' disorders are severe and require rapid correction (i.e., red blood cell transfusion).

PERNICIOUS ANEMIA

Intramuscular cyanocobalamin (vitamin B_{12}) should be given daily for 1 week, then once per week for 4 weeks, and then once per month for life. The dose of each injection is 1000 µg (1 mg).

OTHER COBALAMIN DEFICIENCY STATES

Cobalamin deficiency that does not involve an autoimmune deficiency (i.e., is not pernicious anemia) is often treated with a similar regimen, although some physicians omit the initial daily dosing if neurologic symptoms are absent. If neurologic symptoms are present, some authors favor extending the daily dosing part of the regimen by 1 week.

Treatment with oral cyanocobalamin has been compared with parenteral cyanocobalamin in two trials, but up to 1% of oral cyanocobalamin is absorbed independently of IF. These trials suggested that oral cyanocobalamin may be as effective as parenteral cyanocobalamin if given in high daily doses (1 mg). It is crucial to monitor responses to oral therapy and switch to parenteral therapy if there is inadequate response. Oral therapy may be considered for compliant patients who want to avoid injections.

The expected laboratory response to therapy includes an increase in the number of reticulocytes within the first week. An increase in the hemoglobin concentration is expected within 10 to 14 days after initiation of therapy. Resolution of the anemia is ordinarily expected to occur within 8 to 10 weeks. In addition to hematologic improvement, the concentration of serum cobalamin or folate should improve with therapy, and measurements of homocysteine and methylmalonic acid should also normalize. Neurologic impairments improve much more slowly over time, requiring 6 months or longer in some cases. The severity and chronicity of the cobalamin deficiency are directly related to the amount of time required for neurologic symptoms to resolve.

FOLATE DEFICIENCY

Folic acid is given orally at a dose of 1 mg/day. This amount is often adequate to produce complete resolution of the anemia, even in the presence of malabsorption, although higher doses, from 2 to 5 mg/day,[3] are also used.

Once the underlying cause of the deficiency is corrected, treatment is usually continued for 1 to 4 months to replete folate tissue stores or until resolution of the hematologic abnormalities is noted. Pregnant women and women planning a pregnancy should be encouraged to take folic acid to prevent fetal neural tube defects. The usual dose for prophylaxis ranges from 0.4 mg to 0.8 mg of folic acid daily, although some practitioners advocate higher doses of up to 4 mg/day.[3] If the underlying cause of the deficiency cannot be corrected, then folic acid replacement should continue indefinitely.

A patient's laboratory response to folic acid therapy should mirror the laboratory response to intramuscular cyanocobalamin therapy, as described earlier. Folic acid deficiency does not produce neurologic symptoms, so its replacement should not be expected to produce any neurologic changes. Indeed, although folic acid replacement given to a patient with a megaloblastic anemia caused by cobalamin deficiency and not folate deficiency often corrects the hematologic abnormalities, significant neurologic deficits may develop. It is usually worthwhile to screen for both diagnoses if either is considered likely.

REFERENCES

Antony AC. Megaloblastic anemias. In: Hoffman R, Benz E, Shattil S, et al., Hematology: Basic Principles and Practice. 4th ed. New York: Churchill Livingstone; 2005. p. 519–50.

Aslinia F, Mazza J, Yale S. Megaloblastic anemia and other causes of macrocytosis. Clin Med Res 2006;4:236–41.

Carmel R. How I treat cobalamin (vitamin B12) deficiency. Blood 2008;112:2214–21.

Carmel R. Nutritional anemias and the elderly. Semin Hematol 2008;45:225–34.

Galloway M, Rushworth L. Red cell or serum folate? Results from the National Pathology Alliance benchmarking review. J Clin Pathol 2003;56:924–6.

Klee GG. Cobalamin and folate evaluation: Measurement of methylmalonic acid and homocysteine vs vitamin B(12) and folate. Clin Chem 2000;46:1277–83.

Pruthi R. Pernicious anemia revisited. Mayo Clinic Proc 1994;69:144–50.

Savage D, Lindenbaum J, Stabler S. Sensitivity of serum methylmalonic acid and total homocysteine determinations for diagnosing cobalamin and folate deficiencies. Am J Med 1994;96:239–46.

Toh B, van Driel I, Gleeson P. Pernicious anemia. N Engl J Med 1997;337:1441–8.

Vidal-Alaball J, Butler CC, Cannings-John R, et al. Oral vitamin B12 versus intramuscular vitamin B12 for vitamin B12 deficiency. Cochrane Database Syst Rev 2005;(3) CD004655.

Wickramasinghe SN. Diagnosis of megaloblastic anaemias. Blood Rev 2006;20:299–318.

---

[3]Exceeds dosage recommended by the manufacturer.

Thalassemia

Method of
Sarah A. Holstein, MD, PhD, and Raymond J. Hohl, MD, PhD

Globin Gene Arrangements

Thalassemia syndromes encompass a spectrum of hemoglobin disorders that arise from impaired production of globin chains. The genes that encode globins are located in two clusters: the β gene cluster on chromosome 11 and the α gene cluster on chromosome 16 (Fig. 1). The β gene cluster includes the adult globin genes (β and δ) as well as the fetal Aγ and Gγ genes and the embryonic ε gene. The arrangement of the 5′ to 3′ sequence of these genes parallels the order of their developmental expression. Functional hemoglobin is a tetramer that includes two α and two β globin units. The α gene cluster includes two fetal/adult α genes (α1 and α2) and the embryonic ζ genes. In the embryo, three hemoglobins are found ($\zeta_2\varepsilon_2$, $\alpha_2\varepsilon_2$, and $\zeta_2\gamma_2$). Fetal hemoglobin (HbF) is composed of two α chains and two γ chains ($\alpha_2\gamma_2$). In adults, the predominant hemoglobin is hemoglobin A (HbA), consisting of two α chains and two β chains ($\alpha_2\beta_2$) (see Fig. 106-1). Hemoglobin A2, consisting of two α chains and two δ chains ($\alpha_2\delta_2$), is a normal variant in adults and typically represents less than 3% of the total hemoglobin (see Fig. 1).

In β-thalassemia, there is diminished production of β globin genes, resulting in an excess of α globin chains. Conversely, in α-thalassemia there is impaired production of α globin genes, resulting in an excess of β globin chains. This imbalance of globin production is variable, and the degree of accumulation of unpaired globin chains is directly related to the severity of the disease phenotype. The genetic basis of thalassemia is heterogeneous, and several hundred mutations have been identified. These mutations may affect any level of globin gene expression, including arrangement of the globin gene complex, gene deletion, splicing, transcription, translation, and protein stability. In general, β-thalassemia occurs as a result of mutations, whereas α-thalassemia occurs as a result of gene deletion.

It has been estimated that there are 270 million carriers of thalassemia in the world, including 80 million β-thalassemia carriers. The frequency of β-thalassemia carriers is highest in the malarial tropical and subtropical regions of Asia, the Mediterranean, and the Middle East. The term thalassemia, derived from Greek, refers to the Mediterranean Sea. This distribution is secondary to the selective advantage of heterozygotes against malaria. β-Thalassemia is subdivided into major, intermedia, and minor types (Table 1). α-Thalassemia is classified into four syndromes: α-thalassemia trait 2 (loss of one

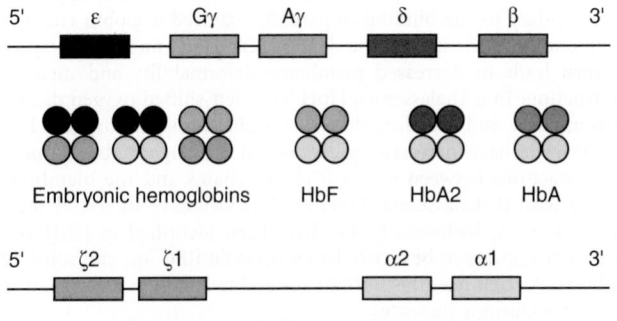

FIGURE 1. Representation of the β and α globin gene clusters. Also shown are the globin tetramers produced during embryonic development.

TABLE 1 Summary of Hematologic and Clinical Features of the Thalassemias

Type	Hematologic Findings	Hemoglobin Electrophoresis Pattern	Clinical Features
β-Thalassemia major	Severe anemia, microcytosis, hypochromia, target cells, nucleated RBCs	Absence of HbA, markedly elevated HbF, elevated HbA2	Splenomegaly, jaundice, skeletal abnormalities, abnormal facies; transfusion dependent
β-Thalassemia intermedia	Mild to moderate anemia, microcytosis, hypochromia	Elevated HbA2, elevated HbF, decreased HbA	Splenomegaly; variable transfusion dependence
β-Thalassemia minor	Mild anemia, microcytosis, target cells	Elevated HbA2	None
Hemoglobin Barts hydrops fetalis	Severe anemia, anisopoikilocytosis, hypochromia, nucleated RBCs	HbBart; absence of HbA, HbA2, and HbF	Death during gestation; fetus with massive hepatosplenomegaly, generalized edema
Hemoglobin H disease	Moderately severe anemia, anisopoikilocytosis, microcytosis, Heinz bodies	Decreased HbA; HbH and HbBart present	Splenomegaly, jaundice; generally transfusion-dependent
α-Thalassemia trait 1	Mild anemia, hypochromia, microcytosis, target cells	Normal	None
α-Thalassemia trait 2	Normal	Normal	None

Abbreviations: Hb = hemoglobin; RBCs = red blood cells.

α globin gene [αα/α−]); α-thalassemia trait 1, also referred to as α-thalassemia minor (loss of two α globin genes [αα/−− or α−/α−]); hemoglobin H (HbH) disease (loss of three alleles [α−/−−]); and hemoglobin Barts hydrops fetalis (loss of all four α globin loci [−−/−−]).

Pathophysiology

The clinical manifestations of thalassemia and their severity are a consequence of the relative excess of unpaired globin chains. In particular, excess α globin chains are unstable and insoluble and therefore precipitate inside the red blood cell (RBC). These inclusions (precipitated hemoglobin) may be visualized as Heinz bodies. The accumulation of α globin chains leads to a variety of insults to the erythrocyte, including changes in membrane deformability and increased fragility. Free β chains are more soluble than free α chains and are able to form a homotetramer (HbH). The hallmark of thalassemia is an anemia that is a consequence of both increased destruction (i.e., hemolysis) and decreased production (i.e., ineffective erythropoiesis). The bone marrow typically displays erythroid hyperplasia.

Oxidant injury is closely linked with the pathology of thalassemia. Under normal conditions, a small amount of methemoglobin (Fe^{3+}) is formed via oxidation and can then be reduced back to hemoglobin (Fe^{2+}). However, isolated globin chains can be oxidized to hemichromes, some forms of which are irreversibly oxidized. The hemichromes can then generate reactive oxygen species, which can oxidize membrane components, leading to cell injury. There is an increase in membrane rigidity in β-thalassemia, and this appears to be secondary to the binding of partially oxidized α globin chains to components of the membrane skeleton. Increased membrane rigidity in turn leads to decreased membrane deformability and increased destruction. In α-thalassemia, HbH has a left-shifted oxygen disassociation curve and therefore does not readily transport oxygen. HbH erythrocytes have increased rigidity, which is thought to be secondary to interactions between excess β globin chains and the membrane. Unlike with β-thalassemia, HbH erythrocytes have increased membrane stability. Inclusion bodies have been identified in HbH cells, and there appears to be a correlation between RBC age and solubility of HbH. As cells age, the amount of soluble HbH decreases, and the level of inclusions increases.

It has also been recognized that there is increased phagocytosis of thalassemia RBCs compared to normal controls. The etiology is not completely understood, but it may be a consequence of reduction in surface levels of sialic acid, increase in surface immunoglobulin G binding, and changes in phosphatidylserine localization.

CURRENT DIAGNOSIS

- Complete blood count: anemia (very severe in β-thalassemia major, mild in β-thalassemia minor and α-thalassemia trait), low mean corpuscular volume, variable leukocytosis, thrombocytopenia (secondary to splenomegaly) or thrombocythemia (after splenectomy)
- Peripheral blood smear: hypochromia, microcytosis, anisocytosis, poikilocytosis, target cells, Heinz bodies, nucleated red blood cells
- Evidence of hemolytic anemia: indirect hyperbilirubinemia, elevated lactate dehydrogenase, decreased haptoglobin
- Hemoglobin electrophoresis pattern:
  β-Thalassemia minor: elevated HbA2 ($\alpha_2\delta_2$)
  β-Thalassemia intermedia: elevated HbA2, elevated HbF ($\alpha_2\gamma_2$), and decreased HbA ($\alpha_2\beta_2$)
  β-Thalassemia major: absence of HbA, markedly elevated HbF, and elevated HbA2
  α-Thalassemia trait: normal
  Hemoglobin H disease: decreased HbA, presence of HbH (β_4) and HbBart (γ_4)
  Hemoglobin Barts hydrops fetalis: HbBart, absence of HbA, HbA2, and HbF
- Timing of symptomatic disease:
  β-Thalassemia minor: asymptomatic
  β-Thalassemia intermedia: variable
  β-Thalassemia major: within first year of life
  α-Thalassemia trait: asymptomatic
  Hemoglobin H disease: symptomatic at time of birth
  Hemoglobin Barts hydrops fetalis: death during gestation

Despite the pronounced hemolysis and marrow erythroid hyperplasia, patients with thalassemia generally do not display the compensatory reticulocytosis that is indicative of the other basis for anemia, ineffective erythropoiesis. Accumulation of α chain aggregates is thought to lead to death of erythrocyte precursors. Furthermore, abnormal assembly of membrane proteins in erythroid precursors has been demonstrated.

Iron overload is one of the primary causes of morbidity. Even without transfusion, the long-standing anemia, however mild, leads to increased iron absorption in the gut and eventual chronic iron overload. Excessive iron deposition causes devastating damage to multiple organs, particularly affecting the heart, liver, and endocrine organs.

β-Thalassemia Major

Symptoms of β-thalassemia major are not present at birth, because HbF ($\alpha_2\gamma_2$) is present. However, as HbF levels decline over the first year, the signs and symptoms of severe hemolytic anemia begin to manifest. Affected individuals display hepatosplenomegaly from expansion of the reticuloendothelial system as well as extramedullary hematopoiesis, pallor, growth retardation, and abnormal skeletal development. If left untreated, 80% of children with β-thalassemia major will die before the age of 5 years.

LABORATORY FEATURES

Thalassemia major is characterized by a severe microcytic anemia. Hemoglobin levels may be as low as 3 to 4 g/dL. The peripheral blood smear is markedly abnormal and is notable for hypochromia, microcytosis, anisocytosis, poikilocytosis, target cells, and tear drop cells. Routine stains show the presence of precipitated α globin chains as Heinz bodies. The reticulocyte count is often low. The white blood cell count is often high but may be artifactually elevated as a consequence of automated inclusion of high numbers of circulating nucleated RBCs. The platelet count is typically normal, but progressive hypersplenism can result in decreased platelet counts. Patients who have undergone splenectomy often have increased white blood cell and platelet counts. Iron studies reveal elevated serum iron, transferrin saturation, and ferritin. Consistent with hemolysis and ineffective erythropoiesis, indirect bilirubin and lactate dehydrogenase levels are increased and haptoglobin levels are low.

CLINICAL FEATURES

Unique to β-thalassemia major is the development of extramedullary erythropoiesis. This may be so severe that the masses of bone marrow lead to broken bones and spinal cord compression. Sites of involvement include the sinuses and the thoracic and pelvic cavities. The expansion of the erythroid bone marrow can lead to a number of skeletal changes. In particular, characteristic changes in the facial bones and skull result in frontal bossing, overgrowth of the maxillae, and malocclusion. This has sometimes been referred to as chipmunk facies. Other bones are also affected, and premature fusion of the epiphyses results in shortened limbs. Compression fractures of the spine may occur. Even if the disease is managed appropriately with transfusions and iron chelation, patients will still suffer from osteopenia and osteoporosis. Possible mechanisms include changes secondary to hypogonadism or increased bone resorption secondary to vitamin D deficiency.

Hepatomegaly and splenomegaly, secondary to extramedullary erythropoiesis and RBC destruction, are prominent. Injury to Kupffer cells and hepatocytes from chronic overload leads to fibrosis and end-stage liver disease. Hepatic iron overload is probably caused in part by comparatively high levels of transferrin receptors. Iron overload, and perhaps other factors, increase susceptibility to viral hepatitis. Laboratory studies show indirect hyperbilirubinemia, hypergammaglobulinemia, and elevated liver markers. The chronic hemolysis leads to formation of bilirubin gallstones, although cholecystitis or cholangitis is not common. Splenic dysfunction results in immune dysfunction. The shortened erythrocyte survival time leaves patients susceptible to aplastic crisis induced by parvovirus B19 infection. Extramedullary hematopoiesis may also affect the kidneys, and patients often have large kidneys. Rapid cell turnover leads to hyperuricemia, and children may develop gouty nephropathy.

A number of endocrine abnormalities are commonly seen in β-thalassemia major, including hypogonadism, growth failure, diabetes, and hypothyroidism. These abnormalities occur even in chronically transfused patients and may be in part related to iron overload.

Endocrine glands, like liver and heart, have high levels of transferrin-receptor and therefore are more susceptible to iron overload. The typical growth pattern for a child with β-thalassemia major is relatively normal until the age of 9 to 10 years. After that time, the growth velocity slows, and the pubertal growth spurt is either absent or reduced. Although secretion of growth hormone does not appear to be altered in thalassemic patients, a reduction in peak amplitude and nocturnal levels of growth hormone has been observed. Amenorrhea is quite common, with 50% of girls presenting with primary amenorrhea. Secondary amenorrhea also develops, particularly in patients who do not receive regular chelation therapy. In males, impotence and azoospermia is common. Primary hypothyroidism typically appears during the second decade of life. The prevalence of diabetes mellitus and impaired glucose intolerance has been estimated at 4% to 20%. Unlike type 1 diabetes mellitus, diabetes associated with thalassemia is rarely complicated by diabetic ketoacidosis. The risk of diabetic retinopathy is lower, but the risk of diabetic nephropathy is higher.

Thalassemic patients suffer from extensive cardiac abnormalities. Chronic anemia causes cardiac dilatation. Although chronic transfusion can help prevent cardiac dilatation, the resulting iron overload leads to cardiac hemosiderosis. Pericarditis, ventricular and supraventricular arrhythmias, and end-stage cardiomyopathy can develop. Ventricular arrhythmia is a common cause of death. Patients may also develop pulmonary hypertension. The degree of iron overload in the heart has traditionally been assessed by cardiac biopsy, but cardiac magnetic resonance imaging (MRI) is increasingly being used.

Vitamin and mineral deficiencies may occur. Folic acid deficiency may develop in patients, presumably as a consequence of increased cell turnover. Although the cause is unknown, patients with β-thalassemia major often have very low serum zinc levels. Serum levels of vitamin E and vitamin C may also be low.

MANAGEMENT OF β-THALASSEMIA MAJOR

Transfusion

The key intervention for the management of β-thalassemia major is chronic transfusion therapy. In particular, during the first decade of life, regular transfusion results in improvements in hepatosplenomegaly, skeletal abnormalities, and cardiac dilatation. Patients typically require 1 to 3 units of packed RBCs every 3 to 5 weeks. The optimal target total hemoglobin level has yet to be determined. Alloimmunization does occur, and some blood centers try to leukodeplete their products, match donors by ethnicity, and limit the donor pool for any particular patient. Although the risk of blood-borne infections is now quite small, regular transfusion of blood products still carries a risk for infections such as HIV and hepatitis C.

CURRENT THERAPY

- Chronic packed red blood cell transfusions for β-thalassemia major (1–3 units of packed leukoreduced erythrocytes every 3–5 weeks) with a target hemoglobin concentration of 9 to 10.5 g/dL; variable transfusion needs for β-thalassemia intermedia and hemoglobin H disease
- Splenectomy with antibiotic prophylaxis and vaccination
- Iron chelation: deferoxamine (Desferal) or deferasirox (Exjade); deferiprone (Ferriprox) does not have FDA approval in the United States
- Osteoporosis management: calcium with vitamin D supplementation; bisphosphonates
- Allogeneic hematopoietic cell transplantation for β-thalassemia major

Splenectomy

The general indication for splenectomy is an increase of more than 50% in the RBC transfusion requirement over the period of 1 year. Splenectomy may initially yield a decrease in the RBC transfusion requirement. It has been noted that thalassemia patients are at higher risk for infection after splenectomy than are those patients splenectomized for other reasons. The bacteria that most frequently cause infections in these patients include *Streptococcus pneumoniae, Haemophilus influenzae, Neisseria meningitidis, Klebsiella, Escherichia coli,* and *Staphylococcus aureus.* The increased susceptibility to infection compared with other splenectomized patients is thought to be a result of greater immune dysfunction secondary to iron overload. In particular, it has been reported that iron-overloaded macrophages lose the ability to kill intracellular pathogens. Antibiotic prophylaxis with penicillin, amoxicillin, or erythromycin is recommended for children up to the age of 16 years. In addition, patients should receive immunizations, including the pneumococcal, influenza, and *Haemophilus influenzae* vaccines.

Iron Chelation Therapy

Because of increased iron absorption and chronic transfusion therapy, iron overload develops. As noted earlier, iron overload causes damage to multiple organs. Because iron is poorly excreted, removal must be accomplished by phlebotomy (not an option in thalassemic patients) or by chelation therapy. Historically, deferoxamine (Desferal) has been the most widely used chelator. This agent may be administered subcutaneously, intramuscularly, or intravenously. The dosing for chronic iron overload is 20 to 40 mg/kg/day SQ or 500 to 1000 mg/day IM + 2 g IV per unit transfused blood. The IV-only route is indicated for patients with cardiovascular collapse. Multiple studies have shown that deferoxamine therapy improves long-term survival. In addition, intensive therapy with deferoxamine has been shown to improve cardiac function in patients with severe iron overload. However, compliance with daily injections has been a particular problem, and, unless regular therapy is given, iron will reaccumulate.

Deferiprone (Ferriprox)[2] was the first orally active chelator to be introduced. It is given three times daily (total of 75 mg/kg/day). Studies have indicated that deferiprone may be as effective as deferoxamine in lowering iron levels. A recent Cochrane Review concluded that deferiprone is indicated in the treatment of iron overload in thalassemia major if deferoxamine therapy is contraindicated or inadequate. Agranulocytosis associated with deferiprone has been reported, and, because of this risk, the drug is currently not available in the United States except through the FDA Treatment Use Program. Deferiprone is available in Europe and Asia. There has also been interest in combined therapy with deferiprone and deferoxamine.

Deferasirox (Exjade) is the first orally active agent approved for use in the United States. Its longer half-life in comparison to deferiprone allows this drug to be given once daily (total of 20–40 mg/kg/day). A phase III trial comparing deferasirox to deferoxamine in patients with thalassemia revealed similar decreases in liver iron concentrations. Side effects include gastrointestinal complaints (abdominal pain, nausea, vomiting, diarrhea) and skin rash. There have been postmarketing reports of acute renal failure, hepatic failure, and cytopenias. It is recommended that serum creatinine, ferritin, and alanine aminotransferase be monitored monthly during therapy.

The gold standard for measurement of liver iron concentration has been liver biopsy with iron measurement by atomic absorption spectrometry. More recently, there has been increasing use of MRI technology to measure liver iron levels. In general, iron content determined by MRI methodology correlates with liver iron concentration determined by biopsy. However, the precision of liver MRI measurement appears to be dependent on iron levels, liver fibrosis, and calibration. Hepatic iron concentration has also been measured using a superconducting quantum interference device (SQUID), although reported consistency has varied and widespread use of this technique has been limited by expense and complexity.

Management of Osteoporosis

Even with calcium and vitamin D supplementation, iron chelation, transfusion therapy, and hormonal therapy, bone loss continues to be a significant problem for thalassemia patients. Recently, there has been interest in the use of bisphosphonates. This class of drugs, which includes clodronate (Bonefos),[2] alendronate (Fosamax), pamidronate (Aredia), and zoledronate (Zometa), inhibit osteoclastic bone resorption and have found extensive use in the management of Paget's disease, osteoporosis, and skeletal metastases. Small studies performed in thalassemia patients have failed to show benefit with clodronate 100 mg IM every 10 days or 300 mg IV every 3 weeks. A very small study using alendronate (Fosamax)[1] 10 mg PO daily revealed an increase in bone mineral density only at the femoral level. Conversely, in a study involving pamidronate (Aredia)[1] 30 or 60 mg IV every month, there was an increase in bone density only at the lumbar level. The most promising results have been achieved with the most potent member of the class, zoledronate. Several trials demonstrated that zoledronate (Zometa)[1] 4 mg IV every 3 or 4 months results in significant improvement in femoral and lumbar bone mineral density and reduces bony pain. Larger, long-term trials are necessary before this agent finds widespread use in the management of thalassemia-induced osteoporosis.

Hematopoietic Cell Transplantation

Hematopoietic cell transplantation is the only curative strategy for patients with hemoglobinopathies. Patients are assigned to a risk class (Pesaro class) based on adherence to regular iron chelation therapy, presence or absence of hepatomegaly, and presence or absence of portal fibrosis. Those children with no or little hepatomegaly, no portal fibrosis, and regular iron chelation therapy (class I) have a better than 90% chance of cure, whereas those with both hepatomegaly and portal fibrosis (class III) have long-term survival rates of about 60% in older studies. More recent reports indicate that class III survival has improved to 80%.

The use of human leukocyte antigen (HLA)-identical sibling donors has been preferred, because the use of HLA-mismatched donors has produced inferior results and is associated with increased graft rejection, graft-versus-host disease, and infection. The use of unrelated donors has been explored, and initial studies showed poorer outcomes. However, more recent data suggest that matched unrelated donors might be a viable option if a suitable sibling donor is lacking, thanks to improved donor selection and transplantation techniques.

Another emerging technique is the use of reduced-intensity conditioning regimens, although long-term success has yet to be achieved.

Gene Therapy

Globin gene therapy, achieved through manipulation of autologous stem cells, is an attractive alternative to allogeneic transplantation. There are three major scientific hurdles that must be overcome: design of vectors that yield therapeutic levels of globin gene expression, ability to isolate and transduce autologous stem cells, and development of transplantation conditions that will permit host repopulation. In addition, the safety of viral and nonviral transfection is an issue. At this point, there has been some success in murine models of β-thalassemia. Likewise, although the use of antisense oligonucleotides to manipulate HbA levels has been attempted in cell cultures, no such approach has been used in humans.

Pharmacologic Induction of Fetal Hemoglobin

Induction of HbF expression has been proposed as a therapeutic strategy. For β-thalassemia, induced γ globin gene expression would be predicted to decrease globin chain imbalance by complexing with free α chains. Hydroxyurea (Hydrea)[1] is an antimetabolite thought to

---

[1]Not FDA approved for this indication.
[2]Not available in the United States.

[1]Not FDA approved for this indication.
[2]Not available in the United States.

interfere with DNA synthesis. It is well established in the management of sickle cell disease, where it has been shown to increase levels of HbF. The use of hydroxyurea in β-thalassemia is much less well established. In the United States, hydroxyurea has been approved for use in sickle cell disease but not for thalassemia. Studies published elsewhere in the world have generally shown improvements in hemoglobin levels in thalassemia intermedia patients, with some patients becoming transfusion independent.

5-Azacytidine (azacitidine [Vidaza]),[1] an inhibitor of DNA methyltransferase, has been shown to induce HbF. However, concerns regarding long-term use have prevented further evaluation in thalassemia. Decitabine (Dacogen),[1] an analogue of 5-azacytidine, has been shown to increase HbF levels in patients with sickle cell disease refractory to hydroxyurea. No data are available for the use of decitabine in thalassemia. Butyrate,[5] an inhibitor of histone deacetylases, is another agent capable of inducing HbF. However, butyrate and its derivatives (arginine butyrate,[5] sodium isobutyramide,[5] and sodium phenylbutyrate [Buphenyl][1]) have failed to show significant clinical benefit in thalassemia patients. Therefore, at this time, no agent has been approved for use in thalassemia patients. A number of hypotheses have been proposed to explain the lack of success of inducers of HbF in thalassemia: there is simply too little γ globin production to significantly affect globin chain balance; these agents decrease expression of partially active β-thalassemia genes; these agents increase expression of α-globin genes; chronic transfusions appear to reduce HbF levels; and these agents suppress erythropoiesis.

Antioxidants

Oxidative damage is believed to be an important cause of tissue damage, and there has been interest in the use of antioxidants in thalassemia patients. A variety of substances have been investigated, including ascorbate,[1] vitamin E,[1] N-acetylcysteine (Mucomyst),[1] flavonoids, and indicaxanthin.[5] A variety of antioxidant effects have been observed in vitro with these agents, but none has been shown to improve anemia in patients with thalassemia.

β-Thalassemia Intermedia

Given the underlying genetic heterogeneity, it is not surprising that the clinical manifestations of β-thalassemia intermedia are also quite varied. Some patients with more mild forms of β-thalassemia intermedia do not require chronic transfusion therapy. There is not a clear consensus as to when chronic transfusion should be initiated. Factors that are considered for children include growth patterns, spleen size, and bone development. Transfusion may be necessary during infection-induced aplastic crises. In some instances, transfusions are begun in childhood to help with growth and then discontinued after puberty. Some adults gradually become more anemic and eventually require transfusion. Some authors have argued that starting transfusions early in life is advantageous, because the prevalence of alloimmunization appears to increase if transfusion is started after the first few years of life.

Splenomegaly usually develops in all patients, including those who do not require transfusion. With progression of splenomegaly and the accompanying sequestration and hemolysis, there is usually worsening of anemia, to the point at which transfusions may be required. Most patients achieve transfusion independence after splenectomy. Gallstones may develop, and a prophylactic cholecystectomy is sometimes performed at the same time as the splenectomy. As with β-thalassemia major patients, intermedia patients are at increased risk for infection and should be appropriately vaccinated.

For reasons that are not entirely clear, there is an increased risk of thromboembolic complications in intermedia patients compared with thalassemia major patients. An Italian study reported that 10% of thalassemia intermedia and 4% of thalassemia major patients experienced a thromboembolic event. Another study reported that

thromboembolism occurred four times more frequently in patients with intermedia versus major disease. This report noted that venous events were more common in the thalassemia intermedia population, whereas arterial events were more common in the thalassemia major population. An even higher rate of venous thrombotic events (29%) was reported in a population of splenectomized patients with thalassemia intermedia. It has been suggested that exposed anionic phospholipids on the surface of damaged RBCs may induce a procoagulant effect. There is no consensus regarding the prophylactic use of antiplatelet agents or anticoagulants in this population.

Patients with thalassemia intermedia may develop iron overload, although it is less severe than in patients with thalassemia major. Even those that are not regularly transfused may develop a degree of iron overload, because there is increased iron absorption. Iron overload may be managed with the iron chelating agents as described earlier. Cardiac toxicity, including congestive heart failure, valvular problems, and pulmonary hypertension (leading to secondary right-sided heart failure), resulting from iron overload is not infrequent in the thalassemia intermedia population.

Bone abnormalities and osteoporosis may develop in thalassemia intermedia patients. In a North American study, the prevalence of fractures in these patients was 12%. Leg ulcers involving the medial malleolus are common and are often difficult to treat. Hypogonadism, hypothyroidism, and diabetes may occur, with frequency related to the severity of anemia and iron overload. Pseudoxanthoma elasticum, a syndrome consisting of skin lesions, angioid streaks in the retina, calcified retinal walls, and aortic valve disease, is more common in thalassemia intermedia than in thalassemia major. Currently, no effective therapy exists, although it has been reported that aluminum hydroxide (Alternagel)[1] reduces skin calcification.

β-Thalassemia Minor

Most patients with β-thalassemia minor are asymptomatic. However, they have an abnormal complete blood count that may sometimes lead to the misdiagnosis of iron deficiency. Although these patients have a microcytic anemia, it is much less severe than in patients with β-thalassemia major. In general, the hematocrit is greater than 30%. The mean corpuscular volume is typically less than 75 fL and the RBC distribution width index is normal, in contrast to iron deficiency, in which the degree of microcytosis is less and the distribution width index is usually increased. The peripheral blood smear shows the presence of target cells. Hemoglobin electrophoresis typically reveals an increase in HbA2. The normal anemia experienced during pregnancy may sometimes be exacerbated in patients with β-thalassemia minor, necessitating transfusion. Otherwise, no long-term effects of β-thalassemia minor have been described, and no interventions are required.

α-Thalassemia

LABORATORY AND CLINICAL FEATURES

Patients with α-thalassemia trait 2 are asymptomatic and have normal laboratory values, including complete blood count, peripheral smear, and hemoglobin electrophoresis. Individuals with α-thalassemia trait 1 are asymptomatic, and the disease resembles β-thalassemia minor. The peripheral smear shows a hypochromic microcytic anemia with the presence of target cells. Hemoglobin electrophoresis is normal.

HbH disease does produce symptoms. Unlike β-thalassemia major, in which HbF production protects the fetus, individuals with HbH disease develop hemolytic anemia during gestation and are symptomatic at birth. This is because α globin production is required for HbF ($\alpha_2\gamma_2$). As with β-thalassemia major, patients with HbH disease suffer from the consequences of chronic hemolytic anemia, although the severity is somewhat less. The transfusion requirements for HbH patients resemble those for patients with β-thalassemia

---

[1]Not FDA approved for this indication.
[5]Investigational drug in the United States.

---

[1]Not FDA approved for this indication.

intermedia, with transfusion support initiated in the second and third decades of life. These patients also develop iron overload, necessitating treatment with chelation therapy.

Hydrops fetalis with hemoglobin Barts is usually fatal in utero. The utter lack of α globin chain production results in absence of HbF. Hemoglobin Barts, a homotetramer consisting of four γ globin genes, is unable to deliver oxygen to tissues. Severe tissue hypoxia develops, leading to widespread tissue ischemia. High cardiac output failure leads to massive edema (hydrops). In most cases, death occurs in the third trimester or late second trimester. There have been reports of live births after intrauterine transfusion, but survival beyond the perinatal period is exceedingly rare. Prenatal diagnosis of hemoglobin Barts hydrops fetalis may be achieved through DNA-based testing using amniocytes from amniocentesis or chorionic villi sampling. Noninvasive testing is under development, including methods that isolate circulating fetal DNA in maternal peripheral blood.

MANAGEMENT

Patients with α-thalassemia 2 and 1 traits do not require treatment. The management of HbH disease is similar to that described for β-thalassemia.

REFERENCES

Angelucci E, Barosi G, Camaschella C, et al. Italian Society of Hematology practice guidelines for the management of iron overload in thalassemia major and related disorders. Haematologica 2008;93:741–52.

Bhatia M, Walters MC. Hematopoietic cell transplantation for thalassemia and sickle cell disease: Past, present, and future. Bone Marrow Transplant 2008;41:109–17.

Borgna-Pignatti C. Modern treatment of thalassemia intermedia. Br J Haematol 2007;138:291–304.

Cohen AR. New advances in iron chelation therapy. Hematology Am Soc Hematol Educ Program 2006;42–7.

Fathallah H, Sutton M, Atweh GF. Pharmacological induction of fetal hemoglobin: Why haven't we been more successful in thalassemia? Ann N Y Acad Sci 2005;1054:228–37.

Gaudio A, Morabito N, Xourafa A, et al. Bisphosphonates in the treatment of thalassemia-associated osteoporosis. J Endocrinol Invest 2008;31:181–4.

Lisowski L, Sadelain M. Current status of globin gene therapy for the treatment of β-thalassemia. Br J Haematol 2008;141:335–45.

Quek L, Thein SL. Molecular therapies in β-thalassemia. Br J Haematol 2006;136:353–65.

Roberts DJ, Brunskill SJ, Doree C, et al. Oral deferiprone for iron chelation in people with thalassaemia. Cochrane Database Syst Rev 2007;(3) CD004839.

Toumba M, Sergis A, Kanaris C, et al. Endocrine complications in patients with thalassaemia major. Pediatr Endocrinol Rev 2007;5:642–8.

Sickle Cell Disease

Method of
Lewis L. Hsu, MD, PhD, and
Griffin P. Rodgers, MD*

Sickle cell anemia is a severe hemoglobinopathy with multisystem complications and is the most common of the hemoglobinopathies worldwide. A single nucleotide substitution in codon 6 of the β globin gene causes the abnormal sickled hemoglobin, HbS. The underlying pathophysiologic mechanism common to all genotypes of sickle cell disease involves the intracellular polymerization of deoxy-HbS. Homozygous HbS is termed *sickle cell anemia* or *sickle cell disease SS*

---

*Adapted from Hsu LL, Rodgers G: Sickle cell disease and other hemoglobinopathies. In Young NS, Gerson SL, High K (eds): Clinical Hematology. Philadelphia: Elsevier, 2006, pp 259–280.

BOX 1   Common Subtypes and Rankings of Disease Severity

Very Mild
SS HPFH
S δβ thalassemia

Milder
Sβ+ thalassemia
SC
SE

Similar to SS
Sβ0 thalassemia
SD^Punjab
SC^Harlem

More Severe than SS
SO^Arab

HPFH = hereditary persistence of fetal hemoglobin.

---

and is the most common type of sickle cell disease, with an incidence of approximately 1 in 360 African Americans and 1 in 1200 Latin Americans in Florida. Coinheriting other abnormal hemoglobins with HbS can produce compound heterozygote types of sickle cell disease (Box 1), even when one parent does not have the sickle trait (an important point during genetic counseling). Incidence of HbC is high in many of the populations with HbS, so that typically one third of the people followed at U.S. sickle cell centers have the sickle cell disease SC. Mutations of the α globin genes can also be coinherited, and α-thalassemia has mixed effects in modulating HbSS: decreased hemolytic anemia, fewer strokes and leg ulcers, but higher risk of osteonecrosis and splenic sequestration.

CURRENT THERAPY—FLUID THERAPY

Renal tubular insufficiency occurs early in childhood in sickle cell disease (SCD), and inability to concentrate urine causes very high susceptibility to dehydration. Dehydration greatly increases sickling of erythrocytes. When a person with SCD cannot take fluids orally (such as before general anesthesia), administer intravenous fluids. In periods of high risk for dehydration, such as the second day after tonsillectomy, a prudent clinician will not shut off IV fluids "to promote thirst." Dehydration also occurs easily in hot weather or dry environments such as airline travel, so that people with SCD should carry their own water. Hydration is fundamental to management of vasoocclusive pain and splenic sequestration. An exception to this principle of liberal hydration is during acute chest syndrome: Parenteral fluid supplements should be moderate (maintenance replacement), to avoid adding pulmonary edema to the region of pneumonitis.

Clinical Features

HEMATOLOGY

Each hemoglobin genotype of SCD has a *likely* range of hematologic values and risks of complications. These are generally most severe in HbSS or HbS β0-thalassemia, less severe for HbSC and HbS β+-thalassemia, and modified by inheritance of other traits such as α-thalassemia and hereditary persistence of fetal hemoglobin (HPFH).

BOX 2 Key Medical History for Sickle Cell Disease and Disease-Specific Review of Systems

Sickle Cell Disease Type and Baseline Key Data

Sickle cell type
Baseline hemoglobin
Reticulocyte fraction
White blood cell count
Pulse oximetry
Spleen size

Potentially Life-Threatening Problems

Allergies
Red blood cell alloantibodies
Transfusion reaction

Sickle Cell Complications (Disease-Specific Review of Systems)

Frequent pain
Recurrent acute chest syndrome
Sepsis
Splenic sequestration
Stroke
Abnormal transcranial Doppler or brain magnetic
   resonance imaging
Priapism
Leg ulcer
Avascular necrosis
Renal insufficiency
Pulmonary hypertension
Iron overload

Past Surgical History

Cholecystectomy
Splenectomy
Central venous line

Subcutaneous port
Hip coring or hip prosthesis
Tonsillectomy

Other Problems

Asthma
Chronic hypoxia
Obstructive sleep apnea
Psychological, psychiatric, family, social

Medical Home

Health care provider
Recent and future appointments

Chronic Transfusion

Latest transfusion
Next transfusion
Percent HbS

Immunizations

Streptococcus pneumoniae conjugate and
   polysaccharide vaccine
Hepatitis B vaccine

Other Long-Term Issues

Plans for surgery
Immunizations or hormone injections due

Individualized Pain Management Plan

Effective medication and nonpharmacologic measures
   for pain management in the hospital, clinic, emergency
   department and home.

However, each individual patient appears to have his or her own baseline anemia or steady-state hemolysis, which can change gradually over the patient's lifetime. These baseline blood counts are crucial (Box 2) for proper evaluation of acute SCD complications. Therefore, empowering SCD patients to know their own blood counts is a major goal of quality medical care. Acute anemia exacerbation (especially dips 2 g/dL below the baseline anemia) should trigger a search for a new acute complication, such as aplastic crisis, splenic sequestration, accelerated hemolysis, or acute chest syndrome (Table 1).

Leukocytosis is common in SCD (baseline can be 10,000 to 30,000/mm^3), which can confuse an evaluation for infection. From this baseline, however, neutrophil counts change acutely as in normal hosts. Severe leukocytosis is also associated epidemiologically with more severe morbidity and mortality. Thrombocytosis is also common.

During acute complications such as splenic sequestration, acute chest syndrome, and sepsis, platelet counts can acutely fall into the thrombocytopenic range. Sickle cell disease and thalassemia share a prothrombotic tendency, so that plasma markers of activated coagulation (D-dimers, prothrombin fragment 1.2 [F1.2], and thrombin–antithrombin [TAT] complex) are often encountered at baseline.

Vasoocclusive pain

The hallmark of sickle cell disease is also its most distressing feature: episodic severe painful vasoocclusion. Triggers for vasoocclusive pain include dehydration, cold temperature or skin cooling, exhaustion or lactic acidosis, infection, weather, emotional stress (including major academic examinations), and menstruation. These triggers appear to be linked to the pathophysiology of increased HbS polymerization, vasoconstriction, and increased endothelial activation. Vasoocclusion often has no objective signs, either on physical examination or laboratory tests. Recognizing one of the characteristic patterns of pain can be the principal clue to diagnosing sickle cell vasoocclusion (Box 3) and spares the patient from unnecessary medical testing. For example, symmetrical bilateral painful hands is probably vasoocclusive dactylitis, but unilateral metacarpal pain may be osteomyelitis. Pain assessment should include a quantitative intensity rating, anatomic location(s), descriptive terms for the pain, time course, aggravating and mitigating factors, and patient self-report about whether this pain feels like previous episodes. Vasoocclusive pain often varies throughout the day and can migrate to different anatomic locations.

TABLE 1 Evaluating a Falling Hematocrit in Sickle Cell Disease

Reticulocyte Fraction	Associated Features	Diagnosis
High	Enlarged spleen or liver, pulmonary infiltrate, decreased platelet count	Splenic sequestration, hepatic sequestration, or acute chest syndrome
Baseline	Hemoglobinuria (Coca-Cola urine), autoantibodies, alloantibodies	Accelerated hemolysis, transfusion reaction
0	Parvovirus B19 exposure, Epstein-Barr virus exposure, excessive oxygen supplementation	Aplastic crisis

---

BOX 3   Patterns of Pain in Differential Diagnosis

Avascular necrosis of femoral head: Recurrent
  vasoocclusive pain, sciatica
Biliary colic: Constipation
Dactylitis: Osteomyelitis, trauma
Hepatic sequestration: Hepatitis, ascending cholangitis
Menstrual trigger: Unexplained recurrent pain
Mesenteric vasoocclusion: Acute surgical abdomen,
  constipation
Priapism: Normal erection, urinary tract infection
Rib infarct: Pulmonary embolism
Skull infarct: Hemorrhagic stroke, skull abscess
Vasoocclusion with joint effusion: Septic arthritis, fracture

---

Infection

Infection dominates sickle cell disease in natural history studies, but comprehensive care and acute interventions have greatly decreased the mortality and morbidity from infectious disease. Research continues on the mechanisms of immunocompromise in sickle cell disease, but the list of mechanisms includes opsonic defect, functional asplenia, complement activation, altered lymphocyte function, impaired antibody response, impaired phagocytosis, and abnormal cytokine production.

Sepsis

Until the 1970s, people with SCD in the United States usually died in childhood of bacterial sepsis, and the childhood fatality rate is still high in the developing world where immunizations and prophylactic antibiotics are not available. Sepsis mortality due to *Streptococcus pneumoniae* was 100- to 400-fold greater in children with SCD than in the general childhood population in historical studies. Sepsis in SCD historically also included other encapsulated bacteria (*Haemophilus influenzae, Neisseria meningitidis*). *Yersinia* sepsis is a particular problem for patients with iron overload, because this family of bacteria has an unusually high requirement for iron.

Pneumonia

Acute chest syndrome is defined as a new infiltrate on chest x-ray in a person with SCD, combined with fever, cough, or chest pain. Acute chest syndrome (ACS) often results in rapid deterioration, with a mortality rate as high as 6%. ACS can have multiple etiologies, but

---

  CURRENT DIAGNOSIS

- In the United States, sickle cell disease is most commonly diagnosed by newborn screening. The public health goal is to confirm the diagnosis of sickle cell disease and start prophylactic antibiotics by 4 to 6 weeks of age to prevent deaths from *Streptococcus pneumoniae* sepsis.

- Diagnosis missed at newborn screening (e.g., new immigrants, errors in the screening program) depends on the alert clinician.

- Anemia, anisocytosis, and reticulocytosis can be detected by automated blood count.

- Sickle deformation is readily seen on the blood smear, and hemoglobin electrophoresis confirms the diagnosis (exceptional compound heterozygotes with unusual hemoglobins can be confusing).

- Infants can present with dactylitis or the life-threatening complications of splenic sequestration or sepsis.

- Later in life, adults may be diagnosed when chronic complications such as gallstones or infarcted vertebral bodies on radiograph.

---

respiratory infection is involved in most episodes of ACS in children. Organisms identified in ACS include typical community-acquired bacterial pneumonia, atypical bacteria such as *Chlamydia pneumoniae* and *Mycoplasma hominis,* and respiratory viruses.

Osteomyelitis and Septic Arthritis

The devitalized ischemic bones in sickle cell disease are more susceptible to bacterial infections of bones and joints than in normal hosts. *Staphylococcus aureus, Salmonella,* and other enteric bacteria are common etiologies for osteomyelitis. However, diagnosing these infections can be extremely challenging because the signs, symptoms, and imaging results of osteomyelitis and septic arthritis overlap with those of sickle cell vasoocclusion.

Parvovirus

One of the ordinary respiratory viruses, parvovirus B19, causes a transient erythroblastopenia (reticulocyte counts are typically zero for 7 to 10 days) that can become aplastic crisis in persons with SCD and other hemolytic anemias. This sudden cessation of erythrocyte production while chronic hemolytic destruction continues can lead to fatal anemia, stroke, or heart failure. In some patients, parvovirus B19 triggers a spectrum of other sickle cell complications (ACS, stroke) and thrombocytopenia, neutropenia, or hemophagocytic syndrome.

RESPIRATORY

Acute chest syndrome is a leading cause of death in sickle cell disease. The most common trigger for ACS in adults is marrow fat embolism and the most common trigger in children is respiratory infection, but multiple etiologies often contribute to ACS: vasoocclusive pain of the chest wall, atelectasis from a splinting respiratory pattern and hypoventilation, and rib infarctions. These problems all lead to hypoxemia and increased sickling, which can then worsen the vasoocclusive contribution to ACS and further compromise respiratory function in a positive feedback loop. ACS can worsen rapidly to include acute respiratory distress syndrome or multi-organ failure syndrome, or both. Other sickle cell complications can accompany ACS, including neurologic complications, splenic or hepatic sequestration, and priapism.

Chronic hypoxemia occurs in a significant fraction of patients with SCD. Abnormally low pulse oximetry in SCD can be caused by complex artifacts in some cases, but true chronic hypoxemia can be determined by arterial blood gas analysis, and this can be a useful part of the patient's record. Obstructive sleep apnea due to adenoidal hypertrophy appears to be more common in children with sickle cell disease than in the general population, but it can be relieved surgically. For unknown reasons, the prevalence of hyperreactive airways is high in sickle cell disease, and pulmonary function testing generally reveals a mixture of restrictive and obstructive dysfunction. Coordinating and optimizing pulmonary and hematologic management can significantly decrease the rate of hospitalizations in children with asthma and SCD.

Pulmonary hypertension has gained recognition as a major concern in sickle cell disease, affecting one third of adults with sickle cell disease SS, with onset in adolescence or earlier. Pulmonary hypertension can be detected by Doppler echocardiogram measurement of a tricuspid regurgitant jet velocity (TRJV) greater than 2.5 m/sec performed when the patient is at steady-state baseline. Although this level of TRJV might be considered trivially mild in patients without hemoglobinopathy, TRJV greater than 2.5 m/sec in patients with SCD is associated with a 10-fold increased rate of mortality in 18 months. The etiology of pulmonary hypertension may be tonic vasoconstriction from low nitric oxide bioavailability due to high hemolysis. Microemboli might also be involved, with significant plexogenic vascular remodeling in the later stages of pulmonary hypertension in autopsy series.

CENTRAL NERVOUS SYSTEM

Cerebrovascular complications are prominent manifestations of SCD vasculopathy, ranging from fatal hemorrhagic stroke to subtle neuropsychological damage, and commonly seen as ischemic changes in children with SCD-SS and SCD-Sβ[0]-thalassemia. Arteries around the circle of Willis are susceptible to focal segments of stenosis with intimal hyperplasia and disrupted elastic lamina. Atherosclerosis is rare in sickle cell cerebrovasculopathy. These stenoses can be detected by magnetic resonance angiography (MRA, with data acquisition adjustments to suppress artifacts of turbulent flow). Infarcts can manifest as major sensory, motor, or cognitive deficits. Infarcts can also be completely silent and detected only by imaging. Small infarcts in the deep white matter are associated with abnormalities of smaller arteries, called *small-vessel disease*, which are not detectable by MRA. Ischemic stroke can occur in association with other sickle cell complications: as a watershed bilateral infarct distribution with transient acute anemia such as splenic sequestration or aplastic crisis or as focal infarcts due to emboli from marrow fat embolism or priapism.

Regular screening of children for high risk of stroke using transcranial Doppler ultrasound is part of the standard comprehensive care of SCD types SS and S-β[0]-thalassemia. A large fraction of ischemic strokes in children with SCD can be prevented by using transcranial Doppler screening to identify a high-risk group and then treating this group with a blood-transfusion program. Without treatment, children with cerebrovascular stenosis are likely to progress to recurrent stroke and the moyamoya pattern of vasculopathy.

Hemorrhagic stroke is more common in adults with SCD than in children, and it is often rapidly fatal. The patient typically complains of "the worst headache of my life," and remarks that the pain is different from sickle cell vasoocclusive pain. The etiology is often an aneurysm, associated with a weakened medial layer of the arterial wall. Multiple aneurysms may be present, and further bleeds may be prevented by vascular clip. Bleeding can also occur from moyamoya collateral vessels.

RENAL

Sickle cells cause renal tubular damage from very early in childhood, causing isosthenuria. As a result, the urine specific gravity is not a reliable sign of hydration status in patients with SCD. Renal tubular damage also leads to nocturia or enuresis, because the urine produced all night is fairly dilute, and the bladder is filled with the larger volume of urine produced by the kidneys during the night. Hematuria is common in SCD, attributable to papillary necrosis from red blood cell (RBC) sickling in the renal medulla.

Proliferative glomerulopathy and microalbuminuria can also begin early in life. By young adulthood, some patients have frank albuminuria and the nephrotic syndrome. Approximately 4% of patients with HbSS and one half as many with HbSC progress to end-stage renal disease requiring hemodialysis.

OTHER COMPLICATIONS

Several other organ systems can suffer complications of sickle cell disease. Proliferative retinopathy can be silent until catastrophic complications like hyphema or retinal detachment occur; a screening ophthalmologic examination can permit early intervention to prevent such problems. Cholelithiasis with pigment stones is present in over one half of adults, but there is a controversy about when to perform elective cholecystectomy on asymptomatic gallstones. Impaired growth and delayed puberty are common, and have been linked to elevated energy expenditure and micronutrient and endocrine abnormalities, but patients usually reach normal adult height eventually.

Leg Ulcers

Leg ulcers occur in patients with SS and S β[0]-thalassemia in the United States with an incidence of 2 to 6 per 100 patient-years, but they are more common in patients living in the tropics. Ulcers typically involve the skin overlying the medial malleoli after trauma, insect bites, or dry skin. Ulcers can be extremely painful and slow to heal, causing functional disability for months to years. Infectious complications can include cellulitis, lymphadenitis, or osteomyelitis. Skin edema can herald recurrence of a leg ulcer. It is controversial whether hydroxyurea therapy worsens leg ulcers.

Bone Infarcts and Osteonecrosis of Femoral and Humeral Heads

Vertebral bone infarcts lead to a characteristic radiographic sign of SCD: the H-shaped vertebral body. Vertebral distortion can lead to nerve compression syndromes. Rib infarcts are significant contributors to ACS pathophysiology.

Osteonecrosis or avascular necrosis causes pain in the hip or shoulder with weight bearing or motion and often aches at night. Avascular necrosis is more common in HbSC and HbS-β[+]-thalassemia. X-rays reveal degeneration of the head of the femur or humerus in advanced cases. MRI is useful in early diagnosis. Bone scan shows decreased uptake early in the course of avascular necrosis, then increased uptake later in the course.

Priapism

Priapism is a prolonged, painful penile erection that probably arises from dysregulated nitric oxide and increased vasoconstrictor tone. Priapism affects more than 30% of male SCD patients at some stage, from early school age to adulthood. Priapism occurs in two patterns: stuttering episodes of 2 to 4 hours, which might precede a major episode, and severe ischemic events that last more than 4 hours and can cause fibrosis and impotence.

Splenic Sequestration

The spleen usually infarcts and involutes, so that normal splenic filtration function is lost in the first years of life in SCD-SS but much later in SCD-SC. Sometimes, however, the spleen enlarges and sequesters a significant fraction of RBCs and platelets, transiently removing them from circulation. Acute splenic sequestration can suddenly drop the hemoglobin level by 2 g/dL, typically accompanied by thrombocytopenia and painful splenomegaly. Simply palpating the acutely enlarged spleen provides the diagnosis of acute splenic sequestration. The patient's activity level decreases as the anemia exacerbates. Additional splenic sequestration can worsen to life-threatening hypovolemic shock and profound anemia exacerbation.

Acute splenic sequestration can resolve spontaneously with intravenous hydration or with blood transfusion. Recurrent acute splenic sequestration can enlarge the spleen again within hours, a pattern called *yo-yo spleen*. Alternatively, the spleen can enlarge gradually over weeks or months without pain, leading to persistently palpable splenomegaly, mild anemia, and thrombocytopenia. This chronic splenomegaly can fluctuate for years and then can spontaneously resolve.

Treatment

COMPREHENSIVE APPROACH TO CARE

Comprehensive care is important in SCD: treating chronic problems, individualizing pain management, screening and preventive care (Table 2 and Box 4). Multidisciplinary comprehensive care is less costly than episode acute care, improves patient satisfaction, and can even be implemented in developing countries. Family education is crucial to significant lifesaving home care (see Table 2) (prophylactic antibiotics for children and spleen palpation), and it can also lay the foundation for home pain management and coping skills. When a patient must receive care at different institutions, key points of the medical history can be given to families as a "health passport" or "travel letter" to promote medical communication and continuity of care (see Box 2).

VASOOCCLUSIVE PAIN

Sickle cell vasoocclusive pain is the leading reason for patients to seek medical care. Vasoocclusion often targets certain sites (Table 3 and Box 5). Patterns often recur in a given patient, and deviations from a previous pattern can be subtle but important in distinguishing vasoocclusive pain from other complications. For example, painful limping could be due to acute vasoocclusion or avascular necrosis of the hip, but painless limp may be due to stroke.

TABLE 2 Comprehensive Care and Family and Patient Education

Care	Newborn	Infant and Toddler	School Age	Adolescent	Adult
Screening	Confirm SCD type	Establish baseline CBC and reticulocytes, pulse oximetry	TCD, hip exam, dental, pulse oximetry, consider gallstones, ECG	Proteinuria, retinopathy, dental care, echocardiogram, pulse oximetry	Proteinuria, retinopathy, ECG, dental care, pulse oximetry
Immunizations	Routine, including conjugated pneumococcal	Routine, including influenza and conjugated pneumococcal	Routine, including influenza, polysaccharide pneumococcal	Routine, including influenza	Routine, including influenza
Education	Fever, spleen palpation prophylactic antibiotics, dactylitis, sickle pathophysiology	Pain prevention and management, stroke symptoms	Pain prevention and management, priapism, academic and career choices	Academic and career choices, HbS genetics and reproduction, personal responsibility, pain management, dependence vs independence, transition to adult health care program	Career and family choices, health insurance, HbS genetics and reproduction, pain management
Prevention	Penicillin prophylaxis	Penicillin prophylaxis, RBC phenotype	Penicillin prophylaxis becomes optional	Healthy habits and hydration	Healthy habits and hydration

CBC = complete blood count; ECG = echocardiogram; Hb = hemoglobin; RBC = red blood cell; SCD = sickle cell disease; TCD = transcranial Doppler.

BOX 4   FARMS

The mnemonic FARMS summarizes major points of self-care for sickle cell disease at every age.

F: Fluids, folic acid.
A: Air. Oxygenation is important to prevent sickling. Avoid smoking. Treat asthma, sleep apnea, and other respiratory diseases.
R: Rest, relaxation. Rest breaks when exercising or working can prevent lactic acidosis, which promotes sickling. Relaxation exercises can help with pain management.
M: Medications, medical care. Know your medications: their names, doses, desired effects and side effects. Communicate with your health care team and try to maintain a medical home to avoid fragmenting care among several medical facilities.
S: Situations, support. Avoid situations that can trigger pain or other problems: dehydration, exhaustion, extremes of temperature, infection, high stress. Seek support from family, friends, and the community.

Pain Management Principles

Pain management in SCD is challenging and sometimes frustrating because the vasoocclusive pain can be episodic, unpredictable, and variable, and it might have no objective signs. However, the basic principles of pain management still apply: quantify the pain, give analgesic combinations to match the intensity of therapy to the intensity of pain, check frequently for response to interventions and adjust therapy. Use the WHO staircase of analgesics strategy (Fig. 1) to add analgesics in a rational sequence. Inflammation plays a large role in SCD, making nonsteroidal antiinflammatory agents (NSAIDs) a rational first choice for pharmacologic intervention. For a patient coming to the emergency department because his or her home pain management was not sufficient, a strong NSAID such as ketorolac can be combined with a parenteral opioid. Maximal analgesia is achieved by combining an NSAID with escalating doses of opioids, plus sometimes other classes of analgesics; however, there have been few clinical trials to determine whether any one combination is superior for vasoocclusive pain. Patient-controlled analgesia (PCA) pumps permit great flexibility of parenteral opioid administration and can be used safely by children as young as 6 years old. Some centers use PCA subcutaneous opioid infusion in patients with poor venous access.

During a hospitalization for sickle cell pain, complications to avoid are acute chest syndrome, constipation, and loss of venous access. Several strategies are available to minimize the adverse effects of parenteral opioids: agonist–antagonist agents such as nalbuphine (Nubain), continuous infusion of a very low dose of antagonist such as naloxone (Narcan), or pharmacologic combinations to manage specific adverse effects (antiemetics for nausea, antihistamine for pruritus, laxatives and stool softeners for constipation, and stimulants for sedation). Incentive spirometry to reduce atelectasis in patients with sickle cell pain in the chest wall has been proved to reduce acute chest syndrome by a factor of 9, and therefore incentive spirometry is part of the standard of care for hospitalized patients with sickle cell pain. Adjunct corticosteroids can provide some benefit for vasoocclusive pain, perhaps with a short steroid taper to avoid rebound pain.

Nonpharmacologic pain management adjuncts can be very important, increasing comfort with little or no adverse effects: warm compresses, cushioned mattress pads, recreational therapy and music for distraction, massage, hydrotherapy, hypnosis, relaxation imagery, and transcutaneous electrical nerve stimulators. Sickle cell centers in Cuba report that laser acupuncture is helpful for pain management.

Improving Hospital Pain Management

Individualized pain management plans can list those combinations that have been effective for the patient (see Table 3), and the patient and continuity doctors can update the list periodically. Vasoocclusive pain intensity and duration of hospitalization can vary widely between and within individual patients. A small subset of patients can have very frequent hospitalizations, and focusing individualized case management on these complex patients may reap a greater economic and clinical impact than broad guidelines for the majority of SCD patients to shorten their already-short hospital stays. Psychosocial staff are vital to the multidisciplinary case management approach. When resources permit sickle cell pain management in a day hospital or a dedicated urgent-care center, 8 hours of parenteral analgesic treatment can provide enough pain relief to allow 80% of patients to avoid admission to the hospital.

TABLE 3 Preventing and Managing Vasoocclusive Pain

Degree	Opioid	NSAID	Adjunct Medications	Nonpharmacologic
Prevention			Influenza prophylaxis: Penicillin VK (Veetids) PO bid *or* Pen G (Bicillin) IM monthly *or* erythromycin PO bid Folic acid Consider hydroxyurea (Droxia)	Maintain good hydration Avoid extremes of temperature Avoid exhaustion and lactic acidosis Reduce stress and epinephrine Avoid hypoxia (treat asthma, sleep apnea)
Mild		Acetaminophen (Tylenol) Ibuprofen (Motrin, Advil) Naproxen (Naprosyn)		
Moderate	Codeine with acetaminophen Oxycodone with acetaminophen	Ketorolac	Laxative ± stool softener Antihistamine	
Severe	Nalbuphine (Nubain) Morphine Hydromorphone (Dilaudid) Oxycodone (OxyContin) Fentanyl (Actiq)	Ketorolac	Low-dose naloxone (Narcan) Antiemetic Antihistamine Laxative ± stool softener	

BOX 5   Mnemonic for Sickle Cell Pain Management: BACK PAIN

Believe the patient
Assess pain
Combine therapy (staircase concept)
Kinetics of medications guide dosing intervals
Primum non nocere
Acute chest syndrome and other complications
Individualize but provide consistency
You are **N**ot alone – involve the patient and team

Home Pain Management

The vast majority of vasoocclusive pain is managed at home. Typically, pain management starts with rest, fluids, and warmth, then adding an NSAID such as ibuprofen (Motrin, Advil), acetaminophen (Tylenol), or naproxyn (Naprosyn). More intense pain may be

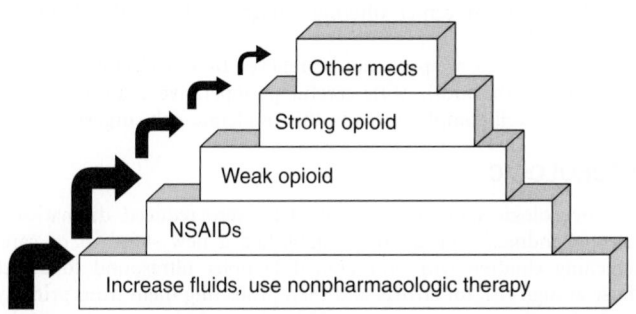

FIGURE 1. Staircase concept for management of vasoocclusive pain. Titrate analgesia upward by adding analgesics of different modalities. Nonpharmacologic measures and increased fluids are fundamental. NSAID = nonsteroidal antiinflammatory drug. (Adapted from Cancer Pain Relief and Palliative Care: Report of a WHO Expert Committee. Geneva, World Health Organization, 1990, p 7–21.)

managed by adding oral opioid combinations such as acetaminophen and codeine or acetaminophen and oxycodone. Prescribing stronger oral opioids for home use might permit patients to avoid some hospitalizations, but other patients find that severe vasoocclusive pain can only be managed with parenteral opioids. Families can prevent some vasoocclusive pain by avoiding triggers of HbS polymerization (see Table 3). Menstruation is a trigger for sickle vasoocclusive pain in some patients, and hormonal regulation to suspend the menses may be offered as a pain-management strategy. Recognizing such pain patterns is important for individualized case management, but many pain episodes have no identifiable trigger. More complete discussion of sickle cell pain management and current analgesic considerations are available in the references.

INFECTION

Sepsis

For patients with SCD and fever, the standard of care is prompt medical evaluation, blood culture, and empiric antibiotics targeting *S. pneumoniae*. Vaccines have successfully reduced sepsis from the bacteria covered by the conjugated vaccines against *S. pneumoniae* and *H. influenzae* type B and the 23-valent polysaccharide vaccine against *S. pneumoniae*. However, vaccinated SCD patients still suffer more cases of *S. pneumoniae* sepsis than the normal population, sometimes with bacteria not covered by the vaccines, and *S. pneumoniae* is becoming increasingly resistant to antibiotics.

Another special consideration arises in patients with SCD and iron overload, due to bacterial avidity for iron. Iron chelators should be withheld temporarily in febrile patients, especially those with abdominal pain, diarrhea and vomiting, or fever and sore throat. The clinician should strongly consider *Yersinia* in an iron-overloaded patient with sepsis and gastrointestinal symptoms.

Acute Chest Syndrome

Because acute chest syndrome often has an infectious etiology, part of the management for acute chest syndrome is empiric antibiotic coverage for both respiratory bacteria and atypical bacteria (e.g., ceftriax-one [Rocephin] or ampicillin-sulbactam [Unasyn], plus a macrolide antibiotic). Antiviral agents are generally not warranted for respiratory infections in sickle cell patients.

Sickle Cell Disease

415

Osteomyelitis

When osteomyelitis is suspected on clinical grounds, sickle cell patients should not be overtreated with antibiotics for osteomyelitis unless infection is proven by bacterial culture, because bone infarction is estimated to be 50 times more likely than osteomyelitis. Note that the erythrocyte sedimentation rate is subject to artifacts from the sickle erythrocytes, and the C-reactive protein may be elevated by vasoocclusive ischemic tissue damage, thus diminishing their value as markers for diagnosing and following osteomyelitis. In patients with culture-proved bone or joint infection, surgical curettage and drainage should be followed by 2 to 6 weeks of antibiotics. Initial empiric antibiotics should cover *Salmonella* and *Staphylococcus* species and then should be adjusted for specific susceptibilities once an organism is isolated. Most patients can be cured with this therapy but, unfortunately, recurrences and refractory infection can occur.

Parvovirus B19

Parvovirus B19 infection usually suppresses erythrocyte production for 7 to 10 days, causing a falling hematocrit and reticulocytopenia. This period of aplastic crisis might be managed by supportive care without transfusion in patients with milder hemolytic anemia and no complications. Deciding whether to give a blood transfusion depends on the severity of anemia (compared with the patient's baseline) and cardiopulmonary compromise, not a specific hematocrit. Additional considerations may include severe RBC alloimmunization or religious objection to transfusion. The patient suspected of parvovirus should be isolated from immunocompromised or pregnant persons, at least until reticulocyte counts begin to rise.

Other Infections

Annual influenza immunization is recommended for persons with sickle cell disease, because influenza can cause acute chest syndrome.

Persons with SCD are quite susceptible to malaria, even though sickle trait confers improved survival with malaria. Malaria treatment should include prompt antimalarials plus fluid supplements to prevent dehydration and splenic sequestration.

The theoretical risk of subacute bacterial endocarditis in SCD patients with hyperdynamic and dilated hearts has led some clinicians to advocate routine antibiotic prophylaxis for dental care of SCD patients. However, the 2007 American Heart Association guidelines indicate that such conditions of turbulent flow no longer require prophylaxis against endocarditis.

RESPIRATORY

Due to the potential for rapid deterioration, patients with ACS should have prompt treatment and initial observation in the hospital. The multiple etiologies of ACS should be addressed by empiric therapy that comprises empiric antibiotics, including a macrolide to cover atypical bacteria, bronchodilators, analgesics, supplemental oxygen, and measures to reduce atelectasis (incentive spirometry, continuous positive airway pressure, or intermittent positive airway pressure). RBC transfusion can produce prompt clinical improvement and should be considered when the patient has hemoglobin dropping by more than 1 g/dL from baseline and pulse oximetry falling below 93% (being cautious not to overtransfuse into hyperviscosity or volume overload). Be moderate with parenteral fluid supplements to avoid adding pulmonary edema to the region of pneumonitis. If the patient requires high supplemental oxygen despite RBC transfusion, consider a double-volume exchange transfusion to reduce the fraction of sickle RBCs below 30%.

Bronchoscopy can provide useful diagnostic information for a patient with worsening ACS, and in rare cases, bronchoscopy has cured ACS by removing bronchial casts from the airway (plastic bronchitis). Severe ACS has many features of acute respiratory distress syndrome and appears to benefit from the same therapies if there is respiratory failure: careful mechanical ventilation, extracorporeal membrane oxygenation, inhaled nitric oxide, and high-frequency ventilation. People with recurrent ACS often have reactive airways disease and benefit from pulmonology consultation.

Pulmonary hypertension in sickle cell disease might respond to antisickling therapy in addition to specific therapy for pulmonary arterial hypertension. Patients can benefit from referral to a pulmonary hypertension center offering clinical trials for this high-risk condition.

Obstructive sleep apnea can be relieved by tonsillectomy or adenoidectomy (or both), with careful perioperative management to avoid sickle cell complications in this moderate-risk surgery.

NEUROLOGIC

The neurologic complications of SCD were reduced dramatically after a landmark clinical trial established a new standard of care: screening children with transcranial Doppler ultrasound to detect those at high risk for stroke, and then protecting them from primary stroke by a long-term program of blood transfusion to maintain the sickle RBC fraction below 30%. After implementing this strategy, California's rate of first stroke in SCD children decreased from 0.88 per 100 person-years to 0.17 per 100 person-years.

In acute stroke, many centers use exchange transfusion to rapidly maintain sickle erythrocytes below 30% to limit the ischemic damage. Acute anticoagulation has not been studied in this setting. Neurology consultation and neurocognitive evaluation can guide a plan

---

CURRENT THERAPY

- Sickle cell disease (SCD) is more than hemolytic anemia and vasoocclusive pain, and the clinician must be alert for complications in nearly every organ system. Multidisciplinary care and a medical home are optimal.
- Diagnosis by newborn screening permits early enrollment in preventive and comprehensive care.
- Much of sickle cell care is based on evidence from randomized clinical trials: transcranial Doppler ultrasound screening for stroke risk, pneumococcal vaccination (Pneumovax) and prophylactic antibiotics, incentive spirometry, extended matching of red blood cell antigens for blood transfusion.
- A patient's baseline hemoglobin level and reticulocytosis are critically important for management, especially for aplastic crisis and splenic sequestration.
- *Streptococcus pneumoniae* is particularly lethal in persons with SCD, so rapid evaluation of the febrile patient and empiric parenteral antibiotics is the current standard of care.
- Acute chest syndrome is potentially fatal, and so an SCD patient with a new radiographic infiltrate and chest symptoms merits close observation.
- Begin acute vasoocclusive pain management with swift assessment and standardized treatment. Subsequent treatment often requires individualized combinations of opioids, nonsteroidal antiinflammatory agents, and nonpharmacologic and pharmacologic adjuncts.
- Extending the transfusion cross-matching to C, E, and Kell antigens can decrease the risk of alloimmunization.
- Environmental triggers for vasoocclusive pain can be mitigated by family and patient education.
- Reduce the risk of leg ulcers by avoiding venipuncture and other trauma to the ankles and avoiding prolonged standing.
- Hydroxyurea (Droxia) can reduce the severity of sickle cell disease, but not all patients respond.
- Sickle cell disease can be cured by hematopoietic stem cell transplantation from an HLA-matched related donor, including sibling umbilical cord–placental blood.

for vigorous rehabilitation therapy, and many neurologic deficits in children are reversible.

After a stroke, a chronic transfusion program to maintain sickle erythrocytes below 30% for at least 3 years reduces the risk of recurrent stroke by as much as 90%. Hydroxyurea appears to confer partial protection against recurrent stroke in children with contraindications to chronic transfusion; a clinical trial is in progress. Hematopoietic stem cell transplantation prevents stroke recurrence and appears to halt cerebrovascular stenosis, and the family should have HLA typing to identify possible related donors.

Intracranial hemorrhage can arise from two features of cerebrovascular disease: aneurysms (which may be in unusual locations) and moyamoya vasculopathy. Patients can present dramatically with severe headache, vomiting, and coma for a subarachnoid hemorrhage. The presentation can have more subtle neurologic deficits for intraparenchymal bleeding. Acute neurologic symptoms should be evaluated with emergent noncontrast head computed tomography (CT) to determine whether neurosurgical intervention is needed. Guidelines for intracranial hemorrhage should be followed, and preoperative transfusion plans may need to be pragmatically modified for the individual circumstances.

If the patient's hemoglobin is less than 10 g/dL, an RBC transfusion should improve cerebral oxygenation, but excessive transfusion to hemoglobin greater than 12 g/dL risks hampering oxygen delivery through hyperviscosity and hypertension. Many clinicians proceed to erythrocytapheresis or manual exchange transfusion to reduce HbS fraction to below 30% to optimize blood flow and oxygenation for the weeks of critical care and recovery ahead. Most clinicians recommend chronic transfusion for a child with severe vasculopathy or unrepaired aneurysm.

RENAL

Enuresis

Desmopressin (DDAVP) and anticholinergics have only modest benefit in children with SCD and enuresis, presumably because the damaged renal tubules have a blunted pharmacologic response. Behavioral training can be effective if applied for at least 3 weeks: reduce fluid intake for a couple of hours before bedtime, urinate just before going to bed, set an alarm and nightlight to wake up and go to the bathroom during the night, and have the child participate in laundering any wet sheets the next day.

Hematuria

An SCD patient with hematuria should be assessed for possible malignancy, infection, and other causes, leaving SCD renal papillary necrosis as the diagnosis of exclusion. The treatment of hematuria in SCD involves bedrest and maintenance of a high urinary flow documented by monitoring of intake and output. If blood loss is significant, iron replacement or blood transfusion, or both, may be indicated.

Glomerulopathy

Microalbuminuria and frank proteinuria are markers of deterioration of glomerular function. Coordinated nephrology and hematology management of patients with renal insufficiency can include angiotensin-converting enzyme inhibitors and hydroxyurea (Droxia), erythropoietin supplementation, and managing the higher risk of thrombotic complications. Renal transplants for people with SCD can be similar to renal transplantation for other end-stage renal disease and might have lower mortality than dialysis.

LEG ULCERS

Leg ulcer treatment requires a consistent, systematic approach to maximize patient compliance over several months: elevation of the legs, meticulous débridement, zinc supplements, antibiotics, and analgesics for chronic pain (see the National Heart, Lung, and Blood Institute guidelines at www.SCInfo.org). Leg ulcers commonly recur. Prevention must be stressed, especially avoiding venipuncture of the lower extremities and avoiding occupations that involve prolonged standing.

BONE INFARCTS AND AVASCULAR NECROSIS

The pain of bone infarcts, sickle arthritis, or other joint complications can persist for weeks, with a waxing and waning course. Physical therapy and NSAIDs are preferable to persistent administration of narcotics, and patients can learn to differentiate the treatment of this chronic pain from treatment of acute pain episodes. During periods of exacerbation of pain in avascular necrosis of the femoral head, for example, non–weight bearing improves the acute problem and can slow progression. Options to reduce the disability caused by avascular necrosis are emerging: early physical therapy, core decompression of the femoral head, and prosthetic hips with improved materials.

PRIAPISM

SCD priapism resulted in impotence in nearly one half of historical cases, but current guidelines for swift intervention aim to reduce this long-term sequela as well as acute suffering. Home therapy may be sufficient to relieve an episode of stuttering priapism: oral fluids, analgesics, urination, moderate exercise, or bathing or showering. Patients with stuttering priapism can be evaluated for priapism prophylaxis using several months of pseudoephedrine (Sudafed),[1] terbutaline (Brethine),[1] or low-dose hydroxyurea (Droxia). Preliminary reports suggest that sildenafil may also be effective prophylaxis for stuttering priapism.

Priapism that fails to resolve within 2 to 4 hours is considered an acute ischemic emergency requiring prompt aspiration of the corpora cavernosa by a urologist, who may also consider intracavernous injection of sympathomimetic drugs and creation of vascular shunts. Intravenous hydration and analgesics are used as in other vasoocclusive pain. The use of exchange transfusion for priapism has become controversial, but it permits further management options that might otherwise trigger vasoocclusion, such as cooling the penis.

Other Therapeutic Issues

PREGNANCY AND CONTRACEPTION

Pregnancy is not contraindicated in women with SCD, but there are increased risks of pregnancy-induced hypertension, vasoocclusive pain, urinary tract infections, hypercoagulability, renal and pulmonary complications, and perinatal mortality. Ideally, managing the pregnancy starts with preconception planning and genetic counseling, gathering a multidisciplinary team with expertise in sickle cell hematology, obstetrics, nutrition, and primary care. Hyperemesis in early pregnancy should be managed early with antiemetics, because dehydration can cause sickle vasoocclusion. Prophylactic transfusions are reserved for women with additional obstetric or hematologic high-risk features. Postpartum care must include screening for SCD in the infant and counseling on plans for future pregnancies.

There is no evidence of increased thrombotic events with modern low-estrogen oral contraceptive formulations in women with SCD. Factors to weigh when choosing contraception include the adverse health effects of pregnancy in SCD and the potential for hormonal therapy to reduce vasoocclusive pain. Men and women on hydroxyurea therapy should use contraceptive methods, because hydroxyurea is well known to be teratogenic in animal models. However, if there is a conception while the patient is taking hydroxyurea, counselors should mention that no birth defects occurred in 14 reported cases of hydroxyurea in human pregnancies.

SURGERY AND PERIOPERATIVE CARE

Coordinated attention to the unique needs of SCD by the anesthesiology, surgery, and hematology teams can significantly reduce the risk of perioperative complications. Older age, regional anesthesia, tonsillectomy, and abdominal surgery are associated with greater risk of SCD-related complications. Sickle cell patients can tolerate major procedures (e.g., neurosurgery, organ transplantation) with preoperative exchange transfusion, perioperative hydration, and close attention to oxygenation

---

[1]Not FDA approved for this indication.

and warmth. For procedures with moderate risk of vasoocclusion, the standard of care is to administer a preoperative RBC transfusion to a hemoglobin level of approximately 10 g/dL instead of exchange transfusion and to administer postoperative respiratory therapy with incentive spirometry. With meticulous supportive care, SCD patients with religious objections to blood transfusion have tolerated low- to moderate-risk surgery without transfusion, sometimes with careful doses of erythropoietin to raise blood counts preoperatively.

BLOOD TRANSFUSION

Transfusion of normal red blood cells has two broad indications in patients with SCD: to improve the oxygen-carrying capacity and to dilute sickled RBCs and prevent extensive sickling in situations of acidosis, hypoxia, or stasis. However, each blood transfusion carries risks (Table 4).

Acute Indications for Transfusion

In various scenarios of acute complications, experts disagree on the indications for transfusion and generally do not fix a standard hemoglobin level that triggers transfusion for all SCD patients. Key considerations are the patient's baseline hemoglobin level and reticulocyte fraction compared with the current levels, the physiologic reserve of cardiorespiratory function, and the likelihood of triggering more sickling with severe acidosis and hypoxemia. Typically, transfusions are given for acute complications like aplastic crisis, splenic sequestration, or acute chest syndrome when the patient's hemoglobin level has fallen by 2 g/dL and symptoms of anemia or hypoxemia emerge.

The typical transfusion goal is to raise the hemoglobin to 10 g/dL, taking care to avoid excessive transfusion to hemoglobin greater than 12 g/dL, where oxygen delivery can be hampered by hyperviscosity and hypertension. Typically, exchange transfusion should be considered when a patient is so physiologically compromised as to require management in an intensive care unit. Exchange transfusion can simultaneously raise the hemoglobin to 10 g/dL and dilute the sickle RBCs to 30%.

Alloimmunization to RBC antigens affects a high percentage of patients with SCD. Extended RBC phenotyping should be done as part of comprehensive care so that whenever possible, RBC units can be matched to the recipient not only for ABO antigens but also C, E, and Kell antigens to decrease the risk of alloantibody formation. Blood banks serving large populations of sickle cell patients often keep a supply of a few RBC units for urgent use that are negative for C, E, and Kell antigens. Hyperhemolysis in an SCD patient receiving transfusions can be life threatening but very difficult to evaluate, because transfusion reaction symptoms overlap with SCD symptoms. Alloimmunized patients who receive transfusions at different medical institutions should be advised to wear medical alert bracelets or to have the blood banks share information about alloantibody history, because routine cross-matching might not detect all alloantibodies.

Chronic Transfusion Programs

Regularly scheduled blood transfusion every 3 or 4 weeks can maintain the sickled RBC fraction at 30%, and this level of dilution of sickled RBCs effectively reduces the risk of stroke and other sickle cell complications. Less intense transfusion programs can prevent recurrence of splenic sequestration or acute chest syndrome. Chronic transfusions should use extended RBC phenotyping and matching of at least antigens C, E, and Kell, to reduce risks of alloimmunization. Complications of chronic transfusion programs include poor venous access, transfusion-transmitted infection, and iron overload. Exchange transfusion, generally by automated erythrocytapheresis, can reduce or eliminate iron overload in a chronic transfusion program. However, erythrocytapheresis has disadvantages: increased exposure to blood donors, need for large-bore venous access, and need for a pheresis team.

Iron overload becomes a concern after about 20 lifetime RBC transfusions. Iron is removed from the body by the chelation medications deferoxamine (Desferal) or deferasirox (Exjade). Patient compliance with deferoxamine is usually poor because it is administered as an overnight subcutaneous infusion. The newer chelator, deferasirox, is administered as an oral solution. Monitoring iron overload and the side effects of the chelators is best coordinated with hematologist and hepatologist consultants.

Hydroxyurea

Hydroxyurea (Droxia), an S-phase cytotoxic drug that raises HbF, is FDA approved as antisickling therapy for adults with severe sickle cell disease complications (see Table 4). HbF modulates the severity of SCD by reducing the concentration of HbS, inhibiting polymerization of HbS, and possibly conferring other beneficial effects on the RBCs. Hydroxyurea daily treatment can reduce the frequency of vasoocclusive pain, acute chest syndrome, hospitalizations, transfusions, and priapism. Hydroxyurea improves longevity and is cost effective. However, some patients do not respond to hydroxyurea. Results of hydroxyurea clinical trials with adolescents and children are similar to those in adults, and an infant study is in progress. Hydroxyurea therapy requires close monitoring for excessive myelosuppression and individualized adjustment of dosage, as well as precautions due to theoretical risks of teratogenicity and leukemia.

TRANSPLANTATION

Curative therapy for sickle cell disease and other hemoglobinopathies is available through hematopoietic stem cell transplantation (HSCT). More than 200 children with severe complications of SCD have had HSCT using HLA-matched related donors through SCD-specific protocols in international consortia of transplant centers. HSCT for children under these conditions is now accepted as a standard care option, with mortality 5% or less, few transplant-related

TABLE 4 Three Major Antisickling Therapies

Therapy	Indications	Contraindications	Advantages	Disadvantages
Bone marrow or cord blood stem cell transplantation	Ischemic CVA Recurrent ACS Frequent pain Avascular necrosis	No matched donor	Curative Prevents further cerebrovascular disease	Risk of procedure-related death, infection, organ failure, GVHD Risk of chronic GVHD
Chronic transfusion	Ischemic CVA Recurrent ACS Splenic sequestration Severe anemia due to renal failure	Multiple RBC alloantibodies Poor venous access	Reduces severity of sickle cell complications Prevents stroke in children	Requires good venous access RBC alloimmunization Iron overload except when using erythrocytapheresis Not curative
Hydroxyurea	Recurrent ACS Frequent pain	Pregnancy	Reduces severity of sickle cell complications Improves longevity Increases Hb Promotes weight gain	Requires monitoring myelosuppression Not curative

ACS = acute chest syndrome; CVA = cerebrovascular accident; GVHD = graft-versus-host disease; Hb = hemoglobin; RBC = red blood cell.

complications, and elimination of sickle-related complications in the majority of patients (see Table 4). In contrast, adults had high mortality rates with HSCT under the same conditions, attributable to age-related impaired organ function, and so new approaches such as reduced-intensity preparative regimens are still in clinical trials for adults with SCD. The major barrier to curing more people through transplantation is the lack of HLA-identical related donors, and additional clinical trials are under way to offer HCT using alternative donors.

REFERENCES

Ballas SK. Sickle Cell Pain. In: Progress in pain research and management, vol. 11. Seattle: IASP Press; 1998.

Benjamin LJ, Dampier CD, Jacox AK, et al. Guideline For the Management of Acute and Chronic Pain in Sickle Cell Disease. Glenview, Ill: American Pain Society; 1999 APS Clinical Practice Guidelines Series no. 1.

Brawley OW, Cornelius LJ, Edwards LR, et al. National Institutes of Health Consensus Development Conference statement: hydroxyurea treatment for sickle cell disease. Ann Intern Med 2008;148(12):932–8.

Castro O, Brambilla DJ, Thorington B, et al. The acute chest syndrome in sickle cell disease: Incidence and risk factors. The Cooperative Study of Sickle Cell Disease. Blood 1994;84(2):643–9.

Davies EG, Riddington C, Lottenberg R, Dower N. Pneumococcal vaccires for sickle cell disease. Cochrane Database Syst Rev 2004;(1) CD003885.

Gladwin MT, Sachdev V, Jison ML, et al. Pulmonary hypertension as a risk factor for death in patients with sickle cell disease. N Engl J Med 2004;350(9):886–95.

Gladwin MT, Vichinsky E. Pulmonary complications of sickle cell disease. N Engl J Med 2008;359(21):2254–65.

Information Center for Sickle Cell and Thalassemic Disorders. Available at http://sickle.bwh.harvard.edu/ [accessed May 16, 2009].

Krishnamurti L. Hematopoietic cell transplantation for sickle cell disease: State of the art. Expert Opin Biol Ther 2007;7(2):161–72.

Lane PA, Buchanan GR, Hutter JJ, Austin RF, et al. Sickle cell disease in children and adolescents: Diagnosis, guidelines for comprehensive care, and care paths and protocols for management of acute and chronic complications. Available at http://www.scinfo.org/protchildindex.htm [accessed May 16, 2009].

National Heart, Lung, and Blood Institute. The Management of Sickle Cell Disease, 4th ed. NIH Publication No. 02-2117. Available athttp://www.nhibi .nih.gov/health/prof/blood/sickle/sc_mngt.pdf [accessed May 16, 2009].

New Jersey Department of Health Sickle Cell. Family Guide, Information For School Personnel. Available at http://nj.gov/health/fhs/sicklecell/index .shtml [accessed May 16, 2009].

Sickle Cell Disease [entire issue]. Hematol Oncol Clin North Am 2005;9 (5):771–987.

Sickle Cell Disease Association of America. Home page. Available at http:// www.sicklecelldisease.org/ [accessed May 16, 2009].

Sickle Cell Information Center. Home page. Available at http://www.SCInfo .org [accessed May 16, 2009].

Steinberg MH. Pathophysiologically based drug treatment of sickle cell disease. Trends Pharmacol Sci 2006;27(4):204–10.

Stuart MJ, Nagel RL. Sickle-cell disease. Lancet 2004;364(9442):1343–60.

Vichinsky EP, Neumayr LD, Earles AN, et al. Causes and outcomes of the acute chest syndrome in sickle cell disease. National Acute Chest Syndrome Study Group. N Engl J Med 2000;342(25):1855–65.

Neutropenia

Method of
Mary Ann Bonilla, MD

Host defense against infection is composed of the humoral and cellular immune systems. B cells provide humoral immunity against extracellular pathogens through antibody production. T cells facilitate antibody production by B cells and also are effectors of antigen-specific cell-mediated immunity that eliminates viruses, mycobacteria, and tumor cells. Phagocytes, such as monocytes and neutrophils, provide protection against invading bacteria and fungi. The neutrophil or polymorphonuclear leukocyte population has two compartments, a marginated pool attached to the vascular endothelium and a circulating pool. In response to an inflammatory stimulus, neutrophils migrate toward the organisms (chemotaxis), ingest them (phagocytosis), and kill them through the process of lysosomal fusion and generation of oxygen radicals.

Neutropenia is defined as an absolute decrease in the number of circulating neutrophils. Normal neutrophil levels are age and race related, with approximately 25% to 50% of persons of African descent and some ethnic groups in the Middle East having lower leukocyte and neutrophil counts without infectious complications (benign ethnic neutropenia). The absolute neutrophil count (ANC) is calculated by multiplying the total white blood cell (WBC) count by the percentage of neutrophils and bands present on the differential: ANC = WBC × (% neutrophils + % bands). An increased susceptibility to infection is proportional to the level of neutropenia. In mild neutropenia (ANC of 1000–1500 cells/mm^3), the patient usually is asymptomatic. In moderate neutropenia (ANC of 500–1000 cells/mm^3), stomatitis or aphthous ulcers, gingivitis, recurrent otitis, or skin infections may be seen. In severe states (ANC <500 cells/mm^3), the risk of pyogenic life-threatening infections increases and includes pneumonias, sinusitis, abscesses, and overwhelming sepsis. Bacteria and fungi that compose the normal oral and enteric flora cause the infections most commonly seen.

The duration of neutropenia influences the risk of infectious complications. Neutropenia may be acute or chronic (lasting >3 months); it may exist as a single cytopenia or as part of a complex disease process; and it may be acquired or congenital. This article provides an approach to the diagnosis, evaluation, and treatment of neutropenia and its complications.

Evaluation of Neutropenia

An accurate and complete clinical history is essential in establishing the onset and possible etiology of the neutropenia. Key points should include the onset, duration, type, frequency, and severity of infections; any exposure to toxins or drugs; and when the neutropenia was first noted by laboratory testing. Obtaining previous complete blood count (CBC) results to document onset can be difficult, because such measurements are not routinely performed in young children, but these data may yield invaluable information.

A detailed physical examination, focusing on adenopathy, splenomegaly, and phenotypic abnormalities including skeletal anomalies, should be performed. Special attention should be given to possible sites of active or chronic infection, especially the oral cavity, gingiva, perirectal area, skin, and sites of chronic infection such as sinuses. Evidence of poor growth suggesting failure to thrive, malabsorption, or nutritional deficiencies must be documented.

Laboratory assays include a CBC with differential and morphologic examination of the peripheral smear for evidence of nutritional deficiency disorders, myelokathexis, Chédiak-Higashi syndrome, or the presence of blasts. Serial blood counts, two to three times weekly, for 4 to 6 weeks are necessary to yield the characteristic 21-day fluctuations in ANC associated with cyclic neutropenia. Viral infections are the most common cause of neutropenia in young children. Titers for hepatitis, Epstein-Barr virus, cytomegalovirus, varicella, influenza, human immunodeficiency virus, and respiratory syncytial virus may be indicated. Assays for T- and B-cell immunophenotyping and function, immunoglobulins, and complement levels may reveal an underlying immunodeficiency.

Positive antineutrophil antibodies detected by agglutination or flow cytometry assays can support the suspected diagnosis of an immune neutropenia. However, a negative result does not exclude this diagnosis, because of the many technical difficulties and reliability of these assays. Gene mutations of ELA2 are commonly seen in cyclic, or non-Kostmann's congenital neutropenias. Genetic studies are commercially

TABLE 1 Congenital Neutropenia

	Inheritance	Chromosome	Gene Mutation
Severe congenital neutropenia	AD	19p13.3	ELA2
	AD	1p22	Gfi
Kostmann's neutropenia	AR	1q21.3	HAX
X-linked neutropenia	X-linked	Xp11.232	WAS
Cyclic neutropenia	AD	19p13.36	ELA2
Shwachman-Diamond syndrome	AR?	7q11	SBDS
Barth's syndrome	X-linked	Xq28	TAZ
Chédiak-Higashi syndrome	AR	1q42.1-q42.2	LYST

Reprinted with permission from Pamblad JE, von dem Borne AE: Idiopathic, immune, infectious, and idiosyncratic neutropenias. Semin Hematol 2002;39(2):113. *Abbreviations:* AD = autosomal dominant; AR = autosomal recessive.

available for other congenital neutropenias as well (Table 1). Additional studies that may be indicated are antinuclear antibodies and complement to screen for collagen vascular disease; and serum copper, vitamin B_{12}, and red blood cell folate levels in adults.

Bone marrow examination is indicated for persistent neutropenia or when more than one lineage abnormality is present, to exclude leukemia, myelodysplasia, metastatic tumor cells, and aplastic anemia. Morphology may reveal a myeloid maturation arrest, or a retention of neutrophils characteristic of a congenital neutropenia. Cytogenetic and fluorescence in situ hybridization (FISH) analysis to detect leukemia or myelodysplastic syndrome–associated abnormalities of chromosomes 5, 7 and 8, should be performed particularly before the initiation of therapy with granulocyte colony-stimulating factor (G-CSF).

Classification

Neutropenia may result from decreased or ineffective marrow production or increased peripheral destruction. A simple classification divides the neutropenias into acquired and congenital forms.

ACQUIRED NEUTROPENIAS

Acquired neutropenias can be caused by infection, drugs, or immune mechanisms, or they may be part of a systemic disorder. The most common cause of acquired neutropenia is infection causing toxic injury or hemophagocytosis. Bacterial infections such as typhoid fever, shigella enteritis, brucellosis, and tularemia are associated with neutropenia. Viral (e.g., hepatitis, Epstein-Barr virus, HIV, cytomegalovirus, herpesvirus-6), rickettsial (e.g., ehrlichiosis) and parasitic (e.g., malaria) infections have been implicated as causative agents. Some drugs (e.g., chemotherapeutic agents) induce neutropenia because of their cytotoxic effects on the bone marrow and the short half-life of neutrophils. Other medications induce neutropenia by idiosyncratic, immune-mediated, or toxic mechanisms. High-risk categories include antithyroid medications, macrolides, and procainamide (Pronestyl). Other agents include antimicrobials (penicillin, cephalosporin, vancomycin [Vancocin]), analgesics and antiinflammatory agents (indomethacin [Indocin], ibuprofen [Advil]), antipsychotics, antidepressants, anticonvulsants (valproic acid [Depakene], phenytoin [Dilantin]), histamine 2 receptor antagonists (cimetidine [Tagamet], ranitidine [Zantac]), and heavy metals (gold, arsenic, and mercury).

Autoimmune neutropenia of childhood (usually diagnosed before 2 years of age) is considered benign because of the low incidence of serious infections and spontaneous resolution of the neutropenia by 5 years of age. Although patients may respond to intravenous immunoglobulin (GammaGard)[1] and G-CSF (filgrastim [Neupogen]), most require no intervention. Idiopathic neutropenia seen in older children and adults is a diagnosis of exclusion when no other etiology can be elicited. There is a female predominance, serious infections are

absent, anemia is occasionally present, splenomegaly is absent, and often there is no spontaneous remission. Other disorders associated with immune-mediated neutropenia include systemic lupus erythematosus, scleroderma, Felty's syndrome, and the inherited autoimmune lymphoproliferative syndrome (ALPS).

CONGENITAL NEUTROPENIA

Although congenital disorders are rare, a family history of neutropenia, severe infection, or sudden death should suggest the diagnosis. Autosomal recessive Kostmann's disease or autosomal dominant non-Kostmann's neutropenia is marked by severe neutropenia (200 cells/mm^3) and a maturational arrest at the promyelocyte level in the bone marrow. Similar features can be seen with a variant of Wiskott-Aldrich syndrome in neutropenic males with monocytopenia, decreased CD4/CD8 ratio, and no eczema. Cardiac or proximal myopathy and hypoglycemia with associated neutropenia (cyclic, chronic, or intermittent) may suggest Barth's syndrome, an X-linked genetic disorder primarily affecting males. Hypoglycemia and neurologic abnormalities manifesting in infancy may reveal metabolic disorders such as glycogen storage disease type 1b. Pancreatic insufficiency resulting in failure to thrive and metaphyseal chondrodysplasia can be signs of Shwachman-Diamond syndrome. Neutropenia in a patient with partial oculocutaneous albinism and giant lysosomes in granulocytes suggest Chédiak-Higashi syndrome. Short stature, thumb abnormalities, or pigment skin anomalies may suggest Fanconi's anemia. The Online Mendelian Inheritance in Man website provides a current comprehensive compendium of human genes and genetic phenotypes of these disorders.

Therapy

TREATMENT OF INFECTION

A diagnosis of neutropenia and fever should be considered a medical emergency. A thorough physical examination, including the ear, nasal, and oral cavities as well as the perirectal areas, is necessary. Imaging of the sinus, mastoids, or lungs may be indicated if symptoms suggest an undocumented infection. A CBC to assess the current ANC and appropriate cultures should be obtained. For patients having an ANC lower than 500 cells/mm^3 and for those who are ill-appearing, broad-spectrum antibiotic therapy should be initiated immediately. Because these patients are at high risk for sepsis from staphylococcal and gram-negative organisms, hospitalization is recommended. Duration of antibiotic therapy is not standardized, but in patients without a focus of infection who subsequently become afebrile and whose cultures are negative, antibiotics may be discontinued after 48 hours of therapy.

TREATMENT OF NEUTROPENIA

In healthy, asymptomatic adults and children, observation alone may be indicated. Offending medications should be withdrawn. The most important preventive measure to avoid infection is good hand

---

[1]Not FDA approved for this indication.

washing and attention to oral hygiene. Regular dental cleaning, daily flossing, and the use of a mouthwash containing peroxide-based (e.g., Colgate Peroxyl 1.5%) or antibacterial (e.g., Biotene Antibacterial Mouthwash) enzymes may alleviate the gingivitis. Despite this, patients still may be symptomatic, and care to avoid dehydration should be taken if aphthous ulcers are present. So-called magic mouthwash solution, containing viscous lidocaine[6] to provide topical relief from oral ulcers, can be employed. Rectal temperature measurements and rectal suppositories should be avoided.

If the patient has severe neutropenia or develops recurrent or persistent infections, growth factor administration should be considered. G-CSF is now considered the standard of care. In patients with congenital neutropenia (e.g., Kostmann's syndrome, Shwachman-Diamond syndrome, glycogen storage disease type 1b), G-CSF may be started at 5 μg/kg/day. Patients with cyclic neutropenia may respond to a lower dose of 3 μg/kg/day. Those occasional patients with idiopathic or immune neutropenia, who develop significant infections, may respond to a lower dose of 1 μg/kg/day. Dosages should be titrated to achieve an ANC between 1000 and 1500 cells/mm^3 and to maintain the patient infection free. If there is no response to increasing doses of G-CSF (seen more commonly in congenital neutropenia), the dose should be increased every 2 to 4 weeks. Neutropenia that fails to respond to doses greater than 100 μg/kg/day are considered refractory. Patients with refractory disease may be candidates for an HLA-matched related stem cell transplantation.

The development of acute myeloid leukemia and sepsis leading to death has been reported in patients with congenital neutropenia. This may be associated with other abnormalities, such as G-CSF receptor mutations. The current recommendation is to monitor with yearly bone marrow studies in congenital neutropenia patients on chronic G-CSF therapy. The Severe Chronic Neutropenia International Registry maintains long-term data regarding this and other outcomes as well as providing a patient and physician referral database and coordinating research efforts.

REFERENCES

Hsieh MM, Everhart JE, Byrd-Holt DD, et al. Prevalence of neutropenia in the U.S. population: Age, sex, smoking status, and ethnic differences. Ann Intern Med 2007;146(7):486.

Online Mendelian Inheritance in Man (OMIM) website. Available at: http://www.ncbi.nlm.nih.gov/sites/entrez?db=omim [accessed June 19, 2009].

Pamblad JE, von dem Borne AE. Idiopathic, immune, infectious, and idiosyncratic neutropenias. Semin Hematol 2002;39(2):113.

Rosenberg PS, Alter BP, Bolyard AA, et al. The incidence of leukemia and mortality from sepsis in patients with severe congenital neutropenia receiving long-term G-CSF therapy. Blood 2006;107:4628.

---

[6]May be compounded by pharmacists.

Hemolytic Disease of the Fetus and Newborn

Method of
Douglas S. Richards, MD

Since the 1960s there has been a marked reduction in the number of fetuses and neonates dying from alloimmune hemolytic anemia. This is primarily because the administration of Rh immune globulin (RhoGAM) to RhD-negative pregnant women has been very effective in preventing sensitization. This article emphasizes measures that ensure adequate prophylaxis and discusses the intensive management that is required for the few women who become sensitized.

The RhD Antigen

In the 1940s the Rh antigen was discovered in Rhesus monkeys, and it was determined that antibodies against this antigen were responsible for most cases of hemolytic disease of the human newborn. Two genes located on the first chromosome determine the Rh type. The *RhD* gene determines the presence or absence of the D antigen, and the *RhCE* gene determines whether the C, c, E, or e antigens will be expressed.

ALLOIMMUNIZATION

Alloimmunization can occur when fetal cells bearing an antigen foreign to the mother enter the maternal circulation. As little as 0.1 mL of RhD-positive blood is sufficient to cause sensitization in an RhD-negative woman. The risk of fetomaternal hemorrhage is low in the first and second trimesters but increases in the third trimester, and at delivery up to 50% of women have sufficient fetomaternal hemorrhage to be at risk for sensitization. Pathologic processes such as abortion and ectopic pregnancy and invasive procedures such as amniocentesis and chorionic villus sampling are associated with an increased risk of fetomaternal hemorrhage and maternal sensitization.

For alloimmunization to occur, the mother must be negative and the fetus must be positive for a particular antigen. The incidence of the RhD negative state varies by ethic origin. Fifteen percent of whites of European ancestry are RhD negative, and 8% of African Americans and Latin Americans from Mexico and Central America are RhD negative. The rate is even lower (<1%) for Native Americans, and persons of Chinese and Japanese ancestries.

PREVENTION OF ALLOIMMUNIZATION

The principle of antibody-mediated immune suppression was first applied to the Rh problem in the 1960s. Postpartum Rh immune globulin administration in Rh-negative pregnant women results in a 10-fold reduction in sensitization rates compared with untreated controls. Consequently, the administration of Rh immune globulin to RhD-negative women after the delivery of RhD positive infants is the standard of care. Administration of Rh immune globulin to RhD-negative women at 28 weeks to prevent third-trimester sensitization is also cost-effective. Although sensitization can rarely occur before 28 weeks, early administration of Rh immune globulin is only indicated when there are complications or procedures that can allow a fetomaternal hemorrhage.

CURRENT DIAGNOSIS

- An antibody screen should be performed in all pregnant women at the time of registration.
- Anti-RhD titers >4 indicate sensitization and require careful follow-up. Titers <16 should be repeated monthly. Titers >16 or the birth of a previous affected child should prompt referral to a maternal–fetal medicine specialist for appropriate fetal surveillance.
- For sensitized women with significant anti-RhD titers, measurement of the middle cerebral artery peak velocity has replaced amniocentesis for ΔOD 450 measurement as the best way to diagnose severe fetal anemia.
- Amniocentesis with determination of the fetal RhD type by polymerase chain reaction techniques allows discontinuation of surveillance when the fetus is found to be RhD negative.
- With sensitization for many of the minor antigens, the father's antigen status should be determined. This is particularly true for the Kell antigen, because only 9% of the population is positive for this antigen. Surveillance can be discontinued when the father is negative for the antigen against which the mother is sensitized.

Treatment

MANAGEMENT OF PREGNANT WOMEN NOT KNOWN TO BE SENSITIZED

A blood type and antibody screen should be performed at the first prenatal visit on all pregnant women. Because of the possibility of laboratory and clerical errors, repeat typing is indicated even if the woman has previously been typed. The antibody screen is performed on all women, even those who are RhD positive, to allow detection of antibodies against other red cell antigens. Patients who are found to be weak RhD positive (previously termed D^u-positive) are not at risk for RhD-alloimmunization and do not require Rh immune globulin.

RhD-negative women with an initial negative antibody screen should have the screen repeated at 28 weeks' gestation. If the antibody screen is still negative, Rh immune globulin, 300 μg, should be given. If anti-RhD antibodies are detected at the time of the repeat screen, the patient is already sensitized, and Rh immune globulin will be of no benefit. Rh immune globulin administration is not harmful in this setting, so it is permissible to administer it before the results of the antibody screen are available.

Because more than 85% of partners of RhD-negative women are RhD positive, and because paternity is not always certain, it is usually best to assume the possibility of an RhD-positive fetus. If a woman declines to receive antepartum Rh immune globulin because she believes the baby's father has RhD-negative blood, I have her sign the following statement in her chart. "I understand that if the father of my baby has RhD-positive blood I should receive Rh immune globulin. Knowing this, I decline to receive Rh immune globulin." Rh immune globulin is also indicated for women who experience induced abortion, spontaneous abortion, vaginal bleeding in pregnancy, ectopic pregnancy, abdominal trauma in pregnancy, or external cephalic version attempt or who undergo chorionic villus sampling or amniocentesis. If there is an indication for Rh immune globulin before 28 weeks, it is generally accepted that repeat doses should be given at least every 12 weeks.

Based on the initial studies with male volunteers, it is recommended that Rh immune globulin be administered within 72 hours of the time of suspected fetomaternal hemorrhage. However, it has never been shown that Rh immune globulin is ineffective if the interval is longer. Therefore, even if there is a delay of greater than 72 hours, Rh immune globulin should be given.

CURRENT THERAPY

- All nonsensitized RhD-negative women should have Rh immune globulin (RhoGAM) administered at 28 weeks' gestation.
- Those whose babies are RhD positive should have Rh immune globulin administered within 72 hours of delivery. A rosette test should be performed to determine whether more than one vial of immune globulin is needed.
- Rh immune globulin should be given to RhD-negative women who experience induced abortion, spontaneous abortion, vaginal bleeding in pregnancy, ectopic pregnancy, abdominal trauma in pregnancy, or external cephalic version attempt or who undergo chorionic villus sampling or amniocentesis. If Rh immune globulin is given before 28 weeks, the dose should be repeated within 12 weeks.
- When a fetus is found to be severely anemic, direct transfusion of packed red cells into the umbilical vein under ultrasound guidance can usually allow safe delay of delivery until after 34 weeks' gestation.
- Fetuses who receive intrauterine transfusions rarely require exchange transfusions after birth.

POSTPARTUM Rh IMMUNE GLOBULIN

Delivery represents the time of greatest risk for fetomaternal hemorrhage. At birth, the antibody screen should be repeated, and the neonatal blood type should be determined. If the baby is RhD positive or weak RhD positive, Rh immune globulin should be given. If the mother received antepartum Rh immune globulin at 28 weeks, low levels of residual passive antibodies are not uncommon. This does not represent sensitization, and Rh immune globulin should be given. If the last dose of antepartum Rh immune globulin was given within 3 weeks of delivery, and there was no large fetomaternal hemorrhage, Rh immune globulin does not need to be repeated.

A standard 300-μg vial of Rh immune globulin is sufficient to cover a fetomaternal bleed of 15 mL of red blood cells (30 mL of whole blood). To avoid sensitization in the 1% of women in whom there is a larger bleed, a screening test for the presence of RhD-positive cells in the maternal circulation is recommended. If the commercially available rosette test (Fetalscreen) is positive, the Kleihauer–Betke test is performed to quantify the fetomaternal hemorrhage. One 300-μg vial should be given to the mother for every 15 mL of fetal red blood cells that have entered the maternal circulation. Because the calculated fetomaternal hemorrhage from the Kleihauer–Betke test is not precise, it is best to be liberal in calculating the Rh immune globulin dose.

MANAGEMENT OF RhD SENSITIZED WOMEN

Antibody Titers

An initial positive antibody screen with a titer of 4 or greater indicates that the patient is sensitized. A titer of 2 may be due to laboratory error, so the screen should be repeated. If the initial titer is less than 16, and there is no history of a previously affected infant, titers should be repeated monthly. When antibody titers are 16 or greater, the fetus should be considered at risk for significant hemolytic disease, and subsequent titers are not helpful. When there has been a prior affected infant, the current fetus is considered to be at risk, and serial titers are not done.

When a woman has significant sensitization, the next step is to determine the father's RhD antigen status and CcEe genotype. If paternity is assured and the father is RhD negative, the fetus is not at risk. If the father is RhD positive, the chance that he is heterozygous can be calculated from his race, his CcEc genotype, and the number of RhD-positive infants he has previously fathered (see the table in Moise 2002).

Amniocentesis

Determination of the fetal RhD antigen status can be determined by polymerase chain reaction (PCR) methods from an amniotic fluid sample. For women with a previously significantly affected baby in whom early intensive surveillance will be required, amniocentesis to determine fetal genotype is usually done at 15 to 16 weeks. If the fetus is found to be RhD negative, no further surveillance is needed. To avoid the small risk of amniocentesis, some sensitized women with lower risk prefer to be followed with noninvasive fetal surveillance as described later. However, amniocentesis is usually indicated to plan the timing of delivery.

Amniocentesis with spectrophotometric analysis of the amniotic fluid is the traditional method of determining the degree of hemolysis in an at-risk fetus. The deviation of optical density reading from the expected value at 450 nm (the ΔOD 450 reading) reflects the amount of bilirubin in the amniotic fluid and is directly related to the severity of hemolysis.

The ΔOD 450 value is plotted on a semilogarithmic graph that has the weeks of gestation on the horizontal axis and the ΔOD 450 on the logarithmic vertical axis. Based on Liley's pioneering work in the 1960s, with subsequent modifications by Queenan, the graph is divided into three zones that describe the degree of fetal risk. Zone I, the lowest zone, indicates mild or no hemolytic disease, and zone III, the upper zone, indicates severe hemolytic disease. Without intrauterine transfusion or delivery, there is a high probability of fetal hydrops and death for fetuses in this zone.

Middle Cerebral Artery Peak Velocity

In recent years, measurement of the middle cerebral artery peak velocity (MCA-PV) in the fetus using Doppler ultrasound has supplanted amniocentesis as the preferred method of fetal surveillance in RhD-sensitized pregnancies. The flow velocity in the middle cerebral artery is increased in severely anemic fetuses as a result of decreased blood viscosity and increased cardiac output. The MCA-PV can be readily and reproducibly measured by a well-trained sonographer. Precise attention to technique is essential for an accurate reading. With an axial view of the fetal head, The MCA is visualized with color Doppler, and the Doppler gate is placed close to its origin at the internal carotid artery, with the angle of insonation as close as possible to 0 degrees. It is important that the fetus is quiescent and apneic.

Not only does MCA-PV measurement avoid the risks of amniocentesis (e.g., rupture of membranes, infection, and worsening fetal sensitization by causing a fetal-to-maternal hemorrhage), it has been proved to be more accurate for predicting severe fetal anemia, especially in the second trimester. The sensitivity of this test is 88%, and an abnormal test (>1.5 multiples of the median for the gestational age) has an 85% predictive value for moderate or severe anemia.

In sensitized patients without a previously affected infant, testing is usually started at 22 to 24 weeks of gestation. Surveillance is begun at 18 weeks if there was a prior fetus with significant hemolysis. The test is usually repeated every 1 to 2 weeks, depending on prior pregnancy outcomes and whether values are approaching the abnormal range.

Fetal Blood Sampling and Intravascular Transfusions

When the MCA-PV is abnormally elevated, ultrasound-guided puncture of the umbilical cord for direct determination of fetal hematocrit is indicated. Intrauterine fetal blood transfusions are begun when the hematocrit falls to less than 30%. Historically, fetal blood transfusions were given into the peritoneal cavity, from which about 50% of the transfused red cells are absorbed. Most practitioners now give the transfusion directly into the umbilical vein.

Intravascular transfusion can be performed as early as 22 weeks' gestation. If the procedure is done at a time when the fetus is potentially viable, intramuscular betamethasone (Celestone; 12 mg IM q24h for 2 doses) is given to the mother in case a transfusion-related complication leads to delivery. An ultrasound estimate of the fetal weight is obtained to aid in the calculation of the required transfusion volume. The blood bank is asked to prepare irradiated, leukocyte-poor, cytomegalovirus-negative, type O-negative blood with a hematocrit of 80% to 85%, cross-matched against the mother.

We perform the procedure in an operating room, observing full sterile technique. Before we begin, we give an intravenous dose of cefazolin (Kefzol 1 g IV) for antimicrobial prophylaxis. Under ultrasound guidance, a 20- or 22-gauge needle is advanced into the umbilical vein at the point that the cord inserts into the placenta. A transplacental approach is often easier with an anterior placenta, but this is avoided because of a greater chance of a fetomaternal hemorrhage, which could augment the mother's immune response.

Once intravascular access is obtained, an aliquot of fetal blood is aspirated for initial determination of hematocrit. The amount of blood to be transfused is calculated, based on the initial fetal hematocrit, the estimated fetal blood volume, the desired final hematocrit, and the hematocrit of the transfused blood. Vecuronium bromide (Norcuron) 0.3 mg/kg is injected directly into the umbilical vein to paralyze the fetus. Once the desired volume is transfused, a fetal blood sample is drawn to check the final hematocrit and to calculate the percentage of circulating red cells that are native fetal cells (the Kleihauer–Betke test).

The fetal hematocrit falls rapidly after the first transfusion, because ongoing hemolysis of the remaining RhD-positive cells occurs and because fetal hematopoiesis slows dramatically. For this reason, the second transfusion is scheduled 2 weeks after the first.

After the second transfusion, the majority of cells in the fetal circulation are RhD negative, so the rate of fall of the hematocrit is governed by the natural senescence of the donor cells. A good general rule is to expect a 1-point drop in the hematocrit per day. Subsequent transfusions are given when the calculated hematocrit falls below 25%. Intervals of 3 to 4 weeks are often possible.

Timing of Delivery

Controversy exists about whether to give a transfusion to a fetus who is due for a final transfusion between 32 and 34 weeks' gestation. Because the chance of extrauterine survival is excellent, one could argue that the risks of prematurity are less at this gestational age than a repeated intrauterine transfusion. I make this determination based on the lecithin-to-sphingomyelin (L/S) ratio, the expected difficulty of performing the transfusion, and the desires of the patient. An intrauterine transfusion would almost never be done after 34 to 35 weeks, so a fetus who reaches this gestational age would be delivered 3 weeks after the last transfusion.

For fetuses in sensitized pregnancies who have not required a transfusion, amniocentesis is performed at 35 weeks' gestation. If not already done, the fetal RhD type is determined. If the fetus is RhD negative, no further special care is needed. The ΔOD 450 value is determined to confirm that the MCA-PV has not been falsely reassuring. Fetal lung-maturity tests are obtained (the FLM test and/or L/S ratio). If the lungs are mature and the ΔOD 450 value or MCA-PV is borderline high, delivery is indicated. If the lungs are mature, delivery at 37 weeks is appropriate even with reassuring testing, because ongoing hemolysis in the last part of pregnancy can lead to hyperbilirubinemia in the baby.

While awaiting the proper time to deliver, the clinician should asses fetal well-being with nonstress testing and daily fetal movement counting. Nonstress tests should be performed at least weekly starting at 34 weeks in all RhD-sensitized women with an RhD-positive baby. The testing can be started earlier and performed more frequently if fetal transfusions have been required.

Neonatal Care

The three greatest problems facing the neonate from an alloimmunized pregnancy are prematurity, hyperbilirubinemia, and anemia. When the management scheme outlined previously is followed, serious problems from prematurity are uncommon, because almost all fetuses can successfully receive transfusions in utero until near term. When there have been two or more intrauterine transfusions, neonatal hyperbilirubinemia is not a serious problem. Most of the circulating red cells are RhD-negative donor cells, and significant hemolysis has long since ceased. Hyperbilirubinemia can usually be managed with phototherapy, and it is uncommon for exchange transfusions to be required.

Hematopoiesis is severely depressed in neonates who have received transfusions in utero. For this reason, these babies should be followed carefully, with weekly hematocrit and reticulocyte counts until normal erythropoetic function returns. It is expected that the postnatal hematocrit will gradually fall, but in order to not further depress hematopoiesis, blood transfusions are given only to symptomatic neonates. In recent years, administration of erythropoietin (Epogen) has proved useful in stimulating neonatal reticulocytosis.

Immunomodulation Therapy

In some cases of RhD sensitization, the disease process is so severe that fetal hydrops and death occur at a gestational age that is earlier than intrauterine transfusion is feasible. Trials including women such as these have shown a benefit of immunomodulation therapy. Treatment has consisted of plasmapheresis three times during the 10th week of gestation, then, after the final plasmapheresis, intravenous immunoglobulin is given weekly until 20 weeks of gestation. In a trial in which this approach was used, all fetuses still required intrauterine transfusions, but the maternal antibody titer was significantly reduced, and all babies survived.

Hemolytic Disease of the Fetus and Newborn from non-RhD Antibodies

Historically, less than 2% of cases of hemolytic disease of the newborn were caused by antigens other than the RhD antigen. With the successful elimination of most cases of RhD sensitization, the so-called minor antigens have assumed a relatively greater importance. Sensitization to these other antigens usually results from a blood transfusion before the current pregnancy. Antibodies against the Lewis, I, and P antigens are not associated with hemolytic disease, because they are of the IgM type and do not cross the placenta. The two most common potentially serious antibody types are anti-Kell, occurring in 10% of sensitized pregnancies requiring intrauterine transfusion, and anti-c, occurring in 3.5%. There are numerous other IgG antibodies that have rarely been reported to cause severe hemolytic disease in the fetus.

Anti-c sensitization is very similar to RhD disease in its propensity to cause hemolytic disease, and affected patients should be followed in the same manner as described earlier. RhC, RhE, and Rhe antibodies are often found in low titers in patients with RhD sensitization, and these antibodies can contribute to fetal hemolysis. When found alone, they rarely cause sufficient hemolysis to require intrauterine treatment.

The Kell antigen system contains many specific antigens. The most concerning of these is the K1 antigen. This antibody not only causes significant hemolysis but also suppresses fetal hematopoiesis. For this reason, fetal surveillance should be started at a lower antibody titer (8), and MCA-PV testing is clearly superior to ΔOD 450 testing of amniotic fluid. This is because the latter test measures bilirubin products from hemolyis and cannot assess the component of fetal anemia that results from impaired red cell production.

REFERENCES

Mari G, Deter RL, Carpenter RL, et al. Noninvasive diagnosis by Doppler ultrasonography of fetal anemia due to maternal red-cell alloimmunization. N Engl J Med 2000;342:9–14.

Moise KJ Jr. Management of rhesus alloimmunization in pregnancy. Obstet Gynecol 2002;100:600–11.

Oepkes D, Seaward PG, Vandenbussche FP, et al. Dopper ultrasonography versus amniocentesis to predict fetal anemia. N Engl J Med 2006;355:156–64.

Ruma MS, Moise KJ Jr, Kim E, et al. Combined plasmapheresis and intravenous immune globulin for the treatment of severe maternal red cell alloimmunization. Am J Obstet Gynecol 2007;196:138.e1–138.e6.

Van Kamp IL, Klumper FJ, Oepkes D, et al. Complications of intrauterine intravascular transfusion for fetal anemia due to maternal red-cell alloimmunization. Am J Obstet Gynecol 2005;192:171–7.

Hemophilia and Related Bleeding Disorders

Method of
Meera Chitlur, MD, and Roshni Kulkarni, MD

Hemophilia A and Hemophilia B

Hemophilia is an X-linked congenital bleeding disorder caused by a deficiency of factor VIII (hemophilia A) or factor IX (hemophilia B). Hemophilia A is the most common severe bleeding disorder and affects 1 in 5000 males in the United States; hemophilia B occurs in 1 in 30,000 males.

PATHOPHYSIOLOGY

The factor VIII gene is one of the largest genes and spans 186 kb of genomic DNA at Xq28. Inversion mutations account for 40% of severe hemophilia A, and deletions, point mutations, and insertions account for the remainder.

Hepatic and reticuloendothelial cells are presumed sites of factor VIII synthesis. Factor VIII is synthesized as a single chain polypeptide with three A domains (A1, A2, and A3), a large central B domain, and two C domains (Fig. 1). The binding sites for von Willebrand's factor (vWF), thrombin, and factor Xa are on the C2 domain, and factor IXa binding sites are on the A2 and A3 domains. The B domain can be deleted without any consequences. vWF protects factor VIII from proteolytic degradation in the plasma and concentrates it at the site of injury.

The factor IX gene is 34kb long and located at Xq26. It is a vitamin K–dependent serine protease composed of 415 amino acids. It is synthesized in the liver and its plasma concentration is about 50 times that of factor VIII. Gene deletions and point mutations result in hemophilia B.

ROLE OF FACTORS VIII AND IX IN COAGULATION

Factor VIII circulates bound to vWF. It is a cofactor for factor IX and is essential for factor X activation. In the classic coagulation cascade, activation of the intrinsic or extrinsic pathway of coagulation results in sufficient thrombin generation. However, this does not explain bleeding in hemophilia, because the extrinsic pathway is intact. This led to the revised cell-based model of coagulation.

The revised pathway incorporates all coagulation factors into a single pathway initiated by FVII and tissue factor. The contact factors (XI, XII, kallikrein, and high-molecular-weight kininogen) are not essential but serve as a backup. Following injury, encrypted tissue factor is exposed and forms a complex with factor VIIa. The tissue factor–factor VIIa complex activates factor IX to IXa (which moves to the platelet surface) and factor X to Xa. This generates small amounts of thrombin that activates platelets, converts platelet factor V to Va and factor XI to XIa, and releases factor VIII from vWF and activates it. The factor XIa activates plasma factor IX to IXa on the platelet surface, which together with factor VIIIa forms the tenase complex (factor VIIIa/IXa) that converts large amounts of factor X to Xa. Factor Xa forms a prothrombinase complex with FVa and converts large amounts of prothrombin to thrombin, called *thrombin burst*. This results in the conversion of sufficient fibrinogen to fibrin to form a stable clot. (An interactive animation on cell-based coagulation is available at http://www.hemostasiscme.org/Activities/CellBasedCoagulation/content/).

In hemophilia, lack of factor VIII or IX produces a profound abnormality. Factor Xa generated by FVIIa and tissue factor is insufficient because it is soon inhibited by tissue factor pathway inhibitor (negative feedback), and factors VIII and IX, which are required for amplifying the production of Xa are absent. The primary platelet plug formation and initiation phases of coagulation are normal. Any clot that is formed (from the initiation phase) is friable and porous.

CLINICAL FEATURES

The diagnosis of hemophilia is often made following a bleeding episode or because of a family history; 30% of cases, however, have no family history. Based on the plasma levels of factor VIII or IX (normal levels are 50%–150%) that correlate with severity and predict bleeding risk, hemophilia is classified as mild (>5%), moderate (1%-5%) and severe (<1%) (Table 1). Approximately 65% of persons with hemophilia have severe disease, 15% have moderate disease, and 20% have mild disease. Most severe disease manifests by 4 years of age; moderate or mild disease is diagnosed later and often following bleeding secondary to trauma or surgery.

Hemophilia can be diagnosed in the first trimester, using chorionic villus sampling and gene analysis. In the second trimester, fetal blood sampling can be performed. Prenatal diagnosis to determine fetal gender can aid in the management of pregnancy and delivery.

The hallmark of severe hemophilia is hemarthrosis, or bleeding into the joint, that can occur spontaneously or with minimal trauma.

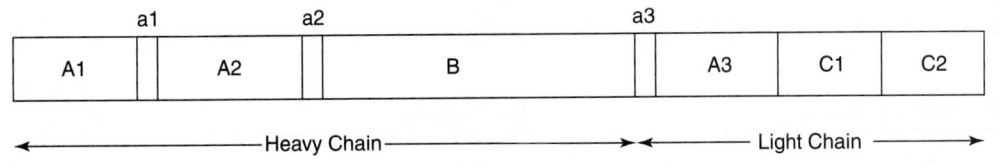

FIGURE 1. Factor VIII protein structure.

Although the immediate effects of a joint bleed are excruciating pain, swelling, warmth, and muscle spasm, the long-term effects of recurrent hemarthrosis include hemophilic arthropathy, which is characterized by synovial thickening, chronic inflammation, and repeated hemorrhages resulting in a target joint. Knees, elbows, ankles, hips, and shoulders are commonly affected. Disuse atrophy of surrounding muscles leads to further joint instability. Limitation of joint range of motion due to hemarthrosis often correlates positively with older age, nonwhite race, and increased body mass index, and it affects quality of life.

Muscle hematomas, another characteristic site of bleeding, can lead to compartment syndrome, with eventual fibrosis and peripheral nerve damage. Iliopsoas bleeds manifest with pain and flexion deformity. Gastrointestinal bleeding and hematuria occur less often.

Central nervous system (CNS) hemorrhage is a rare but serious complication with a 10% recurrence rate and is the leading cause of mortality in hemophiliacs. Although most newborns with severe hemophilia experience an uneventful course following vaginal delivery, vacuum extraction is associated with an increased CNS bleeding risk. The incidence of intracranial hemorrhage in newborns with hemophilia is 1% to 4%.

DIAGNOSIS

Hemophilia A and B are clinically indistinguishable, and specific factor assays are the only way to differentiate and confirm the diagnosis. Both should be differentiated from von Willebrand's disease (vWD). The prothrombin time (PT), platelet function analyzer (PFA-100), and fibrinogen are normal. (PFA, a platelet-function screening test, is replacing bleeding time, because the bleeding time has low sensitivity and specificity and is operator dependent.) The activated partial thromboplastin time (aPTT) is prolonged when the factor levels are below 30%. Table 2 shows the characteristics and differences between the hemophilias and vWD. Female carriers are usually asymptomatic except for those with extreme lyonization resulting in low factor VIII or IX levels. Factor VIII levels increase throughout pregnancy and drop to prepregnancy levels following delivery, but factor IX levels remain constant throughout pregnancy.

TREATMENT

The treatment for hemophilia consists of replacement therapy with intravenous factor VIII or factor IX concentrates produced by purification of donor plasma (plasma derived) or in cell culture bioreactors (recombinant). Careful screening of donors combined with heat treatment and viral inactivation methods have made plasma-derived products safer. Plasma-derived and recombinant products appear to have equivalent clinical efficacy. Recombinant factor concentrates are recommended, but if they are not available, plasma-derived concentrates can be used. Cryoprecipitate is no longer recommended because of concerns regarding pathogen safety.

Treatment administered only during bleeding symptoms is known as *episodic therapy*, and periodic administration of factor concentrates to prevent bleeding is known as *prophylactic therapy*. Response to treatment is more effective when it is administered early. Although prophylaxis prevents the development of joint disease, the high cost of factor replacement coupled with the need for venous access makes it expensive and difficult.

 CURRENT DIAGNOSIS

- The hemophilias and von Willebrand's disease (vWD) account for 80% to 85% of inherited bleeding disorders. Hemophilia A and B are X-linked, whereas vWD and rare bleeding disorders (RBDs) are autosomal disorders.
- The diagnosis of hemophilia and other inherited bleeding disorders should be confirmed by specific assays, because screening tests such as prothrombin time (PT) and activated partial thromboplastin time (aPTT) may be normal. Plasma levels of deficient factor determine clinical severity and management.
- Hemarthrosis is the most common and debilitating complication, and central nervous system bleeding is the most common cause of mortality in hemophilia. Mucosal bleeding and menorrhagia are the most common manifestations of vWD. Bleeding manifestations of RBDs are mild, although homozygotes can present with severe disease.
- Newborns have normal levels of factor VIII; therefore, the diagnosis of hemophilia A can be established at birth. Vacuum delivery should be avoided to prevent head bleeds.
- Women and adolescents with menorrhagia and no underlying pathology should be investigated for a bleeding disorder.

TABLE 1 Hemophilia Severity and Clinical Manifestations

Characteristics	Severe (50%–70%)	Moderate (10%)	Mild 30%–40%
Factor VIII or IX activity (normal 50%–150%)	<1%	1%–5%	>5%
Age of diagnosis	At birth to 2 y	Childhood or adolescence	Adolescence or adult
Bleeding patterns	2–4/mo	4–6/y	Rare
Clinical manifestations	Hemarthroses, muscle, central nervous system, gastrointestinal bleeding, hematuria	Bleeding into joints or muscle following minor trauma, surgical procedure, dental bleeding Rarely spontaneous	Surgical procedures (including dental) and major trauma

TABLE 2 Hemophilias and von Willebrand's Disease: Key Characteristics and Differences

Characteristic	Hemophilia A	Hemophilia B	von Willebrand's Disease
Incidence	1:5000	1:30,000	1%–3% of U.S. population
Abnormality	Factor VIII deficiency	Factor IX deficiency	vWF (qualitative and quantitative defect)
Inheritance	X-linked, affects males Gene at the tip of X-chromosome	X-linked, affects males Gene at the tip of X-chromosome	Autosomal dominant (gene: chromosome 12) Some are recessive or compound heterozygotes
Production site	Unknown, liver endothelium	Liver (vitamin K dependent)	Megakaryocytes and endothelial cells
Function	Cofactor; forms tenase complex with factor IX and activates factor X, leading to thrombin burst that results in conversion of large amounts of fibrinogen to fibrin	Serine protease (inactive form: zymogen) Activated by factor XI or VIIa; forms a tenase complex with factor VIII and activates factor X	Platelet adhesion to site of injury or damaged endothelium Protects factor VIII from proteolysis
Classification (normal levels 50%–150%)	Mild (>5%) Moderate (1–5%) Severe (<1%)	Mild (>5%) Moderate (1–5%) Severe (<1%)	Type 1 Type 2 (2A, 2B, 2M, 2N) Type 3
Clinical presentation	Positive family history (30% new mutation) Hemarthroses, hematomas, hematuria, intracranial hemorrhage, gastrointestinal hemorrhage, etc.	Positive family history (30% new mutation) Milder disease, although identical hemorrhage sites as hemophilia A	Positive family history Mucocutaneous bleeding (epistaxis, menorrhagia, postdental bleeding) Type 3 can manifest as hemophilia A.
PFA, bleeding time	Normal	Normal	May be prolonged
PT	Normal	Normal	Normal
aPTT	Prolonged	Prolonged	Prolonged or normal
Factor VIII assay	Decreased or absent	Normal	Decreased or normal (absent type 3)
Factor IX assay	Normal	Decreased or absent	Normal
vWF antigen	Normal	Normal	Decreased or absent (type 3)
vWF:RCo	Normal	Normal	Decreased or abnormal
vWF multimers	Normal	Normal	Abnormal in types 1, 2A, 2B; absent in type 3
Specific treatment	Recombinant factor VIII (preferred) Pathogen-safe plasma-derived concentrates DDAVP for mild cases	Recombinant factor IX Pathogen-safe plasma-derived concentrates DDAVP ineffective	DDAVP (intranasal or intravenous) vWF concentrates (pathogen-safe plasma derived)
Inhibitor patients	Immune tolerance, recombinant factor VIIa, APCC	Immune tolerance, recombinant factor VIIa	Inhibitors are rare
Adjunct therapy	Antifibrinolytics	Antifibrinolytics	Oral contraceptives, antifibrinolytics

APCC = activated prothrombin complex concentrates; aPTT = activated partial thromboplastin time; DDAVP = desmopressin; PFA = platelet function analyzer; PT = prothrombin time; RCo = ristocetin cofactor; vWF = von Willebrand's factor.

The goal of treatment is to raise factor levels to approximately 30% or more for minor bleeds (hematomas or joint bleeds) and 100% for major bleeds (CNS or surgery). Giving 1 U/kg of factor concentrate raises plasma factor VIII levels by 2% and factor IX levels by 1.5% (except with the recombinant factor IX product, where it increases by 0.8%). The half-life of factor VIII is approximately 8 to 12 hours and that of factor IX is up to 24 hours. Factor concentrates can also be given by continuous infusion (3–4 U/kg/hour). The bolus dose varies from 25 to 50 U/kg depending on the severity, site, and type of bleeding and is dosed to the closest vial because of the cost of the products. Table 3 lists the dosing schedule for various types of bleeds.

For short-term therapy (before dental procedures and minor bleeding episodes) in mild hemophilia A and vWD, the synthetic vasopressin analogue desmopressin acetate (DDAVP [Stimate]) is useful. It increases plasma concentrations of coagulation factor VIII and vWF three- to fivefold by releasing the endothelial stores. A DDAVP trial to determine response is helpful in selecting patients who might benefit from such therapy. For hemostatic purposes, intravenous (0.3 μg/kg in 50 mL of normal saline infused over 15–30 min) or intranasal dose (150 μg) can be used. The intranasal dose is 15 times larger than that recommended for diabetes insipidus. A multidose intranasal spray formulation (Stimate nasal spray) delivers 150 μg per spray. The recommended dosage is one spray for patients who weigh less than 50 kg and two sprays (one in each nostril) for those who weigh more than 50 kg. Desmopressin is ineffective in hemophilia B. Aspirin and aspirin-containing compounds should be avoided in persons with bleeding disorders because they interfere with platelet function and can exacerbate bleeding.

Antifibrinolytics such as ε-aminocaproic acid (Amicar) and tranexamic acid (Cyklokapron) are used as adjunct therapies and in mild hemophilia and can obviate the need for factor concentrates. The recommended dosage for ε-aminocaproic acid is 75 to 100 mg/kg/dose IV or orally every 4 to 6 hours (maximum 30 g/24 hours). The recommended dosage for tranexamic acid is 10 mg/kg/dose IV or 25 mg/kg body weight orally, three times daily.

Type of Bleeding	Desired Factor Level (%)	Factor VIII Dose (U/kg)	Factor IX Dose (U/kg)	Duration of Treatment (Days)	Comments (Dose Factor to the Closest Vial)
Persistent or profuse epistaxis Oral mucosal bleeding (including tongue and mouth lacerations)	20–30	10–15	20–30	1–2	Local pressure, antifibrinolytics, fibrin glue for local control, nosebleed QR for epistaxis Sedation in small children with tongue laceration
Dental procedures	30–50	15–25	30–50	1 h before procedure	Antifibrinolytics for 7–10 d
Acute hemarthrosis, intramuscular hematomas	30–60	15–50	30–60	1–3	Use lower doses if treated early. Non–weight bearing on affected joint.
Physical therapy	30–50	15–25	30–50	Treat before PT	Consider synovectomy (surgical, radioisotope or chemical) for target joints.
Life-threatening bleeding such as intracranial hemorrhage, major surgery, and trauma	80–100	40–50	80–100	10–14 d	Bolus dose followed by continuous infusion (3–4 U/kg/h); may switch to bolus before discharge
Gastrointestinal bleeding	30–50	15–25	30–50	2–3	May use oral antifibrinolytics
Persistent painless gross hematuria	30–50	15–25	30–50	1–2	Increase PO or IV fluids with low-dose antifibrinolytics

PT = physical therapy.

CURRENT THERAPY

- Early and effective treatment and prophylaxis can prevent repeated hemarthrosis and joint destruction in persons with hemophilia. Patients should be tested annually for the presence of inhibitors.
- Wherever available and indicated, recombinant factor concentrates are preferred over plasma-derived products due to potential risk of pathogen transmission. Cryoprecipitate is not recommended. For mild and moderate hemophilia A and von Willebrand's disease, the use of desmopressin coupled with antifibrinolytics can obviate the use of concentrates. Continued vigilance should be implemented for new and emerging bloodborne pathogens.
- All patients with inherited bleeding disorders should be immunized against hepatitis A and B and followed in close collaboration with the local hemophilia treatment center (http://www2a.cdc.gov/ncbddd/htcweb/index.asp). The National Hemophilia Foundation's (www.hemophilia.org) Medical and Scientific Advisory Committee (MASAC) guidelines for updated recommendations and product choice should be followed.

For prophylaxis, factor VIII 25 to 40 U/kg administered every other day or factor IX 25 to 40 U/kg twice weekly (because of the longer half-life of factor IX) is aimed at preventing joint disease. Prophylaxis may begin at 1 to 2 years of age and is continued lifelong. Self-infusion before any planned strenuous activity is recommended. Because of the complications of central venous catheters (infections, thrombosis, and mechanical), use of a peripheral vein is encouraged.

COMPLICATIONS OF TREATMENT

One of the most serious complications of hemophilia treatment is the development of inhibitors or neutralizing antibodies (immunoglobulin [Ig]G) that inhibit the function of substituted factor VIII and factor IX. Approximately 5% to 10% of all hemophiliacs and up to 30%

of patients with severe hemophilia A develop inhibitors. The incidence of inhibitors in hemophilia B is lower (1%–3%). Most factor VIII inhibitors arise after a median exposure of 9 to 12 days in patients with severe hemophilia A. They can be transient or permanent and should be suspected if a patient fails to respond to an appropriate dose of clotting factor concentrate. Inhibitors can exacerbate bleeding episodes and hemophilic arthropathy.

Inhibitor levels, measured using Bethesda units (BU), are classified as high titer (>5 BU) or low titer (<5 BU). In patients with low titer, inhibitors higher than normal doses of factor VIII or IX may be used to treat bleeding. For those with high-titer inhibitors, agents that bypass factor VIII or factor IX are used. These include recombinant activated factor VII and, in the case of hemophilia A, activated prothrombin complex concentrates (APCC) or recombinant porcine factor VIII (currently in prelicensure clinical trials). Immune tolerance induction, a long-term approach designed to eradicate inhibitors, is effective in 70% to 85% of patients with severe hemophilia A; the most important predictor of success of immune tolerance induction is an inhibitor titer of less than 10 BU at the start of immune tolerance induction.

Although inhibitors are rare in hemophilia B, they can result in anaphylaxis with exposure to factor IX–containing products. Immune-tolerance regimens are associated with the nephrotic syndrome and are successful in eradicating the inhibitor only in 40% of cases.

Another important complication of treatment is the transmission of bloodborne pathogens such as hepatitis B and C viruses and HIV. In the 1970s, lyophilized plasma factor concentrates of low purity resulted in the transmission of HIV, causing the deaths of many hemophiliacs. Currently, donor screening for pathogens coupled with viral attenuation by heat or solvent detergent technology make these products pathogen safe. However, nonenveloped virus (parvovirus and hepatitis A) and prions can resist inactivation and can be potentially transmitted.

Patients with bleeding disorders should be encouraged to attend the comprehensive hemophilia treatment centers, where they are educated, trained to self-infuse and calculate dosage, maintain treatment logs, and call for serious bleeding episodes. Hemovigilance at the hemophilia treatment centers is maintained through participation in the Centers for Disease Control and Prevention's (CDC) Universal Data Collection project. The mortality rate among patients who receive care at hemophilia treatment centers is lower than among those who do not: 28.1% versus 38.3%, respectively.

Routine vaccination against hepatitis A and B is recommended. Gene therapy offers promise of a cure but has not yet become reality. Two gene-therapy trials for hemophilia B have shown subtherapeutic or transient expression of factor IX.

Von Willebrand's Disease

von Willebrand's disease (vWD) is an inherited (autosomal dominant) bleeding disorder caused by deficiency or dysfunction of von Willebrand Factor (vWF), a plasma protein that mediates platelet adhesion at the site of vascular injury and prevents degradation of factor VIII. A defect in vWF results in bleeding by impairing platelet adhesion or by decreasing factor VIII.

vWF is synthesized in endothelial cells and undergoes dimerization and multimerization, forming low-, intermediate-, and high-molecular-weight (HMW) multimers. The HMW multimers are most effective in promoting platelet aggregation and adhesion. Circulating HMW multimers are cleaved by the protease ADAMTS13, which is deficient in patients with thrombotic thrombocytopenic purpura.

vWD is the most common bleeding disorder, affecting 1% or more of the population. It occurs worldwide and affects all races. vWD is classified into three major categories: partial quantitative deficiency (type 1), qualitative deficiency (type 2), and total deficiency (type 3). There are several different variants of type 2 vWD: 2A, 2B, 2N, and 2M based on the phenotype. About 75% of patients have type 1 vWD.

CLINICAL PRESENTATION

Mucous membrane–type bleeding (e.g., menorrhagia, epistaxis) and excessive bruising are characteristic clinical features in vWD. Bleeding manifestations vary considerably, and in some cases, the diagnosis is not suspected until excessive bleeding occurs with a surgical procedure or trauma. Although excessive menstrual bleeding may be the initial manifestation, it takes 16 years for a diagnosis of bleeding disorder. It is for this reason that the American College of Obstetrics and Gynecology recommended screening for hemostatic disorders in all adolescents and women presenting with menorrhagia and no pathology and before hysterectomy for menorrhagia. In infants or small children with type 3 (severe) vWD, excessive bruising and even joint bleeding (due to very low levels of factor VIII) can mimic hemophilia A.

DIAGNOSIS

Laboratory evaluation for vWD requires several assays to quantitate vWF and characterize its structure and function. Many variables affect vWF assay results, including the patient's ABO blood type. Persons of blood group AB have 60% to 70% higher vWF levels than those of blood group O. Thus, some laboratories interpret vWF levels referenced to specific normal ranges for blood types.

Clinical conditions and disorders with elevated vWF levels include pregnancy (third trimester), collagen vascular disorders, following surgery, in liver disease, and in disseminated intravascular coagulation. Low levels are seen in hypothyroidism and days 1 to 4 of the menstrual cycle.

Symptoms are modified by medications like aspirin or nonsteroidal antiinflammatory drugs (NSAIDs), which can exacerbate the bleeding; oral contraceptives can decrease the bleeding in women with vWD by increasing vWF levels. vWF levels in African American women are 15% higher than in white women. Clinical symptoms and family history are important for establishing the diagnosis of vWD, and a single test is sometimes not sufficient to rule out the diagnosis.

Initial work-up should include a complete blood count, aPTT, PT, fibrinogen level, or thrombin time. These tests do not rule out vWD but help to rule out thrombocytopenia or factor deficiency as the cause for bleeding. The closure times on the PFA-100, which has replaced the bleeding time as a screening test in some centers, may be prolonged. The aPTT in vWD is only abnormal when factor VIII is sufficiently reduced.

Specific tests for vWD include ristocetin cofactor assay, a factor VIII activity, and vWF antigen (vWF Ag) assay. The Ristocetin cofactor activity measures induced binding of vWF to platelet glycoprotein Ib and is the best functional assay of vWF activity. Multimer analysis is done by agarose gel electrophoresis using anti-vWF polyclonal antibody and is available at reference laboratories.

In type I vWD, the vWF is subnormal in amount, with normal multimer structure. Those with types 2A and 2B vWD lack the HMW multimers. In type 2B, the vWF has a heightened affinity for platelets, often resulting in some degree of thrombocytopenia from platelet aggregation. A useful laboratory test for type 2B is the low-dose ristocetin-induced platelet aggregation (RIPA) assay.

In type 3 (severe) vWD, the affected person has inherited a gene for type I vWD from each parent, resulting in very low levels (3%) of vWF (and low factor VIII, because there is no vWF to protect factor VIII from proteolytic degradation). Less commonly, a person with type 3 is doubly heterozygous. Table 4 provides a quick overview of the laboratory findings in the different variants of vWD.

TREATMENT

In type 1 vWD (with subnormal levels of normally functioning vWF), the treatment of choice is DDAVP, which causes a rapid release of vWF from storage sites. It can be given intravenously or by the intranasal route. The recommended dose for IV use is 0.3 µg/kg, given in saline over 10 minutes. Most persons with type 1 vWD have a two- to four-fold increase in plasma levels of vWF within 15 to 30 minutes following infusion. The IV route is often used for surgical coverage or for a severe bleeding episode requiring hospitalization. When necessary, repeat doses may be given at 12- to 24-hour intervals. Tachyphylaxis is less commonly seen in vWD patients than in hemophilia patients. It is important to monitor free water intake following DDAVP administration because it can cause hyponatremia and seizures.

The concentrated form of desmopressin for intranasal use (Stimate nasal spray) may be used. The recommended dosage is one 150-µg spray for patients who weigh less than 50 kg and two sprays (one in each nostril) for those who weigh more than 50 kg. Some young women with menorrhagia have benefited from its use at the onset of

TABLE 4   Clinical Variants of von Willebrand's Disease

Type	Factor VIII	vWF Ag	Ristocetin Cofactor	RIPA	Multimer
1	↓	↓	↓	↓ or normal	Normal
2A	↓ or normal	↓↓	↓	↓↓	Large and intermediate multimers absent
2B	↓ or normal	↓↓	↓ or normal	↓ to low dose	Large multimers absent
2M	Variably ↓	Variably ↓	↓	Variably ↓	Normal
2N	↓↓	Normal	Normal	Normal	Normal
3	↓↓↓↓	↓↓↓↓	↓↓↓↓	None	Absent
Platelet type	↓ or normal	↓ or normal	↓	↓ to low dose	Large multimers absent

Ag = antigen; RIPA = ristocetin-induced platelet aggregation; vWF = von Willebrand's factor.

TABLE 5 Rare Bleeding Disorders: Inheritance, Clinical Features, and Treatment

Factor	Prevalence	Type	Inheritance	Manifestation and Diagnosis	Treatment	Hemostatic Levels	Half-life
Factor I	1:1,000,000	Afibrinogenemia Dysfibrinogenemia Hypofibrinogenemia	AR AD AD	Mild bleeding CNS, umbilical, joint bleeding Recurrent miscarriage PT, aPTT, TT prolonged Low FI levels Paradoxical thrombosis	FFP 15–20 mL/kg Cryoprecipitate 1 bag/5–10 kg Plasma-derived concentrate[2]* Treatment q3–5d	50 mg–1g/dL	2–5 d
Factor II	1:2,000,000	Type I: hypoprothrombinemia Type II: dysprothrombinemia	AR AR	Hematomas, hemarthroses, menorrhagia CNS, umbilical, postpartum hemorrhage PT abnormal	FFP, PCC 20–30 U/kg for prophylaxis or treatment	20%–30%	3–4 d
Factor V	1:1,000,000	Parahemophilia, labile factor, proaccelerin, Owren's disease	AR	Mucosal bleeding, postpartum hemorrhage, CNS bleeding Platelet factor V deficiency more reflective of bleeding potential Prolonged PT, aPTT Normal TT	FFP Platelet transfusions Antiplatelet antibodies can develop with repeated platelet transfusions	15%–20%	36 h
Factor VII	1:500,000	Proconvertin or stable factor	AR	Menorrhagia; mucosal, muscle, intracranial bleeds (15%–60%); hemarthrosis Prolonged PT Normal aPTT, TT, FI, liver functions	Recombinant factor VIIa, 15–30 µg/kg q2h for major bleeds FFP, PCC 20–30 U/kg for prophylaxis or treatment Plasma-derived factor VII concentrates[2]*	15%–20%	4–6 h
Factor X	1:1,000,000		AR	Menorrhagia; umbilical, joint, mucosal, muscle, intracranial bleeding Prolonged PT, aPTT	FFP, PCCs 20–30 U/kg	15%–20%	24–48 h
Factor XI (common in Ashkenazi Jews)	1:1,000,000		AR	Post-traumatic bleeding, menorrhagia Prolonged aPTT Normal PT	Hemoeleven,[2]* FFP 15–20 mL/kg Inhibitors can occur	15%–20%	
Factor XIII	1:2,000,000		Ar	Intracranial, joint, umbilical bleeding Delayed wound healing Recurrent miscarriages PT, APTT normal ↓FXIII assay	Fibrogammin P[2]† 10–20 U/kg FFP 15–20 mL/kg Cryoprecipitate 1 bag/5–10 kg q3–4wk	2%–5%	11–14 d
Combined factor V and VIII	1:2,000,000			Mucosal bleeding Prolonged PT, aPTT (disproportionately)	Factor VIII concentrates and FFP	15%–20%	
Vitamin K-dependent multiple deficiencies	1:2,000,000			Umbilical stump, intracranial, postsurgical bleeding Skeletal abnormalities Hearing loss	Oral vitamin K, FFP, PCC	15%–20%	

[2]Not available in the United States.
*Available in Europe.
†Compassionate use in the United States.
AD = autosomal dominant; aPTT = activated partial thromboplastin time; AR = autosomal recessive; CNS = central nervous system; FFP = fresh frozen plasma; FI = fibrinogen; PCC = prothrombin complex concentrate; PT = prothrombin time; TT = thrombin time.

menses, with a second dose after 24 hours. Others have used it approximately 45 minutes before invasive dentistry, with good results.

In the type 2 variants (vWF produced is abnormal), desmopressin can cause an increase in abnormal vWF. Although some persons with type 2A might respond, desmopressin is seldom useful in type 2 and might even be contraindicated (as in type 2B, where it can exacerbate the thrombocytopenia).

In type 3 vWD, desmopressin is ineffective because there is no vWF to be released from storage sites. For type 3 patients and in persons with type 1 vWD who do not respond adequately to desmopressin, an intermediate-purity plasma-derived concentrate rich in the hemostatically effective HMW multimers of vWF (such as Humate P) should be used to treat moderately severe or severe bleeding episodes and for before surgery.

As in hemophilia, antifibrinolytics are an effective adjunctive treatment for invasive dental procedures or other bleeding in the oropharyngeal cavity. These may be effective even when used alone in some vWD women with menorrhagia. For epistaxis, Nosebleed QR, a hydrophilic powder, can help.

SPECIAL SITUATIONS

Pregnancy

vWF (and factor VIII) levels increase during the third trimester of pregnancy, and women with type 1 vWD have a decrease in bruising or other bleeding symptoms. However, those with type 2 vWD (abnormal vWF) and type 3 (no vWF) have no change in the bleeding tendency. Even in type 1 vWD, vWF levels fall following delivery, so treatment (with IV desmopressin or Humate P) may be needed.

Acquired von Willebrand's Disease

Acquired vWD occurs in persons who do not have a lifelong bleeding disorder. Conditions associated with acquired vWD include underlying autoimmune disease (lymphoproliferative disorders, myeloproliferative disorders, or plasma cell dyscrasias), valvular and congenital heart disease, Wilms' tumor, chronic renal failure, and hypothyroidism. The mechanism of acquired vWD is unknown. Medications such as valproic acid can also cause vWD. Removal of the underlying condition often corrects the vWF. Desmopressin, Humate P, recombinant factor VIIa, or plasma exchange may be tried, if necessary, to treat bleeding.

Rare Bleeding Disorders

The rare bleeding disorders account for 3% to 5% of inherited coagulation deficiencies, other than factor VIII, factor IX, or vWF deficiencies. They are autosomal recessive and affect both sexes. The prevalence of rare bleeding disorders ranges from 1:500,000 to 1:2 million. Bleeding manifestations are restricted to persons who are homozygotes or compound heterozygotes. Rare bleeding disorders are common in countries such as Iran, where consanguineous marriages are customary. Ashkenazi Jews are particularly affected by factor XI deficiency. Deficiency of factor XII is a risk factor for thrombosis, but not for bleeding. Most cases of rare bleeding disorders are identified by abnormal screening tests coupled with specific factor assays.

Factor concentrates (recombinant or plasma derived) are available for some of the deficiencies (mostly in Europe, but not in the United States). Fibrogammin P, a plasma-derived virally purified factor XIII concentrate, is not yet licensed in the United States but is available under an Investigational New Drug (IND) protocol of the Food and Drug Administration through Dr. Diane Nugent, Children's Hospital of Orange County, 500 S. Main St., Orange County, Calif 92868. The advantages of concentrates are pathogen safety and small volume. The use of antifibrinolytics and fibrin glue as adjunct therapy for bleeding manifestations is encouraged. Table 5 lists the inheritance, frequency, manifestations, and treatments of the rare bleeding disorders.

REFERENCES

Arnold WD, Hilgartner MW. Hemophilic arthropathy. Current concepts of pathogenesis and management. J Bone Joint Surg Am 1977;59(3):287–305.

Bolton-Maggs PH, Pasi KJ. Haemophilias A and B. Lancet 2003;361 (9371):1801–9.

Gill JC, Wilson AD, Endres-Brooks J, Montgomery RR. Loss of the largest von Willebrand factor multimers from the plasma of patients with congenital cardiac defects. Blood 1986;67(3):758–61.

Hoffman M, Monroe 3rd DM. A cell-based model of hemostasis. Thromb Haemost 2001;85(6):958–65.

Miller CH, Dilley AB, Drews C, et al. Changes in von Willebrand factor and factor VIII levels during the menstrual cycle. Thromb Haemost 2002;87 (6):1082–3.

Miller CH, Dilley A, Richardson L, et al. Population differences in von Willebrand factor levels affect the diagnosis of von Willebrand disease in African-American women. Am J Hematol 2001;67(2):125–9.

Mulder K, Llinas A. The target joint. Haemophilia 2004;10(Suppl. 4):152–6.

National Hemophilia Foundation Medical and Scientific Advisory Council (MASAC). MASAC recommendations concerning the treatment of hemophilia and other bleeding disorders (Revised October 2006). Available at http://www.hemophilia.org/NHFWeb/MainPgs/MainNHF.aspx?menuid=57&contentid=693 [accessed May 21, 2008].

Pierce GF, Lillicrap D, Pipe SW, Vandendriessche T. Gene therapy, bioengineered clotting factors and novel technologies for hemophilia treatment. J Thromb Haemost 2007;5(5):901–6.

Soucie JM, Nuss R, Evatt B, et al. Mortality among males with hemophilia; Relations with source of medical care. The Hemophilia Surveillance System Project Investigators. Blood 2000;96(2):437–42.

Veldman A, Hoffman M, Ehrenforth S. New insights into the coagulation system and implications for new therapeutic options with recombinant factor VIIa. Curr Med Chem 2003;10(10):797–811.

Warrier I, Ewenstein BM, Koerper MA, et al. Factor IX inhibitors and anaphylaxis in hemophilia B. J Pediatr Hematol Oncol 1997;19(1):23–7.

Platelet-Mediated Bleeding Disorders

Method of
Suman L. Sood, MD, and Charles S. Abrams, MD

Quantitative and qualitative platelet defects are commonly encountered in clinical practice and can result in bleeding diatheses.

Elements of Platelet Function

The vascular endothelium separates platelets from adhesive substrates in the subendothelial connective tissue. Platelet-mediated hemostasis is initiated by adherence to exposed collagen, fibronectin, and laminin following a breach to the vessel wall. Intracellular signaling cascades lead to secretion of platelet granules, synthesis, and release of thromboxane A_2, and a conformational change in platelet surface glycoprotein IIb/IIIa (GPIIb/IIIa) that enables it to bind soluble fibrinogen or von Willebrand's factor (vWF). Release of thromboxane A_2 and agonists within the secretion granules, such as adenosine diphosphate (ADP) and serotonin, activate neighboring platelets to perpetuate the process.

Fibrinogen binding to GPIIb/IIIa cross-links the platelets into a hemostatic plug, resulting in platelet aggregation and accumulation at the site of injury. Other signaling pathways initiated by agonists such as thrombin, thromboxane A_2, and collagen help promote the process of aggregation. Activated platelet plasma membrane interacts with circulating coagulation factors and provides a surface for assembly and generation of active factor X and thrombin. Secondary hemostasis occurs when the platelet plug is stabilized further by a thrombin-mediated fibrin mesh. The arrest of bleeding in a superficial wound almost exclusively results from the primary hemostatic plug.

Platelet-mediated bleeding disorders are characterized by a prolonged bleeding time, mucocutaneous bleeding, petechiae, and purpura. In contrast, deficiencies in secondary hemostasis result in delayed deep bleeding, such as bleeding into muscles and joints.

Quantitative Bleeding Disorders

Adequate numbers of platelets are required to achieve primary hemostasis. Thrombocytopenia can result from decreased platelet production by bone marrow megakaryocytes, accelerated platelet removal, or platelet sequestration in an enlarged spleen. The clinical context is essential because there is no easy test to differentiate among these possibilities. Most commonly, thrombocytopenia is caused by accelerated platelet removal.

Hemorrhage following trauma or surgery generally does not occur if the platelet count is more than 50,000/μL. In an otherwise hemostatically normal patient, significant spontaneous bleeding usually does not occur with a platelet count greater than 5000 to 10,000/μL. However, there is no absolute threshold for spontaneous bleeding due to thrombocytopenia, and spontaneous bleeding can occur at higher counts when fever, sepsis, severe anemia, and other hemostatic defects are present or when platelet function is impaired by medication. Notably, a prolonged cutaneous bleeding time does not accurately predict clinical bleeding.

THROMBOCYTOPENIA DUE TO DECREASED PLATELET PRODUCTION

Decreased platelet production occurs in primary diseases of the bone marrow such as acute leukemia and aplastic anemia; myelophthisic processes in which marrow is replaced by metastatic carcinoma, fibrosis, or multiple myeloma; following chemotherapy or radiation therapy; with ethanol toxicity; and during infections with viruses such as HIV, cytomegalovirus (CMV), Epstein-Barr virus (EBV), and varicella. Thrombocytopenia also occurs when megakaryocyte proliferation is impaired by myelodysplasia.

Overt bleeding in these disorders, when clearly a result of thrombocytopenia, is treated by platelet transfusion. Prophylactic platelet transfusion, however, is an area of controversy and is complicated by the short life span of platelets (10 days), the 5-day shelf life of stored platelets, and platelet immunogenicity. In patients undergoing treatment for acute leukemia, outcome is unchanged when platelet counts of 5000 to 10,000/μL are used as the threshold for prophylactic transfusion. Single-donor apheresis platelets or platelet donors who are HLA identical to the recipient should be considered to prevent alloimmunization. Preliminary results from the multicenter Platelet Dose trial in patients with malignancy suggest that lower doses of platelets may be safe.

THROMBOCYTOPENIA DUE TO INCREASED PLATELET DESTRUCTION

Nonimmune and immune processes can lead to a shortened platelet life span. Nonimmune causes include sepsis, disseminated intravascular coagulation (DIC), thrombotic thrombocytopenic purpura/hemolytic uremic syndrome (TTP/HUS), preeclampsia and eclampsia, cardiopulmonary bypass, and giant cavernous hemangiomas. The thrombocytopenia resolves with treatment of the underlying disorder, and platelet transfusion is rarely necessary. In TTP/HUS, thrombocytopenia is associated with thrombosis rather than bleeding, and controversial reports exist of clinical deterioration following platelet transfusion.

Immune-mediated platelet destruction can occur due to medication, alloimmune sensitization, or autoimmunity. Medications should always be considered a possible cause of thrombocytopenia. The potential list is long, but drugs with strong evidence of antibody-mediated platelet destruction include quinine (Qualaquin), quinidine, sulfonamides, and gold salts. Besides stopping the offending medication, emergent treatment for severe thrombocytopenia with bleeding includes platelet transfusion, and corticosteroids with or without intravenous immunoglobulin (IVIg).

CURRENT DIAGNOSIS

- Platelet-mediated bleeding disorders are characterized by a prolonged bleeding time, mucocutaneous bleeding, petechiae, and purpura.
- Thrombocytopenia can result from decreased platelet production, accelerated platelet removal, or platelet sequestration in an enlarged spleen.
- In an otherwise hemostatically normal patient, significant spontaneous bleeding generally does not occur until the platelet count declines to <5000–10,000/μL. A prolonged bleeding time does not predict clinical bleeding.
- Medications are common causes of quantitative and qualitative platelet defects.
- Heparin-induced thrombocytopenia must always be considered when thrombocytopenia is detected in a hospitalized patient.
- Idiopathic thrombocytopenic purpura manifests as otherwise unexplained spontaneous mucocutaneous bleeding or asymptomatic thrombocytopenia and is a diagnosis of exclusion.
- Although many medications impair platelet function in vitro, only a few, including aspirin, ticlopidine (Ticlid), clopidogrel (Plavix), and the glycoprotein IIb/IIIa antagonists induce clinically significant bleeding.
- While hereditary disorders of platelet adhesion and aggregation are rare, hereditary disorders of platelet secretion are not uncommon causes of easy bruising, menorrhagia, and excessive postoperative and postpartum blood loss. Platelet aggregation studies are helpful for diagnosis.

Heparin-induced thrombocytopenia (HIT) is a special case of drug-induced thrombocytopenia associated with arterial and venous thrombosis rather than bleeding. HIT occurs in 2% to 5% of patients given unfractionated heparin by any route for 5 to 10 days. Antibodies develop to a heparin–platelet factor 4 (PF4) complex. HIT must always be considered when thrombocytopenia is detected in a hospitalized patient. If a patient has HIT, all heparin administration should be stopped, and alternative anticoagulation such as the direct thrombin inhibitors recombinant hirudin and argatroban should be instituted, at least until the platelet count normalizes. Warfarin (Coumadin) should not be used in acute HIT because of its delayed therapeutic effect and association with a syndrome of venous limb gangrene. Platelet transfusions in this disease are controversial, because some reports suggest that they can precipitate thrombotic complications.

Alloimmune thrombocytopenia due to sensitization to alloantigens such as PIA1 can result from transfusion (post-transfusion purpura, PTP) or maternal sensitization during pregnancy (neonatal alloimmune thrombocytopenia, NAIT). PTP causes profound thrombocytopenia 7 to 10 days after transfusion and can be treated with IVIg or plasma exchange. NAIT can cause severe thrombocytopenia and bleeding in neonates and is treated with platelet transfusion, corticosteroids, and IVIg.

Autoimmune thrombocytopenia, also known as idiopathic thrombocytopenic purpura (ITP), is caused by circulating antiplatelet autoantibodies. An ITP-like picture can also occur in autoimmune diseases such as systemic lupus erythematosus, in patients with low-grade lymphoproliferative disorders such as chronic lymphocytic leukemia, and in patients with HIV infections. ITP can occur at any age in both sexes and manifests with either mucocutaneous bleeding or unexplained asymptomatic thrombocytopenia. The complete blood count (CBC) is otherwise normal, splenomegaly is absent, and peripheral blood smears are only remarkable for a decreased number of platelets, some of which may be larger than normal. Bone marrow examination is usually not necessary in the absence of other findings suggesting myelodysplasia, but it typically shows normal or increased numbers of megakaryocytes.

Management of ITP is guided by symptoms and platelet count. Asymptomatic patients with platelet counts greater than 30,000/μL can be followed without treatment. With bleeding or a platelet count less than 30,000/μL, treatment with prednisone is initiated. Refractory patients may require splenectomy (60%–75% remission rate), other immunosuppressive medications, or new thrombopoiesis-stimulating agents. Emergent presentation with severe thrombocytopenia (<5000/μL) or internal bleeding should be treated with high doses of pulse corticosteroids or IVIg, or both. Platelet transfusion may be given concurrently with the IVIg for critical bleeding. Anti-D immune globulin may be substituted for IVIg in Rh⁺ patients who have not undergone splenectomy; however, occasional patients develop severe autoimmune hemolysis.

THROMBOCYTOPENIA DUE TO HYPERSPLENISM

Approximately 30% of the circulating platelet mass is normally present in the spleen. Additional platelets may be sequestered when the spleen enlarges due to portal hypertension or infiltrative diseases. Platelet counts in patients with hypersplenism generally are not lower than 40,000 to 50,000/μL. Consequently, bleeding due to thrombocytopenia from hypersplenism alone is unusual.

Qualitative Platelet Disorders

ACQUIRED QUALITATIVE PLATELET DISORDERS

Acquired disorders of platelet function are relatively common but are usually asymptomatic or mild. Nonetheless, they can be of substantial clinical importance when engrafted on another hemostatic abnormality. They are subclassified as resulting from drugs, hematologic diseases, and systemic disorders. Drugs are the most common cause of dysfunction, most notably aspirin, which irreversibly inactivates the enzyme cyclooxygenase-1 (COX-1), thus inducing a permanent blockade in platelet prostaglandin synthesis and consequently thromboxane A_2 synthesis. Although the antihemostatic effect is minimal in normal persons, it may be quite prominent in a patient with an underlying bleeding disorder. Nonsteroidal anti-inflammatory drugs (NSAIDs) reversibly inhibit platelet prostaglandin synthesis and generally have little effect on hemostasis. Other medications that interfere significantly with platelet function include clopidogrel (Plavix), ticlopidine (Ticlid), and GPIIb/IIIa receptor antagonists. Numerous other drugs have been implicated in platelet dysfunction in case reports, but the evidence for most of these medications is less well established.

Bone marrow processes that can produce intrinsically abnormal platelets include myeloproliferative disorders, leukemias, myelodysplastic syndromes, and dysproteinemias such as multiple myeloma and Waldenström's macroglobulinemia, in which abnormal plasma proteins impair platelet function. In addition, acquired forms of von Willebrand's disease, a rare disorder that can arise secondary to critical aortic stenosis, multiple myeloma, or other clonal lymphoproliferative disorders, can lead to a bleeding diathesis.

Renal failure is the most prominent systemic disorder associated with abnormal platelet function. The hemostatic defect is generally mild and corrects rapidly with the initiation of dialysis. Intravenous desmopressin (DDAVP), a vasopressin analogue that causes release of von Willebrand factor (vWF) from tissue stores, is helpful in uremia, shortening bleeding time in 50% to 75% of patients. Dosing may be repeated, although tachyphylaxis can occur. Maintaining the hemoglobin greater than 10 g/dL can optimize the efficiency of platelets by enhancing the interactions between platelets and the blood vessel wall. DIC can also lead to impaired platelet function. Thrombocytopenia is a consistent feature of cardiopulmonary bypass surgery, typically secondary to hemodilution, platelet membrane activation from interaction with the bypass circuit, and fragmentation from hypothermia. It generally resolves spontaneously within several days after bypass, but platelet transfusions may be helpful if bleeding persists.

CURRENT THERAPY

- In the absence of bleeding, platelet counts of 5000–10,000/μL are used as the threshold for prophylactic transfusion. Single-donor apheresis platelets should be considered to prevent alloimmunization.
- For hemorrhaging patients or for patients scheduled to undergo delicate operations such as neurosurgery, maintaining the platelet count greater than 75,000 to 100,000/μL is recommended.
- When heparin-induced thrombocytopenia is a possibility, all heparin administration must be stopped and alternative anticoagulation instituted, at least until the platelet count returns to normal.
- Because bleeding in patients with ITP is usually minimal to absent until platelet counts decline to <30,000/μL, asymptomatic patients with platelet counts >30,000 can be followed without treatment.
- Treatment for ITP is initiated with prednisone (1 mg/kg); patients who fail to enter clinical remission are candidates for splenectomy or treatment with immunosuppressive agents including rituximab[1] (Rituxan) and azathioprine[1] (Imuran).
- High doses of corticosteroids (methylprednisolone [Solu-Medrol], 1 g/d for 3 d) or IVIg (1 g/kg/d for 2 d) are indicated for emergency treatment of ITP. Platelet transfusion given concurrently with IVIg can be effective for critical bleeding. Anti-D immune globulin (WinRho) may be used instead of IVIg in Rh⁺ patients, although this treatment can induce clinically significant hemolysis.
- The platelet dysfunction of uremia is usually corrected by dialysis. Maintaining the hemoglobin above 10 g/dL helps minimize bleeding by increasing interactions between platelets and the blood vessel wall. Intravenous desmopressin (DDAVP) given at a dose of 0.3 μg/kg IV over 15 to 30 minutes shortens the bleeding time in most patients with uremia for approximately 4 hours.
- When necessary, treatment of hereditary disorders of platelet adhesion and aggregation usually requires platelet transfusion.

---

[1]Not FDA approved for this indication.
Abbreviations: ITP = idiopathic thrombocytopenic purpura; IVIg = intravenous immunoglobulin.

HEREDITARY QUALITATIVE PLATELET DISORDERS

Bernard-Soulier syndrome (BSS) and Glanzmann's thrombasthenia (GT) are rare autosomal recessive disorders of the platelet membrane glycoproteins GPIb/IX and GPIIb/IIIa, respectively. They manifest with mucocutaneous bleeding in infancy or childhood. Patients with BSS are also thrombocytopenic and have very large platelets that do not agglutinate when exposed to ristocetin. Platelet counts and morphology are normal in GT, but the platelets cannot aggregate in response to ADP or thrombin. Reliable treatment of bleeding in both conditions requires platelet transfusion.

Hereditary disorders of platelet secretion are not uncommon causes of mucocutaneous bleeding and can be due to alpha granule deficiency (gray platelet syndrome), the more common dense granule deficiency (δ storage pool disease [δSPD]), or to aspirin-like defects resulting from abnormalities of the platelet secretory mechanism. δSPD may be associated with albinism (Hermansky-Pudlack and Chédiak-Higashi syndromes) or occur in otherwise normal persons. Patients with δSPD have normal platelet counts with prolonged bleeding times and abnormal platelet aggregation studies with a diagnostic increased adenosine triphosphate-to-adenosine diphosphate (ATP/ADP) ratio due to the absence of platelet dense granule ADP. Although bleeding in patients with secretion disorders can be controlled by platelet transfusion, DDAVP sometimes shortens the bleeding times and improves hemostasis.

REFERENCES

Aster RH, Bougie DW. Drug-induced immune thrombocytopenia. N Engl J Med 2007;357:580–7.

Bolton-Maggs PHB, Chalmers EA, Collins PW, et al. A review of inherited platelet disorders with guidelines for their management on behalf of the UKHCDO. Br J Haematol 2006;135:603–33.

Cines DB, Blanchette VS. Immune thrombocytopenic purpura. N Engl J Med 2002;346:995–1008.

Hedges SJ, Dehoney SB, Hooper JS, et al. Evidence-based treatment recommendations for uremic bleeding. Nat Clin Pract Nephrol 2007;3:138–53.

Lind SE. The bleeding time does not predict surgical bleeding. Blood 1991;77:2547–52.

Mannucci PM. Drug therapy: Treatment of von Willebrand's disease. N Engl J Med 2004;351:683–94.

Nurden AT. Qualitative disorders of platelets and megakaryocytes. J Thromb Hemostasis 2006;3:1773–82.

Nurden AT, Viallard JF, Nurden P. New-generation drugs that stimulate platelet production in chronic immune thrombocytopenic purpura. Lancet 2009;373:1562–9.

Stanworth SJ, Hyde C, Brunskill S, et al. Platelet transfusion prophylaxis for patients with hematological malignancies: Where to now? Br J Haematol 2005;131:588–95.

Warkentin TE. Heparin-induced thrombocytopenia: Pathogenesis and management. Br J Haematol 2003;121:535–55.

Disseminated Intravascular Coagulation

Method of
Eliot C. Williams, MD

Disseminated intravascular coagulation (DIC) is a syndrome characterized by widespread, disorganized, and poorly controlled activation of the coagulation and fibrinolytic systems. DIC almost always occurs as a consequence of a serious, life-threatening underlying illness. In some cases, the coagulation disturbance is asymptomatic. In others, it is manifested by bleeding or widespread tissue injury (purpura fulminans).

Pathophysiology

DIC is usually caused by exposure of blood to excessive amounts of tissue factor. The source of the tissue factor depends on the illness that causes DIC. Subendothelial tissue factor may be exposed to blood as a consequence of diffuse endothelial injury caused by inflammatory cytokines, hypoxia, or other insults. Circulating monocytes express tissue factor in response to stimulation by cytokines. Obstetric accidents cause release of tissue factor–rich amniotic fluid into the blood. Procoagulant platelet- and cell-derived microparticles may be released into the blood as a result of the primary injury or as a secondary phenomenon. The consequences of exposure of blood to large amounts of tissue factor and other procoagulants include consumption of clotting factors, uncontrolled thrombin formation causing increased platelet consumption and formation of soluble fibrin, and a secondary increase in fibrinolytic activity. Consumption of clotting inhibitors such as antithrombin and protein C further diminishes the body's ability to control the coagulopathy. Downregulation of the protein C pathway caused by inflammatory cytokines and consumption of protein C after activation of coagulation increase the susceptibility of endothelial cells to injury by cytokines and hypoxia and thereby promote tissue injury.

Activation of the fibrinolytic system almost always accompanies DIC, because release of tissue-type plasminogen activator (t-PA) from endothelial cells is stimulated by a number of circulating factors whose levels increase during acute illness and because the presence of soluble fibrin in the blood acts as a catalyst for the activation of plasminogen by t-PA. As a general rule, bleeding risk increases with more intense fibrinolysis.

The setting in which DIC occurs has important effects on the course of the coagulopathy. In sepsis or other situations in which there are high levels of inflammatory cytokines, procoagulant pathways are upregulated and profibrinolytic pathways are downregulated. Fibrin formation is therefore favored over fibrinolysis, and accumulation of fibrin in the microcirculation may contribute to tissue injury. In certain malignancies (e.g., acute promyelocytic leukemia, some cases of prostate cancer), malignant cells express profibrinolytic enzymes, resulting in a bleeding disorder in which fibrinolysis plays a dominant role. Liver disease impairs the body's ability to replace clotting factors and inhibitors as they are consumed and so tends to worsen the severity of DIC caused by any given stimulus.

Complications

The two most important complications of DIC are bleeding and tissue injury. Factors that may contribute to bleeding risk include clotting factor and platelet consumption, accelerated fibrinolysis, depletion of inhibitors that normally restrain proteolytic cascades, and tissue injury from underlying disease. Bleeding may be limited to sites of injury, or it may progress to a syndrome characterized by diffuse oozing of blood from mucosal surfaces, sites of catheter insertion, and other sites.

Tissue injury is likewise a complex phenomenon in which the final common pathway is usually severely reduced tissue perfusion. Contributing factors include endothelial injury (exacerbated by downregulation of the protein C pathway), circulatory collapse and shock, fibrin accumulation in small vessels, and, in some cases, the effects of vasopressor drugs. Clinical manifestations include renal failure, respiratory failure, acute adrenal failure, and gangrene of the extremities (purpura fulminans).

Overt thrombosis is relatively uncommon in acute DIC, probably because activation of the clotting system is disorganized and is often accompanied by a vigorous fibrinolytic response. Thrombosis may occur in chronic or smoldering DIC (e.g., in some cases of metastatic cancer) or when catheters or other intravascular devices provide a nidus for thrombus formation.

CURRENT DIAGNOSIS

- Disseminated intravascular coagulation is likely to be present when there is evidence of accelerated consumption of clotting factors and platelets and increased fibrinolytic activity in a patient with a serious underlying illness.

Diagnosis

Scoring systems to diagnose DIC and so-called pre-DIC have been proposed and validated in clinical studies. However, in most cases, a simple rule of thumb will suffice: If the patient has a disease known to cause DIC and there is evidence of clotting factor and platelet consumption as well as increased fibrinolytic activity, DIC is probably present. Useful screening tests include the prothrombin time/international normalized ratio (PT/INR) and the platelet count, the D-dimer or fibrin degradation product level, and a test for soluble fibrin or fibrin monomer. The D-dimer is the most sensitive of these tests, and the fibrin monomer test is the most specific. Rapid increase in the PT/INR and decrease in the platelet count in an appropriate clinical setting is highly suggestive of DIC.

Treatment

Effective treatment of the underlying cause is of paramount importance. If this is not possible, the outcome is likely to be poor regardless of whether the coagulopathy can be successfully controlled. In patients with mild to moderate DIC who are not actively bleeding, it is usually not necessary to treat for DIC per se. However, in more severely coagulopathic patients, particularly in those who have evidence of pathologic bleeding or incipient purpura fulminans, treatment of DIC can sometimes be lifesaving.

Initial treatment of DIC should be directed at replacing clotting factors and platelets and restoring proper balance in the coagulation and fibrinolytic systems by replacing depleted inhibitors. Fresh-frozen plasma is the treatment of choice for clotting factor and inhibitor replacement. The PT/INR should guide administration; an INR of 1.7 to 2.0 is a reasonable target. In patients with very low fibrinogen levels (<75–100 mg/dL), supplementation with cryoprecipitate (10 units for every 2 to 3 units of fresh-frozen plasma) is reasonable. Platelet transfusions (1–2 U/10 kg/day) should be given to patients with severe thrombocytopenia (platelet count <10,000–20,000/mm^3) or patients with moderate thrombocytopenia and active bleeding.

Treatment of DIC with antithrombin concentrate (Thrombate III)[1] has been studied in several trials. These have shown at most a modest benefit from such treatment, and there has been no convincing evidence of improved survival.

Treatment with recombinant human activated protein C (rAPC or drotrecogin alfa [Xigris]) resulted in improved survival in a large, randomized, controlled trial (the PROWESS trial) in patients with severe sepsis. More severely ill patients and those with DIC seemed to derive the most benefit from rAPC treatment. rAPC has anticoagulant effects and increased the risk of bleeding in the PROWESS trial. Active bleeding is therefore considered a contraindication to rAPC treatment.

[1]Not FDA approved for this indication.

CURRENT THERAPY

- Treatment of the underlying disease is critical.
- Patients with severe coagulopathy or bleeding may benefit from administration of fresh-frozen plasma, platelets, and cryoprecipitate.
- Administration of recombinant activated protein C (drotrecogin alfa [Xigris]) is beneficial in patients with severe sepsis.
- Treatment with heparin or antifibrinolytic agents or both should be reserved for carefully selected patients with severe bleeding that persists despite aggressive blood component therapy.

The role of pharmacologic inhibitors of coagulation and fibrinolysis in treating DIC is controversial. Heparin has not been shown to benefit patients with purpura fulminans, probably because factors other than thrombosis are responsible for much of the associated tissue injury. There is anecdotal but convincing evidence of benefit from treatment with unfractionated heparin (UFH) in individual patients with chronic or smoldering DIC. Relatively low doses of UFH (e.g., 5–10 U/kg/hr), given by continuous infusion, may be effective. Administration of full anticoagulant doses of UFH should be reserved for patients with overt thrombosis.

Administration of antifibrinolytic drugs such as epsilon aminocaproic acid (Amicar) to patients with DIC is considered contraindicated by some authorities because of concerns about the potential for thrombosis due to unopposed fibrin formation. However, antifibrinolytic treatment may benefit carefully selected patients with hyperfibrinolytic states who continue to bleed despite aggressive blood component replacement. Depletion of the plasma fibrinolytic inhibitor α_2-antiplasmin is a useful marker to identify patients who may benefit from treatment with Amicar. Administration of Amicar[1] together with low-dose UFH may reduce the chance of thrombosis.

REFERENCES

Aird WC. The role of the endothelium in severe sepsis and multiple organ dysfunction syndrome. Blood 2003;101:3765–77.

Dhainaut JF, Yan SB, Joyce DE, et al. Treatment effects of drotrecogin alfa (activated) in patients with severe sepsis with or without overt disseminated intravascular coagulation. J Thromb Haemost 2004;2:1924–33.

Gando S, Saitoh D, Ogura H, et al. Natural history of disseminated intravascular coagulation based on the newly established diagnostic criteria for critically ill patients: Results of a multicenter, prospective survey. Crit Care Med 2008;36:145–50.

Holland LL, Brooks JP. Toward rational fresh frozen plasma transfusion: The effect of plasma transfusion on coagulation test results. Am J Clin Pathol 2006;126:133–9.

Levi M. Disseminated intravascular coagulation. Crit Care Med 2007;35:2191–5.

Tolti LJ, Swystun LL, Pepler L, Liaw PC. Protective effects of activated protein C in sepsis. Thromb Haemost 2008;100:582–92.

Williams EC. Plasma alpha-2 antiplasmin activity: Role in the evaluation and management of fibrinolytic states and other bleeding disorders. Arch Intern Med 1989;149:1769–72.

Williams EC. Disseminated intravascular coagulation. In: Loscalzo J, Schafer AI, editors. Thrombosis and Hemorrhage. 3rd ed. Baltimore: Lippincott Williams & Wilkins; 2003. p. 781–802.

[1]Not FDA approved for this indication.

Thrombotic Thrombocytopenic Purpura

Method of
Joseph E. Kiss, MD

Thrombotic thrombocytopenic purpura (TTP) is a life-threatening thrombotic disorder in which unrestrained platelet deposition occurs in the microcirculation of many organs, including the brain, kidneys, heart, and abdominal viscera. Thrombocytopenia develops as platelets are progressively consumed. The term microangiopathic hemolytic anemia refers to the fragmentation of red blood cells (schistocytes) during their passage through partially occluded arterioles and capillaries. Therapeutic plasma exchange, the mainstay of therapy, has markedly improved the mortality rate, from more than 90% in the past to 10% to 20% currently. A high index of suspicion for the diagnosis is necessary, because delays in recognizing the disorder can increase treatment failure and death. Because plasma exchange is very effective, it is appropriate to consider TTP as a provisional diagnosis and to initiate therapy when thrombocytopenia and microangiopathic hemolytic anemia are present without another apparent cause.

Classification

A wide variety of disorders can be associated with TTP or can develop TTP-like manifestations. The primary causes and major secondary forms are outlined in Box 1. This classification is based on clinical and laboratory similarities. There is ongoing controversy as to whether certain secondary causes should be considered in this classification and whether they should be treated with plasma exchange. For example, a TTP-like syndrome can occur in the setting of hematopoietic stem cell transplantation, but the efficacy of plasma exchange has been questioned. Experienced clinical judgment may be necessary to decide on the appropriate diagnosis and the best course of therapy.

Pathogenesis

Remarkable progress has been made over the last few years in understanding the pathogenesis of TTP. Defects in ADAMTS13, a key enzyme that normally clips large, sticky multimers of von Willebrand's factor into smaller subunits, have been found in patients with congenital TTP and in patients with idiopathic TTP. Without the enzyme, long strings of ultra-large von Willebrand's factor remain anchored to the surface of endothelial cells, binding platelets and forming occlusive microthrombi throughout many organs, especially the brain and kidneys. A second hit, presumably endothelial cell injury secondary to the stress of infection, surgery, or pregnancy, triggers an acute episode in the setting of ADAMTS13 deficiency.

Dysfunctional enzyme is found in all cases of congenital TTP. Severe ADAMTS13 deficiency (defined as <10% of normal) caused by an immunoglobulin G autoantibody to ADAMTS13 is reported in 30% to 100% of cases of idiopathic TTP. Typical TTP patients have also been described who do not have ADAMTS13 deficiency, suggesting that alternative, unknown mechanisms can also lead to TTP.

Clinical Presentation

Idiopathic TTP often occurs in young, healthy persons. The peak age group is between 20 and 40 years; women are affected twice as often as men. African Americans are disproportionately affected. The classic diagnostic pentad, consisting of thrombocytopenia, microangiopathic anemia, fever, neurologic abnormalities, and renal failure, occurs in only a minority of cases, perhaps because, with increased clinical awareness, the diagnosis is being considered earlier in the course of the disease. Patients might have vague symptoms at first (e.g., malaise, weakness, headache), several days before developing worrisome neurologic complaints including visual disturbances, paresthesias, focal motor weakness, and aphasia (i.e., transient ischemic attacks) or more generalized manifestations such as confusion, seizures, stupor, and coma. The neurologic abnormalities in conjunction with thrombocytopenia and anemia form a common triad that should lead to high diagnostic suspicion. Fever occurs in about 50% of patients at the time of presentation.

Renal injury is associated with rising creatinine and proteinuria and is typically mild in TTP. Cases in which renal failure predominates are termed hemolytic uremic syndrome (HUS). Diarrhea (usually but not always bloody) should prompt consideration of

---

BOX 1   Clinical Classification and Distinguishing Features of TTP and Other Thrombotic Microangiopathies

Primary
Congenital
Caused by mutations in *ADAMTS13* gene
Very rare

Idiopathic
Caused by IgG autoantibody that binds to ADAMTS13
Diagnosed by exclusion of secondary causes
Most common form

Secondary*
Human Immunodeficiency Virus
High response rate reported to plasma infusion and antiretroviral therapy

Collagen Vascular Diseases
Treated in the same way as idiopathic TTP using plasma exchange, immunosuppressants

Drug-Induced Immunologic Disease
Ticlopidine (Ticlid)
Induces antibody to ADAMTS13
Treatment is withdrawing offending drug and performing plasma exchange
Rapid recovery is typical
Related drug, clopidogrel (Plavix), also associated, but the mechanism is uncertain
Quinine also commonly implicated; antiplatelet and antiendothelial antibodies are associated
Must be distinguished from immune thrombocytopenic purpura
ADAMTS13 is not reduced, and efficacy of plasma exchange is questionable

Drug-Induced, Dose-Dependent Toxicity
Associated with cancer chemotherapeutic agents including mitomycin C (Mutamycin) and gemcitabine (Gemzar)
Can develop slowly, sometimes after drug is discontinued
Can also be seen with immunosuppressive agents including cyclosporine (Neoral) and tacrolimus (Prograf)
Treated by stopping drug
Uncertain benefit of plasma exchange

Pregnancy and Postpartum
May be caused by an IgG inhibitor of ADAMTS13
Must be distinguished from HELLP syndrome (HELLP usually occurs during the third trimester of pregnancy or immediately after delivery in association with severe preeclampsia)

Hematopoietic Stem Cell Transplantation–Associated Disease
A TTP-like syndrome that may be caused by infection or graft-versus-host disease
Doubtful benefit of plasma exchange

---

*If laboratory samples are to be drawn to evaluate a possible secondary cause (e.g., systemic lupus erythematosus), it is important to obtain them before plasma exchange therapy is instituted, to avoid a dilution effect.
Abbreviations: HELLP = hemolysis with elevated liver enzymes and low platelets; IgG = immunoglobulin G; TTP = thrombotic thrombocytic purpura.

enterotoxin-associated epidemic HUS. Because of frequent clinical overlap with both neurologic and renal manifestations, it may be difficult to distinguish between TTP and HUS in adults.

Gastrointestinal complaints are also common. Abdominal pain, nausea, vomiting, and diarrhea can reflect the presence of visceral ischemia or pancreatitis. These symptoms, along with mental status changes, elevated bilirubin, and thrombocytopenia, may be mistaken for liver disease, further delaying diagnosis. Chest pain and arrhythmias caused by small-vessel myocardial involvement have been reported in up to 18% of patients in some series. These protean clinical manifestations of TTP reflect its multisystemic pathophysiology.

Diagnosis

The hallmark of microangiopathic hemolytic anemia is the presence of fragmented red blood cells on the blood smear. A number of disorders are known to cause microangiopathic hemolysis and thrombocytopenia, which can mimic the clinical and laboratory features of TTP. These include severe hypertension (persisting blood pressure >200/100 mm Hg with or without papilledema), prosthetic cardiac devices (e.g., left ventricular assist devices, intraaortic balloon pump), hemolysis with elevated liver enzymes and low platelets (HELPP) syndrome with severe preeclampsia, and vasculitis. Disseminated intravascular coagulation may be seen in association with sepsis, and a low-grade form is associated with carcinoma. In contrast to disseminated intravascular coagulation, the fibrinogen level in TTP is normal, and fibrin degradation products are also normal or minimally increased. The direct antiglobulin test is used to exclude immune hemolysis, which can occur concomitantly with thrombocytopenia (Evan's syndrome).

Although measurement of ADAMTS13 is becoming more widely available in clinical laboratories, the usefulness of this test still needs to be validated as a diagnostic and management tool. A number of technical issues affect the analytic sensitivity and specificity of the various assays in use. Therefore, a normal level should not be used to exclude the diagnosis. Severe deficiency of ADAMTS13 has been proposed as a specific test for TTP, but it has also been noted in severe sepsis, disseminated intravascular coagulation, and metastatic malignancy. If these entities can be confidently excluded, a severe deficiency of ADAMTS13 reported by an experienced laboratory strongly supports the diagnosis of TTP.

Treatment

Plasma exchange is the only therapy that has been shown to be effective in a randomized, controlled clinical trial. It is believed to work by replacing ADAMTS13 and by removing inhibitory antibodies to the enzyme. It also appears to be effective in patients who are not deficient in ADAMTS13, so other mechanisms may be involved.

CURRENT DIAGNOSIS

Recommended Diagnostic Tests for Initial Evaluation

- Complete blood count with differential white blood cell, platelet, and reticulocyte count
- Review of peripheral blood smear
- Coagulation studies including fibrinogen and fibrin degradation products
- Lactate dehydrogenase (LDH)
- Blood urea nitrogen, creatinine, electrolytes
- Liver function tests, including direct and indirect bilirubin
- Direct antiglobulin test
- Urinalysis

If there is a delay in instituting plasma exchange, 15 to 30 mL/kg of plasma should be infused, with attention to avoiding volume overload. Cardiac monitoring in the initial stages of management is advisable in light of the relatively high frequency of cardiac involvement. In the absence of serious bleeding, platelet transfusions are contraindicated because of the potential deposition of platelet microthrombi and the risk of serious clinical sequelae (e.g., transient ischemic attack, myocardial infarction). The role of adjuvant therapy, such as corticosteroids, antiplatelet drugs, and other immunosuppressives, is not firmly established in the routine management of TTP.

Between 1 and 1.5 plasma volumes are exchanged daily, using fresh-frozen plasma or alternative products that have been shown to contain ADAMTS13 (e.g., plasma frozen within 24 hours, cryoprecipitate-reduced plasma, thawed plasma). Plasma exchanges are continued daily while the clinical and laboratory responses are assessed (Fig. 1). The platelet count is the single most useful laboratory parameter to follow. Lactate dehydrogenase (LDH), an indicator of tissue ischemia and hemolysis, typically lags behind changes in platelet levels. The therapeutic goal is to induce remission, consisting of a normal platelet count and near-normal LDH (<1.5 times normal levels).

Plasma exchange is usually continued on a daily schedule for 1 to 2 days after remission is achieved. It is not unusual for the disease activity to quickly reappear, leading some to taper the plasma exchanges over a short period (e.g., every other day × 3, then every 3 days × 2, then stop). A study comparing different institutional tapering practices found no differences in exacerbation rates. A total of 10 to 20 procedures may be needed to achieve a durable response.

Although plasma exchange is considered a safe procedure, serious complications, including catheter-related sepsis, venous thrombosis, and death, have been reported. Patients should be observed closely for 30 days after cessation of plasma exchange. This is a critical time for exacerbation of the disease, which occurs in about 20% of patients. In those who do not respond or who respond slowly, the plasma volume may be increased and immunosuppressive therapy may be considered (e.g., prednisone 1 mg/kg/day). Continuation of the daily plasma-exchange regimen (i.e., patience on the part of the treater) is probably the single most important therapeutic strategy.

Patients who remain refractory or who are plasma exchange dependent after several weeks are considered for additional immunosuppressive therapy. Use of the anti-CD20 monoclonal antibody rituximab (Rituxan)[1] has shown very good results, including disease remission in the majority of patients with refractory disease who were treated with it. Relapses occur in 30% to 40% of patients with idiopathic TTP, months to years later, reflecting the relapsing and remitting autoimmune nature of this disorder.

Prognosis

Because of increased recognition and earlier treatment of TTP, most patients achieve remission and go on to complete recovery. More than half of the deaths occur early, within 48 hours after admission to the hospital. A recent clinical analysis found that age older than 40 years, hemoglobin less than 9 g/dL, and temperature higher than 38.5°C at presentation were associated with increased mortality. Outcome cannot be predicted from the severity of the thrombocytopenia or the LDH level. The ADAMTS13 level appears to have prognostic value: Patients with severe ADAMTS13 deficiency have more autoimmune manifestations, lower platelet counts, less renal insufficiency, and a higher risk of relapse. TTP in association with transplantation and malignancy is often resistant to therapy, and novel approaches are needed.

---

[1]Not FDA approved for this indication.

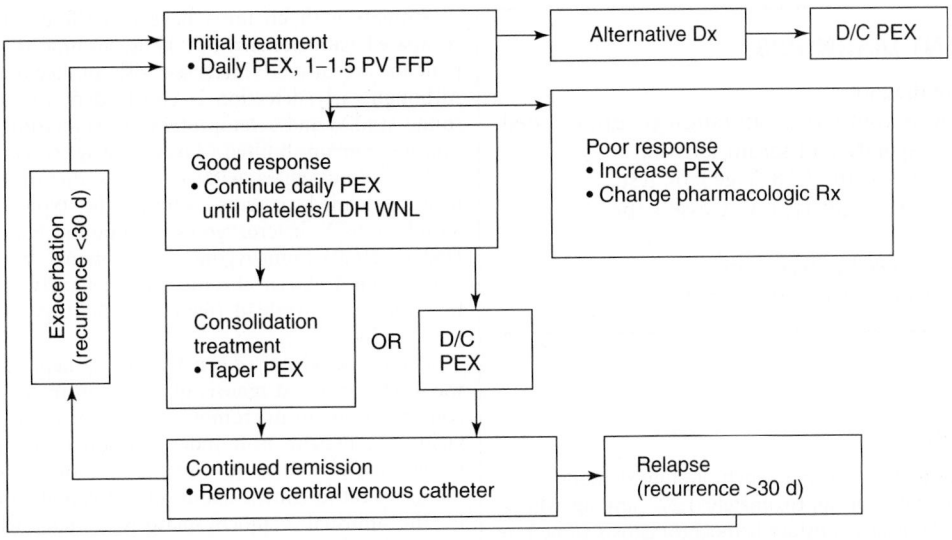

FIGURE 1. Management of thrombotic thrombocytopenic purpura. *Abbreviations:* D/C = discontinue; Dx = diagnosis; FFP = fresh-frozen plasma; LDH = lactate dehydrogenase; PEX = plasma exchange; PV = plasma volume; Rx = prescription; WNL = within normal limits. (Adapted from George JN: How I treat patients with thrombotic thrombocytopenic purpura–hemolytic uremic syndrome. Blood 2000;96:4:1223–29.)

REFERENCES

Allford S, Hunt B, Rose P, et al. Guidelines on the diagnosis and management of the thrombotic microangiopathic haemolytic anemias. Br J Haematol 2003;120:556–73.

Bandarenko N. Members of the United States Thrombotic Thrombocytopenic Purpura Apheresis Study Group (US TTP ASG). Multicenter survey and retrospective analysis of current efficacy of therapeutic plasma exchange. J Clin Apheresis 1998;13:133–41.

Fakhouri F, Vernant JP, Veyradier A, et al. Efficiency of curative and prophylactic treatment with rituximab in ADAMTS13-deficient thrombotic thrombocytopenic purpura: A study of 11 cases. Blood 2005;106:1932–7.

George JN. How I treat patients with thrombotic thrombocytopenic purpura-hemolytic uremic syndrome. Blood 2000;96:41223–9.

Howard MA, Williams LA, Terrell DR. Complications of plasma exchange in patients treated for clinically suspected thrombotic thrombocytopenic purpura-hemolytic uremic syndrome: III. An additional study of 54 consecutive patients. Transfusion 2006;46:154–6.

Moake JL. Thrombotic microangiopathies. N Engl J Med 2002;347:8589–600.

Qu L, Kiss JE. Thrombotic microangiopathy in transplantation and malignancy. Semin Thromb Hemost 2005;31:691–9.

Vesely SK, George JN, Lammle B, et al. ADAMTS13 activity in thrombotic thrombocytopenic purpura-hemolytic uremic syndrome: Relation to presenting features and clinical outcomes in a prospective cohort of 142 patients. Blood 2003;102(1):60–8.

Hemochromatosis

Method of
Paul C. Adams, MD

Hemochromatosis is the most common genetic disease in populations of European ancestry. The diagnosis can be elusive because of the nonspecific nature of the symptoms. With the discovery of the hemochromatosis gene (*HFE*) in 1996 came new insights into the pathogenesis of the disease and new diagnostic strategies.

A fundamental issue that arose after the discovery of the *HFE* gene is whether the disease hemochromatosis should be defined strictly on phenotypic criteria such as the degree of iron overload (i.e., transferrin saturation, ferritin, liver biopsy, hepatic iron concentration, iron removed by venesection therapy), or whether the condition should be defined as a familial disease in Europeans most commonly associated with the C282Y mutation of the *HFE* gene and varying degrees of iron overload. Because the genetic test has been increasingly used as a diagnostic tool, most studies now use a combination of phenotypic and genotypic criteria for the diagnosis of hemochromatosis.

Clinical Features of Hemochromatosis: Liver Disease

Although hemochromatosis is often classified as a liver disease, it should be emphasized that it is a systemic genetic disease with multisystem involvement. The liver is central in both diagnosis and prognosis. Hepatomegaly remains one of the more common physical signs in hemochromatosis, but it is not always present in the young, asymptomatic homozygote. In a study of 717 homozygotes from Australia, 8% of men and 1.7% of women had cirrhosis of the liver at the time of diagnosis. The prevalence of cirrhosis in asymptomatic or screened patients is much lower. It is likely that there are factors other than iron overload that contribute to cirrhosis in hemochromatosis. These can include the effects of alcohol or comodifying genes. The effect of iron depletion therapy is usually stabilization of the liver disease, and fibrosis improves with repeat liver biopsy after iron depletion. This accounts for the relatively small number of C282Y homozygotes that require liver transplantation. The other common clinical manifestations are arthralgias, pigmentation, congestive heart failure, impotence, and fatigue. Several large population studies failed to demonstrate an increase in diabetes compared with a control population. A population-based study estimated that only 28% of male and 1% of female C282Y homozygotes will develop symptoms of iron overload.

Diagnosis of Hemochromatosis

A paradox of genetic hemochromatosis is that the disease is underdiagnosed in the general population and overdiagnosed in patients with secondary iron overload.

CURRENT DIAGNOSIS

- Consider the diagnosis.
- Initial testing is transferrin saturation or unsaturated iron binding capacity and serum ferritin.
- Secondary testing is the C282Y genetic test.
- If the genetic test is not typical, reassess the diagnosis.
- Not all patients need a liver biopsy.
- Siblings are at highest risk in a family study.

UNDERDIAGNOSIS

Preliminary population studies using genetic testing demonstrate a prevalence of homozygotes of approximately 1:227 among whites. The fact that many physicians consider hemochromatosis to be rare implies either a lack of penetrance of the gene (nonexpressing homozygote) or a large number of patients that remain undiagnosed in the community.

DIAGNOSTIC TESTS

Transferrin Saturation

An elevated transferrin saturation has a sensitivity of greater than 90% for hemochromatosis in family studies. The sensitivity of transferrin saturation is much lower in population-screening studies designed to detect C282Y homozygotes (genotypic case definition) and can be in the normal range in young female homozygotes. A large biologic variation in transferrin saturation within an individual patient has also been reported.

Unsaturated Iron Binding Capacity

The measurement of unsaturated iron binding capacity (UIBC) is a one-step colorimetric assay that is used in many reference laboratories to calculate the transferrin saturation. Compared with transferrin saturation, UIBC is inexpensive and performs just as well.

Serum Ferritin

The relationship between serum ferritin and total body iron stores was clearly established by strong correlations with hepatic iron concentration and the amount of iron removed by venesection. However, ferritin can be elevated secondary to chronic inflammation and histiocytic neoplasms. A major diagnostic dilemma in the past was whether the serum ferritin concentration was related to hemochromatosis or to another underlying liver disease, such as alcoholic liver disease, chronic viral hepatitis, or nonalcoholic steatohepatitis. It is likely that most of these difficult cases can now be resolved by genetic testing.

Liver Biopsy

Liver biopsy was previously the gold standard diagnostic test for hemochromatosis; however, it has shifted from a major diagnostic tool to a method of estimating prognosis and concomitant disease. The need for liver biopsy seems less clear now in the young, asymptomatic C282Y homozygote in whom there is a low clinical suspicion of cirrhosis based on history, physical examination, and liver biochemistry. A large study conducted in France and Canada suggested that C282Y homozygotes with a serum ferritin concentration of less than 1000 μg/L, a normal aspartate transaminase (AST) concentration, and no hepatomegaly have a very low risk of cirrhosis. C282Y homozygotes with a ferritin level greater than 1000 μg/L, an elevated AST, and a platelet count of less than 200,000/mm^3 have an 80% chance of having cirrhosis.

Patients with cirrhosis have a 5.5-fold relative risk of death compared with noncirrhotic hemochromatosis patients. Cirrhotic patients are also at increased risk of hepatocellular carcinoma. Although early detection is clearly demonstrated by serial ultrasound studies and α-fetoprotein determination, curative treatment options remain limited. Liver biopsy is considered in typical C282Y homozygotes with liver dysfunction and in potentially iron-overloaded patients without the typical C282Y mutation. Simple C282Y heterozygotes, compound heterozygotes (C282Y/H63D), H63D homozygotes, and patients with other risk factors (e.g., alcohol abuse, chronic viral hepatitis) who have moderate to severe iron overload (ferritin >1000 μg/L) may be considered for liver biopsy.

Before the advent of genetic testing, hepatic iron concentration was useful in the diagnosis of hemochromatosis. The hepatic iron concentration (in micromoles per gram) divided by age (in years) yields the hepatic iron index. Although the hepatic iron index is less useful today, it remains a tool to aid clinicians with their clinical judgment about an individual case. It is most useful in the unusual hemochromatosis patient who is negative by conventional genetic testing but clinically seems to have genetic hemochromatosis.

Genetic Testing

A major advance stemming from the discovery of the hemochromatosis gene is the use of a diagnostic genetic test. Most studies report that more than 90% of typical hemochromatosis patients were homozygotes for the C282Y mutation. A second minor mutation, H63D, was also described in the original report. Compound heterozygotes (C282Y/H63D) and, less commonly, H63D homozygotes resemble C282Y homozygotes with mild to moderate iron overload. Genetic mutations involving ferroportin, hemojuvelin, transferrin receptor 2, ceruloplasmin, and hepcidin are associated with iron overload. It is likely that, as more mutations are found, they will be relevant to only a minority of patients.

Some patients with clinical pictures indistinguishable from genetic hemochromatosis are negative for the C282Y mutation. Most of these are isolated cases, although a few cases of familial iron overload with negative C282Y testing have been reported. A negative C282Y test should alert the physician to question the diagnosis of genetic hemochromatosis and reconsider secondary iron overload related to cirrhosis, alcoholism, viral hepatitis, or an iron-loading anemia. If no other risk factors are found, the patient should begin venesection treatment, similar to any other hemochromatosis patient.

The interpretation of the genetic test in several settings is shown in Box 1. Genetic discrimination is a concern with the widespread use of genetic testing but has been rarely reported in screening studies. In the case of hemochromatosis, the advantages of early diagnosis of a treatable disease outweigh the disadvantages of genetic discrimination.

Family Studies

Once the proband case is identified and confirmed with the genetic test for the C282Y mutation, family testing is imperative. Siblings have a 1 in 4 chance of carrying the gene and should be screened with the genetic test (C282Y and H63D mutation), transferrin saturation, and serum ferritin. A cost-effective strategy now possible with genetic testing is to test the spouse for the C282Y mutation to assess the risk in the children. If the spouse is not a C282Y heterozygote or homozygote, the children will be obligate heterozygotes, assuming paternity and excluding another gene or mutation causing hemochromatosis. This strategy is particularly advantageous if the children are geographically separated or in different health care systems.

BOX 1　Interpretation of Genetic Testing for Hemochromatosis

C282Y Homozygote

This is the classic genetic pattern seen in more than 90% of typical cases. Expression of disease ranges from no evidence of iron overload to massive iron overload with organ dysfunction. Siblings have a 1 in 4 chance of being affected and should have genetic testing. For children to be affected, the other parent must be at least a heterozygote. If iron studies are normal, false-positive genetic testing or a nonexpressing homozygotic state should be considered.

C282Y/H63D Compound Heterozygote

This patient carries one copy of the major mutation and one copy of the minor mutation. Most patients with this genetic pattern have normal iron studies. A small percentage of compound heterozygotes are found to have mild to moderate iron overload. Severe iron overload is usually seen in the setting of another concomitant risk factor (e.g., alcoholism, viral hepatitis).

C282Y Heterozygote

This patient carries one copy of the major mutation. This pattern is seen in approximately 10% of the white population and is usually associated with normal iron studies. In rare cases, the results of iron studies are high, in the range expected in a homozygote rather than a heterozygote. These patients may carry an unknown hemochromatosis mutation, and liver biopsy is helpful to determine the need for venesection therapy.

H63D Homozygote

This patient carries two copies of the minor mutation. Most patients with this genetic pattern have normal iron studies. A small percentage have mild to moderate iron overload. Severe iron overload is usually seen in the setting of another concomitant risk factor (e.g., alcoholism, viral hepatitis).

H63D Heterozygote

This patient carries one copy of the minor mutation. This pattern is seen in approximately 20% of the white population and is usually associated with normal iron studies. This pattern is so common in the general population that the presence of iron overload can be related to another risk factor. Liver biopsy is required to determine the cause of the iron overload and the need for treatment in these cases.

No *HFE* Mutations

If iron overload is present without any mutations in the hemochromatosis gene (*HFE*), a careful history for other risk factors must be reviewed, and liver biopsy can be useful to determine the cause of the iron overload and the need for treatment. Most of these are isolated, nonfamilial cases. There are cases described involving genetic mutations in ferroportin, hemojuvelin, transferrin receptor 2, ceruloplasmin, and hepcidin genes. Genetic tests for these mutations are not widely available.

CURRENT THERAPY

- Iron overload from hemochromatosis is treated by the weekly removal of 500 mL of blood until the serum ferritin is in the low-normal range of approximately 50 µg/L.
- Some but not all patients require maintenance therapy with three to four phlebotomies per year. In some countries, this can be a voluntary blood donation.
- Excess alcohol, high doses of vitamin C, and iron supplementation should be avoided, but strict dietary restrictions are not recommended.
- Siblings and children of patients should be tested for hemochromatosis with transferrin saturation, ferritin, and genetic testing.

Treatment

The treatment of hemochromatosis continues to employ the medieval therapy of periodic bleeding. At our center, patients attend an ambulatory care facility, and the venesections are performed by a nurse using a kit containing a 16-gauge straight needle and collection bag (Blood Pack MR6102, Baxter, Deerfield, IL). Blood is removed with the patient in the reclining position over 15 to 30 minutes. A hemoglobin test is done at the time of each venesection. If the hemoglobin concentration has decreased to less than 10 g/dL, the venesection schedule is modified to 500 mL every other week. Venesections are continued until the serum ferritin concentration is approximately 50 µg/L. The concomitant administration of a salt-containing sport beverage (e.g., Gatorade) is a simple method of maintaining plasma volume during the venesection.

Maintenance venesections after iron depletion, consisting of three to four venesections per year, are performed in most patients, although the rate of iron reaccumulation is highly variable. The transferrin saturation remains elevated in many treated patients and does not normalize unless the patient becomes iron deficient. In some countries, patients with mild iron abnormalities are encouraged to become voluntary blood donors.

Chelation therapy is not recommended for hemochromatosis. Patients are advised to avoid oral iron therapy and alcohol abuse, but there are no dietary restrictions. Patient support groups have been discouraged by the practice of iron fortification of foods, but much of this iron is in an inexpensive form with poor bioavailability.

Population Screening

Early diagnosis and treatment of hemochromatosis lead to a long-term survival rate similar to that observed in the general population. Many prospective and retrospective studies demonstrate that genetic mutations are much more common than clinical illness, and many C282Y homozygotes do not develop progressive iron overload. The natural history of untreated disease remains the most difficult component in an assessment of the cost-effectiveness of screening, and it is unlikely to be resolved because of ethical concerns about withholding therapy.

Large population studies designed to study heart disease and atherosclerosis have demonstrated that many untreated C282Y homozygotes do not develop progressive iron overload. Targeted screening in high-risk groups, improved physician and patient education initiatives, and extended family studies are more likely to be considered than mass population screening.

Hemochromatosis is a common and often underdiagnosed disease. Early diagnosis and treatment result in an excellent long-term prognosis. The development of a diagnostic genetic test has improved the feasibility of the goal of prevention of morbidity and mortality from hemochromatosis.

REFERENCES

Adams PC, Reboussin DM, Barton JC, et al. Hemochromatosis and iron over-load screening (HEIRS) study: Screening in a racially diverse of primary care population. N Engl J Med 2005;352:1769–78.

Adams PC, Reboussin DM, Eckfeldt J, et al. A comparison of the unsaturated iron binding capacity to transferrin saturation as a screening test to detect C282Y homozygotes for hemochromatosis in 101,168 participants in the HEIRS study. Clin Chem 2005;51:1048–52.

Allen KJ, Gurrin LC, Constantine CC, et al. Iron-overload-related disease in HFE hereditary hemochromatosis. N Engl J Med 2008;358:221–30.

Andersen R, Tybjaerg-Hansen A, Appleyard M, et al. Hemochromatosis muta-tions in the general population: Iron overload progression rate. Blood 2004;103:2914–9.

Beaton M, Guyader D, Deugnier Y, et al. Non-invasive prediction of cirrhosis in C282Y-linked hemochromatosis. Hepatology 2002;36:673–8.

Beutler E, Felitti V, Koziol J, et al. Penetrance of the 845G to A (C282Y) HFE hereditary haemochromatosis mutation in the USA. Lancet 2002;359:211–8.

Falize L, Guillygomarch A, Perrin M, et al. Reversibility of hepatic fibrosis in treated hemochromatosis: A study of 36 cases. Hepatology 2006;44:472–7.

Guyader D, Jacquelinet C, Moirand R, et al. Non-invasive prediction of fibrosis in C282Y homozygous hemochromatosis. Gastroenterology 1998;115:929–36.

Pankow JS, Boerwinkle E, Adams PC, et al. HFE C282Y homozygotes have reduced low-density lipoprotein cholesterol: The Atherosclerosis Risk in Communities (ARIC) Study. Transl Res 2008;152:3–10.

Pietrangelo A. Hereditary hemochromatosis: A new look at an old disease. N Engl J Med 2004;350:2383–97.

Wojcik J, Speechley M, Kertesz A, et al. Natural history of C282Y homozygotes for haemochromatosis. Can J Gastroenterol 2002;16:297–302.

Wood MJ, Powell LW, Ramm GA. Environmental and genetic modifiers of the progression to fibrosis and cirrhosis in hemochromatosis. Blood 2008;111:4456–62.

Hodgkin's Lymphoma

Method of
Ralph M. Meyer, MD, and
David C. Hodgson, MD, MPH

Current estimates of the incidence and mortality of Hodgkin's lymphoma in the United States come from American Cancer Society statistics, which predicts approximately 7800 diagnoses and 1800 deaths in 2006. This mortality-to-incidence rate ratio of 0.19 reflects the high potential for cure of this disease and emphasizes that long-term issues of survivorship are important for these patients, but it also demonstrates that curative potential is not achieved in an important fraction of patients. Historically, understandings of the biology and management of Hodgkin's lymphoma have played pivotal roles in developing broader understandings of cancer; this continues to be the case. In this article, we describe these principles and review current management strategies.

Histologic Classification

The diagnosis of Hodgkin's lymphoma requires an adequate tissue biopsy and expert interpretation. The histologic classification of Hodgkin's lymphoma, and lymphomas in general, exemplifies how new understandings of biology, including advances in molecular oncology, require that categorization schema be continuously updated to accommodate new discoveries. Since the initial description of this lymphoma by Thomas Hodgkin in 1832 and the reporting of the hallmark features of the Reed–Sternberg cell in 1902, the classification of Hodgkin's disease has undergone sequential updating. Landmark schemata include those described by Jackson and

Parker in 1943 and Lukes and Butler in 1966. This latter classification system was modified at the 1966 Rye Conference and included four separate entities: lymphocyte predominant, nodular sclerosing, mixed cellularity, and lymphocyte deplete. It is this classification system that has been used in the vast majority of clinical trials that have determined current treatments.

The most current classification schema was determined as part of the Revised European American Lymphoma (REAL) classification of 1994 and was updated in the World Heath Organization classification described in 1997 (Fig. 1). Major changes include recognition of nodular lymphocyte predominant disease as a distinct clinical entity that is separate from the other forms of Hodgkin's lymphoma, which are now grouped under the umbrella term of classic Hodgkin's lymphoma. Within classic Hodgkin's lymphoma are four entities: lymphocyte rich, nodular sclerosing, mixed cellularity, and lymphocyte deplete. As we describe later, the new clinical ramifications of incorporating recent biological findings into the WHO classification system are that an entity that is associated with a different clinical course and might require a different form of therapy has been defined (i.e., nodular lymphocyte predominant disease), and criteria that separate Hodgkin's from non-Hodgkin's lymphomas have been made more explicit. It is crucial that evaluation of biopsy material be performed by an expert pathologist, with necessary ancillary studies such as immunohistochemistry, flow cytometry, and molecular studies completed as appropriate to ensure that the Hodgkin's and non-Hodgkin's lymphomas have been distinguished and that subtypes of lymphoma have been properly characterized.

Staging and Risk Categorization

As with histologic classifications, the variables that determine the extent of disease and prognosis of patients with Hodgkin's lymphoma have evolved to account for new biological understandings and the relevance of these variables within the context of current therapies. Beginning with the initial observations of Peters in 1950, risk categorization of patients with Hodgkin's lymphoma has historically emphasized the anatomic spread of the disease. Subsequently, the Ann Arbor Staging Classification was devised in 1971; this was modified at the Cotswold meeting in 1989. The Cotswold criteria continue to be applied to newly diagnosed cases (Table 1).

Current management strategies for patients with classic Hodgkin's lymphoma involve collapsing the Ann Arbor and Cotswold classifications into two or three categories. These categories include at least limited-stage and advanced-stage disease. In North America, cooperative group clinical trials have defined limited-stage disease as clinical stage I to IIA and an absence of bulky disease. Bulky disease is defined as a mass that is at least 10 cm in diameter or that measures more than one third of the maximum transthoracic diameter on a standard posteroanterior chest radiograph. Other factors that have been considered of potential prognostic importance, such as erythrocyte sedimentation rate (ESR) and histologic subtype within classic Hodgkin's lymphoma, are no longer deemed to be important in defining therapy, because the prognostic properties of these factors have been obviated by current therapies. Patients with stages IIB, III, IV, and bulky disease associated with any stage are considered to have advanced-stage disease. Within this article, these definitions of limited and advanced-stage disease will be used to describe treatment practices. For the purposes of determining prognosis, and for designing clinical trials, patients with advanced-stage disease may be further assessed through use of the International Prognostic Index (IPI), which includes anatomic stage as a variable, but also includes six other parameters that have been shown to be prognostic through evaluation of large databases (Table 2).

Cooperative group practices in Europe use schemata that have considerable overlap with those used in North America. Patients who in North America would be classified in Europe as having limited-stage disease may be classified as having *favorable early-stage* disease. A separate category of *intermediate-stage* or *unfavorable*

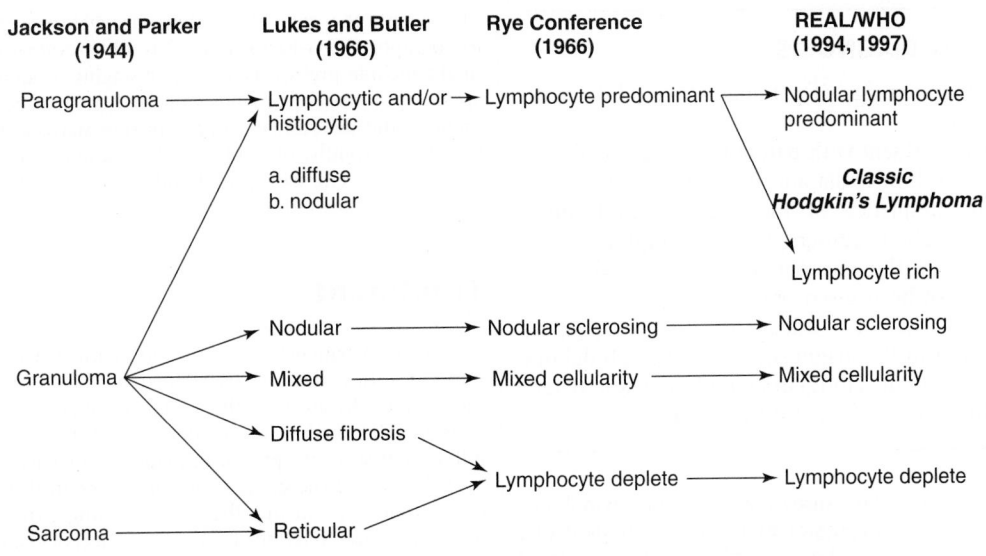

FIGURE 1. Histologic classifications of Hodgkin's lymphoma. REAL = Revised European American Lymphoma; WHO = World Health Organization.

TABLE 1 Ann Arbor Staging System Including Cotswold Modifications

Stage	Disease Involvement
I	Single lymph node region (I) or one extralymphatic site (I$_E$)
II	Two or more lymph node regions, on the same side of the diaphragm (II) or local extralymphatic extension plus one or more lymph node regions on the same side of the diaphragm (II$_E$)
III	Lymph node regions on both sides of the diaphragm (III), which may be accompanied by local extralymphatic extension (III$_E$)
IV	Diffuse involvement of one or more extralymphatic organs or sites
A	No B symptoms
B	Presence of at least one of unexplained weight loss >10% baseline during 6 mo before staging, recurrent unexplained fever >38°C, recurrent night sweats
X	Bulky tumor: either a single mass exceeding 10 cm in largest diameter or a mediastinal mass exceeding one third of the maximum transverse transthoracic diameter measured on a standard posteroanterior chest radiograph

TABLE 2 The International Prognostic Index*

Variable	Risk Level
Serum albumin	<40 g/L
Hemoglobin	<105 g/L
Sex	Male
Stage	Stage IV
Age	≥45 y
White cell count	≥15 × 10^9/L
Lymphocyte count	<0.6 × 10^9/L or <8% of total while cell count

*The number of factors present is totaled.

early-stage disease is used to include patients with stage I, IIA, or IIB disease and presence of one or more predefined risk factors, such as the presence of bulky disease, elevation of the ESR, or an increased number of nodal sites of disease. Advanced stage includes those with stage III or IV disease. Despite these minor variations, these classification systems result in similar stage-related treatment practices in both geographic regions.

Clinical Presentation and Initial Investigations

Patients with Hodgkin's lymphoma are typically young, with the peak incidence of disease occurring in those in late adolescence to their early 40s. The median age observed in most clinical trials is approximately 35 years. Although a bimodal age distribution has been historically described, with a second age peak occurring in elderly patients, recent revisions of lymphoma histologic classification have resulted in changing the diagnosis in many older patients from Hodgkin's disease to non-Hodgkin's lymphoma.

The presentation of patients with Hodgkin's lymphoma typically falls into two major categories: those who present with painless lymphadenopathy and those who present with other symptoms. Usually those with painless adenopathy present with supradiaphragmatic disease, with an enlarged lymph node in the neck or axilla. The lymph nodes are typically described as firm, hard, or rubbery as opposed to the softer or fleshy nodes in patients with lymphadenopathy that is reactive to an inflammatory condition. Nodes that are anatomically asymmetrical (unilateral) and that are present in the posterior triangle of the neck, as opposed to the internal jugular chain, are more suspicious for lymphoma, as opposed to a reactive condition. Only 5% of Hodgkin's lymphoma patients present with disease that is confined to the subdiaphragmatic regions; typically these patients present with adenopathy in the inguinal or femoral region and disproportionately may have the nodular lymphocyte–predominant histologic subtype. Symptoms can relate to local disease or be constitutional. Patients with mediastinal disease may present with chest fullness and cough. Constitutional symptoms often include fatigue, lethargy, or the prognostic B symptoms of fevers, night sweats, or weight loss. Unusual, but potentially distinct, symptoms can include intractable pruritus or pain in a region affected by adenopathy associated with alcohol intake.

CURRENT DIAGNOSIS

- The most common age of patients is late adolescence to the early 40s.
- Many patients present with painless adenopathy that is often in the neck or axilla and is asymmetrical.
- Due to the frequency of mediastinal lymph node involvement, a chest radiograph can be helpful in evaluating patients with persistent symptoms for which an etiology has not been discovered.
- The diagnosis requires an adequate biopsy with expert review to confirm the diagnosis, distinguish Hodgkin's lymphoma from non-Hodgkin's lymphoma, and determine the histologic subtype of the disease.

Evaluation of patients with suspected Hodgkin's lymphoma includes a thorough history and physical examination with particular attention to the presence of the above-described symptoms and of lymphadenopathy, hepatosplenomegaly, or a pleural effusion on physical examination. In patients with chest symptoms, a chest x-ray can be extremely valuable. The definitive diagnosis requires an adequate tissue biopsy; although cytologic evaluations of material obtained from a fine-needle aspirate might suggest a diagnosis of Hodgkin's lymphoma, at present, this technology is not consistently reliable to ensure a correct diagnosis. Material for histologic evaluation obtained from an adequate large-bore core biopsy might, in select circumstances, be sufficient for diagnosis, but in general, an excisional biopsy should be expected to achieve a definitive diagnosis.

Once a diagnosis of Hodgkin's lymphoma is confirmed, patients require systematic evaluation to assess prognostic features that will influence therapy and determine whether complications of the disease are present. Standard investigations are listed in Box 1.

BOX 1   Baseline Investigations for Patients with Hodgkin's Lymphoma

History
Fever
Night sweats
Weight loss

Physical Examination
Hepatosplenomegaly
Lymphadenopathy
Pleural effusion

Laboratory
Complete blood count and white cell differential
Serum bilirubin and liver enzymes
Serum creatinine and calcium
Total protein and albumin

Imaging
Bone marrow: Aspirate and biopsy (can be omitted with limited–stage disease and a normal complete blood count)
Chest radiograph
Computed tomography scanning of the chest, abdomen, and pelvis

Biopsy
Lymph node biopsy with specialized review (see text)

Other
Positron emission tomographic (PET) scanning (see text)
Specialized imaging according to symptoms and signs

At present, the role of ^{18}F-fluorodeoxyglucose positron emission tomography (FDG-PET scanning) is under evaluation. Potential roles might include pretreatment disease staging, evaluation during therapy for purposes of prognosis or prediction of benefit with specific therapy, and determination of remission status at the completion of therapy. Currently, the utility of PET scanning is least well defined as a pretreatment staging tool and cannot yet be considered a standard test for this purpose.

Treatment

Treatment of patients with Hodgkin's lymphoma can be subdivided into categories that are determined by the histologic subtype and the stage of disease with the added potential that risk factors, such as those identified in the Hodgkin's lymphoma IPI, might further influence treatment options. Principles of management include careful balancing of the desire to maximally control the underlying disease, while minimizing the risks of long-term treatment-related toxicities (also referred to as late effects). Late effects include increased risks of developing acute leukemia, which is associated with use of chemotherapy regimens that include alkylating agents or epipodophyllotoxins, and second cancers and cardiovascular events, which are associated with radiation therapy. In addition, chemotherapy regimens that include alkylating agents are associated with dose-dependent risks of gonadal failure and infertility.

LIMITED-STAGE CLASSIC HODGKIN'S LYMPHOMA

The management of patients with limited-stage Hodgkin's lymphoma has changed dramatically over the past 15 to 20 years. As recently as 1990, standard management included a staging laparotomy with splenectomy followed by treatment with subtotal nodal radiation. With this treatment, other prognostic factors were identified and used to refine therapy; these included ESR, number of disease sites, and histologic subtype (e.g., nodular sclerosing vs mixed cellularity). These practices have been improved on by advances in diagnostic imaging and through the availability of more-efficacious and less-toxic systemic chemotherapy. Further improvements should be expected as other technologies, such as PET scanning, become validated.

Based on current data, patients and physicians have two main options for the treatment of limited-stage Hodgkin's lymphoma. These options are associated with specific trade-offs.

The first option is treatment with combined modality therapy that includes two cycles of doxorubicin (Adriamycin), bleomycin (Bleoxane), vinblastine (Velban) and dacarbazine (DTIC-Dome) (ABVD), and radiation therapy to the involved field. The advantage of this approach is that long-term disease control is maximized with initial therapy; this is expected in approximately 95% of patients. The disadvantage relates to use of radiation therapy and the associated risks of late effects such as second cancers and, with mediastinal radiation, cardiovascular events. Advances in radiation technology, such as conformal treatment, use of PET scanning for planning, and limiting the treatment field to the affected nodes as opposed to nodal regions, significantly reduces the radiation dose to normal tissues compared with radiation treatments given in the 1970s to the 1990s. Further data are required before we can confidently conclude that important long-term risks do not remain.

The second option is therapy with four to six cycles of ABVD alone. The advantage of this approach is avoidance of radiation therapy and the associated risks of late effects, with the disadvantage being a decrement in long-term disease control with initial therapy that is estimated to be about 7% (i.e., to approximately 88%). To date, no differences in long-term overall survival have been detected between these options. Ongoing randomized trials that assign use of radiation according to patients' early response to chemotherapy might clarify which patients can be treated with chemotherapy alone without increasing the risk of relapse. In the meantime, balancing these options requires careful discussions with patients about their preferences.

CURRENT THERAPY

Limited Stage Classic Hodgkin's Lymphoma

- Option 1: Combined modality therapy consisting of two cycles of ABVD and involved-field radiation therapy. The advantage is long-term disease control with initial therapy in more than 90% of patients.
- Option 2: Treatment with ABVD (4–6 cycles). The advantage is that, although long-term disease control with initial therapy is about 7% less than with combined modality therapy, the risks of late effects of radiation therapy are avoided.

Advanced Stage Classic Hodgkin's Lymphoma

- Option 1: Treatment with ABVD (6–8 cycles). The advantage is that long-term disease control with initial therapy in at least 65% of patients. Gonadal function and fertility are preserved.
- Option 2: Treatment with escalated BEACOPP. The advantage is that long-term disease control with initial therapy is approximately 10% better than that associated with ABVD, but treatment is associated with more toxicity, including high rates of infertility (see text).

Refractory or Recurrent Classic Hodgkin's Lymphoma

- Usual initial treatment is with high-dose chemotherapy and autologous stem cell transplantation.
- Subsequent treatments require individualized approaches.

Nodular Lymphocyte–Predominant Hodgkin's Lymphoma

- The most common option is involved-field radiation therapy.
- Numerous new options, including use of rituximab and observation have been described.
- Advanced-stage disease is treated the same as classic Hodgkin's lymphoma.

ADVANCED-STAGE CLASSIC HODGKIN'S LYMPHOMA

The management of patients with advanced-stage disease has also evolved over the past 15 to 20 years. In 1990, standard therapy would have included six to eight cycles of nitrogen mustard, vincristine (Oncovin), prednisone, and procarbazine (Matulane) in combination with ABVD (± dacarbazine) (MOPP-ABVD or MOPP-ABV). Recent randomized, controlled trials have demonstrated that these regimens and ABVD all provide long-term disease control in approximately 65% of patients. However, there is less short-term toxicity with ABVD, and importantly, this regimen avoids the long-term risks of infertility and leukemogenesis associated with nitrogen mustard and procarbazine. Treatment with ABVD is therefore considered a standard.

An alternative strategy is to intensify therapy with use of the bleomycin, etoposide (Vepesid),[1] doxorubicin (Adriamycin), cyclophosphamide (Cytoxan), vincristine (Oncovin), prednisone, and procarbazine (BEACOPP) regimen. Use of this regimen, particularly in its escalated-dose form, has been associated with superior disease control and an improvement in overall survival that is in the range of 8% to 10% at 5 years (i.e., 91% with escalated BEACOPP versus 83% with ABVD). In comparison with ABVD, the magnitude of

_____
[1]Not FDA approved for this indication.

disease-control benefits associated with the BEACOPP regimens may be greatest in patients who have more than three IPI risk factors. However, the BEACOPP regimens are associated with more severe toxicities, including more severe myelosuppression and risks of infection during the treatment period, and a greater risk of acute leukemia and myelodysplasia as a late effect. Furthermore, risks of infertility are markedly increased: Preliminary reports suggest that escalated BEACOPP is associated with gonadal failure in 85% to 90% of all men and women who are older than 30 years and in 50% of female patients younger than 30 years.

Another strategy uses weekly chemotherapy that is administered over a shorter time course than ABVD. The prototype of this therapy is the Stanford V regimen. Although this treatment has shown promising results in a phase II trial, in three randomized, controlled trials testing this concept, outcomes were inferior in comparison with ABVD or an equivalent regimen. A large North American Intergroup study has completed accrual to a randomized comparison of Stanford V and ABVD. Until the results of this trial are known, use of regimens based on this concept should be limited to clinical trials testing.

The role of combining radiation therapy with chemotherapy has been studied in a number of randomized trials and an individual patient-data meta-analysis. A summary of these results shows that no differences in overall survival are detected, and particularly in patients with stage III or IV disease who are treated with ABVD or BEACOPP, there are also no differences in disease control. At present, there continues to be a role for combined modality therapy for patients with stage I or II disease who are considered to have advanced-stage disease because of the presence of a bulky mediastinal mass. The need for all of these patients to receive radiation therapy will require reevaluation as the utility of PET scanning is better understood.

Therefore, as with limited-stage disease, practitioners and patients are faced with a decision involving trade-offs as the treatment associated with the best long-term disease control is also associated with the greatest long-term risk. At an individual patient level, the risks of infertility associated with BEACOPP should be regarded as likely. Provided patients are aware of these trade-offs, treatment with either escalated BEACOPP or ABVD is a reasonable option.

RELAPSED OR REFRACTORY DISEASE

Unfortunately, an important number of patients have disease that is refractory to initial therapy or that is associated with subsequent recurrence. The vast majority of these patients present with advanced-stage disease and receive a full course of chemotherapy with ABVD. Based on the results of two randomized trials that have shown significant improvements in progression-free or event-free survival, treatment with high-dose chemotherapy and autologous stem cell transplantation is considered standard. Autologous transplantation is particularly recommended for patients with primary refractory disease and disease that recurs within 1 year of completing initial therapy; it is also a reasonable option for most other patients who experience disease recurrence after a longer disease-free interval. Patients with recurrent disease that includes a site of bulky disease, such as the mediastinum, should also receive radiation therapy to that site following confirmed stem cell engraftment.

Treatment options for recurrent Hodgkin's lymphoma in patients who initially present with limited-stage disease are poorly characterized due to the uncommon occurrence of this event. The choice of therapy is strongly influenced by specifics of the pattern of disease recurrence. Options for patients with recurrent disease after receiving combined modality therapy include receiving a full course of a standard regimen (e.g., ABVD) or, more commonly, stem cell transplantation. For patients whose disease recurs after receiving ABVD alone, and particularly when this recurrence is confined to the initial sites of disease, the option of treatment with combined-modality therapy that includes involved-field radiation is preferred over stem cell transplantation.

The treatment of patients with recurrent disease after stem cell transplantation has been poorly evaluated; there are no randomized, controlled trials. Management must be individualized and should account for the demographic features of the patient, the temporal profile, burden and symptoms associated with the disease, and natures of the previous therapies. A common option includes single-agent vinblastine for purposes of palliation, but additional options can include radiation therapy, including wide-field radiation, use of other standard-dose chemotherapy regimens, and for select patients, observation. For very select patients, the option of allogeneic stem cell transplantation, including with reduced-intensity conditioning regimens, has been described.

NODULAR LYMPHOCYTE–PREDOMINANT HODGKIN'S LYMPHOMA

There are now robust data indicating that nodular lymphocyte–predominant Hodgkin's lymphoma is a distinct biological entity and is associated with a clinical course that differs from classic Hodgkin's lymphoma. Most patients present with limited-stage disease and have an indolent clinical course; extensive mediastinal involvement is rare. An important biological feature is expression by the malignant cell of the CD20 antigen, which raises the opportunity for potential treatment with immunotherapy using the monoclonal antibody rituximab.

The uncommon incidence of this disease means that the clinical trials that inform current practices generally consist of case series, many of which are retrospective, and small subset analyses from larger randomized trials that evaluate patients with all histologic subtypes. From these data, a commonly preferred therapy is with involved-field radiation therapy as a single modality. An alternative option is combined-modality therapy as given for patients with limited-stage classic Hodgkin's lymphoma, but the curative potential of this option is uncertain. Small case series have evaluated observation alone or rituximab treatment, but sufficient data do not yet exist to permit recommending these as standard therapies. Patients with advanced-stage disease should receive the same therapy as patients with classic Hodgkin's lymphoma.

SPECIAL CIRCUMSTANCES

Special circumstances can arise that require modification of these treatment strategies. For each of these circumstances, the data on which current recommendations are based are limited and largely consist of case reports, case series, and generalizations from other diseases or biological principles.

A first circumstance is managing older patients with Hodgkin's lymphoma. As with the therapy of older patients with non-Hodgkin's lymphoma, the treatment plan must initially account for the presence of any comorbidities or specific patient preferences related to individual values. When no additional factors are identified, treatment that incorporates the principles for managing younger patients should be followed. For these patients, the BEACOPP regimens are associated with excessive toxicity and should not be used. For patients with cardiac compromise who cannot receive doxorubicin, treatment with chlorambucil, vinblastine, prednisone, and procarbazine (ChlVPP) may be considered.

A second circumstance is management of female patients in whom Hodgkin's lymphoma is diagnosed during pregnancy. Diagnostic staging of these patients should include replacement of computed tomography with ultrasound examination. Provided that the disease is sufficiently indolent, many patients can be carefully observed until the postnatal period and then complete standard staging tests and therapy. For patients who must receive therapy before delivery, a common option is treatment with single-agent vinblastine, which is not teratogenic, followed by postnatal therapy with a full course of standard chemotherapy. In very select circumstances, patients who have rapidly progressing disease after their first trimester of pregnancy may, after thorough consideration and discussion of options, be treated with ABVD.

A third special circumstance is management of the HIV patient who develops Hodgkin's lymphoma. These patients might not be as profoundly immunosuppressed as HIV patients who develop non-Hodgkin's lymphoma, but unfortunately risks of infection associated with standard chemotherapy are increased. These patients should receive optimal antiretroviral therapy and ideally treatment that is otherwise considered standard for their stage of disease. Due to insufficient data, therapy with BEACOPP is not recommended and these patients should receive ABVD.

Issues of Survivorship

Studies of survivors have shown that delayed morbidity and excess mortality not directly attributable to Hodgkin's lymphoma is an important problem. For patients whose disease was diagnosed in the 1960s to 1980s, deaths from other causes exceeded deaths due to Hodgkin's lymphoma after 15 years of follow-up. A major cause of other deaths is the occurrence of a second cancer. A man whose disease was diagnosed at age 30 and who was treated with historical approaches, the 30-year cumulative incidence of developing a solid-tumor cancer is approximately 15% to 20%, which is 10% higher than expected in the gender- and age-matched general population. Comparable values for a 30-year-old woman include a 30-year cumulative incidence of a subsequent solid cancer of 25%, which is 15% higher than expected. The incremental risk of solid cancers among younger female patients is even more pronounced, largely due to the excess risk of breast cancer related to radiation therapy to the mediastinum.

A second major cause of late morbidity and mortality is cardiovascular diseases. These may be related to doxorubicin, which produces free radicals that are directly toxic to the myocardium, and mediastinal radiation to a field that includes the heart. The cumulative incidence of significant cardiac morbidity 10 years after treatment is approximately 2% to 6% and increases to 15% to 20% by 20 years. This represents a 1.5- to 3-fold increased relative risk and is largely related to the radiation therapy. Technical interventions that reduce the dose of radiation to the heart reduce this risk.

The persistence of symptoms associated with nonfatal complications is also common. Even following modern therapy, many survivors experience persistent fatigue; its cause is uncertain. Although persistent anemia and hypothyroidism are known late effects of treatment, these do not usually provide the reason for fatigue.

Specifically focused follow-up of survivors can reduce the morbidity of late treatment effects. Among patients who receive neck or mediastinal radiation, thyroid function should be evaluated at least annually to detect preclinical hypothyroidism. Female patients treated with mediastinal radiation should undergo annual breast cancer screening beginning 8 years after this treatment or beginning at age 25 years. Due to the suboptimal performance of mammography in women with dense breast tissue, which includes most young women, this screening should include magnetic resonance imaging (MRI) for women younger than 30 years. For women ages 30 to 50 years, mammography can be initiated and the adequacy of mammographic images can guide decisions regarding the appropriate screening modality. For those with good mammographic images (i.e., predominantly fatty breast tissue) mammography alone is recommended, whereas those with dense breast tissue should be screened with MRI plus mammography. Mammographic screening alone is recommended for women older than 50 years.

Recommendations for colorectal cancer screening for patients who have received abdominal radiation therapy are less clear. Some recommendations include initiation of colorectal cancer screening 15 years after treatment, or by age 35 years, whichever comes later. The evidence supporting this recommendation is indirect and there are no data to indicate whether colonoscopy or fecal occult blood testing is superior.

Most cardiac morbidity occurs in survivors who have conventional cardiac risk factors. Consequently, blood pressure and serum lipids should be monitored and, if elevated, treated aggressively.

Similarly, strong efforts should be made to help survivors quit smoking, because the smoking-related risks of heart disease and lung cancer appear to be even greater than among the general population. Young survivors who experience progressive fatigue or chest pain require cardiac evaluation; these symptoms should not be attributed to noncardiac causes until heart disease has been excluded. Preliminary data suggest that screening stress echocardiography can detect clinically important valvular or coronary artery disease among long-term survivors who received mediastinal radiation to doses greater than 35 Gy; future studies are required to clarify the value of routine screening of all asymptomatic patients. Female survivors who become pregnant, however, should undergo cardiac evaluation because of the significant cardiac stress associated with pregnancy and childbirth.

Persistent fatigue among survivors can be a challenging management problem. Depression or dysthymia, hypothyroidism, impaired cardiac function, and anemia should be considered as potential causes. Regular exercise can significantly reduce fatigue and in severe cases, referral to a mental health professional should be considered for cognitive behavior therapy or short-term pharmacotherapy.

Given the nature of these and other survivorship issues, standard oncology clinics might not be well suited to deal with the types of issues that patients who have been otherwise successfully treated for Hodgkin's lymphoma. Specialized clinics for survivors, which focus on these late-effect issues as opposed to the less likely potentials of disease recurrence, are now more common and may be a preferred way to provide this health care.

REFERENCES

Connors JM. State-of-the-art therapeutics: Hodgkin's lymphoma. J Clin Oncol 2005;23(26):6400–8.

Diehl V, Franklin J, Pfreundschuh M, et al. Standard and increased-dose BEACOPP chemotherapy compared with COPP-ABVD for advanced Hodgkin's disease. N Engl J Med 2003;348(24):2386–95.

Duggan DB, Petroni GR, Johnson JL, et al. Randomized comparison of ABVD and MOPP/ABV hybrid for the treatment of advanced Hodgkin's disease: Report of an Intergroup trial. J Clin Oncol 2003;21(4):607–14.

Gospodarowicz MK, Meyer RM. The management of patients with limited-stage classical Hodgkin lymphoma. Hematology 2006;2006(1):253–8.

Harris NL, Jaffe ES, Diebold J, et al. World Health Organization classification of neoplastic diseases of the hematopoietic and lymphoid tissues: Report of the Clinical Advisory Committee Meeting, Airlie House, Virginia, November 1997. J Clin Oncol 1999;17(12):3835–49.

Harris NL, Jaffe ES, Stein H, et al. A revised European–American classification of lymphoid neoplasms: A proposal from the International Lymphoma Study Group. Blood 1994;84(5):1361–92.

Hasenclever D, Diehl V, Armitage JO, et al. A prognostic score for advanced Hodgkin's disease. N Engl J Med 1998;339(21):1506–14.

Hodgson DC, Gilbert ES, Dores GM, et al. Long-term solid cancer risk among 5-year survivors of Hodgkin's lymphoma. J Clin Oncol 2007;25 (12):1489–97.

Lister TA, Crowther D, Sutcliffe SB, et al. Report of a committee convened to discuss the evaluation and staging of patients with Hodgkin's disease: Cotswolds meeting. J Clin Oncol 1989;7(11):1630–6.

Meyer RM, Gospodarowicz MK, Connors JM, et al. Randomized comparison of ABVD chemotherapy with a strategy that includes radiation therapy in patients with limited-stage Hodgkin's lymphoma: National Cancer Institute of Canada Clinical Trials Group and the Eastern Cooperative Oncology Group. J Clin Oncol 2005;23(21):4634–42.

Nogova L, Rudiger T, Engert A. Biology, clinical course and management of nodular lymphocyte–predominant Hodgkin lymphoma. Hematology 2006;2006(1):266–72.

Ralleigh G, Given-Wilson R. Breast cancer risk and possible screening strategies for young women following supradiaphragmatic radiation for Hodgkin's disease. Clin Radiol 2004;59:647–50.

Hodgkin's Disease: Radiation Therapy

Method of
Steve Carpenter, MD, and Ali Mazloom, MD

Hodgkin's disease (HD), or Hodgkin's lymphoma (HL), is an important disease for the primary care physician that was first described by Thomas Hodgkin in 1832. HD has a unique behavior. It usually manifests with painless lymphadenopathy and then spreads in a relatively predictable manner to the adjacent lymphatic regions. Next, the patient may have systemic manifestations such as B symptoms, and only much later does the disease spread to organs beyond the lymph nodes and spleen. HD has a high overall cure rate of greater than 80% for early-stage disease and greater than 50% for advanced-stage disease. In addition, recurrent HD often responds to salvage therapy. HD requires careful follow-up to discover late effects of therapy as well as second malignancies.

Epidemiology

HD is diagnosed in more than 7000 people in the United States each year. HD has a slight male predominance and can occur at almost any age. The incidence has a bimodal distribution, with the largest peak occurring in the third decade and a second peak appearing after the age of 50 years. Epstein-Barr virus infection may predispose to development of HD. Familial or genetic associations may also play a role in the development of this disease. The incidence of HD does not appear to be increased by immunosuppression.

Natural History

Early clinicians characterized the spread of HD from one contiguous nodal region to the next. These observations were enhanced by improvements in imaging modalities and by the systematic use of surgical staging with staging laparotomy. One result was an improved cure rate due to the prophylactic use of irradiation of contiguous uninvolved sites. Hematogenous spread occurs primarily as a late event in stage III disease. Bone marrow involvement is rare, occurring mainly in patients with advanced-stage disease or systemic symptoms, whereas hepatic spread does not usually occur without prior splenic disease.

Some patients report systemic symptoms that are referred to as B symptoms. These include unexplained fevers, drenching night sweats, and weight loss. Other systemic symptoms include fatigue, generalized pruritus, and alcohol-induced pain at affected sites.

The most common sites of disease are the cervical nodes, followed by the mediastinal nodes. Patients with HD also have an increased risk for development of other lymphomas. This can occur before or after the diagnosis of HD.

Pathology

Needle biopsies are not adequate for the diagnosis of HD, and tissue obtained for diagnosis should be from a nodal or mass excision. HD is divided into two types: classic Hodgkin's lymphoma and nodular lymphocyte predominance Hodgkin's lymphoma (NLPHL). NLPHL is a more indolent disease with a unique pattern of involvement that usually spares the mediastinum. NLPHL comprises 5% of HD cases. It usually manifests at an early stage, has a high cure rate with irradiation alone, and only rarely transforms to a diffuse large B-cell lymphoma. The pathologic types of HD, as listed by the World Health Organisation, are given in Box 1.

Immunnophenotyping is used to distinguish HD from other lymphomas and also to distinguish among the subtypes. Some groups have included grading for nodular sclerosis HL, and eosinophilic infiltrate of the specimen may be a high-risk feature. Mixed-cellularity HL more commonly involves the abdomen and spleen. The lymphocyte-depleted type is rare and usually manifests in an advanced stage involving the bone marrow.

Evaluation and Staging

A detailed history should be obtained to evaluate for systemic (B) symptoms. A careful physical examination is performed with attention to nodal areas, Waldeyer's ring, liver, and spleen. Bone marrow

 CURRENT DIAGNOSIS

History

■ Systemic (B) symptoms: unexplained fevers, drenching night sweats, and weight loss (>10% of weight in 6 months)
■ Other symptoms: fatigue, generalized pruritus, alcohol-induced pain at affected sites
■ Performance status

Physical Examination

■ Examine lymphoid regions, spleen, liver

Laboratory Studies

■ Complete blood count with differential
■ Erythrocyte sedimentation rate
■ Lactate dehydrogenase, liver function tests, albumin
■ Blood urea nitrogen, creatinine
■ Pregnancy test for women of childbearing age

Imaging Studies

■ Chest radiography
■ Computed tomography of chest, abdomen, pelvis; computed tomography of the neck if cervical adenopathy is present
■ Positron-emission tomographic scan

Biopsy

■ Excisional biopsy (core needle biopsy and fine-needle aspiration are insufficient)
■ Immunohistochemistry
■ Classic Hodgkin's lymphoma (HL): CD3, CD15, CD20, CD30, CD45
■ Nodular lymphocyte predominance HL: CD3, CD15, CD20, CD21, CD30, CD57

Bone Marrow Biopsy: Stages IB-IIB, III, IV

biopsy is advised for stages IB, IIB, III, and IV. Suspicious extranodal abnormalities may also require biopsy. Radiologic examinations should include chest radiography, computed tomography (CT) of chest and abdomen, and a CT/positron-emission tomographic (PET) scan. A CT of the neck is added if there is cervical adenopathy on examination. Laboratory tests should include a complete blood count, sedimentation rate, and kidney and liver function tests. Any effusion should be sent for cytologic examination.

A clinical stage is assigned based on the findings of these studies. The Ann Arbor Staging Classification has been used for several decades. It has received slight changes with the more recent Cotswold's modification, described in Table 1.

Treatment

The current preferred therapy for nonbulky stage IA and IIA classic HL consists of four cycles of ABVD chemotherapy (doxorubicin [Adriamycin], bleomycin [Bleoxane], vinblastine [Velban], and dacarbazine [DTIC-Dome]) followed by 30 Gy of involved-field irradiation. Involved-field irradiation consists of radiation given to the region of the body initially involved on pretreatment imaging. This includes the discernable tumor as well as the general anatomic area. As an example, for any abnormal lymph node on one side of the neck, involved-field irradiation would include the entire ipsilateral neck (from C1 down to below the clavicle).

Only two cycles of chemotherapy may be sufficient in favorable cases. Restaging is performed after chemotherapy and before irradiation. Two cycles (8 weeks) of the Stanford V regimen (doxorubicin, vinblastine, mechlorethamine [nitrogen mustard, Mustargen], etoposide [Vepesid],[1] vincristine [Oncovin], bleomycin, and prednisone) may be substituted for ABVD. Six cycles of ABVD is a less acceptable alternative to combined-modality therapy (chemotherapy and irradiation).

Bulky disease is defined as any mass greater than 10 cm in diameter. Bulky mediastinal adenopathy can also be defined as a mediastinal mass greater than 35% of the intrathoracic diameter at T5–6 or greater than one third of the maximum intrathoracic diameter (near the level of the diaphragm). Bulky early-stage disease is treated with four to six cycles of ABVD followed by involved-field irradiation. Restaging is performed after four cycles of chemotherapy. Alternatively, Stanford V may given for three cycles (12 weeks), followed by involved-field irradiation.

For stage IB, IIB, III, and IV disease, ABVD chemotherapy is given for six to eight cycles, or an escalated dose of BEACOPP (bleomycin, etoposide,[1] doxorubicin, cyclophosphamide [Cytoxan], vincristine, procarbazine [N-methylhydrazine, Matulane], and prednisone) is given for eight cycles. Involved-field irradiation is given to disease sites greater than 5 cm or to residual abnormalities on PET scan at restaging. Stanford V for three cycles plus involved-field irradiation may also be used. The use of involved-field irradiation (consolidation) for bulky or residual sites in stages III and IV disease is currently being explored in a German Hodgkin's Study Group randomized trial (HD 12).

For those patients who are intolerant of chemotherapy or have medical conditions preventing chemotherapy, subtotal lymphoid irradiation may be used alone with a high cure rate. Subtotal lymphoid irradiation consists of radiation to the nodal sites above the diaphragm (mantle field) followed by radiation to the spleen and paraaortic nodes. Vaccinations for encapsulated organisms are given before irradiation of the spleen.

In NLPHL, radiation therapy alone is given for clinical stages IA and IIA. The literature for chemotherapy alone and for combination therapy is very limited. The mediastinum is usually not included in the radiation fields. For those with B symptoms or advanced stage, a variety of chemotherapy regimens, including ABVD or CHOP (cyclophosphamide, doxorubicin, vincristine, and prednisone), may be used. The regimen should include an alkylating agent. However,

---

[1]Not FDA approved for this indication.

TABLE 1 Cotswolds Staging of Hodgkin's Lymphoma

Stage	Description
I	Involvement of a single lymph node region or lymphoid structure
II	Involvement of two or more lymph node regions on the same side of the diaphragm or involvement of a single extralymphatic organ and one or more lymph node regions on the same side of the diaphragm; the number of sites is given with a numerical subscript
III	Involvement of lymph node regions or structures on both sides of the diaphragm
IV	Involvement of one or more extranodal sites beyond that designated as an E site (diffuse or disseminated)

Additional Designations

III-2	With involvement of paraaortic, iliac, and mesenteric nodes
A	No symptoms
B	Fever (>38°C), drenching night sweats, unexplained loss of >10% body weight within 6 mo
X	Bulky disease
E	Involvement of a single extranodal site that is contiguous or proximal to the known nodal site
CS	Clinical stage
PS	Pathologic stage

some patients have a chronic or indolent course requiring little treatment. A variety of effective second-line chemotherapy regimens exist. High-dose therapy or allotransplantation may be used for relapse or progressive disease, along with radiation to residual sites.

ACUTE EFFECTS OF RADIATION

A variety of acute effects are common and are largely self-limited. Reassurance and occasionally medications are helpful. Fatigue is common but is very rarely severe. Most patients can function normally and work full-time during radiation treatments. Mild exercise programs, increased caloric intake, and extra rest are advised. Xerostomia may occasionally occur to a mild degree if the neck is treated. Significant dryness occurs only with irradiation of very high cervical disease or Waldeyer's fields. Often, the dryness resolves completely

CURRENT THERAPY

Stage IA-IIA

- Four cycles of ABVD + 30 Gy involved-field radiotherapy (IFRT)
- Stanford V for 8 weeks (two cycles) may be used as a substitute for ABVD, followed by IFRT
- Restaging is done with positron-emission tomography/ computed tomography (PET/CT) before administration of IFRT
- ABVD for six cycles without IFRT is a less acceptable alternative

Stage I-II Bulky

- Four to six cycles of ABVD + 30–36 Gy IFRT
- Stanford V for 12 weeks (three cycles) may be used as a substitute for ABVD, followed by IFRT
- Restaging is done with PET/CT after four cycles of chemotherapy with ABVD or completion of therapy with Stanford V

Stage IB-IIB, III-IV

- Six to eight cycles of ABVD + 30–40 Gy IFRT for stage I-II disease and initial bulky disease
- Escalated-dose BEACOPP for eight cycles may be used as an alternative to ABVD, followed by IFRT
- Restaging is done with PET/CT after four cycles of chemotherapy with ABVD or BEACOPP
- IFRT is administered to initial sites >5 cm in diameter

after many months. Chronic dryness predisposes to dental decay, so daily prescription fluoride application and frequent professional cleaning are advised. Mild pharyngitis or dysphagia may occur at about 20 Gy, but this is minimal or absent in many patients. Topical agents are available to minimize and treat these symptoms, which usually resolve soon after irradiation. Hair loss may occur, but only inside the radiation field. Temporary hyperpigmentation or mild erythema of the skin may occur. Sunscreen should be applied during and after radiation therapy.

Pericarditis may occur during or after radiation therapy. Pneumonitis may occur in the first month after irradiation. These effects occur in fewer than 5% of patients and are even rarer with modern techniques and doses. Rare reports of acute pericarditis exist with limited cardiac volumes of radiation after prior exposure to doxorubicin.

Lhermitte's sign is an electrical shock-like sensation that radiates down the legs. It is precipitated by forward flexion of the trunk. This is very uncommon but can be alarming to the patient; the impact can be minimized if the patient is properly educated about the possibility of having these symptoms. It occurs 3 to 12 weeks after radiation and may be related to transient demyelinization of the cord. This syndrome does not predict for any permanent neurologic sequelae and resolves spontaneously after a few months.

Hematologic changes are usually minimal when radiation therapy is given after chemotherapy. These effects can be significant with larger volumes of radiation, especially with the use of irradiation alone with extended fields.

LATE EFFECTS

Pulmonary complications may occur from bleomycin chemotherapy or from excessive radiation volumes. Care should be exercised with radiation volumes after prior treatment with bleomycin. The large mantle fields treated in earlier regimens are rarely used now, so pulmonary toxicity is reduced. Acute symptomatic radiation pnuemonitis typically occurs within 6 to 12 weeks after completion of radiation therapy. A subacute fibrotic phase may occur at 6 months. This acute syndrome is characterized by cough, dyspnea on exertion, and low-grade temperature elevation. The cough can usually be eliminated with oral steroids, but such drugs should be tapered slowly to prevent recurrence of symptoms. Although steroids improve the acute symptoms, they do not prevent the late fibrosis. Fibrotic changes may be seen on chest radiography or lung windows of CT studies without symptoms. The changes usually conform to the pattern of the radiation field.

Chronic cardiomyopathy increases as the dose of doxorubicin accumulates to greater than 400 mg/m^2. The magnitude of the effect of using lower doses and the interactions with radiation are unknown. Irradiation of cardiac vessels probably leads to accelerated arteriosclerosis. Currently used limited radiation fields may treat little or no cardiac vessels compared with previous mantle fields. Additionally, current radiation doses of 20 to 30 Gy may be below a threshold for induction of arteriosclerosis. Chemical hypothyroidism occurs in about one third of patients when the thyroid is included in the radiation field. Patients should routinely be tested for hypothyroidism, and replacement hormone should be given if the thyroid-stimulating hormone concentration is elevated. Herpes zoster (shingles) may occur after radiation therapy. Sepsis may occur with chemotherapy-induced neutropenia or from pneumococcal organisms after splenic irradiation.

Treatment-related secondary malignancies can also occur. Acute myeloid leukemia or myelodysplastic syndrome may occur after chemotherapy. Non-Hodgkin's lymphomas occur more commonly in these patients than in the general population. The incidence of solid tumors is increased after irradiation. Smokers should be advised to discontinue smoking after thoracic irradiation to reduce the increased risk of lung cancer. Breast cancer may be increased after thoracic irradiation in women younger than 30 years of age. The risk is related not only to age but also to the dose and volume of exposed breast. Current progress in lowering the dose of radiation and reducing the field size should dramatically decrease the risk of secondary solid tumors. Women receiving thoracic irradiation should begin breast examinations and mammography at an earlier age. Approximately 5% of patients develop thyroid cancer after exposure to therapeutic levels of radiation to the thyroid gland. This is usually of the well-differentiated type and has a high cure rate.

Infertility may occur after treatment for HD. In males, azoospermia may occur after pelvic irradiation. The magnitude of this effect can significantly be reduced with proper gonadal shielding, allowing for near-complete recovery in most men. Sperm banking is recommended as a precaution for all young men receiving pelvic irradiation. Chemotherapy with MOPP (mechlorethamine, vincristine, procarbazine, and prednisone), MOPP-like regimens that include procarbazine, or BEACOPP causes sterility in most men. Male fertility is usually preserved with ABVD and Stanford V regimens. Elimination of ovarian function often occurs with pelvic irradiation of women older than 30 years of age. Younger women may be protected from pelvic irradiation by oophorpexy, with placement of the ovaries in the midline behind the uterus. Ovarian function is also affected by alkylating agents in women older than 30 years of age.

REFERENCES

DeVita VT, Lawrence TS, Rosenberg SA. DeVita, Hellman, and Rosenberg's Cancer: Principles and Practice of Oncology. 8th ed. Philadelphia: Wolters Kluwer/Lippincott Williams & Wilkins; 2008.

Diehl V, Engert A, Mueller RP, et al. HD 10: Investigating reduction of combined modality treatment intensity in early stage Hodgkin's lymphoma. Interim analysis of a randomized trial of the German Hodgkin Study Group (GHSG). J Clin Oncol 2005;23(16S):561S.

Dores GM. Second malignant neoplasms among long-term survivors of Hodgkin's disease: A population-based evaluation over 25 years. J Clin Oncol 2002;20:3484–94.

Engert A, Franklin J, Eich HT, et al. Two cycles of doxorubicin, bleomycin, vinblastine and dacarbazine plus extended field radiotherapy is superior to radiotherapy alone in early favorable Hodgkin's lymphoma: Final results of the GHSG HD7 trial. J Clin Oncol 2007;25:3495–502.

Engert A, Schiller P, Josting A, et al. Involved-field radiotherapy is equally effective and less toxic compared with extended-field radiotherapy after four cycles of chemotherapy in patients with early-stage unfavorable Hodgkin's lymphoma: Results of the HD8 trial of the German Hodgkin's Lymphoma Study Group. J Clin Oncol 2003;21:3601–8.

Halperin EC, Perez CA, Brady LW. Perez and Brady's Principles and Practice of Radiation Oncology. 5th ed. Philadelphia: Wolters Kluwer Health/Lippincott Williams & Wilkins; 2008.

Hancock SL, Tucker MA, Hoppe RT. Factors affecting late mortality from heart disease after treatment of Hodgkin's disease. JAMA 1993;270:1949–55.

Hoppe RT, Advani RH, Ambinder RF, et al. Hodgkin disease/lymphoma. J Natl Compr Cancer Netw 2008;6:594–622.

NCCN Clinical Practice Guidelines in Oncology. Hodgkin Disease/Lymphoma. Version 2, Available at http://www.nccn.org/professionals/physician_gls/PDF/hodgkins.pdf; 2008 [accessed November 13, 2008].

Acute Leukemia in Adults

Method of
Peter R. Duggan, MD

The acute leukemias are a heterogeneous group of malignancies that arise from the clonal expansion of myeloid or lymphoid blasts. They are characterized by the accumulation of malignant cells in blood, bone marrow, and occasionally other tissues. The common presenting features of leukemia are caused by bone marrow infiltration and failure of normal hematopoiesis. Acute myelogenous leukemia (AML) occurs in all age groups, although the incidence increases with age. The median age at diagnosis is between 65 and 70 years. Acute lymphoblastic leukemia (ALL) occurs mainly in childhood; it accounts for fewer than 20% of the cases of acute leukemia in adults.

Diagnosis of Acute Leukemia

PRESENTATION

The clinical features of acute leukemia at presentation can result from bone marrow failure (anemia, neutropenia, and thrombocytopenia) or organ infiltration. As anemia worsens, patients develop fatigue and lethargy, pallor, palpitations, and dyspnea. Exacerbation of ischemic heart disease, myocardial infarction, and congestive heart failure can occur in patients with underlying heart disease.

Spontaneous bleeding from mucosal membranes, petechiae, easy bruising, and menorrhagia due to thrombocytopenia are common. Concomitant coagulopathy can occur, especially in the setting of promyelocytic leukemia, causing a further increase in bleeding risk. Less commonly, life-threatening gastrointestinal, central nervous system, or other bleeding can occur.

Patients may be predisposed to infections, depending on the severity of the neutropenia. It is uncommon for a patient to present with severe infections, although minor infections often occur.

Leukemia cells can infiltrate any organ outside the bone marrow. Lymphoblastic leukemia commonly causes splenomegaly or lymphadenopathy and can involve the testes and central nervous system, especially at relapse. Large mediastinal masses are a frequent finding in T-cell lymphoblastic leukemia. Skin and gingival involvement is often a feature of acute monocytic leukemia. Myeloid (granulocytic) sarcoma or chloroma is a tumor composed of myeloid leukemia cells. These commonly affect the skin but can be found in any location. Although there is often no other evidence of leukemia when myeloid sarcoma is diagnosed, systemic therapy is required, because bone marrow involvement invariably follows.

Hyperleukocytosis is an uncommon but life-threatening complication of acute leukemia that occurs with higher presenting white blood cell (WBC) counts, usually greater than 100×10^9 cells/L. The lungs and central nervous system are most affected, causing altered level of consciousness, confusion, dizziness, cerebral hemorrhage, visual changes, and other neurologic findings as well as dyspnea and hypoxia. Treatment includes aggressive hydration, urgent initiation of chemotherapy (see later discussion), and leukapheresis to reduce the burden of circulating WBCs.

INVESTIGATION

Diagnosis of acute leukemia requires a combination of morphologic, immunophenotypic, and genetic studies. Assessment by morphology alone is usually inadequate for determining the type of leukemia. Immunophenotypic analysis by flow cytometry is used to determine surface antigen expression by leukemia cells and can identify the leukemia subtype in most cases. Flow cytometry has largely replaced the use of special bone marrow stains for determining AML lineage and classification.

CURRENT DIAGNOSIS

- Complete blood count: Anemia and thrombocytopenia are present in almost all cases; white blood cells are increased in fewer than half of acute leukemia cases.
- Bone marrow aspiration: Aspirate morphology usually differentiates leukemia from other bone marrow disorders. It is not always possible to classify the type of acute leukemia. Aspirate material is usually used for flow cytometry and genetic tests.
- Bone marrow biopsy: can be used for immunophenotyping if marrow cells are not available for flow cytometry.
- Flow cytometry: used to determine immunophenotype of blasts.
- Cytogenetics: Analyze for abnormalities of chromosomes; provides invaluable prognostic information.
- Fluorescence in situ hybridization (FISH): used to detect specific genetic abnormalities with therapeutic or prognostic value.
- Polymerase chain reaction: highly sensitive detection of genetic mutations; can be useful for detecting minimal residual disease.

Genetic studies are becoming increasingly important in the evaluation of acute leukemia. Clonal abnormalities of chromosomes are found in more than half of the cases and can be used to predict response to therapy and survival. Cytogenetic analysis provides important prognostic information and can be useful for diagnosis when leukemia is associated with a specific genetic mutation. Genetic analysis by polymerase chain reaction (PCR) or fluorescent in situ hybridization is used to detect known genetic mutations that can determine diagnosis and affect prognosis. The presence of mutations detectable by sensitive techniques such as PCR can be used to monitor response to therapy and to detect minimal residual disease and early relapses.

CLASSIFICATION

The World Health Organisation (WHO) uses a combination of clinical, morphologic, immunophenotypic, and genetic findings to classify leukemia into distinct entities. The most recent revision of the WHO classification, taking into account growing knowledge of the genetic abnormalities found in cancer, has revised the diagnostic criteria for some diseases and described a number of new entities (Box 1). This revised system is much more expansive than previous classification systems and recognizes diseases not distinguished by the French-American-British (FAB) classification system. Recognition of these distinct entities and their unique genetic or biologic features may open the door for specific and effective therapies in the future. The WHO classification will continue to evolve as new information becomes available.

Prognosis in Acute Leukemia

A number of factors have been identified that affect prognosis in acute leukemia (Table 1). Of these, age and cytogenetic findings appear to be the most important at diagnosis. In AML, remission rates of 70% to 80% and long-term survival rates of 40% are seen for younger patients, but these are less than 25% and 10%, respectively, for patients older than 60 years of age. The survival rate is about 70% for those with good-risk cytogenetics, 30% to 50% with intermediate-risk cytogenetics, and less than 15% with poor-risk cytogenetics. The prognostic findings at diagnosis can be helpful in deciding who should receive intensive therapies such as bone marrow transplantation, investigational therapies, or, in some cases, no

BOX 1 World Health Organisation Classification of Acute Leukemia

Acute Myeloid Leukemia

- AML with recurrent genetic abnormalities
  AML with t(8;21)
  AML with inv(16) or t(16;16)
  Acute promyelocytic leukemia with t(15;17)
  AML with t(9;11)
  AML with t(6;9)
  AML with inv(3) or t(3;3)
  AML (megakaryoblastic) with t(1;22)
  AML with mutated NPM1
  AML with mutated CEBPA
- AML with myelodysplasia-related changes
- Therapy-related myeloid neoplasms
- Acute myeloid leukemia, NOS
  AML with minimal differentiation
  AML without maturation
  AML with maturation
  Acute myelomonocytic leukemia
  Acute monoblastic and monocytic leukemia
  Acute erythroid leukemia
  Acute megakaryoblastic leukemia
  Acute basophilic leukemia
  Acute panmyelosis with myelofibrosis
- Myeloid sarcoma
- Myeloid proliferations related to Down syndrome
  Transient abnormal myelopoiesis
  Myeloid leukemia associated with Down syndrome
- Acute leukemias of ambiguous lineage
  Acute undifferentiated leukemia
  Mixed phenotype acute leukemia with t(9;22)
  Mixed phenotype acute leukemia with t(v;11q23)
  Mixed phenotype acute leukemia B-cell myeloid, NOS
  Mixed phenotype acute leukemia T-cell myeloid, NOS

Precursor Lymphoid Neoplasms

- B lymphoblastic leukemia/lymphoma, NOS
- B lymphoblastic leukemia/lymphoma with recurrent genetic abnormalities
  B lymphoblastic leukemia/lymphoma with t(9;22)
  B lymphoblastic leukemia/lymphoma with t(v;11q23)
  B lymphoblastic leukemia/lymphoma with t(12;21)
  B lymphoblastic leukemia/lymphoma with hyperdiploidy
  B lymphoblastic leukemia/lymphoma with hypodiploidy
  B lymphoblastic leukemia/lymphoma with t(5;14)
  B lymphoblastic leukemia/lymphoma with t(1;19)

T Lymphoblastic Leukemia/Lymphoma

Abbreviations: AML = acute myeloblastic leukemia; CEBPA = CCAAT/enhancer binding protein-α; inv = inversion; NOS = not otherwise specified; NPM1 = nucleophosmin; t = translocation. Modified from Swerdlow SH, Campo E, Harris NL, et al: IARC WHO Classification of Tumours, vol 2: WHO Classification of Tumours of Haematopoietic and Lymphoid Tissues, 4th ed. Geneva, World Health Organisation, 2008. Used with permission.

therapy at all. A number of molecular genetic abnormalities have been described that affect outcome in AML, although for most of these testing is not yet widely available.

Secondary AML occurs in patients who have had previous exposure to chemotherapy, especially alkylating agents and topoisomerase inhibitors, benzene, and radiation. It can also occur as a result of progression of a preexisting hematologic disorder such as myelodysplastic syndrome, myeloproliferative disorder, or aplastic

TABLE 1 Prognostic Factors in Adult Acute Leukemia

Type of Leukemia	Favorable Factors	Intermediate Factors	Unfavorable Factors
Acute megaloblastic leukemia (AML)	Age <60 y t(15;17) t(8;21) inv16, t(16;16) CEBPA mutations	Normal +8, −Y	Age ≥60 y −7, −5 t(6;9) inv 3, t(3;13) Complex karyotype Secondary leukemia FLT3, NPM1, WT1 mutations BAALC, ERG, MN1 expression
Acute lymphoblastic leukemia (ALL)	Age <30 y WBC <30 Hyperdiploidy (>50 chromosomes) t(12;21)		Age ≥30 y WBC ≥30 Hypodiploidy (<44 chromosomes) No remission at 28 d t(9;22), 11q23 abnormalities Complex karyotype

Abbreviations: BAALC = brain and acute leukemia, cytoplasmic gene; CEBPA = CCAAT/enhancer binding protein-α; ERG = ets-related gene; FLT3 = fms-related tyrosine kinase 3; MN1 = meningioma 1 gene; NPM1 = nucleophosmin; WBC = white blood cell count (in cell/m^3); WT1 = Wilms' tumor 1.

anemia. Secondary AML is associated with a higher incidence of unfavorable cytogenetic findings and other adverse prognostic factors, and it has a much poorer outcome compared with de novo AML.

Treatment

SUPPORTIVE CARE

A tunneled central venous catheter is required before therapy is initiated. The use of prophylactic broad-spectrum antibiotic, antifungal, and antiviral medications is controversial and not universally practiced. Low-dose amphotericin (Amphocin, Fungizone)[1] or an azole such as fluconazole (Diflucan),[1] itraconazole (Sporanox),[1] or voriconazole (Vfend)[1] for fungal prophylaxis and acyclovir (Zovirax)[1] or valacyclovir (Valtrex)[1] for viral prophylaxis are the most commonly used agents.

Infection is one of the main causes of death during leukemia therapy. After chemotherapy, patients develop profound neutropenia lasting for several weeks, as well as moderate to severe mucositis, putting them at risk for opportunistic infection. Febrile episodes with or without localizing signs of infection should initiate investigations for the source of infection, including cultures of blood, urine, and sputum; chest radiographs; and other imaging studies as clinically indicated. Broad-spectrum antibiotics with activity against *Pseudomonas*, such as ceftazidime (Ceptaz) 1 g every 8 hours, piperacillin-tazobactam (Zosyn) 2.25 to 4.5 g every 8 hours, or meropenem (Merrem IV) 500 mg to 1 g every 8 hours, should be administered. Ongoing fevers lasting longer than 48 hours despite adequate antibiotic coverage are worrisome for resistant bacterial or fungal infection. Empiric antifungal therapy should be considered in consultation with infectious disease specialists. Both prophylactic and empiric antibiotic use should be tailored to the institution's own patterns of infection occurrence and resistance.

Packed red blood cell and platelet transfusions should be used to keep the hemoglobin concentration greater than 70 to 80 mg/dL and the platelet count greater than 10×10^9/L. Irradiated blood products are indicated for patients who are potential candidates for bone marrow transplantation.

The use of hematopoietic growth factors such as granulocyte colony-stimulating factor (G-CSF [filgrastim, Neupogen]) 300 to 480 μg/day to promote bone marrow recovery after leukemia therapy is not routinely practiced. There is evidence that it results in decreased duration of neutropenia, fewer severe infections, less antibiotic use,

and shorter hospitalizations. There is no increase in relapse rates with use of G-CSF, but there is also no improvement in overall survival.

Evidence of tumor lysis (hyperuricemia, hyperkalemia, hyperphosphatemia, hypocalcemia, rising lactate dehydrogenase concentration) is usually seen within hours after the start of chemotherapy and often before treatment even begins. These biochemical alterations can result in cardiac arrhythmias from severe hyperkalemia or renal failure from uric acid precipitation. Patients should have frequent electrolyte and renal function monitoring. Aggressive hydration should be started before antileukemia therapy is initiated. Allopurinol (Zyloprim) 300 mg PO daily or rasburicase (Elitek) 0.15 to 0.2 mg/kg IV daily for 5 days should be used to control hyperuricemia. The risk of tumor lysis usually resolves 3 to 4 days after treatment begins.

ACUTE MYELOGENOUS LEUKEMIA

Remission Induction

Standard induction regimens for AML consist of cytarabine (Ara-C, Cytosar-U) 100 to 200 mg/m^2/day for 7 days plus an anthracycline, usually daunorubicin (Cerubidine) 45 mg/m^2/day or idarubicin (Idamycin) 12 mg/m^2/day, given as a daily bolus for 3 days. Reported differences in outcome with different anthracycline agents were more likely caused by the use of doses that are not of comparable efficacy rather than by differences in the actual effectiveness of the drugs. Increasing the dose of cytarabine given during induction, or adding or substituting other agents such as etoposide (Toposar),[1] fludarabine (Fludara),[1] mitoxantrone (Novantrone), or G-CSF[1] has not been shown to significantly improve remission rates or long-term survival. A randomized clinical trial evaluating the addition of gemtuzumab ozogamicin (Mylotarg) to standard induction chemotherapy is ongoing.

Consolidation

Although up to 40% of older patients and 80% of young patients achieve remission, all will relapse without further therapy. At least two to three cycles of cytarabine-containing regimens are given. Administration of single-agent high-dose cytarabine (3 g/m^2) twice daily on days 1, 3, and 5 appears to be more effective than regimens containing lower doses of cytarabine, especially if the t(8;21) or inv(16) chromosome rearrangement is present. High-dose cytarabine causes a sterile conjunctivitis that can be prevented with administration of corticosteroid eyedrops during therapy and for 48 hours after the last dose is given. High-dose cytarabine is also

---

[1]Not FDA approved for this indication.

[1]Not FDA approved for this indication.

associated with cerebellar toxicity. This is especially pronounced in the elderly and limits the dose to 1 to 2 g/m^2 in those older than 60 years of age.

Stem Cell Transplantation

A number of clinical trials have compared the outcomes of patients for whom human leukocyte antigen (HLA)-identical sibling is available to treatment with chemotherapy alone or with chemotherapy followed by autologous stem cell transplantation. The results are conflicting, with superiority for both transplant options and chemotherapy seen in different trials. Allogeneic transplantation produces lowest risk of relapse due to an immunologic graft-versus-leukemia effect caused by donor immune cells, but the treatment-related mortality is high, ranging from 20% to 40%, and many recipients suffer the sometimes debilitating effects of graft-versus-host disease. These risks are higher when unrelated or mismatched donors are used. Autologous stem cell transplantation allows the delivery of high-dose chemotherapy without the high treatment–related mortality seen in allogeneic transplantation. However, it does not produce a graft-versus-leukemia effect, and there is a risk that the autologous stem cells may be contaminated by leukemia cells that can contribute to later relapse.

Allogeneic transplantation is clearly indicated for patients with high-risk leukemia, including those with adverse cytogenetic findings, therapy-related AML, and relapsed or refractory disease. In these settings, the results from standard chemotherapy are so poor that transplantation should be pursued if a related or unrelated donor is available. In intermediate-risk disease, allogeneic transplantation with a matched sibling donor is often recommended during first remission, whereas transplantation from unrelated donors is reserved for treatment of relapsed disease in most centers.

Any benefit from the use of allogeneic transplantation in the treatment of AML will be limited, because this is usually an option reserved for younger patients who must have an acceptably HLA-matched donor. The increasing use of unrelated donors allows more patients to proceed to transplantation. The use of less intense, non-myeloablative transplantation regimens in older patients and in those with serious comorbidities also helps extend the use of transplantation in more patients with AML.

ACUTE PROMYELOCYTIC LEUKEMIA

The treatment approach to AML is similar for all subtypes with the exception of acute promyelocytic leukemia (APL). APL is rare, representing 5% to 13% of all cases of AML, and has a number of unique features. The most important of these is a very high response rate to all-*trans*retinoic acid (ATRA [Vesanoid, Tretinoin]), which results in high remission rates and in cure of this leukemia in more than 80% of patients.

APL is characterized by a translocation involving the *PML* gene on chromosome 15 and the retinoic acid receptor-α (*RARA*) gene on chromosome 17 [t(15;17)]. The wild-type *RARA* gene codes for a retinoic acid receptor that acts to inhibit DNA transcription. In the presence of physiologic levels of retinoic acid, this inhibition is lifted. The PML-RARA protein present in APL is a more potent inhibitor of DNA transcription. It is resistant to physiologic levels of retinoic acid but does respond to pharmacologic doses. The PML/RARA protein causes maturation arrest, resulting in a predominance of promyelocytes in the bone marrow of these patients.

A small number of patients with APL (<5%) have translocations involving *RARA* and genes other than *PML,* such as the variant t (11;17), which involves the *PLZF* gene on chromosome 11. APL patients with such translocations have a poorer prognosis, because the disease is resistant to therapy with retinoic acid.

Patients with APL often have evidence of coagulopathy at presentation and have a high risk of life-threatening hemorrhage. If APL is suspected or confirmed, coagulation testing including activated partial thromboplastin time (aPTT), international normalized ratio (INR), fibrinogen, and platelet count should be performed. Coagulopathy should be treated aggressively with plasma and platelet transfusions to maintain the platelet count higher than 50 × 10^9/L and

fibrinogen concentration greater than 1.5 g/L or 150 mg/dL until the coagulopathy resolves, usually within a few days after therapy is started.

Prognosis in APL can be determined from the WBC and platelet counts at presentation, with patients divided into three risk groups: low risk (WBCs <10 × 10^9/L; platelets >40 × 10^9/L), intermediate risk (WBCs <10 × 10^9/L; platelets <40 × 10^9/L), and high risk (WBCs >10 × 10^9/L).

ATRA causes terminal differentiation of APL cells. When used alone, it results in complete remission for most patients, but such remissions are not durable. Relapse rates are also higher in patients treated with chemotherapy alone compared with the combination of ATRA and chemotherapy. Standard induction protocols combine simultaneous ATRA (Vesanoid) 45 mg/m^2 in two divided doses PO daily until morphologic complete remission with an anthracycline (e.g., idarubicin[1] 12 mg/m^2 IV on days 2, 4, 6, and 8). Morphologic complete remission rates of 90% to 95% are reported with this approach. Consolidation with multiple cycles of anthracycline results in molecular remissions and absence of disease by PCR in more than 90% of patients.

The rapid differentiation of leukemia cells that occurs when ATRA therapy is initiated can result in a syndrome of fever, dyspnea, weight gain, pulmonary infiltrates, and pleural effusions that has proved fatal in a small number of patients. Patients with initial WBC counts greater than 10 × 10^9/L or whose WBC count increases above this level after therapy is started are at particular risk. ATRA should be withheld and dexamethasone (Decadron)[1] 10 mg IV given twice daily until symptoms resolve.

Maintenance therapy using intermittent ATRA, with or without methotrexate 20 mg/m^2 weekly and 6-mercaptopurine (Purinethol)[1] 20 mg/m^2 daily, given for up to 2 years, may reduce the risk of relapse, especially in patients with high-risk disease or evidence of minimal residual disease after consolidation. The use of high-dose cytarabine in APL is controversial but may be of benefit as part of consolidation for high-risk patients. Medications such as arsenic trioxide (Trisenox) and gemtuzumab ozogamicin[1] also result in high response rates in APL. Arsenic trioxide, in particular, is frequently used as salvage therapy for relapsed APL. The role of these drugs in induction and consolidation therapy continues to be evaluated in clinical trials.

Relapsed APL is treated with similar approaches, and many patients respond to a repeat course of ATRA. Arsenic trioxide 0.15 mg/kg/day until remission (up to 60 days) is now frequently used for relapsed disease. High-dose chemotherapy with autologous stem cell transplantation is effective salvage therapy, especially for patients who achieve a PCR-negative remission after relapse. Allogeneic transplantation may also be considered for suitable patients.

ACUTE MYELOBLASTIC LEUKEMIA IN THE ELDERLY

Although outcomes have improved for young people with AML, studies continue to show no improvement in survival for older patients. The median survival after a diagnosis of AML in elderly patients is only 2 to 4 months, with fewer than 10% of patients surviving longer than 2 years.

Compared to younger patients, the elderly are more likely to have AML with poor-risk cytogenetics, have higher multidrug resistance gene expression, and are more likely to have secondary leukemia. Older patients are more likely to present with poor performance status and multiple comorbidities, resulting in poor tolerance of intensive chemotherapy. They experience more treatment-related complications and higher treatment-related mortality. Older patients are generally not candidates for bone marrow transplantation, which has had a major impact on outcomes for young patients. The optimal treatment of AML in young people has been extensively evaluated in clinical trials, but relatively few such trials exist for older patients, even though most patients diagnosed with AML are older than 65 years of age.

---

[1]Not FDA approved for this indication.

Most elderly patients with AML are never treated; only 30% of patients over 65 years ever receive therapy. The treatment-related mortality rate is greater than 20%, and remission rates are only 30% to 50%. Age less than 70 years, AML without high-risk cytogenetics, good performance status, and presence of few or no comorbid illnesses predict a better response to therapy and a lower risk of treatment-related mortality. These patients have survival rates of 10% to 20% with chemotherapy, compared to 5% or less for other patients.

For most patients, palliative supportive care is appropriate, and low-dose chemotherapy or investigational agents can be considered. Low-dose chemotherapy with cytarabine (Cytosar-U), mitoxantrone, etoposide,[1] and other agents produces responses but has not been shown to improve survival.

Investigational agents that show some activity in AML and are being evaluated in clinical trials for AML in the elderly include the hypomethylating agents decitabine (Dacogen)[1] and 5-azacytidine (azacitidine [Vidaza]), an anti-sense oligonucleotide oblimersen (Genasense),[5] as well as other agents.

Gemtuzumab ozogamicin, an anti-CD33 monoclonal antibody bound to the chemotherapeutic molecule calicheamicin, when given as a single agent at a dose of 9 mg/m^2 IV on days 1 and 15, produces remissions in about 20% of elderly patients with AML but has not been shown to improve survival.

TREATMENT OF ACUTE LYMPHOBLASTIC LEUKEMIA

Remission Induction

The protocols used in the treatment of adult ALL are based on the highly successful regimens used in children. Despite high remission rates in adults, usually greater than 90%, these regimens have yet to achieve the same long-term initial results in older patients as are seen in childhood disease, and the cure rate in adults is only about 30%.

Treatment usually consists of a remission induction phase, an intensification phase, and a long-term maintenance phase. Although a number of protocols exist, most include vincristine (Oncovin), prednisone, cyclophosphamide (Cytoxan), an anthracycline, and L-asparaginase (Elspar) as part of remission induction. Intensification courses often include thioguanine (Tabloid),[1] 6-mercaptopurine, and drugs such as high-dose methotrexate and cytarabine (Cytosar-U) that penetrate the central nervous system. Central nervous system prophylaxis also includes repeated intrathecal administration of methotrexate 12 to 15 mg and cytarabine 30 to 50 mg. The use of craniospinal radiation can have serious long-term neurocognitive effects, especially in elderly patients.

Maintenance chemotherapy usually consists of monthly IV vincristine (Oncovin) 1.4 mg/m^2, weekly oral methotrexate 20 mg/m^2, daily oral 6-mercaptopurine 60 mg/m^2, and prednisone 60 mg/m^2 for 5 days per month. This regimen is continued for up to 2 years after the diagnosis of leukemia.

Imatinib (Gleevec) 600 to 800 mg/day as a single agent has a high response rate in ALL with t(9;22). Although these responses are very short lived (<3 months on average), ongoing studies will determine whether this or other tyrosine kinase inhibitors may help improve the otherwise poor prognosis when this translocation is present.

There are few studies evaluating the role of allogeneic transplantation in adult ALL. It is unclear whether transplantation is of benefit in low-risk ALL, compared with chemotherapy alone. However, survival seems to be improved in patients with high-risk ALL after transplantation, especially in those with t(9;22). At this time, there does not seem to be a role for autologous transplantation in ALL. As in AML, transplantation is the only curative option for relapsed or refractory disease.

---

[1]Not FDA approved for this indication.
[5]Investigational drug in the United States.

REFERENCES

Forman SJ. Allogeneic transplantation acute lymphoblastic leukemia in adults. In: Thomas ED, Blume KG, Forman SJ, editors. Hematopoietic Cell Transplantation. 2nd ed. London: Blackwell Sciences; 1999. p. 849–58.

Liesveld JL, Lichtman MA. Acute myelogenous leukemia. In: Lichtman MA, Beutler TJ, Kipps TJ, et al., Williams Hematology. 7th ed. New York: McGraw-Hill; 2006. p. 969–76.

Pui C-H. Acute lymphoblastic leukemia. In: Lichtman MA, Beutler E, Kipps TJ, et al, editors. Williams Hematology. 7th ed. New York: McGraw-Hill; 2006. p. 1017–28.

Sanz MA, Grimwade D, Tallman MS, et al. Guidelines on the management of acute promyelocytic leukemia: Recommendations from an expert panel on behalf of the European LeukemiaNet. Blood 2008;113(9):1875–91.

Stockel-Goldstein K, Blume KG. Allogeneic hematopoietic cell transplantation for adult patients with acute myeloid leukemia. In: Thomas ED, Blume SJ, Forman SJ, editors. Hematopoietic Cell Transplantation. 2nd ed. London, Blackwell Sciences; 1999. p. 823–34.

Swerdlow SH, Campo E, Harris NL, et al., editors. WHO Classification of Hematopoietic and Lymphoid Tissues. Geneva: WHO Press; 2008.

Acute Leukemia in Children

Method of
Patrick Brown, MD, and Stephen P. Hunger, MD

The word "leukemia" is derived from the Greek roots *leukos* (white) and *haima* (blood). Leukemia, cancer of the blood-forming cells, is characterized by a marked proliferation of abnormal leukocytes in the bone marrow and blood that may be associated with widespread infiltration in extramedullary sites including the central nervous system (CNS), testes, thymus, liver, spleen, and lymph nodes.

Classification

The first level of classification of leukemia is *acute* versus *chronic*. Acute leukemia is characterized by the predominance of very immature white blood cell precursors, or blasts, and is an aggressive, rapidly fatal disease if left untreated. Chronic leukemia is characterized by proliferation of relatively mature white blood cells and is typically an indolent disease.

The second level of classification is *lymphoid* versus *myeloid*, depending on whether the leukemic cells display characteristics of lymphocyte precursors or myelocyte (granulocyte, erythrocyte, monocyte, or megakaryocyte) precursors. Acute lymphoblastic leukemia (ALL) and acute myeloid leukemia (AML) account for the overwhelming majority of pediatric leukemias. Chronic leukemias are uncommon in pediatrics.

ALL and AML are further subclassified by morphology and expression of cell surface antigens using flow cytometry. For ALL, classification is largely based on cell surface and cytoplasmic marker expression (Table 1). AML cases are classified by characteristic chromosomal abnormalities (if present) or by light microscopic morphology in cases where these specific chromosomal changes are absent (Box 1).

Epidemiology

The incidence of childhood cancer is 14 cases per 100,000 children younger than 16 years of age per year, which translates into approximately 11,000 new cases per year in the United States. Leukemia accounts for approximately 30% of childhood cancers, making it the most common form of childhood cancer. The distribution of the major forms of leukemia is vastly different in children than in adults (Fig. 1). In general, children are far more likely to have acute leukemia,

TABLE 1 Classification of Childhood Acute Lymphoblastic Leukemia

ALL Subtype	Phenotypic Marker				%	Comment
	CD19	CD10	clg	slg		
Pre-pre B	+	–	–	–	5	Mostly infants, poor prognosis, frequent *MLL* 11q23 rearrangements
Early pre-B	+	+	–	–	63	Common ALL, young children, good prognosis
Pre-B	+	+	+	–	16	Older children, good prognosis with intense therapy
B-cell	+	+	+	+	4	Burkitt's leukemia, *MYC/Ig* fusion genes, good prognosis with lymphoma-type therapy
T-cell	–	–	–	–	12	Adolescents, anterior mediastinal mass, CNS involvement, good prognosis with intense therapy

ALL = acute myeloid leukemia; clg = cytoplasmic immunoglobulin; slg = surface immunoglobulin; CNS = central nervous system.

BOX 1   Classification of Childhood Acute Myeloid Leukemia (World Health Organization Criteria)

Acute Myeloid Leukemia with Recurrent Genetic Abnormalities

Acute myeloid leukemia with t(8;21)(q22;q22), *(AML1/ETO)*

Acute myeloid leukemia with abnormal bone marrow eosinophils and inv(16)(p13q22) or t(16;16)(p13;q22), *(CBFβ/MYH11)*

Acute promyelocytic leukemia with t(15;17)(q22;q12), *(PML/RARα)*, and variants

Acute myeloid leukemia with 11q23 *(MLL)* abnormalities

Acute Myeloid Leukemia, Not Otherwise Categorized

Acute myeloid leukemia, minimally differentiated (FAB M0)

Acute myeloid leukemia without maturation (FAB M1)

Acute myeloid leukemia with maturation (FAB M2)

Acute myelomonocytic leukemia (FAB M4)

Acute monoblastic/acute monocytic leukemia (FAB M5)

Acute erythroid leukemia (FAB M6)

Acute megakaryoblastic leukemia (FAB M7)

FAB = French–American–British classification.

---

and ALL is much more common than AML. In adults, most cases of leukemia are chronic, and AML is much more common than ALL.

The incidence of the various forms of leukemia varies by age in both children and adults (Fig. 2). This is especially true for childhood ALL, for which there is a marked incidence peak in the 2- to 4-year-old age group. This ALL age peak is primarily found in children living in industrialized nations, leading to speculation that a common environmental exposure, coupled with age-related immunologic susceptibility, is at least partially responsible for many cases of ALL. Except for a small peak in infants, the incidence of AML is fairly constant in childhood but rises quickly in later adulthood.

Prognosis

One of the most dramatic success stories in modern medicine is the improvement in survival of children with ALL over the past four decades. Leukemia was once a uniformly fatal diagnosis, with less than a 5% to 10% cure rate until the mid to late 1960s. Today, approximately 85% of children with ALL are cured. The improved prognosis is built on pioneering observations on the efficacy of multiagent systemic therapy and the importance of presymptomatic CNS treatment in the late 1960s and early 1970s. Further successive, incremental improvements in outcome have been achieved due to clinical trials conducted by large single centers and national and international cooperative groups that have successfully enrolled a high percentage of eligible children.

Similar approaches have unfortunately not been quite so successful in improving the prognosis of children with AML. Although

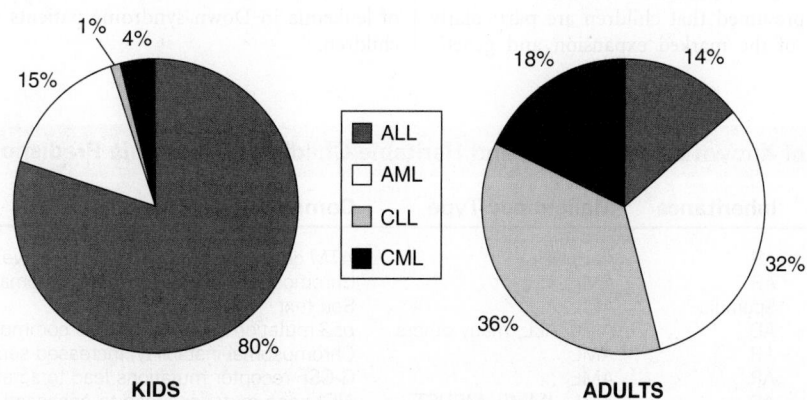

FIGURE 1. Relative incidence of four major leukemia subtypes in children and adults. ALL = acute lymphoblastic leukemia; AML = acute myeloid leukemia; CLL = chronic lymphoblastic leukemia; CML = chronic myeloid leukemia.

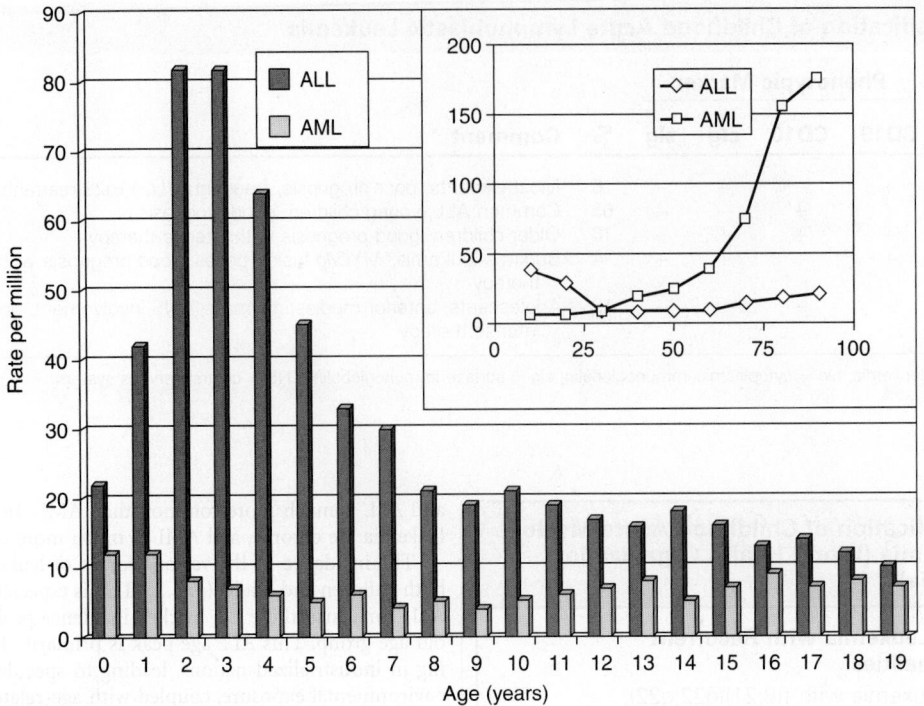

FIGURE 2. Age-specific incidence of acute lymphoblastic leukemia (ALL) and acute myeloid leukemia (ALL) in children and in adults *(inset)*.

approximately one half of children with AML are cured today, this has been accomplished by intensifying therapy to the point that the toxic death rate in the early phases of therapy is about 10%. Current research in AML is therefore focusing on developing novel molecularly targeted agents that hold the promise of improving efficacy and limiting toxicity.

Etiology

The question, "What is the cause of leukemia?" can be considered on a few different levels. First, what is wrong with *this child* that caused the child to develop leukemia? Second, what is wrong with *the leukemia cell* that causes it to behave so badly? Third, what is wrong with *the leukemia cell's genes* that cause the cell to behave that way?

PREDISPOSITIONS

The answer to the first question is unknown in the vast majority of cases. Attempts to correlate various genetic features or environmental or infectious exposures with risk of childhood leukemia have been largely uninformative. It is presumed that children are particularly susceptible to ALL because of the marked expansion and genetic

rearrangement of lymphocytes that occurs during early childhood as the result of exposure to a multitude of immunogenic antigens for the first time. The proliferation required to meet the constant demand for granulocytes, erythrocytes, and platelets is likely a setup for the development of AML in children.

Although a number of constitutional and single-gene disorders are known to confer an increased risk of childhood leukemia (Table 2), in total, these are involved in only a very small minority of cases. The most common of these is Down syndrome. Children with Down syndrome have a 10- to 20-fold increased risk of leukemia, with an approximately equal incidence of ALL and AML. The peak age at onset of leukemia for children with Down syndrome is earlier than for other children. Approximately 30% of Down syndrome children with AML have the megakaryoblastic form (M7AML), a subtype that is extremely rare in children without Down syndrome. In the newborn period, Down syndrome patients can present with transient myeloproliferative disease, a disorder distinguishable from congenital AML primarily by its spontaneous resolution within 3 months. Children with Down syndrome tend to present with biologically favorable subtypes of leukemia, but they also suffer increased toxicity from therapy. On balance, the prognosis of leukemia in Down syndrome patients is similar to that in other children.

TABLE 2 Summary of Known Constitutional and Heritable Childhood Leukemia Predispositions

Disorder	Inheritance	Malignancy Type	Comments
Ataxia-telangiectasia	AR	ALL, NHL	*ATM* gene mutations lead to defective DNA repair
Bloom's syndrome	AR	AML, ALL	Chromosomal instability, sister chromatid exchanges
Down syndrome	Sporadic	AML, ALL	See text
Li-Fraumeni syndrome	AD	AML, ALL, many others	*p53* mutations; leukemias less common than solid tumors
Fanconi's anemia	AR	AML	Chromosomal instability, increased sensitivity to DNA damage
Kostmann's syndrome	AR	AML	G-CSF receptor mutations lead to agranulocytosis
Neurofibromatosis type 1	AD	AML, JMML, MPNST	*NF1* gene mutations lead to enhanced *RAS* signaling

AD = autosomal dominant; ALL = acute lymphoblastic leukemia; AML = acute myeloid leukemia; AR = autosomal recessive; G-CSF = granulocyte colony-stimulating factor; JMML = juvenile myelomonocytic leukemia; MPNST = malignant peripheral nerve sheath tumor; NHL = non-Hodgkin's lymphoma.

The only environmental exposures that are known to predispose to leukemia are ionizing radiation (such as was seen with atomic bomb survivors) and prior exposure to certain chemotherapy drugs (cyclophosphamide [Cytoxan], etoposide [Vepesid]). There is good evidence that in utero exposure to maternal diagnostic radiation also increases the risk of childhood cancer (including leukemia), particularly if the exposure is in the first trimester. Other environmental or infectious exposures remain unproved as risk factors for childhood leukemia, including electromagnetic fields from power lines.

CELLULAR PATHOGENESIS

Three major characteristics of leukemia cells distinguish them from normal hematopoietic cells. They proliferate rapidly, they do not differentiate, and they have defects in apoptosis. This results in a growth advantage for leukemia cells, leading to progressive replacement of the normal bone marrow with a massive clonal population of poorly differentiated leukemic blasts. Another characteristic of leukemia cells is their tendency to spread throughout the body and infiltrate organs other than the bone marrow. This is discussed in more detail in the section on clinical presentation.

MOLECULAR PATHOGENESIS

As is true of most human cancers, development of leukemia is a multihit process. The initiating or permissive mutation (first hit) in childhood ALL often occurs in utero or early infancy, which is the peak of lymphocyte expansion and recombinase activity.

The initiating events are typically chromosomal rearrangements that activate expression of cellular proto-oncogenes by fusing them to transcriptionally active immunoglobulin or T-cell receptor genes or by joining two genes from different chromosomes to create a new fusion gene that encodes a chimeric protein with unique functional properties. The most common of these sentinel chromosomal rearrangements are translocations (exchanges of genetic material between chromosomes), which can serve as a unique marker of the malignant clone. Retrospective studies of blood obtained at birth and preserved on filter paper used for diagnosis of genetic disorders (Guthrie cards) of children who developed leukemia in early childhood have shown that leukemia-associated fusion genes were present at birth in a large percentage of children, including some who did not develop leukemia for one or more years.

In ALL, the promotional mutation (second hit) likely occurs during the proliferative stress generated by immune responses to exogenous antigens. Because these are maximal in the 2- to 4-year-old age group, this is thought to explain the age peak of childhood ALL during these years. The lack of such a peak in AML suggests that the promotional mutations can occur at any time or are not triggered by immune stimulation. Examples of specific genetic hits known to be associated with the development of childhood leukemia are summarized in Table 3.

Clinical Presentation

Most symptoms and signs of childhood leukemia are the result of the propensity of leukemia cells to replace the bone marrow and infiltrate multiple other organs throughout the body. It is estimated that approximately 10^9 (1 trillion) leukemia cells are present in the child's body at diagnosis.

The replacement of normal bone marrow is responsible for the characteristic abnormal blood counts, which in most cases include the triad of neutropenia, anemia, and thrombocytopenia. Depending on the number of circulating leukemic blasts in the peripheral blood, the total white blood cell count may be low, normal, or high. The neutropenia is often profound (absolute neutrophil count $<500/\mu L$), and is associated with an increased risk of serious infection. Blood cultures and broad-spectrum intravenous antibiotic coverage are indicated in any patient with newly diagnosed leukemia and fever. Anemia is often manifested by fatigue, lethargy, headache, pallor, and, in extreme cases, congestive heart failure that may be

TABLE 3 Summary of Common Leukemogenic Genetic Events

Acute Lymphoblastic Leukemia	Acute Myeloid Leukemia
Chimeric Transcription Factors	
t(12;21): *TEL-AML1* fusion	t(8;21): *AML1-ETO* fusion
t(1;19): *E2A-PBX1* fusion	t(15;17): *PML-RAR* α fusion
t(4;11), et al: *MLL* fusions	t(9;11), et al: *MLL* fusions
t(8;14), t(8;22), t(2;8): *Ig-MYC* fusions	inv(16): MYH11-CBFB
T-cell receptor fusions	
Mutationally Activated Oncogenes	
t(9;22): *BCR-ABL* fusion	*FLT3* mutation
PTPN11 mutation	*RAS* mutation
FLT3 mutation	*KIT* mutation
Altered *Rb/p53* Tumor-Suppressor Network	
p16INK4a/p14ARF deletion or silencing	Nucleophosmin mutations
p21CIP1 silencing	p53 mutations
HDM2 overexpression	HDM2 overexpression

precipitated by vigorous transfusion or intravenous hydration. Thrombocytopenia often leads to bruising and petechiae; however, clinically significant hemorrhage is uncommon in industrialized countries. Platelet transfusion is indicated for bleeding or for very low platelet counts ($<10,000–20,000/\mu L$).

Infiltration of organs other than the bone marrow with leukemia cells is responsible for additional presenting clinical features. Box 2 summarizes the organ systems most often involved in leukemia and the typical clinical manifestations.

Medical Emergencies in Childhood Leukemia

Newly diagnosed leukemia in a child is a medical emergency. There are several potentially life-threatening complications that may be present at diagnosis or can develop within a short time after diagnosis. The need to diagnose and treat potential infection in patients who are febrile and neutropenic was discussed earlier.

Tumor lysis syndrome (TLS) is a complication resulting from the rapid lysis of large numbers of tumor cells, releasing intracellular contents. Although TLS is seen most often after initial treatment with chemotherapy, it can also be present before therapy is initiated due to spontaneous lysis. Risk factors include high white blood cell (WBC) count, lymphadenopathy, hepatosplenomegaly, high mitotic index, and a diagnosis of ALL (especially Burkitt's leukemia or lymphoma and T-cell ALL). TLS is characterized by the triad of hyperuricemia (from breakdown of purines by xanthine oxidase), hyperkalemia, and hyperphosphatemia (with secondary hypocalcemia). Renal insufficiency can develop due to the nephrotoxic effects of precipitated urate crystals in the renal tubules; in severe cases, dialysis may be necessary.

Management consists of aggressive hydration to reduce tubular uric acid concentration and alkalinization of urine to promote solubility of urate crystals. The xanthine oxidase inhibitor allopurinol (Zyloprim) is routinely used during the first 3 to 7 days of leukemia treatment to decrease uric acid production. Rasburicase (Elitek) (recombinant urate oxidase) is a new agent used in severe cases of TLS to almost instantaneously convert uric acid to the more soluble allantoin. Frequent electrolyte monitoring with standard management of abnormal levels is essential.

Hyperleukocytosis becomes a potential clinical problem when the WBC count rises above $100,000/\mu L$. Markedly elevated WBCs lead to increased blood viscosity that can produce sludging of blood in the brain, lungs, kidneys, and other organs, causing clinical features such as depressed level of consciousness, stroke, intracranial hemorrhage, respiratory distress, hypoxia, diffuse pulmonary infiltrates, and renal

BOX 2   Summary of Clinical Manifestations of Childhood Leukemia*

Bone Marrow
Pancytopenia, bone pain

Reticuloendothelial System
Lymphadenopathy
Hepatosplenomegaly

Thymus
Anterior mediastinal mass (T-cell leukemia)

Bones
Bone pain is common
Fractures and chloromas are rare

Gums
Gingival hypertrophy (M4 and M5 AML)

Skin
Leukemia cutis and chloromas (M2, M4, and M5 AML, infant ALL)

Central Nervous System
Meningitis
Cranial nerve palsies
Rarely intracranial epidural or orbital chloromas (M4 and M5 AML, T-cell ALL)

Kidneys
Often infiltrated or enlarged
Rarely acute renal failure (except in tumor lysis syndrome)

Genitourinary
Testicular enlargement (T-cell ALL)

*See Box 1 for descriptions of classifications.
ALL = acute lymphoblastic leukemia; AML = acute myeloid leukemia.

insufficiency. The risk of hyperviscosity is higher with AML than ALL, because myelolasts are generally larger and stickier than lymphoblasts (likely due to increased expression of integrins and other mediators of cell–cell adherence on the surface of myeloblasts). Management consists of treating the leukemia as soon as possible and performing exchange transfusion or leukopheresis in cases where symptoms are prominent.

Life-threatening bleeding is another potential complication of leukemia. Although all patients with thrombocytopenia are at risk, patients with concomitant coagulopathy due to disseminated intravascular coagulation (DIC) are at particularly high risk. The leukemia subtype most commonly complicated by DIC and serious bleeding is acute promyelocytic leukemia (APL). This association results from the release of thromboplastin from the cytoplasmic granules in promyelocytic blasts. Aggressive blood product support and early treatment with the differentiation-inducing agent all-*trans* retinoic acid (ATRA) has been shown to decrease the risk of bleeding in APL. Despite these measures, up to 10% of patients die of bleeding complications during the initial weeks of therapy, and additional patients suffer lasting morbidity from retinal hemorrhages and nonfatal central nervous system hemorrhages.

Tracheal compression and superior vena cava syndrome can result from large anterior mediastinal masses, which are commonly present in T-cell ALL but are rare in other forms of leukemia. Patients can present with respiratory distress, cough, orthopnea, headaches,

syncope, dizziness, facial swelling, or plethora. A chest x-ray should be performed to assess the mediastinum in any patient suspected to have ALL. If the mediastinum is enlarged, a CT is indicated to assess airway patency. This evaluation must precede any attempts at sedation for diagnostic procedures, because even light sedation can precipitate acute airway collapse. Diagnostic material should be obtained by the least invasive method possible before treatment. If necessary, emergent airway compromise can be treated with radiation or steroids, or both.

Differential Diagnosis

Although leukemia should be considered in cases of isolated neutropenia, anemia, or thrombocytopenia, the vast majority of leukemia patients present with depressions in more than one cell line. In suspected cases of immune thrombocytopenic purpura (ITP), for example, a careful review of the peripheral blood smear should be performed to rule out the presence of circulating leukemic blasts. Routine bone marrow aspiration is not necessary for children with ITP, but it should be performed in patients with atypical features, such as concomitant anemia or neutropenia, hepatosplenomegaly, bone pain, or significant weight loss. Treatment of ITP with corticosteroids should only be instituted after evaluation by an experienced hematologist.

Pancytopenia can be caused by diseases other than leukemia. Some viral infections have a propensity to suppress bone marrow function and cause low peripheral blood counts, including Epstein-Barr virus (EBV), herpes simplex virus (HSV), influenza, hepatitis viruses, and HIV. Infectious mononucleosis from EBV infection can be particularly difficult to differentiate from leukemia, because patients often have hepatosplenomegaly and circulating atypical lymphocytes (which can appear very similar to leukemic blasts). Pancytopenia on the basis of bone marrow failure (from acquired aplastic anemia or rare inherited bone marrow failure syndromes) can be distinguished from leukemia by bone marrow biopsy for assessment of overall marrow cellularity. Certain solid tumors have a tendency to metastasize to the bone marrow and cause cytopenias, including neuroblastoma, rhabdomyosarcoma, and retinoblastoma, but it is rare for pancytopenia to be the primary presenting feature in these cases.

Joint pain, fever, hepatosplenomegaly, and pallor are common presenting features in both systemic-onset juvenile rheumatoid arthritis (JRA) and leukemia. A bone marrow aspirate should be performed to rule out leukemia before treatment with steroids in suspected cases of systemic-onset JRA.

Risk Stratification

In the last several years, treatment decisions for children with newly diagnosed acute leukemia have been based on the concept of risk stratification. Using factors identified during clinical trials to predict a high or low risk of relapse, patients are separated into risk groups before the start of treatment or at the end of the first month of induction therapy. The treatment plan is then tailored to the degree of risk. The desired result is that patients with relatively low-risk disease can be treated with less toxic therapy without compromising cure rates, and patients with high-risk disease receive more-intensive, potentially toxic therapy. The risk groups are currently defined based on several criteria and differ for ALL and AML. Different centers and cooperative groups typically employ different risk-stratification strategies.

In ALL, the initial risk assessment is based on two simple clinical parameters that are available immediately at the time of diagnosis (the National Cancer Institute [NCI] or Rome criteria): WBC count (>50,000/μL is high risk), and age (<1 year or >9 years is high risk). Further refinement of risk assignment is often based on a combination of leukemia phenotype (B- vs T-lineage), the presence of certain sentinel cytogenetic lesions, and how quickly the patient's leukemia responds to the first few weeks of therapy (rapid clearance of leukemia cells from the blood or marrow is associated with a lower risk of relapse).

Low-risk cytogenetic features include hyperdiploidy (≥50 chromosomes in the leukemia cells) or trisomies of specific chromosomes and the presence of a t(12;21) that results in *TEL/AML1* fusion. High-risk cytogenetic features include hypodiploidy (<44 chromosomes in the leukemia cells) and the presence of either an 11q23 (*MLL* gene) rearrangement or a t(9;22), or Philadelphia chromosome, that creates a *BCR/ABL* fusion gene.

Early response has historically been measured by the response to a prednisone prophase that includes a single dose of intrathecal methotrexate and 7 days of prednisone, or by the percentage of blast cells remaining in the bone marrow after 7 to 14 days of multiagent therapy. Over the past 10 to 15 years, measures of tumor burden remaining in the marrow at the end of induction therapy (minimal residual disease) have been shown to be highly predictive of outcome and have been integrated into risk-stratification schemata of all of the major leukemia cooperative groups.

In AML, risk stratification is based largely on cytogenetics. Low-risk features include a t(8;21), which results in the *AML1/ETO* fusion, and either inv(16) or a t(16;16), both of which create the *CBFβ/MYH11* fusion. High-risk features include monosomy 7 and abnormalities in the long arm of chromosome 5. In addition to these cytogenetic abnormalities, failure to achieve remission with induction chemotherapy is another high-risk feature in AML. All other cytogenetic abnormalities, as well as normal cytogenetics (which are seen in approximately 60% of cases), are considered intermediate risk. More recently, a specific type of genetic mutation in the tyrosine kinase gene *FLT3* has been identified as another high-risk feature. This type of *FLT3* mutation (called an internal tandem duplication [ITD]) occurs in 10% to 15% of childhood AML.

Treatment

There are significant differences in the specific treatments for ALL and AML, so they will be discussed separately. Table 4 summarizes the most salient features of the treatment for each.

ACUTE LYMPHOBLASTIC LEUKEMIA

Treatment for ALL generally occurs in four phases: remission induction, CNS preventive therapy, consolidation, and maintenance. Remission induction in ALL typically lasts 4 to 6 weeks and includes three to five systemic agents. Common to almost all regimens are a corticosteroid (either prednisone [Deltasone] or dexamethasone [Decadron]),

vincristine [Vincasar], and L-asparaginase [Elspar], which compose the three-drug induction. An anthracycline, typically doxorubicin (Adriamycin), is also included in many regimens (four-drug induction), with other agents such as cyclophosphamide (Cytoxan) or etoposide (VePesid) used in a small minority of centers. More than 98% of children enter remission by the end of 4 weeks of induction therapy, and the mortality rate from toxicity during induction therapy is generally less than 2% to 3% in industrialized countries.

The concept that the CNS could be a sanctuary site for leukemia emerged in the mid 1960s when the introduction of multiagent systemic chemotherapy led to high remission rates, but a majority of patients relapsed within 6 to 12 months, with many of these recurrences being limited to the CNS. Routine introduction of presymptomatic CNS radiation in the late 1960s and early 1970s led to substantial increases in cure rates to approximately 50%. Modern CNS preventive therapy includes periodic administration of intrathecal chemotherapy (usually methotrexate) starting at the time of the first diagnostic lumbar puncture. Systemic agents with improved CNS penetration (dexamethasone rather than prednisone, higher doses of intravenous methotrexate) might also play an important role in CNS control. Cranial irradiation is currently reserved for patients at the highest risk for CNS relapse (e.g., those with high diagnostic WBC count or leukemic blasts in CSF at diagnosis). Over time, CNS radiation has been given to fewer and fewer ALL patients; some groups believe that it can be eliminated for all patients. With these modern strategies, the risk of isolated CNS relapse is less than 5%.

Following the induction of remission, patients receive additional chemotherapy designed to consolidate the remission. The intensity and duration of the consolidation phase are risk based, and alternating cycles of non–cross-resistant chemotherapy drugs are typically used. These consolidation or intensification phases typically last about 6 months and often include a reinduction phase similar to the first month of treatment.

It has been clearly demonstrated that the risk of relapse in ALL can be reduced with an extended phase of continuous low-dose chemotherapy (maintenance) that lasts until 2 to 3 years from the time of diagnosis. Oral 6-mercaptopurine (Purinethol) and methotrexate are used universally, with variable administration of intrathecal chemotherapy. Some centers or groups also employ periodic doses of vincristine and 5- to 7-day pulses of prednisone or dexamethasone. The optimal frequency of intrathecal chemotherapy treatments and vincristine and steroid pulses is uncertain and might depend on the intensity of therapy delivered during the induction and consolidation phases.

TABLE 4 Summary of Treatment for Childhood Leukemia

Characteristics	Acute Lymphoblastic Leukemia	Acute Myeloid Leukemia
Remission Induction		
Chemotherapy	4 wk with prednisone or dexamethasone, vincristine, L-asparaginase, doxorubicin (not all cases)	Two courses (6–8 wk) with cytarabine (Ara-C), doxorubicin, others (e.g., etoposide, thioguanine)
Toxic death rate	Low (<3%)	High (>10%)
Remission rate	>98%	75%–85%
CNS Preventive Therapy		
Intrathecal chemotherapy	Methotrexate	Cytarabine
Cranial irradiation	For high risk (blasts in CSF at diagnosis and/or high WBC count)	None
Consolidation		
Chemotherapy	Combinations of various drugs (not cross-resistant) Intensity/duration based on risk stratification	Based on cytogenetic risk group Low risk: 2–3 additional courses Intermediate risk: BMT for patients with HLA-matched related donors High risk: BMT for patients with any suitable donor (including unrelated)
Maintenance		
Chemotherapy	Low-dose oral (6-mercaptopurine and methotrexate) Total duration of therapy 2–3 y	No maintenance therapy (does not improve survival)

BMT = bone marrow transplant; CNS = central nervous system; CSF = cerebrospinal fluid; HLA = human leukocyte antigen; WBC = white blood cell.

ACUTE MYELOID LEUKEMIA

Remission induction in AML typically consists of two courses of very intensive chemotherapy with cytarabine (Tarabine) and doxorubicin, often combined with thioguanine (Tabloid) or etoposide. Remission rates are 75% to 85%, with about one half of the failures due to resistant leukemia and the others to mortality from toxicity (usually infection).

Similar to ALL, CNS preventive therapy in AML begins at diagnosis with intrathecal chemotherapy (usually cytarabine) and continues with additional periodic intrathecal treatments during consolidation. High-dose cytarabine, which is a key component of most AML treatment regimens, also contributes to CNS treatment. Cranial radiation is not typically administered by most groups to children with AML, except for treatment of chloromas (solid masses of leukemia cells) that do not resolve with chemotherapy.

Consolidation in AML is risk dependent. For intermediate-risk patients, most groups have reported the best results using allogeneic bone marrow transplant (BMT) with a histocompatible (i.e., human leukocyte antigen (HLA)-identical or matched) sibling donor. However, only about 25% to 30% of children with AML with have a matched sibling donor. For the remaining intermediate-risk patients, consolidation consists of two to three additional chemotherapy courses that are slightly less intense and usually consist of cytarabine combined with drugs not used in induction such as mitoxantrone (Novantrone) and L-asparaginase. High-risk patients can be identified who have a less than 20% to 25% chance of cure with intensive chemotherapy. Most groups consider these patients to be candidates for BMT. If a matched sibling is unavailable, then alternative donor sources (e.g., matched unrelated bone marrow or umbilical cord blood) are usually offered. For low-risk patients, for whom the cure rate with chemotherapy alone approaches 70%, BMT is usually not offered in first remission, even for patients with a matched sibling donor. In addition, relapses in low-risk patients, unlike relapses in intermediate-risk or high-risk patients, can often be successfully treated with BMT in second remission, justifying reserving BMT for use as a salvage therapy for low-risk patients. Unlike ALL, most groups have found no benefit to extended maintenance therapy in children with AML.

Relapse

The most common site of relapsed leukemia is the bone marrow (with or without concomitant CNS involvement). Less common are isolated extramedullary relapses (CNS or testicular relapse in ALL,

chloromas in AML). For both ALL and AML, a critical determinant of outcome following relapse is the time from diagnosis to relapse.

ALL patients who relapse within 18 months of initial diagnosis have a dismal outcome, with only about one half able to attain a second remission and less than 10% overall cure rate; the outcome is marginally better for those who relapse between 18 and 36 months after diagnosis. ALL patients with such early relapses are typically treated with 3 to 4 months of intensive therapy in an attempt to achieve a second remission and attain further cytoreduction, followed by BMT using a matched sibling or unrelated donor. In contrast, children with ALL who relapse more than 3 years after initial diagnosis have an approximately 95% chance of entering a second remission, and 40% to 45% can be cured with intensive chemotherapy; these patients are generally considered to be candidates for matched sibling, but not unrelated donor, BMT in second remission.

Overall, relapsed AML has a dismal outcome (long-term survival approximately 20%), and the approach is to attempt to reinduce remission and then proceed to BMT or investigational treatments. Even in this setting, there is clearly an improved outcome for patients who relapse after a prolonged initial remission (>12 months from the end of remission-induction therapy) compared with patients who have refractory disease or who relapse after a shorter period of remission.

New treatment strategies are urgently needed for patients with relapsed ALL and AML, because the current regimens produce poor results and are associated with a great deal of toxicity. The major clinical trial groups are testing novel and targeted therapies in these patient populations.

Late Effects

Approximately 70% of children with leukemia are cured of their disease. As the numbers of long-term survivors of childhood leukemia has grown, there has been increasing interest in assessing the late effects of leukemic therapy. In childhood ALL, with cure rates of 85%, a major effort is being made in ongoing clinical trials to reduce the intensity of therapy for lower-risk patients, with the hope of reducing late effects of therapy without compromising high cure rates. The most common late effects of leukemia therapy, with the known treatment-related risk factors and recommended diagnostic approach for each, are summarized in Table 5. Many pediatric oncology centers have developed late-effects programs to conduct surveillance for the development of these problems and provide follow-up care to patients who develop late complications of therapy.

TABLE 5 Summary of Late Effects of Leukemia Treatment

Late Effect	Treatment-Related Risk Factors	Diagnostic Approach
Bone	Avascular necrosis, osteonecrosis	X-ray and/or MRI of major joints for persistent pain
Cardiac dysfunction	Anthracyclines: cardiomyopathy (risk related to cumulative dose, higher risk in AML)	ECG or echocardiogram every 3 y (cardiomyopathy can occur decades after treatment)
Cataracts	CNS RT	Yearly eye exam
CNS and psychosocial	CNS RT, IT chemotherapy: learning problems, neurocognitive dysfunction	Yearly educational assessment, neurocognitive testing
Dental abnormalities	CNS RT	Dental exam at age 5
Endocrine and reproductive	CNS RT: pituitary dysfunction Alkylators: primary gonadal failure	Yearly growth curves, TSH, LH, FSH LH, FSH, estradiol or testosterone, semen analysis
Hepatic dysfunction	Methotrexate, 6-mercaptopurine, 6-thioguanine: late hepatic fibrosis	Yearly LFTs
Secondary neoplasms	CNS RT: brain tumors Alkylators or epipodophyllotoxins: secondary AML	MRI for symptoms Yearly CBC

ALL = acute lymphoblastic leukemia; AML = acute myeloid leukemia; CNS = central nervous system; ECG = electrocardiogram; FSH = follicle stimulating hormone; IT = Intrathecal; LFT = liver function test; LH = luteinizing hormone; MRI = magnetic resonance imaging; RT = radiation therapy; TSH = thyroid stimulating hormone.

REFERENCES

Brown P, Small D. FLT3 inhibitors: A paradigm for the development of targeted therapeutics for paediatric cancer. Eur J Cance 2004;40:707–21.

Gaynon PS, Qu RP, Chappell RJ, et al. Survival after relapse in childhood acute lymphoblastic leukemia: Impact of site and time to first relapse—the Children's Cancer Group Experience. Cancer 1998;82:1387–95.

Gibson BE, Wheatley K, Hann IM, et al. Treatment strategy and long-term results in paediatric patients treated in consecutive UK AML trials. Leukemia 2005;19:2130–8.

Greaves MF, Wiemels J. Origins of chromosome translocations in childhood leukaemia. Nat Rev Cancer 2003;3:639–49.

Hitzler JK, Zipursky A. Origins of leukaemia in children with Down syndrome. Nat Rev Cancer 2005;5:11–20.

Meshinchi S, Alonzo TA, Stirewalt DL, et al. Clinical implications of FLT3 mutations in pediatric AML. Blood 2006;108:3654–61.

Moghrabi A, Levy DE, Asselin B, et al. Results of the Dana—Farber Cancer Institute ALL Consortium Protocol 95–01 for children with acute lymphoblastic leukemia. Blood 2007;109:896–904.

Mrozek K, Heinonen K, Bloomfield CD. Clinical importance of cytogenetics in acute myeloid leukaemia. Best Pract Res Clin Haematol 2001;14:19–47.

Pinkel D, Simone J, Hustu HO, Aur RJ. Nine years' experience with "total therapy" of childhood acute lymphocytic leukemia. Pediatrics 1972;50:246–51.

Pui CH, Cheng C, Leung W, et al. Extended follow-up of long-term survivors of childhood acute lymphoblastic leukemia. N Engl J Med 2003;349:640–9.

Pui CH, Evans WE. Treatment of acute lymphoblastic leukemia. N Engl J Med 2006;354:166–78.

Pui CH, Mahmoud HH, Rivera GK, et al. Early intensification of intrathecal chemotherapy virtually eliminates central nervous system relapse in children with acute lymphoblastic leukemia. Blood 1998;92:411–5.

Pui CH, Sandlund JT, Pei D, et al. Improved outcome for children with acute lymphoblastic leukemia: Results of Total Therapy Study XIIIB at St Jude Children's Research Hospital. Blood 2004;104:2690–6.

Ries LAG, Melbert D, Krapcho M, et al. SEER Cancer Statistics Review, 1975–2004. Bethesda, Md: National Cancer Institute; 2007.

Schrappe M, Reiter A, Zimmermann M, et al. Long-term results of four consecutive trials in childhood ALL performed by the ALL-BFM study group from 1981 to 1995. Berlin–Frankfurt–Munster. Leukemia 2000;14:2205–22.

Stahnke K, Boos J, Bender-Gotze C, et al. Duration of first remission predicts remission rates and long-term survival in children with relapsed acute myelogenous leukemia. Leukemia 1998;12:1534–8.

Wakeford R, Little MP. Risk coefficients for childhood cancer after intrauterine irradiation: A review. Int J Radiat Biol 2003;79:293–309.

Woods WG, Kobrinsky N, Buckley JD, et al. Timed-sequential induction therapy improves postremission outcome in acute myeloid leukemia: A report from the Children's Cancer Group. Blood 1996;87:4979–89.

Woods WG, Neudorf S, Gold S, et al. A comparison of allogeneic bone marrow transplantation, autologous bone marrow transplantation, and aggressive chemotherapy in children with acute myeloid leukemia in remission. Blood 2001;97:56–62.

Chronic Leukemias

Method of
Jorge E. Cortes, MD, Hagop M. Kantarjian, MD, and William Wierda, MD, PhD

Chronic Myeloid Leukemia

CLINICAL FEATURES AND DIAGNOSIS

Chronic myelogenous leukemia (CML) is a clonal myeloproliferative disorder characterized by leukocytosis and the presence of immature white blood cells (WBCs) in the peripheral blood with all maturation stages present. Bone marrow examination reveals a hypercellular marrow with myeloid hyperplasia. The hallmark of the disease is the presence of the Philadelphia (Ph) chromosome, which represents a balanced translocation between the long arms of chromosomes 9 and 22: t(9;22)(q34;q11.2). This juxtaposes the *c-abl* gene located in chromosome 9q34 with the *bcr* gene located in chromosome 22q11.2. The chimeric *BCR-ABL* gene translates into a protein (p210$^{Bcr/Abl}$) that is a tyrosine kinase with increased kinase activity that promotes cellular proliferation and suppresses apoptosis. This kinase activity is critical to the development of CML.

The manifesting features of CML have changed over time. In the past, most patients presented with fatigue, fever, or other features of leukostasis (e.g., headache, priapism) and splenomegaly (e.g., right upper quadrant pain). Now, approximately 70% of patients are asymptomatic and diagnosis is based on a routine blood examination.

CURRENT DIAGNOSIS

Chronic Myeloid Leukemia

- Initial Evaluation
  - History: Visual disturbances, neurologic symptoms, abdominal pain, weight loss, or fever
  - Physical examination: Degree of splenomegaly, signs of leukostasis (visual abnormalities, priapism, focal neurologic deficits), chloromas
  - Peripheral blood: CBC with differential, blood chemistry analysis, molecular ratio (BCR-*ABL*/ *ABL* ratio by real-time PCR), FISH
  - Bone marrow: Morphology, cytogenetics, *BCR-ABL/ABL* ratio
  - The diagnosis of CML is established by the presence of the Philadelphia chromosome and/or the *BCR-ABL* rearrangement
  - Bone marrow aspiration for morphology is necessary for adequate stage classification
  - Follow-up
  - CBC: Every 1–2 weeks until counts stabilize (usually 2–3 mo), then every 6–12 weeks
  - Cytogenetic: Every 3–6 months until CCyR, then every 12 months. After major molecular response, less frequent depending on clinical, hematologic, and molecular findings
  - FISH: Can be used to monitor cytogenetic response until down to 5% to 10% Ph$^+$
  - PCR: Every 3–6 months

Chronic Lymphocytic Leukemia

- Initial Diagnosis
  - Absolute lymphocytosis (>5000 lymphocytes/µL)
  - Well-differentiated, monotonous-appearing lymphocytes
  - <55% blood prolymphocytes
  - Flow cytometry on blood: monoclonal light chain, CD19$^+$, CD23$^+$, CD5$^+$
  - Evaluation of prognostic factors
  - β_2 Microglobulin
  - FISH for 17p del, 11q del, +12, 13q del (sole)
  - IgV$_H$ mutation status
  - ZAP70 expression
  - CD38 expression

CBC = complete blood count; CCyR = complete cytogenetic response; CML = chronic myeloid leukemia; FISH = fluorescence in situ hybridization; Ph = Philadelphia chromosome; PCR = polymerase chain reaction.

NATURAL HISTORY

CML usually runs a biphasic or triphasic course, with an initial chronic phase that, unless adequately treated, eventually transforms into a blastic phase resembling an acute leukemia. An intermediate or accelerated phase precedes the blastic phase in 60% to 80% of patients. Although no definition of these stages is universally accepted, some of the most commonly used criteria are presented in Table 1. Historically, the median survival of patients in chronic, accelerated, and blastic phases was 4 to 5 years, 6 to 18 months, and 2 to 6 months, respectively. Modern therapy with tyrosine kinase inhibitors has significantly improved the outcome, with 95% survival at 5 years for patients in the chronic phase.

Clinical features at diagnosis help segregate patients into different prognostic categories. The most commonly used prognostic system is the Sokal score. In this system, the hazard ratio for death is calculated from baseline characteristics using the following formula:

$$\lambda^i(+)/\lambda_o(t) = \text{Exp}\,0.0116(\text{age} - 43.4) + 0.0345(\text{spleen} - 7.51)$$
$$+0.188[(\text{platelets}/700)^2 - 0.563]$$
$$+0.0887(\text{blasts} - 2.10)$$

Three prognostic groups are identified with hazard ratios of less than 0.8, 0.8 to 1.2, and greater than 1.2, and historical median survivals of 2.5, 3.5, and 4.5 years, respectively.

INITIAL EVALUATION AND TREATMENT OBJECTIVES

The diagnosis of CML requires the documentation of the Philadelphia chromosome or its corresponding gene rearrangement, *BCR-ABL*. In 90% to 95% of patients this is found in a karyotype analysis; in all others it can be identified by polymerase chain reaction (PCR). To properly diagnose and stage CML, all patients need a bone marrow aspiration at the time of diagnosis. In addition, the *BCR-ABL/ABL* ratio should be determined in peripheral blood or bone marrow. Although PCR results obtained from both sources correlate well with each other, it is not recommended to use them interchangeably. Thus, it is better to measure BCR-ABL transcripts in peripheral blood because it is easier to monitor more frequently during therapy.

Conventional chemotherapy with hydroxyurea (Hydrea) or busulfan (Myleran) was used for many years to control the WBC count and splenomegaly (i.e., hematologic response). However, a hematologic response alone does not change the natural history of the disease. With the introduction of interferon (IFN)-α, cytogenetic responses (disappearance of the Philadelphia chromosome) were for the first time achieved in up to 50% to 60% of patients. The response criteria used for patients with CML are detailed in Box 1. Complete cytogenetic response (CCyR) is associated with an improved survival probability of 78% at 10 years compared with 25% to 40% for those with lesser responses. The goal of therapy therefore became to eliminate the malignant clone represented by the Philadelphia

---

> **BOX 1 Response Criteria in Chronic Myelogenous Leukemia**
>
> **Hematologic Remission**
>
> Complete: Normalization of peripheral counts and differential, and disappearance of all signs and symptoms of CML including splenomegaly
>
> **Cytogenetic Remission (Major Cytogenic Response)***
>
> Complete: 0% Ph$^+$ metaphases
> Partial: 1% to 34% Ph$^+$ metaphases
> Minor: 35% to 95% Ph$^+$ metaphases
> None: >95% Ph$^+$ metaphases
>
> **Molecular Remission†**
>
> Complete: Undetectable *BCR-ABL* transcripts
> Major: ≥3-log reduction in *BCR-ABL/ABL* from standardized baseline or a ratio of <0.1 % on a proposed international scale
>
> ---
> * Cytogenetic response is based on a routine karyotype analyzing at least 20 metaphases.
> †Molecular response is based on real-time polymerase chain reaction.
> CML = Chronic myelogenous leukemia.

chromosome (cytogenetic response). In addition, approximately 30% of patients with CCyR after IFN-α had undetectable disease by PCR; none of them has relapsed after a median follow-up of 10 years and are therefore probably cured. With imatinib, most patients can achieve a CCyR, and the achieving molecular response is more likely and might further improve the long-term outcome. Thus, proper monitoring is required during therapy to ensure adequate response and optimize the long-term outcome. An approach to the work-up and management of patients with newly diagnosed CML is summarized in the Current Diagnosis box.

Treatment

The first line of therapy for patients with CML is imatinib 400 mg daily. Patients should be monitored closely with cytogenetics and PCR to ensure that treatment goals are met at specific times. If this is the case, treatment should be continued indefinitely, avoiding unnecessary dose reductions or treatment interruptions. Patients who fail imatinib should be offered therapy with a second-generation

---

TABLE 1 Criteria for Accelerated Phase

Feature	MDACC	IBMTR	WHO
Blasts	15%–29%	10%–29%	10%–19%†
Blasts + promyelocytes	30%	20%	NA
Basophils	20%	20%*	20%
Platelets	<100	Unresponsive increase or persistent decrease	<100 10^9/L, or >1000 10^9/L unresponsive to treatment
Cytogenetics	CE	CE	CE not at the time of diagnosis
WBC	NA	Difficult to control, or doubling in <5 d	NA
Anemia	NA	Unresponsive	NA
Splenomegaly	NA	Increasing	NA
Other	NA	Chloromas, myelofibrosis	Megakaryocyte proliferation, fibrosis

*Basophils plus eosinophils.
CE = clonal evolution; IBMTR = International Bone Marrow Transplant Registry; MDACC = MD Anderson Cancer Center, NA = not applicable; WBC = white blood cell count; WHO = World Health Organization.

tyrosine kinase inhibitor (dasatinib, nilotinib). Stem cell transplantation (SCT) should be considered for patients who have failed imatinib, and in many instances it is considered as third option if a second-generation tyrosine kinase inhibitor has also failed. There is no significant cross-resistance between these agents, so patients who fail imatinib and one second-generation tyrosine kinase inhibitor sometimes respond to a different second-generation inhibitor.

Patients in accelerated-phase CML might still respond well to imatinib. Although responses can be observed in patients in blast phase, these are usually transient, and SCT should be considered after returning to chronic phase.

IMATINIB MESYLATE

Imatinib (Gleevec) is an orally administered tyrosine kinase inhibitor. By inhibiting *BCR-ABL*, it blocks proliferation and induces apoptosis of *BCR-ABL*–expressing cells. Imatinib has become the standard therapy for CML due to its remarkable activity and mild toxicity profile.

The efficacy of imatinib in chronic-phase CML was established in a randomized study in patients with CML in chronic phase compared with the combination of IFN-α (Intron A) and cytarabine (Tarabine). After 5 years of follow-up, the projected CCyR rate with imatinib was 87%, with most responses occurring by 12 months of therapy. Responses are durable, with an event-free survival of 83% at 6 years of follow-up and overall survival of 95%. This compares favorably with the 50% 5-year survival with prior therapies.

Earlier responses are associated with improved outcome. Patients with CCyR or PCyR at 12 months from start of therapy have a 93% to 97% probability of being alive and free from transformation to accelerated or blast phase, compared to 81% for those without CCyR or PCyR. Among patients who achieved a CCyR by 12 months of therapy, 100% of those with a major molecular response (MMR) (*BCR-ABL/ABL* <0.1% on an international harmonized scale, or ≥3-log reduction from a standardized baseline) were alive and free from transformation at 5 years, compared to 95% for those with CCyR but not MMR.

The standard dose of imatinib is 400 mg daily. Among patients who fail imatinib therapy, increasing their dose from 400 mg to 800 mg daily induces a major cytogenetic response in 40% to 50%. Some studies have suggested that initiating therapy with 800 mg daily on diagnosis may be associated with improved outcome. These observations are being confirmed in randomized trials.

Management of Toxicity

Imatinib is overall well tolerated. Although some adverse events occur in 30% to 40% of patients, these are usually mild and manageable. The most commonly encountered side effects and suggestions for management are included in Box 2. Grade 3 or 4 toxicity that is related to imatinib requires treatment interruption. When toxicity resolves to grade 1, treatment should be resumed, usually at a reduced dose, but doses less than 300 mg daily are not recommended. Less than 5% of patients are intolerant to imatinib and require change of therapy.

Myelosuppression is a more common adverse event. Dose interruptions are not recommended unless the patient develops grade-3 neutropenia or thrombocytopenia (neutrophils $<10^9$/L, platelets $<50 \times 10^9$/L). Treatment is restarted when counts recover above these thresholds. If recovery occurs within 2 weeks, treatment is resumed at the same dose. If recovery takes longer than 2 weeks, the dose can be reduced (e.g., from 600 mg to 400 mg, or from 400 mg to 300 mg). Most commonly, myelosuppression occurs within the first 2 to 3 months of therapy, is self-limited, and does not lead to clinical consequences. No interruptions or dose adjustments are usually recommended for anemia.

Monitoring Patients

Adequate monitoring is needed to optimize treatment outcome. The primary goal of therapy is to achieve CCyR. In addition, achieving an MMR can improve the probability of a durable remission and transformation-free survival. However, although achieving

---

BOX 2 Recommended Management of the Most Common Adverse Events Associated with Imatinib

Nausea and Vomiting
Take with food, fluids
Antiemetics

Diarrhea
Loperamide (Imodium)
Diphenoxylate atropine (Lomotil)

Peripheral Edema
Diuretics

Periorbital Edema
Steroid-containing cream

Rash
Avoid sun exposure
Topical steroids
Systemic steroids
(Early intervention is important)

Muscle Cramps
Tonic water or quinine
Electrolyte replacement as needed
Calcium gluconate

Arthralgia, Bone Pain
Nonsteroidal antiinflamatory agents

Elevated Transaminases (uncommon)
Hold therapy and monitor closely
Dose reduction upon resolution

Myelosuppression

Anemia
Treatment interruption and dose reduction are usually not indicated
Erythropoietin (Procrit) or darbepoetin (Aranesp)

Neutropenia
Hold therapy if grade ≥3 (i.e., ANC $<1 \times 10^9$/L)
Consider G-CSF (Neupogen) if recurrent or persistent neutropenia or with sepsis

Thrombocytopenia
Hold therapy if grade ≥3 (platelets $<50 \times 10^9$/L)
Consider IL-11 10 µg/kg 3–7 days/week

ANC = absolute neutrophil count; G-CSF = granulocyte colony-stimulating factor; IL = interleukin.

---

a molecular response is an important objective, failure to achieve MMR or increasing transcript levels should not by itself be considered therapy failure. A description of the techniques and proposed guidelines for monitoring patients is presented earlier and in the Current Diagnosis box.

Imatinib Failure

Despite the favorable results achieved with imatinib, approximately 10% to 15% of patients lose their response after 5 years. Several mechanisms of resistance have been described, including amplification or overexpression of *BCR-ABL* or its protein product, point mutations of the Abl kinase domain, a defective transporter (OCT-1)

CURRENT THERAPY

Chronic Myeloid Leukemia

- Therapy Initiation
    - Initiate imatinib (Gleevec) 400 mg/day as soon as the diagnosis is confirmed
    - Educate patients and family members about objectives of therapy, adequate monitoring, importance of dose, and potential adverse events
- Therapeutic Monitoring
    - Weekly CBC and blood chemistry weekly until counts are stable, then every 4–6 weeks.
    - Monitor for adverse events; identify adverse events early and manage them properly
    - Cytogenetic analysis and bone marrow aspirate every 3–6 months until CCyR, then every 12 months
    - PCR every 3 months in peripheral blood; frequency may be decreased to every 6 months after stable major molecular response is achieved
- Dose Modifications
    - Interrupt imatinib for grades 3–4 nonhematologic toxicities, then resume with dose reduction (i.e., from 800 mg to 600 mg, from 600 mg to 400 mg, from 400 mg to 300 mg).
    - Reduce dose schedule by 25% for grade 2 persistent chronic toxicities.
    - Interrupt imatinib for grades 3–4 hematologic toxicities (i.e., ANC $<10^9$/L, platelets $<50 \times 10^9$/L). Resume therapy once counts recover above these levels. If recovery is within 2 weeks, restart at same dose. Reduce as per nonhematologic toxicity if recovery takes >2 weeks.
- Suboptimal Response
    - Assess compliance and measure imatinib plasma levels
    - Optimize therapy; consider dose increase (i.e., from 300 mg to 600 mg or from 400 mg to 800 mg)
- Failure to Imatinib
    - Assess for mutations of the Abl kinase domain
    - Change therapy to dasatinib (Sprycel) 100 mg daily (70 mg bid for patients in accelerated or blast phase) or nilotinib (Tasigna) 400 mg bid

Chronic Lymphocytic Leukemia

- Initial Evaluation
    - History: Fatigue, weight loss, fever, bleeding, recurrent infections, new adenopathy or change in previously noted adenopathy, prior blood work
    - Physical examination: Extent of lymphadenopathy, degree of splenomegaly and hepatomegaly, signs of infection or anemia
    - Laboratory: CBC with differential, blood chemistry analysis, tests for β_2-microglobulin and LDH levels, immunophenotyping, and HLA typing.
    - Prognostic factors: FISH for 17p del, 11q del, +12, and 13q del; IgV_H gene mutation status; ZAP70 expression; CD38 expression
    - Bone marrow (optional): Morphology, immunophenotyping, metaphase karyotyping
- Initial Management
    - Determine need for therapy (symptoms, stage, lymphocyte doubling time).
    - If WBC count $>2 \times 10^{11}$/L, consider admission, hydration, allopurinol (Zyloprim) therapy, and leukapheresis followed by chemotherapy.
    - Treat patients with autoimmune disorders with corticosteroids.
- Subsequent Management
    - Patients are encouraged to participate in clinical trials.
    - Patients requiring therapy and but who are ineligible for investigational therapy can receive fludarabine-based therapy. A combination of fludarabine plus cyclophosphamide ± rituximab is preferable for younger patients.
    - Patients who have failed fludarabine-based therapy should be offered alemtuzumab.
    - Allogeneic stem cell transplant might be considered for patients who have failed fludarabine-based regimens.

BMT = bone marrow transplantation; CBC = complete blood count; CCyR = complete cytogenetic response; CML = chronic myeloid leukemia; FISH = fluorescence in situ hybridization; HLA = human leukocyte antigen; IgV_{11} = Ig heavy chain variable gene; Ph = Philadelphia chromosome; LDH = lactate dehydrogenase; PCR = polymerase chain reaction; WBC = white blood cell.

---

of imatinib into the cell, overexpression of the multidrug-resistance (MDR) phenotype, and overexpression of Src-related kinases. Among them, mutations in the Abl kinase domain is the most commonly identified, occurring in 40% to 60% of patients who develop resistance to imatinib. More than 50 different mutations have been described. Although some mutations retain relative sensitivity to imatinib, others, particularly T315I, are nearly completely insensitive.

Imatinib failure can be defined based on the response achieved and the time to achieve such response. The current definitions of failure are presented in Table 2. Patients who meet these criteria have a significantly worse outcome, with a median survival of only 5 years in chronic phase and much shorter in the advanced stages. In addition, some patients have a suboptimal response to therapy. These patients have an outcome that is not quite as poor as that of patients with failure, but they do not have the same favorable outcome as those with what would be considered to be an optimal response.

Second-Line Therapy

A second generation of tyrosine kinase inhibitors has been developed to treat patients who develop resistance or intolerance to imatinib. Two agents have been already approved and others are being investigated.

TABLE 2 Definitions of Failure and Suboptimal Response to Imatinib According to the European Leukemianet

Time (mo)	Response	
	Failure	Suboptimal
3	No HR	No CHR
6	No CHR	35% Ph+
	100% Ph+	
12	35% Ph+	5% Ph+
18	5% Ph+	No MMR (<3-log ↓ BCR-ABL/ABL)
Any	Loss of CHR	CE
	Loss of CC_gR	Loss of MMR
	Mutation	Mutation

CC_gR = complete cytogenetic response; CE = clonal evolution; CHR = complete hematologic remission; HR = hematologic remission; MMR = major molecular response; Ph+ = Philadelphia chromosome positive.

Dasatinib (Sprycel) is a dual inhibitor of Abl and Src-related kinases. It is approximately 300 times more potent than imatinib against Abl and inhibits most mutated variants, except T315I. Studies with dasatinib in patients who have failed imatinib have demonstrated significant efficacy. In the chronic phase, nearly 50% of patients have achieved a complete cytogenetic response, with approximately 90% of patients alive and free from progression after 12 months.

Dasatinib is overall well tolerated. Grade 3 neutropenia or thrombocytopenia occurs in approximately 50% of patients. This is usually transient and can be managed with temporary treatment interruptions and, occasionally, dose reductions. Among nonhematologic adverse events, fatigue, headache, diarrhea, dyspnea, and rash are the most common and are usually mild and manageable. Pleural effusions occur in 25% to 35% of patients in the chronic phase, usually grade 1 or 2, and more often in advanced stages. This is best managed with temporary treatment interruptions, diuretics, and occasionally corticosteroids.

Initially, dasatinib was used at a dose of 70 mg twice daily. However, randomized trials in both chronic and advanced-stage disease have suggested that a once-daily dose (100 mg in chronic phase, 140 mg in accelerated phase) may be better tolerated, with decreased incidence of myelosuppression (in chronic phase) and other nonhematologic adverse events such as pleural effusions and gastrointestinal hemorrhage. The approved dose for chronic phase is now 100 mg once daily.

Nilotinib (Tasigna) is a more selective Abl tyrosine kinase inhibitor structurally similar to imatinib. Nilotinib is approximately 30 times more potent than imatinib against Abl, including most of the known mutants, but not more potent against other kinases. Phase II studies with nilotinib after imatinib failure have demonstrated significant activity among patients with resistance or intolerance to imatinib with CCyR in more than 40% of patients. Despite the similar biochemical structure, there is minimal cross-intolerance between imatinib and nilotinib. The standard dose of nilotinib is 400 mg twice daily. Myelosuppression grade 3 or 4 occurs in approximately 30% of patients. Other adverse events include elevation of lipase or bilirubin and hypophosphatemia. All of these are usually transient and asymptomatic.

ALLOGENEIC BONE MARROW TRANSPLANTATION

Allogeneic bone marrow transplantation (BMT) is an established strategy for patients with CML. The best results are reported for young patients (≤30 years) receiving transplants early in chronic phase with a disease-free survival of approximately 70% to 80%. The overall disease-free survival is 40% to 60%, with a 10% to 20% leukemic relapse rate. Allogeneic BMT may be associated with serious morbidity and an early mortality rate of 20% to 30%. Major complications include graft-versus-host disease (GVHD), interstitial pneumonitis, serious viral and fungal infections, organ damage from the conditioning regimen, and bleeding. Improvements in supportive and conditioning regimens (e.g., intravenous busulfan) have decreased the treatment-related mortality but have not affected relapse rates. Today SCT is rarely recommended as first-line therapy in CML and is mostly reserved for second- or third-line therapy.

Chronic Lymphocytic Leukemia

INCIDENCE AND RISK FACTORS

Chronic lymphocytic leukemia (CLL) is the most common type of adult leukemia in the United States and Western Europe. It is most common in persons of European or Russian descent. CLL is a disease of older persons; the median age at diagnosis is 72 years. It is more common in men than women. In contrast to other leukemias, there are no definite environmental exposures associated with this disease. Approximately 10% of cases have a familial association, suggesting a genetic predisposition for some individuals.

DIAGNOSIS

CLL is diagnosed based on finding an absolute blood lymphocytosis consisting of well-differentiated cells with monoclonal immunoglobulin (Ig) light chain expression and expressing CD19, CD5, CD23, and CD20. Chronic lymphoproliferative diseases can be differentiated by morphology, immunophenotype, and cytogenetics. The malignant lymphocytes accumulate in blood and other lymphoid tissues including bone marrow, lymph nodes, spleen, and liver. The differential diagnosis is shown in Table 3.

CLINICAL STAGING AND PROGNOSTIC FACTORS

The original Rai classification characterized CLL into five stages (Table 4). This system was simplified to low-risk (0), intermediate-risk (I and II), and high-risk (III and IV) disease. The Binet system categorizes CLL into three stages: A, B, and C (see Table 4). Both Rai and Binet stages are prognostic for survival, with earlier stages having superior survival.

CLL cells are not rapidly proliferating, making it difficult to generate metaphase chromosome preparations of these cells. Fluorescence in situ hybridization (FISH) is a way to probe interphase cells for specific chromosome abnormalities. Chromosome abnormalities can be identified in leukemia cells of more than 80% of patients with CLL by FISH analysis. A hierarchical categorization was developed in which patients are grouped according to their most unfavorable FISH abnormality in the following order: 17p deletion, 11q deletion, trisomy 12, no abnormality, and 13q deletion (sole).

There are at least four distinct prognostic groups associated with specific chromosome abnormalities. The two noted unfavorable groups are those with the 17p deletion or 11q deletion, with estimated median survivals of 32 and 79 months, respectively. The del (17p) and del(11q) abnormalities are associated with loss of *P53* and *ATM* genes, respectively. Patients with a 13q deletion as a sole abnormality had the best outcome, with an estimated median survival of 133 months.

Normal germinal center B cells can undergo somatic hypermutation, a mechanism to increase the affinity of their antibody for the stimulating antigen. These mutations occur in the Ig heavy chain variable gene (IgV_H), predominantly the CDR3 region. The clonal expressed IgV_H gene can be sequenced, and this sequence compared

TABLE 3 Differential Diagnosis of CLL

Disease	sIg	CD5	CD23	CD10	CD103	Chromosome Abnormality	Morphology
CLL	Weak	++	++	−	−	Varied	Small, well-differentiated
B-PLL	Strong	/+	/+	−	−	Varied	Large, open chromatin, nucleoli
HCL	Strong	−	−	−	++	None	Villous cytoplasmic projections
SLVL	Strong	/+	/+	/+	−	Varied	Short cytoplasmic projections
FL	Strong	−	−	++	−	t(14;18)	Follicular LN architecture
MCL	Strong	++	−	−	−	t(11;14)	Small, irregular nuclei

+ = present; = not present; B-PLL = B-cell prolymphocytic leukemia; CLL = chronic lymphocytic leukemia; FL = follicular lymphoma; HCL = hairy cell leukemia; LN = lymph node; MCL = mantle cell lymphome; sIg = surface immunoglobulin; SLVL = splenic lymphoma with villous lymphocytes.

TABLE 4 Staging of Chronic Lymphocytic Leukemia

Rai Stage	Modified Rai Stage	Description	Binet Stage	Description	Approximate Median Survival (y)
0	Low risk	Lymphocytosis only	A	Two or fewer lymphoid-bearing areas	>10
1	Intermediate risk	Lymphocytosis and lymphadenopathy	B	Three or more lymphoid-bearing areas	8
2		Lymphocytosis and splenomegaly ± lymphadenopathy	—	—	>6
3	High risk	Lymphocytosis and anemia (hemoglobin, <11 g/dL)	C	Anemia (hemoglobin, <10 g/dL) or thrombocytopenia (platelets 10^8/dL)	2
4		Lymphocytosis and thrombocytopenia (platelets <10^8/dL)	—	—	<2

with the expected germline sequence to determine if the leukemia clone has undergone somatic hypermutation. Homology of 98% or greater to germline indicates an unmutated IgV_H gene, and less than 98% homology indicates a mutated IgV_H gene. The mutation status has prognostic importance, particularly for patients with early-stage CLL. IgV_H mutation status is likely static and does not change over time. In retrospective analyses of select patient populations, survival was shorter for patients with an unmutated IgV_H gene compared with those with a mutated IgV_H gene. Surrogate markers for IgV_H mutation status have been sought, owing to the technical complexity of sequencing the IgV_H gene. As a result, expression of ZAP-70 or CD38 were correlated with having an unmutated IgV_H gene and with shorter survival in retrospective studies. Prospective evaluation of all these biomarkers is needed.

TREATMENT

The National Cancer Institute Working Group proposed formal recommendations or criteria in 1996 for initiating therapy for patients with CLL. These indications include bone marrow failure (anemia and thrombocytopenia), symptomatic disease, or rapidly progressing disease. Prognostic factor results are not used as indicators to initiate treatment. For patients with these indications, it is also important to exclude other confounding factors such as infection, immune thrombocytopenic purpura, or hemolytic anemia.

Historically, the approach to treatment was palliation, based on the observations that no treatment was shown to prolong survival and that no standard-dose chemotherapy or regimen results in cure. This approach focuses on improving symptoms and maintains that treatment should be nontoxic and reduce bulk of disease but does not need to result in complete remission. Historical therapy was often initiated with oral chlorambucil, with or without corticosteroids. Patients who progressed on this therapy were then treated with a combination such as cyclophosphamide (Cytoxan), vincristine (Vincasar),[1] and prednisone (Prelone) (CVP), and when this regimen failed, patients would then be treated with cyclophosphamide, doxorubicin (Adriamycin), vincristine, and prednisone (CHOP). Although this paradigm was widely followed, most patients who became refractory to chlorambucil failed to respond to these subsequent treatments.

Clinical research has been aimed at developing new treatments that prolong survival and potentially cure patients with CLL. A response-driven approach is used, based on the observation that patients who achieve complete remission live longer than those who achieve partial remission or those who fail treatment. In general, clinical trials aim to increase the complete remission rate and demonstrate prolonged remission duration with the expectation that this will result in improved survival. New drugs and combinations have

dramatically expanded treatment options and are significantly improving response rates for patients with CLL.

The superiority of purine analogues compared with alkylating agents was confirmed by at least three large randomized trials. The large Intergroup trial demonstrated superior complete remission rate for patients treated with fludarabine (Fludara) (Table 5). In addition, response duration was longer for patients treated with fludarabine. Despite greater activity, no overall survival advantage was demonstrated for treatment with fludarabine.

Cyclophosphamide induces DNA interstrand cross-links as the mechanism of inducing cell death. Leukemia cells, to some extent, can recover from this damage by DNA excision repair. Excision repair is inhibited by fludarabine, thus giving a rationale for combining fludarabine with cyclophosphamide (FC). A similar rationale applies to cladribine (Leustatin)[1] combined with cyclophosphamide. Recently, results from three large randomized trials have demonstrated that patients who received FC had higher complete and overall response rates and longer progression-free survival than those treated with fludarabine alone. None of the trials showed overall survival difference between patient groups (see Table 5).

Alemtuzumab (Campath), the monoclonal antibody (mAb) against CD52, was approved for treatment of fludarabine-refractory patients with CLL. Refractoriness was defined by failure to achieve at least partial remission with the last fludarabine-based regimen or relapse within 6 months of response. In the pivotal trial of alemtuzumab, one third of patients responded (most with partial remission), and the estimated median overall survival was 16 months with alemtuzumab treatment. Higher response rates were seen in a phase II single-arm trial of alemtuzumab for previously treated, but not refractory, patients. Some of these patients were free of minimal residual disease, which correlated with longer overall survival. The highest response rate for single-agent alemtuzumab was reported in previously untreated patients.

Rituximab (Rituxan), the mAb against CD20, has very limited activity at 375 mg/m[2]/week for 4 weeks in patients with CLL. The pivotal trial for rituximab demonstrated an overall response rate of 12% in previously treated patients with IWF (International Working Formulation) A non-Hodgkin's lymphoma, the CLL/SLL equivalent. Dose-intense or dose-dense single-agent rituximab markedly improves response rate over the standard dose and schedule and is well tolerated. Rituximab has been evaluated in a dose-intense regimen of up to 2.25 g/m[2] weekly for 4 weeks and in a dose-dense regimen of 375 mg/m[2] thrice weekly for 4 weeks. These phase II studies showed improved activity compared with that seen with standard-dose single-agent rituximab in the pivotal trial.

Purine analogue-based chemotherapy has been combined with mAbs, referred to as chemoimmunotherapy, for treatment of chemotherapy-naïve, relapsed, and refractory patients with CLL (Table 6).

[1]Not FDA approved for this indication.

[1]Not FDA approved for this indication.

TABLE 5 Randomized Trials of Chemotherapy as Initial Treatment For Chronic Lymphocytic Leukemia

Agent*	No. Pts	% CR	% OR	RD	Survival
Intergroup Study					
F: 20 mg/m² IV d 1–5 plus	123	20	61	NR	55 mo OS
CHL: 20 mg/m² PO d 1 or					
F: 25 mg/m² IV d 1–5 or	170	20	63	25 mo (TTP)	66 mo OS
CHL: 40 mg/m² PO d 1	181	4	37	14 mo (TTP)	56 mo OS
GCLLSG Study					
F: 30 mg/m² IV d 1–3 plus	164	24	95	48 mo (PFS)	80% at 3 y
CYT: 250 mg/m² IV d 1–3 or					
F: 25 mg/m² IV d 1–5	164	7	83	20 mo (PFS)	81% at 3 y
ECOG Study					
F: 20 mg/m² IV d 1–5 plus	137	23	74	32 mo (PFS)	79% at 2 y
CYT: 600 mg/m² IV d 1 or					
F: 25 mg/m² IV d 1–5	132	6	60	19 mo (PFS)	80% at 2 y
UK LRF Study					
F: 25 mg/m² IV d 1–3 plus	182	38	95	43 mo (PFS)	54% at 5 y
CYT: 250 mg/m² IV d 1–3 or					
F: 25 mg/m² IV d 1–5 or	181	15	80	23 mo (PFS)	52% at 5 y
CHL-10 mg/m² PO d 1–7	366	7	72	20 mo (PFS)	59% at 5 y
PALG Study					
CDA: 0.12 mg/kg IV d 1–5 or	166	21	77	24 mo (PFS)	50 mo OS
CDA: 0.12 mg/kg IV d 1–3 plus	162	29	83	22 mo (PFS)	NR
CYT: 650 mg/m² IV d 1 or					
CDA: 0.12 mg/kg IV d 1–3 plus	151	36	80	24 mo (PFS)	NR
CYT: 650 mg/m² IV d 1 plus					
MIT: 10 mg/m² IV d 1					

[1]Not FDA approved for this indication.
*All courses are 28 days.
CDA = cladribine (Leustatin)[1]; CHL = chlorambucil (Leukeran); CR = complete remission; CYT = cyclophosphamide (Cytoxan); ECOG = Eastern Cooperative Oncology Group; F = fludarabine (Fludara); GCLLSG = German CLL Study Group; MIT = mitoxantrone (Novantrone)[1]; NR = not reached; OR = overall response; OS = median overall survival; PALG = Polish Adult Leukemia Group; PFS = median progression-free survival: Pts = patients; RD = median remission duration; TTP = median time-to-progression; UK LRF = United Kingdom Leukaemia Research Fund.

TABLE 6 Chemoimmunotherapy for Patients with Chronic Lymphocytic Leukemia

Treatment	Prior Treatment	No. Evaluable	% CR	% OR
FluCam Regimen (4-wk course)				
F: 30 mg/m² d 1–3, courses 1–6	Yes	36	30	83
A: 30 mg d 1–3, courses 1–6				
MD Anderson Cancer Center Regimen (4-wk course)				
F: 25 mg/m² IV d 2–4, course 1; d 1–3, courses 2–6	No	224	70	95
C: 250 mg/m² IV d 2–4, course 1; d 1–3, courses 2–6	Yes	177	25	73
R: 375–500 mg/m² IV d 1; courses 1–6				
CALGB 9712 Study, Randomized				
Concurrent (4-wk course)				
F: 25 mg/m² IV d 1–5, courses 1–6	No	51	47	90
R: 375 mg/m² IV d 1 and 4, course 1; d1, courses 2–6				
2 months observation, then				
R: 375 mg/m² IV weekly × 4				
Sequential (4-wk course)				
F: 25 mg/m² IV d 1–5, courses 1–6	No	53	28	77
2 months observation, then				
R: 375 mg/m² IV weekly × 4				
Mayo Clinic and Ohio State University Study (3-wk course)				
P: 2 mg/m² IV d 1, courses 1–6	No	64	41	91
C: 600 mg/m² IV d 1, courses 1–6				
R: 375 mg/m² IV d 1, courses 2–6				
Memorial Sloan Kettering Study (3-wk course)				
P: 4 mg/m² IV d 1, courses 1–6	Yes	32	25	75
C: 600 mg/m² IV d 1, courses 1–6				
R: 375 mg/m² IV d 1, courses 2–6				

A = alemtuzumab (Campath); C = cyclophosphamide (Cytoxan); CALGB = Cancer and Leukemia Group B; CR = complete remission; F = fludarabine (Fludara); FluCam = fludarabine phosphate and alemtuzumab; OR = overall response; P = pentostatin (Nipent); R = rituximab (Rituxan).

The phase II randomized CALGB 9712 (Cancer and Leukemia Group B) trial compared concurrent with sequential fludarabine and rituximab and demonstrated a higher complete remission rate with concurrent treatment, indicating potentiation of activity with the combination. Significant activity has been seen with front-line and salvage phase II single-arm trials with chemoimmunotherapy regimens, and randomized phase III controlled clinical trials are ongoing. Overall, management of patients with CLL has changed significantly with the development of new therapeutic agents and combinations.

REFERENCES

Apperley JF. Part I: Mechanisms of resistance to imatinib in chronic myeloid leukaemia. Lancet Oncol 2007;8:1018–29.

Baccarani M, Saglio G, Goldman J, et al. Evolving concepts in the management of chronic myeloid leukemia: Recommendations from an expert panel on behalf of the European LeukemiaNet. Blood 2006;108:1809–20.

Cheson BD, Bennett JM, Grever M, et al. National Cancer Institute—sponsored Working Group guidelines for chronic lymphocytic leukemia: Revised guidelines for diagnosis and treatment. Blood 1996;87:4990–7.

Crespo M, Bosch F, Villamor N, et al. ZAP-70 expression as a surrogate for immunoglobulin-variable-region mutations in chronic lymphocytic leukemia. N Engl J Med 2003;348:1764–75.

Damle RN, Wasil T, Fais F, et al. Ig V gene mutation status and CD38 expression as novel prognostic indicators in chronic lymphocytic leukemia. Blood 1999;94:1840–7.

Dohner H, Stilgenbauer S, Dohner K, et al. Chromosome aberrations in B-cell chronic lymphocytic leukemia: Reassessment based on molecular cytogenetic analysis. J Mol Med 1999;77:266–81.

Druker BJ, Guilhot F, O'Brien SG, et al. Five-year follow-up of patients receiving imatinib for chronic myeloid leukemia. N Engl J Med 2006;355:2408–17.

Hochhaus A, Kantarjian HM, Baccarani M, et al. Dasatinib induces notable hematologic and cytogenetic responses in chronic-phase chronic myeloid leukemia after failure of imatinib therapy. Blood 2007;109:2303–9.

Kantarjian HM, Giles F, Gattermann N, et al. Nilotinib (formerly AMN107), a highly selective Bcr-Abl tyrosine kinase inhibitor, is effective in patients with Philadelphia chromosome–positive chronic myelogenous leukemia in chronic phase following imatinib resistance and intolerance. Blood 2007;110(10):3540–6.

Kantarjian H, Schiffer C, Jones D, Cortes J. Monitoring the response and course of chronic myeloid leukemia in the modern era of BCR-ABL tyrosine kinase inhibitors: Practical advice on the use and interpretation of monitoring methods. Blood 2008;111:1774–80.

Keating MJ, O'Brien S, Albitar M, et al. Early results of a chemoimmunotherapy regimen of fludarabine, cyclophosphamide, and rituximab as initial therapy for chronic lymphocytic leukemia. J Clin Oncol 2005;23:4079–88.

Rai KR, Peterson BL, Appelbaum FR, et al. Fludarabine compared with chlorambucil as primary therapy for chronic lymphocytic leukemia. N Engl J Med 2000;343:1750–7.

Non-Hodgkin's Lymphoma

Method of
Frederick L. Locke, MD, and Sonali M. Smith, MD

Non-Hodgkin's lymphoma (NHL) is an umbrella term encompassing several dozen distinct clinicopathologic lymphoid malignancies. The current World Health Organisation (WHO) pathologic classification identifies almost 60 unique subtypes based on morphologic, immunophenotypic, and genetic differences and clinical behavior. Despite the numerous subtypes, NHL can be broadly divided based on the cell of origin (B-cell or T-cell) or on clinical behavior (indolent, aggressive, or highly aggressive). Most cases of NHL are mature B-cell lymphomas; the most common subtypes and classifications are summarized in Table 1.

In general, indolent lymphomas are slowly progressive but incurable diseases, with a median survival time of 8 to 10 years. Highly aggressive lymphomas, such as Burkitt's and Burkitt-like lymphomas, are rapidly progressive at presentation but curable in 70% to 90% of patients. Aggressive lymphomas are curable in 50% to 90% of patients, with outcome strongly dependent on clinical and biologic features at presentation (see later discussion). A major modern theme in the study of lymphomas is the growing appreciation of biologic heterogeneity within subtypes, as identified by current molecular and immunologic approaches.

Epidemiology and Etiology

NHL is the fifth most common cause of cancer in both men and women. An estimated 70,000 new cases of NHL will be diagnosed in 2009. Although NHL is highly treatable and occasionally curable, it accounts for more than 20,000 deaths in the United States annually. In western Europe and the United States, the overall incidence of NHL increased between the 1970s and the early part of the 21st century, in contrast to the plateau observed in the incidence of Hodgkin's lymphoma. NHL has been described in all age groups, including infants, but the median age at presentation is in the sixth decade of life. Although NHL occurs in all races and ethnicities, the frequencies of various subtypes appear to be geographically influenced. For example, Epstein-Barr virus (EBV)–related Burkitt's lymphoma occurs primarily in sub-Saharan Africa, whereas follicular lymphoma appears primarily in industrialized regions.

The etiology of NHL in most patients remains elusive. NHL is clearly influenced by the immune status of the patient, as reflected by the increased incidence of NHL in patients with iatrogenic immunosuppression (e.g., after solid organ transplantation), acquired immunosuppression (e.g., HIV infection), or a variety of autoimmune disorders (e.g., rheumatoid arthritis, Sjögren's syndrome). Several lymphotrophic viruses have been identified, including EBV, HIV, hepatitis C, human herpesvirus 8 (HHV-8), and human T-lymphotrophic virus 1 (HTLV-1). Bacteria have also been implicated, including *Helicobacter pylori*, which can cause gastric marginal zone lymphoma. Although no clear genetic lesion has been identified, NHL may cluster in families and is increased in a variety of inherited cancer syndromes.

Classification

The current WHO pathologic classification schema for lymphoma recognizes the cell of origin of the neoplasm (B–cell, T–cell, or natural killer [NK] cell) and further categorizes disorders as immature (most acute leukemias and acute lymphoblastic lymphomas) or mature (what is typically referred to as NHL). The separation between leukemia and lymphoma in some cases is arbitrary and dependent on the presence, absence, or combination of malignant cells in the peripheral blood (leukemia) or lymph nodes (lymphoma).

B-cell lymphomas are clonal tumors, and their classification, with a few exceptions, parallels the normal stages of lymphocyte differentiation. Naive B–cells arise in the bone marrow and mature in lymph nodes. Within the lymph nodes, they traverse the germinal center before terminal differentiation into either plasma cells or memory B cells. The various points at which malignant transformation may occur are extensive, leading to almost 60 subtypes of NHL. The two most common B-cell subtypes, diffuse large B-cell lymphoma (DLBCL) and follicular lymphoma (FL), are discussed in detail later in this chapter.

Hodgkin's lymphoma has now been identified as a mature B-cell malignancy (see the chapter on Hodgkin's lymphoma), but because of the independent evolution of treatment approaches, it is usually considered in a distinct manner from NHL. High-throughput gene expression analyses have found strong genetic links between Hodgkin's lymphoma and NHL, and several gray-zone lymphomas sharing features of both disorders are included in the current WHO classification.

Mature T-cell lymphomas and NK-cell lymphomas are less common than B-cell subtypes and comprise only 5% to 10% of NHLs in North America. However, there is geographic variation, and T-cell lymphomas account for up to 20% of NHLs in many parts

TABLE 1 World Health Organisation (WHO) and Clinical Classification of Selected Subtypes of Non-Hodgkin's Lymphoma

WHO Pathologic Category	Clinical Behavior		
	Indolent	Aggressive	Highly Aggressive
Mature B-cell neoplasms	Follicular lymphoma Chronic lymphocytic leukemia/small lymphocytic lymphoma Hairy cell leukemia Extranodal marginal zone lymphoma Lymphoplasmacytic lymphoma/ Waldenstrom's macroglobulinemia* Splenic B-cell marginal zone lymhpoma	Diffuse large B-cell lymphoma, NOS Primary mediastinal large B-cell lymphoma Mantle cell lymphoma	Burkitt's lymphoma
Mature T-cell and NK-cell neoplasms	Mycosis fungoides Sézary syndrome	Hepatosplenic T-cell lymphoma Peripheral T-cell lymphoma, NOS Angioimmunoblastic T-cell lymphoma Anaplastic large cell lymphoma, ALK+ type Anaplastic large cell lymphoma, ALK− type	

Adapted from Jaffe E, Harris NL, Stein H, et al: Introduction and overview of the classification of lymphoid neoplasms. In Swerdlow SH, Campo E, Harris NL, et al (eds): WHO Classification of Tumours of Haematopoietic and Lymphoid Tissues. Lyon, IARC, 2008, pp 158–66.
*Can behave aggressively.
Abbreviations: ALK = anaplastic lymphoma kinase; NK = natural killer; NOS = not otherwise specified; WHO = World Health Organisation.

of Asia. In addition to being more rare, there are dozens of T-cell NHL subtypes, making systematic pathologic and clinical investigations extremely difficult. Many T-cell lymphomas are extranodal in presentation, leading to broad classification into nodal, extranodal, and leukemic categories. T-cell lymphomas are discussed in more detail later.

Clinical Presentation, Diagnosis, and Staging

The clinical features of NHL are highly variable among patients and often reflect the site of involvement. Enlarging lymph nodes are typically painless, and many patients are asymptomatic, with pathologic nodes discovered incidentally in most indolent subtypes. Somatic symptoms may develop as a result of local anatomic effects of enlarging adenopathy or edema caused by altered venous or lymphatic drainage. The presence of constitutional B symptoms at diagnosis directly correlate to prognosis. These symptoms classically include unexplained fevers, night sweats, and unintentional weight loss of greater than 10% of total body weight. In addition, pruritus or malaise may be present. The physical examination often reveals enlarged adenopathy or hepatosplenomegaly.

The marked heterogeneity of NHL subtypes makes acquisition of adequate tissue samples an imperative part of the diagnostic evaluation. Fine-needle aspiration of an accessible, pathologically enlarged lymph node is often the initial diagnostic test obtained and may confirm a clonal B-cell process; however, such aspirates rarely confirm the subtype of lymphoma. Excisional biopsy or multiple core needle biopsies are usually required to provide enough tissue for accurate histologic architecture (or grading) and molecular or cytogenetic studies—information that is important for determining the disease subtype, prognosis, and treatment.

Once a pathologic diagnosis is confirmed, prompt referral to a medical oncologist is warranted. The current staging system for lymphoma is the Ann Arbor system with the Cotswold revision (Table 2). Standard staging evaluation includes imaging of the chest, abdomen, and pelvis with computed tomographic scans and a bone

TABLE 2 Ann Arbor Staging System with Cotswold Revision for Hodgkin's and Non-Hodgkin's Lymphoma

Stage or Modifier	Description
Stage I	One affected lymph node or lymph node region
Stage II	Two or more affected lymph node regions on one side of the diaphragm
Stage III	Affected lymph node regions both above and below the diaphragm
Stage IV	Extralymphatic involvement, such as bone marrow involvement
A	Suffix denoting no B symptoms
B	Suffix denoting the presence of B symptoms such as unexplained weight loss, fever, or drenching night sweats
X	Suffix denoting bulky disease, defined as a mass >10 cm in diameter or a mediastinal mass >1/3 of the chest on a chest radiograph

Adapted from Lister TA, Crowther D, Sutcliffe SB, et al: Report of a committee convened to discuss the evaluation and staging of patients with Hodgkin's disease: Cotswolds meeting. J Clin Oncol 1989;7:1630–36.

marrow aspirate and core biopsy. Some patients may also require a lumbar puncture, depending on the specific NHL subtype and sites of involvement. Increasingly, fluorodeoxyglucose (FDG)-positron-emission tomography (PET) is used for initial staging of lymphomas. Most lymphomas are strongly FDG-PET avid, a feature that allows for more precise staging and more accurate assessment of response after treatment.

Recently, prognostic scoring systems have been validated for some of the more common subtypes of NHL (see later discussion). In order to utilize some of these systems, additional laboratory studies (e.g., lactate dehydrogenase [LDH], β_2-microglobulin) are required before therapy begins.

CURRENT DIAGNOSIS

- A detailed history and physical examination are needed for diagnosis (locating suitable sites for biopsy) and for staging (determination of extent of disease and characterization of B symptoms).
- Serum studies include complete blood count, comprehensive metabolic profile, and lactate dehydrogenase.
- Adequate tissue sampling is necessary, preferably by multiple core needle biopsies or excisional biopsy.
- Pathologic diagnosis requires immunophenotyping and is aided by detailed morphologic description.
- Cytogenetic and molecular studies are helpful in establishing the diagnosis in some forms of non-Hodgkin's lymphoma; examples are *c-myc* (*MYC*) and t(8;14) overexpression in Burkitt's lymphoma and t(11;14) in mantle cell lymphoma.
- The clinical staging work-up includes computed tomographic scans and bone marrow biopsy; in selected cases, lumbar puncture or positron-emission tomographic scanning is included.
- Appropriate clinical prognostic scoring at diagnosis is helpful (e.g., International Prognostic Index for aggressive lymphomas, Follicular Lymphoma International Prognostic Index for follicular lymphoma).

Treatment Principles

Lymphoma is a systemic disorder, and the mainstay of therapy is combination chemotherapy, with the addition of radiation therapy or immunotherapy in selected situations. The anti-CD20 chimeric immunoglobulin G1 monoclonal antibody, rituximab (Rituxan), is often used for B-cell lymphomas and is discussed in some detail later. Surgical intervention is typically limited to establishing the diagnosis. The specifics of treatment are highly variable and are based on the subtype and the stage of disease. Treatment details for the more common subtypes are discussed later under each disease subtype. A general description of treatment modalities and their applicability follows.

Many different chemotherapy combination regimens have been used against NHL. One commonly used regimen (particularly for DLBCL) is R-CHOP. This regimen is typically given on an outpatient basis with all drugs except prednisone given once every 3 weeks for four to six treatment cycles. R-CHOP consists of rituximab, cyclophosphamide (Cytoxan), doxorubicin (hydroxydaunorubicin, Adriamycin), vincristine (Oncovin), and prednisone.

For rare occurrences of localized early-stage FL, external-beam radiation therapy may achieve long-term remission as a single modality. In aggressive lymphomas, craniospinal irradiation may be used to prevent relapse in the central nervous system. Many lymphomas are radiosensitive, and external-beam radiation therapy can be highly beneficial in palliative situations.

Immunotherapies, in particular monoclonal antibodies, have been intensively studied in NHL. CD20 is a surface antigen that is present on both normal and malignant mature B–cells; its exact function is not clearly understood, but monoclonal antibodies targeting CD20 lead to cell death via apoptosis, complement-dependent cytotoxicity, and antibody-dependent cytotoxicity. Rituximab, a chimeric monoclonal antibody against CD20, was the first monoclonal antibody approved for use against human cancers and is widely used to treat B-cell neoplasms. In addition, several radiolabeled anti-CD20 monoclonal antibodies are approved for the treatment of relapsed FL. Denileukin diftitox (Ontak) is recombinant diphtheria toxin conjugated to interleukin 2; it is used for some T-cell lymphomas.

CURRENT THERAPY

- Indolent lymphomas are typically at an advanced stage at initial presentation (stage III or IV) and are slowly growing but incurable. Indolent lymphomas are initially quite chemosensitive, but therapy is not always warranted and can be delayed with a "watch and wait" approach.
- Indications for treatment of indolent lymphomas include systemic symptoms, symptoms related to bulk or location of disease, cytopenias, and transformation to aggressive non-Hodgkin's lymphoma. Stage I disease may show prolonged response to radiation therapy.
- Chemotherapy regimens commonly include alkylating agents (cyclophosphamide [Cytoxan]), nucleoside analogues (fludarabine [Fludara][1]), alkaloids (vincristine [Oncovin]), corticosteroids (prednisone), and monoclonal antibodies (rituximab [Rituxan]). An anthracycline (doxorubicin [Adriamycin]) is often included for aggressive lymphomas.
- Diffuse large B-cell lymphoma is the prototypical aggressive lymphoma and is potentially curable with R-CHOP combination chemotherapy.
- Highly aggressive lymphomas, such as Burkitt's lymphoma, require intensive inpatient chemotherapy on an emergent basis.
- R-CHOP consists of rituximab (**R**), cyclophosphamide (**C**), doxorubicin (**H**ydroxydaunorubicin), vincristine (**O**ncovin), and prednisone (**P**).

[1]Not FDA approved for this indication.

Hematopoietic stem cell transplantation is typically reserved for patients with relapsed lymphoma. High-dose chemotherapy and autologous stem cell rescue can successfully salvage approximately half of patients with relapsed DLBCL, but its use in other lymphoma subtypes remains controversial. Allogeneic transplantation, which capitalizes on a graft-versus-lymphoma effect, can afford long-term disease control in many patients and is usually considered for multiply relapsed patients with a good performance status.

Diffuse Large B-Cell Lymphoma

The most common subtype of NHL is DLBCL, comprising approximately 30% of cases. In general, DLBCL is a chemoresponsive and potentially curable disease, with the outcome strongly dependent on clinical and biologic features at presentation. It is primarily a disease of the elderly (median age at diagnosis, 64 years), and incidence increases with age. DLBCL has several histologic variants (immunoblastic, T–cell rich, centroblastic) and several unique clinical subtypes (primary mediastinal B-cell lymphoma, primary effusion lymphoma, primary intravascular lymphoma). Biologic subtypes that may explain some of the heterogeneity in outcome have been identified with the use of gene expression profiling (see later discussion). Histologically, DLBCL reveals replacement of normal lymph node architecture with large, atypical cells resembling centroblasts or immunoblasts, the cells of origin of this particular lymphoid neoplasm. Immunophenotyping shows common B-cell antigens such as CD19, CD20, and CD22. As with other NHLs, the Ann Arbor staging system is used (see Table 2). Approximately 60% of cases are stage III or IV at diagnosis, and 30% of patients have B symptoms.

An important prognostic tool in DLBCL is the International Prognostic Index (IPI), which was developed by an international task force evaluating more than 2000 patients with newly diagnosed DLBCL who were receiving anthracycline-based chemotherapy.

The IPI assigns 1 point for each of five prognostic factors (age >60 years, performance status >1, LDH elevation, >1 extranodal site, stage III or IV). Lower point scores correlate to complete response rates, relapse-free survival, and overall survival. Because this scoring system is weighted heavily toward older patients, an age-adjusted IPI was released concurrently. It is intended for use with patients younger than 60 years of age and considers only disease stage, LDH level, and performance status. The IPI was developed based on treatment outcomes before the advent of the B cell–specific CD20 monoclonal antibody, rituximab, which has significantly improved outcomes and is the current standard of care. In 2007, a revised version of the IPI, called the R-IPI, was proposed in a population-based study of patients treated with R-CHOP (Table 3). Analysis of patients by the R-IPI shows that, although the overall outcome has improved with R-CHOP, approximately 45% of patients have high-risk disease and continue to have a suboptimal outcome, with only 53% progression-free survival and 55% overall survival at 4 years.

In addition to clinical heterogeneity reflected by the IPI and R-IPI, there is biologic heterogeneity within DLBCL, which has been investigated by gene expression profiling. When de novo DLBCL tumor samples were analyzed for gene expression (messenger RNA), two distinct clusters of gene expression were identified, one resembling normal physiologic germinal center B-lymphocyte expression (termed the GC subtype) and another subset resembling the expression of activated B–lymphocytes (termed the ABC or non-GC subtype). When patients treated with CHOP were evaluated based on these gene expression clusters, those with ABC-like tumors had a reduced probability of overall survival at 5 years of only 16%, compared with 76% for GC patients.

The standard initial therapy for DLBCL is chemoimmunotherapy using both rituximab and an anthracycline, with R-CHOP being the most widely used regimen. The consensus on the utility of CHOP is based on the results of several prospective phase III randomized trials. The addition of rituximab to CHOP clearly produces improved rates of progression-free and overall survival, compared with CHOP alone, in patients with advanced-stage DLBCL. With R-CHOP therapy, 50% to 90% of patients achieve durable remissions, with the outcome highly dependent on the clinical and biologic prognostic factors discussed earlier.

Approximately half of those initially achieving a complete remission eventually relapse and require further therapy. For relapsed patients (or those whose disease is refractory to initial therapy), additional treatment typically consists of a different combination chemotherapy regimen with the goal of proceeding to autologous stem cell transplantation (ASCT). Patients demonstrating a response to so-called salvage regimens are deemed to have chemosensitive disease and are potentially curable with high-dose chemotherapy followed by rescue with ASCT. A superior outcome for ASCT over chemotherapy alone in patients with relapsed DLBCL has been established, with long-term disease control in about 40% to 50% of patients. However, age, performance status, and comorbidities are all factors that influence the success of ASCT. Patients who relapse despite ASCT, and those who are not candidates for ASCT, have a poor prognosis, with average survival of approximately 8 months, although those with a low IPI at relapse may fare better.

Follicular Lymphoma

FL is the prototype of indolent lymphomas and comprises approximately 20% of all lymphomas. FL is generally considered an incurable disorder, but it has a prolonged median survival of 8 to 10 years. Newer advances in therapy have challenged the notion of incurability, and there are accumulating data that the overall survival of patients with FL is improving. FL occurs primarily in elderly patients, with the median age at presentation being in the sixth or seventh decade of life. Histologically, FL is composed mostly of small, mature lymphocytes that maintain a nodular or follicular pattern within the lymph node. The increased presence of large cells often corresponds to the clinical behavior of FL; if sheets of large cells are present, the treatment is usually similar to that for DLBCL. Most FL patients have stage III or IV disease at presentation, with almost 70% having bone marrow involvement. In the natural history of FL, there is usually a period of initial chemosensitivity, followed invariably by relapse and the emergence of drug resistance. Furthermore, FL can transform to DLBCL at a rate of 1% to 2% per year. Patients with transformed FL usually have a poor prognosis, and their disease is often resistant to treatment.

The prognosis of FL is quite variable and appears to be influenced by both clinical and biologic factors. The Follicular Lymphoma International Prognostic Index (FLIPI) is a clinical tool that tallies five risk factors to determine prognosis: age 60 years or older, Ann Arbor stage III-IV, hemoglobin concentration less than 12 g/dL, serum

TABLE 3 International Prognostic Index (IPI), Revised IPI (R-IPI), and Follicular Lymphoma IPI (FLIPI) for Non-Hodgkin's Lymphoma

Risk Factor	Number of Factors	Risk Group	Distribution of Patients (%)	5-Y Overall Survival Rate (%)
IPI				
Age >60 y	0 or 1	Low	35	73
ECOG Performance Status >2	2	Low-intermediate	27	51
Serum LDH > ULN	3	High-intermediate	22	43
>1 extranodal site	4 or 5	High	16	26
Ann Arbor stage III-IV				
R-IPI				
Age >60 y				
ECOG Performance Status >2	0	Very good	10	94*
Serum LDH > ULN	1, 2	Good	45	79*
>1 extranodal site	3, 4, 5	Poor	45	55*
Ann Arbor stage III-IV				
FLIPI				
Age ≥60 y	0 or 1	Low	36	91
Ann Arbor stage III-IV	2	Intermediate	37	78
Hemoglobin level <12 g/dL	3, 4, or 5	High	27	27
Serum LDH > ULN				
>4 nodal sites				

*4-year survival data.
Abbreviations: ECOG = Eastern Cooperative Oncology Group; LDH = lactate dehydrogenase; ULN = upper limit of normal.

LDH greater than the upper limit of normal, and more than four nodal sites. The FLIPI (Table 3) stratifies patients into three risk groups with roughly equal distribution, providing 5- and 10-year overall survival rates of 91% and 71% for low-risk FL (0–1 risk factors), 78% and 51% for intermediate-risk FL (2 risk factors), and 53% and 36% for high-risk FL (3 or more risk factors), respectively. In addition to clinical heterogeneity, gene expression profiling has surprisingly shown that clinical outcome is strongly dependent on genetic signatures of infiltrating *nonmalignant* cells in patients with FL. However, despite the robust prognostic influence, neither the FLIPI nor gene expression profiling currently influences treatment strategies, and numerous studies are under way to determine their optimal use in individual patients.

The current treatment approach to FL is to first determine whether treatment is required, based on the extent of involvement, compromise of normal organs, and patient symptomatology. Patients with stage I disease are usually offered involved-field radiation, but patients with advanced disease (stage II or greater) have a variety of treatment options without a clear standard of care. Because there is no consensus for initial treatment of advanced disease, and because there is no clear survival advantage with any particular chemotherapy regimen, many patients with newly diagnosed FL are observed on a "watch and wait" strategy. Those who require treatment have many options, including monoclonal antibodies, chemotherapy, chemoimmunotherapy, biologic agents, and stem cell transplantation.

A major improvement in the treatment of FL, and many B-cell NHLs, occurred with the advent of monoclonal antibodies against CD20. The combination of rituximab with common chemotherapy regimens for FL, such as CHOP and CVP (cyclophosphamide, vincristine, and prednisone), has been prospectively studied in multiple phase III trials and found to improve event-free and overall survival rates. As a single agent, rituximab has a 70% response rate in patients with FL, although increased overall survival with rituximab as a single agent has yet to be demonstrated. The addition of a radioactive moiety to monoclonal antibodies (i.e., radioimmunotherapy) is also quite promising, and many studies are under way to determine the optimal use of this combination.

Burkitt's Lymphoma

Burkitt's lymphoma is the prototype of highly aggressive lymphomas, although it may manifest as an acute leukemia if circulating cells predominate. The two major clinical forms are the endemic and the sporadic subtypes. The endemic subtype typically involves the bones of the jaw and is common in Africa. Whereas endemic Burkitt's lymphoma is characterized by evidence of EBV infection in all cases, only 20% to 30% of cases of sporadic Burkitt's lymphoma reveal EBV. Sporadic Burkitt's lymphoma is rare and comprises only about 2% of all NHLs in the United States, with children and young adults being primarily affected.

Burkitt's lymphoma originates from the germinal center of lymph nodes and on histologic examination often exhibits a so-called starry-sky appearance. In addition, it has a distinct molecular profile showing evidence of *c-myc* (*MYC*) deregulation, and some histologically atypical cases may be identified and treated accordingly. The disease is highly aggressive, with symptoms often related to the site of rapid growth. Whereas therapy for aggressive lymphomas often involves combination chemotherapy at 3-week intervals, therapy for Burkitt's lymphoma utilizes intensive inpatient induction chemotherapy of short duration coupled with a high degree of supportive care. Subsequent cycles of chemotherapy are usually given as soon as hematopoietic recovery is apparent. Because there is a high potential for progression to the central nervous system, intrathecal methotrexate is used.

Burkitt's lymphoma is potentially curable, with 5-year overall survival rates of 70% to 90%. Any confirmed or highly suspicious pathologic diagnosis of Burkitt's lymphoma is an oncologic emergency and warrants immediate completion of staging and initiation of therapy.

T-Cell and NK-Cell Lymphomas

T-cell lymphomas are an uncommon but complex entity with incidence variable by region and ethnicity and a higher prevalence in Asia. T-cell and NK-cell lymphomas are grouped together and account for approximately 12% of all NHLs. T-cell lymphomas may be associated with EBV or HTLV viral infections. These lymphomas are extremely heterogeneous and can be subdivided into many types based on histology and molecular markers. As with B-cell lymphomas, the clinical progression and natural history are variable depending on subtype. Treatment outcome is typically suboptimal with currently available therapies. Broadly, T-cell and NK-cell neoplasms can be subdivided into leukemic, nodal, and extranodal categories. Extranodal T-cell lymphomas are most commonly cutaneous and include mycosis fungoides and Sézary syndrome. Prognosis is variable by subtype, and therapy may consist of skin-directed therapy, systemic therapy, or a combination of the two. Topically applied drugs include corticosteroids, chemotherapeutic agents (e.g., mechlorethamine [Mustargen]), and retinoids. Disseminated disease limited to the skin may be treated with total skin electron-beam radiotherapy. Systemic therapies include extracorporeal photopheresis, chemotherapeutics, and cytokine therapy (e.g., interferon-alfa [Intron A],[1] denileukin diftitox). Newer agents include histone de-acetylase inhibitors and oral retinoids.

Nodal T-cell lymphomas include peripheral T-cell lymphoma, anaplastic large cell lymphoma, and angioimmunoblastic T-cell lymphoma. The anaplastic lymphoma kinase (ALK)-positive variant of anaplastic large cell lymphoma has a more favorable prognosis than the other subtypes. Leukemic variants of T-cell lymphoma include hepatosplenic γ-δ T-cell lymphoma and T-cell prolymphocytic leukemia. The most commonly used front-line regimen for nodal or systemic disease is CHOP chemotherapy, but the results are suboptimal, with only one third of patients obtaining long-term remission. Some investigators advocate high-dose chemotherapy and ASCT as part of front-line treatment to decrease the relapse rate. Both autologous and allogeneic hematopoietic transplantation are considered at relapse. The ability to develop evidence-based treatment approaches to T-cell lymphomas is substantially hampered by the rarity of each subtype and their aggressive nature, which often precludes participation in a clinical trial.

REFERENCES

Coiffier B, Lepage E, Briere J, et al. CHOP chemotherapy plus rituximab compared with CHOP alone in elderly patients with diffuse large-B-cell lymphoma. N Engl J Med 2002;346:235–42.

Hochster H, Weller E, Gascoyne RD, et al. Maintenance rituximab after cyclophosphamide, vincristine, and prednisone prolongs progression-free survival in advanced indolent lymphoma: Results of the randomized phase III ECOG1496 study. J Clin Oncol 2009;27:1607–14.

Jemal A, Siegel R, Ward E, et al. Cancer statistics, 2008. CA Cancer J Clin 2008;58:71–96.

Kewalramani T, Nimer SD, Zelenetz AD, et al. Progressive disease following autologous transplantation in patients with chemosensitive relapsed or primary refractory Hodgkin's disease or aggressive non-Hodgkin's lymphoma. Bone Marrow Transplant 2003;32:673–9.

Lerner RE, Thomas W, Defor TE, et al. The International Prognostic Index assessed at relapse predicts outcomes of autologous transplantation for diffuse large-cell non-Hodgkin's lymphoma in second complete or partial remission. Biol Blood Marrow Transplant 2007;13:486–92.

Lister TA, Crowther D, Sutcliffe SB, et al. Report of a committee convened to discuss the evaluation and staging of patients with Hodgkin's disease: Cotswolds meeting. J Clin Oncol 1989;7:1630–6.

Pfreundschuh M, Schubert J, Ziepert M, et al. Six versus eight cycles of bi-weekly CHOP-14 with or without rituximab in elderly patients with aggressive CD20+ B-cell lymphoma: A randomised controlled trial (RICOVER-60). Lancet Oncol 2008;9:105–16.

Pfreundschuh M, Trumper L, Osterborg A, et al. CHOP-like chemotherapy plus rituximab versus CHOP-like chemotherapy alone in young patients

[1]Not FDA approved for this indication.

with good-prognosis diffuse large-B-cell lymphoma: A randomised controlled trial by the MabThera International Trial (MInT) Group. Lancet Oncol 2006;7:379–91.

Philip T, Guglielmi C, Hagenbeek A, et al. Autologous bone marrow transplantation as compared with salvage chemotherapy in relapses of chemotherapy-sensitive non-Hodgkin's lymphoma. N Engl J Med 1995;333:1540–5.

Sehn LH, Berry B, Chhanabhai M, et al. The revised International Prognostic Index (R-IPI) is a better predictor of outcome than the standard IPI for patients with diffuse large B-cell lymphoma treated with R-CHOP. Blood 2007;109:1857–61.

Solal-Celigny P, Roy P, Colombat P, et al. Follicular lymphoma international prognostic index. Blood 2004;104:1258–65.

Swerdlow SH, Campo E, Harris NL, et al. WHO Classification of Tumours of Haematopoietic and Lymphoid Tissues. Lyon: WHO Press; 2008.

Multiple Myeloma

Method of

*Rodger E. Tiedemann, MB, ChB, PhD, and
A. Keith Stewart, MB, ChB*

Multiple myeloma is a malignancy of clonal plasma cells that proliferate and accumulate in the bone marrow. The neoplastic plasma cells typically produce a monoclonal immunoglobulin (or M protein) that can be detected in blood or urine. In the United States, myeloma accounts for 15% of hematologic malignancies and for nearly 2% of all deaths due to cancer. The incidence is 4 in 100,000 per year, although African Americans have an incidence twice that of whites. The median age at diagnosis is 65 to 70 years.

Multiple myeloma is often but not always preceded by a premalignant phase known as *monoclonal gammopathy of undetermined significance* (MGUS). MGUS is found in up to 3% of patients older than 50 years, and studies with 30-year follow-ups indicate that approximately 1% of MGUS patients per year progress to myeloma.

Myeloma remains incurable and is associated with a median survival of only 3 to 4 years, although its clinical course can be extremely variable, ranging from indolent disease that progresses only over the space of a decade to aggressive disease causing death within months.

Diagnosis

CLINICAL FEATURES

Bone pain, recurrent infection and symptoms of anemia, renal impairment, or hypercalcemia should raise suspicion of a diagnosis of myeloma. These clinical features can result directly from the mass effect of plasma cells lesions (plasmacytoma) or can arise indirectly from the M-protein or cytokines secreted by plasma cells. Common nonspecific laboratory findings such as an elevated erythrocyte sedimentation rate, normocytic anemia, rouleaux formation, and hypergammaglobulinemia should also prompt consideration of a diagnosis of myeloma, among other possibilities.

INVESTIGATIONS

Laboratory

Patients suspected of having myeloma require careful investigation (Box 1). Most patients (98%) with myeloma have an M protein detectable either by serum or urine protein electrophoresis. Serum electrophoresis alone shows a monoclonal band in 80% of cases. The components of the monoclonal immunoglobulin are identified by immunoelectrophoresis and immunofixation. Sixty percent of

 CURRENT DIAGNOSIS

Multiple Myeloma

- Monoclonal protein in the serum or urine* *and*
- Bone marrow (clonal) plasmacytosis or soft tissue plasmacytoma *and*
- Evidence of related end-organ damage or tissue injury[†]

Smoldering Myeloma

- Serum monoclonal protein $\geq$3.0 g/dL *and/or*
- Bone marrow (clonal) plasma cells $\geq$10% *and*
- *No* related organ or tissue impairment[†]

Monoclonal Gammopathy of Undetermined Significance

- Serum monoclonal protein <3.0 g/dL *and*
- Bone marrow plasma cells <10% *and*
- *No* related organ or tissue impairment[†] *and*
- *No* evidence of other B cell proliferative disorder or amyloidosis

---

*A monoclonal protein is not detected in approximately 1% of MM patients.

[†]Myeloma-elated end-organ damage can consist of hypercalcemia (>2.75 mmol/L or >0.25 mmol/L above normal limits), renal impairment (serum creatinine >173 mmol/L or >1.96 mg/dL), anemia (hemoglobin <10 g/dL or >2 g/dL below normal limits), or bone lesions (lytic lesions or osteopenia with compression fracture), abbreviated to the acronym CRAB. Based on the International Working Group criteria for multiple myeloma (MM), smoldering myeloma (SMM), and monoclonal gammopathy of undetermined significance (MGUS).

myeloma patients have a monoclonal immunoglobulin (Ig)G paraprotein, and 20% have a monoclonal IgA. Isolated monoclonal light chain without identifiable heavy chain is detected in another 15% of myeloma patients (commonly known as *light-chain myeloma* or *Bence Jones myeloma*). Monoclonal IgD and biclonal gammopathies are rarer; each accounts for 1% to 2% of myeloma cases. In 1% of cases, malignant plasma cells synthesize but do not secrete immunoglobulin, and an M protein cannot be detected (nonsecretory myeloma).

BOX 1   Investigations in Multiple Myeloma

- Serum protein electrophoresis
- 24-Hour urine collection for total and Bence Jones protein quantitation
- Immunoelectrophoresis or immunofixation of serum and urine
- CBC with differential and reticulocyte count
- Serum creatinine, calcium, uric acid, electrolytes, lactic acid dehydrogenase, alkaline phosphatase
- Bone marrow aspirate and biopsy
- Cytogenetics and/or FISH [e.g., for del(13) and t(4:14)] recommended
- Skeletal survey
- β_2-microglobulin, C-reactive protein, plasma cell labeling index if available
- If indicated: Biopsy of soft tissue masses
- If hyperviscosity is suspected: Serum viscosity
- If indicated: Cryoglobulins, MRI or CT of affected areas, biopsy for amyloidosis

Abbreviations: CBC = complete blood count; CT = computed tomography; MRI = magnetic resonance imaging; FISH = fluorescence in situ hybridization.

Bone marrow aspiration and biopsy are essential in the diagnostic process and typically show increased numbers of plasma cells (>10%). Aspiration and biopsy might also reveal abnormal plasma cell morphology or amyloid deposition in the marrow space or within blood vessel walls.

Radiology

Plain x-rays of the axial skeleton and long bones are used to survey for skeletal evidence of myeloma and to assess for impending pathologic fracture. Magnetic resonance imaging (MRI) (using T1/T2 settings plus STIR [short T1 inversion recovery] sequences) can also be used and is particularly sensitive in detecting less overt patchy plasma cell involvement of the bone marrow. MRI may be especially useful when plain x-ray films are negative but the index of suspicion for myeloma remains high. In patients with confirmed multiple myeloma, the size and number of lesions on MRI correlate with prognosis. Computed tomography (CT) is less sensitive than MRI but is useful in defining lesions when cord compression is suspected and urgent treatment may be required. Because myeloma lesions are *osteolytic*, a nuclear bone scan, which best detects *osteoblastic* lesions, is not generally useful.

DIAGNOSTIC CRITERIA

Various minimal criteria for the diagnosis of myeloma have been published, most recently those of the International Myeloma Working Group (see the Current Diagnosis box), which has sought to provide standardization.

The presence or absence of myeloma-related end-organ damage and the levels of monoclonal protein and bone marrow involvement by clonal plasmacytosis are keys to distinguishing symptomatic multiple myeloma (MM) from smoldering myeloma (SMM) and MGUS. Myeloma-related end-organ damage can consist of hyper*c*alcemia, *r*enal impairment, *a*nemia, or *b*one lesions (CRAB). Other less common criteria for end-organ damage due to myeloma include symptomatic hyperviscosity or recurrent bacterial infections ($\geq$2 in 12 months).

In most MM patients, plasma cells account for more than 10% of nucleated marrow cells; however, rare symptomatic MM patients can present with plasma cells less than 10%, and a lower limit is not specified in the Working Group criteria. Approximately 1% of patients with symptomatic multiple myeloma do not have a detectable monoclonal protein when highly sensitive techniques are employed.

MGUS may be difficult to distinguish from SMM or early stage MM. Features that help to support a diagnosis of myeloma include depression of the normal immunoglobulin levels and high paraprotein concentration (>30 g/L in serum or >1 g/24 h in urine). Although MGUS and SMM do not usually require immediate therapy, it is nevertheless important to distinguish between the two because the prognoses differ.

Primary or immunoglobulin light chain (AL) amyloidosis is a plasma cell neoplasm related to myeloma that secretes an abnormal immunoglobulin that deposits in tissues in a β-pleated sheet conformation. Notably, 20% of AL amyloid patients have overt myeloma, whereas among myeloma patients nearly 15% develop primary amyloidosis. Amyloidosis should be suspected in myeloma patients who develop progressive neuropathy, cardiac dysfunction with hypotension, enlarged tongue, swollen joints, hepatomegaly, or nephrotic syndrome. A needle biopsy of the involved tissue is the most reliable method to yield a diagnosis, but if involved tissue is inaccessible, blind abdominal fat pad needle aspiration may be helpful. Samples are assessed by Congo red staining for birefringence.

Staging and Prognosis

Several staging systems are in existence. The Salmon/Durie system, developed in 1975, remains widely used and integrates the results of CBC, serum creatinine, calcium, serum and urine M protein

TABLE 1 International Staging System for Myeloma

Stage	Criteria	Median Survival*
1	Serum β$_2$ microglobulin <3.5 mg/dL and serum albumin ≥3.5 g/dL	62 months
2	Serum β$_2$ microglobulin <3.5 mg/dL and serum albumin <3.5 g/dL *or* Serum β$_2$ microglobulin 3.5–5.5 mg/dL (irrespective of serum albumin)	44 months
3	Serum β$_2$ microglobulin >5.5 mg/dL	29 months

*Times reflect median overall survival by International Staging System stage.

levels, and radiology to correlate approximate tumor mass with survival. More recently, the new International Staging System (ISS) has been derived and validated by the International Myeloma Working Group from a cohort of 11,000 patients with newly diagnosed untreated myeloma. The ISS (Table 1) uses a simple combination of serum β$_2$ microglobulin and serum albumin to provide a reproducible and powerful three-stage classification that stratifies patients to groups with median overall survivals of 62, 44, or 29 months.

More sophisticated prognostic tests including tumor cytogenetics and fluorescence-in-situ-hybridization (FISH) are now increasingly recognized as powerful determinants of outcome, and in the near future molecular stratification of tumors may be used to guide therapy. Aberrations such as deletion of chromosome 13, deletion of 17p, or translocation between chromosomes 4 and 14, t(4;14), causing overexpression of fibroblast growth factor receptor 3 (*FGFR3*) and *MMSET* genes, have been associated with significantly poorer survival compared with the absence of any informative abnormality or with t(11;14) translocation or hyperdiploidy.

Therapy

OVERVIEW

Although there are many treatment options for patients with multiple myeloma, at present there is no cure. The disease may remain indolent for many years in some patients, particularly in those with smoldering myeloma or in those with low-level M protein (<30 g/L) and absent bone lesions. There is no evidence that early treatment prolongs survival. Therefore, therapy is generally reserved for patients with symptoms. The decision to begin therapy is based on the patient's symptoms and physical status and results of laboratory and radiographic investigations. Those with smoldering myeloma are not usually treated except within clinical trials. Treatment should be initiated in patients with impending complications (such as renal insufficiency or impending pathologic fracture) even if the patient is not yet symptomatic.

Because multiple myeloma is a systemic disorder from the onset, the primary treatment modality is chemotherapy (Box 2). For eligible patients, the physician should consider a treatment strategy that includes high-dose melphalan combined with autologous peripheral blood stem cell transplantation (ASCT). Four randomized trials comparing high-dose therapy (HDT) plus ASCT with conventional chemotherapy have each shown a survival advantage for HDT, on the order of 5 to 13 months (depending on the alternative treatment strategy provided). These randomized trials were all conducted in patients younger than 65 to 70 years; however, occasional patients older than 70 years might also be candidates for HDT and ASCT on the basis of superior physiologic status.

CURRENT THERAPY

Transplant Candidate (Often ≥65–70 Years)

- Induction therapy:
  - High-dose dexamethasone (HDD), often used in combination with vincristine and doxorubicin (VAD) or with thalidomide (thal/dex). Follow with collection of stem cells
  - High-dose melphalan (HDM) and autologous hematopoietic stem cell transplantation (SCT)
- For relapse or induction failure consider:
  - Thal/dex
  - Lenalidomide (Revlimid)/dexamethasone (rev/dex)
  - Bortezomib (Velcade)/dexamethasone (velcade/dex)
  - Cyclophosphamide/prednisone
- Repeat autologous SCT if first remission is longer than 18–24 months

Not a Transplant Candidate (Often >65–70 Years)

- Melphalan/prednisone (MP) ± thalidomide (MPT)
- For relapse or induction failure consider:
  - MPT or thal/dex, if no prior thalidomide
  - Rev/dex
  - Velcade/dex
  - Cyclophosphamide/prednisone

Select Patients

- Bisphosphonates, particularly for previous or present bone disease: Zoledronic acid (Zometa) 4 mg IV or pamidronate (Aredia) 60–90 mg IV, repeated every 4–6 weeks
- Erythropoietin for Hb <10 g/dL (caution: should not be used together with thalidomide or lenalidomide due to increased venous thrombosis)

HIGH-DOSE THERAPY WITH AUTOLOGOUS STEM CELL TRANSPLANTATION

In patients in whom ASCT is planned, induction therapy is used to control the presenting disease before stem cell harvest. Care must be taken to avoid the use of agents excessively toxic to hematopoietic stem cells (e.g., melphalan). Historically, common induction regimens have included high-dose dexamethasone alone or combined with vincristine and doxorubicin (VAD). VAD is generally given as vincristine 0.4 mg/day IV plus doxorubicin 9 mg/m^2/day IV on days 1 to 4, and dexamethasone 40 mg orally on days 1 to 4, 9 to 12, and 17 to 20. This is usually repeated every 28 days for four cycles. VAD induces partial remission (PR) in approximately 50% to 70% of patients and complete remission (CR) in 5% to 10% of patients. Dexamethasone alone is only mildly less effective and is useful as initial treatment in patients with severe cytopenia, with renal failure, or requiring extensive radiotherapy.

An alternative oral induction regimen consists of thalidomide (Thalomid) 200 mg daily plus dexamethasone (thal/dex). The dexamethasone is given 40 mg/day on days 1 to 4, 9 to 12, and 17 to 20 on odd cycles and days 1 to 4 on even cycles. Thal/dex produces response rates comparable with VAD and superior to dexamethasone alone. Adverse effects include an increased rate of venous thrombosis (15%), which necessitates prophylactic anticoagulation; neuropathy; somnolence; and constipation.

Use of thalidomide within the induction regimen can limit the efficacy of thalidomide-based regimens at relapse. No overall survival advantage is conferred by using this agent upfront instead of as a de novo agent at relapse. In one large study, approximately 50% of 668 myeloma patients were randomly assigned to receive daily

---

BOX 2   Chemotherapy Regimens for Multiple Myeloma

High-Dose Dexamethasone (HDD)
- Dexamethasone (Decadron) 40 mg PO on days 1–4, 9–12, 17–20
- Repeat every 4 weeks

Thal/Dex
- Thalidomide 100–200 mg PO qd, plus HDD
- Prophylactic anticoagulation required (aspirin 325 mg PO qd or full-dose anticoagulation)

Rev/Dex
- Lenalidomide (Revlimid) 25 mg PO on days 1–21, plus HDD
- Repeat every 4 weeks
- Anticoagulation required

VAD
- Vincristine 0.4 mg IV on days 1–4
- Doxorubicin (Adriamycin) 9 mg/m^2/day IV on days 1–4
- HDD days 1–4, 9–12, 17–20 all cycles
- Repeat every 4 weeks (typically × 4) (short-infusional regimen)

High-Dose Melphalan (HDM)
- Melphalan (Alkeran) 200 mg/m^2 IV,[3] followed by SCT

Velcade/Dex
- Bortezomib (Velcade) 1.3 mg/m^2 IV on days 1, 4, 8, and 11, plus HDD
- Repeat every 3 weeks (e.g., × 8)

MP
- Melphalan (Alkeran) 9 mg/m^2 PO on days 1–4
- Prednisone 100 mg PO on days 1–4
- Repeat both every 4–6 weeks

MPT
- Melphalan (Alkeran) 9 mg/m^2 PO on days 1–4
- Prednisone 100 mg/m^2 PO on days 1–7
- Thalidomide 100 mg PO qd, continuous
- Repeat melphalan and prednisone every 4–6 weeks × 12 cycles
- Requires prophylactic anticoagulation

Cyclophosphamide
- Cyclophosphamide (Cytoxan) 300 mg/m^2 weekly PO or IV
- Often given together with prednisone 100 mg PO on alternate days

---

[3]Exceeds dosage recommended by the manufacturer.
Abbreviation: SCT = stem cell transplantation.
Note: Dose reductions may be necessary for side effects, advanced age, frailty, cytopenias, or impaired renal or liver function.

---

thalidomide starting alongside standard HDT plus ASCT therapy. Incorporation of thalidomide into HDT had no effect on overall survival (OS). Use of thalidomide alongside HDT did result in increased event-free survival (EFS). However, this was balanced by substantially shortened survival following relapse and by higher rates of severe peripheral neuropathy and deep venous thrombosis (DVT).

Combination therapies using newer agents such as bortezomib (Velcade) or lenalidomide (Revlimid) are being investigated as induction regimens. These offer the promise of deeper remissions in greater numbers of patients than current induction treatments. However, their benefit on OS following HDT and ASCT remains to be determined.

Following recovery from induction treatment, peripheral blood stem cells are collected from the patient via a cell separator (apheresis) and are frozen until their reinfusion after high-dose chemotherapy. Stem cell mobilization typically requires pretreatment with cyclophosphamide and granulocyte colony-stimulating factor (G-CSF). High-dose melphalan[2] (Alkeran), 200 mg/m^2, is the most common HDT used and in patients younger than 65 years is associated with an upfront mortality rate of approximately 1%.

Unfortunately, many patients continue to have evidence of myeloma after ASCT and all patients eventually relapse. The median time to progression in myeloma patients treated with HDT and ASCT is 18 to 24 months. Pre-relapse maintenance therapy following HDT using various agents (e.g., interferon-α [IFN-α], steroids, thalidomide, or combination chemotherapy) is being tested in several clinical trials; however, evidence of significant benefit in OS is currently lacking.

Tandem sequential ASCTs have been reported to improve OS compared with single ASCT. This benefit was not seen within the first 2 years of follow-up; however, it was subsequently observed up to 7 years after ASCT. The benefits of early tandem transplantation are unlikely to be universal; advantages appear to accrue primarily in patients who fail to achieve satisfactory remission following their first ASCT procedure.

There is no clear standard of treatment following relapse after HDT. Treatment with standard alkylating agents or newer agents, repeat HDT plus ASCT, entry into a clinical trial, or allogeneic transplantation can each be considered.

ALLOGENEIC TRANSPLANTATION

An allogeneic transplant uses stem cells obtained from an HLA-matched donor, usually a sibling, to repopulate the bone marrow following chemotherapy. Allogeneic transplantation can theoretically provide an immunologic graft-versus-myeloma effect that can lead to significant reductions in tumor mass and prolonged remission. However, this potential benefit is balanced by high rates of transplant-related mortality (TRM) and a risk of troublesome graft-versus-host disease (GVHD). Less than 10% of myeloma patients are eligible for intensive myeloablative allogeneic protocols because 90% are aged 50 years or older, and only one third have an HLA-compatible donor. Nonmyeloablative (mini) allogeneic transplantation may be achievable in greater numbers of patients and offers a lower risk of early TRM. However, this approach is again associated with significant risk of GVHD (45% acute GVHD, 55% chronic GVHD reported), and we believe it should be considered primarily in the setting of well-planned clinical trials.

STANDARD ALKYLATING AGENT THERAPY

For elderly patients or those who do not want, or cannot tolerate, aggressive therapy, various oral chemotherapy regimens may be used. Oral melphalan plus predisone (MP), given as melphalan 9 mg/m^2 plus prednisone 100 mg daily for 4 days at 4- to 6-week intervals, is the gold standard in this setting and induces objective responses in 50% to 60% of patients and a median OS of 2 to 3 years. Because melphalan absorption is reduced by food, it should be given in the morning on an empty stomach. Dose reduction should be considered in the elderly and for renal insufficiency. Melphalan doses are titrated to induce mild mid-cycle cytopenia. A mild neutropenic nadir (1.0–1.5 × 10^9/L) or thrombocytopenia (< 100 × 10^9/L) is often targeted to ensure maximal efficacy. Severe cytopenia should be avoided by delaying treatment in weekly increments if significant cytopenias persist at follow-up and by reducing subsequent melphalan dosing in 2-to 4-mg/day decrements. MP is generally continued until maximal reduction in the M protein has occurred plus 2 to 4 months (plateau), or for approximately 1 year. At this point, treatment is stopped because cumulative melphalan exposure can result in late development of myelodysplastic syndrome or leukemia. Objective responses can occur slowly, and unless rapidly progressive disease occurs, treatment should not be abandoned until at least three cycles of treatment can be assessed.

---

[2]Not available in the United States.

Addition of thalidomide to MP (MPT) has recently been shown to improve the results of MP therapy. MPT is given as melphalan 4 mg/m^2 for 7 days, prednisone 40 mg/m^2 for 7 days, and thalidomide 100 mg daily continuously, repeated every 4 weeks for six cycles. Use of MPT in patients older than 65 years resulted in an increased response rate (76%) compared with MP (48%), more complete responses or near-complete responses (28 vs. 7%), and longer EFS (33 vs. 14 months). These gains were balanced, however, by increased toxicity (grade 3–4 toxicity: 49% vs. 25%) and by the need for concurrent anticoagulation (e.g., enoxaparin [Lovenox] 40 mg SC daily). In patients who tolerated six cycles of MPT, there was a trend to survival advantage at 3 years compared with patients treated with similar doses of MP (80 vs. 64%; hazard ratio [HR], 0.68; $P = 0.19$), even when MP patients were permitted to cross over and receive thalidomide following disease progression.

Cyclophosphamide (Cytoxan) can be used as an alternative to melphalan in select patients with a weekly dose of 400 to 500 mg orally or intravenously. Cyclophosphamide is less likely to suppress thrombopoiesis and has less myelosuppressive potentiation in renal failure. It is often administered in conjunction with prednisone 100 mg orally on alternate days.

Multidrug regimens using combinations of vincristine, anthracyclines, melphalan, BCNU [1,3 bis(2-chloroethyl)-1-nitrosourea], cyclophosphamide and corticosteroids can provide a faster onset of action than MP and may be useful in patients with high tumor loads or acute complications. Significantly, however, a large meta-analysis of more than 6000 patients indicates that conventional multiagent chemotherapy regimens do not improve overall survival beyond that achieved with standard MP, even in poor-risk patients.

REFRACTORY MYELOMA AND NOVEL AGENTS

All patients with multiple myeloma who initially respond to treatment subsequently relapse. If relapse occurs more than 6 months after treatment response, a repeat trial of the previous treatment should be considered. Similarly, for patients who have experienced lasting remission (several years) after HDT, repeat HDT and ASCT may be useful. Myeloma patients often continue to show useful responses to prior therapies, although the quality and duration of response generally diminish with repeated exposure.

Patients who become refractory to alkylating agents typically respond poorly to ensuing chemotherapy and traditionally have had a poor prognosis. Dexamethasone often continues to be useful in relapsed patients. Unfortunately, complications of corticosteroids such as depression or agitation, infection, diabetes, hypertension, osteoporosis, and osteonecrosis can limit long-term use.

Importantly, thalidomide has been found to induce response rates of 30% to 35% in patients with relapsed or refractory myeloma when used as a single agent, with a median progression-free survival of 5 months. A greater response rate of approximately 55% is seen when thalidomide is used in combination with corticosteroids, with an improved median time to progression of 12 months and median OS of 27 months, providing a statistically significant advantage over conventional salvage chemotherapy in relapse. Most studies using thalidomide have used a dose of at least 200 mg daily; however, lower doses of 50 to 100 mg daily might also be effective. Adverse effects of thalidomide, which can influence the maximum obtainable dose, include sedation, constipation, and peripheral neuropathy. Rash, venous thrombosis, and the risk of birth defects are also problematic.

Lenalidomide (Revlimid, CC-5013), a derivative of thalidomide with greater potency and less toxicity, has shown promising activity in relapsed or refractory and untreated myeloma. In preliminary studies, lenalidomide 25mg daily on days 1 to 21, repeated every 4 weeks, plus dexamethasone (rev/dex), caused objective responses in 91% of patients with newly diagnosed myeloma, including CR in 6%, and very good PR in 32%. In relapsed patients, rev/dex has been shown to be superior to dexamethasone alone in a multicenter randomized trial of more than 350 patients with progressive myeloma, achieving an overall response rate of 58% (versus 22% for dexamethasone alone) and a median time to progression of 13.1 months (versus 5.1 months for dexamethasone). Other trials have demonstrated lenalidomide efficacy in patients refractory or intolerant to thalidomide. Head-to-head randomized comparisons with thalidomide are awaited at the time of writing.

Bortezomib (Velcade, PS-341), a first-in-class proteosome inhibitor, is an FDA-approved novel antimyeloma agent. When given intravenously at a dose of 1.3 mg/m^2 on days 1, 4, 8, and 11 on a 21-day schedule for eight cycles, followed by a lower intensity 35-day maintenance schedule, bortezomib resulted in objective responses in 46% of relapsed patients, including CR or near CR in 13%. Notably, the APEX (Assessment of Proteasome Inhibition for Extending Remissions) trial has shown bortezomib to be superior to single-agent dexamethasone as a salvage therapy for relapsed patients, 99% of whom have been exposed to prior corticosteroid therapy. Bortezomib provided an OS at 1 year of 80%, versus 66% for dexamethasone ($P = 0.003$), and median time to disease progression of 6.2 months, compared with 3.5 months for dexamethasone. In patients who do not respond to bortezomib alone, cotreatment with dexamethasone can result in additional partial or minimal responses in 15% to 20%. Notable toxicities of bortezomib include fatigue, gastrointestinal disturbance, painful peripheral neuropathy, and thrombocytopenia.

A multitude of clinical trials evaluating thalidomide, lenalidomide, or bortezomib, in combination with conventional therapies or with each other, are now accruing patients worldwide. These might result in rapid changes in the approach to myeloma treatment in coming years.

SUPPORTIVE THERAPY

Renal Failure

Approximately 20% of patients with myeloma have significant renal dysfunction, with serum creatinine >2.0 mg/dL at diagnosis. Common causes include cast nephropathy, dehydration, hypercalcemia, infection, use of nephrotoxic drugs, or amyloid deposition. Cast nephropathy involves deposition of amorphous nonfibrillary material (monoclonal immunoglobulin, usually light chain—thus *light chain deposition disease* or *myeloma kidney*) in the distal tubules and differs from renal amyloidosis in its distribution, absence of β-pleated sheet structure, and absence of Congo red staining. Additionally, the nephrotic syndrome is rare in myeloma kidney and should raise a suspicion of amyloidosis.

Adequate hydration and prompt chemotherapy are pivotal to management and can reverse mild dysfunction in 50% of patients. Allopurinol (Zyloprim) 300 mg daily (or less, according to creatinine clearance) is useful for controlling or preventing secondary hyperuricemia. Nonsteroidal anti-inflammatory drugs (NSAIDs) and nephrotoxic antibiotics should generally be stopped or avoided in the presence of renal impairment. Severe renal failure can require hemodialysis support in order to administer chemotherapy. In addition, plasmapheresis to reduce the plasma M protein can help limit acute renal damage and perhaps reduce the risk of long-term dialysis. However, randomized trials are lacking.

Hypercalcemia

Aggressive hydration with isotonic saline (150–200 mL/h) and steroid therapy (prednisone 100 mg/day) generally leads to rapid resolution of hypercalcemia. Treatment directed at the myeloma should then be instituted. Intravenous bisphosphonates such as pamidronate (Aredia) 60 to 90 mg or zoledronic acid (Zometa) 4 mg, are also commonly employed after resolution of coexisting renal dysfunction and can provide additional bone protection.

Anemia

Most patients with myeloma develop anemia, whose etiology is often multifactorial. Where anemia is caused primarily by marrow infiltration, specific antimyeloma therapy (with or without transfusion) may be beneficial. Recombinant erythropoietin (Eprex)[2] may be helpful in severe anemia (Hb ≤80 g/L), even in the absence of renal failure,

because myeloma patients often have decreased levels or impaired response to endogenous erythropoietin. Doses of 150 U/kg three times weekly have led to hematologic responses in up to 70% of patients. Lower doses may be effective in patients with renal failure.

Skeletal Lesions

Bone lesions causing pain or impending pathologic fracture should be treated early. Skeletal imaging should be performed and repeated at regular intervals if pain develops. Internal fixation of impending long bone fractures (usually indicated when >50% cortical erosion is present) can prevent the significant pain and immobility associated with fracture. Advanced bone lesions that threaten fracture or are painful and unresponsive to systemic chemotherapy are best managed with localized radiation (20–30 Gy). Adequate analgesia is vital and often requires narcotics. Vertebroplasty or kyphoplasty can help decrease pain caused by compression fractures of the spine.

All myeloma patients with active bone disease, including those with significant osteopenia, should be treated with intravenous bisphosphonates unless contraindications exist. Pamidronate 90 mg over 2 hours or zoledronic acid 4 mg over 15 minutes IV every 4 weeks show equal efficacy. Common side effects include flulike symptoms such as fatigue, anorexia, nausea, and bone pain; these can last 3 to 5 days but generally diminish with repeated exposure. More problematic is the recently reported association between prolonged bisphosphonate therapy and osteonecrosis of the mandible. Most cases have been reported in patients also receiving chemotherapy and corticosteroids who had undergone a dental procedure such as tooth extraction. A dental examination with preventive intervention should be considered before bisphosphonate therapy, and invasive dental procedures should, if possible, be avoided in patients receiving bisphosphonate treatment. Because hypocalcemia, renal impairment, and proteinuria can occur in patients receiving bisphosphonates, regular monitoring of serum calcium, electrolytes, creatinine, and urine protein is recommended.

Hyperviscosity Syndrome

Impaired vision, cognitive changes, mucosal bleeding, and congestive heart failure can occur as a consequence of increased serum protein concentration. Symptoms generally do not occur with serum viscosities less than 4.0 Cp (viscosity of water = 1 Cp, normal serum viscosity is 1.4–1.8 Cp), although the relationship between clinical signs and measured viscosity is imprecise. Hyperviscosity is most commonly seen in disorders associated with elevated IgM and is more common in IgA myeloma than in IgG myeloma. Plasmapheresis is used to acutely reduce the level of M protein, and myeloma chemotherapy should be instituted to decrease paraprotein production.

Spinal Cord Compression

Compression of the spinal cord or nerve roots can result from expansion of an extradural soft tissue plasmacytoma or from vertebral collapse and is a medical emergency. Lower back or radicular pain is a typical manifesting symptom. Leg weakness, urinary retention, incontinence, or obstipation can indicate impending cord damage. Urgent MRI or CT scanning is indicated to identify the extent of compression. To prevent permanent paraplegia, high-dose steroids (dexamethasone 16–96 mg/day) should be started immediately to reduce cord edema, and local irradiation (25–30 Gy) should be administered.

REFERENCES

Attal M, Harousseau JL, Facon T, et al. Single versus double autologous stem-cell transplantation for multiple myeloma. N Engl J Med 2003;349:2495–502.

Barlogie B, Tricot G, Anaissie E, et al. Thalidomide and hematopoietic-cell transplantation for multiple myeloma. N Engl J Med 2006;354:1021–30.

Dimopoulos MA, Zervas K, Kouvatseas G, et al. Thalidomide and dexamethasone combination for refractory multiple myeloma. Ann Oncol 2001;12:991–5.

Durie BG, Kyle RA, Belch A, et al. Myeloma management guidelines: A consensus report from the Scientific Advisors of the International Myeloma Foundation. Hematol J 2003;4:379–98.

---

[2]Not available in the United States.

Fonseca R, Blood E, Rue M, et al. Clinical and biologic implications of recurrent genomic aberrations in myeloma. Blood 2003;101:4569–75.

Greipp PR, San Miguel J, Durie BG, et al. International staging system for multiple myeloma. J Clin Oncol 2005;23:3412–20.

Harousseau JL, Attal M. The role of stem cell transplantation in multiple myeloma. Blood Rev 2002;16:245–53.

International Myeloma Working Group. Criteria for the classification of monoclonal gammopathies, multiple myeloma and related disorders. Br J Haematol 2003;121:749–57.

Kyle RA, Therneau TM, Rajkumar SV, et al. A long-term study of prognosis in monoclonal gammopathy of undetermined significance. N Engl J Med 2002;346:564–9.

Palumbo A, Bringhen S, Caravita T, et al. Oral melphalan and prednisone chemotherapy plus thalidomide compared with melphalan and prednisone alone in elderly patients with multiple myeloma: Randomised controlled trial. Lancet 2006;367:825–31.

Rajkumar SV, Hayman SR, Lacy MQ, et al. Combination therapy with lenalidomide plus dexamethasone (rev/dex) for newly diagnosed myeloma. Blood 2005;106:4050–3.

Reece DE. An update of the management of multiple myeloma: The changing landscape. Hematology (Am Soc Hematol Educ Program) 2005;353–9.

Richardson PG, Sonneveld P, Schuster MW, et al. Bortezomib or high-dose dexamethasone for relapsed multiple myeloma. N Engl J Med 2005;352:2487–98.

Polycythemia Vera

Method of
Ike Onwere, MD, and Thorvardur Halfdanarson, MD

Polycythemia vera (PV) is one of the chronic myeloproliferative neoplasms (MPN). The classification of these disorders was recently updated by the World Health Organisation (WHO). Other entities in this group are chronic myelogenous leukemia, chronic neutrophilic leukemia, primary myelofibrosis, essential thrombocythemia, chronic eosinophilic leukemia, hypereosinophilic syndromes, mast cell disease, and unclassifiable MPNs. The hallmark of these disorders is a dysregulation at the multipotent hematopoietic stem cell level. The MPNs manifest as overproduction of one or several lineages of mature blood cells, hypercellular marrow with or without marrow fibrosis, recurrent cytogenetic and molecular abnormalities, thrombotic and hemorrhagic diatheses, and hepatosplenomegaly resulting from extramedullary hematopoiesis. These disorders predispose to a leukemic transformation and have clinical features that may overlap substantially.

In 2005, several groups of investigators reported a specific point mutation in the gene that codes for the Janus kinase 2 (JAK2), a cytoplasmic tyrosine kinase which is a key element in the JAK-STAT pathway of cell growth and differentiation. Mutations of JAK2 lead to constitutive activation of this pathway, causing increased proliferation and survival of hematopoietic precursors in vitro. This mutation has been identified in most patients with PV and in a substantial number of patients with essential thrombocythemia and primary myelofibrosis.

Epidemiology and Prognosis

The reported annual incidence of PV ranges from 0.02 to 2.8 per 100,000 and rises with advancing age. The prevalence of PV in the United States may be in excess of 65,000; the median age at the time of diagnosis is approximately 70 years, and the disorder seems to be more common among males. Genetic factors may play a role, but first-degree relatives of patients with MPN have almost sixfold increased risk of developing PV compared to subjects without a family history of MPN.

The median overall survival time for patients with untreated PV is less than 2 years from the time of diagnosis. Successful treatment greatly improves survival, which now exceeds 10 years, but the life expectancy of treated patients still remains inferior to that of the general population. PV-related causes of death include thrombosis and disease transformation into myelofibrosis and acute myeloid leukemia (AML). The overall mortality rate of patients with PV has been estimated to be 3.7 per 100,000 person-years and is largely related to a moderately increased risk of cardiovascular complications and a greatly increased risk of noncardiac death, mostly transformation to more aggressive hematologic malignancies.

Thromboembolic Complications

Increasing age and a prior history of thromboembolic complications remain the most important predictors of future vascular events. Leukocytosis (white blood cell count $>15 \times 10^6$ cells/μL) has been suggested as a risk factor predicting both thromboembolic events and leukemic transformation, but this factor is currently not routinely considered when making treatment decisions. An association between a higher JAK2 V617F mutation load and higher risk of vascular events has been reported by some investigators.

A simple and widely accepted risk stratification method is shown in Table 1. This stratification scheme is very helpful in assessing the need for therapy in patients with PV.

Clinical Features

Many patients with PV present with symptomatic disease or thromboembolic events, whereas others are diagnosed in the absence of symptoms after being found to have an elevated hematocrit during an evaluation for unrelated conditions. Nonspecific complaints are common and include fatigue, dizziness, and headaches. Excessive perspiration and weight loss may be observed. Aquagenic pruritus (post-bath itching) is frequent and can be ameliorated with selective serotonin reuptake inhibitors and histamine 2 blockers. Nonspecific gastrointestinal complaints such as abdominal discomfort, bloating, and early satiety resulting from massive splenomegaly affect many patients. Some patients have erosive gastroduodenitis. Gouty arthritis is sometimes seen. Dyspnea, angina, and visual disturbances may occur and can result from hyperviscosity related to the high hematocrit.

Erythromelalgia is a well-described complication that manifests as painful and often erythematous digits and may involve the entire hands and feet. Erythromelalgia is thought to result from microvascular thrombosis and occlusion and often responds dramatically to low-dose aspirin therapy. Venous or arterial thromboembolic events are a common complication of PV and may involve the deep veins of the extremities but also unusual sites such as the mesenteric, splenic, or hepatic veins.

On physical examination, patients with PV frequently have splenomegaly, hepatomegaly, and ruddy facial cyanosis. Because more patients are being diagnosed in the asymptomatic phase after routine blood tests, these physical findings may be less prevalent among newly diagnosed patients.

TABLE 1   Risk Stratification in Polycythemia Vera

Risk Category	Age >60 Years or History of Thromboembolism	Cardiovascular Risk Factors
Low	No	No
Intermediate	No	Yes
High	Yes	—

CURRENT DIAGNOSIS

- Elevated hemoglobin (>18.5 g/dL in men, >16.5 g/dL in women) should prompt evaluation for polycythemia vera (PV).
- Secondary polycythemia, such as that caused by chronic hypoxia, needs to be ruled out.
- Low levels of erythropoietin (EPO) suggest PV, but patients with PV can have normal EPO levels.
- High levels of EPO support secondary causes of polycythemia.
- JAK2 mutations are detected in almost all patients with PV and are now an integral part of the diagnostic algorithms.
- A bone marrow examination is still indicated in many patients with suspected PV.

Diagnosis and Differential Diagnosis

Diagnosis of PV has evolved markedly in recent years. Previously, PV was primarily a diagnosis of exclusion, but in the era of JAK2 mutation molecular analysis, the diagnosis can be made with more accuracy. The newly updated diagnostic criteria for PV reflect the improved understanding of its pathogenesis.

The evaluation of PV consists of careful exclusion of secondary causes such as chronic hypoxic states (chronic obstructive pulmonary disease, high altitude, cardiac shunting, chronic smoking, obstructive sleep apnea), erythropoietin (EPO)-producing tumors (renal and hepatic tumors), and familial polycythemic states involving mutations in the von Hippel–Lindau (VHL) gene (Chuvash polycythemia) and the EPO receptor gene and high-affinity hemoglobin (Table 2). It is important, especially in younger patients, to inquire about a family history of polycythemia, because it can on rare occasions be familial. In strength and endurance athletes, androgen abuse and EPO doping should also be excluded.

The JAK2 V617F mutation can be detected in up to 95% of patients with PV, and some of the remaining patients may have a mutation in exon 12 of the *JAK2* gene that is not detected by the commonly used assays for JAK2 mutations. The advent of JAK2 testing has simplified the diagnostic algorithm for PV and necessitated revision of the WHO diagnostic criteria (Table 3). The role of red cell mass measurements as a diagnostic tool has diminished since JAK2

TABLE 2 Classification and Causes of Polycythemia

Primary Polycythemia
Polycythemia vera

Secondary Polycythemia
Congenital
High oxygen-affinity hemoglobin, mutations in the EPO receptor, and so on

Acquired
Hypoxia driven (e.g., COPD, smoking, hypoventilation syndrome, right-to-left cardiopulmonary shunt, renal artery stenosis)
Abnormal EPO production (e.g., hepatocellular carcinoma, renal cell cancer, cerebellar hemangioblastoma)
Drugs (e.g., exogenous EPO [Epogen, Procrit], androgens)

Abbreviations: COPD = chronic obstructive pulmonary disease; EPO = erythropoietin.

TABLE 3 2008 WHO Criteria for Diagnosis of Polycythemia Vera*

Major Criteria
1. Hemoglobin >18.5 g/dL in men or >16.5 g/dL in women or other evidence of increased red cell volume, or
Hemoglobin 17 g/dL in men or 15 g/dL in women if associated with a sustained increase of ≥2 g/dL from baseline that cannot be attributed to correction of iron deficiency, or
Elevated red cell mass >25% above mean normal predicted value
2. Presence of JAK2 V617F or other functionally similar mutation such as JAK2 exon 12 mutation

Minor Criteria
1. Bone marrow biopsy showing hypercellularity for age with trilineage myeloproliferation
2. Subnormal serum erythropoietin level
3. Endogenous erythroid colony formation in vitro

*Diagnosis requires the presence of two major and one minor criterion or the presence of major criterion 1 together with two of the minor criteria.
Abbreviations: JAK2 = Janus kinase 2; WHO = World Health Organisation.
(From Tefferi A, Vardiman JW. Classification and diagnosis of myeloproliferative neoplasms: The 2008 World Health Organization criteria and point-of-care diagnostic algorithms. Leukemia 2008;22:14–22.)

testing became available, and that test is now rarely indicated. Although assays for JAK2 mutations are highly sensitive for the diagnosis of PV, a positive test is not very specific, because JAK2 mutations can also be seen in other MPNs such as primary myelofibrosis and essential thrombocythemia.

A diagnosis of PV is often made in the context of a persistently inappropriately elevated hematocrit as an incidental finding or in the context of a vascular event. Leukocytosis and thrombocytosis may be seen in up to 60% of patients, and levels of vitamin B_{12} can be elevated. Although a bone marrow examination is not a prerequisite for diagnosing PV, the findings can be supportive of the diagnosis, and the presence of trilineage myeloproliferation is a minor criterion for the diagnosis of PV in the 2008 WHO classification. Serum EPO levels are frequently lower than normal in patients with PV, but normal levels may be seen. Elevated EPO levels should prompt evaluation for secondary causes of erythrocytosis. Although elevated EPO levels are seen in acute hypoxia, many patients with secondary polycythemia resulting from chronic hypoventilation and hypoxia have EPO levels within the normal range.

It is important to note that there are racial and gender variations in the reference range of all hematologic indices. The upper limit for hematocrit among whites of Nordic/Anglo-Saxon heritage can be 18.2 g/dL for males and 16.7 g/dL for females, whereas blacks have slightly lower values of 17.9 g/dL for males and 16.3 g/dL for females. In the face of coexisting iron deficiency, the hematocrit might appear normal or even low. A simple diagnostic algorithm for the diagnosis of suspected PV has been proposed (Fig. 1). This approach relies heavily on the measurement of serum EPO levels and assessment of JAK2 mutational status.

Therapy

The primary goal of treatment is to decrease the risk of acute thromboembolic vascular events. Before initiating therapy, patients with PV should be classified into three categories at different risk for vascular complications (low, intermediate, and high) based on age, previous thrombotic events, and the presence of cardiovascular risk factors (see Table 1). No therapy has yet proved to be effective in decreasing leukemic transformation of PV. Alkylating drugs such as chlorambucil (Leukeran)[1] and radioactive phosphorus have been shown to increase the risk of leukemic transformation, and their use is

---

[1]Not FDA approved for this indication.

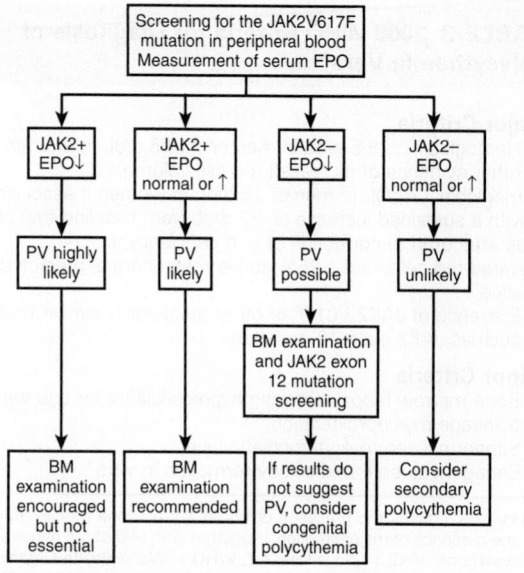

FIGURE 1. Diagnostic algorithm for polycythemia vera (PV). *Abbreviations:* BM = bone marrow; EPO = erythropoietin.

discouraged. There is currently little evidence that hydroxyurea or anelgrelide is leukemogenic.

PHLEBOTOMY

Phlebotomy is currently recommended for all patients with PV and is the only cytoreductive therapy needed in patients who have a low risk for thromboembolic complications. The current recommendation is to keep the hematocrit lower than 45%, but this target has not been defined in prospective studies.

ANTIPLATELET THERAPY

All patients with PV should be considered for therapy with aspirin to decrease vascular events. Only aspirin has been shown in a controlled trial to lower the risk of vascular events. The current recommendation is to use 81 to 100 mg of aspirin daily in patients without contraindications to such therapy. Aspirin should be used with caution in patients with severe thrombocytosis ($>1000 \times 10^9$/L), because such patients can on rare occasions have an acquired von Willebrand's disease and aspirin use can result in hemorrhages.

CYTOREDUCTIVE THERAPY

High risk is inferred in patients older than 65 years of age or in anyone with a previous history of thrombosis regardless of age. Other risk factors for vascular events, such as current smoking, diabetes, hypertension, and dyslipidemia, have uncertain significance in patients with PV. Hydroxyurea (Hydrea)[1] has not been compared with phlebotomy alone in patients with PV in a large randomized trial, but evidence from uncontrolled studies suggest that hydroxyurea can very effectively control cell counts and reduce the risk of vascular events. Therefore, hydroxyurea and low-dose aspirin should be recommended to all patients with intermediate to high risk of thromboembolic complications unless there are contraindications to the use of these agents. Hydroxyurea may also be considered in patients who are not compliant with phlebotomies and in those who have evidence of uncontrolled myeloproliferation resulting in progressive splenomegaly, leukocytosis, or thrombocytosis. Hydroxyurea can be initiated at a dose of 15 to 20 mg/kg daily until the desired goal (i.e., hematocrit <45%) is achieved. The white blood cell count should not be lowered to less than 3×10^9/L, and platelet counts should be kept within the reference range.

CURRENT THERAPY

- The goal of therapy is primarily to prevent thromboembolic complications, which are a major cause of mortality and morbidity.
- No therapy effectively lowers the risk of leukemic transformation that is inherent to polycythemia vera.
- All patients should be stratified based on their risk of thromboembolic events.
- All patients should receive low-dose aspirin if there are no contraindications.
- Patients with low risk can be treated with aspirin and phlebotomy alone, with a hematocrit goal of 45% to 50%.
- Patients with intermediate to high risk should receive cytoreductive chemotherapy in addition to aspirin and phlebotomies, with a hematocrit goal of 45% to 50%. The cytoreductive agent of choice is hydroxyurea (Hydrea),[1] and alkylating agents are to be avoided in most patients.

[1]Not FDA approved for this indication.

Special Considerations

The risk of thrombosis and hemorrhage in patients with PV undergoing surgery is significant, and this risk may be amplified in patients with high leukocyte and platelet counts. Despite adequate cytoreduction, patients with PV still have higher risk of perioperative thrombotic and hemorrhagic complications. The optimal therapy for these patients is not known, but it seems prudent to attempt normalization of their cell counts through cytoreductive therapy before elective procedures are undertaken. Patients should also be treated perioperatively with parenteral anticoagulation as indicated, based on the nature of the surgical procedure.

Pregnancy in women with PV poses certain challenges, because the pregnancy itself increases thromboembolic risk and some of the cytoreductive agents used for PV may be teratogenic. Although there is no clear evidence-based approach for the pregnant woman with PV, a reasonable recommendation is to use phlebotomy to keep the hematocrit lower than 45%. Low-dose aspirin is recommended throughout the pregnancy, and low-molecular-weight heparin has been recommended for 6 weeks after delivery, especially if there is a history of a previous thrombotic event. Cytoreductive agents should be avoided if possible, but if cytoreduction is needed, the safest agent is interferon-alfa 2 (Intron A).[1] Pregnant women with PV should be monitored in specialty clinics throughout the pregnancy, if at all possible.

If elective general surgical procedures are planned, one should consider cytoreductive therapy for 4 to 6 weeks before surgery in nonpregnant and pregnant patients.

REFERENCES

Finazzi G, Barbui T. How I treat patients with polycythemia vera. Blood 2007;109:5104–11.

Finazzi G, Caruso V, Marchioli R, et al. Acute leukemia in polycythemia vera: An analysis of 1638 patients enrolled in a prospective observational study. Blood 2005;105:2664–70.

Fruchtman SM, Mack K, Kaplan ME, et al. From efficacy to safety: A Polycythemia Vera Study group report on hydroxyurea in patients with polycythemia vera. Semin Hematol 1997;34:17–23.

[1]Not FDA approved for this indication.

[1]Not FDA approved for this indication.

James C, Ugo V, Le Couedic JP, et al. A unique clonal JAK2 mutation leading to constitutive signalling causes polycythaemia vera. Nature 2005;434: 1144–8.

Johansson P. Epidemiology of the myeloproliferative disorders polycythemia vera and essential thrombocythemia. Semin Thromb Hemost 2006;32: 171–3.

Kralovics R, Passamonti F, Buser AS, et al. A gain-of-function mutation of JAK2 in myeloproliferative disorders. N Engl J Med 2005;352:1779–90.

Landgren O, Goldin LR, Kristinsson SY, et al. Increased risks of polycythemia vera, essential thrombocythemia, and myelofibrosis among 24,577 first-degree relatives of 11,039 patients with myeloproliferative neoplasms in Sweden. Blood 2008;112:2199–204.

Landolfi R, Marchioli R, Kutti J, et al. Efficacy and safety of low-dose aspirin in polycythemia vera. N Engl J Med 2004;350:114–24.

Marchioli R, Finazzi G, Landolfi R, et al. Vascular and neoplastic risk in a large cohort of patients with polycythemia vera. J Clin Oncol 2005;23:2224–32.

Passamonti F, Rumi E, Pungolino E, et al. Life expectancy and prognostic factors for survival in patients with polycythemia vera and essential thrombocythemia. Am J Med 2004;117:755–61.

Tefferi A. JAK2 mutations in polycythemia vera: Molecular mechanisms and clinical applications. N Engl J Med 2007;356:444–5.

Tefferi A, Vardiman JW. Classification and diagnosis of myeloproliferative neoplasms: The 2008 World Health Organization criteria and point-of-care diagnostic algorithms. Leukemia 2008;22:14–22.

Porphyria

Method of

*Herbert L. Bonkovsky, MD, and
Manish Thapar, MD*

The porphyrias are metabolic disorders caused primarily by inherited defects in heme synthesis (Table 1). They manifest clinically in two major ways: with neurovisceral symptoms and signs (including abdominal pain, constipation, and weakness) and with cutaneous symptoms and signs. In hereditary coproporphyria and variegate porphyria, patients can present with both kinds of symptoms; in the other forms of porphyria, patients have one or the other kind of clinical presentation.

Classification

In considering therapy for the porphyrias, it is useful to classify them into two major categories: acute or inducible porphyrias and chronic cutaneous porphyrias (see Table 1). Regardless of the specific form of acute porphyria or associated enzymatic defect, all of the acute porphyrias produce similar neurovisceral manifestations and should be managed in a similar manner. Management of cutaneous porphyria, although more specific to the particular type, also involves application of some general principles.

Diagnosis

A complete discussion of the diagnosis of porphyria is beyond the scope of this article. However, a correct and definitive diagnosis at the outset is of paramount importance. Box 1 and Table 2 give the recommended approach to diagnosis. Because of the complicated and unfamiliar tests often required for diagnosis, it is recommended that physicians without special training in the porphyrias discuss possible patients with, or refer patients to, physicians who have such expertise. See http://www.porphyriafoundation.com/index.html or call 713-266-9617 for an updated listing. Resources with descriptions on how to diagnose or exclude porphyrias are listed in the references.

Treatment

ACUTE HEPATIC PORPHYRIAS

Management of Acute Attacks

The cardinal symptom of acute porphyria is severe colicky abdominal pain. Nausea, vomiting, constipation, and pain or paresthesias in the extremities are present in about one half of patients. Tachycardia and dark urine are the most common signs. The pathogenesis of acute porphyric attacks involves a deficiency of hepatic heme and induction of hepatic 5-aminolevulinic acid (ALA) synthase by stressors, with resultant overproduction of ALA, which is neurotoxic.

General measures should include parenteral hydration and pain control with meperidine (Demerol) 50 to 150 mg or morphine 3 to 10 mg. Addition of a phenothiazine (e.g., chlorpromazine [Thorazine], 25 to 50 mg) enhances the analgesic and sedative effects of the narcotic. Propranolol (Inderal) may be given for control of severe

TABLE 1 Classification and Major Features of Human Porphyries

Disease	Primary Enzymatic Defect	Autosomal Inheritance	Clinical Features	
			Neurovisceral Symptoms	Photosensitivity Dermatosis
Acute or Inducible Porphyrias				
ALA-D deficiency porphyria	ALA dehydratase	Recessive	+	−
Acute intermittent porphyria	PBG deaminase	Dominant	+	−
Hereditary coproporphyria	Coproporphyrinogen oxidase	Dominant	+	+
Variegate porphyria	Protoporphyrinogen oxidase	Dominant	+	+
Chronic Cutaneous Porphyrias				
Congenital erythropoietic	Uroporphyrinogen III (co)-synthase	Recessive	−	+ +
Hepatoerythropoietic porphyria	Uroporphyrinogen decarboxylase	Recessive	±	+
Porphyria cutanea tarda	Uroporphyrinogen decarboxylase	Dominant (acquired variant exists)	−	+
Protoporphyria	Ferrochelatase	Recessive	−*	+

*A neurovisceral syndrome reminiscent of those observed in the acute porphyrias has been described in a few patients with protoporphyria and hepatic failure around the time of orthotopic liver transplantation.

Abbreviations: ALA = 5-aminolevulinic acid, the first intermediate in the heme biosynthetic pathway; ALA-D = ALA dehydratase; PBG = porphobilinogen, the second intermediate in the heme biosynthetic pathway.

BOX 1 Key to Diagnosis: Screening Tests for Porphyrias

Urinary PBG (porphobilinogen) is substantially elevated in all patients with acute attacks of AIP, HCP, and VP and often during latent periods as well, a finding that occurs in no other medical condition. Urinary PBG offers both sensitivity and specificity in diagnosing the acute porphyrias. PBG is not increased in ADP; diagnosis of this rare condition requires measurement of ALA.

If serum or urine ALA and/or PBG are increased, second-line testing is done to determine the precise disorder of porphyrin metabolism, although treatment (which is the same regardless of the type of acute porphyria) should not be delayed pending these results.

A simple test of considerable value for diagnosis and differential diagnosis of the cutaneous porphyrias is the plasma porphyrin fluorescence pattern. In this test, the fluorescence emission spectrum of diluted plasma is measured. The exciting wavelength is the Soret band (400–410 nm). Uroporphyrin and coproporphyrin, which accumulate in PCT and HCP, have a peak at 618 nm, and protoporphyrin, which accumulates in PP, has a peak at 636 nm. A protein-porphyrin complex unique to VP has a peak at 626 nm. The latter is nearly always present in postpubertal VP patients, and it is the simplest and most reliable method for making a presumptive diagnosis of VP.

Abbreviations: AIP = acute intermittent porphyria; ALA = 5-aminolevulinic acid; CEP = congenital erythopoietic porphyria; EPP = erythopoietic protoporphyria; HEP = hepatoerythopoietic porphyria, HCP = hereditary coproporphyria; PBG = porphobilinogen; PCT = porphyria cutanea tarda; VP = variegate porphyria.

CURRENT DIAGNOSIS

Suspected Acute Porphyria

- In suspected acute porphyria, the screening test of choice is random spot urine for qualitative or quantitative porphobilinogen and creatinine. Urinary porphobilinogen is markedly ($>10 \times$ ULN) increased.
- Mild to moderate increases of urinary porphyrins, with normal urinary ALA and PBG are *not* diagnostic of porphyria but more likely due to secondary porphyrinurias.
- The most useful test for diagnosis of variegate porphyria is the emission fluorescence of plasma excited by the Soret band (excitation wavelength ~ 400 nm). Peak emission at 626 nm is pathognomic of variegate porphyria.

Suspected Cutaneous Porphyria

- Typical skin lesions of CEP, PCT, or HEP are vesicles and bullae on the hands and face.
- Typical skin lesions of EPP are solar urticaria, acute burning and itching.
- The single most useful screening test is plasma porphyrin and fluorescence emission pattern.
- In clinically manifest cutaneous porphyria, plasma porphyrins are increased and the fluorescence emission pattern is helpful in the differential diagnosis (with excitation light of ~ 400 nm, peak emission wavelengths are ~ 618 nm in CEP, HEP, PCT, HCP; 626 nm in VP; and 634 nm in EPP).
- In EPP, urinary porphyrins and porphyrin precursors are completely normal.

Abbreviations: ALA = 5-aminolevulinic acid; CEP = congenital erythopoietic prophyria; EPP = erythopoietic protoporphyria; HCP = hereditary coproporphyria; HEP = hepatoerythopoietic porphyria, PBG = porphobilinogen; PCT = porphyria cutanea tarda; ULN = upper limit of normal; VP = variegate porphyria.

tachycardia or arterial hypertension. The dose should be titrated carefully because of the risk of serious bradycardia and hypotension from propranolol. Frequent checks (every 6 hours) of neuromuscular function, looking for developing weakness of crucial muscles such as the diaphragm, by measuring the vital capacity are recommended.

Specific treatment is directed at correcting the deficiency of hepatic heme and decreasing activity of ALA synthase. The treatment of choice of an acute attack requiring hospital admission is intravenous heme.

Heme is administered intravenously at a dose of 3 to 4 mg/kg/day for 4 days; it is taken up primarily by the liver and replenishes the depleted heme pool. Heme should be started early for most attacks. At this time in the United States, only one FDA-approved form of heme is available: heme hydroxide or hematin (Panhematin, Ovation Pharmaceuticals, Deerfield, IL; www.ovationpharma.com). Each vial of hematin contains 313 mg of heme, supplied as a lyophilized powder that also contains

TABLE 2 Further Testing to Confirm the Diagnosis of Acute Porphyrias

Type of Porphyria	RBC PBGB Deaminase	Urinary Porphyrins	Fecal Porphyrins	Plasma Porphyrins	Peak of Porphyrin Emission Fluorescence (nm)
Acute intermittent (AIP)	Low: <50%	Markedly increased (uroporphyrins)	Normal or slightly increased	Normal or slightly increased	618
Variegate porphyria (VP)	Normal	Markedly increased (coproporphyrins)	Markedly increased (copro- and protoporphyrin)	Markedly increased	626
Hereditary coproporphyria (HCP)	Normal	Markedly increased (coproporphyrins)	Markedly increased (coproporphyrins)	Mostly normal	618
ALA dehydratase porphyria	Normal	Increased (5-aminolevulinic acid and coproporphyrin)	Normal or slightly increased	Increased	618

Abbreviations: PBG = porphobilinogen; RBC = red blood cell.

sodium carbonate. The manufacturer recommends dissolving the powder in sterile water. In this form, the resultant hematin solution is unstable and must be administered within 1 hour of preparation. It is also irritating to veins, often producing thrombophlebitis, and causes a mild coagulopathy due to adverse effects on clotting factors and platelets.

It is now recommended that lyophilized hematin be reconstituted with human albumin (1:1 molar complex), which increases its stability and decreases unwanted side effects. To prepare such a solution, add 132 mL of 25% human serum albumin (33 g) to a vial containing lyophilized hematin and mix gently. Heme given in this form has biochemical and clinical effects on porphyria that appear equivalent to those of freshly prepared aqueous solutions of hematin and are superior to those of aged aqueous solutions of hematin. Hematin can be delivered within a few hours to anywhere in the United States by calling the 24/7 Ovation hotline at 1-888-514-5204.

 CURRENT THERAPY

Acute Porphyria

- Remove inciting factors: Alcohol, drugs, toxins and chemicals (see Box 2)
- Nutritional supplementation: ≥300 g glucose/day may be given enterally if tolerated
- Intravenous heme: 3–5 mg/kg/d for 3–5 days
- Frequent checks of neurologic status: Especially watch for development of paresis of muscles of respiration
- Monitor for hypokalemia, hypomagnesemia, or hyponatremia and treat vigorously, if found
- Parenteral meperidine (Demerol) 50–150 mg or morphine 3–10 mg q4–6h for pain
- Chlorpromazine (Thorazine) 25–50 mg q4–6h for nausea and agitation
- Propranolol (Inderal) 10–40 mg q6h for tachycardia and hypertension
- Magnesium sulfate, gabapentin (Neurontin), and/or vigabatrin (Sabril)[2] for seizures
- All cases should undergo hepatocellular carcinoma screening every 6 months even in the absence of cirrhosis.
- All first-degree family members should be screened for porphyria

Cutaneous Porphyria

- General measures: Protect skin from light and trauma; treat secondary skin infections
- Congenital erythropoietic porphyria: Oral activated charcoal; hypertransfusion to suppress erythropoiesis; heme infusion; splenectomy for hemolysis; glucocorticoid trial for anemia; bone marrow transplantation (gene therapy in the future)
- Hepatoerythropoietic porphyria: Uncertain; probably the same as for congenital erythropoietic porphyria (phlebotomy and antimalarials are not effective)
- Porphyria cutanea tarda: Stop ethanol, estrogen, or other precipitating chemicals; iron depletion by phlebotomy; treat chronic hepatitis C, if present; chloroquine (Aralen)[1] or hydroxychloroquine (Plaquenil)[3]; urinary alkalinization
- Protoporphyria: β-Carotene; adequate iron; oral charcoal; cholecystectomy for gallstones; plasmapheresis; intravenous heme; hypertransfusion; liver transplantation; (gene therapy in the future)

[1]Not FDA approved for this indication.
[2]Not available in the United States.

In some other countries, another effective form of heme is available: heme arginate (Normosang).[2] This preparation consists of heme complexed to arginine and is supplied as a solution that usually is also diluted in approximately 5% human serum albumin just before administration. Usual doses are as for Panhematin.

Another way to decrease ALA synthase is to administer glucose or other readily metabolized carbohydrates, taking advantage of the phenomenon of carbohydrate repression of the enzyme, the so-called glucose effect. This may be used for mild attacks or when awaiting IV hematin. At least 300 g of glucose per day is given, enterally if tolerated or as a 10% infusion. Some patients have elevations of antidiuretic hormone (ADH) and can rapidly develop profound symptomatic hyponatremia and hypomagnesemia, especially when dextrose in water is given intravenously. As a rule, it is best to give dextrose in half-normal saline. Serum electrolytes including magnesium should be checked every 12 hours for the first few days. Hypokalemia or hypomagnesemia should be corrected promptly.

Many drugs and chemicals are known to exacerbate acute porphyrias, and many others are theoretically risky because they induce hepatic cytochrome P-450, deplete hepatic regulatory heme, and induce ALA synthase, especially in animals with a partial block in heme synthesis (Box 2). Among dangerous drugs, the worst offenders are barbiturates, ethanol excess, hydantoins, and sulfonamides. These drugs are absolutely contraindicated in patients with acute porphyric attacks; others, listed in the first two sections of Box 2, should be avoided if possible. The last section of Box 2 lists drugs believed to be safe; however, a wise practice is to use as few systemically absorbed drugs as possible.

Therapy of Seizures in Patients with Acute Porphyria

Treatment of seizures in porphyric patients has been particularly problematic because most of the commonly used anticonvulsants also induce cytochrome P-450 and can precipitate or worsen acute attacks (see Box 2). Seizures in acute attacks can also occur due to hyponatremia or hypomagnesemia. Seizures in patients with acute porphyria have been treated with bromides, which are effective and do not exacerbate porphyria, but they have a narrow therapeutic window. High doses of magnesium sulfate (3 g loading dose; then 1 g/h in 0.15 M NaCl, with or without 5% dextrose) have been of benefit. A suggested therapeutic range for serum magnesium level is 4 to 8 mEq/L. Clonazepam (Klonopin) has helped some patients, but in large doses it has made others worse. High doses of clonazepam must be considered a potential hazard, because it induces cytochrome P-450 and ALA synthase in cultured hepatocytes (see Box 2).

The safety of newer anticonvulsant medications has been studied in cultured liver cells. Phenobarbital, felbamate (Felbatol), lamotrigine (Lamictal), or tiagabine (Gabitril), but not gabapentin (Neurontin) or vigabatrin (Sabril),[2] increased levels of porphyrins and the mRNA of ALA synthase, the first and rate-controlling enzyme of porphyrin synthesis. Vigabatrin[2] or gabapentin is therefore recommended in patients with acute porphyria and seizures. Administration of gabapentin should be individualized; the usual dose range for adults is 900 to 1800 mg/day, given in three divided doses.

Management of Frequent Recurrent Attacks

Some unfortunate women suffer attacks of acute porphyria nearly every month during the luteal phase of their menstrual cycles. Some are helped by oral contraceptives, which are believed to act by interrupting their endogenous cyclic production of sex hormones. However, such therapy is a double-edged sword, because exogenous estrogens and progestogens can induce ALA synthase (see Box 2). Minimal effective doses should be used, and patients should be followed closely, particularly in the first few months. Regular infusions of heme have also been of benefit but require frequent IV access. Also, chronic heme therapy can lead to iron overload, because heme is about 8% iron by weight.

[2]Not available in the United States.

BOX 2 Some Drugs and Chemicals in Acute Hepatic Porphyrias

Reported to Exacerbate Disease

Aminoglutethimide (Cytadren)
Antipyrine
Aminopyrine
Barbiturates
Barbamazepine
Carbamazepine (Tegretol)
Carisoprodol (Soma)
Chloramphenicol (Chloromycetin)
Clindamycin (Cleocin)
Danazol (Danocrine)
Dihydralazine
Diclofenac (Voitaren)
Erythromycin
Estrogens
Ethanol excess
Fosphenytoin (Cerebyx)
Griseofulvin (Grifulvin)
Hydralazine
Hydantoins
Hydroxyzine (Vistaril)
Indinavir (Crixivan)
Ketoconazole (Nizoral)
Ketamine (Ketalar)
Lidocaine
Lynestrenol
Medroxyprogesterone (Provera)
Methyldopa (Aldomet)
Metoclopramide (Reglan)
Norethisterone (Micronor, Aygestin)
Nitrofurantoin (Microdantin)
Oral contraceptives
Orphenadrine (Norflex)
Phenylbutazone
Phenytoin (Dilantin)
Primidone (Mysoline)
Progestogens
Pyrazinamide
Rifampicin (Rifadin)
Sulfonamides
Spironolactone (Aldactone)
Tamoxifen (Nolvadex)
Testosterone
Theophylline and its derivatives
Trimethoprim
Valproic acid (Depakote)

Theoretically Risky

Amlodipine (Norvasc)
Amiodarone (Cordarone)
Amitriptyline (Elavil)
Azathioprine (Imuran)
Amphetamines
Atorvastatin (Lipitor)

Bosentan (Tracleer)
Buspirone (Buspar)
Clonidine (Catapres)
Clonazepam (Klonopin) (large doses)
Ceftriaxone (Rocephin)
Cervistatin (Baycol)
Cetirizine (Zyrtec)
Diazepam (Valium)
Diltiazem (Cardizem)
Diphenhydramine (Benadryl)
Econazole (Spectazole)
Ethosuximide (Zarontin)
Felodipine (Plendil)
Fluconazole (Diflucan)
Fluvastatin (Lescol)
Glibenclamide (Diabeta)
Glipizide (Glucotrol)
Guaifenesin (Robitussin)
Heavy metals
Halothane
Hyoscyamine (Levsin)
Imipramine (Tofranil)
Isoniazid
Itraconazole (Sporanox)
Lansoprazole (Prevacid)
Lamotrigine (Lamictal)
Lamivudine (Epivir)
Metronidazole (Flagyl)
Montelukast (Singulair)
Nortriptyline (Pamelor)
Nifedipine (Adalat)
Oxytetracycline
Oxcarbazepine (Trileptal)
Pioglitazone (Actos)
Probenecid
Quinine (Qualaquin)
Rabeprazole (Aciphex)
Rosiglitazone (Avandia)
Sulfonylureas
Simvastatin (Zocor)
Telithromycin (Ketek)
Tetracycline
Topiramate (Topamax)
Tramadol (Ultram)
Verapamil (Calan)
Voriconazole (VFEND)
All agents known to induce cytochrome P-450 or to increase hepatic heme turnover

Believed to Be Safe

Acetaminophen (Tylenol)
Allopurinol (Zyloprim)
Aspirin

Atropine
Azithromycin (Zithromax)
Bisacodyl (Dulcolax)
Bromides
Cimetidine (Tagamet)
Chlorpromazine
Cephalexin (Keflex)
Ciprofloxacin (Cipro)
Candesartan (Atacand)
Captopril (Capoten)
Dopamine
Digoxin (Lanoxin)
Enalapril (Vasotec)
Ezetimibe (Zetia)
Furosemide (Lasix)
Fondaparinux (Arixtra)
Gabapentin (Neurontin)
Glucocorticoids
Gemfiborzil (Lopid)
Heparin
Hydrochlorothiazide (Microzide)
Ibuprofen (Motrin, Advil)
Insulin
Iron
Irbesartan (Avapro)
Labetalol (Trandate)
Lisinopril (Prinivil, Zestril)
Lithium (Lithobid)
Meperidine (Demerol)
Morphine
Nicotinic Acid (Niaspan)
Nystatin (Mycostatin)
Naproxen (Naprosyn)
Ofloxacin (Floxin)
Ondansetron (Zofran)
Penicillin and its derivatives
Phenylephrine
Phenylpropanolamine
Propranolol (Inderal)
Quinapril (Accupril)
Ramipril (Altace)
Streptomycin
Tetanus toxoid
Thiamine (vitamin B$_1$)
Tobramycin (Tobrex)
Valsartan (Diovan)
Vancomycin (Vancocin)
Vitamins A, B, C, D, and E
Vigabatrin (Sabril)[2]

[2]Not available in the United States.
Refer to http://www.porphyriafoundation.com/ and http://www.porphyria-europe.com/ for more detailed lists.

For most women with cyclic attacks of acute porphyria, the treatment of choice is a luteinizing hormone-releasing hormone (LHRH) analogue. Leuprolide (Lupron)[1] has been used most often. The usual daily dose is 1 mg (0.2 mL), subcutaneously, although higher doses

[1]Not FDA approved for this indication.

are occasionally required. LHRH analogues can produce initial worsening of porphyric symptoms due to partial agonist effects, followed by improvement due to chronic antagonist effects. Therapy with LHRH analogues is usually continued for at least 1 year and sometimes longer. The use of bisphosphonates to minimize development of osteoporosis is advised when prolonged therapy with LHRH analogues is undertaken.

Prevention of Attacks

Patients should be counseled not to use ethanol and avoid drugs not known to be safe (see Box 2). The use of herbal remedies and alternative therapies is also to be discouraged because many such preparations are likely to contain porphyrogenic compounds. Patients should also avoid very-low-calorie diets or prolonged periods of fasting and should receive prompt and vigorous management of intercurrent illnesses or other stressors. Pregnancy does not usually cause acute porphyria to worsen, and termination of pregnancy is not usually indicated on medical grounds, even if both mother and fetus have acute porphyria.

A small fraction of patients with frequent attacks require chronic infusions of heme. In some, the heme needs to be given weekly or even twice weekly. These patients need to be watched for the development of iron overload and can require iron-reduction therapy by therapeutic phlebotomies if serum ferritin exceeds 1000 ng/mL.

Relatives at risk should be evaluated thoroughly and all probands and relatives found to be carriers should be educated and encouraged to wear medical alert bracelets and to carry medical alert cards.

In a rare patient with recalcitrant and unremitting disease, consideration may be given to orthotopic liver transplantation. Liver transplantation has been described in case reports as resulting in biochemical and clinical remission.

Studies have shown a 60- to 70-fold increased prevalence of hepatocellular carcinoma in patients with hepatic porphyrias even in the absence of cirrhosis or steatohepatitis. This lends credence to periodic screening for hepatocellular cancer in this patient population.

CHRONIC CUTANEOUS PORPHYRIAS

Porphyrin accumulations in the skin, red cells, and hepatocytes are responsible for the pathophysiologic changes of the chronic porphyrias. The general principles of therapy of chronic cutaneous porphyrins are to decrease the overproduction and increase the excretion of porphyrins as much as possible. Protection of the skin from light (opaque sunscreens and/or clothing) and physical trauma should also be recommended. Oral activated charcoal or cholestyramine (Questran) can improve symptoms by absorbing porphyrins and hastening their excretion in the urine. In several diseases, the chronic blistering and ulcerating skin lesions are prone to secondary infection, which requires prompt treatment to minimize further damage.

Congenital Erythropoietic Porphyria

Congenital erythropoietic porphyria (CEP; Günther's disease) is a rare autosomal recessive disorder that manifests in infancy with red urine, erythrodontia, anemia, and a severe blistering dermatosis. The marked overproduction of uroporphyrin I characteristic of CEP arises from erythroid precursors. Elevated levels of porphyrins have been improved by large oral doses of activated charcoal (30–60 g every 6 hours), by hypertransfusion, and by infusions of heme. Unfortunately, long-term therapy with any of these is difficult, and chronic transfusions exacerbate iron overload, which is often a pre-existing problem related to ineffective erythropoiesis and increased iron absorption. Some patients with hemolysis have responded to splenectomy, and glucocorticoids have also been reported to improve anemia. Because of the rarity and phenotypic heterogeneity of CEP, a consensus regarding therapy has not emerged. A few patients have been cured by bone marrow transplantation. In the future, gene replacement therapy will deserve serious consideration for treatment of severely affected patients.

Hepatoerythropoietic Porphyria

Hepatoerythropoietic porphyria (HEP) is even rarer than CEP, which it resembles clinically. HEP is due to homozygous or compound heterozygous defects, leading to severe deficiency of uroporphyrinogen decarboxylase. Infants present with severe skin fragility and extensive vesicle and bulla formation, leading to scarring and mutilation of sun-exposed skin. They also present with hypertrichosis, erythrodontia, anemia, and hepatosplenomegaly.

The general and specific measures outlined earlier for therapy of CEP are rational in HEP as well, although none has been shown clearly effective in HEP. HEP shows no response to therapeutic phlebotomy, unlike porphyria cutanea tarda, even though both share a defect in uroporphyrinogen decarboxylase.

Porphyria Cutanea Tarda (PCT)

Porphyria cutanea tarda (PCT) is the most common type of porphyria. It is characterized by an inherited or acquired defect in activity of hepatic uroporphyrinogen decarboxylase. In the common inherited form(s) of PCT, there is a 50% decrease in activity of the decarboxylase, usually identifiable in nonliver tissues as well as in the liver. A defect in the decarboxylase is not sufficient to produce clinical manifestations; other factors, such as iron overload, chronic hepatitis C, ethanol abuse, estrogens, and porphyrogenic toxins, are important pathogenic elements. The typical patient is a middle-aged man with a vesiculobullous eruption on the dorsa of the hands. Patients usually abuse ethanol and have evidence of modest iron overload and liver injury. In some parts of the world, including the United States, most patients with PCT also have chronic hepatitis C.

Patients with mild PCT often respond simply to the general measures and removal of the precipitating agent such as estrogen, ethanol, or halo-aromatic chemical exposure. For those with more severe disease, the treatment of choice is phlebotomy for depletion of hepatic iron stores. The initial treatment regimen should be removal of a pint of blood each week, continued until the patient has developed a mild degree of anemia with decreased serum ferritin, transferrin saturation, and erythrocytic mean corpuscular volume (MCV). Although most patients with PCT have moderate iron overload (~3–4 g), phlebotomy therapy is effective even when hepatic iron stores are not increased.

Unfortunately, the response to iron removal or other therapy of PCT is slow, and evidence of improvement in the skin might not appear for months. It is important to let patients know this and to encourage them to persist in therapy, for it will eventually succeed. Patients should not take medicinal iron and are encouraged to decrease their intake of red meats, which contain relatively large amounts of heme iron, a form of iron particularly well absorbed.

Recent results from our center and others showed that most patients with active PCT also have chronic hepatitis C infection and one or both of the mutations of the HFE gene associated with HLA-linked hereditary hemochromatosis. All patients with PCT should be screened for hepatitis C infection and for HFE gene mutations (C282Y and H63D).

Chloroquine (Aralen)[1] and hydroxychloroquine (Plaquenil)[1] form water-soluble complexes with uroporphyrin, increasing porphyrin removal from tissue stores and excretion in the urine. However, in previously untreated PCT, the doses of these drugs usually used for other disorders can cause acute hepatic injury with fever, jaundice, and right upper quadrant pain. This is due to excessively rapid mobilization of porphyrin from the liver. For this reason, such drugs should be started slowly at low doses (125 mg 2–3 times per week) with gradual increase to 500 mg/day. Monitoring for possible retinal damage is advisable whenever chronic chloroquine or hydroxychloroquine therapy is used.

PCT can occur in association with end-stage renal disease. Because the chloroquine-porphyrin complex is poorly dialyzable, chloroquine is ineffective. Because of anemia, phlebotomy is relatively contraindicated in such patients. However, administration of recombinant human erythropoietin (Epogen, Procrit) stimulates iron mobilization for red cell production sufficient to support therapeutic phlebotomies.

Protoporphyria

Also called erythopoietic protoporphyria (EPP), protoporphyria (PP) is a disorder with highly variable clinical expression. Infants and children develop intense burning pain of sun-exposed skin following brief

---

[1]Not FDA approved for this indication.

exposure in the spring and summer. A few hours later, erythema, edema, and itching become prominent. Vesicles only develop with prolonged exposure. With chronic and repeated exposure, involved skin can become leathery and hyperkeratotic. This is especially prominent in a malar butterfly distribution on the face and over the knuckles of the hands. Diagnosis of PP requires demonstration of increased amounts of protoporphyrin, without increased coproporphyrin, in the stool, red cells, or both. It is the only form of clinically manifested porphyria in which urinary heme precursors are normal. A common complication of PP is development of pigment gallstones, which contain a high content of protoporphyrin. A rare, but serious, complication is development of severe liver disease, due to precipitation of protoporphyrin in hepatocytes and biliary radicles. Such disease can progress and produce liver failure with all its usual complications.

In addition to the usual general measures, PP is treated with β-carotene (Solatene). The usual adult dose is 120 to 180 mg/day. The recommended therapeutic serum β-carotene level is 600 to 800 μg/dL. Drugs or chemicals that can increase protoporphyrin production or decrease its utilization should be avoided. Griseofulvin (Grifulvin) is the most obvious example, because it can cause a protoporphyric condition in mice. Any drug or toxin (e.g., excess alcohol) that produces cholestasis is a risk, because protoporphyrin must be excreted through the bile. Patients should be immunized against hepatitis A and B unless they clearly are immune. Avoidance of iron deficiency is important, because iron deficiency can exacerbate overproduction of protoporphyrin. Oral cholestyramine and activated charcoal have been suggested as treatments to prevent the enterohepatic circulation of protoporphyrin, which appears to be substantial. Patients with symptomatic gallstones are best treated by cholecystectomy, as long as they do not have severe liver disease or other contraindications to surgery.

Patients with evidence of liver disease require regular and frequent monitoring, because decompensation can occur quickly. Those with abnormal liver chemistries or very high red cell (>1500 μg/dL) or plasma (>150 μg/dL) protoporphyrin concentrations should undergo liver biopsy. Patients with liver injury must avoid ethanol or other hepatotoxins that can act synergistically to accelerate liver damage. Liver transplantation is an option for those with advanced liver disease, although it does not correct the biochemical abnormality because ferrochelatase deficiency in the bone marrow persists.

Unfortunately, some patients with PP who have undergone liver transplantation have redeveloped pigmentary fibrosis quite rapidly. Thus, transplantation of bone marrow before, during, or after liver transplantation is considered. In the future, gene therapy (the normal ferrochelatase gene targeted to the bone marrow stem cells) will be a major advance. Transient improvements in PP have been achieved by plasmapheresis followed by intravenous heme infusions. The dose of heme used has been 3 to 5 mg/kg/day. Such therapy is recommended, particularly as a way to stabilize hepatic function while transplantation is awaited or to decrease plasma protoporphyrin concentrations just prior to transplantation. Without such therapy, several patients have suffered severe neuromuscular complications, requiring prolonged and expensive convalescence.

REFERENCES

Anderson KE, Bishop DF, Desnick RJ, Sassa S. Disorders of heme biosynthesis. In: Scriver CR, Beaudet AL, Sly WS, Valle D, editors. The Metabolic and Molecular Bases of Inherited Disease. 8th ed. New York: McGraw-Hill; 2001. p. 2991–3042.

Anderson KE, Bloomer JR, Bonkovsky HL, et al. Recommendations for the diagnosis and treatment of the acute porphyrias. Ann Intern Med 2005;142:439–50.

Anderson KE, Bonkovsky HL, Bloomer JR, Shedlofsky SI. Reconstitution of hematin for intravenous infusion. Ann Intern Med 2006;144:537–8.

Bonkovsky HL, Barnard GF. Diagnosis of porphyric syndromes: A practical approach in the era of molecular biology. Semin Liver Dis 1998;18:57–65.

Bonkovsky HL, Barnard GF. The hepatic porphyrias. In: Brandt L, editor. Clinical Practice of Gastroenterology. Philadelphia: Current Medicine; 1998. p. 947–60.

Bonkovsky HL, Healey JF, Lourie AN, Gerron GG. Intravenous heme-albumin in acute intermittent porphyria: Evidence for repletion of hepatic hemoproteins and regulatory heme pools. Am J Gastroenterol 1991;86:1050–6.

Bonkovsky HL, Poh-Fitzpatrick M, Pimstone N, et al. Porphyria cutanea tarda, hepatitis C, and HFE gene mutations in North America. Hepatology 1998;27:1661–9.

Chemmanur AT, Bonkovsky HL. Hepatic porphyrias: Diagnosis and management. Clin Liver Dis 2004;8:807–38.

McGuire BM, Bonkovsky HL, Carithers RL Jr, et al. Liver transplantation for erythropoietic protoporphyria liver disease. Liver Transpl 2005;11:1590–6.

Therapeutic Use of Blood Components

Method of

Peter A. Millward, MD, and Mark E. Brecher, MD

The transfusion of blood was the first successful transplantation of living tissue in humans. Today, transfusion is so commonplace that it is rarely thought of as a transplant. In 2001, for allogeneic transfusions within the United States alone, it is estimated that 13,898,000 units of whole blood or red blood cells, 2,614,000 units of whole blood–derived platelets, 1,264,000 units of apheresis platelets, and 3,926,000 units of plasma were administered. For red blood cell–containing products alone, this equates to 1 unit transfused every 2.3 seconds. A basic understanding of indications for blood component therapy is essential to optimally treat patients.

Red Blood Cells

Red blood cells are collected via whole blood donation or automated erythrocytapheresis. Both collection techniques employ a sterile closed system for blood collection. The blood is collected into plastic blood bags containing a sufficient formulation of anticoagulant and preservative solution.

The components of the anticoagulant solution determine the maximum shelf life (ranging from 21 to 35 days) of collected blood and blood components. The solution can contain citrate (trisodium citrate and citric acid), dextrose, phosphate (monobasic sodium phosphate), and adenine. Citrate is for anticoagulation, dextrose and adenine are for metabolic energy, and phosphate is for buffering pH.

Shelf life of red cells may be extended to 42 days with the addition of an preservative-additive solution, such as Adsol (AS-1), Nutricel (AS-3), or Optisol (AS-5). This additive solution must be added within 72 hours from primary collection. Additive solution contains dextrose, adenine, and sodium chloride and contains either monobasic sodium phosphate or mannitol.

Even with anticoagulant and preservative-additive solutions, biochemical changes, called storage lesions, develop with stored red blood cells. These biochemical changes are decreased pH, adenosine triphosphate (ATP), and 2,3-diphosphoglycerate (DPG) and increased plasma potassium and plasma hemoglobin (Hb). Even in massively transfused patients, storage lesions do not routinely cause significant clinical consequences when transfused.

The standard collection volume for a whole blood donation is 450 mL ± 45 mL. Because whole blood is rarely indicated, centrifugation is used to separate a whole-blood donation into various components, which maximizes this limited resource. One red blood cell (RBC) unit, also known as *packed RBCs*, is made by removing a significant portion of plasma from a whole-blood donation. Using apheresis technique, one or two RBC units can be specifically collected with each donation. With either technique, an RBC unit volume is approximately 300 mL. Based on the preservative-additive solution used, an RBC unit averages a hematocrit of 60% to 80%.

After initial processing of whole blood, an RBC unit is composed of RBCs, white blood cells (WBCs), platelets, and plasma. An erythrocytapheresis RBC unit is composed of RBCs with decreased platelets and plasma and are *leukocyte reduced* ($<5 \times 10^6$ leukocytes per component) due to intraprocedural leukocyte filtration.

RBC units can be further modified for specific needs of the patient to leukoreduced RBCs, washed RBCs, irradiated RBCs, and frozen deglycerolized RBCs.

LEUKOREDUCED RED BLOOD CELLS

In the United States, a leukoreduced RBC unit must have less than 5 million leukocytes per unit. This decrease in leukocytes is achieved using a leukocyte filter that extracts leukocytes based on their relative larger size and propensity to adhere to certain fiber types. Current leukoreduction filters remove between 3 and 5 log of leukocytes in an RBC unit. Leukocyte filtration can occur during or immediately after collection (prestorage leukocyte reduction) or at the time of transfusion (poststorage leukocyte reduction).

Common indications for leukoreduced RBCs are multiple febrile, nonhemolytic transfusion reactions (FNHTR), prevention of HLA alloimmunization, and reduction of cytomegalovirus (CMV) transmission.

An FNHTR is defined by a greater than $1°C$ ($2°F$) temperature rise occurring up to 2 hours after transfusion and unexplained by the patient's underlying medical condition; it may be accompanied by chills, rigors, nausea, vomiting, malaise, and headache. Two mechanisms of FNHTR with RBC transfusion have been proposed: recipient anti-HLA or antigranulocyte antibodies react with donor leukocytes and induce cytokine release, or donor leukocytes form an antigen-antibody complex resulting in recipient monocytes to release cytokines. Both mechanisms depend on the presence of donor leukocytes, and therefore leukoreduction effectively decreases the incidence of FNHTR associated with red blood cell transfusions.

The formation of HLA antibodies (also known as HLA alloimmunization) can lead to platelet transfusion refractoriness, which is especially problematic for patients requiring substantial platelet transfusion support (e.g., hematology-oncology patients). All potential candidates for bone marrow (BMT) or solid organ transplantation should receive leukoreduced RBCs to minimize the formation of HLA antibodies.

Transfusion-transmitted CMV (TT-CMV) infections in high-risk populations, such as CMV-negative neonates, AIDS patients, and BMT candidates or patients, are associated with considerable mortality and morbidity. CMV is latent in leukocytes, specifically in the monocyte-macrophage lineage. Based on Bowden and colleagues' findings in 1995, leukoreduced RBCs offer a CMV-safe blood product that is an equivalent alternative to providing blood from a CMV-seronegative donor. These findings and other confirming studies led to numerous institutions using leukoreduced RBCs as their sole method for providing CMV-safe blood products and abandoning a CMV-seronegative inventory. Recently, Nicholas and colleagues questioned the equivalence of leukoreduced blood products versus CMV-seronegative blood products and called for further investigation.

WASHED RED BLOOD CELLS

The objective of washing RBCs is to effectively remove 99% of antibodies, plasma proteins, and electrolytes contained within the RBC component. The washing process involves repetitive steps of infusion of normal (0.9%) saline and centrifugation, with final resuspension of washed RBCs in normal saline. Because this process is an open system and the anticoagulant-preservative solution is removed, washed red cells must be transfused within 24 hours. This process can be automated or achieved with a manual technique, leading to up to 20% red cell loss. Approximately 20% to 90% of the platelets and 90% of the leukocytes are removed during this procedure. This decrease in leukocytes is not effective enough to render the component leukoreduced ($<5 \times 10^6$ leukocytes per unit).

Common indications for washed RBCs are recurrent severe allergic reactions not controlled with antihistamines and immunoglobulin A (IgA) deficiency. Washed RBCs also reduce the potassium load of the product. IgA-deficient patients can develop anti-IgA antibodies that react to donor IgA in plasma and lead to anaphylaxis. Potassium accumulates in the plasma during storage of the RBC unit or following irradiation.

IRRADIATED RED BLOOD CELLS

The goal of irradiation is to prevent proliferation of transfused immunocompetent T lymphocytes. This goal is accomplished by using cesium-137 or cobalt-60 as a radiation source, which administers a dose of 2500 cGy (25 Gy or 2500 rad) to the central portion of the RBC unit and a minimum of 1500 cGy to all other areas of the component. Due to decreased survival and viability of the RBCs and increased potassium leakage, irradiated RBCs expire on their original assigned outdate or 28 days after irradiation, whichever occurs first.

The only indication for the irradiated RBCs is to prevent transfusion-associated graft-versus-host disease (TA-GVHD). TA-GVHD is a rare, fatal complication (mortality >90%) caused by the engraftment and proliferation of donor T lymphocytes in the transfused recipient. Irradiated RBCs are indicated for patients receiving hematopoietic stem cell or bone marrow transplantation, patients with congenital immunodeficiency syndromes, intrauterine transfusions, neonates, HLA-matched platelet transfusions, patients with Hodgkin's disease, and patients with chronic lymphocytic leukemia treated with purine analogues (e.g., fludarabine [Fludara]).

Patients receiving transfusions from first-degree relatives require irradiation because of the increased risk of TA-GVHD due to HLA similarity of donor and recipient.

FROZEN RED BLOOD CELLS

The purpose of frozen RBCs is to store units with rare blood types and autologous units for extended periods of time (routinely up to 10 years, but storage may be extended for certain circumstances). Before freezing the RBCs, glycerol, a cryoprotective agent, is added to the system, which allows freezing of the red cells without damage. Based on the concentration of glycerol used ($\sim$20% or $\sim$40%), the storage temperatures vary. Most commonly in the United States, 40% glycerol is used, and therefore the frozen RBCs are stored at $-65°C$.

Frozen RBCs must be deglycerolized before transfusion. Washing the product in saline solutions of progressively decreasing osmolarity achieves glycerol removal. During the process, 99.9% of the plasma along with the vast majority of WBCs and platelets are removed. Depending on the technique used to deglycerolize the RBCs, once deglycerolized, these units have a 24-hour (open system) or 14-day (closed system) shelf life.

Frozen RBCs are indicated for heavily alloimmunized patients (e.g., multiple clinically significant RBC antigens) who require rare phenotypic RBCs for compatible transfusions.

Due to the multiple washing steps in the deglycerolized procedure, these units can be considered equivalent to a washed RBC unit.

INDICATIONS FOR RED BLOOD CELL TRANSFUSION

The purpose of RBC transfusions is to provide oxygen-carrying capacity and to maintain tissue oxygenation when the intravascular volume and cardiac function are adequate for perfusion. In a 70-kg recipient, 1 unit of transfused RBCs should increase the hemoglobin by 1 g/dL and the hematocrit by 3%. To obtain the same expected response in a pediatric patient, the RBC transfusion dose should be 15 mL/kg. RBC transfusions should only be used when time or underlying pathophysiology precludes other management (e.g., iron, erythropoietin, folic acid [folate]).
Criteria for administering RBC transfusions include:

- Hb <8 g/dL in an otherwise healthy patient
- Hb <11 g/dL in cases of increased risk of ischemia (e.g., pulmonary disease, coronary artery disease, cerebral vascular disease)
- Acute blood loss >15% of total blood volume (e.g., 750 mL in 70-kg man) or with evidence of inadequate oxygen delivery (e.g., electrocardiographic signs of cardiac ischemia, tachycardia, cyanosis)

- Symptomatic anemia in a normovolemic patient (e.g., tachycardia, mental status changes, electrocardiographic signs of cardiac ischemia, angina, shortness of breath, lightheadedness or dizziness with mild exertion)
- Regular predetermined therapeutic program for severe hypoplastic or aplastic anemia or for bone marrow suppression for hemoglobinopathies

The post-transfusion hemoglobin should not exceed 11.5 g/dL (12.5 g/dL in cases of increased risk of organ or tissue ischemia). Attempts to increase wound healing or merely to take advantage of available predonated autologous blood without a valid medical indication are not acceptable uses for RBC transfusions.

Platelets

Platelets are often a limited resource because of their relatively short shelf life and the inability to stockpile this product through freezing techniques. Temperature, pH, and gas exchange are critical issues for platelet viability and function, and they all determine the storage shelf life. Platelets remain viable for up to 7 days after collection, but the current 5-day shelf life has been instituted because of increased rates of clinically significant bacterial contamination on days 6 and 7. At a temperature lower than 20°C, platelets can be damaged and become nonfunctional. Platelets must be maintained at room temperature (20°–24°C) with gentle agitation in gas-permeable bags. Gas-permeable bags are required for platelet storage to ensure proper oxygenation and facilitate removal of carbon dioxide buildup. Constant gentle agitation is required to facilitate this gas exchange.

At present, two methods to obtain platelets are employed in the United States. First, platelets may be prepared from whole blood donations via centrifugation separation. These platelets are commonly referred to as *platelet concentrates*, *random donor platelets*, or *whole blood–derived platelets*. One platelet concentrate can be manufactured from a single whole blood donation. This platelet concentrate should have 5.5×10^{10} platelets per unit in 40 to 70 mL of plasma. One platelet concentrate should increase the platelet count by 7 to 10×10^9/L in a 70-kg recipient. Therefore, general platelet-concentrate dosing consists of a pool of 4 to 6 platelet concentrates, also known as a *four-pack* or *six-pack*, respectively. Second, platelets may be prepared using apheresis technology. These products are called *apheresis platelets*, *single-donor platelets*, or *platelet pheresis*.

Due to current apheresis technology, most apheresis platelets are leukoreduced at the time of collection. Apheresis platelets should have 3.0×10^{11} platelets per unit in 300 to 500 mL of plasma. One apheresis unit should increase the platelet count by 40 to 60×10^9/L in a 70-kg recipient.

One apheresis platelet product has an equivalent dose of a six-pack of platelet concentrates. In the United States, the use of apheresis platelets has been increasing annually. In 2004, it was estimated that 77% of all therapeutic doses of platelets transfused were apheresis platelets.

Once a platelet component is collected, it may be further modified in the same manner as RBCs: leukoreduced, washed, or irradiated.

LEUKOREDUCED PLATELETS

As with leukoreduced RBCs, common indications for leukoreduced platelets are multiple FNHTRs, prevention of human leukocyte antigen (HLA) alloimmunization, and reduction of CMV transmission. The proposed mechanisms by which leukoreduction prevents these conditions are discussed in the leukoreduced RBCs section. These mechanisms are the same with one exception. FNHTRs with RBCs are associated with an active release of cytokines induced by leukocyte-antibody interaction. The mechanism of FNHTRs with platelets differs and is due to passively transfused cytokines. At room temperature, residual donor leukocytes release cytokines that accumulate during storage. Therefore, prestorage leukocyte reduction is the only effective way to prevent FNHTR with platelet transfusions because the leukocytes are removed before releasing their cytokines.

It has been determined that cytokine accumulation does not occur if a blood product is refrigerated, which explains why both prestorage and poststorage RBC leukoreductions prevent FNHTRs.

WASHED PLATELETS

As with RBCs, the goal of washing platelets is to effectively remove 99% of antibodies, plasma proteins, and electrolytes contained within the component. The process involves washing platelets with normal saline or saline buffered with ACD-A (acid citrate dextrose) or citrate. This process can be achieved via automated or manual technique, leading to approximately 33% platelet loss. Once a platelet component is washed, it must be transfused within 4 hours because it is now an open system with removed anticoagulant-preservative solution at room temperature. This differs from washed RBCs that have a 24-hour shelf life after washing.

The two most common indications for washed platelets are recurrent severe allergic or anaphylactic reactions and IgA-deficiency in patients with IgA antibodies.

IRRADIATED PLATELETS

As with RBCs, the objective of irradiating platelets is to prevent immunocompetent T lymphocytes from proliferating and leading to TA-GVHD in the transfused recipient. The current dose (2500 cGy to the central portion of the unit and 1500 cGy to other portions of the unit) inactivates the T lymphocytes within the product and achieves this goal without significantly altering platelet function during their maximum shelf life.

Indications for irradiated platelets are the same as for irradiated RBCs: hematopoietic stem cell or BMT patients, congenital immunodeficiency syndrome patients, intrauterine transfusions, neonates, HLA-matched platelet transfusions, Hodgkin's disease patients, and chronic lymphocytic leukemia patients treated with purine analogues (e.g., fludarabine).

Patients receiving transfusions from first-degree relatives require irradiation because of the increased risk of TA-GVHD due to HLA similarity of donor and recipient.

INDICATIONS FOR PLATELET TRANSFUSION

Criteria for instituting a platelet transfusion include:

- Platelet count $<10 \times 10^9$/L for prophylaxis in a stable, nonfebrile patient
- Platelet count $<20 \times 10^9$/L for prophylaxis with fever or instability
- Platelet count $<50 \times 10^9$/L in a patient with documented hemorrhage or rapidly decreasing platelet count or planned invasive or surgical procedure
- Diffuse microvascular bleeding in a patient with disseminated intravascular coagulation or following a massive blood loss (>1 blood volume) with a platelet count not yet available
- Bleeding in a patient with platelet dysfunction

It is unacceptable to empirically transfuse platelets for a massively transfused patient not exhibiting a clinical coagulopathy or for extrinsic platelet dysfunction (e.g., renal failure, hyperproteinemia, or von Willebrand's disease). Platelet transfusion is contraindicated in thrombotic thrombocytopenic purpura (TTP), hemolytic-uremic syndrome (HUS), or idiopathic thrombocytopenic purpura (ITP) unless the patient is experiencing life-threatening bleeding or coagulopathy.

PLATELET REFRACTORINESS

Both nonimmune and immune causes lead to poor platelet increment following transfusion. To accurately assess response to platelet transfusion, a post-transfusion platelet count should be obtained 10 to 60 minutes after the transfusion is complete. If the patient does not respond appropriately, platelet refractoriness must be considered.

Platelet refractoriness is defined as failure to achieve an appropriate post-transfusion response on more than one occasion.

A post-transfusion corrected count increment (CCI) can be calculated to more accurately assess refractoriness. The CCI is calculated as follows:

$$CCI = \frac{(post-transfusion\ count - pretransfusion\ count) \times body\ surface\ area}{platelets\ tranfused \times 10^{11}}$$

where platelet counts are in microliters and body surface area is in square meters. A CCI less than 5000 (using a 10- to 60-minute post-transfusion platelet count) on two separate occasions is consistent with platelet refractoriness.

The most common causes for poor platelet increments are non-immune causes, including splenomegaly, bleeding, fever, sepsis, and disseminated intravascular coagulation (DIC). If refractoriness is determined to be nonimmune in etiology, management often consists of increasing the dose or frequency (or both) of transfused platelets. HLA alloimmunization is the primary cause of immune-mediated platelet refractoriness. Other immune-mediated causes for poor platelet increment are anti–platelet-specific antibodies, drug-induced antibodies, and immune or idiopathic thrombocytopenia purpura (ITP). If HLA alloimmunization is the cause, three common treatment options can be employed:

- Give platelets that are platelet crossmatch compatible with recipient plasma
- Provide HLA antigen-negative platelets (for the identified HLA antibodies)
- Give HLA matched (class I: HLA A and HLA B) platelets

Plasma

FROZEN PLASMA

Platelet-poor plasma is obtained by centrifugation and separation of a whole-blood donation or direct collection with apheresis technique. If this plasma is frozen at $-18°C$ within 8 hours of original collection, the product contains adequate levels of all labile (factor V and factor VIII) and nonlabile coagulation factors and is called *fresh frozen plasma* (FFP). If this plasma is frozen at $-18°C$ for more than 8 hours but within 24 hours from original collection, the product contains adequate levels of all nonlabile and decreased levels of labile coagulation factors and is called *plasma frozen within 24 hours*. Both types of plasma units have a volume of approximately 220 mL, and both can be stored for 12 months at $-18°C$.

These products are indicated for the correction of multiple or specific coagulation factor deficiencies or for the empiric treatment of TTP or HUS. The usual starting dose is 5 to 15 mL/kg (2 to 4 units in a 70-kg recipient).

INDICATIONS FOR PLASMA TRANSFUSION

Criteria for implementing a plasma infusion include:

- Treatment or prophylaxis of multiple or specific coagulation factor deficiencies (PT and/or PTT >1.5 times the mean normal value)
- Congenital coagulation factor deficiencies (antithrombin III; factors II, V, VII, IX, X, and XI; plasminogen; antiplasmin)
- Acquired coagulation factor deficiencies related to warfarin (Coumadin) therapy, vitamin K deficiency, liver disease, massive transfusion (>1 blood volume in 24 h), and disseminated intravascular coagulation
- Patients with a suspected coagulation deficiency (PT/PTT pending) who are bleeding, or at risk of bleeding, from an invasive procedure

Unacceptable criteria are empiric use during massive transfusion in which the patient does not exhibit clinical coagulopathy, nutritional supplementation, or volume replacement. There is little evidence to support prophylactic plasma infusion in patients with mild prolongation of the prothrombin time (<1.5 times the mean normal value).

CRYOPRECIPITATE

Cryoprecipitate is a cold insoluble fraction of FFP that precipitates when FFP is thawed at $4°C$. A unit of cryoprecipitate contains approximately 10 mL, which can be stored for 12 months at $-18°C$. Each unit contains approximately 80 to 100 U of factor VIII and 250 mg of fibrinogen, along with factor XIII, von Willebrand's factor, and fibronectin.

The usual starting dose is one unit per 7 to 10 kg, and therefore multiple units must be pooled for a therapeutic dose. Once pooled, cryoprecipitate must be transfused within 4 hours. In a 70-kg man, 14 units would be expected to raise the fibrinogen 100 mg/dL. Cryoprecipitate (2–4 units) may also be applied topically, with an equal volume of bovine thrombin, taking advantage of its adhesive, hemostatic, and sealant properties.

Appropriate indications for cryoprecipitate include:

- A bleeding patient with congenital or acquired hypofibrinogenemia, dysfibrinogenemia, or afibrinogenemia (fibrinogen <150 mg/dL)
- Treatment or prevention of bleeding associated with certain known or suspected clotting factor deficiencies (factor VIII, von Willebrand's, factor XIII, or factor I)
- Treatment of surface oozing and maintenance of tissues in tight apposition to each other or sealing of leaking spaces (fibrin glue)

Rather than cryoprecipitate, factor concentrates are mostly used to treat hemophilia A and type I von Willebrand's disease. Desmopressin acetate (DDAVP) may be used as an alternative treatment for these patients and for patients with certain platelet dysfunctional disorders.

Granulocytes

Using apheresis techniques, granulocytes contain approximately 20 to 30×10^9 granulocytes per collection, 200 to 400 mL of donor plasma, 10 to 30 mL of donor RBCs, and some donor platelets. Like platelets, this product is stored at room temperature but without agitation. Granulocytes have a 24-hour shelf life, but they should be transfused as soon as possible because of rapid decline of function and viability of the leukocytes.

There are several special considerations for this product. Granulocytes must be ABO compatible with the recipient because of significant RBC contamination. This is an Rh-specific product for female patients of childbearing age. CMV-negative donors must be used for CMV-negative recipients because the product cannot be leukoreduced. It is an HLA-matched product for alloimmunized patients. Granulocytes should be irradiated to prevent TA-GVHD.

Granulocyte infusions are indicated for adult neutropenic patients (granulocyte count <500/μL) who have fever for 24 to 48 hours due to bacterial or fungal sepsis that is unresponsive to appropriate antibiotic or antifungal treatment. In infants, granulocyte therapy should be considered in bacterial septicemic patients with a granulocyte count less than 3000/μL. Daily granulocyte transfusion should be continued until infection resolves or the granulocyte count remains greater than 500/μL for 48 hours.

REFERENCES

Bowden RA, Slichter SJ, Sayers M, et al. A comparison of filtered leukocyter-educed and cytomegalovirus (CMV) seronegative blood products for the prevention of transfusion-associated CMV infection after marrow transplant. Blood 1995;86:3598–603.

Brecher ME. Technical Manual, 15th ed. Bethesda, MD: American Association of Blood Banks; 2005.

British Committee for Standards in Haematology, Blood Transfusion Task Force. Guidelines for the use of platelet transfusions. Br J Haematol 2003;122:10–23.

Development Task Force of the College of American Pathologists. Practice parameters for the use of fresh frozen plasma, cryoprecipitate and platelets. JAMA 1994;271:777.

Goodnough LT, Brecher ME, Kanter MH, AuBuchon JP. Transfusion medicine. First of two parts—blood transfusion. N Engl J Med 1999;340:438–47.

Goodnough LT, Brecher ME, Kanter MH, AuBuchon JP. Transfusion medicine. Second of two parts—blood conservation. N Engl J Med 1999;340:525–33.

Menitove JE, McElligott MC, Aster RH. Febrile transfusion reaction: What blood component should be given next? Vox Sang 1978;5:101–6.

Nichols WG, Price TH, Corey L, Boeckh M. Transfusion-transmitted cytomegalovirus infection after receipt of leukoreduced blood products. Blood 2003;101:4195–200.

Strauss R. Neutrophil (granulocyte) transfusions in the new millennium. Transfusion 1998;38:710–2.

The Trial to Reduce Alloimmunization to Platelets Study Group. Leukocyte reduction and ultraviolet B irradiation of platelets to prevent alloimmunization and refractoriness to platelet transfusions. N Engl J Med 1997;337:1861–9.

Wandt H, Frank M, Ehninger G, et al. Safety and cost effectiveness of a 10×10^9/L trigger for prophylactic platelet transfusions compared with the traditional 20×10^9/L trigger: A prospective comparative trial in 105 patients with acute myeloid leukemia. Blood 1998;91:3601–6.

Adverse Effects of Blood Transfusion

Method of

Chelsea A. Sheppard, MD, and Christopher D. Hillyer, MD

Although blood transfusion is a beneficial and not uncommonly lifesaving therapy, it carries inherent risks or adverse effects. These adverse effects are commonly classified either as *transfusion reactions* (Table 1), which occur immediately or shortly following the transfusion event, or as *transfusion-related complications*, which can occur up to many years following transfusion. These latter complications are commonly divided into *infectious* (Table 2) and *noninfectious*

(Table 3) categories. Indeed, 0.5% to 3% of all transfusions result in an adverse event; however, the majority of these are minor reactions with no long-term sequelae.

Herein we describe a large number of adverse events so that the physician can determine if his or her patient has had an adverse effect from a transfusion, assign a diagnosis, and consider if an intervention is needed. For a complete discussion of all of the adverse events related to transfusion, as well as more detailed references, the reader is referred to *Blood Banking and Transfusion Medicine* (see References).

Transfusion Reactions

When a patient experiences an immediate reaction to a transfusion, the most important question to answer is whether hemolysis is occurring. Thus, transfusion medicine specialists usually classify transfusion reactions as either *hemolytic* or *nonhemolytic*.

Hemolytic reactions are caused by recipient antibodies targeted against donor red cell antigens and the resultant response, which attempts to destroy or clear those foreign cells. These antibodies may be naturally occurring (e.g., a recipient with group A blood has antibodies to B-group red cells) or they can occur after exposure to foreign blood from past transfusion, pregnancy, or transplantation. This process is termed *alloimmunization*.

Nonhemolytic reactions occur via a variety of mechanisms usually involving recipient response to donor leukocytes or their byproducts, including inflammatory cytokines.

HEMOLYTIC TRANSFUSION REACTIONS

Acute Hemolytic Transfusion Reaction

Clinical Description

Arguably, the most devastating transfusion reaction is an acute hemolytic reaction caused by the mistransfusion of ABO incompatible blood. *Mistransfusion* is defined as failure to give the right blood product to the right person at the right time and for the right reason. The severity of the reaction is dose dependent; however, infusion of even a small amount of incompatible blood can cause intravascular hemolysis, resulting in a range of signs and symptoms including pain

TABLE 1 Transfusion Reactions

Type	Frequency	Common Signs and Symptoms	Laboratory Diagnosis	Therapy
Hemolytic				
AHTR	Rare	Pain at the infusion site, back, or flanks Fever, chills, rigors Hemoglobinuria or hemoglobinemia Chest pain Circulatory collapse and shock Vasoconstriction resultant end-organ ischemia Activation of the coagulation system, resulting in microangiopathic thrombosis	Schistocytes on peripheral smear Indirect bilirubinemia and jaundice Decreased haptoglobin Elevated LDH and reticulocyte count	Stop the transfusion Maintain IV fluids (1 L NS over 1–2 h) to maintain urine flow >1 mL/kg/h Diuresis with furosemide or mannitol Support cardiovascular and respiratory function with vasopressors Intubate if necessary
Bacterial contamination	Rare	Fever, chills, rigors Hypotension Intravascular hemolysis	Positive blood cultures Similar organism found in product and recipient	Antibiotics Treat shock if appropriate
DHTR	Rare	Intra- or extravascular hemolysis	Same as AHTR, with spherocytes on peripheral smear if hemolysis is predominantly extravascular	Monitor renal function; forced diuresis or dialysis may be required to support renal function if extravascular hemolysis is severe Transfuse with antigen-negative blood if anemia is symptomatic

Continued

TABLE 1 Transfusion Reactions—Cont'd

Type	Frequency	Common Signs and Symptoms	Laboratory Diagnosis	Therapy
Nonhemolytic				
Allergic	Common	Itching, urticaria, generalized flushing or rash, angioedema Wheezing, cough	No abnormal laboratory tests	Diphenhydramine 25–50 mg PO or IV May premedicate for future transfusions if recurrent
Anaphylactic	Rare	Shortness of breath, vasomotor instability, bronchospasm	No abnormal laboratory tests	Epinephrine 1:1000 0.3 mL IM Secure airway
FNHTR	Common	Fever, chills, rigors Absence of hemolysis	No abnormal laboratory tests R/o hemolysis	Acetaminophen 650 mg PO if not contraindicated May premedicate for future transfusions if recurrent
TA-GVHD	Rare	Fever, mucositis, dermatitis, hepatitis, enterocolitis, pancytopenia	Low blood counts, low reticulocyte count, elevated liver enzymes, elevated inflammatory markers	Treatment is usually ineffective High dose steroids, OKT3, cyclosporine A, and antithymocyte globulin may be helpful Irradiate blood for high-risk patients to prevent TA-GVHD
TRALI	Rare	Noncardiogenic pulmonary edema with dyspnea, acute hypoxemia, hypotension, occasionally fever Bilateral infiltrates on CXR Signs of congestive heart failure (increased jugular venous pressure and/or a third heart sound) absent Normal pulmonary capillary wedge pressure	HLA/HNA antibody or antigen cognates between recipient and donor can support diagnosis	Respiratory support High-dose steroids Avoid diuretics in hypotensive patients

Abbreviations: AHTR = acute hemolytic transfusion reaction; CXR = chest x-ray; DHTR = delayed hemolytic transfusion reaction; FNHTR = febrile nonhemolytic transfusion reaction; HLA = human leukocyte antigen; HNA = human neutrophil antigen; LDH = lactate dehydrogenase; NS = normal saline; OKT3 = muromonab CD3; r/o = rule out; TA-GVHD = transfusion-associated graft-versus-host disease; TRALI = transfusion-related acute lung injury.

Adverse Effects of Blood Transfusion

489

TABLE 2 Infectious Complications of Transfusion

Type	Risk of Transfusion Transmitted Infection from Screened Units
Viruses	
CMV	Leukoreduction has made transfusion transmission rare (~1% remaining risk)
EBV	Rare
HAV	Rare
HBV	~1:200,000
HCV*	~1:2 million
HHV	
HIV*	~1:2 million to 4 million
HTLV	<1:3 million
WNV*	Rare
Parasitic Infections	
Babesia spp.	Rare
Plasmodium spp.	1:4 million
Trypanosoma cruzi	Rare
Prions	
CJD, BSE	Rare

*Risk after nucleic acid testing was implemented.
Abbreviations: BSE = bovine spongiform encephalopathy; CJD = Creutzfeldt-Jakob disease; CMV = cytomegalovirus; EBV = Epstein-Barr virus; HAV = hepatitis A virus; HBV = hepatitis B virus; HCV = hepatitis C virus; HHV = human herpesvirus; HTLV = human T-cell lymphotropic virus; WNV = West Nile virus.

at the infusion site, back, or flank; fever; chills or rigors; hemoglobinuria or hemoglobinemia; chest pain; circulatory collapse or shock; vasoconstriction with resultant end organ ischemia; and activation of the coagulation system, resulting in microangiopathic thrombosis.

The annual incidence of ABO-mismatched transfusion according to observed errors in the New York State database and the FDA database of transfusion-associated fatalities has been reported at between 1 in 12,000 and 1 in 19,000 transfused units. The fatality rate ranges from 1 in 800,000 to 1 in 2,000,000 transfused units. However, these numbers do not take into account the large number of near misses, which have been reported to be as common as 1 in 3000 to 4000 units transfused per year.

Diagnosis

The first signs of an acute hemolytic transfusion reaction (AHTR) are usually fever and pain. However, a decrease in blood pressure, tachycardia, and hemoglobinuria may be the only signs in an anesthetized patient.

Laboratory studies can help confirm a diagnosis of intravascular hemolysis. Red cell abnormalities including schistocytes on peripheral smear, increased indirect bilirubin and jaundice, and decreased haptoglobin are signs of increased red cell destruction. Elevated lactate dehydrogenase (LDH) and reticulocyte count indicate increased red cell turnover. It is important to maintain adequate renal function; therefore, it is necessary to monitor blood urea nitrogen (BUN), creatinine, and urine output.

Occasionally, patients with severe intravascular hemolysis can develop disseminated intravascular coagulation (DIC). Serial

TABLE 3 Noninfectious Complications of Transfusion

Type	Frequency	Common Signs and Symptoms	Laboratory Diagnosis	Therapy
Massive Transfusion Reactions				
Coagulopathy	Common in massive transfusion	Hemorrhage usually described as mucosal bleeding or oozing from suture lines	Prolonged PT, PTT Fibrinogen <100 mg/dL Rapidly decreasing platelet count and antithrombin level	Replace clotting factors with FFP In massive transfusion, RBC/FFP ratio should be 1:1–2 If fibrinogen <100 mg/dL transfuse 1 cryoprecipitate pool and recheck fibrinogen Transfuse platelets if count <50,000/L
Citrate toxicity	Rare	Muscle cramping, shortness of breath secondary to bronchospasm, tetanic contractions, distal extremity numbness, tingling sensations, seizures	Decreased ionized calcium Monitor for hypomagnesemia	Calcium gluconate 2 g/250 mL NS Replete magnesium if indicated
Hyperkalemia	Rare	Generalized fatigue, weakness, paresthesias, paralysis, palpitations ECG changes: peaked T waves, shortened OT interval, ST segment depression	Elevated serum potassium Monitor for evidence of metabolic alkalosis Monitor for ECG changes	Replete with oral or IV potassium preparations if indicated
Iron overload	Rare	Iron deposition with end-organ damage in heart, liver, lungs, pituitary, thyroid, adrenals, exocrine pancreas	Elevated iron, ferritin (~10–20 g in patients with SCD is typical), and transferrin saturation	Phlebotomy or iron chelators if indicated
Transfusion-Related Immunomodulation				
Platelet refractoriness (HLA)	Occasional in highly sensitized patients	FNHTR No response or inadequate response to platelet transfusion	Corrected count increment (see text), flow cytomtery, or ELISA screen for anti-HLA antibodies or platelet-specific antibodies	Consider appropriateness of HLA-matched or crossmatched platelets, contact transfusion medicine specialist
Post-transfusion purpura (HPA)	Rare	Severe thrombocytopenia 5–10 d after transfusion Bruising and petechiae Can result in severe hemorrhage	Flow cytomtery or ELISA screen for anti-platelet-specific antibodies Must r/o other causes of thrombocytopenia, including HIT and DIC	Self-limited IVIg Efficacy of antigen-negative platelets is controversial
Other				
Volume overload	Common	Cardiogenic pulmonary edema with dyspnea, acute hypoxemia, hypertension Bilateral infiltrates on CXR Signs of congestive heart failure, increased jugular venous pressure, and/or absent third heart sound Elevated pulmonary capillary wedge pressure	BNP can help distinguish volume overload from TRALI	Diuresis If transfusion is required, slow the rate

Abbreviations: BNP = brain natriuretic peptide; CXR = chest x-ray; DIC = disseminated intravascular coagulation; ECG = electrorcardiogram; ELISA = enzyme-linked immunosorbent assay; FNHTR = febrile nonhemolytic transfusion reaction; FFP = fresh frozen plasma; HIT = heparin-induced thrombocytopenia; HLA = human leukocyte antigen; HPA = human platelet antigen; IVIg = intravenous immunoglobulin; NS = normal saline; PT = prothrombin time; PTT = partial thromboplastin time; RBC = red blood cells; r/o = rule out; SCD = sickle cell disease; TRALI = transfusion-related acute lung injury.

measurements including prothrombin time (PT), activated partial thromboplastin time (aPTT), D-dimer, fibrinogen, antithrombin, and platelet count can be used to evaluate for the presence of an ongoing consumptive process. After the transfusion is stopped, the unit itself and a post-transfusion sample should be immediately sent to the blood bank for further analysis. The blood bank will perform a clerical check for correct patient identification, look for the presence of visible hemolysis in the post-transfusion plasma, and compare direct Coombs' test results from the pre- and post-transfusion samples for evidence of in vivo antibody adsorption on the red cells.

Treatment and Prevention

If an acute hemolytic transfusion reaction is suspected, the transfusion should be stopped immediately. Intravenous fluids should be given to maintain an adequate blood pressure and to aid the kidneys in expelling circulating hemoglobin. Some experts recommend furosemide (Lasix) or mannitol (Osmitrol) to induce diuresis; however, this has not been studied in a randomized fashion. A patient who develops signs of shock should be treated accordingly. Vasopressors and mechanical ventilation may be required in cases of circulatory collapse and respiratory failure.

Most cases of mistransfusion are the result of human error. More than one half of these errors occur from misidentification of the patient at the bedside. Approximately one third of these errors occur in the blood bank as a result of either a clerical misprint or the misidentification of a specimen. Despite strict transfusion procedures and protocols, the use of hospital identification wrist bands, and multiple redundant check systems, mistransfusions still occur at an alarming rate. Therefore, systems including the use of bar codes, barrier technology (Blood-Loc), and radiofrequency identification (RFID) systems are under investigation.

Delayed Hemolytic Transfusion Reaction

Clinical Description

Red blood cell antibodies acquired through exposure to foreign antigen can cause a delayed hemolytic transfusion reaction (DHTR). These patients can develop signs and symptoms of intra- or extravascular hemolysis approximately 2 weeks after transfusion due to the formation of a de novo alloantibody. Alternatively, symptoms appearing 3 to 4 days after transfusion support previous exposure to the antigen and a robust amnestic response on reexposure to antigen-positive blood.

Diagnosis

Patients with a history of a recent transfusion and signs and symptoms of hemolysis should be evaluated for a possible DHTR. Laboratory studies for intra- and extravascular hemolysis are described earlier. However, in delayed hemolytic transfusion reactions, extravascular hemolysis is more common; thus, spherocytes rather than schistocytes may be the predominant abnormal morphologic red cell type on peripheral smear.

Alloantibodies are usually detected during the antibody screen carried in blood banks as a "type and screen." If the screen is positive, the specificity of the antibody is determined. For patients with multiple antibodies, this can significantly lengthen the time it takes for the pretransfusion work-up. If the patient has not recently received a transfusion, antibody titers may be too low to be detected at the time of screening. However, if the patient is rechallenged with the antigen, an amnestic antibody response can cause destruction of the transfused cells. Intravascular and extravascular hemolysis can be severe and life threatening.

Treatment and Prevention

Treatment of intra- and extravascular hemolysis is discussed under acute hemolytic transfusion reactions.

The inherent immunogenicity of the antigen, antigen concentration per erythrocyte, transfused cell dosage, and individual patient factors determine the rate of alloimmunization. Patients with sickle cell disease are at greater risk, and immunosuppressed patients may be at less risk. Highly immunogenic antigens such as Kell, Duffy, and Kidd are generally associated with more severe reactions. These antigens are also commonly implicated in hemolytic disease of the newborn because these antibodies can cross the placenta.

Antibody screening is required before transfusion in any patient who has received a transfusion or been pregnant in the last 30 days; thus, it is important to take a thorough transfusion history. Additionally, hospitalized patients receiving transfusions should be rescreened every 3 days because antibodies that are initially too low in titer to be detected might be identified later.

Bacterial Contamination of Blood Products

Clinical Description

Bacterial contamination at the time of collection usually occurs through one of three mechanisms: asymptomatic donor bacteremia, introduction of skin flora to the unit, or manufacturing processes and manipulation of the unit. Initially, the amount of bacteria present is low; however, during storage the bacteria can proliferate to levels of 10^6/mL or greater. This amount of bacteria transfused over a short time can result in a spectrum of clinical signs and symptoms including bacteremia, fever, chills, hypotension, nausea, vomiting, diarrhea, and oliguria, which can progress to sepsis and ultimately multisystem organ failure and death.

Pathophysiology

The most common bacteria identified in 70% to 80% of contaminated platelets are gram-positive skin flora introduced to the unit during collection; however, 40% to 80% of fatalities are due to endotoxin-producing gram-negative organisms. The severity of the reaction depends on the species of bacteria present, the inoculum, the rate of bacterial propagation, and patient factors including underlying disease, including leukocyte count, the status of the immune system, and use of concomitant antibiotics in the recipient.

Diagnosis

Blood cultures should be obtained both from the recipient (cultures should not be drawn from the same line used for the transfusion) and from the blood product in question. Confirmation requires that the same organism be cultured from both sites. False negatives can occur in patients taking antibiotics. False-positive cultures are common due to improper collection of the sample.

Additional laboratory tests can help evaluate for end-organ damage including tests of renal and liver function. Endotoxin-induced DIC is a common complication; therefore, serial measurements of the PT, APTT, D-dimer, fibrinogen, antithrombin, and platelet count may be useful in evaluating for the presence of an ongoing consumptive process.

Treatment and Prevention

Sepsis caused by transfusion of a bacterially contaminated unit can be fatal. Antibiotics should be given empirically as soon as symptoms appear. The patient can develop septic shock and should be treated accordingly.

Bacterial contamination is the third most common cause of transfusion-associated fatality reported to the FDA. Improved phlebotomy practices (strict arm preparation standards and diversion of the first 10 mL containing the skin plug), donor questioning for recent illnesses or travel to endemic areas, better materials used in product collection and storage, and implementation of platelet culturing have helped reduce the incidence of fatality as a result of bacterial contamination of blood products. Red cell units and plasma, which are stored refrigerated or frozen, are less often implicated in bacteria-related transfusion reactions. However, platelets, which are stored at room temperature in a large volume of plasma and in a bag that allows oxygen diffusion, are most commonly implicated.

Prior to 2004 and the implementation of American Association of Blood Banks (AABB) Standard 5.1.5.1, which charged blood banks with the responsibility of limiting and detecting bacterial contamination, the infectious risk of receiving a contaminated unit was estimated at 1 in 2000 to 1 in 3000 platelet units per year. Risk of death was 1 in 60,000 to 1 in 85,000 units transfused. Since implementation of the AABB standard, many of the nation's blood collection systems have begun culturing platelet units using automated systems, which detect CO_2 generation or O_2 consumption by bacteria for 24 hours prior to hospital distribution. Despite a marked reduction in the number of cases of transfusion-transmitted bacterial infections, rare fatal consequences have been reported.

Pathogen reduction technology aims at eradicating pathogens without harming the blood cells or generating toxic chemical agents. Several methods under investigation include a number of photodynamic processes that use psoralen-based chemicals, pheno-thiazine dyes (methylene blue [urolene blue]), or riboflavin (vitamin B_2) followed by ultraviolet light to inactivate bacteria and viruses by degrading nucleic acids. Other methods include solvent-detergent treatment and treatment with FRALEs (frangible anchor linker effectors). The appeal of pathogen reduction is that it is proactive and may be able to prevent new and emerging infections. Nonetheless, serious regulatory hurdles remain before these methods are approved for use in the United States.

NONHEMOLYTIC TRANSFUSION REACTIONS

Transfusion-Related Acute Lung Injury

Clinical Description

Transfusion-related acute lung injury (TRALI) has now become the most common cause of transfusion-associated death *reported* to the FDA, with an incidence that ranges widely from 1 case per 432 whole blood units transfused to 1 case per 557,000 red blood cell units transfused. Because it was not until 2004 that standardized criteria were widely accepted for defining and diagnosing TRALI, these previous figures might not reflect current incidence, and thus most authorities agree that the true incidence of TRALI is unknown. Nonetheless, it is becoming increasingly clear that platelets and FFP are the most commonly implicated blood products due to the large plasma volume of these products and the likelihood of alloantibodies being passively transferred (see later).

TRALI is a clinical syndrome characterized by noncardiogenic pulmonary edema with dyspnea, acute hypoxemia, hypotension, and occasionally fever. Bilateral infiltrates in a white-out pattern are commonly described on chest x-ray. Signs of congestive heart failure (increased jugular venous pressure and/or a third heart sound) are usually absent. The pulmonary capillary wedge pressure is typically normal. Symptoms usually appear 1 to 6 hours after transfusion and resolve in 96 hours.

Diagnosis

Until recently, accepted criteria allowing standardized diagnosis of TRALI were lacking, thus complicating the ability to make accurate diagnoses and hindering attempts at determining true incidence rates. In April 2004, a consensus conference convened in Toronto, Ontario, and attempted to further adapt and improve previously proposed definitions of TRALI. The consensus panel recommended criteria for *TRALI* and *possible TRALI*.

TRALI was defined as a new occurrence of acute-onset acute lung injury (ALI) with hypoxemia and bilateral infiltrates on chest x-ray, but no evidence of left atrial hypertension. The ALI cannot have been preexisting, but it must emerge during or within 6 hours of the end the transfusion and have no temporal relation to an alternative ALI risk factor. *Possible TRALI* included cases in which there was a temporal association with an alternative ALI risk factor.

These proposed definitions continue to suffer the limitations inherent in the American-European Consensus Conference definition of ALI (including the subjectivity of certain findings, including chest x-ray and volume status and the influence of PEEP on measurements of the PaO_2/FiO_2 ratio). Brain natriuretic protein (BNP) might help to distinguish cardiogenic from noncardiogenic pulmonary edema.

Pathophysiology

The events and mechanisms that cause TRALI are incompletely understood. They have been described as antibody-mediated and non–antibody-mediated. Antibody-mediated mechanisms implicate alloantibodies directed toward human leukocyte antigen (HLA) or human neutrophil antigen (HNA) on leukocytes or lung tissue, which lead to granulocyte activation and pulmonary injury. In approximately 90% of TRALI cases where antibodies are identified, the antibodies are of donor origin and react with recipient leukocyte epitopes. Multiparous women and recipients of previous transfusions are more likely to be alloimmunized. Many investigators have suggested that a number of hits may be required to cause a full-blown case of TRALI.

The two-hit model of TRALI may be antibody- or non–antibody-mediated. In this model, the first hit is usually described as an underlying illness that primes recipient pulmonary endothelial cells and leukocytes. *Priming* refers to the development of a heightened stage of (cellular) activation. The second hit is delivered by the transfusion, which contains factors (either antibodies or biological response modifiers [BRMs], such as cytokines or certain lipids) capable of inducing complete activation of the presequestered primed neutrophils in the recipient's lungs. This results in the release of cytotoxic compounds

in the pulmonary vasculature, leading to endothelial damage, capillary leak, and noncardiogenic pulmonary edema, namely, TRALI.

Treatment and Prevention

Treatment is primarily respiratory support until the injury resolves (usually in 24–96 hours); however, high-dose intravenous steroids may be beneficial. Approximately 20% of patients with TRALI require 1 week or more to fully recover. Death is estimated to occur in 6% to 23% of cases; survivors have no permanent sequelae.

Without a simple laboratory test to prospectively eliminate high-risk blood products, recommended strategies to prevent TRALI are currently based on deferral of donors implicated in TRALI cases. The United Kingdom has preemptively deferred all women from donating plasma. In the United States, the use of male-only plasma is under consideration, as is the testing of all plasma and platelet units for anti-HLA or anti-HNA antibodies.

Febrile Nonhemolytic Transfusion Reaction

Clinical Description

Febrile nonhemolytic transfusion reaction (FNHTR) is defined as an increase in the recipient's temperature of at least 1°C or 2°F during transfusion in the absence of another cause of fever. Some patients develop chills or rigors. FNHTRs are very common, occurring in 0.1% to 0.5% of all leukodepleted transfusions occurring per year in the United States. The incidence is significantly higher in nonleukoreduced blood products. Additionally, transfusion reactions such as FNHTRs and allergic reactions are believed to be underreported in patients with frequent febrile episodes due to underlying diseases such as cancer and sepsis. Other causes for transfusion-associated fever, including hemolysis or bacterial contamination, must be excluded before a diagnosis of FNHTR can be made.

Pathophysiology

FNHTRS are attributed to white blood cells (WBCs) in blood products that synthesize and release proinflammatory cytokines during storage. Preformed recipient antibodies that target donor WBCs can also lead to cytokine release after transfusion.

Treatment and Prevention

Antipyretics are often used to treat these reactions. Patients prone to FNHTRs can require premedication with antipyretics. Many transfusion medicine services have implemented universal leukoreduction protocols to prevent FNHTRs.

Allergic Reactions

Clinical Description

Allergic transfusion reactions are very common. Allergic reactions are variably severe and result in a spectrum of clinical signs and symptoms. Uncomplicated or simple reactions manifest as itching, urticaria, generalized flushing or rash, or local swelling, also known as *angioedema*. However, recipients can also develop anaphylactoid reactions in which wheezing, cough, shortness of breath, vasomotor instability, and bronchospasm are typically observed. IgA-deficient patients with circulating anti-IgA antibodies can develop life-threatening anaphylaxis and cardiovascular collapse requiring emergent therapy. Most reactions are afebrile. The incidence of uncomplicated allergic reactions is 1% to 3%; however, anaphylactic reactions are very rare (0.002%–0.005% of all transfusions).

Pathophysiology

Simple allergic reactions occur when donor plasma proteins are targeted by preformed IgE antibodies on recipient mast cells, leading to histamine release. More severe reactions have been attributed to antibodies against IgA, C4 determinants, or other nonbiological elements (ethylene oxide used for sterilization of tubing sets). The presence of anti-IgA antibodies in IgA-deficient patients cannot predict the occurrence of allergic reactions.

Treatment and Prevention

Most simple allergic reactions can be treated with antihistamines or anticholinergic medications (e.g., diphenhydramine). Patients with more severe reactions can require IV steroids or epinephrine. Patients with respiratory failure require supportive therapy. In patients with recurrent allergic reactions, prophylactic antihistamine therapy administered 30 minutes before transfusion may be helpful. In patients with simple allergic reactions involving only the skin, the transfusion may be restarted 15 to 30 minutes after the administration of antihistamines; however, transfusions should never be restarted in patients with more severe reactions.

Transfusion-Associated Graft-Versus-Host Disease

Clinical Description

Transfusion-associated graft-versus-host disease (TA-GVHD) is a rare but uniformly fatal complication of blood transfusions in severely immunosuppressed patients in which donor lymphocytes escape immune clearance in the recipient and engraft. Following clonal expansion, these cells cause immune destruction of host tissues including the skin, gastrointestinal (GI) tract, liver, and bone marrow. These patients develop fever, mucositis, dermatitis (starting as a blistering rash on the palms, soles, and face, which then can generalize), hepatitis, enterocolitis with large volumes of secretory diarrhea, and pancytopenia, 1 to 2 weeks after transfusion. Infections are the most common cause of death, which generally occurs within 3 to 4 weeks of the transfusion.

The degree of immunosuppression and the dose of T lymphocytes are factors in determining an individual patient's risk of developing TA-GVHD. Patients with hematologic malignancy, patients with congenital immunodeficiency, premature infants weighing less than 1200 g, bone marrow transplant recipients, and patients receiving fludarabine (Fludara) (see Box 1 for a complete list) are susceptible. Patients with HIV, healthy newborns, and patients who are neutropenic due to sepsis are generally considered to be at low risk. There is a minimally increased risk associated with solid tumor transplants (especially heart and liver) or solid tumor malignancies. There have been reports of TA-GVHD associated with neuroblastomas, rhabdomyosarcomas, bladder tumors, and small cell lung cancer. It is possible that more immunosuppressive and myeloablative chemotherapy protocols are responsible for these cases.

The degree of HLA similarity between the donor and recipient is also an important determinant of a patient's risk of developing TA-GVHD. These patients may be immunocompetent heterozygotes of an HLA haplotype for which the donor is homozygous. Therefore, patients receiving transfusions from first-degree relatives or populations in which there is a great deal of HLA homology (including some Asian populations) might also require irradiated blood products.

Treatment and Prevention

The mortality rate of TA-GVHD approximates 100%. Currently, there is no effective treatment; however, high-dose steroids, muromonab-CD3 (OKT-3), cyclosporine A (Neoral, Sandimmune) and antithy-mocyte globulin (Atgam, Thymoglobin) have been used with few successes.

Prevention of TA-GVHD via irradiation of blood products in at-risk populations is absolutely required. A minimum dose of 25 Gy delivered to the midline of the container (with a minimum of 15 Gy to the distal parts of the bag) cross-links the DNA of T cells, thereby preventing replication and potential engraftment and expansion.

Transfusion-Related Complications

INFECTIOUS COMPLICATIONS

Viral Transmission

Clinical Description

A large number of viruses, including HIV-1 and HIV-2; hepatitis A, B, and C (HAV, HBV, HCV); human T-lymphotrophic viruses (HTLV) 1 and 2; cytomegalovirus (CMV); and West Nile virus can be transmitted via transfusion. These viruses, with the exception of CMV, are acquired from cellular and noncellular blood and blood products including plasma-derived clotting factors, intravenous immunoglobulin (IVIg), and anti-D immunoglobulin. CMV remains latent in monocytes and is essentially therefore transmitted only in cellular products. Other viruses that are potentially transmitted via transfusion are HAV, transfusion-transmitted virus (TTV), Epstein-Barr virus (EBV), human herpesvirus 8 (HHV 8), and parvovirus B19.

Hepatitis

Hepatitis viruses (especially B and C) are readily transfusion transmissible. About 70% of patients infected with HCV develop chronic infections resulting in chronic active hepatitis, cirrhosis, or hepatocellular carcinoma (HCC). A smaller but significant fraction of patients infected with HBV develop chronic disease proceeding to cirrhosis. Hepatitis viruses A and E are rarely transmitted through blood transfusion. Hepatitis G, TTV, and SEN viruses emerged as candidates for non–A to E type post-transfusion hepatitis, but no clear association has been demonstrated.

Human Immunodeficiency Virus

The annual risk of transfusion-transmitted HIV with the addition of nucleic acid testing is reported to be less than 1 in 2,000,000 units in the United States (1:4,000,000 in Canada). However, despite the implementation of this very sensitive testing, cases of transfusion-transmitted HIV have been reported. The average survival after diagnosis for adults and children with transfusion-transmitted HIV is approximately 5.6 months and 13.7 months, respectively.

West Nile Virus and Other Flaviviruses

In 2002, there was an emergence of West Nile virus in the United States, and several cases of transfusion-transmitted disease were identified. Infected elderly and immunocompromised patients developed a severe flulike illness rarely resulting in death. Other flaviviruses including dengue are transfusion transmissible and could threaten the blood supply if an epidemic were to emerge in the United States.

BOX 1	Risk Factors for the Development of TA-GVHD

Significantly Increased Risk
- Bone marrow transplantation
  - Allogeneic and autologous
  - HLA-matched platelet transfusions
  - Hodgkin's disease
  - Intrauterine transfusions
  - Patients treated with purine analogue drugs
  - Transfusions from blood relatives
- Congenital immunodeficiency syndromes

Minimally Increased Risk
- Acute leukemia
- Exchange transfusions
- Non-Hodgkin's lymphoma
- Preterm infants (<1200 g)
- Solid organ transplant recipients
- Solid tumors treated with intensive chemotherapy or radiotherapy

Perceived but No Reported Increased Risk
- Healthy newborns
- Patients with AIDS

Abbreviations: HLA = human leukocyte antigen; TA-GVHD = transfusion-associated graft-versus-host disease. Modified from Schroeder ML: Transfusion-associated graft-versus-host disease. Br J Haematol 2002;117:275–287.

Parvovirus B19

Parvovirus B19 has been transmitted through plasma-derived products including clotting factors. Immunocompromised patients can develop erythema infectiosum, arthralgias, and aplastic crises with chronic anemia after infection with parvovirus B19.

Cytomegalovirus

Transfusion transmission of CMV to immunocompetent patients usually causes an asymptomatic infection or rarely an infectious mononucleosis. However, in seronegative immunocompromised patients, transfusion transmission can lead to lethal CMV disease. Seronegative immunocompromised patients include premature low-birth-weight infants (<1500 g) born to seronegative mothers and seronegative recipients of autologous or seronegative allogeneic bone marrow or peripheral blood stem cell transplantation.

Following primary infection, CMV remains latent and can reactivate, with subsequent production of progeny virus in macrophages. Transfusion-transmitted CMV can be mitigated through the transfusion of leukoreduced or seronegative blood. The rate of infectivity with either leukoreduced or seronegative blood is approximately the same (1%). Box 2 lists the indications for which many hospital blood banks dispense CMV seronegative blood or leukoreduced blood.

Parasitic and Emerging Infections

Clinical Description

Trypanosoma cruzi, Plasmodium spp., and *Babesia* spp. can be transmitted by blood transfusion. *T. cruzi* can cause fatal cardiac and GI disease (Chagas' disease). Malaria, the disease caused by *Plasmodium*, can cause fatal intravascular hemolysis and DIC. Human babesiosis generally causes a mild flulike syndrome, but it can be lethal in the elderly and in immunocompromised patients. At the time of this writing, no agent is tested for in the United States, but it appears likely that tests for *T. cruzi* will commence by early 2007.

TRYPANOSOMA CRUZI

There have been fewer than 10 cases of transfusion-transmitted *T. cruzi* reported in the United States and Canada since 1990. Many of these patients were immunocompromised as a result of hematologic malignancy, AIDS, or bone marrow transplantation. Some of these recipients received platelets only, others received multiple blood products. A majority of the patients developed Chagas' disease. At least one case was fatal. Others did respond to nitrofurtimox[2] (Nifurtimox), interferon-γ[1] (Actimmune), and benznidazole,[1] followed by itraconazole[1] (Sporanox) and fluconazole[1] (Diflucan). In endemic areas, transfusion transmission of Chagas' disease is more common. No screening is currently done for these parasites in blood donors. In the United States, 1 in 25,000 donors are estimated to be seropositive, and as many as one half of these donors are actively parasitemic.

---

[1]Not FDA approved for this indication.
[2]Not available in the United States.

BOX 2   Indications for CMV Seronegative or Leukoreduced Blood

- Intrauterine transfusions
- Premature low-birth-weight infants (<1500 g) born to SN mothers
- SN recipients of autologous bone marrow or peripheral blood stem cell transplantation
- SN recipients of seronegative allogeneic bone marrow or peripheral blood stem cell transplantation
- SN recipients of solid organ transplants from SN donors

Abbreviations: CMV = cytomegalovirus; SN = seronegative.

PLASMODIUM SPECIES AND BABESIA SPECIES

Annually, approximately two cases of transfusion-transmitted *Plasmodium* infections are reported in the United States. Donors who have traveled to malaria-endemic countries are deferred from donation for a period of 1 year. Red cell exchange may be helpful in patients with high parasitemia loads and intravascular hemolysis; however, this is controversial.

There have been more than 50 cases of transfusion-transmitted *Babesia* infections in the world. Currently, there are no licensed tests for screening the blood supply. Human babesiosis is treated with antibiotics.

PRIONS

The agent of variant Creutzfeldt-Jakob disease (vCJD), a novel human prion disease that results in a rare and fatal human neurodegenerative condition, can be transmitted via blood transfusion. Although this agent has no nucleic acids, the transmission results in the conversion of normal prion protein to the abnormal β-sheet amyloid responsible for the clinical disease.

Since 2003, it has been established that prion infection could be transmitted via blood transfusion in animals. Additionally, in 2003 the first case of probable transfusion-transmitted vCJD was reported. The recipient received a transfusion in 1996 from a donor now known to have been incubating vCJD. The recipient died in 1996 from complications of vCJD.

In 2006, the National CJD Surveillance Unit (NCJDSU) and the UK Blood Services (UKBS) released the Transfusion Medicine Epidemiology Review (TMER), a look-back investigation that confirmed three separate incidents of probable transfusion transmission of vCJD infection. Two of these patients died less than 7 years after infection. At this time, sporadic CJD and familial CJD have still not been shown conclusively to be transfusion transmitted.

To date there is no known treatment for transmissible spongiform encephalopathy. The AABB Standard 5.4.1A Requirements for Allogeneic Donor Qualification states that donors with a risk of vCJD as defined by the FDA Guidance for Industry (January 2002) should be indefinitely deferred from giving blood. Currently those donors include anyone who has traveled to or resided in the United Kingdom for a cumulative period of 3 or more months between 1980 and the end of 1996, those with a history of 5 or more years of cumulative residence or travel in France since 1980, and current and former U.S. military personnel, civilian military personnel, and their dependents who were stationed at European bases for 6 months or more between 1980 and 1996.

NONINFECTIOUS COMPLICATIONS

Transfusion-Related Immunomodulation

Clinical Description

Transfusion-related immunomodulation (TRIM) describes the immunosuppression that occurs after transfusion. TRIM was first recognized in the 1960s and 1970s in renal allograft recipients who had less rejection and improved graft survival after receiving blood transfusions from their donors. Since then, TRIM has been implicated in the development of postoperative infections, the recurrence of resected malignancies (especially colorectal cancer), spontaneous abortions, and inflammatory bowel disease. TRIM has been suggested to cause reactivation of latent viruses such as CMV.

Pathophysiology

Most authorities agree that TRIM exists, although the mechanisms and magnitude are unclear. However, it is believed that donor WBCs, BRMs, and soluble HLA antigens that have accumulated during storage exert an effect on cell-mediated immunity. TRIM appears to be dose dependent, and thus conservative transfusion triggers might decrease the incidence.

Treatment and Prevention

There is no known treatment for TRIM. Leukoreduction and washing might reduce the incidence of TRIM.

Alloimmunization

Alloimmunization is the development of an antibody to a foreign donor antigen after exposure through blood transfusion, pregnancy, or transplantation. These antibodies, if directed against RBC antigens, can cause DHTRs and AHTRs. Anti-HLA antibodies can cause FNHTRs and platelet refractoriness. These patients may be difficult to match for bone marrow or solid organ transplants. Thrombocytopenia can result in patients who develop platelet-specific antigens either in utero (neonatal alloimmune thrombocytopenia) or after transfusion (post-transfusion purpura).

Refractoriness to Platelet Transfusions

Patients who become refractory to platelet transfusion can do so by several different mechanisms including immune-mediated and non-immune-mediated mechanisms. Immune-mediated refractoriness occurs in highly sensitized patients with anti-HLA or anti–platelet-specific antibodies to donor-specific antigens. Alternatively, patients with sepsis, DIC, fever, splenomegaly, or portal hypertension and persons taking certain drugs can also appear refractory to platelet transfusion due to the sequestration or accelerated clearance of the transfused platelets.

Diagnosis

The expected corrected count index (CCI) can help distinguish between immune-mediated and non–immune-mediated platelet refractoriness. The CCI is calculated 15 minutes to 1 hour after transfusion using the following equation:

$$CCI = \frac{(Post - transfusion\ platelet\ count - Pretransfusion\ platelet\ count) \times Body\ surface\ area}{Number\ of\ platelets\ tranfused \times 10^{11}}$$

A CCI less than 5000 after two sequential platelet transfusions suggests immune-mediated platelet refractoriness. These patients should be screened for anti-HLA and anti–platelet-specific antibodies if other causes of non–immune-mediated refractoriness have been excluded.

Pathophysiology

HLA antibodies are not routinely tested for in most clinical laboratories and blood banks. Additionally, because platelets are not crossmatched prior to transfusion, the only clue to a significant HLA antibody may be FNHTR or the lack of response to a platelet transfusion. Patients who develop multiple HLA antibodies can become refractory to platelet transfusion. Rarely, patients develop platelet-specific antibodies, causing platelet refractoriness.

Treatment and Prevention

Treatment depends on the etiology of platelet refractoriness. Patients with non–immune-mediated refractoriness (including those with splenic sequestration, sepsis, or DIC) require treatment of the underlying disease. If an immune-mediated mechanism is more likely, HLA-matched or crossmatched platelets can be supplied on request. Leukoreduction can potentially reduce HLA-alloimmunization.

Post-transfusion Purpura

Post-transfusion purpura (PTP) is a rare disorder caused by alloantibodies to platelet-specific glycoprotein, most commonly human platelet antigen (HPA)-1a, resulting in destruction of both transfused platelets and the patient's own platelets, leading to severe thrombocytopenia and risk of life-threatening hemorrhage. Thrombocytopenia can last 1 to 2 weeks after transfusion. IVIg is the first-line treatment. The use of washed antigen-negative platelets is controversial.

Volume Overload

Clinical Description

The development of cardiogenic pulmonary edema and other signs of congestive heart failure after transfusion suggest volume overload. The annual reported incidence in the United States of volume overload secondary to transfusion is greatly variable, anywhere from 1 in 100 to 1 in 15,000 units, and largely depends on patient population. The elderly and newborn, as well as patients with cardiac disease, renal insufficiency, and anemia with expanded plasma volumes, are at greater risk for developing volume overload, especially with massive transfusions.

Diagnosis

Diagnosis depends on establishing a cardiac etiology for the resulting dyspnea and pulmonary edema. Elevated central venous pressures or pulmonary wedge pressures, chest x-ray consistent with pulmonary edema, and response to diuretics are used to confirm the suspected diagnosis. It is important to rule out TRALI and other etiologies of acute respiratory distress syndrome (ARDS). BNP may be a useful adjuvant marker in establishing a diagnosis of volume overload secondary to transfusion.

Treatment and Prevention

Some patients respond simply to slowing the rate of the transfusion. Others require diuretics and supportive therapy.

Massive Transfusion Coagulopathy

Clinical Description

Massive transfusion is usually defined as transfusion of 10 or more units of RBCs in less than 24 hours. Massive transfusion usually occurs in the setting of trauma and can be complicated by coagulopathy secondary to dilution of clotting factors and platelets, hypothermia, and hypofibrinogenemia. Patients often receive crystalloid fluids and numerous uncrossmatched group O packed red cells in transit to the hospital or in the emergency department to correct hypovolemia before receiving plasma (which requires at least 30 minutes' thawing time) or platelets. This results in dilution of platelets, clotting proteins, and fibrinogen. Additionally, as the patient's blood pressure is normalized, bleeding becomes brisker resulting in further losses of platelets and clotting factors.

Treatment and Prevention

Ideally, patients with massive bleeding are transfused with whole blood, thereby minimizing the complications of dilution. Additionally, current guidelines are based on whole-blood transfusion and wash-out equations, simple mathematical models that calculate exponential decay of blood components during bleeding, assuming that the blood volume of the patient is stable and the replacement rates are constant and equal. Blood volumes and bleeding rates are usually quite variable, and replacement tends to lag behind blood loss; therefore, these guidelines and equations tend to underestimate needs. Computer modeling has demonstrated that patients with penetrating traumas have generally lost 2500 mL (or one half the average blood volume) by the time they arrive in the emergency department, 3200 mL (or two thirds the average blood volume) by the start of surgery, and 11,000 mL (or more than two blood volumes) at the end of surgery. PT will be prolonged (>1.5 times normal) after a loss of less than one blood volume. Fibrinogen is next, dropping below 0.8 g/L, in a little over one blood volume. Platelets stay above $50,000 \times 10^9/L$ until after losses of more than two blood volumes.

Various massive transfusion protocols have been reviewed extensively in the literature. Early plasma replacement at higher plasma-to-red cells ratios ($\sim$1:1) is gaining popularity in this clinical setting despite the fear that some patients may be overtransfused. However, there are few studies comparing conservative with liberal plasma and platelet transfusion with regard to outcome.

Hypothermia due to massive transfusion of refrigerated and recently thawed products contributes to the coagulopathy associated with massive transfusion. For this reason, many products are transfused through blood warmers. The use of cryoprecipitate for fibrinogen replacement is often necessary and more efficient than use of plasma.

OTHER ADVERSE EVENTS

Less frequent adverse events of transfusion include hypocalcemia due to large infusions of citrate anticoagulant, hyperkalemia due to RBC leakage during storage, mechanical hemolysis, and iron overload. These events are rare and typically affect infants receiving large amounts of old blood or patients receiving chronic transfusions; thus they are outside of the scope of this article. However, it is important to be aware of their existence and to monitor patients accordingly for signs of their development.

REFERENCES

Allain JP, Bianco C, Blajchman MA, et al. Protecting the blood supply from emerging pathogens: The role of pathogen inactivation. Transfus Med Rev 2005;19(2):110–26.

Blumberg N. Deleterious clinical effects of transfusion immunomodulation proven beyond a reasonable doubt. Transfusion 2005;45(Suppl.):33S–39S.

Blumberg N, Heal JM, Gettings KEJ. WBC reduction of RBC transfusions is associated with decreased incidence of RBC alloimmunization. Transfusion 2003;43:945–52.

Dodd RY, Notari IV, Stramer SL. Current prevalence and incidence of infectious disease markers and estimated window-period risk in the American Red Cross blood donor population. Transfusion 2002;42(8):975–9.

Goldman M, Webert KE, Arnold DM, et al. TRALI Consensus Panel: Proceedings of a consensus conference: Towards an understanding of TRALI. Transfus Med Rev 2005;19(1):2–31.

Hillyer CD, Silberstein LE, Ness PM, et al, editors. Blood Banking and Transfusion Medicine. 2nd ed. Philadelphia: Churchill Livingstone; 2007.

Hirschberg A, Dugas M, Banez E, et al. Minimizing dilutional coagulopathy in exsanguinating hemorrhage: A computer simulation. J Trauma 2003;54:454–63.

Kleinman S, Caulfield T, Chan P, et al. Toward an understanding of transfusion-related acute lung injury: Statement of a consensus panel. Transfusion 2004;44(12):1774–89.

Lee D. Perception of blood transfusion risk. Transfus Med Rev 2006;20(2):141–8.

Linden JV, Wagner K, Voytovich AE, Sheehan J. Transfusion errors in New York State: An analysis of 10 years' experience. Transfusion 2000;40:1207–13.

Luban NC. Transfusion safety: Where are we today? Ann N Y Acad Sci 2005;1054:325–41.

Schroeder ML. Transfusion-associated graft-versus-host disease. Br J Haematol 2002;117:275–87.

Sheppard CA, Roback JD, Hillyer CD. Transfusion-transmitted cytomegalovirus infection: Consideration toward an optimal plan for its mitigation. Blood Ther Med 2005;5(1):6–14.

Zhou L, Giacherio D, Cooling L, Davenport RD. Use of B-natriuretic peptide as a diagnostic marker in the differential diagnosis of transfusion-associated circulatory overload. Transfusion 2005;45:1056–63.

Zou S, Dodd RY, Stramer SL, Strong DM, for the Tissue Safety Group. Probability of Viremia with HBV, HCV, HIV and HTLV among tissue donors in the United States. N Engl J Med 2004;351(8):751–9.

Myelodysplastic Syndromes

Method of
Minoo Battiwalla, MD, and Peiman Hematti, MD

The myelodysplastic syndromes (MDS) are a group of heterogeneous clonal hematopoietic stem cell disorders that are characterized by ineffective hematopoiesis in the bone marrow resulting in low blood counts (cytopenias) and a variable tendency to transform to acute myeloid leukemia.[1] Historically, this group of disorders included the so-called refractory anemias and the preleukemias.

---

[1]Not FDA approved for this indication.

Epidemiology

MDS is typically a disease of older adults; the median age at diagnosis being 65 to 70 years. Incidence is estimated to range between 1 and 10 per 100,000, and in the elderly the rate is several-fold higher. "Anemia of the elderly" should always be considered to have an underlying cause, including unrecognized MDS.

Clinical Manifestations

Patients present with symptoms resulting from cytopenias, usually anemia (80% of cases). Lymphadenopathy and splenomegaly are not associated with MDS. The clinical course is quite variable. Some patients are asymptomatic, and some have mild anemia progressing to transfusion dependence over many years; others exhibit an aggressive course, with multilineage involvement and rapid evolution to acute leukemia.

Diagnostic Evaluation

Examination of peripheral blood and bone marrow (aspiration and biopsy for morphology, flow cytometry, and cytogenetics), often supplemented by specific tests, is needed for diagnosis of MDS and exclusion of other conditions. Minimum diagnostic criteria for MDS require unexplained persistent cytopenia and either evidence of clonality (e.g., a cytogenetic abnormality) or unambiguous dysplastic marrow morphology (e.g., excess blasts, or significant dysplasia in the megakaryocytic lineage).

Prognosis

Life expectancy is significantly shortened, even in patients with low-risk disease; death due to MDS occurs from the complications of cytopenias or progression to AML. Accurate classification and prognosis for this highly heterogeneous disorder are necessary to individualize therapy.

Validated classifications include the French-American-British (FAB), which was expanded in 1982 and is based on morphology (blast count); the WHO classification, and the International Prognostic Scoring System (IPSS). The IPSS is the practical scheme (Table 1), derived from analyses of outcomes in large series of patients treated with supportive care alone, that combines information from cytogenetics, cytopenias, and blast count to generate a prognostic score. These values separate out median survival times for patients with low risk (5.7 years), intermediate-1 risk (3.5 years), intermediate-2 risk (1.2 years), and high-risk (0.4 years) MDS.

Specific subtypes of MDS are associated with well-defined clinical features and prognoses.

5q-SYNDROME

The 5q-syndrome, involving deletion of 5q, most commonly between bands q13 and q33, usually manifests as macrocytic anemia, with or without mild neutropenia and either normal or elevated platelet counts. This syndrome, in contrast to other types of MDS, is most commonly seen in women and carries a relatively good prognosis. Haploinsufficiency of the ribosomal protein gene *RPS14* may account

CURRENT DIAGNOSIS

- Unexplained sustained cytopenia or cytopenias
- Bone marrow dysplastic features
- Evidence of clonality may or may not be present

TABLE 1 International Prognostic Scoring System

Prognostic Variable	Score Value				
	0	0.5	1.0	1.5	2.0
Marrow blasts (%)	<5	5–10	—	11–20	21–30
Karyotype*	Good	Intermediate	Poor		
Cytopenias†	0/1	2/3			

*Karyotypes: Good = normal, −Y, del(5q), del(20q); Intermediate = other karyotypic abnormalities; Poor = complex (≥3 abnormalities) or chromosome 7 abnormalities.
†Cytopenias: Hemoglobin <10 g/dL; absolute neutrophil count <1800 cells/µL; platelets <100,000/µL.

for the phenotype of the 5q syndrome. Complete cytogenetic responses and durable transfusion independence may be seen with lenalidomide (Revlimid), a thalidomide analogue, in patients with del(5q) with or without additional cytogenetic abnormalities.

HYPOCELLULAR MYELODYSPLASTIC SYNDROME

Hypocellular MDS, although not categorized in any schema, clinically resembles aplastic anemia, and patients may respond more favorably to immunosuppression with antithymocyte globulin (ATG).

THERAPY-RELATED MYELODYSPLASTIC SYNDROME

Therapy-related (or secondary) MDS is a vicious subtype, constituting about 15% of cases in most series. This subtype has the highest rate of progression to acute leukemia (75%); it is almost always difficult to treat and rapidly fatal. Almost all patients have recurrent chromosomal abnormalities: deletions in chromosomes 5 and/or 7 occur at a mean interval of 4 to 5 years after exposure to alkylating agents, and 11q23 abnormalities follow in a shorter time period after administration of topoisomerase II inhibitors.

CHRONIC MYELOMONOCYTIC LEUKEMIA

Chronic myelomonocytic leukemia (CMML), although often associated with a dysplastic marrow, is biologically distinct and is now classified as a myeloproliferative disease by the WHO.

Treatment

Strategies combine supportive care, efforts to improve bone marrow function, suppression of the dysplastic clone, and curative attempts with allogeneic blood or marrow transplantation. A judicious approach individualizes therapy, taking into consideration performance, comorbidities, recognition of subtypes that respond favorably to a specific therapy, risk from cytopenias, and the risk of leukemic evolution. Updated guidelines from the National Cancer Center Network are presented in a simplified version in Table 2.

SUPPORTIVE CARE

Supportive care in MDS is influenced by the irreversible nature of the underlying disease and recognition that cytopenias are the single most important contributor to morbidity and mortality. Although it has been the mainstay of therapy for several decades, there are emerging data that conventional supportive care alone may not be the best option and that newer therapies may affect the natural history of MDS.

Even moderate degrees of anemia may not be well tolerated by the elderly, especially in the presence of cardiopulmonary disease, and maintenance of higher hemoglobin levels (>9 g/dL) can improve the quality of life without altering transfusion frequency. Iron chelation for transfusional iron overload is necessary for patients who are expected to have a long duration of transfusion dependence, and it is typically recommended to keep ferritin level lower than 1000 µg/L. The oral iron chelator deferasirox (Exjade) has been a useful advance

TABLE 2 Goal-Based Treatment of Myelodysplastic Syndromes

	Low to Intermediate-1 Risk	Intermediate-2 to High Risk
Clinical problem	Low blood counts	Early mortality
Median survival with supportive care	5.7 and 3.6 y	1.2 and 0.4 y
Relevant endpoints	Hematologic improvement Quality of life	Survival Complete responses Cytogenetic responses
Therapeutic options	Growth factors Lenalidomide (Revlimid) ATG (Thymoglobulin)[1] Demethylating agents	Bone marrow transplantation (if eligible) Demethylating agents

[1]Not FDA approved for this indication.

over subcutaneous infusions of deferoxamine (Desferal). Leukodepletion of blood products and single-donor platelet transfusions reduce the risk of eventual alloimmunization to platelets. If a prophylactic platelet transfusion regimen is adopted, a threshold of 10,000/µL is usually considered adequate. Aminocaproic acid (Amicar)[1] can be a useful adjunct in patients whose disease is refractory to platelet transfusions.

Neutrophils may be dysfunctional in MDS, lowering the threshold for instituting neutropenic precautions. Infections in the setting of neutropenia must be treated aggressively, bearing in mind the combined adverse effects of neutropenia and therapy.

Growth factors are typically used at the lowest doses that maintain a response. Combinations of erythropoietin (Procrit)[1] and granulocyte colony-stimulating factor (Neupogen)[1] are synergistic, even when they fail individually, with hematologic improvements in 40% of patients with low-grade MDS. Helpful algorithms suggest that patients with low erythropoietin serum levels and shorter duration of transfusion dependence may be most responsive. However, growth factors do not appear to enhance survival or progression to leukemia, and they are best considered a part of supportive care.

SPECIFIC THERAPIES

Allogeneic hematopoietic stem cell transplant, which replaces the recipient marrow cells with a suitably human leukocyte antigen (HLA)-matched donor, remains the only curative therapy. Every effort must be made to offer this treatment to eligible patients with a matched donor. In general, patients with IPSS risk of intermediate-2 to high would benefit from allogeneic transplantation as soon as a donor is identified, whereas those with an IPSS risk of low or intermediate-1 would benefit from waiting until progression occurs. Reduced-intensity regimens now offer a transplantation option to carefully selected patients who may not tolerate traditional transplantation due to comorbidity or older age.

Lenalidomide has led to hematologic and cytogenetic responses, particularly in patients with low to intermediate-1 risk and del(5q). Durable red cell transfusion independence was seen in 67% of patients with del(5q) and in 26% of those with non-del(5q) MDS. The precise mechanism of action of this immunomodulatory drug in MDS has not been defined.

Immunosuppressive therapy with antithymocyte globulin (ATG, Thymoglobulin)[1] at 40 mg/kg/day for 4 days, followed by cyclosporine, produces hematologic responses in approximately one third of patients with low-risk MDS. Young age, low-risk disease, and the presence of HLA-DR15 were found to be predictors of response. In the same study, marrow cellularity was not predictive of response. Cyclosporine alone may be effective in T-large granular lymphocyte/MDS patients who are HLA-DR4 positive.

Hypomethylating agents, azacitidine (Vidaza), and 5-aza-2-deoxycytidine (decitabine or Dacogen) belong to the class of epigenetic modulators; at low doses, they induce cellular differentiation by inhibiting DNA methyltransferase, and at higher doses they exert a direct cytostatic effect. Azacitidine is the first agent documented to be superior to supportive care alone in a randomized control trial in patients with MDS; multiple endpoints were used: at 75 mg/m^2/day subcutaneously, delivered for 7 days every 4 weeks, treated patients showed reduction in transfusions, slowed progression to leukemia, and improved quality of life. The optimal dose and schedule of the demethylating agents are under study. A definitive phase III trial showed a significant survival benefit of azacitidine over conventional care regimens for patients with intermediate-2 and high IPSS risk MDS. Demethylating agents should now be considered the standard of care in such patients who are not candidates for transplantation or as a bridge to allogeneic stem cell transplantation. Treatment with demethylating agents may induce significant cytopenias and requires at least 4 to 6 months to produce a benefit; consequently, these are not considered first-line agents in patients with low or intermediate-1 IPSS risk MDS.

The role of cytotoxic chemotherapy in the treatment of MDS remains an area of controversy. Many guidelines have suggested a role for standard chemotherapy to eliminate the neoplastic clone. However, no prospective studies have shown long-term survival benefit. Advanced MDS often demonstrates high response rates to induction chemotherapy, only to be followed by the virtual certainty of relapse (up to 90%). Efforts to eradicate the MDS clone must be balanced against the risk of further reduction of marrow reserve.

FUTURE DEVELOPMENT

There is great interest in therapies directed against cytokine pathways (lenalidomide), epigenetic modulation (demethylating agents and histone deacetylase inhibitors), anti-apoptosis agents, anti-angiogenesis agents, and signal transduction inhibitors, as well as ongoing improvements in supportive care, including the new thrombopoietin receptor c-mpl agonist that stimulates platelets. Developing strategies include a shift in emphasis from eliminating the MDS clone through chemotherapy toward improving the cytopenias; treatments

targeted for distinct syndromes; practical utilization of good prognostic stratification schemes; the adoption of standardized response criteria; and the availability of newer pharmaceutical agents targeting relevant biologic pathways.

CURRENT THERAPY

- Supportive care—transfusions, growth factors, iron chelation, antimicrobials
- Immunomodulatory drugs (lenalidomide [Revlimid])
- Hypomethylating agents (azacitidine [Vidaza], decitabine [Dacogen])
- Immunosuppressive drugs (antithymocyte globulin [Thymoglobulin],[1] cyclosporine [Neoral][1])

---

[1]Not FDA approved for this indication.

REFERENCES

Barrett J, Battiwalla M. Emerging therapeutic strategies for myelodysplastic syndrome. Curr Hematol Rep 2003;2(3):193–201.

Cutler CS, Lee SJ, Greenberg P, et al. A decision analysis of allogeneic bone marrow transplantation for the myelodysplastic syndromes: Delayed transplantation for low-risk myelodysplasia is associated with improved outcome. Blood 2004;104(2):579–85.

Fenaux P, Mufti G, Santini V, Finelli C. Azacitidine (AZA) Treatment Prolongs Overall Survival (OS) in Higher-Risk MDS Patients Compared with Conventional Care Regimens (CCR): Results of the AZA-001 Phase III Study. Presented at 49th annual meeting of the American Society of Hematology, Atlanta, December 8–11, 2007.

Greenberg P, Cox C, LeBeau MM, et al. International scoring system for evaluating prognosis in myelodysplastic syndromes. Blood 1997;89 (6):2079–88.

Kantarjian H, Issa JP, Rosenfeld CS, et al. Decitabine improves patient outcomes in myelodysplastic syndromes: Results of a phase III randomized study. Cancer 2006;106(8):1794–803.

List A, Dewald G, Bennett J, et al. Lenalidomide in the myelodysplastic syndrome with chromosome 5q deletion. N Engl J Med 2006;355(14): 1456–65.

NCCN Clinical Practice Guidelines in Oncology. Myelodysplastic Syndromes V.1. Available at http://www.nccn.org/professionals/physician_gls/PDF/mds.pdf; 2009 [accessed September 14, 2008].

Nimer SD. Myelodysplastic syndromes. Blood 2008;111(10):4841–51.

Raza A, Reeves JA, Feldman EJ, et al. Phase 2 study of lenalidomide in transfusion-dependent, low-risk, and intermediate-1 risk myelodysplastic syndromes with karyotypes other than deletion 5q. Blood 2008;111(1):86–93.

Silverman LR, McKenzie DR, Peterson BL, et al. Further analysis of trials with azacitidine in patients with myelodysplastic syndrome: Studies 8421, 8921, and 9221 by the Cancer and Leukemia Group B. J Clin Oncol 2006;24 (24):3895–903.

Sloand EM, Wu CO, Greenberg P, et al. Factors affecting response and survival in patients with myelodysplasia treated with immunosuppressive therapy. J Clin Oncol 2008;26(15):2505–11.

---

[1]Not FDA approved for this indication.

The Digestive System

Cholelithiasis and Cholecystitis

Method of
Grant R. Caddy, MD

Cholelithiasis

Gallstones affect 10% to 12% of people in Western populations, and the prevalence increases with age. The majority of patients with gallstones (approximately 80%) remain asymptomatic. The risk of complications, mainly that of acute cholecystitis, occurs in around 2% of patients with symptomatic gallstones.

Gallstones can be classified depending on their composition. The commonest stones are cholesterol or cholesterol-predominant stones (mixed stones), which make up around 80% to 85% of all gallstones. Mixed stones can be multiple, of varying sizes, and faceted. Most are radiolucent but 10% are radiopaque. Pure cholesterol stones are commonly solitary but may be multiple and are radiolucent. Pigment stones are less common in Western populations and are associated with hemolytic disorders such as hemolytic anemias, malaria, and cirrhosis.

Risk factors for cholesterol-predominant stone formation are shown in Box 1. Female patients have a 2 to 8 times greater risk of developing gallstones than male patients. This increased risk appears to decline following menopause. High intake of carbohydrate, high

glycemic load, and high glycemic index foods increases the risk of symptomatic gallstone disease by approximately 1.5 times. Other risk factors include a high body mass index (BMI), rapid weight loss (>1.5 kg/week), and history of dieting or gastric bypass surgery. In a 10-year follow-up study, patients who were overweight (defined as BMI >25) were approximately twice as likely to develop gallstones compared with controls. It has also been documented that following antiobesity surgery, 20% to 35% of patients develop gallstones in the postoperative period.

Complications of symptomatic gallstones are shown in Box 2.

Acute Cholecystitis

Acute cholecystitis is suspected when patients present with pain localized to the right upper quadrant (RUQ), pain aggravated by palpation in the RUQ (with or without a positive Murphy's sign), and an inflammatory response (e.g., fever and elevation in white blood cell count, C-reactive protein, and/or erythrocyte sedimentation rate). The exact mechanism of acute cholecystitis is uncertain, but blockage of the cystic duct in addition to irritation to the gallbladder mucosa result in further recruitment of inflammatory mediators such as prostaglandins (PG) I_2 and E_2. Secondary infection develops in approximately 20% of patients, usually with *Escherichia coli*, *Klebsiella* species, or *Streptococcus faecalis*. Mild elevations in bilirubin, aspartate aminotransferase (AST), alkaline phosphatase (ALP), and γ-glutamyl transpeptidase (GGT) are not uncommon (in up to one third of patients), but high levels often indicate concomitant choledocholithiasis, cholangitis, or Mirizzi's syndrome (see later).

DIAGNOSIS

First-line radiologic investigation should be a transabdominal ultrasound (TUS), which has a high specificity for cholecystitis (> 98%). In addition to identifying gallstones, gallbladder thickening

---

BOX 1   Risk Factors for Developing Gallstones

- Age >50 years (relative risk, 2.5; *P* < .001)
- Bile salt loss (e.g., terminal ileal disease)
- Diabetes mellitus
- Female gender
- First-degree relative with symptomatic gallstone disease
- Gallbladder dysmotility and stasis
- Genetic factors
- High intake of carbohydrates and high glycemic load
- Hyperlipidemia
- Overweight and obesity
- Positive family history of previous cholecystectomy in a first-degree family member
- Pregnancy
- Starvation
- Total parenteral nutrition

BOX 2   Complications of Gallstones

- Acalculous cholecystitis
- Acute cholecystitis
- Biliary colic
- Cholecystoenteric fistulas
- Choledocholithiasis ± ascending cholangitis
- Chronic cholecystitis
- Gallstone ileus
- Gallstone pancreatitis
- Gangrenous gallbladder and gallbladder perforation
- Mirizzi's syndrome

CURRENT DIAGNOSIS

- The majority of patients with gallstones (approximately 80%) remain asymptomatic. The risk of complications, mainly acute cholecystitis, occurs in around 2% of patients with symptomatic gallstones.
- Mild elevations in bilirubin, AST, ALP, and GGT occur in approximately one third of patients but high levels often indicate concomitant choledocholithiasis or cholangitis.
- TUS has a high specificity for cholecystitis (>98%). A HIDA scan has a sensitivity of > 95% and a specificity of 90%.
- Approximately 10% to 18% of patients undergoing cholecystectomy have coexisting bile duct stones.
- In choledocholithiasis, TUS is particularly sensitive if there is biliary dilatation (sensitivity is 96%) but is less sensitive in detecting stones within the duct (sensitivity is 63%).
- EUS, MRCP, and ERCP are equivalent in accuracy rates for detecting choledocholithiasis, but because of the complication rate of ERCP, this procedure should be reserved for patients with a high probability of choledocholithiasis.

Abbreviations: ALP = alkaline phosphatase; AST = aspartate aminotransferase; ERCP = endoscopic retrograde cholangiopancreatography; EUS = endoscopic ultrasound; GGT = γ-glutamyl transpeptidase; HIDA = hepatobiliary iminodiacetic acid; MRCP = magnetic resonance cholangiopancreatography; TUS = transabdominal ultrasound.

(>4–5 mm), edema, adjacent pericolic fluid, and tenderness with the transducer strongly suggest cholecystitis. Hepatobiliary iminodiacetic acid (HIDA) scan should be reserved for second-line investigation if the diagnosis remains in doubt. If the cystic duct is patent, HIDA will be taken up by the gallbladder and will be evident on scanning the abdomen after 1 hour. A positive test fails to detect any localization of HIDA within the gallbladder due to obstruction of the cystic duct. The test has a sensitivity of greater than 95% but a specificity of 90%.

TREATMENT

Patients should receive supportive care as first-line treatment with intravenous hydration and analgesia. There is evidence that nonsteroidal anti-inflammatory drugs (NSAIDs) have additional benefits other than their analgesic properties, due to their antagonist effect on prostaglandins, which are central to the inflammation of cholecystitis. NSAIDs reduce intraluminal pressure in the gallbladder, which is increased in acute cholecystitis. In addition, NSAIDs have been shown to reduce the rate of progression of biliary colic to acute cholecystitis. Due to the risk of secondary infection, antibiotics such as cephalosporin (Zinacef) and metronidazole (Flagyl) are generally recommended, but in uncomplicated cholecystitis, the routine use of antibiotics does not appear to reduce the risk of gallbladder empyema.

Laparoscopic cholecystectomy remains the most common surgical treatment for acute cholecystitis and is considered the treatment of choice for most patients. The advantages of laparoscopic cholecystectomy over open cholecystectomy are well documented and include reduced mortality, reduced postoperative pain, better cosmetic result, and a reduction in hospital stay. Studies investigating the optimal timing of laparoscopic cholecystectomy following acute cholecystitis suggest that early cholecystectomy (within 72 hours) compared with delayed cholecystectomy results in a reduction in hospital stay

and readmission rate but no overall differences in operation time, conversion rate, or complication rates. Patient symptom scores (diarrhea, indigestion, and abdominal pain) at 4 weeks are significantly better in patients undergoing early cholecystectomy versus supportive treatment followed by delayed cholecystectomy.

There is evidence supporting mini-laparotomy cholecystectomy (usually defined as open cholecystectomy through an incision of 4 to 7 cm) with similar overall results to laparoscopic cholecystectomy. In one prospective study, laparoscopic cholecystectomy took a longer time to perform but produced a slightly shorter postoperative hospital stay and a smoother postoperative course than mini-laparotomy. The choice of which operation to perform is often determined by the experience of individual surgical centers.

COMPLICATIONS

Emphysematous Cholecystitis

Acute emphysematous cholecystitis is characterized by the presence of gas within the wall or lumen of the gallbladder caused by the gas-forming organisms (e.g., *Clostridium welchii* or *E. coli*). Symptoms can be identical to those of acute cholecystitis. In contrast to acute cholecystitis, emphysematous cholecystitis occurs more commonly in elderly and diabetic patients. Its importance lies in the increased rates of early gangrene and perforation of the gallbladder. Treatment is with empiric antibiotic therapy and early cholecystectomy.

Gangrenous Cholecystitis

Gangrenous cholecystitis occurs in 2% to 20% of patients admitted with acute cholecystitis. The risk factors for gangrenous cholecystitis is increased in male patients older than 50 years; in patients with diabetes, history of cardiovascular disease, or white blood cell count greater than 15,000/mm^3; and in those who delay seeking medical treatment. The risk of gallbladder perforation and mortality is increased with gangrenous cholecystitis. Treatment is with empiric antibiotic therapy and early cholecystectomy.

Gallbladder Perforation

Gallbladder perforation can occur following gangrenous cholecystitis. It is estimated to occur in 3% to 10% of patients with acute cholecystitis. Like gangrenous cholecystitis, patients with gallbladder perforations have similar characteristics including older age and cardiovascular disease. In addition, perforations were associated with more postoperative complications that required more ICU admissions and longer hospital stays. Perforations may be localized, resulting in a pericholecystic abscess, or, less commonly, free perforations may occur into the peritoneum. Diagnosis is often difficult preoperatively.

Acalculous Cholecystitis

Acalculous cholecystitis occurs in 5% to 10% of cases of cholecystitis. It is often associated with critically ill patients, severe trauma, burns, and cardiovascular surgery but is also associated with patients who have diabetes, cardiovascular disease, or AIDS and in patients on total parenteral nutrition or opiates. Without treatment, the mortality rate is 30% to 50%.

Characteristic features on TUS are thickened gallbladder wall, absence of gallstones, gallbladder distention, Murphy's sign induced by probe, and emphysematous cholecystitis with or without perforation. Treatment is initially with supportive therapy with antibiotics and urgent referral for laparoscopic cholecystectomy. In patients with high operative risk, percutaneous cholecystostomy (insertion of a drain into the gallbladder) under radiologic guidance is an alternative treatment.

Other complications of cholelithiasis include gallstone ileus, cholecystoenteric fistulas, and Mirizzi's syndrome (obstruction of the bile duct secondary to extrinsic compression from an impacted stone in the cystic duct).

Acute Cholecystitis in Pregnancy

Overall acute cholecystitis in pregnancy is relatively uncommon. The optimal treatment remains controversial. Conservative management of a pregnant patient results in resolution of symptoms in approximately 90% of patients. However, up to 60% of patients have recurrent symptoms (readmission with acute cholecystitis, biliary colic, and premature delivery). Due to concerns of fetal loss, a conservative approach is often adopted. However, studies have supported the role of laparoscopic cholecystectomy as a safe procedure in pregnant patients with acute cholecystitis, resulting in decreased hospital stay, reduced rate of labor induction, and reduced preterm deliveries.

Chronic Cholecystitis

Chronic cholecystitis refers to recurrent episodes of gallbladder inflammation usually due to stones. These episodes may be asymptomatic but they can also result in recurrent episodes of pain. However, there does not appear to be any correlation of symptoms and degree of fibrosis and thickening of the gallbladder wall. Patients with symptomatic gallstones with recurrent biliary colic should be referred for laparoscopic cholecystectomy.

Biliary Sludge

Biliary sludge is usually diagnosed on ultrasonography. Its appearance on ultrasonography is of layered echoes in the dependent portion of the gallbladder, with no associated acoustic shadows. It is often made up of cholesterol crystals and calcium salts.

Precipitating factors include total parenteral nutrition, rapid weight loss, pregnancy, prolonged fasting, bone marrow and solid organ transplants, and drugs such as octreotide (Sandostatin) and ceftriaxone (Rocephin). In one study, 50% of patients presenting with symptomatic biliary sludge had complete resolution of gallbladder sludge on repeat imaging. In the remaining group, in 50% the sludge remained but patients were asymptomatic and in 50% further symptoms developed.

The management of biliary sludge should be managed similar to gallbladder stones. Asymptomatic sludge should be managed conservatively. Symptomatic patients should be considered for laparoscopic cholecystectomy.

Choledocholithiasis

PRESENTATION

Approximately 10% to 18% of patients undergoing cholecystectomy have coexisting bile duct stones. The symptoms of choledocholithiasis are varied and include biliary colic, jaundice, cholangitis, and pancreatitis. Conversely, a portion of patients with choledocholithiasis are asymptomatic, with a prevalence estimated to be up to 12%. In patients who present with symptoms of retained bile duct stones, the risk of subsequent symptoms is up to 50%, and the risk of complications is up to 25% if the stones are left untreated.

Patients with choledocholithiasis often present with biliary colic—pain that is often located in the RUQ and lasting between 30 minutes and several hours. There is often associated nausea and vomiting. If there is partial or complete obstruction of the common bile duct, then patients develop jaundice with associated pale stools and dark urine. Infection often occurs, resulting in a cholangitis. Approximately three fourths of patients with cholangitis have Charcot's triad of jaundice, fever, and pain. However, in 10% of patients pain may be the only feature of cholangitis. Due to bacterial translocation from the bile duct to the bloodstream, 20% of patients with cholangitis have a bacteremia, usually with gram-negative organisms.

Smaller bile duct stones (up to 8 mm) are more likely to pass spontaneously through the ampulla into the duodenum. However, it is the passage of smaller stones through the ampulla that is more likely to result in gallstone pancreatitis compared with larger stones. For example, one study found that patients who presented with gallstone pancreatitis had a mean stone diameter of 4 mm compared with patients presenting with obstructive jaundice, who had a mean stone diameter of 9 mm.

DIFFERENTIAL DIAGNOSIS

The differential of choledocholithiasis will depend on the clinical presentation. Differentials are shown in Box 3.

DIAGNOSIS

Patients presenting with symptomatic choledocholithiasis often have elevations in serum GGT and ALP (increased in 94% and 91% of cases, respectively). Bilirubin levels may be increased depending on if obstruction of the bile duct has occurred.

BOX 3 Differential Diagnosis of Choledocholithiasis by Presentation

Jaundice with or without Pain
- Alcoholic liver disease
- Benign stricture
- Bile duct injuries
- Drug induced
- Malignant stricture
- Parasitic infection of the biliary tree
- Primary biliary cirrhosis
- Sclerosing cholangitis
- Viral hepatitis

Biliary Colic
- Acute pancreatitis
- Cholecystitis
- Duodenitis
- Esophageal spasm
- Inferior myocardial infarction
- Peptic ulcer disease
- Sphincter of Oddi dysfunction

Pancreatitis
- Appendicitis
- Biliary colic
- Dissecting aneurysm
- Diverticulitis
- Ectopic pregnancy
- Hematoma of abdominal muscles
- Inferior myocardial infarction
- Mesenteric infarction
- Perforated gastric or duodenal ulcer

Cholestatic Liver Function Tests
- Alcoholic liver disease
- Ampullary carcinoma
- Biliary strictures
- Drugs
- Granulomatous hepatitis
- Malignant infiltration of the liver
- Nonalcoholic fatty liver disease (NAFLD)
- Primary biliary cirrhosis
- Sclerosing cholangitis

TUS is the commonest method of imaging the gallbladder and biliary tree in choledocholithiasis. TUS is particularly sensitive if there is biliary dilation (sensitivity up to 96%). It is less sensitive in detecting stones within the duct (sensitivity up to 63%) but has high specificity (specificity 95%). Therefore, a negative TUS does not rule out suspected choledocholithiasis.

Other radiologic investigations include computed tomography (CT), endoscopic ultrasound (EUS), magnetic resonance cholangio-pancreatography (MRCP), and endoscopic retrograde cholangiopancreatography (ERCP). A National Institutes of Health (NIH) consensus statement found that EUS, MRCP, and ERCP were equivalent in accuracy rates. However, due to the risks of ERCP (pancreatitis, bleeding, perforation, infection), ERCP is recommended in patients with a high probability of choledocholithiasis. In patients with an intermediate probability, other imaging modalities, such as MRCP or EUS, should be considered.

TREATMENT

Generally, patients with symptomatic choledocholithiasis should be offered treatment because of the high risk of recurrent symptoms and complications if stones are left in situ as already discussed. In some special circumstances, adopting a conservative approach may be appropriate such as severe end-stage dementia or severe comorbid factors that make removal hazardous.

The two main methods of bile duct stone removal are at ERCP or, in patients with an intact gallbladder, laparoscopic cholecystectomy and bile duct exploration (LC+BDE). Current practice in choosing between the two methods depends on center preference and local expertise in laparoscopic bile duct exploration. A recent Cochrane Database of systematic review comparing LC+BDE and ERCP found that both methods were equally effective, with no significant difference in morbidity and mortality. However, shorter hospital stay was achieved in patients undergoing LC+BDE.

There is a limited role for other techniques, such as extracorporeal shockwave lithotripsy and endoscopic laser lithotripsy, and these techniques should be reserved for bile duct stones that cannot be removed at ERCP or LC+CBE due to technical or safety reasons.

CURRENT THERAPY

- Patients with symptomatic gallstones should undergo laparoscopic cholecystectomy if there is no contraindication.
- For acute cholecystitis, first-line treatment is supportive care with intravenous hydration, analgesia (NSAIDs), and antibiotics. If there are no contraindications, patients should undergo laparoscopic cholecystectomy within 72 hours.
- Percutaneous cholecystostomy is an alternative option in patients with acalculous cholecystitis who are too unwell to undergo cholecystectomy.
- Treatment options for patients with choledocholithiasis include ERCP and stone removal followed by laparoscopic cholecystectomy or, in patients with an intact gallbladder, cholecystectomy and bile duct exploration. Overall, there are no differences in morbidity and mortality between the two procedures.
- There is a limited role for other techniques such as extracorporeal shockwave lithotripsy and endoscopic laser lithotripsy or oral dissolution therapy.

Abbreviation: ERCP = endoscopic retrograde cholangio-pancreatography.

REFERENCES

Al-Waili N, Saloom KY. The analgesic effect of intravenous tenoxicam in symptomatic treatment of biliary colic: A comparison with hyoscine N-butylbromide. Eur J Med Res 1998;3(10):475–9.

Field AE, Coakley EH, Must A, et al. Impact of overweight on the risk of developing common chronic diseases during a 10-year period. Arch Intem Med 2001;161(13):1581–6.

Johansson M, Thune A, Blomqvist A, et al. Impact of choice of therapeutic strategy for acute cholecystitis on patient's health-related quality of life. Results of a randomized, controlled clinical trial. Dig Surg 2004;21 (5–6):359–62.

Lau H, Lo CY, Patil NG, Yuen WK. Early versus delayed-interval laparoscopic cholecystectomy for acute cholecystitis: A meta-analysis. Surg Endosc 2006;20(1):82–7.

Lu EJ, Curet MJ, El-Sayed YY, Kirkwood KS. Medical versus surgical management of biliary tract disease in pregnancy. Am J Surg. 2004;188(6):755–9.

Martin DJ, Vernon DR, Toouli J. Surgical versus endoscopic treatment of bile duct stones. Cochrane Database Syst Rev 2006;(2):CD003327.

Miller K, Hell E, Lang B, Lengauer E. Gallstone formation prophylaxis after gastric restrictive procedures for weight loss: A randomized double-blind placebo-controlled trial. Ann Surg 2003;238(5):697–702.

NIH state-of-the-science statement on endoscopic retrograde cholangiopancreatography (ERCP) for diagnosis and therapy. NIH Consens State Sci Statements 2002;19(1):1–26.

Papi C, Catarci M, D'Ambrosio L, et al. Timing of cholecystectomy for acute calculous cholecystitis: A meta-analysis. Am J Gastroenterol. 2004;99(1): 147–55.

Ros A, Gustafsson L, Krook H, et al. Laparoscopic cholecystectomy versus mini-laparotomy cholecystectomy: A prospective, randomized, single-blind study. Ann Surg 2001;234(6):741–9.

Thornell E, Nilsson B, Jansson R, Svanvik J. Effect of short-term indomethacin treatment on the clinical course of acute obstructive cholecystitis. Eur J Surg 1991;157(2):127–30.

Tsai CJ, Leitzmann MF, Willett WC, Giovannucci EL. Dietary carbohydrates and glycaemic load and the incidence of symptomatic gall stone disease in men. Gut 2005;54(6):823–8.

Cirrhosis

Method of
Harmit Kalia, DO, Priya Grewal, MD, and Paul Martin, MD

Cirrhosis is the 12th most common cause of death in the United States; it is responsible for more than 27,000 deaths and 421,000 hospitalizations annually. Cirrhosis reflects the consequences of chronic hepatic necroinflammatory activity with an incomplete repair response. This involves collagen deposition and nodule formation, leading to disruption of the normal lobular arrangement of hepatocytes, blood vessels, and lymphatics. Although, strictly speaking, the diagnosis of cirrhosis is based on histology, in the absence of a liver biopsy its presence can be inferred in the appropriate setting by complications such as portal hypertension or radiologic appearances consistent with the diagnosis. Cirrhosis can result from any cause of chronic liver disease (Table 1). Most manifestations of advanced cirrhosis, such as portal hypertension and coagulopathy, reflect the consequences of extensive distortion of the hepatic architecture and impaired hepatocellular function. However, some symptoms may also reflect the specific etiology of cirrhosis—most notably, pruritus in patients with cholestasis and malabsorption of fat-soluble vitamins in patients with primary biliary cirrhosis or primary sclerosing cholangitis.

An important distinction among individual patients is whether the cirrhosis is compensated or decompensated. Cirrhosis that remains compensated implies the absence of an index complication such as onset of ascites or variceal hemorrhage, whereas overt hepatic decompensation indicates that a major complication has supervened

TABLE 1 Common Causes of Cirrhosis

Cause	Examples
Infection	Hepatitis B
	Hepatitis C
	Hepatitis D
Toxins	Alcohol, drugs
Cholestasis	Primary biliary cirrhosis
	Secondary biliary cirrhosis
	Primary sclerosing cholangitis
Autoimmune	Autoimmune hepatitis
Vascular	Cardiac cirrhosis
	Budd-Chiari syndrome
	Sinusoidal obstruction syndrome
Metabolic	Hemochromatosis
	Wilson's disease
	α_1-Antitrypsin deficiency
	Nonalcoholic steatohepatitis
Cryptogenic	

and the patient now has evidence of frank hepatic failure. A patient with compensated cirrhosis can continue to have a good prognosis. However, once an initial manifestation of cirrhosis has occurred, the patient's likelihood of long-term survival diminishes in the absence of liver transplantation. The diagnosis of cirrhosis per se does not suggest the need for evaluation for liver transplantation, but transplantation needs to be considered once a major complication such as a variceal hemorrhage, onset of ascites, or hepatic encephalopathy has supervened. Less florid evidence of cirrhosis may include a hyperdynamic circulation reflecting peripheral vasodilation with a resting tachycardia. However, many patients with cirrhosis are completely asymptomatic until a major complication of their liver disease supervenes. Clues to underlying cirrhosis are thrombocytopenia or coagulopathy not related to a primary hematologic disorder or biochemical dysfunction with hyperbilirubinemia and elevated serum aminotransferases or alkaline phosphatase.

In patients with well-compensated cirrhosis, the physical signs of liver disease may be subtle. The liver span may be somewhat diminished on percussion, with a firm edge and with splenic dullness due to splenomegaly. Cutaneous signs of cirrhosis other than jaundice include palmar erythema and spider nevi. In cirrhotic male patients, gynecomastia results from altered metabolism of sex hormones with testicular atrophy; it also reflects the antigonadal effects of alcohol in some patients. The catabolic effects of cirrhosis often result in a diminished muscle mass, obvious on physical examination. More florid evidence of cirrhosis on physical examination includes varying degrees of disturbed mentation along with asterixis, indicative of hepatic encephalopathy. Other key findings include ascites and peripheral edema. Additional physical findings may provide some clues to the underlying etiology of liver disease. For instance, xanthelasmata are frequent in patients with cholestatic liver disease, whereas patients with alcoholic cirrhosis may have other end-organ injury such as peripheral neuropathy.

Laboratory findings suggestive of portal hypertension are a low platelet count and a low leukocyte count due to hypersplenism. Impaired hepatic synthetic and secretory functions are reflected in a diminished serum albumin, elevated serum bilirubin, and prolonged prothrombin time.

Transition from compensated to decompensated cirrhosis occurs at a rate of 5% to 7% per annum. Various models have been developed to predict the likelihood of hepatic decompensation in individual patients. They typically incorporate a combination of routine blood tests, including the platelet count, which is depressed in portal hypertension mainly because of hypersplenism and diminished thrombopoietin. The development of hepatocellular carcinoma (HCC) accelerates the progression of cirrhosis as a result of the tumor mass and vascular invasion, most typically of the portal vein. However, the morbidity and mortality in chronic liver disease are related to a large extent to the severity of portal hypertension.

The median survival time in patients with compensated cirrhosis is 12 years, whereas in those with decompensated cirrhosis it is 1.5 years. Recently, there has been an increasing emphasis on anticipating the complications of cirrhosis, such as variceal hemorrhage (discussed in the chapter on bleeding esophageal varices), HCC, and spontaneous bacterial peritonitis (SBP), in an effort to enhance survival and allow appropriate intervention with liver transplantation.

Cirrhotic patients are immunocompromised and therefore are at increased risk for bacterial infections. The pulmonary complications of cirrhosis are relatively uncommon and include portopulmonary hypertension (PPHTN) and hepatopulmonary syndrome (HPS).

Ascites

Cirrhosis is the underlying cause for ascites in 85% of patients. Ascites is the most common complication of cirrhosis and carries a 2-year survival rate of only 50% after its onset. The pathogenesis of ascites in cirrhosis mainly reflects increased intrahepatic resistance due to fibrosis, which raises portal pressures. Compensatory mechanisms cause splanchnic vasodilation, resulting in a decrease in effective arterial blood volume. This results in a compensatory activation of the neurohumoral (renin-angiotensin) system and increased retention of sodium by the kidneys. The imbalance of elevated hydrostatic pressure due to portal hypertension and decreased oncotic pressure (low albumin) causes ascites. Therefore, sodium retention is key to the development of ascites. Other mechanisms can include disruption of normal lymphatic drainage in the liver due to extensive fibrosis.

Physical examination may reveal a bulging abdomen with shifting dullness; this sign is reliable when the volume of ascites is greater than 1500 mL. Ultrasound of the abdomen is helpful in locating smaller amounts of ascites (as little as 100 mL). Once ascites is found, a diagnostic paracenteses should be performed to determine whether it is exudative or transudative, a determination that narrows the differential diagnosis of ascites (Table 2). The fluid is tested for white blood cell count, culture, and albumin to calculate serum-ascites albumin gradient (SAAG). This must be done on initial paracenteses and accurately distinguishes ascites related to portal versus nonportal hypertensive causes. A SAAG of 1.1 g/dL or higher accurately predicts portal hypertension. Once the diagnosis of ascites is made, it is important to mitigate aggravating factors for fluid retention. Dietary indiscretion, noncompliance with diuretics, therapeutic volume expansion after gastrointestinal bleeding volume expansion, and renal toxicity from use of nonsteroidal antiinflammatory drugs are common causes.

TABLE 2 Diagnostic Tests on Ascites

Test	Comments
Cell count	If PMN ≥250 cells/mm^3, infection is presumed
Culture	High sensitivity if infected
Albumin	Necessary to calculate SAAG
Total protein	Assists in determining cause of ascites
Gram stain	Assists in infectious/inflammatory work-up
LDH	High in malignant ascites
Amylase	Elevated in ascites secondary to pancreatitis
TB smear, culture, PCR	If TB is suspected
Cytology	Assists in diagnosis of malignant ascites
Triglycerides	Chylous ascites if >110 mg/dL
Bilirubin	To confirm leakage of bile in peritoneum

Abbreviations: LDH = lactate dehydrogenase; PCR = polymerase chain reaction; PMN = polymorphonuclear neutrophils; SAAG = serum-ascites albumin gradient; TB = tuberculosis.

The mainstay of management of ascites is sodium restriction and judicious diuresis. Patients should be encouraged to stay on a sodium-restricted diet of 2 g/day. A sodium-to-potassium concentration ratio greater than 1 on a random urine sample correlates well with a 24-hour sodium excretion greater than 78 mmol/day and implies patient compliance with salt restriction. In reality, dietary restriction of sodium is efficacious in only 10% of patients; more typically, diuretics are needed. Mild to moderate ascites is controlled best by the use of diuretics with different modes of action, such as spironolactone (Aldactone) 100 mg (an aldosterone antagonist) and furosemide (Lasix) 40 mg (a loop diuretic) taken once daily. Serum electrolytes need to be monitored to avoid hypokalemia or hyperkalemia. Doses of spironolactone and furosemide can be increased in a 100:40 ratio every 3 to 5 days until an adequate diuresis is achieved. Doses greater than spironolactone 400 mg and furosemide 160 mg are generally not recommended, to lessen the risk of electrolyte imbalance or renal insufficiency. Fluid restriction is recommended if the serum sodium concentration is less than 120 to 125 mmol/L, because hyponatremia in this circumstance reflects an excess of free water rather than sodium depletion. Hospitalized patients can be weighed daily to help guide management. Ideally, the patient should shed about 1 pound of weight every day; failure to do so implies inadequate diuretic dosing or lack of compliance with fluid restriction. Excessive weight loss should also be avoided, to forestall precipitation of hepatorenal syndrome. Diuretic therapy should be withheld if a patient presents with encephalopathy, infection, renal insufficiency, or a serum sodium concentration of 120 mmol/L or greater.

Refractory ascites, defined as inability to obtain a diuresis with high-dose diuretics without inducing renal dysfunction, occurs in 10% of cirrhotic patients with ascites; the resultant 1-year survival rate is only 25%. Serial large-volume paracenteses (LVP) of greater than 5 L of fluid is safe and effective in controlling ascites. Continued dietary restriction of sodium is necessary to avoid overly frequent paracenteses. Patients requiring LVP more frequently than every 2 weeks are probably not complying with a sodium-restricted diet. The use of albumin as colloid replacement is controversial, but it is generally accepted for use with ascitic fluid removal of greater than 5 L, to prevent postparacentesis circulatory dysfunction leading to renal insufficiency.

A patient who requires frequent LVP may be a candidate for a transjugular intrahepatic portosystemic shunt (TIPS). This vascular shunt is placed under fluoroscopic guidance and bridges a branch of the hepatic vein with a branch of the portal vein to reduce portal pressures. It is effective in about 90% of patients with refractory ascites. Diuretic therapy needs to be continued in many patients after institution of TIPS. There is generally no survival advantage for TIPS compared with LVP in cirrhotic patients, although it may simplify patient management by removing the need for large-volume paracenteses.

The Model of End-Stage Liver Disease (MELD) score assesses the severity of liver disease and is based on the natural logarithms (base e) of the concentrations of bilirubin and creatinine (in milligrams per deciliter) and the international normalized ratio (INR):

$$MELD = [3.8 \times ln(\text{Bilirubin})] + [11.2 \times ln(\text{INR})] + [9.6\ ln(\text{Creatinine})]$$

TIPS should be avoided in patients with a MELD score greater than 18 or Child-Pugh grade C disease (Table 3). These patients have a poor outcome because of deterioration in hepatocellular function secondary to this form of therapeutic portosystemic shunting. Not surprisingly, there is a high frequency (up to 40%) of portosystemic hepatic encephalopathy (PSE) after TIPS, which can be disabling and may even necessitate reduction in the shunt diameter to alleviate symptoms. TIPS occlusion was frequent in the past, but with newer covered stents the patency is maintained. As part of the evaluation for TIPS placement, patients should undergo echocardiography to confirm that the cardiac ejection fraction is greater than 60%. This is done to prevent heart failure precipitated by an increased venous return after shunt placement. Since the availability of TIPS, peritoneovenous shunting has fallen out of favor. Given the invasive nature of the procedure, along with its potential complications (disseminated intravascular coagulation, infection of the shunt, bleeding), this intervention is no longer considered in most centers. Despite available modalities for the management of ascites, the presence of ascites implies poor long-term survival, and referral to a transplant center is indicated.

Spontaneous Bacterial Peritonitis

SBP is infection of the ascitic fluid with enteric aerobic organisms in the absence of a primary discrete source of infection such as a perforated viscus. Cirrhotic patients with ascites have a 10% annual incidence of SBP. It is the most common bacterial infection in cirrhotics with ascites, with a mortality rate of 30% in older series. The mortality rises when SBP is complicated by renal failure.

Patients may be asymptomatic (Table 4), and on admission or readmission of a cirrhotic patient with ascites, diagnostic paracentesis is essential to exclude unrecognized SBP. A high index of suspicion is also necessary in cirrhotic patients with unexplained fever, worsening hepatocellular function, nonspecific abdominal pain, or unexplained PSE. SBP is defined as positive ascitic fluid culture (one organism) and a polymorphonuclear neutrophil (PMN) count of 250 cells/mm^3 or higher. Treatment with antibiotics is also indicated if the culture is negative but the PMN count is 250 cells/mm^3 or greater, or if the culture is positive with one organism and the PMN count is 250 cells/mm^3 or greater in a symptomatic patient. Diagnostic paracentesis revealing PMNs greater than 250 cells/mm^3 and multiple enteric organisms suggests secondary bacterial peritonitis, and treatment should include antibiotics with further evaluation to exclude bowel perforation.

TABLE 3 Child-Pugh Classification*

Factor	Points Assigned		
	1	2	3
Ascites	Absent	Slight	Moderate
Bilirubin	<2 mg/dL	2–3 mg/dL	>3 mg/dL
Albumin	>3.5 g/dL (35 g/L)	2.8–3.5 g/dL	<2.8 g/dL
Prothrombin time			
Seconds over control	<4	4–6	>6
International normalized ratio	<1.7	1.7–2.3	>2.3
Encephalopathy	None	Grade 1–2	Grade 3–4

*A total score of 5–6 is considered grade A (well-compensated disease); 7–9 is grade B (significant functional compromise); and 10–15 is grade C (decompensated disease).

TABLE 4 Frequency of Signs and Symptoms in Patients with Spontaneous Bacterial Peritonitis

Sign or Symptom	Frequency (%)
Fever	68
Abdominal pain	49
Abdominal tenderness	39
Rebound	10
Altered mental status	54

Adapted from Feldman M, Friedman LS, Brandt LJ (eds): Sleisenger & Fordtran's Gastrointestinal and Liver Disease, 8th ed. Philadelphia: Saunders Elsevier, 2006.

Treatment of SBP involves the empiric administration of third-generation cephalosporins (e.g., cefotaxime [Claforan]) before the bacterial culture results become available. The organisms most commonly involved are *Escherichia coli*, *Streptococcus* species, and *Klebsiella pneumoniae*. Ascitic fluid cultures are positive in only 50% to 60% of cases. Culture sensitivity is improved by immediate inoculation of aerobic and anaerobic blood culture bottles. For patients with an allergy to cephalosporins, alternatives include amoxicillin-clavulanate (Augmentin) and ciprofloxacin (Cipro). A 5-day antibiotic regimen is used, with resolution in 90% of cases. Repeat paracentesis 48 hours after starting antibiotics is useful to confirm the clinical response of the infection, especially if the initial ascitic white blood cell count was in the thousands. Paracentesis should also be repeated after 5 days of antibiotics to confirm the response before withdrawing antibiotic therapy. If the typical clinical response to antibiotics does not occur, important considerations include secondary bacterial peritonitis, intraabdominal abscess formation, and bacterial resistance. Plasma volume expansion with albumin in addition to antibiotics decreases the incidence of renal dysfunction and improves survival. Albumin, unlike other volume expanders, improves cardiac function by decreasing arterial vasodilation. The recommended dose of albumin is 1.5 g/kg at the time of diagnosis of SBP and 1.0 g/kg after 72 hours of treatment with antibiotics.

After a single episode of SBP, there is a 70%, 1-year cumulative probability of further SBP episodes; therefore, prophylaxis with antibiotics is appropriate. Oral norfloxacin (Noroxin)[1] 400 mg daily or ciprofloxacin[1] 750 mg weekly can reduce the risk of SBP to 20% over 1 year. For patients with a fluoroquinolone allergy, trimethoprim-sulfamethoxazole (one Bactrim DS daily)[1] may be administered. Primary prophylaxis for SBP is beneficial in patients with a low ascitic protein concentration (<1.0 g/dL). Other settings in which antibiotics are helpful include cirrhotic patients admitted with gastrointestinal bleeding. Antiobiotic therapy lowers the infection rate, decreases the rate of further variceal bleeding, and improves survival. Improvements in earlier detection and treatment of this infection have had a major impact on reducing mortality. In addition, prophylaxis against SBP has lowered its incidence in cirrhotics at risk.

Portosystemic (Hepatic) Encephalopathy

PSE is a syndrome of reversible neuropsychiatric dysfunction of varying severity that occurs on a background of portal hypertension with shunting of blood from the portal system into the systemic circulation. Despite its frequency in cirrhotic patients, there is continuing controversy about its exact pathogenesis. Nitrogenous products from the gut are clearly implicated. Pathologically, there may be evidence of swelling of astrocyte cells in the brain. Ammonia and other toxins accumulate in the blood to impair cognitive and motor function.

PSE is classified into three types (Table 5). The most common type has a gradual onset in cirrhotic patients and is referred to as type C. Type A is associated with acute liver failure, and type B is associated with portosystemic bypass (portocaval shunt) in the absence of cirrhosis. The clinical features of type C PSE include a wide range of neuropsychiatric symptoms. Stage 1 is characterized

---

[1]Not FDA approved for this indication.

TABLE 5 Types of Hepatic Encephalopathy

Type	Description
A	Acute liver failure
B	Portosystemic bypass without cirrhosis (portocaval shunt)
C	Chronic liver disease (cirrhosis)

by alterations in consciousness and behavioral changes (inversion of sleep/wake pattern, forgetfulness); stage 2 can include confusion and disorientation; stage 3 includes more profound symptoms, with lethargy and a stuporous state; and stage 4 is frank coma. The physical examination may elicit subtle findings such as mild tremor, as well as the more classic asterixis. Fetor hepaticus is a sweetish breath odor found in some patients with PSE. The diagnosis of PSE remains clinical. Serum ammonia levels correlate poorly with the severity of encephalopathy. An increased level of serum ammonia per se is not an indication to treat a patient with liver disease in the absence of clinical evidence of PSE. Minimal PSE is subclinical and is present in up to 70% of cirrhotics. It is diagnosed by psychomotor and neuropsychological tests only. Its progression to overt PSE seems to be related to deterioration of hepatocellular function.

When a cirrhotic patient presents with overt PSE, management includes identification of a precipitating cause, which is present in more than 80% of cases. Key precipitants include infection, noncompliance with medications, gastrointestinal bleeding, dehydration, electrolyte abnormalities, use of narcotics or sedatives, constipation, TIPS, and increased protein intake. Treatment of the precipitating cause, in addition to inducing a catharsis, is associated with improved cognitive and motor function. Upper gastrointestinal bleeding should be excluded by rectal examination and nasogastric lavage. An absence of improvement in mentation within 48 hours should lead to a further search for unrecognized precipitants (e.g., ongoing sepsis) or a separate neurologic diagnosis (e.g., subdural hematoma). Repeated admissions to hospital with easily reversible PSE suggest noncompliance with lactulose therapy, which remains the mainstay for its treatment.

Available therapies for overt PSE counteract the effects of gut-derived bacterial neuroactive toxins. Therapy for overt PSE includes the induction of a catharsis with lactulose (Cephulac) or lactitol. Lactulose 45 to 90 g/m^3 should be given via nasogastric tube every 2 hours (in severe PSE) until loose bowel movements are observed, and thereafter to obtain two to three loose bowel movements daily. Lactulose enemas may be given in a less alert patient. Cathartics used for PSE have frequent and troublesome common side effects, including abdominal cramping, diarrhea, and flatulence.

Outpatient therapy is initially with lactulose or lactitol titrated to obtain two to three soft bowel movements daily. These medications alter the pH in the colon and may promote ionization of ammonia, making it impossible for the drug to cross the mucous barrier in the colon. A more acidic gut pH always reduces bacterial replication and production of nitrogenous products. The use of spironolactone along with furosemide decreases the incidence of hypokalemia, which increases renal ammonia production. Traditionally, dietary protein restriction has been recommended in cirrhotics, often even in the absence of PSE, but rigorous evidence is lacking to support this strategy. It is more important for a patient with decompensated cirrhosis to maintain adequate nutrition. A nutritional evaluation is key in maintaining muscle mass in these patients.

If the cathartic effects of lactulose are poorly tolerated, nonabsorbable antibiotics can be used to inhibit bacterial toxin production. Neomycin has been used longest, but its ototoxicity and nephrotoxicity limit its long-term use. Other antibiotics, such as metronidazole (Flagyl)[1] and rifaximin (Xifaxan),[1] are now being used to treat PSE. Ongoing clinical trials are attempting to clarify the role of rifaximin. Antibiotics may be used in addition to lactulose if it alone does not improve symptoms.

In patients with intractable and severe post-TIPS PSE, reduction or occlusion of the shunt may be necessary if pharmacologic treatment is not efficacious. Type A PSE associated with acute liver failure does not respond to standard medical therapy, which is futile in this circumstance, and urgent referral for liver transplantation is indicated. Cerebral edema, a frequent and often lethal complication of acute liver failure, may lead to cerebral herniation or intracranial hemorrhage, precluding liver transplantation.

---

[1]Not FDA approved for this indication.
[3]Exceeds dosage recommended by the manufacturer.

Hepatorenal Syndrome

There are several potential explanations for renal dysfunction in patients with cirrhosis. Renal dysfunction can reflect glomerulonephropathy (hepatitis B, hepatitis C, immunoglobulin A nephropathy, diabetes mellitus), whereas the differential for acute renal dysfunction includes hypovolemia (diuretics, gastrointestinal bleed, diarrhea), nephrotoxic drugs (aminoglycosides, nonsteroidal antiinflammatory drugs, contrast dye), sepsis, and hepatorenal syndrome (HRS).

The incidence of HRS in cirrhotic patients with ascites is up to 18% per annum. The pathogenesis of HRS in cirrhosis results from the marked splanchnic and systemic vasodilation and decreased cardiac function, which lead to a decrease in effective arterial blood volume typical of more advanced portal hypertension. Although the renal parenchyma is preserved, there is severe renal arterial vasoconstriction, low renal perfusion, and a decrease in the glomerular filtration rate. Clinically, the diagnosis of HRS is suspected when there is an increase in the creatinine level to greater than 1.5 mg/dL in the absence of shock, dehydration, infection, or nephrotoxic drugs. Clinically, there are two types of HRS (Box 1). Type 1 HRS is defined as a severe, rapidly progressive increase in creatinine to greater than 2.5 mg/dL in less than 2 weeks. It is often precipitated by SBP, alcoholic hepatitis, or gastrointestinal hemorrhage. These patients tend to have floridly decompensated cirrhosis with tense ascites, PSE, and coagulopathy. The median survival time is 2 weeks. Type 2 HRS, with a median survival time of 6 months, is defined as a moderate and steady decline in renal function to a creatinine level greater than 2.5 mg/dL.

Evaluation of renal dysfunction in patients with liver disease should include an ultrasound study to determine the presence of ascites. If ascites is not present, the diagnosis of HRS is unlikely, and prerenal or intrinsic renal causes should be sought. If ascites is present, a work-up for sepsis (urinalysis, diagnostic paracenteses, and blood cultures) is indicated. Discontinuing all diuretics and nephrotoxic agents along with plasma volume expansion (intravenous fluids or albumin) is the initial intervention to correct renal dysfunction in cirrhotic patients. If renal function does not improve, HRS is likely. Additional clues that are helpful in the diagnosis of HRS are urine volume less than 500 mL/day, urine sodium concentration less than 10 mEq/L (despite plasma volume expansion), urine osmolality greater than that of plasma, protein secretion of less than 500 mg/day, and serum sodium concentration less than 130 mEq/L.

Treatment of HRS is mainly limited to establishing whether a reversible component in the renal dysfunction is present. Most data on the efficacy of therapeutic interventions are based on small retrospective and pilot comparative studies. Realistically, patients with severe HRS require either an improvement in liver function or liver transplantation for renal function to recover. Medical therapy may result in modest improvement in renal function. In a small study, combination of an α-agonist, midodrine (ProAmatine),[1]

[1]Not FDA approved for this indication.

BOX 1 Diagnostic Criteria for Hepatorenal Syndrome

Cirrhosis with ascites
Serum creatinine >1.5 mg/dL
No improvement of serum creatinine after at least
  2 days with diuretic withdrawal and volume expansion
Absence of shock
No current or recent treatment with nephrotoxic drugs
Absence of parenchymal kidney disease

Adapted from Salerno F, Gerbes A, Ginès P, et al: Diagnosis, prevention and treatment of hepatorenal syndrome in cirrhosis. Gut 2007;56;1310–1318.

---

with octreotide (Sandostatin)[1] and albumin[1] resulted in improvement in three of five patients with HRS. Another trial of albumin and octreotide infusion failed to show benefit. Vasoconstrictors such as terlipressin (Glypressin)[2] and norepinephrine (Levophed)[1] have been shown to improve renal function, with a decrease in serum creatinine to less than 1.5 mg/dL demonstrated in two thirds of patients with HRS in one study. Albumin has typically been administered with these medications and seems to aid in vasoconstriction as well as plasma volume expansion. A retrospective study suggested improved survival for patients with HRS type 1 who had received terlipressin. However, a meta-analysis of 154 patients indicated no improvement in overall survival. Terlipressin is expensive and is not available for use in the United States.

TIPS has been advocated as a means to improve renal function in patients with HRS. In a small prospective study of 14 patients, 10 patients who had initially responded to medical therapy (midodrine, octreotide, and albumin) and subsequently underwent TIPS had improvement in renal function. This study supported the possible use of this combination. In one study, TIPS was shown to improve survival to an average of 5 months, much better than the otherwise expected survival time of 2 weeks. TIPS may provide short-term benefit, but more studies are needed with TIPS and HRS. TIPS may cause a precipitous deterioration in hepatocellular function in patients with more floridly decompensated liver disease, and its use should be entertained only in collaboration with a liver transplant center.

In patients with confirmed SBP, administration of albumin[1] on days 1 and 3 reduced the incidence of HRS from 33% to 10%. Also, the use of pentoxifylline (Trental)[1] 400 mg three times daily in patients with alcoholic hepatitis reduced the incidence of HRS from 35% to 8%.

Portopulmonary Hypertension

The prevalence of this complication of cirrhosis varies from 2% to 12.5% in candidates awaiting liver transplantation. Before making a diagnosis of PPHTN, other causes of pulmonary arterial hypertension, such as recurrent pulmonary emboli, collagen vascular disease, intracardiac shunts, and medications, need to be excluded. The criteria for diagnosis of pulmonary arterial hypertension by right heart catheterization are mean pulmonary artery pressure greater than 25 mm Hg at rest or greater than 30 mm Hg with exercise; pulmonary capillary wedge pressure lower than 15 mm Hg; pulmonary vascular resistance greater than 120 dynes/sec/cm^5; and transpulmonary gradient (pulmonary arterial diastolic pressure minus pulmonary capillary wedge pressure) greater than 10 mm Hg. The pathogenesis of PPHTN may relate to the effects of vasoconstrictive substances produced in the splanchnic circulation that bypass metabolism by the liver. Candidate substances include serotonin, interleukin 1, glucagon, thromboxane B$_2$, endothelin 1, and vasoactive intestinal peptide. All these have been detected in increased concentrations in patients with PPHTN.

Symptoms of PPHTN include dyspnea on exertion, syncope, chest pain, fatigue, hemoptysis, and orthopnea. On physical examination, an accentuated pulmonic component of the second heart sound, right ventricular heave, and lower extremity edema are common. More than 60% of patients are asymptomatic at the time of diagnosis. Transthoracic echocardiography is used to estimate pressures. Patients who have right ventricular systolic pressures greater than 50 mm Hg or symptoms of right-sided heart failure should undergo right heart catheterization. In one third of these patients, the pulmonary vascular resistance is normal. Treatment should be initiated in those patients who are symptomatic and have mean pulmonary arterial pressure greater than 35 mm Hg and increased pulmonary vascular resistance.

[1]Not FDA approved for this indication.
[2]Not available in the United States.

Several drugs have been used to treat PPHTN with variable success. Epoprostenol (Flolan),[1] a prostacyclin (which directly dilates peripheral vessels), has been frequently used. Other agents have been used, such as bosentan (Tracleer), an endothelin receptor antagonist; sildenafil (Revatio), a phosphodiesterase inhibitor; and iloprost (Ventavis),[1] a vasodilator. β-Blockers should be used cautiously in patients with PPHTN because of the cardiac depressant and pulmonary vasoconstrictive effects of these medications. Anticoagulation therapy should be considered, given the risk of venous stasis and pulmonary vascular thrombosis. These treatments should be attempted in concert with an evaluation for liver transplantation, which can arrest PPHTN. More severe PPHTN is a contraindication to liver transplantation, especially if it does not improve with pharmacologic therapy. Liver transplantation can be delayed if patients have a good clinical response to medical therapy.

Hepatopulmonary Syndrome

In patients with liver disease, hypoxemia (increased alveolar-arterial gradient while breathing on room air) and vascular dilations in the lung suggest the diagnosis of HPS. Its prevalence has been reported to be from 8% to 20% in transplantation candidates. The clinical features of HPS include the insidious onset of dyspnea, platypnea (shortness of breath exacerbated in upright position), orthodeoxia (hypoxemia in upright posture), clubbing, and cyanosis. Cutaneous spider nevi may reflect analogous vascular dilations in the lungs. A widened alveolar-arterial oxygen gradient on room air (>15 mm Hg, or >20 mm Hg in patients older than 64 years of age) should prompt evaluation for HPS in a patient with liver disease. A pulse oximetry reading of less than 97% on room air and an arterial partial pressure of oxygen (PaO_2) lower than 70 mm Hg on blood gas analysis indicate HPS in the absence of intrinsic cardiopulmonary diseases.

The diagnosis of HPS can be confirmed with contrast echocardiography. Agitated saline is injected intravenously, and bubbles are observed in the left side of the heart during the study. Normally, the bubbles from the agitated saline should be visualized on the left side of the heart. Bubbles resulting from vascular dilations in HPS appear 3 to 6 heartbeats after the appearance of contrast in the right side of the heart. If bubbles appear within 3 beats after injection, intracardiac shunting (e.g., atrial septal defect, patent foramen ovale) should be considered. If intrinsic cardiopulmonary disease is present, a technetium-labeled macroaggregated albumin scan can distinguish HPS. Normally, 20 µg of radiolabeled albumin gets trapped in the lung, but in a patient with pulmonary vascular dilations, the tracer escapes to elsewhere in the body. A shunt fraction of greater than 6% confirms the presence of HPS. Pulmonary angiography may be considered to rule out alternative causes of hypoxemia if noninvasive studies are nondiagnostic.

Patients with HPS have a median survival time of 10.6 months, compared with 40.8 months for cirrhotic controls. Therapeutic attempts with various modalities such as acetylsalicylic acid,[1] garlic powder,[7] indomethacin (Indocin),[1] methylene blue,[1] almitrine bismesylate (Duxil),[2] somatostatin analogues (Octreotide),[1] and plasma exchange have been tried, but currently none of these is recommended for use. Results of TIPS have been variable in HRS. Supplemental oxygen therapy has been shown to improve exercise tolerance and quality of life. Patients with HPS should be referred for a liver transplantation evaluation, because transplantation increases survival, with impressive improvement in hypoxemia in about 85% of patients who undergo the procedure. However, resolution of symptoms can take up to 1 year. The 1-year survival after transplantation in HPS is 71%, compared with 90% in patients without HPS.

---

[1]Not FDA approved for this indication.
[2]Not available in the United States.
[7]Available as dietary supplement.

Hepatic Hydrothorax

The manifestation of portal hypertension known as hepatic hydrothorax is defined as a pleural effusion of greater than 500 mL in a cirrhotic patient without evidence of a cardiopulmonary cause. Although patients can tolerate a large amount (>5 L) of ascites before becoming symptomatic, a hepatic hydrothorax greater than 1 L can cause shortness of breath and hypoxemia. It develops on the right side about 85% of the time, is left-sided in 13% of the cases, and is bilateral in 2%. Accumulation of a transudate in the pleural space is caused by portal hypertension with leakage of fluid from the peritoneal space through small defects in the diaphragm. With inspiration, there is an increase in negative intrathoracic pressure, facilitating fluid movement from the peritoneal space to the pleural space.

The clinical presentation includes dyspnea, nonproductive cough, chest discomfort, and even hypoxemia. Ascites is not always present, because it tends to be drawn into the pleural space. Less commonly, patients present dramatically, with severe dyspnea and hypotension, in the presence of tension hydrothorax. In patients with fevers and pleuritic chest pain, infection of the pleural fluid needs to be excluded; its incidence in patients with hepatic hydrothorax is 13%.

Spontaneous bacterial empyema is defined as a PMN count greater than 500 cells/mm^3 or a positive bacterial culture in the absence of parapneumonic effusion. Like most bacterial infections in patients with cirrhosis, It is associated with a high mortality rate of 20% despite therapy. Spontaneous bacterial empyema should be promptly treated with antibiotics (Ceftriaxone 1–2 g daily) to cover organisms such as *E. coli*, *Streptococcus*, *Enterococcus*, *Klebsiella*, and *Pseudomonas*. After an effusion is recognized on chest radiography in a cirrhotic patient, especially when there has been a change in clinical status, a diagnostic thoracentesis should be performed with analysis of fluid cell count, pH, Gram stain, culture, protein, and lactate dehydrogenase. Hepatic hydrothorax is typically transudative in nature. In the absence of infection, white cells should be scarce, fewer than 500 cells/mm^3 (PMNs <250 cells/mm^3); pH greater than 7.4; and total protein less than 2.5 g/dL. If atypical features of hepatic hydrothorax cause concern, such as an exclusively left-sided effusion, other nonhepatic causes of pleural effusion (e.g., pleural infection, congestive cardiac failure) need to be excluded. A confirmatory test for hepatic hydrothorax is the nuclear-tagged colloid albumin study. If hepatic hydrothorax is the source of pleural fluid, the nuclear-tagged albumin injected in the peritoneum should migrate and be identified in the thoracic cavity in the study. Alternative diagnoses should be sought if the tracer does not demonstrate this behavior.

The management of hepatic hydrothorax in essence is similar to management of ascites, as discussed earlier. For severely symptomatic patients and those whose disease is refractory to diuretics, frequent therapeutic thoracentesis is necessary. A need for frequent thoracentesis in a patient who is compliant with medical therapy should lead to consideration of TIPS, which is effective in up to 80% of patients with hepatic hydrothorax. The usual considerations regarding TIPS in any patient need to be addressed.

Indwelling chest tubes should not be used, because they frequently lead to complications, including protein and electrolyte loss, infection, and fistula formation. Pleurodesis is ineffective in ablating the space between the parietal and the visceral pleura in patients with hepatic hydrothorax, and it can be associated with a variety of complications (e.g., fever, empyema, chest pain, pneumonia, incomplete expansion). Surgical repair of diaphragmatic defects has been reported in small case series, but clearly this is a major undertaking in a patient with decompensated cirrhosis.

Hepatocellular Carcinoma

HCC is one of the most common fatal malignancies worldwide, with a rising incidence in the United States reflecting the disease burden of the hepatitis C and B viruses as well as an increasing incidence of

HCC related to nonalcoholic steatohepatitis. The incidence of HCC in patients with cirrhosis is 1% to 4% per year.

The diagnosis is increasingly made radiologically. If two imaging techniques show that a mass in a cirrhotic liver (excluding patients with hepatitis B) has the characteristic features of HCC, with an arterial blood supply and rapid washout, a confident diagnosis can be made. An α-fetoprotein (AFP) level greater than 200 ng/mL is specific for HCC, although AFP is not produced in up to 40% of HCCs, limiting the sensitivity of this test. A radiographically guided biopsy of the mass may be necessary if noninvasive testing is inconclusive.

The prognosis and treatment of HCC are related to tumor stage, liver function, and the patient's performance status. Surgical resection or ablative therapy is an initial option for those with Child-Pugh grade A cirrhosis, a single mass smaller than 5 cm, a normal bilirubin level, and no portal hypertension. Liver transplantation is effective treatment, especially for patients who meet the Milan criteria (HCC with up to three tumors not more than 3 cm in size or one tumor not larger than 5 cm), provided that there is no vascular invasion of the tumors and no metastasis. Transplantation within the Milan criteria results in long-term survival equivalent to that seen in cirrhotic patients without HCC. Although these patients are given priority for liver transplantation, they may be undergo ethanol or radiofrequency ablation if the waiting time will be longer than 6 months, in an effort to prevent tumor progression while awaiting transplantation.

Transarterial chemoembolization may prolong survival in patients who are believed not to be candidates for resection or transplantation, and it can lead to a modest increase in survival time. For symptomatic patients with inoperable tumors and marginal liver function, survival is poor, and systemic chemotherapy is of little value, although sorafenib (a tyrosine kinase inhibitor) has shown some survival benefit compared with supportive care alone.

In order to detect and treat HCC at an early stage, screening and surveillance strategies are recommended. The following groups of patients are at high risk for HCC and should be in a surveillance program (Box 2 and Box 3): Asian males who are carriers of the hepatitis

B virus (HBV) and are 40 years of age or older; Asian female HBV carriers who are 50 years of age or older; all cirrhotic HBV carriers with a family history of HCC or cirrhosis of any etiology. Patients deemed to be at increased risk of HCC should be screened with twice-yearly ultrasound and measurement of AFP. If there is reason to suspect development of an HCC, such as rising AFP levels despite absence of a mass on ultrasound, additional abdominal imaging with magnetic resonance imaging or contrast computed tomography is necessary.

Vaccination

Cirrhotic patients have increased morbidity and mortality if they contract viral or bacterial infections. All patients with chronic liver disease should be vaccinated against hepatitis A virus (HAV), HBV, pneumococcus, and influenza. At initial evaluation for chronic liver disease, total hepatitis A antibody and total hepatitis B core antibody should be ordered to determine preexisting immunity against HAV and HBV, and appropriate vaccines should be administered to nonimmune patients.

Osteopenia

The prevalence of osteopenia is high in patients with chronic liver disease, and there is a particularly high risk of osteoporosis in patients with primary biliary cirrhosis, primary sclerosing cholangitis, hepatitis C, or alcoholic liver disease. Management of osteopenia can reduce morbidity before and after transplantation. All transplantation candidates should undergo screening for bone mineral density by dual-energy x-ray absorptiometry (DEXA), initially and repeated every 1 to 2 years. Hypothyroidism and disordered calcium and vitamin D metabolism should be excluded, and regular exercise should be encouraged. Concern about gastrointestinal irritation and bleeding from use of the oral bisphosphonates can be obviated by parenteral administration.

Liver Transplantation

With improvements in immunosuppression, surgical techniques, anesthesia, prophylaxis of common posttransplantation infections, and patient selection, liver transplantation has become the definitive intervention for decompensated cirrhosis, acute liver failure, and a subset of unresectable hepatic malignancies. Mean 1-year and 3-year survival rates after transplantation in the United States are about 90% and 80%, respectively. Liver transplantation should be considered once a cirrhotic patient has an index complication such as onset of ascites, and a timely referral should be made before the patient becomes debilitated from recurrent complications of cirrhosis.

The most common indication for transplantation is decompensated cirrhosis (Box 4). Other important indications are HCC, acute liver failure, and metabolic liver disease. Most donor organs come from brain-dead donors and are allocated based on the severity of liver disease in the potential recipient. The organ allocation system is now based on the MELD score (see earlier discussion), which ranges from 6 to 40 (Fig. 1). The higher the MELD score, the lower the likelihood that the patient will be alive 3 months later, and the higher the patient's rank on the transplant list. Other determinants regarding allocation of organs are blood type, the patient's weight, and waiting time (for patients with identical MELD scores). Patients with fulminant hepatic failure, posttransplantation primary graft nonfunction, and hepatic artery thrombosis are given highest priority, independent of MELD. Only a few conditions (e.g., HCC HPS) make patients eligible for higher MELD scores (priority), because reduced waiting times for those patients would be likely to increase mortality in other patients due to the finite supply of donor organs. The most frequent example of this situation is the cirrhotic patient with well-preserved hepatocellular function and a low MELD score

---

BOX 2 Surveillance for Hepatocellular Carcinoma in High-Risk Patients: Hepatitis B Carriers*

Asian males ≥40 years of age
Asian females ≥50 years of age
All cirrhotic hepatitis B carriers
Family history of hepatocellular carcinoma
Africans >20 years of age

*For noncirrhotic hepatitis B carriers not listed here, surveillance is based on disease activity and clinical judgment.

BOX 3 Surveillance for Hepatocellular Carcinoma in High-Risk Patients: Non-Hepatitis Carriers

Hepatitis C
Alcoholic cirrhosis
Genetic hemochromatosis
Primary biliary cirrhosis
Consider surveillance based on disease activity and clinical judgment:
  α₁-Antitrypsin deficiency
  Nonalcoholic steatohepatitis
  Autoimmune hepatitis

Adapted from Bruix J, Sherman M; Practice Guidelines Committee, American Association for the Study of Liver Diseases: Management of hepatocellular carcinoma. Hepatology 2005;42:1208–1236.

BOX 4   Indications for Liver Transplantation

Chronic noncholestatic liver disorders (decompensated
   disease)
Chronic hepatitis C
Chronic hepatitis B
Autoimmune hepatitis
Alcoholic liver disease
Cholestatic liver disorders (decompensated disease)
Primary biliary cirrhosis
Primary sclerosing cholangitis
Biliary atresia
Alagille's syndrome
Non-syndromic paucity of the intrahepatic bile ducts
Cystic fibrosis
Progressive familial intrahepatic cholestasis
Metabolic disorders causing cirrhosis
α_1-Antitrypsin deficiency
Wilson's disease
Nonalcoholic steatohepatitis and cryptogenic cirrhosis
Hereditary hemochromatosis
Tyrosinemia
Glycogen storage disease type IV
Neonatal hemochromatosis
Metabolic disorders causing severe extrahepatic
   morbidity
Amyloidosis
Hyperoxaluria
Urea cycle defects
Disorders of branched-chain amino acids
Primary malignancies of the liver
Hepatocellular carcinoma
Hepatoblastoma
Fibrolamellar hepatocellular carcinoma
Hemangioendothelioma
Fulminant hepatic failure
Miscellaneous conditions
Budd-Chiari syndrome
Metastatic neuroendocrine tumors
Polycystic disease
Retransplantation

Adapted from Murray KF, Carithers RL Jr: AASLD practice
guidelines: Evaluation of the patient for liver transplantation.
Hepatology 2005;41:1407–1432.

BOX 5   Contraindications for Liver Transplantation

Absolute:
Irreversible severe cardiopulmonary disease
Extrahepatic malignancy
Active substance abuse
Morbid obesity
Relative (varies by transplant center and experience):
   Age
   HIV
   Irreversible brain damage

whose indication for liver transplant is an HCC that meets Milan criteria. The organ allocation system under these circumstances awards extra MELD points to expedite transplantation, hopefully before metastatic spread has occurred. Specific etiologies of liver disease may be eligible for the highest priority for listing (status 1). An example is Wilson's disease with an acute presentation, because copper chelating therapy is ineffective and may even lead to further deterioration. Any patient with acute liver failure with onset of hepatic encephalopathy within 26 weeks after recognition of liver disease of any etiology is also eligible for status 1.

Expansion of the organ donor pool to reduce deaths on the waiting list for transplantation has been possible with live donor transplantation, in which a healthy adult donates a major portion of his or her liver to another adult (right lobe) or to a child (left lobe). This remains a somewhat controversial approach because of the risk to the donor, especially with right lobe donation, because of the larger volume of hepatic tissue required for an adult patient.

There are several important contraindications in liver transplantation (Box 5). Irreversible brain damage, as frequently occurs due to cerebral edema in acute liver failure, and advanced cardiopulmonary disease are absolute contraindications. PPHTN is not an absolute contraindication unless mean pulmonary pressures are greater than 50 mm Hg. In HPS, a Pa_{O_2} of less than 50 mm Hg and a pulmonary artery shunt fraction greater than 30% are contraindications, because they are associated with a high mortality rate after transplantation. Extrahepatic malignancy or a history of malignancy with a disease-free period of less than 2 years, uncontrolled infection, and active alcohol intake or substance abuse are all contraindications. HIV infection is not a contraindication as long as it is well controlled on antiretroviral therapy. Advanced age is a relative contraindication, but biologic rather than chronologic age is more pertinent, with particular attention to key comorbidities such as cardiovascular disease and diabetes mellitus.

The transplantation evaluation process typically involves a multidisciplinary team. Key components of the evaluation consist of separate medical and surgical evaluations; assessment of the severity of comorbid medical conditions, if any; identification of psychosocial aspects requiring intervention; and determination of financial and insurance status. Other important issues, such as the patient's willingness to undergo transplantation, a history of compliance with medical care, and the availability of a dependable support network, are also evaluated. In patients with a history of drug or alcohol abuse, a commitment to long-term sobriety and a drug-free lifestyle is an important prerequisite for acceptance for transplantation. The management of complications of cirrhosis is challenging. Given the disparity between supply and demand for donor organs, physicians care for increasingly tenuous cirrhotic patients. Anticipation and prevention of complications of end-stage liver disease affect the ability of cirrhotic patients to survive until liver transplantation and to enjoy its benefits.

REFERENCES

Arroyo V, Fernandez J, Ginès P. Pathogenesis and treatment of hepatorenal syndrome. Semin Liver Dis 2008;28(1):81–95.
Boyer TD, Haskal ZJ. The role of transjugular intrahepatic portosystemic shunt in the management of portal hypertension. Hepatology 2005;41(2):386–400.

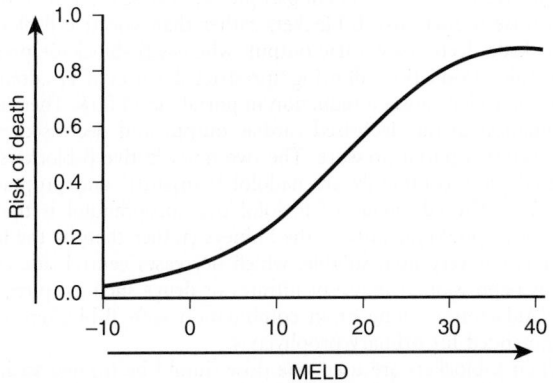

FIGURE 1. The Model for End-State Liver Disease (MELD) score predicts the risk of death over 3 months. See text for details.

Bruix J, Hessheimer AJ, Forner A, et al. New aspects of diagnosis and therapy of hepatocellular carcinoma. Oncogene 2006;25(27):3848–56.

Cárdenas A, Arroyo V. Management of ascites and hepatic hydrothorax. Best Pract Res Clin Gastroenterol 2007;21(1):55–75.

Golbin JM, Krowka MJ. Portopulmonary hypertension. Clin Chest Med 2007;28(1):203–18.

Lopez PM, Martin P. Update on liver transplantation: Indications, organ allocation, and long-term care. Mt Sinai J Med 2006;73(8):1056–66.

Mandell MS. The diagnosis and treatment of hepatopulmonary syndrome. Clin Liver Dis 2006;10(2):387–405.

Morgan MY, Blei A, Grüngreiff K, et al. The treatment of hepatic encephalopathy. Metab Brain Dis 2007;22(3–4):389–405.

Runyon BA. Management of adult patients with ascites due to cirrhosis. Hepatology 2004;39(3):841–56.

Bleeding Esophageal Varices

Method of
Vijay H. Shah, MD, and Patrick S. Kamath, MD

The three major and potentially fatal complications of portal hypertension are gastrointestinal (GI) bleeding from gastroesophageal varices, ascites, and hepatic encephalopathy. Of these, hemorrhage from varices is the most dramatic presentation. The prognosis of patients with variceal bleeding has improved over the past decade, with the risk of mortality at 1 week being approximately 5% to 8% and at 6 weeks approximately 20%.

Variceal Bleeding: Scope of the Problem

Upper GI endoscopy is currently the gold standard used to detect varices. Although computed tomography, ultrasound, and magnetic resonance imaging can detect consequences of portal hypertension and varices, they are currently not accurate enough to detect all large varices. Similarly, platelet counts, splenomegaly, or hypoalbuminemia are unreliable as markers to target patients at risk for large varices. Endoscopic ultrasound is still considered an investigational tool in the diagnosis of portal hypertension.

There are numerous causes of portal hypertension. In the Western world, the most common cause of portal hypertension is cirrhosis but worldwide, schistosomiasis could be the most common cause of portal hypertension. Portal venous thrombosis and idiopathic portal hypertension are more common in the Far East.

Esophageal varices are present in about 40% of patients with cirrhosis. However, in patients with cirrhotic ascites, varices are detected in about 60% of patients. The prevalence of large varices in patients with cirrhosis is approximately 20%, and these patients have a 30% risk of bleeding from varices within 2 years. Because of the high risk of mortality from bleeding varices, it is recommended that all patients with cirrhosis be screened for varices with upper GI endoscopy so that prophylactic therapy can be initiated. If no varices are noted on the initial endoscopy, then a repeat endoscopy should be performed in 2 to 3 years. If small varices are noted at the initial endoscopy, then a repeat endoscopy should be performed in 1 to 2 years.

In the presence of variceal bleeding, spontaneous control is seen in about one half of patients. Hypovolemia that occurs as a result of hypotension and splanchnic vasoconstriction results in a decrease in portal pressure, which results in control of bleeding. Excessive transfusions, therefore, might result in an increased risk of bleeding.

In patients in whom bleeding has been controlled, rebleeding occurs in about one third of patients within the first 6 weeks, and approximately 40% of these episodes occur within the first 5 days. The risk of rebleeding and risk of mortality are related to the degree of liver dysfunction.

CURRENT DIAGNOSIS

- Upper gastrointestinal endoscopy is the gold standard for diagnosis of varices.
- Large esophageal varices that are at risk of bleeding are present in approximately 20% of all patients with cirrhosis.
- Ultrasonography, computed tomography, and magnetic resonance imaging may be less accurate than endoscopy in detecting varices.
- Measurement of portal pressure is the most accurate method of determining which patients are at risk for variceal bleeding.
- Bleeding esophageal varices should be suspected in all patients with gastrointestinal bleeding and jaundice, ascites, and other stigmata of liver disease.

Because of the high risk of morbidity and mortality with a variceal bleed, significant effort needs to be made to prevent initial bleeding (primary prophylaxis), control the acute variceal bleed, and prevent rebleeding from varices (secondary prophylaxis).

Treatment

Portal hypertension results from an increase in resistance to portal blood flow, along with an increase in portal blood flow. Therefore, treatment of portal hypertension is aimed either at reducing portal blood flow with pharmacologic agents like β-blockers or vasopressin and its analogues or by decreasing intrahepatic resistance. At this time, there are no effective drugs that decrease intrahepatic resistance. The major method of reducing intrahepatic resistance is by creating a surgical portosystemic shunt or a radiologic portosystemic shunt (transjugular intrahepatic portosystemic shunt [TIPS]). Bleeding from the varices can be controlled directly by endoscopic methods.

PREVENTION OF FIRST BLEED (PRIMARY PROPHYLAXIS)

Currently, pharmacologic treatment of all cirrhosis patients with the goal of preventing the development of esophageal varices is not recommended. In the absence of such contraindications as significant comorbidity, all patients with large varices—varices larger than 5 mm in diameter on endoscopy—should receive prophylaxis against variceal bleeding. Patients with smaller varices but with more advanced liver disease (Child–Pugh class C) may also receive prophylactic treatment.

The two current modalities used to prevent variceal bleeding are nonselective β-blockers and endoscopic variceal ligation. It is important to use nonselective β-blockers rather than selective β-blockers. $β_1$-blockade decreases cardiac output, whereas $β_2$-blockade prevents splanchnic vasodilation, allowing unrestricted action of $α_1$-adrenergic receptors, which causes a reduction in portal blood flow. Therefore, a combination of the decreased cardiac output and decreased portal flow decreases portal pressure. The two nonselective β-blockers that are used most commonly are nadolol (Corgard)[1] and propranolol (Inderal).[1] The advantage of nadolol over propranolol is that the excretion is predominantly in the kidneys (rather than by the liver), and it is not very lipid soluble, which decreases central side effects such as depression. The use of nitrates or drugs such as spironolactone (Aldactone)[1] alone or in combination with β-blockers is not recommended for primary prophylaxis.

When β-blockers are used, the dose should be titrated such that the resting heart rate decreases by about 25%, or to about 55 to

---

[1]Not FDA approved for this indication.

60 bpm, provided the systolic blood pressure remains greater than 90 mm Hg. Long-acting preparations of propranolol[1] are preferred and may be started in a dose of 60 mg daily. If nadolol[1] is used, the initial dose is 20 mg once daily. The medications are best administered in the evening. The dose of propranolol or nadolol is gradually increased every 3 to 5 days until the target reduction in heart rate is reached. It is possible to increase the dose even further if patients continue to tolerate treatment. The typical dose of long-acting propranolol or nadolol required to reach target heart rates ranges between 40 and 160 mg daily.

In patients on pharmacologic therapy, there is no need for follow-up endoscopy. In general, if only patients with large varices are selected for prophylactic treatment, approximately six patients require treatment to prevent one variceal bleed. However, approximately 22 patients need to be treated to prevent one death. If patients tolerate the medications and have no further bleeding, then the medication is continued indefinitely.

Prophylactic endoscopic injection sclerotherapy is no longer recommended as primary prophylaxis against variceal hemorrhage in view of the significant complications. Endoscopic variceal ligation is the preferred modality and is as effective as β-blockers. Endoscopic variceal ligation is carried out at 2- to 4-week intervals until the varices are obliterated.

Because of ease of use and probable lower costs, pharmacologic therapy with β-blockers is considered the first-line treatment for preventing variceal bleeding. In patients who have contraindications to β-blockers, who are intolerant to β-blockers, or in whom β-blockers are not effective in preventing variceal bleeding, then endoscopic therapy is recommended.

An algorithm on how to approach primary prophylaxis is given in Figure 1.

---

[1]Not FDA approved for this indication.

 CURRENT THERAPY

- Upper endoscopy is recommended to screen for esophageal varices in all patients with cirrhosis who are candidates for prophylactic therapy. If no varices are seen at initial endoscopy, a repeat endoscopy is recommended in 2 to 3 years. If small varices are noted at initial endoscopy, a repeat endoscopy is recommended in 1 to 2 years.
- Patients with large varices and patients with Child–Pugh class C cirrhosis and small varices may be considered for primary prophylactic therapy.
- Either nonselective β-blockers or endoscopic variceal ligation may be used to prevent esophageal variceal bleeding, although β-blockers are preferred (primary prophylaxis).
- Endoscopic therapy combined with vasoactive drugs and antibiotics form the mainstay of treatment of bleeding esophageal varices.
- Patients with acute bleeding require prompt resuscitation. The target for red cell transfusion is a hematocrit of 24%.
- When bleeding cannot be controlled in spite of two sessions of endoscopic therapy, placement of a transjugular intrahepatic portosystemic shunt (TIPS) is recommended.
- Secondary prophylaxis is best carried out with a combination of β-blockers and endoscopic variceal ligation.
- TIPS is carried out when patients continue to bleed in spite of the use of both variceal ligation and β-blockers as secondary prophylaxis.

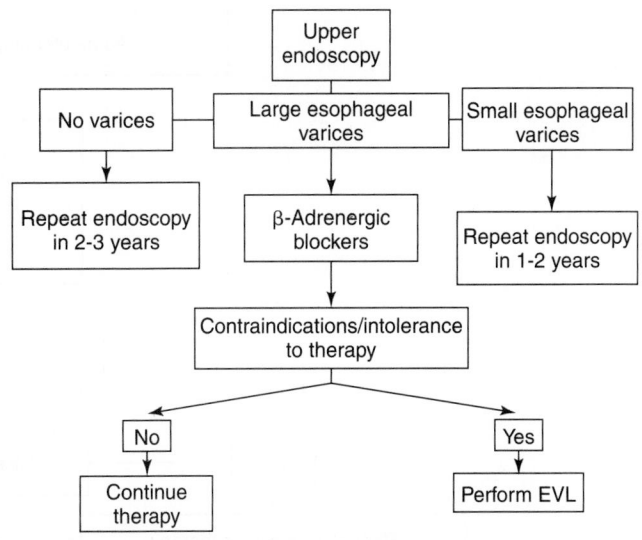

FIGURE 1. Algorithm for primary prophylaxis of esophageal variceal hemorrhage. EVL, endoscopic variceal ligation.

CONTROL OF ACUTE ESOPHAGEAL VARICEAL BLEEDING

It cannot be overemphasized that controlling acute variceal bleeding is a team effort because of the high risk of morbidity and mortality in these patients. Variceal bleeding is ideally carried out by a team of hepatologists, endoscopists, intensive care physicians, radiologists, and hepatobiliary surgeons.

The goals of treatment are to resuscitate the patient, control the acute bleeding episode, prevent complications, and prevent rebleeding. It is recommended that the patient have two large-bore intravenous lines placed immediately on arrival to the emergency department. Red blood cells should be transfused as required to provide a hematocrit of no greater than 24% (hemoglobin of 8 g/dL). Until red blood cells are available for transfusion, normal saline may be used for resuscitation. If there is active bleeding, endotracheal intubation is mandatory.

All patients with cirrhosis and GI bleeding, even in the absence of ascites, should receive prophylactic antibiotics with norfloxacin (Noroxin) 400 mg twice daily for 7 days. If patients have ascites, then a diagnostic paracentesis needs to be carried out before initiating therapy with norfloxacin. This is because some of these patients might have spontaneous bacterial peritonitis, which is better treated with cefotaxime (Claforan) 2 g every 12 hours for 5 days rather than oral norfloxacin. If oral ingestion of antibiotics is not possible, then intravenous antibiotics such as ciprofloxacin (Cipro) or levofloxacin (Levaquin) should be used. The recent reduction in mortality with variceal bleeding is believed to be related to the use of antibiotics.

Pharmacologic therapy should be started as early as possible. Terlipressin[8] is the only vasoactive drug that has been associated with improved survival, but this drug is not currently available in the United States. Octreotide (Sandostatin)[1] is the agent most commonly used in the United States, although the efficacy in such situations is still debatable. It is generally recommended that pharmacologic treatment be continued for up to 5 days to prevent early rebleeding. Octreotide is generally infused intravenously in a dose of 50 μg/hour following a bolus of 50 μg. Side effects with octreotide are few, but hyperglycemia and abdominal discomfort can occur. The most serious side effects are cardiac dysrhythmias, including sinus bradycardia.

Once the vasoactive drug has been infused for about 30 minutes, the patient is hemodynamically stable, and endotracheal intubation has been carried out if the patient has active bleeding, upper endoscopy may be carried out. At upper endoscopy, the actively bleeding

---

[1]Not FDA approved for this indication.
[8]Orphan drug in the United States.

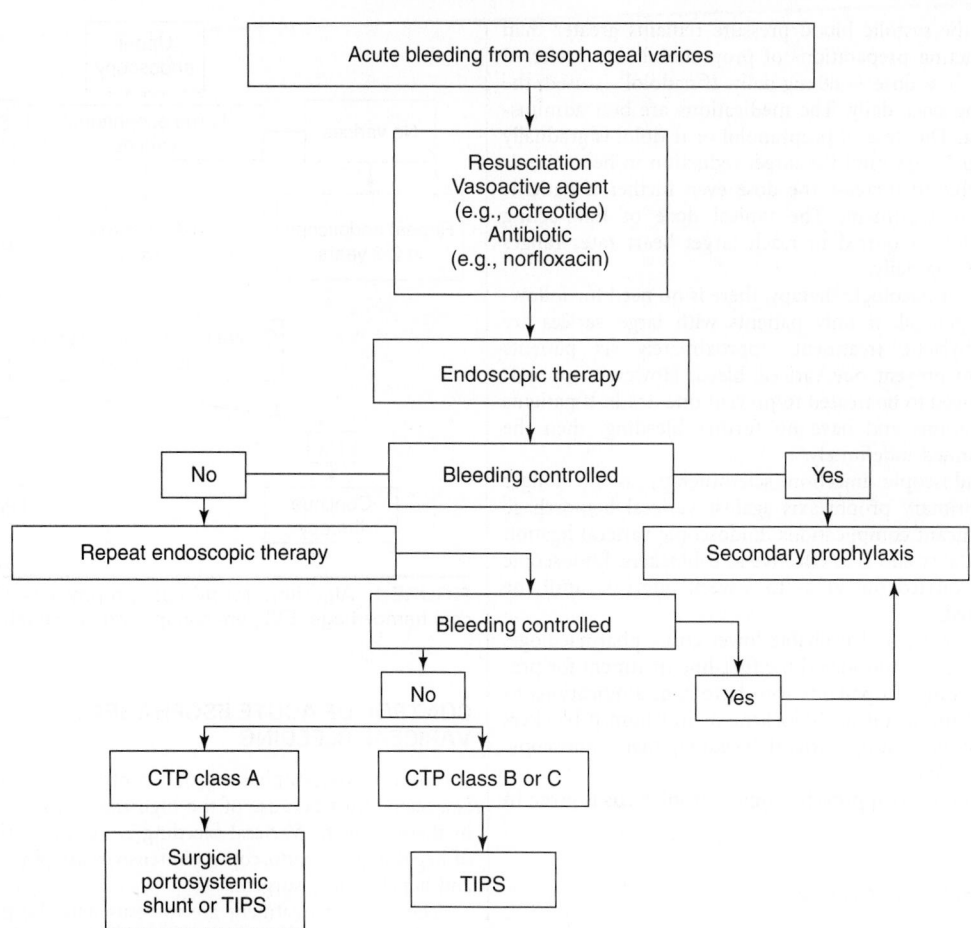

FIGURE 2. Algorithm for managing bleeding esophageal varices. CTP = Child–Turcotte–Pugh, TIPS = transjugular intrahepatic portosystemic shunt.

varix is ligated. Other large varices can also be ligated at the same session. Following endoscopic ligation, most experts use proton pump inhibitors to prevent the development of variceal ligation ulcers, although there are insufficient data to support this recommendation.

In about 10% of patients, bleeding cannot be controlled in spite of all these measures. Failure to control bleeding is defined usually by the requirement of greater than four units of red blood cells to maintain the hematocrit at about 24%. In such patients, a repeat endoscopy may be carried out within 24 hours. However, if in spite of two endoscopic sessions within a 24-hour period bleeding has not been controlled, then a TIPS may be carried out by an interventional radiologist. Unfortunately, mortality in this group is high.

The algorithm for control of acute variceal bleeding is given in Figure 2.

PREVENTION OF VARICEAL REBLEEDING (SECONDARY PROPHYLAXIS)

Initiation of secondary prophylaxis is important, because up to 80% of all patients who have a variceal bleed will rebleed within 2 years without such measures. Patients with a Child–Pugh score of 7 should be referred for evaluation for liver transplantation.

Variceal bleeding can be prevented by using pharmacologic agents, endoscopic therapy, TIPS, or surgical portosystemic shunts.

Usually, a combination of endoscopic therapy (endoscopic variceal ligation and nonselective β-blockers) is initiated to prevent variceal bleeding. The combination is superior to either modality alone.

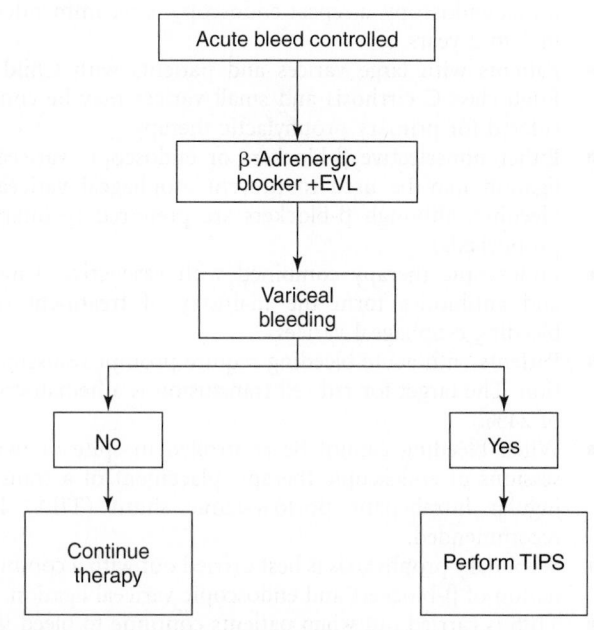

FIGURE 3. Algorithm for preventing recurrent bleeding from esophageal varices (secondary prophylaxis). EVL = endoscopic variceal ligation; TIPS = transjugular intrahepatic portosystemic shunt.

However, endoscopic therapy alone may be used in patients with contraindications or intolerance to β-blockers. The ideal interval between sessions of endoscopic variceal ligation is not clear, but it usually ranges between 2 and 4 weeks. Nonselective β-blockers alone may be used in patients who find it difficult to return frequently for endoscopic treatment. Whereas isosorbide mononitrate (Imdur),[1] when added to β-blockers, can make pharmacologic treatment more effective, it is unusual for most patients to tolerate nitrates after they have been adequately β-blocked.

If patients have variceal rebleeding in spite of receiving a combination of endoscopic and pharmacologic treatments (β-blockers and endoscopic variceal ligation), then a portosystemic shunt is considered. A TIPS is the shunt most widely used because of limited availability of surgical expertise and lower procedure related morbidity. A surgical shunt is recommended only in patients who have good liver function as determined by Child–Pugh class A.

The algorithm for secondary prophylaxis is given in Figure 3.

REFERENCES

D'Amico G, Garcia-Pagan JC, Luca A, Bosch J. Hepatic vein pressure gradient reduction and prevention of variceal bleeding in cirrhosis: A systematic review. Gastroenterology 2006;131(5):1611–24.

Garcia-Pagan JC, Bosch J. Endoscopic band ligation in the treatment of portal hypertension. Nat Clin Pract Gastroenterol Hepatol 2005;2(11):526–35.

Garcia-Tsao G. Portal hypertension. Curr Opin Gastroenterol 2006;22(3):254–62.

Henderson JM. Surgery versus transjugular intrahepatic portal systemic shunt in the treatment of severe variceal bleeding. Clin Liver Dis 2006; 10(3):599–612.

Kamath PS, Shah V. Does nadolol improve the efficacy of endoscopic variceal ligation in the treatment of variceal bleeding? Nat Clin Pract Gastroenterol Hepatol 2005;2(6):254–5.

Longacre AV, Garcia-Tsao G. A commonsense approach to esophageal varices. Clin Liver Dis 2006;10(3):613–25.

Shah VH, Kamath PS. Portal hypertension and gastrointestinal bleeding. In: Feldman LS, Friedman LS, Brandt LJ, editors. Sleisenger & Fordtran's Gastrointestinal and Liver Disease: Pathophysiology, Diagnosis, Management, 8th ed. vol. 2. Philadelphia: Saunders; 2006. p. 1899–934.

Zaman A. Portal hypertension-related bleeding: Management of difficult cases. Clin Liver Dis 2006;10(2):353–70.

Zaman A, Chalasani N. Bleeding caused by portal hypertension. Gastroenterol Clin North Am 2005;34(4):623–42.

---

[1]Not FDA approved for this indication.

Dysphagia and Esophageal Obstruction

Method of
Philip O. Katz, MD, and Girish Anand, MD

Dysphagia refers to a subjective sensation of the delayed passage of food from the mouth through the esophagus to the stomach. It derives its origin from Greek *dys* meaning "difficulty" and *phagia* meaning "eat."

Dysphagia has been reported in about 2% of healthy adults older than 65 years. The incidence increases to 12% to 13% in the hospitalized elderly. Dysphagia has been reported in about 50% to 60% of patients in nursing homes and other chronic care facilities.

There may be associated pain with swallowing (odynophagia) if there is coexistent inflammation. Most patients describe dysphagia as a feeling of food getting "stuck" or "not going down right." The history plays an important role in understanding the anatomic location and the severity of the symptoms. Key questions like the exact location where the food is getting stuck, associated regurgitation, types of foods causing dysphagia, and presence of weight loss or heartburn are crucial in assessing the symptom of dysphagia.

Pathophysiology

In the swallowing process, the oropharyngeal and esophageal phases transport solid or liquid boluses rapidly from the mouth to the stomach. *Primary peristalsis* is the classic coordinated motor pattern of the esophagus, combined with almost simultaneous upper and lower esophageal sphincter relaxation initiated by the act of swallowing. The food bolus is transferred by a progressive pharyngeal contraction through the relaxed upper esophageal sphincter (UES) into the esophagus. The UES closure is followed by a progressive circular contraction beginning in the upper esophagus and proceeding distally along the esophageal body to propel the bolus through the relaxed lower esophageal sphincter (LES), which subsequently closes with a prolonged contraction.

Secondary peristalsis is a progressive contraction in the esophageal body occurring in response to its distention by stimulation of sensory receptors in the esophageal body. It usually begins at or above a level corresponding to the location of the stimulus and is limited to the esophagus. A local intramural mechanism can at times take over as a reserve mechanism to produce peristalsis in the smooth muscle segment of the esophagus. This has been called *tertiary peristalsis*.

Any problem with either the strength or coordination of the musculature causes difficulty with movement of food, leading to obstruction. Similarly, any narrowing in the path of transit causes obstruction and distention of the lumen, leading to the sensation of dysphagia. The motility abnormalities might not be constant, thus giving intermittent dysphagia. The extent of luminal obstruction guides the diagnosis. Partial obstruction might initially give only solid food dysphagia related to large food boluses (e.g., steak). When the extent of obstruction progresses to near total occlusion, the symptoms involve both solid and liquid dysphagia. The extent of associated inflammation (esophagitis) determines whether or not odynophagia is an associated symptom.

Diagnosis

A careful history helps to localize the site of abnormality, and this forms the basis of further work-up. The evaluation of dysphagia begins with a complete history. A problem initiating a swallow and associated coughing or choking indicates a more proximal or oropharyngeal cause for the symptoms. Pure solid food dysphagia suggests a structural lesion, stricture, ring, or malignancy. A problem initially with solids progressing later to liquids suggests a benign or malignant stricture.

Rapidly progressive dysphagia is concerning for malignancy. The presence of other medical problems such as stroke or scleroderma might point to a systemic cause of the symptoms. A careful history of medications is important, because many drugs have been implicated in pill esophagitis and can cause dysphagia as well as odynophagia. The history can also differentiate dysphagia from globus sensation (feeling of a lump in the throat), which has a different evaluation from dysphagia.

Dysphagia for all practical purposes can be classified into oropharyngeal and esophageal dysphagia.

OROPHARYNGEAL DYSPHAGIA

Difficulty in transferring a food bolus from the hypopharyngeal area to the esophageal body across the upper esophageal sphincter gives rise to the suspicion of oropharyngeal or transfer dysphagia. Several clues in the patient's history help to establish the cause.

The onset of symptoms in oropharyngeal dysphagia is almost immediate. The patient describes the feeling of choking or coughing on initiation of swallowing and frequently points to the cervical region as the site of dysphagia. Patients might describe regurgitation of food, aspiration, or halitosis, which can point to a structural abnormality such as a Zenker's diverticulum.

Patients might have to resort to certain physical maneuvers, such as extending their arms and neck and using their fingers to move the bolus. There may be associated speech abnormalities such as hoarseness, nasal quality, or dysarthria, which points to a neuromuscular cause for the oropharyngeal dysphagia. The various causes of oropharyngeal dysphagia are listed in Box 1.

CURRENT DIAGNOSIS

- Differentiate between oropharyngeal and esophageal dysphagia.
- Pure solid food dysphagia implies a mechanical (obstructive) cause.
- Mixed solid and liquid dysphagia suggests functional (motility) abnormality.
- Eosinophilic esophagitis should be considered in any patient with dysphagia.
- Barium swallow (with solid bolus) and endoscopy are complementary.
- Esophageal function testing (manometry) should be performed for nonobstructive dysphagia.

In patients with oropharyngeal dysphagia, the oral cavity, head, and neck should be carefully examined. Special attention should be paid to the neurologic examination, especially the nerves involved in the act of swallowing, namely cranial nerves V, VII, IX, X, XI, and XII. Clues in the physical examination might suggest polymyositis or dermatomyositis as the cause of symptoms.

Video fluoroscopy (barium swallow) is a good first test that permits visualization of the swallowing mechanism. It can identify aspiration, pooling, and abnormal motor activities. This examination concentrates on the cervical esophageal region. A barium swallow can delineate the anatomic anomalies and also can show the remainder of the esophagus. The study starts with liquid barium, progressing to a solid phase. Different consistencies of food are used to assess the oropharynx, UES, and proximal esophagus.

A structural abnormality found on the barium examination generally requires an endoscopy for confirmation or treatment. Endoscopy is not the first test to use to evaluate oropharyngeal dysphagia, because the chances of missing an abnormality in the upper part of esophagus are higher than in the distal esophagus.

A nasopharyngeal laryngoscopy performed by the otolaryngologist provides detailed information of the hypopharynx, larynx, and oropharynx. It also allows a clear visualization of the vocal cords, valleculae, and the pyriform sinuses to assess any pooling of secretions.

Patients with oropharyngeal dysphagia who have an unrevealing barium study or endoscopy might need an esophageal manometry study with careful attention to the UES. Incoordination between UES opening and pharyngeal contractions can cause relaxation (opening) or shortening opening may be associated with dysphagia as well.

Zenker's diverticulum is an outpouching of the mucosa through an area of muscular weakness between the transverse fibers of the cricopharyngeus and the oblique fibers of the lower inferior constrictor. These generally occur in older adults and can show symptoms of pulmonary aspirations, gurgling, or regurgitation. Rarely, they become large enough to manifest as a mass and even cause esophageal obstruction.

ESOPHAGEAL DYSPHAGIA

Esophageal dysphagia occurs either from mechanical or motility causes. The abnormality lies within the body of the esophagus or the lower esophageal sphincter. Patients often complain of symptoms localizing to the upper epigastric region or lower sternum although the association is less significant than in oropharyngeal dysphagia. The type of food producing symptoms and its temporal progression help to identify the cause of symptoms. Dysphagia progressing from solids to liquids usually indicates a mechanical cause, and dysphagia to both solids and liquids from the outset favors a motility disorder. Symptoms of associated heartburn, weight loss, anemia, and regurgitation further narrow the differential diagnosis. Other medical conditions such as radiation therapy and medication use may be associated with dysphagia, as may infectious esophagitis. Both are often associated with odynophagia as well. Opportunistic infections—especially in the setting of HIV disease and AIDS—such as candida, cytomegalovirus, and herpes virus, are the most common and can be managed adequately with medical therapy.

The various causes of esophageal dysphagia are listed in Box 2.

BOX 1 Causes of Oropharyngeal Dysphagia

Structural (Mechanical)
- Carcinoma
- Cervical and proximal esophageal webs
- Cricopharyngeal bar
- Osteophytes and other skeletal abnormalities
- Prior surgery or radiation therapy

Neuromuscular
- Amyotrophic lateral sclerosis
- Brainstem tumors
- Dermatomyositis, polymyositis
- Head trauma
- Idiopathic upper esophageal sphincter dysfunction
- Multiple sclerosis
- Myasthenia gravis
- Myotonic dystrophy
- Paraneoplastic syndromes
- Parkinson's disease
- Postpolio syndrome
- Sarcoidosis
- Stroke

Infection
- Botulism
- Diphtheria
- Lyme disease
- Syphilis

BOX 2 Causes of Esophageal Dysphagia

Structural (Mechanical)
Intrinsic
- Benign tumors
- Carcinoma: Adenocarcinoma and squamous cell cancer
- Diverticula
- Eosinophilic esophagitis
- Esophageal rings and webs: Schatzki's ring
- Foreign body
- Infections: Herpes, CMV, EBV, MAI, *Candida, Pneumocystis*
- Peptic strictures
- Pill esophagitis
- Radiation strictures or esophagitis

Extrinsic
- Cervical osteophytes
- Mediastinal masses
- Vascular compression: Dysphagia lusoria

Motility (Neuromuscular)
- Achalasia
- Diffuse esophageal spasm (DES)
- Hypertensive lower esophageal sphincter
- Ineffective esophageal motility disorder
- Nutcracker esophagus
- Secondary causes like scleroderma, Sjögren's syndrome, Chagas' disease

Functional
- Functional dysphagia

Abbreviations: CMV = cytomegalovirus; EBV = Epstein-Barr virus; MAI = *Mycobacterium avium-intracellulare.*

The most common initial diagnostic approach to esophageal dysphagia is to perform endoscopy. In addition to the diagnostic value, endoscopy affords an opportunity to obtain tissue samples and do therapeutic intervention. A barium swallow with a solid bolus challenge is a reasonable alternative, especially with patients in whom oropharyngeal causes are a possibility or when the history suggests a complex stricture or achalasia. An endoscopy is required if a structural abnormality is discovered on the barium study.

STRUCTURAL CAUSES

Patients reporting only solid food dysphagia typically have a mechanical cause for their symptoms. This can progress to both solid and liquid dysphagia in cases of a high-grade obstruction. These patients tend to develop food impaction and might regurgitate. Benign causes for these symptoms include an esophageal web or a distal esophageal ring. The rings, also called Schatzki's rings, are smooth, thin mucosal structures at the gastroesophageal junction covered by squamous mucosa above and columnar epithelium below. Muscular rings, on the other hand, are characterized by hypertrophic esophageal musculature and are generally located about 2 cm above the gastroesophageal junction. Nonprogressive, episodic dysphagia is a characteristic of esophageal rings. Dysphagia becomes prominent when the diameter is smaller than 13 mm. Rings can manifest with acute dysphagia associated with impaction of a piece of meat, often referred to as "steakhouse syndrome." Esophageal webs, often asymptomatic, have been associated with iron deficiency anemia (Plummer-Vinson syndrome).

Peptic strictures occur in 8% to 10% of patients with symptomatic gastroesophageal reflux disease (GERD). Peptic strictures are associated with a long duration of reflux symptoms, male sex, and older age. Symptoms of dysphagia occur when the luminal diameter narrows to 13 mm or less.

Radiation-related strictures or esophagitis are seen in persons undergoing radiotherapy for thoracic or head or neck tumors. In the acute setting esophagitis is the predominant finding and can progress to fibrosis and strictures in the chronic phase.

Malignancy is the primary concern in patients with rapidly progressive solid food dysphagia associated with weight loss and anorexia. The staging of esophageal cancer involves CT scanning of the chest and abdomen and endoscopic ultrasonography (EUS). EUS provides the most accurate estimate of disease stage and assists with management decisions. The 5-year survival rate for patients with advanced esophageal cancer continues to be less than 5%.

Eosinophilic esophagitis is seen more often as a cause of dysphagia, particularly in young adults. Extensive diffuse eosinophilic infiltration (>15 per high power field), particularly in the proximal esophagus, is seen. The disease can manifest for the first time as a food impaction requiring emergency endoscopic therapy. Feline esophagus, concentric mucosal rings, or ringed esophagus is the classic endoscopic description of eosinophilic esophagitis.

Pill-induced esophagitis has been shown to occur with a variety of medications including bisphosphonates, doxycycline, potassium chloride, quinidine, nonsteroidal antiinflammatory drugs (NSAIDs), aspirin, and iron preparations.

Vascular anomalies such as double aortic arch or aberrant right subclavian artery can cause dysphagia.

MOTILITY CAUSES

Patients reporting both solid and liquid dysphagia are more likely to have a motility disorder. Achalasia is a disease in which there is a loss of peristalsis in the distal esophagus and a failure of LES relaxation. These patients complain of chest pain, regurgitation, heartburn, and weight loss in addition to dysphagia. A barium swallow is the primary screening test when achalasia is suspected and manometry is confirmatory. The characteristic features on manometry include elevated resting LES pressure, incomplete LES relaxation, and aperistalsis.

Spastic motility disorders also manifest with dysphagia and often associated chest pain. The group of spastic motility disorders includes distal esophageal spasm, nutcracker esophagus, and hypertensive LES. The clinical relevance of these abnormalities identified during esophageal manometry is debated, and their management can be challenging.

Treatment

OROPHARYNGEAL DYSPHAGIA

Surgical and endoscopic therapeutic options are available, and these should be based on the patient's age and surgical risk. Surgery has been the mainstay of symptomatic Zenker's diverticulum. These involve cricopharyngeal myotomy with or without diverticulectomy or diverticulopexy. The efficacy of myotomy has been observed to be in excess of 80%. More recently, endoscopic techniques involving coagulation or cutting of the bridge, especially the cricopharyngeal muscle, between the esophagus and the diverticulum have been used. This approach is especially good for patients who are poor surgical risks and is now being used widely by experts in this technique.

Botulinum toxin injection might be an alternative to cricopharyngeal myotomy, although results are variable. Injection is usually performed under electromyographic guidance and has been shown to relieve dysphagia in small trials.

The presence of other structural abnormalities such as proximal strictures, can require endoscopic measures such as dilatation. A neoplasm requires appropriate intervention with surgical resection, chemotherapy, or radiation therapy.

If the oropharyngeal dysphagia is believed to be from nonstructural causes, swallowing rehabilitation may be the best option available. Swallowing rehabilitation is carried out by trained speech and language therapists, who teach patients maneuvers to overcome the risks of aspiration and improve dysphagia. These can involve proper positioning of the head and neck during swallowing, oral motor exercises, and deliberate multiple swallows. Certain diet modifications can improve swallowing and prevent aspirations.

The risk of malnutrition or recurrent aspiration can require placement of gastrostomy tubes for managing long-term nutritional needs.

ESOPHAGEAL DYSPHAGIA

The treatment of peptic strictures can involve dilatation, biopsies to rule out malignancy, and medical therapy for reflux. Proton pump inhibitor therapy has been shown to reduce the development of these strictures and the need for future dilatation.

Radiation-related strictures or esophagitis may be difficult to treat and require frequent esophageal dilatation.

The treatment of esophageal cancer depends on the stage of the cancer at the time of diagnosis. The various options available include surgery, chemotherapy, radiation therapy, palliative intraluminal stenting, and, more recently, photodynamic therapy.

Eosinophilic esophagitis is treated with topical steroid therapy with fluticasone[1] (Flovent), oral methylprednisolone, or montelukast in addition to dietary restrictions. These treatments have been studied in small series and have been shown to be beneficial. Dilatation may be helpful but must be done with care.

Treatment of pill-induced esophagitis involves stopping the offending agent and dilatation of strictures as needed.

Treatment modalities for achalasia include pneumatic dilatation of the LES, laparoscopic myotomy, botulinum toxin injection, and medical therapy with nitrates and calcium channel blockers. Medical therapy should be considered only for people who are not candidates for other modalities. Good to excellent relief of dysphagia can be achieved in patients with achalasia whether treated with pneumatic dilatation or myotomy. Many patients require multiple approaches and should be managed by experts in the field. Minimally invasive (laparoscopic or thoracoscopic) myotomy is gaining popularity, and in some centers it has become the procedure of choice.

Proposed treatments for distal esophageal spasm, nutcracker esophagus, and hypertensive LES include proton pump inhibitors, nitrates, calcium channel blockers, phosphodiesterase inhibitors, and tricyclic antidepressants or selective serotonin reuptake inhibitors.[1] Botulinum toxin[1] application and endoscopic dilatation have been tried in small series with varying results.

[1]Not FDA approved for this indication.

CURRENT THERAPY

- Treat the underlying disorder (e.g., GERD).
- Dilatation and antireflux therapy manage most peptic strictures.
- Multimodality therapy should be considered for malignant dysphagia.
- Achalasia can be effectively treated with pneumatic dilatation or surgery.
- Swallowing rehabilitation is helpful for oropharyngeal dysphagia following stroke.
- Eosinophilic esophagitis may respond to topical corticosteroids.

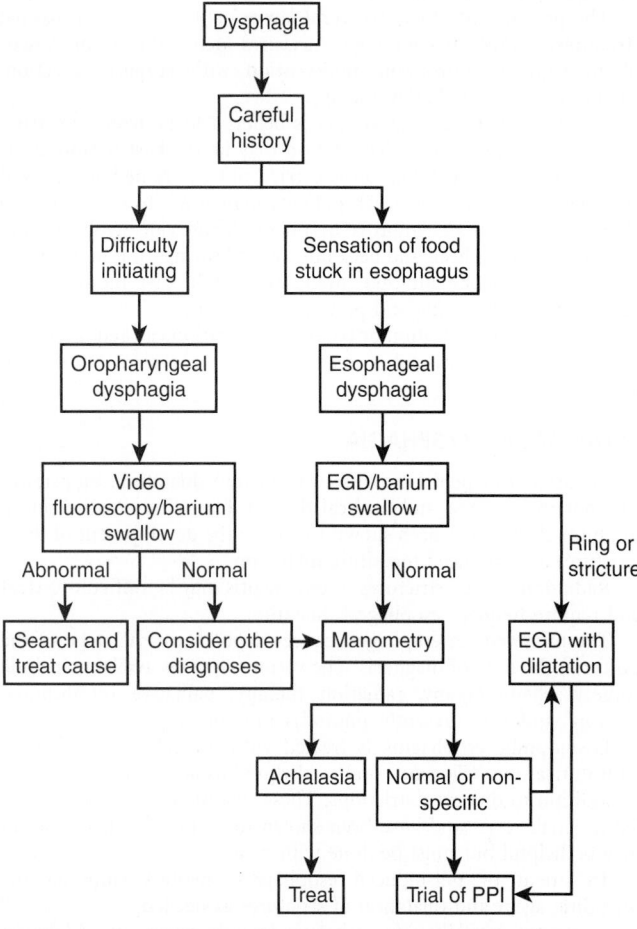

FIGURE 1. Diagnostic algorithm for patients with dysphagia. *Abbreviations:* EGD = esophagogastroduodenoscopy; PPI = proton pump inhibitor.

Summary

This review outlines the various causes and management of dysphagia. A careful history and examination with use of certain diagnostic tests help in establishing the reason for the symptom of dysphagia. Most of the conditions can be managed by medical therapy, endoscopic therapy, or surgery. A possible approach is outlined in Figure 1.

REFERENCES

Cook IJ, Kahrilas PJ. AGA technical review on management of oropharyngeal dysphagia. Gastroenterology 1999;116(2):455–79.

Furuta GT, Liacouras CA, Collins MH, et al. Eosinophilic esophagitis in children and adults: a systematic review and consensus recommendations for diagnosis and treatment. Gastroenterology 2007;133(4):1342–63.

Katz PO, Gilbert J, Castell DO. Pneumatic dilatation is effective long-term treatment for achalasia. Dig Dis Sci 1998;43(9):1973–7.

Khazanchi A, Katz PO. Strategies for treating severe refractory dysphagia. Gastrointest Endosc Clin N Am 2001;11(2):371–86 viii.

Spechler SJ. American Gastroenterological Association medical position statement on treatment of patients with dysphagia caused by benign disorders of the distal esophagus. Gastroenterology 1999;117(1):229–33.

Trate DM, Parkman HP, Fisher RS. Dysphagia: Evaluation, diagnosis and treatment. Prim Care 1996;(3):417–32.

Tutuian R, Castell DO. Esophageal motility disorders (distal esophageal spasm, nutcracker esophagus, and hypertensive lower esophageal sphincter): Modern management. Curr Treat Options Gastroenterol 2006;9(4): 283–94.

Yan BM, Shaffer EA. Eosinophilic esophagitis: A newly established cause of dysphagia. World J Gastroenterol 2006;12(15):2328–34.

Diverticula of the Alimentary Tract

Method of

Alexander Perez, MD, Christopher R. Mantyh, MD, and Danny O. Jacobs, MD, MPH

A diverticulum is an abnormal saccular protrusion from the wall of the intestinal tract. It may be classified as a true diverticulum if the protrusion is composed of all of the layers of the intestinal wall or as a false diverticulum, or pseudodiverticulum, if it lacks the entirety of these layers. Although many diverticula are asymptomatic, some cause symptoms according to their anatomic location and the underlying process (obstruction, inflammation, or bleeding).

Esophagus

ZENKER'S DIVERTICULUM

Zenker's diverticulum, also known as a pharyngoesophageal pseudodiverticulum, is the most common type of esophageal diverticulum. It arises because of muscular discoordination (in the area between the inferior pharyngeal constrictors and the cricopharyngeal muscle) that creates transmural pressure gradients within the esophagus, resulting in mucosal herniation through the esophageal muscular layer. This diverticulum typically manifests in older patients as dysphagia, aspiration, and regurgitation of undigested food. If this pathology is suspected, the diagnosis can be made by barium swallow (Fig. 1). If endoscopy is employed during the work-up, care must be taken to avoid perforation of the diverticulum.

Asymptomatic and incidentally encountered Zenker's diverticula may be managed with observation alone. Patients presenting with symptoms and a diverticulum of 2 cm or larger should undergo surgical resection of the diverticulum and myotomy of the cricopharyngeal muscle; those with smaller symptomatic diverticula may undergo myotomy alone. Patients undergoing surgical management have demonstrated symptomatic improvement more than 90% of the time. Although the diverticulum has traditionally been approached surgically via a cervical incision along the anterior border of the sternocleidomastoid muscle, an endoluminal approach is also available.

EPIPHRENIC DIVERTICULA

Epiphrenic diverticula are rare and are located in the distal third of the esophagus. It is thought that these diverticula are also associated with muscular dysmotility and gastroesophageal reflux. Symptoms include

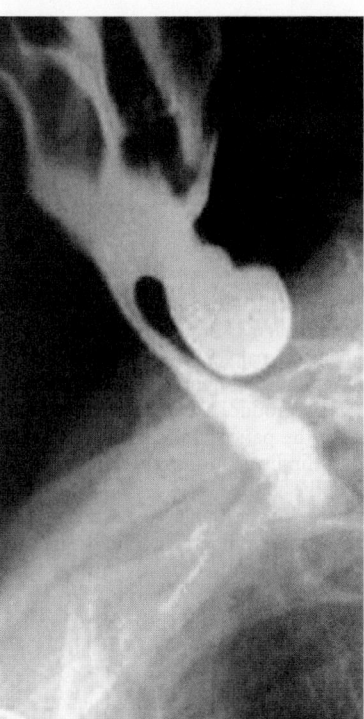

FIGURE 1. Zenker's diverticulum. (Image courtesy of Gastrolab—The Gastrointestinal Site. Available at http://www.gastrolab.net [accessed June 30, 2009].)

dysphagia, spasmodic chest pain, and reflux. The work-up consists of barium swallow, esophageal manometry, upper endoscopy, and 24-hour pH probe studies. Other disease processes, such as malignant obstruction, achalasia, and peptic stricture, should be ruled out.

Management includes resection of the diverticulum together with contralateral myotomy extending proximally through all regions of the esophagus documented to have abnormal motility and distally several millimeters on to the stomach. A partial fundoplication should be employed if reflux is identified during the preoperative work-up. Most recently, a laparoscopic approach has been employed successfully to address this pathology.

TRACTION DIVERTICULUM

A traction diverticulum, which is a true diverticulum (composed of all layers of the esophageal wall), results from inflammation in neighboring lymph nodes during processes such as tuberculosis and histoplasmosis.

These diverticula are usually small and asymptomatic and do not require surgical management. Rare cases of fistulization have been reported and have been managed with excision of the inflammatory mass and closure of the esophageal defect by a thoracotomy.

Stomach

Diverticula of the stomach are rare, with an incidence of 0.02% in autopsy studies. These diverticula may manifest with abdominal pain, dyspepsia, emesis, bleeding, and perforation. Diagnosis is made with an upper gastrointestinal contrast study, endoscopy, or contrast-enhanced computed tomography of the abdomen. Precise localization of the diverticulum is required preoperatively to plan the best operative approach.

Abdominal pain may be controlled with a proton pump inhibitor; however, those patients with persistent symptoms may require resection of the gastric diverticulum. A laparoscopic approach to resection of gastric diverticula is becoming more popular.

Small Intestine

DUODENAL DIVERTICULA

Both true and false diverticula may be found in the duodenum. Most are located in the second portion of the duodenum. Although the majority are asymptomatic, because of their location they may be associated with biliary obstruction or pancreatitis. Associated sphincter of Oddi dysfunction may also be present. Duodenal diverticula may be identified on barium swallow, contrast-enhanced computed tomography, or endoscopic retrograde cholangiopancreatography (Fig. 2).

Incidentally found duodenal diverticula should be left alone. In the rare instance that a duodenal diverticulum produces significant symptoms such as biliary obstruction or bleeding, an approach using endoscopic stenting, angiographic embolization, or surgical resection may be required.

JEJUNAL AND ILEAL DIVERTICULA

Jejunal and ileal diverticula occur throughout the length of the small intestine, predominately on the mesenteric side of the intestine where the blood vessels penetrate the muscular wall of the bowel. They are classified as false diverticula. Many are found incidentally, and some manifest with symptoms secondary to bleeding, obstruction, or infection. These symptoms may be a result of the bacterial overgrowth that occurs within these diverticula. Preoperative diagnosis may be made with a small bowel follow-through contrast study or capsule endoscopy.

Incidentally encountered jejunal and ileal diverticula should not be resected. Bacterial overgrowth may respond to antibiotic and intestinal promotility therapy. Resection may be required for refractory symptomatic diverticula. Laparoscopic approaches are feasible in this setting.

MECKEL'S DIVERTICULUM

A Meckel's diverticulum is a congenital anomaly that results from incomplete obliteration of the vitelline duct. It has a prevalence of approximately 1% to 2% in the population, is usually asymptomatic, is usually located within 2 feet of the ileocecal valve, and may contain ectopic gastric and pancreatic tissue. Symptoms may occur secondary to bleeding or obstruction associated with ectopic gastric mucosa and fibrous attachments to the umbilicus. A technetium 99m (Tc^{99})-pertechnetate scan will identify ectopic gastric mucosa in those presenting with ulceration and bleeding.

Resection of a Meckel's diverticulum is warranted in symptomatic patients. Patients with a Meckel's diverticulum found incidentally should not undergo resection, because there is a significantly higher

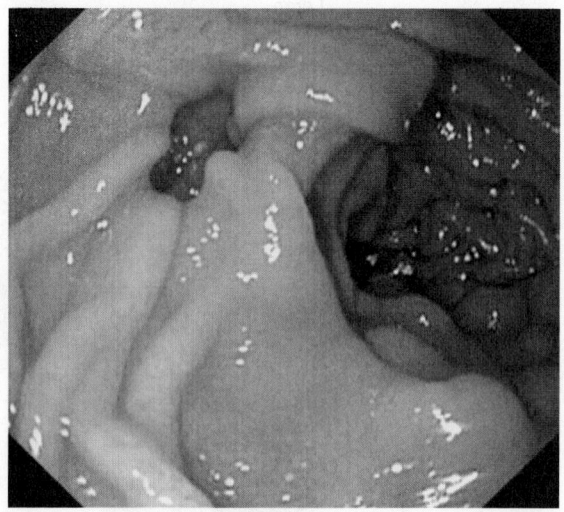

FIGURE 2. Duodenal diverticulum (Image courtesy of Gastrolab—The Gastrointestinal Site. Available at http://www.gastrolab.net [accessed June 30, 2009].)

rate of complications, such as infection and bowel obstruction (5.3% versus 1.3%, $P < 0.0001$), after resection in asymptomatic patients. Some have advocated a selective approach, with resection of incidentally found Meckel's diverticula in male patients, in patients younger than 50 years of age, if the diverticulum is longer than 2 cm, and if the diverticulum contains ectopic tissue.

Colon

The colon is most common site for diverticula of the alimentary tract. Colonic diverticula are of the false type and are composed primarily of mucosa protruding through the intestinal muscular layers (Fig. 3). Their presence is referred to as diverticulosis or diverticular disease. If these diverticula become inflamed or infected, the term diverticulitis is employed. If this acute process progresses to abscess, perforation, fistulization, or stenosis, then the term complicated diverticulitis is used.

Whereas the pathogenesis of diverticulosis remains uncertain, it is clear that its incidence increases with age, with the prevalence after age 80 years estimated to be 50% to 70%. The majority of colonic diverticula are located in the sigmoid colon, but approximately 50% of patients have disease that extends to other segments. The sigmoid is the narrowest portion of the colon and the location at which the highest intraluminal pressure may exist, according to Laplace's Law: $T = (P \times R)/M$, where T = wall tension, P = pressure across the wall, R = wall radius, and M = wall thickness. The pressure across the colonic wall (P) increases as the radius of the wall (R) decreases and the thickness of the wall (M) increases. The sigmoid is the narrowest portion of the colon, and patients with diverticular disease have a striking hypertrophy of the muscular wall that precedes the appearance of the diverticula. These diverticula appear at the site where arterioles penetrate the muscularis on the mesenteric side of the antimesenteric tenia. It is this anatomic relationship and the erosion into these blood vessels that is associated with 50% of all cases of lower gastrointestinal bleeding.

A reason for the predilection of the sigmoid colon to develop diverticula may be its relatively small diameter and increased intraluminal pressure. Other factors that may be associated with the development of diverticula are a low fiber, high fat, and highly refined carbohydrates in the diet.

Evaluation

The clinical presentation of diverticulitis spans the spectrum from mild, predominantly left-sided, lower abdominal pain, fever, and leukocytosis to septic shock with diffuse peritonitis. The disease severity at presentation relates directly to the extent of inflammation, perforation, and the expected response to medical management.

The diagnosis of diverticulitis is made by physical examination, laboratory testing, and imaging. Physical findings may include mild left lower quadrant pain on palpation. However, pain may be elicited at the other sites because of the sigmoid colon's redundancy. If a perforation is present, it may produce signs of localized or generalized peritonitis, depending on the patient's ability to wall off the inflammatory process. Laboratory findings are nonspecific and reflect the degree of inflammation that the patient is experiencing. The most commonly employed imaging studies are plain abdominal radiography, ultrasonography, and computed tomography. The degrees of sensitivity and specificity are almost 100% for computed tomography with the use of intravenous and water-soluble oral contrast. Free air, free fluid, areas of inflammation, and abscesses may be detected with these modalities. Once the acute phase is over, additional modalities, such as colonoscopy and contrast enemas, should be used to establish the extent of disease and rule out the presence of other diseases such as cancer.

Treatment

A mild episode of diverticulitis may be managed on an outpatient basis with oral broad-spectrum antibiotics with coverage of anaerobic microorganisms. More severe episodes require hospitalization and stabilization with bowel rest, analgesia, intravenous fluids, and intravenous broad-spectrum antibiotics.

Localized abscesses may be successfully drained percutaneously under computed tomographic guidance, allowing resolution of symptoms and planning for future elective surgical resection of the involved segment and primary anastomosis of the remaining intestinal ends (Fig. 4). An elective resection should be delayed at least

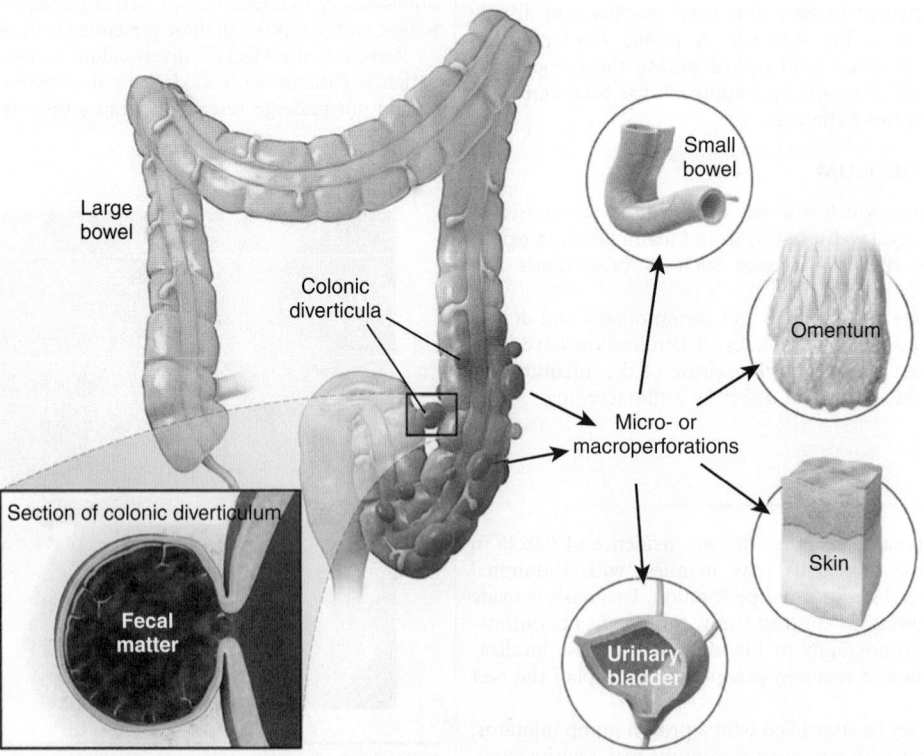

FIGURE 3. Colonic diverticula. Colonic diverticula have narrow necks that can be obstructed by fecal matter. Obstruction may produce distention of the sac, bacterial overgrowth, vascular compromise, and perforation. Some perforations are localized and contained, whereas others may invade the skin or erode into adjacent viscera, causing fistulas. (Image from Jacobs DO: Diverticulitis. N Engl J Med 2007;357:2058, courtesy of New England Journal of Medicine.)

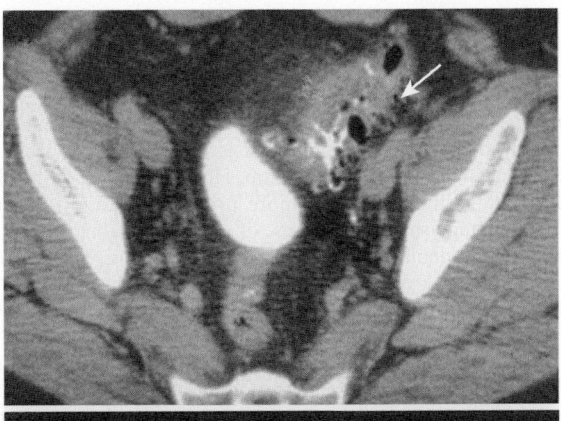

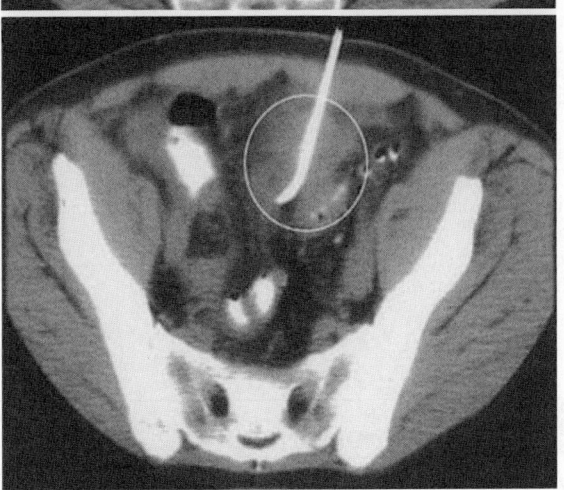

FIGURE 4. Computed tomographic findings of diverticulitis. The upper panel shows evidence of inflammation and wall thickening (*arrow*). The bottom panel shows a diverticular abscess with a percutaneously placed drain. (Images courtesy of Dr. Erik Paulson, Department of Radiology, Duke University Medical Center.)

6 weeks to allow for resolution of inflammation and to lower the likelihood of conversion to an open procedure if a laparoscopic approach is attempted. Elective laparoscopic resection may prove to be superior to the traditional open resection in terms of reduction of morbidity and length of hospital stay.

Emergent surgical intervention may be required if the patient fails to improve or worsens clinically, which occurs approximately 10% of the time. Surgical intervention in this acute setting typically consists of a two-staged procedure beginning with resection of the involved segment, lavage, end colostomy, and oversewing of the distal rectal stump (Hartmann's procedure). During the second stage, the end colostomy is taken down, and intestinal continuity is reestablished in an elective fashion (Fig. 5). It is important that the margin of resection include the entire sigmoid colon, to reduce the risk of recurrence. In long-term quality-of-life studies, surgical management has provided a significant advantage compared with nonsurgical management for complicated diverticulitis.

Special Problems

Special circumstances worthy of further evaluation include diverticulitis in young patients, primary resection and anastomosis (single-stage approach) in cases of perforated diverticulitis, and nonoperative management of recurrent diverticulitis.

Controversy exists as to whether diverticulitis in the younger patient is more virulent than in their older counterparts. Some argue that diverticula in these young patients should be managed more aggressively, with surgical resection, whereas others believe that younger and older patients are at equal risk and should receive equivalent therapy.

Although most surgeons would consider a two-stage approach for perforated diverticulitis, there have been studies showing that a single-stage approach may be feasible in appropriately selected patients.

Controversy exists concerning the need and timing of surgical resection after recurrent diverticulitis. Some advocate elective resection after the second episode; others prefer to wait until after the fourth episode; and still others suggest that surgery can be avoided in uncomplicated recurrent diverticulitis regardless of the number of previous episodes.

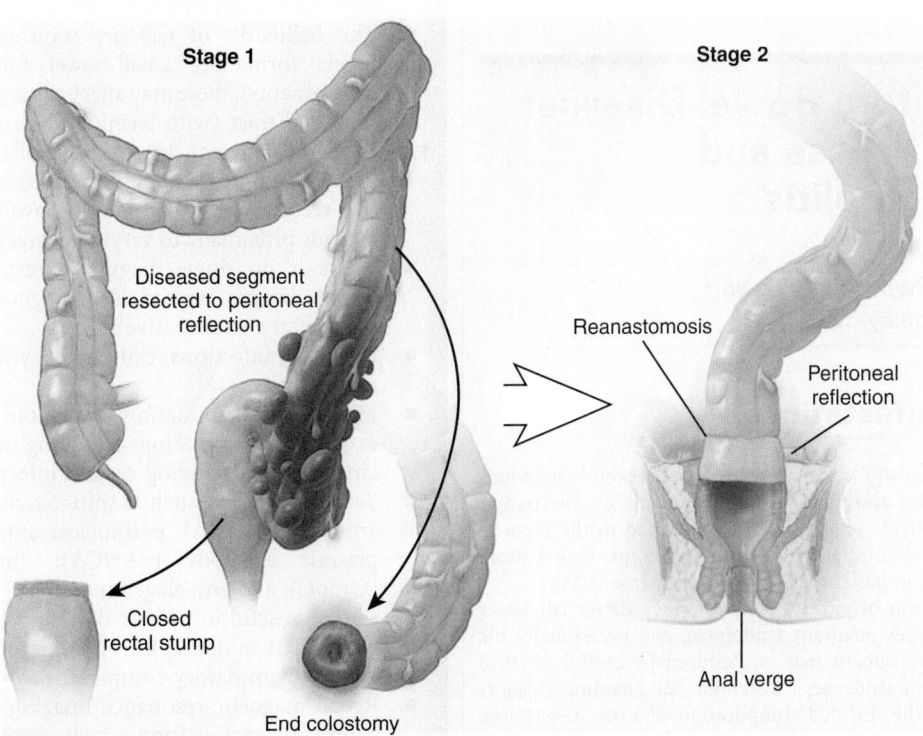

FIGURE 5. Two-staged operative approach to diverticulitis. In stage 1, the diseased segment of bowel is resected, an end colostomy is performed, and the distal rectal stump is oversewn (Hartmann's procedure). In stage 2, performed during a second procedure, colonic continuity is reestablished. (Image from Jacobs DO: Diverticulitis. N Engl J Med 2007;357:2063, courtesy of New England Journal of Medicine.)

REFERENCES

Alves A, Panis Y, Slim K, et al. French multicentre prospective observational study of laparoscopic versus open colectomy for sigmoid diverticular disease. Br J Surg 2005;92(12):1520–5.

Bordeianou L, Hodin R. Controversies in the surgical management of sigmoid diverticulitis. J Gastrointest Surg 2007;11(4):542–8.

Cassivi SD, Deschamps C, Nichols FC 3rd, et al. Diverticula of the esophagus. Surg Clin North Am 2005;85(3):495–503.

Donkervoort SC, Baak LC, Blaauwgeers JL, et al. Laparoscopic resection of a symptomatic gastric diverticulum: A minimally invasive solution. J Soc Laparoendosc Surgeons 2006;10(4):525–7.

Jacobs DO. Clinical practice: Diverticulitis. N Engl J Med 2007;357 (20):2057–66.

Mäkelä JT, Kiviniemi HO, Laitinen ST. Elective surgery for recurrent diverticulitis. Hepatogastroenterology 2007;54(77):1412–6.

Nelson RS, Velasco A, Mukesh BN. Management of diverticulitis in younger patients. Dis Colon Rectum 2006;49(9):1341–5.

Pautrat K, Bretagnol F, Huten N, et al. Acute diverticulitis in very young patients: A frequent surgical management. Dis Colon Rectum 2007;50 (4):472–7.

Richter S, Lindemann W, Kollmar O, et al. One-stage sigmoid colon resection for perforated sigmoid diverticulitis (Hinchey stages III and IV). World J Surg 2006;30(6):1027–32.

Salem L, Veenstra DL, Sullivan SD, et al. The timing of elective colectomy in diverticulitis: A decision analysis. J Am Coll Surg 2004;199(6):904–12.

Scarpa M, Pagano D, Ruffolo C, et al. Health-related quality of life after colonic resection for diverticular disease: Long-term results. J Gastrointest Surg 2008;13(1):105–12.

Schilling MK, Maurer CA, Kollmar O, et al. Primary vs. secondary anastomosis after sigmoid colon resection for perforated diverticulitis (Hinchey Stage III and IV): A prospective outcome and cost analysis. Dis Colon Rectum 2001;44(5):699–703.

Zani A, Eaton S, Rees CM, et al. Incidentally detected Meckel diverticulum: To resect or not to resect? Ann Surg 2008;247(2):276–81.

Zingg U, Pasternak I, Guertler L, et al. Early vs. delayed elective laparoscopic-assisted colectomy in sigmoid diverticulitis: Timing of surgery in relation to the attack. Dis Colon Rectum 2007;50(11):1911–7.

Inflammatory Bowel Disease: Crohn's Disease and Ulcerative Colitis

Method of
Prabhakar P. Swaroop, MD, and
Daniel K. Podolsky, MD

Clinical Manifestations

The cardinal symptom of ulcerative colitis (UC) is bloody diarrhea. Symptoms of tenesmus and the sensation of incomplete evacuation may dominate in patients who have disease limited to the rectum. Although cramping abdominal pain is often present, it is a more prominent symptom in patients with Crohn's disease (CD).

Physical examination of patients with UC may detect left lower quadrant and left upper quadrant tenderness, and occasionally the extent of colonic involvement may be deduced by careful physical examination. Rebound tenderness, distention, or guarding suggests the development of the dreaded complication of toxic megacolon, which may supervene in patients with severe UC.

Patients with CD have more widely varying symptoms as a result of the highly variable sites of involvement and the range of phenotypic forms. Disease manifestations may be dominated by inflammatory activity per se, by fistula formation (fistulizing or perforating disease), or by stricture formation (stricturing disease). Perianal fistulas can be a distressing manifestation and may parallel clinical flares. The symptom complex of right lower quadrant pain, nonbloody diarrhea, and weight loss is most common because of the frequent involvement of the ileum. However, in CD with colonic involvement (with or without more proximal disease), symptoms may be indistinguishable from those of UC. Intestinal narrowing may be caused by edema due to inflammation, fibrosis from chronic inflammation, or a combination of these factors. The presence of a mass in the right lower quadrant suggests inflammatory ileal disease (and probably abscess formation), whereas right lower quadrant pain in conjunction with obstructive symptoms in the absence of a mass may be suggestive of stricture formation. Fistula disease can manifest with especially variable symptoms because of the many anatomic structures that can be involved (e.g., fecaluria and pneumaturia in those with fistulas to the bladder). Rectovaginal fistulas may lead to passage of air from the vagina. Patients with upper gastrointestinal CD may present with dysphagia, early satiety, and fear of food leading to weight loss.

Diarrhea is common but not universal in CD. Inflammation of the ileum or of the colon can cause diarrhea. Occasionally, diarrhea is caused by small intestinal bacterial overgrowth, especially in patients with fistulizing disease, or it may be induced by bile salts in those with ileal disease (or after ileal resection).

CURRENT DIAGNOSIS

- The most common clinical symptom of ulcerative colitis (UC) is bloody diarrhea, which is often associated with cramping abdominal pain.
- Clinical manifestations of Crohn's disease (CD) are highly variable, but the most common constellation is right lower quadrant abdominal pain and nonbloody diarrhea, often accompanied by weight loss and other constitutional symptoms.
- The hallmarks of CD are transmural inflammation, fistula formation, small-bowel fibrosis, and patchy inflammation; these may affect any segment of the gastrointestinal tract (with terminal ileal involvement in two thirds of patients). In contrast, inflammation in UC is limited to mucosa and submucosa and is diffuse, with the rectum most commonly involved. Inflammation extends proximally to varying degrees among patients.
- There is no single diagnostic test for inflammatory bowel disease; instead, the diagnosis is made based on several corroborative features.
- Potential infectious causes of symptoms should be ruled out.
- Endoscopic examination is valuable in establishing the extent of inflammation, obtaining mucosal biopsy specimens, and excluding certain infectious agents.
- Serology studies, such as anti–*Saccharomyces cerevisiae* antibodies (ASCA), perinuclear antineutrophilic cytoplasmic antibody (pANCA), anti-porin antibody (OmpC), and anti-flagellin antibody (CBir1), are occasionally useful to predict disease behavior.
- Computed tomographic enterography can help distinguish inflammatory component from fibrosis.
- Rectal magnetic resonance imaging, endoscopic ultrasound, or examination under anesthesia can be used to fully delineate perianal fistulizing disease.

Diagnosis

Diagnosis of inflammatory bowel disease (IBD) is based on the combination of clinical features, laboratory abnormalities, imaging studies (e.g., upper gastrointestinal series with small bowel follow-through and abdominal computed tomography or magnetic resonance imaging or both), and endoscopic findings including examination of mucosal biopsies. None of these tests alone is diagnostic of IBD. In a patient with new symptoms and in those patients with flares if appropriate, infectious agents should be ruled out. Common pathogens that can mimic IBD are *Salmonella*, *Shigella*, *Aeromonas*, *Campylobacter*, *Yersinia*, *Clostridium difficile*, *Plesiomonas*, and parasites such as *Giardia lamblia* and *Entamoeba*; these should be ruled out. In an immunocompromised host (including patients with established IBD receiving immunosuppressive therapy), viral infections such as cytomegalovirus and herpes simplex virus may cause ulcers suggestive of IBD. Endoscopic imaging is often very useful. The constellation of findings in endoscopy and other studies, together with the histologic and clinical features, usually allows a reliable distinction between UC and CD. However, in as many as 10% of patients, it may not be possible to make the distinction with confidence, and such patients are said to have indeterminate colitis. The distinguishing features of UC and CD are presented in Table 1.

Hematologic abnormalities include evidence of microcytic anemia, elevated white blood cell count in peripheral blood, and thrombocytosis. Markers of inflammation such as erythrocyte sedimentation rate (ESR) and high-sensitivity C-reactive protein (hsCRP) may also be elevated, the latter more commonly in CD than in UC. Very high hsCRP may be associated with infections such as cytomegalovirus or *Clostridium difficile*.

Serologic measurements of perinuclear antineutrophilic cytoplasmic antibody (pANCA), anti–*Saccharomyces cerevisiae* antibodies (ASCA—immunoglobulin G and immunoglobulin A), anti-porin antibody (OmpC), and anti-flagellin antibody (CBir1) are occasionally helpful as corroborative evidence and to help identify patients who are at higher risk for complicating events. They may also be useful in differentiating between CD and UC in patients for whom colectomy is being considered when diagnostic ambiguity remains.

Hypoalbuminemia can be a sign of poor nutritional status, and these patients should be considered for total parenteral nutrition, particularly if surgery is being planned.

Among the imaging modalities commonly used in diagnosis and management of IBD, computed tomography of the abdomen and pelvis can alert physicians to perforation, bowel obstruction, and extent of inflammation. Computed tomographic enterography can

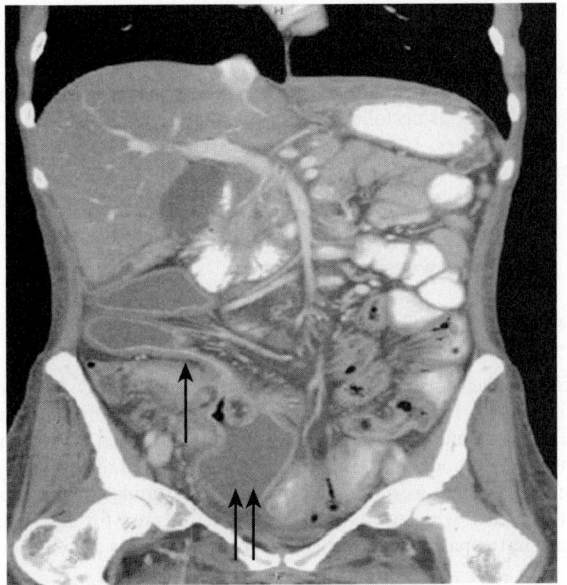

FIGURE 1. Computed tomographic enterography. Mural stratification; ileal wall thickening (*arrow*) suggestive of active inflammation; dilated loops of small bowel (*double arrow*) consistent with partial obstruction; and diffuse increased density of the subcutaneous and intraperitoneal fat compatible with anasarca are seen in this image. (Courtesy of Dr. Cecelia Brewington, MD.)

be used to evaluate the degree and extent of inflammation in the small bowel (Fig. 1). In cases of stenotic lesions of the small bowel, it can be especially helpful in identifying the inflammatory component, as evidenced by mural stranding. Lack of mural stranding in stenotic portions of small bowel suggests fibrosis, and if there is evidence of proximal dilation in a symptomatic patient, resection or strictureplasty should be considered.

Magnetic resonance imaging can be a helpful adjunct, along with examination under anesthesia and rectal endoscopic ultrasonography in cases of perianal fistulizing disease.

Endoscopic examination is helpful to establish the extent of disease and obtain tissue for histologic examination. Esophagogastroduodenoscopy should be done if upper gastrointestinal CD is suspected. Single-balloon and double-balloon enteroscopy have

TABLE 1 Distinguishing Features: Crohn's Disease and Ulcerative Colitis

Features	Crohn's Disease	Ulcerative Colitis
Location	Any part of gastrointestinal tract	Colonic
Inflammation	Transmural	Mucosal/submucosal
Smoking	Smokers higher than expected	Appears to be protective
Risk of colorectal cancer	Elevated in colonic Crohn's	Elevated
Risk of intestinal cancer	Elevated in small-bowel Crohn's disease	NA
hsCRP	Elevation common	Elevation not common
Serology	ASCA, OmpC, CBir1	pANCA
Surgery	Recurrence common	Total proctocolectomy may be curative
Fistulas	Common	Very rare
FDA-approved biologic agents	Infliximab (Remicade), adalimumab (Humira), certolizumab pegol (Cimzia), natalizumab (Tysabri)	Infliximab
Immunomodulator therapy	Azathioprine (AZA, Imuran),[1] 6-mercaptopurine (6MP, Purinethol),[1] methotrexate (MTX, Trexall)[1]	AZA, 6MP, cyclosporine (Sandimmune, Neoral)[1]
Endoscopic features	Skip lesions	Contiguous involvement
Strictures	Common	Colorectal cancer unless proven otherwise
Genetic markers	NOD2, ATG16L1, IRGM, IL23R, IL12B, STAT3, NKX2-3	IL12B, STAT3. NKX2-3

[1]Not FDA approved for this indication.
ASCA = anti–*Saccharomyces cerevisiae* antibodies; CBir1 = anti-flagellin antibody; FDA = U.S. Food and Drug Administration; hsCRP = high-sensitivity C-reactive protein; OmpC = anti-porin antibody; NA = not applicable; pANCA = perinuclear antineutrophilic cytoplasmic antibody.

allowed gastroenterologists to obtain tissue samples from jejunum and proximal ileum. Capsule endoscopy can be a useful alternative, although it does not allow tissue sampling and should not be used if even limited obstruction is suspected. Colonoscopy is helpful in diagnosis and during follow-up to assess response to various therapeutic modalities. It can also be used to obtain biopsy specimens from the colon and terminal ileum to be examined for findings of IBD or potentially confounding processes, including some infections.

Treatment

Once the diagnosis is confirmed, the treatment of IBD is based on manifestation, location, patient history, and severity of symptoms.

Treatment algorithms for IBD are usually divided into management of mild, moderate, and severe disease. The roles of various agents have evolved, and as more data are being accumulated, patients are treated earlier with agents that had been reserved for more severe disease in the past. Treatment goals for these patients are:

- Improving quality of life to as close to normal as possible
- Maintaining remission
- Avoiding surgery
- Minimizing the risk of steroid dependence
- Minimizing the risk of treatment-associated complications

 CURRENT THERAPY

- Mesalamine products in adequate dosage and appropriate formulation can be effective therapy for mild to moderately active ulcerative colitis (UC) and in maintaining remission.
- Mesalamine products may be effective in mild Crohn's disease (CD), and the formulation selected should be determined by disease location.
- Steroids are useful in patients with moderate to severe CD or UC, but their use should be limited as much as possible because of frequent side effects and complications.
- Immunomodulators such as Azathioprine (Imuran)[1] and 6-mercaptopurine (Purinethol)[1] may be used as an adjunct therapy to minimize steroid use in patients who are steroid dependent and to minimize formation of neutralizing antibodies in patients receiving antibody-based biologic agents.
- Anti–tumor necrosis factor (anti-TNF) biologic agents such as infliximab (Remicade) and adalimumab (Humira) are effective in patients with moderate to severe inflammatory CD or UC that is unresponsive to conventional treatments. Certolizumab pegol (Cimzia) may be used to maintain remission. Immunomodulators and biologic agents may be used independently or in combination for treatment of inflammatory bowel disease and for maintaining surgically induced remission in CD.
- The role of antibiotics is limited to septic complications, perianal disease, small intestinal bacterial overgrowth, and pouchitis.
- Nataluzimab (Tysabri), an anti-α_4 agent, is effective in some patients with refractory CD, including those for whom anti-TNF therapy has failed.

[1]Not FDA approved for this indication.

ULCERATIVE COLITIS

In the initial evaluation of UC patients, it is important to establish the extent and degree of inflammation and the concomitant presence of extraintestinal manifestations. Extent and severity of UC are judged on clinical symptoms, basic laboratory parameters (complete blood count and albumin level), and colonoscopic findings. Disease limited to the rectum and distal colon may be treated with local mesalamine therapy, in a suppository (Canasa), foam (Salofalk),[2] or enema (Rowasa) formulation. Newly diagnosed patients with mild to moderate disease activity should be given an appropriate oral formulation of mesalamine (Asacol). Antidiarrheal agents may provide symptomatic relief once infectious causes of colitis have been excluded.

If remission is achieved with a mesalamine formulation, the same dose of mesalamine is continued for maintenance of remission. For an occasional flare suggested by symptoms of recurrence and documented by sigmoidoscopy or colonoscopy, steroids may be used. For patients who have frequent flares (more than two per year), initiation of therapy with a conventional immunomodulator or infliximab (Remicade) should be considered.

For patients with moderate disease unresponsiveness to mesalamine or severe disease, a topical, oral, or intravenous corticosteroid (depending on extent and severity) may be necessary, but it should be used for as short a period as possible, and, if it is not possible to taper and discontinue the steroid within 6 weeks, an immunomodulator should be added.

Surgical intervention should be considered for patients who have no response to therapy with infliximab, steroids, and/or cyclosporine (Neoral).[1] Patients who have high-grade dysplasia or colorectal cancer are also candidates for surgery.

CROHN'S DISEASE

Optimal treatment of CD is based on many factors, including location, severity, specific clinical manifestation and complications, prior clinical course intervention, whether fistulas are present, potential fibrostenotic strictures, history of steroid dependence, history of failure with other agents, and contraindications (e.g., malignancy, opportunistic infections, tuberculosis, intolerance to medications). Before deciding on treatment options, it is important to delineate behavior (fistulizing, stricturing, or inflammatory), location (ileal, colonic, or ileocolonic), and severity and to assess for the presence of extraintestinal complications and nutritional deficiencies.

In patients with mildly active, localized ileocecal disease, treatment has historically begun with a suitable mesalamine product (although effectiveness of this approach remains uncertain).[1] More recently, oral budesonide (Entocort EC, a steroid targeted to the ileum that undergoes extensive first-pass metabolism to minimize systemic steroid effects) has been used. For those with more extensive or severe disease, conventional systemic steroids (prednisone) may be used, but if it is not possible to wean the patient off steroids within 6 weeks, an immunodulatory agent should be started, typically 6-mercaptopurine (Purinethol)[1]/azathioprine (Imuran)[1] or, in those unable to tolerate these agents, low-dose methotrexate (Trexall).[1] For patients with moderate to severe disease, treatment should include an anti-tumor necrosis factor (anti-TNF) agent with or without immunomodulator therapy. Natalizumab (Tysabri), an anti-α_4 integrin, is an alternative and may be used if anti-TNF therapy fails.

Before starting therapy with a biologic agent, patients should have a purified protein derivative (PPD) test and a hepatitis B surface antibody determination. Once biologic therapy begins, patients should continue to have an annual PPD test.

Perianal fistulizing disease, in the absence of abscess, can be treated with a combination of antibiotics, seton placement, immunomodulator therapy, and biologic agents. Complex perianal fistulizing disease may require a diverting ostomy.

[1]Not FDA approved for this indication.
[2]Not available in the United States.

Therapeutic Options

MESALAMINE PREPARATIONS

Aminosalicylate preparations have been used for the treatment of UC and CD. Some data suggest that mesalamine has limited efficacy in patients with CD.

In patients with limited distal UC (e.g., proctitis), treatment may be begun with a mesalamine enema (Rowasa) or suppository (Canasa). For more extensive disease, oral therapy (Asacol) should be used.

Combination therapy (oral administration as well as enemas/suppositories) has been shown to be more effective in inducing remission than either modality alone. In general, the dosage that induces remission is used for maintenance of remission (Table 2).

STEROIDS

The National Co-operative Crohn's Disease Study and the European Co-operative Crohn's Disease Study demonstrated that steroids are efficacious in inducing remission but ineffective in maintaining remission. Among patients who have received steroids, about 26% will have a partial response, and 16% will have no response; among those who have had a complete or partial response, about 28% will become steroid dependent. The requirement for surgery is high in the latter group of patients; about 38% require surgery by the end of 1 year.

The adverse effects of steroids are many and varied and can be classified as early effects and delayed effects associated with prolonged use (>12 weeks). Acne, moon facies, mood changes, sleep disturbances, gastrointestinal intolerance, hyperglycemia, hypertension, weight gain, and ulcers of the gastrointestinal tract can be seen early. Formation of cataracts, aseptic necrosis, suppression of the hypothalamic-pituitary axis, and myopathy are associated with prolonged used. Loss of bone density, previously thought to occur only with chronic use, may be evident in bone density studies after as little as 2 weeks of therapy.

Budesonide (Entocort EC) is used for ileal inflammatory and right-sided colonic CD, reportedly with lower incidences of acne, moon facies, adrenal suppression, and loss of bone mineral density. Alternative therapies (immunomodulators, biologic agents) should be discussed with the patient if there has been no response to steroids in a few weeks.

IMMUNOMODULATORY THERAPY

Azathioprine[1] and 6-mercaptopurine[1] are immunomodulators used as steroid-sparing agents for both CD and UC. Immunomodulators have been shown to modestly reduce the incidence of postsurgical

---

[1]Not FDA approved for this indication.

TABLE 2 Mesalamine Products Indicated for Ulcerative Colitis

Aminosalicylate Product	Daily Dosage	Frequency
Azulfidine (sulfasalazine tablet)	0.5 g–4 g	qid
Asacol (mesalamine delayed-release tablet)	1.6–2.4 g	tid
Pentasa (mesalamine controlled-release tablet)	2–4 g	qid
Colazal (balsalazide capsule)	6.75 g	tid
Dipentum (olsalazine capsule)	1 g	bid
Lialda (mesalamine delayed-release tablet)	2.4–4.8 g	qd
Canasa (mesalamine rectal suppository)*	1 g	qd
Rowasa (mesalamine rectal enema)†	4 g	qd

*Indicated for ulcerative proctitis.
†Indicated for distal ulcerative colitis.

---

recurrence in CD. The onset of action of these agents is slow, up to 3 to 4 months. Some toxicities are associated with genetic variants in the enzymes responsible for catabolism of azathioprine and 6-mercaptopurine, most notably thiopurine methyl transferase (TPMT). A large proportion (89%) of patients have wild-type TPMT (full TPMT enzyme activity), 11% have intermediate enzyme activity, and 0.3% have none. In patients with full TPMT enzyme activity, therapy should be started with 1.5 mg/kg/day of 6-mercaptopurine or 2.5 mg/kg/day of azathioprine; those with intermediate activity should have the dosage reduced by half. Those who do not have any TPMT expression should not be started on these agents because of the high risk of bone marrow toxicity.

Some complications, including pancreatitis, hepatotoxicity, and serum sickness–like syndrome, cannot be predicted. It is recommended that patients starting these medications have a complete blood count and liver function tests performed every other week while their medications are being adjusted. Once they are on a stable dosage, these tests should be done every 2 to 3 months.

Parenteral methotrexate[1] 15 to 25 mg/week can be used to induce remission in patients with CD that has not responded to conventional agents. Once remission has been achieved, oral methotrexate[1] 15 mg can be used to maintain remission. Methotrexate is absolutely contraindicated in pregnancy. Leukopenia, hepatic fibrosis, nausea and vomiting, and hypersensitivity reactions are potential side effects. Risk of hepatic fibrosis is associated with a cumulative dose of more than 1.5 g, diabetes, and concomitant use of alcohol.

CYCLOSPORINE

In patients with severe UC, intravenous cyclosporine (Sandimmune)[1] at a dose of 2 to 4 mg/kg/day has been shown to be effective in inducing remission. A significant proportion of these patients may still require colectomy within 1 year. Those patients who have achieved response and remission on intravenous cyclosporine should be started on oral cyclosporine (Neoral)[1] for a few months, together with prophylaxis against *Pneumocystis jiroveci*. 6-Mercaptopurine or azathioprine can also be used as maintenance agents.

Side effects commonly seen with cyclosporine include renal dysfunction, seizures (particularly in patients with hypocholesterolemia), hypertension, gingival hyperplasia, electrolyte abnormalities, and hirsutism.

BIOLOGIC AGENTS

Infliximab is a chimeric (murine-human) monoclonal anti-TNF antibody that has been approved for induction and maintenance of remission in both CD and UC. It was initially approved for the treatment of fistulizing CD, and subsequent studies showed it to be effective in maintenance therapy as well. In several other studies, it was found to be efficacious in reducing steroid use, length of hospital stay, and surgical intervention and achieving mucosal healing. Infliximab is administered intravenously with or without premedication to avoid allergic reactions.

For induction, infliximab 5 mg/kg is administered at weeks 0, 2, and 6, and maintenance is begun at 5 mg/kg every 8 weeks. Some patients require dose escalation because of diminution of response or failure to maintain remission. In these patients, depending on the clinical scenario, the dose should be increased to 10 mg/kg or the interval reduced to every 6 weeks. In the past, infliximab was routinely used with concomitant immunomodulator therapy to reduce the possibility of infliximab antibodies, but this practice has been associated with a higher risk for a rare hepatosplenic T-cell lymphoma (predominantly in the pediatric population), leading to reconsideration of the need for concomitant immunomodulators in some patients. However, results from the recently released Study of Biologic and Immunomodulator Naive Patients in Crohn's Disease (SONIC) trial demonstrated the superiority of combination therapy over either immunomodulator or infliximab alone, especially in patients with elevated C-reactive protein and ulcers in their baseline colonoscopy. Because reactivation of latent tuberculosis has been

---

[1]Not FDA approved for this indication.

reported, patients should undergo a PPD test and chest radiography before beginning therapy.

OTHER ANTI–TUMOR NECROSIS FACTOR ANTIBODIES

Adalimumab

Recently, adalimumab (Humira), a recombinant fully human immunoglobulin targeting TNF, was approved for use in CD. In the CLASSIC and CHARM trials, adalimumab was demonstrated to be an effective agent in inducing and maintaining remission. It has also been shown to be effective in patients who have lost response to infliximab or are intolerant to it, but it has not yet been approved for treatment of UC. Serious reactions, reactivation of tuberculosis, allergic reactions, lupus-like reactions, and demyelinating diseases are some of the concerns.

For induction, adalimumab 160 mg is given subcutaneously at week 0, 80 mg at week 2, and then, for maintenance of remission, 40 mg every other week.

Certolizumab

Certolizumab (Cimzia) is a polyethylene glycolated Fab fragment of humanized anti-TNF monoclonal antibody approved for use in CD. In the PRECISE 1 and 2 studies, certolizumab was shown to result in modest improvement in response but no clinically significant improvement in remission.

ANTI-α_4 THERAPY

Natalizumab

Natalizumab (Tysabri) is a humanized monoclonal antibody against the α_4 integrin subunit, a molecule involved in cellular adhesion that is required for recruitment of key immune cells to sites affected by IBD. In several studies, it has been shown to be efficacious in inducing remission and maintaining response in CD patients. Enthusiasm has been tempered by the apparent risk for progressive multifocal leukoencephalopathy, a rare but fatal opportunistic infection.

The treatment regimens for UC and CD are summarized in Box 1.

BOX 1 Summary of Treatment Regimen

Ulcerative Colitis
Proctitis
- Initial treatment choices
  - Mesalamine suppositories (Canasa) or enemas (Rowasa) to induce remission
  - Steroid foam enemas (Cortifoam) to induce remission
  - Mesalamine suppositories or enemas to maintain remission
- Second-line treatment choices
  - Oral mesalamine (Asacol) in combination with local therapy
  - Adjunctive treatment with antibiotics: ciprofloxacin (Cipro),[1] metronidazole (Flagyl),[1] or rifaximin (Xifaxan)[1]
  - Probiotics

Left-Sided Colitis
- Initial treatment choices
  - Oral mesalamine product with or without local therapy
- Second-line treatment choices
  - Oral or intravenous steroids
  - Immunomodulator therapy
  - Infliximab (IFX, Remicade)
  - Cyclosporine (Sandimmune)[1] on an inpatient basis (avoid cyclosporine after IFX therapy due to risk of severe immunosuppression)

Pancolitis
- Initial treatment choices
  - Oral mesalamine with a short course of oral or intravenous steroids
- Second-line treatment choices
  - Immunomodulator therapy
  - Infliximab
  - Cyclosporine on an inpatient basis (avoid cyclosporine after IFX therapy due to risk of severe immunosuppression)

Crohn's Disease
Ileocecal Inflammatory Crohn's Disease
- First-line treatment
  - Oral mesalamine (Asacol for ileal disease; Pentasa for more proximal small-bowel disease)[1]
  - Budesonide (Entocort EC) 9 mg PO qd
  - Immunomodulator therapy
  - Biologic agents with or without concomitant immunomodulators

Ileal Stricturing Disease
- No proximal dilation
  - Trial with budesonide or biologic agents (patients with elevated hsCRP are more likely to respond)
- Proximal small-bowel dilation
  - Consider surgical approach

Internally Fistulizing Disease without Intraabdominal Abscess
- Stricture immediately distal to fistula
  - Surgical approach
- No stricture
  - Biologic agents with or without concomitant immunomodulators

Externally Fistulizing Disease without Intraabdominal Abscess
- Biologic agents with or without concomitant immunomodulators

Fistulizing Disease with Intraabdominal Abscess
- Intravenous antibiotics as appropriate
- Percutaneous drainage if appropriate
- Surgical drainage if indicated
- Biologic agents with or without concomitant immunomodulators once infectious process has been treated

Perianal Crohn's Disease without Abscess Formation
- Antibiotics: Ciprofloxacin (Cipro),[1] metronidazole (Flagyl),[1] rifaximin (Xifaxan)[1]
- Immunomodulators
- Biologic agents with or without concomitant immunomodulators
- Seton placement
- Diverting ostomy

Colonic Crohn's Disease
- Oral steroids to induce remission
- Immunomodulator therapy
- Biologic agents with or without concomitant immunomodulator therapy

---

[1]Not FDA approved for this indication.
hsCRP = high-sensitivity C-reactive protein.

REFERENCES

Booya F, Akram S, Fletcher JG, et al. CT enterography and fistulizing Crohn's disease: Clinical benefit and radiographic findings. Abdom Imaging 2008 [Epub ahead of print].

Feagan BG, Panaccione R, Sandborn WJ, et al. Effects of adalimumab therapy on incidence of hospitalization and surgery in Crohn's disease: Results from the CHARM study. Gastroenterology 2008;135(5):1493–9.

Ghosh S, Goldin E, Gordon FH, et al. Natalizumab for active Crohn's disease. N Engl J Med 2003;348(1):24–32.

Hanauer SB, Sandborn WJ, Kornbluth A. Delayed-release oral mesalamine at 4.8 g/day (800 mg tablet) for the treatment of moderately active ulcerative colitis: The ASCEND II trial. Am J Gastroenterol 2005;100(11):2478–85.

Lichtenstein GR, Yan S, Bala M. Infliximab maintenance treatment reduces hospitalizations, surgeries, and procedures in fistulizing Crohn's disease. Gastroenterology 2005;128(4):862–9.

Podolsky DK. Inflammatory bowel disease. N Engl J Med 2002;347(6):417–29.

Thomsen OO, Cortot A, Jewell D, et al. A comparison of budesonide and mesalamine for active Crohn's disease. International Budesonide-Mesalamine Study Group. N Engl J Med 1998;339(6):370–4.

Thukral C, Travassos WJ, Peppercorn MA. The role of antibiotics in inflammatory bowel disease. Curr Treat Options Gastroenterol 2005;8(3):223–8.

Irritable Bowel Syndrome

Method of
Brenda R. Velasco, MD, and
Robert S. Fisher, MD

Epidemiology

Irritable bowel syndrome (IBS) is one of the most common functional gastrointestinal disorders, with a worldwide prevalence estimated to be between 10% and 20%. It is a syndrome characterized by chronic abdominal pain or discomfort and irregular bowel habits that has a significant impact on affected individuals and society. The diagnosis of IBS is based on the absence of detectable structural or biochemical causes and the presence of a constellation of symptoms as outlined by the so-called Rome III criteria (Box 1).

Bloating or visible abdominal distention often is present in patients with IBS but is not considered essential for diagnosis. The Rome III diagnostic criteria divide IBS into subgroups based on stool form and not frequency. Each of the top three IBS subgroups constitutes approximately one third of all IBS patients (Box 2).

Gender differences have been documented in terms of both prominent symptoms and response to treatment. In the community, the ratio of women to men with IBS is estimated to be between 2:1 and 4:1; this difference is greater in the population of IBS patients who seek health care. Women with IBS report greater overall IBS symptom severity, greater intensity of abdominal pain and bloating, greater impact of symptoms on daily life, and lower health-related quality of life, compared to men with IBS. The estimated prevalence of IBS in children is similar to that in adults, and newly diagnosed adults frequently report symptoms of IBS (or other related functional gastrointestinal symptoms) dating back to childhood. The most common age group seen by physicians for treatment of IBS is 20- to 50-year-olds. Patients with a diagnosis of IBS are at increased risk for other, nongastrointestinal functional disorders, such as fibromyalgia, chronic pelvic pain, interstitial cystitis, and migraine headaches.

IBS is associated with substantial economic costs, including the direct costs of excess physician visits, diagnostic testing, medications, hospitalizations, and surgeries and indirect costs from absenteeism and decreased productivity at work (presenteeism). Patients with IBS have been reported to miss three times as many days from work compared to those without bowel symptoms. In 2006, there were at least 2.4 to 3.5 million U.S. physician visits annually for IBS. The annual direct and indirect costs of IBS were recently estimated to be at least $1.6 billion and $19 billion, respectively.

Pathophysiology

The pathophysiology of IBS is multifactorial and complex (Box 3). Altered bowel motility, visceral hypersensitivity, central nervous system effects, and an imbalance in neurotransmitters have all been considered. In addition, roles for infection, small-bowel bacterial overgrowth, abnormal colonic bacterial flora, genetics, and environmental and psychosocial factors have been proposed.

In about 10% of patients the onset of IBS-like symptoms can be attributed to a preceding episode of acute viral or bacterial gastroenteritis that was associated with a significant life stressor. The duration of the infectious gastroenteritis is also a factor in predisposing patients to the development of IBS: the longer the duration of the acute illness, the higher the risk of eventually developing IBS. Altered contractility of the colon and small bowel has been described in patients with IBS and may be related to ingestion of food and

---

BOX 1 Rome III Criteria for the Diagnosis of Irritable Bowel Syndrome

Recurrent abdominal pain or discomfort (with onset at least 6 months before diagnosis) that
- Occurred on at least 3 days per month in the last 3 months, and
- Is associated with two or more of the following:
  - Improvement with defecation
  - Onset associated with a change in frequency of stool
  - Onset associated with a change in form (appearance) of stool

Adapted from Longstreth GF, Thompson WG, Chey WD, et al: Functional bowel disorders. In Drossman DA, Corazziari E, Delvaux M, et al. (eds): Rome III: The functional gastrointestinal disorders, 3rd ed. McLean, VA, Degnon, 2006, pp 487–555.

BOX 2 Subgroups of Irritable Bowel Syndrome (IBS)

- IBS with diarrhea (more common in men)
- IBS with constipation (more common in women)
- IBS with mixed bowel habits (previously known as IBS with alternating bowel habits based on Rome II criteria)
- IBS unsubtyped (not enough stools are abnormal to meet criteria for any other subtype)

Adapted from Longstreth GF, Thompson WG, Chey WD, et al: Functional bowel disorders. In Drossman DA, Corazziari E, Delvaux M, et al. (eds): Rome III: The functional gastrointestinal disorders, 3rd ed. McLean, VA, Degnon, 2006, pp 487–555.

BOX 3 Pathophysiologic Factors of Irritable Bowel Syndrome

- Altered bowel motility
- Visceral hypersensitivity
- Central nervous system effects
- Neurotransmitter imbalance (i.e., serotonin)
- Infection
- Psychosocial factors
- Genetics

CURRENT DIAGNOSIS

- Detailed history and physical examination to elicit red flags and exclude secondary causes
- Appropriate laboratory and imaging studies based on symptoms
- Identification of the subcategory of irritable bowel syndrome that best describes the patient's symptoms

psychological or physical stress. For example, there have been reports of an exaggerated contractile response of the colon (gastrocolic reflex) and small intestine to a high-fat meal.

In addition, pain is more commonly perceived by IBS patients in association with irregular motor activity of the small bowel than by patients with inflammatory bowel disease or normal control subjects. There are documented studies using balloon distention of the rectosigmoid and the ileum that suggest that patients with IBS have a central defect in the ability to process visceral pain, characterized by the perception of pain and bloating at balloon volumes and pressures significantly lower than those required by normal subjects to elicit similar symptoms. Functional magnetic resonance imaging and positron emission tomography of the brain have revealed different levels of activity in the thalamus and the anterior cingulate cortex after balloon distention of the rectum in patients with IBS compared to normal subjects. This phenomenon is referred to as visceral hypersensitivity.

Both altered motility and visceral hypersensitivity could be mediated by imbalances of neurotransmitters. Serotonin has received the most attention given its significant presence in the gastrointestinal tract and its previously reported association with symptoms of nausea, vomiting, abdominal pain, and bloating. Increased concordance of IBS in monozygotic versus dizygotic twins and familial aggregation in IBS may support a genetic component to IBS. As always, the role of nature versus nurture is addressed and the idea that learned behavior plays a part in the manifestation of IBS has been contemplated. It has been observed that children of parents with IBS tend to actively seek medical care for gastrointestinal symptoms more than children of non-IBS patients (hypervigilance). There are reports that IBS is more frequent and more severe in women with a history of physical and/or sexual abuse.

Evaluation

Current clinical guidelines recommend that IBS can generally be diagnosed without additional testing beyond careful history taking, a general physical examination, and routine laboratory studies to exclude other organic causes in patients who have symptoms that meet the Rome criteria and who do not have alarm warning signs (red flags).

The red flags include, but are not limited to, blood in the stool (gross or occult), anemia, weight loss, fever, family history of colon cancer, inflammatory bowel disease or celiac disease, onset of the first symptom after 50 years of age, nocturnal symptoms that awaken the patient from sleep, and a major change in symptoms. Routine laboratory tests have been suggested to include a complete blood count (CBC), thyroid function studies, stool studies for ova and parasites, and a comprehensive metabolic panel. In addition, it has recently been proposed that patients being evaluated for IBS-like symptoms who have a predominance of diarrhea be screened with serologic tests for celiac disease.

CURRENT THERAPY

- Establishment of a strong physician-patient relationship
- Dietary and behavioral modifications
- Pharmacotherapy based on the subcategory of irritable bowel syndrome

---

> **BOX 4   Differential Diagnosis for Irritable Bowel Syndrome**
>
> - Colon malignancy
> - Lymphoma of the gastrointestinal tract
> - Inflammatory bowel disease (Crohn's disease, ulcerative colitis)
> - Diverticulitis
> - Peptic ulcer disease
> - Biliary or liver disease
> - Chronic pancreatitis
> - Celiac disease
> - Small-bowel bacterial overgrowth
> - Parasites
> - Endometriosis
> - Medication-induced symptoms

If the patient meets the Rome III criteria and does not have any red flags, classification of the IBS into one of the subcategories is recommended to guide and facilitate empiric therapy. If a red flag is present, diagnostic tests should be performed as appropriate based on the presenting symptoms, signs, and laboratory findings. The differential diagnosis for IBS-like symptoms is significant and should always be considered when evaluating patients (Box 4).

Treatment

Treatment of IBS involves a multilevel approach. One of the most important components is the establishment of a strong physician-patient relationship; this is done by being nonjudgmental and allowing for a patient-centered interview. Be sure to acknowledge the patient's symptoms, identify whether any of them are stress-related, and determine whether comorbid psychological symptoms exist. Addressing psychosocial factors may improve health status and treatment response. The second component of treatment involves an attempt to identify foods that precipitate or exacerbate symptoms. Recommendations to avoid agents such as caffeine, alcohol, fatty foods, gas-producing vegetables, or products containing sorbitol are valid. In addition, if constipation is a key symptom, it may be beneficial to encourage consumption of 20 to 30 g of fiber per day (as part of the diet or as a supplement). Pharmacotherapy is guided by the predominant symptom; placement of each patient into an IBS subcategory is useful (Table 1). In addition, alternative therapies, including complementary medicines and psychotherapy, are often coupled with the available FDA-approved pharmacotherapy in an effort to treat IBS (Box 5).

Table 1 lists most of the agents that have been employed to treat IBS. Although almost all of these agents have been tested in randomized, controlled studies, only three—alosetron, lubiprostone, and tegaserod—have received FDA approval for treatment of IBS. Alosetron is a serotonin 5-HT_3 antagonist that received FDA approval for treatment of IBS with diarrhea in adult women at a dose of 1.0 mg twice daily. Because of reports of ischemic colitis and bowel perforations, it was removed from the market. It has now been reintroduced for use in patients with refractory disease. The recommended dosing is to begin with 0.5 mg once daily and slowly increase the dose to 1.0 mg twice daily if necessary. Tegaserod, a 5-HT_4 agonist, was approved by the FDA for the treatment of IBS with constipation in adult women at a dose of 6 mg twice daily. It, too, was removed from the market because of cardiovascular side effects. Currently, it is available only in a compassionate use protocol. The third FDA-approved agent for IBS is lubiprostone, which is approved at a dose of 8 mg with breakfast and dinner to treat IBS with constipation in adult women; there are no restrictions on duration of use. Lubiprostone stimulates C-2 chloride channels to secrete chloride into the lumen of the small intestine and the colon.

TABLE 1 Pharmacotherapy for Irritable Bowel Syndrome According to Symptom

Symptom	Initial Dose	Target Dose
Diarrhea		
Loperamide (Imodium)	2 mg/d	2–8 mg/d
Diphenoxylate and atropine (Lomotil)[1]	5 mg	up to 20 mg/d
Alosetron (Lotronex)*	0.5 mg bid	up to 1 mg bid
Constipation		
Fiber (over-the-counter products)		
Laxatives and secretory stimulants		
Polyethylene glycol 3350 (MiraLAX)[1]	17 g/d	up to 34 g bid
Lactulose (Cephulac)[1]	10–20 g/d	up to 40 g/d
Lubiprostone (Amitiza)	8 µg bid	24 µg bid[3]
Osmotic laxatives		
Stimulant laxatives		
Prokinetics		
Tegaserod (Zelnorm)[2]	6 mg bid	
Bloating		
Rifaximin (Xifaxan)[1]		400 mg tid[3]
Probiotics (*Bifidobacterium infantis* 35624; Bifantis)[7]		1 capsule per day
Pain		
Dicyclomine (Bentyl)	10 mg qid	40 mg qid
Hyoscyamine (Levsin)[1]	0.25 mg SL/ PO q4h prn	maximum 1.5 mg/d
Tricyclic antidepressants[1]		
Amitriptyline (Elavil)	10 mg qhs	10–75 mg qhs
Desipramine (Norpramin)	10 mg qhs	10–75 mg qhs
Nortriptyline (Pamelor)	10 mg qhs	10–75 mg qhs
Selective serotonin-reuptake inhibitors[1]		
Paroxetine (Paxil)	10 mg qhs	10–60 mg qhs
Citalopram (Celexa)	5 mg qhs	5–20 mg qhs
Fluoxetine (Prozac)	20 mg qhs	20–40 mg qhs

[1]Not FDA approved for this indication.
[2]Not available in the United States.
[3]Exceeds dosage recommended by the manufacturer.
[7]Available as dietary supplement.
*Available only to physicians enrolled in the Prescribing Program for Lotronex.

BOX 5 Alternative Management of Irritable Bowel Syndrome

Complementary Medicines
- Herbal medicines
- Megavitamins
- Folk remedies
- Microbial food supplements (prebiotics, probiotics, fungi)

Psychotherapy
- Cognitive behavioral therapy
- Relaxation therapy
- Contingency management
- Biofeedback
- Hypnosis

REFERENCES

Gershon MD, Tack J. The serotonin signaling system: From basic understanding to drug development for functional GI disorders. Gastroenterology 2007;132:397–414.

Horwitz BJ, Fisher RS. The irritable bowel wyndrome. N Engl J Med 2001; 344:1846–50.

Longstreth GF, Thompson WG, Chey WD, et al. Functional bowel disorders. In: Drossman DA, Corazziari E, Delvaux M, et al, editors Rome III: The functional gastrointestinal disorders. 3rd ed. McLean, VA: Degnon; 2006. p. 487–555.

Mayer EA. Irritable bowel syndrome. N Engl J Med 2008;358:1692–9.

Park M, Camilleri M. Genetics and genotypes in irritable bowel syndrome: Implications for diagnosis and treatment. Gastroenterol Clin North Am 2005;34:305–17.

Quigley EM, Flourie B. Probiotics and irritable bowel syndrome: A rationale for their use and an assessment of the evidence to date. Neurogastroenterol Motil 2007;19:166–72.

Videlock EJ, Chang L. Irritable bowel syndrome: Current approach to symptoms, evaluation, and treatment. Gastroenterol Clin North Am 2007;36:665–85.

Hemorrhoids, Anal Fissure, and Anorectal Abscess and Fistula

Method of
Dimitrios Christoforidis, MD, and Robert D. Madoff, MD

527

Anatomy and Function of the Anal Canal

The surgical or functional anal canal is 4 to 5 cm long and extends from the anal verge to the top of the external sphincter, or anorectal ring, where the rectal lumen enlarges. The most important anatomic landmark in the anal canal is the dentate line (Fig. 1), which is located approximately 2 cm cephalad from the anal verge. It is formed by a line of anal valves known as crypts, into which the anal glands open. These anal glands (on average, six in number) may become obstructed and secondarily infected, giving rise to perianal abscesses and fistulas. The dentate line is the transition zone for the epithelial lining, the arterial supply, the venous and lymphatic drainage, and the innervation. A rich somatic nerve fiber network makes

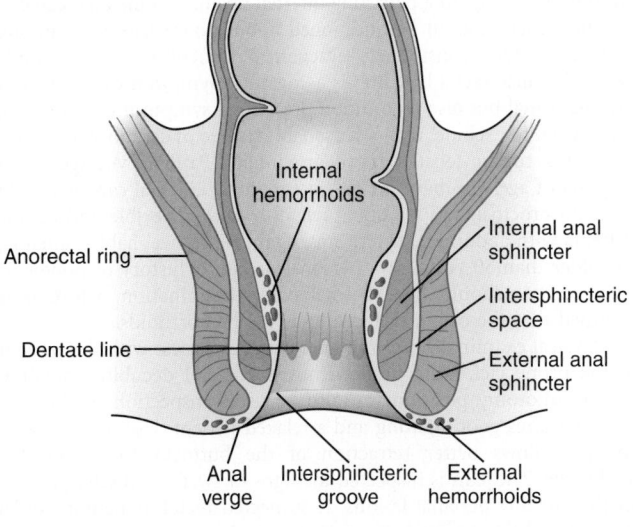

FIGURE 1. Anatomy of the anal canal.

the area below the dentate line very sensitive to pain. In contrast, the area above the dentate line is innervated only by autonomic nerve fibers; its relative inability to sense somatic pain permits such office procedures as rubber band ligation of internal hemorrhoids without anesthesia.

The internal anal sphincter is a thickened continuation of the circular muscle layer of the rectum. It is a smooth muscle with autonomic innervation; its tonic contraction is responsible for resting anal tone and prevents involuntary leakage. Its lower edge ends above the lower edge of the external sphincter, and the intersphincteric groove can be easily palpated, especially when the anal canal is stretched, at approximately 1 cm below the dentate line. The internal and external anal sphincters are separated by the conjoined longitudinal muscle, which is a continuation of the longitudinal outer muscle layer of the rectum mixed with fibers of the levator ani muscle.

The external anal sphincter is a striated cylindrical muscle whose cephalad portion merges with the puborectalis and levator ani muscles to form the pelvic floor. The puborectalis is a sling-shaped muscle that is easily palpable at the posterior anorectal junction on digital rectal examination; it plays an important role in anal continence. The external sphincter is attached posteriorly to the coccyx by the anococcygeal ligament and anteriorly to the perineal body. It contracts voluntarily and by reflex. Although it maintains unconscious resting tone through a reflex arc at the level of the cauda equina, its main function is to permit sphincter contraction as needed to defer defecation.

The external anal sphincter is surrounded by the ischiorectal space laterally. Posteriorly, a distinction is made between the superficial postanal space, below the anococcygeal ligament, and the deep postanal space, located between the anococcygeal ligament and the levator ani muscles.

History and Physical Examination

Patients with all types of anal diseases often present complaining of hemorrhoids. A careful patient history leads to the correct diagnosis in most cases. The differential diagnosis of the most common conditions is based on the following key symptoms: pain, bleeding, discharge, and presence of a lump.

Internal hemorrhoids cause bleeding and discomfort but are usually not painful unless complications occur. More advanced internal hemorrhoids protrude with defecation. External hemorrhoids become symptomatic when thrombosed, causing sudden-onset constant pain but no bleeding and no fever. An anal fissure typically causes severe pain with defecation that may persist for several hours; fissures may also lead to minor, bright red rectal bleeding. A perianal abscess manifests as a painful swelling of the perianal skin and may be accompanied by fever. Purulent discharge results from spontaneous drainage of a perianal abscess or from an anal fistula caused by an abscess that has drained but not healed due to a persisting internal opening in the anal canal.

The patient should be questioned about bowel habits, including frequency, stool consistency, evacuation difficulties, and incontinence. Because rectal bleeding is a common symptom of diseases of the anal canal but also a common presenting symptom of neoplasia, it is crucial to exclude, with a reasonable degree of certainty, the presence of a tumor located more proximally. Patients younger than 50 years of age who have no risk factors for colorectal cancer should undergo proctosigmoidoscopy, preferably with a flexible endoscope. Patients with abdominal symptoms, change in bowel habits, anemia, age older than 50 years, or a personal or family history of polyps or colon cancer should have a total colon examination before it is assumed that the origin of bleeding is the hemorrhoids.

Physical examination of the anorectum is easiest with the patient in the prone jack-knife position but the lateral decubitus position or the lithotomy position can also be used. Inspection of the anal verge requires good lighting and a relaxed patient. Use of two gauze sponges allows better retraction of the buttocks to expose the anal verge. The skin is inspected for signs of swelling, discharge, dermatitis, or any perianal lesions. A suspected rectal or hemorrhoidal prolapse is best seen with the patient seated on a commode, because most patients contract the sphincter for fear of an accident when asked to push in other positions. A digital rectal examination yields information on sphincter tone (both passive and on contraction), the prostate (in men), and the rectovaginal septum (in women), as well as the presence and characteristics of any mass and the type of stool, if present in the rectum. Anoscopy and proctosigmoidoscopy are easy to perform and allow inspection of the anorectal lumen. In the presence of an acute fissure or other painful condition, digital rectal examination, anoscopy, and proctosigmoidoscopy should be postponed until symptoms resolve or performed under anesthesia.

Hemorrhoids

Hemorrhoids are not veins but arteriovenous plexuses. External hemorrhoids lie below the dentate line and are covered by anoderm. Internal hemorrhoids lie above the dentate line and are covered by mucosa. They form submucosal cushions and play an important role in continence by providing a compressible lining that assists the complete closure of the anal canal. Internal hemorrhoids become symptomatic when they enlarge because of loosening and fragmentation of the supportive connective tissue framework, which causes a downward slide of the anal canal lining. Precipitating factors are prolonged straining, constipation or diarrhea, pregnancy, increased intraabdominal pressure with obstruction of venous return, and aging. Large internal hemorrhoids often extend over the dentate line and appear as combined internal and external "mixed" hemorrhoids.

External hemorrhoids become symptomatic when thrombosed, causing sudden-onset, constant, severe pain but no bleeding and no fever. Patients present with one or more hard, blue, perianal lumps covered with skin that may have eroded. The best treatment in the acute setting is incision and evacuation of the clot under local anesthesia. If the patient presents at a subacute stage (i.e., 4–5 days after symptom onset), treatment should be conservative, with sitz baths, pain management, and fiber supplements. Once the acute episode has resolved, the blood clot resorbs, often leaving a painless skin tag that requires no treatment.

The most typical symptom of internal hemorrhoids is bright red bleeding that occurs at the end of defecation; the blood is often described as dripping or squirting in the toilet. More advanced hemorrhoids protrude with defecation. The extent of prolapse should be determined from the history and physical examination and allows staging of the disease (Table 1). Discomfort with burning and itching is common and is caused by irritation of the perianal skin by mucus discharge from the hemorrhoids. Severe pain from internal hemorrhoids alone is rare and indicates thrombosis or incarceration of hemorrhoids or a different, possibly concomitant, pathology, such as a fissure.

The mainstay for the treatment of internal hemorrhoids is optimization of bowel habits. The goals are to achieve formed, soft stools and to minimize the time spent on the commode and the amount of straining. This can be accomplished by dietary modification increasing fruit and vegetable intake, and, most importantly, water intake. In most cases, fiber supplements are needed to reach the recommended dose of 30 to 40 g of fiber per day. Fiber intake should be increased progressively to minimize side effects of bloating and abdominal cramps. Medical therapy with local ointments and suppositories is popular, but there is no strong evidence for the efficacy of this approach. Preparations containing steroids and anesthetics seem to provide symptomatic relief but should not be used for long periods because of local allergic reactions and steroid-induced skin atrophy. Sitz baths (15 minutes in lukewarm water) are harmless and provide valuable symptomatic relief. Oral flavonoids, such as the formulation of micronized purified flavonoid fraction (Daflon), have shown some efficacy in randomized trials.

TABLE 1 Staging of Hemorrhoidal Disease

Grade	Description
I	Protrude only inside the lumen; seen only with the anoscope
II	Protrude during defecation; reduce spontaneously
III	Protrude during defecation; require manual reduction
IV	Permanently prolapsed and irreducible

Several office procedures without anesthesia can be employed to treat hemorrhoids not responding to the simple measures mentioned. Rubber-band ligation is performed by pulling the excessive hemorrhoidal tissue inside the barrel of the ligator, using either suction or a clamp. Firing of the ligator places the rubber band around and at the neck of the hemorrhoid. The strangulated hemorrhoid sloughs off in 5 to 7 days, creating a scar that fixes the tissue. Minor bleeding often occurs when the hemorrhoid sloughs; very occasionally, severe hemorrhage can supervene, especially in anticoagulated patients. As long as the band is placed well above the dentate line, patients do not feel any pain, although they may note some pressure. To avoid excessive discomfort and vasovagal reactions, most authorities place only one band at a time. Shrinkage and scarring of internal hemorrhoids can also be achieved by sclerotherapy (injection of 5% phenol in olive oil or another sclerosant into the hemorrhoid) or by infrared coagulation at the apex of the hemorrhoid.

Surgery is reserved for grade III and IV hemorrhoids that are too extensive for simpler measures or have not responded to them. There are two basic techniques. The classic operation is excision of the hemorrhoidal tissue, with or without suturing of the resulting mucosal and anodermal defect. An alternative method developed in the 1990s uses a specially designed mechanical stapler to excise a circular band of rectal mucosa above the hemorrhoid and staple the defect closed. This operation interrupts the arterial hemorrhoidal flow and lifts the prolapsing hemorrhoid inside the anal canal. A number of randomized trials and systematic reviews have been performed comparing the two techniques. The general consensus is that the stapling technique is less painful and results in a more rapid return to work; the price is a threefold to fourfold higher risk of long-term recurrence (up to 10%) compared with conventional hemorrhoidectomy. In addition, there are reports of rare but severe complications occurring after the stapler operation.

Anal Fissure

Anal fissure is a longitudinal tear of the anoderm, distal to the dentate line. The underlying pathophysiologic mechanism is related to internal sphincter hypertonia, which causes local ischemia. Between 80% and 90% of fissures occur at the posterior midline, where anatomic studies document relatively deficient vascularity. Anterior midline fissures account for 10% to 15% of all fissures and are more common in women. Lateral fissures are rare and should always raise suspicion for other diseases causing anodermal ulcers—in particular, Crohn's disease, anal carcinoma, HIV infection, tuberculosis, and syphilis. Fissures occurring off the midline require biopsy to exclude these diagnoses.

The diagnosis of anal fissure is suggested by a history of painful defecation. The pain is often severe and can persist for hours after defecation. Some patients also complain of passing minor quantities of fresh red blood per rectum. Simple exposure of the anal verge by opposing traction on the buttocks confirms the diagnosis of anal fissure, and further digital examination or anoscopy should be avoided at that time. Chronic fissures (lasting >2–3 months) typically have elevated edges, exposed internal sphincter fibers at the base of the ulcer, and a sentinel skin tag at the distal part.

Most acute fissures heal with conservative treatment consisting of sitz baths and bowel transit regularization with fiber supplements. Recurrence occurs in approximately 20% of the cases. Chronic fissures are more difficult to manage. Besides bowel transit regularization, additional intervention to decrease internal anal sphincter tone is required. This can be accomplished medically with smooth muscle relaxants: 0.2%-0.4% nitroglycerine or 2% diltiazem topical ointment or botulinum toxin injection. The nitroglycerine and diltiazem ointments must be applied two to three times daily for 6 to 8 weeks. Headaches and orthostatic hypotension are frequent side effects with nitroglycerine. Reported healing rates vary from 30% to 100%. Long-term follow-up shows recurrence rates of up to 40%. Botulin toxin injection is reported to have approximately the same healing and recurrence rates as topical sphincter relaxants but is more expensive.

The most effective treatment for chronic anal fissure is surgical sphincterotomy of the internal anal sphincter, and this is the treatment of choice when other measures have failed. Most authors agree that the division of muscle fibers should be made laterally and not at the midline underneath the fissure, to avoid causing a keyhole deformity and stool leakage. There is controversy regarding the appropriate length and depth of the sphincterotomy and whether it should be performed with an open approach (larger incision to expose the internal anal sphincter) or a closed approach (stab incision with blind division of the internal anal sphincter). Generally, a partial-thickness division from the level of the top of the fissure is recommended to minimize the non-negligible risk of minor incontinence that is the main drawback of this treatment.

Anorectal Abscess and Fistula

Anorectal abscesses are common and most often result from obstruction and subsequent infection of the anal glands, which are found in the crypts of the anal canal. Other causes include inflammatory bowel disease, trauma, malignancy, and superficial skin infections such as furuncles and Verneuil's disease (apocrine gland infection). Most anorectal abscesses are located superficially in the subanodermal space or deeper in the ischiorectal fossa. Less frequently, abscesses can form in the intersphincteric space; these cause severe pain but with minimal findings on examination. Supralevator abscesses are rarely related to cryptoglandular infection.

Treatment of acute anorectal abscesses should always be surgical drainage, and there is little, if any, role for antibiotic therapy. Drainage can be performed with the use of local anesthesia for superficial abscesses but requires general anesthesia for deeper or suspected intersphincteric abscesses. Local anesthesia should be injected slowly, starting peripherally, to minimize discomfort; anesthesia administration can be completed after initial decompressing drainage. A cruciate incision, with resection of the resulting skin corners over the summit of the abscess, creates a sufficient opening and avoids premature skin closure. Wound care is based on regular sitz baths until secondary healing has occurred.

Approximately one third of patients with anorectal abscesses ultimately develop an anocutaneous fistula. The internal opening is by definition at the infected crypt at the dentate line, and Goodsall's rule can help locate it. This rule states that if the external opening lies in the anterior perianal hemisphere, the fistula usually forms a straight tract to the dentate line. If the external opening lies in the posterior perianal hemisphere, the fistula is usually curvilinear, and the internal opening is most likely located at the posterior midline. Endorectal ultrasonography and magnetic resonance imaging are useful techniques that are indicated to better characterize complex and recurrent fistula tracts.

For optimal treatment, it is important to determine whether the fistula crosses the anal sphincter, and at which level. Fistulas are classified as superficial, intersphincteric, transsphincteric, suprasphincteric, or extrasphincteric (Fig. 2). The most efficient treatment for fistulas is to unroof and lay open the tract. It is the treatment of choice for the majority of fistulas encountered that are superficial, intersphincteric, or low transsphincteric.

However, fistulotomy is contraindicated in patients with fistulas involving a significant amount of sphincter muscle and in those with other factors that threaten their continence. For such patients, several sphincter-preserving techniques to cure the fistula exist. The first phase is to treat any ongoing sepsis by placing one or more seton drains through the tract. This prevents recurrent abscesses and leads to shrinkage of the tract around the seton. In a second phase, repair of the fistula can be accomplished in various ways. With the cutting seton method, the seton is tightened progressively and cuts through the tract, leaving fibrosis behind. Pain during treatment and continence disturbances are common. The endorectal advancement flap method aims at covering the internal opening with a mucosal flap. The technique is technically demanding, and success rates vary from 50% to 90%. Instillation of fibrin glue into the tract to obliterate it was initially reported to be successful, but long-term results demonstrated a high recurrence rate. More recently, the anal fistula plug was developed, which is made of porcine submucosal connective tissue

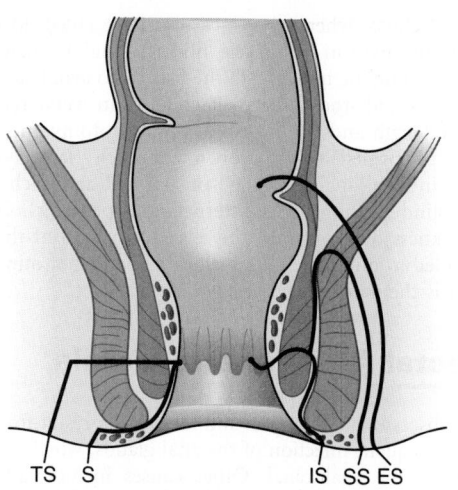

FIGURE 2. Classification of anal fistulas. *Abbreviations:* ES = extrasphincteric; IS = intersphincteric; S = superficial; SS = suprasphincteric; TS = transsphincteric.

and is introduced and anchored in the fistula, providing a collagen scaffold for tissue ingrowth. The early to middle-term success rate with this sphincter-sparing method is approximately 30% to 50%, but long-term efficacy rates are not known.

REFERENCES

Christoforidis D, Etzioni DA, Goldberg SM, et al. Treatment of complex anal fistulas with the collagen fistula plug. Dis Colon Rectum 2008;51:1482–7.

Hamalainen KP, Sainio AP. Cutting seton for anal fistulas: high risk of minor control defects. Dis Colon Rectum 1997;40:1443–6; discussion 1447.

Jayaraman S, Colquhoun PH, Malthaner RA. Stapled versus conventional surgery for hemorrhoids. Cochrane Database Syst Rev 2006(4):CD005393.

Loungnarath R, Dietz DW, Mutch MG, et al. Fibrin glue treatment of complex anal fistulas has low success rate. Dis Colon Rectum 2004;47:432–6.

Nelson R. Non surgical therapy for anal fissure. Cochrane Database Syst Rev 2006(4):CD003431.

Nelson R. Operative procedures for fissure in ano. Cochrane Database Syst Rev 2005(2):CD002199.

Neves Jorge JM, Habr-Gama A. Anatomy and embryology of the colon, rectum, and anus. In: Wolff BG, Fleshman JW, Beck DE, et al, editors. The ASCRS Textbook of Colon and Rectal Surgery. New York: Springer; 2007. pp. 1–22.

Ortiz H, Marzo J. Endorectal flap advancement repair and fistulectomy for high transsphincteric and suprasphincteric fistulas. Br J Surg 2000;87:1680–3.

Parks AG, Gordon PH, Hardcastle JD. A classification of fistula-in-ano. Br J Surg 1976;63:1–12.

Gastritis and Peptic Ulcer Disease

Method of
Sripathi R. Kethu, MD, and Steven F. Moss, MD

Gastritis is by definition a histopathologic diagnosis, and peptic ulcer disease (PUD) is an endoscopic or radiologic diagnosis. Neither of these conditions has a specific symptom complex to help the clinician arrive at a diagnosis. Instead, physicians encounter patients with symptoms of dyspepsia that might or might not be secondary to gastritis or PUD. Thus, for the primary care provider, the discussion of gastritis and PUD must be prefaced by first considering the approach to the patient with dyspeptic symptoms.

Dyspepsia

Dyspepsia refers to pain or discomfort centered in the upper abdomen, which may be intermittent or continuous and might or might not be related to meals. The symptoms may be described by several other terms, including *bloating, fullness, belching,* and *nausea* or simply as *indigestion.*

The prevalence of uninvestigated dyspepsia in the general population is not well documented. However, up to 25% of people in the community each year report chronic or recurrent pain or discomfort in the upper abdomen, and approximately 2% to 5% of family practice consultations are for dyspepsia.

ETIOLOGY AND DIFFERENTIAL DIAGNOSIS

Dyspepsia can result from an identifiable cause such as peptic ulcer disease, malignancy, gastroesophageal reflux, or the use of specific medications. Other rare causes include pancreatic-biliary disease, gastroparesis, celiac disease, lactose intolerance, and parasitic diseases such as giardiasis. Patients who have no definite structural or biochemical explanation for their symptoms are considered to have functional dyspepsia (nonulcer dyspepsia). There is a subset of patients in whom dyspepsia might coexist with a microbiological or structural abnormality such as *Helicobacter pylori* gastritis or duodenitis or with gallstones, but a causal relation between these abnormalities and dyspepsia may be unclear.

The patient's age is one of the most important factors in tailoring the management of patients with dyspepsia because of the very low probability of stomach cancer in younger patients (typically this cut-off is arbitrarily fixed at 55 years). Thus, if a patient older than 55 years presents with new-onset upper abdominal complaints, or patients younger than this age develop alarm symptoms (anemia, anorexia, weight loss > 10% of body weight, early satiety, dysphagia, or gastrointestinal (GI) bleeding either overt or occult), prompt endoscopic evaluation is required to detect the cause before administering empiric therapy.

In a primary care setting, the patient's history is crucial in elucidating the cause of dyspepsia. Peptic ulcer disease is an important consideration in the differential diagnosis of dyspepsia, accounting for up to 15% of cases. Although it is impossible to distinguish gastric and duodenal ulcers by symptoms alone, the pain of gastric and duodenal ulcers is typically epigastric, episodic, and often worse at night. Symptoms are often temporarily relieved with food or antacids in duodenal ulcer; in contrast, food can precipitate gastric ulcer pain. Associated symptoms such as anorexia, nausea, or vomiting can point toward the diagnosis of gastric ulcer or pyloric stenosis. Patients with gastric malignancy, which accounts for less than 2% of all cases of dyspepsia, can also present with similar symptoms.

Gastroesophageal reflux disease (GERD) may be the underlying disorder in 10% to 15% of patients with dyspepsia. Other typical symptoms in GERD include heartburn or a retrosternal burning pain or a feeling of regurgitation of food or acid. However, about 20% of patients with GERD present with epigastric pain alone, thereby creating a diagnostic problem. If medications are responsible for dyspepsia, generally a temporal relationship can be established between the medication intake and the onset of dyspeptic symptoms. Nonsteroidal anti-inflammatory drugs (NSAIDs) are the most common offending agents; other medications that cause dyspepsia are corticosteroids, iron preparations, digitalis, potassium supplements, bisphosphonates, niacin, and antibiotics, particularly erythromycin and ampicillin.

Functional, or nonulcer, dyspepsia accounts for up to 60% of all cases of dyspepsia. Functional dyspepsia and PUD share many symptoms, thus making the distinction by history alone impossible. By definition, the cause of functional dyspepsia is obscure; the putative pathophysiologic abnormalities that have been proposed to cause or to be associated with functional dyspepsia are gastric acid hypersecretion, *H. pylori* infection, gastroduodenal dysmotility, visceral hyperalgesia, and psychological distress including physical or sexual abuse. Although functional dyspepsia is a benign condition, it is the hardest to treat given the uncertain interplay between numerous pathogenic mechanisms.

EVALUATION

Currently the best test in the evaluation of dyspepsia is upper endoscopy. Barium meal radiographs are less sensitive and specific.

In a younger patient (age < 55 years), in the absence of alarm symptoms, and after excluding other causes such as GERD and NSAID use by history, an *H. pylori* test and treat strategy, followed by proton pump inhibitor (PPI) treatment if the patient remains symptomatic or is not infected by *H. pylori*, is the management strategy of choice. The justification for this approach is that among patients with uninvestigated dyspepsia who are *H. pylori* positive, a substantial number have peptic ulcers, and a few without ulcers can improve symptomatically following eradication of *H. pylori*. Whether this strategy is suitable for affluent populations in the United States who have a very low prevalence of *H. pylori* is debatable because it can result in the diagnosis of almost as many false-positive *H. pylori* infections and lead to inappropriate eradication therapy. Furthermore, the cost benefits of the test and treat approach over one with early invasive testing remains unproven in practice. In other populations, noninvasive testing for *H. pylori* either by stool antigen test or urea breath test is reasonable. These tests are relatively less expensive compared with either upper endoscopy or indefinite empiric acid-suppressive therapy and are more accurate than serology.

If symptoms persist after *H. pylori* eradication therapy, or if empiric acid-suppressive therapy in *H. pylori*–negative patients fails, upper endoscopy should be undertaken. Ultrasonography is not recommended as a routine next step unless the history or biochemical tests suggest pancreatic-biliary disease. In patients with diabetes or a history suggesting autonomic neuropathy, a gastric emptying scan (scintigraphy) may be considered to document gastroparesis. Even though functional dyspepsia should be considered a diagnosis of exclusion, clinicians should use their judgment on a case-by-case basis to limit the use of numerous invasive and expensive investigations whenever possible.

MANAGEMENT

Once the cause of dyspepsia is established, management involves treating the underlying cause. The most challenging task is managing patients with functional dyspepsia. *H. pylori* eradication therapy for patients who do not have an ulcer can result in symptomatic improvement in a small minority, approximately in 15% of patients, at best, over placebo. However, most patients remain symptomatic after eradication therapy, thus requiring other therapies.

Reassurance and explanation are important first steps in management. Proving that the symptoms do not represent a malignancy may be sufficient. Patients should be educated to avoid any obvious offending agents, such as coffee, alcohol, smoking, NSAIDs, and spicy and fatty foods; this helps relieve symptoms in some patients. Precipitant psychosocial factors including anxiety and depression should also be explored and treated appropriately. Pharmacologic therapy is not always required, and if required, it should be individualized. No single drug has been clearly shown to be beneficial over the long term, and the results of pharmacologic therapy are disappointing overall.

First-line therapies usually involve a therapeutic trial of either antisecretory agents such as H₂-receptor antagonists (H₂-RAs) or PPIs. A prokinetic agent such as metoclopramide (Reglan) 10 mg 1 hour after meals and at bedtime for 4 to 6 weeks may be useful as an alternative therapy. A drug holiday during therapy can help determine if the medication is still needed. The benefits of individual drugs should be weighed against the side-effect profile and cost. Metoclopramide, for example, is associated with neuropsychiatric complications and therefore cannot be recommended for the long term. Antidepressants such as amitriptyline (Elavil)[1] 150 mg at bedtime or antispasmodics such as dicyclomine (Bentyl)[1] 20 to 40 mg

every 6 hours, can be tried as a next step, but the results are marginal at best. Alternative therapies such as acupuncture, cognitive behavior therapy, and hypnotherapy have been anecdotally reported to be beneficial.

Gastritis

Exposure of the gastric mucosa to various insults can lead to epithelial damage and regeneration with minimal or no inflammation (gastropathy), or the epithelial damage may be associated with significant inflammation (gastritis). For an endoscopist, gastritis usually means petechiae or erosions of the gastric mucosa. These endoscopic findings might not have a good correlation with the presence of inflammatory cells on biopsy. Strictly speaking, gastritis is a histopathologic diagnosis associated with the presence of inflammatory cells. Gastritis and gastropathy can be categorized according to the histologic features and the etiology (Box 1).

ACUTE EROSIVE AND HEMORRHAGIC GASTROPATHY

The most common causes of acute erosive and hemorrhagic gastropathy include NSAIDs, alcohol, and stress due to critical illness. Clinically, the patient might present with nonspecific complaints such as epigastric pain, nausea, or vomiting and occasionally with upper bleeding alone. Upper endoscopy usually reveals erythema or erosions. Histologically, there is usually no or minimal inflammation, hence the term *gastropathy* instead of *gastritis*. Stress gastritis, most likely due to chronic gastric ischemia, can lead to gastric ulceration, usually multiple small ulcers involving the proximal part of the stomach.

Management of symptomatic gastropathy caused by NSAIDs or alcohol involves minimizing or avoiding the offending agents or taking the NSAIDs with food. A short course of H₂-RAs or PPIs is recommended if the patient has persistent symptoms despite conservative measures. Long-term acid-suppression therapy with PPIs may be necessary for patients believed to be at high risk for bleeding but in whom chronic NSAID use is necessary. The development of cyclooxygenase-2 (COX-2) selective NSAIDs has diminished but not eliminated clinically important gastroduodenal bleeding, and the benefit of these agents should be weighed against their reported risk of cardiovascular complications.

Endoscopy is recommended only for patients with risk factors for developing an ulcer (see the section on peptic ulcer disease). Many critically ill hospitalized patients develop superficial erosions ("stress gastritis") from chronic gastric ischemia, but this rarely leads to clinically significant gastric bleeding. Two risk factors that are associated with a high risk of clinically significant bleeding are mechanical ventilation and a coagulopathy. In the absence of these two risk factors, the risk of significant bleeding is less than 0.1%. Preventing stress gastritis and ulcers with the use of acid-suppression medications is strongly recommended in all critically ill patients, particularly if they have the previously mentioned risk factors. The superiority of oral or intravenous PPIs over H₂-RAs in this setting has not been definitely established.

BOX 1   Classification of Gastritis

• Acute erosive and hemorrhagic gastropathy
 • Chronic gastritis
    • *Helicobacter pylori* gastritis (may be atrophic or nonatrophic)
    • Pernicious anemia–associated atrophic gastritis (type A gastritis or autoimmune gastritis)
 • Others
    • Eosinophilic gastritis
    • Infectious (Cytomegalovirus, herpes virus)
    • Granulomatous gastritis (Crohn's disease)
    • Portal gastropathy

---

[1]Not FDA approved for this indication.

CHRONIC *HELICOBACTER PYLORI* GASTRITIS

H. pylori is a gram-negative spiral bacterium acquired in childhood that colonizes the gastric mucosa and usually causes an antral-predominant gastritis. In the developed world, infection is more prevalent in the elderly, the poor, and immigrants from high-incidence regions such as Asia, Africa, and Central and South America.

Inflammation associated with chronic *H. pylori* colonization may be confined to the superficial mucosa or can extend deeper into the gastric glands, leading in some cases to gastric atrophy (atrophic gastritis) and intestinal metaplasia of the gastric epithelium. The majority of all gastric and duodenal ulcers are caused by *H. pylori*; approximately 10% of all patients with chronic gastritis due to *H. pylori* eventually develop peptic ulcer disease.

A more uncommon consequence of *H. pylori* infection is adenocarcinoma of the stomach, typically developing after many decades of infection and after histologic progression from atrophic gastritis through intestinal metaplasia and dysplasia. *H. pylori* infection is associated with a threefold to sixfold increased risk of distal gastric cancer, leading to its designation by the World Health Organization as a carcinogen. It is also a major risk factor for the relatively rare mucosa-associated lymphoid tissue (MALT) gastric B-cell lymphoma. (See the section on peptic ulcer disease for detailed discussion of diagnosis and management of *H. pylori*.)

Factors believed to be important determinants of individual clinical outcome following *H. pylori* infection include host genetics, nutritional and general health status, and specific *H. pylori* virulence genes.

PERNICIOUS ANEMIA–ASSOCIATED ATROPHIC GASTRITIS

Pernicious anemia–associated atrophic gastritis (type A gastritis or autoimmune gastritis) is an autoimmune disorder characterized by antiparietal cell antibodies leading to parietal cell destruction. The disease is more common in women and in persons of northern European descent. Parietal cell destruction in the gastric fundus leads to achlorhydria, and the impaired intrinsic factor production results in vitamin B_{12} malabsorption. Generally, patients are asymptomatic until extreme vitamin B_{12} deficiency causes anemia leading to neurologic syndromes. Patients are at increased risk for developing carcinoid tumors (secondary to prolonged hypergastrinemia) and adenocarcinoma of the stomach. Treatment involves vitamin B_{12} supplementation even if the serum vitamin B_{12} level is not low. The usefulness of periodic endoscopic screening to detect carcinoma or carcinoid tumors is controversial in this condition.

Peptic Ulcer Disease

Peptic ulcer disease is a generic term used to indicate a mucosal defect in the stomach or duodenum. As opposed to an erosion, which is a superficial lesion, an ulcer has a perceivable depth extending through the submucosa. PUD is believed to occur when factors aggressive to the gastric mucosa dominate (such as *H. pylori* infection or gastric acid hypersecretion) or when mucosal defense mechanisms are impaired (by NSAIDs, for example), or both.

The lifetime risk of PUD in the United States is approximately 10%, with a male-to-female ratio of 1.3:1 for a duodenal ulcer and 1:1 for a gastric ulcer. Duodenal ulcer occurs more commonly between ages 25 and 55 years, whereas gastric ulcer affects a slightly older population (ages 40–70 years). NSAID use or *H. pylori* infection increases the peptic ulcer risk by about 20-fold. Cigarette smoking not only increases the ulcer risk (by twofold), but also retards ulcer healing and increases the risk of bleeding. Despite popular beliefs, alcohol and dietary factors have no established relation with the cause of ulcers or their healing. Psychological stress can play some role in idiopathic ulcers.

ETIOLOGY

Depending on their etiology, ulcers can be classified in four groups: *H. pylori*–associated ulcers, NSAID-induced ulcers, idiopathic (non-*H. pylori*, non-NSAID) ulcers, and Zollinger-Ellison syndrome (discussed later). Other less-common causes include ulcers secondary to drugs other than NSAIDs (e.g., potassium chloride, bisphosphonates), stress ulcers due to a critical illness, ulcers of Crohn's disease, and infectious causes (*Cytomegalovirus ulcers* in HIV patients, *herpes simplex*).

Helicobacter pylori–Associated Ulcers

H. pylori infection is responsible for the majority of peptic ulcers. *H. pylori* is believed to be transmitted from person to person, probably via the fecal–oral route. The prevalence of *H. pylori* is between 20% and 50% in the Western world, including the United States. However, *H. pylori* is much more prevalent in developing nations, affecting as many as 90% of the population. In the United States, the prevalence is higher in the elderly, probably reflecting the poor sanitary conditions that existed in the early part of the century, and is more common in those of African American or Latin American ethnicity. *H. pylori* is also more prevalent in persons of low socioeconomic status, possibly related to crowded childhood living conditions.

Initial studies reported that *H. pylori* was present in about 90% of patients with duodenal ulcers and 60% of patients with gastric ulcer. More recent estimates show slightly lower prevalence of *H. pylori* in both duodenal ulcer and gastric ulcer, probably reflecting the relative increase in NSAID-associated ulcers. Approximately 10% of all persons infected with *H. pylori* develop PUD over their lifetime.

The exact pathophysiologic mechanism(s) by which *H. pylori* causes either duodenal or gastric ulcer and why only a minority of infected persons develop clinically overt disease is not known. Generally, duodenal ulcer is a disease of acid hypersecretion and gastric ulcer is associated with states of low acid secretion. *H. pylori* can potentially cause both of these secretory abnormalities. Gastric acid hypersecretion in duodenal ulcer occurs secondary to increased gastric release by a healthy acid-secreting gastric body mucosa (Figure 1). In contrast, when *H. pylori*–associated gastritis affects the proximal stomach too, this results in loss of gastric glands (atrophic gastritis) and hypochlorhydria with impaired mucosal defense, leading to gastric ulceration and even gastric cancer.

NSAID-Induced Ulcers

NSAIDs are among the most prescribed medications in the United States. The incidence of ulcers in chronic NSAID users is approximately 15% to 20%. The risk of NSAID-induced ulcers increases dramatically with the presence of specific risk factors (particularly with age >60 years and a prior history of peptic ulcer) and also with high doses of NSAIDs and concurrent use of either anticoagulants or high-dose corticosteroids. NSAIDs cause gastric ulcers much more commonly than duodenal ulcers. Up to 40% of these persons remain asymptomatic, and patients commonly present with complications.

The most important mechanism by which NSAIDs cause ulcers is by indirectly decreasing prostaglandin production via the inhibition of COX-1. Prostaglandins are important in maintaining mucosal integrity by producing mucus, stimulating bicarbonate production, decreasing acid production, and maintaining mucosal blood flow. The analgesic and anti-inflammatory effects of NSAIDs result from the inhibition of the COX-2 isoenzyme. Nonselective NSAIDs cause inhibition of both COX-2 and COX-1, resulting in considerable GI toxicity. The more recently developed selective COX-2 inhibitors, such as celecoxib (Celebrex), as the name implies, inhibit COX-2 to a much greater extent than COX-1, leading to their better GI safety profile. However, recent reports of cardiovascular complications attributed to COX-2 inhibitors have severely restricted their use.

Idiopathic Ulcers

In a specific subgroup of patients who develop ulcers, all the known etiologic factors are excluded. This subgroup should not be confused with patients who have unexplained ulcers, 60% of whom have a history of surreptitious NSAID use. The true incidence of idiopathic ulcers is hard to assess in various studies as a result of false-negative *H. pylori* tests or surreptitious use of NSAIDs, and the exact pathogenic

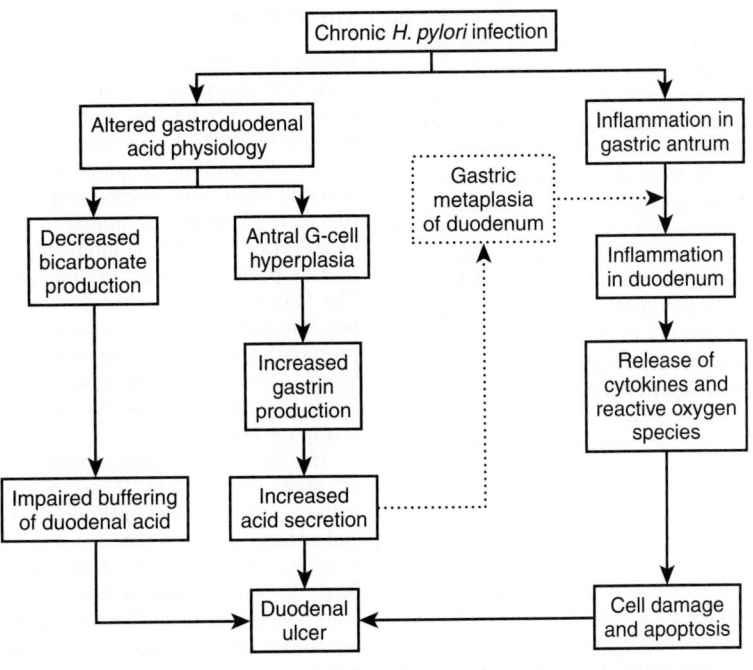

FIGURE 1. Proposed pathogenic mechanisms leading to *Helicobacter pylori*–induced duodenal ulcer.

mechanism that causes these idiopathic ulcers remains unknown. Various abnormalities including genetic predisposition, defective mucosal defense mechanisms, and increased acid production have all been postulated.

CLINICAL FEATURES

Clinical signs and symptoms are unreliable and are not specific enough to make a diagnosis of a peptic ulcer. Upper abdominal pain (dyspepsia) is present in more than 80% of patients; however, only 15% of patients with dyspepsia have PUD. Pain is typically epigastric, described as burning and nonradiating. Food or antacids can relieve duodenal ulcer pain. Nausea or anorexia can occur with gastric ulcers. Nocturnal symptoms awaken patients in two thirds of duodenal ulcer and one third of gastric ulcer cases. Symptoms usually wax and wane over a period of months. The physical examination is usually normal in PUD patients. Epigastric tenderness may be present on palpation, but it is an unreliable sign with a positive predictive value of less than 50%. Stool tests for occult blood may be positive in one third of patients.

DIAGNOSTIC WORK-UP

Routine laboratory studies are not helpful in establishing a diagnosis of PUD. Upper endoscopy is the gold standard in making a diagnosis of peptic ulcer. Endoscopy has the advantage of taking biopsies for the presence of *H. pylori* infection and, in the case of gastric ulcer, to rule out malignancy. However, endoscopy is more expensive and invasive. In the absence of alarm symptoms, double-contrast barium radiography may be a suitable second choice. If barium radiography shows an ulcer (gastric or duodenal), *H. pylori* must be tested noninvasively. Treatment can be instituted with acid-suppression therapy with or without antibiotics depending on the presence of *H. pylori*. Gastric pH and fasting gastrin levels should be obtained only if there is clinical suspicion for gastrinoma (see the section on Zollinger-Ellison syndrome). For gastric ulcers, it is advisable to repeat the endoscopy after 6 to 8 weeks of therapy to confirm the healing of the ulcer and re-biopsy if it is not healed, because 5% of gastric ulcers can be malignant.

Many tests are available for *H. pylori*. Testing for *H. pylori* can be made by either noninvasive or invasive methods (Table 1). An appropriate test should be chosen depending on the clinical situation. For

CURRENT DIAGNOSIS

- In the majority of cases of dyspepsia, no structural abnormality can be identified after investigation.
- Patients with dyspepsia who are older than 55 years or who have alarm symptoms (anemia, anorexia, weight loss, early satiety, dysphagia, or gastrointestinal bleeding) should undergo upper endoscopy.
- *Helicobacter pylori* infection and NSAIDs are the two most common causes of peptic ulcer disease.
- Endoscopic biopsy, urea breath test, and stool antigen testing are the most accurate ways to diagnose active *H. pylori* infection.
- Zollinger-Ellison syndrome should be suspected if there are multiple duodenal ulcers, ulcers that are refractory to treatment, or peptic ulcers associated with diarrhea.

TABLE 1 Diagnostic Tests for *H. pylori*

Diagnostic Test	Sensitivity (%)	Specificity (%)
Noninvasive Tests		
Serum ELISA test for antibody	85	80
Urea breath test (^{14}C or ^{13}C)	95–100	91–98
Stool antigen test	91–98	94–99
Invasive (Endoscopy-Based) Tests		
Rapid urease test	93–97	95–100
Histology	> 95	98–99
Culture	70–80	100

Abbreviation: ELISA = enzyme-linked immunosorbent assay.

example, testing for serologic antibodies against *H. pylori* may be appropriate for the initial testing for *H. pylori* though it is not as accurate as breath or stool tests. Also, serology is not useful to check for eradication after therapy, because it will not distinguish currentactive infection from prior infection that was treated (antibody levels fall slowly and unpredictably). Office-based qualitative antibody tests are cheaper compared with enzyme-linked immunosorbent assay (ELISA) test done in the laboratory but not as accurate, and they have been superseded by stool antigen and breath testing. Patients with alarm symptoms and all patients older than 55 years who have dyspeptic symptoms should undergo endoscopy, at which time *H. pylori* testing can be done by biopsy if an ulcer is found. Confirmation of the eradication of *H. pylori* should be considered after treating this infection in ulcer patients, by either the stool antigen test or the urea breath test, depending on the local resources. Confirmation of eradication by gastric biopsy is only recommended if endoscopy is performed for another reason, for example, to confirm healing of a gastric ulcer.

DIFFERENTIAL DIAGNOSIS

Functional dyspepsia is a major differential diagnostic consideration in all patients with upper abdominal pain (see the section on functional dyspepsia). Other diseases that mimic the symptoms of PUD include cancers of the upper gastrointestinal tract, biliary colic, and mesenteric ischemia.

TREATMENT

Different classes of drugs are available to treat PUD (Table 2). Antacids heal the ulcers and are cheap but are relatively ineffective, are slow to produce healing, and have many side effects. Both PPIs and H_2-RAs block acid secretion, but PPIs inhibit more than 90% of the 24-acid output compared with 65% with H_2-RAs; hence, PPIs heal the ulcer and relieve symptoms faster. Ulcer-healing rates of sucralfate (Carafate) are similar to those for H_2-RAs. The mechanism of action of sucralfate is unknown; it probably coats the ulcer base, thereby promoting ulcer healing, and might have other effects too. The frequent dosing schedule and large tablet size of sucralfate is not conducive to good compliance. Misoprostol (Cytotec) is a prostaglandin analogue approved for preventing NSAID-induced ulcers. Compliance with misoprostol treatment is also a problem, particularly at high doses, owing to its GI side effects of abdominal cramping and diarrhea.

H. pylori eradication is recommended in all ulcer patients who are *H. pylori* positive, but *H. pylori* infection should not be assumed without a documented positive test. *H. pylori* eradication heals ulcers and reduces the ulcer recurrence dramatically, to less than 20% after 2 years. Select *H. pylori* eradication regimens are summarized in Table 3. Confirmation of eradication is mandatory for complicated ulcer associated with bleeding, perforation, or obstruction and is recommended in all ulcer patients receiving *H. pylori* therapy. Treatment of idiopathic ulcers is difficult and often requires indefinite maintenance antisecretory therapy, particularly for a complicated ulcer.

PREVENTION

Ulcers can recur either with continued use of NSAIDs or with *H. pylori* infection that persists after the initial antibiotic course. The incidence of antibiotic resistance to *H. pylori* is rising all over the world. In the United States, approximately 40% of *H. pylori* strains are now resistant to metronidazole (Flagyl), and 10% to 12% are resistant to clarithromycin (Biaxin), which decreases the cure rates by as much as 50% and 37%, respectively. If the patient has persistent symptoms after therapy, eradication failure should be strongly suspected and noninvasive testing for *H. pylori* should be performed. If the initial diagnosis of the ulcer was made by radiography, endoscopy is the next reasonable test. Drugs that are clearly shown to be superior to placebo in preventing NSAID-induced ulcers are PPIs and misoprostol (Cytotec). Double the standard doses of H_2-RAs used for active ulcers are significantly better than placebo in preventing NSAID-induced gastroduodenal ulcers (see Table 2). PPIs are

TABLE 2 Treatment Options for Peptic Ulcers*

Pharmacologic Agent	Active Ulcer (Gastric or Duodenal)†	Prevention of NSAID-Induced Ulcer Recurrence
Antisecretory Agents		
H_2-Receptor Antagonists		
Cimetidine (Tagamet)	400 mg bid or 800 mg qhs	Double the dose indicated for active ulcer[1]
Famotidine (Pepcid)	20 mg bid or 40 mg qhs	
Nizatidine (Axid)	150 mg bid or 300 mg qhs	
Ranitidine (Zantac)	150 mg bid or 300 mg qhs	
Proton Pump Inhibitors		
Esomeprazole (Nexium)	40 mg qd	40 mg qd[1]
Lansoprazole (Prevacid)	30 mg qd	30 mg qd
Omeprazole (Prilosec)	20 mg qd	20 mg qd[1]
Pantoprazole (Protonix)	40 mg qd	40 mg qd[1]
Rabeprazole (Aciphex)	20 mg qd	20 mg qd[1]
Mucosal Protectants		
Misoprostol (Cytotec)	200 µg qid	200 µg qid or 400 µg bid
Sucralfate (Carafate)	1 gm qid	Not effective

[1]Not FDA approved for this indication.
*All patients should be tested for *H. pylori* and treated if positive.
†Duration of treatment for duodenal ulcer is 4 weeks with proton pump inhibitor (PPI) and 6 weeks with H_2-receptor antagonist. Duration of treatment for gastric ulcer is 8 weeks with either PPI or H_2-receptor antagonist.

TABLE 3 Select FDA-Approved *Helicobacter pylori* Eradication Regimens

Drug Combination	Dosing Schedule
PPI* (omeprazole 20 mg or lansoprazole 30 mg) + amoxicillin 1 g + clarithromycin 500 mg	Each bid for 10–14 d
Esomeprazole* 40 mg qd + amoxicillin 1 g bid + clarithromycin 500 mg bid	For 10 d
PPI* (omeprazole 20 mg or lansoprazole 30 mg) + amoxicillin 1 g + metronidazole 500 mg	Each bid for 10–14 d
Rabeprazole* 20 mg + amoxicillin 1 g + clarithromycin 500 mg	Each bid for 7 d
Bismuth subsalicylate 525 mg + metronidazole 250 mg + tetracycline 500 mg†	Each qid for 2 wk plus H_2-RA for 4 wk

*Although not yet approved, pantoprazole (Protonix) can be substituted.
†In patients with penicillin allergy, this regimen can be used. Alternatively, PPI + clarithromycin + metronidazole can be used.
Abbreviations: FDA = U.S. Food and Drug Administration; PPI = proton pump inhibitor.

CURRENT TREATMENT

- In patients with dyspepsia who are younger than 55 years, a *Helicobacter pylori* test-and-treat strategy, followed by PPI treatment (if the patient remains symptomatic or is not infected by *H. pylori*) is the management strategy of choice.
- Long-term acid-suppression therapy with PPIs may be necessary for patients believed to be at high risk for bleeding but in whom chronic NSAID use is necessary.
- PPIs inhibit more than 90% of the 24-acid output compared with 65% with H_2-RAs; hence PPIs heal peptic ulcers and relieve symptoms faster.
- Elderly patients who require long-term NSAID therapy should receive *H. pylori* eradication therapy if they are infected with this bacterium.
- Triple therapy (PPI plus amoxicillin and clarithromycin) is the most widely used treatment strategy for *H. pylori* in the United States.

Abbreviations: H_2-RA = H_2-receptor antagonist; NSAID = nonsteroidal anti-inflammatory drug; PPI = proton pump inhibitor.

---

generally preferred over H_2-RAs given the simplicity of the dosing schedule and comparable cost. Elderly patients who require long-term NSAID therapy should receive *H. pylori* eradication therapy if they are infected with this bacterium.

COMPLICATIONS

Hemorrhage

Gastrointestinal bleeding is the most common complication of PUD. Approximately 10% to 20% of ulcer patients develop significant GI bleeding, with overall mortality of up to 10%. Patients generally present with either melena or hematemesis. Endoscopy is indicated for diagnosis, risk stratification, and therapy in all patients with significant bleeding. High-dose oral or intravenous PPIs should be instituted before endoscopy if upper bleeding is suspected. All *H. pylori*–positive patients must have confirmation of eradication after therapy.

Perforation

Perforations occur in approximately 5% to 7% of ulcer patients. The incidence has not changed in spite of decreasing prevalence of *H. pylori*, because the use of NSAIDs continues to increase. The decision whether to manage operatively or nonoperatively should be made on a case-by-case basis.

Obstruction

Duodenal bulb or pyloric channel ulcers cause scarring and gastric outlet obstruction in approximately 2% of patients with PUD. Patients then present with early satiety, vomiting, and weight loss. Management involves *H. pylori* eradication and acid suppression along with endoscopic dilatation. Surgery is reserved for patients who do not respond to endoscopic therapy.

Zollinger-Ellison Syndrome

Less than 1% of PUD is caused by Zollinger-Ellison syndrome (ZES). This syndrome results from a gastrin-producing neuroendocrine tumor (gastrinoma), two thirds of which are malignant. PUD is caused by increased acid production from very high serum gastrin levels. Most gastrinomas arise in the gastrinoma triangle, bounded

by the porta hepatis, neck of the pancreas, and third portion of the duodenum. The pancreas and the duodenum are the two organs most commonly involved. Approximately one quarter of gastrinomas are part of the multiple endocrine neoplasia type I (MEN-1) syndrome, which is associated with parathyroid hyperplasia, pituitary tumors, and pancreatic endocrine tumors.

Gastrinomas commonly manifest between ages 30 and 50 years and have a male-to-female ratio of 2:1. The clinical features include peptic ulcers (90%), diarrhea (60%), and GERD (20%), all of which are due to gastric acid hypersecretion. The majority of ulcers occur in the duodenum. ZES should be suspected if the ulcers are multiple, in unusual locations, refractory to treatment, or associated with diarrhea.

Diagnosis is made by measuring fasting gastrin levels and gastric pH. If the gastrin levels are elevated to more than 1000 pg/mL in the right clinical setting, the diagnosis of ZES is established. Hypochlorhydria secondary to gastric atrophy from *H. pylori* or autoimmune gastritis, or due to acid suppression therapy by H_2-RAs and PPIs, can increase gastrin levels. Therefore, gastrin levels should be measured after H_2-RAs are held for 24 hours and PPIs for 1 week.

The gastric pH should be measured to distinguish ZES from hypochlorhydria. Gastric pH is less than 2 in ZES, whereas in achlorhydria secondary to gastric atrophy, gastric pH is greater than 2.

Provocative tests, such as the secretin test, can also be used to diagnose gastrinoma. Intravenous administration of secretin can decrease or slightly increase gastrin levels in normal patients and in patients with antral G-cell hyperplasia. In cases of gastrinoma, gastrin levels are significantly increased (>200 pg/mL) from the basal levels.

Tumor localization should be investigated by somatostatin receptor scintigraphy (Octreoscan), computed tomography, magnetic resonance imaging, and endoscopic ultrasound.

Treatment involves medical therapy with a high-dose PPI titrated against symptoms, gastric pH, and endoscopic findings. Surgical resection of isolated hepatic metastasis will decrease symptoms and prolongs survival.

REFERENCES

Chan FK, Graham DY. Review article: Prevention of non-steroidal anti-inflammatory drug gastrointestinal complications: Review and recommendations based on risk assessment. Aliment Pharmacol Ther 2004;19(10):1051–61.

Chan FK, Leung WK. Peptic-ulcer disease. Lancet 2002;360(9337):933–41.

Stollman N, Metz DC. Pathophysiology and prophylaxis of stress ulcer in intensive care unit patients. J Crit Care 2005;20(1):35–45.

Suerbaum S, Michetti P. *Helicobacter pylori* infection. N Engl J Med 2002;347(15):1175–86.

Talley NJ. American Gastroenterological Association. American Gastroenterological Association medical position statement: Evaluation of dyspepsia. Gastroenterology 2005;129(5):1753–5.

Talley NJ, Vakil N. Practice Parameters Committee of the American College of Gastroenterology. Guidelines for the management of dyspepsia. Am J Gastroenterol 2005;100(10):2324–37.

535

Acute and Chronic Viral Hepatitis

Method of
John Garber, MD, and Daniel Pratt, MD

The progress achieved in understanding viral hepatitis over the past decade has been dramatic. There are better diagnostic tools and rapidly evolving therapies, most particularly for hepatitis B. This improved therapy has made it critical that physicians effectively screen for chronic hepatitis B and identify all appropriate candidates for treatment. Hepatitis C therapy is also improving, and a percentage of patients can be cured—a proportion that will only increase as newer drugs become available.

Hepatitis A Virus

Hepatitis A virus (HAV), a member of the Picornaviridae family, exists as a single positive-stranded RNA virus of 7474 nucleotides, which encodes four structural proteins (capsids V1, V2, V3, and V4) and seven nonstructural proteins (e.g., protease, RNA-dependent polymerase). Four distinct genotypes exist. Despite intergenomic sequence variation of up to 20%, the genotypes are immunologically indistinguishable, so infection with one strain of HAV confers lifelong immunity to all strains.

EPIDEMIOLOGY

The virus is extremely stable in the environment and is shed in the stool of infected persons at a very high titer. It spreads within a population predominantly via the fecal-oral route, most commonly through ingestion of contaminated food or water. In the United States, the likelihood of having serologic evidence of past exposure is associated with age; it is approximately 11% at the age of 5 years and increases to almost 75% in those older than 50 years.

DIAGNOSIS

The presence of anti-HAV antibodies of the immunoglobulin M (IgM) class is diagnostic of acute HAV infection. Positive anti-HAV IgG antibodies along with negative anti-HAV IgM antibodies indicates immunity, from either prior infection or vaccination. Clinical laboratories often report the total anti-HAV antibodies, which is a mixture of IgG and IgM. To distinguish acute HAV infection from prior exposure, it is important to specifically test for the presence of anti-HAV IgM.

NATURAL HISTORY

HAV causes an acute hepatitis only; it never results in chronic hepatitis, and lifelong immunity is expected in all patients who recover. Once the virus is orally ingested, it reaches the liver via the portal vein. Viral shedding occurs when the replicating virus is excreted from hepatocytes through the bile duct into the intestine. Shedding continues until the prodromic phase and begins to decline once jaundice develops. However, infectious virions can be detected in the feces up to 2 weeks after the onset of jaundice.

The severity of symptoms associated with HAV depends in part on the age of the patient at the time of exposure: 90% of those infected before 5 years of age are asymptomatic, whereas 70% to 80% of those infected as adults have symptoms. HAV has an incubation period of approximately 25 days. This is followed by a prodromal phase of variable severity, characterized by weakness, anorexia, nausea, abdominal pain, and, less often, fevers, arthralgias, and diarrhea. The levels of the serum aminotransferases are elevated during this time, often to values greater than 500 U/L, and their peak usually coincides with intense nausea, vomiting, and anorexia. Jaundice typically occurs 1 to 2 weeks later and is associated with a lessening of the prodromal symptoms. The serum bilirubin level peaks later than the aminotransferases, rarely exceeds 10 mg/dL, and normalizes more slowly than the aminotransferases. In most patients, jaundice lasts less than 2 weeks. Complete normalization of the serum biochemical abnormalities is observed in 60% of patients by 2 months and in almost 100% by 6 months.

TREATMENT

There is no specific therapy for hepatitis A; treatment is largely supportive. Dehydration is common during the symptomatic phase and requires administration of intravenous fluids. A rare complication of acute HAV is the development of acute liver failure marked by

encephalopathy and coagulopathy. The risk of developing acute liver failure is higher in older patients; those infected after the age of 50 years have a case-fatality rate of 2.7%. Patients with coexisting chronic HBV or HCV infection are also at higher risk for a more severe clinical course. Vaccination for HAV should be offered to all patients who have chronic viral hepatitis or cirrhosis and negative HAV antibodies.

Three vaccines containing inactivated HAV are currently licensed for use: HAVRIX (GlaxoSmithKline), VAQTA (Merck), and TWINRIX (GlaxoSmithKline). All are highly effective at generating antibody responses, with approximately 95% of recipients developing protective levels of anti-HAV antibodies within 1 month after the first dose, and 100% after the second dose. The Advisory Committee on Immunization Practices recommends HAV immunoprophylaxis for all children at the age of 1 year. Vaccination is also recommended for adults who travel to areas of high or intermediate endemicity (Fig. 1), men who have sex with men, people with underlying chronic liver disease, and users of injection drugs.

Passive immunization, in the form of pooled human anti-HAV immunoglobulins (IG; IGIM; GamaSTAN) can be given to patients who have been exposed to HAV. HAV IG is 80% effective in preventing HAV infection if given within 2 weeks after exposure, and a single intramuscular dose of 0.02 mL/kg confers protection for 3 to 5 months. Although the concurrent administration of HAV IG with the first dose of anti-HAV vaccine somewhat reduces the immunogenicity of the vaccine, patients develop antibody levels well above those considered to be protective. There are growing data suggesting that vaccination is as effective as HAV IG for postexposure prophylaxis.

Hepatitis E Virus

Hepatitis E virus (HEV) is an enterically transmitted RNA virus that causes an acute, self-limited hepatitis which varies in severity from an asymptomatic infection to acute liver failure. Its genome consists of a single, positive-stranded RNA that encodes several structural and nonstructural proteins using overlapping open reading frames. As with HAV, there are multiple genotypes but only one serotype. Major protection epitopes are common to all HEV isolates, and exposure to one strain confers immunity to all strains.

EPIDEMIOLOGY

Geographically, endemic regions of high HEV prevalence include Central America, Africa, the Middle East, Southeast Asia, and India. In nonendemic regions, HEV accounts for fewer than 1% of reported cases of acute viral hepatitis, and most of these occur in patients who have recently traveled to endemic areas.

DIAGNOSIS

The diagnosis of HEV is made by serologic detection of anti-HEV IgM and IgG antibodies. Anti-HEV IgM is the hallmark of acute HEV infection. Anti-HEV IgM is usually undetectable by 6 months after infection. Anti-HEV IgG appears during the convalescent phase and is a serologic marker for past infection.

NATURAL HISTORY

Infection with HEV is typically a self-limited disease, and patients are often anicteric. An incubation period of 2 to 8 weeks is followed by a classic prodromal phase. The symptoms usually resolve within 6 weeks. For reasons that are not well understood, women in the second and third trimesters of pregnancy are at risk for a more severe clinical course. Mortality due to acute liver failure from HEV ranges from 20% to 25% in pregnant woman.

TREATMENT

There is no specific treatment for HEV infection; therapy is strictly supportive. There are currently no commercially available vaccines for HEV. Phase II trials of a recombinant anti-HEV vaccine are

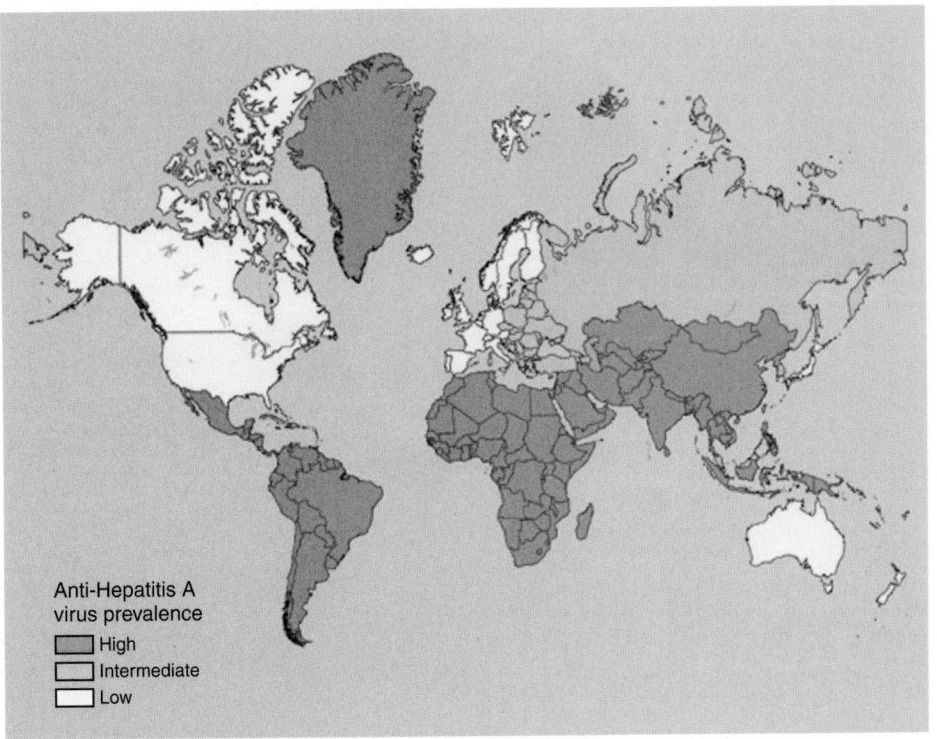

FIGURE 1. Prevalence of antibody to hepatitis A virus, by country, 2006. (From http://wwwn.cdc.gov/travel/yellowBookCh4-HepA.aspx [accessed June 30, 2009].)

under way and have shown promising results. Monoclonal antibodies against HEV have been produced and have proved effective for protecting nonhuman primates from HEV infection, but these preparations are not yet commercially available.

Hepatitis B Virus

Hepatitis B virus (HBV) is a partially double-stranded DNA virus in the Hepadnaviridae family with a 3200 base pair genome that uses multiple overlapping reading frames to encode surface, core, polymerase, and X proteins. Proteins of clinical importance include hepatitis B surface antigen (HBsAg), hepatitis B core antigen (HBcAg), and hepatitis B e antigen (HBeAg). Serum HBsAg is a marker of HBV infection, and HBeAg is a marker of active viral replication.

EPIDEMIOLOGY AND MODE OF TRANSMISSION

HBV infects an estimated 1.25 million people in the United States and 460 million people globally. Areas with a low prevalence of HBV (<2%) include North America, western and northern Europe, Australia, New Zealand, and southern South America; all other parts of the world have an intermediate prevalence (2%–8%) or high prevalence (>8%) in the general population (Fig. 2). Alaska is the only region in the United States considered to have a high prevalence of HBV, with a rate of 6.4% in the native population.

HBV is transmitted more efficiently than either HCV or HIV. The likelihood of transmission increases with the level of HBV DNA in serum. It is transmissible through perinatal, sexual, or percutaneous exposure; close person-to-person contact with open cuts and sores; and sharing of household items such as razors and toothbrushes. In high-prevalence areas, HBV is most often vertically transmitted. In the United States, the route is primarily horizontal; sexual transmission accounts for approximately 30% of cases.

In 2008, the CDC significantly expanded its recommendations for screening for chronic HBV (Box 1) to include all persons from inter-mediate-prevalence areas in addition to those from areas of high

prevalence. Those recommendations also now include patients who require treatment with immunosuppressive medications.

DIAGNOSIS

The presence of HBsAg in serum is the hallmark of infection with hepatitis B. Patients who recover from hepatitis B clear the HBsAg and develop an antibody to it, HBsAb. The presence of HBsAg for longer than 6 months indicates chronic HBV infection. Hepatitis B core antibody (HBcAb) is found in patients with both acute and chronic HBV. The acute illness is marked by the presence of HBcAb of the IgM class, whereas patients with chronic disease have HBcAb of the IgG class.

Appropriate testing for patients with suspected acute hepatitis B includes HBsAg, HBcAb IgM, HBeAg, and HBV DNA. Appropriate testing for patients with suspected chronic HBV includes HBsAg, HBcAb, and HBsAb. Patients found to have chronic HBV should undergo additional testing to assess their viral replication status by checking the levels of HBV DNA, HBeAg, and hepatitis B e antibody (HBeAb). This information allows the physician to determine whether a patient with chronic HBV is a candidate for antiviral therapy.

NATURAL HISTORY

Symptoms of acute HBV infection appear after an incubation period that ranges from 60 to 180 days. The presentation of acute HBV ranges from asymptomatic disease to acute liver failure. Markers of infection and viral replication—HBsAg, HBeAg, and HBV DNA—appear approximately 6 weeks after exposure. Their appearance is followed shortly by a rise in serum aminotransferases; the serum alanine aminotransferase (ALT) level is greater than the serum aspartate aminotransferase (AST) level, and both are generally higher than 500 U/L. During this time, anti-hepatitis B core antibody (HBcAb) of the IgM class, the only marker of acute infection, appears and may persist for many months.

Aminotransferase levels correspond well with the degree of necro-inflammation. The liver injury results from a cytotoxic T lymphocyte–induced apoptosis of virally infected hepatocytes. Acute liver failure occurs when the severity of the injury results in insufficient residual

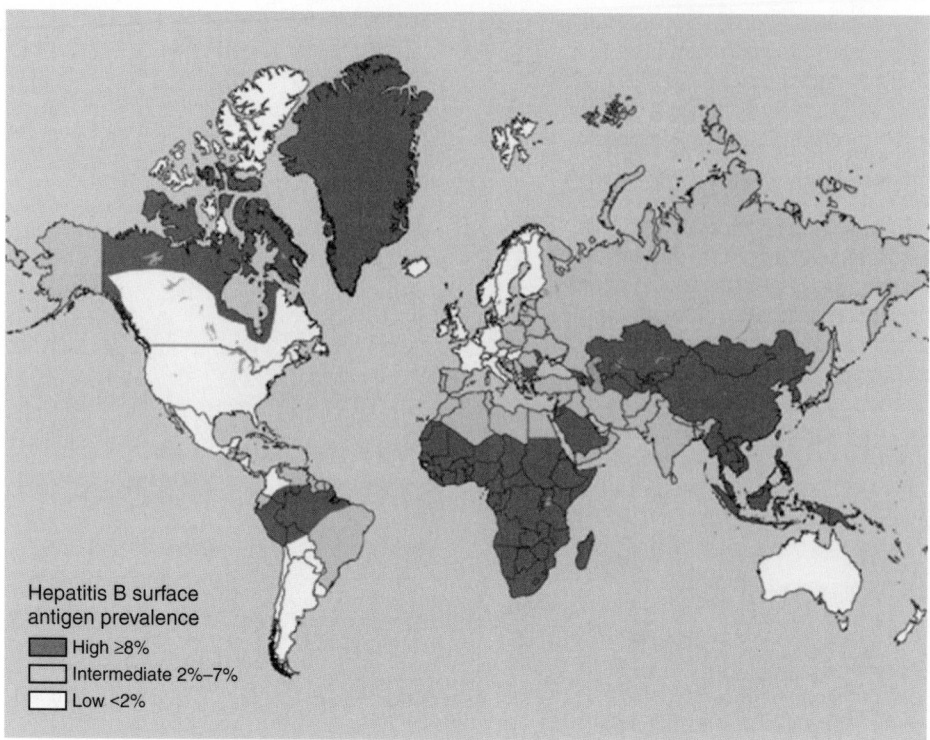

Hepatitis B surface
antigen prevalence

�In High ≥8%

☐ Intermediate 2%–7%

☐ Low <2%

FIGURE 2. Prevalence of chronic hepatitis B virus infection, by country, 2006. (From http://wwwn.cdc.gov/travel/yellowBookCh4-HepB.aspx [accessed June 30, 2009].)

BOX 1   Populations for Whom Screening for Chronic Hepatitis B Virus Infection Is Recommended

- Persons born in areas with intermediate or high disease prevalence (>2%)*
- U.S.-born persons who were not vaccinated at birth and have parents from areas of high disease prevalence
- Injection-drug users*
- Men who have sex with men*
- Persons who require immunosuppressive therapy*
- Persons with unexplained elevation of the serum aminotransferases*
- Hemodialysis patients
- Pregnant women
- Infants born to HBsAg-positive mothers
- Household, needle-sharing, or sex contacts of HBsAg-positive persons
- Persons infected with the human immunodeficiency virus
- Persons who are the source of blood or body fluid exposures who might require postexposure prophylaxis

---

From Recommendations for identification and public health management of persons with chronic hepatitis B virus infection. MMWR Morb Mortal Wkly Rep 2008;57(RR08):1–20. Available at http://www.cdc.gov/mmwr/preview/mmwrhtml/rr5708a1.htm (accessed June 30, 2009).
*New recommendations.
HBsAg = hepatitis B virus surface antigen.

---

hepatic mass and function. Patients who clear the virus have normalization of aminotransferases by 4 months, followed by a slower resolution of hyperbilirubinemia. The likelihood of progression to chronicity (defined as persistence of HBsAg for >6 months) depends on the age at exposure. Whereas 90% of those perinatally infected progress to chronic infection, this rate decreases to 20% to 50% in those infected between age 1 to 5 years, and is less than 5% in persons infected with HBV as an adult.

It is useful to conceptualize the natural history of chronic HBV infection as a spectrum encompassing an immunotolerant stage, an immunoactive stage, an inactive carrier stage, a resolution stage, and an e antigen–negative chronic hepatitis (Fig. 3). This is particularly useful in patients infected via vertical transmission.

In addition to the testing needed to assess viral replication, the serum albumin level and prothrombin time should be checked to assess synthetic function, and a complete blood count should be performed to assess for thrombocytopenia and leukopenia, which are potential indicators of hypersplenism. Careful interpretation of these data allows proper placement of patients with chronic HBV on the natural history continuum and identifies patients who are candidates for therapy.

The immunotolerant stage of disease is characterized by very high HBV DNA levels, normal aminotransferases, and no hepatic necroinflammation. These patients are not currently thought to be candidates for therapy. At an undefined and variable point in time, these immunotolerant patients progress to the immunoactive stage, which is characterized by high serum HBV DNA levels, elevated aminotransferases, and hepatic necroinflammation. They are then at increased risk for disease progression and hepatocellular carcinoma and are candidates for therapy.

The next transition is from the immunoactive stage to the inactive carrier stage; this occurs spontaneously at a rate of 8% to 12% per year. The inactive carrier stage is marked by HBeAg seroconversion (i.e., loss of HBeAg and development of HBeAb). This event carries with it a number of beneficial effects, including a significant reduction in serum HBV DNA levels, resolution of necroinflammation, prevention of histologic progression, reduced risk of hepatocellular carcinoma, and decreased mortality.

Patients in the inactive stage require continued attention, because 20% to 30% will have flares of hepatitis, with or without e antigen reversion. Patients in the inactive carrier stage can develop precore or core promoter mutations that allow for viral replication in the absence of e antigen. Like patients in the immunoactive stage, these patients with e antigen–negative hepatitis have elevated serum

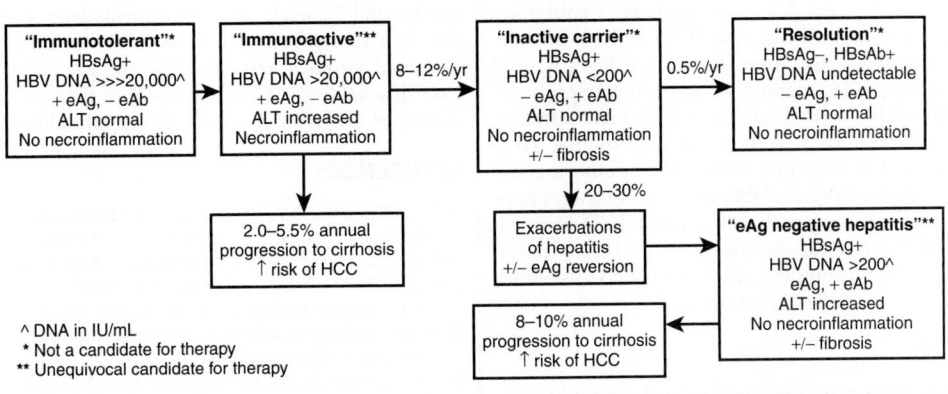

FIGURE 3. Natural history of chronic hepatitis B. ALT = alanine aminotransferase; eAb = hepatitis B e antibody; eAg = hepatitis B e antigen; HBsAb = hepatitis B surface antibody; HBsAg = hepatitis B surface antigen; HBV = hepatitis B virus; HCC = hepatocellular carcinoma. (Adapted from Pratt DS: Evaluation and management of hepatitis B virus infection. J Clin Outcomes Manage 2008;15:147–153.)

aminotransferases levels and necroinflammation on liver biopsy but lower levels of serum HBV DNA, compared with those in the immunoactive stage. They are at increased risk for histologic progression and for hepatocellular carcinoma and are candidates for therapy.

Patients in the inactive stage move into the resolution stage at a rate of 0.5% per year. The resolution stage is marked by surface antigen seroconversion (i.e., loss of surface antigen and development of surface antibody).

TREATMENT

Seven therapies approved by the U.S. Food and Drug Administration (FDA) for the treatment of HBV:

- Interferon: interferon alfa-2b (Intron A) and pegylated interferon alfa-2a (Pegasys)
- Nucleoside analogues: lamivudine (Epivir-HBV), telbivudine (Tyzeka), and entecavir (Baraclude)
- Nucleotide analogues: adefovir (Hepsera) and tenofovir (Viread)

The interferons are prescribed for a defined period (48 weeks), whereas the nucleoside and nucleotide analogues are continued until a specific end point of therapy is reached. The end point of therapy in immunoactive patients is loss of HbeAg and development of HbeAb, which is generally associated with sustained viral suppression. In HBeAg-negative patients, no such marker of treatment success exists, and there is a high likelihood of relapse when therapy is discontinued. These patients are usually treated indefinitely or until surface antigen seroconversion occurs.

Hepatitis D Virus

The hepatitis D virus (HVD) is a subviral particle composed of a single-stranded RNA genome complexed with hepatitis D antigen (HDAg) and enclosed in an outer lipoprotein envelope derived from HBsAg. It is believed that HDV uses some of the same pathways for attachment and entry into host cells as HBV; HDV infection requires the presence of HBV for infectivity. Immunity to HBV also protects against infection with HDV.

EPIDEMIOLOGY

HDV is a blood-borne pathogen with the same modes of transmission as HBV. Co-infection occurs when an individual is infected with both HBV and HDV at the same time. In contrast, HDV infection of a chronically HBV-infected individual is referred to as superinfection and carries a much higher risk of precipitating fulminant hepatic failure. Chronic carriers of both HBV and HDV tend to have more rapid progression of liver disease, compared to those infected with HBV alone. It is estimated that 20 million HBV-infected people also have chronic HDV.

DIAGNOSIS

HDV elicits specific IgM and IgG antibody responses. Anti-HDV IgM is the only specific marker of acute HDV infection, although assays for IgM detection are not in clinical use in the United States. High titers of anti-HDV IgG often characterize chronic infections, but can also be seen in patients with prior infection, and therefore are not useful in distinguishing carriers from those who have cleared the virus. HDV RNA detection via polymerase chain reaction is commercially available in the United States and has a lower limit of detection (10 copies per milliliter). The diagnosis of HDV infection also requires evidence of concurrent HBV infection, and the presence of anti-HBV IgM suggests acute co-infection.

NATURAL HISTORY

HDV infection can produce a broad spectrum of liver injury, ranging from an asymptomatic carrier state to acute liver failure.

TREATMENT

The goal of treatment is suppression of HDV replication. The only drug shown to be of benefit in treating chronic HDV is interferon-alfa.[1] However, although interferon-alfa is capable of suppressing viral replication, its antiviral effect is not sustained after withdrawal of therapy.

Hepatitis C Virus

Hepatitis C virus (HCV) is a single minus-strand RNA virus of 9.6 kb whose genome encodes a core protein, envelope proteins, and several nonstructural proteins.

EPIDEMIOLOGY

Almost 170 million people are chronically infected with HCV worldwide. In the United States, there are an estimated 2.7 million individuals chronically infected, although the number of new cases per year has appreciably declined since 1990.

DIAGNOSIS

The initial test in diagnosing HCV infection is the presence of anti-HCV antibodies. The current serologic test uses a combination of the core protein and several nonstructural proteins in an

[1]Not FDA approved for this indication.

immunoassay that can detect reactive antibodies within 4 to 10 weeks of infection. As a screening test, the detection of anti-HCV antibodies is very sensitive, and it is estimated that only 0.5% to 1.0% of cases will be missed in a low-prevalence population. HCV RNA is used to confirm positive serologic testing and to assess the response to therapy. Measurement of HCV RNA can be either quantitative or qualitative. The quantitative assay is best for determining large changes in viral load and is therefore useful for monitoring the response to therapy; commercially available quantitative assays have a lower limit of detection, approximately 600 copies/mL. In contrast, qualitative tests for HCV RNA can detect as few as 10 copies/mL blood and are useful for confirming the presence of the virus, either when the titer is very low or at the end of therapy.

NATURAL HISTORY

Acute HCV infection is often asymptomatic; patients are rarely diagnosed at this stage. After an average incubation period of 6 weeks, a minority (15%–20%) of patients manifest a clinical syndrome of variable severity. Symptoms include fevers, malaise, nausea and anorexia, abdominal pain, and muscle aches. This period is anicteric, can last for 2 weeks to 3 months, and may be followed by the development of jaundice along with detectable serum HCV RNA. In asymptomatic infection, serum HCV RNA and aminotransferase elevations are usually detectable within 1 to 3 weeks of infection, and anti-HCV antibody becomes positive 3 weeks to 5 months after acute infection.

In approximately 30% of patients, acute HCV infection is self-limited and is followed by the resolution of aminotransferase elevations and disappearance of serum HCV RNA. Most patients who spontaneously clear HCV do so within 12 weeks after infection. Patients who do not clear the acute infection progress to chronic HCV infection, which is most often characterized by an asymptomatic elevation of serum aminotransferases. Approximately 30% of patients with chronic HCV infection have normal ALT levels.

TREATMENT

Because of the high likelihood that acute HCV infection will lead to chronic infection, treatment should be considered in all patients with evidence of acute HCV. Small studies have demonstrated high rates of viral clearance in patients with detectable HCV RNA who are treated within 3 months of infection. Although clear guidelines do not exist for treating this group of patients, a 24-week course of standard-dose pegylated interferon alfa-2b and ribavirin (Rebetol) is an accepted approach.

The decision to treat chronic HCV infection is based on multiple viral and host factors, including viral genotype and load, histology, likelihood of disease progression, and medical comorbidities. Patients with persistently detectable virus and histologic evidence of fibrosis or severe inflammation are at high risk for progression should be treated in the absence of contraindications. The indications for therapy are less clear in patients with no evidence of fibrosis and only minimal inflammation despite many years of infection. These patients have a lower risk of progression and may be observed with monitoring of serum liver enzymes and repeat liver biopsy in 4 to 5 years.

The mainstay of HCV therapy is pegylated interferon alfa-2a or alfa-2b (Intron A)[1] in combination with a weight-based dose of ribavirin. The duration of therapy is determined by the viral genotype: type 1 is treated for 48 weeks and types 2 and 3 for 24 weeks. Response to therapy is monitored by quantitative measurement of HCV RNA after 4 and 12 weeks of therapy. An undetectable HCV RNA level at 4 weeks is defined as a rapid virologic response; a greater than 2 log reduction in viral load at week 12 is defined as an early virologic response (EVR); and an undetectable HCV RNA at week 12 is a complete EVR. A rapid virologic response is the strongest positive predictor of sustained virologic response, which is defined as an undetectable HCV RNA 6 months after completion

---

[1]Not FDA approved for this indication.

---

of treatment. At least an EVR is required to justify continuing therapy beyond 12 weeks, because patients with a less than 2 log reduction in viral load at week 12 have almost no chance of achieving a sustained virologic response. Patients who achieve an EVR but still have detectable virus after 24 weeks of therapy also have a very small chance of achieving SVR and therapy should be discontinued.

REFERENCES

Dalton HR, Brendall R, Ijaz S, Banks M. Hepatitis E: An emerging infection in developed countries. Lancet Infect Dis 2008;8:698–709.
Dienstag JL. Hepatitis B virus infection. N Engl J Med 2008;359:1486–500.
Ghany MG, Strader DB, Thomas DL, Seeff LB. Diagnosis, management, and treatment of hepatitis C: An update. Hepatology 2009;49:1335–74.
Pratt DS. Evaluation and management of hepatitis B virus infection. J Clin Outcomes Manage 2008;15:147–53.
Wasley A, Fiore A, Bell BP. Hepatitis A in the era of vaccination. Epidemiol Rev 2006;28:101–11.
Wrinbaum CM, Williams I, Mast EE, et al. Recommendations for identification and public health management of persons with chronic hepatitis B virus infection, MMWR Morb Mortal Wkly Rep 2008;57(RR08):1–20. Available at http://www.cdc.gov/mmwr/preview/mmwrhtml/rr5708a1.htm [accessed June 30, 2009].

Malabsorption

Method of
Lawrence R. Schiller, MD

Every day the average human being consumes 2000–3000 kcal of food, much of it in the form of polymers or other complex molecules that must be digested and absorbed by the gut. The processes of digestion and absorption are complex and are readily disturbed by pathologic processes. More than 200 conditions have been described that can adversely affect nutrient absorption.

Strictly speaking, *maldigestion* refers to impaired hydrolysis of nutrients, usually due to lack of luminal factors, such as bile acids and pancreatic enzymes, and *malabsorption* refers to impaired mucosal transport. For clinical purposes, "malabsorption" is used to describe both processes.

Malabsorption can be generalized (panmalabsorption) or limited to a specific category of nutrients. Generalized malabsorption is usually due to maldigestion or to extensive mucosal dysfunction. Specific malabsorption occurs when a single transporter is disabled.

The causes of malabsorption can be divided into three categories: impaired luminal hydrolysis, impaired mucosal function (mucosal hydrolysis, uptake, packaging, and excretion), and impaired removal of nutrients from the mucosa (Box 1).

Diagnosis

SYMPTOMS AND SIGNS

Most patients with panmalabsorption have changes in their stools (Box 2). Steatorrhea (excess fat in stools) is characterized by pale color, bulkiness, greasiness, and a tendency to float (probably because of incorporated gas). Occasionally patients with malabsorption present with watery stools due to the osmotic effects of unabsorbed carbohydrates and short-chain fatty acids.

Abdominal distention and excess flatus also commonly occur due to fermentation of unabsorbed carbohydrate by colonic bacteria. This can occur not only with panmalabsorption but also with specific malabsorption of carbohydrate (e.g., lactase deficiency).

Weight loss is typical with severe panmalabsorption, but it might not be very prominent with lesser degrees of malabsorption due to

CURRENT DIAGNOSIS

- Recognize the presence of generalized malabsorption by the combination of typical symptoms: diarrhea, greasy stools, flatulence, weight loss, fatigue, edema.
- Recognize the presence of specific malabsorption by associated symptoms and those symptoms particular to deficiency states of the malabsorbed substance: flatus, diarrhea, anemia, dermatitis, glossitis, neuropathy, paresthesias, tetany, ecchymosis.
- Documentation of generalized malabsorption is best done by stool analysis demonstrating steatorrhea and acid stools (reflecting carbohydrate malabsorption). Diagnosis depends on visualization of the small bowel by endoscopy or radiography and small bowel biopsy. Additional tests may be needed.
- Documentation of specific malabsorption is best done by demonstrating low blood levels of the malabsorbed substance or by tests designed to measure absorption of that substance. Diagnosis depends on studies designed to identify the likely diagnosis for a given situation.

BOX 1   Causes of Malabsorption or Maldigestion

- Impaired luminal hydrolysis or solublization
  - Bile acid deficiency
  - Impaired mucosal hydrolysis, uptake, or packaging
  - Pancreatic exocrine insufficiency
  - Postgastrectomy syndrome
  - Rapid intestinal transit
  - Small bowel bacterial overgrowth
  - Zollinger-Ellison syndrome
- Brush border or metabolic disorders
  - Abetalipoproteinemia
  - Glucose-galactose malabsorption
  - Lactase deficiency
  - Sucrase-isomaltase deficiency
- Mucosal diseases
  - Amyloidosis
  - Chronic mesenteric ischemia
  - Crohn's disease
  - Celiac sprue
  - Collagenous sprue
  - Eosinophilic gastroenteritis
  - Immunoproliferative small intestinal disease (IPSID)
  - Lymphoma
  - Nongranulomatous ulcerative jejunoileitis
  - Radiation enteritis
  - Systemic mastocytosis
- Infectious diseases
  - AIDS enteropathy
  - *Mycobacterium avium-intracellulare*
  - Parasitic diseases
  - Small bowel bacterial overgrowth
  - Tropical sprue
  - Whipple's disease
- After intestinal resection
- Chronic mesenteric ischemia
- Impaired removal of nutrients
  - Lymphangiectasia

BOX 2   Symptoms and Signs of Malabsorption or Maldigestion

- Changes in stool characteristics
  - Floating stools
  - Pale, bulky, greasy stools
  - Watery diarrhea
- Increased colonic gas production
  - Abdominal distention
  - Borborygmi
- Vitamin and mineral deficiencies
  - Anemia
  - Cheilosis
  - Glossitis
  - Dermatitis
  - Neuropathy
  - Night blindness
  - Osteomalacia
  - Paresthesia
  - Tetany
- Ecchymosis
- Fatigue, weakness
- Edema
- Weight loss, muscle wasting

---

compensatory hyperphagia. Weight loss is most prominent early in the course of the illness, but body weight usually stabilizes as calorie absorption and body weight come into balance again. This is in contrast to illnesses like cancer or tuberculosis that produce continuing weight loss. If a patient with malabsorption has continuing weight loss, inflammatory bowel disease or lymphoma should be considered.

Abdominal pain is usually not present with malabsorption, although some cramping may be associated with diarrhea. Severe pain should bring chronic pancreatitis, Zollinger-Ellison syndrome, lymphoma, Crohn's disease, or mesenteric ischemia to mind.

Constitutional symptoms of fatigue and weakness commonly occur, even early in the course. In contrast, appetite is impaired only late in the course of most malabsorption states. Edema is uncommon until late in the course unless protein-losing enteropathy is present.

Vitamin and mineral deficiencies can lead to several symptoms or signs. Glossitis and cheilosis are common in patients with water-soluble vitamin deficiencies. Florid beriberi, pellagra, and scurvy are not commonly seen unless malabsorption has been particularly severe or long-lasting. Fat-soluble vitamin deficiencies also are unlikely to develop except when malabsorption has been long-standing because of substantial body stores.

Miscellaneous findings occasionally seen in patients with malabsorption can provide clues to the diagnosis. Aphthous ulcers in the mouth may be seen with celiac disease, Behçet's syndrome, or Crohn's disease. Hyperpigmentation is seen in Whipple's disease, and dermatitis herpetiformis (pruritic, blistering skin lesions) is seen in celiac disease. Scleroderma can manifest with tight skin, digital ulceration, nail changes, and Raynaud's phenomenon. Chronic sinusitis, bronchitis, and recurrent pneumonia suggest cystic fibrosis or IgA deficiency. Several systemic diseases can be associated with malabsorption syndrome (Box 3).

TESTS

Routine Laboratory Tests

Routine laboratory tests (Box 4) commonly are abnormal in patients with established malabsorption syndrome. Anemia is common but not universal. Iron deficiency anemia may be the only finding in some patients with celiac disease. Microcytic anemia may be present in Whipple's disease (due to occult blood loss) and in lymphomas manifesting with malabsorption. Macrocytic anemia due to folate or vitamin B_{12} deficiency can occur in short bowel syndrome, small bowel bacterial overgrowth, or ileal disease. Lymphopenia may be present in patients with AIDS or lymphangiectasia.

BOX 3   Systemic Diseases Associated with Malabsorption or Maldigestion

Endocrine Diseases

- Addison's disease
- Diabetes mellitus
- Hypoparathyroidism
- Hyperthyroidism, hypothyroidism

Collagen-Vascular and Miscellaneous Diseases

- AIDS
- Amyloidosis
- Scleroderma
- Vasculitis (systemic lupus erythematosus, polyarteritis nodosa)

CURRENT THERAPY

- Once a diagnosis is reached, therapy can be directed toward that specific problem:
  - Gluten-free diet for celiac disease
  - Antibiotics for bacterial overgrowth
  - Lactose-free diet for lactase deficiency

Electrolyte abnormalities may be due to a combination of poor intake and excess loss in stool. Renal function usually is well maintained in malabsorption syndrome, but blood urea nitrogen may be low due to poor protein absorption, and serum creatinine concentration may be low due to depletion of muscle mass. Serum calcium levels may be low due to malabsorption, vitamin D deficiency, or intraluminal complexing of calcium by fatty acids. Hypomagnesemia can produce hypocalcemia or hypokalemia that is resistant to intravenous repletion. Serum phosphorus, cholesterol, and triglyceride levels may be reduced due to poor intake or malabsorption. Liver tests may be abnormal due to fatty liver. Serum protein and albumin levels are well preserved in patients with malabsorption unless protein-losing enteropathy or an acute illness is present.

Prothrombin time is normal unless vitamin K malabsorption (typically associated with steatorrhea), anticoagulant therapy, antibiotic therapy, or colectomy is present.

Assays are available for several potentially malabsorbed substances, including iron, vitamin B$_{12}$, folate, 25-hydroxyvitamin D, and β-carotene. Malabsorption tends to lower blood levels, but substantial body stores of many of these can mitigate the reduction in concentration that otherwise might occur. Thus, the sensitivity and specificity of these assays for malabsorption are poor.

Tests for Malabsorption

Fat Malabsorption

The simplest test for fat malabsorption is a qualitative microscopic examination of stool using a fat-soluble stain, such as Sudan III. The finding of more than 5 stained droplets per high power field is abnormal and correlates well with quantitative measurement of fecal fat excretion. The test is subject to false-positive results with some drugs and food additives, such as mineral oil, orlistat, and olestra.

A more precise estimate of fat absorption is obtained by a quantitative analysis of a timed stool collection (48 or 72 hours). During the collection, a diary of dietary intake should be maintained so that fat excretion can be assessed as a percentage of intake. Normal fat excretion is < 7% of intake when stool weight is normal, but it can be twice as high due to voluminous diarrhea without indicating defective mucosal transport of fat. Thus, fat excretion must be judged against stool weight. Stool fat concentration (grams of fat

BOX 4   Laboratory Tests for Evaluation of Malabsorption or Maldigestion

Routine Blood Tests

- Complete blood count
- Hemoglobin/hematocrit
- Platelet count
- WBC differential count

Biochemistry Tests

- Blood urea nitrogen
- Potassium
- Prothrombin time
- Serum albumin
- Serum calcium
- Serum creatinine

Blood Levels of Potentially Malabsorbed Substances

- Serum iron, vitamin B$_{12}$, folate, 25-OH vitamin D, carotene

Fat absorption

- Qualitative fecal fat
- Quantitative fecal fat

Protein Absorption and Protein-Losing Enteropathy

- α$_1$-Antitrypsin clearance
- Fecal nitrogen excretion

Carbohydrate Absorption

- Osmotic gap in stool water
- Quantitative excretion (anthrone)
- Stool pH < 5.5
- Stool reducing substances
- D-Xylose absorption test
- Oral glucose, sucrose, and lactose tolerance tests
- Breath hydrogen tests

Vitamin B$_{12}$ Absorption

- Schilling test with intrinsic factor

Bile Acid Malabsorption

- ^{14}C-glycocholic acid breath test
- Fecal bile acid excretion
- Radiolabeled bile acid excretion
- ^{75}SeHCAT retention

Small Bowel Bacterial Overgrowth

- ^{14}C-glycocholic acid breath test
- ^{14}C-xylose breath test
- Glucose breath hydrogen test
- Quantitative culture of jejunal aspirate

Exocrine Pancreatic Insufficiency

- Dual-labeled Schilling test
- Secretin/CCK test
- Stool chymotrypsin concentration

Serologic Testing for Celiac Disease

- Anti-tissue transglutaminase antibody (IgA)
- Anti-endomysial antibody (IgA)

Abbreviations: CCK = cholecystokinin; SLE = systemic lupus erythematosus; ^{75}SeHCAT = selenium-75-labeled taurohomocholic acid.

per 100 grams of stool) also is of value. Pancreatic exocrine insufficiency is associated with high fecal fat concentration (>10 g/100 g stool) because unlike hydrolyzed fat, unhydrolyzed fat does not stimulate colonic water and electrolyte secretion that would dilute fecal fat concentration.

Protein Malabsorption

Fecal nitrogen excretion can be employed as a marker of protein malabsorption, but is not often used in clinical medicine because it adds little to the evaluation. If protein-losing enteropathy is suspected, an α_1-antitrypsin clearance study can be done. In this study, *fecal* excretion of α_1-antitrypsin, a serum protein that is relatively resistant to hydrolysis by luminal enzymes, is divided by *serum* concentration of α_1-antitrypsin, and the volume of serum leaked into the lumen can be calculated. Values of more than 180 mL/day are associated with hypoalbuminemia.

Carbohydrate Malabsorption

Carbohydrate malabsorption is difficult to measure directly because fermentation of malabsorbed carbohydrate by colonic bacteria reduces the amount of intact carbohydrate that can be recovered in stool. Indirect estimates of carbohydrate malabsorption can be made by examining fecal pH (<5.5 with carbohydrate malabsorption) or fecal osmotic gap (> 100 mOsm/kg with osmotic diarrhea). Oral carbohydrate tolerance tests may be used to evaluate absorption of sugars, such as lactose or fructose. Following an oral load of a given sugar, blood glucose levels are monitored; failure of blood glucose to increase suggests malabsorption.

Another test for carbohydrate malabsorption is the D-xylose absorption test. In this test, a 25-gram dose of D-xylose is given orally; blood xylose levels are measured 1 and 3 hours later, and urinary excretion of xylose is measured for 5 hours. Failure of blood xylose to rise above 20 mg/dL at 1 hour or above 22.5 mg/dL at 3 hours or failure of urinary excretion to exceed 5 g in 5 hours suggests malabsorption. In addition, because xylose does not require pancreatic enzymes or bile acids for absorption, an abnormal D-xylose test suggests a mucosal problem as the cause for malabsorption. The results of this test can be misleading if the patient is dehydrated or has ascites, if renal function is compromised, or if bacterial overgrowth is present in the upper small bowel.

Breath hydrogen testing is another method to assess carbohydrate absorption. If substrates such as lactose or sucrose are not absorbed in the small intestine, they pass into the colon, where bacterial fermentation produces hydrogen gas. The hydrogen is absorbed into the bloodstream and then is exhaled. The concentration of hydrogen in exhaled breath can be measured easily; a rise of more than 10 to 20 ppm after ingestion of a specific substrate is consistent with malabsorption. False-positive results can be seen in patients with small bowel bacterial overgrowth, and false-negative results can be seen in patients who lack hydrogen-producing flora or who have been on antibiotics recently.

Vitamin B$_{12}$ Malabsorption

The Schilling test can be used to measure vitamin B$_{12}$ absorption. For purposes of a malabsorption evaluation, part II of the Schilling test (measurement of radiolabeled B$_{12}$ absorption *with* intrinsic factor) is all that is needed. Recovery of less than 9% of the radiolabel in the urine is abnormal and suggests ileal dysfunction. The test may be falsely positive in patients with pancreatic exocrine insufficiency, small bowel bacterial overgrowth, or renal failure.

Bile Acid Malabsorption

Tests for bile acid malabsorption are not widely available in the United States. Direct measurement of bile acid excretion has been used mainly in research studies. Retention of a radioactive taurocholic acid analogue (SeHCAT, selenium-75-labeled taurohomocholic acid) is used in Europe to assess bile acid malabsorption. A breath test using ^{14}C-glycocholic acid has been used for evaluating small bowel bacterial overgrowth, but it may have application for assessing bile acid malabsorption as well.

Small Bowel Bacterial Overgrowth

The gold standard method used to test for small bowel bacterial overgrowth in the upper intestine is quantitative culture of jejunal fluid. The sample can be obtained during endoscopy and sent to the laboratory with instructions to quantitate the aerobic and anaerobic flora. Finding more than 10^5 bacteria per mL confirms bacterial overgrowth. Breath tests using glucose, ^{14}C-xylose, and lactulose also have been described for this purpose.

Pancreatic Exocrine Insufficiency

Tests for pancreatic exocrine insufficiency are not commonly used. The gold standard test is a secretin test. This study requires duodenal intubation, injection of secretin, and measurement of bicarbonate output. A tubeless test, the bentiromide test, had average clinical utility; it is no longer available in the United States. Measurement of fecal chymotrypsin or elastase activity is only moderately useful in predicting the presence of exocrine pancreatic insufficiency. For most situations, a therapeutic trial using a high dose of pancreatic enzymes with monitoring of the effect on steatorrhea is the best that can be done.

Evaluation of Suspected Malabsorption

When malabsorption is suspected because of the history, physical findings, and setting, the physician must decide if the malabsorption involves a specific nutrient or represents a generalized process (Figure 1). If the malabsorption seems to be specific, a diet and symptom diary, breath tests using the presumptively malabsorbed substrate, and stool pH to identify acid stools seen with carbohydrate malabsorption are reasonable diagnostic maneuvers.

Suspected generalized malabsorption requires a more intense evaluation. Steatorrhea should be confirmed with either a qualitative fecal fat test (e.g., Sudan stain) or a quantitative stool collection for measurement of fat excretion. If steatorrhea is confirmed, the small bowel should be visualized with either capsule endoscopy or radiography (small bowel follow-through examination or computed

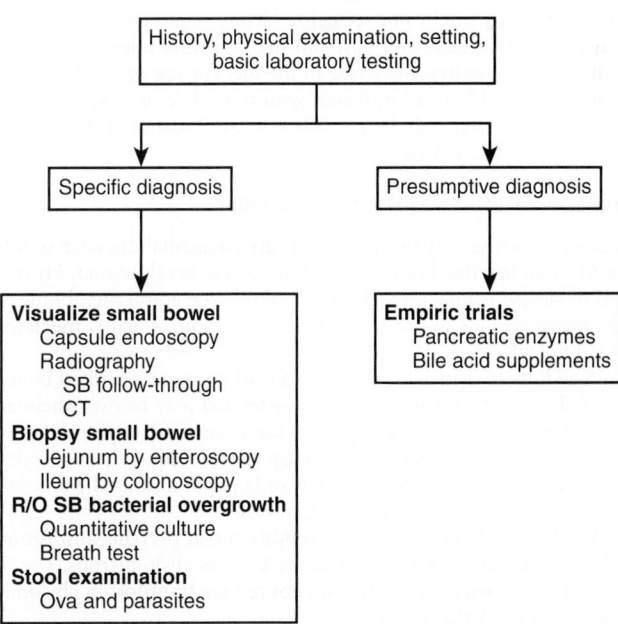

FIGURE 1. Flow chart for evaluation of malabsorption or maldigestion. *Abbreviations:* CT = computed tomography; R/O = rule out; SB = small bowel.

tomography) and biopsied from above by enteroscopy and from below by colonoscopy. During enteroscopy, an aspirate of small bowel contents can be obtained for quantitative culture to look for small bowel bacterial overgrowth. An alternative method to detect small bowel bacterial overgrowth is breath testing (see earlier). Stool samples also should be examined with microscopy or immunoassay for the presence of parasites that may be associated with malabsorption.

This sequence of evaluation often leads to a specific diagnosis. When it does not, empiric trials of pancreatic enzyme replacement or bile acid supplementation can lead to a presumptive diagnosis of pancreatic exocrine insufficiency or bile acid deficiency. Hard endpoints (e.g., quantitative fat excretion) should be used to assess the effectiveness of these empiric trials.

Specific Disorders Associated with Malabsorption

MALABSORPTION OF SPECIFIC NUTRIENTS

Disaccharidase Deficiency

Ingested disaccharides such as lactose and sucrose and starch-digestion products such as maltotriose and α-limit dextrins must be hydrolyzed by brush border enzymes into monosaccharides for abosorption by the mucosa. If these brush border enzymes are not active or if the brush border is damaged, malabsorption of the specific carbohydrate substrate results. This can result in gaseousness or osmotic diarrhea when those substrates are ingested. This rarely occurs on a congenital basis, but it commonly occurs as an acquired disorder.

Lactase deficiency is the most common acquired disaccharidase deficiency. Infant mammals all rely on lactose as the carbohydrate source in milk, but lactase activity is shut off after weaning in most species. Most human populations lose lactase activity during adolescence as a normal part of maturation. Members of the northern European gene pool might maintain lactase activity into adult life, but lactase activity declines gradually in many. At some point the amount of lactose ingested might exceed the ability of the remaining enzyme to hydrolyze it, resulting in lactose malabsorption and symptoms. This also can occur with acute conditions such as gastroenteritis that can disturb the mucosa and temporarily reduce lactase activity. Patients might not recognize lactose ingestion as a cause of their problem because they have not had difficulty tolerating lactose in the past. Restriction of lactose in the diet (or use of products that have predigested lactose) mitigates symptoms. Use of exogenous lactase as a tablet may only be partially effective because of incomplete hydrolysis of ingested lactose.

Transport Defects at the Brush Border

Glucose-galactose malabsorption is a rare congenital disorder resulting from an inactive hexose transporter in the brush border. Hydrolysis of lactose is intact, but transport across the apical membrane of the enterocyte fails to occur. Fructose absorption, which is mediated by a different carrier, is unaffected.

In all human beings the ability to absorb fructose is limited by the availability of carriers in the brush border and may be overwhelmed when excess fructose is ingested. This can occur relatively easily nowadays, because high-fructose corn syrup is used frequently as a sweetener in commercial products such as soda pop. Limiting the amount of fructose ingested will reduce symptoms.

Abetalipoproteinemia is a rare condition that prevents absorption of long-chain fatty acids due to failure to form chylomicrons. Use of medium-chain triglycerides that do not require transport in chylomicrons can bypass this defect.

Pernicious anemia develops when failure to secrete intrinsic factor in the stomach prevents vitamin B_{12} absorption by the ileal mucosa. Parenteral replacement with cyanocobalamin by injection (Cyanoject) or nasal spray (Nascobal) is necessary.

GENERALIZED MALABSORPTION

Celiac Disease

Celiac disease (also known as celiac sprue) is a disorder in which the mucosa of the small bowel is damaged due to activation of the mucosal immune system by ingestion of gluten, a protein component found in wheat, barley, and rye. People who have HLA-DQ2 or DQ8 are susceptible to this condition because these specific antigen-presenting proteins produce particularly strong reactions by interacting with a unique peptide digestion product of gluten. Tissue transglutaminase, an enzyme produced in the mucosa, is an important cofactor in pathogenesis by amplifying the immunogenicity of gluten peptide fragments and is the target of autoantibodies that are characteristic of this disease. The condition produces generalized malabsorption by destroying the villi of the small intestine, reducing the surface area available for absorption.

In addition to malabsorption syndrome with diarrhea and weight loss, celiac disease can produce a host of nonspecific symptoms, including abdominal pain, fatigue, muscle and joint pains, and headaches and seemingly unrelated problems such as iron deficiency anemia, abnormal liver tests, and osteoporosis. These protean manifestations mean that celiac disease must be considered in the differential diagnosis of many conditions. The clinical course is quite variable, with symptoms coming and going. Symptoms can develop during childhood and produce growth retardation or first become manifest in adulthood.

Testing for celiac disease has been simplified by the development of an assay for anti–tissue transglutaminase antibodies. This test largely supplants measurement of antigluten antibodies, although these remain of some use in evaluating adherence to a gluten-free diet. IgA antibodies are the most useful for diagnosis, but IgA deficiency is common enough that an IgA level should be measured concomitantly.

Although serologic tests have high sensitivity and specificity, the implications of adhering to a gluten-free diet are so extreme that the diagnosis of celiac disease should be confirmed whenever possible by small bowel mucosal biopsy, now obtained routinely by endoscopy. An empiric trial of a gluten-free diet may be difficult to interpret because many persons with gastrointestinal symptoms improve with dietary carbohydrate restriction. Wheat starch is particularly hard to digest (due to gluten coating wheat starch granules), and ordinarily 20% of wheat starch are not absorbed by the small bowel and enter the colon.

Treatment of celiac disease at present involves strict lifetime exclusion of gluten from the diet. This is a difficult regimen that excludes most processed foods. Assistance of a dietitian is most helpful. The prognosis with effective treatment is very good. Symptoms should respond to the diet within weeks; failure to do so should prompt an examination of compliance with the diet or reconsideration of the diagnosis. Failure to respond may be seen when lymphoma or adenocarcinoma complicate the course of celiac disease or in cases of "refractory sprue" or "collagenous sprue" which can have a different autoimmune basis from classic celiac disease and which might respond to immunosuppressive drugs such as corticosteroids or azathioprine (Imuran).[1] Persistent diarrhea may be observed in patients with celiac disease who have concomitant microscopic colitis, another condition that is linked to HLA-DQ2 and HLA-DQ8.

Inflammatory Diseases

Diseases that produce extensive mucosal damage by inflammation cause generalized malabsorption by reduction of mucosal surface area, by promotion of small bowel bacterial overgrowth, by ileal dysfunction, or by development of enteroenteral or enterocolic fistulas. Examples include jejunoileitis due to Crohn's disease, nongranulomatous ulcerative jejunoileitis, radiation enteritis, and chronic mesenteric ischemia. With Crohn's disease, previous resection can

---

[1]Not FDA approved for this indication.

add to the problem (see later). Therapy aimed at the underlying process can improve absorption; in some cases (e.g., radiation enteritis) no effective therapy is available for the underlying problem, and symptomatic management is all that is possible. This includes use of antidiarrheal drugs to prolong contact time between luminal contents and the small bowel mucosa, ingestion of a reduced fat diet to reduce steatorrhea, and use of vitamin and mineral supplements to prevent deficiency states.

Infiltrative Disorders

Several conditions involve infiltration of the intestinal mucosa with cells or extracellular matrix that impede absorption or modify mucosal function by secretion of cytokines and other regulatory substances. These include eosinophilic gastroenteritis, systemic mastocytosis, immunoproliferative small intestinal disease (IPSID), lymphoma, and amyloidosis. These conditions are diagnosed by mucosal biopsy, but special stains might have to be employed to identify the infiltrating cells or matrix accurately.

Treatment of the underlying processes can improve absorption, but it is not uniformly effective. For eosinophilic gastroenteritis, a hypoallergenic (elimination) diet and corticosteroids may be useful. Mild systemic mastocytosis is treated with the mast cell-stabilizer sodium chromoglycate, H_1- and H_2-receptor antagonists, and low-dose aspirin. More advanced disease might respond to interferon or cytotoxic chemotherapy. IPSID initially is treated with antibiotics because small bowel bacterial overgrowth may be a causative factor. Once malignant change has occurred, it is treated like lymphoma with cytotoxic chemotherapy. Amyloidosis affecting the gut is not amenable to therapy and is usually fatal.

Infectious Diseases

Small Bowel Bacterial Overgrowth

Small bowel bacterial overgrowth in the jejunum can produce generalized malabsorption. It can occur whenever the mechanisms that reduce overgrowth are compromised. These situations include achlorhydria or hypochlorhydria, motility disorders of the small intestine (e.g., diabetes mellitus or scleroderma), and anatomic alterations (e.g., diverticulosis, gastrocolic fistula, or blind loops postoperatively). Fat malabsorption is attributed to bacterial deconjugation of bile acid. Bacterial toxins or free fatty acids can produce patchy mucosal damage, leading to less efficient carbohydrate and protein absorption. Bacteria also can compete with the mucosa for uptake of certain nutrients such as vitamin B_{12}.

Diagnosis of small bowel bacterial overgrowth can be difficult (see earlier). Treatment consists of antibiotic therapy unless a surgically correctable anatomic defect is discovered. Tetracycline is no longer uniformly effective; amoxicillin–clavulinic acid (Augmentin), cephalosporins, ciprofloxacin (Cipro), metronidazole (Flagyl), and rifaximin (Xifaxan) may be employed. Therapy should be given for 1 to 2 weeks initially and then discontinued. It should be restarted when symptoms recur. If this occurs quickly, longer treatment periods should be considered. Continuous antibiotic therapy is needed rarely.

Tropical Sprue

Tropical sprue is a progressive, chronic malabsorptive condition occurring in both the indigenous population and in visitors residing in certain tropical countries for extended periods. The prevalence of tropical sprue seems to be decreasing for uncertain reasons. The disease starts as an acute diarrheal disease that becomes a persistent diarrhea associated with substantial weight loss and typically megaloblastic anemia. Villi become shortened and thickened (partial villous atrophy), but the flat mucosa of celiac disease is not usually present. Enterocytes have disrupted brush borders and can have megaloblastic changes; the submucosa has a chronic inflammatory infiltrate. Intestinal biopsy is required for diagnosis.

Currently, tropical sprue is believed to represent a form of bacterial overgrowth with organisms that secrete enterotoxins. Most patients have evidence of excessive gram-negative bacterial colonization of the jejunum. The declining prevalence of tropical sprue may be due to improved nutrition, better sanitation, or prompt treatment of acute diarrhea with antibiotics. Treatment consists of pharmacologic doses of folic acid (folate) (5 mg daily[3]), injection of cyanocobalamin (if deficient), and antibiotic therapy for 1 to 6 months. Tetracycline 250 mg four times a day or sulfonamide is the treatment of choice. Newer antibiotics have not been tested extensively in this condition. Improvement should be noted after a few weeks. The prognosis with treatment is excellent; without treatment, tropical sprue can be fatal. Recurrence can occur.

Whipple's Disease

Whipple's disease is a rare chronic bacterial infection with multisystem involvement. The small bowel typically is heavily infiltrated with foamy macrophages containing periodic acid–Schiff (PAS)-positive material, distorting the villi. Small bowel biopsy with special stains or electron microscopy or a specific polymerase chain reaction (PCR) is diagnostic. Foamy macrophages and bacteria can be found outside the intestine in lymph nodes, spleen, liver, central nervous system, heart, and synovium. Accordingly, symptoms are protean. The bacterium has been identified as *Tropheryma whippelii*, a relative of *Acinetobacter*. It does not appear to be very contagious, and no direct person-to-person transmission has been demonstrated. Presumably differences in host resistance allow proliferation within macrophages without clearance of the bacteria.

Whipple's disease occurs mainly in older white men, but women and all ethnic groups are susceptible. Patients can present with malabsorption syndrome or with symptoms related to the extraintestinal disease (arthritis, fever, dementia, headache, or muscle weakness). Gross or occult gastrointestinal bleeding can occur. Protein-losing enteropathy may be present.

Treatment with any of several antibiotics (penicillin, erythromycin, ampicillin, tetracycline, chloramphenicol, or trimethoprim-sulfamethoxazole (TMP-SMX)) produces excellent symptomatic responses within days to weeks, but it should be continued for months to years. Even with protracted courses, relapses are common.

Other Infections

Mycobacterium avium–intracellulare is another chronic bacterial infection that can cause malabsorption, particularly in patients with AIDS. Mucosal biopsy with special stains to distinguish it from Whipple's disease is essential. Antibiotic therapy can reduce the intensity of infection; clearance depends on immunologic reconstitution with antiretroviral therapy. Clarithromycin (Biaxin) and ethambutol (Myambutol) are recommended as initial therapy.

Parasitic diseases can produce malabsorption by competing for nutrients and causing mechanical occlusion of the absorptive surface and epithelial damage. Protozoa that may be associated with malabsorption include *Giardia lamblia*, *Isospora belli*, *Cryptosporidium*, and *Enterocytozoon bieneusi*. Tapeworms associated with malabsorption include *Taenia saginata* (beef tapeworm), *Hymenolepis nana* (dwarf tapeworm), and *Diphyllobothrium latum* (fish tapeworm).

Giardia lamblia is a cosmopolitan parasite acquired from contaminated water or from another person by fecal-oral transmission. Cysts are relatively hardy, and ingestion of as few as 10 cysts is sufficient to establish infection. Patients with dysgammaglobulinemia (especially IgA deficiency) are likely to become infected. Diagnosis depends on finding the organism (cysts or trophozoites) in stool by microscopy (sensitivity ~50% for a single specimen), or detection of giardia antigens by immunologic testing of stool (sensitivity >90%), or discovery of the organism on small bowel biopsy.

Therapy consists of a single dose of tinidazole (Tindamax) (2 g), metronidazole (Flagyl)[1] (250 mg three times a day for a week), nitazoxanide (Alinia) (500 mg twice a day for three days), or quinacrine[2] (100 mg three times a day for a week).

---

[1]Not FDA approved for this indication.
[2]Not available in the United States.
[3]Exceeds dosage recommended by the manufacturer.

Isospora belli and *Cryptosporidium* spp. are coccidia, protozoa that disrupt the epithelium by intracellular invasion (*Isospora*) or by attaching to the brush border, destroying microvilli (*Crptosporidium*). Stool examination or small bowel biopsy can identify the organism. *Cryptosporidium* antigen can be discovered by immunoassay on stool with excellent sensitivity. *Isospora* can be treated with TMP-SMX[1] or furazolidone.[2] *Cryptosporidium* can be treated by nitazoxanide.

Microsporidia are intracellular organisms now believed to be most closely related to fungi and are implicated in diarrhea and malabsorption in patients with AIDS and other immunodeficiency states. Small bowel biopsy can show partial villous atrophy, and electron microscopy displays characteristic changes. Stool examination occasionally is helpful. No treatment is of proven value.

Tapeworms compete with their hosts for nutrients in the lumen. *Diphyllobothrium latum* can produce vitamin B$_{12}$ deficiency. The others can result in more extensive nutritional deficiencies. Diagnosis is based on stool examination, and treatment depends on the particular organism identified.

Luminal Problems Causing Malabsorption

Pancreatic Exocrine Insufficiency

Pancreatic exocrine insufficiency is the most common luminal problem that results in maldigestion. Patients develop symptoms of malabsorption when pancreatic enzyme secretion is reduced by >90%. There are several clinical features that distinguish pancreatic exocrine insufficiency from mucosal disorders, such as celiac disease. When fat is not digested, it is transported through the gastrointestinal tract as intact triglyceride, which can appear as oil in the stool. In contrast, if fat is digested but not absorbed, it is in the form of fatty acids that can produce secretory diarrhea in the colon, resulting in more voluminous, even watery stools. This has two important ramifications: Fecal fat concentration is lower with mucosal disease (typically <9% by weight), and hypocalcemia due to formation of soaps (calcium plus 2 fatty acids) is seen with mucosal disease but not with pancreatic exocrine insufficiency. In addition, patients with mucosal disease tend to have more problems with water-soluble vitamin deficiencies than those with pancreatic exocrine insufficiency. In some patients with pancreatic exocrine insufficiency, carbohydrate malabsorption can produce substantial bloating, flatulence, and watery diarrhea.

Tests to document pancreatic exocrine insufficiency are not widely available or are nonspecific (see earlier), and so diagnosis usually hinges on a consistent history, demonstration of anatomic problems in the pancreas (calcification or abnormal ducts), and documentation of a response of steatorrhea to empiric treatment with a large dose of exogenous enzymes.

Bile Acid Deficiency

Bile acid deficiency is a less common cause of maldigestion, and malabsorption in this setting is limited to fat and fat-soluble vitamins. The usual setting is a patient with an extensive ileal resection (see later), but this also occurs in certain cholestatic conditions in which bile acid secretion by the liver is markedly compromised, such as advanced primary biliary cirrhosis, or complete extrahepatic biliary obstruction. As with pancreatic exocrine insufficiency, stools tend to have high fat concentrations (>9% by weight) when bile acid secretion is limited by hepatic or biliary disorders.

Zollinger-Ellison Syndrome

Zollinger-Ellison syndrome produces several abnormalities that can affect absorption. High rates of gastric acid secretion produce persistently low pH in the duodenum, which precipitates bile acid and inactivates pancreatic enzymes. In addition, excess acid can damage the absorptive cells directly.

---

[1]Not FDA approved for this indication.
[2]Not available in the United States.

Postoperative Malabsorption

Substantial malabsorption can result from gastric surgeries. Weight loss can result from inadequate intake due to early satiety or symptoms of dumping syndrome. Malabsorption can result from impaired mechanical disruption of food, mismatching of chyme delivery and enzyme secretion, rapid transit, or small bowel bacterial overgrowth due to loss of the gastric acid barrier. In addition, gastric surgery sometimes brings out latent celiac disease.

Short intestinal resections are well tolerated, but more extensive resections produce diarrhea and malabsorption of variable severity. When these symptoms are associated with weight loss or dehydrating diarrhea, short bowel syndrome is said to exist. In general, nutrient absorptive needs can be met if at least 100 cm of jejunum is preserved, but fluid absorption will be insufficient and diarrhea may be profuse. The process of intestinal adaptation permits improved absorption with time; it depends on exposure of the absorptive surface to nutrients. Absorption of specific substances, such as bile acids or vitamin B$_{12}$, is reduced permanently by resection of the terminal ileum.

Malabsorption in short bowel syndrome is not due solely to loss of absorptive surface area. Gastric acid hypersecretion, bile acid deficiency, rapid transit (due to loss of the ileal brake), and bacterial overgrowth may be present. These conditions are amenable to treatment and therapy with antisecretory drugs, exogenous bile acids, opiate antidiarrheals, or antibiotics can produce substantial improvement. Injection of growth hormone in combination with glutamine and a special diet has been approved as treatment for short bowel syndrome; it can reduce the volume of parenteral fluid or nutrients required. Results with small bowel transplantation are improving with the use of better immunosuppressive regimens, and it remains the only cure for select patients with postresection malabsorption.

Attention to nutrition is vital in any patient with malabsorption. If adequate nutrition cannot be maintained by oral intake, nutritional therapy is needed. Because of impaired bowel function, success with enteral nutrition may be impossible; parenteral nutrition may be needed. It is important to distinguish between the need for supplemental fluid and electrolytes and the need for nutrients; total parenteral nutrition is not a good choice for patients who only require fluids and electrolytes.

REFERENCES

Bai JC, Mazure RM, Vazquez H, et al. Whipple's disease. Clin Gastroenterol Hepatol 2004;2:849–60.

Culliford AN, Green PH. Refractory sprue. Curr Gastroenterol Rep 2003;5:373–8.

Green PH, Jabri B. Celiac disease. Annu Rev Med 2006;57:207–21.

Gupta V, Toskes PP. Diagnosis and management of chronic pancreatitis. Postgrad Med J 2005;81:491–7.

Horslen SP. Optimal management of the post-intestinal transplant patient. Gastroenterology 2006;130(2 Suppl. 1):S132–7.

Jeejeebhoy KN. Management of short bowel syndrome: Avoidance of total parenteral nutrition. Gastroenterology 2006;130(2 Suppl. 1):S60–6.

Nath SK. Tropical sprue. Curr Gastroenterol Rep 2005;7:343–9.

O'Keefe SJ, Buchman AL, Fishbein TM, et al. Short bowel syndrome and intestinal failure: Consensus definitions and review. Clin Gastroenterol Hepatol 2006;4:6–10.

Petroniene R, Dubcenco E, Baker JP, et al. Given capsule endoscopy in celiac disease. Gastrointest Endosc Clin N Am 2004;14:115–27.

Schiller LR. Nutrition management of chronic diarrhea and malabsorption. Nutr Clin Pract 2006;21:34–9.

Simren M, Stotzer PO. Use and abuse of hydrogen breath tests. Gut 2006;55:297–303.

Singh VV, Toskes PP. Small bowel bacterial overgrowth: Presentation, diagnosis, and treatment. Curr Gastroenterol Rep 2003;5:365–72.

Swallow DM. Genetics of lactase persistence and lactose intolerance. Annu Rev Genet 2003;37:197–219.

Acute and Chronic Pancreatitis

Method of
David C. Whitcomb, MD, PhD

Acute Pancreatitis

The exocrine pancreas normally secretes a variety of digestive enzymes into the duodenum, where they mix with ingested food. In concert, the endocrine pancreas regulates the storage and utilization of the digested and absorbed nutrients through secretion of insulin into the bloodstream. Acute and chronic pancreatitis are disorders of the exocrine pancreas, but, in severe cases, they also affect the endocrine pancreas.

The central location of the pancreas within the body provides significant protection from traumatic injury. Although mechanical injury can occur with pronounced upper abdominal trauma, tissue injury most often is a result of premature activation of digestive enzymes within the pancreatic acinar cells or pancreatic duct. This causes autodigestion of pancreatic tissue, indirect and direct activation of the immune system, and an acute inflammatory reaction. Common etiologic triggers of enzyme activation and acute pancreatitis are listed in Box 1. The risk and severity of acute pancreatitis are amplified or diminished by underlying genetic variants and metabolic factors.

The acute inflammatory reaction to pancreatic injury and injury signals can extend beyond the pancreas and trigger the systemic inflammatory response syndrome (SIRS). Persistent SIRS can lead to a severe and potentially life-threatening condition that can also be triggered by severe trauma and overwhelming sepsis. One of the major complications of SIRS is a vascular leak syndrome that can result in intravascular volume depletion, hemoconcentration, hypotension, renal insufficiency, pulmonary edema, adult respiratory distress syndrome (ARDS), and shock. Multiorgan dysfunction or failure associated with SIRS is a leading cause of morbidity and mortality during the first week of severe acute pancreatitis.

Acute pancreatitis is a dynamic, evolving process, with well-defined events occurring sequentially during the course of the disease. In patients who develop acute pancreatitis after diagnostic endoscopic retrograde cholangiopancreatography (ERCP), the first symptom is pain; then the amylase and lipase rise within the first hour after ERCP, with maximum values seen between 4 and 12 hours. Inflammatory cytokines (e.g., interleukin-6) then begin to increase at 8 to 12 hours, with maximal concentrations reached after 24 to 48 hours. Serum C-reactive protein concentrations increase later, peaking at 72 hours after ERCP. In severe cases, SIRS and organ failure may develop over 12 to 36 hours and continue for several days, with compensatory antiinflammatory response syndrome (CARS) and infections developing after the first week.

DIAGNOSIS OF ACUTE PANCREATITIS

The clinical diagnosis of acute pancreatitis is based on characteristic abdominal pain, elevated serum levels of pancreatic enzymes, and abdominal imaging evidence characteristic of acute pancreatitis. The early diagnosis of acute pancreatitis is critical for implementation of appropriate treatment to ensure an optimal outcome. The major factors determining diagnosis and assessment are given in Box 2.

The pain of gallstone-related acute pancreatitis is typically sudden, epigastric, knife-like, and nauseating and may radiate to the back. In alcoholic pancreatitis, hereditary pancreatitis, and pancreatitis of some metabolic causes, the onset may be less abrupt and the pain poorly localized. The pain is often unbearable and is often associated with severe nausea and vomiting, without postemetic improvement in nausea. Occasionally, the patient experiences minimal pain, in which case the diagnosis must be based on abdominal imaging

---

BOX 1   Risk Factors for Acute Pancreatitis

I. Susceptibility factors

Duct obstruction

- Gallstones
- Parasites
- Tumors
- Anatomic abnormalities
- Endoscopic retrograde cholangiopancreatography (ERCP)

Metabolic

- Hyperlipidemia
- Hypercalcemia
- Acidosis (e.g., diabetic ketoacidosis)

Toxins

- Ethyl alcohol (high doses)
- Organophosphorus insecticides (acetylcholinesterase inhibitors)
- Scorpion toxin (Caribbean and South American varieties)
- Medications* (partial list)
  - Acetaminophen (Tylenol)
  - Azathioprine (Imuran)
  - Erythromycin
  - Estrogen
  - Exenatide (Byetta)
  - Furosemide (Lasix)
  - 6-Mercaptopurine (Purinethol)
  - Metronidazole (Flagyl)
  - Nonsteroidal antiinflammatory drugs (NSAIDs)
  - Pentamidine (Pentam)
  - Stavudine (Zerit)
  - Sulindac (Clinoril)
  - Tetracycline (Sumycin)
  - Valproic acid (Depakene)

Genetic

- Cystic fibrosis gene (*CFTR*)
- Trypsinogen gene (*PRSS1*)
- Pancreatic secretory trypsin inhibitor gene (*SPINK1*), (recurrent disease only)

Alcohol-associated injury
Infectious

- Viruses
- Bacteria

Trauma

- Blunt or penetrating
- Surgical

Ischemia
Idiopathic
II. Modifying factors

- Alcoholism (e.g., >2 drinks per day)
- Obesity (e.g., body mass index >30)
- Genetic factors

---

*Multiple mechanisms exist; usually, reactions are idiosyncratic or linked to hypertriglyceridemia.

---

evidence of acute pancreatitis and elevated pancreatic digestive enzymes in the blood.

Elevated serum pancreatic digestive enzymes levels are one of the most important signs of acute pancreatitis. Most clinical laboratories rapidly measure amylase and lipase, and normal ranges are provided

BOX 2 Admission Documentation and Calculations

Diagnosis

- *Risk factors:* gallstones, alcohol use, trauma, obesity, previous/family history, medication, hypertriglyceridemia, recent ERCP
- *Clinical history:* abdominal pain (onset, nature, location, radiation, nausea, vomiting)
- *Laboratory studies:* amylase, lipase, TAP (if available)

Severity Assessment and Baseline Documentation

Cardiovascular

- *Examination:* pulse rate and blood pressure (supine and standing), thirst, skin turgor, mucus membrane dryness, arterial/venous lactate
- *Laboratory studies:* hematocrit

Pulmonary

- Examination: respiratory rate, dyspnea, rales, effusion
- *Laboratory studies:* pulse-oximeter (ABGs if O_2 saturation is abnormal)
- *Radiology:* chest radiograph

Renal

- *Laboratory studies:* BUN/creatinine

Biliary

- *Examination:* liver tenderness, jaundice
- *Laboratory studies:* ALT, bilirubin (total and conjugated)
- *Radiology:* transabdominal ultrasound

Intestine

- *Examination:* diminished bowel sounds/ileus, distention, nausea and vomiting

Immune

- *Examination:* body temperature
- *Laboratory studies:* WBC, IL-6 (if available), CRP

Special Laboratory Studies

- LDH, serum calcium (for Ranson's score)
- Serum sodium, potassium, bicarbonate (for APACHE II)

Calculations

SIRS — Two or More Features

- Temperature >38°C or <36°C
- Heart rate >90 beats/min
- Respiratory rate >20 breaths/min or Pco_2 < 32 mm Hg
- WBC >12,000 cells/m³ or >10% bands

Multiorgan Failure — two or more organs

- *Respiratory:* Po_2/Fio_2 <400
- *Renal:* creatinine ≥1.4 mg/dL
- *Cardiovascular:* systolic blood pressure <90 mm Hg

ABGs = arterial blood gases; ALT = alanine aminotransferase; APACHE = Acute Physiology, Age, and Chronic Health Evaluation; BMI = body mass index; BUN = blood urea nitrogen; CRP = C-reactive protein; ERCP = endoscopic retrograde cholangiopancreatography; Fio_2 = fractional concentration of oxygen; IL-6 = interleukin 6; LDH = lactate dehydrogenase; Po_2 = partial pressure of oxygen; SIRS = systemic inflammatory response syndrome; TAP = trypsinogen activation peptide; WBC = white blood cell count.

by the laboratories. Based on the observation that mild elevation of these enzymes (less than twice the upper limit of normal) is common in a variety of other acute and chronic conditions, elevation of amylase and lipase more than three times the upper limit of normal is usually required for the diagnosis of acute pancreatitis in clinical studies. There are conditions in which amylase or lipase (usually isolated) can be elevated without acute pancreatitis, but these conditions rarely result in levels higher than the cutoff level of three times the upper limit of normal. Therefore, an elevation of both amylase and lipase is strongly supportive of a diagnosis but is not definitive, and the context of the elevation should be carefully considered. On the other hand, pancreatic enzyme levels may be well below this cutoff value, as can be seen in cases of severe acute pancreatitis with significant pancreatic necrosis, acute pancreatitis superimposed on chronic pancreatitis, and acute pancreatitis after pancreatic resection (i.e., inappropriately normal values when they should be low). More specific but less widely available tests for acute pancreatitis include trypsinogen activation peptide (TAP) and trypsinogen-2 levels.

Abdominal imaging in the setting of acute pancreatitis is usually reserved for the purpose of excluding other abdominal pathologies or identifying, assessing, and managing complications. The primary concern with the use of contrast-enhanced computed tomographic (CT) scanning early in the course of acute pancreatitis (e.g., first 2 days) is that administration of intravenous contrast to a subject with a poorly perfused pancreas has been clearly demonstrated in animal studies to worsen ischemia and extend the region of intrapancreatic cell necrosis. Although this effect has been difficult to demonstrate in human studies, most experts agree that fluid resuscitation (see later discussion) before the use of intravenous contrast and abdominal imaging is very important, and that CT is generally unnecessary within the first 2 days of treatment. Furthermore, the anatomic signs of acute pancreatitis, such as edema and fat stranding, take a number of hours to develop, and 15% to 30% of CT scans appear normal early in the course of acute pancreatitis. On the other hand, abdominal imaging can be invaluable in establishing the diagnosis in complicated cases, as well as in establishing the etiology and identifying important complications.

Diagnosis of Early Complications: Admission

The common complications of acute pancreatitis are listed in Box 3. The risk of various complications evolves with progression of the inflammatory process, so attention to timing relative to the onset of pain and related symptoms is important. The initial evaluation is critical for appropriate triaging and management, but the timing of this evaluation in relation to the time of injury is different in different patients, depending on the delay in seeking medical attention. Patients with more severe acute pancreatitis tend to present earlier in the clinical course, when many of the typical signs and symptoms of established acute pancreatitis (e.g., pancreatic edema) have not yet fully developed. Therefore, frequent reassessment of the patient is warranted during the first 24 hours.

Life-threatening complications are of primary concern, and different problems tend to occur early (first week) and late (>1 week) in the course of acute pancreatitis. Early diagnosis of SIRS and the vascular leak syndrome (VLS) are among the most important diagnostic priorities on admission and during the first 48 hours. In patients with evidence of severe acute pancreatitis, the diagnosis of an impacted gallstone is also important, because it may indicate the need for semiurgent therapeutic endoscopy.

Systemic Inflammatory Response Syndrome

The primary, early, life-threatening complications of acute pancreatitis are systemic rather than intrapancreatic and are tightly linked to the development of SIRS. SIRS defines a group of systemic signs and symptoms that occur with systemic activation of the immune system and can be reproduced experimentally by infusion of tumor necrosis factor-α (TNF-α) or interleukin 1. Thus, SIRS serves as a biomarker of significantly elevated proinflammatory cytokines (see Box 2). Other well-studied and reliable biomarkers used to diagnosis a significant systemic inflammation include serum cytokine interleukin 6 (>400 pg/mL), the leukocyte enzyme polymorphonucleocyte elastase

BOX 3 Common Complications in Acute Pancreatitis

Pancreatic Complications

Ductal

- Duct disruption—with fluid collections
  - Unorganized (previously called a phlegmon)
  - Organized (pseudocysts)
- Duct disruption—with fistula
  - Pancreatic ascites
  - Pleural effusion
  - Cutaneous
- Duct obstruction—pancreatic
  - With up-stream ductal dilation
  - With up-stream fluid leak
- Duct obstruction—biliary
  - Abnormal liver injury tests
  - Bacterial cholangitis

Vascular

- Pancreatic necrosis
- Portal vein thrombosis
- Splenic vein thrombosis
- Hemorrhage (related to pseudoaneurysm)
  - Hemosuccus pancreaticus
  - Pseudocysts
- Retroperitoneal hemorrhage

Inflammatory

- Pancreatic abscess (linked to invasive procedure)
- Postnecrotic inflammatory fluid collections
  - Sterile pancreatic necrosis
  - Infected pancreatic necrosis
- Inflammatory mass

Peripancreatic Complications

- Peripancreatic fat necrosis
- Duodenal stenosis—obstruction
- Colonic stenosis—obstruction
- Abdominal compartment syndrome—intraabdominal pressure of 12 mm Hg or higher

Systemic Inflammatory Complications

- Systemic inflammatory response syndrome (SIRS)
- Compensatory antiinflammatory response syndrome (CARS)
- Infections

Distant Organ Dysfunction or Failure

- Vascular leak syndrome
- Cardiovascular
  - Hypotension
  - Shock
- Pulmonary
  - Pulmonary edema (capillary leak rather than heart failure)
  - Acute lung injury
  - Adult respiratory distress syndrome (ARDS)
- Intestine
  - Ileus
  - Leaky gut syndrome
- Renal
  - Prerenal azotemia
  - Acute tubular necrosis

($>$300 μg/L), and the acute phase protein C-reactive protein ($>$150 mg/L). Interleukin 6 and PMN elastase are elevated early in the course of acute pancreatitis, but these tests are not widely available. C-reactive protein represents an acute phase response of the liver to high levels of proinflammatory cytokines, and it becomes an accurate marker of severe systemic inflammation 48 hours or longer after admission. Other scoring systems measure organ dysfunction rather than the immune response itself and are discussed later.

SIRS can be transient or persistent, depending on the underlying pathologic process. Persistent SIRS, that which lasts longer than 48 hours, is associated with multiorgan failure and a prolonged hospital admission. Therefore, SIRS is important as an early, bedside indication of a high-risk condition leading to systemic organ dysfunction.

The likelihood of SIRS is strongly influenced by preexisting factors. The most important factors are obesity (especially visceral adipose tissue) and chronic alcohol use (e.g., $>$2 drinks per day). Other factors, such as older age, female gender, genetic polymorphisms, metabolic state, and environmental variables, may also be important, but their identity and effects remain under investigation. The effects of obesity, alcohol, and other factors may be additive or multiplicative, so additional vigilance toward the detection of SIRS should be exercised for patients who have one or more of these factors.

Vascular Leak Syndrome

The VLS is an early and serious consequence of SIRS. It occurs with widespread activation of endothelial cells and results in release of injury signals that cause increases in systemic vascular permeability and extravasation of fluid and proteins into the tissues. This process leads to intravascular volume depletion, hemoconcentration, hypotension, renal insufficiency, pulmonary edema, ARDS, and shock. The effects of the VLS may be amplified by patient vomiting and inability to hold ingested fluids. If the VLS is detected early and appropriate therapy is administered, then many of the severe complications can be avoided.

The diagnostic challenge is to identify VLS before the patient develops significant hypovolemia and shock. The visceral organs are at high risk for ischemia and hypoxemia due to hypovolemia because of the high oxygen demands in areas of inflammation and because of reflex shunting of blood away from the viscera for preservation of central blood pressure in the context of injury and pain. Even a short period of ischemia can cause long-term damage and dysfunction. Hypovolemia and shock are associated with pancreatic necrosis, gut mucosal injury (leading to ileus and later to bacterial translocation), and kidney injury. Pulmonary edema and ARDS are also common in VLS and are caused by direct leakage of fluid into the lung.

Hypovolemia

Significant hypovolemia and visceral hypotension may occur before systemic hypotension (e.g., systolic blood pressure $<$90 mm Hg) appears. Indeed, a systolic blood pressure lower than 110 mm Hg may signal significant hypovolemia. The most accurate clinical sign of hypovolemia appears to be abnormal orthostatic vital signs, defined as large postural pulse change on standing ($>$30 beats/min) or severe postural dizziness that prevents vital sign measurement. The patient's pulse when supine should be compared with the pulse after standing for longer than 1 minute (with pulse counted for 30 seconds and multiplied by 2). For patients who are taking cardiovascular medications, those who have renal disease, those who have physical impairments, and those for whom there is concern about monitoring fluid status, continuous monitoring of central venous pressure (which requires an invasive procedure) should be considered. Arterial or venous lactate greater than 4 mmol/L is a sign of occult shock and should trigger rapid fluid resuscitation and expectation of a severe clinical course.

Indirect signs of existing hypovolemia include thirst, dry mouth, altered skin turgor, an elevated blood urea nitrogen (BUN)-to-creatinine ratio ($>$20), and hemoconcentration. Hemoconcentration occurs after plasma extravasation from the vascular system, which leaves red blood cells behind, thereby increasing the hematocrit. Note that hemoconcentration describes the change of hematocrit from baseline (which varies widely) and is a measure of plasma extravasation, whereas an elevated hematocrit (e.g. >44%) is associated with risk of pancreatic necrosis because of hypovolemia (low splanchnic perfusion pressure) and altered rheologic properties of blood (increased viscosity).

Organ Dysfunction

Extrapancreatic organ dysfunction or organ failure is dependent on multiple factors, including the amount of pancreatic injury, the magnitude of the immune response, the development of SIRS, the health of the individual organs, and the physiologic reserve of the major organ systems, which diminishes with age. The primary organs at risk for dysfunction include the cardiovascular system, lungs, kidneys, liver, and intestines. Single-organ dysfunction usually reflects pre-existing disease, and the prognosis is better for these patients than for those with multiple organ failure.

Cardiovascular dysfunction is primarily associated with the VLS (see earlier discussion), but myocardial depressing factors have been described. Altered calcium concentrations in serum (adjusted for albumin) may also affect cardiovascular physiology.

Pulmonary dysfunction is usually linked with pulmonary vascular leak and pulmonary edema and must be carefully assessed and treated. As the acute pancreatitis process evolves, the lungs become susceptible to progressive edema, ARDS, infection, and other complications of seriously ill hospitalized patients. An initial evaluation by pulse oximeter can be helpful, but there should be a low threshold for obtaining arterial blood gas measurements and chest radiographs if dyspnea is present or there is concern for SIRS.

Renal dysfunction is a common complication of acute pancreatitis and is a poor prognostic sign. The etiology may be multifactorial, including prerenal azotemia due to hypovolemia or acute tubular necrosis due to transient ischemia, toxic effects of CT contrast material, or other factors. An elevated BUN or creatinine concentration on admission can be very useful in assessing fluid status, but time is required for either of these levels to rise, so these measurements are tracking earlier conditions.

The liver is the direct recipient of high doses of blood-borne inflammatory signals and other factors that are released from the pancreas in acute pancreatitis via the portal vein or as a result of biliary pathology (common bile duct obstruction and infection). Liver failure is not caused by acute pancreatitis, but evidence of liver injury and dysfunction are detected by altered liver injury tests and change in synthetic function.

Biliary obstruction resulting from a gallstone impacted in the ampulla of Vater predisposes to bacterial cholangitis and worsens the outcome and severity of acute pancreatitis. An elevated alanine aminotransferase (ALT) level in a nonalcoholic patient with pancreatitis is the single best laboratory predictor of biliary pancreatitis. A level greater than three times the upper limit of normal has a positive predictive value of 95% for gallstone pancreatitis. However, normal ALT levels do not reliably exclude biliary pancreatitis. Transabdominal ultrasonography is more sensitive than CT or magnetic resonance imaging (MRI) for identifying stones and sludge in the gallbladder or bile duct dilatation, but it is insensitive for detecting stones in the distal bile duct. Endoscopic ultrasonography (EUS) may be the most accurate test for diagnosis or exclusion of biliary etiologies of acute pancreatitis, and it can guide the use of emergent ERCP, if necessary. However, it is not as widely available as ERCP, and these more invasive procedures are reserved for patients with severe acute pancreatitis (see later discussion).

Intestinal dysfunction is a central pathologic problem in acute pancreatitis. Gut mucosal injury from hypoperfusion and ischemia is a critically important early event because it strongly contributes to persistent SIRS (after the pancreas-generated initiation of SIRS) and is the source of enteric bacteria that cause all types of infections during the later phase of immune paralysis (CARS). The primary sign of intestinal injury is ileus.

Multiorgan Dysfunction

Development and persistence of SIRS and VLS increase the risk of single-organ and multiorgan failure, which in turn increases the likelihood of a prolonged intensive care unit stay and death. Both the Marshall score and the Sequential Organ Failure Assessment (SOFA) score are recommended for assessment of organ dysfunction, although the more cumbersome Acute Physiology, Age, and Chronic Health Evaluation (APACHE II) score, Ranson's score, and others may also be used (see Box 2).

Late Complications

Late complications of acute pancreatitis are the result of damage caused during the early stages of local and systemic injury. The most common problems are fluid collections and pseudocysts, pancreatic necrosis, infections, and nutritional deficits.

Fluid collections are poorly organized and ill-defined collections that occur early in acute pancreatitis, whereas pseudocysts are well-organized fluid collections. Fluid collections are diagnosed by abdominal imaging studies. Persistence of the collections and the presence of high amylase concentrations suggest pancreatic duct disruption.

Pancreatic necrosis is an infarction of the pancreas that is associated with hypovolemia, hemoconcentration, and increased creatinine levels. It is diagnosed by contrast-enhanced CT scan or MRI after 48 hours of supportive treatment.

Bacterial infections are common after the first week of severe acute pancreatitis and are usually caused by enteric flora. Diagnosis is suspected by clinical deterioration, failure to improve, fever, or increasing white blood cell counts. The site of infection should be documented. Infected pancreatic necrosis is a high-mortality infectious complication and is diagnosed by observation of gas collection with the pancreas on imaging studies or by fine-needle aspiration. Definitive diagnosis of an infectious complication is made by culture of the blood, urine, sputum, or aspirates from pancreatic fluid collections or pancreatic necrosis.

TREATMENT OF ACUTE PANCREATITIS

Early, careful assessment and reassessment of the patient with acute pancreatitis and anticipation of complications are essential to maximize the chances for a full and speedy recovery. The primary goals are managing fluid, supplementing oxygen, minimizing ongoing injury (depending on the cause), controlling pain, and addressing complications.

Currently, there are no good models to predict who will develop clinically significant VLS. Therefore, early and aggressive fluid resuscitation is recommended. One approach is to give 1 L of crystalloid solution, followed by intravenous infusion at twice the maintenance rate. The criteria for successful resuscitation remain subjective, and resuscitation may often be inadequate. Input and output should be strictly monitored, and central venous pressure measurements should be used to guide treatment in complicated cases and those predicted to be severe.

If the patient does have VLS and is fluid resuscitated, he or she is likely to develop pulmonary edema. Anticipation of this complication and close monitoring of blood oxygenation are essential. Treatment escalation from supplemental oxygen to mechanical ventilation is determined by clinical conditions.

Therapeutic endoscopy (e.g., ERCP) is often indicated for patients with severe acute pancreatitis resulting from gallstones and in those with biliary complications. An elevated ALT is highly predictive of gallstones, but a normal ALT does not rule them out as an important factor. Early consultation with an experienced endoscopist or transfer to a tertiary care facility may be needed, and this decision should be made as early as possible.

Fluid collections are common, evolve with time, and are usually managed conservatively. If the fluid collections continue to enlarge, cause pain, become infected (as suggested by unexplained fever, leukocytosis, or gas in the fluid collection), or compress adjacent organs, then medical, endoscopic, or surgical interventions may be needed. Asymptomatic pseudocysts may be managed conservatively, whereas symptomatic pseudocysts can often be drained endoscopically or by interventional radiology.

Pancreatic necrosis is thought to develop early in the course of acute pancreatitis, but it becomes a major problem after the first week, when risk of infection is high. If more than 30% of the pancreas is necrotic, then the risk of infection increases; in this situation, prophylactic antibiotics are used by some experts, but not by others. Gut decontamination has also been shown to reduce infections, as has the use of enteral feedings (see later discussion). If infected necrosis does develop, surgery may be needed. If possible, surgery should be delayed for 2 weeks so that the necrotic areas are better defined. Endoscopic and interventional radiology approaches are being used, rather than surgery, in some institutions.

Enteral feeding is the preferred method of providing nutritional support in acute pancreatitis, and it is usually well tolerated, even in patients with ileus. Multiple studies demonstrate that this therapy reduces the duration of SIRS, shortens intensive care unit stay, decreases the infection rate, reduces mortality, and costs less than total parenteral nutrition. The latter may be necessary for patients who cannot tolerate sufficient calories enterally or in whom enteral access cannot be maintained. Elemental or predigested formulas are needed, and about 30% of the minimum daily nutritional requirement is needed to maintain gut integrity.

Discharge Planning

Whenever possible, the cause of pancreatitis should be determined and plans to prevent recurrence developed before hospital discharge. In acute pancreatitis resulting from gallstones, a cholecystectomy should be considered before discharge in mild cases, or within a few months in more severe or complicated cases, to allow inflammatory processes or fluid collections to mature or resolve. ERCP with sphincterotomy is an alternative in patients who are not surgical candidates or for whom surgery must be delayed. If the cause is hypertriglyceridemia, then dietary measures, cessation of alcohol consumption, weight reduction, and possibly medication with gemfibrozil (Lopid) or fenofibrate (Tricor) should be initiated. Identification of hypercalcemia requires attention to the underlying cause. Medications associated with acute pancreatitis should be discontinued.

Patients can be discharged after their pain is controlled with oral analgesics and they are able to eat and drink. Oral feeding may be started when abdominal tenderness is diminishing and the patient is hungry. Patients should be instructed to eat small, low-fat, carbohydrate-protein diets that can be advanced in size over 3 to 6 days as tolerated. Patients who are unable to eat because of persistent pain or gastric compression from a pseudocyst have been successfully managed as outpatients with nasoenteric feeding tubes, surgical jejunal tubes, or total parenteral nutrition.

 CURRENT DIAGNOSIS

Acute Pancreatitis

- Acute pancreatitis requires the presence of two of the following three diagnostic signs:
    - Amylase or lipase higher than 3 times the upper limit of normal values
    - Characteristic sudden-onset abdominal pain
    - Characteristic changes on abdominal imaging
- Early diagnosis of complications is critical for proper management.
- The systemic inflammatory response syndrome (SIRS), when persistent, is the best predictor of early organ failure and can be diagnosed at the bedside.
- Obesity and alcoholism increase the risk of severe acute pancreatitis.
- The Marshal score accurately detects progressive organ failure.
- Hypovolemia is caused by a vascular leak syndrome and is diagnosed on the basis of hypotension, tachycardia, and hemoconcentration. The most sensitive bedside measure is the orthostatic blood pressure, whereas central venous pressure measurements provide accurate monitoring during resuscitation.
- Hypoxia is associated with an adult respiratory distress syndrome (ARDS) and is diagnosed by pulse oximetry or, more accurately, by arterial blood gas measurement.
- Gallstone pancreatitis is common and should be diagnosed on admission by transabdominal or endoscopic ultrasonography (EUS) in severe cases.
- Pancreatic necrosis is an infarction of the pancreas associated with hypovolemia, hemoconcentration, and increased creatinine. It is diagnosed by contrast-enhanced computed tomography (CT) or magnetic resonance imaging after 48 hours of supportive treatment.
- Bacterial infections are common after the first week of severe acute pancreatitis and are usually caused by enteric flora. Diagnosis is suspected on the basis of clinical deterioration, failure to improve, and fever or increasing white blood cell counts. Definitive diagnosis is made by culture of the blood, urine, sputum, or aspirates from pancreatic fluid collections or pancreatic necrosis.
- Infected pancreatic necrosis is also diagnosed by observation of gas collection with the pancreas.
- Fluid collections and pseudocysts are diagnosed by abdominal imaging studies.

Chronic Pancreatitis

- Chronic pancreatitis is defined as an inflammatory syndrome that lasts for longer than 6 months and is associated with permanent damage and complications:
    - Persistent inflammation (e.g., inflammatory mass)
    - Loss of pancreatic exocrine mass (e.g., atrophy)
    - Significant loss of secretory capacity (enzymes or bicarbonate)
    - Pancreatic fibrosis (seen on histology or EUS)
    - Dilated pancreatic ducts
    - Calcifications (ductal or parenchymal)
    - Pain (intermittent or chronic)
- The etiology of chronic pancreatitis is classified using the so-called TIGAR-O system:
    - **T**oxic-metabolic (including alcoholic)
    - **I**diopathic or tropical
    - **G**enetic
    - **A**utoimmune
    - **R**ecurrent and severe acute pancreatitis
    - **O**bstructive
- Severity of chronic pancreatitis is classified by structural and functional criteria:
    - Cambridge classification (CT based)
    - Rosemont classification (EUS based)
    - Functional testing

Chronic Pancreatitis

Recent advances have revolutionized our understanding of chronic pancreatitis. Chronic pancreatitis is a syndrome of inflammation and scarring that is associated with multiple disorders. The chronic pancreatitis syndrome is typically defined as a benign inflammatory process lasting longer than 6 months that is characterized by irreversible changes such as atrophy, fibrosis, calcifications, exocrine and endocrine insufficiency, and pancreatic pain. This definition differentiates chronic pancreatitis from acute pancreatitis, which has a shorter duration of inflammation; from isolated exocrine or endocrine insufficiency without chronic glandular inflammation (e.g., Shwachman-Diamond syndrome, total pancreatectomy, type 1 diabetes mellitus); and from pancreatic cancers that generate a chronic pancreatitis-like desmoplastic reaction.

Alcoholism has been the presumed etiology in the majority of patients diagnosed with chronic pancreatitis, in part because no other common cause was identified. However, more than 95% of alcoholics do not develop chronic pancreatitis, suggesting that other factors are important. Now, careful clinical studies from the United States and Europe have demonstrated that only one third of men and one eighth of women drink alcohol at levels that can be directly associated with chronic pancreatitis. Regression analysis suggests that men must drink more than 5 standard drinks per day as a threshold for development of chronic pancreatitis, although moderate drinking may contribute to disease progression. Furthermore, these studies recognized that smoking is a very important risk factor for chronic pancreatitis, especially in patients who also drink alcohol. The effects of smoking are dose dependent and are potentiated by alcohol consumption, especially heavy consumption.

The 1996 discovery that mutations in the cationic trypsinogen gene (*PRSS1*) cause recurrent acute and chronic pancreatitis significantly affected the understanding of human pancreatic diseases, both in terms of a rare causative mechanism and as a Rosetta stone for many other causes. In a variety of different populations, more than five genes have been observed to increase susceptibility to chronic pancreatitis; in all cases, the mechanism is linked to loss of regulatory control of trypsin inside the pancreas. These discoveries demonstrate that chronic pancreatitis is a complex disorder in which two or more risk factors must be present to cause disease. Modifying factors such as alcohol and smoking alter the response to injury by modifying the immune response and accelerating fibrosis, calcifications, and other complications. Family studies suggest that these complex genetic factors are very common, with the risk of chronic pancreatitis among family members of an affected person being similar to the risk of

inflammatory bowel disease in family members of a person with that disease. Therefore, chronic pancreatitis should be thought of as a complex genetic disorder, similar to inflammatory bowel disease, and not just as a disease of alcoholics.

PATIENT EVALUATION

When chronic pancreatitis is considered as part of the differential diagnosis, two initial questions must be answered: Does the patient have the chronic pancreatitis syndrome (Table 1), and what is the underlying disorder (Table 2). Once the diagnosis has been confirmed, attention is directed toward disease management. Three additional factors (discussed in more detail later) must be considered in monitoring the patient: defining the pathologic stage, minimizing or eliminating the proximal etiologic factors, and choosing biomarkers to assess disease activity and progression. Based on these factors, the treatment should be directed at both the cause of the disease and its symptoms. Chronic pancreatitis may be a symptom of another syndrome, such as atypical cystic fibrosis or autoimmune pancreatitis (AIP), that affects other organs, which also should be evaluated.

EARLY DIAGNOSIS

Early diagnosis of chronic pancreatitis is difficult because most of the primary features develop well into the clinical course, and many of the early features are difficult to measure or are reversible. Furthermore, many of the features are characteristic of other disorders, as noted earlier. Diagnosis requires the detection of complications of chronic pancreatitis that are permanent consequences of inflammation.

The Japanese Pancreas Society divides the diagnosis into definite chronic pancreatitis and probable chronic pancreatitis based on the use of commonly available tests. Definite chronic pancreatitis is diagnosed by any one of the following:

- Pancreatic calcifications diagnosed by ultrasonography or CT scanning
- Irregular dilation of the pancreatic duct or filling defects on ERCP
- Abnormally low bicarbonate levels on the secretin stimulation test
- Histologic evidence on biopsy
- Protein plugs, pancreatic stones, dilatation of the pancreatic duct, hyperplasia and metaplasia of ductal epithelium, and cyst formation, which are observed by other methods.

Probable chronic pancreatitis broadly encompasses abnormalities that do not reach the threshold of definite chronic pancreatitis. Other

TABLE 1 Diagnosis of Chronic Pancreatitis

Diagnostic Test	Abnormal Feature
Functional	
Fecal human elastase	<200 µg/g of stool*
Serum trypsin	<20 ng/mL
Steatorrhea	Positive Sudan stain
Secretin stimulation test	Peak bicarbonate <80 mEq/L
CCK stimulation tests	Peak lipase <300 IU/L
Structural	
CT scan	Parenchymal atrophy/heterogeneity, irregular dilated ducts (>4 mm), thickened duct walls, calcifications
MRI/sMRCP	Pancreatic atrophy, irregular dilated ducts, calcifications
Endoscopic ultrasonography	More than four of the following features: Parenchymal features: hyperechoic foci, hyperechoic, lobularity, cysts, stranding Ductal features: main duct dilation, calcification, irregular contour, hyperechoic walls, visible side ducts
Histology	Chronic inflammatory cells, fibrosis, acinar cell dropout

*Some experts recommend <125 µg/g or <100 µg/g of stool.
CCK = cholecystokinin; CT = computed tomography; MRI = magnetic resonance imaging; sMRCP = secretin-stimulated magnetic resonance cholangiopancreatography.

TABLE 2 Distinct Types of Chronic Pancreatitis

Subtype	Etiology	Age at Onset	Features
CF	Severe *CFTR* mutations	Infancy	Pancreas, lung, intestine, and other organ involvement
Atypical CF	Mild *CFTR* mutations	After age 10 y	May manifest as recurrent acute pancreatitis May have at least one other feature of CF
Hereditary pancreatitis	*PRSS1* mutations	Childhood	Recurrent acute attacks precede chronic pancreatitis Autosomal dominant inheritance
Familial pancreatitis	Multigenic, *SPINK1*	Adolescence	Several affected individuals in same generation
Early-onset ICP (including minimal-change CP)	Multigenic, *SPINK1*, *CFTR*, others	Adolescence to young adulthood	Features similar to familial except only one affected individual; typically more pain and dysfunction than late-onset ICP Some patients, usually young women, are considered to have minimal-change CP
Late-onset ICP (senile CP)	Unknown	After age 35 y	Finding is often incidental on abdominal imaging or work-up for diarrhea Less pain than alcoholic or early-onset ICP
Alcoholic CP	Alcohol plus smoking	After age 20 y	Typically alcoholism (alcohol intake $\geq$50 g/d for >5 y) Almost all patients are smokers Calcifications, dilated ducts, fibrosis, atrophy, and pain are common
Alcohol-associated CP	Alcohol plus genetic, (e.g., *CFTR*)	After age 20 y	An alcohol-consuming subject who does not meet criteria for alcoholic CP (i.e., in amounts not typically considered sufficient to cause pancreatitis) and in whom no other obvious causes are present
Autoimmune CP	Autoimmune	Usually after age 30 y	Diffuse or focal enlargement of the pancreas, duct structuring, IgG$_4$ usually markedly elevated Other organs can be affected, responds to steroids
Autoimmune disease–associated CP	Autoimmune	Usually young	Presentation not typical for autoimmune CP, may be similar to early-onset ICP Associated with other autoimmune diseases such as IBD
Tropical pancreatitis	Gene and environment, *SPINK1*	Childhood	May be painless; enlarged pancreatic duct with large stones Diabetes; possible malnutrition
Postnecrotic CP	Severe acute pancreatitis with necrosis	Any	Severe damage to the pancreas after one or more episodes of acute pancreatitis May include proximal duct strictures, compression, or obstruction
Obstructive CP	Obstruction of main pancreatic duct	Any	Usually associated with a mass, severe mucus plugging, or stricture Fibrosis is typically uniform and bland A subgroup may be caused by pancreas divisum or functional obstruction (e.g., SOD), although this remains controversial
Syndromic CP (e.g., Johanson-Blizzard syndrome, Pearson's marrow-pancreas syndrome, Kearns-Sayre syndrome)	Various (e.g., mutations in *UBR1*, mitochondrial deletions)	Early in life	Associated with complex congenital syndromes Rare

From Whitcomb DC, Cooper S, Raina A, Yadav D: Chronic pancreatitis: Clinical and molecular update. In Carey MC, Dite P, Gabryelewicz A, et al. (eds): Future Perspectives in Gastroenterology: Falk Symposium 161. Dordrecht, The Netherlands, Springer, 2008, pp 176–186.

CF = cystic fibrosis; CP = chronic pancreatitis; IBD = inflammatory bowel disease; ICP = idiopathic chronic pancreatitis; IgG$_4$ = immunoglobulin G type 4; SOD = sphincter of Oddi dysfunction.

groups have attempted to use EUS criteria, or modified secretin or cholecystokinin stimulation tests for early diagnosis, and these approaches appear to be complementary. Newer tests using MRI and other modalities are being developed at major referral centers.

In most cases, the diagnosis of chronic pancreatitis is made by contrast-enhanced spiral CT using a pancreas protocol, which differentiates the arterial and venous phases. Calcifications are readily seen on the precontrast scans, and inflammatory masses, a dilated main pancreatic duct, or parenchymal atrophy seen in the contrast phases usually establishes the diagnosis. Secretin-enhanced MRI (magnetic resonance cholangiopancreatography, or MRCP) is an excellent tool for identifying dilated ducts, strictures, and pseudocysts as well as providing information about the parenchyma and gland function. Because of their diagnostic sensitivity and specificity, CT and MRI/MRCP imaging has generally replaced ERCP for diagnosis of chronic pancreatitis.

Low serum trypsinogen levels are a feature of chronic pancreatitis. Fecal human elastase levels are also valuable for diagnosing moderate to severe pancreatic exocrine insufficiency and are complementary to imaging tests.

DIFFERENTIAL DIAGNOSIS

The age at onset and the environmental context in which signs of chronic pancreatitis develop provide clues to the underlying disease subtype (see Table 2). The earlier the age at onset and the smaller the exposure to environmental stresses, the higher the likelihood of major underlying genetic causes. Patients with gain-of-function *PRSS1* mutations have an autosomal dominant disorder with high penetrance, so family history is important. Patients with atypical cystic fibrosis from mild-variable *CFTR* mutations have disease susceptibility in other organs, including the lung, intestine, and male reproductive tract. Patients with *SPINK1* mutations have a high risk rapid progression to advanced stages of chronic pancreatitis. Genetic testing requires genetic counseling, because these diagnoses will affect the patient's long-term future and have implications for the patient's family as well.

Pancreatic cancer causes a desmoplastic reaction that can mimic chronic pancreatitis, and chronic pancreatitis is a major risk factor for pancreatic cancer. The likelihood of developing pancreatic cancer is increased by focal abnormalities within the pancreas, insidious onset, weight loss without maldigestion or correction with pancreatic enzyme supplements, lack of calcifications, and older age. In addition to typical chronic pancreatitis, there is growing recognition of AIP, which can mimic cancer of the pancreatic head. Early reports that elevated serum immunoglobulin G4 (IgG_4) levels were specific for AIP have been challenged by the discovery of multiple cases of moderately elevated IgG_4 in the presence pancreatic cancer. The best test to differentiate chronic pancreatitis from pancreatic cancer is EUS with fine-needle aspiration, and the diagnostic accuracy is further enhanced by the use of molecular markers. In addition, EUS by an expert endoscopist is highly accurate in predicting resectability.

Main duct intraductal pancreatic mucinous neoplasia (IPMN) can manifest with pain, pancreatic duct dilation, parenchymal atrophy, and pancreatic exocrine insufficiency that mimics chronic pancreatitis. IPMN usually manifests in the fifth or sixth decade of life and is easily diagnosed by ERCP or EUS. There is a significant risk of malignant degeneration of these lesions, and management by an expert is recommended.

 CURRENT THERAPY

Acute Pancreatitis

- Aggressive fluid resuscitation should be initiated on diagnosis of acute pancreatitis, whether or not the clinical course is predicted to be severe.
- Intensive unit monitoring of fluid balance and blood oxygen levels is indicated with early signs of organ dysfunction.
- Early fluid resuscitation and establishment of intravascular fluid balance takes priority over treatment of pulmonary edema with diuresis.
- In cases of pulmonary edema, the use of sedation plus endobronchial intubation and mechanical ventilation may be necessary to maintain optimal arterial blood gas concentrations.
- The treatment of severe gallstone pancreatitis should be done by an expert therapeutic endoscopist.
- Early enteral nutrition is indicated if the hospital course is predicted to last longer than 72 hours. An elemental formula is indicated, and probiotics are contraindicated. Nasogastric and nasojejunal delivery routes are feasible. Total parenteral nutrition may be needed to supplement enteral feedings.
- The prophylactic treatment of infections in severe acute pancreatitis is controversial but may be used if more than 30% of the pancreas is necrotic. If prophylactic treatment is elected, antibiotics that penetrate infected pancreatic necrosis are recommended, and antifungal agents with broad-spectrum antibiotics should be considered.
- The treatment of uncomplicated pancreatic fluid collections or pancreatic pseudocysts is observational. Pseudocysts that are infected, are causing pain, or are compressing other organs (e.g., the stomach) can be treated by endoscopic, transcutaneous, or surgical approaches. This should be done in expert centers.
- The treatment of infected pancreatic necrosis is controversial. There is general agreement that surgery should be delayed for at least 2 weeks from the onset of acute pancreatitis, if possible. Recent studies have demonstrated successful treatment of infected pancreatic necrosis with endoscopic and conservative medical management (i.e., prolonged antibiotics).
- The etiology of an episode of acute pancreatitis should be systematically investigated and the source of pancreatic injury eliminated, if possible. The most common approach is to remove the gallbladder in subjects who have gallstones or likely gallstone pancreatitis.

Chronic Pancreatitis

- Initial therapy is targeted toward the etiologic factors that are driving the inflammatory and fibrotic processes.
- Alcohol cessation can reduce the frequency of recurrent attacks of acute pancreatitis and may improve outcomes. The effects of alcohol are potentiated by smoking.
- Tobacco smoking is one of the most important environmental factors contributing to susceptibility and severity of chronic pancreatitis.
- Hypercalcemia and hyperlipidemia should be aggressively controlled.
- Patients with splenic vein thrombosis and gastric varices may require emergency surgery and splenectomy if major gastrointestinal bleeding occurs.
- Vigilance is needed to detect progression and complications that require intervention.
- Pancreatic exocrine insufficiency should be treated with pancreatic enzyme replacement therapy. The target of therapy is improved nutrition, because diet and symptoms vary greatly. Steatorrhea (fat in the stool) is a late sign and is diet dependent.
- Vitamin B_{12} deficiency in long-standing pancreatic insufficiency should be treated.
- The onset of diabetes mellitus can be insidious. Treatment should be correlated with the treatment of exocrine insufficiency, with pancreatic enzyme replacement to ensure that absorption and disposition of nutrients are correlated.
- Pain is multifactorial and can be mild or severe, intermittent or continuous.
- Pain should be initially managed by relieving duct obstruction or structural problems caused by pseudocysts or other mass lesions.
- Pain associated with meals may be improved by pancreatic enzyme replacement therapy.
- Pain linked with stones may be improved by endoscopic treatments or extracorporeal shock-wave lithotripsy.
- Medical management of pain remains challenging, and severe pain may require the administration of narcotics.
- Surgical treatment may provide long-term pain relief; the type of surgery depends on the size of the pancreatic duct, the presence of an inflammatory mass, and other features.
- Pancreatectomy and islet cell autotransplantation remain treatment options for some patients.

TREATMENT OF THE COMPLICATIONS OF CHRONIC PANCREATITIS

Inflammation of the pancreas results in the destruction of normal tissue, initiation of metaplastic processes, and a variable pain syndrome. The primary complications are listed in Box 4. The development and severity of complications are progressive, so vigilance and continued reassessment are necessary.

Autoimmune Pancreatitis

AIP, also known as lymphoplasmacytic sclerosing pancreatitis, is a treatable form of pancreatitis that is increasingly recognized. AIP is part of a systemic fibroinflammatory syndrome that is IgG$_4$ related, and 40% of patients with AIP have involvement of extrapancreatic organs, especially the bile duct, salivary glands, retroperitoneum, and lymph nodes. Biopsies typically reveal plasmacytes with IgG$_4$-positive staining. AIP is seen in adults of either gender, but it most often affects men older than 50 years of age. Symptoms are nonspecific and can include abdominal pain, obstructive jaundice, diabetes mellitus, weight loss, and maldigestion with or without steatorrhea. On abdominal imaging, the pancreas may appear to have focal or diffuse swelling, which has been described as a sausage shape with a capsule-like peripancreatic rim, and diffuse irregularity and narrowing of the main pancreatic duct. Calcifications and pseudocysts are unusual. AIP can mimic ductal adenocarcinoma, both on clinical criteria (e.g., older patients with painless jaundice and new-onset diabetes mellitus) and radiographically (e.g., focal mass in the head of the pancreas). Most of the reports are from Japan, where the incidence appears to be higher than in the United States or Europe.

Early reports suggested that the diagnosis could be made by detection of elevated IgG$_4$ levels and that the condition was reversed by use of steroids. Although identification of histologic, serologic, radiographic (pancreatic and intrapancreatic), and steroid response features strongly support the diagnosis of AIP, up to 15% of cases do not meet the criteria of any current definitions. A normal IgG$_4$ level is also common, because serum levels fluctuate. Furthermore, up to 7% of pancreatic cancers have moderately elevated IgG$_4$ levels (but <200 mg/dL). For these reasons, careful evaluation and follow-up are very important.

The mainstay of treatment is oral steroids. This treatment should be given if there is a very high suspicion of AIP and low suspicion of, or negative work-up for, pancreatic adenocarcinoma. Patients with AIP often have dramatic improvement in response to steroids, even within 1 to 2 weeks. A typical dose is 40 mg/day of prednisone[1] for 4 weeks, with a taper of 5 mg/week for 12 weeks. If there is no significant improvement in 2 to 4 weeks, then the likelihood of cancer dramatically increases. Although the response to steroids is often dramatic, it may be less in patients with long-standing symptoms, and relapse is common. Patients with biliary involvement have a very high relapse rate. Azathioprine (Imuran)[1] has been used in steroid-refractory disease or as a steroid-sparing agent, but the long-term natural history and response to therapy are poorly documented.

Maldigestion

Maldigestion is inadequate digestion of nutrients of any cause. Symptoms of maldigestion overlap with those of malabsorption and include abdominal bloating, cramping, diarrhea and steatorrhea, and malnutrition. Similar symptoms occur with celiac disease, bile salt depletion, bacterial overgrowth, lactase deficiency, and ingestion of indigestible organic compounds. Maldigestion in chronic pancreatitis occurs with loss of pancreatic enzyme production, delivery, or function relative to nutrients in the intestine. If pancreatic exocrine insufficiency has been diagnosed, three variables must be considered during evaluation and planning of treatment: nutritional needs, residual pancreatic function, and diet (e.g., high- or low-fat diet). In the United States, the quality of pancreatic enzyme replacement is regulated, so the response to treatment can be calibrated to symptoms and to nutritional response (e.g., prealbumin levels). If products without enteric coating are chosen, then gastric acid suppression is required.

Pain

Pain in chronic pancreatitis remains a major challenge. Pain can range from mild to severe and can be intermittent or continuous. Continuous pain is the most difficult to treat and is associated with much worse quality of life. Pain can arise from acute exacerbations, chronic inflammation, pancreatic duct hypertension related to ductal strictures or obstruction, pseudocysts, high tissue pressure linked to fibrosis, tissue ischemia and acidosis, or a complex neuroinflammatory process. If possible, factors contributing to chronic pancreatitis should be controlled, including alcohol use, smoking, hyperlipidemia, and hypercalcemia. If pain occurs at mealtime, a trial of pancreatic enzyme replacement therapy should be undertaken. Some experts also use antioxidants, although strong evidence of their effectiveness is lacking. Medical therapies are listed in Box 5. Endoscopic therapy may be useful if there is a dominant pancreatic duct stricture or stones. Extracorporeal shock-wave lithotripsy can be combined with endoscopic therapy as well. In severe cases, pancreatic surgery may be required to control pain.

Other Complications

Less common and late complications of chronic pancreatitis include diabetes mellitus, splenic vein thrombosis with gastric varices, bile duct obstruction, and the risk of cancer. Some patients with chronic pancreatitis develop type 1 diabetes mellitus, but others with severe exocrine insufficiency and fibrosis do not. Care must be taken to coordinate pancreatic enzyme replacement therapy with hypoglycemia or insulin administration so that absorption of nutrients and clearance of blood sugar are matched. Sudden and severe gastrointestinal bleeding in a patient with chronic pancreatitis may be caused by gastric varices. This medical emergency should be treated with aggressive volume management and may require surgical removal of the spleen. Bile duct obstruction can be initially managed by endoscopic treatment but may require surgical bypass of the obstruction.

> ### BOX 4 Complications of Chronic Pancreatitis
>
> **Pancreatic Exocrine Insufficiency**
> - Steatorrhea
> - Carbohydrate intolerance—bloating, pain, diarrhea
> - Fat soluble vitamin deficiency
> - Vitamin B$_{12}$ deficiency
> - Malnutrition
> - Weight loss
>
> **Pancreatic Endocrine Insufficiency**
> - Glucose intolerance
> - Diabetes mellitus
>
> **Parenchymal Changes**
> - Pseudocysts—pain, pseudoaneurysm
> - Duct strictures
> - Fistulas—retroperitoneal fluid collections, ascites, plural effusions
> - Stone formation—obstruction and pain
> - Ischemia—pain
> - Nerve hypertrophy—pain
> - Splenic vein thrombosis—gastric varices
> - Metaplasia
> - Cancer
>
> **Common Bile Duct Obstruction**
> - Abnormal liver injury tests
> - Jaundice
> - Pain
>
> **Duodenal Stenosis**

---

[1]Not FDA approved for this indication.

BOX 5   Therapies for Chronic Pancreatitis

Malabsorption
- Pancreatic enzyme supplements
  - Enteric coated (e.g., Pancrelipase, Creon)
  - Non–enteric coated with gastric acid suppression (e.g., Pangestyme, Kutrase)
- Vitamin B_{12} injection

Diabetes Mellitus
- Hypoglycemic agents
- Insulin

Autoimmune Pancreatitis
- Prednisone[1]
- Azathioprine (Imuran)[1] for relapses

Pain
- Analgesics
  - Acetaminophen (Tylenol)
  - Narcotics
  - Nonsteroidal antiinflammatory drugs
  - Tramadol (Ultram)
- Antioxidants[1] (with vitamin C, vitamin E, selenium, methionine,[7] and β-carotene[7])
- Pancreatic enzymes[1] (e.g., Pancrease MT, Pancrelipase)
- Octreotide (Sandostatin)[1]
- Tricyclic antidepressants
- Serotonin reuptake inhibitors
- Endoscopic therapy
- Extracorporeal shock-wave lithotripsy
- Nerve blocks
  - Celiac plexus
  - Splanchnic nerve transection
- Surgery
  - Duct drainage
  - Head resection
- Pancreatectomy (with islet cell autotransplantation)

[1]Not FDA approved for this indication.
[7]Available as dietary supplement.

Chronic pancreatitis is a risk factor for pancreatic cancer, especially in patients who smoke. Pancreatic cancer usually manifests 20 to 30 years after the development of chronic pancreatitis; therefore, any changes in symptoms, such as pain or weight loss, could be warning signs.

REFERENCES

Draganov P, Forsmark CE. "Idiopathic" pancreatitis. Gastroenterology 2005;128(3):756–63.

Etemad B. Gastrointestinal complications of renal failure. Gastroenterol Clin North Am 1998;27(4):875–92.

Forsmark CE, Baillie J. AGA Institute technical review on acute pancreatitis. Gastroenterology 2007;132(5):2022–44.

Kamisawa T, Okazaki K, Kawa S. Diagnostic criteria for autoimmune pancreatitis in Japan. World J Gastroenterol 2008;14(32):4992–4.

Mudanna V, Whitcomb DC, Khalid A, et al. Elevated serum creatinine as a marker of pancreatic necrosis in acute pancreatitis. Am J Gastroenterol 2009;104:164–70.

Szmola R, Whitcomb DC. Molecular genetics of chronic pancreatitis. In: Encyclopedia of Life Sciences. Chichester, GB: John Wiley & Sons; 2009.

Whitcomb DC. Mechanisms of disease: Advances in understanding the mechanisms leading to chronic pancreatitis. Nat Clin Pract Gastroenterol Hepatol 2004;1(1):46–52.

Whitcomb DC. Acute pancreatitis. N Engl J Med 2006;354(20):2142–50.

Whitcomb DC, Cooper S, Raina A, Yadav D. Chronic pancreatitis: Clinical and molecular update. In: Carey MC, Dite P, Gabryelewicz A, et al., Future Perspectives in Gastroenterology: Falk Symposium 161. Dordrecht, The Netherlands: Springer; 2008. p. 176–86.

Witt H, Apte MV, Keim V, Wilson JS. Chronic pancreatitis: Challenges and advances in pathogenesis, genetics, diagnosis, and therapy. Gastroenterology 2007;132(4):1557–73.

Yadav D, Hawes RH, Brand RE, et al. Alcohol consumption, cigarette smoking and the risk of recurrent acute and chronic pancreatitis. Arch Intern Med 2009;169(11):1035–45.

Gastroesophageal Reflux Disease

Method of
Jason R. Roberts, MD, and
Donald O. Castell, MD

Gastroesophageal reflux disease (GERD) is a motility disorder of the lower esophageal sphincter (LES). The definition of this disease has evolved over time, reflecting better understanding of the roles that transient LES relaxations and acid/pepsin contact with esophageal mucosa play, as well as the ability to identify these events. The diagnosis of GERD has changed from identification of a hiatal hernia, to identification of erosive esophagitis, to the currently accepted patient-centered definition: any symptom or injury to esophageal mucosa resulting from reflux of gastric contents into the esophagus. GERD should not be confused with physiologic gastroesophageal reflux, which is not associated with symptoms or esophageal mucosal injury.

The prevalence of GERD is difficult to ascertain, although several studies have indicated it to be as high as 50% of adults in Western countries, with 10% to 18% experiencing heartburn on a daily basis. Studies using health care utilization data may underestimate the prevalence because of self-treatment by individuals in the community, whereas population surveys may overestimate it because of inaccurate assessment of symptoms and absence of objective data. Regardless of the real number, the management of this disease costs more than $10 billion annually in the United States. GERD has been called a disease of white males, although recent data suggest increasing prevalence in Asia and Pacific regions.

Pathophysiology

GERD is a motility disorder of the LES characterized by inappropriate or transient relaxations that allow gastric contents to reflux into the esophagus. The LES is a tonically contracted ring of smooth muscle fibers innervated by the vagus nerve. Vagal stimulation during swallowing produces physiologic LES relaxation and is a likely source for transient LES relaxations. Gastroesophageal reflux occurs most frequently during postprandial periods, at a rate of 6 reflux episodes per hour, but averages 2 episodes per hour over the entire day. Increasing frequency of reflux in the postprandial period results from gastric distention after a meal and stimulation of tension receptors in the proximal stomach leading to transient LES relaxations (Box 1). A chronically hypotensive LES is not a major mechanism for GERD in most patients but can be seen in cases of severe erosive esophagitis.

Reflux of acidic gastric contents can lead to injury of the esophageal mucosa, including inflammation, ulceration, stricturing, Barrett's metaplasia, and adenocarcinoma. Peristaltic clearance, tissue resistance, and salivary bicarbonate make up host defense mechanisms that work by clearing reflux and neutralizing the acid residue on the mucosa. Erosive esophagitis or strictures result in the most severe form of GERD, which includes nocturnal reflux with longer acid contact times, decreased salivary production, and lower frequency of swallowing during sleep.

Complications

Acid reflux can lead to significant morbidity if it is not recognized and treated appropriately. Habitual contact of acid and activated pepsin with the stratified squamous epithelium, along with impaired defense mechanisms, results in tissue injury (Box 2). The end result of this process can be ulceration, fibrosis with stricture formation, Barrett's esophagus, or adenocarcinoma. These complications can produce alarm symptoms (Box 3). Patients presenting with alarm symptoms should undergo immediate diagnostic evaluation with an esophagogastroduodenoscopy (EGD).

EROSIVE ESOPHAGITIS

The endoscopic finding of erosive esophagitis is seen in fewer than 50% of patients with heartburn. The severity is stratified according to the Los Angeles Classification of Esophagitis. Treatment with a proton pump inhibitor (PPI) for 4 to 12 weeks heals erosive esophagitis in 78% to 95% of cases. The healing effect of antisecretory therapy, and particularly PPIs, demonstrates the important role of acid reflux in causing tissue injury. The recurrence rates for erosive esophagitis are high after discontinuation of PPI maintenance therapy (75%–92%), necessitating continuation of gastric acid suppression.

STRICTURES

Most strictures caused by GERD are peptic in origin and are located at the squamocolumnar junction. Patients with GERD and strictures, compared to those without strictures, are more likely to have a hypotensive LES, abnormal peristalsis, and prolonged acid clearance time. Stricture formation decreases the luminal diameter, resulting in solid food dysphagia. Dysphagia in these patients is often a combination of decreased luminal diameter and dysmotility of the distal esophageal body with low-amplitude peristalsis. Patients with GERD who develop dysphagia should have immediate barium radiography and an endoscopic evaluation.

BARRETT'S ESOPHAGUS

Barrett's esophagus is a premalignant condition that may evolve into esophageal adenocarcinoma. The histologic abnormality involves intestinal-like metaplasia of the stratified squamous epithelium. Epidemiologic studies show Barrett's to be more common among Caucasians, males, and the elderly (mean age, 60 years). A finding of Barrett's esophagus portends a 30- to 125-fold increased risk of eventual adenocarcinoma, with an incidence of 0.5% per year. Despite the prevalent use of PPIs in the treatment of GERD, the incidence of adenocarcinoma has been increasing. Current guidelines encourage endoscopic surveillance for patients with Barrett's esophagus, yet there are sparse data showing the cost-effectiveness or mortality benefit of this strategy.

ADENOCARCINOMA

Approximately 50% of esophageal cancers are adenocarcinomas. Since the 1970s, the incidence has been rising for reasons that are still unknown. GERD is a risk factor for esophageal adenocarcinoma, and the risk increases with the duration and severity of GERD symptoms. There is a suggestion that cagA strains of *Helicobacter pylori* are protective against development of Barrett's esophagus and adenocarcinoma. The declining incidence of *H. pylori* may be a possible explanation for the rising incidence of adenocarcinoma.

Diagnosis

GERD is largely a clinical diagnosis under the current definition (i.e., any symptom or tissue injury resulting from reflux of gastric contents into the esophagus). Patients with the typical symptoms of heartburn and regurgitation most often associated with meals have a high pretest probability of having GERD. A well-obtained history and symptom questionnaire are usually sufficient to form a presumptive diagnosis and are more cost-effective than ambulatory reflux testing or EGD. An empiric trial of PPI therapy that leads to a significant reduction or resolution of symptoms likely confirms the diagnosis.

The pathophysiology of GERD is much more complex than previously thought. It involves more than acid reflux, because non-acid reflux with a pH greater than 4 can be a common source of symptoms. This entity is unmasked when PPI therapy is found to control gastric acid secretion and impedance-pH testing identifies a temporal relationship between symptoms and episodes of nonacid reflux.

Direct-to-consumer marketing and the availability of over-the-counter PPI medications (Prilosec OTC) have led to self-treatment of GERD-type symptoms and a consequent change in the type of patients seeking medical care for their symptoms. Patients with typical GERD symptoms that do not completely respond to therapy with PPIs, including over-the-counter and prescription PPIs, warrant a more detailed evaluation of their symptoms. A separate population requiring earlier diagnostic evaluation includes patients with exclusively atypical GERD symptoms such as cough, hoarseness, throat clearing, asthma attacks, and chest pain. Less commonly, patients presenting with signs or symptoms of tissue injury, such as solid food dysphagia, should also be more rigorously tested for GERD (Box 4).

Patients who have symptoms associated with GERD, whether typical or atypical, are frequently treated empirically with PPI therapy. With a lack of discrimination regarding symptom types, this population is very heterogeneous and comprises patients with symptoms that are truly associated with GERD, not at all associated with GERD, and a combination of both. The pretest probability of GERD in this group is diluted, and nonresponders to empiric therapy are numerous. Partial responders and nonresponders to PPI therapy should undergo ambulatory reflux testing using combined multichannel intraluminal impedance (MII)-pH or standard pH. MII-pH catheters measure both esophageal pH changes and impedance changes that occur as an ion-rich refluxate passes a pair of ring electrodes, resulting in a drop in the resistance to a low-voltage current between the electrodes. The change in impedance can detect gastroesophageal reflux regardless of the acid content and can distinguish reflux types as liquid, gas, or mixed.

The goals of ambulatory reflux testing are to determine whether the esophageal acid contact time is abnormal, whether there are an abnormal number of reflux episodes, and whether a relationship between reflux and symptoms exists. The advantage of combined MII-pH is its ability to identify both acid and nonacid reflux, so that

testing can be done while the patient is on acid-suppression therapy and the artifact of acidic food or beverage ingestion is eliminated; pH-only testing is affected by both of these conditions. The major disadvantage is that MII-pH testing is less available than conventional pH testing.

EGD is specific for detecting reflux-related tissue injury but is not sensitive, because fewer than 50% of patients with GERD-related heartburn have endoscopic findings of reflux. If erosive esophagitis or Barrett's esophagus is found on endoscopy, aggressive antisecretory therapy with a PPI is warranted.

A barium esophagram is unlikely to add useful diagnostic information in patients with GERD symptoms without dysphagia. It is a useful tool in distinguishing obstructive from nonobstructive dysphagia and may even be more sensitive than EGD in detecting causes of obstructive dysphagia. Achalasia is often mistaken for GERD during the onset of symptoms, and early use of esophagography may help make this diagnosis.

Management

GERD is predominantly a postprandial event involving transient LES relaxations. The primary focus in management of this disease is to eliminate or improve symptoms and prevent tissue injury. In most patients with recurrent GERD symptoms, this can be accomplished by controlling gastric acid secretion with antisecretory therapy. PPIs are the most effective pharmacologic therapy for improving symptoms and preventing tissue injury from acid reflux. Individuals with only occasional heartburn may successfully treat symptoms with a combination of lifestyle modifications and over-the-counter antacids, histamine 2 receptor antagonists, or a PPI.

Patients presenting with typical symptoms and a history consistent with GERD should be given a trial of PPI once daily for at least 4 weeks. A validated GERD symptom assessment questionnaire such as the Reflux Disease Questionnaire should be used as an initial screening tool, because symptom response is the primary outcome measure and subsequent questionnaire responses are useful in comparison with the initial responses for measuring treatment efficacy. If symptoms have not responded or have responded only partially after this trial, then the dosing or frequency of the PPI should be increased over another 4-week period. If the response is still unsatisfactory, diagnostic testing with ambulatory combined MII-pH or pH-only monitoring is indicated.

PPIs are an effective maintenance therapy for most patients with GERD and may be stepped down or used on demand, but GERD is a chronic condition with a high recurrence rate of symptoms without some form of maintenance therapy. This creates a large population of patients on antisecretory therapy for a disease with a low mortality rate, which raises the question of drug safety. There are insufficient data available that would warrant a recommendation against long-term PPI therapy. Clinical judgment in specific patient populations should be used to determine the optimal PPI regimen.

At present, pharmacologic reflux reduction therapy consists solely of the use of baclofen (Lioresal),[1] which has been shown to reduce transient LES relaxations and associated gastroesophageal reflux. The drawback of this medication is its unwanted side effects, which include somnolence and dizziness, limiting its tolerability and clinical utility as a stand-alone therapy.

Antireflux surgery is another alternative that is effective in limiting GERD symptoms in patients with a positive reflux-symptom relationship. Candidates for surgery include younger patients who do not want to continue chronic PPI therapy and patients with symptomatic nonacid reflux. Today, most antireflux surgery is performed laparoscopically with a 360-degree Nissen fundoplication. The associated mortality rate is small (0.5%–1%), and this approach is preferred to open laparotomy. Traditional predictors for surgical success have included the presence of typical symptoms (heartburn

---

> **BOX 4 Clinical Spectrum of Gastroesophageal Reflux Disease–Related Symptoms and Tissue Injury**
>
> **Esophageal**
> *Symptomatic Syndromes*
> - Typical reflux syndrome
> - Reflux chest pain syndrome
>
> *Syndromes with Tissue Injury*
> - Reflux esophagitis
> - Reflux stricture
> - Barrett's esophagus
> - Adenocarcinoma
>
> **Extraesophageal**
> *Established Association*
> - Reflux cough
> - Reflux laryngitis
> - Reflux dental erosions
>
> *Proposed Association*
> - Sinusitis
> - Reflux asthma
> - Pulmonary fibrosis
> - Pharyngitis
> - Recurrent otitis media

---

[1]Not FDA approved for this indication.

and regurgitation), symptom response to a trial of PPIs, and an abnormal ambulatory pH study. These criteria exclude the important group of patients with atypical symptoms or symptoms related to nonacid reflux. However, such patients should be considered candidates for antireflux surgery if a positive reflux-symptom relationship can be demonstrated.

Patients with alarm symptoms and those who are partial responders to PPI therapy should also undergo EGD to aid in determining the cause of the symptoms, such as obstructive dysphagia from peptic strictures, adenocarcinoma, and bleeding esophageal ulcers (which can cause anemia). EGD findings that suggest GERD are a result of acid reflux. However, the incidence of these findings has declined with the use of PPIs.

Nonerosive reflux disease is increasingly common as more patients are converted from acid refluxers to nonacid refluxers with PPI therapy. By definition, these patients have no findings on endoscopy to suggest ongoing GERD. Absence of endoscopic findings does not exclude GERD, however, because tissue injury can occur at the microscopic as well as the macroscopic level. Patients with either erosive esophagitis or nonerosive reflux disease have dilated intercellular spaces on electron microscopy.

As previously discussed, patients with GERD may develop Barrett's esophagus. The metaplastic transformation from normal stratified squamous epithelium to an intestinal-type, columnar-lined epithelium creates a premalignant lesion with a 0.5% per year risk of progression to adenocarcinoma. Screening for Barrett's esophagus remains controversial. There is no evidence that screening results in a mortality benefit due to early detection of esophageal adenocarcinoma. Screening of all patients with GERD for Barrett's esophagus is clearly not cost-effective, but it is reasonable to target the highest-risk populations, such as Caucasian men older than 50 years of age. Current American College of Gastroenterology guidelines recommend surveillance endoscopy in patients with known Barrett's esophagus at intervals determined by the degree of dysplasia. Because there have been no long-term, controlled studies, it is a grade C recommendation.

REFERENCES

Bonino J, Sharma P. Barrett's esophagus. Curr Opin Gastroenterol 2005;21:461–5.

Castell DO, Richter JE. The Esophagus. 4th ed. Philadelphia: Lippincott Williams & Wilkins; 2003.

Frye J, Vaezi M. Extraesophageal GERD. Gastroenterol Clin North Am 2008;37:845–58.

Hila A, Agrawal A, Castell D. Combined multichannel intraluminal impedance and pH esophageal testing compared to pH alone for diagnosing both acid and weakly acidic gastroesophageal reflux. Clin Gastroenterol and Hepatol 2007;5:172–7.

Kahrilas PJ, Shaheen N, Vaezi M. American Gastroenterological Association Institute technical review on the management of gastroesophageal reflux disease. Gastroenterology 2008;135(4):1392–413.

Mainie I, Tutuian R, Agrawal A, et al. Combined multichannel intraluminal impedance-pH monitoring to select patients with persistent gastroesophageal reflux for laparoscopic Nissen fundoplication. Br J Surg 2006; 93:1483–7.

Mainie I, Tutuian R, Castell D. Comparison between the combined analysis and the DeMeester score to predict response to PPI therapy. J Clin Gastroenterol 2006;40:602–5.

Mainie I, Tutuian R, Shay S, et al. Acid and non-acid reflux in patients with persistent symptoms despite acid suppressive therapy: A multicentre study using combined ambulatory impedance-pH monitoring. Gut 2006; 55:1398–402.

Savarino E, Zentilin P, Tutuian R, et al. The role of nonacid reflux in NERD: Lessons learned from impedance-pH monitoring in 150 patients off therapy. Am J Gastroenterol 2008;103:2685–93.

Vakil N, Van Zanten SV, Kahrilas P, et al. The Montreal definition and classification of gastroesophageal reflux disease: A global evidence-based consensus. Am J Gastroenterol 2006;101:1900–20.

Vakil N. Review article: Test and treat or treat and test in reflux disease. Aliment Pharmacol Ther 2003;17(Suppl. 2):57–9.

Wang KK, Sampliner RE. Updated guidelines 2008 for the diagnosis, surveillance and therapy of Barrett's esophagus. Am J Gastroenterol 2008;103: 788–97.

Tumors of the Stomach

Method of
Scott A. Hundahl, MD

Gastric Adenocarcinoma

Thanks to happy accident rather than specific planning, over the past 80 years, gastric adenocarcinoma has changed from the most-common solid organ malignancy in the United States to a relatively uncommon disease. Worldwide, however, it remains a scourge second only to lung cancer.

CLASSIFICATION AND EPIDEMIOLOGY

Several classification schemes exist. Two are commonly used. Bormann's morphologic classification relies on gross characteristics of the tumor. The histologic classification of Lauren, first described by Jarvi and Lauren in 1951, divides gastric adenocarcinomas into intestinal (gland-forming) and diffuse (discohesive) types, based on their microscopic appearance. Several other classification schemes have been proposed, including Broder's classification of differentiation, the WHO (World Health Organization) classification, the Nagayo–Komagome classification, the Ming classification, and the Goseki classification, but none eclipses the Lauren classification.

Epidemiologically, three patterns of disease can be discerned, with *Helicobacter pylori* infection playing an important role in the first two patterns: intestinal-type tumors arising from the lesser curve and distal stomach, related to *H. pylori*–associated atrophic gastritis and intestinal metaplasia; diffuse-type tumors involving the body of the stomach, often associated with intense *H. pylori*–associated inflammation but not associated with significant intestinal metaplasia; and intestinal-type tumors of the gastroesophageal junction.

In high-incidence regions of the world, such as Japan and Korea, up to two thirds of gastric adenocarcinomas are of the first type and are strongly associated with chronic multifocal atrophic gastritis and intestinal metaplasia from chronic *H. pylori* infection. The process usually begins at the antrum–corpus junction along the lesser curvature and predisposes to cancers of the intestinal type occurring in the sixth or seventh decades of life. The second type of gastric adenocarcinoma, also associated with *H. pylori*, afflicts younger persons in the fourth and fifth decades of life. The last type, seen in lower-incidence regions of the world such as the United States, is associated with chronic gastroesophageal reflux and Barrett's esophagitis.

Epidemiologists and public health experts estimate that more than 40% of gastric adenocarcinomas worldwide can be attributed to chronic. *H. pylori* infection. Strains containing the *cagA* gene appear more dangerous. The infection usually starts by the second or third decade, and unless it is successfully treated, it gives rise to chronic inflammation, atrophic gastritis, and eventually intestinal metaplasia, which is a premalignant histologic condition. Dietary factors such as high salt and high nitrates can accentuate this progression as well as the march to cancer. As the condition progresses, acid-producing oxyntic mucosa is progressively wiped out, gastric pH increases, and bacterial overgrowth with non–*H. pylori* bacteria is facilitated. The original *H. pylori*, which requires an acid environment to thrive, often disappears at this point.

Once intestinal metaplasia is established, dietary factors become particularly important in mitigating the risk of cancer development. Protective factors include intake of vitamin C, fresh fruits and vegetables, and antioxidants. The association of *H. pylori* infection with the development of intestinal metaplasia suggests that early detection and elimination of this infection might prevent gastric cancer. Unfortunately, in high-incidence areas, reinfection from contaminated water supply and other sources is common, thus undermining the strategy. Also, in prevention trials to date, benefit appears restricted to the subgroups without preexisting intestinal metaplasia.

RISK FACTORS

Risk factors other than *H. pylori* infection include low socioeconomic status, smoking, a diet deficient in fresh fruits and vegetables or high in salt-preserved high-nitrate foods, previous gastric ulcer, ionizing radiation, family history, and previous gastric resection. Blood group A is associated with higher risk of developing a diffuse-type tumor. Predisposing genetic conditions include the Lynch's syndrome (hereditary nonpolyposis colorectal cancer [HNPCC], a condition with microsatellite instability due to deficient DNA repair enzymes), as well as dominantly inherited germline mutations in the E-cadherin gene.

DIAGNOSIS

In Western populations, by the time gastric cancer causes symptoms, the disease is often relatively advanced. In a large National Cancer Data Base survey of U.S. patients, presenting ascribable symptoms included weight loss (62%), abdominal or epigastric pain (52%), nausea (34%), anorexia (32%), early satiety (32%), dysphagia (26%), and melena (18%).

Mass screening combining upper GI series, endoscopy, and serum pepsinogen I/II ratio have proved beneficial in high-incidence areas such as Japan, but they cannot be justified in the United States, where incidence is low. However, for defined risk groups, such as those with established atrophic gastritis and established intestinal metaplasia, strong family history, and those with HNPCC syndrome, surveillance screening should definitely be considered. For those with hereditary E-cadherin mutations associated with gastric cancer, prophylactic total gastrectomy is recommended.

In the United States, diagnosis is usually made by upper endoscopy. One should be aware that diffuse-type cancers manifesting as linitis plastica are often associated with minimal visible mucosal changes, and deep biopsies are often required for establishing the diagnosis. Furthermore, small, early gastric cancers (defined by the Japanese as in situ and T-1 cancers, with or without node involvement) can be associated with particularly subtle mucosal changes, presenting a challenge for even the most experienced endoscopist. Chromoendoscopy and other sophisticated mucosal imaging techniques have been used to identify such changes but are not yet standard.

Extent-of-disease studies for gastric adenocarcinoma include endoscopic ultrasound (good for estimating depth of tumor and visualizing immediately adjacent nodes), and helical CT scanning, which is good for evaluating extraluminal extent of disease, intraabdominal or mediastinal extension or spread, and liver or lung metastases. Because even high-resolution CT scanning can miss small peritoneal implants, extraregional nodal spread, and small liver metastases, staging laparoscopy or minilaparotomy are valuable adjuncts and should be considered mandatory if any preoperative chemotherapy is considered.

CURRENT DIAGNOSIS

- Intestinal metaplasia, which predisposes to cancer, results from chronic *Helicobacter pylori* infection.
- In the United States, screening studies are reserved for those with definite risk factors.
- Pretreatment staging drives subsequent treatment and involves endoscopy, endoscopic ultrasound, helical computed tomography, and often laparoscopy or mini-laparotomy.
- Mucosal abnormalities can be largely absent in early gastrointestinal stromal tumors, small carcinoids, and even diffuse-type linitis plastica. Deep endoscopic biopsies are required.

CURRENT THERAPY

Adenocarcinoma

- To ensure complete surgical resection, resection should be customized (e.g. gross margin, use of endoscopic mucosal resection for certain mucosal tumors).
- Survival is highest with low Maruyama Index surgery.
- Adjuvant therapy options include preoperative chemotherapy (± postoperative treatment), or postoperative chemoradiation

Gastrointestinal Stromal Tumors

- Node dissection is not indicated.

Gastric Lymphoma

- For aggressive diffuse-type lymphomas, chemotherapy with or without radiation therapy is now the mainstay of treatment. Surgery is reserved for complications such as acute perforation.
- Superficial mucosa-associated lymphoid tissue tumors can sometimes be treated by simply eliminating *Helicobacter pylori* infection. It comes back if reinfection occurs, however.

STAGING

Although a long-established, much-modified Japanese staging system, the General Rules, finds widespread use in many areas of the world, the AJCC/UICC (American Joint Committee on Cancer/International Union Against Cancer) TNM (tumor, nodes, metastases) system is by far the dominant staging system used. T stage is defined a bit differently than that for colorectal cancer: Muscularis propria penetration short of serosal penetration is still considered T2 disease, a serosal breach is required for T3 disease, and a T4 designation requires direct involvement of adjacent structures. Optimally, accurate nodal designation requires that more than 15 nodes be examined by the pathologist. N1 disease means metastases in 1 to 6 regional nodes, N2 disease means metastases in 7 to 15 regional nodes, and N3 disease means metastases in more than 15 nodes. Any N3 disease, any node-positive T4 disease, any M1 distant metastatic disease, and any involved extra-regional M1 nodes translate in the staging matrix to stage IV disease. The reader is referred to the AJCC staging manual referenced at the end of this chapter.

TREATMENT

Curative treatment of gastric cancer involves, as main therapy, complete negative-margin surgical resection of disease. For select tumors, such resection sometimes follows up-front chemotherapy. For localized in situ and select T1 tumors, endoscopic mucosal resection and minimally invasive techniques have been successfully employed. Unfortunately, most tumors in the United States are discovered at a stage where formal open surgery is required.

To secure a histologically negative mural margin of resection, a gross margin of 2 cm is usually adequate for exophytic, noninfiltrating tumors, and a margin of at least 5 to 6 cm of grossly normal tissue is recommended for ulcerated or infiltrating tumors or diffuse histology. Closest mural margins are generally checked by frozen section at the time of surgery to confirm adequacy of resection. Total gastrectomy is not indicated as a routine procedure, except in diffuse-type tumors involving most of the stomach (linitis plastica), but it is warranted whenever required for a negative-margin resection.

Routine splenectomy in the treatment of gastric cancer, as well as routine distal pancreatectomy (performed in the past to clear splenic nodes), should be avoided unless definitely required for complete resection of visible or palpable disease.

The optimal extent of lymph node dissection in this disease has generated—and continues to generate—international controversy. Although several prospective randomized trials to date in non-Asian populations—none perfect—fail to demonstrate that routine extensive lymphadenectomy increases survival, it has also been shown that insufficient lymphadenectomy definitely compromises survival. A prospective randomized single-institution trial in Taipei has documented survival benefit associated with radical lymph node dissection. The adequacy of lymphadenectomy for a given case can be quantified using the Maruyama Index of Unresected Disease. In both a large U.S. adjuvant chemoradiation trial and in a blinded reanalysis of a large Dutch surgical trial, low Maruyama Index score correlates with survival. Moreover, a dose–response effect is seen for the extent of surgical clearance of node groups at risk. Using the Maruyama computer program to predict the extent of nodal spread for a given cancer case before surgery is one way to facilitate a low Maruyama Index operation.

Sentinel node biopsy, an established technique in the treatment of other cancers, has largely failed to win support in cancer of the stomach owing to the organ's lymphatic complexity and relatively high reported false-negative rates.

A large North American prospective randomized trial of postoperative adjuvant 5-fluorouracil–based chemoradiation in completely resected gastric cancer revealed a significant increase in disease-free and overall survival with this treatment. The postoperative nature of this trial thwarted implementation of surgical guidelines, and the extent of node dissection for most patients in the trial was suboptimal. Practitioners in some countries, such as Japan, dismiss the necessity of adjuvant postoperative adjuvant chemoradiation with the (unproved but reasonable) argument that this is only a salvage technique for inadequate surgery. A separate Korean chemoradiation series has shown benefit even for radically treated cases, however. For patients with good postoperative performance status, good organ function, and adequate nutrition, postoperative adjuvant chemoradiation therapy remains the standard in North America.

A recent U.K. study of preoperative plus postoperative ECF (epirubicin [Ellence],[1] cis-platinum, and continuous-infusion 5-fluorouracil [Adrucil]) chemotherapy versus surgery alone has shown encouraging results for ECF, with a significant improvement in survival. Previous preoperative chemotherapy trials, using other regimens, have been negative, however. Preoperative ECF chemotherapy is now recommended by some, and this is especially the case for localized advanced tumors considered borderline resectable.

In Korea, a positive trial of adjuvant perioperative intraperitoneal chemotherapy has been reported. Considerable morbidity and mortality are associated with this adjuvant treatment, however, and it is unlikely it will be implemented without refinement and successful independent duplication of results.

For localized disease deemed not resectable to negative margins, both chemotherapy and chemoradiation have been used to convert such tumors to potentially resectable status. With successful negative-margin resection, some of these patients indeed survive free of disease long term. When localized unresected disease is documented to exist, administering chemoradiation with 5-fluorouracil as a radiation sensitizer can also result in some degree of 5-year survival (per reports, >10%).

Gastrointestinal Stromal Tumors

Gastrointestinal stromal tumors (GISTs) manifest as submucosal spindle cell tumors in the sarcoma family. In contrast to leiomyosarcomas and other spindle cell sarcomas, they express the antigen CD117 and most (>80%) tumors have activating mutations of c-KIT. Formerly considered rare, approximately 5000 of these tumors per year are now diagnosed in the United States. Owing to pattern of growth in the gastric wall, deep to the mucosa, early symptoms

are unusual and these tumors often grow to massive size before mucosal ulceration and hemorrhage (or other major symptoms) finally develop. GISTs are classified as sarcomas. Even low-risk GISTs (< 5 cm and < 1 mitosis per 10 high power fields) can metastasize, and no GIST can be considered truly benign.

Treatment of localized primary GISTs consists of complete surgical resection, and a 2-cm margin of grossly normal tissue usually accomplishes this. Specific lymph node dissection is not indicated for this histology. Surgical series indicate that approximately 50% of primary gastric tumors metastasize and recur within 5 years. For patients with widespread metastases, generally located in the peritoneal cavity or the liver, first-line therapy is now a well-tolerated oral agent, imatinib mesylate (Gleevec or STI-571) at an initial dose of 400 mg daily, which generates partial responses in more than 50% of cases and stable disease in an additional 25% of cases. Side effects are minimal, and 1-year survival in treated patients is approximately 85%. On the basis of a completed American College of Surgeons Oncology Group (ACOSOG) trial, patients who have all disease completely resected should receive postoperative adjuvant therapy for 1 year.

For tumors resistant to imatinib, SU11248, sunitinib malate (Sutent), is now used as effective second-line therapy. Additional targeted biological agents are under active investigation.

Carcinoid Tumors

Carcinoid tumors of the stomach are similar in behavior to small bowel carcinoids. When small (<1 cm), and unassociated with invasion of the muscularis propria, local excision to negative margins is generally deemed sufficient. For such tumors, endoscopic resection has an established role. However, even small tumors can metastasize to lymph nodes. Wider gastrectomy with lymph node dissection is generally recommended for gastric tumors larger than 1 cm. Many of these tumors are associated with serum hypergastrinemia; those without this finding tend to be more aggressive. When metastatic to the liver or other organs, surgical cytoreduction (or other means of tumor ablation) can offer considerable palliation to those with carcinoid syndrome, and this should always be considered. Octreotide therapy is now a palliative mainstay in all patients with carcinoid syndrome.

Gastric Lymphomas

Gastric lymphomas encompass most of the lymphoma subtypes, but low-grade, mucosa-associated B-cell lymphomas (B-cell MALT lymphomas) deserve special mention because they are strongly associated with H. pylori infection. Indeed, localized cases can be controlled simply by treating the H. pylori infection. In such cases, molecular studies indicate persistence of the offending lymphoid clone in about one half of cases. However, and, particularly if H. pylori infection recurs, the lymphoma in such cases returns.

Aggressive high-grade diffuse-type B-cell gastric lymphomas, stage IE and IIE, once treated with multimodal therapy, are now treated with chemotherapy alone as the primary treatment, with or without radiotherapy. Surgical intervention is now reserved for emergencies, such as perforation.

For further information on this and other gastrointestinal lymphomas, please see the chapter on lymphoma.

REFERENCES

Cunningham D, Allum WH, Stenning SP, et al. Perioperative chemotherapy versus surgery alone for resectable gastroesophageal cancer. N Engl J Med 2006;355(1):11–20.

Ferrucci PF, Zucca E. Primary gastric lymphoma pathogenesis and treatment: What has changed over the past 10 years? Br J Haematol 2007;136 (4):521–38.

Hundahl SA, Macdonald JS, Benedetti J, et al. Surgical treatment variation in a prospective, randomized trial of chemoradiotherapy in gastric cancer: The effect of undertreatment. Ann Surg Oncol 2002;9(3):278–86.

---

[1]Not FDA approved for this indication.

Hundahl SA, Peeters KC, Kranenbarg EK, et al. Improved regional control and survival with "low Maruyama Index" surgery in gastric cancer: Autopsy findings from the Dutch D1-D2 Trial. Gastric Cancer 2007;10(2):84–6.

Macdonald JS, Smalley SR, Benedetti J, et al. Chemoradiotherapy after surgery compared with surgery alone for adenocarcinoma of the stomach or gastroesophageal junction. N Engl J Med 2001;345(10):725–30.

Modlin IM, Kidd M, Latich I, et al. Current status of gastrointestinal carcinoids. Gastroenterology 2005;128(6):1717–51.

Siehl J, Thiel E. C-kit, GIST, and imatinib. Recent Results. Cancer Res 2007;176:145–51.

Tumors of the Colon and Rectum

Method of
Pinckney J. Maxwell IV, MD, and
Gerald A. Isenberg, MD

Background, Epidemiology, and Etiology

Colorectal cancer is the third most common cancer in men and women, after prostate and lung/bronchus cancer in men and breast and lung/bronchus cancer in women. The American Cancer Society estimated that there would be 108,070 new diagnoses of colon cancer and 40,070 new diagnoses of rectal cancer in the United States in 2008. The incidence of colorectal cancer has been decreasing since the mid-1980s, with a more dramatic decrease occuring in the most recent decade. This decrease is likely related to an increase in screening with removal of precancerous polyps. The American Cancer Society expected an estimated 49,960 deaths from colorectal cancer in 2008, accounting for 9% of all cancer deaths. The mortality rate of colorectal cancer has similarly decreased since the mid-1980s, again with a sharper decline in the past decade most likely related to improved screening. Colorectal cancer is a highly treatable and frequently curable malignancy when it is detected early, highlighting the need for better screening.

The development of colorectal cancer is related to a number of factors, including age, diet, activity, environmental exposures, family history, and genetics. Ninety percent of colorectal cancers are diagnosed after the age of 50 years, and fewer than 5% of cases are diagnosed before the age of 40. The peak incidence of diagnosis is in the seventh decade of life. Dietary factors play a role in carcinogenesis. Western diets, containing high fat and low fiber, have been associated with increased rates of colorectal cancer, as has the intake of red or processed meats and alcohol. It is likely that the low-fiber Western diet slows transit time, leading to increased exposure to carcinogens. Activity level also can play a role in carcinogenesis: studies have shown an increase in cancer among those with sedentary jobs and a decreased incidence among those who exercise regularly. Exposure to cigarette smoke increases the risk of colorectal adenomas and cancers. The American Cancer Society Cancer Prevention Study II revealed that 12% of colorectal cancer deaths in the general U.S. population can be attributed to smoking. Family history and genetics also play a significant role in carcinogenesis, because approximately 10% of patients diagnosed have a first-degree relative with colorectal cancer.

ADENOMATOUS POLYPS

The progression from normal mucosa to an adenomatous polyp and then to an invasive colorectal cancer proceeds through a well-defined process over many years. Aberrant crypt foci develop into microadenomas and then into adenomatous polyps. Dysplastic cells develop within the polyp, continue to multiply, become a tumor and then break through the subepithelial barrier and invade the layers of the bowel wall, eventually spreading to pericolic tissues or to lymph nodes and distant sites. A number of genes have been implicated in carcinogenesis, including protooncogenes (*KRAS, SRC, MYC*), tumor-suppressor genes (*APC, DCC, TP53, MCC, DPC4*), and DNA-mismatch repair genes (*HMSH2, MLH1, PMS1, PMS2, GTBP*). Sporadic colorectal cancers develop as a result of several cumulative genetic insults involving these genes (Fig. 1).

FAMILIAL COLORECTAL CANCER SYNDROMES

Familial adenomatous polyposis (FAP) is an inherited, non–sex-linked, mendelian dominant disease that accounts for approximately 1% of all colorectal cancers. The high penetrance of FAP means that there is a 50% chance of development of colorectal cancer among members of affected families. However, 20% of FAP patients have no family history, and their cases most likely represent new, spontaneous mutations. The disorder is caused by mutations in the tumor-suppressor *APC* gene, which is located on chromosome 5 (5q21–q22), or in the *MUTYH* gene, which is located on chromosome 1 (1p34.3–p32.1). FAP is characterized by the progressive development of hundreds or thousands of adenomatous polyps located throughout the entire colon. The clinical diagnosis is based on histologic confirmation of at least 100 adenomas. All patients eventually develop colorectal cancer. The adenomas typically appear by the mid-twenties, and cancers by the late thirties.

An attenuated form of FAP is recognized in which fewer adenomas (20–100) are identified. Adenomas and cancers develop somewhat later, at average ages of 44 and 56 years, respectively. FAP also exhibits extracolonic manifestations, including gastric, duodenal, and small-bowel polyps; osteomas and desmoid tumors (Gardner's syndrome); eye lesions (congenital hypertrophy of retinal pigment epithelium [CHRPE]); epidermoid cysts; and brain neoplasms (Turcot's syndrome).

Hereditary nonpolyposis colon cancer (HNPCC), also called Lynch syndrome, is an inherited, non–sex-linked, mendelian dominant disease with virtually complete penetrance. HNPCC is caused by a defect in any of a number of DNA-mismatch repair genes (*MLH1, MSH2, MSH6, PMS, PMS2*) that leads to high-level microsatellite instability (MSI-H). A number of criteria have been generated for the diagnosis of HNPCC, including the Amsterdam I and

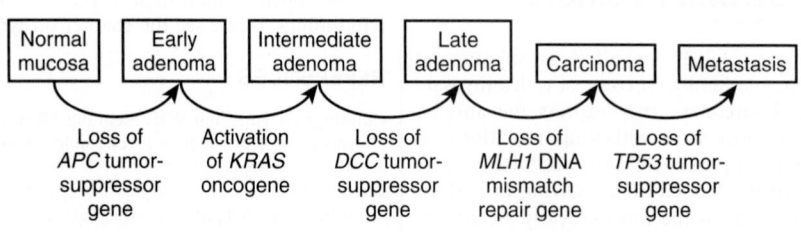

FIGURE 1. Sequence of progression from adenoma to carcinoma.

BOX 1   Diagnosis of Hereditary Nonpolyposis Colon Cancer (HNPCC)

Amsterdam I Criteria, 1990
- Three or more family members with histologically verified colorectal cancer, one of whom is a first-degree relative (parent, child, sibling) of the other two
- Two successive affected generations
- One or more colon cancers diagnosed before age 50 years
- Familial adenomatous polyposis has been excluded.

Amsterdam II Criteria, 1999
- Three or more family members with histologically verified HNPCC-related cancers (endometrium, ovary, stomach, small intestine, hepatobiliary, upper urinary tract, brain, or skin), one of whom is a first-degree relative (parent, child, sibling) of the other two
- Two successive affected generations
- One or more colon cancers diagnosed before age 50 years
- Familial adenomatous polyposis has been excluded.

Revised Bethesda Guidelines, 2002
- Colorectal cancer diagnosed in a patient who is younger than 50 years of age.
- Presence of a synchronous, metachronous colorectal or other HNPCC-related malignancy, regardless of age
- Colorectal cancer with the high-level microsatellite instability (MSI-H) histology diagnosed in a patient who is younger than 60 years of age
  - Presence of carcinoma infiltrating lymphocytes, Crohn's-like lymphocytic reaction, mucinous/signet-ring differentiation, or medullary growth pattern
  - No general consensus based on this age
- Colorectal cancer diagnosed in one or more first-degree relatives with an HNPCC-related neoplasm
  - With one or more neoplasms being diagnosed before age 50 years
- Colorectal cancer diagnosed in two or more first- or second-degree relatives with HNPCC-related malignancies, regardless of age

---

II criteria and the Bethesda guidelines (Box 1). According to the EPICOLON study, the revised Bethesda guidelines are the most discriminating set of clinical parameters for diagnosis of HNPCC.

HNPCC is subdivided into Lynch syndrome types I and II. Lynch type I refers to site-specific nonpolyposis colon cancer, and Lynch type II (formerly called familial cancer syndrome) refers to cancers that develop in the colon and related organs such as the endometrium, ovaries, stomach, pancreas, and proximal urinary tract, among others. Lynch syndrome differs from sporadic colorectal cancer in a number of important ways. It has an autosomal dominant inheritance, a predominance of proximal lesions (75% are found in the right colon), an excess of multiple primary colorectal cancers (18%), an early age at onset (average, 44 years), a significantly improved survival rate with right-sided lesions (53% at 5 years, compared with 35% for distal colorectal cancer in family members), and an increased risk for development of metachronous lesions (24%). Patients and family members of those diagnosed with HNPCC or FAP should undergo genetic testing to help improve future diagnosis and treatment options.

 ### CURRENT DIAGNOSIS

- Screening of asymptomatic, average-risk patients should begin at 50 years of age.
- Colonoscopy should be performed if any screening test result is positive.
- Colonoscopy should be performed for any patient with signs or symptoms of colorectal cancer.
- Screening of high-risk patients—those with inflammatory bowel disease, familial adenomatous polyposis, or hereditary nonpolyposis colorectal cancer) and those with a significant positive family history—should begin at an earlier age and occur more frequently.

INFLAMMATORY BOWEL DISEASE

Both Crohn's disease and ulcerative colitis are associated with an increased risk of colorectal cancer; with the latter conferring approximately double the risk of the former. The duration and severity of Crohn's disease and the duration and extent (left-sided colitis versus pancolitis) of ulcerative colitis contribute to cancer risk in patients with inflammatory bowel disease. Cancer in Crohn's disease typically occurs in a stricture or bypassed segment. Neoplasia in ulcerative colitis does not follow the adenoma-carcinoma development sequence seen in sporadic colorectal cancer, and this has important screening and treatment implications.

Evaluation

SCREENING AVERAGE-RISK PATIENTS

Patients with no personal history of colorectal polyps or cancers, no personal history of inflammatory bowel disease, no symptoms suspicious for colorectal cancer, no family history of colorectal polyps or cancers, and no evidence of a familial or genetic syndrome may be screened as having average risk. The two main categories of screening tests are those that detect adenomatous polyps and cancers (flexible sigmoidoscopy, colonoscopy, double-contrast barium enema, and computed tomographic [CT] colonography) and those that primarily detect cancer (fecal occult blood testing, fecal immunohistochemical testing, and stool DNA testing). The goal of screening is to reduce mortality by reducing the incidence of advanced disease. It seems intuitive that tests that detect polyps, the premalignant phase of colorectal cancer, would be preferred to tests that detect only cancers. However, testing for polyps and cancers is usually procedure related, whereas testing for only cancers can be conducted on stool samples alone. Screening with simple stool samples has the potential to more easily increase overall screening.

Regardless of the method employed, testing in the average-risk, asymptomatic patient should begin at age 50 years. A total colonoscopy is required only every 10 years but involves oral bowel preparation and carries a small risk of perforation (approximately 1/1000). A flexible sigmoidoscopy is required every 5 years, in combination with annual fecal occult blood testing. Flexible sigmoidoscopy requires only enemas for preparation and carries a lower risk of perforation. Air-contrast barium enemas may be used for screening every 5 years, but they also require oral bowel preparation and are only diagnostic. CT colonography is an evolving method for screening every 5 years and offers the opportunity for more accessible screening; however, the procedure is limited in regard to identification of polyps smaller than 1 cm, also requires oral bowel prepation, and is only diagnostic. Fecal occult blood testing and fecal immunohistochemical testing are done annually. The interval for stool DNA testing is uncertain, and it tests only for a limited number of mutations. The most complete screening test, which allows removal of any precancerous lesions that are identified, remains the total colonoscopy.

SCREENING HIGH-RISK PATIENTS

High-risk patients include those with a personal history of colorectal polyps or cancers, a family history of colorectal cancer in a first-degree relative, Crohn's disease or ulcerative colitis, or a personal or family history of FAP or HNPCC. Screening in these patients has been adjusted for changes in incidence and age at onset of neoplasia (Table 1).

CURRENT THERAPY

- Patients with familial adenomatous polyposis or hereditary nonpolyposis colorectal cancer should undergo early, prophylactic colon resection.
- Colon tumors should be treated with segmental laparoscopic or open resection.
- Chemotherapy is offered for colon cancers with locally advanced, nodal (stage III), or metastatic (stage IV) disease.
- Rectal tumors that are small (<3 cm), involve <25% of the rectal circumference, are superficial (Tis or T1), lack nodal involvement, and have favorable pathologic characteristics should be removed by transanal techniques.
- Rectal tumors that are larger, are locally invasive, or have nodal involvement should be removed by formal open resection, with sphincter-preservation if possible.
- Combination chemotherapy and radiation therapy is offered for advanced (stage II), nodal (stage III), or metastatic (stage IV) rectal cancer.
- Postoperative surveillance includes frequent office evaluations, measurements of carcinoembryonic antigen, endoscopy, and imaging.

TABLE 1   Screening High-Risk Patients for Colorectal Cancer

Risk Category	Age to Begin	Recommended Test	Comment
Personal history of <3 adenomas with low-grade dysplasia	5–10 y after the initial polypectomy	Colonoscopy	Exam interval should be based on other clinical factors, such as prior findings, family history, or endoscopist or patient preference.
Personal history of 3–10 adenomas, or 1 adenoma >1 cm, or any adenoma with villous features or high-grade dysplasia	3 y after the initial polypectomy	Colonoscopy	Adenomas require compete excision. If the follow-up is normal, the next examination should be in 5 y. Presence of >10 adenomas should raise suspicion of a familial syndrome.
Personal history of colorectal cancer	1 y after resection	Colonoscopy	Patients should undergo high-quality preoperative clearance. Follow-up after normal examinations should be extended to 3 y and then to 5 y.
Family history of adenomas or cancer in a first-degree relative <60 y of age or in 2 first-degree relatives at any age	Age 40 y, or 10 y before the age at onset of youngest affected family member	Colonoscopy	Every 5 y
Family history of adenomas or cancer in a first-degree relative >60 y of age or in 2 second-degree relatives with cancer	Age 40 y	Colonoscopy	Screening should be initiated at an earlier age. Intervals are based on findings or on the average-risk patient
FAP or suspected FAP	Age 10–12 y	Annual FS, counseling for genetic testing if showing polyps	Colectomy should be considered for positive genetic testing
HNPCC or risk for HNPCC	Age 20–25 y, or 10 y before the age at onset of youngest affected family member	Colonoscopy, counseling for genetic testing	Every 1–2 y. Genetic testing should be offered to first-degree relatives of persons with a known DNA-mismatch repair gene defect or with 1 of the first 3 Bethesda criteria
IBD, Crohn's disease, or chronic UC	8 y after the onset of pancolitis, or 12–15 y after the onset of left-sided colitis	Colonoscopies with random four-quadrant biopsies every 10 cm for dysplasia	Screening should be offered every 1–2 y, and patients are best referred to a center with experience in the surveillance and management of IBD.

FAP = familial adenomatous polyposis; FS = flexible sigmoidoscopy; HNPCC = hereditary nonpolyposis colorectal cancer; IBD = inflammatory bowel disease.

SYMPTOMS AND DIAGNOSIS

Symptoms of colorectal cancer include bleeding (85%), a change in bowel habits, abdominal pain, malaise, and obstruction. Frequently, anemia is the only sign a patient exhibits. Patients with symptoms suspicious for colorectal cancer should undergo a colonoscopy. An anorectal source of bleeding should not preclude a complete colonic evaluation.

Management

PREOPERATIVE MANAGEMENT

Before operative intervention is undertaken, a complete evaluation should occur, including a careful history and physical examination, routine laboratory testing, and measurement of the level of carcinoembryonic antigen. A complete evaluation of the colon is essential, including colonoscopy with biopsy, or barium enema or CT colonography if colonoscopy is incomplete. Bowel preparation is no longer indicated as a routine preoperative measure for colonic surgery.

Preoperative staging should be undertaken for colorectal cancers. CT scanning of the abdomen and pelvis are indicated to aid in evaluating the extent of localized or metastatic disease and the presence of enlarged lymph nodes. Staging of rectal cancers includes determining the distance from the anal verge, frequently with the use of a rigid proctoscope; the depth of invasion; and the presence of enlarged lymph nodes, using endorectal ultrasound or endoanal coil magnetic resonance imaging. Metastatic disease mandates neoadjuvant chemotherapy in the absence of acute symptoms of obstruction or exsanguination. Rectal cancers with evidence of local invasion into perirectal fat or adjacent structures or evidence of enlarged metastatic lymph nodes may benefit from neoadjuvant chemotherapy and irradiation. Preoperative staging allows for the application of neoadjuvant therapy in selected candidates, which can downstage and downsize tumors and can decrease rates of local recurrence in rectal cancer. Neoadjuvant therapy can also allow for sphincter-preserving procedures in patients with previously bulky or very low rectal tumors.

SURGERY FOR COLONIC TUMORS

The primary therapy for tumors of the colon is operative. The basic principles of surgery for colon cancer are the following:

- Exploration: adequate visual, tactile, and potentially intraoperative hepatic ultrasound staging at the time of primary resection
- Removal of the entire cancer with enough proximal and distal bowel to encompass the possibility of submucosal lymphatic tumor spread
- Removal of the regional mesenteric pedicle, including draining lymphatics, based on the predictable lymphatic spread of the disease and the potential for regional mesenteric involvement without concurrent distant involvement
- En bloc resection of involved structures (T4 tumors).

Segmental colonic resections (right, transverse, left, or sigmoid colectomy) are undertaken based on the tumor location and blood supply with lymphatic drainage; specifically the ileocolic, middle colic, and left colic arteries. These arteries define a convenient anatomic boundary for standard colonic resection and also provide for adequate regional lymph node clearance, because the major draining lymphatics follow these blood vessels in the mesentery. Locally invasive tumors (T4) require en bloc resection of involved structures. Metastatic colonic tumors (M1) may require neoadjuvant chemotherapy before resection or palliation.

Numerous studies have verified that laparoscopic surgery is appropriate, and perhaps preferred, for colon cancer in experienced hands. The landmark Clinical Outcomes of Surgical Therapy (COST) trial in 2004 established that laparoscopic resection is equivalent to open resection for colon cancer.

SURGERY FOR RECTAL TUMORS

Two approaches for rectal tumors are local excision and formal rectal resection. Local excision is the treatment of choice for a select, small group (3%–5% of all patients diagnosed with rectal cancer). Tumors amenable to transanal excision are small (<3 cm), involve less than 25% of the rectal circumference, are confined to the mucosa or submucosa (Tis or T1), lack nodal involvement by preoperative imaging, and have favorable pathologic characteristics (well or moderately differentiated with no lymphovascular invasion). Tumors in the lower or middle third of the rectum are accessible by simple transanal excision, but tumors of the upper rectum require the use of transanal endoscopic microsurgery (TEMS) techniques for resection. Local excision requires a 1-cm normal margin, but the defect usually does not require closure.

Tumors staged at T2 or greater require a formal resection, the type of which depends on the location of the tumor. Upper and middle rectal tumors can usually be managed with a low or very low anterior resection. Lower rectal tumors frequently require a proctectomy with coloanal anastomosis or an abdominoperineal resection. The goal of resection is to obtain a 5-cm distal margin, but lower tumors can be managed with a 2-cm distal margin. Very low tumors and those involving the sphincter mechanism require an abdominoperineal resection.

Rectal tumors with greater depth of rectal wall invasion (T3), evidence of fixation or local invasion (T4), or evidence of lymph nodal (N1–2) or metastatic (M1) disease mandates neoadjuvant chemoradiation therapy. Proctectomy requires a specimen-appropriate total mesorectal excision. This involves complete excision of all mesorectal tissue located behind the rectum with no carcinoma at the lateral or circumferential margins. The goal is to remove all malignant tissue, so as to reduce or eliminate the possibility of locally recurrent disease.

Locally advanced rectal tumors may preclude an effective or safe resection. Some indications for likely inoperability include extensive pelvic disease, invasion of ileofemoral vessels, extensive lymphatic involvement or significant lower extremity lymphedema, bony involvement, and life expectancy less than 3 to 6 months.

Laparoscopy is being performed for rectal malignancies in advanced centers, and studies are under way to verify the efficacy and safety of laparoscopic rectal resection in comparison with traditional open resection.

COMPLICATED DISEASE

Colorectal tumors may manifest with complications such as obstruction, perforation, or significant bleeding. These presentations are generally related to more advanced disease and may preclude a complete staging work-up or potential neoadjuvant therapy. Unless patients are unstable or critically ill or the tumor is unresectable, the tumor should be appropriately resected. An ostomy is usually performed, whether as an end ostomy or as a proximal loop diversion for a primary anastomosis. Colonic stenting is an attractive option for obstructing lesions as palliation or as a bridge to resection after medical stabilization and staging for potential neoadjuvant therapy.

SURGERY FOR HIGH-RISK CONDITIONS

High-risk conditions for the development of colorectal malignancies include FAP, HNPCC, and chronic ulcerative colitis. Surgical management may be prophylactic or possibly therapeutic after a malignancy has been diagnosed. The mainstay of operative management in FAP and chronic ulcerative colitis is a total proctocolectomy. Reconstructive options include an ileal pouch–anal anastomosis, a continent ileostomy (Kock pouch), or an end ileostomy. A total abdominal colectomy with ileorectal anastomosis may be performed for temporary preservation of rectal function in selected cases of chronic ulcerative colitis with rectal sparing and FAP with few rectal polyps, but this requires aggressive surveillance of the remaining rectal mucosa because of the risk of malignancy. Patients with HNPCC should also undergo subtotal colectomy with ileorectal anastomosis; because of the prevalence of associated gynecologic malignancies, a total hysterectomy with bilateral salpingo-oophorectomy should be offered to women as well.

TABLE 2 Pathologic Staging Systems for Colorectal Cancer

Pathologic Features	Stage	TNM	Dukes	Astler-Coller	5-yr Survival (%)
Depth of Invasion					
Lamina propria, muscularis mucosa	0	T0/Tis	A		>90
Submucosa	I	T1	A	B1	
Muscularis propria	I	T2	A	B1	
Subserosa, pericolic fat	II	T3	B	B1	70–85
Adjacent organs, perforation	II	T4	B	B2	55–65
Lymph Nodal Involvement					
None		N0			
1–3 nodes	III	N1	C	C1, C2	45–55
>3 nodes	III	N2	C	C1, C2	20–30
Distant Metastatic Disease					
Absent		M0			
Present	IV	M1	D		<5

TNM = tumor-node-metastasis system.

PATHOLOGIC STAGING AND ADJUVANT THERAPY

Excellent pathologic sampling and review of the operative specimen provide important prognostic and therapeutic information. Current standards recommend that at least 12 lymph nodes be removed for adequate staging of colon cancer. The decision for adjuvant chemotherapy or radiation therapy or both is based on the pathologic staging. This information also provides prognostic information in terms of survival for the patient and family. A number of staging systems have been developed, but the tumor-nodes-metastasis (TNM) system is the one most commonly used in the United States (Table 2).

Chemotherapy is offered for patients who have colorectal cancers with locally advanced, nodal (stage III), or metastatic (stage IV) disease. The combination of chemotherapy and radiation therapy for advanced rectal cancer (stage II–IV) has decreased local recurrence and increased survival. Numerous protocols are available for treatment, with the standard of care being FOLFOX: oxaliplatin (Eloxatin), 5-fluorouracil (5-FU, [Adrucil]), and leucovorin. Elderly patients and those with multiple comorbidities who may not be able to tolerate full-dose chemotherapy may be candidates for capecitabine (Xeloda) or 5-FU and leucovorin. Numerous study protocols are available at specialized centers evaluating other medications. Newer technologies continue to evolve, such as antiangiogenesis agents and immunomodulatory agents.

METASTATIC DISEASE

Surgical therapy is also available for metastatic disease in certain situations. Metastatic liver lesions amenable to resection can be addressed at the time of colon resection or after the patient has healed from colectomy. The lesions could be resected or treated with radiofrequency ablation, a newer technology that allows in situ destruction of liver lesions. Similarly, selected pulmonary metastases can be resected, possibly with the use of minimally invasive thoracoscopic techniques.

SURVEILLANCE

Surveillance for colon and rectal cancer is a lifelong process. Patients are seen and examined in the office every 3 months for 2 years, then every 6 months for 3 years, and then yearly for 5 years. Levels of carcinoembryonic antigen are measured at each office visit, but current literature recommends obtaining levels every 3 months for 3 years as a marker for tumor recurrence in stage II–III patients. Colonoscopy should be performed at 1 year postoperatively, assuming a high-quality preoperative study has cleared the rest of the colon. A normal colonoscopy at one year postoperatively would allow the next surveillance colonoscopy to be performed three years later. If that one is normal, subsequent examinations should be performed every 5 years.

After the examination at 1 year postoperatively, the subsequent intervals should be shortened if there is evidence of HNPCC or if additional adenomas are found. As an addition to formal colonoscopies, flexible sigmoidiscopies are performed with each office visit for patients with rectal cancer. Routine imaging utilizing CT scans of the chest, abdomen, and pelvis is performed annually for 3 years in patients with colorectal cancer. Patients with increased or rising CEA levels, as noted by routine surveillance checks, or evidence of recurrent disease, as noted by history and physical examinations or routine surveillance imaging studies, can be evaluated with the use of positron emission tomography (PET), an emerging sensitive test for tumor recurrence.

REFERENCES

American Cancer Society. Cancer Facts and Figures 2008, Atlanta, GA: American Cancer Society; 2008. Available at: http://www.cancer.org/downloads/STT/2008CAFFfinalsecured.pdf [accessed June 30, 2009].

Beart RW, Steele Jr GD, Menck HR, et al. Management and survival of patients with adenocarcinoma of the colon and rectum: A national survey of the Commission on Cancer. J Am Coll Surg 1995;181:225–36.

Bentrem DJ, Okabe S, Wong WD, et al. T1 Adenocarcinoma of the rectum: Transanal excision or radical surgery? Ann Surg 2005;242:472–9.

Clinical Outcomes of Surgical Therapy Study Group. A comparison of laparoscopically assisted and open colectomy for colon cancer. N Engl J Med 2004;350:2050–9.

Desch CE, Benson AB 3rd, Somerfield MR, et al. Colorectal cancer surveillance: 2005 update of an American Society of Clinical Oncology Practice Guideline. J Clin Oncol 2005;23(33):8512–9.

Floyd ND, Saclarides TJ. Transanal endoscopic microsurgical resection of pT1 rectal tumors. Dis Colon Rectum 2005;49:164–8.

Lan Y-T, Lin J-K, Li AFY, et al. Metachronous colorectal cancer: Necessity of post-operative colonoscopic surveillance. Int J Colorectal Dis 2005;20:121–5.

Levin B, Lieberman DA, McFarland B, et al. Screening and surveillance for the early detection of colorectal cancer and adenomatous polyps, 2008: A joint guideline from the American Cancer Society, the US Multi-Society Task Force on Colorectal Cancer, and the American College of Radiology. For the American Cancer Society Colorectal Cancer Advisory Group, the US Multi-Society Task Force, and the American College of Radiology Colon Cancer Committee. Gastroenterology 2008;134:1570–95.

Maetani I, Tada T, Ukita T, et al. Self-expandable metallic stent placement as palliative treatment of obstructed colorectal carcinoma. J Gastroenterol 2004;39:334–8.

Pinol V, Castells A, Andreu M, et al. Accuracy of Revised Bethesda Guidelines, microsatellite instability, and immunohistochemistry for the identification of patients with hereditary nonpolyposis colorectal cancer. JAMA 2005;293:1986–94.

Rex DK, Kahi CJ, Levin B, et al. Guidelines for colonoscopy surveillance after cancer resection: A consensus update by the American Cancer Society and the US Multi-Society Task Force on Colorectal Cancer. Gastroenterology 2006;130:1865–71.

Sauer R, Becker H, Hohenberger W, et al. for the German Rectal Cancer Study Group: Preoperative versus postoperative chemoradiotherapy for rectal cancer. N Engl J Med 2004;351:1731–40.

Stipa F, Chessin DB, Shia J, et al. A pathologic complete response of rectal cancer to preoperative combined-modality therapy results in improved oncological outcome compared with those who achieve no downstaging on the basis of preoperative endorectal ultrasonography. Ann Surg Oncol 2006;13(8):1047–53.

Winawer SJ, Zauber AG, Fletcher RH, et al. Guidelines for colonoscopy surveillance after polypectomy: A consensus update by the US Multi-Society Task Force on Colorectal Cancer and the American Cancer Society. CA Cancer J Clin 2006;56:143–59.

Intestinal Parasites

Method of

Nathan Thielman, MD, MPH, and
Elizabeth Reddy, MD

Intestinal parasites are a diverse group of pathogens with local and global significance. Immigration, international adoption, travel, and the frequency of HIV, AIDS, and other immune-compromising conditions (e.g., malignancy, organ transplantation) have all contributed to a need for ongoing or increased awareness of parasitic infections in the United States. Persons who reside in chronic care facilities, children in daycare, and persons whose sexual practices increase the likelihood of fecal–oral contact are also at risk for acquiring intestinal parasitic infection.

Globally, intestinal parasites are responsible for an enormous burden of disease. Although these pathogens are rarely fatal, ongoing exposure to intestinal parasites among persons in endemic areas exacerbates malnutrition, carries multiple morbidities, and causes stunting of growth and development in children, all of which have far-reaching consequences.

Patients who present with diarrheal illness (especially prolonged or travel-associated), unexplained eosinophilia, or expulsion of worms should be evaluated for intestinal parasites. In such cases, a careful history should focus on the patient's country of origin, detailed travel and recreational activities, dietary habits and new or unusual food exposures, occupation, sexual history, sick contacts, and risks for or known immunodeficiency. Some specialists advocate obtaining a complete blood count with differential to assess eosinophil count in all international adoptees and immigrants from areas where parasitic infections are common. If eosinophilia is present, antibody testing for schistosomiasis and strongyloidiasis—two chronic parasitic infections with potentially serious consequences—should be performed, and appropriate therapy should be administered if infection is discovered. For key features of common intestinal parasitic infections, see the Current Diagnosis box.

Diagnosis of intestinal parasites has improved recently with the advent of quick, simple, and accurate stool antigen tests for some major pathogens, such as *Entamoeba*, *Giardia* and *Cryptosporidium* species. However, the fecal examination for ova and parasites is still the mainstay of diagnosis in many cases. Whenever possible, stool specimens should be sent to a laboratory with clinical expertise in parasitology, where wet preparation, concentration, or staining can identify most pathogens. Evaluation of fresh specimens and repeated examinations improve diagnostic sensitivity. Key diagnostic points are summarized in the Current Diagnosis box.

This review focuses on basic understanding, recognition, diagnosis and treatment of common intestinal parasites in the United States and throughout the world. Within each section, parasites are listed in order of relative clinical significance.

Protozoa: Amoebae, Flagellates, Ciliates

ENTAMOEBA HISTOLYTICA

Entamoeba histolytica, the cause of amoebic dysentery and amebic liver abscess, is a worldwide pathogen of major clinical significance. Approximately 10% of the world's population and up to 60% of children in highly endemic areas show serologic evidence of infection, and *E. histolytica* is estimated to cause 100,000 deaths per year globally. In the United States, infection is almost exclusively found among returned travelers, immigrants from endemic areas (especially Mexico and Central and South America), men who have sex with men (MSM), and institutionalized persons. *E. histolytica* exists in only two forms, the hardy cyst characterized by four nuclei, and the trophozoite, which has a single nucleus and survives poorly outside the human body. It is important to note that *Entamoeba dispar* and *Entamoeba moshkovskii*, which are morphologically identical to *E. histolytica* in stool microscopy, are now known to be non-pathogenic species. Other *Entamoeba*, including *Entamoeba hartmanni*, *Entamoeba coli*, *Entamoeba polecki* and others can be individually identified on microscopy but are of uncertain pathogenicity and thought to be benign.

E. histolytica infection is acquired by ingestion of cysts in contaminated water or food or by fecal–oral contact, as can occur in chronic care facilities or with anal–oral sexual practices. Acquisition of the parasite can result in asymptomatic infection (most common), diarrheal illness, or extraintestinal infection, the latter most commonly manifest as amebic liver abscess. An appropriately robust layer of colonic mucin may be protective against symptomatic infection, whereas attachment to intestinal epithelium results in penetration of the organism into the submucosal layer, where extensive tissue destruction can take place in the form of apoptosis and lysis of cells, hence the name "histolytica."

Symptoms of classic amebic dysentery begin insidiously 1 to 2 weeks after infection. Diarrhea is almost universal and typically consists of numerous small-volume stools that can contain mucous or frank blood, or both. Stools are almost always heme positive if not grossly bloody. Abdominal pain and tenesmus are common; fever is present in approximately 30% of cases. Some persons have a chronic course characterized by weight loss, intermittent loose stools, and abdominal pain. Rare presentations of amebic dysentery include amebomas, which can mimic malignancy, and perianal ulcerations or fistulae. Severe disease can occur in the form of fulminant colitis or toxic megacolon; the latter almost universally requires colectomy. Young age, pregnancy, and corticosteroid use predispose to severe infection. Although persons with HIV infection or AIDS can develop invasive disease, *E. histolytica* does not appear to be a common opportunistic infection, and infection is curable in this population.

Amebic liver abscess is the most common extraintestinal complication of *E. histolytica*; cerebral and ocular amebiasis have also been reported. Amebic liver abscess affects children of both sexes equally, but it is up to nine times more common in men, indicating that hormonal milieu likely plays a role. Amebic liver abscess almost always manifests within 3 to 5 months of initial infection, but it can surface years later. Illness is characterized by fever and abdominal tenderness that worsen over several days to weeks. Weight loss, jaundice, and cough from diaphragmatic irritation can also occur. Symptoms of dysentery usually are not present, and diarrhea is reported in less than one third of cases. Laboratory abnormalities include leukocytosis, transaminitis, elevated alkaline phosphatase, and elevated sedimentation rate. Chest radiograph often demonstrates elevation of the right hemidiaphragm, and pleural effusion may be present. Rupture of the abscess can occur into the abdomen or pleuropulmonary space, manifesting as acute abdomen or empyema.

Diagnosis of intraintestinal *E. histolytica* infection has classically relied on stool microscopy, and this remains the only available method in much of the world. At least three stool specimens should be examined to improve sensitivity. Cysts visualized in stool might or might not indicate active infection and cannot be distinguished from *E. dispar* and *E. moshkovskii*. Presence of trophozoites with ingested red blood cells on stool preparation is diagnostic of dysentery secondary to *E. histolytica*, as are mobile amebae if seen within freshly examined biopsy material.

Diagnosis of *E. histolytica* infection has improved greatly with the advent of antigen tests, now available as enzyme-linked immunosorbent assays (ELISAs) and immunoflorescent probes. The Techlab ELISA antigen test is highly sensitive and specific and can be used on a freshly passed stool specimen, serum, or hepatic abscess material. It becomes positive with onset of symptomatic disease and resolves on treatment of infection. Other available antigen tests appear to function well but have not been as rigorously studied. Aspirate of liver abscess material may be necessary to distinguish from pyogenic liver abscess; a negative stool examination for *E. histolytica* does not preclude amebic liver abscess. In a patient at high risk for amebic liver abscess (e.g., young male immigrants), a trial of antimicrobial therapy can help in diagnosis because infection typically responds rapidly.

All patients who have confirmed *E. histolytica* infection and reside in nonendemic areas should be treated regardless of whether they are symptomatic, because invasive disease can develop in the future. Asymptomatic cyst passers may be treated with an intralumnal agent alone, such as paromomycin (Humatin) or iodoquinol (Yodoxin). In the United States, the most readily available effective treatment for patients with amebic colitis or liver abscess is metronidazole (Flagyl). It can be given intravenously for patients unable to tolerate oral medications. Experts recommend that a course of therapy with an intraluminal agent be given following the completed course of the systemic agent for all cases of invasive *E. histolytica*. See Table 1 for medications and doses.

CURRENT DIAGNOSIS

Signs and Symptoms

- Watery diarrhea—Most protozoal infections: *Giardia, Blastocystis, Dientamoeba, Cryptosporidium, Cyclospora, Isospora, Microsporidia*
- Dysentery—Most commonly *Entamoeba histolytica*; less commonly *Balantidium coli, Trichuris trichuria* (whipworm)
- Eosinophilia—Throughout chronic infection: *Strongyloides*, schistosomiasis, *Isospora*; usually only in early infection: *Ascaris*, hookworm, whipworm
- Prolonged or severe diarrhea in HIV infection—Spore-forming protozoal infections: *Cryptosporidium, Cyclospora, Isospora, Microsporidia*
- Visible worms passed in stool—*Ascaris, Taeniasis, Diphyllobothrium*

Diagnosis of Parasitic Infections

- Stool antigen assay—*Entamoeba histolytica, Giardia, Cryptosporidium*
- Serology*—Strongyloides, schistosomiasis
- Stool for ova and parasites—All intestinal parasites. Sensitivity increased with repeat exams if necessary. Concentration, preservation, and staining improve diagnosis of certain pathogens.

Note: Key features of intestinal parasitic infection may overlap with other conditions, including non-parasitic infections, and extra-intestinal parasites.

*Optimal method of diagnosis in returned travelers and immigrants from endemic to nonendemic areas. Does not distinguish between active and resolved infections.

GIARDIASIS

Giardia lamblia, also known as *Giardia intestinalis* or *Giardia duodenalis*, is the most commonly identified diarrheal parasitic infection in the United States, with an estimated 100,000 to 2.5 million cases per year. It is globally distributed and found in fresh water throughout mountainous regions of the United States and Canada. The organism is a flagellated aerotolerant anaerobe that exists in a cyst and trophozoite form. Cysts can survive for several weeks in cold water. Contaminated food and water are the most common sources of infection, but the organism can also be passed by person-to-person contact. In the United States, giardiasis is primarily diagnosed among international travelers, persons with recreational water exposure, institutionalized persons and children in day care, and persons with anal–oral sexual practices.

Illness can result from ingestion of as few as 10 to 25 cysts, which transform into trophozoites in the small intestine and attach to and damage the small bowel wall. Symptomatic disease begins insidiously over approximately 2 weeks in 25% to 50% of persons who ingest *Giardia* cysts. Others become asymptomatic cyst passers (5%–15%) or have no signs of infection (35%–50%). Hallmarks of infection are watery diarrhea, bloating, gas, abdominal pain, and weight loss; less commonly, patients have nausea, vomiting, or low-grade fever. Steatorrhea and malabsorption, particularly secondary to *Giardia*-induced lactase deficiency, can be observed. Chronic *Giardia* infection should be considered in the differential diagnosis for a long-standing diarrheal illness, especially if there is history of exposure to possibly contaminated water. Patients with common variable immune deficiency, X-linked agammglobulinemia, and IgA deficiency syndromes are at risk for fulminant and sometimes incurable disease, suggesting a significant role for humoral immunity in control of infection. Persons with HIV infection or AIDS have symptoms similar to those in patients without HIV and typically can be cured of infection with standard therapy.

Diagnosis of giardiasis is made by examination of fresh or preserved stool or by stool antigen assays. In the case of fecal examination, trophozoites may be directly visualized in fresh liquid stool; semiformed and preserved stool should be stained before examination. Currently, there are immunochromographic, direct fluorescence antibody, and ELISA tests for diagnosis of *Giardia*, including the ImmunoCard STAT! Cryptosporidium/Giardia Rapid Assay (Meridian Bioscience, Cincinnati, Ohio), which tests for both pathogens simultaneously. Although it is rarely necessary, the diagnosis can sometimes be made on duodenal biopsy.

For details of treatment options, see Table 1. Metronidazole is the most commonly prescribed treatment in the United States and should be given for a 10-day course. Tinidazole (Tindamax), recently approved in the United States, appears to have excellent efficacy and improved tolerability over metronidazole. Nitazoxanide (Alinia) has also been shown to eradicate infection well and can be used as an alternative or in patients who fail a first course of treatment. Patients who fail first-line therapy might have a persistent source of infection (contaminated water source, close contact with an infected person), immune deficiency predisposing to difficult eradication, or persistence of cysts. Once possible sources of reinfection have been investigated and eliminated, relapsed infections should either be re-treated with a longer course of therapy (21–28 days) or treated with a different agent. Patients who fail more than one course of therapy should undergo immunologic work-up.

Prevention of *Giardia* infection, as with other parasitic infections, involves primarily close attention to personal hygiene, hand washing, and avoidance of ingestion of fresh unfiltered water. Boiling water or use of a 0.2- to 1-µm water filter offer optimal protection against *Giardia* and other parasitic pathogens, although such filters still might not protect against *Cryptosporidium*.

BLASTOCYSTIS HOMINIS

Blastocystis hominis is a protozoan with worldwide distribution found most commonly in tropical regions; it is present in humans and several other animals. In temperate regions, *B. hominis* is detected at a

TABLE 1 Pharmacologic Treatment of Major Protozoan Infections

Clinical Situation	Drug	Adult Dose	Pediatric Dose	Comments
Amebiasis				
Entamoeba histolytica				
Asymptomatic	Recommended: Paromomycin (Humatin) *or*	25–35 mg/kg/d in 3 doses × 7 d	25–35 mg/kg/d in 3 doses × 7 d	
	Iodoquinol (Yodoxin)	650 mg tid × 20 d	30–40 mg/kg/d (max 2 g) in 3 doses × 20 d	
	Alternative: Diloxanide furoate (Furanmide)[2,*]	500 mg tid × 10 d	20 mg/kg/d in 3 doses × 10 d	
Mild to moderate intestinal disease	Recommended: Metronidazole (Flagyl) *or*	500–750 mg tid × 7–10 d	35–50 mg/kg/d in 3 doses × 7–10 d	Treatment should be followed by a course of iodoquinol or paromomycin in the dosage used to treat asymptomatic amebiasis.
	Tinidazole (Tindamax)[§]	2 g once daily × 3 d	50 mg/kg once daily (max 2 g) × 3 d	
Severe intestinal or extraintestinal disease*	Metronidazole *or*	750 mg tid × 7–10 d	35–50 mg/kg/d in 3 doses × 7–10 d	
	Tinidazole	2 g once daily × 5 d	50 mg/kg once daily (max 2 g) × 5 d	A nitroimidazole similar to metronidazole, tinidazole is FDA approved and appears to be as effective and better tolerated than metronidazole. It should be taken with food to minimize GI adverse effects. For children and patients unable to take tablets, a pharmacist may crush the tablets and mix them with cherry syrup. The syrup suspension is good for 7 d at room temperature and must be shaken before use. Ornidazole, a similar drug, is also used outside the United States.
Balantidiasis				
Balantidium coli				
Symptomatic and asymptomatic disease	Recommended: Tetracycline[1,†,‖]	500 mg qid × 10 d	40 mg/kg/d (max 2 g) in 4 doses × 10 d[5]	
	Alternatives: Metronidazole[1]	750 mg PO tid × 5 d	35–50 mg/kg/d in 3 doses × 5 d	
	or Iodoquinol[1]	650 mg tid × 20 d	30–40 mg/kg/d (max 2 g) in 3 doses × 20 d	
Blastocystis hominis				
Symptomatic disease only				Organism's pathogenicity is uncertain.[‡]
Cryptosporidiosis				
Cryptosporidium parvum				
Immune competent	Nitazoxanide	500 mg bid × 3 d	1–3 y: 100 mg bid × 3 d 4–11 y: 200 mg bid × 3 d	FDA approved as a pediatric oral suspension for treating Cryptosporidium in immunocompetent children <12 y and for *Giardia*. It might also be effective for mild to moderate amebiasis. Nitazoxanide is available in 500-mg tabs and an oral suspension; it should be taken with food.
HIV-infected	No optimal therapy available			All HIV-infected patients with cryptosporidiosis should receive HAART whenever possible. Limited data suggest nitazoxanide might have some benefit in patients with CD4 counts >50. Recent meta-analysis showed no efficacy over placebo for any antiparasitic therapy for cryptosporidiosis.
Cyclosporiasis				
Cyclospora cayetanensis	Recommended: TMP-SMX (Bactrim, Septra)[1]	160 mg TMP, 800 mg SMX (1 DS tab) bid × 7–10 d	5 mg/kg TMP, 25 mg/kg SMX bid × 7–10 d	In immunocompetent patients, usually a self-limited illness. Immunosuppressed patients might need higher doses, longer duration (TMP-SMX qid × 10 d, followed by bid × 3 wk) and long-term maintenance. For isosporiasis in sulfonamide-sensitive patients, pyrimethamine, 50–75 mg qd in divided doses (*plus* leucovorin 10–25 mg/d) is effective.

Continued

TABLE 1 Pharmacologic Treatment of Major Protozoan Infections—Cont'd

Clinical Situation	Drug	Adult Dose	Pediatric Dose	Comments
Dientamoebiasis *Dientamoeba fragilis* Symptomatic disease only	Iodoquinol[1] *or*	650 mg tid × 20 d	30–40 mg/kg/d (max 2g) in 3 doses × 20 d	
	Paromomycin[1] *or*	25–35 mg/kg/d in 3 doses × 7 d	25–35 mg/kg/d in 3 doses × 7 d	
	Tetracycline[1] *or*	500 mg qid × 7–10 d	40 mg/kg/d (max 2g) in 4 doses × 10 d[5]	
	Metronidazole	500–750 mg tid × 10 d	20–40 mg/kg/d in 3 doses × 10 d	
Giardiasis *Giardia lamblia* All symptomatic disease and asymptomatic carriage in nonendemic areas	Recommended: Metronidazole[1] *or* Nitazoxanide *or*	250 mg tid × 5–7 d 500 mg bid × 3 d	15 mg/kg/d in 3 doses × 5 d 1–3 y: 100 mg bid × 3 d 4–11 y: 200 mg bid × 3 d	
	Tinidazole	2 g once	50 mg/kg (max 2 g) once	Treatment should be followed by a course of iodoquinol or paromomycin in the dosage used to treat asymptomatic amebiasis.
	Alternatives: Quinacrine[1],* *or*	100 mg tid × 5 d	2 mg/kg/d (max 300 mg/d) tid × 5 d	Albendazole, 400 mg daily × 5 d alone or in combination with metronidazole may also be effective. Combination treatment with standard doses of metronidazole and quinacrine for 3 wk is effective for a small number of refractory infections. In one study, nitazoxanide was used successfully in high doses to treat a case of *Giardia* resistant to metronidazole and albendazole.
	Furazolidone (Furoxone) *or*	100 mg qid × 7–10 d	6 mg/kg/d in 4 doses × 10 d	
	Paromomycin[1]	25–35 mg/kg/d in 3 doses × 7 d	25–35 mg/kg/d in 3 doses × 7 d	Nonabsorbed luminal agent; may be useful for treating giardiasis in pregnancy
Isosporiasis *Isospora belli*[‡]	Recommended: TMP-SMX[1]	160 mg TMP, 800 mg SMX bid × 7–10 d	5 mg/kg TMP, 25 mg/kg SMX bid × 7–10 d	
Microsporidiosis ***Enterocytozoon bineusi*** Diarrheal or disseminated disease	Fumagillin[2]	60 mg/d PO × 14 d		Oral fumagillin (Sanofi Recherche, Gentilly, France) is effective in treating *E. bieneusi* but is associated with thrombocytopenia. HAART can lead to microbiological and clinical response in HIV-infected patients with microsporidial diarrhea. Octreotide (Sandostatin) has provided symptomatic relief in some patients with large-volume diarrhea.
Encephalocytozoon intestinalis Diarrheal or disseminated disease	Albendazole[1]	400 mg bid × 21 d		

Adapted from Drugs for parasitic infections. Med Lett Drug Ther, Volume 5 (Suppl) 2007.

[1]Not FDA approved for this indication.

[2]Not available in the United States.

[5]Investigational drug in the United States.

*The drug is not available commercially, but as a service it can be compounded by Panorama Compounding Pharmacy, 6744 Balboa Blvd., Van Nuys, CA 91406 (800-247-9767) or Medical Center Pharmacy, New Haven, CT (203-688-6816).

[†]An approved drug, but considered investigational for this condition by the FDA.

[‡]Clinical significance of these organisms is controversial; metronidazole 750 mg tid × 10 d, iodoquinol 650 mg tid × 20 d, or TMP-SMX11 double-strength tab bid × 7 d are effective. Metronidazole resistance may be common. Nitazoxanide is effective in children.

[§]Dosing recommendations only available for children > or = to 3 y.

[‖]Contraindicated in pregnant and breastfeeding women and children < 8 y.

DS = double strength; GI = gastrointestinal; HAART = highly active antiretroviral therapy; max = maximum; tab = tablet; TMP-SMX = trimethoprimsulfamethoxazole.

high rate among men who have sex with men. *B. hominis* was long thought to cause only asymptomatic colonization, but there is some evidence to suggest a role in human disease, although this remains controversial. Ongoing molecular analysis might elucidate subtypes of *B. hominis* with varying degrees of pathogenicity in humans.

B. hominis has four forms: vacuolated, ameba-like, granular, and cyst, the latter of which is likely to be the infectious form. It appears to be transmitted via the fecal–oral route, possibly from waterborne sources.

As suggested previously, the majority of infections appear to be entirely asymptomatic, and number of organisms does not appear to accurately predict severity of illness. Symptoms consist mainly of watery diarrhea, bloating, and abdominal cramps. There are typically no pathologic findings on colonoscopy and there are no reports of invasive disease. Infection is diagnosed by stool microscopy with use of a trichrome or hematoxylin-stained preserved specimen. The organism is susceptible in vitro to numerous antimicrobials. Bactrim[1] or metronidazole is the treatment of choice; details are listed in Table 1.

DIENTAMOEBA FRAGILIS

Dientamoeba fragilis was originally classified as an amoeba, but it is more closely related to the flagellates such as *Trichomonas vaginalis*. It is distributed worldwide, including in Western nations, and has only recently been recognized as a clinically significant pathogen, possibly because it is difficult to visualize without specific staining techniques. Illness has commonly been found in travelers and MSM, but it can affect anyone.

The parasite exists only in the trophozoite form. Despite its genetic relationship to the flagellates, *D. fragilis* does not have a flagellum and is immotile. Trophozoites range in size from 4 to 20 μm and are binucleate. Patients in the United States who have *D. fragilis* were found in some studies to harbor other intestinal parasites as well, such as *E. vermicularis* and *B. hominis*, and in general *D. fragilis* is more prevalent in areas of the world with limited public sanitation. These features support a fecal–oral mode of transmission for *D. fragilis*.

Most patients are asymptomatic; however, numerous case reports and small series describe patients with no other organisms identified to cause their symptoms who improve significantly after treatment and documented clearance of *D. fragilis* from their stool. Illness is typically subacute to chronic, characterized by abdominal pain, watery diarrhea, anorexia, fatigue, and malaise. Diagnosis can be difficult, because the parasite is fastidious. If *D. fragilis* is suspected, stool should be preserved with polyvinyl alcohol and quickly stained with iron–hematoxylin and trichrome. Polymerase chain reaction (PCR) has been used for diagnosis as well, but it is not readily available for use in most clinical settings.

For full treatment information, see Table 1. Iodoquinol (Yodoxin) and metronidazole have both been used successfully to treat *D. fragilis*.

BALANTIDIUM COLI

Balantidium coli is the largest protozoan that infects humans, and the only ciliate. Balantidiasis is a relatively rare cause of illness and is found primarily in rural agrarian communities in Southeast Asia, Central and South America, and Papua New Guinea. *B. coli* is highly associated with animal farming, in particular, pigs; humans are incidental hosts. The parasite is transmitted by direct contact with animals or on ingestion of water or food contaminated by animal excrement. Persons with malnutrition or immune deficiency are particularly susceptible to infection.

B. coli invades the intestinal mucosa from the terminal ileum to the rectum. About one half of infections are asymptomatic; the other one half result in a subacute or chronic diarrheal illness with abdominal cramping, nausea, vomiting, weight loss, and occasional low-grade fever. Fewer than 5% of patients present with severe or even fulminant dysentery, and rare cases of colonic penetration with peritonitis, mesenteric lymphadenitis, or hepatic infection have been reported.

Diagnosis is made by visualization of trophozoites in fresh stool specimens or preserved and permanently stained samples. The trophozoite is large and ciliated; cysts are difficult to distinguish. It displays a distinct spiraling motility that can be seen under low power. On stained sample, visualization of *B. coli*'s characteristic macronucleus and spiral micronucleus can help confirm the diagnosis. All patients should be treated regardless of symptoms. Tetracycline (Sumycin) is the therapy of choice; the infection also responds to metronidazole[1]; see Table 1 for dosing information.

Spore-Forming Protozoa and Microsporidia

CRYPTOSPORIDIOSIS

Cryptosporidium is a pathogen with worldwide distribution that is endemic to the United States. Humans are most commonly infected by the recently reclassified *Cryptosporidium hominis*, but *Cryptosporidium parvum*, primarily a bovine pathogen, also causes human disease. *Cryptosporidium* has caused multiple waterborne out-breaks in the United States and can be acquired secondary to recreational water exposure (e.g., swimming pools, water parks). The best-known outbreak occurred secondary to heavy rains that brought farm runoff into the drinking water supply in Wisconsin in 1984. It resulted in 430,000 documented cases of cryptosporidiosis and contributed to the deaths of dozens of persons with advanced HIV infection or malignancy.

Cryptosporidium is a coccidian, part of a group of spore-forming protozoa with a complex life cycle and a structure that allows mechanical penetration into host cells. *Cryptosporidium* can mature and reproduce entirely within human hosts, thereby enabling infection to occur both from environmental sources and by direct person-to-person contact. Its oocysts, the source of infection on ingestion, are markedly hardy; they can withstand heavy chlorination, survive for months in cold water, and are small enough to occasionally evade even the smallest available water filtration systems.

All persons are susceptible to infection, which usually is self-limited. Fulminant or chronic infection, or both, can be seen among patients with immune compromise secondary to HIV infection or AIDS (especially those with CD4 < 50), in patients with malignancy, and in malnourished children. As few as 100 oocysts can cause infection, which results when the parasite penetrates small bowel epithelium and replicates just beneath its surface. Villous flattening and small bowel wall edema are seen on pathologic examination from infected persons.

Asymptomatic infections occur but are relatively rare. Symptoms begin within several days to 1 week of ingestion of oocysts. The hallmark of infection is explosive watery diarrhea, which can be so voluminous as to resemble cholera and can cause significant dehydration and electrolyte imbalance. Abdominal discomfort, nausea, vomiting, fever, malaise, and myalgia can also be present, and weight loss is common. Illness lasts 1 to 2 weeks, but a substantial percentage of patients report a relapse of symptoms after initial improvement. The biliary tract can be involved, particularly in patients with HIV infection, and infection at other distant sites, such as the lungs, has rarely been reported.

Diagnosis of *Cryptosporidium* has improved dramatically in recent years with the advent of antigen tests, which are highly sensitive and specific and can be used on a single sample of fresh stool. The ImmunoCard STAT! Cryptosporidium/Giardia Rapid Assay is useful because it can detect both pathogens. When such tests are not available, stools submitted for examination should be fixed in formalin and stained for trophozoites or cysts; multiple stool specimens improves the diagnostic sensitivity. Luminal fluid or biopsy specimens obtained during endoscopy can also reveal the organism.

Infection with *Cryptosporidium* is typically a self-limited illness in otherwise healthy persons, but symptoms can be improved and the course shortened with the antiparasitic nitazoxanide. *Cryptosporidium* remains an extremely challenging and potentially devastating infection in immunocompromised patients, especially those with HIV and a low CD4 count (counts < 200 increase risk of severe illness, and counts < 50 markedly increase risk). Although anticryptosporidial therapies in this population have shown very limited efficacy, restoration of immune function with HAART often effects cure. Limited data suggest a trial of nitazoxanide may be reasonable in this circumstance as well. Appropriate supportive measures are also crucial in all patients with *Cryptosporidium*, including fluid and electrolyte replacement; avoiding lactose products is likely to be beneficial during the first 2 weeks after infection as the brush border regenerates. Appropriate treatment doses for nitazoxanide are listed in Table 1.

Prevention of *Cryptosporidium* infection requires a highly developed public water purification system including flocculation, sedimentation, and filtration. Use of 0.2- to 1-μm personal water filters for campers and hikers greatly reduces but does not eliminate risk of infection, whereas boiling water before drinking kills oocysts. Close attention to hygiene and avoidance of fecal–oral contact is the mainstay of prevention in the settings of institutional and community outbreaks.

CYCLOSPORA SPECIES

Cyclospora cayetanensis is a coccidian with structure similar to that of *Cryptosporidium*. Unlike *Cryptosporidium*, *C. cayetanensis* requires a period of development outside the human body, thereby eliminating the possibility of close person-to-person contact as a means of acquiring the infection. *C. cayetanensis* is distributed worldwide, most commonly in the tropics and subtropics where infection tends to exhibit seasonality. It has also been associated with food (e.g., raspberries) and waterborne outbreaks in temperate regions, including the United States, and in recent years it has become increasingly recognized as a cause of infectious diarrhea in returned travelers.

All persons are susceptible to infection, but those with HIV are at risk for more severe and prolonged disease, as seen with cryptosporidiosis and isosporiasis. Symptomatic disease appears to be most common in adults who do not have previous exposure to *Cyclospora*, such as travelers or persons who have relocated to endemic areas. Illness begins about a week after ingestion of sporulated oocysts and is characterized by watery diarrhea, abdominal cramping, bloating, anorexia, and weight loss. Low-grade fever can occur; marked fatigue is common and can last weeks or even months, and untreated infections can relapse after apparent resolution. Biliary involvement can occur in patients with HIV coinfection, as with cryptosporidiosis. Cyclosporiasis, similar to infection with other coccidians, causes damage to the small bowel epithelium, with resultant crypt flattening, edema, and inflammatory infiltrate. Lactose deficiency can remain for months following initial infection.

Diagnosis is made by stool examination. As with diagnosis of other parasitic infections, multiple stool specimens improve sensitivity. In the case of *Cyclospora*, concentration of the stool specimen also increases yield. If cyclosporiasis is suspected, specific testing should be requested, because the organism exhibits unique properties. Organisms are about two times the size of *Cryptosporidium* and can be seen with Kinyoun acid-fast stain. They also autofluoresce and can be visualized under ultraviolet microscopy. Currently there is no stool antigen assay, but PCR testing has been used in experimental and limited clinical settings to assist in diagnosis.

Cyclosporiasis is best treated with trimethoprim-sulfamethoxazole (Bactrim)[1]; ciprofloxacin[1] may be effective for patients who have a sulfa allergy. Patients with HIV infection can require longer courses of treatment or chronic suppressive therapy; appropriate antiretroviral therapy is also important in the treatment of severe or relapsing infections. See Table 1 for details.

ISOSPORA SPECIES

Isospora belli is a large coccidian native to tropical areas. Similar to *Cyclospora*, it requires a period of maturation outside the human body and therefore cannot be spread directly from person to person. It appears to cause largely asymptomatic or mild infection in tropical areas to which it is endemic; the exception is among patients coinfected with HIV and particularly those with AIDS, in which it is a very common cause of chronic diarrhea in the Caribbean and Central America. Currently in wealthy countries it is found primarily in travelers returning from endemic areas.

Illness is typically mild and self-limited, consisting primarily of watery diarrhea. However, some immunocompetent persons can develop a chronic spruelike syndrome with malabsorption, and those with HIV infection or AIDS often have severe and prolonged diarrhea. *Isospora* can invade to the lamina propria and can cause eosinophilia, which is different from other coccidian infections.

Diagnosis is made by observation of cysts in stool. As with *Cyclospora*, they can be visualized with acid-fast stains or ultraviolet microscopy. Stool may also contain Charcot–Leiden crystals. Infection in immunocompetent hosts responds well to antimicrobials; persons coinfected with HIV can require longer courses of therapy or chronic suppression, and appropriate antiretroviral therapy may be helpful as well. Trimethoprim-sulfamethoxazole[1] is the treatment of choice. Ciprofloxacin (Cipro)[1] or pyrimethamine (Daraprim)[1] may be used in cases of sulfa allergy. Doses are listed Table 1.

MICROSPORIDIOSIS

Microsporidia are eukaryotic organisms that have been recently reclassified as fungi based on molecular genotyping. They are distributed globally, and more than 100 genera have been identified, seven of which contain species known to be pathogenic in humans: *Encephalitozoon*, *Enterocytozoon*, *Trachipleistophora*, *Pleistophora*, *Nosema*, *Vittaforma*, and *Microsporidium*. These pathogens cause a wide variety of systemic and focal illness throughout the world.

Many immunocompetent patients in wealthy nations exhibit positive serology for certain types of microsporidial infections without a history of disease or travel. Microsporidia are most commonly associated with systemic infection in immunosuppressed persons, particularly those with HIV and a CD4 count of less than 100 or patients with organ transplants. Mode of transmission is not entirely clear, but the pathogen likely is spread both from water sources and possibly from close household contact.

Encephalitozoon intestinalis and *Enterocytozoon bieneusi* are responsible for intestinal microsporidial infections. *E. bieneusi* has been associated with self-limited diarrheal illness; *E. intestinalis* is commonly found in stool specimens throughout the developing world, but its pathogenicity is often not certain. Symptomatic infections, most often in patients coinfected with HIV, typically include a gradual onset of watery diarrhea, which may be worse in the morning and after oral intake. Significant volume and electrolyte depletion can occur, as well as fatigue, anorexia, weight loss, and malabsorption. *E. intestinalis* can disseminate and cause acute abdomen with peritonitis, cholangitis, nephritis, and keratoconjunctivitis, and *E. bieneusi* infection can result in cholangitis and nephritis as well as rhinitis, bronchitis, and wheezing. Other microsporidia are implicated in a wide variety of illness both in previously healthy and immunosuppressed hosts and include several ocular pathogens.

Diagnosis of microsporidiosis is attained by visualization of spores in stool or in tissue specimens. As suggested by their name, microsporidial spores are much smaller than those produced by spore-forming protozoal infections; most are approximately 1 μm in length and can easily be confused with bacteria or debris on slides. Special staining techniques have been described, but electron microscopy is required for species identification. See Table 1 for details of treatment. Albendazole (Albenza)[1] is the treatment of choice for *Encephalocytozoon intestinalis*.

---

[1]Not FDA approved for this indication.

[1]Not FDA approved for this indication.

Treatment of *Enterocytozoon bieneusi* is more challenging. Although some response to albendazole has been reported, oral fumagillin[2] may have more efficacy. Unfortunately, it is not currently commercially available in the United States. Use of appropriate antiretroviral therapy is perhaps the most important treatment for patients with HIV infection or AIDS and chronic microsporidial infections.

Helminths

NEMATODES

Nematodes (roundworms) are cylindrical nonsegmented organisms that are found throughout the world both as free-living species and as human and animal pathogens. Nematodes are the most common type of human parasitic infestation, found in approximately one quarter of the world's population; often susceptible hosts carry multiple different pathogenic nematodes. There are at least 60 species that have been shown to infect humans and 10 times that many that cause disease in other animals, but a few pathogens account for the bulk of human infections, in particular *Ascaris*, hookworm, and whipworm. These three organisms all require a period of maturation outside the human body—typically in warm, moist soil—underscoring the fact that repeated contact with fecally contaminated soil or food and water is necessary to sustain the cycle of infestation. *Strongyloides* and *Enterobius* are unique in that they can both complete their life cycle on or within human hosts and therefore can cause chronic infection and be transmitted directly by close person-to-person contact where there is the possibility of fecal–oral contamination.

Ascaris

Ascaris lumbricoides, the most common human helminthic infection, is estimated to affect 20% to 25% of the world's population. Up to 80% of community members are infected in heavily endemic areas, namely in Africa, Asia, and Central and South America. Cases of *Ascaris* infestation are also seen in rural areas in the southeastern United States. *A. lumbricoides* are white to pinkish worms that range from 10 to 40 cm in length; the infectious eggs are oval white bodies with an adherent mucopolysaccharide capsule that clings to multiple surfaces and aids in transmissibility of the parasite. Eggs are also remarkably durable, capable of surviving up to 6 years in moist soil and able to weather brief droughts and periods of freezing.

Fecal contamination of water, food, and environmental surfaces such as doorknobs and countertops provide the means of transmission for *Ascaris*, and recurrent infection occurs as long as living conditions that predispose people to infection remain unchanged. Lack of adequate public sanitation, use of human feces as fertilizer (night soil), and frequent contact with soil or shared contaminated surfaces among close household members are risk factors for infection. Persons who move to environments with improved sanitation typically lose their infection within 2 years as all the adult worms die. Eggs excreted by an infected person must mature outside the human body for approximately 2 weeks. On ingestion by a susceptible host, mature eggs hatch in the small intestine and release larvae, which penetrate the intestinal wall and travel through the venous circulation to the lungs, where they are coughed up and swallowed. They then undergo maturation into adult worms in the intestine and produce eggs by 2 to 3 months after initial infection, which are excreted in the feces and mature outside the body to continue the cycle.

Most persons with *Ascaris* infection are asymptomatic. Approximately 15% of people have morbidity as a result of infection, which is associated with young age, large burden of worms, coinfection with other intestinal parasites, and genetic predisposition. In children, infection contributes to malabsorption of protein, fat, and vitamins A and C, and treatment of heavily infected children can improve their nutritional status. *Ascaris* infection can also cause intestinal, pancreatic, or biliary obstruction as a result of worm mass or worm migration. Despite the low incidence of obstructive complications

per infected person, the *Ascaris*-related acute abdomen is a significant problem on a global level given the enormous number of people infected. Some patients with intestinal *Ascaris* infection report vague abdominal complaints, such as abdominal discomfort, nausea, vomiting or diarrhea, but these are relatively rare. Pulmonary migration of a large quantity of worms can produce Loeffler's syndrome, or eosinophilic pneumonitis.

Diagnosis is easily attained with standard saline stool preparation, and large numbers of eggs are typically seen. Larvae or worms can also sometimes be seen in sputum or stool samples. In cases of intestinal obstruction, worms may be visualized on upper gastrointestinal series, computed tomography, and even ultrasound. Eosinophilia with *Ascaris* infection is found only during the larval migratory phase, but not at all times. Chronic eosinophilia in an at-risk person suggests another parasitic infection, often *Strongyloides*.

All persons documented to carry *Ascaris* who have migrated to nonendemic areas should be treated to prevent complications in the future; in endemic areas, adults need only be treated if they are symptomatic. Children have been shown to benefit from intermittent anthelminthic therapy in heavily affected areas of the world.

For patients with intestinal obstruction, bowel rest and intravenous hydration are usually sufficient to relieve the obstruction, at which time anthelminthic therapy can be administered. In such cases, gastroenterology consultation should be obtained. In rare cases, surgical intervention is required. Treatment of pulmonary infection is controversial; however, most experts recommend steroid therapy for severe infections followed 2 to 3 weeks later (at the time full-grown worms will have migrated to the intestine) by administration of anthelminthic therapy.

The benzimadazoles (mebendazole [Vermox], albendazole,[1] levamisole,[2] and pyrantel [Pin-X]) all exhibit excellent activity against *Ascaris*. Doses and other options are listed in Table 2. Although albendazole and mebendazole carry a pregnancy class B label, they have been used in pregnant women, adolescent girls, and women of reproductive age without demonstrable effects on fetuses; most experts recommend holding treatment until the second trimester whenever possible.

Sanitary conditions that allow for proper management of human feces are crucial in control and prevention of *Ascaris* infection; boiling water kills the eggs.

Whipworm (Trichuriasis)

Trichuris trichuria has become recognized in recent years as a worldwide pathogen with a scope similar to that of *Ascaris*. Sanitary conditions that predispose to ingestion of food and water contaminated with human feces place people at risk for infection; in many communities infection is hyperendemic, with almost universal carriage of the pathogen.

The adult organism is a small worm about 4 cm in length with a unique whip-like structure that allows its thin tail to become embedded in colonic crypts. Whipworm eggs have a characteristic barrel shape with mucous plugs at either end. Infection is acquired by ingesting *Trichuris* eggs that have undergone embryonation in the soil for 2 to 4 weeks after excretion from a previous host. Larvae emerge from eggs in the intestine and migrate into crypts, where they begin to mature. Egg production begins approximately 3 months later.

Most persons with whipworm carry few worms (approximately 20) and are asymptomatic. As with many other intestinal parasites, children are at greater risk for symptomatic infection, which can cause failure to thrive, anemia, clubbing, inflammatory colitis, and rectal prolapse. Adults with a high worm burden can also experience inflammatory colitis characterized by frequent—often bloody—diarrhea and tenesmus. Infection has been shown to result in production of tumor necrosis factor (TNF)-α by lamina propria cells in the colon, which can contribute to poor appetite and wasting that can be seen with significant infection.

---

[2]Not available in the United States.

[1]Not FDA approved for this indication.
[2]Not available in the United States.

TABLE 2 Pharmacologic Treatment of Nematode, Trematode, and Cestode Infections

Clinical Situation	Drug	Adult Dose	Pediatric Dose	Comments
Anisakiasis *Anisaka* spp. or *Pseudoterranova decipiens*	No recommended medical therapy Surgical or endoscopic removal of worm	—	—	Successful treatment of a patient with *Anisakiasis* with albendazole has been reported
Ascariasis *Ascaris lumbricoides*	Albendazole (Albenza)[1,†] *or*	400 mg once	400 mg PO × 1	
	Mebendazole* (Vermox) *or*	100 mg bid × 3 d or 500 mg once	100 mg bid × 3 d or 500 mg once	
	Ivermectin[1] (Stromectol)	150–200 µg/kg once	150–200 µg/kg once	In heavy infection, therapy may be given for 3 d
Enterobiasis (Pinworm) *Enterobius vermicularis*	Pyrantel pamoate *or*	11 mg/kg base (max 1 g) once; repeat in 2 wk	11 mg/kg base (max 1 g) once; repeat in 2 wk	Because all family members are usually infected, treatment of the entire household is recommended.
	Mebendazole* *or*	100 mg once, repeat in 2 wk	100 mg once, repeat in 2 wk	
	Albendazole[1]	400 mg once, repeat in 2 wk	400 mg once, repeat in 2 wk	
Hookworm *Ancylostoma duodenale, Necator americanus*	Albendazole[1] or Mebendazole or	400 mg once 100 mg bid × 3 d or 500 mg once	400 mg once 100 mg bid × 3 d or 500 mg once	
	Pyrantel pamoate[‡]	11 mg/kg (max 1 g) × 3 d	11 mg/kg (max 1 g) × 3 d	
Schistosomiasis *Schistosoma haematobium, Schistosoma mansoni*	Praziquantel *or*	40 mg/kg/d in 2 doses × 1 d	40 mg/kg/d in 2 doses × 1 d	
S. mansoni only	Oxamniquine[2]	15 mg/kg once	20 mg/kg/d in 2 doses × 1 d	Effective in some patients in whom praziquantel is less effective Contraindicated in pregnancy
Schistosoma japonicum, Schistosoma mekongi	Praziquantel	60 mg/kg/d in 3 doses × 1 d	60 mg/kg/d in 3 doses × 1 d	
Strongyloidiasis	Recommended: Ivermectin	200 µg/kg/d × 2 d	200 µg/kg/d × 2 d	In immunocompromised patients or in patients with disseminated disease, it may be necessary to prolong or repeat therapy or use other agents Veterinary parenteral and enema formulations of ivermectin are used in severely ill patients unable to take oral medications
	Alternative: Albendazole[1]	400 mg bid × 7 d	400 mg bid × 7 d	
Tapeworm *Taenia solium* (intestinal disease), *Taenia sanguinata, Diphyllobothrium latum*	Praziquantel[1,‡] (Biltricide) *or*	5–10 mg/kg once	5–10 mg/kg once	
	Niclosamide[‡] (Yomesan)	2 g once	50 mg/kg once	Available in the United States only from the manufacturer
Trichuriasis (Whipworm) *Trichuris trichuria*	Recommended: Mebendazole	100 mg bid × 3 d or 500 mg once	100 mg bid × 3 d or 500 mg once	
	Alternatives: Albendazole *or*	400 mg daily × 3 d	400 mg daily × 3 d	
	Ivermectin	200 µg/kg daily × 3 d	200 µg/kg daily × 3 d	

Adapted from Drugs for parasitic infections. Med Lett Drug Ther, August 2004.
[1]Not FDA approved for this indication.
[2]Not available in the United States.
*The drug is not available commercially, but as a service it can be compounded by Panorama Compounding Pharmacy, 6744 Balboa Blvd., Van Nuys, CA 91406 (800-247-9767) or Medical Center Pharmacy, New Haven, CT (203-688-6816).
[†]An approved drug, but considered investigational for this condition by the FDA.
[‡]Limited or no availability in the United States.
max = maximum.

Diagnosis is made by standard stool microscopy without a need to concentrate stool, because large numbers of eggs are excreted. Worms can also be seen on colonoscopy, or they can be visualized grossly in cases of rectal prolapse. Eosinophilia may be seen.

Treatment of symptomatic infections can be accomplished with mebendazole, albendazole,[1] or ivermectin (Stromectal)[1]; see Table 2 for details.

Hookworm (*Necator americanus* and *Ancylostoma duodenale*)

Like other helminthic infections, hookworm affects a substantial portion of the world's population, particularly in rural subtropical and tropical communities where human feces is used as a component of fertilizer. Infection results primarily from parasite penetration into the skin; therefore persons with an agrarian lifestyle and significant soil contact are at greatest risk.

Two species are responsible for the majority of human hookworm: *Necator americanus* and *Ancylostoma duodonale*. *Ancylostoma braziliense*, a canine intestinal pathogen, causes cutaneous larval migrans in humans because the pathogen cannot penetrate the human dermis. Of the two common forms of human hookworm, *N. americanus* is smaller and a less aggressive pathogen with a longer life span than *A. duodenale*. Both parasites are found in warm climates throughout the world; *A. doudenale* exists in smaller pockets, whereas *N. americanus* is widely distributed throughout impoverished rural areas of the tropics in the Americas, Asia, and Africa.

Hookworms are small helminths, between 0.5 and 1 cm in length. Infection results from larval penetration of the skin on contact with contaminated soil. An intensely pruritic, erythematous, papulovesicular rash called *ground itch* can develop at the site of entry. Parasites then enter the venous or lymphatic circulation and travel to the lungs, at which point an urticarial rash with cough can develop. The larvae are swallowed and migrate to the small intestine, where they attach to the bowel wall with teeth or biting plates and take a continuous blood meal by sucking with strong esophageal muscles. As the hookworms lodge in the small intestine, peripheral eosinophilia peaks, and gastrointestinal discomfort with or without diarrhea can result. Large oral ingestion of *A. duodenale* can cause Wakana syndrome, characterized by cough, shortness of breath, nausea, vomiting, and eosinophilia. The most important clinical manifestation of hookworm infection is iron-deficiency anemia, which can be mild or severe and may be accompanied by malabsorption of protein in hosts with heavy burden of disease. Infants and pregnant women can become extremely ill or even die as a result of the anemia.

Hookworm may be difficult to diagnose because light infections often do not produce enough eggs to be readily seen on stool examination; stool should therefore be concentrated if infection is suspected. Eggs do not appear in stool until approximately 2 months after infection, so patients with pulmonary complaints will not yet have a positive stool examination.

Hookworm infection can be eradicated with benzimidazole anthelminthics; see Table 2 for details. Prevention of hookworm infection, as with other parasites, lies in improved sanitary conditions; wearing shoes is especially important because the majority of infections are acquired through the skin. Mass anthelminthic treatment campaigns have shown some efficacy in reducing disease in children; however, reinfection and concern for development of resistance continue to present significant challenges. Candidate vaccines are currently under investigation.

Strongyloides

Strongyloides stercoralis is a global pathogen that is estimated to affect as many as 100 million people, mostly in tropical regions of the world. In recent years, it has become more commonly recognized

---

[1]Not FDA approved for this indication.

in the United States among immigrants as a cause of chronic eosinophilia as well as symptomatic infection.

Strongyloides infection results when filariform larvae dwelling in fecally contaminated soil penetrate the skin or mucous membranes of a susceptible host. Larvae move to the lungs and subsequently to the trachea, where they are coughed up and swallowed. Females, about 2 cm in length, lodge in the lamina propria of the duodenum and proximal jejunum where they begin to oviposit. Rhabtidiform larvae emerge from these eggs and either repenetrate the intestinal wall or are passed in the feces, at which point they can begin a free-living cycle and reproduce sexually, or can molt directly into an infectious form ready to enter a subsequent susceptible host.

Persons infected with *Strongyloides* are typically asymptomatic. Those who have symptoms might report abdominal discomfort, diarrhea alternating with constipation, or rarely blood-tinged stool. Severe intestinal infections can occur and are manifest by chronic watery or mucousy diarrhea. In such cases, colonoscopy reveals excessive bowel wall thickening and copious secretions, or edema (catarrhal enteritis or edematous enteritis). Parasite migration through the dermis can manifest as serpiginous, erythematous, and pruritic patches along the buttocks, perineum, and thighs, known as *larvae currens*.

Strongyloides appear to attain a balanced state in their host, with similar numbers of adult worms throughout the many years of infection. During periods of host immunocompromise, in particular in patients taking corticosteroids, *Strongyloides* can enter into a state of rapid autoinfection and rampant reproduction called *hyperinfection syndrome*, which results in devastating illness. Persons with HIV infection do not seem to be at particular risk for symptomatic disease or hyperinfection, but hyperinfection has been linked to HTLV-1 infection. *Strongyloides* has also caused hyperinfection in organ-trans-plant patients whose donor had been infected asymptomatically with the parasite. Although it has long been thought that steroid-induced immune compromise was the major trigger for hyperinfection, growing evidence suggests that steroids themselves may be the culprit by directly inducing the accelerated life cycle in the parasite.

The hyperinfection syndrome is characterized by systemic illness with fever, cough, hypoxia, patchy or diffuse pulmonary infiltrates with alveolar microhemorrhages, and dermatitis; it can include myocarditis, hepatitis, splenic abscess, meningitis and cerebral abscess, and endocrine organ involvement. Larvae migrating out of the intestines can drag bacteria with them, resulting in gram-negative or polymicrobial sepsis. The prognosis of *Strongyloides* hyperinfection syndrome is grave even with highly effective anthelminthic treatment given the diffuse nature of this disease. However, earlier recognition and intensive supportive care can result in cure.

Diagnosis of uncomplicated *Strongyloides* infection in endemic areas can be challenging because few larvae are passed in stool, and numerous examinations may be necessary to detect them. ELISA is available and is highly sensitive, but it does not distinguish between active and past infections. It is, however, the test of choice for persons who have migrated to nonendemic areas, and all persons in this setting should be treated. Ivermectin is the treatment of choice; see Table 2 for dosing. During the first days of treatment, patients can experience intense dermal pruritis as parasites die. Eosinophilia and positive ELISA can persist for months even after effective therapy.

Enterobius vermicularis

Human pinworm infection, caused by the thread-like nematode *Enterobius vermicularis*, is found throughout the world and continues to be diagnosed commonly in the United States, especially in children. Its persistence is likely related to the fact that pinworm does not require a period of maturation outside the human body, and autoinfection or transmission by very close contact sustains the parasite within communities. *E. vermicularis* is at maximum 1 cm long with a tapered tail, and dwells in the cecum, appendix, and adjacent colon. At night, female worms travel to the anus and lay small (25–50 μm), double-walled oval eggs in the perianal skin. Within 6 hours, the eggs embryonate within their capsule and are infectious. In scratching the perianal area and subsequently bringing his or her hand to the mouth, the host ingests the embryos, which then hatch in the bowel about 2 months later and continue the cycle of infection. Embryonated eggs can also attach to bedclothes, thereby placing other household members with close contact at risk for infection. In family groups, infection is associated with close living quarters, poor hand washing, and infrequent washing of clothes and sheets. It can also be prevalent in among institutionalized persons.

Infection is often asymptomatic, but it can cause perianal itching, which helps to facilitate persistent infection by encouraging frequent touching of the perianal area. Rarely, worms migrate into ectopic foci and produce painful genitourinary tract disease with granulomatous inflammation; pinworm infection rarely results in pain that mimics acute appendicitis.

Pinworm infestation is best diagnosed by the classic Scotch tape test, which involves placing and immediately removing a piece sticky tape firmly across the perianal area early in the morning when the eggs have been deposited. The tape can then be brought into a physician's office or laboratory, where it is placed sticky-side down for microscopic examination to detect the eggs. Three specimens should be examined if necessary to improve the sensitivity. It is also sometimes possible to see the worms directly on the perianal region, although they are so small that they may easily be mistaken for residual bits of toilet paper. E.vermicularis is susceptible to standard anthelminthic therapies as listed in Table 2. All household contacts should be empirically treated with the same regimen to avoid reintroducing infection from family members who may be asymptomatically carrying the parasite. Careful laundering of all bedclothes is recommended as well.

Anisakiasis

Anisakiasis is a descriptive term for human infection with parasites of two distinct genuses: *Anisakis* and *Pseudoterranova*. Humans are incidental hosts for these roundworms that inhabit multiple species of fish and other marine animals (tuna, mackerel, hake, cod, sardines, and cephalopods) as intermediate hosts, and marine mammals such as whales, seals, sea lions, and walruses as final hosts. Humans acquire the parasite in its larval stage by eating raw fish (e.g., sushi, ceviche), and therefore the condition predominates in cultures where uncooked fish is consumed. Cases are most commonly reported from Japan but are seen throughout the world in other coastal nations and among restaurateurs.

On consumption of fish with anisakid larvae embedded in its musculature, humans can experience immediate symptoms in the form of itching or burning in the throat, which can provoke coughing that expels the parasite. If the parasite is swallowed, the larva attempts to embed in the gastric musculature at the pylorus. This can produce acute, short-lived epigastric abdominal pain and possibly immediate vomiting, at which point the parasite might again be ejected. If the larva does manage to penetrate gastric tissue, it dies because it is incapable of further tissue invasion in humans. An intense inflammatory response to the dead pathogen can then result, with gastric pain, nausea, and occasionally diarrhea with blood or mucus if a gastric ulcerative lesion has resulted.

Rare cases have been reported in which the larva penetrates the peritoneum, causing focal peritonitis and abscess formation. *Pseudoterranova* appears to cause milder symptoms and less tissue invasion, and the worm might simply be vomited several days after initial ingestion and presented to a physician, often by an alarmed patient. Because the vast majority of infections are caused by a single organism, vomiting of the parasite results in a definitive cure and patients can be reassured. Diagnosis in patients with ongoing symptoms related to an embedded parasite is ultimately endoscopic. Effective cure results on endoscopic or surgical removal of the worm.

TREMATODES

Schistosomiasis

Schistosomes are freshwater pathogens with areas of endeminicity in Africa, South America, Southeast Asia, and parts of the Middle East. These small trematodes cause varied, often chronic infections that can carry significant morbidity, although some species cannot invade beyond the dermis in humans and result strictly in cercarial dermatitis or swimmer's itch. There are five species of schistosomes known to cause disease in humans: *Schistosoma haematobium*, found through much of Africa and parts of the Middle East; *Schistosoma mansoni*, also native to Africa and the Middle East as well as Latin America; *Schistosoma japonicum*, present in China, Southeast Asia, and the Philippines; *Schistosoma mekongi*, found only in the Mekong River basin in Southeast Asia; and *Schistosoma intercalatum*, endemic only in West Africa.

All persons who come in contact with schistosomes are at risk for infection, even after only very brief exposure to fecally contaminated freshwater in which the intermediate hosts of the pathogen (snails) reside. Frequency and degree of infection tend to be highest in children in endemic areas and then levels off in the early teenage years, likely secondary to level of environmental exposure and possibly to host immunity. S. hematobium causes disease in the genitourinary system; the others cause intestinal, hepatic, and sometimes pulmonary diseases.

Infection is acquired rapidly on contact with freshwater (including brief swims or by repeated splashing, as can occur during river rafting), when free-living fork-tailed schistosomal larvae penetrate human skin and lose their tail. These schistomorulae can cause intense itching and a papulovesicular, pruritic rash at the site of penetration, swimmer's itch. Invasive schistomorulae then enter the venous bloodstream and ultimately lodge in gut mesenteric and portal venules, where maturation occurs, and male and female forms join and mate for life. Females begin to oviposit, and the resultant inflammatory response to the eggs can cause either acute illness or chronic fibrosis and granulomatous inflammation of the tissues in which they reside.

Acute illness, called *Katayama fever*, is more common among hosts who have not been previously exposed to the organism and can be quite severe, even fatal. Katayama fever begins 4 to 8 weeks after exposure to the schistosomes, with fever, cough, abdominal pain, hepatomegaly, and lymphadenopathy. Eggs might not yet be present in the stool at the time of diagnosis. Chronic schistosomiasis is a slowly progressive illness. S. haematobium infection is manifest by gross or microscopic hematuria, urinary symptoms, and chronic bacterial urinary tract infections; ultimately ureteral fibrosis, hydronephrosis, and granulomatous genital lesions also can ensue. In infection with other invasive schistosomes, chronic illness can manifest as abdominal pain and diarrhea, which is often bloody, with associated iron-deficiency anemia. Hepatomegaly is often the first clinical finding in chronic intestinal schistosomiasis. Over many years, hepatic congestion and fibrosis can result in liver failure, and the pulmonary vasculature can be involved as well, which causes pulmonary hypertension and cor pulmonale.

Diagnosis of schistosomiasis is by observation of eggs in stool (intestinal disease), urine (urinary tract disease), or biopsy specimens, or by serum antibody testing. Concentration of stool may be necessary to detect the pathogen. The eggs of the three most common species of schistosomes can be readily identified microscopically: S. haematobium has an inferior spine, S. mansoni an inferolateral spine, and S. japonicum lacks a spine. Eosinophilia is a hallmark of chronic infection and is a common cause of asymptomatic eosinophilia among immigrants from schistoendemic regions of the world. Serology is highly sensitive and specific but cannot distinguish acute, chronic, or cleared infection; it is very useful when attempting to diagnose infection in returned travelers.

All patients with schistosomiasis should be treated, and those with chronic manifestations might experience significant regression of even late-stage organ-specific disease. Treatment of choice is with praziquantel; see Table 2 for details.

Prevention of schistosomiasis involves improving access to treated water and exploration of avenues to eliminate the intermediate snail hosts. Host immunity does appear to occur, and efforts are under way to better understand and induce such immunity in the form of a vaccine.

CESTODES

Taeniasis

Human tapeworm infection has long been implicated in North American oral folklore as a cause of insatiable appetite and excessive weight loss. In reality, despite their impressive size of up to 12 meters, tapeworm infection tends to be minimally symptomatic.

Taenia solium, pork tapeworm, and *Taenia sanguinata*, beef tapeworm, are the two most common flatworm infections of humans worldwide and occur in any setting in which raw or undercooked meat is served and cattle and pigs have access to feed contaminated with human feces. *T. sanguinata* is still found in areas of North America and Europe, as well as in Central and South America and Africa; *T. solium* is common throughout Mexico, Central and South America, Africa, China, and the Indian subcontinent. Although humans are the definitive hosts for both parasites, *T. solium* is best known for its pathogenicity in the form of cysticercosis. Cysticercosis is not an intestinal parasitic infection.

Domesticated animals acquire infection on ingestion of eggs excreted by humans; the eggs mature in their musculature and develop a scolex. When humans consume infected meat, the scolex attaches in the small intestine, and the adult tapeworm develops over approximately 2 months. Adult tapeworms are made up of hundreds to thousands of gravid proglottids and can live for up to 25 years. Symptoms tend to be mild or absent but can include nausea, abdominal pain, loose stools, anal pruritus, and occasionally weakness or increased appetite, especially in children. Serious illness rarely results when a tapeworm becomes lodged in the biliary or pancreatic ducts or is coughed up and aspirated. Some patients come to medical attention when the worm is noted emerging from the anus or on extrusion of proglottids in the stool.

Diagnosis of taeniasis can be made on visualizing the round eggs in stool; however, the species cannot be determined unless a segment of the worm is examined. Serum antibody and antigen tests, as well as stool PCR, have been developed for diagnosis but are not widely used in clinical practice. Eosinophilia and elevated IgE levels may be present. Single dose praziquantel[1] (see Table 2) is curative in almost all cases, but infectious eggs can still be released in the feces for a time; ingestion of these could result in the subsequent development if cysticercosis, so patients should be counseled to avoid fecal–oral contact.

Proper cooking of meat is the mainstay of prevention; disposal of human waste away from animals would also be effective in interrupting the life cycle.

Diphyllobothriasis

Diphyllobothrium latum is the longest parasite known to infect humans (10 to 12 m). It is found in freshwater lakes in areas of the Americas, Northern Europe, Africa, China, and Japan and has a complex life cycle involving two intermediate hosts: crustaceans and small fish. Humans and other fish-eating mammals are the definitive hosts and acquire the infection on ingestion of raw fish or roe.

The organism attaches within the small intestine, and hosts are usually asymptomatic. Infected persons might complain of increased appetite, nausea, or abdominal discomfort. Many present after passage of portions of the tapeworm in stool, as with taeniasis; in others, diagnosis is on stool examination done for other purposes or during screening colonoscopy. As with other worms, the parasite occasionally migrates into biliary ducts or causes intestinal obstruction. Attachment of the parasite higher in the intestine can result in decreased levels of vitamin B_{12}. Rarely, pernicious anemia develops as a result (tapeworm anemia).

Diagnosis is made either by seeing eggs in unconcentrated stool or by encountering the adult worm. Eosinophilia is present in a minority of cases. Treatment with praziquantel[1] is curative; see Table 2. Vitamin B_{12} supplementation is necessary in cases of severe or symptomatic deficiency, but it will not recur once the tapeworm is eliminated. Prevention involves not ingesting undercooked fish.

REFERENCES

Abubakar I, Aliyu SH, Hunter PR, Usman NK. Prevention and treatment of cryptosporidiosis in immunocompromised patients. Cochrane Database Syst Rev 2007;(1):CD004932.

Bethony J, Brooker S, Albonico M, et al. Soil-transmitted helminth infections: Ascariasis, trichuriasis, and hookworm. Lancet 2006;367(9521):1521–32.

Boggild A, Yohanna S, Keystone J, Kain K. Prospective analysis of parasitic infections in Canadian travelers and immigrants. J Travel Med 2006;13:138–44.

Boulware DR, Stauffer WM, Hendel-Paterson RR, et al. Maltreatment of Strongyloides infection: Case series and worldwide physicians-in-training survey. Am J Med 2007;120:545.e1–545.e8.

Concha R, Hartington W Jr, Rogers AI. Intestinal strongyloidiasis: Recognition, management, and determinants of outcome. J Clin Gastroenterol 2005;39(3):203–11.

Drugs for parasitic infections. The Medical Letter [serial online]. 2004;46. Available at: www.medicalletter.org [Accessed June 17, 2007].

Goodgame RW. Understanding intestinal spore-forming protozoa: Cryptosporidia, microsporidia, isospora, and cyclospora. Ann Intern Med 1996;124(4):429–41.

Guerrant R, Walker D, Weller P, editors. Tropical Infectious Diseases: Principles, Pathogens, and Practice. Philadelphia: Churchill Livingstone; 1999.

Huang DB, White AC. An updated review on Cryptosporidium and Giardia. Gastroenterol Clin North Am 2006;35:291–314.

Mandell G, Bennett J, Dolin R, editors. Mandell, Douglas and Bennett's Principles and Practice of Infectious Diseases. 5th ed. Philadelphia: Churchill Livingstone; 2005.

Pardo J, Carranza C, Muro A, et al. Helminth-related eosinophilia in African immigrants, Gran Canaria. Emerg Infect Dis 2006;12(10):1587–9.

Stark D, Beebe N, Marriott D, et al. Dientamoebiasis: Clinical importance and recent advances. Trends Parasitol 2006;22(2):92–6.

---

[1]Not FDA approved for this indication.

[1]Not FDA approved for this indication.

Metabolic Disorders

Diabetes Mellitus in Adults

Method of
Anthony L. McCall, MD, PhD, and
J. Terry Saunders, PhD

Epidemiology

The Centers for Disease Control and Prevention (CDC) estimated that in 2007 the prevalence of diabetes in the United States was 23.6 million. Diabetes is diagnosed in 17.9 million persons and undiagnosed in 5.7 million. Type 2 diabetes mellitus (T2DM) is 90% to 95% of prevalent diabetes, and type 1 diabetes (T1DM) is about 5% to 10%. There are fewer persons with secondary or monogenic forms of diabetes, called *maturity-onset diabetes of the young* (MODY). About 57 million people in the United States are believed to have prediabetes.

The focus of this article is T2DM because it is the most prevalent form and is increasing rapidly in the United States and worldwide. A few comments are made on adult T1DM. This chapter emphasizes both lifestyle and pharmacologic treatments.

Diagnosis and Classification of Diabetes and Prediabetes

DIAGNOSIS

Most diabetes is diagnosed by random or fasting glucose (Table 1). Symptoms should be present if random glucose criteria are used, but surprisingly, many people with diabetes are relatively asymptomatic. In the elderly, cognitive changes can occur and atypical symptoms such as prostatism can appear. The American Diabetes Association (ADA) screening recommendations suggest screening every 3 years starting at age 45 for the general population, but they suggest earlier and more frequent screening in those with high risk. Recently, a case has been made for using elevated A1c as an adjunct combined with glucose measurement or as a sole criterion when >7% for screening and diagnosis of diabetes.

Patients from diabetes-prone ethnic groups (e.g., Latin Americans, African Americans, Native Americans) or with a strong family history, polycystic ovary syndrome (PCOS), or gestational diabetes should have early and frequent screenings. High-risk persons include those with prediabetes (impaired glucose tolerance, impaired fasting glucose) or who meet the National Cholesterol Education Program (NCEP) criteria for the metabolic syndrome or its individual components (dyslipidemia, hypertension, central obesity, prediabetes). The metabolic syndrome as defined by the NCEP is criticized as flawed,

but such critique does not reduce the importance of fully documenting and treating cardiometabolic risk components in those with or at risk for T2DM in a targeted manner (see Box 1). The metabolic syndrome concept is useful to teach patients and clinicians about these risks and the response of the overweight and sedentary to a healthier lifestyle.

CLASSIFICATION

The classification of diabetes into its two most prominent types (T1DM and T2DM) seems straightforward in theory but in practice is increasingly confusing as more Americans become overweight. Although T1DM patients are traditionally lean, many now are overweight and some have metabolic syndrome characteristics. About 80% to 90% of persons with T2DM are overweight or have metabolic syndrome characteristics, but some are leaner and more active and do not have the metabolic syndrome. C-peptide measurements are not very helpful for those who are difficult to classify, but measuring three antibodies—including IA-2 (islet cell antigen 512), anti-GAD$_{65}$ (glutamic acid decarboxylase), and anti-insulin antibodies in high titers—can clarify a diagnosis of latent autoimmune diabetes. Younger age at onset, lean body habitus, severe loss of glycemic control with or without ketonemia, and weight loss all suggest insulin deficiency but might not be definitive.

Pathophysiology

The primary causes of most adult diabetes are insulin resistance and lack of compensatory insulin secretion. Insulin resistance is typically longstanding and begins at a young age because of heredity combined with environmental causes (sedentary lifestyle and calorie overconsumption with resultant overweight). Insulin secretory defects usually start about 10 years before diagnosis, and no therapy is proven so far to prevent progressive loss of insulin secretion. A few patients develop diabetes associated with malnutrition, but this is much less common. Longstanding insulin resistance is associated with dyslipidemia, central obesity, hypertension, and hyperglycemia. This long prodrome accounts for the common coexistence of cardiovascular disease and diabetes.

CARDIOVASCULAR RISK MANAGEMENT

Cardiovascular risk management in diabetes starts with lifestyle counseling and education. It is paramount that patients understand the intimate and direct links among diabetes, glycemic control, and cardiovascular disease. Drug interventions are ultimately needed for glycemia, lipid risks, and blood pressure in most patients. Women have higher relative risk and similar overall risk as men and are often undertreated. Specific recommended targets of therapy for diabetes in glycemia, blood pressure, dyslipidemia, and lifestyle are shown in Box 1.

TABLE 1 Diagnosis and Classification of Diabetes and Prediabetes

Diagnosis	Glucose Test	Diagnostic Level	Comments
Diabetes	Random	≥200 mg/dL	Plus classic symptoms*
Diabetes	Fasting	≥126 mg/dL	8-hour fast; need confirmation
Diabetes	Postglucose load (75 g in nonpregnant adults)	≥200 mg/dL at 2 h	Need confirmation
Prediabetes IFG	Fasting	≥100 mg/dL	Decreased insulin secretion
Prediabetes IGT	Postglucose load (75 g)	140–199 mg/dL at 2 h	Increased insulin resistance

*Polyuria, polydipsia, unexplained weight loss.
Abbreviations: IFG = impaired fasting glucose; IGT = impaired glucose tolerance.

BOX 1 Summary of Goals for Treatment

Lifestyle
Medical Nutrition Therapy (individualized)
- Appropriate calories
- Low saturated and *trans* fats
- Moderate, consistent carbohydrates (whole grains, vegetables, fruits)
- Healthy fats and proteins (decreased saturated and trans fats, increased monosaturated fat; reduced consumption of animal protein)

Activity
- Consistent, regular activity tailored to complications and safety (ECG or stress test may be needed before starting an exercise program)

Glycemia
- Best possible without frequent or severe hypoglycemia
- HbA1c <7% minimally; 6% or less if possible in selected patients early in disease course

Self-Monitored Blood Glucose
- Preprandial 90–130 mg/dL; <110 ideally
- Postprandial (1 to 2 h) <180 minimal; <140 ideally

Lipids
- LDL <100 mg/dL; optional <70 mg/dL (ACS, clinical ASCVD)
- Non-HDL <130 mg/dL; optional <100 mg/dL
- HDL >40 mg/dL (men); >50 mg/dL (women)
- Triglycerides <150 mg/dL

Blood Pressure
- Systolic <130 mm Hg
- Diastolic <80 mm Hg

Abbreviations: ACS = acute coronary syndrome, ASCVD = atherosclerotic cardiovascular disease (also multiple severe risk factors that are difficult to control); HDL = high-density lipoprotein; LDL = low-density lipoprotein.

DOCUMENTING AND FOLLOWING COMPLICATIONS

Patients should have a thorough examination and evaluation for complications at the time of diabetes diagnosis. About one half of patients with newly diagnosed T2DM have established chronic complications, indicating delayed recognition of this disorder.

Neuropathy and circulatory signs and symptoms on foot examination should be assessed. Risk of ulcer and amputation can be gauged by 10-g Semmes-Weinstein monofilaments that test for severe neuropathy and attendant risk of ulceration. Retina examinations

---

CURRENT DIAGNOSIS

- Screening for diabetes should be done in high-risk populations, especially:
  - Those with prediabetes or the metabolic syndrome.
  - High-risk ethnic groups (e.g., Native American, Latino American, African American).
  - Gestational diabetes.
  - Patients might present with atypical symptoms.
  - Most diabetes is type 2 in adults, but type 1 does occur in adults, and delayed diagnosis is common.
- Cardiovascular risk should be aggressively screened for and treated.
- Complications should be documented and tracked.
  - Check fasting lipids.
- Check renal function and albuminuria yearly.
  - Have a low threshold for stress testing, with imaging for all patients.
  - Refer for yearly eye examinations.
  - Check feet for sensation, deformity, and circulation at regular visits.
- All patients should receive an educational assessment and training in self-management and self-monitoring of blood glucose.
- Take a diet history; this is especially important for patients on insulin.
- Get a baseline HbA1c and repeat 2 to 4 times per year (twice yearly if at glycemic goal).

---

should be done by skilled eye professionals likely to pick up significant eye disease. High-risk patients (poor glycemic control, established retinopathy, especially if preproliferative or worse) should be referred promptly to an eye specialist. Pregnancy counseling should be given to all women of childbearing age with diabetes. Microalbumin-to-creatinine ratio in the urine should be assessed and kidney function (serum creatinine and blood urea nitrogen [BUN]) should be tracked yearly.

Home glucose monitoring should be taught to patients so they understand the effects of food, stress, and exercise on glycemic patterns. Diabetes education should be arranged for all patients, preferably by a diabetes educator. Diabetes is unique in being a self-managed condition where patient knowledge and skills are critical to avoiding complications.

Treatment

BEHAVIORAL SELF-MANAGEMENT

Self-management of behavioral factors, including eating, physical activity, and psychological stress, is essential to good diabetes self-care. Ideally, professional support for behavioral self-management should

CURRENT THERAPY

- Diabetes requires nutrition and behavioral self-management counseling as well as drug therapy.
- Repeatedly encourage healthy eating and an active lifestyle.
- Prediabetes diagnosis represents an opportunity for behavioral and drug interventions.
- Metformin (Glucophage) is usually the first drug therapy.
- Don't expect one drug to do the job for very poorly controlled glycemia.
- Dual defects (insulin resistance and secretion) should be addressed in most patients.
- Very insulin resistant patients might need a dual insulin resistance strategy.
- Therapy goals for both HbA1c and self-monitored blood glucose can be achieved in most patients.
- Cardiovascular risk reduction therapy is a very high priority.
- When patients have not met goals on dual oral agent therapy, basal insulin is often the most appropriate choice, particularly when patients are not near glycemic goals.
- For oral agent therapy, add don't switch unless side effects require it.
- When adding basal insulin, continue oral agent therapies.
- Threatening patients with insulin therapy is counterproductive.
- Follow the 3F rule: Fix the fasting glucose first, especially in patients with poor glycemic control.
- Prompt recognition of the need for meal insulin is critical to achieve glycemic goals.
- Balance meal and basal insulin.

be a coordinated, multidisciplinary effort involving expertise appropriate to a given patient from the areas of nutrition, nursing, exercise training, and behavioral counseling. The provider should develop a referral network of available multidisciplinary resources and make regular use of any appropriate community-based resources (e.g., weight loss programs, fitness programs, diabetes support groups). Unfortunately, multidisciplinary resources are often in short supply or difficult to pay for. Therefore, it is essential that the provider develop basic skills and techniques for working with patients on behavior change.

Behavior change is slow and is inherently a multisession activity. Quick, one-shot interventions seldom change longstanding patterns of behavior. Initial sessions should be scheduled closely together (1–2 weeks), then further apart as the patient gains momentum and confidence. If multiple one-on-one sessions are impossible, other options such as group meetings, telephone support, or e-mail messaging should be considered.

Behavior change interventions should be highly individualized and specific. General advice about diet and exercise does not address the life experience or problems of a given patient and is often perceived as insensitive or unhelpful. Arriving at individualized objectives for behavior change can be accomplished using a simple three-step process composed of initial assessment, setting behavioral objectives, and follow-up and reassessment.

Initial Assessment

Initial assessment includes identifying salient features of social and family history that can affect efforts to change behavior. A nutrition assessment should be performed, including an appraisal of usual food intake, the patient's perception of problem eating behavior, and

weight history. A physical activity assessment should also be conducted, focusing on past and current physical activity, preferences, perceived barriers, and general attitudes. Readiness to make changes in behavior should be assessed by asking how important a patient thinks it is to change a given area of behavior and how confident she or he is that she or he can succeed in making changes (on a 1 to 10 scale). Discussion of specific objectives for behavioral change should occur in areas where the patient indicates a definite readiness to begin. Other areas of change should be discussed, but not forced or driven by the provider. Finally, ask patients about current levels and sources of stress. Because depression is common with diabetes, patients should be screened for possible depression.

Behavioral Objectives

Setting behavioral objectives is initiated and facilitated by the provider, but the patient is responsible for selecting his or her own behavioral objectives. Resist the temptation to take over responsibility for this function. Objectives should be FIRM: *few* (1–3 at a time is plenty), *individualized* to the patient's specific behavioral challenges, *realistic* (beware of trying to make big strides quickly), and *measurable*. For measurement, the patient should be given a tracking form (such as the example in Figure 1) to use in recording daily progress on each objective. Note that although the patient might have long-term goals in the areas of weight loss, calorie intake, or general fitness, specific behavioral objectives such as eating a bowl of cereal for breakfast or walking one-half hour on five mornings each week are the means to achieving those outcomes. The primary focus of provider-patient discussions of progress should be on behavioral objectives, not outcomes. The ADA offers a web-based continuing medical education program to assist health care professionals in acquiring more detailed knowledge and skills in setting behavioral objectives for lifestyle change.

Follow-up and Reassessment

Follow-up and reassessment occur during each return visit, following a period of patient efforts to carry out mutually agreed on behavioral objectives. Reassessment focuses on the behavioral records kept by patients as well as on their verbal reports of difficulties and successes. Praise and encouragement are the order of the day. Efforts to initiate behavior change are highly responsive to external positive reinforcement, and the patient will need maximum external reinforcement until new behavior becomes self-sustaining. After review and discussion of patient records, new behavioral objectives or incremental changes in existing objectives are selected by mutual agreement, with the patient taking the lead.

A modest weight loss of 5% to 10% has a positive impact on cardiovascular risk factors and progression of diabetes. Reassure patients that medical goals for weight loss are achievable and worth the effort.

When discussing changes in eating with patients, distinguish dieting from gradual behavioral changes that result in a lasting pattern of healthy eating. Diets are impermanent and run the risk of large weight losses followed by even larger weight gains. Gradual behavioral changes offer the possibility of permanent lifestyle changes.

Prohibiting or demonizing foods is counterproductive. It leads patients to think of food in moral extremes (e.g., "sugar is bad for my diabetes") rather than along a continuum of nutritional benefit and blood glucose control. Food prohibition also casts the provider as withholding and overly controlling. These traps can be avoided by exploring very small changes that are not perceived as significant losses.

Patients may be extremely confused about the role of carbohydrates in weight loss and weight maintenance because of popular myths about sugar and the controversy surrounding low-carbohydrate diets. Low-carbohydrate diets (<130 g/day) are not recommended as an approach to weight loss. Carbohydrates should be included as an important part of a healthy diet for people with diabetes. Recommendations for achieving consistent, appropriate carbohydrate intake at meals are based on controlling postprandial blood glucose (<180 mg/dL 1 to 2 hours after beginning a meal). Carbohydrate counting and blood glucose pattern management are complicated and time consuming to teach. Referral to a dietitian for medical nutrition therapy (MNT) or nutrition education through an ADA-recognized diabetes patient education program is recommended.

My Behavioral Goals

To take better care of my diabetes and improve my health, I will:
(Write your behavioral goal in the blank spaces below and track your daily progress in the boxes on the tracking form. Make notes about your successes and challenges.)

Walk for 30 minutes, 5 days per week

Circle the day you will start and mark your progress every day with a check or number.

Monday	Tuesday	Wednesday	Thursday	Friday	Saturday	Sunday
		20	10	25	30	25
0	30					

Date	My Successes
11/30	Finally did 30 minutes on Saturday!
	My Challenges

FIGURE 1. Example of a behavioral goals tracking form.

The best place to begin setting behavioral objectives for nutrition and exercise is where the patient is currently. Obtaining a 3-day food record (2 work days and one nonwork day) and a baseline for activity (we generally use a week of daily steps measured with a pedometer) provide a solid baseline for setting objectives.

An irregular pattern of eating often underlies unhealthy food choices. For example, staying up late encourages late-night snacking, which in turn can suppress interest in eating breakfast. Eating tends to be deferred to the afternoon or evening, perpetuating the cycle.

A modest reduction in caloric consumption of around 250 to 500 kcal/day and moderate physical activity on the order of at least 150 minutes a week are the recommended approaches to weight loss. Reducing calories through decreased food consumption is more effective for weight loss than increasing energy expenditure through physical activity. Box 2 contains a checklist of healthy eating behaviors that can be used to stimulate patients' thinking about places they might like to make changes. Physical activity plays an important role in weight maintenance, but higher levels of activity (200 min/week) may be required to prevent long-term weight regain. Box 3 lists ways that patients can become more active. It is worth repeating that the point of these and other suggestions is not to direct patients but to expand their thinking about what might work for them.

Stress reduction is important in controlling blood glucose, but it can also play a role by helping patients achieve a mental focus on their behavior-management efforts. We encourage patients to sit calmly for a period of 5 to 10 minutes each day, focusing on slow deep breathing and muscle relaxation. Activities such as yoga or tai chi also reduce stress and support awareness of body and mind. Box 4 contains suggestions for coping behaviors that may be useful to patients in dealing with stress.

PHARMACOLOGIC THERAPY

Overview

Eventually, most patients with T2DM require drug treatment, often with multiple agents (combination therapy). Progressive insulin secretory loss probably is the primary explanation for the need to advance treatment. A resultant general rule with all therapies is *add, don't switch.* Table 2 lists major types of pharmacotherapeutic interventions with their usual hemoglobin (Hb) A1c lowering, balance of preprandial versus postprandial effects, and some comments on their actions and side effects. Table 3 lists classes of drugs, commonly used agents, and typical doses.

Recently the ADA and European Association for the Study of Diabetes (EASD) have issued a joint consensus algorithm on controlling hyperglycemia in T2DM. In our practice, we similarly initiate behavioral self-management along with medication, typically metformin unless there are contraindications or intolerance. Commonly, ineffective early attempts by physicians to change behavior (e.g., giving general advice) lead to abandonment of this therapy. A second oral medication may be initiated if patients cannot achieve glycemic goals. Commonly, we favor insulin secretagogues especially glimepiride (Amaryl) or extended-release glipizide (Glucotrol XL) for their relatively low risk of hypoglycemia, convenient once-daily dosing, and low expense. An alternative treatment strategy for heavier, more insulin-resistant patients is use of a thiazolidinedione, effectively a dual insulin-resistance strategy (see thiazolidinediones).

More reliably effective is the use of basal insulin treatment as a second agent to achieve control. Insulin initiation should be preceded by an open discussion of the patient's attitudes, beliefs, and possible fears regarding insulin. Insulin therapy should never be used as a

---

BOX 2   Checklist of Healthy Eating Behaviors

☑ **Eat meals and snacks at set times to promote health.**
Examples:

- I will eat breakfast within 1 hour of getting up.
- I will not skip meals.
- Other: ....
....

☑ **Eat healthy carbohydrates.**
Examples:

- I will avoid regular soft drinks and choose water or diet soft drinks instead.
- I will eat 5–7 servings of fruits and vegetables every day.
- I will choose whole-grain breads and cereals.
- Other: ....
....

☑ **Decrease serving sizes.**
Examples:

- I will keep a record of the food I eat and drink.
- I will know what counts as a serving size.
- When I am eating out, I will share or split an entrée and eat a salad.
- Other: ....
....

☑ **Eat less fat and choose healthy fats.**
Examples:

- I will bake, broil, roast, grill, or boil instead of fry food.
- I will have a meatless meal at least once a week.
- I will choose fried or high-fat foods no more than once a week.
- I will drink fat-free or low-fat milk.
- I will use healthy oils (olive oil, canola oil) and buy tub margarine.
- Other: ....
....

☑ **Make other healthy choices.**
Examples:

- I will drink plenty of fluids (at least 8 glasses of water or low-calorie fluid per day).
- I will limit how much alcohol I drink. (Women should drink no more than 1 alcoholic drink per day. Men should drink no more than 2 alcoholic drinks per day.)
- Other: ....
....

Unpublished source: Virginia Center for Diabetes Professional Education, University of Virginia; Virginia Diabetes Council.

threat or possible negative consequence for failure to carry out behavioral management. Many patients associate insulin with serious diabetes complications and mortality. A positive attitude about the value of insulin therapy and a reassuring, educational approach can help to reduce initial fears enough to begin. Self-demonstration of injection technique using saline is also useful in overcoming fear of injections. Improvement in blood glucose control with insulin generally makes patients feel better, which further reinforces its perceived value. Use of insulin pens may increase acceptance of insulin treatment, patient convenience, and dosing accuracy.

Oral Agents

Secretagogues

These drugs enhance insulin secretion. There are first- and second-generation oral sulfonylureas; the latter are most commonly used. They are inexpensive, are moderately effective, and often can be dosed once daily. First-generation agents such as tolbutamide, chlorpropamide (Diabenese), and tolazamide (Tolinase) are less often used than the second-generation agents glyburide (Diabeta, Glynase), glipizide (Glucotrol), and glimepiride (Amaryl).

BOX 3   Checklist for Physical Activity

☑ **Do something that you enjoy.**
Examples:

- I will take the stairs.
- I will park my car farther away and walk.
- I will walk.
- I will swim or do water exercises.
- I will ride a bike.
- I will use an exercise video.
- I will do yoga.
- Other: ....
....

☑ **How often?**
Examples:

- ❏ Every day
- ❏ 3x/week
- ❏ 5x/week
- ❏ ....

☑ **How long?**
Examples:

- ❏ 10 minutes
- ❏ 15 minutes
- ❏ 20 minutes
- ❏ 30 minutes
- ❏ 60 minutes
- ❏ ___ minutes

☑ **Limit inactivity.**
Examples:

- I will watch no more than 1 hour of television per day.
- I will spend no more than 2 hour(s) per day on the computer.
- Other: ....
....

Unpublished source: Virginia Center for Diabetes Professional Education, University of Virginia; Virginia Diabetes Council.

BOX 4 Checklist of Coping Behaviors

Examples:

- Talk about how you feel to people you trust.
- Decide one small way to change your mood or old habit, and do it.
- Write down 10 good things about your life and think about and appreciate them.
- Organize your day with a To Do list.
- Learn how to relax through yoga, meditation, biofeedback, tai chi, deep breathing, or visual imagery.
- Take 30 minutes each day to relax through music, yoga, bath, writing, etc.
- Take time to have fun every day by exploring a new interest, watching a funny movie, going shopping, playing with a pet, etc.
- Get in touch with your spiritual side to help you feel better about yourself.
- Keep a stress diary to see what triggers your stress and discover better ways to react.
- Exercise every day to help you focus your energy on a more positive path.
- Keep your sleep cycle as regular as possible.
- Develop a favorite hobby.
- Other:

....

....

Unpublished source: Virginia Center for Diabetes Professional Education, University of Virginia; Virginia Diabetes Council.

The dose-response characteristics of sulfonylureas suggest that one half the approved maximum dose achieves maximum HbA1c lowering, typically 1 to 1.5 percentage points. If the patient is not at goal with half-maximum doses, it is more effective to add a second agent than raise the dose. Common side effects include hypoglycemia, weight gain of about 2 kg, and, more rarely, hematologic or skin reactions.

TABLE 3 Dosing Used for Various Agents

Agent	Dose
Thiazolidinediones	
Pioglitazone (Actos)	15, 30, 45 mg
Rosiglitazone (Avandia)	2, 4, 8 mg
α-Glucosidase inhibitors	
Acarbose (Precose)	25, 50, 100 mg ac
Miglitol (Glycet)	25, 50 mg ac
Biguanides	
Metformin (Glucophage) IR	500, 850, 1000 mg
Metformin SR	500, 750 mg
Glinides	
Nateglinide (Starlix)	60–120 mg ac
Repaglinide (Prandin)	0.5–4 mg ac
Sulfonylureas (Second Generation)	
Glimepiride (Amaryl)	1–4 mg
Glipizide (Glucotrol) IR	2.5–20 mg
Glipizide SR	2.5–10 mg
Glyburide (Glynase)	1.25–10; 1.5–6 mg
Incretins	
Exenatide (Byetta)	5, 10 μg
Sitagliptin (Januvia)	25, 50, 100 mg*
Vildagliptin (Galvus)[4]	50, 100 mg
Amylin Agonists	
Pramlintide (Symln)	15, 30, 60, 90, 120 μg
Insulin	
Aspart (Novolog)	No dose limit
Detemir (Levemir)	No dose limit
Glargine (Lantus)	No dose limit
Glulisine (Apidra)	No dose limit
Inhaled powder insulin (Exubera)	No dose limit
Lispro (Humalog)	No dose limit
NPH	No dose limit
Regular	No dose limit

[4]Not yet approved for use in the United States.
*Based on renal function.
Abbreviations: ac = before meals; IR = immediate release; NPH = neutral protamine Hagedorn; SR = sustained release.

TABLE 2 Overview and Characteristics of Therapy Interventions

Drug Type	HbA1c Lowering (Percentage Points)	Effect on Glycemia Levels Preprandial	Postprandial	Actions	Side Effects
SUs and non-SU rapid secretagogues**	1.5–2*	++	+	Direct and indirect secretagogue	Hypoglycemia, weight gain
Biguanides	1.5–2*	+++	0	↓ hepatic glucose output	GI, lactic acidosis, weight neutral
Thiazolidinediones	0.7–1.5	+++	0	↓ muscle insulin sensitivity	Edema, CHF, fractures
Incretin agonists	0.9–1.1	+	++	Strong GLP-1 effects ↑ insulin ↓ glucagon	Nausea, vomiting, weight loss
DPP-4 inhibitors	0.6–0.8	+	++	Moderate GLP-1 effects ↑ insulin ↓ glucagon	Weight neutral
Basal insulin	1.5–2.5	+++*	0*	↓ hepatic glucose output, ↑ muscle glucose disposal	Hypoglycemia, weight gain
Meal insulin	1.0–2.0	0–+*	++*	↓ hepatic glucose output, ↑ muscle glucose disposal	Hypoglycemia, weight gain
Pramlintide	0.5–0.7	0–+	++	↑ insulin ↓ glucagon	Nausea, vomiting
Colesevalem	0.4–0.8	+	+	Unknown	Constipation, hypertriglyceridemia

*Older drugs may be less effective in well-controlled patients.
**Rapid secretagogues have more postprandial effects and less preprandial effects.
Abbreviations: CHF = congestive heart failure; DPP = dipeptidyl peptidase; GI = gastrointestinal; GLP = glucagon-like peptide; Hb = hemoglobin; PFT = pulmonary function test; SU = sulfonylurea.

Rapid secretagogues, the glinides (repaglinide [Prandin] and nateglinide [Starlix]), are more expensive and should be considered for patients who are sulfonylurea allergic, extremely erratic in eating, or at high risk for hypoglycemia.

Biguanides

Metformin is the only available agent in this class. It is useful in both obese and normal weight T2DM patients. HbA1c lowering is typically about 1.5 percentage points in monotherapy or in combination therapy. Maximum efficacy is achieved with 2000 mg daily. The sustained-release preparation will last 24 hours if given with the evening meal.

Metformin's hypoglycemic mechanism is primarily by reduction of liver glucose production. It is cleared by the kidney, and the risk of lactic acidosis, a rare side effect with 50% mortality, may be increased in renal dysfunction. Serum creatinine should be less than 1.4 mg/dL in women and less than 1.5 mg/dL in men, and glomerular filtration rate (GFR) should be assessed in patients 80 years and older. It is also an increased lactic acidosis risk in patients with drug-treated congestive heart failure (CHF) or respiratory insufficiency. Intravascular contrast administration should prompt holding the drug for 24 to 48 hours until renal function is assured to be adequate. GI side effects are common initially and are dose dependent but wane; they can require gradual titration. Sustained-release preparations have fewer GI side effects. Weight gain is less with this drug than with many others for diabetes. The United Kingdom Prospective Diabetes Study (UKPDS) found that risk of MI and death was reduced, making it a first choice for pharmacotherapy in most patients.

Thiazolidinediones

Two drugs of the thiazolidinedione (TZD) class are available, rosiglitazone (Avandia) and pioglitazone (Actos). Both have similar glycemic-lowering effects and side effects. These drugs work by increasing the sensitivity of muscle tissue and fat to insulin action, probably through action of adipokines like adiponectin and muscle effects on adenosine monophosphate–activated protein kinase (AMPK), a fuel sensor enzyme. HbA1c lowering varies considerably, dependent on whether patients are very insulin resistant (central adiposity, often hypertriglyceridemia) and whether there is adequate endogenous insulin secretion (short diabetes duration or secretagogues) or insulin is given.

Diabetes may be prevented with rosiglitazone, and this is being tested for pioglitazone. Both TZDs can precipitate edema, weight gain due to obesity, and occasionally congestive heart failure even absent a prior heart failure history. It is thus wise to track weight in all patients and limit it to 5 or 6 pounds. The risk of heart failure is increased when TZDs are combined with insulin. Both TZDs have beneficial effects on some lipid parameters, but pioglitazone appears more effective in reducing hypertriglyceridemia. Recent analyses suggest, but do not prove, increased coronary ischemic events with rosiglitazone. Pioglitazone studies suggest reduced ischemic risk (stroke or myocardial infarction). Both medicines may increase heart failure, and new studies suggest more self-reported fractures in women, which will need further study.

Incretins

Incretins are gut hormones that enhance food-induced insulin secretion. Incretin drugs either are receptor agonists (e.g., exenatide) for glucagon-like peptide-1 (GLP-1), perhaps the most important incretin, or they enhance endogenous levels for both GLP-1 and gastrointestinal insulinotropic polypeptide (GIP).

Exenatide (Byetta) is the only available GLP-1 receptor agonist. Its actions increase meal insulin, decrease meal hyperglucagonemia, decrease rate of stomach emptying, and suppress appetite, which may cause a moderate weight loss. It works rapidly on injection. It has substantial GI side effects including nausea, vomiting, and diarrhea in a large minority of patients. Despite this, many patients favor it, probably because the side effects generally wane within weeks and

there can be substantial weight loss in some very overweight patients. Typically, exenatide is given in doses of 5 μg twice daily at meals, advancing after a month to 10 μg twice daily. Patients might report that nausea is more tolerable if they have a little food in their stomach at the time of dosing. Pancreatitis may rarely occur (case reports).

Because incretin drugs all have a glucose-dependent insulin secretion and glucagon suppression, there is little tendency for hypoglycemia used alone or when they are combined with metformin and TZDs in comparison with sulfonylureas. HbA1c lowering with exenatide has been 0.9 to 1.1 percentage points.

Dipeptidyl Peptidase-4 Inhibitors

Dipeptidyl peptidase-4 (DPP-4) is the peptidase that normally rapidly degrades the incretins GLP-1 and GIP to inactive proteolytic products. Inhibitors of DPP-4 have been shown to enhance GLP-1 and GIP levels to high physiologic levels and thereby reduce HbA1c concentrations, typically about 0.6 to 0.8 percentage points. At this writing, one of two drugs, sitagliptin (Januvia), has been approved and appears to be effective in doses of 100 mg once daily. This drug is excreted by the kidney largely unchanged and therefore should be given in lower doses (50 mg once daily) for those with moderate renal insufficiency (GFR 30–50 mL/min) and further reduced (25 mg) for those with severe renal dysfunction (GFR <30 mL/min).

Because DPP-4 inhibitors are oral, they may be preferred to the injectable exenatide. The side effects for these drugs are relatively minor and cause little nausea, vomiting, or diarrhea. They also do not cause significant weight loss but, like metformin, appear to be weight neutral. Recently, rare but serious allergic reactions such as angioedema and Stevens-Johnson syndrome have been reported in a few patients.

Amylin Agonists

Insulin is cosecreted with another beta cell hormone called amylin. The effects of amylin appear to be to help lower glycemia, reduce excess glucagon levels, curb appetite, and possibly reduce the rate of gastric emptying. A synthetic analogue of amylin, pramlintide (Symlin), is available as an injectable agent for treating both T1DM and T2DM as an adjunct to insulin. It lowers HbA1c about 0.5 to 0.7 percentage point. It also appears to have some weight loss effect, typically around 1 to 2 kg. Its action primarily controls glucose postprandially. Nausea and vomiting can occur in patients with either T2DM or T1DM but are worse in T1DM patients who require low doses at first (15 μg or less with meals) and slower titration. Those with T2DM usually start with 60 μg and can usually advance to 90 to 120 μg at meals.

Insulin

Barriers to Insulin Use

Insulin deficiency underlies the genesis of both T1DM and T2DM. Progression of therapy to use of insulin typically with oral agents in T2DM also seems predicated on progressive loss of insulin secretion. Nonetheless, it is often started too late, and patients often are in very poor control when this is done. Reluctance by patients and physicians alike might underlie this. Physicians should understand that exogenous insulin in T2DM is needed, does not negatively alter life quality, and is more likely to achieve therapeutic targets. Moreover, exogenous insulin does not worsen insulin resistance, does not cause excess cardiovascular disease, and has a low frequency of severe hypoglycemia, especially when used relatively early in the disease. Table 4 lists common insulin preparations and some notes about kinetics and timing.

Starting Insulin: Use of Basal Insulin in Type 2 Diabetes

How should insulin be started? Practitioners should use temporary insulin for patients whose glycemia is initially poorly controlled or when patients temporarily have worse control due to illness or

TABLE 4 Insulin Preparations

Insulin Type	Pharmacokinetics			Comments
	Onset (h)	Peak (h)	Duration (h)	
Basal Insulin				
NPH (Humulin N, Novolin N)	0.5	4–10	18	Kinetics is dose dependent Peak effects exert meal action
Glargine† (Lantus)	2–4	none	24*	Dose at breakfast, bedtime, supper* Up to 1/3 of C-peptide-negative T1DM need bid administration Dose can be given at any time of day if consistent
Detemir† (Levemir)		Less peak activity than NPH		Kinetics is dose dependent Dose at breakfast, bedtime, supper*
Meal Insulin				
Regular (Humulin R, Novolin R)	15–30	2–3	5–8	Give 1/2 hour before meals
Lispro (Humalog)	0.1–0.2	1.5–2.0	4	Dose at mealtime or immediately after
Aspart (Novolog)	0.1–0.2	1.5–2.0	4	Dose at mealtime or immediately after
Glulisine (Apidra)	0.1–0.2	1.5–2.0	4	Dose at mealtime or immediately after
Mixed Preparations				
NPH/regular (Humulin, Novolin)	70/30 dual kinetics based on components			Dosing 1/2 hour before meals Should not be dosed at bedtime
Lispro/NPLispro (Humalog Mix 75/25)	25/75 dual kinetics			Dosing at mealtime; should not be dosed at bedtime
Lispro/NPLispro Humalog Mix 50/50	50/50 dual kinetics			Dosing at mealtime, should not be dosed at bedtime
Aspart/NPAspart (NovoLog Mix 70/30)	30/70 dual kinetics			Dosing at mealtime; should not be dosed at bedtime

*Bedtime dosing may be preferred for some patients, especially those on low doses.
†Should not be mixed with other insulins or used in the same syringe that other insulin has been in.
Abbreviation: NPH = neutral protamine Hagedorn.

medications, such as glucocorticoids. It is unwise to use insulin as a threat because it creates a sense of personal failure and dread of insulin use. When therapy progresses but there is failure to achieve glycemic goals after one or two oral medications, use of basal insulin is often the best way to achieve euglycemia, especially if patients are much more than 1 percentage point from HbA1c goal (< 7%).

The Treat-to-Target Trial offers a good example of how to initiate insulin therapy. In this study, as often in our practice, patients start with a basal insulin either with NPH insulin or insulin glargine (Lantus). Insulin detemir (Levemir) represents another new option to be used similarly. Insulin is instituted as 10 U once daily, commonly in the evening near bedtime, followed by weekly increases between 2 and 8 units depending on proximity to glucose goals, focusing on the fasting glucose.

This strategy is sometimes called the *fix the fasting first* rule. Average doses in that study were around 45 to 50 units for patients whose BMI was about 31 kg/m². An alternative initial dosing might be 0.2 U/kg body weight, but whatever the starting dose, a forced titration guided by patient self-monitoring with clear communication of target fasting glucose (90–130 mg/dL), size of increment (or decrement in case of hypoglycemia; usually 10%–20% of dose), and frequency of change (every 3–7 days) is necessary to get most patients to overall glycemic (HbA1c) goal. This strategy is referred to as *pattern management*. The intent is to use monitoring to adjust the insulin dose likely to affect the fasting glucose for basal insulin therapy. NPH and detemir usually can be used once daily, typically at bedtime. Patients using glargine may choose any time of the day as long as it is reasonably consistent, usually within an hour. Occasionally, twice-daily NPH or detemir is used.

At some point, basal insulin therapy alone may be insufficient for glycemic control for T2DM patients. Usually this is a consideration in patients whose HbA1c values are over 9% to 9.5% or where the fasting goal is met but HbA1c or daytime glycemia remains elevated. The need for meal insulin is particularly likely to occur with larger meals, such as supper. Diagnostically, what is important is to have patients check either both before and after large meals or, if they are unwilling to check frequently, simply check about 2 to 3 hours after meals. Self-monitored glucose values that exceed even minimum postprandial glycemic guidelines (<180 mg/dL) indicate the need for meal insulin. A common mistake made in practice is to treat fasting hyperglycemia only with increases in basal insulin, when in some patients, the cause is overeating or lack of meal insulin the previous evening. This can be discerned by observing the pattern of glycemia, with lows often between meals or overnight and highs occurring after meals or at bedtime.

FIXED-RATIO COMBINED INSULINS

A commonly employed strategy is to use fixed-ratio combination short-acting (either regular or rapid analogue) insulin combined with intermediate insulin (NPH or neutral protamine modified rapid analogue that mimics NPH timing). Examples of these preparations include 70/30 NPH and regular insulin, 75/25 neutral protamine lispro and lispro insulin (Humalog), and 70/30 neutral protamine aspart and aspart insulin (Novolog). These have the advantage of being able to achieve control very conveniently in T2DM patients who have quite poor control (HbA1c of 9.5% or more) with a simple twice-daily injection regimen. They also offer the advantage of greater dosing accuracy, especially when used with insulin pens. Important to the success of these formulations is consistent eating and carbohydrate intake with meals. Unfortunately, when such consistency is not advised or followed, patterns of glycemia can be erratic and hypoglycemia can be significantly increased due to both components of the combination. Patients who skip meals are poor candidates for such treatments and should either switch to individual dosing of an insulin mixture or, even safer, use a basal bolus insulin regimen.

Colesevelam hydrochloride (WelChol) in doses of 3.8 g/day altogether or in divided doses has been shown to reduce hyperglycemia when compared with placebo in patients with type 2 diabetes mellitus. A1c reductions range from 0.4% to 0.8% in comparison with placebo when used alone, with patients on metformin alone or in combination with other oral agents, with sulfonylureas, on sulfonylureas and other oral agents and when used with insulin and other oral agents. Although this drug has already been approved for hyperlipidemia, it is now FDA approved also for type 2 diabetes. It has the potential, however, to increase triglycerides, and thus baseline fasting lipid values should be obtained and tracked, especially in hypertriglyceridemic patients. There is little reason to justify its use alone or with thiazolidinediones but may be appropriate for some patients with type 2 diabetes not at goal on other therapies.

ADULTS WITH TYPE 1 DM

A significant minority of patients with a diagnosis of T2DM actually have a late onset of T1DM and typical autoimmunity (IA-2 antibodies, GAD-65 antibodies, and insulin antibodies). The diagnosis should certainly be suspected in patients who rapidly fail combination oral agent therapy. Nonobese body habitus, marked weight loss, extremely elevated glucose values, or a family or personal history of autoimmune disease (e.g., Hashimoto's or Graves' thyroid problems) should lead to diagnostic evaluation for such signs of autoimmunity.

T1DM patients need combined mealtime and basal insulin therapy. Although it is tempting to do so in a convenient fashion with combined preparations such as those with analogue fixed ratios, it usually is far preferable to use a better basal insulin, such as glargine or detemir combined with a rapid-acting analogue (separately injected) before meals. Sometimes an insulin pump is the best way for patients who have frequent hypoglycemia or marked variability to achieve good glycemic control safely. T1DM patients should preferably be seen by an endocrine specialist or other practitioner with extensive experience in T1DM management. Ready access to diabetes educators is an important key to success with both T1DM and T2DM.

ADULTS WITH TYPE 2 DM

Many T2DM patients eventually need mealtime insulin. For those on insulin alone, incretin mimetics[1] can be successfully used for mealtime control, because they effectively lower prandial hyperglycemia. If using exenatide, then additional injections will be required at the two major meals of the day. If using an incretin-enhancer drug such as sitagliptin, injections are not required. There are no published data yet to provide guidelines for this strategy, but we have occasionally used this approach with exenatide in patients who need to lose weight, who gain considerable weight with meal insulin, or who experience poor control despite attempts to regulate meal glycemia with short-acting insulins.

REFERENCES

American Diabetes Association. Diagnosis and classification of diabetes mellitus. Diabetes Care 2006;29(Suppl. 1):S43–8.

American Diabetes Association. Facilitating Behavior Change: Key Strategies for Empowering Your Patients. http://www.facilitatingbehaviorchange.org/2009.

Diabetes Prevention Program Research Group. The Diabetes Prevention Program (DPP): Description of lifestyle intervention. Diabetes Care 2002;25:2165–71.

Grundy SM, Cleeman JI, Daniels SR, et al. Diagnosis and management of the metabolic syndrome. An American Heart Association/National Heart, Lung, and Blood Institute Scientific Statement. Executive summary. Circulation 2005;112:2735–52.

Kahn R, Buse J, Ferrannini E, Stern M. The metabolic syndrome: Time for a critical appraisal. Joint statement from the American Diabetes Association and the European Association for the Study of Diabetes. Diabetes Care 2005;8:2289–304.

Knowler WC, Barrett-Connor E, Fowler SE, et al. Reduction in the incidence of type 2 diabetes with lifestyle intervention or metformin. N Engl J Med 2002;346:393–403.

Monnier L, Lapinski H, Colette C. Contributions of fasting and postprandial plasma glucose increments to the overall diurnal hyperglycemia of type 2

diabetic patients: Variations with increasing levels of HbA1c. Diabetes Care 2003;26:881–5.

Nathan DM, Buse JB, Davidson MB, et al. Management of hyperglycemia in type 2 diabetes: A consensus algorithm for the initiation and adjustment of therapy. A consensus statement from the American Diabetes Association and the European Association for the Study of Diabetes. Diabetes Care 2006;29:1963–72.

Nathan DM, Buse JB, Davidson MB, et al. Medical management of hyperglycemia in type 2 diabetes: A consensus algorithm for the initiation and adjustment of therapy. Diabetes Care 2009;32:193–203.

Nesto RW, Bell D, Bonow RO, et al. Thiazolidinedione use, fluid retention, and congestive heart failure. A consensus statement from the American Heart Association and American Diabetes Association. Diabetes Care 2004;27:256–63.

Pihoker C, Gilliam LK, Hampe CS, Lernmark A. Autoantibodies in diabetes. Diabetes 2005;54:S52–61.

Riddle MC, Rosenstock J, Gerich J. The treat-to-target trial: Randomized addition of glargine or human NPH insulin to oral therapy of type 2 diabetic patients. Diabetes Care 2003;26:3080–6.

Saudek CD, Herman WH, Sacks DB, et al. A new look at screening and diagnosis of diabetes mellitus. J Clin Endocrinol Metab 2008; May 6, [epub ahead of print].

Diabetes Mellitus in Children and Adolescents

Method of
Lori M. B. Laffel, MD, MPH, and
Jamie R. S. Wood, MD

Diabetes mellitus is a group of metabolic disorders that have hyperglycemia as a common feature caused by inadequate insulin secretion, insulin action, or both. Chronic hyperglycemia and its numerous downstream effects lead to micro- and macrovascular complications involving the eyes, kidneys, nerves, and blood vessels. Childhood and adolescent years are periods of rapid physical growth and psychosocial change, and these two factors make the care of children and adolescents with diabetes both challenging and rewarding. The health care professional must balance the important goals of optimal glycemic control and normal growth and development along with the risks of hypoglycemia and the challenges of expected glycemic excursions during childhood. Multidisciplinary care is the hallmark of successful diabetes management for the child and adolescent with diabetes and for family members.

The American Diabetes Association (ADA) classifies diabetes mellitus into four main types: type 1 diabetes (T1D), type 2 diabetes (T2D), other specific types, and gestational diabetes mellitus (Table 1). T1D is caused by insulin deficiency, which results from the autoimmune destruction of the pancreatic β cells. There are multiple genetic loci in the major histocompatibility region of chromosome 6 that predispose (DR 3/4, DQ 0201/0302, DR 4/4, and DQ 0300/0302) or protect against (DQB1*0602, DQA1*0102) the development of T1D. T2D is caused by the combination of insulin resistance and relative insulin deficiency.

Genetic forms of diabetes include maturity-onset diabetes in the young (MODY), mitochondrial diabetes, and certain syndromes of insulin resistance. MODY is characterized by young age of onset, autosomal dominant inheritance, the lack of association with obesity, and a variable phenotype. The most common disease of the exocrine pancreas that causes diabetes in children and adolescents is cystic fibrosis. Glucocorticoids used in the treatment of systemic illnesses are also commonly associated with hyperglycemia and diabetes. Certain genetic syndromes, such as Down syndrome, Klinefelter's syndrome, and Turner's syndrome, increase the risk for diabetes.

[1]Not FDA approved for this indication.

TABLE 1 Classification of Diabetes Mellitus*

Type 1 diabetes
Type 2 diabetes
Other specific types:
- Genetic defects of β-cell function
  - MODY 1: chromosome 20, HNF-4α
  - MODY 2: chromosome 7, glucokinase
  - MODY 3: chromosome 12, HNF-1α
  - MODY 4: chromosome 13, IPF-1
  - MODY 5: chromosome 17, HNF-1β
  - MODY 6: chromosome 2, NeuroD1
  - Mitochondrial diabetes
- Genetic defects in insulin action
  - Leprechaunism
  - Rabson-Mendenhall syndrome
- Diseases of the exocrine pancreas
  - Pancreatitis
  - Cystic fibrosis
  - Pancreatectomy
- Endocrinopathies
  - Acromegaly
  - Cushing's syndrome
  - Glucagonoma
  - Pheochromocytoma
- Drug or chemical induced
  - Glucocorticoids
- Infections
  - Congenital rubella
  - Cytomegalovirus
- Other genetic syndromes associated with diabetes
  - Down's syndrome
  - Klinefelter's syndrome
  - Turner's syndrome
Gestational diabetes mellitus (GDM)

*Table is not all inconclusive and gives examples of each subtype of diabetes mellitus. For complete list, see American Diabetes Association: Diagnosis and classification of diabetes mellitus. Diabetes Care 2005;28 (Suppl 1):S37–S42.
Abbreviations: MODY = maturity-onset diabetes in the young.

CURRENT DIAGNOSIS

ADA Recommendations for the Diagnosis of Diabetes

- Symptoms (polyuria, polydipsia, unexplained weight loss) and a casual plasma glucose (any time of day without regard to time since last meal) ≥200 mg/dL (11.1 mmol/L) *or*
- Fasting (no caloric intake for at least 8 h) plasma glucose ≥126 mg/dL (7.0 mmol/L) *or*
- 2-hour plasma glucose ≥200 mg/dL (11.1 mmol/L) during an oral glucose tolerance test (glucose load of 75 g anhydrous glucose dissolved in water or 1.75 g/kg body weight if weight <43 kg).

Note: Criteria 2 and 3 should be confirmed on a second day if child/adolescent is asymptomatic. The OGTT is not recommended for routine clinical use and should be reserved for the asymptomatic child with incidental glucosuria/hyperglycemia or in the child with suspected diabetes but normal fasting plasma glucose.

Adapted from American Diabetes Association: Care of children and adolescents with type 1 diabetes. Diabetes Care 2005;28(1):186–212.

Initial Management

The goals of initial management of the child or adolescent newly diagnosed with diabetes mellitus are to correct fluid and electrolyte imbalances, reverse hepatic gluconeogenesis and ketogenesis by halting lipolysis with insulin replacement, and begin the process of diabetes education. The location of this initial management depends on the severity of the clinical presentation, the age of the patient, the psychosocial assessment of the child or adolescent and caregiver, and the diabetes-related resources available in the family's geographic location (availability of an outpatient education program).

Diagnosis

The diagnosis of T1D in children and adolescents is typically straightforward. The classic symptoms of polyuria, polydipsia, polyphagia, and weight loss over a several-week period are common. A thorough history and physical exam may reveal perineal candidiasis or thrush. Such symptoms may be followed by nausea, abdominal pain, vomiting, lethargy, and Kussmaul respirations if diabetic ketoacidosis (DKA) and lactic acidosis develop. The presentation of T2D in children and adolescents can be more subtle and sometimes even clinically silent. However, approximately a third of adolescents with T2D have ketosis and a quarter have ketoacidosis at presentation.

The Current Diagnosis box outlines the diagnosis of diabetes mellitus. In the asymptomatic child or adolescent, diabetes is diagnosed when a fasting plasma glucose is 126 mg/dL or more, a 2-hour plasma glucose during an oral glucose tolerance test (OGTT) is 200 mg/dL or more, or a random plasma glucose is 200 mg/dL or more with confirmation on a second day. The symptomatic child or adolescent with a random plasma glucose of 200 mg/dL or more does not need repeat testing to confirm the diagnosis. Measurement of islet cell autoantibodies consistent with T1D (GAD, insulin, IA2) at diagnosis may help distinguish between type 1 and T2D. Care must be taken to avoid delay in the diagnosis and initiation of treatment because of the risk of rapid metabolic deterioration with insulin deficiency.

Diabetic Ketoacidosis

Approximately 30% of children with newly diagnosed T1D present with diabetic ketoacidosis (DKA). Children who are younger (less than 4 years), without a first-degree relative with T1D, and from a family of lower socioeconomic status are at higher risk of DKA at onset of T1D. The majority of DKA episodes occur in patients with established diabetes, not in those newly diagnosed. Children or adolescents with established T1D are at higher risk for DKA if they are in poor metabolic control, have had a previous episode of DKA, are peripubertal/adolescent girls, have a psychiatric disorder, or are from a disadvantaged background.

Management of DKA in children and adolescents is based on the same principles used in adults and therefore is covered in a separate chapter in this book. The development of cerebral edema, however, warrants discussion because this complication is seen primarily in children and is associated with both high morbidity and mortality. Risk factors for the development of cerebral edema include lower initial partial pressure of carbon dioxide, higher initial serum urea nitrogen concentrations, treatment with bicarbonate, and an attenuated rise in measured serum sodium concentrations during therapy. In addition, children who are younger (less than 5 years), have new-onset T1D, and longer duration of symptoms may also be at an increased risk. A high index of suspicion is needed with mannitol (Osmitrol) at the bedside to allow for timely intervention.

Initiation of Insulin Replacement Therapy

Subcutaneous insulin is initiated in the patient who does not present in DKA or following intravenous insulin therapy in the child with resolved DKA who is tolerating oral intake (pH of $\geq$7.3, tCO_2 $\geq$18, anion gap 12 ± 2 mEq/L). The starting dose of insulin replacement therapy depends on the age, weight, and pubertal status of the patient, as well as the presence or absence of DKA. For the prepubertal child without DKA, the starting dose is usually 0.25 to 0.5 U/kg/day. For the prepubertal child with resolved DKA, the usual starting dose is 0.5 to 0.75 U/kg/day. For the pubertal child without DKA, the starting dose is 0.5 to 0.75 U/kg/day and for the pubertal child with resolved DKA, 0.75 to 1 U/kg/day. This total daily dose (TDD) of insulin is typically divided into either two or three injections per day, with the latter the preference toward implementation of intensive therapy (Figure 1). The twice-daily regimen may be selected for the younger (less than 4 years) child or if the psychosocial assessment determines that fewer injections per day would be beneficial. The use of an insulin pump at diagnosis remains within the research realm currently.

When the patient is metabolically stable, the focus turns to the psychosocial assessment of the child or adolescent and caregiver(s) and the initiation of diabetes education. A licensed social worker or other mental health professional evaluates each family and screens for circumstances that might complicate diabetes management: family composition, alternative caregiver(s), financial concerns, lack of health insurance, psychiatric or medical illness in a family member, or severe emotional distress of caregiver secondary to the diabetes diagnosis.

Diabetes education is provided by a certified diabetes nurse educator (DNE) and focuses on the set of essential skills needed to keep a child or adolescent with diabetes safe at home and school. These survival skills include techniques of blood glucose monitoring, urine or blood ketone measurement, drawing up and administration of subcutaneous insulin and glucagon, recognition and treatment of hypoglycemia and hyperglycemia, basics of sick day management, and indications for and methods of contacting the child's diabetes team. In addition to the survival skills, the child or adolescent and family should meet with a registered dietician who will assist them in developing an individualized meal plan and introduce the family to the concept of carbohydrate counting or exchanges. Once the child or adolescent (if developmentally appropriate) and caregiver(s) demonstrate the knowledge and skills needed, they are discharged with the expectation of daily phone contact with a member of their diabetes team to further titrate insulin doses and answer questions. When available and clinically indicated, a visiting nurse may assist with ongoing home-based education and support in the short term.

Outpatient Diabetes Care

The management of children and adolescents with diabetes requires a multidisciplinary team approach. Members of this team include either a pediatric endocrinologist or pediatrician with training in diabetes, a pediatric DNE, a dietician, and a mental health professional (social worker and psychologist). Members of this team need to be easily accessible to the family in times of illness or metabolic crisis. Another member of the child/adolescent's team is a pediatrician or family doctor who will continue to provide routine well child care including anticipatory guidance, immunizations, and general medical care.

In the first few months of outpatient diabetes care, patients are seen frequently by members of the diabetes team to assess the family's adaptation to the new diagnosis, reinforce skills and knowledge learned during the first few days, and expand on the skills and knowledge needed for intensive diabetes management. Patients are subsequently seen at a minimum frequency of every 3 months, alternating between their DNE and their pediatric endocrinologist. Visits with the dietician are recommended yearly or more frequently if circumstances warrant (e.g., young child or toddler, desired weight loss, initiating pump therapy, etc.).

Diabetes Education

Diabetes education is an ongoing process with continuous need for review of previously learned material and introduction of new concepts as the family develops a more sophisticated understanding of intensive diabetes management. The educator should evaluate the patient and his or her caregiver's knowledge and skills regularly. In addition, age-appropriate issues need to be discussed as the patient matures (e.g., driving guidelines, issues related to alcohol and smoking, etc.). Diabetes education needs to be tailored to each family taking into account their educational level and cultural practices. The educator must be sensitive to the age and developmental stage of the child or adolescent, and shift his or her educational efforts from the caregiver(s) to the adolescent when it is developmentally appropriate. Continued parental involvement and supervision of the adolescent with diabetes is crucial to good metabolic control.

The health care provider should complete a focused interval history at each visit that includes recent illnesses, visits to the emergency department, hospitalizations, medications prescribed other than insulin, types of insulin and current doses, daily routine including meal plan and activity level, self-care behaviors and identifying who performs them, episodes of hypoglycemia and their precipitants, school performance, emotional health, and a review of systems focusing on symptoms of hyperglycemia (polyuria, polydipsia, polyphagia,

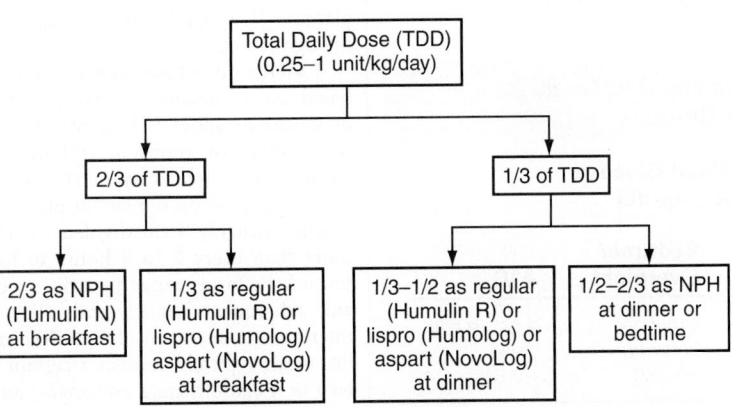

FIGURE 1. Initiation of Insulin Replacement Therapy. Two thirds of the total daily dose (TDD) is given at breakfast and further divided into NPH (two thirds) and short/rapid-acting insulin (one third). The remaining one third is either given in one injection at dinner (in a twice-daily regimen) or divided between dinner and bedtime (in a thrice-daily regimen), and should also be divided into NPH (two thirds) and short/rapid-acting insulin (one third). Short/rapid-acting insulin can be regular (Humulin R), lispro (Humalog), or aspart (NovoLog).

weight loss, candidal infections) and the possible development of other autoimmune disorders. If appropriate, a history of tobacco, alcohol, recreational drugs, and sexual activity should be elicited. A focused physical examination that includes measurement of blood pressure and heart rate, weight, height, body mass index (BMI), and examination of the thyroid gland, sites of blood glucose monitoring, and insulin injections should be completed at each visit. A more thorough physical examination including Tanner staging should be performed once per year or more frequently if indicated.

The hemoglobin A1C, the fraction of hemoglobin that has glucose attached to it, is a measure of the average level of blood glucose over the preceding 2 to 3 months. It should be measured every 3 months and serves as an objective measure of blood glucose control. A discrepancy between the hemoglobin A1C and the average blood glucose levels from self-monitoring records suggests that the patient needs to monitor at different times of day, may benefit from a review of blood glucose monitoring technique and equipment, or there may be fabrication of results. Obtaining computer downloaded data helps eliminate the latter possibility.

Goals of Therapy

The Diabetes Control and Complications Trial (DCCT) demonstrated that the incidence of microvascular complications was reduced with improved blood glucose control (hemoglobin A1C approximately 7%). The reduction in complications, however, was accompanied by an increased risk of severe hypoglycemia. Because young children are more vulnerable to hypoglycemia (reduced catecholamine response to hypoglycemia, decreased ability to communicate symptoms of hypoglycemia, and risk for neuropsychologic impairment from hypoglycemia), the ADA has developed age-specific glycemic targets (Table 2).

Insulin Therapy

The ideal insulin replacement therapy would be one that mirrors the basal and prandial insulin secretion in individuals without diabetes. Numerous insulin preparations are available that vary in time to onset, peak, and duration of action (Table 3). No single regimen is superior to another; thus individualization of the insulin regimen to the child or adolescent and family remains a major determinant. Important factors for consideration include blood glucose monitoring frequency, number of daily injections the family can perform, the need for flexibility in meal planning, and the unique family schedule. Regimens range in intensity from twice-a-day injections with a set dose of premixed insulin to intensive diabetes management with multiple injections per day of two or more types of insulin or use of an insulin pump (continuous subcutaneous insulin infusion [CSII]).

TABLE 2 Blood Glucose and A1C Goals for Type 1 Diabetes by Age Group

| Age Group | Plasma Blood Glucose Range (mg/dL) | | |
	Before Meals	Bedtime/ Overnight	A1C
<6 y	100–180	110–200	7.5%–8.5%
6–12 y	90–180	100–180	<8%
13–19 y	90–130	90–150	<7.5%

Adapted from American Diabetes Association: Care of children and adolescents with type 1 diabetes. Diabetes Care 2005;28(1):186–212.
Goals should be individualized; lower goals may be reasonable and achievable without hypoglycemia.
Goals should be higher in patients with frequent hypoglycemia or hypoglycemia unawareness.

CURRENT THERAPY

Examples of Insulin Regimens

Injections bid:
- Insulin mixtures (70/30, 75/25) given at breakfast and dinner
- NPH and rapid- or short-acting insulin given at breakfast and dinner

Injections tid:
- NPH and rapid- or short-acting insulin given at breakfast, rapid- or short-acting insulin given at dinner, and NPH given at bedtime
- NPH and rapid- or short-acting insulin given at breakfast, rapid- or short-acting insulin given at dinner, and NPH or glargine (Lantus) given at bedtime

Injections qid:
- NPH and rapid-acting insulin given at breakfast, rapid-acting insulin given at lunch and dinner, and rapid-acting insulin and NPH given at bedtime
- NPH and rapid-acting insulin given at breakfast and lunch, rapid-acting insulin given at dinner, and NPH given at bedtime
- Rapid-acting insulin given at breakfast, lunch, and dinner, and glargine (Lantus) given at breakfast, dinner, or bedtime

Continuous subcutaneous insulin infusion (CSII)
- Rapid-acting insulin given for basal requirements and as bolus at every meal/snack and periodically to correct hyperglycemia (no more frequent than q2–3h)

The typical regimen that children or adolescents begin at diagnosis was described previously (Figure 1). Some centers initiate a basal-bolus regimen in which insulin is replaced in a manner that attempts to mimic physiologic insulin release. Basal-bolus regimens include the insulin pump and glargine (Lantus) given once a day with rapid-acting insulin (lispro [Humalog] or aspart [NovoLog]) before each meal/snack and as needed for correction of hyperglycemia. The school-age child who hopes to avoid an injection at lunch often benefits from a regimen of glargine (Lantus) at dinner or bedtime, along with NPH (Humulin N) and a rapid-acting insulin at breakfast, plus a rapid-acting insulin at dinner. The peak of the NPH covers carbohydrate intake at lunch. The use of basal insulin analogue glargine (Lantus) in the evening is associated with less nocturnal hypoglycemia.

Patients on a basal-bolus regimen determine their insulin doses based on an insulin-to-carbohydrate ratio and a correction factor or sensitivity index (CF or SI). The insulin-to-carbohydrate ratio is the number of grams of carbohydrate covered by 1 U of insulin (roughly 450 divided by TDD) for each meal and snack. The CF/SI is the expected decrement in glucose following 1 U of rapid-acting insulin (roughly 1650 divided by TDD). The CF/SI is applied no more than every 2 to 3 hours to lower an elevated blood glucose toward the target range to avoid so-called stacking of insulin action and subsequent hypoglycemia. For patients on a combination of intermediate-acting insulin (NPH) and rapid- or short-acting insulin, meals typically contain a certain amount of carbohydrates (e.g., 60 g or 4 carbohydrate exchanges) and require consistency in timing to avoid hypoglycemia.

The CSII, otherwise known as insulin pump therapy, comes the closest to mimicking the basal and prandial insulin secretion of an individual without diabetes. The insulin pump is steadily becoming a commonly used method to replace insulin, especially in the pediatric population. There are many advantages to the insulin pump

TABLE 3 Insulin Analogues

Insulin Preparation	Onset of Action	Peak Action	Effective Duration
Rapid Acting			
Insulin lispro	5–15 min	30–90 min	2–4 h
Insulin aspart	5–10 min	60–180 min	3–5 h
Insulin glulisine*	5–15 min	30–90 min	3–5 h
Short Acting			
Regular (soluble insulin)	30–60 min	2–3 h	3–6 h
Intermediate Acting			
Lente (insulin zinc preparation)†	3–4 h	4–12 h	12–18 h
NPH (isophane insulin)	2–4 h	4–10 h	10–16 h
Long Acting			
Ultralente (extended insulin zinc preparation)†	4–6 h	8–20 h	20–24 h
Insulin glargine	1.1 h	None	24 h
Insulin detemir*	2–3 h	6–14 h	16–24 h
Insulin Mixtures			
70/30 human mix‡	30–60 min	dual	10–16 h
(70% NPH, 30% regular)			
70/30 aspart analogue mix	5–15 min	dual	10–16 h
(70% intermediate, 30% aspart)‡			
75/25 lispro analog mix‡ (75% intermediate, 25% lispro)	5–15 min	dual	10–16 h
50/50 human mix (50% NPH, 50% regular)	30–60 min	dual	10–16 h

In many countries, including the United States, insulin preparations contain 100 U/mL and are referred to as U-100 insulin. Highly concentrated U-500 short-acting insulin is available and used primarily in adults with severe insulin resistance.

Profiles for each insulin preparation are reasonable estimates only, based on data from adult study participants. There is variation between individuals, and time of onset, peak, and duration are also affected by size of dose, site and depth of injection, dilution, exercise, and temperature.

*FDA approved for adult use only.

†Recently discontinued by manufacturer (Lilly); estimated to be available until end of 2005.

‡Typically used in fixed doses in twice-a-day insulin regimens.

including the elimination of multiple daily injections, increased flexibility in meal planning, ease of decreasing insulin for physical activity, fewer hypoglycemic events, and the ability to deliver very small amounts of insulin. The disadvantages are more frequent blood glucose monitoring, always being tethered to the pump, and increased risk for the development of DKA. Because only rapid-acting insulin (lispro [Humalog] or aspart [NovoLog]) is used in the insulin pump, discontinuation of insulin delivery can result in ketone production within hours. Increased vigilance, therefore, is necessary to ensure proper functioning of the insulin pump with frequent blood glucose monitoring and checking for ketones if hyperglycemia develops.

Self-Monitoring

One of the main goals of diabetes education is to teach and empower the patient and family in the self-management of diabetes. Self-management of diabetes includes measuring blood glucose and blood/urine ketone levels, recording the results along with amount of carbohydrate intake and amount of insulin administered, and the ability to make insulin dosing decisions based on the interpretation of these records. Monitoring blood glucose four or more times daily is recommended in children with T1D. Additional monitoring may be necessary postprandially, overnight, or during periods of increased physical activity to help optimize control and prevent severe hypoglycemia. Preschool or early school-age children may require more frequent monitoring because of their inability to recognize symptoms or to communicate during episodes of hypoglycemia. In addition, children and adolescents using the insulin pump typically check their blood sugar six or more times per day. Ketone measurements should be done whenever the blood glucose is greater than 250 to 300 mg/dL and/or if the patient is ill, especially with nausea, vomiting, or abdominal pain. Ketones can be measured either in the urine (acetoacetate and acetone) or blood (β-hydroxybutyric acid). Measurement of blood ketones is now available on a home meter and is the preferred method in the current era stressing blood glucose monitoring. The key to successful intensive diabetes management is frequent blood glucose monitoring, good record keeping, and communication of these results with the diabetes team at frequent intervals so that timely modifications can be made to the insulin regimen and/or meal plan.

Medical Nutrition Therapy

The meal plan remains an important component of management aimed at good glycemic control, although it is often the most difficult aspect of intensive diabetes management for families. A dietician trained in pediatric nutrition and diabetes should meet with the family at the time of T1D diagnosis and periodically thereafter. The dietician should help develop a meal plan that is individualized to the patient's daily schedule, food preferences, cultural influences, and physical activity. The meal plan is more likely to be successful if it is designed to fit into the family's already established schedule and preferences. The patient and family should also be instructed on carbohydrate counting so that either carbohydrate exchanges or insulin-to-carbohydrate ratios can be used. Like the child without diabetes, the total number of recommended calories follows the child's growth requirements along with consideration of the need for weight gain or loss. Growth velocity, weight gain, and BMI should be monitored at every visit to ensure that the meal plan is sufficient to meet the energy requirements of the patient. Unexpected weight loss or poor weight gain should prompt consideration of suboptimal metabolic control, as well as eating disorders, thyroid dysfunction, or gastrointestinal disease.

The ADA does not have pediatric specific guidelines for medical nutrition therapy, but the recommendations for adults can be extrapolated to children. The ADA recommends that carbohydrates provide 45% to 65% of total calories, with protein and fat contributing 15% and 30%, respectively. The patient and family should be educated to avoid foods high in cholesterol, saturated fat, and concentrated sweets and select foods high in complex carbohydrate and dietary fiber.

All children and adolescents are recommended to have three meals per day. If they receive intermediate-acting insulin preparations, they should also receive three snacks per day (morning, afternoon, and bedtime) to match anticipated peaks of insulin action. If the child or adolescent is on a basal-bolus regimen, snacks are optional and require insulin coverage based on insulin-to-carbohydrate ratios.

Exercise

Exercise, or periods of sustained physical activity, can be beneficial to the patient by contributing to a sense of well-being, helping achieve the recommended BMI, improving glycemic control (exercise enhances insulin sensitivity), improving the lipid panel (increasing HDL), and lowering blood pressure and improving cardiovascular fitness. All children and adolescents, especially those with diabetes, should be encouraged to participate in routine physical activity.

The child or adolescent with diabetes needs to take precautions to avoid hypoglycemia during periods of increased physical activity. The patient and family need to check blood glucose before the initiation of activity, every hour during sustained activity, and at the completion of physical activity. For the first several days of increased activity, the child should also check his or her blood sugar frequently during the 12-hour postexercise period because there is often a delayed drop in the blood glucose following exercise (i.e., the lag effect). Some children require additional carbohydrate before, during, and after activity; lower insulin doses on the days of increased physical activity; or both. It is suggested that the child take 5 to 15 g of carbohydrates, depending on age and exercise intensity, before exercise if the blood sugar is below target, and repeat the 5 to 15 g of carbohydrate for every 30 minutes of sustained activity. Rapid-acting carbohydrate should be readily available, and coaches and trainers should be aware of the diagnosis of diabetes and trained in the treatment of hypoglycemia.

Psychosocial Support

The mental health professional is an important member of the diabetes team. A thorough family assessment generally accompanies the diabetes diagnosis with appropriate referrals for additional services as needed. Thereafter, children or adolescents should be referred back to a mental health professional if social, emotional, or economic barriers to the achievement of good glycemic control are identified. Family conflict, especially conflict over diabetes care, can be associated with deterioration in glycemic control. Encouragement of ongoing family teamwork in the management of childhood diabetes promotes successful outcomes with respect to glycemic control, reducing diabetes-specific conflict, and preventing acute complications and emergency assessments.

Sick Day Management

The goals for the management of children and adolescents during sick days are never omit insulin, prevent dehydration and hypoglycemia, monitor blood glucose frequently (every 2 to 4 hours), monitor for ketosis, provide supplemental rapid- or short-acting insulin doses (5% to 20% of TDD) depending on degree of hyperglycemia and ketosis, treat underlying illness, and have frequent contact with the diabetes team. The majority of DKA among children or adolescents with established diabetes is caused by insulin omission or errors in administration of insulin. Inadequate insulin therapy in the context of an intercurrent illness accounts for the remaining small percentage. Although it is more common for children to require more insulin during illnesses, some children require a reduction of the basal and/or rapid-acting insulin dose if he or she is unable to eat and the blood glucose is less than 200 mg/dL.

Families need to be educated about symptoms that warrant immediate medical attention, including signs of dehydration (dry mouth, sunken eyes, cracked lips, weight loss, dry skin), persistent vomiting for more than 2 to 4 hours, persistence of blood glucose levels greater than 300 mg/dL or ketones for more than 12 hours, or symptoms of DKA (nausea, abdominal pain, chest pain, vomiting, ketotic breath, hyperventilation, or altered consciousness). It is helpful for the diabetes team to review sick day management annually with the family (can accompany flu immunization) to avoid metabolic decompensation during intercurrent illness.

Hypoglycemia

Fear of hypoglycemia can be a common occurrence in the management of childhood diabetes, especially among caregivers, and can be a barrier to optimal glycemic control. Recognition and treatment of hypoglycemia are important topics for diabetes education. Families are trained to treat hypoglycemia with 10 to 15 g of rapid-acting carbohydrate, recheck blood glucose in 15 minutes, repeat treatment with 10 to 15 g if blood sugar remains below target, and follow with a protein-containing snack if a meal will not follow within 1 to 2 hours. This technique avoids the natural tendency to overtreat low blood glucose levels. Caregivers should also receive glucagon training (20 to 30 μg/kg; maximum 1 mg) for severe hypoglycemia and low-dose glucagon (1 U on an insulin syringe for every year of life up to 15 years) for impending hypoglycemia, for example, in the context of a gastrointestinal illness or inadvertent insulin administration (lispro given instead of NPH). A member of the diabetes team should assess frequency, treatment, awareness, and circumstances of hypoglycemia at each visit.

Screening for Diabetes-Related Complications

Patients, families, and caregivers worry about the risk of diabetes-related complications, and therefore the diabetes team must educate families and screen for complications with sensitivity and optimism, emphasizing prevention of complications and the maintenance of health. Screening for nephropathy, hypertension, dyslipidemia, and retinopathy are indicated.

Microalbuminuria (MA) is the first sign of diabetic nephropathy, and patients who develop persistent MA are at increased risk of progression to macroalbuminuria. Poor glycemic control, smoking, and a family history of essential hypertension are risk factors for the development of MA and nephropathy. Identification of persistent MA provides an opportunity for intervention and prevention of progressive renal disease through improvements in glycemic control and/or therapy with angiotensin-converting enzyme (ACE) inhibitors. There are currently no pediatric data on the use of angiotensin receptor blockers (ARBs). Table 4 outlines definitions, screening recommendations, and treatment.

Hypertension is an important predictor of the progression of diabetic nephropathy to end-stage renal disease. Hypertension in children and adolescents may go unrecognized because providers are not familiar with the gender-, age-, and height-specific definitions. Blood pressure should be measured every 3 months with standardized technique, using the proper size cuff. If elevated blood pressures are detected and confirmed, the first step is to exclude causes not related to diabetes. Table 4 outlines the definitions, screening recommendations, and treatment.

Dyslipidemia and diabetes are established risk factors for cardiovascular disease, and recent research suggests that a significant proportion of adolescents with diabetes already have evidence of atherosclerosis. Low-density lipoprotein (LDL) cholesterol is most closely associated with cardiovascular disease, and therefore, the ADA has developed guidelines for LDL cholesterol. Screening may be delayed until puberty if family history is negative for cardiovascular disease. A lipid profile should be performed on prepubertal children with diabetes who are older than 2 years if there is a positive family history of cardiovascular disease or if the family history is unknown. If the LDL cholesterol is less than 100 mg/dL, screening

TABLE 4 Screening for Diabetes-Related Complications

Complication	How to Screen	Definition	When to Screen	Therapy
Microalbuminuria	Spot urine sample timed overnight or 24-h collection	Spot urine albumin/creatinine ratio 30–299 µg/g or AER 20–199 µg/min from timed collection	Annual screening begins at 10 y or after ≥5 y duration of diabetes	Optimize glucose control, smoking cessation, normalize BP
Persistent microalbuminuria		2/3 of urine samples meet above criteria		Above, plus addition of ACE inhibitor
High-normal BP	Manual BP measurement with standard technique	Systolic or diastolic BP within the 90th–95th percentile for age, gender, and height	At every clinic visit	Dietary intervention, weight control, and exercise; if target BP not reached within 3–6 mo, then initiate pharmacologic therapy
Hypertension		Systolic or diastolic BP above the 95th percentile for age, gender, and height, or >130/80 on ≥3 occasions (whichever is lower)		Above, plus pharmacologic therapy titrated to achieve target BP

Note: Urine collection should not be performed following vigorous exercise, during an acute infection, during a female patient's menstrual cycle, or following an episode of severe hypoglycemia. Once angiotensin-converting enzyme (ACE) inhibitor is started, microalbumin excretion should be monitored q3–6 mo. Target BP is <130/80 or <90th percentile for age, gender, and height. Initial drug treatment is ACE inhibition.
Abbreviations: AER = albumin excretion rate; BP = blood pressure.

can be repeated every 5 years. The mainstay of therapy for dyslipidemia is dietary management (saturated fat less than 7% of calories and less than 200 mg/day of cholesterol). Children with levels between 130 and 159 mg/dL should be started on medication if diet and lifestyle modification are unsuccessful after 6 months or if the child has additional risk factors for cardiovascular disease, such as obesity or hypertension. Pharmacotherapy is recommended if the LDL cholesterol is more than 160 mg/dL. The LDL goal for children with diabetes is less than 100 mg/dL.

Diabetic retinopathy is a feared complication because it is the leading cause of vision loss. According to the ADA, the first ophthalmologic exam should be requested when the child is 10 years or older and has had diabetes for more than 3 to 5 years. Examinations with an eye care professional with expertise in diabetic retinopathy should occur early.

Screening for Other Autoimmune Diseases

Children and adolescents with T1D are at an increased risk for other autoimmune diseases and should be screened accordingly. Approximately 15% of patients with T1D also have autoimmune thyroid disease. All children and adolescents should be screened for autoimmune thyroid disease at the time of diabetes diagnosis once metabolic control is established. TSH measurement is a useful initial screen, with and without measuring the presence of thyroid autoantibodies. Screening should be repeated yearly or if there is any clinical suspicion of thyroid disease (abnormal growth rate, symptoms of hypo- or hyperthyroidism, goiter on examination, erratic blood glucose control).

Another commonly associated disorder is celiac disease. Nearly 6% of patients with T1D have elevated levels of circulating autoantibodies to tissue transglutaminase. Celiac disease can cause diarrhea, weight loss or failure to gain weight, abdominal pain, fatigue, and unexplained hypoglycemia or erratic blood glucose secondary to malabsorption. Patients with T1D should be screened with circulating IgA autoantibody to tissue transglutaminase. A quantitative serum IgA level should be drawn at the same time to rule out IgA deficiency as a cause for falsely low IgA tissue transglutaminase levels. Positive antibodies should be confirmed with a second measurement, and if positive, a referral should be made to a gastroenterologist for small bowel biopsy. If the diagnosis is confirmed, celiac disease is treated with a gluten-free diet with recommendations and support from a registered dietician with pediatric expertise in diabetes and celiac management.

Type 2 Diabetes Mellitus in Youth

With the increasing prevalence of childhood obesity during the last two decades, there is an increased occurrence of T2D in youth. Based on National Health and Nutrition Examination survey data, the prevalence of overweight children (defined as a body mass index greater than the 95th percentile for children and youth) increased from 5% in the 1970s to more than 15% by 1999. The epidemic of obesity follows the increased consumption of fast foods, increased consumption of soft drinks, increased sedentary behavior with more television watching, and decreased physical activity. Mirroring this epidemic of childhood obesity is the occurrence of T2D in children and adolescents. Before 1990, T2D in youth was a rare occurrence. By 2000, between 8% and 45% of all newly diagnosed cases of childhood diabetes were caused by T2D. T2D occurs most commonly in those with a family history of T2D; individuals from certain racial and ethnic minority groups including Native Americans, Hispanics, African Americans, and Asian and Pacific Islanders; those with obesity falling above the 85th percentile for BMI based on age and gender; and in association with markers of insulin resistance (Table 5). Markers of insulin resistance include the occurrence of acanthosis nigricans and polycystic ovarian syndrome (PCOS). In addition, other well-known risk factors include hypertension and hyperlipidemia.

As noted earlier, the diagnosis of T2D is based on fasting plasma glucose (FPG), 2-hour glucose value during an OGTT, or a casual glucose level. Because T2D often goes without symptoms, individuals who are overweight, have a positive family history of T2D, come from one of the high-risk racial and ethnic minority groups, and/or have markers of insulin resistance warrant screening for T2D. Screening can be performed with a FPG or OGTT when clinical concerns are high and the FPG is normal.

Currently one oral medication is approved for the treatment of T2D in youth. This medication is metformin (Glucophage), which is also available in a liquid formulation. The maximum recommended daily dose of metformin (Glucophage) in youth is 2000 mg/day divided as 1000 mg twice daily. Often patients with

Diabetes Mellitus in Children and Adolescents

TABLE 5 Risk Factors and Screening for Type 2 Diabetes in Children

Criteria	Age of Initiation	Frequency	Method
Overweight (BMI >85th percentile for age and gender), weight for height >85th percentile, or weight >120% of ideal for height Plus 2 of the following risk factors: Family history of T2D in 1st- or 2nd-degree relative Race/ethnicity (American Indian, African American, Hispanic, Asian/ Pacific Islander) Signs of or conditions associated with insulin resistance (acanthosis nigricans, PCOS, HTN, dyslipidemia)	10 y or at pubertal onset if puberty occurs at a younger age	q2y	Fasting plasma glucose

Adapted from American Diabetes Association: Type 2 diabetes in children. Diabetes Care 2000;23(3):381–389.
Note: Clinical judgment should be used to test for diabetes in high-risk patients who do not meet these criteria.
Abbreviations: BMI = body mass index; T2D = type 2 diabetes; HTN = hypertension; PCOS = polycystic ovarian syndrome.

TABLE 6 Medications to Treat Type 2 Diabetes

Class	Mechanism of Action	Adverse Effects
Biguanides (metformin)*	Decrease hepatic glucose production Increase peripheral glucose disposal	Gastrointestinal upset Lactic acidosis
Sulfonylureas (glimepiride, glyburide, glipizide)	Insulin secretagogues	Hypoglycemia Weight gain
Meglitinides (repaglinide, nateglinide)	Insulin secretagogues	Hypoglycemia Weight gain
α-Glucosidase inhibitors (acarbose)	Decrease gut carbohydrate absorption	Gastrointestinal upset
Thiazolidinediones (rosiglitazone and pioglitazone)	Decrease hepatic glucose production Increase peripheral glucose disposal	Weight gain Edema Increased liver enzymes Anemia

*Metformin (Glucophage) is the only medication with FDA approval for use in children.

T2D present in ketoacidosis and require initial insulin therapy. The goal of management of the child with T2D is initial stabilization often with insulin therapy, metformin (Glucophage) directed at managing the insulin resistance, and education. Once glucose levels are stabilized, insulin dosage may be lowered along with continued treatment with metformin (Glucophage) and approaches to lifestyle management. Lifestyle management involves a healthy diet, increasing exercise, and decreasing sedentary behaviors.

Other medications used to treat T2D include second-generation sulfonylureas, meglitinides, thiazolidinediones, and α-glucosidase inhibitors, none of which is currently approved for use in pediatric patients. There is ongoing studies to assess the efficacy and safety of these medications (Table 6).

REFERENCES

American Diabetes Association. Diagnosis and classification of diabetes mellitus. Diabetes Care 2005;28(Suppl 1):S37–42.
American Diabetes Association. Type 2 diabetes in children. Diabetes Care 2000;23(3):381–9.
Barroso I. Genetics of type 2 diabetes. Diabet Med 2005;22:517–35.
Dunger DB, Sperling MA, Acerini CL, et al. ESPE/LWPES consensus statement on diabetic ketoacidosis in children and adolescents. Arch Dis Child 2004;89:188–94.
Fox LA, Buckloh LM, Smith SD, et al. A randomized controlled trial of insulin pump therapy in young children with type 1 diabetes. Diabetes Care 2005;28:1277–81.
Glaser N, Barnett P, McCaslin 1, et al. The Pediatric Emergency Medicine Collaborative Research Committee of the American Academy of Pediatrics. N Engl J Med 2001;344(4):264–9.
Goodwin G, Volkening LK, Laffel LM. Younger age at onset of type 1 diabetes in concordant sibling pairs is associated with increased risk for autoimmune thyroid disease. Diabetes Care 2006;29(6):1397–8.
Hannon TS, Rao G, Arslanian SA. Childhood obesity and type 2 diabetes mellitus. Pediatrics 2005;116(2):473–80.
Hirsch IB. Insulin analogues. N Engl J Med 2005;352:174–83.
Laffel LM, Vangsness L, Connell A, et al. Impact of ambulatory, family-focused teamwork intervention on glycemic control in youth with type 1 diabetes. J Pediatr 2003;142(4):409–16.
Rosenbloom AL. Cerebral edema in diabetic ketoacidosis and other acute devastating complications: Recent observations. Pediatr Diabetes 2005;6:41–9.
Silverstein J, Klingensmith G, Copeland K, et al. American Diabetes Association: Care of children and adolescents with type 1 diabetes. Diabetes Care 2005;28(1):186–212.
Wysocki T, Harris MA, Mauras N, et al. Absence of adverse effects of severe hypoglycemia on cognitive function in school-aged children with diabetes over 18 months. Diabetes Care 2003;26(4):1100–5.

Diabetic Ketoacidosis

Method of
*Isaiah D. Wexler, MD, PhD, and
David Zangen, MD*

Diabetic ketoacidosis (DKA) and the hyperglycemic hyperosmolar state (HHS) are two acute life-threatening complications associated with diabetes mellitus (DM). The mortality for DKA is declining, but it remains high for HHS. The morbidity and mortality are also higher at the extremes of age, possibly because of the delay in diagnosis or because of the presence of comorbid conditions, especially among the elderly.

Classically, DKA was considered a complication of type 1 DM (T1DM) and HHS of type 2 DM (T2DM). However, there is significant overlap, and children and adults with T2DM can present with DKA (especially among the nonwhite population), and HHS can occur in those with T1DM. Both DKA and HHS may be the presenting manifestation of new-onset diabetes.

Diagnosis

The diagnosis of DKA and HHS is laboratory based, but there are clinical manifestations that suggest the diagnosis. For both HHS and DKA, there are signs of dehydration and hypovolemia. However, as the dehydration in these entities is hypertonic, signs such as significant tachycardia and low blood pressure may only be prominent in advanced DKA and HHS. In DKA, there is a fruity or acetone smell to the breath, emesis, and abdominal pain, and when the pH is especially low (<7.1), the breathing pattern may be aberrant (Kussmaul breathing). Mental status changes can occur in both DKA and HHS, and patients may be frankly obtunded and even comatose. In HHS, the changes in sensorium may be gradual, and the index of suspicion for HHS should be high, especially in elderly or moribund patients with unexplained changes in mental status.

The diagnostic criteria for DKA and HHS are based on blood glucose, osmolarity, pH, serum bicarbonate, and the presence of significant ketosis as manifested by high levels of serum or urine ketones. The presence of acidosis defined as an arterial blood pH less than 7.3 and or serum bicarbonate less than 15 mmol, or both, in children and adults distinguish DKA from HHS. When the bicarbonate is in the range of 15 to 18 mmol, other criteria including the degree of ketonemia and ketonuria assist in the diagnosis of DKA. Serum bicarbonate is often a more accurate indication because the arterial pH is also affected by the ventilatory rate. For a diagnosis of HHS, the blood glucose must be greater than 600 mg/dL and the effective serum osmolality greater than 320 mOsm/L (which can be calculated by the formula $2 \times$ serum Na [mEq/L] + serum glucose [mg/dL]/18). In HHS, the fluid and electrolytes losses are often more severe than in DKA. The presence of ketones in the urine does not negate the diagnosis of HHS.

Treatment

PRECIPITATING CAUSES

Key elements in the treatment of DKA and HHS are the identification of precipitating causes and stabilization of the patient. The pathophysiologic basis of hyperglycemic crisis is insulinopenia and elevation of counter-regulatory stress hormones including catecholamines, cortisol, and growth hormone. Among patients with an established diagnosis of DM, infection (even mild) and noncompliance with the medical regimen are the leading causes of DKA and HHS. As the use of insulin pumps is increasing, pump malfunction or misuse has also become a more common cause of DKA. A source of infection should be sought in any patient presenting with DKA.

Abdominal pain, which is often attributed to ketosis, may be a manifestation of acute appendicitis or pelvic inflammatory disease. Conversely, the diagnosis of DKA may be delayed because abdominal pain is attributed to an acute abdominal process.

Other factors associated with DKA and HHS include cardiovascular disease and the use of medications such as corticosteroids, thiazides, and sympathomimetic agents. DKA and HHS have also been associated with the use of atypical (second-generation) antipsychotic agents. Cocaine use has been found to precipitate DKA.

HHS can often occur in obtunded or intellectually limited persons whose fluid intake is restricted. Fluid restriction can precipitate dehydration and decreased renal function, leading to both hyperglycemia and hyperosmolarity.

Identification and treatment of the precipitating cause of DKA and HHS are extremely important because it is often difficult to stabilize the patient if the precipitant is not dealt with appropriately.

MANAGEMENT

The management of DKA and HHS is based on repairing the fluid deficit and correcting the metabolic derangements. The mainstay of DKA management is fluid replacement and insulin administration. Other supporting interventions include providing potassium and, when clinically indicated, phosphate and bicarbonate. Most patients respond well to treatment if it is instituted in a timely fashion. Pitfalls associated with the treatment of hyperglycemic crises include excessive fluids; inappropriate administration of insulin, bicarbonate, or potassium; and iatrogenically induced hypoglycemia.

In recent years, the American Diabetic Association, the Lawson Wilkins Pediatric Endocrine Society, and the European Society for Pediatric Endocrinology have developed consensus evidence-based protocols for treating DKA and HHS. These protocols are summarized in Tables 1 to 3. The basis for these protocols is discussed below.

Fluids

Patients with DKA and HHS often have a fluid deficit of 100 to 200 mL/kg of body weight. Patients with hyperglycemic crises can present with severe hypovolemic shock, and if signs of shock are present, patients should be given resuscitation fluids, usually with a 0.9% sodium chloride solution (normal saline). Normal saline is continued until the hemodynamic status is stabilized. Subsequently, 0.45% NaCl is substituted for normal saline to prevent sodium overload, especially in older patients who might have compromised cardiac function.

The rate of fluid administration is designed to correct the fluid deficits over 48 hours. In children, this means providing fluid at a rate that approximates 1.5 times the daily fluid maintenance requirement. For adults, the rate of fluid administration should be based on the hemodynamic and hydration status of the patient as determined by vital signs, the physical examination, urine output, and repeated measurements of renal function.

In patients with diminished cardiac or renal function, the rate of fluid administration might have to be modified, and in these situations, hemodynamic monitoring is appropriate. Caution needs to be exercised in terms of the amount of fluid administered, especially during the early hours of treatment, because excessive fluid administration has been associated with cerebral edema in children and adolescents, and it can cause fluid overload states or rapid osmotic shifts.

Insulin

Administration of insulin corrects hyperglycemia and the metabolic acidosis and ketosis of DKA. Many different modes of insulin administration have been used. Most authorities prefer providing insulin as an intravenous drip because this mode of delivery is easily regulated; there is a more-rapid attainment of pharmacologic levels of insulin in the blood. Intravenous administration of insulin is not associated with problems of absorption that can occur with insulin that is administered intramuscularly or subcutaneously, especially in states of dehydration and poor perfusion. Regular insulin has been the insulin of choice for treating hyperglycemic crises, but recent studies indicate that rapid-acting insulin analogues administered subcutaneously may be equally effective in the treatment of DKA in children and adults.

Optimally, the rate of decline for serum glucose levels should be between 50 and 75 mg/dL/hour so as to avoid rapid osmotic shifts. In some cases, serum glucose might not fall appropriately. This may be due to mistakes in preparing the insulin drip or failure to prime the tubing of the intravenous administration setup. Alternatively, the patient might have severe insulin resistance, excessive hepatic glucose production related to stress, or compromised renal function. In these situations, the insulin drip can be increased stepwise until the desired rate of serum glucose reduction is achieved. Too rapid a decline in the level of serum glucose may be the result of excessive fluid administration.

TABLE 1 Management of Diabetic Ketoacidosis and Hyperglycemic Hyperosmolar State in Children and Adolescents

Treatment	Precautions
Fluids	
Initial Treatment	
NS, 10–20 mL/kg during the first h	Amount of fluid administered depends on hydration status
	For a patient in shock, continue NS, 20 mL/kg/h until vital signs are stable
Subsequent Treatment	
Continue intravenous NS, 10 mL/kg/h for 1 h, then correct estimated fluid deficit over 48 h with 0.45% NaCl (usually at a rate equal to 1.5–2 times the daily maintenance requirement based on hydration status)	Overhydration must be avoided
	Do not exceed 3.5 L/m^2/24 h
	Use NS if patient has hyponatremia
Dextrose and Insulin	
Dextrose	
Add dextrose (5%) to 0.45% NaCl when serum glucose declines to ≤250 mg/dL	Maintain serum glucose at 150–250 mg/dL
	Might need to increase dextrose concentration to 10% if serum glucose is less than target levels
Insulin	
Intravenous regular insulin drip at a rate of 0.1 U/kg/h	If continuous intravenous insulin administration is not feasible, an
When pH is >7.25 and HCO$_3$ >15 mEq/L, lower insulin infusion to 0.05 U/kg/h until SC insulin therapy is begun	alternative is to give SC or IM rapid-acting insulin or short-acting analogues at a dose of 0.1 U/kg/h after an initial insulin bolus of 0.3 U/kg
Electrolytes	
Potassium	
Starting K$^+$ concentration in intravenous fluids 40 mEq/L	If serum K$^+$ <2.5 mEq/L, hold insulin drip, and administer KCl,
Maintain K$^+$ concentration at 3.5–5 mEq/L	1 mEq/kg over 1 h; continue until serum K$^+$ ≥2.5 mEq/L
If necessary, adjust K$^+$ concentrations in infusate to 20–40 mEq/L	If serum K$^+$ > 5 mEq/L, do not add KCl
	Some authorities recommend using both the chloride and phosphate salts of K$^+$ at a ratio of 2:1
Bicarbonate	
Only consider administering HCO$_3$ if pH <7.0	Do not administer HCO$_3$ if pH ≥7.0
HCO$_3$ 75 mEq should be added to a liter bag containing 0.45% NS and given at a rate that does not exceed 2 mEq/kg/h of HCO$_3$	
Monitoring	
Monitor vital signs and perform frequent neurologic examinations, including fundoscopic evaluation	Monitor blood gases, serum glucose, and serum electrolytes more frequently if pH < 7.0 or is not rising appropriately, serum glucose
Initially obtain blood gases, serum electrolytes including BUN and creatinine, glucose, and urinary ketones	is <150 mg/dL or declining at a rapid rate, and/or serum K$^+$ is <3.5 mEq/L or >5 mEq/L
ECG monitoring in severe DKA	Check neurologic signs for evidence of cerebral edema (e.g.,
Monitor fluid input, urine output, blood gases, electrolytes, and serum glucose every 2–4 h until stable	headache, drowsiness)

BUN = blood urea nitrogen; DKA = diabetic ketoacidosis; ECG = electrocardiogram; NS = normal saline.

Dextrose

A major challenge in the treatment of hyperglycemic crises is the prevention of treatment-induced hypoglycemia, which can lead to changes in the level of consciousness due to reduced glucose delivery to the brain. When serum glucose levels reach target levels as listed in the tables, dextrose as a 5% solution is added to the intravenous fluids. Sometimes, especially in children, 5% dextrose is not adequate to maintain serum glucose in the target range, and it may be necessary to increase the concentration of dextrose in the administered intravenous fluids. A common mistake made in managing DKA is to lower the rate of insulin administration as a means of regulating the serum glucose. The fallacy of this approach is that the reduction in insulin administration slows the correction of acidosis and ketosis.

Potassium

During DKA and its treatment, there are significant shifts in total body and serum potassium. Before treatment, there is significant depletion of total body potassium associated with polyuria, but at the same time, the acidosis associated with DKA causes cellular extrusion of potassium into the blood, leading to an increase in serum potassium. During treatment of DKA, both insulin

administration and correction of the acidosis drive potassium back into cells, thereby lowering serum potassium. Because changes in serum potassium may be difficult to predict, it is important to monitor serum potassium at the time of admission and frequently during treatment. Potassium should not be administered when the serum potassium is too high, and potassium replacement should be given simultaneously with insulin if serum potassium is low or even in the normal range (see Tables 1 and 2 for specific guidelines). Electrocardiogram monitoring is useful for early detection of potentially symptomatic hyperkalemia or hypokalemia.

Phosphate

Similar to serum potassium, there is a significant depletion in cellular phosphate as a result of acidosis and derangements associated with hyperglycemic crises, and serum phosphate declines during treatment. Phosphate is an important molecule for energy metabolism, and severe hypophosphatemia is associated with muscle weakness, diminished cardiac contractility, and respiratory insufficiency. Reduced 2,3-diphosphoglycerate concentrations resulting from hypophosphatemia can impair tissue oxygenation. Repletion of phosphate remains a theoretical benefit because no clinical trials have conclusively shown a benefit to phosphate administration for treating hyperglycemic crises. However,

TABLE 2 Management of Diabetic Ketoacidosis in Adults

Treatment	Precautions
Fluids	
Initial Treatment	
NS, 1 L/h for 1 h or until hemodynamically stable	Hemodynamic monitoring if evidence of cardiogenic or severe hypovolemic shock
	Rate of fluid administration may have to be modified in patients with cardiac compromise
Subsequent Treatment	
Patients with high or normal serum Na^+ should receive 0.45% NaCl at a rate of 250–500 mL/h depending on hydration status	Use NS in place of 0.45 NaCl if patient has hyponatremia
Continue fluid therapy until patient's hydration status is stabilized and the patient can take oral feeds	
Dextrose and Insulin	
Dextrose	
Add dextrose (5%) to 0.45% NaCl when serum glucose declines to ≤200 mg/dL	Maintain serum glucose at 150–200 mg/dL by adjusting the rate of fluid infusion (150–250 mL/h) and insulin administration (0.05–0.1 U/kg/h)
Insulin	
Intravenous regular insulin drip is initially administered as a bolus of 0.1 U/kg and then continued at a rate of 0.1 U/kg/h	An alternative is to give SC rapid-acting insulin short-acting analogues with an initial bolus of 0.2 U/kg
Monitor serum glucose hourly and if rate of glucose decline is <50–75 mg/dL, double rate of insulin infusion every h until the glucose falls at a rate of 50–75 mg/dL/h	Subsequently, the patient is given SC or IM regular or short-acting analogue insulin at a rate of 0.1 U/kg every hour
Continue insulin and glucose intravenous treatment until metabolic stability is achieved (glucose <200 mg/dL, pH >7.30, and HCO_3 >18 mEq/L) and the patient can begin SC insulin treatments	Monitor serum glucose hourly and if rate of glucose decline is <50–75 mg/dL, double the dose of the hourly insulin injection
Electrolytes	
Potassium	
K^+ concentration in intravenous fluids is 20–30 mEq/L	If serum K^+ is <3.3 mEq/L, hold insulin and administer KCl, 20–30 mEq/h; continue until serum K^+ is ≥3.3 mEq/L
Maintain serum K^+ concentration at 4–5 mEq/L	If serum K^+ is >5.3 mEq/L, do not add K^+
	Some authorities recommend giving both the chloride and phosphate salts of K^+ at a ratio of 2:1
Bicarbonate	
Only consider administering HCO_3 if blood pH is ≤7.0	Do not administer HCO_3 if pH is >7.0
If pH is <6.9, give $NaHCO_3$ 100 mmol diluted in 400 mL of H_2O at a rate of 200 mL/h. For pH 6.9–7.0, administer $NaHCO_3$ 50 mmol in 200 mL of H_2O at a rate of 100 mL/h	
Continue administering HCO_3 until pH is >7.0	
Monitoring	
Monitor vital signs and perform frequent neurologic examinations, including fundoscopic evaluation	Monitor blood gases, serum glucose, and serum electrolytes more frequently if the pH is <7.0 or is not rising appropriately, serum glucose is <150 mg/dL or the rate is not falling appropriately, and/or serum K^+ is ≤3.3 or ≥5.3 mEq/L
Initially obtain blood gases, serum electrolytes, including BUN and creatinine, glucose, urinary ketones, and an ECG	Check hemodynamic, respiratory, and neurologic status for signs of overhydration
Monitor fluid input, urine output, blood gases, serum electrolytes, and serum glucose every 2–4 h until stable	

BUN = blood urea nitrogen; ECG = electrocardiogram; NS = normal saline.

it seems prudent to administer phosphate as a potassium salt (as detailed in the tables) to patients in whom the impact of hypophosphatemia may be significant, such as those with cardiac or pulmonary disease. If phosphate is administered, serum calcium should be monitored.

Bicarbonate

Significant controversy surrounds the use of bicarbonate in DKA. There is little evidence supporting a beneficial effect of bicarbonate administration in terms of improved outcomes, and there is some evidence from both clinical studies and animal models that the treatment of acidosis with bicarbonate might even be deleterious. Current recommendations are to not administer bicarbonate if the pH is 7.0 because insulin administration is sufficient to correct the acidosis. For cases in which the pH is less than 7.0, recommendations are less clear. If bicarbonate is to be administered, it should be done slowly, and by the methods listed in Tables 1 and 2.

MONITORING

The treatment of DKA and HHS is based on physiology, and with appropriate treatment, most patients will respond. Difficulties in the management of DKA and HHS usually result from too-aggressive treatment with fluids, electrolytes, insulin, or bicarbonate. To prevent such problems, it is very important to monitor the clinical and biochemical status of the patient. Clinically, the neurologic status of patients must be monitored closely. The sudden development of lethargy, obtundation, or headache can herald cerebral edema in pediatric patients. Respiratory difficulties, signs of congestive heart failure, or mental status changes can indicate fluid overload or rapid osmotic shifts. Biochemically, it is important to monitor response to treatment in terms of correcting the acidosis and lowering serum glucose. Patients are also at risk for electrolyte abnormalities and hypoglycemia, and frequent measurement of serum glucose and electrolytes, including phosphate, should be performed. Because the

TABLE 3 Management of Hyperglycemic Hyperosmolar State in Adults

Treatment	Precautions
Fluids	
Initial Treatment	
NS, 1 L/h for 1 h or until hemodynamically stable	Hemodynamic monitoring if evidence of cardiogenic or severe hypovolemic shock Rate of fluid administration might have to be modified in patients with cardiac compromise
Subsequent Treatment	
Patients with high or normal serum Na^+ should receive 0.45% NaCl at a rate of 250–500 mL/h depending on the hydration status Continue fluid therapy until patient's hydration status is stabilized, the serum osmolality is ≤315 mOsm/L, and the patient's mental status has returned to baseline	Use NS in place of 0.45 NaCl if patient has hyponatremia
Dextrose and Insulin	
Dextrose	
Add dextrose (5%) to 0.45% NaCl when serum glucose declines to ≤200–250 mg/dL	Maintain serum glucose at 150–200 mg/dL by adjusting the rate of fluid infusion (150–250 mL/h) and insulin administration (0.05–0.1 U/kg/h)
Insulin	
Intravenous regular insulin drip is initially administered as a bolus of 0.1 U/kg and then continued at a rate of 0.1 U/kg/h Monitor serum glucose hourly, and if rate of glucose decline is <50 mg/dL, double rate of insulin infusion every h until the serum glucose falls at a rate of 50–75 mg/dL/h When serum glucose falls under 300 mg/dL, reduce insulin infusion to 0.05–0.1 U/kg/h to maintain the serum glucose at 250–300 mg/dL Continue insulin and glucose IV treatment until serum glucose is stabilized at 250–300 mg/dL and the patient can begin SC insulin therapy	Monitor serum glucose frequently to avoid hypoglycemia. Clinical signs of hypoglycemia may be unapparent due to obtunded state and underlying neurologic disease
Electrolytes	
K^+ concentration in intravenous fluids is 20–30 mEq/L Maintain serum K^+ concentration at 4–5 mEq/L	If serum K+ is <3.3 mEq/L, hold insulin and administer KCl 20–30 mEq/h; continue until serum K+ is >3.3 mEq/L If serum K+ is >5 mEq/L, do not add K^+ Some authorities recommend giving both the chloride and phosphate salts of K^+ at a ratio of 2:1
Monitoring	
Initially obtain arterial blood gas, CBC, serum electrolytes including BUN and creatinine, glucose, urinalysis, and an ECG Obtain serum or calculated osmolality Monitor electrolytes, serum glucose, serum osmolality, fluid input, and urine output every 2–4 h until stable	Monitor more frequently if serum glucose is <250 mg/dL or the rate is not falling appropriately and/or serum K+ is ≤3.3 or ≥5.3 mEq/L Check hemodynamic, respiratory and neurologic status for signs of overhydration

BUN = blood urea nitrogen; CBC = complete blood count; ECG = electrocardiogram.

management of DKA and HHS is fairly complicated, it is imperative that there be a bedside flowchart in which vital signs, central nervous system status, fluid input, type of fluid, urine output, and laboratory values are recorded as a function of time.

Complications

Many of the complications of DKA, including hypoglycemia and hypokalemia, have been addressed.

A significant complication, most prevalent among the pediatric population, is cerebral edema. Cerebral edema developing during the course of treatment of DKA is a major cause of morbidity and mortality in children with DKA. The causes of cerebral edema are unclear, but studies suggest that it may be due to excessive fluid administration, especially during the early course of treatment, severity of the initial presentation, rapid osmotic shifts, or administration of bicarbonate. In cases in which cerebral edema is suspected (e.g., headache, lethargy, confusion), the rate of fluid administration should be decreased immediately and the patient should be carefully monitored. If there are clinical signs of cerebral edema (e.g., posturing, changes in papillary reflexes, Cushing's triad), mannitol

(Osmitrol) should be administered at a dose of 0.25 to 1.0 g/kg over 20 minutes. Alternatively, hypertonic saline (3%) can be given at a dose of 5 to 10 mL/kg over 30 minutes. The decision to intubate and hyperventilate patients with cerebral edema should be based on the clinical situation and in consultation with medical intensivists.

Adults should be monitored for pulmonary edema, cerebral edema, vascular accidents related to thrombotic conditions, hyperviscosity, and disseminated intravascular coagulation.

Summary

DKA and HHS, in most cases, remain preventable. Compliance with treatment, frequent monitoring, and close contact with a physician or diabetes health professionals during times of illness can reduce the frequency of DKA and HHS. Early consultation with a diabetologist is warranted at the beginning of an intercurrent illness and can often prevent development of DKA or HHS at the earliest stages. Patient education regarding the appropriate use of insulin, sick day management, early signs of DKA and HHS, drug interactions, and the dangers of certain recreational drugs will continue to have a major role in reducing the incidence of recurrent DKA or HHS.

REFERENCES

Dunger DB, Sperling MA, Acerini CL, et al. ESPE/LWPES consensus statement on diabetic ketoacidosis in children and adolescents. Arch Dis Child 2004;89:188–94.

Kitabchi AE, Nyenwe EA. Hyperglycemic crises in diabetes mellitus: Diabetic ketoacidosis and hyperglycemic hypersosmolar state. Endocrinol Metab Clin N Am 2006;35:725–51.

Kitabchi AE, Umpierrez GE, Murphy MB, Kreisberg RA. Hyperglycemic crises in adult patients with diabetes: A consensus statement from the American Diabetes Association. Diabetes Care 2006;29:2739–48.

Wolfsdorf J, Craig ME, Daneman D, et al. Diabetic ketoacidosis. ISPAD clinical practice consensus guidelines 2006–2007. Pediatric Diabetes 2007;8:28–43.

Hyponatremia

Method of

Beejal Shah, MD, and Susan L. Samson, MD, PhD

Homeostasis maintains the concentration of sodium in the serum between 138 and 142 mEq/L (normal, 135–145 mEq/L) despite variations in water intake. Hyponatremia is defined as a serum sodium concentration of less than 135 mEq/L. It is one of the most common electrolyte abnormalities found in the inpatient setting, occurring in up to 2.5% of patients, and it is a significant marker for mortality, associated with a 60-fold higher risk of death. It is not clear whether hyponatremia itself is the cause of a more adverse prognosis or whether it echoes the degree of stress caused by illness. In the outpatient setting, chronic hyponatremia is most prevalent among the elderly and nursing home residents. The approach to management of hyponatremia is highly dependent on the underlying process. Establishing the correct etiology is critical, because inappropriate treatment can worsen hyponatremia. Therapy must be administered judiciously because of the risk of severe neurologic sequelae, including central nervous system demyelination. However, with a systematic approach to the differential diagnosis of hyponatremia, the correct diagnosis can be made and therapy initiated.

Clinical Presentation

Acute hyponatremia is defined as hyponatremia of less than 48 hours in duration. Mild symptoms include headache, nausea, vomiting, confusion, and weakness, which usually occur with a sodium level of less than 129 mEq/L. More severe neurologic manifestations—seizure and coma—are seen usually below a threshold of 120 mEq/L, although there currently is no evidence-based critical sodium level above which neurologic sequelae do not occur. The neurologic manifestations of acute or recurrent symptomatic hyponatremia can be delayed, so continued monitoring is important.

In contrast, patients with chronic hyponatremia more often are asymptomatic or have blunted symptoms. In elderly patients with mild chronic hyponatremia, subtle neurocognitive manifestations can occur, with decreased balance, lowered reaction speed, memory loss, and directed gait. Mild hypoosmolar hyponatremia is not independently associated with increased morbidity and mortality. Even so, the underlying etiology needs to be determined because of the potential for other factors (e.g., new medications, dehydration, occult illness) to contribute to the development of more severe hyponatremia with its potential for neurologic injury.

Regulation of Water Balance

Approximately two thirds of total body water is contained in the intracellular fluid (ICF) and one third as extracellular fluid (ECF). Plasma osmolality is tightly regulated between 280 and 290 mOsm/kg and reflects the osmolality of the ECF. A change in plasma osmolality results in a shift of total body water between the ECF and the ICF to maintain their osmolar equivalence. Because sodium is the major osmole in the ECF, hyponatremia most often is a manifestation of decreased osmolality, so-called hypoosmolar or hypotonic hyponatremia.

RENAL HANDLING OF WATER

The major osmoregulatory hormone is arginine vasopressin, also called antidiuretic hormone, which is synthesized in the paraventricular and supraoptic nuclei of the hypothalamus. It is transported along axons to the posterior pituitary, where it is processed and stored in vesicles. Vasopressin secretion is regulated by osmotic and nonosmotic stimuli. Secretion occurs with a 1% to 2% rise in osmolality (>288 mOsm/kg), as detected by receptors in the anterolateral walls of the hypothalamus adjacent to the third ventricle. Vasopressin secretion is inhibited when the plasma osmolality is lower than 280 mOsm/kg. The major nonosmotic stimulus is a decrease in effective circulating volume, which is detected by baroreceptors in the aortic arch and carotid sinuses. Although this mechanism requires a large drop (10%-15%) in blood pressure, the secretory response is more robust than for increases in osmolality. As such, acutely lowered blood pressure can override the inhibitory signal of low osmolality because of the need to maintain perfusion. Other physiologic nonosmotic stimuli include catecholamines and angiotensin II, but there is a long list of hormones and pharmacologic agents that induce or repress vasopressin secretion (Table 1).

The renal site of action of vasopressin is the V_2 receptors on the basolateral membrane of collecting duct cells in the distal nephron. The hormone-receptor interaction initiates intracellular signaling via cyclic adenosine monophosphate–dependent pathways, resulting in translocation of cytoplasmic aquaporon-2 channels to the surface of the collecting duct luminal membrane. These channels allow movement of water back into the cell for later reabsorption into the circulation. This results in a net concentration of urine and decreased plasma osmolality.

TABLE 1 Molecules That Regulate Vasopressin Secretion

Stimulate Vasopressin Release	Inhibit Vasopressin Release
Hormones and Neurotransmitters	
Acetylcholine (nicotinic)	Atrial natriuretic peptide
Histamine (H_1)	γ-Aminobutyric acid
Dopamine (D_1 and D_2)	Opioids (κ receptors)
Glutamine	
Aspartate	
Cholecystokinin	
Neuropeptide Y	
Substance P	
Vasoactive inhibitory peptide	
Prostaglandin	
Angiotensin II	
Pharmacologic Agents	
Vincristine (Oncovin)	Ethanol
Cyclophosphamide (Cytoxan)	Phenytoin (Dilantin)
Tricyclic antidepressants	Low-dose morphine
Selective serotonin reuptake inhibitors	Glucocorticoids
Nicotine	Fluphenazine (Prolixin)
Adrenaline (epinephrine)	Haloperidol (Haldol)
High-dose morphine	Promethazine (Phenergan)
	Butorphanol (Stadol)

RENAL HANDLING OF SODIUM

In addition to renal water handling, sodium reabsorption and excretion are important for maintenance of water homeostasis. The renin-angiotensin-aldosterone system is activated by reduced arterial perfusion pressure sensed by the juxtaglomerular apparatus of the afferent renal arteriole. Reduced arteriole effective volume (low or perceived) is sensed by the juxtaglomerular apparatus, which secretes renin, activating the renin-angiotensin system. This cascade of events ultimately stimulates aldosterone secretion, which acts at the distal nephron to cause reabsorption of filtered sodium via Na^+,K^+-adenosine triphosphatase (ATPase)–dependent sodium channels.

Central Nervous System Response to Hyponatremia/ Hypoosmolality

Osmolar equivalence between the ECF and ICF is closely maintained by shifts in water between the two compartments. The major symptoms and signs of hyponatremia are neurologic in nature and are a clinical manifestation of swelling of the cells in the central nervous system, which results in cerebral edema. The most devastating consequence is herniation due to anatomic limitations on brain volume within the confines of the skull. Premenopausal women are at the highest risk for brain injury from hyponatremia.

A major compensatory mechanism in the central nervous system is the extrusion from the cells of intracellular solutes, which prevents further water influx. In the first few hours, inorganic ions (potassium, sodium, chloride) move out of the cell. After a few days of persistent hypoosmolality, the cells further compensate by extruding organic osmoles (glutamate, taurine, inositol). The clinician must be aware of this protective adaptation, because it necessitates a slower time course of correction during treatment. A rapid rise in plasma osmolality from aggressive treatment causes water to rapidly shift out of the cells, resulting in demyelination of neurons. In the past, this was termed pontine demyelinosis, but it has also been reported for extrapontine neurons and is now referred to as osmotic demyelination. The sequelae are permanent and devastating. There is clinical progression from lethargy to a change in affect, to mutism and dysarthria, and finally to spastic quadriparesis and pseudobulbar palsy.

Classification and Differential Diagnosis of Hyponatremia

Initial evaluation of hyponatremia requires a systematic and sequential approach. First, a thorough history and physical examination are required. It is important to identify any history of brain injury,

CURRENT DIAGNOSIS

- Perform a thorough history and physical examination with focus on the accurate assessment of volume status, neurologic symptoms and signs, current medications, and concurrent illnesses.
- Classify the hyponatremia as hypovolemic, euvolemic, or hypervolemic.
- Determine whether the hyponatremia is acute or chronic, based on the history and the clinical manifestations.
- Order the key laboratory tests, including a basic metabolic panel (serum sodium, glucose, blood urea nitrogen, and creatinine), plasma osmolality, urine osmolality, and urine sodium.

stroke, mental illness, or chronic illness and the patient's current medication usage. On examination, special attention should be paid to mental status and neurologic abnormalities; manifestations of cardiac, hepatic, or renal disease; and signs of adrenal insufficiency or hypothyroidism. From the assessment of volume status, the hyponatremia should be classified as hypervolemic, euvolemic, or hypovolemic; each of these conditions leads in a different direction for diagnosis and treatment of the underlying cause (Figs. 1 and 2). Finally, it should be determined whether the hyponatremia is acute (<48 hours) or chronic, because this can determine the time course of treatment.

For the laboratory work-up, essential basic tests are the serum sodium and potassium levels, renal function tests with blood urea nitrogen (BUN) and creatinine, and liver function tests. It is likely that these tests have already been performed, motivating the assessment of hyponatremia. After this, the plasma osmolality (P_{Osm}), urine osmolality (U_{Osm}), and urine sodium concentration are key diagnostic tests. P_{Osm} is directly measured in the laboratory and also can be calculated. Calculated osmolality is the sum of the concentrations of the known major osmoles—sodium and glucose—in the ECF and the BUN:

$$P_{Osm} = (2 \times Na) + (glucose) + (BUN)$$

The calculation is done in SI units. For sodium, mEq/L is the same as the SI unit, mmol/L; if glucose and BUN values were reported in mg/dL, they must be divided by 18 and 2.8, respectively, to convert to SI units (mmol/L). The directly measured osmolality should be within 10 to 12 mOsm/kg of the calculated value; an increased osmolar gap compared with the calculated value points toward the presence of additional osmoles in the plasma that are causing hypertonicity.

Because hyponatremia usually is a reflection of plasma osmolality, most patients also have a low P_{Osm}, and the clinician often can proceed to the differential diagnosis of hypoosmolar (or hypotonic) hyponatremia after excluding pseudohyponatremia (which usually has normal osmolality) and hyperosmolar hyponatremia. Pseudohyponatremia can occur if the plasma lipid or protein content is greatly increased in the plasma (usually to >6%–8% of volume), as in extreme hypertriglyceridemia and paraprotein disorders. These extra components decrease

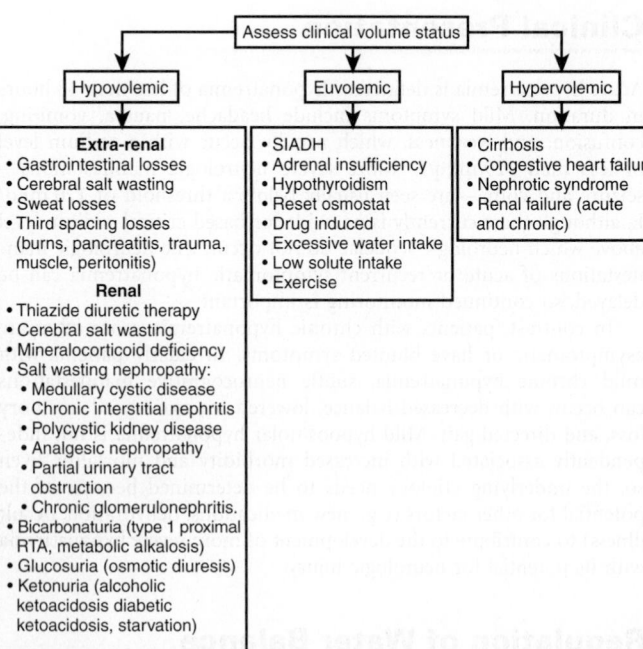

FIGURE 1. The differential diagnosis of hypoosmolar hyponatremia. *Abbreviations:* RTA, renal tubular acidosis; SIADH, syndrome of inappropriate antidiuretic hormone.

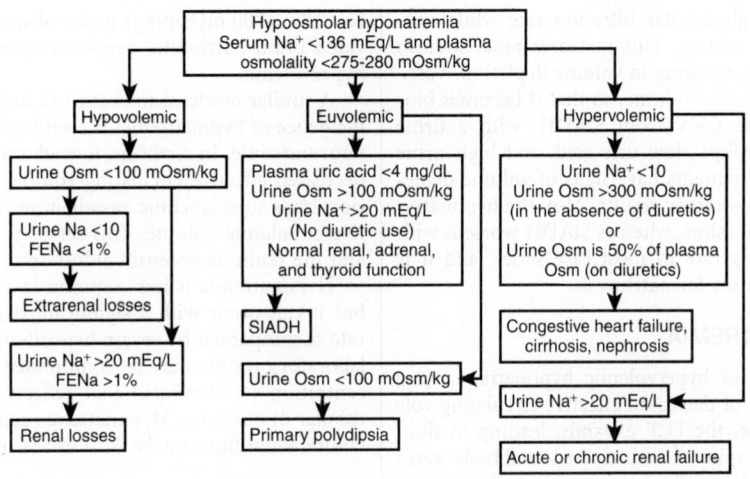

FIGURE 2. Laboratory findings in hypoosmolar hyponatremia. *Abbreviations:* FENa, fractional excretion of sodium; Osm, osmoles; SIADH, syndrome of inappropriate antidiuretic hormone.

the aqueous portion of the plasma volume and thereby interfere with the laboratory measurement of sodium by dilutional, indirect methods such as flame photometry. Most laboratories now use direct measurement of sodium to avoid this problem.

Hyperosmolar hyponatremia can occur if there are additional osmoles present that cause water movement from the ICF into the ECF, resulting in ECF expansion and dilutional hyponatremia. Overall, the total body water and total body sodium are unchanged in this situation. An important clinical example occurs with hyperglycemia, and the reported sodium value should be corrected for high glucose by the clinician, by adding 1.6 mEq/L to the measured Na for every 100 mg/dL rise in glucose above 200 mg/dL. Because glucose is included in the calculation of osmolality, there will be no significant osmolar gap.

Other osmotically active solutes encountered clinically are mannitol, which is used to manage increased intracranial pressure, and glycine, which is used for irrigation in urologic procedures. Mannitol and glycine are retained in the ECF and are not part of the calculated osmolality, so their presence results in an osmolar gap. High levels of alcohol or ethylene glycol also increase the osmolality, but these substances are so quickly metabolized that an osmolar gap may not be apparent by the time testing is performed.

Once pseudohyponatremia and hypertonicity have been ruled out, the diagnosis is narrowed to hypoosmolar hyponatremia. The combined physical examination and laboratory results allow classification of the patient as having hypervolemic hyponatremia with excess total body sodium, hypovolemic hyponatremia with a deficit of total body sodium, or euvolemic hyponatremia with near-normal total body sodium.

HYPOVOLEMIC HYPONATREMIA

The causes of hypovolemic hyponatremia can be classified as extrarenal or renal (see Fig. 1). Signs of volume contraction are apparent on examination, including poor skin turgor, skin tenting (forehead), decreased or undetectable jugular venous pressure, dry mucous membranes, and orthostatic changes in blood pressure and pulse rate. If the volume status is not completely clear from the examination, laboratory values can be helpful (see Fig. 2), but they need to be interpreted in the context of renal function tests. If the urine osmolality is less than maximally concentrated (<500 mOsm/kg), an infusion of 0.5 to 1 L of isotonic saline over 24 to 48 hours may help with differentiation. With hypovolemia, the sodium will begin to correct and the patient should improve clinically. Conversely, if the patient is actually euvolemic, such as with syndrome of inappropriate antidiuretic hormone (SIADH), discussed later, the serum sodium level will remain constant or decrease due to retention of free water with a concomitant increase in urinary sodium.

Extrarenal causes of hyponatremia include gastrointestinal losses and third-space losses such as in severe burns and pancreatitis. In the volume-depleted state, with intact renal function, the urine sodium is low (<10 mEq/L) reflecting a normal response by the kidney to maximally reabsorb sodium in response to volume depletion.

The renal causes of hypovolemic hyponatremia involve the inappropriate loss of sodium into the urine, and this is reflected by a urine sodium concentration of greater than 20 mEq/L.

Thiazide diuretics cause renal sodium loss, so the urine sodium is high. However, they also impair the kidney's diluting capacity, decreasing free water excretion and concentrating the urine. Only certain patients may be susceptible to hyponatremia while on thiazides. These patients may have an abnormally sensitive thirst response to the mild hypovolemia induced by the diuretics, causing increased water intake. Elderly women are the most susceptible, and hyponatremia can occur within days after initiation of thiazide therapy. Additional laboratory results reveal hypokalemia and a metabolic alkalosis. It is appropriate to stop the diuretic and restore potassium levels and volume status. Patients often have a recurrence of hyponatremia if rechallenged with thiazides. Loop diuretics, such as furosemide, are a less frequent cause of hyponatremia, which occurs only after long-term therapy.

In the absence of diuretic use, a urine sodium concentration greater than 20 mEq/L with hypovolemia is evidence for underlying renal pathology. Patients with salt-wasting nephropathy, from a number of causes (see Fig. 1), usually have significant renal failure, with a creatinine value in the range of 3 to 4 mg/dL. Because of the large net sodium loss, this condition is treated with salt tablets. Renal tubular acidosis causes bicarbonaturia, which requires a compensatory excretion of urinary cations, mainly Na$^+$ and K$^+$, to maintain electroneutrality. Similarly, excretion of ketones into the urine also demands additional electrolyte losses in spite of ECF volume depletion, leading to a loss of sodium.

Cerebral salt wasting (CSW), although it could be considered an extrarenal cause, also involves the renal loss of sodium (>20 mEq/L). The biochemical presentation is very similar to that of SIADH, but the diagnosis of CSW is restricted to cases involving extreme central nervous system pathology. CSW is most commonly associated with subarachnoid hemorrhage but also has been reported with stroke, brain trauma, infection, metastases and after neurosurgery. Onset of CSW is usually within first 10 days after the neurologic event.

CSW may be a protective mechanism against increased intracranial pressure. The proposed pathophysiologic mechanism of CSW is controversial, but one hypothesis is that the initiating event is a primary natriuresis, with renal loss of sodium, caused by the secretion of natriuretic peptides. Clinical studies have found both increased brain natriuretic peptide and increased atrial natriuretic peptide in neurosurgical patients with hyponatremia. Both hormones are vasodilators that increase the glomerular filtration rate while suppressing the renin-angiotensin system. This increases renal sodium losses as well as water excretion, resulting in volume depletion. Vasopressin levels rise in response to low volume, so that it becomes biochemically difficult differentiate CSW from SIADH, with a urine sodium level greater than 20 mEq/L, low uric acid, and high urine osmolality. It is helpful if CSW patients have signs of volume depletion in combination with the laboratory results. Also, the hyponatremia of CSW responds to normal saline, whereas SIADH worsens with normal saline. CSW is relatively rare in most case series, and it is important to rule out other causes for natriuresis.

HYPERVOLEMIC HYPONATREMIA

There are a variety of causes of hypervolemic hyponatremia (see Fig. 1), all of which are a result of decreased effective circulating volume. To correct this imbalance, the ECF expands, leading to fluid retention and hyponatremia. In spite of the increased total body water and low serum sodium on testing, all of these patients have some degree of total body sodium excess. In many cases, volume overload is clinically evident from the presence of subcutaneous edema, ascites, elevated jugular venous pressure, or pulmonary edema.

In congestive heart failure (CHF), patients can develop hyponatremia with only 2 to 3 L of fluid intake per day despite normal renal function. The decreased filling pressures and cardiac output of CHF are perceived as volume depletion, detected by the baroreceptors. This stimulates vasopressin secretion, overriding the signal of low osmolality detected by the hypothalamic osmoreceptors. This lack of inhibition of vasopressin secretion is believed to be the most important contributing factor to the development of hyponatremia. In addition, decreased right atrial pressures result in inhibition of secretion of atrial natriuretic peptide, contributing to the water and sodium gain. With the low perfusion pressure, there is a decrease in the glomerular filtration rate, which is sensed by the juxtaglomerular apparatus, causing neurohumoral activation of the renin-angiotensin system and sympathetic nervous system. This leads to increased circulating levels of catecholamines, angiotensin II, and aldosterone, further stimulating tubular sodium and water reabsorption. In the absence of diuretics, the urine sodium level is very low (<10 mEq/L) in patients with CHF because of activation of the renin-angiotensin-aldosterone system and maximal tubular reabsorption of sodium. Also, there is less than maximally dilute urine

(usually >300 mOsm/kg) in the absence of diuretic therapy. An elevated brain natriuretic peptide concentration helps to confirm the hypervolemia.

A similar mechanism is at work in cirrhotic patients, in whom the incidence of hyponatremia is even higher and is a strong predictor of poor outcome. In cirrhosis, low albumin results in third-spacing and decreased effective circulating volume. In addition, portal hypertension leads to splanchnic vasodilation, which also decreases the effective circulating volume. This serves to activate vasopressin secretion and the renin-angiotensin-aldosterone system.

Hyponatremia is less common in acute and chronic renal failure, but it can occur with a significant decrease in glomerular filtration rate accompanied by severe hypoalbuminemia. Interpretation of the laboratory results may be confounded by a high urine sodium concentration (>20 mEq/L) that reflects the concomitant presence of tubular dysfunction. Hyponatremia can develop in stage IV or V renal failure when fluid intake is in excess of 3 L/day.

EUVOLEMIC HYPONATREMIA

Euvolemic hyponatremia is caused by impaired excretion of free water by the kidney. The differential diagnosis is more limited (see Fig. 1) and the majority of cases are due to SIADH (Table 2). However, this often is a diagnosis of exclusion, and hypothyroidism and adrenal insufficiency must be ruled out clinically or biochemically in patients with euvolemic hyponatremia.

Hypothyroidism leads to reduced glomerular filtration rate and decreased flow to the distal nephron, causing maximal reabsorption of water to maintain arterial volume. Hypothyroidism has to be severe to cause hyponatremia and usually is obvious on examination. However, in the elderly population, apathetic hypothyroidism may be difficult to diagnose. Hypothyroidism can be confirmed by the presence of a high level of thyroid-stimulating hormone and a low level of free T_4 (thyroxine). Treatment involves thyroid hormone replacement and supportive care.

In primary adrenal insufficiency (Addison's disease), the concomitant aldosterone deficiency results in hyponatremia combined with hyperkalemia, prerenal azotemia, a urine sodium concentration greater than 20 mEq/L, and a urine potassium level lower than 20 mEq/L. In secondary or central adrenal insufficiency, the adrenal zona glomerulosa remains intact for the secretion of aldosterone. However, glucocorticoid deficiency still causes impaired water

TABLE 2 Causes of SIADH

CNS Disorders	Pulmonary Disorders	Medications	Other
Mass lesions	Viral/bacterial pneumonia	Vasopressin analogues	Pain
Tumors	Positive-pressure ventilation	(Desmopressin [DDAVP])	Nausea
CNS abscess	Bronchogenic carcinoma	NSAIDs	AIDS
Intracranial hemorrhage or hematoma	(small cell)	Tricyclic antidepressants	Prolonged exercise
Stroke	Acute respiratory failure	Phenothiazines	Idiopathic
CNS infections or inflammatory diseases	COPD	Butyrophenones	
Spinal cord lesions	Tuberculosis	SSRIs	
Acute psychosis	Aspergillosis	Morphine	
Pituitary stalk lesions	Pulmonary abscess	Opiates	
Hydrocephalus		Chlorpropamide (Diabinese)	
Dementia		Clofibrate (Atromid-S)[2]	
Guillain-Barré syndrome		Cyclophosphamide (Cytoxan)	
Head trauma		Vincristine (Oncovin)	
		Nicotine	
		Tolbutamide (Orinase)	
		Barbiturates	
		Acetaminophen (Tylenol)	
		ACE inhibitors	
		Carbamazepine (Tegretol)	
		Omeprazole (Prilosec)	

[2]Not available in the United States.
Abbreviations: ACE, angiotensin-converting enzyme; AIDS, acquired immunodeficiency syndrome; CNS, central nervous system; COPD, chronic obstructive pulmonary disease; NSAIDs, nonsteroidal antiinflammatory drugs; SSRIs, selective serotonin reuptake inhibitors.

excretion, which can lead to dilutional hyponatremia. Vasopressin release may be stimulated by the nausea, vomiting, and orthostatic hypotension that occurs with adrenal insufficiency. Finally, corticosteroids normally inhibit vasopressin release, so their deficiency leads to enhanced vasopressin release, causing retention of free water that further contributes to the hyponatremia. The appropriate diagnostic test is a 250-µg ACTH (cosyntropin, Cortrosyn) stimulation test, although an extremely low 8 AM cortisol level (<3 µg/dL) can be diagnostic. Treatment consists of glucocorticoid replacement.

Syndrome of Inappropriate Antidiuretic Hormone

SIADH is the most common cause of euvolemic hypoosmolar hyponatremia. Edema, ascites, and orthostasis are absent, and thyroid, adrenal, and renal functions are normal. Recent diuretic use should be ruled out. The primary event is the release of vasopressin, which results in water retention. The increased intravascular volume stimulates a natriuresis, which actually is appropriate, but the resulting loss of sodium compounds the hyponatremia. There is an extensive list of causes of SIADH, usually involving pulmonary or central nervous system pathology (see Table 2). A number of medications also are known to stimulate vasopressin release or to potentiate its antidiuretic properties at the level of the kidney (see Tables 1 and 2).

The diagnosis of SIADH is suggested by a low P_{Osm} (<280 mOsm/kg) with a high U_{Osm} (>100 mOsm/kg), confirming water retention and an inappropriately concentrated urine. A spot urine sodium level will be greater than 20 mEq/L, and usually greater than 30 mEq/L. Other helpful laboratory findings include low plasma uric acid (<4 mg/dL) which has a positive predictive value of 73% to 100% for SIADH in this setting. In complicated cases confounded by use of diuretics, the fractional excretion of uric acid has a positive predictive value of 100% for SIADH when the calculated excretion is greater than 12%.

Reset osmostat can be considered a form of SIADH, but the hyponatremia is usually chronic, mild, and asymptomatic. Vasopressin release continues to be regulated, but at a lower threshold of plasma osmolality. The thirst threshold may be altered as well. Interventions to raise the sodium usually have short-lived effects, and the sodium resets at its previous value over time. Therefore, treatment is not recommended if the sodium level is stable and the patient is asymptomatic. A physiologic example of reset osmostat is seen in pregnancy, when the normal sodium range is lowered by 5 mEq/L.

Other Causes of Euvolemic Hypoosmolar Hyponatremia

Primary or psychogenic polydipsia should be considered in patients presenting with hyponatremia and a history of psychiatric illness and treatment. Almost 6% to 7% of psychiatric inpatients are at risk for hyponatremia from increased water intake. The polydipsia may be related to a lowered osmolar threshold for thirst, below the threshold of suppression of vasopressin secretion. This can be further complicated by the side effect of dry mouth caused by many psychiatric medications, which compounds the increased thirst and water intake. Because the kidney is capable of excreting up to 15 to 20 L/day of dilute urine, the fact that hyponatremia develops in these patients may point toward an additional and inappropriate increase in vasopressin release or sensitivity. These patients are clinically euvolemic because of renal excretion of the excess water and have otherwise normal laboratory results except for a dilute urine (<100 mOsm/kg), which is caused by vasopressin suppression and helps differentiate primary polydipsia from SIADH. However, some patients have mildly concentrated urine (>100 mOsm/kg), in which case the psychiatric history helps with the diagnosis.

Exercise-induced hyponatremia (e.g., from marathon running) is a form of euvolemic hypoosmolar hyponatremia primarily caused by excessive fluid intake during exercise. Vasopressin levels also may be inappropriately high, secondary to pain or the use of NSAIDs, which remove prostaglandin inhibition of vasopressin release. Low solute intake combined with high fluid intake also can cause hyponatremia, as is with beer potomania or a low-protein "tea and toast" diet in elderly patients. In both cases, the lack of solute in the urine

CURRENT THERAPY

- Severe and symptomatic hyponatremia should be treated with hypertonic saline (3%) at 1 to 2 mL/kg per hour. Neurologic status and serum sodium should be monitored every 2 to 4 hours. The objective is to raise sodium by 2 mEq/L per hour (or to >125 mEq/L) until deleterious neurologic symptoms improve. After this, the rate of infusion should be titrated to increase the serum sodium by 0.5 to 1.0 mEq/L per hour, with a maximum increase of 10 to 12 mEq/L over 24 hours and no more than 18 mEq/L over 48 hours, to avoid precipitating osmotic demyelination.

- As a general rule, the treatment of hyponatremia should be adjusted so that the serum sodium increases by 0.5 to 1.0 mEq/L per hour with a maximum increase of 10 to 12 mEq/L over 24 hours and no more than 18 mEq/L over 48 hours. Acute hyponatremia (<48 hours) may be treated more rapidly than chronic hyponatremia if dictated by neurologic findings. Treat SIADH with fluid restriction, medications, or observation; rule out adrenal insufficiency and hypothyroidism.

- Most cases of euvolemic hyponatremia are caused by the syndrome of inappropriate antidiuretic hormone (SIADH), which usually can be managed with fluid restriction, salt tablets, and demeclocycline (Declomycin)[1] in refractory cases.

- Discontinue thiazide diuretics in all cases of hypoosmolar hyponatremia.

- Hypovolemic and hypervolemic hyponatremia require therapy to correct the underlying cause (e.g., heart failure) and restore status to euvolemia.

- Conivaptan (Vaprisol) is a vasopressin receptor antagonist that is approved for inpatient management of euvolemic and hypovolemic hyponatremia. The same parameters apply for rate of sodium correction and monitoring as in conventional therapy.

[1]Not FDA approved for this indication.

does not allow retention of water in the filtrate, so the excess water is not excreted.

Hyponatremia also is common after pituitary surgery (transsphenoidal or by craniotomy) and may be a result of damage to the hypothalamic-pituitary tract that causes release of preformed vasopressin from damaged neurons. Often, hyponatremia occurs as the second phase of the classic triphasic response: transient diabetes insipidus, transient SIADH, followed by permanent diabetes insipidus. Hyponatremia can be delayed up to 1 week postoperatively, and sodium should be monitored during the second week as well. Contributions by central adrenal insufficiency and hypothyroidism also are considerations after pituitary surgery, although with these conditions there will be obvious clinical manifestations in addition to the hyponatremia.

Management

The major considerations for choosing the type and time course of treatment for hyponatremia are the duration of hyponatremia (acute or chronic) and the presence of neurologic signs and symptoms, especially severe manifestations such as altered mental status or seizure (see Table 2). Treatment options for hyponatremia include fluid restriction, saline infusion (hypertonic or isotonic), vasopressin receptor antagonists (Conivaptan, [Vaprisol]), and demeclocycline (Declomycin).[1] Also, treatment of the underlying abnormality, such as CHF or salt wasting, and correction of volume status are important for hypovolemic or hypervolemic patients. Autocorrection may occur after initiation of therapy, especially in cases of hypovolemia, adrenal insufficiency, or thiazide use. Once treatment is started, the contribution of the nonosmotic stimulation of vasopressin secretion is removed, and the patient is able to raise the sodium level by 2 mEq/L per hour over 12 hours.

ACUTE SEVERE SYMPTOMATIC HYPONATREMIA

Acute severe hyponatremia is defined as a rapid fall in sodium in less than 48 hours to less than 120 mEq/L. Under these circumstances, most patients develop neurologic symptoms because of the rapid fluid shifts between the ECF and the ICF in the brain. If left untreated, it can result in irreversible neurologic damage and death. Because of the acute drop in sodium, initial rapid correction is acceptable and should not lead to osmotic demyelination. Treatment is aimed at raising the sodium enough to resolve the neurologic signs and symptoms. The goal is to raise the serum sodium by 1 to 2 mEq/L per hour or to greater than 125 mEq/L until symptoms resolve. Hypovolemic patients will respond to infusion of isotonic saline (normal saline 0.9%), especially if the urine sodium concentration is less than 30 mEq/L. If the neurologic findings are severe, hypertonic saline (3%) may be infused at rate of 1 to 2 mL/kg per hour, or even up to 4 to 6 mL/kg per hour if the imbalance is life-threatening. A loop diuretic can be combined with the saline to enhance solute-free water excretion. Sodium levels should be monitored every 2 to 4 hours in patients undergoing hypertonic infusion. Once symptoms resolve, the rate of correction should be reduced to 0.5 to 1 mEq/hour, and the total rise in sodium should not exceed 8 to 12 mEq in 24 hours and no more than 18 mEq in 48 hours. No benefit has been observed for faster rates of correction of hyponatremia, whether acute or chronic. Useful formulas to determine the rate of infusion for fluids is provided in Figure 3. The formulas can only estimate the rate of correction, and sodium should be measured frequently.

---

[1]Not FDA approved for this indication.

CHRONIC HYPONATREMIA

Chronic hyponatremia is defined as a gradual fall in sodium over more than 48 hours. By this time, the brain has begun to compensate for hypoosmolality by extrusion of solutes. However, the patient is at risk of osmotic demyelination if hyponatremia is treated too aggressively. If the duration of hyponatremia is unknown, the recommendation is to assume that it is chronic. However, as with acute hyponatremia, severe neurologic symptoms and signs need to be treated with hypertonic saline until they resolve, after which the rate of correction can be slowed to 0.5 to 1 mEq/L per hour. Most cases of osmotic demyelination occur with correction rates of greater than 12 mEq/L in 24 hours, but there are cases reported with increases of 9 or 10 mEq/day. Asymptomatic hyponatremia can be treated with an infusion of isotonic saline calculated to raise the sodium by 0.5 to 1 mEq/hour. If the patient has a dilute urine (<200 mOsm/kg), water restriction may be sufficient.

SYNDROME OF INAPPROPRIATE ANTIDIURETIC HORMONE

The mainstays of treatment of SIADH are fluid restriction and treatment of the underlying cause. Mild SIADH usually can be controlled with fluid restriction alone.

In most cases of SIADH, the degree of fluid restriction required can be calculated. It is dependent on three factors: the daily osmolar load, the minimum U_{Osm}, and the patient's maximum urine volume. A typical diet has a daily osmolar load of 10 mOsm/kg of body weight. For a 70 kg person, this would be 700 mOsm/day. With SIADH, the urine osmolality is held constant for that particular patient, as revealed by a spot U_{Osm}. If the U_{Osm} is 500 mOsm/kg and the solute load is 700 mOsm, the fluid load has to be less than 700/500 or 1.4 L/day just to maintain the serum sodium level. Fluid intake above this amount will cause the sodium to decrease.

When needed, salt tablets (sodium chloride tablet 1 g taken once to three times daily) can help to make up for renal loss of sodium in SIADH. With symptoms and severe hyponatremia, short-term use of hypertonic saline may also be instituted to restore sodium to the ECF compartment. Loop diuretics (e.g., furosemide [Lasix]) can increase free water clearance when given with solute (e.g., hypertonic saline or salt tablets). In refractory cases, demeclocycline (300–600 mg PO twice daily) can be used. Demeclocycline

---

Symptomatic hyponatremia with severe neurologic symptoms (acute <48 hours or chronic >48 hours)
1. Correct serum Na to 125 mEq/L in the first 24 hours at a rate of 1–2 mEq/L per hour or until symptoms have resolved
2. Correct Na at a rate of 0.5 to 1 mEq/L per hour

Acute hyponatremia with mild symptoms
1. Correct at rate of 0.5 to 1 mEq/L per hour

Chronic hyponatremia with mild symptoms or asymptomatic
1. Correct at rate of 0.5 mEq/L per hour with fluid restriction
2. Treat underlying cause

Parameters for acute or chronic hyponatremia:
3. Do not increase serum Na by more than 10 to 12 mEq/L in 24 hours, or 18 mEq/L in 48 hours

Calculation of the rate of infusion of saline to correct hyponatremia
1. Change in serum sodium per liter infusate (# mEq/L) = $\dfrac{\text{Infusate [sodum]} - \text{Serum [sodium]}}{\text{TBW} + 1}$

2. # L required in 24 hours =
$\dfrac{\text{Desired change in sodium over 24 hours}}{\text{\# mEq/L}}$

3. Rate of infusate (x mL/h) to raise serum Na by approximately 1 mEq/h

$\dfrac{\text{\#mEq/L}}{1 \text{ mEq}} = \dfrac{1000\text{mL/h}}{X \text{ mL/hour}}$

4. (simplified) Hypertonic saline infused at 1–2 mL/kg per hour

Monitoring:
1. Monitor for improvement or worsening of symptoms
2. If on hypertonic saline or severely symptomatic, check sodium q2–4h

Infusate	Infusate [Na] mEq/L
5% sodium chloride in water	855
3% sodium chloride in water	513
Isotonic saline (0.9%)	154
Ringer's Lactate solution	130
0.45% sodium chloride in water	77
0.2% sodium chloride in water	34
5% dextrose in water	0

Total Body Water (TBW) is equal to 60% of body weight in young adult men and 50% in young adult women. Older patients have less TBW. In elderly males, TBW is equal to 50% of body weight and in elderly females it is 45%.

FIGURE 3. Treatment of hyponatremia. *Abbreviation:* TBW, total body water.

(Declomycin)[1] antagonizes the actions of vasopressin by inhibiting formation of cyclic adenosine monophosphate in the collecting duct. Long-term use is limited by the side effect of photosensitivity and by nephrotoxicity in patients with underlying liver disease. The vasopressin receptor antagonist, conivaptan (Vaprisol), is an important new adjunct treatment (see later discussion). A less favored treatment is urea (powder or capsules)[1,6] which causes an osmotic diuresis and increased free water excretion.

CEREBRAL SALT WASTING

Management of CSW involves treatment of the underlying neurologic problem as well as volume replacement. CSW often is difficult to differentiate biochemically from SIADH, but the rise in vasopressin in CSW is secondary to volume depletion. As a result, CSW responds to volume replacement with isotonic saline, suppressing release of vasopressin, whereas SIADH worsens with this therapy. The recommended correction rate is 0.7 to 1.0 mEq/L per hour, with a maximum of 8 to 10 mEq per 24 hours. Salt tablets may also be given to replete total body sodium. Fludrocortisone (Florinef[1] 0.05 to 0.1 mg every 12 hours), an aldosterone receptor agonist, is a third-line treatment to encourage volume expansion and sodium retention, but the potassium concentration and blood pressure should be monitored. Fluid restriction is inappropriate for CSW and should be avoided, especially in patients with subarachnoid hemorrhage, because volume depletion can exacerbate cerebral vasospasm and cause infarction. The duration of CSW is usually 3 to 5 weeks.

VASOPRESSIN RECEPTOR ANTAGONISTS

Vasopressin receptor antagonists, or vaptans, are a new class of nonpeptide drugs that have great potential for the treatment of dilutional hyponatremia. They block the binding of vasopressin to its receptors in the distal nephron, thereby inhibiting the insertion of aquaporin-2 channels into the membrane, increasing excretion of solute-free water by the kidneys, and resulting in a rise in serum sodium content. Currently, conivaptan (Vaprisol) is FDA approved for clinical use in euvolemic and hypervolemic hyponatremia in hospitalized patients, with the exception of patients with CHF or cirrhosis. Obviously, it is contraindicated in hypovolemic hyponatremia because of the water excretion that is induced. Conivaptan is given intravenously with a bolus of 20 mg over 30 minutes in 100 mL of 5% dextrose in water (D5W). After this, the drug (20 mg in 100 mL of D5W) is infused over 24 hours. Sodium is monitored every 2 to 4 hours, and the dose may be titrated to 40 mg per 24 hours to obtain an increase in sodium of 0.5 to 1.0 mEq/L per hour. During Vaprisol treatment, fluid restriction is liberal at 1.5 to 2.0 L/day. There are no documented cases of osmotic demyelination with conivaptan, but the same precautions about the rate of rise of sodium are in place as for more conventional treatments of hyponatremia. Conivaptan is used with caution in patients with renal or hepatic impairment. Inhibitors of the cytochrome P-450 3A4 isoenzyme (CYP3A4) are contraindicated, including ketoconazole (Nizoral), itraconazole (Sporanox), clarithromycin (Biaxin), ritonavir (Norvir), and indinavir (Crixivan).

Summary

Hyponatremia is a common electrolyte abnormality and is usually caused by decreased plasma osmolality. Accurate assessment of volume status is a key to determining the underlying cause and choosing the correct treatment approach. The biggest risk of hyponatremia and its treatment is the possibility of severe neurologic sequelae, including fatal cerebral edema and osmotic demyelination. Therefore, more aggressive initial treatment is needed in patients with neurologic manifestations (hypertonic saline), but a more conservative approach (e.g., fluid restriction) is needed for less symptomatic patients. The

new availability of the vasopressin receptor antagonist, conivaptan, for euvolemic (SIADH) or hypervolemic hyponatremia is a welcome step forward for the treatment of hyponatremia in the inpatient setting.

REFERENCES

Androgué HJ. Consequences of inadequate management of hyponatremia. Am J Nephrol 2005;25:240–9.

Androgué HJ, Madias NE. Hyponatremia. N Engl J Med 2000;342(21):1581–9.

Cerdà-Esteve M, Cuadrado-Godia E, Chillaron JJ, et al. Cerebral salt wasting syndrome: Review. Eur J Intern Med 2008;19:249–54.

Ellison DH, Berl T. Clinical practice: The syndrome of inappropriate antidiuresis. N Engl J Med 2007;356:2064–72.

Fenske W, Störk S, Koschker A. Value of fractional uric acid excretion in differential diagnosis of hyponatremia patients on diuretics. J Clin Endocrinol Metab 2008;93:2991–7.

Hew-Butler T, Jordaan E, Stuempfle KJ. Osmotic and nonosmotic regulation of arginine vasopressin during prolonged exercise. J Clin Endocrinol Metab 2008;93:2072–8.

Palm C, Pistrosch F, Herbrig K, Gross P. Vasopressin antagonists as aquaretic agents for the treatment of hyponatremia. Am J Med 2006;119(Suppl. 1): S87–93.

Vaprisol conivaptan hydrochloride injection: Prescribing information. Deerfield, Ill: Astellas Pharma US, Inc; 2007.

Verbalis JG, Goldsmith SR, Greenberg A, et al. Hyponatremia treatment guidelines 2007: Expert panel recommendations. Am J Med 2007;120(11 Suppl. 1):S1–21.

Zada G, Liu CY, Fishback D, et al. Recognition and management of delayed hyponatremia following transphenoidal pituitary surgery. J Neurosurg 2007; 106:66–71.

Hyperuricemia and Gout

Method of
Beth K. Rubinstein, MD, and
Christopher M. Wise, MD

Gout is a common cause of inflammatory arthritis typically affecting middle-aged men. However, women and men older than 65 years are affected equally. Gout classically evolves through various stages, starting with a period of asymptomatic hyperuricemia and progressing to a period during which episodes of acute intermittent gouty arthritis occur. Over many years, attacks become more frequent and prolonged, and chronic tophaceous gout develops.

Asymptomatic hyperuricemia is associated with an increased risk of gout. The annual incidence increases from 0.1% to 5% with rising serum urate levels (<7 mg/dL to >9 mg/dL). The cumulative incidence of gouty arthritis reaches 22% in 5 years with serum uric acid levels greater than 9 mg/dL. Risk factors for hyperuricemia and gout include elevated serum creatinine, obesity, insulin resistance, elevated blood pressure, diuretic use, alcohol consumption, and higher meat and seafood intake. Higher intake of dairy products might decrease the risk. Hyperuricemia and gout are now considered elements of the metabolic syndrome, and gout may be an independent risk factor for myocardial infarction.

Diagnosis

Acute gouty arthritis, a mono- or oligoarthritis escalating over a 6- to 12-hour period with pain, swelling, and erythema, is usually easily recognized, but the presence of fever, chills, or leukocytosis broadens the differential diagnosis to include infection and pseudogout.

---

[1]Not FDA approved for this indication.
[6]May be compounded by pharmacists.

A definitive diagnosis of gout can be accomplished by arthrocentesis of a symptomatic joint and identification of monosodium urate crystals in the joint fluid. Aspiration of an asymptomatic joint can reveal crystals even between attacks.

In many patients, a gradual transition from acute intermittent gout to chronic tophaceous gout occurs over the next 10 to 20 years. Tophi and erosions form due to the deposition of urate crystals in the subcutaneous tissue and articular cartilage, respectively. Eventually, joint destruction and deformity occur, which can mimic rheumatoid arthritis.

Treatment

ACUTE GOUT

Acute gouty arthritis tends to resolve spontaneously, but attacks can be quite painful and disabling, necessitating early therapeutic intervention. Nonsteroidal antiinflammatory drugs (NSAIDs), colchicine, and intraarticular or systemic corticosteroids are used most often to terminate an acute gout attack. NSAIDs have a relatively rapid onset of effect and low toxicity profile in the acute setting but their use may be limited by the potential for gastric ulceration and gastritis, acute or chronic renal failure, fluid retention, exacerbation of congestive heart failure, interference with antihypertensive therapy, and alteration of mentation in the elderly. Indomethacin (Indocin) has been the most widely used NSAID, but other agents in the same class are comparable in efficacy and may be better tolerated.

Colchicine begins to relieve symptoms of acute gout within 12 to 24 hours. It is often administered in oral dosages of 0.6 to 1.2 mg initially, followed by 0.6 mg every 2 hours until improvement, but most patients experience gastrointestinal symptoms with these dosages. More serious toxicities, including bone marrow suppression, renal and hepatic injury, central nervous system (CNS) dysfunction, or neuromyopathy can occur if an inappropriately high cumulative dose is given acutely, in the elderly, or in patients with renal or hepatic insufficiency. Low doses of colchicine (0.6 mg bid) may be effective in milder attacks and are less toxic. Intravenous colchicine has been used in the past for treating acute attacks, but it is currently not widely available and is seldom used given its potential to reach toxic levels if not used judiciously.

Corticosteroids have become more widely used to treat acute gout, particularly in patients with contraindications to NSAIDs and colchicine. Intraarticular steroid injection can be done after arthrocentesis and usually provides rapid relief of pain in patients with monoarticular attacks. Systemic corticosteroids (intramuscular or oral) are very useful in patients with polyarticular involvement. Oral prednisone can be given as a taper starting at doses of 40 to 60 mg daily, with gradual decreases in the dose over a period of 7 to 14 days to prevent rebound flares in the first several days after therapy. A single intramuscular injection of triamcinolone (Kenalog) (40–60 mg) has been shown to be comparable to NSAIDs in efficacy and may be preferable in patients who have difficulty taking oral medications.

INTERCRITICAL GOUT

After the initial attack of gout resolves, management should be aimed at preventing further attacks, assessing the baseline serum urate level (with or without urinary urate excretion), and determining the need for long-term urate-lowering therapy. There is a general correlation between the serum urate levels and frequency of subsequent attacks, although serum urate levels can vary and may be falsely low in the setting of an acute attack. Measurements of serum urate levels during asymptomatic periods, therefore, can provide a more accurate assessment of chronic hyperuricemia.

Patients are at increased risk for a recurrent attack of gout for several weeks after an initial attack, although 40% of patients might not have another attack within the next year. During this intercritical period, prophylaxis with small doses of NSAIDs or colchicine (0.6 mg once or twice daily) should be used for most patients and will prevent recurrences in about 85% of patients if used for 6 to 12 months after the last attack.

INDICATIONS FOR URATE-LOWERING THERAPY

Not all patients with hyperuricemia need to be treated with urate-lowering therapy. Some patients with gout never have another attack and will not develop renal stones or renal damage. However, most patients have microscopic evidence of synovial urate deposition (microtophi) at the time of the first attack. Indications for urate-lowering therapy are listed in Box 1. Patients should only be started on urate-lowering therapy if they are willing to comply with a long-term regimen and accept the cost and potential risks of such therapy.

CHRONIC HYPERURICEMIA

Urate levels can be lowered by agents that either decrease production or increase renal excretion of urate. Most patients with gout are underexcretors of urate; therefore, drugs that increase urate excretion can be used to lower serum levels. However, these agents promote urate nephrolithiasis and should only be considered for patients who have normal renal function (glomerular filtration rate >50–60 mL/min), have no history of nephrolithiasis, have a 24-hour urate excretion of less than 700 mg/day, and are willing to drink at least 2 L of fluid daily and maintain good urine flow. Probenecid (1–2 g/day) is the most commonly used agent in this class, although sulfinpyrazone (Anturane) (up to 400–800 mg/day) may also be used. Gastrointestinal side effects and rash can occur.

Allopurinol (Zyloprim), an inhibitor of xanthine oxidase, reduces serum urate levels in nearly all compliant patients and eventually prevents further attacks and promotes resorption of tophi. The dose of allopurinol should be titrated up as frequently as every 2 to 3 weeks to achieve a serum urate level of less than 6 mg/dL. Allopurinol is well tolerated except for occasional skin rashes, which are seen in about 2% of patients, and gastrointestinal symptoms. Other rare but serious reactions include bone marrow suppression, alopecia, and the allopurinol hypersensitivity syndrome. This syndrome, which has a mortality rate of up to 25%, is manifested by rash, fever, eosinophilia, hepatic injury, and renal failure. Allopurinol should be discontinued in any patient who experiences an unexplained rash or fever and should be restarted only if the rash is mild. Allopurinol hypersensitivity can be overcome through desensitization protocols if needed.

Urate-lowering therapy should generally not be initiated during an acute gout attack, but it may be started 2 to 3 weeks after an acute attack has resolved. In addition, urate-lowering therapy should not be stopped in the setting of an acute flare, even if the serum urate level

---

> ### BOX 1 General Indications for Hypouricemic Therapy
>
> Tophaceous gout
> Destructive arthropathy attributable to gout
> Marked overproduction of urate (>1000 mg urate excretion daily)
> History of nephrolithiasis (urate or other)
> Chronic urate nephropathy (due to deposition of monosodium urate crystals in the renal medulla and pyramids)
> Gout with renal insufficiency
> Frequent attacks of acute gout (>2/year)
> Patients *without* documented gout should be treated or considered for treatment:
> Acute uric acid nephropathy (acute renal failure seen in tumor lysis syndrome from chemotherapy or rapidly proliferating lymphomas/leukemias)
> Asymptomatic hyperuricemia with marked (>1000 mg/day) hyperuricosuria or serum urate level >10 mg/dL
> Hyperuricemia associated with heritable disorders of purine metabolism leading to urate overproduction (hypoxanthine-guanine phosphoribosyltransferase [HGPRT] deficiency, Phosphoriboxyl-pyrophosphate synthetase polypeptide [PRPP] synthetase superactivity)

TABLE 1 Adult Maintenance Dosages of Allopurinol and Colchicine Based on Creatinine Clearance

Creatinine Clearance (mL/min)	Maintenance Dose of Allopurinol (mg)	Maintenance Dose of Colchicine (mg)
≧100	300–600 qd	0.6 bid-tid
80	250 qd	0.6 bid
60	200 qd	0.6 bid
40	150 qd	0.6 qd
20	100 qd	0.6 q2–3d
10	100 qod	Contraindicated
<10	50–100 q3d	Contraindicated

appears to be at goal. Prophylactic agents, such as NSAIDs and low-dose colchicine, may be started a few weeks before, and given concomitantly with, urate-lowering therapy to prevent attacks during initiation of such therapy, and it should be continued until the serum urate level is less than 6 mg/dL and the patient has been free of attacks for at least 6 months. Chronic colchicine use can be associated with neuromyopathy and bone marrow suppression in patients with renal or hepatic insufficiency. Maintenance doses of both allopurinol and colchicine should be adjusted according to renal function (Table 1).

Other agents that appear to have modest urate-lowering effects include fenofibrate (Tricor),[1] losartan (Cozaar),[1] amlodipine (Norvasc),[1] and vitamin C[1] (500 mg daily). Dietary adjustments such as decreasing the intake of purine-rich foods (organ meats, shellfish, anchovies) and alcohol, especially beer and distilled spirits, should be part of a urate-lowering regimen, and medications known to decrease urate excretion (cyclosporine [Neoral], nicotinic acid [Niaspan], furosemide [Lasix], thiazide diuretics, ethambutol [Myambutol], pyrazinamide, and aspirin) should also be switched or dose-adjusted if possible.

ELDERLY PATIENTS

Gout is the most common inflammatory arthritis affecting the elderly, but it may be difficult to recognize in this population. The incidence of gout increases in postmenopausal women when the level of estrogen, which has uricosuric effects, decreases. Women can also get gouty arthritis in atypical joints such as the distal interphalangeal (DIP) joints of the hands. The treatment of gout in the elderly is the same as that in younger patients; however, the doses of medications used should be decreased to avoid potential toxic effects. Joint aspiration and corticosteroids may be safer alternatives for some patients. Analgesics can also be used alone when other agents are contraindicated because acute attacks are usually self-limited.

RESISTANT GOUT

Most patients treated for acute gouty arthritis respond to initial therapy with NSAIDs or colchicine; however, an occasional patient responds poorly. In this circumstance, one should consider an alternative diagnosis, such as infectious arthritis, and perform arthrocentesis and culture of the synovial fluid. In the absence of an infection, a corticosteroid (systemic or intraarticular) can be added to achieve a therapeutic response. In a patient with polyarticular involvement who has had inadequate response to an intramuscular corticosteroid, it is not unreasonable to repeat injection 2 to 3 days later. When giving oral corticosteroids for acute gout, one should ensure that the length of therapy is sufficient to prevent rebound attacks.

Patients receiving urate-lowering therapy who continue to have frequent attacks are usually found to have persistently elevated serum urate levels (>6 mg/dL). Medication noncompliance can explain the lack of efficacy of urate-lowering agents; however, urate levels also remain elevated in compliant patients if the dose of the urate-lowering medication is not adjusted to achieve goal urate levels.

---

[1]Not FDA approved for this indication.

CURRENT DIAGNOSIS

- Definitive diagnosis of gout depends on the finding of intracellular monosodium urate crystals in synovial fluid or from tophaceous deposits.
- Even in acute settings where gout is the most likely diagnosis, alternative diagnoses such as infection and pseudogout should be considered.
- Chronic polyarticular gout can mimic rheumatoid arthritis.
- Most patients with gout have elevated serum urate levels at some point during their clinical course, but hyperuricemia alone is not diagnostic of gout.

CRITICALLY ILL PATIENTS

Acute gouty arthritis often occurs in hospitalized or critically ill patients due to fluctuations in the urate levels related to trauma, surgery, or serious infections. This usually occurs in patients with established gout, but initial gout attacks are also seen in this setting. Treatment of gout is often difficult in these patients due to hemodynamic instability, renal or hepatic dysfunction, or altered oral intake status. Intraarticular corticosteroid injections may be the safest treatment if a single joint or small number of joints are involved and provide an opportunity to aspirate the joint fluid to exclude infection, which can coexist with gout. If multiple joints are involved and oral medication is contraindicated, then intramuscular corticosteroids may be preferable. Urate-lowering therapy should not be initiated in a hospitalized or critically ill patient.

TRANSPLANT PATIENTS

Organ transplant patients have typically been more susceptible to the development of gout within a few years of the transplant due to the interference of urate excretion by certain immunosuppressive medications, but use of these agents (cyclosporine) is less common in recent years and can, in turn, decrease the incidence of gout in this patient population. In addition, allopurinol interferes with the metabolism of other immunosuppressive medications (azathioprine [Imuran] and 6-mercaptopurine [Purinethol]), necessitating a decrease in the dose of these medications or a switch to another medication such as mycophenolate mofetil (Cellcept).

CURRENT THERAPY

- The goals of gout treatment include termination of the acute attack, prevention of further attacks, identification and management of associated conditions and risk factors, and consideration of long-term urate-lowering therapy.
- NSAIDs, colchicine, and corticosteroids remain the mainstay of treatment of acute gouty arthritis.
- A serum uric acid level of 6 mg/dL is the initial target when using urate-lowering therapy.
- Urate-lowering medications should not be stopped (or started) during an acute gout flare.
- Prophylactic agents such as colchicine or NSAIDs should be administered when initiating urate-lowering therapy for a period of 3 to 12 months.
- Lifestyle changes, dietary adjustments, and medication alterations may be useful in preventing acute gout and its progression to chronic tophaceous gout.

NSAID = nonsteroidal antiinflammatory drug.

NEW AND OTHER POTENTIAL THERAPIES

Until recently, no new urate-lowering agents had become available since 1964. The US FDA recently approved Febuxostat (Uloric), a nonpurine selective xanthine oxidase inhibitor. Febuxostat has been shown to lower urate levels at least as effectively as allopurinol, and it might have an advantage over allopurinol in patients with renal insufficiency or in those who have had hypersensitivity reactions to allopurinol. The starting dose of Febuxostat is 40 mg daily; if uric acid levels have not reached the goal of less than 6 mg/dL after two weeks, then the dose is increased to 80 mg daily. Side effects were found to include elevated transaminases and diarrhea. Other agents have also been studied and may have potential efficacy in treating gout. Recombinant uricase (rasburicase [Elitek]), which is primarily used in malignancy-associated hyperuricemia, has been shown to rapidly lower serum urate levels and resorb tophi when given intravenously, but it has a short half-life and may be associated with allergic reactions and anaphylaxis. Subcutaneous and intravenous forms of polyethylene glycol–modified uricase[5] have been studied and found to greatly reduce serum urate levels in patients with severe or refractory gout, but acute gout flares occurred commonly.

REFERENCES

Becker MA, Schumacher HR Jr, Wortmann RL. Febuxostat compared with allopurinol in patients with hyperuricemia and gout. N Engl J Med 2005; 353:2450–61.

Campion EW, Glynn RJ, DeLabry LO. Asymptomatic hyperuricemia: risks and consequences in the Normative Aging Study. Am J Med 1987;82:421–6.

Choi HK, Atkinson K, Karlson EW, Curhan G. Obesity, weight change, hypertension, diuretic use, and risk of gout in men: The health professionals follow-up study. Arch Intern Med 2005;165:742–8.

Choi HK, Liu S, Curhan G. Intake of purine-rich foods, protein, and dairy products and relationship to serum levels of uric acid: The Third National Health and Nutritional Examination Survey. Arthritis Rheum 2005;52: 283–9.

Hoskison KT, Wortmann RL. Management of gout in older adults: Barriers to optimal control. Drugs Aging 2007;24:21–36.

Keith MP, Gilliland WR. Updates in the management of gout. Am J Med 2007;120:221–4.

Krishnan E, Baker JF, Furst DE, Schumacher HR. Gout and the risk of acute myocardial infarction. Arthritis Rheum 2006;54:2688–96.

Lee SJ, Terkeltaub RA, Kavanaugh A. Recent developments in diet and gout. Curr Opin Rheumatol 2006;18:193–8.

Pascual E, Sivera F. Therapeutic advances in gout. Curr Opin Rheumatol 2007;19:122–7.

Sundy JS, Ganson NJ, Kelly SJ, et al. Pharmacokinetics and pharmacodynamics of intravenous PEGylated recombinant mammalian urate oxidase in patients with refractory gout. Arthritis Rheum 2007;6:1021–8.

Vogt B. Urate oxidase (rasburicase) for treatment of severe tophaceous gout. Nephrol Dial Transplant 2005;20:431–3.

---

[5]Investigational drug in the United States.

Dyslipoproteinemias

Method of
Kerem Ozer, MD, and Lawrence Chan, MD

All cells need lipids to survive, and lipids are essential for maintenance of tissue structure and function. Lipids comprise an essential component of biologic membranes, and molecular communication within and between cells relies heavily on lipids. Not surprisingly, an imbalance in lipid metabolism has the potential to cause serious malfunction in multiple systems. In addition, abnormal accumulation of excess lipids in cells or tissues can lead to a severe disruption of normal structure and function. Among the many organ systems that are affected by lipid excess and imbalance, the cardiovascular system is the most susceptible; specifically, atherosclerotic cardiovascular disease continues to exert a heavy toll on human health. Indeed, atherosclerosis and its complications are the foremost causes of death and disability for men and women in the Western world. Atherosclerosis is a chronic, multifactorial disease with a complex pathogenesis. Insulin resistance and dyslipidemia are predominant risk factors in many patients with atherosclerosis. High among these risk factors are disorders of lipid and lipoprotein metabolism. Such dyslipoproteinemias encompass a wide spectrum of monogenic and polygenic conditions that are strongly modulated by environmental factors.

Dynamics of Lipid Metabolism and Its Contribution to Atherosclerosis

Lipids have two main points of entry into the circulation: the gut (exogenous pathway) and the liver (endogenous pathway). The exogenous and endogenous pathways are further interconnected by intermediate pathways (reverse cholesterol transport pathway and others). These pathways are outlined in Figure 1.

EXOGENOUS PATHWAY

Dietary fat constitutes the sole source of exogenous lipids to the body. Triglycerides in food are hydrolyzed by pancreatic lipases within the intestinal lumen. They are then incorporated into micelles through interaction with bile acids acting as emulsifiers. Cholesterol, monoglycerides, free fatty acids, and phospholipids are absorbed through the intestinal brush border via carriers on the enterocyte membrane. Cholesterol molecules are turned into cholesteryl esters in intestinal epithelial cells by the addition of a fatty acid. Long-chain fatty acids (>12 carbons) are esterified to triglycerides and packaged with apolipoprotein (Apo) B48, cholesteryl esters, phospholipids, and cholesterol into the largest-sized lipoprotein particles, known as chylomicrons (>100 nm in diameter, more than 98% lipids, 1%–2% protein), which are secreted into intestinal lymph and delivered to the systemic circulation. Here, they function as a major source of lipids for cells. At the peripheral cell level, chylomicrons are acted on by lipoprotein lipase, which hydrolyzes the triglycerides, releasing the free fatty acids that are taken up by tissues for further metabolism or storage. Apo CII is an important cofactor for lipoprotein lipase. During their transit through the bloodstream, chylomicrons continue to lose lipids, and they also transfer cholesterol and phospholipids to high-density lipoproteins (HDL); they shrink in size and finally are taken up by the liver through chylomicron remnant receptors that

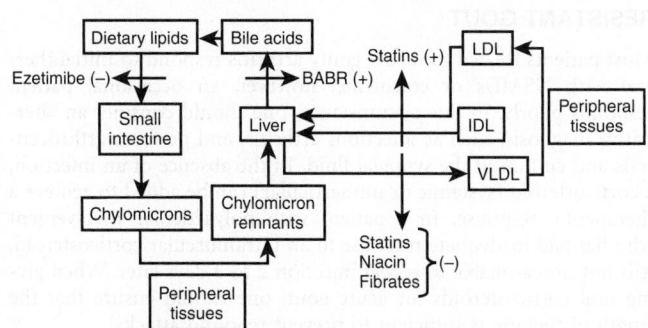

FIGURE 1. Overview of lipid metabolism showing points of therapeutic intervention by available pharmaceutical agents. High-density lipoprotein (HDL) is not shown because there is no approved agent that directly targets HDL, which can be raised indirectly by aerobic exercise, weight loss, and niacin. (+), stimulate; (−), inhibit; BABR, bile acid–binding resins; IDL, intermediate-density lipoprotein; LDL, low-density lipoprotein; VLDL, very-low-density lipoprotein.

use Apo E as a ligand. As a result of this extremely efficient process, normally within hours of eating, chylomicrons are no longer detectable in the circulation.

ENDOGENOUS PATHWAY

The endogenous pathway starts in the liver, which produces another species of triglyceride-rich lipoprotein particles called very-low-density lipoproteins (VLDL), which have a diameter of 30 to 70 nm and contain 85% to 90% lipids and 10% to 15% protein. The major apolipoprotein in VLDL is Apo B100. These particles also contain E and C apolipoproteins. Especially in muscle and adipose tissue, VLDL, like chylomicrons, undergo processing by lipoprotein lipase, which also hydrolyzes VLDL triglycerides, releasing free fatty acids. Catabolism of VLDL by lipoprotein lipase produces smaller particles, known as intermediate-density lipoprotein (IDL), which are enriched in cholesterol. The liver removes about half of the IDL (also known as VLDL remnants) through the action of apo E. The remaining IDL is further processed into low-density lipoproteins (LDL) by hepatic lipase. This process involves further triglyceride hydrolysis. All apoproteins except Apo B100 are removed and transferred to other lipoproteins, and LDL become further enriched in cholesterol. Normally, LDLs carry about 70% of the cholesterol in circulation. Liver cells recognize Apo B100 on LDL, which is taken up via the LDL receptor.

REVERSE CHOLESTEROL TRANSPORT

A major control mechanism by which the body maintains lipid homeostasis in mammals is reverse cholesterol transport. Because all cells synthesize cholesterol but only hepatocytes can metabolize and excrete it, excess cholesterol needs to be carried from peripheral tissues to the liver, where it can be eliminated by secretion into bile after conversion into bile acids. HDLs are the major lipoproteins involved in the transport of cholesterol from peripheral tissues back to the liver. HDLs are synthesized by both hepatocytes and enterocytes, initially in the form of small discoidal particles containing Apo AI and phospholipids. Nascent HDL rapidly accumulates unesterified cholesterol and phospholipids through the action of the membrane protein ABCA1 and the enzyme lecithin-cholesterol acyl transferase (LCAT). As additional lipids are transferred from VLDL to HDL, the latter become more spherical. HDLs are taken up directly in the liver by class B type I scavenger receptor (SR-BI) molecules. Lipids are also transported to the liver via Apo B–containing lipoproteins through the action of cholesteryl ester transfer protein.

PLASMA LIPIDS AND ATHEROSCLEROSIS

Although the physiologic function of the cholesterol-rich lipoproteins, IDL and LDL, is to deliver cholesterol to peripheral tissues, high circulating levels of these particles have long been known to be associated with an increased risk of atherosclerosis. These lipoproteins can pass through endothelial barriers and therefore have the potential to accumulate in the subendothelial space. Once trapped in the extracellular space of the intima, their lipid components are susceptible to biochemical modifications, including oxidation, the products of which become molecular targets for macrophages within the subendothelial space. Macrophages undergo upregulation of their scavenger receptors and take up and accumulate lipids, turning into lipid-engorged macrophages or foam cells, which are key constituents of fatty streaks, the earliest phase of the atherosclerotic plaque. Such early fatty streak plaques may regress, or they may progress to more advanced lesions. Macrophage activation leads to the recruitment of other inflammatory cells, with secretion of inflammatory cytokines initiating a vicious cycle of inflammatory cells and mediators culminating in lesion progression and instability.

As opposed to the atherogenic potential of IDL and LDL, HDL particles are protective against atherosclerotic plaque formation; high HDL levels are associated with a lower incidence of coronary artery disease. This is a result of the capacity of HDL to act in clearing cholesterol from peripheral tissues to the liver for elimination and locally as antiinflammatory and antioxidative mediators.

CURRENT DIAGNOSIS

- Dyslipidemia encompasses a wide range of inherited and acquired conditions.
- The initial diagnosis should be followed by a complete fasting lipid profile and a thorough search to identify and treat secondary causes of dyslipidemia, such as hypothyroidism, alcoholism, diabetes mellitus, and nephrotic syndrome.
- The importance of early recognition and treatment of dyslipidemia lies in its role as a major risk factor for atherosclerosis and for pancreatitis (with high triglycerides).
- A comprehensive global risk assessment for cardiovascular disease should be carried out to stratify risk and guide treatment.

Assessment of the Patient with Dyslipoproteinemia

Given the strong epidemiologic evidence, supported by animal and cell experiments, for a proatherogenic role of VLDL, IDL, and LDL and a protective role of HDL in atherosclerotic cardiovascular disease risk in numerous populations, various societies and professional organizations have established clinical guidelines to aid the physician in reducing risk in people without heart disease (primary prevention) and to treat patients with known atherosclerotic disease (secondary prevention). Among the most widely used set of recommendations is the National Cholesterol Education Program (NCEP) Adult Treatment Panel III (ATP III) guidelines.

The NCEP ATP III defined stratified risk levels and treatment goals for each level. Risk stratification is based on consideration of cardiovascular risk factors. Smoking, HDL cholesterol (abbreviated HDL) concentration less than 40 mg/dL, hypertension or use of antihypertensive agents, family history of premature coronary artery disease, and age greater than 45 years in men or 55 years in women are positive risk factors, whereas an HDL level greater than 60 mg/dL is considered to be a negative risk factor. If two or more risk factors are present, a Framingham risk score is calculated (http://hp2010.nhlbihin.net/atpiii/calculator.asp?usertype=prof [accessed June 30, 2009]). The National Heart, Lung and Blood Institute (NHLBI) has provided this and other excellent clinical tools online to calculate risk and guide treatment. For purposes of primary prevention, the presence of zero or only one risk factor is defined as low risk for atherosclerotic vascular disease; two or more risk factors constitute moderate risk, and higher numbers constitute high risk. In patients with moderate risk, a 10-year risk for CHD of >20% qualifies one as "high risk." An optimal LDL cholesterol (abbreviated LDL) goal is 100 mg/dL for all patients. Also of note is the introduction of LDL 100 mg/dL as a goal for people with known coronary artery disease. More recently, the committee has added consideration of 70 mg/dL as a goal for LDL in patients with very high risk (recent acute coronary syndrome or multiple poorly controlled risk factors, especially diabetes mellitus).

Using these goals as guidelines, a practicing physician aims to achieve therapeutic targets through early and consistent implementation of lifestyle changes along with pharmacologic therapy in appropriately selected patients according to the following general principles.

Lifestyle Changes

All patients with dyslipidemia should be counseled on lifestyle modifications. Dietary modification is an essential component, given that the main source of lipids is exogenous dietary fat. In a patient with dyslipidemia, dietary intake of saturated fatty acids should be limited,

CURRENT THERAPY

- Dyslipidemia is a modifiable risk factor and one of the major risk factors for atherosclerotic cardiovascular disease.
- First-line therapy is therapeutic lifestyle modification.
- Therapy depends on risk stratification, as does the timing of initiation of treatment with pharmacologic agents in addition to lifestyle changes.
- Therapy should be guided based on goals which are in turn based on risk stratification.
- The main problem should be identified as high cholesterol (high LDL), high triglycerides, or a combined lipid problem.
    - High LDL: start with statin add ezetimibe (Zetia) if necessary.
    - High triglycerides: start fibrates; consider adding orlistat (Xenical, Alli)[1]; also, limit fat intake.
    - High LDL and triglycerides: consider combining statins and fibrates.
- Manage all other risk factors appropriately.

[1]Not FDA approved for this indication.

and a reduction in dietary total lipids is necessary. Other important goals include weight loss in overweight patients. Exercise and the use of plant stanols (e.g., Benecol) or omega-3 fatty acids may also be helpful. The dietary component to be restricted depends also in the component of lipid profile that is high. Patients with triglyceride levels in the >1000 mg/dL range should severely limit total fat intake, not only to reduce cardiovascular risk but also to prevent acute pancreatitis. In patients for whom the goal is to achieve LDL reduction, dietary changes emphasizing certain fatty acid classes, as detailed later, provide a better starting point. The addition of soy products to the diet also may contribute to lowering of LDL.

The American Heart Association heart-healthy diet recommendations are commonly used to guide patients in their dietary practices. The previously used step I and step II dietary recommendations have given way to the therapeutic lifestyle change (TLC) diet, which can be summarized as follows:

- Total dietary fat should be limited to 25% to 35% of total caloric intake, and saturated fats should constitute less than 7% of this fraction.
- Polyunsaturated fats should be less than 10% of energy intake, whereas monounsaturated fats (mainly olive and canola oil) may constitute up to 20% of energy intake.
- Carbohydrates are allocated 50% to 60% and proteins approximately 15% of energy intake.
- Cholesterol intake should be limited to less than 200 mg/day.
- Total caloric intake should balance energy intake and expenditure to maintain desirable body weight and prevent weight gain.

If present, obesity should be aggressively treated. Treatment of obesity has a favorable effect on lipid levels. Obese patients who succeed in losing weight tend to show a decrease in triglycerides and LDL and an increase in HDL. The benefit of TLC usually becomes measurable within 6 to 12 months. There is a large amount of heterogeneity in the response to lifestyle changes, which is in part genetically based. Referral to a dietitian may lead to greater success in the short term. The benefits attained by dietary modifications tend to be short-lived in most patients, and diet compliance tends to decrease over time, especially after 1 year. Therefore, the physician should be ready to institute drug therapy concurrent with starting dietary modifications in patients who fulfill criteria for pharmacologic interventions (Table 1) and should be ready to add lipid-lowering agents for patients who have not responded to TLC or who display worsening lipid levels.

Drug Therapy for Dyslipoproteinemia

GENERAL CONSIDERATIONS

The decision to initiate pharmacotherapy should be based on a patient's risk status. The approach used in this chapter is largely based on the NCEP ATP III recommendations and as outlined in Table 1. The main goal in lipid reduction in most cases is to reduce the risk of atherosclerotic cardiovascular disease. The currently available lipid-lowering agents can be classified based on their structure and mechanism of action into statins (3-hydroxy-3-methylglutaryl coenzyme A [HMG-CoA] reductase inhibitors), cholesterol absorption inhibitors such as ezetimibe (Zetia), fibric acid derivatives (fibrates), bile acid sequestrants, and nicotinic acid (niacin). These classes differ with regard to degree and type of lipid lowering, and drugs within each group may differ in efficacy and side effects. Conventional dosing regimens and common adverse effects are summarized in Table 2. The choice of drug depends on the specific lipid abnormality and concurrent medical conditions.

Statins are usually the first choice in patients with high cholesterol levels for reduction of primary or secondary cardiovascular risk. If the LDL goal cannot be reached with statins only, addition of an agent from another class should be considered. The recommended goals for treatment are summarized in Table 1. For patients who cannot tolerate one specific statin because of myopathy, it may be appropriate to try pravastatin (Pravachol), which has a lower risk of myopathy. For patients who cannot tolerate statins, a combination of other agents can be started, and the patient can be referred to a lipid specialist.

STATINS

Statins have been in clinical use for more than 2 decades. They work through inhibition of HMG-CoA reductase, the rate-limiting enzyme in cholesterol biosynthesis. Among all lipid-lowering agents, statins achieve the highest degree of LDL reduction. In addition to decreasing cholesterol biosynthesis, statins also increase the clearance of IDL and LDL by upregulation of LDL receptors on hepatocytes. Stimulation of Apo AI expression and increased hepatic HDL secretion have also been observed. In addition to their direct effects on lipid homeostasis, statins have been reported to have other, largely beneficial

TABLE 1 LDL-Cholesterol Goals and Levels for Initiating Lifestyle and Pharmacologic Interventions (NCEP ATP III)

Risk Category*	LDL Goal (mg/dL)	LDL Level at Which To Initiate TLC (mg/dL)	LDL Level at Which To Initiate Drug Therapy (mg/dL)
CAD or CAD risk equivalents (risk >20%)	<100	≥100	≥130 (>100 optional)
2+ risk factors (risk 10%–20%)	<130	≥130	≥130
2+ risk factors (risk 5%–10%)	<130	≥130	≥160
0–1 risk factor (risk 0%–5%)	<160	≥160	≥190

*Number of risk factors and 10-year risk for atherosclerotic cardiovascular disease.
Abbreviations: CAD, coronary artery disease; LDL, low-density lipoprotein; NCEP ATP III, National Cholesterol Education Program Adult Treatment Panel III guidelines; TLC, therapeutic lifestyle changes.

TABLE 2 Major Drugs for Management of Dyslipidemia

Drug	Indications	Dose (Starting-Maximum)	Mechanism	Side Effects
Statins				
Atorvastatin (Lipitor)	Elevated LDL	10–80 mg qhs	Decreased cholesterol synthesis, increased hepatic LDL receptors, decreased VLDL release	Myalgias Arthralgias High liver enzymes Dyspepsia
Fluvastatin (Lescol)		20–80 mg qhs		
Lovastatin (Mevacor)		20–80 mg daily		
Pravastatin (Pravachol)		40–80 mg qhs		
Rosuvastatin (Crestor)		10–40 mg qhs		
Simvastatin (Zocor)		20–80 mg qhs		
Cholesterol Absorption Inhibitors				
Ezetimibe (Zetia)	Elevated LDL	10 mg daily	Decreased intestinal cholesterol absorption	High liver enzymes
Bile Acid Sequestrants				
Cholestyramine (Questran)	Elevated LDL	4–32 g daily	Increased bile acid excretion, increased LDL receptors	Bloating Constipation Elevated triglycerides
Colestipol (Colestid)		5–40 g daily		
Colesevelam (Welchol)		3750–4375 mg daily		
Fibrates				
Fenofibrate (Tricor)	Elevated TG Elevated remnants	160 mg daily 50–160 mg daily	Increased LPL activity, decreased VLDL synthesis	Dyspepsia, myalgia, gallstones, high liver enzymes
Gemfibrozil (Lopid)		600 mg bid		
Other				
Niacin (Niaspan, generic)	Elevated LDL, low HDL, elevated TG	100 mg-2g tid (rapid tab) 0.5–2 g qhs (ER tab, Niaspan)	Decreased VLDL synthesis	Flushing, high glucose, uric acid, liver enzymes
Fish oils (omega-3 fatty acids,[7] omega-3 acid ethyl esters [Lovaza])	Severely elevated TG	3–12 g daily 4 g daily (Lovaza)	Decreased chylomicron	Dyspepsia

[7]Available as dietary supplement.
Abbreviations: ER, extended release; LDL, low-density lipoprotein; LPL, lipoprotein lipase; TG, triglycerides; VLDL, very-low-density lipoprotein.

pleiotropic effects, which are thought to involve reductions in a wide range of atherogenic events (e.g., reduced formation of reactive oxygen species, inhibition of platelet reactivity, decreased vasoconstriction).

Statins are the only class of lipid-lowering agents that have been shown in multiple randomized clinical trials to have a direct effect on, and to produce clear improvement in, overall mortality in primary and secondary prevention. Statins decreased rates of myocardial infarction, stroke, coronary mortality, and all-cause mortality in both primary and secondary prevention studies. Furthermore, risk reduction was apparent in a wide range of patients, including men, women, smokers, patients with diabetes, and those with hypertension, as well as in older populations.

Atorvastatin (Lipitor) and rosuvastatin (Crestor) are the most potent statins. They cause an LDL reduction of 60% at doses of 80 and 40 mg/day, respectively. These agents also have the advantage of decreasing triglyceride levels. Rosuvastatin increases HDL cholesterol levels better than atorvastatin, simvastatin (Zocor), or pravastatin (Pravachol).

Statins are well tolerated, and usually they are taken in tablet form once daily. Potential common side effects include nonspecific gastrointestinal side effects such as dyspepsia. Headaches, fatigue, and muscle or joint pain have also been reported. Two important, albeit rare, side effects about which the patient should be informed are myopathy and hepatitis; the physician should monitor for these effects. Myopathy risk is increased in patients with renal insufficiency and in those who are taking multiple agents because of drug interactions. Commonly used drugs that can decrease statin metabolism include erythromycin, antifungal agents, immunosuppressive agents, and fibrates.

The risk of hepatotoxicity is less than 1%, and that of myopathy is less than 0.1%. Patients should be advised to report muscle pain of unexplained origin, and creatine kinase (CK) should be measured. Patients who develop muscle pain and CK elevations 10 times the

upper limit of normal should be taken off the statin. CK elevations that are between 3 and 10 times the upper limit of normal require close clinical and biochemical monitoring. It is therefore valuable to determine a baseline CK level at initiation of therapy; however, serial CK measurements are of limited value, because myopathy and rhabdomyolysis can occur suddenly without antecedent CK elevation. The potential for hepatotoxicity does require follow-up of liver transaminases (alanine and aspartate aminotransferase) before the start of treatment, at 2 months, and every 6 months thereafter. Substantial elevation (>3 times the upper limit of normal) should prompt discontinuation. Severe elevations are very rare and resolve after discontinuation of the drug. When using statins in combination with a fibrate, especially in patients with elevations in both cholesterol and triglycerides, it is advisable to use lower doses of the statin.

EZETIMIBE

Ezetimibe (Zetia) is the first in a new class of agents that act through inhibition of absorption of sterol transporters in the gut lumen. LDL reduction is approximately 15% when the drug is used as monotherapy. Ezetimibe may be considered a good agent to add to statin therapy in a patient not achieving goal levels. As an added benefit, it may be possible to use a lower dose of statin and reduce potential statin toxicity. A recent study raised the issue of ezetimibe effectiveness in reducing adverse cardiovascular events; this should be resolved by ongoing research on this relatively new medication.

BILE ACID–BINDING RESINS

This class of agents has been in clinical use for many decades. They work by binding to bile acids in the intestine and promoting their fecal excretion. This causes the liver to integrate more cholesterol into bile acid synthesis, so as to maintain a stable bile acid pool. The consequent decrease in hepatic cholesterol causes LDL receptor upregulation and enhances LDL clearance from the plasma, leading to a net decrease in LDL levels. LDL can decrease 15% to 30%, and HDL can go up 3% to 5%. HMG CoA synthase activity can increase, so combination therapy with statin would be synergistic, especially in patients with a suboptimal response.

Available agents are colestipol (Colestid), cholestyramine (Questran), and colesevelam (Welchol). Most side effects involve the gastrointestinal tract, with constipation and bloating being the most common. These agents may interfere with the absorption of warfarin (Coumadin), phenobarbital, levothyroxine (Synthroid), and digoxin (Lanoxin), among other medications. Patients on multiple medications should be advised to take bile acid–binding resins 1 hour before or 4 hours after their other medications.

Because these drugs are not systemically absorbed, they may be preferred when systemic absorption is to be avoided, such as during pregnancy or lactation.

FIBRATES

Fibrates are effective in lowering plasma triglyceride levels; they are especially valuable in patients who have a combination of high triglycerides and low HDL. The Veterans Affairs High-Density Lipoprotein Intervention Trial (VA-HIT), one of the early secondary prevention lipid-lowering studies, showed that men with coronary artery disease and low HDL who were treated with gemfibrozil (Lopid) experienced a 6% increase in HDL and a 31% decrease in triglycerides, with no change in LDL, compared with similar subjects treated with placebo; there was also a 22% decrease in all-cause mortality and nonfatal myocardial infarction. Fibrates have multiple favorable metabolic effects, including activation of peroxisome proliferator–activated receptor-α (PPARα) (which contributes to the regulation of both lipid and carbohydrate metabolism), stimulation of lipoprotein lipase (increasing triglyceride hydrolysis), and downregulation of Apo CIII (improved lipoprotein remnant clearance, because Apo CIII inhibits lipoprotein lipase). An enhanced VLDL-to-LDL conversion may lead to mild LDL elevation in some patients. This effect may decrease over weeks as LDL receptor upregulation occurs.

Fibrates are generally well tolerated. The most common side effect is dyspepsia. Other side effects include low rates of myopathy and hepatic enzyme elevation. Fibrates increase the risk of gallstones, and patients on warfarin may need dose adjustment. Monitoring of liver enzymes is recommended every 6 months.

Patients with high triglycerides should start with a low-fat diet and a fibrate. Patients, especially those with familial high triglycerides, may benefit from the addition of orlistat ([Xenical, Alli],[1] a pancreatic lipase inhibitor that decreases fat digestion and absorption, or omega-3 fatty acids,[7] or both.

NIACIN

Niacin or nicotinic acid (Niaspan, generic) is a B_3 vitamin that effectively increases HDL levels by blocking HDL uptake by the liver. Hepatic VLDL secretion is decreased due to inhibition of flux from adipocytes to the liver and inhibition of diacylglyceryl acyl transferase in the liver. It also increases Apo B100 catabolism. In the HDL Atherosclerosis Study (HATS), high-dose niacin combined with statins decreased cardiovascular mortality.

Patient education and monitoring of therapy are key to successful treatment with niacin. The most common side effect is flushing. This can be avoided or improved by initiating therapy with a low dose of niacin, taking an aspirin 1 hour before niacin, and avoiding hot foods or beverages at the time the niacin is taken. Other side effects include pruritus and increased uric acid levels. Mild elevations in liver enzymes can occur in 15% of subjects and rarely require discontinuation of the niacin.

[1]Not FDA approved for this indication.
[7]Available as dietary supplement.

REFERENCES

Ballantyne CM. Treatment of dyslipidemia to reduce cardiovascular risk in patients with multiple risk factors. Clin Cornerstone 2007;8(Suppl. 6):S6–13.
Ballantyne CM, Grundy SM, Oberman A, et al. Hyperlipidemia: Diagnostic and therapeutic perspectives. J Clin Endocrinol Metab 2000;85:2089–112.
Broedl UC, Geiss HC, Parhofer KG. Comparison of current guidelines for primary prevention of coronary heart disease. J Gen Intern Med 2003; 18:190–5.
Grundy SM, Balady GJ, Criqui MH, et al. When to start cholesterol-lowering therapy in patients with coronary heart disease: A statement for healthcare professionals from the American Heart Association Task Force on Risk Reduction. Circulation 1997;95:1683–5.
Jones P, Kafonek S, Laurora I, et al. for the CURVES investigators: Comparative dose efficacy study of atorvastatin versus simvastatin, pravastatin, lovastatin, and fluvastatin in patients with hypercholesterolemia. Am J Cardiol 1998;81:582–7.
Otvos JD, Collins D, Freedman DS, et al. Low-density lipoprotein and high-density lipoprotein particle subclasses predict coronary events and are favorably changed by gemfibrozil therapy in the Veterans Affairs High–Density Lipoprotein Intervention Trial. Circulation 2006;113:1556–63.
Probstfield JL, Hunninghake DB. Nicotinic acid as a lipoprotein-altering agent: Therapy directed by the primary physician. Arch Intern Med 1994; 154: 1557–9.
Randomised trial of cholesterol lowering in 4444 patients with coronary heart disease: The Scandinavian Simvastatin Survival Study (4S). Lancet 1994; 344:1383–9.
Sacks FM, Pfeffer MA, Moye LA, et al. The effect of pravastatin on coronary events after myocardial infarction in patients with average cholesterol levels: Cholesterol And Recurrent Events trial investigators. N Engl J Med 1996; 335:1001–9.
Shepherd J, Cobbe SM, Ford I, et al. Prevention of coronary heart disease with pravastatin in men with hypercholesterolemia. N Engl J Med 1995;33:1301–7.
Third Report of the National Cholesterol Education Program (NCEP) Expert panel on detection, evaluation and treatment of high blood cholesterol in adults (Adult Treatment Panel III). Circulation 2002;106:3143–421.
Wilson PW. Established risk factors and coronary artery disease: The Framingham Study. Am J Hypertens 1994;7(7 Pt 2):7S–12S.

Obesity

Method of
Nicole Nader, MD, and Seema Kumar, MD

Epidemiology

Obesity is a complex disease that represents a growing epidemic in the United States and worldwide. According to current estimates, more than 33.5% of adult men, 35.3% of adult women, and 16.3% of children and adolescents age 2 to 19 years in the United States are obese. Between 1976–1980 and 2003–2004, the prevalence of obesity among adults almost doubled. There are disparities in the prevalence of obesity between ethnic groups, especially among women. In the United States, the prevalence of obesity is highest in non-Hispanic black women. Obesity is no longer a cosmetic issue; it has been found to be associated with several comorbidities and increased mortality.

Diagnosis

Obesity is a condition marked by the accumulation of excess body fat. The body mass index (BMI) is the most practical way to evaluate the degree of excess weight. It is calculated from the weight (in kilograms) and the square of the height (in meters), as follows:

$$BMI = Weight \div Height^2$$

TABLE 1 Classification of Overweight and Obesity by BMI, Waist Circumference, and Associated Health Risk

Classification	BMI (kg/m²)	Disease Risk* Waist ≤102 cm (≤40 in) in men or ≤88 cm (≤35 in) in women	Disease Risk* Waist >102 cm (>40 in) in men or >88 cm (>35 in) in women
Underweight	<18.5	—	—
Normal†	18.5–24.9	—	—
Overweight	25.0–29.9	Increased	High
Obesity—class I	30.0–34.9	High	Very high
Obesity—class II	35.0–39.9	Very high	Very high
Extreme obesity—class III	≥40	Extremely high	Extremely high

Reproduced from Clinical Guidelines on the Identification, Evaluation, and Treatment of Overweight and Obesity in Adults: The Evidence Report. National Institutes of Health. Obes Res 1998;6(Suppl 2):51S-209S.
*Disease risk for type 2 diabetes, hypertension, and cardiovascular disease relative to normal weight and waist circumference.
†Increased waist circumference can also be a marker for increased risk even in persons of normal weight.

The World Health Organisation (WHO) and National Institutes of Health (NIH) define overweight as BMI between 25 and 24.9 kg/m² and obesity as a BMI greater than 30 kg/m² (Table 1). These guidelines apply to whites, Hispanics, and blacks. Because Asians can have higher percentage of body fat at a lower BMI, overweight for this particular ethnic group is a BMI between 23 and 29.9 kg/m², and obesity is a BMI equal to or greater than 30 kg/m². Because BMI normative values are age and gender specific during childhood, BMI values greater than or equal to the 95th percentile for age and sex are used to define obesity in children and adolescents. The BMI correlates with percentage of body fat and body fat mass, as well as with mortality. However, for a given BMI, the degree of body fatness tends to be higher in women compared with men, and it is higher in older compared with younger people. Additionally, the BMI may overestimate the degree of body fat in athletes. The relationship between BMI and mortality appears to form a J- or U-shaped curve, with the lowest mortality rate seen in those with a BMI of about 25 kg/m² (Fig. 1).

Because people with abdominal (central) adiposity are more likely to develop many of the health conditions associated with obesity, waist circumference is an important adjuvant measurement to obtain when screening for obesity. Waist circumference is measured at the level of the top of the iliac crest with the measuring tape snug against the skin. A waist circumference of more than 102 cm (40 in) in men or 88 cm (35 in) in women is considered high and confers an increased risk for comorbidities such as type 2 diabetes, hypertension, and coronary heart disease (see Table 1). More precise measurement of abdominal fat can be made with abdominal computed tomography or magnetic resonance imaging. Alternative methods to assess body composition and degree of fatness include measurements of skin fold thickness, hydrostatic weighing, bioelectric impedance, and scanning by dual-energy x-ray absorptiometry (DEXA). These methods require specialized equipment and trained personnel, and they are not used routinely in clinical practice.

CURRENT DIAGNOSIS

- Body Mass Index (BMI) is calculated as weight in kilograms divided by height in meters squared (kg/m²). BMI is currently the preferred method for determining whether a patient is obese.
- Patients with a BMI of 30 or greater are considered obese.
- Abdominal circumference should also be measured when screening for obesity.
- A waist circumference of greater than 102 cm (40 in) in men or 88 cm (35 in) in women is considered indicative of abdominal obesity.

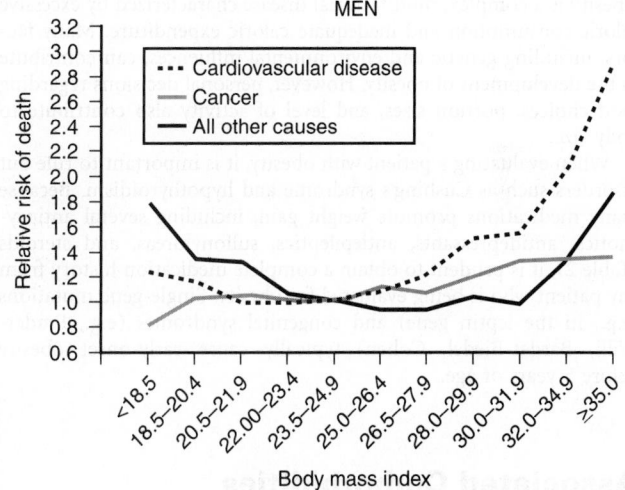

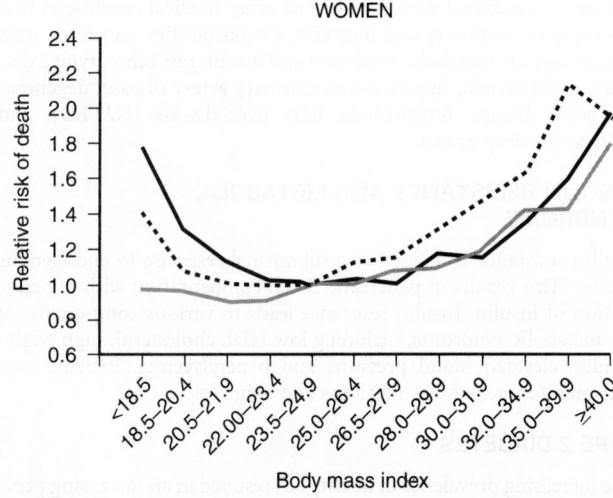

FIGURE 1. Correlation between mortality risk and increasing body mass index. (Data from Calle EE, Thun MJ, Petrelli JM, et al: Body-mass index and mortality in a prospective cohort of U.S. adults. N Engl J Med 1999;341:1097–1105.)

TABLE 2 Medications That May Promote Weight Gain

Drug Class	Examples
Antipsychotics	Risperidone (Risperdal), olanzapine (Zyprexa), clozapine (Clozaril)
Antidepressants	Imipramine (Tofranil), amitriptyline (Elavil), doxepin (Sinequan), tranylcypromine (Parnate)
Lithium	
Anticonvulsants	Valproic acid (Depakene), carbamazepine (Tegretol)
Antidiabetics	Insulin, rosiglitazone (Avandia), pioglitazone (Actos), glipizide (Glucotrol), glyburide (Diabeta, Micronase), glimepiride (Amaryl)
Antihistamines	Diphenhydramine (Benadryl)
α-Blockers	Doxazosin (Cardura), prazosin (Minipress), terazosin (Hytrin)
Steroids	Glucocorticoids
β-Blockers	Propranolol (Inderal), metoprolol (Lopressor), atenolol (Tenormin)

Etiology and Pathophysiology

Obesity is a complex, multifactorial disease characterized by excessive caloric consumption and inadequate caloric expenditure. Many factors, including genetic and environmental influences, can contribute to the development of obesity. However, personal decisions regarding food choices, portion sizes, and level of activity also contribute to body size.

When evaluating a patient with obesity, it is important to rule out disorders such as Cushing's syndrome and hypothyroidism. Because many medications promote weight gain, including several antipsychotics, antidepressants, antiepileptics, sulfonylureas, and steroids (Table 2), it is prudent to obtain a complete medication history from any patient who is being evaluated for obesity. Single-gene mutations (e.g., in the leptin gene) and congenital syndromes (e.g., Prader-Willi, Bardet-Biedel, Cohen) typically cause early-onset obesity before 5 years of age.

Associated Comorbidities

Obesity is associated with a variety of other medical conditions that can increase morbidity and mortality. Comorbidities associated with obesity include metabolic syndrome and insulin resistance, type 2 diabetes, dyslipidemia, hypertension, coronary artery disease, degenerative joint disease, nonalcoholic fatty liver disease (NAFLD), and obstructive sleep apnea.

INSULIN RESISTANCE AND METABOLIC SYNDROME

Insulin resistance is defined as a subnormal response to endogenous insulin. This results in pancreatic B-cell compensation with hypersecretion of insulin. Insulin resistance leads to various components of the metabolic syndrome, including low HDL cholesterol, high triglycerides, elevated blood pressure, and hyperglycemia. Patients may also manifest acanthosis nigricans and skin tags.

TYPE 2 DIABETES

The increasing prevalence of obesity has resulted in an increasing prevalence of type 2 diabetes as well. More than 80% of type 2 diabetes can be attributed to obesity, but other factors, such as family history, are also involved. Criteria for diagnosis of type 2 diabetes include a fasting glucose level greater than 125 mg/dL or glucose levels greater than 200 mg/dL during a 2-hour oral glucose tolerance test.

HYPERTENSION

Hypertension is a common chronic disease, and it has been estimated that obesity is associated with approximately 30% to 50% of the cases of hypertension in the United States. Hypertension is associated with an increased risk for stroke, myocardial infarction, heart failure, and kidney disease. Even a modest weight loss (5%–10% of initial weight) can lead to a significant fall in blood pressure and, often, decreased need for antihypertensive medications.

DYSLIPIDEMIA

A variety of blood lipid abnormalities are seen frequently in obese patients. These include elevated levels of total cholesterol, LDL cholesterol, and triglycerides and decreased levels of HDL cholesterol. Patients with central adiposity are at particularly high risk for the development of hypertriglyceridemia and low HDL. Screening for dyslipidemia should be done with a fasting lipid profile. However, if the testing opportunity is nonfasting, the total cholesterol and HDL values can still be measured.

CORONARY HEART DISEASE

Comorbidities associated with obesity such as hypertension, insulin resistance, type 2 diabetes, and dyslipidemia lead to increased risk of cardiovascular disease in obese adults. Obesity is also associated with increased risk of coronary heart disease, heart failure, cardiovascular mortality, and all-cause mortality.

RESPIRATORY ABNORMALITIES

Obstructive sleep apnea is the most important respiratory problem associated with obesity. It is often underrecognized and inadequately treated. Patients may present with snoring, apneic episodes, excessive daytime somnolence, fatigue, irritability, and erectile dysfunction. Consequent nocturnal hypoxemia may result in arrhythmias, pulmonary hypertension, and right-sided heart failure. Treatment includes weight loss and use of continuous positive airway pressure at night.

HEPATOBILIARY DISEASE

Obesity increases the risk of cholelithiasis and of NAFLD. The spectrum of NAFLD ranges from steatosis with mild disruption of the liver architecture by fat to steatohepatitis with varying degrees of fibrosis and cirrhosis. Increased liver transaminase levels and findings of steatosis on ultrasonography are both suggestive of NAFLD in obese patients. However, the definitive diagnosis remains histologic.

OSTEOARTHRITIS

The incidence of osteoarthritis is increased in obese subjects. Osteoarthritis commonly develops in the knees and ankles but can also affect non–weight-bearing joints. Weight loss results in decreased risk of osteoarthritis.

CANCER

For both men and women, increased BMI is associated with increased mortality from several cancers, such as those of the esophagus, colon and rectum, liver, gall bladder, pancreas, kidney, as well as non-Hodgkin's lymphoma and multiple myeloma. Additionally, obese men are at increased risk of death from stomach and prostate cancer, and obese women are at increased risk of death from cancers of the breast, uterus, cervix, and ovary.

Treatment

Patients must undergo a detailed history and physical examination before a treatment plan is initiated. Secondary causes of obesity, such as Cushing's syndrome and hypothyroidism, should be considered in

CURRENT THERAPY

- Treatment of patients with obesity requires a multidisciplinary team approach.
- Lifestyle modifications, including dietary changes and increased physical activity, remain first-line treatment for patients with obesity.
- Adjuvant pharmacotherapy may be considered for patients with a BMI greater than 30 kg/m^2 or a BMI of 27 to 30 kg/m^2 with concomitant weight-related complications.
- Bariatric surgery should be considered for patients with a BMI of 40 kg/m^2 or greater and for those with a BMI of 35 kg/m^2 or greater who have significant comorbidities such as severe diabetes, sleep apnea, or joint disease after nonsurgical weight loss attempts have failed.

the evaluation. A complete medication history is crucial to determining whether any medications may have promoted weight gain.

Laboratory studies should be directed at ruling out secondary causes in selected patients and ruling out comorbidities (fasting glucose, lipid profile, liver function tests). It is important that practitioners assess each patient's willingness to change and expectations for weight loss. Treatment should be based on the patient's BMI, risk factors, and willingness to lose weight (Fig. 2). Patients who are in the precontemplative phase (i.e., in the early stages of thinking about it) are not likely to be successful despite appropriate counseling. Health care providers must enforce the idea that even a modest weight loss improves complications associated with obesity.

Treatment of obesity requires a multidisciplinary team approach. Lifestyle modifications, including dietary change and increased physical activity, represent first-line treatment for patients with obesity. Self-efficacy, which is a feeling of being able to perform the behaviors required, and positive coping skills are associated with improved success. Pharmacotherapy and bariatric surgery may be used as adjuvant therapies in certain patients.

The goal of treatment is to prevent the complications of obesity. The initial target goal of weight loss therapy is to decrease body weight by 10%. Once this target is achieved, further weight loss can be attempted if indicated. The rationales for this initial goal of moderate weight loss are that:

- It can decrease the severity of obesity-associated risk factors.
- It can set the stage for further weight loss, if indicated.
- It is realistic and can be achieved and maintained over time.

A reasonable timeline for a 10% reduction in body weight is 6 months of therapy. A period of weight maintenance should then occur. Further weight loss may be considered if the initial goal is achieved and then maintained for at least 6 months. It is important to inform patients that it is preferable to maintain a moderate amount of weight loss over time than to lose more weight but later regain it.

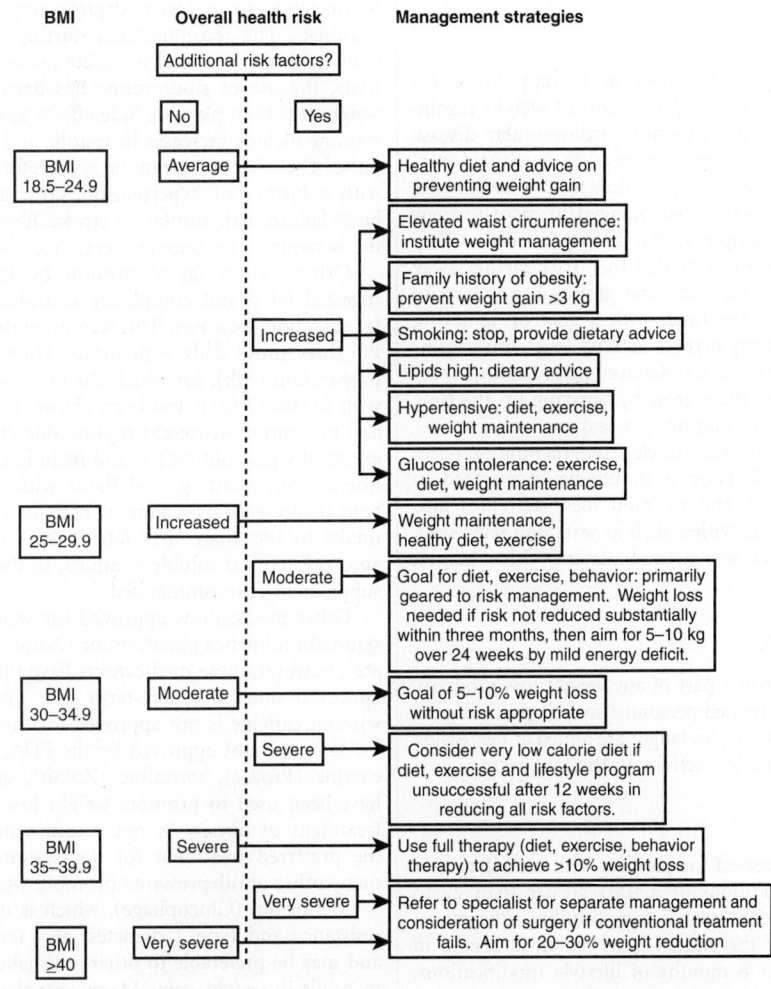

FIGURE 2. Assessment of health risk and management of obesity. BMI, body mass index. (Reproduced with permission from World Health Organisation: Obesity: Preventing and managing the global epidemic. Report of a WHO consultation. World Health Organ Tech Rep Ser 2000;894: i. Copyright 2000 World Health Organisation.)

DIETARY THERAPY

Obese patients should be counseled to follow a hypocaloric and balanced meal plan. These typically provide 1200 to 1800 calories per day, with 20% to 30% of calories from fat, 50% to 55% from carbohydrates, and 15% to 20% from protein. In general, women should be advised to consume approximately 1000 to 1200 kcal/day and men 1200 to 1600 kcal/day during the weight loss phase of treatment. It has been recommended that total fat intake not exceed 30% of total daily calories, that saturated fat account for not more than 8% to 10% of total calories, and that cholesterol intake be limited to 300 mg/day. A healthy diet should also contain 20 to 30 g of fiber daily. Patients should be counseled to avoid unnecessary calories from alcohol and sugary beverages such as soda and juice. These diets result in losses of approximately 1 to 2 lb per week or 4 to 8 lb per month.

Several alternative diets have been tried over the years. Recent data suggest that the so-called Mediterranean diet and low-carbohydrate diets may represent effective alternatives to the low-fat diet for weight loss. The long-term efficacy and safety of these diets remains unknown at this time.

Very-low-calorie diets contain less than 800 kcal/day and are usually administered in the form of liquid supplements. Although these diets do produce significant and rapid weight loss, results are difficult to maintain in the long term. These diets require close monitoring by a health care professional. Side effects associated with very-low-calorie diets include fatigue, constipation, hair loss, and gallstones. These diets are strictly contraindicated in children and in pregnant and lactating women and are generally reserved for patients who require rapid weight loss for a specific purpose such as surgery.

PHYSICAL ACTIVITY

Physical activity is an integral component of therapy for obese patients and is most important in the prevention of weight regain. Physical activity also decreases the risks for cardiovascular disease and type 2 diabetes. Sedentary obese patients need to start their exercise program slowly and may require supervision from a health care professional. Initially, patients may be encouraged to increase their activities of daily living. For example, it may be suggested that they take the stairs instead of the elevator or that they park farther away from work or shopping. The intensity and duration of exercise should be increased gradually over time, with a goal of achieving 150 minutes of moderate-intensity aerobic activity (e.g., brisk walking) or 75 minutes of vigorous-intensity exercise (e.g., running) every week. It is acceptable to achieve these goals by breaking up the time into smaller chunks of at least 10 minutes per session.

Ideally, adults should also perform muscle strengthening exercises on two or more days per week. Patients should be encouraged to choose activities that they enjoy and to build these activities into their daily schedule. Sedentary activities, such as watching television, sitting in front of a computer screen, and playing video games, should be discouraged.

BEHAVIOR MODIFICATION

Behavior modification is an integral part of any weight loss program. This requires the availability of trained personnel such as psychologists and therapists. The behavioral strategies taught are aimed at decreasing caloric intake and increasing physical activity in the long term.

PHARMACOTHERAPY

Pharmacotherapy is usually reserved for patients with a BMI greater than 30 kg/m^2 without complications or a BMI greater than 27 to 30 kg/m^2 with concomitant weight-related complications. Pharmacotherapy typically is initiated if the patient has been unsuccessful in attaining goal weight loss after 6 months of lifestyle modifications, but it must be used in conjunction with a program that includes dietary changes and physical activity. In general, the use of medication promotes only a modest weight loss, in the range of 2 to 10 kg. The effects are generally maximal during the first 6 months of therapy.

TABLE 3 Drugs Approved by the FDA for Treatment of Obesity

Drug	Trade Names	Dosage
Pancreatic Lipase Inhibitor Approved for Long-Term Use		
Orlistat	Xenical	120 mg tid before meals
Norepinephrine-Serotonin Reuptake Inhibitor Approved for Long-Term Use		
Sibutramine	Meridia Reductil[2]	5–15 mg/d
Noradrenergic Drugs Approved for Short-Term Use		
Phentermine	Adipex	15–37.5 mg/d
	Ionamin (slow-release resin)	15–30 mg/d
Diethylpropion	Tenuate	25 mg tid
	Tenuate Dospan	75 mg every morning
Benzphetamine	Didrex	25–50 mg tid
Phendimetrazine	Bontril	17.5–70 mg tid
	Prelu-2	105 mg/d

[2]Not available in the United States.

The two medications most commonly prescribed for weight loss are sibutramine (Meridia) and orlistat (Xenical) (Table 3). Sibutramine is an anorexiant medication that inhibits norepinephrine, serotonin, and, to a lesser degree, dopamine reuptake into nerve terminals. The recommended starting dose in adults is 10 mg PO daily, with the potential to titrate up to 15 mg PO daily. In multiple trials, the use of sibutramine has been shown to result in greater weight loss than placebo. Side effects associated with the use of sibutramine include increases in systolic and diastolic blood pressure and pulse. The use of sibutramine is therefore contraindicated in patients with a history of hypertension, coronary heart disease, congestive heart failure, arrhythmias, or stroke. Regular blood pressure monitoring is required for patients receiving sibutramine.

Orlistat alters fat absorption by inhibiting pancreatic lipases. Ingested fat is not completely hydrolyzed to fatty acids, and fecal fat excretion increases. The recommended dose for adults is 120 mg PO three times daily with meals. There is also an over-the-counter preparation (Alli), for which the dose is 60 mg PO three times daily with meals. Orlistat has been shown to be effective for weight loss and prevention of weight regain. Side effects associated with orlistat are mostly gastrointestinal and include cramping, flatus, fecal incontinence, oily spotting, and flatus with discharge. These side effects tend to decrease over time as patients learn to restrict their dietary intake to less than 30% fat. Orlistat may also interfere with the absorption of fat-soluble vitamins, so the use of a daily multivitamin supplement is recommended.

Other medications approved for weight loss therapy include the sympathomimetics phentermine (Adipex) and diethylpropion (Tenuate); however, these medications have the potential for abuse and are approved only for short-term use. The use of ephedra[2] with or without caffeine is not approved for the treatment of obesity.

Although not approved by the FDA, antidepressants such as fluoxetine (Prozac), sertraline (Zoloft), and bupropion (Wellbutrin) have been used to promote weight loss. The use of these drugs for treatment of obesity is not recommended; however, they may be the preferred treatment for depression in obese patients, because many other antidepressants promote weight gain.

Metformin (Glucophage), which is used for treatment of insulin resistance and type 2 diabetes, also tends to promote weight loss and may be preferable to other antidiabetic medications, which tend to result in weight gain. Many over-the-counter dietary and herbal

[2]Not available in the United States.

supplements are also available to obese patients. However, there are limited efficacy and safety data to support their use, and they are generally not recommended.

BARIATRIC SURGERY

Bariatric surgery should be considered for patients with a BMI greater than 40 kg/m^2 or a BMI greater than 35 kg/m^2 with significant comorbid conditions. Patients should be well informed and motivated and have failed a trial of nonsurgical weight loss. They should also be of acceptable risk for surgery. Contraindications to bariatric surgery include untreated major depression, binge eating disorders, active drug or alcohol abuse, and a history of noncompliance. A comprehensive preoperative evaluation and close extended follow-up after surgery are required. Bariatric surgery has been shown to result in a significant and sustained weight loss, as well as resolution of many obesity-related complications, in most patients. Patients may lose more than 60% of their excess weight after bariatric surgery.

Bariatric surgery for children and adolescents remains highly controversial. However, surgery on patients between 12 and 18 years of age who had significant medical problems related to their obesity (diabetes mellitus, obstructive sleep apnea, reactive airway disease, steatohepatitis, metabolic syndrome) resolved their comorbidities.

Bariatric procedures can be divided into three types: restrictive procedures, which decrease gastric volume and limit food intake; malabsorptive procedures, which alter digestion of food and decrease the effectiveness of nutrient absorption; and mixed procedures, which have components of both restriction and malabsorption. Currently, the most common procedures performed in the United States are the Roux-en-Y gastric bypass (a mixed procedure) and the laparoscopic adjustable band (a restrictive procedure) (Fig. 3).

Roux-en-Y Gastric Bypass

A Roux-en-Y bypass is performed by making a small pouch at the superior portion of the stomach. The pouch is then connected to the jejunum, bypassing the duodenum, where the majority of calories are absorbed. Roux-en-Y bypasses are now being performed laparoscopically at several centers. The mortality rate associated with gastric bypass is low (<1%), but patients can have significant postoperative complications, including pulmonary emboli, deep vein thromboses, leaks from the gastrointestinal tract, gastric remnant distention, stomal stenosis, ulcers, gallstones, and hernias. Patients are required to take lifelong vitamin and mineral supplementation, because absorption of iron, vitamin B_{12}/folate, and others are affected.

Laparoscopic Adjustable Gastric Band

The vertical-banded gastroplasty was the restrictive procedure performed routinely in the past (see Fig. 3). It is not routinely performed any longer and has been superceded by the laparoscopic adjustable band. An adjustable band is placed around the entrance to the stomach. The band is connected to an infusion port that is placed in the subcutaneous tissue. The port can be accessed with a needle and syringe, and injection or removal of saline into the port may be used to manipulate the size of the band diameter, leading to greater or lesser degrees of restriction. Although weight loss with banding tends to be slower than with other weight loss procedures, the procedure is popular because it is performed laparoscopically and is reversible. The band is currently not approved by the FDA for adolescents younger than 18 years of age. Laparoscopic banding can also be associated with side effects such as stomal obstruction; band erosion, slippage, or prolapse; port malfunction, pouch or esophageal dilation; and infection.

Future Directions

Many genes, gene products, and hormones such as leptin,[5] peptide YY, and melanocortin 4 receptors that potentially have a role in the development of obesity have been identified. These discoveries point to potentially novel therapies for obesity.

In conclusion, obesity is a growing public health problem that has significant short- and long-term consequences. Lifestyle modification with or without adjuvant therapies should be used to achieve a goal of modest weight loss. With modest weight loss, patients experience a decreased risk of mortality and improvement of obesity-related complications.

---

[5]Investigational drug in the United States.

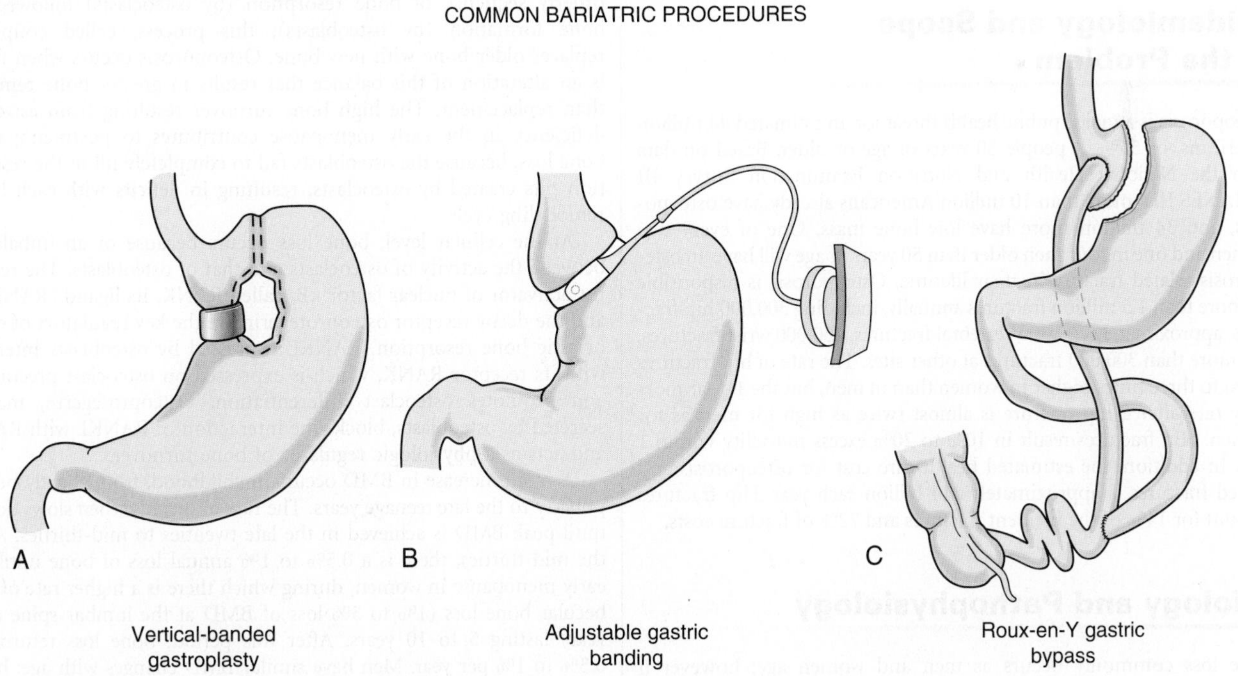

COMMON BARIATRIC PROCEDURES

FIGURE 3. Techniques commonly used for the surgical treatment of obesity: vertical-banded gastroplasty (**A**), adjustable laparoscopic band (**B**), Roux-en-Y gastric bypass (**C**).

A — Vertical-banded gastroplasty

B — Adjustable gastric banding

C — Roux-en-Y gastric bypass

REFERENCES

Apovain C. The medical management of obesity and the role of pharmaco-therapy: An update. Nutr Clin Pract 2000;15:5–12.

Aronne LJ. Classification of obesity and assessment of obesity-related health risks. Obes Res 2002;10:105S–115S.

Buchwald H, Avidor Y, Braunwald E, et al. Bariatric surgery: A systematic review and meta-analysis. JAMA 2004;292(14):1724–37.

Hedley AA, Ogden CL, Johnson CL, et al. Prevalence of overweight and obesity among US children, adolescents, and adults, 1999–2002. JAMA 2004;291:2847–50.

National Institutes of Health; National Heart, Lung and Blood Institute: North American Association for the Study of Obesity. The Practical Guide to the Identification, Evaluation, and Treatment of Overweight and Obesity in Adults. Bethesda, Md: National Institutes of Health; 2000. Available at http://www.nhlbi.nih.gov/guidelines/obesity/ob_home.htm [accessed June 30, 2009].

Yanovski SZ, Yanovski JA. Obesity. N Engl J Med 2002;346:591–602.

Osteoporosis

Method of
Ramaswami Nalini, MBBS

Osteoporosis is the most common bone disease in humans and is a serious public health issue. It is a systemic skeletal disease characterized by low bone mass and microarchitectural deterioration, compromised bone strength, and skeletal fragility resulting in an increased risk of fracture. Bone strength reflects the integration of bone density and bone quality. Osteoporosis is a silent disease until fracture occurs. Fractures contribute to pain, deformity, loss of height, and disability. The World Health Organization (WHO) defines osteoporosis as a bone mineral density (BMD) at the hip or spine less than or equal to 2.5 standard deviations below the young normal mean reference population (see later discussion).

Epidemiology and Scope of the Problem

Osteoporosis is a major public health threat for an estimated 44 million Americans, or 55% of people 50 years of age or older. Based on data from the National Health and Nutrition Examination Survey III (NHANES III), more than 10 million Americans already have osteoporosis, and 34 million more have low bone mass. One of every two women and one in four men older than 50 years of age will have an osteoporosis-related fracture in their lifetime. Osteoporosis is responsible for more than 1.5 million fractures annually, including 300,000 hip fractures, approximately 700,000 vertebral fractures, 250,000 wrist fractures, and more than 300,000 fractures at other sites. The rate of hip fractures is two to three times higher in women than in men, but the 1-year mortality rate after a hip fracture is almost twice as high for men as for women. Hip fractures result in 10% to 20% excess mortality within 1 year. In addition, the estimated health care cost for osteoporosis and related fractures is approximately $14 billion each year. Hip fractures account for 14% of the incident fractures and 72% of fracture costs.

Etiology and Pathophysiology

Bone loss commonly occurs as men and women age; however if optimal peak bone mass is not achieved during childhood and adolescence, osteoporosis may develop without the occurrence of accelerated bone loss. The bone mass of an individual in later life is

TABLE 1 Secondary Causes of Osteoporosis

Endocrine Disorders	Lifestyle Factors
Hyperparathyroidism	Vitamin D and calcium deficiency
Hyperthyroidism	Excess vitamin A
Cushing's syndrome	Immobilization
Hypogonadism	Inadequate physical activity
Diabetes mellitus	
Hyperprolactinemia	**Medications**
Adrenal insufficiency	Glucocorticoids
	Cancer chemotherapy
Gastrointestinal Disorders	Immunosuppressants
Celiac disease	Anticonvulsants
Gastric bypass/gastrectomy	Heparin
Malabsorption	Depot medroxyprogesterone (Depo-Provera)
Liver disease	GnRH agonists and antagonists
Inflammatory bowel disease	**Hematologic Disorders**
Pancreatic insufficiency	Multiple myeloma
	Leukemia and lymphomas
Rheumatologic Disorders	Mastocytosis
Rheumatoid arthritis	Sickle cell disease
Lupus	**Miscellaneous**
	Alcoholism
Genetic Factors	Renal disease
Osteogenesis imperfecta	Organ transplantation
Idiopathic hypercalciuria	
Hypophosphatasia	

Abbreviation: GnRH, gonadotropin-releasing hormone.

a result of the peak bone mass accrued by age 18 to 25 years and the subsequent rate of bone loss. Peak bone mass is largely determined by genetic factors, with contributions from nutrition, endocrine status, physical activity, and health during growth.

Osteoporosis can be further characterized as primary or secondary. Primary osteoporosis can occur at any age but often follows menopause in women and occurs later in life in men. Secondary osteoporosis is the result of medications, other conditions, or disease (Table 1).

Continuous bone remodeling maintains a healthy skeleton by an orderly sequence of bone resorption (by osteoclasts) followed by bone formation (by osteoblasts); this process, called coupling, replaces older bone with new bone. Osteoporosis occurs when there is an alteration of this balance that results in greater bone removal than replacement. The high bone turnover resulting from estrogen deficiency in the early menopause contributes to postmenopausal bone loss, because the osteoblasts fail to completely fill in the resorption pits created by osteoclasts, resulting in deficits with each bone remodeling cycle.

At the cellular level, bone loss occurs because of an imbalance between the activity of osteoclasts and that of osteoblasts. The receptor activator of nuclear factor κB, called RANK, its ligand (RANKL), and the decoy receptor osteoprotegerin are the key regulators of osteoclastic bone resorption. RANKL expressed by osteoblasts interacts with its receptor RANK, which is expressed on osteoclast precursors and promotes osteoclast differentiation. Osteoprotegerin, mainly secreted by osteoblasts, blocks the interaction of RANKL with RANK and acts as a physiologic regulator of bone turnover.

A rapid increase in BMD occurs in childhood, from shortly before puberty to the late teenage years. The rate of increase then slows down, until peak BMD is achieved in the late twenties to mid-thirties. After the mid-thirties, there is a 0.5% to 1% annual loss of bone until the early menopause in women, during which there is a higher rate of trabecular bone loss (1% to 3% loss of BMD at the lumbar spine each year) lasting 5 to 10 years. After this period, bone loss returns to 0.5% to 1% per year. Men have similar BMD changes with age; however, they do not have the accelerated bone loss that women do during menopause. Men have higher BMD values and larger diameters of their bones, resulting in less fracture risk compared to women (Fig. 1).

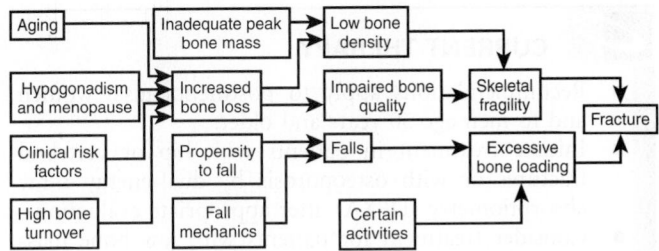

FIGURE 1. Pathogenesis of osteoporosis-related fractures. (Adapted from Cooper C, Melton LJ: Epidemiology of osteoporosis. Trends Endocrinol Metab 1992;3(6):224–229, with modification in National Osteoporosis Foundation: Clinician's Guide to Prevention and Treatment of Osteoporosis. Available at: http://www.nof.org/professionals/Clinicians_Guide.htm [accessed July 3, 2009].)

Risk Factors

A distinction must be made between risk factors that affect bone metabolism and risk factors for fracture. Risk factors associated with osteoporosis are supported by evidence that includes large prospective studies.

Predictors of low bone mass include female gender, older age, estrogen deficiency, Caucasian or Asian race, low body weight and low body mass index, family history of osteoporosis or fracture, smoking, and history of prior fracture. Late menarche, early menopause, nulliparity, and low endogenous estrogen levels are also associated with low BMD. In addition, environmental factors including low nutritional levels of calcium and vitamin D, alcohol use, lack of regular physical activity, and a high-protein, high-caffeine, high-sodium diet can increase the risk of bone loss. Measures of physical function and activity, including grip strength and current exercise level, have been associated with increased bone mass.

Although low BMD is an important predictor of future fracture risk, evidence indicates that clinical risk factors related to the risk of falling also serve as important predictors of fracture. Fracture risk is associated with a history of falls, low physical function (e.g., slow gait speed, decreased quadriceps strength), impaired cognition, impaired vision, and the presence of environmental hazards such as throw rugs. The risk of a fracture occurring with a fall is also increased in tall persons and in falls to the side and may be influenced by attributes of bone geometry such as hip axis and femur length.

Several of these risk factors have been included in the WHO 10-year fracture risk model (Box 1). Combined use of these risk factors in multivariate models allows prediction of the 10-year probability of hip or other fractures. The WHO Fracture Risk Algorithm (FRAX) was derived from large prospective cohort studies conducted around the world and was calibrated to U.S. fracture and mortality rates with the assistance of the National Osteoporosis Foundation. The Foundation also performed an economic analysis to find a threshold above which treatment is cost-effective. This analysis confirmed the previously established threshold to diagnose and treat osteoporosis; namely, a T-score of −2.5 or lower at the hip or spine (see later discussion) or a history of prior hip or spine fracture.

The new guidelines establish a threshold for treating patients who are classified as having osteopenia. Treatment should be considered for those with low bone mass and a 10-year probability of a hip fracture equal to or greater than 3% or a 10-year probability of a major osteoporosis-related fracture equal to or greater than 20%, calculated based on the FRAX algorithm. This long-awaited and clinically useful WHO instrument has some limitations. Certain important risk factors, such as poor muscle strength, gait imbalance, history of falls, and other risk factors for falls, have not been rigorously validated in large prospective cohort studies and therefore were not included in the WHO model. In addition, this model can be applied only to treatment-naive individuals. The thresholds established are only guidelines; the ultimate treatment decisions lie with the physicians and their patients.

BOX 1   Risk Factors Included in the WHO Fracture Risk Assessment Model

- Current age
- Gender
- A prior osteoporotic fracture (including morphometric vertebral fracture)
- Femoral neck BMD
- Low body mass index (kg/m^2)
- Oral glucocorticoids ≥5 mg/d of prednisone for ≥3 mo (ever)
- Rheumatoid arthritis
- Secondary osteoporosis
- Parental history of hip fracture
- Current smoking
- Alcohol intake (≥3 drinks per day)

Data from Kanis JA; on behalf of the WHO Scientific Group: Assessment of Osteoporosis at the Primary Health Care Level. Technical Report. Sheffield, UK, World Health Organisation Collaborating Centre for Metabolic Bone Diseases, University of Sheffield, 2008.
Abbreviations: BMD, bone mineral density; WHO, World Health Organization.

Evaluation

The first step in the evaluation for osteoporosis in a patient considered to be at risk is the measurement of BMD to establish the diagnosis of osteoporosis. This is followed by establishing the fracture risk and making decisions on choosing therapy. Secondary causes should be ruled out by a detailed history and physical examination, and relevant

CURRENT DIAGNOSIS

- Measure bone mineral density (BMD) by dual-energy x-ray absorptiometry (DEXA) in women age 65 years and older, men age 70 years and older, postmenopausal women, and men age 50 to 69 years with risk factors.
- Osteoporosis is defined as a T-score of ≤ −2.5 (i.e., 2.5 standard deviations below the young normal mean reference population); low bone density (osteopenia) is defined as a T-score between −1.0 and −2.5.
- Consider vertebral fracture assessment imaging of the thoracic and lumbar spine using DEXA.
- Establish fracture risk using the World Health Organisation absolute fracture risk model (FRAX algorithm)

Initial Laboratory Tests

- Complete biochemistry profile (including serum total calcium, serum phosphorus, serum alkaline phosphatase, liver function tests, and serum creatinine)
- Complete blood count
- Serum parathyroid hormone
- Serum 25-hydroxy-vitamin D
- 24-Hour urine calcium, sodium, and creatinine

Additional Laboratory Tests Based on Suspicion of Specific Secondary Causes

- Serum thyroid-stimulating hormone
- Serum protein electrophoresis
- 24-Hour urine free cortisol
- Celiac screen

blood and urine studies should be obtained. A history of fragility fractures (unrelated to substantial trauma) in a postmenopausal woman strongly supports the diagnosis of osteoporosis, regardless of BMD.

BONE MINERAL DENSITY

BMD has been shown to correlate strongly with load-bearing capacity of the hip and spine, and it is an excellent predictor of future risk of fracture. The WHO selected BMD measures to establish criteria for the diagnosis of osteoporosis. BMD assessments are measured by dual-energy x-ray absorptiometry (DEXA) in absolute terms (grams of mineral per square centimeter scanned) and expressed in relation to two norms: the expected BMD for the patient's age and gender (Z-score) and the mean for young normal adults of the same gender (T-score).

According to the WHO definition, osteoporosis is present if the T-score is ≤ -2.5 (i.e., 2.5 standard deviations below the mean of the reference population) or lower, and low bone density (osteopenia) is present if the T-score is between -1.0 and -2.5. The WHO BMD diagnostic classification should not be applied to premenopausal women, men younger than 50 years of age, or children. The International Society for Clinical Densitometry has recommended that, instead of T-scores, Z-scores adjusted for ethnicity or race should be used, with Z-scores of -2.0 or lower deemed to represent either "low bone mineral density for chronological age" or "below the expected range for age" and those higher than -2.0 being "within the expected range for age." For every 1.0 standard deviation decrease in BMD below the mean for young adults of the same gender and ethnicity, the fracture risk roughly doubles at the spine and hip. FRAX was developed to calculate the 10-year probability of a hip fracture or a major osteoporotic fracture, taking into account femoral neck BMD and certain clinical risk factors.

Indications for bone mineral density testing are the following:

- Women age 65 years and older and men age 70 years and older, or younger postmenopausal women and men age 50 to 69 years with risk factors
- Adults with an osteoporotic fracture after age 50 years
- Monitoring osteoporosis therapy with an FDA-approved drug
- Primary hyperparathyroidism
- Individuals who are receiving or planning to receive long-term glucocorticoid therapy in a daily dose of 5 mg or more of prednisone or equivalent for 3 months or longer

Because radiographically confirmed vertebral fractures are a strong predictor of new vertebral fractures and other fractures, vertebral fracture assessment imaging of the thoracic and lumbar spine using DEXA scanning should be considered at the time of BMD assessment, when the presence of a vertebral fracture not previously identified may influence clinical management.

LABORATORY EVALUATION

Serum calcium, phosphorus, alkaline phosphatase, thyroid-stimulating hormone, creatinine, serum protein electrophoresis, parathyroid hormone (PTH), and 25-hydroxy-vitamin D should be assessed as appropriate to rule out secondary causes. Measurement of 24-hour urinary excretion of calcium, sodium, and creatinine helps rule out idiopathic hypercalciuria.

Biochemical markers of bone turnover, such as *N*-telopeptide or osteocalcin, are not useful in the diagnosis of osteoporosis. However, they may give a clue to the pathogenesis of osteoporosis, predict the risk of future fracture (independently of bone loss), and predict and monitor the response to therapy.

Management

Bone mass attained in early life is perhaps the most important determinant of lifelong skeletal health. Although genetic factors exert a predominant influence on peak bone mass, environmental and modifiable lifestyle factors can also play a significant role. Management of

 CURRENT THERAPY

- Recommendations apply to postmenopausal women and to men age 50 years and older.
- Initiate treatment in patients with hip or vertebral fractures or with osteoporosis by dual-energy x-ray absorptiometry (DEXA) after appropriate evaluation.
- Consider treatment for patients with low bone mass (i.e., osteopenia, T-score between -1.0 and -2.5) and a 10-year probability of hip fracture of 3% or greater, or a 10-year probability of major osteoporosis-related fracture of 20% or greater, calculated based on the WHO FRAX algorithm.

Nonpharmacologic Therapies

- Adequate calcium and vitamin D nutrition
- Regular weight-bearing and muscle-strengthening exercise
- Avoidance of smoking and excessive alcohol intake
- Fall prevention

Pharmacologic Therapies

- Bisphosphonates: alendronate (Fosamax), risedronate (Actonel), ibandronate (Boniva), and zoledronic acid (Reclast)
- Estrogen agonist/antagonists or selective estrogen receptor modulators (Raloxifene [Evista])
- Estrogen therapy or hormone (estrogen + progesterone) therapy
- Teriparatide (Forteo)
- Nasal calcitonin (Miacalcin)

osteoporosis starts with prevention, that is, maximizing acquisition of bone mass during childhood and young adulthood and minimizing bone loss after peak bone mass is attained.

NONPHARMACOLOGIC THERAPY

Adequate Calcium and Vitamin D Nutrition

Lifelong adequate calcium intake is necessary for the acquisition of peak bone mass and subsequent maintenance of bone health. Calcium supplementation should be adjunctive treatment for all women with osteoporosis and must be part of any preventive strategy for bone loss. Controlled clinical trials have demonstrated that a combination of supplemental calcium and vitamin D can reduce the risk of fracture. A total calcium intake of 1200 to 1500 mg/day (through diet, supplements, or both) is recommended for all postmenopausal women. Vitamin D is important for calcium absorption, bone health, muscle strength, balance, and decreasing the risk of falls. The National Osteoporosis Foundation recommends 800 to 1000 IU of vitamin D per day for adults age 50 years and older.

Physical Activity

Regular weight-bearing and muscle-strengthening exercise reduces the risk of falls and may reduce the risk of fractures. In addition, exercise can modestly increase bone density. Weight-bearing exercise includes walking, jogging, dancing, and similar activities; muscle-strengthening exercise includes weight training and other resistive exercises.

Avoidance of Smoking and Excessive Alcohol Intake

Smoking and alcohol intake (≥ 3 drinks per day) are detrimental to bone health and have been linked to greater fracture risk. Counseling on smoking cessation and reduction of excessive alcohol intake is routinely warranted.

Fall Prevention

Strategies to reduce the risk of falls include maintaining adequate vitamin D levels and physical activity, checking and correcting vision and hearing, evaluating neurologic problems, reviewing prescription medications for side effects that may affect balance, and providing a checklist for improving safety at home.

Hip protectors reduce trauma during a fall and have been reported to reduce the risk of hip fracture when used properly. They may be considered for patients who have a high fall risk or previous hip fracture.

PHARMACOLOGIC THERAPY

Postmenopausal women with established osteoporosis (T-score ≤ -2.5 or lower) or a fragility fracture (hip or vertebral) should be treated with a pharmacologic agent to decrease fracture risk and improve quality of life. Pharmacologic therapy is also suggested for high-risk postmenopausal women with T-scores between -1.0 and -2.5 at the femoral neck or spine and a calculated 10-year probability of hip fracture of 3.0% or greater or a 10-year probability of combined major osteoporotic fracture of 20% or greater (based on FRAX). The two main groups of drugs are antiresorptives, which inhibit osteoclast-mediated bone resorption, and anabolic agents, which stimulate osteoblast-mediated bone formation (Table 2).

Bisphosphonates are considered first-line therapy for the treatment of postmenopausal osteoporosis. They suppress osteoclastic activity and slow the remodeling cycle, increasing mineralization of the bone matrix. Less than 1% of a dose of an oral bisphosphonate is normally absorbed via the gut. Alendronate (Fosamax), risedronate (Actonel), and ibandronate (Boniva) are the oral bisphosphonates that are approved by the FDA for treatment of osteoporosis. The first two reduce the risk of vertebral, nonvertebral, and hip fractures, whereas for ibandronate there are data only for reduction of vertebral fractures. Alendronate and risedronate are also approved for prevention and treatment of osteoporosis in men and for glucocorticoid-induced osteoporosis. They must be taken on an empty stomach, first thing in the morning, with 8 ounces of water; patients should wait 30 to 60 minutes before eating or drinking and should remain upright during that time.

Ibandronate (Boniva 3 mg by IV injection every 3 months) and zoledronic acid (Reclast 5 mg IV given over 15 minutes annually) are the FDA-approved intravenous bisphosphonates. They are used for patients who cannot tolerate the oral bisphosphonates or cannot follow the dosing requirements. Zoledronic acid is the only intravenous bisphosphonate that has demonstrated efficacy for fracture prevention, and it is the preferred choice for intravenous therapy. However, long-term safety data (>3 years) in patients with osteoporosis is lacking for zoledronic acid. The common side effect of bisphosphonates is esophagitis, and a destructive rare side effect with high doses of intravenous bisphosphonates in cancer patients is osteonecrosis of the jaw.

TABLE 2 Medications Approved by the FDA for Treatment and Prevention of Postmenopausal Osteoporosis*

Drug	Method of Administration and Dose	Reduction in Risk of Fracture	Side Effects	FDA Approval
Bisphosphonates				
Alendronate (Fosamax)	35–70 mg PO weekly 5–10 mg PO daily	Vertebral, nonvertebral, hip	Esophagitis, myalgias, concern for ONJ[†]	Treatment and prevention
Risedronate (Actonel)	30–35 mg PO weekly 5 mg PO qd 150 mg PO monthly[‡]	Vertebral nonvertebral, hip	Same as above	Treatment and prevention
Ibandronate (Boniva)	150 mg PO monthly 2.5 mg PO qd 3 mg IV q3mo[§]	Vertebral	Same as above First dose: myalgias, joint aches, flu-like symptoms	Treatment and prevention
Zoledronic acid (Reclast)	5 mg IV yearly infusion	Vertebral, nonvertebral, hip	Same as above Flu-like symptoms, mild transient hypocalcemia, atrial fibrillation	Treatment only
Selective Estrogen Receptor Modulator				
Raloxifene (Evista)	60 mg PO qd	Vertebral	Hot flashes, nausea, DVT, leg cramps	Treatment and prevention
Anabolic Agent				
PTH (1–34) (Teriparatide, Forteo)	20 µg SQ qd	Vertebral, nonvertebral	Hypercalcemia, nausea, leg cramps	Treatment only (for severe osteoporosis)
Calcitonin (Miacalcin)	100 IU SQ qod 200 IU intranasal qd	Vertebral	Nasal stuffiness, nausea	Treatment only
Estrogen				
Conjugated equine estrogens (Premarin)	0.30–1.25 mg PO qd	Vertebral, nonvertebral, hip (at dose of 0.625 mg/d)	Risk of DVT, cardiovascular disease, breast cancer	Prevention only
17β-Estradiol (Estrace, Estraderm)	0.5 mg PO qd 0.025–0.10 mg TD twice weekly	No data from RCTs	Same as above	Prevention only
	Ultra-low-dose: 0.014 mg TD weekly	No data available	Same as above	Prevention only

Modified from Rosen CJ: Postmenopausal osteoporosis. N Engl J Med 2005;353:595–603.

*All agents approved for treatment have been shown to have fracture reduction efficacy in RCTs. The use of calcitonin (Miacalcin) is generally not recommended.

[†]Risk factors for development of ONJ include intravenous bisphosphonates, cancer and anticancer therapy, duration of exposure, and preexisting dental disease.

[‡]Risedronate (Actonel) may be given as 150 mg once a month or as 75 mg on two consecutive days each month; the efficacy is similar for increasing spine and hip BMD as daily administration of 5 mg.

[§]There are no direct fracture efficacy data on intravenous ibandronate (Boniva).

Abbreviations: DVT, deep vein thrombosis; FDA, U.S. Food and Drug Administration; IV, intravenous; ONJ, osteonecrosis of the jaw; PTH, parathyroid hormone; PO, oral; qod, every other day; qd, every day; RCTs, randomized, controlled trials; SQ, subcutaneous; TD, transdermal.

Raloxifene (Evista 60 mg/day) is a selective estrogen receptor modulator and is approved for the prevention and treatment of osteoporosis. It has been shown to reduce vertebral fractures but not hip fractures. It can worsen the vasomotor symptoms, and it increases clotting risk; therefore, it is contraindicated in patients with a history of deep vein thrombosis. It has some extraskeletal benefits such as decreasing the risk of breast cancer and decreasing total and LDL cholesterol, although it has not been shown to decrease the risk of coronary artery disease.

Calcitonin nasal spray (Miacalcin 200 IU per day) is approved for treatment of postmenopausal osteoporosis. It has been shown to reduce the risk of vertebral fractures (but not nonvertebral fractures) and to reduce fracture-associated pain. However, it is considered preferable to treat osteoporosis with more potent agents than calcitonin and to treat pain separately. The main side effect is rhinitis.

Combined estrogen and progestin therapy is no longer a first-line approach for the treatment of osteoporosis in postmenopausal women because of the increased risk of invasive breast cancer, stroke, venous thromboembolism, and myocardial infarction reported by The Women's Health Initiative study. The risk-benefit profile in the estrogen-only arm of that trial was different. The FDA has approved estrogen/progestin therapy in postmenopausal women with persistent vasomotor symptoms or vulvovaginal atrophy and for prevention of osteoporosis. The FDA advises using the lowest effective doses for the shortest duration to meet treatment goals. The Women's Health Initiative found that both combined estrogen/progestin (Prempro) and unopposed estrogen (Premarin) reduced the risks of hip fracture and vertebral fracture.

Parathyroid Hormone

Teriparatide (Forteo) is a recombinant human parathyroid hormone analogue with a different mechanism of action than the antiresorptive agents already described. It is a potent anabolic agent that is administered by daily subcutaneous injection. It is approved by the FDA for the treatment of osteoporosis in postmenopausal women who are at high risk for fracture. It significantly decreases the risk of vertebral fractures and nonvertebral fractures. It is also indicated for men with primary or hypogonadal osteoporosis and high risk of fracture. It is used for a maximum of 2 years. It is common practice to follow teriparatide treatment with a bisphosphonate to maintain and further increase BMD, but teriparatide is not used in combination with a bisphosphonate, because the combination is less effective than teriparatide alone. Side effects include dizziness and nausea; it is contraindicated in patients with a history of osteosarcoma, Paget's disease of the bone, unexplained hypercalcemia, or history of skeletal radiation and in those younger than 18 years of age.

Combination Therapy

The combination of hormone therapy and bisphosphonates (alendronate) can provide small additional increases in BMD compared with monotherapy alone. However, the fracture risk reduction is not known. Estrogen plus calcitonin, estrogen plus androgen, estrogen plus etidronate (Didronel),[1] and alendronate plus raloxifene also appear to act synergistically on bone density. However, fracture data are unavailable for these combinations.

Use of PTH with bisphosphonates (alendronate) results in no additional benefit for spine or hip BMD compared with PTH alone, and the addition of alendronate may even attenuate the increase in BMD with PTH. Therefore, concurrent PTH-bisphosphonate therapy is not recommended. However, raloxifene does not appear to suppress PTH effects on the bone.

The other investigational agents include denosumab,[5] an investigational humanized monoclonal antibody against RANKL that reduces osteoclastogenesis; strontium ranelate (Protelos)[2]; tibolone[2]; fluoride[1];

oral calcium-sensing receptor antagonists; sclerostin inhibitors; integrin antagonists; and cathepsin K inhibitors.

Response to therapy is monitored by measurement of BMD (DEXA) every 2 years, or more frequently if the clinical situation warrants. Suppression of biochemical markers of bone turnover measured after 3 to 6 months of antiresorptive therapy may predict greater BMD response.

REFERENCES

Cooper C, Melton LJ. Epidemiology of osteoporosis. Trends Endocrinol Metab 1992;3(6):224–9.

Kanis JA. on behalf of the WHO Scientific Group. Assessment of Osteoporosis at the Primary Health Care Level. Technical Report. Sheffield, UK: World Health Organisation Collaborating Centre for Metabolic Bone Diseases, University of Sheffield; 2008.

National Institutes of Health Consensus Development Panel. Osteoporosis prevention, diagnosis, and therapy. JAMA 2001;285:785–95.

National Osteoporosis Foundation. Clinician's Guide to Prevention and Treatment of Osteoporosis, Available at: http://www.nof.org/professionals/Clinicians_Guide.htm [accessed July 3, 2009].

Rosen CJ. Postmenopausal osteoporosis. N Eng J Med 2005;353:595–603.

Sambrook P, Cooper C. Osteoporosis. Lancet 2006;367:2010–8.

Paget's Disease of Bone

Method of
Ian R. Reid, MD

Paget's disease is a focal skeletal condition in which one or more bones has a clearly circumscribed area of increased turnover (Fig. 1A). Either osteoblasts or osteoclasts may predominate at a given time, resulting in sclerosis or lysis, respectively. Areas that are initially lytic often become sclerotic later, and it is common to see both changes within the same bone (see Fig. 1B). Unaffected areas of the skeleton are completely normal, in marked contrast to some rare congenital conditions which are sometimes (inappropriately) referred to as early-onset or juvenile Paget's disease. Such conditions (e.g., familial expansile osteolysis, idiopathic hyperphosphatasia) have different etiologies, clinical presentations, and responses to treatment when compared to Paget's disease.

Etiology

Within pagetic bone, there is a loss of the usual tight control of bone cell function, and the bone-resorbing cells (osteoclasts) and bone-forming cells (osteoblasts) both exhibit overactivity. In the case of osteoclasts, this leads to local areas of bone loss, which can result in deformity or fracture. Osteoblast overactivity leads to the random laying down of new bone, which is disorganized in its structure, mechanically inadequate, and prone to deformity. Osteoblast overactivity can also lead to bone expansion, resulting in bone pain, premature arthritis (if it affects articular surfaces), and nerve compression (e.g., in the spine or skull). Figure 1B shows the effects of osteoblast and osteoclast overactivity on the structure of an affected tibia. The disease progresses along a long bone at a rate of about 1 cm per year, so most patients have had active disease for 1 or more decades before presentation. Typically, the disease progresses until the entire bone is involved. However, Paget's disease does not spread from one bone to another, so the number of affected bones remains constant throughout the disease course.

Paget's disease sometimes runs in families, and about 10% of patients are reported to have an affected relative. This observation has led to much work seeking genetic associations of the condition.

---

[1]Not FDA approved for this indication.
[2]Not available in the United States.
[5]Investigational drug in the United States.

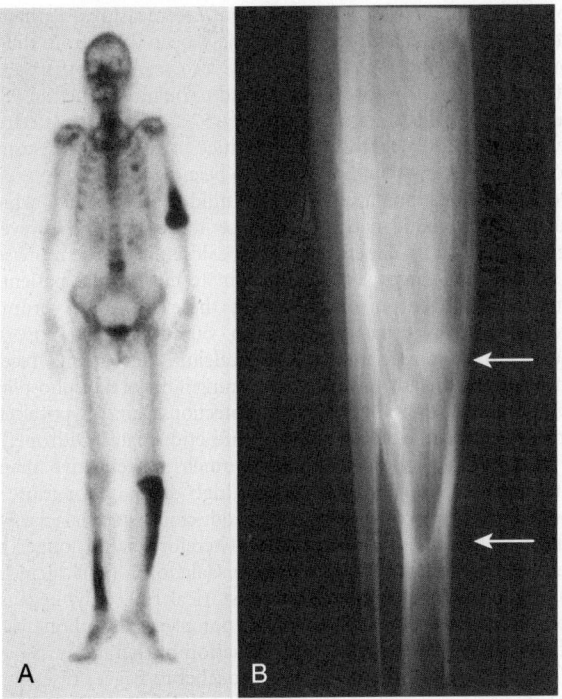

FIGURE 1. A, Bone scintigram in a patient with Paget's disease, demonstrating the multifocal nature of the condition and the presence of normal bone at other sites. **B,** Tibia affected by Paget's disease. The upper tibia is of increased density and width as a result of osteoblast overactivity, whereas the lower part of the affected bone shows a lytic region (*between arrows*) resulting from osteoclastic bone resorption. Below this, the bone is normal. (Copyright I. R. Reid, used with permission.)

It is now apparent that mutations of the gene for sequestosome 1 are associated with Paget's disease in some families. Other research has focused on possible environmental causes, and a slow viral infection has been suggested. Evidence that the prevalence of Paget's disease has decreased in recent decades would be consistent with altered exposure to an environmental agent. However, both the genetic and environmental hypotheses fail to account for the focal nature of the condition, which in some ways resembles a benign neoplasm.

Altered gene expression in osteoblasts and bone marrow stromal cells from pagetic bone has been demonstrated recently, including increased levels of dickkopf-1, interleukin-1, and interleukin-6. These changes are likely to result in stimulation of osteoclast proliferation and inhibition of osteoblast growth, leading to development of the characteristic lytic bone lesions. This work suggests that the key abnormality may reside in the osteoblast, rather than the osteoclast, as was assumed in the past. Uncertainties remain regarding the primary abnormality giving rise to this condition.

Epidemiology

Paget's disease is classically a condition of older adults, most patients being older than 60 years of age at diagnosis. There is a male preponderance in some studies. It is overwhelmingly a condition of individuals with European forebears, particularly from the United Kingdom and Western Europe (excluding Scandinavia), where about 6% to 7% of the older population is affected. Among older white Americans, the prevalence is about 2%. There is some evidence that prevalence and disease severity are both declining, possibly reflecting change in an environmental etiologic factor. It is extremely uncommon in individuals with predominantly Asian or Polynesian ancestry, although it is observed in some black populations.

 CURRENT DIAGNOSIS

- Suspect the presence of Paget's disease in those patients with bone pain, bone deformity, isolated elevation of alkaline phosphatase, or lytic/sclerotic lesions on radiographs.
- Paget's disease is diagnosed from plain radiographs.
- Bone scintigraphy identifies the affected bones and allows some assessment of disease activity.
- Biochemical markers of bone turnover allow more precise assessment of turnover and response to therapy.
- Serum total alkaline phosphatase activity is the most cost-effective marker, although bone-specific alkaline phosphatase and procollagen type I N-terminal propeptide (PINP) are marginally more sensitive.

Clinical Presentation

The most common symptoms attributable to Paget's disease are bone and joint pain. The bone pain is typically worse at rest and may trouble patients particularly at night. With skull involvement, pounding headaches can result. If Paget's disease leads to deformity of joint surfaces, premature arthritis occurs. This is particularly common at the hips. Deformity in long bones can occur, and involvement of the radius or weight-bearing bones of the lower limb often manifests in this way. Microfractures, which can be very painful, sometimes occur over the convexity of a deformed, weight-bearing bone. These can progress to complete fractures. Fractures can also occur through an area of active lytic disease in a weight-bearing bone.

Deafness is a common manifestation of Paget's disease and is caused by involvement of the bones of the middle ear or compromise of the eighth cranial nerve. More rarely, other neurologic syndromes can arise from nerve entrapment, including paraplegia as a result of spinal cord involvement.

Some pagetic patients are asymptomatic and are diagnosed because of an incidental finding of elevated circulating levels of alkaline phosphatase. The diagnosis may also result from an incidental radiographic finding, such as in studies of the urinary tract. Commonly, only one or two bones are involved, although disease may be more widespread. The pelvis, vertebral bodies, long bones, and skull are the most common sites, but almost any bone can be involved.

Diagnosis

Serum alkaline phosphatase, the most widely available marker of osteoblast activity, is usually elevated; however, if only one bone is involved, this test can be normal. In any patient with an elevation of alkaline phosphatase, it is important to determine whether this is coming from liver or bone. This question is usually addressed by measuring other liver function tests, although assays of bone-specific alkaline phosphatase and of other osteoblast-specific markers (e.g., procollagen type I N-terminal propeptide [PINP]) are available. If the elevation of alkaline phosphatase is bony in origin, it is important to rule out other bone conditions such as metastatic cancers (e.g., breast, prostate). This is usually done by identifying the sites of skeletal abnormality on a bone scintigram and then obtaining plain radiographs of the abnormal areas.

Paget's disease has a characteristic appearance on plain radiographs, showing either bony rarefaction or sclerosis (depending on whether the osteoclastic or osteoblastic phase is predominating), disorganization of trabecular architecture, and the other abnormalities already discussed (e.g., deformity). Bone biopsy is not usually necessary to confirm the diagnosis.

Other biochemical markers of osteoblast or osteoclast activity, such as breakdown products of bone collagen, have been used in

CURRENT THERAPY

- Zoledronate (zoledronic acid, Reclast) 5 mg given as a single infusion over 15 minutes; retreatment is seldom required within 5 years.
- Alendronate (Fosamax) 40 mg/day for 6 months; retreatment may be required between 2 and 6 years.
- Risedronate (Actonel) 30 mg/day for 2 months; retreatment may be required between 1 and 5 years.

Paget's disease. Total alkaline phosphatase, bone alkaline phosphatase, PINP or N-terminal telopeptide of type I collagen (NTX) identified more than 95% of pagetic subjects in one cohort of pagetic subjects, although the poorer precision of NTX reduced its utility in monitoring the effects of treatment. Osteocalcin, C-telopeptide of type I collagen, and urinary free deoxypyridinoline are less useful for assessment of baseline activity and monitoring response to therapy. Total alkaline phosphatase remains the most widely used test because of its low cost and wide availability.

Treatment

Treatment of Paget's disease almost always relies on the potent bisphosphonates. These compounds have a very high affinity for the bone surface, where they remain for years. They are ingested by osteoclasts when bone is resorbed and inhibit a key enzyme in the mevalonate pathway, farnesyl pyrophosphate synthase. This results in disruption of the osteoclast cytoskeleton and cell death. Bisphosphonates are preferentially taken up at sites of high bone turnover, which accounts for their utility as bone scintigraphy agents, and therefore target active pagetic bone.

The injectable bisphosphonate pamidronate (Aredia) has been used for many years in the treatment of Paget's disease. It is typically given as a series of infusions of 60 to 90 mg, each administered over a period of 1 to 2 hours. Pamidronate produces partial or complete remissions of disease activity that last for up to several years. The first administration of the drug may be accompanied by mild flu-like symptoms, which settle over 24 to 48 hours and usually do not recur. Their resolution can be hastened by the use of paracetamol (acetaminophen, Tylenol) or similar agents.

More recently, potent oral bisphosphonates such as alendronate (Fosamax) and risedronate (Actonel) have become widely used. These are administered daily over periods of 2 to 6 months and produce good disease control. The duration of treatment chosen in the pivotal clinical trials was arbitrary to some extent, and individual patients may require longer or shorter initial courses to achieve remission. Oral bisphosphonates have a very low bioavailability. Therefore, they must be taken in a fasting state, with a glass of water, and at least 30 minutes before consumption of food or other fluids. Positively charged ions (including calcium supplements, antacids, and mineral supplements) bind avidly to bisphosphonates and impair their absorption, so they must be taken at a different time of day. Potent bisphosphonates can cause irritation to the upper gastrointestinal tract and should not be prescribed to patients with inflammation or ulceration in that region. Patients should remain upright for 30 minutes after taking oral bisphosphonates to minimize the risk of reflux and associated esophagitis or ulceration.

The latest addition to the therapeutic armamentarium in managing Paget's disease is the more potent intravenous bisphosphonate zoledronate (Reclast), which is administered in a single dose of 5 mg over 15 minutes. It was recently compared with the standard 2-month course of risedronate in two randomized, controlled trials. At 6 months, 96% of patients receiving zoledronate had a therapeutic response, compared with 74% of those randomized to risedronate ($P < 0.001$). Alkaline phosphatase levels normalized in 89% of patients in the zoledronate group and in 58% of those in the risedronate group ($P < 0.001$). Zoledronate showed a more rapid onset of

action and superior effects on quality-of-life measures. Perhaps the most impressive data with zoledronate have been those from the open follow-up of responders in these studies. Two years after drug administration, therapeutic response was found to be maintained in 98% of those receiving zoledronate but in only 57% of risedronate-treated patients. Therefore, zoledronate produces much more sustained responses to therapy than have hitherto been possible.

Potent bisphosphonates can cause mild hypocalcemia, which is usually asymptomatic and not a cause for concern. However, in patients with vitamin D deficiency, hypocalcaemia can be more severe and sustained. Therefore, it is important to ensure that patients are vitamin D sufficient before receiving these drugs—a serum 25-hydroxyvitamin-D level greater than 50 nmol/L is more than adequate. Many physicians prescribe calcium to patients receiving bisphosphonate therapy (given in the evening if the oral bisphosphonate is given in the morning), as a further protection against hypocalcemia.

In the past, the weak bisphosphonate etidronate (Didronel) was used to treat Paget's disease. This is much less effective than the agents discussed previously. If used in high doses or for more than a few months, it carries the risk of producing osteomalacia, which can lead to bone pain and fractures. Therefore, it no longer has a place in the treatment of Paget's disease. Calcitonin (Miacalcin Injection) has also been relegated to an historical role only, because its efficacy is much less than that of the potent bisphosphonates, and its effects are rapidly reversed after cessation of therapy.

There are several philosophical approaches to Paget's disease management, none of which is strictly evidence based. There is general agreement that patients with symptoms attributable to Paget's disease should receive treatment. This is clear-cut in patients who have bone pain at the site of a pagetic lesion, but it is a common observation that antipagetic drugs can produce variable degrees of improvement in pain from joints adjacent to pagetic bone. Patients with neurologic complications from spinal cord or other nerve entrapments also improve with antipagetic therapy.

Treatment aimed at preventing complications of Paget's disease is variably endorsed, because there is no clinical trial evidence that treatment prevents the progression of deformity, the development of pagetic symptoms, or fracture. However, it is clear that treatment leads to a restoration of normal bone histology (Fig. 2) and

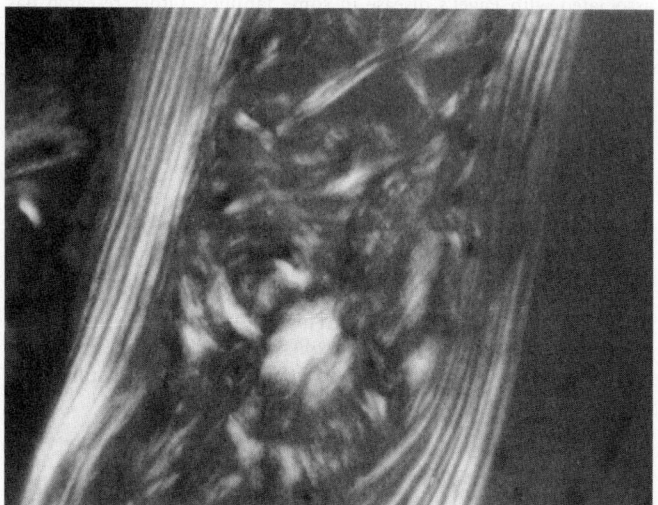

FIGURE 2. Section of a bone trabecula affected by Paget's disease, viewed under polarized light to show orientation of lamellae. In the center of the trabecula, the collagen fibers are chaotically laid down (woven bone), consistent with active Paget's disease. Over the outer surfaces, collagen is organized in parallel lamellae, indicating the restoration of normal bone microarchitecture after treatment with alendronate. (Reprinted with permission from: Reid IR, Nicholson GC, Weinstein RS, et al: Biochemical and radiologic improvement in Paget's disease of bone treated with alendronate: A randomized, placebo-controlled trial. Am J Med 1996;101:341–348.)

radiographic healing of lytic lesions and that, in the absence of such intervention, both bone lysis and deformity progress. It seems unreasonable to withhold safe therapies that are able to halt histologic and radiologic disease progression. Therefore, many experienced physicians endorse the provision of antipagetic therapy for individuals with lytic lesions in long bones, lesions at sites that are likely to lead to neurologic complications, arthritis or deformity, or involvement of the skull that could compromise hearing. Expert opinion also supports the use of antipagetic therapy before elective surgery on pagetic bone, because this approach reduces the vascularity of pagetic bone and results in less perioperative blood loss. On the other hand, Paget's disease in asymptomatic patients whose future risk of complications is thought to be low (e.g., with involvement of the ilium) is commonly managed without specific pharmaceutical intervention, although the availability of a safe, single-dose treatment with zoledronate is increasing the inclination to treat.

When providing treatment targeted at these goals, it is important to consider how adequacy of therapy can be judged. In the case of patients with pain, maximal relief of pain is an important endpoint. Lytic lesions should be treated and monitored with sequential radiographs until healing is apparent. Activity at other sites can be assessed indirectly with biochemical markers of bone turnover, although these are much less sensitive in patients with monostotic disease. In this context, there can be considerable residual activity at a single affected site without the markers' being abnormal. Bone scintigrams provide the most sensitive method of assessing local disease activity.

In the past, Paget's disease caused substantial morbidity in the elderly population. However, it is now possible to achieve adequate and sustained disease control with use of the potent bisphosphonates. Prompt use of these agents, when indicated, can be expected to halt disease progression and to effectively prevent the development of significant complications from this condition.

REFERENCES

Kanis JA. Pathophysiology and Treatment of Paget's Disease of Bone. London: Martin Dunitz; 1991.

Lyles KW, Siris ES, Singer FR, et al. A clinical approach to diagnosis and management of Paget's disease of bone. J Bone Miner Res 2001;16:1379–87.

Miller PD, Brown JP, Siris ES, et al. A randomized, double-blind comparison of risedronate and etidronate in the treatment of Paget's disease of bone. Am J Med 1999;106:513–20.

Ralston SH, Langston AL, Reid IR. Pathogenesis and management of Paget's disease of bone. Lancet 2008;372:155–63.

Reid IR, Davidson JS, Wattie D, et al. Comparative responses of bone turnover markers to bisphosphonate therapy in Paget's disease of bone. Bone 2004;35:224–30.

Reid IR, Miller P, Lyles K, et al. Comparison of a single infusion of zoledronic acid with risedronate for Paget's disease. N Engl J Med 2005;353:898–908.

Reid IR, Nicholson GC, Weinstein RS, et al. Biochemical and radiologic improvement in Paget's disease of bone treated with alendronate: A randomized, placebo-controlled trial. Am J Med 1996;101:341–8.

Selby PL, Davie MWJ, Ralston SH, et al. Guidelines on the management of Paget's disease of bone. Bone 2002;31:366–73.

Parenteral Nutrition in Adults

Method of
Elaine B. Trujillo, MS, RD, and
Malcolm K. Robinson, MD

Since the inception of parenteral nutrition (PN) in the 1960s, the science of PN has matured in a number of ways. The initial excitement of being able to feed basic nutrients, vitamins, and trace elements intravenously has been tempered by the realization that indiscriminant use of PN can be harmful. Although PN can still be lifesaving,

it is imperative that it be used judiciously and only as long as necessary. This chapter discusses the current use of PN in adult patients.

Indications and Contraindications

Enteral nutrition is the preferred method of nutrition support, primarily because it is associated with fewer infectious and metabolic complications. However, total PN (TPN), which is the provision of all nutrient requirements intravenously, may be indicated when feeding through the gastrointestinal (GI) tract is not possible. PN may be appropriately initiated in those who cannot receive enteral nourishment and are malnourished or at risk for developing malnourishment. Malnourishment can be defined as unintentional loss of more than 10% of usual body weight or greater than 7 to 10 days of inadequate nutrient intake. The body stores of well-nourished persons are generally sufficient to provide the essential nutrients, resist infection, promote wound healing, and support other necessary physiologic functions for this time period. In patients who are anticipated not to be able to receive adequate enteral nutrition for longer than 10 days, it is not necessary to wait 10 days before initiating PN. This may include patients with short-bowel syndrome and others who are expected to have prolonged GI dysfunction.

According to the American Society of Parenteral and Enteral Nutrition guidelines, enteral nutrition is contraindicated in conditions such as diffuse peritonitis, intestinal obstruction, early stages of short-bowel syndrome, intractable vomiting, paralytic ileus, severe GI bleeding and severe diarrhea and malabsorption syndromes. Other relative contraindications to enteral nutrition include pancreatitis and enterocutaneous fistulae, although depending on the clinical circumstances, enteral nutrition may be indicated. PN and enteral nutrition may be provided concomitantly, although in patients who are critically ill, PN should not be started until all strategies to maximize enteral feeding (such as the use of postpyloric feeding tubes and motility agents) have been attempted. PN support is unlikely to benefit a patient who will be able to take enteral nutrition within 4 or 5 days after the onset of illness or who has a relatively minor injury (Fig. 1).

There are four key steps to consider before initiating PN, including assessing nutritional status, determining energy needs, evaluating GI function, and estimating the length of time a patient will require PN (Box 1).

Assessment of Nutritional Status

Nutrient depletion is associated with increased morbidity and mortality, and the prevalence of malnutrition in hospitalized patients is approximately 50%. Therefore, it is imperative to identify patients who have or are at risk for developing protein-energy malnutrition or specific nutrient deficiencies. A patient's risk of developing malnutrition-related medical complications needs to be quantified, and it is necessary to monitor the adequacy of nutritional therapy.

Nutrition assessment begins with a thorough history and physical examination in conjunction with select laboratory tests aimed at detecting specific nutrient deficiencies in patients who are at high risk for future abnormalities. The nutrition assessment should establish whether the patient will need maintenance therapy or nutrition repletion and should assess the status of the patient's GI tract, especially if nutrition support will be required.

A thorough history includes an assessment of recent weight changes, dietary habits, GI symptoms, and changes in exercise tolerance or physical abilities that would indicate functional capacity deficiencies. The physical examination includes inspecting for a loss of subcutaneous fat and muscle wasting, which indicate a loss of body energy and protein stores; edema and ascites, which can also indicate altered energy demands or decreased energy intake; and signs of vitamin and mineral deficits such as dermatitis, glossitis, cheilosis, neuromuscular irritability, and coarse, easily pluckable hair.

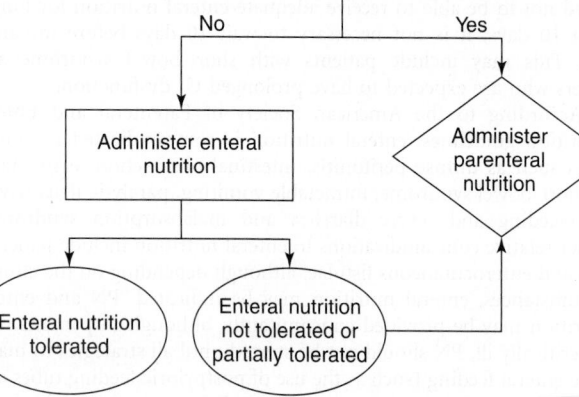

Consider nutritional support if any are present:
Patient has been without nutrition for 7 days.
Expected duration of illness is >10 days.
Patient is malnourished (unintentional weight
loss of >10% body weight).

Initiate nutritional support only if tissue perfusion
is adequate and PO₂, PCO₂, electrolytes, and
acid–base balance are near normal.

Is there a contraindication to enteral feeding, such as:
diffuse peritonitis
intestinal obstruction
early stages of short bowel syndrome
intractable vomiting
paralytic ileus
severe gastrointestinal bleeding
severe diarrhea and malabsorption syndromes

No   Yes

Administer enteral
nutrition

Administer
parenteral
nutrition

Enteral nutrition
tolerated

Enteral nutrition
not tolerated or
partially tolerated

FIGURE 1. Determining route of feeding.

Several laboratory measurements have been used as nutritional biomarkers to aid the nutritional assessment. The serum proteins prealbumin, transferrin, and retinol binding protein have a rapid turnover rate and short half-lives and therefore may be used as indicators of recent nutritional intake. However, these proteins are affected by the metabolic responses to stress and illness, as well as other conditions, including iron status (transferrin) and renal status (retinol binding protein, prealbumin). This can limit their usefulness during acute illness states.

Prealbumin is least affected by fluctuations in hydration status and by liver and renal function compared with other plasma proteins. However, prealbumin levels drop in acute inflammatory conditions during which the liver switches to acute phase protein production and decreases prealbumin synthesis. A rise in C-reactive protein, a protein synthesized by the liver as part of the acute-phase response, indicates inflammatory states. Thus, C-reactive protein, when measured along with prealbumin, can help differentiate a low prealbumin due to nutritional inadequacy versus low prealbumin due to an acute-phase response.

The serum albumin concentration has traditionally been used as an indicator of nutritional status. Although it is a good preoperative predictor of outcome for patients undergoing surgery, it is affected by too many variables in the acute care setting to make it a reliable marker of nutritional status under such conditions or in the immediate postoperative period.

A simple and practical index of malnutrition is the degree of weight loss. Unintentional weight loss of greater than 10% within the previous 6 months indicates protein-energy malnutrition and is a good prognosticator of clinical outcome. Weight can also be compared with an ideal or desirable weight, or an index of body weight relative to height. The body mass index (BMI) is the best known such index and can be used to detect both undernutrition and overnutrition: BMI equals weight in kilograms divided by height in meters squared. This index is independent of height, and the same standards apply to both men and women. A BMI of 18.5 to 25 is considered normal, 25 to 29.9 is considered overweight, and greater than 30 is considered obese. Patients with a normal or high BMI can still have nutrient deficiencies and therefore can be malnourished if they have recently lost a significant amount of weight. In addition, a BMI of 18 kg/m² or less in an adult indicates moderate malnutrition and a BMI less than 15 kg/m² is associated with increased morbidity.

Another practical tool for evaluating nutritional status is the subjective global assessment (SGA) that encompasses historical, symptomatic, and physical parameters. The SGA technique determines if nutrient assimilation has been restricted because of decreased food intake, maldigestion, or malabsorption; if any effects of malnutrition on organ function and body composition have occurred; and if the patient's disease process influences nutrient requirements. The findings of the history and physical examination are subjectively weighted to rank patients as being well-nourished, moderately malnourished, or severely malnourished and are used to predict their risk for medical complications (Box 2).

Estimating Nutritional Requirements

Historically, TPN often provided nutrients in excess of actual requirements. This was based on the assumption that patients requiring nutritional intervention were severely depleted and required aggressive repletion, hence the misnomer "hyperalimentation." Overfeeding is associated with increased carbon dioxide production and difficulty weaning from a ventilator as well as metabolic complications, such as hyperglycemia, which can lead to increased infection, morbidity, and mortality. Thus, nutritional support should be titrated to match actual metabolic requirements.

ENERGY REQUIREMENTS

There are four components of daily energy requirement. The first component is the basal metabolic rate (BMR), which is the amount of energy expended under complete rest, shortly after awakening and in a fasting state (12–14 hours). BMR varies with age, sex, and body size, correlates roughly with body surface area, and is proportional to lean tissue mass. This relationship holds true even among persons of different ages and sexes. Resting metabolic rate or resting

---

BOX 1   Decision-Making Steps When Initiating Parenteral Nutrition

Assess the patient's nutritional status. Nutrition support (PN and/or EN) should not be initiated in well-nourished patients unless they have received a suboptimal diet for more than 7 days.

Determine if the patient has extreme energy needs (hypermetabolism) that warrant the early use of nutrition support (PN and/or EN) within 7 days of injury or illness. These are typically critically ill patients who have suffered severe burns or trauma.

Evaluate the function of the GI tract; if it is intact and can be used safely, PN should be avoided. PN support is indicated until enteral access is established and the patient can meet nutrient needs via tube feedings.

Estimate how long the patient will require PN support. If GI function is expected to return within 5 days, there is no known benefit of initiating PN.

EN = enteral nutrition; GI = gastrointestinal; PN = parenteral nutrition.

BOX 2 Subjective Global Assessment

Select the appropriate category with a checkmark, or enter a numeric value where indicated by #.

History

1. Weight change
   Overall loss in past 6 months: amount = # _____ kg; %loss = # _____.
   Change in past 2 weeks: _____ increase, _____ no change, _____ decrease.
2. Dietary intake change (relative to normal)
   _____ No change
   _____ Change _____ duration = # _____ weeks.
   _____ Type: _____ suboptimal solid diet, _____ full liquid diet, _____ hypocaloric liquids, _____ starvation.
3. Gastrointestinal symptoms (that persisted for >2 weeks)
   _____ None, _____ nausea, _____ vomiting, _____ diarrhea, _____ anorexia.
4. Functional capacity
   _____ No dysfunction (e.g., full capacity),
   _____ Dysfunction _____ duration = # _____ weeks.
   _____ Type: _____ working suboptimally, _____ ambulatory, _____ bedridden.
5. Disease and its relation to nutritional requirements
   Primary diagnosis (specify)
   Metabolic demand (stress): _____ no stress, _____ low stress, _____ moderate stress, _____ high stress.

Physical (for each trait specify: 0 = normal, 1+ = mild, 2+ = moderate, 3+ = severe)

_____ Loss of subcutaneous fat (triceps, chest)
_____ Muscle wasting (quadriceps, deltoids)
_____ Ankle edema
_____ Sacral edema
_____ Ascites

SGA Rating (select one)

_____ A = Well nourished
_____ B = Moderately (or suspected of being) malnourished
_____ C = Severely malnourished

Reprinted with permission from Detsky AS, McLaughlin JR, Baker JP, et al: What is subjective global assessment of nutritional status? JPEN 1987;11:8–13.

---

energy expenditure (REE) represents the amount of energy expended 2 hours after a meal under conditions of rest and thermal neutrality. However, although it is often used synonymously with BMR, the REE is typically 10% higher.

The second component of daily energy expenditure is the thermic effect of exercise or the energy used in physical activity. The contribution of this component increases markedly during intense muscular work, and admission to a hospital generally results in a marked decrease in physical activity. Hospital activity in ambulatory patients accounts for a 20% to 30% increase in BMR. Critically ill patients who are on a ventilator generally have low activity levels (BMR increases by only 5% to 10%) because the ventilator performs the work of breathing, and they are not ambulatory.

The third component of energy expenditure is dietary thermogenesis, the increase in BMR that follows food intake. The digestion and metabolism of exogenous nutrients, whether delivered to the gut or vein, result in an increase in metabolic rate. The magnitude of the thermic effect of food varies depending on the amount and composition of the diet and accounts for approximately 10% of daily energy expenditure.

Finally, acute illness adds an additional stress factor to the daily energy expenditure and correlates with disease severity. For example, a patient's metabolic rate increases by 10% to 30% after a major fracture, from 20% to 60% with severe infection, and from 40% to 110% with a severe third-degree burn. In addition, fever accelerates chemical reactions and the BMR rises approximately 10% for each degree Celsius increase in temperature. Alternatively, cooling of febrile patients produces a reduction in BMR of approximately 10% per degree Celsius.

The first step of estimating calorie requirements is to estimate the BMR. This is usually accomplished using one of several predictive equations. The most commonly used method is based on the predictive equations reported by Harris and Benedict in 1909. The Harris–Benedict equations are as follows:

$$\text{BMR (men)} = 66.47 + 13.75(W) + 5.0(H) - 6.76(A)$$
$$\text{BMR (women)} = 655.1 + 9.56(W) + 1.85(H) - 4.68(A)$$

where W is weight in kg, H is height in cm, and A is age in years.

After the BMR is calculated, it is adjusted for the level of stress induced by injury or the disease process (Fig. 2) and activity level. Activity factors for hospitalized patients are 1.0 to 1.1 for intubated patients, 1.2 for patients confined to bed, and 1.3 for patients out of bed. Therefore, the patient's energy requirements (total energy expenditure [TEE]) are finally calculated:

$$\text{TEE} = \text{BMR} \times \text{Activity factor} \times \text{Stress factor}$$

The thermic effect of feeding is generally not included in the calculation of energy requirements for hospitalized patients.

Alternatively, some clinicians estimate energy requirements based on actual body weight. Thus, 20 to 25 calories (kcal)/kg is administered to the critically ill intubated patient and 30 kcal/kg is given to nonventilated patients in whom excessive intake is not a major concern.

Predicting energy expenditure in obese patients can be difficult, because using predictive formulas with current body weight can lead to high TEE and potentially to overfeeding. A factor of 18 to 21 kcal/kg has been validated in obese patients, and the Harris–Benedict equation using the average of actual and ideal weight and a stress

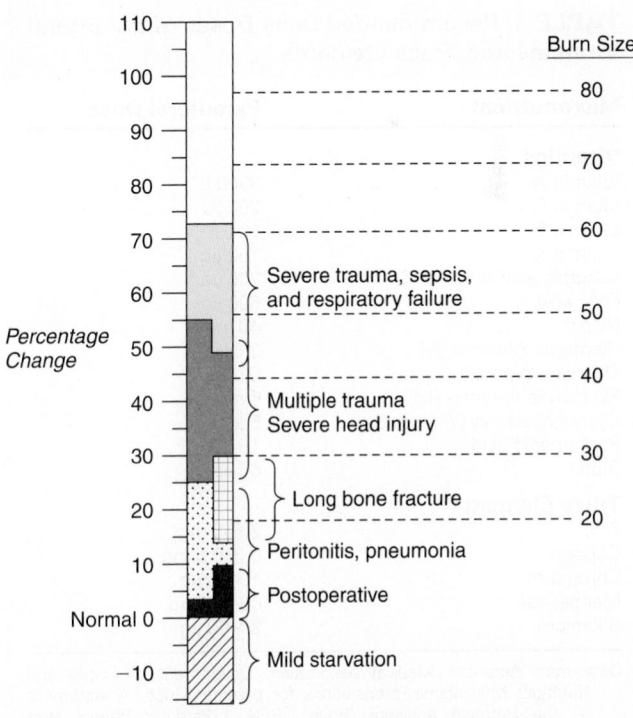

FIGURE 2. Percentage change in metabolic rate due to injury. (Adapted from Wilmore DW: The Metabolic Management of the Critically Ill, New York: Plenum Medical Books, 1977.)

factor of 1.3 accurately predicts REE in acutely ill obese patients with a BMI of 30 to 50 kg/m².

Indirect calorimetry is a more precise, clinically practical and individualized method to determine energy expenditure, particularly in patients in whom estimating requirements through predictive equations are difficult, such as those who continue to lose weight despite what appears to be an adequate caloric intake, who are critically ill, or who have rapidly changing energy needs.

Indirect calorimetry measures changes in oxygen consumption and carbon dioxide production to calculate the REE. Including a stress factor to account for injury is not necessary with indirect calorimetry because the measured energy expenditure accounts for the effects of disease state, stress, and trauma. However, the measurement occurs at rest, and therefore an activity factor of 1.0 to 1.3, depending on whether the patient is intubated, bedridden, or ambulatory, must be applied.

NUTRIENT REQUIREMENTS

The recommended daily protein allowance for most healthy persons who are not hospitalized is 0.8 g/kg or about 60 to 70 g of protein each day. The stressed, critically ill patient generally needs a higher dose of protein in the range of 1.0 to 1.5 g/kg/day. For most patients, providing protein beyond 1.5 g/kg/day is not beneficial. In fact, providing excess protein does not enhance uptake and can lead to increased ureagenesis, which can cause renal injury in some patients.

The calorie-to-nitrogen ratio for most PN solutions typically is around 150:1, with an acceptable range of 100:1 to 180:1. Nitrogen content is used as a marker for protein, and hence the two terms are used interchangeably. Usually, 6.25 g of protein is equal to 1.0 g of nitrogen. The conversion factor is slightly higher (6.4) for PN solutions, such as those with higher concentrations of crystalline amino acids.

Vitamin and mineral requirements are altered in certain disease states due to increased losses, greater use or both. Guidelines for parenteral vitamin and trace elements, developed by the Nutrition Advisory Group of the American Medical Association, were approved by the U.S. Food and Drug Administration (FDA) in 1979 and amended in 2000 (Table 1).

TABLE 1 Recommended Daily Doses of Parenteral Vitamins and Trace Elements

Micronutrient	Parenteral Dose
Vitamins	
Vitamin A	3300 IU
Vitamin D	200 IU
Vitamin E	10 IU
Vitamin K	150 µg
Ascorbic acid (Vitamin C)	200 µg
Folic acid	600 µg
Niacin	40 mg
Riboflavin (Vitamin B$_2$)	3.6 mg
Thiamine (Vitamin B$_1$)	6 mg
Pyridoxine (Vitamin B$_6$)	6 mg
Cyanocobalamin (Vitamin B$_{12}$)	5 µg
Pantothenic acid	15 mg
Biotin	60 µg
Trace Elements	
Zinc	2.5–5 mg
Copper	0.3–0.5 mg
Chromium	10–15 µg
Manganese	60–100 µg
Selenium	20–60 µg

Data from American Medical Association, Department of Foods and Nutrition: Multivitamin preparations for parenteral use. A statement by the Nutrition Advisory Group, JPEN J Parenter Enteral Nutr 1979;3:258–262; Food and Drug Administration: Parenteral multivitamin products: Drugs for human use: Drug efficacy study implementation: Amendment, Federal Register 2000;65(77):21200–21201.

Composition of Central and Peripheral Venous Solutions

Central venous access is required for providing TPN because of the hypertonicity of the formulas infused (1900 mOsm/kg). The infusion of a hypertonic solution into a peripheral vein, known as *peripheral parenteral nutrition* (PPN), can result in thrombophlebitis and venous sclerosis unless the PN is drastically diluted to lower the tonicity. To minimize the hypertonicity of PPN solutions, dextrose is limited to 5% to 10% and amino acids are limited to 2.5% to 3.5%. Lipids are isotonic and therefore provide a significant portion of the caloric substrate of PPN formulas.

Central venous solutions, which are prepared by the hospital's pharmacy, typically combine carbohydrate in the form of dextrose, protein as crystalline amino acids, and lipids from polyunsaturated long-chain triglycerides such as soybean oil or a safflower/soybean oil mixture. Vitamins, electrolytes, and trace elements are added to the formulation as needed. Typical substrate profiles of carbohydrate, protein, and lipids in central PN are shown in Table 2. A usual PN prescription administers 1 to 2 L of a solution each day. Administration of 500 mL of a 20% fat emulsion 1 day each week is sufficient to prevent essential fatty acid deficiency. Alternatively, if additional calories from lipids are needed on a daily basis, they can be administered as a separate infusion or most commonly as part of the mixture of dextrose and amino acids, a technique known as *triple mix* or *three-in-one*.

Including intravenous fat emulsion into a parenteral admixture changes the conventional nutritional solution into an emulsion. Various electrolytes and micronutrients can adversely influence emulsion stability, and therefore their concentration in three-in-one solutions is limited to prevent cracking of the TPN solution, in which microscopic or macroscopic precipitates are formed. The higher the cation valence, the greater the destabilizing influence to the emulsifier. Therefore, trivalent cations such as ferric ion (iron dextran) are more disruptive than divalent cations such as calcium or magnesium ions, which are more disruptive than monovalent cations such as sodium or potassium. No concentration of iron dextran is safe in triple-mix formulations. In-line filtration is necessary for all PN solutions, including triple-mix solutions because it is impossible to visually detect precipitates until they are grossly incompatible and unsafe for infusion.

Once the basic solution is created, electrolytes are added as needed (Table 3). Sodium or potassium salts are given as chloride or acetate depending on the patient's requirements. Normally, equal amounts of chloride and acetate are provided. However, if chloride losses from the body are increased, such as can occur in patients who have nasogastric tubes, then most of the salts should be given as chloride. Similarly, more acetate should be given to patients when additional base is required because acetate generates bicarbonate when it is metabolized. Sodium bicarbonate is incompatible with PN solutions and so cannot be added to the mixture. Phosphate

TABLE 2 Central Versus Peripheral Parenteral Nutrition

Property	Central Nutrition	Peripheral Nutrition
Daily calories	2000–3000	1000–1500
Protein	Variable	56–87 g
Volume of fluid required	1000–3000 mL	2000–3500 mL
Duration of therapy	≥7 d	5–7 d
Route of administration	Dedicated central venous catheter	Peripheral vein or multi-use central catheter
Substrate profile	55%–60% carbohydrate 15%–20% protein 25% fat	30% carbohydrate 20% protein 50% fat
Osmolarity	~2000 mOsm/L	~600–900 mOsm/L

TABLE 3 Electrolyte Concentrations in Parenteral Nutrition

Electrolyte	Recommended Central PN Doses	Recommended Peripheral PN Doses	Usual Range of Doses
Potassium (mEq/L)	30	30	0–120 (CVL) 0–80 (PV)
Sodium (mEq/L)	30	30	0–150
Phosphate (mmol/L)	15	5	0–20
Magnesium (mEq/L)	5	5	0–16
Calcium (mEq/L) (as gluconate)	4.7	4.7	0–10
Chloride (mEq/L)	50	50	0–150
Acetate (mEq/L)	40	40	0–100

CVL = central venous line; PN = parenteral nutrition; PV = peripheral vein.

may be given as the sodium or potassium salt. Lipid emulsions contain an additional 15 mmol/L of phosphate.

Commercially available preparations of fat-soluble and water-soluble vitamins, minerals, and trace elements are added to the nutrient mix unless they are contraindicated. Adequate thiamine is essential for patients receiving PN and can be provided separately. Vitamin K is not a component of any of the vitamin mixtures formulated for adults. Maintenance requirements can be satisfied by adding 10 mg of vitamin K weekly in the PN solution for patients who are not receiving anticoagulants such as warfarin (Coumadin).

Trace element preparations that include zinc, copper, manganese, and chromium are added to the PN solution in amounts consistent with the American Medical Association guidelines (Table 1). Manganese accumulation can be toxic, and overexposure can lead to progressive neurodegenerative damage. Manganese is usually supplied in the PN solution at a daily dose of 0.5 mg as part of a multiple trace element additive. Because manganese is primarily eliminated via biliary excretion, patients with biliary obstruction or cholestasis can accumulate potentially toxic levels of manganese. Hence, manganese should be removed from the PN of patients with hyperbilirubinemia. Higher doses, 10 to 15 mg/day, of zinc are provided to patients with excessive GI losses.

Iron is not a part of commercial additive preparations because it is incompatible with triple mix solutions and can cause anaphylactic reactions when it is given intravenously. Patients who need this trace element should receive it orally or by injection. Iron is not given to patients who are critically ill because hyperferremia can increase bacterial virulence, alter polymorphonuclear cell function, and increase host susceptibility to infection.

PPN is less commonly used than central PN or TPN and can be disadvantageous. Because of the low concentration of dextrose, greater volumes ($\geq$2 L/day) are required to provide sufficient calories, which might not be feasible in fluid-restricted patients. PPN generally does not approximate a patient's energy needs, because PPN provides only 1000 to 1500 kcal/day and a large percentage of the calories (50%) are derived from fat. High-fat infusions are undesirable because they are associated with impaired reticuloendothelial system function and are potentially immunosuppressive. There is no evidence that IV lipids improve outcomes or significantly decrease nitrogen losses. Generally, PPN should be avoided unless it is combined with enteral feeding in patients who can not tolerate full enteral feeding, patients who cannot get a central venous catheter, or patients with low body weights in whom PPN can meet at least two thirds of estimated needs.

Administration and Venous Access

Typically, central PN solutions are administered into the superior vena cava. Access to this vein can be achieved by cannulation of the subclavian or internal jugular veins. Peripherally inserted central venous catheters (PICC) (typically inserted via an antecubital vein and advanced into the superior vena cava) are the most commonly used central venous access devices for providing PN. PICC placement offers the advantage of central venous access while avoiding the risks associated with accessing the subclavian or jugular veins, such as hemothorax, pneomothorax, and arterial injury.

Tunneled catheters or catheters with indwelling ports should be considered for patients who will need prolonged central venous nutrition (e.g., >6 weeks). Patients who will be using their catheters solely for daily central PN and who require home IV feeding may be best served by a tunneled catheter rather than an indwelling port. Tunneled catheters may be more easily manipulated and cared for, which can minimize the risk of infection.

Inserting a dedicated line for infusing hypertonic solutions requires strict aseptic technique or maximal barrier protection: Hat, mask, gown, and gloves must be worn. The position of the catheter tip in the superior vena cava is confirmed by chest x-ray before any concentrated solutions are administered. Once the position of the tip has been confirmed, the line should be used exclusively for administering the hypertonic nutrient solution based on the Centers for Disease Control and Prevention (CDC) guidelines.

Multiple-lumen central venous catheters are most commonly used. Although at least one lumen is dedicated to the infusion of the PN solutions, the other(s) may be used for monitoring, blood drawing, or medication. The rate of catheter sepsis associated with multiple-port catheters may be the same as or slightly greater than the rate associated with the use of single-port catheters. However, multiple-port PICCs are used to infuse PN solutions for a shorter time, which can minimize their inherent risk. Multiple-port catheters should be carefully maintained, including dressing changes, maintaining the dedicated lumen, careful handling of the other lumens, and removing the catheter as soon as it is no longer needed.

Infusion and Patient Monitoring

It is advisable to start with 1 L of central PN and increase the volume as needed, depending on the patient's metabolic stability. Blood sugar levels should be closely monitored and maintained at 80 to 110 mg/dL, tissue perfusion should be adequate, and Po_2, Pco_2, electrolytes (especially potassium, phosphate, and magnesium) and acid–base balance should be near normal before starting or advancing to the goal solution. The solutions should be administered using a volumetric pump set at a constant rate. It is important not to modify the infusion rate during any given day to try to compensate for excess or inadequate administration of the PN solution, such as when the PN solution arrives later than expected. A cyclic schedule (10–16 h/day) for patients requiring long-term PN can be initiated once the patient is metabolically stable. In situations when the central PN solution must be suddenly discontinued, a 10% dextrose solution may be given at the same infusion rate as was used for the PN unless the patient is severely hyperglycemic. PN solutions may be administered at one half the infusion rate to patients who are undergoing surgical procedures because circulating glucose and electrolyte levels are easier to control.

In addition to hyperglycemia, metabolic complications include hyper- and hypophosphatemia, hyper- and hypokalemia, hyper- and hypomagnesemia, and hyper- and hypocalcemia. Thus, it is important to monitor the patient's serum electrolytes closely, especially when initiating TPN. Once the patient has stabilized on the individual nutritional prescription, serum chemistries should be obtained at least twice weekly to measure chloride, CO_2, potassium, sodium, blood urea nitrogen, creatinine, calcium, and phosphate levels and once weekly for a full profile that includes liver function, magnesium, and triglyceride levels.

Patients with Special Needs

GLUCOSE INTOLERANCE

Hyperglycemia is the most common metabolic complication related to PN, and glucose regulation may be especially difficult in patients who have diabetes mellitus or who develop insulin resistance in response to severe stress or infection. Control of blood glucose levels is important for all patients who receive PN because uncontrolled hyperglycemia may be associated with complications such as fluid and electrolyte disturbances and increased infection risk due to impairment of host defenses, including decreased polymorphonuclear leukocyte mobilization, chemotaxis, and phagocytic activity. Evidence suggests that maintaining tight blood glucose concentrations between 80 and 110 mg/dL decreases morbidity and mortality in critically ill surgical patients. Intensive insulin therapy minimizes derangements in normal host defense mechanisms and modulates release of inflammatory mediators.

Patients with difficult glycemic control may best be managed by continuous insulin infusion, which is safe, effective, and more timely than subcutaneous insulin therapy. Hypoglycemia that occurs during this type of infusion generally is short lived and more easily corrected than hypoglycemia resulting from subcutaneous insulin administration. A separate IV insulin infusion can be used rather than adding incremental doses of insulin to the PN bag every 24 hours in patients in whom glycemic control is difficult. Many intensive care units (ICUs) have an insulin drip infusion protocol in which there are frequent checks of serum glucose and adjustments of the insulin infusion drip (e.g. every 1–2 hours) to maintain tight control of glucose levels. The conventional approach of using sliding scale insulin to cover high blood glucose levels may be unsafe and ineffective, and repetitive doses of subcutaneous insulin in the edematous patient can have a cumulative effect leading to prolonged hypoglycemia. In addition, adjusting insulin in the TPN bag every 24 hours might not achieve the desired rapid correction of hyperglycemia deemed appropriate based on the literature, which indicates worse outcomes for those with poor glucose control. See Table 4 for guidelines for managing hyperglycemia in critically ill patients receiving PN.

Abrupt discontinuation of PN can lead to hypoglycemia and should be avoided. Instead, it is recommended to decrease the PN infusion rate by one half before discontinuation to prevent rebound hypoglycemia.

PANCREATITIS

Most cases of pancreatitis are mild, and nutritional support is not needed. However, 10% to 20% of patients with pancreatitis develop severe disease that results in a hypermetabolic, hyperdynamic, systemic inflammatory response syndrome that creates a highly catabolic stress state. Although the usual care of pancreatitis had been gut rest, with or without PN, an evidence-based review found a trend toward reductions in the adverse outcomes of acute pancreatitis after administration of enteral nutrition. Hence, if feasible, enteral nutrition should be used in patients with pancreatitis because it is associated with a significant reduction in infectious morbidity and hospital length of stay compared with PN.

Initiation of PN should be delayed in patients with acute pancreatitis who cannot tolerate enteral nutrition even though they might eventually require PN. Providing PN within 24 hours of admission

TABLE 4 Management of Hyperglycemia in Critically Ill Patients Receiving Parenteral Nutrition

Blood Glucose	Treatment
Before Parenteral Nutrition or Insulin Infusion	
>220 mg/dL	Start insulin infusion at 2–4 U/h
110–220 mg/dL	Start insulin infusion at 1–2 U/h
<110 mg/dL	Do not start insulin infusion
	Check BG every 4 h
During Insulin Infusion	
Above Normal Range	
>140 mg/dL	Increase insulin infusion by 1–2 U/h
	Monitor BG every 1–2 h until in normal range
110–140 mg/dL	Increase insulin infusion by 0.5–1 U/h
	Monitor BG every 1–2 h until in normal range
Normal Range	
80–110 mg/dL	No change
	Monitor BG every 4 h
Below Normal Range	
60–80 mg/dL	Reduce insulin dosage
	Monitor BG every 4 h
	Recheck BG within 1 h
40–60 mg/dL	Stop insulin, ensure adequate baseline glucose intake
	Recheck BG within 1 h
<40 mg/dL	Stop insulin, ensure adequate baseline glucose intake, give 10 g IV glucose bolus
	Recheck BG within 1 h
Steeply Falling	
Any	Reduce insulin dosage by one half
	Monitor BG every h

Adapted from Butler SO, Btaiche IF, Alaniz C: Relationship between hyperglycemia and infection in critically ill patients. Pharmacotherapy 2005;5(7):963–976.
BG = blood glucose.

has been shown to worsen outcome, and providing PN after resuscitation and abatement of the acute inflammatory process appears to improve outcome compared with standard therapy. Consequently, if enteral nutrition is not feasible, the initiation of PN should be delayed for at least 5 days after admission to the hospital, when the peak period of inflammation has abated.

ACUTE RENAL FAILURE

Acute renal failure (ARF) is associated with severe nutritional deficits. Most patients with ARF are catabolic and have energy requirements of 50% to 100% greater than resting requirements, likely the result of other coexisting conditions such as sepsis, trauma, and burns. Calories are provided to patients with ARF in sufficient quantities to minimize protein degradation, generally in the range of 25 to 35 kcal/kg/day. Lipid emulsions can be used as a source of concentrated energy in patients who are on fluid restriction.

Protein loss is accelerated and protein synthesis is impaired in patients with ARF. Loss of amino acids in the dialysate and renal replacement therapies add to the protein deficit and increase individual protein needs. Approximately 10 to 12 g of amino acids are lost with each dialysis therapy, depending on the type of dialyzer membrane, blood flow rate, and dialyzer reuse procedure, and approximately 10 to 16 g/day of amino acids are lost through continuous renal replacement therapies (CRRT). The provision of protein 1.0 to 1.4 g/kg/day and 1.5 to 2.5 g/kg/day is recommended for ARF patients receiving hemodialysis and CRRT, respectively.

Protein is provided with a standard solution containing both essential and nonessential amino acids. Traditionally, formulas designed for renal failure contained predominantly essential amino acids. These formulas often were insufficient in calories and protein for metabolic needs and further compromised the patient's nutritional status. They also increase the risk for hyperammonemia and metabolic encephalopathy when used for longer than 2 to 3 weeks. The current recommendations are to provide adequate protein while treating the patient aggressively with dialysis to prevent the accumulation of nitrogenous waste products.

Fluid and electrolyte balance are often impaired in patients with ARF. The amount of fluid from the PN might need to be adjusted daily, depending on the phase of ARF, whether the patient is receiving dialysis, and whether dialysis is continuous or intermittent. Serum potassium and phosphate levels typically rise in patients with ARF until dialysis is initiated, at which time levels might drop, especially with the provision of PN. Potassium, phosphate, and magnesium levels need close monitoring and adjusting to correct imbalances. Acetate salts of potassium or sodium can be administered to help correct a metabolic acidosis.

Standard doses of the water-soluble vitamins and additional folic acid (1 mg/day total) and pyridoxine (vitamin B_6) (10 mg/day) might need to be added to the solution for patients who are being dialyzed because these vitamins are lost from the body in the dialysate bath. The dose of vitamin C might need to be restricted to 100 mg/day to prevent oxalate deposits. The supplementation of fat-soluble vitamins is usually not required, especially in patients who also are eating, because excretion of fat-soluble vitamins is reduced in renal failure. For example, serum vitamin A levels may be elevated in ARF due to enhanced hepatic release of retinol and retinol-binding protein, decreased renal catabolism, and decreased degradation of vitamin A transport protein by the kidneys. Vitamin D levels may be decreased because of impaired activation of 1,25-dihydroxycholecalciferol in the kidneys. In anuric patients, trace elements may be withheld from the PN solution; however, for prolonged PN, trace elements and fat-soluble vitamins should be monitored and replaced accordingly.

Patients with chronic renal failure (CRF) also have nutritional deficits due to anorexia, amino acid losses into the dialysate, concurrent illness, metabolic acidosis, and endocrine disorders. However, unlike those suffering from ARF, patients with CRF have normal energy requirements. Protein intake generally is restricted in predialysis patients to 0.5 to 0.6 g/kg/day but required in higher amounts in patients on dialysis, depending on the type of dialysis (1.2 g/kg/day for hemodialysis; 1.2 to 1.5 g/kg/day for peritoneal dialysis). Predialysis patients who become acutely ill should be given protein 1.2 to 1.5 g/kg/day even if this precipitates the need for dialysis. Starvation from insufficient calories or protein in the patient with renal dysfunction increases the risk of nutritionally related complications and should be avoided in the severely ill patient regardless of the potential need for dialysis.

Intradialytic PN is the provision of IV amino acids, carbohydrates, and fat directly into the venous drip chamber of the hemodialysis unit during treatment. It is a method of providing additional calories and protein in malnourished chronic hemodialysis patients. It is associated with significant increases in body weight and serum albumin in patients with chronic renal failure. However, intradialytic PN is expensive and the benefits have not been fully elucidated. A typical solution contains about 1100 kcal and 50 g of protein, which is provided three times per week with dialysis. For example, intradialytic PN provides a patient with energy and protein requirements of 2500 kcal and 70 g of protein/day, respectively, only 20% of the weekly calorie and 30% of the weekly protein needs. Thus, intradialytic PN is reserved for patients with CRF who cannot ingest sufficient nutrients by mouth and who are not candidates for nutritional support via enteral nutrition on PN due to GI intolerance or venous access problems or for other reasons. Appropriate use of intradialytic PN should be limited to a very small fraction of people who are on dialysis.

HEPATIC DYSFUNCTION AND LIVER FAILURE

Hepatic dysfunction is associated with a variety of abnormalities including metabolic abnormalities, malabsorption, maldigestion, anorexia, and early satiety due to ascites. Dietary restrictions also can contribute to malnutrition.

Protein intake in patients with stable chronic liver disease depends on the patient's nutritional status and protein tolerance. Nutritionally depleted patients can require as much protein as 1.5 g/kg estimated dry weight. In a minority of patients who have protein-sensitive hepatic encephalopathy, protein intake might need to be decreased to 0.5 to 0.7 g/kg/day and gradually increased to 1.0 to 1.5 g/kg/day, as tolerated. These patients have deranged plasma amino acid profiles, with increased concentrations of aromatic amino acids (phenylalanine, tyrosine, and tryptophan) and methionine and decreased branched-chain amino acids (valine, leucine, and isoleucine). Randomized, controlled trials that provided parenteral or enteral formulas enriched with branched-chain amino acids have been inconsistent and have had results including no benefit, improved morbidity, no change in mortality, and improvement in encephalopathy. These specialty products should be reserved for patients with disabling encephalopathy who do not tolerate standard proteins and have not responded to other therapies, such as lactulose or neomycin administration.

Energy requirements are difficult to predict in patients with liver failure. Whereas most patients have a normal metabolic rate, up to one third may be hypermetabolic. Although providing 25 to 30 kcal/kg/day is a guideline for providing energy needs, basing requirements on indirect calorimetry is often recommended.

Fluid restriction due to ascites and edema often necessitates increasing the dextrose concentration in the PN so as to maintain sufficient calories in a restricted volume. Sodium is reduced in the formula because liver-failure patients excrete nearly sodium-free urine. Vitamin and mineral deficiencies often occur as a result of suboptimal nutrient intake, decreased absorption, decreased storage, and in some cases alcohol use, which decreases thiamine (vitamin B_1) and folate absorption. Copper and manganese may be contraindicated because a major route of excretion for these substances is the biliary system. Zinc deficiency is common in cirrhotic patients, and supplementation of this mineral may be necessary, especially if there are excessive GI losses.

ACUTE RESPIRATORY DISTRESS SYNDROME

Patients with protein-calorie malnutrition have an increased incidence of pneumonia, respiratory failure, and acute respiratory distress syndrome (ARDS). Nutritional support is indicated in patients with ARDS, and underfeeding and overfeeding can be detrimental to pulmonary function.

Overfeeding calories, and particularly glucose, can lead to increased minute ventilation, increased dead space, and increased carbon dioxide production and ultimately to difficulty weaning from a ventilator. Hypercapnia from increased carbon dioxide production is the result of glucose combustion causing more carbon dioxide production and excess calories triggering lipogenesis. A healthy person increases ventilation in response to increased calories and thus avoids hypercapnia. However, patients with compromised ventilatory status might not be able to compensate with increased ventilation and can develop respiratory distress, acute respiratory failure, and difficulty weaning from mechanical ventilation. Thus, the use of indirect calorimetry measurements to determine respiratory quotient and energy expenditure is imperative in patients with ARDS.

OTHER CONDITIONS AND NUTRITIONAL TREATMENTS

The catabolic response to major surgery, trauma, burn, and sepsis is characterized by a net breakdown of body protein stores to provide substrates for gluconeogenesis and acute-phase protein synthesis. Adequate nutrition can attenuate whole-body catabolism but rarely, if ever, prevents or reverses the loss of lean body mass during the acute phase of injury. Several strategies to prevent the loss of lean body mass have been investigated, including growth hormone, growth factors, and conditionally essential amino acids, such as glutamine.

Growth hormone is a potent anabolic agent, and administration to humans increases the rate of wound healing, decreases rates of wound infection, and decreases the catabolism and muscle wasting of critical illness. However, a large European trial found increased morbidity and mortality in patients with prolonged critical illness who received high doses of growth hormone. Thus, the use of growth hormone in patients who are in the acute phase of critical illness is not recommended.

Alternative anabolic agents, such as oxandrolone (Oxandrin) and testosterone[1] are being pursued to induce positive nitrogen balance and enhance wound healing in critically ill patients. These anabolic steroid hormones increase protein synthesis and can reduce the rate of protein breakdown. In a study of patients with alcoholic hepatitis, administration of oxandrolone was associated with lower mortality compared with patients receiving placebo. The patients receiving oxandrolone had improvements in the severity of their liver injury and the degree of malnutrition. Several studies have demonstrated a benefit of oxandrolone use in the burn patient population. Other anabolic steroid hormones, such as methandieone and nandrolone decanoate, have been shown to increase protein anabolism and nitrogen balance in hospitalized patients.

Growth factors should be reserved for patients with major burns and documented impaired healing, patients who have large wounds or enterocutaneous fistulae and who have impaired healing, and patients with muscle wasting and weakness associated with AIDS, other failure to thrive conditions, and in general, patients who have not responded to aggressive nutritional support but whose underlying disease processes are controlled. Growth factors have not been shown to decrease length of time on a respiratory

_____
[1]Not FDA approved for this indication.

in ICU patients. In fact, such factors can increase ventilator time and worsen outcome.

Glutamine-supplemented PN solutions administered to trauma or stressed patients can improve overall nitrogen balance, enhance muscle protein synthesis, improve intestinal nutrient absorption, decrease gut permeability, improve immune function, and decrease hospital stays and costs in some patient populations. A review of 14 randomized trials in surgical and critically ill patients found that glutamine supplementation was associated with reduced mortality, lower rates of infectious complications, and a decreased hospital stay. The greatest benefit was in patients receiving high-dose (>0.29 g/kg/day) parenteral glutamine.

Patients with intestinal dysfunction requiring PN, such as those with short bowel syndrome, mucosal damage following chemotherapy, irradiation, or critical illness might benefit from glutamine-containing PN. Glutamine-containing PN might also be beneficial in patients with immunodeficiency syndromes, including AIDS, immune-system dysfunction associated with critical illness, and bone marrow transplantation; patients with severe catabolic illness, such as major burns; patients with multiple trauma; and patients with other diseases associated with a prolonged ICU stay. Glutamine-supplemented solutions should not yet be considered routine care and should not be used in patients with significant renal insufficiency or in patients with significant hepatic failure.

TABLE 5 Possible Etiologies and Treatment of Common Complications of Central Parenteral Nutrition

Problem	Possible Etiology	Treatment
Glucose		
Hyperglycemia, glycosuria, hyperosmolar nonketotic dehydration, or coma	Excessive dose or rate of infusion, inadequate insulin production, steroid administration, infection	Decrease the amount of glucose given, increase insulin, administer a portion of calories as fat
Diabetic ketoacidosis	Inadequate endogenous insulin production and/or inadequate insulin therapy	Give insulin Decrease glucose intake
Rebound hypoglycemia	Persistent endogenous insulin production by islet cells after long-term high-carbohydrate infusion	Give 5%–10% glucose before parenteral infusion is discontinued
Hypercarbia	Carbohydrate load exceeds the ability to increase minute ventilation and excrete excess CO_2	Limit glucose dose to 5 mg/kg/min Give greater percentage of total caloric needs as fat (up to 30%–40%)
Fat		
Hypertriglyceridemia	Rapid infusion Decreased clearance	Decrease rate of PN infusion Allow clearance (~12 h) before testing blood
Essential fatty acid deficiency	Inadequate essential fatty acid administration	Administer essential fatty acids in doses of 4%–7% of total calories
Amino Acids		
Hyperchloremia metabolic acidosis	Excessive chloride content of amino acid solutions	Administer Na^+ and K^+ as acetate salts
Prerenal azotemia	Excessive amino acids with inadequate caloric supplementation	Reduce amino acids Increase the amount of glucose calories
Miscellaneous		
Hypophosphatemia	Inadequate phosphorus administration with redistribution into tissues	Give 15 mmol phosphate/1000 IV kcal Evaluate antacid and Ca^{2+} administration
Hypomagnesemia	Inadequate administration relative to increased losses (diarrhea, diuresis, medications)	Administer Mg^{2+} (15–20 mEq/1000 kcal)
Hypermagnesemia	Excessive administration; renal failure	Decrease Mg^{2+} supplementation
Hypokalemia	Inadequate K^+ intake relative to increased needs for anabolism; diuresis	Increase K^+ supplementation
Hyperkalemia	Excessive K^+ administration, especially in metabolic acidosis; renal decompensation	Reduce or stop exogenous K^+ If ECG changes are present, treat with calcium gluconate, insulin, diuretics, and or Kayexalate
Hypocalcemia	Inadequate Ca^{2+} administration; reciprocal response to phosphorus repletion without simultaneous calcium infusion	Increase Ca^{2+} dose
Hypercalcemia	Excessive Ca^{2+} administration; excessive vitamin D administration	Decrease Ca^{2+} and/or vitamin D administration
Elevated liver transaminases or serum alkaline phosphatase and bilirubin	Enzyme induction secondary to amino acid imbalances or overfeeding	Reevaluate nutritional prescription Cycle TPN Avoid overfeeding calories Consider administering carnitine

ECG = electrocardiogram; PN = parenteral nutrition; TPN = total parenteral nutrition.

Common Complications and Management

CATHETER SEPSIS

Central venous catheter–related bloodstream infection ranges from 3% to 20% in hospitalized patients and is the most common complication of central venous catheters. The migration of microorganisms along the external surface of the catheter is likely the most common cause, followed by intraluminal contamination from manipulation of the catheter hub or IV connectors. The most common organisms associated with catheter-related bloodstream infections include *Staphylococcus epidermidis, Staphylococcus aureus, Enterococcus* spp, *Candida albicans,* and *Enterobacter* spp as well as resistant strains such as methicillin-resistant *S. aureus* and vancomycin-resistant enterococci. Primary catheter sepsis occurs when there are signs and symptoms of infection and the indwelling catheter is the only anatomic focus of infection. Secondary catheter infections are associated with another focus or multiple infectious foci that cause bacteremia and seed the catheter.

Management of patients with catheter infection depends on their clinical condition. With extremely ill patients with high fevers who are hypotensive or who have local signs of infection around the catheter site, the catheter should be removed, its tip cultured, and peripheral and central venous blood cultures obtained. The organisms that grow from the catheter tip are the same as the ones that are identified in the peripheral blood culture and typically greater than 10^3 organisms are grown from cultures of the catheter tip.

Specific therapy should be initiated against the primary source in patients in whom a source of infection, other than the catheter tip, is present. Peripheral blood cultures should be obtained and blood cultures should not be taken from the central venous catheter port dedicated for PN because this increases the risk of contaminating the line. If the infection resolves, central venous feedings can be continued. If a secondary source is not identified and the symptoms persist, the catheter should be removed and its tip should be cultured. If the culture of the catheter tip returns positive or if the index of suspicion is high, appropriate antibiotic therapy is initiated. Central venous feeding can be resumed, maintaining euglyemia.

Occasionally, the situation arises in which a site of infection, other than the catheter, is identified, but signs and symptoms persist despite what is assumed to be adequate therapy. Again, if blood cultures are positive, the safest course of action may be to remove the catheter. If peripheral blood cultures are negative, the catheter may be changed over a guidewire and the catheter tip cultured to determine if it was contaminated. Central venous feedings may be continued during this interval if the patient is stable. If the catheter tip returns positive, a new catheter should be inserted at a different site. Changing the central venous catheter over a guidewire can also facilitate the diagnosis of primary catheter infections. Changing the site of catheter location, rather than guidewire exchange, is recommended in patients in whom infection is suspected.

OTHER COMPLICATIONS

Common complications, their etiologies, and treatments are outlined in Table 5. Prolonged administration of PN can result in altered hepatic function and changes in liver pathologic conditions that can lead to liver failure. One to 2 weeks after initiating PN, transaminases may be elevated, but this often resolves without any change in the composition of PN or rate of administration. However, in patients receiving long-term PN (>20 days), prolonged elevations of alkaline phosphatase followed by elevated levels of serum transaminases can occur, even after therapy is discontinued.

Serum levels of alkaline phosphatase and bilirubin initially remain normal, but they rise in many patients who receive long-term PN. Patients who do not receive lipids in the PN solution have more frequent and severe hepatic abnormalities, most likely due to higher carbohydrate loads. Excess glucose increases insulin secretion, which stimulates hepatic lipogenesis and results in hepatic fat accumulation. Fatty infiltration is the initial histopathologic change; it is

---

BOX 3 Management of Parenteral Nutrition–Related Liver Dysfunction

Have the patient eat, if possible.
Avoid administering large amounts of glucose or protein calories.
Supply lipid emulsions (up to 30% of total calories).
Cycle the parenteral nutrition, infusing for 10–12 hours per day.
Reevaluate caloric needs; reduce caloric intake if liver dysfunction persists.

---

readily reversible and might not be accompanied by altered liver function tests.

Longer PN therapy may be associated with cholestasis, cholelithiasis, steatosis, and steatohepatitis and can progress to active chronic hepatitis, fibrosis, and eventual cirrhosis. The management of PN-related liver dysfunction is summarized in Box 3.

Complications are minimized and nutritional therapy maximized when the care of patients who require specialized nutritional support is supervised by a nutrition support team. Ideally, the nutrition support team consists of a pharmacist, dietitian, nurse, and physician.

REFERENCES

ASPEN Board of Directors. Guidelines for the use of parenteral and enteral nutrition in adult and pediatric patients. JPEN J Parenter Enteral Nutr 2002;26(1 Suppl.):1SA–138SA.

Bistrian BR, McCowen KC. Nutritional and metabolic support in the adult intensive care unit: Key controversies. Crit Care Med 2006;34:1525–31.

Butler SO, Btaiche IF, Alaniz C. Relationship between hyperglycemia and infection in critically ill patients. Pharmacotherapy 2005;25:963–76.

Heyland DK, Dhaliwal R, Drover JW, et al. Canadian clinical practice guidelines for nutrition support in mechanically ventilated, critically ill adult patients. JPEN J Parenter Enteral Nutr 2003;27:355–73.

Heyland DK, Dhaliwal R, Suchner U, Berger MM. Antioxidant nutrients: a systematic review of trace elements and vitamins in the critically ill patient. Intensive Care Med 2005;31:327–37.

Heyland DK, MacDonald S, Keefe L, Drover JW. Total parenteral nutrition in the critically ill patient: A meta-analysis. JAMA 1998;280:2013–9.

Kochevar M, Guenter P, Holcombe B, et al. ASPEN statement on parenteral nutrition standardization. JPEN J Parenter Enteral Nutr 2007;31:441–8.

McClave SA, Chang W-K, Dhaliwal R, Heyland DK. Nutrition support in acute pancreatitis: A systematic review of the literature. JPEN J Parenter Enteral Nutr 2006;30:143–56.

Novak F, Heyland DK, Avenell A, et al. Glutamine supplementation in serious illness: A systematic review of the evidence. Crit Care Med 2002;30:2022–9.

O'Grady NP, Alexander M, Dellinger EP, et al. Guidelines for the prevention of intravascular catheter-related infections. MMWR Recomm Rep 2002;51 (RR-10):1–29.

Parenteral Fluid Therapy for Infants and Children

Method of
*Jeremy N. Friedman, MB, ChB, and
Carolyn E. Beck, MD, MSc*

One could dedicate an entire textbook to the subject of parenteral fluid therapy for infants and children. For the purposes of this article we have chosen to focus on three main issues that confront us, as clinicians, on a daily basis. The first question is what types of intravenous fluids are most appropriate to provide maintenance requirements in children? The second question is how best to assess dehydration. This is extremely common in pediatrics and absolutely critical if appropriate fluid therapy is to be instituted. Finally, when and how should intravenous fluid be used in the management of the dehydrated patient? Unfortunately, many of these issues remain controversial and have not been satisfactorily resolved. As general pediatricians we provide you with some practical, simple, and general principles to guide your approach to parenteral fluid therapy.

Maintenance Fluids

FLUID REQUIREMENTS

Hospitalized children often require intravenous fluids, necessitating that physicians have an approach to their requirements—both fluid composition and volume—at their fingertips. While seemingly second nature to many clinicians, the prescription of IV fluids is in fact complex and requires a solid foundation for safe and effective practice.

Maintenance fluid requirements are deep-rooted in pediatric history, dating back to calculations proposed by Holliday and Segar in 1957. These requirements are based on their study of caloric expenditure in healthy children, resulting in the "100/50/20" rule (closely approximated by the "4/2/1" rule) commonly cited today (Table 1). Applying these rules, a 12-kg toddler requires 1100 mL per day by the 100/50/20 rule, or 44 mL per hour by the 4/2/1 rule, values which are almost equivalent.

Maintenance fluids are designed only to replace, or input, naturally occurring output when oral fluids are contraindicated or not tolerated. Output includes urinary losses, in addition to insensible water loss from the skin and lungs. If renal function is abnormal, maintenance fluids by definition do not apply; in this case, fluid requirement is better estimated by calculating insensible water loss (Table 2) and adding it to urine output and any other significant losses (e.g., diarrhea, nasogastric suction). Similarly, factors such as raised body temperature increase insensible water losses and need to be considered when determining appropriate fluid volume.

TABLE 1 Maintenance Fluid Requirements*

Weight (kg)	100/50/20 Rule (Daily Requirements)	4/2/1 Rule (Hourly Requirements)
0–10	100 mL/kg/d	4 mL/kg/h
11–20	1000 mL + 50 mL/kg/d for every kg 11–20	40 mL + 2 mL/kg/h for every kg 11–20
>20	1500 mL + 20 mL/kg/d for every kg >20	60 mL + 1 mL/kg/h for every kg >20

*Assuming normal renal function and usual insensible losses.

TABLE 2 Insensible Fluid Losses by Body Surface Area

Insensible Losses	Body Surface Area (m²)
400 mL/m² BSA/d (spontaneously breathing) 300 mL/m² BSA/d (ventilated) 500–600 mL/m² BSA/d (neonates)	$\sqrt{\dfrac{\text{Height (cm)} \times \text{Weight (kg)}}{3600}}$

Abbreviation: BSA = body surface area.

ELECTROLYTE REQUIREMENTS

Sodium

In the same 1957 paper, Holliday and Segar proposed maintenance sodium requirements for children to be 30 mmol/L. This requirement translates to the use of a hypotonic saline solution for maintenance fluids, equivalent to 0.2% NaCl in 5% dextrose in water (D_5W). Although this solution, or similar hypotonic composites, continues to be widely used in pediatric practice, there is good reason to question its appropriateness.

Holliday's water requirements were based on caloric expenditure in healthy children, and electrolyte composition was derived from that of human and cow's milk. The recommended sodium concentration is less than the average dietary salt intake, and the guideline fails to account for impaired water excretion, an important factor in hospitalized children. Several case reports have raised concern about the routine use of hypotonic solutions in hospitalized children, because reports of potentially fatal hyponatremia have come to light. Factors implicated in the development of hyponatremia include the action of antidiuretic hormone (ADH) preventing water excretion as well as the input of electrolyte-free water (EFW).

There are several reasons for ADH secretion to be elevated in hospitalized children. Apart from osmotic forces, stimuli for ADH release include malignancies, central nervous system disorders (including meningitis), pulmonary disorders (including pneumonia), and several medications, including commonly used drugs such as morphine sulfate (morphine). Additionally, nonspecific symptoms such as pain, nausea, and stress, as well as a postoperative state and hypovolemia, all result in an increase in ADH. Given the illness of hospitalized children in the 21st century, it is rare to care for a patient who does not have at least one of these risk factors for elevated ADH, making water retention an essential consideration in the prescription of IV fluids.

With respect to EFW, the routine use of hypotonic maintenance fluids provides the major source for hospitalized patients. There is 154 mmol/L of sodium in 0.9% NaCl (normal saline), which is isotonic with respect to the cell membrane. Ringer's lactate provides a similar sodium concentration. Solutions with less sodium content are hypotonic (Table 3). Holliday's historic prescription of 0.2% NaCl contributes a large degree of EFW (78%). This contribution of free water via IV fluids, compounded by an impaired ability to excrete water, place the hospitalized child at risk for developing acute hyponatremia. Consequently, IV solutions that are less hypotonic, or even isotonic, are starting to be used in pediatric hospital wards.

Potential risks of using isotonic fluids as maintenance solutions include fluid overload in children with an impaired ability to excrete sodium and hypernatremia in patients with renal concentrating defects, significant water loss, or prolonged fluid restriction. In the absence of these factors, the risks of isotonic fluids are largely theoretical.

Potassium

Maintenance potassium requirements have similarly been derived at 20 mmol/L. In most clinical situations, maintenance potassium should be added to the IV solution. Exceptions include uncertainty regarding the patient's renal function, poor urine output, or any other risk factors for hyperkalemia. In these scenarios, the addition of potassium is not advised, and renal function and electrolytes

TABLE 3 Source of Electrolyte-Free Water

IV Solution	Tonicity	Na (mmol/L)	EFW (%)
D_5W/0.9% NaCl	Isotonic	154	0
D_5W/0.45% NaCl	Hypotonic	77	50
D_5W/0.2% NaCl	Hypotonic	34	78

Abbreviation: EFW = electrolyte-free water.

should be closely monitored. Ongoing losses of potassium (e.g., diarrheal losses) or other reasons for hypokalemia (e.g., prolonged use of albuterol (salbutamol [Ventolin]) can require higher concentrations of potassium, along with appropriate electrolyte monitoring.

GLUCOSE

Dextrose should routinely be added to maintenance fluids as a carbohydrate source when children are in a fasting state in order to provide some calories (albeit minimal) and prevent ketosis. Generally, a child with normal glucose metabolism requires a 5% dextrose solution (D_5W), which can be safely combined with either hypotonic or isotonic solutions. Unlike sodium, glucose can freely cross the cell membrane and thus does not contribute to the osmotic force.

METHOD FOR PRESCRIBING MAINTENANCE FLUIDS: A PRACTICAL APPROACH

No prospective studies have evaluated the risks or benefits of hypotonic versus isotonic IV fluids. Clearly, the routine use of 0.2% saline requires reconsideration, and it is likely inappropriate for use in pediatric wards. A case-control study by Hoorn and colleagues, the most rigorous on the topic to date, recommends that isotonic fluids be used perioperatively as well as in children with a plasma sodium less than 138 mmol/L.

Practically, a decision regarding IV fluid composition must be made on a case-by-case basis. The choice may be viewed as a prescription, taking details about the patient, the clinical scenario, and the baseline laboratory values into account, and monitoring and reevaluating the child's fluids and electrolytes on a regular basis. Rather than following strict rules, judgment is required for each patient. The following scenarios provide some guidance about IV fluid composition.

A normal sodium value ($\geq$136 mmol/L) in a patient who is relatively well should lead one to consider half-normal saline (0.45% NaCl) in D_5W a good choice. This solution provides more sodium (and contributes less EFW) than 0.2% saline while still providing the patient with some free water. A second patient with the same sodium value, however, might require a different fluid prescription. For example, a child with a low-normal sodium of 137 mmol/L in the clinical context of severe pain, meningitis, or pneumonia—all risk factors for elevated ADH—is likely a good candidate for an isotonic solution such as 0.9% NaCl in D_5W. If this same patient presented with a sodium of 132 mmol/L, 0.9% NaCl in D_5W should almost certainly be instituted. In any of these solutions, 20 mmol/L of potassium could be added provided that the patient's urine output is appropriate and no other risk factors for hyperkalemia are present.

With respect to the surgical patient, the recent literature would suggest that isotonic fluids (0.9% NaCl in D_5W, Ringer's lactate) be routinely used in the perioperative period. Postoperatively, approximately 1% of patients develop a serum sodium less than 130 mmol/L. The development of hyponatremia in this clinical context is not surprising, given the multiple factors placing these patients at risk for increased ADH secretion, namely, pain, nausea, stress, narcotic medications, and volume depletion.

A NOTE ABOUT VOLUME

Provided that a patient has normal renal function and usual insensible losses, maintenance fluid guidelines may be followed, estimated by the rules noted in Table 1. It is crucial to note, however, that in studies examining the question of IV fluids in children, excess fluid volume—greater than maintenance requirements—was an important factor associated with development of acute hyponatremia. Often clinicians prescribe maintenance IV fluids when the child is unwell and not taking anything by mouth. In most cases, when the patient's clinical condition improves, oral intake is initiated. Be mindful that oral fluid is hypotonic and can add significantly to the patient's free water load. To prevent the development of hyponatremia and its significant clinical consequences in these children, IV fluid prescriptions should be reevaluated on a regular basis, taking oral intake into account and adjusting the IV volume to maintain an appropriate total fluid intake.

Rehydration

ASSESSMENT OF DEHYDRATION

Gastroenteritis and Dehydration

Acute gastroenteritis accounts for more than 1.5 million outpatient visits, 10% of all pediatric hospitalizations (200,000), and approximately 300 deaths per year in the United States. This pales in comparison with the estimated 30% of worldwide deaths among infants and toddlers, amounting to 8000 children younger than 5 years dying per day, from diarrhea and dehydration in the developing world. Young children with diarrhea are more prone to dehydration than older children and adults because of their higher body surface–to–volume ratio, a higher metabolic rate, and smaller fluid reserves. In addition, they are often dependent on others to provide fluid. Viruses, primarily rotavirus, are responsible for 70% to 80% of infectious diarrhea in the developed world. There are also many other causes of dehydration not involving diarrhea, including poor oral intake (e.g., stomatitis), increased insensible losses (e.g., fever, tachypnea), and renal losses (e.g., diabetes mellitus, diabetes insipidus).

Classification of Dehydration

The American Academy of Pediatrics (AAP) classifies dehydration as mild (3%–5% fluid deficit), moderate (6%–9%), and severe ($\geq$10%). The first signs of dehydration are believed to appear when the fluid deficit is 3% to 4%. Dehydration can be further classified based on the serum sodium concentration. Isotonic dehydration (Na 130–150 mmol/L) accounts for the vast majority, and hypotonic (Na <130 mmol/L) and hypertonic (Na > 150 mmol/L) dehydration account for less than 5% of the total cases. Inaccurate assessment of dehydration can result in permanent injury and death if fluid deficits are underestimated, and overestimation likely leads to unnecessary interventions and inappropriate use of resources.

Accuracy of Historic Factors and Physical Examination

Traditional teaching regarding the assessment of dehydration is empiric and based on clinical experience (Table 4). The gold standard for measuring dehydration is considered to be acute body weight change over the course of the illness. Unfortunately, this information is seldom available due to a lack of an accurate pre-illness weight.

Steiner and colleagues recently performed a systematic review of the literature on the precision and accuracy of history, physical examination, and laboratory tests in identifying dehydration in children younger than 5 years. They found that historic factors have only moderate sensitivity as a screening test for dehydration. Duration, frequency, and quantity of vomiting, diarrhea, and urination only give a rough estimate of the risk of dehydration. Signs of dehydration (see Table 4) on physical examination are generally imprecise and tend to show only fair to moderate agreement among examiners. Capillary refill time had the best measurement properties, with a sensitivity of 0.60 (95% CI, 0.29–0.91) and specificity of 0.85 (95% CI, 0.72–0.98) for detecting 5% dehydration. The absence of sunken eyes and dry mucous membranes was also found to be potentially clinically useful in decreasing the likelihood of 5% dehydration.

A prospective cohort study by Gorelick and colleagues in an urban U.S. pediatric emergency department evaluated 10 clinical signs of dehydration and found that any two or more of four factors:

- Capillary refill >2 sec
- Dry mucous membranes
- Absent tears
- Abnormal general appearance

indicate a fluid deficit of at least 5%. This subset of four factors predicted dehydration as well as the entire set.

In addition, a clinical dehydration scale has been developed by Friedman and coworkers using formal measurement methodology. A score of 0 reflects no dehydration, and a maximum score of 8 reflects severe dehydration as per Table 5.

TABLE 4 Signs Associated with Dehydration

Symptom	Minimal or No Dehydration (<3% Loss of Body Weight)	Mild to Moderate Dehydration (3%–9% Loss of Body Weight)	Severe Dehydration (≥10% Loss of Body Weight)
General appearance	Normal	Thirsty, restless or lethargic, but irritable when touched	Drowsy, limp, cold, sweaty ± comatose
Urine output	Normal	Decreased	Minimal
Breathing	Normal	Normal to increased	Deep and increased
Heart rate	Normal	Increased	Increased
Systolic blood pressure	Normal	Normal or low	Low
Mucous membranes	Moist	Sticky	Dry
Eyes	Normal	Slightly sunken	Very sunken
Tears	Normal	Decreased	Absent
Skin turgor	Instant recoil	<2 sec	>2 sec
Capillary refill	Normal	Normal to prolonged	Prolonged >2 sec

Eliciting Signs of Dehydration

As is true in the physical examination of any young child, *opportunism* is the operative word! Start with the least-invasive part, which involves observing the child's overall appearance and interaction with the caregiver. This also allows you to record the respiratory rate over a 30-second period, looking for hyperpnea suggesting a metabolic acidosis. To assess capillary refill time, sufficient pressure should gradually be applied to blanch the palmar surface of the distal fingertip, and then immediately released. Less than 1.5 to 2 seconds for restoration of normal color is considered normal. The examining room should be at a warm ambient temperature. Autonomic nervous system abnormalities or extremes in patient temperature can affect measurement. Dryness of the mucous membranes is best assessed by examination of the tongue because the lips are often dry in mouth breathers and in children with conditions other than dehydration. If the child does not cry during your examination, the presence of tears may need to be inquired about on history. Skin turgor is usually assessed by pinching a small skin fold on the lateral abdominal wall at the level of the umbilicus. This is then released, and return to its normal position is classified as immediate, slightly delayed, or prolonged. False negatives can be seen in hypernatremia and obese children, and malnutrition can cause false positive results. Although decreased blood pressure and severe tachycardia should be examined for, they are late signs and only tend to become evident in severe dehydration.

Remember that the degree of dehydration may be underestimated in hypertonic dehydration as a result of the movement of water from the intracellular to the extracellular space, which helps to preserve the intravascular volume. In hypotonic dehydration the opposite occurs, and an overestimation of dehydration can result.

Usefulness of Blood Tests

There is a tendency to want to use blood test results to help in the assessment of dehydration because they are perceived to be more reliable than the features on history and physical examination. Unfortunately their usefulness has not been supported by data in the

literature. In his systematic review, Steiner reviewed six studies that looked at blood urea nitrogen (BUN), BUN-to–serum creatinine ratio, and acidosis in children. The only laboratory measurement that seemed to be helpful was serum bicarbonate. A normal serum bicarbonate concentration of more than 17 mEq/L reduced the likelihood of 5% dehydration.

Why are the laboratory findings so unhelpful? A number of reasons have been suggested. In cases of isolated vomiting or nasogastric drainage, either a metabolic alkalosis can result from gastric acid losses or a metabolic acidosis can result from volume contraction and lactic acidosis. Volume depletion without renal insufficiency should cause a disproportionate rise in the BUN with little or no change in creatinine. This is caused by increased passive reabsorption of urea in the proximal tubule as a result of appropriate renal conservation of sodium and water. But BUN results may be misleading because children with gastroenteritis can have decreased protein intake during their illness, which can cause hypouremia. Not knowing the child's baseline BUN means that it could double but still remain in the normal range. Finally, if dehydration is rapid, BUN, which is a waste product that builds up gradually with decreased renal excretion, might not have the chance to increase significantly.

What Are the Lessons for the Clinician?

Acute change in weight is the best indicator of dehydration. If a child was seen the day before with a weight of 10 kg and returns the next day with a weight of 9 kg, then by definition the child is 10% dehydrated. Unfortunately, this information is not often available, and based on current data, the empiric classification systems suggested in the past are not particularly accurate or reliable. There are more than 30 different potential tests for assessing dehydration but no conclusive way to approach this.

A general classification of a child's dehydration status as none (<3% fluid deficit), some (mild to moderate—3%–9% fluid deficit), or severe (≥10%) is a useful starting point. Having some awareness of the diagnostic usefulness of individual tests allows you to focus on those that have been shown to correlate best with the presence (or absence) of dehydration. Signs of dehydration start to become evident at 3% to 4% fluid deficit. As a single sign, delayed capillary refill seems to have the highest predictive value but can be influenced by a number of factors, including the examination technique and ambient temperature. Groups of signs can simplify and even improve diagnostic precision. For example, any two out of abnormal capillary refill, abnormal general appearance, dry mucous membranes, and reduced tears increase the likelihood of moderate dehydration sixfold.

Commonly obtained laboratory tests are generally not particularly helpful and therefore not usually indicated unless severe dehydration is suspected or other diagnoses requiring testing are being entertained. Of the laboratory tests, a serum bicarbonate greater than 17 mEq/L is the most useful because it means that the child is approximately one fifth as likely to have moderate dehydration. Intuitively, it makes sense that blood tests (e.g., bicarbonate, electrolytes,

TABLE 5 A Dehydration Score

Characteristic	0	1	2
General appearance	Normal	Thirsty, restless, lethargic, but irritable when touched	Drowsy, limp, cold, sweaty, ± comatose
Eyes	Normal	Slightly sunken	Very sunken
Mucous membranes (tongue)	Moist	Sticky	Dry
Tears	Present	Decreased	Absent

BUN, creatinine, glucose) should be drawn at the time of IV placement in children with dehydration sufficiently severe to require IV rehydration or in those whose assessment or diagnosis remains unclear after a complete history and physical examination, when they can be used as an adjunctive tool. Current AAP guidelines do not recommend blood tests as part of the assessment of children with diarrhea and mild dehydration.

FLUID MANAGEMENT OF THE DEHYDRATED CHILD

A number of decisions need to be made by the clinician once the degree of dehydration has been assessed. The first decision is whether to try oral rehydration therapy (ORT) or move immediately to placement of an IV line for parenteral therapy. The next decision is exactly how much fluid and how fast to give it. Finally, if using parenteral therapy, which is the most appropriate solution?

Does the Child Require Intravenous Therapy?

Quantifying the extent of a child's dehydration accurately is critical in deciding whether the child is safe to be managed at home, requires observation during ORT, or needs to receive immediate IV fluid therapy. Mild or moderate dehydration caused by gastroenteritis can be treated with ORT if the child is able to orally replace fluid losses. Parenteral fluid therapy (or on occasion, ORT by nasogastric tube) is recommended for children with severe dehydration or those who cannot replace the estimated fluid deficit or ongoing losses orally, for example, because of ongoing vomiting. Although ORT is the recommended treatment for acute gastroenteritis with dehydration, it is used in less than 30% of cases in the United States for which it is indicated. Three quarters of pediatric emergency medicine providers, who classified themselves as very familiar with the AAP recommendations for ORT, reported nearly exclusive use of IV fluids for moderately dehydrated children. Some feel that ORT is too time consuming in a busy outpatient setting, and others feel that rapid IV rehydration therapy might break the vomiting cycle more quickly, allowing more rapid discharge home.

Management with Oral Rehydration Therapy

Absorption of water in the small bowel is mediated by the cotransport of sodium and glucose. Different varieties of ORT are available, based on slight variations in the composition of sodium, chloride, carbohydrate, and osmolality. They have been shown in numerous randomized, controlled trials to be as effective as IV rehydration and to have fewer complications in the management of children with diarrhea and dehydration. Fruit and bubblegum flavors have been added to combat the salty taste, and frozen flavored ice pops are also available. Vomiting is not a contraindication to the use of ORT, and children who are truly dehydrated seldom refuse to drink it.

Children who have no or minimal signs of dehydration can continue with their regular age-appropriate diet, with ORT to compensate for ongoing diarrhea or vomiting losses. Using ORT in mildly to moderately dehydrated children requires 50- to 100 mL/kg given quickly over 3 to 4 hours until the child appears clinically rehydrated. Fluid can be given by spoon, syringe, or cup beginning with 5 mL every few minutes and gradually increasing as tolerated. Gut rest is not indicated, with the goal to quickly return the child to an age-appropriate unrestricted diet after rehydration has been accomplished. Breast-feeding should not be interrupted, and full-strength formula is usually tolerated. Fluid losses from vomiting and diarrhea need to be recorded and replaced on an ongoing basis. An empiric amount of 5 to 10 mL/kg for each watery stool or 2 mL/kg for each emesis has been suggested.

The nasogastric route is an option that should be considered if a slow, steady rate would be helpful (e.g., if the child is vomiting) or if there is refusal to drink (e.g., stomatitis). Children who are not improving with ORT and those who have extremely high losses need to be reassessed carefully on an ongoing basis and remain under careful observation. These children and those who do not tolerate

CURRENT DIAGNOSIS

- Acute change in weight is the best indicator of dehydration, hence the importance of frequent monitoring of weight in children with potential dehydration.
- Signs of dehydration are generally imprecise but start to become evident at 3% to 4% fluid deficit.
- Delayed capillary refill (>2 seconds) seems to have the highest predictive value for dehydration. Any two or more out of delayed capillary refill, dry mucous membranes, absent tears, and abnormal general appearance increases the likelihood of moderate dehydration sixfold.
- Laboratory values are generally unhelpful in assessing dehydration and are not indicated unless IV rehydration is necessary. Of the laboratory tests, the most useful is the serum bicarbonate; a normal bicarbonate (>17 mEq/L) decreases the likelihood of moderate dehydration approximately fivefold.

ORT, have a poor suck, have depressed mental status, or are severely dehydrated group require IV rehydration.

Studies of mortality caused by acute diarrhea in the United States have identified prematurity, young maternal age, black race, and rural residence as risk factors for suboptimal outcome. This should be factored in when deciding on length and degree of observation before discharge.

Intravenous Therapy for Dehydration: How Much and How Fast?

The total volume of fluid required has three components: rehydration requirements to replace the deficit of salt and water, maintenance requirements to maintain euvolemia, and replacement of ongoing losses.

Rehydration Requirements (Deficit Therapy)

Step 1 is to restore cardiovascular stability with a rapid bolus of 20 mL/kg over 10 to 30 minutes. Different from providing maintenance fluids, rehydration should always be achieved using isotonic fluids (normal saline or Ringer's lactate), to effectively restore the extracellular fluid volume. Always remember to order fluid on a per-kilogram basis, which differs from the practice in adults, where it may be safe to order by the liter. The child with mild dehydration might not need a bolus, but the severely dehydrated child might require multiple boluses until the pulse, perfusion, and mental status return to normal. Generally, if a child is continuing to show signs of dehydration after 60 mL/kg of isotonic fluid resuscitation, a critical care unit should be consulted and the institution of inotropic therapy considered. Serum electrolytes, bicarbonate, BUN, creatinine, and glucose are usually drawn at the time of the IV start, although rehydration should commence immediately because the laboratory results will not change the initial fluid management.

Step 2 is to calculate the child's fluid deficit based on weight loss or your clinical assessment of dehydration (see previous section). AAP guidelines recommend using a formula of 50 mL/kg deficit for mild dehydration (3%–5% fluid deficit) and 100 mL/kg for moderate dehydration (6%–9% fluid deficit). Subtract the amount of fluid given by bolus from the total amount of rehydration fluid required in 24 hours. In isotonic (Na 130–150 mmol/L) and hypotonic (Na < 130 mmol/L) dehydration, you can give one half of this volume divided over 8 hours, with the other one half over the next 16 hours, or simply divide the total amount required by 24 for a simplified continuous IV rate. Either way, you should aim to rehydrate over 24 hours. As an example, a 10-kg infant who is believed to be 10% dehydrated will require 1000 mL over 24 hours. The baby receives 200 mL as a bolus and then needs 400 mL over the next 8 hours and

CURRENT THERAPY

- Individualize IV orders for children based on the clinical scenario, baseline laboratory results, and frequent reassessments, with particular attention to the concentration of sodium in your prescribed solution. The traditional use of 5% dextrose in 0.2% NaCl is increasingly being questioned, with consideration required for the use of 5% dextrose in half-normal saline or normal saline in certain scenarios.
- Mild or moderate dehydration can be treated with oral rehydration therapy (ORT), which is currently underused in this setting in the United States.
- Appropriate IV therapy for dehydration requires separate consideration of rehydration and maintenance requirements, as well as replacement of ongoing losses.
- IV fluid therapy calculations are really just approximations, and the child's clinical response is far more important. It is therefore imperative to have regular monitoring of clinical signs, urine output, weight, overall fluid balance, and in certain cases serum electrolytes.

a further 400 mL over the following 16 hours to account for the rehydration requirement.

For most patients, half-normal saline in D_5W with KCl 20 mEq/L is an appropriate fluid to use. Potassium is usually not included in the intravenous fluids until the child voids. In the less common scenario of hypertonic dehydration (Na > 150 mmol/L), the rehydration period should be extended over 48 hours so as not to decrease the serum sodium concentration by more than 0.5–1 mmol/hour, to minimize the risk of cerebral edema. Repeated serum sodium measurements will initially be required every 4 to 6 hours until normalizing.

Maintenance Requirements

Step 3 is to calculate maintenance requirements as described earlier and add to the rehydration requirement to come up with an hourly rate. As an example, the 10-kg child previously described requires 40 mL/hour of maintenance fluids, which would be added to the initial rehydration requirement of 50 mL/hour (400 mL over 8 hours) for a total of 90 mL/hour in the first 8 hours. For the next 16 hours this is decreased to 40 mL/hour plus 25 mL/hour (400 mL over 16 hours) for a total of 65 mL/hour. Following return to a euvolemic state, and assuming no ongoing losses, normal maintenance fluid volume may be resumed. Remember to account for oral fluid intake as the patient improves.

Replacement Requirements

Step 4 is to calculate replacement requirements. If ongoing stool losses are a factor, they must be accounted for in the IV fluid prescription. Volume of stool loss is normally about 5 mL/kg/day. With diarrhea this can increase dramatically to 200 mL/kg/day or more. It is easy to see how rapidly a small infant can become dehydrated if these ongoing losses are not being consistently recorded and replaced. If possible, the stool losses should be measured by weighing the diaper and replacing with 1 mL of fluid for each 1 mL of stool. If this is not possible to record, then an estimate of 5 to 10 mL/kg per stool has been suggested as a rough guide. Depending on how rapidly the losses are occurring, this can be calculated every 4 to 6 hours. As an example, if our dehydrated child had three stools over 4 hours for a total of 200 mL, then a further 50 mL/hour (200 divided by 4) is added to the 90 mL/hour (which comprises the rehydration and maintenance components) for a total of 140 mL/hour.

A Note on Rapid Rehydration

The preceding approach to the dehydrated child requiring IV fluids adheres to classic pediatric teaching, where circulation is restored via an isotonic fluid bolus, and electrolyte abnormalities are corrected and deficits replaced over a 24-hour period. There is an increasing interest in an alternative approach, termed *rapid rehydration*. The principle here is to rapidly and fully restore the extracellular fluid volume, usually using 40 to 60 mL/kg of an isotonic solution over a few hours. Theoretically, hospital admission is averted because the patient is discharged home with oral feedings successfully resumed in an 8- to 24-hour period. Although potentially an important method, rapid rehydration has not yet been prospectively studied and should be used with appropriate caution. Its safety and efficacy, including patients' urine and serum electrolytes, hydration, and accompanying clinical status, have yet to be determined. Further study is needed to clarify the optimal rapid rehydration regime, as well as its safety.

Monitoring Requirements

It is essential to remember that the fluid therapy calculations for maintenance IV therapy, rehydration, and replacement are all approximations. There is no formula that works in all cases, so therapy must be individualized. The clinical response to therapy is far more important than any calculations, and there is no substitution for frequent clinical and laboratory monitoring. Regular monitoring of any patient on IV fluids should include:

- General appearance, signs of dehydration, heart rate, respiratory rate, blood pressure
- Urine output, urine specific gravity
- Overall fluid balance
- Daily weights
- Electrolytes (if initially abnormal or at risk, e.g., significant ongoing losses)

Euvolemic patients receiving maintenance fluids should maintain their weight and urine output, achieve a balanced fluid status, and have normal electrolytes, with particular attention to the serum sodium.

A previously dehydrated child who is clinically improving demonstrates weight gain, a positive fluid balance, and increasing urine output with decreasing urine specific gravity. In this patient, consideration should be given to decreasing the intravenous fluids and moving toward ORT and normalizing the diet. Conversely, if the steps are followed as outlined and the child still looks dehydrated, continues to lose weight, remains in negative fluid balance, or has poor urine output, then consider further bolus therapy and increasing the intravenous fluid rate.

REFERENCES

Centers for Disease Control and Prevention. Managing acute gastroenteritis among children: Oral rehydration, maintenance, and nutritional therapy. MMWR Recomm Rep 2003;52(No. RR-16):1–8.

Friedman JN, Goldman RD, Srivastava R, Parkin PC. Development of a clinical dehydration scale for use in children between 1 and 36 months of age. J Pediatr 2004;145:201–7.

Gorelick MH, Shaw KN, Murphy KO. Validity and reliability of clinical signs in the diagnosis of dehydration in children. Pediatrics 1997;99(5):E6.

Halberthal M, Halperin ML, Bohn D. Acute hyponatraemia in children admitted to hospital: Retrospective analysis of factors contributing to its development and resolution. BMJ 2001;322:780–2.

Holliday MA, Segar WE. The maintenance need for water in parenteral fluid therapy. Pediatrics 1957;19:823–32.

Hoorn EJ, Geary D, Robb M, et al. Acute hyponatremia related to intravenous fluid administration in hospitalized children: An observational study. Pediatrics 2004;113:1279–84.

Steiner MJ, Dewalt DA, Byerley JS. Is this child dehydrated? JAMA 2004;291:2746–54.

The Endocrine System

Acromegaly

Method of
Moises Mercado, MD

Acromegaly is a disorder resulting from an excessive secretion of growth hormone (GH), with a prevalence of 40 to 60 cases per million and an annual incidence of 3 to 4 per million.

Physiology, Biochemistry and Regulation of the GH/IGF-1 Axis

GH secretion is regulated at the hypothalamus (Fig. 1). The pulsatile secretion of GH-releasing hormone (GHRH) stimulates somatotroph proliferation and GH gene transcription, whereas somatostatin, which is secreted tonically, inhibits GH synthesis. These two hypothalamic signals result in the pulsatile secretion of pituitary GH, with most pulses occurring during the night. GH is also stimulated by ghrelin, a hypothalamic and gastrointestinal orexigenic hormone that binds specific receptors in the somatotroph known as GH-secretagogue receptors. GH exerts its actions through a specific membrane receptor located predominantly in the liver and cartilage. One molecule of GH interacts with two molecules of GH receptor, resulting in functional dimerization and conformational changes that lead to the phosphorylation of several kinases and eventually the interaction with target genes such as the insulin-like growth factor (IGF)-1 gene.

IGF-1 is closely related to proinsulin and circulates in plasma bound to six binding proteins (IGFBPs) that are synthesized and released by the liver. IGFBP3 is the most important of these binding proteins and is also GH dependent; it forms a heterotrimeric complex composed of BP3, IGF-1, and the acid-labile subunit (ALS). IGF-1 is responsible for most of the trophic and growth-promoting effects of GH. Blood levels of IGF-1 are increased during puberty, coinciding with the acceleration of somatic growth, and decline with aging. Malnutrition, poorly controlled type 1 diabetes, hypothyroidism, and liver failure all result in diminished IGF-1 concentrations. IGF-1 is the main player in GH negative feedback regulation and it acts at both the pituitary and the hypothalamic levels. Glucose regulates GH release by increasing (hypoglycemia) or decreasing (hyperglycemia) somatostatin synthesis in the hypothalamus. Exercise and amino acids such as arginine also stimulate GH secretion.

Etiopathogenesis of Growth Hormone–Secreting Tumors

The molecular pathogenesis of pituitary tumors includes the inactivation of tumor suppressor genes, the activation of oncogenes, and the trophic effect of factors such as the hypothalamic releasing hormones. Approximately 40% of GH-producing tumors in whites harbor somatic point mutations of the α subunit stimulatory G protein coupled to the GHRH receptor (GSPα mutations). This molecular alteration causes constitutive activation of the GHRH receptor, resulting in an increased transcription of the GH gene and the promotion of somatotroph proliferation. Acromegalic patients whose tumors harbor GSPα mutations usually have a more benign clinical course and appear to be more susceptible to management with somatostatin analogues. Nonwhite acromegalic populations, including persons of Japanese, Korean, and Mexican heritage, have a much lower prevalence of GSPα mutations.

Other molecular events should be present in GSPα-negative somatotrophinomas. Menin is a protein encoded by a tumor suppressor gene located on the short arm of chromosome 11. Inactivating mutations of menin are the molecular basis of type 1 multiple endocrine neoplasia (MEN1); however, GH-secreting tumors occurring out of this context do not have such genetic abnormalities. Inactivating mutations of other putative tumor-suppressor genes located relatively close to the menin locus have been described in several kindreds with familial acromegaly; however they do not seem to play an important oncogenic role in the sporadic form of the disease. Other genetic alterations such as underexpression of GADD 45γ (growth arrest and DNA damage-inducible protein) and overexpression of the securing molecule PTTG (pituitary tumor transforming gene) have also been shown to be involved in the molecular pathogenesis of acromegaly. Although hereditary acromegaly is rare (less than 2% of the cases) familial somatotrophinomas account for 30% of the tumors seen in the syndrome of familial isolated pituitary adenomas. Patients with isolated familial somatotrophinomas are younger and usually have more aggressive tumors than subjects with sporadic acromegaly. Affected members do not show any molecular alterations in the MEN1 gene. However, 15% of 73 tested families harbor inactivating, germline mutations of the AIP gene (Aryl Hydrocarbon Interacting Protein) located on chromosome 11q13.3.

In more than 90% of cases, acromegaly is caused by a sporadic pituitary adenoma. In approximately 70% of these patients, these benign epithelial neoplasms are larger than 1 cm in diameter and are known as *macroadenomas*, whereas one third of the patients harbor lesions smaller than 1 cm or *microadenomas*. One third of the patients have tumors that cosecrete GH and prolactin (PRL) (mammosomatoroph cell adenomas). Real pituitary GH-secreting carcinomas, with

639

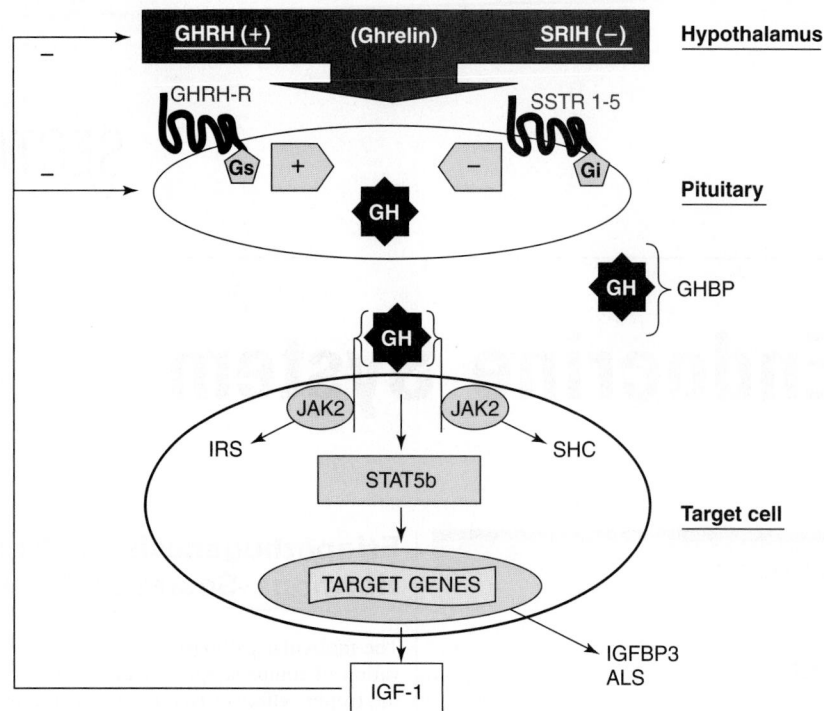

FIGURE 1. GH is regulated positively by GHRH and negatively by somatostatin. Fifty percent of circulating GH is bound to the GH binding protein, which represents the extracellular portion of the GH receptor. One molecule of GH dimerizes two molecules of GH receptor, and the ensuing signal transduction results in IGF-1 synthesis and secretion, which exerts negative feedback on GH secretion at the hypothalamic and pituitary levels. ALS = acid-labile subunit; GH = growth hormone; GHRH = growth hormone–releasing hormone; IGF = insulin-like growth factor; IGFBP3 = insulin-like growth factor binding protein 3; IRS = insulin receptor S; SRIH = somatostatin; SSTR = somatostatin receptor.

documented metastasis as the irrefutable malignancy criterion, are exceedingly rare. On rare occasions, acromegaly results from GHRH-secreting neuroendocrine tumors, usually located in the lungs, thymus, or endocrine pancreas. In this scenario, the ectopically produced GHRH leads to hyperplasia of the somatotroph, with the consequent excessive production of GH. Even less common are GH-secreting tumors arising in ectopic pituitary tissue, usually located in the sphenoid sinus. A case of GH-secreting lymphoma has been reported.

Clinical Manifestations

Acromegaly develops insidiously over many years. An 8- to 10-year delay in diagnosis has been estimated from the beginning of the first symptom. Clinical characteristics are often attributed to aging. Symptoms and signs can be divided into those resulting from the compressive effects of the pituitary tumor and those that are a consequence of the GH and IGF-1 excess.

LOCAL TUMOR EFFECTS

Headache results from an increase in intracranial pressure and from the effects of GH itself; it is usually described as a dull pain that persists throughout the day. Occasionally, large tumors invading laterally into the cavernous sinuses give rise to cranial nerve syndromes, usually third and sixth. Visual field defects are relatively common with macroadenomas extending superiorly and compressing the optic chiasm. This usually results in different combinations of bitemporal homonymous hemianopia or quadrontopia.

CONSEQUENCES OF THE GH/IGF-1 EXCESS
Skeletal Growth and Skin Changes

A GH excess developing before the pubertal closure of epiphyseal bone leads to an acceleration of linear growth, and this results in gigantism. Once the patient is in adulthood, the GH/IGF-1 excess results in acral enlargement, which is manifested by increases in ring and shoe sizes as well as enlargement of the nose, supracilliary arches, frontal bones and mandible. There is thickening of soft tissues of the hands and feet; hands are fleshy and bulky and the heel pad is increased. The skin is thickened due to the deposition of glycosaminoglycans and excessive collagen production. Hyperhidrosis and seborrhea occur in 60% of patients; skin tags (previously associated with colon cancer) and acanthosis nigricans are common.

Musculoskeletal System

Generalized arthralgias are present in the majority (80%) of patients. Degenerative osteoarthritis is more common than in the general population. Paresthesias of the hands and feet and a proximal painful myopathy are often reported. Nerve entrapment syndromes such as the carpal tunnel syndrome occur in nearly one half of patients.

Cardiovascular System

Arterial hypertension is found in 30% of patients, and when associated with diabetes it contributes to the increased mortality rate of the disease. Hyperaldosteronism with low renin levels and the resulting sodium retention play an important role in the pathogenesis of hypertension, but other contributors such as an increased sympathetic tone are also present. Echocardiographic findings include left ventricular and septal hypertrophy with varying degrees of diastolic dysfunction. Symptomatic cardiac disease develops in 15% of patients and is usually due to coronary artery disease, heart failure, and arrhythmias. Although the existence of an acromegalic cardiomyopathy is still controversial, there are patients without hypertension and with angiographically normal coronaries, who develop severe congestive heart failure, in whom histologic evidence of subendocardial, subepicardial and myocardial fibrosis and necrosis has been documented.

Respiratory Abnormalities

The majority of patients with acromegaly are affected by loud snoring. A significant fraction of these have sleep apnea (with both central and obstructive components) with significant drops in oxygen saturation, which can be complicated by arrhythmias, daytime somnolence, and chronic fatigue.

Abnormalities in Glucose Metabolism

Chronic GH hypersecretion creates a state of insulin resistance, and glucose intolerance has been reported in 30% to 50% of patients with acromegaly; the percentage with fasting hyperglycemia can be close to 30%, depending on the population. Hyperglycemia has correlated with GH concentrations in some studies and with IGF-1 levels in others.

Abnormalities in Lipid Metabolism

The classic lipid profile consists of diminished total cholesterol, along with elevated triglyceride concentrations. Intermediate-density lipoprotein (IDL) particles and Lipoprotein(a) might also be elevated, and there is a higher percentage of the more atherogenic type II low-density lipoprotein (LDL).

Bone and Calcium Metabolism

Acromegaly is associated with hypercalciuria and hyperphosphatemia. High serum 25-hydroxyvitamin D_3 and urinary levels of hydroxyproline can be found, reflecting a state of increased bone turnover. Cortical bone mineral density is elevated, whereas trabecular bone mass is diminished.

Neoplasia

Retrospective studies suggested that colonic adenomatous polyps and adenocarcinoma were more frequent in acromegalic patients than in the general population. Prospective studies have demonstrated that the risk, albeit smaller than previously thought, is real and probably justifies screening colonoscopy in these patients. Patients with uncontrolled acromegaly have a higher risk of recurrence of premalignant polyps and a higher mortality rate from colon cancer compared with subjects with biochemically controlled disease and the general population.

Associated Endocrine Abnormalities

A euthyroid goiter is often found but seldom requires specific treatment. Hypopituitarism occurs variably, depending on the size and extension of the tumor and whether the patient has undergone surgery or radiation therapy. Hypogonadotropic hypogonadism is the most common pituitary deficiency, occurring in 20% of patients. A decreased libido is a common presenting complaint in both male and female patients with acromegaly; women often have menstrual and ovulatory disturbances and men complain of impotence.

Although an elevated PRL is common, it does not always reflect cosecretion of this hormone by the somatotrophinoma, but rather an interruption of the descending dopaminergic tone by the tumor compressing the pituitary stalk. Central hypocortisolism and hypothyroidism are less common.

GH-secreting pituitary adenomas are the second, after prolactinomas, pituitary tumor occurring in the context of MEN1 (multiple parathyroid adenomas, pituitary adenoma, and pancreatic islet cell tumors). Acromegaly can also develop in patients with the McCune–Albright syndrome (polyostotic fibrous dysplasia, café au-lait-spots, and endocrinopathies such as sexual precocity and autonomous thyroid nodules).

Mortality

Life expectancy in patients with acromegaly is decreased by about 10 to 15 years, and the standardized mortality ratio is 1.5 to 2. Most patients die of cardiovascular causes, followed by cerebrovascular events, respiratory abnormalities, and neoplastic diseases. Hormonal control has a definite impact on survival. Lowering serum GH to less than 2.5 ng/mL results in reduction of the mortality rate to levels comparable with the general population. These safe GH levels were obtained using old radioimmunoassays, and there are no equivalent studies using ultrasensitive GH assays. IGF-1 levels have not been as good as GH as independent predictors of mortality. Other factors associated with an increased mortality include advanced age and the presence of hypertension and diabetes. A recent meta-analysis including 16 series from 1970 to 2005 reveals a 72% increase in all-cause mortality in patients with acromegaly. Although the mortality rate has decreased in the past decade, likely due to modern treatment strategies, there is still a 32% increase in mortality risk.

Biochemical Diagnosis

Due to the pulsatile nature of GH secretion, random determinations of this hormone are not useful in the diagnosis of acromegaly. The gold standard for the diagnosis is the measurement of GH after an oral glucose load of 75 g; current guidelines state that suppression to less than 0.3 ng/mL (using ultrasensitive assays), reliably excludes the diagnosis. Situations associated with decreased suppression of GH by glucose include puberty, pregnancy, use of oral contraceptives, uncontrolled diabetes, and renal and hepatic insufficiency.

IGF-1 levels reflect the integrated concentrations over 24 hours of GH and correlate well with clinical activity. Blood IGF-1 concentrations decrease with age, reflecting the parallel decline of the somatotropic axis. There is a gender difference in IGF-1 (premenopausal women have lower levels than age-matched male subjects). Other conditions that lower IGF-1 levels include malnutrition, uncontrolled diabetes, and hepatic and renal failure. Normal ranges for IGF-1 should be established in each particular center based on age and sex. The determination of other GH-dependent peptides such as IGFBP3 and ALS has not proved to be superior to IGF-1.

Imaging

Pituitary magnetic resonance imaging (MRI) with gadolinium enhancement allows visualization of lesions as small as 2 or 3 mm in diameter. High-resolution computed tomography (CT) is a reasonable alternative, although it is much less sensitive. An ectopic source of GHRH should be suspected when the MRI is completely normal. In these rare cases, serum GHRH should be measured and the ectopic tumor should be sought, usually with high-resolution CT of the chest and abdomen.

Treatment

The decision as to what therapeutic modality should be used has to take into account medical issues (cardiopulmonary comorbidities, size, and extension of the tumor) as well as the local characteristics of the treating center. The latter refers to the availability of pituitary surgeons and radiotherapeutic technologies as well as the economic feasibility of pharmacologic therapy.

SURGERY

Transsphenoidal surgery has been the traditional treatment for acromegaly and achieves biochemical cure (normalization of IGF-1 and a glucose-suppressed GH <1 ng/mL) in 80% to 90% of microadenomas. Cure rates for macroadenomas are much lower (40%–50%), and invasive lesions have a very slight chance (<10%) of being cured by surgery. Even though surgery often fails to achieve a full biochemical cure, debulking the pituitary adenoma relieves optic chiasm compression and can result in a sufficient decrement of tumor mass (and therefore of GH production) to allow better results with either pharmacologic or radiotherapeutic regimens.

CURRENT DIAGNOSIS

Clinical

- Headaches, visual field defects
- Coarse features, increased size of hands (rings) and feet (shoes)
- Thick, oily skin, skin tags, acanthosis nigricans
- Arthralgias, osteoarthritis
- Paresthesias, carpal tunnel syndrome
- Hypertension, arrhythmia, heart failure
- Glucose intolerance, diabetes, hypertrygliceridemia
- Snoring, sleep apnea
- Risk of colon polyps or colon cancer

Biochemical

- Glucose-suppressed growth hormone >0.3 ng/mL by ultrasensitive assays or >1 ng/mL by old radio-immunoassays
- Elevated age- and sex-matched insulin-like growth factor 1
- Other growth hormone–dependent peptides: insulin-like growth factor binding protein 3, acid-labile subunit

Imaging

- Computed tomography
- Magnetic resonance imaging

CURRENT THERAPY

- If a pituitary surgeon is available: Transsphenoidal surgery for microadenomas, intrasellar macroadenomas, and debulking or decompressing surgery in invasive macroadenomas
- Somatostatin analogues as secondary treatment for patients failing surgery or waiting for radiotherapy effect to occur and as a primary treatment for patients with inaccessible lesions, contraindications for surgery, or preference
- Dopamine agonists: Bromocriptine (Parlodel) is ineffective; cabergoline (Dostinex)[1] may be added to patients resistant to somatostatin analogues
- Growth hormone receptor antagonists: Pegvisomant (Somavert) for patients resistant or intolerant to somatostatin analogues and who have tumors >5 mm from the optic chiasm
- Radiotherapy for patients resistant or intolerant to pharmacologic therapy, with clinically and biochemically active disease and a tumor remnant on MRI
- Radiosurgery might be better than external-beam radiotherapy

[1]Not FDA approved for this indication.

PHARMACOLOGIC THERAPY

Somatostatin analogues are the most commonly used medical treatment for acromegaly. Somatostatin inhibits GH secretion and somatotroph cell growth via its interaction with five different somatostatin receptor (SSTR) subtypes. The development of long-acting somatostatin analogues such as octreotide (Sandostatin) and lanreotide (Somatuline) overcame the pharmacologic difficulties of native somatostatin (short half-life, rebound GH secretion, and need for IV administration) and resulted in a more potent inhibition of GH secretion. The most commonly used preparations are intramuscular octreotide LAR (long-acting repeatable) and subcutaneous lanreotide autogel, which are administered every 4 weeks. Doses of octreotide-LAR range from 10 to 40 mg and those of lanreotide autogel from 60 to 120 mg, both administered every 4 weeks; although in specific patients the interval of injection can be increased to every 6 or even 8 weeks, thus diminishing the cost of therapy. Octreotide and lanreotide have very high affinities for SSTR-2 and to a lesser extent SSTR-5, which are precisely the most commonly expressed somatostatin receptors in GH-secreting adenomas.

When used after surgery has failed, somatostatin analogues can achieve a safe and a normal IGF-1 in 50% to 60% of patients. Primary treatment with somatostatin analogues is increasingly being used in patients with invasive tumors, when cardiopulmonary contraindications are present, and more recently as a result of the patient or treating physician's preference. In these settings, biochemical success rates (achievement of safe GH levels and normalization of IGF-1) have ranged between 50% and 80%, and more than 80% report significant relief of symptoms. Tumor shrinkage occurs in 70% of primarily treated patients. Overall, treatment success is directly related to the abundance of SSTR-2 and SSTR-5 in the tumor. Lower pretreatment GH levels are also associated with a better response to somatostatin analogues. Side effects of somatostatin analogues, including nausea, abdominal pain, alopecia, and biliary sludge, occur in 20% of subjects.

Pegvisomant is a GH mutant that prevents functional dimerization of the GH receptor, thus acting as an antagonist. Its use results in normalization of IGF-1 in more than 90% of patients, while increasing GH levels. Concern about adenoma growth due to the abolition of IGF-1 negative feedback on the tumoral somatotroph, prevents its use in patients with very large lesions in close proximity to the optic chiasm. Transient elevations of liver aminotransferases can occur, although this seldom requires drug discontinuation. Pegvisomant does not compromise insulin secretion, as somatostatin analogues do. GH-receptor antagonists are expensive and should not be used as primary treatment; they are currently indicated in patients who are intolerant or have failed somatostatin analogue therapy.

Few patients respond marginally to difficult-to-tolerate large doses of bromocriptine. Newer dopamine agonists, such as cabergoline, are better tolerated and more efficacious, particularly in tumors that cosecrete PRL. Combination treatment with cabergoline and octreotide appears to be promising in cases resistant to somatostatin analogues.

RADIATION THERAPY

Both external-beam radiotherapy and radiosurgery are indicated in patients with persistent disease and a demonstrable tumor remnant who are either intolerant or resistant to pharmacologic treatment. Biochemical success occurs in 20% to 60% and requires many years to become apparent. Hypopituitarism, involving at least two axes, develops in more than 50% of patients within 10 years. Serious adverse effects such as brain necrosis and optic nerve damage seldom occur with the currently used techniques that minimize radiation to the normal surrounding tissues.

Novel pharmacologic therapies are being developed, some of which will likely become useful particularly in patients who do not respond to current somatostatin analogues. These include the so-called "universal" somatostatin analogue pasireotide, which is capable of interacting not only with the sstrs 2 and 5, but also with subtypes 1 and 3. At earlier stages of development are "chimeric" compounds which behave as somatostatin analogues and dopamine agonists at the same time.

REFERENCES

Beckers A, Daly AF. The clinical, pathological and genetic features of familial isolated pituitary adenomas. Eur J Endocrinol 2007;157:371–82.

Bevan JS. Clinical review: The antitumoral effects of somatostatin analog therapy in acromegaly. J Clin Endocrinol Metab 2005;90:1856–63.

Colao A, Ferone D, Marzullo P, Lombardi G. Systemic complications of acromegaly: Epidemiology, pathogenesis and management. Endocr Rev 2004;25:102–52.

Dekkers OM, Biermasz NR, Pereira AM, et al. Mortality in acromegaly: A metaanalysis. J Clin Endocrinol Metab 2008;93:61–7.

Espinosa-de-Los-Monteros AL, Sosa E, Cheng S, et al. Biochemical evaluation of disease activity after pituitary surgery in acromegaly: A critical analysis of patients who spontaneously change disease status. Clin Endocrinol 2006;64:245–9.

Freda P. Current concepts in the biochemical assessment of the patient with acromegaly. Growth Horm IGF Res 2003;13:171–84.

Freda P, Katznelson L, van der Lely AJ, et al. Long-acting somatostatin analog therapy of acromegaly: A meta-analysis. J Clin Endocrinol Metab 2005;90:4465–73.

Growth Hormone Research Society. Pituitary Society. Biochemical assessment and long term monitoring in patients with acromegaly: statement from a joint consensus conference of the Growth hormone Research Society and the Pituitary Society. J Clin Endocrinol Metab 2004;89:3099–102.

Holdaway IM, Rajasoorya RC, Gamble GD. Factors influencing mortality in acromegaly. J Clin Endocrinol Metab 2004;89:667–74.

Kopchick JJ, Parkinson C, Stevens EC, Trainer PJ. Growth hormone receptor antagonists: Discovery, development, and use in patients with acromegaly. Endocr Rev 2002;23:623–46.

Melmed S. Acromegaly. N Engl J Med 2006;355:2558–73.

Melmed S, Colao A, Barkan A, et al. Guidelines for acromegaly management: An update. J Clin Endocrinol Metab 2009; February, published ahead of print.

Vance ML, Laws ER. Role of medical therapy in the management of acromegaly. Neurosurgery 2005;56:877–85.

Adrenocortical Insufficiency

Method of
Joseph M. Hughes, MD

Adrenocortical insufficiency, also referred to as Addison's disease, is an uncommon endocrine disorder. The presentation varies from the nonspecific symptoms of anorexia, nausea, and weight loss to the dramatic hypotensive crisis. The original description by Thomas Addison in 1849 was of a patient with adrenocortical destruction, and the term Addison's disease typically is reserved for those with primary adrenocortical failure. The challenge for the clinician is to establish not only the diagnosis but also the etiology. Patients may present with either primary adrenocortical failure or secondary adrenal insufficiency—disruption of hypothalamic-pituitary function. The long-term treatment with glucocorticoids and mineralocorticoids is effective but differs depending on the etiology. Finally, special attention must be given to the unique problem of patients with potential adrenal insufficiency from chronic pharmacologic doses of glucocorticoids.

Clinical Presentation

The presenting symptoms are often nonspecific, which frequently delays the diagnosis. The clinician often thinks of patients with adrenal insufficiency as presenting in crisis with vomiting, diarrhea, dehydration, and life-threatening hypotension. However, most patients have had a chronic course with symptoms present for a prolonged period. The prominent ones are anorexia, weight loss, fatigue, nausea, diarrhea, and abdominal pain. The symptoms, when associated with physical findings and laboratory clues, should prompt evaluation.

There may be a paucity of findings on physical examination. The clinician may be struck when reviewing the vital signs by weight loss and hypotension, particularly orthostatic hypotension. Examination of the skin may help to distinguish primary from secondary causes. The patients with primary causes, resulting from increased levels of plasma corticotropin (ACTH) and the subsequent stimulation of melanocytes, are described as having bronzing of the skin and increased pigmentation of the buccal mucosa, gingiva, palmar creases, scars, and pressure points (e.g., the elbows). A further clue to the etiology may be the finding of vitiligo, which is associated with autoimmune adrenalitis.

There are characteristic findings on routine laboratory testing—electrolytes, blood urea nitrogen, glucose, creatinine, and hematology profile—which further suggest the diagnosis to the clinician. The most common of these is hyponatremia, which is seen in both primary and secondary forms, although the etiology is different. With secondary causes, excess antidiuretic hormone has been proposed as an explanation; with primary causes, because of the destruction of the adrenal cortex, there is aldosterone deficiency. The finding of hyperkalemia due to hypoaldosteronism often prompts the investigation for adrenal insufficiency and is specific for primary adrenal insufficiency. Azotemia develops because of dehydration. Hypercalcemia is reported. Hypoglycemia is uncommon and is most often seen with secondary forms. The complete blood count demonstrates eosinophilia in up to 20% of patients. Less common findings are anemia and neutropenia.

Evaluation

The diagnosis can usually be made by three tests: random cortisol levels, plasma ACTH levels, and the synthetic corticotropin stimulation test. The random cortisol can be a helpful test as a first step. A value less than the lower limit of normal may be diagnostic and provides enough data to initiate therapy in patients with clinical signs and known pathology (e.g., a hypothalamic-pituitary lesion). The converse is also true: a random cortisol level greater than 20 μg/dL, unless the patient's presentation is highly suspicious for adrenal insufficiency, makes the diagnosis unlikely. It is important to remember that patients with adrenal insufficiency can have a random cortisol level within the laboratory's normal range, and further testing would be required to establish the diagnosis.

The rapid synthetic corticotropin stimulation test is the principal investigation for the diagnosis of adrenal insufficiency. Synthetic tetracosactrin (Synacthen,[2] cosyntropin [Cortrosyn]) contains the the first 24 amino acids of the human ACTH sequence. The traditional dose has been 250 μg given intravenously or intramuscularly. Plasma cortisol levels are measured at time 0 and at 30 and 60 minutes and can be drawn at any time during the day. Various criteria have been used to determine a normal response. Typically, the baseline, the peak, and the delta from baseline to peak have been used. However, careful study by various authors has shown that a peak level at any time greater than 20 μg/dL is a normal response. Lower levels indicate adrenal insufficiency but do not distinguish between primary and secondary failure.

There has been a great deal of discussion recently about the recommended dose of tetracosactrin. There is agreement that the standard dose, 250 μg, delivers pharmacologic concentrations. Newer protocols have advocated the use of 1 μg, a more physiologic concentration. The hypothesis is that a low-dose protocol allows the diagnosis of borderline or mild cases of adrenal insufficiency. Previously, when only the high-dose test was used, some patients with normal tests became adrenally insufficient, especially during times of extreme stress. This is a concern, especially if the etiology is secondary adrenal insufficiency. The experience with both tests at our hospital shows that normal patients can have inadequate stimulation with the low-dose test. Our protocol is to use the high-dose test almost exclusively, except in the special situation in which one expects possible borderline secondary adrenal insufficiency.

The clinician is simultaneously diagnosing and establishing the etiology. The now-accurate measurement of plasma ACTH levels

---

[2]Not available in the United States.

has proved to be very helpful in distinguishing primary from secondary failure. In primary failure, the pituitary is intact, and one anticipates elevated ACTH levels, typically greater than 100 pg/mL. ACTH levels should be low in patients with secondary failure. However, the concentrations may also be in the normal range in these patients.

After it is determined that the patient has either primary or secondary insufficiency, radiologic studies provide important information. With primary failure, the computed tomography scan may show atrophied adrenal glands in autoimmune adrenalitis. Enlarged glands with high-density areas or calcification suggest hemorrhage, granulomatous disease, or neoplasm. The magnetic resonance scan of the hypothalamic-pituitary region in patients with secondary insufficiency is often diagnostic.

Infrequently, other studies can be helpful if the diagnosis of adrenal insufficiency or the cause is in question. The gold standard for diagnosing secondary adrenal insufficiency is the insulin tolerance test. Because the patient must become hypoglycemic and the test has, rarely, been implicated in fatalities, it is best performed by those familiar with the protocol. Several prolonged ACTH protocols to distinguish primary from secondary insufficiency have been published. Finally, with the availability of corticotropin-releasing hormone (CRH) for testing, measurement of ACTH levels after CRH localizes secondary insufficiency to a lesion in either the hypothalamus or the pituitary.

Etiology

After the diagnosis of primary adrenal insufficiency has been established, the clinician is confronted by multiple possible causes (Table 1). The most common (80%–90% of patients) is autoimmune adrenalitis, which is often associated with other autoimmune diseases (Box 1). Evidence of these diseases should be sought and may be present at the time of diagnosis or may appear months or years later. The diagnosis of autoimmune adrenalitis may be the first finding in a patient with an autoimmune polyendocrine syndrome. Tuberculosis has been reported as the second most common cause of primary adrenal insufficiency. Although they are rare, adrenoleukodystrophy and adrenomyeloneuropathy should be considered in a young man who presents with adrenal insufficiency.

Secondary adrenal insufficiency may also be caused by a number of diseases (Box 2), but it is most commonly a result of chronic glucocorticoid therapy, pituitary tumors, or iatrogenic causes. Radiation-induced adrenal failure may present 5 or more years after

TABLE 1 Causes of Primary Adrenal Insufficiency

Type	Examples
Autoimmune	
Infectious	Tuberculosis, histoplasmosis, blastomycosis, coccidioidomycosis, cryptococcosis, HIV, cytomegalovirus
Hemorrhage	Sepsis, anticoagulation
Metastatic disease	Lung, breast
Drugs	Ketoconazole (Nizoral), aminoglutethimide (Cytadren)
Infiltrative diseases	Sarcoid, hemochromatosis, amyloidosis
Familial	Adrenoleukodystrophy, adrenomyeloneuropathy, familial glucocorticoid deficiency
ACTH resistance syndromes	
Congenital adrenal hypoplasia	

Abbreviation: ACTH, adrenocorticotropic hormone (corticotropin).

BOX 1 Autoimmune Diseases Associated with Adrenal Insufficiency

Thyroid disease (Hashimoto's thyroiditis or Graves' disease)
Type 1 diabetes mellitus
Pernicious anemia
Primary ovarian or testicular failure
Vitiligo
Gastrointestinal (celiac disease, inflammatory bowel disease, chronic hepatitis)
Rheumatologic (Sjögren's syndrome)
Alopecia
Neurologic (multiple sclerosis)
Hypoparathyroidism
Chronic candidiasis

---

therapy. If the patient is found to have secondary adrenal insufficiency, other hypothalamic-pituitary hormonal deficiencies should be sought, because isolated ACTH deficiency is rare. Initiation of therapy for growth hormone deficiency or hypothyroidism may uncover previously clinically inapparent adrenal insufficiency.

Treatment

When considering the treatment of adrenal insufficiency, one must understand the management of adrenal crisis, long-term glucocorticoid and mineralocorticoid therapy, and stress-dose glucocorticoids at the time of acute illness. In adrenal crisis, the goal is to reverse the hypovolemia with normal saline, 2 to 3 L infused rapidly, and to administer parenteral glucocorticoids. The choice of glucocorticoid is critical. If the diagnosis of adrenal insufficiency has not been established and diagnostic testing is required, then 4 mg of dexamethasone (Decadron) should be given intravenously every 12 hours. Dexamethasone does not interfere with the cortisol assay, and corticotropin stimulation can be performed as the patient is receiving dexamethasone. Preferably, the ACTH level is obtained and the corticotropin stimulation tests are performed close to the time of initiation of therapy. If the diagnosis and etiology of adrenal insufficiency are known, then either dexamethasone or hydrocortisone (Solu-Cortef) 100 mg IV every 6 to 8 hours may be used. Intravenous glucocorticoid on a tapering dose may be required for several days until oral replacement therapy is begun. Mineralocorticoids are not required for acute management. After the patient is stable, oral therapy is initiated.

All patients with adrenal insufficiency require glucocorticoids. I usually prescribe hydrocortisone (Cortef). Even though the plasma concentrations rise and fall rapidly after oral administration, most patients respond well to a single morning dose and a second dose

---

BOX 2 Causes of Secondary Adrenal Insufficiency

Steroid therapy
Iatrogenic (pituitary or adrenal adenoma surgery, radiation therapy)
Pituitary tumors, adenoma, craniopharyngioma, Rathke cleft cyst
Infiltrative (sarcoid)
Pituitary infarction
Lymphocytic or granulomatous hypophysitis
Isolated corticotropin (ACTH) deficiency
Metastasis
Tuberculosis

in the early afternoon. Individualizing the dose is important to prevent long-term complications from overreplacement. The calculation, 12 mg/m^2/day, is helpful in determining the total dose of hydrocortisone. For example, if the total daily calculated dose is 25 mg, then 20 mg could be given in the morning and 5 mg in the early afternoon. In the long term, the patient may find that only the morning dose is required.

Some experts prescribe the longer-acting preparations prednisone or dexamethasone. The rationale is a more prolonged pharmacologic effect as opposed to what is seen with hydrocortisone or cortisone acetate (Cortone). The usual doses are 5 mg for prednisone and 0.5 mg for dexamethasone. Because of the prolonged action and an attempt to mimic the circadian rhythm, these medications are given in the morning or at bedtime.

Patients with primary adrenal failure are unable to produce aldosterone. In patients with secondary adrenal insufficiency, the renin-angiotensin-aldosterone system is intact, and aldosterone is infrequently required. Mineralocorticoid is prescribed as fludrocortisone (Florinef); the usual dose is 0.1 mg/day. The patient should obtain a medical alert bracelet and be instructed in the use of stress-dose steroid at times of acute illness. For example, the patient may double or triple the dose of glucocorticoids for 3 days if he or she has a febrile illness. There is no need to taper the dose. If vomiting or profuse diarrhea occurs, the patient should be instructed to seek emergency care. Some patients are capable of giving intramuscular injections of glucocorticoids (Decadron, Solu-Cortef) at home in an attempt to prevent the need for an emergency department visit. For outpatients having procedures, administration of 50 to 100 mg of hydrocortisone (Solu-Cortef) IV beforehand, then converting to oral stress doses afterward, is appropriate. The adrenal cortex is also a source of androgens. For patients, especially women, with decreased libido and persistent fatigue, dehydroepiandrosterone (DHEA)[7] 25 to 50 mg daily may be added.

After glucocorticoids and mineralocorticoids have been prescribed, the clinician constantly monitors the adequacy of the treatment. There is equal concern for insufficient as for excessive doses, particularly glucocorticoids. Through the history, the clinician learns about symptoms of low-grade adrenal insufficiency, particularly fatigue and orthostatic hypotension. On examination, one looks for evidence of Cushing's syndrome, particularly weight gain, striae, and facial plethora, indicating possible overreplacement. Osteoporosis is always a concern. On laboratory testing, the sodium and potassium levels and the plasma renin or plasma renin activity levels should be normal if the patient is receiving adequate doses of fludrocortisone. Finally, by its inhibitory effects on release of arginine vasopressin and renal effects, glucocorticoid treatment may uncover quiescent central diabetes insipidus.

Adrenal Suppression and Chronic Glucocorticoid Therapy

Chronic glucocorticoid (prednisone) therapy causes secondary adrenal insufficiency. There is generalized consensus about the doses and duration of prednisone therapy that cause suppression. If prednisone at doses greater than 20 mg/day for more than 3 weeks is prescribed, then the dose of prednisone should be tapered. Also, patients who have required prednisone at doses greater than 5 mg/day for months to years are presumed to be suppressed. If there is a question about the integrity of the hypothalamic-pituitary-adrenal axis in patients taking prednisone 5 mg/day or less, then a corticotropin stimulation test can be helpful. After suppression is established, a prolonged taper is required, because 6 to 12 months is needed for the axis to recover.

The tapering of prednisone must be gradual, especially after the 5-mg dose is reached. An approach to the patient on high-dose prednisone is to decrease the dose by increments of 5 to 10 mg every

[7]Available as dietary supplement.

2 weeks until the 20-mg dose is reached. Afterward, the dose should be adjusted by 5 mg or less every 2 weeks until the 5-mg dose is established. At that point, decreasing the dose by 1 mg per month is a conservative approach. After the patient reaches the dose of 1 or 2 mg/day, a corticotropin stimulation test can be helpful. Also, a fasting cortisol measurement before the dose of prednisone that is greater than 10 ng/dL usually predicts normal adrenal function. Often, the limitation in tapering prednisone is the activity of the underlying disease, not the integrity of the hypothalamic-pituitary-adrenal axis. Stress-dose steroids for major illness, surgery, or trauma should be provided for the first year after a patient has successfully stopped prednisone.

REFERENCES

Barbetta L, Dall'Asta C, Re T, et al. Comparison of different regimens of glucocorticoid replacement therapy in patients with hypoadrenalism. J Endocrinol Invest 2005;28:632–7.
Crown A, Lightman S. Why is the management of glucocorticoid deficiency still controversial: A review of the literature. Clin Endocrinol 2005;63:483–92.
Hughes J, Whelan MA, Deringer P. Adrenoleukodystrophy: An important cause of adrenal insufficiency. Endocrinologist 2000;10:271–6.

Cushing's Syndrome

Method of
Vijay Yechoor, MD

Cushing's syndrome is the manifestation of prolonged exposure to inappropriately elevated free glucocorticoids (referred to generically as hypercortisolism). The signs and symptoms of Cushing's syndrome mimic, to an exaggerated degree, the extensive physiologic effects of glucocorticoids on the various tissues. Despite the rarity of this syndrome (incidence of 5–6 cases per million), delay in diagnosis of Cushing's syndrome has severe consequences because of the high morbidity and mortality (50% at 5 years) of this disease if it is left untreated. Some broad consensus guidelines have been developed that facilitate the diagnosis and management, although individualized therapy is essential.

Clinical Features

The full-blown syndrome with its classic features (centripetal obesity, hirsutism, moon facies, reddish-purple striae, and plethora) is easy to diagnose but is rarely seen nowadays, because patients present in an earlier stage to their primary care provider. The spectrum of symptoms and signs can be extensive (Table 1) and can vary significantly at presentation; to make matters difficult, the symptoms and signs also overlap with those of other conditions that are common in the general population, such as obesity, diabetes, metabolic syndrome, and polycystic ovarian disease. Hence, it is important to have a high index of suspicion, especially in the presence of more discriminatory features such as reddish-purple striae, plethora, proximal muscle weakness, bruising without trauma, and unexplained osteoporosis. In addition, in patients with multiple and progressive features or features that are unusual for age (e.g., osteoporosis, hypertension), in children with increasing weight and decreasing height percentiles, and in the presence of an adrenal incidentaloma, especially one that is consistent with an adenoma on imaging, evaluation for Cushing's syndrome needs to be carried out.

TABLE 1 Clinical Features of Cushing's Syndrome*

System	Feature
General	Obesity (centripetal, except in children), with moon facies, buffalo hump, and supraclavicular fat pad; fatigue; vellus hirsutism
Eye	Glaucoma, chemosis
Psychiatric	Depression, psychosis
Cardiovascular	Hypertension, thromboembolism.
Infections	Tuberculosis, fungal infections, wound infections
Reproductive	Menstrual irregularities, hypogonadism, loss of libido
Metabolic	Diabetes mellitus, impaired glucose tolerance, hyperlipidemia, metabolic syndrome, hypokalemic alkalosis
Skin	Hirsutism, easy bruisability secondary to skin thinning, acne, facial plethora, striae (>1 cm and reddish-purple)
Muscle/Bone	Muscle weakness, proximal myopathy, poor linear growth (in children), osteoporosis and fractures, hypercalcemia and renal stones

*Presence of multiple features, especially the underlined ones (which have a higher discriminatory value) and especially if progressive, should evoke a high index of suspicion.

Etiology

The causes of Cushing's syndrome (Box 1) dictate the diagnostic algorithm that is described here. Iatrogenic Cushing's syndrome due to exogenous glucocorticoids is the most common cause and is often easy to exclude with a careful medication history. A specific drug history should include exposure via all routes, including inhalational, topical, injected, and oral. Surreptitious use, often of performance-enhancing drugs, needs to be kept in mind.

BOX 1 Classification and Etiology of Cushing's Syndrome

Exogenous
Endogenous
- ACTH dependent
  - Pituitary adenomas (Cushing's disease), either solitary or as part of MEN-1 syndrome
  - Ectopic ACTH/CRH producing tumors
- Small cell lung carcinoma
- Carcinoids (pancreatic, lung, other)
- Islet tumors
- Medullary carcinoma of thyroid
- Pheochromocytoma
  - Macronodular adrenal hyperplasia
- ACTH independent
  - Adrenal adenoma
  - Adrenal carcinoma
  - Primary pigmented nodular adrenal hyperplasia (as part of Carney's syndrome)
  - McCune-Albright's syndrome
  - Aberrant expression of G protein–coupled receptor (for GIP, IL-10, vasopressin V_{1a}, α_2 adrenergic, LH)

Abbreviations: ACTH = adrenocorticotropic hormone (corticotropin); CRH = corticotropin-releasing hormone; IL-10 = interleukin-10; LH = luteinizing hormone; MEN-1 = multiple endocrine neoplasia type 1.

CURRENT DIAGNOSIS

- A high index of suspicion is necessary to diagnose Cushing's syndrome, because many of its features are nonspecific and overlap with those of numerous common disorders, including obesity, polycystic ovarian disease, and metabolic syndrome.
- The most discriminative clinical features are those that are progressive (see Table 1), which include combinations of centripetal obesity, menstrual irregularity, hirsutism, easy bruisability, violaceous striae more than 1 cm wide, and proximal myopathy. In children, poor linear growth with increasing weight should prompt a work-up for Cushing's syndrome.
- A stepwise approach is critical in the work-up of Cushing's syndrome, because the same test has a different predictive value if the steps are done out of order, leading to erroneous diagnosis and unnecessary investigations. The first step is to establish autonomous hypercortisolism, allowing the diagnosis of Cushing's syndrome. The second step is to establish whether this condition is adrenocorticotropic hormone (ACTH) dependent or ACTH independent. Only then is a determination made as to whether the ACTH-dependent Cushing's syndrome is of pituitary or ectopic origin.
- The combination of a 1-mg overnight dexamethasone suppression test (O/N DST) and a urinary free cortisol (UFC) test is sufficient to establish a diagnosis, but vigilance needs to be exercised in cases of pseudo-Cushing's syndrome, for which an additional test, the low-dose dexamethasone suppression test (LDDST) with corticotropin-releasing hormone (CRH) stimulation, is necessary.
- A suppressed ACTH (<9 pg/mL) at 0900 hours is sufficient to establish ACTH-independent disease, and the work-up can proceed to imaging of the adrenals.
- Because pituitary incidentalomas are common (incidence of approximately 10% in the general population), magnetic resonance imaging evidence alone is not sufficient to indicate surgery; suppressability in a high-dose dexamethasone suppression test (HDDST) or a positive gradient on bilateral inferior petrosal sinus sampling (BIPSS) is also needed.
- Ninety-five percent of patients with ectopic Cushing's syndrome have a hypokalemic alkalosis, but fewer than 10% of those with Cushing's syndrome of pituitary origin have it.
- BIPSS remains the gold standard to establish an ACTH origin from a pituitary source.

It is important to note that hypercortisolism may be present in conditions without Cushing's syndrome (Box 2), some of which frequently are lumped together as pseudo-Cushing's syndrome. It is imperative to specifically exclude these conditions before embarking on an expensive and often invasive but futile work-up to explain the hypercortisolism.

Diagnosis

The evaluation and diagnostic work-up of Cushing's syndrome must be done in a stepwise fashion. There are no diagnostic tests with 100% specificity and sensitivity in all populations. For this reason,

BOX 2   Nonautonomous Hypercortisolism (Not Cushing's Syndrome)

With Some Features of Cushing's Syndrome (Pseudo-Cushing's Syndrome)
- Pregnancy
- Depression
- Alcohol dependence
- Morbid obesity
- Poorly controlled diabetes mellitus
- Glucocorticoid resistance

With No Features of Cushing's Syndrome
- Physical stress (surgery, infections etc.)
- Malnutrition, anorexia nervosa
- Hypothalamic amenorrhea
- Cortisol-binding globulin excess

the positive (or negative) predictive value of a test depends on the likelihood of the disease (pretest probability). As one goes down the diagnostic tree (Fig. 1), the probability of the disease increases, and so does the predictive value. If the tests are done out of order, as frequently happens, they are inconclusive and often lead to erroneous conclusions.

The first step addresses whether the patient has Cushing's syndrome, and the next two steps address the cause by determining whether the source of the hypercortisolism is ACTH dependent (pituitary or ectopic source) or ACTH independent (adrenal source) (see Box 1). This allows the correct sequence for evaluation of the existence and source of pathologic hypercortisolemia.

STEP 1: DIAGNOSING CUSHING'S SYNDROME

The diagnosis of pathologic hypercortisolemia rests on establishing either an increase in the production rates of cortisol, a disruption in normal regulation of the hypothalamic-pituitary-adrenal (HPA) axis, or a disruption of the normal circadian rhythm of cortisol. The diagnostic algorithm that incorporates these principles is shown in Figure 1. It is important to note that there is no place for a screening 8 AM cortisol measurement in the diagnosis of Cushing's syndrome.

24-Hour Urine Free Cortisol

The 24-hour urine free cortisol (UFC) test measures the unbound free cortisol in the urine integrated over a 24-hour period. Because it measures the unbound fraction, it is not affected by the conditions that increase cortisol-binding globulin (and, consequently, the measured serum cortisol), such as use of oral contraceptives in women. The collection needs to be adequate (assessed by measuring creatinine in the same sample) and should be repeated at least two times if normal. This is a good screening test in most conditions, and to achieve a good sensitivity, we recommend using the upper limits of normal of the assay as the criterion for a positive test, even though most Cushing's syndrome patients have a threefold to fourfold increase in UFC. False-positive elevations may be seen with excessive fluid intake (>5 L/day) or with any of the conditions listed in Box 2. False-negative tests may result from renal insufficiency (creatinine clearance <60 mL/min) or from intermittent cortisol production (as may be seen with adrenal adenomas). Therefore, it is important to confirm positive results with the overnight dexamethasone suppression test (O/N DST).

1-mg Overnight Dexamethasone Suppression Test

The O/N DST measures the normal suppressability of the HPA axis by means of a supraphysiologic dose of glucocorticoids. For this test, 1 mg of oral dexamethasone (Decadron) is given to the patient between 2300 and 2400 hours, and the serum cortisol concentration

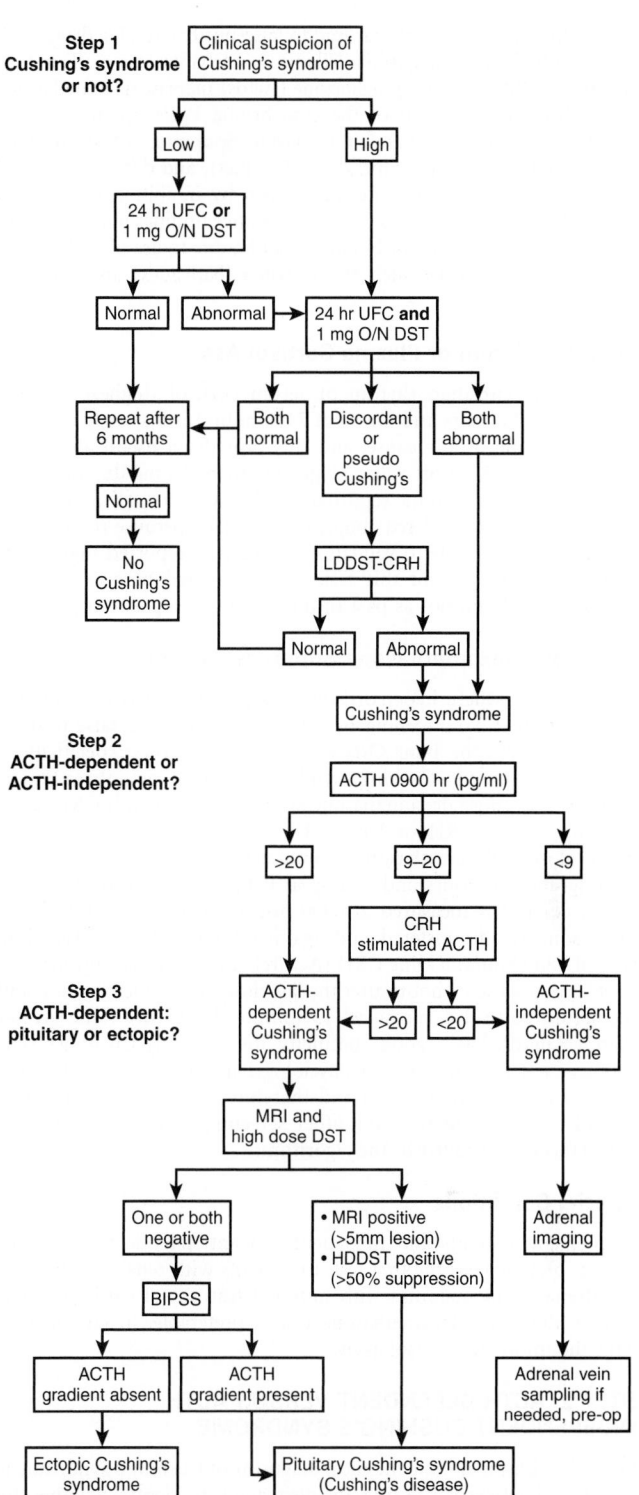

FIGURE 1. Evaluation and diagnostic work-up of Cushing's syndrome. *Abbreviations:* ACTH = adrenocorticotropic hormone; BIPSS = bilateral inferior petrosal sinus sampling; CRH = corticotropin-releasing hormone; DST = dexamethasone suppression test; HDDST = high-dose dexamethasone suppression test; LDDST = low-dose dexamethasone suppression test; MRI = magnetic resonance imaging; O/N = overnight; UFC = urine free cortisol.

is measured the next morning, between 0800 and 0900 hours. A serum cortisol level of less than 1.8 μg/dL is considered normal and has a good sensitivity to rule out Cushing's syndrome. Use of a higher cutoff value of 5 μg/dL may miss a significant proportion of patients with ACTH-dependent Cushing's syndrome of pituitary origin and therefore is discouraged. Altered metabolism of dexamethasone in the liver may lead to false-positive results: drugs such as phenobarbital, phenytoin (Dilantin), carbamazepine (Tegretol), rifampicin (Rifadin), and pioglitazone (Actos) increase dexamethasone metabolism by induction of the cytochrome P-450 isoenzyme 3A4 (CYP3A4). On the other hand, itraconazole (Sporanox), ritonavir (Norvir), fluoxetine (Prozac), cimetidine (Tagamet), and diltiazem (Cardizem) decrease dexamethasone metabolism by inhibition of CYP3A4 and lead to false-negative results. False-negative findings may also result from an increase in cortisol-binding globulin due to use of oral contraceptives or other drugs such as tamoxifen (Nolvadex) and mitotane (Lysodren).

Midnight Serum or Plasma Cortisol Assay

The normal circadian rhythm of serum cortisol (highest between 0700 and 0900 hours and lowest at 2400 hours) is lost early in Cushing's syndrome of any cause, and this provides a useful alternative screening test. A cutoff value of greater than 7.5 mg/dL for serum or a value greater than the reported normal range for salivary cortisol at 2400 hours is considered abnormal. However, because recent studies have not been able to validate the originally reported high sensitivity and specificity of this test, it is presented here as a useful alternative test and not as part of the diagnostic algorithm.

Low-Dose Dexamethasone Suppression Test

In conditions where hypercortisolism is present but is not autonomous (see Box 2), screening by UFC may produce a false-positive result. Similarly, the 1-mg O/N DST may have a lower specificity in patients with pseudo-Cushing's syndrome. To overcome these limitations, the low-dose dexamethasone suppression test with CRH stimulation (LDDST-CRH or Dex-CRH) is used. This test employs a higher dose of dexamethasone (0.5 mg every 6 hours for eight doses, starting at 1200 hours and ending at 0600 hours 2 days later); the serum cortisol is measured at 0900 hours on the day before dexamethasone is administered and again 2 hours after the last dose (i.e., at 0800 hours). Ovine CRH (Acthrel) 1 µg/kg IV is administered at 0800 hours (i.e., 2 hours after the last dose of dexamethasone), and the serum cortisol is measured 15 minutes later. Any value greater than 1.8 µg/dL has a good specificity for detecting Cushing's syndrome, even in patients with physiologic hypercortisolism. Because this test is more complicated and therefore more prone to error, it should be combined with the other screening tests, in specific circumstances, as detailed in the algorithm.

Special Conditions

In pregnant patients and in patients on antiepileptic medications, UFC is preferable as the first test. In patients with renal insufficiency or adrenal incidentalomas with minimal features of Cushing's syndrome, the 1-mg dexamethasone test is preferable, in conjunction with the midnight cortisol assay.

STEP 2: ACTH-DEPENDENT VERSUS ACTH-INDEPENDENT CUSHING'S SYNDROME

Once the clinical and biochemical diagnosis of Cushing's syndrome is established with step 1 testing, the next step is to identify whether the hypercortisolism is ACTH dependent or independent. A cortisol-producing lesion (adrenal source) is ACTH independent and leads to a complete suppression of pituitary ACTH, which would be undetectable, whereas an ACTH- or CRH-producing lesion (pituitary or ectopic source) leads to hypercortisolemia by stimulating the adrenal glands (ACTH-dependent) and is manifested by inappropriately normal (with respect to the elevated cortisol) or elevated ACTH levels. Therefore, although it is difficult to obtain in the outpatient setting, a detectable midnight plasma ACTH level is strongly suggestive of ACTH-dependent disease, as is an 0900-hour ACTH level that is greater than 20 pg/mL. If the plasma ACTH is less than 9 pg/mL, the likelihood of adrenal disease is very high and adrenal imaging is mandated. However, if the plasma ACTH level is between 9 and 20 pg/mL, the overlap between ACTH-dependent and ACTH-independent diseases necessitates another test. If administration of

CRH (1 µg/kg or a single 100-µg dose of IV ovine CRH) stimulates plasma ACTH (measured 15 and 30 minutes after CRH injection) to a level greater than 20 pg/mL, further work-up of ACTH-dependent disease is indicated; if not, adrenal imaging is in order. For all patients with ACTH-independent Cushing's syndrome, we prefer high-resolution, nonenhanced computed tomography, followed by a delayed contrast-enhanced study with thin cuts (3–5 mm) to look for adrenal lesions; however, T1- and T2-weighted magnetic resonance imaging with chemical shift imaging is also an alternative.

STEP 3: PITUITARY VERSUS ECTOPIC SOURCE OF ACTH-DEPENDENT CUSHING'S SYNDROME

To avoid inconclusive results with erroneous interpretations, further work-up should be undertaken only after ACTH-dependent Cushing's syndrome has been confirmed with step 1 and step 2 testing. More than 90% of these cases are of pituitary origin (usually microadenomas >5 mm). A feature that is helpful, although not diagnostic, is that 95% of patients with ectopic Cushing's syndrome have hypokalemic alkalosis, in contrast to fewer than 10% of those with Cushing's syndrome of pituitary origin. However, there exists a significant overlap of biochemical values, including plasma ACTH, between Cushing's syndrome of pituitary origin and that from an ectopic source.

The most specific test to distinguish a pituitary from an ectopic source is demonstration of ACTH secretion from the pituitary by bilateral inferior petrosal sinus sampling (BIPSS). Because this is an invasive test, we recommend adopting a combination of tests to distinguish these entities before BIPSS is attempted. Magnetic resonance imaging of the pituitary with enhancement is a reliable way to identify pituitary microadenomas. However, false-positive results are possible due to pickup of incidentalomas that may be present in up to 10% of the general population, although these are mostly smaller than 5 mm. To minimize the false-positives, a cutoff of greater than 6 mm is recommended for any adenoma in this setting, to achieve a high specificity. We also recommend performing a standard high-dose dexamethasone suppression test (HDDST), in which 2 mg of dexamethasone is given orally every 6 hours for eight doses, and the serum cortisol levels before and after dexamethasone administration are compared. A 50% suppression has a high specificity for a pituitary source. More importantly, the cutoff of greater than 50% suppression virtually excludes an ectopic source.

If one or both of these two tests are negative, then BIPSS needs to be undertaken. BIPSS should be performed in a tertiary care center that routinely does these procedures, because the complication rate is low in experienced centers. In this test, samples are collected simultaneously from the bilateral inferior petrosal sinuses, into which the pituitary veins drain, and from a peripheral vein; these measurements are then repeated at 3, 5, and 10 minutes after an IV injection of ovine CRH (100 µg in a single dose or 1 µg/kg). A ratio of petrosal sinus-to-peripheral ACTH greater than 2 at baseline or greater than 3 after CRH is highly suggestive of a pituitary source. Some studies have looked at high jugular sampling as an alternative with lower cutoffs, but, unless more studies are done with these tests, BIPSS remains the gold standard.

Once a pituitary source has been excluded by these tests, the search for an ectopic source of ACTH is undertaken, including detailed radiologic evaluations of the thorax and abdomen. Occasionally, scanning with an indium 111–labeled octreotide (Sandostatin)[1] may be beneficial for localizing the source if computed tomography or magnetic resonance imaging is not conclusive. A confirmation with specific venous sampling may be indicated in selected cases of identified lesions.

Treatment

The mainstay of treatment is to achieve normal cortisol levels as quickly and safely as possible, because there is a significant increase in cardiovascular-related mortality among patients with Cushing's

---

[1]Not FDA approved for this indication.

syndrome. In addition, attention needs to be directed toward managing the complications of Cushing's syndrome, such as hypertension, glucose intolerance, cardiovascular complications, osteoporosis, psychiatric manifestations, and other hormonal abnormalities, because they affect the morbidity, mortality, and quality of life significantly.

EXOGENOUS CAUSES OF HYPERCORTISOLEMIA

Although the best treatment in these cases is to slowly decrease and then discontinue the exogenous glucocorticoids, this is not practical in several circumstances; for example, in severe autoimmune conditions and after transplantation, a decrease in steroid dosing would exacerbate the underlying condition or lead to rejection of the transplant. However, every effort needs to be made to decrease the exogenous steroids. The steroids need to be tapered in a structured fashion, with close clinical monitoring to pick up early symptoms and signs of adrenal insufficiency.

ENDOGENOUS HYPERCORTISOLEMIA

Treatment of endogenous Cushing's syndrome is primarily surgical and depends on the etiology.

Primary Adrenal Etiology

Adrenal adenomas are cured by unilateral adrenalectomy after appropriate localization. Currently, a laparoscopic approach has replaced open laparotomy in most tertiary surgical centers, because it results in a shorter hospital stay. Bilateral adrenalectomy may be indicated in cases of macronodular hyperplasia or rare bilateral adenomas. Adrenal carcinomas are frequently diagnosed late in the course, and surgical cure is infrequently achieved; often, a combination of surgical and medical therapy is required.

Primary Pituitary Etiology

Transsphenoidal resection of an identified adenoma is the standard of care for all pituitary microadenomas causing Cushing's syndrome. It achieves a remission in 65% to 90% of cases, with 10% to 20% recurrence after 10 years of follow-up. For patients with no identified discrete adenomas, a partial or total hypophysectomy may be indicated. In cases of macroadenomas with suprasellar extension or cavernous sinus invasion, an open craniotomy may become necessary, leading to significantly lower remission rates and higher recurrences.

After the procedure, all patients should be closely observed in an intensive care unit to ensure that there is no disruption of vasopressin release (excess leading to syndrome of inappropriate antidiuretic hormone [SIADH], or deficiency leading to diabetes insipidus). All patients should be monitored with a morning (0800 hours) cortisol measurement during the first postoperative week, to assess for remission. This testing should be done after the glucocorticoids are withheld the previous evening if the patient is in hospital, or while the patient is on low-dose dexamethasone if the assessment is done in an outpatient setting. Persistent morning serum cortisol levels greater than 5 µg/dL require further evaluation and are associated with higher recurrence rates. A 24-hour UFC test may also be used, and values lower than 20 µg in 24 hours are associated with remission.

All patients after surgery require chronic replacement of glucocorticoids (12–15 mg/m^2 of hydrocortisone [Cortef] or equivalent), to avoid the secondary adrenal insufficiency induced by the prolonged preoperative hypercortisolism. Most patients recover the HPA axis during the first year after surgery, and the replacement dose can be stopped if the morning cortisol or the cortisol response after cosyntropin (Cortrosyn) is greater than 18 µg/dL. In addition, all patients should be monitored after discharge with testing of all the other hormonal axes, including the thyroid axis (thyroid-stimulating hormone and free thyroxine), the gonadal axis (testosterone in men; follicle-stimulating hormone and luteinizing hormone in women with a detailed menstrual history), and the growth hormone axis (insulin-like growth factor 1).

Primary Ectopic Etiology

The main determinant of success in treating ectopic Cushing's syndrome is identification of the source and the feasibility of its surgical removal. For example, an identified carcinoid source may be cured by its removal, in contrast to the difficulty in managing a paraneoplastic Cushing's syndrome with disseminated small cell lung cancer. In the absence of surgical removal of the source, medical therapy is often adopted to ameliorate the hypercortisolism.

Recurrent Cushing's Syndrome

Recurrence of adrenal adenomas is rare after surgical removal. A recurrence may occur with partially resected adrenal carcinomas, which overall have a grim prognosis. A return of hypercortisolism usually occurs with incomplete surgical removal of pituitary adenomas or with a recurrence. With longer follow-ups, this is being recognized as more common than previously reported. A repeat transsphenoidal surgery, if possible, is usually indicated, although the overall rate of success is lower than with the first surgery, and there is a higher incidence of hypopituitarism. If this is not feasible, pituitary irradiation by fractionated external-beam radiation or stereotactic radiosurgery may be undertaken. Control of hypercortisolism may be achieved in up to 60% of patients within 3 to 5 years, although hypopituitarism is a very common consequence. For uncontrolled Cushing's syndrome, bilateral adrenalectomy may occasionally be considered as a treatment of last resort. For these patients, close follow-up is essential to identify a sudden rapid increase in the pituitary adenoma (Nelson's syndrome).

MEDICAL MANAGEMENT

Medical management of Cushing's syndrome is directed primarily toward management of complications resulting from the consequences of chronic hypercortisolemia. This encompasses a close attention to identifying and treating hypertension, glucose intolerance, hyperlipidemia, osteoporosis, menstrual irregularities, and depression and other psychiatric manifestations.

 CURRENT THERAPY

- The primary treatment for Cushing's syndrome is surgical.
- Adrenalectomy cures adrenal adenoma–related adrenocorticotropic hormone (ACTH)-dependent Cushing's syndrome. A laparoscopic approach is preferred.
- Transsphenoidal adenomectomy for identified pituitary lesions is the surgery of choice; it has a low rate of complications and a long-term remission rate of 65% to 90%.
- All patients after transsphenoidal resection should receive replacement doses of steroids until they have been tested for adequate cortisol response off replacement steroids. This may take up to 1 year in some patients.
- Repeat surgery or pituitary irradiation for recurrence has a high incidence of associated panhypopituitarism.
- Medical therapy aimed toward hypercortisolism has a limited adjunctive role in inoperable or recurrent cases. It also serves in a preparatory role preoperatively in severe cases of Cushing's syndrome. Newer drugs with better therapeutic-to-side effect profiles are in clinical trials.
- Medical management of the complications of Cushing's syndrome (e.g., hypertension, diabetes mellitus, osteoporosis) is critical to decrease the associated morbidity and mortality.

Medical therapy directed toward ameliorating the hypercortisole-mia is not very effective, and the medications used have numerous side effects. Hence, medical therapy has been relegated to a secondary option in cases of failed surgical therapy, for patients who are not surgical candidates, or as a preoperative preparatory measure in severe hypercortisolism.

The medications that target hypercortisolemia can be broadly classified into three groups. The first group comprises inhibitors of adrenal steroid biosynthesis and can potentially be used in all cases of hypercortisolism. Metyrapone (Metopirone)[1] blocks 11β-hydroxylase enzyme and is most commonly used as an adjunct in preparation for surgery or with pituitary irradiation. Ketoconazole (Nizoral),[1] the other commonly used drug of this class, blocks multiple CYP-dependent enzymes in the steroidogenesis pathway. Other, less commonly used and more toxic drugs include aminoglutethimide (Cytadren) and mitotane (Lysodren), which may be used in patients with refractory adrenal carcinoma. The goal in administering these drugs is to titrate the dose so as to return the UFC to normal values while minimizing side effects.

The second class of drugs inhibits ACTH secretion, with cabergoline (Dostinex),[1] a dopamine agonist, showing promise. However, these drugs need to be evaluated in larger trials before they are used as primary agents or as adjuvants for surgical management.

The third class is glucocorticoid receptor blockers, which limit the deleterious effects of hypercortisolemia. Mifepristone (Mifeprex)[1] is the one that has been tried, and its efficacy is currently being investigated in a large clinical trial (the SEISMIC study). The combined use of drugs from the first group (e.g., metyrapone, ketoconazole) and mifepristone may have additional benefits in severe cases and needs to be further evaluated in clinical trials.

REFERENCES

Arnaldi G, Angeli A, Atkinson AB, et al. Diagnosis and complications of Cushing's syndrome: A consensus statement. J Clin Endocrinol Metab 2003;88:5593–602.

Biller BM, et al. Treatment of adrenocorticotropin-dependent Cushing's syndrome: A consensus statement. J Clin Endocrinol Metab 2008;93:2454–62.

Pecori GF, et al. Specificity of first-line tests for the diagnosis of Cushing's syndrome: Assessment in a large series. J Clin Endocrinol Metab 2007;92:4123–9.

---

[1]Not FDA approved for this indication.

Diabetes Insipidus

Method of
Jennifer Kelly, DO, and Arnold M. Moses, MD, FACP, FACE

General Principles of Treating Central (Neurogenic) Diabetes Insipidus

The hormonal treatment of diabetes insipidus is accomplished using the synthetic nanopeptide desmopressin (1-deamino [8-D-arginine] vasopressin; DDAVP). Arginine vasopressin (AVP) is the natural hormone of humans. Desmopressin is a synthetic analogue of AVP that does not constrict smooth muscle and has a longer antidiuretic action than does the natural hormone. Because of its lack of vasoactivity, desmopressin can be used without precipitating angina, abdominal cramps, or headaches. It can also be used to treat diabetes insipidus during pregnancy because it resists inactivation by placental

CURRENT DIAGNOSIS

Central diabetes insipidus (DI) can be diagnosed as follows:

1. Ensure urine volume is increased to ≥3 L/day in adults.
2. Rule out glycosuria (dipstick will suffice).
3. Measure serum sodium concentration during ad libitum fluid intake.
4. If the serum sodium concentration is *above* normal while urine osmolality is *less than* 300 mOsm per kilogram of water, injection of desmopressin (DDAVP) at least doubles the urine osmolality in patients with central DI. If the urine osmolality response is less, the patient may have nephrogenic DI.
5. If the serum sodium concentration is *normal* while urine osmolality is *less than* 300 mOsm per kilogram of water, additional procedures, including a water deprivation or saline infusion test, may be required. Refer to an experienced specialist.
6. Magnetic resonance imaging to detect the presence or absence of the pituitary hyperintense signal may be helpful in differentiating central DI from primary polydipsia. Plasma arginine vasopressin levels do *not* differentiate these two polyuric conditions.

---

vasopressinase. The available preparations of vasopressin are listed in the table above. The durations of antidiuretic responses to the different preparations are listed in Table 1.

For most patients with diabetes insipidus, the treatment of choice is intranasal desmopressin (100 μg/mL). Two delivery systems are available: a nasal (rhinal) tube, which the patient uses to blow measured amounts (0.05–0.2 mL) into the nose, and a compression pump system, which delivers 0.1 mL (see Current Therapy). Treatment is usually initiated with 10 μg of intranasal desmopressin. Patients are instructed to repeat this dose when polyuria recurs. Some patients respond better if the hormone is administered on a more defined schedule. The dose administered can be increased or decreased in accordance with the patient's response. Patients should be told to drink only when they are thirsty.

Some patients prefer to start therapy with oral desmopressin; others can be switched to the oral preparation when absorption of the intranasal form is decreased in the presence of nasal congestion.

TABLE 1 Mean Time That Urine Remains Hypertonic in Adults with Diabetes Insipidus*

Route of Administration	Amount Administered	Mean Duration of Action (hr)
Intranasal desmopressin	10 μg (0.1 mL)	12
	15 μg (0.15 mL)	16
	20 μg (0.2 mL)	20
Subcutaneous or intravenous desmopressin	0.5 μg	10
	1.0 μg	14
	2.0 μg	18
	4.0 μg	22
Oral desmopressin	0.1 mg	6–8
	0.2 mg	8–12
	0.4 mg	16–20
Subcutaneous arginine vasopressin	5 U	4

* Note: Onset of antidiuretic action of subcutaneous or intravenous preparation is 30–45 minutes. Onset of antidiuretic effect of tablets is about 60 minutes.

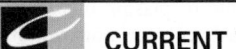
Trade Name	Chemical Composition	Concentration	Size	Pharmaceutical Company
Intranasal Preparations				
Desmopressin Rhinal Tube	Desmopressin acetate	100 μg/mL	2.5-mL bottle with rhinal tube delivering sprays of 10–20 μg	Ferring
DDAVP Rhinal Tube	Desmopressin acetate	100 μg/mL	2.5-mL bottle with rhinal tube delivering sprays of 10–20 μg	Aventis
DDAVP Nasal Spray	Desmopressin acetate	100 μg/mL	5.0-mL bottle with spray pump delivering 50 sprays of 10 μg each	Aventis
Oral Preparation				
DDAVP Tablets	Desmopressin acetate	Not applicable	0.1-mg, 0.2-mg tablets	Aventis
Injectable Preparations (Subcutaneous, Intravenous)				
DDAVP Injection	Desmopressin acetate	4 μg/mL	1.0, 10.0 mL/vials	Aventis
Pitressin Injection	Arginine vasopressin	20 U/mL	1 mL/vial	Monarch
Arginine Vasopressin Injection	Arginine vasopressin	20 U/mL	0.5, 1, and 10 mL/vials	American Regent

Caution: Stimate Nasal Spray (desmopressin acetate) is marketed by Aventis Pharmaceuticals in a 2.5-mL nasal spray bottle. It is designed for treating bleeding disorders and contains 1.5 mg/mL desmopressin. Stimate can be confused easily with the less concentrated preparations of desmopressin acetate that are used for treating diabetes insipidus.

The starting dose of the tablet is usually 0.05 mg (half of a 0.1-mg tablet) twice per day. The maintenance dose is gradually adjusted to provide an adequate limitation of water turnover. The daily oral dose may range from 0.1 to 1.2 mg in divided doses. We do not currently recommend the use of nonhormonal agents such as chlorpropamide (Diabinese),[1] clofibrate,[1,2] or carbamazepine.[1]

In the uncooperative or unconscious patient with diabetes insipidus, desmopressin should be injected subcutaneously, usually starting with 0.5 or 1.0 μg (see Table 1 for duration of action). Subcutaneous AVP is sometimes used in patients with acute onset of diabetes insipidus after head trauma or neurosurgical procedures. Its short duration of action might help prevent water intoxication in patients receiving poorly monitored intravenous fluids. As with desmopressin, it is safest to administer subsequent doses of AVP when polyuria reappears.

As long as untreated patients with diabetes insipidus are conscious, retain normal thirst, and have enough fluid to drink, they seldom become dehydrated. However, severe dehydration with extremely high serum sodium concentrations may occur acutely when patients with untreated diabetes insipidus do not receive adequate fluids (orally or intravenously).

The most common and important problem in the hospitalized patient with diabetes insipidus is iatrogenic hyponatremia. Particularly when it occurs rapidly, hyponatremia may cause severe neurologic problems. Hyponatremia in this setting is caused by overhydration (only rarely does sodium loss contribute) in patients receiving vasopressin and can be prevented by allowing patients to self-regulate their oral intake of fluids whenever possible. When such self-regulation is not feasible because the patient is obtunded, has a defective thirst mechanism, or cannot drink, extreme care must be taken in ordering intravenous fluids to prevent hyponatremia. The patient can be maintained in an antidiuretic state by giving vasopressin when the urine becomes dilute. The intravenous fluid should consist largely of 5% dextrose in water with amounts of normal saline gauged to replace daily urinary sodium losses. The volume of intravenous fluid for every 8-hour period should replace 8-hour urine volumes plus estimated 8-hour insensible losses and fluid losses through perspiration and other routes. The amount of intravenous fluid should be adjusted according to plasma sodium, blood urea nitrogen, and creatinine levels. If hypernatremia occurs, the amount of intravenous fluids should be increased accordingly.

If a major decrease in serum sodium concentration occurs, intravenous fluids should be temporarily discontinued, and, if necessitated by clinical manifestations, the patient should be given 200 to 300 mL of 3% saline, perhaps with 40 mg of furosemide (Lasix) intravenously. Temporary discontinuation of vasopressin should also be considered. To emphasize, the patient with central diabetes insipidus whose fluid intake is maintained intravenously presents a major medical problem and must be followed up carefully to maintain normonatremia.

Pregnancy is associated with significant alterations in water metabolism. The osmotic threshold for secretion of vasopressin is lowered and the threshold for thirst reduced, with a resulting decrease in plasma osmolality by about 10 mOsm per kilogram of water. A deficiency of plasma vasopressin can also result from increased degradation of the hormone by placental vasopressinase. This disorder is referred to as *gestational diabetes insipidus* because the symptoms of diabetes insipidus occur only during pregnancy and remit soon after delivery. An underlying subclinical deficiency in vasopressin secretion may also be involved. Gestational diabetes insipidus is treated successfully with desmopressin, which is not degraded by vasopressinase. The dose of desmopressin should be about the same as that used in the nonpregnant state, but the normal range for serum sodium is about 5 mEq/L lower.

Principles of Treating Specific Problems

THE ALERT PATIENT WITH INTACT THIRST

When antidiuretic therapy is initiated in the alert patient with diabetes insipidus, the patient must consciously avoid excessive drinking for at least several days. By that time, the thirst mechanism usually

---

[1]Not FDA approved for this indication.
[2]Not available in the United States.

adapts to the more normal urine volume. However, some patients must be reminded to avoid excessive drinking, which causes the syndrome of inappropriate antidiuresis. Thirst may be perceived with normal or low serum sodium concentration because of a dry mouth, as might occur with mouth breathing, anticholinergic drugs, β-adrenergic blockers, or cigarette smoking. An occasional patient is hyperdipsic because of increased circulating angiotensin II levels or from hypothalamic involvement, as may occur with sarcoidosis involving the hypothalamus. Use of ice instead of liquids may help limit fluid intake.

THE ALERT PATIENT WITH ADIPSIA

The alert patient with adipsia presents a difficult management problem in the hospital and particularly after the patient is discharged from the hospital. Because of the loss of thirst perception, normal serum sodium concentration is maintained only with great difficulty. The patient and family must closely and continuously monitor the patient's intake and output of fluids, body weight, and vital signs. Serum sodium concentration and blood urea nitrogen, uric acid, and creatinine levels should be checked often. Such a patient must always relate fluid intake to volume of urine plus fluid losses through perspiration and the gastrointestinal tract. Failure to properly monitor these patients may allow their condition to go unrecognized until they develop severe dehydration. This may require the infusion of normal saline to restore pulse and blood pressure and then water orally or dextrose in water intravenously. Appropriate antidiuretic therapy should be instituted along with the fluids.

THE CONFUSED, OBTUNDED, OR UNCONSCIOUS PATIENT

When confused, obtunded, or unconscious, such as postoperatively or after head trauma, the patient with diabetes insipidus is monitored in the same ways described for the alert patient with adipsia. The only major difference is that vasopressin must be given by injection or infusion and the fluids given intravenously. In the presence of hypernatremia and associated hypovolemia, normal saline is required to help restore pulse and blood pressure to normal. Otherwise, patients with hypernatremia should be treated with dextrose in water (see later) while antidiuretic therapy is instituted and maintained.

Postoperative hypernatremia should be prevented by the early recognition of diabetes insipidus before, during, and after surgery and by avoidance of osmotic diuretic use during surgery. The patient should be switched to oral fluids as soon as possible, and the adequacy of the patient's thirst mechanism to control fluid intake appropriately should be evaluated. Diabetes insipidus that occurs postoperatively or after head trauma may be variable (biphasic or triphasic), and frequently the diabetes insipidus is transient. Therefore, hormonal treatment should be withheld periodically to determine whether the symptoms of diabetes insipidus recur. After 6 months of diabetes insipidus, remission is very unlikely.

Special Problems of Fluid Balance

THE HYPERNATREMIC PATIENT

Hypernatremia in patients with diabetes insipidus is usually associated with normal total body sodium. The hypernatremia is due to loss of free water by way of the kidneys, but losses from the skin and lungs can aggravate the problem. Alterations in the composition of water and solutes in the brain cells may contribute to the symptoms of hypernatremia. An abrupt increase in plasma sodium concentration causes more severe symptoms than does a gradual rise to the same sodium level.

The goal of treating hypernatremia in patients with diabetes insipidus is restoration of normal plasma volume and tonicity. Desmopressin should be injected to maintain concentrated urine. If the patient has circulatory disturbances due to hypovolemia, isotonic saline should be given until systemic hemodynamics are stabilized.

In fact, isotonic saline is relatively hypotonic to plasma in patients with severe hypernatremia and simultaneously corrects both volume and water deficits. After volume deficits are corrected, the hypernatremia can be treated intravenously with 5% dextrose in water, or water can be given by mouth if the patient is able to drink.

The water deficit in these patients can be calculated on the basis of the serum sodium concentration and on the assumption that 60% of body weight is water. For example, if the patient's usual weight is 75 kg, total body water would normally be 75 kg × 0.6 = 45 L. If the serum sodium value is 154 mEq/L, the patient has a 10% deficit of water (154 − 140) ÷ 140 and theoretically requires 4.5 L of water to correct the deficit. Continuing losses of water must also be replaced. Despite inaccuracies, including the assumption that body water is always 60% of the body weight and the postulate that water is lost uniformly throughout all body cells, this approach provides an approximate value that can be used in planning therapy. The major problem is determining the appropriate rate at which to lower serum sodium concentration to normal. Because seizures or even fatal cerebral edema may occur when serum sodium concentration is lowered rapidly, the best recommendation is to correct the hypernatremia over 48 to 72 hours and at a rate not exceeding 0.5 to 2.0 mEq/L/hr. As total body water expands, the serum sodium concentration may fall proportionally. Serum electrolyte values should be monitored frequently to ensure an appropriate response.

Treatment of the hypernatremia due to water loss, as occurs in untreated patients with diabetes insipidus, must also address associated electrolyte abnormalities and underlying medical and surgical conditions. An example is the patient with diabetes insipidus with coexisting hyperglycemia. In this case, the "corrected" serum sodium concentration should be used to calculate the water deficit. Slightly low or abnormal serum sodium concentrations in the presence of high serum glucose often result, when corrected, in hypernatremic values. The corrected serum sodium concentrations can be calculated by increasing the sodium concentration by 1.5 mEq/L for every 100 mg/dL increment in the serum glucose concentration above 100 mg/dL. For example, in a patient with a sodium level of 138 mEq/L and a glucose level of 700 mg/dL, the corrected serum sodium concentration is 138 + (1.5 × 6), or 147 mEq/L.

THE HYPONATREMIC PATIENT

Hyponatremia in diabetes insipidus occurs almost exclusively in patients who are overhydrated orally or parenterally while they are being treated with desmopressin. The severity of hyponatremia correlates closely with the magnitude of fluid overload. The amount of excessive body water can be calculated using the same approach as described for hypernatremia. Rarely, the hyponatremia is aggravated by large amounts of sodium in the urine, probably related to increased levels of atrial natriuretic peptide and glomerular filtration rate and inhibition of aldosterone. The hyponatremia due to natriuresis in the water-overloaded patient can be corrected only partially with saline infusions, because the natriuresis continues until the hypervolemic state is corrected. Hyponatremia can be caused or aggravated by adrenal or thyroid insufficiency.

A large body of literature on the appropriate rate at which to correct hyponatremia is available. Rapidly occurring (acute) and marked hyponatremia can be lethal and should be treated urgently. Under these conditions, and when neurologic symptoms are severe, initial therapy should raise the serum sodium concentration by 1 to 2 mEq/L/hr regardless of the duration of the electrolyte abnormality. Most authorities agree that the rate of change in serum sodium concentrations should not exceed 12 to 20 mEq/L/day. However, in patients with chronic hyponatremia, correction of serum sodium concentration approximating this rate occasionally causes serious, even fatal complications by inducing central pontine myelinolysis.

Fluid restriction is adequate for treatment of the asymptomatic mildly hyponatremic patient. Urine should be analyzed every 4 to 8 hours for volume and osmolality, and fluid replacement should be ordered in relation to *urine volume*. Remember that insensible fluid losses of about 600 mL of free water per day occur in the usual adult. *It is NOT appropriate to write for a fixed amount of fluid replacement.* Plasma sodium concentration should be checked frequently and fluid replacement adjusted accordingly. The complaint of thirst by a water-restricted patient should not be ignored. Long-term management is usually less disrupted by adjusting fluid intake than by discontinuing hormonal therapy and allowing the patient to "break through." Alternatively, when the patient has symptomatic or severe hyponatremia (serum sodium concentration <115 mEq/L in chronic hyponatremia or 125 mEq/L in acute hyponatremia), intravenous furosemide (Lasix), may help by causing the excretion of urine that is slightly hypotonic or isotonic. After injection of 40 mg or more of furosemide, 100 mL of 3% saline should be infused in the first hour. This rate should be decreased or discontinued subsequently if symptoms have ameliorated or if the plasma sodium concentration has increased by more than 2 mEq/L in that hour. Infusion of more than a total of 250 mL of 3% saline is rarely necessary.

PREPARATION FOR DIAGNOSTIC TESTS OR TREATMENT

Special care must be taken when patients with treated diabetes insipidus are subjected to certain "standard protocols" associated with many diagnostic and therapeutic procedures. These protocols require the patient to be either fluid restricted, as for preparation for intravenous pyelography, or hydrated, as for intravenous administration of chemotherapy. Tests requiring that a patient receiving no oral fluids should be performed with adequate intravenous hydration matched to the patient's urine output. Intravenous fluids should be started from the time the patient is no longer able to take oral fluids and can be discontinued when oral fluids are again allowed. In contrast, patients receiving antidiuretic therapy for diabetes insipidus should not be made to "force fluids" beyond the amounts determined by thirst or be subject to hydration orders at rates not related to urine output. If high urine flow rates are needed, the patient's antidiuretic therapy must be discontinued. Oral or intravenous fluids can then be given to match the large urine volumes. Sometimes, it may be appropriate (to obtain more precise timing of a diuresis) to continue antidiuretic therapy and administer intravenous furosemide. Close monitoring of serum sodium levels will greatly assist in determining the status of fluid balance in these situations.

Nephrogenic Diabetes Insipidus

Nephrogenic diabetes insipidus is characterized by resistance of the kidney to the antidiuretic action of vasopressin. This disorder is often hereditary, caused by inactivating mutations of the V2 receptor or of the vasopressin-regulated water channel protein aquaporin 2. Standard doses of desmopressin or AVP do not decrease the polyuria. The urine volume can be decreased by 25% to 40% by severe solute restriction and by further inducing hypovolemia with thiazide diuretics. Rarely, very high doses of desmopressin may be effective in females. Occasionally, acquired nephrogenic diabetes insipidus resolves by eliminating the underlying cause (i.e., treating the hypercalcemia or hypokalemia or discontinuing lithium therapy). Nephrogenic diabetes insipidus due to long-term lithium therapy may persist after discontinuation of lithium. Treatment of lithium-induced nephrogenic diabetes insipidus is limited to a low-sodium diet and possibly diuretics. Treatment may reduce urine volume by up to 30% or 40%. Caution must be taken because solute restriction, especially with a diuretic, may lead to lithium toxicity.

REFERENCES

Adrogue HJ, Madias NE. Hypernatremia. N Engl J Med 2000;342:1493–9.
Gross P. Treatment of severe hyponatremia. Kidney Int 2001;60:2417–27.
Moses AM, Clayton B, Hochhauser L. Use of T1-weighted MR imaging to differentiate between primary polydipsia and central diabetes insipidus. AJNR Am J Neuroradiol 1992;13:1273–7.
Moses AM, Moses LK, Notman D, Springer J. Antidiuretic responses to injected desmopressin, alone and with indomethacin. J Clin Endocrinol Metab 1981;52:910–3.
Moses AM, Scheinman SJ, Oppenheim A. Marked hypotonic polyuria resulting from nephrogenic diabetes insipidus with partial sensitivity to vasopressin. J Clin Endocrinol 1984;59:1044–9.
Rose BD, Post TW. Clinical Physiology of Acid-Base and Electrolyte Disorders. 5th ed. New York: McGraw-Hill; 2001, pp 716–9, 764–75.

Primary Hyperparathyroidism and Hypoparathyroidism

Method of
John P. Bilezikian, MD

Primary Hyperparathyroidism

INCIDENCE AND GENERAL CHARACTERISTICS

Primary hyperparathyroidism (PHPT) is a relatively common endocrine disease with an incidence as high as 1 in 500 to 1 in 1000. The high visibility of PHPT today marks a dramatic change from several generations ago when it was considered rare. The increased incidence is undoubtedly due to widespread use of the multichannel autoanalyzer. PHPT occurs in individuals of all ages but occurs most frequently in the sixth decade of life. Women are affected more often than men by a ratio of 3:1. PHPT in children is an unusual event. It might be a component of one of several endocrinopathies with a genetic basis, such as multiple endocrine neoplasia (MEN), type I or II. PHPT is caused by excessive secretion of parathyroid hormone (PTH) from one or more parathyroid glands. A benign, solitary adenoma is found in 80% of patients. Less commonly, in 15% to 20% of subjects, all four glands are hyperplastic. Four-gland parathyroid disease may occur sporadically or in association with the MEN syndromes. The most uncommon presentation of PHPT is parathyroid cancer, occurring in less than 0.5% of patients with PHPT.

DIFFERENTIAL DIAGNOSIS

The major diagnostic distinction to be made is between PHPT and malignancy, the other most common cause of hypercalcemia. These two etiologies account for more than 90% of all patients with hypercalcemia (Table 1). A much longer, complete list of potential causes of hypercalcemia is considered after these two etiologies are ruled out or if there is reason to believe that a different cause is likely. Today, PHPT presents most often as an asymptomatic disorder. In contrast, malignancy-associated hypercalcemia is usually found at a

TABLE 1 Differential Diagnosis of Hypercalcemia

Primary hyperparathyroidism
Malignancy
Other endocrinopathies
  Hyperthyroidism
  Pheochromocytoma
  Adrenal insufficiency
  VIPoma
Medications
  Lithium
  Thiazides
  Thyroid hormone
  Vitamin D
  Vitamin A
Granulomatous diseases
Familial hypocalciuric hypercalcemia
Immobilization

later stage of the malignant process and is associated with symptoms. Besides a major difference in clinical presentation between these two most common causes of hypercalcemia, the PTH immunoassay is a helpful distinguishing point. In patients with PHPT, the PTH level will be elevated or in the upper range of normal, whereas in malignancy, the PTH level is invariably suppressed.

PATHOPHYSIOLOGY, MOLECULAR GENETICS, AND PATHOLOGY

The pathophysiology of PHPT relates to the loss of normal feedback control of PTH by extracellular calcium. Why the parathyroid cell loses its normal sensitivity to calcium is not known. Genetic abnormalities that could be linked to sporadic parathyroid tumors have been described. A rearrangement of the cyclin D1/(PRAD1) proto-oncogene has been seen in some patients with PHPT. The rearrangement associates the PTH gene with the growth promoter cyclin D1. Only a small number of parathyroid tumors have been demonstrated to harbor this defect. Tumor suppressors, such as the gene associated with MEN-I, have generated interest, as have potential abnormalities in the gene for the calcium-sensing receptor. Although the gene for the calcium receptor has been implicated in familial hypocalciuric hypercalcemia and neonatal severe hyperparathyroidism, there is little evidence for this genetic abnormality in the sporadic form of PHPT. Even the vitamin D receptor has been implicated in pathogenetic abnormalities associated with parathyroid neoplasia.

The typical parathyroid adenoma is an enlarged, oval-shaped, smooth, red-brown gland. A visible rim of normal yellow-brown parathyroid tissue is sometimes seen. The typical parathyroid adenoma is between 300 and 500 mg, much larger than a normal gland that generally weighs 35 to 50 mg. Microscopically, the parathyroid adenoma consists of a network of cells arranged alongside a capillary network, resembling classic endocrine microanatomy. Fat cells are reduced or absent. The form of PHPT characterized by four-gland hyperplasia is seen grossly as enlarged glands that may be of equal size. Microscopically, solid masses of chief cells are seen in the absence of fat cells. In contrast to the adenoma, in which a rim of normal tissue can sometimes be seen, normal tissue is absent in hyperplastic disease.

SIGNS AND SYMPTOMS

PHPT is associated classically with skeletal and renal complications. In severe cases, the skeleton can be involved in a process called *osteitis fibrosa cystica*. Subperiosteal resorption of the distal phalanges, tapering of the distal clavicles, a "salt and pepper" appearance of the skull, bone cysts, and brown tumors of the long bones are all overt manifestations of hyperparathyroid bone disease. This form of hyperparathyroid bone disease is now most unusual, occurring in fewer than 5% of patients with PHPT. Much less severe, but nevertheless significant, skeletal involvement in PHPT is detected by dual energy x-ray absorptiometry (see later). Similar to the reduced incidence of gross skeletal disease, the kidney is also involved in PHPT much less commonly than before. From an incidence of approximately 33% in the 1960s, most series place the incidence of nephrolithiasis now to be no more than 15% to 20%. Nephrolithiasis, nevertheless, is still the most common complication of PHPT. Other renal features of PHPT include diffuse deposition of calcium–phosphate complexes in the parenchyma (nephrocalcinosis). The frequency of this complication is unknown. Hypercalciuria (daily calcium excretion of >250 mg in women or >300 mg in men) is seen in 30% to 40% of patients. PHPT may be associated with a reduction in creatinine clearance, in the absence of any other cause. Classic associations exist between PHPT and other organs, such as the neuromuscular system, the gastrointestinal tract, and the cardiovascular and articular systems, but such panopleistic features of PHPT are rarely seen today. More vexing are nonspecific elements associated with PHPT, such as easy fatigability, a sense of weakness, and a feeling that the aging process is advancing faster than it should be. This is sometimes accompanied by an intellectual weariness and a sense that cognitive faculties are less sharp. Whether these nonspecific features of PHPT are truly part of the disease process, reversible upon successful parathyroid surgery, remains under active investigation.

CLINICAL FORMS OF PRIMARY HYPERPARATHYROIDISM

Asymptomatic PHPT with serum calcium levels within 1 mg/dL above the upper limits of normal is the most common clinical presentation. Most patients do not have specific complaints and do not show evidence of any target organ complications. In parts of the world where severe vitamin D deficiency is common, more symptomatic PHPT is seen. Unusual clinical presentations of PHPT include MEN-I and MEN-II, familial PHPT not associated with any other endocrine disorder, familial cystic parathyroid adenomatosis, jaw tumor syndrome, and neonatal PHPT. Another presentation of PHPT is being described, namely, in individuals with normal serum calcium concentrations but elevated PTH levels. Potential secondary causes of elevated PTH levels are considered but have not been found. It is considered likely that these patients represent the earliest stage of PHPT, when there is glandular overproduction of hormone, before hypercalcemia becomes evident.

DIAGNOSIS AND EVALUATION

Hypercalcemia and elevated levels of PTH establish the diagnosis. The serum phosphorus concentration tends to be in the lower range of normal. Serum alkaline phosphatase activity may be elevated. More specific markers of bone formation (bone-specific alkaline phosphatase, osteocalcin) and bone resorption (urinary deoxypyridinoline, *N* or *C*-telopeptide of collagen) tend to be in the upper range of normal. In some patients, the actions of PTH in altering renal acid-base handling leads to a small increase in the serum chloride concentration and a concomitant small decrease in the serum bicarbonate concentration. Urinary calcium excretion, when elevated, is not generally excessively high. The circulating 25-hydroxyvitamin D concentration is low, and the 1,25-dihydroxyvitamin D concentration is high in some patients.

ROLE OF BONE MASS MEASUREMENT

Dual-energy x-ray absorptiometry shows a pattern of skeletal involvement that is consistent with the physiologic actions of PTH, that of eroding cortical bone while sparing cancellous sites. The typical patient with PHPT shows reductions in bone density that are most marked in the distal third of the forearm, a cortical site, with much less involvement of the lumbar spine, a cancellous site. The hip region, a mixture of cortical and cancellous bone, shows changes that are intermediate between changes in the forearm and the lumbar spine.

   CURRENT DIAGNOSIS

Primary Hyperparathyroidism

- Most common cause of hypercalcemia.
- Diagnosis established by elevated serum calcium concentration and parathyroid hormone level that is frankly elevated or is in the upper range of normal.
- In some patients, the parathyroid hormone level is elevated but the serum calcium concentration is normal.

Hypoparathyroidism

- Much less common than primary hyperparathyroidism.
- Most often due to autoimmune destruction or removal of the parathyroid glands.
- Diagnosis is established by hypocalcemia and low parathyroid hormone levels.

CURRENT THERAPY

Primary Hyperparathyroidism

- When symptoms are present, parathyroid surgery is indicated.
- In the absence of symptoms, surgery is recommended if any one of four criteria is met (see Table 2).
- Preoperative localization testing prior to surgery has become routine.
- Medical management is reserved generally for those who do not meet surgical criteria in whom it is intended to lower the serum calcium or to increase the bone mineral density.
- Prudent use of calcium and vitamin D is recommended, and ambulation is encouraged.
- Pharmacologic agents, such as bisphosphonates and calcimimetics, show promise.

Hypoparathyroidism

- Acute management of hypocalcemia is a medical emergency and requires intravenous administration of calcium.
- Chronic treatment is based upon adequate calcium, vitamin D, and, in some cases, the active vitamin D metabolite 1,25-dihydroxyvitamin D.

TREATMENT

Localization Tests Prior to Surgery

Imaging of abnormal parathyroid tissue is accomplished most accurately with technetium-99m sestamibi. Sestamibi is taken up by both thyroid and parathyroid tissue, but it persists in the parathyroid glands. Various approaches to the use of technetium-99m sestamibi include using the imaging agent alone, and thereby depending upon a difference in uptake kinetics between thyroid and parathyroid tissue, or in combination with iodine 123 (^{123}I). Some believe that use of dual isotopic methods provides better definition of the thyroid from which the image obtained with sestamibi can be subtracted. Even more sophisticated approaches have been developed using sestamibi imaging with single-photon emission computed tomography. Ultrasound, computed tomography, and magnetic resonance imaging are also used to localize abnormal parathyroid tissue. Invasive localization tests with arteriography and selective venous sampling for PTH are used when noninvasive studies have not been successful. In the past, parathyroid imaging was reserved for patients who had undergone neck surgery. With greater success in parathyroid imaging and the increasing popularity of minimally invasive parathyroid surgery, preoperative imaging is becoming routine in all patients.

Guidelines for Surgical Management of Primary Hyperparathyroidism

The Third International Workshop on the Management of Asymptomatic Primary Hyperparathyroidism was held in 2008, the proceedings of which were published in 2009. The Workshop reviewed new data since the previous workshop in 2002 and suggested revised guidelines for surgical management (Table 2). The major changes are summarized here. Since the urinary calcium excretion does not predict stone disease in patients with primary hyperparathyroidism who do not have nephrolithiasis or nephrocalcinosis, it has been removed as a guideline. However, the collection of a 24-hour urine for calcium determination is routinely performed and still recommended. The other major change in the guidelines relates to the cut-point of creatinine clearance below which surgery is recommended. A creatinine clearance <60 mL/min

TABLE 2 2008 Guidelines for Parathyroid Surgery in Asymptomatic PHPT

Measurement	Surgery Recommended if
Serum calcium	>1.0 mg/dL (0.25 mmol/L) above normal
Creatinine clearance (calculated)	Reduced to less than 60 mL/min/1.73 m³
Bone mineral density	T score less than −2.5 SD at spine, hip (total or femoral neck), and radius (distal 1/3 site predominantly cortical bone) or presence of fragility fracture
Age	Patient age less than 50 years

is associated with an increase in PTH levels in individuals without primary hyperparathyroidism. In primary hyperparathyroidism, therefore, if the creatinine clearance is reduced to below this level, it seems likely that PTH levels will increase further. The Workshop Panel recommends that surgery be considered in these individuals.

SURGERY

PHPT is cured when abnormal parathyroid tissue is removed. Asymptomatic patients are advised to have surgery if they meet current guidelines (see Table 2). Symptomatic patients are always advised to undergo parathyroid surgery. At the present time, a number of different surgical procedures can be performed. The standard four-gland parathyroid gland exploration is performed under general or local anesthesia. The single adenoma is removed, and the other glands are ascertained to be normal but not removed. In the case of multiglandular disease, the approach is to remove all tissue except for a remnant that is left in situ or autotransplanted in the nondominant forearm. A popular recent advance in parathyroid surgery is the minimally invasive parathyroidectomy. This procedure depends upon preoperative localization by an imaging technology and confirmation of the success of parathyroid surgery with intraoperative PTH measurements. The circulating PTH level should fall to less than 50% of the preoperative value within minutes after removal of the parathyroid adenoma. Minimally invasive parathyroid surgery, this latter approach, has become a standard for many parathyroid surgeons now.

MEDICAL MANAGEMENT

In patients who do not meet surgical guidelines or who, for other reasons, will not undergo parathyroid surgery, the following medical principles apply. Adequate hydration and ambulation are always encouraged. Thiazide diuretics are to be avoided because they may lead to worsening hypercalcemia. Dietary intake of calcium should be moderate, avoiding both high- and low-calcium diets. Low-calcium diets theoretically could fuel abnormal parathyroid tissue to secrete more PTH. High-calcium diets could be detrimental by worsening hypercalcemia, especially if the 1,25-dihydroxy vitamin D level is elevated. Monitoring with annual measurements of the serum calcium and annual or every-other-year measurements of bone mass by dual-energy x-ray absorptiometry are recommended. In patients whose 25-hydroxyvitamin D level is low, careful replacement seems reasonable. The serum calcium concentration must be monitored to guard against the potential for worsening hypercalcemia in some patients.

Oral phosphate will lower the serum calcium concentration in PHPT by approximately 0.5 to 1 mg/dL, but concerns about ectopic calcium–phosphate deposition limit its utility. Prior to the results of the Women's Health Initiative, estrogen was an option in postmenopausal women. The serum calcium concentration would fall by about 0.5 mg/dL; estrogens are no longer advised for this specific reason. Preliminary observations suggest that raloxifene, a selective estrogen receptor modulator, may have calcium-lowering effects similar to those of estrogen in postmenopausal women with PHPT.

The bisphosphonate alendronate (Fosamax) has shown promise in patients with PHPT. Lumbar spine bone density improves by as much as 5% in the first year of therapy. Neither the serum calcium concentration nor the PTH level falls significantly. Patients who will not undergo parathyroid surgery but in whom lumbar spine bone density is reduced may benefit from bisphosphonate therapy.

An early clinical experience with hyperparathyroid postmeno-pausal women has shown that, in principle, a calcimimetic can significantly reduce PTH and serum calcium levels in patients with the disease. By binding to a site on the calcium-sensing receptor, the calcimimetic increases the affinity of the calcium receptor for extracellular calcium. The result is an increase in intracellular calcium and thus reductions in PTH synthesis and secretion. Even though the drug has not yet been approved for use for PHPT in the United States, early data are promising. The serum calcium concentration typically becomes normal and remains within normal limits for as long as the drug is used. Interestingly, the serum PTH level falls only modestly and continues to be elevated despite correction of the hypercalcemia by the drug.

Hypoparathyroidism

Hypoparathyroidism is much more uncommon than is PHPT. It results from the destruction, removal, or dysfunction of all parathyroid tissue.

ETIOLOGY

The most common causes of hypoparathyroidism are neck surgery and an autoimmune process (Table 3). Surgical hypoparathyroidism can follow the operation by many years and can occur after any neck surgery. Autoimmune destruction of the parathyroid glands can occur in an isolated fashion or in connection with a variety of polyglandular syndromes. The two major forms are type I (multiple endocrine gland failure along with candidiasis, pernicious anemia, and/or alopecia) and type II (with adrenal or thyroid failure and/or diabetes mellitus). Activating mutations of the calcium-sensing receptor or of the parathyroid gene itself can be associated with hypoparathyroidism. Parathyroid gland destruction is rarely due to infiltration of the glands by iron, copper, granulomas, or malignancy. In severe magnesium deficiency, parathyroid secretion is impaired along with a peripheral resistance to the actions of PTH. Mild hypoparathyroidism can become symptomatic in the presence of a potent bisphosphonate such as alendronate.

TABLE 3 Causes of Hypoparathyroidism

Parathyroid gland destruction
  Postsurgical
  Autoimmune
    Sporadic
    Polyglandular syndromes
  Activating antibodies against the calcium-sensing receptor
  Infiltration
    Iron, copper
    Malignancy
    Granulomatous
Genetic
  Activating mutations of the calcium-sensing receptor
  Inactivating mutations in the PTH gene
  DiGeorge syndrome
Impaired secretion and/or action of PTH
  Hypomagnesemia
Pseudohypoparathyroidism

Abbreviation: PTH = parathyroid hormone.

CLINICAL FEATURES

Increased neuromuscular irritability is the clinical hallmark of hypoparathyroidism. Features of hypoparathyroidism can range from mild paresthesias around the mouth, fingers, and toes to muscle cramping, and, at their worst, carpal, pedal, or laryngospasm. Central nervous system seizure activity is also seen as a severe manifestation of hypocalcemia. These symptoms are due, in part, to the actual serum calcium level but also to the rate at which the serum calcium level falls. Rapid declines in the serum calcium concentrations are more likely to be associated with symptoms than to situations in which the serum calcium concentration has fallen gradually. If respiratory or metabolic alkalosis is present, symptoms can worsen because the partition between bound and free calcium is shifted to the bound state when the blood pH rises. Signs of hypocalcemia include the Chvostek sign (evoked facial nerve irritability), the Trousseau sign (carpal spasm when the blood pressure cuff is inflated to pressures above systolic), and a prolonged QT interval on the electrocardiogram. When severe hypocalcemia is present, impaired cardiac contractility, unresponsive to inotropic agents until the hypocalcemia is corrected, has been reported. Pseudopapilledema and subcapsular cataracts can be seen. In some individuals, hypoparathyroidism is detected only by an asymptomatic reduction in the serum calcium concentration. Pseudohypoparathyroidism is a group of genetic disorders of the PTH receptor/G-protein transduction system responsible for PTH action. In the type I variant, subjects have a classic phenotype (Albright's hereditary osteodystrophy) with short stature, brachydactyly, subcutaneous and basal ganglia calcifications, rounded facies, shortened neck, seizures, and below-average intelligence. Other endocrine glands, such as the thyroid and gonads, can also be dysfunctional. In the type II form of pseudohypoparathyroidism, PHT resistance is present in the absence of the clinical phenotype.

DIAGNOSIS

Hypocalcemia and an elevated serum phosphorus concentration in association with absent PTH levels confirm the diagnosis of hypoparathyroidism. In pseudohypoparathyroidism, PTH levels are elevated, reflecting the PTH-resistant state, but otherwise the biochemical findings of hypocalcemia and hyperphosphatemia are similar to those of hypoparathyroidism. The urinary calcium concentration is usually not elevated because the filtered load of calcium is low, but actually renal handling of calcium is impaired in this setting because of the lack of PTH. Such individuals have an increase in urinary calcium for the given filtered calcium load, even though the actual amount of urinary calcium excretion might not be excessive.

TREATMENT

The goals of treatment are to establish a serum calcium concentration that is not associated with symptoms or signs and to prevent long-term complications of hypocalcemia. Acute, symptomatic hypocalcemia is a medical emergency and must be treated urgently. The management of chronic hypocalcemia follows a different set of guidelines.

Acute Management

The initial approach is to infuse intravenously 1 to 2 ampules of calcium gluconate (90–180 mg of elemental calcium), diluted in 50 to 100 mL of 5% dextrose over a 10- to 15-minute period. If the acute symptoms are not quickly ameliorated, another 1 to 2 ampules can be administered. To raise the serum calcium concentration further, but more gradually, an infusion of 15 mg/kg of calcium gluconate in 1 L of 5% dextrose over 8 to 10 hours will raise the serum calcium concentration by 2 to 3 mg/dL. Because 1 ampule of calcium gluconate contains 90 mg of elemental calcium, 9 to 11 ampules of calcium gluconate are required for an average-size adult (60–70 kg). The serum calcium concentration should be monitored frequently. If the hypocalcemia is due to magnesium deficiency, these measures are also appropriate while magnesium is being replaced. Acute administration of magnesium without calcium will not immediately correct hypocalcemia because peripheral resistance to PTH, one component of hypocalcemia induced by magnesium deficiency, is not corrected for several days. Intravenous replacement of magnesium is 2.4 mg/kg, up to 180 mg, over a 10-minute period or a continuous infusion of 576 mg of magnesium over 24 hours.

Chronic Management

Oral calcium supplementation is required in virtually all patients. The amount varies but is generally in the range of 1 to 3 g in divided doses. The carbonate or citrated form of calcium is most commonly used. Calcium carbonate is generally preferred because it contains the highest amount of elemental calcium. When calcium preparations are given with meals, both the carbonate and the citrated form of calcium are equally bioavailable. The presence of food obviates the need for gastric acid when calcium carbonate is used.

Most patients also require vitamin D. The amount of ergocalciferol (vitamin D_2) or cholecalciferol (vitamin D_3) ranges from 25,000 to 200,000 IU daily (1.25–10 mg). These large amounts are required because the absence of PTH and hyperphosphatemia both limit the amount of vitamin D that ultimately is converted to 1,25-dihydroxy-vitamin D, the active metabolite in the kidney. Because activation of vitamin D is impaired, much more vitamin D is required. There is no impairment of the first activation step in the liver, namely, from vitamin D to 25-hydroxyvitamin D, the storage form. Because there is no impairment in this step, large amounts of 25-hydroxyvitamin D can accumulate in fat tissues. At times and unpredictably, these stores can be mobilized and lead to hypercalcemia. Sometimes, the hypercalcemia is severe, requiring emergent treatment. Other times, a simple adjustment in the amount of calcium and/or vitamin D is sufficient. In any event, patients receiving large doses of vitamin D should always be regularly monitored for serum calcium concentrations approximately every 3 to 6 months.

Although many patients with hypoparathyroidism can be adequately managed with oral calcium and vitamin D, other patients also require therapy with 1,25-dihydroxyvitamin D, the active metabolite of vitamin D. 1,25-Dihydroxyvitamin D is used in addition to, but not in place of, vitamin D because 1,25-dihydroxyvitamin D alone does not provide for smooth control. Perhaps this is because 1,25-dihydroxyvitamin D is not stored to any appreciable extent in fat tissue. The half-life of 1,25-dihydroxyvitamin D is as short as 6 hours. Therefore, patients managed without parent vitamin D but with 1,25-dihydroxyvitamin D as the only source of vitamin D are more likely to have unpredictable fluctuations in serum calcium concentration. The amount of 1,25-dihydroxyvitamin D ranges from 0.5 to 1.0 μg/day. Some patients require more. Enhanced gastrointestinal absorption of calcium with 1,25-dihydroxyvitamin D can lead to hypercalciuria because in hypoparathyroidism there is no PTH to facilitate calcium reabsorption in the renal tubule. Urinary calcium should be checked on a regular basis. If hypercalciuria occurs, the dose of 1,25-dihydroxyvitamin D and/or vitamin D should be adjusted downward. In this situation, a thiazide diuretic such as hydrochlorothiazide[1] can be used to reduce urinary calcium excretion. In pseudohypoparathyroidism, hypercalciuria is less likely to occur because PTH is present and does have some renal effects in reabsorbing filtered calcium.

Another reason for variability in the control of serum calcium concentration in hypoparathyroidism is a change in medications. For example, if a thiazide or loop diuretic is started for hypertension, the serum calcium concentration may increase or decrease, respectively. Glucocorticoids can lead to a reduction in the serum calcium concentration because glucocorticoids interfere with vitamin D action in the gastrointestinal tract. Bile-sequestering resins can interfere with vitamin D absorption. Midcycle changes in estrogen levels in premenopausal women can lead to altered control.

Hypoparathyroidism is one of the few endocrine disorders for which the replacement hormone, namely, PTH, is not yet available, but it is being studied in some clinical trials.

---

[1]Not FDA approved for this indication.

REFERENCES

Arnold A, Shattuck TM, Mallya SM, et al. Molecular pathogenesis of primary hyperparathyroidism. J Bone Miner Res 2002;17(Suppl. 2):N30–6.

Bilezikian JP, Khan AA, Potts JT Jr. 2009 Guidelines for the Management of Asymptomatic Primary Hyperparathyroidism: Summary Statement from the Third International Workshop. J Clin Endocrinol Metab 2009;94:335–9.

Bilezikian JP, Silverberg SJ. Primary hyperparathyroidism. In: Rosen C, editor. Primer on the Metabolic Bone Diseases and Disorders of Calcium Metabolism. 7th ed. Am Soc Bone Min Research. 2008. p. 302–6.

Eastell R, Arnold A, Brandi ML, et al. 2009 Diagnosis of Asymptomatic Primary Hyperparathyroidism: Proceedings of the Third International Workshop. J Clin Endocrinol Metab 2009;94:340–50.

Grey A, Lucas J, Horne A, et al. Vitamin D repletion in patients with primary hyperparathyroidism and coexistent vitamin D insufficiency. J Clin Endocrinol Metab 2005;90:2122–6.

Khan AA, Bilezikian JP, Kung AWC, et al. Alendronate in primary hyperparathyroidism: a double-blind, randomized, placebo-controlled trial. J Clin Endocrinol Metab 2004;89:3319–25.

Lowe H, McMahon DJ, Rubin MR, et al. Normocalcemic primary hyperparathyroidism: further characterization of a new clinical phenotype. J Clin Endocrinol Metab 2007;92:3001–5.

Marx SJ. Hyperparathyroid and hypoparathyroid disorders. N Engl J Med 2000;343:1863–75.

Peacock M, Bilezikian JP, Klassen PS, et al. Cinacalcet hydrochloride maintains long-term normocalcemia in patients with primary hyperparathyroidism. J Clin Endocrinol Metab 2005;90:135–41.

Rubin MR, Bilezikian JP, McMahon DJ, et al. The natural history of primary hyperparathyroidism with or without parathyroid surgery after 15 years. J Clin Endocrinol Metab 2008;93:3462–70.

Rubin MR, Dempster DW, Zhou H, et al. Dynamic and structural properties of the skeleton in hypoparathyroidism. J Bone Miner Res 2008;23:2018–24.

Silverberg S, Bilezikian JP. The diagnosis and management of asymptomatic primary hyperparathyroidism. Nat Clin Practice Endocrinol Metab 2006;2:494–503.

Silverberg SJ, Lewiecki EM, Mosekilde L, et al. 2009 Presentation of Asymptomatic Primary Hyperparathyroidism: Proceedings of the Third International Workshop. J Clin Endocrinol Metab 2009;94:351–65.

Primary Aldosteronism

Method of
Beejal Shah, MD, and Lawrence Chan, MD

Primary Aldosteronism

Aldosterone was first discovered in 1952, and Jerome W. Conn described the first case of primary aldosteronism (PA) in 1954. PA is a state of excess aldosterone secreted autonomously of the renin-angiotensin system. It is the most common cause of secondary hypertension, and recent reports suggest that 5% to 20% of hypertensive patients have PA, a result of increased awareness and screening. It is a curable form of hypertension but, if left untreated, can result in renal, cardiovascular, and cerebrovascular morbidity greater than that seen in age-matched controls with essential hypertension.

CAUSES OF PRIMARY ALDOSTERONISM

The most common cause of PA is an adrenal adenoma autonomously producing aldosterone or hyperfunctioning adrenal nodules (usually bilateral) producing aldosterone. Less common causes of PA are listed in Box 1.

CLINICAL PRESENTATION

The classic clinical presentation of a patient with PA in the past was hypertension and hypokalemia; however, most patients with PA (60%) are hypertensive and normokalemic with inappropriate

Most Common
- Aldosterone-producing adenoma
- Bilateral adrenal hyperplasia or idiopathic hyperaldosteronism

Less Common
- Unilateral hyperplasia or primary adrenal hyperplasia
- Familial hyperaldosteronism type 1 or glucocorticoid remedial aldosteronism
- Familial hyperaldosteronism type 2
- Aldosterone-producing adrenocortical carcinoma
- Ectopic aldosterone-secreting tumor (ovary, kidney)
- Multiple endocrine neoplasia type 1

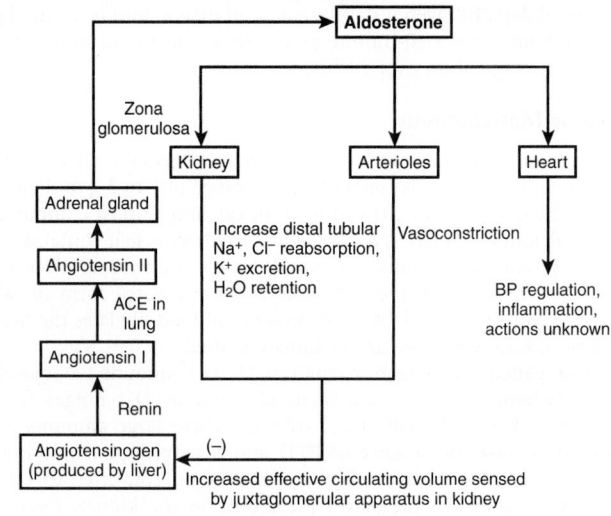

FIGURE 1. The renin-angiotensin-aldosterone system (RAAS). *Abbreviations:* ACE = angiotensin-converting enzyme; BP = blood pressure.

aldosterone excess. All patients with PA have hypertension, which can be severe but is rarely malignant. If a patient does present with hypokalemia, then aldosterone excess may be severe and the patient may have symptoms of hypokalemia (if <2.5 mEq/L), such as muscle weakness and disorientation. Patients with PA usually do not develop edema, because there is preserved hormonal balance of sodium wasting with sodium retention (mineralocorticoid escape). Less often, patients present with left ventricular hypertrophy, albuminuria, or retinopathy. PA patients have greater cardiovascular morbidity and mortality than patients with essential hypertension; however, once their condition is appropriately treated, they have no excess cardiovascular risk beyond the general population.

PATIENT SCREENING CRITERIA

Any patient who fulfills any of the following profiles should be screened for PA (reported prevalence included when known):

- Joint National Commission (JNC) 7 stage 2 hypertension (≥160–179 mm Hg systolic, ≥100–109 mm Hg diastolic), prevalence 8%
- JNC 7 stage 3 hypertension (≥180/110 mm Hg), prevalence 13%
- Drug-resistant hypertension, prevalence 17% to 23%
- Hypertension and spontaneous or diuretic-induced hypokalemia
- Hypertension and family history of early-onset hypertension or cerebrovascular accident at a young age (<40 years)
- Family members with PA
- Adrenal incidentaloma and hypertension, median prevalence 2%

Patients with essential hypertension who are not included in these criteria should not be routinely screened for PA.

PATHOPHYSIOLOGY

Aldosterone is a hormone produced by the zona glomerulosa in the adrenal gland. It is part of the renin-angiotensin-aldosterone system (RAAS). Normally, low plasma volume, reduction in effective circulation volume, or a low glomerular filtration rate (GFR) is sensed by the zona glomerulosa and stimulates renin production, which initiates the RAAS cascade (Fig. 1). Aldosterone acts at the distal nephron, where it stimulates sodium reabsorption and potassium excretion. Mineralocorticoid receptors are present at high levels in the distal nephron, but they also occur in other tissues, including the heart.

A negative feedback mechanism exists in the kidney at the juxtaglomerular apparatus, which responds to volume expansion and vasoconstriction by decreasing renin secretion and consequently decreasing aldosterone production. PA is therefore a low-renin state, as opposed to secondary aldosteronism, which is a high-renin state as seen in cases of renovascular hypertension and diuretic therapy. Under abnormal physiology, there is autonomous adrenal production of aldosterone despite an appropriately suppressed renin, which results in excess sodium reabsorption, hypokalemia, water retention, and hypertension.

HYPOKALEMIA

The prevalence of hypokalemia in PA is vastly overestimated. It is found in fewer than 40% of patients with PA, with APA being the subtype majority. The etiology of hypokalemia in PA is threefold. First, hyperaldosteronism causes potassium secretion from principal cells into the lumen of the cortical collecting tubule, resulting in urinary potassium wasting. Second, increasing sodium intake exacerbates hypokalemia, because the associated volume expansion does not appropriately suppress aldosterone production. Third, many PA patients are not hypokalemic under basal conditions, probably because a new steady state may occur wherein the potassium-wasting effect of hyperaldosteronism (due to increasing sodium absorption) is counterbalanced by the physiologic potassium-retaining effect of hypokalemia itself. PA also causes metabolic alkalosis, mild hypernatremia, hypomagnesemia, and increased urinary albumin excretion, which in two case series resolved with treatment of PA but not in patients with essential hypertension.

BIOCHEMICAL TESTS

An early-morning (8–9 AM) plasma aldosterone level is most accurate. Measurement of urine aldosterone excretion over 24 hours (from 8–9 AM to the next morning) is also useful. The aldosterone secretion rate has many drawbacks and therefore is not clinically useful.

Renin cleaves circulating angiotensinogen into angiotensin and is measured in terms of this enzymatic activity, called plasma renin activity (PRA). Current assays are very sensitive; the normal range is laboratory dependent but usually very low. All normal ranges for any assay are dependent on hydration, posture, and salt intake. Angiotensin I and II assays are neither sensitive nor specific and are rarely used.

Screening Test for Primary Aldosteronism

A quick and inexpensive screening test for PA is the ratio of plasma aldosterone concentration (PAC) to the PRA. A positive test is a PAC/PRA ratio equal to or greater than 20, or 30 for greater specificity. The PAC should be greater than 15 ng/dL to avoid a false-positive result, because the PRA is almost always very low or undetectable, which can raise the PAC/PRA ratio. If the PRA is greater than 1 ng/mL/hour, then PA is very unlikely.

The sensitivity of the PAC/PRA ratio is about 87%, and the specificity is 75%, when the patient is off medications that affect the ratio. There is no consensus on cutoff values for PRA, PAC, or the PAC/PRA ratio, so the sensitivity and specificity of this test change

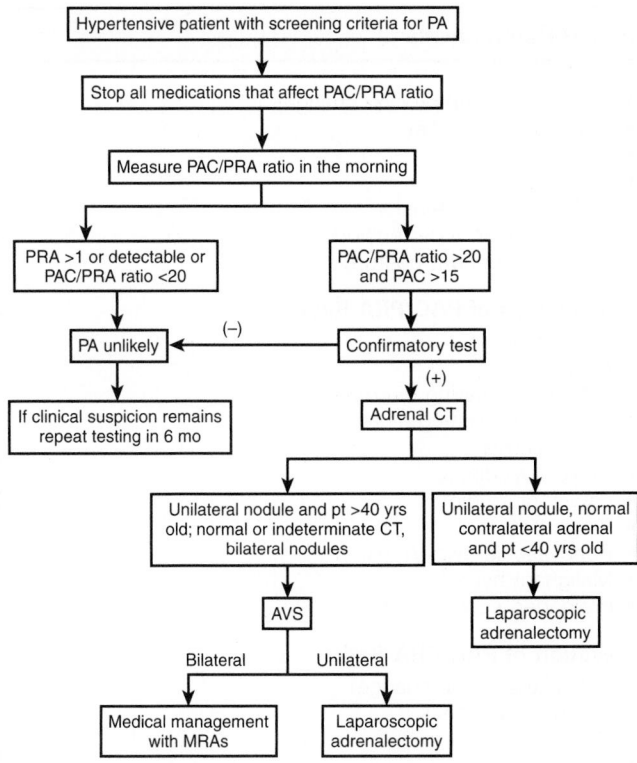

FIGURE 2. Evaluation of primary aldosteronism (PA). *Abbreviations:* AVS = adrenal vein sampling; CT = computed tomography; MAs = mineralocorticoid receptor antagonists; PAC = plasma aldosterone concentration; PRA = plasma renin activity; pt = patient.

depends on the cutoff values used. Inconclusive results should be repeated, and once a positive screening test establishes hyperaldosteronism, a confirmatory test should be performed (Fig. 2).

Protocol for the PAC/PRA Screening Test

Performing the screening test under correct conditions is the most important step in establishing the diagnosis of PA. The following drugs should be withdrawn at least 4 weeks, and ideally 6 weeks, before testing: spironolactone (Aldactone), eplerenone (Inspra), amiloride (Midamor), triamterene (Dyrenium), potassium-losing diuretics, and licorice-derived products.[7] Angiotensin-converting enzyme inhibitors (ACEIs), angiotensin receptor blockers (ARBs), and renin inhibitors should be withdrawn 2 weeks before testing. If ACEIs, ARBs, or diuretics are continued, the PRA will be falsely elevated. In this situation, a detectable PRA or a low PAC/PRA ratio does not exclude PA. However, if the PRA is undetectable while the patient is on ACEIs, ARBs, or diuretics, suspicion of PA is increased. If needed, hypertensive medications that do not affect the RAAS system can be substituted (Box 2).

Before testing, the hypokalemia is corrected and liberal salt intake is encouraged. Hypokalemia decreases aldosterone levels, and a low salt diet increases aldosterone levels. For utmost accuracy, PAC and PRA should be measured between 8 and 10 AM (because aldosterone has a diurnal variation), with the patient ambulatory just before the venipuncture and recumbent for the blood draw. If the PAC/PRA is nondiagnostic, the test is repeated with the following drugs also withdrawn for at least 1 to 2 weeks: β-blockers, central α₂-agonists, nonsteroidal antiinflammatory drugs, and dihydropyridine calcium channel blockers.

Imperative to diagnostic testing and its interpretation is understanding of the factors that can affect the aldosterone and renin levels (see Box 2). All medications that affect the ratio should be stopped.

Low sodium intake and upright posture increase PRA and increase PAC, whereas high sodium intake and supine posture decrease both PRA and PAC.

The elimination of factors that affect the PAC/PRA ratio pertains most to patients who in actuality do not have PA despite clinical suspicion. A false-positive or false-negative result can lead to diagnostic and therapeutic misadventures. In patients with PA, the aldosterone secretion is autonomous from RAAS, regardless of influencing factors, so the PAC/PRA ratio should remain high despite elimination of such factors. However, because the physician does not know which patients ultimately have true disease, the screening protocol must be followed.

Confirmatory Testing for Primary Aldosteronism

The confirmatory test is aimed at suppressing aldosterone, which rules out PA. However, there is no gold standard confirmatory test. To confirm PA, patients undergo an oral salt loading test, a saline suppression test, or, more rarely, a fludrocortisone (Florinef)[1] suppression test or a captopril (Capoten)[1] challenge test.

Oral Sodium Loading Test

PROTOCOL

The protocol for the oral sodium loading test is as follows:

1. Hold all pertinent blood pressure medications (see Box 2).
2. Place the patient on a high-sodium diet (2 g NaCl tablets every 6 hours) for 3 days.
3. Replace potassium to compensate for the kaliuresis induced by the high-sodium diet.
4. Collect a 24-hour urine sample (morning to morning) for determination of aldosterone, sodium, and creatinine. The urine collection is adequate if the urine sodium over 24 hours is greater than 200 mmol/day.

INTERPRETATION OF RESULTS

PA is confirmed if the 24-hour urine aldosterone concentration is greater than 33 nmol or 12 to 14 μg. PA is ruled out if the 24-hour urine aldosterone is less than 10 ng, and the test is equivocal if the value falls in between 10 and 12 ng/24 hr. This test has a sensitivity of 96% and a specificity of 93%. Alternatively, an 8 AM aldosterone level can be determined in place of a 24-hour urine collection on the morning of day 3, and a cut off value of 7 ng/dL or higher confirms PA. An 8 AM aldosterone level greater than 7 ng/dL has a sensitivity of 88% and a specificity of 100% if the screening PAC/PRA ratio is greater than 40, although this varies.

PRECAUTION

Do not perform this test in patients with severe uncontrolled hypertension, renal failure, cardiac failure, cardiac arrhythmias, or severe hypokalemia.

Intravenous Saline Infusion Test

PROTOCOL

1. Hold all pertinent blood pressure medications (see Box 2).
2. Place the patient supine 1 hour before drawing blood for morning baseline fasting levels of renin, aldosterone, cortisol, and potassium.
3. Start an infusion of 2 L 0.9% sodium chloride over 4 hours, keeping the patient supine.
4. Monitor for increased blood pressure and heart rate.
5. After 4 hours, draw a blood sample for measurement of renin, aldosterone, cortisol, and potassium.

INTERPRETATION OF RESULTS

PA is ruled out if the PAC is suppressed to less than 5 ng/dL or 139 pmol/L. PA is biochemically confirmed if the PAC after saline infusion is greater than 10 ng/dL or 277 pmol/L. If the PAC falls between these values, the test is equivocal.

---

[7] Available as dietary supplement.

[1] Not FDA approved for this indication.

BOX 2 Medications and Factors That Affect Aldosterone and Renin Levels

Decrease Renin Level
- β-Blockers
- Central α₂-agonists
- NSAIDs
- Renin inhibitors (when renin is measured as PRA)
- Potassium loading (or no change)
- High-sodium diet
- Aging (>65 y)
- Renal failure
- Prolonged supine posture

Increase Renin Level
- Potassium-wasting diuretics
- ACE inhibitors
- ARBs
- Dihydropyridines (mild elevation)
- Hypokalemia (or no change)
- Pregnancy
- Low-sodium diet
- Renovascular hypertension
- Malignant hypertension
- Prolonged upright posture

Decrease Aldosterone Levels
- β-Blockers
- Central α₂-agonists
- NSAIDs
- ACE inhibitors
- ARBs
- Dihydropyridines (or no change)
- Renin inhibitors
- Hypokalemia
- High-sodium diet
- Aging (>65 y)
- Prolonged supine posture

Increase Aldosterone Levels
- Potassium-wasting diuretics (or no change)
- Potassium-sparing diuretics

- Dihydropyridones (or no change)
- High-potassium diet
- Low-sodium diet
- Pregnancy
- Malignant hypertension
- Renovascular hypertension
- Prolonged upright posture

Suppression of PAC/PRA Ratio
- ACE inhibitors
- ARBs
- Potassium-sparing diuretics
- Potassium-wasting diuretics
- Hypokalemia
- Dihydropyridines
- Low-sodium diet
- Pregnancy
- Renovascular hypertension
- Malignant hypertension
- Prolonged supine posture

Elevation of PAC/PRA Ratio
- β-Blockers (or no change)
- Central α₂-agonists
- NSAIDs
- Renin inhibitors
- High-potassium diet
- High-sodium diet
- Renal failure
- Upright posture
- Aging (>65 y)

Minimal Effect on PAC/PRA Ratio
- Verapamil slow release (Calan SR)
- Hydralazine (Apresoline)
- Prazosin (Minipress)
- Doxasozin (Cardura)
- Terazosin (Hytrin)

Abbreviations: ACE = angiotensin converting enzyme; ARBs = angiotensin receptor blockers; NSAIDs = nonsteroidal antiinflammatory drugs; PAC = plasma aldosterone concentration; PRA = plasma renin activity.

PRECAUTION

Do not conduct this test in patients with severe uncontrolled hypertension, renal failure, cardiac failure, cardiac arrhythmias, or severe hypokalemia.

Fludrocortisone Suppression Test

PROTOCOL

1. Give 0.1 mg fludrocortisone (Florinef)[1] every 6 hours for 4 days, with the potassium level checked every 6 hours to be sure that it is greater than 4 mmol/L. Encourage a liberal sodium diet to keep urinary sodium excretion greater than 3 mmol/kg/day.
2. On day 4, draw blood for an upright 7 AM plasma cortisol level and a 10 AM upright plasma aldosterone, renin, and cortisol levels.

INTERPRETATION OF RESULTS

PA is confirmed if the 10 AM PAC is greater than 6 ng/dL, as long as PRA is less than 1 ng/mL/hour and the plasma cortisol at 10 AM is less than at 7 AM.

PRECAUTION

Because of its risky nature, the test may require hospitalization. Risks include severe hypokalemia, QT changes on electrocardiography, worsening of left ventricular function, hypertension, and consequences of the frequent blood draws for potassium levels.

Captopril Challenge Test

PROTOCOL

1. The patient remains upright throughout the test.
2. Give 25 to 50 mg captopril (Capoten)[1] after the patient has been upright for 1 hour.
3. Draw blood for measurement of plasma renin, aldosterone, and cortisol at time 0, at 1 hour, and at 2 hours.

INTERPRETATION OF RESULTS

Normally, captopril suppresses PAC by more than 30% from baseline. PA is confirmed if there is no suppression of PAC. The false-negative rate for this test is high, because suppression occurs in more than

---

[1]Not FDA approved for this indication.

[1]Not FDA approved for this indication.

CURRENT DIAGNOSIS

- Screen patients with the following criteria: Joint National Commission (JNC) 7 stage 2 or 3 hypertension, young age, hypertension and spontaneous or diuretic-induced hypokalemia, significant family history for hypertension or primary aldosteronism (PA), or adrenal incidentaloma and hypertension.

- Measure a morning plasma aldosterone concentration (PAC, in ng/dL) and plasma renin activity (PRA, in ng/mL/hour) with the patient in a sodium- and potassium-repleted state and off spironolactone (Aldactone), eplerenone (Inspra), amiloride (Midamor), triamterene (Dyrenium), potassium-losing diuretics, and licorice-derived products[7] for at least 4 to 6 weeks.

- A positive screening test result is a PAC/PRA ratio equal to or greater than 20 to 40 with a PRA <1 ng/mL/hr and a PAC equal to or greater than 15 ng/dL.

- Perform a confirmatory test for PA with a saline suppression, oral salt loading, fludrocortisone (Florinef)[1] suppression, or captopril (Capoten)[1] challenge test.

- If the confirmatory test is positive, proceed to computed tomography (CT) of the adrenal glands to subtype the PA, which most often is caused by an aldosterone-producing adrenal adenoma or bilateral adrenal hyperplasia, and to exclude adrenal cortical carcinoma.

- Perform adrenal vein sampling on all patients with biochemically confirmed PA unless the patient is younger than 40 years of age and has a CT-confirmed adrenal nodule larger than 1 to 2 cm and a normal contralateral adrenal on imaging.

---

[1]Not FDA approved for this indication.
[7]Available as dietary supplement.

30% of PA patients. A slight decrease in aldosterone can suggest bilateral adrenal hyperplasia or idiopathic hyperaldosteronism (a subtype of PA). Overall, this is a poor confirmatory test because of the high proportion of false-negative or equivocal results.

Summary of Confirmatory Tests

In summary, there is insufficient evidence-based data to support one PA confirmatory test over another. Therefore, factors such as cost, accessibility, feasibility, patient compliance, local expertise, and accuracy of assay testing at the institution should play a role in determining which test is best.

DETERMINING THE CAUSE OF PRIMARY ALDOSTERONISM

The two most common causes of PA are BAH, also known as idiopathic hyperaldosteronism, and aldosterone-producing adenomas (APAs). These entities cannot be differentiated biochemically or clinically. The next step in the workup of biochemically positive PA is adrenal imaging to determine the etiology or subtype of PA.

Imaging Studies

Computed Tomography and Magnetic Resonance Imaging

Radiologic studies are critical to differentiate unilateral from bilateral adrenal nodules or APA from BAH. The next test after a positive confirmatory test for PA is computed tomography (CT). In most institutions, CT is the test of choice for reasons of cost and availability,

compared to magnetic resonance imaging (MRI). CT can confirm an adrenal adenoma and can place BAH as a diagnosis of exclusion, but there is significant variation in sensitivity with both imaging modalities. The sensitivity of adrenal CT is only 53% to 73%, whereas MRI has a sensitivity of 70% to 100%. The lack of sensitivity in CT is a result of the 5-mm cuts, which often miss very small adenomas. Up to 20% of adenomas in series of 143 cases were smaller than 1 cm. Specificity is limited because of a high prevalence of adrenal incidentalomas, the possibility of a dominant nodule in macronodular BAH, and increasing adrenal nodularity with age and hypertension.

The results of a CT or MRI scan of the adrenals can lead to one of five conclusions: normal adrenals, unilateral macroadenoma (>1 cm), minimal unilateral adrenal limb thickening, unilateral microadenoma (≤1 cm), and bilateral macroadenomas and/or microadenomas. Adenomas are typically smaller than 2 cm, and BAH exhibits either normal or nodular adrenals on CT. However, adrenal hyperplasia could be misread as microadenomas, which could lead to an unnecessary surgery. Also, nonfunctioning unilateral adrenal adenomas are radiologically indistinguishable from APA on CT. Although imaging criteria exist for an adrenal adenoma, no study has conclusively established specific criteria that differentiate a nonfunctioning from a hyperfunctioning adenoma.

One study using CT or MRI suggested measurement of mean adrenal limb width as a differentiating criterion for BAH. Mean adrenal limb width was found to be larger in BAH compared with APA and normal adrenals. Lingam and colleagues recently proposed that a measured mean adrenal limb width of 5 mm or greater confirms BAH regardless of whether a nodule was seen on imaging. If the CT or MRI showed a nodule and the mean adrenal limb width is 3 mm or less, APA is confirmed. If the mean adrenal width is between 3 and 5 mm, then adrenal vein sampling (AVS) should be done, regardless of the presence of a nodule on imaging. In Lingam's study, this algorithm had a 100% specificity and 100% sensitivity for BAH. However, it was a small study, most patients still required AVS, and the results need confirmation by larger studies.

NP-59 Adrenal Scintigraphy

The NP-59 (iodocholesterol) nuclear medicine scan assesses adrenal hyperfunction, but its use should only be supplementary to CT, MRI, and AVS in difficult cases, to differentiate functioning from nonfunctioning adenomas, or if there are bilateral nodules on CT. After stopping all pertinent medications and 7 days before the scan, dexamethasone (Decadron) suppression (1 mg every 6 hours) is given to enhance sensitivity. Adrenal imaging begins on day 4 and can continue to day 10, until the NP-59 is taken up by the adrenal glands. Early (<5 days) unilateral uptake is consistent with APA. Symmetrical early uptake (<5 days) suggests BAH, whereas symmetrical late uptake (>5 days) suggests normal adrenal glands. A negative adrenal scintigraphy scan does not rule out BAH or APA. Sensitivity of the test for functional adenomas varies widely, and smaller adenomas (<1.5 cm) can be missed by NP-59, because its uptake correlates with adrenal volume.

Summary of Imaging

A multimodality approach can be used to diagnose the cause of PA; however, to date no specific imaging algorithm has established proven superiority.

Adrenal Vein Sampling

AVS is the gold standard for diagnosing the cause of PA and is often essential, given the limited sensitivity and specificity of imaging. In more recent years, its popularity and usefulness have dramatically increased due to greater operator skill. It should be performed only by physicians experienced with AVS. Complications of AVS include adrenal hemorrhage, adrenal infarction, adrenal vein perforation, and adrenal vein thrombosis, which all occur only rarely in the hands of a skilled physician.

Indications for Adrenal Vein Sampling

It is important to include patients who would otherwise have unnecessary adrenalectomies without AVS, as well as those who otherwise would be excluded from surgery if CT or the biochemical work-up pointed toward BAH. Debate still exists as to whether bilateral AVS should be performed on all patients. The only situation in which a PA patient can go directly to adrenalectomy without AVS is if the patient meets all of the following criteria: solitary, unilateral, small, hypodense macroadenoma (>1 cm); normal contralateral adrenal on CT; and age less than 40 years.

AVS should be performed only after biochemical confirmation of inappropriate aldosterone excess. There are several indications for AVS, including CT/MRI scan showing normal adrenals, unilateral nodules smaller than 1 cm, bilateral macronodules, minimal unilateral adrenal limb thickening on CT/MRI, and age older than 40 years (because older patients have a higher incidence of nonfunctioning adrenal adenomas).

Performing the Adrenal Vein Sampling Test

RECOMMENDED PROTOCOL

1. After both adrenal veins have been cannulated, draw baseline samples for PAC, adrenocorticotropic hormone (ACTH), cortisol, and PRA from the inferior vena cava (IVC), right adrenal vein, and left adrenal vein.
2. Inject 250 µg ACTH (cosyntropin, Cortrosyn) after cannulation, or infuse 50 µg cosyntropin per hour beginning 30 minutes before adrenal vein cannulation. This reduces stress-related fluctuations in aldosterone and cortisol values and augments the biochemical gradients. This step is optional but is recommended.
3. Draw blood for aldosterone and cortisol levels at 5, 15, and 30 minutes from the peripheral site and each adrenal vein.

INTERPRETATION OF RESULTS

The use of cosyntropin stimulation is still controversial, and some believe that it has no effect on AVS accuracy. If cosyntropin stimulation is performed, a ratio of aldosterone to stimulated cortisol is used to confirm proper cannulation and stimulation. If cosyntropin is not used, then AVS should be done in the morning, after overnight recumbency, to avoid postural changes in the aldosterone level and to obtain benefit from circadian aldosterone secretion.

Interpreting the Results of Adrenal Vein Sampling

First, determine whether the procedure was done correctly. If cosyntropin was given, the adrenal vein-to-IVC cortisol ratio should be greater than 10:1. Without cosyntropin, the adrenal vein-to-IVC cortisol ratio should be greater than 3:1. If the ratios are significantly less than these, improper cannulation is implied. Next, divide the PAC values for the right and left adrenal veins by their respective cortisol values; this is termed the cortisol-corrected aldosterone (A/C) ratio.

RESULTS THAT CONFIRM UNILATERAL ALDOSTERONE EXCESS

If the cosyntropin-stimulated A/C ratio in the vein of the affected side is at least fourfold higher than the ratio for the contralateral gland, or if the contralateral gland has a suppressed ratio, unilateral excess or APA is confirmed. The mean A/C ratio for APA is 18:1.

If cosyntropin stimulation was not done, unilateral aldosterone excess is confirmed if the A/C ratio on one side is 2.5-fold higher than in the periphery and the contralateral side is not higher than the periphery, indicating suppression of the contralateral side (Table 1).

RESULTS THAT CONFIRM BILATERAL ALDOSTERONE EXCESS

BAH is confirmed if the A/C ratio in each adrenal vein is greater than the A/C ratio in the IVC. If cosyntropin stimulation was used, an A/C ratio of less than 3:1 (i.e., the higher adrenal gland value is less than 3 times that of the lower adrenal gland) is suggestive of BAH. The mean comparison from the high to the low side is 1.8:1. If the comparison ratio is between 3:1 and 4:1, then it is unclear whether aldosterone excess production is bilateral or unilateral.

Without cosyntropin stimulation, a comparison of A/C ratios from the high side to the low side of less than 2:1 confirms BAH (see Table 1).

INTERPRETATION OF RESULTS WITH ONE ADRENAL VEIN CATHETERIZED

AVS results can still be interpreted if only one adrenal vein was catheterized. If the A/C ratio of the catheterized adrenal vein divided by the IVC A/C ratio is less than 1 or suppressed, an APA or primary adrenal hyperplasia on the contralateral side (noncatheterized side)

TABLE 1   Interpretation of Dynamic Testing

Test	Findings
Screening Test	
PAC/PRA ratio	Positive if >20–30 with PAC >15 ng/dL and PRA <1 ng/mL/h
Confirmatory Test for PA	
Oral sodium loading test	Positive if 24-h urine aldosterone excretion is >12–14 µg
Saline infusion test	Positive if PAC after infusion is >10 ng/dL
Fludrocortisone (Florinef)[1] suppression test	Positive if upright PAC is >7 ng/dL on day 4 at 10 AM
Captopril (Capoten)[1] challenge test	Positive if PAC does not decrease by 30% and PRA remains suppressed
Adrenal Vein Sampling	
After cosyntropin (Cortrosyn) stimulation	A/C ratio from high to low side >4:1: unilateral aldosterone excess
	A/C ratio 3:1 to 4:1: overlap zone
	A/C ratio <3:1: bilateral aldosterone excess
Without cosyntropin stimulation	A/C ratio in one adrenal vein is 2.5 times higher than in the peripheral vein (and in the contralateral adrenal vein is less than in the periphery): unilateral aldosterone excess
	A/C ratio from high to low side is <2:1: bilateral aldosterone excess
Diagnostic Tests if AVS Is Equivocal	
Recumbent 18-hydroxycorticosterone	A level >100 ng/dL is consistent with APA
Postural stimulation test	PAC falls or fails to rise by 30%: consistent with APA
	PAC increases by at least 33%: consistent with BAH
NP-59 iodocholesterol scintigraphy	Unilateral early uptake (<5 d): consistent with unilateral excess
	Bilateral early uptake (<5 d): consistent with bilateral aldosterone excess
	Negative scan does not rule out either etiology

[1]Not FDA approved for this indication.
Abbreviations: A/C ratio = cortisol-corrected aldosterone ratio; APA = aldosterone-producing adenomas; BAH = bilateral adrenal hyperplasia; PA = primary aldosteronism; PAC = plasma aldosterone concentration; PRA = plasma renin activity.

is confirmed. If the result is greater than 1, an adenoma or hyperplasia on the ipsilateral side or on both sides is confirmed. In the setting of only one catheterized vein, AVS results are not 100% accurate and should be placed in the context of the prior findings from the biochemical and imaging work-up.

FOLLOW-UP OF INCONCLUSIVE RESULTS

If the AVS results are inconclusive, there are three options: repeat AVS, treat medically, or obtain another diagnostic test, such as the postural stimulation test or a plasma 18-hydroxycorticosterone level.

Postural Stimulation Test. The postural stimulation test is a supplementary test for diagnosing the cause of PA. Aldosterone levels in APA have a preserved diurnal variation because APAs are ACTH responsive, but APA is not affected by angiotensin II. In contrast, BAH has increased sensitivity to angiotensin II that occurs with standing, causing a rise in the aldosterone level.

The protocol for the postural stimulation test is as follows:

1. With the patient supine, draw blood for measurement of 8 AM cortisol, renin, and aldosterone.
2. Ambulate the patient for 4 hours.
3. After 4 hours, with the patient upright, draw blood for measurement of upright plasma cortisol, renin, and aldosterone.

APA is diagnosed if the aldosterone level falls or fails to rise by 30% after 4 hours of ambulation. An aldosterone level that increases with standing (usually by 33%) is consistent with BAH.

The postural stimulation test has some important shortcomings. This test is valid only if the cortisol decreases between 8 AM and 12 PM, and its sensitivity is only 65% to 85% for APA. Moreover, some APAs are also angiotensin II sensitive, and some cases of BAH exhibit diurnal variation in aldosterone.

Plasma 18-Hydroxycorticosterone Level. Measured plasma 18-hydroxycorticosterone level can be a useful blood test if the results of prior testing are equivocal. 18-Hydroxycorticosterone is an immediate precursor of aldosterone or an end product formed after 18-hydroxylation of corticosterone.

A recumbent plasma 18-hydroxycorticosterone level greater than 100 ng/dL at 8 AM is consistent with APA. A level lower than 100 ng/dL is consistent with BAH. Again, the accuracy is less than 80%.

CHARACTERISTICS OF APA VERSUS BAH

Besides testing there are a few characteristic features of each disease that can be helpful towards establishing the cause of PA.

Patients with APA tend to be younger (<40 years), are predominantly female, are very hypertensive with marked hypokalemia (<3 mmol/L), have a very high PAC (>25 mg/dL), and have no change in the PAC after 4 hours of standing. Pathologically, APAs are distinct. They are typically yellowish, round, and smaller than 2 cm. It is important to pursue high specificity for diagnosing APA, to minimize false positive findings and subsequent unnecessary surgery. Unilateral primary adrenal hyperplasia is biochemically like unilateral adenoma but histologically like nodular hyperplasia. Both APA and primary adrenal hyperplasia are treated surgically.

In BAH, patients are older (>40 years), are moderately hypertensive with mild hypokalemia and modest elevations of aldosterone (<25 mg/dL), and their aldosterone level increases after 4 hours of standing. In BAH, the saline infusion test is more likely to be indeterminate. The adrenal glands are grossly enlarged and can be smooth, micronodular, or macronodular. Given this variability, some experts suggest that there is a spectrum to PA, with a solitary adrenal nodule at one end and BAH at the other end. In most cases, diagnosis is not straightforward and requires a combination of tests and imaging to confirm the source of PA.

TREATMENT OF PRIMARY ALDOSTERONISM

Treatment of PA is more straightforward than establishing its diagnosis. APA and unilateral adrenal hyperplasia are managed surgically with an adrenalectomy of the respective side, and BAH is managed medically with mineralocorticoid receptor antagonists (MRAs).

CURRENT THERAPY

- If the adrenal vein sampling (AVS) result lateralizes, with a cortisol-corrected aldosterone ratio (A/C ratio) from the high to the low side greater than 4:1, perform a laparoscopic adrenalectomy.
- If there is no lateralization on AVS, treat medically with a mineralocorticoid receptor antagonist, spironolactone (Aldactone), or eplerenone (Inspra).[1]
- Spironolactone: 12.5 to 25 mg/day titrated to a maximum dose of 400 mg/day to achieve normokalemia. Side effects are increased serum creatinine, gynecomastia, menstrual irregularities, erectile dysfunction, and hyperkalemia.
- Eplerenone: 25 mg once or twice daily titrated to a maximum dose of 100 mg/day to achieve normokalemia. Side effects are increased creatinine, hyperkalemia, hypertriglyceridemia, increased liver enzymes, headache, and fatigue.
- Other useful antihypertensive agents include thiazide diuretics, triamterene (Dyrenium),[1] and amiloride (Midamor).[1] The Ca^{+2} channel blockers, angiotensin-converting enzyme inhibitors, and angiotensin receptor blockers have not been as effective in lowering aldosterone levels but are an option for blood pressure control.

[1]Not FDA approved for this indication.

Aldosterone-Producing Adenomas and Unilateral Adrenal Hyperplasia

Adrenalectomy, usually laparoscopic, is the only successful treatment for APA and unilateral adrenal hyperplasia, but surgery alone is often not totally curative. After adrenalectomy, blood pressure improves in all patients, but 30% to 60% of patients have persistent hypertension.

MRAs, mainly spironolactone and eplerenone,[1] can be used to control blood pressure in patients awaiting adrenalectomy. Preoperatively, the patient should be normokalemic, and MRAs should be discontinued. Postoperatively, all MRAs, potassium supplements, and intravenous fluids should be discontinued. Also postoperatively, the serum potassium level should be kept at 3 mmol/L or higher and monitored weekly for 4 weeks. The patient is kept on a generous sodium diet to avoid hyperkalemia of hypoaldosteronism due to chronic suppression of the axis.

To confirm a biochemical cure, the PAC and PRA are checked every 3 to 5 days after surgery. If the surgery is successful and the patient indeed had an APA and not some element of BAH, the hypertension should resolve in 1 to 3 months. Risk factors for persistent hypertension after adrenalectomy include older age, duration of hypertension (>5 years), use of two or more antihypertensive agents preoperatively, blood pressure higher than 165/100 mm Hg, low PAC/PRA ratio preoperatively, low urine aldosterone, poor response to spironolactone preoperatively, family history of more than one first-degree relative with hypertension, and a raised serum creatinine concentration.

A few cases of successful CT-guided ablation and transarterial embolization of a presumed aldosteronoma have been reported. Side effects can be serious and include transient increase in blood pressure, fever, flank pain, pneumothorax, adrenal hematoma, and adrenal infarction. Also, in both procedures, the ablated lesion cannot be confirmed histologically.

Bilateral Adrenal Hyperplasia

Antihypertensive medications are the only treatment modality for BAH. However, there have been no randomized, double-blinded, placebo-controlled trials to evaluate the efficacy of drugs in the treatment of PA. The mainstay of treatment is MRAs.

[1]Not FDA approved for this indication.

Spironolactone is the most widely used MRA. It is very effective in decreasing blood pressure in PA. The medication is dosed initially at 12.5 to 25 mg daily and can be titrated to 400 mg/day, with most patients needing at least 200 mg daily. The patients should attain normokalemia without use of potassium supplements. Use of spironolactone is limited by side effects. In men, its antiandrogenic effects can cause gynecomastia, decreased libido and energy, galactorrhea, and hyperkalemia. In women, its progesterone effect can cause menstrual irregularities and hyperkalemia. Spironolactone increases the half-life of digoxin and should be taken separately from salicylates, because the latter decrease the effectiveness of spironolactone.

Eplerenone[1] is a steroid-based antimineralocorticoid that is competitive and selective for the aldosterone receptor; it was approved by the FDA in 2003 for children and adults. It has lower binding affinity to androgen and progesterone receptors than spironolactone. This leads to less antiandrogenic and progestational side effects. However, there are no trials comparing eplerenone with spironolactone. Dosing is started at 25 mg twice daily, with a maximum dose of 100 mg/day. Blood pressure, potassium, and creatinine are monitored. Possible side effects include dizziness, headache, fatigue, diarrhea, hypertriglyceridemia, and elevated liver enzymes. All MRAs are contraindicated in patients with hyperkalemia, a creatinine concentration greater than 2.0 mg/dL in men or 1.8 mg/dL in women, diabetes with microalbuminuria, or concomitant administration of strong cytochrome P-450 isoenzyme 3A4 inhibitors such as ketoconazole (Nizoral) or itraconazole (Sporanox).

Other useful antihypertensive agents are amiloride,[1] which is dosed at 10 to 20 mg PO daily in divided doses to normalize potassium. Side effects are dizziness, fatigue, and impotence. Triamterene (Dyrenium)[1] is dosed at 200 to 300 mg PO daily in divided doses, and its side effects are mainly dizziness and nausea. Patients with BAH may have hypervolemia, and addition of a thiazide diuretic (12.5–50 mg daily) is helpful. If blood pressure remains uncontrolled, other antihypertensive agents may be used. Potassium levels should be maintained at the upper limits of normal, with supplementation used only if MRAs are unable to maintain normokalemia. Potassium levels are monitored frequently the first 4 to 6 weeks after initiation of treatment, especially in renal and diabetic patients.

Nonpharmacologic treatment for both subtypes of PA includes aerobic exercise, smoking cessation, weight loss, and a low-sodium diet (<100 mEq/day).

Diagnosis and Treatment of Less Common Causes of Primary Aldosteronism

Glucocorticoid remedial aldosteronism (GRA) is a rare disease caused by a mutation of the aldosterone synthase gene. In GRA, aldosterone is ectopically produced in the zona fasciculata and regulated by ACTH (as opposed to normal production in the zona glomerulosa and regulation by angiotensin II). Clinically, most patients present with childhood hypertension, and 50% are normokalemic; the morning cortisol level is elevated, but patients are not cushingoid. Biochemically, elevated serum 18-hydroxycortisol and 18-oxocortisol concentrations are diagnostic for GRA. Genetic testing for GRA is recommended for PA patients who are younger than 20 years of age or have a family history of PA or stroke at a young age. Treatment for GRA is physiologic cortisol replacement in children, usually as a long-acting glucocorticoid given at bedtime to suppress morning ACTH, and MRAs can be given in place of steroids to avoid disruption of growth. The target blood pressure is age specific in children.

Familial hyperaldosteronism II is another rare cause of PA. It is an autosomal dominant, possibly genetically heterogeneous, disease. The aldosterone level does not suppress with dexamethasone, and the GRA mutation is absent. Patients with familial hyperaldosteronism II are clinically indistinguishable from those with APA or BAH.

---

[1]Not FDA approved for this indication.

REFERENCES

Auchus RJ, Chandler DW, Singeetham S, et al. Measurement of 18 hydroxysterone during adrenal vein sampling for primary aldosteronism. J Clin Endocrinol Metab 2007;92:2648–51.

Funder JW, Carey RM, Fardella C, et al. Case detection, diagnosis, and treatment of patients with primary aldosteronism: An Endocrine Society clinical practice guideline. J Clin Endocrinol Metab 2008;93:3266–81.

Ganguly A. Primary aldosteronism. N Engl J Med 1998;339:1828–34.

Lau JH, Drake W, Matson M. The current role of venous sampling in the localization of endocrine disease. Cardiovasc Intervent Radiol 2007;30:555–70.

Mulatero P, Bertello C, Rossato D, et al. Roles of clinical criteria, computed tomography scan, and adrenal vein sampling in differential diagnosis of primary aldosteronism subtypes. J Clin Endocrinol Metab 2008;93:1366–71.

Mulatero P, Milan A, Fallo F, et al. Comparison of confirmatory tests for the diagnosis of primary aldosteronism. J Clin Endocrinol Metab 2006;91:2618–23.

Patel SM, Lingam RK, Beaconsfield TI, et al. Role of radiology in the management of primary aldosteronism. Radiographics 2007;27:1145–57.

Schirpenbach C, Reinke M. Primary aldosteronism: Current knowledge and controversies in Conn's syndrome. Nat Clin Pract Endocrinol Metabol 2007;3:220–7.

Tiu SS, Choi CH, Shek CC, et al. The use of aldosterone-renin ratio as a diagnostic test for primary hyperaldosteronism and its test characteristics under different conditions in blood sampling. J Clin Endocrinol Metab 2005;90:72–8.

Young WF. Primary aldosteronism: Renaissance of a syndrome. Clin Endocrinol 2007;66:607–18.

Hypopituitarism

Method of

Erica V. Gonzalez, MD, and Susan L. Samson, MD, PhD

The Function of the Pituitary

The pituitary gland often is referred to as the master gland because of its central role in the function of the hypothalamic-pituitary-endocrine axis. It is housed in the sella turcica ("Turkish saddle") at the base of the skull. The anterior pituitary (adenohypophysis or pars anterior) develops as an upward evagination from the ectoderm of the oropharynx (Rathke's pouch) to meet the developing posterior pituitary (neurohypophysis or pars posterior), which descends from the hypothalamus and third ventricle. As a result of this process, there is intimate anatomic, neurologic, and vascular communication between the hypothalamus and pituitary via the neurons and vasculature of the pituitary stalk.

The hypothalamus produces releasing factors that induce secretion of pituitary hormones, and the hormone-rich blood then drains into the cavernous sinuses and the venous circulation to travel to target glands and organs (Fig. 1).

- Pulsatile release of gonadotropin-releasing hormone (GnRH) signals the pituitary to release gonadotropins, called luteinizing hormone (LH) and follicle-stimulating hormone (FSH), that target the ovaries and testes.
- Thyrotropin-releasing hormone induces secretion of thyroid-stimulating hormone (TSH, or thyrotropin), which results in increased thyroid hormone production and release.
- Corticotropin-releasing hormone induces secretion of adrenocorticotrophic hormone (ACTH), which signals the release of cortisol from the adrenal gland.
- Growth hormone (GH) secretion is regulated, in part, by growth hormone–releasing hormone (GHRH) and hypothalamic somatostatin. Circulating GH can have direct effects on peripheral targets,

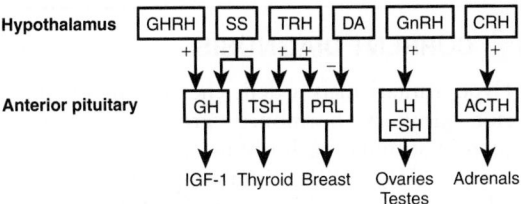

FIGURE 1. The hypothalamic-pituitary axis. *Abbreviations*: ACTH = adrenocorticotropic hormone; CRH = corticotrophin-releasing hormone; DA = dopamine; FSH = follicle-stimulating hormone; GH = growth hormone; GHRH = growth hormone–releasing hormone; GnRH = gonadotropin-releasing hormone; IGF-1 = insulin-like growth factor 1; LH = luteinizing hormone; PRL = prolactin; SS = somatostatin; TSH = thyroid-stimulating hormone; TRH = thyrotropin-releasing hormone.

affecting bone density and fat distribution, or it can induce the hepatic production of insulin-like growth factor 1 (IGF-1, or somatomedin-C), which then mediates GH effects.

Of course, both the hypothalamus and pituitary are subject to negative feedback by the hormones produced in the periphery. The lactation hormone prolactin is regulated through tonic neural inhibition by dopamine produced by the neurons that extend down from the hypothalamus through the pituitary stalk. In addition to the anterior pituitary hormones, the posterior pituitary produces arginine vasopressin (antidiuretic hormone), which regulates osmolality and water balance, and its deficiency leads to diabetes insipidus.

Causes of Hypopituitarism

Hypopituitarism is a deficiency of one or more of the anterior pituitary hormones (i.e., GH, TSH, LH, FSH, and ACTH); depending on the degree or type of injury to the pituitary stalk and posterior pituitary, it also may be accompanied by elevated prolactin, from a lack of dopaminergic inhibition, or diabetes insipidus, caused by vasopressin deficiency.

Hypopituitarism is rare, with an incidence of approximately 4 cases per 100,000 and a prevalence of 45 per 100,000 in one series. Known causes of hypopituitarism are listed in Table 1, but essentially any injury to the pituitary or hypothalamus can manifest with partial or complete hypopituitarism. Most cases are acquired, because congenital hypopituitarism is very rare.

The pituitary gland is highly vascularized, with a blood flow of 0.8 mL/g per minute, so that any event which disrupts or decreases the blood supply can result in hypopituitarism due to infarction of the gland. Sheehan's syndrome is a result of peripartum hypotension. Pituitary apoplexy is caused by hemorrhage into the sella, usually associated with a pituitary adenoma. Patients with traumatic brain injury also are at risk, with 25% to 40% developing chronic hypopituitarism, most commonly manifested as GH deficiency (15%–18%) and hypogonadism (14%), whereas the adrenal and thyroid axes appear to have greatest resilience.

The rich blood supply also makes the gland susceptible to hematogenous infiltration by infectious agents, granulomatous disease, and metastatic (e.g., breast cancer) or hematologic (e.g., lymphoma or leukemia) neoplasms (see Table 1). In these situations, the pituitary stalk also can be affected, so a finding of diabetes insipidus in the absence of major anatomic injury to the area should prompt consideration of infiltrative disease as part of the differential diagnosis. Lymphocytic hypophysitis involves infiltration of lymphocytes into the gland and stalk and may have an autoimmune component, affecting women more frequently than men. It most often manifests during pregnancy or the postpartum period as an enlarged pituitary with local signs, such as severe headache and visual disturbance. The lymphocytic infiltration can eventually lead to fibrosis of the gland.

TABLE 1 Causes of Hypopituitarism

Cause	Examples
Vascular insult	Sheehan's syndrome
	Pituitary apoplexy
	Stroke
Iatrogenic (surgery)	External beam irradiation (sellar, head and neck)
	Craniotomy for sellar or suprasellar pathology
	Transsphenoidal resection of pituitary adenoma
Infiltrative (granulomatous, infectious, autoimmune, neoplastic, other)	Sarcoidosis
	Eosinophilic causes
	Langerhans' cell histiocytosis
	Fungal causes
	Tuberculous meningitis
	Cytomegalovirus meningitis
	Lymphocytic hypophysitis
	Lymphoma or leukemia
	Metastatic carcinoma
	Hemochromatosis
Mass lesions/neoplasms (pituitary, hypothalamic, other)	Pituitary adenoma
	Pituitary cyst (Rathke's cleft, epidermoid, dermoid, arachnoid)
	Craniopharyngioma
	Germinoma
	Meningioma
	Hamartoma
Congenital (multiple deficiencies, single deficiency)	Mutations of pituitary developmental transcription factors (see Table 2)
	Kallmann's syndrome (hypogonadism)
	Growth hormone 1
	Growth hormone–releasing hormone receptor
	Pro-opiomelanocortin
Trauma	Traumatic brain injury
	Basal skull injury
Other	Empty sella

The pituicytes are sensitive to compressive pressure in the sella from mass lesions, such as a pituitary macroadenoma. This may be a direct result of decreased blood flow or neural signaling. The somatotrophs (GH) are the most sensitive, followed by the corticotrophs (ACTH) and gonadotrophs (LH and FSH). The least likely to be affected are the thyrotrophs. Pituitary tumors account for more than 10% of intracranial neoplasms and have a high prevalence; they are found in up to 35% of autopsies and in up to 40% of patients undergoing magnetic resonance imaging, depending on the series. Prolactinomas and nonfunctioning (gonadotroph) tumors account for the majority of pituitary adenomas. Most are microadenomas (<1 cm), which will not become clinically significant, but a portion (approximately 0.2%) are macroadenomas, which can cause substantial effects on pituitary function. Cystic lesions also can cause compressive effects; examples are Rathke's cleft, dermoid, epidermoid, and arachnoid cysts. Disruption of the hypothalamus or the pituitary stalk by a suprasellar neoplasm (e.g., craniopharyngioma) also can cause hypopituitarism from the lack of hypothalamic releasing hormones. Hypopituitarism due to mass effect also has been reported secondary to local meningiomas, hamartomas, and germinomas.

A hierarchy of pituicyte resilience also is seen after external beam irradiation of the head for intrasellar lesions, head and neck or skull tumors, or leukemia. Decreased blood flow is one possible cause, but there also is evidence of a decrease in hypothalamic releasing factors. The hormone deficiencies often develop in a sequential manner over

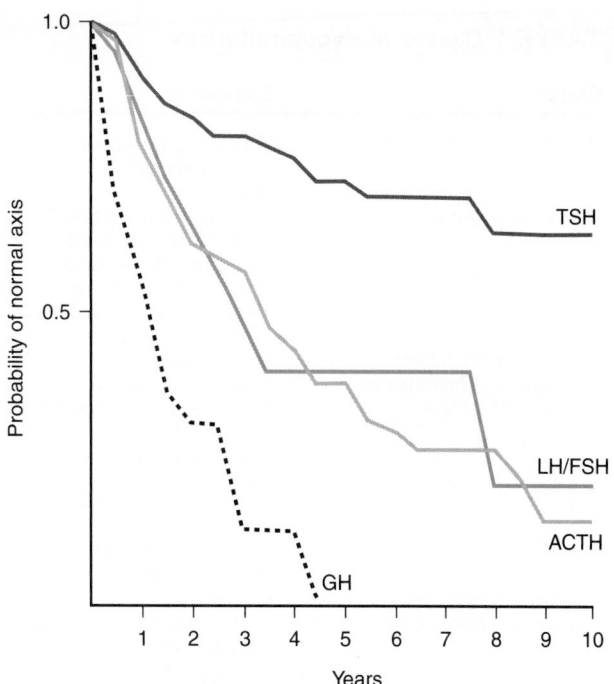

FIGURE 2. Time course of pituitary hormone deficiencies after external beam radiotherapy. *Abbreviations:* ACTH = adrenocorticotropic hormone; FSH = follicle-stimulating hormone; GH = growth hormone; LH = luteinizing hormone; TSH = thyroid-stimulating hormone. (Reprinted with permission from Littley MD, Shalet SM, Beardwee GC, et al: Hypopituitarism following external radiotherapy for pituitary tumours in adults. Q J Med 1989;70:145.)

several years, usually with an initial loss of the GH axis, followed by loss of gonadotroph and corticotroph function (Fig. 2). Thyrotropin deficiency develops later and in a smaller proportion of patients. Younger patients appear to be more vulnerable to the effects of radiation on pituitary function, and the degree of damage is dependent on the grays delivered. Some of the pituitary effects can be diminished with proper shielding of the sella.

Congenital hypopituitarism is a rare condition that usually occurs secondary to genetic mutations affecting the function of key transcription regulators in pituitary development, including POU1F1, PROP1, HESX1, and LHX4. The hormone-specific pituicytes differentiate from a multipotent precursor cell through the sequential expression of developmental transcription factors (Fig. 3). Depending on the temporal placement of the affected factor during development, there are variable anterior pituitary hormone deficits which can be accompanied by additional phenotypic abnormalities (Table 2). For example, PROP1 is active early in pituitary development, and an inactivating mutation will cause panhypopituitarism. Mutations of the

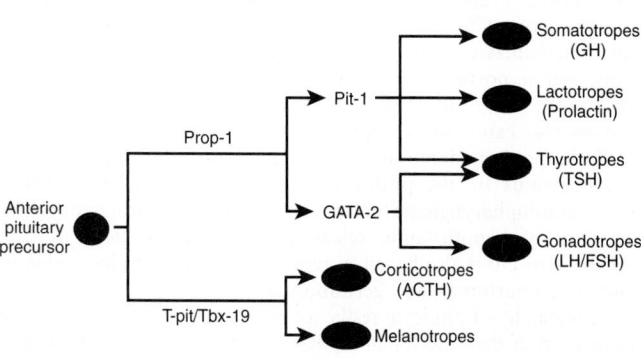

FIGURE 3. Pituitary cell differentiation from a single precursor cell type.

 CURRENT DIAGNOSIS

- Hypopituitarism is a deficiency of one or more anterior pituitary hormones—growth hormone (GH), thyroid-stimulating hormone (TSH), luteinizing hormone (LH), follicle-stimulating hormone (FSH), or adrenocorticotropic hormone (ACTH)—with or without elevated prolactin and diabetes insipidus.
- The initial laboratory tests are LH, FSH, TSH, free thyroxine (T_4), insulin-like growth factor 1 (IGF-1), prolactin, estrogen in females, and testosterone in males. The adrenal axis can be assessed with an ACTH stimulation test using cosyntropin (Cortrosyn)[1] 1 µg IV or 250 µg IM or IV, but a morning cortisol measurement can be helpful if the levels are less than 3 to 4 µg/dL or greater than 18 to 20 µg/dL.
- Patients with a pituitary hormone deficiency require assessment by magnetic resonance imaging of the sellar and suprasellar regions.
- Random GH levels are not useful for the diagnosis of GH deficiency. Dynamic testing with insulin-induced hypoglycemia or other provocative reagents such as arginine 10% (R-Gene 10), L-dopa (Levodopa),[1] or glucagon (GlucaGen)[1] is performed in a specialized endocrine testing clinic. However, the presence of three or four other pituitary hormone deficiencies or an IGF-1 below the age-specific lower limit of normal has a positive predictive value of 95% for GH deficiency.
- Testing for GH deficiency in adults should be performed only if there is a high pretest probability, such as in patients with known sellar or suprasellar lesions, a history of head and neck irradiation, deficiency of another pituitary hormone, or childhood- or adolescent-onset GH deficiency.
- In the absence of a large injury or mass lesion involving the hypothalamus or pituitary stalk, the finding of diabetes insipidus should increase suspicion for an infiltrative process such as granulomatous disease, lymphocytic hypophysitis, infection, metastatic carcinoma, or a hematologic neoplasm.

[1]Not FDA approved for this indication.

downstream factor PIT1 (POU1F1) will affect only somatotroph (GH), mammotroph (prolactin), and thyrotroph differentiation.

Other mutations have been reported that cause more isolated deficiencies (see Table 2), such as hypogonadotropic hypogonadism with Kallmann's syndrome. In these cases, the neurons that produce GnRH fail to migrate to the hypothalamus during development because of a deficiency in the cell adhesion molecule, anosmin-1 (X-linked) or in fibroblast growth factor receptor 1 (autosomal dominant). Isolated GH deficiency with short stature is seen with mutations of the genes encoding the GHRH receptor and the GH peptide itself. Mutations of the pro-opiomelanocortin gene cause abnormal processing of the prohormone, resulting in ACTH deficiency and obesity.

Clinical Presentation, Diagnostic Testing, and Treatment

The need to assess a patient for hypopituitarism may be obvious based on the initial presentation (e.g., known sellar or suprasellar mass lesion). Other patients may not have an obvious clinical or

TABLE 2 Mutations Causing Congenital Hypopituitarism

Gene	Function	Inheritance	Hormone Deficiency	Phenotype
POU1F1 (PIT1)	Pituitary developmental transcription factor	AD, AR	GH, TSH, PRL	Severe hypopituitarism
PROP1	Pituitary developmental transcription factor	AR	GH, TSH, PRL, LH, FSH	ACTH deficiency may develop with age
HESX1	Pituitary developmental transcription repressor	AD, AR	GH deficiency to panhypopituitarism	Septo-optic dysplasia Anterior pituitary hypoplasia Ectopic posterior pituitary
LHX3	Pituitary developmental transcription factor	AR	GH, TSH, PRL, LH, FSH	Anterior pituitary hypoplasia Elevated and anteverted shoulders with limited neck rotation
LHX4	Pituitary developmental transcription factor	AR	GH, TSH, ACTH	Anterior pituitary hypoplasia Ectopic posterior pituitary
SOX2	Transcription factor (SRY high-mobility group box) family	De novo	LH, FSH	Hypogonadism Microphthalmia or anophthalmia Developmental delay Esophageal atresia Sensorineural hearing loss
GHRHr	G protein–coupled receptor on somatotrophs	AR	GH	Short stature Anterior pituitary hypoplasia
GH1	GH peptide	AR	GH	Short stature Abnormal facies
KAL1	Anosmin-1 cell adhesion molecule	XL	GnRH, FSH, LH	Hypogonadotropic hypogonadism Arrested puberty Anosmia Synkinesis Renal agenesis
FGFR1 (KAL2)	Fibroblast growth factor receptor	AD	GnRH, FSH, LH	Hypogonadotropic hypogonadism Arrested puberty
POMC	Pro-opiomelanocortin	AR	ACTH	Adrenal hypoplasia Adrenal insufficiency Obesity
GPR54	G protein–coupled receptor	AR	FSH, LH	Absent or delayed puberty
DAX1	Orphan nuclear receptor	AR, XL	FSH, LH	Severe neonatal adrenal insufficiency Absent, arrested, or delayed puberty

Modified from Toogood AA, Stewart PM: Hypopituitarism: Clinical features, diagnosis and management. Endocrinol Metab Clin North Am 2008;27:235.
Abbreviations: ACTH = adrenocorticotropic hormone; AD = autosomal dominant; AR = autosomal recessive; FSH = follicle-stimulating hormone; GH = growth hormone; GHRHr = growth hormone–releasing hormone receptor; LH = luteinizing hormone; PRL = prolactin; TSH = thyroid-stimulating hormone; XL = X-linked.

anatomic reason for hypopituitarism and may present with vague, nonspecific symptoms. As a result, hypopituitarism can go unrecognized, such as with infiltrative disease or after traumatic brain injury or occult pituitary apoplexy. If a single hormone deficiency is suspected from the clinical presentation or laboratory tests, the remaining anterior pituitary hormones should be measured as well. These patients also should be evaluated by magnetic resonance imaging (pituitary protocol with gadolinium enhancement) to assess the anatomy of the sella and suprasellar regions.

ADRENOCORTICOTROPIN DEFICIENCY

Central or secondary adrenal insufficiency can manifest with nonspecific symptoms of fatigue, lethargy, decreased appetite, weight loss, and vague abdominal discomfort. A subtle clinical finding in patients with complete ACTH deficiency is that of decreased skin pigmentation or even a sallow or alabaster complexion, which likely is caused by lack of ACTH activation of the melanocyte-stimulating hormone receptors. Unlike primary adrenal insufficiency (Addison's disease), aldosterone secretion from the adrenal zona glomerulosa is intact, and hypotension and orthostasis are unusual findings unless there is extreme physiologic stress from a serious illness or surgery. Corticosteroids are needed, in part, to potentiate the vasoconstrictive

action of catecholamines so as to maintain effective circulating volume.

The hypothalamic-pituitary-adrenal (HPA) axis has a diurnal rhythm, with a peak in the early morning and a nadir at about midnight. An early-morning serum cortisol measurement that is greater than 18 to 20 μg/dL (500–550 mmol/L) or less than 3 to 4 μg/dL (83–110 mmol/L) generally can confirm adequacy or deficiency, respectively. However, if the serum cortisol level is between these values, dynamic testing is required. The ACTH (Synacthen[2] or Cosyntropin [Cortrosyn]) stimulation test is performed by administering 1 μg intravenously or 250 μg IV or intramuscularly with measurement of serum cortisol at 0, 30, and 60 minutes. The 1-μg test should cause an increase in cortisol to greater than 18 to 20 μg/dL at 30 minutes. The cutoff for the 250-μg test is 20 to 22 μg/dL at 30 or 60 minutes. Although the 1-μg test has moderately increased sensitivity for secondary adrenal insufficiency in some studies, a systematic review did not support its superiority. Also, many endocrinologists avoid ordering the 1-μg test because it is more prone to error (e.g., with dilution of the ACTH). Because the stimulation test relies on atrophy of the adrenals, it is valid only in adrenal

[2]Not available in the United States.

insufficiency of long standing (weeks or longer) once the adrenals have atrophied. In acute secondary adrenal insufficiency, such as with pituitary apoplexy, the adrenals still are able to respond to ACTH, and the test will be falsely reassuring. Empiric corticosteroid coverage should be given in these cases, or the axis can be tested with the use of insulin-induced hypoglycemia or metyrapone (Metopirone), because both of these tests rely on intact ACTH secretion.

The gold standard for evaluation of the HPA axis is the insulin tolerance test (ITT). Subcutaneous insulin is given (0.1 to 0.25 units per kg, depending on predicted insulin resistance) to induce hypoglycemia and a counterregulatory response, with secretion of ACTH and cortisol. The glucose levels should drop to less than 40 mg/dL (2.2 mmol/L) for a successful test, and the cortisol should increase to greater than 18 to 20 μg/dL with an ACTH level greater than 150 pg/mL. One advantage of performing an ITT is that the GH axis also can be assessed, because GH should rise to 3.3 to 5.1 μg/L. However, there are obvious inherent dangers in inducing hypoglycemia, and the test must be performed under a physician's supervision, with a ready source of glucose (10% dextrose IV or orange juice PO). It is contraindicated in patients with a seizure history, in the aged (>60–65 years old), and in patients with significant cardiovascular disease (e.g., unstable angina).

The metyrapone test also can assess central adrenal insufficiency, although it is used less frequently because most physicians are more comfortable if the patient is admitted overnight. Metyrapone blocks the final enzyme in cortisol synthesis (11β-hydroxylase) so that cortisol levels drop and feedback inhibition on the hypothalamus and pituitary is lost. As a result, ACTH secretion is stimulated and morning 11-deoxycortisol levels rise to greater than 7 μg/dL if pituitary function is normal. A low cortisol level (<5 μg/dL) indicates appropriate inhibition of 11β-hydroxylase by metyrapone, so that the clinician can be confident with the results.

With a diagnosis of adrenal insufficiency, glucocorticoid replacement is mandated. Hydrocortisone (Cortef) is considered the most physiologic agent, compared with synthetic corticosteroids. It is given at 8 AM (two thirds of the total daily dose) and 4 PM (one third of the total dose) to mimic the diurnal rhythm of cortisol. Dosing is usually 15 to 30 mg of hydrocortisone in the morning and 10 to 15 mg in the afternoon. Some patients need more frequent hydrocortisone, in three divided doses, because of its short half-life. Alternative glucocorticoid regimens include prednisone 5.0 mg AM and 2.5 mg PM and dexamethasone (Decadron) 0.5 mg at bedtime. The patient should be monitored for symptoms or signs of excess replacement (e.g., cushingoid features, hypertension, elevated glucose). Patients starting on GH replacement therapy may need an additional 5 mg of hydrocortisone per day due to increased cortisol clearance. The replacement dose also should be increased in pregnancy by approximately 50%, starting in the late second or early third trimesters. Patients should be instructed to triple the dose should they become ill, and they should obtain a medic alert bracelet to identify them as having adrenal insufficiency. For surgical procedures or during hospitalization for an acute illness, patients should receive hydrocortisone (Solu-Cortef) 50 to 100 mg IV every 8 hours, to be tapered after they are improved.

GROWTH HORMONE DEFICIENCY

The symptoms of GH deficiency in adults often are nonspecific and can include decreased energy, vitality, and poor sleep. However, more objective measures have shown that GH-deficient adults have altered protein, fat, and carbohydrate metabolism which manifest as changes in body composition, with increased fat mass and decreased lean mass. The visceral fat depot is affected most, and this can lead to insulin resistance. Bone density is decreased, possibly because of slowed mineralization, and there is an increased risk of fracture. Patients who are GH deficient before reaching peak bone mass (at approximately 30 years old) can have the most severe deficits, with bone density in the osteoporotic range and a relative risk of fracture twofold to threefold higher than in age-matched controls. With regard to cardiovascular health, there is increased low-density lipoprotein cholesterol, sometimes combined with decreased high-density lipoprotein cholesterol, and

elevation of other markers associated with cardiovascular risk (homocysteine, C-reactive protein, and interleukin-6). Left ventricular function also appears to be reduced. These findings may contribute to the twofold increase in cardiovascular mortality that is observed in adults with hypopituitarism.

These manifestations of GH deficiency are more difficult to isolate from general hypopituitarism itself, but they have been shown to improve with GH replacement. Treatment results in decreased fat mass along with increased muscle mass and strength. GH also has an anabolic effect on bone, although the benefit may not be apparent until after 24 months of treatment if measured by densitometry. For young patients who are in transition to adult clinics, continuation of GH replacement beyond the attainment of height potential provides added benefit for bone density. There are no long-term, prospective data to confirm decreased cardiovascular morbidity or mortality with GH replacement at this time, but clearly there are improvements in known cardiovascular risk factors. Standardized quality-of-life measurements have shown improvement in a subset of studies. Overall, it seems that the patients who have the worst baseline measurements for these parameters benefit the most from GH replacement therapy, so the decision should be made on a case-by-case basis.

Testing for GH deficiency in adults should be undertaken only in patients with a moderate to high pretest probability, such as those with a history of pituitary or hypothalamic disease, neurosurgery, or cranial radiation and a subset of patients with traumatic brain injury. Also, patients who were treated with GH in childhood and adolescence should be retested. Idiopathic GH deficiency in childhood may resolve as the patient reaches adulthood, but if there was a known cause, the deficiency is likely to persist. Because of large fluctuations of GH in normal subjects throughout the day, random GH levels are not useful. Measurements of IGF-1 (somatomedin-C) are helpful if the patient has known sellar disease and an IGF-1 value lower than the normal age-specific range. In one study, an IGF-1 value lower than 77 μg/L had a positive predictive value of 95% for GH deficiency. However, some patients with high pretest probability of deficiency have an IGF-1 value in the normal range and require provocative testing. Established tests include insulin-induced hypoglycemia (ITT) and stimulation by glucagon (GlucaGen), arginine (Arg, R-Gene 10), L-dopa (Levodopa), Arg-L-dopa, and Arg-GHRH. The GH cutoffs for each of these tests differ depending on the stimulus and the desired sensitivity and specificity. Dynamic tests like these should be performed in a specialized clinic by a trained endocrine nurse, with the results interpreted by an endocrinologist. ITT is the gold standard, and the cutoffs used for the peak GH levels are determined by the need for sensitivity (95% at GH 5.1 μg/L) or specificity (95% at 3.3 μg/L). The age of the patient also is a consideration, and the GH threshold should be higher than 6.1 μg/L in adolescents and young adults. The ITT is the least preferred test among patients and is contraindicated in some groups (e.g., seizure disorders, cardiovascular disease, age >65 years), so clinicians may prefer to use one or even two of the other stimulation tests if ITT is not performed. A deficiency of three or four pituitary hormones other than GH has a positive predictive value of 95% for GH deficiency, and some patients in this category do not require expensive dynamic testing, especially if IGF-1 is below normal.

The starting dose for recombinant GH (somatropin) replacement (Genotropin or Humatrope) in adults is 2 to 5 μg/kg/day, much lower than in children with GH deficiency (40 μg/kg/day), with additional considerations for age and gender. The dose is titrated every few weeks to attain an IGF-1 in the age-specific normal range. Side effects of GH therapy can be similar to those seen with acromegaly, including fluid retention as well as musculoskeletal complaints such as myalgias, arthralgias, and even carpal tunnel syndrome. In such cases, the dose of GH should be reduced. Doses of thyroid and adrenal replacement drugs may need to be increased with initiation of GH therapy, because GH replacement leads to more rapid clearance of these hormones. Women generally require higher doses than men due to the blunting of GH effects by estrogen. Patients with history of primary brain tumor should undergo surveillance scans at baseline, at 12 months, and thereafter according to accepted protocols or change in clinical symptoms. However, there is no clear-cut evidence that GH replacement induces recurrence or progression of residual sellar (e.g., pituitary adenoma) or suprasellar (e.g., craniopharyngioma) masses.

THYROTROPIN DEFICIENCY

Hypothyroid symptoms are similar to those classically seen with primary hypothyroidism. However, they are likely to be milder, because there usually is some residual TSH secretion and basal thyroxine (T_4) production. Secondary hypothyroidism is diagnosed by low or inappropriately normal serum TSH with a low free T_4 level. Levothyroxine (T_4, Synthroid) replacement (1.3 to 1.6 μg/kg) is titrated to maintain an upper-normal level of free T_4. Lower doses should be used in elderly patients who have a significant cardiovascular history (e.g., angina) or risk factors. Monitoring of the TSH is not helpful for T_4 titration in hypopituitarism. Triiodothyronine (T_3, liothyronine [Cytomel]) replacement or the combination of T_3 with T_4 (Thyrolar) has not been shown to improve patients' health or quality of life.

PROLACTIN

Prolactin may be either increased or decreased in hypopituitarism, and the serum prolactin level should be interpreted in the context of other pituitary hormone levels. A large prolactinoma can have compressive effects on the rest of the pituitary, causing deficiencies of other pituitary hormones. Because elevated prolactin also causes secondary hypogonadism due to inhibition of GnRH secretion, the presence of low LH and FSH can occur secondary to the prolactin itself or compressive effects on the gonadotrophs. Increased prolactin levels also may be seen if there is disruption of, or pressure on, the pituitary stalk, which causes decreased dopaminergic inhibition. In these cases, prolactin is usually only moderately elevated (20–200 ng/mL). Even so, this can cause clinically significant symptoms including amenorrhea and galactorrhea in women and decreased libido and erectile dysfunction in men. Decreased or absent prolactin is an indicator of significant hypopituitarism, but there are no major known clinical sequelae except for an inability to lactate in the postpartum period. As such, there is no treatment for low prolactin.

HYPOGONADISM IN MALES

Congenital gonadotropin deficiency in males can manifest with cryptorchidism and microphallus (<2.5 standard deviations below normal for age) due to decreased androgen production in the third trimester of pregnancy. In prepubertal males, gonadotropin deficiency is associated with failure to initiate puberty or to progress normally through the Tanner stages. Although secondary sexual hair may be present from the effect of adrenal androgens, testicular androgen deficiency decreases the growth of secondary sexual hair, and the pubic hair may assume a female distribution. Patients with isolated gonadotropin deficiency have growth of the long bones caused by secretion of GH, but failure of epiphyseal fusion will occur in the absence of testosterone (aromatized to estrogen). The result is a tall stature with a so-called eunuchoid habitus, in which the arm span is more than 2 cm greater than the height and the pubis-to-floor distance is more than 2 cm greater than the length from the crown of the head to the pubis. Children and adolescents with gonadotropin deficiency should be managed by a pediatric endocrine specialist because of the delicate balance between maintaining growth velocity and inducing sexual maturity.

Androgen deficiency in adult males is most often brought to the clinician's attention because of decreased libido and sexual dysfunction. Other manifestations are less specific and can include fatigue, sleep problems, and mild muscle weakness with decreased exercise capacity. On examination, there usually is maintenance of secondary sexual hair, unless the deficiency is severe and long-standing. With FSH deficiency, testes may become soft and decreased in size secondary to atrophy of the seminiferous tubules. Over time, there is

thinning of the skin, and fine wrinkles develop. There is a decrease in bone density with increased fracture risk. Total testosterone levels are measured in the morning (9 AM) and may be confirmed with a second total testosterone measurement on a different day or with a bioavailable (free and weakly bound) testosterone measurement if a low level of sex hormone–binding globulin is suspected (e.g., with obesity).

There are many different testosterone preparations available for replacement therapy. The clinical goal of androgen replacement is to improve vitality and sexual function. Depot testosterone esters (testosterone cypionate [Depo-Testosterone] and enanthate [Delatestryl]) are injected intramuscularly at a dose of 100 mg per week or 200 mg every 2 weeks. Levels may be supraphysiologic 2 to 3 days after injection, but the mid-interval testosterone level should be in the mid-normal range (700 ng/dL), and the nadir level before the next dose should be in the low-normal range (300 ng/dL). Longer-term depot injections (testosterone undecenoate [Andriol[2]] 1000 mg at 6 weeks and then every 12 weeks) produce less fluctuation but require injection of a large volume (4 mL). Testosterone pellets (Testopel) may be implanted to achieve steady-state levels for 4 to 6 months, but this requires a surgical incision.

Transdermal delivery provides more constant levels. The biochemical goal is to maintain testosterone levels in the mid-normal range (700 ng/dL). The testosterone patch (Androderm) is applied daily (5–10 mg), and the dosing is adjusted based on the testosterone levels at 3 to 10 hours after application. Testosterone gel (AndroGel) 5 to 10 g (50–100 mg testosterone) is applied to the skin. Testosterone levels reach steady state after 1 week, and the dose can be adjusted based on the testosterone levels achieved. However, care must be taken, because testosterone gel can be transferred on contact with other family members. Other available transdermal systems are buccal tablets (Striant) and the scrotal patch (Testoderm).[2] Oral replacement is not recommended because of first-pass hepatic metabolism, which decreases the dose delivered to the circulation and can cause liver test abnormalities.

Adverse effects include gynecomastia, erythrocytosis, and prostate problems. Patients are monitored at 3 months and then yearly. Patients with risk of prostate cancer should be assessed for prostatic symptoms and should undergo digital rectal examination. A urologic consultation is obtained if the annual prostate-specific antigen measurement is greater than 4 ng/mL or if it increases more than 1.4 ng/mL in 1 year. Laboratory testing also should include a hematocrit, and the testosterone should be discontinued or reduced if the hematocrit is greater than 54%.

HYPOGONADISM IN FEMALES

Gonadotropin deficiency in prepubertal females manifests with delayed breast development and primary amenorrhea. If the gonadotropin deficiency is isolated, GH secretion allows normal growth velocity during childhood until adolescence, when the expected growth spurt fails to occur. Sex steroid replacement in adolescent females should be managed by a pediatric endocrinologist.

Adult women with acquired gonadotropin deficiency present with oligomenorrhea or secondary amenorrhea. Additionally, there can be symptoms of estrogen deficiency such as vaginal dryness, dyspareunia, vasomotor instability (hot flushes), and breast atrophy. Laboratory testing reveals low estradiol levels with low or inappropriately normal FSH and LH. Postmenopausal women, who normally have high levels of FSH and LH, also show low or inappropriately normal levels.

For women with gonadotropin deficiency before menopause, hormone replacement is necessary to improve symptoms of estrogen deficiency and to optimize bone health. Most endocrinologists continue replacement until the usual time of menopause. The therapeutic options are a birth control pill or hormone replacement therapy (e.g., Premarin, Provera), with the dose titrated to alleviate symptoms.

---

[2]Not available in the United States.

CURRENT THERAPY

- Secondary adrenal insufficiency is treated with glucocorticoids. One widely used regimen is hydrocortisone (Cortef), with a two-thirds dose (e.g., 20 mg) given in the morning and a one-third dose (e.g., 10 mg) in the afternoon, to mimic diurnal cortisol levels.
- Secondary hypothyroidism is treated with levothyroxine (T4, Synthroid), with the dose titrated to maintain free T_4 levels in the normal range combined with clinical euthyroidism on history and examination. Monitoring of thyroid-stimulating hormone levels is not useful in secondary hypothyroidism.
- Treatment of secondary hypothyroidism should be initiated only after assessment of the hypothalamic-pituitary-adrenal axis, or with empiric adrenal replacement, because thyroid hormone increases clearance of cortisol and can precipitate an adrenal crisis.
- Growth hormone (GH) replacement in adults is administered at a lower dose than in GH-deficient children (e.g., 10% of the latter) and is titrated to maintain a normal age-specific level of insulin-like growth factor 1. Use of GH therapy in adults is controversial and should be determined on a case-by-case basis, with consideration for body composition, dyslipidemia, and bone density. Patients who have the worst baseline values tend to benefit the most from therapy.

Conclusion

Patients with hypopituitarism have twofold increased mortality compared with age-matched controls, so a goal of treatment is to restore the quality of life and prognosis to normal. Replacement therapy for the thyroid and adrenal axes is necessary and life-sustaining. However, the initiation of GH or sex steroid replacement requires that patient-specific factors be taken into account.

REFERENCES

Biller BMK, Samuels MH, Zagar A, et al. Sensitivity and specificity of six tests for the diagnosis of adult GH deficiency. J Clin Endocrinol Metab 2002;87:2067–9.

Darzy KH, Shalet SM. Hypopituitarism following radiotherapy revisited. Endocr Dev 2009;15:1–24.

Molitch ME, Clemmons DR, Malozowski S, et al. Evaluation and treatment of adult growth hormone deficiency: An Endocrine Society clinical practice guideline. J Clin Endocrinol Metab 2006;91:1621–34.

Littley MD, Shalet SM, Beardwee GC, et al. Hypopituitarism following external radiotherapy for pituitary tumours in adults. Q J Med 1989;70:145–60.

Owens G, Balfour D, Biller BMK, et al. Clinical presentation and diagnosis: Growth hormone deficiency in adults. Am J Manag Care 2004;10(13 Suppl.):S424–30.

Rupp D, Molitch M. Pituitary stalk lesions. Curr Opin Endocrinol Diabetes Obes 2008;15:339–45.

Schneider HJ, Aimeretti G, Kreitschmann-Andermahr I, et al. Hypopituitarism. Lancet 2007;369:1461–70.

Bhasin S, Cunningham GR, Hayes FJ, et al. Testosterone therapy in adult men with androgen deficiency syndromes: An Endocrine Society clinical practice guideline. J Clin Endocrinol Metab 2006;91:1995–2010.

Toogood AA, Stewart PM. Hypopituitarism: Clinical features, diagnosis and management. Endocrinol Metab Clin North Am 2008;37:235–61.

Hyperprolactinemia

Method of
Morali Sharma, MD

Physiology of Prolactin Secretion

Prolactin (PRL) is secreted by the lactotrophs in the anterior pituitary gland. Its secretion is regulated by hormones synthesized by tuberohypophyseal neurons. PRL secretion is stimulated by prolactin-releasing factor and other peptides, including thyrotropin-releasing hormone and arginine vasopressin. Central serotonergic and endorphinergic pathways also increase PRL secretion.

The hypothalamus releases a prolactin release–inhibitory factor, which is mainly dopamine and to a lesser extent γ-aminobutyric acid (GABA). These peptides are transmitted from the hypothalamus to the anterior pituitary by the hypothalamo-hypophyseal portal system located along the pituitary stalk. Any disruption of the stalk causes a decrease in dopamine secretion, resulting in PRL elevation.

PRL secretion increases in response to some external stimuli, which include suckling, mating, emotional and physical stress, and sleep. Estrogens also increase PRL secretion. A high level of PRL in the hypothalamus inhibits luteinizing hormone–releasing hormone, which results in hypogonadism.

Clinical Manifestations

The causes of hyperprolactinemia are presented in Box 1.

High PRL causes suppression of gonadotropin secretion, resulting in hypogonadism. Women with hyperprolactinemia present with oligomenorrhea or amenorrhea, galactorrhea, and infertility. Low estrogen causes symptoms of menopause (e.g., hot flashes, vaginal dryness, low bone density).

Men with hyperprolactinemia complain of decreased libido, erectile dysfunction, and infertility. Gynecomastia and galactorrhea can also occur but are rare. Low testosterone causes fatigue, low bone density, decreased muscle mass, and decreased body hair.

Patients with macroprolactinoma can present with symptoms related to a pituitary mass lesion, such as headache and visual disturbance.

Diagnosis of Prolactinoma

The finding of elevated PRL should be confirmed by repeating the test. A history and physical examination, comprehensive metabolic panel, thyroid function tests, and pregnancy test will exclude all causes except hypothalamic-pituitary disease. If these screening tests do not reveal the etiology of the hyperprolactinemia, magnetic resonance

CURRENT DIAGNOSIS

- A prolactin level lower than 100 ng/mL suggests microadenoma, stalk compression from a nonfunctioning pituitary macroadenoma, or other causes of hyperprolactinemia (see Box 1).
- A prolactin level greater than 100 ng/mL is more likely to be from a prolactinoma, and a level greater than 200 ng/mL suggests a macroprolactinoma. Magnetic resonance imaging of the pituitary gland and hypothalamus should be performed in a patient with a prolactin level greater than 100 ng/mL or with visual field defects.

BOX 1 Causes of Hyperprolactinemia

- Physiologic: pregnancy (PRL ranges from 100 to 500 ng/dL) and lactation, nipple stimulation, stress, exercise, and sleep
- Pituitary disease: PRL-secreting tumor (prolactinoma), mixed tumor secreting growth hormone and PRL
- Drugs: neuroleptics (including some atypical antipsychotics), metoclopramide (Reglan), antidepressants, estrogens, opiates, verapamil (Calan), cimetidine (Tagamet), methyldopa (Aldomet)
- Primary hypothyroidism increases PRL by increasing secretion of TSH
- Renal failure
- Hypothalamic disease: craniopharyngioma, histiocytosis X, sarcoidosis
- Pituitary stalk compression
- Neurogenic: chest wall injury
- Polycystic ovarian disease
- Cirrhosis of liver
- Idiopathic
- Macroprolactinemia*

---

*This is a benign clinical condition and does not cause symptoms of hyperprolactinemia. The normal PRL molecule is 23 kDa, whereas macroPRL, a glycosylated form, is 25 kDa. This larger peptide molecule results in decreased renal clearance and higher serum prolactin levels. MacroPRL can be separated from normal PRL by gel filtration or PEG precipitation. Approximately 10% of patients with high PRL levels have macroPRL.
Abbreviations: PEG = polyethylene glycol; PRL = prolactin; TSH = thyroid-stimulating hormone.

imaging of the pituitary and hypothalamus with contrast should be performed to rule out a tumor. Visual-field examination should also be performed in all patients with macroadenomas.

Some giant prolactinomas can manifest with inappropriately normal or only mildly high PRL levels, as a result of the so-called hook effect. Measurement of PRL involves a two-sided immunochemiluminometric assay (ICMA) which involves formation of a sandwich complex. Very high PRL levels can prevent sandwich formation, resulting in falsely low PRL measurements. This artifact can be overcome by serial dilutions of the serum.

Treatment of Nontumoral Hyperprolactinemia

Treatment of primary hypothyroidism normalizes PRL production. Drug-induced hyperprolactinemia resolves upon discontinuation of the offending drug. If the drug treatment cannot be discontinued, the patient should be evaluated for hormone replacement therapy to correct symptoms of hypogonadism.

Treatment of Prolactinoma

MEDICAL THERAPY

Dopamine receptor agonists are the first line of treatment of prolactinomas.

Bromocriptine (Parlodel) is the standard dopaminergic agonist, but cabergoline (Dostinex), a long-acting agonist of the D_2 receptor, has been more commonly used in recent years. Cabergoline exhibits greater efficacy and fewer side effects than bromocriptine in

patients with tumoral and nontumoral hyperprolactinemia. Cabergoline binds the D_2 receptors in the pituitary with greater affinity and has a longer half-life, which makes it more effective in correcting hypogonadism. Dopamine agonists normalize PRL in 80% to 85% of patients and cause significant reduction in tumor size. More than 1 year after treatment with a dopamine agonist, greater than 50% reduction in tumor size occurs in 50% to 60% of patients with prolactinoma; and a 25% to 50% reduction in size occurs in 10% to 15% of patients; tumor shrinkage of 10% to 25% can be expected in 20% to 30% of patients. About 5% to 10% of patients with prolactinoma are resistant to dopamine agonists, and this is thought to be caused by a decrease in number of dopamine receptors in the tumor.

Common adverse reactions to dopamine agonists are nausea, vomiting, orthostatic hypotension, and nasal congestion. Treatment with a dopamine agonist should be closely monitored in a patient who has a large prolactinoma, because it has been reported to precipitate pituitary apoplexy.

Cardiac side effects such as valvular regurgitation are rare and occur with high doses. The average cabergoline dose used to treat prolactinomas is 1 to 2 mg/week. Doses exceeding 3 mg/day, used to treat parkinsonism, have been reported to cause significantly higher risk of valvular regurgitation.

TRANSSPHENOIDAL SURGERY

Efficacy of treatment with transsphenoidal surgery depends on the experience of the surgeon. The cure rate of microadenomas is 70% to 80%, whereas that of macroadenomas is only 10% to 50%. Complications of surgery include hypopituitarism and diabetes insipidus, which is usually transient but can be permanent (1% of cases). The postoperative tumor recurrence rate is about 20%.

IRRADIATION

Prolactinomas that do not respond to dopamine agonists or are inoperable can be treated with radiation therapy. The efficacy of radiation therapy is low, normalization of PRL occurs in fewer than 25% of cases, and the time to normalization varies from 5 to 15 years. Adverse effects include hypopituitarism, memory defects, and increased risk of cerebrovascular events.

Treatment of hyperprolactinemia is recommended as long as fertility is desired. Once the PRL level normalizes, the dose can be decreased to the lowest effective dose that controls symptoms. Women not desiring fertility can be treated with estrogen replacement (oral contraceptives). Patients with macroprolactinoma require continued treatment to maintain tumor shrinkage. Asymptomatic postmenopausal women with hyperprolactinemia need not be treated.

 CURRENT THERAPY

- Dopamine agonists are the first line of treatment of prolactinoma. If the hyperprolactinemia is secondary to a nonsecreting pituitary macroadenoma causing stalk compression, surgical resection is recommended. Drug-induced hyperprolactinemia generally resolves after discontinuation of the drug. Treatment with a dopamine agonist should be avoided in patients who have hyperprolactinemia induced by neuroleptics, because it may reverse the antipsychotic effect of these drugs, resulting in exacerbation of the underlying psychiatric condition.
- Treatment of hyperprolactinemia is recommended as long as fertility is desired. Once the prolactin level normalizes, the dose can be decreased to the lowest effective dose that controls symptoms.

Natural History of Prolactinoma

Follow-up of women with prolactinoma over 15 years has shown a significant fall in PRL levels after discontinuation of treatment for 3 to 5 years in about 50% of patients and normalization of PRL in 15%. Studies have also shown that hyperprolactinemia can be self-limited in 20% to 30% of the cases.

Prolactinoma and Pregnancy

In women desiring fertility, bromocriptine is given to normalize PRL and restore normal ovulation. Once pregnancy is established, bromocriptine can be discontinued in patients with microprolactinoma, and the patient can be monitored clinically for signs of tumor growth. Microprolactinomas rarely enlarge during pregnancy. About 25% of patients with macroprolactinoma develop symptoms such as headaches and visual disturbance during pregnancy. Prepregnancy surgical decompression should be considered for patients with large prolactinomas. Bromocriptine may be continued throughout pregnancy in those patients with large prolactinomas. The safety of bromocriptine treatment during pregnancy has been demonstrated in more than 6000 pregnancies, whereas data for safety of cabergoline exist from about 300 pregnancies.

REFERENCES

Casanueva FF, Molitch ME, Schlechte JA, et al. Guidelines of the Pituitary Society for the diagnosis and management of prolactinomas. Clin Endocrinol (Oxf) 2006;65:265–73.

Colao A, Vitale G, Cappabianca P, et al. Outcome of cabergoline treatment in men with prolactinoma: Effects of a 24-month treatment on prolactin levels, tumor mass, recovery of pituitary function, and semen analysis. J Clin Endocrinol Metab 2004;89:1704–11.

Ferrari CI, Abs R, Bevan JS, et al. Treatment of macroprolactinoma with cabergoline: A study of 85 patients. Clin Endocrinol (Oxf) 1997;46:409–13.

Gillam MP, Molitch ME, Lombardi G, Colao A. Advances in the treatment of prolactinomas. Endocr Rev 2006;27:485–534.

Molitch ME. Medical treatment of prolactinomas. Endocrinol Metab Clin North Am 1999;28:143–69.

Pellegrini I, Rasolonjanahary R, Gunz G, et al. Resistance to bromocriptine in prolactinomas. J Clin Endocrinol Metab 1989;69:500–9.

Verhelst J, Abs R, Maiter D, et al. Cabergoline in the treatment of hyperprolactinemia: A study in 455 patients. J Clin Endocrinol Metab 1999;84:2518–22.

Webster J, Piscitelli G, Polli A, et al. A comparison of cabergoline and bromocriptine in the treatment of hyperprolactinemic amenorrhea. N Engl J Med 1994;331:904–9.

Hypothyroidism

Method of
Mona Shimshi, MD, and Terry F. Davies, MD

Hypothyroidism

NORMAL THYROID HORMONE PHYSIOLOGY

The major active thyroid hormone is triiodothyronine (T_3), which is produced either directly by the thyroid gland or peripherally from thyroxine (T_4) by a process of deiodination. Thyroid hormone synthesis and secretion is under the pituitary control of thyroid-stimulating hormone (TSH). Serum T_4 and T_3 exert negative feedback at the anterior pituitary thyrotroph cell, thus controlling TSH release.

In the normal thyroid gland, the ratio of T_4 to T_3 is approximately 15:1, but in the peripheral circulation the amount of T_3 is very much increased. The majority of this additional T_3 is produced in a wide variety of peripheral tissues, particularly the liver and muscles, by the conversion of T_4 to T_3 by a family of deiodinase enzymes. Type 1 $5'$-monodeiodinase is responsible for most of the T_3 in the circulation and also converts T_4 to rT_3 (reverse T_3). The Type 2 $5'$-deiodinase enzyme is primarily responsible for local and intracellular production of T_3, especially within the thyrotroph, and maintains a constant level of intracellular T_3 so important, for example, to the central nervous system. A reduction in circulating T_4 causes an increase in the type 2 enzyme in order to maintain this constant level of T_3. The type 3 $5'$-deiodinase enzyme is the major T_3 and T_4 inactivating enzyme. It protects the tissues from local thyroid hormone excess and is the enzyme primarily responsible for catalyzing the inner ring deiodination of T_4 and T_3. These enzymes are polymorphic and their efficiency varies from person to person.

Thyroid hormones, particularly T_4, are bound to serum proteins such as thyroxine-binding globulin and, therefore one should measure the total or the active free hormone levels. Note that the half-life of T_4 is approximately 6 to 7 days, whereas the half-life of T_3 is only 1 day.

DIAGNOSIS OF THYROID FAILURE

Reference ranges for individual serum total T_4 and T_3 levels are narrow, compared with significantly wider group reference ranges for a population, making the measurement of thyroid hormone levels a relatively insensitive tool for detecting abnormalities. This also applies to measurement of the free thyroid hormones. In contrast, the response of pituitary TSH to minor changes in thyroid hormone levels in a given person is logarithmic, indicating that serum TSH assessment is a superior tool for detecting changes in thyroid hormone output. Hence, an increase in serum TSH is a highly sensitive indicator of hypothyroidism and a decrease in serum TSH is a highly sensitive indicator of hyperthyroidism.

One of the difficulties in discussing hypothyroidism is the definition of the normal TSH range. Since the advent of improved immunoassay techniques for measuring TSH levels, the concern has changed from accurately reproducing the TSH level to greater concern over the normal TSH range. In a population that contains persons at risk for developing hypothyroidism, for example by including patients with antibodies to thyroid peroxidase and a family history of hypothyroidism, the upper limit of TSH was defined as 4.5 or 5.5 µU/mL. However, when one uses a population that does not include such persons known to be at increased risk for developing thyroid disease, the upper limit of TSH is 3.0 µU/mL. The 3.0 µU/mL is now considered by some to be the upper limit of normal in young healthy individuals. TSH, like many pituitary hormones, exhibits a diurnal variation in its pattern of secretion. It is at its lowest level between 9 AM and noon and at its highest level from 8 PM until midnight. In some euthyroid persons, the differences are significantly different, and in patients with any degree of hypothyroidism the differences may become even more exaggerated. Therefore, it is helpful if TSH levels are checked at similar times, and preferably between 9 AM and noon, when they are at their lowest levels.

ETIOLOGY

Hypothyroidism is most commonly due to a primary decrease in production of thyroid hormone by the thyroid gland itself (Box 1). An obvious cause would be that the patient has had thyroid surgery or received radioiodine ablation therapy. However, iodine deficiency remains the most common cause of primary hypothyroidism worldwide, especially in the developing world.

In the United States, autoimmune thyroid disease (AITD), in the form of Hashimoto's thyroiditis, is the most common cause of hypothyroidism. Autoimmune hypothyroidism is due to T cell–mediated apoptosis of thyroid cells. Tissue damage is reflected by the development of serum thyroid peroxidase antibodies (anti-TPO) and thyroglobulin antibodies (anti-Tg), which can themselves be cytotoxic and contribute to the further destruction of the thyroid cells. This results in the subsequent elevation of serum TSH levels. The presence of thyroid autoantibodies is a useful clinical marker of susceptibility to clinical thyroid failure, which progresses at a rate of 2% to 5% per year when TSH levels are borderline. Autoimmune thyroid disease can also be associated with other autoimmune diseases, including other endocrine diseases, such as type 1 diabetes mellitus, Addison's disease, and the polyglandular autoimmune syndromes.

BOX 1 Example Causes of Hypothyroidism

Primary Hypothyroidism
Autoimmune (Hashimoto's thyroiditis)
Iodine deficiency (primarily Asia, Africa, Latin America)
Congenital causes: Organ defects, thyroid hormone
  resistance, TSH receptor defects

Thyroid Ablation
Radioiodine treatment
Surgery
External irradiation

Transient Hypothyroidism
Subacute thyroiditis
Postpartum thyroiditis
Sick euthyroid syndrome

Central Hypothyroidism (Hypothalamic or Pituitary)
Tumors: Pituitary adenoma, craniopharyngioma
Pituitary apoplexy
Radiation
Infiltrative diseases: Sarcoidosis, tuberculosis
Hypophysitis

Medications
Inhibition of synthesis: Antithyroid drugs (e.g.,
  methimazole [Tapazole]) or propylthiouracil
Iodine excess
Amiodarone (Pacerone, Cordarone)
Lithium (Lithobid)
Inhibition of thyroid hormone action: Anticonvulsants in
  susceptible people
Precipitation of autoimmune thyroid disease: Interferons
Sunitnib chemotherapy agent
Changes in thyroid-binding globulin levels:
• Increased: Estrogens, tamoxifen (Soltamox),
  methadone (Dolophine), heroin
• Decreased: Androgens, glucocorticoids
Changes in T_4 absorption
Calcium, iron, aluminum hydroxide gels, sulcrafate (Carafate),
  resin binders, e.g., cholestyramine (Questran)
Diets high in soy

TSH = thyroid-stimulating hormone.

BOX 2 Signs and Symptoms of Hypothyroidism

Metabolic
Mild weight gain
Elevated cholesterol
Increased sensitivity to insulin
Sleepiness

Cardiovascular
Slowed heart rate
Decreased cardiac output

Muscular (Skeletal)
Muscle weakness
Decreased energy
Increased fatigability

Skin
Dry, scaly skin
Loss of hair

Psychiatric
Impaired concentration
Depression
Fatigue
Lethargy

Gynecologic
Irregular menses
Infertility
Menorrhagia

Gastrointestinal
Constipation
Iron-deficiency anemia
Macrocytic anemia

Ears, Nose, and Throat
Hoarseness of voice
Deepening of voice

Severe Hypothyroidism
Accumulation of hyaluronic acid and water resulting in
  nonpitting edema
Pericardial and pleural exudative effusions
Periorbital edema

A number of medications are known to affect thyroid function, either by increasing or decreasing thyroid hormone clearance, presenting high iodine loads, or inducing thyroid-specific T cells and antibodies (see Box 1). Transient hypothyroidism can occur due to subacute thyroiditis or postpartum Hashimoto's disease and during the recovery phase of the sick euthyroid syndrome. Rarely, secondary hypothyroidism may be due to pituitary or hypothalamic disorders that can result in TSH or TSH-releasing hormone (TRH) deficiency.

PREVALENCE

Up to 25 million Americans have an underactive thyroid gland, which remains undiagnosed in almost one half of these people. Women are six to eight times more likely than men to develop such thyroid failure. AITD also runs in families, and the incidence of hypothyroidism increases with age. By age 60 years, as many as 20% of women and 9% of men will have developed an underactive thyroid.

SIGNS AND SYMPTOMS

Thyroid hormones are the primary regulator of the body's metabolism. The signs and symptoms of hypothyroidism are, therefore, multisystemic and are summarized in Box 2.

TREATMENT

T_4 Therapy

The treatment that most closely mimics normal thyroid physiology is replacement using levothyroxine (T_4) (Synthroid, Levoxyl). The absorbed T_4 is then converted by the deiodinase enzymes to the active hormone T_3. A normal TSH level is the target of this replacement. As discussed earlier, the definition of a normal TSH level varies. For replacement patients we use 0.5 to 3.0 µU/mL, and we generally teach patients that their TSH level should be 1.0.

The average T_4 full-replacement dose for adults is 1.6 µg/kg/day. However, the degree of remaining thyroid reserve greatly influences the required amount of T_4 and can change considerably with time. Patients who are otherwise healthy and without concurrent illnesses or risk factors for coronary artery disease (CAD) can be started near the full calculated replacement dose. Patients who are elderly or who have CAD or other comorbid risk factors should not be started at dosages greater than 12.5 to 25 µg/day. Therapy is then guided by evaluation of the TSH level at 4- to 6-week intervals.

Replacement in patients who are older than 65 years should be calculated using a more cautious algorithm irrespective of their medical history. Checking T_4 levels sooner than 4 weeks can be helpful in confirming that the patient is taking and absorbing the T_4 replacement medication but will not be helpful in assessing the final dose needed for adequate replacement, because it takes 4 weeks for TSH to normalize on a new thyroid dose.

Patients who are pregnant might need an increase in preconception T_4 intake as high as 50%, and women who initiate estrogen as an oral contraceptive or in the postmenopausal period, while taking T_4, might also require an increase in dose.

T_4 supplements should be taken on an empty stomach 1 hour before or 2 hours after a meal, and 1 hour before or 3 to 4 hours after taking other medications. Many medications and nutrients affect absorption of T_4 (see Box 1). Note, therefore, that intravenous replacement of T_4 in patients who cannot take oral medications should contain only 70% to 80% of the calculated oral dose.

Alternatives to T_4 Therapy

The majority of clinical studies have failed to show a physiologic or clinical benefit to using T_3 (Cytomel) alone or in adding T_3 to T_4 supplementation in hypothyroid patients. Thyroid hormone preparations that contain T_3 or the addition of T_3 supplements to T_4 therapy are, therefore, currently not recommended. T_3 has a short half-life and causes early peaks and then plummets in the same day, requiring twice-or thrice-daily dosing. T_4 supplementation and its subsequent conversion to T_3 provides physiologically stable levels of both T_4 and T_3.

Thyroid hormone should also not be replaced with dessicated thyroid preparations (e.g., Armour Thyroid, Nature-Throid, Westhroid, Bio-Throid). These compounds are made from beef or pork thyroid glands and contain thyroglobulin and both T_4 and T_3. The ratio of T_4 to T_3 is variable from one preparation to the next and reflects the intrathyroid ratio rather than that of the peripheral circulation. These preparations are, therefore, highly unnatural although they claim otherwise, and patients often run low TSH levels and intermittent high T_3 values.

Thyroid Hormone Bioequivalency

In October 2006, the Endocrine Society, the American Association of Clinical Endocrinology, and the American Thyroid Association (ATA) presented to the FDA their concerns about the methods used for testing the bioequivalence of different commercial thyroid hormone preparations.[4] Many patients and practitioners noticed over the years that switching from one T_4 brand to another, which was considered equivalent by their standards of bioequivalency testing, led to failures in treating patients with hypothyroidism. Hormones would become either underreplaced or overreplaced, as judged by serum TSH levels, on doses of thyroid hormones that had previously controlled the levels very well. The only difference was a change in the brand. The FDA does not incorporate the TSH level into its pharmacokinetic testing when declaring different brands of T_4 replacement bioequivalent, and as of the date of writing has so far refused to do so. Therefore, we recommend that all patients should be maintained on the same brand of T_4 replacement and not subjected to different brands or different generic preparations. Using generic versions of T_4, or changing commercial brands, in our experience creates unstable replacement regimens requiring costly re-equilibration and retesting strategies.

Subclinical Hypothyroidism

DEFINITION

Subclinical hypothyroidism is defined as an elevated TSH level associated with total and free T_4 and T_3 levels within the normal range. Usually the TSH in such patients falls between 4.0 and 10.0 µU/mL.[5]

PREVALENCE

The prevalence of patients in the general population with TSH levels between 4.0 and 10.0 µU/mL is typically 5% to 10%. With advancing age this increases, and in women older than 60 years, it can be greater than 20% of the population. Numerous studies have shown that once the diagnosis of subclinical hypothyroidism is made, and TPO antibodies are present, patients develop overt hypothyroidism at the rate of about 5% per year.

SCREENING

In the controversial meetings of the Consensus Panel on Subclinical Hypothyroidism convened, but not endorsed, by the Endocrine Societies and the American Thyroid Association, there were differences in opinions on whom should be screened for this condition within the general population, whether or not all women contemplating pregnancy or in their first trimester of pregnancy should be screened, and whether or not patients with TSH levels less than 10.0 µU/mL should be treated.

The ATA now recommends screening of both men and women beginning at age 35 years and then every 5 years afterward. The American College of Physicians only recommends screening women older than 50 years who present with symptoms consistent with subclinical hypothyroidism. These approaches totally ignore the pregnant population.

TREATMENT

During the Consensus Panel Meeting on Subclinical Hypothyroidism, there were also differences of opinion on which patients should be treated, and no consensus exists to this day. Much of this controversy arises from the quality of the outcomes data related to the treatment of such patients. Although such data remain incomplete, we interpret the evidence as sufficient to warrant treatment of these patients. We believe that once the diagnosis of subclinical hypothyroidism is confirmed by repeat testing within 1 to 3 months, and that causes such as subacute thyroiditis and recovery from nonthyroidal illness have been ruled out as causes of the elevated TSH levels, it is appropriate and safe to treat many such patients to a normal TSH level of 1.0 µU/mL.

OUTCOMES

Two important studies have become available concerning the impact of subclinical hypothyroidism. The first is a prospective study of 3121 cardiac patients with subclinical hypothyroidism, subclinical hyperthyroidism, and low T_3 syndrome. These patients were followed for a mean follow-up of 32 months. Hazard ratios (HRs) for cardiac death were higher in subclinical hypothyroidism (HR, 2.40; 95% confidence interval [CI], 1.36–4.21; $P = 0.02$). Survival from cardiac events was lower, and overall mortality was higher in patients with subclinical hypothyroid patients than in euthyroid patients. In a second report of a prospective study, patients with subclinical hypothyroidism, followed for 12 years, with a TSH level of 10 to 20 mU/L, had a significantly higher incidence of heart failure than patients who were euthyroid or had TSH levels between 4.5 mU/L and 9.9 mU/L. These studies strongly suggest that subtle thyroid failure can have deleterious cardiac effects.

Because thyroid function affects Ca^{2+} influx to the myocardium, it stands to reason that treatment might improve function. In fact, the majority of studies, although small in patient number, have shown clinical improvement in surrogate markers of cardiac function: improvement in actual ventricular function, endothelial function, and lipid profiles. In terms of the effects on mortality, the data remain unclear, although a Japanese population showed a survival advantage in treated men with subclinical hypothyroidism. However, one study of patients older than 85 years has also suggested that such elderly patients with subclinical hypothyroidism who were untreated might actually have an advantage in terms of survival.

Hence, except for patients with an unstable cardiac status, or the very elderly, we feel that subclinical hypothyroidism should be treated, because the treatment of a reliable patient is unlikely to have any harmful effects. In patients with an unstable cardiac status, subclinical hypothyroidism may be watched carefully.

Special Situations

SECONDARY HYPOTHYROIDISM

Secondary hypothyroidism often occurs in the setting of damage to the pituitary gland or hypothalamus. TSH elevation and reduction in this setting are not reliable measures of adequate T_4 replacement. The free T_4 must be corrected to the normal range, ignoring the TSH value. In this setting it is imperative to be certain that the patient does not have coexisting glucocorticoid deficiency. Often it is important to treat with replacement glucocorticoids in order to avoid adrenal insufficiency because the cortisol clearance is enhanced when thyroid hormone is supplemented.

MYXEDEMA COMA

Myxedema coma is a medical emergency. Even with prompt diagnosis the mortality can be as high as 30%. The mean age of patients is approximately 75 years.

Myxedema coma can be precipitated by hypothermia, infection, myocardial infarction, respiratory depression, or blood loss. Often patients have undiagnosed hypothyroidism or have discontinued their medication. Physical signs of hypothyroidism are usually obvious. Usually a high-dose treatment regimen is used in such patients, such as T_4 300 to 500 µg IV followed by 100 µg daily. Some practitioners advocate T_3 10 to 20 µg IV every 4 hours.

Respiratory support and slow rewarming are also essential. Signs of infection may be obscured. Treatment of hyponatremia and hypoglycemia may be necessary as well. Adrenal replacement of hydrocortisone (Cortef) with 50 to 100 mg every 8 hours is advocated.

PREGNANCY

Screening

Only confused recommendations have appeared for screening women planning pregnancy and during the first trimester of pregnancy, except in populations known to be at high risk for developing hypothyroidism, such as in patients with type 1 diabetes mellitus or other autoimmune diseases. However, we recommend screening all pregnant and prepregnant patients for hypothyroidism. A recent study showed that patients at high risk for developing hypothyroidism during their first trimester will be identified if screened, but if the entire population is not screened, then 30% of patients who develop primary hypothyroidism during their first trimester will be missed.

The Endocrine Society has published their recommendations for screening of thyroid dysfunction in pregnancy. This states that although the benefits of universal screening for thyroid dysfunction (primarily hypothyroidism) might not be justified by the current evidence, we recommend case finding among the following groups of women at high risk for thyroid disease by measurement of TSH:

- Women with a history of hyperthyroid or hypothyroid disease, postpartum thyroiditis, or thyroid lobectomy
- Women with a family history of thyroid disease
- Women with a goiter
- Women with thyroid antibodies (when known)
- Women with symptoms or clinical signs suggesting thyroid underfunction or overfunction, including anemia, elevated cholesterol, and hyponatremia
- Women with type 1 diabetes
- Women with other autoimmune disorders
- Women with infertility who should have screening with TSH as part of their infertility work-up
- Women with previous therapeutic head or neck irradiation
- Women with a history of miscarriage or preterm delivery

Postpartum thyroid studies are recommended at 3 and 6 months for patients at risk for thyroid disease.

Treatment

Pregnancy increases the dosage requirements of T_4 replacement for several different reasons. Estrogen causes an increase in the serum thyroxine-binding globulin level, which increases T_4 binding requirements; there is an increased transfer of T_4 to the fetus; and T_4 clearance itself is increased. During the first trimester, normal TSH levels are low or may be suppressed, and the upper limit if normal TSH in pregnancy is considered to be 2.5 µU/mL.

Hypothyroidism in pregnancy is associated with increased obstetric and fetal risks. A recent study suggests that T_4 supplementation starting in the first trimester in patients who have positive TPO antibodies regardless of the baseline TSH level had reduced obstetric complications, miscarriages, and premature deliveries.

For normal intellectual development of the child, it is also essential that the mother be euthyroid during the pregnancy. Therefore, thyroid status in the woman treated with T_4 replacement should be monitored each month. In contrast to the nonpregnant woman, the treatment of subclinical hypothyroidism in pregnancy is endorsed by all clinical societies.

TRANSIENT HYPOTHYROIDISM

Postpartum thyroiditis (a variant transient form of Hashimoto's thyroiditis) and subacute thyroiditis, typically manifests with hyperthyroidism as the thyroid cells undergo apoptosis, and this is then followed by a transient hypothyroid state. Postpartum thyroiditis might affect 10% of all pregnancies. At particular risk are patients with thyroid antibodies in the first trimester of pregnancy, patients with type 1 diabetes mellitus, and patients with a previous history of postpartum thyroiditis.

Postpartum thyroiditis typically develops 3 to 12 months following delivery. Most cases of hypothyroidism following the hyperthyroid phase are transient. Whether or not to treat the hypothyroidism is often, therefore, a clinical decision based on how symptomatic the person is. If one chooses to treat, one may choose to treat with a lower than full replacement dose, making it easier to monitor recovery to the euthyroid state. If one treats with a complete replacement dose, the thyroid supplement has to be stopped completely after 6 to 8 weeks to see if there is recovery.

In people with painful or painless subacute thyroiditis, the treatment scenario is essentially the same. Following the hyperthyroid phase, transient hypothyroidism typically develops. Whether or not to treat the person with a T_4 supplement and at what dose is a clinical decision depending on symptoms.

EUTHYROID SICK SYNDROME

A variety of metabolic abnormalities contribute to a syndrome of abnormal thyroid function tests commonly observed in sick patients. Typically the serum T_3 levels are low as an isolated observation, but the T_4 levels can also fall dramatically as the condition of the patient deteriorates. Serum TSH may be normal or modestly suppressed or even increased. A strong case has been made for the treatment of such patients with thyroid hormone replacement. However, this view is controversial, has not been satisfactorily subjected to controlled trials, and is a view we do not share at this time.

REFERENCES

Abalovich M, Amino N, Barbour LA, et al. Management of thyroid dysfunction during pregnancy and postpartum: An Endocrine Society Clinical Practice Guideline. J Clin Endocrinol Metab 2007;92:S1–47.

American Thyroid Association; Endocrine Society; American Association of Clinical Endocrinologists. Joint statement on the U.S. Food and Drug Administration's decision regarding bioequivalence of levothyroxine sodium. Thyroid 2004;14(7):486.

Andersen S, Pedersen KM, Bruun NK, Laurberg P. Narrow individual variations in serum T4 and T3 in normal subjects: A clue to the understanding of subclinical thyroid disease. J Clin Endocrinol Metab 2002;87:1068–72.

Andersen S, Bruun NH, Pedersen KM, Laurberg P. Biologic variation is important for interpretation of thyroid function tests. Thyroid 2003;13:1069–78.

Casey BM. Subclinical hypothyroidism and pregnancy. Obstet Gynecol Surv 2006;61:415–20.

de Groot LJ. Nonthyroidal illness syndrome is a manifestation of hypothalamic–pituitary dysfunction, and in view of current evidence, should be treated with appropriate replacement therapies. Crit Care Clin 2006;22:57–86 vi.

De Jong FJ, Peeters RP, Den HT, et al. The association of polymorphisms in the type 1 and 2 deiodinase genes with circulating thyroid hormone parameters and atrophy of the medial temporal lobe. J Clin Endocrinol Metab 2007;92:636–40.

Gussekloo J, Van EE, De Craen AJ, et al. Thyroid status, disability and cognitive function, and survival in old age. JAMA 2004;292:2591–9.

Iervasi G, Molinaro S, Landi P, et al. Association between increased mortality and mild thyroid dysfunction in cardiac patients. Arch Intern Med 2007;167:1526–32.

Imaizumi M, Akahoshi M, Ichimaru S, et al. Risk for ischemic heart disease and all-cause mortality in subclinical hypothyroidism. J Clin Endocrinol Metab 2004;89:3365–70.

Negro R, Formoso G, Mangieri T, et al. Levothyroxine treatment in euthyroid pregnant women with autoimmune thyroid disease: Effects on obstetrical complications. J Clin Endocrinol. Metab 2006;91:2587–91.

Rodondi N, Cappola A, Cornuz J, et al. Subclinical thyroid dysfunction, cardiac function, and the risk of congestive heart failure: The Cardiovascular Health Study American Thyroid Association Annual Meeting. Thyroid 2007;17(Suppl. 1):S1–73.

Surks MI, Ortiz E, Daniels GH, et al. Subclinical thyroid disease: Scientific review and guidelines for diagnosis and management. JAMA 2004;291:228–38.

Vaidya B, Anthony S, Bilous M, et al. Detection of thyroid dysfunction in early pregnancy: Universal screening or targeted high-risk case finding? J Clin Endocrinol Metab 2007;92:203–7.

Wartofsky L, Van ND, Burman KD. Overt and "subclinical" hypothyroidism in women. Obstet Gynecol Surv 2006;61:535–42.

676

Hyperthyroidism

Method of
Peter A. Singer, MD

Hyperthyroidism encompasses a heterogeneous group of disorders, all of which have two features in common. Firstly, all of the types of hyperthyroidism include a β-adrenergic-mediated symptom complex of varying degrees of severity characterized by symptoms of nervousness, heat intolerance, irritability, palpitations, and increased bowel motility, with frequency of movements. Secondly, hyperthyroidism is associated with the catabolic effects of excess circulating levels of thyroid hormone; such effects can include weight loss, fatigue, muscle weakness, increased appetite, and bone loss. The symptoms and signs of hyperthyroidism depend on a number of variables, including levels of circulating thyroid hormone, duration of disease, the age of the patient, and concurrent illnesses.

Hyperthyroidism can be classified according to the capacity of the thyroid gland to trap radioactive iodine (Box 1). Disorders with increased radioiodine uptake have thyroid gland autonomy (with the exception of thyroid-stimulating hormone [TSH]-secreting pituitary tumors) and require specific treatment, whereas those with suppressed radioiodine uptake include conditions that are usually self-limited and might require only symptomatic treatment.

Physical examination of the hyperthyroid patient generally reveals a person who is somewhat anxious and has a rapid pulse. In the elderly, atrial fibrillation is common, and many elderly patients have widened pulse pressure, warm skin, and palpable thyroid gland findings, depending on the underlying etiology. Examination of the eyes in all types of hyperthyroidism might show eyelid retraction, which is mediated by β-adrenergic stimulation. Infiltrative ophthalmopathy is seen almost exclusively in patients with thyrotoxic Graves' disease.

BOX 1 Causes of Hyperthyroidism*

Hyperthyroidism with Elevated RAIU
- Graves' disease
- Toxic multinodular goiter
- Toxic adenoma
- TSH-secreting pituitary tumor
- Hydatidiform mole
- Choriocarcinoma
- Pituitary resistance to thyroid hormone

Hyperthyroidism with Low RAIU
- Factitious
- Subacute granulomatus thyroiditis
- Subacute lymphocytic (postpartum or sporadic)
- Amiodarone-induced thyroiditis
- Iodine-induced hyperthyroidism
- Radiation-induced thyroiditis
- Metastatic functioning follicular tumor
- Struma ovarii

*In probable decreasing order of frequency.
Abbreviations: RAIU = radioactive iodine uptake; TSH = thyroid-stimulating hormone.

Diagnosis

Because many of the symptoms of hyperthyroidism may be compatible with some nonthyroid disorders, such as anxiety or the perimenopausal state, TSH, should be measured in patients in whom hyperthyroidism is suspected. TSH suppressed in hyperthroidism, although in patients with rare TSH-secreting pituitary tumors, TSH

 CURRENT DIAGNOSIS

Symptoms of Graves' Hyperthyroidism
- Emotional lability
- Eye irritation, photophobia, diplopia
- Fatigue
- Heat intolerance
- Increased appetite
- Increased frequency of bowel movements
- Increased perspiration
- Menstrual irregularities
- Muscle weakness
- Nervousness
- Palpitations
- Shortness of breath
- Sleep disturbances
- Weight loss

Signs of Graves' Hyperthyroidism
- Diffuse goiter
- Eye stare
- Hyperreflexia
- Infiltrative dermopathy (~5%)
- Proptosis
- Proximal muscle weakness
- Systolic hypertension
- Tachycardia
- Thyroid bruit
- Warm, smooth skin
- Widened pulse pressure

levels may be normal or even slightly elevated. TSH levels may be suppressed in hospitalized patients, especially those who are seriously ill or who are receiving pharmacologic doses of glucocorticoids or dopamine, thus limiting the usefulness of serum TSH measurements in such patients.

A suppressed TSH level in patients suspected to have hyperthyroidism should be complemented with a serum free thyroxine (T_4) or its estimate to confirm the diagnosis. Patients with normal thyroid hormone levels and suppressed TSH concentrations have what is termed *subclinical hyperthyroidism*, a disorder usually free of overt symptoms of hyperthyroidism.

After the diagnosis of hyperthyroidism is confirmed, its etiology should be determined by obtaining a thyroid radioactive iodine uptake. Patients with obvious Graves' disease (such as those with infiltrative ophthalmopathy or large goiters with bruits), may forgo the radioactive iodine uptake test. It is important, however, to differentiate between Graves' disease and low radioactive iodine uptake conditions, which usually are self-limited.

In addition to the radioactive iodine uptake, a scan may be helpful in establishing the diagnosis in patients with suspected toxic multinodular goiter, a condition encountered more commonly nowadays due to increasing immigration into the United States from endemic goiter regions.

Treatment

Because approximately 80% of patients with hyperthyroidism in the United States have thyrotoxic Graves' disease, most of the comments in this article pertain to that disorder. Among patients with high radioactive iodine-uptake hyperthyroidism, only Graves' disease may be associated with remission following the use of thionamide drugs.

DEVELOPING A TREATMENT STRATEGY

General Measures and Patient Education

Essential in the early management of Graves' hyperthyroidism is emphasizing to the patient that strict adherence to the treatment regimen is essential in alleviating symptoms and restoring health. Persons with hyperthyroidism commonly tend to be impatient, likely due to their symptoms, and it must be stressed that compliance with treatment advice is essential for a successful outcome. If family members or friends accompany the patient to the appointment, it is helpful to make them familiar with the treatment plan as well.

Initial Treatment of Symptoms

Because many of the symptoms of hyperthyroidism are related to enhanced β-adrenergic stimulation, I routinely employ β-adrenergic-blocking drugs, although mild symptoms might not warrant their use. I prefer propranolol (Inderal),[1] even though it must be given approximately every 6 hours to be completely effective. Propranolol's relatively short half-life makes this agent preferable, because patients learn to titrate their own medication, depending on their symptoms. As patients improve during the course of thionamide therapy (see later), they can omit more doses of propranolol.

The usual starting dose of propranolol[1] is between 20 and 40 mg approximately every 6 hours (or four times a day), and the desired target heart rate is approximately 80 beats per minute. Some physicians prefer longer acting β-blockers, such as atenolol (Tenormin),[1] which may be given as a single daily dose. In patients in whom compliance may be problematic, or in those who prefer once-daily dosing, atenolol 50 to 100 mg a day is an excellent alternative. Other long-acting β-blockers are nadolol (Corgard)[1] and metoprolol (Lopressor).[1] Long-acting β-blockers are cardioselective and are not contraindicated in patients with coexisting asthma, as propranolol is.

---

[1]Not FDA approved for this indication.

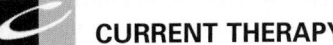

CURRENT THERAPY

Treatment Modality	Advantages	Disadvantages
Thionamide drugs	Chance of remission	Relapse (40%)
	Relatively inexpensive	Side effects (5–10%)
Surgery	Rapid, permanent cure	Surgical complications (hypocalcemia, recurrent nerve injury ~1%–3%)
		Hypothyroidism
Radioactive iodine	Permanent cure	Expensive
		Hypothyroidism

In my experience, patients who are treated with adequate doses of β-adrenergic blocking drugs have significant relief of symptoms within a few days after the medication is initiated.

Reduction of Serum Thyroid Hormone Levels

Unfortunately, there have been few advances in the management of hyperthyroidism in recent years. Treatment basically consists of lowering the concentrations of serum thyroxine (T_4) and triiodothyronine (T_3), which may be accomplished either with thionamide drugs or with ablative therapy, either radioiodine or surgery. In the United States, radioiodine ablation with ^{131}I is the preferred method of treatment of most practicing endocrinologists. Indeed, in a survey of thyroid experts completed in 1991, 69% of respondents chose radioiodine as the primary form of therapy for a prototypic 43-year-old woman with uncomplicated Graves' disease. Only 1% of physicians recommended surgery, and 30% selected thionamide drugs as the primary form of therapy. The responses were in sharp contrast to thyroid experts in both Europe and Japan, where a similar survey revealed that the majority of physicians favored thionamide drugs as the primary form of therapy. The rationale provided by physicians in the United States who selected radioiodine therapy was the fact that the remission rate following 1 to 2 years of thionamide drugs was only approximately 30%.

Before recommending a specific type of therapy for a patient with Graves' disease, it is essential that the patient be aware of the benefits and pitfalls of each type of treatment.

THIONAMIDE DRUG THERAPY

Initial Treatment

Currently, there are two thionamide drugs available for clinical use in the United States, methimazole (MMI, Tapazole) available in 5-mg and 10-mg tablets, and propylthiouracil (PTU) available in 50-mg tablets. Both agents inhibit the synthesis of thyroid hormone by blocking organification of iodine. PTU also inhibits peripheral conversion of T_4 to T_3, although clinically this may be more of a theoretical than a practical advantage.

I generally prefer MMI, rather than PTU, because of its longer biological half-life and its potency. For uncomplicated hyperthyroidism, MMI may initially be given 2 to 3 times a day in a total dose of 20 to 30 mg, whereas PTU is usually administered 3 to 4 times a day in a total dose of 300 to 400 mg. When biochemical euthyroidism is achieved, usually after 6 to 8 weeks of therapy, MMI may be given once a day, or PTU twice a day, and the total dose may be halved. The relative simplicity of using MMI versus PTU can render it more suitable for patients in whom compliance may be difficult. It must be stressed to the patient that omitting medication doses can result in a rebound of the hyperthyroid state, because the intrathyroid deficiency of iodine produced by thionamide drugs results in more avid trapping of exogenous iodine.

In general, I obtain serum T_4 and T_3 levels about 6 to 8 weeks after initiating thionamide drug therapy to ensure adequacy of treatment response. If there has been little clinical or biochemical improvement, the likeliest scenario is that doses of medication are being omitted. A serum TSH provides no additional information at this point, because TSH suppression is common for up to 3 or 4 months after euthyroidism has been achieved. Patients with very large goiters and fairly severe hyperthyroidism often take somewhat longer than 6 to 8 weeks to become euthyroid and can require larger doses of MMI (e.g., 40 mg/day) or PTU (e.g., 400–600 mg/day).

I stress to patients that any improvement with thionamide drugs can take several weeks, and I recommend that they defer, if possible, making definitive decisions regarding long-term thionamide versus ablative therapy until they have improved to the extent that they are better able to make more reasoned choices. I always discuss the various forms of treatment of hyperthyroidism with patients during our first appointment, however, and reiterate the options after they have improved.

Although the overall remission rate of patients treated with thionamide drugs in the United States is approximately 30%, some patients are more likely than others to go into remission. Patients with mild hyperthyroidism, small goiters, and a negative family history for hyperthyroidism are more likely to respond favorably, as are patients who respond quickly to thionamide drugs in terms of thyroid gland shrinkage and biochemical improvement. Conversely, patients with severe thyrotoxicosis and those with a strong family history of Graves' disease infrequently go into remission. Some clinicians have advocated serologic markers, such as thyroid-stimulating immunoglobulin or anti-TPO antibodies, to predict the likelihood of remission, but there has been no confirmation of their usefulness for such a purpose.

Continuing Treatment

I reevaluate patients taking thionamide drugs approximately every 3 months, and in addition to the clinical examination, I obtain a serum free T_4 (estimate) and TSH. If hypothyroidism occurs while on medication, I often add levothyroxine (Synthroid) rather than reduce the dose of thionamide drug. Most patients can be maintained euthyroid on 20 mg of MMI and 0.1 mg of levothyroxine taken in a single daily dose. If PTU is employed, it usually must be given twice daily.

Combined therapy with thionamide drugs and levothyroxine resulted in a considerable amount of controversy several years ago, following the publication of an article from a Japanese group of researchers who reported that 98% of patients taking both MMI and levothyroxine achieved remission. The researchers maintained serum TSH levels in the suppressed range and theorized that TSH inhibition with levothyroxine resulted in less stimulation of antigen release. Unfortunately, their findings have not been confirmed in subsequent studies, either in Japan or elsewhere. Some physicians, however, have reported improved remission rates following longer durations of thionamide administration, of up to 10 years. The practical aspects of such prolonged therapy however, might be open to question.

Side Effects of Thionamide Drugs

The most common allergic side effects of thionamide drugs range from mild maculopapular rashes to urticarial eruptions and occur in approximately 5% of patients. Allergic reactions usually do not occur until 2 to 4 weeks after initiation of therapy. Mild symptoms may be managed with antihistamines, although complete resolution of itching and rash is uncommon. Therefore, I routinely switch patients from the type of medication they are taking (e.g., MMI) to PTU. Approximately 20% of patients are also allergic to the other thionamides, preventing their continued use.

The most serious side effect of thionamide drugs is agranulocytosis, and although it is rare (0.2%–0.5% of patients), it is potentially fatal. It is usually manifested by fever and symptoms of infection, such as a severe sore throat. Patients must be instructed that if they develop fever and signs and symptoms of infection, they must stop the thionamide drug and call their physician immediately. A white blood cell count and differential must be performed, and, if agranulocytosis is diagnosed, hospital admission is required. Successful reversal of agranulocytosis, sometimes employing granulocyte colony stimulating factor (G-CSF), should occur within a few days to a week.

Some physicians obtain periodic white blood cell (WBC) counts, although this practice is probably unnecessary because the WBC does not predict agranulocytosis. Nevertheless, before initiating therapy with thionamide drugs, it is helpful to have a baseline WBC because leukopenia is common in patients with Graves' disease, and if a subsequent WBC is obtained, it is useful for comparison.

Other potential side effects of antithyroid drugs include arthralgias and, rarely, hepatitis. Hepatitis is also potentially fatal.

Stopping Antithyroid Drug Therapy

If therapy with thionamide drugs is used to induce remission, an endpoint of therapy should be determined. I usually treat for 12 to 18 months and then discontinue the thionamide agent. Patients are reevaluated approximately 4 to 6 weeks later, and a serum TSH is obtained. If the serum TSH is suppressed during thionamide therapy, the likelihood of remission is poor. If the patient is euthyroid at 4 to 6 weeks, the next visit is scheduled for approximately 3 months later and at increasing intervals thereafter, but at intervals no longer than 1 year.

Most relapses of hyperthyroidism occur within the first year after stopping thionamide drugs, but they can occur at any time. If relapse occurs, a second course of thionamide drugs does not appear to increase the likelihood of remission, and ablation with radioiodine is then recommended. Some patients, however, prefer to take antithyroid drugs for several, or even many years and often can be maintained on a very small dose of thionamide drug (e.g., 2.5–5 mg/day of MMI). Although such extended therapy is not my preference, there is no absolute contraindication to it. Patients on such a regimen need to be instructed that periodic follow-up, perhaps every 3 to 6 months, is necessary.

RADIOACTIVE IODINE THERAPY

Therapy with radioiodine (^{131}I) is the preferred method of treatment for hyperthyroidism among other thyroid specialists practicing in the United States. Radioiodine has distinct advantages: It is effective, relatively inexpensive, and predictable, and it appears to be free of side effects other than the development of hypothyroidism. Radioiodine has been used to treat hyperthyroidism for approximately 45 years in the United States, and careful follow-up has failed to show an increased incidence of cancer in patients so treated or in genetic defects in offspring of ^{131}I-treated patients. Radioiodine is contraindicated during pregnancy, which should be ruled out in women of childbearing age before its administration. In addition, women who are breast-feeding should not be treated with radioiodine, because the isotope can recirculate in breast milk for up to several weeks after administration.

Selection of Radioiodine Dose

Some clinicians advocate administering a ^{131}I dose that is sufficient to control hyperthyroidism without resulting in hypothyroidism. Various strategies have been employed over the years in an effort to achieve this goal, but they generally have failed. Therefore, I prefer administering a dose large enough to result in hypothyroidism, which usually occurs within 3 to 6 months after ^{131}I administration. A dose of 15 mCi of ^{131}I is usually sufficient to achieve this goal, but the appropriate dose depends on the radioactive iodine uptake and size of the thyroid gland. A 24-hour radioactive iodine uptake should be measured before the treatment dose is administered to ensure that adequate quantities of ^{131}I will be absorbed by the thyroid. A dose of 100–150 fCi/g of thyroid tissue is generally an adequate ablative dose. Some patients are resistant to an initial dose of ^{131}I and require a second or even third treatment. In my experience, male patients, Asians, and patients with large goiters appear to require larger or additional doses. If patients continue to be hyperthyroid 6 months after an initial treatment with ^{131}I, a second dose is administered.

Before administering radioiodine, I usually pretreat patients with thionamide drugs until they are euthyroid, because depletion of thyroid hormone from the thyroid prevents release of excess of thyroid hormone from the gland, thereby preventing exacerbation of hyperthyroidism. This is especially important for older patients or those with cardiovascular risk factors. Antithyroid drugs should be discontinued 3 to 5 days before radioiodine treatment. Patients receiving ^{131}I without having been pretreated with antithyroid drugs (for example, patients who are allergic to thionamides) benefit from administration of propranolol[1] or other β-blockers after treatment, because their underlying hyperthyroidism may be transiently exacerbated by ^{131}I-induced thyroiditis.

Follow-up after Radioiodine Treatment

I usually evaluate patients approximately 6 weeks following radioiodine administration in order to assess the clinical and biochemical responses. If the thyroid gland has not decreased in size by 6 weeks, a beneficial response from radioiodine is unlikely. If patients are euthyroid at 6 weeks, they return 4 to 6 weeks later, and if they are hypothyroid by that time, levothyroxine therapy is begun. If patients are still euthyroid (or hyperthyroid) 3 months after therapy, they are reevaluated in another 3 months. Nearly all patients are hypothyroid by 6 months after radioiodine treatment, and those who are still hyperthyroid require another treatment dose.

As experience with radioiodine has increased over the years, age limits for patients believed to be appropriate for treatment have decreased. It appears to be safe to treat teenagers with radioiodine, although I defer treatment in those who have not completed linear growth. There is little concern for developing thyroid nodularity in teenagers following ^{131}I treatment provided ablative doses are administered.

Radioiodine Treatment and Graves' Ophthalmopathy

Some clinicians think the administration of ^{131}I to patients with Graves' ophthalmopathy can worsen the eye disease and administration of pharmacologic amounts of glucocorticoids for a period of one month to 6 weeks following radioiodine treatment will lessen the likelihood of this occurrence. The data concerning efficacy of steroids are not conclusive, however. I believe that patients with moderate symptoms and signs of eye disease should be evaluated by an ophthalmologist with expertise in Graves' ophthalmopathy before administration of [131]I. Indeed, it is often helpful to involve the ophthalmologist in the care of patients with ophthalmopathy, regardless of the type of treatment for hyperthyroidism.

SURGERY

Surgery for Graves' hyperthyroidism is infrequently employed in the United States. Candidates for such treatment include children and teenagers, especially those who have difficulty complying with antithyroid drugs. Other indications include patients with very large goiters, especially those likely to be resistant to radioiodine because of large goiter size. In addition, surgery is the only choice for patients who are allergic to thionamide drugs and who refuse to take radioiodine. Surgery is also indicated for pregnant patients who are allergic to thionamide drugs (see later). Patients who have a coexistent thyroid nodule suspicious for cancer on fine-needle aspiration should be treated surgically.

Before surgery, it is preferred to render the patient euthyroid with thionamide drugs. Some surgeons prefer to administer exogenous iodides for 10 days before surgery. Exogenous iodides produce benefit both by inhibiting thyroid hormone release and by decreasing thyroid gland vascularity. Potassium iodide or Lugol's solution, 10 drops in a glass of water daily for 10 days, is sufficient.

Patients electing to undergo thyroidectomy should be made aware that permanent hypothyroidism will most likely result and that they will require the same type of follow-up as those treated with radioiodine. If insufficient thyroid tissue is removed, persistent or recurrent hyperthyroidism will result, which will necessitate radioiodine ablation.

---

[1]Not FDA approved for this indication.

Although surgery has the advantage of being rapidly curative, it also has potential complications. One is injury to the recurrent laryngeal nerve and the other is the possibility of permanent hypoparathyroidism. In skilled hands, these complications occur no more than 1% to 3% of the time, yet these potential risks must be explained fully to the patient beforehand.

Other Forms of Hyperthyroidism

TOXIC NODULAR GOITER

Toxic multinodular goiter increases in prevalence with increasing age. In elderly persons it is a more common cause of hyperthyroidism than is Graves' disease. The diagnosis should be documented with a radioactive iodine uptake and thyroid scan. Patients with toxic multinodular goiter will not go into remission on thionamide drugs, limiting definitive treatment to either radioiodine or surgery.

Before radioiodine is employed in elderly patients, thionamide drugs should be administered to minimize the risk of exacerbating hyperthyroidism. Radioiodine is the treatment of choice for most patients with toxic multinodular goiter, although surgery may be preferred for patients with especially large glands or with symptoms of compression who are good operative risks. If radioiodine is used for treatment of toxic nodular goiter, the dose required is usually greater than that employed for Graves' disease.

A single thyroid nodule producing hyperthyroidism occurs much less often than toxic multinodular goiter, and it generally occurs in persons younger than those with multinodular goiter. Although radioiodine is commonly employed for such patients, surgery is usually recommended for patients younger than 25 to 30 years.

HYPERTHYROIDISM AND PREGNANCY

Hyperthyroidism during pregnancy can lead to adverse outcomes both for mother and fetus. Adequate control of hyperthyroidism during pregnancy is essential. Either MMI or PTU may be used during pregnancy, but most clinicians favor PTU because it does not cross the placenta as easily as does MMI. For hyperthyroidism that is difficult to control, or if the patient is allergic to antithyroid drugs, thyroidectomy should be performed during the second trimester. β-Adrenergic blocking agents may be given safely during pregnancy to control symptoms.

Patients who continue to be treated with thionamide drugs during pregnancy should have a thyroid-stimulating immunoglobulin level drawn during the last trimester to predict the possible occurrence of neonatal hyperthyroidism. Hyperthyroid pregnant patients should be followed carefully at least every 4 to 6 weeks, and close communication should be maintained between the endocrinologist and obstetrician. It is advisable to use the lowest dose of thionamide drug that maintains maternal euthyroidism.

THYROID STORM

Thyroid storm (or crisis) is characterized by severe manifestations of hyperthyroidism, fever, and altered mental status. The disorder is usually precipitated by a concurrent illness.

Early recognition and treatment of thyroid storm are essential because it is life threatening. Patients must be managed in the intensive care unit, and, in addition to general supportive measures and treatment of concurrent illness, aggressive pharmacologic management of the hyperthyroidism is necessary. Either MMI or PTU may be used, although PTU has the potential advantage of reducing production of T_3 from T_4. A dose of 150 mg of PTU every 6 hours or 15 to 20 mg of MMI every 8 hours is usually sufficient. For patients unable to take medication orally, MMI may be crushed and given by nasogastric tube or may be prepared by the pharmacy as a rectal suppository.

In addition to thionamide drugs, exogenous iodides should be administered. Iopanoic acid may be used for this purpose, because it not only inhibits thyroid hormone release but also has the advantage of being a potent inhibitor of T_4 to T_3 conversion. A dose of

500 mg to 1 g orally daily is sufficient. However it is not currently available in the United States. Alternatively, iodine can be administered in the form of Lugol's solution or saturated solution of potassium iodide, 10 drops in water three times daily, or sodium iodide, 500 mg intravenously every 12 hours. It is essential to administer the first dose of thionamide drug a few hours before administration of iodides to prevent further organification of iodide with resultant additional thyroid hormone production. Some clinicians also use pharmacologic doses of glucocorticoids to further inhibit T_4 to T_3 conversion, although the clinical efficacy of this treatment has not been shown convincingly.

β-Blocking agents, preferably propranolol,[1] are essential in the management of thyroid storm and may be given either orally or intravenously. If the latter route is used, 1 mg every 5 to 10 minutes is given intravenously until the heart rate is less than 100 bpm. Once adequate control of the heart rate is achieved, oral propranolol may be given, and doses of 160 mg or more every 6 hours are not uncommon. Heart failure, which may be due in part to uncontrolled tachycardia, must be treated with adequate digitalis. If diuretics[1] are used, they must be administered very cautiously, because patients with thyroid storm are peripherally vasodilated and can suffer vascular collapse if conventional doses of diuretics are given. Plasmapheresis has been described as a treatment for thyroid storm, although I have neither used it nor seen it employed.

REFERENCES

Auer J, Scheibner P, Mische T, et al. Subclinical hyperthyroidism is a risk factor for atrial fibrillation. Am Heart J 2001;142:838–42.

Baldini M, Gallazzi M, Orsatti A, et al. Treatment of benign nodular goiter with mildly suppressive doses of L-thyroxine: Effects on bone mineral density and on nodule size. J Intern Med 2002;251:407–14.

Bauer DC, Ettinger B, Nevitt MC, Stone KL. Risk for fracture in women with low serum levels of thyroid-stimulating hormone. Ann Intern Med 2001;134:561–8.

Charkes ND. The many causes of subclinical hyperthyroidism. Thyroid 1996;5:391–6.

Cooper DS. Antithyroid drugs. N Engl J Med 1984;311:1353–62.

Cooper DS. Antithyroid drugs and radioiodine therapy: A grain of (iodized) salt. Ann Intern Med 1994;121:612–4.

Cooper DS. Treatment of thyrotoxicosis. In: Braverman LE, Utiger RD, editors. Werner and Ingbar's The Thyroid: A Fundamental and Clinical Text. 7th ed. Philadelphia: Lippincott-Raven; 1996. p. 708–34.

Cooper DS. Antithyroid drugs for the treatment of hyperthyroidism caused by Graves' disease. Endocrinol Metab Clin North Am 1998;27:225–47.

Franklyn JA. The management of hyperthyroidism. N Engl J Med 1994;130:1731–8.

Franklyn JA. Drug therapy: The management of hyperthyroidism. N Engl J Med 1994;330:1731–8.

Klein I, Becker D, Levey G. Treatment of hyperthyroid disease. Ann Inter Med 1994;121:281–8.

Klein I, Ojamaa K. Cardiovascular manifestations of endocrine disease. J Clin Endocrinol Metab 1992;75:339–42.

McIver B, Morris JC. The pathogenesis of Graves' disease. Endocrinol Metab Clin North Am 1998;27:73–89.

Mestman JH. Hyperthyroidism and pregnancy. Best Pract Res Clin Endocrinol Metab 2004;18:267–88.

Motomura K, Brent GA. Mechanisms of thyroid hormone action. Endocrinol Metab Clin North Am 1998;27:1–23.

Papi G, Pearce EN, Braverman LE, et al. A clinical and therapeutic approach to thyrotoxicosis with thyroid-stimulating hormone suppression only. Am J Med 2005;118:349–61.

Roti E, Minelli R, Salvi M. Management of hyperthyroidism and hypothyroidism in the pregnant woman. J Clin Endocrinol Metab 1996;81:1679–82.

Sawin CT. Thyroid dysfunction in older persons. Adv Intern Med 1991;37:223–49.

Sawin CT, Geller A, Wolf P, et al. Low serum thyrotropin concentrations as a risk factor for atrial fibrillation in older persons. N Engl J Med 1994;331:1249–52.

Singer PA, Cooper D, Levy E, et al. Treatment guidelines for patients with hyperthyroidism and hypothyroidism. JAMA 1995;273:808–12.

Surks MI, Chopra I, Mariash C, et al. American Thyroid Association guidelines for use of laboratory tests in thyroid disorders. JAMA 1990;263:1529–32.

Torring O, Tallstedt L, Wallin G, et al. Graves' hyperthyroidism: Treatment with antithyroid drugs, surgery, or radioiodine a prospective, randomized study. J Clin Endocrinol Metab 1996;81:2986–93.

Wing DA, Millar LK, Koonings PP, et al. A comparison of propylthiouracil versus methimazole in the treatment of hyperthyroidism in pregnancy. Am J Obstet Gynecol 1994;170:90–5.

Thyroid Cancer

Method of
Richard A. Prinz, MD, and Emery Chen, MD

Thyroid cancer is the most common malignancy of the endocrine system. It affects more women than men by a ratio of 3:1. The National Cancer Institute (NCI) estimates that in 2009, 37,200 new cases of thyroid cancer were diagnosed in the United States and 1630 patients will die of thyroid cancer.

From 1997 to 2006, the incidence of thyroid cancer has increased by about 6% per year. This may be due, in part, to the frequent use of imaging modalities that have been detecting increasing numbers of incidental thyroid nodules. The mortality associated with thyroid cancer has not increased appreciably despite its rising incidence. The biological behavior of thyroid cancers, as a group, covers a broad spectrum. The overall 5- and 10-year survival rates of patients with papillary thyroid cancer, the most common type, remain approximately 97% and 90% respectively. Patients with anaplastic thyroid cancer, the least common type, rarely survive beyond 1 year.

The five subtypes of thyroid cancer are papillary, follicular, Hürthle cell, medullary, and anaplastic. Surgery is the initial treatment for all of these; however, the extent of surgery and subsequent adjuvant therapy depend on the clinical features and characteristics of each type.

Causes and Risk Factors

The causes of most sporadic forms of thyroid cancer remain unclear. Persons who have a family history of thyroid cancer or are older than 40 years are at greater risk for developing the disease. The incidence of malignancy in thyroid nodules is higher in children than adults, varying from 15% to 20% versus 5% to 6%, respectively.

The link between prior radiation exposure of the thyroid gland and cancer is clear. In the past, children and adults were sometimes treated with radiation for acne, fungal infections of the scalp, enlarged thymus, tonsils and adenoids, and other benign conditions. Numerous studies have linked these treatments to a higher risk of developing thyroid cancer, especially in patients with a thyroid nodule where the likelihood may be as high as 30% to 50%. Population studies of those affected by the Chernobyl accident showed a dramatic spike in the incidence of thyroid cancer, especially in children. Radiation exposure in adulthood carries a lesser risk of developing thyroid cancer than in children but it is still higher than in the general population.

A diet low in iodine is a risk factor for follicular thyroid cancer, the most common type of thyroid cancer in parts of the world where iodine deficiency is endemic. A low-iodine diet also seems to increase the risk of papillary thyroid cancers in those exposed to radiation.

---

[1]Not FDA approved for this indication.

Diagnosis

Most patients with thyroid cancer present with a nodule, which is extremely common in the general population. Sonographic screening of populations without thyroid disease shows that 33% of adults have at least one thyroid nodule. The number of detected nodules increases with age, with the highest prevalence in the seventh decade. Cancer is rare, occurring in 5% to 6% of those with a palpable thyroid nodule.

The best way to determine the nature of a thyroid nodule is by fine needle aspiration (FNA) for cytology. Some cancers are diagnosed after surgical excision for presumed benign disease (an indeterminate nodule, symptomatic multinodular goiter, or Graves' disease). These occult thyroid cancers are of uncertain biological behavior. Retrospective studies with long-term follow-up suggest that death resulting from papillary or follicular thyroid cancers detected in this fashion is uncommon with appropriate treatment.

Evaluation of a patient with a thyroid nodule (Box 1) should include a detailed review of their risk factors and symptoms, and a thorough neck examination that notes the characteristics of the nodule, and the presence or absence of cervical lymphadenopathy. Serum thyroid stimulating hormone (TSH) level should be measured to determine the patient's thyroid function. If the patient is euthyroid or hypothyroid by clinical evaluation or by having a normal or high TSH level, we proceed directly to FNA biopsy. We also start these patients on a TSH-suppressive dose of levothyroxine (Synthroid), beginning with 25 µg daily and titrating it to a TSH level just below 1 mIU/L to halt or reverse the growth of the nodule. However, there is no consensus as to the effectiveness of this approach. If the TSH level is suppressed below normal, a thyroid scan can determine if the nodule is a hyperfunctioning adenoma. Increased isotope uptake confirms a toxic or hot nodule. The risk of a hot nodule harboring a malignancy is less than 1%. We recommend thyroid lobectomy for definitive treatment of toxic adenomas; others favor radioiodine if the adenoma is less than 4 cm in diameter.

FNA biopsy is the gold standard test to separate benign disease from malignant disease. This can be guided by direct palpation of the nodule or with ultrasound to increase accuracy. It is a rapid, safe, sensitive, and inexpensive test that can be performed in the office and is well tolerated by patients. Its false-positive rate of 1% to 2% and false-negative rate of 2% to 5% have been well validated.

There are four possible cytopathologic results from an FNA biopsy specimen: malignant, benign, suspicious or indeterminate, and nondiagnostic. Treatment options for the first two possibilities are clear. Malignant lesions mandate thyroidectomy. Benign lesions should be followed unless they are associated with symptoms or growth while under observation. In addition, we recommend a second FNA biopsy in 6 to 12 months to decrease the possibility of a false-negative result.

BOX 1 Risk Factors, Signs, and Symptoms Associated with Thyroid Cancer

Risk Factors
Head and neck irradiation
Family history of thyroid cancer
Low-iodine diet

Signs
Hard, fixed mass in a thyroid lobe
Cervical lymphadenopathy
Rapidly enlarging thyroid mass

Symptoms
Generally asymptomatic except in advanced disease
New onset of dysphonia, dyspnea, or dysphagia
Pressure or pain is unusual

CURRENT DIAGNOSIS

- A history of thyroid irradiation or family history of thyroid cancer increases the likelihood that a patient with a thyroid nodule will have thyroid cancer.
- Thyroid nodules in children are more likely to be cancers.
- Plasma thyroid-stimulating hormone level should be measured to assess thyroid function.
- A hyperfunctioning thyroid nodule is unlikely to harbor a malignancy.
- Ultrasound evaluation of the thyroid and neck can aid in the diagnosis and treatment of thyroid cancer.
- Fine needle aspiration (FNA) biopsy is the gold standard diagnostic test to detect most thyroid cancers.
- Follicular and Hürthle cell neoplasms require thyroid lobectomy because histopathologic evidence of capsular or vascular invasion is required to diagnose malignancy.

Suspicious or indeterminate lesions are mainly follicular and Hürthle cell neoplasms. These encapsulated tumors can be either benign or malignant. The differentiation cannot be made on the cytologic appearance of individual or even clusters of cells. The diagnosis of malignancy can only be made by finding direct tumor invasion into the capsule or vasculature. Therefore, thyroid lobectomy with definitive histologic examination of the specimen is recommended. There is conflicting evidence about the accuracy of intraoperative frozen section evaluation to guide surgical treatment. We use it because it is available and can be helpful when the pathologist makes a diagnosis of malignancy, but quite often the diagnosis must be deferred to permanent sections. If the final pathologic diagnosis reveals malignancy, a second procedure for completion thyroidectomy is recommended. For Hürthle and follicular neoplasms larger than 4 cm, total thyroidectomy is advised because of the greater risk of cancer. If the FNA is nondiagnostic, a repeat aspiration should be performed under ultrasound guidance. Patients with nodules that continue to yield nondiagnostic results should be offered thyroidectomy to clarify the diagnosis.

Histologic Classification, Treatment, and Prognosis

Cytology and management of thyroid tumors are shown in Table 1.

PAPILLARY CANCER

Papillary thyroid cancers are the most common form of thyroid cancer, accounting for approximately 80% of thyroid malignancies. They typically appear as hard, white nodules on gross examination. They are characterized microscopically by cuboidal cells with intranuclear cytoplasmic inclusions, nuclear grooves, prominent nuclei with marginated chromatin (Orphan Annie eyes), and round collections of calcium (psammoma bodies). Generally, the tumors are not encapsulated, but if they are, it is usually a good prognostic sign. Multicentric disease is common in papillary cancers, occurring in up to 85% of patients.

The cancer spreads early within the thyroid gland and through the lymphatics of the central and lateral neck. Cervical lymph node metastases occur in 30% to 40% of patients. Hematologic spread to the lungs and bones is usually found only in advanced disease.

The best treatment for papillary thyroid cancer is total thyroidectomy followed by radioiodine ablation and TSH suppression. Central and lateral modified radical neck dissections should be performed when there are nodal metastases in these compartments. Some

TABLE 1 Fine Needle Aspiration Cytology and Associated Management

FNA Cytology Result	Diagnosis	Treatment
Benign	Benign nodule	Observation with repeat FNA in 6–12 mo
Malignant	Papillary, medullary, or anaplastic thyroid cancer	Total thyroidectomy with TSH suppression and ± adjuvant radioiodine
Indeterminant or suspicious	Follicular or Hürthle cell neoplasm	Thyroid lobectomy; return to surgery for completion thyroidectomy if final pathology shows cancer
Nondiagnostic	N/A	Repeat FNA with ultrasound guidance Lobectomy if still nondiagnostic

FNA = fine needle aspiration; N/A = not applicable; TSH = thyroid-stimulating hormone.

surgeons advocate routine central compartment lymph node sampling or dissection, which can upstage papillary thyroid cancers without substantially increasing operative morbidity. External beam radiation is reserved for those rare patients who cannot tolerate an operation, have recurrent disease not amenable to resection or who do not concentrate radioiodine, or for treatment of bony metastases. Overall 10-year survival after suitable treatment is greater than 90%.

FOLLICULAR CANCER

Follicular thyroid cancers macroscopically appear as a firm, solitary nodule that is usually encapsulated. Microscopically, they have a well-formed follicular structure composed of well-differentiated cells that are indistinguishable from their benign counterpart, follicular adenoma.

 CURRENT THERAPY

- Total thyroidectomy is the initial treatment for most thyroid cancers.
- Therapeutic neck dissections are performed when evidence of lymph node involvement exists.
- Radioactive iodine and thyroid-stimulating hormone suppression are effective adjuvant therapies in patients with well-differentiated thyroid cancers.
- When final pathology proves a follicular or Hürthle cell neoplasm to be malignant, completion thyroidectomy is recommended if only a lobectomy has been performed.
- Patients with medullary thyroid cancer should be screened for pheochromocytoma, which should be treated before thyroidectomy.
- External beam irradiation and multidrug chemotherapy are adjuvant therapies for patients with anaplastic thyroid cancer.
- Most thyroid cancer patients require long-term follow-up after treatment.

Diagnosis of malignancy requires histologic confirmation of vascular or capsular invasion. Metastases are hematogenous, and lymphatic spread develops late in the disease.

The optimal management for a preoperative diagnosis of follicular neoplasm smaller than 4 cm is thyroid lobectomy and isthmusectomy. If there is histologic evidence of malignancy at operation, a total thyroidectomy should be performed followed by radioactive iodine therapy and TSH suppression. If the diagnosis must be deferred to permanent sections and the final pathology identifies a follicular thyroid cancer, a second procedure for a completion thyroidectomy followed by radioiodine is usually recommended. Lymph node dissection is rarely indicated and is reserved for patients with clinical evidence of nodal metastases. The 10-year survival rate following appropriate treatment is approximately 75% to 85%.

HÜRTHLE CELL CANCER

The American Thyroid Association and the World Health Organization classify Hürthle cell carcinomas, which account for up to 5% of thyroid malignancies, as a subtype of follicular thyroid cancer. Hürthle cell cancers are often more aggressive than the typical follicular cancer, with an increased likelihood of multicentricity and lymphatic spread and a decreased tendency to concentrate radioactive iodine. Microscopically, the eosinophilic granular cytoplasm, large clear nuclei, and trabecular architecture distinguish them from typical follicular thyroid cancers.

Treatment is the same as that described for follicular thyroid cancers. Some surgeons recommend routine central-compartment lymph node sampling or dissection due to the tumor's propensity for lymphatic spread, but there is no consensus on this because good evidence of benefit is lacking. The overall 10-year survival is approximately 60% to 70% following treatment.

MEDULLARY CANCER

Medullary thyroid carcinomas (MTCs) arise from the parafollicular C-cells. These neuroendocrine cells typically secrete calcitonin and can also secrete carcinoembryonic antigen (CEA), which can be used as tumor markers for both diagnosis and monitoring response to treatment. MTCs make up approximately 5% of thyroid cancers.

Grossly, MTC appears as a hard, unencapsulated nodule in the thyroid gland. Microscopically, the tumor's round, polyhedral, and spindle-shaped cells form a variety of patterns that range from trabecular to glandlike. Sheets of amyloid are also commonly found. MTCs tend to metastasize early through the lymphatics but can also spread through the bloodstream to the liver and lungs.

MTC is usually sporadic but approximately 25% are familial. Familial MTC is an autosomal dominant disorder due to mutations in the RET (rearranged during transfection) proto-oncogene. Identification of RET mutations in family members should prompt consideration for early prophylactic thyroidectomy to avert the certain development of medullary thyroid cancer. This is usually done between the ages of 6 months and 10 years, depending on the aggressiveness of the specific RET mutation.

MTC is also one of the endocrinopathies, along with pheochromocytoma and hyperparathyroidism, that make up the multiple endocrine neoplasia (MEN) type 2 syndromes. Patients with MTC should be screened for pheochromocytoma before thyroidectomy. If pheochromocytoma is present, it should be removed before thyroidectomy.

There is widespread agreement that total thyroidectomy with routine central compartment lymph node dissection is the best treatment for MTC. A lateral neck dissection is reserved for patients with clinically involved lymph nodes in the jugular chain. Radioiodine therapy is not an option because parafollicular cells do not take up iodine. Therapy with tyrosine kinase receptor inhibitors that selectively target pathways for tumor growth and angiogenesis is under investigation.

The overall 10-year survival after treatment is approximately 70% to 80% when the disease is confined to the thyroid gland and 30% to 40% when distant metastases are present.

ANAPLASTIC CANCER

Anaplastic thyroid cancers are exceptionally aggressive and lethal. They result in more than one half the deaths attributed to thyroid malignancy every year. They are rare, accounting for up to 2% of all thyroid cancers.

Anaplastic thyroid cancers arise from dedifferentiation of papillary thyroid cancer and usually manifest as a rapidly growing central neck mass. Most patients are elderly, with locally advanced disease and nodal and distant metastases at presentation.

The three main conditions that can occur in a similar fashion are Riedel's thyroiditis, thyroid lymphoma, and parapharyngeal sarcoma. FNA cytology is often insufficient to establish a firm diagnosis and early open wedge biopsy may be needed.

Aggressive therapy with surgery, radiation, and chemotherapy is recommended. However, complete surgical resection is usually not possible, and there is no effective chemotherapy. Tracheostomy should be considered for impending obstruction rather than prophylaxis. Prognosis is poor, and median survival varies from 2 to 12 months. One-year survival after multimodality therapy is less than 3%.

Follow-up

Papillary, follicular, and Hürthle cell thyroid cancers are grouped together and referred to as *well-differentiated thyroid cancers* (WDTC). They are all derived from thyroid follicular cells, respond well to surgical and adjuvant therapies, and are associated with generally favorable outcomes (Table 2). A small minority of patients, however, eventually succumbs to WDTC.

Many prognostic factors have been used to classify patients with WDTC into high-risk and low-risk groups. They include the patient's age and sex, tumor size and extent of invasion or metastasis, and completeness of surgical resection. Using these prognostic factors, several scoring systems were devised to reliably predict individual patient prognosis. Among the first was the AGES scoring system (*age*, histologic *grade* of the tumor, *extrathyroidal invasion and distant metastases*, tumor *size*), which was later refined to the MACIS scoring system (*metastases*, *age*, *completeness of resection*, extrathyroidal *invasion*, tumor *size*). The DeGroot classification consists of class I (intrathyroidal), class II (cervical node metastases), class III (extrathyroidal extension), and class IV (distant metastases) groups. The AMES system (*age*, *metastases*, *extrathyroidal invasion*, primary tumor *size*) is easy to use, but does not accurately distinguish low-risk from high-risk patients with FTC. Arguably the most widely used

is the TNM staging system (*tumor* size, *nodal* status, distant *metastases*). None of the scoring systems can be used to guide the extent of surgical resection because the only factors known preoperatively are age and sex.

The rate of recurrence in low-risk patients with WDTC is about 10%, whereas in high-risk patients it is about 45%. Among the low-risk patients who have a recurrence, 33% to 50% die from their disease. Traditionally, radioactive iodine whole body scans (WBS) have been performed every 6 to 12 months to detect recurrent disease. However, the usefulness of serum thyroglobulin assays combined with routine neck ultrasound has decreased the need for frequent WBS.

Serum thyroglobulin is a useful marker for follow-up of patients with WDTC, because most of these tumors synthesize thyroglobulin. After successful treatment, thyroglobulin levels should be undetectable. Thyroglobulin levels that are elevated more than 10 ng/mL in the absence of thyroglobulin antibodies indicate residual thyroid tissue or persistent or recurrent thyroid cancer. Further imaging studies are then used to localize the residual tissue or cancer. For medullary thyroid cancer, elevated serum calcitonin or CEA levels after thyroidectomy should prompt appropriate imaging studies to localize persistent or recurrent disease. Persistent and recurrent disease that is detectable with imaging should be resected if it can be done with minimal morbidity.

There are no useful tumor markers for anaplastic thyroid cancer.

Summary

Thyroid cancer is increasing in frequency. The majority of thyroid cancers are slow growing and indolent, but a small minority can be aggressive and fatal. Thyroid cancer treatment depends on the characteristics of each histopathologic type. FNA biopsy can be useful in detecting the presence and type of thyroid cancer prior to the initiation of therapy. Thyroidectomy is the first step in the successful treatment of most thyroid cancers; however, the extent of surgery and subsequent adjuvant therapy varies with the subtype of thyroid cancer. Serial measurement of tumor markers coupled with neck imaging studies is useful in the long-term follow-up of patients treated for thyroid cancer.

REFERENCES

Ball DW. Medullary thyroid cancer: Therapeutic targets and molecular markers. Curr Opin Oncol 2007;19:18–23.

Chabre O, Piolat C, Dyon JF. Childhood progression of hereditary medullary thyroid cancer. N Engl J Med 2007;356:1583–4.

Cooper DS, Doherty GM, Haugen BR, et al. Management guidelines for patients with thyroid nodules and differentiated thyroid cancer. Thyroid 2006;16:109–42.

D'Avanzo A, Ituarte P, Treseler P, et al. Prognostic scoring systems in patients with follicular thyroid cancer: A comparison of different staging systems in predicting the patient outcome. Thyroid 2004;14:453–8.

Fialkowski EA, Moley JF. Current approaches to medullary thyroid carcinoma, sporadic and familial. J Surg Oncol 2006;94:737–47.

Kebebew E, Clark OH. Differentiated thyroid cancer: "Complete" rational approach. World J Surg 2000;24:942–51.

Kim AW, Maxhimer JB, Quiros RM, et al. Surgical management of well-differentiated thyroid cancer locally invasive to the respiratory tract. J Am Coll Surg 2005;201:619–27.

Lang BH, Lo CY. Surgical options in undifferentiated thyroid carcinoma. World J Surg 2007;31:969–77.

Mazzaferri EL, Robbins RJ, Spencer CA, et al. A consensus report of the role of serum thyroglobulin as a monitoring method for low-risk patients with papillary thyroid carcinoma. J Clin Endocrinol Metab 2003;88:1433–41.

Pacini F, DeGroot LJ. Thyroid neoplasia. In: DeGroot LJ, Jameson JL, editors. Endocrinology. 5th ed. Philadelphia: Saunders; 2006. p. 2147–80.

Phitayakorn R, McHenry CR. Follicular and Hürthle cell carcinoma of the thyroid gland. Surg Oncol Clin N Am 2006;15:603–23.

Sanders Jr EM, Livolsi VA, Brierley J, et al. An evidence-based review of poorly differentiated thyroid cancer. World J Surg 2007;31:934–45.

TABLE 2 Long-Term Follow-Up

Type	Tumor Marker(s)	Imaging	Frequency
WDTC	Tg (basal and stimulated with ↑TSH levels)	Neck U/S, ^{131}I whole body scan	6–12 mo or when Tg > 10 ng/mL
Medullary	Calcitonin, CEA	CT of neck, thorax, abdomen; consider PET scan	6–12 mo or when calcitonin is newly elevated
Anaplastic	None	Neck U/S	1–3 mo

CEA = carcinoembryonic antigen; CT = computed tomography; PET = positron emission tomography; Tg = thyroglobulin; TSH = thyroid stimulating hormone; U/S = ultrasound; WDTC = well-differentiated thyroid cancer.

Pheochromocytomas

Method of
Pierre-François Plouin, MD

Pheochromocytomas (PHs) and functional paragangliomas (PGLs) are neoplasms of chromaffin tissue that synthesize catecholamines. Most of these tumors appear in the adrenal medulla (PH proper), but 10% to 20% arise in extra-adrenal chromaffin tissue (PGL). In descending order of frequency, functional PGL can develop in the Zuckerkandl body (located at the root of the upper mesenteric artery), the sympathetic plexus of the urinary bladder, the kidneys, and the heart, sympathetic ganglia in the mediastinum, the head, or the neck. Most head and neck PGLs are nonfunctional. Patients with familial diseases can have bilateral PH or PH plus functional or nonfunctional PGL.

The prevalence of PH and functional PGL is about 0.1% in patients with hypertension and 4% in patients with incidentally discovered adrenal masses or incidentalomas. Their incidence in the general population is less than 1 per 100,000 persons per year. The lifetime incidence of PH and PGL is high in familial syndromes affected by these tumors: 1% to 5% in neurofibromatosis type 1 (NF1), 15% to 20% in von Hippel–Lindau (VHL) disease, 30% to 50% in multiple endocrine neoplasia type 2 (MEN-2), and probably more than 50% in *SDHB* and *SDHD* gene mutation carriers.

Presentation

The increase in catecholamine production in patients with PH and functional PGL causes symptoms (mainly headaches, palpitations, and excessive sweating) and signs (mainly hypertension, weight loss, and diabetes) that reflect the effects of catecholamines on α- and β-adrenergic receptors. Signs and symptoms are varying and often paroxysmal due to the variable and disorderly release of catecholamines by the tumor. The typical presentation is a combination of variable hypertension with paroxysmal symptoms, either occurring spontaneously or provoked by abdominal pressure during anteflexion, micturition, or defecation.

The diagnosis of PH or PGL can be delayed for several reasons. First, these tumors are rare. Second, hypertension may be absent for long periods because active catecholamines can be converted into biologically inactive metanephrines within the tumor. Third, the symptoms and signs are nonspecific and are common to both the tumoral (in PH and PGL) and neuronal (during stress) release of catecholamines. For these reasons, the mean time from the onset of hypertension, when present, to diagnosis of the tumor exceeds 3 years. Indeed, the tumor is often discovered fortuitously during diagnostic testing for symptoms or clinical conditions not related to adrenal disease.

Presymptomatic diagnosis during the exploration of incidentalomas currently accounts for 25% of all cases. Presymptomatic diagnosis is also possible in patients with phenotypic evidence or a family history of a genetic disease associated with PH or PGL.

Diagnosis

LABORATORY TESTING

Biochemical investigation for PH or PGL is offered to hypertensive patients reporting bouts of headaches, palpitations, and sweating, those with hypertension resistant to treatment, and those with incidentalomas or with a familial disease conferring a predisposition to PH or PGL (Figure 1). The positive diagnosis of PH and functional PGL is based on the quantification of plasma or urinary

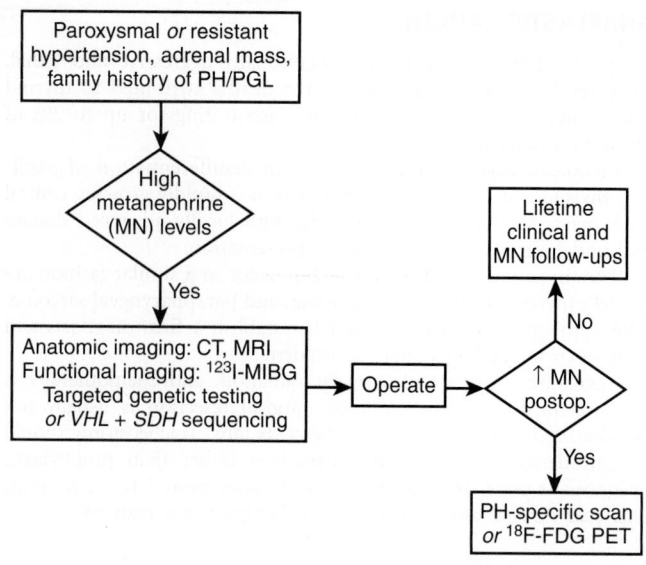

FIGURE 1. Algorithm for the initial management and long-term follow-up of patients with pheochromocytomas (PH) and secreting paragangliomas (PGL). *Abbreviations:* CT = computed tomography; ^{18}F-FDG PET = ^{18}F-fluorodeoxyglucose positron-emission tomography; MIBG = ^{123}I-metaiodobenzylguanidine; MRI = magnetic resonance imaging.

metanephrines (metanephrine itself and normetanephrine), because this test is more sensitive than the quantification of urinary vanillylmandelic acid excretion or plasma concentrations of catecholamines, neuropeptide Y, or chromogranin A. The relative merits of the various determinations of plasma and urinary metanephrines are summarized in Table 1.

Patients undergoing biochemical tests for PH or PGL should be given instructions enabling them to obtain an accurate 24-hour sample of acidified urine (for urine testing) and should be told to avoid tricyclic antidepressants and acetaminophen (paracetamol, Tylenol) for 5 days, because these drugs can cause false-positive results in plasma metanephrine tests. Because accurate plasma or urinary metanephrine assays are readily available, there is no need to subject patients to the hazards of pharmacologic provocative or suppression tests.

IMAGING

Preoperative imaging tests are designed to locate the tumor and to determine whether it is single or multiple, adrenal or ectopic, benign or malignant, and isolated or present with other neoplasms in the context of familial syndromes. The combination of anatomic imaging studies based on computed tomography (CT) or magnetic resonance imaging (MRI) and radionuclide imaging studies yields a sensitivity of almost 100% for the diagnosis of catecholamine-producing tumors. CT is the most commonly used anatomic imaging technique, but MRI is preferred for children and pregnant patients.

Functional imaging with ^{123}I-metaiodobenzylguanidine (MIBG) should be carried out when possible, because ^{131}I-MIBG scintigraphy is less sensitive. Labetalol (Trandate, Normodyne) and antipsychotic drugs should be withdrawn for several days before the investigations because they reduce MIBG uptake. If no MIBG uptake is observed, mostly in cases of nonfunctional PGL, additional investigations by scintigraphy with nonspecific ligands such as somatostatin receptor scintigraphy or ^{18}F-fluorodeoxyglucose positron-emission tomography (^{18}F-FDG PET) should be carried out.

In addition to the primary tumor, imaging tests can disclose lymph node, bone, liver, or pulmonary metastases, thereby establishing the presence of malignant PH or PGL.

TABLE 1 Advantages and Limitations of Determining Metanephrine and Normetanephrine in Urine or Plasma

Determinations*	Advantages	Limitations
Urinary-free and conjugated MN and NMN	Easy determination, widely available Integration of 24-h secretion Sensitivity enhanced by use of the MN+NMN-to-creatinine ratio	Need for an acidified 24-h urine collection
Plasma-free and conjugated MN and NMN	Long half-life, high concentration (25 × higher than free MN and NMN)	Includes sulfate-conjugated MN and NMN produced in the GI tract High in cases of renal failure
Plasma-free MN and NMN	Reflects tumor release of MN and NMN and the conversion of epinephrine and norepinephrine into MN and NMN	Unstable, low concentration, technically demanding
	Provides the best combination of sensitivity and specificity	Acetaminophen-containing drugs can give false-positive results

*All these tests have sensitivities exceeding 90%.
Abbreviations: GI = gastrointestinal; MN = metanephrine; NMN = normetanephrine.

Differential Diagnosis

Catecholamine-secreting tumors mimic paroxysmal conditions with hypertension or cardiac rhythm disorders, particularly panic attacks, in which sympathetic activation linked to anxiety reproduces the signs and symptoms of PH. Plasma and urinary metanephrine concentrations are usually normal in these conditions. Acute cardiovascular events, such as myocardial infarction, pulmonary edema, and stroke, also induce an increase in catecholamine levels that may be sustained for several days and are associated with an increase in plasma or urinary metanephrine concentration. The diagnosis of PH or secreting PGL is excluded in these cases by the normalization of metanephrine levels 10 days after the onset of the event.

Genetic Counseling

Before 2000, three different familial and syndromic diseases were known to result in PH or PGL: MEN-2 due to *RET* gene mutations, VHL disease due to *VHL* gene mutations, and NF1 due to *NF1* mutations. The overall incidence of familial PH or PGL was estimated at 10%. The recent identification of mutations in the *VHL*, *SDHB*, and *SDHD* genes in patients with apparently sporadic tumors has increased estimates of the incidence of an underlying genetic disease in patients with PH or PGL to 20% to 25%. Familial cases are more likely to be bilateral and recurrent than sporadic cases. Carriers of *SDHB* mutations have a high risk of malignant primary tumor or metastatic recurrence. Genetic screening should therefore be offered to most patients with PH or PGL (Figure 2).

Targeted genetic testing should be offered to patients with phenotypic signs consistent with or a family history of MEN-2, VHL

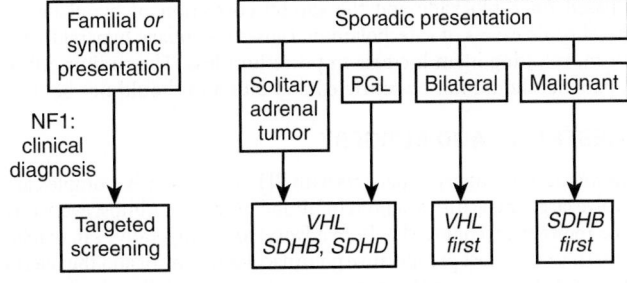

FIGURE 2. Suggested genetic screening in patients with pheochromocytomas (PH) and secreting paragangliomas (PGL). *Abbreviation*: NF1 = neurofibromatosis type 1.

disease, or hereditary PGL. Phenotypic signs of MEN-2 include medullary thyroid cancer and hyperparathyroidism, signs of VHL disease include hemangioblastomas and renal or pancreatic tumors, and signs of hereditary PGL include head and neck PGLs and family history in the paternal branch. In patients with an apparently sporadic PH or PGL, priority should be given to analysis of the *VHL*, *SDHB*, and *SDHD* genes. In patients with bilateral PH, the *RET* and *VHL* should be analyzed first. Identification of a causative mutation in one affected patient should lead to presymptomatic genetic testing of the family, because early detection of small tumors in persons deemed to be at risk can reduce the morbidity of the disease. Screening for *NF1* gene mutations is feasible but rarely carried out, because the NF1 phenotype (multiple café-au-lait spots, neurofibromas, Lisch nodules, and axillary and inguinal freckling) is sufficiently clear for diagnosis of the condition in adults.

Treatment

TREATMENT OBJECTIVES

PH and functional PGL carry risks of hypersecretion and tumor growth. Surgery aims to eliminate both risks. The consequences of hypersecretion should be carefully managed before and during surgery. Primary tumor resection does not eliminate the risk of tumor persistence (in malignant tumors) or tumor recurrence (mostly in genetic diseases).

PREOPERATIVE MANAGEMENT

Blood pressure (BP) should be normalized, whenever possible, before surgery, because the incidence of perioperative complications has been consistently linked to preoperative BP. Given the variability of BP in PH or PGL, it may be useful to determine 24-hour ambulatory BP. Antihypertensive regimens aim to reduce mean office BP to less than 140/90 mm Hg or 24-hour ambulatory BP to less than 125/80 mm Hg. However, the total abolition of hypertensive paroxysms is not currently possible, and patients should undergo surgery after 1 to 2 weeks of preparation.

BP control requires α- and β-adrenergic antagonists. Because most PHs and PGLs secrete predominantly norepinephrine, an α-agonist, α-adrenergic antagonists are the cornerstone of hypertensive control. Noncompetitive α-blockers, such as phenoxybenzamine (Dibenzyline), bind covalently to α-receptors, causing an irreversible blockade. They allow stable BP control, but they increase the risk of hypotension during tumor removal and the immediate postoperative period. Competitive α-blockers, such as prazosin (Minipress) are more suitable. The initial dose of prazosin can induce a sharp drop in BP, so the dose should be gradually increased from 0.5 to 5 mg three times a day. α-Adrenergic blockade generally gives rise to tachycardia secondary to catecholamine β-receptor stimulation. This requires the subsequent addition of a β-blocker, such as 25 to 100 mg atenolol (Tenormine) daily.

If adrenergic blockade proves insufficient to control BP, then a dihydropyridine may also be administered. Arrhythmia prevention is based on β-blockade and the careful correction of hypokalemia: The chronic excess of catecholamine causes secondary hyperaldosteronism, resulting in an increase in potassium loss. The sodium intake of patients should not be restricted and diuretics should not be used.

ANESTHESIA AND SURGERY

Anesthesia and surgery in patients with PH or PGL may be complex and involve large and acute variations in BP and heart rate. Almost every possible anesthetic technique has been advocated. Perioperative safety relies primarily on correct preoperative pharmacologic control and the referral of patients to centers with extensive experience in treating the disease.

Large variations in BP and heart rate can occur during induction, intubation, peritoneal incision, and tumor handling and devascularization. Radial artery pressure and the electrocardiogram (ECG) should be monitored continuously. I generally use intravenous infusions of nicardipine (Cardene) 0.1 to 1[3] mg/min to control BP and intravenous esmolol (Brevibloc) loading infusion of 0.5 mg/kg/min over 1 minute to control arrhythmia.

Laparoscopic surgery has supplanted open surgery in the management of most cases of PH and intra-abdominal PGL. Adrenal cortex–sparing surgery may be carried out by laparoscopy in patients with hereditary forms of PH.

Postoperative and Long-term Follow-up

Plasma or urinary metanephrine concentration should be determined 10 days after surgery, to check for normalization. If metanephrine concentrations remain high, ^{123}I-MIBG scintigraphy should be performed. This technique can detect distant metastases whose MIBG uptake was masked by the primary tumor's higher metabolic activity before surgery. No MIBG uptake might occur in dedifferentiated metastases, and nonspecific radionuclide imaging may be required (see Figure 1).

---

[3]Exceeds dosage recommended by the manufacturer.

CURRENT DIAGNOSIS

- Most patients with symptomatic PH or functional PGL are hypertensive. Blood pressure typically rises when symptoms are present (mostly headaches, palpitations, and sweating).
- Presymptomatic diagnosis has become common in patients with incidentally discovered adrenal masses (incidentalomas) and in relatives of patients with symptomatic PH.
- The diagnosis of PH or functional PGL is based on the determination of metanephrines.
- Most catecholamine-secreting tumors arise in the adrenal glands (PH proper) and are easily detected by computed tomography or magnetic resonance imaging. Patients might also harbor extra-adrenal primary tumors (PGL) or distant metastases. Adrenal imaging should therefore be combined with whole-body meta-iodobenzylguanidine scintigraphy.
- One in four patients with PH or PGL has germline mutations conferring a predisposition to catecholamine-secreting tumors. The identification of a causative mutation should lead to presymptomatic genetic testing in the family.

Abbreviations: PGL = paraganglioma; PH = pheochromocytoma.

CURRENT THERAPY

- Patients with catecholamine-secreting tumors should be referred to centers with extensive experience in the anesthetic and surgical management of the disease.
- Blood pressure should be normalized before surgery, using α-adrenergic and possibly β-adrenergic antagonists.
- Most PHs and many PGLs can be resected laparoscopically.
- Adrenal cortex–sparing surgery is feasible in patients with bilateral PH.
- PH and PGL can recur. Patients should be subject to lifelong follow-up, with checkups at least yearly, including blood pressure measurement and metanephrine determination.

Abbreviations: PGL = paraganglioma; PH = pheochromocytoma.

Because PH and PGL can recur, patients undergoing surgery for PH or PGL should have lifelong follow-up, with checkups at least once yearly, including BP measurement and plasma or urinary metanephrine determination. In a cohort of patients undergoing surgery for PH or PGL, the 10-year probability of recurrence—defined as the reappearance of the disease after eradication of the tumor had been confirmed by negative biochemical and imaging tests—was 16%. Patients with recurrences were younger, had larger tumors, and were more likely to have familial disease or bilateral or extra-adrenal PGL than patients with no recurrence. Recurrences were malignant in one in two patients.

Malignant PH or PGL is compatible with prolonged survival, with symptom-free intervals lasting from months to decades. In 54 patients with malignant PH or PGL followed at my center, the 5-year and 10-year probabilities of survival were 0.75 and 0.52, respectively.

In cases of small recurrences with an accessible vascular pedicle, surgical excision may be preceded or replaced by therapeutic embolization. In cases in which soft-tissue or skeletal metastases are too widespread for surgery or embolization, several palliative therapies may be considered. Pharmacologic treatment aimed at the long-term blockade of catecholamine synthesis with α-methyl-*p*-tyrosine (Demser) 1 to 4 g/day in divided doses can improve the patient's quality of life, but it has no effect on tumor progression. Conventional radiotherapy can provide effective palliation in cases of painful metastases. Metabolic radiotherapy with ^{131}I-MIBG and chemotherapy can provide clinical, hormonal, and, in some cases, tumoral improvement.

REFERENCES

Diner EK, Franks ME, Behari A, et al. Partial adrenalectomy: The National Cancer Institute experience. Urology 2005;66:19–23.

Eisenhofer G, Bornstein SR, Brouwers FM, et al. Malignant pheochromocytoma: Current status and initiatives for future progress. Endocr Relat Cancer 2004;11:423–36.

Itias I, Pacak K. Current approaches and recommended algorithm for the diagnostic localization of pheochromocytoma. J Clin Endocrinol Metab 2004;89:479–91.

Lenders JW, Pacak K, Walther MM, et al. Biochemical diagnosis of pheochromocytoma: Which test is best? JAMA 2002;287:1427–34.

Plouin PF, Duclos JM, Soppelsa F, et al. Factors associated with perioperative morbidity and mortality in patients with pheochromocytoma: Analysis of 165 operations at a single center. J Clin Endocrinol Metab 2001;86:1480–6.

Plouin PF, Gimenez-Roqueplo AP. The genetic basis of pheochromocytoma: Who to screen and how? Nat Clin Pract Endocrinol Metab 2006;2:60–1.

Prys-Roberts C. Phaeochromocytoma: Recent progress in its management. Br J Anaesth 2000;85:44–57.

Thyroiditis

Method of
Anthony P. Weetman, MD, DSc

Thyroiditis simply means inflammation of the thyroid gland, and it arises from a number of different causes. Clinically these are best classified by the tempo of inflammation: acute, subacute, or chronic. Mild to moderate focal thyroiditis, in which there is a patchy infiltration of the thyroid gland by lymphocytes, is so common (in ~15% of all autopsy specimens) that it has little clinical significance; in only a small fraction of such patients does disease progress to a chronic thyroiditis and destruction of thyroid tissue. Similarly, a focal thyroiditis is often found adjacent to (or even within) benign or malignant neoplasms of thyroid.

Acute Thyroiditis

BACKGROUND

Acute (suppurative) thyroiditis is a rare condition caused by a suppurative infection of the thyroid through the bloodstream, lymphatics, trauma, a persistent thyroglossal duct, or most commonly, extension from nearby infection. The latter typically arises through the piriform sinus, an anomalous remnant of the fourth branchial pouch, usually on the left side. This is the main cause of acute thyroiditis in children and young adults; a long-standing goiter, degeneration in a carcinoma, and immunosuppression are additional risk factors.

Virtually any bacterium can cause acute thyroiditis. The most common are *Staphylococcus aureus*, *Streptococci* species, *Klebsiella pneumoniae*, and *Escherichia coli*. In immunosuppressed patients, including those with AIDS, unusual organisms can invade the thyroid, including *Aspergillus*, *Candida*, and *Coccidioides* species and *Pneumocystis jiroveci*. In rare instances, tuberculosis can affect the thyroid, but the picture then is usually one of subacute thyroiditis.

The dominant clinical features are pain in the thyroid radiating to the ear, tenderness and erythema over the gland, fever, dysphagia, respiratory symptoms, and malaise. Features of septicemia may be present, as may lymphadenopathy and a local thrombophlebitis. The differential diagnosis for thyroid pain includes subacute and, rarely, chronic thyroiditis, hemorrhage into a cyst, and lymphoma. Clinical features help in the diagnosis, and simple investigations usually confirm the clinical suspicion.

TREATMENT

Treatment is with high-dose antibiotics selected on the basis of the microbiology results from fine-needle aspiration biopsy. Surgical drainage of any abscess is indicated when pus cannot be fully removed by aspiration. Complications of acute thyroiditis include tracheal obstruction, retropharyngeal abscess, mediastinitis, and internal jugular venous thrombosis. Any piriform sinus should be located (usually by barium swallow study 2 months after the acute episode) and excised to prevent a recurrence; a thyroid lobectomy is usually needed for this.

Subacute Thyroiditis

BACKGROUND

Subacute thyroiditis (de Quervain's, viral, or granulomatous thyroiditis) has a variable incidence, depending on region. In North America the incidence is 5 cases per 100,000 population per year. It is possible that it is overlooked in areas of apparently low incidence. Three times more women are affected than men, with a median incidence around the age of 45 years, and HLA-B35 is a predisposing genetic factor.

Many viruses have been implicated, especially Coxsackievirus, influenza, measles, mumps, and Epstein-Barr virus. There is no need to attempt identification serologically.

The main clinical features are a painful and tender goitrous thyroid with fluctuating thyroid hormone levels. The pain can be in one or both thyroid lobes. Occasionally, a nodular form can be detected on palpation.

Patients usually have a phase of thyrotoxicosis (caused by release of stored hormone from the damaged gland) lasting up to 4 weeks, followed by a phase of hypothyroidism of 1 to 3 months and then recovery. Many patients describe a prodromal phase of systemic upset or upper respiratory tract infection. The diagnosis is confirmed by the high erythrocyte sedimentation rate (ESR) and low isotope uptake.

TREATMENT

Mild cases do not require treatment except analgesics, usually nonsteroidal antiinflammatory drugs. Severe disease (around one third of cases) warrants treatment with prednisolone at a dose of 30 to 40 mg/day initially. Depending on the clinical response and sedimentation rate, this is gradually tapered after 1 to 2 weeks so that steroids are stopped after 4 to 6 weeks. Patients' thyroid function should be monitored closely (every 1 to 2 weeks).

During a phase of symptomatic thyrotoxicosis, propranolol (Inderal),[1] 20 to 40 mg three to four times a day, is useful for controlling the symptoms. Antithyroid drugs (methimazole [Tapazole], propylthiouracil [PTU]) are not effective in this situation. Subsequent symptomatic hypothyroidism is treated with levothyroxine (Synthroid, Levothroid, Levoxyl) 50 to 100 μg/day, but this should be withdrawn after 6 to 8 weeks because the phase is typically transient.

---

[1]Not FDA approved for this indication.

CURRENT DIAGNOSIS

- Thyroiditis can be classified as acute, subacute, or chronic, with pain as a hallmark of the first two types.
- Silent thyroiditis occurs after pregnancy or following drug treatment.
- A combination of thyroid function testing and thyroid peroxidase antibody measurement, supplemented by erythrocyte sedimentation rate and thyroid radionuclide uptake is sufficient to establish a diagnosis in most cases.
- Thyrotoxicosis in patients with thyroiditis is transient, and subsequent hypothyroidism should be anticipated.

CURRENT THERAPY

- Antibiotics and subsequent surgery are generally required for acute bacterial thyroiditis.
- Most patients with subacute thyroiditis can be managed with nonsteroidal antiinflammatory drugs; around one third require a short course of prednisolone.
- Thyrotoxicosis following destructive thyroiditis is treated with propranolol (Inderal)[1]; antithyroid drugs are useless in this setting.
- Levothyroxine (Synthroid, Levoxyl) remains the treatment of choice for chronic thyroiditis associated with hypothyroidism.

---

[1]Not FDA approved for this indication.

However, patients with preexisting thyroid abnormalities can develop permanent hypothyroidism after subacute thyroiditis (5%–10% of cases), and therefore full recovery of thyroid function must be established by testing.

Recurrences occur in around 5% of cases and are dealt with in the same way as the initial attack, although prolonging prednisolone treatment by 2 to 4 weeks may be useful.

Silent Thyroiditis

A similar pattern of subacute thyroid dysfunction without thyroid pain is called *silent thyroiditis*. This has an autoimmune etiology and occurs most distinctly 3 to 6 months after pregnancy in women with thyroid peroxidase antibodies before delivery. Treatment for thyroid dysfunction is again with propranolol for thyrotoxicosis and levothyroxine for the usually transient hypothyroidism; steroids are not needed. Thyroxine treatment is discontinued 1 year after delivery and the TSH is checked after 6 weeks to verify the patient is euthyroid.

Postpartum thyroiditis is a risk factor for the development of future permanent hypothyroidism. Affected women should therefore be screened annually for this and should be warned that the disease may well recur in future pregnancies. The appropriateness of screening all pregnant women for thyroid peroxidase antibodies in the first trimester is not yet clear except in women with type 1 diabetes mellitus, who are at particular risk of developing postpartum thyroiditis. In such women, the presence of thyroid antibodies before delivery should lead to careful monitoring of postpartum thyroid function.

Chronic (Autoimmune) Thyroiditis

BACKGROUND

Hypothyroidism caused by autoimmunity affects approximately 1% of women and 0.1% of men. However, there is a much higher prevalence of subclinical autoimmune thyroiditis shown by the presence of sustained, elevated circulating thyroid-stimulating hormone (TSH) levels with normal free thyroxine levels, with or without accompanying thyroid peroxidase or thyroglobulin antibodies. This condition often comes to light during screening for nonspecific symptoms such as fatigue or weight gain.

Some patients have a goiter of variable size that is usually hard and often irregular (bosselated); this is Hashimoto's, or goitrous, thyroiditis. At the opposite end of the pathologic spectrum is atrophic thyroiditis or primary myxedema in which the thyroid is replaced by fibrous tissue and the only clinical sign of the destructive process is the development of hypothyroidism. These patients may have antibodies that block the TSH receptor, but these are neither frequent nor unique in atrophic thyroiditis.

TREATMENT

Overt hypothyroidism resulting from chronic thyroiditis is treated with levothyroxine. There is no role normally for thyroid extract or for liothyronine (triiodothyronine, T_3) supplementation (Thyrolar, liotrix) or substitution (Cytomel), inasmuch as levothyroxine is converted smoothly and physiologically to T_3, whereas the short half-life of liothyronine leads to peaks and troughs of circulating T_3. Several recent trials have failed to confirm initially promising results from the addition of triiodothyronine to levothyroxine, and such current formulations of treatment can lead to excessive T_3 levels, with the potential for adverse effects on bone and the heart.

In otherwise healthy patients younger than 60 years with overt hypothyroidism, I start levothyroxine at 50 to 100 μg a day, but in those older than 60 years or with ischemic heart disease, the usual starting dose is 12.5 to 25 μg a day, increasing every 2 weeks by 25-μg increments. In all cases, the aim is to normalize the TSH level, although rarely this proves impossible in patients whose angina is worsened by thyroxine replacement. Propranolol[1] or other β-blockers help minimize this adverse effect.

If the TSH is maintained in the reference range, there are no adverse effects. I check TSH levels only 2 to 3 months after changing dose because it can take this length of time for symptoms and TSH levels to normalize. The same applies if the commercial preparation of levothyroxine is changed. Once the desired dose is achieved, TSH levels need to be checked only annually. It is unusual for patients to need more than 200 μg of levothyroxine a day. In my experience an elevated (and usually fluctuating) TSH level in patients taking higher doses usually indicates poor compliance, although malabsorption syndromes and certain drugs—such as colestipol (Colestid), cholestyramine sucralfate (Questran), ferrous sulfate (Feosol), aluminum hydroxide (Amphojel), phenytoin (Dilantin), activated charcoal (CharcoAid), rifampicin (rifampin, Rifadin), and hormone replacement therapy—can interfere with absorption or metabolism.

There is controversy about the optimal management of subclinical hypothyroidism. The risk of progression to overt hypothyroidism is highest in patients with both an elevated TSH and positive thyroid antibodies, and in my view it is worth treating these patients and those whose TSH is higher than 10 mU/L with levothyroxine (usually 25–50 μg initially) from the outset. In those with an elevated TSH but no thyroid antibodies, one option is a 3-month trial of levothyroxine, and if any symptomatic improvement occurs, to continue with this. If there is no improvement or the patient chooses not to have treatment, an annual check of thyroid function should be arranged to deal with the risk of progression to overt hypothyroidism.

The goiter of Hashimoto's thyroiditis usually shrinks with levothyroxine. Surgery is only rarely needed to control the goiter. Any focal irregularity in the goiter raises the suspicion of malignancy; such hard nodules are sometimes found in Hashimoto's thyroiditis and should be investigated, initially by aspiration biopsy. Pain suggests lymphoma, which is a rare complication of autoimmune thyroiditis. Very rarely is the thyroid tender in uncomplicated Hashimoto's thyroiditis, and this may be associated with an elevated ESR. Corticosteroids may be used but are sometimes unhelpful, and surgery may be needed in extreme cases.

Drug-Induced Thyroiditis

Autoimmune thyroiditis can be precipitated by lithium, excess iodide, or recombinant cytokines such as interferon (IFN)-α, interleukin-2, and granulocyte-macrophage colony-stimulating factor (GM-CSF). Such patients usually have thyroid peroxidase and other thyroid antibodies before treatment, and screening for these, as well as measuring serum TSH, should be undertaken before starting these drugs. Regular monitoring of TSH thereafter is also indicated.

Thyroxine replacement should be given and adjusted to maintain a normal TSH level. Treatment with amiodarone (Cordarone), lithium, and IFN-α can be continued. Amiodarone can cause both hypothyroidism, readily managed by levothyroxine, and thyrotoxicosis, the latter resulting either from a destructive process or from excess iodide supply that precipitates hyperthyroidism. Amiodarone-induced thyrotoxicosis can be very difficult to manage and necessitates specialist advice. Corticosteroids, potassium perchlorate, antithyroid drugs, and even surgery might be needed to control the disease, whereas stopping amiodarone has no immediate impact because of the long half-life of the drug. A painful but transient thyroiditis can occur 1 to 2 weeks after radioiodine for hyperthyroidism. It responds to simple analgesics, or corticosteroids if severe.

Riedel's Thyroiditis

Riedel's thyroiditis is a rare condition of unknown etiology that is caused by fibrosis of the thyroid, leading to a woodlike, hard mass often extending outside the thyroid and involving any of the adjacent structures. There is an association with idiopathic fibrosis

---

[1]Not FDA approved for this indication.

elsewhere (retroperitoneum, orbit, mediastinum, biliary tree, lung). The condition is often detected because of suspicion of thyroid malignancy. Aspiration biopsy typically yields no specimen, and diagnosis requires open biopsy. Thyroxine is useful only if there is hypothyroidism, and corticosteroids are ineffective. The condition runs an unpredictable course, with a slow progression in many cases, and surgery should be reserved only for patients with esophageal or tracheal compression. Tamoxifen (Soltamox)[1] treatment 20 mg twice daily has been successful in individual cases; due to the rarity of the disease, there have been no controlled trials of treatment.

---

[1]Not FDA approved for this indication.

REFERENCES

Basaria S, Cooper DS. Amiodarone and the thyroid. Am J Med 2005;118:706–14.

Escobar-Morreale HF, Botella-Carretero JI, Escobar del Rey F, Morreale de Escobar G. Treatment of hypothyroidism with combinations of levothyroxine plus liothyronine. J Clin Endocrinol Metab 2005;90:4946–54.

Fatourechi V, Aniszewski JP, Fatourechi GZ, et al. Clinical features and outcome of subacute thyroiditis in an incidence cohort: Olmsted County, Minnesota, study. J Clin Endocrinol Metab 2003;88:2100–5.

Jung YJ, Schaub CR, Rhodes R, et al. A case of Riedel's thyroiditis treated with tamoxifen: Another successful outcome. Endocr Pract 2004;10:483–6.

Nicholson WK, Robinson KA, Smallridge RC, et al. Prevalence of postpartum thyroid dysfunction: A quantitative review. Thyroid 2006;16:573–82.

Surks MI, Ortiz E, Daniels GH, et al. Subclinical thyroid disease: Scientific review and guidelines for diagnosis and management. JAMA 2004;291:228–38.

Weetman AP. The thyroid gland and disorders of thyroid function. In: Warrell TM, Cox TM, Firth JD, Benz EJ, editors. Oxford Textbook of Medicine, vol. 2. Oxford: Oxford University Press; 2003. p. 209–24.

Thyroiditis

689

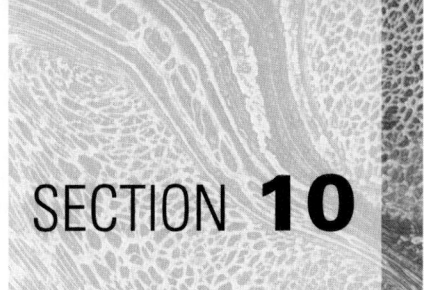

The Urogenital Tract

Bacterial Infections of the Male Urinary Tract

Method of
John N. Krieger, MD

Urinary tract infections (UTIs) include a wide clinical spectrum whose common denominator is bacterial invasion of the genitourinary organs and tissues. Any portion of the urinary tract may be involved from the renal cortex to the urethral meatus. UTI can predominate at a single site, such as the bladder (cystitis), prostate (prostatitis), epididymis (epididymitis), kidneys (pyelonephritis), or perinephric space (perinephric abscess). When any of its parts has become infected, the entire urinary tract is placed at risk for bacterial invasion.

The great majority of UTIs occur by the ascending route. Bacteria from the fecal flora colonize the perineum and then ascend via the urethra to involve the bladder, the ureter, and the kidneys. On occasion, hematogenous dissemination can result in bacterial seeding of the urinary tract. Classic examples of such hematogenous infection are genitourinary tuberculosis or staphylococcal infection of a renal cyst (historically known as a *renal carbuncle*). On rare occasions, the urinary tract may be involved by infection from contiguous structures. For example, patients with diverticulitis or appendicitis occasionally develop abscesses or fistulae that involve the urinary tract.

Distinguishing Complicated from Uncomplicated Infections

The first step in evaluating a patient is to distinguish uncomplicated (medical) infections from complicated (surgical) infections. An uncomplicated UTI occurs in the absence of underlying structural, functional, or neurologic disorders of the urinary tract. Uncomplicated UTIs usually respond promptly to appropriate antimicrobial therapy. Anatomic evaluation and imaging studies are seldom indicated in patients with uncomplicated UTIs.

In contrast, complicated UTIs occur when the urinary tract has been repeatedly invaded by bacteria, leaving residual inflammation or—in cases accompanied by obstruction—stones, foreign bodies, or neurologic conditions that interfere with urinary drainage. Antimicrobial therapy alone is markedly less effective in complicated UTIs than in uncomplicated UTIs. Managing patients with complicated infections often requires anatomic evaluation and imaging studies. An important differential point is that patients with complicated UTIs tend to have persistence of bacteria within the urinary tract in the face of antimicrobial agents to which the bacteria appear to be sensitive in laboratory tests. Often, it is necessary to correct an underlying obstructive lesion or voiding problem to clear the infection.

The ideal goal of UTI therapy is total elimination of the infecting organism from the urinary tract. This is a realistic goal for patients with uncomplicated UTIs. However, achieving this goal can prove difficult in patients with complicated UTIs whose underlying abnormalities cannot be corrected. For example, it is often impossible to achieve long-standing resolution of bacteriuria in patients who require indwelling catheters or who have functional obstruction of their voiding mechanisms. In such cases, resolution of symptoms directly related to UTI is the only practical therapeutic goal.

Natural History

During infancy, the incidence of symptomatic UTIs is higher in boys than in girls. In part, this has been related to male circumcision status. It appears that bacteria can adhere to the prepuce of uncircumcised boys, providing access to the urinary tract. Neonatal circumcision appears to reduce the UTI rate in boys by about 90%. After the neonatal period, symptomatic UTIs in boys and men are distinctly uncommon until middle age. This contrasts dramatically with UTI rates in girls and women, who experience increasing rates of both symptomatic and asymptomatic infections with a marked increase following initiation of sexual activity, then a continued gradual rise with increasing age. Asymptomatic bacteriuria is also distinctly unusual in male patients compared with female patients.

Well-documented UTIs in boys mandate thorough urologic investigation. This is because of the high prevalence of structural urinary tract abnormalities in boys with UTIs. Often, UTI represents the key diagnostic presentation for major abnormalities of the urinary tract. For example, vesicoureteral reflux of urine, posterior urethral valves, and other major structural abnormalities often manifest initially with bacterial UTIs. Early diagnosis and appropriate therapy offer the best chance for preservation of maximal renal function. Unfortunately, the developing kidneys are very susceptible to continued renal scarring, which may be progressive despite appropriate treatment.

Structural urinary tract abnormalities remain a major cause of renal failure in children. Morbidity may be minimized by appropriate evaluation and therapy. Our choice for evaluation of a boy with a urinary tract infection is the combination of renal ultrasound to evaluate the upper urinary tract plus a voiding cystourethrogram to evaluate the lower urinary tract. Voiding cystourethrography should be obtained after resolution of the initial infection, because dilation of the upper urinary tract may be exaggerated after a recent UTI.

Because UTIs are unusual in young men, there are few well-done natural history studies in this population. In young men with UTIs who have no obvious neurologic or structural abnormalities, sexual intercourse, particularly among homosexual men or heterosexual men who practice insertive anal intercourse, may be a risk factor. The overall contribution of these practices to bacterial UTIs in men is uncertain.

Traditional urologic teaching is to carry out a thorough evaluation for structural abnormalities in such patients, including radiographic studies and cystourethroscopy. However, our published experience suggests that previously healthy college-age men with well-documented UTIs have a low rate of structural genitourinary tract abnormalities. A uroflow study and postvoid residual urine determination by ultrasound are adequate to screen for structural abnormalities in young men whose UTIs resolve. We reserve cystoscopy for patients whom we determine to be at risk for significant abnormalities on the basis of these screening studies and a thorough physical examination. The other major risk factors for UTIs in men are instrumentation of the urinary tract and bacterial prostatitis.

Diagnosis and Localization

Accurate diagnosis is prerequisite for appropriate UTI therapy. Therefore, we recommend culture and sensitivity testing of urine specimens from any male patient with symptoms or signs suggesting a UTI. In patients who do not have obstructive lesions, stasis, stones, or foreign bodies, recurrent and persistent bacterial UTIs are often related to bacterial prostatitis. Segmented localization cultures can be used to differentiate cystitis and urethritis from bacterial prostatitis. The procedure should be carried out at a time when the patient does not have bacteriuria.

My procedure for lower urinary tract localization is outlined briefly. After cleaning the glans with sterile water, the first-void urine (initial 5–10 mL of voided urine) is collected in a sterile container. Next, a midstream specimen is obtained. The patient is asked to stop voiding. Prostatic fluid is expressed by digital rectal prostate massage. The post–prostate massage urine (next 5–10 mL voided after the massage) is then collected. Culture and sensitivity testing are then carried out on each of these four specimens. It is critical to ensure that the clinical microbiology laboratory is aware of the purpose of these studies so that they will evaluate low concentrations of uropathogens that may be present in the localization cultures.

Diagnosis of chronic bacterial prostatitis can be made if the post–prostate massage urine specimen or the expressed prostatic secretion contains a 10-fold or greater increase in the concentration of the uropathogen compared with that in the first-void urine specimen. In patients with well-documented bacterial prostatitis, the causative organism is identical to the uropathogen causing recurrent UTI episodes.

It is important to recognize that only a small minority of men presenting with symptoms of prostatitis fit into the acute or chronic bacterial prostatitis categories. The great majority of patients with symptoms of prostatitis are classified in the chronic prostatitis/chronic pelvic pain category. In contrast to the recognized benefit of therapy for patients with acute and chronic bacterial prostatitis, the role of antimicrobial therapy and other treatments has not been defined for men with symptoms of chronic prostatitis/chronic pelvic pain syndrome.

Treatment

There are three keys to successful UTI therapy. First, eliminate or control predisposing factors, if possible. For example, we are often asked to manage resistant urinary infections in long-term care patients with indwelling catheters. One approach is to change their bladder management from a chronic indwelling catheter to an intermittent self- or assisted-catheterization program. Other examples include removal or correction of obstructing lesions, stones, or strictures to improve drainage of the urinary tract. These measures may be successful in eliminating the focus of infection, even with no antimicrobial therapy. Second, eradicate the infection as soon as possible to prevent colonization of the prostate and other structures. Third, ensure resolution of the UTI by obtaining cultures during or immediately after therapy and at follow-up 1 to 2 months after therapy.

UNCOMPLICATED INFECTIONS

Uncomplicated infections generally manifest with symptoms of bacterial cystitis, such as the combination of urinary frequency, urgency, dysuria, nocturia, suprapubic discomfort, low-back pain, or hematuria. Systemic symptoms of fever, chills, and rigor are absent. Urine culture confirms the diagnosis, with *Escherichia coli* being the most common pathogen. Uncomplicated infections, including those introduced by a single or short course of indwelling urethral catheterization, generally respond promptly to a short course of antimicrobial therapy. The infection can persist and become difficult to eradicate if the prostate becomes colonized or if the patient has a stone or structural abnormality of the urinary tract. Thus, an effort should be made to eliminate predisposing factors while routine therapy is guided by in vitro susceptibility tests.

I prefer oral therapy with one of the agents listed in Table 1. In the Pacific northwest, bacteria causing urinary tract infections have developed substantial resistance to trimethoprim-sulfamethoxazole (Bactrim). Therefore, I usually initiate empiric therapy with a quinolone. Nitrofurantoin (Macrodantin) remains highly effective and is an attractive alternative drug. In general, I recommend that the duration of therapy be at least 2 weeks, although only limited data address this point in male patients.

CURRENT DIAGNOSIS

- UTIs include a wide clinical spectrum.
- Infection at any site in the urinary tract places the entire system at risk.
- The critical clinical issue is to distinguish uncomplicated (medical) from complicated (surgical) infections.
- Anatomic evaluation and imaging studies are seldom indicated for patients with uncomplicated UTIs.
- Well-documented UTIs in boys require thorough urologic investigation because of the high prevalence of structural urinary tract abnormalities.
- We recommend culture and sensitivity testing of urine specimens for any male patient with symptoms or signs suggesting a UTI.
- In contrast, we discourage routine screening urine cultures in long-term care patients who have no localizing signs or symptoms suggesting a UTI.

UTI = urinary tract infection.

CURRENT THERAPY

- The optimal goal of therapy is to eliminate the infecting organism from the urinary tract.
- Antimicrobial therapy alone is less effective for patients with complicated UTIs than for patients with uncomplicated UTIs.
- Managing patients with complicated UTIs often requires anatomic evaluation and imaging studies.
- For patients with complicated UTIs it is often necessary to eliminate or control predisposing factors.
- Rapid eradication of the infection can limit the potential for infection of adjacent structures.
- Ensure elimination of the infection by repeating urine cultures.
- A prolonged course of antimicrobial therapy may prove necessary for patients with persistent infections.

UTI = urinary tract infection.

TABLE 1 Oral Antimicrobial Agents Prescribed for Urinary Tract Infections In Men

Agent	Dosage
Fluoroquinolones	
Ciprofloxacin (Cipro)	250–500 mg bid
Ciprofloxacin (CiproXR)	500–1000 mg qd
Lomefloxacin (Maxaquin)	400 mg qd
Levofloxacin (Levaquin LEVA-pak)	500–750 mg qd
Ofloxacin (Floxin)	200–400 mg bid[3]
Norfloxacin (Noroxin)	400 mg bid
Combination Agents	
Trimethoprim-sulfamethoxazole (Bactrim, Septra, Bactrim DS, Septra DS)	160 mg trimethoprim, 800 mg sulfamethoxazole bid
Amoxicillin-clavulanate (Augmentin)	500–875 mg amoxicillin, 125 mg clavulonate bid
Other Antimicrobials	
Nitrofurantoin (Macrobid)	50–100 mg bid
Nitrofurantoin (Macrodantin)	50–100 mg qid

[3]Exceeds dosage recommended by the manufacturer.

COMPLICATED INFECTIONS

Patients with systemic signs or those with a history of structural or neurologic abnormalities merit anatomic and functional investigation of the urinary tract. Antimicrobial therapy alone might fail to cure infection and urosepsis can develop unless there is specific management of the underlying problem. My initial choice for evaluating these patients is either computed tomography (CT) with contrast or an excretory urogram with postvoid film. If a renal or retroperitoneal abscess is suspected, computed tomographic scanning has proved superior to the other modalities for diagnosis. In contrast, I prefer transrectal ultrasound for evaluation of possible prostatic abscesses.

Prolonged courses of therapy are indicated for patients with persistent infections, Often, I have used 3 to 4 months of therapy in this situation. In patients with chronic bacterial prostatitis, elderly patients, or those in nursing homes, continuous therapy may be necessary to suppress bacteriuria, even though eradication can prove impossible. Thus, for patients with recurrent or complicated infections, I recommend an attempt to eradicate the focus of infection, following thorough evaluation of the urinary tract. The therapy is usually with the drugs listed in Table 1. My first choice for curative therapy is usually a quinolone. For patients with persistent or frequently relapsing infections, I consider long-term therapy (months or years) using low dosages of antimicrobial drugs for prophylaxis or suppression. In this situation, my choice is usually either trimethoprim-sulfamethoxazole (Bactrim) or nitrofurantoin (Macrodantin).

PROSTATITIS

Acute and chronic bacterial prostatitis can manifest with local urinary tract symptoms characteristic of bacterial cystitis or with systemic signs and symptoms. Acute bacterial prostatitis can manifest with the sudden onset of chills, fever, malaise, and low back and perineal pain, as well as difficulty with urination. On rectal examination, the prostate is tense and exquisitely tender. Excessive palpation can induce septicemia.

For patients who require hospitalization, my initial choice is the combination of a β-lactam drug and an aminoglycoside until the results of antimicrobial sensitivity testing are available. Following parenteral therapy, the patient is managed with continued antimicrobial therapy for at least 4 weeks, usually employing a quinolone. Patients with acute bacterial prostatitis usually respond well to a variety of antimicrobial agents that penetrate an acutely inflamed prostate. Many of these agents are not effective in chronic bacterial prostatitis.

In contrast to acute bacterial prostatitis, chronic bacterial prostatitis is often insidious in onset. Patients usually have recurrent symptomatic UTIs and, sometimes, recurrent episodes of acute prostatitis. Between symptomatic episodes, patients may be totally asymptomatic. Diagnosis depends on the localization cultures described earlier. Treatment must be prolonged, because diffusion of many antimicrobial agents into the uninflamed prostate is poor.

My initial choice is usually a quinolone, with trimethoprim-sulfamethoxazole (Septra, Bactrim) as a second-choice agent. Carbenicillin indanyl sodium (Geocillin) is also approved for this indication, but it has not been particularly effective in my hands.

It is important to avoid confusing bacterial prostatitis with chronic prostatitis/chronic pelvic pain syndrome. This is the most common category of symptomatic prostatitis. A critical distinguishing point is that patients with chronic prostatitis/chronic pelvic pain syndrome do not have bacteriuria and they have negative bacterial localization cultures.

LONG-TERM CARE PATIENTS

My approach to managing UTI differs in long-term care patients, including those with incontinence and indwelling urinary catheters or other devices. In such patients, chronic asymptomatic bacterial colonization should not be treated. It is impossible to sterilize the urine permanently in such men. Furthermore, resistant organisms will likely emerge, making subsequent therapy difficult. I treat such patients only if they develop acute symptoms referable to the urinary tract or before genitourinary tract procedures. I strongly recommend against obtaining screening cultures in long-term care patients because these cultures often lead to unnecessary therapy that selects resistant bacterial flora. Further, there is evidence that bacterial colonization with relatively benign strains can inhibit establishment of symptomatic infections caused by more virulent bacteria.

REFERENCES

Abarbanel J, Engelstein D, Lask D, et al. Urinary tract infection in men younger than 45 years of age: Is there a need for urologic investigation? Urology 2003;62:27–9.

Andrews SJ, Brooks PT, Hanbury DC, et al. Ultrasonography and abdominal radiography versus intravenous urography in investigation of urinary tract infection in men: Prospective incident cohort study. BMJ 2002; 324:454–6.

Bjerklund Johansen T. Diagnosis and imaging in urinary tract infections. Curr Opin Urol 2002;12:39–43.

Craig JC, Knight JF, Sureshkumar P, et al. Effect of circumcision on incidence of urinary tract infection in preschool boys. J Pediatr 1996;128:23–7.

Griebling TL. Urologic diseases in America project: Trends in resource use for urinary tract infections in men. J Urol 2005;173:1288–94.

Hummers-Pradier E, Ohse AM, Koch M, et al. Urinary tract infection in men. Int J Clin Pharmacol Ther 2004;42:360–6.

Johansen TE. The role of imaging in urinary tract infections. World J Urol 2004;22:392–8.

Krieger JN, Nyberg L, Nickel JC. NIH consensus definition and classification of prostatitis. JAMA 1999;282:236–7.

Krieger JN, Ross SO, Simonsen JM. Urinary tract infections in healthy university men. J Urol 1993;149:1046–8.

Naber KG. Levofloxacin in the treatment of urinary tract infections and prostatitis. J Chemother 2004;16(Suppl. 2):18–21.

Nicolle LESHEA Long-Term-Care Committee. Urinary tract infections in long-term-care facilities. Infect Control Hosp Epidemiol 2001;22:167–75.

Sunden F, Hakansson L, Ljunggren E, et al. Bacterial interference—is deliberate colonization with Escherichia coli 83972 an alternative treatment for patients with recurrent urinary tract infection? Int J Antimicrob Agents 28 Suppl 2006;1:S26–9.

Ulleryd P, Zackrisson B, Aus G, et al. Selective urological evaluation in men with febrile urinary tract infection. BJU Int 2001;88:15–20.

Wagenlehner FM, Naber KG. Current challenges in the treatment of complicated urinary tract infections and prostatitis. Clin Microbiol Infect 2006;12(Suppl 3):67–80.

Urinary Tract Infections in Women

Method of
Burke A. Cunha, MD

General Concepts

Urinary tract infections (UTIs) are common in adult women. The two major clinical manifestations of UTIs in adult women are cystitis or pyelonephritis. Young adult women may also present with so-called dysuria pyuria syndrome (abacteriuric cystitis), previously known as acute urethral syndrome, as outpatients. Hospitalized compromised female hosts with cystitis may be complicated by bacteremia or ascending infection. Renal abscess may complicate pyelonephritis in normal or compromised female hosts.

Cystitis Versus Pyelonephritis

The therapeutic approach to UTIs in adult women depends on accurate localization of the site of infection in the urinary tract. The most common clinical problem is differentiating cystitis from pyelonephritis. Patients with acute bacterial cystitis present with dysuria and frequency, which may or may not be accompanied by suprapubic discomfort or lower back pain. The fever accompanying cystitis is ≤ to 38.9°C (102°F) and is not usually associated with chills. The clinical manifestation of cystitis is confirmed by finding pyuria and significant bacteriuria, (i.e., ≥10⁶ CFU/mL) in such patients. The urinalysis in acute cystitis is not usually accompanied by microscopic hematuria.

Staphylococcus saprophyticus is the only uropathogen in the ambulatory setting that is responsible for the majority of cases of UTIs accompanied by microscopic hematuria. Microscopic hematuria in a urinalysis in a patient with an apparent UTI should be carefully observed and should disappear after therapy of the UTI. If the microscopic hematuria disappears, then the physician can safely assume it was related to the UTI. Particularly in elderly patients, if the microscopic hematuria persists after eradication of the UTI, then the patient should be investigated for a bladder or renal source of the microscopic hematuria.

Dysuria-Pyuria Syndrome

In sexually active young women, dysuria-pyuria syndrome manifests with the symptoms of cystitis but with negative urine cultures, or if organisms are cultured, they are present in low numbers (i.e., *E. coli*) (≤10³ CFU/mL). Most cases of dysuria-pyuria syndrome are caused by *Chlamydia trachomatis*. In patients with dysuria-pyuria syndrome, if the urine is cultured for *Chlamydia*, cultures are frequently positive.

Catheter-Associated Bacteriuria (CAB)

Hospitalized patients with indwelling Foley catheters often acquire bacteriuria as a function of time that the Foley catheter is in place. Pyuria is often in the urine of patients with indwelling Foleys because the catheter elicits inflammation of the urinary tract. The presence of pyuria and bacteriuria in a patient with an indwelling Foley suggests either UTI or CAB. The majority of such patients are asymptomatic and afebrile. More than 95% of the time these patients have colonization of the urinary tract without infection. The urinalysis in patients with indwelling Foley catheters is helpful if either bacteria without pyuria or pyuria without bacteria is demonstrated. Bacteriuria without pyuria signifies colonization of the urinary tract, whereas pyuria without bacteriuria indicates inflammation of the urinary tract. In non–Foley catheter patients, the presence of pyuria plus significant bacteriuria is diagnostic of a UTI. This is not the case with CAB. In normal hosts with a Foley catheter, CAB, i.e., bacteriuria plus pyuria, represents colonization and not a UTI.

Benign Bacteriuria of the Elderly

In elderly female patients, varying degrees of relaxation of the pelvic musculature are common. Patients often have varying degrees of cystocele of rectocele, which changes anatomic relationship and the angularity of the urethra as it enters the bladder and predisposes to colonization of the bladder urine by the introital flora, such as coliform flora derived from the colon. For this reason, elderly female patients often have bacteriuria with few or no symptoms of a UTI. The presence of bacteriuria/pyuria is often discovered on a routine urinalysis obtained as part of either admission laboratory work or an outpatient workup/screening test battery. The presence of bacteriuria/pyuria in an elderly female patient without underlying genitourinary (GU) disease or impaired host defenses has been appropriately termed *benign bacteriuria of the elderly*, it has been shown that these patients do not go on to have symptomatic UTIs, ascending infection (e.g., pyelonephritis/renal abscess), or bacteremia from the urinary tract.

Recurrent Urinary Tract Infections: Reinfection Versus Relapse

Most UTIs in women are acute. CAB is often incorrectly considered a chronic UTI because in most cases it represents colonization rather than infection. Recurrent UTIs are chronic in the sense that they persist over a long period of time, but are really episodic infections. However, the approach to recurrent UTIs is based on determining whether the recurrence is on the basis of reinfection or relapse. The reinfection variety of recurrent UTIs is defined as a recurrent UTI because of different organisms being cultured during each UTI episode. The relapse form of recurrent UTIs is defined as demonstrating the same organism during repeated bouts of UTIs. The reinfection form of recurrent UTIs is usually because of rapid colonization of the vaginal introitus/entry into the urethra, usually following sexual intercourse. The relapse variety of recurrent UTI by the same organism recovered during each episode suggests an underlying structural abnormality of the GU tract. The correct diagnostic approach to recurrent UTIs because of relapse is a thorough investigation of the GU tract from the urethra to the kidneys, which determines a possible source for the focus for the organisms to periodically reappear as a relapsing UTI. Relapse UTIs cannot be successfully approached therapeutically without correcting the underlying condition predisposing to relapse (i.e., bladder calculi, kinked ureters, renal stones, renal abscesses).

Acute Pyelonephritis

Acute pyelonephritis is most common in pregnancy and as a complication of an ascending infection from cystitis/GU instrumentation. An acute episode of pyelonephritis may occur in patients who have chronic pyelonephritis; the acute episode is superimposed on the chronic condition. Renal abscess may complicate acute and chronic pyelonephritis. Renal cortical abscesses are often caused by gram-positive cocci (e.g., staphylococci acquired hematogenously), whereas medullary abscesses are usually caused by aerobic gram-negative bacilli (e.g., coliforms or enterococci).

Acute pyelonephritis may be differentiated from cystitis by the presence of unilateral costovertebral angle (CVA) tenderness (otherwise unexplainable) and a temperature of $\geq 38.9°C$ (102°F). Bilateral pyelonephritis is unusual, and the presence of bilateral CVA tenderness should suggest an alternative diagnosis. Pyelonephritis is often bilateral pathologically, but clinically it is almost always unilateral in its presentation with CVA tenderness. The urinalysis in pyelonephritis is the same as in cystitis, for example with significant pyuria/bacteriuria in addition to the findings suggestive of pyelonephritis. The clinical presentation of renal abscess may resemble pyelonephritis if CVA tenderness is present, but this is not an invariable finding. The urinalysis in renal abscess may reveal pyuria and bacteria if the abscess is medullary but only pyuria if the renal abscess is cortical. Renal imaging studies are usually unnecessary in cystitis or pyelonephritis. If there is confusion regarding the presence or absence of chronic pyelonephritis, then a computed tomography/magnetic resonance imaging (CT/MRI) scan of the abdomen or renal ultrasound is appropriate.

Chronic Pyelonephritis

Chronic pyelonephritis results in shrunken and distorted kidneys with a distorted collecting system. If the patient presents with *chronic pyelonephritis* and has kidneys of normal or large size, then an alternate explanation should be sought. The only way to diagnose a renal abscess with certainty is with renal imaging studies. For this purpose, the CT/MRI of the kidneys is vastly superior in picking up small lesions than is the renal ultrasound. For the purposes of excluding a renal abscess, a negative renal ultrasound should never be used to rule out the diagnosis. A negative renal ultrasound should always be followed with a renal CT/MRI of the kidneys if a renal abscess is in the differential diagnosis.

 CURRENT DIAGNOSIS

- Acute uncomplicated cystitis is the most common type of UTI in adult women.
- The initial peak incidence of cystitis occurs with sexual intercourse and gradually increases through adulthood.
- Cystitis may occur as a single event or may be recurrent because of reinfection or relapse.
- Cystitis is usually caused by coliform or enterococci from the fecal flora or by *Staphylococcus saprophyticus* from the skin flora.
- Clinically, cystitis is marked by low-grade fever ($\leq 38.9°C$ [102°F]) with lower abdominal/suprapubic discomfort, and/or dysuria.
- *Staphylococcus aureus, Streptococcus pneumoniae*, groups A, C, G streptococci, and *Bacteroides fragilis* are not uropathogens in cystitis.
- In elderly women, *cystitis* manifests as pyuria and bacterluria without fever or dysuria, which is termed *benign bacteriuria of the elderly.*
- A variant of cystitis, the so-called *dysuria/pyuria syndrome*, is also known as *abacteriuric cystitis.*
- Dysuria/pyuria syndrome, most common in young adult women, manifests as cystitis, but urine cultures are negative for bacteria or uropathogens such as *Escherichia coli* are present in low numbers. *Chlamydia trachomatis* is frequently isolated if the urine is cultured for *Chlamydia.*
- Pyelonephritis in women may occur as an uncommon complication of cystitis or during pregnancy.
- It is not possible to predict the uropathogen of cystitis from clinical features except for *S. saprophyticus.*
- *S. saprophyticus* cystitis is characterized by a fishy urine odor, microscopic hematuria, and an alkaline urinary pH.
- Cystitis with alkaline urine suggests infection secondary to *S. saprophyticus, Ureaplasma urealyticum*, or a struvite stone with associated infection caused by a urea-splitting organism such as *Proteus.*
- Microscopic hematuria is common with *S. saprophyticus* cystitis but is uncommon with other uropathogens. If a patient with cystitis and microscopic hematuria fails to promptly resolve with antimicrobial therapy, work up the patient for a bladder/renal neoplasm or renal TB.

- The diagnosis of cystitis in women is made by demonstrating pyuria and significant bacteriuria ($\geq 10^6$ col/mL) in the setting of cystitis symptoms.
- Cystitis symptoms with gross hematuria should suggest a viral hemorrhagic cystitis or a renal lesion.
- Pyuria without bacteriuria indicates urinary tract inflammation. Persistent pyuria without bacteriuria should suggest interstitial cystitis or renal TB.
- With cystitis, the specific gravity of the urine is not decreased in contrast to pyelonephritis where the specific gravity is decreased.
- Urinary concentration returns to normal with treatment in pyelonephritis.
- Pyelonephritis may be differentiated from cystitis by the presence of fever $\geq 38.9°C$ (102°F) and otherwise unexplained unilateral CVA tenderness.
- The urine analysis/culture findings in pyelonephritis and cystitis are the same. Bacteremia frequently occurs with pyelonephritis but is not a feature of cystitis in normal hosts.
- Nonleukopenic compromised hosts, such as diabetes mellitus, systemic lupus erythematosus, multiple myeloma, cirrhosis, and so on, with cystitis may be complicated by pyelonephritis or bacteremia.
- Pyelonephritis is caused by the same uropathogens that cause cystitis; however, *S. saprophyticus* occurs only in cystitis.
- Acute pyelonephritis clinically improves unless complicated by renal abscess.
- Clinically, pyelonephritis is almost always unilateral, but pathophysical findings may be bilateral.
- Bilateral CVA tenderness should suggest an alternate diagnosis.
- In pyelonephritis, radiologic studies typically show unilateral renal involvement characterized by cortical scarring, medullary abnormalities, and renal shrinkage.
- Bilateral, normal-sized, or enlarged kidneys should suggest an alternate diagnosis to pyelonephritis.

Abbreviations: CVA = costovertebral angle; TB = tuberculosis; UTI = urinary tract infection.

CURRENT THERAPY

- Virtually all cases of initial uncomplicated cystitis will resolve spontaneously with or without treatment. No urine analysis/culture is needed with the initial episode of cystitis.
- For the dysuria of cystitis, phenazopyridine (Pyridium), which has no antibacterial properties but relieves pain and relative urinary obstruction from muscle spasm, may be used. Relief of spasm promptly clears the bacteriuria.
- Recurrent cystitis of the reinfection variety is because of different uropathogens with each episode that the urine is cultured. Reinfection is related to vaginal introital colonization following sexual intercourse and may be treated with a postcoital/HS of an appropriate antibiotic.
- Although the initial attack of cystitis resolves in virtually all patients without treatment, those who prefer to treat may use single-dose therapy with nitrofurantoin (Macrodantin), TMP-SMX (Bactrim), or amoxicillin (Amoxil).
- Cystitis in a nonleukopenic compromised host (discussed previously) should be treated for 1 to 2 weeks to prevent bacteremia/ascending infection, such as pyelonephritis/renal abscess.
- Ampicillin should be avoided because of its high resistance potential. Amoxicillin should be used instead, which has not been associated with resistance and is effective against the common coliforms and enterococci (*Enterococcus faecalis*).
- Nitrofurantoin has no resistance potential, is effective against all common uropathogens and all enterococci, such as *E. faecalis* (non-VRE) and *Enterococcus faecium*

- (VRE). Nitrofurantoin (Macrodantin) is useful in cystitis or catheter-associated bacteremia but is not to be used in pyelonephritis/bacteremia.
- Recurrent UTI of the relapse variety is caused by the same uropathogen with each occurrence. The problem in relapse UTIs is not therapeutic but diagnostic. Relapsing UTIs have an underlying structural abnormality or ureteral shunts that do not permit antimicrobial therapy to be effective.
- The treatment of pyelonephritis is with IV or PO antibiotics, depending on the severity of the clinical manifestation. Treatment is for 2 to 4 weeks with an effective antibiotic.
- For pyelonephritis, parenteral agents useful against coliforms are cephalosporins, aztreonam (Azactam), aminoglycosides, TMP-SMZ (Bactrim), or renally eliminated quinolones. Against enterococci (most of which are non-VRE), parenteral ampicillin, antipseudomonal penicillins, and meropenem (Merrem) are useful.
- Oral antibiotics useful against coliform causes of pyelonephritis include renally eliminated quinolones, amoxicillin (Amoxil), antipseudomonal penicillins, or TMP-SMZ (Bactrim).
- Linezolid (Zyvox) may be used for pyelonephritis caused by enterococci (non-VRE), amoxicillin (Amoxil), or for VRE.
- Patients with acute pyelonephritis become afebrile/nearly afebrile within 72 hours with or without treatment. Persistence of high fevers for greater than 72 hours should be considered as representing a renal abscess until proved otherwise.

Abbreviations: HD = half dose; IM = intramuscular; IV = intravenous; TMP-SMZ = trimethoprim-sulfamethoxazole; UTI = urinary tract infection; VRE = vancomycin-resistant *Enterococcus*.

Therapeutic Considerations

ACUTE CYSTITIS

The initial episode of acute complicated cystitis in a normal host without GU abnormalities/preexisting renal disease need not be treated with antimicrobial therapy. Usually treatment with phenazopyridine (Pyridium), which has no antibacterial effect, is sufficient to relieve bladder spasm and the relative urine obstruction because of the bladder spasm, and the bacteria will spontaneously clear itself without antimicrobial therapy. Repeated episodes of acute cystitis should have appropriate diagnostic studies, for example, a urinalysis and urinary culture with sensitivities with each episode to differentiate reinfection from relapse. If cystitis occurs in a nonleukopenic compromised host (e.g., with diabetes mellitus, systemic lupus erythematosus, multiple myeloma, cirrhosis, etc.), then a 7-day course of therapy is recommended with an oral agent such as nitrofurantoin (Macrodantin), trimethoprim-sulfamethoxazole (TMP-SMX) (Bactrim), fosfomycin (Monurol), or amoxicillin (Amoxil). Ampicillin should be avoided because of its resistance potential with coliform bacteria.

DYSURIA-PYURIA SYNDROME

The dysuria-pyuria syndrome because of *Chlamydia* should be treated with a 2-week course of doxycycline (Vibramycin). Patients unable to tolerate doxycycline (Vibramycin) may be treated with a

macrolide for the same period of time. A grossly hemorrhagic cystitis suggests a viral etiology for which no specific therapy is available. Patients with cystitis and microscopic hematuria are often infected with *S. saprophyticus*.

Fortunately, *S. saprophyticus* is susceptible to a wide range of antibiotics and virtually any agent selected to treat a UTI will be effective. Antimicrobial resistance has not been a problem in *S. saprophyticus* UTIs. Chronic interstitial cystitis is not an infectious disorder and therefore antimicrobial therapy is unnecessary.

CATHETER-ASSOCIATED BACTERIURIA

CAB in hospitalized patients who are normal hosts without structural abnormalities need not be treated, because virtually all of these patients are colonized and not infected. CAB in nonleukopenic compromised hosts (with diabetes mellitus, systemic lupus erythematosus, multiple myeloma, cirrhosis, and so forth) should be treated to prevent ascending infection/bacteremia from the lower urinary tract. Such individuals should be treated with an oral agent such as amoxicillin (Amoxil), nitrofurantoin (Macrodantin), or TMP-SMX (Bactrim) for 1 to 2 weeks.

Nonleukopenic compromised hosts with enterococci CAB are best treated with oral nitrofurantoin (Macrodantin), which is effective against enterococcal strains such as *E. faecalis* (non-vancomycin-resistant *Enterococcus* [non-VRE]) as well as *E. faecium* [VRE]). *Enterococcus faecalis* strains may also be treated with oral amoxicillin (Amoxil). These instances represent prophylaxis/early therapy because the majority of patients who are nonleukopenic-compromised hosts will have colonization of the urinary tract prior to catheterization or rapidly develop it soon thereafter. Therefore, prevention of ascending infection/bacteremia is the primary aim of therapy in patients with CAB who are compromised on the basis of their host defenses or GU tract abnormalities (e.g., ureteral stents).

ACUTE PYELONEPHRITIS

Acute pyelonephritis may be caused by aerobic gram-negative bacilli, such as coliforms or enterococci (almost always *E. faecalis*). The empirical treatment of pyelonephritis is based on a Gram stain of the urine, which, if the diagnosis is pyelonephritis, will show significant pyuria and a single predominant organism. In a patient with presumed pyelonephritis, the absence of bacteria in the Gram stain of the urine in an acutely ill patient essentially eliminates the diagnosis of pyelonephritis from further consideration, and an alternate explanation for the patient's fever and CVA tenderness should be sought (e.g., renal imaging studies).

Because acute pyelonephritis is often accompanied by bacteremia (urosepsis), parenteral agents may be used initially followed by oral agents; or in mild-to-moderate cases, oral agents may be used for the entire course of therapy. The parenteral agents useful in the treatment of acute pyelonephritis because of aerobic gram-negative bacilli include aminoglycosides, aztreonam (Azactam), antipseudomonal penicillin (e.g., ticarcillin [Ticar]), piperacillin (Pipracil), or a renally excreted respiratory quinolone. Patients presenting with acute pyelonephritis, who have streptococci in the Gram stain of the urine indicating enterococci, may be treated empirically with ampicillin and antipseudomonal penicillin, ticarcillin (Ticar), piperacillin (Pipracil), or meropenem (Merrem). In the rare instance where there is enterococcal urosepsis complicating acute pyelonephritis because of VRE, then linezolid (Zyvox), quinupristin-dalfopristin (Synercid), or daptomycin (Cubicin) may be used. In patients presenting with acute pyelonephritis where a Gram stain is unobtainable or unavailable, then empirical coverage for both aerobic gram-negative bacilli and enterococci (*E. faecalis*), may be achieved with antipseudomonal penicillins, nonrenally eliminated respiratory quinolones, or meropenem (Merrem). After the organism responsible for the pyelonephritis is subsequently identified by urine/blood culture, then the patient may be switched to one of the agents mentioned. Similarly, if the patient is shown to have enterococci as the cause of the urosepsis, it may be treated initially as non-VRE, as indicated previously in the article. Patients with pyelonephritis are usually treated for 1 to 2 weeks.

Particularly in critically ill patients, initial therapy is often started parenterally. Patients may be switched to an oral agent as soon as the patient clinically defervesces or treated entirely by an oral agent for the duration of therapy. The ideal oral antibiotic has the same spectrum as its parenteral counterpart and has excellent bioavailability; blood/tissue levels are approximately the same after intravenous/oral (IV/PO) administration. For example, by giving 1 g of amoxicillin (Amoxil) every 8 hours, the same blood/tissue levels are achieved as by giving ampicillin by intramuscular injection (IM). Nonrenally eliminated respiratory quinolones, such as levofloxacin (Levaquin) and gatifloxacin (Tequin), achieve the same blood and tissue levels when given either by the IV or PO route. This permits completion of therapy at home and does not require 2 to 4 weeks of inpatient hospitalization for intravenous drug therapy. There is some rationale for treating acute pyelonephritis for an extended period, such as 2 to 4 weeks, to prevent chronic pyelonephritis.

CHRONIC PYELONEPHRITIS

Patients with chronic pyelonephritis are a therapeutic challenge because of the distorted intrarenal architecture and decreased blood supply to the kidney, which limits access of white blood cells (WBCs), impairs host defenses, and limits penetration of the antibiotic into the infected/diseased areas of the kidney. Treatment of chronic pyelonephritis should be based on susceptibility testing of the isolates that are present in the urine. In chronic pyelonephritis, bacteriuria is intermittent but is present over a long period of time and will persist after short or inadequate treatment. The antibiotic selected should be effective against the isolate recovered from the urine in patients with chronic pyelonephritis and possess the ability to penetrate into diseased kidneys. The ideal oral agents for therapy are TMP-SMX (Bactrim), doxycycline (Vibramycin), or a nonrenally eliminated respiratory quinolone.

RENAL ABSCESS

Acute pyelonephritis treated appropriately results in a rapid defervescence of temperature and decrease in CVA tenderness within 72 hours. If the temperature does not decrease after 72 hours of appropriate therapy, suggest a renal abscess until proved otherwise. Renal abscesses should be treated for the presumed organism based on the location of the abscess by renal imaging studies. If sensitivities from an isolate available from the urine or percutaneous aspiration of the abscess are unavailable, then empirical treatment directed against aerobic gram-negative bacilli for medullary abscesses is indicated. Treatment is the same as for pyelonephritis except is more prolonged and should be given until the abscess is drained or it resolves. For cortical abscesses in the absence of culture and sensitivity data, antibiotic therapy should be directed against *Staphylococcus aureus* and *E. faecalis*, and treated in the same manner as pyelonephritis but for an extended period of time. Acute pyelonephritis with or without acteremia is usually treated for 7 days.

RECURRENT UTIs

Reinfection may be treated with nitrofurantoin (Macrodantin), TMP-SMX (Bactrim), or amoxicillin (Amoxil) as a single postcoital dose. Therapeutic approach to relapse is to remove the underlying condition responsible for perpetuating the bacteriuria. Antimicrobial therapy may be selected based on the susceptibility of the organism, but antimicrobial therapy alone will not eradicate the relapsing form of recurrent UTI.

REFERENCES

Cunha BA. Clinical concepts in the treatment of urinary tract infections. Antibiotics for Clinicians 1999;3:88–93.

Cunha BA. Nosocomial catheter-associated urinary tract infections. Hosp Physician 1986;22:13–6.

Cunha BA. *Staphylococcus saprophyticus* urinary tract infections. Intern Med 1985;19:35–7.

Cunha BA. Urosepsis in the Critical Care Unit. In: Cunha BA, editor. Infectious Diseases in Critical Care Medicine. 3rd ed. New York, NY: Informa Healthcare USA, Inc.; 2009.

Cunha BA. Antibiotic Essentials. 8th ed. Sudbury, MA: Jones and Bartlett; 2009.

Cunha BA. Urinary tract infections: Therapy. Postgrad Med 1981;70:149–57.

Hooton TM. The current management strategies for community-acquired urinary tract infection. Infect Dis Clin North Am 2003;17:303–32.

Kahan E, Kahan NR, Chinitz DP. Urinary tract infection in women—Physician's preferences for treatment and adherence to guidelines: A national drug utilization study in a managed care setting. Eur J Clin Pharmacol 2003;59:663–8.

Kraft JK, Stamey TA. The natural history of symptomatic recurrent bacteriuria in women. Medicine (Baltimore) 1977;56:55.

Meiland R, Geerlings SE, Hoepelman LI. Management of bacterial urinary tract infections in adult patients with diabetes mellitus. Drugs 2002;62: 1859–68.

Miller LG, Tang AW. Treatment of uncomplicated urinary tract infections in an era of increasing antimicrobial resistance. Mayo Clin Proc 2004;79: 1048–53.

Nicolle LE. Urinary tract infection: Traditional pharmacologic therapies. Am J Med 2002;113(Suppl. 1A):35S–44S.

Nicolle LE, Ronald AR. Recurrent urinary tract infection in adult women: Diagnosis and treatment. Infect Dis Clin North Am 1987;1:793.

Ronald AR, Conway B. An approach to urinary tract infection in women. Infection 1992;20(Suppl. 3):S203.

Schaeffer AJ, Stuppy BA. Efficacy and safety of self-start therapy in women with recurrent urinary tract infections. J Urol 1999;161:207.

Wong ES, McKevitt M, Running K, et al. Management of recurrent urinary tract infections with patient administered single-dose therapy. Ann Intern Med 1985;102:302.

Urinary Tract Infections in Infants and Children

Method of
Ellen R. Wald, MD

The urinary tract is the most common site for serious bacterial infections in infants and young children. Urinary tract infections (UTIs) are more common than bacterial meningitis, bacterial pneumonia, and bacteremia.

Infection of the urinary tract may involve only the bladder, or only the kidney, or both. In general, infections of the bladder (cystitis), while causing substantial morbidity, are not regarded as serious bacterial infections. In contrast, infections that involve the kidney (pyelonephritis), can cause acute morbidity and lead to scarring with the consequences of hypertension, preeclampsia, and chronic renal disease.

Diagnosis

The diagnosis of UTI may be suggested by certain signs and symptoms, but culture of the urine is the gold standard. Because culture results are not available for at least 24 hours, there has been considerable interest in evaluating tests that may predict the results of urine culture, so that appropriate therapy can be initiated at the first encounter with the symptomatic patient. The tests that have received the most attention are urine microscopy for white cells and bacteria and biochemical analysis of leukocyte esterase and nitrite, which can be assessed rapidly by dipstick.

Several studies have concluded that both the presence of any bacteria on Gram staining of an uncentrifuged urine sample and dipstick analysis for leukocyte esterase and nitrite perform similarly in children from birth through 12 years of age and are helpful in identifying individuals with UTI. Other recent studies done involving young infants (<2 months of age) and older infants (<12 months and 1–24 months) concluded that a hemocytometer white blood cell count of 10 or more cells per microliter provides the most valuable cutoff point for identifying infants for whom urine culture is warranted.

The definition of a positive urine culture depends on the method used to collect the specimen. This variable definition reflects the fact that urine which has passed through the urethra may be contaminated by bacteria present in the distal urethra. If the urine is obtained by the clean-catch method, a positive culture is defined as equal to or greater than 10^5 colony-forming units (CFU)/mL. If the specimen is obtained by catheterization of the urethra, a positive culture is defined as equal to or greater than 5×10^4 CFU/mL. Finally, if a urine culture is obtained by suprapubic aspiration, a method that bypasses the potential source of contamination, a positive culture is defined as recovery of any bacteria from the urine.

Imaging

Imaging studies have been the standard of care for young children with a first UTI for the past decade. Commonly, a renal ultrasound study is performed to evaluate the gross anatomy of the urinary tract (size and shape of the kidneys, duplication or dilatation of the ureters). A voiding cystourethrogram (VCUG) is done to determine whether vesicoureteral reflux is present. This practice has rested on the unproven assumption that continuous prophylactic antimicrobial therapy is effective in reducing the incidence of reinfection of the kidney and renal scarring that may occur in children with vesicoureteral reflux. Until such time as a definitive study is undertaken to dispel this assumption, most clinicians will perform VCUGs and prescribe prophylaxis for children with any degree of reflux.

Treatment

In general, there are many choices for the antibiotic treatment of UTIs in children. If a child is toxic in appearance or vomiting (thereby precluding oral antimicrobials), admission to the hospital for parenteral therapy is appropriate. Many would recommend a third-generation cephalosporin, such as ceftriaxone (Rocephin) 50 mg/kg/day given once daily or cefotaxime (Claforan) 50 mg/kg/dose every 6 hours, until the emesis has resolved and the patient can be treated orally. Otherwise, children, even those with presumed pyelonephritis, do well on oral therapy.

For the child who is to receive oral therapy, the choices are amoxicillin potassium clavulanate (Augmentin) 30 mg/kg/dose given every 12 hours[3]; a second- or third-generation cephalosporin such as cefuroxime (Ceftin) 50 mg/kg/dose twice daily,[3] cefpodoxime (Vantin)[1] 5 mg/kg/dose given twice daily, cefdinir (Omnicef)[1] 7 mg/kg/dose given twice daily, or cefixime (Suprax)[1] 10 mg/kg/dose once daily[3]; or sulfamethoxazole-trimethoprim (Bactrim) 6 mg/kg/day[3] or trimethoprim given once daily. There has been a tendency during the past several years for the prevalence of antimicrobial resistance to increase. The overall resistance to antibiotics varies geographically, and it is essential for the practitioner to be familiar with local antibiotic resistance patterns. In patients with suspected acute pyelonephritis, amoxicillin (Amoxil), cephalexin (Keflex), and sulfamethoxazole-trimethoprim should be avoided because of the potentially high rate of antibiotic resistance.

The optimal duration of therapy for children with UTI has been somewhat controversial. If the diagnosis of pyelonephritis is known or suspected, 10 days of treatment is conventional. Shorter courses of therapy have been successful in adult women with infection of the lower urinary tract. A recent meta-analysis conducted by the Cochrane Database of Systematic Reviews evaluated 10 trials (652 children) with lower-tract UTI. There was no significant difference in frequency of positive urine cultures between short-term (2–4 days) and standard (7–14 days) duration of oral antibiotic therapy for cystitis in children, either early after treatment or at 1 to 15 months after treatment. Furthermore, there was no difference between groups in the development of resistant organisms at the end of treatment or in the incidence of recurrent UTIs. Accordingly, in cases in which the diagnosis of cystitis is assured, 4 days of antimicrobial therapy is sufficient.

Voiding Dysfunction

Voiding dysfunction is a broad term indicating a voiding pattern that is abnormal for the child's age. This is a condition that should be considered in all children who are diagnosed as having a UTI after toilet training has been accomplished. Constipation plays a significant role in some children with voiding dysfunction, and attention to this comorbidity sometimes results in resolution of recurrent UTIs.

Prophylaxis

For children who are considered to be at risk for recurrent UTIs and potential scarring, prophylactic treatment with sulfamethoxazole-trimethoprim or nitrofurantoin (Macrodantin) is recommended. These groups include children with vesicoureteral reflux, those with frequent and closely spaced UTIs without reflux, and, occasionally, those who have urologic abnormalities or who have just sustained an episode of acute pyelonephritis.

The latest Cochrane Review of the effectiveness of long-term antibiotics for preventing recurrent UTIs in children indicated that most published studies to date have been poorly designed without proper blinding. There is no question of the biologic plausibility of

[1]Not FDA approved for this indication.
[3]Exceeds dosage recommended by the manufacturer.

prophylactic antimicrobial therapy in preventing recurrent UTI; however, adverse effects and difficulties with long-term adherence to prophylactic strategies present barriers to effectiveness.

REFERENCES

Gorelick MH, Shaw KN. Screening tests for urinary tract infection: A meta-analysis. Pediatrics 1999;104:e54.

Hellerstein S, Linebarger JS. Voiding dysfunction in pediatric patients. Clin Pediatr 2003;42:43–9.

Hellerstein S, Nickell E. Prophylactic antibiotics in children at risk for urinary tract infection. Pediatr Nephrol 2002;17:506–10.

Hoberman A, Charron M, Hickey RW, et al. Imaging studies after a first febrile urinary tract infection in young children. N Engl J Med 2003;348:195–202.

Hoberman A, Wald ER, Hickey RW, et al. Oral versus initial intravenous therapy for urinary tract infections in young febrile children. Pediatrics 1999;104:79–86.

Hoberman A, Wald ER, Reynolds EA, et al. Pyuria and bacteriuria in urine specimens obtained by catheter from young children with fever. J Pediatr 1994;124:513–9.

Huicho L, Campos-Sanchez M, Alamo C. Metaanalysis of urine screening tests for determining the risk of urinary tract infection in children. Pediatr Infect Dis J 2002;21:1–11, 88.

Lin D-S, Huang F-Y, Chui N-C, et al. Comparison of hemocytometer leukocyte counts and standard urinalyses for predicting urinary tract infection in febrile infants. Pediatr Infect Dis J 2000;19:223–7.

Michael M, Hodson EM, Craig JC, et al. Short versus standard duration oral antibiotic therapy for acute urinary tract infection in children. Cochrane Database Syst Rev 2009;(1):CD003966 [First published in 2003].

Williams GJ, Wei L, Lee A, Craig JC. Long-term antibiotics for preventing recurrent urinary tract infection in children. Cochrane Database Syst Rev 2003;(2):CD001534 [First published in 2001].

Childhood Incontinence

Method of
Walid Farhat, MD, and Kristin Kozakowski, MD

Urinary incontinence is defined by the International Continence Society as "involuntary loss of urine, objectively demonstrable, and constituting a social or hygienic problem." In contrast to adults, in whom incontinence is always considered pathologic, pediatric urinary incontinence must be evaluated in the context of the child's developmental age.

An infant voids approximately 20 times a day via a vesicovesical reflex mechanism mediated by the spinal cord. As the child develops, the neural pathways in the spinal cord mature. In the first 18 to 24 months of life, this primitive voiding reflex is gradually inhibited, bladder capacity increases, and voiding becomes less frequent. Eventually, the more complex voiding reflex develops, and the coordination of voiding control becomes mediated by the pons and midbrain, the pontine micturition center. By the age of 2 years, children become consciously aware of bladder fullness, which leads to the ability to postpone voiding.

Although most children are toilet trained by 3 years of age, there can be a wide variation. Bloom and associates found that the mean age ranged from 0.75 to 5.25 years, with girls being trained earlier (2.25 years) than boys (2.56 years). In two other studies, Wnydaele and colleagues found that 12% of Belgian schoolchildren aged 10 to 14 years had incontinence episodes, and Dahm and colleagues found that 29% of 7- to 8-year-old Danish children had symptoms of underdeveloped bladder control. However, by the age of 5 years and entry into school, children can be expected to have developed volitional urinary control. Therefore, urinary incontinence after age 5, specifically daytime urinary incontinence, is a matter of both social and clinical concern.

Classification of Pediatric Urinary Incontinence

Clinical management of pediatric urinary incontinence is often complicated by a lack of standardized definitions as to what exactly constitutes different types of incontinence in children. This stems from the fact that a large percentage of wetting in children is sporadic and can be considered a variation of normal behavior. Parents and children are often embarrassed or desensitized to the incontinence and fail to bring it to their doctor's attention. It is also important to recognize that urinary incontinence is frequently related to an underlying disease process (organic urinary incontinence). This is distinct from functional urinary incontinence, in which no anatomic or neurologic abnormality is present. Organic incontinence is subdivided into structural and neurologic causes. Structural incontinence includes all congenital, traumatic, and iatrogenic factors that interfere with the bladder's ability to store and empty urine. Neurologic causes include congenital or acquired conditions that interfere with the innervation of the bladder and urinary sphincter (Fig. 1).

To address this problem, the International Children's Continence Society (ICCS) published a report in 1997 that attempted to standardize and define lower urinary tract dysfunction in children; this was updated in 2006. They defined incontinence as the uncontrollable leakage of urine, which can be broadly classified as continuous or intermittent (Fig. 2). Continuous urinary incontinence is constant urine leakage with no dry periods. This is almost exclusively associated with organic urinary incontinence. Intermittent incontinence is urine leakage in discrete amounts, which can occur day or night and is applicable to children older than 5 years of age. Bedwetting, also termed "enuresis", is intermittent incontinence that occurs at night. Accidents that occur during the day are classified as daytime incontinence. Patients with both daytime incontinence and bedwetting have two separate diagnoses; the term "diurnal incontinence" is now obsolete.

ENURESIS

Enuresis, often termed "nocturnal enuresis", is a normal void that occurs while the child is sleeping, usually without the child's being aroused by the wetting. Bedwetting is usually not considered pathologic before the age of 7 years, and it is an extremely common occurrence. In a recent large-scale, longitudinal study, at least 20% of children in the first grade occasionally wet the bed, and 4% wet the bed two or more times per week. Bedwetting is more common in boys and can often show a familial tendency. The ICCS subdivides enuresis into two types: monosymptomatic enuresis (no other lower urinary tract symptoms) and non-monosymptomatic enuresis (other lower urinary tract symptoms are present). Primary enuresis means that the child never had any dry periods at night; children who had at least 6 months of nighttime dryness are said to have secondary enuresis.

Most cases of enuresis resolve with time and when the child becomes more focused on changing the behavior. The treatment of enuresis begins with behavioral modification, including reducing evening fluid intake, increasing daytime voiding frequency, and the use of alarm therapy to condition the child to awaken with wetting. Pharmacologic therapy with desmopressin (DDAVP), which reduces overnight production of urine, is usually reserved for situations such as overnight visits and summer camp; this is no longer considered acceptable as a

COMMON CAUSES OF ORGANIC INCONTINENCE

Structural	Neurologic
Ectopic ureter	Spina bifida
Exstrophy/epispadias complex	Tethered cord
Posterior urethral valves	Sacral agenesis
	Cerebral palsy
	Spinal cord injury

FIGURE 1. Common causes of organic incontinence.

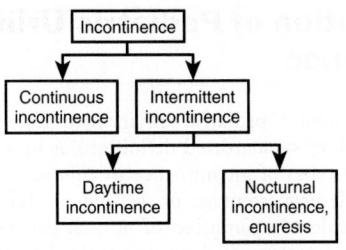

FIGURE 2. Terminology of lower urinary tract function in children and adolescents. (Reprinted with permission from Nevéus T, von Gontard A, Hoebeke P, et al: The standardization of terminology of lower urinary tract function in children and adolescents: Report from the Standardisation Committee of the International Children's Continence Society. J Urol 2006;176:314–324.)

first-line agent or for regular usage. Tricyclic antidepressants are no longer used because of their adverse side-effect profiles.

DAYTIME WETTING CONDITIONS

The classification of daytime wetting conditions is difficult, because children often have overlapping symptoms that can change as they age. The ICCS recommends that clinicians focus on four symptom parameters when assessing children with wetting accidents: incontinence (presence, absence, and frequency), normal voiding frequency, voided volumes, and fluid intake. There are several recognized syndromes that affect the pediatric population, and incontinence may occur in any of them.

Overactive Bladder and Urge Incontinence

The hallmark symptom of overactive bladder is urgency, the imperative urge to void is usually accompanied by holding maneuvers such as squatting and often results in the socially inappropriate loss of urine. Urgency is caused by overactive detrusor contractions early in the bladder filling phase; these are then countered by voluntary pelvic floor contractions or maneuvers to compress the urethra. In these children with overactive bladder, normal voiding frequency may be high, and bladder capacity is often small for age. This type of incontinence occurs more commonly in girls and can progress to a very severe form of dysfunctional voiding.

Urge incontinence is treated with a combination of behavioral therapy, specifically timed voiding programs, and anticholinergic agents such as oxybutynin (Ditropan), which can help to reduce bladder overactivity. Oxybutynin can have side effects such as constipation, dry mouth, drowsiness, and flushing, which lead to discontinuation of its use in approximately 10% of children.

Voiding Postponement

Children who continuously postpone the urge to urinate at normal voiding intervals experience wetting accidents because they do not void unless their bladder is full and contracts involuntarily due to overcapacity. These children infrequently void and are often observed performing holding maneuvers. Children who routinely postpone the need to void often do so because of aversion to public bathrooms or because of not being allowed to use the bathroom during class. These children also may have comorbid psychological or behavioral disturbances.

Management consists of behavioral modification, and specifically of strictly timed voiding bladder retraining programs. In extreme cases in which the child refuses to void, clean intermittent catheterization becomes necessary to empty the bladder.

DYSFUNCTIONAL VOIDING

Dysfunctional voiding patterns, specifically staccato and fractionated voiding, involve some form of overactivity of pelvic floor musculature during voiding, with an uncoordination between the detrusor and the musculature of the external sphincter or pelvic floor or both. These children habitually contract the urethral sphincter during

voiding, but the condition is not related to any dysfunction of bladder storage.

Staccato voiding is a pattern characterized by periodic contractions of the pelvic floor musculature during voiding and interruptions in the flow of urine, leading to prolonged voiding time and residual urine. Fractionated voiding is characterized by small voided volumes with incomplete bladder emptying and an underactive detrusor muscle. Some children augment this voiding pattern with Valsalva maneuvers. These patients usually have large-capacity bladders and detrusor hypoactivity. Dysfunctional voiding can have serious long-term consequences, including high-pressure voiding, chronic urinary tract infections, vesicoureteral reflux, and decompensation of the detrusor muscle.

These dysfunctional voiding patterns are often very difficult to treat. Behavioral modification and biofeedback therapy are the most useful tools.

UNDERACTIVE BLADDER

Children with underactive bladder typically void only once or twice per day. They have increased bladder capacity and diminished bladder sensation to void and carry a high postvoid residual. They also typically need to strain to urinate and show decreased detrusor activity. The leakage that occurs is due to overflow incontinence.

The first line of therapy for these patients is timed-voiding and double-voiding bladder retraining programs. If this treatment fails, clean intermittent catheterization must be used to empty the bladder.

NON-NEUROGENIC NEUROGENIC BLADDER SYNDROME

Non-neurogenic neurogenic bladder, also called Hinman-Allen syndrome, is the most severe form of dysfunctional voiding. This occurs when there is chronic voluntary tightening of the external sphincter during an overactive detrusor contraction, resulting in learned failure to relax the external sphincter during voluntary voiding. This pattern results in bladder-sphincter dyssynergy and eventually leads to detrusor decompensation. These children present with symptoms of daytime and nighttime wetting, overflow and urge incontinence, and recurrent urinary tract infections, and their bladders show severe trabeculations and high postvoid residuals. Often, they have acquired vesicoureteral reflux and hydronephrosis from the decreased bladder compliance. Despite the abnormal findings, they are neurologically normal.

The treatment for these children is a combination of behavioral modification, biofeedback therapy, and possibly prophylactic antibiotics and anticholinergic medications. These patients need aggressive treatment.

GIGGLE INCONTINENCE

Giggle incontinence, which occurs most commonly in girls, is a large-volume loss of urine that happens exclusively with laughter. Patients have no other voiding symptoms, and their bladder is otherwise completely normal.

Treatment is a combination of timed-voiding programs and use of anticholinergic medications to suppress the bladder contraction. For patients in whom excessive muscle relaxation is thought to be the cause, α-sympathomimetic agents or methylphenidate (Ritalin)[1] has been used.

VAGINAL VOIDING

Patients with vaginal reflux present with urine leakage that occurs within 10 minutes after voiding, usually after standing up; foul-smelling urine; and frequent nonfebrile urinary tract infections. It occurs because of urine backflow into the vagina caused by labial fusion or failure to adequately separate the legs while voiding due to obesity or improper voiding posture.

---

[1]Not FDA approved for this indication.

Vaginal voiding is treated by mechanical or pharmacologic (hormonal cream) separation of labial fusion or by adjusting the voiding position.

CONSTIPATION

Treatment of underlying constipation is vital in the management of pediatric urinary incontinence. The combination of a high-fiber diet and agents such as polyethylene glycol (MiraLax) has been shown to maintain a regular bowel routine and help in addressing urinary incontinence.

Clinical Assessment

MEDICAL HISTORY

In addition to a thorough overall medical history, the focused voiding history should include information about urinary frequency, urgency, wetting accidents, urinary tract infections, dysuria, voiding postures, and, importantly, associated constipation. Patients should be asked to keep a voiding diary and to record urinary frequency, bowel activity, wetting accidents, and fluid intake. It is also important to ask about any developmental delay, impaired motor skills, traumatic birth history, prenatal diagnoses, and mental disorders. In addition, a family history of voiding dysfunction, particularly enuresis, and any stressful social situation, whether at home or at school, is very useful in the assessment of pediatric incontinence.

PHYSICAL EXAMINATION

A focused physical evaluation should include examination of the abdomen, genitalia, perineum, and spine and a directed neurologic examination of the lower pelvis and extremities. Specifically, the abdomen is palpated for a full bladder or possible fecal impaction. The female perineum must be examined for possible labial adhesions, ectopic ureter, vaginal irritation, and abnormal position of the urethral meatus. The male genitalia should be examined for possible phimosis or abnormal urethral meatus. The lower back must be inspected for a sacral dimple or hair tuft, absence of the sacrum, or asymmetry.

LABORATORY AND IMAGING STUDIES

A basic urinalysis can provide valuable information about the presence of infection, hematuria, glucose, and protein and urine concentrating ability.

A renal and bladder ultrasound study provides information about possible structural abnormalities of the urinary tract, thickness of the bladder wall, and the presence of kidney or bladder stones. Based on a history of febrile urinary tract infections or structural abnormality found on ultrasonography, a voiding cystourethrogram may be indicated. Spinal radiography or magnetic resonance imaging may be necessary to diagnose a suspected underlying neurologic abnormality. Basic uroflowmetry and measurement of postvoid residuals provides information about voided volumes, strength of flow, and whether the bladder can empty—all indirect ways of investigating bladder and sphincter function. More invasive urodynamic testing is reserved for complex cases such as non-neurogenic neurogenic bladder syndrome.

REFERENCES

Bauer SB. Special considerations of the overactive bladder in children. Urology 2002;60:43–9.

Bloom DA, Seely WW, Ritchey ML, McGuire EJ. Toilet habits and continence in children: An opportunity sampling in search of normal parameters. J Urol 1993;149:1087–90.

Butler RJ, Heron JA. The prevalence of infrequent bedwetting and nocturnal enuresis in childhood: A large British cohort. Scand J Urol Nephrol 2008;42:257–326.

Chin-Peuckert L, Pippi Salle JL. A modified biofeedback program for children with detrusor-sphincter dyssynergia: 5 year experience. J Urol 2001;166:1470–5.

Feldman AS, Bauer SB. Diagnosis and management of dysfunctional voiding. Curr Opin Pediatr 2006;18:139–47.

Hinman Jr F. Nonneurogenic neurogenic bladder (the Hinman syndrome): 15 years later. J Urol 1986;136:769–77.

Loening-Baucke V. Urinary incontinence and urinary tract infection and their resolution with threatment of chronic constipation in childhood. Pediatrics 1997;100:228–32.

Nevéus T, von Gontard A, Hoebeke P, et al. The standardization of terminology of lower urinary tract function in children and adolescents: Report from the Standardisation Committee of the International Children's Continence Society. J Urol 2006;176:314–24.

Nijman RJM. Role of antimuscarinics in the treatment of nonneurogenic daytime urinary incontinence in children. Urology 2004;63:45–50.

Norgaard JP, van Gool JD, Hjalmas K, et al. Standardization and definitions in lower urinary tract dysfunction in children. Br J Urol 1998;81(Suppl. 3):1–16.

Sher P, Reinberg Y. Successful treatment of giggle incontinence with methylphenidate. J Urol 1996;156:656–8.

Urinary Incontinence

Method of
E. Ann Gormley, MD

Urinary incontinence is a significant problem that affects millions of Americans. Patients may not report incontinence to their primary care providers because of embarrassment or misconceptions regarding treatment. Because incontinence is often treatable, it behooves the health care professional to identify patients who might benefit from treatment. Given that the treatment of incontinence varies depending on the etiology, the aim of evaluation is to identify the etiology.

Etiology

Urinary incontinence is generally the result of either bladder or urethral dysfunction (Table 1). Incontinence also may result from a non-urologic cause and is usually reversible when the underlying problem is treated (Table 2). More uncommon causes of incontinence are urinary fistulae and ectopic ureteral orifices.

BLADDER DYSFUNCTION

Bladder dysfunction causes urge or overflow incontinence. *Urge incontinence* occurs when the bladder pressure is sufficient to overcome the sphincter mechanism. Elevated bladder or detrusor pressure tends to

---

TABLE 1 Etiology of Incontinence

Bladder Dysfunction
1. Urge incontinence
   - Detrusor overactivity
     - Idiopathic
     - Neurogenic origin
   - Poor compliance
2. Overflow incontinence

Urethral Dysfunction
3. Stress incontinence
   - Anatomic
   - Intrinsic sphincter deficiency

TABLE 2 Transient Causes of Incontinence *(DIAPPERS)*

Cause	Comment
Delirium	Incontinence may be secondary to delirium and will often stop when acute delirium resolves.
Infection	Symptomatic infection may prevent a patient from reaching the toilet in time.
Atrophic vaginitis	Vaginitis may cause the same symptoms as an infection.
Pharmacologic	
• Sedatives	Alcohol and long-acting benzodiazepines may cause confusion and secondary incontinence.
• Diuretics	A brisk diuresis may overwhelm the bladder's capacity and cause uninhibited detrusor contractions, resulting in urge incontinence.
• Anticholinergics	Many nonprescription and prescription medications have anticholinergic properties. Side effects of anticholinergics include urinary retention with associated frequency and overflow incontinence.
• α Adrenergics	Tone in the bladder neck and proximal sphincter is increased by α-adrenergic agonists and can cause urinary retention, particularly in men with prostatism.
• α Antagonists	Tone in the smooth muscles of the bladder neck and proximal sphincter is decreased with α-adrenergic antagonists. Women treated with these drugs for hypertension may develop or have an exacerbation of stress incontinence.
Psychological	Depression may be occasionally associated with incontinence.
Excessive urine production	Excessive intake, diabetes, hypercalcemia, congestive heart failure, and peripheral edema can all lead to polyuria, which can lead to incontinence.
Restricted mobility	Incontinence may be precipitated or aggravated if the patient cannot get to the toilet quickly enough.
Stool impaction	Patients with impacted stool can have urge or overflow urinary incontinence and may also have fecal incontinence.

From Resnick NM: Urinary incontinence in the elderly. Med Grand Rounds 1984;3:281–290.

open the bladder neck and urethra. An elevation in detrusor pressure may occur from intermittent bladder contractions (detrusor overactivity) or because of an incremental rise in pressure with increased bladder volume (poor compliance). Detrusor overactivity may be idiopathic, or it may be associated with a neurologic disease (detrusor overactivity of neurogenic origin). Detrusor overactivity is common in the elderly and may be associated with bladder outlet obstruction. Poor bladder compliance results from loss of the viscoelastic features of the bladder or because of a change in neuroregulatory activity. The patient with urge incontinence may appreciate a sudden sensation to void but then is unable to suppress the urge fully. In severe cases, the patient may not be aware of the sensation of needing to void until he or she is actually leaking. The amount of leakage in patients with urge incontinence is variable, depending on the patient's ability to suppress the contraction. Patients with urge incontinence will often have frequency and nocturia in addition to urgency and urge incontinence. They may also have nocturnal enuresis.

Overactive bladder is a newer term that describes patients with frequency and urgency with or without urge incontinence.

Overflow incontinence occurs at extreme bladder volumes or when the bladder volume reaches the limit of the bladder's viscoelastic properties. The loss of urine is driven by an elevation in detrusor pressure. Overflow incontinence is seen in the case of incomplete bladder emptying caused by either obstruction or poor bladder contractility. Obstruction is rare in women but can result from severe pelvic prolapse or following surgery for stress incontinence. Patients with overflow incontinence complain of constant dribbling, and they may also describe extreme frequency.

URETHRAL-RELATED INCONTINENCE

Urethral-related incontinence, or *stress incontinence,* occurs because of either urethral hypermobility or intrinsic sphincter deficiency (ISD). Incontinence associated with urethral hypermobility has been called *anatomic incontinence* because the incontinence is due to malposition of the sphincter unit. Displacement of the proximal urethra below the level of the pelvic floor does not allow for transmission of abdominal pressure that normally aids in closing the urethra. Some women with mobility of the bladder neck or urethra do not experience incontinence. ISD was initially believed to occur after failure of one or more operations for stress incontinence. Other causes of ISD include myelodysplasia, trauma, and radiation. Some authors have theorized that all incontinent patients must have an element of ISD in order to actually leak. The patient with stress incontinence leaks urine with any sudden increase in abdominal pressure. In patients with severe ISD, the increase in abdominal pressure required to cause leakage is small, so patients may leak urine with minimal activity.

Evaluation of the Incontinent Patient

The evaluation of the incontinent patient includes a history, physical examination, laboratory tests, and possibly urodynamic testing. The onset, frequency, severity, and pattern of incontinence should be sought, as well as any associated symptoms such as frequency, dysuria, urgency, and nocturia. Incontinence may be quantified by asking the patient if he or she wears a pad and how often the pad is changed. Obstructive symptoms, such as a feeling of incomplete emptying, hesitancy, straining, or weak stream, may coexist with incontinence, particularly in males and in female patients with previous incontinence procedure, cystoceles, or poor detrusor contractility. Female patients should be asked about symptoms of pelvic prolapse, such as recurrent urinary tract infection, a sensation of vaginal fullness or pressure, or the observation of a bulge in the vagina. All incontinent patients should be asked about bowel function and neurologic symptoms. Response to previous treatments, including drugs, should be noted. Important features of the history include previous gynecologic and urologic procedures, neurologic problems, and past medical problems. A list of the patient's current medications, including over-the-counter medications, should be obtained.

Although the history may define the patient's problem, it may be misleading. Urge incontinence may be triggered by activities such as coughing, so according to the patient's history, he or she seems to have stress incontinence. A patient who complains only of urge incontinence may also have stress incontinence. Mixed incontinence is very common; at least 65% of patients with stress incontinence have associated urgency or urge incontinence.

A complete physical examination is performed, with emphasis on the neurologic assessment and on the abdominal, pelvic, and rectal examinations. In females, the condition of the vaginal mucosa and the degree of urethral mobility are determined. Simple pelvic examination with the patient supine is sufficient to determine if the urethra moves with straining or coughing. The degree of movement is not as important as the determination of whether movement occurs. The presence of associated pelvic organ prolapse should be noted because it can contribute to the patient's voiding problems and may have an impact on diagnosis and treatment. A rectal examination in both males and females includes the evaluation of sphincter tone and perineal sensation.

A urinalysis is performed to determine if there is any evidence of hematuria, pyuria, glucosuria, or proteinuria. A urine specimen is sent for cytologic examination if there is hematuria and/or irritative voiding symptoms. The urine is cultured if there is pyuria or bacteriuria. Infection should be treated prior to further investigations or interventions. Hematuria consisting of more than three red cells per high-power field warrants further investigation.

CURRENT DIAGNOSIS

Urge Incontinence

Symptoms
- Urgency
- Frequency
- Nocturia
- Unable to reach the toilet with urge

Stress Incontinence

Symptoms
- Leakage with physical activity

Signs
- Bladder neck mobility
- Positive stress test

Mixed Incontinence

Symptoms
- Urgency
- Frequency
- Nocturia
- Unable to reach the toilet with urge
- Leakage with physical activity

Signs
- Bladder neck mobility
- Positive stress test

Overflow Incontinence

Symptoms
- Frequency
- Nocturia
- Urgency
- Leakage with physical activity

Signs
- High postvoid residual

A postvoid residual (PVR) should be measured either with pelvic ultrasound or directly with a catheter. A normal PVR is less than 50 mL, and a PVR greater than 200 mL is abnormal. A significant PVR urine may reflect either bladder outlet obstruction or poor bladder contractility. The only way to distinguish outlet obstruction from poor contractility is with urodynamic testing.

Urodynamic testing is used to accurately diagnose the etiology of a patient's incontinence; however, many patients can be successfully treated without urodynamic testing. The purpose of urodynamic testing is to examine compliance, diagnose stress incontinence, and rule out obstruction as a cause of either overflow or urge incontinence. Urodynamic testing should ideally be performed prior to invasive therapies and certainly in patients who are undergoing repeat procedures following failed procedures.

Treatment of Urinary Incontinence

URGE INCONTINENCE

Patients with urge incontinence need to understand that they leak urine because their bladder contracts with little or no warning. The first line of treatment is timed voiding. Often, reminding patients to void every 1 to 2 hours during the day, before they get an urge to void, will result in them staying dry. Other behavioral interventions, such as modification of fluid intake, avoidance of bladder irritants, and bladder retraining, where the patient attempts to

consciously delay voiding and to increase the interval between voids, may also have a role in the treatment of urge incontinence.

Anticholinergics are the mainstay of medical therapy in achieving continence. The side effects of anticholinergics include urinary retention, dry mouth, constipation, nausea, blurred vision, tachycardia, drowsiness, and confusion. They are contraindicated in patients with narrow-angle glaucoma. Anticholinergics are also used to decrease bladder pressure in patients with poor compliance. Anticholinergics are combined with clean intermittent catheterization in patients who have a significant PVR prior to treatment and in patients who develop retention while taking anticholinergics.

Patients with intractable detrusor overactivity may require surgical intervention, consisting of neuromodulation with a sacral nerve stimulator or various forms of bladder augmentation.

The primary goal in caring for the patient with poor compliance is treating the high bladder pressure. Complete bladder emptying with clean intermittent catheterization combined with anticholinergics will often lower bladder pressure to a safe range. Some patients may require a combination of anticholinergics and α agonists. Bladder augmentation is required when medical management fails.

OVERFLOW INCONTINENCE

Overflow incontinence is treated by emptying the bladder. If the cause of overflow is obstruction, then relieving the obstruction should lead to improved emptying. Anatomic obstruction in males derives from either urethral stricture disease or prostatic obstruction. Depending on the severity of urethral stricture disease, the patient may require urethral dilation, internal urethrotomy, or urethroplasty. Prostatic obstruction may be treated in a variety of ways, but transurethral resection remains the gold standard. If a woman is obstructed from previous surgery or from pelvic prolapse, she may benefit from urethrolysis or surgical correction of the prolapse. Clean intermittent catheterization is an option in the obstructed patient who does not want or could not tolerate further surgery.

The patient with overflow incontinence secondary to poor detrusor contractility is best treated with clean intermittent catheterization.

Indwelling catheters are not an optimum treatment modality for treatment of incontinence. All patients with indwelling catheters will have infected urine, which predisposes them to bladder calculi and ultimately to squamous cell carcinoma of the bladder. Any foreign object in the bladder can cause or exacerbate elevated bladder pressure that is associated with hydronephrosis, ureteral obstruction, renal stones, and eventually renal failure.

STRESS INCONTINENCE

The amount of incontinence and how it affects the patient often determines the aggressiveness of treatment. The patient who is severely restricted because of severe leakage with minimal movement may not want to try medical therapy but may opt for surgical treatment, whereas the patient who leaks small amounts infrequently may choose conservative treatment. Pelvic floor exercises can improve anatomic stress urinary incontinence by augmenting closure of the external urethral sphincter and by preventing descent and rotation of the bladder neck and urethra. To benefit from the exercises, women must be taught to do the exercises properly, and they must do them. Adjuncts to learning pelvic floor exercises include weighted vaginal cones, a perineometer, and electrical stimulation.

α Agonists such as phenylpropanolamine[1] and pseudoephedrine (Sudafed)[1] can be used for treatment of stress incontinence. The bladder neck and proximal urethra have abundant α receptors. Activation of these receptors by α agonists leads to an increase in smooth muscle tone. The usual dose is twice daily, but some women who are incontinent with exercise may benefit from taking an α agonist 1 hour before exercise. Tricyclic antidepressants, such as imipramine (Tofranil),[1] have both α-agonist and anticholinergic properties.

---

[1]Not FDA approved for this indication.

CURRENT THERAPY

Urge Incontinence

Behavioral Changes
- Avoidance of bladder irritants
- Timed voiding
- Pelvic muscle exercises

Anticholinergics—Antimuscarinics—Nonselective for M3 Receptor
- Propantheline (Pro-Banthine)[1] 7.5 to 30 mg orally, three to five times daily
- Tolterodine (Detrol LA) 4 mg orally, daily
- Trospium (Sanctura) 20 mg orally, two times daily
- Solifenacin (Vesicare) 5–10 mg orally, daily

Anticholinergics—Antimuscarinics—Selective for M3 Receptor
- Darifenacin (Enablex) 7.5–15 mg orally, daily

Anticholinergics—Antimuscarinics/Smooth Muscle Relaxants
- Oxybutynin
- Regular (Ditropan) 2.5–5 mg orally, one to three times daily
- Extended-release (Ditropan XL) 5–30 mg orally, daily
- Transdermal (Oxytrol) 3.9-mg patch, twice per week
- Hyoscyamine (Levsin) 0.125–0.375 mg orally, two to four times daily

Anticholinergics/α Agonists—For Urge or Mixed Incontinence
- Imipramine (Tofranil)[1] 10–25 mg, once to three times daily

Stress Incontinence

Behavioral Changes
- Weight loss
- Quitting smoking
- Pelvic muscle exercises

α Agonists
- Pseudoephedrine (Sudafed)[1] 30–60 mg, up to four times daily

Surgery
- Anatomic
  - Retropubic suspensions
    - Burch
    - Marshall-Marchetti-Krantz
  - Slings
  - Pubovaginal
  - Midurethral
  - Obturator
- Intrinsic Sphincter Deficiency
  - Slings
    - Pubovaginal
    - Midurethral
    - Obturator
  - Artificial sphincter
  - Submucosal Injections with Bulking Agents
  - Collagen (Contigen)
  - Carbon-coated zirconium oxide beads (Durasphere)
  - Ethylene vinyl alcohol copolymer (Tegress)

[1]Not FDA approved for this indication.

BOX 1   Overview of Treatments

Behavioral Changes
- Avoidance of bladder irritants
- Weight loss
- Quitting smoking
- Pelvic muscle exercises

Medical Therapy
- α Agonists
  - Stress incontinent patients
  - Mixed incontinent patients
- Anticholinergics
  - Urge incontinent patients
- Anticholinergics/α agonists
  - Mixed incontinent patients

Surgical Therapy
- Stress incontinent patients
- Rare patients with urge incontinence

Surgical therapy for stress incontinence is indicated when a patient does not wish to pursue nonsurgical therapy, or if such therapy has failed. The type of surgical therapy depends on the diagnosis. Patients who have anatomic stress incontinence can benefit from a variety of surgical repairs that restore the bladder neck to its normal retropubic position or improve urethral support. Patients with ISD usually have a well-supported bladder neck. These patients require a procedure that will close or coapt the proximal urethra. Coaptation may be achieved with a variety of bulking agents that are injected into the bladder neck or proximal urethra. A pubovaginal sling is the ideal procedure for the patient with both ISD and anatomic stress incontinence, as a sling will coapt the proximal urethra and restore the bladder neck to its normal location.

Synthetic midurethral slings are ideal for the patient with anatomic stress incontinence who wishes surgery with minimal recovery time. In one of the rare randomized surgical trials for stress incontinence, the result with tension-free vaginal tape has been shown to be comparable to that of a Burch colposuspension at 6, 12, and 24 months. The newest sling is a transobturator sling that is placed transversely underneath the urethra from one obturator foramina to the other. The advantage of this sling is that the retropubic space is avoided, with low risk of bladder, bowel, and major vessel injury.

Randomized trials comparing midurethral or transobturator slings to pubovaginal slings have not been performed.

MIXED INCONTINENCE

Stress and urge incontinence often coexist. Burgio et al. advocate pelvic muscle exercises with biofeedback for treatment of stress and urge incontinence. Behavioral therapy can result in a reduction in incontinence episodes and patient-perceived improvement.

Imipramine (Tofranil)[1] is beneficial in patients with mixed (stress and urge) incontinence. The recommended dose is 10 to 25 mg, three times daily.

Seventy percent of patients with combined incontinence (stress and urge) will be relieved of urge incontinence following a procedure for stress incontinence. Patients whose urge incontinence does not respond to anticholinergics preoperatively may have a good response to anticholinergics once their stress incontinence is treated. Box 1 provides an overview of treatments.

REFERENCES

Blaivas JG, Groutz A. Urinary incontinence: Pathophysiology, evaluation, and management overview. In: Walsh PC, Retik AB, Vaughan Jr ED, Wein AJ, editors. Campbell's Urology. 8th ed., vol. 2. Philadelphia: WB Saunders; 2002. p. 1027.

---

[1]Not FDA approved for this indication.

Burgio KL, Locher JL, Goode PS, et al. Behavioral vs drug treatment for urge urinary incontinence in older women: A randomized controlled trial. JAMA 1998;280:1995–2000.

Leach GE, Dmochowski RR, Appell RA, et al. Female Stress Urinary Incontinence Clinical Guidelines Panel summary report on surgical management of female stress urinary incontinence. The American Urological Association. J Urol 1997;158:875.

Ward KL, Hilton P. A randomized trial of colposuspension and tension-free vaginal tape (TVT) for primary genuine stress incontinence: 2 year followup. Int Urogynecol J Pelvic Floor Dysfunct 2001;12(Suppl. 2): S7–8.

Epididymitis

Method of
John N. Krieger, MD

Epididymitis is the inflammatory reaction of the epididymis to infection or to local trauma. Epididymitis causes major morbidity, accounting for more than 600,000 visits to physicians per year in the United States. Acute epididymitis is responsible for more days lost from military service than any other disease and is responsible for 20% of urologic admissions in the military. A survey of ambulatory patients documented epididymitis as a cause of 1 in 345 visits (0.3%), representing the fifth most common urologic condition, after prostatitis, urinary tract infections, urinary stones, and sexually transmitted infections.

Clinical Presentation

Painful swelling of the scrotum is the characteristic clinical presentation. In most patients the pain and swelling are unilateral. The onset may be acute over 1 or 2 days or more gradual. Pain can radiate along the spermatic cord or into the lower abdomen. Symptoms of cystitis or urethritis are common. Dysuria or irritative lower urinary tract symptoms are characteristic. Many sexually active men have a urethral discharge. Thus, particular attention should be directed to eliciting a history of genitourinary tract disease or sexual exposure. Some men may have only a nonspecific finding of fever or other signs of infection. This is especially common in hospitalized men who have had urinary tract manipulation or catheterization and may be obtunded by medication.

Tender swelling can occur in the posterior aspect of the scrotum. Usually, the swelling is unilateral and is often accompanied by erythema of the scrotal skin. Early in the course, swelling may be localized to one portion of the epididymis. However, the swelling often progresses to involve the ipsilateral testis, producing an epididymoorchitis. At this point it is difficult to distinguish the testicle from the epididymis within the inflammatory mass. Scrotal examination reveals the characteristic inflammatory hydrocele caused by secretion of fluid between the layers of the tunica vaginalis. Urethral discharge may be apparent on inspection or on stripping of the urethra.

Ideally, evaluation for urethritis should be done before the patient voids because micturition can make mild urethritis difficult or impossible to detect. The nursing staff should be taught to instruct patients with urogenital tract complaints not to void until after the physical examination. This is a common problem when we are asked to consult on patient management in the emergency department or in primary care settings. Patients with no sexual risk factors or evidence of urethritis should have microscopic evaluation of their midstream urine.

Pathogenesis

Acute epididymitis occurs when uropathogens overcome the host defenses of the male lower genitourinary tract to establish infection of the epididymis. Most cases result from retrograde ascent of organisms through the urethra, prostate, ejaculatory duct, and vas deferens to reach the epididymis. Structural or functional abnormalities of the lower urinary tract increase the risk of epididymitis.

The risk factors for epididymitis vary substantially in different patient populations. In children and older men, anatomic abnormalities are critical risk factors for development of epididymitis. These include congenital anatomic abnormalities, such as an ectopic ureter draining into the vas deferens in children, and acquired anatomic abnormalities, such as bladder outflow obstruction in older men. In contrast, most sexually active younger men with epididymitis have normal urinary tracts. Thus, urologic investigations are indicated in children and older men with epididymitis but are seldom needed for management of epididymitis in young sexually active men.

Infections of the urethra, bladder, or prostate are important risk factors for development of epididymitis. In children and older men, the most common organisms are the typical bacteria that cause urinary tract infections, especially *Escherichia coli*, other enterics, and pseudomonads. In sexually active men, the most common pathogens are *Chlamydia trachomatis* and *Neisseria gonorrhoeae*. Men who practice insertive anal intercourse are also at risk for epididymitis caused by *E. coli* and other enteric bacteria. In addition to the usual causative organisms, immunocompromised patients are at higher risk for epididymitis caused by mycobacteria and fungi.

Diagnosis and Treatment

ACUTE EPIDIDYMITIS

Most patients with acute epididymitis can be considered in two categories, nonspecific bacterial epididymitis or sexually transmitted epididymitis. Unusual patients develop epididymitis after genital trauma or with disseminated infections.

 CURRENT DIAGNOSIS

History

- Exposure to sexually transmitted infection
- Urologic abnormalities or genitourinary tract instrumentation
- Symptoms of dysuria or urethral discharge

Physical Examination

- Pain or swelling on palpation of the epididymis
- Inflammatory hydrocele
- Scrotal skin erythema
- Urethral discharge
- Abnormal genitourinary tract anatomy
- Elevated temperature

Laboratory Studies

- Urethral swab specimen or first-void urine for pyuria
- Midstream urine for evidence of bacteriuria or pyuria
- Urine culture and sensitivity testing
- Samples for evaluation of sexually transmitted infections, as appropriate
- Doppler scrotal ultrasound may be helpful to differentiate epididymitis from testicular torsion or tumor

---

CURRENT THERAPY

Age Younger Than 35 Years with No History of Allergy

- Ceftriaxone (Rocephin) 250 mg IM once *plus*
- Doxycycline (Vibramicin) 100 mg PO bid for 10 days *or*
- Azithromycin (Zithromax) 1 g PO as a single dose

Age Older Than 35 Years or Patient with a History of Allergy to Cephalosporins or Tetracyclines

- Ofloxacin (Floxin) 300 mg PO bid for 10 days *or*
- Levofloxacin (Levaquin) 500 mg PO qd for 10 days

All Patients

- Antiinflammatories
- Decreased activity
- Scrotal elevation
- Pain control

Follow-up

- Failure to improve within 3 days: Reevaluate initial diagnosis and therapy
- For persistent swelling and tenderness after therapy, consider:
  - Testicular tumor
  - Abscess
  - Testicular infarction
  - Tuberculosis
  - Fungal epididymitis

Clinical evaluation begins with a history, with specific attention to eliciting recognized risk factors, and a thorough physical examination. Initial laboratory tests include urinalysis, culture, and sensitivity testing for men with presumed nonspecific bacterial epididymitis. Men at risk for sexually transmitted epididymitis should also have a gram-stained urethral smear, culture for *N. gonorrhoeae*, and testing for *C. trachomatis*. In the latter group, serologic testing is also recommended for syphilis and for HIV infection.

NONSPECIFIC BACTERIAL EPIDIDYMITIS

Infection with coliform or *Pseudomonas* species is the most common cause of epididymitis in men older than 35 years. In most series, gram-negative rods caused more than two thirds of cases of bacterial epididymitis. However, gram-positive cocci are also important pathogens and constituted the most common organisms in other reports.

Patients with bacterial epididymitis often have underlying urologic pathology or have a history of genitourinary tract manipulation. Epididymitis can occur weeks or rarely months after genitourinary tract surgery or urethral catheterization. Epididymitis constitutes a special risk for men who undergo urinary tract surgery or instrumentation while they are bacteriuric. Acute and chronic bacterial prostatitis represent other important predisposing conditions for development of bacterial epididymitis.

Medical management is appropriate for most patients with bacterial epididymitis. Typical patients are managed as outpatients. Initial empiric treatment is initiated with agents appropriate for both gram-negative rods and gram-positive cocci pending urine culture and sensitivity results. Fluoroquinolones represent our first choice for management of nonspecific epididymitis in outpatients. Agents of choice include ofloxacin (Floxin) and levofloxacin (Levaquin). Ciprofloxacin (Cipro) represents a reasonable alternative quinolone. In areas where the rate of bacterial resistance is low, trimethoprim-sulfamethoxazole (TMP-SMX; Bactrim, Septra) represents another reasonable alternative. Initial empiric therapy may be changed, if necessary, after culture results are available. A standard course of therapy is 10 days. More prolonged therapy may be needed for select patients such as those with evidence of bacterial prostatitis, whose antimicrobial therapy is continued for 6 to 12 weeks.

Indications for hospitalization include systemic symptoms, such as leukocytosis and fever, complications, or associated medical conditions. In these severe cases, parenteral antimicrobial therapy is used until the patient defervesces. Choices for empiric therapy of severe cases include the combination of an aminoglycoside plus either a β-lactam agent or a third-generation cephalosporin. After resolution of the acute systemic infection, therapy is continued with oral agents, guided by the culture and sensitivity results.

Nonspecific measures are worthwhile, including bedrest, scrotal elevation, analgesics, and local ice packs. A spermatic cord block with bipuvicaine (Marcaine) may be helpful for managing severe pain. We recommend urologic evaluation, because structural or functional abnormalities are common among men and boys with nonspecific bacterial epididymitis.

SEXUALLY TRANSMITTED EPIDIDYMITIS

Sexually transmitted epididymitis is most common in young men. *C. trachomatis* and *N. gonorrhoeae* are the major pathogens. In most series, *Chlamydia* was identified as the most common cause of epididymitis in younger, sexually active populations. For example, in our institution, *C. trachomatis* infections were documented in 17 (50%) of 34 cases of epididymitis in men younger than 35 years but in only 1 (6%) of 16 cases of epididymitis in men older than 35 years. In the past, these patients were considered to have "idiopathic" nonspecific epididymitis. Sexually transmitted *E. coli* infection also occurs among men who are the insertive partners during anal intercourse.

Often patients with chlamydial epididymitis do not complain of urethral discharge. However, 11 (65%) of 17 patients with epididymitis caused by *Chlamydia* had demonstrable discharge. In most cases, the discharge was scant and watery, characteristic of nongonococcal urethritis. The median interval from the last sexual exposure was 10 days and ranged from 1 to 45 days. Thus, urethral *C. trachomatis* may be carried for long periods before overt epididymitis develops.

In the preantibiotic era, epididymitis occurred in 10% to 30% of men with gonococcal urethritis. However, in current series, *N. gonorrhoeae* was identified in 16% of men with epididymitis in military populations and in 21% of men with epididymitis in civilians younger than 35 years. Many patients with epididymitis do not have a history of urethral discharge, and a discharge may be demonstrable in only 50% of such patients. Diagnosis depends on a high index of clinical suspicion, evaluation for presence of urethritis (which may be asymptomatic), appropriate cultures, or antigen detection tests.

Empiric therapy is recommended before culture results are available. Appropriate therapy includes coverage for both *N. gonorrhoeae* and *C. trachomatis* infections. The first choice regimen is the combination of ceftriaxone (Rocephin) plus doxycycline (Vibramycin) for 10 days. Allergic patients are treated with one of the quinolone regimens described earlier. Alternatives for coverage of *N. gonorrhoeae* include cefixime (Suprax), ciprofloxacin, ofloxacin, levofloxacin, or spectinomycin (Trobicin). Azithromycin (Zithromax) represents an effective alternative for coverage of *C. trachomatis*. Nonspecific measures are helpful, including bedrest, scrotal elevation, analgesics, and local ice packs. A spermatic cord block with bipuvicaine can reduce the need for analgesics in men with severe pain.*

Patients should be evaluated for other sexually transmitted infections, and treatment of sexual partners is important. Patients should be instructed to avoid intercourse until symptoms have resolved completely and to refer all sex partners within the previous 60 days for evaluation and treatment. Underlying genitourinary tract abnormalities are uncommon in this population. Thus, a complete urologic work-up is indicated rarely for patients with uncomplicated sexually transmitted epididymitis.

---

*Because of recent increases in resistance rates, the CDC now recommends parenteral regimens only for treatment of gonococcal infections in the United States.

UNCOMMON CAUSES

Tuberculous epididymitis is the most common manifestation of genital tuberculosis in men, with orchitis and prostatitis less common. The usual symptom is heaviness or swelling. Scrotal swelling with bead-like enlargement of the vas deferens is characteristic. Chronic draining scrotal sinuses can occur. The systemic mycoses rarely cause epididymitis; blastomycosis is the most common pathogen and can also cause a draining sinus through the scrotal wall. Men with HIV infection and uncomplicated epididymitis should receive the same treatment as those without HIV. However, fungal and mycobacterial causes of epididymitis are more common among patients who are immunocompromised.

In the pediatric population, epididymitis can occur with congenital anatomic abnormalities, such as ectopic ureter or posterior urethral valves. Epididymitis occasionally occurs after testicular trauma. Many of these men have evidence of genitourinary tract infections with organisms outlined earlier, but occasional men develop traumatic epididymitis that is not associated with positive cultures or inflammation. We also described an unusual syndrome of noninfectious epididymitis associated with amiodarone (Cordarone) therapy for refractory ventricular arrhythmias. Rare patients develop epididymitis as a complication of collagen vascular disorders, such as Wegener's granulomatosis or Behçet's disease.

Differential Diagnosis

Severe inflammation can lead to an enlarged indurated epididymis that is indistinguishable from the testicle. This can present difficulties in the differential diagnosis of epididymitis from testicular torsion or testicular cancer. Normally, the epididymis lies posterior to the testis. This demarcation is often preserved in cases of epididymitis. Reactive hydrocele formation can render palpation of intrascrotal structures difficult. Although transillumination often identifies hydroceles, color-flow Doppler ultrasonography is my preferred imaging study when the diagnosis is in doubt.

Acute epididymitis must be distinguished from testicular torsion at the initial evaluation because uncorrected torsion results in testicular death within 24 hours. Men with swelling and tenderness that persist after completing therapy should be reevaluated for testicular cancer, tuberculosis, or fungal epididymitis.

Complications

Most patients experience relief of their symptoms within 48 hours. However, swelling and discomfort can persist for weeks or months following eradication of the infecting organism. In some cases, the epididymis remains enlarged or indurated indefinitely. Such men can develop chronic epididymitis, which is characterized by pain and occasionally by recurrent swelling.

Bacterial epididymitis may be an important focus of organisms causing both local morbidity and bacteremia in men with indwelling transurethral catheters. Genitourinary tract complications of acute epididymitis include testicular infarction, scrotal abscess, pyocele of the scrotum, a chronic draining scrotal sinus, chronic epididymitis, and infertility. Ultrasonography, particularly color-flow Doppler ultrasonography, is useful for the differential diagnosis of complicated cases. Surgery may be necessary for complications of acute epididymal infections.

REFERENCES

Centers for Disease Control and Prevention. Sexually transmitted diseases treatment guidelines, 2006. MMWR Morb Mortal Wkly Rep 2006; 55:1–94.

Collins MM, Stafford RS, O'Leary MP, Barry MJ. How common is prostatitis? A national survey of physician visits. J Urol 1998;159:1224–8.

Furuya R, Takahashi S, Furuya S, et al. Is seminal vesiculitis a discrete disease entity? Clinical and microbiological study of seminal vesiculitis in patients with acute epididymitis. J Urol 2004;171:1550–3.

Karmazyn B, Steinberg R, Kornreich L, et al. Clinical and sonographic criteria of acute scrotum in children: A retrospective study of 172 boys. Pediatr Radiol 2005;35:302–10.

Krieger JN. Sexually transmitted diseases. In: Tanagho EA, McAninch JW, editors. Smith's Urology. 16th ed. New York: Lange Medical Books/McGraw-Hill; 2004. p. 245–55.

Mittemeyer BT, Lennox KW, Borski AA. Epididymitis: A review of 610 cases. J Urol 1966;95:390–2.

Naber KG, Bergman B, Bishop MC, et al. EAU guidelines for the management of urinary and male genital tract infections. Urinary Tract Infection (UTI) Working Group of the Health Care Office (HCO) of the European Association of Urology (EAU). Eur Urol 2001;40:576–88.

Nickel JC, Siemens DR, Nickel KR, Downey J. The patient with chronic epididymitis: Characterization of an enigmatic syndrome. J Urol 2002;167:1701–4.

Nickel JC, Teichman JM, Gregoire M, et al. Prevalence, diagnosis, characterization, and treatment of prostatitis, interstitial cystitis, and epididymitis in outpatient urological practice: The Canadian PIE Study. Urology 2005;66:935–40.

Stehr M, Boehm R. Critical validation of colour Doppler ultrasound in diagnostics of acute scrotum in children. Eur J Pediatr Surg 2003;13:386–92.

Primary Glomerular Diseases

Method of
Manuel Praga, MD, and Enrique Morales, MD

Clinical Presentation and Diagnosis

The clinical manifestations of primary glomerular diseases are very variable, ranging from asymptomatic urinary abnormalities to severe forms of rapidly progressive glomerulonephritis. The different clinical presentations are summarized and defined in Box 1.

Most milder forms of glomerular diseases are diagnosed by a positive dipstick test for microhematuria or proteinuria. All these patients should have quantitative estimations of proteinuria (24-hour proteinuria or protein-to-creatinine ratio in a random sample of urine), urinary microscopic examination, and serum creatinine. Glomerular disorders can be the renal manifestation of systemic diseases of different causes (e.g., malignancies, infections, autoimmune disorders), as discussed later. Therefore, medical history and physical examination should carefully investigate data suggesting such diseases. In addition to general laboratory analysis and assessment of renal morphology (renal echography), more specific determinations should be performed in all patients with suspected glomerular diseases: protein electrophoresis, serum levels of immunoglobulins, serum complement fractions C3 and C4, antinuclear antibody (ANA), anti-DNA antibodies, antineutrophilic cytoplasmic antibodies (ANCA), and tests for hepatitis B virus (HBV), hepatitis C virus (HCV), and HIV infections.

Renal biopsy is the conclusive method for establishing the diagnosis and classification of primary glomerular disorders. Indications for renal biopsy include the nephrotic syndrome in adults (except cases attributed to diabetic nephropathy) and steroid-resistant nephrotic syndrome in children, rapidly progressive nephritis, persistent nephritic syndrome with deteriorating renal function, and, usually, recurrent macroscopic hematuria. The need for renal biopsy in patients with asymptomatic urinary abnormalities should be individualized. The most characteristic pathologic findings of the main primary glomerulonephritis are summarized in Box 2, and their commonest clinical presentations are summarized in Box 3.

BOX 1 Clinical Presentations of Glomerular Diseases

Nephrotic Syndrome
- Proteinuria >3.5 g/d in adults and >40 mg/h/m² in children
- Hypoalbuminemia
- Hyperlipidemia
- Edema

Nephritic Syndrome
- Hypertension
- Oliguria
- Edema
- Hematuria (usually macroscopic)
- Red cell casts
- Non-nephrotic proteinuria
- Mild and nonprogressive GFR decrease

Rapidly Progressive Glomerulonephritis
- Acute or subacute progressive worsening of renal function
- Hematuria (usually macroscopic)
- Red cell casts
- Proteinuria (usually <3.5 g/d)
- Blood pressure often normal

Persistent Asymptomatic Urinary Abnormalities
- Non-nephrotic proteinuria (<3.5 g/d in adults and <40 mg/h/m² in children)
- Persistent microscopic hematuria

Recurrent Macroscopic Hematuria
- Bouts of gross hematuria, usually triggered by infections
- Persistent microhematuria between the episodes of gross hematuria

Chronic Renal Insufficiency
- Persistent proteinuria and/or microhematuria
- Hypertension
- Small kidneys

Hypocomplementemia
The C3 and C4 fractions of serum complement are characteristically reduced in some types of glomerular diseases. This is an important clue for diagnosis.

Abbreviation: GFR = glomerular filtration rate.

BOX 2 Main Histologic Findings of Primary Glomerular Diseases

Minimal Change Disease
- Normal glomeruli on light microscopy
- Negative immunofluorescence and diffuse effacement of epithelial foot processes on electron microscopy

Focal and Segmental Glomerulosclerosis
- Focal (some glomeruli) and segmental (parts of affected glomeruli) scarring of the glomerular tuft

Membranous Nephropathy
- Thickening of glomerular capillary walls with projections of glomerular basement membrane ("spikes")
- Subepithelial immune deposits detected by immunofluorescence and electron microscopy

Membranoproliferative Glomerulonephritis
- Increase of mesangial cells and mesangial matrix
- Widening (double contoured appearance) of capillary loops
- IgG, C3, and IgM on immunofluorescence and subendothelial (type I) or intra-GBM (type II) deposits on electron microscopy

IgA Nephropathy
- Predominant deposition of mesangial IgA on immunofluorescence
- Proliferation of mesangial cellularity and mesangial matrix on light microscopy
- Mesangial electron-dense deposits on electron microscopy

Acute Postinfectious (Diffuse Proliferative) Glomerulonephritis
- Marked hypercellularity due to mesangial and endothelial cell proliferation and glomerular influx of neutrophils
- Hump-like subepithelial dense deposits on electron microscopy

Crescentic Glomerulonephritis
- Cellular or fibrocellular crescents in a variable percentage of glomeruli
- Immunofluorescence pattern distinguishes the main three types:
- Type I: Linear IgG staining of the GBM (anti-GBM disease)
- Type II: Granular deposits along GBM (immune complex deposition)
- Type III: Negative immunofluorescence (pauci-immune glomerulonephritis)

Abbreviations: GBM = glomerular basement membrane; Ig = immunoglobulin.

 CURRENT DIAGNOSIS

- Clinical presentations of glomerular diseases range from asymptomatic urinary abnormalities (proteinuria, microhematuria) to severe forms of rapidly progressive glomerulonephritis (gross hematuria, edema, acute renal function worsening, hypertension).
- Secondary causes of glomerular disease should be excluded by means of history, physical examination, and appropriate laboratory tests.
- Renal biopsy establishes the diagnosis and classification of primary glomerular diseases.

Treatment

CONSERVATIVE THERAPY

Hypertension is a common finding in patients with primary glomerulonephritis. Current guidelines recommend blood pressure targets lower than 130/80 mm Hg in these patients and lower than 125/75 mm Hg in patients with proteinuria greater than 1 g/24 hours. Any antihypertensive drug or drug combinations are useful, and they should be selected on the basis of the patient's characteristics.

BOX 3 Commonest Presentations of the Main Primary Glomerular Diseases

Minimal Change Disease
- Nephrotic syndrome

Focal and Segmental Glomerulosclerosis
- Nephrotic syndrome in more than two thirds of patients
- Non-nephrotic proteinuria in the remaining patients
- Renal insufficiency (20%–40%), hypertension (50%), and microhematuria (40%)

Membranous Nephropathy
- Nephrotic syndrome in >80% of patients
- Non-nephrotic proteinuria in the remaining patients

Membranoproliferative Glomerulonephritis
- Nephrotic syndrome in 50%
- Nephritic syndrome in 20%–30%
- Asymptomatic urinary abnormalities in 20%–30%
- Hypocomplementemia is common.

IgA Nephropathy
- Asymptomatic urinary abnormalities (microhematuria ±proteinuria) in >75%
- Intercalated recurrent or isolated episodes of macroscopic hematuria in >40%
- Nephritic or nephrotic syndrome in <10%

Acute Postinfectious Glomerulonephritis
- Nephritic syndrome
- Hypocomplementemia

Crescentic Glomerulonephritis
- Rapidly progressive glomerulonephritis

Abbreviation: Ig = immunoglobulin.

CURRENT THERAPY

- Appropriate treatment should be instituted as early as possible.
- Blood pressure should be lower than 130/80 mm Hg (<125/75 mm Hg in patients with proteinuria >1 g/24h).
- Angiotensin-converting enzyme inhibitors and angiotensin receptor blockers are indicated in most cases of chronic proteinuric glomerular diseases due to their antiproteinuric, antihypertensive, and renoprotective effects.
- Specific therapy of primary glomerular diseases includes steroids, anticalcineurinic agents, and cytotoxics. Due to the potential risks of these therapies, the likelihood of progression and the presence of chronic irreversible parenchymal damage must be carefully assessed.
- Primary or idiopathic glomerular diseases comprise a wide variety of glomerular histologic lesions, with different clinical presentations and variable prognosis. Although some entities portend a favorable long-term prognosis, a considerable fraction of untreated patients who have other glomerular entities reach end-stage renal failure.

However, blockade of the renin-angiotensin system either with an angiotensin-converting enzyme inhibitor (ACEI) or an angiotensin receptor blocker (ARB) should be the main basis of antihypertensive treatment because of their demonstrated renoprotective effect (slowing or preventing loss of renal function) in patients with chronic renal diseases. The beneficial effects of ACEIs and ARBs appear to be similar and are also observed in proteinuric patients with normal blood pressure. Renal protection induced by ACEIs and ARBs is closely related to the significant reduction in proteinuria that these agents induce. The level of proteinuria is the best way to monitor the efficacy of ACEIs and ARBs. Recent studies in primary glomerular diseases have shown that a combination of ACEI and ARB is more beneficial in terms of proteinuria decrease than either drug alone. Aldosterone antagonists (spironolactone, eplerenone) have also shown a remarkable antiproteinuric efficacy. Nevertheless, serum creatinine and potassium should be monitored after ACEI, ARB, or antialdosteronic agents are initiated, particularly in patients with reduced renal function.

Hyperlipidemia is a common finding in patients with glomerular diseases, particularly in those with the nephrotic syndrome. Prospective clinical studies have demonstrated that treatment of hyperlipidemia decreases proteinuria and prevents renal function loss. Statins such as atorvastatin (Lipitor) (10–40 mg after the evening meal) are the most commonly used lipid-lowering drugs. A level of LDL cholesterol lower than 100 mg/dL is recommended. Weight loss in obese patients induces a significant reduction in proteinuria, and smoking should be strictly forbidden, because smoking is associated with a more rapid progression toward renal failure in any type of renal disease.

All these measures (blood pressure lowering, treatment with ACEIs and ARBs, treatment of hyperlipidemia, weight loss, cessation of smoking) are also beneficial for the global cardiovascular risk that is significantly higher in proteinuric patients (mainly in those with renal insufficiency) than in the normal population.

The complications of the nephrotic syndrome require specific treatment. Edema is usually managed with a low-sodium diet plus furosemide (Lasix) in doses carefully adjusted to the severity of edema. Daily weight measurement is very important, because excessive diuretic doses can lead to volume depletion and functional worsening of renal function. In resistant cases, combinations of different types of diuretics (furosemide plus a thiazide diuretic, or furosemide plus a potassium-sparing diuretic such as spironolactone [Aldactone] in patients with hypokalemia) are needed. More severe cases require albumin infusions followed by high-dose intravenous furosemide (although intravenous albumin [Albuminar][1] increases proteinuria) or even removal of fluids by hemodialysis. Nephrotic patients are at increasing risk for thrombotic events. Prophylactic treatment (subcutaneous low-molecular-weight heparin) is indicated in conditions of high risk, such as immobilization.

SPECIFIC THERAPY

Box 4 summarizes the immunosuppressive treatment of primary glomerular diseases.

Minimal Change Disease

Minimal change disease (MCD) is most common in children but also causes 10% to 15% of nephrotic syndrome in adults. Corticosteroid therapy is a very effective treatment for MCD. For children, the dose of prednisone is 60 mg/m²/day and for adults 1 mg/kg/day (up to 80 mg/day). About 75% of patients respond (complete proteinuria disappearance) within 2 weeks, and more than 90% respond within 8 weeks, but adults show in general a slower response than children. Initial steroid dose is continued for 4 weeks and then changed to alternate-day prednisone (40 mg/m² on alternate days) or to daily prednisone, slowly tapering off over 6 to 10 weeks. Keeping patients on steroids for more than 3 months is associated with a lower 1-year relapse rate.

---

[1]Not FDA approved for this indication.

BOX 4 Immunosuppressive Treatment of Primary Glomerular Disease

Minimal Change Disease
First Line
- Steroids

Second Line
- Cytoxics (frequent relapsers)
- Anticalcineurinics or mycophenolate mofetil (CellCept)[1] (steroid-dependent)

Focal Segmental Glomerulosclerosis
First Line
- Steroids
- ACEIs
- ARBs

Second Line
- Anticalcineurinics
- Mycophenolate mofetil[1]

Membranous Nephropathy
First Line
- Anticalcineurinics
- Steroids plus cytoxics
- ACEIs
- ARBs

Second Line
- Mycophenolate mofetil
- Intramuscular ACTH (Synacthen)[1,2]
- Rituximab (Rituxan)[1]

Membranoproliferative Glomerulonephritis
- Steroids
- ACEIs
- ARBs

IgA Nephropathy
First Line
- ACEIs
- ARBs

Second Line
- Steroids
- Fish oil
- Cytoxics

Acute Postinfectious Glomerulonephritis
- Conservative therapy

Crescentic Glomerulonephritis
Type I (anti-GBM)
- Steroids
- Cyclophosphamide (Cytoxan)[1]
- Plasmapheresis

Type II and III
Induction
- Steroids
- Cyclophosphamide[1]
- Plasmapheresis in severe acute renal failure

Maintenance
- Low-dose steroids
- Azathioprine (Imuran)[1]

[1]Not FDA approved for this indication.
[2]Not available in the United States.
Abbreviations: ACEI = angiotensin-converting enzyme inhibitor; ACTH = adrenocorticotropic hormone; ARB = angiotensin receptor blocker; GBM = glomerular basement membrane; Ig = immunoglobulin.

Up to 75% of children and many adults have nephrotic syndrome relapses. Isolated relapses are re-treated with steroids as in the first episode. Frequent relapsers (two or more relapses within a 6-month period) are treated with a low-dose steroid course plus cyclophosphamide (Cytoxan) (1.5–2 mg/kg/day) or chlorambucil (Leukeran)[1] (0.1–0.2 mg/kg/day) in an 8-week course. After these short-term cytotoxic courses, a considerable fraction of patients remain free of proteinuria for prolonged periods, with a low rate of serious complications. Longer or repeated courses can induce severe side effects and are not recommended.

The response of steroid-dependent patients (reappearance of the nephrotic syndrome during or immediately after steroid withdrawal) to cytotoxics is poorer than that of frequent relapsers. Steroid-dependent patients and frequent relapsers unresponsive to cytotoxics are commonly treated with cyclosporine (Neoral)[1] given in an initial dose of 3–4 mg/kg in two divided doses, then adjusting for serum levels of 100–175 ng/mL. Most steroid-dependent patients transform into cyclosporine-dependent, and the risk of cyclosporine-induced nephrotoxicity should be considered. Mycophenolate mofetil (MMF, CellCept)[1] (600 mg/m²/12 h in children, 500–1000 mg/12 h in adults) is a very useful alternative. Rates of response and relapse are similar to those of cyclosporine, but tolerance is better and there

is no risk of nephrotoxicity. Therapy with cyclosporine or MMF if the patient responds is continued for up to 12 months before slow and careful tapering.

Less than 10% of MCD patients are steroid resistant. Because most of them subsequently have focal segmental glomerulosclerosis (FSGS) on biopsy, their therapeutic approach is the same as for FSGS.

Focal and Segmental Glomerulosclerosis

Causes of secondary FSGS (obesity, reflux nephropathy, reduction in renal mass) should be carefully excluded. Treatment with an ACEI or ARB (or both) is the first option in patients with non-nephrotic proteinuria or in patients with nonaggressive nephrotic syndrome (proteinuria <5 g/day, serum albumin >3 g/dL, normal renal function), mainly if hypertension coexists. Patients with severe nephrotic syndrome or nephrotic proteinuria after ACEI or ARB introduction should be treated with prednisone 1 mg/kg/day. Several retrospective studies have shown that steroid treatment maintained for at least 6 months is followed by more than 50% partial or complete remissions. However, in responsive patients, proteinuria starts to decrease after 2 to 3 months of treatment.

If proteinuria did not show significant changes within this period, introduction of an anticalcineurinic agent together with steroid tapering is recommended. Cyclosporine (doses and blood levels as in MCD) has been the most commonly used drug, and prospective studies have

[1]Not FDA approved for this indication.

shown more than 70% partial or complete remission after 6 months of treatment. Tacrolimus (Prograf)[1] (0.05–0.10 mg/kg/day in two divided doses, then adjusted for serum levels of 4–7 ng/mL) is proved to be effective in some cyclosporine-resistant FSGS cases.

In patients with complete or partial response to cyclosporine or tacrolimus, these drugs should be maintained at the lowest effective doses for at least 1 year before slowly tapering off. In some patients resistant to steroids and cyclosporine, or in those with mild degrees of renal insufficiency, MMF[1] (same doses as in MCD) has decreased proteinuria and stabilized renal function for prolonged periods. Sirolimus (Rapamune)[1] has induced complete (19%) or partial (38%) remission in a series of patients, although other studies have failed to confirm these beneficial effects and have shown a remarkable number of serious side effects.

About 20% to 25% of children with aggressive forms of FSGS have mutations in the genes coding for several podocyte proteins, mainly podocin. Most of these patients are unresponsive to any kind of treatment.

Membranous Nephropathy

More than one third of MGN patients have a spontaneous remission, and most remissions take place during the first 2 years of the disease. Conservative therapy should be maintained during the first 9 to 12 months, unless renal function starts to deteriorate. ACEIs or ARBs, or both, can induce partial remission (non-nephrotic proteinuria) in a considerable percentage of cases.

In patients with an aggressive presentation (massive nephrotic syndrome and deteriorating renal function) a 6-month course of alternating monthly prednisone 0.5 mg/kg/day with a month of chlorambucil[1] 0.2 mg/kg/day is recommended. Other clinicians simultaneously use prednisone starting with 1 mg/kg/day and tapering off over 6 months plus chlorambucil 0.15 mg/kg/day for 14 weeks. Another regimen is prednisone 0.5 mg/kg/day every other day for 6 months plus cyclophosphamide[1] 1.5 mg/kg/day for 12 months.

In patients maintaining normal renal function and persistent nephrotic proteinuria beyond 9 to 12 months, immunosuppressive therapy should be initiated, mainly in the presence of markers of poor outcome, which include male gender, older age, and proteinuria persistently higher than 8 g/day after ACEI or ARB treatment. Alternating prednisone and chlorambucil (as indicated earlier), prednisone and cyclophosphamide, and cyclosporine[1] 3–4 mg/kg/day, targeting blood levels of 100–175 ng/mL are beneficial, inducing complete or partial remission in most patients.

Side effects (diabetes, bone necrosis, infections) are more serious with steroids plus cytotoxic treatments; trimethoprim-sulfamethoxazole (TMP-SMX, Bactrim) (80 mg/400 mg/day) should be concurrently administered for *Pneumocystis jiroveci* prophylaxis. Cyclosporine, administered for 6 months, is followed by approximately 50% of recurrences after drug withdrawal.

No studies comparing anticalcineurinic and cytotoxics have been published for MGN. Tacrolimus,[1] another anticalcineurinic agent, can also induce partial response in more than 80% of treated patients, although recurrence after withdrawal is the same (50%) as with cyclosporine. A recent randomized pilot trial reported that tetracosactide (Synacthen),[1,2] an analogue of ACTH (1 mg IM twice a week for 1 year) induced remissions in the same percentage as a regimen of steroids plus cyclophosphamide.

Uncontrolled studies reported that MMF[1] (1000–2000 mg/day) reduced proteinuria and stabilized renal function in some MGN patients unresponsive to other therapies. Rituximab (Rituxan),[1] a monoclonal antibody against CD20-lymphocytes, has induced complete (15%–20%) or partial (35%–40%) remission in several series of patients, although no prospective controlled studies have been published. On the other hand, rituximab has been effective to avoid nephrotic syndrome relapse after tacrolimus withdrawal in patients successfully treated with this drug but showing anticalcineurin dependence.

Membranoproliferative Glomerulonephritis

The incidence of idiopathic membranoproliferative glomerulonephritis (MPGN) has progressively decreased over the last decades, being currently an uncommon disease in developed countries. Most cases of MPGN are now secondary to HCV infection and concurrent cryoglobulinemia. No prospective studies about the treatment of idiopathic MPGN have been carried out in the last several years. Uncontrolled series of patients suggested that prolonged (>2 years) prednisone treatment is beneficial in terms of proteinuria reduction and renal survival. Prospective randomized trials with aspirin[1] and dipyridamole (Persantine)[1] showed a significant reduction in proteinuria some decades ago, but later analysis did not demonstrate long-term benefits on renal survival.

Conservative therapy, including ACEIs and ARBs, should be prescribed in all cases. In patients with the nephrotic syndrome after an observation period or in those with more aggressive presentations (deteriorating renal function, crescents), a 6- to 12-month course of prednisone could be indicated. Some small series of patients suggested that cyclophosphamide[1] is effective in aggressive cases of MPGN, but conclusive evidence is lacking.

Immunoglobulin A Nephropathy

As in all types of primary glomerular diseases, the aggressiveness of therapeutic approaches in patients with immunoglobulin A (IgA) nephropathy should be graded according to the severity of the presentation. In patients with microhematuria and normal renal function, only regular follow-up is required. If slowly increasing proteinuria appears, an ACEI or ARB, or a combination of both drugs, should be started, even in the absence of hypertension, targeting for proteinuria less than 1 g/day and blood pressure lower than 125/75 mm Hg.

In patients with increasing proteinuria greater than 1–1.5 g/day in spite of these measures, other therapies should be contemplated. Steroids were proven to be beneficial in patients with normal renal function and proteinuria greater than 1 g/day in a prospective randomized trial: methylprednisolone (Solu-Medrol) pulses, 1 g/day for 3 days in the beginning of months 1,3, and 5, and oral prednisone 0.5 mg/kg every other day for 6 months reduced proteinuria and increased renal survival in comparison with untreated patients.

Treatment with fish oil supplements[1] in this type of patient remains controversial. Although eicosapentaenoic acid (1.8 g/day) or docosahexaenoic acid (1.2 g/day) demonstrated beneficial effects in some trials, these effects were not reproduced in others.

In patients with more aggressive presentations (proteinuria and deteriorating renal function), a prospective trial demonstrated that prednisone 40 mg/day tapering to 10 mg/day within 2 years plus cyclophosphamide[1] 1.5 mg/kg/day for 3 months followed by azathioprine (Imuran)[1] 1.5 mg/kg/day for at least 2 years significantly improved renal survival in comparison with untreated patients.

After initial suggestions of the benefits of MMF[1] 1000 to 2000 mg/day in IgA nephropathy patients unresponsive to other therapies, recent prospective and controlled trials have failed to demonstrate these good results, although the number of study subjects was small and many of them had advanced renal insufficiency.

Acute Postinfectious (Diffuse Proliferative) Glomerulonephritis

As in MPGN, the incidence of diffuse proliferative glomerulonephritis has drastically decreased in recent years in developed countries. The prognosis is generally good, and signs and symptoms of the disease (nephritic syndrome) resolve sporadically within 2 to 6 weeks in a great majority of cases. Treatment should be focused on adequate control of blood pressure, salt restriction, and diuretics to prevent fluid excess and the risks of cardiac failure. The triggering infection should be investigated and treated if it has not disappeared spontaneously.

---

[1]Not FDA approved for this indication.
[2]Not available in the United States.

---

[1]Not FDA approved for this indication.

Some patients present with more aggressive courses, developing progressive renal insufficiency. In these cases, crescents involving a large proportion of glomeruli can be observed in a second biopsy. No controlled studies have been carried out in these aggressive cases, but some series of patients recommend high-dose intravenous pulse steroid, followed by oral prednisone 1 mg/kg/day, tapering off over 2 to 3 months. There is no evidence that more aggressive immunosuppressive therapy is beneficial.

Crescentic Glomerulonephritis

Treatment of crescentic glomerulonephritis (CGN) should be promptly instituted because of the rapid transformation of cellular crescents into irreversible fibrotic crescents that collapse the glomerular tufts. Prognosis of type I (anti-GBM disease) CGN is poorer than that of types II and III, particularly in the presence of oligoanuria, dialysis requirement, or a large fraction of glomeruli with crescents.

Treatment of type I CGN includes steroids, cyclophosphamide,[1] and plasmapheresis. Pulse intravenous methylprednisolone (500–1000 mg daily for 3–4 days) is followed by oral prednisone (1 mg/kg/day for 3–4 weeks, then slowly tapering off over 6 months). Oral cyclophosphamide (2 mg/kg/day) is usually maintained for 2 to 3 months. Plasmapheresis (daily or alternate-day 4-liter exchanges) using albumin as replacement fluid or fresh frozen plasma if bleeding risk is high, is usually performed for 2 to 3 weeks. The duration of plasmapheresis, as well as the intensity and the duration of immunosuppressive therapy, should be guided by the clinical status and the titers of anti-GBM antibodies. In patients without pulmonary hemorrhage and with very advanced renal involvement (massive presence of glomerular fibrotic crescents), aggressive immunosuppression is not indicated.

The precise etiology of type II CGN (e.g., systemic lupus erythematosus, cryoglobulinemia) should be identified and the therapy guided by the diagnosis. If no apparent diagnosis is available, treatment is similar to that for type III (pauci-immune) CGN.

Induction treatment of type III CGN consists of steroids (oral prednisone, 1 mg/kg/day for 3–4 weeks, slowly tapered to a maintenance dose of 10–20 mg), and intravenous monthly pulses of cyclophosphamide (initial dose 0.5 to 1 g/m^2, adjusted for renal function and age), which has proved to be as effective and less toxic than oral administration. Once remission is achieved (recovery of renal function, absence of extrarenal symptoms), usually within 3 to 6 months, cyclophosphamide is replaced by azathioprine[1] 1 to 2 mg/kg/day for 12 to 18 months plus prednisone 5 to 10 mg daily or every other day. Positive titers of ANCA, particularly p-ANCA, can indicate more prolonged, low-dose, maintenance treatment, because the risk of recurrence is high. Plasmapheresis (similar to that in type I CGN) is proven to add benefits in type III CGN manifesting with severe renal failure. Although not tested in prospective trials, MMF[1] (1500–3000 mg/day) has been shown effective and well tolerated, even as induction therapy in some series of patients.

REFERENCES

Cattran DC, Appel GB, Hebert LA, et al. A randomized trial of cyclosporine in patients with steroid-resistant focal segmental glomerulosclerosis. Kidney Int 1999;56:2220–6.

Cattran DC, Appel GB, Hebert LA, et al. Cyclosporin in patients with steroid-resistant membranous nephropathy: A randomized trial. Kidney Int 2001;59:1484–90.

Jayne D, Rasmussen N, Andrassy K, et al. A randomized trial of maintenance therapy for vasculitis associated with antineutrophil cytoplasmic autoantibodies. N Engl J Med 2003;349:36–44.

Nakao N, Yoshimura A, Morita H, et al. Combination treatment of angiotensin-II receptor blocker and angiotensin-converting-enzyme inhibitor in non-diabetic renal disease (COOPERATE): A randomized controlled trial. Lancet 2003;361:117–24.

Ponticelli C, Altieri P, Scolari F, et al. A randomized study comparing methylprednisolone plus chlorambucil versus methylprednisolone plus cyclophosphamide in idiopathic membranous nephropathy. J Am Soc Nephrol 1998;9:444–50.

Pozzi C, Bolasco PG, Fogazzi GB, et al. Corticosteroids in IgA nephropathy: A randomised controlled trial. Lancet 1999;13:883–7.

Praga M, Gutiérrez E, González E, et al. Treatment of IgA nephropathy with ACE inhibitors: A randomized and controlled trial. J Am Soc Nephrol 2003;14:1578–83.

Torres A, Domínguez-Gil B, Carreño A, et al. Conservative versus immunosuppressive treatment of patients with idiopathic membranous nephropathy. Kidney Int 2002;61:219–27.

Pyelonephritis

Method of
Patricia D. Brown, MD

Acute pyelonephritis (APN) is a urinary tract infection (UTI) that involves the renal parenchyma, also referred to as *upper tract UTI*. Most episodes of APN occur as a result of ascending infection from the bladder; patients with APN might or might not have symptoms of concomitant cystitis. Rarely, pyelonephritis occurs secondary to hematogenous seeding of the kidney as a result of infection elsewhere, most commonly endocarditis due to *Staphylococcus aureus* or disseminated fungal infection.

Epidemiology

Surprisingly little is known about the epidemiology of APN. Similar to cystitis, APN (and hospitalization for APN) is more common in women than men; men have been reported to have higher in-hospital mortality. In contrast to cystitis, risk factors for pyelonephritis are not well defined. One recent study of nonpregnant women 18 to 49 years of age found risk factors for APN included factors known to be risk factors for acute cystitis, including frequency of sexual intercourse, recent UTI, diabetes, and maternal UTI history. The incidence of bacteremia in patients with APN is reported to be 11% to 53% in various studies; risk factors for bacteremia are not well established.

Similar to lower UTI, APN can be further classified into complicated or uncomplicated infection. The factors that make an episode of APN a complicated UTI are outlined in Box 1.

BOX 1 Factors Associated with Complicated Pyelonephritis

- Diabetes
- Foreign body (catheter, stent)
- Health care–associated infections
- Immunocompromise
- Incomplete voiding (detrusor muscle dysfunction due to neurologic disease or medications)
- Infections due to multidrug-resistant pathogens
- Obstruction (including stones)
- Pregnancy
- Recent history of instrumentation
- Renal transplant recipient
- UTI in a male patient
- Vesicoureteral reflux

Abbreviation: UTI = urinary tract infection.

---

[1]Not FDA approved for this indication.

Clinical Presentation

The classic presenting features of APN include abrupt onset of fever, flank pain, and costovertebral angle tenderness with or without symptoms of lower UTI including dysuria, urgency, and frequency. Unfortunately, there is no single constellation of signs or symptoms that is pathognomonic for APN. When localization studies have been performed on patients with symptoms of acute cystitis, 30% to 50% have been shown to have APN. Women who present with symptoms that have been present more than 7 days and those with a recent history of UTI are more likely to have APN. Flank pain is reported in approximately one half of patients with APN but also occurs in almost 20% of patients with cystitis. Fever is present in one half of patients with APN, but less than 5% of patients with cystitis. Nausea, vomiting, and diarrhea occur commonly in patients with APN, and gastrointestinal (GI) symptoms can dominate the presenting complaints.

In general, patients who present with lower urinary tract symptoms or laboratory evidence of urinary tract infection accompanied by fever, flank pain or tenderness, or signs of systemic toxicity, such as GI symptoms, should be treated for APN.

The diagnosis can be particularly challenging in the frail elderly patient, because symptoms such as frequency, urgency, and incontinence are often chronic in this patient population and unrelated to active UTI. Change in mental status may be the only presenting complaint. Because the prevalence of bacteriuria in this patient population is high, particularly among those with chronic indwelling catheters, UTI must be a diagnosis of exclusion.

Acute pelvic inflammatory disease can have a presentation similar to APN. Pelvic examination should be performed on all sexually active women to exclude this diagnosis.

The differential diagnosis of APN is outlined in Box 2.

Diagnosis

Urinalysis, ideally with microscopic examination, using a clean-catch, midstream specimen, should be performed in all patients with suspected APN. Pyuria is a key finding in the diagnosis of UTI, and the absence of pyuria is strong evidence against a diagnosis of APN. Direct microscopic examination under high power of the urinary sediment from a centrifuged specimen should reveal more than 10 leukocytes per high-powered field. The presence of white blood cell (WBC) casts is highly specific for localization of the infection to the kidney, but it is inadequately sensitive to exclude the diagnosis of APN. The dipstick test for leukocyte esterase is used as a rapid screening test to detect significant pyuria; the sensitivity is reported to be 75% to 96%, with a specificity of 94% to 98%. Because of the lower range of the reported sensitivity of the dipstick test, microscopic examination to exclude significant pyuria should be obtained in patients with suspected APN.

BOX 2   Differential Diagnosis of Acute Pyelonephritis

- Appendicitis
- Cholecystitis
- Diverticulitis
- Gastroenteritis
- Herpes zoster
- Musculoskeletal pain, including vertebral disorders
- Ovarian cysts, tumors
- Pancreatitis
- Perforated viscus
- Pelvic inflammatory disease
- Pneumonia
- Renal stones, renal vein thrombosis, renal infarction

 CURRENT DIAGNOSIS

- Abrupt onset of fever, flank pain, and costovertebral angle tenderness with or without symptoms of cystitis are classic presenting features.
- Patients with lower UTI symptoms or laboratory evidence of UTI accompanied by flank pain, fever, or signs of systemic toxicity such as GI complaints should be managed as having APN.
- Urinalysis with microscopic examination should be performed in all patients with suspected APN. Absence of pyuria is strong evidence against the diagnosis.
- A urine culture should be obtained in all patients with APN. Blood cultures should be obtained in those who are hospitalized.
- Patients should be categorized into those with uncomplicated and those with complicated infections.

Abbreviations: APN = acute pyelonephritis; GI = gastrointestinal; UTI = urinary tract infection.

The presence of nitrite in the urine, detected by a dipstick test, has a reported sensitivity of 35% to 85% and a specificity of 92% to 100% for UTI. Microscopic examination of a Gram-stained, centrifuged urine specimen revealing at least one bacterium per oil-immersion field correlates with more than 10^5 colony-forming units (cfu)/mL of bacteria, with a sensitivity of 95%. Although this is the standard definition of significant bacteriuria, it has been shown that women with UTI can have levels of bacteriuria as low as 10^2 cfu/mL.

Although the microbiology of APN has remained predictable, significant changes in antimicrobial susceptibility patterns have occurred. Therefore, in contrast to recommendations for acute uncomplicated cystitis, a urine culture should be obtained in all patients with suspected APN. The need to obtain blood cultures has been debated, because blood cultures rarely yield a pathogen different from what was isolated from the urine. Bacteremia has been reported in 11% to 53% of patients hospitalized with APN. Bacteremic patients have a longer length of stay, and one recent report suggests that this is due to a longer time to resolution of fever. Many experts continue to recommend that blood cultures be obtained as part of the diagnostic evaluation of patients who are ill enough to require hospitalization; blood cultures are not necessary for those who will be managed as outpatients.

The role of diagnostic imaging in the management of APN is discussed later. In some cases with an atypical presentation, imaging may be helpful to confirm the diagnosis of APN. In this setting, pre- and postcontrast computed tomography (CT) is the imaging procedure of choice in adults.

Microbial Etiology

Most cases of APN are caused by *Escherichia coli*. Other enterobacteriaceae, including *Klebsiella* species and *Proteus* species, are also occasionally implicated. Other gram-negative pathogens such as *Pseudomonas, Serratia, Enterobacter,* and *Acinetobacter* should be considered in health care–associated infections. *Enterococcus* is an uncommon pathogen in community-acquired infections, but it must be considered in health care–associated infections, including vancomycin-resistant enterococci. Other gram-positive pathogens include *Streptoccocus agalactiae* and *Staphylococcus* species. Although a common cause of acute cystitis in young women, *Staphylococcus saprophyticus* is a rare cause of pyelonephritis; the finding of *Staphylococcus aureus* in a urine culture should always prompt a search for an extrarenal source of infection that might have served as a source of hematogenous seeding. A Gram stain of the urine is a simple and rapid test to exclude a gram-positive pathogen as the etiology of APN and guide the initial selection of empiric therapy.

The emergence of resistance to trimethoprim-sulfamethoxazole (TMP-SMX [Bactrim]) among *E. coli* has had a major impact on the approach to initial empiric antimicrobial therapy for APN. It is clear that the prevalence of resistance varies depending on geographic region, and clinicians often do not have access to meaningful local resistance data. Recent reports of increasing fluoroquinolone resistance among uropathogens are of great concern, although overall resistance rates in North America remain low.

Treatment

The first decision in the management of patients with APN is whether or not the patient requires hospitalization. Although prospective randomized trials are lacking, several retrospective studies as well as several prospective nonrandomized trials suggest that outpatient management is safe for many patients. Hospitalization should be considered for patients who cannot tolerate oral intake or who have severe pain or signs of severe sepsis. A strategy of initial management in the emergency department or an observation unit with an initial dose of parenteral antibiotic therapy, intravenous fluids, and symptomatic treatment of nausea and pain may be used in select patients to avoid hospital admission. Patients who will be treated as outpatients should have a stable social situation and the ability to contact the physician and return promptly if their symptoms worsen. Hospitalization is generally recommended for patients with complicated infections. Most experts believe that pregnant women with APN should always be hospitalized.

There are surprisingly few prospective randomized trials of the treatment of pyelonephritis. For patients who require hospitalization, parenteral therapy with an aminoglycoside, a third-generation cephalosporin, or a fluoroquinolone is recommended. At my institution, we discourage fluoroquinolones for this indication because there are other effective alternatives and we wish to minimize the use of these very broad-spectrum agents in the hospital setting. Although resistance to TMP-SMX among uropathogenic *E. coli* appears to have leveled off and might actually be decreasing, this agent should not be used for empiric therapy of APN.

If a gram-positive pathogen is suspected or suggested by the results of urine Gram stain, ampicillin or ampicillin-sulbactam (Unasyn) with or without an aminoglycoside can be used. Patients should receive intravenous therapy until they are clinically improving and able to reliably tolerate oral intake; oral therapy can be chosen based on the results of urine culture and susceptibility data. TMP-SMX, a fluoroquinolone, and ampicillin are all potential candidates for oral switch therapy. The narrowest spectrum, least expensive agent to which the isolated pathogen is susceptible should be chosen. Despite in vitro susceptibility data, first- and second-generation cephalosporins have a poor track record in the treatment of APN and are generally not recommended, with the exception of pyelonephritis in pregnancy.

CURRENT THERAPY

- Hospitalization is recommended for patients unable to tolerate oral intake, those with severe pain, and those with signs of severe sepsis. Hospitalization is generally recommended for patients with complicated infections and for all pregnant women.
- Parenteral regimens for hospitalized patients include an aminoglycoside, third-generation cephalosporin, or fluoroquinolone, with oral switch therapy selected on the basis of culture and susceptibility data.
- Initial empiric therapy for outpatients is a fluoroquinolone.
- Imaging is not recommended for patients with uncomplicated infections. Pre- and postcontrast computed tomographic scans should be obtained in those who fail to respond within 72 hours to appropriate antibiotic therapy.

BOX 3   Antimicrobial Therapy for the Management of Acute Pyelonephritis

Parenteral Regimens
- Ampicillin 2 g q4h–q6h
- Ampicillin-sulbactam (Unasyn) 3 g q6h
- Ceftriaxone (Rocephin) 1–2 g q24h
- Ciprofloxacin (Cipro) 400 mg q12h
- Gentamicin (Garamycin) 3–5 mg/kg q24h
- Levofloxacin (Levaquin) 250–500 mg q24h

Oral Regimens
- Amoxicillin 500 mg q8h
- Ciprofloxacin 500 mg q12h
- Ciprofloxacin XR 1000 mg q24h
- Levofloxacin 250 mg q24h
- Trimethoprim-sulfamethoxazole DS (Bactrim DS) 160/800 mg q12h

Bacteremic patients might take longer to respond but do not require more prolonged parenteral therapy. The total duration of therapy for pyelonephritis is generally 14 days. Seven days of therapy with a fluoroquinolone for uncomplicated APN has been shown to be effective. Longer courses of therapy may be required for select patients with complicated pyelonephritis. For outpatients, initial empiric therapy with a fluoroquinolone is recommended, with adjustment of therapy, if needed, based on the results of urine culture. All of the currently available fluoroquinolones can be used, with the exception of moxifloxacin (Avelox), which does not achieve adequate levels in the urine. Although it is useful in the treatment of cystitis, norfloxacin (Noroxin) is not recommended for the treatment of APN because it does not achieve sustained tissue or serum levels. Suggested antimicrobial dosing regimens for APN are outlined in Box 3.

Imaging

Imaging is generally not needed in patients with uncomplicated APN. For patients with complicated infections (e.g., history of stones, prior renal surgery), renal ultrasound with abdominal plain films is considered an acceptable alternative to excretory urography. For patients with diabetes or other immunocompromise and for patients who fail to respond after 72 hours of appropriate antibiotic therapy, pre- and postcontrast CT is the imaging procedure of choice.

Follow-up

Most patients will respond to appropriate antibiotic therapy. Follow-up urine cultures to document microbiological response are not recommended in patients who have responded clinically.

REFERENCES

Foxman B, Klemstine KL, Brown PD. Acute pyelonephritis in US hospitals in 1997: Hospitalization and in-hospital mortality. Ann Epidemiol 2003; 13:144–50.

Pappas PG. Laboratory in the diagnosis and management of urinary tract infections. Med Clin North Am 1991;75:313–25.

Sandler CM, Amis ES Jr, Bigongiari LR, et al. Imaging in acute pyelonephritis. American College of Radiology. ACR appropriateness criteria. Radiology 2000;215(Suppl):677–81.

Scholes D, Hooton TM, Roberts PL, et al. Risk factors associated with acute pyelonephritis in healthy women. Ann Intern Med 2005;142:20–7.

Talan DA, Stamm WE, Hooton TM, et al. Comparison of ciprofloxacin (7 days) and trimethoprim-sulfamethoxazole (14 days) for acute uncomplicated pyelonephritis in women: A randomized trial. JAMA 2000;283:1583–90.

Warren JW, Abrutyn E, Hebel JR, et al. Guidelines for antimicrobial treatment of uncomplicated acute bacterial cystitis and acute pyelonephritis in women. Clin Infect Dis 1999;29:745–58.

Trauma to the Genitourinary Tract

Method of
Sean P. Elliott, MD, and Bahaa S. Malaeb, MD

The genitourinary tract is involved in 3% to 10% of trauma cases. The kidney, followed by the bladder and urethra, are the most commonly involved genitourinary organs. In most cases, injury to the genitourinary tract is not isolated, and the initial evaluation of the urologic injuries should emphasize the context of the patient's associated injuries that might be more pressing or life-threatening. Still, early involvement of the urologist is prudent to help plan further interventions. The spectrum of genitourinary injuries is widespread, and management can range from immediate repair to temporization with delayed reconstruction. The goal of a urologist in the trauma setting is to establish urinary drainage in order to optimize kidney function, minimize hemorrhage, and control urinary extravasation to reduce associated complications such as infection or ileus.

Renal Trauma

Renal injury occurs in 1% to 5% of all trauma cases. Blunt impact accounts for the majority of renal injuries (90%–95%) and causes damage secondary to direct organ injury or disruption of the kidney from its attachments (e.g., renal hilum and ureteropelvic junction). Penetrating trauma most commonly is caused by stabbing or gunshot wounds. The damage from penetrating injury can be limited to the tract of the stab wound, or it can be more extensive secondary to necrosis from energy transfer and the blast effect of high-velocity bullets. The history is crucial in the diagnosis of renal injury and should include the mechanism of trauma as well as any preexisting kidney disease or condition that might contribute to worsening renal function. Hematuria has a very poor correlation with degree of injury, because disruption of the ureteropelvic junction, arterial disruption or thrombosis, and other severe injuries can exist in a setting with no hematuria.

The American Association for the Surgery of Trauma (AAST) classifies renal injuries into five grades (Figs. 1 and 2):

- Grade 1: Nonexpanding subcapsular hematoma/contusion with absence of parenchymal injury

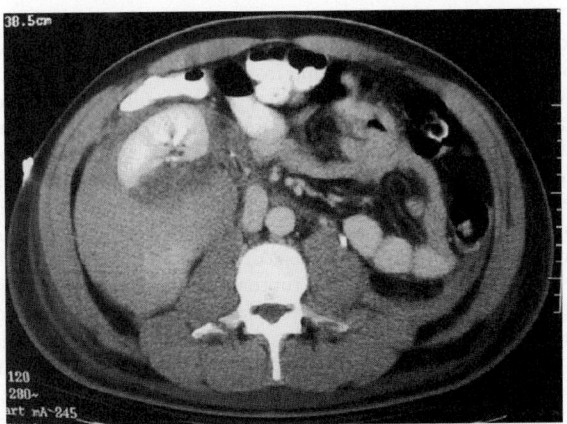

FIGURE 1. Computed tomography scan demonstrating large right perirenal hematoma and thrombosed posterior segmental artery. This was classified as a grade IV renal injury.

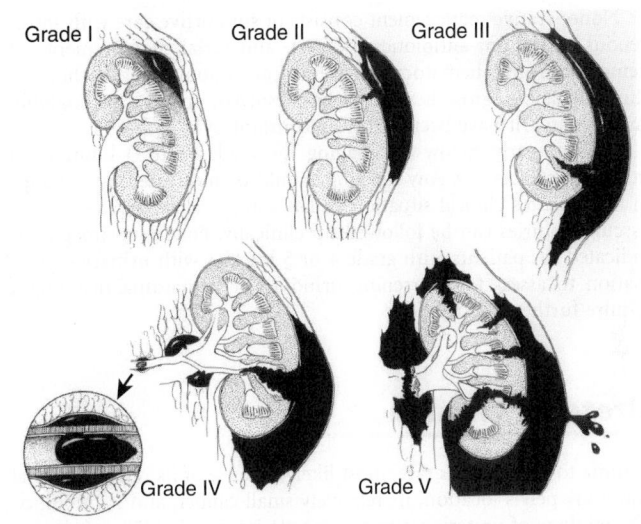

FIGURE 2. American Association for the Surgery of Trauma grading system for traumatic renal injuries: grade I, renal contusion and subcapsular hematoma; grade II, cortical laceration and perirenal hematoma; grade III, laceration into medulla or segmental renal artery thrombosis without a parenchymal injury; grade IV, laceration involving the collecting system, with or without a devascularized segment and contained vascular injury; grade V, renal artery thrombosis, avulsion of the renal pedicle, and shattered kidney (From McAninch JW [ed]: Traumatic and Reconstructive Urology. Philadelphia, WB Saunders, 1996.)

- Grade 2: Less than 1 cm laceration into the renal cortex, not extending into the collecting system, with a nonexpanding hematoma confined to the perirenal fascia
- Grade 3: Greater than 1 cm laceration, extending through the renal cortex and medulla but not the collecting system
- Grade 4: Laceration extending to the collecting system with urinary extravasation or a segmental vascular injury with contained hematoma; renal artery thrombosis
- Grade 5: Shattered kidney or renal pedicle avulsion

Renal injury should be suspected in any trauma patient who has a penetrating injury with gross or microscopic hematuria (>2 red blood cells per high-power field), a blunt injury with gross hematuria, or a blunt injury with microscopic hematuria and shock (systolic blood pressure <90 mm Hg). In addition, imaging of the urinary tract should be obtained in children who have more than 50 red blood cells per high-power field even in the absence of hypotension.

In a stable patient, radiographic evaluation should consist of computed tomographic (CT) scanning with intravenous contrast and delayed images showing opacification of the collecting system and ureters. In the absence of a CT scan in a patient who is transported directly to the operating room for exploration, an intraoperative single-film intravenous pyelogram can be performed to confirm that two functioning kidneys are present; however, the poor quality of the images makes them unreliable for staging purposes.

Kidney exploration is indicated for the unstable patient in whom renal injury is thought to be the reason for a life-threatening and persistent hemorrhage. Another absolute indication for renal exploration and revascularization is renal artery hilar avulsion or renal artery thrombosis, if bilateral or in a solitary kidney. In patients undergoing exploratory laparotomy for associated injuries, renal exploration should be performed only in the presence of an expanding or pulsatile hematoma. Exploration of a nonexpanding, nonpulsatile hematoma is associated with a higher rate of nephrectomy and should be avoided. Almost all other injuries can be managed conservatively or with minimally invasive methods.

Nonoperative management consists of supportive care with intravenous hydration, antibiotics, bedrest, and serial measurements of hemoglobin and hematocrit. Patients can ambulate after they are clinically stable, gross hematuria has resolved, and the hemoglobin and hematocrit have been relatively constant over 24 hours.

Routine early follow-up imaging for grades 1 to 3 blunt renal injury is unnecessary. Any imaging should be motivated by a change in the patient's clinical situation or laboratory values. Grade 4 renovascular injuries can be followed up clinically. Follow-up imaging is indicated for patients with grade 4 or 5 injuries with urinary extravasation to assess for worsening urinoma or hematoma that might require further intervention.

Ureteral Trauma

Trauma to the ureter is rare, most likely because of its retroperitoneal and bony pelvis location, its relatively small caliber, and its mobility. The etiology of ureteric trauma is mostly iatrogenic (75% of all ureteric injuries); 73% of iatrogenic injuries occur secondary to gynecologic procedures, and the remainder are divided between general surgery and urologic procedures. Ureteral injury should be suspected in all cases of penetrating trauma to the abdomen, especially with high-velocity projectiles, because of the blast effect.

The AAST has classified ureteric injuries into five grades of severity:

- Grade 1: Hematoma only
- Grade 2: Injury involving less than 50% of the circumference of the ureter
- Grade 3: Injury involving more than 50% of the circumference of the ureter
- Grade 4: Complete transsection with less than 2 cm of devascularization
- Grade 5: Complete transsection with more than 2 cm of devascularization

The diagnosis usually is made intraoperatively if a high suspicion of ureteric injury is present or postoperatively by imaging obtained for investigation of fistula formation or clinical signs of upper tract obstruction. For noniatrogenic injuries, imaging should be obtained in patients who had rapid deceleration or penetrating injuries to the flank. Imaging modalities used are usually intravenous pyelography, CT scanning with intravenous contrast and delayed images, and retrograde pyelography. Findings indicative of ureteral injury include contrast extravasation, ureteral narrowing, and delayed peristalsis (Fig. 3). Alternatively, the ureters may be interrogated intraoperatively by using direct inspection, by injecting intravenous methylene blue[1] and watching for leakage of dye, or by passing a ureteral catheter (if it passes easily, an injury is unlikely).

Grade 1 and 2 injuries can be managed initially by placement of a ureteral stent. If grade 2 or 3 injuries are identified immediately during exploration for a suspected ureteric injury, they can be managed by primary closure of the ureteric injury over an internal stent and placement of a nonsuction abdominal drain, as long as there is no associated thermal injury or necrosis. Grade 3 to 5 injuries usually require débridement of nonviable ends with reanastomosis over an internal ureteral stent or more complicated surgical procedures involving mobilization of the bladder and reimplantation of the ureter into the bladder. The type of ureteral repair depends on the amount of devitalized tissues and the location of the injury (proximal, middle, or distal ureter). Ureteroureterostomy, transureteroureterostomy, ureterocalicostomy, renal autotransplantation, ureteroneocystostomy with or without Boari flap or psoas hitch, and bowel interposition are all treatment options for various degrees of ureteral injuries.

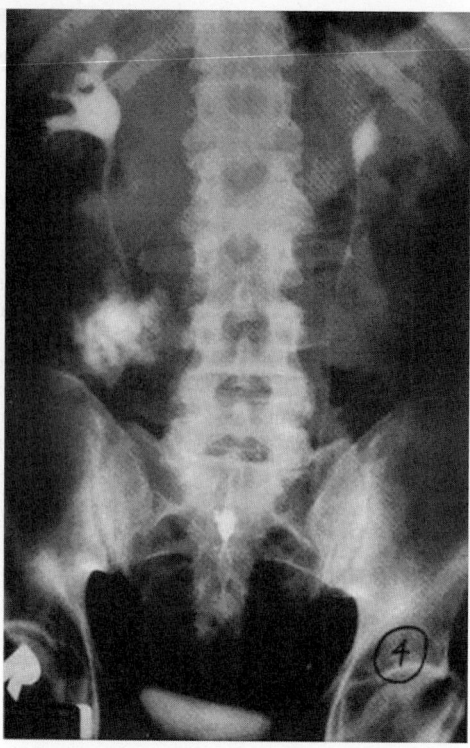

FIGURE 3. Intravenous pyelogram demonstrating extravasation of urine from right mid-ureter.

Bladder Trauma

Blunt trauma accounts for 67% to 86% of bladder injuries resulting from external trauma, and up to 97% of those patients have associated pelvic fractures. The most common cause of blunt trauma is motor vehicle crashes. Penetrating trauma accounts for 14% to 33% of traumatic bladder injuries. The incidence of iatrogenic injury varies by procedure but is highest for hysterectomy and other obstetric and gynecologic procedures (up to 61 per 1000 cases). In cases of blunt trauma, injury should be suspected in patients who have pelvic fractures, suprapubic pain and inability to void, ileus, absent bowel sounds, or abdominal distention. For iatrogenic injuries, any urine in the field, visible laceration in bladder, or gas distention of the urinary drainage bag in laparoscopic surgery warrants further investigation. It is important to delineate whether a bladder injury involves intraperitoneal or extraperitoneal rupture. Intraperitoneal rupture occurs at the level of the bladder dome, where the muscular support is weakest (Figs. 4 and 5).

The diagnostic test of choice is a CT cystogram, in which the bladder is filled with contrast to capacity (350–400 mL instilled by gravity). In children, the volume instilled is 60 mL plus 30 mL per year of age up to a maximum of 300 mL. Passive filling of the bladder by clamping of the catheter is associated with unacceptably high rates of false-negative tests. Plain film cystography is an alternative, but a single anteroposterior film is insufficient; postdrainage films and, preferably, oblique views should be obtained as well. In both settings, retrograde urethrography should be performed, if there is a suspicion of urethral injury, before placement of a Foley catheter.

Most extraperitoneal bladder ruptures can be managed with Foley catheter drainage for 7 to 10 days. Bladder neck involvement, concomitant vaginal or rectal injuries, presence of bone fragments in the bladder, or bladder wall entrapment necessitates surgical intervention. Intraperitoneal ruptures should be managed with surgical exploration because of the associated ileus and peritonitis caused by urine leak. In contrast, all penetrating bladder injuries should be explored and repaired because of the risk of necrosis and nonhealing. Bladder repair is performed with a multiple-layer closure and catheter drainage for 7 to 10 days.

---

[1]Not FDA approved for this indication.

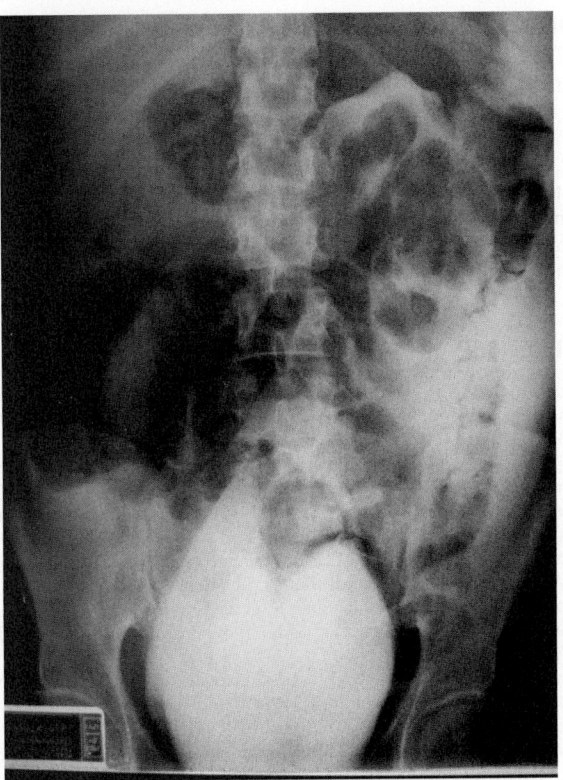

FIGURE 4. Intraperitoneal bladder rupture. Note contrast extravasating from the dome of the bladder and outlining the small intestine as well as the left colon.

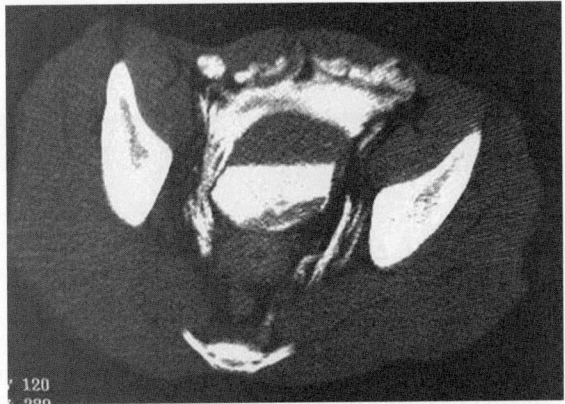

FIGURE 5. Extraperitoneal bladder rupture seen on computed tomographic cystogram.

Urethral Trauma

Traumatic injury to the urethra occurs in 10% of patients who sustain a pelvic fracture. Female urethral injuries are very rare. The male urethra is anatomically divided into a posterior part (prostatic and membranous urethra) and an anterior part (bulbous urethra, penile/pendulous urethra, and fossa navicularis). Injury to the anterior urethra occurs mostly from blunt trauma, penetrating injuries, or instrumentation. Posterior urethral injuries are usually associated with pelvic fractures but can occur secondary to blunt, penetrating, or iatrogenic injury.

Classic signs of urethral injury include blood at the meatus, a high-riding prostate on rectal examination, and perineal or scrotal

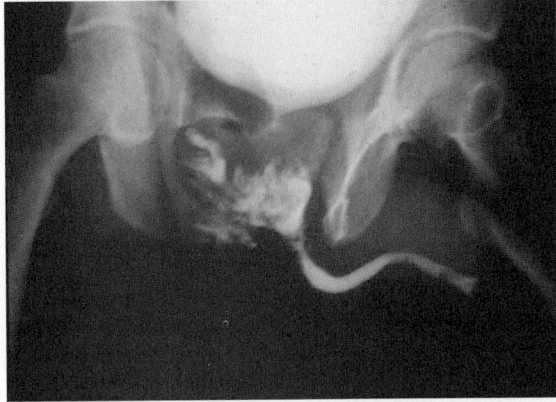

FIGURE 6. Retrograde urethrogram diagnostic of partial bulbar urethral transaction resulting from straddle injury.

ecchymosis. Imaging is indicated with any of these signs. The imaging study of choice is a retrograde urethrogram, and it should be performed before placement of a urethral catheter is attempted. In the absence of any signs, the diagnosis is most frequently made when retrograde urethrography is performed to investigate difficulty with urethral catheter placement (Fig. 6).

The AAST grading system does not distinguish between anterior or posterior injury but classifies urethral injuries as follows:

- Grade 1: Contusion and blood at the meatus with normal urethrogram
- Grade 2: Stretch injury with no extravasation of contrast
- Grade 3: Partial disruption with contrast extravasating at the injury site but still reaching the bladder
- Grade 4: Complete disruption with contrast not reaching the bladder; urethral defect of less than 2 cm
- Grade 5: Complete disruption with urethral defect greater than 2 cm or complex injury involving the bladder neck, prostate, rectum, or vagina

Grade 1 and 2 injuries can be managed conservatively by placement of a urethral catheter. Management of grade 3 urethral injury should initially emphasize stabilization of the patient, because extensive bleeding could be present in cases of severe injury to the pelvis. Placement of a catheter may be attempted even if there is a suspicion of partial urethral injury. If this is met with difficulty, a suprapubic tube may be placed.

In cases of complete disruption, evidence supports early endoscopic realignment performed within the initial hospitalization if the patient is stable. This involves endoscopic passage of a guidewire across the defect and placement of a catheter over the guidewire, with the purpose of reestablishing urethral continuity. An alternative method is placement of a suprapubic tube and delayed reconstruction; the latter approach is associated with a 100% rate of stricture formation. Early endoscopic alignment has been shown to decrease the rate of stricture formation and the severity of strictures when they do occur, compared with suprapubic tube placement and delayed urethral reconstruction. Immediate open repair is rarely indicated unless complex injury extends into the bladder, rectum, or vagina and the patient is undergoing surgery for associated injuries. Immediate exploration is recommended for anterior urethral injuries associated with penetrating trauma or penile fractures.

Trauma to the External Genitalia

Injury to the scrotum is most frequently secondary to blunt trauma and can cause subcutaneous hematoma, hematocele, or testicular injury. Scrotal swelling and patient discomfort can make separation of testicular injury from extratesticular scrotal trauma difficult on

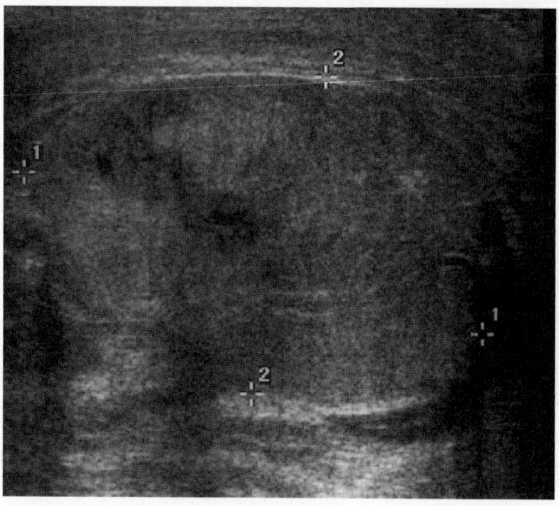

FIGURE 7. Testis ultrasound image demonstrating heterogeneous architecture characteristic of testicular rupture.

physical examination. Therefore, one should have a low threshold for further investigation with ultrasound. A heterogeneous echo pattern in the testicular parenchyma on ultrasonography suggests testicular injury (Fig. 7). Visualization of a tear in the tunica albuginea is less accurate. Ultrasound studies additionally provide information about any compromise in testicular blood flow.

Scrotal exploration should be performed whenever testicular injury is suspected. If the tunica is ruptured and there is extrusion of seminiferous tubules, the extruded tubules should be débrided, hemorrhage controlled, and the tunica closed. Testicular salvage rates are high (90%) when the scrotum is explored acutely but drop by half if exploration is delayed. Another indication for scrotal exploration is a large hematocele; evacuation of the hematoma can decrease the morbidity associated with protracted recovery and resolution of the hematoma and can occasionally identify a manageable source of bleeding. Scrotal exploration should also be performed in cases of inconclusive ultrasound findings or whenever the clinical suspicion for testicular injury is high.

Trauma to the penis can range in severity from a contusion to complete amputation. In cases of penile amputation, stabilization of the patient is important, and the need for transfusion should be addressed. Immediate microreimplantation is the management technique of choice if available. Penile fracture occurs after blunt injury to the erect penis, usually incurred during sexual intercourse. Patients often report a "crack" or a "pop" followed by severe pain and detumescence. Penile fractures involve rupture of the tunica albuginea. The hematoma is usually limited to the penis, unless the injury also involves Buck's fascia, causing ecchymosis and bruising that involves the scrotum as well. It is important to rule out associated urethral injury, which occurs in 10% of the cases. Surgical exploration, closure of the fascial defect, and repair of any associated urethral injury should be done acutely.

In females, blunt trauma to the vulva is rare. Injuries to genitalia can be associated with sexual assault and must be evaluated in that context. Consequently, vaginal smears should be taken, and the vagina should be thoroughly inspected with a speculum and with the patient under anesthesia.

Trauma resulting in skin loss, such as burns, large abrasions, and avulsions, the lesions should be explored and débrided in an effort to stage the injury and decrease the risk of complications such as Fournier's gangrene and urinoma. Delayed reconstruction can be performed after stabilization and proper delineation of viable versus nonviable tissues. The reconstruction options include mobilization of local flaps or skin grafts.

Conclusion

An understanding of the mechanism of injury is important to establish clinical suspicion of urologic trauma. Radiologic imaging is essential in making the correct diagnosis and managing it appropriately. Early diagnosis minimizes patient morbidity.

Studies of prospective design are clearly lacking for urologic trauma. Consolidation of the experience of major trauma institutions nationwide in a consortium for multi-institutional protocols could be the answer to this lack of prospective data.

REFERENCES

Brandes S, Coburn M, Armenakas N, McAninch J. Diagnosis and management of ureteric injury: An evidence-based analysis. BJU Int 2004;94 (3):277–89.

Chapple C, Barbagli G, Jordan G, et al. Consensus statement on urethral trauma. BJU Int 2004;93(9):1195–202.

Gomez RG, Ceballos L, Coburn M, et al. Consensus statement on bladder injuries. BJU Int 2004;94(1):27–32.

Lynch TH, Martínez-Piñeiro L, Plas E, et al. European Association of Urology: EAU guidelines on urological trauma. Eur Urol 2005;47(1):1–15.

Malcolm JB, Derweesh IH, Mehrazin R, et al. Nonoperative management of blunt renal trauma: Is routine early follow-up imaging necessary? BMC Urol 2008;8:11.

Morey AF, Metro MJ, Carney KJ, et al. Consensus on genitourinary trauma: External genitalia. BJU Int 2004;94(4):507–15.

Phonsombat S, Master VA, McAninch JW. Penetrating external genital trauma: A 30-year single institution experience. J Urol 2008;180 (1):192–5; discussion 195–196.

Santucci RA, Fisher MB. The literature increasingly supports expectant (conservative) management of renal trauma: A systematic review. J Trauma 2005;59(2):493–503.

Santucci RA, Wessells H, Bartsch G, et al. Evaluation and management of renal injuries: Consensus statement of the renal trauma subcommittee. BJU Int 2004;93(7):937–54.

Prostatitis

Method of

Andrea Gallina, MD, Umberto Capitanio, MD, and Pierre I. Karakiewicz, MD

The clinical entity termed *prostatitis* affects 2% to 10% of men during their lifetime. Moreover, prostatitis symptoms are the most common cause for urologic consultation in men 50 years of age. The definition of prostatitis includes a large variety of clinical and nonclinical entities with a common underlying background. To standardize the diagnostics and the therapeutic approaches, the National Institutes of Health (NIH) proposed a classification system of prostatitis syndromes. It consists of four categories that reflect the wide variety of clinical manifestations of this syndrome (Box 1).

Category I: Acute Bacterial Prostatitis

Acute bacterial prostatitis affects 2% to 5% of prostatitis patients. It typically represents an ascending infection of the prostate with uropathogenic bacteria (*Escherichia coli, Klebsiella* spp., *Enterobacter* spp., *Serratia marcescens, Pseudomonas aeruginosa*). The classic presentation includes systemic (fever, chills and malaise) and local symptoms. Local symptoms consist of dysuria and perineal and prostatic pain, and they may be associated with complete or partial bladder outlet obstruction (urinary frequency, incomplete emptying, urgency, hesitancy, or retention). The onset may be sudden. The severity of systemic symptoms determines the need for hospitalization.

On history, recent urinary tract infections and urologic instrumentation (e.g., prostate biopsies, urinary catheters) should be ruled out. A gentle digital rectal examination (DRE) (to avoid local or systemic exacerbation of symptoms) assesses the extent of tenderness (acute infection), and rules out masses (abscess formation or associated prostatic or nonprostatic lesions). Postvoid residual is best assessed ultrasonically, because passage of catheters should be avoided. Presence of significant residual (>20% of voided volume) represents a relative indication for catheter drainage. Size 14 F or smaller catheters represent a valid alternative for suprapubic drainage. Urinalysis, midstream specimen for urine culture, and blood cultures (if systemic symptoms are present) complete the assessment.

Patients with systemic symptoms usually require hospitalization. Intravenous antibiotics (ampicillin and gentamicin) and hydration represent the mainstay of therapy. Ciprofloxacin and levofloxacin are alternatives if allergies or other contraindications exist. Once the patient is afebrile for 24 hours or according to blood culture results, oral fluoroquinolones or trimethoprim-sulfamethoxazole (TMP-SMX) may be initiated. Persistent fever and symptoms after 48 hours of IV antibiotic therapy can indicate an abscess formation, which may be identified with computed tomography (CT), magnetic resonance imaging (MRI), or transrectal ultrasonography. Antibiotic-refractory prostatic abscesses might require drainage with transurethral prostatic resection. Periprostatic abscesses may be drained transrectally.

Category I prostatitis represents a complicated urinary tract infection (UTI). Once symptoms have subsided and antibiotic therapy has been completed, a careful investigation of the upper and lower urinary tract is in order to identify any potentially predisposing causes. Imaging studies (ultrasound, CT, MRI), cystoscopy, and urodynamic studies can reveal an underlying cause, such as prostatic hypertrophy with urinary retention, bladder stone or diverticulum, or urethral stricture, among others.

Category II: Chronic Bacterial Prostatitis

NIH category II prostatitis is defined as a chronic or persistent pathogenic infection (culture proven) of the prostate without systemic symptoms. It accounts for 2% to 5% of patients with prostatitis. It is characterized by intermittent episodes of cystitis-like urinary symptoms, which only rarely involve appreciable discomfort or pain. Recurrent infectious episodes are highly suggestive of chronic bacterial prostatitis, especially if the same pathogen is documented in either a midstream urine specimen or a postprostatic massage urine specimen. *E. coli* (which represents 80% of the infectious agents), *Klebsiella* species, *P. aeruginosa*, and *Proteus* species represent the most commonly seen pathogens.

History and physical and laboratory examinations are virtually the same as those for category I prostatitis. The more protruded nature of category II prostatitis requires 4 to 8 weeks of antimicrobials (fluoroquinolones or TMP-SMX). This therapy is effective in 60% to 80% of patients. However, in cases of recurrent infections, long-term (3–6 months) antibiotic therapy is an alternative treatment. Other modalities have been investigated (for example intraprostatic injection of antibiotics) but have met with limited success.

Category III: Chronic Nonbacterial Prostatitis/Chronic Pelvic Pain Syndrome

Category III prostatitis (CP/CPPS) accounts for 90% to 95% of prostatitis cases and is the most challenging subgroup. Symptoms include pelvic or perineal (or both) pain or discomfort, as well as urinary or ejaculatory symptoms. Pain may be perineal, suprapublic, coccygeal, rectal, urethral, or testicular or scrotal. Urinary frequency, dysuria, urgency, or incomplete emptying and ejaculatory pain affect a significant proportion of patients. Ejaculatory pain suggests worse prognosis. Presence or absence of inflammatory cells in the ejaculate distinguishes between category IIIA (inflammatory) and category IIIB (noninflammatory) prostatitis. However, the clinical presentation and therapeutic approaches are the same for these two groups, and the reliability of this distinction is suboptimal. Only in up to 5% of patients is a pathogen successfully isolated from urine or semen.

The clinical heterogeneity of category III prostatitis and the absence of a diagnostic marker add complexity to the classification and treatment of this syndrome. A multifactorial etiology, which includes infectious, traumatic, inflammatory, hormonal, neurologic, and psychological triggers, is the most likely cause.

DIAGNOSIS

The evaluation of patients with category III prostatitis should include a detailed history (focusing on previous infections, trauma, surgery, or neurologic problems). It should be complemented with the NIH Chronic Prostatitis Symptom Index (NIH-CPSI) questionnaire, which is a standardized assessment of the type and severity of symptoms. Physical examination should include the same elements as in categories I and II prostatitis. Urine analysis and midstream culture are mandatory. Urinary cytology is recommended to rule out irritative symptoms of bladder cancer. Urine flow rate and residual urine determination can also help in the diagnostic work-up. In rare instances, abdominal, pelvic, or neurologic imaging, urodynamic studies, cystoscopy, or prostate-specific antigen testing may be useful.

In most men, the disease has a protracted natural history. Symptom severity predicts recurrence in 30% of men, and previous symptoms predict recurrence in 50% of men. Unfortunately, in most category III prostatitis patients, the cause of pelvic pain cannot be identified. Thus, the diagnosis of CP/CPPS remains a diagnosis of exclusion.

TREATMENT

Several treatments have been investigated and studied for category III prostatitis, with mixed results (Figure 1). These include α-blockers, antibiotics, nonsteroidal anti-inflammatory drugs (NSAIDs), and pentosan polysulfate, among others.

Mehik's group tested the efficacy of an α-blocker, alfuzosin (Uroxatral)[1] 5 mg, against placebo for symptom relief in 70 patients. At 6 months, the pain score was lower in the alfuzosin group ($P = 0.02$). Similar results were obtained by Cheah and colleagues in a cohort of 86 patients treated with terazosin (Hytrin),[1] with dose escalation from 1 to 5 mg/day compared with placebo. The α-blocker significantly improved the quality of life and significantly reduced pain at 14 weeks ($P = 0.03$). Nickel and colleagues randomized 58 men younger than 55 years to 0.4 mg tamsulosin (Flomax)[1] or placebo. At 45 days, tamsulosin significantly reduced symptoms. However, these benefits were not always replicated, especially in pretreated men.

---

[1]Not FDA approved for this indication.

CURRENT DIAGNOSIS

Category I (Acute Bacterial Prostatitis)

- History
- Physical examination (including gentle DRE)
- Urinalysis
- Urine culture
- Blood cultures (if systemic symptoms are present)
- Postvoid residual

Category II (Chronic Bacterial Prostatitis)

- History
- Physical examination
- Urinalysis
- Urine culture
- Postprostatic massage urine culture
- Evaluation of complicated UTI (optional)

Category III (Chronic Pelvic Pain Syndrome)

- History
- Physical examination
- NIH-Chronic Prostatitis Symptom Index (NIH-CPSI) questionnaire
- Urinalysis
- Midstream culture
- Optional tests (cytology, urine flow, postvoid residual, etc.)

Category IV (Asymptomatic Inflammatory Prostatitis)

- No further evaluation

Abbreviations: DRE = digital rectal examination; NIH = National Institutes of Health; UTI = urinary tract infection.

CURRENT THERAPY

Category I (Acute Bacterial Prostatitis)

- Admission
- Intravenous antibiotics (ampicillin or gentamicin)
- Bladder drainage, if urinary retention
- Oral antibiotics for 3 to 4 weeks (fluoroquinolones or TMP-SMX)

Category II (Chronic Bacterial Prostatitis)

- Outpatient treatment
- Antibiotics for 4 to 8 weeks (fluoroquinolones or TMP-SMX)
- Long-term antibiotic therapy

Category III (Chronic Pelvic Pain Syndrome)

- Antibiotics for 4 to 6 weeks (fluoroquinolone or TMP-SMX)
- α-Blockers (e.g., tamsulosin [Flomax],[1] alfuzosin [Uroxatral],[1] terazosin [Hytrin][1])
- Anti-inflammatory medications
- Finasteride (Proscar),[1] pentosan polysulfate (Elmiron),[1] and phytotherapies (e.g., cernilton,[7] quercetin[7])
- Nonpharmacologic therapies (biofeedback, pelvic floor training, thermal treatments)
- Repeat treatment if relief is noted.
- Combine therapies if partial relief is noted.

Category IV (Asymptomatic Inflammatory Prostatitis)

- No treatments

[1]Not FDA approved for this indication.
[7]Available as dietary supplement.
Abbreviation: TMP-SMX = trimethoprim-sulfamethoxazole.

A 4- to 6-week trial of antibiotics is one of the key management options for patients with category III prostatitis, despite absence of benefit in placebo-controlled trials. Lack of efficacy at 6 and 12 weeks was shown by Nickel's group, who randomized 80 patients with category III prostatitis to either levofloxacin or placebo for 6 weeks. Alexander's group recapitulated these findings with ciprofloxacin.

NSAIDs were tested in a placebo-controlled trial of 161 patients, Rofecoxib (Vioxx) (50 mg) significantly improved pain and NIH-CPSI scores. It has been withdrawn from the market.

Pentosan polysulfate (Elmiron)[1] was tested in a placebo-controlled, randomized trial of 100 men. Three daily 100-mg doses of Elmiron for 16 weeks resulted in a significant improvement in NIH-CPSI quality-of-life scores.

[1]Not FDA approved for this indication.

Several other therapeutic approaches are available. These include prostatic massage, which should be considered once or twice weekly, in men who report some degree of symptom relief. Finasteride (Proscar)[1] 5 mg daily and phytotherapy (e.g., cernilton[7] and quercetin[7]) showed some, albeit limited, efficacy. Tricyclic antidepressants (amitriptyline [Elavil][1]), anticholinergics (oxybutynin [Ditropan][1]), anticonvulsants, lifestyle changes (e.g., nutrition, stress reduction), biofeedback, pelvic floor training, and thermal therapy reduced symptoms in some category III prostatitis patients. The use of

[1]Not FDA approved for this indication.
[7]Available as dietary supplements.

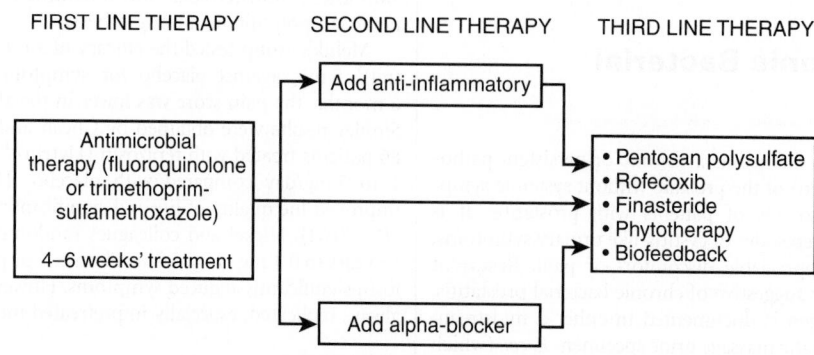

FIGURE 1. Management of NIH category III prostatitis.

allopurinol has been reported to alleviate symptoms of CP, but further evaluation is required. Similarly, biofeedback, acupuncture, electromagnetic stimulation, immune and neuromodulating agents, muscle relaxants and pudendal nerve modulation have been suggested. Although invasive procedures have been advocated for CP/CPPS patients, surgery (including transurethral resection, microwave thermotherapy, or needle ablation) should be considered only as last therapeutic options. The multitude of trials addressing CP/CPPS patients emphasizes the high failure rate (~66%) of sequential monotherapy. It suggests the need for structured assessment of multimodality approaches.

Category IV: Asymptomatic Inflammatory Prostatitis

Category IV prostatitis is defined as incidental observation of leukocytes in prostatic secretions or tissue obtained during evaluation for other disorders, (e.g., leukocytes noted in prostate biopsies performed for elevated prostate-specific antigen (PSA]). Epidemiologic studies estimate the prevalence of category IV prostatitis to be as high as 32.2% in a population of men with elevated PSA levels. Category IV prostatitis needs no further evaluation or treatment.

Acknowledgments

Pierre I. Karakiewicz is partially supported by the Fonds de la Recherche en Santé du Québec, the Centre hospitalier de l'Université de Montréal (CHUM) Foundation, the Department of Surgery, and Les Urologues Associés du CHUM.

REFERENCES

Clemens JQ, Meenan RT, O'Keeffe-Rosetti MC, et al. Prevalence of prostatitislike symptoms in a managed care population. J Urol 2006;176(2): 593–6.

Dimitrakov JD, Kaplan SA, Kroenke K, et al. Management of chronic prostatitis/chronic pelvic pain syndrome: an evidence-based approach. Urology 2006;67(5):881–8.

Fowler JE Jr. Antimicrobial therapy for bacterial and nonbacterial prostatitis. Urology 2002;60(6 Suppl):24–6.

Habermacher GM, Chason JT, Schaeffer AJ. Prostatitis/chronic pelvic pain syndrome. Annu Rev Med 2006;57:195–206.

Krieger JN, Egan KJ, Ross SO, et al. Chronic pelvic pains represent the most prominent urogenital symptoms of "chronic prostatitis." Urology 1996;48 (5):715–21.

Krieger JN, Nyberg L Jr, Nickel JC. NIH consensus definition and classification of prostatitis. JAMA 1999;282(3):236–7.

Krieger JN, Ross SO, Riley DE. Chronic prostatitis: Epidemiology and role of infection. Urology 2002;60(6 Suppl.):8–12.

Litwin MS, McNaughton-Collins M, Fowler FJ Jr, et al. The National Institutes of Health chronic prostatitis symptom index: Development and validation of a new outcome measure. Chronic Prostatitis Collaborative Research Network. J Urol 1999;162(2):369–75.

Nickel JC. Treatment of chronic prostatitis/chronic pelvic pain syndrome. Int J Antimicrob Agents 2008;31:S112–6.

Pontari MA, Ruggieri MR. Mechanisms in prostatitis/chronic pelvic pain syndrome. J Urol 2004;172(3):839–45.

Rothman I, Stanford JL, Kuniyuki A, Berger RE. Self-report of prostatitis and its risk factors in a random sample of middle-aged men. Urology 2004;64 (5):876–9.

Schaeffer AJ, Datta NS, Fowler JE Jr, et al. Overview summary statement: Diagnosis and management of chronic prostatitis/chronic pelvic pain syndrome (CP/CPPS). Urology 2002;60(6 Suppl):1–4.

Wagenlehner FM, Weidner W, Sorgel F, Naber KG. The role of antibiotics in chronic bacterial prostatitis. Int J Antimicrob Agents 2005;26(1): 1–7.

Benign Prostatic Hyperplasia

Method of
Gopal H. Badlani, MD, and Matthew E. Karlovsky, MD

Epidemiology

Bladder outlet obstruction (BOO) secondary to benign prostatic hyperplasia (BPH) is one of the most common medical conditions in older men and represents up to a 40% clinical risk for urinary retention in a man's lifetime. It is the most prevalent condition in the aging male, affecting 14 million men in the United States, with an annual cost of $4 billion to treat. Age and normal androgenic function are two of the better established risk factors. Whereas BPH is rare before the age of 40, the prevalence of histologic BPH at autopsy is 50% by 60 years of age and 90% by 85 years of age. Approximately 40% of males 70 years of age or older have lower urinary tract symptoms (LUTS) secondary to BPH, and with age, the prevalence increases. Symptomatically, approximately 25% of 55-year-old men experience decreased urinary flow rate and other symptoms of BPH. By 75 years of age, the appearance of this symptom increases to 50%. Age, however, is not a causative factor of BOO. Although the risk for developing symptoms from BPH doubles for each decade of life between 60 and 90 years of age, clinical symptoms of the individual patient do not necessarily progress with age. BPH is more commonly diagnosed because of increased life expectancy and a greater tendency today to seek medical advice at an earlier disease stage.

Normal androgenic function is required for development of BPH. Both androgenic and estrogenic hormonal stimulation can induce prostatic hypertrophy. Other factors, such as race, sexual activity, smoking, socioeconomic status, vasectomy, alcohol intake, and diet, have been implicated in BPH development. Identifying men at clinical risk for BPH and its progression has clinical usefulness in selecting the appropriate intervention when necessary.

Pathophysiology

The pathophysiology of BPH is poorly understood because no direct correlation can be made between prostatic glandular enlargement and the symptomatology of BPH. Because the condition is rare in those younger than 40 years of age and does not develop in castrated men, it is accepted that BPH development requires aging and functional testes for androgen production. BPH is believed to originate in the transitional zone of the prostate, which surrounds the prostatic urethra between the bladder neck and the verumontanum, and is progressive.

Both a static and a dynamic component are involved in BPH development. The static component relates to epithelial and stromal cell proliferation in the prostatic transitional zone (TZ); enlargement is evident as median or lateral lobe hypertrophy. Proliferation is induced by testosterone and its biologically active conversion product, dihydrotestosterone. Conversion of testosterone to dihydrotestosterone occurs via the enzyme 5α-reductase. Two forms of this enzyme have been described, type 1 and type 2. Type 1 is present in liver, skin, and other organs. Type 2 is present in urogenital tissues. Individuals lacking 5α-reductase type 2 do not develop genitalia and prostates.

Conversely, the dynamic component relates to prostatic smooth muscle. High concentrations of α_1-adrenergic receptors occur in the prostatic capsule and bladder neck. An increase in smooth muscle tone is responsible for increased urethral resistance and pressure. Pharmacologic blockade with α_1 antagonists blocks prostatic smooth muscle contraction and decreases urethral resistance and pressure, subsequently relaxing the dynamic component of BPH.

Symptoms

The diagnosis of BPH is presumptive, based on symptoms. These symptoms, commonly referred to as lower urinary tract symptoms (LUTS), are not specific for BPH. LUTS include frequency, retention, intermittency, decreased force of stream (FOS), straining, urgency, and nocturia. Individuals with LUTS should be carefully assessed to determine the cause, to confirm diagnosis of BPH, and to exclude other bladder and prostate processes. Normal prostate size on digital rectal examination (DRE) does not rule out a diagnosis of BPH because palpable prostate size does not correlate with degree of obstruction or severity of LUTS. However, the odds of having moderate to severe symptoms are five times higher for men with enlarged prostates compared with those with normal prostates. Symptoms of BPH are difficult to assess and quantify, yet they are the keys to proper diagnosis and treatment. Because the vast majority of procedures performed for BPH are to provide symptomatic relief, it is necessary to quantify the level of interference in the quality of life of the patient. Assessment of interference on quality of life can be reliably accomplished using the well-validated International Prostate Symptom Score (IPSS) (Figure 1). Symptoms based on overall score are classified as mild (0 to 7), moderate (8 to 19), and severe (20 to 35). The subjective impact of these symptoms on overall quality of life must also be taken into account. The patient with a severe-range IPSS may feel the symptoms are less bothersome than a patient with a lower IPSS, and this subjective impact on quality of life can direct therapeutic options.

Name: _____   Date: _____

	Not at all	Less than 1 time in 5	Less than half the time	About half the time	More than half the time	Almost always	Your score
Incomplete emptying Over the past month, how often have you had a sensation of not emptying your bladder completely after you finish urinating?	0	1	2	3	4	5	
Frequency Over the past month, how often have you had to urinate again less than two hours after you finished urinating?	0	1	2	3	4	5	
Intermittency Over the past month, how often have you found you stopped and started again several times when you urinated?	0	1	2	3	4	5	
Urgency Over the past month, how difficult have you found it to postpone urination?	0	1	2	3	4	5	
Weak stream Over the past month, how often have you had a weak urinary stream?	0	1	2	3	4	5	
Straining Over the past month, how often have you had to push or strain to begin urination?	0	1	2	3	4	5	

	None	1 time	2 times	3 times	4 times	5 times or more	Your score
Nocturia Over the past month, how many times did you most typically get up to urinate from the time you went to bed until the time you got up in the morning?	0	1	2	3	4	5	

Total IPSS score	

Quality of life due to urinary symptoms	Delighted	Pleased	Mostly satisfied	Mixed—about equally satisfied and dissatisfied	Mostly dissatisfied	Unhappy	Terrible
If you were to spend the rest of your life with your urinary condition the way it is now, how would you feel about that?	0	1	2	3	4	5	6

FIGURE 1. International Prostate Symptom Score (IPSS).

Diagnosis

Diagnosis of BPH relies on an accurate medical history eliciting the specific voiding complaints, as well as quantification of these symptoms using the IPSS. Other possible causes of LUTS also must be ruled out, including urinary tract infection (UTI), urolithiasis, diabetes, urethral stricture, overactive or neurogenic bladder, prostate/bladder cancer, or congestive heart failure. Medications that can exacerbate obstructive symptoms include tricyclic antidepressants, anticholinergic agents, diuretics, narcotics, and first-generation antihistamines and decongestants. Physical examination should include DRE for prostatic abnormalities, such as palpable nodules, induration or irregularities of malignancy, or infection. On DRE, the posterior lobes, not the transition zone, are palpable. Abdominal examination may detect a suprapubic or low abdominal mass in a patient with BPH-induced retention. The American Urological Association and the American Cancer Society recommend all men older than age 50 receive an annual prostate-specific antigen (PSA) serum level to screen for prostate cancer. In black men or men with a family history of prostate cancer in a first-degree relative, PSA screening should begin at 40 years of age or younger. The normal range for PSA is up to 4.0 µg/mL. Other valuable laboratory data include urinalysis to rule out infection or hematuria, a serum creatinine level to determine renal function, and urine cytologic studies if irritative voiding symptoms are present. More sophisticated studies, such as urinary flow rate, postvoid residual, and pressure flow urodynamic studies, are appropriate for evaluation of men with more severe symptoms (IPSS >8) or with more complex comorbidities. These tests are often used to determine baseline function prior to initiation of therapy or to determine subsequent response to therapy. In patients who fail medical therapy, urodynamic pressure-flow studies and cystoscopy may be appropriate to evaluate the need for operative intervention and to rule out other urologic pathologies. Cystoscopy is also reserved for situations in which invasive treatment is strongly considered. If watchful waiting or noninvasive therapies are appropriate, invasive diagnostic tests are usually not necessary. The variables of importance of disease progression in an artificial neural network analysis were PSA, obstructive symptom score, and transitional zone volume. The Olmsted County study showed risk progression of acute urinary retention (AUR) with age. Overall, a 60-year-old man has a 23% chance of AUR if he survives the next 20 years. The average annual change in prostate volume was 1.6% for all ages. The annual increase was not significantly related to baseline age but was significantly related to baseline prostate volume.

Treatment

WATCHFUL WAITING

Indications for treatment of BPH rely, in large part, on the subjective nature of the symptoms. For the majority of patients with BPH, symptoms are not severe or bothersome enough to warrant long-term medical or surgical intervention. Men with an IPSS of less than 8 are usually treated with expectant management. Advising the patient toward lifestyle modifications, such as minimizing evening fluid intake, avoiding caffeine, and avoiding decongestants, anticholinergics, and other medications that impair voiding, often provides an effective resolution of symptoms. In a study of 556 men with moderate symptoms of BPH comparing outcomes following transurethral resection of the prostate (TURP) with watchful waiting for more than 3 years, 8% of men randomized to TURP and 17% of men with watchful waiting failed treatment. Treatment failure with watchful waiting was mostly because of high postvoid residuals and significant increases in IPSS symptoms. Patients who respond poorly to watchful waiting have multiple medical and surgical options for treatment of BPH.

α_1-ADRENERGIC BLOCKING AGENTS

The α_1-adrenergic antagonists have been shown in numerous randomized placebo-controlled trials to be safe and effective in the treatment of BPH. The most commonly prescribed α_1-adrenergic blockers appear to have similar safety profiles and clinical efficacy and are the common first approach for urologists. Terazosin (Hytrin) and doxazosin (Cardura) were the first α antagonists available for treatment of BPH; however, orthostatic hypotension was a significant concern, requiring careful dose titration. Tamsulosin (Flomax), a highly selective α-blocker, does not induce orthostatic hypotension and so does not require dose titration. Overall, the most common side effects include headaches, dizziness, asthenia, and drowsiness. Sexual side effects are limited to retrograde ejaculation. Alfuzosin (Uroxatral), a newer nonspecific α-blocker, has minimal vasoactive or retrograde ejaculation side effects. Table 1 provides a list for medication dosing and schedules.

5α-REDUCTASE INHIBITION

Finasteride (Proscar) and dutasteride (Avodart) are 5α-reductase inhibitors (type 1 and type 1/2, respectively) that block conversion of testosterone to dihydrotestosterone, the androgen involved in development of BPH. These medications represent the paradigm for androgen suppression of BPH. They have their greatest therapeutic effect in men with prostates greater than 40 g, and treatment for 6 months or more is usually required for a clinical response. The first randomized, multicenter, double-blind, placebo-controlled trial investigating the efficacy of finasteride demonstrated significant improvements in maximum flow rate and decreased prostatic volume. Since then, further studies have confirmed a reduced risk of acute urinary retention and surgical intervention with finasteride use. Finasteride can reduce BPH-associated hematuria. It is effective as adjuvant therapy, following other treatments, and as neoadjuvant therapy prior to minimally invasive therapy. Adverse effects include decreased libido, ejaculatory dysfunction, and gynecomastia. In the patient being monitored for prostate cancer with PSA testing, finasteride therapy must be taken into account when interpreting PSA values; finasteride decreases PSA values by 50%, leading to a false-negative result.

Efficacy of Medical Therapy

The Medical Therapy of Prostate Symptoms (MTOPS) study evaluated the efficacy of doxazosin and finasteride to determine if medical therapy delays or prevents disease progression. At 4 years, combination therapy was most effective for reducing risk of clinical

TABLE 1 Common Medications for Benign Prostatic Hyperplasia

Medication	Class	Dose	Schedule
Alfuzosin (Uroxatral)	α-1 Blocker	10 mg	Once daily
Doxazosin (Cardura)	α-1 Blocker	1–8 mg, titrated	Once daily at bedtime
Tamsulosin (Flomax)	α-1a Blocker	0.4 mg	Once daily
Terazosin (Hytrin)	α-1 Blocker	1–10 mg, titrated	Once daily at bedtime
Dutasteride (Avodart)	5-α Reductase inhibitor	0.5 mg	Once daily
Finasteride (Proscar)	5-α Reductase inhibitor	5 mg	Once daily

progression (AUR) and improving symptom score and urinary flow rate. Finasteride and combination therapy significantly reduced the risk of AUR and invasive therapy over 4 years. Monotherapy with either medication reduced symptom score and improved flow significantly, but to a lesser degree than combination therapy. Doxazosin delayed time to progression of AUR and invasive therapy but not the risk. Without treatment, the risk of BPH progression was 20% more during the trial. Risk factors for progression include baseline prostate volume (>40 g) and higher serum PSA value (>2 μg/mL).

Phytotherapy

Saw palmetto (*Serenoa repens*)[1,2] extract is the most popular phytotherapeutic agent. Its likely mechanism is inhibition of 5α-reductase. A recent meta-analysis of numerous randomized trials using saw palmetto described a mild to moderate improvement in flow and LUTS; however, because of small study sample, varying products, short treatment times, and varying outcomes, these study conclusions are difficult to interpret. Other popular preparations are African plum (*Pygeum africanum*)[1,2] and South African star grass (*Cynodon nlemfuësis*).[1,2] The former has been shown to have several in vitro effects, such as antiestrogen effects, leukotriene blockade, and inhibition of fibroblast growth factors. The latter has been shown in vitro to increase plasminogen activators, as well as to stimulate release of transforming growth factor-β, an inducer of apoptosis, yet these in vitro effects have not been shown to occur in vivo. A meta-analysis of four clinical trials of South African star grass extract, β-sitosterol, concluded that β-sitosterol improved urologic symptoms and flow rates in men.

There is no standard of care for management of patients using phytotherapy. Nor have the long-term safety effects been established. Patients should be cautioned that doses, efficacy, side effects, and drug interactions with phytotherapy are unknown. For the patient refusing medical therapy of α-blockers and 5α-reductase inhibitors, phytotherapy may be attempted as long as the patient understands the limitations of these agents. If retention, UTI, calculi, or decreased renal function occurs, phytotherapy should be discouraged and more aggressive medical and surgical management undertaken.

Minimally Invasive Therapies

The most commonly employed surgical procedure, and the gold standard for BPH, is transurethral resection of the prostate (TURP), involving endoscopic resection of the obstructive component of the prostate. TURP is highly effective, improving symptoms in up to 95% of patients. Common complications include inability to void postoperatively, clot retention, incontinence, impotence, and retrograde ejaculation. A number of new minimally invasive therapies have been developed to reduce the complications associated with TURP, as well as provide alternatives for the unfavorable surgical candidate. Most minimally invasive therapies use energy, such as radio waves, laser, ultrasound, microwaves, or electrical current.

Transurethral incision of the prostate (TUIP) involves endoscopic placement of one to two incisions into the prostate and capsule to reduce urethral constriction. This procedure is highly effective on prostate glands less than 30 g and is well documented and safe, with efficacy comparable with TURP. TUIP is associated with a 78% to 83% improvement of symptoms. Because TUIP is associated with fewer retrograde ejaculations, less morbidity, and a reoperation rate of less than 1% in 10 years, this procedure is the treatment of choice for small gland BPH in men concerned with fertility and ejaculation.

In transurethral needle ablation (TUNA), low-level energy is transferred by radiofrequency to the prostate, creating a well-defined necrotic lesion within the prostatic parenchyma while preserving the urethral mucosa. A cystoscope-like instrument with two needles set at 90 degrees from each other ablates tissue in 3 to 5 minutes when needles reach temperatures of 27° to 38°C (80° to 100°F). Urethral and rectal temperatures are also vigorously monitored as the device adjusts. Preliminary studies show an increase in peak flow and a decrease in symptom score following TUNA, with no major complications. Transient urinary retention is reported in 10% to 40% of patients. In a prospective study, TURP was superior to TUNA in increasing flow rates but demonstrated comparable improved symptoms at 1 year postoperatively. Transurethral microwave thermotherapy (TUMT) heats prostatic transitional zone tissue to between 60° and 80°C (140° to 176°F), inducing tissue damage. Thermotherapy preferentially destroys smooth muscle by coagulative necrosis while water-conductive cooling of the urethral mucosa preserves periurethral tissues. Although prospective studies indicate that TURP produces more pronounced urinary improvements versus TUMT, thermotherapy consistently improves symptom scores by 75% and increases peak flow rates by 75%. Furthermore, TUMT is a procedure done under local anesthesia. Retrograde ejaculation and urinary retention with prolonged catheterization occurs in greater than one third of patients.

Ultimately, therapeutic decisions depend in large part on symptom scores. Men with low symptom scores without bother are appropriately managed through watchful waiting. As scores increase, or if progression with clinical morbidity develops, more aggressive management is appropriate.

REFERENCES

Bhargava S, Canda AE, Chapple CR. A rational approach to benign hyperplasia evaluation: Recent advances. Curr Opin Urol 2004;14:1–6.

Djavan B, Waldert M, Ghawidel C, Marberger M. Benign prostatic hyperplasia progression and its impact on treatment. Curr Opin Urol 2004;14:45–50.

Fong YK, Milani S, Djavan B. Role of phytotherapy in men with lower urinary tract symptoms. Curr Opin Urol 2005;15:45–8.

Hoffman RM, MacDonald R, Monga M, Wilt TJ. Transurethral microwave thermotherapy vs. transurethral resection for treating benign prostatic hyperplasia: A systematic review. BJU Int 2004;94:1031–6.

Walsh PC, Retik A, Vaughan D, editors. Campbell's Urology. 8th ed Philadelphia: Saunders Elsevier Science; 2002.

Erectile Dysfunction

Method of
Luciano Kolodny, MD

The term *erectile dysfunction* (ED) is relatively new, having replaced *impotence* approximately a decade ago. ED is defined as the "inability of the male to attain or maintain an erection sufficient for satisfactory sexual intercourse." ED affects millions of men worldwide with implications that go far beyond sexual activity alone. ED is now recognized as a sentinel event in cardiovascular disease, diabetes mellitus (DM), and depression. It can also be damaging to interpersonal relationships and self-esteem.

Epidemiology

The Massachusetts Male Aging Study is one of the pivotal studies on the prevalence of ED. Between 1987 and 1989, men between the ages of 40 and 70 years received questionnaires inquiring about several aspects of their sexual health. Of the 1790 men who received the questionnaires, 1290 responded. They revealed that 52% of them had some degree of dysfunction, 17% with minimal, 25% with

---

[1]Not FDA approved for this indication.
[2]Available as a dietary supplement.

moderate, and almost 10% with complete absence of erectile function. It also showed the extremely detrimental link between coronary artery disease (CAD), DM, and ED. A few years later another group used the same patient database and followed up on these subjects. The risk of ED was 26 cases per 1000 men annually, which increased with age, lower education, DM, heart disease, and hypertension.

Physiology of Erection

The penile erection requires intact vascular, neuronal, and hormonal systems. The intricate details of this process are beyond the scope of this article, but in summary, after any sensorial stimulation, which can be visual, tactile, auditory, or olfactory, nitric oxide (NO) and other neurotransmitters are released at the cavernous nerve terminals. The endothelial cells then release vasoactive relaxing factors, which lead to vasodilatation of the penile blood vessels and increased blood flow. As blood flow increases, compression of the subtunical venular plexuses will substantially decrease venous outflow and finally cause the penis to change from flaccid to erect (Figure 1).

NO is the principal neurotransmitter involved in penile erection, but other vasoactive substances such as vasoactive intestinal peptide, neuropeptide Y, calcitonin gene-related peptide (CGRP), substance P, and serotonin also play roles. High levels of intrapenile NO facilitate the relaxation of intracavernosal trabeculae, thereby maximizing blood flow and penile erection. Nonadrenergic, noncholinergic neurons have been found to release NO, leading to increased production of cyclic guanosine monophosphate (cGMP). Through a series of reactions, cGMP will lead to relaxation of the smooth muscle, directly impacting the ability to go from a flaccid to an erect penile state. The return from erect to flaccid requires the hydrolysis of cGMP to guanosine monophosphate (GMP) by phosphodiesterase 5 (PDE5) (see Figure 1).

Testosterone and Erectile Function

Testosterone provides intrapenile nitrous oxide synthase (NOS), which has an important role in enhancing the production of NO, subsequent local vasodilatation, and penile erection. There is no correlation between serum testosterone levels and the degree of ED. However, hypogonadal men may experience significantly reduced libido. Hypogonadism is associated with decreased self-esteem, depression, osteoporosis, insulin resistance, increased fat mass, decreased lean body mass, and cognitive dysfunction.

Pathophysiology of Erectile Dysfunction

ED can be classified as psychogenic, organic (hormonal, vascular, drug-induced, or neurogenic), or mixed psychogenic and organic. Up to 80% of ED cases have an organic origin. The most common cause of ED is vascular disease (Box 1).

Atherosclerosis is the most common cause of vasculogenic ED, whereas endothelial damage is the most common mechanism. Aging is a well-known risk factor for ED, and it is hypothesized that there are alterations in the levels of NO that occur as a consequence of the aging endothelium. Additionally, chronic illness, depression, and lack of a sexual partner are all prevalent in this age population.

Chronic tobacco use is a major risk factor for the development of vasculogenic ED because of its effects on the vascular endothelium. Additionally, blood nicotine levels rise after smoking, which increases sympathetic tone in the penis and leads to nicotine-induced, smooth-muscle contraction in the cavernosal body. Chronic smoking also leads to decreased penile NOS activity and neuronal NOS content.

DM is a major risk factor for ED. In the Massachusetts Male Aging Study, the diabetic subset had a threefold increased prevalence of ED compared with nondiabetic subjects (28% versus 9.6%). In the same study, the overall incidence rate of ED was 26 cases per 1000 man-years in nondiabetics and 50 cases per 1000 man-years in the diabetic population. The pathogenesis of ED in the diabetic patient is related to accelerated atherosclerosis, alterations in the corporal erectile tissue, and neuropathy.

Hypertension is another major risk factor for ED. Whether ED in patients with hypertension is related to the disease itself or to the use of antihypertensive medications has been debated for years. In a study looking at 104 subjects, the differences in incidence or severity of ED were minor between distinct types of antihypertensive medications or the number of agents being used simultaneously. This favors the concept that antihypertensive agents as well as the disease itself contribute to the appearance of ED. There are, however, classes of antihypertensive medications that are notorious for their negative impact on erectile function such as thiazides and β-blockers. The only β-blocker not associated with significant incidence of ED is carvedilol (Coreg).

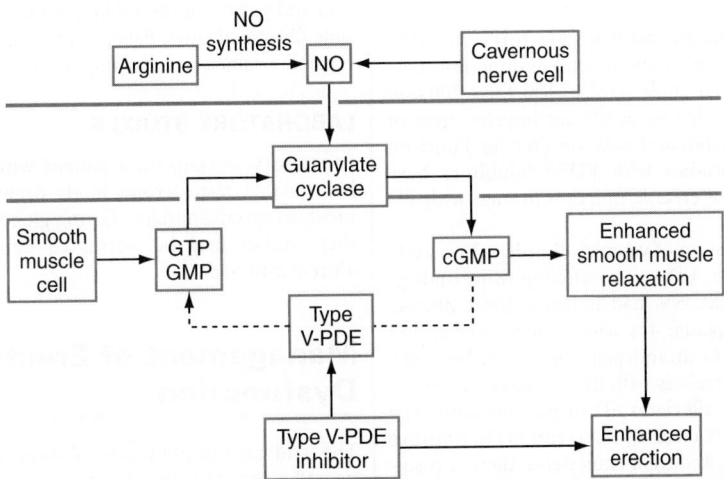

FIGURE 1. The biochemical process involved in erections and the mechanism of action of sildenafil citrate (Viagra). The cavernous nerves (S2-S4) innervate the penis and release NO. NO stimulates the production of cGMP in the smooth muscle cells of the penis. cGMP is directly responsible for increasing smooth muscle relaxation, which leads to increased arterial inflow and an erection. When cGMP is metabolized by PDE5, the penis undergoes detumescence. Sildenafil citrate (Viagra) inhibits PDE5 and increases the available cGMP, thereby leading to an enhanced erection. cGMP = cyclic guanosine monophosphate; NO = nitric oxide; PDE5 = phosphodiesterase 5.

BOX 1   Classification of Erectile Dysfunction

Endocrine
- Hypogonadism
- Hyperprolactinemia

Drug Induced
- β-Blockers
- Calcium channel blockers
- Alcohol
- Nicotine
- Antiandrogens
- Cocaine
- Heroin
- Marijuana
- Cimetidine
- Metoclopramide
- Antidepressant medications
- Antipsychotic medications

Vascular
- Coronary artery disease
- Peripheral vascular disease
- Hypertension
- Diabetes mellitus

Psychogenic
- Depression
- Performance anxiety

Neurogenic
- Spinal cord injury
- Neuropathy (diabetic, hypertensive)
- Cerebrovascular disease
- Radical prostatectomy
- Pelvic surgery

Multifactorial
- Aging
- End-stage renal disease
- Pelvic trauma (neurogenic and vasculogenic)
- Diabetes mellitus (neurogenic, vasculogenic, drug induced)

Hyperlipidemia is another etiologic factor for ED. It is believed to contribute to ED by its relationship to endothelial dysfunction. One study showed that decreasing total cholesterol to less than 200 mg/dL by using atorvastatin (Lipitor) led to significant improvement of ED as measured by the International Index of Erectile Function (IIEF). A number of clinical studies with PDE5 inhibitors have shown significant improvement of erectile function in men with ED and hyperlipidemia.

ED may be a sentinel manifestation of vascular disorders. In a study of 980 subjects seeking ED advice, 18% were suffering from undiagnosed hypertension, 16% had DM, 5% had ischemic heart disease, 15% had benign prostatic hyperplasia, 4% had prostate cancer, and 1% had depression. ED can itself be an independent marker for CAD. In addition, the extent of CAD correlates with the prevalence of ED.

Cardiovascular risk reduction alleviates ED in patients with type 2 DM. In a study in which patients received interventions to improve hemoglobin A1C, blood pressure, and total cholesterol, there was significant improvement in the International Index of Erectile Function-5 (IIEF-5), suggesting that improved glycemic control in men with diabetes may lead to an improvement in ED. A study by Thompson revealed significant trends regarding the association of ED and subsequent cardiovascular disease in a retrospective analysis of data from 9457 men. A study published in 2009 looked at the association between ED and the long-term risk of CAD. Results showed that when ED occurred in a younger man, it was associated with a marked increase in the risk of future cardiac events, whereas in older men it appeared to be of little prognostic significance.

Quantification of the Severity of Erectile Dysfunction and Improvement

There are several tools designed to assess the severity of ED, as well as to measure the efficacy of different treatments. We discuss three different measures, the IIEF, the Sexual Encounter Profile (SEP), and the Global Assessment Question (GAQ) (Box 2).

PATIENT HISTORY

When assessing sexual dysfunction, it is important to inquire about a number of issues:

1. Differentiate between decreased libido and ED: assess whether the patient has one or both
2. Tobacco use: type, amount, duration
3. Alcohol intake
4. History of depression or anxiety disorder
5. Presence of social/relationship stressors
6. Ability to have erections while masturbating versus when with partner
7. List of all prescription, over-the-counter, and herbal medications
8. Knowledge of whether nocturnal erections are present
9. History of drug use: marijuana, cocaine, other recreational drugs
10. History of genitourinary trauma
11. History of prostatic disease, or possible related symptoms
12. History of hypertension, hyperlipidemia, CAD, peripheral vascular disease, cerebrovascular disease
13. History of DM
14. History of spinal cord injury
15. History of penile plaques: possible Peyronie's disease
16. Frequency of intercourse or attempted intercourse
17. Ability to ejaculate

PHYSICAL EXAMINATION

The physical examination should include a careful testicular examination to assess testicular size, asymmetries, presence of hernias, or varicoceles. Additionally, a digital rectal examination to assess the prostatic size, consistency, and presence of nodules is warranted. Penile inspection and palpation should be performed, with special attention to possible fibrotic plaques. Palpation and auscultation of femoral arteries for possible bruits is another important part of the examination.

LABORATORY STUDIES

Laboratory workup on a patient with ED should include total and bioavailable testosterone levels drawn in the morning, prolactin, prostate-specific antigen, fasting glucose, and fasting lipid panel. Further studies may be warranted depending on the results of the aforementioned.

Management of Erectile Dysfunction

The landscape of ED was revolutionized with the introduction of sildenafil citrate (Viagra), the first oral medication for the treatment of this condition. Since then, oral agents have become the preferred mode of treatments by patients in surveys worldwide. There are three oral agents that inhibit PDE5 currently on the market:

1. Sildenafil citrate (Viagra)
2. Vardenafil (Levitra)
3. Tadalafil (Cialis)

BOX 2 Tools Used to Quantify Erectile Dysfunction Severity

Tools used in the quantification of the severity of erectile dysfunction (ED) include the International Index of Erectile Function (IIEF), the Sexual Encounter Profile (SEP), and the Global Assessment Question (GAQ).

International Index of Erectile Function

The IIEF is a standardized questionnaire designed to measure ED and detect treatment-related changes. It is a 15-item questionnaire addressing five different domains: erectile function, orgasmic function, sexual desire, intercourse satisfaction, and overall satisfaction. The IIEF is the most frequently used efficacy measurement employed in ED drug trials. Using a scale from 1 (never/almost never) to 5 (almost always/always), men grade each domain. It is very sensitive and specific, and has been validated in 20 languages to assess treatment-related changes in sexual function. The questions 1–5 and 15 are used to quantify erectile dysfunction severity and are as follows:

1. How often were you able to get an erection during sexual activity?
2. When you had erections with sexual stimulation, how often were your erections hard enough for penetration?
3. When you attempted sexual intercourse, how often were you able to penetrate (enter) your partner?
4. During sexual intercourse, how often were you able to maintain your erection after you had penetrated (entered) your partner?
5. During sexual intercourse, how difficult was it to maintain your erection to completion of intercourse?
6. How do you rate your confidence that you could get and keep an erection?

And it is scored as follows:

26–30	Normal ED
22–25	Mild ED
17–21	Mild to moderate ED
11–16	Moderate ED
≤10	Severe ED

Sexual Encounter Profile

SEP is a five-question survey provided to patients with ED in clinical studies of oral therapies. The survey is completed after each sexual attempt. The questions are as follows:

1. Were you able to achieve at least some erection?
2. Were you able to insert your penis into your partner's vagina?
3. Did your erection last long enough to have successful intercourse?
4. Were you satisfied with the hardness of your erection?
5. Were you satisfied with the overall sexual experience?

Answers to questions 2 and 3 are the ones most often used in the literature.

Global Assessment Questions

GAQ is usually administered at the end of the treatment period during efficacy studies.
Question 1: Has the treatment taken during the study improved your erections?
Question 2: If yes, has the treatment improved your ability to engage in sexual activity?
This is very subjective, and its responses tend to be valued less than SEP and IIEF.

All three drugs work by inhibiting PDE5, which maintains intracavernosal levels of cGMP, subsequently producing vasodilatation and penile erection (see Figure 1).

SILDENAFIL CITRATE (VIAGRA)

Sildenafil citrate (Viagra) is an orally active, potent, and selective inhibitor of cGMP-specific PDE5. The predominant phosphodiesterase isoform in the penile tissue is type 5. The selectivity of sildenafil citrate (Viagra) for PDE5 is approximately 4000-fold greater than its selectivity for phosphodiesterase 3 (PDE3), the isoform involved in the control of cardiac contractility. Sildenafil citrate (Viagra) is absorbed rapidly after oral administration, with an absolute bioavailability of 40%. The time of maximal (T-max) plasma after oral dosing in the fasting state is between 30 and 120 minutes. A high-fat meal increases the time to peak plasma concentration by 60 minutes and reduces the peak plasma concentration by 29%. The half-life of the drug is from 3 to 5 hours. Sildenafil citrate (Viagra) is metabolized by hepatic microsomal cytochrome P450 isoenzyme 3A4 for the most part. Cytochrome P450 3A4 inhibitors, cimetidine (Tagamet), erythromycin, ketoconazole (Nizoral), and protease inhibitors may retard the metabolism of sildenafil citrate (Viagra).

The recommended dose is from 25 to 100 mg as needed approximately 1 hour before sexual activity. In some individuals, the onset of activity may be seen as early as 11 to 19 minutes, but this is not the norm. The usual starting dose is 50 mg.

The maximum recommended dose is 100 mg, and the maximum dosing frequency is once daily. A starting dose of 25 mg can be considered for patients older than age 65 years as well as for patients with severe hepatic cirrhosis or severe renal impairment.

There are more than two dozen, randomized, double-blind, placebo-controlled studies involving this agent. It produces positive results regardless of the etiology of ED. It has been studied in patients with DM, CAD, postcoronary artery bypass graft (post-CABG), spinal cord injury, depression, hypertension, prostate cancer post-prostatectomy, benign prostate enlargement post-transurethral resection of the prostate (TURP), patients on hemodialysis, as well as recipients of renal transplants. Results vary according to the underlying condition causing ED in the first place, ranging from 50% to 85%.

The most common side effects of sildenafil citrate (Viagra) include vasodilatory effects such as headaches, flushing, and nasal congestion caused by hyperemia of the nasal mucosa, as well as dyspepsia. Up to 30% of patients may get at least one side effect. Another side effect that presents on occasion is blurred or blue-green vision because of inhibition of phosphodiesterase 6 (PDE6) in the retina. It is absolutely contraindicated in men taking long-acting or short-acting nitrate drugs, and men taking any form of nitrates should be informed about the dangerous interaction.

Do not prescribe sildenafil citrate (Viagra) to patients with unstable CAD who need nitrates. Assess the need for ordering treadmill testing in select patients. Initial monitoring of blood pressure (BP) after the administration of sildenafil citrate (Viagra) may be indicated in men with complicated congestive heart failure (CHF). α-Blockers should not be used in combination with sildenafil citrate (Viagra) because of possible orthostatic hypotension.

VARDENAFIL (LEVITRA)

Vardenafil (Levitra) is a highly potent inhibitor of PDE5. It was approved for use in the United States in late 2003. It is a more selective PDE5 inhibitor than sildenafil citrate (Viagra). The absorption of vardenafil (Levitra) is delayed by a fatty content of more than 30% in a meal. However, that does not seem to affect its effectiveness in different trials. The half-life of vardenafil (Levitra) is 4.4 to 4.8 hours, and the clinical effectiveness may be as long as 12 hours. The time for maximum plasma concentration is between 42 and 54 minutes. The first trial using the agent included 580 patients, excluding patients with spinal cord injury, radical prostatectomy, hypogonadism, thyrotoxicosis, or DM.

The successful rates of intercourse were 71% to 75% on patients taking 5 or 10 mg at a time. Those taking 20 mg had a success rate of 80%. The placebo groups had an average success rate of 30%.

Vardenafil (Levitra) has been tested in patients with type 2 DM; 452 patients were enrolled in a double-blind, placebo-controlled trial. The success rate in the vardenafil (Levitra) group ranged from 57% to 72%.

In a different study involving 736 subjects including men with DM and stable CAD, the success rates were 28% for the placebo group, 65% for those taking 5 mg, 80% for those taking 10 mg, and 85% for the 20-mg group.

Patients who were unresponsive to sildenafil citrate (Viagra) at a dose of 100 mg on several attempts were given vardenafil (Levitra) in doses of 10 and 20 mg (proved in trial). Vardenafil (Levitra) produced statistically and clinically significant results compared with placebo in men who were historically unresponsive to sildenafil citrate (Viagra). The dose that offers the best clinical results is 20 mg. It should not be taken more than once every 24 hours. Safety studies have shown no deleterious effects with long-term daily use of this drug for up to 12 months.

The most common side effects include headaches (10% to 21%), flushing (5% to 13%), rhinitis (9% to 17%), and dyspepsia (1% to 6%) because vardenafil (Levitra) does not inhibit PDE6. Unlike sildenafil citrate (Viagra), it does not produce problems of blurred vision or blue-green visual disturbances. The same warning regarding the use of nitrates as sildenafil citrate (Viagra) applies to vardenafil (Levitra). Patients taking vardenafil (Levitra) may use α-blocking agents with caution.

TADALAFIL (CIALIS)

The third oral agent of this class is tadalafil (Cialis). It has a half-life of 17.5 hours, with two thirds of patients experiencing clinical benefits of this drug up to 36 hours after its use. The clinical onset of action occurs in less than 1 hour. There is no interaction between food and alcohol on the absorption of the drug.

There have been numerous phase II and III studies in Europe, Canada, and the United States using doses of 2, 5, 10, and 25 mg of the drug in comparison with placebo. The average success rates on these studies averaged 17% for placebo, 51% for the 2-mg dose, and 80% for the other doses, as well as up to 88% on the 25-mg dose in one study. In one study looking at 216 subjects with type 2 DM, improved erections were reported in 56% to 64% of the patients.

A recent article looking at all the previously published patient data showed that among 2102 men studied in 11 randomized placebo-controlled trials lasting 12 weeks, each mean improvement in IIEF at 20 mg of tadalafil (Cialis) was 8.6. Mean positive Sexual Encounter Profile Diary Question 3 (SEP3) response was 68% versus 31% in placebo groups. Mean GAQ was 84% versus 33% in placebo group.

In a multicenter, randomized, double-blind, crossover study looking at 181 men who received either sildenafil citrate (Viagra) or tadalafil (Cialis), 73% (132) preferred tadalafil (Cialis) at 20 mg instead of sildenafil citrate (Viagra) at 50 or 100 mg.

The most clinically effective dose of tadalafil (Cialis) is 20 mg. It should be taken at least 30 minutes before intercourse. It may be used with caution in patients using α-blocking agents. Nitrates are absolutely contraindicated for use in patients taking tadalafil (Cialis). The most common side effects include headaches, dyspepsia, back pain, rhinitis, and flushing. There are no visual side effects reported. Tadalafil has most recently been studied for use on a daily basis, with doses ranging from 2.5 to 5 mg, and showed favorable results.

Use of PDE5 Inhibitors and Cardiovascular Safety

The safety and efficacy of the three currently available PDE5 inhibitors (sildenafil, tadalafil, vardenafil) have been evaluated extensively in patients with ED and concomitant CVD, hypertension, hyperlipidemia, or diabetes, with or without additional risk factors. Overall, these studies have shown similar efficacy for the three agents, resulting in significant improvement of erectile function in patients with any of these comorbid conditions, and there was no evidence of cardiovascular risk from using any of these agents. However, because ED is known to be a harbinger of cardiovascular events in some men, the presence of ED should prompt investigation and intervention for cardiovascular risk factors.

APOMORPHINE (UPRIMA)[1]

Apomorphine (Uprima)[1] is a potent emetic that acts on central dopaminergic receptors. The stimulation of central dopaminergic receptors transmits excitatory signals down the spinal cord to the sacral parasympathetic nucleus, stimulating activity of the sacral nerves supplying the penis. It has been used successfully in up to 67% of patients when administered through a sublingual preparation. Subcutaneous injections[2] of apomorphine (Uprima)[1] produce almost a 100% erectile response, but nausea and vomiting are limiting factors to this mode of administration.

The most common side effects are headache, nausea, and dizziness. Rare syncopal episodes have been reported.

PHENTOLAMINE (REGITINE)

Phentolamine (Regitine) is an α_1- and α_2-adrenergic receptor antagonist.

The sympathetic system via the release of noradrenaline (NA) is the primary determinant of cavernosal smooth muscle contraction and detumescence. A relative predominance of NA-induced contraction over NO-induced smooth muscle relaxation may contribute to ED.

In large phase III studies, 55% to 59% of patients receiving 40 and 80 mg were able to achieve vaginal penetration. Adverse effects include nasal congestion (10%), headaches (3% to 5%), dizziness (3% to 5%), tachycardia (3%), and nausea.

TRAZODONE (DESYREL)[1]

Trazodone (Desyrel)[1] is a serotonin reuptake inhibiting agent. Its action in ED is believed to be the result of central serotonergic and peripheral α-adrenolytic activity. The efficacy of trazodone is poorly demonstrated; however, it may have a place in those with performance anxiety. Side effects include drowsiness, insomnia, headaches, and weight loss.

DIETARY SUPPLEMENTS AND ERECTILE DYSFUNCTION

Yohimbine[1] is an α_2-adrenoreceptor antagonist with short duration of action. It is administered orally, and it is believed to have a central effect at adrenergic receptors in brain centers associated with libido and penile erection. A meta-analysis of seven studies established that it is superior to placebo, although results can be very erratic. Side effects include palpitations, tremors, and anxiety. Yohimbine should *not* be recommended as part of the management of ED.

A study with 60 patients who had failed papaverine[1] injections (50 mg or less) were treated with an extract of *Ginkgo biloba*, 60 mg for 12 to 18 months. After 6 months, 50% of the patients reported improvement in erectile function. A placebo-controlled randomized trial using 240 mg of *Ginkgo biloba* extract daily for 24 weeks in patients with vasculogenic ED did not demonstrate significant differences between the groups.

L-Arginine[1] is an amino acid that is the precursor to NO. Three small studies are looking at this drug. There are encouraging results in one study.

Zinc is found in high concentrations in seminal fluid. Anecdotal reports of improvement in ED.

ALPROSTADIL (PROSTAGLANDIN E1, CAVERJECT, MEDICATED URETHRAL SYSTEM FOR ERECTION)

Prostaglandin E1 (PGE_1) exerts a number of pharmacologic effects including systemic vasodilatation, inhibitory actions on platelet aggregation, and relaxation of smooth muscle. PGE_1 binds to PGE receptors and causes a relaxation response mediated by cyclic adenosine monophosphate (cAMP). It can be administered intracavernosally or intraurethrally.

---

[1]Not FDA approved for this indication.
[2]Not available in the United States.

It has been used in combination with papaverine,[1] and the combination was superior to PGE_1 alone. The intracavernosal administration seems to be more effective than transurethral (medicated urethral system for erection [MUSE]). MUSE should be administered in 1-mg doses, applied intraurethrally. Responses to intracavernosal injections (Caverject) as high as 80% may be expected in patients with organic ED with a dose of 20 μg, and much lower to MUSE (35% to 43%). Injections are given with 27- to 30-gauge needles. The administration of PGE_1 is usually relegated as an alternative in patients who have contraindications to the use of phosphodiesterase 5 (PDE5) inhibitors. The possible side effects include penile fibrosis, priapism, urethral bleeding, hypotension, or syncopal episodes.

Papaverine[1] is a nonspecific phosphodiesterase inhibitor that increases cAMP and cGMP levels in penile erectile tissue. It produces smooth muscle relaxation and vasodilatation. It decreases the resistance to arterial inflow and increases the resistance to venous outflow. It is highly effective in psychogenic and neurogenic ED but not vasculogenic. It has been commonly used in combination with phentolamine (Regitine). Major side effects include priapism, corporeal fibrosis, and possible elevation of liver transaminases.

Moxisylyte chlorohydrate[2] is an α-blocking agent. In a study where 156 subjects received either alprostadil or moxisylyte in a dose-escalating fashion, alprostadil had much better success rates (46% versus 81%).

Chlorpromazine (Thorazine)[1] is useful when given in combination with alprostadil or papaverine. It has α-blocking properties, and it is cheaper than phentolamine (Regitine).

Decreased concentration of vasoactive intestinal polypeptide (VIP)* has been reported in the penile tissue of men with ED. VIP is believed to play a role in the erectile process. It is ineffective when administered alone but can be quite effective in combination with phentolamine (Regitine). In a small study of 52 subjects with organic ED, 100% of them achieved an erection sufficient for intercourse. Further studies into the effectiveness of VIP may be needed.

PENILE PROSTHESES

This surgical approach used to be quite common before the advent of oral agents. The use of prostheses is still a suitable alternative for those who are unresponsive to less invasive treatments. Prostheses can be classified as rod, one-piece inflatable, two-piece inflatable, and three-piece inflatable. Postsurgical infections and malfunctions are the most common complications. Patients are usually satisfied with the results of prosthetic placement.

---

[1]Not FDA approved for this indication.
[2]Not available in the United States.
*Investigational drug in the United States.

 ## CURRENT DIAGNOSIS

- The risk factors for ED include tobacco, alcohol, and drug use, as well as DM, hypertension, hyperlipidemia, and prostate disease.
- ED is widely prevalent, and incidence sharply increases with age.
- ED is a cardiovascular sentinel event, and its occurrence warrants a cardiac workup.
- The workup of ED should include checking testosterone levels, prolactin, glucose, and lipid levels.
- First-line therapies include the use of PDE5 inhibitors such as sildenafil citrate (Viagra), vardenafil (Levitra), and tadalafil (Cialis).

Abbreviations: DM = diabetes mellitus; ED = erectile dysfunction; PDE5 = phosphodiesterase 5.

 ## CURRENT THERAPY

- PDE5 inhibitors
  Sildenafil citrate (Viagra) 25–100 mg
  Vardenafil (Levitra) 10–20 mg
  Tadalafil (Cialis) 10–20 mg
- Alprostadil (PGE_1) intracavernosal injections
  (Caverject) 20 μg
  Intraurethral application (MUSE) 1-mg pellet
- Papaverine injections [1] 30–60 mg
- Agents not yet approved for use by the FDA:
  Apomorphine (Uprima)[1] 3, 4, 6 mg
  Phentolamine (oral)[1] 40, 60, 80 mg

---

[1]Not FDA approved for this indication.
Abbreviations: MUSE = medicated urethral system for erection; PDE5 = phosphodiesterase 5; PGE_1 = prostaglandin E1.

Vacuum Constrictive Device

Vacuum constrictive device is a plastic cylinder that is placed over the penis and connected to a pump that creates a partial vacuum. After achieving penile rigidity, a band is placed around the base of the penis to maintain the erection. This is a safe, noninvasive, and effective method of treating ED. It requires an understanding partner and the quality of the erection is not ideal, but patients are usually satisfied.

Testosterone

Patients who have low testosterone levels may benefit substantially from replacement. Men may expect significant improvements in libido, self-esteem, and overall energy levels. Additionally, testosterone is necessary for NO generation in the penile tissue.

The different testosterone preparations include injections such as testosterone enanthate (Delatestryl), cypionate (Depo-Testosterone) given as an intramuscular (IM) injection in doses of 100 to 200 mg, every 2 weeks on average. They also include transdermal testosterone patches (Androderm and Testoderm, 5 mg/d) or transdermal gel (AndroGel 5-g packets, one daily; or Testim 1% testosterone gel, one packet daily). Testosterone gel preparations provide physiologic replacement of testosterone and are preferred more than depot IM injections.

REFERENCES

Archer SL. Potassium channels and erectile dysfunction. Vascul Pharmacol 2002;38:61–71.

Burchardt M, Burchardt T, Baer L, et al. Hypertension is associated with severe erectile dysfunction. J Urol 2000;164(10):1188–91.

Carson CC, Rajfer J, Eardley I, et al. The efficacy and safety of tadalafil: An update. BJU Int 2004;93:1276–81.

Crowe SM, Streetman DS. Vardenafil treatment for erectile dysfunction. Ann Pharmacother 2004;38:77–85.

Donatucci CF, Wong DG, Giuliano F, et al. Efficacy and safety of tadalafil once daily: Considerations for the practical application of a daily dosing option. Curr Med Res Opin 2008;24(12):3383–92.

Feldman HA, Goldstein I, Hatzichristou DG, et al. Impotence and its medical and psychosocial correlates: Results of the Massachusetts Male Aging Study. J Urol 1994;151(1):54–61.

Inman BA, St. Sauver JL, Jacobson DJ, et al. A population-based, longitudinal study of erectile dysfunction and future coronary artery disease. Mayo Clin Proc 2009;84(2):108–13.

Jackson G, Betteridge J, Dean J, et al. A systematic approach to erectile dysfunction in the cardiovascular patient: A consensus statement—Update 2002. Int J Clin Pract 2002;56(9):663–71.

Jaynat D, Shepherd MD. Evaluation and treatment of erectile dysfunction in men with diabetes mellitus. Mayo Clin Proc 2002;77(3):276–82.

Johannes CB, Araujo AB, Feldman HA, et al. Incidence of erectile dysfunction in men ages 40 to 69 years old: Longitudinal results from the Massachusetts Male Aging Study. J Urol 2000;163(2):460–3.

Khatana SAM, Taveira TH, Miner MM, et al. Does cardiovascular risk reduction alleviate erectile dysfunction in men with type II diabetes mellitus? Int J Impotence Res 2008;20:501–6.

Kirby M, Jackson G, Betteridge J, et al. Is erectile dysfunction a marker for cardiovascular disease? Int J Clin Pract 2002;55(9):614–8.

Lue TF. Drug therapy: Erectile dysfunction. N Engl J Med 2000;342 (24):1802–13.

Michelakis E, Tymchak W, Archer S. Sildenafil: From the bench to the bedside. CMAJ 2000;163(9):1171–5.

Nehra A. Erectile dysfunction and cardiovascular disease: Efficacy and safety of phosphodiesterase type 5 inhibitors in men with both conditions. Mayo Clin Proc 2009;84(2):139–48.

NIH Consensus Development Panel on Impotence. Impotence (NIH Consensus Conference). JAMA 1993;270(1):83–90.

Padma-Nathan H. Intra-urethral and topical agents in the management of erectile dysfunction. In: Carson CC III, Kirby RS, Goldstein I, editors. Textbook of Erectile Dysfunction. Oxford: Isis Medical Media; 1999. p. 323–6.

Rhoden EL, Teloken C, Mafessoni R, et al. Is there any relation between serum levels of testosterone and the severity of erectile dysfunction? Int J Impot Res 2002;14:167–71.

Shokeir AA, Alserafi MA, Mutabagani H. Intracavernosal versus intraurethral alprostadil: A prospective randomized study. BJU Int 1999;83:812–5.

Spahn M, Manning M, Juenemann KP. Intracavernosal therapy. In: Carson RS III, Kirby RS, Goldstein I, editors. Textbook of Erectile Dysfunction. Oxford: Isis Medical Media; 1999. p. 345–53.

Sullivan ME, Thompson CS, Dashwood MR, et al. Nitric oxide and penile erection: Is erectile dysfunction another manifestation of vascular disease? Cardiovasc Res 1999;43:658–65.

Thompson IM, Tangen CM, Goodman PJ, et al. Erectile dysfunction and subsequent cardiovascular disease. JAMA 2005;294(23):2996–3002.

730

Acute Renal Failure

Method of
Kevin Schroeder, MD

Epidemiology and Definitions

Acute renal failure (ARF), increasingly called acute kidney injury, is a clinical syndrome that can include decreased urine output, retention of nitrogenous metabolic waste products normally excreted by the kidney, retention of sodium and extracellular fluid resulting in peripheral and sometimes central edema, and various electrolyte and acid-base disturbances that may be associated with elevations in the blood urea nitrogen (BUN) and serum creatinine concentrations. Typically these changes occur rapidly over hours to days. Acute renal failure may further be described by the decrement in urine output: polyuric failure, indicating greater than 3 L urine output per 24 hours; nonoliguric failure, indicating 0.4 to 3L urine output per 24 hours; oliguric failure, indicating less than 400 mL urine output per 24 hours; and anuric failure, with less than 50 mL urine output per 24 hours.

Currently accepted definitions of ARF include a rise in the serum creatinine concentration by more than 0.5 mg/dL or a relative increase in the serum creatinine concentration by more than 25% for patients with preexisting chronic kidney disease (CKD) and a reduction in the glomerular filtration rate (GFR) by 50%. Note that these definitions are very operational and based on laboratory data readily available to practicing physicians, but consensus regarding a single, more sensitive measure of ARF is lacking.

Traditionally, ARF has been subclassified mechanistically into three categories. *Prerenal azotemia* refers to conditions that cause a fall in GFR because of reduced glomerular perfusion pressure. *Intrinsic renal*

failure refers to conditions that directly damage any of the four main structural components of the kidney, including the afferent and efferent arterioles, glomeruli, tubules, and interstitium. *Postrenal failure* commonly refers to any condition that causes obstruction of either the upper or lower urinary tract. From a practical standpoint, clinicians must also consider the situation in which ARF occurs (in an ambulatory patient, at hospital admission, during hospitalization, or after discharge) and the rapidity of deterioration, because some diagnoses are more likely depending on the clinical context.

The reported incidence of ARF varies by clinical situation and patient population, occurring in about 2% of all inpatient admissions. Varying definitions of disease and methodologic characteristics of epidemiologic studies also affect the reported incidence. General surgical patients undergoing nonemergent, noncardiac surgery had ARF at a reported incidence of 0.8%, and critically ill surgical patients undergoing noncardiac surgery experienced ARF at a rate nearly 80 times higher. Several scoring systems have been developed to predict the risk of ARF in patients undergoing cardiac surgery, which can vary from 5% to 25%. General medicine patients can experience ARF during a hospitalization at a rate of up to 7%, but the incidence may be in the 30% to 50% range for patients in critical care units. It may be possible that the true incidence of ARF in the United States will increase substantially as the baby boom generation enters its seventh decade.

Despite advances in medical technology, pharmacotherapeutics, and dialysis modalities in the critical care setting, mortality associated with ARF remains largely untouched at 20% to 80%. Recent studies have detected an increased mortality with even a slight rise in serum creatinine (increase <0.5 mg/dL). ARF adds to length of stay by about 4 days and can easily increase the cost of admission by more than $10,000.

Classification

Causes of ARF (Box 1) are elucidated chiefly from the history and physical examination. In particular, the history should focus first on symptoms causing volume depletion, second on symptoms relating to obstruction, and third on systemic symptoms including unexplained malaise, weight loss, fever, sinopulmonary bleeding, joint pain or swelling, rashes, myalgias, and neuropathies. All these factors must be considered in light of the patient's comorbid conditions, especially cardiovascular disease, hypertension, diabetes, liver disease, and peripheral vascular disease. Medications including antihypertensives, diuretics, analgesics, and over-the-counter supplements should be reviewed carefully. The physical examination serves to confirm the patient's volume status (e.g., frank hypotension or orthostatic change in blood pressure with tachycardia), to identify signs of cardiovascular disease and cardiopulmonary decompensation, to assess the status of the urinary bladder, and to detect signs of systemic disease. In addition to routine serum chemistries, BUN, and serum creatinine levels, all patients with nonanuric ARF must have a urinalysis. The clinician must observe the urine sediment for the presence of protein, blood, dysmorphic red cells, and cellular and noncellular casts. Finally, for oliguric patients, calculation of the fractional excretion of sodium (FE_{Na}) might prove useful. Serologic testing regarding acute glomerulonephritis should be obtained when the history and physical examination suggest sufficient pretest probability.

PRERENAL AZOTEMIA

Prerenal azotemia is the most common cause of ARF among patients admitted to general medicine services. It is commonly observed in cases of volume depletion or decreased effective arterial blood volume. These include profuse emesis or diarrhea, hemorrhage, and overzealous diuresis, especially in the face of poor oral intake. In these cases, peripheral and central edema is often absent. Decompensated CHF, decompensated cirrhosis leading to the hepatorenal syndrome, and the nephrotic syndrome all lead to effective decreases in circulating arterial volume. Commonly, patients with these conditions have peripheral edema and sometimes central edema with

BOX 1 Causes of Acute Renal Failure

Prerenal Azotemia
Effective Arterial Blood Volume and Hypotension
Emesis or diarrhea
Hemorrhage
Nephrotic syndrome
Sepsis
Third spacing
- Acute abdomen
- Bowel infarct
- Burns
- Cirrhosis or hepatorenal syndrome
- *Clostridium difficile* colitis
- Pancreatitis
- Peritonitis
- Postoperative abdomen

Pump Failure
- Acute myocardial infarction
- Congestive heart failure
- Tamponade

Overmedication
- Anesthetics
- Diuretics
- Nonsteroidal antiinflammatory drugs (including cyclooxygenase-2 inhibitors)

Intrinsic Acute Renal Failure
Acute Tubular Necrosis
Toxins
- Aminoglycosides
- Cyclosporine (Neoral)
- Ethylene glycol
- Heavy metals
- Hemoglobinuria
- Iodinated dye
- Myoglobinuria
- Nonsteroidal antiinflammatory drugs (including cyclooxygenase-2 inhibitors)
- Pentamidine (Pentam)
- Tumor lysis syndrome
Ischemia
- Cardiovascular surgery
- Dissection
- Embolism

- Severe hypotension
- Trauma
Septic
- Gram-positive or gram-negative sepsis

Interstitial Nephritis
Allopurinol (Zyloprim)
Antibiotics
- Cephalosporins
- Penicillins
- Rifampin (Rifadin)
- Sulfonamides
Diuretics
Nonsteroidal antiinflammatory drugs
Phenytoin (Dilantin)

Macrovascular Disease
Atheroembolic disease
Malignant hypertension

Microvascular Disease
HELLP syndrome
Hemolytic-uremic syndrome and thrombotic thrombocytopenic purpura
Hepatorenal syndrome
Rapidly progressive glomerulonephritis
Vasculitis

Postrenal Obstruction
Intratubular Obstruction
Crystals
Myeloma casts

Ureteral Obstruction
Ligation
Retroperitoneal fibrosis
Stones/papillae
Tumor compression

Bladder Outlet Obstruction
Anticholinergic medicines
Benign prostatic hyperplasia
Diabetic autonomic dysfunction
Stones and papillae
Urethral valves

HELLP = hemolysis, elevated liver enzymes, low platelets.

---

low albumin states. In the former case, diuretics often improve not only the heart failure but also the renal dysfunction concomitantly. Recalling the principles of vascular autoregulation (Fig. 1), the clinician must realize that the kidneys of elderly patients and patients with chronic hypertension are especially susceptible to intravascular volume changes. This is particularly true when patients are medicated with angiotensin converting enzyme inhibitors and angiotensin receptor blockers, nonsteroidal antiinflammatory drugs and cyclooxygenase-2 inhibitors, and calcineurin inhibitors, all of which effectively paralyze the kidney's ability to regulate glomerular perfusion.

Typical laboratory findings in prerenal azotemia include an elevated BUN:creatinine ratio (>20:1) and a FE_{Na} of less than 1%. However, if the patient had been taking diuretics, the FE_{Na} may be falsely elevated. Metabolic alkalosis and hypokalemia might or might not be present. The urinalysis is expected to show a high specific gravity with no blood,

no protein, and bland sediment except may be a few hyaline casts. Clinically, pure prerenal azotemia often responds quickly to restoration of euvolemia with increased urine output and a falling creatinine within 24 hours. Therapy for prerenal azotemia should be aimed at restoring clinical euvolemia and eliminating the cause of the azotemia. Infusion of isotonic saline is the norm, with supplemental oral rehydration where possible, and use of colloids or blood products when needed. In the case of decompensated left heart failure with pulmonary embarrassment, it is often necessary to employ an inotrope (e.g., dobutamine [Dobutrex]) in combination with a diuretic, whereas with hepatorenal syndrome, combinations of midodrine (Proamatine)[1] and octreotide (Sandostatin)[1] have been employed with some success.

---

[1]Not FDA approved for this indication.

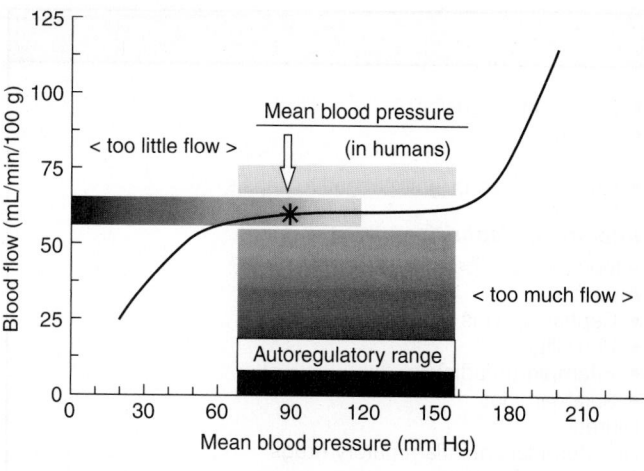

FIGURE 1. Principle of vascular autoregulation.

Intrinsic renal failure may be subdivided into diseases that affect the renal microvasculature, glomeruli, tubules, and interstitium. Although the pharmacologic effects of certain medications (e.g., angiotensin-converting enzyme inhibitors [ACEIs] and nonsteroidal antiinflammatory drugs [NSAIDs]) directly affect the renal microvasculature, renal dysfunction associated with their use physiologically produces a prerenal picture. However, cholesterol emboli syndrome and small vessel vasculitis represent two diseases whose impact on the renal microvasculature is pathologic. In the former case, cholesterol-laden debris dislodged from the abdominal aorta or aortic arch showers distal vascular beds. The classic scenario involves a patient who, having recently undergone an endovascular procedure, presents with abdominal colic, ARF, livedo reticularis, and evidence of ischemic toes. Depending on the size of the embolus, the patient can have frank intestinal or renal infarction or an acutely ischemic lower extremity, necessitating emergent intervention. Eosinophiluria and hypocomplementemia may be noted. The elevation in creatinine can progress in a stepwise fashion for several days to weeks after the original event. Magnetic resonance imaging (MRI) can show evidence of wedge-shaped infarcts in the renal parenchyma. Optimal therapy with regard to antiplatelet agents versus anticoagulants remains uncertain.

GLOMERULAR DISEASE

Glomerular disease accounts for roughly 10% of ARF among hospitalized patients. The hallmarks of rapidly progressive acute glomerulonephritis (RPGN) include an active urine sediment (dysmorphic red blood cells (RBCs) and cellular casts), hypertension, some edema, and a rapid decline in renal function over days. World Health Organization (WHO) class IV systemic lupus erythematosus (SLE) nephritis, anti-neutrophil cytoplasmic antibodies (ANCA)-mediated disease, and anti-GBM (glomerular basement membrane) disease are examples. Serologic testing is often useful, but a renal biopsy is almost always indicated for definitive diagnosis. Treatment usually involves some combination of corticosteroids and cytotoxic medications. Because of the severe increase in morbidity and mortality when these diseases are untreated, RPGN should be considered a medical emergency, with prompt attempts to diagnose and treat. It is important to recognize that whereas diseases that primarily manifest as the nephritic syndrome commonly cause ARF, entities associated more with a nephrotic-syndrome picture—including membranous disease, minimal change disease, or focal sclerosis—can certainly produce ARF as well. This usually occurs in the setting of massive nephrotic-range proteinuria (10–20 g/24 hours) and associated marked hypoalbuminemia.

ACUTE TUBULAR NECROSIS

Acute tublar necrosis (ATN) accounts for fully 50% of ARF among hospitalized patients; depending on the scenario, this figure can rise to as much as 75%. ATN has three common causes: ischemic, toxic, and septic. ATN has been described by its phases: Injury, during which time the insult causes direct damage to the tubules, is manifested as a progressive increase in the serum creatinine and possibly the development of oliguria. In the plateau phase, the creatinine, urinary output, and volume status are relatively stable. Recovery is marked by a spontaneous decline in serum creatinine and increase in urinary output, perhaps even into a polyuric range. The time course of ATN from injury to recovery is variable. Depending on the severity of the injury and the preexistence of renal disease, ATN can reverse within 1 to 3 weeks, although a small percentage of patients with ATN remain dialysis dependent after months. ATN is typically associated with a loss of urinary concentration, elevated urinary sodium excretion, and an elevated FE_{Na} of greater than 2%. The BUN and creatinine tend to rise proportionally. The urinary sediment can reveal tubular epithelial cell casts that have a coarsely granular or muddy brown appearance.

Ischemic ATN typically occurs during periods of prolonged hypotension and represents an evolution of prerenal azotemia. Ischemic ATN is commonly observed to varying degrees after cardiovascular and major orthopedic or trauma surgery. Careful attention must be paid to urine output and volume status. High-dose diuretics may be employed to avoid pulmonary edema, and if a suboptimal response is seen, the dosage should be doubled after the first dose. Patients who rapidly become oliguric have a high mortality rate, which is unaffected by diuretics and can therefore require early initiation of dialysis. Specific risk factors for developing ischemic ATN in the postoperative setting include advanced age (older than 70 years), preexisting CKD, diabetes, emergent surgery, preexisting vascular disease, and the need for valvular, particularly aortic valve, heart surgery in addition to bypass grafting. The degree and duration of intraoperative hypotension as well as time spent on cardiopulmonary bypass can also play roles.

Toxic ATN is proximal tubular cell death as a consequence of drugs or other endogenous chemicals. Drugs that classically cause toxic ATN include aminoglycosides, amphotericin B (Fungizone), radiocontrast, platinum-based chemotherapy, and NSAIDs. Endogenous chemicals known to cause toxic ATN include uric acid, myoglobin, and heme. Clinically, it is worthwhile noting that although the onset of ATN after a single dose of NSAID or iodinated radiocontrast material may be rapid (24–72 hours) especially in volume-depleted patients, in the case of aminoglycosides the onset of injury may be a bit slower, consistent with cumulative dose exposure. In general, ATN is best avoided by limiting the dose of potentially toxic medications (e.g., once-daily dosing of aminoglycosides), maintenance of adequate volume status, and close attention to the serum creatinine and urinary output.

In the case of radiocontrast agents, low osmolar and isosmolar agents are thought to be less toxic, and dose limitation (or elimination) to less than 100 mL are helpful strategies. Although prospective randomized, controlled trial data are inconclusive, and meta-analyses are equivocal, in cases of elective contrast exposure it remains common practice at many centers to administer N-acetylcysteine (Mucomyst)[1] in a dosage of 600 mg orally every 12 hours on the day before and the day of exposure. This, along with intravenous fluid administration for up to 6 hours before elective procedures (some authors use bicarbonate-containing solutions) seem to be reasonably safe, low-cost measures that can offer some protection against ATN in patients with known renal disease. After contrast-enhanced procedures, serum creatinine should be measured daily in hospitalized patients and at 48 hours after the procedure in outpatients.

Septic ATN often manifests in the critical care setting in patients with multisystem organ failure. Patients are typically hypotensive with either gram-positive or gram-negative bacteremia and anuria, often with severe acidemia. Unlike patients with prerenal azotemia whose urine output responds to volume resuscitation, patients with septic ATN do not produce urine in response to substantial volume resuscitation (Table 1). The clinical picture is difficult to distinguish from ischemic ATN because the two disease processes can coexist. Clinically, ischemic and toxic ATN are thought to show signs of

---

[1]Not FDA approved for this indication.

TABLE 1 Laboratory Differentiation of Prenatal Azotemia from Acute Tubular Necrosis

	Result	
Test	Prerenal Azotemia	Acute Tubular Necrosis
U_{Na}	<10–20	>40
FE_{Na}	<1	>1
Urine SG	>1.020	<1.010
BUN:Cr	>20:1	≈10:1
Fe_{Ur}	>60:1	<20:1
$U_{Cr}:P_{Cr}$	>40:1	<10:1

BUN = blood urea nitrogen; Cr = creatinine; FE_{Ur} = fractional excretion of urea; FE_{Na} = fractional excretion of sodium; SG = specific gravity; $U_{Cr}:P_{Cr}$ = ratio of urine creatinine to serum creatinine; U_{Na} = urine sodium.

 CURRENT DIAGNOSIS

- Prerenal azotemia may be associated with a BUN-to-creatinine ratio >20:1 and a FE_{Na} <1%.
- Intrarenal ARF (ATN) may be associated with a BUN-to-creatinine ratio <20:1 and a FE_{Na} >1%.
- Postrenal ARF can manifest with frank anuria.
- Follow the trends of serum chemistries, BUN, creatinine, and urine output on a daily basis.

ARF = acute renal failure; ATN = acute tubular necrosis; BUN = blood urea nitrogen; FE_{Na} = fractional excretion of sodium.

resolution within 14 days of removal of the insult, whereas the sequelae of septic ATN can persist for one or several months after the infection requiring prolonged hospitalization and dialysis support. Mortality in this setting can be as high as 80%, and patients who survive their initial illness are particularly susceptible to nosocomial infections, catheter-related bacteremia, and malnutrition.

INTERSTITIAL DISEASE

Interstitial disease represents the third most common cause of ARF among hospitalized patients after prerenal azotemia and ATN. Acute interstitial nephritis is usually the effect of either drugs or pyelonephritis. In the case of medications, key diagnostic points include a delayed onset after medication exposure, as much as 7 days, and the co-incidence of fever and a central rash in about 30% of patients. The diagnosis may be suspected in the presence of sterile pyuria, eosinophiluria, and eosinophilia. Because the disease is of nonglomerular and nontubular origin, the urine sediment should be relatively bland, with minimal hematuria or proteinuria. Renal biopsy confirming the presence of increased numbers of eosinophils in the interstitium remains the gold standard. Antibiotics that are particularly notorious for causing acute interstitial nephritis include penicillins, particularly methicillin (Staphcillin); sulfa-containing drugs; rifampin (Rifadin); and quinolones. Typically, cessation of the suspected agent results in improved renal function within 5 days; however, in severe, prolonged cases, a course of corticosteroids can hasten improvement. Importantly, if the patient is re-exposed to the offending agent, acute interstitial nephritis can develop much more rapidly.

OBSTRUCTIVE DISEASE

Obstructive renal disease, although relatively uncommon, should be highly suspected in any patient with otherwise unexplained anuria, especially in those with a known pelvic malignancy or recent pelvic surgery. Obstruction of the lower tract and bladder outlet is more prevalent among elderly men with prostatic hypertrophy and diabetics with autonomic nervous dysfunction. Upper-tract obstruction can be seen in cases of retroperitoneal fibrosis, uroepithelial malignancy, and nephrolithiasis. Certain systemic processes including tumor lysis syndrome, myeloma cast nephropathy, and ethylene glycol overdose can all cause an intratubular obstruction due to massive crystal and cast deposition within the kidney.

Clinically, obstruction of the bladder outlet may be diagnosed and treated via placement of a Foley catheter. Bladder scans, ultrasounds, and measurement of the pre- and postvoid residual bladder volumes are also important but not always immediately necessary. Bilateral upper tract obstruction requires intervention in the form of bilateral percutaneous nephrostomy tubes or internal double-J stent placement via cystourethroscopy. Patients with severe obstruction may be significantly hyperkalemic at presentation, requiring prompt treatment. Fortunately, if the obstruction is relieved in a timely fashion, the hyperkalemia usually dissipates without emergent dialysis.

Treatment

Management of hospitalized patients is generally supportive. Specific measures include a thorough daily review of the medication list to ensure that all possible toxic medications have been eliminated and that all drugs excreted via the kidneys have been dose adjusted for the level of renal dysfunction. The patient's volume status should be assessed frequently, with appropriate adjustments in intravenous fluids or diuretics. Similarly, electrolytes, BUN, and creatinine should be checked daily. In general, hospitalized patients should remain hospitalized until the clinical course has at least stabilized and close outpatient follow-up is ensured. Outpatients with acute renal failure can require urgent hospitalization if the cause is not immediately apparent and reversible, or if significant hyperkalemia or volume overload exists, or if the patient has significant comorbidities.

The decision to initiate renal replacement therapy is made by the nephrologist on a patient-by-patient basis. Some absolute clinical indications for dialysis exist, such as severe hyperkalemia; peaked T waves or prolongation of the QRS complex by electrocardiogram; volume overload or acidosis refractory to medical therapy; certain intoxications or electrolyte abnormalities; and symptomatic uremia with pericarditis, neurologic changes, or bleeding diatheses. Depending on the clinical setting, the two most common are hyperkalemia and volume overload; rarely will the nephrologist let ARF with either of these conditions progress to the point of cardiac arrhythmia or intubation undialyzed.

Patients who require urgent or emergent dialysis can typically be dialyzed via standard intermittent hemodialysis. This method is more effective for acute correction of electrolyte, toxin, and acid–base aberrations as well as pulmonary edema. Controversy exists as to the proper dose of dialysis for patients with ARF, particularly those in the critical care setting. Clinical practice varies by center, but studies have shown a survival benefit favoring daily hemodialysis to keep the BUN less than 100 mg/dL.

Continuous renal replacement therapy (CRRT) or continuous veno-venous hemofiltration is usually reserved for critically ill patients, particularly those with hypotension requiring vasopressor support or those with sufficiently poor cardiac performance and volume overload who cannot tolerate acute intravascular volume shifts associated with conventional hemodialysis.

Acute peritoneal dialysis, although certainly a viable modality, is practiced much less commonly in the United States partly due to the widespread availability of hemodialysis.

Emerging Issues

In clinical practice, the diagnosis and treatment of ARF rest on the ability to recognize it in a timely fashion. The two universally available indicators—urinary output and serum creatinine measurement—are limited in their sensitivity and specificity; however, new urinary and

CURRENT THERAPY

- Hemodynamic support and maintenance of euvolemic state
- Correction of electrolyte and acid–base imbalances
- Removal of all offending agents and correction of underlying causes
- Adjustment of all medications for decreased glomerular filtration rate
- Renal replacement when needed on an individual basis

plasma biomarkers are emerging that can allow earlier identification of ARF. Urinary neutrophil gelatinase–associated lipocalin (NGAL), kidney injury molecule-1 (KIM-1), and interleukin-18 (IL-18), in combination with plasma NGAL and cystatin C measurements, are all currently being evaluated in ARF clinical trials. These assays hold the promise of earlier detection and perhaps more specific anatomic localization of the injury within the kidney. Whether these biomarkers are used alone, serially, or in combination as an acute kidney injury panel remains to be seen as they transition from primarily clinical trial–based application to widespread clinical use. Questions regarding their ability to help predict which patients with ARF will spontaneously recover renal function and which will require dialysis remain to be answered.

Nephrotoxicity associated with gadolinium-containing contrast media has risen to the front of discussion among radiologists and nephrologists. Originally thought to be non-nephrotoxic, gadolinium has been implicated in a number of well-documented cases. Perhaps more striking are the mounting reports of gadolinium-related nephrogenic systemic fibrosis, which is characterized by brawny epidermal fibrotic plaques developing over several weeks after exposure. It is important to recognize that other organs including the subcutaneous tissues, skeletal musculature, lungs, and heart may be involved. Although the pathogenesis of this disease has not been fully elucidated, epidemiologically, 90% of cases have been described among end-stage renal disease patients requiring dialysis, and fully 10% have occurred among patients with CKD stages 3 and 4. Because there is no cure for this disease and its clinical consequences are potentially devastating, clinicians now must consider the risk-to-benefit ratio of exposing a patient to gadolinium-enhanced MRI procedures and weigh that risk against the well-established risk of iodinated contrast used in CT scans.

REFERENCES

Coca SG, Peixoto AJ, Garg AX, et al. The prognostic importance of a small acute decrement in kidney function in hospitalized patients: A systematic review and meta-analysis. Am J Kidney Dis 2007;50(5):712–20.

Dennen P, Parikh CR. Biomarkers of acute kidney injury: Can we replace serum creatinine? Clin Nephrol 2007;68(5):269–78.

Devarajan P. Proteomics for biomarker discovery in acute kidney injury. Semin Nephrol 2007;27(6):637–51.

Eachempati SR, Wang JC, Hydo LJ, et al. Acute renal failure in critically ill surgical patients: Persistent lethality despite new modes of renal replacement therapy. J Trauma 2007;63(5):987–93.

Greenberg A, Cheung A, Coffman T, et al. editors. Primer on Kidney Diseases. 2nd ed. San Diego: Academic Press; 1998.

Johnson J, Feehally J. Comprehensive Clinical Nephrology. 1st ed. St Louis: Mosby; 2000.

Kheterpal S, Tremper KK, Englesbe MJ, et al. Predictors of postoperative acute renal failure after noncardiac surgery in patients with previously normal renal function. Anesthesiology 2007;107(6):892–902.

Nagle PC, Warner MA. Acute renal failure in a general surgical population: Risk profiles, mortality, and opportunities for improvement. Anesthesiology 2007;107(6):869–70.

Rakel R, Bope E, editors. Conn's Current Therapy 2007. Philadelphia: Elsevier; 2007.

Chronic Renal Failure

Method of
Jeffrey A. Kraut, MD

Chronic renal failure is defined as a reduction in glomerular filtration rate (GFR) below the normal values of approximately 120 to 130 mL/minute developing over months to years. Its incidence has increased significantly over the last several years, but this probably reflects more accurate estimations of GFR. However, there is an increased prevalence of type II diabetes mellitus, a frequent cause of renal disease, in Western societies that could contribute to a higher incidence of chronic renal failure. When renal failure is severe (GFR <10 mL/minute), renal replacement therapy, either dialysis or renal transplantation, is required to preserve life. However, even before several renal failure ensues, the presence of chronic renal failure has an important impact on organ function and can contribute to the development of significant electrolyte derangements, important hormonal abnormalities, and anemia. Also, its presence can alter the metabolism and therefore the blood concentrations and tissue concentrations of drugs administered for the treatment of various diseases. Moreover, a reduced GFR is associated with an increased risk of death, increased incidence of cardiovascular events, and hospitalizations independent of known risk factors or a history of cardiovascular diseases. Finally, the mortality of several surgical procedures is substantially increased by the presence of chronic renal failure. Therefore, detecting and treating patients with chronic renal failure is extremely important.

Causes of Chronic Renal Failure

Many disorders can cause chronic renal failure. However, epidemiologic studies indicate that diabetes mellitus and hypertension account for the majority of cases (>60%). Chronic glomerulonephritis, polycystic kidney disease, obstructive uropathy, and ischemic nephropathy caused by atherosclerotic renal artery stenosis are less common, but important causes of renal impairment. The latter disorder is postulated to be more frequent than previously believed and is an important undiagnosed cause of chronic renal impairment.

Recent studies have indicated that a reduction in GFR occurs with aging in the absence of factors known to produce renal injury such as hypertension or diabetes. Indeed, the average GFR of subjects in the 8th decade of life in one large study was 40 to 50 mL/minute. Pathologic examination of these individuals, when available, may reveal only benign nephrosclerosis.

Importantly, because a majority of individuals older than 60 years of age have lower muscle mass, the reduced GFR is not accompanied by a rise in serum creatinine concentration. Therefore, renal failure is not detected unless the physician considers other variables such as the patient's age and muscle mass in assessing GFR (see the following section).

Approach to the Diagnosis of Chronic Renal Failure

The first step in the diagnosis of chronic renal failure is, of course, to detect a reduction in GFR. In the past, estimations of GFR were based on the measurement of serum creatinine concentration alone. In adults, the normal serum creatinine ranges between 0.6 and 1.3 mg/dL. Individuals with values greater than this are said to have renal failure. However, there is a wide range of normal values. Also, creatinine production, which is dependent on muscle mass, is a critical variable affecting serum creatinine concentration. Thus, a large group of individuals with reduced muscle mass can have serum creatinine values within the normal range, but a decreased GFR. The most common situation in which this paradox is encountered is in the elderly and in individuals with malignancy or chronic liver disease.

Precise measurement of GFR is accomplished by calculating the clearance of creatinine in a timed urine collection, generally 24 hours in duration:

$$\text{Creatinine clearance (mL/minute)} = Ucr \text{ (mg/dL)} \times \text{volume (mL)}/Scr \text{ (mg/dL)}/1440.$$

where Ucr = urine creatinine concentration,
　　　 Scr = plasma creatinine concentration

However, timed urine collections are often inaccurate because of errors in collection. Moreover, as renal function progresses and serum creatinine rises, or in the presence of nephrotic range proteinuria, GFR tends to be overestimated by creatinine clearance. Most recently, formulas derived from studies of large groups of patients—such as those by Cockroft and Gault and the Modification of Diet in Renal Disease (MDRD) in which GFR was correlated with other factors (e.g., body weight, age, and serum albumin)—are sufficiently accurate to use for clinical purposes:

$$\text{Cockroft} - \text{Gault:CrCl (mL/minute)} = \{(140 - age) \times wt \times [1 - (0.15 \times gender)]\}/(0.814 \times Scr)$$

$$\begin{aligned}\text{MDRD:GFR} = 170 &\times [PCr]^{-0.999} \times [Age]^{-0.176} \\ &\times [0.762 \text{ female}] \times [1.180 \text{ if patient is black}] \\ &\times [SUN]^{-0.170} \times [Alb]^{+0.318}\end{aligned}$$

Once renal function is depressed, the physician determines whether this represents acute or chronic renal failure, When previous measurements of GFR are available, it is relatively easy to determine if the renal failure is chronic in nature. However, if these studies are not available, demonstration that the kidneys are small in size (less than 8 to 9 cm when they are normally approximately 10 to 12 cm) by renal ultrasound will confirm the chronicity of the disease. Evidence of increased echogenicity reflecting augmented fibrous deposits is also suggestive of chronic disease. However, several disorders associated with chronic renal failure have normal kidney size such as diabetes mellitus, polycystic kidney disease, and amyloidosis. Therefore, normal kidney size does not exclude chronic renal failure. If individuals have normal kidney size, the presence of anemia and/or certain abnormalities of divalent ion metabolism can also suggest the disease is chronic in nature.

Once impaired renal function is recognized, measurements of blood urea nitrogen (BUN), sodium, potassium, chloride, bicarbonate, hemoglobin and hematocrit, and calcium and phosphorus are obtained. A urinalysis is obtained looking for increased excretion of protein, presence of blood in the urine, and abnormal cellular elements. In patients with diabetes, studies to find microalbuminuria (albumin urine concentrations less than 300 mg per day) are important to detect the early stages of renal disease. A 24-hour or spot urine protein and creatinine determination to assess the urine's protein-to-creatinine ratio is obtained to quantitate the amount of protein being excreted. Urine protein excretion in excess of 3.5 g daily indicates the presence of glomerular pathology, whereas interstitial disease is characterized by values below 2 g. However, urine protein excretion can vary with glomerular disease so values below 3.5 g are still consistent with this diagnosis. Assessment of urine protein excretion is important for diagnostic purposes, but also because urine protein excretion is often followed to assess effectiveness of therapy.

Obstruction uropathy, an important cause of chronic renal failure and exacerbation of renal failure, can be excluded in the majority of cases by ultrasound of the kidneys. Doppler ultrasound of the renal arteries performed at the same time is helpful in excluding obstruction of the renal arteries. The necessity of obtaining other diagnostic studies such as measurement of serum complement, blood and urine eosinophils, serum and urine and protein electro-phoresis, antiglomerular basement membrane antibodies, anti–double-stranded DNA (dsDNA) antibodies, hepatitis B and C antibodies, sedimentation rate, and HIV studies depends on the context of the renal failure.

CURRENT DIAGNOSIS

The following lists the optimal care of patients with chronic kidney disease:

- Test for albuminuria and estimate glomerular filtration rate using MDRD formula yearly for early diagnosis and stratification of CKD.
- If possible, determine cause of kidney disease.
- Initiate treatment to delay or prevent progression of disease including use of converting enzyme inhibitors and/or angiotensin receptor blockers to reduce BP to less than 130/80 mm Hg and urine protein excretion to as low as possible but at least less than 1 g/24 hours.
- Control or prevent biochemical or clinical abnormalities including those of serum potassium, serum bicarbonate, serum phosphorus, parathyroid hormone, and hemoglobin.
- Evaluate patients for presence of and treat important co-morbid conditions, particularly heart disease.
- If the GFR is less than 30 mL/min, consider referral to a nephrologist.

Abbreviations: BP = blood pressure; CKD = care of patients with chronic kidney disease; GFR = glomerular filtration rate; MDRD = modification of diet in renal disease.

Finally, a renal biopsy may be required in certain situations to make a definitive diagnosis. Because treatment of specific diseases can vary, making a precise pathologic diagnosis can be extremely important for proper management. Unfortunately, once the renal failure is moderate to severe in nature, renal pathologic examination may not always be helpful in determining the cause.

Clinical and Laboratory Abnormalities in Chronic Renal Failure

Because the kidney plays a critical role in the regulation of the serum concentrations of sodium, potassium, bicarbonate, chloride, calcium, and phosphorus as well as the levels of hemoglobin and hematocrit, blood pressure and extracellular volume, chronic renal injury can lead to derangements in these parameters as summarized in Table 1.

TABLE 1 Clinical and Electrolyte Abnormalities Noted with Chronic Renal Failure

Clinical or Laboratory Disorder	GFR or Stage of Renal Failure*
Hypertension	GFR <60 mL/min (stage 3)
Hyponatremia or hypernatremia	GFR <30 mL/min (stage 4)
Hyperkalemia*	GFR <30 mL/min (stage 4)
Hyperphosphatemia*	GFR <30 mL/min (stage 4)
Metabolic acidosis	GFR <30 mL/min (stage 4)
Anemia	GFR <60 mL/min (stage 3)
Uremic symptoms	GFR <15 mL/min (stage 5)
Nausea, vomiting, disturbances in sleep	

*Descriptions of the various stages are presented in the text. These electrolyte abnormalities can be seen at higher levels of GFR.
Abbreviation: GFR = glomerular filtration rate.

HYPONATREMIA AND HYPERNATREMIA

The kidney plays an essential role in excreting water by producing a dilute urine (less than 1/6 plasma osmolality) or retaining water by producing a concentrated urine (three to four times plasma osmolality). The ability to concentrate or dilute the urine in the majority of cases is usually retained until GFR falls to less than 30% of normal, and therefore hyponatremia or hypernatremia are uncommon until that time. If the disease is primarily interstitial in nature, alterations in urine concentrating ability can appear prior to significant reductions in GFR. However, even with higher levels of GFR the patient can be at risk for either of these electrolyte abnormalities should they ingest large quantities of fluid or be deprived of appropriate fluid intake.

HYPERKALEMIA

The kidney plays the most critical role in the regulation of potassium balance. Adaptive changes in renal tubular function and possible colonic function enable the kidney to maintain serum potassium within the normal range until GFR falls below 20% to 25% of normal (serum creatinine of 4 mg/dL or greater). Recent studies indicate a tendency for elevations in serum potassium to appear at even modest reductions in GFR (<60 mL/min). When disease of the kidney involves the medullary portion or hormonal derangements such as hyporeninemic hypoaldosterinism are present, hyperkalemia can be observed prior to significant declines in GFR. In addition, patients with even moderate renal failure have a reduced reserve to eliminated potassium and therefore can develop hyperkalemia if potassium load is increased dramatically.

METABOLIC ACIDOSIS

A fall in plasma bicarbonate concentration in association with a reduced blood pH (metabolic acidosis) is frequently observed when GFR falls below 20% to 25% of normal. The acidosis results from acid excretion falling below acid production leading to positive proton balance. Recent studies have documented that a tendency to the development of metabolic acidosis can be seen with mild reductions in GFR (<60 mL/min).

The electrolyte pattern seen with the metabolic acidosis of renal failure is often of the high anion gap variety, but frequently a hyperchloremic (normal anion gap) or combined anion gap and hyperchloremic pattern can be observed. The degree of acidosis is usually mild to moderate with plasma bicarbonate concentration ranging from 12 to 22 mEq/L. Of interest, at any given level of GFR, the acidosis is often not progressive, but plasma bicarbonate concentration remains stable unless renal function declines further or there is an increment in acid production.

ABNORMAL DIVALENT IN METABOLISM

Serum phosphorus is regulated by the kidney but in most cases remains within the normal range until GFR falls below 20% to 25% of normal. This stabilization of serum phosphorus is attributed to increased tubular excretion of phosphorus as a result of increased parathyroid hormone secretion. As with potassium and bicarbonate, recent studies demonstrate a tendency for elevation in serum phosphorus to be observed with mild renal failure (<50 to 60 mL/min). Serum calcium is usually in the normal range, but varies receiprocally with serum phosphorus. Because of derangements in divalent ion metabolism bone disease with increased tendency to fractures and disordered soft tissue structures can be observed.

Hyperparathyroidism is a common occurrence in patients with renal failure, the values usually being higher with a greater degree of renal impairment. The elevated PTH values are usually induced by hypocalcemia, although increased serum phosphorus concentrations independent of serum calcium values can also play a role. The increased parathyroid hormone levels can induce damage to bone and soft tissue structures, but also may affect other functions such as cardiac function and the production of red blood cells.

ANEMIA

The kidney is the source of erythropoietin, the hormone that regulates bone marrow production of red blood cells. Thus, with the development of renal impairment, there is a fall in red blood cell production. A fall in red cell survival also contributes to development of anemia. Anemia generally appears when GFR falls below 60 mL/minute. There is a rough correlation between the severity of renal failure and the degree of anemia: the more severe the renal failure the greater the degree of anemia. However, this relationship is not invariable, and many patients have only mild reductions in hemoglobin and hematocrit.

Anemia initially was believed to contribute only to changes in oxygen delivery. However, recent studies show that anemia can contribute to the genesis of left ventricular hypertrophy and other cardiomyopathies noted with chronic renal failure and can raise mortality in patients with chronic renal failure.

HYPERTENSION

Recent studies emphasize the importance of the kidneys in the regulation of blood pressure, and the bulk of patients with diabetes or other glomerular disease will develop hypertension in the course of their renal failure. In many instances, hypertension does not develop until GFR is below 40% to 50% of normal. The type of renal disease underlying chronic renal failure appears to be important, as hypertension is less common with pyelonephritis. Hypertension might be observed earlier in the course of renal failure, however, in patients with polycystic kidney disease or ischemic nephropathy. Because hypertension is one of the most critical factors in the genesis of cardiovascular disease and can accelerate the progression of renal failure, careful attention of control of hypertension is important.

VOLUME OVERLOAD

Salt retention often accompanies chronic renal failure even when GFR is not severely compromised. The degree of salt retention can be profound if significant albuminuria with resultant hypoalbuminemia is seen and is more severe as GFR falls below 20% to 25% of normal. Salt retention is a critical factor in the development of hypertension and can promote congestive heart failure.

Symptoms and Signs of Renal Failure

Patients with chronic renal failure are often asymptomatic with little evidence of disease other than laboratory abnormalities until late in the course of renal failure. If anemia is present, patients may complain of fatigue; and if significant elevations in parathyroid hormone levels are noted, bone pain, ruptured tendons or other disorders of soft tissue structures can be noted. Once moderate to severe renal failure appears, symptoms of the electrolyte abnormalities can be observed. Hyperkalemia, if severe, can lead to arrhythmias or heart block and muscle weakness. Metabolic acidosis can contribute to fatigue. Anemia can contribute to fatigue and changes in mentation and physical stamina. Weight loss related to metabolic acidosis and or retention of various uremic toxins may occur. Sexual dysfunction characterized by reduced libido and reduced fertility are common with moderate to severe renal failure.

Once severe renal failure develops (stage 4 or 5), the uremic syndrome can be observed characterized by a decreased appetite, nausea, vomiting, and subtle changes in mental status including changes in sleep patterns. However, even with severe renal failure many patients feel surprisingly well.

Management of Chronic Renal Failure

STAGING OF CHRONIC RENAL FAILURE

As noted earlier, within the last several years, a great deal of effort has been expended into developing guidelines for the evaluation, monitoring, and treatment of patients with chronic renal failure. To this end, experts working with the National Kidney Foundation have divided chronic renal failure into different states based on measurements or estimations of GFR. The value of staging to the physician is that the studies necessary to monitor patients and the complications of chronic renal failure are often different depending on the stage of renal failure.

Stage 0 (GFR Greater Than 90 mL/Minute with Risk Factors for Renal Disease)

Patients at stage 0 have increased risk for development of chronic renal failure, such as those with diabetes or hypertension but who have GFR greater than 90 mL/minute in the absence of proteinuria or urinary sedimentary abnormalities. These patients should have their blood pressure and diabetes controlled. Estimates of GFR should be obtained approximately every 6 months from measurement of serum creatinine, and qualitative tests for urine protein excretion should be obtained. In diabetics measurement of microalbumin should also be obtained. Because control of disease may forestall progression glycosylated hemoglobin (HbA1C) values should also be obtained.

Stage 1 (GFR Greater Than 90 mL/Minute with Albuminuria)

Once evidence of renal damage is obtained, as reflected by microalbuminuria or proteinuria, but GFR is either normal or increased, patients are said to be in stage 1. These individuals should be monitored more closely and strict attention must be given to maintain blood pressure below 130/80. Furthermore, angiotensin converting enzyme inhibitor (ACEI) or angiotensin receptor blocker (ARB) should be given to prevent evolution of microalbuminuria to full-blown proteinuria (see the following). No clinical or laboratory abnormalities are observed at this stage.

Stage 2: Mild Renal Failure (GFR 60 to 90 mL/Minute)

When GFR is mildly reduced to values from 60 to 90 mL/minute, patients are in stage 2. These patients should also be carefully monitored and blood pressure tightly controlled. If diabetes is present, strict attention to maintaining HbA1C within recommended guidelines should be given. Again, it is rare at this stage for any significant clinical abnormalities other than hypertension to be present.

Stage 3: Moderate Renal Failure (GFR 30 to 59 mL/Minute)

When GFR ranges between 30 to 59 mL/minute, patients are in stage 3. At this point hypertension might appear, mild abnormalities in serum phosphorus might be observed, and anemia can be seen. Also in some patients an elevation in serum potassium can be noted, particularly if they are ingesting a relatively high potassium diet. These patients need to be followed more closely, and it is recommended that patients at the lower end of this stage (i.e., close to 30 mL/min) be monitored by a nephrologist.

Stage 4: Moderate to Severe (GFR from 15 to 29 mL/Minute)

Once GFR falls to values from 15 to 29 mL/minute, patients have severe renal failure, or stage 4 disease. At this level of GFR, significant electrolyte abnormalities such as metabolic acidosis, hyperkalemia, and hyperphosphatemia are frequent. Anemia is common and the patient may begin to note reductions in appetite and have a fall in muscle mass. However, there is great variability in the appearance of symptoms or laboratory derangements.

Stage 5: Severe (GFR Less Than 15 to 29 mL/Minute)

When GFR falls below 15 mL/minute, severe electrolyte abnormalities are often present, anemia is common. Clinical symptoms can develop. Renal replacement therapy, either dislysis or transplantation, is usually required at this stage.

Recommendations for treatment of patients are summarized below. The frequency of patient visits, of course, largely depends on the complications of renal disease present and co-morbid conditions. Therefore, these are only general recommendations for frequency of examination.

When patients are in stage 0, they should be seen once per year for renal evaluation. When GFR remains normal or elevated, but proteinuria is present, renal evaluation should be performed every 6 months. When stage 3 develops, we usually repeat renal evaluation every 3 months. Patients in stage 4 are seen more frequently, usually at the minimum of once per month. Patients with end-stage disease require renal replacement therapy.

GENERAL APPROACH TO TREATMENT OF CHRONIC RENAL FAILURE

Treatment of chronic renal failure can be divided into the modalities that are specific to the underlying disorder and those that are used to treat all patients with chronic renal failure. Thus, patients with systemic lupus erythematosus or other immune-mediated or inflammatory disease may benefit from treatment with steroids and immunosuppressive agents. Treatments specific for individual disorders are beyond the scope of this article.

The physician treating the patient with renal failure has two goals: preventing or delaying progression of renal failure, and alleviating the electrolyte and hormonal abnormalities that can lead to symptoms or complications of the disease. Understanding the methods to accomplish the former requires knowledge of those factors that are integral to progression of the disease.

FACTORS CAUSING PROGRESSION OF CHRONIC RENAL FAILURE

It has been recognized for several years that once renal failure has developed, renal function can decline at a predictable rate in the absence of further insults to the kidney. Essential to the optimal approach used to treat chronic renal failure, therefore, is an understanding of those factors that can cause progression of renal failure, including:

- Systemic and intraglomerular hypertension
- Glomerular hypertrophy
- Intrarenal precipitation of calcium and phosphorus
- Hyperlipidemia
- Altered metabolism of prostanoids
- Metabolic acidosis
- Anemia
- Tubulointerstitial disease
- Proteinuria

Intraglomerular Hypertension and Glomerular Hypertrophy

As nephrons are lost, changes are induced in the kidney to preserve GFR such as renal vasodilatation, an increase in glomerular capillary pressure, and an increment in size of individual glomeruli raising wall stress. These adaptive mechanisms probably induce damage by causing endothelial cell damage with detachment of epithelial cells allowing enhanced flux of water and solutes that might cause narrowing of capillary lumens. Also, strain on mesangial cells causes them to produce cytokines and extracellular matrix with resultant expansion of the mesangium and glomerular sclerosis.

Proteinuria

Although proteinuria has traditionally been a marker of glomerular injury, with greater amounts of urinary protein excretion being associated with more severe injury, recent studies indicate that proteinuria, can induce mesangial and tubular damage. Therefore, treatments to reduce proteinuria, may be beneficial in limiting further renal damage.

Tubulointerstitial Disease

Some component of tubulointerstitial disease is generally found in individuals with chronic renal failure even when the primary process affects the glomerulus. It has been postulated that the tubulointerstitial disease can produce atrophy of tubules or obstruction destroying individual nephrons. Even when tubular inflammation is treated, progressive scarring can continue unabated. Thus, treatments designed to reduce interstitial fibrosis may be important for preventing progression of disease. At present, only experimental drugs not available for human use have been examined for this purpose.

Hyperlipidemia

Hyperlipidemia is frequently observed in disorders associated with nephrotic range proteinuria, but is also noted in a large percentage of the general population without renal disease. Experimental evidence obtained from animal studies shows hyperlipidemia can promote progression of renal failure. Thus, loading with cholesterol augments renal injury and treatment with cholesterol-lowering drugs slows the rate of progression. This effect is synergistic to that achieved by lowering blood pressure.

The mechanisms underlying the effects of lipids are not well understood, but possible explanations include mesangial lipid deposition leading to glomerular injury or tubular injury. A few studies performed in human subjects have demonstrated benefit from lipid lowering on the progression of renal injury, although they are not conclusive. Because patients with chronic renal failure have a high prevalence of cardiovascular disease, it is reasonable to initiate therapy with statin drugs to lower serum cholesterol and lipid levels.

Calcium-Phosphate Deposition

A rise in serum phosphorus, usually seen at the later stages of renal failure, can lead to precipitation of calcium phosphate in the renal interstitium. The deposits can then induce an inflammatory response producing interstitial fibrosis and tubular atrophy. Some have indicated that the deposits may form prior to detectable elevations in serum phosphorus concentrations.

Increased Glomerular Prostaglandin Production

An increment in glomerular prostaglandin production has been found in several studies of chronic renal failure. The increased prostanoids produce renal vasodilatation and a rise in intraglomerular pressure, factors that augment progression of disease.

METABOLIC ACIDOSIS

Metabolic acidosis commonly develops in the course of chronic renal failure. In response to the acidosis, ammonia production per residual functioning nephron is augmented. It has been postulated that the increased local production of ammonia in some way induces tubulointerstitial damage. This issue remains controversial, as some studies do not support this possibility.

SPECIFIC TREATMENT MEASURES

Treatment of patients with chronic renal failure should be designed to ameliorate those factors that can cause progression of renal injury, treat or prevent important complications, and normalize important laboratory abnormalities that contribute to symptoms of the disease.

Measures Designed to Reduce the Rate of Progression of Renal Failure

CONTROL OF SYSTEMIC AND INTRAGLOMERULAR HYPERTENSION

Experimental and human studies demonstrate that control of systemic hypertension can slow the rate of progression of renal disease substantially. Recent evidence indicates that target blood pressure levels should be lower than recommended for the general population (<130/80). Control of hypertension with the use of myriad agents can benefit the patient with renal failure. However, as indicated

previously, reduction in intraglomerular hypertension may be the most important factor underlying the benefits from blood pressure control. Therefore, when possible, treatment with ACEIs, ARBs, or the combination of these agents should be first-line antihypertensive therapy in these patients. Patients who do not tolerate these drugs might benefit from administration of non-dihydropyridine calcium channel blockers. In patients with proteinuria, even if blood pressure is controlled or they are normotensive, the doses of ACEIs or ARBs should be raised to levels even greater than recommended to reduce urine protein excretion to levels less than 500 mg. This reduction in proteinuria is the most optimal in protecting the kidney.

Potentially serious complications with ACEIs or ARBs include acute reduction in GFR and hyperkalemia. If these complications occur, a reduction in dose or even discontinuation of these agents might be required. It is recommended that these agents be continued even when GFR is less than 20 mL/min. Given the potential severity of these complications, patients should be monitored closely.

PROTEIN RESTRICTION

The benefits of protein restriction in preventing progression are unclear, but it has suggested that reducing protein intake to 0.8 to 1.0 g/kg body weight of high biologic value is beneficial. Others have indicated that 0.6 g/kg body weight should be used. In patients with substantial proteinuria, the quantity of protein recommended will have to be adjusted to prevent hypoalbuminemia. Once patients reached later stage 4, protein restriction may be useful to prevent expression of uremic symptoms. Reducing protein intake will have the added benefit of decreasing acid, potassium, and phosphate production.

CONTROL OF LIPIDS

Control of cholesterol with statins may help prevent progression and should reduce the burden of cardiovascular disease, which remains the most lethal disorder for patients with chronic renal failure. Adherence to the newly proposed aggressive recommendation appears reasonable.

Measures Designed to Treat Significant Laboratory Abnormalities

ANEMIA

Patients with renal anemia should be treated with erythropoietin (Procrit). Although this requires subcutaneous injection once per week, newer, long-lasting forms (darbepoetin [Aranesp]) enable patients to be treated every 3 weeks. Because iron stores need to be repleted for anemia to be successfully treated, these should be monitored and iron given. Because of the vagaries of ferritin measurements, we use serum iron and iron binding capacity with the goal of maintaining saturation above 20% and near 30%. At present, the target hemoglobin and hematocrit vary between 11 mg/dL and 12 mg/dL 33 and 36, respectively. Given the recent concern about vascular complications with EPO therapy, the clinican must be vigilant in preventing Hg values from exceeding 12 gm/dL.

METABOLIC ACIDOSIS

Controversy exists as to the target value of bicarbonate for patients with chronic renal failure. Some experts recommend raising plasma bicarbonate to levels above 20 mEq/L, whereas others recommend complete normalization of plasma bicarbonate. To properly raise plasma bicarbonate concentration, the deficit should be calculated from the formula:

Desired − prevailing level of plasma bicarbonate
$$\times\ 50\%\ \text{body weight} = \text{Total bicarbonate deficit}$$

The deficit should be corrected slowly over several days.

CURRENT THERAPY

The recommendations for the treatment of patients with renal failure is as follows:

Recommendation	Goal
Control BP.	130/80 mm Hg
Reduce proteinuria by administering angiotensin converting enzyme inhibitors or angiotensin receptor blockers. In some cases both agents may have to be given concomitantly.	Decrease urine protein excretion as low as possible but at least less than 1 g per day.
Control phosphate concentrations with phosphate binders with noncalcium containing binders when possible.	Serum phosphate <4.5 mg/dL
Maintain vitamin D by administration of ergocalciferol.	Maintain 25 OH D levels at 30 ng/mL by administration of ergocalciferol
Prevent hyperparathyroidism with vitamin D or calcimimetics.	Maintain PTH <150 pg/mL
Correct anemia with erythropoietin and iron replacement as needed.	Maintain Hg between 11 and 12 mg/dL
Administer diuretics to control hypertension and volume overload.	Maintain euvolemia when possible
Control serum potassium with dietary restriction, diuretics, and/or potassium exchange resin as necessary.	Maintain serum potassium <5.0 mEq/L
Keep protein intake at 0.6 to 0.8 g/kg body weight per day.	Slow progression of renal disease while preventing protein depletion
Control metabolic acidosis with administration of sodium citrate (Citra pH).	Maintain serum HCO_3 >20 mEq/L

Abbreviations: BP = blood pressure; HCO_3 = bicarbonate; Hg = mercury; PTH = parathyroid hormone.

Because patients experience gas when the base is given as bicarbonate, the base is usually administered as Shohl's solution sodium citrate,* the citrate being metabolized to bicarbonate in the liver. Each milliliter of Shohl's solution represents 1 mEq of the base.

DIVALENT ION METABOLISM

Serum phosphorus is controlled by administration of phosphate binders usually starting with calcium citrate (Citracal) or acetate (PhosLo). If these are not successful or if patients have elevated serum calcium levels, then sevelamar (Renagel) or lanthanum (Fosrenol) can be used alone or in combination with calcium binders. Physicians should aim to maintain serum phosphorus levels below 5 mg/dL and keep serum calcium phosphorus product below 60.

Parathyroid hormone (PTH) levels should be maintained below 150 pg/mL, or less depending on stage; levels associated with proper

---

*Investigational drug in the United States.

bone remodeling but not to values observed in patients without kidney disease. Suppression of parathyroid hormone secretion can be achieved by administration of various vitamin D analogues. The recent recognition of the calcium-sensing receptor and development of calcimimetic drugs that are extremely effective in lowering PTH secretion may make using vitamin D compounds obsolete in the future.

Low 25 OH D levels have been documented in a large number of individuals both with and without renal failure. In patients with renal impairment this can contribute to the abnormal 1,25 OH vitamin D levels. Measurement of 25-hydroxy vitamin D levels should be obtained in all patients with CKD and EGFR <60 mL/min. If levels are below 30 ng/mL they should be supplemented with ergocalciferol sufficient to maintain levels above this level.

HYPERKALEMIA

As this is the most serious electrolyte disorder encountered, patients should be monitored closely. Serum potassium concentrations should be maintained below 5 mEq/L. If hyperkalemia develops during treatment with ACEIs or ARBs, the doses of these agents should be reduced or discontinued. Diuretic administration, often given for control of hypertension, can help control hyperkalemia, but if it should develop, particularly when GFR falls below 20% of normal, it can be treated with the potassium exchange resin, sodium polystyrene sulfonate (Kayexalate).

ELEVATED BLOOD UREA NITROGEN CONCENTRATION

The precise solutes that are retained, which are important for the pathogenesis of the uremic syndrome, are not clear. However, BUN is a marker for other retained solutes and is roughly correlated with development of uremic symptoms. When the BUN is greater than 100 mg/dL and serum creatinine concentration is greater than 8 mg/dL uremic symptoms may develop. These symptoms will often abate merely with protein restriction and reduced production of these compounds. Protein restriction is usually not instituted until GFR is less than 15% to 20% of normal. Prior to that time, it is important to maintain protein intake to keep serum albumin within the normal range.

VOLUME OVERLOAD

Because salt retention is an essential component of the development of hypertension and underlies volume overload, diuretic administration is usually necessary in the treatment of chronic renal failure. Thiazides frequently used in the treatment of hypertension or volume overload in subjects with normal renal function may not be efficacious once GFR is less than or equal to 33% of normal. Therefore, loop diuretics, such as furosemide (Lasix) or a combined loop and proximal tubule diuretic such as metolozone (Zaroxolyn), are generally indicated. Because the effectiveness of both agents requires access to the tubule lumen, the effective dose is often higher than in those with normal renal function. Once patients are in stage 4 renal failure, use of diuretics is hampered by worsening of renal failure and often must be used cautiously.

REFERENCES

Beco JA, Bansal VK. Medical nutrition therapy in chronic kidney failure: Integrating clinical practice guidelines. J Am Diet Assoc 2004;104:404–9.

Clase CM, Garg AX, Kiberd BA. Prevalence of low glomerular filtration rate in nondiabetic Americans: Third National Health and Nutrition Examination Survey (NHANES III). J Am Soc Nephrol 2002;13.

Cleveland DR, Jindal KK, Hirsch DJ, et al. Quality of pre-referral care in patients with chronic renal insufficiency. Am J Kidney Dis 2002;40:30–6.

Curtin RB, Becker B, Kimmel PL, Schatell D. An integrated approach to care for patients with chronic kidney disease. Semin Dial 2003;16:399–402.

Djamali A, Kendziorski C, Brazy PC, Becker BN. Disease progression and outcomes in chronic kidney disease and renal transplantation. Kidney Int 2003;64:1800–7.

KDOQI. Clinical practice guidelines and clinical practice recommendations for diabetes and chronic kidney disease. Am J Kidney Dis 2007;49:S1–154.

Kopple JD. National Kidney Foundation K/DOQ1 clinical practice guidelines for nutrition in chronic renal failure. Am J Kidney Dis 2001;37:S66–S70.

Maschio G, Alberti D, Janin G, et al. Effect of the angiotensin-converging-enzyme inhibitor benazepril on the progression of chronic renal insufficiency. N Engl J Med 1996;334:939–45.

Tonelli M, Gill J, Pandeya S, et al. Slowing the progression of chronic renal insufficiency. Can Med Assoc J 2002;166:906–7.

Malignant Tumors of the Urogenital Tract

Method of
Peter E. Clark, MD

Carcinoma of the Prostate

Prostate cancer is the most common noncutaneous solid malignancy among men in the United States, and it is second only to lung cancer with respect to cancer-related mortality. In 2008, there were an estimated 186,320 new cases of prostate cancer and 28,660 deaths due to this disease. Because prostate cancer is predominantly a disease of the elderly, its incidence may be expected to rise over time as the U.S. population ages.

There is a familial predisposition to prostate cancer, which is more common among those with a first-degree relative who also has the disease, and it appears to be more common among African American men than among Caucasian men. Environmental factors that have been associated with an increased risk of prostate cancer include a high-fat Western-style diet, as compared with a high-soy Asian diet, and low levels of vitamin D.

Hereditary prostate cancer is relatively rare but may account for up to 40% of tumors among young men with the disease. One of several genes found in families with hereditary prostate cancer is hereditary prostate cancer 1 (*HPC1*), which is located on the long arm of chromosome 1. Translocations leading to fusion of two genes (TMPRSS2:ERG gene fusion) has also been implicated in a large number of sporadic prostate cancers.

DIAGNOSIS

The vast majority of prostate cancers are adenocarcinomas. There is a large discrepancy between the risk of finding incidental prostate cancer at autopsy (estimated to be as high as 75% by age 80 or older) and the risk of having the disease clinically diagnosed (lifetime risk, approximately 1 in 6). Most men with early-stage prostate cancer diagnosed in the modern era have no specific disease-related symptoms. Benign prostatic hypertrophy is often found in association with prostate cancer and is also more common in men as they age, but there is no known causal relationship between the two. Prostate cancer can rarely manifest with pelvic pain, bladder outlet obstruction, or ureteral obstruction from locally advanced disease or with bone pain from distant metastatic disease.

The advent and widespread use of the serum prostate-specific antigen (PSA) test as a screening tool for prostate cancer has resulted in a stage migration, with most men now diagnosed with early-stage disease. This has been associated with better recurrence-free survival rates after definitive local therapy. Certain groups, such as the American Urologic Association and the American Cancer Society, have advocated that physicians offer annual screening with a serum PSA determination and digital rectal examination for all men older than 50 years of age and for African American men and those with a family history of prostatic cancer starting at age 40 years. However, these recommendations are not uniformly accepted; the U.S. Preventive Services Task Force continues to state that the available evidence is insufficient to recommend routine screening with PSA for prostate cancer. It is generally accepted that the decision to screen for prostate cancer should be made in individuals with at least 10 years of life expectancy.

Serum PSA is specific for the prostate but is not specific for cancer. It is secreted by both benign and malignant prostatic epithelial cells. The PSA may be elevated in men with a variety of prostate-related conditions, such as prostatitis, benign prostatic hypertrophy, urinary tract infection, or prostatic cancer. Until recently, a PSA level lower than 4.0 ng/mL was considered normal, and in younger men a value of greater than 2.5 ng/mL could perhaps be considered abnormal. More recently, it has become clear that there is no true cutoff value for PSA. Instead, the association between PSA and prostate cancer risk is a continuum. Even at a PSA of essentially zero, there is still a 6% chance of having prostate cancer on biopsy.

The majority of the serum PSA is bound to protease inhibitors such as α_1-antichymotrypsin, whereas a fraction is unconjugated or free. The relative proportion of free serum PSA can be used to improve the specificity of PSA for diagnosis of prostate cancer by biopsy. Benign prostatic hypertrophy is associated with a higher proportion of free PSA, and patients with greater 25% free serum PSA are less likely to harbor prostate cancer. The precise cutoff point associated with prostate cancer is controversial and ranges from 10% to 20% or higher. Development of new tests to improve PSA specificity, such as measurement of complexed PSA or early pro-forms of PSA, is an area of ongoing investigation.

The most common method used to diagnose prostate cancer is a transrectal ultrasonography (TRUS)-guided prostate biopsy. TRUS allows for accurate localization of the zonal anatomy of the prostate and can accurately measure its size. It therefore acts as a guide for the biopsy, because prostatic cancers typically reside in the peripheral zone, and biopsies are concentrated within that zone. Although prostate cancer can manifest as hypoechoic lesions on TRUS, the tumors usually are not visible. TRUS lacks both sensitivity and specificity and should not be used as a screening test.

The most common grading system used to estimate the degree of tumor differentiation is the Gleason grading system. The two most common Gleason grade patterns (on a scale of 1 to 5) are summed to give a score between 2 and 10. Tumors with Gleason scores between 2 and 6 are well differentiated and have a better prognosis, whereas those with Gleason scores between 8 and 10 are poorly differentiated and have a worse prognosis. Gleason score 7 is associated with intermediate differentiation and prognosis. The majority of cancers found in the modern era are well to intermediately differentiated (Gleason score 5 to 7).

Staging of prostatic cancer defines the local, regional, and distant extent of disease. The tumor-node-metastasis (TNM) staging system is the most commonly used method. The most common clinical stage in the modern era is that of nonpalpable tumors detected because of a concerning PSA result (stage T1c). The primary staging modality for local disease is the digital rectal examination. This may be supplemented by pelvic magnetic resonance imaging in selected cases where there is significant concern for locally advanced disease based on the digital rectal examination. Although PSA only roughly correlates with the overall disease burden, bone metastasis is quite uncommon among patients whose PSA value is less than 20 ng/mL. Therefore, a radionucleotide bone scan in the absence of symptoms is not required routinely if the PSA value is less than 10 ng/mL and the Gleason sum is 7 or less. Computed tomography (CT) scanning is not routinely used, because grossly positive nodes are detected rarely with a clinically localized tumor.

Lymph node staging is important in selecting patients for therapy. CT scanning may show enlarged lymph nodes in patients with high-volume or high-grade primary tumor but has poor sensitivity and specificity. Laparoscopic pelvic lymphadenectomy can provide adequate sampling of the pelvic lymph nodes in those patients not selecting surgery. More commonly, lymph node dissection is performed concomitantly at the time of radical prostatectomy.

TREATMENT

There is no one optimal treatment for clinically localized prostatic cancer, so therapy must be individualized. Among men with a life expectancy of less than 10 years, observation alone may be appropriate. Carefully selected men with low-risk prostate cancer may choose active surveillance rather than curative treatment but must be rigorously monitored for evidence of worsening disease.

Surgery and radiation therapy are the most commonly used curative modalities. For low-risk, organ-confined tumors, the 15-year disease-free survival rates are greater than 90% among patients treated with surgery. Moreover, the survival outcome is similar after radiation therapy and after surgery. However, properly done prospective, randomized comparisons among similarly staged patients have not been done. Radiation therapy can be delivered as external-beam radiotherapy or as brachytherapy using radioactive seeds (iodine 125 or palladium 103) implanted directly into the prostate. Cryotherapy (i.e., freezing of the prostate) is another approved treatment for men with prostatic carcinoma that is becoming more widely accepted as an alternative treatment option.

Radical prostatectomy, or surgical removal of the prostate, may be performed via an open incision or by a laparoscopic technique. Traditionally, an open surgery is performed through an anterior, retropubic approach or, less commonly, through a perineal incision. Laparoscopic and, in particular, robot-assisted radical prostatectomy is being performed with increasing frequency. The benefits of a robot-assisted approach may include reduced blood loss, sooner return to normal function, and possibly better functional outcomes and better surgical margin rates (although the latter two have not been definitively demonstrated to this point). In patients who were sexually active before therapy, preservation of the neurovascular bundles is often undertaken in an attempt to maintain postoperative sexual function. For patients with organ-confined disease, the prognosis is excellent, with a life expectancy similar to that of men without prostatic cancer. For those patients with positive surgical margins or positive lymph nodes on final pathology, consideration can be given to delivering, respectively, adjuvant irradiation or androgen-deprivation therapy (ADT).

Serum PSA should rapidly become undetectable after radical prostatectomy, because, in theory, all PSA-producing tissue has been removed. After radiation therapy or cryotherapy, the PSA is expected to reach low levels over time and then remain stable. An increasing serum PSA is evidence of tumor recurrence. There is controversy about when to initiate ADT in men with a rising PSA level after treatment.

Prostatic cancer, at least initially, is an androgen-sensitive disease. Therefore, the primary first-line treatment for metastatic prostate cancer is ADT. Suppression of serum testosterone can be achieved by orchiectomy (i.e., surgical castration). Alternatively, medical castration may be considered. Luteinizing hormone–releasing hormone analogues effectively suppress testosterone to the castrate range within 1 month after administration by suppressing central nervous system secretion of luteinizing hormone. There is increasing awareness that ADT can be associated with significant long-term morbidity, including vasomotor reflex changes (hot flushes), loss of libido, erectile dysfunction, osteoporosis, anemia, muscle wasting, gynecomastia, and possibly cognitive changes and increased risk of cardiovascular disease. The choice to use ADT must, therefore, be carefully balanced based on the individual patient's overall risk of prostate cancer–related morbidity and mortality versus ADT-related morbidity.

Most patients with metastatic disease initially respond to ADT, but almost inexorably the disease progresses despite ongoing ADT, to become castrate-resistant prostate cancer (CRPC). At that point, the median survival time is less than 2 years. The standard chemotherapy for CRPC is docetaxel (Taxotere) plus prednisone, and prospective randomized trials have demonstrated a modest survival benefit among patients so treated. Another approved drug is mitoxantrone (Novantrone) for palliative relief of symptomatic bone pain from CRPC. Radiation therapy can be used effectively to palliate focal sites of bone metastases. The mechanisms by which prostatic carcinoma escapes hormonal control and becomes castrate resistant represent an area of ongoing intensive research.

Tumors of the Renal Parenchyma

Malignant tumors of the renal parenchyma are of either primary or metastatic origin. Primary renal tumors may be benign or malignant. The most common tumor is primary renal cell carcinoma (RCC);

other tumor types, such as papillary, chromophobe, collecting duct, and medullary carcinomas and sarcomas, occur infrequently. The most common benign renal tumors are angiomyolipomas and oncocytomas. The latter, in particular, are generally indistinguishable from malignant lesions on radiographic imaging. Metastatic lesions (e.g., from lung, breast, melanoma, or ovary) may occur, and primary lymphoma may be present in the kidney.

RENAL CELL CARCINOMA

RCC is the most common primary neoplasm of the kidney, accounting for more than 85% of all primary renal tumors. There were an estimated 54,390 newly diagnosed cases of RCC in the United States in 2008, and an estimated 13,010 people died of this disease. RCC represents approximately 3% of all adult malignancies and usually manifests between 40 and 60 years of age, although it can be found in younger age groups. It has a 2:1 male-to-female preponderance and in both sporadic and familial forms is associated with aberrations of the von Hippel–Lindau (VHL) gene and protein.

RCC is thought to arise from cells of the proximal convoluted tubule. The most consistent genetic aberration found in most cases of sporadic, conventional RCC are aberrations in the *VHL* gene. No specific agent has been implicated as the cause of RCC, although tobacco products are associated with an approximately twofold increased risk of being diagnosed with the disease. Patients, and particularly younger patients, with end-stage renal disease who develop acquired cystic disease of the kidney also have an increased risk of RCC. Between 1% and 2% of these patients develop RCC, so annual renal ultrasonography is reasonable as a screening tool in this population, with confirmatory studies such as CT for complex or suspicious lesions.

Diagnosis

The most common sign associated with RCC in 29% to 60% of cases is hematuria. The classic triad of flank pain, hematuria, and a palpable abdominal mass is relatively rare, occurring in fewer than 10% of cases. Other common symptoms and signs include fever, anemia, hypercalcemia, thrombocytosis, and elevated erythrocyte sedimentation rate, lactate dehydrogenase, or alkaline phosphatase. Currently, there are no reliable, commercially available tumor markers for RCC. Most often, these tumors are incidentally diagnosed on radiographic imaging performed for unrelated or nonspecific purposes.

The most commonly used staging system for RCC is the TNM staging system. It allows for a distinction between venous involvement and nodal invasion and stratifies the extent of each stage. RCC can involve the renal vein and vena cava and may even extend into the right atrium. Locally, it can directly invade surrounding structures such as the adrenal gland and colon. Five-year survival rates range from 80% to 90% for stages T1 N0 M0 (<7 cm) and T2 N0 M0 (>7 cm), 40% to 60% for stage T3 N0 M0, and 10% to 20% for N1–3 and M1 disease.

Treatment

Surgical excision of the tumor is the primary treatment for RCC. The classic procedure was a radical nephrectomy, in which the kidney was removed en bloc within Gerota's fascia and the ipsilateral adrenal gland and lymph nodes. This was routinely performed as an open procedure (flank, transabdominal, or thoracoabdominal incision). Adrenalectomy is now generally reserved for upper-pole tumors, very large tumors, or lesions that directly extend into the adrenal gland. Although these operations are increasingly performed through a laparoscopic approach, an open approach is usually preferred if there is extensive involvement of the inferior vena cava. In rare cases with supradiaphragmatic tumor extension within the cava, cardiopulmonary bypass may be required for tumor extraction.

A partial nephrectomy has become a standard approach for surgical excision of renal parenchymal tumors, particularly for individuals with solitary kidneys, those with bilateral masses, and those with compromised renal function. It has become the preferred operation for patients who have lesions of 4 cm or smaller and a normal contralateral kidney, because local recurrence rates are less than 5%, and partial (rather than radical) nephrectomy is associated with a lower long-term risk of chronic renal failure. As with radical nephrectomy, there is a growing experience with laparoscopic approaches to partial nephrectomy. There are also several investigational, minimally invasive approaches that are being explored including radiographically guided, percutaneous thermal tumor ablation using radiofrequency ablation or cryotherapy. Final acceptance of these modalities awaits more long-term data on their oncologic efficacy.

Up to 25% of patients initially present with metastatic disease. Sites of metastasis of RCC, in decreasing frequency of occurrence, include lung, lymph nodes, liver, bone, and adrenal gland. Chemotherapy and irradiation have little to no survival benefit, with radiation therapy only palliating painful metastases. The mainstay of treatment in the past was immunotherapy, with 5-year survival rates of 10% to 20%. Modern therapies for advanced or metastatic RCC now include the so-called targeted therapies, such as the oral tyrosine kinase inhibitors, sunitinib (Sutent) and sorafenib (Nexavar), and the mammalian target of rapamycin (mTOR) inhibitor, temsirolimus (Torisel). Evidence suggests improved survival among those patients who undergo nephrectomy before systemic immunotherapy.

BENIGN RENAL TUMORS

Although they are not as frequent as malignant tumors, benign solid masses are also seen in the kidney. Angiomyolipomas can often be diagnosed radiographically based on the appearance of fat by CT scan. They can occur sporadically or as part of an inherited familial syndrome, tuberous sclerosis. The latter entity is characterized by mental retardation, benign tumors of the cerebellum, epilepsy, adenoma sebaceum, and angiomyolipomas. Approximately 50% of patients with tuberous sclerosis develop angiomyolipomas, most of which are bilateral and multifocal. The management of angiomyolipoma is controversial and should be individualized. Asymptomatic tumors smaller than 4 cm can generally be observed with annual radiographic imaging. Symptomatic lesions (bleeding, pain, rapid growth) and lesions larger than 4 cm should be considered for surgical excision, although angioembolization is another option. Acute hemorrhage from an angiomyolipoma can often be managed or at least stabilized by angioembolization.

Oncocytomas are the most common solid, benign renal tumors and account for 5% to 10% of solid renal lesions. Although these lesions tend to have a more uniform density than RCC and can have a characteristic central scar or spoke-wheel appearance on CT, there is no radiographic feature that reliably distinguishes an oncocytoma from a malignant renal lesion. Oncocytoma is therefore a diagnosis that should be made only on histologic analysis. The tumors characteristically exhibit eosinophilic, granular cells packed with mitochondria. Oncocytomas are thought to arise from the distal portion of the renal tubule.

METASTATIC RENAL LESIONS

The most common primary malignancy to metastasize to the kidney is lung cancer, although cancers of the ovary, breast, or bowel, melanoma, and lymphoma can do so as well. Lymphoma of the kidney is almost always a manifestation of systemic disease. The management is therefore grounded in systemic chemotherapy, with surgery reserved for palliative symptom relief. However, approximately 15% of renal lymphomas manifest with a solitary renal mass as the sole radiographic manifestation. These lesions can be challenging to manage and difficult to distinguish from RCC preoperatively.

Tumors of the Renal Pelvis and Ureter

Approximately 10% of all renal tumors originate in the renal pelvis rather than the renal parenchyma. These account for 5% of all urothelial carcinomas (the majority of which arise in the bladder). Of the upper tract urothelial carcinomas, approximately one fourth arise in the ureter and the remainder in the renal pelvis. Urothelial carcinoma of the upper urinary tract is more common in men than in women and more common in whites than in blacks. Environmental exposures associated with

a higher risk of developing upper tract urothelial carcinoma include analgesic abuse, cyclophosphamide (Cytoxan), and a strong association with tobacco abuse.

Among patients with bladder cancer, approximately 3% to 5% develop upper tract urothelial carcinoma. This can increase to as high as 20% among those with carcinoma in situ (CIS) or high-grade disease. Conversely, approximately 30% to 70% of patients with a history of upper tract urothelial carcinoma go on to develop bladder cancer. As a consequence, these patients require ongoing periodic cystoscopic surveillance. The incidence of bilateral upper tract tumors is 2% to 5%. Other histologic tumor types that can manifest in the upper urinary tract include squamous cell carcinoma (SCC) and adenocarcinoma. Although they are rare, the risk is increased among patients with a history of recurrent, refractory urinary tract infections or staghorn calculi.

DIAGNOSIS

The most common presenting symptom for upper tract urothelial tumors is hematuria. For patients with adequate renal function, the evaluation for hematuria includes CT urography, urinary cytology (or another urinary-based tumor marker), and cystoscopy. Urinary cytology has a high specificity but a generally poor sensitivity, particularly for low-grade disease. Other urinary tumor markers, such as NMP-22, and fluorescent in situ hybridization approaches typically have better sensitivity but are not as specific. A retrograde ureteropyelogram may be helpful in patients with poor renal function who cannot receive intravenous contrast agents. In general, if a suspicious mass is seen on CT or other imaging, a ureteroscopy is typically performed with biopsy or brushings to establish the diagnosis. The TNM system is the standard for staging.

TREATMENT

Disease isolated to the distal ureter is most often managed with distal ureterectomy and ureteroneocystostomy. High-grade or high stage disease and multifocal disease isolated to one side are optimally managed in most cases by excision of that upper tract system via a radical nephroureterectomy, including excision of the distal portion of the ureter and complete excision of the ureteral orifice together with a cuff of bladder. Traditionally, these procedures were done via open incisions (one or two separate incisions, depending on the surgeon), but laparoscopy is increasingly being used to decrease patient morbidity and improve surgical recovery. In selected patients who have low-grade, low-stage disease with a small overall disease burden, an endoscopic approach using laser or electrocautery to destroy the tumors may be considered. This is also a strong consideration for those patients with bilateral disease or involvement of a functionally solitary renal unit. Most often, retrograde endoscopic approaches via ureteroscopy are employed, although in highly selected cases antegrade percutaneous approaches have been reported.

Carcinoma of the Bladder

UROTHELIAL CARCINOMA OF THE BLADDER

Bladder carcinoma is the fifth most common malignancy in the United States, with more than 68,810 new cases diagnosed annually. It is almost three times more common in men than in women, in whom it is the fourth most common cancer. Because of its propensity to recur, particularly in patients with superficial disease, it is the second most prevalent cancer. High-grade bladder cancer is a deadly disease and is the fifth most common cause of cancer deaths among men. There is a well-established relationship between the development of bladder cancer and a variety of carcinogens. Perhaps the most widespread factor is tobacco abuse. Cigarette smoking is thought to account for up to half of all bladder cancers in men. Bladder cancer is also associated with other, less frequent occupational exposures, such as in the rubber and oil refinery industries. It is also associated with exposure to the chemotherapeutic agent, cyclophosphamide (Cytoxan); exposed patients have up to a ninefold increased risk of developing bladder cancer, most likely related to a urinary metabolite of cyclophosphamide, acrolein.

Carcinoma of the Prostate

- Average-risk patients are offered screening with prostate-specific antigen (PSA) testing and digital rectal examination (DRE) at 50 years of age, high-risk patients with a strong family history, and African American patients at age 40 years.
- Patients with an elevated PSA or abnormal DRE are referred for discussion regarding risks, benefits, and alternatives to biopsy of the prostate.
- Diagnosis is made with transrectal ultrasound-guided biopsy of the prostate.
- Staging with bone scan is done for patients with high-grade tumors (Gleason grade 4 or 5), PSA levels greater than 20 µg/mL, elevated alkaline phosphatase levels, or bone pain.

Renal Cell Carcinoma

- Hematuria is the single most common sign, occurring in up to 60% of cases. Flank pain and a palpable mass can also occur, but the classic triad of hematuria, flank pain, and a palpable abdominal mass is present in only 10% of cases. Other common signs and symptoms are fever, anemia, thrombocytosis, hypercalcemia, and an elevated sedimentation rate.
- Most tumors are asymptomatic and are detected incidentally on radiographic imaging (renal ultrasonography, computed tomography [CT] scanning, or magnetic resonance imaging).

Benign Renal Tumors

- Angiomyolipomas have a characteristic appearance of fat within the lesion on CT scans.
- Angiomyolipomas may occur sporadically or as part of the tuberous sclerosis complex.
- Tuberous sclerosis is characterized by benign tumors within the cerebellum, mental retardation, epilepsy, and adenoma sebaceum. Angiomyolipomas occur in half of these patients and are typically bilateral and multifocal, making management more challenging.
- Oncocytomas are benign renal tumors that account for 5% to 10% of solid renal lesions.
- Oncocytomas can be more round and of uniform density, or they may have a central scar or spoke-wheel appearance on CT scan. However, no feature can reliably distinguish these tumors from a malignant renal tumor.
- Oncocytomas should be diagnosed only histologically; they are characterized by eosinophilic granular, mitochondria-laden cells.
- In general, a non–fat-containing, solid renal mass should be considered malignant until proven otherwise.

Tumors of the Renal Pelvis and Ureter

- Tumors arising in the renal pelvis account for 10% of all renal tumors and approximately 5% of all urothelial carcinomas.
- Ureteral tumors account for 25% of upper tract urothelial carcinomas.
- These tumors are more common in men than in women.
- Cigarette smoking is strongly associated with an increased risk, as are analgesic abuse and cyclophosphamide (Cytoxan).
- The most common presenting symptom is hematuria.

- Diagnostic work-up usually includes CT urography, urinary cytology, and cystoscopy.
- Cytologic examination of the urine has a high specificity but poor sensitivity, particularly for low-grade lesions.
- Between 3% and 5% of patients with bladder cancer have associated upper tract urothelial carcinoma. This risk is increased in patients with carcinoma in situ (CIS) or high-grade disease, in whom the risk can be as high as 20%.
- Patients with upper tract urothelial carcinoma have a 30% to 70% risk of developing bladder cancer.

Urothelial Carcinoma of the Bladder

- Painless, gross hematuria is the most common presenting symptom.
- Twenty percent of patients present with only microscopic hematuria.
- Irritative voiding symptoms such as frequency, urgency, or dysuria may also suggest a malignancy, particularly CIS.
- Patients with suspected bladder cancer should undergo an evaluation of their upper tracts (typically by CT), cystoscopy, and cytologic examination of the urine (or another urine-based tumor marker study).
- Transurethral biopsy or resection confirms the diagnosis.
- Ninety percent of bladder cancers are urothelial carcinoma, and 75% are non–muscle-invasive (superficial) at presentation.

Urethral Carcinoma

- Urethral carcinoma is the only urologic malignancy that is more common in females than in males.
- Fifty percent of cases are associated with urethral stricture.
- Urethral carcinoma may manifest as hematuria, obstructive voiding, or a palpable mass.
- Transurethral biopsy is usually required for diagnosis.

Penile Cancer

- Squamous cell carcinoma of the penis occurs most commonly in the sixth decade of life.
- Symptoms are related to ulceration, necrosis, suppuration, and hemorrhage of the penile lesion.
- The diagnosis is established by biopsy.
- Clinical evaluation of patients with penile cancer includes physical examination with palpation of the inguinal region, chest radiography, CT of the abdomen and pelvis, and bone scan.

Testicular Cancer

- Testicular cancer is relatively rare overall, but it is the most common malignancy in men between the ages of 15 and 35 years, with 8090 new cases occurring annually.
- Testicular cancer often manifests as a painless, enlarging testicular mass.
- Malignant tumors of the testis can be divided into those originating from the germinal cells (seminomatous and nonseminomatous germ cell tumors), rare tumors from the supporting cells (Leydig cells and Sertoli cells), and rare metastases from another primary site.
- Ninety-five percent of tumors originating in the testis are germ cell tumors. Fewer than 10% of all germ cell tumors arise from extragonadal primary sites such as the mediastinum or retroperitoneum.
- Human β-chorionic gonadotropin and α-fetoprotein are accurate and relatively specific tumor markers for testicular cancer.

Approximately 90% of bladder malignancies are urothelial carcinomas. Of these, the majority (70%) are papillary, 10% are sessile, and 20% demonstrate mixed morphology. Although roughly three quarters of bladder cancer patients present with superficial disease, approximately 20% to 25% progress to muscle invasion over time. Nevertheless, 80% to 90% of patients with muscle-invasive disease had it at initial presentation. A strong correlation exists between tumor grade and stage; most well-differentiated tumors are superficial, and most poorly differentiated tumors are invasive. CIS is a poorly differentiated urothelial carcinoma that grows as a sheet confined to the urothelium. CIS may be found as a solitary or multifocal process and is associated with invasive carcinoma in 25% of cases, where it portends a poor prognosis. Between 10% and 20% of patients treated with cystectomy for diffuse or refractory CIS are found to have microscopic muscle-invasive disease.

Diagnosis

Gross painless hematuria is the most common presenting sign of bladder cancer. However, approximately 1 in 5 patients have only microscopic hematuria. Other symptoms that can be indicative of urothelial carcinoma (in particular, CIS) include irritative voiding symptoms such as frequency, urgency, and dysuria. Patients who present with symptoms and signs concerning for urothelial carcinoma should undergo an evaluation that includes cystoscopy, urinary tumor marker study (typically, urinary cytology), and evaluation of the upper tracts (typically by CT urography). The diagnosis is usually confirmed at the time of transurethral resection or biopsy.

Treatment

The management options for urothelial carcinoma are heavily dependent on the stage and grade of disease. The TNM system is recommended for staging. For most superficial, low-grade tumors, transurethral resection, with or without a single, immediate instillation of a chemotherapeutic agent such as mitomycin-C (Mutamycin),[1] is all that is required. This must then be followed by careful, ongoing surveillance by cystoscopy, urinary tumor studies (typically cytology), and periodic upper tract imaging. For patients with high-grade disease (including CIS) and tumors that superficially invade the lamina propria (stage T1) or are rapidly recurrent tumors, adjuvant treatment with intravesical agents such as thiotepa (Thioplex), doxorubicin (Adriamycin), and mitomycin-C (Mutamycin)[1] or intravesical bacillus Calmette-Guérin (Tice BCG) may be indicated. In the United States, the most frequently used agent for this purpose, particularly for CIS, is intravesical BCG.

Patients with superficial disease must undergo regular surveillance, because the recurrence rate is as high as 50% at 5 years. Surveillance protocols vary but typically include cystoscopy and urinary tumor studies (usually urinary cytology) every 3 months for 2 years, then every 6 months for 3 years, and annually thereafter. Periodic evaluation of the upper tracts, typically by CT urography, is warranted, because there is a 3% to 5% incidence of development of upper tract urothelial carcinoma among patients with bladder urothelial carcinoma.

The risk of disease progression in patients with low-grade, low-stage (Ta) urothelial carcinoma is less than 5% to 10%. This risk increases as the stage and grade of the tumor increase. Patients who have muscle-invasive disease (stage T2 or higher), either at presentation or with progression after therapy for superficial disease, are best treated by radical cystectomy and urinary diversion. A thorough pelvic lymphadenectomy should be performed at the time of surgery. The precise limits of dissection for the lymphadenectomy remain somewhat controversial, although the latest data suggest that patients who have more lymph nodes removed fare better.

High-grade bladder cancer is a potentially lethal disease. There are an estimated 14,100 deaths due to bladder cancer annually. Among patients with organ-confined (pT2a-pT2b), muscle-invasive disease

who undergo cystectomy, the 5-year recurrence-free survival rates are between 60% and 85%. For patients undergoing radical cystectomy who have extravesical extension of their disease (pT3-pT4 disease), the 5-year recurrence-free survival rates are lower, 40% to 60%. Patients with lymph node–positive disease fare the worst, with 5-year recurrence-free survival rates of 20% to 30%.

Patients with muscle-invasive bladder cancer should be considered for multimodal therapy (i.e., chemotherapy in addition to surgery). The standard regimen over the past decade has been MVAC: methotrexate (Trexall),[1] vinblastine (Velban),[1] doxorubicin (Adriamycin), and cisplatin (Platinol). This can be delivered either before surgery (neoadjuvant) or in the postsurgery setting (adjuvant). There is level 1 evidence to support MVAC chemotherapy combined with cystectomy for muscle-invasive bladder cancer, although the survival benefit across studies is only on the order of 5% to 10%. Newer agents, such as gemcitabine (Gemzar)[1] along with cisplatin, appear to offer similar response rates and reduced toxicity and are often used currently in lieu of MVAC. Cytotoxic chemotherapy produces response rates of 50% to 70% in patients with advanced or metastatic disease; however, the durable, long-term, complete response rates at 5 years are no more than 15% across series.

Urinary diversion may be accomplished after cystectomy in several ways, but the fundamental categories are incontinent and continent forms. Incontinent forms of diversion include ileal and colon conduits, both of which require that the patient wear an external collection appliance. Continent forms of diversion include the continent cutaneous diversion, which requires creation of a low-pressure reservoir (often of colon) and a catheterizable efferent limb with an associated valve mechanism to prevent urine leakage. More recently, emphasis has shifted to continent diversions in which the low-pressure reservoir is anastomosed to the native urethra. These orthotopic neobladders may be crafted from colon or ileum and offer the opportunity to avoid any external collection devices and, usually, any need for catheterization. Such devices may improve patients' quality of life after surgery, although this has not been formally demonstrated in a randomized trial.

ADENOCARCINOMA OF THE BLADDER

Adenocarcinomas account for fewer than 2% of bladder cancers. They can be found in three settings: as primary lesions in the bladder, as metastases or local extensions from another site, or as primary urachal carcinomas. They are typically invasive and poorly differentiated and carry a poor prognosis. Adenocarcinomas may be found in association with bladder augmentation cystoplasties and are the most common form of bladder cancer in patients born with bladder exstrophy. The treatment of choice is typically radical cystectomy, pelvic lymphadenectomy, and urinary diversion.

SQUAMOUS CELL CARCINOMA OF THE BLADDER

SCC accounts for approximately 6% of bladder cancers in the United States but more than 75% of bladder cancers in Egypt. SCC is associated with chronic bladder inflammation from a variety of sources. These include chronic indwelling Foley catheters, recurrent or refractory bladder infections, and bladder diverticula or stones. In Egypt, approximately 80% of SCCs are associated with *Schistosoma haematobium* infestation. These bilharzia-associated SCCs of the bladder tend to occur in patients 10 to 20 years earlier than in the United States.

SCC of the bladder often carries a poor prognosis and is usually best treated by radical cystectomy. After surgery, this form of bladder cancer has a higher propensity for local recurrence, compared with urothelial carcinomas. SCC of the bladder is typically resistant to cytotoxic chemotherapy, particularly the regimens frequently used for urothelial carcinoma. The benefit of neoadjuvant radiation therapy before cystectomy remains to be proven, at least for the non-bilharzial SCC typically found in the United States.

---

[1]Not FDA approved for this indication.

[1]Not FDA approved for this indication.

Urethral Carcinoma

DIAGNOSIS

Urethral carcinoma is unusual in that it is more common in women than in men. It is a disease of the elderly, typically occurring after 60 years of age. The etiology remains to be determined, but approximately half of the cases are associated with urethral stricture disease. In women, there is an association with urethral malakoplakia and urethral caruncles. The usual presenting symptom in this circumstance is a papillary or fungating urethral mass and hematuria. A number of scenarios warrant a more thorough evaluation for possible urethral carcinoma, including a palpable urethral mass, an obstruction that does not respond to conventional management, development of a urethral abscess or fistula, presence of microscopic or gross hematuria, and the development of inguinal adenopathy.

TREATMENT

The primary treatment of urethral carcinoma is most often surgical excision, with the approach and the extent of surgery driven by both gender and the location of the mass relative to the sphincteric complex (likelihood of postoperative continence). For example, cystectomy with en bloc urethrectomy and anterior vaginectomy along with pelvic lymphadenectomy is usually required for tumors located in the proximal urethra or tumors with extension into adjacent structures. In selected cases, radiation therapy can provide local control. In locally advanced disease, multimodality treatment with chemotherapy and either surgical excision or radiation therapy provides the optimal chance for long-term cure, although there is no standard regimen to date.

Penile Cancer

DIAGNOSIS

Penile cancer is relatively rare in the United States. Penile carcinoma has been associated with retained phimotic foreskin and poor personal hygiene. It is rare among men who are circumcised before puberty and occurs most commonly in the sixth decade of life. The symptoms relate directly to the mass itself and can include ulceration, pain, necrosis, foul odor, hemorrhage, and suppuration of the lesion. The clinical evaluation of patients with penile cancer involves a thorough physical examination including of the phallus and careful attention to palpation of the inguinal lymph nodes. Additional studies include radiographic testing with chest radiography, CT scan of the abdomen and pelvis, and bone scan.

TREATMENT

Treatment is usually dictated by the tumor stage (TNM system), size, and location. Small tumors that are confined to the prepuce can often be managed by circumcision alone. Smaller tumors on the distal shaft can be treated by partial penectomy, provided that a 1-cm normal tissue margin can be achieved and there is enough penile length remaining to permit voiding in the standing position. Among patients treated by partial penectomy, the 5-year recurrence-free survival rate is 70% to 80%. Large lesions and tumors on the proximal shaft may require total penectomy and perineal urethrostomy to achieve adequate local tumor control. If there is involvement of local structures such as the scrotum or pubis, radical en bloc resection may be required. Achieving negative margins is critical, because local recurrence of the disease can rarely be salvaged by radiation or chemotherapy.

Although many patients have inguinal lymphadenopathy at presentation, inguinal lymph node enlargement before excision of the primary tumor may be the result of infection and not metastatic disease. Clinical assessment of the inguinal region is therefore typically delayed for 4 to 6 weeks, during which time the patient receives antibiotic treatment. Lymphadenopathy that persists or develops de novo raises the strong possibility of lymph node metastases, and an ilioinguinal lymphadenectomy should be performed. If inguinal lymphadenopathy resolves on antibiotics, prophylactic lymph node dissection may not be necessary. It is often necessary to perform bilateral inguinal lymphadenectomy, particularly in patients with high-risk disease, for whom this should be considered regardless of the presence or absence of palpable nodes. Radiation of the primary tumor and regional lymph nodes is an alternative to surgery in carefully selected patients with small ($\leq$2 cm), low-stage tumors. Similarly, Mohs' surgery is an option for small tumors, particularly ones at the base that otherwise might require a total penectomy.

Testicular Cancer

Malignant tumors of the male gonads can be divided into neoplasms originating from the germinal cells, rare tumors from the supporting cells (Leydig cells and Sertoli cells), and rare metastases from another primary site. The germinal neoplasms include seminomatous and nonseminomatous germ cell tumors (NSGCTs). Ninety-five percent of tumors originating in the testis are germ cell tumors. Fewer than 10% of all germ cell tumors arise from extragonadal primary sites such as the mediastinum and retroperitoneum. Testicular cancer is relatively rare overall, but it is the most common malignancy in men between the ages of 15 and 35 years, with 8090 new cases occurring annually.

Testicular cancer represents one of the great success stories in modern medicine. The mortality rates for testis cancer have decreased from more than 50% before the 1970s to less than 10% in the modern age. This is the result of a variety of advances, including more effective multiagent chemotherapy, improved surgical techniques, and better methods to diagnose and monitor the disease (e.g., CT scans, tumor markers). Testicular cancer currently serves as a paradigm for the multimodal treatment of malignancies.

Germ cell tumors are substantially more prevalent in Caucasians than in African Americans, by a margin of at least 5:1. Indeed, a report from the U.S. military indicated a relative incidence of 40:1. The exact etiology of germ cell tumors is not fully understood. Familial clustering has been demonstrated, particularly among siblings. Two conditions associated with a higher risk for germ cell tumors are cryptorchidism and Klinefelter's syndrome, the latter associated with disease arising from the mediastinum. Orchidopexy for cryptorchidism does not appear to reduce the risk of neoplasia, but it does improve the ability to monitor the testis.

DIAGNOSIS

A painless testicular mass in a patient of the appropriate age group should be considered a primary testicular tumor until proven otherwise. A substantial number of testicular tumors manifest with less specific symptoms, including diffuse testicular pain, swelling, hardness, or some combination of these findings. A tumor can be difficult to distinguish from an infectious epididymo-orchitis. However, because the latter is more common than a testicular tumor, a short trial of antibiotics is often undertaken. If symptoms do not abate or the findings do not revert to normal within 2 to 4 weeks, testicular sonography is indicated to identify any underlying testicular mass. A radical inguinal orchiectomy with early, high ligation of the spermatic cord at the internal ring is required for all patients with a suspected testicular tumor.

Testicular cancers typically first spread to regional, retroperitoneal lymph nodes below the level of the renal vessels. The primary nodal landing zone for right-sided tumors lies between the aorta and the inferior vena cava (interaortocaval nodes), whereas for left-sided tumors it is lateral to the aorta (para-aortic). Other frequent sites of metastases include the left supraclavicular lymph nodes and the lungs. Standard initial metastatic evaluation should include a CT scan of the abdomen and pelvis and chest radiography.

Enlarged lymph nodes (>1–2 cm) in the primary lymphatic drainage areas (landing zones) of the affected side are involved by metastatic disease in approximately 70% of cases. CT imaging of the chest is required if mediastinal, hilar, or lung parenchymal disease is suspected. Serum tumor markers should be measured before orchiectomy and should include human β-chorionic gonadotropin (β-hCG), α-fetoprotein (AFP), and the less specific marker, lactate dehydrogenase.

TREATMENT

All suspected testicular tumors should be treated with a radical orchiectomy through an inguinal approach and early, high ligation of the spermatic cord. β-hCG and AFP are relatively specific tumor markers for testicular cancer. They have substantially improved the ability to monitor the disease and to intervene early in the event of recurrence. They, along with lactate dehydrogenase, should be measured before orchiectomy. AFP production is restricted to NSGCTs, specifically tumors that contain at least a component of embryonal carcinoma or yolk sac tumor. Patients with an increased AFP and pure seminoma on pathologic examination of the orchiectomy specimen are still considered to have an NSGCT. Increased serum β-hCG can occur with seminomatous and nonseminomatous tumors. Increased concentrations of β-hCG are seen in 40% to 60% of patients with metastatic NSGCT and in 15% to 20% of patients with metastatic seminomas. Lactate dehydrogenase is less specific but has independent prognostic value in patients with advanced germ cell tumors. Serum lactate dehydrogenase is increased in approximately 60% of patients with NSGCT and in 80% of those with seminomatous germ cell tumors.

Persistently elevated concentrations of AFP and β-hCG, even in the absence of radiographic or clinical findings, implies active disease and is sufficient cause to initiate systemic therapy, provided that false-positive elevations have been ruled out. The serum half-life of β-hCG is 5 to 7 days, and that for AFP is 30 hours. A slow decrease in serum levels after orchiectomy also implies metastatic disease.

Seminoma is the most common histologic form of germ cell tumor and generally carries a better prognosis than other variants. Standard therapy for low-stage (T1, 2a, or 2b) disease is orchiectomy with consideration of radiation therapy to the retroperitoneal and possibly the ipsilateral pelvic lymph nodes. Relapse is relatively rare, occurring in 4% of patients with stage 1 and 10% of patients with stage 2 disease. Relapses after radiation therapy can be salvaged in more than 90% of cases by systemic chemotherapy. The long-term cure rate for low-stage seminoma is approximately 99%.

NSGCTs include embryonal cell carcinomas, choriocarcinomas, yolk sac carcinomas, teratomas, and mixed germ cell tumors. As with pure seminoma, the cure rate is high (>95%) in patients with stage 1 disease. Retroperitoneal lymphatic metastases may be found in 20% of patients who have no lymphatic or vascular invasion or invasion into the tunica albuginea, spermatic cord, or scrotum at the time of orchiectomy, even if CT scans are negative for lymphadenopathy. There are two options for low-stage NSGCT after orchiectomy in the absence of radiographic evidence of lymphadenopathy and with normalized serum tumor markers: surveillance and nerve-sparing retroperitoneal lymph node dissection (RPLND). Patients with clinical stage 1 disease but embryonal histology or the presence of lymphovascular invasion or extension beyond the tunica albuginea have a higher risk of relapse (>30%) with surveillance and should be considered for primary RPLND.

Although RPLND is a major abdominal operation, it offers the best way to control disease within the retroperitoneum. Lymph nodes are removed from the level of the renal hilum caudad to the level of the aortic bifurcation. The lateral margins are the ureters. Historically, this operation was associated with loss of ejaculatory function due to ligation of the sympathetic nerve fibers in the region. With modern, nerve-sparing techniques, ejaculatory function can be preserved in more than 95% of patients. Patients with persistently elevated AFP or β-hCG after orchiectomy most likely have metastatic disease, even in the absence of radiographically detectable lesions.

These patients usually should go on to systemic chemotherapy first, rather than RPLND.

Clinical stage 2 NSGCTs can be managed by either RPLND or primary chemotherapy, depending on several factors. Those patients who are without marker elevation, are asymptomatic, and have small-volume retroperitoneal-only disease can be offered primary RPLND. Those with persistently elevated tumor markers, symptomatic disease, or more bulky retroperitoneal disease usually undergo systemic chemotherapy. Local recurrence in the retroperitoneum after a properly performed RPLND is rare (<10%).

Adjuvant chemotherapy after RPLND should be considered if any lymph node is more than 2 cm in diameter, if six or more nodes are involved, or if there is extranodal invasion. Cure rates are not different in those who do or do not receive adjuvant chemotherapy, but the former group require fewer cycles of chemotherapy and fewer additional surgeries.

Approximately one third of patients require up-front chemotherapy. Those patients with clinical stage 2c disease (or higher), primary retroperitoneal germ cell tumor, or mediastinal seminomas treated with radiation therapy should all undergo systemic, cisplatin-based, multiagent chemotherapy.

Postchemotherapy RPLND for seminoma is typically reserved for patients with residual masses more than 3 cm in size. For NSGCT, this issue is more controversial. Some groups reserve this treatment for patients who do not have substantial tumor shrinkage (>90% shrinkage of retroperitoneal nodes and no residual nodes >1.5 cm) and for those with teratomatous elements in the primary tumor. Others advocate surgery for all patients with initial bulky retroperitoneal disease, regardless of the response to chemotherapy. All agree that a clear residual mass after chemotherapy in the setting of NSGCT warrants a postchemotherapy RPLND.

The first successful combination chemotherapy regimens for testicular cancer included cisplatin, vinblastine, and bleomycin (Blenoxane) and resulted in complete remission in 70% to 80% of patients with metastatic disease. Studies have shown that prolonged maintenance chemotherapy is unnecessary, and etoposide (VePesid) has largely replaced vinblastine (because it is less toxic and probably more efficacious). Serious adverse effects of chemotherapy include neuromuscular toxic affects, myelosuppression, bleomycin-induced pulmonary fibrosis, Raynaud's phenomenon, and secondary malignancy.

Leydig cell tumors are generally benign tumors that make up between 1% and 3% of all testicular tumors. The majority of cases occurs in men aged 20 to 60 years old, although roughly one fourth are diagnosed before puberty. After radical orchiectomy, the prognosis is usually good, with recurrences rarely reported.

Gonadoblastoma is a rare tumor that occurs almost exclusively in patients with a history of gonadal dysgenesis. They account for fewer than 1% of all testicular neoplasms and can occur at any age from infancy to beyond 70 years, although most patients are diagnosed before age 30. Initial management is with radical orchiectomy. Because of a 50% incidence of bilateral disease, a contralateral gonadectomy is generally warranted. The prognosis after orchiectomy is usually excellent.

Lymphoma is the most common secondary neoplasm of the testicle and the most common testicular neoplasm in men older than 50 years of age, with a median age at presentation of 60 years. Although survival is often poor for patients with bilateral disease and those presenting with lymphoma at other sites who later experience a testicular relapse, the prognosis is substantially better for patients presenting with primary testicular lymphoma confined to the testicle.

Disclaimer

The views expressed in this article are those of the author and do not reflect the official policy or position of the United States Army, the Department of Defense, or the U.S. government.

CURRENT THERAPY

Carcinoma of the Prostate

- Potentially curative treatment is generally offered to men with at least a 10-year life expectancy.
- Treatment options for clinically localized T1c and T2 tumors include active surveillance/watchful waiting, radiation therapy (external irradiation and brachytherapy), cryotherapy, and surgery (open and laparoscopic).
- Treatments for locally advanced tumors (T3/T4) or high-risk cancer patients include surgery and external irradiation in combination with androgen-deprivation therapy (ADT).
- Treatment for patients with metastatic disease (N1–2 or M1) is generally palliative with ADT.
- Follow-up includes history, physical examination, and monitoring of prostate-specific antigen at least every 6 months for 2 years and then annually. Any abnormalities may be more fully evaluated with appropriate imaging.

Renal Cell Carcinoma

- Treatment for localized masses is almost always surgical excision via radical or partial nephrectomy. Both operations may be performed with an open or a laparoscopic approach.
- Partial nephrectomy should be attempted in patients who have a solitary kidney, bilateral disease, or renal insufficiency. Partial nephrectomy is the preferred operation for patients who have lesions 4 cm or larger and a normal contralateral kidney, with local recurrence rates of less than 5%.
- Minimally invasive approaches including percutaneous radiofrequency ablation and cryotherapy are under investigation, although more long-term data are needed.
- Up to 25% of patients have metastatic disease at diagnosis. Sites of metastasis, in decreasing frequency, include lungs, lymph nodes, liver, bone, and adrenal gland.
- Chemotherapy and radiation therapy provide little to no survival benefit, with radiation only palliating painful metastases.
- The mainstay of treatment in the past was immunotherapy, with 5-year survival rates of 10% to 20%.
- Modern therapies for advanced or metastatic RCC include targeted therapies such as the oral tyrosine kinase inhibitors, sunitinib (Sutent) and sorafenib (Nexavar), and the mammalian target of rapamycin (mTOR) inhibitor, temsirolimus (Torisel).
- Evidence suggests improved survival for those undergoing nephrectomy before systemic immunotherapy for metastatic disease.

Benign Renal Tumors

- For angiomyolipomas, management should be individualized. With asymptomatic lesions smaller than 4 cm, observation with annual imaging is reasonable.
- For patients with a symptomatic angiomyolipoma or one larger than 4 cm, surgical excision should be considered, although angioembolization is another option. Angioembolization can be used to stabilize a patient with acute hemorrhage secondary to an angiomyolipoma.

Tumors of the Renal Pelvis and Ureter

- Distal ureteral tumors can be managed with distal ureterectomy and ureteroneocystostomy.
- High-grade, multifocal, or high-stage tumors are optimally treated by nephroureterectomy with removal of a cuff of bladder at the ureteral orifice.
- Laparoscopic (with or without hand assist) nephroureterectomy is the preferred surgical approach, allowing for complete tumor removal and often quicker convalescence.
- Carefully selected patients, especially those who have bilateral disease or a functionally solitary kidney, can be managed with endoscopic tumor ablation.

Urothelial Carcinoma of the Bladder

- Treatment depends on tumor stage.
- Superficial (Ta) low-grade cancers are managed with transurethral resection, with or without a single, immediate postresection instillation of a chemotherapeutic agent, typically mitomycin-C (Mutamycin).
- Carcinoma in situ or high-grade stage Ta tumors that involve the lamina propria (stage T1) and recurrent tumors are managed with transurethral resection and intravesical agents such as thiotepa (Thioplex), doxorubicin (Adriamycin), and mitomycin-C[1] or intravesical bacillus Calmette-Guérin (Tice BCG).
- Bladder surveillance is mandatory, because the recurrence rate in the bladder can be as high as 50% at 5 years.
- Surveillance protocols vary but typically include cystoscopy and urinary tumor studies (usually cytology) every 3 months for the first 2 years, semiannually in years 3 to 5, and annually thereafter.
- Periodic evaluation of the upper tracts should be performed, usually by computed tomographic (CT) urography.
- Superficial disease that progresses or is refractory to conservative management, as well as tumors that invade the bladder muscle (stages T2–4), is best managed by radical cystectomy and urinary diversion.
- Urinary diversion may be either incontinent (conduit) or continent (orthotopic or continent cutaneous).
- Five-year recurrence-free survival rates are 60% to 85% after cystectomy for organ-confined disease (stages T2a–T2b). For extravesical disease (stages T3a to T4), the 5-year survival decreases to 40% to 60%, for node-positive disease it is less than 30%.
- Patients with T2–T4 disease should be strongly considered for combination therapy with surgery plus chemotherapy, either in the neoadjuvant or the adjuvant setting. Recent randomized trials have suggested an approximately 5% survival advantage for neoadjuvant chemotherapy plus surgery, compared with surgery alone.
- Patients with M1 disease are usually treated with chemotherapy.
- The standard regimen over the past decade has been MVAC: methotrexate (Trexall),[1] vinblastine (Velban),[1] doxorubicin (Adriamycin), and cisplatin (Platinol); however, durable complete response rates are less than 15%.
- Newer agents such as gemcitabine (Gemzar)[1] along with cisplatin appear to offer similar response rates and reduced toxicity.

---

[1]Not FDA approved for this indication.

Urethral Carcinoma

- Treatment of the primary tumor is surgical excision and varies based on the location and stage of the tumor.
- In men, urethrectomy can be performed via a perineal incision.
- Proximal tumors of the bulbar urethra are often managed with cystoprostatectomy and en bloc urethrectomy.
- Among women, for tumors of the proximal urethra and tumors with extension into adjacent structures, cystectomy with en bloc urethrectomy and anterior vaginectomy along with pelvic lymphadenectomy is usually required.
- Radiation therapy is also reported to provide local control in selective cases.

Penile Cancer

- Small penile cancers limited to the prepuce can be treated by circumcision alone.
- Partial penectomy with at least a 1-cm margin of normal tissue is used to treat smaller (2–5 cm) distal penile tumors. The remaining penis should be long enough to permit voiding in the standing position. The 5-year cure rate for patients treated with partial penectomy is 70% to 80%.
- Larger distal penile lesions and proximal tumors require total penectomy and perineal urethrostomy. If the scrotum, pubis, or abdominal wall is involved, radical en bloc excision may be necessary.
- Many patients have inguinal lymphadenopathy at presentation. However, inguinal lymph node enlargement before excision of the primary tumor may be the result of infection and not metastatic disease. Therefore, clinical assessment of the inguinal region should be delayed 4 to 6 weeks, during which time the patient is treated with antibiotics.
- If inguinal lymphadenopathy persists or develops, there is a high likelihood of metastatic disease, and ilioinguinal lymphadenectomy should be performed. The procedure is performed on the contralateral side if the initial side contains tumor and could be simultaneously performed or staged.
- Irradiation of the primary tumor and regional lymph nodes is an alternative to surgery in patients with small (≤2 cm), low-stage tumors.
- Mohs' surgery is another alternative for small lesions (≤2 cm).

Testicular Cancer

- All patients with suspected testicular tumors should undergo a radical orchiectomy through an inguinal approach and early, high ligation of the spermatic cord.
- Serum tumor markers should be measured before surgery and are used for disease staging and to monitor for recurrence.
- Radiographic staging should include, at a minimum, a CT scan of the abdomen and pelvis and chest radiography.
- Seminoma is the most common histologic form of germ cell tumor and generally carries a better prognosis than other variants. Standard therapy for low-stage (T1, 2a, or 2b) disease is orchiectomy with consideration of radiation therapy to the retroperitoneal and possibly the ipsilateral pelvic lymph nodes. Relapse is relatively rare, occurring in 4% of patients with stage 1 and 10% of patients with stage 2 disease. Relapses after radiation therapy can be salvaged in more than 90% of cases through systemic chemotherapy. The long-term cure rate for low-stage seminoma is approximately 99%.
- Nonseminomatous germ cell tumors (NSGCTs) include embryonal cell carcinomas, choriocarcinomas, yolk sac carcinomas, teratomas, and mixed germ cell tumors. As with pure seminoma, the cure rate for low-stage NSGCTs is high (>95%) in patients with stage 1 disease.
- Surveillance and retroperitoneal lymph node dissection (RPLND) are both standard treatment options for stage 1 NSGCT. Twenty percent of these patients have lymph node involvement, and those with vascular invasion or predominance of embryonal cell carcinoma are at increased risk (>30%).
- RPLND is a major abdominal operation in which lymph nodes from the retroperitoneum are removed, from the renal hilum down to the level of the common iliac artery, with lateral margins being confined by the ureters.
- Adjuvant chemotherapy after RPLND should be considered if any lymph node is larger than 2 cm in diameter, if at least six nodes are involved, or if there is extranodal invasion.
- Patients with persistently increased concentrations of α-fetoprotein, human β-chorionic gonadotropin, or both but without other clinical evidence of disease after orchiectomy usually have systemic disease and are treated with chemotherapy.
- Approximately one third of patients require up-front chemotherapy. Those with clinical stage 2c disease (or higher), primary retroperitoneal germ cell tumors, or mediastinal seminomas treated with radiation therapy should undergo systemic, cisplatin-based, multiagent chemotherapy.
- Postchemotherapy RPLND for seminoma is typically reserved for patients with residual masses larger than 3 cm. For NSGCT, some groups reserve postchemotherapy RPLND for patients who do not have substantial tumor shrinkage (>90% shrinkage of retroperitoneal nodes and no residual nodes >1.5 cm) and those with teratomatous elements in the primary tumor. Others advocate surgery for all patients with initial bulky retroperitoneal disease. All agree that a clear, residual mass after chemotherapy in the setting of NSGCT warrants postchemotherapy RPLND.
- Multimodal therapy has allowed 90% to 95% of testicular cancer patients to be cured, even in the face of metastatic disease.

REFERENCES

Barocas DA, Clark PE. Bladder cancer. Curr Opin Oncol 2008;20:307–14.

Damber JE, Aus G. Prostate cancer. Lancet 2008;371:1710–21.

Flechon A, Rivoire M, Droz JP. Management of advanced germ-cell tumors of the testis. Nat Clin Pract Urol 2008;5:262–76.

Jemal A, Siegel R, Ward E, et al. Cancer statistics, 2008. CA Cancer J Clin 2008;58:71–96.

Rini BI, Rathmell WK, Godley P. Renal cell carcinoma. Curr Opin Oncol 2008;20:300–6.

Urethral Strictures

Method of
Brian J. Flynn, MD, and David Hadley, MD

Urethral stricture occurs when scar tissue in the epithelium contracts and subsequently narrows the urethral lumen. The scarring process is induced by trauma, inflammation, or ischemia, with more severe strictures involving progressive fibrosis into the corpus spongiosum (spongiofibrosis). By definition, urethral strictures may involve the anterior urethra (fossa navicularis, pendulous urethra, and bulbous urethra), the posterior urethra (membranous or prostatic urethra), or both. Anterior urethral injuries commonly result from direct penile or perineal trauma, instrumentation, catheterization, infections, or lichen sclerosis. Posterior urethral strictures may represent an actual defect in the membranous urethra after a distraction injury or a complication from prostate cancer treatment (surgery, irradiation, cryosurgery, or brachytherapy).

The prevalence of urethral strictures has been reported to be as high as 0.6% in the male population, and they have been a recognized problem throughout history, usually in relation to trauma and infection. Antibiotics for gonococcal urethritis have significantly reduced the incidence of strictures after infection, but iatrogenic injuries from urologic instrumentation and urethral catheterization have significantly increased as a cause of urethral stricture disease.

Evaluation and Diagnosis

Men with a urethral stricture may present acutely in the emergency department with urinary retention or may be referred to the clinic with chronic obstructive voiding symptoms. Patients complain of decreased force of the urinary stream, hesitancy, inability to empty, nocturia, postvoid dribbling, and difficulty emptying the bladder. Irritative symptoms can also occur, including frequency, urgency, and dysuria. Patients are typically 16 to 40 years of age and tend to live an active lifestyle (e.g., mountain biking, riding motorcycles or all-terrain vehicles, horseback riding), which may cause chronic perineal trauma. Often a hallmark event such as urethral trauma or urethral instrumentation resulting in blood per urethra occurs immediately before the onset of symptoms.

CURRENT DIAGNOSIS

- Retrograde urethrography is essential in the diagnosis and management of urethral stricture disease.
- Obstructive voiding complaints are the most common presentation in patients with urethral stricture disease.
- Patients with recurrent urinary tract infections, prostatitis, or epididymitis should be evaluated for urethral stricture.

Physical examination should include a standard genital examination for any abnormalities, specifically evaluating the meatus for stenosis and the penile shaft for any fibrosis or stigmata of lichen sclerosis. Laboratory evaluation should include urinalysis, urine culture for infection, and a basic metabolic panel for renal function. Basic urodynamic studies, including simple uroflowmetry and measurement of the postvoid residual with ultrasound, can assess for obstruction and ability to empty. Inability to pass a catheter should further raise suspicion for a urethral stricture and prompt an evaluation of the urethra with endoscopy and retrograde urethrography.

Retrograde urethrography remains the gold standard for diagnosis and evaluation of urethral strictures, defining the length, location, caliber, and number of strictures. A voiding cystourethrogram (VCUG) obtained by means of a suprapubic cystostomy tube should outline the proximal urethra in cases of complete urethral occlusion. Alternative imaging modalities include magnetic resonance imaging and ultrasonography. These studies are better able to image a urethral cancer or diverticulum.

Cystourethroscopy complements the radiologic findings, confirming the anatomic location of the stricture and its caliber, and can rule out other urethral pathology such as stones, necrosis, fistula, or cancer. Urethral dilation, if planned, can also be performed by initially placing a wire under direct vision across the stricture and into the bladder.

Management

Once the diagnosis has been made, the first step is to treat the acute issues such as urinary retention and concomitant genitourinary infections. Urinary retention is treated with urethral catheterization or with a suprapubic cystostomy tube if urethral catheterization is unsuccessful. Once the acute issues are resolved, future management is based on the length, location, degree, and cause of the stricture and patient preference. Absolute indications for intervention include urinary retention, azotemia, recurrent infections, stone formation, and pain.

URETHROTOMY AND DILATION

Urethral dilation or urethrotomy is often the initial treatment, because it is less invasive than open surgical management. Dilation may be performed with filiforms and followers, serial dilators, or a balloon in the clinic or the emergency room. Urethrotomy is performed in the operating room with the patient under general regional anesthesia, with the use of an endoscopic knife or a laser to incise the scar under direct vision.

Strictures amenable to dilation are short (<1.0 cm) and are associated with minimal spongiofibrosis. Typically, dilation is performed initially, and urethrotomy is reserved for denser strictures in the bulbar or posterior urethra. In general, there is no statistical difference in success rate between dilation and urethrotomy. Recurrent strictures, long strictures, and those associated with significant fibrosis reoccur in more than 80% of cases and therefore require self-dilation or open urethral reconstruction (urethroplasty).

STENTS

Urethral stents such as the UroLume (American Medical Systems, Minnetonka, MN) are made with titanium and are considered permanent. Introduced with much enthusiasm, stents have fallen out of favor secondary to problems of migration, encrustation, postvoid dribbling, and perineal and penile pain. Overall, long-term success is less than 30%, and these devices are best reserved for patients who are not candidates for open reconstruction.

OPEN RECONSTRUCTION

Surgical excision of the diseased segment with primary anastomosis (EPA) remains the gold standard for short strictures in the bulbous or posterior urethra, with long-term success rates greater than 95% in most studies. Keys to a successful repair include complete excision of the spongiofibrosis and a widely spatulated, tension-free anastomosis. Typically, strictures smaller than 2 cm are amenable to EPA, although longer stricture repair has been reported, especially in the

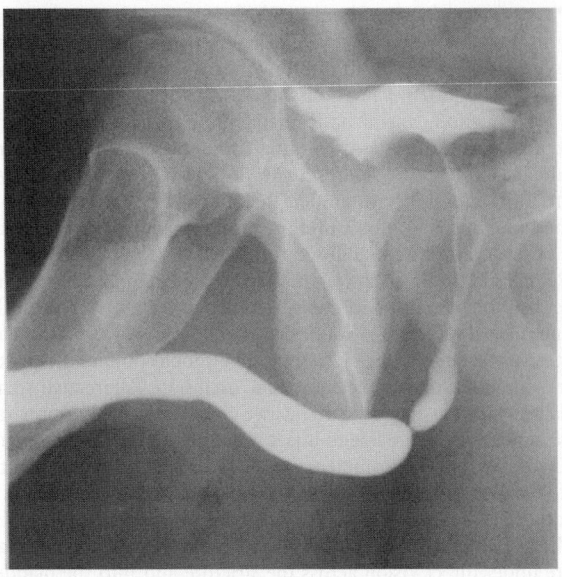

FIGURE 1. Retrograde urethrogram demonstrating a short bulbar urethral stricture amenable to excision with primary anastomosis.

posterior urethra (Fig. 1). Whereas significant bulbar urethral mobilization can create length in men with longer strictures, this may compromise penile length and cosmesis.

If the stricture is located in the pendulous urethra or its length exceeds the limits of EPA (>2 cm), substitution urethroplasty with a graft or a flap may be performed (Figs. 2 and 3). The graft or flap is onlayed ventrally or dorsally after a longitudinal incision is made in the diseased segment, thereby increasing the urethral caliber. A hybrid technique involves stricture excision of the worst disease with onlay to the less severe adjacent segments. If there are long obliterative segments, a two-stage repair is necessary.

Multiple sources of graft material have been successfully used in urethroplasty, including preputial skin, split-thickness skin from the thigh, bladder epithelium, rectal mucosa, and buccal mucosa. Buccal mucosa has emerged as the graft of choice, with excellent short-term results. Buccal mucosa has the ideal histologic characteristics, is non–hair bearing, leaves no visible scar, and is water resistant and hence does not appear to have has much contracture as other graft materials.

Posterior urethral distraction injuries are a result of pelvic fracture and occur in up to 10% of cases. At the time of pelvic fracture, if there

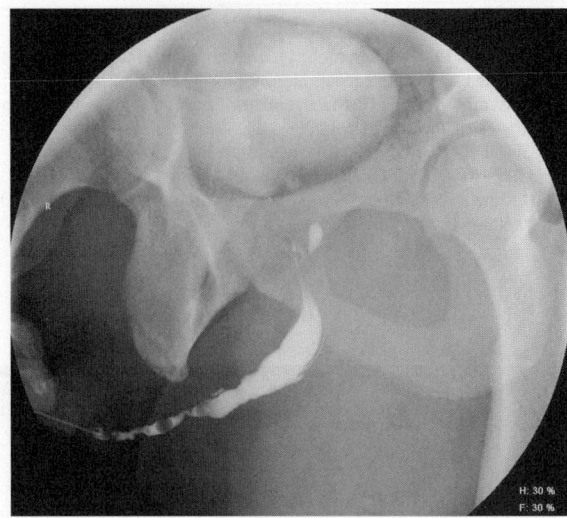

FIGURE 3. Retrograde urethrogram showing a panurethral stricture from lichen sclerosis. These may be repaired with complex staged reconstruction or perineal urethrostomy.

is blood at the meatus, a high index for suspicion, or inability to void, a RUG should be performed (Fig. 4). In some cases, a partial disruption may have occurred, with a small portion of epithelium left intact. An endoscopically placed urethral catheter can facilitate stricture-free healing. If complete transection has occurred or a urethral catheter cannot be placed, the patient can be taken to the operating room, where a suprapubic cystotomy tube is placed. An antegrade-retrograde two-team approach using cystoscopy and fluoroscopy is then performed in an effort to place a catheter across the defect. Recent literature has suggested that early realignment decreases the need for subsequent urethroplasty without compromising erectile or sphincter function. However, if a primary realignment is not feasible, a suprapubic catheter is used for drainage, and delayed repair (3 months after the injury) is indicated. A progressive perineal anastomotic repair in these cases has a success rate of more than 95%. Complex posterior urethral injuries (e.g., with a concomitant bladder neck injury, rectal injury, or fistula) usually require an abdominal-perineal approach.

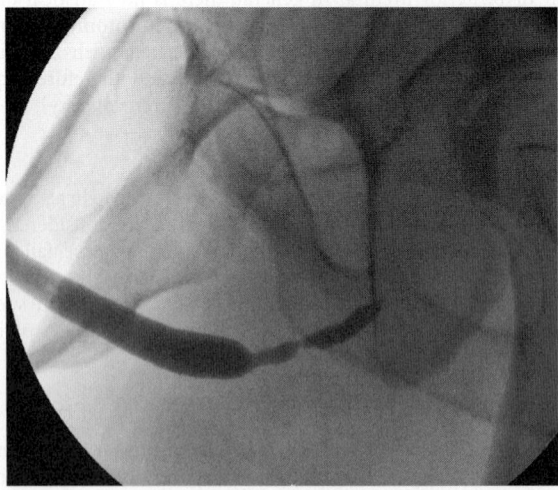

FIGURE 2. Retrograde urethrogram demonstrating a longer bulbar urethral stricture requiring excision of the most significant area of stricture and onlay of the remaining stricture: the excisional, augmented anastomotic urethroplasty.

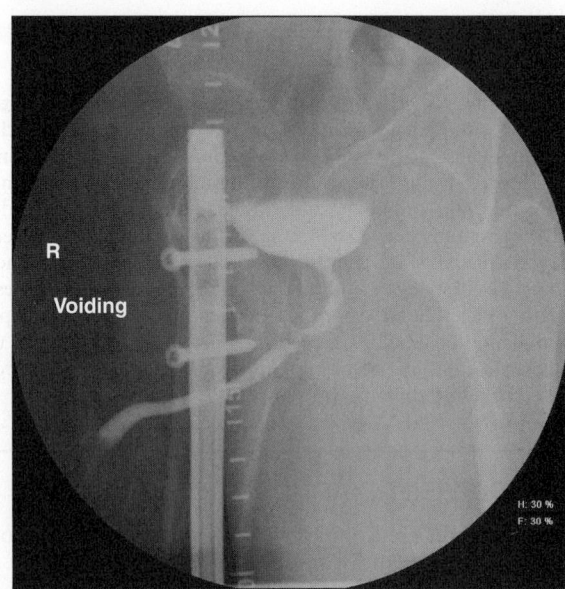

FIGURE 4. Retrograde urethrogram may be combined with a voiding cystourethrogram (the bladder is filled via a suprapubic catheter) to demonstrate a posterior urethral disruption due to pelvic fracture. These defects are usually amenable to excision with primary anastomosis.

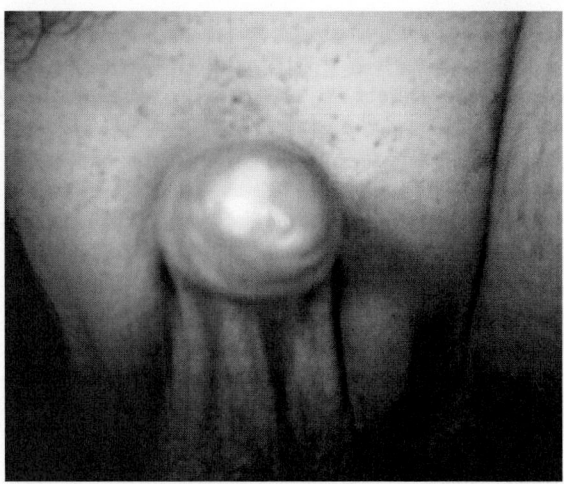

FIGURE 5. Picture of the glans penis afflicted with lichen sclerosis.

 CURRENT THERAPY

- The patient and doctor should have a good understanding of the goals, limitations, and definitions of success before treatment of urethral stricture disease is undertaken.
- Office-based dilation is the most common and accepted initial treatment for urethral strictures.
- Dilation and urethrotomy are equivalent in terms of long-term success and are more likely to succeed in short, bulbar strictures with minimal fibrosis.
- Open surgical therapy is based on the length, location, and cause of the urethral stricture.

A variant of lichen sclerosis, balanitis xerotica obliterans, is an idiopathic, lymphocyte-mediated inflammatory skin disease that affects the anogenital region. A sclerotic white ring around the prepuce or glans penis is diagnostic in the early stage (Fig. 5) and can lead to phimosis or meatal stenosis and urethral stricture in as many as 20% of patients. The use of genital tissue for reconstruction is contraindicated because it has a failure rate of more than 90%. Surgical options include a two-stage repair with buccal mucosa or extended meatotomy and perineal urethrostomy for more severe disease. In some cases, penile biopsy for diagnosis and to rule out squamous cell carcinoma is necessary preoperatively.

REFERENCES

Abouassaly R, Angermeier KW. Augmented anastomotic urethroplasty. J Urol 2007;177(6):2211–5; discussion 2215–16.

Armitage JN, Cathcart PJ, Rashidian A, et al. Epithelializing stent for benign prostatic hyperplasia: A systematic review of the literature. J Urol 2007;177(5):1619–24.

Dubey D, Vijjan V, Kapoor R, et al. Dorsal onlay buccal mucosa versus penile skin flap urethroplasty for anterior urethral strictures: Results from a randomized prospective trial. J Urol 2007;178(6):2466–9.

Eltahawy EA, Virasoro R, Schlossberg SM, et al. Long-term followup for excision and primary anastomosis for anterior urethral strictures. J Urol 2007;177(5):1803–6.

Flynn BJ, Webster GD. Urethral stricture and disruption. In: Graham SD, Keane J, Glenn J, editors. Glenn's Urologic Surgery. 6th ed. Philadelphia: Lippincott Williams & Wilkins; 2003. p. 394–407.

Heyns CF, Steenkamp JW, Kock MLSD, et al. Treatment of male urethral strictures: Is repeated dilation of internal urethrotomy useful? J Urol 1998;160 (2):356–8.

Jordan GH. Imaging of the penis and male urethra. AUA Update Series 2008;27: [Lesson 23].

Jordan GH, Schlossberg SM. Surgery of the penis and urethra. In: Wein AJ, Kavoussi L, et al., editors. Campbell-Walsh Urology. 9th ed. Philadelphia: Saunders/Elsevier; 2007. p. 1054–87.

Levine LA, Strom KH, Lux MM. Buccal mucosa graft urethroplasty for anterior urethral stricture repair: Evaluation of the impact of stricture location and lichen sclerosis on surgical outcome. J Urol 2007;178(5):2011–5.

Mouraviev VB, Coburn M, Santucci RA. The treatment of posterior urethral disruption associated with pelvic fractures: Comparative experience of early realignment versus delayed urethroplasty. J Urol 2005;173(3):873–6.

Pugliese JM, Morey AF, Peterson AC. Lichen sclerosis: Review of the literature and current recommendations for management. J Urol 2007;178 (6):2268–76.

Santucci RA, Joyce GF, Wise M. Male urethral stricture disease. J Urol 2007;177(5):1667–74.

Renal Calculi

Method of
Vahan Vartanian, BS, and Sangtae Park, MD, MPH

In the United States, upper urinary tract stones are responsible for significant morbidity, loss of work, and medical cost. The prevalence of urinary stone disease is estimated at 5% to 12%, and the lifetime chance of being diagnosed with a stone is 1 in 8. In the United States, the annual medical expenditure for a diagnosis of nephrolithiasis approaches $2.1 billion. Furthermore, long-term effects such as renal function loss are significant. A recent study of more than 1300 new cases of end-stage renal disease requiring dialysis found that, in 3.2% of the cases, renal failure was a direct result of stone disease.

In addition to the morbidity of an acute stone event, at least 50% of patients ultimately require surgical intervention. As such, the goal of medical treatment is to prevent disease progression and recurrence and, potentially, to reduce stone burden. Nonetheless, the recurrence rate of urinary calculi is roughly 50% within 5 years.

Epidemiology

Most kidney stones occur in patients between 20 and 50 years old, with peak onsets of disease between the third and fifth decades of life. Kidney stones are more prevalent in Caucasians, Latinos, and Asians than in African Americans or Native Americans. Men are more commonly affected with kidney stones than women, by a ratio of 2:1. Geographic analysis demonstrates that stones are more common in hot and dry areas.

Pathophysiology

Calcareous stones, including calcium oxalate, calcium apatite, and brushite stones, represent approximately 75% of upper tract stones, and the remaining 25% are struvite, cystine, uric acid, and other stones (Table 1). Supersaturation of urine by urinary constituents such as calcium, oxalate, and uric acid is necessary for stone formation. Supersaturation is defined as concentration of an ion to a level beyond which it is not soluble.

HYPERCALCIURIA

Hypercalciuria is classified as absorptive, renal, or resorptive based on the underlying pathophysiologic abnormality. Absorptive hypercalciuria is caused by intestinal overabsorption of calcium. It is classified as type II if urinary calcium normalizes with dietary calcium

TABLE 1   Classification of Nephrolithiasis

Condition	Metabolic or Environmental Defect	Prevalence (%)
Hypercalciuria		
Absorptive hypercalciuria	Increased gastrointestinal calcium absorption	20–40
Renal hypercalciuria	Impaired renal calcium reabsorption	5–8
Resorptive hypercalciuria	Primary hyperparathyroidism	3–5
Hyperuricosuric calcium nephrolithiasis	Dietary purine excess, uric acid overproduction	10–40
Hypocitraturic calcium stone		10–50
Chronic diarrhea	Gastrointestinal alkali loss	
Distal RTA	Impaired renal acid excretion	
Thiazide-induced	Hypokalemia and intracellular acidosis	
Hyperoxaluric calcium stone		2–15
Primary hyperoxaluria	Genetic oxalate overproduction	
Dietary hyperoxaluria	Excessive dietary intake	
Enteric hyperoxaluria	Increased gastrointestinal oxalate absorption	
Gouty diathesis	Low urinary pH	15–30
Cystinuria	Impaired renal cystine reabsorption	<1
Infection stones	Urinary infection with urease-producing bacteria	1–5

restriction or type I if it is unresponsive to diet. In renal hypercalciuria, impaired renal tubular reabsorption of calcium results in elevated urinary calcium levels. Resorptive hypercalciuria is an uncommon abnormality that is most often associated with primary hyperparathyroidism and calcium resorption from bone stores.

HYPERURICOSURIA

Hyperuricosuria is present in up to 10% of calcium stone formers. Hyperuricosuria predisposes to calcium or uric acid stone formation by causing supersaturation of the urine with respect to monosodium urate. At urinary pH values lower than 5.5, the undissociated form of uric acid predominates, leading to uric acid stone formation. At pH values greater than 5.5, sodium urate formation promotes development of calcium oxalate stones through heterologous nucleation. The most common cause of hyperuricosuria is increased dietary purine intake because uric acid is the end product of purine metabolism. However, acquired and hereditary diseases, such as gout and hematologic disorders, can cause hyperuricosuria.

CYSTINURIA

Cystinuria is an autosomal recessive disorder characterized by a defect in intestinal and renal tubular transport of dibasic amino acids, resulting in excessive urinary excretion of cystine. Cystine is poorly soluble in urine, so its precipitation and subsequent stone formation occur at physiologic urine conditions.

INFECTION STONES

Struvite stones (magnesium ammonium phosphate) occur only in association with urinary infection by urea-splitting bacteria. Under these conditions, urinary urea is hydrolyzed to ammonia by bacterial urease, resulting in alkaline urine that further promotes phosphate dissociation and allows formation of the stones.

Diagnosis

Patients with urinary calculi can present with pain, fever, dysuria, or hematuria. Nonobstructive intrarenal calculi do not usually cause pain, in contrast to ureteral calculi. As ureteral calculi move distally through the ureter, pain migrates from the flank to the abdomen, then to the groin, and finally to the scrotal or labial area. Staghorn calculi are kidney stones that occupy the renal pelvis and calyceal system. These stones are often asymptomatic, and if they do manifest, it is usually with hematuria and infection rather than acute onset of pain.

During history-taking, it is important to ask about the presence of fever, nausea, or vomiting and the location and duration of pain. A history of recurrent urinary tract infections, previous renal calculi,

medications, a family history of calculi, and the presence of a solitary or transplanted kidney are informative.

On physical examination, the patient is usually in significant distress, and costovertebral angle tenderness is common. Patients do not present with peritoneal signs. The presence of fever, tachycardia, or hypotension is a sign of impending or frank urosepsis from an obstructing calculus, and this is a bona fide surgical emergency requiring ureteral stenting or percutaneous nephrostomy tube placement.

Laboratory and Radiographic Studies

All patients should be evaluated with urinalysis, urine culture, a complete blood count, and a chemistry profile. Urinalysis assesses for pH, microhematuria, and crystalluria. An elevated white blood cell count may reflect renal or systemic infection. The chemistry profile, including measurements of serum electrolytes, creatinine, calcium, parathyroid hormone, and uric acid, assesses the patient's renal and metabolic function. Patients who are recurrent stone formers and those who are high-risk first-time stone formers (age <30 years, multiple bilateral calculi, pediatric calculi, intestinal disease, or solitary or transplanted kidney) warrant a more extensive laboratory evaluation, including 24-hour urine collections. Elevation of the 24-hour excretion of calcium, oxalate, or uric acid indicates predisposition to stone formation. Decreased urinary volume and a decreased urinary citrate level suggest stone-forming propensity, because citrate is the most common stone inhibitor.

The plain abdominal radiograph is mandatory in assessing total stone burden and the size, shape, and location of urinary calculi. Although the sensitivity and specificity are in the range of 70% to 80%, radiography is a cheap and simple means of monitoring the course of the stone if it is visible. Ultrasonography is useful for detecting hydronephrosis and hydroureter but is limited because of the inability to visualize ureteral calculi and small intrarenal calculi. Intravenous pyelography is an historical study that has been replaced by the current diagnostic gold standard test, the noncontrast abdominopelvic computed tomography scan.

Treatment

MEDICAL CARE

Once renal colic has been diagnosed, pain is usually well controlled with nonsteroidal anti-inflammatory drugs such as ketorolac (Toradol) and opiates. Outpatient management is possible if none of the

TABLE 2 Summary of Medical Expulsive Therapy for Distal Ureteral Calculi

Medicine	Dose
Nifedipine extended-release (Procardia XL)[1]	30 mg PO daily
Tamsulosin (Flomax)[1]	0.4 mg PO daily
Terazosin (Hytrin)[1]	5–10 mg PO daily

[1]Not FDA approved for this indication.

following clinical signs and symptoms exists: fever, intractable nausea and vomiting, uncontrolled pain, solitary kidney, acute renal failure, or sepsis. Outpatient medical care includes the use of analgesics, antinausea medications, and expulsive therapy (α-blocker or calcium channel blocker) for small (<5 mm) distal ureteral calculi. Urologic follow-up is critical to prevent obstructive renal failure from untreated renal or ureteral calculi. Medical expulsive therapy (Table 2) has been shown to be effective in randomized controlled trials for α-blockers such as tamsulosin (Flomax)[1] and calcium channel blockers such as nifedipine (Procardia).[1]

For prevention of stone recurrence, randomized clinical trials have demonstrated that the most important factor is increased fluid intake so that urine output is more than 2 L/day. Excessive intakes of salt, oxalate, and animal protein should be avoided. Empiric dietary restriction of calcium is not necessary in most patients, and it can have adverse effects on bone mineralization, especially in women and in patients with osteoporosis.

SURGICAL CARE

Endoscopic surgery is the mainstay of treatment for nephrolithiasis. Indications for surgery are intractable pain, active infection, and obstruction. Renal obstruction lasting longer than 1 month leads to permanent renal dysfunction; for this reason, medical expulsive therapy should be limited to that period, with surgical therapy instituted thereafter. Treatment for most renal calculi is noninvasive (e.g., extracorporeal lithotripsy), and open or laparoscopic surgical excision is limited to rare, atypical cases. In an obstructed and infected collecting system secondary to a stone, emergent relief of obstruction is necessary by ureteral stenting or percutaneous nephrostomy placement.

---

[1]Not FDA approved for this indication.

Almost 85% of kidney and ureteral stones requiring intervention are treated with extracorporeal shock-wave lithotripsy (ESWL) under general anesthetic or monitored anesthetic care. Shocks are generated and are focused on the calculus. As the stone is hit by the shockwave, it breaks into smaller fragments that can pass in the urine. ESWL is less successful if the stone is larger than 1.5 cm or is in the lower pole of the kidney. Absolute contraindications to ESWL include pregnancy, ureteral obstruction distal to the stone, and uncorrected coagulopathy.

Ureteroscopic management is the second most common management option. With the patient under anesthesia, a flexible 7F or rigid scope is passed through the bladder and up the ureter to visualize the stone. The stone is either extracted with a stone basket or fragmented with the use of a Holmium laser. Complete ureteral and renal endoscopy is performed to ensure stone-free status and to treat any concomitant obstructive disease. Percutaneous nephrostolithotomy is reserved for stones larger than 2 cm. In this operation, a percutaneous nephrostomy tract is created, followed by insertion of a sheath 1 cm in diameter. Ultrasonic or pneumatic lithotripsy is performed under direct vision of the calculi. Because of the rather invasive nature of this operation, morbidity can reach 20%; therefore, this modality is reserved for large, infectious stones that are not appropriate for ESWL or ureteroscopy.

REFERENCES

Borghi L, Meschi T, Amato F, et al. Urinary volume, water and recurrences in idiopathic calcium nephrolithiasis: A 5-year randomized prospective study. J Urol 1996;155:839–43.

Borghi L, Schianchi T, Meschi T, et al. Comparison of two diets for the prevention of recurrent stones in idiopathic hypercalciuria. N Engl J Med 2002;346:77–84.

Clark JY, Thompson IM, Optenberg SA. Economic impact of urolithiasis in the United States. J Urol 1995;154:2020–4.

Grover PK, Ryall RL. Urate and calcium oxalate stones: From repute to rhetoric to reality. Miner Electrolyte Metab 1994;20:361–70.

Jungers P, Joly D, Barbey F, et al. ESRD caused by nephrolithiasis: Prevalence, mechanisms, and prevention. Am J Kidney Dis 2004;44:799–805.

Ng CS, Streem SB. Contemporary management of cystinuria. J Endourol 1999;13:647–51.

Pak CY. Kidney stones. Lancet 1998;351:1797–801.

Pak CY, Britton F, Peterson R, et al. Ambulatory evaluation of nephrolithiasis: Classification, clinical presentation and diagnostic criteria. Am J Med 1980;69:19–30.

Rahman NU, Meng MV, Stoller ML. Infections and urinary stone disease. Curr Pharm Des 2003;9:975–81.

Shekarriz B, Stoller ML. Uric acid nephrolithiasis: Current concepts and controversies. J Urol 2002;168:1307–14.

The Sexually Transmitted Diseases

Chancroid, Granuloma Inguinale (Donovanosis), and Lymphogranuloma Venereum

Method of
Michele Van Vranken, MD

Patients presenting with anogenital ulcerative lesions should be evaluated for sexually transmitted infections. Although most patients with genital ulcers have genital herpes or syphilis, chancroid, granuloma inguinale (donovanosis), and lymphogranuloma venereum (LGV) also are important sexually transmitted infections to consider in the differential diagnosis.

Epidemiology

Chancroid, granuloma inguinale, and LGV predominantly occur in tropical regions and in developing countries, and they sporadically occur in outbreaks throughout the industrialized world. Chancroid is an infection caused by *Haemophilus ducreyi*. Granuloma inguinale is caused by *Klebsiella granulomatis* (formerly known as *Donovania granulomatis* and *Calymmatobacterium granulomatis*). Lymphogranuloma venereum is caused by *Chlamydia trachomatis* serovars L1, L2, or L3. Although its prevalence was rare in North America and Europe before 2003, sporadic outbreaks have occurred among men who have sex with men in Belgium, France, the United Kingdom, Sweden, Germany, and Spain and in the cities of Atlanta, San Francisco, and New York in the United States.

Diagnosis

The initial lesion of chancroid is usually a small, tender papule that occurs at the site of inoculation approximately 3 to 10 days after infection. The papule may progress to a pustular lesion, followed by an ulcer over the next 24 to 48 hours; vesicles are never seen.

Classically, the ulcers are painful, and the bases are necrotic with a purulent exudate. Painful inguinal adenitis occurs in approximately 40% to 50% of cases and is usually unilateral.

The first manifestation of granuloma inguinale is a small, firm nodule, which later ulcerates. The painless, progressive ulcerative lesions are highly vascular and have a beefy red appearance. They bleed easily on contact. Rarely, there are hypertrophic, necrotic, or sclerotic variants. Unlike chancroid and LGV, granuloma inguinale usually is not associated with lymphadenopathy.

LGV is a systemic infection with three stages of disease. The primary stage consists of a small, nonpainful papule that may quickly ulcerate. Unlike the sharp and demarcated chancre of syphilis, this ulcer usually has ragged, irregular borders. The ulcer heals rapidly and without a scar, and it may go unnoticed by a patient. The secondary stage includes lymphadenitis with bubo formation (the inguinal syndrome) or proctitis with rectal pain and discharge, depending on the site of inoculation. If the inguinal and femoral lymph nodes are involved, they may be separated by the inguinal ligament, creating the pathognomonic groove sign (in 20% of patients with LGV). Subsequent bubo formation is usually unilateral and begins as a firm, painful mass that enlarges and becomes fluctuant over 1 to 2 weeks. This pattern is different from that of the lymphadenitis of syphilis, which remains firm, is nontender, and is usually bilateral. Bubo due to LGV subsequently ruptures in about one third of patients. Most patients recover after this secondary stage without complications, but without treatment, a longer-term inflammatory response (third stage) is possible that can lead to fistulas and strictures in the anogenital region.

Success in the laboratory diagnosis of chancroid, granuloma inguinale, and LGV has been limited. Gram-negative coccobacilli identified on a Gram stain of an ulcer's exudate suggest chancroid, but isolating *H. ducreyi* is difficult. Microscopy of freshly crushed granulomatous tissue stained with Wright or Giemsa stain may show Donovan bodies (intracellular bacilli), which are diagnostic for granuloma inguinale, but no further serologic or polymerase chain reaction (PCR) test exists. *Chlamydia* serology can support a diagnosis of LGV if titers are more than 1:64, but this has not been validated as a diagnostic tool. Ultimately, clinical suspicion remains a primary means of identifying chancroid, granuloma inguinale, and LGV. A probable diagnosis can often be made if syphilis is ruled out by darkfield examination or serology (at least 7 days after the onset of ulcer), if the result of the herpesvirus evaluation of the exudate is negative, and if the clinical manifestation of the ulcer or adenopathy suggests disease (Table 1).

TABLE 1 Clinical Features of Chancroid, Granuloma Inguinale, and Lymphogranuloma Venereum

Characteristic	Chancroid	Granuloma Inguinale	Lymphogranuloma Venereum
Incubation period	1–14 d	1–4 wk	3 d–6 wk
Primary lesion	Papule	Papule	Papule, pustule, or vesicle
Pain	Very tender	Uncommon	Variable
Base	Purulent, easily bleeds	Red and velvety, bleeds easily	Nonvascular, variable
Lymphadenopathy	Usually unilateral, tender, may suppurate	Uncommon	Usually unilateral, tender, may suppurate

Treatment

Multiple treatment recommendations exist for chancroid. Patients should be evaluated 3 to 7 days after treatment. If clinical improvement has not occurred during that time, other diagnoses, co-infection, drug resistance, or poor compliance should be considered.

CURRENT DIAGNOSIS

Chancroid

- A small, tender papule occurs at the site of inoculation 3 to 10 days after infection, progresses to a pustular lesion, and then forms an ulcer over the next 24 to 48 hours.
- The base of the painful ulcer is necrotic, and the lesion has a purulent exudate.
- Unilateral, painful inguinal adenitis occurs in 40% to 50% of cases.
- Gram-negative coccobacilli identified on a Gram stain of an ulcer's exudate suggest chancroid.

Granuloma Inguinale

- Initial lesions are small, firm nodules, which later ulcerate.
- The painless ulcers are highly vascular (beefy red appearance) and bleed easily on contact.
- Hypertrophic, necrotic, or sclerotic variants may be seen, but granuloma inguinale usually is not associated with lymphadenopathy.
- Microscopic examination of granulomatous tissue stained with Wright or Giemsa stain may show Donovan bodies, which are diagnostic for granuloma inguinale.

Lymphogranuloma Venereum

- The initial small, nonpainful papule may quickly ulcerate.
- The ulcer usually has ragged, irregular borders and heals rapidly and without a scar.
- Second-stage LGV includes lymphadenitis with bubo formation, often with proctitis, rectal pain, and discharge, depending on the site of inoculation.
- Involved inguinal and femoral lymph nodes may be separated by the inguinal ligament, creating the pathognomonic groove sign.
- Subsequent bubo formation begins as a firm, painful, typically unilateral mass that enlarges and becomes fluctuant over 1 to 2 weeks; the bubo subsequently ruptures in about one third of patients.
- Without treatment, a longer-term inflammatory response can lead to fistulas and strictures in the anogenital region.
- *Chlamydia* serology can support a diagnosis of LGV if titers are more than 1:64, but clinical suspicion remains a primary means of identifying LGV.

CURRENT THERAPY

Chancroid

- Azithromycin (Zithromax) 1 g PO in a single dose
- Ceftriaxone (Rocephin) 250 mg IM in a single dose
- Ciprofloxacin (Cipro) 400 mg PO twice daily for 3 days (if not pregnant or lactating)
- Erythromycin base (Ery-Tab) 500 mg PO three times daily for 7 days.

Granuloma Inguinale

- Doxycycline (Vibramycin) 100 mg PO twice daily for a minimum of 3 weeks or until all lesions have healed
- Azithromycin (Zithromax) 1 g PO weekly
- Ciprofloxacin (Cipro) 750 mg PO twice daily
- Erythromycin base (Ery-Tab) 500 mg PO four times daily
- Trimethoprim-sulfamethoxazole (Bactrim) one double-strength tablet PO twice daily for at least 3 weeks and until all lesions have healed

Lymphogranuloma Venereum

- Doxycycline 100 mg PO twice daily for 3 weeks
- Erythromycin base 500 mg PO four times daily
- Needle aspiration or incision and drainage of a bubo (optional)

The recommended treatment for granuloma inguinale is doxycycline. Prolonged treatment is usually required, and relapses of symptoms can occur 6 to 18 months later, even after effective treatment. If a patient cannot tolerate doxycycline, alternative regimens are available. Of the antibiotic options, only azithromycin and erythromycin should be used during pregnancy.

One of the primary goals of treatment of LGV is prevention of long-term complications, such as strictures and fistulas in the anogenital region. Recommended therapy includes doxycycline, but erythromycin base can be used if the patient is pregnant or does not tolerate doxycycline. Needle aspiration or incision and drainage of a bubo may be required for symptomatic relief, but it is not routinely recommended for treatment because it may delay the healing process.

In addition to the treatment of chancroid and LGV, all sexual partners within the previous 60 days should be notified and presumptively treated. Sexual contacts of patients with a diagnosis of granuloma inguinale also need to be evaluated, but the value of empiric therapy has not been established.

REFERENCES

Ballard R. Genital ulcer adenopathy syndrome. In: Holmes K, editor. Sexually Transmitted Diseases. 3rd ed. New York: McGraw-Hill; 1999. p. 887–92.

Centers for Disease Control and Prevention. Sexually transmitted treatment guidelines. 2006. Available at http://www.cdc.gov/std/treatment/2006/genital-ulcers.htm (accessed May 2, 2009).

Kaliaperumal K. Recent advances in management of genital ulcer disease and anogenital warts. Dermatol Ther 2008;21:196–204.

O'Farrell N. Donovanosis. In: Holmes K, editor. Sexually Transmitted Diseases. 3rd ed. New York: McGraw-Hill; 1999. p. 525–9.

Perine P. Lymphogranuloma venereum. In: Holmes K, editor. Sexually Trans-
mitted Diseases. 3rd ed. New York: McGraw-Hill; 1999. p. 423–31.
Richardson D, Goldmeier D. Lymphogranuloma venereum: An emerging cause
of proctitis in men who have sex with men. Int J STD AIDS 2007;18:11–5.
Ronald A. Chancroid and *Haemophilus ducreyi*. In: Holmes K, editor. Sexually
Transmitted Diseases. 3rd ed. New York: McGraw-Hill; 1999. p. 515–21.

Gonorrhea

Method of
Khalil G. Ghanem, MD, PhD

Gonorrhea is caused by the gram-negative diplococcus *Neisseria
gonorrhoeae*, an obligate parasite of humans that has no other natural
host and to which no animal is naturally susceptible. In 2007,
355,991 cases were reported to the Centers for Disease Control and
Prevention (CDC). This number is likely an underestimate because
many cases are asymptomatic and others go unreported. Rates of
gonorrhea in the United States declined sharply starting in the
1970s after the institution of gonorrhea control programs. It remains,
however, the second most commonly reported communicable disease. Worldwide, more than 60 million new cases are estimated to
occur every year.

In 2007 in the United States, the gonorrhea rate among women
was 123.5 and the rate among men was 113.7 cases per 100,000 people in the general population; the rate among African Americans was
19 times greater than the rate for whites, although this is a decrease
from 2001, when there was a 26-fold difference. Risk factors for
infection include young age, unprotected intercourse, multiple sexual
partners, new sexual partners, and sexual activity associated with
illicit drug use. Gonococcal infection increases the rate of HIV transmission fivefold.

N. gonorrhoeae infects noncornified epithelia, including urethral,
endocervical, rectal, oropharyngeal, and conjunctival cells. It is transmitted through contact with infected secretions, most often sexually,
although vertical transmission from mother to infant is well
described. Sexual transmission is efficient; a man who has intercourse
2.5 times with an infected female partner has a 22% chance of
becoming symptomatically infected. The transmission from men to
women is thought to be even more efficient.

Clinical Manifestations

Asymptomatic urethral infections occur in at least 10% of men and
asymptomatic cervical infections occur in about 40% to 50% of
women. More than 50% of rectal and up to 90% of pharyngeal gonorrhea in men and women may be asymptomatic. These numbers
highlight the importance of a thorough sexual history in all at-risk
patients that focuses on a history of exposure rather than symptoms.

In men, urethritis is the most common manifestation of gonococcal infection. Urethral discharge and dysuria are the most frequent
signs occurring 2 to 5 days after exposure. Acute epididymitis manifesting as unilateral scrotal pain is the most common local complication. In young men, 30% of cases of acute epididymitis are caused by
N. gonorrhoeae. Rarely, cellulitis, lymphangitis, or periurethral
abscesses may complicate local infections. Differential diagnosis of
urethritis in men includes *Chlamydia trachomatis*, *Mycoplasma genitalium*, and *Trichomonas vaginalis* infections.

Among women, the most common manifestation of local
gonococcal infection is cervicitis, which tends to occur 5 to 10 days
after exposure. When patients are symptomatic, common complaints
include a vaginal discharge, dysuria, and genital itching. Concomitant infection of the urethra may occur in up to 90% of women
and accounts for some of these symptoms. *N. gonorrhoeae* may
also infect Skene's and Bartholin's glands. The differential diagnosis

of cervicitis includes infection with *C. trachomatis*, *T. vaginalis*,
M. genitalium, or herpes simplex virus and bacterial vaginosis. An
important complication of gonococcal infections in women is pelvic
inflammatory disease (PID). PID is the result of ascending infection
involving the uterus, fallopian tubes, ovaries, or peritoneum.
Sequelae of PID include infertility, ectopic pregnancy, and chronic
pelvic pain. All women presenting with cervicitis should undergo a
bimanual examination. The diagnosis of PID is made when one or
more of the following signs are present: uterine tenderness, cervical
motion tenderness, or adnexal tenderness.

Among men and women with rectal gonorrhea, those who are
symptomatic may complain of rectal discharge, pain, and tenesmus.
Most cases of rectal gonorrhea in men result from receptive anal
intercourse; some cases in women may result from perineal contamination. The differential diagnosis includes *C. trachomatis* (including
lymphogranuloma venereum strains), *Treponema pallidum*, and herpes simplex virus infections. Most cases of pharyngeal gonorrhea
are asymptomatic; when present, signs and symptoms may include
acute pharyngitis, tonsillitis, and cervical lymphadenopathy.

The pharynx may be the only infected site in up to 10% of
patients. A careful history, including past oral-genital contact, is
mandatory. Conjunctivitis is rare in adults and usually is a result of
self-inoculation from anogenital infections.

Disseminated gonococcal infections may occur in up to 2% of
untreated patients. Certain gonococcal strains are more likely to
cause disseminated gonococcal infections. Although patients are bacteremic, many appear nontoxic. Symptoms and signs may include
fevers, myalgias, arthralgias, asymmetrical polyarthritis, and a characteristic dermatitis consisting of a small number (<30) of skin lesions
on the distal extremities that begin as papules and progress to pustules and ulcerations. Rarely, meningitis and endocarditis may occur.

Vertical transmission to neonates may result in ophthalmia neonatorum, sepsis, arthritis, meningitis, rhinitis, vaginitis, urethritis,
and inflammation at the sites of fetal monitoring. Gonococcal infections diagnosed in preadolescent children usually indicate sexual
abuse.

Diagnosis

Gram's stain of urethral discharge among symptomatic men is 90%
sensitive and 95% specific. It is only 70% sensitive in asymptomatic
men. Endocervical Gram's stain is only 50% to 70% sensitive, and
anal swabs are only 60% sensitive. Culture (usually on Thayer-Martin
medium) is 95% sensitive in symptomatic men but is less so for
asymptomatic men and women (80%–90%). The sensitivity of culture in detecting gonococcal infections from urine is low. Culture is
the most common test used to diagnose pharyngeal and rectal infections (despite low sensitivity) and is the only FDA-approved test to
diagnose gonococcal infections in children. Antibiotic susceptibility
testing can be performed only on cultured specimens.

Definitive diagnosis of gonorrhea by culture from any genital or
extragenital site requires confirmation of isolates by biochemical,
enzymatic, serologic, or nucleic acid testing (e.g., carbohydrate use,
rapid enzyme substrate tests, serologic methods such as coagglutina-
tion or fluorescent antibody tests) supplemented with additional tests
that can ensure accurate identification of isolates or a DNA probe
technique for confirmation. After the culture is submitted, this type
of identification is usually performed by the laboratory without
requesting it, and when these methods are used, there should be no
pitfalls in interpreting the extragenital culture data.

Nonamplified molecular tests (e.g., GenProbe Pace II) are the
most common tests used in the United States. The sensitivity is
85% to 90%, and the specificity is more than 95%. The tests can
be performed only on urethral or endocervical specimens. Nucleic
acid amplification tests (e.g., polymerase chain reaction, transcription-
mediated amplification) are the most sensitive (>95%) and specific
(>95%), and most can be performed on urethral or cervical specimens in addition to urine and self-collected vaginal swabs. They
are not FDA cleared for pharyngeal and rectal specimens, although
data increasingly suggest that some are far more sensitive than culture in detecting gonococcal infections at these sites. Serologic tests

CURRENT DIAGNOSIS

- Gonorrhea is caused by the gram-negative diplococcus *Neisseria gonorrhoeae*.
- Asymptomatic genital gonococcal infections are common in men and women.
- Most cases of rectal and pharyngeal infections are asymptomatic.
- Culture and molecular tests are available for diagnosis, depending on the specimen type and anatomic site tested.
- All patients diagnosed with gonorrhea should be tested for other sexually transmitted infections, including HIV.

CURRENT THERAPY

- Ceftriaxone (Rocephin) 125 mg IM × 1 *or* cefixime (Suprax) 400 mg PO × 1 is the first-line treatment for gonorrhea.
- In the United States, fluoroquinolones should no longer be used to treat gonorrhea.
- Patients treated for gonorrhea also should be treated for concomitant *Chlamydia trachomatis* infection.

have been used for epidemiologic studies, but they should not be used for diagnosis. All patients tested for gonorrhea should also be tested for *Chlamydia trachomatis*, syphilis, and HIV.

ANTIMICROBIAL RESISTANCE AND THERAPY

For 40 years, penicillin was the drug of choice for treating gonorrhea. Tetracyclines were also highly effective. By the 1980s, widespread resistance to both of these drug classes rendered them all but useless. Subsequently, drug resistance to aminoglycosides, spectinomycin,[2] macrolides, trimethoprim-sulfamethoxazole (Bactrim),[1] and fluoroquinolones has made the treatment of gonorrhea more challenging.

Fluoroquinolone-resistant *N. gonorrhoeae* (FQRNG) strains emerged in the 1990s, and high rates have been reported in Asia, Africa, and the Middle East. In April 2007, the CDC recommended that fluoroquinolones not be used to treat gonococcal infections in the United States.

Table 1 summarizes the current CDC recommendations for treating uncomplicated and complicated gonococcal infections. Since 1997,

[1]Not FDA approved for this indication.
[2]Not available in the United States.

TABLE 1   Centers for Disease Control and Prevention 2006 Treatment Recommendations for Complicated and Uncomplicated Gonorrhea

Disease	Treatment
Uncomplicated infections of the cervix, urethra, and rectum*	Ceftriaxone (Rocephin) 125 mg IM × 1 *or* Cefixime (Suprax) 400 mg PO × 1 *plus* Treatment for *Chlamydia trachomatis* if not ruled out: Azithromycin (Zithromax) 1g PO × 1 *or* Doxycycline (Vibramycin) 100 mg PO bid × 7 d
Infections of the pharynx	Ceftriaxone (Rocephin) 125 mg IM × 1 *plus* Treatment for *Chlamydia trachomatis* if not ruled out
Epididymitis	Ceftriaxone (Rocephin) 250 mg IM × 1 *plus* Doxycycline (Vibramycin) 100 mg PO bid × 10 d
Gonococcal conjunctivitis	Ceftriaxone (Rocephin) 1g IM × 1
Disseminated gonococcal infections†	Ceftriaxone (Rocephin) 1g IM or IV q24h

*Alternate agents include spectinomycin 2 g IM × 1, if available.
†Should be treated with a parenteral regimen until 24 hours after clinical improvement; can complete a 7-day course of therapy with oral cefixime.

there have been no reports of ceftriaxone-resistant strains in the United States. Cephalosporins are the most reliable and only recommended first-line agents to treat gonorrhea. Ceftriaxone (Rocephin) is given intramuscularly and is effective for infections at all sites. Cefixime (Suprax) is effective for anogenital infections, but it may have lower efficacy than ceftriaxone for pharyngeal infections. Cephalosporins are safe to use in pregnancy. Patients should be treated for presumed *C. trachomatis* co-infection unless it is ruled out. All sexual contacts in the preceding 60 days of index patients should also be treated.

For penicillin-allergic patients, treatment of gonorrhea has become more challenging. Initially, spectinomycin was recommended as a second-line agent. Spectinomycin has a more than 80% efficacy in treating pharyngeal gonococcal infections. However, spectinomycin is no longer available in the United States.

Alternate agents include a single dose of azithromycin (Zithromax) 2 gm PO. The gastrointestinal side effects associated with this high dose and concern about increasing drug resistance resulted in the CDC dropping it as a second-line agent in its 2006 treatment guidelines. However, if tolerated by the patient, this regimen has excellent activity against anogenital and pharyngeal infections. Azithromycin has been used in pregnant women without evidence of teratogenicity.

To prevent gonococcal ophthalmia neonatorum, 1% silver nitrate aqueous solution, 0.5% erythromycin ophthalmic ointment (Ilotycin), or 1% tetracycline ophthalmic ointment[1] should be instilled into the eyes of all newborns. Treatment of gonococcal ophthalmia requires hospitalization, evaluation for evidence of disseminated infection, and ceftriaxone (Rocephin) 25 to 50 mg/kg IM or IV × 1 dose.

Several drugs are being tested for the treatment of gonorrhea. They include cefpodoxime (Vantin), ertapenem (Invanz),[1] telithromycin (Ketek),[1] tigecycline (Tygacil),[1] and newer-generation fluoroquinolones (e.g., gemifloxacin [Factive][1]). None is currently recommended by the CDC.

Prevention and Screening

Abstinence from sexual intercourse is the single most reliable method of preventing infection. Male condoms, when used correctly and consistently, are highly effective in preventing infection. Diaphragms may help prevent gonococcal infections in women. There have not been any successful vaccine candidates.

The CDC does not recommend universal screening for *N. gonorrhoeae*. High-risk women (e.g., multiple sexual partners, illicit drug use, history of gonorrhea or other sexually transmitted infection, commercial sex worker, inconsistent condom use) should be screened. Up to 20% of heterosexual men and women diagnosed

[1]Not FDA approved for this indication.

with gonorrhea become reinfected in the next few months. High-risk pregnant women should be screened during the first prenatal visit. Repeat testing during the third trimester for those at continued risk is recommended.

REFERENCES

Centers for Disease Control and Prevention. Update to CDC's sexually transmitted diseases treatment guidelines, 2006: Fluoroquinolones no longer recommended for treatment of gonococcal infections. MMWR Morb Mortal Wkly Rep 2007;56(14):332–6.

Newman LM, Moran JS, Workowski KA. Update on the management of gonorrhea in adults in the United States. Clin Infect Dis 2007;44: S84–101.

Schachter J, Moncada J, Liska S, et al. Nucleic acid amplification tests in the diagnosis of chlamydial and gonococcal infections of the oropharynx and rectum in men who have sex with men. Sex Transm Dis 2008;35 (7):637–42.

Workowski KA, Berman SM, Douglas Jr JM. Emerging antimicrobial resistance in *Neisseria gonorrhoeae*: Urgent need to strengthen prevention strategies. Ann Intern Med 2008;148(8):606–13.

Workowski KA, Berman SM. for the Centers for Disease Control and Prevention. Sexually transmitted diseases treatment guidelines, 2006. MMWR Morb Mortal Wkly Rep 2006;55(RR-11):1–94.

Nongonococcal Urethritis

Method of
John N. Krieger, MD

Urethritis is defined as inflammation of the urethra and is commonly caused by urogenital infection. Urethritis is classified as either gonococcal, in patients whose inflammation is caused by *Neisseria gonorrhoeae*, or nongonococcal (NGU), in patients with inflammation that is not related to infection with *N. gonorrhoeae*.

Clinical Presentation

More than 4 million NGU cases are estimated to occur among men in the United States every year. Urethritis is characterized by symptoms of urethral discharge and dysuria, often accompanied by increased urinary frequency or pruritis. Signs of urethritis include urethral discharge that can occur spontaneously or after stripping of the urethra, erythema, and urethral tenderness.

Although the clinical presentation varies, the incubation of NGU averages 7 to 14 days from exposure to an infected partner. Typically the onset is gradual, with mild dysuria and mucoid discharge. In some high-risk populations, up to 50% of infections are asymptomatic.

Etiology

NGU should be considered infectious until proven otherwise. Most infectious cases of urethritis are sexually transmitted.

Chlamydia trachomatis remains the most important pathogen, accounting for 15% to 40% of NGU cases. The prevalence of *C. trachomatis* is lower in older patients and in referral populations. Other infectious causes of NGU include *Mycoplasma genitalium*, *Trichomonas vaginalis*, and herpes simplex virus. The etiologic roles are less well defined for other infectious agents including *Ureaplasma urealytimum*, enteric bacteria, anaerobes, and *Candida* species.

CURRENT DIAGNOSIS

- Documenting urethral inflammation is critical for diagnosis of urethritis. One or more of the following techniques can provide documentation:
  - Physical examination showing urethral discharge, either present spontaneously at the meatus or after stripping the urethra. This discharge may be either mucoid or purulent in character.
  - Gram stain of urethral exudate showing five or more WBCs per oil immersion field (×1000). The Gram stain is the preferred rapid diagnostic test.
  - Urine leukocyte esterase dip stick test positive on first-void urine
  - First-void urine sediment microscopic examination demonstrating 10 or more WBCs per high-power field (×400).

Abbreviation: WBC = white blood cell.

Occasionally, patients with other urologic conditions (e.g., prostatitis, urethral stricture disease, or, rarely, bacterial urinary tract infection) present with symptoms of NGU. Other unusual causes of NGU include chemical, allergic, and autoimmune processes.

Diagnosis

It is important to document the presence of urethral inflammation. This may be done by finding mucoid or mucopurulent discharge on physical examination or by diagnostic testing. The Gram stain is the preferred rapid diagnostic test. Urethral inflammation may also be documented by a positive leukocyte esterase test on first-void urine or by finding pyuria on microscopic examination of the first-void urine sediment.

Diagnostic testing for both *N. gonorrhoeae* and *C. trachomatis* organisms is strongly recommended. Specific etiologic diagnosis may guide therapy and can improve compliance and partner notification. These infections are both reportable to state health departments. Patients at risk for *N. gonorrhoeae* and *C. trachomatis* should receive appropriate counseling and should receive testing for HIV and syphilis. Clinical evaluation and treatment of sex partners are critical for preventing complications and interrupting sexual transmission. Pathogens responsible for NGU are associated with cervicitis, pelvic inflammatory disease, and tubal infertility.

The Gram stain is the preferred rapid diagnostic test for evaluating urethritis because it provides high sensitivity and specificity. Gonococcal infection can be established by documenting the presence of white blood cells (WBCs) containing intracellular gram-negative diplococci. Presence of gram-negative rods should raise the suspicion for enteric bacteria.

Confirmatory tests should be employed to identify a specific etiology. *N. gonorrhoeae* and *C. trachomatis* can be detected using culture, DNA hybridization tests on a urethral specimen, or nucleic acid amplification tests on a urethral or urine specimen. Because of their increased sensitivity, nucleic acid amplification tests are recommended for diagnosing chlamydial infection. For urine testing, 10 to 15 mL of first-void urine is collected then evaluated using nucleic acid amplification testing.

Diagnostic tests for the genital mycoplasmas (*M. genitalium*, *U. urealyticum*, and other genital mycoplasmas) are available in research settings. Such tests are usually unavailable for routine clinical use. *T. vaginalis* may be cultured, but specific media are necessary for isolation. To increase sensitivity, cultures of both a urethral swab sample and a urine specimen are recommended.

Treatment

If gonorrhea cannot be ruled out by Gram stain of urethral secretions, potentially noncompliant patients should be treated for both gonorrhea and chlamydial infection. Both azithromycin (Zithromax) and doxycycline (Vibramycin) are highly effective for treating chlamydial NGU. Azithromycin also provides convenient single dosing and the opportunity for directly observed therapy. Doxycycline is inexpensive but requires twice-daily dosing for a full week. Alternatives include erythromycin and fluoroquinolone regimens.

For patients with erratic health care–seeking behavior in whom poor compliance is anticipated, azithromycin offers the easiest administration. Further, *M. genitalium* appears to respond better to macrolides than to tetracyclines. Patients should be advised to abstain from sex until therapy is completed, symptoms have resolved, and sex partners have been treated.

Follow-up

Routine follow-up is not recommended for patients whose symptoms resolve after therapy. Patients with persistent or recurrent symptoms should return for reevaluation.

Symptoms alone should not prompt a second course of therapy unless the patient has documented urethritis or a positive test for a urogenital pathogen. Patients should return for evaluation and treatment if their symptoms persist or recur after completion of therapy. Patients with NGU should refer all sex partners in the past 60 days for evaluation and treatment.

Chronic Urethritis

Chronic urethritis is defined as persistent or recurrent urethritis within 6 weeks following treatment. An estimated 20% to 40% of NGU cases do not respond to first-line therapy. Although up to 20% of men with chlamydial NGU develop chronic urethritis, up to 50% of men with nonchlamydial NGU develop chronic urethritis. Noncompliance and reinfection are important considerations. Other causes include organisms that do not respond to the standard treatment regimens, such as *T. vaginalis*, tetracycline-resistant mycoplasmas, viral etiologies, and other bacteria.

CURRENT THERAPY

Recommended Regimens

- Azithromycin (Zithromax) 1 g PO in a single dose
- Doxycycline (Vibramycin) 100 mg PO bid × 7 days

Alternative Regimens

- Erythromycin base (E-Mycin, ERYC, E-Base) 500 mg PO qid × 7 days
- Erythromycin ethylsuccinate (EES) 800 mg PO qid × 7 days
- Ofloxacin (Floxin) 300 mg PO bid × 7 days
- Levofloxacin (Levaquin)[1] 500 mg PO qd × 7 days
- If an erythromycin regimen is the only possibility and the patient cannot tolerate high-dose schedules, then one of the following regimens should be considered.
- Erythromycin base (E-Mycin, ERYC, E-Base) 250 mg PO qid × 14 days
- Erythromycin ethylsuccinate (EES) 400 mg PO qid × 14 days

---

[1]Not FDA approved for this indication.

Up to 30% of NGU has no identifiable infectious etiology. These cases can involve allergy and postinfectious immunologic responses. Before administering therapy, presence of urethral inflammation should be documented. Patients with persistent or recurrent urethritis who did not comply with therapy or who had exposure to an untreated sex partner should be re-treated with the initial drug regimen. Otherwise, recommended treatment regimens include metronidazole (Flagyl),[1] 2 g orally in a single dose, plus either erythromycin base (E-Base), 500 mg orally four times a day for 7 days, or erythromycin ethylsuccinate (EES), 800 mg orally four times a day for 7 days.

Complications

For infected men, complications of untreated NGU include epididymitis in less than 3% of cases and, rarely, Reiter's syndrome. Patients with a history of NGU also appear to be at increased risk for developing chronic prostatitis/chronic pelvic pain syndrome.

Female sex partners are at risk for pelvic inflammatory disease, tubal infertility, and ectopic pregnancy. Prompt and appropriate therapy and treatment of sexual partners decrease the risk of complications substantially.

REFERENCES

Aydin D, Kucukbasmaci O, Gonullu N, Aktas Z. Susceptibilities of *Neisseria gonorrhoeae* and *Ureaplasma urealyticum* isolates from male patients with urethritis to several antibiotics including telithromycin. Chemotherapy 2005;51:89–92.

Bradshaw CS, Tabrizi SN, Read TR, et al. Etiologies of nongonococcal urethritis: Bacteria, viruses, and the association with orogenital exposure. J Infect Dis 2006;193:336–45.

Centers for Disease Control and Prevention. Screening tests to detect *Chlamydia trachomatis* and *Neisseria gonorrhoeae* infections. MMWR Recomm Rep 2002;51(RR-15):3–19.

Centers for Disease Control and Prevention. Sexually transmitted disease treatment guidelines 2002. MMWR Recomm Rep 2002;51(RR-6):30–42.

Deguchi T, Yoshida T, Miyazawa T, et al. Association of *Ureaplasma urealyticum* (biovar 2) with nongonococcal urethritis. Sex Transm Dis 2004;31:192–5.

Falk L, Fredlund H, Jensen JS. Symptomatic urethritis is more prevalent in men infected with *Mycoplasma genitalium* than with *Chlamydia trachomatis*. Sex Transm Infect 2004;80:289–93.

Geisler WM, Yu S, Hook EW 3rd. Chlamydial and gonococcal infection in men without polymorphonuclear leukocytes on Gram stain: Implications for diagnostic approach and management. Sex Transm Dis 2005;32:630–4.

Jensen JS. *Mycoplasma genitalium:* The aetiological agent of urethritis and other sexually transmitted diseases. J Eur Acad Dermatol Venereol 2004;18:1–11.

Kaydos-Daniels SC, Miller WC, Hoffman I, et al. The use of specimens from various genitourinary sites in men, to detect *Trichomonas vaginalis* infection. J Infect Dis 2004;189:1926–31.

Leung A, Eastick K, Haddon LE, et al. *Mycoplasma genitalium* is associated with symptomatic urethritis. Int J STD AIDS 2006;17:285–8.

O'Mahony C. Adenoviral non-gonococcal urethritis. Int J STD AIDS 2006;17:203–4.

Ozgül A, Dede I, Taskaynatan MA, et al. Clinical presentations of chlamydial and non-chlamydial reactive arthritis. Rheumatol Int 2006;26:879–85.

Pontari MA, McNaughton-Collins M, O'Leary P, et al. A case-control study of risk factors in men with chronic pelvic pain syndrome. BJU Int 2005;96:559–65.

Swygard H, Sena AC, Hobbs MM, Cohen MS. Trichomoniasis: Clinical manifestations, diagnosis and management. Sex Transm Infect 2004;80:91–5.

Taylor SN. *Mycoplasma genitalium.* Curr Infect Dis Rep 2005;7:453–7.

Taylor-Robinson D, Gilroy CB, Thomas BJ, Hay PE. *Mycoplasma genitalium* in chronic non-gonococcal urethritis. Int J STD AIDS 2004;15:21–5.

Yasuda M, Maeda S, Deguchi T. In vitro activity of fluoroquinolones against *Mycoplasma genitalium* and their bacteriological efficacy for treatment of *M. genitalium*–positive nongonococcal urethritis in men. Clin Infect Dis 2005;41:1357–9.

---

[1]Not FDA approved for this indication.

Syphilis

Method of
Mrunal Shah, MD

One of the oldest infections known, syphilis dates back more than 500 years. It was known as "The Great Pox" because of its skin manifestations; in contrast to the "small pox" seen around the same time. Studies were done before the use of antibiotics, which is where most of our natural history information comes from. The most recent epidemic occurred in 1990 (20.3 cases per 100,000 population) and has fallen steadily each year since. In the year 2000, the rate was at an all time low of 2.2 cases per 100,000 population. This was a 9.6% drop since 1999. The Centers for Disease Control and Prevention (CDC) hopes to eradicate the disease completely by 2005, but this may be difficult.

Peak ages are 30 to 39 years of age in men and 20 to 24 years of age in women. African Americans have always had higher incidences than whites. In the 1990s, it was 60:1, but the incidence has since declined to 30:1.

Microbiology

Treponema pallidum is the bacterium responsible for causing syphilis. It is very small and cannot be detected by ordinary microscopy, a feature that complicates diagnosis. The organism can be seen with dark-field microscopy, a technique that uses a special condenser to cast an oblique light. This allows visualization of a corkscrew-shaped organism with tightly wound spirals. This organism is extremely sensitive to penicillin, as is discussed later in the article. It has a very slow doubling rate, therefore requiring longer courses of treatment.

Pathophysiology

T. pallidum initiates infection when it gains access to subcutaneous tissues through microabrasions that can occur during sexual intercourse. Even though it has a slow doubling time (30 hours), it escapes host immune defenses and leads to the initial ulcerative lesion, the chancre. These can be seen anywhere around the genitalia including the cervix, perianal and rectal areas, and the oral mucosa. Regional lymphadenopathy also can be seen. As the host immune system fights the initial infection, *T. pallidum* is disseminated throughout the host. This is known as latency, as the patient will have no symptoms. There is also vertical spread in utero or during delivery, which is why prenatal panels include screening tests for syphilis.

Clinical Manifestations

The initial clinical manifestation is also called *primary* syphilis. This usually consists of a painless chancre at the site of inoculation. Primary syphilis represents a local infection, but it quickly becomes systemic with widespread dissemination of the spirochete. Because it is painless, most people do not seek medical attention. Even without treatment, the chancre will resolve in 4 to 6 weeks. It is this painlessness that helps separate it from herpes simplex virus (genital herpes) and *Haemophilus ducreyi* (chancroid).

In approximately weeks to months after the resolution of the chancre, patients will develop *secondary* syphilis, which includes systemic symptoms of rash, fever, headache, malaise, anorexia, and diffuse lymphadenopathy. The rash typically involves the palms and soles but can also include mucosal surfaces. Many patients do not realize that they had these lesions. These symptoms usually resolve spontaneously but can relapse for up to 5 years.

After symptoms resolve, and for up to many years later, the disease goes into *latent* syphilis, which is characterized by a lack of symptoms but seropositive test results. This can be separated into early and late latent phases based on being potentially infectious in the early phase. This is defined by the United States Public Health Service (USPHS) as infection of 1 year's duration or less. Anything longer is late latent.

Finally, for the next 1 to 30 years, untreated patients have a 25% to 40% risk of developing *late* or *tertiary* syphilis. It may involve many tissue types, so the spectrum of disease can be very confusing. Moreover, patients need not have had symptoms of primary or secondary syphilis prior to developing late syphilis. Tissues involved include cutaneous (gumma formation), cardiovascular (aortic disease), and central nervous system (CNS) (tabes dorsalis, meningitis, neurosyphilis) diseases (Table 1).

Diagnosis

The quickest, most direct method of diagnosing primary and secondary syphilis is direct visualization of the spirochete of moist lesions by means of darkfield microscopy. This is difficult and requires using laboratories that perform a high volume of sexually transmitted disease analyses. In general, a moist lesion should be cleaned with saline

TABLE 1 Clinical Manifestations and Treatment of Syphilis

Stage	Clinical Manifestation	Treatment
Primary	Painless ulcer (chancre), adenopathy	Benzathine penicillin G (Bicillin LA), 2.4 million U IM × 1
Secondary (weeks to months)	Rash, mucocutaneous lesions, adenopathy, hepatitis, arthritis, glomerulonephritis, condyloma lata	Benzathine penicillin G, 2.4 million U IM × 1
Latent	Asymptomatic	
Early (<1 year)		Benzathine penicillin G, 2.4 million U IM × 1
Late		Benzathine penicillin G, 2.4 million U IM weekly × 3
Tertiary (late) 1–30 years		
Cutaneous	Gummatous lesions	Benzathine penicillin G, 2.4 million U IM weekly × 3
Cardiovascular	Aortic aneurysm, aortic insufficiency, neurosyphilis, tabes dorsalis, Argyll-Robertson pupils, paresis, seizures, subtle psychiatric manifestations, dementia; may be asymptomatic	Benzathine penicillin G, 2.4 million U IM weekly × 3
CNS		Aqueous crystalline penicillin G, 18–24 million U/d given as 3–4 million units IV q4h for 10–14 days or Procaine penicillin (Wycillin), 2.4 million U qd with probenecid 500 mg PO qid for 10–14 days

Adapted from the CDC: Guidelines for the treatment of STDs. MMWR Morb Mortal Wkly Rep 2002;51(RR-06):1–80.
Abbreviations: CNS = central nervous system; IM = intramuscularly; IV = intravenously; PO = orally; qd = daily; qid = 4 times per day.

(not iodine because of bactericidal effect). Then, using gauze, the lesion should be unroofed. Any serosanguineous material should be collected on a dry slide for examination.

More common is serologic testing that can be done in most laboratories. The two most common screening tests are rapid plasma reagin (RPR) and the Venereal Disease Research Laboratory (VDRL) test. These tests are designed to test for IgM and IgG antibodies against a cardiolipin-cholesterol-lecithin antigen. Positive tests are reported as a dilutional titer. False positives are less than 1:4, whereas higher titers (1:16 to 1:128) are found in secondary and early latent syphilis. This titer is important as a benchmark to follow treatment. Lack of expected decreases in titer indicate inadequate treatment, false-positive result, re-infection, or late-stage therapy.

Before treatment, a positive screening test needs to be confirmed with specific *T. pallidum* antigen testing, such as the fluorescent treponemal antibody absorption test (FTA-ABS). These tests are expensive and have a high false-positive rate, making them unsuitable as screening tests. They also remain positive for life in most people.

Newer molecular tests include the use of polymerase chain reaction (PCR), which can be used to detect multiple organisms. It has high sensitivity and specificity and can distinguish among *H. ducreyi*, herpes simplex virus, and *T. pallidum*. This test is very expensive and is likely to be available only in specialized laboratories, for now.

The most significant morbidity of syphilis occurs during the tertiary phase and includes neurosyphilis. *T. pallidum* can be found in the cerebrospinal fluid (CSF) during primary and secondary phases, but it usually resolves on its own. Those patients who have an abnormal CSF during the latent phase are at higher risk for symptomatic neurosyphilis, making it helpful to distinguish asymptomatic neurosyphilis. The CDC recommends that CSF testing be done whenever there is clinical evidence of neurosyphilis or vision changes, active tertiary syphilis, treatment failure, or HIV infection. CSF-VDRL is highly specific, but, unfortunately, very insensitive (as low as 30%) and therefore can rule in but cannot exclude neurosyphilis.

Although the HIV epidemic showed a resurgence of syphilis, it is controversial as to what diagnostic changes occurred in testing. Several studies show contradictory information; one shows that there was an increase in the false-positive rates, whereas a second study showed a decrease in true-positive rates, and a third study showed higher false negatives. In any case, testing should still be performed as in non-HIV patients and followed accordingly.

Pregnancy poses only increased risk, including perinatal death, premature delivery, low birth weight, congenital anomalies, and active congenital syphilis of the neonate. Physical examination and serologic testing should be performed in any female considering pregnancy or during initial antepartum testing at least. Treatment, discussed below, should be given as if the patient is not pregnant.

Treatment

In all stages, the main reason for treatment is to prevent progression and spread of the disease. Historic treatments included mercury, salvarsan (an arsenic derivative), fever therapy, and malarial injection. Today's treatment has been in use since 1943, since the introduction of penicillin. Because there has been no reported resistance, penicillin remains the treatment of choice, so much so that penicillin-allergic patients have undergone desensitization therapy in order to receive it. Although penicillin G, given parenterally, is the preferred drug, the preparation used (benzathine, procaine, crystalline), dosage, and duration of therapy depend on stage and clinical manifestations (see Table 1). Oral penicillin is not considered appropriate for treatment. Alternative treatments could include doxycycline (Vibramycin), tetracycline, erythromycin, or ceftriaxone (Rocephin).[1]

Once treatment is started, physicians should be aware of a potential complication called the Jarisch-Herxheimer reaction. It is an

---

[1]Not FDA approved for this indication.

acute, febrile reaction accompanied by headache and myalgias, which represents treponemal cell death and release of toxins. It peaks within 2 hours and subsides within 24 hours, and is most common in primary and secondary disease.

Follow-up of Treated Patients

Any patient with syphilis diagnosed at any stage should get testing for HIV and should be retested in 3 to 6 months if a member of a high-risk population. After treatment, repeat serologic testing should be done at 6 and 12 months and titers at 24 months. If there is not at least a fourfold decrease in 6 months, there is likely treatment failure. A lumbar puncture should be done to rule out neurosyphilis, and retreatment with three weekly injections of 2.4 million units of benzathine penicillin (Bicillin LA) is recommended unless there is evidence of neurosyphilis.

Partners of patients with syphilis should also be notified and treated. In primary disease, any partner within the previous 3 months should be identified. Empiric treatment is recommended unless there is good follow-up and serologic surveillance.

Contraception

Method of
Emily J. Herndon, MD

More than 15% of all primary care visits to an internist or family physician is for contraceptive counseling and care. Compared with the financial costs and mortality of pregnancy-related births and abortions, contraception saves money and lives. Despite these facts, 49% of the pregnancies in the United States are unintended, with almost one half of these ending in an elective abortion. In a study of women who had had an unintended pregnancy, 41% believed that they could not get pregnant at the time of conception. These statistics demonstrate the need for primary care providers educating patients regarding contraception.

The ideal contraceptive is one that is safe, highly effective, and rapidly reversible; provides good cycle control; and protects against sexually transmitted infections (STIs). Patients want a method that is user-friendly, is easily accessible, and has minimal side effects. Although no single contraceptive provides all these characteristics, primary care providers need to be aware of all the methods to help a patient choose one that is medically appropriate and best suits his or her needs.

Contraceptives can be categorized as hormonal and nonhormonal, as reversible or permanent, and as precoital or postcoital. The reversible, nonhormonal methods include the copper intrauterine device (IUD) (ParaGard), barrier methods, spermicides, withdrawal, abstinence, fertility awareness, and lactation amenorrhea (Table 1). Of these, male condoms are the most widely used reversible, nonhormonal method, with 18% of couples choosing this method for contraception. All other methods combined are used less frequently (<10% of choices).

Combined Hormonal Methods

The hormonal methods of contraception can be divided into two categories: those with combined estrogen and progesterone and those with progesterone only. The combined estrogen and progesterone methods all work by suppressing ovulation and thickening the cervical mucus, and only their delivery systems are different. The estrogen and progesterone methods available in the United States include combined oral contraceptive pills (COCPs), the vaginal ring, and the contraceptive patch.

TABLE 1 Reversible Nonhormonal Methods of Contraception

Method	Percent Failure (%)*	Advantages	Disadvantages	Comments
Abstinence	0 (unknown)	Can be started or restarted at any time; decreases risk of STIs and cervical cancer; no cost	Requires commitment, self-control, and communication between patient and partner	Patient needs to establish ground rules and be aware of back-up methods if changes mind
LAM	0.5 (2)	No cost; helps postpartum weight loss; decreases risk of ovarian and endometrial cancers	Contraindicated if patient is HIV+; offers no protection against STIs; return of ovulation unpredictable	Effectiveness sharply decreases after 6 mo; return of fertility often precedes menses
Withdrawal	4 (2.7)	No cost	Not adequate protection against STIs; contraindicated if history of premature ejaculation; male partner must be very disciplined	Couples must be able to communicate during intercourse, and men must be able to predict ejaculation in time
FAM	1–9 (25)	May be only method acceptable to couples for religious or cultural reasons	Not useful if patient's periods are irregular; no protection against STIs; need good discipline and documentation of cycles	Use back-up form of contraception during fertile times
Barriers				Consider having EC at home
Condom, male	2 (15)	Low cost and easily available; protects against STIs	Need to use consistently; may interrupt love making	Third most common method used in the United States
Condom, female	5 (21)	Same as for male condom	More difficult to use than male condom	
Diaphragm	6 (16)	Can insert several hours earlier; no need to remove for multiple acts of intercourse up to 24 h	Needs a doctor visit and prescription; does not protect against HIV; may increase risk of UTIs; patient must be comfortable with inserting and removing device	Contraindicated in cases of latex allergy
Cervical cap	9–26 (16–32)	Same as for diaphragm; can stay in for 48 h	Same as for diaphragm	Two cervical caps available in the United States; both types latex free
Cervical sponge	18 (29)	Easily available; relatively low cost	Same as for diaphragm	Made of polyurethane foam prefilled with spermicide
Spermicide	15 (29)	Easily available and easy to use	N-9 contraindicated if at high risk for HIV	Some studies suggest increased risk of HIV transmission with N-9
Copper IUD	0.6 (0.8)	Highest level of user satisfaction; long duration of action; rapidly reversible	Requires office procedure; may increase cramps and menstrual bleeding; no protection against STIs	Most cost-effective reversible method; increased infection risk in first 20 d after insertion

*Percent failure is defined as the percentage of women experiencing an unintended pregnancy in the first year, when the method is used perfectly (% with typical use).
Abbreviations: CA = cancer; EC = emergency contraception; FAM = fertility awareness combined with periodic abstinence; HIV = human immunodeficiency virus; IUD, intrauterine device; LAM = lactation amenorrhea; N-9 = nonoxynol-9 spermicide; STI = sexually transmitted infection; UTI = urinary tract infection.

The noncontraceptive benefits of combined hormonal therapy include excellent cycle control[1] and decreased rates of ectopic pregnancy,[1] pelvic inflammatory disease,[1] and endometrial and ovarian cancer.[1] They are also used to treat dysfunctional uterine bleeding,[1] dysmenorrhea,[1] mittelschmerz,[1] ovarian cysts,[1] and acne[1] (except Ortho Tri-Cyclen and Estrostep). Likewise, the side effect profile and contraindications are similar and usually result from the estrogen component of the methods. Higher estrogen doses are associated with nausea, headache, breast tenderness, and chloasma, whereas breakthrough bleeding occurs more commonly with the lower estrogen methods. With the exception of chloasma, most of these side effects are seen in the first few cycles, and they tend to improve with time. Combined hormonal methods should not be used if the patient has a history of liver or breast cancer or has a significant history of liver or gallbladder disease. Because estrogen can interfere with lactation, it is also contraindicated in the first 6 months after delivery if a woman is breast-feeding.

The most serious concerns about using combined hormonal methods are the potential cardiovascular complications. Although rare, the use of estrogen has been associated with the development of deep vein thrombosis, myocardial infarction, hypertension, and stroke. Combined hormonal methods are contraindicated if the patient has a history of any of these conditions or has other factors that may increase the risk of these complications. Factors include age older than 35 years combined with smoking, uncontrolled hypertension, coronary artery disease, having diabetes for more than 20 years, having a positive family history of deep vein thrombosis, or having a known hypercoagulable condition. Studies have also shown that patients who have a history of migraine headaches associated with focal neurologic findings or auras are at higher risk for stroke when using combined hormonal methods.

COMBINED ORAL CONTRACEPTIVE PILLS

Of the hormonal therapies, COCPs are the most widely used, with 31% of all couples choosing this method. COCPs have a failure rate of 0.3% with perfect use and 8% when used typically. The difference in these rates largely results from incorrect use of the pills. Patients must take the COCP daily, ideally at the same time each day. If the patient accidently misses a pill, she should take the missed pill as soon as possible. If she misses two or more pills, the patient should

---
[1]Not FDA approved for this indication.

double up on the pills daily until the missed tablets are taken and use a backup form of contraception for 7 days.

COCPs come in monophasic (i.e., same dose of hormones in each active tablet) and multiphasic (i.e., active tablets with different doses) combinations, and they are available in various cycle lengths. A 28-day cycle, with 21 active tablets and 7 placebo tablets, is the most commonly used form. Extended cycle forms (84 active pills and 7 placebo pills) are monophasic, and they are ideal for patients who have problems associated with menstruation such as endometriosis, dysmenorrhea, or menstrual headaches. Patients should be warned that breakthrough bleeding is more likely with extended cycles. COCPs that contain drospirenone as the progesterone component (Yaz) have an antimineralocorticoid-like activity with decreased rates of bloating and premenstrual weight gain. Potassium levels should be monitored if these patients are also taking other potassium-sparing drugs.

Intermenstrual spotting is a common problem for COCP users, and it may lead to discontinuation of the pill by patients. Patients should be counseled that spotting is more likely in the first two cycles and that 70% to 90% of women have no further breakthrough bleeding by the third cycle. Because incorrect or inconsistent use of the pill is one of the most common reasons for intermenstrual bleeding, the patient must be instructed on how to take the pill and what she should do and expect if a pill is missed. Other causes of vaginal bleeding, such as pregnancy, cervicitis, vaginitis, and medications that interfere with the hormones, should be ruled out. If persistent spotting continues after 2 or 3 months, changing to a different formulation of pill may help. Patients who report spotting before they complete their active pills usually need higher progesterone levels, and changing to a different monophasic pill or to a triphasic formulation, which usually has a higher progesterone content in the last active pills, is a good option. Patients who report continued bleeding after their normal withdrawal bleeding usually need a higher estrogen-to-progesterone ratio. Options for these patients include changing to a higher-dose estrogen pill or changing to a formulation that has lower progesterone levels in the early part of the cycle.

CONTRACEPTIVE PATCH

The contraceptive patch (Ortho Evra) delivers 20 μg of ethinyl estradiol and 150 μg of progesterone (norelgestromin) per day and is ideal for patients who want to avoid daily pill taking. It has a failure rate similar to COCP, although it is much less effective in women weighing more than 90 kg. The patch is applied weekly on the same day of the week (i.e., the patch change day) for 3 weeks, followed by a patch-free week. Recommended application sites include the upper arms, buttocks, lower abdomen, and upper torso, excluding the breasts. Patients should be told to rotate the application site to decrease the risk of pigment changes or skin irritation, an uncommon side effect that occurs in 1% of women. Adhesion rates are very reliable, with less than 2% of patches completely detaching. If a patch detaches and has been off for less than 24 hours, patients should apply a new patch but keep the previous patch change day. If it detaches and has been off for 24 hours or more, patients should apply a new patch, change the patch change day to that day, and use a backup form of contraception for 7 days. Because the patch has enough medicine to last for 9 days, the patient has 2 extra days during which it remains effective if left on too long. However, the patient should *not* extend the patch-free interval. If the patient has a late restart (≥9 days), she should apply a new patch and use a backup form of contraception for 7 days.

The average estrogen concentration in women using the patch was higher than in those taking COCPs, raising the possibility of an increased risk of deep vein thrombosis and cardiovascular events. Epidemiologic data show conflicting results, and further studies are pending, but patients should be adequately counseled regarding this potential risk.

VAGINAL RING

The vaginal ring (NuvaRing) releases 15 μg of ethinyl estradiol and 120 μg of etonogestrel per day, and, in studies, it had the lowest steady-state level of hormones compared with other methods, making it ideal for patients who want good cycle control but are worried about estrogen-related side effects. The ring is placed in the vagina and left there for 3 weeks; it is then removed for 1 week to allow for withdrawal bleeding. Unlike barrier methods, the ring does not have to be in any particular position because transmucosal hormone absorption occurs as long as the ring is in the vagina. Like the patch, the ring also has enough medicine to last longer than the time recommended for use (up to 35 days for the ring), allowing some flexibility regarding insertion and removal times. Although not recommended, patients may take the ring out during intercourse, as long as the ring-free time is less than 3 hours/day. Although douching is discouraged, there are no contraindications to using intravaginal topical agents (e.g., antifungal creams) at the same time as the ring.

The rate of adverse effects that led to discontinuation of the ring was low (3.6%), and they included foreign body sensation, coital problems, and device expulsion. The ring should not be exposed to high temperatures outside the body for prolonged periods because this can activate premature release of the hormones. It may be stored for up to 4 months at room temperature or can be refrigerated if stored for longer periods.

Progesterone-Only Methods

For women who would like to use a hormonal method of contraception but cannot take estrogen, progesterone-only methods are an excellent choice. These methods provide a steady dose of progesterone daily, and they work by thickening the cervical mucus, thinning the endometrial lining, and inhibiting ovulation. Because there is no hormone-free interval, menstrual periods are often irregular, and amenorrhea is common. Like combined hormonal methods, progesterone-only methods have been shown to decrease dysmenorrhea and menstrual bleeding. Progesterone-only methods include mini-pills (Micronor), injections, the intrauterine system, and implants.

PROGESTERONE-ONLY PILLS

Mini-pills or progesterone-only pills have a failure rate similar to that for COCPs. On average, the cost of mini-pills is slightly more than that for COCPs. Because the dose of progesterone in each pill is very close to the therapeutic level needed for contraception, it is important to take the tablets at the same time each day. A backup form of contraception should be used if there is a delay of more than 3 hours in taking the pills or if the pill is missed altogether.

PROGESTERONE INJECTIONS

Depot medroxyprogesterone acetate (DMPA) injections are one of the most popular progesterone-only methods. The intramuscular injection (Depo-Provera) is given every 12 weeks and has a perfect-use failure rate of 0.3% and a typical-use failure rate of 3%. A lower dose of DMPA (104 mg in Depo-SubQ Provera 104) has been approved for subcutaneous injection and has the potential advantage of allowing the patient to administer the injection in the privacy of her home. Noncontraceptive benefits of DMPA include improvement of endometriosis and decreased rates of sickle cell crisis in patients with sickle cell anemia. It is also an ideal choice for women who are on anticonvulsants because there is no potential decrease in the contraceptive's effectiveness as there is with COCPs.

Disadvantages of DMPA injections include spotting, weight gain, a delayed return of fertility (average of 10 months), and a decrease in bone mineral density. The average weight gain is 5.4 pounds in the first year and 16.5 pounds at 5 years. The effect on bone mineral density was unique to DMPA, with an average decrease of 5% to 7% after 2 years of continuous use. This decrease returned to baseline by 2 to 3 years after stopping DMPA in women who were not menopausal. All women who use DMPA should be counseled to stop smoking, participate in weight-bearing exercise at least three times per week, and take 1000 to 1200 mg/day of calcium in the diet or as a supplement.

PROGESTERONE INTRAUTERINE SYSTEM

A levonorgestrel-releasing intrauterine system (Mirena) has been available in the United States since 2001. The device is effective for 5 years and has a failure rate of 0.1%. Unlike the copper IUD, which has side effects of dysmenorrhea and menorrhagia, the levonorgestrel-releasing intrauterine system decreases the incidence of both effects. Approximately 20% of women have reversible amenorrhea after 1 year of use, and that number increases to 47% at 5 years. Because of the bleeding pattern, the levonorgestrel-releasing intrauterine system is being studied as a treatment for other conditions that cause dysfunctional uterine bleeding.

Disadvantages of the system include a risk of expulsion (similar to that for the copper IUD) and increased rates of headache, acne, and breast tenderness during the first few months of use. The cost is also significantly higher compared with the copper IUD, which is the most cost-effective contraceptive over a 5-year period.

PROGESTERONE IMPLANTS

Subdermal implants have a long duration of action and are therefore very convenient and appealing to many patients. Both two-rod (Jadelle)[2] and single-rod systems (Implanon) are FDA approved, although only the single-rod system is marketed in the United States. The single-rod system releases etonogestrel at a rate of 60 μg/day in the first year, decreasing to 30 μg/day by the end of the third year, at which time it is removed and replaced. It has a failure rate of 0.2% with typical use and was well accepted, with a continuation rate of 87% after 2 years in one study. The rod is 4 cm long and 2 mm in diameter, and it is easily placed under the skin of the nondominant arm using a 16-gauge, disposable inserter. Removal is much easier than with the previous six-rod system, with an average removal time of 3 minutes. Irregular bleeding, although common, has not been as heavy as with the six-rod system (Norplant),[2] and amenorrhea occurs in 18% of women at 1 year. Patients should be counseled before insertion of the implant that these side effects are normal and to be expected while the implant is in place.

Initiating Hormonal Methods of Contraception

Traditionally, all hormonal methods of contraception were initiated after delivery, on the first Sunday of a patient's menses, or on the first day of her cycle. This made it less likely that she would be pregnant,

---

[2]Not available in the United States.

---

and if her periods had been regular, it allowed her to continue her usual cycle.

The quick-start method of initiating hormonal contraception has been gaining popularity. If a woman is reasonably sure that she is not pregnant and an in-office pregnancy test confirms this, she can begin the hormonal method on the same day as her office visit, as long as she uses a backup form of contraception for the next 7 days. The quick-start method is especially useful for women with oligomenorrhea and for women who may have trouble correctly remembering initiation instructions with a delayed start.

Emergency Contraception

Emergency contraception should not be used regularly as a form of contraception. It is meant to be used if unplanned intercourse occurs or a condom breaks. Worldwide, progesterone-only pills, COCPs, and copper IUDs have been used for emergency contraception. In the United States, progesterone-only pills are most commonly used and have the least side effects.

In 2006, the FDA ruled that Plan B, which contains two 750-μg pills of levonorgestrel and is packaged specifically for emergency contraception, could be sold without a prescription to women 18 years old or older. These pills should be taken as soon as possible after unplanned intercourse or condom breakage. The contraceptive effectiveness of this method is better if the first pill is taken before 12 hours, but it can be used as late as 120 hours. The second pill can be taken at the same time as the first pill or 12 hours later. Use of emergency contraception has not been shown to decrease compliance with other first-line methods. Plan B One-Step, a single progesterone-only emergency contraceptive is also available without a prescription for women 17 years or older.

Permanent Birth Control Methods

Permanent birth control methods include vasectomy and female sterilization by various procedures. Female sterilization is the second most popular form of birth control after COCPs, with 27% of all couples choosing this form. Male sterilization is chosen by 9% of couples. Each sterilization procedure has advantages and disadvantages that should be considered by the patient before choosing which one to use (Table 2).

TABLE 2 Permanent Birth Control Methods

Procedure	Percent Failure (%)*	Advantages	Disadvantages	Comments
Male sterilization	0.1 (0.15)	Office procedure; simpler, safer, and more cost-effective than female sterilization; allows man to take part in contraception	Short-term postoperative discomfort, bruising, and swelling; back-up method needed until confirmation of no sperm	No increased risk of postoperative sexual dysfunction, cancers, tumors, or masses; 1% of men choose reversal later

Female sterilization
  PP partial salpingectomy
  Bands or clips
  Bipolar cautery
	0.5 (0.5)	Ease of surgery; does not extend hospital stay
		Easiest female method to reverse
			Counseling must be done before onset of labor
			
			Higher risk of ectopic pregnancy
				PP women most likely to regret sterilization

Transcervical tubal occlusion		Does not require an incision; can be done in an outpatient setting under local anesthesia; recovery time much faster	Requires back-up method for first 3 months; requires hysterosalpingogram to confirm blockage; not reversible	Bilateral placement successfully achieved after first attempt in 86%; only 4.6% unable to rely on the device

*Percent failure for male and female sterilization is defined as the percentage of women experiencing an unintended pregnancy in the first year when the method is used perfectly (% with typical use).
Abbreviation: PP = postpartum (within 48 hours of delivery).

- Combined estrogen and progesterone methods (e.g., pills, patch, ring) provide excellent cycle control and decreased rates of ectopic pregnancy, pelvic inflammatory disease, and endometrial and ovarian cancer.
- Although rare, the use of estrogen has been associated with the development of deep vein thrombosis, myocardial infarction, hypertension, and stroke, and it should not be used in smokers older than 35 years; patients who have diabetes for more than 20 years; patients with uncontrolled hypertension, coronary artery disease, or migraines with aura; and patients with a family history of deep vein thrombosis or a known hypercoagulable condition.
- Combined oral contraceptive pills come in extended-cycle forms for patients who desire or for medical reasons need to have fewer periods (i.e., those with endometriosis, dysmenorrhea, or menstrual migraines).
- The patch (Ortho Evra) and ring (NuvaRing) work the same way as combined oral contraceptive pills, but they have a longer duration of action, making it easier for patients to adhere to the correct regimen.
- The patch is less effective in women weighing more than 90 kg.
- Progesterone-only methods (i.e., mini-pills [Micronor], intrauterine device [Mirena], and subdermal implants) do not have any estrogen-related side effects, but they are associated with irregular periods and amenorrhea.

- Depot medroxyprogesterone acetate is available as an intramuscular or subcutaneous injection, and its use is associated with mild weight gain and a reversible decrease in bone mineral density.
- The single-rod subdermal progesterone implant (Implanon) is effective for 3 years and is easier to insert and remove than the six-rod system used previously.
- Patients can initiate hormonal methods on the same day as the office visit (i.e., quick-start method) if they are reasonably sure they are not pregnant and are willing to use a backup form of contraception for the first week.
- Emergency contraception (Plan B One-Step) in the form of one progesterone-only pill, can be sold without a prescription to anyone 17 years old or older, and it can be used any time during the first 120 hours after unplanned intercourse or condom breakage.
- Transcervical tubal occlusion offers an outpatient alternative for female patients desiring permanent sterilization. A follow-up hysterosalpingogram should be done 3 months after the procedure, and a backup method must be used during that interval.
- Contraceptive counseling includes helping patients choose a method that is medically appropriate and educating them about its correct use. The only effective contraception is one that a patient is willing to use consistently and correctly.

Contraceptive Counseling

Although patients may not be concerned about contracting an infection as much as they are about preventing pregnancy, this is an ideal time to evaluate and discuss behavior that may put them at higher risk for disease. The contraceptives with the greatest efficacy for preventing pregnancy provide no protection against STIs, and the contraceptives that best protect against STIs have larger contraceptive failure rates for typical users. For patients at highest risk for STIs, it is prudent to stress barrier methods, specifically condoms, alone or in combination with another method.

When counseling patients about their contraceptive choices, it is important that providers are aware of their own biases. The only effective contraceptive is one that a patient is willing to use consistently and correctly, and the choice of contraception is ultimately the patient's decision. Providers must educate patients regarding the advantages and disadvantages of each method that is medically appropriate for them. If patients are not candidates for their first contraceptive choice, the physician should help them decide on another method that is medically appropriate and discuss how to correctly use it. Educational handouts should be given and reviewed, and counseling should be documented in the medical record.

REFERENCES

Bensyl DM, Iuliano D, Carter M, et al. Contraceptive Use—United States and Territories, Behavioral Risk Factor Surveillance System 2002. MMWR Surveill Summ 2005;18, 54(6):1–72.

Hatcher RA, Trussell J, Nelson A, et al. Contraceptive Technology. New York: Ardent Media; 2007.

Herndon EJ, Zieman M. New contraceptive options. Am Fam Physician 2004;69:853–60.

Scholle S, Chang J, Harman J, McNeil M. Trends in women's health services by type of physician seen: Data from the 1985 and 1997–98 NAMCS. Womens Health Issues 2002;12(4):165–77.

Nettleman MD, Chung H, Brewer J, et al. Reasons for unprotected intercourse: Analysis of the PRAMS Survey. Contraception 2007;75:361–6.

Van den Heuvel MW, van Bragt AJM, Alnabawy AK, Kaptein MC. Comparison of ethinylestradiol pharmacokinetics in three hormonal contraceptive formulations: The vaginal ring, the transdermal patch and an oral contraceptive. Contraception 2005;72:168–74.

Westhoff C, Heartwell S, Edwards S, et al. Initiation of oral contraceptives using a quick start compared to a conventional start: A randomized controlled trial. Obstet Gynecol 2007;109(6):1270–6.

World Health Organization (WHO). Medical eligibility criteria for contraceptive use, Available at http://www.who.int/reproductive-health/publications/mec/mec.pdf (accessed May 12, 2009).

Zieman M, Hatcher RA, Cwiak C, et al. A Pocket Guide to Managing Contraception. Tiger, GA: Bridging the Gap Foundation; 2007.

Diseases of Allergy

Anaphylaxis and Serum Sickness

Method of
Stephen F. Kemp, MD

Anaphylaxis

Anaphylaxis, an acute and potentially lethal multisystem allergic reaction, is virtually unavoidable in medical practice. Health care professionals must be able to recognize the signs of anaphylaxis, treat an episode promptly and appropriately, and be able to provide preventive recommendations. Epinephrine, which should be administered immediately, is the drug of choice for acute anaphylaxis.

Anaphylaxis is not a reportable disease, and both its morbidity and mortality are probably underestimated. A variety of statistics on the epidemiology of anaphylaxis have been published, but the lifetime risk per person in the United States is presumed to be 1% to 3%, with a mortality rate of 1%.

There is no universally accepted definition of anaphylaxis. An international and interdisciplinary group of representatives and experts from thirteen professional, governmental, and lay organizations proposed the following working definition: "Anaphylaxis is a serious allergic reaction that is rapid in onset and may cause death." Clinically, anaphylaxis is considered likely to be present if any one of the following three criteria is satisfied within minutes to hours: Acute onset of illness with involvement of skin, mucosal surface, or both, and at least one of the following: respiratory compromise, hypotension, or end-organ dysfunction; two or more of the following occurring rapidly after exposure to a likely allergen: involvement of skin or mucosal surface, respiratory compromise, hypotension, or persistent gastrointestinal symptoms; hypotension develops after exposure to a known allergen for that patient: age-specific low blood pressure or decline of systolic blood pressure of greater than 30% compared with baseline. In clinical practice, however, waiting until the development of multiorgan symptoms is risky because the ultimate severity of anaphylactic reaction is difficult to predict from the outset.

Anaphylaxis has varied clinical presentations, but respiratory compromise and cardiovascular collapse cause the most concern because they are the most frequent causes of fatalities. Urticaria and angioedema are the most common manifestations (more than 90% in retrospective series) but may be delayed or absent in rapidly progressive anaphylaxis. The previous severity of anaphylaxis is not predictive of the severity of a future reaction. The more rapidly anaphylaxis occurs after exposure to an offending stimulus, the more likely the reaction is to be severe and potentially life threatening.

Anaphylaxis often produces signs and symptoms within 5 to 30 minutes, but reactions sometimes may not develop for several hours.

PATHOPHYSIOLOGY

The chemical mediators that cause anaphylaxis are preformed and released from granules (histamine, tryptase, and others) or are generated from membrane lipids (prostaglandin D_2, leukotrienes, and platelet-activating factor) by the activated mast cell or basophil.

Tryptase is concentrated selectively in the secretory granules of all human mast cells. Its plasma levels during mast cell degranulation correlate with the clinical severity of anaphylaxis but need not be elevated in all forms of anaphylaxis (e.g., food-associated anaphylaxis).

Histamine exerts its pathophysiologic effects via both H_1 and H_2 receptors. Erythema (flushing), hypotension, and headache are mediated by both H_1 and H_2 receptors, whereas tachycardia, pruritus, bronchospasm, and rhinorrhea are associated with H_1 receptors alone.

Increased vascular permeability during anaphylaxis can produce a shift of 35% of intravascular fluid to the extravascular space within 10 minutes. This shift of effective blood volume causes compensatory catecholamine release, activates the renin-angiotensin-aldosterone system, and stimulates production of endothelin-1.

Mast cells accumulate at sites of coronary plaque erosion and rupture and they may contribute to coronary artery thrombosis. Because antibodies attached to mast cells can trigger mast cell degranulation, some investigators suggest that anaphylaxis may promote plaque rupture.

AGENTS THAT CAUSE ANAPHYLAXIS

Cause and effect often is confirmed historically in subjects who experience recurrent, objective findings of anaphylaxis upon inadvertent reexposure to the offending agent. Diagnostic testing, where appropriate, may confirm the presence of specific IgE and/or the degranulation of mast cells and basophils.

CURRENT DIAGNOSIS

- Cutaneous: urticaria, angioedema, diffuse erythema, generalized pruritus
- Respiratory: tachypnea, bronchospasm, laryngeal or tongue edema, dysphonia
- Cardiovascular: tachycardia, bradycardia, hypotension, angina, cardiac arrhythmias
- Gastrointestinal: nausea, emesis, diarrhea, abdominal cramps, dysphagia
- Other: rhinitis, conjunctivitis, uterine cramps, headache, dizziness, syncope, blurred vision, seizure

TABLE 1 Representative Agents That Cause Anaphylaxis

IgE dependent:
- Foods (such as peanuts, tree nuts, and crustaceans)
- Medications (such as antibiotics)
- Venoms (fire ants, yellow jackets, others)
- Allergen extracts
- Latex
- Exercise (where food or medication dependent)
- Hormones

IgE independent:
- Nonspecific degranulation of mast cells and basophils
  - Opioids
  - Muscle relaxants
  - Idiopathic
  - Physical factors
    - Exercise
    - Cold, heat
- Disturbance of arachidonic acid metabolism
  - Aspirin and other nonsteroidal anti-inflammatory drugs (NSAIDs)
- Immune aggregates
  - Intravenous immunoglobulin
- Cytotoxic
  - Transfusion reactions to cellular elements (IgM, IgG)
- Multimediator complement activation/activation of contact system
  - Radiocontrast media
  - Angiotensin-converting enzyme (ACE) inhibitor administered during renal dialysis with selected dialysis membranes
  - Protamine (possibly)

Modified and abridged from Kemp SF, Lockey RF: Anaphylaxis: A review of causes and mechanisms. J Allergy Clin Immunol 2002;110:341–348.

Virtually any agent capable of activating mast cells or basophils may potentially precipitate anaphylactic or anaphylactoid reactions. Table 1 lists common causes of anaphylaxis classified by pathophysiologic mechanism. Idiopathic anaphylaxis, anaphylaxis with no identifiable cause, has accounted for approximately a third of cases in most retrospective studies of anaphylaxis. However, of 601 patients evaluated more than two decades in a university-affiliated practice (the largest retrospective series), 59% of subjects were deemed to have idiopathic anaphylaxis.

Idiopathic anaphylaxis remains a diagnosis of exclusion, however. Serial histories and diagnostic tests for foods, spices, and vegetable gums occasionally identify a specific culprit in subjects previously presumed to have idiopathic anaphylaxis. The most common identifiable causes of anaphylaxis are foods, medications, insect stings, and immunotherapy injections. Anaphylaxis to peanuts and/or tree nuts causes the greatest concern because of its life-threatening severity, especially in subjects with asthma, and the tendency for subjects to develop lifelong allergic responsiveness to these foods.

RECURRENT ANAPHYLAXIS

Depending on the report, recurrent (biphasic) anaphylaxis occurs in 1% to 20% of subjects who experience anaphylaxis. Signs and symptoms experienced during the recurrent phase of anaphylaxis may be equivalent to or worse than those observed in the initial reaction and may occur 1 to 72 hours (most within 8 hours) after apparent remission. Thus, it may be necessary to monitor subjects up to 24 hours after apparent recovery from the initial phase. Observation periods after apparent recovery from the initial phase should be individualized and based on such factors as comorbid conditions and distance from the patient's home to the closest emergency facility, particularly because there are no reliable predictors of biphasic anaphylaxis.

DIFFERENTIAL DIAGNOSIS

Several systemic disorders share clinical features with anaphylaxis. The vasodepressor (vasovagal) reaction probably is the condition most commonly confused with anaphylactic reactions. In vasodepressor reactions, however, urticaria is absent, dyspnea is generally absent, the blood pressure is usually normal or elevated, and the skin is typically cool and pale. Tachycardia is the rule in anaphylaxis. Bradycardia may be underrecognized in anaphylaxis, however. Brown and others conducted sting challenges in 19 subjects known to be allergic to jack jumper ants (*Myrmecia*). All eight subjects who became hypotensive developed bradycardia after an initial tachycardia.

Systemic mastocytosis, a disease characterized by mast cell proliferation in multiple organs, usually features urticaria pigmentosa (brownish macules that transform into wheals upon stroking them) and recurrent episodes of pruritus, flushing, tachycardia, abdominal pain, diarrhea, syncope, or headache. Other diagnostic considerations include myocardial dysfunction, pulmonary embolism, foreign body aspiration, acute poisoning, seizure disorder, and psychogenic manifestations (no objective findings observed or documented).

MANAGEMENT OF ANAPHYLAXIS

Table 2 outlines a sequential approach to management. Assessment and maintenance of airway, breathing, circulation, and mentation are necessary before proceeding to other management steps. Subjects are monitored continuously to facilitate prompt detection of any treatment complications. The recumbent position is strongly recommended. In a retrospective review of prehospital anaphylactic fatalities in the United Kingdom, the postural history was known for 10 individuals. Four of the 10 were associated with assumption of an upright or sitting posture and postmortem findings consistent with "empty heart" and pulseless electrical activity.

Epinephrine is the treatment of choice for acute anaphylaxis. Aqueous epinephrine 1:1000 dilution, 0.2 to 0.5 mL (0.01 mg/kg in children; maximum dose, 0.3 mg) administered intramuscularly every 5 minutes, as necessary, should be used to control symptoms and sustain or increase blood pressure. Comparisons of intramuscular injections to subcutaneous injections during acute anaphylaxis are not available. However, absorption is more rapid and plasma levels are higher in asymptomatic individuals who receive epinephrine intramuscularly in the anterolateral thigh.

All subsequent therapeutic interventions depend on the initial response to epinephrine and the severity of the reaction. Development of toxicity or inadequate response to epinephrine injections indicates that additional therapeutic modalities are necessary.

The α-adrenergic effect of epinephrine reverses peripheral vasodilation, which alleviates hypotension and also reduces angioedema and urticaria. It may also minimize further absorption of antigen from a sting or injection. The β-adrenergic properties of epinephrine increase myocardial output and contractility, cause bronchodilation, and suppress further mediator release from mast cells and basophils.

Fatalities during witnessed anaphylaxis usually result from delayed administration of epinephrine and from severe respiratory and/or cardiovascular complications. *There is no absolute contraindication to epinephrine administration in anaphylaxis.*

Oxygen should be administered to subjects with anaphylaxis who require multiple doses of epinephrine, receive inhaled β_2 agonists, have protracted anaphylaxis, or have preexisting hypoxemia or myocardial dysfunction.

Antihistamines (H_1 and H_2 antagonists) support the treatment of anaphylaxis. However, these agents act much slower than epinephrine and should never be administered alone as treatment for anaphylaxis. Antihistamines thus should be considered as *second-line* treatment.

Systemic corticosteroids have no role in the acute management of anaphylaxis because even intravenous administration of these agents may have no effect for 4 to 6 hours after administration. Although corticosteroids traditionally are used in the management of anaphylaxis, their effect has never been evaluated in placebo-controlled trials. Corticosteroids administered during anaphylaxis might provide additional benefit for patients with asthma or other conditions recently treated with corticosteroids.

TABLE 2 Management of Anaphylaxis

Immediate intervention:
- Assessment of airway, breathing, circulation, and adequacy of mentation.
- Administer aqueous epinephrine 1:1000 dilution, 0.2–0.5 mL (0.01 mg/kg in children; maximum dose, 0.3 mg) *intramuscularly* q5 min, as necessary, to control symptoms and blood pressure.

Possibly appropriate, subsequent measures depending on response to epinephrine:
- Place subject in recumbent position and elevate lower extremities.
- Establish and maintain airway.
- Administer oxygen.
- Establish venous access.
- Use normal saline IV for fluid replacement.

Specific measures to consider after epinephrine injections, where appropriate:
- An epinephrine infusion might be prepared. Continuous hemodynamic monitoring is essential (see reference for specific details).
- Diphenhydramine (Benadryl). Note: In the management of anaphylaxis, a combination of diphenhydramine and ranitidine (Zantac)[1] is superior to diphenhydramine alone.
- For bronchospasm resistant to epinephrine, use nebulized albuterol (Proventil).
- For refractory hypotension, consider dopamine (Intropin), 400 mg in 500 mL D$_5$W, administered IV at 2–20 µg/kg/min titrated to maintain adequate blood pressure. Continuous hemodynamic monitoring is essential.
- Where use of β-blockers complicates therapy, consider glucagon,[1] 1–5 mg (20–30 µg/kg; maximum: 1 mg in children), administered IV over 5 min followed by an infusion 5–15 µg/min. Aspiration precautions should be observed.
- For patients with a history of asthma and for those who experience severe or prolonged anaphylaxis, consider methylprednisolone (Solu-Medrol) (1.0–2.0 mg/kg/d).
- Consider transportation to the emergency department or an intensive care facility.

Interventions for cardiopulmonary arrest occurring during anaphylaxis:
- High-dose epinephrine and prolonged resuscitation efforts are encouraged, if necessary, because efforts are more likely to be successful in anaphylaxis where the subject (often young) has a healthy cardiovascular system (see reference for specific details).

Observation and subsequent outpatient follow-up:
- Observation periods after apparent resolution must be individualized and based on such factors as the clinical scenario, comorbid conditions, and distance from the patient's home to the closest emergency department. After recovery from the acute episode, patients should receive epinephrine syringes (EpiPen or TwinJect) and be instructed in proper technique. Everyone postanaphylaxis requires a careful diagnostic evaluation in consultation with an allergist-immunologist.

Modified from Lieberman P, Kemp SF, Oppenheimer J, et al (chief eds). Joint Task Force on Practice Parameters. The diagnosis and management of anaphylaxis: An updated practice parameter. J Allergy Clin Immunol 2005;115:S483–S523.
[1]Not FDA approved for this indication.
Abbreviation: IV = intravenous.

Numerous cases of unusually severe or refractory anaphylaxis are reported in subjects receiving β-blocking agents. Greater severity of anaphylaxis observed in usual doses of epinephrine administered during anaphylaxis to subjects taking β-blockers may not produce the desired clinical response. In such situations, both isotonic volume expansion and glucagon[1] administration are recommended. Glucagon may potentially reverse refractory hypotension and bronchospasm because it bypasses the β-adrenergic receptor and directly activates adenyl cyclase.

[1]Not FDA approved for this indication.

Persistent hypotension despite epinephrine injections should first be treated with intravenous crystalloid solutions. Saline is generally preferred. One to 2 L of normal saline might need to be administered to adults at a rate of 5 to 10 mL/kg in the first 5 minutes. Children should receive up to 30 mL/kg in the first hour. Large volumes (e.g., 7 L) are often required.

Vasopressors should be administered if epinephrine injections and volume expansion fail to alleviate hypotension. Dopamine (Intropin) frequently increases blood pressure while maintaining or enhancing renal and splanchnic perfusion. These agents would not be expected to work as well in patients already maximally vasoconstricted by their internal compensatory response to anaphylaxis.

PREVENTION OF ANAPHYLAXIS

Table 3 outlines the basic principles for the prevention of future anaphylactic episodes in high-risk individuals. An allergist-immunologist can provide comprehensive professional advice on these matters.

All subjects at high risk for recurrent anaphylaxis should carry epinephrine syringes and know how to administer them. An EpiPen (Dey Laboratories) is a spring-loaded, pressure-activated syringe with a single 0.3 mg dose (1:1000 dilution) of epinephrine. It is easy to use and injects through clothing. An EpiPen Jr, which delivers 0.15 mg (1:2000 dilution) epinephrine, is appropriate for children weighing less than 30 kg. The TwinJect (Sciele Pharma) is a pre-filled, pen-sized, epinephrine auto-injector with two doses of either 0.3 or 0.15 mg.

Serum Sickness

Serum sickness is a clinical syndrome of fever, malaise, and urticarial and/or morbilliform cutaneous eruption that is often preceded by generalized erythema and pruritus. Arthralgias or arthritis (mainly

TABLE 3 Preventive Measures for Subjects with Anaphylaxis

General measures:
- Obtain thorough history to diagnose life-threatening food or drug allergy.
- Identify cause of anaphylaxis and those individuals at risk for future attacks.
- Provide instruction on proper reading of food and medication labels, where appropriate.
- Patient should avoid exposure to antigens and cross-reactive substances.
- Manage asthma and coronary artery disease optimally.
- Employ a waiting period of 30 minutes after injections
- Consider office waiting period of 2 hours for oral medication patient has not taken previously.

Specific measures for high-risk subjects:
- Individuals at high risk for anaphylaxis should carry self-injectable syringes of epinephrine (EpiPen or TwinJect) at all times and receive instruction in proper use with placebo trainer.
- Individuals should wear a Medic Alert bracelet or chain.
- Other agents for β-adrenergic antagonists, angiotensin-converting enzyme (ACE) inhibitors, tricyclic antidepressants, and monoamine oxidase inhibitors should be substituted whenever possible.
- Agents suspected of causing anaphylaxis should be administered slowly, supervised, and orally if possible.
- Where appropriate, use specific preventive strategies, including pharmacologic prophylaxis, short-term challenge and desensitization and long-term desensitization.

Modified from Kemp SF: Office approach to anaphylaxis: sooner better than later. Am J Med 2007;120:664–668.

TABLE 4 Representative Agents That Cause Serum Sickness

Medications: β-lactam antibiotics, sulfonamides, ciprofloxacin (Cipro), metronidazole (Flagyl), rifampin (Rifadin), allopurinol (Zyloprim), carbamazepine (Tegretol), phenytoin (Dilantin), fluoxetine (Prozac), bupropion (Wellbutrin), methimazole (Tapazole), propylthiouracil, thiazide diuretics, captopril (Capoten), propranolol (Inderal), verapamil (Calan), streptokinase (Streptase), others.

Heterologous (animal-derived) antisera:
- Horse: snake and spider venom, tetanus, botulism, diphtheria
- Horse or rabbit: anti-lymphocyte globulin
- Mouse: monoclonal antibodies (muromonab-CD3 [Orthoclone OKT3], rituximab [Rituxan], infliximab [Remicade])

Homologous (human-derived) antisera: cytomegalovirus, hepatitis B, rabies, tetanus, perinatal $RH_0(D)$

large joints), neuropathy, lymphadenopathy, nephritis, abdominal pain (emesis or melena are possible), or vasculitis (cutaneous or systemic) may occur in some cases. Cutaneous vasculitis, also known as hypersensitivity vasculitis, is often manifested by palpable purpura, which most commonly are found on the lower extremities of ambulatory individuals or on the sacral or gluteal region of patients with restricted mobility. These purpura reflect vascular leakage from inflamed postcapillary venules. Systemic vasculitis may occur in association with autoimmune diseases, infection, or malignancy.

Many agents may produce serum sickness or serum sickness–like reactions (Table 4). *Serum sickness* classically refers to the immune complex syndrome caused by immunization with heterologous serum proteins (often equine or murine). The most frequent cause is immune complex-mediated drug hypersensitivity. A serum sickness–like drug reaction generally develops 6 to 21 days after the culprit medication is started, but it can occur within 12 to 48 hours in previously sensitized individuals.

PATHOGENESIS AND LABORATORY ABNORMALITIES

Healthy individuals regularly generate low levels of circulating immune complexes, which are either excreted by the kidneys or extracted in the liver and spleen by monocytes and macrophages. It is hypothesized that serum sickness results when a drug (hapten) binds to plasma protein and antibodies are generated in response to the drug-protein complex. Complement activation occurs when large quantities of soluble antigen-antibody (immune) complexes fix to vascular endothelial receptors. Complement fragments attract and activate neutrophils, which release proteases that induce tissue injury. The urticaria in serum sickness probably results from immune complex necrotizing vasculitis and complement activation that induces mast cell degranulation. IgE-dependent mechanisms likely are also contributory in some individuals. Laboratory abnormalities include elevated erythrocyte sedimentation rate, leukopenia (acute phase), occasional plasmacytosis, and decreased total hemolytic complement (CH50), C3, and C4. Slight albuminuria, hyaline casts, and microscopic hematuria may also occur.

TREATMENT

Stoppage of the culprit agent, when identified, is recommended. Serum sickness is usually self-limited and rarely life threatening when the offending drug or protein is stopped or removed. Symptoms generally improve over 2 to 4 weeks as patients clear their immune complexes. Evidence-based treatment recommendations for serum sickness are very limited. Long-acting, less-sedating H_1 antihistamines such as cetirizine (Zyrtec), desloratadine (Clarinex), fexofenadine (Allegra), or loratadine (Claritin) generally control urticaria. Systemic corticosteroids (e.g., prednisone, 0.5 to 1.0 mg/kg/day)

may help severe symptoms. Fever and arthralgias typically resolve within 48 to 72 hours of treatment, and the formation of new cutaneous eruptions usually ceases within the same time frame. Antihistamine therapy is continued for 1 week after apparent resolution of symptoms and then slowly discontinued. Skin testing with heterologous antisera is performed routinely to avoid anaphylaxis to future administration of heterologous serum.

REFERENCES

American Heart Association in collaboration with International Liaison Committee on Resuscitation. 2005 American Heart Association guidelines for cardiopulmonary resuscitation and emergency cardiovascular care. Anaphylaxis. Circulation 2005;112(Suppl. 4):143–5.

Brown SGA, Blackman KE, Stenlake V, Heddle RJ. Insect sting anaphylaxis: Prospective evaluation of treatment with intravenous adrenaline and volume resuscitation. Emerg Med J 2004;21:149–54.

Kemp SF, Lockey RF, Simons FE. World Allergy Organization Ad Hoc Committee on Epinephrine in Anaphylaxis. Epinephrine: The Drug of Choice for Anaphylaxis. A statement of the World Allergy Organization. Allergy 2008;63:1061–70.

Kemp SF, Palmer GW. Anaphylaxis. emedicine from WebMD. Updated April 29, 2009. Available at http://emedicine.medscape.com/article/135065-overview.

Lieberman P. Biphasic anaphylactic reactions. Ann Allergy Asthma Immunol 2005;95:217–26.

Lieberman P, Kemp SF, Oppenheimer J, et al., chief editors. Joint Task Force on Practice Parameters. The diagnosis and management of anaphylaxis: An updated practice parameter. J Allergy Clin Immunol 2005;115:S483–523.

Project Team of the Resuscitation Council (UK). Emergency medical treatment of anaphylactic reactions. J Accid Emerg Med 1999;16:243–7.

Pumphrey RSH. Fatal posture in anaphylactic shock. J Allergy Clin Immunol 2003;112:451–2.

Pumphrey RSH. Fatal anaphylaxis in the UK, 1992–2001. Novartis Found Symp 2004;257:116–28.

Sampson HA, Muñoz-Furlong A, Campbell RL, et al. Second symposium on the definition and management of anaphylaxis: Summary report—second National Institute of Allergy and Infectious Disease/Food Allergy and Anaphylaxis Network symposium. J Allergy Clin Immunol 2006;117:391–7.

Simons FER, Gu X, Simons KJ. Epinephrine absorption in adults: Intramuscular versus subcutaneous injection. J Allergy Clin Immunol 2001;108:871–3.

Simons FER, Roberts JR, Gu X, Simons KJ. Epinephrine absorption in children with a history of anaphylaxis. J Allergy Clin Immunol 1998;101:33–7.

Wener M. Serum sickness and serum sickness-like reactions. In: Rose BD, editor. UpToDate. www.uptodateonline.com, Version 17.1 (current through January 2009). Wellesley, Ma.

Asthma in Adolescents and Adults

Method of
Michael Schatz, MD, MS

Asthma is an extremely common chronic medical condition that causes substantial morbidity among its sufferers. In addition to discomfort, asthma can cause sleep disruption, missed school and work, limitations of recreational activities, and acute episodes requiring emergency hospital care. Although the past 30 years have seen the introduction of increasingly effective and convenient medications, recent surveys continue to suggest that asthma remains suboptimally controlled in the majority of patients. The purpose of this article is to describe an approach to assessment and therapy that leads to optimal asthma control. It is based on the recently released National Asthma Education and Prevention Program (NAEPP) Expert Panel Report 3: Guidelines for the Management of Asthma (http://www.nhlbi.nih.gov/guidelines/asthma/asthgdln.pdf).

Diagnosis

The first step in evaluating a patient with asthma is to confirm the diagnosis. This is particularly important in patients with atypical symptoms or a poor response to asthma therapy. Asthma is confirmed by the demonstration of reversible airways obstruction, which most commonly is an increase in forced expiratory volume in 1 second (FEV_1) by 12% or more and at least 200 cc after an inhaled bronchodilator. For some patients, 2 to 4 weeks of chronic inhaled asthma therapy or 2 weeks of oral corticosteroid therapy is necessary to demonstrate reversibility. The latter is particularly important in adults with a history of smoking in whom chronic obstructive pulmonary disease (COPD) is a diagnostic consideration. In patients with normal pulmonary function, asthma can also be confirmed by means of methacholine (Provocholine) or exercise challenge.

Particularly important masqueraders of asthma include vocal cord dysfunction, panic attacks, hyperventilation, and cough due to postnasal drip, reflux, or angiotensin-converting enzyme (ACE) inhibitor therapy. All of these can also coexist with asthma, so their presence does not exclude asthma. Even when these conditions coexist with asthma, their diagnosis and appropriate therapy usually reduce the patient's respiratory symptoms.

Assessment

Assessment of asthmatic patients involves assessment of past severity, identification of aggravating factors, and definition of current status regarding treatment and clinical severity or control.

PAST SEVERITY

Asthma can be a mild, infrequent illness or a daily severe one. Certain severity markers identify patients who are more likely to experience severe exacerbations or to have symptoms that are more difficult to control and who thus require more careful surveillance. These include histories of asthma hospitalization, especially requiring intensive care or intubation, past requirement for oral corticosteroids, and exacerbation by aspirin or other NSAIDs. In patients with prior severe exacerbations, the rapidity of the onset of the exacerbation should be ascertained.

AGGRAVATING FACTORS

Factors that appear to trigger asthma symptoms should be assessed because they may be targets for avoidance therapy. Certain aspects of the patient's *environment* that can contribute to asthma triggering should be specifically ascertained, including occupational exposures, age of the home, pets, carpeting, visible mold, passive smoke, and cockroach exposure. Patients with persistent asthma should have in vitro or skin tests to identify *allergic sensitization* to pollens, house dust mites, mold spores, animal dander, and cockroaches that can contribute to the maintenance of asthma inflammation or can trigger episodes. The presence of *comorbidities* that can aggravate asthma, including cigarette smoking, obesity, rhinitis, sinusitis, reflux, and COPD, should be identified and treated. Finally, *psychosocial factors* to assess include a history or symptoms of anxiety or depression, attitudes toward asthma and asthma therapy, adherence to therapy, and social support. These may be targets for therapy or may be necessary to understand in order to create an effective therapeutic plan and therapeutic alliance.

CURRENT STATUS

Assessment of the current therapy the patient is actually taking is necessary for understanding the asthma's severity and to appropriately initiate or change therapy. It is particularly important to determine if the patient is taking long-term control medications, such as inhaled corticosteroids, long-acting β-agonists, leukotriene modifiers, cromolyn (Intal), nedocromil (Tilade), or theophylline (Theo-Dur). If the patient is not taking controllers, *severity* should be assessed,

CURRENT DIAGNOSIS

- Confirm the diagnosis by demonstrating an increase in FEV_1 by 12% or more after asthma therapy.
- Assess past severity by a history of exacerbations requiring hospitalization, intubation, or oral corticosteroids.
- Identify environmental exposures, allergic sensitization, and comorbidities that may be aggravating asthma.
- Assess current *severity* in patients not taking long-term control medications and assess *control* in patients who are taking long-term control medications based on symptom frequency, nocturnal awakenings, rescue therapy use, activity limitation, spirometry, and recent exacerbation history.

Abbreviation: FEV_1 = forced expiratory volume in 1 second.

---

as described in Table 1, based on symptom frequency, nocturnal awakenings, rescue therapy use, activity limitation, spirometry, and exacerbation history. If the patient is already taking controllers, *control* should be assessed (Table 2). Normal FEV_1/FVC (forced vital capacity) by age is shown in Table 3.

Long-Term Management

The goals of long-term management are to achieve and maintain well-controlled asthma. Both nonpharmacologic and pharmacologic therapy must be considered.

NONPHARMACOLOGIC THERAPY

The first tenet of nonpharmacologic therapy in the long-term management of asthma is *education*. Patients need to understand the inflammatory pathophysiology of asthma and the relationships among airway inflammation, bronchospasm, and symptoms. Patients should be informed that the cause of asthma is unknown and there is no cure but that triggers can be identified and asthma can be controlled. They should receive education regarding self-assessment, either based on symptoms or peak flow monitoring, and regarding the recognition of early signs of an impending exacerbation.

The next step is to discuss and agree on the *goals of therapy*. The NAEPP has defined the following goals:

- Prevent chronic and troublesome daytime and nighttime symptoms.
- Maintain optimal pulmonary function for that patient.
- Maintain normal activity, including work, school, leisure activity, and exercise.
- Prevent recurrent exacerbations, especially those requiring urgent medical visits.
- Provide pharmacotherapy with minimal or no adverse effects.
- Achieve patient and family satisfaction with asthma care.

The physician should let the patient know that these are the expectations of optimal management and confirm that those are the patient's goals as well.

A very important component of nonpharmacologic therapy is reduction of relevant *environmental triggers*. Information should be given regarding environmental control of pollen, mite, mold, animal dander, and cockroach antigens (Box 1) that appear to be relevant based on the history and results of skin or in vitro specific IgE tests. Inhalant allergen *immunotherapy* should be considered for patients who have persistent asthma when there is clear evidence of a relationship between symptoms and exposure to an allergen to which the patient is sensitive.

TABLE 1 Classifying Asthma Severity and Initiating Treatment in Patients 12 Years and Older Not Currently Taking Long-Term Control Medications

| | | Classification of Severity* | | |
| | | | Persistent | | |
Components of Severity	Intermittent	Mild	Moderate	Severe
Impairment				
Symptoms	≤2 d/wk	>2 d/wk but not daily	Daily	Throughout the d
Nighttime awakenings	≤2 ×/mo	3–4 ×/mo	>1 ×/wk but not nightly	Often 7 ×/wk
Short-acting β₂-agonist use for symptom control (not prevention of EIB)	≤2 d/wk	>2 d/wk but not daily, and not more than 1 time on any d	Daily	Several times per d
Interference with normal activity	None	Minor limitation	Some limitation	Extremely limited
Lung function†	Normal FEV₁ between exacerbations FEV₁ > 80% predicted FEV₁/FVC normal	FEV₁ >80% predicted FEV₁/FVC normal	FEV₁ >60% but <80% predicted FEV₁/FVC reduced 5%	FEV₁ <60% predicted FEV₁/FVC reduced >5%
Risk				
Exacerbations requiring oral systemic corticosteroids	0–1/y‡	≥2/y‡		

← Consider severity and interval since last exacerbation. →
Frequency and severity may fluctuate over time for patients in any severity category.

Relative annual risk of exacerbation may be related to FEV₁.

Recommended Step for Initiating Treatment§				
Initiation	Step 1	Step 2	Step 3¶	Step 4 or 5¶
Follow-up	In 2–6 wk, evaluate level of asthma control and adjust therapy accordingly.			

Data from the National Asthma Education and Prevention Program (NAEPP) Expert Panel Report 3: Guidelines for the Management of Asthma.

*Level of severity is determined by assessment of both impairment and risk. Assess impairment domain by patient's/caregiver's recall of previous 2–4 weeks and spirometry. Assign severity to the most severe category in which any feature occurs.

†See Table 3 for normal FEV₁/FVC.

‡At present, there are inadequate data to correspond frequencies of exacerbations with different levels of asthma severity. In general, more frequent and intense exacerbations (e.g., requiring urgent, unscheduled care, hospitalization, or ICU admission) indicate greater underlying disease severity. For treatment purposes, patients who had ≥2 exacerbations requiring oral systemic corticosteroids in the past year may be considered the same as patients who have persistent asthma, even in the absence of impairment levels consistent with persistent asthma.

§See Table 6 for treatment steps. The stepwise approach is meant to assist, not replace, the clinical decision making required to meet individual patient needs.

¶And consider short course of oral systemic corticosteroids.

Abbreviations: EIB = exercise-induced bronchospasm; FEV₁ = forced expiratory volume in one second; FVC = forced vital capacity; ICU = intensive care unit.

Finally, *psychosocial* issues should be considered and addressed. For many patients, the education and therapeutic alliance described earlier adequately addresses psychosocial concerns. For other patients, poor past adherence requires identifying the barriers to adherence and finding solutions together. Resources for patients with poor social support should be identified. Clinically significant anxiety or depression that can make asthma harder to control should be treated.

PHARMACOLOGIC STEP THERAPY

The main principle of asthma pharmacologic step therapy is to add therapy in steps until control is achieved (step up) and decrease therapy in reverse steps (step down) to established the lowest effective dose necessary to maintain control.

There are two types of asthma medications: quick-relief medications (Table 4) and long-term control medications (Table 5). Systemic corticosteroids can be used either short-term to treat an exacerbation (see Table 4) or as long-term maintenance therapy for patients with severe disease (see Table 5). The generally recommended steps of pharmacologic therapy are shown in Table 6. Definitions of low, medium, and high dose inhaled corticosteroids for each of the available preparations are given in Table 7. At each therapeutic step level, the NAEPP Expert Panel has indicated *preferred* medications, which generally identify medications with the best balance of efficacy and

safety in clinical trials for patients at that level of severity. However, these recommendations are based on population data and must be tailored to individual patient needs, circumstances, and responsiveness to therapy.

All patients with asthma should have an action plan that describes their pharmacologic self-management. Aspects of pharmacologic self-management include the maintenance medication schedule, rescue therapy doses for increased symptoms, when and how to increase control medication therapy, when and how to use prednisone, how to recognize a severe exacerbation, and when and how to seek urgent or emergency care. Control medications should be increased with an upper respiratory infection or with symptoms requiring more than two doses of rescue therapy in 12 hours. Although doubling the dose of inhaled corticosteroids does not appear to generally be sufficient to provide clinical benefit under these circumstances, higher-fold increases may be effective (e.g., three- or fourfold increases). The increased dose of control medications should be maintained at least until increased symptoms resolve. Prednisone is usually needed for patients with incomplete or temporary responses to adequate doses of β-agonists (4 puffs with a spacer, waiting at least 1 minute between puffs), substantial interference with sleep every night, requirement for 12 or more puffs of β-agonist in a 24-hour period, or a peak flow less than 60% predicted. Home treatment of exacerbations is further discussed later.

TABLE 2 Assessing Asthma Control and Adjusting Therapy in Patients 12 Years and Older

Components of Control	Classification of Control*		
	Well Controlled	Not Well Controlled	Very Poorly Controlled
Impairment			
Symptoms	≤2 d/wk	>2 d/wk	Throughout the d
Nighttime awakenings	≤2 ×/mo	1–3 ×/wk	≥4 ×/wk
Short-acting β₂-agonist use for symptom control (not prevention of EIB)	≤2 d/wk	>2 d/wk	Several times per d
Interference with normal activity	None	Some limitation	Extremely limited
FEV₁ or peak flow	>80% predicted or personal best	60%–80% predicted or personal best	<60% predicted or personal best
Validated Questionnaires[b]			
ACQ	≤0.75[†]	≥1.5	N/A
ACT	≥20	16–19	≤15
ATAQ	0	1–2	3–4
Risk			
Exacerbations requiring oral systemic corticosteroids	0–1/y	≥2/y[a] ⟶	
Progressive loss of lung function	Evaluation requires long-term follow-up care		
Treatment-related adverse effects	Medication side effects can vary in intensity from none to very troublesome and worrisome. The level of intensity does not correlate to specific levels of control, but it should be considered in the overall assessment of risk.		
Recommended action for treatment[‡]	Maintain current step Regular follow-up at every 1–6 mo to maintain control Consider step down if well controlled for ≥3 mo	Step up 1 step and reevaluate in 2–6 wk For side effects, consider alternative treatment options	Consider short course of systemic oral corticosteroids Step up 1–2 steps and reevaluate in 2 wk For side effects, consider alternative treatment options

Data from the National Asthma Education and Prevention Program (NAEPP) Expert Panel Report 3: Guidelines for the Management of Asthma.

[a]At present, there are inadequate data to correspond frequencies of exacerbations with different levels of asthma control. In general, more frequent and intense exacerbations (e.g., requiring urgent, unscheduled care, hospitalization, or ICU admission) indicate poorer disease control. For treatment purposes, patients who had ≥2 exacerbations requiring oral systemic corticosteroids in the past year may be considered the same as patients who have not-well-controlled asthma, even in the absence of impairment levels consistent with not-well-controlled asthma.

[b]Validated questionnaires for the impairment domain (the questionnaires do not assess the risk domain). Minimal important difference. 0.5 for the ACQ, 1.0 for the ATAQ, not determined for the ACT.

*The level of control is based on the most severe impairment or risk category. Assess impairment domain by patient's recall of previous 2–4 weeks and by spirometry or peak flow measures. Symptom assessment for longer periods should reflect a global assessment, such as inquiring whether the patient's asthma is better or worse since the last visit.

[†]ACQ values of 0.76–1.4 are indeterminate regarding well-controlled asthma.

[‡]See Table 6 for treatment steps. The stepwise approach is meant to assist, not replace, the clinical decision making required to meet individual patient needs. Before a step up in therapy, review adherence, inhale technique environmental control, and comorbid conditions. If an alternative treatment option was used in a step, discontinue it and use the preferred treatment for that step.

Abbreviations: ACQ = Asthma Control Questionnaire; ACT = Asthma Control Test; ATAQ = Asthma Therapy Assessment Questionnaire; EIB = exercise-induced bronchospasm; FEV₁ = forced expiratory volume in one second; N/A = not applicable.

For patients not on long-term control medications, assess *severity* and select the level of treatment that corresponds to the patient's level of severity (see Table 1). Persistent asthma is most effectively controlled with daily long-term control medications, specifically anti-inflammatory therapy. For patients receiving long-term control medications, identify their current *step of therapy*, based on what they are actually taking (see Table 6), and their level of *control* (see Table 2). In general, step up one step for patients whose asthma is not well controlled. For patients with very poorly controlled asthma, consider increasing by two steps, a course of oral corticosteroids, or both. Before increasing pharmacologic therapy, consider adverse environmental exposures, poor adherence, or comorbidities as targets for intervention. For patients with troublesome or debilitating side effects from asthma therapy, explore a change in therapy.

TABLE 3 Normal FEV₁/FVC by Age*

Age Range (y)	Normal FEV₁/FVC (%)
8–19	85
20–39	80
40–59	75
60–80	70

Data from the National Asthma Education and Prevention Program (NAEPP) Expert Panel Report 3: Guidelines for the Management of Asthma.
*Doses listed apply to all preparations.
Abbreviations: FEV₁ = forced expiratory volume in one second; FVC = forced vital capacity.

Follow-up

Patients whose asthma is not controlled should be seen every 2 to 6 weeks (depending on their initial level of severity or control) until control is achieved. Once control is achieved, follow-up contact at 1- to 6-month intervals is recommended. These checkups should ensure continued control, identify other changes in the patient's status, and update the patient's action plan.

When well-controlled asthma has been maintained for at least 3 months, a step down in therapy can be considered to determine the minimal amount of medication required to maintain control or reduce the risk of side effects. Reduction in therapy should be gradual

BOX 1   Measures to Control Environmental Factors That Can Make Asthma Worse

ALLERGENS

Reduce or eliminate exposure to the allergen(s) the patient is sensitive to:

Animal Dander

- Remove animal from house or, at a minimum, keep animal out of the patient's bedroom and keep the bedroom door closed.

House-dust Mites

- Recommended
  - Encase mattress in a special dust-proof cover
  - Encase pillow in a special dust-proof cover or wash it weekly in hot water.
  - Wash sheets and blankets on the patient's bed in hot water weekly. Water must be hotter than 130°F to kill the mites. Cooler water used with detergent and bleach can also be effective.
- Desirable
  - Reduce indoor humidity to 60% or less.
  - Remove carpets from the bedroom.
  - Avoid sleeping or lying on cloth-covered cushions or furniture.
  - Remove carpets that are laid on concrete.

Cockroaches

- Keep all food out of the bedroom.
- Keep food and garbage in closed containers.
- Use poison baits, powders, gels or paste (e.g., boric acid). Traps can also be used.
- If a spray is used to kill cockroaches, stay out of the room until the odor goes away.

Pollens (from Trees, Grass, or Weeds) and Outdoor Molds

- Try to keep windows closed
- If possible, stay indoors, with windows closed, during periods of peak pollen exposure, which are usually during the midday and afternoon.

Indoor Mold

- Fix all leaks and eliminate water sources associated with mold growth.
- Clean moldy surfaces.
- Dehumidify basements if possible.

TOBACCO SMOKE

- Advise patients and others in the home who smoke to stop smoking or to smoke outside the home.
- Discuss ways to reduce exposure to other sources of tobacco smoke, such as from daycare providers and the workplace.

INDOOR AND OUTDOOR POLLUTANTS AND IRRITANTS

- If possible, do not use a wood-burning stove, kerosene heater, fireplace, unvented gas stove, or heater
- Try to stay away from strong odors and sprays, such as perfume, talcum powder, hair spray, paints, new carpet, or particle board.

Data from the National Asthma Education and Prevention Program (NAEPP) Expert Panel Report 3: Guidelines for the Management of Asthma.

---

because asthma can deteriorate at a highly variable rate and intensity. Doses of inhaled corticosteroids may be reduced about 25% to 50% every 3 months to the lowest dose possible to maintain control. Most patients with persistent asthma relapse if inhaled corticosteroids are totally discontinued.

Patients should be encouraged to contact their asthma physician for signs of loss of asthma control, such as nocturnal symptoms, increasing β-agonist use, or activity limitation. The Expert Panel recommends consultation with an asthma specialist if the patient has difficulties achieving or maintaining control of asthma, immunotherapy or omalizumab (Xolair) is being considered, the patient requires step 4 care or higher, or the patient has had an exacerbation requiring hospitalization.

Treatment of Exacerbations

Asthma exacerbations are acute or subacute episodes of progressively worsening shortness of breath, cough, wheezing, or chest tightness associated with decreases in expiratory airflow.

HOME MANAGEMENT

Patients' action plans should direct their home therapy of asthma exacerbations according to the following recommendations.

Initial therapy should be with inhaled short-acting β-agonists (2–6 puffs by metered-dose inhaler [MDI] or nebulizer). This may be repeated in 20 minutes. With a good response (minimal or no symptoms and peak expiratory flow (PEF) $\geq$80% predicted or personal best), the patient may continue β-agonists every 3 to 4 hours for 24 to 48 hours. If repeated β-agonists are needed, a short course of oral corticosteroids should be considered.

With an incomplete response to initial therapy (persistent wheezing and dyspnea and PEF 50% to 79% predicted or personal best), oral corticosteroids should be added, β-agonists should be repeated, and the clinician should be contacted that day.

With a poor response (marked wheezing and dyspnea at rest, PEF <50% predicted or personal best), oral corticosteroids should be added, the β-agonist should be repeated immediately, and the patient should call the clinician and usually proceed to the emergency department. For signs of severe distress (e.g., difficulty talking in full sentences, diaphoresis, drowsiness, confusion, or cyanosis), 911 should be called. Patients with histories of rapid-onset severe exacerbations should have self-injectable epinephrine (Epipen)[1] at home to use at the onset of increased symptoms.

---

[1]Not FDA approved for this indication.

CURRENT THERAPY

- Nonpharmacologic therapy includes asthma education (especially regarding inhaler technique, self-monitoring, and self-management), reduction in environmental triggers, addressing any relevant psychosocial issues, and immunotherapy for select patients.
- Preferred step therapy for long-term asthma management is (in order): low-dose inhaled corticosteroids; medium-dose inhaled corticosteroids or low-dose inhaled corticosteroids plus long-acting β-agonists; medium-dose inhaled corticosteroids plus long-acting β-agonists; high-dose inhaled corticosteroids plus long-acting β-agonists; and oral prednisone.
- Asthma exacerbations should be treated with high-dose inhaled β-agonists and early use of systemic corticosteroids.

TABLE 4 Usual Dosages for Quick-Relief Medications for Patients 12 Years and Older

Medication	Dosage Form	Adult Dose	Comments
Inhaled Short-Acting β₂-Agonists (SABA)		*Applies to all four SABAS*	
Metered-Dose Inhaler			
Albuterol CFC	90 μg/puff, 200 puffs/canister	2 puffs 5 min before exercise	An increasing use or lack of expected effect indicates diminished control of asthma.
Albuterol HFA (Proventil, Ventolin)	90 μg/puff, 200 puffs/canister		Not recommended for long-term daily treatment. Regular use exceeding 2 d/wk for symptom control (not prevention of EIB) indicates the need for additional long-term control therapy.
Pirbuterol CFC (Maxair)	200 μg/puff, 400 puffs/canister	*or* 2 puffs q4–6h prn	Differences in potencies exist, but all products are essentially comparable on a per puff basis.
Levalbuterol HFA (Xopenox)	45 μg/puff, 200 puffs/canister		May double usual dose for mild exacerbations. For levalbuterol, should prime the inhaler by releasing 4 actuations prior to use. For HFA, periodically clean HFA activator, as drug may block/plug orifice. Nonselective agents (epinephrine [Primatene Mist], isoproterenol [Isopro Aerometer], metaproterenol [Alupent]) are not recommended due to their potential for excessive cardiac stimulation, especially in high doses.
Nebulizer Solutions			
Albuterol (Accuneb, Proventil)	0.63 mg/3 mL 1.25 mg/3 mL 2.5 mg/3 mL 5 mg/mL (0.5%)	1.25–5 mg in 3 mL saline q4–8h prn	May mix with budesonide (Pulmicort) inhalant suspension, cromolyn (Intal) or ipratropium (Atrovent) nebulizer solutions. May double the dose for severe exacerbations.
Levalbuterol (R-albuterol) (Xopenex)	0.31 mg/3 mL 0.63 mg/3 mL 1.25 mg/0.5 mL 1.25 mg/3 mL	0.63 mg–1.25 mg q8h prn	Compatible with budesonide (Pulmicort) inhalant suspension. The product is a sterile-filled, preservative-free, unit-dose vial.
Anticholinergics			
Metered-Dose Inhalers			
Ipratropium HFA (Atrovent)	17 μg/puff, 200 puffs/canister	2–3 puffs q6h	Multiple doses in the emergency department (not hospital) setting provide additive benefit to short-acting beta agonists. Treatment of choice for bronchospasm due to beta blocker. Dose not block EIB Reverses only cholinergically mediated bronchospasm; does not modify reaction to antigen. May be alternative for patients who do not tolerate short-acting beta-agonist. Evidence is lacking for anticholinergics producing added benefit to β₂ agonists in long-term control asthma therapy.
Ipratropium with albuterol (Combivent)	18 μg/puff of ipratropium bromide and 90 μg/puff of albuterol 200 puffs/canister	2–3 puffs q6h	
Nebulizer Solutions			
Ipratropium bromide	0.25 mg/mL (0.025%)	0.25 mg* q6h	
Ipratropium bromide with albuterol (DuoNeb)	0.5 mg/3 mL ipratropium bromide and 2.5 mg/3 mL albuterol	3 mL q4–6h	Contains EDTA to prevent discoloration of the solution. This additive does not induce bronchospasm.
Systemic Corticosteroids			
Methylprednisolone (Medrol)	2, 4, 6, 8, 16, 32 mg tab	Short course (burst): 40–60 mg/d as single or 2 divided doses for 3–10 d	Short courses (bursts) are effective for establishing control when initiating therapy or during a period of gradual deterioration. Action may be begin within an hour. The burst should be continued until symptoms resolve. This usually requires 3–10 d but can require longer. There is no evidence that tapering the dose following improvement prevents relapse in asthma exacerbations.
Prednisolone (Delta-Cortef, Prelone)	5 mg tabs; 5 mg/5 mL, 15 mg/5 mL		
Prednisone (Deltasone, Orasone)	1, 2.5, 5, 10, 20, 50 mg tabs; 5 mg/mL, 5 mg/5 mL		
Repository Injection			
Methylprednisolone acetate (Depo-Medrol)	40 mg/mL 80 mg/mL	240 mg[3†] IM once	May be used in place of a short burst of oral steroids in patients who are vomiting or if adherence is a problem.

Data from the National Asthma Education and Prevention Program (NAEPP) Expert Panel Report 3: Guidelines for the Management of Asthma.
[3]Exceeds dosage recommended by the manufacturer.
*0.5 mg per package insert.
[†]80–120 mg per package insert.
Abbreviations: CFC = chlorofluorocarbon; EIB = exercise-induced bronchospasm; HFA = hydrofluoroalkane; PEF = peak expiratory flow; tab = tablet.

TABLE 5 Usual Dosages for Long-Term Control Medications for Patients 12 Years and Older

Medication	Dosage Form*	Adult Dose	Comments
Systemic Corticosteroids			
Methylprednisolone (Medrol)	2, 4, 8, 16, 32 mg tab	7.5–60 mg qd in a single dose in AM or qod as needed for control	For long-term treatment of severe persistent asthma, administer single dose in AM either daily or on alternate d (alternate-day therapy may produce less adrenal suppression).
Prednisolone (Delta-Cortef, Prelone)	5 mg tab 5 mg/5 mL, 15 mg/5 mL	Short-course (burst) to achieve control, 40–60 mg/d as single or 2 divided doses for 3–10 d	Short courses (bursts) are effective for establishing control when initiating therapy or during a period of gradual deterioration. There is no evidence that tapering the dose following improvement in symptom control and pulmonary function prevents relapse.
Prednisone (Deltasone, Orasone)	1, 2.5, 5, 10, 20, 50 mg tab 5 mg/mL, 5 mg/5 mL		
Inhaled Long-Acting β2-Agonists			Should not be used for acute symptoms relief or exacerbations. Use only with ICS.
Salmeterol (Serevent)	DPI 50 μg/blister	1 blister q12h	Decreased duration of protection against EIB may occur with regular use.
Formoterol (Foradil)	DPI 12 μg/single-use capsule	1 cap q12h	Each cap is for single use only; additional doses should not be administered for at least 12 h. Caps should be used only with the Aerolizor inhaler and should not be taken orally.
Inhaled Combined Medications			
Fluticasone and salmeterol (Advair)	DPI 100 μg/50 μg, 250 μg/50 μg, or 500 μg/50 μg HFA 45 μg/21 μg 115 μg/21 μg 230 μg/21 μg	1 inhalation bid; dose depends on level of control	100/50 DPI or 45/21 HFA for patients not controlled on low-to-medium dose ICS. 250/50 DPI or 115/21 HFA for patients not controlled on medium-to-high dose ICS.
Budesonide and formoterol (Symbicort)	HFA MDI 80 μg/4.5 μg 160 μg/4.5 μg	2 inhalations bid; dose depends on level of control	80/4.5 for patients not controlled on low-to-medium dose ICS. 160/4.5 for patients not controlled on medium-to-high dose ICS.
Inhaled Cromolyn and Nedocromil			
Cromolyn (Intal)	MDI 0.8 mg/puff	2 puffs qid	One dose before exercise or allergen exposure provides effective prophylaxis for 1–2 h. Not as effective for EIB as SABA.
	Nebulizer	1 amp qid	4–6 wk trial of cromolyn or nedocronil may be needed to determine maximum benefit. Dose by MDI may be inadequate to affect hyperresponsiveness.
Nedocromil (Tilade)	20 mg/ampule MDI 1.75 mg/puff	2 puffs qid	Once control is achieved, the frequency of dosing may be reduced.
Leukotriene Modifiers			
Leukotriene Receptor Antagonists			
Montelukast (Singulair)	4 mg or 5 mg chewable tab 10 mg tab	10 mg qhs	Montelukast exhibits a flat dose-response curve. Doses >10 mg do not produce a greater response in adults.
Zafirlukast (Accolate)	10 or 20 mg tab	40 mg/d (20 mg tab bid)	For zafirlukast: Administration with meals decreases bioavailability; take at least 1 h before or 2 h after meals. Zafirlukast is a microsomal p450 enzyme inhibitor that can inhibit the metabolism of warfarin. Doses of this drug should be monitored accordingly. Monitor for signs and symptoms of hepatic dysfunction.
5-Lipoxygenase Inhibitor			
Zileuton (Zyflo)	600 mg tab	2400 mg daily (600 mg qid)	Monitor hepatic enzymes (ALT). Zileuton is a microsomal p450 enzyme inhibitor that can inhibit the metabolism of warfarin and theophylline. Doses of these drugs should be monitored accordingly.

Continued

TABLE 5 Usual Dosages for Long-Term Control Medications for Patients 12 Years and Older—Cont'd

Medication	Dosage Form*	Adult Dose	Comments
Methylxanthines			
Theophylline (Slophyllin, Theobid, TheoDur)	Liquids, sustained-release tab, cap	Starting dose 10 mg/kg/d up to 300 mg max Usual max 800 mg/d	Adjust dosage to achieve serum concentration of 5–15 µg/mL at steady-state ($\geq$48 h on same dosage). Due to wide interpatient variability in theophylline metabolic clearance, routine serum theophylline level monitoring is essential. Patient should be told to discontinue if they experience symptoms of toxicity. Various factors (diet, food, febrile illness, age, smoking, and other medications) can affect serum concentration.
Immunomodulators			
Omalizumab (Anti-IgE)	Subcutaneous (SQ) injection 150 mg/1.2 mL following reconstitution with 1.4 mL sterile water for injection	150–375 mg SQ every 2–4 wk, depending on body weight and pretreatment serum 1 gE level	Do not administer more than 150 mg per injection site. Monitor patient following injections; be prepared and equipped to indentify and treat anaphylaxis that may occur. Whether patients will develop significant antibody titers to the drug with long-term administration is unknown.

Data from the National Asthma Education and Prevention Program (NAEPP) Expert Panel Report 3: Guidelines for the Management of Asthma.
*See Table 7 for estimated comparative daily dosages for inhaled corticosteroids.
Abbreviations: ALT = alanine aminotransferase; amp = ampule; cap = capsule; DPI = dry powder inhaler; EIB = exercise-induced bronchospasm; HFA = hydrofluoroalkane; ICS = inhaled corticosteroid; LABA = long-acting β$_2$-agonist; max = maximum; MDI = metered-dose inhaler; SABA = short-acting β$_2$-agonist; tab = tablet.

TABLE 6 Stepwise Approach For Managing Asthma in Patients 12 Years and Older[a]

Step	Preferred Therapy	Alternative Therapy
1	Short-acting β-agonist prn	—
2	Low-dose ICS	Cromolyn (Intal), LTRA, nedocromil (Tilade), theophylline (Theo-Dur)
3	Low-dose ICS *plus* LABA *or* Medium-dose ICS	Low-dose ICS *plus* LTRA *or* theophylline *or* zileuton (Zyflo)
4	Medium-dose ICS *plus* LABA	Medium-dose ICS *plus* LTRA *or* theophylline *or* zileuton
5	High-dose ICS *plus* LABA Consider omalizumab (Xolair) for patients who have allergies	—
6	High-dose ICS *plus* LABA *plus* oral corticosteroid[b] Consider omalizumab for patients who have allergies	—

Data from the National Asthma Education and Prevention Program (NAEPP) Expert Panel Report 3: Guidelines for the Management of Asthma.
[a]The stepwise approach is meant to assist, not replace, the clinical decision making required to meet individual patient needs.
[b]In step 6, before oral corticosteroids are introduced, a trial of high-dose ICS + LABA + either LTRA, theophylline or zileuton may be considered, although this approach has not been studied in clinical trials.
Abbreviations: ICS = inhaled corticosteroid; LABA = long-acting β agonist; LTRA = leukotriene receptor antagonist.

TABLE 7 Estimated Comparative Daily Dosages for Inhaled Corticosteroids for Patients 12 Years and Older

Drug	Dosage Form	Daily Dose		
		Low (µg)	Medium (µg)	High (µg)
Beclomethasone HFA (QVAR)	40 or 80 µg/puff	80–240	>240–480	>480
Budesonide DPI (Pulmicort)	90, 180, or 200 µg/inhalation	180–600	>600–1200	>1200
Ciclesonide*	80 or 160 µg/actuation	80–240	>240–480	>480
Flunisolide (AeroBid)	250 µg/puff	500–1000	>1000–2000	>2000
Flunisolide HFA (AeroSpan)	80 µg/puff	320	>320–640	>640
Fluticasone-HFA (Flovent HFA, Flovent Diskus)	MDI: 44, 110, 220 µg/puff DPI: 50, 100, 250 µg/inhalation	88–264 100–300	>264–440 >300–500	>440 >500
Mometasone DPI (Asmanex)	200 µg/inhalation	200	400	>400
Triamcinolone acetonide (Azmacort)	75 µg/puff	300–750	>750–1500	>1500

Data from the National Asthma Education and Prevention Program (NAEPP) Expert Panel Report 3: Guidelines for the Management of Asthma.
*Available since release of Expert Panel Report 3. Doses estimated based on package insert information.
Abbreviations: DPI = dry powder inhaler; HFA = hydrofluoroalkane.

Asthma in Adolescents and Adults

777

EMERGENCY DEPARTMENT AND HOSPITAL MANAGEMENT

Assessment should rapidly determine the severity of the exacerbation based on intensity of symptoms, signs (heart rate, respiratory rate, use of accessory muscles, chest auscultation), peak flow (unless the patient is too dyspneic to perform), and pulse oximetry. Treatment should begin immediately following recognition of an exacerbation severe enough to cause dyspnea at rest, peak flow less than 70% predicted or personal best, or pulse oximetry oxygen saturation less than 95%. While treatment is being given, a brief focused history and physical examination pertinent to the exacerbation can be obtained.

In patients with *mild-moderate exacerbations* (PEF >40% predicted), initial therapy is oxygen to achieve oxygen saturation greater than 90% and inhaled short-acting β-agonist by nebulizer or MDI (4–8 puffs) with holding chamber, which may be repeated up to three times in the first hour. Oral corticosteroids (prednisone 40–80 mg) are recommended if there is no immediate response to therapy or if the patient had been recently treated with oral corticosteroids.

In patients with *severe exacerbations* (PEF <40% predicted), initial therapy is oxygen as above, inhaled high-dose short-acting β-agonist (e.g., albuterol 5 mg) and ipratropium (0.5 mg) by nebulizer every 20 minutes or continuously for 1 hour, and oral or intravenous corticosteroids (prednisone or methylprednisolone 80 mg).

Repeated assessments of symptoms, signs, PEF, and oxygen saturation determine the responsiveness of the exacerbation to therapy. Such assessments should be made in patients presenting with severe exacerbations after the initial bronchodilator treatment and in all patients after three doses of bronchodilator therapy (60–90 min after initial treatment). In patients who are improving, short-acting β-agonists may be repeated every hour until a good response is achieved (no distress, PEF >70%). When this response is sustained at least 60 minutes after the last treatment, the patient may usually be discharged on a course of oral corticosteroids (generally prednisone 40–60 mg for 5–10 days), initiation or continuation of medium-dose inhaled corticosteroids, and arrangement for outpatient follow-up.

In patients who are not improving with the above therapy, adjunctive therapy, such as with intravenous magnesium sulfate[1] (2 g) or heliox, may be considered. Intubation and mechanical ventilation may be required for patients with respiratory failure in spite of treatment.

Summary

Asthma is a very common problem with the potential to cause substantial interference with quality of life. Although there is no cure for asthma, asthma can be well controlled in the majority of patients with proper management and an effective patient-physician relationship. I hope that the method described herein for assessing and managing asthma will help physicians help their patients to achieve well-controlled asthma.

---

[1]Not FDA approved for this indication.

Asthma in Children

Method of
Gerald B. Kolski, MD, PhD

Asthma is the most common cause of significant childhood morbidity. This includes school absenteeism, hospitalizations, emergency department visits, and acute care visits. Its prevalence has been increasing throughout the 1990s and into this century. An estimated 5 million children younger than 15 years have asthma as identified by the National Health Interview Survey of 2003. According to this survey, the prevalence of asthma in the general population is somewhere between 6% and 10%. Prevalence in inner-city populations and especially in African Americans is closer to 14% to 15%. Pediatricians and family practitioners are often reluctant to make the diagnosis because of difficulty with giving prognostic information to parents. Wheezing during the first few years of life can often be associated with acute viral infections, especially respiratory syncytial virus (RSV) and rhinovirus (RV). Longitudinal studies suggest there are three patterns to wheezing in children. There are a group of children who wheeze during infancy associated with viral infections, a second group that wheeze during infancy and also as they get older, and a third group that only develops wheezing later after sensitization with allergens. Because of these groups it is oftentimes difficult to give prognostic information to parents until you have seen the pattern that a child will follow.

Despite tremendous improvement in medications and treatments for asthma, deaths from asthma continue to occur. Most recently, however, the mortality rates seem to have leveled off or decreased slightly.

One theory for the high prevalence of asthma is the "hygiene hypothesis." Studies done in homogeneous populations in Europe and Scandinavian countries have noted less asthma and allergies in rural populations versus those that live in urban environments. Attempts have been made to correlate this with endotoxin exposure during infancy and/or infections during this period of time that turn on immune responses that do not promote allergies. This concept favors an immune response, which postulates that certain infections and endotoxin exposure promote a T_H1 T cell response in which interferon gamma and interleukin(IL)-2 predominate, whereas a lack of these infections promotes a T_H2 response where there is an IL-4, IL-13, and IL-5 predominance with increased IgE production.

Pathophysiology

Over the last several decades the idea that reversible bronchoconstriction is the main element in asthma has changed. It has become apparent that in addition to bronchoconstriction there is considerable inflammation involving increased mucus production, inflammatory cell infiltrates, and airway thickening. With longitudinal studies it has become apparent that there may in fact be some fibrosis that leads to "airway remodeling." The increased inflammatory infiltrates lead to increasing airway reactivity characterized by hyperresponsiveness to various stimuli. The inflammatory cell infiltrates can include eosinophils, lymphocytes, basophils, neutrophils, and macrophages depending on the stimulus. Unchecked inflammation is believed to be the cause of the fibrosis. Clearly it is important to try and identify the triggers in an individual patient that are causing the inflammation as well as treating the inflammation.

Differential Diagnosis

Determining the cause of wheezing in infancy can often be difficult. During the first year of life if the wheezing is associated with a viral infection, a diagnosis of bronchiolitis is often made. A clinical response to bronchodilators might be helpful in assessing whether this is going to be a child with asthma. Recurrent wheezing in an atopic child with a strong family history of asthma would strongly suggest that the child has underlying asthma. An association with eczema and/or other allergic manifestations might also be suggestive of asthma. Because of the difficulty in doing pulmonary functions during the first few years of life, clinical assessment is the key. In addition to asthma, Table 1 lists the other diagnoses that have to be considered. Cystic fibrosis, gastroesophageal reflux disease, and foreign body aspiration probably are the most common diagnoses that have to be entertained. Recurrent infiltrates should make you worry about immune deficiencies including hypogammaglobulinemia and ciliary defects such as immotile cilia syndrome.

TABLE 1 Differential Diagnosis of Wheezing

Infants	Older Children
Laryngomalacia	Asthma
Tracheomalacia	Cystic fibrosis
Vascular rings	Gastroesophageal reflux disease
Subglottic stenosis	Foreign body aspiration
Airway congenital masses	Airway tumors
Gastroesophageal reflux	Viral infections (RSV, adenovirus)
Bronchiolitis	Tuberculosis
Pneumonia	

Abbreviation: RSV = respiratory syncytial virus.

BOX 1 Asthma Triggers

- Allergies: perennial or seasonal
- Viral infections
- Irritants, especially cigarette smoke and air pollution
- Exercise
- Weather changes
- Gastroesophageal reflux
- Medications including aspirin and nonsteroidal anti-inflammatory drugs (NSAIDs)
- Sinusitis

Diagnostic tests such as a sweat test, immunoglobulins, skin or radioallergosorbent assay test (RAST), barium swallow, bronchoscopy, or chest radiograph may be indicated.

In older children asthma may be diagnosed by doing pulmonary functions. Spirometry can often be done in the office and can be a reproducible way to measure the extent of airway disease in known asthmatics as well as diagnostic by looking at pre- and postbronchodilator responses. The forced expiratory volume at 1 second (FEV_1) is often thought to be a measure of large airway obstruction. The FEF_{25-75} or expiratory flow between the 25th and 75th percentile of the forced vital capacity (FVC) is often thought to be a measure of small airway disease. A 15% increase in FEV_1 pre- and postbronchodilator or 25% increase in FEF_{25-75} is thought to be diagnostic of asthma. Inhalation challenges with methacholine (Provocholine) or histamine are often used to measure airway reactivity in experimental studies. Bronchoconstriction with these inhalation challenges can determine the degree of airway hyperreactivity. Similar results can also be obtained with exercise challenges or cold air challenges. These tests are often used to diagnose asthma in children whose pulmonary functions at baseline are not significantly depressed. In children with asthma, peak expiratory flow rates (PEFRs) are often used to monitor the asthma as well as the management. This test is effort dependent.

Key Diagnostic Points Consistent with Asthma

- Recurrent wheezing responding to bronchodilators
- Coughing or wheezing shortly after exercise
- Pulmonary functions that show obstruction responding to bronchodilators
- Strong family history of asthma
- Associated allergic symptoms including seasonal rhinitis, eczema, or urticaria

History

Once a diagnosis of asthma is made, it is important to determine the trigger for this individual's asthma symptoms or exacerbations. The history is very important in determining treatment. Box 1 lists the most common causes for asthma exacerbations.

The most common perennial allergens are dust mites, cockroaches, mold, and pets. In the inner cities, cockroaches and dust mites are very common causes for allergic sensitization. They are extremely common and very difficult to control. Dust mites need moisture and thus are much more common in humid areas. With increased humidity, molds also can play a significant role. Children are often treated with humidifiers or vaporizers for upper respiratory infections, which may exacerbate dust mite and mold exposure. In drier climates, pets, especially indoor animals, are often exacerbating causes. Recent studies have indicated that more than two or three pets decreased the likelihood of sensitization, whereas an isolated pet is more likely to be associated with the development of allergy. This may have to do with endotoxin and the previously discussed hygiene hypothesis.

Children who only have difficulty with their asthma in the spring and fall may have sensitization to the pollens. This is very regional and often associated with being outdoors. Pollination and dissemination is most problematic with dry windy days. Keeping the windows closed at night as well as air conditioning may benefit individuals with seasonal allergies. These children may need medications at particular times of the year but not throughout the year. Airway reactivity often continues even 4 to 6 weeks after the allergen is no longer present.

Children who have trouble with viral infections may also have increased reactivity from perennial or seasonal exposures that exacerbate the asthma with infection. It is often helpful to reduce allergy exposure in these individuals so as to reduce their response to viral infections. Parents may be alerted to signs of upper respiratory infection so that they can increase asthma treatment at those times.

At all times cigarette smoke causes increased mucus production as well as decreases mucociliary clearance. Children with asthma thus are especially prone to having difficulty around cigarette smoke. During infancy, cigarette smoke exposure is associated with a two- to threefold increase in risk of asthma as well as upper respiratory infections, ear infections, and pneumonia. Smoking during pregnancy is also associated with a sustained decrease in infant pulmonary functions. Smoke is a form of indoor air pollution. Outdoor air pollution, especially small particles, ozone, nitrogen dioxide, and sulfur dioxide, all can be exacerbating factors in asthma.

Exercise is associated with asthma exacerbations because of the inhalation of cold dry air. Exercise is often associated with mouth breathing. The nose normally moisturizes, filters, and warms the air. Nasal congestion secondary to allergies, viral infections, or nasal obstruction can all lead to more difficulty with exercise as well as with breathing cold dry air at any time.

Weather changes are often a problem secondary to what is in the air or the changes in temperature of the air. Children who have trouble with weather changes are often responding to changes in pollen distribution or other allergens or irritants.

Children who have reflux as the exacerbating cause of their asthma often have difficulty at night when they lie down, shortly after meals, or when ingesting very acidic substances. Often there will be

 CURRENT DIAGNOSIS

- Always focus on the ABCs (airway, breathing, and circulation).
- Start prescription early and aggressively (titrate β-agonist to effect).
- Reevaluate frequently (try to avoid intubation at all cost).
- Lack of wheezing is not always a good thing.
- Plan ahead in case things go bad.
- Ensure adequate hydration.

considerable coughing and if the child is old enough to talk some significant heartburn. Reflux is often worse when the asthma is a problem because the lower esophageal sphincter tone decreases with hyperinflation at that time.

Children with sensitivity to aspirin or nonsteroidal anti-inflammatory drugs (NSAIDs) often have associated sinusitis, nasal polyps, and profuse rhinorrhea with aspirin exposure. It often goes undiagnosed until adulthood. Nasal polyps should always raise this possibility in addition to a diagnosis of cystic fibrosis.

Sinusitis can be associated with significant exacerbations of asthma. Often treating the sinusitis treats the asthma exacerbation. Purulent nasal discharge for 5 to 7 days associated with significant coughing and maxillary tenderness may be suggestive of underlying sinusitis. In children with allergic rhinitis, complications of sinusitis often occur.

In all children with asthma it is very important that you try and assess severity of disease. There should be questions asked about whether the patient has ever been intubated or had an intensive care unit admission. In addition questions about recent use of oral corticosteroids should be asked to determine the recent course of asthma. Children with underlying seizure disorders are also important to identify because they are at greater risk for mortality. Signs of mental illness or depression should also be noted because this predisposes children to significant morbidity and mortality.

Physical Examination

In examining a patient with asthma, the complete physical is extremely helpful. Children with skin findings of eczema or hives associated with an exacerbation of asthma may often lead to a search for an allergy exposure that is responsible for symptoms. Nasal examination may show boggy turbinates suggestive of allergy or erythematous turbinates suggestive of infection. Purulent discharge associated with sinus tenderness may suggest sinusitis. Nasal polyps should also be looked for to ascertain whether the patient may have underlying cystic fibrosis or aspirin-sensitive asthma. Enlarged tonsils and adenoids may predispose to mouth breathing and exacerbate underlying asthma. Examination of the chest may show whether there is a pectus suggesting chronic disease or whether there is hyperinflation with a barrel chest. Supraclavicular, intercostal, and subcostal muscular activity give information as to the work of breathing. The cardiac examination should focus on heart rate as well as any sign that might indicate this is cardiac wheezing instead of asthma. Abdominal examination is important to evaluate any signs of liver or spleen enlargement that might indicate evidence of pulmonary hypertension or cardiac disease. Examination of the extremities is important to look for clubbing and/or cyanosis. The neurologic exam is especially important acutely to ascertain whether the patient is having any change in mental status secondary to hypoxia.

Treatment

Treatment for asthma has changed considerably since the mid 1990s. The chronic management of asthma has focused on assuring that the patient functions as normally as possible with the following goals of asthma management:

- No nocturnal asthma
- Full exercise activity
- No emergency department visits or hospitalizations
- No lost time from school or work
- No or minimal side effects from medication

Asthma treatment has focused on the anti-inflammatory nature of the disease to eliminate long-term damage to the lungs. Asthma treatment has followed the National Heart, Lung, and Blood Institute (NHLBI) guidelines with assessment of asthma severity and management based on the classifications (Table 2). We developed a color-coded questionnaire that gives an indication of asthma control. The new guidelines for 2008 put out by NHLBI focus on asthma control and asthma control questionnaires.

Medications

Asthma medications are classified according to medications that are used for acute relief of symptoms called *relievers* and those that are used for chronic control of symptoms characterized as *controllers*. This classification was established to give patients a better understanding of the role of their individual medications. It is also a better way to educate patients as to why they have to continue to take medications even when they are not having symptoms. It is important to discuss these individual classifications and medications for both acute and chronic management.

RELIEVERS

Various bronchodilators are used for acute management of asthma. These bronchodilators are predominantly β-agonists such as albuterol (Proventil), pirbuterol (Maxair), levalbuterol (Xopenex), and terbutaline (Brethine) that are selective for β₂-receptors. Table 3 gives the generic as well as trade names for these medications. The short-acting β-agonists are used for acute relief in most circumstances. In children anticholinergics such as ipratropium bromide (Atrovent) are often used in the emergency department and hospital setting acutely but are rarely given chronically. Chronic use of β-agonists is avoided because of a decrease in effectiveness as well as an increase in airway reactivity with their chronic use. With chronic use there is also a decrease in both the number and affinity of β-receptors for these bronchodilators. The affinity as well as number of β-receptors is increased with the use of corticosteroids.

In the management of acute episodes of asthma, an algorithm is used (see Current Therapy box). β-agonists are given either by nebulizer or inhaler. In addition to albuterol, a selective stereoisomer levalbuterol (Xopenex) is also available but is more expensive. This isomer may cause fewer side effects and have a slightly longer duration of action. In the acute setting, treatments are often given every 20 minutes times three and then are continued every 2 to 3 hours for hospitalized patients. In critical situations, albuterol may also be given continuously. It is during the acute situation where ipratropium bromide is beneficial for the first 24 to 48 hours of treatment. It can be given by nebulizer every 4 to 6 hours.

Injectable epinephrine is still recommended especially in the acute attack if it is thought to be secondary to allergies or anaphylaxis. It also can be used in the acute situation to make sure that inhaled drugs can reach the lower airway.

Magnesium sulfate[1] is used intravenously in severe asthmatics for its bronchodilator properties to prevent intubation or respiratory failure. This is outlined again in the acute management algorithm (Current Therapy box).

Theophylline (Theolair) was often the mainstay of asthma management in the 1980s, but its toxicity and the difficulty in having to monitor levels has reduced its use. Nausea, vomiting, abdominal pain, and an increase in hyperactivity often lead to noncompliance. With the selective β-agonists their use has been minimal. They can be used for chronic management in patients to decrease corticosteroid need.

Oral or systemic corticosteroids are always indicated in acute management of episodes of asthma exacerbation. The usual recommended starting dose is 2 mg/kg and should be continued during the episode. Prolonged use of corticosteroids may require a taper, but a short course of 4 to 5 days does not usually require a taper. Any patient who was admitted for an acute exacerbation of asthma should go home on a controller with an action plan for future attacks.

---

[1]Not FDA approved for this indication.

CURRENT THERAPY

- **Severe:** ABCs, oxygen, monitors, POX, IV, isotonic fluids to maintain volume.

Start with (consider SC epinephrine if really tight):

- Albuterol, 0.5% inhalation solution, 0.5 mL (<20 kg), 0.75 mL (>20 kg) q20min × 3 (may give as mini-Nebs or start continuous at 2–3 mL/h). After initial stabilization patient will likely need q2h Nebs or continuous albuterol.
- Methylprednisolone (Solu-Medrol), 2 mg/kg IV (maximum, 125 mg) then start 1 mg/kg q6h (maximum, 80 mg/dose).
- Ipratropium bromide (Atrovent), 250 µg (<5 y), 500 µg (>5 y) × 2, then q4h.

If minimal improvement:

- Magnesium sulfate,[1] 45 mg/kg IV over 20 min (maximum, 2 g).

If still severe, consider terbutaline drip:

- Terbutaline (Brethine), 2–10 µg/kg loading dose, then start infusion at 0.1–0.4 µg/kg/min (maximum, 6 µg/kg/min). **Needs pediatric intensive care unit (PICU).**

At any time if minimal air entry, use:

- Epinephrine (1:1000), 0.01 mL/kg SC (maximum, 0.3 mL) or
- Terbutaline, 0.01 mg/kg SC (maximum, 0.25 mg)

Note: Adequate volume can be critical in maintaining circulatory volume (preload), so use volume freely. Also buffering with THAM for severe acidosis can be useful. These two strategies may help you avoid intubation.

If you really need to intubate (impending respiratory failure), use atropine, 0.02 mg/kg IV (minimum), 0.1 mg (maximum, 1 mg); ketamine (Ketalar), 1–2 mg/kg IV; or vecuronium (Norcuron), 0.1–0.2 mg/kg IV.

- **Moderate:** ABCs, POX, oxygen, monitors. ± IV

Start with

- Albuterol, 0.5 mL (<20 kg), 0.75 mL (>20 kg) q20 min × 3 (may start with mini Nebs or continuous). Then patient will likely need q2h Nebs or continuous albuterol (2 mL/h <10 kg, 3 mL/hr >10 kg)
- Ipratropium bromide, 250 µg (<5 y), 500 µg (>5 y) × 2, then q4h
- Prednisone, 2 mg/kg (maximum, 80 mg) if tolerating PO or
- Methylprednisolone, 2 mg/kg (maximum, 80 mg) (continue steroids for 5 d, 2 mg/kg/d)

If minimal improvement:

Consider magnesium sulfate as above.

- **Mild:** ABCs, POX

Start with

- Albuterol Nebs or MDI with spacer q2–4h
- Prednisolone, 2 mg/kg loading dose (maximum, 80 mg), then 2 mg/kg/d divided bid × 5 d

For mild to moderate exacerbation, discharge home may be considered if patient shows good improvement, is no longer dyspneic or hypoxic, tolerates Nebs q4h, and has good supervision at home.

CXR: Consider for a first-time wheezer; a condition other than asthma (i.e., FB); a febrile child with clinical signs of pneumonia; or no clinical improvement or worsening condition (pneumothorax, pneumomediastinum).

Continuous albuterol: To calculate the total amount of albuterol and normal saline, remember that the total amount of solution per hour must equal 30 mL.

Example: For a child >10 kg, the albuterol dose for continuous Nebs is 3 mL/h so you need to add 27 mL of NSS to run for 1 h (to set it up for 4 h, total mL = 120 with 12 mL albuterol + 108 mL NSS).

---

[1]Not FDA approved for this indication.

Abbreviations: ABCs = airway, breathing, and circulation; CXR = chest radiograph; FB = foreign body; IV = intravenous; Nebs = nebulization; NSS = normal saline solution; POX = pulse oximeter; SC = subcutaneous; THAM = tromethamine.

In the chronic management of asthma, albuterol is still the mainstay of acute attacks, pre-exercise, and for any reduction in peak flow or pulmonary functions. Albuterol (Proventil or Ventolin) is usually given by metered-dose inhaler and for most patients it is recommended that it be given with a spacer. Spacers increase the deposition in the lower airway and increase the effectiveness of inhaled drugs. In the chronic management of asthma, the NHLBI guidelines recommend that if albuterol is being used more than two or three times a week a step up in controller medications is suggested (Table 2).

CONTROLLERS

Inhaled corticosteroids are established as the mainstay of chronic management of asthma. Various preparations are available either by dry powder inhaler or metered-dose inhaler. Table 2 outlines the doses and route. Side effects of growth suppression and decreases in bone mineralization are dose related as well as preparation dependent. Individuals on any of the corticosteroids need to have their growth monitored and also to have instructions on mouth rinsing after inhalation to reduce fungal colonization in the oropharynx.

Leukotriene antagonists are available in oral preparations. These offer some advantage in pediatric patients in that they do not require good inhalation technique and can be given once a day. This may improve compliance and offer benefit in asthma as well as allergic rhinitis. They are not as effective as inhaled corticosteroids but offer some benefit in mild disease or as an adjunct to inhaled corticosteroids.

Cromolyn (Intal) and nedocromil (Tilade) are available as inhaled medications. Both of these drugs are mast cell stabilizers and appear to be most effective in allergic patients. These drugs should be taken three to four times a day, which makes their compliance more difficult. There are no significant side effects to these medications, however, and they are used in children because of their safety profile. They are used primarily in the mildest of patients and as pretreatment before allergy exposure.

Long-acting β-agonists are characterized as controllers, but these medications cannot be taken as anti-inflammatory agents. They have an increased risk of mortality when taken alone. For this reason only the preparations that are in combination with inhaled corticosteroids should be used in children. The drug preparations contain varying doses of inhaled corticosteroid with one standard dose of long-acting β-agonist.

TABLE 2 Stepwise Approach for Managing Asthma in Children

Classify Severity: Clinical Features Before Treatment or Adequate Control			Medications Required to Maintain Long-Term Control
	Symptoms/Day	*PEF or FEV₁*	
	Symptoms/Night	*PEF Variability*	*Daily Medications*
Step 4 Severe persistent	Continual Frequent	<60% >30%	**Preferred treatment:** • High-dose inhaled corticosteroids, *and* • Long-acting inhaled β_2-agonists (combination preferred) *and,* if needed, • Corticosteroid tablets or syrup long term (2 mg/kg/d, generally do not exceed 60 mg/d). (Make repeat attempts to reduce systemic corticosteroids and maintain control with high-dose inhaled corticosteroids.)

Step 3
Moderate persistent
	Daily
	>1 night/wk
		>60% – <80%
		>30%
			• **Preferred treatment:**
			  • Low- to medium-dose inhaled corticosteroids.
			• **Alternative treatment** (listed alphabetically):
			  • Increase inhaled corticosteroids within medium-dose range
			  or
			  • Low to medium–dose inhaled corticosteroids and either leukotriene modifier or theophylline.
			
			If needed (particularly in patients with recurring severe exacerbations):
			• **Preferred treatment:**
			  • Increased inhaled corticosteroids within medium-dose range and add long-acting inhaled β_2-agonists (combination inhaler preferred).
			• **Alternative treatment** (listed alphabetically);
			  • Increase inhaled corticosteroids within medium-dose range, and add either leukotriene modifier or theophylline.

Step 2
Mild persistent
	>2/wk but <1/d
	>2 nights/mo
		>80%
		20% – 30%
			• **Preferred treatment:**
			  • Low-dose inhaled corticosteroids.
			• **Alternative treatment** (listed alphabetically):
			  • Cromolyn (Intal).
			  • Leukotriene modifier.
			  • Nedocromil (Tilade) *or* sustained-release theophylline (Slo-bid Gyrocaps) to serum concentration of 5–15 µg/mL.

Step 1 Mild intermittent	<2d/wk <2 nights/mo	>80% <20%	• **No daily medication needed.** • Severe exacerbations may occur, separated by long periods of normal lung function and no symptoms. A course of systemic corticosteroids is recommended.

Note: Children <5 y cannot do adequate peak flows.

Quick relief
All patients

- Short-acting bronchodilator: 2–4 puffs short-acting inhaled β_2-agonists as needed for symptoms.
- Intensity of treatment depends on severity of exacerbation; up to 3 treatments at 20-min intervals or a single nebulizer treatment as needed. Course of systemic corticosteroids may be needed.
- Use of short-acting β_2-agonists >2 times/wk in intermittent asthma (daily, or increasing use in persistent asthma) may indicate the need to initiate (increase) long-term-control therapy.

↓ **Step down**
Review treatment q1–6 mo; a gradual stepwise reduction in treatment may be possible.

↑ **Step up**
If control is not maintained, consider step up.
First, review patient medication technique, adverse effects from medications.

Notes:
The stepwise approach is meant to assist, not replace, the clinical decision making required to meet individual patient needs.
Classify severity: Assign patient to most severe step in which any feature occurs (PEF is percentage of personal best; FEV₁ is percentage predicted).
Gain control as quickly as possible (consider a short course of systemic corticosteroids); then step down to the least medication necessary to maintain control.
Minimize use of short-acting inhaled β_2-agonists. Overreliance on short-acting inhaled β_2-agonists (e.g., use of approximately 1 canister/mo even if not using it every day) indicates inadequate control of asthma and the need to initiate or intensify long-term control therapy.
Provide education on self-management and controlling environmental factors that make asthma worse (e.g., allergens and irritants).
Refer to an asthma specialist if there are difficulties controlling asthma or if step 4 care is required. Referral may be considered if care at level step 3 is required.

Continued

TABLE 2 Stepwise Approach for Managing Asthma in Children—Cont'd

Usual Dosages for Long-Term-Control Medications

Medication	Dosage Form	Child Dose
Systemic Corticosteroids		
Methylprednisolone (Medrol)	2-, 4-, 8-, 16-, 32-mg tablets	0.25–2 mg/kg daily in single dose in AM or qod as needed for control
Prednisolone (Prelone) (Orapred)	5-mg tablets 5 mg/5 mL, 15 mg/5 mL	Short-course "burst": 1–2 mg/kg/d, maximum
Prednisone (Orasone)	1-, 2.5-, 5-, 10-, 20-, 50-mg tablets: 5 mg/5 mL, 5 mg/mL	60 mg/d for 3–10 d
Long-Acting β₂-agonists		
(Do not use for symptom relief or for exacerbations.)		
Salmeterol (Serevent)	DPI 50 µg/blister	1 blister q12h
Formoterol (Foradil)	DPI 12 µg/single-use capsule	1 capsule q12h
Combine Medication		
Fluticasone/ salmeterol (Advair)	DPI 100, 250, or 500 µg/50 µg	1 inhalation bid; dose depends on severity of asthma
Budesonide/ formoterol	80 or 160/4.5	
Mast Cell Stabilizer		
Cromolyn (Intal)	MDI 800 µg/puff Nebulizer 20 mg/ampule	1–2 puffs tid–qid 1 ampule tid–qid
Nedocromil (Tilade)	MDI 1.75 mg/puff	1–2 puffs bid–qid
Leukotriene Modifiers		
Montelukast (Singulair)	4- or 5-mg chewable tablet 10-mg tablet	4 mg qhs (2–5 y) 5 mg qhs (6–14 y) 10 mg qhs (>14 y)
Zafirlukast (Accolate)	10- or 20-mg tablet	20 mg daily (5–11 y) (10-mg tablet bid)
Methylxanthines		
(Serum monitoring is important.)		
Theophylline (Slo-Phyllin)	Liquids, sustained-release tablets and capsules	Starting dose 10 mg/kg/d; usual maximum: <1 y: 0.2 (age in wks) + 5 = mg/kg/d >1 y: 16 mg/kg/d

Estimated Comparative Daily Dosages for Inhaled Corticosteroids

Drug	Low Daily Dose	Medium Daily Dose	High Daily Dose
Beclomethasone HFA (QVAR) 40 or 80 µg/puff	80–160 µg	160–320 mcg	>320 µg
Budesonide DPI (Pulmicort) 200 µg/inhalation	200–400 µg	400–800 mcg	>800 µg
Budesonide inhalation suspension for nebulization (Pulmicort Respules)	0.5 mg	1.0 mg	2.0 mg
Flunisolide (AeroBid) 250 µg/puff	500–750 µg	1000–1250 µcg	1250 µg
Fluticasone (Flovent)	88–176 µg	176–440 µg	>440 µg
MDI: 44, 110, or 220 µg/puff	100–200 µg	200–400 µg	>400 µg
DPI: 50, 100, or 250 µg/inhalation			
Triamcinolone acetonide (Azmacort) 100 µg/puff	400–800 µg	800–1200 µg	>1200 µg
Mometasone fumarate (Asmanex) 220 mg	220 µg	440 µg	880 µg

Abbreviations: DPI = daily permissible intake; FEV₁ = forced expiratory volume at 1 second; MDI = metered-dose inhaler; PEF = peak expiratory flow (rate).

Oral corticosteroids have been used for asthma since they were developed. They were used for patients with severe or chronic asthma before inhaled steroids were available. Because oral corticosteroids have significant side effects they should be used with caution. Prolonged use of systemic steroids leads to adrenal suppression, osteoporosis, and growth suppression. With prolonged use the dose should be reduced gradually. Inhaled corticosteroid effects can be similar to the systemic corticosteroids, especially if they are used at doses higher than recommended.

OMALIZUMAB

Omalizumab (Xolair) is a monoclonal antibody that is humanized and was developed against IgE. It is expensive and requires monthly injections. It is most effective when allergies are the main trigger for

asthma. It is also used in patients with severe anaphylaxis.[1] It is indicated for children with moderate to severe persistent asthma that is exacerbated by significant documented allergies. Because it is nonspecific it does not reduce specific allergies and cannot be used in patients who have no significant atopy.

IMMUNOSUPPRESSIVE AGENTS

Various experimental studies in patients with chronic steroid-dependent asthma have used immunosuppressive agents such as methotrexate[1] (Trexall), IV gammaglobulin[1] (Gamimune N), and anti-inflammatory

---

[1]Not FDA approved for this indication.

TABLE 3 Medications for the Acute Relief of Symptoms

Generic β-agonist	Brand Name*
Albuterol	Ventolin, Ventolin HFA, Proventil HFA, Proventil
Pirbuterol	Maxair, Maxair Autohaler
Terbutaline	Brethaire, Brethine, Bricanyl
Metaproterenol	Alupent
Levalbuterol	Xopenex

Albuterol is also available in an inhaler in combination with ipratropium bromide (Combivent).

*Many of these drugs are available in liquid, tablet, inhalation aerosol, as well as metered-dose inhalers.

monoclonal antibodies against cytokines. None of these produced dramatic results, and none is available or can be recommended at this time.

IMMUNOTHERAPY

Specific injections of extracts of allergens to which the patient is allergic is effective for allergic rhinitis that is secondary to certain allergens. Therapy with allergy extracts is effective for pollens, and by reducing allergic rhinitis symptoms it can affect nasal breathing and therefore benefit asthma. Because of the risk of reactions to immunotherapy it should be used cautiously when the patient is having significant asthma symptoms at the time of injection. Studies in Europe suggest that in the future sublingual immunotherapy may be effective. Well-documented studies in this country have not been done and it is not approved as an FDA procedure.

Education and Environmental Control

Education of the individual asthmatic is important. Action plans in which treatment of acute episodes is outlined is recommended. Parents and patients should be taught about the patient's triggers as well as steps they should take to increase or decrease their medications depending on symptoms. Environmental precautions such as dust mite avoidance, focusing on reducing humidity, and limiting tobacco smoke exposure have had some success. Pet avoidance has not worked unless the pet is totally eliminated.

The NHBLI Guidelines as put forth in NAEPP Expert Panel 3 has been updated. It focuses on asthma control and uses asthma control questionaries.[1] In addition, it recommends that asthmatics on being discharged from the hospital or after being seen by their primary care physician be sent home with an action plan. In addition to assessing severity of asthma and outlining an action plan, a risk assessment is suggested with an emphasis on removing triggers, controlling the environment, and assessing comorbidities. The characteristic of the new guidelines focuses on the severity at the initial assessment, but in subsequent evaluations focuses on assessing control. The recommendation is to step up treatment if there is inadequate control and step down on treatment if it can be achieved with continued excellent control. Periodic assessment and monitoring are recommended, especially using spirometry, when possible.

REFERENCES

Castro-Rodriguez JA, Holberg CJ, Wright AL, Martinez FD. A clinical index to define risk of asthma in young children with recurrent wheezing. Am J Respir Crit Care Med 2000;162:1403–6.

National Institutes of Health/National Heart, Lung, and Blood Institute. NAEPP expert panel report 2: Guidelines for the diagnosis and management of asthma. Publication no. 97–4051. Bethesda, Md: The Institutes; 1997.

National Institutes of Health/National Heart, Lung, and Blood Institute. NAEPP expert panel report 3: Guidelines for the diagnosis and management of asthma. Publication no. 08–4051Bethesda, Md: The Institutes; 2007.

O'Connor GT. Allergen avoidance in asthma: What do we do now? J Allergy Clin Immunol 2005;116:26–30.

Romagnani S. Immunologic influences on allergy and the TH1/TH2 balance. J Allergy Clin Immunol 2004;113:395–400.

Spahn JD, Szefler SJ. Childhood asthma: New insights into management. J Allergy Clin Immunol 2002;109:3–13.

---

[1]Not FDA approved for this indication.

Allergic Rhinitis Caused by Inhalant Factors

Method of
David M. Quillen, MD

Rhinitis is characterized by one or more of the following nasal symptoms: congestion, anterior and posterior rhinorrhea, sneezing, and nasal itching. Rhinitis has significant morbidity and is not a trivial disease. Rhinitis has several causes (Box 1). The most common form is allergic rhinitis (AR), which is rhinitis caused primarily by inhaled allergens. The three main AR subgroups are *seasonal* (i.e., hay fever), *perennial* (i.e., chronic allergic rhinitis), and *occupational*. Among the atopic diseases of AR, asthma, and dermatologic reactions, AR is the most common. Depending on the source of information, AR affects between 10% and 30% of all adults and as many as 40% of children (40 million Americans). Most patients who present with rhinitis symptoms have AR, but several other causes should be considered as part of the evaluation (see Box 1).

Pathophysiology and Morbidity

AR involves inflammation of the upper respiratory tract mucosa (i.e., nasal mucosa, eustachian tubes, and sinuses) and eyes. In severe cases, patients can also have systemic symptoms. Complex interactions among inhaled allergens and irritants, immunoglobulin E (IgE), and inflammatory mediators are the cause of the inflammation. Genetics play a role in the tendency for an individual to develop atopic disease such as AR and asthma. AR usually develops in childhood and is slightly more common in boys than girls. By adulthood, the incidence is equal between men and women. Susceptible individuals produce specific IgEs in response to inhaled proteins. The IgEs cause the mast cells to release a variety of mediators, such as histamine, tryptase, chymase, kinins, leukotrienes, prostaglandins, and heparin. The inflammatory mediators cause immediate vasodilatation, nasal congestion, sneezing, and itching. The mediators also cause recruitment of other inflammatory cells (i.e., macrophages, eosinophils, neutrophils, and lymphocytes), which lead to a delayed response that can last for hours or days and occasionally include systemic symptoms (e.g., malaise, fatigue).

AR is not a life-threatening disease, but the effects on an individual's quality of life are high. Societal costs from AR are also high and have been estimated at more than $5 billion per year in lost productivity, time away from work, and other expenses. AR predisposes affected individuals to otitis media and sinusitis. Those with AR frequently have associated atopic conditions (e.g., asthma, atopic dermatitis, nasal polyps), and there is some evidence that poorly controlled AR can worsen asthma.

BOX 1 Differential Diagnosis of Rhinitis Symptoms

Allergic rhinitis
  Seasonal
  Perennial
  Episodic
  Occupational (may be nonallergic)
Nonallergic rhinitis
  Infectious
    Acute (usually viral)
    Chronic (rhinosinusitis)
  Nonallergic rhinitis with eosinophilia syndrome (NARES)
  Perennial nonallergic rhinitis (vasomotor rhinitis)
  Other types
    Ciliary dyskinesia syndrome
    Atrophic rhinitis
    Hormone induced
      Hypothyroidism
      Pregnancy
      Oral contraceptives
      Menstrual cycle
    Exercise induced
    Drug induced
      Rhinitis medicamentosa
      Oral contraceptives
      Antihypertension medications
      Aspirin
      Nonsteroidal antiinflammatory drugs
    Reflux induced
      Gustatory rhinitis
      Chemical or irritant
      Postural reflexes
      Nasal cycle
      Emotional cause
    Occupational (may be allergic)
Conditions that may mimic symptoms of rhinitis
  Structural or mechanical causes
    Deviated septum
    Hypertrophic turbinates
    Enlarged adenoids
    Foreign bodies
    Choanal atresia
  Inflammatory or immunologic
    Wegener's granulomatosis
    Midline granuloma
    Sarcoidosis
    Systemic lupus erythematosus
    Sjögren's syndrome
    Nasal polyposis
  Cerebrospinal fluid rhinorrhea

Modified from Dykewicz MS, Fineman S, Skoner DP, et al: Diagnosis and management of rhinitis: Complete guidelines of the Joint Task Force on Practice Parameters in Allergy, Asthma and Immunology. American Academy of Allergy, Asthma, and Immunology. Ann Allergy Asthma Immunol 1998;81(Pt 2):478–518.

Diagnosis

DIFFERENTIAL DIAGNOSIS

Differentiating AR from the other forms of rhinitis is important. Nonallergic rhinitis (NAR) is a common cause of rhinitis and can be difficult to differentiate from AR. The ratio of AR to NAR is approximately 3:1. However, preliminary data suggest that up to two thirds of patients with AR may have mixed rhinitis, a combination of AR and NAR. Understanding that many patients have some component of NAR explains why many have mixed symptoms.

In many cases, a thorough history suggests the diagnosis. Infectious causes of rhinitis (i.e., viral upper respiratory infections, influenza, or sinusitis) usually produce more acute symptoms with limited durations, unlike the more chronic nature of AR and NAR. Vasomotor rhinitis and NAR usually do not have historical triggers or seasonal patterns. Endocrine and hormonal conditions such as hypothyroidism and pregnancy can cause chronic congestion, as can a variety of medications. Systemic disease such as Wegener's granulomatosis, Sjögren's syndrome, and nasal polyposis can also cause similar symptoms. Unilateral symptoms suggest an obstruction, and, particularly in children, a foreign body must be excluded.

PATIENT EVALUATION

A comprehensive history usually suggests the correct diagnosis. Occasionally, the diagnosis may be elusive because of the many different causes of rhinitis (Fig. 1). Areas to focus on include symptoms (i.e., duration, exposures, magnitude of reaction, patterns, and chronicity), triggers, seasonal variation, environmental influences, history of allergies, medical history, and family history. Eighty percent of patients with AR first develop symptoms before the age of 20 years. Eliciting a positive family history is helpful, because allergic symptoms and asthma tend to run in families. The success of past and current treatments can help to identify the cause and help to direct future treatment.

A focused physical examination should follow the history. Patients with chronic allergic symptoms may have dark circles under the eyes (i.e., allergic shiners) or be obvious mouth breathers. Conjunctivitis and an acute viral upper respiratory infection may be components of AR. A careful examination of the nose is important to identify structural abnormalities, obvious polyps, mucosal swelling, and discharge. Examining the pharynx for enlarged tonsils and postnasal drip can help support viral causes or chronic drainage from chronic rhinitis. Lymphadenopathy with associated symptoms can help support the diagnosis of viral or bacterial rhinitis, and findings of other atopic diseases (e.g., wheezing from asthma, eczema) support an allergic cause.

In most cases, the history and physical examination provide enough information to make the diagnosis or at least initiate a treatment program with periodic follow-up. Specific testing should be used when the diagnosis is in question or attempts are being made to tailor therapy. The two most common tests are percutaneous skin testing and allergen-specific IgE antibody testing (i.e., radioallergosorbent test [RAST]). Intradermal skin testing is less common.

CURRENT DIAGNOSIS

- Appropriate history
  - Perennial or seasonal symptoms
  - Identified triggers
  - History of asthma or eczema
  - Supported by family history of atopy
  - Previous response to treatment
- Nonallergic causes
  - Hormones
  - Medications
  - Systemic disease
  - Obstruction
  - Nonallergic rhinitis
- Physical examination
  - Rhinorrhea
  - Nasal congestion
  - Allergic facial changes
- Diagnostic testing
  - Percutaneous test (prick test)
  - Radioallergosorbent test (RAST)
  - Allergen-specific IgE antibody testing

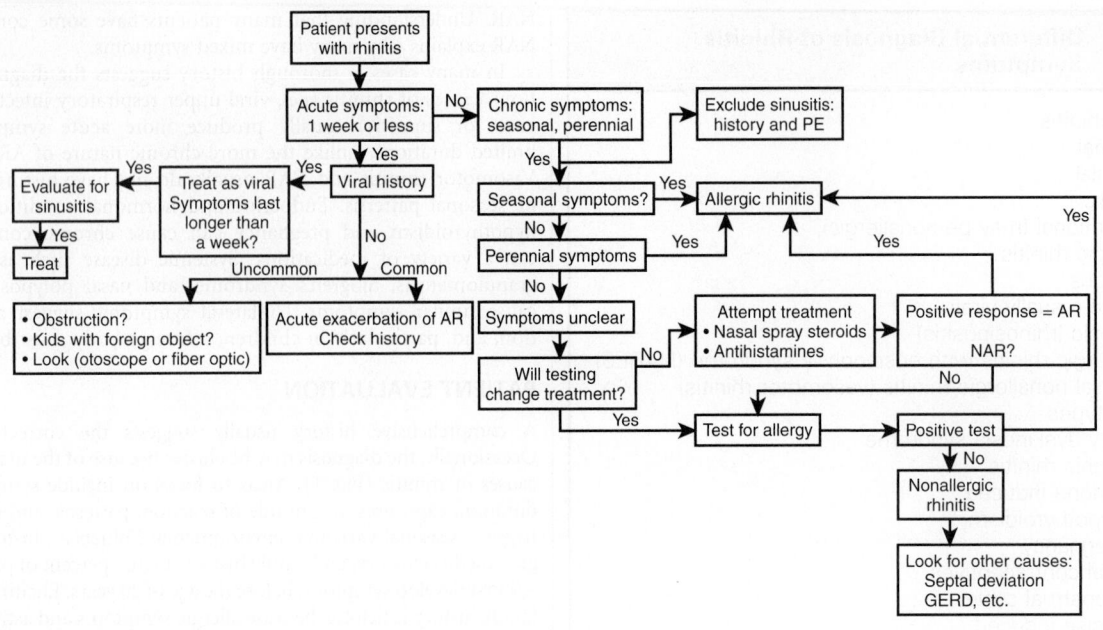

FIGURE. 1. Rhinitis algorithm. *Abbreviations:* AR = allergic rhinitis; GERD = gastroesophageal reflux; NAR = nonallergic rhinitis; PE = physical examination.

Percutaneous skin testing (i.e., prick test) is specific and cost effective, but it is not always available and may require referral. RAST testing, a blood test, usually is available and is useful for common allergens, such as pet dander, dust mites, grass pollen, and common molds, but is not very specific for food, venom, or drug allergies. Intradermal skin testing is an alternative option and historically considered to be more sensitive but with a lower specificity. Controversy remains about which test is superior, but there does appear to be increased safety concerns with intradermal testing. If available, we recommend percutaneous testing and RAST testing to local allergens.

Treatment

Treatment for allergic rhinitis is relatively straightforward (Box 2). General principles include using the minimum medication for relief, combination treatment (i.e., nasal spray steroids and antihistamines work better together than either alone), and continuously reevaluating

---

BOX 2 Treatment Strategy for Allergic Rhinitis

- Confirm the diagnosis with a history and physical examination; if in doubt, consider allergy testing.
- Reduce exposure to allergens.
- Start an oral antihistamine; use a second-generation drug before a first-generation drug if possible or use nasal spray steroid for a 2-week trial.
- Select a second agent, an antihistamine or nasal spray steroid, if relief has been inadequate.
- If results are not satisfactory, consider testing (if not already done).
- Consider a leukotriene receptor antagonist.
- Treat ocular symptoms with a nonsteroidal antiinflammatory drug, antihistamine, or mast cell stabilizer (use one at a time).
- Other options include use of a nasal spray antihistamine, a nasal spray mast cell stabilizer, or a nasal spray anticholinergic.
- If relief is inadequate, consider testing to confirm sensitivity to specific allergens and institution of immunotherapy.

---

when treatment is not working. Testing is not required initially if the history and physical examination findings are consistent. However, if standard treatment is not working, testing is important to eliminate the many other diagnoses that cause rhinitis symptoms.

Pharmacotherapy, environmental modification, and immunotherapy are the primary treatment modalities. Pharmacotherapy is usually tried first, and oral antihistamines are the most commonly selected agent. Oral antihistamines have been around for more than 50 years and are used in numerous over-the-counter (OTC) cold and allergy preparations. Overall efficacy of the oral antihistamines is good, but they are not as effective as nasal spray steroids.

The older first-generation antihistamines (H_1-blockers) are effective against the symptoms of rhinorrhea, itching, and sneezing. There are many OTC first-generation antihistamines available in generic form. The antihistamines are not very effective against congestion, which is why many OTC preparations are combined with an oral decongestant (pseudoephedrine or phenylephrine). Common side effects of antihistamines include sedation and anticholinergic effects, and they require dosing several times per day.

Second-generation H_1-blockers include loratadine (Claritin, Alavert), fexofenadine (Allegra), and cetirizine (Zyrtec). All are available as generic preparations, and loratadine and cetirizine are available OTC. All three have less anticholinergic and sedative side effects than first-generation antihistamines. All can be taken once daily. Cetirizine is the active metabolite of the first-generation H_1-blocker hydroxyzine (Atarax). Of the three second-generation H_1-blockers, cetirizine has more potential for sedation.

Topical treatments include nasal spray antihistamines, nasal spray mast cell stabilizers, ophthalmic antihistamines, ophthalmic nonsteroidal antiinflammatory drugs (NSAIDs), nasal spray anticholinergics, and nasal spray steroids. Azelastine (Astelin) is an H_1-antagonist, and it can be used in a nasal spray twice daily for nasal symptoms and in an ophthalmic solution (Optivar) for allergic conjunctivitis. Patient acceptance is limited because of the bitter taste associated with the nasal spray. Many types of ophthalmic drops can be used for ocular symptoms associated with AR or for allergic conjunctivitis alone. Olopatadine (Patanol) is an H_1-antagonist that is approved for allergic conjunctivitis. Ketorolac (Acular 0.5%) is an NSAID and available in an ophthalmic solution for allergic conjunctivitis, although only the 0.5% drop is approved for this indication.

Cromolyn is a specific mast cell stabilizer that inhibits degranulation. For AR, cromolyn is available in a nasal spray (Nasalcrom) and in an ophthalmic solution (Crolom).[1] It is well tolerated and has minimal side effects; however, its efficacy is limited due to frequency of administration (3–6 times daily). Ipratropium (Atrovent nasal spray) is the only available anticholinergic for nasal administration, and it produces a localized parasympatholytic effect on the nasal mucosa. Ipratropium antagonizes the action of acetylcholine by blocking muscarinic cholinergic receptors, which reduces watery hypersecretion from mucosal glands of the nose. This provides symptomatic relief by reducing rhinorrhea associated with the common cold or allergic or nonallergic perennial rhinitis.

Topical or nasal spray steroids are by far the most effective single medication for AR, and they are effective for long-term and short-term treatment. Corticosteroids exhibit antiinflammatory, antipruritic, and vasoconstrictive properties. Early antiinflammatory effects of topical corticosteroids include the inhibition of macrophage and leukocyte activity in the inflamed area and reversal of vascular dilation and permeability. Nasal spray steroids are generally well tolerated; however, side effects may include epistaxis, headaches, sinus infection, coughing, musculoskeletal pain, and dysmenorrhea. Rare reports of nasal septum perforation are most likely related to improper dosing or administration techniques. Results of clinical trials have not supported concerns about long-term exposure to nasal steroids and growth retardation in children.

Available nasal spray preparations include fluticasone (Flonase), budesonide (Rhinocort Aqua), mometasone (Nasonex), beclomethasone (Beconase), flunisolide (Nasalide [available only as a generic]), and triamcinolone (Nasacort). Although there are variations in potency and systemic bioavailability among the different preparations, most differences are not clinically important.

The practice of using oral or intramuscular injections of steroids to manage AR is not advised. The efficacy, side effects, and potential risks do not justify the treatment.

The leukotriene receptor antagonist montelukast (Singulair) has been FDA approved for AR. Its efficacy is comparable to that of antihistamines, but it is less effective than the nasal spray steroids. The expense of this treatment is a major drawback, but it is well tolerated and has few side effects. The addition of montelukast to the treatment regimen is probably best done after a trial of antihistamines or nasal spray steroids, or both.

There is evidence that topical saline wash is beneficial in the treatment of the symptoms of chronic rhinorrhea and rhinosinusitis when used as a sole modality or for adjunctive treatment. When to use this treatment for patients with AR is unclear. The side effects and risks of saline washes are minimal, and they therefore can be used at any point in a treatment plan.

Avoiding specific allergens can be difficult and impractical. The most common allergic triggers are pollens, molds, dust mite excrement, furry animal dander, and insect emanations (e.g., cockroaches). The types of pollen responsible for rhinitis symptoms vary widely with locale, climate, and introduced plantings. Depending on the region of the United States or world, pollen seasons vary in length and by time of year. Fungi and molds can produce clinically important allergens. Reduction of indoor fungi requires removal of moisture sources and replacement of contaminated materials. The use of dilute bleach solutions on nonporous surfaces can help. Humidity control helps to retard mold and fungus growth and can help to control dust. Dust mite control requires covers for bedding, high-efficiency particulate air (HEPA) filter vacuuming of carpeting or removal to nonporous floors. Avoidance is the most effective way to manage sensitivity to animals. Cockroaches are a significant cause of nasal allergy, particularly in inner-city populations and warm climates.

For patients who fail to get adequate results with medications and avoidance measures, allergen injection immunotherapy is an effective treatment for AR. Exactly how injection therapy works is unclear. High doses of systemic allergens are thought to change humeral and cellular components of the immune process, resulting in modulation of the immune response. Successful injection therapy can result in up to a 50% reduction in symptom scores and an 80% reduction in medication use. The effects of injection treatment can persist for at least 3 years after discontinuation of treatment. However, there are reports of severe systemic reactions, including a few fatalities. Weekly injection treatments with observation up to an

---

[1]Not FDA approved for this indication.

CURRENT THERAPY

- Allergen avoidance
- Nasal spray steroids (most effective single agent, less patient acceptance than antihistamines)
  - Triamcinolone (Nasacort AQ)
  - Fluticasone (Flonase)
  - Budesonide (Rhinocort Aqua)
  - Mometasone (Nasonex)
  - Flunisolide (Nasalide)
  - Beclomethasone (Beconase AQ)
- Oral antihistamines (first-line or second-line agent after nasal spray steroids)
  - Cetirizine (Zyrtec) (nonsedating second generation)
  - Fexofenadine (Allegra) (nonsedating second generation)
  - Loratadine (Claritin, Alavert) (nonsedating second generation)
  - Diphenhydramine (Benadryl)
  - Hydroxyzine (Atarax)[1]
  - Chlorpheniramine (Chlor-Trimeton)
  - Many other generics
- Topical antihistamines (add-on treatment)
  - Azelastine (Astelin intranasal spray)
- Topical ophthalmic drops (allergic conjunctivitis symptoms)
  - Antihistamines (e.g., azelastine [Optivar], olopatadine [Patanol])
  - NSAIDs (e.g., ketorolac [Acular 0.5%])
  - Mast cell stabilizer (e.g., cromolyn [Crolom][1])
- Oral leukotriene receptor antagonist (add-on treatment, confirm AR with testing)
  - Montelukast (Singulair)
- Nasal saline irrigation (add-on therapy)
- Oral decongestants (better for congestion rather than rhinorrhea)
  - Pseudoephedrine* (Sudafed and combined with many antihistamines)
  - Phenylephrine (alone or combined with antihistamines)
- Immunotherapy (requires testing)
  - Injection therapy
  - Sublingual therapy

---

[1]Not FDA approved for this indication.
*Federal and state restrictions limit the purchase of pseudoephedrine to discourage illegal conversion to methamphetamine.

---

hour afterward make injection therapy time consuming and expensive. Because of the risks and expense associated with injection therapy, alternate routes of treatment have been investigated.

Immunotherapy by nasal spray and sublingual administration has been investigated, with sublingual immunotherapy being the most successful route. Meta-analysis of 22 studies of sublingual administration has demonstrated efficacy. The buildup process (i.e., increasing dose over time) appears to be faster than injection. The availability of sublingual immunotherapy is limited partially because of insurance coverage taking time to catch up to clinical science.

Management Overview

AR is a common condition that has a significant negative impact on the quality of life for those who suffer. Diagnosis is usually straightforward with the option for specific testing if needed. Treatment is usually pharmacologic, and antihistamines and nasal spray steroids are the most commonly used agents. Making lifestyle changes to avoid specific allergens can help. Second-generation antihistamines have fewer anticholinergic side effects and require less frequent dosing than first-generation antihistamines. Combination therapy using nasal spray steroids with antihistamines works better than either medication alone. For patients who do not get adequate relief, there are other medication options, and reevaluating to confirm diagnosis should be explored. Immunotherapy can help those with severe disease who do not respond to standard treatments.

REFERENCES

Agency for Healthcare Research and Quality. Evidence report/technology assessment no. 54. Management of allergic and nonallergic rhinitis, May 2002. Available at http://www.ahrq.gov/clinic/tp/rhintp.htm (accessed June 3, 2009).

Plaut M, Valentine MD. Clinical practice. Allergic rhinitis. N Engl J Med 2005;353:1934–44.

Quillen DM, Feller DB. Diagnosing rhinitis: Allergic vs. nonallergic. Am Fam Physician 2006;73(9):1583–90.

Settipane RA, Lieberman P. Update on nonallergic rhinitis. Ann Allergy Asthma Immunol 2001;86:494–507.

Wallace DV, Dykewicz MS, Bernstein DI, et al. The diagnosis and management of rhinitis: An updated practice parameter. J Allergy Clin Immunol 2008;122(2 Suppl.):S1–84.

Wilson DR, Lima MT, Durham SR. Sublingual immunotherapy for allergic rhinitis: Systematic review and meta-analysis [review]. Allergy 2005;60(1):4–12.

Allergic Reactions to Drugs

Method of
Donald McNeil, MD

Drug allergic reactions fall under the broader category of adverse drug reactions (ADRs), which also include toxic drug effects, drug interactions, drug intolerance, and, finally, allergic (or immunologic) drug reactions. Adverse drug reactions are common and often result in only trivial consequences. Some may be severe and life-threatening, and may result from both allergic and nonallergic causes.

The incidence of adverse drug effects is unknown but estimates of 20% of hospital admissions are not unreasonable. A skin rash is the most common manifestation; more importantly, however, severe life-threatening reactions occur, of which only a small portion have an allergic etiology. Most drug reactions are the result of unknown mechanisms. Drug intolerance, drug overdose, and side effects of drugs, as well as drug interactions, all play a significant role. These reactions should be considered both common and predictable.

Although allergic drug reactions are potentially severe, they are also the least common and least predictable. Allergic drug reactions are given particular attention because of the unpredictable, costly, and severe consequences that occasionally arise.

Several mechanisms may play a role in the underlying etiology of immunologic drug reactions. Immediate IgE-mediated reactions represent the classic allergic reaction. This is well characterized and the best understood, but other mechanisms also exist, for example, a cytotoxic reaction in which drug-induced antibodies result in hemolytic anemia. Another example is immune complex formation resulting in organ damage. This is commonly referred to as a "serum sickness" reaction and is characterized by fever, rash, and arthralgia beginning 2 to 4 weeks after initiation of drug. Finally, a delayed-type hypersensitivity reaction occurs when drug-specific T-lymphocytes react. This completes the picture of the four types of immunologic-mediated drug reactions according to the original Gell and Coombs classification. These are referred to as Type I, II, III, or IV reactions, respectively.

Cutaneous reactions comprise the most frequent type of allergic drug reaction. Approximately 94% cause a morbilliform rash and only 5% cause an urticarial reaction. Idiosyncratic reactions are still the most likely cause for a rash and occur much more frequently than a true drug-induced allergic reaction. Ampicillins in conjunction with a viral hepatitis or sulfa drugs taken in the AIDS population are common examples.

Both allergic and nonallergic reactions are known to be associated with severe reactions, including fatalities. Contrast media agents, allergic extracts, anesthetics, and antibiotics are the most commonly implicated drugs. Penicillin remains the most common cause of fatal drug reactions and accounts for up to 75% of these severe drug reactions in the United States.

An allergy to penicillin is the most frequently reported, but as many as 90% of patients labeled "penicillin allergic" are able to tolerate penicillin. This allergy is often mislabeled because of underlying illness or interaction between antibiotic and illness. Unfortunately one third to half of vancomycin (Vancocin) prescriptions in hospitals are given because of a history of "penicillin allergy." This raises the incidence of drug-resistant bacteria because of broad-spectrum antibiotic overuse. The economic impact of treating antibiotic-resistant infections is roughly $4 billion annually.

Pathophysiology

Some drugs are capable of reacting in the body without further alteration in chemical structure, whereas others must first be metabolized to become immunogenic. Many drugs are too small to be immunogenic alone and are incapable of eliciting an immune allergic response. These drugs require binding to a high-molecular-weight protein followed by antigen processing and presentation by the macrophage in the presence of major histocompatibility complex (MHC)-specific antigen to appropriate T-cell receptors.

Penicillin is capable of inducing an allergic reaction in more than one manner. Benzylpenicilloyl, the major penicillin determinant, is able to produce a strong antigenic response. A commercially available product, benzylpenicilloyl-polylysine (PPL) (Pre-Pen), provides the means to reproduce the same allergic response by simple skin testing. Minor determinants are metabolic derivatives of penicillin that may also produce an immune response. The diagnostic capabilities of a penicillin allergy are strengthened by including some measure of the allergic response to the minor determinants when skin testing is conducted for penicillin (Figure 1).

Patients with a history of penicillin allergy but negative skin testing to PPL and the minor determinants rarely experience allergic reactions on re-exposure. If they should occur, these are not fatal, but rather mild and self-limited.

PPL alone will potentially miss a significant percentage of allergic reactions to penicillin. Allergy testing with fresh benzylpenicillin G, aged penicillin (reconstituted more than 24 hours) as well as skin testing with the specific penicillin in question will greatly enhance the likelihood of uncovering of penicillin allergy in a patient with a positive history.

Cephalosporins do not provide the same degree of certainty with respect to an allergic evaluation. Cross-reactivity with penicillin allergy patients is known to exist, and although uncommon, it is also unpredictable. To err on the side of safety, a patient with a known penicillin allergy should not be treated with a cephalosporin. A patient with a previous cephalosporin reaction with a negative penicillin skin test cannot safely receive penicillin or another cephalosporin unless further diagnostic measures are taken. This patient may be allergic to a side chain on the cephalosporin that has not been identified by penicillin skin testing. Others recommend a graded oral challenge using a cephalosporin with a different side chain. The latter should be done realizing that standardized procedures have not been developed for this and therefore false negative results may occur.

Successful desensitization to penicillin has permitted a similar approach with other drugs. If the drug in question is required, either intravenous or oral drug administration is possible by incremental doses given usually every 15 minutes. A 10,000-fold dilution of the initial dose is usually sufficient to begin, followed by higher doses,

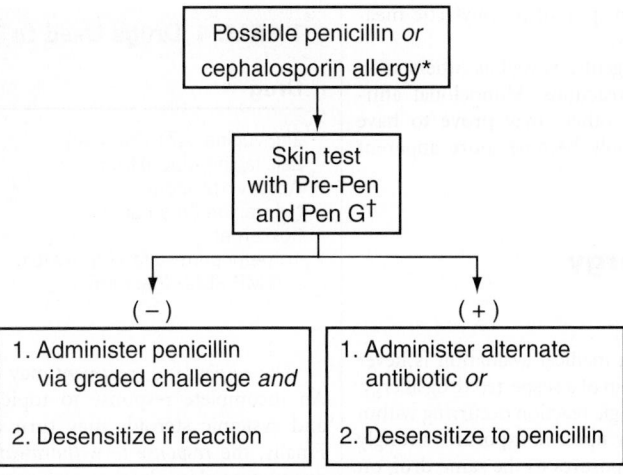

*Only 10%–20% of patients who report a penicillin allergy are actually allergic.
†Benzylpenicilloyl-polylysine (Pre-Pen) and penicillin G (Pen G) will not include all potential penicillin derivatives. The additional benefit of testing with the minor determinant mixture is impractical and usually not available.

FIGURE 1. Penicillin allergy evaluation.

2-fold or greater. The vital signs are monitored throughout the procedure with timely medical intervention if problems arise.

Sulfonamides typically cause cutaneous reactions, infrequently in healthy individuals but extremely common in AIDS patients. Reactions may be relatively benign in nature such as urticaria or fixed-drug eruption, but may also cause more serious reactions (Stevens-Johnson syndrome, toxic epidermal necrolysis). A variety of mechanisms may exist, alone or in combination, using IgE antibody response, T-lymphocytes, and inflammatory cytokines. Because of our inadequate understanding of these mechanisms, there are no universally acceptable means of evaluating sulfonamide hypersensitivity. Unless there has been previously severe reaction, a graded challenge with the drug in question is considered a reasonable alternative (Box 1). Although a theoretical risk exists between sulfonamides and drugs with sulfonamide derivatives (diuretics, COX-2 inhibitors), little data show this is actually true.

Radiographic contrast media (RCM) produce an anaphylactoid reaction by an unknown mechanism. Conventional RCM is hypertonic. The newer nonionic RCM with lower osmolarity are associated with fewer anaphylactoid or allergic-like reactions. Complement system activation, which is capable of causing histamine release, is thought to be the method by which this reaction occurs.

In the continuum of adverse drug effects with suspected hypersensitivity, exposure to *aspirin* and other nonsteroidal anti-inflammatory drugs (NSAIDs) rarely exhibits features that are IgE mediated and allergic in nature, and are more often nonimmunologic mediated. A non-IgE-mediated event must still be approached with caution because the consequences are potentially life-threatening.

BOX 1   Graded Challenge

1. Cautious administration of medications to patient not likely allergic to drug.
2. Not to be considered equivalent to desensitization.
3. Used when insufficient evidence available to exclude drug allergy.
4. Medication administered in incremental doses beginning at 1:100 dilution of final dose.
5. Adequate medical resources exist to treat allergic reaction.

More commonly, NSAIDs are associated with the asthma triad syndrome associated with nasal polyps or rhinitis, and severe asthma. This is not an allergic drug reaction, but it represents a largely unrecognized subpopulation of asthmatics who will benefit by avoiding the use of NSAIDs.

The antibiotic *vancomycin* (Vancocin) causes a reaction referred to as *red man syndrome*. Histamine and other mast cell mediators are released, but not through vancomycin-induced IgE antibody (rare cases have been reported). Most, but not all, cases of the red man syndrome are related to the rate of the infusion, and most will subside once the medication is stopped. A graded challenge with the drug or a full course of desensitization usually permits resumption of treatment.

Angiotensin-converting enzyme (ACE) inhibitors are well known to be associated with cough and angioedema, but like NSAIDs, the mechanism is unknown. Newer ACE inhibitors have been described to cause similar reactions but at a much lower incidence. The symptoms of cough and angioedema may continue to recur for several months and up to a year after the discontinuation of the drug.

As seen from the discussion above, IgE-mediated allergic drug reactions represent only a portion of immune-mediated drug reactions. To assist in the diagnosis, a 7- to 10-day delay in the appearance of the drug reaction after initial treatment or immediate reactivation on re-exposure suggests an immunologic etiology. Oftentimes, only the history will provide this index of suspicion. Confirmation by positive skin testing with the drug in question is highly predictive of IgE-mediated hypersensitivity.

Attempts to label reactions as either IgE- or non-IgE-mediated may prove to be costly, time-consuming, and of no immediate benefit. Non-IgE reactions are capable of eliciting changes in vital signs, pulmonary function, and cutaneous effects similar to anaphylaxis and are referred to as anaphylactoid. These need to be regarded with the same degree of caution as IgE-mediated reactions. Narcotics, radiographic contrast media, and chemotherapeutic agents may directly affect mast cell mediator release with the consequences listed above. Antihistamines and corticosteroids given prior to administration of these drugs are usually sufficient to prevent a reoccurrence, or at least to minimize these reactions.

Drug desensitization is indicated for those patients with positive skin tests who must receive the drug, but should not be assumed to be universally safe or protective. Some chemotherapeutic agents, such as etoposide (VePesid) and teniposide (Vumon), have a much higher incidence of anaphylactoid reactions. Readmimistration of these drugs in the face of a previous reaction and in spite of prophylactic measures often leads to disappointing results.

Current biologic response modifier agents, as well as others soon to arrive, are associated with adverse reactions. Monoclonal antibodies, T- and B-cell inactivators, and others may prove to have adverse immunologic effects that will only become more apparent with the experience of increased use.

Evaluation of Drug Allergy in Practice

The importance of a reliable history in a medical evaluation is never more evident than during the initial workup of a suspected drug allergy. The timing of exposure, with the first allergic reaction occurring within days of the priming dose or immediately upon re-exposure, strongly points to an allergic etiology. Multiple exposures to the same drug on previous occasions do not preclude an allergic reaction de novo. Similarly, a previous history of an allergic drug reaction does not by itself predict a reoccurrence on re-exposure. The allergic diathesis may wane over time for drugs just as it may occur for other allergens.

Armed with this suggestive drug history and clinical findings such as a rash, fever, bronchospasm, or anaphylaxis, the evaluation becomes more straightforward. In the appropriate clinical setting, eosinophilia will also support a drug-allergic reaction.

Avoiding the implicated drug may be the simplest approach because confirmation of the diagnosis with appropriate skin testing is often unavailable. (Standardized skin testing exists only for penicillin, but even this does not provide 100% reliability.) Skin testing with the drug is questionable, but using both a positive and negative control of histamine and saline may still provide useful information. A positive skin test would certainly discourage use of this drug unless adequate precautions were taken.

If a non-life-threatening history of a reaction exists and the drug cannot be appropriately substituted, the option exists for a graded oral challenge to confirm the diagnosis. This should not be considered to be the same as desensitization because it involves higher doses and exposure over a shorter period of time than would be considered safe in a truly allergic individual. A challenge such as this should be conducted in suitable medical facilities under close medical supervision.

If the drug in question has been shown to cause an allergic reaction but still must be used, then a carefully monitored drug desensitization program should be considered. Under medical supervision, the drug should be administered orally or intravenously beginning with doses that are tenfold more dilute than the final strength. Incrementally higher doses of the drug should be administered every 15 minutes, increasing the dose twofold each time.

Drug-induced skin reactions are common and warrant particular attention. Early recognition is necessary to avoid an incorrect diagnosis and to institute appropriate interventional measures as soon as possible.

The following points will assist the physician in arriving at a correct diagnosis. The *timing of the onset* of the reaction in relation to the time the drug was given provides an important clue. Often signs and symptoms develop 1 to 2 weeks after time of initial drug exposure. Symptoms may develop rapidly on repeat exposure. *Pruritic urticarial lesions* strongly suggest an adverse drug reaction. A *symmetrical or truncal distribution* or a rash that occurs only in sun-exposed areas (polymorphous light eruption) also supports an ADR finding. The morphology of the reaction is helpful, although many types occur (lichenoid, morbilliform, eczematous). The histopathology of the lesion on skin biopsy may reveal eosinophils, which may also be detected in the peripheral blood.

Drugs that commonly cause ADRs tend to be antibiotics. The most common is the morbilliform rash when ampicillin is given in the presence of a viral infection such as infectious mononucleosis or cytomegalovirus. Rarely is this IgE mediated and it should not be regarded as a basis for a history of penicillin allergy. It should also be noted that not all ADRs are caused by prescription medications. A patient may fail to disclose over-the-counter medications that might be responsible (e.g., St. John's wort).

TABLE 1 Drugs Used to Treat AIDS/HIV

Drug	Reaction
Zidovudine, AZT (Retrovir)	Hyperpigmentation
Zalcitabine, ddC (Hivid)	Oral ulcers
Abacavir (Ziagen)	Severe rash/anaphylaxis
Nevirapine (Viramune)	Toxic epidermal necrolysis
Foscarnet	Urethral ulceration
Trimethoprim-sulfamethoxazole (TMP-SMX) (Bactrim)	Morbilliform rash or erythema multiforme

The *response to treatment* may aid in the recognition of an ADR. An incomplete response to topical steroids is typical of an ADR and systemic steroids may turn out to be the therapy of choice. Finally, the *response to withdrawal* of drug may range from a rapid recovery to slow clearing over many weeks, but a favorable response nonetheless.

Table 1 lists several drugs used to treat AIDS/HIV that are worthy of mention. Not all should be considered to be an allergic cause of ADR.

A careful and systematic approach to the patient with a suspected drug allergy will provide valuable information for both the immediate and the long-term management of the patient. A suspected drug allergy that is disproved will facilitate good medical care because unnecessary expense and the risk of further sensitizing the patient to a new medication will be spared if the patient is not allergic. On the other hand, a positive screen for a suspected drug allergy will result in a safe alternative. It should be emphasized, however, that neither a family history of a drug allergy nor a patient requesting a "test" for a possible drug allergy without other reason is an indication for further drug allergy evaluation because of the risk of false-negative results.

Allergic Reaction to Stinging Insects

Method of
Theodore M. Freeman, MD

Most stinging insects belong to the order Hymenoptera. They include species of bees (genus *Apis*, including honey bees and bumblebees), wasps (genus *Polistes*), yellow jackets (genus *Vespula*), hornets (genus *Dolichovespula*), and fire ant (genus *Solenopsis*).

Diagnosis

There are two important historical points to ascertain when seeing a patient with an allergic reaction to a stinging insect. The first is the type of insect that caused the sting. The physician may not rely on the patient's identification. Clues about the type of insect can be obtained from the circumstances of the sting.

Bees are herbivores and not aggressive. Stings from these insects often occur in fields with flowering plants when a barefoot patient steps or accidently sits on them. Bees have a barbed stinger and attached venom sac, which may be left in place after a sting. These should be removed immediately with a scraping motion; any pinching of the sac may inject additional venom.

Yellow jackets are aggressive scavengers and are found wherever food is left in the open. Stings from these insects usually occur in picnic areas or around open garbage containers. Like bees, yellow jackets occasionally leave a stinger in place, so this historical feature is not definitive. Wasps usually are not aggressive, except in defense of their nests. However, they tend to build these nests under the eaves and overhangs of our homes, and people stung by wasps are usually entering or exiting their homes.

Hornets are not aggressive, except in defense of their nest. Because the nests are built in trees, stings by these insects are rare.

Fire ants are very aggressive in defense of their nests, which are low mounds built above ground with extensive tunnels beneath the surface. In endemic areas (mostly southeastern United States), they swarm and attack as a group when disturbed. Patients stung by fire ants are usually outdoors and accidently stand in a mound or disturb a mound while working or playing in their yard or garden. Fire ant workers do not fly. They bite only to get a grip and then sting from the abdomen and inject a toxic alkaloid venom. Because they attack as a group, they are usually seen and clearly identified by the patient. The size of the fire ants means their venom is injected less deeply than that of other hymenoptera, which leads to the usual development of a pseudopustule about 24 hours after a sting. These pseudopustules contain necrotic cellular material but are sterile because fire ant venom has antibiotic properties that can kill bacteria and fungi. The pseudopustules should be left alone; opening and draining them only increases the risk of secondary infection.

The second historical point is the type of reaction by the patient to the sting. The active venom components produce immediate swelling, redness, and tenderness with fairly intense pain at the site of the sting that slowly resolves over several hours. Sometimes, the immediate reaction progresses, and swelling (>10 cm) continues for 1 to 2 days and extends across several contiguous joints from the site of the sting. This large local reaction may take 5 to 10 days to fully resolve, and it may be difficult to differentiate this from a secondary infection. Large local reactions peak in 1 to 2 days and then slowly recede, whereas secondary infections continue to get worse. Large local reactions do not cause systemic fever or lymphangitis, which should be treated with antibiotics if they occur.

The reaction of most concern is anaphylaxis. Unfortunately, many of the symptoms are similar to those of anxiety, which also may occur in a concerned patient: feelings of impending doom, a rapid heartbeat, shortness of breath, and nausea. Other symptoms that should not be seen in anxiety include a metallic taste, pruritus, and abdominal or uterine cramping. Signs of anaphylaxis include flushing, urticaria, angioedema, vomiting, diarrhea, bronchospasm, hypotension, and shock. Involvement of the upper airway and cardiopulmonary systems is associated with death, and hymenoptera stings are the cause of about 40 deaths per year in the United States. Documentation of the type of reaction is essential for future risk assessment and determination of whether prophylactic therapy should be offered.

The risk for a systemic reaction after hymenoptera sting in the general population is estimated to be 3% to 5%. In patients who have a documented large local reaction to an insect sting, the risk of systemic reactions increases slightly to about 10%. Patients suffering large local reactions may be referred to a specialist for specific IgE testing. For patients who have suffered anaphylaxis, the risk of systemic reactions after a sting is 50% to 60%. However, children (<16 years old) who have only cutaneous signs and symptoms of anaphylaxis (e.g., pruritus, flushing, urticaria, angioedema) do not seem to have a tendency for life-threatening anaphylaxis, and their risk for more than cutaneous anaphylaxis is only about 10%. If a patient has suffered an anaphylactic event after a hymenoptera sting and has specific IgE to that hymenoptera as determined by in vivo (skin testing) or in vitro methods and is then placed on immunotherapy for that insect, the risk of systemic reaction after another sting is only 2% to 3%. Immunotherapy entails the use of specific venom products for each species, with the exception of fire ants. Because of the difficulty in extracting venom from fire ants, the only commercially available product for fire ants is the whole-body extract. Although whole-body extract is not effective therapy for other hymenoptera, it has been shown to be effective for fire ants.

 CURRENT DIAGNOSIS

- Determine the insect involved by recording circumstances of sting event.
- Determine the type of reaction: usual (expected), large local, or systemic (anaphylaxis).

Treatment

Immediate therapy for insect stings depends on the type of reaction. For the expected short-duration local reaction, treatment includes cold compresses; antihistamines, such as diphenhydramine (Benadryl 25 to 50 mg for adults; 1 mg/kg [up to 50 mg] for children) or cetirizine (Zyrtec 10 mg for adults and children older than 6 years; 5 mg for children younger than 6 years); and analgesics, such as acetaminophen (Tylenol) or ibuprofen (Motrin). Avoidance of future stings may be discussed with the patient. Recommendations include the following:

- Avoid looking or smelling like a flower—avoid flower-printed clothing and flowery or fruity colognes and perfumes.
- Remove wasps' nests from around the home, especially near doorways.
- Avoid areas near open garbage.
- Do not leave open food or drinks during outdoor eating.
- Wear shoes, socks, and work gloves when working in the yard or garden.

Large local reactions may be treated as described for short-duration local reactions, with the addition of a short course (5–7 days) of oral steroids (e.g., Medrol dose pack), especially if there is significant morbidity associated with the site of the reaction. For instance, if a hand or foot is involved, a patient may not be able to write, work, or walk for up to a week. Avoidance measures should be discussed. Epinephrine autoinjectors (e.g., EpiPen, EpiPen Jr, Twinject) may be given, depending on the patient's anxiety about future stings. Epinephrine autoinjectors are simple devices with instructions clearly printed on them, but mistakes in usage do occur. The most common include "bouncing" the injector off the leg, which ejects the epinephrine onto the leg instead of delivering it intramuscularly, and putting the thumb over the end of the injector, which if the injector is reversed leads to no delivery of epinephrine and thumb trauma. Demonstration pens and videos of proper technique may be obtained from the manufacturers (e.g., Dey, Sciele).

The primary treatment of anaphylaxis is epinephrine (1:1000 concentration), with 0.3 to 0.5 mL given intramuscularly in adults or 0.01 mL/kg in children every 5 to 15 minutes as needed. The patient should be placed in a recumbent position with the feet elevated. Supplemental therapy includes antihistamines (i.e., H_1-receptor antagonists); H_2-blockers (e.g., ranitidine [Zantac[1]] 150 mg PO) for cutaneous signs and symptoms; β-adrenergics (e.g., albuterol [Proventil, AccuNeb]) administered by metered-dose inhaler or nebulizer for bronchoconstriction; oxygen for hypoxia; intravenous fluids and possibly vasopressors for hypotension; and intubation for compromise of the upper airway.

Physicians must avoid the tendency to treat cutaneous-only anaphylaxis with antihistamines alone, because cutaneous signs and symptoms often develop rapidly into life-threatening events. The appropriate therapy, even for only cutaneous signs and symptoms, is epinephrine. Most anaphylaxis responds quickly to a single dose of epinephrine, although up to 30% of anaphylaxis cases require two or more doses. Because anaphylaxis may be prolonged and last hours and epinephrine has a short duration of action (1 hour), patients should be observed for 4 to 6 hours after the last epinephrine dose. They should remain symptom free during that time before being released from the clinic or emergency department. In 3% to 20% of patients, a biphasic reaction occurs with recurrence of signs and symptoms 4 to 6 hours (range, 1 to 72 hours) after the initial reaction. For patients with prolonged or severe reactions, which are more often associated with a recurrence, overnight admission for observation should be considered.

---

[1]Not FDA approved for this indication.

CURRENT THERAPY

- Treatment for usual reactions
  - H$_1$-antihistamines, analgesics, cold compresses
  - Discussion of avoidance measures
- Treatment of large local reactions
  - H$_1$-antihistamines, analgesics, cold compresses
  - Discussion of avoidance measures and possible prescription of epinephrine autoinjectors (e.g., EpiPen, Twinject)
- Treatment of systemic reactions
  - Epinephrine
  - Supplemental therapy, including antihistamines, β-adrenergics, oxygen, intravenous fluids, and perhaps vasopressors
  - Patients on β-blockers may require glucagon (e.g., Glucagon Emergency Kit, GlucaGen HypoKit)
  - Discussion of avoidance measures, medical alert accessories, prescription for epinephrine autoinjectors
  - Referral to allergist-immunologist to evaluate for specific IgE and possible institution of immunotherapy

Oral (prednisone 1 mg/kg up to 50 mg daily) or intravenous (methylprednisolone [Solu-Medrol] 1 to 2 mg/kg every 6 hours) steroids are sometimes given to minimize recurrences. Many patients are on β-blocking agents, which may make patients suffering anaphylaxis refractory to treatment with epinephrine. In this case, glucagon (e.g., GlucaGen HypoKit, Glucagon Emergency Kit[1]) at a dose[3] of 1 to 5 mg (20 to 30 μg/kg [maximum 1 mg] in children) may be tried intravenously over 5 minutes, followed by infusions (5 to 15 μg/min)[3] titrated to clinical response. Patients who have suffered anaphylaxis must be given instructions on avoidance of future stings, epinephrine pen autoinjectors (EpiPen), and information on medical alert accessories (e.g., necklaces, bracelets). They should also be referred to an allergist-immunologist to evaluate them for the presence of specific IgE, counseling, and consideration of immunotherapy, which may significantly reduce their future risk.

REFERENCES

Freeman TM, Hylander RD, Ortiz AA, Martin MF. Imported fire ant immunotherapy: Effectiveness of whole body extracts. J Allergy Clin Immunol 1992;90:210–5.

Freeman TM. Hypersensitivity to hymenoptera stings. N Engl J Med 2004;351:1978–84.

Hunt KJ, Valentine MD, Sobotka AK, et al. A controlled trial of immunotherapy in insect hypersensitivity. N Engl J Med 1978;299:157–61.

Moffitt JE, Golden DBK, Reisman RE, et al. Stinging insect hypersensitivity: A practice parameter update. J Allergy Clin Immunol 2004;114:869–86.

Sampson HA, Munoz-Furlong A, Campbell RL, et al. Second symposium on the definition and management of anaphylaxis: Summary report—Second National Institute of Allergy and Infectious Disease/Food Allergy and Anaphylaxis Network symposium. J Allergy Clin Immunol 2006;117:391–7.

Schuberth KC, Lichtenstein LM, Kagey-Sobotka A, et al. Epidemiologic study of insect allergy in children. II. Effects of accidental stings in allergic children. J Pediatr 1983;102:361–5.

[1]Not FDA approved for this indication.
[3]Exceeds dosage recommended by the manufacturer.

Diseases of the Skin

Psychocutaneous Medicine

Method of
Ladan Mostaghimi, MD

Psychocutaneous medicine explores the interactions between mind and skin. The spectrum of patients ranges from those who are delusional and refuse to see a psychiatrist to those who are depressed because of chronic disfiguring skin problems. The relationship between chronic skin diseases and psychological factors has been known for many years. In the first reference to it from 1200 BC, the physician to the Prince of Persia speculated that his patient's skin disease (possibly psoriasis based on the description) was related to his anxiety about succeeding his father. Research in psychoneuroimmunology has better defined the relationship between skin and mind. This chapter discusses common psychodermatologic disorders and their treatment.

Classification

The five general categories of psychocutaneous medicine, as adapted from *Psychocutaneous Medicine*, are as follows:

- Psychophysiologic disorders: Emotional factors can exacerbate a skin disorder, such as psoriasis.
- Primary psychiatric disorders: Patients have no primary skin disorder, and the cutaneous signs are self-induced, such as delusions of parasitosis.
- Secondary psychiatric disorders: A chronic, disfiguring skin disorder causes psychological problems.
- Cutaneous sensory disorders: Patients have a purely sensory complaint, such as pruritus, burning, stinging, or biting, without a visible primary skin disease or an underlying medical condition.
- Use of psychotropic medications for dermatologic conditions such as urticaria or postherpetic neuralgia.

Another way to classify psychocutaneous conditions is based on the underlying psychopathology, such as depression, anxiety, delusional disorders, and impulse control disorders. Standardized self-rating questionnaires are available for different conditions. These questionnaires can be administered and rated by office staff before the appointment with the physician. This classification system can also help with treatment choices and follow-up plans.

Delusions of Parasitosis

Delusions of parasitosis falls under the *Diagnostic and Statistical Manual of Mental Disorders*, fourth edition, text revision (DSM-IV-TR),

category of delusional disorder, somatic type. These patients have false fixed beliefs that they are infested by parasites. To meet the diagnostic criteria, the problem should last at least for a month, and it should not be part of schizophrenia manifestations. Apart from the impact of the delusions, the patient's functioning is not markedly impaired, and behavior is not always odd or bizarre. Other delusional disorders for which a patient would seek dermatologic advice are delusion of bromhidrosis (i.e., patients are convinced they have a foul odor that no one else can perceive) and the delusion of dysmorphosis (i.e., patients are convinced that they have a defect in appearance that no one else can appreciate).

Another group of patients with delusions of parasitosis are those with psychotic mood disorders such as depression or bipolar disorder and false fixed somatic beliefs. If the patient has mood symptoms in addition to delusional symptoms, treatment of the mood problem may correct the delusional beliefs. For about 12% of patients, the delusion of parasitosis is shared by a family member or significant other. This condition is called folie à deux (i.e., madness of two) or folie partagé (i.e., shared delusions).

The patient with delusions of parasitosis usually has multiple superficial excoriations due to manipulating the skin to try to remove the parasites. Patients come to the clinic with many boxes and bags of skin samples, which is known as the matchbox sign. They can become very agitated when the physician denies presence of any infestation after physical examination or assessment of the samples collected and brought in.

Physicians should rule out substance abuse disorders. Some substances, especially amphetamines, cocaine, and phencyclidine (PCP), can cause formication and organic delusional syndrome in some patients. Organic reasons such as temporal lobe epilepsy or other brain pathology, neurosyphilis, pernicious anemia, hypothyroidism or hyperthyroidism, and systemic lupus erythematosus should be investigated, especially in older patients and if any neurologic symptoms are identified during the physical examination.

Treatment consists of antipsychotic or neuroleptic medications. For patients with psychotic mood disorder, treatment of the mood disorder usually improves the delusional symptoms. Depending on the amount of distress that the delusions are causing, treatment may start with combination of a neuroleptic medication and an antidepressant and later taper off the neuroleptic and continue only the antidepressant. To facilitate acceptance of the treatment, it is important for the physician to have a good rapport with patients and address their concerns; at the same time, the physician must not accept or feed into their delusions by giving the impression that the delusion is believed to be real. Statements such as the following may help to encourage patients to accept treatment: "I'll be very honest with you; what you are telling me is very unusual. In most cases of infectious diseases, the doctors are able to easily identify the culprit. In your case, we have not found anything. Although we will keep looking to find the culprit, I know it is difficult to live with this condition, and we have medications that can help to alleviate the symptoms you are experiencing."

TABLE 1 Recommended Monitoring for Patients on Atypical Antipsychotics According to the American Diabetic Association Consensus Statement on Diabetes Care, 2004

Characteristic	Baseline	4 Weeks	8 Weeks	12 Weeks	Quarterly	Annually	Every 5 Years
Personal and family history	+					+	
Weight (BMI)	+	+	+	+	+		
Waist circumference	+					+	
Blood pressure	+			+		+	
Fasting plasma glucose	+			+		+	
Fasting lipid profile	+			+			+

Modified with permission from The American Diabetes Association. Diabetic Care 2004;27:596–601. Copyright 2004 American Diabetes Association.

CURRENT DIAGNOSIS

Delusions of Parasitosis

- The patient has false fixed beliefs about being infested.
- Look for the matchbox sign: Many samples of excoriated pieces of skin, scabs, clothing lint, or other debris are kept in plastic wrap, on adhesive tape, or in matchboxes by the patient and brought to the physician's office for examination to detect suspected parasites.
- Determine the type of delusional disorder: primary or secondary, such as mood disorder with delusional features.
- Determine possible causes and contributing factors, such as substance abuse, organic brain pathology, pernicious anemia, hypothyroidism or hyperthyroidism, and systemic lupus erythematosus.
- Determine the extent of damage to the skin and history of skin infections.

Dermatitis Artefacta, Neurotic Excoriations, and Acne Excoriée

- Determine the type of problem: need to assume sick role (dermatitis artefacta), secondary gain (malingering), impulsive skin picking (neurotic excoriations and acne excoriée).
- Assess the degree of scarring, which requires intensive treatment.

Prurigo Nodularis and Lichen Simplex Chronicus

- Hard nodules that are 1 to 5 cm in diameter with hyperpigmentation and warty or excoriated surface in prurigo nodularis
- Lichenification (thickening) of the skin in lichen simplex chronicus
- Different histopathology for prurigo nodularis and lichen simplex chronicus

- Complete blood cell count to rule out lymphoma and polycythemia rubra vera
- Renal function tests (BUN, creatinine, and electrolytes) to rule out renal failure
- Liver function tests to rule out chronic obstructive biliary disease
- Serology for hepatitis
- Test for diabetes mellitus
- Levels of thyroid and parathyroid hormones
- Total serum IgE levels for atopy
- Patch test if allergies are suspected
- HIV test and PPD (if indicated)
- Skin biopsy and direct and indirect immunofluorescence assays to rule out immunobullous diseases
- Stool check for parasites
- Gastrointestinal testing to rule out malabsorption and gluten sensitivity
- Psychological evaluation

Trichotillomania

- Hair loss is caused by repeated hair pulling, producing oddly shaped patches of alopecia with broken hair and no signs of inflammation.
- Other areas beside the scalp may be affected.
- The age of onset and underlying psychopathology should be determined.
- If patient denies hair pulling, rule out other causes of alopecia.

Cutaneous Sensory Disorders

- Patients have a sensation of burning and itching in different areas of skin and mucous membranes, with no signs and symptoms of inflammation.

Pimozide (Orap)[1] is a first-generation antipsychotic that dermatologists have traditionally used for delusions of parasitosis. However, most antipsychotic medications can help this condition. Physicians should be familiar with the first- and second-generation antipsychotics (Table 2) and their side effect profile to select the treatment that is best tailored to each patient. Please notice the FDA warning about increased risk of stroke with the use of neuroleptics in elderly patients with Alzheimer's disease.

---

[1]Not FDA approved for this indication.

Dermatitis Artefacta, Neurotic Excoriations, and Acne Excoriée

DERMATITIS ARTEFACTA OR FACTITIOUS DERMATITIS

Dermatitis artefacta (i.e., factitious dermatitis) refers to intentional production of skin lesions to satisfy a psychological need. This may be achieved by different methods, such as excoriation, burning, or injection of toxic substances. Patients usually deny the self-induced nature of the problem. If the motivation for production of skin lesions is unconscious (e.g., assuming sick role), it falls under the category of factitious disorder. If the motivation is apparent and

CURRENT THERAPY

Delusions of Parasitosis

- Treatment of main problem in cases of secondary delusional disorder helps to clear the delusions.
- Psychosocial intervention is warranted; work with families, and provide a good support system.
- Evaluate and monitor safety for the patient, family members, and health care providers.
- Some patients may try to get rid of parasites by burning their belongings or their body or by using toxic substances to treat parasites, damaging their skin and causing serious toxicity, which must be treated.
- Treatment may include psychoeducation and cognitive-behavioral therapy (CBT).
- Neuroleptic and antipsychotic medications may be used: Pimozide (Orap)[1] is a first-generation antipsychotic frequently used by dermatologists.
  There are case reports of second-generation antipsychotics working well in these situations.
- Treatment must be customized based on each patient's profile and the medications' side effects.

Dermatitis Artefacta, Neurotic Excoriations, and Acne Excoriée

- For dermatitis artefacta and malingering, the patient should be confronted in a nonjudgmental, empathetic way. Provide supportive dermatologic care for the skin and refer the patient for appropriate psychological interventions.
- For acne excoriée and neurotic dermatitis, rule out underlying psychopathology, and use a combination of therapy (cognitive-behavioral therapy or behavioral therapy) and medications that help impulsive behavior, such as selective serotonin reuptake inhibitors (SSRIs), serotonin-norepinephrine reuptake inhibitors (SNRIs), buspirone (Buspar),[1] anticonvulsants, naltrexone (ReVia),[1] and neuroleptics, depending on the extent of the problem and scarring.
- There are no FDA-approved medications for these impulse control problems, and use of the suggested medications should be based on the risk-benefit assessment for each patient.

Prurigo Nodularis and Lichen Simplex Chronicus

- Topical antipruritic creams

- Topical steroids
- Topical capsaicin (Zostrix)[1]
- For lichen simplex chronicus, some reports of efficacy of tacrolimus (Protopic)[1]
- Narrow-band ultraviolet B (UVB) light
- Psychosocial and therapy interventions to break the itch/scratch cycle
- Psychotropic medications to help with itching and sleep: mirtazapine (Remeron),[1] doxepin (Sinequan),[1] or trazodone (Desyrel)[1]
- In resistant cases, other treatments such as naltrexone (ReVia,)[1] cyclosporine (Sandimmune),[1] or thalidomide (Thalomid)[1]

Trichotillomania

- In children, trichotillomania is usually self-limited, and parents should be reassured. Psychotherapeutic interventions are helpful.
- In adolescents and adults, first-line treatment is psychotherapy: cognitive-behavioral therapy or behavioral therapy and habit reversal. Improving coping mechanisms with stress is helpful.
- Case reports and small double-blind studies have shown the efficacy of clomipramine (Anafranil)[1] and SSRIs.
- Depending on the extent of the problem, augmentation with neuroleptics can be considered, but because of the important side effects profile of these medications, their risks and benefits should be carefully considered.
- Before using antidepressants, patients should be screened for a family history of bipolar disorder or personal history of previous manic episodes.

Cutaneous Sensory Disorders

- Rule out possible causes of abnormal sensations: infection, allergic reactions (e.g., dental fillings), vitamin and minerals deficiencies, diabetes, Sjögren's syndrome, nerve injuries, medications, and neoplasia.
- Treat the primary cause of the abnormal sensation if found.
- In cases of idiopathic abnormal sensations, some medications may help: Tricyclic Antidepressant, gabapentin (Neurontin),[1] pregabalin (Lyrica),[1] SNRIs, and SSRIs.

---

[1]Not FDA approved for this indication.

conscious (e.g., legal gain, disability), it falls under the category of malingering. Clinically, the lesions are located in reachable areas of the skin and can mimic any skin disease.

Factitious dermatitis usually occurs in patients with underlying psychopathology. After a diagnosis is made, the physician needs to discuss it with the patient in a nonjudgmental, empathetic way. Supportive dermatologic care should be provided for wounds, and the patient should be referred for psychological evaluation. Antidepressant and antianxiety medications can help to treat underlying depression and anxiety. Supplementary therapies include biofeedback, relaxation, acupuncture, hypnosis, cognitive behavioral therapy, and behavioral therapy.

ACNE EXCORIÉE AND NEUROTIC EXCORIATIONS

Patients with acne excoriée create excoriations by repetitive scratching or skin picking. Women are affected more than men. Patients scratch and pick at their acne, an inset bite, or other bumps or rough spots on the skin, and any part of the skin that is not smooth can be a target. However, the patient may inflict neurotic excoriations without the trigger of any skin pathology because the condition is a psychological process with dermatologic manifestations. Patients usually have ritualistic picking habits and report building of tension before picking and release of tension afterward.

For any self-injurious behavior, patients must be screened for underlying psychopathologies such as personality disorders. However, in many patients, the behavior results from an impulse control problem.

In addition to treating the underlying psychopathology, treatment includes a combination of behavioral therapy and medications that help with impulsive behavior. The success of treatment depends on patients' motivation to avoid scarring and to replace the self-injurious behavior with better behavior, including gentle skin care. Patients need to replace picking with other relaxing behaviors that are not harmful to skin, such as breathing relaxation or using a stress

TABLE 2 Medications Used in Psychocutaneous Disorders

Drug Class	Drug Name	Dosage Range*	Side Effects to Monitor
Neuroleptics			
First-generation neuroleptics	Pimozide (Orap)[†]	1 mg daily in divided doses, gradually increase up to maximum dose of 10 mg/d	Multiple drug-drug interactions due to metabolism through CYP-450 1A2 and CYP 3A4; prolonged QT interval; torsades de pointes; GI, hematologic, hepatic, and neurologic (tardive dyskinesia, neuroleptic malignant syndrome, extrapyramidal symptoms, akathisia) effects; drug-induced SLE and priapism
	Haloperidol (Haldol)[†]	0.5–3 mg bid or tid	Neurologic side effects; QT prolongation; drug-drug interactions
Second-generation neuroleptics	Olanzapine (Zyprexa)[†] Risperidone (Risperdal)[†] Aripiprazole (Abilify)[†] Quetiapine (Seroquel)[†] Ziprasidone (Geodon)[†]	2.5–max 20 mg/d 1–4 mg/d, max 8 mg/d 2–max 30 mg/d 25–max 800 mg/d in divided doses 20–80 mg bid	QT prolongation; neurologic side effects (extrapyramidal symptoms, tardive dyskinesia, neuroleptic malignant syndrome) less with second-generation neuroleptics (least for quetiapine) but still exist; metabolic syndrome (needs regular monitoring; see Table 1); drug-drug interactions, blood dyscrasias
Antidepressants and Antianxiety Medications			
Antidepressants/ antianxiety SSRIs	Sertraline (Zoloft)[†] Citalopram (Celexa)[†] Escitalopram (Lexapro)[†] Fluoxetine (Prozac)[†] Paroxetine (Paxil)[†] Fluvoxamine works best in OCD	50–200 mg/d 20–60 mg/d 10–20 mg/d 20–60 mg/d 20–50 mg/d 50–300 mg/d in divided doses (bid)	Each SSRI has own side effect profile (e.g., fluoxetine may prolong QT interval, Luvox may cause Stevens-Johnson syndrome); watch for sweating, GI symptoms, sexual side effects, myalgia, sleep problems, tremor, dizziness, bleeding tendencies, hyponatremia (rare), seizure (rare), manic episode, and suicidal ideation and suicide (rare); watch for drug-drug interactions
Antidepressants/ antianxiety SNRIs (help for peripheral neuropathies)	Venlafaxine (Effexor),[†] extended-release form available	37.5–225 mg/d	Hypertension, sweating, GI symptoms, blurred vision, sexual side effects, hyponatremia, bleeding tendencies, neuroleptic malignant syndrome, serotonin syndrome, hepatitis (rare), drug-drug interactions
	Duloxetine (Cymbalta), also for treatment of fibromyalgia	30–120 mg/d[‡]	Sweating, GI symptoms, sleep problems, bleeding tendencies, hepatotoxicity, fatigue, drug-drug interactions
Antidepressants/ antianxiety other	Trazodone (Desyrel), helps insomnia[†] and sometimes itching[†]	50–400 mg/d	Sweating, weight change, GI symptoms, neurologic symptoms, blurred vision, hypertension, hypotension (rare), cardiac dysrhythmia (rare), priapism, seizure, drug-drug interactions
	Mirtazapine (Remeron), helps insomnia[†] and itching[†] with higher affinity for histamine receptors than doxepin (Sinequan)	15–45 mg/d	Increased appetite, hyperlipidemia, somnolence, neurologic disorders, agranulocytosis and neutropenia (rare), seizure, drug-drug interactions
	Bupropion (Wellbutrin),[†] sustained-release and extended-release forms available	100–450 mg/d in divided doses	Hypertension, tachycardia, arrhythmia, pruritus, urticaria, GI symptoms, arthralgia, myalgia, neurologic symptoms, agitation, anger outbursts, menstrual problems, Stevens-Johnson syndrome, anaphylaxis, drug-drug interactions
	Buspirone (BuSpar), works for anxiety problems	5–60 mg/d in divided doses	Nausea, blurred vision, nervousness, angry behavior, neurologic symptoms, CHF (rare), MI (rare), CVA (rare), drug-drug interactions
Tricyclic antidepressant for pruritus	Doxepin (Sinequan)	10–300 mg/d single and divided doses for depression 10–25 mg/d for pruritus[†]	Weight gain, GI symptoms, neurologic symptoms, blurred vision, urinary retention, arrhythmia (rare), blood pressure changes, bleeding tendencies, hematologic changes, drug-drug interactions
Tricyclic antidepressant for trichotillomania	Clomipramine (Anafranil)[†]	25–250 mg/d	Weight gain or loss, GI symptoms, blurred vision, neurologic symptoms, urinary retention, MI, orthostatic hypotension, hematologic side effects, hepatotoxicity
Neuropathic Pain Treatments			
Tricyclic antidepressant	Amitriptyline[†]	10–150 mg/d	Weight gain, GI symptoms, neurologic symptoms, blurred vision, cardiac dysrhythmia, hematologic symptoms, hepatic symptoms, CVA, drug-drug interactions
Antiepileptic medications	Gabapentin (Neurontin), for postherpetic neuralgia	100 mg at night, gradually increase to up to 1800 mg daily in divided doses if needed	Myalgia, peripheral edema, neurologic symptoms, angry behavior, mood swings, problems with thinking, Stevens-Johnson syndrome, seizure, drug-drug interactions
	Pregabalin (Lyrica), for postherpetic neuralgia and treatment of fibromyalgia	50 mg tid, with gradual increase up to 600 mg/d in divided doses	Peripheral edema, weight gain, GI symptoms, ataxia, somnolence, blurred vision, euphoria, problems with thinking, angioedema

Continued

TABLE 2 Medications Used in Psychocutaneous Disorders—Cont'd

Drug Class	Drug Name	Dosage Range*	Side Effects to Monitor
	Carbamazepine (Tegretol), for trigeminal neuralgia Screen patients for HLA-B*1502 allele prior to treatment§	50–1200 mg/d in divided doses for blood levels of 4–12 μg/mL	Hyponatremia, severe blood dyscrasias (rare but needs regular CBC monitoring), toxicity over therapeutic ranges, atrioventricular block, cardiac dysrhythmia, CHF, syncope, hypertension or hypotension, GI symptoms, hepatitis, SLE, rash, Stevens-Johnson syndrome, TEN, psoriasis, acne, angioedema, nephrotoxicity, drug-drug interactions
	Lamotrigine (Lamictal), helps impulsive behavior† and neuropathic pain†	25–400 mg/d in divided doses; do not increase to more than 50 mg/wk Needs dose adjustment if used with valproate or enzyme-inducing AEDs	Headaches, sleep problems, diplopia, ataxia, GI symptoms, rhinitis, photosensitivity, rash, Stevens-Johnson syndrome, TEN, angioedema, hypersensitivity reactions, neutropenia, DIC, hematologic problems, hepatic failure, pancreatitis, rhabdomyolysis, teratogenicity, drug-drug interactions
Various treatments for intractable pruritus	Thalidomide (Thalomid),† also used in Behçet's syndrome†	50–400 mg/d	Severe birth defects in pregnancy, edema, skin rash, GI symptoms, leukopenia, thrombotic disorder, peripheral neuropathy, Stevens-Johnson syndrome, TEN, seizure, pulmonary embolism, hypocalcemia, tremor, somnolence, drug-drug interactions
	Naltrexone (ReVia)†	50 mg/d	GI symptoms, headaches, anxiety, hepatic damage, opioid withdrawal (rare), drug-drug interactions
	Cyclosporine (Sandimmune)†	4–5 mg/kg/d	Hirsutism, pruritus in some patients, GI symptoms, neurologic symptoms, hepatotoxicity, nephrotoxicity, infectious disease, hyperkalemia, hypomagnesemia, hypertension, anaphylaxis, lymphoproliferative disorder, drug-drug interactions
Benzodiazepines (sometimes used for burning mouth syndrome)	Clonazepam (Klonopin)†	0.25 mg at night, with gradual increase to 1 mg at night if needed	Sialorrhea, ataxia, dizziness, somnolence, impaired cognition, aggravation of seizure, depression, behavioral problems, respiratory depression

Note the FDA black box warning suggesting an increased risk of mortality with use of antipsychotics in the elderly, suicidality with antidepressants in those under age 25, and increased suicidality with antiepileptic medications.

*Because of a lack of clinical trials in psychocutaneous disorders, these medications do not have specific FDA approval for these disorders, and their use is based on case reports and my experience. The dosage in the table is adult dosing. For pediatric dosing and for a complete list of side effects, consult other medication databases such as the *Physicians' Desk Reference* (PDR). Always begin with the smallest dose and increase gradually. After the symptoms are controlled, decrease the dose to the minimum effective dose for maintenance. Give each dose 1–2 weeks before increasing.

†Not FDA approved for this indication.

‡Exceeds dosage recommended by the manufacturer.

§Strong association between severe dermatologic reaction and HLA-B*1502 allele.

Abbreviations: AED = antiepileptic drugs; CBC = complete blood cell count; CHF = congestive heart failure; DIC = disseminated intravascular coagulopathy; FDA = U.S. Food and Drug Administration; GI = gastrointestinal; MI = myocardial infarction; OCD = obsessive-compulsive disorder; SLE = systemic lupus erythematosus; SNRI = serotonin-norepinephrine reuptake inhibitor; SSRI = selective serotonin reuptake inhibitor; TEN = toxic epidermal necrolysis.

797

ball, Chinese exercise balls, Greek worry beads, stuffed animals, or Silly Putty. In finding appropriate replacement behavior, the physician should remember that tactile stimulation is important for these patients' anxiety relief.

There is no FDA-approved medication for this condition, and the use of different classes of medications is mostly based on case reports. The first step is to use an SSRI, such as fluoxetine (Prozac),[1] sertraline (Zoloft),[1] paroxetine (Paxil),[1] or citalopram (Celexa),[1] or use an SNRI, such as venlafaxine (Effexor)[1] or duloxetine (Cymbalta).[1] Dosage and side effect profiles are provided in Table 2. If this is insufficient, the physician can add antianxiety medications, such as buspirone (Buspar),[1] and some of the newer anticonvulsant medications, such as lamotrigine (Lamictal).[1] In the case of severe picking, multiple infections, and scarring, such as in patients with Prader-Willi syndrome, other medications such as the opioid antagonist naltrexone (ReVia)[1] and sometimes the use of neuroleptics such as aripiprazole (Abilify)[1] and quetiapine (Seroquel)[1] can help to break the cycle of scratching and give time for behavioral treatments to take effect. After the patient has improved, medications can be tapered and discontinued, but he or she may need to stay on a maintenance dose of medications.

Prurigo Nodularis and Lichen Simplex Chronicus

PRURIGO NODULARIS

Clinically, prurigo nodularis (i.e., chronic circumscribed nodular lichenification or picker's nodules) is a chronic, severe itch accompanied by 1- to 5-cm, hard nodules with smooth or warty surfaces surrounded by hyperpigmentation. The new lesions are usually red and inflamed, whereas old lesions are pigmented. The lesions may also be excoriated. The lesions are mostly located in extensor surfaces of limbs, but they can be located on the face and trunk. Histopathologic evaluation shows lichenification, a dense infiltrate in dermis and neural hyperplasia, and proliferation of Schwann cells.

Computed tomography scans and chest radiographs are obtained if lymphoma is suspected.

Topical treatments with antipruritic creams are not very helpful. Potent topical steroids such as betamethasone dipropionate (Diprosone)[1] ointment under occlusion or intralesional injection of steroids such as triamcinolone acetonide (Kenalog-10)[1] may be successful, but they have the risk of skin atrophy. Topical capsaicin (0.025 to 0.1% Zostrix),[1] a component of red pepper, can help in the early stages.

[1]Not FDA approved for this indication.

[1]Not FDA approved for this indication.

For diffuse and resistant forms of prurigo nodularis, broadband and narrowband ultraviolet B (UVB) and ultraviolet A (UVA) can be effective. Narrowband UVB is more effective and has fewer side effects than UVA.

For resistant forms, cyclosporine (Sandimmune)[1] at the dosage of 4 mg/kg/day can help. It should be continued at least for 6 months (see Table 2).

Thalidomide (Thalomid)[1] at the dose of 200 to 400 mg in different studies has been an effective treatment for prurigo nodularis. It is difficult to obtain because of its teratogenicity, and it does have serious side effects, such as irreversible peripheral neuropathies. Naltrexone (ReVia),[1] an opioid antagonist, at the dosage of 50 mg/day is effective in some cases. Another treatment that had some success was the synthetic retinoid etretinate (Tegison), but it was removed from the U.S. market because of the high risk of birth defects.

Psychological intervention is important in breaking the itch/scratch cycle. Help can be obtained with techniques such as biofeedback, in which patients learn how to consciously control their autoimmune responses; hypnosis; cognitive-behavioral therapy; and supportive counseling.

Some psychotropic medications can help with excessive itching and compulsive scratching, including doxepin[1] (10 mg at bedtime, which can be increased up to 25 mg; the recommended dose for pruritus is lower than the dose for the treatment of depression, anxiety, or alcoholism, in which case it can be increased up to a maximum of 300 mg daily in divided doses); mirtazapine (Remeron)[1] (15 to 45 mg at night); and trazodone (50 to 400 mg at night). Doxepin is a tricyclic medication, and because it has the potential to cause cardiac arrhythmias, it should not be used in patients with recent myocardial infarction. Patients need to have periodic cardiovascular evaluations if they use tricyclic medications long term. Antidepressants should not be used in patients with bipolar disorder without a mood stabilizer because of the risk of triggering a manic episode.

LICHEN SIMPLEX CHRONICUS

Lichen simplex chronicus (i.e., circumscribed neurodermatitis) is characterized by lichenification of skin due to chronic, excessive scratching. Clinically, it appears as plaques of thickened skin with hyperpigmentation and accentuated skin lines. The most commonly affected areas are the occipital scalp, sides of the neck, ankles, genital areas, and extensor forearms. Itching is the main symptom. The histopathologic pattern in lichen simplex chronicus is different from that of prurigo nodularis and does not show the neural hyperplasia.

The physician must rule out underlying diseases that may cause pruritus. The treatment for lichen simplex chronicus is similar to that for prurigo nodularis. In addition to other treatments, topical tacrolimus (Protopic)[1] has been effective in some cases of lichen simplex chronicus.

Trichotillomania

Trichotillomania is partial hair loss caused by repeated hair pulling. Clinically, the patient has patches of alopecia with broken hair and different hair lengths without any inflammation of the scalp. The affected area has an unusual shape. A hair pull test result is negative. It can involve areas other than the scalp, and patients may pull hair in many sites. Trichotillomania occurs in any age group. In children, it is usually benign and self-limited, but in adults, it usually accompanies other psychopathologies and requires psychological intervention.

Trichotillomania is classified with impulse control disorders in the DSM-IV-TR. If a patient denies hair pulling, other causes of alopecia, especially alopecia areata, need to be ruled out.

In children, trichotillomania may occur during periods of increased stress, such as the arrival of a new sibling or parent's divorce. It is usually self-limited, and parents should be reassured.

In preadolescents and young adults, the diagnosis needs to be established first, followed by psychotherapeutic interventions; behavioral modification usually works well. Psychopharmacologic treatments should be reserved for last. Because of the FDA black box warning about the increased risk of suicide and suicidal behavior with use of antidepressants in children, adolescents, and young adults, these patients should be referred to a psychiatrist for medication, if needed.

In adults, trichotillomania often accompanies other psychopathology, and the treatment of the underlying illness helps to resolve the condition. Habit reversal therapy usually works better than negative feedback. Habit reversal therapy teaches the patient to monitor the behavior and the triggering factors and to replace the harmful habit with another habit. Working on increasing coping strategies for stress is also helpful. Relaxation and other stress-relief techniques are helpful, especially in patients with underlying anxiety. The Trichotillomania Learning Center (www.trich.org) is a good source of information for patients.

Psychotropic medications can be used if psychotherapy alone is not enough. Most reports of effective medications are based on open-label studies. Clomipramine (Anafranil)[1] at a dosage of 180 mg to 250 mg/day in a small, double-blind comparison with desipramine (Norpramin)[1] showed greater efficacy with a significant decrease in symptoms. There have been some open-label studies showing efficacy of fluoxetine (Prozac),[1] but this result was not reproduced in double-blind, placebo-controlled trials. Other SSRIs, such as sertraline (Zoloft),[1] fluvoxamine (Luvox),[1] and paroxetine (Paxil),[1] have shown efficacy in case reports and open-label studies. In some augmentation trials, adding haloperidol (Haldol),[1] pimozide (Orap),[1] or olanzapine (Zyprexa)[1] has been beneficial for patients taking fluoxetine or clomipramine. Small studies on using haloperidol or lithium (Eskalith) have shown some efficacy. Because of important side effects such as tardive dyskinesia with haloperidol and the narrow therapeutic window with lithium, it is best to leave these treatments to psychiatrists. Before these patients use antidepressants, it is important to screen them for bipolar disorder.

Cutaneous Sensory Disorders

Cutaneous sensory disorders are part of chronic pain syndromes, with pain occurring in different parts of the skin or mucous membranes. Disorders include burning mouth syndrome and vulvodynia (i.e., burning and itching of the vagina).

Burning mouth syndrome is a burning sensation that happens more frequently in middle-aged women. It affects the tongue more frequently, but other parts of the mouth also may be affected. It can be associated with dry mouth and a metallic taste in the mouth.

The physician should rule out local problems (e.g., dental disorders, allergic reactions, infection) and systemic problems (e.g., vitamin B, folate, iron, and zinc deficiencies; diabetes; autoimmune problems such as Sjögren's syndrome; nerve injury; problems related to antiretrovirals, antiseizure medications, hormones, and angiotensin-converting enzyme [ACE] inhibitors). The diagnosis needs a thorough physical examination and laboratory work-up, as well as screening for depression and anxiety. Mood problems may result from chronic pain issues.

The primary cause is treated. In idiopathic cases, therapy to help relaxation, instruction on coping skills, and biofeedback may help. There is no FDA-approved medication for this condition, but medications used to treat neuropathies may help. Gabapentin[1] can be started at 100 mg at night, for 3 days and gradually increased to 100 mg three times a day. The dosage can be adjusted to 300 to 600 mg three times a day as tolerated up to a maximum of 1800 mg. Tricyclics such as amitriptyline (Elavil) (10 to 35 mg PO at bedtime[1]) may increase every week to a maximum dosage of 150 mg/day. SNRIs such as venlafaxine (Effexor extended-release capsule)[1] can be given at a dosage of 37.5 mg in the morning with a gradual weekly increase to the maximum of 225 mg daily, and duloxetine (Cymbalta)[1] can be given as 60 mg daily. Clonazepam (Klonopin)[1] given

---

[1]Not FDA approved for this indication.

[1]Not FDA approved for this indication.

in small doses at night may help in some cases. Up to two thirds of patients report spontaneous partial recovery within 6 to 7 years of onset.

Vulvodynia is burning and pain in vulvar area. It should be evaluated by a gynecologist. Infectious, neoplastic, and inflammatory causes need to be ruled out. Depression and the impact on quality of life should be evaluated. Biofeedback and gabapentin[1] or amitriptyline[1] have been helpful in some cases. Depression and anxiety lower the pain threshold, and their treatment can help patients with chronic pain syndromes to better cope with their pain and have a higher pain threshold.

Medications for Pain and Itching

Some of the psychotropic medications can be used for various dermatologic conditions, such as urticaria or postherpetic neuralgia. The older tricyclic medications have specific effects on pain or itching.

When itching is the main symptom, doxepin[1] has a much higher affinity for histamine receptors than conventional antihistamines. It has a long half-life, and taking it once at night can control daytime itching. The effective antipruritic dosage is usually 10 to 25 mg at night, but it can be increased at weekly intervals as needed. Amitriptyline (Elavil)[1] works best for disorders with pain as the main symptom, such as burning mouth syndrome or postherpetic neuralgia. The usual dosage is 10 to 35 mg taken orally at bedtime, but it may be increased every week to a maximum dosage of 150 mg/day. Because tricyclic medications can affect cardiac conduction, patients need to have stable cardiovascular status and a normal electrocardiogram. Periodic testing is required during long-term treatment. These drugs should not be used with other medications that prolong the QT interval, such as cisapride (Propulsid).[2] They should not be prescribed during the immediate recovery period after myocardial infarction, and they should not be used at the same time as monoamine oxidase inhibitors. Patients need to be instructed to avoid driving due to drowsiness side effects of tricyclics.

Other medications can help with pain symptoms:

- Gabapentin is started at 100 mg at night, increased every 3 days to 300 mg at night, and then increased weekly to 900 to 1800 mg daily in three to four divided doses as tolerated.
- Pregabalin is started with 50 mg taken orally three times daily and increased to 100 mg three times daily within 1 week based on efficacy and tolerability. If patients with postherpetic neuralgia do not experience sufficient pain relief in 2 to 4 weeks and are tolerating the medication well, the dosage can be increased to 300 mg twice daily or 200 mg three times daily (600 mg/day).
- SNRIs such as duloxetine (60 mg daily) have FDA approval for diabetic neuropathy and fibromyalgia.[1]
- Venlafaxine,[1] which has a mechanism of action similar to that of duloxetine at the dosage of 37.5 mg in the morning, with a gradual weekly increase to the maximum of 225 mg daily, may help pain symptoms, but it is not FDA approved for pain treatment.
- There are some reports that SSRIs can help pain symptoms.

REFERENCES

Epocrates database. Available at http://www.epocrates.com [accessed September 19, 2009].
Grant JE, Odlaug BL, Kim SW. Lamotrigine treatment of pathologic skin picking: An open-label study. J Clin Psychiatry 2007;68:1384–91.
Koo JY, Lee CS. Psychocutaneous Medicine. New York: Marcel Dekker; 2003.
Koo JY, Lee CS. Psychocutaneous diseases. In: Bolognia JL, Jorizzo JL, Rapini RP, editors. Dermatology. 2nd ed. Philadelphia: Elsevier; 2008.
Koo JY. Psychotropic agents in dermatology. Dermatol Clin 1993;11:215–24.
Lotti T, Buggiani G, Prignano F. Prurigo nodularis and lichen simplex chronicus. Dermatol Ther 2008;21:42–6.
Micromedex database. Available at http://www.micromedex.com/products/ under Physicians Drugdex® System [accessed May 13, 2009].
Sah DE, Koo J, Price V. Trichotillomania. Dermatol Ther 2008;21:13–21.

---

[1]Not FDA approved for this indication.
[2]Not available in the United States.

Shafii M, Shafii SL. Exploratory psychotherapy in the treatment of psoriasis. Twelve hundred years ago. Arch Gen Psychiatry 1979;36:1242–5.
Shah M. Burning mouth syndrome. In: Ferri FF, editor. Ferri's Clinical Advisor. St Louis: Mosby; 2009.

Acne Vulgaris and Rosacea

Method of
Steven R. Feldman, MD, PhD, and
Alan B. Fleischer, Jr., MD

Acne and rosacea are common conditions that share a propensity to cause red follicular papules of the face. Nonetheless, they are distinct disorders.

Acne is associated with comedones, a noninflammatory plugging of follicular orifices. Comedones may become inflamed, at least partially due to the inflammatory activity induced by the action of bacterial skin flora (*Pityrosporum* species) on lipids produced by sebaceous glands. There is a distinct tendency toward development of acne nodules with scarring.

The pathogenesis of rosacea is less well understood. Vascular dilatation and inflammation are important components of the process, with prominent flushing and blushing. Although telangiectasia can become permanent, scarring is rare. Another feature distinguishing rosacea from acne is a tendency for ocular involvement.

Acne Vulgaris

CLINICAL FEATURES

Acne is a common disorder of teenagers and young adults but occurs in middle age as well. The manifestations of acne are diverse. The face is characteristically involved, and the upper trunk is involved in some patients. The individual lesions can consist of comedones, inflammatory papules, pustules, and deeper inflammatory nodules mistakenly termed *cysts*. There might or might not be resulting scarring. Genetics contributes to the pattern of involvement. Environmental exposures seem less important, although some oil-based cosmetic products can induce acne comedones.

TREATMENT

Treatments for acne address several different components of the pathogenesis of the disorder. Topical retinoids appear to have a primary effect on normalizing keratinization of the follicular ostia, reducing comedones and inflammatory papules and pustules. Topical and oral antibiotics reduce bacteria counts on the skin and can have intrinsic anti-inflammatory activity. Hormonal treatments in women reduce the production of sebaceous gland lipids. Oral retinoids (isotretinoin in particular), the most effective therapy for acne, reduces sebaceous gland activity as well.

There are no well-established evidence-based guidelines for acne treatment. There are, however, generally accepted patterns of treatment based on the type and extent of the clinical lesions. At its simplest, topical retinoids are the foundation of treatment because of their effect on comedones, the primary lesion of acne, as well as their effect on inflammatory acne papules and pustules. With increasing microbial resistance, retinoid agents work independently of direct effects on skin flora and are excellent long-term agents. Topical antibiotics, prescribed singly, in combination with antimicrobial products, or in combination with topical retinoids, are used for superficial inflammatory lesions. Oral antibiotics are used when the inflammation and potential scarring are more severe. Hormonal treatment (in the form of oral contraceptives) is used for female patients when the acne is unresponsive to both topical retinoids and topical and oral antibiotics or if there are menstrual abnormalities that suggest the acne is secondary to a primary hormonal process.

Topical Retinoids

Topical retinoids are used for nearly all patients with acne because of their comedolytic effect and their activity on papules and pustules, as well as to spare the use of antibiotics in an age of growing antibiotic resistance. The first topical retinoid was topical tretinoin (Retin-A). It is available in cream, gel, solution, and newer slow-release particle vehicles. The main side effect of topical retinoids is the potential for drying and irritation of the skin. This is less of a problem with lower strengths of topical tretinoin (0.025% and 0.05% cream) and more of a problem with the stronger strengths (0.01% and 0.025% gel and the 0.1% cream). The drying effect may be beneficial for patients who feel their skin is too oily.

Topical tretinoin is easily oxidized and photodegraded. With the growing use of benzoyl peroxide as an anti-acne treatment, there is greater concern about the lability of topical tretinoin. Stabilized tretinoin in the form of microsphere (Retin A Micro 0.04% and 0.1%) and in the combination with clindamycin 1.2% (Ziana) have both been demonstrated to be stable in the presence of benzoyl peroxide. Topical adapalene (Differin) gel or cream can be used as an alternative. It is equally effective as tretinoin, but it has far less potential to cause irritation. Less irritation can lead to greater compliance. It also is a robust molecule that is stable when combined with other agents, including benzoyl peroxide. Topical tazarotene (Tazorac) is another retinoid that is more effective than tretinoin and adapalene, but it is much more irritating than the other agents.

Adapalene and tazarotene may be used at any time of the day, but tretinoin should be used at night because of its photodegradation. This recommendation probably started with topical tretinoin because of the potential for photoinactivation of tretinoin.

Topical Antimicrobial Agents

The most widely used topical antimicrobial agent is benzoyl peroxide. This biocide is available in a wide variety of inexpensive and expensive over-the-counter and prescription acne products. Benzoyl peroxide is very effective at reducing bacterial counts on the skin, and it is probably far more effective than the traditional topical antibiotics such as erythromycin (Akne-Mycin), clindamycin (Cleocin), and sulfacetamide (Klaron).

Benzoyl peroxide (in 2.5%–10% formulations) is often used in conjunction with topical retinoids or with other topical antibiotics. Combined use of benzoyl peroxide with topical erythromycin (Benzamycin) or clindamycin (BenzaClin) helps prevent development of bacterial strains resistant to the antibiotics. A combined benzoyl peroxide–erythromycin product was once widely used, but it needed to be kept refrigerated, and had a short shelf life. Newer benzoyl peroxide–clindamycin preparations (Acanya, Benzaclin, Duac) are more stable, can be used once or twice daily, and have excellent efficacy. A combination of 2.5% benzoyl peroxide plus 0.1% adapalene (Epiduo Gel) is more effective than either of its components and provides an option for simplifying the treatment regimen in patients who would otherwise require separate topical antimicrobial and retinoid products.

All benzoyl peroxide products bleach clothing, bed linens, and towels. Not all vehicles are appropriate for all patients, and excellent vehicle choices can enhance compliance and clinical outcomes.

Topical azelaic acid is a useful adjunct, especially in the 15% gel formulation (Finacea). It is antimicrobial and antiinflammatory, and it can promote pigmentary normalization. Azelaic acid can be simultaneously combined with many other agents and does not appear to be subject to microbial resistance.

A combination clindamycin–tretinoin product is now available in the United States (Ziana). Topical dapsone (Aczone) (has also been approved by the FDA but is not currently marketed) has recently entered the market as the first new molecule approved for treating acne. In an elegant and nonirritating vehicle this product is a useful antiinflammatory adjunct to other treatment. Sulfacetamide is occasionally used and many forms are available (e.g., Klaron), either alone or combined with precipitated sulfur. Sulfacetamide and dapsone chemically react with benzoyl peroxide, and these two agents should not be used simultaneously with a stay on benzoyl peroxide preparation.

Oral Antibiotics

Oral antibiotics remain widely used for acne, sometimes for short courses, other times for more prolonged periods. There are growing efforts to limit the course of these drugs in order to limit side effects and antibiotic resistance. Commonly used antibiotics include tetracycline (Sumycin), doxycycline (Doryx), minocycline (Dynacin), and erythromycin.

Of these, minocycline may be the most effective, although it has potential for uncommon and rare side effects. Common side effects include vestibular symptoms; rare ones include altered cutaneous pigmentation and lupus-like syndromes. Minocycline, in extended-release tablets (Solodyn), is the only FDA-approved antibiotic for acne treatment and has fewer vestibular side effects than other agents. This agent has an established dose-response relationship and is most effective with least toxicity at 1 mg/kg/day. It is available in 45-mg, 90-mg, and 135-mg doses.

None of the tetracycline agents should be used during pregnancy or in children younger than 12 years, because tetracycline can stain developing teeth. Erythromycin may be used in these situations; however, there are often poor gastrointestinal tolerance and marginal efficacy. Other antibiotics such as cephalexin (Kelex),[1] ampicillin,[1] or trimethoprim-sulfamethoxazole (Bactrim)[1] are alternatives that are occasionally used.

Birth Control Pills

Oral contraceptives are somewhat effective antiacne treatments that can be used in women. Three products (Tri-Cyclen, Estrostep, and Yaz) are FDA approved for the treatment of acne. The former two are combinations of norethindrone acetate and ethinyl estradiol, although other formulations are probably also effective. Yasmin and Yaz, for instance, have an effective antiandrogenic agent, drospirenone, combined with the ethinyl estradiol. Oral contraceptives should be considered as a treatment for moderate to severe acne in women (along with topical agents and oral antibiotics) before isotretinoin is used. If effective, it can spare the need to expose a woman of childbearing potential to the teratogenic isotretinoin. If this approach is not effective, the woman will already be taking an oral contraceptive when isotretinoin is started.

Isotretinoin

Isotretinoin (Accutane, Sotret, and others) is a highly effective oral agent that can cure even very severe acne. It is given in doses of 0.5 to 2.0 mg/kg/day for 4 to 5 months. It is a potent teratogen and must be used with great caution in women of childbearing potential. Although evidence is lacking, it has been reported to cause depression in rare instances, and true informed consent is required. Other potential side effects include hair loss, decreased night vision, xerophthalmia, epistaxis, cheilitis, xerosis, arthralgias, hepatic dysfunction, and elevated cholesterol and triglycerides. Oral retinoids should not be used in conjunction with tetracycline agents because of the possible increased risk of pseudotumor cerebri.

Behavioral Issues

Perhaps the most important environmental exposure affecting acne is behavioral: patients' tendency to pick at their acne lesions, resulting in excoriation, infection, and scarring. Psychological fixation on facial appearance is not uncommon. Patients often perceive that their follicular ostia (pores) are too large. They can manipulate their skin,

---

[1]Not FDA approved for this indication.

resulting in excoriated lesions that mimic acne. This type of acne is not uncommon and is termed acne excoriée. The severity and extent of the lesions vary. Some patients have few lesions, others have many with considerable scarring.

Treatment of acne excoriée is difficult. Some patients respond to the suggestion that they "are spreading the infection by manipulating the skin," For other patients with more severe psychological issues, oral psychotropic medication and psychotherapy may be warranted.

Another key factor affecting outcomes of acne treatment is adherence. Patients' adherence to even short-term oral medication regimens is often poor. Adherence to topical treatment is generally worse, and adherence to chronic topical treatment is probably severely limited. Involvement of the patient in treatment planning, choosing regimens of limited complexity, and psychological interventions to promote better adherence can lead to improved treatment outcomes. Whenever possible, agents that can be administered in combination and may be used once daily are likely to promote compliance and increase efficacy.

Rosacea

DIAGNOSIS AND DIFFERENTIAL DIAGNOSIS

Rosacea is a common cause of a red face in adults. It must be distinguished from other conditions causing a red face, particularly seborrheic dermatitis, irritant dermatitis, and lupus. Seborrheic dermatitis, another common condition, is typically more scaly than rosacea. Seborrheic dermatitis involves the scalp (a cause of dandruff), eyebrows, nasal bridge, nasolabial and melolabial folds, and central chest. Rosacea does not typically have scale or scalp involvement of seborrhea and typically involves the cheeks and nose, sparing the fold in between. Irritant dermatitis may be confused as well, because rosacea patients report burning and stinging. Lupus is a far less common disorder and may be associated with scarring lesions of the face or a malar pattern of erythema.

CLASSIFICATION

Rosacea is divided into four subtypes, papulopustular, erythematotelangiectatic, phymatous, and ocular. Papulopustular rosacea responds best to topical and oral therapies, ocular disease responds best to oral therapy, and erthematotelangiectatic and phymatous types respond best to physical modalities. None of these subtypes or treatment modalities is mutually exclusive. Rosacea patients with papulopustular and erythematotelangiectatic subtypes should receive counseling about gentle cleansing and use of moisturizers and sunscreens, because these improve outcomes.

TREATMENT

Topical Antibiotics

Most patients with papulopustular rosacea benefit from topical antibiotic therapies. There are three agents in widespread use: metronidazole, azelaic acid, and sodium sulfacetamide and sulfur preparations. Metronidazole is widely used and is available in gel, lotion (Metrolotion), and cream (Metrocream) for twice-daily use at 0.75%, and cream (Noritate) and gel (Metrogel) for once-daily use at 1%. The gel vehicle is likely the preferred for facial use, and this is a generally well-tolerated agent. The 1% product offers the advantage of single daily dosing. Some patients report mild irritation from the use of these agents. Topical azelaic acid 15% (Finacea) gel is more effective than metronidazole gel 0.75%, but appears to be equal in effectiveness to metronidazole 1% gel. Like metronidazole, it can cause mild irritation and appears slightly more irritating than metronidazole.

Sodium sulfacetamide and sulfur compounds are available as washes and topical gels and may be additional agents that can improve outcomes in treating rosacea. One product, with sodium sulfacetamide 10% and 5% sulfur with sunscreen (Rosac) was found to be at least as effective as metronidazole cream 0.75%. Small reports of the efficacy of topical clindamycin and erythromycin appear in the dermatology literature.

As with acne therapy, combinations of topical agents are more effective than monotherapy. Thus, combinations of metronidazole, azelaic acid, and sodium sulfacetamide and sulfur compounds in various combinations and permutations improve outcomes. Most patients, when counseled about appropriate use of combinations of products, with good soap-free cleansing and moisturizing products, can tolerate these agents.

Oral Antibiotics

Oral tetracycline agents are commonly used to treat rosacea. Some employ antimicrobial doses such as tetracycline 500 mg twice daily or doxycycline 100 mg twice daily. Then the dose is tapered to the lowest dose that maintains control of the disease. A sub-antimicrobial dose doxycycline product (Oracea) has been FDA approved as a rosacea treatment. This product reduces the inflammation of rosacea and can help prevent development of organisms resistant to the antibiotic. When oral therapies are employed, efficacy of topical therapies is increased, which can decrease the need for or duration of the systemic agent.

Isotretinoin

Isotretinoin is an effective agent in treating papulopustular rosacea, and lower doses than those employed for acne can be highly effective. With increasing difficulty in using isotretinoin due to the iPLEDGE program, physicians might find other therapeutic alternatives more appealing.

Physical Modalities

Although there has been a report of a series of patients with erythematotelangiectatic rosacea responding well to azelaic acid 15% gel, most patients are likely to require optical vascular destructive modalities, including vascular laser or intense pulsed light. These approaches often require multiple treatment sessions, but they do decrease erythema, flushing and blushing, and telangiectasia. Phymatous disease responds well to surgical approaches, including use of high-frequency electrosurgery with a wire loop, CO_2 laser, or scalpel surgery.

REFERENCES

Gollnick H, Cunliffe W, Berson D, et al. Global Alliance to Improve Outcomes in Acne: Management of acne: A report from a Global Alliance to Improve Outcomes in Acne. J Am Acad Dermatol 2003;49(1 Suppl.):S1–37.

James WD. Clinical practice. Acne. N Engl J Med 2005;352(14):1463–72.

Leyden JJ, Shalita A, Thiboutot D, et al. Topical retinoids in inflammatory acne: A retrospective, investigator-blinded, vehicle-controlled, photographic assessment. Clin Ther 2005;27(2):216–24.

Leyden JJ, Thiboutot DM, Shalita AR, et al. Comparison of tazarotene and minocycline maintenance therapies in acne vulgaris: A multicenter, double-blind, randomized, parallel-group study. Arch Dermatol 2006;142(5):605–12.

Margolis DJ, Bowe WP, Hoffstad O, Berlin JA. Antibiotic treatment of acne may be associated with upper respiratory tract infections. Arch Dermatol 2005;141(9):1132–6.

Ozolins M, Eady EA, Avery AJ, et al. Comparison of five antimicrobial regimens for treatment of mild to moderate inflammatory facial acne vulgaris in the community: Randomised controlled trial. Lancet 2004;364 (9452):2188–95.

Sanchez J, Somolinos AL, Almodovar PI, et al. A randomized, double-blind, placebo-controlled trial of the combined effect of doxycycline hyclate 20-mg tablets and metronidazole 0.75% topical lotion in the treatment of rosacea. J Am Acad Dermatol 2005;53(5):791–7.

Thevarajah S, Balkrishnan R, Camacho FT, et al. Trends in prescription of acne medication in the U.S.: Shift from antibiotic to non-antibiotic treatment. J Dermatolog Treat 2005;16(4):224–8.

Diseases of the Hair

Method of
Shannon Harrison, MBBS, MMed, Melissa Piliang, MD, and Wilma Bergfeld, MD

Hair loss can involve hair shedding by the root (Table 1), hair fragility and breakage (Table 2), and thinning or loss of density of the scalp hair (Table 3). Other symptoms of hair disease include scalp pruritus, erythema, scaling, and burning. Hair diseases can affect hair at body sites other than the scalp. The diagnosis of a hair disease requires an accurate and detailed patient history and clinical examination. The clinician must be familiar with normal hair biology to correctly understand hair loss disorders.

TABLE 1 Main Causes of Diffuse Hair Loss or Shedding

Acute telogen effluvium
Chronic telogen effluvium
Early pattern hair loss
Alopecia areata*
Anagen hair loss
    Chemotherapeutic agents
    Heavy metal or chemical poisoning

*Can have telogen or anagen hair loss.

TABLE 2 Main Causes of Hair Fragility and Breakage

Acquired trichodystrophies
Inherited trichodystrophies
Traction alopecia
Trichotillomania
Tinea capitis
Central centrifugal cicatricial alopecia

TABLE 3 Main Causes of Hair Thinning

Pattern hair loss
Telogen effluvium
Anagen effluvium
Alopecia areata
Traction alopecia
Trichotillomania
Scarring alopecias
Tinea capitis

Hair Growth

Normally, 80% of the scalp hair follicles are in an active growth phase called anagen, which lasts 2 to 8 years unless a disease process intervenes. At the end of the anagen, the hair follicles involute during the catagen phase and then enter telogen, the resting phase. Telogen has a duration of 2 to 3 months, and approximately 100 hairs per day are shed normally. With each new anagen phase, hair stem cells form the new hair follicle. The hair stem cells are found in the permanent region of the hair follicle called the bulge. Injury or inflammation to the stem cells leads to a permanent cicatricial (scarring) alopecia. Other types of hair loss are nonscarring (noncicatricial), such as telogen effluvium, pattern hair loss, and alopecia areata.

CURRENT DIAGNOSIS

- Hair shedding
- Hair thinning
- Hair fragility and breakage
- Scarring versus nonscarring patterns
- Diffuse versus localized areas of loss
- Other hair-bearing sites affected
- Inflammatory versus noninflammatory changes
- Associated acne, seborrhea, and hirsutism
- Associated skin or nail abnormalities

CURRENT THERAPY

- Observation is needed for anagen hair loss.
- Identification and removal or correction of the trigger is essential in telogen effluvium.
- For male pattern hair loss, topical minoxidil 5% (Rogaine Extra Strength for Men) twice daily and finasteride (Propecia) 1 mg daily are the treatment options.
- For female pattern hair loss, topical minoxidil 2% (Rogaine) twice daily is the only FDA-approved therapy, but off-label treatments include spironolactone (Aldactone) and cyproterone acetate (Androcur).[2]
- Treatment options for alopecia areata include topical and intralesional corticosteroids. Topical therapies such as minoxidil 5%[1] and anthralin[1] are available, and the topical sensitizer diphenylcyclopropenone (DPCP)[4] has been used.
- Topical and intralesional corticosteroids are the mainstay of treatment for most scarring alopecias.
- Damaging hair care practices should be avoided in cases of hair shaft disorders and traction alopecia.
- Some patients may require referral for hairpieces, wigs, or hair transplantation.

[1]Not FDA approved for this indication.
[2]Not available in the United States.
[4]Not yet approved for use in the United States.

Hair Disorders

ANAGEN EFFLUVIUM

Anagen hair shedding results from the sudden reduction of division of the hair follicle matrix during anagen, leading to narrowing and breakage of the hair with hair loss. The hair loss occurs several days to weeks after injury to the hair. Irradiation and antimitotic agents used in chemotherapy can precipitate anagen effluvium. The scalp hair is usually most affected, but body hair can be involved. Heavy metal and boric acid ingestion can manifest with anagen hair loss. Alopecia areata also can manifest as anagen hair loss and is important to recognize. Anagen hair loss manifests with diffuse scalp alopecia, and hair growth starts again within weeks of cessation of the injury. Treatment of anagen effluvium is usually observation because the cause will be clear from the patient's history, and removal of the cause leads to regrowth.

TELOGEN EFFLUVIUM

Telogen hair shedding results from disruption in the normal hair cycle. A trigger or stress prompts rapid conversion of a group of anagen hairs to prematurely enter telogen, and these hairs shed 2 to 3 months later. Up to 300 hairs per day can be shed, and diffuse scalp hair thinning can be seen. The hair pull test can be positive for telogen hairs. Possible triggers include childbirth, surgery, crash dieting, serious illness, stress, and hormonal imbalance. Certain medications and local scalp inflammation can also precipitate telogen hair shedding. If telogen hair shedding persists for longer than 6 months, it is called *chronic telogen effluvium*. Chronic systemic diseases, thyroid disease, and nutritional deficiencies can cause chronic telogen hair shedding. Any repetitive or ongoing trigger can cause chronic telogen hair loss. Idiopathic chronic telogen effluvium is chronic, diffuse telogen hair shedding without identifiable triggers and with no widening of the midline scalp part, and it requires exclusion of other causes of chronic telogen hair loss.

Blood tests are needed to exclude other causes and identify contributing causes of hair loss (Table 4). A complete blood cell (CBC) count, a comprehensive metabolic panel, and iron studies (including

TABLE 4 Hair Loss Investigations

Men	Women
Complete blood cell count	Complete blood cell count
Iron studies	Iron studies
Ferritin level	Ferritin level
TSH level	TSH level
T_4 level	T_4 level
Thyroid autoantibodies*	Thyroid autoantibodies*
Zinc level*	Zinc level
DHEAS level*	Testosterone level
DHT level*	DHEAS level
	SHBG level
CMP*	CMP
	ANA level*
Syphilis serology*	Syphilis serology*

*If clinically warranted.
Abbreviations: ANA = antinuclear antibody; CMP = comprehensive metabolic panel; DHEAS = dihydroepiandrostenedione sulfate; DHT = dihydrotestosterone; SHBG = sex hormone–binding globulin; T_4 = thyroxine; TSH = thyroid-stimulating hormone.

a ferritin level) can identify iron deficiency anemia, renal disease, or liver disease. Determinations of thyroid-stimulating hormone (TSH) and thyroxine (T_4) levels can diagnose thyroid disease, and a zinc level can define zinc deficiency. Histologic assessment shows no miniaturization of the scalp hair follicles but does show an increase in telogen hair follicles.

If the trigger of acute telogen effluvium is corrected, shedding is self-limited. A detailed medical history is essential to accurately identify the triggers. Any underlying systemic disease should be treated. A multivitamin[1] and biotin[7] and zinc supplementation[7] can support hair regrowth. Topical minoxidil 2% (Rogaine)[1] or 5% (Rogaine Extra Strength for Men)[1] may be helpful for promoting hair regrowth.

PATTERN HAIR LOSS

Pattern hair loss (PHL), or androgenetic alopecia, occurs in men and women. It is thought that genetically susceptible hair follicles miniaturize under the influence of androgens and that the duration of anagen decreases, leading to an overall reduction in hair density. In women, the role of androgens is uncertain. Some patients (men more than women) have a family history positive for PHL. Patients complain of a thinning hair density, and particularly in women, telogen hair shedding can herald PHL. In men, PHL occurs over the bifrontotemporal and vertex areas. Rarely, men experience a female type of PHL. In women, the hair loss is a diffuse thinning over the crown in a pattern with or without frontal accentuation. Women can infrequently experience a male-type pattern of loss with frontal and bitemporal recession. Associated signs of androgen excess should be identified in women.

The diagnosis of male PHL is usually straightforward. If clinically warranted, thyroid function tests and a CBC count should be performed. In some men with early-onset PHL, dihydroepiandrostenedione sulfate (DHEAS) and dihydrotestosterone levels may be elevated (Bergfeld WF, personal communication, 2009) and may reflect a gene carrier state for polycystic ovarian syndrome (see Table 4). In women with PHL, screening blood tests should include a CBC count; comprehensive metabolic panel; levels of TSH, T_4, and zinc; and iron studies with a ferritin level. Androgen levels should be determined, including the total or free testosterone level, sex hormone–binding globulin concentration, and DHEAS level, to exclude androgen excess disorders (see Table 4). Two 4-mm scalp

[1]Not FDA approved for this indication.
[7]Available as a dietary supplement.

biopsies with horizontal and vertical sectioning are sometimes needed to confirm the diagnosis of female PHL and exclude chronic telogen effluvium and diffuse alopecia areata. Histologic assessment of PHL demonstrates miniaturization of terminal hairs into vellus hairs.

Tinted powders, wigs, hairpieces, and hair transplantation are PHL treatment options. Pharmacologic treatment of PHL in men consists of the FDA-approved therapies of topical 5% minoxidil twice daily or finasteride (Propecia) 1 mg daily. Neither therapy corrects baldness, but treatment is aimed at maintaining the density of the remaining hair. Long-term use is needed to maintain this benefit, and 12 months is required to determine response to treatment.

For women, the only FDA-approved treatment for PHL is topical 2% minoxidil applied twice daily. The 5% minoxidil is not FDA-approved for women, but it is more effective and more likely to cause facial hypertrichosis. Antiandrogens are also used as off-label treatments in women with PHL. The treatment response to antiandrogens may be different for women with biochemical evidence of androgen excess and those with PHL without androgen excess, but studies are limited. Spironolactone (Aldactone)[1] is an antiandrogen that can be used at 100 to 200 mg daily for treatment of female PHL. Potassium levels should be monitored with spironolactone use. Cyproterone acetate (Androcur)[2] is available in Europe as an antiandrogen for female PHL. Finasteride[1] has not been shown to be effective in postmenopausal women with female PHL. With any antiandrogen treatment, women of childbearing years must be using an effective contraceptive method because of the risk of feminization of a male fetus. Oral contraceptive pills with low levels of androgenic progestins such as gestodene[2] and norgestimate (Ortho-Cyclen)[1] or oral contraceptives containing drospirenone (Yaz, Yasmin)[1] are useful for female PHL (Harrison S, unpublished data, 2008).

ALOPECIA AREATA

Alopecia areata is thought to be a multifactorial autoimmune disease. Some patients report a positive family history. Alopecia areata also clusters with other autoimmune conditions such as Hashimoto's thyroiditis, vitiligo, and diabetes mellitus. The common presentation is a single, round patch of alopecia with visible follicular openings reflecting the nonscarring nature of this type of hair loss. It may affect any hair-bearing area of the body. Alopecia areata can progress and involve multiple patches or cause total scalp (i.e., alopecia totalis) and body hair loss (i.e., alopecia universalis). The hair pull test result may be positive at the patch margin, and exclamation mark hairs may be seen. Some patients have nail changes such as pitting or trachyonychia. Blood testing can identify possible autoimmune associations (see Table 4).

No cure exists for alopecia areata. Treatment for a single patch or multiple patches of alopecia areata is a potent topical corticosteroid or intralesional corticosteroid. Intralesional injections are not preferred in patients younger than 10 to 12 years because of the pain of injection. Intralesional steroid suspension (triamcinolone acetonide [Kenalog-10] 10 mg/mL) can be placed in small injections (0.1 mL) into each active site every 6 to 8 weeks. The maximum intralesional corticosteroid should not exceed a total of 10 to 20 mg per visit. With more severe disease, topical anthralin 0.5% or 1.0% (Dritho-scalp 0.5%, Drithocreme 1%)[1] or topical 5% minoxidil[1] may be useful. Topical anthralin as a short contact therapy is especially helpful in children younger than 10 years. Application is done daily for 10 to 30 minutes, increasing the time slowly over 2 weeks until a mild erythema and pruritus are achieved. Topical minoxidil has obtained cosmetically acceptable regrowth in some patients. Use of diphenylcyclopropenone (DPCP),[1] the topical contact sensitizer, is also effective in some patients, with reported hair growth rates of 4% to 85%. At the initial visit, the patient is sensitized to 2% DPCP. After 2 weeks, a low concentration of 0.001% is applied to the scalp. This concentration is incrementally increased slowly over time until mild erythema and pruritus are obtained. Adverse side effects with DPCP therapy are contact allergic dermatitis, pruritus, and

lymphadenopathy. Systemic treatment with oral corticosteroids or cyclosporine is arguable because of their side effect profiles. Biologic therapies have been unsatisfactory.

TRACTION ALOPECIA

Repetitive traction forces on the hair from tight braiding, ponytails, or rollers can cause hair loss and breakage. The repeated hairstyle should be ceased.

TRICHOTILLOMANIA

Trichotillomania is a compulsive disease of hair pulling. Incomplete linear areas of alopecia occur with broken hairs of different lengths. Psychotherapy and psychiatric medication are needed.

TINEA CAPITIS

Tinea capitis is a fungal infection of the hair follicles with *Trichophyton* or *Microsporum*. It manifests as a scaly, pruritic patch of scalp hair loss or, rarely, as a kerion. Diagnosis is made by microscopy of scalp scrapings and hair clippings with potassium hydroxide (KOH) and fungal culture. A systemic antifungal agent is required along with an antifungal shampoo. Griseofulvin (Grifulvin V) is the only FDA-approved treatment for tinea capitis, and absorption is increased with a fatty meal. Micronized griseofulvin 20 to 25 mg/kg/day[1] or ultramicronized griseofulvin (Gris-PEG)[3] 15 to 20 mg/kg/day (off-label doses) is the treatment of tinea capitis for 6 to 8 weeks. Other antifungal agents, such as terbinafine (Lamisil) and itraconazole (Sporanox), have been used off-label.

CICATRICIAL ALOPECIAS

Scarring (cicatricial) alopecias result in permanent hair loss, and hair follicle openings are no longer visible on the scalp. Primary scarring alopecias have been classified by the North American Hair Research Society.

Lichen planopilaris (LPP) is thought to be an autoimmune disease. It manifests with erythematous patches of scarring alopecia with scaling, follicular plugging, and burning or pruritus. LPP is associated with other autoimmune diseases. Discoid lupus erythematosus manifests as scarring areas of hair loss with erythema, dyspigmentation, telangiectasia, scale, and follicular plugging. Treatment for both conditions involves potent topical corticosteroids, such as clobetasol 0.05% (Olux Topical Foam)[1] twice daily or serial intralesional corticosteroids. Antidandruff and antifungal shampoos such as 1% zinc pyrithione (e.g., Selsun Salon Shampoo) and 1% ketoconazole (Nizoral A-D Shampoo) can be used to remove scale. Off-label use of tetracycline, retinoids, and antimalarials has been reported.

Central centrifugal cicatricial alopecia in African American women is likely related to traumatic hair care practices. Treatment involves avoidance of these practices and the use of potent topical corticosteroids daily or serial intralesional corticosteroids weekly for 6 to 8 weeks (Harrison S, unpublished data, 2008).

Folliculitis decalvans and dissecting folliculitis of the scalp manifest with inflammatory papules, pustules, and scarring with a tufted folliculitis. Treatment involves long-term antibiotics, and off-label isotretinoin (Accutane) can be helpful. Folliculitis keloidalis manifests with alopecia, papules, pustules, and hypertrophic scarring. Treatment involves topical or intralesional corticosteroids. Off-label isotretinoin and laser hair removal have been effective in some cases. Secondary causes of scarring alopecia can include infections and malignancies. Any new area of scarring hair loss with an infiltrated plaque requires a biopsy.

HAIR SHAFT DISORDERS: TRICHODYSTROPHIES

Hair shaft disorders may be hereditary or acquired conditions. Hereditary hair shaft disorders are uncommon. Acquired trichodystrophy is commonly seen in women who use perming, coloring,

---

[1]Not FDA approved for this indication.
[2]Not available in the United States.

---

[1]Not FDA approved for this indication.
[3]Exceeds dosage recommended by the manufacturer.

and straightening procedures, damaging the hair shafts and causing fragile hair that is prone to breakage. Nonforceful handling and conditioners are important, as is avoidance of detrimental hair practices.

Acknowledgment

Dr. Harrison was funded by the F. C. Florance Bequest, administered by the Australasian College of Dermatologists for 2008.

REFERENCES

Bergfeld WF, Elston DM. Cicatricial alopecia. In: Olsen EA, editor. Disorders of Hair Growth: Diagnosis and Treatment. 3rd ed. New York: McGraw-Hill; 2003. p. 363–98.

Bergfeld WF. Telogen effluvium. In: McMichael MK, Hordinsky M, editors. Hair and Scalp Diseases: Medical, Surgical and Cosmetic Treatments. New York: Informa Healthcare; 2008. p. 119–35.

Carey AH, Chan KL, Short F, et al. Evidence for a single gene effect causing polycystic ovaries and male pattern baldness. Clin Endocrinol 1993; 38:653–8.

Cotsarelis G, Millar S, Chan EF. Embryology and anatomy of the hair follicle. In: Olsen EA, editor. Disorders of Hair Growth: Diagnosis and Treatment. 3rd ed. New York: McGraw-Hill; 2003. p. 23–48.

Fiedler VC, Gray AC. Diffuse alopecia: Telogen hair loss. In: Olsen EA, editor. Disorders of Hair Growth: Diagnosis and Treatment. 3rd ed. New York: McGraw-Hill; 2003. p. 303–20.

Harries MJ, Sinclair RD, MacDonald-Hull S, et al. Management of primary cicatricial alopecias: Options for treatment. Br J Dermatol 2008;159: 1–22.

Headington JE. Telogen effluvium—New concepts and review. Arch Dermatol 1992;129:356–63.

Kligman AM. Pathologic dynamics of human hair loss, I. Telogen effluvium. Arch Dermatol 1961;83:175–98.

Loo DS. Systemic antifungal agents: An update of established and new therapies. Adv Dermatol 2006;22:101–24.

Madani S, Shapiro J. Alopecia areata update. J Am Acad Dermatol 2000;42:549–66.

Olsen EA, Messenger AG, Shapiro J, et al. Evaluation and treatment of male and female pattern hair loss. J Am Acad Dermatol 2005;52:301–10.

Olsen EA, Bergfeld WF, Cotsarelis G, et al. for the Workshop on Cicatricial Alopecia. Summary of North American Hair Research Society (NAHRS)–sponsored Workshop on Cicatricial Alopecia, Duke University Medical Center, February 10 and 11, 2001. J Am Acad Dermatol 2003; 48:103–7.

Paus R, Cotsarelis G. The biology of hair follicles. N Engl J Med 1999;341:491–7.

Price VH, Roberts JL, Hordinsky M, et al. Lack of efficacy of finasteride in postmenopausal women with androgenetic alopecia. J Am Acad Dermatol 2000;43:768–76.

Price VH, Hordinsky MK, Olsen EA, et al. Subcutaneous efalizumab is not effective in the treatment of alopecia areata. J Am Acad Dermatol 2008;58:395–402.

Roberts JL, DeVillez RL. Infectious, physical and inflammatory causes of hair and scalp abnormalities. In: Olsen EA, editor. Disorders of Hair Growth: Diagnosis and Treatment. 3rd ed. New York: McGraw-Hill; 2003. p. 87–122.

Rook A, Dawber R. Diffuse alopecia: Endocrine, metabolic and chemical influences on the follicular cycle. In: Rook A, Dawber R, editors. Diseases of the Hair and Scalp. Oxford, UK: Blackwell Science Publications; 1982. p. 115–45.

Sah DE, Koo J, Price V. Trichotillomania. Dermatol Ther 2008;21:13–21.

Sinclair R, Grossman KL, Kvedar JC. Anagen hair loss. In: Olsen EA, editor. Disorders of Hair Growth: Diagnosis and Treatment. 3rd ed. New York: McGraw-Hill; 2003. p. 275–302.

Strober B, Siu K, Alexis A, et al. Etanercept does not effectively treat moderate to severe alopecia areata: An open label study. J Am Acad Dermatol 2005;52:1082–4.

Wasserman D, Guzman-Sanchez DA, Scott K, et al. Alopecia areata. Int J Dermatol 2007;46:121–31.

Whiting DA. Chronic telogen effluvium: Increased scalp hair shedding in middle-aged women. J Am Acad Dermatol 1996;35:899–906.

Whiting DA. Traumatic alopecia. Int J Dermatol 1999;38:34–44.

Whiting DA. Hair shaft defects. In: Olsen EA, editor. Disorders of Hair Growth: Diagnosis and Treatment. 3rd ed. New York: McGraw-Hill; 2003. p. 123–75.

Cancer of the Skin

Method of
Yaohui G. Xu, MD, PhD, Humza Ilyas, MD, and Stephen N. Snow, MD

Nonmelanoma skin cancer (NMSC), mainly composed of basal cell carcinoma (BCC) and squamous cell carcinoma (SCC), is the focus of discussion of this chapter; melanoma is covered elsewhere. NMSC is the most common cancer in humans. The exact incidence of NMSC is difficult to obtain because of inconsistent data collection. Nevertheless, the incidence continues to increase worldwide, which surpasses the annual incidence of all other cancers combined. More than 1 million cases of NMSC are diagnosed in the United States each year, and approximately one of five Americans will develop NMSC in their lifetime.

Ultraviolet (UV) radiation exposure superimposed on genetic predisposition plays the most important role in the development of BCC and SCC. BCC is related to intermittent, recreational sun exposure, and SCC is associated with cumulative UV exposure. The gene most often altered in BCC is the tumor suppressor gene *PTCH1*, followed by *TP53*, another tumor suppressor gene. Mutations in *TP53* are the most common genetic abnormalities in SCC. Fitzpatrick skin type (e.g., pale skin that is highly subject to burns) and the status of the host immune system are other well-recognized risk factors for both cancers. In lightly pigmented populations, BCC accounts for approximately 80% of all NMSCs. Among darkly pigmented individuals, the incidence of BCC and SCC is almost equal. Compared with the general population, organ transplant recipients on long-term immunosuppression therapy have a 40- to 250-fold and 5- to 10-fold greater incidence of developing SCC and BCC, respectively. Less common risk factors for SCC include exposure to ionizing radiation (e.g., radiation therapy), chronic ulcers, burn scars, exposure to arsenic and coal tar derivatives, and several oncogenic strains of human papillomavirus (HPV), most commonly HPV-16, -18, -31, and -33.

Patients with certain genetic disorders, in whom an essential repair mechanism to correct UV damage at the molecular level is missing, have an increased incidence of NMSC, with numerous lesions occurring at a young age. Examples include basal cell nevus syndrome, albinism, xeroderma pigmentosa, and epidermolysis bullosa. Like organ transplant recipients, these patients are extremely challenging to manage.

Clinical Characteristics and Diagnosis

CLINICAL FEATURES OF BASAL CELL CARCINOMA

BCC, the most common type of skin cancer with an unknown precursor lesion, has a predilection for the sun-exposed, follicle-bearing skin, most commonly on the face. It is often an asymptomatic, slow-growing lesion. As it grows and ulcerates, it may manifest with tenderness or bleeding.

Many subtypes of BCC exist, but nodular BCC is the most common variant, accounting for 60% of all BCCs. A nodular BCC typically manifests as a pearly, translucent papule or nodule with overlying telangiectasia, a central hemorrhagic crust, and a rolled border. A pigmented variant of nodular BCC may resemble melanoma. Superficial BCC is the second most common subtype, and it occurs more often on the trunk and extremities. It manifests as an erythematous and scaly macule, patch, or thin plaque that is clinically inseparable from actinic keratosis, early SCC, or a dermatitis-like inflammatory lesion. Less common subtypes of BCC include morpheaform (often with increased collagen deposition that clinically resembles a scar), cystic (often a bluish gray papule with a clear,

BOX 1 High-Risk Tumors Indicated for Mohs Micrographic Surgery

- Large tumor size (>2 cm at a low-risk site, such as the trunk and extremities; >1 cm at a medium-risk site such as the cheeks, forehead, neck, and scalp)
- Tumor of any size in a high-risk site or in functionally and cosmetically unique areas (e.g., nose, ears, eyelids, lips)
- Aggressive histologic subtype (e.g., morpheaform, micronodular, or basosquamous subtypes of basal cell carcinoma; invasive squamous cell carcinoma >4 mm deep)
- Poor clinical margins
- Recurrent lesions
- Tumors with increased risk of distant metastasis (e.g., squamous cell carcinoma at the site of ulcer, scar, or chronic inflammation)
- Positive perineural, perifollicular, or perivascular invasion

mucin-filled center), fibroepithelioma of Pinkus (often a pedunculated, pink plaque), basosquamous, and micronodular forms. The latter two subtypes are diagnosed histologically rather than clinically.

BCC tends to grow very slowly and has an extremely low metastatic rate (<0.005%). However, if not treated appropriately, it can cause local destruction of subcutaneous fat, muscle, nerve, cartilage, and bone. BCC should be stratified as a high-risk or low-risk tumor for optimized management (Box 1).

CLINICAL FEATURES OF SQUAMOUS CELL CARCINOMA

SCC, the second most common type of skin caner, is derived from keratinocytes. SCC in situ is also known as Bowen's disease, which may arise de novo or from a precancerous lesion of actinic keratosis. It most commonly manifests as an erythematous and scaly patch or as a thin plaque that is sometimes crusted and keratotic. It typically develops on the sun-damaged skin of the head, neck, upper trunk, and extremities, and it can be difficult to distinguish clinically from BCC. A helpful hint for differentiating SCC from BCC is that SCC usually appears more solid than translucent and does not have a pearly border with overlying telangiectasia. SCC also tends to develop in the background of actinic keratosis.

As SCC in situ evolves into invasive SCC, it becomes an erythematous, ulcerated nodule or plaque with a hyperkeratotic crust that often bleeds with minor friction. Variants of SCC include a pigmented form and a verrucous form. Bowenoid papulosis refers to a lesion of condyloma acuminata that shows histologic features of SCC in situ. Erythroplasia of Queyrat is SCC in situ, and it is found on the uncircumcised penis as a bright red, eroded plaque with well-defined borders. Marjolin's ulcer is a term used when SCC occurs in a chronic ulcer or scar. Keratoacanthoma is a sharply circumscribed, erythematous nodule

CURRENT DIAGNOSIS

- Nonmelanoma skin cancers (NMSCs), mainly basal cell carcinomas (BCCs) and squamous cell carcinomas (SCCs), commonly occur on sun-exposed skin.
- NMSCs often have characteristic clinical features. BCC typically is described as a pearly, telangiectatic papule with a central ulceration and rolled border; SCC often is described as an erythematous, scaly, keratotic patch or thin plaque.
- Histopathologic examination of a skin biopsy specimen is essential for confirming the diagnosis and for optimizing management.

or tumor with a central keratotic crater that has rapidly formed over a few weeks. Lesions of keratoacanthoma may regress spontaneously over weeks to months. However, some may continue to grow, and rare examples of metastasis have been reported. Keratoacanthoma is best viewed as a well-differentiated subtype of SCC and is managed as such.

Although the overall risk of metastasis for SCC is low (≈2%), it often progresses more quickly and has an increased risk for distant metastasis compared with BCC. As with BCC, high-risk lesions of SCC need to be recognized and evaluated for an appropriate treatment choice (see Box 1).

Management of Nonmelanoma Skin Cancer

Management of NMSC is schematically illustrated in Figure 1. A high index of clinical suspicion is encouraged when lesions resembling BCC or SCC are identified. The examiner should consider pertinent history, such as the rate of growth of the lesion, prior therapy, prior cancer, sunburn history, family history of cancer, local neurologic symptoms, and evidence of immunosuppression.

A thorough skin examination focuses on the patient's skin type and the lesion's size, location, border (well delineated or poorly defined), and possible connection to underlying structures and adjacent skin. Skin biopsy is essential for confirming the diagnosis and optimizing management. Skin biopsy with a shave technique or a deep shave (i.e., saucerization) is usually sufficient to obtain adequate depth for histologic examination. If the area is flat or depressed, as with morpheaform BCC, a punch biopsy may be preferred to sample sufficient depth.

Local and regional lymph nodes should be routinely examined in patients with NMSC, particularly in patients with high-risk tumors of SCC (see Box 1). Lymph nodes are the most common sites of metastasis. Clinically enlarged lymph nodes should be further investigated by imaging tests or fine-needle aspiration, or both, as deemed necessary.

Many treatments are known to be effective for NMSC. A careful assessment of the relative risk of recurrence for an individual lesion is helpful in selecting treatment. Tumors are stratified as high- and low-risk lesions (see Box 1). Lower-risk tumors usually can be treated with topical therapy, destructive modalities, and excision, whereas high-risk tumors are better suited for Mohs micrographic surgery and radiation therapy. Options such as intralesional interferon

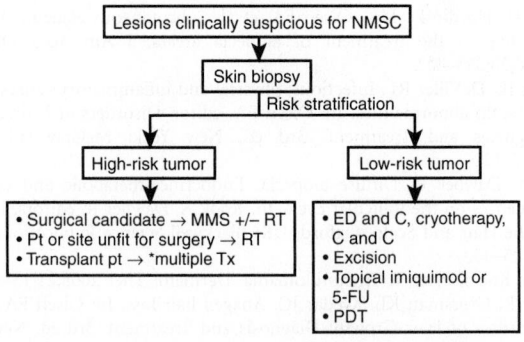

FIGURE 1. Simplified diagram of the management of nonmelanoma skin cancer. A multidisciplinary approach (*multiple Tx) and combinational therapies are often needed for transplant patients (pt). Systemic retinoids can be used to reduce the risk of nonmelanoma skin cancer (NSMC); topical therapy with imiquimod or 5-fluorouracil (5-FU) or photodynamic therapy (PDT) to reduce the tumor burden; electrodesiccation and curettage (ED&C), curettage and cryotherapy (C&C), or excision for individual low-risk tumors; and Mohs micrographic surgery (MMS) or radiation therapy (RT), or both, for individual high-risk tumors.

CURRENT THERAPY

Topical Therapy

- Imiquimod (Aldara) and fluorouracil (Efudex 5%) are noninvasive modalities that provide excellent cosmesis.
- Topical modalities are appropriate for small, superficial basal cell carcinomas and squamous cell carcinomas in situ that are not in areas at high risk for disease recurrence.

Destructive Methods

- Electrodesiccation and curettage, cryotherapy with liquid nitrogen, and curettage and cryotherapy are methods of blind destruction that are fast, inexpensive, and highly effective for treating low-risk nonmelanoma skin cancers (NMSCs) on the trunk and extremities.
- Tumor debulking by curettage is combined with topical imiquimod or photodynamic therapy for increased efficacy.

Surgical Excision

- Standard elliptical excision with predetermined (4- to 5-mm) margins is an ideal choice for low-risk tumors.
- Mohs micrographic surgery has the highest cure rate for NMSCs and is recommended for high-risk tumors.

Photodynamic Therapy

- Topical photodynamic therapy using 5-aminolevulinic acid (ALA) is used for low-risk, superficial NMSCs or for high-risk lesions when more effective modalities are contraindicated or unacceptable to patients.
- Photodynamic therapy has limited efficacy for thicker tumors and is associated with a high recurrence rate in these cases.

Radiation Therapy

- Side effects and cost limit the usefulness of radiation therapy to high-risk NMSCs in patients who are older than 50 years and not surgical candidates.
- Radiation is used as adjuvant therapy after surgery for aggressive NMSCs with perineural invasion or nodal metastases.
- Radiation therapy is contraindicated for recurrent NMSCs arising in previously irradiated areas.

alfa-2b (Intron A)[1] injection and ablative laser for low-risk NMSC offer no real advantage and therefore are not commonly employed. Common treatment methods are described in the following sections.

TOPICAL THERAPY

5-Fluorouracil

Topical 5-fluorouracil (5-FU) is an antimetabolite that causes tumor death by interfering with DNA synthesis in actively dividing cells. Topical 5-FU (Efudex 2% solution, 5% solution or 5% cream, and Carac 0.5% cream) is primarily indicated for actinic keratoses. The 5% strength (Efudex 5% cream or solution) is an effective noninvasive treatment for superficial BCCs when conventional methods are impractical, such as with multiple lesions, sites with difficult accessibility for surgery, or patients unable to tolerate more aggressive procedures. 5-FU is used off-label for SCC in situ in similar circumstances. Typically, it is used twice daily for 3 to 6 weeks. It may take 10 to 12 weeks to eliminate the lesion. Small case series have

demonstrated that this regimen provides a histologic clearance rate of about 92%. Patients need to be counseled on expected local irritation and inflammation, including erythema, erosions, itching, burning, soreness, scaling, and swelling. The treated area typically heals without scarring a few weeks after treatment.

Imiquimod

Imiquimod (Aldara 5% cream) is a topical immunomodulator that is effective against virus-infected cells and cancer cells. It mainly promotes innate and acquired immune responses through binding to cell surface toll-like receptors TLR7 and TLR8. Imiquimod has been approved by the FDA for the treatment of external genital warts, actinic keratoses, and superficial BCC. It is indicated for small (<2 cm), primary, superficial BCC in immunocompetent patients, excluding lesions on the face, anogenital skin, hands, and feet. The recommended dosing for superficial BCC is application for 5 days per week for 6 weeks, and studies have proved that this regimen provides an 88% histologic clearance rate. As with topical 5-FU, patients should be counseled regarding expected local irritation and inflammation, and rest periods are recommended if there is excessive inflammation.

Imiquimod has also been tested off-label for other types of NMSCs, including SCC in situ and nodular BCC. Monotherapy of imiquimod for nodular BCC is not recommended because of its inferior success rate (mid-70% range). However, it has demonstrated effectiveness as an adjuvant therapy after debulking curettage. The use of 5-FU and imiquimod for superficial NMSCs is summarized in Table 1.

PHOTODYNAMIC THERAPY

Photodynamic therapy is a novel and minimally invasive topical modality that shows promise in managing actinic keratoses, superficial BCC, and SCC in situ. A topically administered photosensitizing compound such as the porphyrin 5-aminolevulinic acid (ALA) or the methyl ester of ALA (mALA) preferentially accumulates within the tumor cell, subsequently is activated by a proper light source in the 450- to 750-nm wavelength range, and generates reactive oxygen species, causing apoptosis and cell death. Patients experience stinging, burning, and itching. Cosmesis after healing is usually excellent. The depth of penetration of the photosensitizing agent has limited its effectiveness against thicker tumors and the recurrence rate with this technique is high, necessitating close clinical follow-up.

DESTRUCTIVE METHODS

Cryotherapy Using Liquid Nitrogen

Liquid nitrogen is a cryogen with a boiling point of $-196°C$. When administered using a cryogen-spray device, cell death occurs through rapid crystal formation intracellularly and extracellularly. Melanocytes are very sensitive to freezing, which explains why cryotherapy often results in hypopigmentation. Rapid cooling and slow thawing cycles have proved to be more effective. As a blind destructive method with no histologic examination, cryotherapy is typically used for benign growths and premalignant lesions. It is also used for low-risk NMSCs with well-defined borders in elderly or debilitated patients when cosmesis is less of a concern. To be effective, the tumor tissue must reach a temperature of $-50°C$, which can be ensured by using a thermocouple device inserted into the center of the tumor. Local anesthetic is often needed. Patients must be informed that scarring and hypopigmentation often result from this treatment. The reported 5-year cure rates for BCC and SCC treated by cryosurgery are 93% and 96%, respectively.

Electrodesiccation and Curettage

Electrodesiccation and curettage provide another method of blind destruction under local anesthesia and are typically used to treat superficial NMSCs with a low risk of recurrence on the trunk and extremities. This is feasible because of a textural difference between tumor cells and the surrounding normal tissue. A curette is used to scrape in three directions over the lesion plus a 3-mm margin until

---

[1]Not FDA approved for this indication.

TABLE 1 Topical Treatments for Selected Superficial Basal Cell Carcinoma and Squamous Cell Carcinoma In Situ

Drug (Brand Name)	Mechanism	Application	Side Effects	Special Care Measures	Contraindication
5-Fluorouracil (Efudex 5%)	Topical chemotherapy	bid × 3–6 wk, may need 10–12 wk	Local irritation and inflammation	Wash hands after use. Use petrolatum or topical corticosteroid if too inflamed.	Allergic reaction, pregnancy, DPD deficiency
Imiquimod (Aldara)	Topical immunomodulator	Superficial BCC: 5 ×/wk × 6 wk SCC in situ: qd × 16 wk	Local irritation and inflammation	Wash hands after use. Apply to lesion plus 1-cm margin. Use overnight for 8 h.	Allergic reaction

Abbreviations: DPD = dihydropyrimidine dehydrogenase enzyme; NMSC = nonmelanoma skin cancer.

the friable tumor tissue is removed. The wound bed is then electrodesiccated to cause necrosis of cells. The same process is repeated for a total of three cycles, and the wound is allowed to heal by second intention, which occasionally results in a hypertrophic scar. This method is not suitable for tumors extending into the fat because the textural difference is lost, for tumors with a high risk of recurrence, and for patients with pacemakers or defibrillators. Overall, the 5-year cure rates for primary BCC and SCC treated with electrodesiccation and curettage are 92% and 96%, respectively.

Curettage and Cryotherapy

Modified from electrodesiccation and curettage, treatment with curettage and cryotherapy refers to the method in which cryotherapy instead of electrodesiccation is used after debulking tumor tissue with a curette.

SURGICAL TREATMENT

Standard Elliptical Excision

Standard surgical excision with a predetermined margin and performed under local anesthesia is the most common treatment for NMSCs. Tissue is submitted in formalin for histopathologic examination. It is best suited for primary lesions with well-defined borders and a low risk of recurrence. Usually, the tumor is removed with a 4–5-mm margin, and 95% of primary low-risk tumors are adequately excised by this method. The wound is closed in an elliptical fashion for best cosmesis. This typically creates a scar two to three times longer than the size of original tumor. Recurrent tumors are best treated with Mohs micrographic surgery, because the cure rates offered by standard surgical excision decrease to 83% and 77% for recurrent BCC and SCC, respectively.

Mohs Micrographic Surgery

Mohs micrographic surgery provides the highest cure rate and best tissue preservation, and it is recommended for high-risk NMSCs, as summarized in Box 1. Using the Mohs technique, the excised tumor tissue is mapped, immediately processed by frozen section in an en face fashion, and analyzed microscopically. Contiguous tumor spread, as occurs in BCC and SCC, is a prerequisite for using this technique. In contrast to traditional vertically orientated histopathology sections, which assess less than 1% of the tumor margin, 100% of peripheral and deep margins of the specimen are examined by the surgeon using the Mohs method. The tumor is removed layer by layer. Any area with remaining tumor indicated by tissue mapping is removed precisely, until a tumor-free plane is reached with the greatest degree of tissue sparing. With confidence, the surgeon can repair the wound with appropriate reconstructive methods, including primary closure, flaps, or grafts. In complicated cases in which deeper structures are involved, the patient may be referred to a plastic surgeon for reconstruction.

Mohs micrographic surgery remains the most effective method for removing NMSCs, with a 5-year recurrence rate of 1% for BCC and 3% for SCC, compared with recurrence rates of 5.3% and 8%, respectively, for standard excision. Although the cost of Mohs micrographic surgery is higher than standard excision, a reduction in tumor recurrence decreases the total cost associated with potential repeat treatment.

RADIATION THERAPY

Several factors have limited the use of radiation therapy to highly selected NMSC cases, such as elderly individuals (>50 years old) who are unable to withstand extensive surgery or when a large wound from surgical excision would be too disfiguring. It also provides adjuvant therapy for surgery in cases of aggressive NMSC with perineural invasion or nodal metastases. Radiation is usually delivered in fractionated doses over a period of several weeks. It is time consuming and is five to eight times more expensive than standard excision. Patients may develop acute radiation dermatitis and late side effects of depigmentation, atrophy, and telangiectasia. Ionizing radiation is also a known risk factor for SCC. Patients with tumors with ill-defined borders; those with tumors on the lower legs, feet, hands, or genitalia; those with tumors arising in previously irradiated areas; and patients with genodermatoses such as basal cell nevus syndrome or xeroderma pigmentosa are unsuitable for radiation therapy. Recurrent and infiltrative NMSCs show decreased responsiveness to radiation therapy. The 5-year cure rates for primary, small (<2 cm) BCC and SCC are 90% to 93%, which is comparable to responses to other treatment methods.

PROPHYLACTIC THERAPY IN TRANSPLANT RECIPIENTS

Oral retinoids, represented by acitretin (Soriatane),[1] are derivatives of vitamin A that are used as chemopreventative agents in reducing the risk of NMSC in transplant recipients or other selected high-risk patients. They function primarily through induction of apoptosis and stimulation of cell differentiation. Another promising treatment is the new generation of immunosuppressants, represented by sirolimus (Rapamune), formerly known as rapamycin.[1] Unlike cyclosporine (Sandimmune, Neoral), which increases the incidence of NMSC in transplant recipients, sirolimus inhibits skin carcinogenesis and reduces the incidence of NMSC in these patients.

Follow-up and Prevention

All patients with a history of NMSC deserve close clinical follow-up for possible recurrence or new lesions at 6 to 12 months after treatment. A shorter follow-up period may be tailored to individual

---

[1]Not FDA approved for this indication.

patients at high risk for recurrence or those with the need for repeat therapy. Patients need to be educated on self-examination of the skin and about sun precautions, which can be achieved by avoiding intense UV exposure, wearing sun-protective clothing and a hat, and applying broad-spectrum sunscreen effective for both UVB and UVA radiation.

REFERENCES

Cox NH, Eedy DJ, Morton CA. Guidelines for management of Bowen's disease, 2006 update. Br J Dermatol 2007;156:11–21.

National Comprehensive Cancer Network (NCCN). Clinical practice guidelines in oncology for basal cell and squamous cell skin cancers, V.I, Available at: http://www.nccn.org/professionals/physician_gls/PDF/nmsc.pdf [accessed May 20, 2009].

Neville JA, Welch E, Leffell DJ. Management of nonmelanoma skin cancer in 2007. Nat Clin Pract Oncol 2007;4:462–9.

Telfer NR, Colver GB, Morton CA. Guidelines for the management of basal cell carcinoma. Br J Dermatol 2008;159:35–48.

Cutaneous T-Cell Lymphomas, Including Mycosis Fungoides and Sézary Syndrome

Method of
Gary S. Wood, MD

Cutaneous T-Cell Lymphomas

CLASSIFICATION

Virtually every subtype of T-cell lymphoma involves the skin primarily or secondarily. The principal types of primary cutaneous T-cell lymphomas (CTCLs) recognized in the World Health Organization and European Organization for Research and Treatment of Cancer classification include mycosis fungoides (MF) and its leukemic variant, the Sézary syndrome (SS); CD30$^+$ large cell lymphoma; CD30$^-$ large cell lymphoma; and pleomorphic CD4$^+$ small or medium cell variants (Table 1). All other primary CTCLs comprise only a few percent of the total. This discussion focuses on MF and SS because they account for up to 75% of primary cutaneous cases.

TABLE 1 Classification of Primary Cutaneous T-Cell Lymphomas

CTCL Type	Proportion of Primary CTCLs (%)	5-Year Survival Rate (%)
MF and variants	70	85
SS	<5	<50*
CD30$^+$ large cell	13	90
CD30$^-$ large cell	7	15
Pleomorphic small/medium cell	4	60
Miscellaneous	<1	Variable

*The 5-year survival rate depends on the criteria used to define SS, and it may be as low as 10%.
Abbreviations: CTCL = cutaneous T-cell lymphoma; MF = mycosis fungoides; SS = Sézary syndrome.

CURRENT DIAGNOSIS

For Cutaneous T-cell Lymphomas, Obtain the Following:

- History: duration and pace of lesion development
- Skin examination: extent of patches, plaques, tumors, and ulcers
- Extracutaneous examination: status of lymph nodes, liver, and spleen
- Laboratory: complete blood cell count, differential, and lesional biopsy results
- Imaging: CT or fused PET/CT scans of the chest, abdomen, and pelvis (not needed for early stage mycosis fungoides)

Standard Diagnosis and Staging Methods

The evaluation of CTCL patients begins with a thorough clinical history and physical examination. Key elements of the history include the pace and nature of disease development, the presence or absence of spontaneous regression of lesions, prior therapy, and ingestion of drugs (e.g., anticonvulsants, antihistamines, other agents with antihistaminic properties) that have been associated with pseudolymphomatous skin eruptions that can mimic CTCLs. The review of systems should establish the presence of lymphoma-associated constitutional symptoms (e.g., fever of unknown origin, night sweats, weight loss, fatigue). In addition to general aspects, the physical examination should document the type and distribution of skin lesions and whether there is lymphadenopathy, hepatosplenomegaly, or edema of extremities (i.e., potential sign of lymphatic obstruction).

Histopathologic analysis of representative lesional skin biopsy specimens is the primary means of confirming the clinical diagnosis. Biopsy specimens should be deep enough to include the deepest portions of the cutaneous lymphoid infiltrates because these areas often exhibit the most diagnostic features. Putative extracutaneous involvement should be confirmed by biopsy if it is relevant to clinical management.

Routine blood tests include a complete blood cell count, differential review, and general chemistry panel. A "Sézary prep" is used to assess peripheral blood involvement.

Internal nodal and visceral involvement by lymphoma usually is assessed with chest radiography, computed tomography (CT), or combined positron emission tomography and CT (PET/CT) scans of the chest, abdomen, and pelvis. These radiologic studies usually are not needed for patients with early forms of MF (i.e., nontumorous skin lesions without evidence of extracutaneous involvement assessed by physical examination); however, they are usually obtained during the work-up of other types of CTCLs. The role of immunopathologic and molecular biologic assays in the diagnosis and staging of CTCLs is discussed later.

An algorithm for the diagnosis of early MF has been proposed by the International Society for Cutaneous Lymphomas (ISCL) (see Pimpinelli et al. in References). It relies on a combination of clinical, histopathologic, immunopathologic, and clonality criteria. This differs from former approaches that have been based primarily on histopathologic criteria.

Mycosis Fungoides, Sézary Syndrome, and Variants

CLINICAL FEATURES

MF classically manifests as erythematous, scaly, variably pruritic, flat patches or indurated plaques, often favoring the most sun-protected areas. The patches or plaques may progress to cutaneous tumors and involvement of lymph nodes or viscera, although this usually does not occur as long as the skin lesions are reasonably well controlled by therapy. SS manifests as total-body erythema and scaling (i.e., erythroderma), generalized lymphadenopathy, hepatosplenomegaly, and leukemia. Large-plaque parapsoriasis is essentially the prediagnostic patch phase of MF. Lesions may exhibit poikiloderma (i.e., atrophy, telangiectasia, and mottled hyperpigmentation and hypopigmentation) and have then been referred to as *poikiloderma atrophicans vasculare*.

Follicular mucinosis refers to a papulonodular eruption in which hair follicles are infiltrated by T cells and contain pools of mucin. In hairy areas, this may result in alopecia. Follicular mucinosis may exist as a lesional variant of MF (i.e., follicular MF) or as a clinically benign entity (i.e., alone or associated with other lymphomas).

Granulomatous slack skin is a variant of MF that manifests with pendulous skin folds in intertriginous areas. Lesional skin biopsy specimens contain atypical T cells in a granulomatous background.

Pagetoid reticulosis manifests as a solitary or localized, often hyperkeratotic plaque containing atypical T cells that are frequently confined to a hyperplastic epidermis. Some authorities regard it as a variant of unilesional MF, whereas others think it is a distinct entity.

Other variants of MF include hypopigmented, palmoplantar, bullous, and pigmented purpuric forms. The latter form shows clinicopathologic overlap with the pigmented purpuric dermatoses. *Tumor d'emblée* MF is an outmoded concept used in the past to refer to supposed cases of MF that manifested as cutaneous tumors in the absence of patches or plaques. Most experts now prefer to classify such cases as other forms of CTCL, depending on their histopathologic features.

HISTOPATHOLOGIC AND CYTOLOGIC FEATURES

A well-developed plaque of MF contains a bandlike, cytologically atypical lymphoid infiltrate in the upper dermis that infiltrates the epidermis as single cells and cell clusters known as Pautrier's microabscesses. The atypical lymphoid cells exhibit dense, hyperchromatic nuclei with convoluted, cerebriform nuclear contours and scant cytoplasm. The term *cerebriform* comes from the brainlike ultrastructural appearance of these nuclei. In more advanced cutaneous tumors, the infiltrate extends diffusely throughout the upper and lower dermis and may lose its epidermotropism. In the earlier patch phase of the disease, the infiltrate is sparser, and lymphoid atypia may be less pronounced. In some cases, it may be difficult to distinguish early patch-type MF from various types of chronic dermatitis. The presence of lymphoid atypia and absence of significant epidermal intercellular edema (i.e., spongiosis) help to establish the diagnosis of early MF.

Involvement of lymph nodes by MF begins in the paracortical T-cell domain and may progress to complete effacement of nodal architecture by the same types of atypical lymphoid cells that infiltrate the skin. These cells can be seen in low numbers in the peripheral blood of many MF patients; however, those with SS develop gross leukemic involvement, usually defined as at least 1000 tumor cells/mm^3. These cells are known as Sézary cells, and they are traditionally detected by manual review of the peripheral blood smear (the so-called Sézary prep). They may also be defined by various immunophenotypic criteria.

IMMUNOPHENOTYPING

Cellular antigen expression is usually assessed by immunoperoxidase methods for tissue biopsy specimens and by flow cytometry for blood specimens. Almost all cases of MF or SS begin as phenotypically and functionally mature CD4$^+$ T-cell neoplasms of skin-associated lymphoid tissue (SALT). They express the SALT-associated homing molecule cutaneous lymphocyte antigen (CLA) and most mature T-cell surface antigens, with the exceptions of CD7 and CD26, which are often absent. As disease progresses, the tumor cells often dedifferentiate and lose one or more mature T-cell markers, such as CD2, CD3, or CD5.

Cases typically express the α/β form of the T-cell receptor. At least in advanced cases, the cytokine profile is consistent with the T$_H$2

subset of CD4$^+$ T cells (i.e., production of interleukin [IL]-4, IL-5, and IL-10 rather than T$_H$1 cytokines such as IL-2 and interferon-γ). Expression of the high-affinity IL-2 receptor (CD25, TAC) ranges widely, with most cases showing a variable minority of lesional CD25$^+$ cells. Tumor cells can be induced to express a regulatory T-cell phenotype (Treg) in vitro. MF cases that express CD8$^+$ or other aberrant phenotypes occur occasionally but behave like conventional cases. They should not be confused with rare aggressive CTCLs exhibiting cytotoxic T-cell differentiation.

In addition to tumor cells, MF and SS lesions contain a minor component of immune accessory cells (i.e., Langerhans cells and macrophages) and CD8$^+$ T cells with a cytolytic phenotype. This presumed host response correlates positively with survival and tends to decrease as lesions progress. A favorable response to therapy such as photopheresis appears to correlate with normal levels of circulating CD8$^+$ cells.

MOLECULAR BIOLOGY

Well-developed MF or SS is a monoclonal T-cell lymphoproliferative disorder. Southern blotting or polymerase chain reaction (PCR) assays demonstrate monoclonal T-cell receptor gene rearrangements. The greater sensitivity of PCR assays allows the demonstration of dominant clonality in many early patch-type lesions of MF. These assays sometimes detect dominant clonality in lesional skin showing only chronic dermatitis histopathologically. These cases are called *clonal dermatitis* and may represent the earliest manifestation of MF because several have progressed to histologically recognizable MF within a few years. However, some cases of clinicopathologically defined early-phase MF lack a detectable monoclonal T-cell population until later in their clinical course.

In addition to aiding initial diagnosis, gene rearrangement analysis has facilitated staging and prognosis. Because some patients without MF or SS can have low levels of circulating Sézary-like cells and because not all cases of peripheral blood involvement in MF or SS exhibit morphologically recognizable tumor cells, the demonstration of dominant clonality that matches the clone in lesional skin has proved to be a useful diagnostic adjunct. The same holds true for assessing lymph node involvement. T-cell receptor gene rearrangement analysis of MF and SS lymph nodes is more sensitive than histopathology and possesses at least some prognostic relevance.

TNMB STAGING

Although several proposed methods have used a weighted extent approach to more accurately determine the MF or SS tumor burden, the preferred approach is the TNMB system, which is detailed in Tables 2 and 3. The original tumor (skin), lymph nodes, and metastasis (visceral organs) version of this system has been modified by the ISCL to incorporate the extent of blood involvement (B classification) into the staging process. Table 2 shows the TNMB classification relevant to MF and SS, and Table 3 shows how this information is used to determine the stage of disease. The prognostic relevance of this staging system has been supported by numerous studies, and use of the TNMB helps to guide the selection of therapies. For example, early-stage MF is the most amenable to control with topically directed treatments, whereas advanced MF or SS with extracutaneous involvement usually requires systemic therapies or topical plus systemic combinations.

TREATMENT

Rather than cure, which is attained in less than 10% of cases, the goal of MF and SS therapy is to reduce the impact of the skin disease on quality of life. For most patients, this is achieved by reducing pain, itch, and infection and improving clinical appearance. Appearance is affected by the disfigurement of the eruption and by the profound degree of scale shedding in some patients. Because the natural history of early-stage MF predicts a virtually normal life span, the goal of treatment must be directed at quality of life. For more advanced stages, prolongation of life expectancy may be a reasonable treatment goal.

TABLE 2 TNMB Classification of Mycosis Fungoides and Sézary Syndrome

Skin (T)

T1	Patches and/or plaques; <10% body surface area
T2	Patches and/or plaques; ≥10% body surface area
T3	Tumors with/without other skin lesions
T4	Generalized erythroderma

Lymph Nodes (N)

N0	Not clinically enlarged; histopathology not required
N1	Clinically enlarged; histopathologically negative
N2	Clinically enlarged; histopathologically equivocal
N3	Clinically enlarged; histopathologically positive

Visceral Organs (M)

M0	No involvement
M1	Involvement

Peripheral Blood (B)

B0	Atypical cells ≤5% of leukocytes
B1	Atypical cells >5% of leukocytes
B2	Atypical cells ≥1000/mm^3

TABLE 3 TNMB Staging System for Mycosis Fungoides and Sézary Syndrome

Stage	Skin	Lymph Nodes	Viscera	Blood
IA	T1	N0	M0	B0–1
IB	T2	N0	M0	B0–1
IIA	T1–2	N1–2	M0	B0–1
IIB	T3	N0–2	M0	B0–1
IIIA	T4	N0–2	M0	B0
IIIB	T4	N0–2	M0	B1
IVA-1	T1–4	N0–2	M0	B2
IVA-2	T1–4	N3	M0	B0–2
IVB	T1–4	N0–3	M1	B0–2

Modified from Olsen E, Vonderheid E, et al: Revisions to the staging and classification of mycosis fungoides and Sézary syndrome: A proposal of the International Society for Cutaneous Lymphomas (ISCL) and the cutaneous lymphoma task force of the European Organization of Research and Treatment of Cancer (EORTC). Blood 2007;110(6):1713–1722.

Regardless of presentation, relief of symptoms should be addressed early. For dryness and scaling, the use of emollient ointments is indicated. These include petrolatum, Aquaphor, and commercially available shortening such as Crisco (an inexpensive alternative).[1] For modest dryness, creams (e.g., Nivea, Cetaphil, Eucerin) can be adequate and more acceptable to patients. Mild superfatted soaps such as Dove and Oil of Olay are recommended. Soap substitutes such as Cetaphil are also acceptable. Pruritus can be addressed with oral agents such as hydroxyzine (Atarax) or diphenhydramine (Benadryl)[1] 2 to 5 mg/kg/day and divided into four daily doses. Antipruritics work better when used on a regular basis rather than on an as-needed basis. Nonsedating antihistamines tend to be less effective. Measures to reduce dryness also help to reduce pruritus. Secondary infection needs to be treated with appropriate antibiotics. Their selection is guided by results of skin cultures but usually involves coverage of gram-positive organisms.

Phototherapy

Two main phototherapeutic regimens are used to treat CTCLs. Ultraviolet B radiation (290–320-nm broad band or 311-nm narrow

band) can be used for patients with patches but not those with well-developed plaques or tumors. Seventy percent of patients achieve total clinical remission, usually within about 3 to 5 months. Another 15% achieve partial remission. Narrow-band UVB usually is more effective than broadband UVB and achieves maximal responses more rapidly.

Psoralen–ultraviolet A (PUVA) photochemotherapy uses oral 8-methoxypsoralen (8-MOP)[1] 0.6 mg/kg as a photosensitizer before UVA (320–400 nm) exposure. Sixty-five percent of patients with patch or plaque disease achieve complete remissions, and 30% have partial responses to this modality. For most patients, maximal responses are achieved within 3 months, and after 5 months, it is unlikely that further improvement will be gained. Limitations of these modalities include actinic damage, photocarcinogenesis, retinal damage (if eyes are not protected), and the inconvenience of getting to phototherapy centers. PUVA also has the risk of nausea and a theoretical risk of cataract induction without proper eye protection.

During the clearing phase of treatment, phototherapy treatments usually are administered three times per week. After resolution of skin lesions, treatment frequency is usually tapered gradually to once weekly for UVB and once every 4 to 6 weeks for PUVA. These maintenance regimens are often continued for months to years because abrupt cessation of phototherapy is commonly associated with rapid relapse, which is probably related to the persistence of microscopic disease after clinical clearing.

Topical Therapy

Like phototherapeutic regimens, topical therapies are appropriate for disease confined to the skin (stage I). Topical corticosteroids are frequently used for CTCLs, often before diagnosis. Low-potency formulations are useful on the face and skin folds. Medium-potency preparations are appropriate for the trunk and extremities. High-potency formulations are useful for recalcitrant lesions; however, prolonged use of such potent agents can cause local atrophy and adrenal suppression. Roughly one half of patients achieve complete remissions, and most others have partial remissions. Response duration varies widely with the individual pace of disease and patient compliance. Topical corticosteroids are particularly useful as a means to relatively quickly ameliorate severe signs and symptoms and as an adjuvant therapy in combination with other primary treatments.

Mechlorethamine (nitrogen mustard, HN$_2$, Mustargen)[1] is applied topically in an aqueous solution or in an ointment, such as Aquaphor. The aqueous form is prepared at home and involves a daily dose totaling 10 mg in 60 mL water. The ointment form is prepared by a pharmacist in 1-pound lots at a concentration of 10 mg of mechlorethamine per 100 g of ointment. Only the amount of ointment needed to apply a thin layer is used. Either formulation is usually applied at bedtime to lesional skin for limited disease or to the entire skin surface (excluding the head unless it is also involved) for more extensive disease. It is then showered off every morning using soap and water. Results are similar to those from PUVA. Advantages include therapy at home and availability in all regions of the country. Disadvantages are daily preparation (aqueous form only), daily application, and possible allergic contact dermatitis (more common with the aqueous preparation). Maximal efficacy is expected within 6 months. Mild flares of disease may occur during the first few months of treatment and probably represent inflammation of subclinical skin lesions, analogous to the clinical accentuation of actinic damage during topical therapy with 5-fluorouracil (Efudex). As with phototherapy, topical mechlorethamine is tapered gradually after remission is achieved in an effort to delay clinical relapse.

Carmustine (BCNU, BiCNU)[1] is applied to the total skin surface as an alcohol/aqueous solution (10 to 20 mg in 60 mL).[6] Complete responses are seen in 85% of patients with stage IA disease (<10% involvement) and 50% of patients with stage IB disease (>10% involvement). Another 10% of patients obtain partial responses.

[1]Not FDA approved for this indication.

[1]Not FDA approved for this indication.
[6]May be compounded by pharmacists.

Advantages include those described for nitrogen mustard and reports of success with application only to lesional skin. Disadvantages include skin irritation followed by telangiectasia formation and possible bone marrow suppression necessitating blood monitoring.

A topical gel formulation of the retinoid X receptor (RXR)–specific retinoid, bexarotene (Targretin), is useful for localized or limited skin lesions. The principal side effect is local irritation.

Radiotherapy

Conventional radiotherapy for mycosis fungoides therapy has been used for approximately 100 years. It is useful in the treatment of isolated, particularly problematic lesions such as recalcitrant tumors or ulcerated plaques. In addition to benefit from the photons delivered by radiotherapy, electron beam therapy (0.4 Gy per week for 8 to 9 weeks) is also useful for CTCL therapy. An approximately 85% complete response rate of skin disease with a median duration of 16 months is expected with electron beam therapy. An advantage is an excellent rate of complete response. Disadvantages include limited access to required equipment and expertise and cutaneous toxic effects, such as alopecia, sweat gland loss, radiation dermatitis, and skin cancers. As with other skin-directed therapy, the benefit for internal disease is limited. Cumulative toxicity also limits the number of courses a patient may receive. Localized electron beam therapy is also useful for treating cases of limited-extent MF and in treating selected problematic MF lesions in patients who are otherwise responding to therapy. After completion of total-skin electron beam therapy, patients require maintenance therapy such as topical mechlorethamine[6] or phototherapy to prolong remission.

Apheresis-Based Therapy

Leukapheresis and particularly lymphocytapheresis (6000 to 7000 mL of blood treated tiw initially, then according to response) have been used in the treatment of SS patients. Benefit has been reported in several case reports and small case series; however, response rates are not possible to determine. Photopheresis (i.e., extracorporeal photochemotherapy) describes an apheresis-based therapy in which circulating lymphocytes are first exposed to a psoralen (orally or extracorporeally) and then exposed to UVA extracorporeally. In contrast to leukapheresis, in which leukocytes are discarded, all cells are returned to the patient's circulation during photopheresis. Response rates in erythrodermic patients are 33% to 50%, and median survival for SS patients is prolonged from 30 months to more than 60 months. In recent years, extracorporeal photochemotherapy has been used increasingly in conjunction with one or more systemic therapies to enhance efficacy. The toxicity of the systemic agents is diminished because they are often used in combination at reduced doses.

Cytokine Therapy

Interferon alfa-2a (Roferon-A) or alfa-2b (Intron-A)[1] (1 to 100 × 10^6 units) is given subcutaneously or intralesionally every other day to once weekly. A standard starting dose is 3×10^6 units three times per week. Response rates are approximately 55%, with complete responses occurring in 17% of patients. Advantages include the relative ease of delivery. Disadvantages include anorexia, fever, malaise, leukopenia, and risk of cardiac dysrhythmia. Interferon alfa-2a or alfa-2b combined with narrow-band UVB or PUVA is effective for many patients with generalized skin lesions unresponsive to phototherapy alone.

Tumor-Associated Antigen-Directed Therapies

Various specific tumor-associated antigens have been targeted with antibody-based therapy. The response rate typically is low, and response durations are short. Less specific targets are CD4, CD5, and IL-2 receptors. Of this class of agent, the most promising is denileukin diftitox (Ontak, DAB389 IL-2) (9 to 18 μg per/kg/day IV

on 5 consecutive days, every 3 weeks). This agent is a fusion protein combining IL-2 and diphtheria toxin. Cells bearing the IL-2 receptor (in the lesions of at least one half of MF patients) bind and internalize the drug. The drug also may destroy Treg cells that are CD25$^+$ and suppress immune responses. Inside the cell, the toxin portion of the molecule disrupts protein synthesis, leading to cell death. Approximately 10% of patients achieve complete responses, and total response rates of near 40% have been reported. One half of responders and 20% of nonresponders experienced decreased pruritus. Adverse events include capillary leak syndrome, flulike symptoms, and allergic reactions. Combination therapy with denileukin diftitox and multiagent chemotherapy is being explored for advanced disease. Alemtuzumab (Campath)[1] is an antibody directed against CD52. It has shown benefit in advanced-stage disease. This agent can be used alone or in conjunction with multiagent chemotherapy.

Systemic Chemotherapy

Various regimens of single-agent and multiagent chemotherapy have been used in the treatment of MF and SS. Oral methotrexate, chlorambucil (Leukeran)[1] with or without prednisone,[1] and etoposide (VePesid)[1] have shown therapeutic activity. The best response has been in erythrodermic patients treated with methotrexate (5 to 125 mg weekly),[3] who have shown a 58% response rate.

The use of multiagent regimens is controversial because of the small number of patients treated with any given regimen. There is even some evidence that for some populations of CTCL patients, survival may be reduced. For individual patients with advanced disease, however, cyclophosphamide (Cytoxan),[1] doxorubicin (Adriamycin),[1] vincristine (Oncovin),[1] and prednisone[1] (CHOP regimen) can provide some short-term palliation. In some cases, CHOP has successfully eradicated large cell transformation of MF and returned patients to their more clinically indolent patch or plaque baseline disease. Idarubicin (Idamycin)[1] in association with etoposide, cyclophosphamide, vincristine, prednisone, and bleomycin (Blenoxane)[1] (VICOP-B regimen) has demonstrated response rates of 80% (36% complete response rate) for patients with stage II through IV disease and 84% for MF patients, with a median duration of response longer than 8 months. Other regimens have been used with more modest success.

Several purine nucleoside analogues have been used for CTCL treatment, including erythrodermic variants. These include 2-chlorodeoxyadenosine (cladribine [Leustatin],[1] with a response rate of 28%), 2-deoxycoformycin (pentostatin [Nipent],[1] with a response rate of 39%), and fludarabine (Fludara).[1] Toxicities include pulmonary edema, bone marrow and immune suppression, and neurotoxicity.

Retinoids

Retinoids have therapeutic activity against MF and SS alone and in combination with other therapies, such as interferon alfa or PUVA (the latter combination is called Re-PUVA). Arotinoid,[5] acitretin (Soriatane),[1] and 13-*cis*-retinoic acid (isotretinoin [Accutane])[1] have various degrees of efficacy, and they typically are used in conjunction with other modalities. A newer RXR-specific retinoid, bexarotene, has an overall response rate of about 40% and can be used alone or in combination with phototherapy and other systemic agents such as interferon alfa-2. Disadvantages of bexarotene therapy include signs of hypothyroidism and vitamin A toxicity, particularly hyperlipidemia.

Enzyme Inhibitors

Vorinostat (Zolinza) is the first histone deacetylase inhibitor to be FDA approved for MF and SS. The overall response rate approaches 40% using a standard oral dose of 400 mg/day. Side effects include gastrointestinal symptoms, thrombocytopenia, and cardiac conduction

---

[1]Not FDA approved for this indication.
[6]May be compounded by pharmacists.

---

[1]Not FDA approved for this indication.
[3]Exceeds dosage recommended by the manufacturer.
[5]Investigational drug in the United States.

abnormalities. Other histone deacetylase inhibitors such as romidepsin[5] are undergoing clinical trials in the United States. Forodesine[5] is a purine nucleoside phosphorylase inhibitor that preferentially affects T cells because they contain relatively high concentrations of this enzyme. Forodesine is undergoing clinical trials for MF and SS in the United States and appears to have a response rate of about 40%.

Miscellaneous Therapies

Various other therapies have been tried for MF and SS with modest success. Nonmyeloablative allogeneic stem cell transplantation has led to favorable responses in some patients; however, the total number treated is small. Cyclosporine (Sandimmune)[1] has been used for MF and SS. Transient improvement is followed by worsened survival due to immunosuppression, and it is not a recommended therapy. Thymopentin[5] has given excellent results in SS patients (i.e., 40% complete response rate and 35% partial response rate, with a median duration of response of 22 months). The lack of follow-up reports in recent decades leaves the status of this therapy in question.

Selection of Therapy

Initial choices among conventional treatments for MF and SS depend on the types of lesions and the stage of disease. Disease subsets are followed by recommended initial treatments in parentheses: unilesional or localized MF (local radiation therapy), patch MF (broad- and narrow-band UVB, PUVA, mechlorethamine), patch/plaque MF (PUVA, mechlorethamine), thick plaque/tumor MF (electron beam radiation therapy, interferon alfa-2, bexarotene, vorinostat), erythrodermic MF/SS (photopheresis), and nodal or visceral MF or SS (interferon alfa-2, bexarotene, vorinostat, denileukin diftitox, experimental systemic therapies, systemic chemotherapy).

Second-line therapeutic choices often involve interferons, retinoids, or histone deacetylase inhibitors, usually in combination with primary modalities. Multimodality combinations, often at reduced doses, are used commonly to treat patients with stage IIB or more advanced disease. Medium-potency topical corticosteroids, such as 0.1% triamcinolone cream or ointment (Kenalog),[1] are useful adjuncts to many different therapies. The optimal use of newer therapeutic agents in various subtypes and stages of MF and SS is still being established.

---

[1]Not FDA approved for this indication.
[5]Investigational drug in the United States.

 CURRENT THERAPY

Guidelines Are Primarily for Mycosis Fungoides and Sézary Syndrome:

- Stages IA-IIA: skin-directed therapy with potent topical corticosteroids, topical mechlorethamine (Mustargen),[1] or phototherapy; radiation therapy or topical bexarotene (Targretin) in selected cases
- Stages IIB-IVB: skin-directed therapy plus one or more systemic therapies, such as interferon alfa-2a (Roferon-A) or alfa-2b (Intron A),[1] bexarotene (Targretin), vorinostat (Zolinza), denileukin diftitox (Ontak), or methotrexate; photopheresis for erythrodermic cases
- Combination therapies are often used in intermediate- and advanced-stage disease.
- Multiagent chemotherapy is usually not an effective long-term treatment strategy.

---

[1]Not FDA approved for this indication.

Lymphoproliferative Disorders Associated with Mycosis Fungoides and Sézary Syndrome

TYPES AND CLINICAL FEATURES

Patients with MF or SS are at increased risk for large T-cell lymphomas, lymphomatoid papulosis, and Hodgkin's disease. Molecular biologic analysis has shown that these disorders and MF often share the same clonal T-cell receptor gene rearrangement when they arise in the same individual. As a consequence, they are considered to be subclones of the original MF tumor clone. The development of large T-cell lymphoma in a patient with MF or SS is referred to as *large cell transformation of MF*. This occurs in up to 20% of cases in some series and is associated with a median survival of only 1 to 2 years. One half of these large T-cell lymphomas are CD30[+]; however, the generally favorable prognosis of primary cutaneous CD30[+] anaplastic large cell lymphoma does not extend to these secondary forms of CD30[+] lymphoma. These patients are usually treated with systemic chemotherapy such as CHOP or with experimental systemic therapies appropriate for advanced-stage CTCL.

Lymphomatoid papulosis manifests as recurrent, usually generalized crops of spontaneously regressing, erythematous papules that can exhibit crusting or vesiculation before resolution. It is the clinically benign end of a disease continuum that has primary cutaneous CD30[+] anaplastic large cell lymphoma at its other extreme. Intermediate forms of disease can occur. Histopathologically, lesions contain a mixed-cell infiltrate, including large, atypical T cells that resemble Reed-Sternberg cells and their mononuclear variants (so-called type A) or large MF-type cells (so-called type B). Type A cells are CD30[+]. A type C form is also recognized. It has sheets of type A cells histologically mimicking CD30[+] large T-cell lymphoma but is different from it clinically. Patients with lymphomatoid papulosis sometimes respond to tetracycline or erythromycin (500 mg PO bid), presumably on the basis of antiinflammatory activity. Most cases improve within 1 month with low-dose methotrexate (10 to 20 mg PO every week). PUVA and narrow-band UVB given three times per week are other therapeutic options.

TREATMENT

In most cases, non-MF/SS CTCLs are treated with radiation therapy (with or without complete surgical excision) if they are localized or with various multiagent systemic chemotherapy regimens if they are generalized. The roles of other agents remain to be defined, except that studies have proved that methotrexate (10 to 40 mg PO every week) is effective therapy for most cases of primary cutaneous CD30[+] anaplastic large cell lymphoma. Therapies being investigated for this lymphoma include anti-CD30 antibodies, alone or conjugated to toxins. Denileukin diftitox has been reported to be effective against some subcutaneous panniculitic T-cell lymphomas.

REFERENCES

Olsen E, Vonderheid E, et al. Revisions to the staging and classification of mycosis fungoides and Sézary syndrome: A proposal of the International Society for Cutaneous Lymphomas (ISCL) and the cutaneous lymphoma task force of the European Organization of Research and Treatment of Cancer (EORTC). Blood 2007;110(6):1713–22.

Pimpinelli N, Olsen EA, Santucci M, et al. Defining early mycosis fungoides. J Am Acad Dermatol 2005;53(6):1053–63.

Richardson SK, Lin JH, Vittorio CC, et al. High clinical response rate with multimodality immunomodulatory therapy for Sézary syndrome. Clin Lymphoma Myeloma 2006;7(3):226–32.

Vonderheid EC, Bernengo MG, Burg G, et al. Update on erythrodermic cutaneous T-cell lymphoma: Report of the International Society for Cutaneous Lymphomas. J Am Acad Dermatol 2002;46(1):95–106.

Willemze R, Jaffe ES, Burg G, et al. WHO-EORTC classification for cutaneous lymphomas. Blood 2005;105(10):3768–85.

Wood GS, Greenberg HL. Diagnosis, staging, and monitoring of cutaneous T-cell lymphoma. Dermatol Ther 2003;16(4):269–75.

Papulosquamous Eruptions—Psoriasis

Method of
David Puchalsky, MD

Psoriasis is one of the papulosquamous (i.e., red, scaly, and noninfectious) skin diseases. The onset of psoriasis can occur at any age from birth to old age, but it usually occurs between the ages of 20 and 30 years. Both sexes are affected equally. The incidence is 2% to 3% of the population in North America. Psoriasis is chronic, and treatment controls but does not cure. The severity of untreated psoriasis tends to vary only slightly around each patient's baseline, which is established soon after onset. The appearance of psoriasis and its clinical variants are characteristic enough that a biopsy is usually not needed for diagnosis.

When a biopsy is needed, it is more often diagnostic if done to nonmanipulated and nontreated involved skin. Patients tend to have one dominant clinical variant, although some have more than one or shift from one to another. The cause of psoriasis is unknown, although certain genes are found to cluster in affected families and about 40% have a known family history of the disease. Symptoms of untreated psoriasis include itch, although this is severe in less than 50% of patients and often only when the skin is dry; discomfort, especially in the palms and soles when they are fissured or pustular; irritation, especially in skin folds; pain and stiffness in joints, ligaments, and tendons; and perception of social stigma.

Treatment

Current therapy is summarized in Figure 1. All psoriasis patients should be reassured that psoriasis is noncontagious and not cancerous. They should be informed that it is chronic and incurable but fortunately controllable. Baseline severity can be most safely reduced by a basic management approach (Box 1) that maximizes topical

---

CURRENT DIAGNOSIS

- Sharply demarcated, red, symmetrical plaques have a silvery scale (unless in skin folds).
- There are five clinical variants:
  - Plaque: silvery scale–topped, round or oval plaques on extensor surfaces, the torso, and often on the scalp
  - Guttate: <1-cm scaly papules, often occurring in children or young adults and often after streptococcal infection
  - Inverse: little scale, located in skin folds, often occurring in the obese, and occasionally occurring with secondary infection
  - Pustular: frank pustules with little scale, often localized to palms or soles or may be generalized, and often occurring with secondary infection
  - Erythrodermic: covering almost all of the skin
- Fifty percent of patients have nail findings, such as surface pits, lifting of the nail plate from the nail bed, and yellow discoloration under the nails, called *oil spots*.
- About 15% of patients develop psoriatic arthritis, most commonly asymmetrical oligoarthritis of the small joints of the hands and feet but rarely rheumatoid-like or spondylitis-like disease.

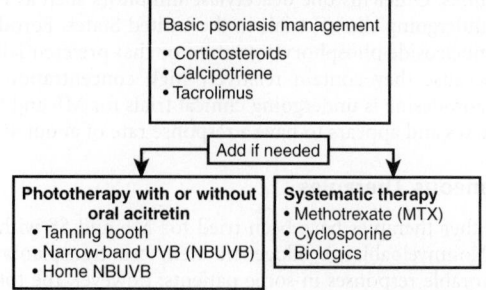

FIGURE 1. Algorithm for psoriasis management, including topical therapies (see Box 1).

treatment and that should be continued long term, even if more aggressive treatment is added.

The objective and subjective severity of psoriasis should be carefully assessed to guide treatment choices. Objective severity for research purposes is assessed with a psoriasis area and severity index (PASI) score, which is a composite of measures of area involved as a percentage of the total-body surface area (TBSA) and severity (i.e., elevation, redness, and scale) of lesions in particular regions of the skin. In clinical practice, objective severity is more quickly assessed as a combination of percent of TBSA involved and general intensity of inflammation. TBSA involvement is often estimated using the patient's total hand and finger area as an approximation of 1% of the TBSA. Lesion inflammation is usually described in terms of degree of redness, elevation, scale, and the presence of pustules.

Subjective severity is best measured with a quality-of-life (QOL) tool (Box 2). Objective and subjective severity should be measured regularly to guide treatment decisions. A hypothetical patient can help make this point. Assume the presenting patient has a TBSA of 15% with moderately inflamed but nonpustular lesions and a QOL score of 80 of 110. If he has not been on any type of topical or other basic management, it would be reasonable to start such management alone. However, if on follow-up the TBSA is greater than 10%, lesions are still mildly inflamed, and the QOL score is higher than 50 despite reasonable compliance with basic psoriasis management (BPM), ultraviolet (UV) or systemic treatment should be strongly considered.

Compliance is difficult for psoriasis patients, as it is in any patient with a chronic disease. One study showed that primary adherence (i.e., filling prescriptions) is lower for psoriasis patients than for those with other common skin diseases. Compliance with topical

---

> ### BOX 1 Basic Psoriasis Management
>
> - Educate and support the patient (requires frequent visits).
> - Reduce skin injury (koebnerization):
>   No scratching, picking, or rubbing
>   As-needed application of menthol or camphor creams
>   Oral sedating antihistamines 2 hours before bed to
>   decrease itch and scratch cycle
> - Reduce or eliminate other exacerbating factors:
>   Streptococcal and other infections
>   Stress
>   Alcohol consumption
>   Smoking
>   Obesity
> - Use certain medicines (e.g., lithium, β-blockers, antimalarials).
> - Repair dry skin or microinjury (see Box 3).
> - Monitor for joint, tendon, and ligament involvement.
> - Maximize topical therapy.
> - Urge patient to seek natural sun exposure but avoid burning.

BOX 2 Quality-of-Life Tool

	Not at All				Somewhat				Very Much	
1. How much does psoriasis affect your *social life*?	0	1	2	3	4	5	6	7	8	9	10
2. How *helpless* do you feel because of your psoriasis?	0	1	2	3	4	5	6	7	8	9	10
3. How *embarrassed* do you feel because of your psoriasis?	0	1	2	3	4	5	6	7	8	9	10
4. How *angry or frustrated* are you about your psoriasis?	0	1	2	3	4	5	6	7	8	9	10
5. How *unsightly* is your psoriasis?	0	1	2	3	4	5	6	7	8	9	10
6. How much does psoriasis affect your *clothing choices*?	0	1	2	3	4	5	6	7	8	9	10
7. How much does psoriasis impact your *overall life enjoyment*?	0	1	2	3	4	5	6	7	8	9	10
8. How much does your psoriasis *itch*?	0	1	2	3	4	5	6	7	8	9	10
9. How much does your psoriasis *irritate or chafe*?	0	1	2	3	4	5	6	7	8	9	10
10. How much does your psoriasis *hurt or cause pain*?	0	1	2	3	4	5	6	7	8	9	10
11. I would be willing to take stronger medications that could carry significant risks to *control but not cure* my skin psoriasis.	0	1	2	3	4	5	6	7	8	9	10

Total points: _____/110

medications is especially poor, falling off soon after each visit and then rising before the next visit. I suggest frequent visits, good patient rapport, prescribing less-expensive generic medications, having the patient bring in unused medications to each visit, and carefully assessing compliance at each visit as methods to improve compliance and therefore treatment response.

TOPICAL THERAPY

Topical steroids are the first-line therapy for all psoriasis patients. They should be continued long term along with all other aspects of BPM. Adherence to BPM can lessen the required doses and therefore the toxicity of any added UV or systemic treatment. Topical steroids work on inflammation and hyperproliferation, the two key elements of psoriasis pathology. Topical steroid ointment preparations are preferable, because ointment vehicles repair the skin surface cracking, which perpetuates inflammation (i.e., the Koebner phenomenon). Petroleum jelly (Vaseline) alone improves psoriasis, whereas alcohol vehicles (in topical steroid solutions for scalp use) worsen psoriasis, and cream vehicles are often neutral. Ointments are the simplest vehicles, requiring fewer inactive ingredients that have the potential for irritation or contact sensitization. Ointment does not rub into the skin, and the patient should be instructed to apply the ointment gently in a thin film. The prescription amount should be based on the area treated, knowing that 20 g of ointment covers the entire skin once. For example, 4 g can cover 20% of TBSA once, and a 120-g tube of topical steroid ointment for once-daily use is a 30-day supply.

The timing of topical steroid application is important. To maximize efficacy and compliance, application should be done once daily after a hydrating bath in the evening (Box 3). After application, soft cotton clothing can be worn to keep the ointment from soiling home surfaces such as upholstery and sheets. Daytime application, although messy, is tolerated by many patients, and it can provide some additional control. Because steroid receptors are saturated at twice-daily applications, topical steroids can be applied more frequently without harm. One strategy is to allow patients to use topical steroids any time to help stop scratching behavior, because scratching is counterproductive and can be more of a habit than a response to a true itch. Alternatively, less messy nonsteroidal anti-itch creams can be used in this manner.

The potency of topical steroids is an important issue. Because psoriasis is a chronic disease, a safe but maximal potency is favored for each skin zone. Potency needs to match the thickness of the skin in each zone. There are seven potency groups, from group 1 (ultrapotent) to group 7 (least potent), and five skin-thickness zones. Box 4 provides the recommended generic topical steroid for each zone. Tachyphylaxis to topical steroids probably is minimal, with apparent decrease in potency over time resulting from declining compliance.

The physician should monitor for side effects, including adrenal suppression (avoid by following Box 4), skin thinning with prominent surface capillaries or stretch marks, infections, and rosacea-like facial eruptions. Topical steroids (even group 7) should be avoided near the eyelids, because they can increase risk of cataracts and glaucoma.

Occasionally, steroids can be injected intralesionally into resistant body plaques. This is best done by experienced clinicians. Triamcinolone typically is used at concentrations of 5 to 10 mg/mL (Aristospan Intralesional 5 mg/mL, Kenalog-10 10 mg/mL). Side effects are atrophy and secondary infection.

BOX 3 Evening Bath and Dry Skin Repair

- Take a *bath*—better than a shower.
- *Evening* bath is best so ointments can be applied generously.
- Use *warm* water, not hot, and do not use additives.
- Use only *mild* soap (near the end of the bath) only on skin folds and other necessary areas.
- *Do not scrub or scrape skin* (e.g., do not use a loofa, washcloth, or brush).
- Rinse soap off *thoroughly*.
- Pat dry—*no rubbing*.
- When skin is still slightly damp, apply medicated ointments to psoriasis.
- Apply plain Vaseline or plain mineral oil (may be warmed by prior immersion of bottle in bath water) to entire dry areas and psoriasis-prone areas.
- Wear loose-fitting cotton clothes (e.g., long johns, socks, gloves) after moisturizing and overnight.

BOX 4 Recommended Topical Steroids for Skin Thickness Zones*

- Palms or soles: group 1 ointment
  Clobetasol (Temovate), augmented betamethasone dipropionate (Diprolene)
  May be occluded under plastic for increased potency
- Body <30% TBSA: group 2 ointment
  Fluocinonide 0.05% (Lidex), desoximetasone 0.25% (Topicort)
- Body >30% TBSA: group 3 ointment
  Betamethasone valerate 0.1% (Valisone)
- Scalp: group 2 solution
  Fluocinonide 0.05% (Lidex)
- Folds: group 4 or 5
  Triamcinolone (Kenalog) 0.1% ointment or cream
- Face: group 7 ointment
  Hydrocortisone (Hytone) 1% or 2.5% (avoid eyelids)

TBSA = total body surface area.

Another major topical treatment in the armamentarium for psoriasis is calcipotriene (Dovonex), a vitamin D analogue. Unfortunately, it is available only in a cream vehicle, but it may be available soon as a generic drug and in the more effective ointment vehicle. It has no steroid side effects. Although it is not impressive as monotherapy, it does have additive efficacy with topical steroids, which can lower the mild irritancy of calcipotriene. Calcipotriene can be applied immediately before topical steroid ointments to all zones, although calcipotriene can occasionally be too irritating to use on the face. Use should be less than 400 g per month because of the risk of hypercalcemia. Calcipotriene is available in a very expensive, premixed combination with a group I steroid (i.e., betamethasone dipropionate), marketed as Taclonex ointment. Calcipotriene should not be used within 2 or 3 hours before UV treatment, because it decreases UV penetration.

Calcineurin inhibitors can be useful for psoriasis. Of the two available, tacrolimus, available only as brand-name Protopic,[1] is more effective because it is in an ointment vehicle. The 0.1% strength is more effective than the 0.03%. Tacrolimus ointment can be used on the face and even on the eyelids without fear of steroid side effects. Potency of tacrolimus 0.1% is somewhat unclear for psoriasis, but it is probably equivalent to a group 5 or 6 topical steroid. The FDA has put a black box warning on calcineurin inhibitors. This warning was based on giving mice and rats large systemic quantities and finding that lymphoma was more common and observing that tacrolimus did get absorbed through the skin in some pediatric patients with genetic deficiencies in skin barrier function. Most dermatologists think that calcineurin inhibitors are safe, although most avoid use in infants and toddlers and in patients with skin barrier function defects.

Many other topical medications have been used to treat psoriasis. Tazarotene (Tazorac) is a topical retinoid that has proved to be too irritating for routine use, except in some cases of localized pustular palm or sole psoriasis. Anthralin (Dritho-Scalp 0.5%, Psoriatec 1%) is also very irritating and stains surfaces, and it is rarely used. Tar (DHS Tar, Doak Tar) is of mostly historical interest because of poor efficacy, odor, and messiness, although it has mild efficacy in shampoos.

Topical adjuncts can be very useful. Camphor and menthol are ingredients that occupy skin temperature receptors and give an immediate cooling sensation that can provide instant relief of psoriasis pruritus. These products (e.g., Sarna Original Lotion, Eucerin, or Aveeno Anti-Itch Lotion) can be applied any time as a substitute behavior for scratching.

Topical antihistamines, such as those containing pramoxine (Prax),[1] can be helpful, although topical diphenhydramine (Benadryl)[1] can be sensitizing, as can topical doxepin (Zonalon[1]), which can also cause sedation. Oral sedating antihistamines taken before bed are preferred (see Table 1).

PHOTOTHERAPY AND ACITRETIN

Phototherapy with or without acitretin (Soriatane) is a natural next step if BPM is not effective enough. BPM must be continued to decrease the doses and toxicity of phototherapy. Phototherapy ages the skin and can cause skin cancer. Patients should be examined for precancerous or cancerous lesions before, during, and forever after this approach to controlling their psoriasis. Natural sun, which contains UV radiation in the range of 320 to 400 nm (UVA) and in the range of 280 to 320 nm (UVB), can be helpful. However, burning can trigger a flare of psoriasis through the Koebner phenomenon. In some climates, natural sun is practical only in summer or on vacation. Tanning booths, which emit largely UVA light (which tends not to burn but which causes tanning and some cutaneous immunosuppression) can help psoriasis but not as much as UVB light. UV therapy is not necessarily contraindicated by risk factors for skin cancer, including a history of skin cancer itself. First, improving the patient's

psoriasis by any means allows earlier detection of precancerous and cancerous growths, especially those in the nonmelanoma lineage, which can occasionally blend in with the psoriasis because they are also erythematous and often scaly. Second, systemic treatments are a concern because of their carcinogenicity, including that of the skin. The exception is acitretin, which has antineoplastic effects and is often paired with UV treatment.

Choice of provider-administered UV treatment has become simpler. First, narrow-band UVB (NBUVB) with a wavelength of 311 nm (the UVB wavelength most effective for psoriasis) has replaced broad-spectrum UVB. Second, NBUVB has largely replaced PUVA (i.e., psoralens PO [8 MOP, Oxsoralen-Ultra] or topically [Oxsoralen lotion] plus UVA). NBUVB is associated with easier compliance, better tolerance, reduced risk of burning, reduced risk of ocular damage, and equal or near-equal efficacy.

The NBUVB initial dose is based usually on an estimate of the patient's minimal erythematous dose and then steadily but carefully increased (e.g., by 5%) each treatment to achieve a mild and transient erythema the day after each treatment. Maximal treatment is usually four times per week. A consent form should be employed. It reviews risks and benefits of treatment and gives some responsibility to the patient to keep health care providers apprised of medication changes that could change the tendency to burn. Natural sun exposure should be limited because added UV can cause burning, and depending on the timing, a suntan can limit efficacy of the NBUVB. Most patients improve by 80% to 90% after 2 months of maximal treatment. Psoriasis clears completely in very few patients, except some who have guttate psoriasis. The scalp and skin fold areas are particularly resistant.

Many patients benefit from a maintenance protocol with a reduction of treatment to twice and then once per week after improvement is near-maximal. Most maintenance protocols hold the dose steady at an amount 50% to 75% of the maximal dose achieved. The dose is held steady because patients do not build an increasing tolerance to the NBUVB with less frequent treatments. One efficient approach in geographic locations with pronounced seasons is to treat aggressively in the winter, go to a maintenance protocol in the spring, and then consider maintenance with natural sun in the summer.

A home NBUVB unit is recommended for some patients who are experienced with provider-administered NBUVB, are located far from facilities, and are reliable about follow-up appointments.

Acitretin is a systemic treatment that can improve natural sun, tanning booth, or NBUVB efficacy. This oral retinoid does not cause immunosuppression, nor is it carcinogenic. It can reduce the number and the dose of UV treatments required for near-clearing efficacy. At the usual dose of 25 mg/day with food, this agent tends to be well tolerated. The minimal side effects include a slight and reversible increase in triglyceride or cholesterol levels, rare and mild increase in the levels of liver transaminases, and manageable mucocutaneous drying.

Acitretin does not work well without UV treatment, unless used for pustular psoriasis, in which case it works well for generalized or localized forms. Acitretin is a teratogen, and use is not advised in fertile women. The agent is stored in fat as a teratogenic metabolite for at least 3 years after the last dose. Storage may be increased with alcohol consumption. Alcohol consumption should be limited when using acitretin.

OTHER SYSTEMIC AGENTS

Systemic treatment of psoriasis is undergoing a constant evolution, especially with new biologic agents becoming available every few years. Although very expensive, these agents can help control moderate to severe psoriasis, and some work for psoriatic arthritis. Topical agents and the rest of BPM need to be continued to keep doses and toxicities low. These agents are to some extent immunosuppressive and thereby increase the risk of infection and neoplasia. Certain agents seem to increase the risk of some infections more than others or certain forms of cancer more than others. This is a controversial and evolving area as postmarketing studies continue to collect data.

---

[1]Not FDA approved for this indication.

Each agent has specific risks in addition to immunosuppression. The advisability of written informed consent when using these agents cannot be overstated. Systemic agents usually are reserved for those who fail to improve well enough on BPM and have other issues. These issues include inability to get UVB treatment because of distance from facilities; lack of candidacy for UV treatment because of UV-induced disease, such as lupus; resistance to UV treatment, such as severe skin fold psoriasis; long history of poor response to previous UV treatment; and significant psoriatic arthritis, preferably diagnosed by a rheumatologist.

Methotrexate (MTX; Trexall) is the systemic agent with the longest record of use. It is effective for all variants of psoriasis and helps psoriatic arthritis, although not as well for the spinal type. MTX is a dihydrofolate reductase inhibitor and has been found to work as an immune modulator. The major potential toxicity is hepatic. It is metabolized by the kidney, and renal dysfunction can increase the risk of hepatotoxicity. This drug is contraindicated in pregnancy; for patients with liver disease, renal dysfunction, some types of immunodeficiency or immunosuppression, and acute or chronic infection; and for those with malignancy. Alcohol abuse (>1 drink/day) is not allowed while on this hepatotoxic agent. Sulfa drugs cannot be used simultaneously, and nonsteroidal antiinflammatory drugs can be used only at low doses. Because of the rare but devastating possibility of agranulocytosis, MTX is often given at a low 5- to 7.5-mg test dose, followed by a complete blood cell (CBC) count before dose progression.

This systemic agent is relatively inexpensive, because it is available generically. The least expensive option is to use injection solution MTX.[1] It can be given in preloaded syringes that patients can squirt into orange juice. Folic acid 1 g/day decreases nausea experienced by some and oral ulcerations experienced by few, and it does not decrease efficacy. Intramuscular weekly dosing rather than oral dosing is an option for those with gastrointestinal intolerance or poor efficacy because this mode of administration bypasses the portal circulation and some metabolism that occurs.

Monthly laboratory monitoring is best done 6 to 7 days after a weekly dose and should include levels of liver enzymes and creatinine, a CBC count with a differential, and any tests for infection that may be suggested by the patient's history. Patients should be checked monthly for efficacy as the dose is increasing. Doses start at 7.5 mg and can be steadily increased to 30 mg in a single once-weekly dose. After near-clearing has occurred, the dose can usually be held steady or decreased, and patients can be seen and blood tests drawn every 3 months.

Liver enzymes are not completely sensitive for MTX-induced liver damage. A liver biopsy done under ultrasound guidance is required at 1.5 g of cumulative MTX and should be done sooner if there are liver abnormalities. Some patients prefer not to get a liver biopsy, despite the documented excellent safety and tolerance of this procedure. They must be switched from MTX to another agent or approach. If the liver biopsy interpreted by an experienced pathologist shows no significant fibrosis, MTX can be continued up to another 3 g (cumulative) with monitoring until a repeat liver biopsy is advised. Even with a second normal liver biopsy result, I recommend a switch to another agent after 6 g of cumulative MTX. Patients can be switched to UV, if a candidate, or a nonhepatotoxic systemic agent. For example, at the common dose of 25 mg of MTX per week, this occurs at 5 years of treatment.

Oral cyclosporine (Neoral) is a potent immunosuppressive agent that has been used for the past 20 years for psoriasis. Its greatest strength is its speed in improving the skin. However, it has no significant effect on the symptoms or signs of psoriatic arthritis. It predictably raises blood pressure and decreases renal function, even in the low doses (≤4 mg/kg/day) used for psoriasis. It is contraindicated if there is known renal disease and dysfunction, hypertension that is newly diagnosed or under poor control, immunodeficiency or immunosuppression, infection, or malignancy. The creatinine level must be checked twice before starting the medication, and blood pressure should be monitored closely in the first few weeks. Ultimately, blood pressure and creatinine levels should be checked at least once each month.

Cyclosporine is used mostly as an emergency drug to quickly decrease moderate to severe psoriasis over 1 to 3 months. It is a way to bridge to another approach that can maintain the improvement in a safer manner. Systemic steroids are never used for this purpose because they can cause a rebound severe or even pustular flare of psoriasis. This has been reported even after a relatively short course or a relatively long taper.

BIOLOGICALS

Biologic agents for psoriasis are proteins produced by recombinant DNA technology. There are four FDA-approved biologic agents for psoriasis: etanercept (Enbrel), adalimumab (Humira), infliximab (Remicade), and alefacept (Amevive). Efalizumab (Raptiva)[2] was withdrawn from the U.S. market as of June 8, 2009, because of the risk of progressive multifocal leukoencephalopathy. These are expensive and powerfully marketed agents. Most insurance carriers do not cover these biologicals unless patients have failed treatment with UV and MTX. Efficacy for the skin usually is no greater than that of MTX, cyclosporine, or NBUVB (especially NBUVB combined with acitretin). However, the tumor necrosis factor (TNF) blockers etanercept, adalimumab, and infliximab are as effective or more effective than MTX for psoriatic arthritis. Rheumatologists have much experience with the TNF blockers, and FDA approval has followed for moderate to severe skin psoriasis even without psoriatic arthritis.

Etanercept is a recombinant human TNF-α receptor (p75) protein fused with the Fc portion of IgG1 that binds to soluble and membrane-bound TNF-α. It is prescribed in a subcutaneous autoinjector that is easy to use for most patients. Dosage is 50 mg twice each week for the first 3 months, followed by once-weekly dosing thereafter.

Adalimumab binds specifically to soluble and membrane-bound TNF-α and blocks TNF-α interactions with the p55 and p75 cell surface TNF receptors. A dose of 80 mg is given by subcutaneous autoinjector, followed by 40 mg the next week and then every 2 weeks thereafter. Written consent forms should be used when prescribing adalimumab or etanercept. Both are contraindicated in patients with active infections or malignancy. Tuberculosis testing should be performed before starting them, because they can reactivate the disease. They should not be used with live vaccines. There may be an increased risk of lupus, multiple sclerosis, and new onset or worsening of congestive heart failure. Hepatitis B reactivation has been reported, and patients should be screened for hepatitis. Patients not uncommonly report injection-site reactions. Rarely, skin psoriasis can flare even after months of excellent control. Etanercept or adalimumab can be overlapped with MTX when there is a rotation from MTX to a TNF blocker or if rotating from TNF blocker to MTX. Long-term combined use may be needed for refractory severe disease. In these cases, there is added concern about infection and neoplasia plus the usual concern about MTX hepatotoxicity.

The third TNF blocker infliximab has been used more by gastroenterologists than by rheumatologists because it is used for inflammatory bowel disease. It is a chimeric antibody composed of a mouse variable region and a human IgG1-α constant region. It binds to the soluble and the transmembrane TNF-α molecules. Administration is by intravenous infusion of 5 mg/kg over 2 to 3 hours at weeks 0, 2, and 6 and then every 8 weeks for psoriasis and psoriatic arthritis. Infliximab has a rapid response and may work slightly better than other TNF blockers. However, some patients develop infusion reactions and serum sickness. Infusion reactions may need to be ameliorated by concurrent administration of MTX. Infliximab shares the

---

[1]Not FDA approved for this indication.

[2]Not available in the United States.

same list of potential side effects as etanercept and adalimumab, including infection and malignancy. All of the TNF blockers are pregnancy category B drugs.

Alefacept is less useful for a few reasons. The efficacy is probably somewhat less than that for the TNF blockers; medical experience is less because it has no activity against psoriatic arthritis or colitis; and it has some potential side effects that are worrisome. Alefacept binds to CD2 on memory-effector T lymphocytes, depleting these T cells. The lymphocytes must be measured before treatment and monitored every other week, with the medication withheld if the CD4 count falls below 250 cells/mL. The marketing claim for longer remissions than those from other biologicals is not convincing.

Only a very experienced dermatologist should prescribe biologic agents. Some patients are reluctant or unwilling to rotate off these medications and back to UV light or MTX. It is unknown whether these agents have some cumulative side effects. For etanercept and adalimumab, we have the rheumatologists' longer experience, but they tend to use the agents in lower doses for rheumatoid arthritis, and there may be some differences in the patient populations (e.g., psoriatic arthritis patients may have more side effects).

There is promise for future biologic agents directed against interleukins, which are involved in psoriasis inflammation. At least eight chromosomal loci have been identified as significantly linked to psoriasis. There is hope that identifying gene products will help the understanding of psoriasis and the development of better biologic treatments.

In summary, BPM has not been emphasized enough in treating patients with psoriasis, despite our knowledge that this is a chronic disease with no cure. Compliance has not been emphasized, with the result that many patients who would not need treatment beyond BPM are placed on more potentially harmful treatment. There are still many patients with good compliance with BPM who have severe enough skin psoriasis (measured objectively and subjectively) or who have significant psoriatic arthritis that requires more potent treatment. UV treatment, particularly NBUVB, is favored for skin disease before going to systemic treatment, but systemic treatment is needed for significant psoriatic arthritis. These patients still need BPM to minimize the doses and toxicities of their systemic agents. Patients should be followed especially carefully for side effects, many of which are arguably worse than the psoriasis itself. Long-term risks of biologic agents are still not clear, but the TNF blockers have established themselves as bona fide options and have probably replaced cyclosporine, even for skin psoriasis alone, except when cyclosporine is used for only 1 or 2 months to quiet a severe flare.

REFERENCES

Brown KK, Rehmus WE, Kimball AB. Determining the relative importance of patient motivations for nonadherence to topical corticosteroid therapy in psoriasis. J Am Acad Dermatol 2006;55(4):607–13.

Carroll CL, Feldman SR, Camacho FT, et al. Better medication adherence results in greater improvement in severity of psoriasis. Br J Dermatol 2004;151 (4):895–7.

Feldman SR, Koo JY, Menter A, et al. Decision points for the initiation of systemic treatment for psoriasis. J Am Acad Dermatol 2005;53(1):101–7.

Gottlieb A, Korman NJ, Gordon KB, et al. Guidelines of care for the management of psoriasis and psoriatic arthritis: Section 2. Psoriatic arthritis: Overview and guidelines of care for treatment with an emphasis on the biologics. J Am Acad Dermatol 2008;58(5):851–64.

Gutman AB, Kligman AM, Sciacca J, et al. Soak and smear: A standard technique revisited. Arch Dermatol 2005;141(12):1556–9.

Menter A, Gottlieb A, Feldman SR, et al. Guidelines of care for the management of psoriasis and psoriatic arthritis: Section 1. Overview of psoriasis and guidelines of care for the treatment of psoriasis with biologics. J Am Acad Dermatol 2008;58(5):826–50.

National Psoriasis Foundation. About psoriasis and treatment overview for medical providers, Available at: http://www.psoriasis.org/NetCommunity/Page.aspx?pid=798 [accessed May 24, 2009].

Storm A, Andersen SE, Benfeldt E, et al. One in 3 prescriptions are never redeemed: primary nonadherence in an outpatient clinic. J Am Acad Dermatol 2008;59(1):27–33.

Autoimmune Connective Tissue Disease

Method of
Molly Hinshaw, MD, and Susan Lawrence-Hylland, MD

Lupus Erythematosus

Lupus erythematosus is an autoimmune connective tissue disease that may localize to the skin or involve several organ systems. A complete review of systems with evaluation of positive findings is necessary to thoroughly assess patients for signs of systemic lupus as defined by the American Rheumatism Association. Cutaneous lupus erythematosus manifests in chronic, subacute, and acute forms. A punch biopsy from within an erythematous lupus lesion is useful for confirming the diagnosis.

CLINICAL FEATURES

Discoid lupus and tumid lupus are the two forms of chronic cutaneous lupus erythematosus. Discoid lupus lesions are tender or pruritic, erythematous to violaceous, scaly plaques that typically occur on sun-exposed skin. The lesions resolve with scarring, and when the lesions affect the scalp, they cause scarring alopecia. Tumid lupus manifests as pruritic, erythematous to violaceous, nonscaly plaques that typically preferentially affect the face and trunk.

The lesions of subacute cutaneous lupus erythematosus occur as erythematous to violaceous, scaly macules and as annular or polycyclic patches. These lesions are commonly located on sun-exposed skin and heal without scarring.

Acute cutaneous lupus erythematosus is exemplified by malar erythema (i.e., butterfly rash) and by poikiloderma (i.e., hyperpigmentation, telangiectasias, and epidermal atrophy). It is a manifestation of systemic lupus erythematosus (SLE). Cutaneous lesions may be widespread. In addition to the American Rheumatism Association criteria, patients with SLE may also develop Raynaud's phenomenon, hypercoagulability, and overlap syndromes with Sjögren's disease, dermatomyositis, and other conditions.

Hydrochlorothiazide (HydroDIURIL), terbinafine (Lamisil), minocycline (Minocin), procainamide (Pronestyl), hydralazine (Apresoline), and isoniazid (Nydrazid) are a few of the pharmaceutical agents that cause drug-induced lupus. This disease manifests with synovitis, photosensitivity, and positive serology results, and it may have cutaneous lesions that do not necessarily abate with cessation of the medication.

MANAGEMENT

Prevention

All patients with lupus erythematosus should be counseled on photoprotection, including protecting skin from sunlight and avoiding sun exposure during peak hours (i.e., between 10 AM and 2 PM). Ultraviolet A and B wavelengths may cause lupus to flare. Broad-spectrum sunscreen with an SPF of 30 or higher and that contains titanium, zinc, Mexoryl (L'Oreal), or Helioplex (Neutrogena) should be used whenever patients are outdoors. Photoprotective clothing that is available from multiple vendors is useful for limiting sun exposure.

Patients with lupus are relatively immunosuppressed by their disease. Vaccinations should be kept up to date, although there is a debate about the necessity and safety of vaccination against meningococcal disease (*Neisseria meningitidis*) (Menactra, Menomune), varicella-zoster virus (Zostavax), and *Streptococcus* (Pneumovax).

Treatment of Cutaneous Lupus Erythematosus

Medium-potency topical corticosteroids should be used for lupus localized to the skin, and they are used as adjunct treatment for patients with systemic lupus. Use of triamcinolone 0.1% cream (Flutex) for lesions on the head and neck until symptoms subside or up to 2 weeks continuously is an appropriate starting strength. Ointment-based vehicles are useful for lesions on the trunk and extremities. They are also the vehicles of choice on the scalp of patients of African American descent. Foam or liquid- or lotion-based corticosteroids work well in the scalp of other ethnic groups and can be used on the trunk and extremities. If lesions persist, the corticosteroid can be occluded, or intralesional injections with triamcinolone can be repeated monthly as needed. Intralesional triamcinolone acetonide at concentrations of 5 mg/mL (Kenalog) can be injected into lesions on the face or neck and doses of 10 to 20 mg/mL (Kenalog-10, Kenalog) into lesions on the trunk or extremities. Intralesional corticosteroids may cause mild discomfort, atrophy of the skin or subcutis, or stretch marks. Topical calcineurin inhibitors such as pimecrolimus (Elidel)[1] or tacrolimus (Protopic)[1] may be used for maintenance treatment but are not recommended for new or active lesions because they do not work quickly. Recurrent or refractory cutaneous lesions require systemic treatment.

Treatment of Systemic Lupus Erythematosus

Antimalarials, including hydroxychloroquine (Plaquenil),[1] are disease-modifying agents that limit the progression of lupus. Hydroxychloroquine, chloroquine (Aralen),[1] and quinacrine[2] (at compounding pharmacies) raise the pH of inflammatory cells, inhibiting inflammatory pathways that cause end-organ damage in patients with SLE.

Hydroxychloroquine is typically used first at 200 mg daily for 2 weeks and then increased to 400 mg daily. Patients need laboratory monitoring and a baseline and then yearly eye examination because the medication may be deposited in the retina over time. Hydroxychloroquine exerts its effects within 2 to 3 months of beginning treatment. Its effects are diminished in smokers.

Depending on end-organ involvement in SLE, immunosuppression with systemic corticosteroids such as prednisone at doses of 1 mg/kg/day is appropriate. Steroid-sparing drugs such as methotrexate (Rheumatrex),[1] acitretin (Soriatane),[1] or mycophenolate mofetil (CellCept)[1] are added. After signs of inflammation subside, prednisone is tapered.

Treatment of Musculoskeletal Manifestations

Arthralgia is a common complaint that can usually be managed with acetaminophen or nonsteroidal antiinflammatory drugs (NSAIDs). For true arthritis unresponsive to the previously described measures, hydroxychloroquine[1] 200 mg twice daily can be added. After that, treatments similar to those used for rheumatoid arthritis can be added, although the antitumor necrosis factor agents usually are avoided in lupus. Methotrexate[1] 7.5 to 25 mg PO once weekly may be used along with folic acid[1] 1 mg daily to help limit side effects. Routine toxicity monitoring includes frequent complete blood cell counts and liver tests. Azathioprine (Imuran)[1] 0.5 to 2 mg/kg can be used with frequent monitoring of complete blood cell counts and liver tests. A sample for testing the thiopurine methyltransferase activity level should be drawn before initiating therapy because a genetic deficiency can lead to severe pancytopenia. Leflunomide (Arava)[1] 10–20 mg PO once daily can be used with frequent blood cell counts and liver tests. Low-dose glucocorticoids (prednisone 5 to 10 mg/day) may be used as a bridge to steroid-sparing therapy and to treat intermittent flares.

Treatment of Hematologic Manifestations

Autoimmune cytopenias are common and are often a defining feature of SLE. Lymphopenia (absolute lymphocyte count <1500 cells/

microliter) does not require therapy. Hemolytic anemia in SLE is the result of antierythrocyte antibodies that activate complement, and it is treated with prednisone at a dose based on clinical severity. Typically, 1 mg/kg/day, or approximately 60 mg, is used for 4 to 6 weeks, with gradual tapering as long as the response is maintained. For severe hemolytic anemia, pulse methylprednisolone (Solu-Medrol) 1 g IV for 3 consecutive days can be tried, followed by the previously described standard dosing. For patients who do not respond to glucocorticoids or are unable to taper prednisone to low doses, other treatments can be used. They may include azathioprine[1] 1.5 to 2.5 mg/kg/day, mycophenolate mofetil[1] 1000 to 2000 mg/day in divided doses, danazol (Danocrine)[1] 300 to 600 mg/day in divided doses, intravenous immunoglobulin,[1] or rituximab (Rituxan)[1] 375 mg/m^2 weekly for four doses.

Immune thrombocytopenia results from antiplatelet antibodies that identify platelets for early destruction. Treatment is indicated when patients have signs or symptoms of spontaneous bleeding or when the platelet count drops below 50,000/mL. The initial treatment approach with glucocorticoids is similar to that used for hemolytic anemia. For patients with chronic thrombocytopenia or for those who cannot achieve an acceptable long-term dose of prednisone, steroid-sparing agents, including azathioprine,[1] mycophenolate mofetil,[1] danazol,[1] rituximab,[1] and intravenous immunoglobulin[1] can be used in doses similar to those used for hemolytic anemia. Dapsone,[1] cyclosporine (Sandimmune, Neoral),[1] and cyclophosphamide (Cytoxan)[1] have also been used.

Thrombotic thrombocytopenia purpura may occur in SLE, and it must be differentiated from immune thrombocytopenia because treatment requires emergent plasmapheresis. Manifestations of thrombotic thrombocytopenia purpura include fever, microangiopathic hemolysis, and central nervous system and renal abnormalities.

Antiphospholipid antibodies include the lupus anticoagulant, anticardiolipin antibodies, and β_2-glycoprotein. They are associated with coagulopathy, thrombocytopenia, late-trimester miscarriage, and heart valve abnormalities. Antiphospholipid antibodies that can be determined with blood testing but are not associated with thromboembolism do not require treatment. Low-dose aspirin[1] may be considered but has not been shown to prevent future thrombosis. Hydroxychloroquine[1] 200 mg twice daily has been shown to reduce the risk. Patients with antiphospholipid antibodies who develop thromboembolism need lifelong treatment with warfarin (Coumadin). A goal international normalized ratio (INR) remains controversial because different studies advocate for high-intensity warfarin (INR >3) or low-intensity therapy (INR >2). For women who have suffered a miscarriage determined to be related to antiphospholipid antibodies, low-dose aspirin and heparin 5000 units SQ twice daily may increase the likelihood of a successful pregnancy.

Treatment of Renal Manifestations

Many patients with SLE have mild to severe renal involvement. Diagnosis by renal biopsy is important to establish the type of kidney involvement. Lupus nephritis is considered one of the more severe manifestations of the disease, and treatment is aimed at preventing renal failure. Treatment should be coordinated with a rheumatologist or nephrologist.

Class I disease requires no specific therapy. The class IIb pattern with more than 1 g of proteinuria can be treated with moderate-dose prednisone (20 mg/day for 6 weeks to 3 months), followed by tapering. Class III and IV patterns of disease have the same prognosis and are treated similarly with high-dose prednisone (1 mg/kg/day) for at least 6 weeks before tapering based on clinical response by 10 mg a week to a maintenance of 10 to 15 mg/day. In addition to prednisone, cytotoxic therapy is initiated with cyclophosphamide[1] 0.5 to 1 g/m^2 of body surface area monthly for 6 months and tapered to every 3 months based on clinical response for a total of 2 to 3 years. Cyclophosphamide has serious toxicities, including hemorrhagic cystitis, bone marrow suppression, infertility, teratogenicity, and

---

[1]Not FDA approved for this indication.
[2]Not available in the United States.

---

[1]Not FDA approved for this indication.

increased risk of malignancy. 2-Mercaptoethane sulfonate sodium (Mesna)[1] can be given with each infusion to minimize bladder toxicity. Class V disease can be treated with prednisone alone, similar to class IIb disease, unless there are coexisting features of class III or IV disease, for which treatments outlined previously should be implemented.

An acceptable alternative to cyclophosphamide for class III and IV disease is mycophenolate mofetil[1] 2 to 3 g/day in divided doses combined with corticosteroids (dosing outlined earlier). This appears to be an effective therapy with fewer side effects than traditional therapy.

Treatment of Nervous System Manifestations

Neuropsychiatric involvement is common in patients with lupus. Symptoms can range from mild to severe and include headache, aseptic meningitis, neuropathy, myelopathy, cognitive dysfunction,

---

[1]Not FDA approved for this indication.

CURRENT DIAGNOSIS

Lupus Erythematosus

- The erythematous-violaceous and variably pruritic, tender, or scaly eruption is photosensitive.
- Mild to moderate systemic involvement may include arthritis and pleurisy.
- Severe systemic involvement may include nephritis, cerebritis, vasculitis, and severe cytopenias.
- Associated findings include antiphospholipid antibodies associated with thromboembolism or stroke, Raynaud's phenomenon, and sicca symptoms.

Dermatomyositis and Polymyositis

- Photosensitive, violaceous-erythematous, poikilodermatous, and variably scaly patches occur around eyes, on extensor extremities (especially over joints), upper back, scalp, and dystrophic nail folds with prominent telangiectasias.
- Patients may have or develop myositis or pulmonary involvement.
- Age-appropriate cancer screening is required for adults.

Scleroderma

- Patients have firm, variably pruritic, and indurated plaques.
- Localized scleroderma (i.e., morphea or asymmetric sclerotic plaques) may be seen.
- Limited systemic sclerosis is characterized by symmetric sclerosis of distal extremities, and patients may have systemic disease.
- Diffuse systemic sclerosis is characterized by symmetric sclerosis of the trunk and proximal extremities, and patients may have systemic disease.
- Sclerodactyly (i.e., thickening of skin of digits) may occur in patients with systemic sclerosis.
- Pulmonary, cardiac, and gastrointestinal screening should be done for patients with systemic sclerosis.
- Patients with systemic sclerosis should be evaluated and monitored for renal crisis.
- Raynaud's phenomenon may develop in patients with systemic sclerosis.

---

seizures, cerebritis, and stroke. A thorough evaluation is necessary to define the cause of nervous system dysfunction and differentiate it from a medication side effect. For seizures, antiepileptic therapy is used, preferably in coordination with a neurologist. Lupus cerebritis and transverse myelitis are two of the more serious manifestations that need to be treated emergently with aggressive immunosuppression in coordination with a rheumatologist or neurologist. Treatment includes high-dose corticosteroids and cyclophosphamide,[1] similar to treatment for lupus nephritis.

Dermatomyositis and Polymyositis

CLINICAL FEATURES

Dermatomyositis may affect skin and muscle. Cutaneous dermatomyositis manifests with violaceous erythema of characteristic areas, including the periorbital skin (i.e., heliotrope rash), upper back (i.e., shawl sign), dorsal hands (i.e., Gottron's papules), scalp, lateral thighs (i.e., holster sign), and periungual skin, where dilated capillary loops and erythema are observed. Patients may report muscle weakness. As in lupus, a punch biopsy of an actively inflamed cutaneous lesion shows characteristic features.

Evaluation of patients with cutaneous dermatomyositis is not complete without assessment for systemic involvement. Serum aldolase is the most specific marker for myositis, and it can be used as a measure of response to treatment. Creatinine kinase and alanine aminotransferase levels may be elevated but are not specific indicators. An electromyogram shows dampening of signals, and a muscle biopsy shows a characteristic pattern of myositis. Inflammatory lung disease, diagnosed by the characteristic pattern on chest computed tomography, bronchoalveolar lavage, or biopsy, may be life limiting and therefore should be treated aggressively, similar to lung disease in scleroderma. Adult patients should have age-appropriate cancer screening because dermatomyositis is a paraneoplastic phenomenon in 10% to 50%.

Some patients present with characteristic cutaneous dermatomyositis but no systemic involvement (i.e., dermatomyositis sine myositis). The risk of concurrent or subsequent cancer development is thought to be increased. These patients require monitoring for systemic involvement that may develop over time.

TREATMENT

Patients with dermatomyositis need photoprotection similar to patients with lupus. Periodic evaluation by clinical examination and review of systems allows for early intervention for developing visceral or muscle involvement.

Cutaneous dermatomyositis is treated the same as lupus (see earlier). Dermatomyositis with systemic involvement is initially treated with immunosuppression using prednisone at doses of 1 mg/kg/day. Steroid-sparing agents are incorporated early in the disease and include antimalarials, methotrexate,[1] azathioprine,[1] and mycophenolate mofetil[1] at doses that are used in treating lupus.

Scleroderma

CLINICAL FEATURES

Scleroderma is a sclerosing condition of skin or viscera, or both. The cause is unknown, but transforming growth factor-β plays a role. Type I and III collagens are excessively produced, as are other substances, including glycosaminoglycans, tenascin, and fibronectin.

Cutaneous scleroderma without Raynaud's phenomenon or clinically relevant systemic involvement is also known as *morphea*. Morphea has different distribution patterns, including guttate, linear,

---

[1]Not FDA approved for this indication.

CURRENT THERAPY

Lupus Erythematosus

- Patients should be counseled on photoprotection measures.
- Localized cutaneous disease is treated with medium- to high-potency topical corticosteroids, and intralesional triamcinolone acetonide 10 mg/mL (Kenalog-10) is added if needed.
- Mild to moderate systemic involvement is treated with low- to medium-potency prednisone 5 to 20 mg/day and with antimalarials.
- Severe disease is treated with prednisone 1 mg/kg/day with a taper based on clinical response. Steroid-sparing agents include azathioprine (Imuran),[1] mycophenolate mofetil (CellCept),[1] methotrexate (Rheumatrex),[1] and cyclophosphamide (Cytoxan).[1]
- Thromboembolism or stroke is treated by anticoagulation with warfarin (Coumadin), aspirin, or heparin.
- Sicca syndrome is treated with frequent water intake, saliva replacement, artificial tears, routine dental care, and pilocarpine (Salagen).

Dermatomyositis and Polymyositis

- Patients should be counseled on photoprotection measures.
- Medium-potency topical corticosteroids and calcineurin inhibitors are used for cutaneous disease.
- Prednisone 1 mg/kg/day is first-line therapy for muscle or pulmonary disease.
- Methotrexate[1] 10 to 25 mg/week is a steroid-sparing agent used for muscle involvement.
- Hydroxychloroquine (Plaquenil)[1] 200 mg/day is used for persistent skin involvement.

Scleroderma

- For localized scleroderma, UVA[1] 20 to 60 J/cm^2 or psoralen plus UVA (PUVA) is used to resolve established lesions; high-potency corticosteroids and calcipotriene (Dovonex)[1] may help to reduce pruritus and inflammation in new lesions; and systemic prednisone[1] or methotrexate[1] may be used for rapidly progressive new lesions.
- Treatment of systemic sclerosis is primarily aimed at limiting complications.
- Physical therapy is used for contractures.
- Systemic sclerosis is treated with cyclophosphamide (Cytoxan),[1] mycophenolate mofetil (CellCept),[1] methotrexate[1] 10 to 25 mg/week, and photopheresis.
- Renal crisis is treated with captopril (Capoten)[1] 6.25 mg three to six times/day and titrated to effect.
- Raynaud's is treated with warming techniques, calcium channel blockers, antiadrenergic agents, antiplatelet drugs, and topical vasodilators.

---

[1]Not FDA approved for this indication.
[2]Not available in the United States.

---

segmental, or diffuse distribution, but it is always characterized by indurated plaques that are inflammatory initially, have an advancing inflammatory ("lilac") border as they progress, and then become hyperpigmented. The cutaneous lesions may restrict movement of joints and can cause restricted growth of underlying structures, particularly when they develop in childhood.

Systemic sclerosis may affect the respiratory, renal, cardiovascular, genitourinary, and gastrointestinal systems and vascular structures. Raynaud's phenomenon may be the first presenting symptom of systemic sclerosis, and it can be severe, leading to digital ulcerations and autoamputation. The American College of Rheumatology has defined criteria for the diagnosis.

Tests for antinuclear antibodies are positive in approximately 95% of patients, who typically present with a homogeneous or speckled pattern. A nucleolar pattern is more specific for systemic sclerosis. Anticentromere antibodies are present in 60% to 90% of patients with limited disease but are rare in diffuse disease. Topoisomerase I (Scl-70) antibodies are positive in 30% of patients with diffuse disease and are associated with pulmonary fibrosis. Anti-PM-Scl antibodies are present in overlap syndromes and are associated with myositis and renal involvement.

TREATMENT

Treatment of Limited Scleroderma

For limited scleroderma, treatment with topical medium-potency corticosteroids such as triamcinolone 0.1% ointment (Kenalog) plus calcipotriene (Dovonex)[1] 0.005% cream or intralesional triamcinalone[1] 20 mg/mL may slow progression of active lesions or improve the pruritus and cutaneous stiffness that typify cutaneous scleroderma. For rapidly evolving disease, prednisone[1] 1 mg/kg/day and methotrexate[1] 15 to 20 mg/week may help slow progression of disease. UVA[1] given over 36 treatments at doses of 30 to 60 mJ/cm^2 or PUVA (oral methoxsalen [8-MOP] 10 mg taken 2 hours before treatment with UVA light) can soften the existing plaques of morphea.

Treatment of Systemic Sclerosis: Raynaud's Phenomenon

First-line treatment for Raynaud's phenomenon is preventive, with cold avoidance and the use of warming techniques. If pharmacotherapy is required, extended-release calcium channel blockers such as nifedipine (Procardia XL)[1] starting at 30 mg/day or amlodipine (Norvasc)[1] starting at 5 mg/day may be useful. If this is not helpful, the α-blocker prazosin (Minipress)[1] 1 mg three times daily or the angiotensin receptor blocker losartan (Cozaar)[1] 50 mg daily may be helpful. Antiplatelet therapy with low-dose aspirin[1] (81 mg/day) or dipyridamole (Persantine)[1] 50 to 100 mg three or four times daily may be useful. Topical vasodilators such as nitroglycerin ointment (Nitro-Bid)[1] applied to the base of the affected finger three times daily can be helpful in refractory disease. Digit-threatening ischemia may be treated with an intravenous prostaglandin such as alprostadil (Prostin VR)[1] or iloprost (Ilomedine),[5] which require peripheral or central access. Patients with severe recurrent digital ischemia may ultimately benefit from surgical sympathectomy.

Treatment of Gastrointestinal Manifestations

The most common gastrointestinal manifestation is esophageal reflux caused by esophageal dysmotility. Proton pump inhibitors such as omeprazole (Prilosec)[1] 20 mg twice daily should be used and may prevent the development of esophageal strictures. Prokinetic drugs such as metoclopramide (Reglan)[1] 10 mg four times daily can be helpful. Erythromycin[1] 500 mg three or four times daily can help esophageal and gastric hypomotility. Small bowel hypomotility can lead to bacterial overgrowth, resulting in malabsorption and diarrhea. Rotating antibiotics that include metronidazole (Flagyl),[1] ciprofloxacin (Cipro),[1] and amoxicillin/clavulanate (Augmentin)[1] can be used.

Treatment of Pulmonary Manifestations

Inflammatory lung disease occurs commonly in patients with scleroderma and can be life limiting. Cyclophosphamide[1] at doses of up to 2 mg/kg/day for up to 2 years may slow progression of pulmonary

---

[1]Not FDA approved for this indication.
[5]Investigational drug in the United States.

disease. Pulmonary hypertension occurs more commonly in limited systemic sclerosis than in diffuse disease. Symptomatic patients may receive treatment with prostacyclin analogues, which require continuous infusions. The endothelin receptor antagonist bosentan (Tracleer)[1] can be given orally starting at 62.5 mg twice daily. Liver tests should be monitored frequently. At this point, care is typically coordinated with a cardiologist to monitor disease progression and treatment response. Anticoagulation for pulmonary hypertension may improve survival because of the frequent occurrence of pulmonary arterial thrombosis.

Treatment of Renal Manifestations

Angiotensin-converting enzyme (ACE) inhibitors (e.g., captopril [Capoten[1]] beginning at 6.25 mg three to six times daily and titrated for blood pressure control) have dramatically reduced the incidence of renal failure and death due to renal crisis. Avoidance of prednisone at doses greater than 15 mg/day is also important in reducing the risk of renal crisis.

REFERENCES

Atzeni F, Bendtzen K, Bobbio-Pallavicini F, et al. Infections and treatment of patients with rheumatic diseases. Clin Exp Rheumatol 2008;26(Suppl. 48):S67–73.

Dziadzio M, Denton CP, Smith R. Losartan therapy for Raynaud's phenomenon and scleroderma. Arthritis Rheum 1999;42(12):2646–55.

Ginzler EM, Dooley MA, Aranow C, et al. Mycophenolate mofetil or intravenous cyclophosphamide for lupus nephritis. N Engl J Med 2005;353 (21):2219–28.

Iorizzo LJ, Jorizzo JL. The treatment and prognosis of dermatomyositis: An updated review. J Am Acad Dermatol 2008;59:99–112.

Matucci-Cerinic M, Steen VD, Furst DE, et al. Clinical trials in systemic sclerosis: Lessons learned and outcomes. Arthritis Res Ther 2007; 9(Suppl. 2):S7.

Nihtyanova SI, Denton CP. Current approaches to the management of early active diffuse scleroderma skin disease. Rheum Dis Clin North Am 2008;34:161–79.

Pisoni CN, Sanchez FJ, Karim Y, et al. Mycophenolate mofetil in systemic lupus erythematosus: Efficacy and tolerability in 86 patients. J Rheumatol 2005;32:1047–52.

Steen VD. The many faces of scleroderma. Rheum Dis Clin North Am 2008;34:1–15.

Subcommittee for Scleroderma Criteria of the American Rheumatism Association Diagnostic and Therapeutic Criteria Committee. Preliminary criteria for the classification of systemic sclerosis (scleroderma). Arthritis Rheum 1980;23:581–90.

Tan EM, Cohen AS, Fries JF, et al. The 1982 revised criteria for the classification of lupus erythematosus. Arthritis Rheum 1982;25:1271–2.

Wallace DD. Lupus Erythematosus. 7th ed. Philadelphia: Lippincott Williams & Wilkins; 2006.

---

[1]Not FDA approved for this indication.

Cutaneous Vasculitis

Method of
Manisha J. Patel, MD, and
Joseph L. Jorizzo, MD

Vasculitis refers to inflammation and necrosis of blood vessels. It can be local or systemic and may be primary or secondary to another disease process. In patients with systemic involvement, the kidneys, gastrointestinal (GI) tract, or peripheral nerves may be involved. The classic cutaneous manifestation of small-vessel vasculitis is palpable purpura; the clinical manifestation greatly depends on the size and type of the vessel affected.

Clinical Presentation

The typical primary skin lesion of small-vessel cutaneous vasculitis (CV) is palpable purpura with lesions ranging in size from 1 mm to several centimeters (Figure 1). The lesions arise as a simultaneous *crop* and result from the exposure to an inciting stimulus. Usually macular in the early stages, lesions may progress to wide array of lesions including, papules, nodules, vesicles, plaques, bullae, or pustules. Secondary findings include ulceration, necrosis, and postinflammatory hyperpigmentation. Other cutaneous findings include livedo reticularis, edema, and urticarial lesions. Lesions most commonly occur on dependent areas, such as ankles and lower legs or other areas prone to stasis.

Although normally asymptomatic, local symptoms may include pruritus, pain, or burning. Systemic symptoms including fever, arthralgias, myalgias, anorexia, or GI pain should raise the suspicion that the CV may be associated with a systemic vasculitis.

Typically 50% of all patients with CV experience an acute or transient course, 30% develop chronic disease, and 20% experience relapsing disease. The percentage of patients with CV who have systemic involvement of one or more systems depends on the subspecialty of the series authors and the definition of systemic involvement. Most patients presenting to dermatologists do not have significant systemic involvement, excluding arthralgias, myalgias, fever, and serum sickness-like symptoms. It is best to consider that every patient with small-vessel CV may have systemic disease; this mandates a careful history, physical examination, and laboratory evaluation. Table 1 summarizes the key steps in evaluating suspected small-vessel CV and highlights the assessment for possible systemic involvement.

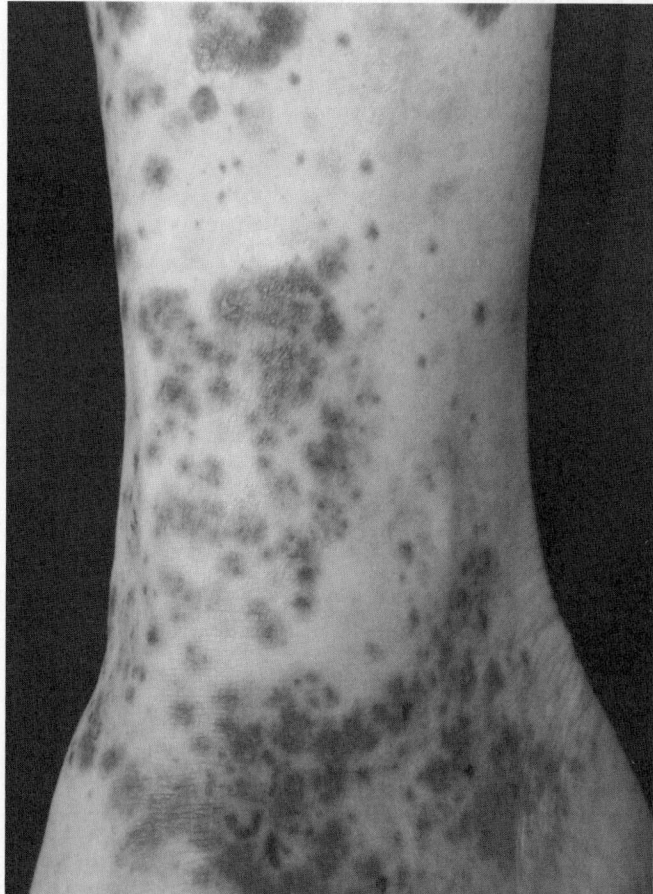

FIGURE 1. Small-vessel cutaneous vasculitis. Palpable purpura and early central necrosis are seen on the distal lower extremity. (Courtesy of Dr. Kelly Barham, Wake Forest University School of Medicine, Winston-Salem, NC.)

TABLE 1 Evaluation of Suspected Small Vessel Cutaneous Vasculitis

Confirming Histopathologic Correlation	Assessing the Extent of the Disease	Establishing Etiology
Punch biopsy early lesion	General • Myalgia • Arthralgia • Fever	Infection • Bacterial • Viral • Fungal • Acid-fast bacilli • Other
Incisional biopsy for suspected larger vessel vasculitis	Renal involvement (acute and chronic renal failure) • Proteinuria • Hematuria Nervous system • Central or peripheral • Diffuse or local findings	Drugs Diseases associated with immune complexes • Connective tissue/autoimmune diseases • Malignancy (especially myelodysplastic) • Inflammatory bowel disease Idiopathic (50%)
	Musculoskeletal involvement • Nonerosive polyarthritis Gastrointestinal system • Abdominal pain (colicky, nausea, vomiting, diarrhea) • Gastrointestinal bleeding (melena or hematemesis) Pulmonary involvement • Pleural effusion • Pleuritis • Hemoptysis Pericardial involvement (myocardial angiitis or pericarditis) • Pericardial effusion Ocular involvement (retinal vasculitis) • Conjunctivitis • Keratitis Other	

Modified from Barham KL et al: Rook's Textbook of Dermatology, 7th ed. Oxford, Blackwell Publishing, 2004.

Histopathology

The hallmark histopathologic pattern of small-vessel CV is leukocytoclastic vasculitis. The histologic specimen shows an infiltration of neutrophils within and around blood vessel walls; leukocytoclasia (degranulation and fragmentation of neutrophils leading to the production of nuclear dust); fibrinoid necrosis of the damaged vessel walls; and necrosis, swelling, and proliferation of the endothelial cells. New clinical lesions should be selected for biopsy because specimens taken too late (i.e., older than 48 hours) may show the pathology of repair more than of the initial injury. Direct immunofluorescence microscopic studies on fresh lesions frequently demonstrate perivascular deposits of IgM or activated third component of complement (C3) in the superficial dermal papillary vessels. One exception is the deposition of IgA in patients with Henoch-Schönlein purpura. Documenting leukocytoclastic vasculitis in biopsy specimens is essential to confirming the diagnosis.

Etiology

Small-vessel CV is considered to be an aberrant immune complex response that is usually triggered by an infection, exposure to a drug, or association with an autoimmune disease; most etiologic factors identified have been incriminated by association rather than by direct demonstration. Between 50% and 60% of patients have no identifiable cause. Of the approximately 50% of patients in whom a cause is identifiable, 20% are associated with infections; and another 20% are thought to be triggered by an exposure to a drug. Bacterial

infections associated with CV include streptococcus, staphylococcus, and gram-negative organisms. Several viral agents include HIV, hepatitis B and C, herpes simplex virus (HSV), and influenza. Suspected medications include antibiotics (penicillins, sulfonamides), anticonvulsants, isoniazid (Laniazid), oral contraceptives, and thiazides. Less than 5% of patients have underlying connective tissue disease. There have been patients with small-vessel CV reported rarely in patients with malignancies, especially Hodgkin's disease, mycosis fungoides, and adult T-cell lymphoma.

Differential Diagnosis

Not all dermatoses associated with purpura are a result of vasculitis. In the differential diagnosis of vasculitis, be aware of disorders that may present with livedo or infarcted lesions secondary to vascular occlusion disorders. Some examples of vaso-occlusive disorders include cryoglobulinemia, cholesterol emboli, Sneddon's syndrome, septic emboli, and malignant atrophic papulosis (Degos' disease). The histopathology in these disorders results from either initially occlusive or mediation by antiphospholipid antibodies, and therefore, falls into the category of microvascular occlusion. The differential diagnosis also includes trauma, coagulopathies, and thrombocytopenia. Purpuras secondary to coagulopathies and thrombocytopenia are noninflammatory and often nonpalpable; they can be distinguished promptly on histologic and laboratory testing.

Given the wide array of systemic diseases that can be associated with small-vessel CV, it is important to carefully evaluate each patient for coexistent disease; the first manifestation of large-vessel vasculitis is often small-vessel disease.

CURRENT DIAGNOSIS

- Clinical spectrum of lesions ranging from purpura to palpable purpura, urticarial lesions, or ulcers: concentrated on dependent areas
- Small-vessel CV involves postcapillary venules only
- Histologic finding: leukocytoclastic vasculitis
- Pathogenesis: circulating immune complexes, neutrophils, cytokines, and adhesion molecules

Abbreviation: CV = cutaneous vasculitis.

HENOCH-SCHÖNLEIN PURPURA

Henoch-Schönlein purpura (HSP) deserves specific mention given its history and frequent occurrence. Heberden first described a single patient with HSP in 1801. Johann Schönlein and Eduard Henoch elucidated features in the mid-19th century as a tetrad of palpable purpura, arthritis, and GI and renal involvement. Henoch-Schönlein purpura is defined by the Chapel Hill Consensus Conference as a vasculitis affecting small vessels, involving deposition of IgA immune complexes that characteristically involves the skin, GI system, and glomeruli with or without arthralgia or arthritis. Approximately 30% of cases follow an upper respiratory infection. The clinical outcome is excellent with fewer than 10% of patients developing chronic disease. A small percent of patients will develop persistent renal or GI disease requiring systemic immunosuppressive therapy.

URTICARIAL VASCULITIS

Another important subtype of small-vessel CV is urticarial vasculitis. Urticarial vasculitis is a chronic disorder consisting of episodic urticarial and/or angioedematous lesions lasting longer than 24 hours that histologically manifest features of leukocytoclastic vasculitis.

Urticarial vasculitis may range from patients with only urticarial skin lesions to those with urticarial vasculitis associated with hypocomplementemia with some systemic features; this meets criteria for systemic lupus erythematosus. Patients with urticarial vasculitis may also have underlying autoimmune connective tissue diseases, infections (hepatitis B and C), neoplastic processes, or medications as underlying etiologic factors. Treatment is directed at underlying etiologies and/or follows the same therapeutic ladder as for small-vessel CV (Table 2).

Treatment

Because small-vessel CV is generally self-limited, treatment is often unnecessary except for symptomatic relief. When possible, identification and removal of a causative agent (e.g., infection, drug, chemicals, food) should be accomplished. Removal of an inciting agent is occasionally followed by rapid resolution of the lesions and no other treatment is indicated; otherwise, local and systemic therapies are recommended. Symptomatic improvement may be achieved with leg elevation, gradient support stockings, nonsteroidal anti-inflammatory drugs, and antihistamines.

Small-vessel CV with persistent palpable purpura without significant internal organ complications may respond to treatment with oral colchicine[1] in doses of 0.6 mg two to three times daily. Dosing is limited by GI symptoms. This therapy is supported by anecdotal reports, but a statistically significant difference was not confirmed in a randomized controlled trial. Dapsone[1] (50 to 200 mg per day) has also been used in patients only having skin involvement.

Systemic treatment is advised for patients with small-vessel CV who have significant systemic manifestations or significant cutaneous ulceration. However, almost no double-blind, placebo-controlled prospective trials exist. Table 2 describes a therapeutic ladder for

---

[1]Not FDA approved for this indication.

TABLE 2 Therapeutic Ladder for Small-Vessel Cutaneous Vasculitis

	Double-Blind Studies	Case Series	Case Reports
Skin lesions alone	Colchicine[1]	Nonsteroidal anti-inflammatory drugs Dapsone[1]	Supportive therapy • Antihistamines • Pentoxifylline (Trental)[1] • Hydroxychloroquine (Plaquenil)[1] • Thalidomide (Thalomid)[1] • Low-dose weekly methotrexate (Rheumatrex)[1]
Ulcerative skin lesions alone		Prednisone[1]	
Systemic disease	Interferon-α and ribavirin (Rebetron) (if associated with hepatitis C) 3 million units 3/wk and 1000 mg/d, respectively	Prednisone[1] Azathioprine (Imuran)[1] 1–2.5 mg/kg/d PO as single dose or divided in half Cyclophosphamide (Cytoxan)[1] pulsed dosing regimen, 40–50 mg/kg IV in divided doses over 2–5 d *or* 10–15 mg/kg IV q 7–10 d *or* 3–5 mg/kg IV 2/wk	Mycophenolate mofetil (CellCept)[1] 500–2000 mg PO bid Cyclosporine (Neoral, Sandimmune)[1] 2.5 mg/kg/d PO divided in half qd; after 4 wk, dose may be increased 0.5 mg/kg/d at 2-wk intervals; maximum of 4 mg/kg/d • IV gammaglobulin (Gammagard)[1] • Extracorporeal immunomodulation • Biologic agents: infliximab (Remicade),[1] etanercept (Enbrel)[1] (TNF-α inhibitors) • Rituximab (Anti-CD20)[1]
	Methotrexate (Trexall)[1] 7.5–15 mg once a week*		

Modified from Barham KL et al: Rook's Textbook of Dermatology, 7th ed. Oxford, Blackwell Publishing, 2004.
*There is no study associated with this drug.
[1]Not FDA approved for this indication.
Abbreviations: IV = intravenously; TNF-α = tumor necrosis factor-α.

CURRENT THERAPY

- Small-vessel CV is generally self-limited; treatment is often unnecessary except for symptomatic relief, which may be achieved with leg elevation, gradient support stockings, nonsteroidal anti-inflammatory drugs, and antihistamines.
- Skin manifestations alone may be managed with agents such as colchicine and dapsone.
- Systemic treatment is advised for patients with significant systemic manifestations or those with significant cutaneous ulceration.

Abbreviation: CV = cutaneous vasculitis.

small-vessel CV. The medications discussed in Table 2 have not been FDA approved for this indication. Oral corticosteroids (Prednisone[1] 0.5 to 1 mg/kg per day) are indicated for progressive, symptomatic nodular, vesicular, or ulcerating purpura as well as systemic involvement. Once the patient's symptoms have stabilized, prednisone should be tapered gradually over 3 to 6 weeks because a rapid taper can lead to clinical disease rebound.

Small-vessel CV can manifest clinically with a spectrum of cutaneous lesions; palpable purpura is the classic presentation. The hallmark histologic appearance is a leukocytoclastic vasculitis. There is a presumed immune complex mediated pathogenesis. The therapeutic approach requires elimination of the cause (drugs, chemicals, infection) when possible. In most patients, only the skin is involved and can be treated with supportive measures. The most important step in evaluation is the full workup to find etiology and extent (systemic involvement) of the disease process. Skin manifestations alone may be managed with nonsteroidal anti-inflammatory drugs, gradient support stockings, colchicine, and dapsone. Systemic treatment is advised in small-vessel CV with significant systemic manifestations or those with significant cutaneous ulceration.

REFERENCES

Fiorentino DF. Cutaneous vasculitis. J Am Acad Dermatol 2003;48(3):311–40.
Gonzalez-Gay MA, Garcia-Porrua C, Pujol RM. Clinical approach to cutaneous vasculitis. Curr Opin Rheumatol 2005;17(1):56–61.
Lamprecht P. TNF-alpha inhibitors in systemic vasculitides and connective tissue diseases. Autoimmun Rev 2005;4(1):28–34.
Lotti T, Ghersetich I, Comacchi C, Jorizzo JL. Cutaneous small-vessel vasculitis. J Am Acad Dermatol 1998;39(5 Pt 1):667–87.

[1]Not FDA approved for this indication.

Diseases of the Nails

Method of
Nathaniel Jellinek, MD, and Ralph C. Daniel, MD

Overview

The nail plate in humans has many functions. It facilitates scratching; it is used as a tool, a weapon, and a form of adornment (to the cost of approximately $6 billion per year in the United States); and most importantly it supports the underlying distal phalanx and soft tissue to maximize fine touch and manual dexterity.

The nail unit consists of the nail plate, an underlying nail bed, a germinative nail matrix, proximal and lateral nail folds, a cuticle

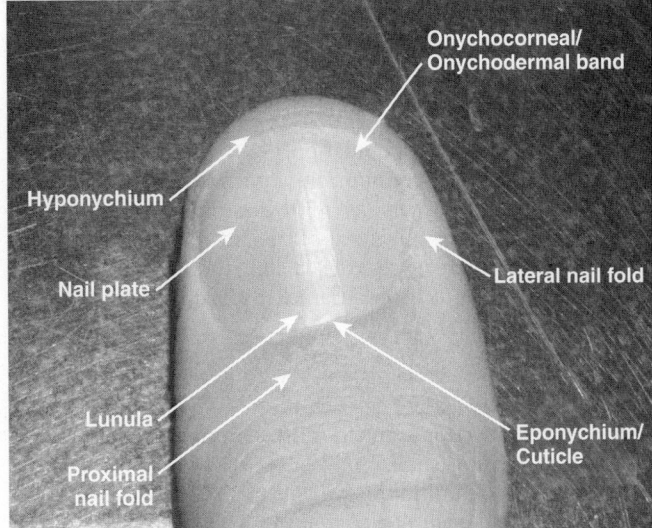

FIGURE 1. Surface anatomy of the nail.

and distal hyponychium (Fig. 1). The matrix exists under the proximal nail fold, beginning just distal to the insertion of the dorsal extensor tendon, and extends distally under the nail plate beyond the cuticle as the crescent-shaped lunula. The lunula is usually most apparent on the thumbnail, less so on each consecutive finger. The nail bed is contiguous with the matrix, tightly adherent to the overlying plate, to which it is connected in a tongue-and-groove pattern, ending distally at the onychocorneal (or onychodermal) band, the distal-most attachment point between the bed and plate. The onychocorneal band region provides the ventral barrier of the nail unit. When it is breached, onycholysis results.

Dorsally and laterally, the nail folds provide an anatomic barrier to the nail unit. When they are breached, moisture, yeast, bacteria, and contact irritants and allergens penetrate the normal barrier and cause paronychia, acute and chronic.

An understanding of normal nail anatomy facilitates comprehension of the pathology discussed here.

Lichen Planus

CLINICAL FEATURES AND DIAGNOSIS

Lichen planus is an inflammatory disorder that can involve the skin, hair, nails, and mucous membranes. Nail disease can accompany skin or mucosal disease or can manifest as isolated nail disease. It is characterized histologically by lichenoid inflammation and can involve any or all of the nail subunits. Onychorrhexis, longitudinal striations in the nail plate, and nail plate thinning or fragility, result from nail matrix involvement. Onycholysis (nail lifting) and nail thickening are caused by hyponychium and nail bed involvement. Nail pain can herald the onset of bullous lichen planus of the nail. This represents an urgent problem, because permanent scarring of the nail bed and matrix can result, manifesting clinically as dorsal pterygium. It is crucial to check all patients with suspected nail lichen planus with a complete skin and oral mucosal examination for lesions.

TREATMENT

Overt, repetitive, and incidental trauma to the nail apparatus worsens the nail disease and makes it more resistant to treatment (the Koebner phenomenon.) The Koebner and Koebner-like phenomena are important in the diathesis of lichen planus. Therefore, trauma, contact irritants, and moisture must be minimized or avoided. The nails should be kept short. Intralesional triamcinolone 2.5 to 5 mg/mL monthly for several months and occasionally systemic corticosteroids may be required in more severe cases or with scarring.

CURRENT DIAGNOSIS

Brittle Nails

- Brittle nails are present in approximately 20% of the North American population.
- They are more common in women, those who use nail cosmetics, and persons >50 years old.
- Diagnose with subjective complaint of brittle nails with observation of onychorrhexis (longitudinal nail plate ridging) and onychoschizia (lamellar splitting of nail plate).

Onychomycosis

- Make an objective diagnosis with KOH, culture or clipping for periodic acid–Schiff.
- Onychomycosis is much more common on the toenails than the fingernails.
- The most common organisms are *Trichophyton rubrum* or *Trichophyton mentagrophytes.*
- *Candida* only rarely causes onychomycosis. It is primarily a colonizer in the setting of barrier breakdown of the nail apparatus.
- Nondermatophyte molds (such as *Aspergillus, Fusarium, Penicillium* spp) are unusual causes of onychomycosis in the United States. Repeat tests showing the same organisms and ruling out other causes are mandated before initiating treatment.

Primary Onycholysis and Chronic Paronychia

- Primary onycholysis and chronic paronychia are diagnoses of exclusion. Onychomycosis, psoriasis, lichen planus, and drug reactions all must be ruled out before diagnosis.
- Both are more common on the fingernails than the toenails, in women, in adults, in those who use nail cosmetics, or and those who have recurrent exposure to moisture or chemicals.
- Both primary onycholysis and chronic paronychia represent breakdown in the normal barrier of the nail apparatus. Onycholysis results from breakdown of the onychocorneal band or nail bed–nail plate connection. Chronic paronychia results from breakdown of the cuticle and nail folds.
- In both scenarios, moisture, contact irritants, contact allergens, colonizing yeast, and bacteria invade the exposed nail apparatus and contribute to a cycle of inflammation.

Ingrown Nails

- Common risk factors include incorrect nail cutting, wide feet, narrow-toed shoes, lateral plate malalignment, and lateral nail fold hypertrophy.
- Neonates and infants demonstrate distal nail ingrowing, which is separate in pathogenesis and treatment from the disease in adolescents and adults.
- Ingrown nails can be graded on a scale from I to III, with I being erythema and swelling with drainage from the nail fold and III being associated with exuberant overgrowth of granulation tissue over and around the ingrown nail plate.

CURRENT THERAPY

Brittle Nails

- Treatment is frustrating and represents the limitations in our understanding of disease pathogenesis.
- Oral biotin, 2–3 mg (2000–3000 μg) (Appearex) daily, dosed for 4–6 months and then discontinued, is a reasonable trial. Patients will notice an effect during this period if it has helped, then may continue to treat if it is helpful.
- Topical moisturizers (petrolatum) or humectant agents (12% ammonium lactate, 20% urea) might help those with hard brittle nails.

Onychomycosis

- Topical treatment is disappointing, except in cases of superficial white onychomycosis.
- Oral treatment should be reserved for patients with symptomatic disease or who are at risk for complications (diabetics, immunosuppressed, at risk of secondary bacterial cellulitis).
- Oral treatment is more successful than topical treatment. Terbinafine (Lamisil) 250 mg PO qd × 90 days in adults is the first-line treatment. Itraconazole (Sporanox), dosed daily or pulsed 1 week per month, is the next most successful agent.
- Patients are at high risk for recurrence. Post-treatment prevention of tinea pedis is important to prevent reinfection.

Primary Onycholysis and Chronic Paronychia

- It is important not to misdiagnose the presence of yeast (especially *Candida*) as a primary infection or pathogen. It almost always represents a colonizer. Treatment of the yeast is therefore secondary.
- Avoidance is the mainstay of treatment. Avoid all wet work and exposure to acids, bases, and chemicals by wearing cotton gloves under heavy-duty vinyl gloves. Avoid all nail cosmetics and nail manipulation except for regular plate trimming. No nail salon. Keep the plate trimmed to its proximal-most attachment point. Avoid obvious triggers and traumas to the nail apparatus.
- It can take up to 6 months for the nail apparatus to normalize.

Ingrown Nails

- Infantile disease: Warm soaks followed by massage of the nail and distal phalangeal tuft.
- Adolescent and adult disease: Correct nail plate cutting and shoes. For mild disease, twice daily cold soaks, topical steroids, 20% to 40% topical urea cream (Keralac, Carmol), and cotton wisps or dental floss under the aggravating part of the lateral nail plate will decrease inflammation, improve symptoms, and normalize the nail plate without surgery.
- For more advanced cases, twice-daily warm soaks, oral antibiotics (with signs of infection), followed by lateral plate avulsion and lateral matricectomy (either chemical or surgical).

Onychomycosis

CLINICAL FEATURES AND DIAGNOSIS

Approximately one half of all doctor visits relating to nail complaints are for onychomycosis. It is not only the most common nail diagnosis, however; it is also the most common misdiagnosis, and even experienced nail clinicians might not make an accurate diagnosis up to 50% of the time. It is therefore crucial to confirm the diagnosis by potassium hydroxide, fungal culture, or clipping for periodic acid–Schiff analysis before initiating any therapy, with its inherent risks and costs.

In the United States, 80% to 90% cases of onychomycosis are caused by dermatophyte fungi, most commonly *Trichophyton rubrum* or *Trichophyton mentagrophytes*. The tendency to acquire these infections appears to be inherited in an autosomal dominant fashion with incomplete or variable penetrance. The infection usually begins with tinea pedis; the nail barrier between plate and hyponychium or nail fold is compromised, often through repetitive trauma, and fungus enters the nail apparatus.

There are four main types of onychomycosis: distal and lateral subungual onychomycosis (DLSO, most common), occasionally leading to total dystrophic onychomycosis (TDO), superficial white onychomycosis (SWO), and proximal subungual onychomycosis (PSO). SWO is the most straightforward to diagnose; scraping the surface yields abundant fungi for examination. DLSO and TDO are best diagnosed by acquiring the proximal-most area of involved nail plate and subungual debris; this occasionally involves aggressive paring by the practitioner to remove the distal nail plate and debris, with lower diagnostic yield. PSO may be a marker for systemic immunosuppression and is therefore important to diagnose. A nail plate punch biopsy is the most direct and accurate way to make this diagnosis of the latter.

Candida only rarely causes onychomycosis. This fact is widely misunderstood, probably because *Candida* is commonly found as a colonizing organism in conditions such as primary onycholysis and chronic paronychia. The unusual situation of primary *Candida* onychomycosis is limited to those with inherited chronic mucocutaneous candidiasis or severe immunosuppression. The presence of this organism in the setting of onychomycosis should arouse doubt rather than confirm the diagnosis. In most cases, it is a colonizer rather than a pathogen.

The presence of an underlying disease with nail manifestations (such as psoriasis or lichen planus) does not rule out the concomitant presence of onychomycosis and can cause barrier breakdown of the nail apparatus, facilitating secondary fungal infection.

TREATMENT

Oral treatment should be reserved for patients who have symptomatic disease or who are at risk for complications, such as diabetics and immunocompromised patients, who are at risk for secondary bacterial cellulitis.

Confirm the diagnosis. The presence of *Candida* or nondermatophyte mold is unusual in the United States. Tests should be repeated and other diagnoses should be entertained before diagnosing onychomycosis and initiating treatment. If a dermatophyte is found, systemic terbinafine (Lamisil) offers the best systemic choice. Systemic itraconazole (Sporanox) is the next most effective agent and can be dosed in a pulsed fashion (off label) or daily like terbinafine. Topical ciclopirox (Loprox) clears the nails in less than 10% of cases; other topical agents are equally ineffective.

Because a person is often genetically predisposed to acquire onychomycosis, once the disorder is cleared by a systemic agent, then topical agents must be used indefinitely, with the goal being to avoid subsequent cases of tinea pedis. Powders and lotions are available over the counter and may be used on a regular basis.

Brittle Nails

CLINICAL FEATURES AND DIAGNOSIS

A simplistic view, but perhaps representing the best of our understanding about brittle nails, is that hard brittle nails are caused and worsened by too little moisture, and that soft brittle nails are associated with too much moisture. Both may be worsened by irritants. Older persons tend to have dry brittle nails, analogous to skin in the aging population. Although up to 20% of North Americans have brittle nails, our understanding of the pathogenesis is limited.

Brittle nails are diagnosed when subjective and objective criteria are met. Patients must complain of nail fragility and easy breaking with clinical signs of onychorrhexis (longitudinal ridging), onychoschizia (lamellar splitting), and occasionally dull, lusterless plate appearance.

TREATMENT

Biotin (vitamin H or B_7) 2 to 3 mg (often dosed as 2000–3000 µg) [gkuo2][3,7] taken once daily improves brittleness in some cases. It is helpful to have the patient take this water-soluble vitamin for 4 to 6 months, then discontinue it for a several months to evaluate for improvement, worsening, or no change. This initial trial therapy can prevent continued cost to the patient if he or she notices no improvement and then worsening when taking and discontinuing the vitamin, respectively. Irritant avoidance is also helpful. Application of petrolatum at bedtime under light white cotton gloves (apply ointment after soaking the nail in water for 5 minutes) increases the moisture content of the nail plate. Topical humectant agents include over-the-counter 12% ammonium lactate cream and 10% to 20% urea preparations.

Ingrown Nails

CLINICAL FEATURES AND DIAGNOSIS

Ingrown nails represent a foreign body reaction of the nail plate in the lateral nail fold. It is more common on toenails, particularly the great toenails, than fingernails. Predisposing factors include wide feet, ill-fitting or narrow-toed or high heeled shoes, lateral plate malalignment, hypertrophic lateral nail folds, cutting the nails incorrectly in a half-circle instead of straight across, and possibly hyperhidrosis. Secondary infection can occur after the plate pierces the nail fold skin.

In adolescents and adults, the nail fold embedding and spicule formation tends to be lateral, whereas in neonates and young children the embedding tends to be distal. The former group is predisposed to multiple episodes of ingrowing; procedural treatment is recommended and often required. The latter group often responds to conservative treatment; surgery is only occasionally required.

TREATMENT

Correct nail cutting and appropriate shoes are the main treatment. For mild disease, use of twice-daily cold soaks, topical steroids, 20% to 40% topical urea cream, and cotton wisps or dental floss under the aggravating part of the lateral nail plate can decrease inflammation, improve symptoms, and normalize the nail plate without requiring surgery. For more advanced cases, twice-daily warm soaks, oral antibiotics (with signs of infection), followed by lateral plate avulsion and lateral matricectomy (either chemical or surgical) represent standard of care. Infantile disease responds to warm soaks followed by massage of the nail and distal phalangeal tuft.

Subungual Hematoma

CLINICAL FEATURES AND DIAGNOSIS

Blood under the nail plate can appear red or black. Because the physiologic blood-metabolizing enzymes are not found in the nail plate, blood trapped between the plate and bed is not metabolized to the

---

[3]Exceeds dosage recommended by the manufacturer.
[7]Available as a dietary supplement.

same evolving brown- and green-colored metabolites in the nail, and instead stays red-black and grows out with the nail plate. Nail plate growth is slow, approximately 3 mm/month for fingernails and about one half that rate for toenails, so that growing out of the hematoma will take several months and may be difficult to appreciate without photographs or serial measurements.

Diagnosis is usually straightforward. In ambiguous presentations, a urinalysis reagent strip efficiently and accurately tests for subungual blood. However, nail tumors are often preceded or first recognized after trauma, and they might even bleed spontaneously. Therefore, the presence of blood does not rule out a concomitant neoplasm.

TREATMENT

Any hematoma involving more than 50% of the nail plate carries a significant risk of underlying distal phalangeal fracture, and an x-ray should be ordered. For relief of acute symptomatic subungual hematomas, digital anesthesia followed by trephination using a sterilized hot paper clip, punch, #11 blade, or nail drill provides rapid relief and confirms the diagnosis. For most cases, however, no treatment is indicated, and the blood will grow out distally with the nail plate, albeit slowly.

Psoriasis

CLINICAL FEATURES AND DIAGNOSIS

Psoriasis commonly involves the nails in patients with cutaneous disease and occasionally occurs as a disease isolated to the nail unit. In those with psoriatic arthritis, nail disease is over-represented, and may be present up to 90% to 95% of the time. Like lichen planus, psoriasis can involve any part of the nail unit; hyponychium and nail bed involvement manifest as onycholysis and subungual hyperkeratosis and a red nail bed or oil drop (salmon patch) change.

Nail pitting occurs from proximal matrix psoriasis, where parakeratotic columns lose attachment from the superficial plate, leaving a narrow depression behind in the nail plate. Any patient with these signs should have a detailed history (looking for family history) and complete skin examination, with particular attention given to the scalp, external auditory meatus, postauricular crease, umbilicus, intergluteal fold, groin, and flexural areas. Even without these helpful cutaneous signs, the combination of three nail signs is highly suggestive of nail psoriasis. In ambiguous cases, a nail clipping or nail bed biopsy can provide additional diagnostic information.

TREATMENT

Overt, repetitive, and incidental trauma to the nail apparatus worsens the nail disease and makes it more resistant to treatment (the Koebner phenomenon.) Therefore, it is important to keep the nails trimmed short, use no nail cosmetics or artificial nails, and avoid aggressive nail manicuring or débridement of nail bed hyperkeratosis.

Topical treatment may be applied with a variety of agents, many of which represent off-label uses: corticosteroids, 5-fluorouracil (Efudex, Carac),[1] calcipotriene (Dovonex), tazarotene (Tazorac), cyclosporine (Sandimmune), and urea (Keralac, Carmol). Topical treatment is low risk but generally disappointing. Intralesional injection of triamcinolone 2.5 to 5 mg/mL is effective and can be dosed on a monthly basis and gradually tapered until the nails are free of disease; this therapy can provide a period of remission from nail disease. Systemic agents (methotrexate [Trexall], cyclosporine, or injectable therapies) used for severe psoriasis and psoriatic arthritis are inappropriate to use off label for isolated nail disease; however, in the case of widespread disease, they often improve concomitant nail psoriasis. Systemic corticosteroids, as with all forms of psoriasis, are contraindicated and can provoke an outbreak of widespread pustular (von Zumbush) psoriasis.

---

[1]Not FDA approved for this indication.

Primary (Simple) Oncholysis

CLINICAL FEATURES AND DIAGNOSIS

Onycholysis means separation of nail plate from nail bed or nail folds and represents a ventral or lateral break in the normal nail barrier. It can be graded from stage 1 (minimal involvement) to stage 4 or 5 (maximal involvement). The longer onycholysis is present, the less likely it is to resolve as the nail bed can pathologically cornify and develop a granular layer.

The most common causes are trauma and contact irritants or moisture. Other causes include psoriasis and onychomycosis; whereas onychomycosis tends to involve the toenails only and manifests with yellow nails, onycholysis nearly always involves the fingernails and demonstrates classic physical signs. Primary onycholysis usually involves the fingernails, and might involve only one nail. Women, those who use nail cosmetics, and persons with prolonged irritant or moisture contact, are all at highest risk.

Monodactylous onycholysis should always raise the possibility of an underlying neoplasm. Yeast is commonly cultured but is usually an opportunistic colonizer rather than a pathogenic organism. Hence the presence of *Candida* does not mean a diagnosis of onychomycosis, but secondary colonization in the setting of onycholysis.

TREATMENT

Nails must be kept short. Patients must practice a strict irritant and moisture avoidance regimen, including avoidance of all nail cosmetics and artificial nails. They should use heavy cotton gloves for dry work and light cotton gloves under vinyl gloves for wet work. A topical antifungal solution, lotion, or lacquer may be added as an adjuvant agent but is considered secondary after the avoidance regimen. For monodactylous cases, x-ray and biopsy should always be considered.

Primary (Simple) Chronic Paronychia

CLINICAL FEATURES AND DIAGNOSIS

Chronic paronychia may be defined as inflammation of one or more nail folds, usually the proximal fold, lasting 6 weeks or longer. It represents a dorsal or lateral (or both) barrier breakdown of the nail unit, compared with onycholysis on the ventral of the nail plate. In both situations, irritants and moisture contribute to a chronic irritant contact dermatitis and yeast colonization. Women, persons who use nail cosmetics or work in the food industry, and persons with prolonged irritant or moisture contact are at risk. As with onycholysis, patients with single-digit involvement or refractory cases who fail to respond to treatment should bring to mind the possibility of an underlying neoplasm, and a biopsy is warranted.

TREATMENT

The same principles apply to treatment of chronic paronychia as for onycholysis. An irritant and moisture avoidance regimen, combined with an antifungal solution as an adjuvant, is central to therapy. Nail cosmetics and nail manipulation, with an orange stick, for example, are forbidden. A topical corticosteroid agent may be used to decrease inflammation for 3 to 4 weeks initially, combined with the avoidance regimen. Refractory cases might respond to intralesional corticosteroids 2.5 to 5 mg/mL or occasionally a surgical saucerization of the proximal nail fold.

REFERENCES

Daniel CR 3rd, Daniel MP, Daniel J, et al. Managing simple chronic paronychia and onycholysis with ciclopirox 0.77% and an irritant-avoidance regimen. Cutis 2004;73(1):81–5.

de Berker D. The physical basis of cosmetic defects of the nail plate. J Cosmet Dermatol 2002;1(1):35–42.

de Berker D. Management of nail psoriasis. Clin Exp Dermatol 2000;25 (5):357–62.

Gupta AK, Tu LQ. Onychomycosis therapies: Strategies to improve efficacy. Dermatol Clin 2006;24(3):381–6.

Haneke E. Ingrown and pincer nails: evaluation and treatment. Dermatol Ther 2002;15:148–58.

Rounding C, Bloomfield S. Surgical treatments for ingrowing toenails. Cochrane Database Syst Rev 2005;(2):CD001541.

Tosti A, Piraccini BM. Treatment of common nail disorders. Dermatol Clin 2000;18(2):339–48.

van de Kerkhof PC, Pasch MC, Scher RK, et al. Brittle nail syndrome: A pathogenesis-based approach with a proposed grading system. J Am Acad Dermatol 2005;53(4):644–51.

Keloids

Method of

Rungsima Wanitphakdeedecha, MD, MA, MSc, Papapit Tuchinda, MD, and Tina S. Alster, MD

Patients with keloids commonly present for dermatologic consultation because of functional and cosmetic disfigurement. Various degrees of pruritus, pain, dysesthesia, ulceration, secondary infection, restricted range of motion, and psychological distress may be associated with these scars. The upper arms, back, chest, shoulders, cheeks, earlobes, head, and neck are the predominant regions in which these scars occur. Black and Hispanic populations have a higher incidence of keloid development, but keloids can occur in members of any ethnic group. Men and women are at equal risk for scarring, and those between the ages of 10 and 30 years are most commonly affected. Several different types of skin injuries, including surgery, burns, piercing, lacerations, abrasions, tattoo placement, vaccinations, insect bites, and inflammatory reactions (e.g., varicella, folliculitis) can provoke a proliferative scar response.

Clinical Features

Keloids should be differentiated from hypertrophic scars. The most important distinction is that hypertrophic scars remain within the confines of the original area of dermal injury, whereas keloids transgress beyond the original wound borders and are associated with high rates of treatment resistance and recurrence (Figs. 1 and 2). Keloids appear months to years after injury and tend to proliferate without spontaneous regression.

Treatment

Because there is no universally accepted method to treat or cure keloids, the best strategy is prevention. If patients are predisposed to development of these proliferative scars, elective surgical procedures should be avoided, particularly in body regions that are more prone to scarring.

CURRENT DIAGNOSIS

- Keloids transgress beyond the original wound borders and have high rates of treatment resistance and recurrence.
- Keloids appear months to years after an injury and tend to proliferate without spontaneous regression.

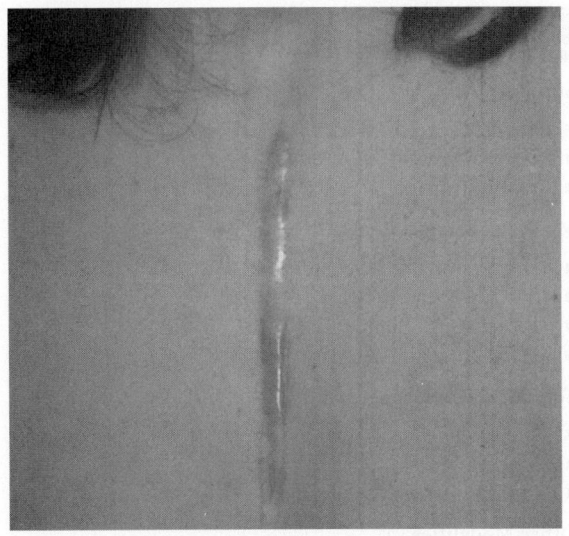

FIGURE 1. Hypertrophic scar.

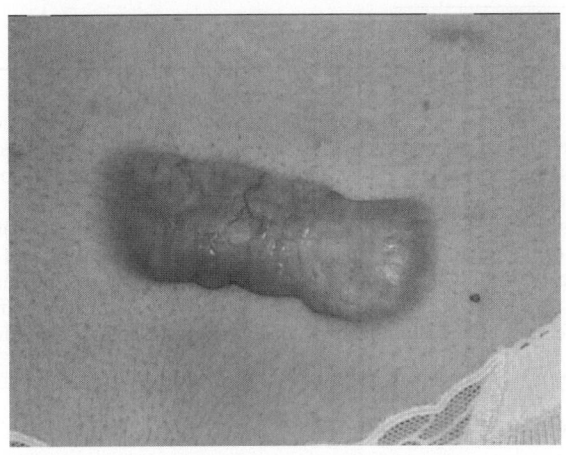

FIGURE 2. Keloid.

SURGICAL THERAPIES

Surgical Excision with or without Grafting

If used as monotherapy, lesions recur in 45% to 100% of patients with surgically excised scars. Because the excision exposes the tissue to the same forces as the original wound, additional collagen synthesis is stimulated. The keloid recurs, and it often becomes larger. Surgical closure techniques using intradermal monofilamentous sutures impose the least amount of injury to the tissue and have been shown to be somewhat helpful in reducing keloid formation.

Cryosurgery

Cryosurgery, which involves two to three consecutive freeze-thaw cycles of 30-second durations, induces ischemia of the skin due to vascular damage and reduced microcirculation. Anoxia and eventual tissue necrosis ensue when treatments are delivered at 3- to 4-week intervals. Facial keloids and scars older than 1 year do not significantly improve with this modality. Permanent hypopigmentation due to irreversible melanocyte destruction may result, making cryosurgery a less feasible option for patients with darker skin.

Laser Surgery

Advances in laser technology have made vascular-specific laser therapy one of the most effective treatments for keloids. Whereas older vaporizing lasers (e.g., carbon dioxide) demonstrated no advantage

CURRENT THERAPY

Surgical Therapies

- Surgical excision and/or grafting
- Cryosurgery
- Laser surgery

Medical Therapies

- Intralesional corticosteroids
- 5-Fluorouracil (5-FU [Adrucil])[1]
- Bleomycin (Blenoxane)[1]
- Interferon alfa-2b (Intron A)[1]

Topical Therapies

- Imiquimod (Aldara)[1]
- Silicone gel
- Onion extract (Mederma)

Other Modalities

- Pressure therapy
- Irradiation

[1]Not FDA approved for this indication.

over scalpel excision and were associated with high rates of scar recurrence, the newer nonablative pulsed-dye lasers (PDLs) have shown marked improvement in scar erythema, texture, height, and pliability without scar worsening or recurrence after two or three treatment sessions on a bimonthly basis. The clinical effectiveness of PDL irradiation on keloids presumably results from controlled tissue heating and hypoxia, with subsequent diminution of cellular function and inflammation. The ease of PDL treatment and lack of significant side effects render nonablative laser therapy a suitable choice in children and adults.

MEDICAL THERAPIES

Intralesional Corticosteroids

Intralesional corticosteroids have long been considered the gold standard for treatment of keloids. Corticosteroids suppress collagen synthesis by decreasing gene expression within the scar and suppress glycosaminoglycan synthesis and fibroblast proliferation. Corticosteroids also reduce transforming growth factor β (TGF-β) and insulin-like growth factor type 1 (IGF-1), which are involved in the would-healing process. Prophylactic use of corticosteroids has prevented scar development in scar-prone patients. Scar recurrence rates drop to below 50% when corticosteroids are used in conjunction with surgical excision. They have also been used in combination with other therapies, such as 5-fluorouracil (5-FU [Adrucil]),[1] cryotherapy, and laser treatment.

One of the most commonly administered drugs used for intralesional injection is triamcinolone acetonide (Kenalog), which can be diluted with lidocaine to reduce the discomfort associated with dermal injection. Injections using concentrations of 10 to 40 mg/mL, depending on the site and size of the scars, are typically administered at 2- to 4-week intervals. Complications of treatment include pain at the injection sites, skin atrophy, telangiectasia, and long-term hypopigmentation.

5-Fluorouracil

5-FU[1] is a pyrimidine analogue with antimetabolite activity. Limited studies have shown that intralesional 5-FU injection can improve scars by decreasing keloid fibroblast proliferation. Injections are typically administered weekly at concentrations of 40 to 50 mg/mL and are often combined with other treatments, including corticosteroids or laser therapy. Side effects include severe pain during injection, purpura at sites of injection, and localized superficial tissue slough.

[1]Not FDA approved for this indication.

Bleomycin

Bleomycin (Blenoxane),[1] a chemotherapeutic agent, exerts cellular effects by inhibition of the cell cycle and degradation of cellular RNA and DNA. Intralesional injection or multiple punctures of bleomycin have induced regression of keloids. Complications include hyperpigmentation and skin atrophy.

Interferon Alfa-2b

Interferons (e.g., interferon alfa-2b [Intron A][1]) are cytokines with antiproliferative and antifibrotic properties. Because of their ability to decrease type I and III collagen synthesis and induce apoptosis, they have been studied in the treatment of keloids. Although amelioration rates as high as 50% have been reported, evidence suggests that the performance of interferons as an adjuvant to surgical excision is inferior to postoperative intralesional corticosteroid injections. Adverse systemic effects, such as dose-dependent flulike symptoms, reduce the practicality of this treatment in clinical practice.

TOPICAL THERAPIES

Imiquimod

Imiquimod,[1] an immune response modifier, induces local cytokine production, which leads to down-regulation of collagen synthesis. An 8-week study in which 5% imiquimod cream was applied after surgical keloid excision demonstrated no recurrence for 11 of the 13 keloids at 24 weeks' follow-up. Another small study of four patients with eight large, pedunculated earlobe keloids showed that a combination of tangential excision and topical imiquimod cream resulted in no recurrence after 12 months' follow-up. Using an alternate-night application of 5% imiquimod cream for 8 weeks in 45 patients produced a recurrence rate of 28.6% after 7.9 months. Side effects are limited to local skin irritation, abrasion, and mild hyperpigmentation.

Silicone Gel

It has been hypothesized that the mechanism of action of silicone gel sheeting applied over scars has more to do with hydration than with the pressure applied or the silicone in the dressing. Hydration can lead to fibroblast modification, and the dressing serves as a protective barrier, mimicking the stratum corneum. Clinical studies have shown that 12 hours' daily application of silicone sheeting for 2 to 4 months results in scar softening and reduced pruritus. The lack of significant adverse effects of this treatment makes it a popular therapeutic option, particularly in the pediatric population.

Onion Extract

Studies of onion extract in vitro have demonstrated fibroblast-inhibiting properties. Further research has shown reduced proliferative activity and decreased production of substances in the extracellular matrix, but the exact mechanism of action by which the onion extract exerts its effect remains unclear. In addition to its known antibacterial properties, the flavonoids (i.e., quercetin and kaempferol) in onion extract are thought to account for its fibroblast inhibition and other antiproliferative effects. Mederma gel is prescribed for use on new scars with twice-daily application for 3 to 4 months. Scar erythema and discomfort are typically diminished, although some patients develop mild pruritus after its application.

OTHER THERAPEUTIC MODALITIES

Pressure Therapy

Although the mechanism of action of compression therapy is not completely understood, it has been hypothesized that pressure induces tissue ischemia, leading to decreased tissue metabolism and increased collagenolysis. For maximum effectiveness, 24 to 40 mm Hg of pressure should be exerted, and the pressure garment should be worn for at least 18 hours daily for 6 months. Because many patients find pressure dressings cumbersome and uncomfortable, treatment compliance is irregular, limiting the ultimate benefits of treatment.

[1]Not FDA approved for this indication.

Irradiation

Radiation therapy can be used as monotherapy, but it is most often delivered after surgical scar excision, effectively decreasing recurrence rates to 10% to 20%. Radiation exposure damages fibroblasts, hindering their proliferation and neoangiogenesis. Within 10 days of surgery, at least 1500 Gy is delivered in divided doses. Because of associated carcinogenicity, radiation treatment is controversial, and caution must be exercised when treating children or radiosensitive regions such as the breast or neck (i.e., thyroid gland).

Management Overview

A multitude of medical and over-the-counter treatments are available for scar treatment. Although several in-office scar therapies, such as corticosteroid injections and laser irradiation, have shown marked clinical efficacy, many common over-the-counter products purported to treat scars are based on anecdotal evidence and unsubstantiated claims. Individual differences in scar response to treatment make it difficult to reach consensus on the best therapeutic modality. Combination treatment regimens, including laser or surgical excision and corticosteroid injections, have significantly reduced rates of keloid recurrence. As research is directed toward controlling aberrant collagen formation, novel and more efficacious treatments are anticipated for this difficult problem.

REFERENCES

Al-Attar A, Mess S, Thomassen JM, et al. Keloid pathogenesis and treatment. Plast Reconstr Surg 2006;117(1):286–96.

Alster TS, Tanzi EL. Hypertrophic scars and keloids. Etiology and management. Am J Clin Dermatol 2003;4(4):235–43.

Alster T, Zaulyanov L. Laser scar revision: A review. Dermatol Surg 2007; 33:131–40.

Atiyeh BS, Costagliola M, Hayek SN. Keloid or hypertrophic scar: The controversy: Review of the literature. Ann Plast Surg 2005;54:676–80.

Butler PD, Longaker MT, Yang GP. Current progress in keloid research and treatment. J Am Coll Surg 2008;206:731–41.

Chuangsuwanich A, Gunjittisomram S. The efficacy of 5% imiquimod cream in the prevention of recurrence of excised keloids. J Med Assoc Thai 2007;90:1363–7.

Durani P, Bayat A. Levels of evidence for the treatment of keloid disease. J Plast Reconstr Aesthet Surg 2008;61:4–17.

Fujiwara M, Muragaki Y, Ooshima A. Keloid-derived fibroblasts show increased secretion of factors involved in collagen turnover and depend on matrix metalloproteinase for migration. Br J Dermatol 2005;153:295–300.

Naeini FF, Najafian J, Ahmadpour K. Bleomycin tattooing as a promising therapeutic modality in large keloids and hypertrophic scars. Dermatol Surg 2006;32:1023–9.

Roques C, Téot L. The use of corticosteroids to treat keloids: A review. Int J Low Extrem Wounds 2008;7:137–45.

Stashower ME. Successful treatment of earlobe keloids with imiquimod after tangential shave excision. Dermatol Surg 2006;32:380–6.

Yamamoto T. Bleomycin and the skin. Br J Dermatol 2006;155:869–75.

Warts (Verruca)

Method of
Anne E. Rosin, MD

Warts are a nuisance. For the most part, they are benign and harmless skin growths caused by one of the more than 80 saprophytic human papillomaviruses (HPVs). These viruses are ubiquitous and spread by contact with an infected person or indirectly through fomites such as wet towels, swimming pools, and locker room floors. The conventional thinking is that the epidermis must be defective at the site of inoculation.

CURRENT DIAGNOSIS

- Common warts: rough, hyperkeratotic, firm papules on the hands, legs, or feet
- Flat warts: small, flat-topped, pink or flesh-colored papules on the face, arms, or legs
- Plantar and palmar warts: hard, thickened, callus-like lesions that disrupt skin lines
- Mosaic warts: large clusters of warts
- Filiform warts: small, finger-like lesions on the face
- Differential diagnoses: seborrheic keratoses, keratoacanthoma, squamous cell carcinoma, callus, and corns

Clinical Features

Nongenital warts affect 10% of the population and are among the three most common reasons for dermatologic visits. Warts are more common in adolescents and in immunosuppressed persons because of immature or compromised immune systems.

Several types of warts occur with variations in appearance, the site affected, and the virus involved. Common warts (i.e., verrucae vulgaris) are rough, hyperkeratotic, firm papules that most often occur on the hands and legs and that are caused by HPV types 1, 2, or 4. Flat warts (i.e., verrucae planae), caused by HPV 3 or 10, are small, flat-topped, and flesh-colored growths that occur in large numbers on the face, arms, or legs. Plantar and palmar warts (i.e., verrucae plantares et palmares) are hard, thickened, callus-like lesions that disrupt skin lines on the soles or palms. Mosaic warts are larger clusters of these warts. Filiform warts are small, digitate or finger-like lesions most commonly seen on the face, especially around the eyelids, nose, and mouth. Periungual warts are common warts impinging on and growing under finger- or toenails. Genital warts are discussed in a separate chapter.

Differential diagnoses include seborrheic keratoses, keratoacanthoma, squamous cell carcinoma, callus, and corns. Paring the stratum corneum (outer layer of the skin) may reveal thrombosed or bleeding capillaries seen as black dots.

The manifestation of viral warts and various modes of therapy have been referenced throughout history. The word *condyloma* is of Greek origin and means "knuckle or knob"; *verruca* is Latin for "little hill." Warts are mentioned in early Hippocratic writings and in the Old and New Testaments of the Bible. In Arthurian legend, King Arthur was known by the diminutive nickname *wart* until he proved his royalty by pulling Excalibur from a stone. Chaucer described a distinctive wart on the Miller's nose in his *Canterbury Tales*. Shakespeare invokes warts as the result of a curse in *Hamlet*. The phrase "warts and all" is attributed to Oliver Cromwell, who gave specific instructions to his portraitist. Tom Sawyer was afflicted with common warts from "playing with frogs" (obviously not possible because HPV is species specific). Even "The King," Elvis Presley, had a wart removed from his right hand. It now resides in a velvet-lined box in a museum in Hawaii.

Treatment

ALTERNATIVE AND STANDARD APPROACHES

Because 40% of warts will spontaneously disappear within 2 years in healthy individuals, treatment is not always necessary. As a corollary, treatment of warts does not guarantee their complete resolution. Many patients are compelled to seek treatment of their warts because of the social embarrassment or physical discomfort that warts can cause. Patients with compromised immune systems due to immunodeficiency or immunosuppression are at higher risk for numerous warts, and treatment to prevent their progression to squamous cell carcinoma is important.

Popular reports and the medical literature are replete with descriptions of successful methods for treating warts. Whether anecdotal or evidence based, reports are largely without the support of randomized, controlled trials. No one therapy is always effective, and warts resolve, recur, shrink, or grow despite therapy. It is likely that all wart therapies work by triggering an immune response to the presence of papillomavirus in the skin.

Treatment methods fall into several broad categories, which include folk remedies, over-the-counter (OTC) treatments, and office-based therapies. Office-based treatments include destructive methods, surgical or laser procedures, immunologic intervention, and combination therapy.

Folk remedies for curing warts are espoused by Tom Sawyer and Huck Finn more than once in Mark Twain's classics. Tom recommended rubbing the warts with a split potato and then burying the potato, whereas Huck was certain that swinging a dead cat over his head and then burying it trumped the potato. They recited the wart chant:

Barley-corn, barley-corn, injun meal shorts,
Spunk-water, spunk-water, swaller these warts.

Both agreed that the wart chant spoken at midnight in the middle of the woods was the superior method, although neither was brave enough to prove the hypothesis.

The many alternative folk cures include transference, various prayers and incantations, hypnosis, and applications of garlic extract,[7] tea tree oil,[7] bacon fat, blood or entrails of various animals, and saliva of a loved one. Duct tape[1] application has received much attention. One study comparing cryotherapy with duct tape occlusion of common warts showed resolution in 85% of the children treated by occlusion, compared with 60% in the liquid nitrogen group. Another study found no statistically significant difference between duct tape and moleskin for the treatment of warts in an adult population.

Treatment of warts is often initiated by the patient, who most often uses one of the OTC salicylic acid products available. These keratolytic products, when used consistently and as directed, can be quite successful. Unfortunately, salicylic acid treatment, which destroys the infected epidermis and causes an immune reaction, can be irritating and tedious, prompting many patients to seek medical care.

Office-based treatments are largely destructive or immunomodulating, or both. The first line of therapy in the physician's office is usually cryotherapy. Liquid nitrogen is −196°C in the canister, and when applied by cotton-tipped application or cryospray, it effects a freeze that far surpasses a Wisconsin winter's frostbite. It is painful, unfortunately. Another destructive physician-applied treatment is cantharidin (Cantharone),[1,6] a chemical derived from blister beetles. It is painless on application and well tolerated by children. Acids, including bichloroacetic and trichloroacetic (Tri-Chlor), have risks, including pain on application, ulceration, and scarring.

Other destructive methods of wart removal usually are reserved for resistant or multiple lesions. Surgical removal followed by electrodesiccation and curettage is effective for large, solitary common warts but requires local anesthesia and results in scarring. Laser therapy, most often with pulsed-dye (PDL) or carbon dioxide (CO_2) lasers, has its place for selected patients. The PDL method is less aggressive and less painful than CO_2 vaporization, which is reserved for resistant common or plantar warts, multiple warts in immunosuppressed patients, or genital warts.

Immune modulation alone or in combination with destructive methods is helpful in treating resistant warts. The newest immunomodulator in the wart warrior's armamentarium is imiquimod (Aldara),[1] which was initially approved for treatment of genital warts but has since received FDA approval for treatment of nonmelanoma skin cancers. It is also frequently used to treat flat warts, acting through immune system modulation by inducing cytokines, including interferon-α. Other topical immunomodulators, such as squaric acid dibutylester (SADBE)[1,6] or diphencyprone[1,6] are contact sensitizers that induce an allergic dermatitis through type IV hypersensitivity

reactions. Treatment with SADBE is well tolerated and a good choice for recalcitrant warts in children, although it is time consuming.

Intralesional immunotherapy by *Candida* antigen injection (Candin)[1] is effective in improving or clearing warts in up to 74% of patients. It is considered a first-line therapy in children with large or multiple warts and second-line therapy for warts resistant to standard therapies. It is well tolerated. Intralesional interferon alfa-2b (Intron A)[1] has been used successfully to treat genital warts and warts that have not responded to conventional therapies.

Oral immunomodulation with high-dose cimetidine (Tagamet)[1] has been proposed as a helpful adjunctive therapy in the treatment of multiple warts in children and adults. It is postulated to enhance cell-mediated immune response. Studies comparing cimetidine with placebo have not been convincing, but cimetidine is well tolerated, and anecdotal reports of its usefulness abound.

Other topical products available for off-label treatment of warts include retinoids, formaldehyde compounds, and 5-fluorouracil (Efudex).[1] These agents interfere with epidermal proliferation, effect a nonspecific antiviral action, or inhibit mitosis, leading to keratinocyte and therefore viral death.

Because photodynamic therapy (PDT) with 20% 5-aminolevulinic acid (ALA [Levulan Kerastick])[1] is all the rage in dermatology for the treatment of actinic keratoses, acne, nonmelanoma skin cancers, and aging, why not add warts to the list? Studies have shown various success rates, but most demonstrated improvement or resolution of recalcitrant warts treated by ALA-PDT.

Family medicine physicians, internists, and dermatologists are asked to treat warts on a regular basis. Almost 50% of visits to a dermatologist are for wart treatment. The choice of therapeutic modality depends on the wart, the patient, and the practitioner. As Lempriere stated in his treatise on the treatment of warts: "Of all the futile disorders of the skin, it would be hard to find any that are regarded with greater contempt by the lay public and yet capable of resisting a greater variety of treatment than the group of papillary lesions commonly known as warts."

The American Academy of Dermatology has established guidelines for the treatment of warts:

- Desire of the patient for therapy
- Symptoms of pain, bleeding, itching, or burning
- Disabling or disfiguring lesions
- Large numbers or large size of lesions
- Desire to prevent spread to unblemished skin of the patient or others
- Immunocompromised condition

The goal of all therapy, including treatment of the pesky wart, should be "First, do no harm." To ensure resolution and nonrecurrence of warts, however, the patient and practitioner must often make compromises that include inconvenience, discomfort, and scarring. Treatment choices depend on the patient's age and level of pain tolerance; the location, type, and size of the warts; and the comfort level of the practitioner with the specific treatment.

---

[1]Not FDA approved for this indication.
[6]May be compounded by pharmacists.

CURRENT THERAPY

- Keratolytics such as salicylic acid
- Cantharidin (Cantharone)[1,6]
- Cryotherapy
- Surgical removal
- Pulsed-dye laser
- Immunotherapy: topical imiquimod (Aldara)[1], intralesional *Candida* antigen (Candin)[1]
- Photodynamic therapy

---

[1]Not FDA approved for this indication.
[6]May be compounded by pharmacists.

---

[1]Not FDA approved for this indication.
[6]May be compounded by pharmacists.
[7]Available as a dietary supplement.

SELECTED TREATMENT METHODS

Over the years, I have used most of the office methods mentioned previously, often asking the patient to incorporate OTC methods as well. Simple methods are appropriate for warts that are small and few. In children, painless methods are preferred and usually successful. I tend to combine modalities of destruction and immune stimulation, such as cantharidin,[1,6] and cimetidine[1] in children or use liquid nitrogen and *Candida* antigen injection[1] in more mature patients.

Keratolytics, which are 40% salicylic acid plaster pads (OTC Mediplast), are an excellent first-line therapy for common hand warts and plantar warts in motivated patients. Repeated application, with pumice stone or callus file use, results in cure rates of up to 80%. This method can cause irritation if the pad slips out of place (patients should try duct tape over the plaster) and can take several weeks to work.

Cantharidin[1,6] in a 0.7% colloidal solution can induce a painless blister after application and occlusion for 8 hours. It is applied in the office and repeated every 4 weeks. It is useful for treatment of common, periungual, and plantar warts in children, and the cure rate approaches 80%. Unfortunately, an occasional "donut wart," a ring of new warts surrounding the cleared original, occurs.

Cryotherapy uses liquid nitrogen applied by cotton applicator or, better, by a cryospray gun, and it is the most commonly used office-based treatment. The wart and a 1- to 2-mm margin around it should be frozen for 10 to 20 seconds. The freeze should be repeated once after a thaw of 20 seconds. If the warts are thick, they can be pared first. The patient is told that a blister (sometimes hemorrhagic) will result and should be left intact if possible. Treatment should be repeated every 3 to 4 weeks until normal skin markings return. If warts persist beyond 3 months of therapy, another method of treatment should be selected.

Surgery is used for large warts. Large common warts of the hands or extremities are more easily treated if they are debulked. If the wart is solitary, this method is more direct and often more successful than others. The wart should be anesthetized, removed at its base using a blade, and then curetted and cauterized. This method is not recommended for plantar warts because of scarring.

Pulsed-dye lasers (585- to 595-nm wavelength) can provide selective photothermolysis of blood vessels within the wart, which compromises blood supply and results in necrosis. This technique results in destruction of blood vessels within the wart but minimal damage to normal skin. It is generally well tolerated, but local anesthesia can be used if necessary. I use the following parameters: 7-mm spot size, pulse duration of 1.5 msec, and fluence of 10 to 12 J/cm^2, with double pulses applied to achieve purpura. This method is useful for recalcitrant flat, periungual, common, and plantar warts and has a success rate of 50% to 90%.

Immunotherapy is an effective method of treating some patients. I often add oral cimetidine[1] at daily doses of 30 to 40 mg/kg to other painless therapies for wart treatment in children. If the patient tolerates injections, I am a fan of *Candida* antigen[1] as monotherapy in patients with multiple warts or in combination with a destructive method such as cryotherapy or PDL. I choose the largest wart and inject 0.2 to 0.3 mL of a commercially available 1:1000 dilution of *Candida* antigen directly into the wart using a 30-gauge needle and tuberculin syringe. Pretesting is unnecessary, side effects are minimal, and more than 75% of patients treated with a series of three injections have clearing of the injected and distant warts. Imiquimod[1] is effective as monotherapy for genital warts, and I agree with anecdotal reports of its efficacy in flat warts. However, it is expensive (gram for gram it costs as much as platinum), and I have not found it useful except as adjunctive therapy for common warts. Treatment protocol is a thin coat of imiquimod cream applied three times weekly and combined with cryotherapy or salicylic acid.

Photodynamic therapy is useful for patients with multiple recalcitrant warts, especially patients who are immunosuppressed due to organ transplantation and anti-rejection therapy or human immunodeficiency virus (HIV) disease. PDT, which involves a topically applied photosensitizer that is activated by visible light, results in tissue destruction, and studies of this method for treatment of warts have been promising. My protocol includes a 60-minute incubation of affected lesions with topically applied ALA[1] followed by a 15-minute exposure to blue light, repeated every 4 weeks as needed. Transplant recipients I have treated, who typically present with many warts and early squamous cell cancers, have shown remarkable improvement in their skin lesions.

Warts are a bane and frustration to the patient and the physician who treats them. The myriad treatments available are for the most part supported by anecdotal evidence rather than randomized control trials. There are few inclusive reviews of successful treatment methods, and until an effective HPV vaccine is developed for all strains that cause warts, we will have to limp along using methods that are comfortable and have produced results. Each treatment should be tailored to fit the wart, the patient, and the practitioner.

REFERENCES

Bigby M, Gibbs S, Harvey I, Sterling J. Warts. Clin Evid 2005;14:2091–103.

Drake LA, Ceilley RI, Cornelison RL. Guidelines of care for warts: Human papillomavirus. J Am Acad Dermatol 1995;32:98–103.

Gibbs S, Harvey I, Sterling J, Stark R. Local treatments for cutaneous warts: Systematic review. Br Med J 2002;325:461.

Johnson SM, Roberson PK, Horn TD. Intralesional injection of mumps or *Candida* skin test antigens: A novel immunotherapy for warts. Arch Dermatol 2001;137:451–5.

Leman JA, Benton EC. Verrucas. Guidelines for management. Am J Clin Dermatol 2000;1:143–9.

Lempriere WW. Treatment of warts. Aust J Dermatol 1951;1:34–8.

Massing AM, Epstein WL. Natural history of warts. A two-year study. Arch Dermatol 1963;87:306–10.

Oster-Schmidt C. Imiquimod: A new possibility for treatment-resistant verrucae planae. Arch Dermatol 2001;137:666–7.

Robson KJ, Cunningham NM, Kruzan KL, et al. Pulsed-dye laser versus conventional therapy in the treatment of warts: A prospective randomized trial. J Am Acad Dermatol 2000;43:275–80.

Stender IM, Na R, Fogh H, et al. Photodynamic therapy with 5-aminolaevulinic acid or placebo for recalcitrant foot and hand warts: Randomized double-blind trial. Lancet 2000;355:963–6.

Sterling JC, Handfield-Jones S, Hudson PM, for the British Association of Dermatologists. Guidelines for the management of cutaneous warts. Br J Dermatol 2001;144:4–11.

Yelverton CB. Warts. In: Arndt KA, Hsu JT, editors. Manual of Dermatologic Therapeutics. 7th ed. Philadelphia: Lippincott Williams & Wilkins; 2006. p. 233–40.

---

[1]Not FDA approved for this indication.

Condyloma Acuminata (Genital Warts)

Method of
Athena Daniolos, MD

Etiology

Genital warts or condylomata acuminata are the result of cutaneous human papillomavirus (HPV) infection. HPV is a member of the Papillomaviridae family. This virus is a non-enveloped DNA virus with an icosahedral capsid that is 50 to 55 nm in diameter and contains 72 capsomeres. More than 90 different types of HPV have been

---

[1]Not FDA approved for this indication.
[6]May be compounded by pharmacists.

described, based on the results of DNA sequencing studies. This virus is epidermotropic, and different HPV types appear to have predilections for different anatomic sites.

Epidemiology and Pathogenesis

The Centers for Disease Control and Prevention (CDC) estimated the incidence of genital HPV infection to be 1% to 2% in the United States. This incidence appears to be increasing and is probably underestimated. The peak age of occurrence is between 15 and 29 years. The disease is primarily transmitted through sexual contact, and based on available data, the virus is easily transmitted. Condylomata acuminata are often caused by HPV genotypes 6 or 11. Viral infection of the squamous epithelial cells results in an increase in the epithelium and keratin production, ultimately producing a clinically evident wart. Anogenital HPV infection with the high-risk HPV genotypes (e.g., 16, 18, 31, 33, 35, 45) is associated with vulvar, vaginal, cervical, penile, and anorectal intraepithelial neoplasia and with invasive squamous cell carcinoma.

Clinical Presentation

Most anogenital warts are asymptomatic on presentation, although localized irritation, itching, or bleeding may occur. Typically, the flesh-colored, pink, brown, or whitish gray lesions are flat to exophytic "cauliflower" papules or plaques. The lesions may be single or multiple, and the size may range from 1 mm to several centimeters in diameter. The presence of anogenital condylomata externally

CURRENT DIAGNOSIS

- Mucocutaneous disease may affect the perineum, external genitalia, anus, perianal area, vagina, or urethra.
- Flat to raised lesions may be skin colored, pink, brown, or whitish gray.

should prompt an examination of the urethral meatus, vagina, cervix, anus, and oral mucosa, based on the patient's clinical and sexual history. Flat HPV lesions may not be grossly visible. Application of dilute acetic acid solution (5% acetic acid) to the skin surface with a Q-tip or applied with a 5- to 10-minute gauze soak may help to detect subtle HPV lesions. Acetic acid screening may have up to a 25% false-positive rate because other keratinized skin lesions may appear "aceto-white," including dermatitis, lichen planus, psoriasis, and local infections (e.g., *Candida*, herpes simplex virus).

Diagnostic Tests

When the clinical appearance of the lesions is typical, no other confirmatory tests or investigations may be necessary. Pap smears of samples from the lesions may demonstrate degenerative cytoplasmic vacuolization and koilocytosis in the virus-infected epithelial cells. Tissue biopsy can provide histopathologic confirmation of the diagnosis. Although rarely indicated in the routine evaluation of an HPV-infected patient, HPV identification and DNA genotyping

TABLE 1 Treatments for Human Papillomavirus Infections Recommended by the CDC

Treatment	Mechanism of Action	Methods		Adverse Reactions	Studies
		Patient Applied	**Provider Applied**		
Podophyllotoxin 0.5% gel or solution (Condylox)	Antimitotic agent; secondary cell necrosis	2×/d for 3 d, then 4 d off; repeat up to 4–6 cycles		Erythema, pain, erosion	CDC, Von Krogh, et al
Imiquimod 5% cream (Aldara)	Interferon-α and cytokine induction; cytolysis	3×/wk at bedtime, wash off in 6–10 h; can apply qhs if tolerated; repeat up to 16 wk		Erythema, pain, erosion, infection	CDC, Von Krogh, et al, Wiley, et al
Cryotherapy	Thermal injury, inflammatory reaction, and cell necrosis		Apply liquid nitrogen with cotton-tipped applicator; freeze time of 10–20 sec, depending on wart thickness; two freeze-thaw cycles; treat every 1–2 wk	Pain, blistering, scarring, pigmentary changes, infection	Beutner, et al, CDC
Podophyllin resin 10%–25% in tincture of benzoin (Podocon 25)	Antimitotic agent; secondary cell necrosis		Apply small amount; wash off in 4 h; treat every 1–2 wk	Erythema, pain, erosion, rare systemic toxicity	CDC, Von Krogh, et al, Wiley, et al
TCA (Tri-Chlor 80%) or BCA 80%–90%	Caustic chemical ablation and cell necrosis		Apply small amount every 1–2 wk	Pain, erythema, blistering, erosion, ulceration, pigmentary changes	CDC, Von Krogh, et al
Surgical—excision, curettage, electrosurgery	Physical removal or destruction		Office procedure	Pain, scarring, infection	CDC, Von Krogh, et al
Interferon, intralesional (Intron A)	Immunomodulatory cytokine		Injection 1–3×/wk, for up to 4 wk	Pain, flulike symptoms	CDC, Wiley, et al
Laser surgery	Physical ablation		Office procedure	Pain, scarring, pigmentary changes, infection	CDC, Von Krogh, et al

Abbreviations: CDC = Centers for Disease Control and Prevention; BCA = bichloroacetic acid; TCA = trichloroacetic acid.

TABLE 2 Other Treatments for Human Papillomavirus Infection

Treatment	Mechanism of Action	Methods Patient Applied	Methods Provider Applied	Adverse Reactions	Studies
5-Fluorouracil 5% cream (Efudex)[1]	Fluorinated pyrimidine antimetabolite; inhibits DNA and RNA synthesis	Thin coat at bedtime, 1–3×/wk as tolerated; repeat up to 6 wk		Pain, erythema, erosion, ulceration	Wiley, et al
5-Fluorouracil, intralesional (Adrucil)[1]	Fluorinated pyrimidine antimetabolite; inhibits DNA and RNA synthesis		Injection weekly for up to 6 wk	Pain, erythema, erosion, ulceration	Beutner, et al
Retinoids, oral— acitretin (Soriatane)[1] or isotretinoin (Accutane)[1]	Modify cell keratinization and proliferation	0.5–1 mg/kg/d PO for up to 12 wk		Erythema, xerosis, photosensitivity, teratogen, hypervitaminosis A syndrome	Cardamakis, et al, Tsambaos, et al
Cidofovir 1% gel or ointment[5]	Acyclic nucleoside phosphonate; broad anti-DNA virus activity	Thin coat daily for 5 d, every other week; repeat up to 12–16 wk		Erythema, pain, erosion	Snoek, et al
Photodynamic therapy (ALA-PDT, Levulan Kerastick)	Laser-induced photochemical cytotoxicity with free radical–mediated local cell destruction		Office procedure	Pain, erythema, pigmentary changes	Ross, et al

[1]Not FDA approved for this indication.
[5]Investigational drug in the United States.
Abbreviations: ALA = 5-aminolevulinic acid; PDT = photodynamic therapy.

by polymerase chain reaction in situ hybridization is the most sensitive technique available.

Treatment and Management

The 2006 CDC guidelines state that treatment for subclinical HPV infections, in the absence of dysplasia, is not necessary. None of the current treatments for condylomata acuminata is specifically antiviral, and none of these interventions can eradicate the virus from the host. The ultimate therapeutic goal is to treat and clear all clinically apparent HPV disease. Two clinically relevant areas are the treatment of sexual partners and the prevention of HPV disease.

The factors to consider when deciding on treatment include wart size and location, the patient's tolerance of the therapy, cost, and the clinician's preference and training. Data regarding the efficacy

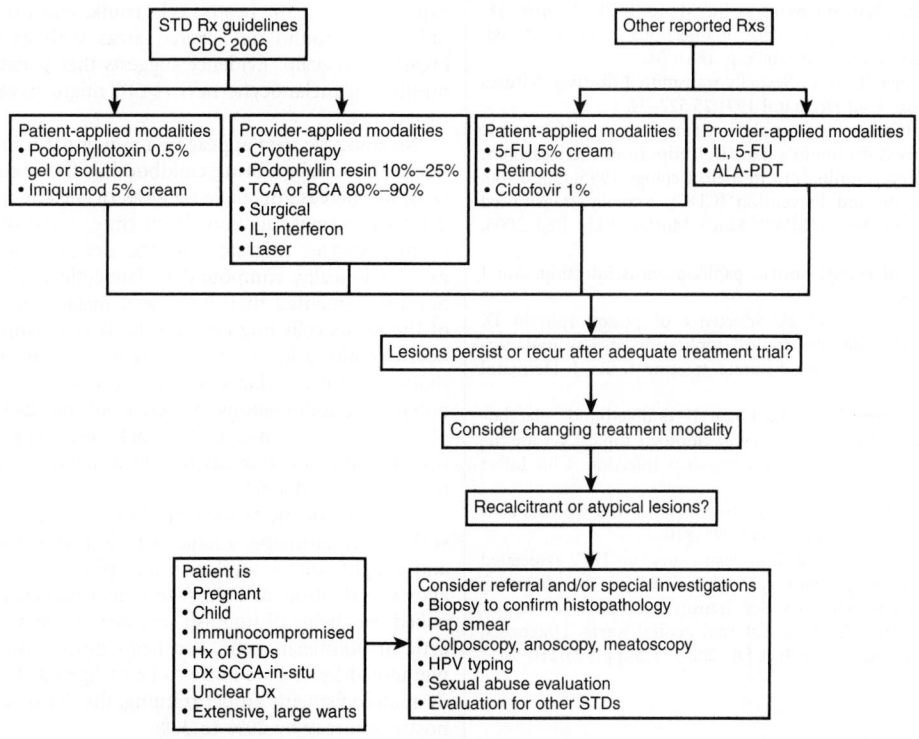

FIGURE 1. Algorithm for the treatment of anogenital warts. *Abbreviations:* ALA = 5-aminolevulinic acid; BCA = bichloroacetic acid; CDC = Centers for Disease Control and Prevention; Dx = diagnosis; 5-FU = 5-fluorouracil; HPV = human papillomavirus; Hx = history; IL = interleukin; PDT = photodynamic therapy; Rx = treatment; STD = sexually transmitted disease; TCA = trichloroacetic acid.

CURRENT THERAPY

- Treatment of subclinical HPV disease is not recommended by the 2006 STD Treatment Guidelines from the Centers for Disease Control and Prevention.
- No specifically antiviral and curative therapy exists for HPV infection.
- Recommended therapies include podophyllotoxin (podofilox [Condylox]), podophyllin resin (Podocon-25), imiquimod (Aldara), cryotherapy, trichloroacetic acid (TCA) or bichloroacetic acid (BCA), standard or laser surgery, and intralesional interferon alfa-2b (Intron A).

of using more than one treatment at a time are lacking. However, it is not uncommon for health care providers to combine more than one treatment modality when managing HPV-infected patients. Various therapeutic approaches are summarized in Tables 1 and 2.

Referral for consultation with a specialist should be considered in certain situations, as indicated in the treatment algorithm (Fig. 1). Advances in the treatment of HPV disease could include the development of a therapeutic HPV vaccine to boost the patient's antiviral immune response. Potential complementary medicine approaches may use green tea polyphenols.[7]

Counseling should be part of the comprehensive management of these patients. Education regarding the nature of HPV disease, prevention strategies, and screening of sexual partners are important components of quality health care.

REFERENCES

Baker GE, Tyring SK. Therapeutic approaches to papillomavirus infections. Dermatol Clin 1997;15:331–40.

Beutner KR, Ferenczy A. Therapeutic approaches to genital warts. Am J Med 1997;102(5A):28–37.

Bonnez W, Reichman RC. Papillomaviruses. In: Mandell GL, Bennett JE, Dolin R, editors. Principles and Practice of Infectious Diseases. 6th ed. Philadelphia: Churchill Livingstone; 2005. p. 1841–51.

Buntin DM, Rosen T, Lesher JL, et al. Sexually transmitted diseases: Viruses and ectoparasites. J Am Acad Dermatol 1991;25:527–34.

Cardamakis E, Kotoulas IG, Relakis K, et al. Comparative study of systemic interferon alfa-2a plus isotretinoin versus isotretinoin in the treatment of recurrent condyloma acuminatum in men. Urology 1995;45:857–60.

Centers for Disease Control and Prevention (CDC). Sexually transmitted diseases treatment guidelines. MMWR Morb Mortal Wkly Rep 2006; 55:14–30.

Koutsky L. Epidemiology of genital human papillomavirus infection. Am J Med 1997;102(5A):3–8.

Ross EV, Romero R, Kollias N, et al. Selectivity of protoporphyrin IX fluorescence for condylomata after topical application of 5-aminolaevulinic acid: Implications for photodynamic treatment. Br J Dermatol 1997; 137:736–42.

Snoeck R, Bossens M, Parent D, et al. Phase II double-blind, placebo-controlled study of the safety and efficacy of cidofovir topical gel for the treatment of patients with human papillomavirus infection. Clin Infect Dis 2001;33:597–602.

Tsambaos D, Georgiou S, Monastirli A, et al. Treatment of condylomata acuminata with oral isotretinoin. J Urol 1997;158:1810–2.

Von Krogh G, Lacey CJ, Gross G, et al. European course on HPV associated pathology: Guidelines for primary care physicians for the diagnosis and management of anogenital warts. Sex Transm Infect 2000;76:162–8.

Wiley DJ, Douglas J, Beutner K, et al. External genital warts: Diagnosis, treatment, and prevention. Clin Infect Dis 2002;35(Suppl. 2):210–24.

[7]Available as a dietary supplement.

Melanocytic Nevi

Method of
**Jane M. Grant-Kels, MD, and
Michael Murphy, MD**

Melanocytic nevi, or moles, are benign neoplasms composed of melanocytes. Melanocytic nevus cells are derived from melanocytes. Compared with melanocytes, nevus cells are not dendritic, are larger, and contain more abundant cytoplasm, often with coarse melanin granules. Nevus cells tend to aggregate into groups or nests. Melanocytic nevi are extremely common and can be found on almost everyone, anywhere on the cutaneous surface. This article discusses the most common types of melanocytic nevi: acquired melanocytic nevi, recurrent melanocytic nevi, halo melanocytic nevi, congenital melanocytic nevi, blue nevi, Spitz nevi, and dysplastic melanocytic nevi.

Acquired Melanocytic Nevi

Acquired melanocytic nevi are subdivided into junctional, compound, and intradermal types based on the location of the nevus cells. By definition, these lesions are not present at birth but can begin to appear in early childhood, usually after 6 to 12 months of age. Peak ages of appearance of melanocytic nevi are 2 to 3 years of age in children and 11 to 18 years in adolescents. Although nevi can appear at any age, it is relatively unusual for new melanocytic nevi to develop in middle-aged or older adults. With time, nevi can spontaneously regress. Consequently, patients in their ninth decade of life usually demonstrate few melanocytic nevi. An average white adult has 10 to 40 melanocytic nevi, but African Americans have far fewer, averaging only 2 to 8.

The number and location of melanocytic nevi have been shown to be associated with sun exposure, immunologic factors, and genetics. Consequently, melanocytic nevi are most numerous on the sun-exposed skin of the head, neck, trunk, and extremities, but they are only rarely found on covered areas such as the buttocks, female breasts, and scalp. Evidence suggests that patients with an increased number of melanocytic nevi (>50) might have an increased risk of melanoma.

Melanocytic nevi appear in a sequential fashion. Junctional melanocytic nevi arise during childhood as flat, dark macules. Histologically, an increase in single or nests of melanocytes are located at the dermoepidermal junction. With time, some of the junctional nests of melanocytes migrate into the dermis (compound melanocytic nevi). Clinically, compound melanocytic nevi are elevated and less heavily pigmented than junctional melanocytic nevi. Ultimately, all of the nevus cells migrate into the dermis (intradermal melanocytic nevi), resulting in the development of a tan or skin-colored dome-shaped papule. Melanocytic nevi can be flat or elevated and even polypoid, papillomatous, or verrucous and can demonstrate a range of color from skin-tone to black, but they are characteristically uniform in color, symmetrical, well marginated, and usually smaller than 6 mm in diameter.

All melanocytic lesions of clinical concern should be examined with a dermatoscope, a hand-held instrument with a magnified lens and a light source similar to an ophthalmoscope. This instrument allows evaluation of colors and microstructures not visible to the naked eye, helps distinguish whether pigmented lesions are melanocytic or nonmelanocytic, and helps distinguish whether melanocytic pigmented lesions are likely to be malignant. Used by an experienced dermatologist with proper training, the dermatoscope improves diagnostic accuracy by 20% to 30%.

It is unnecessary to surgically remove all melanocytic nevi because they are benign neoplasms of melanocytes. However, indications for removal include ABCD (*a*symmetry, irregular *b*order, variegation or change in *c*olor, or change in *d*iameter), symptoms (e.g., pruritus), evidence of inflammation or irritation, cosmetic issues, and patient anxiety. Melanocytic nevi on acral, genital, or scalp skin that appear benign do not require surgical removal. Shave biopsies are appropriate therapy for lesions considered clinically benign. However, if a lesion is being removed because of concern regarding the possibility of malignancy, an excisional biopsy (biopsy of choice) or incisional biopsy (including punch or deep scoop) that extends to the subcutaneous tissue is indicated. All melanocytic lesions should be submitted to a dermatopathologist for histologic review. A history of recent sun exposure or trauma should be conveyed to the dermatopathologist because such external trauma can induce reactive atypical histologic findings.

Recurrent Melanocytic Nevi

Recurrent melanocytic nevi are melanocytic nevi that have previously been incompletely removed (either iatrogenically or traumatically) and have recurred weeks to months later. Irregular brown pigmentation is clinically noted within the scar site. If the original biopsy demonstrated a benign melanocytic nevus, re-treatment is unnecessary unless the aforementioned indications are present. However, these nevi can demonstrate pseudomelanomatous histologic features. Therefore, if the repigmented area is excised, the dermatopathologist should be notified of the clinical history and, if possible, the slides from the original biopsy should be obtained and reviewed to ensure that the lesion is not histologically misdiagnosed.

Halo (Melanocytic) Nevi

Halo (melanocytic) nevi are melanocytic nevi in which a white rim or halo has developed. This phenomenon most commonly occurs around compound or intradermal nevi and is histologically associated with a dense, bandlike inflammatory infiltrate. The white halo area is histologically characterized by diminished or absent melanocytes and melanin. Approximately 20% of patients with halo nevi also exhibit vitiligo.

Although a halo can develop around many lesions in the skin, the most important differential diagnosis is between a halo nevus and melanoma with a halo. The halo and the central melanocytic nevus of halo nevi are symmetrical, round or oval, and sharply demarcated. Halo nevi most commonly occur in adolescence as an isolated event, but approximately 25% to 50% of affected persons have two or more.

The clinical course of halo nevi is variable. With time, the halo can repigment while the central nevus persists. Alternatively, the melanocytic nevus can regress completely and leave a depigmented macule that can persist or repigment over months or years.

Halo nevi do not require surgical excision unless atypical clinical features suggest the possibility of an atypical melanocytic lesion. It is advisable (particularly in adults, in whom halo nevi are less

CURRENT DIAGNOSIS

Benign Melanocytic Lesions

- Symmetrical
- Sharply demarcated border
- Uniform color
- Diameter usually ≤6 mm and stable

Malignant Melanocytic Lesions

- Asymmetrical
- Poorly circumscribed border
- Variegated in color
- Diameter often ≥10 mm and increasing (changing or evolving)

common) to perform a complete cutaneous examination with and without the aid of a Wood's lamp to rule out any associated atypical pigmented or regressed lesions. All patients should be warned to use sunscreens or protective clothing because of the increased risk of sunburn in the depigmented halo region.

Congenital Melanocytic Nevi

By definition, congenital melanocytic nevi are present at birth. Arbitrarily, they have been classified into small (<1.5 cm), medium (1.5–20 cm) and large (>20 cm) lesions. Terms such as *bathing trunk* or *garment-type* nevi refer to CMN that cover a significant portion of the cutaneous surface.

The approximate incidence of small congenital nevi is 1% of all live births. Large congenital nevi are rare and reported in only 1 in 20,000 births. Histologically, some congenital nevi have distinguishing histologic features (melanocytic nevi cells that extend into the deeper dermis as well as the subcutis and melanocytic nevi cells arranged periadnexally, angiocentrically, within nerves, and interposed between collagen bundles). However, these features have been identified in some acquired melanocytic nevi and are absent in some congenital nevi (especially small ones). In addition, the history obtained from the patient or their parents is often inaccurate. Consequently, it can be very difficult in some cases to distinguish a small congenital nevus from an acquired nevus.

Congenital nevi can give rise to dermal or subcutaneous nodular melanocytic proliferations. The vast majority of these lesions, particularly in the neonatal period, are biologically benign, despite a worrisome clinical presentation and atypical histologic features. Genetic analysis has shown that benign melanocytic proliferations within congenital nevi express aberrations qualitatively and quantitatively different from those seen in melanoma.

The primary significance of congenital nevi is related to the potential risk for progression to melanoma. Essentially, the larger the nevus, the greater the risk of progression to melanoma. Historically, even small nevi were estimated to exhibit a lifetime melanoma risk of 5%. However, recent prospective studies suggest that small and medium congenital nevi are associated with a low risk that may approximate the risk of acquired nevi. Conversely, large congenital nevi have a lifetime risk of melanomatous progression of approximately 6.3%.

CURRENT THERAPY

- Acquired melanocytic nevus: No treatment is required unless the lesion is asymmetrical or has an irregular border, change or variegated in color, or change in diameter. Symptomatic lesions should be biopsied.
- Recurrent melanocytic nevus: No treatment required if the original biopsy was benign.
- Halo melanocytic nevus: No treatment, but excision is recommended if atypical clinical features are identified.
- Congenital melanocytic nevus: Removal based on melanoma risk, cosmetics, and functional outcome. If not excised, routine follow-up with the use of photography, dermoscopy, and computer assistance is recommended.
- Blue nevus: No treatment, but excision is recommended if atypical clinical features are identified.
- Spitz nevus: If clinically unusual, a complete excisional biopsy is recommended.
- Dysplastic nevus: If only one lesion is present, excision is recommended. Patients with many dysplastic nevi require close surveillance with removal of any lesion suspicious for melanoma.

Up to two thirds of melanomas that arise in these giant congenital nevi have a nonepidermal origin, thus making clinical observation for malignant change difficult. Approximately 50% of these melanomas occur in the first 5 years of life, 60% in the first decade, and 70% before 20 years of age. Patients with large congenital nevi, especially those that involve posterior axial locations (head, neck, back, or buttocks) and are associated with satellite congenital nevi, are at increased risk for neurocutaneous melanosis (melanosis of the leptomeninges).

For large congenital nevi that involve a posterior axial location, magnetic resonance imaging (MRI) is indicated. If clinical symptoms or MRI indicate neurocutaneous melanosis, excision of the large nevus should be postponed until 2 years of age (the median age of neurologic symptoms). Patients with neurocutaneous melanosis have a greater than 50% mortality rate within 3 years. The risk and morbidity of multiple, staged excisions of a large congenital melanocytic nevus is not appropriate in patients with symptomatic neurocutaneous melanosis. All other large congenital melanocytic nevi are candidates for excision as soon as general anesthesia is considered a relatively safe risk. Other issues that need to be considered before undertaking staged excisions include cosmetic issues, functional outcome, and psychosocial issues. The staged excisions are usually started after 6 months of age for nevi on the trunk and extremities and later for those on the scalp to allow closure of the fontanelle. If removal is not undertaken, follow-up with monthly self-examination, photography, dermoscopy, confocal laser microscopy, and computer assistance are recommended.

For small congenital nevi, routine excision is not always recommended because the risk of melanoma is lower, and if it occurs, it usually arises within the epidermis after puberty. If the lesions are not excised, follow-up by alternating visits to a dermatologist and primary care physician along with serial photography are indicated. Inasmuch as small congenital nevi typically enlarge with the growth of the child and can change in appearance with time, educating families on benign, predictable changes in contradistinction to potentially alarming changes is extremely important. If a lesion enlarges or changes suddenly or if parental anxiety or cosmetic issues arise, excision should then be contemplated for even small congenital nevi. Elective excision is best done when the patient is approximately 8 years old. With the use of topical anesthetic cream EMLA (eutectic mixture of local anesthetics: 2.5% lidocaine plus 2.5% prilocaine) or topical 4% lidocaine (ELA-Max), children of this age are usually cooperative and unscathed by the procedure.

Blue Nevi

Blue nevi occur primarily on the face and scalp, in addition to the dorsal surfaces of the hands and feet, as well-circumscribed, slightly raised or dome-shaped bluish papules that are usually less than 1 cm in diameter. Although these lesions are usually acquired in childhood and adolescence, rare congenital lesions have been reported. Histologically, blue nevi demonstrate a combination of intradermal spindle or dendritic melanin-pigmented melanocytes and melanophages with dermal fibrosis. The blue appearance of these lesions is a function of both the depth of the melanin in the dermis and the Tyndall phenomenon: longer wavelengths of light penetrate the deep dermis and are absorbed by the lesional melanin, and shorter wavelengths (e.g., blue) are reflected back. Blue nevi that are clinically stable and that do not demonstrate atypical features do not require removal.

Spitz Nevi

Nevi of large spindle and epithelioid cells (Spitz nevi) are relatively uncommon. In Australia, an annual incidence of 1.4 per 100,000 people has been recorded. Most Spitz nevi are noted in children and adolescents: One third occur before the age of 10 years, one third between the ages 10 to 20 years, and one third past the age of 20 years. Rarely, lesions can occur in patients older than 40 years. Seven percent of SN have been reported as congenital.

Four clinical types of SN are recognized: light-colored soft Spitz nevi that can resemble a pyogenic granuloma; light-colored hard Spitz nevi that can resemble a dermatofibroma; dark Spitz nevi that must be distinguished from other melanocytic lesions, including melanoma; and disseminated or agminated Spitz nevi. Spitz nevi are typically smaller than 6 mm in diameter and dome shaped, with a smooth pink or tan surface and sharp borders. Although they can occur anywhere on the cutaneous surface except mucosal or palmoplantar areas, they are most commonly seen on the face (especially in children) and legs (especially in women). Spitz nevi in adults are usually more heavily melanized than those in children.

Dermatoscopy or epiluminescent microscopy (examination of lesions with enhanced light and a dermatoscope) helps magnify the images in vivo and can assist in establishing the clinical diagnosis of some Spitz nevi. Histologically, the lesion can demonstrate features similar to those of melanoma, which earned the lesion its original designation by Sophie Spitz as a melanoma of childhood. Because Spitz nevi can be histologically difficult to distinguish from melanoma, if a biopsy is performed on a lesion because of parental, cosmetic, or transitional concern, complete excision with clear margins is recommended. Spitz nevi show fundamental genomic differences compared with MM, consistent with the generally benign behavior of these lesions. Spitz nevi typically demonstrate no or only a very restricted set of chromosomal aberrations (i.e., 11p gain in a subset of Spitz nevi).

Dysplastic Melanocytic Nevi

Dysplastic melanocytic nevi, or Clark's nevi, or nevi with architectural disorder and cytologic atypia can occur sporadically as an isolated lesion or lesions or as part of a familial autosomal dominant syndrome. When such lesions occur sporadically, they are considered a marker for a patient who is at increased risk of melanoma (6% risk versus an approximate 0.6% risk in the normal white population in the United States). In association with a family history or personal past medical history of melanoma, patients with dysplastic melanocytic nevi should be considered to have a significant risk of melanoma. One first-degree family member with melanoma is associated with a lifetime risk of melanoma of 15% for the patient with dysplastic melanocytic nevi. Two or more first-degree family members with melanoma place a patient with dysplastic melanocytic nevi at a lifetime risk of developing melanoma that approaches 100%. Less commonly, dysplastic melanocytic nevi can progress to melanoma. Such progression has been documented by serial photography. However, these data are confounded by the fact that clinically and histologically, dysplastic melanocytic nevi may be difficult to distinguish from an early melanoma.

Dysplastic melanocytic nevi are clinically distinguished from common acquired melanocytic nevi by a diameter usually larger than 6 mm, irregular border, asymmetry, and variable color with possible shades of brown, red, pink and black; DMN can be flat with or without a raised center (fried egg appearance). The lesions begin to appear in mid-childhood and early adolescence. New lesions can appear throughout the patient's life. In addition to the back and extremities, these lesions can occur on sun-protected areas, including the scalp, buttocks, and female breasts. Dysplastic melanocytic nevi can be few or numerous, with hundreds of lesions.

Histologically, dysplastic melanocytic nevi show both architectural disorder: extension of the junctional component beyond the dermal component (shouldering); bridging between adjacent rete ridges; papillary dermal concentric and lamellar fibroplasia; and a variable lymphocytic infiltrate with vascular ectasias. They also show cytologic atypia of melanocytes: increased nuclear size, hyperchromasia, dispersion or variation of nuclear chromatin patterns, and presence of nucleoli. Although there is some discordance in the histologic grading of dysplastic melanocytic nevi among expert dermatopathologists, there is some evidence to support the use in clinical practice of a two-tier grading system: Grade A are dysplastic melanocytic nevi with mild or moderate cytologic atypia and grade B are dysplastic melanocytic nevi with severe cytologic atypia. The probability of having a personal history of melanoma in any given dysplastic melanocytic nevi patient correlates with the grade of cytologic atypia in dysplastic melanocytic nevi. In addition, the presence of severe cytologic atypia in dysplastic melanocytic nevi correlates with a significantly greater risk of melanoma development (19.7%) compared with moderate (8.1%) or mild (5.7%) cytologic atypia.

Management of these patients is difficult. Dysplastic melanocytic nevi are not uncommon. Reportedly, as many as 4.6 million people in the United States have one or more sporadic dysplastic melanocytic nevi. Familial dysplastic melanocytic nevi are estimated to involve 50,000 patients in the United States. The risk of melanoma for these patients is probably on a continuum and correlated with their family history of melanoma or dysplastic melanocytic nevi, personal history of melanoma, number of acquired melanocytic and dysplastic lesions, and history of sun exposure. Removal of all dysplastic melanocytic nevi is inappropriate inasmuch as the chance of any single lesion becoming malignant is small and, in addition, the melanoma can arise de novo.

Management includes patient education and total body photography for comparison at future skin examinations. Patients should avoid the sun and use sun screens and protective clothing. These patients should have regular biannual or quarterly examinations of the entire integument, including the oral, genital, and perianal mucosa, the scalp, and an ophthalmologic examination. Comparison with the previous total body photographs and use of the dermatoscope can be helpful. Any lesions that are suspicious for melanoma should be excised. Examination of first-degree family members (parents, siblings, and children) of patients with melanoma or dysplastic melanocytic nevi is recommended to identify other persons at high risk.

REFERENCES

Arumi-Uria M, McNutt NS, Finnerty B. Grading of atypia in nevi: Correlation with melanoma risk. Mod Pathol 2003;16:764–71.

Bauer J, Bastian BC. Distinguishing melanocytic nevi from melanoma by DNA copy number changes: Comparative genomic hybridization as a research and diagnostic tool. Dermatol Ther 2006;19:40–9.

Bett BJ. Large or multiple congenital melanocytic nevi: Occurrence of cutaneous melanoma in 1008 persons. J Am Acad Dermatol 2005;52:793–7.

de Snoo FA, Kroon MW, Bergman W, et al. From sporadic atypical nevi to familial melanoma: Risk analysis for melanoma in sporadic atypical nevus patients. J Am Acad Dermatol 2007;56:748–52.

Ferrara G, Soyer HP, Malvehy J, et al. The many faces of blue nevus: A clinicopathologic study. J Cutan Pathol 2007;34:543–51.

Kinsler VA, Chong WK, Aylett SE, Atherton DJ. Complications of congenital melanocytic naevi in children: Analysis of 16 years' experience and clinical practice. Br J Dermatol 2008;159:907–14.

Krengel S, Hauschild A, Schafer T. Melanoma risk in congenital melanocytic naevi: A systematic review. Br J Dermatol 2006;155:1–8.

Margoob AA, Borrego JP, Halpern AC. Congenital melanocytic nevi: Treatment modalities and management options. Semin Cutan Med Surg 2007; 26:231–40.

Naeyaert JM, Brochez L. Dysplastic nevi. N Engl J Med 2003;349:2233–40.

Park HK, Leonard DD, Arrington JH 3rd, Lund HZ. Recurrent melanocytic nevi: Clinical and histologic review of 175 cases. J Am Acad Dermatol 1987;17:285–90.

Melanoma

Method of
George T. Reizner, MD, and
Mark R. Albertini, MD

Melanoma is the least frequently diagnosed but deadliest of the three most common skin cancers. In 2008, an estimated 116,500 patients were diagnosed with melanoma in the United States. Of these, 62,480 (34,950 men and 27,530 women) had invasive melanoma, and more than 8420 were projected to die of the disease. For comparison, more than a million diagnoses of basal cell and squamous cell carcinomas of the skin were predicted for the same year. Melanoma rates are increasing faster than any other malignancy for men and are second only to lung cancer for women. For a boy born in 2000, the lifetime risk of developing melanoma is projected to be as high as 1 in 41, and for women, the projected rate is 1 in 61. The median age at diagnosis is 45 to 55 years, and melanoma ranks second overall behind adult leukemia in terms of lost years of productivity.

Risk factors for melanoma include a positive personal or family history of melanoma, multiple atypical or dysplastic nevi, light complexion, history of sunburns, or an inability to tan. The lesions are typically found in sun-exposed skin, with the most common location on the trunk and back of men and the lower legs and back of women. However, melanoma can occur on any skin surface, including areas with little or no history of sun exposure, mucous membranes, in the eyes, as metastatic disease without a clear primary site, and in any ethnic group or skin type.

Diagnosis

Early diagnosis is essential for good patient outcomes. Even melanomas with 1 mm of thickness at the time of diagnosis carry a significant risk of recurrence and death. The clinician should have a low threshold for evaluation and removal of changing lesions. Clinical features that help guide early identification include *asymmetry* (A), irregular or notched *borders* (B), irregular distribution of *color* (C), *diameter* of 6 mm or greater (D), and new *elevation, erosion,* or ulceration (E). An experienced physician can be aided in making the diagnosis using any or all of the following: epiluminescent microscopy, dermoscopy, or the comparison of prior photographic images.

Early detection and surgical removal remain the cornerstone of care. The initial biopsy should be carefully planned to remove, if possible, the entire lesion. The pathologic analysis of this specimen is important for management decisions, including the wide excision width, whether a sentinel lymph node biopsy is recommended, adjunct therapy, and potential stratification for clinical trials.

Ideally, a suspected lesion should be removed by excisional biopsy, including elliptical, punch, or saucerization techniques, with 1 to 3 mm of clinically normal margins. The full thickness of the questioned lesion should be included in this initial biopsy. Wider margins should be avoided, and if possible, the surgical orientation should minimize lymphatic disruption in anticipation of later lymphatic mapping. If complete initial removal is impractical because of anatomic considerations or lesion size, a subtotal punch or incisional biopsy can be taken from the thickest or darkest areas. A shave biopsy should not be performed if the lesion being removed is considered to be a possible melanoma.

CURRENT DIAGNOSIS

- The ABCDEs should be used to evaluate pigmented or any unusual skin lesions:
  - *A*symmetry of sides, which do not match and are unequal
  - *B*orders that are irregular and may be notched or scalloped
  - *C*olor that is variegated or changing and can include a variety of shades (e.g., black, brown, white, red)
  - *D*iameter greater than 6 mm (about the size of a pencil eraser) or a diameter that is increasing
  - *E*levated, ulcerated, or bleeding lesions
- Diagnostic aids include epiluminescence, dermoscopy, and comparison with prior photographic images.
- Proper biopsy technique is an excisional biopsy with 1.0-mm margins or an incisional biopsy of the most nodular-appearing area of larger lesions.

The pathology report should be interpreted by a physician experienced in the diagnosis of melanoma, with attention to the Breslow depth, ulceration, Clark's level (particularly for lesions less than 1 mm thick), histologic subtype, deep and lateral margins, mitotic rate, lymphatic or vascular invasion, neurotropism, satellitosis, inflammatory infiltrate, and regression.

Treatment

STAGING AND SURGICAL THERAPY

Staging and prognosis are determined by the thickness of the melanoma at the time of diagnosis and the absence or presence of distant disease. The prognostic importance of tumor depth is emphasized by two stages being dedicated to patients with local disease: stage I–II (i.e., localized disease without evidence of metastases); stage III (i.e., regional disease); and stage IV (i.e., distant metastatic disease). These stages are further divided based on additional clinical information (Table 1).

Most patients present with localized disease in the skin of 1 mm or less and have a predicted long-term survival of more than 90%. For lesions greater than 1 mm, long-term survival drops to between 50% and 90%. If regional lymph nodes are involved, these rates are approximately cut in half. However, there can be wide variation, with 5-year survival ranging from approximately 20% to 60% and depending heavily on the amount to nodal involvement. As a group, patients with distant metastatic disease have a less than 10% 5-year survival rate.

Patients with intermediate-depth lesions (1 to 4 mm) and patients with melanomas deeper than 4 mm are candidates for sentinel lymph node biopsy. Selected patients with lesions with an initial depth of less than 1 mm and adverse features may also be considered for this procedure. Although the impact on patient survival remains contested, this technique is widely practiced and is a valuable tool to help identify patients at greater risk for recurrence and to stratify individuals in clinical trials. The procedure uses a blue dye and radioactive isotopes injected around the initial biopsy site. Nuclear imaging is used to determine the site of regional lymph node drainage. An incision overlying this site is made, and a handheld detector and the blue dye guide the surgeon to the correct location and identification of the lymph node in question. If this node is histopathologically positive for disease, a completion lymph node dissection can be undertaken and adjuvant therapy considered. Clinically palpable lymph nodes present at the time of initial diagnosis should be biopsied and removed if they demonstrate metastatic disease. Lymph node involvement is a key determinant in the patient's management and prognosis.

TABLE 1 Clinical Staging of Melanoma

Stage 0	Melanoma in situ
Stage Ia	≤1 mm, Clark's* level II or III, with or without some adverse features†
Stage Ib	≤1 mm, with ulceration or Clark's level IV or V; or 1.01–2.0 mm, no ulceration
Stage IIa	1.01–2.0 mm, with ulceration or 2.01–4.0 mm without ulceration
Stage IIb	2.01–4.0 mm, with ulceration or >4.0 mm without ulceration
Stage IIc	>4.0 mm with ulceration
Stage III	Any depth with in-transit disease or lymph node involvement
Stage IV	Distant metastasis

*Clark's levels are based on penetration of tumor through anatomic levels in the skin.
†Adverse features include a positive deep margin, lymphvascular invasion, or a mitotic rate ≥1 mitoses/mm².

TABLE 2 Surgical Margins and Recommendation for Sentinel Lymph Node Biopsy

Depth	Margins*	Sentinel Node Biopsy
In situ	0.5 cm	No
≤1 mm	1 cm	No†
1.01–2 mm	1–2 cm	Yes
>2 mm	≥2 cm	Yes (if nodes not clinically noted)

*Margins may need to be modified because of anatomic or functional considerations.
†Reasons for sentinel lymph node biopsy at this depth include ulceration, a positive deep margin on initial biopsy, extensive regression, and mitotic rate greater than zero.

The wide local excision can be performed at the same time as the sentinel lymph node biopsy, but whenever possible, it should not be performed before the lymph drainage has been determined. The width of this excision is based on the initial thickness of the melanoma and reflects the risk of local metastases to the surrounding tissue. An elliptical, full-thickness removal of underlying fascia is typically performed, and the specimen is sent for pathologic confirmation of adequate negative margins (Table 2).

ADJUVANT SYSTEMIC THERAPY AFTER SURGERY FOR HIGH-RISK DISEASE

The FDA-approved adjuvant therapy after resection of high-risk (stage IIC and stage III) melanoma is interferon alfa-2b (IFN-α-2b, Intron A), which is given intravenously at 20 MU/m²/day for 5 days each week for 4 weeks, followed by subcutaneous administration three times weekly at 10 MU/m²/day for 48 weeks. This dose and schedule of IFN-α-2b has been tested in large, prospective, randomized trials and compared with observation and with a GM2 vaccine.[5] Although a consistent benefit in terms of relapse-free survival has been demonstrated for this IFN-α-2b regimen, the impact on overall survival is less clear. Some data suggest that clinical manifestations of autoimmunity during IFN-α-2b therapy may be associated with improved survival. Unfortunately, substantial clinical toxicities, including hepatotoxicity, myelotoxicity, and significant flulike symptoms, are frequently seen with IFN-α-2b therapy.

Several studies have evaluated various alternate doses and schedules of interferon as adjuvant therapy for patients with resected melanoma. Although some preliminary results suggested possible benefit, no consistent improvement in overall survival or relapse-free survival has been demonstrated for high-risk melanoma patients after low- or intermediate-dose adjuvant interferon regimens. High-dose IFN-α-2b remains the only systemic adjuvant treatment with confirmed activity against melanoma after resection of stage IIC or III disease. Although there is agreement regarding the confirmed benefit of this treatment on relapse-free survival, the extent of the impact on overall survival is less clear. Consensus does not exist regarding the standard use of high-dose IFN-α-2b, and improvements are clearly needed in our adjuvant treatment of patients with resected, high-risk melanoma.

Alternate systemic therapies have been evaluated for patients with resected, high-risk melanoma. Although controlled studies have suggested benefit for adjuvant therapy with granulocyte-macrophage colony stimulating factor (GM-CSF, sargramostim [Leukine]),[1] this benefit remains unproven and is receiving additional clinical testing. Numerous other adjuvant therapies, including vaccines, other immunotherapies, and chemotherapy, have been evaluated and shown to have limited or no benefit in randomized and nonrandomized adjuvant therapy trials enrolling melanoma patients. Participation in clinical trials should be encouraged for patients with resected, high-risk melanoma.

---

[1]Not FDA approved for this indication.
[5]Investigational drug in the United States.

CHEMOTHERAPY FOR ADVANCED DISEASE

The success of various chemotherapy strategies for patients with metastatic melanoma has been limited. The use of single-agent dacarbazine (dimethyl-triazeno-imidazole carboxamide [DTIC]) has been a standard treatment and remains the only FDA-approved cytotoxic drug for metastatic melanoma patients. However, its response rate of 15% to 20%, median response duration of 4 to 6 months, and complete response rate of less than 5% leaves ample room for improvement.

Many other drugs have been evaluated for single-agent activity against melanoma. Although the results from several single-agent, phase II chemotherapy studies appear better than single-agent DTIC, none has been confirmed as superior in a prospective, randomized, phase III study. Temozolomide (Temodar)[1] is used instead of DTIC by many oncologists because it has a mechanism of action similar to that of DTIC with the additional benefit of being an oral agent with penetration into the central nervous system.

Combination-chemotherapy regimens that combine agents with distinct single-agent activity or add novel agents as a means to enhance activity have also been investigated. One of the more promising regimens was the combination of cisplatin (Platinol-AQ),[1] dacarbazine (DTIC-Dome), carmustine (BCNU),[1] and tamoxifen (Nolvadex)[1] (CDBT regimen, also known as the Dartmouth regimen), which had been suggested for many years to have significant activity for patients with metastatic melanoma. However, a prospective, randomized trial compared CDBT with single-agent DTIC therapy and found no difference in overall survival with either of these treatments. Several phase II studies have suggested potential benefit for combination chemotherapy over single-agent chemotherapy, but results from subsequent phase III testing have been disappointing.

IMMUNOTHERAPY FOR ADVANCED DISEASE

Many cytokines and other immune activators are being evaluated as therapy for patients with metastatic melanoma. Measurable responses are occasionally seen with interferon therapy for melanoma patients with advanced metastatic disease. Unfortunately, most of these responses are transient and last only a few months.

The FDA has approved high-dose bolus interleukin-2 (IL-2, aldesleukin [Proleukin]) treatment for patients with metastatic melanoma. For some melanoma patients, measurable shrinkage of grossly evident tumor metastases can be induced by IL-2 treatment. Approximately 6% of patients achieved complete remission, and 10% of patients achieved partial remission in numerous phase II studies using high-dose bolus IL-2. The approved regimen is administration of IL-2 at 600,000 to 720,000 IU/kg every 8 hours, up to a maximum of 15 doses, on days 1 through 5 and 15 through 19 of a treatment course. This IL-2 therapy has a dose-dependent toxicity profile and has significant toxicity when administered in the approved high-dose bolus regimen. Use of high-dose IL-2 should therefore be restricted to specialized centers with expertise in managing this toxicity.

Studies involving administration of lymphokine-activated killer (LAK)[5] cells and tumor-infiltrating lymphocytes (TILs)[5] together with IL-2 have not demonstrated sufficient additional activity to support noninvestigational use of these approaches. Other approaches, including combining IL-2 therapy with tumor-reactive monoclonal antibodies[5] and using antibody-cytokine fusion proteins[5] to target IL-2 directly to tumor cells, are being investigated.

Immunotherapy has been combined with chemotherapy in an attempt to enhance antitumor activity. Several nonrandomized, single-institution, phase II studies have evaluated combination chemotherapy given with IL-2 and IFN-α as biochemotherapy for patients with metastatic melanoma. Inpatient and outpatient regimens have been evaluated, and response rates of 40% to 60% and durable response rates up to 10% were reported. Unfortunately, subsequent prospective, randomized clinical trials did not confirm

the earlier observations. Although addition of immunotherapy to combination chemotherapy may occasionally increase antitumor activity, it also significantly increases toxicity without having an impact on overall survival. Biochemotherapy is therefore not a standard therapy for metastatic melanoma patients.

NOVEL INVESTIGATIONAL APPROACHES

Numerous advances in molecular biology and immunology have provided new opportunities for the design and analysis of novel therapies for melanoma patients. Identification of distinct genetic pathways in the development of melanoma and the elucidation of signaling pathways provide opportunities for targeted therapies. Examples of the approaches being tested clinically include the combination of chemotherapy with the antisense BCL2 oligonucleotide[5] to inhibit antiapoptotic pathways and the combination of chemotherapy with novel agents such as RAF kinase inhibitors.[5] Sorafenib (Nexavar)[1] is a targeted agent that blocks BRAF and tyrosine kinases, and it has demonstrated antitumor activity when combined with several chemotherapy agents in phase II studies. A phase III study testing carboplatin (Paraplatin)[1] and paclitaxel (Taxol)[1] combined with sorafenib or a placebo as first-line therapy for metastatic melanoma has completed accrual. Novel targeted therapies will receive increased testing in upcoming clinical trials.

Increased understanding of the immunobiology of human melanoma provides many opportunities for translational clinical trials. Clinical testing of antibodies to immunoregulatory molecules, most notably anti-CTLA4,[5] demonstrated antitumor activity in several clinical trials, and additional studies are in progress. Several studies are examining immunogenicity and the antitumor activity of novel melanoma vaccine[5] constructs. Approaches being studied also include the use of nonmyeloablative chemotherapy before adoptive transfer of cloned T cells and high-dose IL-2 therapy. The appreciation of regulatory T-cell interactions in melanoma provides additional opportunities for translational immunotherapy clinical trials. It is anticipated that combination immunotherapy clinical trials will receive expanded testing for patients with advanced melanoma. It is also anticipated that expanded clinical testing of novel agents will occur in the setting of minimal residual disease, a setting predicted to most likely be of benefit based on preclinical models of melanoma.

---

[1]Not FDA approved for this indication.
[5]Investigational drug in the United States.

CURRENT THERAPY

- Early diagnosis and surgical removal with the recommended margins remain the foundation of treatment.
- A sentinel lymph node biopsy is recommended for lesions of 1 mm or greater depth and for lesions with less than 1 mm depth with adverse features.
- Palpable regional lymph nodes should be biopsied and managed surgically.
- Consider adjuvant therapy with interferon alpha-2b (Intron A) or clinical trial participation after resection of stage IIC or stage III disease. There is no standard adjuvant therapy for stage I or stage II (A, B) disease.
- Consider surgery for patients with a single site of distant metastasis.
- Consider clinical trial participation as an important option for patients with stage IV disease. FDA-approved standard treatments include high-dose IL-2 (Proleukin) and dacarbazine (DTIC).

---

[1]Not FDA approved for this indication.
[5]Investigational drug in the United States.

Miller AJ, Mihm Jr MC. Melanoma. N Engl J Med 2006;355:51–65.
Morton DL, Thompson JF, Cochran AJ, et al. Sentinel-node biopsy or nodal observation in melanoma. N Engl J Med 2006;355:1307–17.
National Comprehensive Cancer Network (NCCN). Clinical Practice Guidelines in Oncology. Available at http://www.nccn.org. version v.2, 2009.
Vence L, Palucka AK, Fay JW, et al. Circulating tumor antigen-specific regulatory T cells in patients with metastatic melanoma. Proc Natl Acad Sci U S A 2007;104:20884–9.

TABLE 3 Frequency of Follow-up Examinations of Melanoma Patients

Stage	Recommended Follow-up Intervals
Stage 0 (in situ)	At least annual examinations for life
Stage Ia	3–12 months for 5 years, then annually for life
Stage Ib and above	3–6 months for 2 years, then 3–12 months for 3 years, then annually for life

Patient Follow-up

Lifetime follow-up for all patients with a history of melanoma is important. This includes monthly self-examinations, including lymph node palpation, by the patient using the ABCDE principles previously described. Photographs can help selected patients track pigmented lesions, and a spouse, family member, or trusted friend can be employed to check difficult-to-see areas, such as behind the ears, on the scalp, and on the back. Patients should also be thoughtful about their sun exposure and use sun blocks and sun-protective clothing.

Regular, comprehensive skin examinations with appropriate review of systems and lymph node evaluations by a health care provider are also important. Patients with a diagnosis of an invasive melanoma should be considered for a chest radiograph and laboratory studies, including a lactate dehydrogenase (LDH) determination, and other liver function studies at baseline. These tests are then obtained at intervals of 3 to 6 months for patients with stage II and higher-stage melanoma for the first 2 years and then every 6 to 12 months for years 3 to 5. Additional imaging, including baseline computed tomography (CT) scans and a baseline positron emission tomography (PET) scan, is often considered for patients with resected stage IIB or higher-stage disease or patients with specific signs and symptoms. However, intensive radiologic follow-up does not have demonstrated benefit. The use of molecular markers in the blood as predictors of disease recurrence is being investigated. A reasonable frequency of follow-up examinations of melanoma patients is outlined in Table 3.

Acknowledgments

Dr. Mark Albertini thanks Ann's Hope Foundation, the Gretchen and Andrew Dawes Charitable Trust, the Steve Leuthold Family Foundation (Jay Van Sloan Memorial), and Kathy Eagle (Tim Eagle Memorial) for gifts to the University of Wisconsin Carbone Cancer Center supporting our research on melanoma immunotherapy. The authors thank Melinda Baker for assistance with manuscript preparation.

REFERENCES

Albertini MR, Hank JA, Sondel PM. Native and genetically engineered anti-disialoganglioside monoclonal antibody treatment of melanoma. Cancer Chemother Biol Response Modif 2005;22:789–97.
Albertini MR, Longley BJ, Harari PM, et al. Cutaneous melanoma. In: Chang AE, Ganz PA, Hayes DF, et al., editors. Oncology: An Evidence-Based Approach. New York: Springer-Verlag; 2005. p. 1073–92.
Balch CM, Buzaid AC, Soong SJ, et al. Final version of the American Joint Committee on Cancer staging system for cutaneous melanoma. J Clin Oncol 2001;19:3635–48.
Carlson JA, Ross JS, Slominski A, et al. Molecular diagnostics in melanoma. J Am Acad Dermatol 2005;52:743–75; quiz 775–8.
Curtin JA, Fridlyand J, Kageshita T, et al. Distinct sets of genetic alterations in melanoma. N Engl J Med 2005;353:2135–47.
Gogas H, Ioannovich J, Dafni U, et al. Prognostic significance of autoimmunity during treatment of melanoma with interferon. N Engl J Med 2006;354:709–18.
Jemal A, Siegel R, Ward E, et al. Cancer statistics, 2008. CA Cancer J Clin 2008;58:71–96.
Middleton MR, Grob JJ, Aaronson N, et al. Randomized phase III study of temozolomide versus dacarbazine in the treatment of patients with advanced metastatic malignant melanoma. J Clin Oncol 2000;18:158–66.

Premalignant Cutaneous and Mucosal Lesions

Method of
Juliet Gunkel, MD

Identification and clinical monitoring of premalignant skin lesions can reduce the morbidity and mortality of skin cancer for many patients with diverse histories and exposures. The link between precancerous and cancerous lesions and ultraviolet (UV) light exposure has been studied extensively. Some patients do not understand the importance of or choose not to adhere to sun-protection precautions and the prudent use of sunscreens. The cause of premalignant lesions also includes human papillomavirus (HPV) disease, arsenic exposures, and degeneration of benign nevi, birthmarks, and neoplasms.

Although certain exposures and conditions are associated with premalignant lesions, some groups of patients are at higher risk for precancerous and cancerous lesions. In many cases, these cancers are rapidly progressive, high grade, and aggressive. Patients who are at high risk are immunocompromised due to human immunodeficiency virus infection or acquired immunodeficiency syndrome, have heritable immunodeficiencies, have had effective immunosuppression of chronic lymphocytic leukemia, have undergone organ transplantation, or are on immunosuppressive medications. An increased susceptibility to infection with oncogenic HPV types may be important in the pathogenesis of malignancies in these patients. Genodermatoses associated with a higher risk of skin cancer include xeroderma pigmentosa, oculocutaneous albinism, Bazex syndrome, and nevoid basal cell carcinoma syndrome. A history of UV exposure and cigarette smoking further compounds the risk for many of these patients.

A variety of dermatoses and neoplasms have a demonstrated association with development of malignancies, although these benign conditions or lesions are not necessarily precancerous. In certain long-standing skin diseases, persistence or progression of characteristic lesions despite apparent appropriate treatment may herald development of skin cancer. Similarly, atypical appearance of or change in the classic lesion of a skin condition or in a previously stable neoplasm is suspicious. These conditions include Zoon balanitis or vulvitis, discoid lupus erythematosus, lichen planus, lichen sclerosus, lymphedema, and chronic radiodermatitis. The neoplasms include nevus sebaceus, plexiform neurofibromas, and leukoplakia or erythroplakia. Scars, epitomized by the persistent scarring seen in dystrophic epidermolysis bullosa, and nonhealing wounds (e.g., burns, chronic ulcers) also may provide sites for malignant growth.

By recognizing these risk factors, predispositions, special populations, and associations, the practitioner can identify premalignant lesions in at-risk patients and recommend appropriate follow-up evaluation and treatment. This approach is essential for prevention and early detection of various types of cancers of cutaneous and mucosal surfaces. Lesions that progress, become symptomatic, become locally destructive or disfiguring, do not respond to appropriate treatment, or change their clinical appearance or behavior should be evaluated for malignancy. Biopsy and referral to a dermatologist are recommended.

Actinic Keratoses or Cheilitis

CLINICAL MANIFESTATIONS

Precursors to squamous cell carcinoma in situ (SCCIS) and squamous cell carcinoma (SCC) can develop on cutaneous and mucosal surfaces subjected to intense, intermittent, or frequent sun exposure. They manifest as flesh-colored, red, or pigmented papules and plaques. Some are rather firm and indurated with a hard scale; others are thin and friable, with a more delicate scale or without scale, appearing shiny and atrophic.

Clinical diagnosis is facilitated by light palpation of sun-exposed sites with the fingertips because the characteristic, gritty, sandpaper-like scale can be very prominent. Involvement can range from multiple or few discrete lesions to an ill-defined zone or field. Occurrence on the lip, often exclusively the lower lip, may be associated with pain, swelling, and fissures. Most lesions remain stable for years without progression or degeneration. The absolute risk is not known but is estimated at 1 case in 1000 lesions per year. Lesions that persist after treatment or show rapid progression should raise suspicion for malignant degeneration. Suspicion should be elevated if mucosal lesions are ulcerated, and biopsy is recommended.

TREATMENT

Limited mechanical removal of discrete lesions is possible with curettage. Liquid nitrogen applied with a cotton-tipped applicator or spraying device is a common and effective treatment for cutaneous and mucosal lesions. Lesions can be treated until they appear white or frozen for 8 to 10 seconds on the lip and other delicate tissues. Thicker skin and thicker lesions require freeze times of 20 seconds or to the patient's tolerance. After this, a second cycle may be used immediately. Some lesions may require two or three such treatments separated by 4 to 12 weeks before resolution. Posttreatment pain, swelling, and blistering can be limiting. Because this modality is nonselective, normal and atypical cells are affected equally.

Treatment of individual lesions with chemical peeling agents such as glycolic acid 20% (e.g., Biomedic MicroPeel Solution)[1] and trichloroacetic acid 10% to 30%[1] can be effective and repeated as needed. These nonselective agents can also be applied to a wider field of involvement for broader effect (i.e., field treatment).

Field treatment also is available as a patient-delivered topical chemotherapy. Topical 5-fluorouracil (available as 0.5% [Carac], 1% [Fluoroplex], and 5% cream [Efudex] for cutaneous surfaces and 1% [Fluoroplex], 2% [Efudex], and 5% solution [Efudex] for mucosal surfaces) can be applied in various regimens, once or twice daily for 2 to 6 weeks as the patient tolerates. More delicate mucosal tissues should be treated once or twice daily for 1 to 3 weeks. Use is limited by development of irritation, pain, and skin breakdown. Because this is a selective chemical treatment, affected cells are targeted, and a more vigorous response should lead to more significant improvement. Inflammatory response is individual, and for patients who are not tolerating treatment well, application can be reduced to once to three times weekly. Breaks or time off during a treatment course can be introduced. The treatment course can be abbreviated if needed. An effective treatment course also may treat early or in situ lesions of SCC or basal cell carcinoma (BCC) in the field.

Other topical chemotherapeutic field treatments include diclofenac sodium 3% gel (Solaraze) applied once or twice daily for 8 to 12 weeks. The inflammatory response is attenuated and therefore may be better tolerated by patients. Concomitantly, improvement is less dramatic. Imiquimod 5% cream (Aldara) may be applied daily for 3 to 6 weeks or twice daily for 3 days per week for 4 to 8 weeks. Another regimen is once or twice application per week for 4 to 8 months, used continuously or in alternating 1-month cycles. The daily dosing schedule and treatment course should be decreased by about one half for mucosal surfaces. The disadvantage is unpredictability of response. However, imiquimod also may treat early or in situ lesions of SCC and BCC in the field.

---

[1]Not FDA approved for this indication.

Photodynamic treatment is another selective treatment for individual lesions or field treatment. Application of 20% 5-aminolevulinic acid (ALA [Levulan Kerastick]) to affected areas is followed by activation by a light source. Treatment can be completed by the practitioner in 1 day. Before ALA application, scale should be removed with acetone, chemical peel, or microdermabrasion. Alternatively, the patient can apply 5-fluorouracil cream or solution for 5 days or any topical retinoid (tretinoin [Retin-A],[1] adapalene [Differin],[1] or tazarotene [Tazorac][1]) for 1 month. ALA is available as a stick or swablike applicator, and application is challenging on larger areas. After ALA application, absorption or incubation is required: 1 to 2 hours for the face and lips, 3 to 4 hours for the chest and upper extremities, and 5 to 24 hours for the lower extremities. The light source for activation can be laser (585 or 595 nm), intense pulsed light (560 to 1200 nm), or blue light (412 to 422 nm). Only the blue light source is conducive for field treatment. Like 5-fluorouracil and imiquimod, photodynamic therapy may treat early or in situ lesions of BCC or SCC in the field.

Topical (tretinoin, adapalene, or tazarotene) and oral (acitretin [Soriatane][1]) retinoids can decrease development of actinic keratoses and nonmelanoma skin cancer in at-risk individuals. Efficacy is relatively mild, but any topical retinoid can be used each night indefinitely as tolerated by the patient. Acne and early signs of aging improve with this regimen. Oral retinoids can be used daily or every other day at the lowest dose (acitretin 10 mg) producing clinical improvement. The dose should be titrated up (to 50 mg maximum) as needed and as tolerated. Benefits are conferred only with maintenance of retinoid therapy.

---

[1]Not FDA approved for this indication.

CURRENT DIAGNOSIS

Actinic Keratoses or Cheilitis

- Flesh-colored, red, or pigmented lesions with thick or delicate keratotic scale
- Swelling, fissures, and scaling on lower lip
- Sun-exposed sites

Arsenical Keratoses

- Punctate, hyperkeratotic lesions of palms and soles
- Exposure to contaminated well water or medications

Porokeratoses

- Lesions with atrophic center and peripheral grooved ridge of hyperkeratosis
- Large and solitary; diffuse, small, and annular on sun-exposed sites; linear, segmental, or generalized; punctate on palms and soles without ridge

Human Papillomavirus Disease

- Verrucous, hyperkeratotic lesions on palms and soles
- Fleshy, hyperkeratotic lesions or shiny, atrophic lesions or erosions in the anogenital region
- White, adherent, keratotic lesions on mucosal surfaces; may become verrucous and exophytic

Atypia in Melanocytic Nevi

- "Fried egg" appearance with a papular center on a macular base
- Asymmetry, ill-defined borders, variegated color, diameter larger than 6 mm, ulceration, bleeding, pain, or pruritus in a new or previously stable pigmented lesion

Arsenical Keratoses

CLINICAL MANIFESTATIONS

The small, punctate, hyperkeratotic lesions of arsenical keratoses are seen on the palms and soles of patients exposed to arsenic through contaminated well water and various medications. Carcinoma may develop after 10 to 20 years and evolve from precancerous keratoses or on any skin surface.

TREATMENT

Although acute toxicity can be treated with chelation, it has little value in chronic exposure. As for actinic keratoses, treatment of arsenical keratoses includes cryotherapy, topical chemotherapy, photodynamic therapy, and retinoids.[1] Discrete lesions can be treated with surgery or curettage.

Porokeratoses

CLINICAL MANIFESTATIONS

The classic porokeratosis has a smooth, atrophic center surrounded by a grooved ridge of hyperkeratosis called a *cornoid lamella*. The plaque form (i.e., Mibelli's porokeratosis) is large and progressive, often appearing early in life. The disseminated superficial type favors sun-exposed sites and manifests as numerous, small, annular papules. The linear type may be generalized or segmental and often manifests very early in life. Only the punctate keratotic papules seen in *porokeratosis palmaris, plantaris et disseminate* have no clinically evident cornoid lamellae. Malignant transformation occurs mostly commonly in the linear type, followed by the Mibelli type. It is rare in the disseminated type and has not been reported in the punctate type.

TREATMENT

Treatment modalities include those described for actinic keratoses. Other destructive modalities may be beneficial for discrete lesions, including curettage, surgical excision, dermabrasion, and ablative lasers such as carbon dioxide (CO_2) and erbium yttrium-aluminum-garnet (Er:YAG) lasers.

Human Papillomavirus Disease

CLINICAL MANIFESTATIONS

The clinical manifestations of precancerous HPV infection on cutaneous and mucosal surfaces are diverse. The initial appearance and clinical behavior of verrucous carcinoma (i.e., Buschke-Lowenstein tumor on the genitals and oral florid papillomatosis) is as plantar, genital, and mucosal HPV disease; verrucous hyperkeratotic papules and plaques on the plantar surface; fleshy or hyperkeratotic papules in the anogenital region; and white, adherent keratotic plaques or leukoplakia of the mucosal surfaces. The clinically benign appearance and behavior change may signal malignant degeneration. Lower-risk types HPV-6 and -11 or high-risk HPV-16 may be implicated.

HPV-8, -16, -31, and -33 may be the causative agents in premalignant anogenital squamous intraepithelial lesions. The preferred terms *vulvar intraepithelial lesions/neoplasia* (VIL/N), *anal intraepithelial lesions/neoplasia* (AIL/N), and *penile intraepithelial lesions/neoplasia* (PIL/N) have replaced the confusing terminology Bowen's disease, erythroplasia of Queyrat, and bowenoid papulosis for these anogenital lesions. Dermatologists reserve the term *bowenoid papulosis* for discrete, fleshy, red-brown papules with a better prognosis that are seen in younger patients. Clinical appearance includes verrucous keratotic plaques, erosions, bowenoid-papulosis–type lesions, erosions, and erythematous, well-demarcated plaques, which may be shiny on the glans penis.

[1]Not FDA approved for this indication.

CURRENT THERAPY

Actinic Keratoses or Cheilitis

- Physical methods: curettage, liquid nitrogen
- Nonselective topical chemical agents: glycol acid 20%,[1] trichloroacetic acid 10% to 30%[1]
- Selective topical chemical agents: 5-fluorouracil (Carac, Efudex), diclofenac sodium (Solaraze), imiquimod (Aldara), 5-aminolevulinic acid (Levulan Kerastick) activated by a light source, and retinoids, including tretinoin (Retin-A),[1] adapalene (Differin),[1] and tazarotene (Tazorac)[1]
- Oral agents: retinoids[1]

Arsenical Keratoses

- Surgery and modalities used for actinic keratoses

Porokeratoses

- Surgery, dermabrasion, lasers (CO_2 and Er:YAG)
- Modalities for actinic keratoses

Human Papillomavirus Disease

- Blistering agents: liquid nitrogen, Cantharone (0.7% cantharidin),[1,6] podophyllin 25% in tincture of benzoin (Podocon-25), purified podophyllotoxin 0.5% solution or gel (Condylox)
- Keratolytics: topical salicylic acid products (e.g., Compound W, Wart-Off, Dr. Scholl's, Duofilm, Salactic, Mediplast, Sal-Acid), topical retinoids,[1] and topical urea 10% to 40% (Carmol, Gordon's)
- Physical methods: curettage, liquid nitrogen, surgery, ablative laser, electrofulguration, occlusive tapes such as duct tape
- Immunotherapy: imiquimod (Aldara), intralesional candida or mumps antigen injections[1]
- Oral agents: cimetidine (Tagamet)[1]

Atypia in Melanocytic Nevi

- Close clinical observation and mole mapping
- Surgery, curettage, ablative laser

[1]Not FDA approved for this indication.
[6]May be compounded by pharmacists.

Progressive verrucous leukoplakia may appear as benign leukoplakia early—hyperplastic, thin, white plaques of the mucosal surface. These slowly progress to verrucous exophytic masses, many of which degenerate to SCC. HPV-16 infection has been associated with this multifocal premalignant condition.

Epidermodysplasia verruciformis (EDV) is a rare, inherited condition that predisposes to infection with the less common viral types of HPV-5, -8, -9, -12, -14, -15, -17, -19, -25 through -36, and -38 and with the more common types of HPV-3 and -10. This leads to flat verrucous papules on the extremities, face, and neck, which may be numerous and may coalesce. Lesions similar to tinea versicolor may develop over the trunk. SCC develops in 30% to 60% of these patients, and HPV-5, -8, and -47 are identified in 90% of the lesions.

TREATMENT

Eradication of HPV infection is challenging and often requires months of treatment. Observation may be reasonable for certain lesions with clinically benign appearance and behavior, and spontaneous resolution may occur.

Lesions of nonmucosal sites, including the plantar feet, can be treated by freezing with liquid nitrogen for 10 to 30 seconds for two cycles. This may need to be repeated every 3 to 6 weeks until resolution. Another blistering agent, Cantharone (0.7% cantharidin [Canthacur][1,6]), can be applied under occlusion for 6 to 24 hours. The advantage is painless application, but individual responses are unpredictable. Hyperkeratotic lesions, such as those on the plantar surface, require more aggressive use of these modalities. Imiquimod (Aldara)[1] applied daily can be beneficial, but it may require 6 months of treatment. Constant use of occlusive tapes such as duct tape has demonstrated efficacy and may be combined with any treatments. Between liquid nitrogen treatments or as adjunctive therapy, use of keratolytics such as topical salicylic acid products (e.g., liquid [Compound W, Wart-Off, Dr. Scholl's, Duofilm], film [Salactic], plaster [Mediplast, Duofilm, Sal-Acid], compounded in ointment), topical retinoids, and topical urea 10% to 40% (Carmol, Gordon's), as well as mechanical paring, can reduce the size of the lesion. This approach is rarely effective as monotherapy. Oral cimetidine (Tagamet)[1] 30 to 40 mg/kg/day may be a helpful adjunctive therapy. In those demonstrating sensitivity, cure rates of 60% to 80% can be achieved with intralesional candidal (*Candida albicans* skin test antigen [Candin])[1] or mumps antigen (mumps skin test antigen)[1] injections. Surgical treatment, including excision, curettage, and ablative CO_2 laser, have relatively low efficacy and may result in painful scars.

For treatment of lesions in the anogenital region, liquid nitrogen may be used less aggressively. Imiquimod (Aldara) applied twice daily for 3 days of the week for 10 to 16 weeks is about 50% effective. Adjunctive treatment with cimetidine (Tagamet)[1] has a role as described earlier. Physician-applied podophyllin 25% in a tincture of benzoin (Podocon-25) is placed for 4 to 8 hours each week for 6 weeks. Alternatively, purified podophyllotoxin 0.5% solution or gel (podofilox [Condylox]) is applied by the patient over 3 consecutive days for 4 to 6 weeks. Electrofulguration may be the most effective treatment, with a cure rate of 70% at 3 months. Surgical treatment, including excision, curettage, and ablative CO_2 laser, have relatively low efficacy and may result in painful scars.

Lesions of the oral mucosa are best treated with cryotherapy as for anogenital lesions, curettage, surgical excision, electrofulguration, and ablative CO_2 laser.

Treatment recommendations for lesions of EDV include those for lesions on nonmucosal surfaces as described earlier. Although there is no particular treatment for patients with EDV, prevention (i.e., UV protection and smoking cessation) is important, as it is for all patients.

Atypia in Melanocytic Nevi

CLINICAL MANIFESTATIONS

Because almost one half of melanomas arise in benign, preexisting melanocytic nevi, these nevi can be considered premalignant lesions. Nevi manifest as acquired pigmented macules and papules in the first 3 decades of life. Dysplastic nevi are clinically and histologically atypical and therefore likely represent a higher risk. They have a "fried egg" appearance, with a papular center on a macular base, and they are 5 to 12 mm in diameter, larger than common nevi. Their shape is often irregular with indistinct borders and variegated tan, brown, and pink coloration.

The incidence of melanoma arising in a giant congenital melanocytic nevus (CMN) is 2% to 15%. Other associated sarcomas are rare. Giant CMN are pigmented plaques larger than 20 cm in diameter in adults. They often cover most of an extremity, the trunk, the scalp, or even the entire dorsal surface in the neonate. They grow with the individual but do not spread. Often, satellites or smaller nevi are seen beyond the border of the primary lesion.

TREATMENT

Pigmented lesions should be monitored for changes such as development of asymmetry, irregular borders, change or variegation in color, and growth, especially greater than 6 mm. Ulceration, bleeding,

---

[1]Not FDA approved for this indication.
[6]May be compounded by pharmacists.

pain, or pruritus can signal malignant degeneration. On a given individual, identification of the pigmented lesion clinically dissimilar to the others is known as the ugly duckling sign. Changes in a giant CMN or a satellite such as nodularity are worrisome. In these cases, biopsy or very close monitoring, including use of clinical photographs called mole mapping, is essential. For giant CMNs, in theory, decreasing the number of nevus cells should decrease the risk of malignant degeneration, and partial or serial excision using tissue expanders, curettage, and ablative laser treatment may be beneficial.

REFERENCES

Bolognia JL, Jorizzo J, Rapini RP, editors. Dermatology. New York: Mosby; 2003.
James WD, Berger TG, Elston DM, editor. Andrews' Diseases of the Skin—Clinical Dermatology. 10th ed. Philadelphia: WB Saunders; 2006.
McKenna WG, editors. Abeloff's Clinical Oncology. 4th ed. Philadelphia: Churchill Livingstone; 2008.
Morton CA, McKenna KE, Rhodes LE, et al. Guidelines for topical photodynamic therapy: Update. Br J Dermatol 2008;159:1245–66.
Robinson JK, Hanke CW, Sengelman RD, Siegel DM, editors. Surgery of the Skin—Procedural Dermatology. New York: Mosby; 2005.
Wood GS, Gunkel J, Stewart D, et al. Nonmelanoma skin cancers. In: Abeloff JO, Armitage JO, Niederhuber JE, Kastan MB, editors. Abeloff's Clinical Oncology. Philadelphia, 2008.

Bacterial Diseases of the Skin

Method of
Dennis L. Stevens, MD, PhD

The spectrum of bacterial diseases of the skin ranges from superficial, localized, easily recognized, and treated skin eruptions to deep, aggressive, gangrenous, or necrotizing infections that may appear innocuous at first but quickly become life threatening. The prompt recognition and treatment of these infections are paramount in limiting morbidity and mortality. A healthy respect for the aggressiveness of gangrenous and necrotizing infections of the skin and soft tissues is developed by first harboring a high index of suspicion to provide early recognition and appropriate treatment before overwhelming clinical infection occurs.

Common Infections

IMPETIGO

Impetigo is the most common bacterial infection of the skin. It is highly contagious and can occur at any age from infancy to adulthood, but it is most common in preschool-age children. There are two classic forms of impetigo: nonbullous and bullous. Both forms have a predominantly staphylococcal cause, but they manifest with different morphologic characteristics.

Nonbullous (crusted) impetigo can be recognized by the development of a serous, yellow-brown exudate, which dries into a golden crust. Lesions rarely elicit pain but can be associated with erythema and pruritus. They are most common on exposed areas such as the hands, feet, face, and legs and are often associated with a minor traumatic event such as an insect bite, abrasion, or laceration. Crusted impetigo is usually caused by a heavy mixed flora of staphylococci and streptococci. Streptococcal impetigo has been associated with the postinfectious sequelae of post-streptococcal glomerulonephritis.

The bullous variety usually manifests as a rapidly spreading papule, which may progress to a thin-walled vesicle if the lesion is infected with *Staphylococcus aureus*, an organism that produces an exfoliative toxin. These lesions occur most often in warm, moist areas of the body. Predisposing factors include warm ambient temperatures, humidity, poor hygiene, and crowded living conditions.

TABLE 1 Suggested Antibiotic Therapy for Gram-Positive Bacterial Isolates

Isolate	Oral	Parenteral
GABHS	Penicillin G or V Erythromycin First-generation cephalosporin	Penicillin G Ampicillin/sulbactam (Unasyn) First-generation cephalosporin
Staphylococcus aureus (methicillin sensitive)	Penicillinase-resistant synthetic penicillin (Oxacillin)	First-generation cephalosporin Clindamycin (Cleocin) Oxacillin
Staphylococcus aureus (methicillin resistant)	Linezolid (Zyvox)	Vancomycin (Vancocin) Daptomycin (Cubicin) Linezolid (Zyvox)
Clostridial species	Penicillin G or V Clindamycin (Cleocin) Metronidazole (Flagyl)	Penicillin G Clindamycin Metronidazole

Abbreviation: GABHS = group A β-hemolytic *Streptococcus.*

Treatment of impetigo begins with eradication or with the environmental factors thought to be influential in its development. Aggressive lesion débridement with mesh gauze sponges or brushes and antibacterial soap is encouraged. Special attention to hygiene and disinfection of towels and bedding are also necessary. Topical antibiotic treatment with mupirocin (Bactroban) or bacitracin[1] has been effective in mild to moderate cases. In more extensive cases, oral antibiotic therapy with a penicillinase-resistant synthetic penicillin (oxacillin) is the treatment of choice (Table 1). However, a high percentage of methicillin-resistant strains of *S. aureus* (MRSA) are isolated in institutional and community settings. Patients should be treated for at least 5 to 7 days. If no improvement is seen, lesions should be cultured and antibiotics adjusted appropriately.

Systemic complications from impetigo are very uncommon. Cellulitis has occurred but is usually susceptible to systemic antibiotic therapy. Septicemia and staphylococcal scaled skin syndrome are rare complications of impetigo. When they occur, systemic therapy is indicated.

FOLLICULITIS

Folliculitis is a pyoderma that arises within a hair follicle. The process is known as a furuncle (boil) when the infection extends beyond the hair follicle. These lesions occur most frequently in the moist areas of the body and in areas subject to friction and perspiration. Host factors known to predispose one to folliculitis include obesity, blood dyscrasias, defects in neutrophil function, immune deficiency states (e.g., diabetes, transplantation-related immunosuppression, acquired immunodeficiency syndrome [AIDS]), and treatment with corticosteroids or cytotoxic agents. The offending organism in most immunocompetent patients is *S. aureus*; however, when immunosuppression impairs host defenses, gram-negative organisms (*Klebsiella, Enterobacter,* and *Proteus* species) can be involved. *Pseudomonas* species such as *aeruginosa* or *cepacia* are associated with hot-tub folliculitis, which involves numerous hair follicles. It is usually self-limited, resolving in 7 to 10 days.

Successful treatment of folliculitis depends on correcting the predisposing factors that promote the development of this condition. For patients with localized disease, topical wound care including antibiotics such as mupirocin (Bactroban) is effective. Patients with furunculosis or multiple lesions with surrounding erythema of more than 2.5 cm should be treated with orally administered systemic antibiotics that are effective against *S. aureus*. Any fluctuant nodules or abscesses should be incised and drained. Patients with recurrent furunculosis should have their nares cultured for methicillin-susceptible *Staphylococcus aureus* (MSSA) or MRSA because nose rubbing and self-inoculation are the

usual means of developing infection. This not only determines which type of *Staphylococcus* is causing the infection, but illustrates to the patient the importance of self-inoculation. Intranasal bacitracin or mupirocin (Bactroban) and daily baths with chlorhexidine (Hibiclens) or hexachlorophene (PHisoHex) (adults only) may break the cycle of nasal colonization and reinfection.

CELLULITIS

Cellulitis is an acute infection of the skin and underlying soft tissues. It commonly begins as a hot, red, edematous, sharply defined eruption and may progress to lymphangitis, lymphadenitis, or in severe cases, necrotizing fasciitis and gangrene. Cellulitis usually occurs in local skin trauma caused by insect bites, abrasions, surgical wounds, contusions, or other cutaneous lacerations. Immunosuppressed patients are particularly susceptible to the progression of cellulitis to regional or systemic infections, and these patients should be treated aggressively with systemic antibiotics, drainage, and débridement when indicated. Cellulitis is 20-fold more common in patients with chronic venous stasis or lymphedema. Recurrent cellulitis may occur in patients at the exact site of saphenous donor site surgery.

Initial presentation is that of a rapidly expanding, tender, erythematous, indurated area of skin. An ascending lymphangitis may be present, especially in cellulitis involving an extremity often associated with regional lymphadenopathy. Systemic signs and symptoms can eventually evolve and when present, mandate hospitalization and treatment with systemic antibiotics. Offending organisms are most commonly group A β-hemolytic *Streptococcus* (GABHS) species and *S. aureus*. Cellulitis caused by *S. aureus* usually is associated with localized abscess, furuncles, or carbuncles. In diabetic patients, cellulitis can be caused by group B *Streptococcus*.

Localized processes are treated with oral antibiotics (see Table 1). If fever, septicemia, or other signs of advancement to deeper tissues are present, the patient should be admitted to the hospital for blood and wound cultures, parenteral antibiotics (see Table 1), and observation. If a prompt response is not observed after parenteral antibiotic treatment, surgical exploration of the involved area may be indicated to establish an etiologic diagnosis and rule out the presence of necrotic or gangrenous tissue. Immunosuppressed patients or patients with recurrent cellulitis should be extensively examined to exclude chronic sources of infection, and these patients should be treated with parenteral antibiotics until the cellulitis resolves, followed by 5 to 7 days of oral antibiotics.

ABSCESS

Local skin signs and symptoms such as pain (dolor), redness (rubor), warmth (calor), and swelling (tumor) often denote an abscess. Loss of function associated with fluctuation may also indicate abscess formation. Localization of purulent fluid necessitates surgical drainage and local wound care. The administration of oral or parenteral antibiotic therapy should not be used routinely after incision and drainage of localized abscesses. They should be administered only when clinically indicated, and antibiotic therapy should be based on culture and sensitivity testing.

CURRENT DIAGNOSIS

- Most infections are superficial and local and not associated with systemic toxicity.
- Deeper infections may involve many layers of the soft tissues, including fascia and muscle.
- Systemic toxicity is always present in deeper infections.
- Rapid advancement of the local infection with areas of necrosis indicates more serious infections, including necrotizing and gangrenous processes.
- Streptococci and clostridial microorganisms are the cause of most gangrenous infections.
- Mixed aerobic and anaerobic microflora cause most necrotizing infections.

---

[1]Not FDA approved for this indication.

Life-Threatening Infections

GROUP A β-HEMOLYTIC STREPTOCOCCAL GANGRENE

Group A β-hemolytic streptococcal gangrene is an extremely rapidly progressing skin and soft tissue infection commonly caused by *Streptococcus pyogenes*. These organisms secrete hemolysins and streptolysins O and S, which are cardiotoxic, leukocytic, and responsible for the characteristic hemolysis. Gangrene results when the cutaneous blood vessels thrombose, a finding that is often associated with intense local pain. The involved skin is initially erythematous and indurated and quickly evolves to hemorrhagic blebs with focal necrotic zones. The potential for extensive tissue loss and mortality exists, especially if treatment is delayed. Prompt, aggressive tissue débridement and antibiotic therapy are necessary for a favorable outcome (see Table 1).

SYNERGISTIC NECROTIZING CELLULITIS

Synergistic necrotizing cellulitis (SNC) is an extremely aggressive, often lethal, polymicrobial infection of the skin and soft tissues, which exhibits progressive invasion superficial to fascial planes. This condition may initially begin as a benign process with scant indication of its impending severity. The initial lesion is typically an erythematous, tender pustule or abscess with a small area of necrosis. The benign appearance of this lesion belies the widespread and aggressive tissue destruction that has occurred beneath it.

Direct inspection through skin incisions reveals extensive gangrene of the superficial tissues and fat that rarely involves the underlying fascia and muscles. These lesions characteristically exude a thin, brown, malodorous discharge, which manifests mixed flora with abundant polymorphonuclear leukocytes with a Gram stain. Crepitus, which is caused by the accumulation of gas in the tissue produced by facultative or obligate anaerobes, can be palpated in 25% of patients, and it mandates immediate surgical attention.

The most common site of involvement is the perineum, which is involved in 50% of patients with SNC. Predisposing factors include perirectal abscess and ischiorectal abscess, both of which may track to the deeper structures of the pelvis, leading to abscess formation and subsequent septicemia. The thigh and leg are involved in approximately 40% of patients. This infection can occur after amputation and is usually associated with diabetes mellitus (75% of cases) or peripheral vascular disease (50% of cases). The relative immunosuppression and poor circulation that accompany these significant causes of morbidity are also responsible for upper extremity and neck SNC, which account for the remaining 10% of cases.

Synergistic necrotizing cellulitis is commonly caused by mixed flora originating in the gastrointestinal tract. Coliforms are the most prevalent aerobes (*Escherichia coli*, *Klebsiella*, *Proteus*), and anaerobic flora include *Bacteroides*, *Peptostreptococcus*, *Clostridium*, and *Fusobacterium*. The primary treatment modality is aggressive débridement of nonviable skin and subcutaneous tissues. This may involve several operations and dressing changes under general anesthesia, which should be performed until all necrotic tissue is removed. Rotation or free myocutaneous flaps and split-thickness skin grafting may cover areas of tissue loss when necessary. If the perineum is involved, fecal diversion by colostomy may be necessary to facilitate healing. Empiric parenteral antibiotics effective against polymicrobial gram-positive and gram-negative aerobic and anaerobic flora are also a mainstay of therapy. However, antibiotic coverage must be modified as soon as culture and susceptibility testing reveal specific offending organisms (Table 2) to reduce the emergence of resistant organisms.

CLOSTRIDIAL MYONECROSIS

Clostridial myonecrosis (i.e., gas gangrene) is a destructive infectious process of muscle associated with infections of the skin and soft tissues. It is often associated with local crepitus and systemic signs of toxemia, which are caused by the anaerobic, gas-forming bacilli of the *Clostridium* species. This infection most often occurs after abdominal operations on the gastrointestinal tract; penetrating trauma, such as gunshot wounds, and frostbite can also expose muscle, fascia, and subcutaneous tissues to these organisms. Common to all these conditions is an environment containing tissue necrosis, low oxygen tension, and sufficient amounts of amino acids and calcium to allow germination of clostridial spores and production of the lethal α toxin.

Clostridia are gram-positive, spore-forming, obligate anaerobes that are widely found in soil contaminated with animal excreta. They have also been isolated in the human gastrointestinal tract and skin, most importantly in the perineum and oropharynx. *Clostridium perfringens* is the most common isolate (in 80% of cases) and is among the fastest growing clostridial species, having a generation time under ideal conditions of approximately 16 minutes. This organism produces collagenases and proteases that cause widespread tissue destruction and produces α toxin, which is associated with the high mortality rate of clostridial myonecrosis. The α toxin, a phospholipase C, causes platelet-neutrophil complexes, vascular obstruction, and extensive compromised vascular perfusion, leading to necrosis of the muscle and overlying fascia, skin, and subcutaneous tissues.

Historically, clostridial myonecrosis was a disease associated with battle injuries, but 60% of current cases occur after trauma: 50% after automobile accidents and the remainder after crush injuries, industrial accidents, and gunshot wounds. Mortality can be the result of a failure to recognize that clostridial infection is under way, which leads to a delay in the débridement of devitalized tissues. Patients often complain of a sudden onset of pain at the site of trauma or surgical wound, which increases rapidly in severity and extends beyond the original borders of the wound. The skin initially exhibits tense edema, but its pale appearance progresses to a magenta hue. Hemorrhagic bullae and a thin, watery, foul-smelling discharge are common. A Gram stain examination of wound discharge reveals abundant gram-positive rods with a paucity of leukocytes.

The diagnosis of gas gangrene is based on the appearance of the muscle on direct visualization by surgical exposure, because many changes are not apparent when inspected through a small traumatic wound. Initially, the muscle is pale, edematous, and unresponsive to stimulation. As the disease process continues, the muscle becomes frankly gangrenous, black, and extremely friable. This occurs as a late event and is often accompanied by septicemia and shock. Despite profound hypotension and impending organ failure, these patients may be remarkably alert and extremely sensitive to their surroundings. They feel their impending doom and often panic just before slipping into toxic delirium and eventually into coma.

The clinical features should arouse suspicion early in the course, so the disease can be recognized and treated with aggressive surgical débridement. Gas in the wound is a relatively late finding, and by the time crepitation is observed, the patient may be near death. Approximately 15% of blood cultures are positive, but this is also a late finding. Serum creatinine kinase levels, although relatively nonspecific, are always elevated in cases with muscle involvement.

The mortality rate for gas gangrene is as high as 60%. It is highest in cases involving the abdominal wall and lowest in those affecting the extremities. Among the signs that prognosticate a poor outcome are leukopenia, thrombocytopenia, hemolysis, and severe renal failure. Myoglobinuria is common and can contribute significantly to worsening renal function. Frank hemorrhage may also be present and indicates disseminated intravascular coagulation.

Successful treatment of this life-threatening infection depends on early recognition and débridement of devitalized and infected tissues. Hyperbaric oxygen and systemic antibiotics are important adjuncts. Surgical intervention should include wide débridement of all necrotic tissue and amputation if extremities are involved. Hyperbaric oxygen (100% O_2 at 3 atm) has been reported to reduce associated tissue loss and mortality; however, core treatment is surgical débridement, and it should never be delayed to arrange for hyperbaric oxygen treatments. In animal studies of gas gangrene, hyperbaric oxygen was not efficacious, whereas clindamycin (Cleocin) treatment had dramatic effects in reducing mortality. A parenteral antibiotic is directed toward the offending organism (see Table 1). Clindamycin is the treatment of choice because of its ability to suppress toxin production. Cardiovascular collapse mandates careful monitoring of intravenous fluid resuscitation, which may require large volumes. Failure to adequately resuscitate these patients compromises therapy by limiting oxygen delivery and antibiotic distribution to the affected tissues and may promote progression to multisystem organ failure.

A less life-threatening form of this disease is known as clostridial cellulitis. In this process, the bacterial tissue invasion is primarily superficial, extending to the fascial layer without muscle involvement. Prompt recognition and treatment can reduce morbidity and mortality. Spontaneous gas gangrene caused by *Clostridium septicum* can occur in the absence of trauma in patients with gastrointestinal lesions such as carcinoma of the colon.

NECROTIZING FASCIITIS

Necrotizing fasciitis is an aggressive soft tissue infection involving the fascia with extensive undermining and tracking along anatomic planes. This process usually occurs in patients with significant comorbidity, such as diabetes mellitus or peripheral vascular disease, but it is also seen in obese or malnourished patients and intravenous drug abusers. Cellulitis is a frequent occurrence, and progressive necrosis to subcutaneous tissue results from thrombosis of the perforating vessels. Necrotizing fasciitis can be caused by single organisms such as GABHS and staphylococci (MRSA), *Vibrio vulnificus* or *Aeromonas hydrophila*, or a combination of a variety of organisms, including aerobic streptococci, staphylococci, and coliforms, as well as anaerobic *Peptostreptococcus* and *Bacteroides*. Ninety percent of these infections have a polymicrobial cause, and it is common to culture up to five organisms from the fascial planes involved with this infection.

Polymicrobial necrotizing fasciitis most commonly evolves from a benign-appearing skin lesion (80% of cases). Minor abrasions, insect bites, injection sites, and perirectal abscesses have been implicated. Rare cases have been reported in women with Bartholin's gland abscess, from which the infection has spread to fascial planes of the perineum and thigh. The remaining 20% of patients have no visible skin lesion. Surgical procedures, especially bowel resections, and penetrating trauma can be complicated by superficial wound infections that evolve into necrotizing fasciitis. The infection commonly involves the buttocks and perineum, which results from untreated perirectal abscesses or decubitus ulcers; intravenous drug abusers commonly participate in *skin popping*, which leads to infections of the upper extremities.

Fifty percent of group A streptococcal necrotizing fasciitis patients have a portal of entry such as an insect bite, slivers, surgical procedures, or burns, whereas the other 50% have no portal of entry, and the infection begins at the exact site of nonpenetrating trauma, such as a muscle strain or bruise. This idiopathic form, commonly known as spontaneous necrotizing fasciitis, is particularly dangerous because of the frequent delay in diagnosis.

For those with a portal of entry, the initial presentation is a slowly advancing cellulitis that progresses to a firm, tense, woody feel of the subcutaneous tissues. This entity may be distinguished from other aggressive anaerobic soft tissue infections (e.g., SNC) by the brawny, pale, erythematous appearance of the skin overlying subcutaneous tissues that are unyielding, making fascial planes and muscle groups indistinguishable during palpation. Often, a broad, erythematous tract along the route of

TABLE 2 Suggested Parenteral Antibiotic Therapy for Mixed Infections

Organisms	Primary Choice
Aerobic (must include an agent effective against anaerobic organisms)	Amikacin (Amikin) Aztreonam (Azactam) Ceftriaxone (Rocephin) Ciprofloxacin (Cipro) Gentamicin (Garamycin) Levofloxacin (Levaquin) Tobramycin (Nebcin)
Anaerobic (must include an agent effective against aerobic organisms)	Clindamycin (Cleocin) Metronidazole (Flagyl)
Aerobic and anaerobic coverage	Ampicillin/sulbactam (Unasyn) Imipenem/cilastatin (Primaxin) Meropenem (Merrem) Piperacillin/tazobactam (Zosyn) Tigecycline (Tygacil)

the underlying fascial plane can be discerned through the skin. If an open wound exists, probing the edges with a blunt instrument permits ready dissection of the superficial fascia well beyond the wound margins, and this is the most important diagnostic feature of necrotizing fasciitis. On direct inspection, the fascia is swollen and dully gray in appearance, with stringy areas of fat necrosis. A thin, brown exudate can be expressed from the wound, but frank purulent drainage is rare. These wounds are remarkably insensate when found and mandate immediate débridement.

As with other gangrenous soft tissue infections, the most important component of the treatment plan is aggressive, total débridement of all devitalized and necrotic tissue. This often necessitates frequent operations and dressing changes. Wide débridement and parenteral antibiotics have a profound effect on survival, and limited or staged débridement has no place in the treatment of this very aggressive, life-threatening infection. Parenteral antibiotics (see Table 2) should be directed against the polymicrobial aerobic and anaerobic microorganisms isolated from these infections. Every effort should be made to quickly identify the offending organisms, and antibiotic therapy should be changed accordingly.

In patients with no defined portal of entry, severe pain at the site of previous nonpenetrating trauma is common. Early in the course, there may be no cutaneous evidence of infection. Severe pain and fever may be the only presenting symptoms. These patients usually have a slightly elevated white blood cell count with a left shift and an elevated pulse. Later, erythema, induration, and warmth occur and may rapidly progress to violaceous skin, ecchymosis, and blister formation. A markedly elevated creatine phosphokinase levels in a patient with any erythematous rash may suggest a necrotizing process. By the time these late cutaneous findings are present, most patient have evidence of shock and organ failure. Misdiagnosis and delay in diagnosis are common and associated with significant morbidity and mortality. Surgical exploration with débridement of infected and necrotic tissue in addition to systemic antibiotic therapy directed toward the aerobic *Streptococcus* organism can result in decreased morbidity and mortality (see Table 1).

Special Circumstances

FOURNIER'S GANGRENE

Fournier's gangrene is a necrotizing fasciitis that originates as a necrotic black area on the scrotum of male patients or the labia of female patients, and it most often has a cryptogenic origin. In my experience, Fournier's gangrene occurs more commonly without a predisposing event or after routine, uncomplicated hemorrhoidectomy. Less commonly, this condition has occurred after urologic manipulation or as a late complication of deep anorectal suppuration.

CURRENT THERAPY

- Local care and oral antibiotics chosen for the suspected or culture-proven pathogens are the usual treatment for most limited skin infections.
- Infections that show evidence of rapid advancement associated with bullae, blebs, crepitus, or necrosis require parenterally administered antibiotics and prompt surgical débridement.
- Morbidity and mortality rates associated with the deeper infections increase with delays in antibiotic therapy and surgical débridement.
- Antibiotic therapy should be guided by clinical presentation and changed if necessary when culture and sensitivity studies are available.

Fournier's gangrene is characterized by necrosis of the skin and soft tissues of the scrotum or perineum and is associated with a fulminant, painful, and severely toxic infection. Definitive diagnosis is made by identification of a necrotic black area on the scrotum associated with local and systemic signs of infection. Left untreated, death ensues from uncontrolled, severe systemic sepsis and multiple-organ failure. Prompt recognition and treatment can minimize tissue loss, especially the skin and soft tissues of the scrotum, labia, and perineum, and may prevent complete loss of genitalia.

The infection is often polymicrobial, as with necrotizing fasciitis, with several species of aerobic and anaerobic bacteria predominating. Successful treatment is based on early recognition and vigorous surgical débridement, occasionally including diversion of the fecal stream. Empiric treatment is appropriate until results of culture and susceptibility testing are available (see Table 2). The therapeutic benefit of hyperbaric oxygen treatments has not been proved and, it should be used only as an adjunct to surgical débridement.

ECTHYMA GANGRENOSUM

Occasionally, hospitalized patients with overwhelming pseudomonal septicemia develop a patchy dermal and subcutaneous necrosis. Although sepsis caused by *Pseudomonas aeruginosa* is often indistinguishable from other types of gram-negative sepsis, a characteristic skin lesion may develop with erythematous macular eruptions that quickly become bullous with central ulceration and necrosis. This lesion may resemble a decubitus ulcer with the characteristic black eschar. There are usually multiple lesions occurring in different stages of development. They may concentrate on the extremities or the gluteal region. These lesions may be distinguished from the lesions of pyoderma gangrenosum (a noninfectious dermatosis) by their association with clinical signs of infection (i.e., fever and leukocytosis) in addition to the isolation of *P. aeruginosa* from culture of the lesion.

Treatment is primarily administration of antimicrobial therapy effective against the *Pseudomonas* organism and by débridement of the multiple lesions. This may lessen the bacterial burden, perhaps allowing greater antibiotic efficacy.

SEA AND FRESH WATER INFECTIONS

Infections caused by *V. vulnificus* and *A. hydrophilia* can be extremely aggressive, with necrosis often occurring within hours and necessitating rapid, wide débridement. Although infections caused by these organisms cannot be differentiated from those caused by mixed infections, a history of exposure to sea water (*V. vulnificus*) or fresh water (*A. hydrophila*) and the rapidity with which the infection spreads often suggest the cause of the infection. The antibiotics of choice for *V. vulnificus* infection are doxycycline (Vibramycin) or tetracycline and an aminoglycoside. In patients with impaired renal function, chloramphenicol (Chloromycetin) may be used. *A. hydrophila* is susceptible to cephalosporins such as ceftazidime (Fortaz), cefuroxime (Ceftin), and fluoroquinolones such as levofloxacin (Levaquin) and ciprofloxacin (Cipro).

Conclusions

The many types of soft tissue infections caused by bacteria may be distinguished by their presenting signs, symptoms, and body location and by the time course of the pathologic processes unique to each. Early recognition is of paramount importance to the effective treatment plan, which most often includes aggressive surgical débridement and specific antimicrobial therapy. This approach can often minimize tissue damage and promote recovery.

REFERENCES

Adinolfi MF, Voros DC, Moustoukas NM, et al. Severe systemic sepsis resulting from neglected perineal infections. South Med J 1983;76:746–9.
Craig ML, Hardin Jr WD, Fox LS, et al. Ecthyma gangrenosum: A deadly complication. Hosp Physician 1987;23:65–71.
Moustoukas NM, Nichols RL, Voros D. Clostridial sepsis: Usual clinical presentations. South Med J 1985;78:440–5.
Nichols RL, Florman S. Clinical presentations of soft-tissue infections and surgical site infections. Clin Infect Dis 2001;33(Suppl. 2):84–93.
Nichols RL. Postoperative infection in the age of drug-resistant gram-positive bacteria [review]. Am J Med 1998;104(Suppl. 5A):11S–16S.
Stevens DL, Bisno AL, Chambers HF, et al. Practice guidelines for the diagnosis and management of skin and soft-tissue infections. Clin Infect Dis 2005;41:1373–406.
Stevens DL. Necrotizing infections of the skin and fascia, UpToDate 2009;9.2. Available at: www.uptodate.com [accessed June 2009].

Viral Diseases of the Skin

Method of
Rosella Creed, MD

Many virus families have cutaneous manifestations, but some of the most common cutaneous viral infections encountered by physicians include herpes simplex virus type 1 and 2 (HSV-1 and HSV-2), varicella-zoster virus, human papillomavirus (HPV), and molluscum contagiosum. These infections are typically limited to the skin, and the following discussion focuses on the diagnosis and treatment of these diseases.

Herpesviruses

HERPES SIMPLEX

Clinical Manifestations

HSV-1 is responsible for most cold sores and some genital herpes. More than 85% of people in the general population are seropositive for HSV-1. Persons in developing countries and in lower socioeconomic groups are more likely to become seropositive for HSV-1 at an earlier age than persons living in developed countries and those of the upper or middle class, but the prevalence becomes similar by the age of 40 years.

HSV-2 is typically responsible for most cases of genital herpes and some cold sores. Genital herpes is one of the most common sexually transmitted diseases. In the United States, approximately 22% of people 12 years old or older are seropositive for HSV-2. Most seropositive individuals are unaware of their status. Between 10% and 25% of seropositive individuals report having signs and symptoms of genital herpes. It is estimated that 70% of HSV infections are contracted from patients having viral shedding without any clinical evidence of infection. Some evidence suggests that the HSV-1 seropositivity may provide partial protection of individuals against HSV-2. However, those who are infected with both HSV-1 and HSV-2 are more likely to have asymptomatic shedding of the HSV-2 virus.

Transmission of the virus occurs through fluid from active vesicular lesions, saliva, semen, and cervical fluid. The virus initially replicates in the skin to produce a primary infection and then travels in a retrograde fashion to the dorsal root ganglia. HSV-1 usually establishes latency in the trigeminal ganglia, whereas HSV-2 establishes latency in the sacral sensory ganglia. During a recurrence, the virus travels down the sensory nerve and manifests as skin or mucosal lesions. Recurrence of herpes simplex infections has been associated with stress, fever, ultraviolet (UV) light exposure, nerve or tissue damage, menses, and fatigue.

Primary herpes lesions are typically seen on the gingival and buccal mucosa. Primary herpetic gingivostomatitis (PHGS) is most commonly seen in young children. Recurrences tend to occur as herpes labialis appearing at the vermillion border. Patients with primary and recurrent infection often have a prodrome of localized tingling or burning pain, paresthesias, lymphadenopathy, and constitutional symptoms such as headache, fatigue, fever, and anorexia. In about 75% of cases, the prodrome is followed by the development of papules, vesicles, and eventually ulcerations and erosions. HSV-1 and HSV-2 produce the same clinical symptoms of herpes labialis, but HSV-2 is less likely than HSV-1 to cause recurrences. The differential diagnosis of PHGS includes hand-foot-mouth disease, herpangina, erythema multiforme, pemphigus vulgaris, and acute necrotizing ulcerative gingivitis.

Primary herpes genitalis has an incubation period of about 3 to 14 days. Women may develop lesions on the vulva, vagina, cervix, perineum, perianal region, buttocks, and thigh; men develop lesions on the glans penis, the shaft of the penis, perineum, buttocks, and thigh. Homosexual men also can have perianal lesions. Transmission is four times more likely to occur from a man to a woman than from a woman to a man. Constitutional symptoms occur in almost 80% of primary infections, especially in women. A prodrome of localized pain and tingling also occurs.

Recurrent herpes genitalis often results in less pain, fewer lesions, less viral shedding, and faster healing than during the primary infection. Recurrence is most common in the first year after the primary infection. Herpes genitalis due to HSV-1 is often milder and less likely to recur than that caused by HSV-2. It has also been suggested that HSV-1 has a greater predilection for the genitals than HSV-2 does for the orolabial area.

A diagnosis of herpes labialis or herpes genitalis is often made clinically, but Tzanck smears, viral culture, serologic testing, and polymerase chain reaction (PCR) techniques can be used in atypical cases to diagnose herpes.

Treatment

Antiviral therapy cannot cure HSV infections, but it can prevent viral shedding, decrease transmission, decrease the healing time of herpetic lesions, and suppress recurrences from even starting. Early treatment is important. Antiviral drugs administered during the prodrome of a herpes infection can prevent lesions from forming.

Topical, oral, and intravenous therapies are available. Topical agents include docosanol 10% cream (available over-the-counter as Abreva), penciclovir 1% cream (Denavir), and acyclovir 5% cream (Zovirax), which are approved for the treatment of recurrent herpes simplex labialis.

Oral therapies for herpes genitalis and herpes labialis include acyclovir, valacyclovir (Valtrex), and famciclovir (Famvir). These drugs are nucleoside analogues that inhibit the replication of the virus but do not have activity against latent viruses. Acyclovir, a guanosine analogue, is the most familiar drug of this class. Because it is activated by the thymidine kinase of the virus, it works only in cells that have the virus. It has been shown to be effective in reducing pain and healing time, but the main drawback is that the low bioavailability necessitates frequent dosing. Valacyclovir, the prodrug of acyclovir, has an excellent safety profile and a better bioavailability than acyclovir, which results in less frequent dosing. Famciclovir, the oral prodrug of penciclovir, also has a higher bioavailability than acyclovir. These drugs can be used for treatment of primary genital herpes and recurrent genital herpes and for suppressive therapy (Tables 1 and 2).

Several vaccines for HSV have been tested in clinical trials, but there are no FDA-approved HSV vaccines on the market.

VARICELLA-ZOSTER

Clinical Manifestations

The varicella-zoster virus ((human herpesvirus 3) is responsible for primary varicella (chickenpox) and herpes zoster recurrence (shingles). Almost all cases of chickenpox are in children 14 years old or younger, but adults occasionally present with primary varicella. The virus is spread by respiratory droplets or from vesicular fluid of patients with primary varicella or herpes zoster. The average incubation period is 2 weeks. Adults and adolescents usually have 1 to 2 days of prodromal fever, headache, anorexia, and malaise before the development of the rash; children tend to develop the constitutional symptoms simultaneously with the rash. The rash is pruritic and progresses from macules to papules to vesicles to crusts in a matter of 24 to 48 hours. New lesions may form as older lesions heal. Adults are more likely to have complications of varicella, the most common of which is pneumonia. After the primary varicella infection has resolved, the varicella-zoster virus travels to the dorsal root ganglia or cranial root ganglia, where it becomes latent.

TABLE 1 Dosing Regimen for Herpes Genitalis

Use	Drug	Dosage	Course
Primary episode	Acyclovir (Zovirax)	200 mg PO 5 × daily	7–10 d
		Alt dose: 400 mg PO tid	7–10 d
	Valacyclovir (Valtrex)	1 g PO bid	7–10 d
	Famciclovir (Famvir)[1]	250 mg PO tid	5–10 d
	Immunocompromised hosts		
	Acyclovir	200–400 mg PO 5 × daily or	10 d
		5 mg/kg IV over 1 h, then q8h	5 d
Recurrent episode	Acyclovir	200 mg PO 5 × daily	5–10 d
		Alt dose: 400 mg PO tid	5 d
	Valacyclovir	500 mg PO bid	3–5 d
	Famciclovir	125 mg PO bid	5–10 d
		Alt dose: 1 g PO bid	1 d
	Acyclovir	IH: 400 mg PO tid or	5–10 d
		5 mg/kg IV over 1 h, then q8h	7–10 d
		(children <12 years old: 250 mg/m² of BSA)	
	Valacyclovir	IH: 1 g PO bid	5–10 d
	Famciclovir	IH: 500 mg PO bid	5–10 d
Suppression	Acyclovir	400 mg PO bid	
	Valacyclovir	1000 mg PO daily if ≥10 episodes/y	
		500 mg PO daily if <10 episodes/y	
	Famciclovir	250 mg PO bid	
	Acyclovir	IH: 400–800 mg PO bid to tid	
	Valacyclovir	IH: 500 mg PO bid	
	Famciclovir	IH: 500 mg PO bid	

[1]Not FDA approved for this indication.
Abbreviations: Alt dose = alternative dosage; BSA = body surface area; IH = immunocompromised hosts.

TABLE 2 Dosing Regimen for Herpes Labialis

Use	Drug	Dosage	Course
Primary episode	Acyclovir (Zovirax)	200 mg PO 5 × daily	7–10 d
		Alt dose: 400 mg PO tid	7–10 d
	Valacyclovir (Valtrex)	1 g PO bid	7–10 d
	Famciclovir (Famvir)[1]	500 mg PO bid	7–10 d
	Acyclovir	IH: 5 mg/kg IV over 1 h, then q8h	7 d
		(children <12 years old: 250 mg/m^2 of BSA)	
Recurrent episode	Acyclovir	400 mg PO 5 × daily	5 d
	Valacyclovir	2 g PO bid	1 d
	Famciclovir	1500 mg PO (one-time dose)	1 d
	Acyclovir	IH: 400 mg PO 5 × daily or	5–10 d
		5 mg/kg IV over 1 h, then q8h	7–10 d
		(children <12 years old: 250 mg/m^2 of BSA)	
	Valacyclovir	IH: 1 g PO bid	5–10 d
	Famciclovir	IH: 500 mg PO bid	5–10 d
Suppression	Acyclovir	400 mg PO bid	
	Valacyclovir	500 mg PO qd	
		Alt dose: 1 g PO qd	
	Famciclovir	500 mg bid	
	Acyclovir	IH: 400–800 mg PO bid to tid	
	Valacyclovir	IH: 500 mg PO bid	
	Famciclovir	IH: 500 mg PO bid	

[1]Not FDA approved for this indication.
Abbreviations: Alt dose = alternative dosage; BSA = body surface area; IH = immunocompromised hosts.

When the virus reactivates, it manifests as shingles, a painful, unilateral, vesicular rash of a dermatomal distribution. Patients most at risk for developing zoster infection are older patients and immunocompromised patients. Advancing age, lymphoma, chemotherapy, steroid treatment, human immunodeficiency virus (HIV) infection, and physical or emotional stress lower cell-mediated immunity, leading to the reactivation. Patients may have a prodrome of pain or paresthesias 1 to 3 days before the rash becomes evident. Lesions begin as erythematous macules and papules and progress to vesicles and then crusts. Herpes zoster infection of the first branch of the trigeminal nerve can cause herpes zoster ophthalmicus, which can lead to sight impairment if not treated. The most common complication of shingles is postherpetic neuralgia (PHN), in which patients can be left with excruciating pain for weeks to years after the rash has gone. Older age is a risk factor for the development of PHN. Less than 5% of patients have a second episode of zoster because immunity is usually boosted sufficiently after the first episode.

Treatment

The treatment of varicella and shingles uses the same antivirals used for HSV infections (Table 3). Children with varicella are often treated symptomatically, but antiviral therapy can reduce the duration of the infection and allow the child to return to school earlier. Adults and immunocompromised patients should always be treated because of the risk of complications. Acyclovir is FDA approved for the treatment of varicella. Valacyclovir and famciclovir are approved for zoster therapy; they are often used to treat primary varicella, and valacyclovir is indicated for treatment of varicella in children. Antiviral therapy must be instituted within the first 24 to 48 hours of rash, because this is when the virus is replicating. Immunocompromised patients usually are treated with intravenous acyclovir.

In shingles therapy, these antivirals have been shown to decrease the healing time of the zoster rash and decrease the level of zoster-related pain. Studies have shown that antiviral therapy is effective when given within the first 72 hours after rash onset. Antiviral therapy decreases viral shedding and reduces the duration and amount of acute pain. The main benefit, however, is that it also may reduce the amount of PHN. Prednisone[1] has been used alone or with antivirals to treat zoster and to reduce the likelihood of having PHN. However, studies have shown that the combination of steroids and acyclovir was no different from acyclovir monotherapy in improving PHN. Some of the most common options for treatment of PHN include gabapentin (Neurontin), pregabalin (Lyrica), and lidocaine patches (Lidoderm). Tricyclic antidepressants,[1] capsaicin (Zostrix), opiates, and nerve blocks are sometimes used.

[1]Not FDA approved for this indication.

TABLE 3 Regimen for Varicella-Zoster Virus Infection

Use	Drug	Dosage	Course
Primary varicella (children)	Acyclovir (children >2 years old and <40 kg)	20 mg/kg PO qid	5 d
		(max dose: 800 mg PO qid)	
	Acyclovir (children >40 kg)	800 mg PO qid	5 d
Primary varicella (adults)	Acyclovir	800 mg PO 5 × daily	7–10 d
	Valacyclovir*	1 g PO tid	7 d
	Famciclovir*	500 mg PO tid	7 d
Herpes zoster treatment	Acyclovir	800 mg PO 5 × daily	7–10 d
	Valacyclovir	1 g PO tid	7 d
	Famciclovir	500 mg PO tid	7 d
Immunocompromised hosts	Acyclovir	10 mg/kg IV over 1 h, then q8h	7–10 d
	Acyclovir (children <12 years old)	500 mg/m^2 of BSA IV over 1 h, then q8h	7–10 d

*Off-label treatment for adolescents and adults.
Abbreviation: BSA = body surface area.

CURRENT DIAGNOSIS

- HSV-1 causes recurrent herpes labialis, which manifests as vesicles at the vermillion border. HSV-2 causes genital herpes, which manifests as vesicular lesions in the genital region.
- Varicella results in a diffuse, pruritic rash that progresses from macules and papules to vesicles and to crusts.
- Herpes zoster, the recurrence of the varicella-zoster virus, results in a painful, dermatomal, vesicular rash.
- HPV is responsible for verrucous papules seen in verruca vulgaris (common warts) and condyloma acuminatum (genital warts).
- Molluscum contagiosum manifests as umbilicated papules in children. It is often a sexually transmitted disease in adolescents and adults.

CURRENT THERAPY

- Acyclovir (Zovirax), valacyclovir (Valtrex), and famciclovir (Famvir) are used to treat herpes simplex virus and varicella-zoster virus infections.
- HPV and molluscum contagiosum treatments include cryotherapy, curettage, electrosurgery, cantharidin (Cantharone),[1,6] imiquimod (Aldara), trichloroacetic acid (Tri-Chlor), and podophyllotoxin (Condylox).
- Vaccines are available for the prevention of varicella (Varivax), herpes zoster (Zostavax), and HPV (Gardasil).

---

[1]Not FDA approved for this indication.
[6]May be compounded by pharmacists.

A vaccine to prevent primary varicella (Varivax) was approved in the United States in 1995, and a quadrivalent form, ProQuad (including measles, mumps, and rubella), was approved in 2005. A two-dose regimen is recommended to prevent breakthrough disease. This was followed in 2006 by the FDA approval of a vaccine (Zostavax) to prevent zoster for people 60 years old or older.

Human Papillomavirus

VIRUS TYPES AND TRANSMISSION

More than 100 types of human papillomaviruses (HPVs) have been discovered. Common benign cutaneous lesions include plantar warts, which are caused by HPV type 1, common warts (verruca vulgaris) caused by HPV types 2, 4, and 29, and flat warts caused by HPV types 3, 10, 28, and 49. These types are not thought to be associated with malignant transformation. Transmission occurs by direct contact or by contact with contaminated objects. Epidermodysplasia verruciformis is an inherited disease in which persons with a defect in their cell-mediated immunity develop skin cancers in sun-exposed areas. HPV types 5 and 8 are commonly associated with this disorder.

ANOGENITAL HUMAN PAPILLOMAVIRUS INFECTIONS

Clinical Manifestations

One of the most common sexually transmitted diseases in the world is condyloma acuminatum (i.e., anogenital warts). HPV types 6 and 11 are associated with anogenital warts that have a low potential for malignant transformation. HPB types 16 and 18 are associated with 70% of cervical cancers and are associated with squamous cell carcinomas of the penis, anal canal, and vulva. PCR testing has shown that HPV DNA is present in 99.7% of cervical cancers. HPV types 31, 33 39, 42 through 45, and several others are associated with malignancy.

Anogenital warts can manifest as asymptomatic, flesh-colored, pink, or brownish papules that can coalesce as they enlarge. They can also results in sessile, smoother papules, which may resemble condyloma lata. Lesions can become large, exophytic, cauliflower-like growths, particularly in immunocompromised individuals. These larger lesions may cause pain, pruritus, and bleeding. Clinical evidence of infection usually appears 1 to 8 months after the initial infection. Cervical warts are more difficult to diagnosis and may require 5% acetic acid solution to become visible. Cervical dysplasia is typically asymptomatic and is usually identified on a Pap smear.

Treatment

Nongenital warts can be treated with topical salicylic acid or lactic acid, cantharidin (Cantharone),[1,6] or several other keratolytic compounds. Salicylic acid therapy is effective but requires many weeks of treatment time. Cryotherapy is a common first-line treatment that is effective but is probably best reserved for older children and adults because of the pain involved. Repeat treatments are frequently needed. Intralesional bleomycin (Blenoxane),[1] surgical excision, curettage, and cautery are considered an option for resistant warts that have not responded to other therapies. Data on the efficacy of most treatment modalities are limited.

A variety of therapies exist for the symptomatic treatment of condyloma. Antiproliferative agents include podophyllotoxin (podofilox [Condylox]) and 5-fluorouracil cream (Efudex).[1] Podophyllin (Podocon-25) was used in the past but contains two mutagens, has a risk of toxicity, is not a standardized compound, and is physician applied. It has been largely replaced by podophyllotoxin, which can be applied by the patient at home.

Destruction of genital warts can be done with cryotherapy, trichloroacetic acid (Tri-Chlor), electrocautery, or carbon dioxide laser. Cryotherapy is commonly done but frequently requires multiple treatments. Warts can be excised, but recurrence rates are high, and there is a risk of scarring.

Immunomodulation includes imiquimod 5% cream (Aldara), which is used three times per week for 16 weeks. Imiquimod activates the toll-like receptor 7 on antigen-presenting cells and induces cytokines. The main adverse effect is a local skin reaction. Studies have shown that it is associated with a lower rate of recurrence that other treatment modalities. Like podophyllotoxin, imiquimod can be applied by the patient at home.

In June 2006, a quadrivalent vaccine (Gardasil) offering protection against HPV types 6, 11, 16, and 18 was licensed in the United States. It is approved for females between 9 and 26 years old, but the recommendation from the Centers for Disease Control and Prevention (CDC) is for vaccination at 11 to 12 years of age, before the onset of sexual activity. It is a preventative measure and is not recommended as a treatment for women who already have genital warts or cervical dysplasia. The efficacy of the vaccine in men is still being studied.

Molluscum Contagiosum

Clinical Manifestations

This poxvirus infection manifests as smooth, 3- to 5-mm, flesh-colored or white, umbilicated papules. It commonly affects immunocompetent children and immunocompromised hosts. Atopic dermatitis and Darier's disease are also predisposing conditions.

---

[1]Not FDA approved for this indication.
[6]May be compounded by pharmacists.

Most immunocompetent patients have between 11 and 20 papules. Molluscum contagiosum is transmitted by fomites, autoinoculation, and direct contact with infected individuals. Lesions in children can be on any part of the body but most commonly are found on the groin, axillae, antecubital fossa, and popliteal fossa. Adolescents and adults can have lesions on the lower abdomen or genital region due to sexual transmission. HIV-positive patients may be affected with nodules larger than 1 cm in diameter or may have hundreds of small papules. Their lesions are often refractory to standard therapies and are in unusual locations such as the face and neck.

Treatment

Without any treatment, immunocompetent individuals will clear the infection within 6 months to 4 years. Destructive therapies can be used to hasten the clearance of the lesions, but because of the long incubation period (14 days to 6 months), new lesions may still form after previous lesions have been treated. The most common treatments include simple incision with expression of the molluscum body, cryotherapy, curettage, electrosurgery, cantharidin,[1,6] and 5% imiquimod cream.[1] Less commonly, physicians may use trichloroacetic acid,[1] podophyllin,[1] podophyllotoxin,[1] topical retinoids, or laser therapy. Topical cidofovir (Vistide)[1,6] and imiquimod[1] have shown promise in treating the resistant lesions of HIV patients.

REFERENCES

Ahmed AM, Madkan V, Tyring SK. Human papillomaviruses and genital disease. Dermatol Clin 2006;24:157–65, vi.

Brentjens MH, Yeung-Yue KA, Lee PC, Tyring SK. Human papillomavirus: A review. Dermatol Clin 2002;20:315–31.

Brown J, Janniger CK, Schwartz RA, Silverberg NB. Childhood molluscum contagiosum. Int J Dermatol 2006;45:93–9.

Chen TM, George S, Woodruff CA, Hsu S. Clinical manifestations of varicella-zoster virus infection. Dermatol Clin 2002;20:267–82.

Dworkin RH, Johnson RW, Breuer J, et al. Recommendations for the management of herpes zoster. Clin Infect Dis 2007;44(Suppl. 1):S1–26.

Fatahzadeh M, Schwartz RA. Human herpes simplex virus infections: Epidemiology, pathogenesis, symptomatology, diagnosis, and management. J Am Acad Dermatol 2007;57:737–63.

Heininger U, Seward JF. Varicella. Lancet 2006;368:1365–76.

Ting PT, Dytoc MT. Therapy of external anogenital warts and molluscum contagiosum: A literature review. Dermatol Ther 2004;17:68–101.

Tyring SK. Molluscum contagiosum: The importance of early diagnosis and treatment. Am J Obstet Gynecol 2003;189:S12–6.

Weinberg JM. Herpes zoster: Epidemiology, natural history, and common complications. J Am Acad Dermatol 2007;57:S130–5.

Wu JJ, Pang KR, Huang DB, Tyring SK. Advances in antiviral therapy. Dermatol Clin 2005;23:313–22.

Yeung-Yue KA, Brentjens MH, Lee PC, Tyring SK. Herpes simplex viruses 1 and 2. Dermatol Clin 2002;20:249–66.

[1]Not FDA approved for this indication.
[6]May be compounded by pharmacists.

Parasitic Diseases of the Skin

Method of
*Andreas Katsambas, MD, PhD, and
Clio Dessinioti, MD, MSc*

Diseases Caused by Protozoa

CUTANEOUS AMEBIASIS

Intestinal amebiasis is caused by *Entamoeba histolytica*, which may rarely invade the skin and cause cutaneous amebiasis. The disease is transmitted by ingestion of food or water contaminated with cyst forms of the parasite and through fecal exposure during sexual contact.

CURRENT DIAGNOSIS

Parasitic diseases are a common cause of morbidity and mortality, particularly in tropical and developing countries. They may be caused by protozoa, helminths, or arthropods. Because of the immigration of persons from tropical and subtropical countries worldwide and the travel of people from industrialized to tropical regions, parasitic diseases may be found in temperate climates. Skin lesions may provide important diagnostic clues for parasitic infections, and they are reviewed in the following sections, along with updated treatment guidelines.

Cutaneous amebiasis develops at the site of the invasion of the parasites into the skin from an underlying amebic abscess, usually at the perianal area or the abdominal wall. Cutaneous findings include purulent, foul-smelling nodules, cysts, and sinuses, which are associated with regional adenopathy and dysentery. Skin lesions grow rapidly and may lead to death if left untreated.

Diagnosis of cutaneous amebiasis is confirmed by microscopic identification of *E. histolytica* in the stool and in aspirates or biopsy samples obtained during colonoscopy, during surgery, or from the border of an ulcer. Treatment of choice for extraintestinal amebiasis is oral metronidazole (Flagyl) 750 mg PO three times daily for 7 to 10 days or tinidazole (Tindamax). Tinidazole was FDA approved in 2004 for the treatment of intestinal amebiasis in adults (2 g/day for 3 days) and children older than 3 years, and it appears to be as effective as and better tolerated than metronidazole. Either treatment should be followed by iodoquinol (Yodoxin) 650 mg PO three times daily for 20 days or paromomycin 25 to 35 mg/kg/day PO divided in three doses for 7 days.

LEISHMANIASIS

Leishmaniasis results from the infection with intracellular protozoan parasites belonging to the genus *Leishmania*. Leishmania parasites are transmitted to humans and other mammalian hosts (e.g., dogs, rodents) during feeding by infected female phlebotomine sandflies that serve as vectors. The parasites exist as promastigotes in the midgut of sandflies and as amastigotes (i.e., Leishman-Donovan bodies) within macrophages of humans and other mammals. Based on the extent and the severity of involvement in the human host, leishmaniasis may be clinically classified as cutaneous leishmaniasis, diffuse cutaneous leishmaniasis, mucocutaneous leishmaniasis, and visceral leishmaniasis.

Cutaneous leishmaniasis (New World or Old World form) begins as a small erythematous papule at the site of the bite of the sandfly, which evolves into an ulcerated nodule with a raised and indurated border (i.e., volcano sign) (Fig. 1). The lesions gradually heal with a depressed scar. Diffuse cutaneous leishmaniasis is characterized by widespread cutaneous involvement without visceralization. Mucocutaneous leishmaniasis (known as espundia in South America) affects the skin, the mucosa, and the cartilages of the upper respiratory tract (especially the nose and the larynx) and may result in severe disfigurement. Visceral leishmaniasis results from the involvement of the bone marrow, spleen, and the liver, and it may lead to death if left untreated. It manifests with fever, splenomegaly, pancytopenia, and wasting. Post–kala azar dermal leishmaniasis may appear within a year after visceral disease independent of treatment, and it is characterized by macules, papules, and nodules, which are usually hypopigmented.

Diagnosis of leishmaniasis is based on finding the parasites in the skin from the lesion aspirate or biopsy by direct examination or culture. The leishmanin (Montenegro) skin test shows past and current infections, and it detects the inflammatory response in the skin after injection of phenol-killed parasites into the dermis. A past or current infection is also documented by an in vitro lymphocyte proliferation assay that requires a drop of blood from a finger prick. Polymerase chain reaction (PCR) techniques may be used to identify different

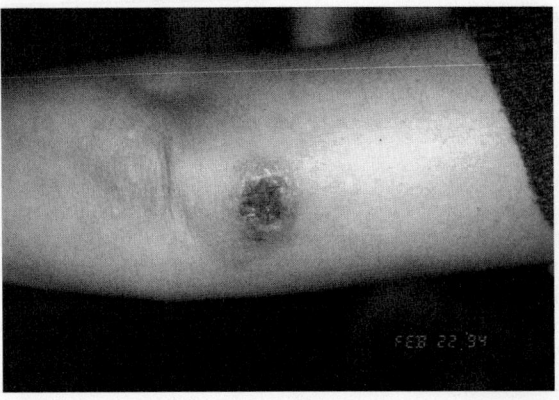

FIGURE 1. Cutaneous leishmaniasis is characterized by an ulcerated nodule with a raised and indurated border (i.e., volcano sign).

Leishmania species. Circulating antibody levels are not considered a useful diagnostic sign.

Cutaneous leishmaniasis is usually self-limited and may not require treatment. Treatment of cutaneous leishmaniasis is indicated in case of numerous lesions or when lesions affect the face to avoid scarring. Therapies include sodium stibogluconate (Pentostam)[10] 20 mg/kg/day IV or IM for 20 days. Meglumine antimoniate (Glucantime)[2] 20 mg/kg/day IV or IM for 20 days or miltefosine (Impavido)[2] 2.5 mg/kg/day PO (up to 150 mg/day) for 28 days may be used. Alternatively, intralesional injections of antimonials 1 mg/kg once weekly, cryotherapy, local heat, oral ketoconazole (Nizoral),[1] topical amphotericin B,[2] pentamidine (Pentam)[1] 2 to 3 mg/kg IV or IM daily or every second day for four to seven doses, or topical paromomycin[6] (applied twice daily for 10–20 days) may be used.

The production of antileishmanial antibodies does not correlate with resolution of the disease. Infection and recovery are associated with lifelong immunity to reinfection by the same species of *Leishmania*, although interspecies immunity may also exist.

TRYPANOSOMIASIS

There are three types of trypanosomiasis:

- American trypanosomiasis or Chagas' diseases, caused by *Trypanosoma cruzi*
- East African sleeping sickness, caused by *Trypanosoma brucei rhodesiense*
- West African sleeping sickness, caused by *Trypanosoma brucei gambiense*

American trypanosomiasis (i.e., Chagas' disease) is caused by the parasite *T. cruzi*, and it is endemic in Central and South America. The disease is transmitted by the bite of infected "cone-nosed" insects, by transfusion of infected blood, by organ transplantation, and across the placenta. During the acute stage, Chagas' disease manifests with a painful erythematous nodule, known as chagoma, which is associated with regional adenopathy. The chronic stage manifests with cardiomyopathy, megaesophagus, and megacolon. Diagnosis is confirmed by microscopic identification of the parasite in fresh anticoagulated blood, in blood smears, by lymph node biopsy or skin biopsy, or by culture. Treatment includes benznidazole (Radanil, Rochagan)[2] 5 to 7 mg/kg/day PO in two doses for 60 to 90 days or nifurtimox (Lampit)[10] 8 to 10 mg/kg/day PO in three or four doses for 90 to 120 days.

African trypanosomiasis (i.e., East and West sleeping sickness) occurs in Africa and is transmitted by the bite of infected male and female tsetse flies. It manifests with a highly inflammatory, painful,

red or violaceous, indurated nodule surrounded by an erythematous halo, called trypanosome chancre, at the site of the inoculation of the parasites. There is regional adenopathy. Later, the chancre resolves spontaneously, and the patient has fever, malaise, a generalized pruritic eruption with erythematous annular plaques or urticarial lesions, and central nervous system (CNS) involvement with personality changes, apathy, somnolence, coma, and death. Diagnosis is based on the identification of trypanosomes by microscopic examination in chancre fluid, affected lymph node aspirates, blood, bone marrow, or in the late stages of infection, cerebrospinal fluid.

Treatment of East African sleeping sickness consists of suramin (naphthylamine sulfonic acid, Germanin)[10] 100 to 200 mg (test dose) IV and then 1 g IV on days 1, 3, 7, 14, and 21. For late disease with CNS involvement, melarsoprol B (a trivalent organic arsenical, Mel-B)[10] is used in the following dosage regimen: 2 to 3.6 mg/kg/day IV for 3 days; after 7 days, 3.6 mg/kg/day for 3 days; and the latter repeated after 7 days. For West Africa sleeping sickness, treatment of choice is pentamidine isethionate (Pentam 300)[1] 4 mg/kg/day IM for 10 days or suramin (Germanin) as used for East African sleeping sickness. For late disease with involvement of the CNS, eflornithine (Ornidyl)[2] 400 mg/kg/day IV in four doses for 14 days is used.

CUTANEOUS TOXOPLASMOSIS

Systemic toxoplasmosis (congenital or acquired) is caused by the parasite *Toxoplasma gondii*, and it usually is transmitted from contact with infected cats. The disease may also be acquired by eating raw or undercooked meats from infected animals. Cutaneous involvement is rare. It manifests with punctate macules or ecchymoses in the congenital form, and the acquired form manifests with roseola and erythema multiforme lesions, urticaria, prurigo-like nodules, and maculopapular lesions. Diagnosis of cutaneous toxoplasmosis is confirmed by isolation of the parasite in the skin. Treatment is not needed for healthy nonpregnant patients because symptoms resolve in a few weeks. Treatment for pregnant women or immunocompromised patients includes pyrimethamine (Daraprim) 25–100 mg/d PO for 3–6 wks together with sulfadiazine[1] 1–15 g PO qid for 3–6 wks. Leucovorin should be taken with each dose of pyrimethamine.

Diseases Caused by Helminths

ASCARIASIS

Ascariasis is caused by *Ascaris* species, mainly *Ascaris lumbricoides*. It is transmitted by the ingestion of eggs in soil contaminated with human feces. Skin involvement of ascariasis manifests with urticaria. Diagnosis is based on finding the adult worm or eggs in the feces. Treatment includes albendazole (Albenza)[1] 400 mg PO once or mebendazole (Vermox) 100 mg PO twice daily for 3 days (or 500 mg once) or ivermectin (Stromectol)[1] 150 to 200 μg/kg PO once.

CUTANEOUS LARVA MIGRANS

Cutaneous larva migrans is also known as creeping eruption, with the first term describing a syndrome and the second a clinical sign found in various conditions. The syndrome cutaneous larva migrans is caused when various nematode larvae (i.e., hookworms, such as *Ancylostoma braziliense*, *Ancylostoma caninum*, *Bunostomum phlebotomum*) of dogs, cats, and other mammals penetrate and migrate through the skin. Cutaneous larva migrans is transmitted by skin contact to soil contaminated with animal feces. In humans, larvae are unable to reach internal organs and eventually die. Cutaneous larva migrans manifests with intensely pruritic, papular lesions, which evolve as the larvae migrate to a characteristic linear, minimally elevated, serpiginous tract that moves forward in an irregular pattern. Diagnosis is easily made clinically and is supported by a travel history or by possible exposure in an endemic area.

---

[1]Not FDA approved for this indication.
[2]Not available in the United States.
[6]May be compounded by pharmacists.
[10]Available in the United States from the Centers for Disease Control and Prevention.

---

[1]Not FDA approved for this indication.
[2]Not available in the United States.
[10]Available in the United States from the Centers for Disease Control and Prevention.

CURRENT DIAGNOSIS

Cutaneous Amebiasis

- Purulent, foul-smelling nodules, ulcers, cysts, sinuses
- Microscopic identification of *Entamoeba histolytica* in stool or biopsy samples
- Molecular methods

Cutaneous Leishmaniasis

- Ulcerated nodule (i.e., volcano sign)
- Identification of *Leishmania* parasites by direct examination or culture from the lesion aspirate or biopsy
- Montenegro skin test
- In vitro lymphocyte proliferation assay
- Polymerase chain reaction

Trypanosomiasis

CHAGAS' DISEASE

- Chagoma: painful erythematous nodule
- Regional adenopathy
- Cardiomyopathy, megaesophagus, megacolon
- Microscopic examination of *Trypanosoma cruzi* in blood, lymph node biopsy, or skin biopsy or culture

AFRICAN SLEEPING SICKNESS

- Trypanosome chancre: painful, inflammatory nodule
- Regional adenopathy
- Fever, generalized pruritic eruption with erythematous annular plaques
- Central nervous system involvement
- Microscopic identification of *Trypanosoma brucei* in chancre fluid, lymph node aspirates, blood, bone marrow, cerebrospinal fluid

Cutaneous Toxoplasmosis

- Roseola, urticaria, prurigo-like nodules
- Isolation of *Toxoplasma gondii* in the skin

Ascariasis

- Urticaria
- Identification of adult worm or eggs in stool

Cutaneous Larva Migrans

- Creeping eruption
- Intense pruritus

Cysticercosis

- Subcutaneous nodules
- Isolation of *Taenia solium* in skin lesion
- Serologic tests

Dracunculiasis

- Ruptured blister with prolapsing worm

Filariasis

LYMPHATIC FILARIASIS

- Fever with lymphangitis and lymphadenitis
- Chronic pulmonary infection
- Progressive lymphedema leading to massive tissue thickening, especially of the legs and scrotum (i.e., elephantiasis)
- Microscopic identification of microfilariae in blood

ONCHOCERCIASIS (RIVER BLINDNESS)

- Subcutaneous nodules, dermatitis, "leopard skin," "lizard skin," lymphedema
- Identification of microfilariae in skin snips
- Blindness

LOIASIS (CALABAR SWELLINGS)

- Pruritus, localized subcutaneous swellings
- Serpiginous lesion on the conjunctivae
- Microscopic identification of microfilariae in blood

Schistosomiasis (Snail Fever)

- Pruritic papules, edema
- Fever, lymphadenopathy, diarrhea
- Bilharziasis cutanea tarda: pruritic, grouped papules
- Identification of the eggs in stool, urine, biopsy of affected tissues
- Enzyme-linked immunosorbent assay (ELISA) tests

Cercarial Dermatitis (Swimmer's Itch)

- Extremely pruritic erythematous macules, papules, vesicles on body areas exposed to infested water

Human Scabies

- Pruritus worsening at night
- Papules, excoriations, nodules, burrows on genitals, interdigital spaces, axillae, wrists
- Microscopic identification of mites or eggs or feces from burrows or papules

Pediculosis

PEDICULOSIS CAPITIS

- Intense pruritus of the scalp
- Nape dermatitis
- Identification of lice and nits on the hair

PEDICULOSIS CORPORIS (VAGABOND'S ITCH)

- Intense pruritus, erythema, urticarial lesions, papules, nodules, and excoriations
- Identification of lice and nits on clothing

PEDICULOSIS PUBIS

- Pruritus
- Blue macules
- Identification of lice and nits on pubic hair

Treatment of choice consists of ivermectin (Stromectol)[1] at a single dose of 200 µg/kg. In case of treatment failure, a second dose usually suffices. Ivermectin has an excellent safety profile, without any notable adverse events, and it has been used in millions of individuals in developing countries during onchocerciasis and filariasis control operations. It is contraindicated in children who weigh less than 15 kg (or are younger than 5 years) and in pregnant or breast-feeding women. Alternatively, repeated courses of oral albendazole (Albenza)[1] 400 mg daily for 3 days may be used. Treatment with oral thiabendazole (Mintezol) 50 mg/kg daily for 2 to 4 days has been associated with adverse events such as dizziness, nausea, vomiting, and intestinal cramps, and it is therefore not recommended. In the absence of multiple or widespread lesions, topical treatments may be considered, such as topical thiabendazole[6] 10% to 15%, applied three times daily for 5 to 7 days, which has similar efficacy with oral ivermectin and no adverse events.

---

[1]Not FDA approved for this indication.

[6]May be compounded by pharmacists.

CYSTICERCOSIS

Cysticercosis is caused by the larval stage (i.e., cysticerci) of the pork tapeworm *Taenia solium*, and it is the most common helminthic infection of the CNS. It is transmitted by ingesting eggs in food, water, or on hands contaminated with human feces. Cutaneous manifestations are subcutaneous nodules that occur mainly on the extremities and trunk. There may be involvement of the CNS (i.e., seizures), the eye, the intestines, the skeletal muscle, heart, kidneys, lung, and liver. Diagnosis is confirmed by isolation of the parasite in a nodule and by serologic tests.

Treatment options include surgery, albendazole (Albenza) 400 mg PO twice daily for 8 to 30 days, or praziquantel (Biltricide)[1] 100 mg/kg/day PO in three doses for 1 day and then 50 mg/kg/day in three doses for 29 days. Any cysticercocidal drug may cause irreparable damage when used in the presence of ocular or spinal cysts.

DRACUNCULIASIS

Dracunculiasis is caused by the nematode *Dracunculus medinensis*. It is transmitted by drinking water with copepods (i.e., tiny aquatic arthropods) infected with the larvae of *D. medinensis*. In the human stomach, copepods release the larvae that mature and migrate to the skin, causing an erythematous papule or blister. The blister ruptures, and the female worm can often be seen prolapsing through the skin. Treatment includes extraction of the worm combined with wound care. Metronidazole (Flagyl)[1] 250 mg PO three times daily for 10 days may be efficacious and facilitates removal of the worm.

FILARIASIS

Filariasis is caused by nematodes (i.e., roundworms) that inhabit the lymphatics and subcutaneous tissues. The most common filarial infections include lymphatic filariasis, onchocerciasis, and loiasis.

Lymphatic Filariasis

Lymphatic filariasis is caused by *Wuchereria bancrofti*, *Brugia malayi*, and *Brugia timori*, and it is transmitted by mosquitoes. Adult worms result in a chronic inflammatory cell infiltrate around lymphatic vessels, causing their dilatation, hypertrophy, and obstruction. Many patients are asymptomatic, but some may develop fever with lymphangitis and lymphadenitis, chronic pulmonary infection, and progressive lymphedema leading to massive tissue thickening, especially of the legs and scrotum (i.e., elephantiasis). The overlying skin is thickened. Diagnosis is based on microscopic identification of the microfilariae in the blood and affected tissues.

Treatment consists of diethylcarbamazine (DEC, Hetrazan)[10] in the following regimen: 50 mg on day 1, 50 mg three times daily on day 2, 100 mg three times daily on day 3, and 6 mg/kg in three doses on days 4 through 14. Prophylaxis with DEC 500 mg/day for 2 days each month is effective against *W. bancrofti* infection for travelers in endemic areas.

Onchocerciasis

Onchocerciasis (i.e., blinding filariasis) is caused by the filarial nematode *Onchocerca volvulus*, which is transmitted by the blackflies *Simulium*. It may manifest with subcutaneous onchocercid nodules, acute or chronic dermatitis, depigmentation (i.e., leopard skin), and skin atrophy (i.e., lizard skin), and in later stages, it may manifest with lymphadenopathy and lymphedema. The microfilariae have a predilection for the eyes, and the infection can lead to blindness (i.e., river blindness). Diagnosis is based on identification of microfilariae in skin snips.

Treatment consists of ivermectin (Stromectol) 150 µg/kg PO every 6 to 12 months until asymptomatic. DEC is contraindicated as it may lead to blindness.

Loiasis

Loiasis (i.e., Calabar swellings) is caused by the parasite *Loa loa*, which is transmitted by deerflies (*Chrysops*). Cutaneous manifestations include pruritus, urticaria, and Calabar swellings, which are erythematous, warm, subcutaneous swellings associated with the migration of the worm through the subcutaneous tissues. Occasionally, there is subconjunctival migration of the adult worm, producing a migrating serpiginous lesion on the conjunctivae. Diagnosis is confirmed by identification of microfilariae in the blood by microscopic examination.

DEC[10] is the treatment of choice in the following regimen: 50 mg on day 1, 50 mg three times daily on day 2, 100 mg three times daily on day 3, and 9 mg/kg/day in three doses on days 4 through 14. Ivermectin (Stromectol)[1] may cause encephalopathy in patients with a heavy *L. loa* infection. Prophylaxis with DEC is effective for *L. loa* in adults who travel in endemic areas.

SCHISTOSOMIASIS

Schistosomiasis (i.e., snail fever) in humans is caused mainly by the trematodes *Schistosoma haematobium*, *Schistosoma japonicum*, and *Schistosoma mansoni*. All trematodes have a life cycle that involves the snail as an intermediate host. The infective cercariae leave the snail, swim, and penetrate the human skin, causing a pruritic papular dermatosis. The disease is transmitted by exposure to contaminated water with live cercariae or by drinking infested water. Skin findings of acute schistosomiasis include pruritic schistosomal dermatitis due to a hypersensitivity response to the cercariae and edema of the face, extremities, genitals, and trunk. Schistosomal fever (i.e., Katayama fever), lymphadenopathy, and diarrhea may also develop. Late skin findings (i.e., bilharziasis cutanea tarda) appear in patients with visceral disease and include firm, pruritic, grouped papules. Secondary infection, ulceration, and development of squamous cell carcinoma may follow. Diagnosis is confirmed by identification of the eggs in the urine or stool, by biopsy of affected tissues, or by enzyme-linked immunosorbent assay (ELISA).

Treatment includes praziquantel (Biltricide)[3] 40 mg/kg/day in two doses for 1 day (for *S. haematobium* and *S. mansoni*) or 60 mg/kg/day in three doses for 1 day (for *S. japonicum*).

CERCARIAL DERMATITIS

Cercarial dermatitis (i.e., swimmer's itch) is caused by cercariae (i.e., larvae) of nonhuman schistosomes that penetrate the skin and die without invading other tissues. It is transmitted by contact with fresh or salt water contaminated with cercariae. It manifests with extremely pruritic, erythematous macules of sudden onset, which evolve into papules, vesicles, and urticarial lesions located on parts of the body directly exposed to the water, while sparing clothed areas. Cercarial dermatitis is a self-limited disease, and treatment is symptomatic with topical steroids and oral antihistamines.

Diseases Caused by Arthropoda

HUMAN SCABIES

Scabies is a common skin infestation caused by the mite *Sarcoptes scabiei*, which is an obligate human parasite. Scabies is transmitted by direct contact with an infested individual or by contact with bedding and clothing. The incubation period for scabies is about 3 weeks, and reinfestation results in symptoms within 1 to 3 days. Scabies is characterized by pruritus that usually worsens at night. Papules, nodules, excoriations, and burrows may be found. Lesions are usually located on interdigital spaces, wrists, ankles, axillae, waist, and genitals. Scabies manifests as red-brown nodules that represent a hypersensitivity response. In adults, the head is usually spared, whereas the involvement of the scalp, palms, and soles is common in infants.

---

[1]Not FDA approved for this indication.
[10]Available in the United States from the Centers for Disease Control and Prevention.

---

[1]Not FDA approved for this indication.
[3]Exceeds dosage recommended by the manufacturer.
[10]Available in the United States from the Centers for Disease Control and Prevention.

CURRENT THERAPY

Cutaneous Amebiasis

- Metronidazole (Flagyl) 750 mg PO three times daily for 7 and 10 days, or
- Tinidazole (Tindamax) 2 g once PO daily for 5 days, followed by iodoquinol (Yodoxin) 650 mg PO three times daily for 20 days or paromomycin (Humatin) 25 to 35 mg/kg/day PO in three doses for 7 days

Cutaneous Leishmaniasis

- Sodium stibogluconate (Pentostam)[10] 20 mg/kg/day IV or IM for 20 days, or
- Meglumine antimoniate (Glucantime)[2] 20 mg/kg/day IV or IM for 20 days, or
- Miltefosine (Impavido)[2] 2.5 mg/kg/day PO (up to 150 mg/day) for 28 days, or
- Topical paromomycin, a formulation of 15% paromomycin and 12% methylbenzethonium chloride in soft white paraffin (Lesheutan)[1,6] applied twice daily for 10 days or
- Pentamidine (Pentam 300)[1] 2 to 3 mg/kg IV or IM daily or every second day for four to seven doses

Trypanosomiasis

CHAGAS' DISEASE (AMERICAN TRYPANOSOMIASIS)

- Nifurtimox (Lampit)[10] 8 to 10 mg/kg/day PO in three or four doses for 90 to 20 days, or
- Benznidazole (Radanil, Rochagan)[2] 5 to 7 mg/kg/day PO in two doses for 60 to 90 days

EAST AFRICAN SLEEPING SICKNESS

- Suramin (Germanin)[10] 100 to 200 mg (test dose) IV, then 1 g IV on days 1, 3, 7, 14, 21
- For late disease with involvement of the central nervous system, melarsoprol (Mel-B)[10] 2 to 3.6 mg/kg/day IV for 3 days; after 7 days, 3.6 mg/kg/day for 3 days; repeat after 7 days

WEST AFRICAN SLEEPING SICKNESS

- Pentamidine (Pentam 300)[1] 4 mg/kg/day IM for 10 days,[1] or
- Suramin (Germanin)[10] 100 to 200 mg (test dose) IV, then 1 g IV on days 1, 3, 7, 14, 21
- For late disease with involvement of the central nervous system, melarsoprol (Mel-B)[10] 2.2 mg/kg/day IV for 10 days, or
- For late disease with involvement of the central nervous system, eflornithine (Ornidyl)[2] 400 mg/kg/day IV in four doses for 14 days

Cutaneous Toxoplasmosis

- Self-limited disease; treatment not needed in healthy, nonpregnant persons
- For pregnant women or immunocompromised patients: pyrimethamine (Daraprim) 25 to 100 mg/day PO for 3 to 4 weeks (plus leucovorin 10 to 25 mg with each dose of pyrimethamine) and sulfadiazine[1] 1 to 1.5 g PO four times daily for 3 to 4 weeks

Ascariasis

- Albendazole (Albenza)[1] 400 mg PO once, or
- Mebendazole (Vermox) 100 mg PO twice daily for 3 days or 500 mg once, or
- Ivermectin (Stromectol)[1] 150 to 200 µg/kg PO once

Cutaneous Larva Migrans

- Ivermectin (Stromectol)[1] 200 µg/kg PO once; a second dose may be needed, or
- Albendazole (Albenza)[1] 400 mg daily PO for 3 days
- Topical thiabendazole[6] 10% to 15% applied three times daily for 5 to 7 days for a limited number of lesions

Dracunculiasis

- Slow extraction of the worm, which is facilitated by metronidazole (Flagyl)[1] 250 mg PO three times daily for 10 days

Filariasis

LYMPHATIC FILARIASIS

- Diethylcarbamazine (DEC, Hetrazan)[10] 6 mg/kg/day PO in three doses for 12 days, or
- Ivermectin (Stromectol)[1] 200 g/kg PO once together with albendazole (Albenza)[1] 400 mg PO once; kills only the microfilaria, not the adult worms
- For patients with microfilaria in the blood, DEC as follows: day 1: 50 mg; day 2: 50 mg three times daily; day 3: 100 mg three times daily; days 4 through 14: 6 mg/kg in three doses

ONCHOCERCIASIS

- Ivermectin (Stromectol) 150 µg/kg PO once for 6 to 12 months, until asymptomatic
- DEC: contraindicated because it may lead to blindness

LOIASIS

- DEC[10] 6 mg/kg/day PO in three doses for 12 days
- For patients with microfilaria in the blood, DEC as follows: day 1: 50 mg; day 2: 50 mg three times daily; day 3: 100 mg three times daily; days 4 through 14: 9 mg/kg in three doses

Schistosomiasis

- Praziquantel (Biltricide) 40 mg/kg/day[3] in two doses for 1 day (S. haematobium and S. mansoni) and 60 mg/kg/day[3] in three doses for 1 day (S. japonicum, S. mekongi)

Human Scabies

- Permethrin (Acticin, Elimite) 5% cream rinse, applied for 10 hours; a second application 7 to 10 days later, or
- Benzyl benzoate 25% solution[6] applied topically; second application 7 to 10 days later, or
- Crotamiton 10% (Eurax) applied twice daily for 2 days; second application 7 to 10 days later
- Sulfur 6% to 10% ointment in petrolatum[6]
- Ivermectin (Stromectol)[1] 200 µg/kg PO once: treatment of choice for crusted scabies

Pediculosis

PEDICULOSIS CAPITIS

- Malathion (Ovide) 0.5% lotion, applied for 8 to 12 hours before being washed off; approved for children older than 6 years, or
- Permethrin (Nix) 1% lotion, applied to shampooed hair and washed off after 10 minutes; second application 7 to 10 days later; approved for children older than 2 years
- Pyrethrins with piperidyl butoxide (RID) applied for 10 minutes

- Benzyl benzoate 25% solution[6]
- Lindane shampoo: for recalcitrant disease, not to be used in children
- Ivermectin (Stromectol)[1] 200 μg/kg on days 1, 2, and 10[1]

---

[1]Not FDA approved for this indication.
[2]Not available in the United States.
[3]Exceeds dosage recommended by the manufacturer.
[6]May be compounded by pharmacists.
[10]Available in the United States from the Centers for Disease Control and Prevention.

PEDICULOSIS CORPORIS

- Disinfection of clothes

PEDICULOSIS PUBIS

- Same treatment as pediculosis capitis: three times daily

Crusted or Norwegian scabies manifests with hyperkeratotic papules or plaques of the hands and feet (often with nail involvement) and an erythematous scaly eruption on the face, neck, scalp, and trunk. Because pruritus is often absent, this disease can be misdiagnosed as psoriasis, eczema, or an adverse drug reaction. Lesions contain thousands of mites and are highly contagious. Crusted scabies mainly affects immunocompromised patients (e.g., patients with human immunodeficiency virus infection), mentally retarded persons, or debilitated patients.

Diagnosis is based on the microscopic identification of mites or their eggs or feces from burrows or papules. Treatment should be applied from the neck down in adults, and in infants, application should include the scalp and face (avoiding the eyes and mouth).

Treatment includes 5% permethrin (Elimite) applied for 10 hours and repeated after 1 week. A 25% benzyl benzoate solution[6] is also efficacious in adults, and because of low toxicity, it is recommended in a lower concentration (10%) for children older than 4 months and for women during pregnancy. Sulfur ointments in petrolatum[6] at concentrations of 6% to 10% may be used for scabies in children and pregnant women. Alternative treatments for scabies include crotamiton 10% (Eurax) applied once daily for 2 days, or ivermectin (Stromectol)[1] as a single- or two-dose regimen of 200 μg/kg/dose can be used. Aggressive treatment with ivermectin at a single dose of 200 μg/kg, repeated after 2 weeks with or without topical 5% permethrin cream (two applications, 1 week apart) and keratolytics (5% salicylic acid ointment[1] applied twice daily) is the treatment of choice for crusted scabies. All sexual and close personal and household contacts within the preceding 6 weeks should be treated simultaneously. Bedding and clothing should be decontaminated (i.e., machine washed and dried using the hot cycle or dry cleaned) or removed from body contact for at least 3 days, because the mite dies when separated from the human host.

PEDICULOSIS

Pediculosis (i.e., lice) is a contagious dermatosis, caused by lice, which are blood-sucking, wingless insects and are obligate human parasites. Two species of lice infest humans causing three clinical forms of infestation: *Pediculus humanus capitis* (i.e., head louse), *Pediculus humanus corporis* (i.e., body louse), and *Phthirus pubis* (i.e., pubic louse). The body louse is the only louse that can carry human disease, including rickettsioses and epidemic typhus.

Pediculosis Capitis

Pediculosis capitis is caused by *P. humanus capitis*, and it is transmitted by close contact or by fomites with combs, brushes, towels, and hats. It manifests with pruritus (due to the saliva of the louse), excoriations, nape dermatitis, secondary bacterial infection, and cervical and suboccipital lymphadenopathy. Diagnosis is based on identification of lice and eggs or nits on the hair and on fluorescence of nits with Wood's light. Visible nits are deposited on the hair shaft, close

to the scalp. After adequate treatment, nits found at 1.0 to 1.5 cm from the scalp are not alive.

Treatment includes malathion (Ovide) 0.5% lotion applied for 8 to 12 hours or permethrin (Nix) 1% cream rinse applied to shampooed hair for 10 minutes. A second application with permethrin is recommended 1 week later to kill hatching progeny. Alternatively, pyrethrins with piperidyl butoxide (RID) can be applied and washed off after 10 minutes. Benzyl benzoate 25% solution[6] is mainly a scabicide, but it may also be used as a pediculicide. Ivermectin (Stromectol)[1] can be used at a dose of 200 μg/kg on days 1, 2, and 10. Vinegar[1] may be used to facilitate nit removal from the hair shaft, using a fine-toothed comb. Bedding, clothing, and headgear should be decontaminated (as for scabies) or removed from body contact for 2 weeks. Information for managing head lice can be found at the National Pediculosis Association Web site (http://www.headlice.org).

Pediculosis Corporis

Pediculosis corporis (i.e., vagabond's itch) is caused by *P. humanus corporis*, which lives and reproduces in the lining of clothes and leaves the clothing only for feeding from the skin. This disease is usually found among vagabonds. Transmission occurs mainly through contact with contaminated clothing or bedding. Clinical manifestations include pruritus, excoriations, and small, red macules that usually occur on the back. Clothes should be examined carefully for lice.

Treatment is the same as for pediculosis capitis. Dry heat or washing in hot water followed by ironing is effective in killing the lice and their ova in clothing. Items that cannot be washed should be removed from body contact for 2 weeks.

Pediculosis Pubis

Pediculosis pubis is caused by *P. pubis* and affects the pubic hair. However, if left untreated, it may also affect very hairy regions of the chest, abdomen, axillary region, and especially in children, the eyelashes, edge of the scalp, and eyebrows. Patients present with pruritus. Useful diagnostic signs include small, blue-gray macules on the trunk, thighs, and axillae (i.e., taches bleuâtres or maculae ceruleae) due to conversion of bilirubin to biliverdin by the saliva of the louse and a brown "dust" found on underclothing due to the excreta of the insects. *P. pubis* is transmitted mainly by sexual contact, but it also may be transmitted by clothing or from parents to children.

Patients with pubic lice should be evaluated for other sexually transmitted diseases. Treatment of pediculosis pubis is the same as for pediculosis capitis. Bedding and clothing should be decontaminated (as for scabies) or removed from body contact for 2 weeks. Attention should be paid to treating sexual partners within the previous month because they are a common cause of reinfestation. For infested eyelashes and eyebrows, ophthalmic-grade petrolatum ointment may be used two to four times daily for 10 days, and lice and nits should be carefully removed from the eyelashes with forceps.

---

[1]Not FDA approved for this indication.
[6]May be compounded by pharmacists.

---

[1]Not FDA approved for this indication.
[6]May be compounded by pharmacists.

REFERENCES

Centers for Disease Control (CDC). Disease exposure while traveling. Available at: http://www.cdc.gov/travel/ [accessed June 2009].

Gorkiewicz-Petkow A. Scabicides and pediculicides. In: Katsambas AD, Lotti TM, editors. European Handbook of Dermatological Treatments. 2nd ed. Berlin: Springer; 2003. p. 775–9.

Goyal NN, Wong GA. Psoriasis or crusted scabies. Clin Exp Dermatol 2008;33:211–2.

Heukelbach J, Feldmeier H. Epidemiological and clinical characteristics of hookworm-related cutaneous larva migrans. Lancet Infect Dis 2008; 8:302–9.

Klaus SN, Frankenburg S, Dhar AD. Leishmaniasis and other protozoan infections. In: Freedeberg IM, Eisen AZ, Wolff K, et al., editors. Fitzpatrick's Dermatology in General Medicine. 6th ed. New York: McGraw-Hill; 2003. p. 2215–24.

Lucchina LC, Wilson ME. Cysticercosis and other helminthic infections. In: Freedeberg AZ, Eisen AZ, Wolff K, et al., editors. Fitzpatrick's Dermatology in General Medicine. 6th ed. New York: McGraw-Hill; 2003. p. 2225–59.

Paller AS, Mancini AJ. Bites and infestations. In: Hurwitz Clinical Pediatric Dermatology. 3rd ed. Philadelphia: WB Saunders; 2006. p. 479–501.

Stone SP. Scabies and pediculosis. In: Freedeberg IM, Eisen AZ, Wolff K, et al., editors. Fitzpatrick's Dermatology in General Medicine. 6th ed. New York: McGraw-Hill; 2003. p. 2283–9.

Tsoureli-Nikita E, Campanile G, Hautmann G, et al. Pediculosis. In: Katsambas TM, Lotti TM, editors. European Handbook of Dermatological Treatments. 2nd ed. Berlin: Springer; 2003. p. 775–9.

Cutaneous Fungal Infections

Method of
William Aughenbaugh, MD

Cutaneous fungal infections are caused by dermatophytes, yeasts, and saprophytes. Infections are classified according to depth of penetration: superficial, subcutaneous, and deep. Superficial mycoses involve the stratum corneum, nail plate, and hair shaft. These may arise from human (anthropophilic), animal (zoophilic), or soil (geophilic) sources. Subcutaneous fungal infections involve dermis or subcutaneous tissue and are typically caused by traumatic implantation. Deep (systemic) fungal infections result from local invasion or hematogenous spread. This chapter focuses on superficial mycoses.

Cutaneous Dermatophyte Infections

Dermatophytes are divided into three genera: *Microsporum*, *Trichophyton*, and *Epidermophyton*. These organisms cause the most commonly encountered superficial fungal infections, which are classified according to the site of involvement: tinea capitis (head), tinea faciei (face), tinea barbae (beard), tinea corporis (body), tinea cruris (inguinal folds), tinea manuum (hands), tinea pedis (feet), and tinea unguium (nails).

Tinea corporis manifests with round or annular plaques with central clearing and scaling at the periphery. Coalescence may result in large plaques with serpiginous borders. The eruption may produce vesicles or pustules, particularly when the dermatophyte is zoonotic in origin.

Tinea capitis is most common among children and may manifest as black dots on the scalp because of endothrix involvement of the hair shaft or as scaling patches of alopecia when ectothrix organisms are involved. Severe inflammation may cause pustules, fluctuant nodules, serous crusting, and widespread alopecia.

Dermatophytes may invade the hair follicle in the case of tinea barbae and Majocchi's granulomas. Tinea barbae infections are characterized by severe inflammation, pustules, and overlying serous crust

with alopecia. Systemic antifungal agents are required for treatment because topical agents do not adequately penetrate the dermis.

Tinea cruris manifests with erythema with or without scale. It classically spares the scrotum.

Tinea pedis occurs in several forms: interdigital, pustular, moccasin distribution, and two feet–one hand disease. Interdigital tinea pedis involves the web spaces of the toes with associated maceration. Pustular tinea pedis is intensely pruritic and involves the instep with vesicles and pustules. The moccasin distribution covers the entire plantar foot, with extension to the lateral and dorsal foot. Two feet–one hand disease produces inflammatory tinea pedis with scaling of one palm. The inflammation of the hand results from an 'id' reaction (a cutaneous response distant from the primary inflammatory process) and does not represent active infection at that site. Tinea pedis has a high rate of recurrence despite adequate treatment.

Tinea incognito is caused by the application of topical steroids, which reduces cutaneous inflammation. A high index of suspicion is required because the area of involvement may be more extensive and erythema reduced.

Onychomycosis may manifest as yellow, subungual hyperkeratosis or as superficial white dystrophy. Involvement of fingernails may suggest underlying immunosuppression.

Nondermatophyte Cutaneous Infections

Pityriasis (tinea) versicolor is typically asymptomatic and involves the trunk and proximal extremities. In the summer months, the patches appear hypopigmented because of tanning of the surrounding skin. As the tan fades, the patches take on a salmon-colored hue. The scale is characteristically fine, white, and branny, and it may be detected by gentle scraping of the skin. *Malassezia furfur* is the causative organism. The differential diagnosis includes pityriasis alba, postinflammatory hypopigmentation, vitiligo, atopic dermatitis, seborrheic dermatitis, pityriasis rosea, and secondary syphilis.

Superficial infections with *Candida* species demonstrate a broad range of clinical presentations. These infections are supported by warm, moist environments and therefore involve inframammary skin folds, abdominal pannus, and inguinal folds. Additional risk factors include immunosuppression, diabetes mellitus, hyperhidrosis, occlusion, and use of oral antibiotics.

Intertrigo manifests with erythematous papules that coalesce into plaques. Erosions may be present. The hallmark is inflammatory, satellite papules and pustules. Chronic infections may itch or burn and may be associated with a foul odor. The scrotum may be involved, in contrast to the pattern of dermatophyte infections.

Oral candidiasis manifests with an adherent, white material with or without glossitis. Perlèche (i.e., angular cheilitis) is characterized by fissures of the lateral commissure of the mouth. Secondary *Candida* infection may impede healing.

Pityrosporum folliculitis demonstrates uniform, erythematous papules of the trunk and extremities. *Pityrosporum orbiculare* is the cause of this pruritic eruption.

Differential Diagnosis

Cutaneous fungal infections are classified as papulosquamous disorders that are characterized by papules and plaques with overlying scale. The differential diagnosis includes atopic dermatitis, seborrheic dermatitis, contact dermatitis, psoriasis, lichen planus, granuloma annulare, drug eruptions, sarcoid, secondary syphilis, and lupus erythematosus. Atopic dermatitis may be distinguished by the patient having an atopic diathesis, flexural predominance, and chronic remitting course.

Psoriasis favors extensor surfaces and demonstrates a thick, white scale. Nail pitting may help support a diagnosis of psoriasis. Inguinal involvement (inverse psoriasis) is sharply demarcated, brightly erythematous, and macerated without satellite papules.

Tinea barbae may mimic acne vulgaris, bacterial folliculitis, actinomycosis, and herpesvirus infections. A potassium hydroxide (KOH) examination or culture may help distinguish these conditions. Alopecia areata may be distinguished from tinea capitis by the absence of scale and identification of exclamation point hairs at the periphery of the involved patch.

Diagnosis

The KOH test helps to confirm the diagnosis of tinea or *Candida* infections. This test is performed by gently scraping the advancing edge of an annular plaque or the roof of a vesicle with a no. 15 blade scalpel or edge of a glass slide. The collected material is placed on a glass slide, and a drop of KOH is applied. A cover slip is placed, and the slide is gently heat-fixed over a flame, carefully avoiding boiling the solution. The slide is examined at 4× power to identify hyphae or pseudohyphae, which are used to diagnose dermatophyte and *Candida* infections, respectively. Care must be exercised when performing a KOH examination that overlapping cell walls are not erroneously read as hyphae.

Pityriasis versicolor demonstrates short hyphae and clusters of spores, commonly referred to as "spaghetti and meatballs." False-negative results may arise from prior application of a topical antifungal agent.

Onychomycosis may be diagnosed with fungal culture or histopathologic examination of a nail clipping. Placement of clippings over dermatophyte test medium (DTM) identifies dermatophyte infections when the indicator turns red.

 CURRENT DIAGNOSIS

Tinea Capitis

- Scalp erythema, scale, and alopecia: pustules may be present.

Tinea Corporis

- Pruritic, annular, erythematous, scaling patches with central clearing

Tinea Cruris

- Erythema and scale of the medial thighs and inguinal folds
- Scrotum is spared.

Tinea Pedis

- Interdigital maceration and scale, plantar scaling, vesicles, and pustules of the instep
- An 'id' reaction may be present with scaling of one palm (i.e., two feet–one hand disease).

Tinea Unguium (Onychomycosis)

- Yellow, subungual hyperkeratosis or superficial, white dystrophy

Pityriasis (Tinea) Versicolor

- Pink patches with fine, white scale in the absence of a tan
- Hypopigmented patches with fine, white scale with tanned skin
- Truncal involvement is most common.

Cutaneous Candidiasis

- Erosive, erythematous papules and plaques with satellite papules and pustules
- May involve the scrotum

Pityrosporon Folliculitis

- Uniform, pink papules of the trunk and proximal extremities

Therapy

TOPICAL ANTIFUNGAL AGENTS

Superficial fungal infections are typically amenable to topical therapies. Topical allylamines include terbinafine (Lamisil) and naftifine (Naftin). They are effective against dermatophytes, but minimally effective against *Candida* species. Studies reveal superior efficacy of allylamines over imidazoles in the treatment of dermatophyte infections. Naftifine is also effective against some saprophytes, which are uncommon causes of superficial fungal infections.

Topical imidazoles, including clotrimazole (Lotrimin), econazole (Spectazole), miconazole (Micatin,[1] Monistat), and ketoconazole (Nizoral), demonstrate efficacy against dermatophytes, *Candida albicans*, and *Malassezia furfur* infections. Twice-daily application for 2 to 4 weeks is recommended for topical antifungal agents. Patients with a moccasin distribution of tinea pedis may require chronic daily dosing to minimize the risk of recurrence.

Nystatin (Mycostatin) is effective against *Candida* yeast and has demonstrated fungistatic and fungicidal properties in vitro. Nystatin is not effective against dermatophytes.

Ciclopirox olamine (Loprox) has a unique mechanism of action and is effective against dermatophytes, yeasts, some saprophytes, and gram-positive and gram-negative bacteria. The cream may be used to treat superficial cutaneous mycoses. The nail lacquer 8% formulation (Penlac) penetrates the nail plate and may be effective in the treatment of onychomycosis after 48 weeks.

Selenium sulfide is available in a 1% (Selsun Blue) and 2.5% lotion (Selsun) formulation. It is indicated for seborrheic dermatitis and tinea versicolor.

The choice of vehicle may maximize compliance with topical therapy. Creams are most commonly used for cutaneous sites. Sprays may be used for widespread truncal or inguinal involvement. Powders may reduce maceration associated with intertrigo, but abrasive clumps may result. Nystatin is available as an oral troche (Mycostatin Pastilles) and is effective in the treatment of oral candidiasis.

ORAL ANTIFUNGAL AGENTS

Oral antifungal agents are typically reserved for severe inflammatory or widespread involvement. Onychomycosis responds to oral terbinafine and imidazoles, including ketoconazole[1] and itraconazole (Sporanox). Treatment regimens include continuous dosing terbinafine 250 mg daily for 12 weeks for toenails and 6 weeks for fingernails. Pulse treatment with terbinafine 250 mg twice daily for 1 week per month for 3 months or with itraconazole 200 mg twice daily for 1 week per month for 3 months has proved effective in the treatment of onychomycosis but at a lower cost. The pulse schedule is an off-label dosing regimen for terbinafine and itraconazole (toenails).

Tinea capitis, tinea barbae, and Majocchi's granulomas require systemic antifungal therapy. Treatment duration is 2 to 4 weeks for tinea corporis and cruris and 2 to 6 weeks for tinea pedis. Tinea capitis typically requires 6 to 12 weeks of treatment with griseofulvin (Grifulvin V, Gris-PEG) and 4 to 6 weeks of treatment with itraconazole[1] and terbinafine.[1] Concomitant use of topical antifungal shampoos may help reduce the risk of recurrence.

Oral imidazoles are effective in the treatment of widespread pityriasis versicolor and dermatophyte infections. Ketoconazole is rapidly absorbed and detected in sweat. In the treatment of extensive pityriasis versicolor, patients are instructed to take 400 mg of ketonconazole,[1] wait 1 hour after ingestion, exercise to the point of sweating, and rinse the skin after 4 hours. This regimen may be repeated after 1 week. The risk of idiopathic hepatotoxicity is discussed with all patients taking oral imidazoles. Drug interactions must be considered with oral antifungals. Oral itraconazole is metabolized by the hepatic cytochrome P-450 enzymes, and the risk of toxicity is therefore increased with concomitant use of terfenadine (Seldane),[2] Cisapride (Propulsid),[2] statin lipid-lowering agents, benzodiazepines, warfarin (Coumadin), and other agents.

---

[1]Not FDA approved for this indication.
[2]Not available in the United States.

CURRENT THERAPY

Dermatophyte Infections

TINEA CORPORIS, TINEA CRURIS, TINEA MANUUM, AND TINEA PEDIS

- Terbinafine (Lamisil) 1% cream twice daily
- Clotrimazole (Lotrimin) 1%, econazole (Spectazole) 1%, ketoconazole (Nizoral) 2% cream twice daily for 2 to 4 weeks
- Naftifine (Naftin) 1% cream twice daily × 2 weeks
- Ciclopirox (Loprox) 0.77% cream twice daily × 4 weeks
- Systemic therapy as for tinea capitis; treatment duration is 2 to 4 weeks for tinea corporis or cruris and 2 to 6 weeks for tinea pedis

TINEA CAPITIS AND TINEA BARBAE

- Griseofulvin microsize (Grifulvin V)[3] 20 to 25 mg/kg/day × 6 to 12 weeks
- Griseofulvin ultramicrosize (Gris-PEG)[3] 10–15 mg/kg/day × 6 to 12 weeks
- Terbinafine (Lamisil)[1] 62.5 mg/day (<20 kg), 125 mg/day (20–40 kg), 250 mg/day (>40 kg) × 4 weeks
- Itraconazole (Sporanox)[1] 200 mg/day (>40 kg) × 4 weeks

TINEA UNGUIUM (ONYCHOMYCOSIS)

- Terbinafine 250 mg/day × 6 weeks (fingernails) and × 12 weeks (toenails) *or* terbinafine pulse therapy (off-label schedule) with 250-mg tablet twice daily for 1 week each month; treat for a total of two cycles (fingernails) or three cycles (toenails)
- Itraconazole 200 mg/day *or* itraconazole pulse therapy (off-label schedule) 200 mg twice daily for 1 week each month; 6 wks or continuous two pulse cycles (fingernails) and 12 wks or continuous three pulse cycles (toenails)[1]
- Ciclopirox 8% lacquer (Penlac) daily to nails; file off after 7 days and repeat for 48 weeks

Nondermatophyte Infections

CUTANEOUS CANDIDIASIS

- Clotrimazole (Lotrimin) 1%, econazole (Spectazole) 1%, ketoconazole (Nizoral) 2% cream twice daily × 2 weeks
- Nystatin cream or powder (Mycostatin) twice daily × 2 weeks
- Naftifine (Naftin)[1] 1% cream twice daily × 2 weeks
- Fluconazole (Diflucan) 150 mg one-time dose for vaginal candidiasis
- Itraconazole (Sporanox)[1] 200 mg daily × 2 weeks for cutaneous candidiasis

PITYRIASIS (TINEA) VERSICOLOR

- Selenium sulfide 2.5% lotion (Selsun) twice daily
- Clotrimazole 1% cream (plus other azole antifungals) twice weekly × 4 weeks
- Ketoconazole 200 mg 2 tablets PO (off-label dose); wait 1 hour, and exercise to point of sweating; rinse after 4 hours; and repeat in 1 week

PITYROSPORUM FOLLICULITIS

- Treatment is the same as for pityriasis versicolor (off-label indication).

---

[1]Not FDA approved for this indication.
[3]Exceeds dosage recommended by the manufacturer.

Griseofulvin remains the only FDA-approved treatment for tinea capitis. The ultramicronized formulation (Gris-PEG) is dosed[3] at 15 to 20 mg/kg/day in children. Treatment duration is between 6 and 12 weeks. An increasing body of evidence supports the safety and efficacy of oral terbinafine[1] in the treatment of tinea capitis in the pediatric population. Dosing for terbinafine is weight-based: 62.5 mg/day (<20 kg), 125 mg/day (20–40 kg), or 250 mg/day (>40 kg). Itraconazole[1] 200 mg/day may be used in individuals weighing more than 40 kg. Duration of treatment is 4 weeks. Careful observation is recommended because the risk of recurrence is high.

REFERENCES

Gupta AK, Cooper EA, Bowen JE. Meta-analysis: Griseofulvin in the treatment of tinea capitis. J Drugs Dermatol 2008;7(4):369–72.

Gupta AK, Cooper EA. Update in antifungal therapy of dermatophytosis. Mycopatholgica 2008;166(5–6):353–67.

Huang DB, Osktrosky-Zeichner L, Wu JJ, et al. Therapy of common superficial fungal infections. Dermatol Ther 2004;17(6):517–22.

Wolverton S. Comprehensive Dermatologic Drug Therapy. Philadelphia: WB Saunders; 2001.

---

[1]Not FDA approved for this indication.
[3]Exceeds dosage recommended by the manufacturer.

Diseases of the Mouth

Method of
Gary C. Coleman, DDS, MS

The numerous diseases that affect the oral cavity can pose difficult diagnostic and therapeutic challenges. Some simplification can be attained by dividing oral diseases into three groups based on management perspective. The first group includes conditions such as dental caries and periodontitis that are directly associated with the teeth and are the dentist's treatment responsibility. The second group consists of conditions that do not cause symptoms, present little risk of adverse consequences, or are so rarely encountered that they represent more of a novelty than a clinically significant consideration. The third group consists of a relatively short list of conditions that produce pain or pose the risk of serious complications and require treatment other than dental care. The diseases of this third group are compared in the Current Diagnosis box and were selected to frame this therapeutic overview because patients may seek treatment from the physician rather than the dentist.

Disseminated Odontogenic Infection

With few exceptions, disseminated bacterial infections of odontogenic origin represent a dramatic, acute exacerbation of a chronic, asymptomatic infection. A variety of dental conditions are possible causes, such as a periodontal abscess, an abscess within the supportive bone resulting from the pulpal necrosis of a carious tooth, or an infection of the gingiva surrounding a partially erupted third molar. The patient often describes a history of one or more prior acute episodes of bacterial infection symptoms from the site followed by resolution. The degree of swelling, lymphadenopathy, pain, and fever is proportional to the risk of potential complications such as septicemia. Of particular concern is evidence of rapid progression of diffuse swelling into the floor of the mouth and neck because of the risk of respiratory distress (i.e., Ludwig's angina) or superiorly from the anterior portion of the maxilla because of the possibility of cavernous sinus thrombosis.

Definitive dental treatment to eliminate the underlying infectious source is the treatment goal after the acute, disseminated infection has been controlled. Penicillin is still considered the empiric antibiotic choice for disseminated odontogenic bacterial infections in individuals with no history of adverse reaction, and clindamycin (Cleocin) is used for those hypersensitive to penicillin. Many patients mistakenly assume that empiric antibiotic treatment can eliminate the infection in the same sense that antibiotic treatment can cure bacterial sinusitis or pharyngitis. The patient should be informed that improvement of an acute odontogenic infection after antibiotic treatment is not curative and that dental care to eliminate the underlying cause is necessary. One or more courses of antibiotics without elimination of the source increase the probability of the emergence of more virulent, antibiotic-resistant pathogens. More aggressive treatment, including intravenous antibiotics and surgical drainage in a hospital setting, must be considered in cases of rapid progression or extensive swelling, particularly if the anterior maxilla or submandibular areas are involved and in instances of compromised host resistance.

Suspicion of Oral Cancer

Primary malignant neoplasms originating from virtually every tissue type found in the oral cavity have been reported. However, more than 90% of intraoral malignancies are squamous cell carcinoma (SCC) originating from the lining oral epithelium. The typical features and clinical course of oral SCC heavily influence the differential diagnostic assessment of any oral lesions if malignant neoplasia is suspected. Careful consideration is critical because the 5-year survival probability for oral SCC is approximately 50%, and early diagnosis is one of the few favorable prognostic factors.

Several features that strongly correlate an eventual diagnosis of oral SCC are summarized in Table 1. The two most significant etiologic factors for intraoral SCC are the habitual use of tobacco and alcoholic beverages. Other potential causative factors, such as exposure to virulent human papillomavirus (HPV) subtypes, have shown some positive correlation, but by far the probability of oral cancer is greatest among heavy drinkers and smokers. The carcinogenic effect of the two substances appears to be synergistic. This process typically requires decades for the emergence of clinical lesions, as is shown by the observation that the initial diagnosis of more than 90% of oral SCCs is made after age 40, with a peak incidence in the sixth decade of life.

SCC of the exposed lower lip surface usually is included in oral cancer statistics, but important differences in cause and prognosis compared with intraoral SCC affect diagnosis and management. SCC of the exposed lower lip is primarily caused by actinic cellular damage and is comparable to actinic skin lesions in terms of appearance, a more positive prognosis, and low probability of metastasis. As with actinic skin cancers of the face, the possibility of SCC of the lower lip is greatest during the sixth or seventh decade for fair-skinned individuals with a vocation or avocation associated with prolonged sun exposure.

Premalignant dysplastic lesions and early intraoral SCC may manifest as a superficial white or red patch compared with the typical appearance of the mucosa. However, routine frictional irritation or incidental abrasion is the much more common cause of this appearance, and this is by far the most likely cause in areas prone to friction, such as the buccal mucosa. A white or red lesion of the soft palate or floor of the mouth is much more suspicious. Oral SCC may manifest primarily as an ulcer, although most oral ulcers are inflammatory. In contrast to asymptomatic white or red mucosal patches, the patient's history reveals valuable awareness of the duration and course of oral ulcers because of the pain they cause. Intraoral ulcers of SCC tend to be of long duration and much less painful compared with inflammatory ulcers of similar size. Palpation tends to demonstrate an indurated periphery to the malignant oral ulcer.

Most oral enlargements are benign neoplasms or inflammatory in origin. Enlargements that are benign tend to be sharply delineated and of long duration (many months or years) and have a normal surface appearance. Chronic inflammatory enlargements are somewhat tender and compressible to palpation with a shorter duration (days or weeks) or vary in size with time. The combination of induration, altered surface appearance, lack of tenderness to palpation, and progressive enlargement over a period of weeks or months suggests malignancy.

Definitive diagnosis of most oral lesions requires a biopsy, and this is indicated if oral SCC is considered a significant differential diagnostic possibility. Exfoliative cytology is much less reliable as a screening method in the assessment of malignant and premalignant oral disease compared with lesions of the uterine cervix. The harsh nature of the oral environment from food, tobacco use, and other habits limits the appreciation of cytologic features. The diagnosis of oral candidiasis and some viral lesions can be made by exfoliative cytology. Table 1 lists features that prompt increased suspicion of oral cancer and the need for definitive diagnosis by biopsy. As with any differential diagnosis, one or two corresponding features may not be compelling unless dramatic. A greater number of findings that suggest oral SCC indicate a stronger justification for biopsy. The decision to obtain a biopsy of an oral lesion should be made with consideration of the substantial positive impact that early detection has on a disease with an otherwise unfavorable prognosis.

Necrotizing Ulcerative Gingivitis

Necrotizing ulcerative gingivitis (NUG) is a characteristic, potentially destructive infection of the dental supportive tissues caused by a predominance of fusiform bacteria and spirochetes. Some combination of psychologic stress, compromised immune function, malnutrition, or other condition of diminished host resistance dramatically increases the risk of NUG. This is suggested by the colloquial phrase *trench mouth* used to refer to this infection, because it was frequently observed among debilitated soldiers during World War I. It has also been called Vincent's infection and acute NUG (ANUG).

TABLE 1 Clinical Suspicion Factors for Oral Squamous Cell Carcinoma

Feature	More Suspicious	Less Suspicious
Causative factors	Alcohol and tobacco use	Frictional cause (e.g., sharp tooth)
Age	>40 years (younger much less likely)	<40 (probability increases if immunocompromised)
Surface appearance	Altered and heterogeneous	Unaltered or homogeneous
Peripheral delineation	Vague borders	Sharp borders
Distribution	Isolated	Multifocal
Pain (ulcers)	Painless or less pain than expected for lesion size	Pain (inflammatory)
Location	Tongue, oropharynx, floor of mouth	Gingiva, hard palate, buccal mucosa (less likely)
Palpation	Indurated, nontender	Compressible, tender
Clinical course	Unchanging (weeks), progressive (months)	Variable (within weeks), static (months or years)

Acute onset of poorly localized, severe dental pain and a putrid taste are typically the patient's chief complaints. Onset usually corresponds with a significant alteration in the general health or emotional status, although a more chronic course of variably pronounced symptoms can be expected with protracted conditions such as acquired immunodeficiency syndrome (AIDS). Visual features of NUG include necrotic deterioration of the gingiva with pronounced peripheral erythema and a superficial pseudomembrane. The tissue around the mandibular anterior teeth is most severely affected in most cases, and the gingiva often appears "punched out" from between the teeth. The gingival necrosis produces the characteristic fetid breath that is far more pungent than that caused by typical gingivitis. The putrid odor in combination with the acute onset and poor localization of pain is usually a more reliable basis for diagnosis than visual findings. Additional features, such as fever and cervical lymphadenopathy, are proportional to the severity of the oral findings.

CURRENT DIAGNOSIS

High-Risk Conditions

- Acute exacerbation of odontogenic infections: rapid onset, swelling, purulence, obvious dental origin
- Suspicion of oral cancer: mucosal surface color change, nonhealing ulcer, enlargement, asymptomatic or incidental finding, use of tobacco and alcohol

Opportunistic Infections and Dry Mouth

- Necrotizing ulcerative gingivitis (trench mouth): compromised host resistance, generalized dental pain, usually acute onset, fetid odor
- Oral candidiasis: compromised host resistance, chronic or recurring course, poorly localized "burning" soreness, superficial change in mucosal appearance
- Salivary dysfunction (xerostomia): patient's perception of dry mouth, causative condition or associated findings

Acute-Onset Oral Ulcers with Focal Pain

- Aphthous stomatitis: recurring episodes, formation of one or more superficial oral ulcers, located on nonbound mucosa, healing in approximately 7 to 10 days
- Primary herpetic gingivostomatitis: acute onset of systemic viral infection features, including fever and multiple oral vesicles degenerating into ulcers, resolution in 7 to 10 days
- Recurrent herpes: recurring episodes, acute formation of vesicles collapsing to ulcers, located on exposed lip or bound mucosa, healing in 7 to 10 days
- Erythema multiforme: acute onset of oral ulcers, triggering event, mild systemic features such as fever, characteristic skin lesions, resolution in 2 to 4 weeks

Chronic Oral Ulcers

- Erosive lichen planus and lichenoid reaction: reticular appearance at periphery of ulcers, buccal mucosa affected, may cause desquamative gingivitis, skin lesions possible
- Mucous membrane pemphigoid: typically desquamative gingivitis presentation, possible eye and genital ulcers, skin lesions unlikely
- Pemphigus vulgaris: ulcers of irregular shape and jagged peripheral contour, possible skin lesions

Treatment of NUG consists of the combination of supportive care, antimicrobial measures, and improvement in the underlying compromising health conditions. Supportive care is nonspecific and includes rest, fluid intake, and a soft but nutritious diet. Warm saline, dilute hydrogen peroxide, and chlorhexidine gluconate (Peridex) are effective antimicrobial rinses. Penicillin and metronidazole (Flagyl) are the empiric systemic antibiotics of choice. Ultimately, the most effective antimicrobial treatment is the combination of thorough dental cleaning of the teeth with débridement of the necrotic soft tissue and improved oral hygiene. Resolution of NUG, including complete healing of the gingival tissue, is strikingly rapid in most instances if this is accomplished and underlying health status improves. Persistence or recurrence of NUG after débridement suggests the possibility of human immunodeficiency virus (HIV) infection or another undiagnosed compromising condition.

Oral Candidiasis

Oral candidiasis is a superficial fungal infection of the oral mucosa that is clinically similar to vaginal candidiasis in many respects. With isolated exceptions, the infection is caused by the fungus *Candida albicans*, which can be identified in the mouths of approximately 50% of healthy adults. The risk of oral candidiasis is increased by one or more factors of compromised host resistance: decreased local resistance, compromised immune function, or uncontrolled systemic disease. Frequently encountered examples of decreased local resistance include poor oral hygiene, xerostomia, wearing dentures that provide an organism reservoir or limit hygiene, and recent antibiotic therapy that has altered the normally competitive oral bacteria. The combination of one or more of these local factors with a systemic condition that causes compromised immune status or constitutional compromise dramatically increases the risk of clinical apparent infection. Common examples include AIDS, corticosteroid therapy, severe anemia, and poorly controlled diabetes mellitus.

Oral candidiasis lesions can have four distinct appearances. The most characteristic form is the pseudomembranous, curdlike globules of thrush that wipe off with cotton gauze, leaving a sore, erythematous mucosal surface. The erythematous or atrophic form of oral candidiasis produces a thin, "beefy" appearance often affecting the dorsum of the tongue or mucosa that supports a denture. The third type of lesion is the formation of fissures similar to those of tinea pedis that usually are at the corners of the mouth and are referred to as angular cheilitis. The fourth is a hyperplastic form that produces a patchy, white thickening of the surface epithelium that does not rub off and that appears similar to the hyperkeratosis of chronic frictional irritation. Oral candidiasis often produces more than one lesion form simultaneously in different areas of the mouth, which may be a confirmational finding. Patients often describe little discomfort or only a mild burning sensation from affected sites.

The clinical course of the infection may be acute, chronic, or cyclic in severity, depending on the nature of the underlying causes. The combination of clinical appearance, suspected compromised host status, and improvement after empiric treatment provides an adequate basis for the diagnosis. Exfoliative cytology provides definitive evidence of the infection in more equivocal situations.

Antifungal treatment eliminates oral candidiasis in most instances, but recurrences or a chronic, subclinical course can be expected if the predisposing condition remains unchanged. This implies that treatment of superficial oral candidiasis may not be justified in such instances if the affected individual is asymptomatic, because the only realistic treatment goal is elimination of symptoms. That decision must be weighed against the possibility of spread to the esophagus.

Options for routine topical treatment of oral candidiasis include clotrimazole (Mycelex) troches or nystatin (Mycostatin) pastilles, and use should continue for 1 week after resolution of symptoms. Several considerations can complicate effectiveness. Patients with xerostomia have difficulty dissolving the troches or pastilles and prefer a nystatin rinse. Concurrent management of the dry mouth (discussed later) increases the effectiveness of topical antifungal treatment for candidiasis. Limiting the *Candida* organism reservoir in the denture acrylic for those who wear dentures can be accomplished by soaking overnight in most commercial denture soaking solutions, mouthwashes such as Listerine, or chlorhexidine gluconate. These products are adequately fungicidal, and keeping the denture out overnight disrupts adherence and colonization of candidal organisms. Some patients are more compliant about managing the denture problem by applying a thin layer of nystatin ointment[1] or clotrimazole cream (Lotrimin)[1] to the denture before wearing. Direct application of these preparations also promotes rapid resolution of angular cheilitis. Systemic administration of ketoconazole (Nizoral) or fluconazole (Diflucan) is an alternative for patients who cannot manage topical treatment or for severely immunocompromised individuals in the interest of controlling oral symptoms and minimizing the risk of spread to the esophagus.

Xerostomia

Xerostomia is defined by the patient's subjective perception of "dry mouth" rather than by any objective parameter. The amount of saliva is decreased, and its character typically is altered to a more viscous, ropey consistency. The condition is common because salivary function is adversely affected by so many routinely encountered influences, including many frequently prescribed medications, smoking, methamphetamine abuse, several common systemic diseases, and tumoricidal irradiation exposure. In addition to these influences, primary Sjögren syndrome is characterized by chronic dry eyes and dry mouth caused by autoimmune-mediated acinar degeneration. Secondary Sjögren syndrome is defined as oral and ocular dryness concurrent with an autoimmune connective tissue disorder such as rheumatoid arthritis.

The subjective response of different individuals to a mild or moderate degree of oral dryness varies considerably. Many patients who appear to produce adequate saliva complain of dryness, whereas others who seem unusually dry during oral examination have no complaints. Most patients with an advanced degree of dryness find the continual "cotton mouth" sensation and other consequences to be a significant quality-of-life issue. Decreased saliva production causes difficulty chewing and swallowing, as well as painful abrasion of the mucosa by coarse foods. Beyond the physical irritation, limited saliva alters the sense of taste and the enjoyment of food. Saliva contributes to oral health by providing antimicrobial components such as lactoperoxidase and IgE antibodies, and it has a significant flushing and cleansing function. Xerostomia causes a rampant and rapidly progressive pattern of dental decay that is particularly destructive even for previously caries-resistant individuals. This is compounded if the patient compensates for the dryness by drinking sucrose-rich soft drinks or sucking on hard candy. Similarly, periodontitis tends to progress rapidly despite normally effective treatment if saliva production is limited. Xerostomia is also associated with complaints of generalized soreness of the mouth caused by frequent and persistent episodes of oral candidiasis.

Management of xerostomia is challenging and often frustrating for the patient and the clinician. The treatment for severe, irreversible xerostomia, as in cases of head and neck radiotherapy, is essentially symptomatic. Different patients prefer different combinations of compensation methods. Sipping water throughout the day is the single most effective and simplest way to counter loss of saliva. Some patients report additional improvement with the use of commercially available saliva substitutes, although many do as well with water and ice chips. Most patients soon learn to avoid abrasive foods, irritating commercial mouth rinses that contain alcohol, and highly flavored toothpastes in favor of less irritating alternatives. Use of a humidifier at night is often beneficial. Comprehensive dental treatment should be recommended to limit the progression and severity of dental caries and periodontitis. Smoking and compensation by drinking sucrose-rich soft drinks, sports drinks, drinks that contain caffeine, and highly acidic citric juices should be discouraged.

Additional options beyond the previous recommendations are available for those who have some residual salivary function. Drinking ample water moistens the mucosa and maintains general hydration, which maximizes the residual saliva production. Sugar-free gum or hard candy significantly stimulates saliva flow. Alternate medications may be substituted in some cases to treat conditions such as hypertension that are equally effective therapeutically but are less likely to cause xerostomia.

Several cholinergic sialologs are available, including cevimeline (Evoxac), pilocarpine (Salagen), and bethanechol (Urecholine).[1] Titration of dosage is usually necessary to optimize saliva flow while minimizing frequent adverse effects such as excessive sweating and gastritis. Many patients discontinue treatment because of these and less common side effects that become more troublesome than the xerostomia. Contraindications such as glaucoma and the risk of serious complications such as arrhythmia must also be considered.

Aphthous Stomatitis

Recurrent aphthous stomatitis, colloquially known as *canker sores*, is a common condition of complex immune-mediated pathogenesis. Patients describe recurring episodes of painful ulcers that often follow triggering events such as minor tissue abrasion, eating certain foods, or episodes of emotional stress. The phrase *minor aphthous stomatitis* differentiates the most common, mild form of the disease from the more severe *major* and *herpetiform variations*. Most authorities believe these categorizations are somewhat artificial distinctions within a continuum of a single process. Similar ulcers are a feature of Behçet's syndrome but are of minor diagnostic and treatment significance compared with the other manifestations of this rare, multisystem condition.

The clinical features of minor recurrent aphthous stomatitis are characteristic. One or more painful ulcers develop soon after a short prodromal period of burning or itching at the affected site. The superficial ulcers exhibit a uniform, yellowish white, pseudomembranous surface with an erythematous peripheral halo at the sharply delineated ulcer margin. Typical size is 1 to 2 cm, and lesions affect only unbound oral mucosal surfaces of the lips, cheeks, floor of the mouth, or soft palate. This distribution specifically excludes the bound surfaces of the gingiva, hard palate, and the dorsum of the tongue. This feature is valuable for differentiating aphthous stomatitis from the intraoral recurrent herpetic lesions (discussed later) that affect only bound surfaces.

Aphthous lesions typically heal within 7 to 10 days, and most patients describe a long clinical course of symptom-free periods of various durations interrupted by episodes of ulcer formation. Lesion-free periods of weeks, months, or even years typically distinguish recurrent aphthous stomatitis from autoimmune conditions such as erosive lichen planus (discussed later) that produce a continuous course of oral ulcers.

The major form of recurrent aphthous stomatitis produces ulcers of similar appearance, but the lesions are larger, require a longer healing time, often heal with scarring, and form so frequently that at least one ulcer is usually present. The herpetiform variant is characterized by a cluster of numerous smaller (1–3 mm) ulcers that often coalesce into a single, large lesion, and the ulcers are described as exceptionally painful. The clustering distribution explains the somewhat misleading herpetiform designation for this nonviral condition. This form of aphthous stomatitis may affect keratinized and nonkeratinized surfaces, which in addition to the clustering distribution may lead to confusion with recurrent herpes simplex lesions.

Minor recurrent aphthous stomatitis is more irritating than serious, and treatment beyond symptomatic management is usually not justified. Patients soon learn to avoid their particular trigger event as much as possible, and many find relief during outbreaks from over-the-counter preparations such as Orabase with benzocaine 20% or by rinsing with soothing, coating products such as bismuth subsalicylate (Kaopectate).[1] Rinses containing a variety of ingredients, such as

---

[1]Not FDA approved for this indication.

[1]Not FDA approved for this indication.

tetracycline,[1] aloe,[7] and chlorhexidine gluconate,[1] have been reported to promote ulcer healing in some cases. Treatment with corticosteroids (see Current Therapy box), however, is more consistently effective and is justified for major and herpetiform variants, as well as for particularly severe or frequent outbreaks of minor aphthous lesions.

Orofacial Herpes Simplex Infection

Most herpes simplex infections of the oral mucosa are caused by herpes simplex virus type 1 (HSV-1). A much smaller proportion of oral cases results from the type 2 herpes simplex virus that typically causes genital lesions. Transmission occurs by direct contact or contaminated saliva, and serologic studies demonstrate that as much as 90% of the population has been infected by age 50.

The initial infection, referred to as acute herpetic gingivostomatitis or primary herpes, usually affects children and causes acute onset of cervical lymphadenopathy, chills, and fever similar to many acute viral infections. The distinguishing manifestation is the formation of multiple, painful oral vesicles that rapidly rupture. The resulting ulcers most prominently affect the gingiva, lips, and tongue but may occur on any oral surface. Primary herpes in adults is more likely to cause complaints of pharyngitis rather than oral ulcers, which makes distinguishing it from other systemic viral infections unlikely. The severity of primary herpes varies from virtually subclinical or indistinguishable from nonspecific viral infections to debilitating. The distinguishing oral lesions are probably seen only in severe cases because relatively few seropositive individuals recall the oral ulcers of the primary infection when questioned. Symptoms resolve within 5 days to 2 weeks, depending on the severity of the manifestations, and significant complications such as encephalitis or keratoconjunctivitis are rare.

The HSV-1 virus becomes latent within the sensory neurons that supply the primary infection site. Episodes of recurrent lesions may develop after the primary infection, a pattern similar to the recurring genital lesions caused by HSV-2. The frequency, severity, and course of these outbreaks vary widely among individuals, and at least one half of HSV-1–seropositive individuals rarely or never suffer recurrent lesions. Those who do often associate occurrence with causative events, such as sun exposure of the exposed lip, abrasion of the surface, or an illness such as a nonspecific viral infection. This explains the colloquial terms *cold sore* and *fever blister* used to describe the most common presentation affecting the exposed lip, which is referred to as herpes labialis.

The typical episode begins with a prodromal sensation of burning or itching at the site near the vermillion border, followed by formation of one or more vesicles within 24 hours. The vesicles soon rupture, forming a coalesced crust that heals after 7 to 10 days. A few individuals suffer similar recurrent herpes lesions of the intraoral mucosa. Intraoral herpes lesions produce features of pain, onset, recurrent course, and healing time that are similar to those for aphthous stomatitis, which may present some differential diagnostic uncertainty. The diagnosis can be made in most cases based on the affected surface. Aphthous lesions are usually limited to the unbound mucosa of the lips, cheeks, soft palate, and floor of the mouth, whereas the intraoral ulcers of recurrent herpes simplex infection are limited to the bound mucosa of the gingiva and hard palate.

Treatment of primary herpes simplex infection for immunocompetent individuals is supportive and symptomatic, as for any acute systemic viral infection. In cases of significant oral discomfort, a rinse consisting of a 1:1 mixture of diphenhydramine (Benadryl)[1] elixir 12.5 mg/5 mL and Kaopectate[1] used as needed provides some relief by coating the ulcers. The FDA recommends that systemic antiviral medication such as acyclovir (Zovirax)[1] and valacyclovir (Valtrex)[1] be reserved for immunocompromised individuals, with the goal of decreasing the duration and severity of symptoms. Administration of the antiviral agent must be started during the initial stage of the infection to be effective.

Most individuals affected by secondary herpes lesions suffer relatively few episodes, and no treatment is warranted. Patients prone to frequent lip lesions after sun exposure soon learn the preventive value of sunscreen lip balms, but the advice may be helpful to those who have not made the association. For patients who experience numerous secondary herpetic episodes, topical antiviral treatment with penciclovir (Denavir) cream or docosanol 10% (Abreva) cream may limit the severity and duration of the lesions, but applications must begin during the prodromal stage to be effective. Systemic administration of valacyclovir (Valtrex) can be used therapeutically during the prodromal stage or prophylactically.[1] FDA recommendations limit the use of systemic acyclovir[1] for recurrent orofacial herpetic lesions to immunocompromised patients for prophylaxis and treatment of individual outbreaks at the onset of prodromal symptoms.

Erythema Multiforme

Erythema multiforme, which is discussed in greater detail elsewhere in this textbook, is characterized by shallow oral ulcers and characteristic "target" skin lesions. Outbreaks of secondary herpetic lesions have been implicated as a frequent trigger for erythema multiforme. A prodrome of mild fever, malaise, sore throat, and headache may precede the appearance of the oral ulcers and skin lesions. The shallow oral ulcers usually affect the lips, tongue, or soft palate and are less likely to develop on the gingiva or hard palate. Ulcers gradually heal after 2 to 4 weeks, and approximately 20% of affected individuals experience multiple episodes. Certain medications, especially antibiotics, have also been implicated as triggers for erythema multiforme. Medication exposure is the typical stimulus for the onset of Stevens-Johnson syndrome and toxic epidermal necrolysis, which by similar allergic mechanisms produce much more extensive, generalized epithelial sloughing.

Treatment of the oral lesions of erythema multiforme is somewhat controversial. Topical and systemic corticosteroids have been recommended in the past based largely on the presumed pathogenesis of the lesions. However, little evidence exists to demonstrate the effectiveness of this approach. Supportive care usually is adequate and includes a less abrasive diet, maintaining hydration, use of analgesics, and use of a soothing, coating rinse (1:1 mixture of Benadryl elixir and Kaopectate).[1] Patients who experience recurring episodes may benefit from herpes simplex virus suppression with acyclovir or valacyclovir. More extensive epithelial sloughing or rapid progression suggesting Stevens-Johnson syndrome or toxic epidermal necrolysis requires hospitalization.

Erosive Lichen Planus and Similar Autoimmune Ulcerative Conditions of the Oral Mucosa

Several diseases cause oral ulcers by autoimmune-mediated degeneration at or near the epithelial–connective tissue interface. In some patients, painful oral ulceration is the only presenting feature of the disease. For other patients, the oral pain is only an occasional or secondary complaint. With few exceptions, however, a chronic course of oral pain for months or years without complete remission is described by the patient. The location and severity may change over time with cyclic formation of new ulcers and concurrent healing of others, but the dominant trend is a chronic, protracted, or progressive course with little or no complete relief. This continuous course distinguishes the ulcers caused by autoimmune diseases from those of other conditions, such as aphthous stomatitis, which characteristically have an episodic pattern of occurrence. As with autoimmune diseases in general, the demographic pattern tends toward middle-aged women. Definitive diagnosis typically relies on biopsy results, but the differential diagnosis is often narrowed by the appreciation of additional findings, such as lesions of the skin or other mucous membranes, and by laboratory tests, such as obtaining an antinuclear antibody (ANA) titer.

Diseases of the Mouth

---

[1]Not FDA approved for this indication.
[7]Available as a dietary supplement.

---

[1]Not FDA approved for this indication.

Most patients presenting with a chronic course of oral ulcers are suffering from one of three conditions: erosive lichen planus (ELP), mucous membrane pemphigoid (MMP), or pemphigus vulgaris (PV). Because ELP is relatively common and the oral ulcers are a prominent feature of the condition, it is described in some detail. The clinical features that are of differential diagnostic value in distinguishing similar diseases are briefly compared.

The characteristic skin manifestations of lichen planus are a pruritic, papular eruption of flexor surfaces of the limbs and linear hyperkeratotic lesions known as Wickham's striae. These findings combined with the chronic course typically provide an adequate basis for the clinical diagnosis. Approximately 1% of the adult population is affected by lichen planus or the clinically indistinguishable adverse reaction to certain medications referred to as *lichenoid reaction*. Oral lesions affect a significant proportion of patients with skin lesions, and many individuals exhibit oral lesions without skin abnormalities. The oral lesions appear as a lacy network of white, hyperkeratotic lines that bilaterally affect the buccal mucosal surfaces, although any intraoral surface may be affected. This is referred to as the *reticular presentation* of oral lichen planus, and no treatment is warranted because the white lesions are asymptomatic. The erosive form of lichen planus is less common but is of greatest therapeutic concern because affected patients seek pain relief. Ulcers tend to form in the same oral sites for a given patient and cyclically vary in severity as ulcers concurrently heal somewhat in some areas and progress elsewhere. Buccal mucosa and gingiva are the typically affected sites, but any intraoral surface may be affected.

One helpful distinguishing visual feature of ELP lesions from other autoimmune oral ulcers is that the zone between the ulcer and unaffected mucosa often exhibits a fine pattern of white lines that suggests the reticular form of the disease. This appearance is enhanced by drying the saliva with cotton gauze. The term *desquamative gingivitis* is used to describe the clinical presentation if the erosive lesions most dramatically affect the gingiva, which is often the case. The gingiva appears uniformly erythematous and delicately thin, with isolated ulcers. Bulla formation after lateral pressure on this atrophic surface (i.e., Nikolsky's sign) results from the compromised epithelial–connective tissue interface. The patient often complains of sore, bleeding "gums," but the atrophic appearance and Nikolsky's sign are helpful in distinguishing similar complaints from the much more commonly encountered gingivitis and periodontitis caused by poor oral hygiene.

MMP has also been referred to as *cicatricial pemphigoid* and *benign MMP*. The typical presentation of MMP is a chronic course of primarily gingival vesicles and bullae that rapidly degenerate into ulcers that fit the desquamative gingivitis description, although any intraoral area may be affected. The white, hyperkeratotic striations seen at the periphery of the ulcers caused by ELP are absent or less conspicuous with MMP. In contrast to ELP, if nonoral lesions of MMP are present, they affect the conjunctiva and genital mucous membrane surfaces rather than the skin. Occurrence of ocular lesions eventually approaches nearly 25% of affected individuals during the protracted disease course, and these lesions may cause blindness in severe cases.

Of the four characteristic forms of pemphigus, only PV causes oral lesions to any clinically significant degree. Approximately one half of patients develop oral ulcers before the appearance of skin lesions. Oral ulcers may affect any intraoral surface and appear superficial with an irregular shape. Initial vesicle or bulla formation is unusual with oral PV, in contrast to MMP, and the peripheral striations described with ELP are absent. The oral ulcers caused by PV tend to show slow progression without healing over time, in contrast to the cyclic variation of concurrent healing and lesion formation characteristic of ELP and MMP.

Several less common conditions can cause oral ulcers with a protracted clinical course. Bullous pemphigoid typically develops after age 60, but the condition is uncommon, skin lesions are the prominent feature, and less than one third of patients exhibit oral lesions. Lupus erythematosus can cause oral ulcers very similar to those of ELP, but this occurs infrequently and only well into the course of the disease after the diagnosis has been established. Approximately 20% of individuals affected by erythema multiforme experience recurrences, but the course of oral lesions is much more episodic than continuous, and the characteristic target skin lesions often suggest the diagnosis. Graft-versus-host disease produces oral lesions similar to those of ELP, but the cause is obvious.

The oral ulcers caused by all of the conditions in this group respond to corticosteroid medications in the recommended therapeutic approach as described in the Current Therapy box. Several pivotal issues about these conditions and treatment with corticosteroids are important for successful management:

- The possibility of candidiasis and recurrent herpes simplex infection should be excluded on the basis of clinical course and features before empiric treatment of oral ulcers because corticosteroids worsen these infectious conditions.
- The patient should understand that the therapeutic goal is to control the oral ulcers rather than to cure the disease. Optimal treatment for ELP using corticosteroids, for example, converts the ulcers to the asymptomatic reticular form. Neither the patient nor the clinician should expect treatment to yield a completely normal tissue appearance.
- Oral candidiasis is a frequent complication of corticosteroid treatment, and this risk is increased with any concurrent condition such as xerostomia. Candidiasis can be detected early with periodic recall evaluation and by exfoliative cytology in suspected situations. Understanding the typical oral candidiasis symptoms increases the patient's awareness of the need to return for treatment.
- Empiric topical corticosteroid treatment should be discontinued for 2 weeks if a biopsy becomes necessary for a definitive diagnosis.

Every effort should be made to identify and discontinue use of causative or irritating agents. Examples such as the link of acidic foods with aphthous ulcers are obvious to the patient, but many are more subtle. One example is cinnamon flavoring agents in many foods and toothpastes. Others are irritating to the mucosa but are mistakenly perceived as beneficial. Hydrogen peroxide, phenol preparations, and alcohol-based mouth rinses that "seem to be doing some good" because they are painful and consequently assumed to be killing bacteria are examples, and they should be avoided by patients with oral ulcers.

Corticosteroid Treatment of Immune-Mediated Oral Ulcers

Corticosteroid management of oral ulcers is similar to the approach for immune-mediated skin lesions. The therapeutic goal is lesion and symptom control, because disease cure or spontaneous remission is unlikely. This should be understood by the patient to avoid unreasonable expectations. Healing of ulcers should be achieved with as little corticosteroid medication as possible. Topical corticosteroids should be tried first, limiting systemic administration to "bursts" as needed to control outbreaks of refractory ulcers followed by maintenance with topical treatment. Long-term systemic corticosteroid administration should be considered only as a last resort. The severity of lesions in these conditions typically varies with time, which means that the need for treatment beyond topical control also varies. Understanding several issues unique to the oral cavity can increase treatment effectiveness:

- Application of the topical corticosteroid after eating and at bedtime and avoiding frequent snacks promote adherence, absorption, and effectiveness.
- Application of preparations with a cotton swab minimizes the risk of onychomycosis from routine application with the fingers.
- Low- and intermediate-potency topical corticosteroid preparations such as hydrocortisone (Hytone) and betamethasone valerate (Valisone) tend to be less than optimally effective in the oral environment. Initial trial with a higher-potency preparation is justifiable because significant systemic absorption through the oral mucosa is minimal. The use of ultrapotent topical corticosteroids is reserved for persistent ulcers if some systemic absorption is acceptable.

CURRENT THERAPY

Initial Management with Potent Corticosteroid Preparations

- Fluocinonide (Lidex)[1] gel 0.05%: apply thin film to affected area as needed after meals and at bedtime to control oral ulcers
- Dexamethasone (Decadron)[1] elixir 0.5 mg/5 mL: rinse with 1 teaspoon for 2 minutes and spit out after meals and at bedtime to control oral ulcers

Management of Resistant Ulcers with Ultrapotent Corticosteroid Preparations

- Clobetasol propionate (Temovate)[1] 0.05%
- Halobetasol propionate (Ultravate)[1] 0.05%

Management of Ulcers That Cannot Be Controlled with Topical Preparations

- Prednisone 5- to 20-mg tablets concurrent with topical preparations: as needed to control ulcers and then taper and maintain control with topical corticosteroids
- Prednisone minimum dose: alternate-day concurrent with topical preparation as needed to control ulcers

[1]Not FDA approved for this indication.

REFERENCES

Coleman GC. Oral cancer suspicion factors. Tex Dent J 2003;120(6):486–94.

Goldberg MH, Topazian RG. Odontogenic infections and deep fascial space infections of dental origin. In: Topazian RG, Goldberg MH, Hupp KR, editors. Oral and Maxillofacial Infections. 4th ed. Philadelphia: WB Saunders; 2002. p. 158–87.

Greenberg MS, Glick M. Burket's Oral Medicine Diagnosis & Treatment. 10th ed. Ontario, BC Decker, Hamilton; 2003.

Neville BW, Damm DD, Allen CM, Bouquot JE. Oral and Maxillofacial Pathology. 3rd ed. St Louis: Saunders Elsevier; 2009.

Silverman S, Eversole LR, Truelove EL. Essentials of oral medicine. Ontario, BC Decker, Hamilton; 2002.

Venous Ulcers

Method of
Zuleika L. Bonilla-Martinez, MD, and
Robert S. Kirsner, MD, PhD

Ulcers resulting from venous insufficiency are the most common cause of leg ulceration. Many definitions exist for a chronic wound, which ultimately reflect the demographics, incidence, and prevalence data available. For example, although sometimes referred to as stasis ulcers, patients actually have increased blood flow locally. The Wound Healing Society classifies wounds as *acute* if they sustain restoration of anatomic and functional integrity in an orderly and timely process and *chronic* if they do not. Some of the biologic events that affect the "orderly" process include inflammation, angiogenesis (i.e., new blood vessel formation), matrix regeneration, and remodeling. The "timely" process is affected by the environment, age, pathologic process, wound location, and other factors.

Epidemiology

Venous disease affects approximately 5% of the world's population, and about 2% of the American population. It was once thought to be a disease affecting solely the elderly. The incidence increases from middle age onward. Seventy percent of all leg ulcers result solely from venous disease, and an additional 20% of patients have mixed arterial and venous disease. The other 10% of leg ulcers result from a variety of causes, including neuropathy, prolonged pressure, and infectious, malignant, and inflammatory causes.

The high prevalence of venous disease directly affects patients' quality of life. Family history of venous disease, obesity, smoking, high cost of treatment, time off work, prolonged standing, and hypertension are among the factors that contribute to a strong socioeconomic impact of a country's health care. A retrospective study from Cleveland Clinic Foundation showed the average cost per month of care was approximately $2400, and the mean total cost per patient was between $9685 and $14,136 U.S. dollars.

PATHOPHYSIOLOGY

In the lower extremities, the venous system comprises the deep and superficial veins, which are connected by the perforating venous system. Blood flows from the superficial to the deep veins through the communicating veins to ultimately reach the heart. Veins contain valves that prevent blood reflux and allow the unidirectional flow. When a healthy individual contracts the calf muscles, a high pressure develops in the deep vein system, allowing blood flow to go from the deep to the superficial veins. During calf muscle relaxation, the pressure difference (high pressure in the superficial veins) allows blood flow from the superficial to deep veins. Venous ulcers are associated with venous hypertension, which is defined as sustained elevated venous pressures during ambulation. Venous hypertension results from failure of the calf muscle pump, which normally assists in venous return. Blood reflux from the deep to superficial veins creates the sustained high pressure in the superficial vein system and therefore increased cutaneous blood flow. Valvular incompetence, vein distention, muscular weakness, and a decreased in the range of motion of the ankle may lead to calf muscle pump failure. Alterations in the microcirculation because of calf muscle pump failure ultimately lead to ulceration.

How does the skin ulcerate in patients with venous insufficiency? The mechanism of cutaneous ulceration as a consequence of venous insufficiency remains unknown. Several hypotheses have been reported since the beginning of the 20th century. In the early 1980s, Browse and Burnard suggested that venous hypertension could lead to endothelial distention, causing extravasation of fibrinogen into the interstitial fluid, which results in "pericapillary fibrin cuff" formation around the capillary vessels. Fibrin cuffs act as a barrier to diffusion of oxygen and nutrients, causing ischemia and ulcer formation. A few years later, Coleridge and colleagues suggested that venous hypertension could lead to decreased capillary perfusion, resulting in leukocyte trapping. The trapped leukocytes release proteolytic enzymes, which result in free radical formation and capillary damage. The increased capillary permeability causes extravasation of fibrinogen and other metabolites, which leads to formation of a fibrin cuff around the capillaries and ultimately ischemia.

Further studies supported the presence of increased levels of monocyte aggregation. Claudy and colleagues showed that leukocyte activation caused release of tumor necrosis factor alpha (TNF-α), ultimately leading to pericapillary fibrin cuff formation. In 1993, Falanga and Eaglstein observed that fibrin cuffs were discontinuous around capillaries and therefore did not form a barrier to oxygen and nutrients causing ischemia. They also postulated the "trap" hypothesis, which suggests that venous hypertension causes endothelial cell distention leading to extravasation of macromolecules (i.e., α_2-macroglobulin and fibrinogen) into the dermis. Moreover, α_2-macroglobulin can bind to growth factors, such as TNF-α and transforming growth factor beta (TGF-β), making them unavailable for wound repair. Patients with venous disease may have other factors that contribute to venous ulcer formation, such as systemic alteration in fibrinolysis and arteriovenous shunting. Despite all previously conducted studies and hypotheses, further research is needed to explain the mechanism of cutaneous ulceration resulting from venous insufficiency.

Evaluation and Diagnosis

The typical location for a venous ulcer is around the medial aspect of the lower extremity near the ankle (medial malleolus) or the gaiter area. The ulcer usually begins as a blister or erosion on the skin. Ulcer borders are irregular and usually smooth. The base of the ulcer may be covered with granulation tissue or yellow slough, or both.

Venous ulcers are associated with presence of pigmentation, erythema, dermatitis, edema, and induration (i.e., lipodermatosclerosis) of the surrounding skin and with varicose veins in the lower leg. Hemosiderin deposition resulting from red blood cell extravasation causes the surrounding hyperpigmentation. Lipodermatosclerosis, commonly known as an inverted bottle shape, is caused by sclerosis of the dermis and subcutaneous tissue. The presence of lipodermatosclerosis has been associated with a greater impairment of fibrinolysis in patients with venous ulcers and may be a poor prognostic factor for restriction of leg movement. Other known prognostic factors are duration and size of the ulcer and history of venous surgery. Ulcers present for longer than 6 months and larger than 5 cm^2 in diameter tend to be more refractory to therapy. Duration (27 months) and size (15.9 cm^2) were reported as poor prognostic factors.

A diagnosis of venous ulcers may be based on clinical presentation. The findings of a lower leg ulcer associated with lipodermatosclerosis or varicose veins, or both, suggest a venous ulcer. Other common findings include atrophie blanche (i.e., porcelain white scars with telangiectasia and dyspigmentation) and dermatitis. Venous dermatitis is associated with erythema, eczema, pruritus, and scaling of the skin. Contact dermatitis surrounding the ulcer may result from the use of topical agents.

Venous disease can be confirmed by a variety of techniques, including duplex ultrasound or plethysmography. However, it is critical that arterial disease be excluded because treatment with compression bandages is the mainstay of therapy and should be used cautiously in patients with arterial disease. A simple, noninvasive measurement to assess peripheral vascular disease is the ankle brachial index (ABI). This value is calculated by dividing the systolic pressure in the ankle by the systolic pressure in the arm. An ABI of less than 0.9 indicates peripheral vascular disease and represents an independent risk factor for vascular disease in other vascular beds, such as the coronary arteries. Care must be taken with diabetic or elderly patients who may have a falsely negative ABI value. All patients with an abnormal ABI value should be further evaluated. Consider a vascular consultation, magnetic resonance angiography (MRA), angioplasty, and stent bypass.

To aid in the exclusion of any underlying disease (e.g., hematologic disease, diabetes), initial laboratory tests should include complete blood cell (CBC) count with a differential count, chemistry panel, hemoglobin A_{1C}, prealbumin and albumin determinations, liver function tests, and levels of homocysteine, protein C and S, antithrombin III, and factor V Leiden.

Several vascular studies help in the diagnosis and severity of venous disease. Color duplex ultrasound is usually the initial study done to assess venous reflux in the lower extremities. Continuous-wave Doppler studies may yield false-negative results because it may be difficult to differentiate between the superficial and deep venous system. Air plethysmography and photoplethysmography are helpful in evaluating venous reflux and calf muscle dysfunction. Invasive venography is the gold standard to assess venous reflux, but it is used only as a last resort because of its invasive properties.

The CEAP classification was developed in 1994 by the American Venous Forum (AVF) to standardize the diagnosis and treatment of venous disease. It was based on clinical manifestations (C), etiologic factors (E), anatomic distribution of disease (A), and underlying pathophysiologic findings (P).

 CURRENT DIAGNOSIS

- Venous ulcers are the most common cause of lower extremity ulceration, affecting up to 8% of the world's population.
- Valvular incompetence, vein distention, muscular weakness, or a decrease in the range of motion of the ankle may lead to calf muscle pump failure.
- The mechanism of cutaneous ulceration resulting from venous insufficiency remains unknown.
- The typical location for a venous ulcer is around the medial malleolus.
- Complications of chronic venous ulcers are osteomyelitis and squamous cell carcinoma.
- Compression is the gold standard of treatment of venous disease.

Complications

Main complications of long-term or chronic venous ulcers are osteomyelitis and squamous cell carcinoma. A finding of exposed tendon or bone, in addition to suggesting an underlying osteomyelitis, suggests an ulcer with a nonvenous cause.

Radiographs and biopsy for histology and culture are appropriate first steps in evaluation. Consult an orthopedic surgeon for further analysis and treatment, which may include a bone biopsy and bone débridement.

Treatment

Compression is the gold standard of treatment of venous disease. After arterial disease has been excluded, reversal of the effects of venous hypertension through compression bandages and leg elevation is the cornerstone of therapy.

The goal of compression therapy is to deliver sustained graded compression with 30 to 40 mm Hg at the ankle. These bandages are applied circumferentially from the toes to the knees (involving the heel) with the foot dorsiflexed. The optimal method to deliver this pressure is through multilayered elastic compression dressings. Elastic compression dressings deliver compression during ambulation (i.e., walking) and at rest, accommodate to reduction in edema, and are superior to single-layered dressings. Inelastic compression (short-stretch compression) may deliver similar results but appear to require greater sophistication by those applying them to accomplish this. Inelastic bandages, which do not deliver compression at rest, may be advantageous in patients with arterial disease or patients who do not tolerate full compression (e.g., elderly). Patients with associated lymphatic damage may also benefit from pneumatic compression.

 CURRENT THERAPY

- Compression therapy is used to deliver a graded compression of 30 to 40 mm Hg at the ankle. Exclude arterial disease before using compression.
- Systemic medications as adjuvant therapy to compression bandages include aspirin,[1] pentoxifylline (Trental), or micronized purified flavonoid fraction (Daflon 500).[2]
- Other treatments, along with compression, include engineered skin, skin graft, electrical stimulation, locally derived growth factors, and venous surgery.
- The lifelong use of elastic compression stockings (30–40 mm Hg) is the mainstay of therapy.

[1]Not FDA approved for this indication.
[2]Not available in the United States.

Systemic medication as adjuvant therapy to compression bandages, such as pentoxifylline (Trental 400 to 800 mg three times daily[3]), aspirin,[1] or micronized purified flavonoid fraction (MPFF, Daflon 500[2] [diosmin[7] 90% and hesperidin[7] 10%]) may be superior to compression bandages alone with regard to the rate of healing. The use of pentoxifylline as adjuvant therapy to compression in venous ulcers has been shown to be very beneficial.

Wound bed preparation was proposed as a way to help the healing process. It is a multistep process that improves the wound bed by removing necrotic and fibrinous wound tissue, increasing the amount of granulation tissue, and decreasing edema, chronic wound fluid (i.e., exudate), and bacterial burden.

Local care is best accomplished with occlusive dressings. Occlusive dressings provide a moist environment for healing. A variety of types of occlusions may be used, and the choice depends on several factors, including the location of the wound and the amount of fibrinous slough and exudate present. A fear of excessive infection with the use of occlusive dressings is unfounded. Topical antiseptics and cleansing agents should be used with caution because they may prolong healing. Topical agents such as cadexomer iodine (Iodosorb), silver-impregnated dressings, and topical anesthetics are alternatives that do not prolong healing, but they should be applied directly to the wound because they may lead to skin sensitization.

Up to 50% of venous ulcers may be refractory to compression therapy alone. This refractory subset may be predicted by baseline characteristics (size and duration) and by a decrease in size with 2 to 4 weeks of treatment (Fig. 1). Other available treatments include tissue-engineered skin, autologous skin, electrical stimulation, treatment with locally delivered growth factors, and venous surgery. Three categories exist for skin grafts: autograft, allogeneic (cultured), and artificial (tissue-engineered skin). Two types of autografts are full-thickness (FTSG) and split-thickness (STSG) skin grafts. The latter is commonly used by expanding it with a meshing technique.

Apligraf, a bilayered engineered living skin composed of keratinocytes and fibroblasts from neonatal foreskin, is approved by the FDA

---

[1]Not FDA approved for this indication.
[2]Not available in the United States.
[3]Exceeds dosage recommended by the manufacturer.
[7]Available as a dietary supplement.

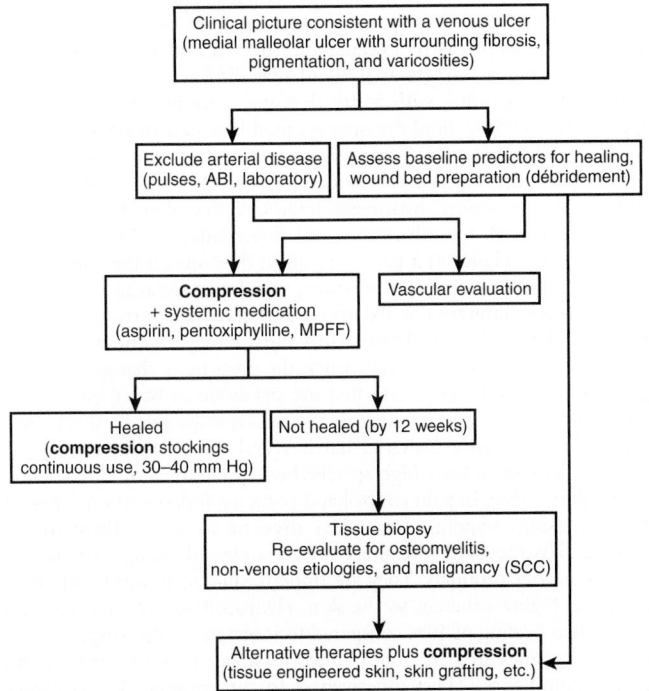

FIGURE 1. Simplified algorithm for the diagnosis and treatment of patients with venous ulcers. *Abbreviations*: ABI = ankle-brachial index; MPFF = micronized purified flavonoid fraction.

for treatment of venous leg and diabetic neuropathic foot ulcers. Surgical treatment of incompetent superficial and perforator veins along with standard of care (i.e., compression) reduce the risk of recurrence.

After healing occurs, patients with venous insufficiency are at risk for recurrence. The lifelong use of elastic compression stockings (30–40 mm Hg) is the mainstay of therapy, but early intervention after recurrence is critical. Health professionals need to understand the importance of further research to ultimately minimize the psychological, physical, and socioeconomic impact that ulcers caused by venous insufficiency have on patients and society.

REFERENCES

Abbade LP, Lastória S. Venous ulcer: Epidemiology, physiopathology, diagnosis and treatment. Int J Dermatol 2005;44:449–56.
Browse NL, Burnand KG. The cause of venous ulceration. Lancet 1982;2:243–5.
Claudy AL, Mirshahi M, Soria C, et al. Detection of undegraded fibrin and tumor necrosis factor alpha in venous leg ulcers. J Am Acad Dermatol 1991;25:623–7.
Coleridge-Smith PD, Thomas P, Scurr JH, et al. Causes of venous ulceration: A new hypothesis? Br Med J 1988;296:1726–7.
Falanga V, Eaglstein WH. The trap hypothesis of venous ulceration. Lancet 1993;341:1006–8.
Jull A, Arroll B, Parag V, Waters J. Pentoxyphilline for treating venous leg ulcers. Cochrane Database Syst Rev 2007;(3):CD001733.
Kirsner R. Wound bed preparation. Ostomy Wound Manage 2003;(Feb, Suppl.):2–3.
Kirsner RS, Falanga V. Techniques of split-thickness skin grafting for lower extremity ulcerations. J Dermatol Surg Oncol 1993;19:779–83.
Kirsner RS, Pardes JB, Eaglstein WH, Falanga V. The clinical spectrum of lipodermatosclerosis. J Am Acad Dermatol 1993;28:623–7.
Lazarus GS, Cooper DM, Knighton DR, et al. Definitions and guidelines for assessment of wounds and evaluation of healing. Arch Dermatol 1994;130:489–93.
Olin JW, Beusterien KM, Childs MB, et al. Medical costs of treating venous stasis ulcers: Evidence from a retrospective cohort study. Vasc Med 1999;4:1–7.
Phillips TJ, Machado F, Trout R, et al. Prognostic indicators in venous ulcers. J Am Acad Dermatol 2000;43:627–30.
Trent JT, Falabella A, Eaglstein WH, Kirsner RS. Venous ulcers: Pathophysiology and treatment options. Ostomy Wound Manage 2005;51:38–54.

Pressure Ulcers

Method of
David R. Thomas, MD

A pressure ulcer is the visible evidence of pathologic changes in blood supply to the dermal and underlying tissues, usually because of compression of the tissue over a bony prominence.

A differential diagnosis of ulcer type is critical to treatment. Chronic ulcers of the skin include arterial ulcers, venous stasis ulcers, diabetic ulcers, and pressure ulcers. Pressure ulcers generally appear in soft tissue over a bony prominence. A classic presentation aids the diagnosis. For example, arterial ulcers occur in the distal digits or over a bony prominence, diabetic ulcers occur in regions of callus formation, and venous stasis ulcers occur on the lateral aspect of the lower leg. However, atypical presentations may occasionally obscure the etiology. The treatment of these various etiologies differs considerably. This discussion is limited to the treatment of pressure ulcers and should not be used to treat other types of ulcers.

Seven principles of management guide treatment of pressure ulcers. The chief cause of these ulcers is pressure applied to the tissues that compromises blood flow. Therefore, the first treatment principle is to relieve pressure. Pressure relief can be obtained by positioning the patient frequently at a fixed interval to relieve pressure over the compromised area. Turning and positioning may be difficult to achieve because of a patient's self-positioning or medical treatments that interfere with the ability to position the patient. Because of this difficulty, a number of medical devices are designed in an attempt to relieve

CURRENT DIAGNOSIS

- Differentiate among pressure, diabetic, venous stasis, and arterial ulcers.

pressure. These devices can be classified as static or dynamic. Static devices include air-, gel-, or water-filled containers that reduce the tissue–surface interface. Dynamic devices use a power source to fill compartments with air that support the patient's weight or alternate the pressure on different areas of the body. Choose a static device when the patient has good bed mobility. Choose a dynamic device when the patient cannot self-position in bed.

At the present time, results of reported clinical trials do not favor one device over another. The choice should be based on durability, ease of use, and patient comfort. A simple check for so-called bottoming out should be done for all devices. Your hand should be inserted palm upward under the patient's sacrum between the device and the bed surface. If there is not an air column between the patient and the bed surface, the device is ineffective and should be changed. No device is effective in reducing heel pressure, the second most common site for pressure ulcers. Bridging with pillows is effective in reducing heel pressure in immobile patients; patients with high bed mobility may require boot devices to elevate the heel off the bed surface. Patients who fail to improve or who have multiple pressure ulcers should be considered for a dynamic-type device, such as a low-air-loss bed or air-fluidized bed.

Studies in turning and positioning suggest an optimum interval of 4 hours while on a pressure-reducing device. More frequent turning schedules, including the often-suggested 2-hour interval, have not been demonstrated to prevent pressure ulcers.

The second principle of pressure ulcer therapy is to assess pain. Pressure ulcers do not always result in pain, particularly in insensate patients. However, some pressure ulcers do result in pain and should be treated aggressively. Oral or parenteral pain medications should be used to control symptoms.

The third principle of ulcer therapy is to assess nutrition and hydration. Pressure ulcers occur in sicker individuals in whom nutrient intake may be reduced by coexisting illness. Increased intake of protein (1.2 to 1.5 g/kg/day) is associated with higher healing rates. Achievement of high protein intake may be difficult because of anorexia of aging or anorexia associated with coexisting diseases. Adequate calories, adjusted for stress (30 to 35 kcal/kg/day), should be prescribed. Adequate dietary intake should provide adequate vitamins and minerals. No difference in healing rates is associated with supratherapeutic doses of vitamin C or zinc. If adequate dietary intake is compromised, a supplemental vitamin/mineral prescription at RDA (recommended daily allowance) doses should be considered. Adequate hydration can be maintained by 30 mL/kg/day of water. The decision to institute enteral feeding in patients with pressure ulcers who are unable to maintain adequate oral intake should not be undertaken lightly. The decision to use enteral feeding must consider the patient's wishes, overall goal of care, and the complications of enteral feeding. In several studies, the long-term result of enteral feeding was associated with poorer outcomes in patients with pressure ulcers.

CURRENT THERAPY

Seven Principles of Pressure Ulcer Therapy

- Relieve pressure.
- Assess pain.
- Assess nutrition and hydration.
- Remove necrotic debris.
- Maintain a moist wound environment.
- Encourage granulation and epithelial tissue formation.
- Control infection.

The fourth principle of pressure ulcer management requires removing necrotic debris. Phagocytosis removes necrotic debris naturally. Accelerating the rate of removal may shorten healing time. Options include sharp surgical débridement, mechanical débridement with gauze dressings, application of exogenous enzymes, or autolytic débridement under occlusive dressings. Choose surgical débridement if the ulcer is infected. Surgical débridement is the fastest method but may remove some viable tissue, cause discomfort, and is the most expensive method, especially if done in an operating room. Applying moist gauze that is allowed to adhere to the ulcer bed by drying is a form of débridement. When the dry dressing is removed, nonselective tissue removal occurs. This method can be associated with discomfort, may delay healing while débridement is in progress, and is often defeated when the dressing is remoistened before removal. Enzymatic débridement can digest necrotic material. Only one enzymatic preparation is currently available in the United States: collagenase. Enzyme preparations are nonselective, possibly resulting in some damage to fibroblasts, epithelial cells, or granulation tissue. Enzymatic débridement is slower, can be associated with discomfort, and should be limited in duration until a clean wound bed is obtained. Autolytic débridement is achieved by allowing autolysis under an occlusive dressing. Both enzymatic and autolytic débridement may require 2 to 6 weeks to achieve a clean wound bed. A total of five clinical trials did not show that enzymatic agents increased the rate of complete healing in chronic wounds compared to control treatment. Unless clinically infected, heel ulcers are better left undébrided because they occur in poorly vascularized tissues.

The fifth principle of pressure ulcer management is to maintain a moist wound environment. Maintaining a moist wound environment is associated with more rapid healing rates compared to dressings that are allowed to dry. Continuously moist saline gauze is the historical standard dressing for stage II through IV pressure ulcers. Care must be taken to change the gauze frequently to prevent drying because this may delay healing. Newer wound dressings provide a low moisture vapor transmission rate (MVTR), a measure of how quickly the dressing allows drying. A MVTR of less than 35 g of water vapor per square meter per hour is required to maintain a moist wound environment. Woven gauze has a MVTR of 68 g/m²/hour, and impregnated gauze has a MVTR of 57 g/m²/hour. By comparison, hydrocolloid dressings have a MVTR of 8 g/m²/hour. Dressings with low MVTR provide a healing environment that encourages granulation tissue formation and epithelialization.

The use of occlusive-type dressings is more cost effective than gauze dressings primarily because of a decrease in nursing time for dressing changes. A meta-analysis of five clinical trials comparing a hydrocolloid dressing with a dry dressing demonstrated that treatment with a hydrocolloid dressing resulted in a statistically significant improvement in the rate of pressure ulcer healing (odds ratio: 2.6).

Occlusive dressings can be divided into broad categories of polymer films, polymer foams, hydrogels, hydrocolloids, alginates, and biomembranes. Each has advantages and disadvantages. No single agent is perfect. The choice of a particular agent depends on the clinical circumstances. Nonpermeable polymers can be macerating to normal skin. Polymer films are not absorptive and may leak, particularly when the wound is highly exudative. Most films have an adhesive backing that may remove epithelial cells when the dressing is changed. Hydrogels are hydrophilic polymers that are insoluble in water but absorb aqueous solutions and are available in amorphous gels or sheet dressings. They are poor bacterial barriers and are nonadherent to the wound. Because of their high specific heat, these dressings are cooling to the skin, aiding in pain control and reducing inflammation. Most of these dressings require a secondary dressing to secure them to the wound. Hydrocolloid dressings are complex dressings similar to ostomy barrier products. They are impermeable to moisture and bacteria and highly adherent to the skin. Hydrocolloid dressings have an accelerated healing of 40% compared to moist gauze dressings. Hydrocolloid dressings are particularly suited for areas subject to urinary and fecal incontinence. Their adhesiveness to surrounding skin is higher than some surgical tapes, but they are nonadherent to wound tissue and do not damage epithelial tissue in the wound. The adhesive barrier is frequently overcome in highly exudative wounds. Hydrocolloid dressings should be used cautiously over tendons or on wounds with eschar formation. Alginates are complex polysaccharide dressings that are highly absorbent in exudative wounds. This high absorbency is particularly suited to exudative wounds. Alginates are nonadherent to the wound, but if the wound is allowed to dry, damage to the epithelial tissue may occur with removal. Alginates may be used under other dressings to absorb exudate. The biomembranes are very expensive and not readily available.

Stages I and II pressure ulcers can be managed with a polymer film or hydrocolloid dressing. Stages III and IV pressure ulcers may be treated with a film or hydrocolloid dressing. In addition, some stage III and IV wounds with dead space or tunneling may require a wound filler, such as a calcium alginate or an amorphous hydrogel, to obliterate dead space and decrease potential for anaerobic colonization.

Vacuum-assisted closure is used in both acute and chronic wounds. Only two randomized, controlled trials in pressure ulcers are reported. In both trials, vacuum-assisted closure was not superior to treatment with a hydrogel or moistened gauze, at a higher cost.

Electrotherapy is used for stages III and IV pressure ulcers unresponsive to conventional therapy. Several clinical trials suggest that electrotherapy is likely to be marginally effective. Hyperbaric oxygen, ultrasound, infrared, ultraviolet, and low-energy laser irradiation have insufficient data to recommend their use currently. No data support the use of a systemic vasodilator, hemorheologics, serotonin inhibitors, or fibrolytic agents in the treatment of pressure ulcers. Topical agents such as zinc, phenytoin,[1] aluminum hydroxide,[1] honey, sugar, yeast, aloe vera gel, or gold[1] were not effective in clinical trials.

Because the theory of augmenting ulcer healing under the newer dressings suggests that wound fluid contains favorable healing factors, it is important not to change the dressings too frequently. Unless the wound fluid seeps from under the dressing, it should not be changed more often than every 3 to 7 days.

The sixth principle of pressure ulcer treatment is to encourage granulation tissue formation and promote reepithelialization. Growth factors show promising early results, but the data do not suggest accelerated healing of pressure ulcers. It is important not to affect granulation and epithelial tissue negatively. A number of wound cleaners and antiseptics are toxic to fibroblasts and epithelial tissues, including benzalkonium chloride, povidone-iodine solution (Betadine), Dakin's solution, hydrogen peroxide, Granulex, Hibiclens, and pHisoHex. The use of these agents in a pressure ulcer should be limited to use in infected ulcers and strictly limited in duration.

The seventh principle of pressure ulcer management is to control infection. Quantitative microbiology alone is a poor predictor of clinical infection in chronic wounds. All pressure ulcers are colonized with bacteria, usually from skin or fecal flora. The presence of microorganisms alone (colonization) does not indicate an infection in pressure ulcers. The diagnosis of infection in chronic wounds must be based on clinical signs: erythema, warmth, pain, edema, odor, fever, or purulent exudate. In the presence of clinical signs of infection, enteral or parenteral antibiotics should be used. In ulcers that are not progressing toward healing, an empirical trial of topical antimicrobials may be considered, although the data are inconclusive.

REFERENCES

Thomas DR. The role of nutrition in prevention and healing of pressure ulcers. Geriatr Clin North Am 1997;13:497–512.

Thomas DR. Are all pressure ulcers avoidable? J Am Med Dir Assoc 2001;2:297–301.

Thomas DR. Improving the outcome of pressure ulcers with nutritional intervention: A review of the evidence. Nutrition 2001;17:121–5.

Thomas DR. Issues and dilemmas in managing pressure ulcers. J Gerontol Med Sci 2001;56:M238–340.

Thomas DR. Prevention and management of pressure ulcers. Rev Clin Gerontol 2001;11:115–30.

Thomas DR. The promise of topical nerve growth factors in the healing of pressure ulcers. Ann Intern Med 2003;139:694–5.

Thomas DR. Management of pressure ulcers. J Am Med Dir Assoc 2006;7:46–59.

Thomas DR. Managing pressure ulcers: Learning to give up cherished dogma. J Am Med Dir Assoc 2007;8:347–8.

Thomas DR. Prevention and management of pressure ulcers. Clin Rev Gerontol 2008;17:1–17.

Atopic Dermatitis

Method of
Peck Y. Ong, MD

Atopic dermatitis (AD) is a chronic inflammatory skin disease that is characterized by itch and a predilection of eczema on extensor areas in young infants or flexural areas in older children and adults. In the United States, AD affects about 15% of children and 2% of adults. For more than 85% of patients, AD begins during the first 5 years, but 50% of the children with AD improve significantly or outgrow the disease by age 7. The persistence of AD depends on various factors: early onset, severity, family history of AD, personal history of asthma, and food or inhalant allergies.

The itch associated with AD causes significant discomfort in these patients and often leads to sleep loss and to poor school or work performance. The quality of life of children with generalized AD is worse than that for children with diabetes, epilepsy, asthma, cystic fibrosis, or renal disease. The maternal stress in taking care of children with moderate to severe AD is equivalent to that associated with care of children with diabetes, Rett syndrome, profound deafness, or the need for enteral feeding.

Pathophysiology

AD is caused by a combination of genetic and environmental factors. Patients with AD have a defective skin barrier. This leads to a loss of skin hydration and susceptibility to environmental triggers. There is evidence that the skin barrier defects of AD are caused by genetic mutations. Studies have shown that many AD patients carry a genetic mutation in filaggrin, a protein with important barrier function.

Potential external triggers of AD include microbial pathogens and environmental allergens. Almost 100% of AD skin lesions are colonized by *Staphylococcus aureus*, which may produce toxins that trigger immune response in the skin. As a result, AD patients produce an increased amount of pro-allergic cytokines, such as interleukin-4 (IL-4), IL-5, and IL-13 in their skin. These cytokines lead to an increased infiltration of inflammatory T cells and eosinophils. IL-4 and IL-13 also are important for the production of serum IgE, the level of which is elevated in AD patients.

Diagnosis and Clinical Assessment

Most AD patients can be diagnosed by clinical history and physical examination. Typical presentation includes itch, dryness, flexural dermatitis, early age of onset, and atopy such as multiple food allergies. Patients with generalized eczema or adult-onset eczema can present as a diagnostic challenge. The differential diagnosis includes immunodeficiency (e.g., hyper-IgE syndrome, Omenn syndrome), malignancy (e.g., cutaneous T-cell lymphoma), zinc deficiency (i.e., acrodermatitis enteropathica), and celiac-associated dermatitis (i.e., dermatitis herpetiformis) (Table 1). AD children seldom present with failure to thrive, unless they are under severe dietary restriction.

Atopic Dermatitis

TABLE 1   Differential Diagnoses of Atopic Dermatitis

Disease Category	Differential Diagnoses
Dermatologic diseases	Contact dermatitis, seborrheic dermatitis, psoriasis, dyshidrotic eczema, eosinophilic pustular folliculitis, ichthyosis vulgaris
Neoplastic diseases	Cutaneous T-cell lymphoma, Langerhans cell histiocytosis
Immunodeficiencies	Hyper-IgE syndrome, severe combined immunodeficiency, Omenn syndrome, IPEX (immune dysregulation, polyendocrinopathy, enteropathy X-linked) syndrome
Infectious diseases	Scabies, cutaneous candidiasis, tinea versicolor
Nutritional deficiencies	Acrodermatitis enteropathica (zinc deficiency), essential fatty acid deficiency, biotin deficiency
Multisystemic disorders	Netherton syndrome, dermatitis herpetiformis

Failure to thrive should therefore prompt further investigation. Punch skin biopsies may be needed when the diagnosis is still unclear.

The prevalence of mild, moderate, and severe AD is 80%, 18%, and 2%, respectively. Most patients with mild to moderate disease have flexural, extensor, or facial involvement, whereas patients with severe disease often present with total-body involvement with or without erythroderma (Fig. 1). Validated scales for assessing the severity of AD include Scoring of Atopic Dermatitis (SCORAD) and Eczema Area and Severity Index (EASI). These scoring systems or a simplified diagram documenting the extent of dermatitis are useful for more objective follow-up of the patient's progress.

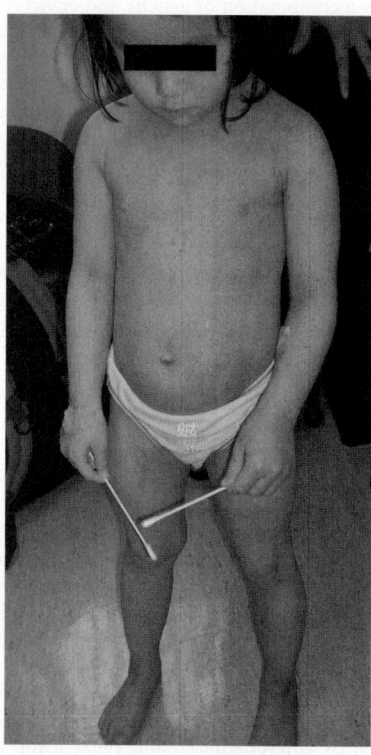

FIGURE 1. Generalized atopic dermatitis.

CURRENT DIAGNOSIS

- Itch must be present for the diagnosis of atopic dermatitis. In addition, the diagnosis must include three or more of the following criteria (U.K. Working Party's Diagnostic Criteria for Atopic Dermatitis):
  - History of generalized dry skin
  - Visible flexural dermatitis
  - Onset of the skin condition before 2 years (not used for patients younger than 4 years)
  - History of itchy skin involving the following areas: elbows, behind knees, front of ankles, or around the neck
  - History of asthma or allergic rhinitis (or for children younger than 4 years, history of atopic disease in a first-degree relative)

Management of Atopic Dermatitis and Associated Conditions

DAILY MAINTENANCE CARE

Changes in humidity can adversely affect AD symptoms. Dry conditions lead to increased transepidermal water loss and dry AD skin. Extreme heat, humidity, and sweating may lead to irritation of AD skin. AD patients are at increased risk for contact or irritant dermatitis, which may occur with over-the-counter topical skin medications that contain multiple ingredients. Wool or synthetic acrylic fabrics may also be irritating to AD skin.

To improve barrier function, AD patients should bathe or shower for 10 to 20 minutes once or twice daily, followed immediately by gently drying the skin and applying an emollient on the unaffected areas and a topical antiinflammatory medication on the affected areas. A petrolatum-based emollient is recommended in infants and young children because of its occlusive property. In older children and adults, the ointment may not be tolerated well because of its greasy feel, and another emollient or moisturizer may be chosen based on the patient's preference or experience.

Itch may continue to be a problem even if the rash has improved. The mechanisms of itch in AD are not fully understood but do not appear to be mediated solely by histamine. The use of first-generation antihistamines (diphenhydramine [Benadryl] and hydroxyzine [Vistaril]) in AD largely depend on their sedative effects and are best used at bedtime. The second-generation, nonsedating antihistamines such as loratadine (Claritin)[1] and cetirizine (Zyrtec)[1] have not proved helpful in treating AD.

TOPICAL AND SYSTEMIC MEDICATIONS

The first-line medication for AD is a topical corticosteroid (TCS). For mild AD, a TCS with group VI and VII potency (Table 2) may suffice. However, for moderate to severe AD, a TCS with at least group III to V potency is chosen to increase efficacy and to shorten the duration of need for these medications.

The use of TCS is confronted with various obstacles, including rare side effects such as skin atrophy, but mostly with patients' or parents' misunderstanding of TCS. Studies have shown that twice-daily use of fluticasone propionate (Cutivate) 0.05% cream (group V) and desonide (DesOwen, Tridesilon) 0.05% ointment or aqueous gel (group V and VI, respectively) continuously up to 1 month in young children with AD resulted in no significant adverse effect. It is therefore important to clarify for patients or parents the safety and side effects based on the potency of the TCS.

[1]Not FDA approved for this indication.

TABLE 2 Classification of Topical Corticosteroids Based on Potency

Group	Topical Corticosteroids
I (most potent)	Clobetasol propionate 0.05% (Temovate) (cream, ointment, gel), betamethasone dipropionate, augmented 0.05% (Diprolene) (cream, ointment), diflorasone diacetate 0.05% (Psorcon) (ointment)
II	Amcinonide 0.1% (Cyclocort) (ointment), betamethasone dipropionate 0.05% (Diprosone) (ointment), mometasone furoate 0.1% (Elocon) (ointment), halcinonide 0.1% (Halog) (cream), fluocinonide 0.05% (Lidex) (gel, cream, ointment), desoximetasone (Topicort) (0.05% gel, 0.25% cream, 0.25% ointment)
III	Fluticasone propionate 0.005% (Cutivate) (ointment), amcinonide 0.1% (Cyclocort) (lotion, cream), diflorasone diacetate 0.05% (Florone) (cream), betamethasone valerate 0.1% (Valisone) (ointment)
IV	Flurandrenolide 0.05% (Cordran) (ointment), mometasone furoate 0.1% (Elocon) (cream), triamcinolone acetonide 0.1% (Kenalog) (cream), fluocinolone acetonide 0.025% (Synalar) (ointment), hydrocortisone valerate 0.2% (Westcort) (ointment)
V	Flurandrenolide 0.05% (Cordran) (cream), fluticasone propionate 0.05% (Cutivate) (cream), hydrocortisone butyrate 0.1% (Locoid) (cream), fluocinolone acetonide 0.025% (Synalar) (cream), desonide 0.05% (Tridesilon) (ointment), betamethasone valerate 0.1% (Valisone) (cream), hydrocortisone valerate 0.2% (Westcort) (cream), prednicarbate 0.1% (Dermatop) (cream)
VI	Alclometasone dipropionate 0.05% (Aclovate) (cream, ointment), fluocinolone acetonide 0.01% (Synalar) (solution, cream) (Derma-Smoothe/FS Oil), Desonide 0.05% (Tridesilon) (cream and aqueous gel)
VII (least potent)	Hydrocortisone 1%/2.5% (lotion, cream, ointment).

Data from Stoughton RB: Vasoconstrictor assay—specific applications. In Maibach HI, Surber C (eds): Topical Corticosteroids. Basel, Switzerland: Karger, 1992, p 42–53.

Topical calcineurin inhibitors (TCI) (pimecrolimus [Elidel] 1% cream and Protopic/tacrolimus ointment) are alternative nonsteroidal antiinflammatory medications for AD. Elidel is indicated for mild to moderate AD in patients older than 2 years, whereas 0.03% and 0.1% Protopic are indicated for moderate to severe AD in patients 2 to 15 years old and in patients 16 years old or older, respectively. Both Elidel and Protopic have an FDA black box warning saying that their long-term use may be associated with cancer risk. It is recommended that these medications be used on a short-term and as-needed basis in minimal amounts. They continue to be useful alternatives for skin areas that are prone to atrophy, including the face, axillae, and groins.

A new class of topical medications (so-called barrier creams) emphasize skin barrier repair. These medications include Atopiclair, MimyX, Eletone, and EpiCeram. Only EpiCeram has been compared directly with TCS. It was shown to be as effective as fluticasone propionate 0.05% cream in children with moderate to severe AD in a preliminary study. Atopiclair and MimyX may be effective for patients with mild to moderate AD. There is no published study on Eletone. These barrier creams have no age limitations, but they require a prescription because they have been approved as a medical device by the FDA.

Wet-wrap treatment, phototherapy, and systemic immunosuppressive therapies (e.g., cyclosporine [Sandimmune, Neoral],[1] azathioprine [Imuran],[1] methotrexate [Trexall],[1] and mycophenolate mofetil [Cell-Cept][1]) are reserved for severe AD patients. Because of the potential serious adverse effects associated with these treatments, referral to an allergist or dermatologist is recommended before their initiation.

Systemic corticosteroids usually are not recommended for AD because of their known adverse effects, including stunted growth in children, adrenal suppression, osteoporosis, and cataracts. A rebound of AD symptoms is common after the medication is stopped. If a systemic corticosteroid is used, it should be tapered over a short period (e.g., a week) while topical antiinflammatory treatment is intensified.

[1]Not FDA approved for this indication.

The efficacy and side effects of the following medications have not been established in AD: intravenous immunoglobulin (IVIG), anti-IgE (omalizumab [Xolair][1]), probiotics,[7] montelukast (Singulair),[1] Chinese medicinal herbs,[7] and fish oils.[1]

FOOD ALLERGIES

At least 30% of children with moderate to severe AD have one or more food allergies, compared with 4% to 6% of the general population. Accurate diagnosis of food allergies in AD patients is crucial, because it can prevent life-threatening anaphylaxis or unnecessary food restriction.

The diagnosis of food allergy involves one or more of the following: history taking, skin tests, serum-specific IgE tests, and food challenge. History taking is helpful in the diagnosis of food allergy in most patients. It is often useful to begin by asking the patients whether they have any problems or reactions with any of the seven food allergens: milk, egg, peanut, wheat, soybean, seafood, and tree nuts. These foods account for more than 90% of food allergies. Almost all food allergic reactions occur in the first hour. AD patients may complain of immediate worsening of itching after ingestion. Symptoms of anaphylactic reactions include throat-clearing, cough, shortness of breath, vomiting, dizziness, fainting, and headache, which may be attributed to hypotension. Most food allergic reactions also manifest with skin symptoms, including hives, swelling, or generalized itching.

Skin tests are useful in the context of negative test results because they have a negative predictive value of more than 95%. A positive test result has only a 50% positive predictive value.

Quantitative serum-specific IgE antibodies (ImmunoCAP, Phadia) have become useful in the diagnosis of food allergies because of their high positive predictive values (Table 3). These tests are also

[1]Not FDA approved for this indication.
[7]Available as a dietary supplement.

TABLE 3 Predictability of ImmunoCAP-Specific IgE

Reaction*	Milk	Soy	Egg	Wheat	Peanut	Fish	Tree Nuts
Reaction highly probable	>15 kU/L	>60 kU/L	>7 kU/L	>80 kU/L	>14 kU/L	>20 kU/L	>15 kU/L
Reaction highly probable (young children)	>5 kU/L (<1 y)		>2 kU/L (<2 y)				

*Because of their high positive predictive values, quantitative serum-specific IgE antibodies are used in the diagnosis of food allergies.

useful for deciding whether a food challenge is necessary to confirm the diagnosis.

Although history, skin tests, and serum-specific IgE values are useful in the diagnosis of food allergy, a double-blind, placebo-controlled food challenge remains the gold standard in diagnosing food allergy. Food challenge should be done in consultation with an allergist because of the risk of anaphylaxis.

Patients with confirmed food allergy should avoid any amount of the food allergen. Parents or patients should be instructed to read food allergen labels carefully. All packaged foods in the United States are required to label the contents of milk, eggs, peanuts, wheat, soybeans, fish, shellfish, or tree nuts. Organizations, such as the Food Allergy and Anaphylaxis Network, can provide patients and parents with useful information on potential hidden food allergens and alternative food sources.

AD children often have multiple food allergies, including cow's milk and soy, and the use of a hydrolyzed or amino acid–based formula can provide an alternative source of nutrition. For these patients, consultation with a dietitian can be helpful in managing food avoidance and nutrition needs.

Patients or parents of children with anaphylactic reactions should be prescribed and instructed on the use of an epinephrine autoinjector (EpiPen or Twinject: 0.15 mg for patients who weigh more than 15 kg but less than 30 kg; 0.3 mg for patients who weigh 30 kg or more).

Delaying highly allergic foods in early childhood remains controversial. However, for infants who are at high risk for food allergy (e.g., children with AD and multiple food allergies), it is recommended that they avoid eggs, peanuts, tree nuts, fish, and shellfish in the first 3 years, unless there are major issues such as nutrition or social hindrance. Further studies are needed to confirm the role of this practice in preventing food allergies.

INFECTIONS

Most AD patients are colonized by *S. aureus* on their skin lesions or in their nostrils. The frequency of colonization increases with AD severity. Exacerbation of AD is frequently associated with secondary *S. aureus* skin infections. Other common skin pathogens in AD include group A β-hemolytic *Streptococcus* and herpes simplex virus (HSV), which causes eczema herpeticum (Fig. 2). Many reports have documented invasive *S. aureus* infections such as bacteremia, septic arthritis, osteomyelitis, and endocarditis in AD patients. Persistent fever or focal limb pain should alert the physician to the possibility of these infections.

The reasons for the high rate of bacterial colonization and skin infections in AD are not completely understood. A defective skin barrier and decreased cutaneous innate immunity (i.e., deficiency in natural skin antibiotics) likely contribute to the frequency of skin infections in patients with AD.

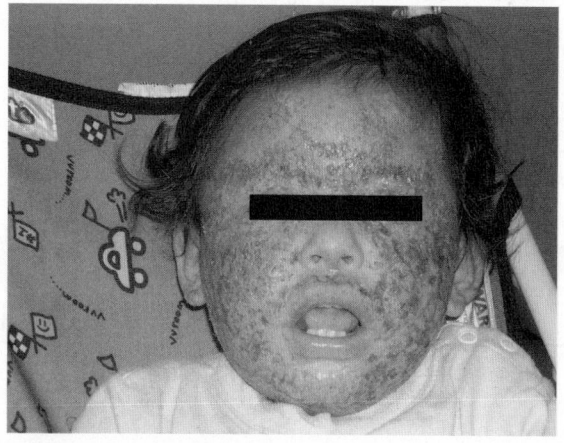

FIGURE 2. Eczema herpeticum.

CURRENT THERAPY

- Bathe or shower for 10 to 20 minutes daily and pat dry gently.
- Follow immediately by applying an emollient on unaffected areas and an antiinflammatory medication on affected areas.
- Use topical corticosteroids as a first-line antiinflammatory medication; alternative medications are topical calcineurin inhibitors or barrier creams.
- Avoid environmental triggers such as extreme heat, humidity, or dryness.
- Avoid food allergens that may cause anaphylaxis. Consult an allergist regarding the interpretation of serum-specific IgE tests or food challenge.
- Treat skin infection only when clinical signs are present (e.g., oozing, impetigo).
- Severe, generalized infection or vesicular lesions may indicate herpes simplex virus infection; persistent fever may indicate invasive *S. aureus* infection.

Because of the concern about increasing bacterial resistance, antibiotics are not recommended for treating *S. aureus* colonization in patients with AD. An area of active research involves the use of silver-coated fabrics or antimicrobial-coated silk fabrics to reduce *S. aureus* colonization and improve symptoms in AD patients.

INHALANT ALLERGIES AND ASTHMA

Eighty-five percent of AD infants have concurrent respiratory allergies or are at risk for allergic rhinitis or asthma. However, whether inhalant allergens lead to a worsening of AD remains controversial. Randomized, double-blind, placebo-controlled studies have shown positive and negative effects of house dust mites (HDM) as a trigger for AD symptoms. Because there is no serious side effect associated with the use of HDM-proof bed and pillow encasings, unless cost is an issue, these encasings are recommended for AD patients with HDM sensitization. Further research is needed to confirm the role of inhalant allergens, including furry pets and pollens as triggers for AD.

Investigational Treatments for Atopic Dermatitis

Because of the concern about potential side effects associated with existing therapies of AD, several agents are being investigated for the treatment of AD. They include a topical nuclear factor-κB decoy, phosphodiesterase 4 inhibitors, urocanic acid oxidation products, vitamin B[12],[1] *Vitreoscilla filiformis*, alefacept (Amevive),[1] and pitrakinra (Aerovant).[5] Subcutaneous and sublingual allergen immunotherapy may also be helpful in a subgroup of patients with HDM sensitization. Topical opioid receptor antagonists, systemic chymase inhibitors, and cannabinoid receptor agonists are potential anti-itch medications for AD.

REFERENCES

Beattie PE, Lewis-Jones MS. A comparative study of impairment of quality of life in children with skin disease and children with other chronic childhood diseases. Br J Dermatol 2006;155:145–51.
Bewley A. Dermatology Working Group: Expert consensus: Time for a change in the way we advise our patients to use topical corticosteroids. Br J Dermatol 2008;158:917–20.
Bock SA. Diagnostic evaluation. Pediatrics 2003;111:1638–44.

[1]Not FDA approved for this indication.
[5]Investigational drug in the United States.

Boguniewicz M, Zeichner JA, Eichenfield LF, et al. MAS063DP is effective monotherapy for mild to moderate atopic dermatitis in infants and children: A multicenter, randomized, vehicle-controlled study. J Pediatr 2008;152:854–9.

Eichenfield LF, Basu S, Calvarese B, et al. Effect of desonide hydrogel 0.05% on the hypothalamic-pituitary-adrenal axis in pediatric subjects with moderate to severe atopic dermatitis. Pediatr Dermatol 2007;24:289–95.

Elias PM. Barrier-repair therapy for atopic dermatitis: Corrective lipid biochemical therapy. Expert Rev Dermatol 2008;3:441–52.

Faught J, Bierl C, Barton B, Kemp A. Stress in mothers of young children with eczema. Arch Dis Child 2007;92:683–6.

Friedlander SF, Hebert AA, Allen DB. for the Fluticasone Pediatrics Safety Study Group: Safety of fluticasone propionate cream 0.05% for the treatment of severe and extensive atopic dermatitis in children as young as 3 months. J Am Acad Dermatol 2002;46:387–93.

Ong PY. Emerging drugs for atopic dermatitis. Expert Opin Emerg Drugs 2009;14:165–79.

Ong PY, Leung DYM. Immune dysregulation in atopic dermatitis. Curr Allergy Asthma Rep 2006;6:384–9.

Sampson HA. The evaluation and management of food allergy in atopic dermatitis. Clin Dermatol 2003;21:183–92.

Sugarman J, Parish L. A topical lipid-based barrier repair formulation (EpiCeram) cream is highly effective monotherapy for moderate-to-severe pediatric atopic dermatitis. J Invest Dermatol 2008;128(Suppl. 1):S54 [Abstract].

Erythema Multiforme, Stevens-Johnson Syndrome, and Toxic Epidermal Necrolysis

Method of
Erin Vanness, MD

Erythema multiforme (EM), Stevens-Johnson syndrome (SJS), and toxic epidermal necrolysis (TEN) were previously thought to represent a spectrum of one disorder and therefore have been traditionally grouped together. Current understanding of these disease entities allows us to separate EM from the latter two disorders. EM usually represents a hypersensitivity reaction to human herpes simplex virus type 1 or 2 (HSV-1, HSV-2) reactivation. SJS and TEN are severe, life-threatening drug hypersensitivity reactions that represent a spectrum of mucosal and cutaneous involvement. Exceptions are discussed in the following paragraphs.

Erythema Multiforme

DIAGNOSIS

EM is an abrupt, self-limited, but often recurrent eruption of symmetrically distributed papules, plaques, and targetoid erythematous to dusky red lesions that are fixed and have a predilection for the extensor and acral surfaces. Many patients also have oral erosions or targetoid lesions. Vesicles and bullae may evolve from the target lesions. Eye or genital involvement is not typical. Symptoms may include burning or pruritus. The skin heals without scarring, but transient hyperpigmentation is commonly seen.

Young adults are most commonly affected. EM is rare in the young and elderly. There should not be a prodrome or systemic illness associated with the eruption, although some patients report vague flulike symptoms. The eruption most commonly follows clinical or subclinical HSV-1 or HSV-2 reactivation. EM can uncommonly be associated with mycoplasma, histoplasmosis, or Epstein-Barr virus infection. An EM-like drug eruption and other similar clinical entities exist.

 CURRENT DIAGNOSIS

Erythema Multiforme

- Acute, symmetric, primarily extensor and acral eruption
- Oral lesions sometimes present
- Papules, plaques, targets, and blisters
- Preceding herpes simplex virus episode
- Young adults

Stevens-Johnson Syndrome and Toxic Epidermal Necrolysis

- Severe, potentially life-threatening hypersensitivity reactions
- Erythema and tenderness of skin and mucosa
- Subsequent extensive denudation of epithelium
- Associated prodrome and systemic illness

The clinician should consider the following in the differential diagnosis: subacute cutaneous lupus erythematosus; urticaria and urticarial vasculitis; gyrate erythema; multiple, fixed drug eruptions; granuloma annulare; polymorphous light eruption; and multiple forms of acute cutaneous small vessel vasculitis. Although EM is a clinical diagnosis, skin biopsy with interpretation by a dermatopathologist and appropriate laboratory work-up are helpful when indicated.

TREATMENT

Patients with isolated episodes or first episodes of erythema multiforme should be treated symptomatically, reassured, and educated about HSV and EM. HSV reactivation typically precedes the onset of EM by 3 to 14 days; antiviral medications are not beneficial after the eruption has commenced.

Symptomatic measures to reduce burning and pruritus include oral antihistamines (diphenhydramine [Benadryl] 25 to 50 mg PO every 6 hours as needed, weight-based dosage in children) and mid-potency topical corticosteroids (triamcinolone acetonide cream [Kenalog] 0.1% twice daily applied to affected skin; avoid the face). For oral involvement, gentle oral hygiene (saline rinses, very soft toothbrush, 0.2% chlorhexidine gluconate [Corsodyl] or the 0.12% concentration [Peridex] in the United States) and topical anesthetics (2% viscous lidocaine [Xylocaine Viscous] applied as pea-sized amount every 2 hours as needed) can help alleviate symptoms. A short burst of oral corticosteroids may be helpful for severe involvement of the oral mucosa (prednisone 0.5 to 1 mg/kg/day for 4 to 5 days).

 CURRENT THERAPY

Erythema Multiforme

- First episode: symptomatic care
- Recurrent episodes: prophylaxis with antivirals

Stevens-Johnson Syndrome and Toxic Epidermal Necrolysis

- Discontinue offending agents immediately
- Supportive care in intensive care unit or burn unit
- Skilled wound care (minimize manipulation, avoid débridement)
- Avoid and monitor for infection
- Pain control
- Ophthalmology consultation for eye involvement
- Consider intravenous immune globulin (IVIG, Baygam)[1] and cyclosporine (Sandimmune, Neoral)[1]

[1]Not FDA approved for this indication.

Patients who suffer from multiple recurrences of EM may be treated prophylactically with oral antiviral medications. When patients can identify the onset of the preceding HSV reactivation, episodic treatment initiated at the onset of the HSV prodrome may significantly reduce the severity and duration of the following EM. Treat with valacyclovir (Valtrex) 500 mg twice daily for 7 days. When patients have multiple recurrences (>6 per year) or cannot identify the preceding HSV activation, treat with valacyclovir 500 mg daily or acyclovir (Zovirax) 400 mg twice daily for at least 6 months. Some patients may achieve a remission at this point, and some may require further suppressive therapy.

Stevens-Johnson Syndrome and Toxic Epidermal Necrolysis

DIAGNOSIS

SJS and TEN are rare, severe, potentially fatal drug hypersensitivity reactions characterized by extensive denudation of skin or mucosal epithelium, or both, and they are accompanied by systemic illness. These entities are best considered on a diagnostic spectrum: SJS has less than 10% body surface area (BSA) with epidermal detachment and two or more mucosal surfaces involved; SJS/TEN overlap has 10% to 30% BSA with detachment and mucosal surfaces typically involved; and TEN has more than 30% detachment, and mucosal surfaces are usually involved. SJS is characterized by an EM-like eruption of the skin of variable severity (see earlier description of EM) and extensive mucosal erosions of at least two sites (i.e., lips or oral tissue, ocular tissue, and genital mucosae). TEN has a skin eruption characterized by dusky red plaques that rapidly progress to denuded, coalescing plaques with a shiny red base. Epidermal detachment can be elicited by placing lateral pressure on a dusky plaque (i.e., Nikolsky's sign).

The accompanying systemic illness usually correlates with the severity of the overall clinical picture. SJS or TEN has an initial flulike prodrome followed by various degrees of fever, lymphadenopathy, systemic toxicity with dehydration and electrolyte imbalance, toxic hepatitis, leukocytosis, anemia, proteinuria, and microscopic hematuria. Less commonly, there is involvement of the nasal, esophageal, pulmonary, and gastrointestinal mucosae; arthritis; myocarditis; and nephritis.

A causal drug can usually be identified. The eruption follows drug exposure by 1 week to 2 months. It is crucial that all potential causative drugs be discontinued immediately (Box 1). Other factors are thought to less frequently induce SJS (Box 2).

The clinician should consider autoimmune bullous disease (i.e., pemphigus, pemphigoid, paraneoplastic pemphigus, and linear IgA bullous dermatosis [LABD]), staphylococcal scalded skin syndrome (SSSS), bullous lupus Kawasaki disease, acute generalized exanthematous pustulosis, and acute graft versus host disease in the differential diagnosis. Biopsy of early lesional skin (with epidermis still attached) may reveal necrolysis and interface dermatitis and can help to rule out SSSS. Biopsy of perilesional, noninvolved skin for direct immunofluorescence can help to rule out autoimmune bullous disease.

TREATMENT

It is essential to immediately identify the offending agent and discontinue it. If several possible agents exist, they must all be immediately discontinued. Prompt discontinuation is associated with a 35% reduction in mortality per day (Table 1).

Supportive care is the mainstay of treatment of SJS or TEN. If systemic illness is significant or if the BSA involved exceeds 10% to 20%, the patient should be cared for in an intensive care unit or burn unit setting whenever possible.

Essential supportive care includes thermoregulatory equipment, monitoring, and replacement of fluid and electrolytes as indicated. A controlled-pressure thermoregulated bed is helpful. All care should be performed under sterile conditions, and isolation precautions are necessary to reduce infection risk. Wound care should be performed under the supervision of a dermatologist or burn specialist. Goals of wound care are to minimize manipulation and further denudation of skin, promote healing, reduce infection risk, and increase comfort. Isotonic saline can be used to cleanse involved skin once daily. Silicon or biologic dressings or skin equivalents may be left in place, but the surfaces and surrounding skin should be cleansed. Vaseline gauze may be used for limited BSA and in pressure sites. Mucosal surfaces,

---

BOX 2 Reported Causes of Stevens-Johnson Syndrome

- Drugs
- Bacterial infections
- Mycobacterial and mycoplasma infections
- Fungal infections (e.g., histoplasmosis, coccidioidomycosis)
- Viral infections
- Radiation therapy
- Inflammatory bowel disease
- Vaccines

BOX 1 Drugs Commonly Associated with Stevens-Johnson Syndrome and Toxic Epidermal Necrolysis*

- Sulfonamide antibiotics (trimethoprim-sulfamethoxazole [Bactrim])
- Aminopenicillins
- Quinolones
- Cephalosporins
- Tetracyclines
- Acetaminophen (Tylenol)
- Carbamazepine (Tegretol)
- Phenobarbital
- Valproic acid (Depakene)
- Nonsteroidal anti-inflammatory drugs (NSAIDS, oxicam group)
- Allopurinol (Zyloprim)
- Corticosteroids

*Many other drugs are reported to induce Stevens-Johnson syndrome and toxic epidermal necrolysis.

TABLE 1 SCORTEN: Predicted Mortality In Stevens-Johnson Syndrome and Toxic Epidermal Necrolysis

Prognostic Factor	Present	Absent
Age >40 y	1	0
Heart rate >120 beats/min	1	0
Malignancy present	1	0
Day 1 BSA >10%	1	0
Serum urea >10 mmol/L	1	0
Serum HCO_3 <20 mmol/L	1	0
Serum glucose >14 mmol/L	1	0
SCORTEN sum*		

SCORTEN Value	Predicted Mortality
0–1	3.7%
2	12.1%
3	35.8%
4	58.3%
5 or higher	90%

*SCORTEN is a severity-of-illness score developed for toxic epidermal necrolysis (TEN).

orifices, and crusts should be cleansed with saline several times daily, and mupirocin (Bactroban) ointment should be placed around orifices and in macerated areas twice daily.

An ophthalmologist should be consulted to manage ocular involvement and help prevent adhesions and scarring. Eyelids should be cleansed three times daily with saline and antibiotic ointment subsequently applied to the lids. Antibiotic drops should be instilled to protect the cornea. Gentle oral care with 0.2% chlorhexidine gluconate (0.12% in the United States) should be administered three to four times daily.

Pain control and nutritional support are imperative. Lines should be placed through noninvolved skin when possible and changed every 3 days with culture of the catheter tips. Routine cultures from involved skin and sputum can help to monitor for infection and guide treatment when necessary. Clinical infection should be treated quickly and aggressively.

There are no generally accepted evidence-based standards for specific therapy for SJS or TEN. When patients are stable with limited skin and mucosal involvement and do not seem to be progressing to worse disease, supportive care with close observation is most appropriate. If the patient has extensive or rapidly progressing disease, immunosuppressive therapy should be considered, weighing the risks and benefits, and started without delay if it is to be pursued.

Evidence from several case series and other reports supports the use of intravenous immunoglobulin (IVIG)[1] in TEN, but there also exists contradictory evidence from limited controlled trials that IVIG is not beneficial. If used, it should be started as early as possible in an attempt to halt progression to further BSA involvement. A dose of 1 g/kg for 3 consecutive days is recommended. Some case reports and a case series support the use of cyclosporine (Sandimmune, Neoral)[1] to reduce disease progression, but no randomized trials have been conducted to prove its efficacy. Although IVIG would usually be the drug of choice under current practice standards, cyclosporine may also be considered. Conflicting reports about the use of corticosteroids exist, and some evidence points to increased mortality associated with their use. However, evidence to the contrary was found in a retrospective analysis that showed reduced mortality associated with corticosteroid use. The rarity of SJS or TEN combined with the variability in patient and institutional factors and the bias inherent in retrospective studies has resulted in a paucity of evidence to support any specific therapy. Ultimately, treatment decisions must be made on an individual basis.

REFERENCES

Bachot N, Revuz J, Roujeau JC. Intravenous immunoglobulin treatment for Stevens-Johnson syndrome and toxic epidermal necrolysis; a prospective noncomparative study showing no benefit on mortality or progression. Arch Dermatol 2003;139:33–6.

Bastuji-Garin S, Fouchard N, Bertocchi M, et al. SCORTEN: A severity-of-illness score for toxic epidermal necrolysis. J Invest Dermatol 2000;115:149–53.

Craven N. Toxic epidermal necrolysis and Stevens-Johnson syndrome. In: Lebwohl M, et al., editors. Treatment of Skin Disease. London: Mosby; 2002. p. 633–6.

French LE, Prins C. Toxic epidermal necrolysis. In: Bolognia JL, et al., editors. Dermatology. Edinburgh: Mosby; 2003. p. 323–31.

Prins C, Kerdel FA, Padilla S, et al. Treatment of Toxic epidermal necrolysis with high-dose intravenous immunoglobulins: Multicenter retrospective analysis of 48 consecutive cases. Arch Dermatol 2003;139:26–32.

Roujeau JC, Kelly JP, Naldi L, et al. Medication use and the risk of Stevens-Johnson syndrome or toxic epidermal necrolysis. N Engl J Med 1995; 333:1600–7.

Schneck J, Fagot J, Sekula P, et al. Effects of treatments on the mortality of Stevens-Johnson syndrome and toxic epidermal necrolysis: A retrospective study on patients included in the prospective EuroSCAR Study. J Am Acad Dermatol 2008;58:33–40.

Schofield JK, Tatnall FM, Leigh IM. Recurrent erythema multiforme: Clinical features and treatment in a large series of patients. Br J Dermatol 1993;128:542–5.

Weston WL. Erythema multiforme and Stevens-Johnson syndrome. In: Bolognia J, et al., editors. Dermatology. Edinburgh: Mosby; 2003. p. 313–21.

[1]Not FDA approved for this indication.

Bullous Diseases

Method of
Craig N. Burkhart, MD, MS, David S. Rubenstein, MD, PhD, and Luis A. Diaz, MD

Bullous Pemphigoid

OVERVIEW

Bullous pemphigoid is an autoimmune blistering disease in which basal keratinocyte hemidesmosomal proteins are targeted by immunoglobulin (Ig)G autoantibodies, resulting in complement activation and neutrophil recruitment. Neutrophil proteases lead to subepidermal vesicles. Bullous pemphigoid is most commonly a generalized cutaneous disease affecting persons in the sixth to seventh decade. Nevertheless, localized, mucosal, pediatric, and young adult cases have been described.

Before pursuing treatment, the clinician must distinguish bullous pemphigoid from other blistering dermatoses such as erythema multiforme, epidermolysis bullosa acquisita, bullous systemic lupus erythematosus, and linear IgA disease. This is accomplished by histology, direct and indirect immunofluorescence, antigen-specific enzyme-linked immunosorbent assay (ELISA) and clinical history.

TREATMENT

Localized and Nonaggressive Disease

Less-aggressive, localized forms of bullous pemphigoid are amenable to conservative therapy. For instance, ultrapotent topical corticosteroids, such as clobetasol (Temovate) cream or ointment two or three times daily, can control localized disease without any systemic medications. Dapsone[1] may be used when topical corticosteroids are ineffective (Table 1). Therapy is begun at 50 mg/day for the first week. If no significant drop in the red or white blood cell count is detected, the dose is increased at weekly intervals by 50 mg a day until the disease responds or a maximum of 200 mg/day (100 mg twice daily) is reached. Once the disease is under control (as evidenced by the absence of new blister formation), the dapsone dose is decreased to the minimum that allows disease control. If no response is achieved within 6 weeks of reaching the maximum dose, then the patient is considered unresponsive to dapsone as a single agent.

[1]Not FDA approved for this indication.

CURRENT DIAGNOSIS

- All bullous diseases are diagnosed by combining clinical, histologic, and immunologic findings.
- The pemphigoid group is characterized by subepidermal bullae and autoantibodies to hemidesmosomal and hemidesmosome-related proteins.
- The pemphigus group is characterized by intraepidermal bullae and autoantibodies to desmosomal proteins.
- Clinical features such as scarring, mucosal involvement, pattern of cutaneous disease, and systemic findings are used to subclassify disease within the pemphigoid and pemphigus groups.

TABLE 1 Steroid-Sparing Agents

Medication	Contraindications	Baseline Labs	Initial Dose	Titration	Renal Dosing	Maximum Dose	Routine Labs	Important Side Effects	Long-Term Risks
Dapsone[1]	G6PD deficiency Sulfonamide allergy	G6PD, CBC with differential, LFTs, BUN, creatinine	50 mg PO qd	Increase every wk by 50 mg	Data not available	200 mg/d	CBC with differential Weekly × 1 mo Monthly × 5 mo Then q6mo	Hemolysis Methemoglobinemia Gastric distress Agranulocytosis Dapsone hypersensitivity syndrome Hepatitis	Peripheral neuropathy
Azathioprine (Imuran)[1]	TPMT deficiency	TPMT level, CBC with differential, LFTs, BUN, creatinine	50–100 mg PO qd	Increase every 4–6 wk by 0.5 mg/kg/d	Cl_{Cr} 10–50 mL/min: 75% of normal dose Cl_{Cr} <10 mL/min: 50% of normal dose	2.5 mg/kg	CBC with differential, LFTs, BUN, creatinine Weekly × 1 mo Biweekly × 1 mo Then bimonthly	Gastric distress Myelosuppression Hepatitis pancreatitis	Hematologic malignancy
Cyclophosphamide (Cytoxan)[1]	Neutropenia Active infection Bladder cancer History of hemorrhagic cystitis Pregnancy	CBC with differential, BUN, creatinine, urinalysis	1–2 mg/kg/d	Increase every 4–6 wk	Cl_{Cr} <10 mL/min: 75% of normal dose	2.5 mg/kg/d	CBC with differential, BUN, creatinine urinalysis Biweekly	Hemorrhagic cystitis, myelosuppression	Transitional cell carcinoma of the bladder
Mycophenolate mofetil (Cellcept)[1]	Active peptic ulcer disease HGPT deficiency (Lesch–Nyhan syndrome) Pregnancy	CBC with differential, BUN, creatinine, urine pregnancy test	500–1000 mg PO bid	Increase every 2–4 wk	Cl_{Cr} <25 mL/min: avoid dosing >2000 mg/d	3000 mg/d	CBC with differential Weekly × 1 mo Biweekly × 2 mo Then monthly	Myelosuppression Gastric distress	Lymphoma
Methotrexate[1]	Cirrhosis Active hepatitis Alcoholism Severe renal disease	CBC with differential, LFTs, BUN, creatinine	2.5 mg PO × 1	Increase every 2–4 wk by 2.5 mg	Cl_{Cr} 51–80 mL/min: 70% of dose Cl_{Cr} 10–50 mL/min: 30% of dose Cl_{Cr} <10 mL/min: avoid	15 mg/wk	CBC with differential, LFTs, BUN, creatinine Weeks 1, 2, 4, 8, and 12 Then q3mo	Gastric distress Myelosuppression Pneumonitis	Cirrhosis Lymphoma

[1]Not FDA approved for this indication.
BUN = blood urea nitrogen; CBC = complete blood count; Cl_{Cr} = creatinine clearance; G6PD = glucose-6-phosphate dehydrogenase; HGPT = hypoxanthine–guanine phosphoribosyltransferase; LFT = liver function test; TPMT = thiopurine methyltransferase.

Tetracycline (Sumycin)[1] and niacinamide[1] can also be effective for a nonaggressive or localized bullous pemphigoid, although in our hands its use has been unrewarding. Therapy is begun with tetracycline 500 mg four times daily and niacinamide 500 mg three times daily. If no new lesions develop after 1 month, the medications are slowly tapered. Baseline liver function tests (LFTs) should be obtained before and 1 month after initiation of therapy. Patients should be clinically monitored for signs of pseudotumor cerebri, photosensitivity, and hepatotoxicity. Gastric distress from tetracycline can be managed by decreasing its dose or changing to doxycycline (Doryx)[1] or minocycline (Dynacin).[1] Gastric distress and flushing from niacinamide require reducing its dose.

Aggressive and Generalized Disease

Because of their rapid onset of action, systemic corticosteroids are the first-line treatment of choice for aggressive, generalized bullous pemphigoid. Prednisone is begun at 1.0 mg/kg every morning and increased incrementally to 2.0 mg/kg in nonresponding patients. After 2 to 4 weeks in which no new blisters develop, the daily prednisone dose can be tapered by 5 mg every 2 to 4 weeks. At 30 mg/day, switch to alternate-day dosing by reducing the first day's dose by 2.5 mg every 2 weeks while maintaining the second day's dose at 30 mg/day. In the absence of recurrence, tapering of the second day's dose is then continued by 2.5 mg every 2 weeks. Patients on chronic prednisone should be followed for signs of infection, adrenal suppression, hypertension, diabetes, glaucoma, atherosclerosis, peptic ulcer disease, and osteoporosis.

Adjunctive therapies are initiated when bullous pemphigoid fails to respond rapidly to systemic prednisone and to limit side effects from chronic systemic corticosteroid use. The most commonly used agents are dapsone,[1] azathioprine (Imuran),[1] cyclophosphamide (Cytoxan),[1] mycophenolate mofetil (CellCept),[1] and methotrexate[1] (see Table 1). These agents are coadministered with systemic corticosteroids. Once disease has been under control for 6 weeks, the steroid-sparing agent is maintained at its current dose, and the systemic corticosteroid is tapered as above. After the corticosteroid taper is complete, the patient should remain on adjuvant therapy for an additional 3 to 6 months before discontinuing therapy.

Azathioprine and mycophenolate mofetil are excellent first-line adjuvants due to their great effectiveness and low toxicity when compared with other agents. Thiopurine methyltransferase (TPMT) levels may be helpful in guiding initial dosing (Table 2). If TPMT levels are not available, initiating therapy at a low dose (50 mg/day) and rechecking a complete blood count (CBC) with differential with every dosage increase (see Table 1) reduces the risk of severe myelosuppression. The most common side effect of mycophenolate mofetil, gastric distress, may be avoided by initiating therapy at 500 mg/day before titrating to its effective dose. Gastric distress can also occur with methotrexate and is minimized by supplementing folate (1 mg/day) on the 6 days of the week that methotrexate is not dosed.

---

[1]Not FDA approved for this indication.

 CURRENT THERAPY

- Localized nonscarring disease may be managed with topical corticosteroids alone.
- Progressive, scarring, or generalized disease requires early institution of systemic immunosuppressants.
- Close follow-up is required because all forms of immunosuppression are commonly complicated by side effects.
- Response to therapy is guided primarily by clinical findings.

Additional therapeutic options in treatment-resistant patients include plasmapheresis, intravenous immunoglobulin (IVIg),[1] and tumor necrosis factor α (TNF-α) antagonists.[1] All TNF-α antagonists should be avoided in patients with a personal or family history of demyelinating central nervous system disorders, uncontrolled congestive heart failure, or active infections. IVIg (400 mg/kg/day) appears effective, is relatively safe, and has few side effects; however, prohibitive cost can prevent its widespread use.

Cicatricial Pemphigoid

OVERVIEW

Also known as *mucous membrane pemphigoid*, cicatricial pemphigoid is a group of chronic, progressive, scarring autoimmune diseases that result from subepidermal blisters of mucosal surfaces or skin, or both. Pathogenic autoantibodies attach to hemidesmosomal proteins or proteins that link the hemidesmosome to anchoring fibrils. Cicatricial pemphigoid typically manifests with painful mucosal erosions and ulcerations of the oral cavity or irritation and scarring of the eyes. Involvement of other mucosal epithelia, including nasal, laryngeal, esophageal, urogenital, and anogenital, can cause significant morbidity from scarring and stenosis. Cicatricial pemphigoid can be clinically distinguished from bullous pemphigoid, which less commonly involves mucosal surfaces and does not cause scarring, and epidermolysis bullous acquisita, which occurs on trauma-prone surfaces and heals with scars and milia. Before initiating therapy, a diagnosis of cicatricial pemphigoid should be confirmed by histology and by direct and indirect immunofluorescence studies.

TREATMENT

The high morbidity associated with scarring in cicatricial pemphigoid requires an aggressive approach. Patients should be screened for signs and symptoms of ocular (conjunctivitis or burning, gritty, or dry sensations), laryngeal (hoarseness or dysphonia), and esophageal (dysphagia) involvement. If any of these signs or symptoms are present, early referral to the appropriate specialist (ophthalmologist, otolaryngologist, or gastroenterologist) is warranted.

Localized Cutaneous and Oral Disease

Disease localized to the skin or oral mucosa alone is occasionally controlled with local therapies. Ultrapotent corticosteroids (clobetasol), in an ointment or cream for application to the skin or in a gel or orabase for application to the oral mucosa, may be effective when applied two or three times daily. Alternatively, perilesional triamcinolone (usually 5–10 mg/mL suspension) to a maximum dose of 40 mg/mL can be injected every 4 weeks.

Unresponsive, Ocular, and Systemic Disease

Patients who fail to respond to local measures or who present with ocular or systemic disease require systemic therapy. Dapsone[1] is a highly effective first-line agent for cicatricial pemphigoid (see Table 1). If no response is obtained within 4 to 6 weeks, or if there are signs or symptoms of disease progression, systemic corticosteroids (1–2 mg/kg/day) should be initiated. Adjunctive agents (see Table 1) are added to gain better control of the disease and to aid in weaning from systemic corticosteroids. When these modalities fail, other modalities such as plasmapheresis and IVIg[1] may be tried.

Surgical repair of ocular deformities, laryngeal stenosis, or esophageal stenosis should be delayed until the disease is under good control to prevent further, surgically induced scarring. Increasing the dose of immunosuppressive medications in the perioperative period can also improve surgical outcomes.

---

[1]Not FDA approved for this indication.

TABLE 2 Recommended Azathioprine Dosing

TMPT Level (U/mL of RBC Lysates)	Azathioprine Dose
<5.0	None
5.0–13.7	0.5 mg/kg
13.7–19.0	1.5 mg/kg
>19.0	2.5 mg/kg

RBC = red blood cell; TPMT = thiopurine methyltransferase.

Pemphigus Vulgaris

OVERVIEW

Pemphigus is a group of autoimmune blistering diseases in which autoantibodies against desmoglein 3 (desmosomal glycoprotein) induce loss of cell–cell adhesion in the epidermis (acantholysis). The two major variants are pemphigus vulgaris and pemphigus foliaceous. Pemphigus vulgaris produces suprabasal splitting and pemphigus foliaceous produces upper epidermal splitting. The mechanism by which pemphigus vulgaris IgG induces blister formation is incompletely understood, but it might include proteinase activation, steric hindrance, or activation of transmembrane signaling.

The typical clinical presentation is a middle-aged (40 to 60 years) individual with painful erosions in the mouth. Patients can have coexistent cutaneous blisters and erosions or involvement of other mucosal surfaces (pharyngeal, laryngeal, esophageal, ocular, anal, or genital). Pemphigus vulgaris limited to mucosa is termed *mucosal pemphigus vulgaris*. Pemphigus vulgaris affecting the mucosa and skin is termed *mucocutaneous pemphigus vulgaris*. Before initiating treatment, the diagnosis of pemphigus vulgaris should be confirmed by histology, direct and indirect immunofluorescence, and antigen-specific ELISAs.

TREATMENT

Treatment of pemphigus vulgaris is guided in the short term by clinical findings and in the long term by laboratory findings. Systemic therapy should be initiated immediately alone or in combination with immunosuppressive agents. Once blistering stops and erosions have healed, indirect immunofluorescence titers are used to guide steroid and immunosuppressant tapering. Immunosuppression should only be tapered when patients are clinically in remission and indirect immunofluorescence titers are stable or decreasing. As a practical rule, we must educate the patient that the therapy will last for several months or years and that the response to therapy in individual patients is unpredictable.

Systemic corticosteroids (prednisone 1.0–2.0 mg/kg/day) are used first. If the disease fails to respond rapidly to systemic steroids (no new bullae or erosions within 1–2 weeks), adjuvant therapy should be initiated (see Table 1). As with bullous pemphigoid, azathioprine[1] and mycophenolate mofetil[1] are first-line adjuvants and titrated in the same manner as described for bullous pemphigoid. Azathioprine and mycophenolate mofetil are also effective as monotherapy in mild cases. As opposed to bullous pemphigoid, however, methotrexate,[1] tetracycline[1] plus niacinamide[1], and single-agent dapsone[1] are ineffective for pemphigus vulgaris. Tapering steroids and immunosuppressive agents should be very slow and gradual, we find the schedule described for bullous pemphigoid therapy is very useful in our patients.

Adjuvant IV immunoglobulins, TNF-α antagonists (etanercept [Enbrel][1] 50 mg subcutaneously twice weekly with prednisone), IVIg, plasmaphoresis, and rituximab (Rituxan)[1] (anti-CD20 chimeric monoclonal antibody) may be tried. In the future, medications targeting specific intracellular signaling events important in cell–cell adhesion may be used. For example, several p38 mitogen-activated protein kinase (MAPK) inhibitors are currently in phases II and III clinical trials for other inflammatory disorders and might show promise in the treatment of pemphigus vulgaris.

Pemphigus Foliaceus

OVERVIEW

Pemphigus foliaceus is a form of pemphigus in which superficial epidermal vesicles form as a result of the binding of pathogenic IgG autoantibodies against desmoglein 1, a desmosomal glycoprotein. Due to the superficial location of epidermal splitting, patients usually present with crusted, scaling plaques on the face, scalp, and upper trunk of middle-aged adults. Unlike pemphigus vulgaris, mucosal surfaces are uninvolved and patients generally have a better prognosis. As with all bullous diseases, histology, direct and indirect immunofluorescence, and confirmatory antigen-specific ELISA should be obtained before initiating therapy.

TREATMENT

Pemphigus foliaceous is managed in a very similar manner to pemphigus vulgaris. Due to the generally milder and more insidious course, topical corticosteroids (clobetasol ointment twice daily) are often used as first-line agents for localized disease. Nevertheless, disease that is widespread or resistant to local therapy requires systemic prednisone combined with steroid-sparing agents at the same dosing as used for bullous pemphigoid and pemphigus vulgaris (see Table 1).

Acknowledgment

This work was supported in part by National Institutes of Health grants T32 AR007369, RO1 AR32081, and RO1 AR32599 (Luis A. Diaz) and RO1 AI49427 (David S. Rubenstein).

REFERENCES

Berkowitz P, Hu P, Liu Z, et al. Desmosome signaling. Inhibition of p38MAPK prevents pemphigus vulgaris IgG-induced cytoskeleton reorganization. J Biol Chem 2005;280(25):23778–84.

Berkowitz P, Hu P, Warren S, et al. p38MAPK inhibition prevents disease in pemphigus vulgaris mice. Proc Natl Acad Sci U S A 2006;103(34): 12855–60.

Korman NJ. Bullous pemphigoid. The latest in diagnosis, prognosis, and therapy. Arch Dermatol 1998;134:1137–41.

Liu Z, Diaz LA, Troy JL, et al. A passive transfer model of the organ-specific autoimmune disease, bullous pemphigoid, using antibodies generated against the hemidesmosomal antigen, BP 180. J Clin Invest 1993;92: 2480–8.

Mutasim DF. Management of autoimmune bullous diseases: Pharmacology and therapeutics. J Am Acad Dermatol 2004;51(6):859–77.

Nousari HC, Griffin WA, Anhalt GJ. Successful therapy for bullous pemphigoid with mycophenolate mofetil. J Am Acad Dermatol 1998;39:497–8.

Snow JL, Gibson LE. The role of genetic variation in thiopurine methyltransferase activity and the efficacy and or side effects of azathioprine in dermatologic patients. Arch Dermatol 1995;131:193–7.

Yosipovitch G, Hoon TS, Leok GC. Suggested rationale for prevention and treatment of glucocorticoid-induced bone loss in dermatologic patients. Arch Dermatol 2001;137:477–81.

[1]Not FDA approved for this indication.

Contact Dermatitis

Method of
Rita Lloyd, MD

Contact dermatitis can be caused by irritant exposure (80% of cases) or allergens (20%). *Irritants* include soap, water, astringents, strong acids, strong bases, and solvents. These substances are more likely to cause dermatitis when the concentration of exposure is high, the occurrence of exposure is frequent, or the skin barrier is impaired by previous dermatitis, including atopic dermatitis. The symptoms are usually burning, stinging, or pain, with itch being a minor component. The rash usually corresponds to the site of contact, without spread beyond.

Allergens are usually small molecules that combine with a skin protein to create a complete allergen. Many chemicals, including preservatives, rubber additives, plant secretions, and metals, are potential sensitizers; the most well-known example of this dermatitis is a poison ivy rash. Itch is the main symptom. The rash may extend beyond the site of immediate contact with the chemical. Much of the time, the sensitizer is not a new exposure, but rather a new and persistent reaction to an old exposure.

Diagnosis

It is important to differentiate irritant from allergic contact dermatitis. Allergens must be avoided completely to prevent the dermatitis, whereas irritant exposures can continue in smaller amounts or concentrations, and healing may occur.

Patch testing is the procedure that identifies delayed-type hypersensitivity to contact allergens; prick testing, intradermal testing, and radioallergosorbent assay test (RAST) have a role in diagnosing immediate-type, IgE-mediated hypersensitivity (which usually manifests as allergic rhinitis, not dermatitis). A screening panel of patch test allergens is available, sold as the TRUE test (Allerderm, Petaluma, CA). This panel can identify up to one third of relevant allergens; more extensive panels of allergens have greater sensitivity in identifying relevant allergens in the home and workplace.

Treatment

IRRITANT CONTACT DERMATITIS

In addition to decreasing the frequency or concentration of exposure to irritants, cream- or ointment-based emollients can help to restore a normal skin barrier (Vaseline ointment, Aquaphor ointment, Cetaphil Cream, Eucerin Cream). Lotions are less effective in restoring the skin barrier. Topical steroids (mid-strength such as triamcinolone [Kenalog] cream or ointment 0.1%) may be used in the acute phase of treatment, but they have a less important role than in allergic contact dermatitis.

CURRENT DIAGNOSIS

Irritant Contact Dermatitis

- Subjective symptoms: burning, stinging, pain
- Rash corresponds to exposure site
- Irritants have additive effect and include chemicals (e.g., soap, water, solvents) and environmental factors (e.g., temperature, humidity).

Allergic Contact Dermatitis

- Subjective symptom: itch
- Rash may extend beyond the exposure site.
- Allergens are often "old," not new exposures.
- Patch testing is usually necessary to identify the allergen.

ALLERGIC CONTACT DERMATITIS

Patch testing is usually necessary to identify contact allergens, and the allergens must be avoided completely for recovery to occur. This sometimes requires protective wear and even changes in occupation for some individuals.

The dermatitis responds to topical or systemic steroids. Localized acute severe dermatitis can be treated with ultrapotent topical steroids (clobetasol propionate [Temovate] cream or ointment), except on the face or body folds. Use should be limited to no more than 2 weeks because of the risk of steroid atrophy.

A milder steroid (triamcinolone [Kenalog] 0.1% cream or ointment) may be used after the acute dermatitis has improved or for less severe nonfacial dermatitis. Products such as desonide (DesOwen), hydrocortisone butyrate (Locoid), or alclometasone dipropionate (Aclovate) ointments are appropriate for treating severe facial dermatitis. Hydrocortisone 1% or 2.5% cream or ointment (Hycort), pimecrolimus (Elidel)[1] cream, or tacrolimus (Protopic)[1] ointment is appropriate for more chronic or milder facial dermatitis.

If the provider is concerned about allergy to the topical steroid, desoximetasone (Topicort) cream or ointment 0.25% is appropriate for nonfacial use because it is an infrequent sensitizer; mometasone (Elocon) cream or ointment is appropriate for short-term facial use under the same circumstances.

Systemic steroids should be reserved for more diffuse or severe dermatitis and should be tapered over 3 weeks. Starting doses are often 60 mg, or 1 mg/kg/day.

Emollients and skin care products that avoid the most common sensitizers are advised when allergic contact dermatitis is suspected; Pharmaceutical Specialties (Rochester, MN) makes products that are free of fragrance, formaldehyde-related preservatives, and lanolin (sold with the brand name Vanicream or Free and Clear).

The impaired skin is more vulnerable to infection, and obtaining a culture and treating the secondary infection (often *Staphylococcus aureus*) with the appropriate antibiotic (often cephalexin [Keflex] 500 mg twice daily for 10 to 14 days) is frequently necessary for complete clearing of irritant contact dermatitis or allergic contact dermatitis.

When gloves are necessary to protect from irritants or allergens, the choice depends on whether the patient needs protection from physical factors (e.g., heat, friction), chemicals (e.g., hydrophobic, hydrophilic, small or large molecules), or microbes (e.g., virus, bacteria, fungus). Whether the exposure is brief, continuous, or by means of immersion or splash is also important. Dexterity is an important factor in choosing a glove compatible with completing a task accurately and safely. For some patients, it may be the glove itself that is the irritant or allergen. For all these reasons, it is not possible to make a global recommendation for glove wear.

---

[1]Not FDA approved for this indication.

CURRENT THERAPY

Irritant Contact Dermatitis

- Decrease frequency or concentration of irritant exposure.
- Use cream- or ointment-based emollients.
- Mid-strength topical steroids have a minor role in healing.
- Identify and treat secondary infection.

Allergic Contact Dermatitis

- Identify allergens; patch testing may be necessary.
- Advise patient about allergen avoidance.
- Advise patients about personal care products of low allergy potential until patch testing is feasible.
- Use topical steroids for dermatitis; strength depends on the location of dermatitis and whether it is acute or chronic.
- Save systemic steroids for severe, generalized dermatitis, and taper dose over 3 weeks.
- Identify and treat secondary infection.

The examination-type disposable glove least likely to contain allergens is vinyl; this avoids exposure to the latex protein and the most common rubber accelerator allergens, which may be present in synthetic rubber gloves (nitrile) and latex gloves. Household-weight, reusable gloves are also available in vinyl.

Powder in gloves is infrequently an allergen and makes gloves easier to don. However, it may be an irritant for some individuals, and it is a carrier of latex protein, and aerosolizing more of this protein is important for those who have immediate-type hypersensitivity to latex.

Conclusions

Diagnosis is often the challenge in treating contact dermatitis, because the clinical picture of irritant contact dermatitis, allergic contact dermatitis, atopic dermatitis, dyshidrosis, hyperkeratotic hand dermatitis, and psoriasis is similar, with many shared subjective and objective features. If dermatitis fails to respond to the measures outlined previously or requires frequent intervention with systemic treatment, consultation with a dermatologist for evaluation, including patch testing to a robust panel of allergens, is advised.

REFERENCES

Boman A, Estlander T, Wahlberg J, Maibach H. Protective Gloves for Occupational Use. Boca Raton, FL: CRC Press; 2005.

Hunt LW, Kelkar P, Reed CE, Yunginger JW. Management of occupational allergy to natural rubber latex in a medical center: The importance of quantitative latex allergen measurement and objective follow-up. J Allergy Clin Immunol 2002;110(Suppl.):S96–106.

Mark Jr JG, Elsner P, DeLeo VA. Allergy and ICD. In: Contact and Occupational Dermatology. 3rd ed. Philadelphia: Mosby; 2002. p. 3–15.

Rietschel RL, Fowler JF. Reactions to topical corticosteroids. In: Fisher's Contact Dermatitis. 5th ed. Philadelphia: Lippincott Williams & Wilkins; 2001. p. 203–10.

Saripalli YV, Achen F, Belsito DV. The detection of clinically relevant contact allergens using a standard screening tray of twenty-three allergens. J Am Acad Dermatol 2003;49:65–9.

Wilkinson SM, Beck MH. Fluticasone propionate and mometasone furoate have a low risk of contact sensitization. Contact Dermatitis 1996;34:365–6.

Anogenital Pruritus

Method of
*Lynette Margesson, MD, FRCPC, and
F. William Danby, MD, FRCPC*

Anogenital pruritus is a common symptom that affects the genitals or anus, or both. Pruritus ani affects 1% to 5% of the population and is more common in men. Pruritus vulvae is a common vulvar complaint affecting up to 10% of women. Genital pruritus in men is less common. Pruritus in these areas can be acute or chronic, and it can range from minor to debilitating.

Finding the cause of the pruritus is of utmost importance to manage these patients effectively. The most common causes are outlined in Box 1. Because the cause of pruritus is often multifactorial, always consider a combination of conditions.

In the vulvar area, the most common cause is acute candidiasis. Irritant contact dermatitis is next and often results from overzealous cleansing habits or exposure to topical irritants such as urine, feces, sweat, and topical medications. Among the chronic conditions, the most common causes are lichen simplex chronicus and lichen sclerosus. Psoriasis and lichen planus are seen less often. Patients may have a combination of infection, contact dermatitis (usually irritant), and dermatoses. Pruritus of the penis alone is unusual, and the most common causes are scabies and monilial balanitis. Scrotal itch may result from a primary irritant

---

BOX 1   Causes of Anogenital Pruritus

Acute Pruritus
Infections
- *Candida*, dermatophytosis
- Herpes simplex virus, human papillomavirus, molluscum contagiosum
- *Staphylococcus aureus, Streptococcus*

Dermatoses
- Contact dermatitis (irritant, allergic)
- Atopic dermatitis/eczema
- Psoriasis

Chronic Pruritus
Dermatoses
- Lichen simplex chronicus
- Contact dermatitis (irritant or allergic)
- Lichen sclerosus
- Lichen planus
- Psoriasis

Neuropathy
Malignancy
- Vulvar and anal intraepithelial neoplasia
- Squamous cell carcinoma, extramammary Paget's disease

Anal-Specific Causes
- Dietary factors
- Hemorrhoids
- Anal fissures and fistulae
- Proctitis
- Inflammatory bowel disease

(often in atopics) or allergic contact dermatitis, scabies, and tinea cruris, even though the dermatophyte rarely involves the scrotum itself. Pubic lice cause pruritus of the entire hairy genital area.

In the anal area, dietary factors (through irritant contact dermatitis from fecal soiling) account for most cases of anal pruritus. As in the vulva, this is confounded by excessive cleansing and irritation and less frequently by allergic reactions to topical medications. Underlying anorectal diseases should be sought. Dermatologic diseases, infections, and infestations need to be considered. Concurrent conditions can confuse the picture. Anxiety and depression can further confuse the diagnosis.

Evaluation and Diagnosis

A complete history and careful full-surface physical examination of the skin is needed. The examiner should adequately detail information about all hygiene practices and all topical products (prescribed and proprietary) used. For vulvar pruritus, a complete vulvar and vaginal examination is essential. Telephone diagnosis is unacceptable. For anal pruritus, a digital examination with anoscopy, proctoscopy, or colonoscopy may be indicated. Consider appropriate potassium hydroxide (KOH) preparations, cultures, skin biopsies, and patch testing as indicated (Box 2).

Management

Support and education of the patient are important (Box 3). All irritants must be eliminated, particularly overwashing. Unnecessary topical agents must be stopped. Infection control is important. Use oral antibiotics, and for women, add fluconazole (Diflucan)[1] to prevent secondary yeast infection. Topical anesthetics such as lidocaine 5% ointment

---

[1]Not FDA approved for this indication.

BOX 2   Investigations for Anogenital Pruritus

- Culture—bacteria, *Candida*, dermatophyte
- Wet prep of vaginal secretions for *Candida*, bacterial vaginosis, trichomoniasis
- Culture all balanitis for yeast and bacteria
- Adhesive tape testing for pinworms
- Potassium hydroxide testing of skin and vaginal secretions for yeast, scabies, dermatophytes
- Patch testing for allergic contact dermatitis
- Skin biopsy for dermatoses, tumors
- Anal or gastrointestinal disease—anoscopy, proctoscopy, colonoscopy
- Prostate cancer—prostate-specific antigen (PSA) and digital rectal examination (DRE)

BOX 3   Treatment of Anogenital Pruritus

Non-Specific Measures
- Patient support and education
- Stop all irritants (e.g., overwashing, scratching, infection, unnecessary topical preparations)
- Topical anesthetics (e.g., 5% lidocaine ointment bid to qid [may sting]), avoid benzocaine (Vagisil).
- Cool compresses, soaks, gel packs (not frozen); keep in refrigerator in self-sealed plastic bag.
- Bland emollients (plain petrolatum or zinc oxide) ointment to soothe open fissured or eroded tissue.

Specific Measures
- Eliminate local secondary bacterial and yeast infection
- Stop scratching—use nighttime sedation (hydroxyzine [Vistaril]/doxepin [Sinequan] 10–100 mg)/citalopram (Celexa) 20–40 mg each morning
- Reduce inflammation—topical corticosteroid ointments once infection is controlled

Mild disease: 1 to 2.5% hydrocortisone ointment with or without pramoxine (Pramasone)
Moderate disease: triamcinolone 0.1% (Kenalog) ointment
Severe pruritus or thick skin areas: superpotent clobetasol (Temovate) or halobetasol (Ultravate) 0.05% ointment
For very severe pruritus—systemic prednisone or IM triamcinolone (Kenalog-40) 1 mg/kg up to maximum 80 mg/dose

- As steroid sparer, consider calcineurin inhibitors 1% pimecrolimus cream (Elidel) or 0.03% to 1% tacrolimus ointment (Protopic)
- Manage anxiety and depression

Specific for Pruritus Ani
- Implement dietary changes
- Control fecal leakage and constipation

Specific for Pruritus Vulvae
- Treat vaginitis
- Manage urinary incontinence and contributory menstrual flow

For Neuropathic Pruritus
- Amitriptyline (Elavil) 10–150 mg qhs
- Gabapentin (Neurontin) up to 3600 mg per day
- Venlafaxine (Effexor) up to 150 mg per day

---

can help ease the need to scratch. Avoid benzocaine (Vagisil), because it can be a very strong irritant and allergen. Cooling the area is helpful, and this can be done with Sitz baths, gel packs (cold but not frozen), or compresses. Keep the gel packs or cool, moist clothes in self-sealing bags in the refrigerator. Ice can cause frostbite of the area.

For anal pruritus, dietary factors may be important. Avoid foods, beverages, and medications that can exacerbate symptoms. Address dietary changes to improve bowel function. It is essential to control fecal leakage and constipation. Consider the possibility of rectal or prostatic pathology. Use bland emollients such as plain petrolatum or zinc oxide ointment to coat eroded, fissured skin after careful cleansing.

For genital pruritus, manage urinary incontinence and any contributing irritation from menstrual flow. Adjustments can be made to minimize flow with medications. Consider tampons rather than pads.

Gentle hygiene is important. The patient should use a hypoallergenic cleansing bar with hands only and avoid washcloths and wipes. Use a small amount of mineral oil or Albolene cleanser on a tissue to remove fecal material. Scratching must be controlled with nighttime sedation such as hydroxyzine (Vistaril) or doxepin (Sinequan).[1] These patients have a tendency to scratch at night. They may be unaware of this. These medications assist with a deeper sleep to help stop the scratching. This is imperative for healing. Daytime sedation with citalopram (Celexa)[1] or fluoxetine (Prozac)[1] may be necessary.

Inflammation must be addressed. Classically, topical corticosteroid ointments are used. For mild disease, mild-potency hydrocortisone (Hycort) 1% to 2.5% ointment may be all that is necessary. A 1% hydrocortisone/1% iodoquinol cream (Vytone) used topically as an antimicrobial with mild antiinflammatory action can be effective for perianal pruritus and skin fold areas such as labiocrural and inguinal folds and the gluteal cleft. For more severe pruritus, especially if the skin is thickened with lichen simplex chronicus or lichen sclerosus or is severely involved with lichen planus, a superpotent corticosteroid is needed. Lichen sclerosus is treated with a superpotent steroid one or two times daily for 8 to 12 weeks and then three times per week, gradually decreasing to a maintenance regimen of one or two applications per week for the long term. Lichen simplex chronicus responds to superpotent steroid twice daily for 2 weeks, once daily for 2 weeks, and then three times per week. Consider switching to a calcineurin inhibitor such as pimecrolimus (Elidel)[1] or tacrolimus (Protopic)[1] twice daily as a steroid sparer. Ointments are suggested because they are more effective and less allergenic than creams. Use as a thin, invisible film. There is controversy about the use of calcineurin inhibitors in the treatment of lichen sclerosus and lichen planus. Calcineurin inhibitors can cause a burning sensation.

For severe intractable pruritus, a limited course of systemic corticosteroid may be indicated, using intramuscular triamcinolone acetonide (Kenalog 40), 1 mg/kg up to a maximum dose of 80 mg, or prednisone tapered over a three week course.

For perianal pruritus, a mild 1% to 2.5% hydrocortisone ointment may be all that is necessary. Because the skin is thin, strong corticosteroids should be used only for a limited time. The calcineurin inhibitors can be very helpful. For patients with intractable anal symptoms, cautious local injections of methylene blue (Urolene Blue)[1] have been beneficial.

For patients with neuropathy, management is like that for chronic pain conditions, with amitriptyline (Elavil),[1] gabapentin (Neurontin),[1] venlafaxine (Effexor),[1] or combinations of these drugs. Anxiety and depression need to be addressed in all of these patients.

Itching in these areas can be chronic and recurrent, and long-term follow-up will be needed. Treatment regimens must be used long enough to get adequate healing and completely break the itch, scratch, itch cycle. Otherwise, relapse is common.

REFERENCES

Al-Ghnaniem R, Short K, Pullen A, et al. 1% Hydrocortisone ointment is an effective treatment of pruritus ani: A pilot randomized controlled crossover trial. Int J Colorectal Dis 2007;22(12):1463–7.

Bohl TG. Overview of vulvar pruritus through the life cycle. Clin Obstet Gynecol 2005;48(4):786–807.

---

[1]Not FDA approved for this indication.

Farage MA, Miller KW, Berardesca E, Maibach HI. Incontinence in the aged: Contact dermatitis and other cutaneous consequences. Contact Dermatitis 2007;57(4):211–7.

Koca R, Altin R, Konuk N, et al. Sleep disturbance in patients with lichen simplex chronicus and its relationship to nocturnal scratching: A case control study. South Med J 2006;99(5):482–5.

Kranke B, Trummer M, Brabek E, et al. Etiologic and causative factors in perianal dermatitis: Results of a prospective study in 126 patients. Wien Klin Wochenschr 2006;118(3–4):90–4.

Lynch PJ. Lichen simplex chronicus (atopic/neurodermatitis) of the anogenital region. Dermatol Ther 2004;17(1):8–19.

Margesson LJ. Contact dermatitis of the vulva. Dermatol Ther 2004;17 (1):20–7.

Mentes BB, Akin M, Leventoglu S, et al. Intradermal methylene blue injection for the treatment of intractable idiopathic pruritus ani: Results of 30 cases. Tech Coloproctol 2004;8(1):11–4.

Weichert GE. An approach to the treatment of anogenital pruritus. Dermatol Ther 2004;17(1):129–33.

Weisshaar E. Successful treatment of genital pruritus using topical immuno-modulators as a single therapy in multi-morbid patients. Acta Derm Venereol 2008;88(2):195–6.

Urticaria and Angioedema

Method of
Joyce M. C. Teng, MD, PhD

Urticaria, or hives, is a common cutaneous eruption that occurs in up to 25% of the general population sometime during their lives.[1] It is characterized by transient, circumscribed, pruritic, erythematous papules or plaques, often with central pallor. Individual lesions often coalesce into large wheals on the trunk and extremities that may resolve over a few hours without leaving any residual skin changes. The process is mediated by mast cells in the superficial dermis.

Angioedema is a similar process occurring in deep dermis or subcutaneous tissue. Angioedema may occur independently, accompanied by urticaria, or as a component of anaphylaxis. It is characterized by localized swelling that develops over minutes to hours and resolves within 24 to 48 hours. Common locations of angioedema include the mucosa and areas with loose connective tissue, such as the face, eyes, lips, tongue, and genitalia. Patients usually do not have pruritus, but they may have pain and a sensation of warmth. Angioedema is usually a benign process that resolves without sequelae unless it involves the larynx. African Americans are disproportionately affected, representing up to 40% of the hospital admissions for angioedema.[2]

Classification

Urticaria can be classified as acute or chronic, depending on the duration. Acute urticaria usually lasts for less than 6 weeks and is commonly triggered by infection, medication, insect bite, and food (Table 1). The chronic form, lasting more than 6 weeks, accounts for approximately 30% of cases of urticaria, and no clear causes can be identified in more than 80% of these cases. A significant number of patients with chronic urticaria may have persistent symptoms for more than 10 years.[3] Approximately 40% of patients with chronic urticaria have associated angioedema, although the incidence of laryngeal edema is low.

[1]Not FDA approved for this indication.
[2]Not available in the United States.
[3]Exceeds dosage recommended by the manufacturer.

TABLE 1 Mechanisms in Urticaria and Angioedema

Disorder	Causes
Immunoglobulin-mediated urticaria	Ig-E mediated: food, medication, insect bites, contact allergen, aeroallergens, other causes Urticaria associated with autoimmunity: antinuclear antibodies (ANAs), thyroid autoantibodies, other causes
Direct activation of mast cell degranulation	Physical stimuli: exercise, heat, cold, pressure, aquagenic, solar radiation, etc. Other agents: opiates, antibiotics (e.g., vancomycin [Vancocin]), radiocontrast, ACTH (Cortrosyn), muscle relaxants
Complement-mediated	Viral infections, parasites, blood transfusion
C1 inhibitor deficiency	Genetic and acquired angioedema, paraproteinemia
Reduced kinin metabolism	Angiotensin-converting enzyme (ACE) inhibitors
Reduced arachidonic acid metabolism	Aspirin

CURRENT DIAGNOSIS

- Acute and chronic urticaria have the same features, including erythematous, edematous papules or wheals with central pallor that last less than 24 to 48 hours.
- Laboratory assessments are not recommended for acute urticaria in the absence of evidence suggesting underlying systemic illness.
- Limited laboratory studies are indicated for chronic urticaria.
- Serum measurements of C4 and C1 are the recommended initial tests if hereditary or acquired angioedema are suspected.
- Skin biopsy should be considered to rule out urticarial vasculitis if an individual lesion is painful and persists for more than 2 to 3 days with accompanying ecchymosis or petechiae.

Diagnosis

Urticaria is diagnosed clinically in most cases. A detailed history, physical examination, and complete review of systems are essential for diagnosing patients with urticaria and angioedema. The history should include the distribution and characteristics of lesions (e.g., pain, pruritus), duration of skin eruption, accompanying angioedema, airway involvement and other associated systemic symptoms (e.g., fever, arthralgia, swelling joints, refusal to walk by children). Patients should also be questioned about changes in dietary habits, recent exposures, infection, and newly administered medications, including antibiotics, over-the-counter analgesia, and hormones.

Laboratory assessment is usually not helpful in diagnosing patients with acute urticaria who lack any history or clinical findings to suggest an underlying disease process. A limited number of diagnostic tests are indicated in the evaluation of patients with chronic urticaria, such as a complete blood cell count with differential white blood cell count, an erythrocyte sedimentation rate (ESR) or C-reactive protein (CRP) determination, a thyroid-stimulating hormone (TSH) level, antithyroglobulin and antimicrosomal antibodies, antinuclear antibodies (ANA), and hepatitis B and C serologies. A detailed review of systems may help to narrow the focus of the screening test.

CURRENT THERAPY

- Primary treatment of urticaria and angioedema is removal of triggering factors and initiation of therapy for symptomatic relief.
- Oral antihistamines are the cornerstones of therapy. The application of first-generation H_1-antihistamines may be limited by central nervous system and anticholinergic side effects.
- Nonsedating second-generation antihistamines are often used in combination and can be as effective as first-generation agents.
- Systemic corticosteroids and immunosuppressive therapy, especially cyclosporine (Neoral),[1] have been used successfully in cases that are refractory to the maximum dose of antihistamines.
- Fresh-frozen plasma infusions along with standard airway precautions have been recommended for angioedema patients with laryngeal edema.

[1]Not FDA approved for this indication.

A skin biopsy of an early lesion should be performed to rule out urticarial vasculitis if the affected individual has skin lesions that are painful and last for more than 2 to 3 days with residual ecchymosis or petechiae. In patients with angioedema, prominent edema of the interstitial tissue may be demonstrated by biopsy. Serum measurements of C4 and C1 are recommended initial tests if hereditary or acquired angioedema is suspected. A C1q level should be obtained to screen for the acquired form of angioedema if the affected individual is middle-aged.[3]

Treatment

More than two thirds of cases of urticaria are self-limited. Spontaneous remission of chronic urticaria and angioedema is also common. The primary objective of management is to identify and discontinue the offending trigger. A patient presenting with angioedema must first be assessed for signs of airway compromise. Medical therapy is indicated for those who are symptomatic.

Antihistamines remain the first-line therapy for most patients with urticaria, because the primary complaint of pruritus is predominantly mediated by histamine released from mast cells.[5,6] First-generation antihistamines such as hydroxyzine (Atarax or Vistaril 25 to 50 mg every 6 hours), diphenhydramine (Benadryl 25 to 50 mg every 6 hours), cyproheptadine (Periactin 4 mg three times daily), and chlorpheniramine (Chlor-Trimeton 4 mg every 6 hours) are potent and have the quickest onset of action. However, the treatments are often limited by their sedating and anticholinergic side effects. Many first-generation antihistamines are available over the counter, providing accessible first-line therapy for patients. Patients with urticaria that lasts for several days should be considered for treatment using second-generation antihistamines such as loratadine (Claritin[1] 10 mg twice daily[3]), desloratadine (Clarinex 5 mg twice daily[3]), cetirizine (Zyrtec 10 mg twice daily[3]), levocetirizine (Xyzal 5 mg daily), and fexofenadine (Allegra 180 mg twice daily[3]). Doxepin (Sinequan),[1] an H_1- and H_2-receptor antagonist, is seven times more potent than hydroxyzine in suppression of wheal and flare responses. Because of its central nervous system side effects, combined use of doxepin with a first-generation antihistamine should be restricted.

[1]Not FDA approved for this indication.
[3]Exceeds dosage recommended by the manufacturer.
[5]Investigational drug in the United States.
[6]May be compounded by pharmacists.

Topical 5% doxepin cream (Zonalon)[1] may help to suppress pruritus in patients with localized urticaria.

Systemic prednisone at 30 to 40 mg in a single morning dose is sufficient to suppress urticaria in adults. Tapering should be gradual over a 3- to 4-week period by decreasing the dosage 5 mg every 3 to 5 days to minimize rebound. Alternate-morning dosing when reaching 20 mg daily may help to minimize the steroid side effects. Methylprednisolone (Solu-Medrol 40 mg) should be given intravenously as initial therapy to patients with angioedema. This may be followed by a tapering oral course. Three months of treatment with cyclosporine (Neoral)[1] at 3 to 5 mg/kg can be given safely to patients who are refractory to corticosteroid therapy or have difficulty tapering their therapy. Close monitoring for hypertension and renal insufficiency is necessary during the treatment.

Leukotriene inhibitors such as zileuton (Zyflo[1] 600 mg four times daily), zafirlukast (Accolate[1] 20 mg twice daily), and montelukast (Singulair[1] 10 mg once daily) may be effective for patients with autoimmune urticaria. Successful treatment of chronic urticaria with anti-IgE (omalizumab [Xolair][1]) has been reported but is not yet approved by the FDA.

Proper management of underlying autoimmune thyroid disease or autoimmune collagen vascular diseases has been beneficial for patients with associated urticaria. Life-threatening angioedema triggered by angiotensin-converting enzyme (ACE) inhibitors has been successfully treated with infusion of fresh-frozen plasma. Treatments with warfarin (Coumadin),[1] plasmapheresis, and intravenous immunoglobulin (Baygam)[1] have been reported for severe, refractory[1] urticaria. These treatments are administered only by specialists on an individual basis.

REFERENCES

Bailey E, Shaker M. An update on childhood urticaria and angioedema. Curr Opin Pediatr 2008;20(4):425–30.
Champion RH, Roberts SO, Carpenter RG, Roger JH. Urticaria and angioedema. A review of 554 patients. Br J Dermatol 1969;81(8):588–97.
Joint Task Force on Practice Parameters. The diagnosis and management of urticaria: A practice parameter. Part II. Chronic urticaria/angioedema. Ann Allergy Asthma Immunol 2000;85(2):521–44.
Kaplan AP, Joseph K, Maykut RJ, et al. Treatment of chronic autoimmune urticaria with omalizumab. J Allergy Clin Immunol 2008;122(3):569–73.
Lin RY, Cannon AG, Teitel AD. Pattern of hospitalizations for angioedema in New York between 1990 and 2003. Ann Allergy Asthma Immunol 2005;95 (2):159–66.
Nizami RM, Baboo MT. Office management of patients with urticaria: An analysis of 215 patients. Ann Allergy 1974;33(2):78–85.
Powell RJ, Du Toit GL, Siddique N, et al. BSACI guidelines for the management of chronic urticaria and angio-oedema. Clin Exp Allergy 2007;37(5):631–50.

---

[1]Not FDA approved for this indication.

Pigmentary Disorders

Method of
Robert A. Schwartz, MD, MPH, and
Camila K. Janniger, MD

Cutaneous pigmentation protects humans from harmful ultraviolet light radiation. It results from many factors, including carotenoids and hemoglobin, with the number, size, type, and distribution pattern of melanosomes being an important determinate. Melanin produced in epidermal melanocytes is the principal pigment of concern, although the lipochrome carotene, when ingested in excessive amounts, can produce a yellow-orange coloration that can be mistaken for jaundice. However, hypothyroidism, diabetes mellitus, hepatic diseases, anorexia nervosa, and renal diseases can produce carotenemia unassociated with the ingestion of carotene. Similarly, deposition of some medications or their metabolites produce discoloration. A correct diagnosis is mandatory.

Pigmentary disorders represent a wide variety of diseases, including tinea versicolor, acanthosis nigricans, Addison's disease, melanoma, onchocerciasis, mycosis fungoides, tuberous sclerosis and leprosy, the latter a reason for the social stigma of depigmentation in much of the world.

Superficial melanin tends to be seen as tan or brown, whereas deeper deposits often produce a gray or blue-gray hue due to the Tyndall light-scattering effect. Wood's lamp examination can aid in this distinction, showing epidermal melanin, which absorbs it, to appear darker than dermal melanosis, in which light scattering makes the patches less prominent. In general, epidermal melanosis is more amenable to therapy. Both types may be present. In addition, the Wood's lamp long wavelength ultraviolet blacklight examination may be valuable for hypopigmentation in separating total pigment loss from partial forms, detecting the yellowish-green fluorescence of some patches of tinea versicolor, and visualizing 1- to 10-cm depigmented spots (Fitzpatrick patches) on light-complexioned babies with tuberous sclerosis.

Patient education and realistic expectations are critical. All skin products should be first tested by limited application to noncosmetically sensitive normal skin and evaluated at 24 and 48 hours. In addition, effective sunscreens or sunblocks should be employed whenever tretinoin, psoralens, or hydroquinone is used. Therapy for the disorders discussed here is usually directed at improvement rather than cure. Thus, the results may be modest but are usually not permanent, and repeat courses of therapy may be necessary.

The risk of side effects needs to be stressed. Tretinoin and hydroquinone can produce irritant or allergic dermatitis. Hydroquinone has recently come under regulatory scrutiny, in part because it can induce exogenous ochronosis, a permanent blue-black hyperpigmentation at the site of application after prolonged and extensive use, which should be avoided. Some hydroquinone products contain sodium metabisulfite, a sulfite that can cause allergic reactions, sometimes life-threatening, which are more common in asthmatics than in nonasthmatics.

New medications are being developed for hyperpigmentation, in part as a response to concern about the safety of hydroquinone. They include kojic acid, mandelic acid, azelaic acid, bearberry extract, licorice extract, mulberry extract, and arbutin. Kojic acid is a chelation agent produced by several species of fungus, especially *Aspergillus oryzae*, and normally used as a food additive and preservative, a skin-whitening agent in cosmetics, a plant-growth regulator, and a chemical intermediate. It can be employed alone or in combination with hydroquinone. However, kojic acid can be problematic in terms of its chemical stability and its potential negative effects on the skin.

Hyperpigmentation Disorders

MELASMA

Clinical Findings

Melasma (chloasma) is a common cutaneous disorder characterized by patchy hyperpigmentation of the face, occasionally the neck, and rarely the forearms. There are three main patterns: centrofacial, malar, and mandibular. It occurs most commonly in women taking oral contraceptives or in those who are pregnant (mask of pregnancy) and rarely in women with ovarian tumors, but it can also be evident in adolescent girls, boys in puberty, men, and nonpregnant women. Hormonal and genetic factors are important; people of lineages from South Asia, China, and Latin America have a propensity for melasma. It tends to darken on solar exposure and fade during winter without it. Hydantoin use can induce a similar eruption.

Treatment

In melasma, epidermal pigmentation, often tan and appearing to darken on Wood's lamp examination due to epidermal melanin absorption, tends to respond to hydroquinone, whereas bluish gray dermal pigmentation is much less responsive. Tri-Luma cream (fluocinolone acetonide 0.01%, hydroquinone 4%, tretinoin 0.05%) is a good approach. It needs to be used together with an appropriate sunscreen, ideally a sunblock such as Lydia O'Leary's Covermark. Tri-Luma cream is indicated for short-term and intermittent long-term treatment of moderate to severe melasma. A combination of hydroquinone 4% cream containing sunscreen (Solaquin Forte) applied twice daily and 0.05% tretinoin emollient cream (Renova)[1] applied at night for 4 to 6 months can produce substantial lightening, but also can cause irritation, especially when first applied. A similar product is hydroquinone 4% and retinol, EpiQuin Micro, a high-technology effort that is worth trying. Another combination formulation is AlphaquinHP (hydroquinone 4% cream with glycolic acids and sunscreens).

Tretinoin 0.1% cream alone can fade the spots somewhat, but treatment is often protracted. Applying tretinoin cream every other night for the first 2 to 3 weeks and then increasing the frequency of application to nightly can minimize the irritation. Azelaic acid (Azelex)[1] 20% cream applied twice daily with or without 0.05% tretinoin cream for 6 months may also bleach the patches. It can also be combined with hydroquinone 4% cream, both agents to be applied twice daily. The value of azelaic acid for melasma may be enhanced by the use of sequential therapy with it and a potent topical steroid.

It is critical that hormonal therapy, if in use, be discontinued and sun exposure be avoided diligently during therapy. Some hydroquinone products, such as Solaquin Forte, contain sunscreens. All patients with melasma should also use an additional sunscreen agent after treatment. The product should have a sun protection factor (SPF) of at least 15. Water-resistant products are preferred in those who exercise outdoors or sweat heavily (Table 1). If not otherwise contraindicated, oral vitamins C and E supplements may be slightly beneficial.

SOLAR LENTIGO

Clinical Findings

Solar lentigines (also called senile lentigines or liver spots) occur in most elderly light-complexioned persons of European or East Asian heritage. A majority by age 60 years may be affected, although lentigines often occur in younger people with marked solar exposure. They begin as tiny macules on the face, shoulders, or dorsal hands, expanding and coalescing into uniformly brown patches, often with an irregular configuration. Solar lentigo has no malignant potential, but it takes clinical experience to distinguish it from lentigo maligna, an early melanoma.

---

[1]Not FDA approved for this indication.

TABLE 1 Sunscreens

Brand Name	Sunscreen Type	Characteristics
Bull Frog QuikGel	Chemical sunscreen	Greaseless vehicle, waterproof
Coppertone Sport	Chemical sunscreen	Waterproof, reduced eye stinging
Durascreen 30	Combination chemical and physical sunscreen	Wide spectrum of UV protection, thicker vehicle
Olay Complete	Chemical sunscreen, physical blocker	Elegant vehicle, wide spectrum of UV protection
Ombrelle 30	Chemical sunscreen	Water-resistant, fragrance-free, wide spectrum of UV protection

Treatment

Tretinoin 0.05% emollient cream (Renova)[1] applied sparingly once daily, might gradually work. Bleaching creams containing hydroquinone or azelaic acid[1] function slowly and incompletely in most cases. The addition of tretinoin cream can improve the results somewhat. Tri-Luma cream[1] (flucinolone acetonide 0.01%, hydroquinone 4%, tretinoin 0.05%) is more effective, but it needs to be used together with an appropriate broad-spectrum sunscreen of SPF 30 or higher. A combination of mequinol 2% and tretinoin 0.01% has been FDA approved for solar lentigines, marketed as Solagé. It should not be used in women of childbearing potential or in patients using other potentially phototoxic oral or topical medications. A comprehensive ultraviolet light avoidance plan needs to be employed. Another combination formulation is AlphaquinHP (hydroquinone 4% cream with glycolic acid and sunscreen).

Liquid nitrogen cryotherapy is effective using a superficial freeze (light pressure with dipped cotton swab for 5–7 seconds), but posttherapy hypopigmentation can occur. Mid-depth trichloroacetic acid or glycolic acid chemical peels can lighten or eradicate multiple lesions in a single sitting. The Nd-YAG laser, Q-switched ruby laser, photodynamic therapy, or resurfacing CO_2 laser, can also be effective.

DRUG-INDUCED HYPERPIGMENTATION

Clinical Findings

Many medications can produce abnormal skin, nail, or oral pigmentation as a result of either deposition of the drug or its metabolites or a drug-induced stimulation of epidermal melanogenesis (Table 2). Some reactions require or are enhanced by ultraviolet light exposure. These color alterations range from tan to slate gray to blue-black. Drugs such as 5-fluorouracil (Adrucil), gold, silver, and amiodarone (Cordarone) produce preferential darkening in sun-exposed sites. Other medications such as zidovudine (Retrovir), bleomycin (Blenoxane), doxorubicin (Adriamycin), chloroquine (Aralen), and cyclophosphamide (Cytoxan) also cause pigmented bands in the nails. Minocycline (Minocin; Dynacin) can produce brown-gray discoloration in old acne scars, hyperpigmented patches on the anterior legs, and a generalized brown-gray discoloration.

Treatment and Prevention

In most instances, the dyspigmentation that appears with drugs slowly fades in months to years after the drug has been discontinued. However, certain medications such as gold and topical hydroquinone

---

[1]Not FDA approved for this indication.

TABLE 2 Medication-Induced Pigmentary Abnormalities

Medication	Clinical Characteristics
Amiodarone (Cordarone)	Gray discoloration in sun-exposed sites
Busulfan (Myleran)	Generalized increased skin color resembling Addison's disease
Doxorubicin (Adriamycin)	Pigmented nail bands and palmar creases
Estrogen (Premarin)	Melasma
5-Fluorouracil	Increased pigment in sun-exposed sites
Gold (Myochrysine)	Permanent blue-gray color in sun-exposed areas
Hydroxychloroquine (Plaquenil)	Brown or gray discoloration of the shins, trunk
Levodopa plus carbidopa (Sinemet)	Diffuse hyperpigmentation
Minocycline (Minocin)	Gray pigment in old scars and/or on the legs or a generalized muddy color
Zidovudine (AZT) (Retrovir)	Nail pigmentation, diffuse Addison's-like pigmentation

can be responsible for irreversible color changes. The use of sunscreens is encouraged in patients with photo-enhanced drug-induced hyperpigmentation to minimize additional pigment production.

POSTINFLAMMATORY HYPERPIGMENTATION

Clinical Findings

This is probably the most common cause of altered skin coloration. This acquired excess of pigment represents the sequelae of a variety of skin disorders, traumas, therapeutic interventions, infections, allergic reactions, mechanical injuries, burns, reactions to medications, phototoxic reactions, and inflammatory diseases, and requires that the underlying process be effectively treated. This results in melanin being released into the dermis, where it is phagocytized by macrophages. This pigment can remain indefinitely and cause macular hyperpigmentation. Superficial melanin tends to be seen as tan or brown, whereas deeper deposits often produce a gray or blue-gray hue.

Treatment

One should attempt to effectively treat underlying skin disorders, avoiding the inciting reaction, regardless of etiology. This includes manual manipulation when applicable. Topical tacrolimus 0.03% ointment (Protopic)[1] or pimecrolimus 1% cream (Elidel)[1] twice a day for 3 months is now our first choice, because it is also therapy for many of the underlying concerns. Patients should avoid cosmetics. Topical tretinoin 0.05% cream may be effectively employed every other day for 2 weeks and continued nightly as tolerated.

If the pigment is superficial, the areas can be lightened somewhat with the agents noted earlier for melasma. They do not work well in deep dermal melanosis. A combination of hydroquinone 4% cream containing sunscreen (Solaquin Forte) applied twice daily and 0.1% tretinoin gel (Retin-A)[1] applied at night for 4 to 6 months can produce substantial lightening. Daily use of sunscreens with a sun protection factor of 15 or greater is essential. Tri-Luma cream (flucinolone acetonide 0.01%, hydroquinone 4%, tretinoin 0.05%) is another option, which needs to be used together with an appropriate sunscreen. Other choices are hydroquinone 4% cream combined with hyaluronic acid, 10% glycolic acid, and the sunscreens avobenzone, oxybenzone, and octocrylene as Glyquin-XM. The combination can cause irritation when first used. Applying tretinoin cream every other night for the first 2 to 3 weeks and then increasing the frequency of application to a nightly treatment program can minimize the irritation. Tretinoin alone can fade the spots somewhat, but treatment is often protracted. Laser therapy is ineffective in most cases. Sunscreens are helpful to minimize increased pigmentation in sites that are already too dark.

A common concern in the dark complexioned acne vulgaris patient is postinflammatory acne hyperpigmentation, often accentuated by manipulating the papules or pustules. The naturally occurring dicarboxylic acid, azelaic acid, in a 20% cream (Azelex) applied as a thin film twice a day, is a good choice for moderately severe comedonal and inflammatory acne and for the hyperpigmentation itself. However, for both purposes its onset of action is somewhat slow. In addition, it can cause annoying stinging, itching, and burning which usually desists with continued use. Its adverse effects include hypopigmentation and the possible initiation of vitiligo. It is a pregnancy category B drug, and safety in patients younger than 12 years is not established.

ACRAL ACANTHOTIC ANOMALY

Acral acanthotic anomaly, a distinct entity viewed by some as a distal form of acanthosis nigricans, is a disorder seen relatively commonly as velvety hyperpigmented plaques in dark-complexioned persons. It is particularly prominent over the elbows, knees, knuckles, and dorsal surfaces of the feet in otherwise healthy persons. Axillae and other intertriginous regions appear normal. Tretinoin cream at bedtime alone can fade the eruption somewhat after prolonged treatment.

---

[1]Not FDA approved for this indication.

Hypopigmentation Disorders

VITILIGO

Clinical Findings

Milk white patches of idiopathic vitiligo affect about 1% to 2% of the general population worldwide without racial, sexual, or regional differences. However, they are more pronounced and easily visualized in darker-complexioned people, and visibility is enhanced by a tendency of some patches to be surrounded by borders of hyperpigmentation. Because vitiliginous patches do not tan, ultraviolet light exposure also emphasizes them when adjacent skin tans normally.

Vitiligo reflects total destruction of all melanocytes within the affected epidermis. The hair within vitiligo becomes white if hair bulb melanocytes are destroyed. Vitiligo is most often seen on the face, backs of the hands and wrists, in the axillae and umbilicus, and on the genitalia. It tends to be especially prominent around body orifices: eyes, nostrils, mouth, nipples, umbilicus and genitalia. It begins as small patches and enlarges peripherally, with new lesions appearing occasionally. It can coalesce into large patches or remain localized. Evolving lesions may be hypopigmented initially, especially in dark complexioned persons. Vitiligo can also appear on the arms, elbows, and knees at sites of trauma or sunburn (Koebner's phenomenon). Striking generalized vitiligo after dermatitis medicamentosa might also reflect this circumstance in a predisposed patient.

Nonsegmental vitiligo is about three times more common than segmental vitiligo; the latter is generally more common in children. Segmental vitiligo tends to have an early onset, spreads rapidly into the involved dermatome, stabilizes within 2 years, and persists throughout life. The initial involvement is usually solitary. The face is the most common site; trigeminal is the commonest dermatome. Nonsegmental vitiligo typically has new patches appearing throughout life and shows a persistent degree of symmetry in early as well as advanced lesions. Patients should also be evaluated for possible coexisting thyroid disease, as well as for a wide range of other occasionally associated autoimmune disorders. Some consider the white halo surrounding the halo nevus and the halo melanoma to represent a type of vitiligo. Halo nevi are not unusual in adolescent girls using birth control pills.

Chemical-induced vitiligo may be caused by industrial germicidal phenolic cleansers, rubbers, and plastics. Therapy must begin by terminating such exposure.

Treatment

There are multiple options but no reliable therapy. Patients might find a psychological benefit from cosmetic cover-ups, such as Dermablend or Covermark, even if no therapy is desired after patient education that vitiligo will not go away spontaneously and that medical therapy might not be effective. Topical dyes and self-tanning products, such as Vitadye stain and sun-free tanning products containing dihydroxyacetone, such as Chromelin Complexion Blender, are also good. Regardless, sunscreen use, if it is not already incorporated into one of these agents, is important, because skin with vitiligo is more likely to sunburn than skin with normal pigmentation, and can ultimately develop skin cancer.

Successful therapy is initially reflected by perifollicular repigmentation after about 3 months, which enlarges as melanocytes migrate laterally. Thus, if vitiligo is on the vermilion borders of the lips, distal fingers, or penile shaft, or has white hair extruding from it, the patient should be advised that medical therapy will not be successful. In that case, surgical repigmentation techniques such as thin-split section grafts or minigrafts of autologous skin or autologous cultured melanocytes into large vitiliginous dermabraded patches would be necessary for stable vitiligo, although the Koebner phenomenon might limit this approach.

Topical tacrolimus 0.03% ointment (Protopic)[1] or pimecrolimus 1% cream (Elidel)[1] twice a day for 3 months is now our first choice, because cutaneous atrophy and telangiectasia are a risk with topical steroids. For a child with localized vitiligo, our next approach is a topical steroid. In children younger than 10 years, hydrocortisone valerate 0.2% cream daily on the face or desonide 0.05% cream daily to the trunk or extremities may be good. For facial and genital vitiligo, use 0.05% fluorcinonide cream (Lidex).[1] Elsewhere, clobetasol propionate cream (Temovate)[1] has been employed in patients as young as 5 years of age, with the best results in facial lesions of dark-complexioned patients, in whom progressive repigmentation continues after discontinuing therapy. Vitiligo might respond on the face but rarely does so on the hands, elbows, and knees. One can use this steroid for 3 to 4 months, evaluating monthly and stopping if there is evidence of cutaneous atrophy or telangiectasia.

Photochemotherapy for vitiligo is sometimes beneficial in the highly motivated, because response is often partial and can take years. For localized vitiligo, the topical psoralen methoxsalen (Oxsoralen lotion 0.01%) is applied 30 minutes before UVA exposure (PUVA), although blistering can be a problem. Widespread vitiligo requires oral methoxypsoralen 0.6 mg/kg administered 90 minutes before UVA exposure three times a week for 3 to 4 months before perifollicular spots become evident. We do not recommend phototherapy for children younger than 12 years. Vitiligo might respond on the face but rarely does so on hands, elbows, and knees. Narrowband UVB by itself is another option and is photochemotherapy using natural sunlight. Patients should be warned that phototherapy has hazards, including the risk of cancer.

If vitiligo involves more than 50% to 75% of the skin, a permanent depigmentation (chemical vitiligo) may be induced, to provide uniform coloration. Generalized permanent bleaching can be achieved with monobenzyl ether of hydroquinone 20% cream (Benzoquin) twice a day for 6 to 12 months or longer for adults with generalized vitiligo. Hyperpigmentation from acquired ochronosis is a risk with this therapy, potentially exacerbating the cosmetic problem.

IDIOPATHIC GUTTATE HYPOMELANOSIS

Clinical Findings

Idiopathic guttate hypomelanosis is a common benign condition of unknown etiology in which asymptomatic oval or angular 2- to 3-mm or larger white macules develop. They are persistent, are most numerous on the anterior lower extremities, and tend to increase in incidence with age so that elderly persons can have hundreds of them.

Treatment

Therapy is usually unsatisfactory. Tretinoin 0.1% gel used for 4 to 6 months can partially restore skin color in affected areas. Cryotherapy with liquid nitrogen may be tried; a gentle 5-second light freeze is sometimes beneficial. Intralesional triamcinolone acetonide 3 mg/mL occasionally is beneficial.

PITYRIASIS ALBA

Clinical Findings

Pityriasis alba is a relatively common disorder of hypopigmented macules that appears most commonly on the faces of preadolescent children and occasionally young adults. It may be the manifesting complaint or an incidental finding. It is a benign, chiefly cosmetic defect that is more prominent in, and problematic for, dark-skinned persons. The etiology of pityriasis alba is not known precisely, although it has been linked with atopy, and it is thought by some to be a postinflammatory reaction in atopic dermatitis. It is usually evident as round to oval hypopigmented macules, 0.5 to 5 cm or more in diameter, with generally well defined but irregular borders. Macules are chiefly on the face (forehead and malar ridges) but occasionally on the shoulders, upper arms, or legs. There are often two or three, but this can vary from one to twenty or more. Some become confluent.

---

[1]Not FDA approved for this indication.

[1]Not FDA approved for this indication.

Initially there is a pink patch with an elevated, slightly erythematous border, which may be slightly pruritic. After a few weeks the erythema fades, leaving a whitish macule, which may be covered with a fine, adherent scale. The late stage is a smooth hypopigmented macule. Repigmentation usually occurs in months to years. Macules in all three stages can occur simultaneously, or all may be in the same stage. The lesions are often most apparent in summer, due to tanning of the surrounding skin. On rare occasions, mycosis fungoides has hypopigmented macules resembling pityriasis alba. Therefore, longstanding patches unresponsive to therapy might require biopsy.

Treatment

An emollient or bland lubricant, such as petrolatum, may be useful in masking scale; no therapy is overwhelmingly successful. Repigmentation can be sometimes accelerated by the use of a mild to medium strength nonfluorinated topical steroid such as hydrocortisone 1% cream or desonide 0.05% cream. Mild peeling agents may be used with or without these topical steroids. More-potent steroids, such as triamcinolone acetonide 0.1% cream and hydrocortisone valerate 0.2% cream, are recommended for nonfacial lesions. Topical tretinoin 0.05% cream applied every other evening may also be useful.

REFERENCES

Huggins RH, Janniger CK, Schwartz RA. Childhood vitiligo. Cutis 2007; 79:277–80.
Lacz NL, Vafaie J, Kihiczak NI, Schwartz RA. Postinflammatory hyperpigmentation: a common and often troubling disorder. Int J Dermatol 2004; 43:362–5.
Schwartz RA. Acral acanthosis nigricans (acral acanthotic anomaly). J Am Acad Dermatol 2007;56:349–50.
Schwartz RA, Fernández G, Kotulska K, Józwiak S. Tuberous sclerosis complex: advances in diagnosis, genetics, and management. J Am Acad Dermatol 2007;57:189–202.
Schwartz RA, Kihiczak NI. Postinflammatory hyperpigmentation. eMedicine Dermatology [Journal serial online]. Available at: http://emedicine.com/derm/topic876.htm; 2009 [Last accessed May 15, 2009].
Sinha S, Schwartz RA. Juvenile acanthosis nigricans. J Am Acad Dermatol 2007;57:502–8.

Sunburn

Method of
Warwick L. Morison, MD

Sunburn is a common problem, particularly in fair-skinned white persons, caused by excessive exposure to ultraviolet (UV) radiation from sunlight or artificial sources such as sunlamps. When induced by sunlight, it is mainly due to UVB (280–320 nm) radiation plus a smaller contribution from UVA (320–400 nm) radiation. Sunburn is also described as erythema and it appears 3 to 4 hours after exposure, reaches a maximum at 12 to 18 hours, and usually settles after 72 to 96 hours. In severe reactions with blistering, complete resolution can take a week or more.

Sunburns are graded as pink, red, and blistering. In contrast, thermal burns are graded by degree (first, second, and third), but this classification should not be applied to sunburns because thermal burns have quite different sequelae, such as scarring and death, which are extremely rare consequences of a sunburn. Keratoconjunctivitis, or ocular sunburn, can also be caused by UV radiation and it follows a similar time course.

There are two facets to management of sunburn: prevention and treatment. Because there is no effective treatment for an established sunburn, most emphasis should be placed on prevention.

CURRENT DIAGNOSIS

- Sunburn appears 3 to 4 hours after exposure to sunlight or an artificial source of UV radiation such as a sunlamp.
- The redness of skin is diffuse and continuous, unlike rashes, which are often discontinuous.
- Sunburns are graded as pink, red, and blistering.

Prevention

Skin color and the capacity of a person to tan will determine how important it is for an individual person to take preventive measures. However, even dark-skinned people can sunburn provided the exposure dose is sufficiently high. Skin color, past history of sunburn, and likely exposure should therefore be used as a guide in advising people about protection. Protection from sunlight is often equated with use of sunscreens, but this approach is too narrow, and protection should consist of a package of measures: avoiding overexposure to sunlight, using sunscreens, and wearing protective clothing.

AVOIDANCE OF EXPOSURE

Simple avoidance of excessive exposure to a threshold dose of UV radiation is often the best advice for fair-skinned people. Scheduling outdoor activities for before 10 AM and after 4 PM will avoid the peak UV irradiance period and still permit enjoyment of the outdoors. This advice should be accompanied by several warnings. Sitting in the shade or under a beach umbrella only reduces exposure by about 70%. A cloudy day is often the setting for the worst sunburns because even complete white cloud cover reduces UV exposure by only about 50%.

Clothing is not always an effective protector. If it is possible to see through a fabric, UV radiation can also penetrate to a significant extent. The geographic location of exposure must also be considered because UV radiation may be twice as intense at the equator as compared with much of continental North America.

SUNSCREENS

There is now a great number of sunscreens on the market, and they contain numerous active ingredients. If this is not enough to cause confusion, some are not even labeled as sunscreens: sunblocks and tanning lotions are other terms. However, the informed physician need only know four properties of a sunscreen: the sun protection factor (SPF), the spectrum of protection, the base, and whether or not it is water resistant.

The SPF is a index of the amount of protection provided by the sunscreen. For example, a fair-skinned person who normally begins to sunburn after a 10-minute exposure to sunlight should be able to tolerate up to 150 minutes of exposure after application of an SPF 15 sunscreen.

There are several provisos for this statement. To provide the stated protection, a sunscreen must be applied 10 minutes before exposure to allow binding to skin proteins to occur, and it must be applied in an adequate amount. Several studies have shown that under ideal circumstances in which sunscreen is supplied freely and the subject is observed while making the application, most people only use one half the required amount. Ordinary use probably provides much less protection. As a rough guide, one ounce of sunscreen is necessary to cover a 70-kg adult in a bathing suit; in other words, a four ounce bottle of sunscreen only provides four applications.

Sunscreens vary in the amount of the solar spectrum for which they provide protection. All sunscreens provide protection against UVB radiation and the shorter end of UVA radiation. Some sunscreens claim to provide broad-spectrum protection against UVB and UVA radiation and contain avobenzone or titanium dioxide to protect against the longer wavelengths in the UVA spectrum. Ecamsule

CURRENT THERAPY

- Prevention is the best approach to management and consists of a package of measures: avoiding over-exposure, using sunscreens, and wearing protective clothing.
- Treatment of a sunburn consists of cool baths and use of moisturizing creams.
- Topical and systemic corticosteroids do not alter the course of a sunburn.

(Mexoryl SX), a recently approved sunscreen active, provides good absorption in the middle of the UVA spectrum so that a sunscreen containing this, avobenzone, and octocrylene, an absorber of UVB radiation, provides very good broad-spectrum protection.

The base of a sunscreen is also important because it often determines whether or not a sunscreen will be used. Men usually prefer alcohol-based lotions because they dry quickly and leave a dry and nongreasy film. Women usually prefer lotions or creams because they give a moisturizing feel to the skin.

Finally, a sunscreen may be labeled water resistant or very water resistant. Because almost all outdoor pastimes involve perspiring or contact with water, a very water-resistant sunscreen should be selected.

A fair-skinned person should always use a sunscreen with an SPF 15 or higher. People who tan well and never burn are probably adequately protected with an SPF of 8 to 10. People with black or brown skin probably do not need sunscreens except for extreme occupational or social exposure.

A few myths should be dismissed. There is no effective oral sunscreen. Many have been tested and all have failed. Self-tanning preparations are not sunscreens. They do provide the appearance of a tan and are safe to use but they provide no significant protection against UV radiation.

PROTECTIVE CLOTHING

There has been significant progress in recent years in the development, testing, and classification of UV-protective clothing. Akin to the SPF for sunscreens, such clothing is labeled with an ultraviolet protective factor (UPF), and a fabric with a UPF of 50 blocks transmission of 98% of UV radiation. A hat with a 3-inch brim all around completes the package of protection.

PROTECTIVE TANNING

The proliferation of suntan parlors has generated a lot of interest in protective tanning, with much misinformation provided by the commercial interests involved. Little scientific information is available to provide a guide as to whether protective tanning is of any value in preventing the long-term hazards of excessive exposure to sunlight, namely skin cancer and premature aging of the skin. Certainly, preventive tanning using multiple suberythemal doses of UV radiation can prevent sunburn, but the cost in terms of chronic damage is unknown.

Most tanning salons claim to use only UVA radiation in their tanning beds, but this claim is false. All so-called UVA tanning beds emit some UVB radiation, the most damaging wavelengths, and in addition, UVA radiation, especially in large doses can produce the same damaging effect as UVB radiation. Furthermore, a UVA-induced tan is not very protective and at most has an SPF of 6 to 8.

A person who tans well and never burns might gain some protection from sunlight by preventive tanning without incurring too much damage. However, the risk-to-benefit ratio for people who do sunburn is probably very unfavorable.

Treatment

When a person has a sunburn, general supportive measures are the only approach to treatment. Cold compresses and cool baths with bath oil provide some relief. Frequent application of moisturizing creams help alleviate dryness. Blistering of the skin can lead to secondary infection and require use of an antibiotic cream. Rarely, an extremely severe sunburn necessitates hospitalization and management as a thermal burn.

Topical corticosteroids reduce erythema by causing vasoconstriction, but this effect is temporary and does not reduce epidermal damage. Systemic corticosteroids, even in very large doses, do not alter the course of a sunburn. Nonsteroidal antiinflammatory drugs, if given at the time of exposure or beforehand, reduce the degree of erythema over the first 24 hours but do not change epidermal damage. Of course, few people lying on the beach anticipate an excessive exposure, so they are unlikely to embark on such preventive measures.

The Nervous System

Alzheimer's Disease

Method of
Edmond Teng, MD, PhD, and Mario F. Mendez, MD, PhD

Dementia is an acquired impairment in cognitive abilities that results in significant functional decline. The most common dementing illness is Alzheimer's disease (AD), which accounts for 50% to 70% of demented patients. Globally, AD affects approximately 26.6 million people, and the annual worldwide societal costs of AD and other dementias are estimated to be $315.4 billion. The prevalence of AD is strongly associated with increasing age. The rapidly growing elderly populations in the United States and other industrialized countries suggest that AD may continue to consume a disproportionate share of health care resources and expenditures in the coming years.

Neuropathology

AD is a neurodegenerative disorder characterized by insidious onset and gradual progression. The underlying neuropathologic changes begin to develop many years before cognitive, behavioral, or functional deficits become clinically apparent and are typically quite advanced by the time a diagnosis is made.

The amyloid cascade hypothesis postulates that AD pathogenesis begins with the accumulation of β-amyloid (Aβ), which is derived from amyloid precursor protein (APP). β-Secretase and γ-secretase proteases sequentially cleave APP to produce neurotoxic $A\beta_{40}$ and $A\beta_{42}$ peptides, which subsequently aggregate into oligomers and fibrils that form extracellular amyloid plaques. These *senile plaques* are among the neuropathologic hallmarks of AD. Many experimental therapeutic agents for AD being evaluated in clinical trials target specific mechanisms along the Aβ pathway.

Although Aβ accumulation appears to be one of the earliest steps in the pathogenesis of AD, the extent of Aβ plaque deposition does not consistently correlate with clinical severity. These findings suggest that additional pathology precipitated by Aβ accumulation contributes to the progressive synaptic dysfunction, neuronal loss, and neurotransmitter deficits that produce the clinical symptoms of AD. These Aβ-induced pathologic changes include the hyperphosphorylation of tau protein to form intracellular neurofibrillary tangles (NFTs) and increased levels of inflammation, oxidative stress, and excitotoxicity.

Neuropathologic criteria for AD focus on plaque and NFT deposition, which is primarily seen in medial temporal lobe structures such as the entorhinal cortex and the hippocampus in the earliest stages of the disease. With disease progression, these changes extend to neighboring limbic structures, with later widespread deposition in other cortical regions. These microscopic changes are reflected by similar patterns of increasing regional brain atrophy.

Epidemiology

Epidemiologic studies have identified several genetic and environmental risk factors for AD. Increasing age is the strongest of these factors. Most patients are older than 60 years. By age 65, approximately 1% of the general population meets diagnostic criteria for AD. The prevalence roughly doubles with every 5 years thereafter, with estimates as high 35% to 40% for individuals older than 90 years.

A family history of AD is another major risk factor. Individuals with at least one first-degree relative diagnosed with AD are four times more likely to develop the disease themselves than people without a family history of AD. Genetic studies indicate that much of this increased risk may depend on apolipoprotein E (ApoE) genotype. Relative to the more common ApoE3 allele, the ApoE4 allele is associated in a copy-dependent fashion with a greater prevalence of AD and an earlier age of onset. Other variables associated with increased risk for AD include female gender, low levels of education, cardiovascular risk factors, and history of head trauma.

Clinical Presentation

The clinical presentation of AD is heterogeneous and related to disease severity. The primary symptoms fall into three categories: cognitive, behavioral, and functional. In mild cognitive impairment (which often represents incipient AD) or in mild AD, defined as a Mini-Mental Status Examination (MMSE) score >20, cognitive deficits are commonly seen in episodic memory, primarily for recall and recognition of recent events and other newly learned information, and in word-finding abilities. Behavioral abnormalities such as apathy, depression, and irritability start to emerge. In mild cognitive impairment, functional abilities remain essentially intact, but in mild AD, difficulties with employment and other complex instrumental activities of daily living (ADLs), such as finances and driving, begin to develop.

With moderate AD (MMSE score of 11–20), patients begin to experience increasing difficulty with remote memory, verbal communication, and getting around without getting lost. Agitation, aggression, and anxiety are frequently reported. They are no longer able to independently perform their instrumental ADLs, and they may need increasing assistance with some basic ADLs, such as dressing, bathing, and toileting.

With severe AD (MMSE score ≤10), patients have widespread deterioration in all cognitive domains, including near-mutism, which limits formal assessment. Agitation continues to worsen, and aberrant motor activity (i.e., pacing, restlessness, and wandering) becomes a major issue. They are no longer able to perform their basic ADLs and may develop urinary and fecal incontinence.

Diagnosis

The two most commonly used diagnostic criteria for AD, the *Diagnostic and Statistical Manual of Mental Disorders*, fourth edition (DSM-IV), and the National Institute of Neurological and Communicative Disorders and Stroke-Alzheimer's Disease and Related Disorders Association (NINCDS-ADRDA) criteria, share a common emphasis on gradual symptom onset and progression, impairments in memory and at least one additional cognitive domain, deficits in ADLs, and exclusion of delirium and other medical or psychiatric conditions as the primary cause of these deficits. Factors that make a diagnosis of AD less likely include sudden onset or the presence of focal neurologic or extrapyramidal signs, seizures, gait abnormality, and behavioral disturbances early in the disease course. The DSM-IV and NINCDS-ADRDA criteria exhibit accuracy ranging from 65% to 90% in clinicopathologic studies, but may be relatively insensitive to incipient AD. More recently proposed criteria focus on deficits in episodic memory supported by genetic, imaging, or cerebrospinal fluid biomarkers.

A diagnostic evaluation for AD should start with a comprehensive history, obtained from the patient and a knowledgeable informant, that focuses on the time course and progression of cognitive, behavioral, and functional symptoms; relevant medical history; and medication use. Mental status examination to confirm subjective cognitive deficits should be performed with instruments such as the MMSE, the Memory Impairment Screen, the Clock Drawing Test, or other brief screening tools. Patients with more subtle cognitive deficits or higher levels of premorbid functioning may perform well on these assessments and should be referred for formal neuropsychological testing if a clinical suspicion of cognitive impairment persists. Physical and neurologic examination results are typically normal aside from parkinsonism or frontal release signs that can be seen with more advanced disease.

Although there are no laboratory tests of sufficient accuracy to independently confirm a diagnosis of AD, several tests can rule out other conditions that can cause or contribute to the presenting symptoms: complete blood cell count, serum chemistries, glucose, thyroid function, vitamin B_{12}, rapid plasma reagin, and liver function. Structural neuroimaging by computed tomography (CT) or magnetic resonance imaging (MRI) can assess medial temporal lobe atrophy and rule out other potential etiologies. Additional assessments that are not routinely indicated but may be useful in more complicated cases include positron emission tomography (PET) to assess for glucose metabolism in temporal, parietal, and posterior cingulate regions; cerebrospinal fluid levels of $A\beta_{42}$ and tau; and genetic testing for early-onset autosomal dominant forms of AD. ApoE testing has no current diagnostic utility, but it may become more useful in the future; research is emerging that suggests genotype-specific responses to various therapeutic interventions.

Differential diagnosis for AD includes other common dementing conditions: vascular dementia (15% to 25% of dementia cases), dementia with Lewy bodies (10% to 20%), depression (5% to 10%), and frontotemporal lobar degeneration (5%). Vascular dementia can manifest with abrupt symptom onset, stepwise deterioration, focal neurologic signs or symptoms, multiple cardiovascular risk factors, and neuroimaging abnormalities consistent with cerebrovascular disease. Vascular dementia can be difficult to distinguish from AD because these conditions share similar risk factors and a significant proportion of vascular dementia cases exhibit comorbid AD pathology. The core features that distinguish dementia with Lewy bodies include spontaneous parkinsonism, visual hallucinations, and fluctuations in alertness and cognition. Severe depression can cause cognitive deficits in elderly patients, particularly on tasks that emphasize attention, information-processing speed, or effort. Depression-related dementia can resemble AD or vascular dementia because depressive symptoms are commonly seen in these conditions. Frontotemporal lobar degeneration results in prominent social, behavioral, and language impairment early in the course of the disease, and in most cases, manifests before age 65. Referral to a memory disorders specialist is appropriate if the patient exhibits atypical clinical features, rapid progression, or poor response to AD therapeutics.

CURRENT DIAGNOSIS

- Memory and other cognitive domains (e.g., language, visuospatial, executive, motor skills) are impaired.
- Declines are noticed in social or occupational function or in performance of usual activities of daily living.
- Symptoms are insidious in onset and exhibit a gradual and continuing progression.
- Symptoms do not occur solely in the context of a delirium syndrome.
- Symptoms are not better explained by other neurologic conditions (e.g., stroke, subdural hematoma, normal pressure hydrocephalus, brain tumor, traumatic brain injury, other neurodegenerative conditions); other systemic medical conditions (e.g., vitamin B_{12} deficiency, hypothyroidism, neurosyphilis, human immunodeficiency virus infection, sleep apnea, medication effects); or other psychiatric disorders (e.g., depression, bipolar disorder, schizophrenia, substance abuse).
- Factors suggesting other causes include sudden onset or prominent early neurologic signs, seizures, gait abnormality, and behavioral disturbances.
- Diagnosis may be supported by findings from structural neuroimaging (i.e., medial temporal lobe atrophy on MRI or CT); functional neuroimaging (i.e., reduced glucose metabolism in temporal, parietal, or posterior cingulate regions on PET); and cerebrospinal fluid biomarkers (i.e., decreased $A\beta_{42}$ and increased total and phosphorylated tau).

Treatment

At preclinical and clinical stages of drug development, investigators are assessing a plethora of pharmacologic interventions that target key steps in the pathophysiology of AD, including $A\beta$ and tau synthesis, aggregation, and deposition into plaques and NFTs. Although these strategies have shown much potential in animal and in vitro models of AD, several putative disease-modifying agents have produced disappointing results in phase III clinical trials.

Four FDA-approved medications are available for the treatment of AD (Table 1). Three are cholinesterase inhibitors (ChE-I): donepezil (Aricept), galantamine (Razadyne), and rivastigmine (Exelon). The fourth, memantine (Namenda), is an *N*-methyl-D-aspartate (NMDA) receptor antagonist. These medications demonstrate modest effects on slowing the progress of cognitive, behavioral, and functional symptoms of AD, but they do not appear to reverse or arrest the underlying neurodegenerative processes associated with the disease.

ChE-I therapy addresses the relative depletion of acetylcholine (ACh) levels in AD brains by preventing its metabolism and potentiating ACh-related neurotransmission. The utility of ChE-I therapy appears to be most robust in mild to moderate AD, although there appears to be some benefit with donepezil (Aricept) among subjects with incipient or severe AD. Although the ChE-Is that are available have slightly different enzymatic specificities, their overall efficacy appears to be similar. Treatment responses appear to be dose related, and dosing should be gradually titrated up every 4 weeks to the maximum recommended dosages or until limited by side effects. ChE-Is are reasonably well tolerated, and side effects are typically transient and dose dependent. The most common adverse reactions are gastrointestinal, such as nausea, vomiting, and anorexia. Other frequently encountered side effects include dizziness, bradycardia, insomnia, and vivid dreams. The use of once-daily oral or transdermal patch (Exelon Patch) formulations may minimize the incidence of these adverse effects. Oral formulations of galantamine or rivastigmine should be administered with food. Responses to ChE-Is are often

TABLE 1 First-Line Pharmacologic Treatments for Alzheimer's Disease

Feature	Donepezil (Aricept)	Rivastigmine (Exelon)	Galantamine (Razadyne*)	Memantine (Namenda)
Mechanisms	AChE-I	AChE-I BuChE-I	AChE-I Nicotinic receptor modulator	NMDA receptor antagonist
Disease severity	Mild to moderate	Mild to moderate	Mild to moderate	Moderate to severe
Initial dose	5 mg daily	1.5 mg bid (oral) 4.6 mg daily (patch)	4 mg bid (standard) 8 mg daily (ER)	5 mg daily
Maximum dose	10 mg daily	6 mg bid (oral); 9.5 mg daily (patch)	12 mg bid (standard) 24 mg daily (ER)	10 mg bid
Plasma $t_{1/2}$	70 h	1.5 h	7 h	70 h
Common side effects	Nausea, vomiting, anorexia, diarrhea, bradycardia, syncope, insomnia, vivid dreams	Nausea, vomiting, anorexia, diarrhea, bradycardia, syncope, insomnia, vivid dreams	Nausea, vomiting, anorexia, diarrhea, bradycardia, syncope, insomnia, vivid dreams	Dizziness, headache, confusion, constipation
Significant drug-drug interactions	Bethanechol (Urecholine), ketoconazole (Nizoral), quinidine, succinylcholine (Anectine)	None	Amitriptyline (Elavil), fluoxetine (Prozac), fluvoxamine (Luvox), paroxetine (Paxil), ketoconazole, quinidine	Carbonic anhydrase inhibitors, cimetidine (Tagamet), ranitidine (Zantac), quinidine, hydrochlorothiazide (HCTZ), sodium bicarbonate

*Previously Reminyl.
Abbreviations: AChE-I = acetylcholinesterase inhibitor; BuChE-I = butyrylcholinesterase inhibitor; NMDA = N-methyl-D-aspartate; bid = twice daily; ER = extended release.

idiosyncratic, and patients who report poor efficacy or tolerability on one medication may achieve better results when switched to another.

Memantine blocks NMDA receptor ion channels, but how this mechanism translates into clinical efficacy remains uncertain. Studies suggest that it is most effective for the treatment of moderate to severe AD, although weaker evidence also supports its use in mild AD. The starting dose is 5 mg daily, and it is typically titrated up by 5 mg per week to a final dose of 10 mg twice daily in patients with normal renal function and 5 mg twice daily for those with creatinine clearance rates less than 30 mL/min. Adverse events are less frequently reported with memantine than with the ChE-Is, and include dizziness, headache, confusion, and constipation. Memantine can be used as monotherapy, particularly in patients who cannot tolerate ChE-I therapy, but it may be more effective when administered in tandem with a ChE-I.

Earlier work indicated that high doses of vitamin E[1] (2000 IU/day) administered to patients with moderate AD significantly delayed progression to a composite end point of death, institutionalization, loss of basic ADLs, or severe AD. However, a later trial of this dosage of vitamin E in incipient AD showed no benefit, and a meta-analysis revealed that doses >400 IU/day result in an increase in all-cause mortality. The role of vitamin E in the treatment of AD therefore remains uncertain. Smaller studies of dietary supplements such as gingko biloba[1,7] and huperzine A[1,7] conducted in Europe and China demonstrate benefits similar to the ChE-Is, but larger studies in the United States have shown no benefit (gingko biloba) or are in progress (huperzine A). Likewise, other potential interventions such as coenzyme Q10,[1,7] selegiline (Eldepryl),[1] nonsteroidal antiinflammatory drugs (NSAIDs), statins, and hormone replacement therapy have yet to consistently demonstrate significant benefits in the treatment of AD and should not be routinely recommended for this purpose.

Although cognitive complaints are the most common presenting symptoms of AD, behavioral symptoms are often the most problematic for caregivers, particularly with disease progression. Treatment with a ChE-I or memantine demonstrates modest reductions in many of the behavioral abnormalities associated with AD. However, adjunctive pharmacologic or nonpharmacologic therapy may be necessary. The wide spectrum of AD-related neuropsychiatric disturbances necessitates specific treatment strategies that are tailored to each patient's symptoms.

Nonpharmacologic approaches should be pursued before pharmacologic interventions. Although many such treatments have been proposed and investigated, most studies are not rigorously blinded or controlled, which limits the scope of evidence-based recommendations. Agitation and aggression may be most amenable to nonpharmacologic strategies, such as maintaining a consistent and predictable daily routine, providing frequent reassurance and reorientation to time and place, minimizing insufficient or excessive sensory and social stimulation, simplifying instructions and tasks, and distraction or redirection when such behaviors occur.

Adjunctive pharmacologic treatments that have demonstrated efficacy for treating behavioral disorders in AD include antipsychotics, anticonvulsants, anxiolytics, and antidepressants (Table 2). Studies investigating the use of these medications for AD-related psychopathology have not been uniformly supportive, and for some patients, the risks posed by their potential adverse effects may outweigh the expected therapeutic gains. To reduce risks associated with prolonged use of these psychotropic medications, treatments initiated for specific target symptoms should be administered at the lowest effective doses and discontinued on sustained symptom resolution.

Antipsychotics have demonstrated some utility for ameliorating agitation, aggression, psychosis, and insomnia. The most effective agents appear to be risperidone (Risperdal),[1] olanzapine (Zyprexa),[1] and to a lesser extent, quetiapine (Seroquel).[1] For acute agitation and aggression in patients who are unable or unwilling to take oral medications, intramuscular forms of olanzapine (Zyprexa IntraMuscular)[1] and haloperidol (Haldol)[1] are available. However, antipsychotic use in elderly dementia patients has been associated with a small increase in all-cause mortality. The FDA has issued a black-box warning highlighting this risk, and it emphasizes that the use of typical and atypical antipsychotics for behavioral symptoms in this population is not formally approved. Nevertheless, short-term use of these agents may be warranted in patients with behavioral disturbances of appropriate severity that have not responded to other therapies and after a careful discussion of risks and benefits with the patient and the caregivers.

[1]Not FDA approved for this indication.
[7]Available as dietary supplement.

[1]Not FDA approved for this indication.

TABLE 2 Adjunctive Pharmacologic Therapies for Behavioral Symptoms

Medication	Symptoms	Dose	Side Effects	Safety Issues
Antipsychotics				
Risperidone (Risperdal)[1]	Agitation, aggression, psychosis, insomnia	0.25–2 mg daily	Extrapyramidal symptoms, sedation, confusion, headache, weight gain	FDA black box warning for increased all-cause mortality when used in demented elderly patients
Olanzapine (Zyprexa)[1]	Agitation, aggression, psychosis, insomnia	2.5–10 mg daily (oral), 2.5–5 mg daily (IM)	Extrapyramidal symptoms, sedation, confusion, weight gain, psychosis	FDA black box warning for increased all-cause mortality when used in demented elderly patients
Quetiapine (Seroquel)[1]	Agitation, aggression, psychosis, insomnia	25–200 mg daily	Sedation, weight gain, dizziness, urinary symptoms	FDA black box warning for increased all-cause mortality when used in demented elderly patients
Haloperidol (Haldol)[1]	Agitation, aggression, psychosis, insomnia	0.25–1 mg daily (IM)	Hypotension, somnolence, extrapyramidal symptoms, tardive dyskinesia	FDA black box warning for increased all-cause mortality when used in demented elderly patients
Anticonvulsants				
Carbamazepine (Tegretol)[1]	Agitation, aggression	300–600 mg daily	Sedation, confusion, dizziness, ataxia, confusion, nausea, vomiting	Many drug-drug interactions
Anxiolytics				
Lorazepam (Ativan)	Anxiety, agitation,[1] aggression[1]	0.5–2 mg daily	Sedation, confusion, dizziness	Short-term use for acute symptoms only
Antidepressants				
Citalopram (Celexa)	Depression, anxiety,[1] irritability,[1] agitation,[1] aggression[1]	10–40 mg daily	Sedation, nausea, vomiting, dry mouth, diarrhea, sexual dysfunction	
Sertraline (Zoloft)	Depression, anxiety,[1] irritability,[1] agitation,[1] aggression[1]	25–150 mg daily	Sedation, insomnia, nausea, vomiting, dry mouth, dizziness, tremor, sexual dysfunction	Reduce dosing in patients with hepatic impairment
Mirtazapine (Remeron)	Depression, insomnia,[1] anorexia[1]	15–45 mg daily	Sedation, dizziness, headache, increased appetite, weight gain, edema	Rare agranulocytosis

[1]Not FDA approved for this indication.
Abbreviation: IM = intramuscular.

Alternatives to antipsychotics for the treatment of agitation and aggression include anticonvulsants and anxiolytics. Many studies indicate that the severity of these symptoms can be reduced with carbamazepine (Tegretol).[1] Factors that may limit the use of carbamazepine include the potential for side effects such as ataxia, dizziness, and sedation and drug-drug interactions caused by induction of hepatic enzymes. The efficacy of valproic acid (Depakene)[1] has been evaluated in other studies, but the results have been less encouraging. Anxiolytics, particularly benzodiazepines, may be indicated for short-term management of acute agitation and anxiety. However, prolonged use can be associated with tolerance, dependence, somnolence, and exacerbation of cognitive impairment.

Antidepressants also have a role in the management of a range of behavioral pathology in AD. Serotonin-specific reuptake inhibitors (SSRIs) such as citalopram (Celexa) or sertraline (Zoloft) significantly reduce mood symptoms such as depression, anxiety,[1] and irritability[1] with relatively few adverse effects or drug-drug interactions. Mirtazapine (Remeron), which blocks presynaptic α_2-adrenergic receptors and increases norepinephrine and serotonin release, is another attractive option, particularly because it exhibits antihistaminergic effects that can help address other common neuropsychiatric symptoms seen in AD, such as insomnia,[1] anorexia,[1] and weight loss.[1] Although its potential efficacy in this population is suggested by small preliminary studies, it has yet to be evaluated by more rigorous clinical trial methodologies. Treatment with citalopram has been associated with reductions in agitation[1] and aggression,[1] suggesting that the benefits of antidepressants in this population may extend beyond the treatment of mood disorders.

Community Support Services

Dedicated caregivers are an essential component for optimizing quality of life for AD patients. In particular, caregivers can encourage continued physical, mental, and social activities. Unfortunately, caregiver

CURRENT THERAPY

First-line pharmacologic treatments

■ Cholinesterase inhibitors, including donepezil (Aricept), rivastigmine (Exelon), or galantamine (Razadyne [previously Reminyl]), which are primarily indicated for mild to moderate AD

■ NMDA receptor antagonists, including memantine (Namenda), which are primarily indicated for moderate to severe AD; better efficacy when used in conjunction with a cholinesterase inhibitor

Adjunctive therapies for behavioral symptoms

■ Nonpharmacologic interventions are used with emphasis on reorientation, reassurance, and redirection.

■ Pharmacologic interventions include atypical antipsychotics for agitation, aggression, psychosis, or insomnia; anticonvulsants for agitation or aggression; anxiolytics for agitation, aggression, or anxiety; and antidepressants for depression, anxiety, or irritability.

Early referral to community organizations such as the Alzheimer's Association and Leeza's Place for additional caregiver support resources

[1]Not FDA approved for this indication.

stress and burnout often increases with disease severity. Early referral to community organizations such as the Alzheimer's Association (www.alz.org) or Leeza's Place (www.leezaplace.org) may help minimize caregiver distress and frustration and improve patient care and safety. These organizations frequently sponsor educational programs and support groups targeted toward caregivers of patients at various stages of the disease. Consultation is often available to assist with advance planning, such as establishing advance directives, durable power of attorney, and other legal considerations. As the disease progresses and patients become more difficult to manage, these organizations can provide referrals for additional support services, including adult day care programs, professional in-home caregivers, and assisted living or skilled nursing facilities.

REFERENCES

Buschke H, Kuslansky G, Katz M, et al. Screening for dementia with the memory impairment screen. Neurology 1999;52:231–8.

Cummings JL. Alzheimer's disease. N Engl J Med 2004;351:56–67.

Dubois B, Feldman HH, Jacova C, et al. Research criteria for the diagnosis of Alzheimer's disease: Revising the NINCDS-ADRDA criteria. Lancet Neurol 2007;6:734–46.

Farlow MR, Miller ML, Pejovic V. Treatment options in Alzheimer's disease: Maximizing benefit, managing expectations. Dement Geriatr Cogn Disord 2008;25:408–22.

Folstein MF, Folstein SE, McHugh PR. "Mini-mental state." A practical method for grading the cognitive state of patients for the clinician. J Psychiatr Res 1975;12:189–98.

Herrmann N, Lanctot KL. Pharmacologic management of neuropsychiatric symptoms of Alzheimer disease. Can J Psychiatry 2007;52:630–46.

Holsinger T, Deveau J, Boustani M, Williams Jr JW. Does this patient have dementia? JAMA 2007;297:2391–404.

McKhann G, Drachman D, Folstein M, et al. Clinical diagnosis of Alzheimer's disease: Report of the NINCDS-ADRDA Work Group under the auspices of Department of Health and Human Services Task Force on Alzheimer's Disease. Neurology 1984;34:939–44.

Sink KM, Holden KF, Yaffe K. Pharmacological treatment of neuropsychiatric symptoms of dementia: A review of the evidence. JAMA 2005;293:596–608.

US Food and Drug Administration. Information for healthcare professionals: Antipsychotics. Available at http://www.fda.gov/Drugs/DrugSafety/Postmarket DrugSafetyInformationforPatientsandProviders/DrugSafetyInformationfor HealthcareProfessionals/ucm084149.htm#note [accessed September 2009].

Sleep Disorders

Method of
David N. Neubauer, MD

In recent years there has been increasing recognition of the high prevalence and significant consequences of sleep disorders and the effects of insufficient sleep. The National Sleep Foundation estimates that about 70 million Americans have problems with their sleep. Research has documented various medical and psychiatric comorbidities with sleep disorders and how sleep disturbances can increase the risk of other disorders. While the number of sleep specialists and sleep disorder centers continue to grow, primary care medicine remains the frontline in the clinical evaluation and treatment of sleep disorders. This chapter provides a broad overview of the common sleep disorders encountered in clinical practice. Sleep-disordered breathing is covered in greater detail in the chapter on Sleep Apnea.

The foundation of understanding sleep disorders is an appreciation of the two primary processes normally regulating the sleep-wake cycle. A *homeostatic* sleep drive determines the amount of sleep we need for alertness and vigilance during our waking hours. For most individuals, a daily sleep total of approximately 8 hours is ideal. Insufficient sleep, whether acute or chronic, leads to increased sleepiness. The ability to achieve sufficient sleep at night and subsequent

wakefulness throughout the daytime and evening is optimized by the *circadian* process, which is coordinated through the suprachiasmatic nucleus in the anterior hypothalamus with input from the photoperiod. The circadian process generates maximum arousal in the evening to offset the homeostatic sleepiness that evolves throughout the day. These two processes together promote sustained wakefulness for about 16 hours and sleep for about 8 hours in synchrony with the day-night cycle.

The homeostatic and circadian processes describe the normal pattern of alertness and sleepiness, but they also may help explain clinical problems associated with insufficient sleepiness (insomnia) and excessive sleepiness. Daytime or evening napping reduces the homeostatic sleep drive available to promote sleep onset and maintenance during a desired nighttime sleep period. This may lead a patient to complain of insomnia. Difficulty falling asleep and remaining asleep also may result from attempts to sleep outside the normal photoperiod-reinforced circadian zone of increased sleep propensity. Sleep difficulty associated with shift work is a typical example.

Symptoms of Sleep Disorders

The evaluation of patients with sleep difficulties should begin with a thorough history of their sleep-related symptoms. How long has it been a problem? Is it intermittent, or a daily or nightly problem? What time of the day or night do the symptoms occur? Are there obvious precipitants or consequences? Is there impairment in normal functioning? What have been the typical sleep-wake hours for the individual, and what is the current pattern? Are there medical or psychiatric disorders or medications that might be influencing the sleep-related symptoms? Input from a bed partner or other informant can be invaluable. Having patients maintain sleep logs can offer a concise view of the patterns of their sleep disturbances and help demonstrate the effects of treatment strategies. Questionnaires and scales (e.g., Epworth Sleepiness Scale, Pittsburgh Sleep Quality Index) can be useful for screening patients for possible sleep disturbances.

Symptoms of sleep disorders may include an inability to sleep at desired times (insomnia), an inability to remain fully awake and attentive at desired times (excessive sleepiness), snoring and fluctuations in breathing patterns during sleep, uncomfortable sensations prior to sleep onset, abnormal movements before and during sleep, and abnormal behaviors emanating from sleep (parasomnias). Although insomnia, excessive daytime sleepiness, and parasomnias are the primary symptom clusters, individual patients may experience overlapping symptoms. For instance, sleep-disordered breathing can be associated with disrupted nighttime sleep and excessive daytime sleepiness.

Insomnia

Insomnia is difficulty falling asleep or remaining asleep when people expect to be able to sleep and when there is an opportunity for them to be in bed sleeping. An insomnia disorder persists for at least 1 month and is associated with daytime impairment. Insomnia affects about 30% of the general adult population intermittently and about 10% on a chronic basis. Insomnia is a problem for more than half of patients with chronic medical conditions. Insomnia may occur idiopathically or may result from distressing circumstances; psychological conditioning; environmental factors; jet lag and shift work schedules; medication effects; and medical, psychiatric, and sleep disorders.

Treatment of insomnia may require multiple strategies that involve correction of sleep hygiene problems, bedtime routine and schedule modifications, cognitive and other psychotherapeutic techniques, strategically timed exposure to bright light, and use of medications. Additionally, optimizing the management of comorbid conditions (e.g., major depression, chronic pain, sleep-disordered breathing, and congestive heart failure) may be necessary for sleep quality improvements. General sleep hygiene recommendations are listed in Table 1. Delaying bedtime may help patients spending excessive frustrating wakeful time in bed. Cognitive therapy techniques

TABLE 1 Sleep Hygiene Recommendations

- Try to maintain a regular sleep-wake schedule.
- Avoid afternoon or evening napping.
- Allow yourself enough time in bed for adequate sleep duration (e.g., 11 PM to 7 AM).
- Develop a relaxing evening routine for the hours approaching bedtime.
- Spend some idle time reflecting on the day's events before going to bed. Make a list of concerns and how some might be resolved.
- Reserve the bed for sleep and sex. Do not do homework, pay bills, or engage in serious domestic discussions in bed.
- Avoid evening alcohol.
- Avoid caffeine in the afternoon and evening.
- Minimize annoying noise, light, or temperature extremes.
- Consider a light snack before bedtime.
- Exercise regularly, but not late in the evening.
- Do not try harder and harder to fall asleep. If you are unable to sleep, do something else out of bed and in another room, if possible.
- Avoid smoking.

may be especially helpful for the patients who catastrophize about their sleep problems.

Significant advances in the pharmacologic treatment of insomnia have been made in recent years. Patients may experience improved sleep with sedating medications prescribed for comorbid conditions (e.g., antidepressants). The medications indicated for treatment of insomnia (Table 2) include both traditional benzodiazepines and newer nonbenzodiazepine hypnotics. All of these hypnotics function through enhancing the inhibitory responses of γ-aminobutyric acid (GABA)-A receptors. The newer medications have pharmacokinetic and pharmacodynamic characteristics that improve their safety profile. Ramelteon (Rozerem), a nonsedating, selective melatonin receptor agonist that targets activity of the circadian system, also is approved for treatment of insomnia.

The duration of action of the newer generation hypnotics ranges from the very short-acting zaleplon (Sonata) to the progressively longer-acting zolpidem (Ambien), extended-release zolpidem (Ambien CR), and eszopiclone (Lunesta). The pattern of patients' sleep disturbances influences the selection of hypnotics. Exclusive sleep-onset difficulty may be treated adequately with a very short-acting medication; however, most insomnia patients have combined difficulty falling asleep and maintaining sleep. Accordingly, moderately short-acting medications that do not cause residual morning sedation generally are optimal.

TABLE 2 Medications Indicated for Treatment of Insomnia

Medication	Available Doses (mg)	Duration of Action
Hypnotic		
Benzodiazepines:		
Estazolam (ProSom)	1, 2	Intermediate-long
Flurazepam (Dalmane)	15, 30	Long
Quazepam (Doral)	7.5, 15	Long
Temazepam (Restoril)	7.5, 15, 22.5, 30	Intermediate
Triazolam (Halcion)	0.125, 0.25	Short-intermediate
Nonbenzodiazepines:		
Eszopiclone (Lunesta)	1, 2, 3	Intermediate
Zaleplon (Sonata)	5, 10	Very short
Zolpidem (Ambien)	5, 10	Short
Zolpidem (Ambien CR) extended-release	6.25, 12.5	Short-intermediate
Melatonin Receptor Agonist		
Ramelteon (Rozerem)	8	Short

Until recently, all prescription sleep-promoting medications were approved for short-term treatment of insomnia; however, beginning in 2005 the FDA began approving sleep-promoting agents simply for treatment of insomnia without the implied short-term restriction. Whereas the majority of patients taking hypnotic medications require help with their sleep only for limited periods of time, others with chronic insomnia have experienced continued improvement in nighttime sleep and daytime functioning with longer-term nightly or intermittent hypnotic use. All of the currently approved benzodiazepine receptor agonist hypnotics remain Schedule IV controlled substances. In contrast, ramelteon (Rozerem) is not classified as a controlled substance.

Circadian Rhythm Disorders

Although the circadian system typically promotes nighttime sleep from approximately 10 to 11 PM until about 6 to 7 AM, many individuals have long-standing tendencies to experience either earlier or later sleep propensity zones. An individual's circadian phase can contribute to complaints of insomnia or excessive sleepiness, although this influence often is not recognized. Adolescents and young adults are more likely to have later sleep propensities, whereas elderly individuals tend to have an earlier onset and offset of sleepiness. People with an *advanced sleep phase* are early birds; they become sleepy earlier in the evening and then are unable to sleep later in the morning. They may complain of persistent early morning awakening as well as daytime fatigue and sleepiness. Night owls with a *delayed circadian phase* have difficulty falling asleep early and tend to sleep later in the morning. This can represent a significant clinical problem. Patients may report sleep-onset insomnia or excessive daytime sleepiness, particularly during the morning hours. Melatonin receptor agonists given prior to bedtime also may help advance and stabilize the sleep onset and morning awakening times for delayed sleep phase patients. Evening bright light exposure may help patients with a long-term predisposition for early evening sleepiness and bothersome early morning awakening. Conversely, bright light exposure upon awakening may help those with a night-owl pattern.

Excessive Daytime Sleepiness

Excessive sleepiness during waking hours is a major public health problem most evident in associated workplace and vehicular accidents, injuries, and fatalities. Excessively sleepy patients typically complain of sleepiness for major portions of the day and report a high propensity for falling asleep during sedentary activities. In severe cases, patients may fall asleep while driving, conversing, or attending important meetings. Chronic sleepiness may lead to educational, occupational, and social difficulties. The most common cause of excessive sleepiness is insufficient sleep, whether due to work schedules or lifestyle choices. Sedating medications and other substances can lead to excessive sleepiness. Emerging evidence suggests that sleep deprivation may contribute to metabolic and immune impairment, even in healthy young individuals.

Patients complaining of difficulty remaining awake during the daytime should be evaluated at a sleep center unless there is an obvious and reversible cause. Sleep laboratory testing includes the standard nighttime polysomnography and possibly a series of daytime nap opportunities that objectively assess sleep onset latency and sleep stages. The key sleep disorders associated with excessive daytime sleepiness are narcolepsy, hypersomnolence disorders, and sleep-disordered breathing. To a limited extent, insomnia and other disorders causing frequent arousals and awakenings, or awakenings with difficulty returning to sleep, may contribute to daytime sleepiness. The latter might include restless legs syndrome, periodic limb movement disorder, and parasomnias.

Narcolepsy

Although *narcolepsy* is the classic disorder of excessive sleepiness, it affects only about 0.05% of the population. It is characterized by persistent sleepiness and difficulty maintaining attention. Symptoms typically begin to evolve by the late teens and continue through life. In addition to disturbed daytime wakefulness and nighttime sleep, narcolepsy patients have symptoms reflecting dysregulation of the characteristics of rapid eye movement (REM) sleep. *Cataplexy* is the loss of postural muscle tone that occurs during waking and is precipitated by heightened emotion, such as anxiety or laughter. The effects may range from a barely noticeable jaw drop to the patient lying on the ground awake but unable to move for up to several minutes. *Sleep paralysis* occurs at the transition to sleep when a person becomes aware of a complete inability to move any muscles voluntarily. It resolves spontaneously within minutes. Cataplexy and sleep paralysis both involve the intrusion of the normal paralysis that accompanies REM sleep; however, it occurs at an abnormal time. Narcolepsy patients also are more likely to experience *hypnagogic hallucinations*, which are dreamlike experiences occurring at sleep onset. Sleep laboratory testing confirms the diagnosis.

Treatment of narcolepsy begins with the establishment of therapeutic goals, typically including maximizing attention and alertness during certain hours of the day, along with the elimination of cataplexy. Narcolepsy patients should be careful to allow sufficient hours for nighttime sleep, as sleep deprivation will exacerbate their symptoms. Scheduled brief naps and periods of increased physical activity during the daytime may be very helpful. Most narcolepsy patients will require pharmacotherapy to enhance daytime alertness. Modafinil (Provigil) may be adequate for some patients; however, many will respond best to amphetamine medications. Antidepressants (e.g., venlafaxine[1] [Effexor]) may reduce cataplexy. Sodium oxybate (Xyrem), which is taken in two nighttime doses, has been shown to improve nighttime sleep, reduce cataplexy, and increase daytime alertness in narcolepsy patients.

Hypersomnolence Disorders

In addition to narcolepsy, various central nervous system processes can cause persistent sleepiness that interferes with daytime functioning. Patients with hypersomnolence may sleep for extended periods and nap during the day, but they still never feel fully alert and refreshed. This condition may be idiopathic, or it may be related to head trauma, viral infections, encephalitis, tumors, and neurodegenerative disorders. As with narcolepsy, stimulants represent the primary treatment approach but often are less reliable in providing significant benefit for these patients.

Sleep-Disordered Breathing

This topic is covered in greater detail in the article on Sleep Apnea. *Sleep-disordered breathing* involves fluctuations in airflow during sleep. Most commonly it is due to an obstructive process involving an abnormal collapsibility of the upper airway, which may result in recurrent episodes of hypopneas and apneas. Alternately, it may involve a decreased respiratory drive associated with central mechanisms, as can occur with congestive heart failure with a prolonged circulation time. Sleep apnea can cause frequent arousals that undermine sleep quality and lead to excessive sleepiness during the daytime.

Restless Legs Syndrome and Periodic Limb Movements

Although the primary discomfort of restless legs syndrome (RLS) occurs prior to sleep, it is considered a sleep disorder because it is associated with delayed and disrupted sleep and because the irresistible urge to move the legs follows a circadian pattern with increasing symptoms as bedtime approaches. As the condition worsens over time,

- Patient should be screened routinely for problems associated with sleep and wakefulness.
- Ask patients and bed partners about difficulty falling and staying asleep, movements and behaviors during sleep, and snoring and breathing irregularities during sleep.
- The most common sleep disorders encountered in primary care settings are insomnia, sleep-disordered breathing, and restless legs syndrome. Parasomnia, narcolepsy, and other hypersomnolence disorders are relatively uncommon.
- Excessive sleepiness is a potentially dangerous condition that should be evaluated aggressively. Sleep laboratory testing is appropriate for cases not easily explained by sleep deprivation.

the sense of restlessness may begin earlier in the afternoon or morning. The discomfort is most bothersome when patients are at rest. Moving the legs offers only very brief relief. In severe cases, patients often experience such intense restlessness that they are unable to sleep for long periods and often will pace until exhaustion finally allows sleep. During sleep, about 80% of RLS patients exhibit periodic limb movements. In some patients, these involuntary jerking movements occur frequently and cause arousals that further undermine sleep quality. Occasionally patients have periodic limb movements during sleep without the pre-sleep restlessness.

Although RLS often occurs idiopathically, there also is a significant familial component. Other risk factors are iron deficiency, peripheral neuropathies, renal failure, and use of certain medications, including most antidepressants, sedating antihistamines, and centrally acting dopamine antagonists. Pregnancy may be associated with a temporary worsening of symptoms.

Iron supplementation may be beneficial for RLS patients with low ferritin levels (<50 ng/mL). Otherwise, the first-line approach consists of dopamine agonists, such as ropinirole (Requip) and pramipexole (Mirapex). Selected patients may benefit from opiates (e.g., propoxyphene[1] [Darvon] and methadone[1] [Dolophine]), benzodiazepines (e.g., clonazepam[1] [Klonopin]), or gabapentin[1] (Neurontin).

Parasomnias

Behaviors and other symptoms emanating from sleep are considered *parasomnias*. Although most parasomnias are relatively benign, occasionally injuries to patients or bed partners result from these behaviors. Evaluation of patients with parasomnias should include a consideration of sleep-disordered breathing as a possible precipitant to the abnormal behaviors. Most parasomnias can be categorized according to their association with non-REM or REM sleep.

Slow-wave sleep, classified as non-REM stages 3 and 4, generally occurs during the first few hours of sleep. Children have the most slow-wave sleep, and the amount declines with age. Compared with other sleep stages, it is most difficult to awaken from these stages. *Sleep terrors, sleepwalking, sleep-related eating disorder,* and *confusional arousals* all represent incomplete awakenings. Often people experiencing these parasomnias have no recollection of them the following morning. These parasomnias may be exacerbated by sleep insufficiency when there is an increase in slow-wave sleep intensity during recovery sleep. Sleep terrors may be especially dramatic. When they are frequent or involve dangerous behaviors, then treatment with a benzodiazepine receptor agonist may be appropriate.

CURRENT THERAPY

- Patients with persistent insomnia may benefit from improved sleep hygiene measures, cognitive-behavioral therapy, and pharmacologic agents.
- Sleep-promoting medications approved by the Food and Drug Administration include benzodiazepine and nonbenzodiazepine hypnotics, and a selective melatonin receptor agonist.
- Iron supplementation may benefit patients with restless legs syndrome and low ferritin levels. Otherwise, dopamine agonists are the first-line treatment.
- Narcolepsy can be treated with central nervous system stimulants, rapid eye movement suppressants, and sodium oxybate (Xyrem).
- Parasomnia behaviors should be treated when they frequently disrupt sleep or represent a danger to the patient or bed partners.

REM sleep is associated with the most intense dreaming experiences and markedly decreased skeletal muscle tone. It occurs intermittently throughout the night but for the longest periods during the last few hours of the night. *Nightmares* are distressing awakenings from REM sleep with the awareness of frightening dream content. *REM sleep behavior disorder*, which is more common among elderly individuals, involves an incomplete muscle paralysis during REM sleep leading patients to move during REM sleep. Patients seem to be acting out intense dream experiences. The results can be dangerous because patients may thrash about in bed, fall out of bed, or even attack bed partners before awakening. Bedtime clonazepam[1] (Klonopin) has been the standard treatment; however, recent studies suggest melatonin[1] also may be beneficial.

Summary

Sleep disorders can have a significant impact on a patient's quality of life and on comorbid conditions. Initial screening for sleep-wake cycle disturbances is as simple as asking patients how they are sleeping and whether they feel awake and alert throughout the daytime. Most sleep disorders can be identified with a thorough history in a primary care setting; however, consultation with a sleep specialist and sleep laboratory testing may be helpful in the evaluation and management of complex insomnia, hypersomnia, and parasomnia patients.

REFERENCES

The International Classification of Sleep Disorders. Diagnostic & Coding Manual, ICSD-2. 2nd ed. Westchester, IL: American Academy of Sleep Medicine; 2005.

Chokroverty S. Sleep Disorders Medicine: Basic Science, Technical Considerations, and Clinical Aspects. Boston: Butterworth-Heinemann; 1994.

Earley CJ. Clinical practice: Restless legs syndrome. N Engl J Med 2003;348:2103–9.

Kryger MH, Roth T, Dement WC. Principles and Practice of Sleep Medicine. 4th ed. Philadelphia: Elsevier/Saunders; 2005.

Mahowald MW, Bornemann MC, Schenck CH. Parasomnias. Semin Neurol 2004;24:283–92.

Neubauer DN. Understanding Sleeplessness: Perspectives on Insomnia. Baltimore: Johns Hopkins University Press; 2003.

Reid KJ, Zee PC. Circadian rhythm disorders. Semin Neurol 2004;24:315–25.

Thorpy M. Current concepts in the etiology, diagnosis and treatment of narcolepsy. Sleep Med 2001;2:5–17.

[1]Not FDA approved for this indication.

Intracerebral Hemorrhage

Method of
J. Claude Hemphill III, MD, MAS

Spontaneous nontraumatic intracerebral hemorrhage (ICH) accounts for 10% to 15% of acute stroke in most case series. It is consistently associated with a high mortality rate (usually around 40%) and is more likely to result in death or major disability than cerebral infarction or subarachnoid hemorrhage (SAH). Currently, without an approved treatment of proven benefit, recent clinical trials have helped to define surgical indications and suggest new interventions for ICH.

Epidemiology and Etiology

Of the 700,000 strokes occurring annually in the United States, more than 70,000 are ICH (Box 1). ICH is more common among minority groups, including Asians and African Americans. Whether this represents a genetic predisposition or a result of less access to preventive health care is not completely clear. The average age of ICH patients is younger than for ischemic stroke, and only 20% of ICH patients are functionally independent a year after their stroke.

HYPERTENSION

Hypertension remains the most common, and most treatable, cause of acute ICH. At least 60% of ICH is caused by the chronic effects of hypertension on the small penetrating arteries of the brain. Typical sites of hypertensive ICH are the basal ganglia (especially the putamen), the thalamus, the pons, and the cerebellum. An ICH occurring in other locations (e.g., lobar ICH) or in a young person without a prior history of hypertension should prompt a diagnostic evaluation for other causes of ICH. Aggressive treatment of hypertension prevents a substantial portion of ICH from occurring in the first place, and this is the mainstay of primary and secondary prevention for ICH.

CEREBRAL AMYLOID ANGIOPATHY

Cerebral amyloid angiopathy (CAA) is an increasingly recognized cause of primary intracerebral hemorrhage, especially lobar ICH. Occurring almost exclusively in patients older than 65 years, CAA is associated with dementia and recurrent lobar ICH, especially in carriers of the apolipoprotein E ε4 gene allele. Magnetic resonance imaging (MRI) using gradient echo sequences and demonstrate prior microhemorrhages and is a useful diagnostic test in the setting of lobar hemorrhage in older patients. There is currently no treatment for CAA.

BOX 1   Etiologies of Primary Intracerebral Hemorrhage

Common
Arteriovenous malformations
Cerebral amyloid angiopathy
Chronic hypertension
Coagulopathy (warfarin-related)
Drugs of abuse (cocaine, methamphetamine)

Rare
Cerebral vasculitis
Coagulopathy (von Willebrand's)
Moyamoya syndrome

COAGULOPATHY, VASCULAR MALFORMATIONS, AND DRUGS OF ABUSE

Warfarin (Coumadin)-related ICH is increasing in incidence and accounts for 5% to 15% of ICH. Mortality from warfarin-related ICH is substantially higher than for noncoagulopathic ICH. Additionally, hematoma expansion is even more common in the setting of an elevated international normalized ratio (INR) (<1.4) and can continue for up to a day after ICH onset unless coagulopathy is corrected back to normal.

Vascular malformations are a relatively uncommon cause of ICH, but they account for a substantial portion of young patients with ICH and for ICH in patients without hypertension. Arteriovenous malformations (AVMs), cavernous malformations, dural arteriovenous fistulas (dAVFs), and saccular aneurysms can all cause acute ICH.

Diagnostic evaluation with MRI and magnetic resonance angiography (MRA) is recommended in patients with lobar hemorrhage and in patients younger than 45 years without an obvious other cause. CT angiography (CTA) is increasingly being used instead of MRA. Diagnostic catheter angiography remains the gold standard for AVMs and dAVF, but it does not detect cavernous malformations. Because the ICH hematoma can obscure a small vascular anomaly, delayed MRI after hematoma resorption (2–3 months) may be necessary. Primary and metastatic tumors can bleed, mimicking primary ICH, and therefore a delayed MRI is useful if there is no other systemic evidence of a tumor.

Sympathomimetic drugs of abuse are an increasing cause of ICH, especially in younger patients. A urine toxicology screen for cocaine and methamphetamine should be a routine part of the ICH work-up in all patients. A positive toxicology screen is not necessarily ultimately diagnostic because these drugs can precipitate hemorrhage from an underlying vascular anomaly such as an AVM or aneurysm.

Numerous other less common etiologies of ICH exist, including cerebral vasculitis, moyamoya syndrome, and secondary hemorrhage into an arterial or venous infarct. Many times the pattern of hemorrhage on head CT scan or other associated findings on physical or laboratory examination provides clues to one of these less common etiologies.

Diagnosis

Patients with ICH present with what appears to be an acute stroke, although level of consciousness is often more diminished than with ischemic stroke. An urgent head CT scan is an essential part of the diagnostic evaluation of all acute stroke patients. Noncontrast head CT scanning has traditionally been performed, but recent studies suggest that the addition of contrast may be useful, because contrast extravasation predicts mortality, likely due to hematoma enlargement. Also, CTA can be performed concurrently to evaluate for an underlying vascular anomaly.

A rapid coagulation panel (prothrombin time [PT], INR, and partial thromboplastin time [PTT]) should be obtained in all patients, as should a urine toxicology screen. Because history may be limited at the time of initial evaluation, these laboratory tests can provide unexpected clues as to etiology and identify urgent interventions needed.

CURRENT DIAGNOSIS

- Obtain an emergency head CT scan immediately on hospital arrival.
- Extravasation on contrast CT might predict hematoma expansion.
- Check INR and determine if the patient is on anticoagulant therapy.
- Obtain history: Check for hypertension, dementia, prior stroke.
- MRI, MRA, CTA, or angiography for patients younger than 45 years or with lobar ICH.

Abbreviations: CT = computed tomography; ICH = intracerebral hemorrhage; INR = international normalized ratio; MRA = magnetic resonance angiography; MRI = magnetic resonance imaging.

The importance of early hematoma expansion is now recognized in ICH. Previously, enlargement of an ICH was believed to indicate systemic coagulopathy or underlying AVM, but it is now recognized that a significant portion of all ICH patients will suffer early hematoma expansion. Hematoma expansion tends to happen early in the clinical course, with hematomas enlarging by at least one third in 30% to 40% of patients who present within 3 hours of symptom onset. Hematoma expansion to this degree is usually associated with neurologic deterioration.

Numerous studies have identified a range of clinical and neurologic imaging factors that predict outcome. The ICH Score (Table 1) is one simple clinical grading scale that can be used to risk stratify patients for 30-day mortality based on age, Glasgow Coma Scale score, hematoma volume and location, and presence of intraventricular hemorrhage on CT scan.

Treatment

The revised 2007 guidelines from the Stroke Council of the American Heart Association address numerous aspects of ICH management, with the recognition that there is limited evidence to guide many of these treatments (Table 2).

INITIAL EVALUATION AND TRIAGE

Because level of consciousness is often diminished in acute ICH patients, early attention to airway protection is essential to avoid aspiration and hypoxia. Intubation may be necessary. Most patients with acute ICH should be managed in an intensive care unit for at least 24 hours.

BLOOD PRESSURE MANAGEMENT

Most patients with ICH are acutely hypertensive, sometimes to very extreme levels. The 2007 ICH guidelines recommend lowering the blood pressure to achieve a mean arterial pressure (MAP) less than 110 mm Hg or a combined blood pressure less than 160/90.

TABLE 1 The ICH Score

Component	ICH Score Points
Glasgow Coma Scale Score*	
3–4	2
5–12	1
13–15	0
ICH Volume (mL)†	
≥30	1
<30	0
Intraventricular Hemorrhage‡	
Yes	1
No	0
Infratentorial Origin of ICH	
Yes	1
No	0
Age (years)	
≥80	1
<80	0
Total	**0–6**

*GCS score on discharge from the emergency department.
†ICH volume on the initial CT scan was calculated using the ABC/2 method, where A is the greatest diameter of the hemorrhage (by CT scan), B is the diameter 90 degrees to A, and C is the CT slice thickness (cm) times the approximate number of CT slices that include hemorrhage.
‡Presence of any intraventricular hemorrhage on initial CT.
Abbreviations: CT = computed tomography; GCS = Glasgow Coma Scale; ICH = intracerebral hemorrhage.

CURRENT THERAPY

- Remember the ABCs (airway, breathing, circulation).
- Reverse warfarin (Coumadin) coagulopathy immediately with a prothrombin complex concentrate or recombinant factor VIIa (NovoSeven); also give fresh-frozen plasma and vitamin K.
- Lower blood pressure to mean arterial pressure less than 110 mm Hg or combined blood pressure less than 160/90.
- Surgery for cerebellar hemorrhage and possibly lobar hemorrhage.
- Clinical monitoring for re-bleeding or neurologic worsening for the initial 24 hours.
- Do not use corticosteroids.

The guidelines also recommend maintaining a cerebral perfusion pressure (CPP) of 60–80 mm Hg in patients with elevated intracranial pressure (ICP). Lowering blood pressure to limit hematoma expansion is intuitively appealing, but studies of the influence of high blood pressure on hematoma expansion have had conflicting results. Prior concerns that blood pressure lowering might create perihematoma ischemia appear largely unfounded. Clinical trials are currently under way in the United States and Australia to determine whether acute blood pressure lowering improves outcome after ICH.

SURGICAL HEMATOMA EVACUATION

Prior studies of ICH hematoma evacuation have included no more than 100 patients. Thus, the recent completion and publication of the results of the STICH (Surgical Trial in Intracerebral Haemorrhage) study represent a major step both in understanding the role of surgical hematoma evacuation and in demonstrating that large clinical trials in intracerebral hemorrhage can be undertaken.

The STICH study was a randomized, controlled trial designed to test the hypothesis that early surgical evacuation in supratentorial spontaneous intracerebral hemorrhage was superior to initial conservative treatment. Overall, 1033 patients from 27 different countries were randomized. About one half of patients had lobar intracerebral hemorrhage and one half had deep (thalamic or basal ganglia) hemorrhages. At 6 months, there was no difference in the fraction of patients with good functional outcome (early surgery 26%, initial conservative treatment 24%; $P = 0.4$) and no difference in mortality (early surgery 36%, initial conservative treatment 37%; $P = 0.7$). However, 26% of the patients randomized to initial conservative treatment underwent surgical hematoma evacuation later in their hospital course based on the discretion of their treating surgeon. The subgroup of STICH patients with lobar hematomas within

1 cm of the cortical surface had a strong trend toward better outcome with surgical evacuation, and the new STICH II trial is examining surgical evacuation in this group of patients.

STICH included only patients with supratentorial ICH. Cerebellar hemorrhages are considered by most to be surgically appropriate lesions, despite the lack of a randomized trial studying this group of patients. The 2007 ICH guidelines recommend surgery for deteriorating patients with cerebellar hemorrhages larger than 3 cm.

PREVENTING HEMATOMA EXPANSION

The safety and efficacy of recombinant factor VIIa (NovoSeven)[1] were tested in a randomized, blinded, placebo-controlled phase II study of patients with acute ICH. Hematoma growth (the primary study outcome measure) was significantly less in the patients who received recombinant factor VIIa (pooled across three doses tested, $P = 0.01$). Three-month mortality (secondary outcome) was significantly less in those treated with recombinant factor VIIa (18% vs. 29%; pooled $P = 0.02$), and functional outcome was better as well. However, a recently completed phase III trial of recombinant factor VIIa in ICH did not demonstrate clinical benefit despite less hematoma growth compared with placebo.

COAGULOPATHY-RELATED INTRACEREBRAL HEMORRHAGE

Because of the especially high risk of ongoing hematoma expansion and increased morbidity and mortality in the setting of warfarin-related ICH, immediate correction of coagulopathy (to an INR ≤ 1.4) is absolutely essential. Studies have demonstrated that protocols that use only fresh-frozen plasma (FFP) and vitamin K (Phytonadione) might not reverse coagulopathy sufficiently fast. International guidelines recommend prothrombin complex concentrate (PCC) in addition to FFP and vitamin K. There are also reports of the successful use of recombinant factor VIIa in this setting.

OTHER MANAGEMENT ISSUES

The use of prophylactic anticonvulsants is controversial. Some advocate administration in all ICH patients or just in lobar hemorrhage, and others treat with anticonvulsants only after a seizure. Prior small trials of corticosteroids in ICH suggested no benefit and an increase in systemic complications. Deep venous thrombosis prophylaxis is essential. Use of sequential compression devices (SCDs) and stockings should be instituted at hospital admission; subcutaneous heparin or heparinoids are likely safe to administer 72 to 96 hours after ICH onset, unless the patient has an intracranial pressure monitor in place, in which case they may be deferred in favor of SCDs.

REFERENCES

Becker KJ, Baxter AB, Bybee HM, et al. Extravasation of radiographic contrast is an independent predictor of death in primary intracerebral hemorrhage. Stroke 1999;30:2025–32.
Broderick J, Connolly S, Feldmann E, et al. Guidelines for the management of spontaneous intracerebral hemorrhage in adults: 2007 update: A guideline from the American Heart Association/American Stroke Association Stroke Council, High Blood Pressure Research Council, and the Quality of Care and Outcomes in Research Interdisciplinary Working Group. Stroke 2007;38:2001–23.
Brott T, Broderick J, Kothari R, et al. Early hemorrhage growth in patients with intracerebral hemorrhage. Stroke 1997;28:1–5.
Hemphill JC 3rd, Bonovich DC, Besmertis L, et al. The ICH score: A simple, reliable grading scale for intracerebral hemorrhage. Stroke 2001;32:891–7.
Kothari RU, Brott T, Broderick JP, et al. The ABCs of measuring intracerebral hemorrhage volumes. Stroke 1996;27:1304–5.
Mayer SA, Brun NC, Begtrup K, et al. Recombinant activated factor vii for acute intracerebral hemorrhage. N Engl J Med 2005;352:777–85.
Mendelow AD, Gregson BA, Fernandes HM, et al. Early surgery versus initial conservative treatment in patients with spontaneous supratentorial intracerebral haematomas in the international surgical trial in intracerebral haemorrhage (STICH): A randomised trial. Lancet 2005;365:387–97.
Qureshi AI, Tuhrim S, Broderick JP, et al. Spontaneous intracerebral hemorrhage. N Engl J Med 2001;344:1450–60.

TABLE 2   Highlights of the 2007 Intracerebral Hemorrhage Treatment Guidelines

Management Issue	Recommendations
Blood pressure	Maintain MAP < 110 mm Hg or BP < 160/90
Surgical hematoma evacuation	Cerebellar ICH > 3 cm. Consider lobar ICH in young patient if deteriorating. Structural lesions (e.g., AVM)
Intracranial pressure (ICP) monitoring	Treat elevated ICP with analgesia and sedation, osmotic diuretics, CSF drainage. Maintain CPP 60–80 mm Hg.
Anticonvulsants	Consider prophylaxis
Glucocorticoids	No
Temperature	Maintain normothermia

Abbreviations: AVM = arteriovenous malformation; GCS = Glasgow Coma Scale; ICH = intracerebral hemorrhage; MAP = mean arterial pressure.

[1]Not FDA approved for this indication.

Ischemic Cerebrovascular Disease

Method of
Alvaro Cervera, MD, and Geoffrey A. Donnan, MD

Treatment of ischemic stroke has improved significantly in the past few years, and mortality and disability rates due to this condition have decreased. The demonstration of efficacy of thrombolysis in the management of patients in stroke units has been crucial in this achievement. Control of vascular risk factors has decreased the number and severity of events. Improved management has included high-quality rehabilitation, which is started as soon as possible to improve the recovery (i.e., functional independence) of stroke survivors.

The multidisciplinary management of stroke can be improved with specific educational programs aimed at increasing awareness of stroke in the general population and among professionals. The concept of *time is brain* has a great value in emphasizing that stroke is an emergency. Because the window for the available time-dependent treatments is very narrow, avoiding delay is the major goal in the prehospital phase of acute stroke care. All stroke patients must be transported as soon as possible to the closest hospital with a stroke unit. In rural or remote areas with no stroke unit facilities, telemedicine has proved to be a valid alternative.

Prevention

Lifestyle modification can be a major contributor to reducing the risk of ischemic stroke. Strategies to achieve this protection include avoiding smoking and excessive alcohol consumption, keeping a low-normal body mass index, practicing regular exercise, and having a diet low in salt and saturated fat, high in fruit and vegetables, and rich in fiber. There is no need to add vitamin supplements to the diet because they have not been found to affect stroke prevention.

Regular assessment of vascular risk factors (e.g., hypertension, diabetes, hypercholesterolemia) is important because their control can reduce significantly the incidence of vascular events. Blood pressure should be managed with diet and pharmacologic therapy, aiming at normal levels of 120/80 mm Hg. After an ischemic stroke, blood pressure should be lowered even in patients with normal blood pressure. Diabetes should be managed with lifestyle modification and pharmacologic therapy as required, and blood pressure needs to be more tightly controlled in these patients (<130/80 mm Hg). The best antihypertensive treatments for diabetics are angiotensin-converting enzyme (ACE) inhibitors or angiotensin receptor antagonists. Hypercholesterolemia should be managed with lifestyle modification and a statin. After a noncardioembolic ischemic stroke, statins are beneficial in all patients for secondary prevention.

Postmenopausal hormone replacement therapy should be avoided for the primary or secondary prevention of stroke because it can increase the risk of new vascular events. Other strategies to prevent stroke include the treatment of obstructive sleep apnea with continuous positive airway pressure (CPAP) breathing.

ANTITHROMBOTIC THERAPY

Low-dose aspirin can be used for the primary prevention of stroke in women or myocardial infarction. Nevertheless, its effect is very small, and it cannot be recommended on a population-wide basis. Aspirin is beneficial for the prevention of stroke in patients with asymptomatic carotid stenosis.

In patients with atrial fibrillation, aspirin can prevent ischemic events in those younger than 65 years and free of vascular risk factors. In patients older than 65 years, anticoagulation is the first option, although aspirin is an alternative for those younger than 75 years without other risk factors (Table 1). In all patients with atrial

TABLE 1 Prevention of Stroke In Patients with Atrial Fibrillation

Prevention	Therapy
Primary prevention	
No risk factors	<65 years old: aspirin
	65–75 years old: aspirin or warfarin
	>75 years old: warfarin
Risk factors*	All age groups: warfarin
Secondary prevention	All groups: warfarin

*Previous systemic embolism, high blood pressure, or poor left ventricular function.

fibrillation who have suffered a stroke, anticoagulation should aim for an international normalized ratio (INR) of 2.0 to 3.0. Patients with prosthetic heart valves should also receive anticoagulation, and the target INR depends on the prosthesis type.

After ischemic stroke, all patients should receive antithrombotic therapy. Antiplatelet agents are the first choice unless anticoagulation is required. The most effective regimen is aspirin and extended-release dipyridamole combined (Aggrenox). However, after the PRoFESS trial failed to show the noninferiority criteria for aspirin plus dipyridamole compared with clopidogrel (Plavix), this superiority is not clear. Aspirin plus dipyridamole, clopidogrel, or aspirin alone are acceptable therapies for secondary stroke prevention. Triflusal[2] is another alternative. The combination of aspirin and clopidogrel is not recommended after stroke, except if there is an association with unstable angina or non-Q-wave myocardial infarction, or there has been a recent stenting.

Anticoagulation is usually indicated for secondary prevention if the stroke cause is cardioembolic and in specific situations such as aortic arch atheroma, fusiform aneurysms of the basilar artery, cervical artery dissection, or patent foramen ovale in the presence of proven deep venous thrombosis. However, level one evidence is lacking for these approaches.

Management of Carotid Stenosis

In patients with asymptomatic carotid stenosis ($\geq$60%), surgery is indicated only if the risk of stroke is high. Endarterectomy is the treatment of choice if the stenosis is symptomatic (i.e., has been associated with an ipsilateral stroke or transient ischemic attack) and severe (70% to 99%). Surgery should be performed in centers with a perioperative complication rate of less than 6% and as soon as possible after the last ischemic event.

Endarterectomy may be indicated for certain patients with moderate stenosis (50% to 69%), although it should be performed only in centers with a perioperative complication rate of less than 3% to be effective. In cases of symptomatic carotid lesions, angioplasty plus stenting is recommended only for selected patients because trials of efficacy versus endarterectomy are ongoing. If stenting is performed, a combination of clopidogrel and aspirin is required immediately before the procedure and for at least 1 month to prevent stent thrombosis.

In patients with intracranial atheromatosis and stroke recurrences despite appropriate antiplatelet therapy, endovascular treatment may be a reasonable choice.

Management of Acute Ischemic Stroke

All stroke patients should be treated in a stroke unit, because this is associated with a reduction of death, dependency, and the need for institutional care. This effect is seen for all types of patients, irrespective of gender, age, stroke subtype, and stroke severity. Patients with

---

[2]Not available in the United States.

stroke should have a careful clinical assessment, including a neurologic examination. The use of a stroke rating scale, such as the National Institutes of Health Stroke Scale (NIHSS), provides important information about the severity of stroke.

Urgent cranial computed tomography (CT) is mandatory after an ischemic stroke before starting any therapy. Alternatively, magnetic resonance imaging (MRI) can be performed and can provide additional information about the selection of patients for thrombolytic therapy beyond 3 hours. However, there is not enough evidence to recommend its routine use in the acute stroke setting.

For the detection and early management of the medical complications of stroke, neurologic status, pulse, blood pressure, temperature, and oxygen saturation should be monitored. Similarly, serum glucose levels need to be monitored and hyperglycemia treated with insulin accordingly. Normal saline is recommended for fluid replacement during the first 24 hours after stroke. If the patient has fever, treatment with paracetamol (acetaminophen) may be used while sources of infection are being sought. Reducing blood pressure is recommended only in patients with extremely high blood pressure or when indicated by other medical conditions. Blood pressure should be lowered gradually, avoiding abrupt changes.

THROMBOLYSIS

All patients with an ischemic stroke within 3 hours of onset should receive thrombolytic treatment with intravenous tissue plasminogen activator (tPA [Activase]) unless contraindicated, because it is effective in improving stroke outcome (Box 1). The ECASS III clinical trial showed that this effect could also be obtained over a longer period (4.5 hours). Based on the available evidence, thrombolysis with tPA can be given in ischemic stroke within 4.5 hours of onset, provided that it is approved by the local regulatory authorities. There is also evidence from phase II trials (e.g., EPITHET) that selecting patients with MRI to assess the penumbra can be an appropriate tool to extend the time to more than 3 hours, because tPA was associated with increased reperfusion in these patients and a trend toward better outcomes. Nevertheless, increasing the time window does not mean that treatment can be delayed. As evidenced by pooled analysis, earlier treatment results in a better outcome. There is little evidence that thrombolysis is effective in patients older than 80 years, but the available information indicates that it is safe.

Intraarterial administration of a thrombolytic agent within a 6-hour time can be an alternative therapy. Another treatment, which has been approved by some regulatory authorities, is the MERCI device. It mechanically removes the thrombus, which can be associated with thrombolytic therapy. However, no evidence for the clinical efficacy of mechanical devices has been derived from randomized clinical trials.

BOX 1   Treatment of Acute Ischemic Stroke: Intravenous Administration of Tissue Plasminogen Activator

- Infuse 0.9 mg/kg (maximum dose 90 mg) of tissue plasminogen activator (tPA) over 60 minutes, with 10% of the dose given as a bolus over 1 minute.
- Admit the patient to a stroke unit for monitoring. Perform neurologic assessment and blood pressure measurement every 15 minutes during the infusion, every 30 minutes thereafter for the next 6 hours, and then hourly until 24 hours after treatment. Administer antihypertensive medications to maintain systolic blood pressure ≤180 and diastolic ≤105.
- If intracranial hemorrhage is suspected, discontinue the infusion, and obtain an emergency CT scan.
- Obtain a follow-up CT scan at 24 hours before starting anticoagulants or antiplatelet agents.

ANTITHROMBOTIC DRUGS

All patients should receive a low dose of aspirin daily, and this should be started within 48 hours after stroke onset. The use of other antiplatelet agents during the acute phase of stroke cannot be recommended based on available evidence. Similarly, early administration of unfractionated heparin, low-molecular-weight heparin, or heparinoids is not indicated in acute ischemic stroke patients.

TREATMENT OF STROKE COMPLICATIONS

Brain edema develops between the second and fifth day after stroke onset and is the cause of early deterioration and death. In the case of a malignant infarction of the middle cerebral artery, the mortality rate is 80%. In patients younger than 60 years with this pattern of cerebral infarction, hemicraniectomy has been effective in reducing mortality and severe disability, as shown in the pooled analysis of the DECIMAL, DESTINY, and HAMLET trials. Surgery needs to be performed within 48 hours after symptom onset. Surgical decompression is also indicated in the case of large cerebellar infarctions that compress the brainstem.

Stroke-associated infections require appropriate antibiotics, but prophylactic administration is discouraged. Venous thromboembolism is a frequent complication after stroke, but its incidence can be reduced with appropriate hydration and graded compression stockings. If the risk of deep venous thrombosis or pulmonary embolism is high, the use of subcutaneous heparin or low-molecular-weight heparins is beneficial. Early mobilization is an effective way of preventing complications such as aspiration pneumonia or pressure ulcers. Anticonvulsants are administered only to prevent recurrent seizure but are not used prophylactically.

In stroke patients at risk for falls, hip fracture can be prevented with bisphosphonates. In case of urinary incontinence, specialist assessment and management are recommended. Dysphagia is common after stroke and is associated with a higher incidence of medical complications and increased mortality. Malnutrition also predicts a poor functional outcome and increased mortality, and it is important to assess the swallowing capacity and the nutritional status of the patient.

Rehabilitation should be started after admission to the stroke unit. The optimal timing of first mobilization is unclear, but mobilization within the first few days appears to be well tolerated. The AVERT study demonstrated that very early mobilization (i.e., within 24 hours of symptom onset) is safe and feasible. An ongoing study is assessing its efficacy and cost-effectiveness. It is important to assess cognitive deficits and depression during the patient's hospital stay, because this may require specific intervention, although evidence about the type is lacking.

REFERENCES

Adams Jr HP, del Zoppo G, Alberts MJ, et al. Guidelines for the early management of adults with ischemic stroke: A guideline from the American Heart Association/American Stroke Association Stroke Council, Clinical Cardiology Council, Cardiovascular Radiology and Intervention Council, and the Atherosclerotic Peripheral Vascular Disease and Quality of Care Outcomes in Research Interdisciplinary Working Groups: The American Academy of Neurology affirms the value of this guideline as an educational tool for neurologists. Stroke 2007;38:1655–711.

Bernhardt J, Dewey H, Thrift A, et al. A very early rehabilitation trial for stroke (AVERT): Phase II safety and feasibility. Stroke 2008;39:390–6.

Davis SM, Donnan GA, Parsons MW, et al. Effects of alteplase beyond 3 h after stroke in the Echoplanar Imaging Thrombolytic Evaluation Trial (EPITHET): A placebo-controlled randomised trial. Lancet Neurol 2008;7:299–309.

European Stroke Organisation (ESO). Executive Committee; ESO Writing Committee: Guidelines for management of ischaemic stroke and transient ischaemic attack 2008. Cerebrovasc Dis 2008;25:457–507.

Hacke W, Kaste M, Bluhmki E, et al. Thrombolysis with alteplase 3 to 4.5 hours after acute ischemic stroke. N Engl J Med 2008;359:1317–29.

Kent DM, Thaler DE. Stroke prevention—Insights from incoherence. N Engl J Med 2008;359:1287–9.

Sacco RL, Diener HC, Yusuf S, et al. Aspirin and extended-release dipyridamole versus clopidogrel for recurrent stroke. N Engl J Med 2008;359:1238–51.

Vahedi K, Hofmeijer J, Juettler E, et al. Early decompressive surgery in malignant infarction of the middle cerebral artery: A pooled analysis of three randomised controlled trials. Lancet Neurol 2007;6:215–22.

Rehabilitation of the Stroke Patient

Method of

*Marlís González-Fernández, MD, PhD, and
Dorianne Feldman, MD, MSPT*

According to the national center for health statistics, 5.6 million Americans live with the disability caused by a previous stroke. Stroke is the leading cause of permanent disability in adults. Conservative estimates suggest that about 45% of stroke patients have moderate to severe disabilities requiring rehabilitation.

The goals of stroke rehabilitation are to maintain and optimize medical management, to maximize functional recovery, to minimize disability, and to improve quality of life and participation in society. The rehabilitative approach endeavors to provide patient-centered care that is organized, comprehensive, and specific to the needs of the stroke patient. The concerted efforts of the patient, family, and the rehabilitation team are essential for achieving these goals. Recovery after stroke can be a long and challenging process for the patient and the family. Although functional gains occur most rapidly in the first year after a stroke, additional motor recovery is possible beyond 1 year when patients are involved in targeted rehabilitation programs.

The rehabilitation team is composed of rehabilitation physicians (physiatrists), other physicians such as neurologists and neurosurgeons, rehabilitation nurses, occupational therapists, physical therapists, speech and language pathologists, rehabilitation neuropsychologists, social workers, case managers, nutritionists, vocational counselors, and pharmacists. A goal of the acute inpatient rehabilitation team is discharging the patient to the least restrictive environment, ideally home. To accomplish this goal, it is critical to evaluate family support and the home environment.

Rehabilitation should start as part of the acute stroke inpatient stay. The decision-making process to determine the appropriate rehabilitation setting after discharge is described in Figure 1. Speech-language pathologists, physical therapists, and occupational therapists evaluate deficits in cognition, communication, deglutition, mobility, and activities of daily living. The severity of deficits in these major areas and the ability of the patient to tolerate therapy determine the appropriate rehabilitation setting.

Stroke patients with mild deficits are able to return home with home or outpatient therapy services. Patients with moderate to severe strokes benefit from more intensive therapy in an institutional setting. Comprehensive inpatient rehabilitation is suitable for patients with moderate to severe deficits who can tolerate intensive rehabilitation (3 hours/day). If the severity of deficits or medical comorbidities limits the ability of the patient to participate in intensive therapy, alternate settings can be considered.

During the inpatient rehabilitation stage, medical management focuses on secondary stroke prevention: diet, exercise, smoking cessation, and reducing complications, including optimizing blood pressure control while maintaining cerebral perfusion, preventing and treating lipid disorders, and managing post-stroke pain, depression, and abnormal muscle tone. During this stage, much of the rehabilitation effort is directed toward educating stroke survivors about complications and the importance of adherence to medical recommendations.

Medical complications such as deep venous thrombosis and related thromboembolism, pneumonia (usually related to aspiration), skin breakdown, and urinary infections can hinder a patient's recovery. Early identification of these complications is necessary to maintain progress in the rehabilitation effort. Other complications, such as seizures and cardiac decompensation, are possible and should be monitored.

Stroke often causes significant impairment and activity limitations. Deficits in strength, swallowing, vision, balance, muscle tone, communication, comprehension, cognition, attention, sensory perception, and bladder function are common and can cause difficulty completing activities of daily living, walking, transferring to and from different surfaces, and getting in and out of the bed. Post-stroke depression, fatigue, and pain are common and should be addressed to maximize participation in rehabilitative efforts.

Transition to the chronic phase begins after the patient is medically stable and inpatient therapy goals are met. Outpatient therapy services are initiated in conjunction with physiatric, primary care, and neurologic follow-up.

Hemiparesis

Hemiparesis, or one-sided weakness, is one of the most frequent complications after stroke. Recovery of motor function varies. Often, it is limited by muscle atrophy, co-contraction of agonists and antagonists, and abnormal tone. Usually, motor recovery is preceded by the development of patterned muscle movements, or synergies. Synergies occur when select muscles contract in a predictable manner. In the paretic upper extremity, a flexion synergy pattern (i.e., humeral adduction, internal rotation, elbow flexion, forearm pronation, and wrist and finger flexion) is common. In the lower extremity, extension synergies (i.e., hip internal rotation, adduction, extension, knee extension, and ankle extension and inversion) predominate. These patterns can be regarded as functional and nonfunctional. For instance, extension synergy patterns of the lower limb can augment rehabilitation because this position fosters early ambulatory therapy. Conversely, flexion synergy patterns in the upper extremity can significantly impair arm function.

Rehabilitation of the patient with hemiparesis should concentrate on maintaining range of motion and improving strength and posturing. Exercise programs should incorporate functional use of the hemiparetic limb and weight bearing to promote limb recognition, better alignment, muscle elongation, and muscle tone reduction.

Hemiparesis can lead to contracture, particularly when profound weakness is present. and contracture occurs most commonly in the wrist and ankle. Resting hand splints and solid ankle-foot orthoses can be used to maintain the limb in a neutral position. These devices can be used to prevent loss of motion, control muscle tone, and aid in positioning, particularly when wheelchairs are necessary.

Functional electrical stimulation (FES) has gained increasing interest as a means of enhancing functional movement and strength. Muscle contraction is induced with electrical stimulation. Many products on the market incorporate FES technology for the treatment of footdrop and hand weakness.

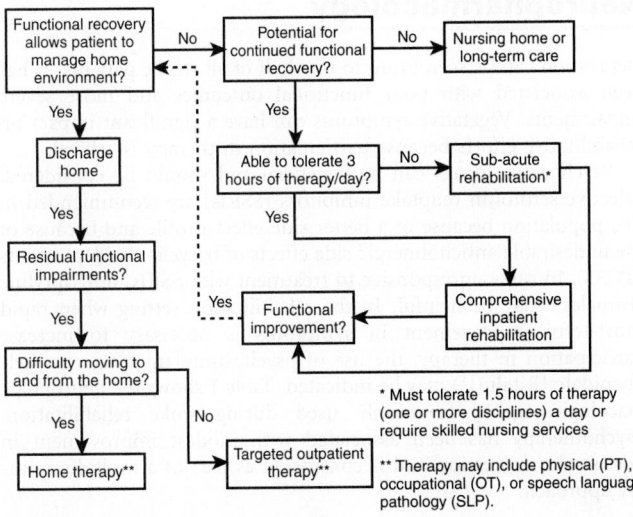

FIGURE 1. Determination of rehabilitation needs of patients being discharged after an acute stroke.

Preservation of scapulohumeral positioning is a critical component of rehabilitation. With shoulder weakness, the scapula becomes downwardly rotated, causing the glenoid fossa to move vertically and resulting in humeral subluxation. Traditionally, shoulder slings have been prescribed for the hemiplegic shoulder, but their effectiveness in preventing subluxation is questionable.

FES has been used to augment motor return in the hemiplegic shoulder and prevent subluxation. Despite advances in the treatment of the hemiplegic shoulder, it is still unclear which therapeutic interventions should constitute the standard of care.

Constraint-induced therapy, a therapeutic approach in which the nonparetic limb is restrained, can improve functional movement of the paretic upper extremity in patients with residual hand and wrist movement, even in patients more than 1 year after a stroke.

Dysphagia

Dysphagia after stroke occurs acutely in approximately 50% of stroke patients. Identifying dysphagia in this population is essential for preventing associated morbidity and mortality. Stroke patients with dysphagia are at risk for dehydration, malnutrition, and aspiration pneumonia. As allowed by their overall clinical status and consciousness level, stroke patients should be evaluated as early as possible during their acute hospital stay. Trained clinicians (most commonly speech-language pathologists) should evaluate the patient to make recommendations regarding further dysphagia evaluation or testing and the need for diet modifications or dysphagia rehabilitation.

Hemiplegic Shoulder Pain

Stroke survivors with residual hemiparesis or weakness are at risk for pain syndromes (particularly in the upper extremity), which can significantly limit rehabilitation efforts. These pain syndromes are usually multifactorial. In the rehabilitation setting, prevention of shoulder pain is key, and interventions should focus on proper positioning, handling, and transfer techniques.

In severe cases, shoulder pain can be accompanied by hand swelling, tenderness, skin changes, erythema, hyperhidrosis, and allodynia. When this occurs, it is referred to as shoulder-hand syndrome, a subtype of complex regional pain syndrome (CRPS). Although the mechanism and cause are unclear, it has been suggested that this process is the result of an overreaction to a neurologic insult and may be inflammatory in nature. In some cases, the pain is severe, resulting in decreased and guarded movements of the limb that limit functional use. Shoulder pathology such as rotator cuff strains or tears, bicipital tendonitis, subacromial and subdeltoid bursitis, and glenohumeral subluxation or dislocation contribute to post-stroke shoulder pain and should be treated.

Nonpharmacologic treatment focuses on desensitization techniques, gentle range-of-motion exercises, and physical modalities (e.g., heat, cold, transcutaneous electrical nerve stimulation [TENS], functional electrical stimulation). Pharmacologic management includes medications typically used for neuropathic pain syndromes, such as anticonvulsants, tricyclic antidepressants, nonsteroidal antiinflammatory drugs, topical agents (e.g., lidocaine [Xylocaine],[1] clonidine [Catapres-TTS],[1] capsaicin [Zostrix][1]), and injections of steroid or local anesthetics. Antispasmodic medications have been used. When pain relief is not achieved with conservative treatment, sympathetic blocks can be considered. Sympathectomies and spinal cord stimulators can be considered as last resorts.

Spasticity

Spasticity after stroke can significantly impact rehabilitation. The classic upper extremity flexor synergy pattern (i.e., adducted shoulder with flexed elbow, wrist, and fingers) can markedly interfere with

function of the affected arm. Conversely, the classic lower extremity extensor synergy pattern (i.e., extended hip and knee and ankle plantar flexion) can be advantageous for ambulation if plantar flexion can be controlled by physical or pharmacologic agents. If untreated, these patterns can lead to abnormal positioning and contracture.

Treatment of spasticity after stroke should address positioning and exacerbating factors. Splinting or bracing, appropriate wheelchair sitting position, and physical therapy techniques are important to prevent contracture and promote motor recovery. Painful or noxious stimuli can exacerbate spasticity. Shoulder pain, pressure sores, deep venous thrombosis, bladder distention, and constipation are examples of stimuli that can exacerbate spasticity. Pharmacologic treatment should take into account the presence of these triggers because spasticity is likely to improve after the stimuli are resolved or relieved.

Pharmacologic treatment of post-stroke spasticity presents some challenges. Effective antispasticity agents such as baclofen (Lioresal) or tizanidine (Zanaflex) can cause somnolence or weaken unaffected muscles, which can significantly affect rehabilitation. Localized treatments such as botulinum toxin injections[1] or phenol[1] blocks can be useful, because treatment can be directed toward muscles that are affecting functional use of the limbs. Surgical interventions can be used for patients with severe spasticity limiting functional positioning or for those with the potential for functional grip if tendon lengthening or transfer can be considered.

Cognitive Dysfunction

Stroke patients can experience many cognitive deficits, including visuospatial neglect, cognitive-linguistic deficits, apraxia, memory loss, and attention deficits. Cognitive rehabilitation should concentrate on treatment of the specific deficits of the patient. Visuospatial rehabilitation (including scanning training) is recommended for deficits associated with visual neglect after right stroke. Cognitive-linguistic therapies are recommended for left hemispheric stroke patients with language deficits. Treatment of apraxia should include specific gestural and strategy training.

The use of medications that may impair cognitive function should be limited. Medications that are commonly considered during a stay in a rehabilitative facility that may have a significant impact on cognition and rehabilitation are highlighted in Table 1.

Depression and Neuropharmacology

Depression can be seen in up to one half of all stroke patients. It has been associated with poor functional outcomes and more severe impairments. Vegetative symptoms can have a significant impact on rehabilitative efforts because participation in therapy is critical.

Psychoactive drugs can be beneficial and should be considered. Selective serotonin reuptake inhibitors (SSRIs) are recommended in this population because of a better side effect profile and because of the undesirable anticholinergic side effects of tricyclic antidepressants (TCAs). In cases unresponsive to treatment with SSRIs, nortriptyline (Pamelor) may be helpful. In the rehabilitation setting when rapid short-term improvement in symptoms is necessary to increase participation in therapy, the use of psychostimulants (e.g., methylphenidate [Ritalin][1]) may be indicated. Table 1 shows the neuropharmacologic agents commonly used during stoke rehabilitation. Psychotherapy has been associated with modest improvement in post-stroke depression and is considered as part of a multidisciplinary approach.

---

[1]Not FDA approved for this indication.

[1]Not FDA approved for this indication.

TABLE 1 Neuropharmacologic Agents Commonly Used During Stroke Rehabilitation

Drug Class	Drug Name	Indication	Potential Problems
Benzodiazepines	Diazepam (Valium)	Agitation,[1] spasticity	Sedation, confusion, sundowning
	Lorazepam (Ativan)	Agitation,[1] seizures	Sedation, paradoxical reactions, confusion, sundowning
Tricyclic antidepressants (TCAs)	Nortriptyline (Pamelor)	Depression, neuropathic pain,[1] central pain[1]	Anticholinergic effects, sedation
Selective serotonin reuptake inhibitors (SSRIs)	Sertraline (Zoloft) Escitalopram (Lexapro) Citalopram (Celexa)	Depression, stimulation[1]	Long titration period, suicidal ideations, serotonin syndrome, syndrome of inappropriate antidiuretic hormone (SIADH), somnolence, seizures
Stimulants	Modafinil (Provigil) Methylphenidate (Ritalin)	Drowsiness,[1] decreased alertness,[1] impaired concentration,[1] diminished attention[1]	Arrhythmia, seizures, hepatotoxicity, blood pressure changes

[1]Not FDA approved for this indication.

Bladder Dysfunction

Bladder dysfunction after stroke depends on the stroke's location. During the rehabilitation phase, the most common problem is urinary incontinence and urgency associated with uninhibited bladder contraction. Ultrasound bladder scans (usually every 4 hours and after voiding) should be ordered to detect bladder distention and urinary retention. It is standard practice to intervene when bladder volumes are greater than 500 mL. If volumes exceed this cutoff point, intermittent catheterization should be started. Intermittent catheterization is preferable to indwelling catheters because the risk of urinary tract infection is higher with the latter. Bladder scans are usually discontinued when post-voiding residual volumes at 3- to 4-hour intervals are low (<150 mL) for a period of 24 to 48 hours.

Mobility and Use of Adaptive Equipment

Activity limitations vary among stroke survivors and can include difficulties with bed mobility, wheelchair propulsion, transfers, gait, stairs, and basic activities of daily living. The goal of physical therapy and occupational therapy is to maximize functional independence. Addressing mobility limitations is fundamental in stroke rehabilitation because it is related to long-term care needs and independence.

Transfer training comprises learning how to maneuver from one surface or height to another. Ideally, patients should learn to roll and transfer toward the involved and uninvolved sides; however, early mobility efforts are directed to the uninvolved side to minimize the risk of injury.

CURRENT THERAPY

- Stroke rehabilitation improves functional outcomes.
- A comprehensive rehabilitation team composed of physicians, nurses, therapists, and community reintegration professionals can achieve the best outcomes.
- Early evaluation of family support and the home environment is critical to prevent unnecessary institutionalization.
- Evaluation and management of modifiable stroke risk factors, such as smoking, hypertension, and diabetes, are imperative during stroke rehabilitation to prevent stroke recurrence.
- Rehabilitation of the stroke patient can be hindered by conditions such as pneumonia (usually caused by aspiration), deep venous thrombosis, urinary tract infections, shoulder pain, depression, and spasticity. Early identification and treatment of these conditions are necessary to maximize functional outcomes.

Gait deviations are common after stroke and interfere with safety and efficiency of locomotion. If an assistive device is needed, the goal of physical therapy is to progress to the least restrictive device possible. Hemiwalkers and wide-based quad canes provide the most stability. An ankle-foot orthosis may be indicated for patients with decreased ankle control and footdrop.

Instruction in ascending or descending stairs depends on assistive device requirements. With weakness, stairs are ascended by initiating movement with the uninvolved or stronger lower extremity. This process is reversed when descending.

For some stroke survivors, functional ambulation is not a realistic goal. In these cases, the wheelchair becomes the primary means of locomotion. Wheelchair prescription requires considerable skill and training and must take into account posturing, body habitus, cognition, physical fitness level, and the home environment. An appropriate wheelchair prescription is required to maximize mobility and prevent complications such as shoulder pain. Physical and occupational therapists should evaluate the patient to provide wheelchair recommendations to vendors.

Hemi-wheelchairs (i.e., wheelchairs situated closer to the ground) and one-arm drive wheelchairs allow hemiplegic patients to use the uninvolved side for wheelchair propulsion. Lap boards with arm supports can be added to improve hemiparetic arm posturing and sitting symmetry.

For some stroke survivors, the ability to return to driving is considered one of the most important long-term rehabilitation goals. Formal driving rehabilitation programs are available to evaluate and improve driver safety. Driver rehabilitation specialists perform vision, cognitive, and perceptual examinations. Perception tests assess reaction times to visual and auditory stimuli. Values for vision and reaction times are standardized and state dependent. Specialists should also perform a behind-the-wheel assessment, beginning in a parking lot and progressing to negotiation of more complex traffic situations. Many modifications can increase independence and assist with return to driving, including a spinner knob, which can be attached to the steering wheel to allow one-arm control; hand controls for acceleration and braking; left foot pedals to substitute for right foot impairment; and wheelchair lifts.

Adaptive equipment, including bracing, shoe modification, and other tools, increase independence through completion of activities of daily living (e.g., long-handled sponge, reacher, shoe horn, mirror, sock aids) and are extremely beneficial for those with moderate to severe strokes, particularly if hemiparesis is dense (Fig. 2). Silverware, pens, and other utensils can be modified for easier maneuverability. Multipodus boots can be used to prevent plantar flexion contracture development in the hemiparetic limb.

Falls

Falls are common after moderate to severe strokes. In rehabilitation settings, fall prevention usually requires a multimodal approach. Strategies include use of bed-chair alarms, placing those at risk close

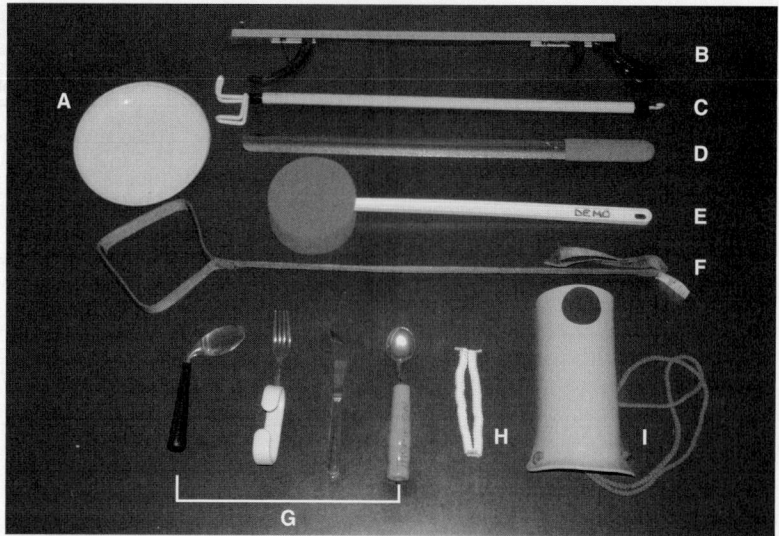

FIGURE 2. Adaptive equipment commonly used during stroke rehabilitation. The tapered front scoop dish (A) has non-skid feet to keep the plate from sliding. The curved edge simplifies scooping food. The dish is especially suited for individuals who have limited flexibility, have decreased motor coordination, or feed using one hand, such as a hemiparetic stroke patient. The reacher (B) is used to get items from the floor. The long-handled dressing aid (C) is used to reach clothes on the floor or to bring clothes up the paretic side. The long-handled shoe horn (D) aids with slipping into shoes. The long-handle sponge (E) is used for reaching the involved side while bathing or when the shoulder range of motion does not allow reaching. The leg lifter (F) and the sound upper limb can be used to assist in moving the paretic lower limb. Adapted feeding utensils (G) are used for patients with grip weakness or difficulties with upper limb range of motion; *left to right*: bent-handle spoon, no-grip fork, rocker bottom knife, and thick-handle spoon. No-tie laces (H) are elastic shoelaces that do not require tying. When using the sock-donning aid (I), the sock slides onto the plastic portion of the device, and the strap is used to pull the sock with the device on the foot.

to the nursing station, wearing skid socks, limiting or refraining from polypharmacy, eliminating slick or irregular floors, and in some cases, providing a sitter for closer monitoring. Physical and occupational therapists must include general safety and fall recovery as part of the treatment plan.

Visual Impairment

Depending on the location of the stroke, the visual system may be involved. One of the most debilitating visual impairments is visuospatial neglect, a complication of right hemisphere strokes. Left-sided stimuli are not attended to or recognized, and affected individuals must learn to deal with this deficit. Other complications include gaze weakness or paralysis, diplopia, visual field loss, ptosis, tracking disorders, decreased visual acuity, and cortical blindness.

Screening for primary visual skills, including visual acuity, visual fields, and visual tracking, should be done by physiatrists, neurologists, and occupational therapists. If problems are identified, patients should be referred to neuro-ophthalmologists and low-vision rehabilitation programs. Visual acuity problems often can be addressed by incorporating the use of glasses into the therapy session or by changing the prescription. Eye movement disorders and visual field deficits usually lessen as time elapses and may respond to treatment with prisms, head positioning, and unilateral eye occlusion with tape or a patch technique. Those with continued visual field impairment should be taught eye movement techniques to expand the visual area.

Conclusions

Stroke rehabilitation requires the concerted efforts of the patient, family, and medical professionals. A multidisciplinary team with training to address the particular impairments and functional limitations of the stroke patient is critical. The physician's efforts should

focus on preventing complications and treating stroke sequelae with the primary goal of improving overall function and participation in society.

REFERENCES

Bhakta BB. Management of spasticity in stroke. Br Med Bull 2000;56:476.

Cicerone KD, Dahlberg C, Malec JF, et al. Evidence-based cognitive rehabilitation: Updated review of the literature from 1998 through 2002. Arch Phys Med Rehabil 2005;86:1681.

Hackett ML, Anderson CS, House A, et al. Interventions for treating depression after stroke. Cochrane Database Syst Rev 2008;(4):CD003437.

Jones SA, Shinton RA. Improving outcome in stroke patients with visual problems. Age Ageing 2006;35:560.

Kelly-Hayes M, Beiser A, Kase CS, et al. The influence of gender and age on disability following ischemic stroke: The Framingham Study. J Stroke Cerebrovasc Dis 2003;12:119.

Lannin NA, Cusick A, McCluskey A, et al. Effects of splinting on wrist contracture after stroke: A randomized controlled trial. Stroke 2007;38:111.

Legg L, Drummond A, Leonardi-Bee J, et al. Occupational therapy for patients with problems in personal activities of daily living after stroke: Systematic review of randomised trials. BMJ 2007;335:922.

Pertoldi S, Di Benedetto P. Shoulder-hand syndrome after stroke. A complex regional pain syndrome. Eura Medicophys 2005;41:283.

Poole D, Chaudry F, Jay WM. Stroke and driving. Top Stroke Rehabil 2008;15:37.

Starkstein SE, Mizrahi R, Power BD. Antidepressant therapy in post-stroke depression. Expert Opin Pharmacother 2008;9:1291.

Stein J. Stroke. In: Frontera WR, Silver JK, editors. Essentials of Physical Medicine and Rehabilitation. Philadelphia: WB Saunders; 2002. p. 778–83.

Stein J, Harvey RL, Macko RF, et al, editors. Stroke Recovery & Rehabilitation. New York: Demos Medical Publishing; 2009.

Umphred DA. Neurological Rehabilitation. St Louis: Mosby Elsevier Health Science; 1995.

van Wijk I, Algra A, van de Port IG, et al. Change in mobility activity in the second year after stroke in a rehabilitation population: Who is at risk for decline? Arch Phys Med Rehabil 2006;87:45.

Wolf SL, Winstein CJ, Miller JP, et al. Effect of constraint-induced movement therapy on upper extremity function 3 to 9 months after stroke: The EXCITE randomized clinical trial. JAMA 2006;296:2095.

Seizures and Epilepsy in Adolescents and Adults

Method of
Erik K. St. Louis, MD, and Mark A. Granner, MD

Epilepsy is a common public health problem afflicting approximately 2.5 million Americans and 30 million persons worldwide. Epilepsy is equally prevalent between the sexes until older age, where the increased incidence of epilepsy in elderly men mirrors that of cerebrovascular disease.

Epilepsy was recognized in antiquity, described by Hippocrates as "the falling sickness." The etymology of epilepsy stems from the Greek *epilepsia*, "to be seized or taken hold of," derived from the erroneous belief and unfortunately persistent stigma that epileptic seizures result from supernatural or spiritual, rather than medical causes. Such historical misunderstandings, coupled with limited availability of effective treatments, have instilled fear of epilepsy for centuries in patients, their families and caregivers, and society. Fortunately, an evolving medical understanding of epilepsy and its many causes and imitators has enabled improved diagnostic testing and an ever-expanding palette of effective, tolerable antiepileptic drug and surgical therapies over the last three decades. All clinicians should be familiar with epilepsy not only because of its prevalence, but because its treatments are increasingly adopted for a wide variety of neurologic and psychiatric conditions including migraine, pain, and mood disorders.

Seizures and Epilepsy Defined

An epileptic seizure is a sudden, transient alteration in behavior caused by an abnormal, excessive neuronal discharge in the cerebral cortex. Everyone has a seizure threshold and holds the potential to have a seizure. Only a small subset of the population, however, experiences spontaneous seizures or develops epilepsy. The lifetime prevalence of experiencing a single seizure is approximately 10%, but only approximately 30% of incipient seizures recur and become epilepsy.

Seizures are most often provoked by an extrinsic (systemic) or intrinsic (brain) factor. Table 1 lists the causes of provoked seizures. An individual may have recurrent provoked seizures without developing epilepsy. In most cases, a provoked seizure does not recur when the provoking factor is successfully corrected, avoided, or removed. The tendency toward recurrent provoked seizures speaks either to the root cause (e.g., recurrent episodes of alcohol withdrawal seizures) or to a heightened sensitivity to seizures in the individual (e.g., a lower than average seizure threshold).

Epilepsy is characterized by recurrent, unprovoked seizures. The prevalence of epilepsy in the general population is approximately 1%. The principal clinical symptoms and signs of epilepsy include ictal (during a seizure), postictal (immediately following seizure termination), and interictal (between seizure episodes) manifestations. Behavioral alterations accompanying epileptic seizures are diverse, ranging from subjective feelings reported by the patient, to objectively witnessed behavioral arrest, unresponsiveness, or involuntary movements. The nature of the ictal behavioral disturbance depends on the location of seizure onset in the brain and its pattern of propagation.

Diagnosis of Seizure Type and Epilepsy Syndrome

A seizure is only a symptom of brain dysfunction, and the seizure type is not in itself an etiologic diagnosis. A diversity of underlying causative pathologies may result in identical phenotypes of clinical seizure behavior and electroencephalographic (EEG) manifestations. The patient's prognosis and treatment are directed by a diagnosis of the underlying

TABLE 1 Common Causes of Provoked Seizures

Drugs of Abuse
Alcohol
- Severe acute alcohol intoxication
- Alcohol withdrawal

Amphetamine and methamphetamine
Cocaine
Lysergic acid diethylamide (LSD)
Phencyclidine

Iatrogenic (Prescription Drugs)
Antibiotics
- High-dose intravenous penicillin
- Imipenem

Antiarrhythmic agents
- Lidocaine (Xylocaine)
- Procainamide (Pronestyl)
- Propafenone (Rythmol)

Insulin overdose
Pain medications
- Opiate analgesics, especially meperidine (Demerol)
- Tramadol (Ultram)

Psychotropic drugs
- Antidepressants
  - Clomipramine (Anafranil)
  - Bupropion (Wellbutrin)
- Antipsychotics
  - Clozapine (Clozaril)

Stimulants
- Amphetamines mixed (Adderall), methylphenidate (Ritalin)

Infection
Brain abscess
Cerebritis
- Lyme disease
- Neurosyphilis

Encephalitis
- Cytomegalovirus
- Herpes simplex virus type 1
- Varicella-zoster virus
- West Nile virus

Acute meningitis
- Bacterial
- Fungal
- Viral

Metabolic Disorders
Hypocalcemia
Hypoglycemia
Hyperglycemia
- Nonketotic hyperosmolar state
- Diabetic ketoacidosis

Hypomagnesemia
Hyponatremia
Hypernatremia
Hypophosphatemia

Herbal Products
Guarana
Ma Huang

epilepsy syndrome, which incorporates an understanding of the cause of the seizures as well as the clinical and EEG characteristics. Epilepsy syndromes are regarded as idiopathic, symptomatic, or cryptogenic.

The International League Against Epilepsy (ILAE) has created consensus terminology defining different seizure types and, in parallel, descriptions of epilepsy syndromes. Diagnosis of ILAE seizure type and epilepsy syndrome is based on electroclinical criteria, including the description of seizure behavior and EEG manifestations. Most experts now also use neuroimaging to diagnose the most likely seizure type and epilepsy syndrome. The seizure type and epilepsy syndrome diagnoses are crucial steps in the approach to the patient with epilepsy because this information determines the patient's prognosis, which type of antiepileptic drug (AED) therapy is indicated, and whether surgical therapies can potentially be offered if AEDs are ineffective.

CURRENT DIAGNOSIS

- Seizures may be partial (focal or localization-related) or generalized in onset. Clinical history, EEG, and imaging data assist the clinician in determining the seizure type and epilepsy syndrome.
- The most important initial diagnostic tests for evaluating new-onset epilepsy in adolescents and adults are high-resolution brain magnetic resonance imaging and EEG.
- In refractory epilepsy or spells of an uncertain type, the patient should be referred for video-EEG monitoring to document and localize the seizure type.

The two principal varieties of epileptic seizures are partial (also known as focal or localization-related) and generalized seizures. Partial seizures begin in one brain region, whereas generalized seizures have their onset simultaneously in both cerebral hemispheres. Differentiating epileptic seizure type and syndrome is often difficult in new-onset epilepsy. Many partial seizures present clinically as a secondarily generalized tonic–clonic seizure without focal features, and patients usually present for evaluation after only one or a few seizures have occurred, so the full spectrum of their epilepsy is not yet apparent.

Partial seizures are subclassified as simplex, complex, and secondarily generalized seizures. A simple partial seizure is restricted at onset to one focal cortical region and does not impair consciousness. Simple partial seizures are synonymous with the term *aura* and involve autonomic, gustatory, cognitive, somatosensory, or involuntary motor activity depending on where they begin in the brain. When a simple partial seizure propagates beyond the initial seizure focus, it may evolve into a complex partial or secondarily generalized seizure. A complex partial seizure is defined by the feature of altered consciousness (although often not full loss of consciousness) and may involve behavioral arrest, blank staring, oral automatisms such as chewing or swallowing, limb automatisms including aimless fumbling movements of the hands, and amnesia. A complex partial seizure may or may not be preceded by an aura, and it may propagate to the whole brain to become a generalized tonic–clonic seizure. There may be considerable variability of behavioral characteristics between different patients with partial seizures or even within a given patient (although a patient's personal seizures tend to be rather monomorphic). Table 2 provides a summary of characteristic auras and behavioral manifestations of

partial seizures according to the region of seizure onset. An EEG during a partial seizure usually demonstrates focal rhythmic activity overlying the region of seizure onset.

Generalized seizures involve simultaneous seizure onset in both cerebral hemispheres. By definition, consciousness is impaired from seizure onset, although myoclonic seizures may be too brief to detect an alteration in consciousness. Absence seizures, frequently confused with complex partial seizures because both were previously (and unfortunately) referred to as petit mal seizures, are brief episodes (typically less than 10 seconds) of behavioral arrest, staring with unresponsiveness, and oral or limb automatisms. Absence seizures lack an aura or postictal state. Tonic seizures involve symmetric tonic posturing of the extremities and, if prolonged, may have prominent autonomic instability. Atonic (also known as astatic) seizures involve loss of tone and may lead to falls. Generalized tonic–clonic seizures involve an initial phase of tonic posturing, generally lasting less than 20 seconds, followed by symmetric clonic movements of the limbs for 1 to 3 minutes. Ictal EEG during generalized seizures demonstrates generalized epileptiform patterns of repetitive spike-wave discharges, polyspikes, or background attenuation.

The accurate diagnosis of an epilepsy syndrome in each patient is an important tenet in epilepsy care; whereas diagnosis of the habitual seizure type describes the ictal seizure characteristics, an epilepsy syndrome diagnosis reaches further, inferring knowledge of the underlying etiology and therefore determining the prognosis and most appropriate therapy. Despite rigorous diagnostic testing, many times the epilepsy syndrome remains ambiguous in new-onset epilepsy cases.

Partial seizures and their associated epilepsy syndromes are most common in adolescents and adults, representing approximately 70% of all epilepsy in these age groups. Most partial epilepsy is related to known acquired etiologies such as head injury, cerebrovascular disease, or tumors. Conversely, idiopathic or cryptogenic partial epilepsies and idiopathic generalized epilepsies are often inherited. The basis of inherited epilepsies is a rapidly evolving field. Many of the known gene effects relate to ion channelopathies.

The Differential Diagnosis of Paroxysmal Spells

The differential diagnosis of epilepsy is wide. Numerous paroxysmal non-neurologic and neurologic disorders may closely mimic the behavioral alterations of an epileptic seizure. Table 3 differentiates commonly confused seizure types and nonepileptic paroxysmal spells by behavioral characteristics, duration, and usual ictal EEG findings. Although most of these conditions are reviewed elsewhere in this text, psychological mimicry of epilepsy is particularly common. Psychogenic nonepileptic spells (also known as pseudoseizures) are most often an expression of a conversion disorder with subconsciously motivated spells of behavioral unresponsiveness or unusual movements that may closely resemble epileptic seizures. Psychogenic spells, however, frequently involve behavioral characteristics of eye closure, nonphysiologic patterns of movements, prominent pelvic thrusting, prolonged duration (often over 5 to 10 minutes), lack of stereotypy between episodes, and failure to respond to antiepileptic drugs. Because true epileptic seizures may also share all of these characteristics, the diagnosis of psychogenic nonepileptic spells is necessarily a diagnosis of exclusion and requires diagnostic ictal video-EEG monitoring for confirmation.

Clinical Approach to the Patient with Seizures

The fundamental goals in epilepsy care are both diagnostic and therapeutic: to understand the underlying cause of epilepsy and determine the epilepsy syndrome when possible; to strive for seizure freedom without adverse side effects of treatment whenever feasible

TABLE 2 Typical Partial Seizure Characteristics According to Region of Seizure Onset

	Simple Partial	Complex Partial	Secondary Generalized
Frontal	Focal clonic motor or none	Amnestic Automatisms Hypermotor common	Frequent

Temporal	Mesial (none possible)
	• Autonomic
	• Dysmnesic
	  • Déjà vu
	  • Jamais vu
	  • Gustatory
	Lateral/posterior neocortical
	Auditory
	Complex visual
		Amnestic Automatisms
		
		Amnestic Automatisms
			Less frequent

Parietal	Somatosensory or none	Amnestic Automatisms	Frequent
Occipital	Simple visual or none	Amnestic Automatisms	Frequent

TABLE 3 Differentiating Epileptic Seizures from Nonepileptic Spells

	Premonitory Symptoms	Behavioral Characteristics	Duration	Postictus Symptoms	Ictal EEG Findings
Absence seizure	None	Staring, automatisms	<10 sec	None	Generalized 3-Hz spike wave
Partial complex seizure	Aura variable; if sensory march, brief over 10–30 sec	Staring, automatisms, posture often preserved	30–180 sec	Common; amnesia, aphasia, sleepiness, ± incontinence	Focal rhythmic activity
Generalized tonic–clonic seizures	Aura variable	Sequence of tonic limb posturing for 10 sec, then clonic movements	1–3 min	Invariable; frequently amnesia, sleep, incontinence, tongue biting	Repetitive spikes (tonic phase); spike wave (clonic phase)
Psychogenic nonepileptic spells (pseudoseizures)	Variable	Variable; behavioral unresponsiveness Nonstereotypy, and unusual movements common	Variable; may be prolonged (>10 min)	Variable; often none	None, other than movement artifact
Syncope	Common; lightheadedness	Falling, eye closure, variable convulsive movements, incontinence	Minutes	None to brief confusion; no postical amnesia	Suppression
Migraine	Prolonged; sensory march over minutes	"Positive" symptoms (e.g., tingling paresthesias)	20–30 min	None	Slowing/ suppression
Transient ischemic attack (TIA)	Sensory march rapid (<10 sec)	More often "negative" (e.g., anesthetic numbness, weakness)	Variable; <1 h	None	Slowing/ suppression
Sleep disorders: Cataplexy	Emotional provocation	Behavioral sleep	Minutes	None	REM stage sleep
Parasomnias	None	Arousal from sleep, confusion, dream enactment	Minutes	Brief confusion	Onset in REM/ NREM sleep

Abbreviations: EEG = electroencephalogram; NREM = nonrapid eye movement (sleep); REM = rapid eye movement (sleep).

909

(or, at the very least, to minimize disabling, injurious seizures and limit adverse effects); and to identify and treat interictal comorbidities in epilepsy.

THE INTERICTAL STATE IN SEIZURES AND EPILEPSY

Recent studies have shown that quality of life in epilepsy is largely determined by the interictal state. Although reducing seizure burden is an integral determinant of patient quality of life, interictal mood disorders such as depression or bipolar affective disorder, cognitive impairments, and adverse effects of antiepileptic drugs more often affect how patients feel on a daily basis between their seizure episodes, and have great impact on perceived quality of life. Physicians should thus proactively inquire regarding altered mood and adverse affects in patients with epilepsy. The approach to new-onset seizures and chronic care of the patient with established epilepsy is now considered.

THE SINGLE SEIZURE AND NEW-ONSET EPILEPSY

The focus during the approach to new-onset seizures is different than in chronic epilepsy. The emphasis for new-onset seizures is prompt diagnosis of the underlying cause because it is imperative to ensure there is no symptomatic etiology requiring further diagnosis or therapy (e.g., brain mass or vascular malformation). Diagnostic tests also help determine the epilepsy syndrome diagnosis and judge the prognosis for future seizure recurrence.

After an apparent single seizure, the physician should take a detailed history from the patient and any available collateral historians about the presenting event. Although serum laboratory values are frequently obtained after a first seizure, these tests actually have little value in the diagnosis of most uncomplicated first seizures in adolescents and adults. Electrolytes and complete blood count may

assure overall general health and serve as a baseline prior to contemplation of antiepileptic drug therapy. A serum or urine drug screen is often appropriate to exclude drug abuse or intoxication as a cause of provoked seizures in adolescents and adults.

The two most important diagnostic tests in the initial evaluation of new-onset seizures are a magnetic resonance image (MRI) of the brain and an EEG; the former provides a measure of structure and the latter a complementary measure of function. A computed tomography (CT) of the head is insufficient to disclose subtle epileptogenic pathology in the brain. The only reason to obtain a head CT after a new-onset seizure is for emergency exclusion of acute neurologic catastrophes requiring urgent attention, such as cerebral hemorrhage or infarction. If a patient has recovered to baseline and neurologic examination is normal, head CT can often be deferred if a definitive brain MRI and neurologic consultation may be obtained promptly (i.e., within 1 week following the seizure). If there is a question of head or neck trauma, head CT should be performed emergently, and cervical radiographs may be necessary. EEG is particularly valuable when brain MRI is normal because it may disclose functional evidence for a heightened epileptogenic potential by demonstrating interictal epileptiform discharges that help determine risk of seizure recurrence after a single seizure or diagnose the epilepsy syndrome when there have been recurrent spells.

Additional diagnostic studies such as ictal video-EEG monitoring, positron emission tomography (PET) of the brain, magnetoencephalography (MEG), and neuropsychological testing may be used later in the course of a patient's evaluation if empirical medical therapy is unsuccessful and if surgical candidacy is questioned, but they are of generally limited value in new-onset seizure disorders. V-EEG is appropriate when psychogenic nonepileptic spells are the suspected diagnosis to exclude epilepsy and to allow prompt triage to appropriate psychological care, thereby sparing the patient from an errant diagnosis and the potential risks of unnecessary antiepileptic drug therapy.

The risk of seizure recurrence following a single seizure is approximately 30% when both MRI and EEG are normal. Multiple seizures occurring over a single day should still be considered as a single seizure episode. The risk of recurrence following a second remote seizure is variable, ranging from roughly 50% to 80%. Evidence is conflicting on the precise prognostic value of an abnormal EEG following a first seizure, but most experts consider EEG abnormalities to raise the risk of seizure recurrence substantially, especially when the EEG shows generalized epileptiform discharges.

Following a second unprovoked seizure, most experts diagnose epilepsy and recommend treatment. Treatment may be considered even following a first seizure if a structural cortical lesion is found because the risk of seizure recurrence is more than 50% in such instances, or if the patient leads a lifestyle where a second seizure would be highly undesirable (such as dependency on driving or a risky occupation).

All patients with new-onset epilepsy must be counseled regarding safety and driving. All patients with consciousness-impairing seizures should be instructed to avoid work, hobbies, or sports activities exposing them to heightened risk of personal injury until seizures are controlled for at least 3 to 6 months. Driving is a critical personal and public safety concern with legal implications to both patient and physician. Because laws vary between states, clinicians must ensure intimate familiarity with the law governing epilepsy in their own jurisdiction and counsel patients appropriately, then document their discussion in the medical record. A few states require physicians to report epilepsy patients.

CHRONIC EPILEPSY CARE AND DETERMINATION OF REFRACTORY EPILEPSY

The approach to the patient with chronic epilepsy is to determine whether the epilepsy is benign or refractory (also known as medically intractable, pharmacoresistant). Following from the tenet in new-onset epilepsy evaluation, determination of the patient's epilepsy syndrome directs the choice of AED therapy most likely to control seizures successfully and allows prognosis for future remission or commitment to long-term AED therapy. Symptomatic or cryptogenic partial or generalized epilepsies and juvenile myoclonic epilepsy rarely remit and usually require long-term AED treatment. Idiopathic partial epilepsy or unclassified epilepsy syndromes more frequently remit after 2 to 5 years of treatment, suggesting future AED withdrawal is worth considering. Drug withdrawal is a complicated decision that is best made in consultation with a neurologist.

Determination of the epilepsy syndrome is more readily achieved during longitudinal continuity of care, given information derived from observations of seizure episodes and further opportunities to obtain interictal or ictal EEG recordings. With repeated or prolonged interictal EEG recording, the yield of identifying interictal epileptiform discharges increases. However, even after repeated outpatient EEGs, or with intensive inpatient V-EEG recording, approximately 20% of those with eventually proven epilepsy lack definite interictal EEG abnormalities. It is important to realize that the diagnosis of epilepsy remains at heart a clinical determination. The absence of abnormalities on MRI or interictal laboratory EEGs does not exclude an epilepsy diagnosis. If MRI or EEG has not been performed prior to evaluation, it is helpful to begin with these investigations to determine the patient's epilepsy syndrome and to exclude symptomatic pathology. Inpatient V-EEG is the gold standard for establishing a diagnosis of epilepsy and should be considered when patients are refractory to one to two empirical AED treatment trials. Even if a patient has infrequent seizures while maintained on AED therapy, admitting patients to an epilepsy monitoring unit allows an opportunity for withdrawal of medication in a safe, carefully supervised environment with a goal of increasing seizure frequency so that one or more habitual clinical seizures may be recorded. Ambulatory EEG or outpatient V-EEG are also available at many centers but have lower yield, given limitations of the inability to withdraw AEDs safely, to conduct behavioral testing or capture video, and to accomplish a technically adequate recording.

Patients continuing to experience breakthrough seizures may have refractory epilepsy. Just more than 10% of patients who have an efficacy failure on their first AED ever become seizure free during future AED trials, suggesting the need for vigilance toward achieving the clinical goals of seizure freedom without AED side effects. If a patient fails to achieve seizure freedom following one to two AED monotherapy trials, referral to a comprehensive epilepsy center should be strongly considered to permit appropriate seizure classification and consideration of surgical options.

Approximately one third of those with epilepsy, or about 750,000 in the United States, have medically refractory epilepsy (i.e., epilepsy that is resistant to AEDs with continued breakthrough seizures and intolerable AED adverse effects). Those afflicted with refractory epilepsy consistently report lower quality of life for multiple reasons, including lost productivity at work or school, inability to drive, self-injury, and the fear of living with the constant uncertainty of when their next seizure may occur. Even more alarming, growing evidence indicates that patients with refractory epilepsy are at a heightened risk for mortality from sudden unexplained death in epilepsy (SUDEP). Even in patients who are well controlled on their drug treatment, approximately half of those surveyed are not satisfied with their current regimen of AEDs, in most instances because of unpleasant or disabling drug-related side effects. A determination of refractory epilepsy from breakthrough seizures or intolerable AED adverse effects should be made relatively early in the course of treatment to permit other potentially more effective care options to be considered. Because of the limitations of current AEDs, both patients and their physicians may be lulled into a dangerous complacency by the desperation of chronic refractory epilepsy, perhaps figuring that any further efforts toward improvement of the situation will prove futile. However, given the severe morbidity and potential mortality of refractory epilepsy, clinicians must aspire beyond the status quo of a so-called acceptable seizure burden and educate their patients that intensive evaluation may lead to more effective treatment for their seizures. Patients who may benefit from referral to a comprehensive epilepsy center include those with these situations:

- An uncertain diagnosis of spells (i.e., the diagnosis of epilepsy is still in question)
- Failure to achieve complete seizure control
- Adverse effects on current AED therapy
- Injury from their seizures
- Lost productivity at work or school because of seizures or adverse effects
- A complicated regimen of concurrent medications and/or other confounding medical, psychiatric, or psychosocial conditions

Epilepsy Therapies

The goals of all epilepsy therapies are to achieve seizure freedom without adverse effects of treatment. Choosing between the numerous options available for epilepsy treatment can be daunting for physicians and patients alike. The last two decades have seen the release of a number of newer AEDs into clinical use, many of which offer improved tolerability and safety profiles. Another advent is vagus nerve stimulation (VNS), the first device using the novel approach of electrical stimulation in epilepsy approved by the Food and Drug Administration (FDA). Centers offering expert evaluation for epilepsy surgery have also become more widely available.

Guidelines for choosing among epilepsy therapies are currently lacking. Until evidence-based guidelines are developed, optimal therapeutic triage must be highly individualized by synthesizing available data, clinical wisdom, and the patient's preference.

All AEDs have the potential to cause dose-related neurotoxic adverse effects. Fortunately, these may be obviated in most patients by dose reduction or substituting for a better tolerated AED.

ANTIEPILEPTIC DRUG THERAPY

Table 4 itemizes specific AEDs with accompanying information on clinical spectrum of uses, typical dosing and blood levels, and cardinal adverse effects. There are currently no clear evidence-based algorithms to guide the temporal sequencing of different AED trials.

TABLE 4 Properties of the AEDs

	Spectrum of Effect	Daily Adult Dosage/Interval	Usual Level (μg/mL)	Adverse Effects	Idiosyncratic Toxicities	Interactions
Older AEDs						
Carbamazepine (Tegretol)	Partial	400–1600+ mg (bid-qid)	4–12+	Diplopia, dizziness, ataxia, hyponatremia	Yes	Bidirectional (AEDs, OC, AC, many)
Ethosuximide (Zarontin)	Absence	500–1500+ mg (bid)	40–100+	Nausea, sedation	Yes	Undirectional
Phenobarbital	Partial	90–180+ mg (qd)	15–40	Sedation, psychomotor slowing	Yes	Bidirectional (AEDs, OC, AC, many)
Phenytoin (Dilantin)	Partial	200–400+ mg (qd–bid)	8–20+	Sedation, dizziness, ataxia, gingival hyperplasia	Yes	Bidirectional (AEDs, OC, AC, many)
Primidone (Mysoline)	Partial	500–1500+ mg (bid-tid)	5–12 (measure phenobarbital)	Sedation, psychomotor slowing	Yes	Bidirectional (AEDs, OC, AC, many)
Valproate (Depakene, Depakote)	Broad	750–2500+ mg (qd–tid)	50–100+	Nausea, tremor, hair loss, weight gain	Yes	Bidirectional (AEDs)
Newer AEDs						
Felbamate (Felbatol)	Broad	1800–4800+ mg (bid–tid)	30–100+	Irritability insomnia, weight loss	Yes	Bidirectional (AEDs, OC, AC)
Gabapentin (Neurontin)	Partial	900–3600+ mg (tid-qid)	4–20++	Sedation, dizziness, weight gain	No	None
Lacosamide (Vimpat)	Partial (? Broad)	200–600 mg	?	Sedation, fatigue	? (None in clinical trails)	None known
Lamotrigine (Lamictal)	Broad	300–600+ mg (qd–bid)	1–20+	Dizziness, rash	Yes	Bidirectional (AEDs, OC)
Levetiracetam (Keppra)	Broad	1000–3000++ mg (bid)	5–40++	Sedation, dizziness	No	None
Oxcarbazepine (Trileptal)	Partial	600–3600+ mg (bid)	10–40+ (MHD)	Sedation, dizziness	Yes	Bidirectional (AEDs, OC)
Pregabalin (Lyrica)	Partial	150–600+ mg (bid)	2–10	Sedation, dizziness weight gain	No	None
Retigabine	Partial	600–1200+	?	Dizziness, somnolence, confusion, incoordination	?	?
Rufinamide (Banzel)	Broad	400–3200 mg/d	?	Sedation, diarrhea	?	Bidirectional
Tiagabine (Gabitril)	Partial	16–64 mg (bid-tid)	100–300 μg/mL	Sedation, weight gain	No	Unidirectional
Topiramate (Topamax)	Broad	100–600+ mg (qd–bid)	10–20+	Sedation, cognitive complaints, paresthesias, weight loss, rare nephrolithiasis	Glaucoma-like reaction	Bidirectional (AEDs, OC at high doses)
Vigabatrin (Sabril)	Partial/ infantile spasms	2000–4000+ mg/d	?	Somnolence, fatigue, weight gain, behavioral disturbances	Visual field deficit	Unidirectional
Zonisamide (Zonegran)	Broad	100–600+ mg (qd–bid)	10–40+	Sedation, paresthesias, weight loss, rare nephrolithiasis	Yes	Unidirectional

Notes: AED = antiepileptic drug; + = higher doses/levels often additionally effective, as tolerated; ++ = considerably higher doses/levels sometimes additionally effective in intractable patients, as tolerated; MHD = 10, 11 Monohydroxy derivative active metabolite of oxcarbazepine. Interactions: Unidirectional indicates that other AEDs or drugs may affect this AED; bidirectional indicates that other drugs may affect this AED, and this AED affects other drugs; OC = oral contraceptives; AC = anticoagulants; many = many other non-AEDs.
? = Available information incomplete and based on pre-marketing published data from clinical trials.

Nonetheless, common treatment principles underlie the choosing, dosing, sequencing, and monitoring of AED therapy in epilepsy care. Here are several basic principles:

- Choose AED therapy appropriate for the epilepsy syndrome.
- Consider patient characteristics and co-morbidities when choosing AEDs.
- Employ AED monotherapy at the lowest effective dosage to achieve seizure freedom.

- Reserve AED polytherapy (combining two or more AEDs) for refractory patients and minimize total drug load to limit adverse effects.
- Treat according to the patient's clinical response, not the AED level.
- Monitor for long-term complications of older AED therapy and consider withdrawal of therapy when appropriate.
- Choose affordable AED therapy.

Choosing an AED appropriate for the patient's epilepsy syndrome is an important tenet of epilepsy care. AEDs have different spectrums of efficacy for various seizure types within epilepsy syndromes. Some AEDs are narrow in their spectrum of efficacy, whereas others are broader, treating a variety of different seizure types well. Broad-spectrum AEDs may be favored when the epilepsy syndrome diagnosis is ambiguous because they offer potential efficacy against most seizure types and have less potential to aggravate some epilepsy syndromes. To some degree, the spectrum of efficacy of an AED is related to its postulated mechanism of action. AEDs that chiefly antagonize sodium channel ionophores or promote γ-aminobutyric acid (GABAergic) neurotransmission are generally most effective in partial-onset seizures, whereas drugs that combine these and other mechanisms of action may have broader efficacy in primary generalized seizure types.

Evidence from prospective, blinded, randomized clinical trials is only available for certain AEDs for monotherapy use. Gabapentin (Neurontin), oxcarbazepine (Trileptal), and lamotrigine (Lamictal) possess randomized controlled trial evidence for monotherapy treatment of partial-onset seizures, and topiramate (Topamax) has evidence for monotherapy use in new-onset epilepsy. All older AEDs and other newer AEDs have either comparator trial or anecdotal monotherapy evidence. All marketed newer AEDs have randomized controlled trial evidence for use as adjunctive treatment in partial-onset seizures, whereas older AEDs have comparator trial evidence.

Patient characteristics and co-morbidities may affect the choice of an AED. For example, weight is an important consideration. Valproate (Depakene, Depakote), pregabalin (Lyrica), and carbamazepine (Tegretol) may contribute to weight gain, whereas topiramate (Topamax) and zonisamide (Zonegran) may include weight loss among their adverse effect profile. The patient with both epilepsy and migraine might favor topiramate or valproate, drugs that are efficacious for both conditions.

In general, AED monotherapy is just as effective—or more effective—than polytherapy. Monotherapy limits the potential for adverse effects and drug interactions. AED dosing must be individualized to achieve optimal results. Our strategy is to titrate the AED toward a target dose that has proven effective for most individuals in clinical studies and in our experience. Dose adjustment can then be made in the event of adverse drug reactions or recurrent seizures. If the endpoint of seizure freedom is preserved, maintaining a lower but clinically therapeutic AED dosage is entirely acceptable. If a patient continues to experience breakthrough seizures, raising the AED dose to the maximal dose tolerated is sometimes necessary, although recent evidence demonstrates that only a minority of patients become seizure free when dosed above the usual therapeutic range, so a practical viewpoint of treatment futility should be realized when patients experience frequent breakthrough seizures despite adequate AED dosages. Therapeutic change should be made when seizure freedom is not maintained at AED doses effective for most patients. Overlapping AEDs in transitional polytherapy (where the baseline AED is maintained at the current dose to limit breakthrough seizures, the newly added AED is titrated to a protective dose, then the original drug is tapered and discontinued) is the preferred method when introducing a new AED monotherapy. Abruptly stopping the existing AED increases the risk of seizures (and perhaps status epilepticus), whereas introducing the new AED too rapidly may induce adverse effects that taint the patient's perception of what could be an effective therapy.

Many medically refractory epilepsy patients require chronic polytherapy. Overall, only a small minority of refractory patients can be rendered seizure free with AED polytherapy, but they may benefit substantially by reduction of seizure burden. Although no good evidence for specific AED polytherapy combinations exists, augmenting monotherapy with an AED offering a different or complementary mechanism of action may be considered. Great care must be taken to avoid excessive drug dosing and drug–drug interactions. Initiating and maintaining AED polytherapy is difficult and requires oversight by a neurologist with extensive knowledge of clinical pharmacology.

AED dosing should be adjusted to achieve the clinical goals of seizure freedom without adverse effects. This may indeed be a delicate balancing act for some patients because all AEDs have the potential to cause dose-related "neurotoxic" adverse effects. Fortunately, adverse effects may be obviated in most patients by dose reduction or substituting for a better tolerated AED.

Philosophies on the use of AED blood level monitoring differ, but most agree that blood levels should in most cases be considered only a guideline to treatment. AED levels should not be perceived as an absolute indication for altering AED dosing, divorced from clinical judgment of the patient's seizure control or adverse effects. Blood-level monitoring can help guide therapy, but so-called therapeutic levels are derived from treatment of populations. An individual patient may require a lower or higher intensity of AED therapy to achieve optimal results. For example, some patients develop breakthrough seizures even at supratherapeutic or toxic levels, others may experience adverse effects within the usual therapeutic range, whereas some patients become seizure-free on levels in a subtherapeutic range. The danger of overreliance on AED blood levels is twofold: levels may lead both physicians and patients to a false sense of therapeutic adequacy or may lead to errant manipulation of AEDs in patients who require no adjustments. Typical clinical scenarios where clinicians should obtain AED levels include the following:

1. After reaching steady-state administration of an AED, to establish a patient's individual personal baseline against which future comparisons can be made in event of breakthrough seizures.
2. While titrating individual AEDs in complex polypharmacy regimens, when drug interactions may influence either the new adjunctive AED or baseline antiepileptic and other medications.
3. Adjusting for alterations in AED metabolism during aging, disease states, and during each trimester of pregnancy when AED levels can fluctuate substantially based on altered drug absorption, metabolism, protein binding, and clearance. With some heavily protein-bound drugs, especially phenytoin (Dilantin), obtaining free drug levels is necessary to discern the biologically active fraction of the drug, especially in chronically or critically ill patients.
4. When trying to determine the AED responsible for adverse effects in a patient receiving polytherapy.

In summary, AED levels are most useful when testing a clinical hypothesis. We discourage the use of routine or scheduled levels, an exception being chronic phenytoin therapy in institutionalized patients (where zero-order kinetics from nonlinear hepatic metabolism may lead to drug accumulation and toxicity) and during pregnancy when altered AED absorption, metabolism, and elimination may lead to declining drug concentrations during successive trimesters.

With chronic AED therapy, intermittent blood testing for monitoring of liver function tests and hematologic functions is reasonable although not of proven value. The highest risk of idiosyncratic reactions associated with AEDs such as serious rash, hepatotoxicity, and hematologic dyscrasias is during the first 6 to 12 months of therapy and extremely rare thereafter. Recently, the FDA has recommended assessing the HLA-B*1502 genotype prior to initiating carbamazepine (Tegretol) in patients of Asian ethnicity, given that patients of Han Chinese ancestry carrying this allele have demonstrated a heightened risk of severe allergic rash, including Stevens-Johnson syndrome or toxic epidermal necrolysis, and the drug should be avoided in such patients. It seems likely that expanded screening of selected patient populations will prove necessary as knowledge concerning heightened vulnerability for severe idiosyncratic reactions continues to grow through further research in the fields of pharmacogenomics and pharmacoepidemiology.

There is mounting concern that patients on chronic maintenance therapy with older AEDs are at risk for osteopenia and osteoporosis. Any enzyme-inducing AED (carbamazepine [Tegretol], phenytoin [Dilantin], phenobarbital, primidone [Mysoline], and oxcarbazepine [Trileptal]) has the potential to decrease bone density. Valproate (Depakote) may also lead to decreased bone density. Chronic phenytoin exposure is of particular concern, given its rare association with cosmetic adverse effects including gingival hyperplasia (which may be severe enough to warrant repeated gingivectomies), peripheral neuropathy, and irreversible cerebellar ataxia. Considering AED withdrawal in appropriate candidates or transition to another newer AED therapy without such untoward effects is often reasonable.

AED cost is a crucial social issue that may trump all other medical principles in selection and maintenance of AED therapy in patients who lack adequate medical insurance. Choosing expensive AEDs that a patient cannot afford may erode the patient's adherence to treatment and trust in the physician. Insurance and financial status must therefore be considered, so that available resources (i.e., indigent federal- or state-sponsored insurance or corporate pharmaceutical assistance programs) can be summoned if a prohibitively expensive newer AED is the best therapeutic choice. Of the newer AEDs, gabapentin, lamotrigine, levetiracetam, oxcarbazepine, topiramate, and zonisamide are available as generic formulations. Because evidence regarding the pharmacokinetic and therapeutic equivalence of these generic formulations in epilepsy patients is not available, caution is advisable prior to switching between different AED formulations. Although there is no evidence to guide clinicians in switching between AED formulations, obtaining a baseline AED level prior to a contemplated switch between AED formulations and rechecking levels once the new formulation is adjusted to its target dosage is a reasonable precaution to avoid breakthrough seizures or inadvertent toxicity.

Withdrawal from chronic AEDs is a difficult consideration in the older adolescent or adult with epilepsy because seizure recurrence may impact driving and work abilities. In general, it is worthwhile to consider an attempt at withdrawing AED therapy when the patient has been seizure free for an arbitrary period between 2 and 5 years. Available data suggest that approximately 25% to 70% of patients experience seizure recurrence with AED withdrawal. The decision to withdraw AED therapy must be discussed in the context of the patient's lifestyle and responsibilities because driving and work considerations may be paramount and trump the medical prognosis. Neurologic consultation should be strongly considered when AED withdrawal is contemplated.

EPILEPSY SURGERY

Evaluation for epilepsy surgery should be strongly considered in patients with refractory partial epilepsy. A syndrome particularly amenable to surgical intervention is mesial temporal-lobe epilepsy (MTLE), characterized by medically refractory complex partial seizures, often a history of complex febrile seizures in infancy, and hippocampal sclerosis on brain MRI.

Resective surgery for epilepsy has been performed for over a century, and advances in EEG and neuroimaging have increased the widespread application of epilepsy surgery. A pivotal clinical trial established the clear superiority of anterior temporal lobectomy over medical therapy for chronically refractory MTLE in carefully selected patients.

Identification of potential candidates for epilepsy surgery remains the biggest challenge for tertiary care epilepsy centers. Some have estimated that nearly 75,000 potential surgical candidates in the United States remain under care in primary care settings with ongoing seizures, yet only 3000 or fewer surgical procedures for epilepsy are performed annually.

Potential candidates for resective epilepsy surgery have refractory epilepsy with ongoing seizures that have been resistant to at least two to three appropriately administered AEDs. The precise seizure burden meriting an aggressive, invasive approach remains a subject of conjecture, but even one to two consciousness-impairing seizures annually may be highly disabling in patients who aspire to work and drive.

The basic approach in epilepsy surgery involves identification and precise localization of the epileptogenic zone, the region of the brain that is necessary and sufficient to cause clinical seizures; determining whether the patient possesses appropriate functional reserve for safe removal of that seizure focus; and subsequent operative resection of this area.

A variety of investigations must be performed at specialized comprehensive epilepsy centers to determine if epilepsy surgery would be effective and safe for an individual patient. The most useful and important initial investigations are a high-resolution volumetric brain MRI (with thin cut coronal plane acquisition perpendicular to the hippocampal long axis) and inpatient prolonged ictal V-EEG monitoring that permits intimate correlation and offline, post hoc detailed analysis of the ictal behavior and EEG to localize the patient's habitual clinical seizures. Additional techniques that help localize the epileptic focus preoperatively include functional imaging techniques such as single photon emission computed tomography (SPECT) and PET, magnetoencephalography, and neuropsychological testing. An intracarotid sodium amytal test is necessary in most patients to lateralize memory

functions accurately and estimate functional reserve prior to surgery. In some cases, invasive EEG recording with surgically implanted subdural or parenchymal strips or grids of electrodes is necessary to confirm the seizure focus precisely and allow mapping of eloquent functional cerebral cortex to reduce operative morbidity.

When a structural epileptogenic mesial temporal brain lesion evident on MRI is concordant with well-localized habitual clinical seizures by ictal V-EEG, there is a 60% to 90% chance that surgery will produce seizure freedom. Resection in neocortical epilepsies offers a 30% to 80% chance of achieving a seizure-free outcome, depending largely on whether a MRI lesion concordant with the seizure focus is present. Surgical efficacy contrasts with a 5% or less chance that additional AED therapy will render the refractory patient seizure free. Favorable seizure outcome must be balanced with a 3% or less risk of major morbidity (i.e., hemorrhage, infection, stroke, memory, language, or hemianopic visual field deficit) incurred by surgery. Risk may be higher in extratemporal epilepsy surgery for postoperative motor, sensory, and visual deficits, depending on the location of the seizure focus. Memory or language deficits may occur in temporal lobe operations.

OTHER ALTERNATIVE THERAPIES

Some patients with refractory partial epilepsy are not suitable epilepsy surgical candidates because of diffuse or unlocalizable epileptic foci, whereas others may choose not to undergo brain surgery despite suitable candidacy. In these cases, other options may still exist.

The vagus nerve stimulator (VNS) is the only electrical device currently approved as an adjunctive treatment for partial-onset seizures. A battery-operated generator and programmable computerized stimulator are placed surgically in a subcutaneous pocket on the left anterior chest. The device looks much like a cardiac pacemaker and has electrical leads connected to the left vagus nerve in the neck. Once implanted, the device is programmed by means of a radiofrequency wand in the physician's office and provides a small electrical current to the nerve at preset intervals and amounts. The patient also has the opportunity to trigger a stronger current to attempt to abort or lessen an oncoming seizure by means of a magnet that is passed externally over the device.

The efficacy of VNS for seizure reduction is roughly comparable to that of AEDs; approximately 40% of patients experience a 50% or greater reduction in their seizures, and up to 15% of patients become seizure free. Although there are no current evidence-based guidelines for the best timing of VNS placement, we reserve VNS for patients who are not resective surgery candidates or who refuse surgery and those who have failed most older and newer AEDs. In addition to reducing seizure burden, VNS may improve a patient's quality of life by improving alertness, mood, and memory. Predictors of which patients are most likely to benefit from VNS, and the optimal dosing of the device once it is implanted, are yet to be defined in prospective clinical trials. A recently completed large, randomized controlled trial of deep brain stimulation in refractory partial epilepsy has demonstrated that 60% of patients responded with a 50% or greater seizure reduction and nearly 20% of patients achieved 90% seizure reduction during long-term follow-up. Additional neurostimulation therapies are being evaluated, including cortical stimulation and transcranial magnetic stimulation. Two recent randomized controlled trials of transcranial magnetic stimulation (TMS) have yielded conflicting findings concerning efficacy; one study targeting patients with MRI-visible cortical malformations demonstrated TMS efficacy for seizure reduction.

Specialized diets may be a useful adjunctive treatment for epilepsy. The best studied of these is the ketogenic diet, a high-fat, low-protein, low-carbohydrate diet that induces systemic ketosis, which has an antiepileptogenic effect on the brain. The ketogenic diet is most often successfully used in children, but it may also be tried in adolescents and adults. Unfortunately, unless rigid compliance is assured, the ketogenic diet produces little benefit and, in general, most adolescents and adults have limited tolerance of the diet. However, highly motivated and desperately refractory epilepsy patients may benefit from the ketogenic diet. An alternative that is often more tolerable, but not yet robustly studied, is the modified Atkins diet, a high-fat, moderate-protein, low-carbohydrate diet that induces mild ketosis.

Identifying and treating seizure aggravators is an important consideration. Recent studies have suggested that obstructive sleep apnea (OSA) is a frequent co-morbidity in refractory epilepsy, and nasal continuous-positive airway pressure in patients with refractory epilepsy and co-morbid OSA may lead to seizure reduction. Primary sleep disorders such as restless legs syndrome and periodic limb movements disorder may fragment sleep and worsen seizure burden in patients with refractory epilepsy. If a primary sleep disorder is suspected, a diagnostic polysomnogram should be ordered, and aggressive treatment for the sleep disorder should be initiated.

Although most complementary and alternative therapies in epilepsy have not been rigorously studied, a variety of behavioral stress reduction techniques, meditation, yoga, or naturopathic treatments may be considered. Most of these therapies have few risks and occasionally benefit individual patients. Botanical extracts for epilepsy therapy that possess potent in vitro antiepileptogenic properties and wide therapeutic windows are currently being investigated as another avenue of therapy for refractory patients.

STATUS EPILEPTICUS: IDENTIFICATION AND MANAGEMENT

Status epilepticus is a prolonged, unremitting epileptic seizure that constitutes a medical emergency. Until the past decade, status epilepticus was defined as a seizure lasting 30 minutes or longer (from onset through the end of the ictal period, exclusive of the postictal recovery phase that may in itself last well over 30 minutes). However, more recent data suggest that most seizures that self-terminate do so by 3 minutes after onset, indicating that longer lasting seizures are unlikely to stop without intervention.

Status epilepticus may be convulsive or nonconvulsive. Status epilepticus frequently begins with a prolonged generalized tonic–clonic or partial motor seizure, followed by a minimally convulsive or nonconvulsive phase with or without subtle motor features such as facial or eyelid twitching, or nystagmus. Status epilepticus thus evolves in a manner analogous to a lethal cardiac dysrhythmia, proceeding from clinically overt convulsive movements toward an eventual electromechanical dissociative state where the epileptic seizure continues as a subclinical electrographic discharge evident only during EEG monitoring.

Management of status epilepticus begins with securing the airway, respiration, and circulation and placement of two large-bore intravenous catheters for drug administration and fluid resuscitation. Obtaining a stat glucose is appropriate before rapid administration of thiamine, followed by intravenous dextrose (to avoid Wernicke encephalopathy in malnourished patients). If intravenous access is not readily available, rectal diazepam (Diastat) or intramuscular fosphenytoin (Cerebyx) can be used. Rectal diazepam is also useful in the out-of-hospital treatment of prolonged seizures or seizure clusters in adolescents and adults, potentially obviating escalation into status epilepticus and preventing an emergency department visit.

Initial pharmacotherapy of status epilepticus begins with intravenous lorazepam (Ativan) given at 2 mg/minute to a goal of 0.1 mg/kg (or 8 mg total) with cautious respiratory monitoring, then loading with phenytoin (Dilantin) at 20 mg/kg, given no faster than 50 mg/minute to avoid hypotension, with ECG and hemodynamic monitoring. Phenytoin should be given through a dedicated peripheral intravenous line because of potential for cardiotoxicity and to avoid precipitation by other drugs. Intravenous phenytoin, a highly insoluble alkaline solution, may lead to substantial soft-tissue toxicity (including the much feared purple-glove phenomenon). An alternative is fosphenytoin, which may be administered at up to 150 mg/min, and is not associated with tissue injury if extravasation occurs.

The success of treatment of status epilepticus can be measured clinically, but if the patient remains unresponsive after the convulsive movements stop, an urgent EEG may be needed to exclude nonconvulsive status epilepticus. Refractory status epilepticus can be treated with midazolam (Versed),[1] pentobarbital (Nembutal), sodium pentothal (Thiopental), or phenobarbital.[1] Case series reports suggest that intravenous valproate, lacosamide, and levetiracetam may

also be effective. An advantage of short-acting agents such as midazolam is the rapidity with which pharmacologically induced coma can be reversed to examine the patient, whereas valproate, lacosamide, and levetiracetam offer the advantage of avoiding hemodynamic or respiratory complications. Although propofol (Diprivan)[1] was also a favored therapy for the adjunctive treatment of refractory status epilepticus, recent reports have led to declining use for this application given that fatal propofol infusion syndrome (characterized by irreversible metabolic acidosis, bradycardia, myocardial and/or renal failure, rhabdomyolysis, and cardiopulmonary arrest) may be an underrecognized complication. An expanding therapeutic armamentarium for acute seizures and status epilepticus is expected, given that several non-oral treatments are currently being developed, including an intravenous form of carbamazepine, as well as intravenous, intramuscular, and intranasal forms of novel investigational AEDs.

Conclusion

Epilepsy is characterized by recurrent, spontaneous seizures. Epilepsy has many causes and represents a collection of syndromes that have varying natural histories and responses to therapy. Diagnosis is based on the history and may be supported by physical examination. The two most important investigations in initial evaluation of the patient with new-onset seizures or epilepsy are high-resolution brain MRI and EEG. There are many mimickers of epilepsy requiring careful differential diagnosis. When confronted with spells of an uncertain type, evaluation with VEEG may secure the correct diagnosis.

The past decade has seen tremendous expansion in available AED therapies, many of which are more tolerable and safer for long-term use. Choice of AED in an individual patient depends on the epilepsy syndrome, consideration of available efficacy evidence, patient characteristics and co-morbidities, and cost. AED monitoring should reinforce, and not replace, clinical judgment. Chronic complications of certain older AEDs may include osteopenia, adverse cosmetic effects, weight gain, and neuropathy. Withdrawal of AEDs in selected seizure-free patients or transition to AEDs without chronic toxicities should be considered in such instances.

Unfortunately, despite advances in available AEDs, more than a third of patients with epilepsy are refractory. Early determination of refractory epilepsy and triage to intensive diagnostic and therapeutic resources at a comprehensive epilepsy care center is critical. Epilepsy surgery may render carefully selected patients seizure free, and VNS is a viable alternative when surgery is not possible, leading to reduced seizure burden and improved quality of life. Physicians should approach their patients with epilepsy with enthusiasm and hope for effecting an improvement in their condition.

---

[1]Not FDA approved for this indication.

REFERENCES

French JA, Kanner AM, Bautista J, et al. Efficacy and tolerability of the new antiepileptic drugs: I. Treatment of new-onset epilepsy: Report of the Therapeutics and Technology Assessment Subcommittee and Quality Standards Subcommittee of the American Academy of Neurology and the American Epilepsy Society. Neurology 2004;62(8):1252–60.

French JA, Kanner AM, Bautista J, et al. Therapeutics and Technology Assessment Subcommittee of the American Academy of Neurology; Quality Standards Subcommittee of the American Academy of Neurology; American Epilepsy Society. Efficacy and tolerability of the new antiepileptic drugs: II. Treatment of refractory epilepsy: Report of the Therapeutics and Technology Assessment Subcommittee and Quality Standards Subcommittee of the American Academy of Neurology and the American Epilepsy Society. Neurology 2004;62(8):1261–73.

Kwan P, Brodie MJ. Early identification of refractory epilepsy. N Engl J Med 2000;342(5):314–9.

St. Louis EK, Gidal BE, Henry TR, et al. Conversions between monotherapies in epilepsy: Expert consensus. Epilepsy and Behavior 2007;11(2):222–34.

Wiebe S, Blume WT, Girvin JP, Eliasziw M. A randomized, controlled trial of surgery for temporal-lobe epilepsy. N Engl J Med 2001;345:311–8.

---

[1]Not FDA approved for this indication.

Epilepsy in Infants and Children

Method of
Mary Zupanc, MD

Epilepsy is defined as two or more unprovoked seizures. A seizure is the result of an abnormal synchronous depolarization of a group of neurons. The clinical manifestations of a seizure depend on where in the brain the discharges begin and how they spread.

Epilepsy is a common medical condition, occurring in 0.5% to 1% of all children. Each year 150,000 children and adolescents in the United States have a single unprovoked seizure. One fifth of those, or 30,000, eventually develop epilepsy. The highest incidence of epilepsy is during the first year of life.

Appropriate classification of epilepsy is the cornerstone of therapy. Most children with epilepsy are seizure-free with the use of one antiepileptic drug (AED) without side effects. Some epileptic children, approximately 15%, have medically refractory seizures.

Classification

In any evaluation of a child who might have had a seizure, the first job of the physician is to determine whether the event was indeed an epileptic seizure or some other paroxysmal event. The history is the key to differentiating between these episodes and epileptic seizures.

There are many different types of paroxysmal events in children that can mimic seizures (Box 1). For example, pallid or cyanotic breath-holding spells can result in brief generalized tonic–clonic seizures. Pallid breath-holding spells are precipitated by excitement, surprise, or trivial head trauma, resulting in an exaggerated vasovagal event with concomitant bradycardia and central nervous system (CNS) ischemia. If the event is sufficiently prolonged, the child might have a brief seizure. Cyanotic breath-holding spells, on the other hand, are prolonged crying episodes, often stimulated by frustration or anger, resulting in an involuntary inability to breathe, with concomitant cyanosis, decreased oxygen concentration, and hypercapnia. This is typically followed by a brief loss of consciousness; sometimes a brief generalized tonic–clonic seizure follows. These episodes must be distinguished from the unprovoked seizures characteristic of epilepsy. Breath-holding spells do dissipate in the preschool years and do not need to be treated with AEDs.

Other paroxysmal events that can resemble seizures include motor tics; vasovagal syncope; shuddering attacks, a rare condition associated with tremor or shuddering of the upper trunk and shoulders with no alteration of consciousness, occurring in young toddlers

and preschoolers; confusional migraines, which can mimic complex partial seizures; sleep disturbances; gastroesophageal reflux, which sometimes produces tonic posturing and can resemble tonic seizures (Sandifer's syndrome); and paroxysmal choreoathetosis or dystonia. There are also patients who have pseudoseizures. Their events can mimic seizures; sometimes they cannot be distinguished from clinical epileptic seizures without performing closed-circuit television electroencephalographic monitoring. Children with pseudoseizures often have complex psychosocial situations and may be victims of either physical or sexual abuse.

If it is determined that a child most likely has epilepsy, the primary physician must determine the appropriate seizure classification and epilepsy syndrome in order to make intelligent decisions with respect to diagnostic studies, treatment, and prognosis. The International League Against Epilepsy has established the International Classification of the Epilepsies and Epileptic Syndromes. This system is used as the foundation for decision making.

In the classification of epilepsy, seizures are divided into two categories, generalized and partial (Box 2). *Generalized seizure* indicates that the clinical seizure does not contain any focal features. Electrographically, the electroencephalogram (EEG) demonstrates generalized spike, polyspike, or sharp wave discharges (or some combination of these) without localizing features over both hemispheres. Clinical seizures of this type are myoclonic, tonic (episodes of tonic posturing), atonic (drop attacks), absence (formerly petit mal), and tonic–clonic (old terminology, grand mal). On the other hand, *partial seizures* are events that begin focally in one part of the brain. The clinical manifestations depend on where in the brain the epileptic discharge begins. A simple partial seizure is a seizure in which there is no associated alteration of consciousness. A simple partial seizure can constitute the aura that patients often refer to before they have more recognizable clinical seizures. As the electrical discharges progress, simple partial seizures typically transform into complex partial seizures. Complex partial seizures are defined as focally generated seizures that are associated with an alteration of consciousness. These seizures can, and often do, generalize to become generalized tonic–clonic seizures. Examples of simple partial seizures include olfactory hallucination, abdominal queasiness, déjà vu, jamais vu, or a tingling sensation in the hands. An example of a complex partial seizure is a paroxysmal episode that begins with staring, drooling, lip smacking automatism, and confusion, lasting 1 to 2 minutes.

BOX 1   Nonepileptic Events That Can Be Mistakenly Diagnosed as Epilepsy in Children

Benign paroxysmal vertigo
Breath-holding spells
- Classic (cyanotic)
- Pallid
Paroxysmal choreoathetosis or dystonia
Syncope
Migraine, especially acute confusional
Pseudoseizures
Shuddering spells
Sleep disorders
Tics

BOX 2   Classification of Epileptic Seizures

Partial Seizures
Simple partial seizures
- With motor signs, such as focal clonic activity
- With somatosensory or special-sensory symptoms such as lateralized numbness, tingling, visual or auditory hallucinations, abnormal odors or smells
- With automatic symptoms or signs such as tachycardia, diaphoresis
- With psychic symptoms such as fear, anxiety, déjà vu, jamais vu, confusion
Complex partial seizures
- With simple partial seizures (aura) at onset
- With impairment of consciousness at onset
Partial seizures evolving to secondarily generalized seizures

Generalized Seizures
Absence seizures
Myoclonic seizures
Clonic seizures
Tonic seizures
Tonic–clonic seizures
Atonic seizures

In addition to seizure classification, the clinician should be aware of the International Classification of Epilepsy Syndromes. The epilepsy syndromes are determined by further classifying epileptic seizures on the basis of age at onset; seizure type; family history; risk factors for epilepsy; associated neurodevelopmental delays; neuroimaging results; EEG data, both ictal and interictal; other diagnostic tests, such as lumber puncture and metabolic testing; and physical examination. This information can more specifically identify an epileptic condition, resulting in more appropriate management and predictions with respect to prognosis.

Epilepsy Syndromes

The classification of epilepsy syndromes differentiates generalized, localization-related, and undetermined epileptic syndromes, in addition to special syndromes (Box 3). These syndromes are classified into *idiopathic*, implying normal neurologic status and a genetic predisposition; *symptomatic*, implying an underlying lesion or other CNS pathologic condition; and *cryptogenic*, implying that the epileptic condition is probably symptomatic but the exact cause cannot be pinpointed.

GENERALIZED EPILEPSY SYNDROMES

Examples of idiopathic generalized epilepsy syndromes include childhood absence epilepsy, juvenile absence epilepsy, and juvenile myoclonic epilepsy. Childhood absence epilepsy is probably genetically linked to juvenile absence epilepsy and juvenile myoclonic epilepsy. These epilepsy syndromes are most likely different phenotypic expressions of the same gene. These children have normal neurologic examinations and tend to have above-average intelligence. Depending on the age at onset, children and adolescents with these epilepsy syndromes can have a varied clinical manifestation: absence, myoclonic, or generalized tonic–clonic seizures.

BOX 3   Classification of Epileptic Syndromes

Localization Related (Focal, Local, Partial)
Benign rolandic epilepsy
Benign occipital epilepsy
Idiopathic
Symptomatic

Generalized
Idiopathic, Age Related
Benign idiopathic convulsions
Benign myoclonic epilepsy in infancy
Benign neonatal familial convulsions
Childhood absence epilepsy
Epilepsy with tonic–clonic seizures on awakening
Juvenile absence epilepsy
Juvenile myoclonic epilepsy

Idiopathic and/or Symptomatic
Epilepsy with myoclonic–astatic seizures
Epilepsy with myoclonic absences
Infantile spasms (West's syndrome)
Lennox–Gastaut syndrome
Symptomatic: early myoclonic encephalopathy

Focal or Generalized (Not Known)
Acquired epileptic aphasia (Landau–Kleffner syndrome)
Epilepsy with continuous spike waves during slow-wave sleep
Neonatal seizures
Severe myoclonic epilepsy in infancy

Childhood and Juvenile Epilepsy

Childhood absence epilepsy accounts for 2% to 8% of all cases of childhood epilepsy. The age at onset is during elementary school age, and the peak is at 6 to 7 years of age. The seizure semiology is characterized by absence seizures, which are brief episodes of staring, often accompanied by eyelid fluttering, facial clonic activity, or upper extremity myoclonus. These seizures are very brief, lasting only 2 to 10 seconds, occurring multiple times per day and without a concomitant postictal phase. Absence seizures can be induced by hyperventilation. If the epilepsy begins before 9 years of age, the risk of having comorbid generalized tonic–clonic seizures is only 16%. If the epilepsy begins later, the risk of generalized tonic–clonic seizures is close to 50%. Myoclonic seizures are rare.

Juvenile absence epilepsy is associated with absence seizures and generalized tonic–clonic seizures. The age at onset is prepubertal, usually between 10 and 15 years of age. Absence seizures occur in all patients; generalized tonic–clonic seizures occur in almost 80%.

With juvenile myoclonic epilepsy, the age at onset is typically during adolescence, between 12 and 18 years of age. The characteristic clinical symptom is early morning sudden myoclonic jerks of the shoulders and arms. Ninety percent of patients have generalized tonic–clonic seizures, and 33% have absence seizures.

The interictal EEG in all cases demonstrates generalized spike and slow-wave discharges. With the earlier onset, the generalized spike and slow-wave discharges are at 3 cycles per second (cps). With juvenile myoclonic epilepsy, the generalized discharges consist of generalized polyspike, spike, and slow-wave discharges at 4 to 5 cps.

The treatment for these three epilepsy syndromes is similar. Valproate (Depakote) is the drug of choice for patients with both absence and generalized tonic–clonic seizures, except in girls of reproductive age (see later). Ethosuximide (Zarontin) can be used if the patient is having only absence seizures. There recently has been an NIH multicenter study that compared the efficacy of valproate, ethosuximide, and lamotrigine in the treatment of childhood absence epilepsy. It was a double-blinded, placebo-controlled study. It demonstrated that valproate and ethosuximide (as monotherapy treatments) are significantly more effective than lamotrigine monotherapy in the treatment of childhood absence epilepsy. Lamotrigine is approved as adjunctive therapy for generlized tonic–clonic seizures in children older than 2 years. It has been successfully used in the treatment of juvenile myoclonic epilepsy, as add-on therapy. Topiramate (Topamax) also shows promise in treating generalized tonic–clonic seizures and myoclonus but not with absence seizures. Levetiracetam (Keppra)[1] is also being studied to determine its efficacy with respect to absence seizures. Levetiracetam is approved as adjunctive therapy for myoclonic seizures in juvenile myoclonic epilepsy in adolescents 12 years and older. Levetiracetam is also approved as adjunctive therapy for primary generalized tonic clonic seizures in the idiopathic generalized epilepsy syndromes in children and adolescents 6 years and older.

The prognosis varies, depending on the age at onset. Juvenile myoclonic epilepsy requires lifelong treatment because of the high rate of relapse when AED therapy is discontinued. On the other hand, childhood absence epilepsy has a much better prognosis, with more than 50% of patients outgrowing their epilepsy by the age of puberty.

Infantile Spasms

Another generalized epilepsy syndrome is infantile spasms. The incidence of infantile spasms is 1 in 4000 to 6000 live births. The peak age at onset is 4 to 6 months. The seizures are characterized by flexor or extensor (or both) myoclonic spasms, usually occurring in clusters after the infant awakens in the morning or from a nap.

Infantile spasms can be divided into three categories: symptomatic, cryptogenic, and idiopathic. Improvements in neuroimaging and metabolic testing now enable better identification of a specific etiology for infantile spasms. Some of the most common causes of symptomatic infantile spasms include tuberous sclerosis (approximately 25% of patients with tuberous sclerosis have infantile spasms); malformations

---

[1]Not FDA approved for this indication.

of cortical development, such as Aicardi's syndrome or malformations in the posterior quadrants of the brain; chromosomal abnormality, one of the most common abnormalities is trisomy 21; inborn errors of metabolism, aminoacidopathies, or mitochondrial cytopathies; asphyxia; meningitis or encephalitis; and trauma.

Interictally, the EEG demonstrates a hypsarrhythmia pattern. This is a markedly abnormal pattern with high amplitude slowing at 1 to 3 cps and multifocal polyspike, spike, and slow-wave discharges.

According to the new practice parameter published by the American Academy of Neurology, the mainstay of treatment for infantile spasms in the United States is corticotropin (ACTH [HP Acthar]).[1] It demonstrates "probable" efficacy, using current evidence-based medicine. The mechanism of action for ACTH remains unclear, but this drug does affect CNS concentration of various biogenic amines and increases γ-aminobutyric acid (GABA)-receptor affinity. It also reduces corticotropin-releasing hormone (CRH), which is elevated in patients with infantile spasms and is a potent proconvulsant. In Europe and Canada, vigabatrin (Sabril),[5] a structural analogue of GABA, is the drug of choice in treating infantile spasms, particularly in children with tuberous sclerosis. Vigabatrin appears to be about 89% to 90% effective in eliminating infantile spasms in children with tuberous sclerosis and infantile spasms. Vigabatrin has not been approved by the FDA because of reports of retinal changes and peripheral visual constriction after long-term use of this drug. Other drugs that have questionable efficacy (due to inadequate evidence) in treating infantile spasms include the benzodiazepines, valproate, zonisamide (Zonegran),[1] topiramate,[1] lamotrigine,[1] and felbamate (Felbatol).[1] The principal deterrent in the use of valproate in these children is the risk of hepatotoxicity.

Lennox–Gastaut Syndrome

Lennox–Gastaut syndrome (LGS) is another generalized epilepsy syndrome, predominantly confined to children. The criteria for the diagnosis of LGS include generalized, multiple seizure types, including tonic, atonic, absence, and myoclonic seizures; an electrographic signature of generalized slow spike and wave discharges at 1½ to 2½ cps; and cognitive impairment. The degree of cognitive impairment is correlated with the underlying substrate of epilepsy and seizure control. As with infantile spasms. LGS can be divided into categories of symptomatic, cryptogenic, and idiopathic. In 30% of patients, infantile spasms evolve to LGS. Therefore, it follows that the two epileptic syndromes have similar underlying etiologies. This epileptic syndrome is often medically intractable.

Relatively few AEDs have been shown to be effective in treating LGS. The ketogenic diet is one of the oldest known treatments for pediatric epilepsy and status epilepticus. It remains a reasonable alternative therapy for LGS. The ketogenic diet consists of a high ratio of fats to carbohydrates and protein. Every piece of food must be carefully weighed and measured for fat, carbohydrate, and protein content so that the proper ratios are maintained. Any deviation from the diet can result in a loss of ketosis and renewed seizures. The exact mechanism by which the ketogenic diet provides seizure control remains unknown. It is presumed that the ketones have anticonvulsant properties. One third to one half of children with LGS have an excellent response to the ketogenic diet, with either a significant reduction in or complete elimination of seizures. Phenobarbital[1] and phenytoin (Dilantin),[1] in part because of their sedative effects, have never been shown to be effective in treating LGS.

The introduction of valproate in the late 1970s provided one of the first effective antiepileptic drugs in treating LGS, based on empiric evidence. There has never been a double-blind, placebo-controlled trial of valproate in treating LGS. The AEDs that have evidence to support their use in treating LGS are felbamate, topiramate, lamotrigine, and the newly FDA-approved drug, rufinamide. Rufinamide is very effective in treating the tonic and atonic seizures associated with LGS, but it can cause nausea, vomiting, and somnolence. Felbamate, released

in 1993, showed great promise in treating LGS. Unfortunately, it has been associated with an increased risk of aplastic anemia and liver failure. The risk of aplastic anemia is now known to be highest in women with known autoimmune disorders; it has never been reported in a child younger than 13 years. The collective risk is 20 to 207 per million patients treated with this drug. The risk of hepatotoxicity is no greater than that of any of the other AEDs. Felbamate is reserved for patients with severe, intractable epilepsy. It is probably the most effective AED in treating LGS. The benzodiazepines are occasionally helpful in patients with LGS, but only if given intermittently to abort seizure clusters. Otherwise they are too sedating, and many patients develop tachyphylaxis.

LOCALIZATION-RELATED EPILEPSIES

The localization-related epilepsies can also be divided into two categories: symptomatic and idiopathic. The symptomatic localization-related epilepsies are the result of an underlying CNS abnormality, such as tumor, stroke, encephalomalacia from head trauma, hemorrhage, or malformation of cortical development. It is thought that the idiopathic epilepsies have an underlying genetic predisposition.

The most common epilepsy syndrome of childhood is an idiopathic localization-related epilepsy (benign rolandic epilepsy or benign epilepsy of childhood) associated with central-temporal spikes (BECTS). It accounts for 24% of all epileptic seizures in children between the ages of 5 and 14 years. It is genetically determined, probably autosomal dominant with variable penetrance and age-limited expression. The children are neurologically normal. The seizure semiology is characterized by sensorimotor symptoms and clonic activity in the face, arm, or leg, usually with associated hypersalivation and speech arrest. The seizure frequency varies, but typically seizures are rare. They are usually nocturnal, occurring in children in the early morning hours before they awaken or soon after they fall asleep. One known precipitating factor is sleep deprivation.

In benign rolandic epilepsy, the interictal EEG demonstrates drowsiness and sleep-activated central temporal spikes that can be asymmetrical or have a wide field spread. AEDs are seldom used in patients with rare seizures. They may be indicated for patients who are experiencing more frequent seizures that disrupt sleep, school performance, or psychosocial well-being. This epilepsy condition is outgrown in virtually 100% of patients by the time of adolescence.

SPECIAL SYNDROMES

Neonatal Seizures

Neonatal seizures are commonly the result of hypoxic–ischemic injury, hypoglycemia, or hypocalcemia in the perinatal period. Sepsis can also result in seizures. Three rare causes of neonatal seizures include pyridoxine dependency, folinic acid deficiency, and glucose transporter deficiency.

Pyridoxine dependence causes seizures unresponsive to AEDs. It is related to an insufficient production of GABA, a primary inhibitory neurotransmitter. The glucose transporter deficiency is characterized by a low cerebrospinal glucose concentration. There is an enzymatic defect in glucose transport that disrupts facilitative diffusion of glucose across the blood–brain barrier. The seizure semiology is different from that in older children and adolescents. Because of the primitive synaptic network, neonatal seizures can be quite subtle. Examples of neonatal seizures include eye deviation with apnea or multifocal clonic activity. Neonates do not have generalized tonic–clonic seizures, although they can have tonic seizures. There is controversy over whether or not the bicycling movements and lip-smacking seen in neonates are subtle seizures or "brainstem release" phenomena.

The most important therapeutic intervention in neonatal seizures is recognition of the underlying cause, followed by its prompt treatment. This can, in itself, abort any further seizure activity without the use of chronic AEDs. A pyridoxine[1] challenge and treatment with folinic acid (Leucovorin)[1] should be given to any neonate with intractable seizures. For status epilepticus in neonates, the most

---

[1]Not FDA approved for this indication.
[5]Investigational drug in the United States.

---

[1]Not FDA approved for this indication.

effective initial therapy is 20 mg/kg of phenobarbital given twice if necessary. Fosphenytoin (Cerebyx)[1] [mcl] at 20 mg/kg can also be used if the phenobarbital is ineffective. However, even when both of these medications have been given for neonatal status epilepticus, the success rate is only 67%. Preliminary studies indicate that intravenous lidocaine (Xylocaine)[1] may be effective for refractory neonatal seizures. The benzodiazepines are less effective in neonates than in older infants and children because the GABA receptors are excitatory in neonates, not inhibitory.

Febrile Seizures

Febrile seizures denote a special developmental seizure disorder that is not highly correlated with the development of epilepsy. By definition, a febrile seizure is a generalized tonic–clonic seizure occurring in a child between the ages of 6 months and 5 years and associated with a high fever not related to an underlying CNS infection. Simple febrile seizures carry a low risk of epilepsy (only 1%–2%) compared with the general population's risk of 0.5% to 1%. There is an underlying genetic predisposition, with a positive family history in one third of first-degree relatives. The risk of febrile seizure recurrence is quite high, with 33% of children having at least one recurrence. If a child is younger than 12 months at the time of the first febrile seizure, the risk of recurrence is 50%.

If the history is clear, no diagnostic studies need to be performed, with the exception of a lumbar puncture in infants younger than 18 months. The physician should design the work-up in response to the most likely cause of the fever. If meningitis is suspected at all, a lumbar puncture should be performed. This is particularly true in infants younger than 18 months who present with high fever, because they might not have reliable clinical signs and symptoms of meningismus.

Although phenobarbital[1] was once used to prevent febrile seizure recurrence, this is no longer the standard of care. There is no evidence to suggest that phenobarbital treatment decreases the risk of the development of epilepsy. Furthermore, the side effects of phenobarbital in these children are significant, with more than 40% exhibiting hyperactivity, aggressive behavior, impulsivity, poor attention and concentration, or sleep disturbance. Oral or rectal diazepam (Valium, Diastat) therapy can be given to prevent recurrence of febrile seizures in predisposed children. The dosage of oral diazepam[1] is 0.33 mg/kg every 8 hours during the course of the febrile illness. This medication can produce side effects including sedation and irritability. The dosage of rectal diazepam for patients 2–5 years of age is 0.5 mg/kg. It is usually reserved for febrile seizure recurrence and prolonged febrile seizure (>5 min).

The prognosis for febrile seizures is excellent. Very few children develop epilepsy (1%–2%). Those who have a greater risk for developing epilepsy include children with focal or prolonged febrile seizures, children with a family history of epilepsy, and children with developmental delays and abnormal neurologic examinations. These risk factors suggest that an underlying substrate of epilepsy already exists and that the seizure threshold was simply lowered by the fever.

Landau–Kleffner Syndrome

Landau–Kleffner syndrome (acquired epileptic aphasia) is a poorly understood syndrome that is characterized by a regression in expressive and receptive language in association with an epileptiform EEG, either focal or multifocal. Overt clinical seizures occur in more than 70% of patents; in the remaining 30%, the only ictal manifestation is the deterioration in speech and language. The diagnosis of Landau–Kleffner syndrome is determined solely on the basis of clinical symptoms and EEG finding. Twenty-four-hour EEG monitoring may be helpful in establishing the diagnosis because there is generally activation of the epileptiform discharges during sleep.

The underlying pathophysiology of Landau–Kleffner syndrome remains unknown. The treatment of this syndrome is controversial, in part related to our poor understanding of this disorder. The goal of therapy is normalization of the EEG and improvement in speech

and language, although it has still not been determined if the epileptiform discharges produce the symptoms of Landau–Kleffner syndrome or if they simply represent an epiphenomenon. AEDs are used, particularly valproate (Depacon). Steroid therapy has also been tried with some reported success. In refractory cases, multiple subpial transections have been performed over the epileptogenic zone, with only a few reported cases in the literature. A multicenter, double-blind, placebo-controlled treatment trial is needed to determine appropriate and effective therapies. The prognosis for this disorder is variable.

Some clinicians have broadened the definition of Landau–Kleffner syndrome to include children with developmental aphasia and underlying epileptiform EEGs. As a result, some children with autism have been treated with AEDs and even steroids to see whether there would be an improvement in clinical symptoms. This remains an area of considerable controversy. Again, are the epileptiform discharges producing the clinical symptoms or are the epileptiform abnormalities merely an epiphenomenon pointing to an underlying, poorly understood CNS disorder?

Assessment

Appropriate classification of a paroxysmal event is the initial step in the evaluation of a child with a suspected seizure. The history is the key to the diagnosis. Care must be taken to elicit possible precipitating factors and risk factors for epilepsy. Precipitating factors that result in provoked seizures include an underlying CNS infection or head trauma. With breath-holding spells, as mentioned earlier, frustration, anger, surprise, excitement, or trivial head trauma can provoke a spell sometimes followed by a brief generalized tonic–clonic seizure. The risk factors for epilepsy include history of encephalitis or meningitis; history of significant head trauma–associated loss of consciousness, concussion, skull fracture, prolonged coma, or penetrating injury; history of a prolonged febrile seizure lasting longer than 20 minutes; developmental delays; abnormal neurologic examination; and history of asphyxia.

The seizure semiology and its evolution are also very helpful in determining the portion of the brain where the epileptogenic focus resides. Specifically, if the patient typically senses a funny taste or feels queasy before the episode of staring, drooling, and lip smacking automatism, one can surmise that the epileptogenic zone probably resides in either one of the temporal lobes. If the epileptogenic focus is near the sensorimotor cortex, the patient might first experience numbness and tingling in the contralateral extremity followed by rhythmic clonic activity of this same extremity as the epileptogenic discharges spread. Forced head version is a reliable indicator of a contralateral frontal epileptogenic focus.

Home videos of paroxysmal events have proved helpful in appropriately classifying both epileptic and nonepileptic events. An EEG—both awake and asleep—is especially helpful. The presence of focal or generalized epileptiform discharges in the context of an appropriate clinical history is usually sufficient for making the appropriate diagnosis. However, a normal awake and asleep EEG does not exclude the diagnosis of epilepsy, particularly in the face of a compelling history. If the epileptiform discharges are infrequent or deep-seated in the mesial temporal structures, the EEG might not reflect the underlying epileptogenic zone. Untreated generalized epilepsies, however, almost invariably are associated with generalized spike and slow-wave discharges on routine EEGs. Prolonged closed-circuit television EEG monitoring is reserved for patients whose diagnosis is unclear or whose seizures are sufficiently intractable to warrant an evaluation for epilepsy surgery.

If epilepsy is confirmed, depending on the nature of the epilepsy syndrome, further diagnostic studies may be necessary. If the diagnosis is clearly a known benign generalized epileptic syndrome such as childhood absence epilepsy, no further tests are needed and the child can begin AED therapy. If the diagnosis is a localization-related epilepsy, a neuroimaging study is indicated, preferably magnetic resonance imaging (MRI). Computed tomography is inadequate for

---

[1]Not FDA approved for this indication.

detecting the underlying substrates of epilepsy. If the epilepsy is thought to be the result of an underlying encephalopathy, metabolic testing and a chromosomal analysis might also need to be performed. In addition, the neurocutaneous syndromes, particularly tuberous sclerosis, are associated with epilepsy. In 25% of patients with tuberous sclerosis, the initial apparent symptom is infantile spasms.

Treatment

Epilepsy is a condition characterized by recurrent seizures. It is not necessary to treat the patient after the first seizure. The chance of seizure recurrence after the first seizure is approximately 30% to 40%. If the EEG demonstrates temporal epileptiform discharges or generalized spike and slow-wave discharges, the chance of recurrence is much higher, bordering on 90%. If a child has a second seizure, the risk of continued seizures is also much higher. Antiepileptic medication is generally recommended after a second seizure. There are exceptions to this, particularly if a benign epilepsy syndrome is identified (e.g., benign rolandic epilepsy). There are also epilepsy syndromes that are malignant. When these are identified, treatment should begin without delay, regardless of the seizure frequency.

When antiepileptic drug therapy is discussed, it is important to recognize the seizure type as well as the epileptic syndrome. This is the single most important criterion in making a decision about antiepileptic medication. There are basic principles to remember in choosing AED therapy:

- AED monotherapy is effective in most patients and avoids undesirable drug interactions.
- AEDs should be titrated slowly and only to the point of seizure control, if possible.
- Seizure control should not be achieved without trying to avoid side effects. If side effects develop, attempts should be made to reduce the dosage, change to a sustained-release formulation, or change AEDs.
- Drug compliance is enhanced when medication is given once or twice daily. Therefore, sustained-release medication should always be considered.
- Therapeutic blood levels are determined on the basis of trough levels and represent a statistical range of efficacy. They are not absolute levels.

The past few years have seen a rapid escalation in the marketing of AEDs. The drugs of choice for partial seizures now include a broad range of AEDs, including carbamazepine (Tegretol; Carbatrol [extended-release formulation]), oxcarbazepine (Trileptal), gabapentin (Neurontin), lamotrigine, topiramate, valproate, levetiracetam, zonisamide (not approved for children <16 years), phenobarbital, and phenytoin (Tables 1 and 2). The new AEDs have all been approved by the FDA as adjunctive therapy in treating partial seizures in adults. Topiramate has received approval for treating partial seizures in children as young as 2 years. Lamotrigine has been approved for treating both partial seizures and generalized tonic–clonic seizures, as adjunctive therapy, in children ages 2 or older. Levetiracetam is approved as adjunctive therapy for partial seizures and for myoclonic seizures. Phenobarbital and phenytoin are not currently being prescribed by pediatric neurologists nearly as often as they were in the past 10 years.

ANTIEPILEPTIC DRUGS

Carbamazepine

Carbamazepine is still the most widely used AED in treating partial seizures. Its mechanism of action is similar to that of phenytoin. Both drugs work by inhibiting the high-frequency repetitive firing of voltage-dependent sodium channels. Carbamazepine is generally tolerated well but should be introduced slowly. This reduces the risk of toxicity and enhances compliance. Autoinduction of carbamazepine metabolism via the cytochrome P-450 enzyme system occurs within the first month of therapy, often necessitating an increase in the total dosage of carbamazepine. If at all possible, once the dosage has been adjusted, attempts should be made to change to a sustained-release preparation. Carbamazepine is available in a liquid formulation, chewable tablets, tablets, a sustained-release preparation, and sustained-release sprinkle capsules.

The toxic side effects of carbamazepine include dizziness, diplopia, sedation, ataxia, and nausea. Rare idiosyncratic reactions include aplastic anemia and hepatic dysfunction. Transient leukopenia occurs in 10% of children, usually during the first month of therapy. Allergic rash occurs in about 8% to 10% of patients; cases of Stevens-Johnson syndrome have been reported. Other rare side effects include irritability and dystonia. The antibiotic erythromycin alters the kinetics of carbamazepine, resulting in significant increases in carbamazepine levels.

Before carbamazepine therapy is initiated, a baseline complete blood cell count with differential and liver function tests should be obtained. These studies should be repeated monthly for the first 3 months of therapy or if there are signs or symptoms of liver dysfunction or blood dyscrasias.

Oxcarbazepine

Oxcarbazepine is related to carbamazepine and is approved as adjunctive therapy in treating localization related epilepsy. It does not induce the cytochrome P-450 enzyme system and is not metabolized to 10,11-epoxide, the known metabolite of carbamazepine thought to be responsible for teratogenicity and for many of carbamazepine's toxic side effects. It is formulated as a liquid (300 mg/5 mL suspension) or in pills (150 mg; 300 mg; 600 mg). It can be given twice daily. It has the same mechanism of action as carbamazepine and can produce the same side effects with toxicity. Patients can develop hyponatremia with this medication.

Valproate

Valproate is a broad-spectrum AED demonstrating efficacy for both partial and generalized seizures. Its mechanisms of action include reduction of T-type calcium channel currents, modulation of sodium channels, and, possibly, enhancement of GABA activity, the primary inhibitory neurotransmitter. Valproate comes in several formulations, including the liquid valproic acid, sodium divalproex tablets; and sodium divalproex sprinkle capsules.

The most common side effects of valproate include an increase in appetite with concomitant weight gain and tremor. Rarely, valproate causes an encephalopathy with sedation and cognitive impairment. Occasionally, this is due to hyperammonemia. At other times, the exact mechanism remains unclear. With high doses, tremor, transient alopecia, and thrombocytopenia (with easy bruising and bleeding) can occur. Another rare side effect of valproate is pancreatitis.

The most publicized and serious side effect of valproate is hepatotoxicity. There have been fatalities. The highest risk group is children younger than 2 years who have developmental delays and abnormal neurologic examination and who are on multiple AEDs. The risk of hepatic failure in these children is estimated at 1 in 500. The hepatotoxicity is an idiosyncratic reaction, is not dose related, and occurs in the first 6 months of therapy. The initial signs and symptoms of liver dysfunction are sedation, nausea, vomiting, and anorexia. Most pediatric neurologists and researchers agree that these cases of fatal hepatotoxicity probably occur in children with an underlying defect in the β-oxidation of fatty acids. Carnitine is an essential cofactor in this process. Therefore, carnitine supplementation[1] at 30 to 100 mg/kg/day is recommended for any child younger than 2 years. It is thought that carnitine provides protection against liver toxicity, aiding β-oxidation by bringing fatty acids across the mitochondrial membrane and binding to toxic valproate metabolites.

Literature has implicated valproate in the development of polycystic ovary syndrome. This syndrome is associated with infertility, dyslipidemia, and insulin-resistant diabetes mellitus. The exact mechanism by which this occurs is still being investigated, but the risk of polycystic

---

[1]Not FDA approved for this indication.

TABLE 1   Summary of Commonly Used Antiepileptic Drugs (Established Drugs)

Drug	Indications	Maintenance Dosage (mg/kg/d)	Starting Dosage	Half-Life (h)	Therapeutic Range (μg/mL)	Common Side Effects	Serious Idiosyncratic Side Effects
Carbamazepine (Tegretol)	Partial Partial w/secondary general, primary general, tonic-clonic	10–20	5–10 mg/kg/d	8–25	8–12	Diplopia, lethargy, blurred vision, ataxia, incoordination	Rashes, hepatic dysfunction, pancreatitis, aplastic anemia, leukopenia
Ethosuximide (Zarontin)	Absence	15–40; most children require 15–20	<6 y: 10 mg/kg/d >6 y: 250 mg/d	25–40	40–100	Gastrointestinal distress, hiccups, lethargy	Rashes, leukopenia, pancytopenia, systemic lupus erythematosus
Phenobarbital	Partial Partial w/secondary general, primary general, tonic-clonic	<1 y: 5–6 >1 y: 4–6 Teenagers, adults: 1–3	Same as maintenance	40–70	15–40	Irritability, hyperactivity, lethargy	Rashes
Phenytoin (Dilantin)	Partial Partial w/secondary general, primary general, tonic-clonic	5 (might need higher doses in children <5–6 y)	Same as maintenance	Depends on concentration	10–20	Lethargy, dizziness, ataxia, gingival hypertrophy, hirsutism	Rashes, hepatic dysfunction, lymphadenopathy, blood dyscrasias
Primidone (Mysoline)	Partial Partial w/secondary general, primary general, tonic-clonic	12–25	<6 y: 50 mg qhs <12 y: 100 mg qhs[3] >12 y: 100–125 mg qhs[3]	5–8 (phenobarbital 40–70)	5–12	Irritability, hyperactivity, lethargy, nausea	Rashes
Valproic Acid (Depakene)	Partial Partial w/secondary general, primary general, tonic-clonic Absence Myoclonic Tonic Atonic	15–60	5–15 mg/kg/d; incr by 10–15 mg/kg/d every 2 wk Max dosage 60 mg/kg/d	4–14	60–100	Lethargy, weight gain or loss, hair loss, tremor	Hepatic dysfunction, pancreatitis, anemia, thrombocytopenia

[3]Exceeds dosage recommended by the manufacturer.

TABLE 2 Summary of Commonly Used Antiepileptic Drugs (New Drugs)

Drug	Indications	Maintenance Dosage (mg/kg/d)	Starting Dosage	Half-Life (h)	Therapeutic Range (mg/mL)	Common Side Effects	Serious Idiosyncratic Side Effects
Felbamate (Felbatol)	Partial Partial w/secondary general Tonic Atonic	30–45, max 90[3]	15 mg/kg/d; incr in 10-mg/kg increments to 60 mg/kg/d[3] if necessary	13–24	30–100 (not well established)	Anorexia, insomnia, somnolence, tics	Aplastic anemia, hepatoxicity, rashes
Gabapentin (Neurontin)	Partial Partial w/secondary general	20–60[3]	10 mg/kg/d, incr in 5-mg/kg increments	5–8	Not established 2–6	Lethargy, dizziness, irritability	None
Lamotrigine (Lamictal)	Partial Partial w/secondary general Generalized tonic–clonic	5–15[3], dosage depends on other drugs used: w/ enzyme inducers, use 10–15: w/valproate, use 2–3	12.5–25 mg/d, incr slowly; be cautious in patient on valproate	15–60 (highly dependent on concomitant AEDs)	Not established 5–15	Rashes, lethargy, irritability, movement disorder	Rashes
Levetiracetam (Keppra)	Partial Partial w/secondary general Myoclonic	30–60	10 mg/kg/d, incr in 10-mg/kg increments	6–8	3–40	Agitation, behavioral disinhibition	None
Oxcarbazepine (Trileptal)	Partial Partial w/secondary general	30–60	15 mg/kg/d[3], incr by 10–15 mg/kg increments	8–10	10–35	Hyponatremia, somnolence, lethargy, dizziness, blurred vision	Rash
Rufinamide (Banzel)	Partial (See footnote.)	45 mg/kg/day	10 mg/kg/day	6–10	Not established	Nausea, vomiting, somnolence	None
Tiagabine (Gabitril)	Partial Partial w/secondary general (approved for ≤12 y)	0.5–1; dosage depends on other drugs used: w/ enzyme inducers, use 0.7–1.5; w/o enzyme inducers, use 0.3–0.4	0.1 mg/kg/d; incr weekly by 0.1 mg/kg/d	3–13	Not established 5–70 ng/mL	Lethargy, confusion, mental dullness, difficulties with concentration	None
Topiramate (Topamax)	Partial Partial w/secondary general	5–10[3]	1–2 mg/kg/d; incr weekly by 1 mg/kg/d	12–60	5–20	Irritability, hyperactivity, cognitive slowing, weight loss, renal stones, metabolic acidosis, oligohidrosis	Rash
Zonisamide (Zonegran)	Partial Partial w/secondary general (approved for ≤16 y)	5–10	2 mg/kg/d, incr by 1–2 mg/kg	48–65	10–40	Irritability, cognitive slowing, weight loss, renal stones, oligohidrosis	Rash

Banzel is approved as adjunctive therapy for the tonic and atonic seizures associated with Lennox–Gastaut syndrome.
[3]Exceeds dosage recommended by the manufacturer.
AED = antiepileptic drug; incr = increase.

Epilepsy in Infants and Children

ovaries, hyperandrogenism, and anovulatory menstrual cycles is definitely increased in women with epilepsy who are taking valproate. In addition, because of these findings and its teratogenic effects (increased risk of neural tube defects and possible neurocognitive effects in the fetus), the American Academy of Neurology and the American Epilepsy Society have both stated that valproate is relatively contraindicated in women with epilepsy who are in the reproductive age.

A baseline complete blood cell count with differential and liver function studies should be obtained before initiating valproate therapy. During the first 6 months of therapy; these blood parameters should be followed monthly or more often if signs and symptoms warrant a closer check.

Gabapentin

Gabapentin is one of the newer AEDs that is sometimes used in treating partial seizures. Its mechanism of action remains largely unknown although it is structurally related to GABA. Gabapentin has not been shown to be effective in treating generalized epilepsies. Gabapentin does not come in a chewable tablet but is available in an oral solution and in tablet and capsule form.

One of the biggest advantages of gabapentin is the lack of drug interactions. It is generally safe and tolerated well. There are no known fatal side effects. In the pediatric population, irritability, aggressiveness, agitation, and other behavioral side effects have been reported, particularly in children with underlying encephalopathy.

Unlike other AEDs, gabapentin is not metabolized by the liver, does not induce the cytochrome P-450 enzyme system, and is not highly protein bound. It is excreted via the kidneys.

Lamotrigine

Lamotrigine was released in 1994. The best known mechanisms of action for lamotrigine include an inhibition in the release of glutamate and an effect on voltage-sensitive sodium channels. It has been approved as adjunctive therapy for treating partial seizures and for treating generalized tonic–clonic seizures. It is probably another broad-spectrum AED, effective in treating partial and generalized seizures. Clinical research is ongoing to determine its efficacy in treating generalized epilepsies. Lamotrigine comes in several formulations including tablets and chewable dispersible tablets.

Lamotrigine has been associated with an allergic rash. Patients who take a combination of valproate and lamotrigine are at highest risk for an allergic rash. Valproate inhibits the metabolism of lamotrigine, resulting in an increase in the half-life from 12 to 72 hours. Therefore, the level of lamotrigine escalates considerably if valproate is added; the required dosage of lamotrigine when taken in combination with valproate is only 2 to 3 mg/kg/day as opposed to 4.5–7.5 mg/kg/day.[3] When lamotrigine therapy is initiated, the dosage must be increased very slowly, especially when it is used in combination with valproate. If a rash is reported, the patient should be seen immediately because the rash can progress rapidly. Patients who have reported skin allergies to other drugs, especially to carbamazepine, are also at high risk for an allergic rash from lamotrigine.

Other less common side effects of lamotrigine include dizziness, headaches, diplopia, sedation, and movement disorders, including choreoathetosis and dystonia. Positive behavioral side effects, including antidepressant effects, have been reported with lamotrigine.

Topiramate

Topiramate is another broad-spectrum AED. Topiramate appears to have a variety of mechanisms of action, including inhibition of voltage-sensitive sodium channels, enhancement of the inhibitory action of GABA, modest inhibitory effects on glutamate receptors, and weak inhibition of carbonic anhydrase. Drug interactions are minimal. It comes in several formulations including tablets and sprinkle capsules.

The major side effect of topiramate is cognitive dysfunction, including dysnomia, slowing of cognitive processing, and poor memory. These side effects can be minimized by a slow titration process, waiting to increase the dosage until habituation has taken place. Rare patients have an idiosyncratic reaction to topiramate, becoming encephalopathic on very small dosages of this medication. Topiramate can also cause renal stones, probably a result of its inhibition of carbonic anhydrase. Therefore, it should be used with caution in patients who are on the ketogenic diet or who have kidney dysfunction. Patients should be kept well hydrated.

Tiagabine

Tiagabine (Gabatril) is another antiepileptic drug that has been approved as adjunctive therapy by the FDA for treating partial seizures (for those ≤12 years of age). Its mechanism of action is via the inhibition of GABA reuptake in the synaptic cleft. There are no known drug interactions. It is formulated in pills only.

The major side effects of tiagabine include lethargy, irritability, aggressive behavior, dizziness, headache, and tremor. It is 96% protein bound and is metabolized by the liver.

Levetiracetam

Levetiracetam is also one of the newer antiepileptic medications. It has a novel mechanism of action that probably involves the synaptic vesicle protein. Levetiracetam has been approved as adjunctive therapy for partial seizures in children and adolescents 4 years and older, for myoclonic seizures in juvenile myoclonic epilepsy in adolescents 12 years and older, and for generalized tonic–clonic seizures in primary generalized epilepsy in children and adolescents 6 years and older.

Levetiracetam has no drug interactions; it is not toxic to the bone marrow or to the liver. It is excreted via the kidneys. Its major side effect is irritability and agitation. This is most prominent in those children who are already behaviorally disinhibited. Levetiracetam comes in a liquid preparation (500 mg/5 mL) or in tablets of 250 mg, 500 mg, 750 mg, or 1000 mg.

Zonisamide

Zonisamide is related to topiramate, with respect to its mechanisms of action. It is approved as adjunctive therapy in partial seizures in children and adolescents at least 16 years of age. In Japan, it is commonly used for myoclonic seizures associated with mitochondrial disorders. Preliminary studies indicate possible efficacy with infantile spasms,[1] myoclonic seizures,[1] and absence seizures.[1]

Its major side effects include lethargy, irritability, cognitive slowing, renal stones, and oligohidrosis. Therefore, it should be used with caution in patients who are on the ketogenic diet or who have kidney dysfunction. Patients should be kept well hydrated. Zonisamide comes in 25-mg, 50-mg, and 100-mg capsules.

ALTERNATIVES TO ANTIEPILEPTIC DRUGS

The ketogenic diet as a treatment for epilepsy has been known since biblical times. It was rediscovered in the modern era by Dr. Haddow Keith from the Mayo Clinic, who observed in a 1921 newsletter that children with status epilepticus usually experienced cessation of seizure activity once they were in ketosis. The ketogenic diet again fell out of favor with the advent of phenobarbital and phenytoin as AEDs. It has recently been repopularized by the Johns Hopkins Medical Center.

In appropriately chosen cases, the ketogenic diet can eliminate seizures in one third of patients and can decrease seizure frequency by more than 50% in another third, but it lacks efficacy in the final third. Patients with LGS have the best chance of responding to this diet. The diet requires that every piece of food and medicine be analyzed with respect to fat, carbohydrate, and protein content. All food and drink must be weighed and measured with respect to calories and type of food. The diet can be very difficult for children who already have dietary preferences.

---

[3]Exceeds dosage recommended by the manufacturer.

[1]Not FDA approved for this indication.

The vagal nerve stimulator (VNS) has been approved by the FDA for use as adjunctive therapy in treating medically refractory, localization-related epilepsy in adults and children older than 12 years. The vagal nerve stimulator is a pacemaker, implanted in the chest pocket below the clavicle, that delivers pulses from a bipolar electrode connected to the vagus nerve. The exact mechanism of action remains an enigma. The VNS influence over the EEG is probably mediated by the solitary tract nucleus–parabrachial nucleus ceruleus–thalamic pathways with concomitant cortical projections. High stimulation of the vagus nerve appears to result in EEG desynchronization, with the full effects gradually being seen over 6 months to 1 year.

Side effects include bleeding, infection, voice alteration or hoarseness when the VNS cycles on, cough, throat pain, dyspepsia, and nausea. There are no reports of cardiac arrhythmias with this device.

Preliminary research on the VNS in patients with symptomatic generalized epilepsies such as LGS indicates significant efficacy, especially over time.

IMMUNOTHERAPY

Immunotherapy has been used in treating a variety of rare and unusual epileptic syndromes, such as Rasmussen's syndrome and Landau–Kleffner syndrome. Rasmussen's syndrome is characterized by progressive hemiparesis, associated cognitive decline, and epilepsia partialis continua. Studies have suggested that autoimmune mechanisms play a role in the pathogenesis of Rasmussen's syndrome. The syndrome affects only one hemisphere. Immunotherapy appears to result in a transient improvement in seizure control.

Steroids are also used in treating infantile spasms and Landau–Kleffner syndrome, as described earlier.

EPILEPSY SURGERY

The five most important questions that must be asked before the consideration of a presurgical evaluation are as follows: is this an epileptic syndrome that is most likely going to continue without resolution? Are the epileptic seizures having a significant impact on the child's development or quality of life? Have the seizures been intractable to a variety of AEDs? Is the epileptogenic zone identifiable? Can the epileptogenic zone be resected without unacceptable neurologic deficits?

Certain children are possible candidates for epilepsy surgery. It can be effective for children with nonlesional localization-related epilepsy in whom standard AED therapy—two to three AEDs—has failed and in children with lesional localization-related epilepsy—the presence of a tumor or other structural lesion, whether or not controlled with AEDs. Children with catastrophic epilepsies in whom the continuation of the epileptic encephalopathy and clinical seizures would result in substantial morbidity in terms of development and quality of life can benefit from surgery. Examples include patients with infantile spasms; Sturge–Weber syndrome with progressive hemiparesis and intractable seizures; Rasmussen's syndrome with progressive encephalopathy, seizures, and hemiparesis; and malformations of cortical development (e.g., hemimegalencephaly). Surgery can be effective for children with medically refractory generalized or multifocal epilepsies in whom the clinical presentation, seizure semiology, EEG findings, MRI of the brain, or other ancillary tests suggest an underlying focal generator for the epileptic condition. Children with intractable generalized epilepsy who have tonic or atonic seizures may be candidates for corpus callosotomy.

The presurgical evaluation must consist of a multidisciplinary approach. The concept of convergence is very important. The identification of the epileptogenic zone requires the confluence of data accumulated by the medical history, seizure semiology, physical examination, EEG interictal and ictal MRI of the brain, and the newer neuroimaging techniques. One technique is MRI of the brain with thin contiguous cuts and FLAIR sequencing (fluid-attenuated inversion recovery technique, i.e., T2-weighted imaging with the cerebrospinal fluid signal subtracted out). Ictal SPECT scan determines cerebral blood flow using radiotracers. These compounds rapidly cross the blood–brain barrier and record the cerebral blood flow at the time of injection. Observations made a century ago document that there is increased cerebral blood flow at the site of the epileptogenic focus during an ictal event. The SPECT scan can, therefore, provide one with a snapshot of the epileptogenic zone. It becomes increasingly accurate if the ictal SPECT scan is subtracted from the interictal SPECT scan and coregistered with the MRI study, a technique termed SISCOM. Interictal positron-emission tomography (PET) scan is another noninvasive functional imaging technique used to identify cerebral metabolic rates using a radioisotope designed to measure glucose metabolism. Interictally, the epileptogenic zone is hypometabolic. Other experimental technologies include MRI (looking at dynamic metabolism of the brain), magnetoencephalography (looking at the flux of magnetic fields in the brain), and functional MRI mapping.

The type of epilepsy surgery performed depends on the localization of the epiletogenic zone. Some of the more common surgical procedures include temporal lobectomy with amgydalohippocampectomy, focal cortical resection, hemispherectomy, implantation of a VNS, corpus callosotomy, and multiple subpial transaction (a technique employed over eloquent cortex that one chooses not to resect because of the potential loss of functional tissue).

Epilepsy surgery can be very effective in eliminating seizures in carefully chosen patients. For example, if a patient has mesial temporal sclerosis and seizures emanating from the temporal lobe, the chance of surgery's producing a seizure-free outcome is as high as 85% to 90%.

REFERENCES

Baumann RJ, Duffner PK. Treatment of children with simple febrile seizures: The AAP practice parameter. Pediat Neurol 2000;23(1):11–7.

Donat JF. The age-dependent epileptic encephalopathies. J Child Neurol 1992;7:7–21.

Dreifuss FE, Rosman NP, Cloyd JC, et al. A comparision of rectal diazepam gel and placebo for acute repetitive seizures. N Engl J Med 1998;26:1869–75.

Freeman JM, Vining EP, Pillas DJ, et al. The efficacy of the ketogenic diet-1998: A prospective evaluation of intervention in 150 children. Pediatrics 1998;102(6):1358–63.

Genton P, Dravet C. Lennox–Gastaut syndrome and other childhood epileptic encephalopathies. In: Engel J Jr, Pedley TA, editors. Epilepsy: A Comprehensive Textbook, vol. 3. Philadelphia: Lippincott-Raven; 1997. p. 2355–66.

Glauser TA, Pellock JM, Bebin EM, et al. Efficacy and safety of levetiracetam in children with partial seizures: An open-label trial. Epilepsia 2002;43(5):518–24.

Hirtz D, Berg A, Bettis D, et al. Practice parameter: Treatment of the child with a first unprovoked seizure. Neurology 2003;60:166–75.

Levisohn PM. Safety and tolerability of topiramate in children. J Child Neurol 2000;15(Suppl. 1):S22–6.

Loiseau P. Benign focal epilepsies of childhood. In: Wyllie E, editor. The Treatment of Epilepsy: Principles and Practice. Philadelphia: Lea and Febiger; 1993. p. 503–12.

Mackay MT, Weiss SK, Adams-Webber T, et al., for the American Academy of Neurology and Child Neurology Society. Practice parameter: medical treatment of infantile spasms. Report of the American Academy of Neurology and the Child Neurology Society. Neurology 2004;62(10):1668–81.

Messenheimer J, Ramsay RE, Willmore LJ, et al. Lamotrigine therapy for partial seizures: A multicenter, placebo-controlled, double-blind, cross-over trial. Epilepsia 1994;35:113–21.

Morrell MJ. Reproductive and metabolic disorders in women with epilepsy. Epilepsia 2003;44(Suppl. 4):11–20.

Murphy JV. Pediatric VNS Study Group. Left vagal nerve stimulation in children with medically refractory epilepsy. J Pediatr 1999;134:563–6.

Nordli DR, Bazil CW, Sheuer ML, Pedley TA. Recognition and classification of seizures in infants. Epilepsia 1997;38:553–60.

Shinnar S, Pellock JM, Berg AT, et al. Short term outcomes of children with febrile status epilepticus. Epilepsia 2001;42(1):47–53.

Tharp BR. Neonatal seizures and syndromes. Epilepsia 2002;43(Suppl 3):2–10.

Trevathan E. Seizures and epilepsy among children with language regression and autistic spectrum disorders. J Child Neurol 2004;19(Suppl 1):S49–57.

Zupanc ML. Infantile spasms. Expert Opin Pharmacother 2003;4(11):2039–48.

Zupanc ML. Early Onset Epilepsy. Pediatric Neurology Continuum: Lifelong Learning in Neurology. Philadelphia, Pennsylvania: American Academy of Neurology, Lippincott Williams and Wilkins; 1999.

Zupanc ML. Neuroimaging in the evaluation of children and adolescents with intractable epilepsy. I: MRI and substrates of epilepsy. Pediatr Neurol 1997;17:19–26.

Attention-Deficit/ Hyperactivity Disorder

Method of
Harris Strokoff, MD, and Craig L. Donnelly, MD

Attention-deficit/hyperactivity disorder (ADHD) is among the most commonly diagnosed illnesses in pediatric medicine. Approximately 4% to 8% of children are diagnosed with ADHD. ADHD is most commonly diagnosed in children between the ages of 6 and 12 years, but it is also diagnosed and treated in children as young as age 3. Although previously thought to largely abate in adolescence and adulthood, ADHD is now considered to be a chronic condition. More than 60% of children with ADHD have impairing symptoms well into adolescence and adulthood. ADHD can cause social problems, academic and learning problems, emotional problems, delinquency, and increased risk-taking behavior, including substance abuse.

ADHD is highly heritable. Approximately 10% to 35% of immediate family members of children with ADHD have ADHD themselves, and approximately 30% of siblings of children with ADHD also have the disorder. Parents of children with ADHD are at high risk for ADHD themselves, and appropriate assessment and potential treatment of ADHD in the parents can improve the child's environment. ADHD is thought to reflect decreased dopamine and norepinephrine transmission in the brain. Maternal smoking and alcohol use, low birth weight, and lead exposure are associated with increased rates of ADHD. Social factors are not thought to play a major role in the development of ADHD.

Diagnosis

Children with ADHD tend to have profound difficulties in maintaining or sustaining attention, and/or they are hyperactive or impulsive. The core inattentive and hyperactive/impulsive symptoms of ADHD are defined by the *Diagnostic and Statistical Manual of Mental Disorders*, fourth edition (DSM-IV). ADHD is classified according to three subtypes: predominantly inattentive type, predominantly hyperactive/impulsive type, and combined type, which is the most common subtype.

The predominantly inattentive type of ADHD is characterized by at least six of the inattention core symptoms but fewer than six of the hyperactive/impulsive symptoms (see Current Diagnosis box). The predominantly hyperactive/impulsive type of ADHD involves six of

CURRENT DIAGNOSIS

- Patients with ADHD have several impairing inattentive symptoms or hyperactive/impulsive symptoms, or both.
- The DSM-IV inattentive core symptoms of ADHD include difficulty sustaining attention, making careless mistakes, increased distractibility, forgetfulness, not seeming to listen when spoken to, not following through on instructions, difficulties with organization, reluctance to engage in schoolwork, and a tendency to lose things.
- The DSM-IV hyperactive/impulsive core symptoms of ADHD include being fidgety; running or climbing excessively; having difficulty awaiting a turn, staying seated, or being quiet; acting as if "driven by a motor"; talking excessively, blurting out answers, and interrupting others.

CURRENT THERAPY

- Stimulant medications (e.g., methylphenidate [Ritalin, Methylin, Concerta] and amphetamine preparations) and atomoxetine (Strattera) are the primary treatments for ADHD in children and adults.
- Medication should be implemented collaboratively, with the child's parents and teachers providing feedback about treatment efficacy and tolerability.
- Psychosocial therapies can add benefit to pharmacotherapy and may be necessary for patients who cannot use pharmacotherapy due to intolerability or preference.

nine hyperactive/impulsive symptoms but fewer than six of the inattention symptoms. If a patient has at least six of the inattention and six of the hyperactive/impulsive symptoms, the diagnosis is combined-type ADHD. These symptoms must also cause significant impairment in the child's life in more than one domain (e.g., in school and home settings) to meet the criteria for ADHD. Symptoms of ADHD must have been present before the age of 7 years to meet the full criteria, although lack of this specifier alone should not preclude treatment.

ADHD is diagnosed by clinical interviews of the child and parents and from information from outside sources, especially from the child's school or daycare. Standardized assessment tools and rating scales, such as the Medium SNAP IV (developed by Swanson, Nolan, and Pelham), the Behavior Assessment System for Children (BASC), the Achenbach Child Behavior Checklist (CBCL), the Achenbach Teacher Report Form (TRF), the Achenbach Youth Self-Report (YSR), and the Connor's rating scale are useful for the diagnosis of ADHD, for monitoring of symptoms over time, and as broader indicators of psychopathology in children and adolescents with ADHD. It is important to rule out underlying conditions (e.g., absence seizures, sleep apnea, learning disorder, anxiety) when making a diagnosis of ADHD.

Comorbidity is the rule in childhood ADHD. It is estimated that only 30% of children with ADHD have the disorder alone. Up to 60% of children with ADHD may have learning disorders, 30% to 40% of children with ADHD also have oppositional defiant disorder or conduct disorder, approximately 30% of children with ADHD have a comorbid anxiety disorder, and approximately 25% of these children have a comorbid major depressive disorder. ADHD is typically diagnosed three or four times more often in boys than in girls, and girls tend to have more predominant inattentive symptoms that may not be noticed as easily in classroom or home settings.

In adults with ADHD, hyperactivity commonly found in children tends to change into a sense of internal restlessness, and impaired attention and distractibility tend to evolve into difficulties with organization and planning. An estimated 4.4% of adults in the United States meet the diagnostic criteria for ADHD. Adults with ADHD tend to be underdiagnosed and have a higher incidence of criminal behavior, injuries, accidents, and employment and marital difficulties compared with adults without ADHD. Untreated symptoms of inattention or hyperactivity often cause or exacerbate anxious and depressive disorders, which may manifest in adulthood in complex comorbid patterns along with ADHD.

Treatment

The gold standard for treatment of ADHD is pharmacotherapy. Treatment with a stimulant medication or atomoxetine (Strattera) is most effective for ADHD, regardless of ADHD subtype. Psychosocial interventions can be a useful adjunct in many children with ADHD, especially those for whom poor tolerability or comorbid diagnoses could be better addressed with psychotherapy.

STIMULANTS

For approximately 75% of children with ADHD, treatment with stimulants decreases their symptoms. As a class, stimulants are fast acting (i.e., improvements are usually evident in the first few days of treatment) and usually well tolerated. Several types of stimulant medications are available. No stimulant has consistently proved to be more effective than another. Choice of a first stimulant medication for the treatment of ADHD is typically based on the desired duration of effect, frequency of dosing, percentage of short-acting medication versus long-acting medication, and the desired delivery system.

The two major classes of stimulant medications are methylphenidate (e.g., Ritalin, Methylin, Concerta) and amphetamine-type preparations. Figure 1 summarizes the medications FDA approved for the treatment of ADHD. Because the data equally support short-acting (immediate-release) and longer-acting stimulant preparations, most clinicians begin with longer-acting preparations, which are thought to offer a smoother level of medication effect and need to be dosed only once daily, which tends to improve compliance. Reasons to consider a shorter-acting medication include wanting to give a test dose before beginning a longer-acting stimulant, wanting to use a very low dose (e.g., in very young children or children with a pervasive developmental disorder), or attempting to minimize potential side effects, such as insomnia and anorexia. Stimulants given twice daily are typically given once in the morning and once at lunchtime. Stimulant medications are available in tablet, capsule, liquid, chewable, and transdermal patch forms.

Like all medications, stimulants have side effects. Stimulants commonly cause appetite suppression, which can lead to weight loss. Stimulants also can decrease linear growth rates, and children with ADHD who are managed with stimulant medication over time may have decreases in projected maximum height of approximately 0.4 to 1 inch. However, after stimulant pharmacotherapy is discontinued, children's linear growth velocity usually accelerates. In the past, drug holidays (e.g., having a child with ADHD off medication for the summer) were common, but it is currently thought that these holidays interrupt optimal treatment and that untreated symptoms during drug holidays can be difficult for the child psychologically and socially. If weight loss and decreased linear growth velocity remain concerns despite attempts at optimizing the psychopharmacologic regimen, drug holidays could be considered.

Stimulants can cause or exacerbate vocal and motor tics. Stimulants may also cause insomnia. α-Blocking agents such as clonidine (Catapres)[1] or guanfacine (Tenex)[1] are sometimes used in addition to stimulant medication to treat the side effects of insomnia or tics. Insomnia can sometimes be managed by decreasing the dose of the stimulant, changing the timing of the dose, or changing to a different stimulant preparation. Melatonin[1,7] is commonly used as an adjunct therapy for the treatment of stimulant-induced insomnia.

Headaches and stomachaches are side effects of stimulants, although they are usually transient in nature. In some patients, stimulants can cause or worsen anxiety in patients with comorbid anxiety disorders, and in these cases, switching to a more anxiety-neutral ADHD treatment (e.g., atomoxetine) or the addition of a selective serotonin reuptake inhibitor (SSRI) should be considered. Rarely, stimulants can cause mood changes and psychotic reactions.

Stimulant treatment in preschool-age children (3–5.5 years old) with ADHD is effective, but it is not as effective as using stimulants to treat school-age children with ADHD. Side effects commonly include emotional lability and aggression in this population, and stimulants should be dosed lower and monitored carefully.

Stimulants have the potential to exacerbate preexisting cardiac conditions, and children should be screened for cardiac disease and a history of premature cardiac death in the family. Patients on stimulant medication should have their heart rate and blood pressure monitored, although the average predictable increases in heart rate (1–2 beats/min) and blood pressure (3–4 mm Hg) are thought to be clinically insignificant. In April 2008, the American Heart Association (AHA) released a statement recommending that children receiving stimulant treatment for ADHD receive screening electrocardiograms (ECGs), and in May 2008, the AHA released a clarification stating that screening ECGs for patients with ADHD are reasonable to consider but not mandatory. In summary, children on stimulants should have their height, weight, blood pressure, and heart rate monitored while receiving therapy.

Stimulants are potential drugs of abuse and are class II schedule medications. Stimulant abuse can cause euphoria, enhance academic and athletic performance, cause weight loss, and induce desired insomnia. ADHD alone is associated with increased rates and severity of substance abuse, and most studies show no change in substance abuse rates in adolescents with ADHD treated with stimulants compared with those left untreated. Longer-acting and alternative formulations (e.g., patch, prodrug, osmotic pump mechanism) stimulants are more difficult to abuse (e.g., intranasally, intravenously) than are immediate-release agents.

NONSTIMULANTS

Atomoxetine is an FDA-approved medication used to treat children, adolescents, and adults with ADHD. Although the degree of effect tends to be somewhat lower than those found with stimulant treatments of ADHD, it is typically effective and well tolerated. Atomoxetine works less quickly than stimulants (peak effectiveness usually apparent around weeks 4 to 6), but it may provide longer duration (i.e., 24-hour) coverage. Atomoxetine is less likely to exacerbate anxiety or cause tics compared with stimulant medications. Atomoxetine has no abuse liability and is not a controlled substance.

Side effects include increased heart rate and blood pressure, and it should be used with caution in children with structural or conductive cardiac abnormalities. Atomoxetine carries an FDA black box warning recommending monitoring for the potential emergence of suicidality in patients taking this medication. Atomoxetine can markedly elevate hepatic enzymes and bilirubin, although hepatic failure is thought to be a rare event. Patients who exhibit symptoms such as jaundice or other indices of liver disease should stop taking this medication and receive medical work-up. Other potential side effects of atomoxetine include agitation, gastrointestinal upset, and headaches, although overall, this medication is thought to be well tolerated.

α-Adrenergic agonists such as clonidine[1] and guanfacine[1] are antihypertensive medications that have been used off-label for many years for the treatment of ADHD, lacking FDA approval for this purpose. Although these medications can improve functioning in patients with ADHD, clinical response is usually less robust than with stimulants. Clonidine and guanfacine are potentially useful in the treatment of hyperactive/impulsive symptoms and are most commonly used adjunctively with stimulants in children with ADHD to treat stimulant-induced tics and insomnia. Clonidine requires three to four doses throughout the day, and guanfacine is typically dosed twice daily. These medications should be used with caution because they carry risks of sedation, orthostasis, potential cardiac side effects, and rare reports of sudden cardiac death with overdose. They should be started at low doses and then titrated slowly. These medications should not be discontinued without a gradual taper over the course of 1 to 2 weeks because of the potential of rebound hypertension and irritability.

Certain antidepressant medications are used to treat children and adults with ADHD, although they do not carry FDA approval for this purpose. Some studies have shown that the antidepressant bupropion (Wellbutrin)[1] improves symptoms of ADHD in children and adults, and it is efficacious in treating depression and ADHD in children and adults who suffer from these comorbid conditions. Potential side effects of bupropion include increases in pulse and blood pressure and potential lowering of a person's seizure threshold. Bupropion, like all antidepressants, carries an FDA black box warning about the potential of these medications to increase suicidality in youths and young adults.

Although rarely used for this purpose and not FDA approved, the tricyclic antidepressants desipramine (Norpramin),[1] imipramine (Tofranil),[1] and nortriptyline (Pamelor)[1] are thought to have some efficacy in the treatment of ADHD. These medications are used less commonly because of significant side effects such as ECG changes (prolonged QTc), sedation, and risk of sudden cardiac death with overdose.

Attention-Deficit/Hyperactivity Disorder

---

[1]Not FDA approved for this indication.
[7]Available as dietary supplement.

---

[1]Not FDA approved for this indication.

Drug	Dosing	Typical starting dose	Comments
Methylphenidate preparations			
Methylphenidate (generic name)			
(Brand name formulations)			
Ritalin	bid to tid	5 mg bid	
Methylin	bid to tid	5 mg bid	available in both liquid and chewable tablet forms
Methylin ER	once daily	10 mg qam	capsule can be opened and contents can be sprinkled into food, longer-acting formulation
Metadate ER	once daily	10 mg qam	capsule can be opened and contents can be sprinkled into food, longer-acting formulation
Metadate CD	once daily	20 mg qam	
Ritalin SR	once daily	10 mg qam	
Ritalin LA	once daily	20 mg qam	capsule can be opened and contents can be sprinkled into food, longer-acting formulation
Concerta	once daily	18 mg qam	uses osmotic pump mechanism, longer-acting formulation
Daytrana patch	apply once daily, then remove at end of the day	10 mg patch	
D-methylphenidate (generic name)			
(Brand name formulations)			
Focalin	bid to tid	2.5 mg bid	
Focalin XR	once daily	5 mg qam	capsule can be opened and contents can be sprinkled into food, longer-acting formulation
Amphetamine preparations			
Mixed amphetamine salts [D-amphetamine and amphetamine] (generic name)			
(Brand name formulations)			
Adderall	qd to bid	3–5 y: 2.5 mg qam ≥6 y: 5 mg qd to bid	
Adderall XR	once daily	≥6 y: 10 mg qam	capsule can be opened and contents can be sprinkled into food, longer-acting formulation
D-amphetamine (generic name)			
(Brand name formulations)			
Dexedrine	qd to bid	3–5 y: 2.5 mg qam ≥6 y: 5 mg qd to bid	capsule can be opened and contents can be sprinkled into food
Dextrostat	qd to bid	3–5 y: 2.5 mg qam ≥6 y: 5 mg qd to bid	capsule can be opened and contents can be sprinkled into food
Dexedrine Spansule	qd to bid	≥6 y: 5–10 mg qd to bid	capsule can be opened and contents can be sprinkled into food, longer-acting formulation
Lisdexamphetamine (generic name)			
(Brand name formulations)			
Vyvanse	once daily	30 mg qam	is a pro-drug, thus must be enzymatically cleaved in the gastrointestinal tract in order to yield active D-amphetamine. Not thought to be abusable intranasally
Non-stimulant medication			
Atomoxetine (generic name)			
(Brand name formulations)			
Strattera	once daily (also can be given divided bid)	patients <70 kg: 0.5 mg/kg/day for 4 days; then 1 mg/kg/day for 4 days; then 1.2 mg/kg/day	less likely to exacerbate anxiety in some children, not thought to be abusable

FIGURE 1. Medications commonly used to treat ADHD. *Abbreviations:* bid = twice daily; ER = extended release; LA = long acting; qam = every morning; qd = once daily; SR = sustained release; tid = three times daily; XR = extended release.

Modafinil (Provigil)[1] is FDA approved for the treatment of narcolepsy, shift-work sleep disorder, and obstructive sleep apnea/hypopnea syndrome, and it is thought to improve vigilance and decrease distractibility. It is sometimes used to treat ADHD. Modafinil is not thought to be as easily abused as the stimulant medications.

Stimulant pharmacotherapy should be the initial treatment for most cases of ADHD. Formal dosing guidelines of stimulants should be followed. Titration of the dose until sufficient improvement is gained or limiting side effects emerge is the best way to optimize stimulant treatment outcome. There is sufficient evidence to suggest switching to another stimulant if treatment with the initial agent is suboptimal (e.g., switching from an amphetamine preparation to a methylphenidate preparation), and if the second stimulant trial fails, consideration should be given to a third stimulant trial. If there is a partial response to a stimulant trial, consider augmentation with atomoxetine or the addition of an α-blocking agent if insomnia or tics are mitigating side effects.

Although ADHD tends to be a chronic condition, not all children with ADHD progress to become adults with ADHD. Children who are being treated for ADHD should be reassessed yearly to determine if treatment for ADHD is still indicated. In the treatment of adults with ADHD, the same treatment strategies apply, although adults may require higher doses of medication. Stimulants and atomoxetine are the primary treatments for adults with ADHD. Because of higher rates of substance abuse comorbidities in adults, the risks of potential stimulant abuse and diversion may be higher in this population.

PSYCHOSOCIAL TREATMENTS

Psychosocial therapies can be a useful and sometimes necessary adjunct to pharmacotherapy for the treatment of ADHD. Behavior therapy can be effective in helping to manage symptoms of ADHD, and parents and teachers are essential for implementing behavioral strategies and for continually assessing ADHD symptoms and treatment side effects. Parent training groups are effective at maximizing children's compliant behaviors, and several books (e.g., Barkley's *Your Defiant Child*, Forehand and Long's *Parenting the Strong-Willed Child*) are available for training parents and clinicians to teach and reinforce behavioral therapy.

Classroom management techniques are an important part of any psychosocial approach to the treatment of ADHD in children and adolescents. Teachers of students with ADHD have found it helpful to increase the structure in classrooms, use consistent rewards and punishments, and use daily report cards to communicate school performance to parents at home.

Psychosocial interventions alone are not highly effective for the treatment of children with ADHD. For children with uncomplicated ADHD, psychosocial interventions may not significantly add benefit to pharmacotherapy alone. Because of the high rates of comorbidity in children and adolescents with ADHD, additional psychotherapies (and sometimes pharmacotherapies) may be necessary to treat these more complex presentations.

REFERENCES

Adler LA. From childhood into adulthood: The changing face of ADHD. CNS Spectr 2007;12(Suppl. 23):12.

American Academy of Pediatrics/American Heart Association. Clarification of statement on cardiovascular evaluation and monitoring of children and adolescents with heart disease receiving medications for ADHD. Available at http://americanheart.mediaroom.com/index.php?s=43&item=422 [accessed July 2009].

American Psychiatric Association Task Force on DSM-IV. Diagnostic and Statistical Manual of Mental Disorders: DSM-IV-TR. Washington, DC: American Psychiatric Association; 2000.

Barkley R. Attention-Deficit Hyperactivity Disorder: A Handbook for Diagnosis and Treatment. 3rd ed. New York: Guilford Press; 2006.

Clinical Pharmacology Online Version 8.06. Drug and toxicology information. Available at http://www.clinicalpharmacology.com [accessed July 2009].

Gilchrist RH, Arnold EL. Long-term efficacy of ADHD pharmacotherapy in children. Pediatr Ann 2008;37:46.

---

[1]Not FDA approved for this indication.

Greenhill L, Kollins S, Abikoff H, et al. Efficacy and safety of immediate-release methylphenidate treatment for preschoolers with ADHD. J Am Acad Child Adolesc Psychiatry 2006;45:11.

Jensen PS, Arnold LE, Swanson JM, et al. 3-Year follow-up of the NIMH MTA study. J Am Acad Child Adolesc Psychiatry 2007;46:8.

Kessler RC, Adler L, Barkley R, et al. The prevalence and correlates of adult ADHD in the United States: Results from the National Comorbidity Survey Replication. Evid Based Ment Health 2006;9:116.

Newcorn JH. Nonstimulants and emerging treatments in adults with ADHD. CNS Spectr 2008;13(Suppl. 13):9.

Palumbo DR, Sallee FR, Pelham WE. Clonidine for attention-deficit/hyperactivity disorder. I. Efficacy and tolerability outcomes. J Am Acad Child Adolesc Psychiatry 2008;47:2.

Pliszka S. AACAP Work Group on Quality Issues: Practice parameter for the assessment and treatment of children and adolescents with attention-deficit/hyperactivity disorder. J Am Acad Child Adolesc Psychiatry 2007;46:7.

Towbin K. Paying attention to stimulants: Height, weight, and cardiovascular monitoring in clinical practice. J Am Acad Child Adolesc Psychiatry 2008;47:9.

Gilles de la Tourette Syndrome

Method of
Steve W. Wu, MD, and Donald L. Gilbert, MD, MS

Gilles de la Tourette syndrome, or Tourette syndrome, was named after French neurologist Georges Gilles de la Tourette, who in 1885 described a series of nine patients with chronic tics. Tourette syndrome is a neuropsychiatric illness that begins in childhood. It is characterized by multiple motor and vocal tics that last for longer than 1 year (see Current Diagnosis box). The prevalence of Tourette syndrome varies greatly among epidemiologic studies, ranging from 0.1% to 3.8%. The prevalence of tic disorders is even higher, especially in children requiring special education.

Simple motor tics are sudden, brief, patterned movements such as eye blinking, facial grimace, head jerk, or shoulder shrug. Complex motor tics can involve a series of simple tics or a seemingly purposeful action, such as jumping, touching, or copropraxia (i.e., performing obscene gestures). Simple vocal tics consist of sounds such as throat clearing, sniffing, and coughing. Patients with complex vocal tics may exhibit echolalia (i.e., repeating others' words), palilalia (i.e., repeating their own words), or coprolalia (i.e., utterance of foul language).

Older children and adolescents often describe a premonitory urge before their tics. Tics can usually be transiently suppressed and are often diminished during focused mental or physical activities. Unlike myoclonus or chorea, tics usually do not affect activities of daily living or occupational or recreational activities. After the brief suppression, the release of the tic often brings relief to the patient. Tic severity commonly worsens during times of emotional stress. Fatigue or illness may also increase tics. Parents often notice more tics when the child is bored or unoccupied with an activity. Tics can occur during light sleep and rapid eye movement (REM) sleep.

Clinical Course

The onset of tics can occur after children are 3 years old, but they usually begin in children 6 to 7 years old. Children often present with motor tics first, followed by the development of vocal tics. Tics often wax and wane in the course of Tourette syndrome. During the early school years, tics often can go unnoticed or be mislabeled as a habit. If tics are noticed by fellow students, bullying is typically not an issue at this age. However, when parents notice the tics, they are often distressed and frequently tell their children to stop the movements.

Tic severity usually increases in the later elementary school years and into adolescence. This is the time when social interference such as bullying begins to occur. By late adolescence and early adulthood, most patients with Tourette syndrome have minimal tics, and some may "outgrow" tics. Because of this pattern, most individuals presenting for medical attention for tics are children.

Patients with Tourette syndrome frequently present with comorbid attention-deficit/hyperactivity disorder (ADHD) and obsessive-compulsive disorder (OCD). They also tend to have more sleep problems, anxiety, and mood disorders.

Diagnosis and Differential Diagnosis

Diagnosis of tic disorders depends on correctly recognizing that the abnormal movements are tics by means of a careful history and thorough physical examination. Laboratory and imaging studies are rarely needed.

Tics may resemble other abnormal movements, such as stereotypy, chorea, ballism, dystonia, and myoclonus. *Stereotypies* are repetitive, simple movements that are suppressible and that usually occur when a child is excited. Stereotypies usually start when the child is younger than 3 years. *Chorea* consists of a sequence of random, continual, involuntary, nonpurposeful, nonrhythmic movements. Choreic movements often flow from one body part to another. *Ballism* is a large-amplitude choreic movement affecting the proximal limb. *Myoclonus* is an involuntary, sudden, shocklike movement. Chorea, ballism, and myoclonus cannot be volitionally suppressed. *Dystonia* is produced by co-contraction of agonist and antagonist muscles, leading to abnormal postures, and its twisting movements typically are slower than tics.

Vocal tics may sometimes lead to the misdiagnosis of asthma, chronic cough, or allergic rhinitis. Other primary tic disorders include transient tic disorder, chronic motor or vocal tic disorders, and tic disorder not otherwise specified. Persons with autistic spectrum disorders often have tics.

Tics are nonspecific and may occur in drug-induced movement disorders, after head trauma, and in a variety of neurodevelopmental and neurodegenerative disorders. Complex or atypical cases with multiple comorbidities or multiple abnormalities identified on a general or neurologic examination should be referred for specialist consultation.

A controversial diagnosis in which tics or OCD may occur is called pediatric autoimmune neuropsychiatric disorders associated with streptococcal infections (PANDAS). Criteria for this diagnosis classically include abrupt appearance in prepubertal children of tics or OCD on two or more occasions after documented group A β-hemolytic streptococcal (GABHS) infections. The paradigm for this diagnosis is rheumatic (Sydenham's) chorea; however, PANDAS has no arthritis, carditis, or nephritis and is not thought to be a rheumatic disease. Epidemiologic studies of PANDAS show mixed findings, with stress and other types of infections appearing to trigger exacerbations. The following interventions are not routinely recommended: diagnostic throat cultures and antistreptococcal antibody tests; therapeutic or preventive antibiotics; and immune-modulating therapies such as steroids, intravenous immunoglobulins, or plasmapheresis. Specialty consultation should be considered.

Treatment

There are many factors to consider when treating a patient with Tourette syndrome, including the presence of common symptoms such as inattentiveness, hyperactivity, obsessive or compulsive behaviors, depression, and anxiety (Box 1). When deciding to treat the patient, it is important to prioritize all the neuropsychiatric

---

CURRENT DIAGNOSIS

- Multiple motor and one or more vocal tics have been present for some time during the illness, although not necessarily concurrently.
- The tics occur many times per day (usually in bouts) almost every day or intermittently throughout a period of more than 1 year. During this time, there is not a tic-free period of more than 3 consecutive months.
- The disturbance causes marked distress or significant impairment in social, occupational, or other important areas of functioning.
- Onset occurs before age 18 years.
- The disturbance is not caused by the direct physiologic effects of a substance or a general medical condition.

BOX 1   Therapeutic Approach for Tourette Syndrome

- Educate the patient and family about tics and how tics often diminish spontaneously. Long-term reductions in tics may occur in the late teens, irrespective of pharmacologic therapy.
- Rank the tics, attention-deficit hyperactivity disorder (ADHD), obsessive-compulsive disorder (OCD), anxiety, mood problems, learning problems, and behavior problems in order of the patient's or the family's perception of severity.
- Consider nonpharmacologic and pharmacologic treatment for each symptom in the order of perceived severity or impairment.
- Provide information to educate teachers and classmates to reduce social impairment.
- If the patient has learning problems, encourage formal assessment through the school or a psychologist. These children may qualify for modified educational methods.
- If ADHD is the most concerning problem, consider treating with clonidine (Catapres),[1] guanfacine (Tenex),[1] atomoxetine (Strattera), or methylphenidate (Ritalin). Stimulants are *not* absolutely contraindicated in patients with Tourette syndrome. However, if symptoms of OCD, anxiety, or pervasive developmental disorder are present, ticcing or compulsions may escalate on stimulants. If a patient has done well for months to years on stimulants for ADHD before an exacerbation of tics, it usually is not necessary to discontinue stimulants.
- If behavior problems are the most concerning problem or if a first-degree family member has a bipolar or psychotic disorder, refer the patient to a psychologist or psychiatrist.
- Anxious parents often worsen tic severity. If the family's anxiety is excessive, refer family members to a psychologist.
- If OCD or generalized anxiety disorder is the most severe problem, treatment with a selective serotonin reuptake inhibitor may be considered.
- Do not begin treatment with more than one central nervous system drug simultaneously. Start one, wait 2 to 4 weeks, and then reassess all symptoms before starting the next medication.
- Monitor the benefits and side effects at regular intervals.
- Maintain stable dosing during the school year; consider tapering medications in the summer.
- Consider weaning tic-suppressing medications in the middle to late teen years if tics wane.

---

[1]Not FDA approved for this indication.

symptoms and provide accurate educational information. Tics may not always need to be treated medically, and if treatment is needed, tics may not be the first symptom to manage. Daily tic-suppressing medication is considered when there is functional interference, social interference, pain, or classroom or occupational disruption.

The first step in treating Tourette syndrome is educating the patient, parents, and other adult caregivers. Parents, teachers, and other adult caregivers are discouraged from telling the child to stop ticcing because this produces emotional anxiety that may worsen the tics. Educational materials for teachers often promote a conducive environment for the child at school. The patient is encouraged to openly talk about his or her disorder to classmates to promote understanding and minimize bullying. Newer cognitive-behavioral treatments for tic suppression appear to be helpful for children and adolescents, and they should be considered.

Clinical trials enrolling patients with Tourette syndrome are usually small and show small effect sizes. Most commonly used tic-suppressing medications belong to two classes: α_2-adrenergic agonists and dopamine receptor blocking agents (Table 1). Other agents may show modest benefit. Because Tourette syndrome is a chronic, nonfatal disorder, it is prudent to start treatment with medications that carry the least side effects. For this reason, α_2-adrenergic agonists are usually the first-line treatment. Although it is unclear what the second-line agents should be, it is reasonable in many cases to restrict dopamine receptor blocking agents to the most severe cases.

α_2-ADRENERGIC AGONISTS

Clonidine (Catapres)[1] and guanfacine (Tenex)[1] are α_2-adrenergic agonists often used to treat tics. Several randomized trials have shown that these agents reduce tic and ADHD symptoms. The main side effects are sedation and lightheadedness due to mild hypotension. Sedation is more common with clonidine. The clonidine patch (Catapres-TTS)[1] may produce less peak sedation, but it commonly produces local skin irritation.

DOPAMINE RECEPTOR BLOCKING AGENTS

Typical and atypical neuroleptics are dopamine receptor blocking agents that can be used to treat tics. Neuroleptics can be very effective in tic suppression, but they can cause acute akathisia, dystonic reactions, cognitive blunting, acute anxiety with somatizations and school refusal, sedation, weight gain, metabolic syndrome, and QT prolongation. Monitoring for tardive dyskinesia is also important. Some experts recommend baseline electrocardiograms, particularly for individuals with personal or family history of cardiac arrhythmias. Weight gain and metabolic syndrome should be considered when starting neuroleptics, particularly risperidone (Risperdal).[1]

[1]Not FDA approved for this indication.

Some experts recommend obtaining baseline values for weight, blood pressure, fasting glucose, and lipid profile, with follow-up monitoring every 3 months to detect drug-induced metabolic syndrome. Diet modification, routine exercise, or medical therapy may be needed.

OTHER TIC-SUPPRESSING MEDICATIONS

Several small, controlled studies show benefit for dopamine agonists, baclofen (Lioresal),[1] benzodiazepines, and botulinum toxin type A (Botox) injections for focal, strong tics. Tetrabenazine (Xenazine),[1] a drug approved by the FDA for use in Huntington disease, has been reported to reduce tics.

EVOLVING THERAPIES

A new form of cognitive-behavioral/habit reversal therapy, in which the patient learns to increase self-awareness of tics and premonitory urges and to apply antagonistic movements to compete with the tics, has shown early beneficial results. Transcranial magnetic stimulation therapy and deep brain stimulation have been reported anecdotally to reduce tics.

TREATMENT OF COMORBID CONDITIONS

ADHD and OCD are common comorbid conditions in Tourette syndrome. These comorbid symptoms are often more debilitating than the tics. Concern about stimulant therapy worsening tics was addressed by the Tourette Syndrome Study Group in the landmark Treatment of ADHD in Children with Tics (TACT) study. In this study, children treated with methylphenidate (Ritalin) had, on average, reduced tic severity, contrary to the widely held belief that stimulants exacerbate tics.

Medical treatment options for ADHD include psychostimulants and the selective norepinephrine reuptake inhibitor atomoxetine (Strattera). OCD management includes cognitive-behavioral therapy, clomipramine (Anafranil), and any of the selective serotonin reuptake inhibitors.

Summary

Tourette syndrome is a complex neuropsychiatric illness with many potential symptoms that may need medical and nonmedical therapies. Cooperation among the primary care physician, neurologist, psychiatrist, and psychologist is imperative for the comprehensive care of severely affected patients. If a patient has mild tics and few or no comorbid symptoms, medical therapy may not be needed. However, if the tics are severe in the presence of many neuropsychiatric symptoms, it is reasonable to refer patients to specialists.

[1]Not FDA approved for this indication.

TABLE 1 Therapy for Tics in Tourette Syndrome

Medication	Starting Dose	Titration	Goal Dose
Clonidine (Catapres)[1]	0.05 mg qhs	0.05 mg every 3–7 d	0.05–0.1 mg tid
Clonidine patch (Catapres-TTS)[1]	Catapres TTS-1 weekly*	Weekly as needed	Catapres TTS-1, -2, or -3 weekly*
Guanfacine (Tenex)[1]	0.5 mg qhs	0.5 mg every 3–7 d	1–4 mg divided bid
Baclofen (Lioresal)[1]	10 mg qhs	10 mg every 3–7 d	40–90 mg/d divided bid/tid
Clonazepam (Klonopin)[1]	0.5 mg qhs	0.5 mg every wk	1–2 mg bid
Pimozide (Orap)	1 mg qhs	1 mg every 3–5 d	1–4 mg/d divided daily or bid
Haloperidol (Haldol)	0.25–0.5 mg qhs	0.25–0.5 mg every 5–7 d	1–4 mg/d divided daily or bid
Fluphenazine (Prolixin)[1]	0.5 mg qhs	0.5 mg every 3–5 d	1–4 mg/d divided daily or bid
Risperidone (Risperdal)[1]	0.5 mg qhs	0.5 mg every 3–5 d	1–4 mg/d divided daily or bid
Ziprasidone (Geodon)[1]	20 mg qhs	20 mg every wk	20–80 mg/d divided daily or bid
Botulinum toxin type A (Botox)[1]	Not applicable	Not applicable	30–300 units in one or more focal sites, injected once every 3 mo

[1]Not FDA approved for this indication.
*The system areas are 3.5 cm^2 (Catapres-TTS-1), 7.0 cm^2 (Catapres-TTS-2), and 10.5 cm^2 (Catapres-TTS-3), and the amount of drug released is directly proportional to the area.

REFERENCES

Gilbert DL. Treatment of children and adolescents with tics and Tourette syndrome. J Child Neurol 2006;21:690–700.

Kurlan R, Johnson D, Kaplan EL. Streptococcal infection and exacerbations of childhood tics and obsessive-compulsive symptoms: A prospective blinded cohort study. Pediatrics 2008;121:1188–97.

Scahill L, Erenberg G, Berlin Jr CM, et al. Contemporary assessment and pharmacotherapy of Tourette syndrome, NeuroRx 2006;3:192–206. Available for medical and allied professionals at http://www.tsa-usa.org [accessed July 2009].

Tourette Syndrome Study Group. Treatment of ADHD in children with tics: A randomized controlled trial. Neurology 2002;58:527–36.

Zinner SH. Tourette syndrome: Much more than tics. Contemp Pediatr 2004;21:22–49.

Headache

Method of
R. Michael Gallagher, DO

Headache is a disturbing and sometimes fearsome affliction that has plagued humankind throughout recorded history. It often is debilitating and particularly disturbing to the sufferer because the pain is located in the head, the very center of the body's cognitive and control functions. With its accompanying pain and debilitating symptoms, stress can mount and the headache can become all consuming.

Headache is experienced by all age groups from young children to the elderly. It is more common than asthma, diabetes, mental illness, and rheumatoid arthritis. In fact, the World Health Organization identifies severe migraine, along with psychosis and quadriplegia, as "one of the most debilitating chronic conditions." Although the majority of Americans experience tension-type headaches at some time in their lives, approximately 30 million experience migraine headache: 13% of women and 6% of men, predominantly in their most productive years between the ages of 13 and 55 years. Prepubescent boys and girls suffer equally; however, boys often outgrow their migraine attacks as they mature, and they are less subjected to hormonal influences. Smaller percentages of people, by comparison, suffer with other chronic headaches, such as cluster headache and chronic daily headache.

No sure diagnostic tests are available to differentiate headache types. The headache condition can progress over time in frequency, severity, and debilitation. Each sufferer can be different and may require a detailed evaluation and individualized treatment plan; more frequent or prolonged attacks often necessitate a more comprehensive treatment plan. Thus, the headache problem can be a challenge for both the sufferer and the clinician.

During the 20th century, dramatic advancements were made in medicine. Longevity and quality of life improved for many individuals. Unfortunately, for headache sufferers, most of these advances were for maladies that killed or maimed rather than for non–life-threatening conditions. It was not until the 1960s that even a reasonable preventive medication, propranolol (Inderal), was introduced, and by the 1980s only a handful of medications were available for wide use. Physicians had to improvise with medications and treatments that were originally designated for other medical conditions.

In the late 1980s and 1990s, epidemiologic, psychosocial, and pharmacologic research resulted in an increase in available headache information and treatment possibilities. The development of the triptans, serotonin agonists, brought a new awareness to both physicians and sufferers. Today, seven triptans and two relatively new preventive medications are available. In spite of this, a minority of migraine sufferers use these options, and more than 50% continue to self-treat without benefit of professional care.

In the past, patients wanted the physician to believe their headache problem was real. They hoped that they would be taken seriously and that the physician would make a sincere attempt to help them. The headache patient has changed. The headache sufferer who seeks treatment today is more knowledgeable and interested in rapid relief and tolerability of medication.

Evaluation and Diagnosis

An accurate diagnosis is essential for effective management of patients with the more commonly encountered headaches. Because no biologic markers or diagnostic tests exist to determine headache type, the history is the single most important element in the evaluation of the headache patient. Various headache types sometimes have similar initial presentations, or patients may suffer with more than one type of headache (e.g., migraine and tension-type headache), which can be confusing at first, but the careful history usually differentiates the headache type. In general, little in the way of diagnostic testing is needed unless a physical cause is suspected. Some physicians prefer to perform simple laboratory tests to establish a baseline for medication toleration and monitoring as necessary (Table 1).

The headache complaint on occasion can be a sign of a more serious medical condition, such as a tumor, infection, or aneurysm. For this reason, the clinician always must be cautious and diligent in establishing an accurate and timely diagnosis. Certain so-called red flags in the history require immediate attention. These include any complex of symptoms or history that does not fit a typical headache type; report of a significant neurologic deficit; significant or prolonged neurologic deficit with aura; late-onset migraine (patient older than 30 years); sudden onset of a new head pain without history of similar headaches; changes in headache character; headache associated with elevated temperature; or completely unresponsive attacks in the absence of analgesic or caffeine overuse. When any of these symptoms are present or physical examination reveals significant findings, further diagnostic evaluation with imaging studies and consultation is imperative.

The appropriate headache patient evaluation includes a thorough history, physical examination with special attention to the head and the neurologic, cardiovascular, and musculoskeletal systems, and

TABLE 1 Current Diagnosis

Symptoms	Frequency	Duration
Tension-Type Headache		
Bilateral variable pain	Variable	Hours to days
Squeezing or bandlike	Often related to	
Tightness of head and	known	
shoulders	precipitant	
Migraine Headache		
Unilateral mostly	1–6 mo	Hours to days
Throbbing or constant pain	Sometimes cyclic	
Nausea, vomiting		
Photophobia/phonophobia		
Fluid disturbances		
Mood changes		
Can be associated with		
aura		
Cluster Headache		
Unilateral severe boring	Multiple daily	45–90 min
pain		
Ipsilateral lacrimation,	Near-daily	Cycles of
scleral injection,		attacks
rhinorrhea		
Eyelid droop		
Restlessness		

diagnostic tests when appropriate. The history should include headache onset, location, pain character (e.g., pressure, throb), frequency, duration, associated symptoms, aura or prodrome, triggers, previous treatment, and family history. Certain clues in the history may lean toward the diagnosis of migraine, such as motion sickness, absence of headache during pregnancy, and headache relationship to menses, sun glare, oversleep, fatigue, fasting, foods, or alcohol.

Various diagnostic screening questionnaires and tools have been developed over the years to assist busy clinicians in establishing the diagnosis of migraine. Most are long and cumbersome and do not easily become a part of routine patient evaluation. A simple three-question screener for migraine is helpful for generalist clinicians. A "yes" answer to all three questions indicates a strong possibility of the migraine diagnosis:

1. Do you experience headaches severe enough to see a physician?
2. Are your headaches accompanied by other symptoms?
3. Are your headaches intermittent (i.e., nondaily)?

Note: This screener should not be substituted for a complete history; it should be used only for screening purposes.

TENSION-TYPE HEADACHE

Tension-type headache (TTHA) is the most common of headaches and first was believed to be caused by sustained muscle contraction of the neck, jaw, scalp, or facial muscles. However, it is now thought that the sustained muscle contraction can, in fact, be an epiphenomenon to possible central disturbances rather than a primary process. Evidence suggests that altered levels of serotonin, substance P, and neuropeptide Y in the serum or platelets of patients with TTHA are responsible.

TTHA is characterized by intermittent or persisting bilateral pain, usually described as a squeezing pressure or a bandlike sensation around the head. Most patients experience their symptoms in the frontal, temporal, or occipital areas of the head. Location frequently varies with the attack, and tightness of the neck and shoulders is common. Intensity varies greatly. The attacks can last from hours to days, and in some extreme cases they may last for months. Aura, nausea, photophobia and phonophobia, and incapacitation are not typically associated with TTHA.

Many TTHA sufferers easily recognize the origin of their attacks. TTHA typically results from emotional upset, periods of stress, and major life changes. Anxiousness, poor adaptation skills, and anxiety and depression often are present. Physical causes, such as degenerative joint disease, trauma to the head or neck, poor posture, or temporomandibular joint dysfunction, also can precipitate attacks. Persons older than 50 years are prone to excessive muscle contraction because of arthritis of the neck and jaw, poor posture, or stress. TTHA that is consistently precipitated by tension or pathology of the neck frequently is referred to as a *cervicogenic headache*. In contrast to migraine headache, TTHA is more likely to begin in later life.

MIGRAINE HEADACHE

Migraine headache is a familial disease characterized by unilateral or bilateral paroxysmal headache lasting hours to days. Adult women experience attacks more than men by a ratio of 3:1. Children and the elderly experience migraine equally. Attacks occur from as infrequently as one or two per year to several times weekly. Associated symptoms usually occur and frequently include throbbing, nausea, vomiting, photophobia, phonophobia, fluid retention, and mood changes.

The two basic types of migraine headache are *migraine with aura* (previously called classic migraine) and *migraine without aura* (previously called common migraine). Migraine with aura is preceded by an aura, a transient neurologic symptom that usually is visual, such as scotoma, teichopsia, tunnel vision, or visual field deficit, lasting 10 to 30 minutes. However, aura can manifest as any neurological deficit. Migraine without aura is more commonly experienced and comes on gradually or is present on awakening from sleep. In some patients, these headaches are associated with a nonspecific prolonged prodrome, such as mood changes, food cravings, or fluid retention hours before the pain.

BOX 1   Migraine Dietary Triggers

- Dairy: Ripened cheese (cheddar, brie, camembert, half-cup of sour cream)
- Meats: Processed lunch meats, hot dogs, sausage, bologna, salami, chicken liver
- Fish: Pickled or dried herring
- Grains: Sourdough bread
- Fruits: Bananas, raisins, figs, avocado, half-cup limit of citrus
- Vegetables: Broad and fava beans, onions, snow peas
- Other: Chocolate, nuts, peanut butter, pickled foods, Chinese food with monosodium glutamate (MSG)
- Beverages: Most wines and alcohol, 200-mg daily limit of caffeine
- Additives: MSG, soy sauce, meat tenderizers, aspartame, sulfites, garlic

---

The underlying cause of migraine headache is not clearly established, and various theories are proposed. Migraine appears to be of genetic origin and to be an inflammatory disease that causes disturbances in serotonin use and activity. Strong evidence indicates the migrainous attack originates in the central nervous system by stimulation of the locus ceruleus and dorsal raphe nuclei. Resultant changes alter cerebral and extracranial blood flow, activate the trigeminovascular system, and cause vascular dilation, neurogenic inflammation, and pain. Various precipitants are known, and many sufferers report that migraine attacks frequently are associated with menstruation or are triggered by foods containing vasoactive amines, strong odors, too much or too little sleep, sun glare, stress, altitude, weather changes, exertion, or fasting (Boxes 1 and 2, Table 2).

Some physicians classify migraine according to its precipitant or description (e.g., menstrual migraine, exertional migraine, coital migraine, cervicogenic migraine, cyclic migraine, acephalic migraine). Regardless, the fundamentals of evaluation and treatment are the same.

CLUSTER HEADACHE

The cause of cluster headache is unknown, and little credible research is available. Various possibilities or theories are suggested and include, but are not limited to, disturbances in histamine production or use; hypothalamic biorhythm dysfunction; or serotonin and neurotransmitter mechanisms similar to those of migraine. Some authorities consider cluster headache one of the most severe pain conditions known to humankind.

Cluster headache predominantly affects men, with a male-to-female ratio of 6:1. It occurs in well under 0.5% of the population. Onset later in life (after age 30 years) is common, and patients

---

BOX 2   Migraine Triggers

- Altitude
- Alcohol
- Caffeine withdrawal
- Fluorescent or flickering lights
- Sun glare
- Weather changes
- Stress, stress letdown
- Foods
- Skipping meals
- Smoky environment
- Noisy environment
- Strong odors
- Lack of sleep, oversleep
- Exertion
- Hormonal changes

TABLE 2 Current Therapy

Headache Type	PRN	Prophylaxis
Tension	OTC*	Stress/precipitant avoidance
	NSAIDs	Stretching
	Muscle relaxants	Warm packs
	Combination analgesics	Relaxation techniques
		NSAIDs
		Muscle relaxants
		Antidepressants
Migraine	NSAIDs*	Biofeedback
	Triptans*	β-Blockers*
	Ergotamine*	Divalproex sodium*
	Dihydroergotamine*	
	Isometheptene*	Topiramate*
	Combination analgesics	TCA antidepressants
		Calcium channel blockers
Cluster	Oxygen	No alcohol
	Triptans	Calcium channel blockers
	Dihydroergotamine	Divalproex sodium
	Ergotamine	NSAIDs
		Lithium
		Steroids

*FDA indication.
Abbreviations: NSAID = nonsteroidal antiinflammatory drug; OTC = over-the-counter; TCA = tricyclic antidepressant.

sometimes report head injury or a traumatic event occurring months before onset. Attacks occur on a daily or near-daily basis for weeks or months at a time and mysteriously disappear for months to years regardless of treatment, only to recur and cycle again. Although nonspecialist physicians only occasionally encounter the patient with cluster headaches, it is important to consider cluster headaches in the differential diagnosis.

The typical patient with a cluster headache experiences relatively brief attacks (45–90 minutes) of horrible unilateral head pain associated with ipsilateral lacrimation, scleral injection, rhinorrhea, or eyelid droop. The hallmark of the syndrome is its associated symptoms and its severe and intense pain. During attacks, most cluster patients move about, trying unsuccessfully to get more comfortable, similar to renal colic, in contrast to migraine sufferers, who prefer to lie quietly in a dark quiet room. Few triggers are identified, and alcohol almost always precipitates an attack during a cluster "on" cycle. A rare form of cluster headache, chronic cluster, does not cycle and continues on a daily or near-daily basis without cessation.

Treatment

The doctor–patient relationship frequently is the key to successful treatment in the headache patient. Although to some this statement seems an obvious truism, its importance cannot be overemphasized. Patients who experience frequent, near-daily, or daily headaches invariably require a comprehensive treatment program that necessitates good communication. Anxious patients sometimes do not comprehend medical explanations or instructions; busy doctors sometimes do not have or take the time to ensure that the patient understands.

The two elements of headache treatment are *abortive treatment*, directed at attacks once they have begun, and *prophylactic treatment*, directed at preventing or reducing the frequency of attacks. In general, the abortive approach is used for patients who suffer infrequent attacks and for those who experience breakthrough attacks while undergoing prophylactic therapy. Prophylactic therapy should be instituted when headaches are frequent, when headaches are unresponsive to abortive medication, or when there are contraindications to abortives (Table 2).

Headache treatment can include nonpharmacologic measures, such as physical exercise, stretching, stress avoidance, relaxation exercises, biofeedback, manipulation, massage, or cold/warm packs. Pharmacologic therapies can include a vast array of medicaments from over-the-counter (OTC) drugs to prescription drugs such as triptans, other vasoconstrictors, β-blockers, antiepileptic agents, antidepressants, nonsteroidal antiinflammatory drugs (NSAIDs), analgesics, muscle relaxants, anxiolytics, and others.

Treatment, whether prophylactic or abortive, should follow a definite plan incorporating the clinician and patient into a team focused on reducing the headache frequency, severity, and disability. As mentioned earlier, impressions and physical findings should be explained to the patient in as much detail as necessary to ensure the patient's complete understanding. The complexity of the headache condition needs to be explained, emphasizing its chronicity, rather than its curability, and that the goal of treatment is disease control.

The comprehensiveness of the treatment plan depends on the frequency of the patient's attacks. The more frequent and severe the attacks, the more detailed plan may be necessary. Patients experiencing infrequent attacks (e.g., once or twice monthly) may require only an abortive medication and little else. Patients with more frequent attacks may benefit from dietary restrictions, psychosocial intervention, biofeedback relaxation training, manipulation, and physical modality intervention, in addition to medication.

TENSION-TYPE HEADACHE TREATMENT

TTHA often is associated with emotional stress and muscle strain or tension of the shoulders and neck. Simple self-administered measures, such as stress avoidance, stretching, warm packs, or relaxation techniques, can be helpful in reducing or relieving attacks. More comprehensive professional intervention, such as manipulation, physical therapy, local injections, or biofeedback training, are considerations for more frequent or severe cases.

Prophylactically, the use of OTC or prescription medications can be considered in addition to nonmedicinal measures for reducing the frequency and duration of attacks. NSAIDs, muscle relaxants, or antidepressants (tricyclic antidepressant [TCA], selective serotonin reuptake inhibitor [SSRI]), at the lowest effective doses, are more commonly used.

Daily use of the longer-acting NSAIDs, such as naproxen[1] (Naprosyn) or celecoxib[1] (Celebrex), in the appropriately screened patient over a 2- to 3-week period, can be an effective preventative. TCAs, such as nortriptyline[1] (Pamelor) or amitriptyline[1] (Elavil), in low doses at night over 1 to 3 months, are frequently effective, especially in patients with anxiety or mild depression. The SSRI drugs, such as fluoxetine[1] (Prozac) or sertraline[1] (Zoloft), similarly can be useful. The muscle relaxant cyclobenzaprine[1] (Flexeril), at low doses, with a similar mechanism to the TCAs, can be administered at night for limited periods. Other muscle relaxants occasionally can be effective. Potential side effects can limit the use of NSAIDs (gastrointestinal irritation) and the TCAs (fatigue and weight gain).

Abortive or symptomatic treatment of TTHA can include simple OTC medications (e.g., aspirin or acetaminophen), NSAIDs (short-acting), muscle relaxants, combination analgesics, and, in some cases, opioid or opioidlike drugs. Caution should be exercised in prescribing potentially habituating drugs. Daily or near-daily use of analgesics can lead to analgesic rebound headache, Medication Overuse Headache, which can compound the patient's headache problem.

Botulism toxin[1] (Botox) reportedly is helpful in the treatment of tension-type and migraine headache, but controlled studies are limited. In this treatment, a diluted solution of botulism toxin is injected into various muscles of the face, scalp, neck, or shoulders. Because this treatment frequently is used in headache specialty and pain centers, simultaneous comprehensive measures and medication may contribute to positive results. Side effects from botulism toxin are low when injected properly.

---

[1]Not FDA approved for this indication.

MIGRAINE TREATMENT

Migraineurs are unique individuals, and the effectiveness and tolerance of medications can vary from patient to patient. Medication changes, combinations of medications, and trial and error may be necessary in the early stages of treatment.

Nonmedicinal measures for migraine sufferers include biofeedback stress reduction, caffeine and dietary restrictions, regimentation of meals and sleep, rest, exercise, stretching, and avoidance of work or activity overload. Limiting caffeine to less than 200 mg/day is important to prevent the caffeine headache (rebound headache) in most patients. Elimination of vasoactive foods, such as chocolate, aged cheese, and processed meats, and avoidance of fasting for more than 4 hours can be helpful for patients with more frequent attacks (Table 3). Regular exercise and stretching, planned relaxation, regular sleep schedules, and following a healthy lifestyle are frequently included in a comprehensive treatment regimen. In some patients, especially children and adolescents, biofeedback stress reduction or psychotherapeutic intervention may be necessary.

The more commonly used medications for prophylaxis are β-blockers, calcium channel blockers, antiepileptics (neurostabilizers), and the antidepressants. Treatment should be continued for a 4- to 8-week trial before discontinuation for ineffectiveness. Determination of which medication to use depends on comorbidities, interactions with concomitant medications, and tolerability.

β-Blockers such as propranolol (Inderal) and timolol (Blocadren) are nonselective and are approved by the Food and Drug Administration (FDA) for migraine prevention. Other β-blockers, such as nadolol[1] (Corgard), metoprolol[1] (Lopressor), and atenolol[1] (Tenormin), also can be effective. The mechanism of action in migraine is not wholly understood, but it is thought to involve anxiolytic effects as well as vascular changes and stabilization. The usual dosage is recommended (e.g., timolol 10–30 mg/day, propranolol 120–160 mg/day), and many consider the nighttime dose the more significant.

Calcium channel antagonists are well tolerated in general and can be as effective as the β-blockers. They are believed to alter serotonin release and inhibit platelet serotonin uptake and release within the brain. Verapamil[1] (Calan) is considered the more effective and is commonly recommended to patients. Dosage can vary from 120 to 480 mg/day. Nimodipine[1] (Nimotop) is equally effective, but it is rarely used in the United States because of its high cost.

Antiepileptic medications such as phenytoin[1] (Dilantin) and carbamazepine[1] (Tegretol) have been prescribed for migraine prevention over the years, with mixed results. Their use is now limited with the advent of newer, more easily tolerated agents, such as divalproex sodium (Depakote) and topiramate (Topamax).

Divalproex sodium is effective in reducing migraine attacks and is particularly useful in patients with coexisting head injury, seizure dis-

---

[1]Not FDA approved for this indication.

TABLE 3 Triptans

Medication	Brand Name	Half-Life	Form/Strength
Sumatriptan	Imitrex	1.5 hr	Oral: 25, 50, 100 mg; NS: 20 mg; injection: 6 mg, 4 mg
Naratriptan	Amerge	6 hr	Oral: 2.5 mg
Zolmitriptan	Zomig	3 hr	Oral: 2.5, 5 mg; Melt: 2.5, 5 mg; NS: 5 mg
Rizatriptan	Maxalt	2–3 hr	Oral: 5, 10 mg; Melt: 10 mg
Almotriptan	Axert	3–4 hr	Oral: 6.25, 12.5 mg
Frovatriptan	Frova	25 hr	Oral: 5 mg
Eletriptan	Relpax	4 hr	Oral: 20, 40 mg

Abbreviations: Melt = oral disintegrating; NS = nasal steroid.

---

orders, and bipolar disorders. It is thought to improve inhibitory and excitatory amino acid imbalance in the brain. It is best to start with a lower dose and to gradually increase as needed and tolerated. The dosage of 500 to 1000 mg/day is more frequently prescribed. A commonly experienced side effect is sedation, which can sometimes be used to the patient's advantage when anxiolytic effects are needed.

Topiramate is the most recent preventive medication approved by the FDA for migraine prophylaxis. It has multiple mechanisms of action, but its exact mechanism in migraine headache is unknown. Its effectiveness is believed to involve sodium ion channel stabilization, calcium ion channels, GABA (γ-aminobutyric acid) receptors, and neuronal membrane stabilization. The average daily dose is variable and ranges from 30 to 100 mg/day. A most unusual side effect of weight loss or appetite suppression can be used to the patient's advantage in preventing weight gain, which frequently accompanies migraine prophylactic medications.

The TCAs can be useful in patients who experience frequent attacks and in those who experience anxiety and depression. The TCAs inhibit synaptic reuptake of serotonin, thereby reducing neuron firing and release of neurotransmitters. Starting with a low dose in the evening and titrating up to efficacy and tolerability is recommended. Significant anticholinergic and sedation effects sometimes limit their use. The SSRIs[1] are reported helpful in some patients, but their use in migraine prevention is limited.

In general, prophylactic medications should be taken for 6 to 8 weeks to determine efficacy. If effective, a course of 4 to 6 months is recommended before an attempt is made to discontinue medication.

A variety of abortive treatment options are available for migraine sufferers. Although the triptans (Table 3) have generated much interest and are frequently prescribed, other medications continue to be used, including ergotamine and its derivatives, isometheptene, and NSAIDs. Many of the abortive medications carry significant prescribing limitations that must be taken into consideration. Vasoconstrictor medications are contraindicated in patients with cardiovascular or peripheral vascular disease. NSAIDs should not be used in those with gastrointestinal or bleeding disorders. As with all medications, the clinician must consider appropriate prescribing, contraindications, and side-effect information.

The vasoconstrictor ergotamine is available in oral, rectal (Ergocaff PB), and sublingual forms (Ergomar). Ergotamine has a relatively long half-life and duration of action (up to 3 days) and should be used no more frequently than every 4 to 5 days to avoid ergotamine rebound headache. The ergot derivative dihydroergotamine (DHE-45, Migranal NS) is available for intramuscular (IM), subcutaneous (SC), intravenous (IV), and intranasal use. IV dihydroergotamine (DHE-45) sometimes is used for intractable migraine (status migrainosus) in emergency departments and inpatient settings. The intranasal form (Migranal) is an effective treatment when administered correctly by the patient. Unfortunately, dihydroergotamine is not absorbed by the gastrointestinal tract, and, unlike other abortive nasal sprays, any swallowed medication will be wasted. Dihydroergotamine has a low headache recurrence rate of approximately 12%. All forms of ergotamine and dihydroergotamine are more effective when taken early in attacks.

Isometheptene is used in combination with dichloralphenazone and acetaminophen (Midrin, Duradrin). It is slow acting and more effective when taken early in attacks and when used for attacks preceded or accompanied by stress and muscle tension of the neck. Although isometheptene is considered less potent than ergotamine and triptans, it is preferred by many patients whose headaches have features of both migraine and TTHA.

At the present time, seven serotonin agonists (triptans) are approved for abortive migraine treatment in the United States (see Table 3). As a category, the triptans are approximately 65% to 70% effective in published clinical trials. Their similarities are greater than their differences, but each triptan is not necessarily effective for all patients, and familiarity with their differences can be helpful to the treating physician. Half-life, onset and duration of action, adverse

---

[1]Not FDA approved for this indication.

events, tolerability, recurrence of headache, and routes of administration may vary and allow the physician to match the medication to the individual patient. For example, a slower onset of action and longer-lasting triptan may be appropriate for slow-onset, longer-lasting migraine attacks.

Like other treatments, oral triptan tablets are more effective in the early phases of migraines. It is thought that peripheral sensitization—allodynia—is a sign of later phase migraine, and treating the attack before this phenomenon occurs is important. When treatment is delayed or the patient awakens with severe migraine, the injection, nasal spray, or rapidly acting triptans may be more beneficial. Although triptans as a group are very effective, recurrence of headache, after initial relief, requiring retreatment is common and can be as high as 40%. The recurrence rate tends to be less with triptans having a longer half-life.

The ergots and triptans are contraindicated in patients with ischemic heart disease, uncontrolled hypertension, and cerebrovascular disease. Physicians initially were extremely cautious about recommending triptans to their patients when the triptans were first introduced in the United States. However, significant human exposure to the triptans has revealed that catastrophic myocardial infarction or serious ischemia is rare. Chest pain following triptan use affects a small percentage of patients, and because the significance of this finding is not clear, refraining from future triptan use in these patients is recommended.

Sumatriptan (Imitrex), the first triptan approved in the United States, is available in nasal spray (20 mg), SC (6 mg, 4 mg), and oral formulations (25, 50, 100 mg). Its half-life is approximately 1.5 hours, and its duration of action is less than 4 hours. The injectable form produces rapid relief in 70% to 80% of patients, and it appears to be the most effective of all the available triptan forms. Conversely, it appears to cause the most side effects, and, for this reason, it should be used only for the more severe attacks. The oral forms are more favorable with regard to adverse effects, and their effectiveness is similar to that of other triptans (approximately 65%). Because of sumatriptan's short half-life and duration of action, recurrence of headache is common, necessitating repeat dosing.

Zolmitriptan (Zomig) is available in 2.5- and 5-mg oral and oral disintegrating tablets (ZMT) and as a 5-mg nasal spray. The efficacy of oral zolmitriptan is approximately 65% and that of the nasal form is 70%. The half-life of oral zolmitriptan is 3 hours, and its duration of action is longer than the nasal form, which improves on the need to re-medicate. The nasal spray has a biphasic absorption curve, which accounts for its favorable adverse effect profile over the 5-mg oral tablet.

Naratriptan (Amerge) was the first to be approved of the gradual-onset, longer-acting triptans. It is available as oral 2.5-mg tablets and has a half-life of 6 hours. Naratriptan is well tolerated by patients and often is used by patients with slow-onset migraine. Some specialists prescribe daily naratriptan for limited periods for treatment of menstrual or intractable migraine attacks.

Rizatriptan (Maxalt) is available as oral 5- and 10-mg tablets and as an oral disintegrating form (MLT). It has a relatively rapid onset of action and a favorable one-dose 2-hour response rate. Patients who are undergoing concomitant treatment with propranolol should take the lesser 5-mg rizatriptan dose because of higher resultant rizatriptan plasma levels.

Almotriptan (Axert) is available in 6.25- and 12.5-mg tablets. It has a half-life of 3.5 hours and, because of a broad T_{max} (time of maximal concentration) range of 1.4 to 3.8 hours, a relatively rapid onset of action. Almotriptan has favorable adverse effect and headache recurrence profile. Chest pain symptoms after almotriptan use are similar to placebo in clinical trials.

Frovatriptan (Frova) is a long-acting triptan available in 2.5-mg oral tablets. It has the longest half-life of 25 hours and a favorable recurrence rate. Frovatriptan is frequently used for treatment of menstrual migraine and for attacks of longer duration. Some specialists prescribe daily frovatriptan for a limited period for menstrual and prolonged migraine attacks.

Eletriptan (Relpax) is the most recently approved triptan. It is available in 20- and 40-mg oral tablets and has a half-life of nearly 5 hours. Eletriptan has a relatively rapid onset but a longer duration of action and a favorable recurrence rate. In studies, some patients who were unresponsive to other triptans responded to eletriptan.

Various attempts have been made to compare triptans. Head-to-head trials mostly have compared one triptan to sumatriptan. A meta-analysis of 53 clinical trials published in 2001 compared the efficacy, recurrence, duration of action, and tolerability of all available triptans. Almotriptan and eletriptan were rated favorably across the major parameters of onset of action, efficacy, adverse events, and recurrence. In spite of efforts to adjust for variations in protocols and placebo response, specialists reached no clear consensus as to the validity or value of the meta-analysis or the preferability of one triptan over another.

NSAIDs frequently are recommended for treatment of acute migraine and can be effective when taken early. Their effects on the physiology of pain, inflammation, and platelets are believed to be the mechanisms responsible. Some physicians recommend taking a NSAID with the first dose of a triptan for added efficacy. Various agents are used, but none of the rapid-acting NSAIDs appears to have significant efficacy superiority. OTC ibuprofen (Motrin) and aspirin, in combination with caffeine and acetaminophen (Excedrin Migraine), is approved by the FDA for treatment of migraine.

Symptomatic treatment of pain may be necessary in patients who do not respond to recommended abortive treatment. Any effective analgesic can be appropriate, provided it is used infrequently and not on a daily or near-daily basis. In general, the more effective analgesics have anti-inflammatory and sedative properties.

CLUSTER HEADACHE TREATMENT

Cluster headache is one of the more unusual pain conditions occasionally encountered by physicians. Pain onset is rapid, and the duration of the attack is brief. For this reason, prophylactic treatment usually is the most practical. Abortive prescriptions frequently are given, but, for the most part, the cluster attack is resolving by the time medication is absorbed.

Nonmedicinal prophylactic measures are extremely limited. The reduction of cigarette smoking, the addressing of individual stress and hostility issues when appropriate, and the complete cessation of alcohol consumption during cluster periods should be part of any treatment program. Prophylactic medications include the calcium channel blockers verapamil[1] (Calan) and nimodipine[1] (Nimotop), the neurostabilizers valproate[1] (Depakote) and topiramate[1] (Topamax), various NSAIDs, ergotamine,[1] lithium[1] (Eskalith), cyproheptadine (Periactin) and, in extreme cases, short intervals of steroids.[1] These medications are used in average therapeutic doses, and combinations of medications are commonly needed (Table 4). The preventatives should be used during the cluster cycle and discontinued during off-cycle periods.

---

[1]Not FDA approved for this indication.

TABLE 4   Cluster Headache Prophylactic Medications

Medication	Brand	Average Daily Dose
Verapamil[1]	Calan, Isoptin, Verelan	240–420 mg
Divalproex[1]	Depakote	500–1500 mg
Topiramate[1]	Topamax	50–200 mg
Indomethacin[1]	Indocin	100–150 mg
Naproxen[1]	Naprosyn	1000–1500 mg
Lithium[1]	Lithobid	600–1200 mg*
Ergotamine[1]	Bellergal[1]	1 tablet bid†
Prednisone[1]	—	100 mg, decrease to 0
Cyproheptadine	Periactin	8–16 mg

[1]Not FDA approved for this indication.
*With serum level monitoring.
†Ergotamine 0.6 mg with phenobarbital 40 mg and 0.2 mg L-alkaloids of belladonna.

Abortive treatment is less preferred for cluster headache, as noted previously. However, inhalation oxygen via facial mask at 6 L terminates cluster attacks in 75% to 80% of sufferers within 12 minutes. Other possibilities include sumatriptans (Imitrex) SC or nasal spray,[1] zolmitriptan (Zomig ZMT) nasal spray,[1] ergotamine (Ergomar) sublingual, or dihydroergotamine injection (DHE-45) or nasal spray[1] (Migranal). The occasional patient reports relief with the oral triptans or analgesics. When triptans, ergotamine, or analgesics are used, appropriate prescribing and frequency guidelines should be followed. In general, with the exception of oxygen, daily as-needed medications should be avoided.

Headache continues to present a challenging problem for clinicians as well as for suffering patients. In spite of recent treatment advances and more public awareness, millions continue to needlessly endure pain and debilitation. At first glance, the headache problem appears complex and difficult when, in actuality, most sufferers experience straightforward, easily diagnosed headaches. The interested generalist or specialist who takes the time to elicit a careful history can establish the headache diagnosis and direct a simple treatment plan that can make a tremendous difference in the headache sufferer's life.

REFERENCES

Astin JA, Ernst E. The effectiveness of spinal manipulation for the treatment of headache disorders: A systematic review of randomized clinical trials. Cephalalgia 2002;22:617–23.

Diamond ML, Dalessio DJ, editors. Diamond and Dalessio's The Practicing Physician's Approach to Headache. 5th ed. Philadelphia: WB Saunders; 1999.

Ferrari MD, Roon KI, Lipton RB, et al. Oral triptans (serotonin 5HT-IB/ID-agonists) in acute migraine treatment: A meta-analysis of 53 trials. Lancet 2001;358:1668–75.

Gallagher RM, Kunkel R. Migraine medication attributes important for patient compliance: Concerns about side effects may delay treatment. Headache: J Head Face Pain 2003;43:36–43.

Goadsby PJ, Lipton RB, Ferreri MD. Migraine current understanding and treatment. N Engl J Med 2002;346:257–70.

Silberstein SD, Lipton EB, Dalessio DJ. Wolff's Headache and Other Head Pain. 7th ed. New York: Oxford University Press; 2001.

Vernon H, McDermaid C, Hagino C. Systematic review of randomized clinical trials of complementary/alternative therapies in the treatment of tension-type and cervicogenic headache. Complement Ther Med 1999;7:142–55.

[1]Not FDA approved for this indication.

Viral Meningitis and Encephalitis

Method of
Mark J. Abzug, MD

Viral meningitis is the most common cause of aseptic meningitis, an inflammatory process involving the meninges in which usual bacterial etiologies cannot be identified. Encephalitis is an inflammatory process that affects the brain parenchyma, typically producing more severe illness. Many viral infections of the central nervous system produce inflammation of both the meninges and brain tissue (meningoencephalitis). Encephalitis may result from acute viral invasion of the brain and a concomitant inflammatory response or from a postinfectious, autoimmune process characterized by demyelination following a viral illness or vaccination (acute disseminated encephalomyelitis). The majority of the approximately 8000 to 13,000 cases of aseptic meningitis and approximately 20,000 cases of encephalitis reported annually in the United States are caused by viral infections.

Clinical Features

Regardless of etiology, most cases of viral meningitis present similarly. Infants and young children display nonspecific symptoms, such as fever, irritability, lethargy, anorexia, and emesis. More specific findings suggestive of meningeal inflammation, such as nuchal rigidity, bulging fontanelle, and photophobia, are often absent. In older children and adults, nuchal rigidity and photophobia, along with fever, headache, and emesis, are more frequent. Focal neurologic findings and seizures are uncommon presenting findings in viral meningitis, although approximately 10% of children hospitalized with viral meningitis may develop acute complications such as obtundation, seizures, increased intracranial pressure, and inappropriate antidiuretic hormone secretion. Illness can last up to 1 to 2 weeks, with protracted headache not uncommon in adults.

Encephalitis is distinguished from meningitis by a change in sensorium and/or by focal neurologic findings. In younger children, encephalitis typically presents with irritability and/or lethargy, often after a febrile illness. Older children may manifest headache, disorientation, unusual behavior, abnormal speech, bizarre movements, and disorientation in addition to fever, nausea, emesis, myalgias, and photophobia. Generalized or, less commonly, focal neurologic abnormalities, including seizures and motor deficits, may be present. Progression to extreme lethargy, stupor, or coma may ensue.

Etiology

In recent studies, a specific etiologic agent was identified in 55% to 70% of presumed cases of viral meningitis and in only 25% to 65% of cases of encephalitis despite thorough investigation. The list of implicated viruses is extensive (Table 1). Enteroviruses (EVs) are the most common cause of both viral meningitis and encephalitis of proven etiology. Other important agents include arboviruses (transmitted by arthropod vectors such as mosquitoes or ticks), herpes simplex virus (HSV), influenza virus, Epstein-Barr virus, varicella-zoster virus, adenovirus, and rabies virus.

Diagnosis

Important diagnostic clues may come from history (respiratory or gastrointestinal symptoms, family exposures, seasonality, prevalent diseases, travel, animal and insect exposure, and recreational activities) and physical examination (see Table 1). The presence of a rash may suggest specific agents, such as varicella-zoster virus or EVs. Whereas identification of a mucocutaneous vesicle in a neonate may be key to the diagnosis of HSV infection, cold sores in older children and adults are *not* predictive of HSV encephalitis. The combination of findings of encephalitis and myelitis in the same patient is suggestive of infection with an EV (especially EV 71), West Nile virus, or Japanese encephalitis virus. Although focal signs are present in the majority of older children and adults with HSV encephalitis, the positive predictive value of focal findings for HSV is low.

Examination of the cerebrospinal fluid (CSF) is indicated in suspected meningitis or encephalitis unless contraindicated by concern for a space-occupying lesion or increased intracranial pressure. CSF in viral meningitis typically has a low-grade pleocytosis (100–1000 white blood cells [WBCs]/mm^3, range <100 to ≥2000 WBC/mm^3). Polymorphonuclear leukocytes may predominate early, with the profile becoming mononuclear within 8 to 48 hours In general, CSF protein is normal or slightly increased, and the glucose concentration is normal or slightly decreased, although exceptions occur. The CSF in encephalitis typically has a predominantly mononuclear pleocytosis, increased protein, and normal glucose, although CSF may be normal in 3% to 5% or more of cases, especially early in the course. Certain viruses, including influenza and parvovirus B19, typically cause encephalopathies characterized by the absence of pleocytosis.

Imaging and electroencephalography (EEG) are useful adjuncts, particularly for encephalitis. Magnetic resonance imaging generally

TABLE 1   Epidemiology and Clinical Features of Viral Meningitis and Encephalitis

Enteroviruses
Epidemiology
- Most common proven cause of viral meningitis and encephalitis (up to 85%–95% of viral meningitis and 80% of viral encephalitis).
- Majority of meningitis and encephalitis occurs in children <1 year old; incidence of meningitis exceeds that of encephalitis.
- Epidemic in warm seasons in temperate climates.
- Poliovirus infection decreased with widespread immunization.
- Enterovirus 71 frequently occurs in regional outbreaks, e.g., Asia since the late 1990s. Severe disease occurs primarily in children <5 years old.

Clinical Features
- Meningitis and severe encephalitis more common in younger children, especially neonates. Encephalitis may be part of multisystem illness in newborns.
- Encephalitis typically generalized, although focal seizures and other abnormalities may occur, especially in neonates.
- May have biphasic febrile course; meningeal and encephalitic symptoms occur during second phase.
- Rash (macular, maculopapular, petechial, vesicular), enanthem, conjunctivitis, respiratory symptoms, pleurodynia, pericarditis, myocarditis, diarrhea, myalgias may accompany.
- Chronic meningoencephalitis with waxing and warning neurologic symptoms and high fatality rate occur in hypogammaglobulinemic patients.
- Enterovirus 71 associated with hand-foot-and-mouth disease, herpangina, and neurologic disease (meningitis, brainstem encephalitis, myelitis/acute flaccid paralysis, Guillain-Barré syndrome).
  - Signs of brainstem encephalitis include myoclonic jerks, tremors, ataxia, cranial nerve palsy, limb weakness, altered consciousness, seizures, increased intracranial pressure.
  - Imaging reveals high-intensity lesions in the midbrain, brainstem, and spinal cord anterior horn cells and ventral roots.
  - Pulmonary edema/hemorrhage, cardiac failure, shock may develop rapidly.

Herpes Simplex Virus
Epidemiology
- ~1%–3% of viral meningitis.
  - Predominantly associated with primary type 2 HSV genital infection and less frequently with primary type 1 HSV genital infection, nonprimary HSV genital infection (either type), or without recent genital disease.
  - Mollaret's meningitis (recurrent, benign aseptic meningitis) mostly associated with type 2 infection without signs of genital infection and occasionally with type 1 HSV or with Epstein-Barr virus.
- ~10%–20% of encephalitis in the United States.
  - Encephalitis primarily due to type 2 HSV in neonates and type 1 HSV in older age groups.
  - Encephalitis occurs in ~50% of neonatal HSV infections.
  - ~33%–50% of non-neonatal HSV encephalitis is caused by primary HSV infection and ~50%–67% is caused by HSV reactivation.
  - Most common focal viral encephalitis in nonepidemic settings; most common sporadic fatal encephalitis.

Clinical Features
- Neonatal encephalitis characterized by seizures (focal and generalized), lethargy, irritability, tremors, anorexia, temperature instability, bulging fontanelle.
  - Central nervous system–only disease frequently begins in temporal lobe and then becomes bitemporal.
  - Encephalitis with disseminated disease more commonly is diffuse.
- Non-neonatal encephalitis characterized by fever and focal encephalitis with necrosis and hemorrhage.
  - Tropism for temporal lobe: Aphasia, anosmia, temporal lobe seizures, other focal findings.
  - Findings include headache, emesis, altered consciousness, bizarre behavior, personality changes, disorientation, ataxia, hallucinations, hemiparesis.
  - Focal findings are not always present; bilateral disease, widespread disease, or brainstem encephalitis may occur.
  - Elevated red blood cell count may be present in CSF; CSF protein levels may be normal early and increase over time.
  - Focal abnormalities on imaging studies, especially involving one or both temporal lobes, are suggestive of HSV disease. However, focal disease may occur with other viruses, other regions of the brain may be affected by HSV, and imaging may be normal in early HSV.
  - Temporal lobe focality on electroencephalography, especially with periodic lateralizing epileptiform discharges, is characteristic of HSV but is not specific.
  - Rapid progression is common; however, atypical and mild, slowly progressive cases are increasingly being reported.

Arboviruses
Epidemiology
- ~5% of viral meningitis and important cause of encephalitis.
- Prevalent during warm and/or wet seasons; incidence related to mosquito or tick exposure.
- Leading agents in the United States:
  - West Nile virus: U.S. outbreaks since late 1990s; July to December predominance. Lower incidence and severity in children. Risk factors for severe neurologic disease include older age and immune compromise.
  - La Crosse virus: Central, eastern United States. Incidence of encephalitis approximately equal to that of meningitis; affects children more than adults.
- St. Louis encephalitis virus: Central, western, southern United States. Incidence of encephalitis less than that of meningitis; lower incidence and severity of encephalitis in children.
- Japanese encephalitis virus: Most common cause of epidemic encephalitis worldwide; causes encephalitis more than meningitis. Prevalent in Asia and Australia; affects children more than adults.
- Other important viruses
  - Eastern equine encephalomyelitis virus: Causes encephalitis more than meningitis.
  - Western equine encephalomyelitis virus: Causes encephalitis more than meningitis.
  - Venezuelan equine encephalomyelitis: Causes encephalitis more than meningitis.
  - Colorado Tick Fever virus: Rocky Mountains; tickborne. Meningitis in up to 18% of cases; encephalitis uncommon.
  - Powassan, Rocio, Murray Valley, Kyasuma Forest, Jamestown Canyon, California encephalitis, tickborne encephalitis, Ilheus, Snowshoe Hare, Rift Valley viruses.

Continued

TABLE 1 Epidemiology and Clinical Features of Viral Meningitis and Encephalitis—Cont'd

Clinical Features
- West Nile virus
  - ~20% of infections are symptomatic; West Nile fever in majority of these infections.
  - Neurologic illness in ~1/150 infected; of these, meningitis in ~30% and encephalitis in ~65%. Neurologic manifestations also include acute asymmetrical flaccid paralysis, polyradiculitis, transverse myelitis, Guillain-Barré syndrome, optic neuritis, and chorioretinitis.
  - Encephalitis is characterized by altered consciousness, cranial nerve palsies (brainstem involvement), generalized or focal motor deficits (weakness, tremor, myoclonus), movement disorders, sensory deficits, and ataxia. Focal temporal lobe disease may mimic HSV. Case fatality rate ~10%.
  - Fever, emesis, maculopapular rash (especially in children) frequently accompany neurologic disease.
- Japanese and Eastern equine encephalitides
  - Thalamic, midbrain, basal ganglia, brainstem lesions characteristic.

Influenza Virus
Epidemiology
- Rare cause of meningitis.
- Cause of 8%–10% of encephalitis.
  - More commonly associated with influenza A than with influenza B.
  - Encephalitis may be acute or postinfectious.
  - Acute necrotizing encephalopathy reported primarily in 1- to 5-year-old children in Asia since the late 1990s.
- Neurologic spectrum includes Reye's syndrome (influenza B), myelitis, Guillain-Barré syndrome.

Clinical Features
- Acute necrotizing encephalopathy
  - Fever, altered consciousness, prolonged seizures; rapid progression to coma.
  - Elevated CSF protein, usually without pleocytosis.
  - Magnetic resonance imaging: Bilateral thalamic lesions and multifocal symmetrical lesions (brainstem, putamina, medulla, periventricular white matter, cerebellum).
  - Mortality ~30%; severe sequelae among survivors.

Varicella-Zoster Virus
Epidemiology and Clinical Features
- Chickenpox associated with cerebellar ataxia, meningitis, encephalitis, postinfectious encephalitis/ADEM, transverse myelitis, Guillain-Barré syndrome.
- Zoster associated with encephalitis, granulomatous hemiparesis, myelitis, cranial neuritis (including Bell's palsy). Neurologic complications may occur with rash, weeks to months after rash or without rash (especially in immune-compromised patients).

Epstein-Barr Virus
Epidemiology and Clinical Features
- Neurologic complications occur in 1%–5% of primary infections.
- Etiology of 2%–5% of acute viral encephalitis.
- Spectrum includes meningitis, encephalitis, ADEM, cranial nerve palsy (including Bell's palsy), transverse myelitis, and Guillain-Barré syndrome. Alice in Wonderland syndrome, consisting of visual seizures with metamorphopsia, may accompany encephalitis.
- Neurologic disease more frequent in immune-compromised hosts.
- Typical features of infectious mononucleosis, atypical lymphocytosis, and heterophile antibody often absent in Epstein-Barr virus neurologic syndromes.

Cytomegalovirus
Epidemiology and Clinical Features
- Encephalitis primarily in congenitally infected neonates and immune-compromised hosts.
- Insidious progression.

Human Herpesvirus 6
Epidemiology and Clinical Features
- Meningoencephalitis occasionally occurs with primary infection.
- Increased incidence of encephalitis in immune-compromised hosts.
- Confusion, headache, seizures may accompany encephalitis; disease may be focal and mimic HSV encephalitis.

Adenovirus
Epidemiology and Clinical Features
- Neurologic spectrum includes acute encephalitis, postinfectious encephalitis, Reye's syndrome-like encephalopathy, and transient encephalopathy.
  - Acute encephalitis is characterized by seizures, CSF pleocytosis, and severe disease.
  - Transient encephalopathy is characterized by obtundation, normal CSF, and complete recovery within several days.

Lymphocytic Choriomeningitis Virus
Epidemiology and Clinical Features
- Transmission by rodent secretions.
- Meningitis and encephalitis more commonly occur in developing countries.
- Spectrum includes encephalitis, hydrocephalus, transverse myelitis.

Human Immunodeficiency Virus
Epidemiology and Clinical Features
- Transient meningitis and, more rarely, encephalitis may accompany primary infection (acute retroviral syndrome).
- Chronic infection may be associated with subacute encephalopathy (loss of developmental milestones in young children, dementia).
- Acute encephalitis may accompany treatment failure during chronic infection (uncommon).

Continued

TABLE 1 Epidemiology and Clinical Features of Viral Meningitis and Encephalitis—Cont'd

Rabies Virus
Epidemiology and Clinical Features
- Relatively uncommon in United States; major sources are bats, raccoons, foxes, skunks.
- Important cause of encephalitis in developing countries; important sources are dogs and cats.
- Incubation period can vary from weeks to months to years. Pain, pruritus, or paresthesias at bite wound is followed by prodromal fever and anxiety and then by encephalitis.

Measles, Mumps, Rubella Viruses
Epidemiology and Clinical Features
- Meningitis occurs in ~30% of measles infections; measles also causes acute encephalitis, postinfectious encephalitis, and delayed subacute sclerosing panencephalitis.
- Mumps was the leading cause of meningitis in the prevaccine era.
- Meningitis and encephalitis due to each virus dramatically decreased with widespread immunization in developed countries.

Other Viral Agents
- Parainfluenza virus, respiratory syncytial virus, human metapneumovirus, rhinovirus, coronavirus, parvovirus B19, rotavirus, encephalomyocarditis virus, hepatitis C virus simian herpes B virus, human T-lymphotropic virus, JC virus, Lassa fever virus, yellow fever virus, Hendra virus, Nipah virus, Australian bat Lyssavirus.

Acute Disseminated Encephalomyelitis
Epidemiology
- Implicated in 10%–15% of cases of encephalitis in the United States.
- Increased incidence in infants and children.
- Onset days to weeks after respiratory tract infection (influenza, enteroviruses, measles, mumps, rubella, *Mycoplasma pneumoniae*, and others), gastroenteritis (rotavirus), and other infections (HSV, Epstein-Barr virus, varicella-zoster virus, human herpesvirus 6, cytomegalovirus).
- History of preceding infection or vaccination elicited in up to two thirds of cases.
- Winter–spring predominance in some series.

Clinical Features
- Diffuse, often multifocal symptoms reflecting regions of brain affected. Spectrum includes motor deficits, cranial nerve palsies, optic neuritis, cerebellar ataxia, altered consciousness, psychosis, seizures, transverse myelitis, peripheral neuritis.
- Multifocal, asymmetrical demyelinating lesions in imaging studies, with predilection for white matter.
- CSF cytology may be normal or show pleocytosis; CSF protein elevated in 50%–70%.
- Typically monophasic; occasionally relapses occur.
- Acute hemorrhagic leukoencephalitis is a rare entity representing the fulminant end of the spectrum. It primarily affects young adults and is characterized by seizures, coma, cerebral edema, and a rapid, often fatal course.

Abbreviations: ADEM = acute disseminated encephalomyelitis; CSF = cerebrospinal fluid; HSV = herpes simplex virus.

---

has better sensitivity than does computed tomography, especially early in disease. Characteristic imaging findings may suggest specific pathogens (see Table 1), and imaging can exclude alternative diagnoses; for example, a parameningeal focus or tumor. EEG is the most sensitive tool for confirming encephalitis and can distinguish infection from metabolic encephalopathy.

Viral culture, polymerase chain reaction (PCR), and serology are the major techniques for specific virologic diagnosis. Sensitivity of CSF viral culture is better for meningitis than for encephalitis. Sensitivity reaches 65% to 75% for EVs, and CSF culture may be positive in young infants lacking pleocytosis. CSF culture is positive in 25% to 40% of neonates with HSV encephalitis but in less than 2% of older children and adults. CSF PCR is generally more sensitive than culture in both meningitis and encephalitis. CSF PCR for EVs has greater than 95% sensitivity and specificity. Sensitivity and specificity of CSF PCR for HSV are between 75% and 100% in neonatal HSV encephalitis and 91% and 98% in older children and adults with HSV encephalitis. Importantly, HSV PCR may be falsely negative within the first 3 to 4 days of illness in up to 25% of cases; repeat testing 4 to 7 days later is generally positive. In many viral encephalitides, viral cultures, antigen detection tests, and PCR of non-CSF specimens have better yields than do CSF culture and PCR (e.g., throat and stool/rectum for EV 71, for which CSF culture and PCR are more often negative, and respiratory specimens for influenza, adenovirus, and other respiratory viruses). Detection of serum and CSF antibodies can be performed for many viruses (e.g., most arboviruses and lymphocytic choriomeningitis virus), frequently requiring acute and convalescent specimens. Serum and CSF IgM assays can be diagnostic for West Nile virus, Japanese encephalitis virus, Epstein-Barr virus, and EV 71. A brain biopsy should be considered in a patient with symptoms that are progressive or do not improve, with an uncertain diagnosis, and with a focal, accessible lesion.

Treatment

The mainstay of therapy for viral meningitis and encephalitis is supportive care. In patients in whom there is difficulty distinguishing between bacterial and viral meningitis (e.g., young children, especially those younger than 1 year), hospitalization and parenteral antibiotics (e.g., vancomycin [Vancocin] plus a third-generation cephalosporin such as cefotaxime [Claforan] or ceftriaxone [Rocephin]) are administered until bacterial cultures are negative and/or an alternative diagnosis is made. Additionally, newborns or other immune-compromised patients with EV meningitis may require supportive therapy for severe disseminated disease (e.g., hepatitis, coagulopathy, or myocarditis). A presumptive diagnosis of viral meningitis can often be made in older children and adults who are not very ill based on clinical and CSF examination (low-grade pleocytosis with mononuclear predominance initially or 8–24 hours later, normal to slightly depressed glucose concentration, normal to slightly increased protein level). Lumbar puncture may alleviate symptoms such as headache, irritability, and emesis. Therefore, in older children and adults, hospitalization and/or empirical antibiotic treatment are indicated for patients who appear ill, including those requiring parenteral hydration and/or analgesics, those in whom viral and bacterial infection cannot be readily distinguished, and those who manifest findings of encephalitis. Presumptive therapy for *Mycobacterium tuberculosis* may be indicated if the exposure history, clinical presentation, CSF examination, and imaging findings are suggestive of this agent.

There are few proven specific antiviral therapies for meningitis and encephalitis. Acyclovir[1] (Zovirax) can hasten recovery from HSV meningitis, although HSV meningitis without encephalitis generally has an excellent outcome without antiviral treatment. Valacyclovir[1] (Valtrex) and famciclovir[1] (Famvir) are also available for oral therapy of HSV meningitis associated with genital HSV in immune-competent patients.

---

[1]Not FDA approved for this indication.

CURRENT DIAGNOSIS

Differential diagnosis of viral meningitis and encephalitis is broad and includes:

- Bacteria: *Streptococcus pneumoniae, Neisseria meningitidis, Haemophilus influenzae, Listeria monocytogenes, Mycobacterium tuberculosis, Borrelia burgdorferi, Mycoplasma pneumoniae, Mycoplasma hominis, Bartonella henselae*, syphilis, leptospirosis, brucellosis, rickettsial and ehrlichial infections
- Parasites: Neurocysticercosis, toxoplasmosis, amebic encephalitis
- Fungi: *Cryptococcus neoformans, Coccidioides immitis*
- Parameningeal focus: Brain abscess or subdural or epidural empyema
- Kawasaki disease
- Sarcoidosis
- Autoimmune disease: Systemic lupus erythematosus, cerebral vasculitis, Wegener's granulomatosis, Hashimoto's disease
- Medication-induced meningitis: Nonsteroidal anti-inflammatory drugs, sulfa antibiotics, immune globulin, cytosine arabinoside (Cytarabine), muromonab-CD3 (Orthoclone OKT3), carbamazepine (Tegretol)
- Metabolic derangements: Inborn errors of metabolism, leukodystrophy, uremia, hepatic encephalopathy, Reye's syndrome
- Cerebrovascular hemorrhage and/or infarct
- Malignancy
- Drug toxicity (e.g., neuroleptic malignant syndrome)
- Toxins

Historical information may suggest specific etiologic viruses:

- Respiratory symptoms: Influenza virus, adenovirus, other respiratory viruses
- Gastrointestinal symptoms: Rotavirus
- Family exposure: Influenza virus, EV
- Seasonality and prevalent diseases in the community: EV, West Nile virus, other arboviruses, influenza virus, other respiratory viruses
- Travel to areas with endemic or epidemic disease: West Nile virus, EV 71, Japanese encephalitis virus, other arboviruses
- Animal exposure: Rabies virus, lymphocytic choriomeningitis virus
- Mosquito exposure: West Nile virus, other arboviruses
- Tick exposure: Colorado tick fever virus, Powassan virus
- Recreational activities: Spelunking-associated bat exposure and rabies infection, hiking-associated mosquito and tick exposure and arbovirus infection

Useful laboratory evaluations for viral meningitis and encephalitis include CSF examination, imaging (especially magnetic resonance imaging), and electroencephalography. Imaging abnormalities may suggest certain pathogens (see Table 1). CSF PCR, serum and CSF IgM assays, and viral culture/antigen detection/PCR of mucosal specimens are especially useful specific diagnostic tests.

- CSF PCR is a more sensitive technique than viral culture for detection of viruses such as EVs; HSV; varicella-zoster virus, cytomegalovirus, human herpesvirus 6, Epstein-Barr virus, and JC virus in immune-compromised patients; measles virus; parvovirus B19; and human immunodeficiency virus. CSF PCR for other viruses, such as adenovirus, influenza virus, and arboviruses (including West Nile virus), has low or variable sensitivity. PCR of saliva has high sensitivity for rabies virus (other testing includes immunostain of a nape of neck biopsy, corneal impression, buccal mucosa, or brain tissue and serology).
- The etiology of encephalitis is elusive in many cases. Extensive investigations ultimately are able to identify a specific etiologic agent in only 25% to 65% of cases.

Abbreviations: CSF = cerebrospinal fluid; EV = enterovirus; PCR = polymerase chain reaction.

For children and adults with encephalitis, empirical therapy with acyclovir (30 mg/kg/day up to 45–60 mg/kg/day intravenously divided every 8 hours) should generally be initiated pending diagnostic studies, particularly in the presence of fever and any evidence of focal neurologic abnormality (clinical examination, imaging, or electroencephalography). Treatment for 14 to 21 days* is indicated if HSV infection is confirmed or if clinical and diagnostic findings are strongly suggestive in the absence of other proven etiologies; a 21-day course is generally favored for more severe disease. Acyclovir (60 mg/kg/day intravenously divided every 8 hours) should be presumptively administered to newborns with encephalitis with focal or generalized findings. Treatment of proven or highly suspect neonatal HSV encephalitis is generally continued for 21 days and until an end-of-therapy CSF PCR is negative, although proof that extending therapy until the PCR is negative is beneficial is lacking. Whether higher doses (60 mg/kg/day) or longer courses (21 days) confer additional benefit and are safe outside the neonatal period is not established. Relapse within the first 1 to 3 months after therapy of neonatal and childhood/adult HSV encephalitis has been reported with variable incidence, in some cases correlated with lower daily dose and treatment duration. Whether relapses reflect active viral replication or an immune-mediated phenomenon is controversial, although CSF PCR positivity in some cases suggests the former.

Whether encephalitis associated with varicella-zoster virus is due more often to direct viral infection or an immune-mediated parainfectious process is not established. Thus, although acyclovir is frequently used for varicella-zoster virus encephalitis, including cerebellar ataxia, the role of antiviral therapy is unproven. Ganciclovir (Cytovene) and foscarnet (Foscavir) are used for meningoencephalitis in immune-compromised hosts caused by cytomegalovirus and human herpesvirus 6.

Pleconaril (Picovir) is an experimental agent that has been studied for treatment of EV meningitis and encephalitis, including chronic meningoencephalitis in hypogammaglobulinemic patients, with some evidence of benefit; however, the agent is not currently available. Intraventricular, intrathecal, and intravenous administration of immune globulin[1] have been used to suppress or stabilize chronic EV meningoencephalitis in immune-compromised patients. The mainstays of management of severe EV 71 neurologic disease are close monitoring, fluid restriction, osmotic diuretics, and cardiorespiratory support. Various agents, including pleconaril, interferon α,[1] intravenous immune globulin, and corticosteroids have been tried, but none has been proven to be effective.

---

*Exceeds duration recommended by the manufacturer.

[1]Not FDA approved for this indication.

CURRENT THERAPY

- General supportive measures for patients with severe meningitis or encephalitis include:
  - Analgesics for headache, antiemetics, intravenous fluids and medications for patients with depressed consciousness, anticonvulsants for seizures, provision of a quiet environment
  - Intensive care for severely ill patients, including tracheal intubation for airway protection, respiratory support, cardiorespiratory monitoring
  - Mild fluid restriction for cerebral edema or inappropriate antidiuretic hormone secretion
  - Head of bed elevation, hyperventilation, osmotic (mannitol) and loop diuretics, and control of temperature, pain, and seizures for increased intracranial pressure
- Specific antiviral agents available for meningoencephalitis include acyclovir (Zovirax) for HSV and varicella-zoster virus, ganciclovir (Cytovene) for cytomegalovirus and human herpesvirus 6, foscarnet (Foscavir) for cytomegalovirus and human herpesvirus 6, amantadine (Symmetrel) for susceptible influenza A, rimantadine (Flumadine) for susceptible influenza A, and oseltamivir (Tamiflu) for susceptible influenza A and B.
- Rehabilitative therapy and neurodevelopmental follow-up are frequently necessary after the acute phase of encephalitis regardless of the etiologic agent.
- Prognosis for viral meningitis is generally favorable without long-term sequelae, although fatigue, decreased concentration, and irritability may last for several weeks.
- Prognosis for viral encephalitis is variable and may be difficult to predict, especially early in the course of illness. In general, a worse prognosis is associated with extremes of age (infants <1 year and older adults), specific etiologies (HSV, enterovirus 71, West Nile virus, Japanese encephalitis virus, rabies), more severe illness (lower Glasgow Coma Scale) and extensive brain involvement, and, in the case of HSV, longer duration prior to initiation of treatment.

Abbreviation: HSV = herpes simplex virus.

Influenzal encephalitis is frequently treated with oral antivirals, including amantadine (Symmetrel) for influenza A (if susceptible), rimantadine (Flumadine) for influenza A (if susceptible), and oseltamivir (Tamiflu) for influenza A (if susceptible), and B; corticosteroids and immune globulin[1] have also been tried. However, none of these agents has been proven to be effective for influenzal encephalitis. A combination of antiviral treatment, corticosteroids, and intravenous immune globulin has been suggested to reduce mortality due to influenzal acute necrotizing encephalopathy. There currently are no established therapies for West Nile virus encephalitis. Ribavirin (Rebetol),[1] interferon, high-titer immune globulin, and corticosteroids have been used, and therapeutic trials are currently ongoing. No specific therapies have been proven to be effective for encephalitis due to other arboviruses or for rabies; successful use of coma-inducing therapy plus the antivirals ribavirin and amantadine was reported in one patient with rabies encephalitis. Corticosteroids, intravenous immune globulin, and plasmapheresis have been used for acute disseminated encephalomyelitis, but efficacy trials have not been performed.

[1]Not FDA approved for this indication.

REFERENCES

Beaman MH, Wesselingh SL. Acute community-acquired meningitis and encephalitis. Med J Aust 2002;176:389–96.

Chang L, Hsia S, Wu C, et al. Outcome of enterovirus 71 infections with or without stage-based management: 1998–2002. Pediatr Infect Dis J 2004;23:327–31.

Glaser CA, Gilliam S, Schnurr D, et al. In search of encephalitis etiologies: Diagnostic challenges in the California encephalitis project, 1998–2000. Clin Infect Dis 2003;36:731–42.

Huang C, Morse D, Slater B, et al. Multiple-year experience in the diagnosis of viral central nervous system infections with a panel of polymerase chain reaction assays for detection of 11 viruses. Clin Infect Dis 2004;39:630–5.

Kennedy PGE. Viral encephalitis: causes, differential diagnosis, and management. J Neurol Neurosurg Psychiatry 2004;75(Suppl 1):i10–5.

Kimberlin DW. Herpes simplex virus infections of the central nervous system. Semin Pediatr Infect Dis 2003;14:83–9.

Rotbart HA. Viral meningitis. Semin Neurol 2000;20:277–92.

Watson JT, Gerber SI. West Nile virus: A brief review. Pediatr Infect Dis J 2004;23:355–8.

Weitkamp J, Spring MD, Brogan T, et al. Influenza A virus-associated acute necrotizing encephalopathy in the United States. Pediatr Infect Dis J 2004;23:259–63.

Whitley RJ, Gnann JW. Viral encephalitis: Familiar infections and emerging pathogens. Lancet 2002;359:507–14.

Willoughby RE Jr, Tieves KS, Hoffman GM, et al. Survival after treatment of rabies with induction of coma. N Engl J Med 2005;352:2508–14.

Multiple Sclerosis

Method of
Robert J. Fox, MD

Multiple sclerosis (MS) is a recurrent, chronic demyelinating disorder affecting the central nervous system (CNS): the brain, spinal cord, and optic nerves. MS affects approximately 400,000 people in the United States and 2.5 million worldwide.

The pathology of MS classically has been thought to involve primarily CD4+ helper T cells directed against the myelin sheath around axons. However, recent studies have suggested an important role of CD8+ cytotoxic T cells, monocytes, and even antibody-producing B cells in the pathogenesis of MS. MS was originally thought to only affect the myelin sheath that surrounds and protects nerve fibers, but studies have identified significant neuronal injury and atrophy early in the disease course.

The accumulation of tissue injury over time makes MS the most common nontraumatic cause of neurologic disability among young adults. The development of effective therapies that slow the progression of tissue damage and physical disability emphasizes the importance of accurate diagnosis and early treatment.

Symptoms and Classification

There are two general types of clinical symptoms associated with MS: clinical relapses and gradual progression of disability. Clinical relapses are subacute in onset, typically developing over several days or weeks and stabilizing or resolving over several weeks to months. Symptoms can include any neurologic function but typically involve blurry or double vision, numbness, weakness, or dyscoordination. Relapses usually have no precipitants, although infections are sometimes associated with relapses. Clinical relapses herald the onset of the relapsing-remitting form of MS (RRMS), which accounts for about 85% of MS patients.

After 10 to 20 years of RRMS, clinical relapses become relatively infrequent, being replaced by gradually progressive neurologic symptoms (Fig. 1). This form of the disease most commonly manifests as a

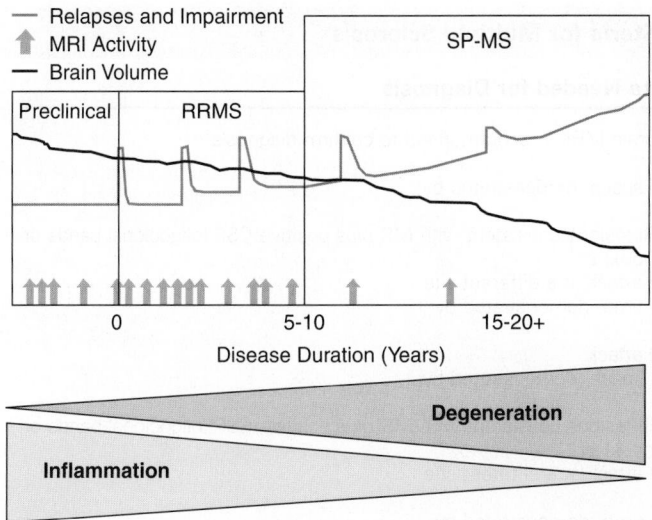

FIGURE 1. Typical clinical and MRI course of multiple sclerosis. MRI activity (*vertical arrows*) indicates an inflammatory lesion measured on brain MRI. MRI activity typically is more frequent than clinical relapses (*spikes* in clinical disability). Loss of brain volume, or atrophy, is measured on MRI and indicates permanent tissue damage. The early inflammatory activity is thought to be replaced later by a neurodegenerative process. MRI = magnetic resonance imaging; MS = multiple sclerosis; SP = secondary progressive; RR = relapsing-remitting. (Adapted from Fox RJ, Bethoux F, Goldman MD, Cohen JA: Multiple sclerosis: Advances in understanding, diagnosing, and treating the underlying disease. Cleve Clin J Med 2006;73(1):91–102.)

myelopathy involving the legs and later the arms, with progressive weakness, numbness, spasticity, and lack of coordination. This later stage of MS is called *secondary progressive MS* (SPMS), indicating that it has followed an initial relapsing-remitting form of the disease. SPMS is thought to represent an accelerated degenerative process, initiated during the relapsing-remitting stage of the disease. Current disease-modifying therapies are most effective in the RRMS stage, with little efficacy in SPMS.

Gradually progressive symptoms may also be the initial manifesting symptoms of the disease, a form of disease called *primary progressive MS* (PPMS). PPMS accounts for about 10% of MS patients and, similar to SPMS, has limited treatment options to slow progressive disability.

In about 2% to 4% of patients, inflammation is limited to the optic nerves and spinal cord and is called neuromyelitis optica, or Devic's disease. Brain involvement is unusual in this form of the disease, appearing as large, atypical lesions extending from the surface of the ventricles. Spinal cord involvement extends over many segments, sometimes involving the entire length of the spinal cord. Pathology shows necrotic destruction of nervous tissues, which explains the significant residual neurologic disability persisting after clinical episodes. Recent studies have identified the aquaporin-4 water ion channel as the autoimmune target in neuromyelitis optica, and many clinicians now differentiate neuromyelitis optica as a disease separate from MS.

Diagnosis

The diagnosis of MS is made through an assimilation of clinical history, neurologic examination, and paraclinical studies. Diagnostic criteria have shifted over time, but the basic elements remain unchanged: identification of multiple episodes of demyelination, disseminated in both time and space throughout the central nervous system, with other etiologies excluded. The most basic scenario is two episodes of demyelination affecting two different areas of the central nervous system and leaving findings on neurologic examination.

CURRENT DIAGNOSIS

Recurrent CNS Demyelination, Disseminated in Time and Space

- Dissemination demonstrated clinically or on MRI
- Typical lesions on brain or spine MRI
- Inflammatory CSF (when needed)
- Visual evoked potentials (when needed)

MRI Lesions

- Periventricular
- Perpendicular to the lateral ventricle
- Corpus callosum
- Subcortical white matter
- Deep white matter (nonspecific)
- Hypointense on T1 images
- Gadolinium-enhancing lesions
- Posterior fossa, particularly cerebellum
- Spinal cord

CNS = central nervous system; CSF = cerebrospinal fluid; MRI = magnetic resonance imaging.

For example, transverse myelitis (inflammation of the spinal cord) and optic neuritis (inflammation of the optic nerve), the onset of each separated by at least 1 month, would fulfill the diagnostic criteria if objective findings were observed during the episodes or afterward. Transverse myelitis can leave hyperreflexia, and optic neuritis can leave disc pallor on fundoscopy or delayed visual evoked potentials. Two episodes of optic neuritis or transverse myelitis also fulfill criteria, so long as the two episodes involve different eyes or different regions of the spinal cord.

Current diagnostic criteria also allow the diagnosis to be made after a single episode of demyelination, often called a clinically isolated syndrome (Table 1). Dissemination can be fulfilled through magnetic resonance imaging (MRI) studies, with different requirements for dissemination in time and space. Dissemination in space requires a minimum number of lesions seen on brain and spine MRI. Dissemination in time requires an MRI 3 months or more after the onset of the clinically isolated syndrome showing either a gadolinium-enhancing lesion at a location different from the location of the initial event or a new T2 lesion (seen on T2-weighted MRI scan) compared with an MRI done at least 1 month after the initial event.

Brain MRI has taken on an increasingly important role in both the diagnosis and management of MS. Typical MS lesions are located in the periventricular white matter, as well as the subcortical white matter and posterior fossa (cerebellum) (Figs. 2 and 3). Lesions involving the deep white matter are also typical of MS, but they are relatively nonspecific, being seen commonly in patients with vascular risk factors, migraine, or even just normal aging. MS lesions are typically round or ovoid and often oriented perpendicular to the lateral ventricles—Dawson's fingers. These perpendicular lesions are best seen on sagittal T2-weighted imaging, such as fluid-attenuated inversion recovery (FLAIR) MRI. Also adding to the specificity of MS diagnosis is gadolinium enhancement and lesions in the spinal cord, although there are no pathognomonic findings on MRI for MS (Fig. 4).

The diagnosis of PPMS requires 1 year of progressive symptoms and a combination of MRI findings and inflammatory cerebrospinal fluid studies. Proposed diagnostic criteria for neuromyelitis optica require optic neuritis, acute myelitis, and two of the following three supportive criteria: contiguous spinal cord lesion extending at least 3 vertebral segments, brain MRI not meeting diagnostic criteria for MS, and positive neuromyelitis optica immunoglobulin G (NMO-IgG) serology.

Evaluation of cerebrospinal fluid used to be an essential element in the diagnostic evaluation of MS, but its limited sensitivity and specificity and the widespread availability of MRI have reduced the importance of cerebrospinal fluid studies. Currently, cerebrospinal

TABLE 1 2005 Revision to the McDonald Diagnostic Criteria for Multiple Sclerosis

Clinical Presentation	Additional Data Needed for Diagnosis
Two or more attacks; objective clinical evidence of two or more lesions	None, although brain MRI is recommended to confirm diagnosis
Two or more attacks; objective clinical evidence of one lesion	Dissemination in space, demonstrated by: MRI* *or* Two or more MRI lesions consistent with MS *plus* positive CSF (oligoclonal bands or elevated IgG index) *or* A second clinical attack at a different site
One attack; objective clinical evidence of two or more lesions	Dissemination in time, demonstrated by: MRI† *or* A second clinical attack
One attack; objective clinical evidence of one lesion (clinically isolated syndrome)	Dissemination in space, demonstrated by: MRI* *or* Two or more MRI lesions consistent with MS *plus* positive CSF (oligoclonal bands or elevated IgG index) *or* A second clinical attack at a different site *plus* Dissemination in time, demonstrated by: MRI† *or* A second clinical attack
Insidious neurologic progression suggesting MS (primary progressive MS)	One year of neurologic progression and two of the following: Positive brain MRI (9 T2 lesions or ≥4 T2 lesions with positive visual evoked potentials) Positive spinal cord MRI (≥2 focal T2 lesions) Inflammatory CSF (oligoclonal bands or elevated IgG index)

Adapted from Polman CH, Reingold SC, Edan G et al: Diagnostic criteria for multiple sclerosis: 2005 revisions to the "McDonald Criteria." Ann Neurol 2005;58:840–846.

*MRI criteria for dissemination in space require three of the following: ≥1 gadolinium-enhancing lesion or ≥9 T2 hyperintense lesions in the brain or spine; ≥1 one infratentorial brain lesion or spine lesion; ≥1 juxtacortical lesion; ≥3 periventricular lesions.

†MRI criteria for dissemination in time requires either gadolinium-enhancing lesion ≥3 months after the onset of the initial clinical event and in a different site corresponding to the initial event *or* a new T2 lesion compared with a reference scan done at least 30 days after the onset of the initial clinical event.

CSF = cerebrospinal fluid; IgG = immunoglobulin G; MRI = magnetic resonance imaging; MS = multiple sclerosis.

fluid is useful when there are only a few lesions on brain MRI or in the diagnosis of primary progressive MS.

Evoked potential studies are used to evaluate neural transmission, which is impaired within demyelinated tissue. Visual evoked potentials are useful in either confirming previous optic neuritis or identifying a previous subclinical episode of optic neuritis. Auditory brainstem and somatosensory evoked potentials can also detect impaired neural transmission, but their poor sensitivity and specificity significantly reduce their usefulness.

Although MS is a diagnosis of exclusion, the recognition of classic MRI changes have helped improve diagnostic accuracy. Many symptoms of MS overlap with other disorders, such as the fatigue, numbness, paresthesias, and pain seen in fibromyalgia and chronic fatigue syndrome. In contrast to MS, these nonspecific symptoms tend to wax and wane over hours and days and to migrate through different parts of the body. The diagnosis of MS should be made only with extreme caution in patients with these relatively nonspecific symptoms, particularly in the absence of objective neurologic findings.

Similarly, T2 hyperintensities on brain MRI are relatively common, being seen in up to 7% of healthy adults. These nonspecific lesions are typically located in the deep frontal and parietal white matter, sparing the periventricular region, corpus callosum, cerebellum, temporal lobe,

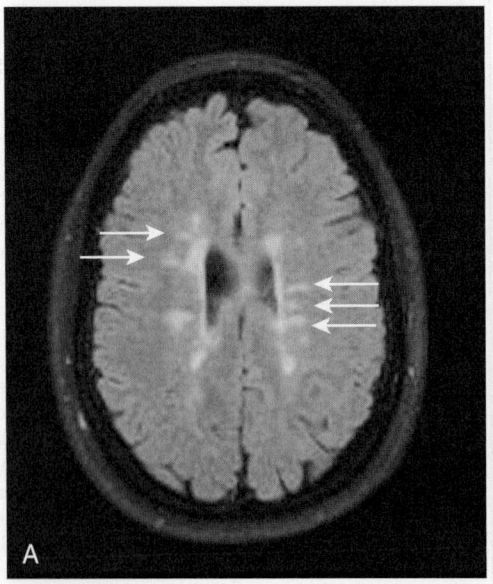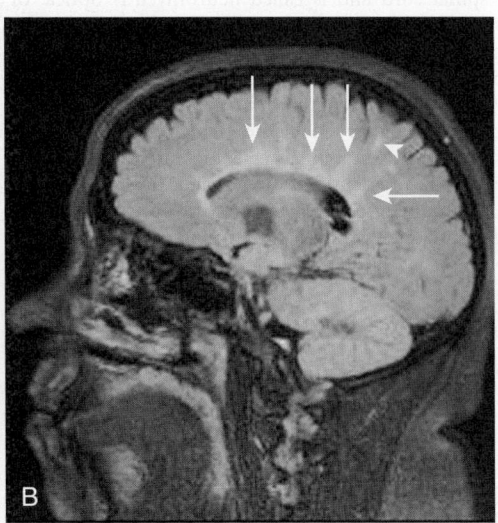

FIGURE 2. Axial (**A**) and sagittal (**B**) FLAIR MR images of the brain, illustrating the periventricular nature of demyelinating lesions (*arrows*), often perpendicular to the lateral ventricle. A subcortical lesion can also be seen (*arrowhead* in **B**). FLAIR = fluid-attenuated inversion recovery.

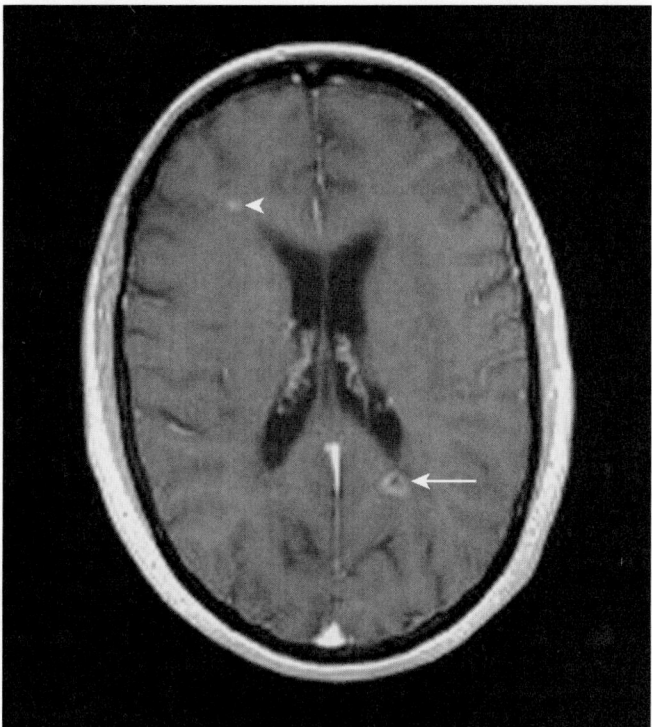

FIGURE 3. Axial post-gadolinium T1 MRI of the brain, illustrating areas of active inflammation. The *arrow* indicates a ring-enhancing lesion, which usually represents reactivation of an old multiple sclerosis lesion. The *arrowhead* indicates a homogeneous enhancing lesion, which usually represents a new focus of inflammation.

and spinal cord. Brain MRIs from patients with vascular risk factors (smoking, hypertension, diabetes) and migraine headaches commonly have these nonspecific findings. Despite their commonness, radiology reports typically include demyelination in the differential diagnosis, which leads to needless referrals and work-ups. In a patient without specific neurologic symptoms or findings on neurologic examination, these nonspecific findings need no further evaluation.

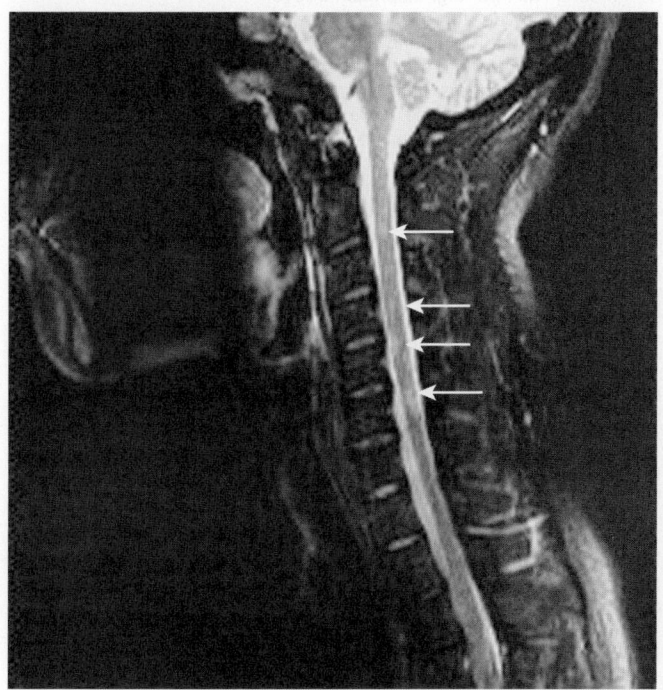

FIGURE 4. Sagittal short tau inversion recovery (STIR) MRI of the cervical spinal cord, illustrating demyelinating lesions (*arrows*).

Differential Diagnosis

When MS manifests in a classic fashion—multiple discrete episodes of CNS inflammation, disseminated in time and space, with periventricular T2 lesions and gadolinium enhancement—the differential diagnosis is very limited. There are no required exclusionary tests, although many clinicians would consider blood tests for antinuclear antibodies (ANA), vitamin B$_{12}$, and (where geographically indicated) Lyme serology. When the presentation is atypical, the differential diagnosis is extremely broad, including a wide variety of other inflammatory disorders, infections, metabolic disorders, and neoplastic disorders. Atypical presentations of MS should be a red flag that prompts careful consideration of other etiologies. MS remains a diagnosis of exclusion, requiring continuing vigilance for alternative diagnoses. Recognition of neuromyelitis optica is important because its long-term treatments are different from those for typical RRMS.

Treatment

Treatment of MS can be divided into three broad categories: treatment of relapses, long-term disease-modifying medications, and symptomatic management. These three treatment pathways should be considered in parallel, with the clinical picture driving the priority for different pathways. Treatment of progressive MS is limited and typically focuses on symptomatic management, optimizing current neurologic functioning. Devic's disease also requires a different treatment approach.

RELAPSES

The development of acute or subacute neurologic symptoms suggests active inflammation within the CNS. Most clinical relapses recover spontaneously, regardless of treatment. Two lines of evidence argue for treating clinical relapses with corticosteroids. First, controlled trials have found that treatment with corticosteroids hastens recovery from relapse, although final level of clinical recovery is not improved with corticosteroids. Second, pathologic studies have found more than 10,000 transected axons/mm^3 in areas of active inflammation. This irreversible axonal injury argues for aggressive curtailment of inflammation to minimize permanent tissue injury.

Therefore, most clinicians treat a clinical relapse with a course of corticosteroids. A typical relapse treatment regimen is 3 days of 1 g/day intravenous methylprednisolone (Solu-Medrol), with or without an oral prednisone taper. Treatments of up to 5 days are sometimes used with severe relapses or when a second course is needed for the same relapse. Typical side effects include emotional lability (particularly irritability), fluid retention, increased appetite, and metallic taste. Hypokalemia and hyperkalemia are also occasionally seen. Corticosteroids are relatively well absorbed and tolerated when orally administered, although comparator trials with intravenous formulations have not yet been reported.

 CURRENT THERAPY

Clinical Relapse

- Evaluate for infections
- Methylprednisolone (Solu-Medrol)

Long-Term Disease Therapy

- Interferon-β-1
- Glatiramer acetate (Copaxone)
- Mitoxantrone (Novantrone)
- Natalizumab (Tysabri)

Symptomatic Therapy

- Medications
- Physical therapy
- Assistive devices
- Psychotherapy

Low or moderate doses of oral corticosteroids are used by some clinicians, particularly for mild relapses. The Optic Neuritis Treatment Trial suggested that low-dose steroids were associated with a shorter interval to the next attack, compared with placebo. Accordingly, high-dose corticosteroids are preferred wherever possible. Oral administration of high doses of corticosteroids is a reasonable administration option for patients in whom intravenous administration is not possible.

Treatment of a relapse should also include evaluation and treatment of infection. Infections can precipitate a relapse and can prevent later recovery. Bladder infections are the most common infection needing treatment. Patients reporting an incomplete response to a treatment with corticosteroids should also be evaluated for infection.

Recovery from a clinical relapse usually starts within a couple days of corticosteroid initiation and continues for many months. When relapses do not respond sufficiently to corticosteroid treatment, plasma exchange or immune globulin (Gammagard)[1] should be considered.

Relapse treatment has traditionally targeted clinical symptoms. However, active inflammation is sometimes observed as multiple gadolinium-enhancing lesions on MRI in patients without any symptoms. The severe tissue injury observed in pathologic studies of active

---

[1]Not FDA approved for this indication.

---

inflammation suggest that this MRI relapse would benefit from a course of corticosteroids.

LONG-TERM DISEASE

Currently, there are six long-term disease-modifying therapies approved throughout the world for the treatment of relapsing forms of MS, as well as several other treatments that have some data supporting their efficacy. All of these treatments are only partially effective when assessed in large groups of patients, although in individual patients, disease may be completely controlled by any of these therapies. All approved treatments are given by either injection or infusion, and each has its own specific side effects. The four injection therapies (three interferon-β-1 preparations, and glatiramer acetate [Copaxone]) are standard first-line treatments for RRMS. The chemotherapy mitoxantrone (Novantrone) and the monoclonal antibody natalizumab (Tysabri) are reserved for patients who fail or are intolerant to the injectable therapies (Table 2).

INTERFERON-β-1

The same endogenous cytokine made by the body to fight viral infections is produced in vitro for exogenous administration in MS. Originally used when MS was hypothesized to be caused by a viral infection, its precise mechanism of action in MS is not fully

---

TABLE 2 Side Effects and Complications of Common Therapies Used in Multiple Sclerosis

Side Effects and Complications	Comments
Corticosteroids	
Insomnia	Over-the-counter sleep aids, short-acting benzodiazepines
Altered mood: irritability, restlessness, rarely mania	
Fluid retention	Minimize salt intake
Potassium depletion (rare)	Increase dietary potassium (bananas, orange juice)
Indigestion	H_2-blockers; avoid NSAIDs
Metallic taste	Candy might help
Interferon-β1	
Flulike symptoms (myalgias, chills, fever, headache)	Start at low (Rebif) of partial (Avonex, Betaseron) dose and gradually escalate to full dose over 1–2 mo
	Long-acting NSAIDs, e.g., naproxen (Aleve)
	Changing to powder formulation (Avonex preparation only)
Hepatic and bone marrow irritation	Periodic blood test monitoring
Skin reactions (subcutaneous preparations only)	Allow medication to warm to room temperature before injection
	Witch hazel (Hamamelis water) or diphenhydramine cream (Benadryl)
	Lidocaine 2.5% + prilocaine 2.5% cream (EMLA)
	Ice site before and after injection
	Occasionally causes abscess
Worsened preexisting conditions, such as depression, spasticity, pain	Targeted symptomatic management
	Consider changing to non-interferon therapy
Glatiramer Acetate (Copaxone)	
Skin reactions, pain	Allow medication to warm to room temperature before injection
	Witch hazel or diphenydramine cream
	Lidocaine 2.5% + prilocaine 2.5% cream (EMLA)
	Ice site before and after injection
	Administer after a hot shower
Self-limited postinjection systemic reaction: chest tightness, dyspnea, palpitations, flushing, anxiety	Always self-limited
	Does not need treatment discontinuation
Mitoxantrone (Novantrone)	
Cardiotoxicity	Monitor with echocardiogram or MUGA scan before every dose
Leukemia	May be seen years after treatment is discontinued
Natalizumab (Tysabri)	
Hypersensitivity reaction: rash, pruritus, dyspnea	May be seen up to 1 h after infusion is complete
	Immediately and permanently discontinue treatment
Progressive multifocal leukoencephalopathy	Clinical vigilance for changes in personality or cognition, weakness, ataxia
	Further evaluate with brain MRI and cerebrospinal fluid, if indicated

EMLA = eutectic mixture of local anesthetics; MRI = magnetic resonance imaging; MUGA = multiple uptake gated acquisition; NSAID = nonsteroidal antiinflammatory drug.

understood. Three interferon-β-1 therapies are available. All three were found in phase III clinical trials to similarly reduce the rate of clinical relapses by 31% to 32% compared with placebo. All three preparations led to a robust reduction in new lesions on brain MRI. Where properly powered placebo-controlled trials were performed, sustained progression of disability was also reduced by interferon-β-1 treatment.

Common side effects of interferon-β-1 therapy include flulike symptoms and transient transaminitis and bone marrow suppression. Flulike symptoms are relieved by nonsteroidal antiinflammatory drugs (NSAIDs). Interferon therapies are given in the evening, so that patients can sleep through the flu symptoms. The long-acting NSAID naproxen (Aleve) is particularly helpful, because its dosing schedule provides full overnight efficacy. Periodic monitoring of liver and bone marrow function is recommended but rarely leads to discontinuation of interferon therapy. Other possible side effects include depression and worsening of preexisting weakness, spasticity, pain, and headaches.

One interferon-β-1 preparation is given by intramuscular injection: interferon-β-1a (Avonex), taken once weekly. The other two interferon-β-1 preparations are given by subcutaneous injection: interferon-β-1a (Rebif), given thrice weekly; and interferon-β-1b (Betaseron), given every other day. Injection site reactions can be seen with the subcutaneous preparations, rarely leading to abscess formation.

GLATIRAMER ACETATE

Glatiramer acetate is a random polypeptide 80 to 120 amino acids in length, derived using the four amino acids contained in brain proteins thought to be an common autoimmunogenic target in MS. First developed to induce an animal model of MS, its surprising protective effect led to successful clinical trials in MS. Similar to the interferon therapies, glatiramer acetate therapy is associated with a 29% reduction in the rate of clinical relapses and significant reduction in new brain lesions on MRI.

Common side effects of glatiramer acetate are primarily injection-site reactions. There are no associated flulike symptoms or hepatic or bone marrow disturbance. About 10% of patients treated with glatiramer acetate report a systemic reaction involving transient flushing, chest pain, palpitations, anxiety, and dyspnea shortly after injection. This reaction usually lasts only several minutes and is not thought to be related to cardiac ischemia. The reaction is always self-limited, and treatment discontinuation is not necessary.

OPTIMAL INITIAL TREATMENT

As suggested by their similar efficacy in separate placebo-controlled trials, open-label comparison studies have generally found the four injectable therapies to have relatively comparable efficacies. A few head-to-head studies suggested that the more frequently administered subcutaneous interferon-β-1 preparations might have slightly greater efficacy than the less frequently administered intramuscular interferon-β-1 preparations. In one trial, this advantage was limited to the first 6 months of therapy, after which the efficacies were similar. The lack of difference among therapy results after 6 months may be explained by the development of anti-interferon antibodies, which are much more common with subcutaneous interferon-β-1 (25%–35%) than intramuscular interferon-β-1 (2%–4%). These antibodies typically develop in the first 6 to 24 months of treatment and have been shown to abrogate both the biological effect and therapeutic benefit of interferon-β-1. In addition, bone marrow and hepatic toxicity is greater in subcutaneous interferon-β-1 preparations, most likely due to their higher amount of administered interferon.

Early MRI studies suggested that interferon-β-1 therapy had a greater reduction in the development of new brain lesions than glatiramer acetate, leading many clinicians to suspect greater clinical efficacy from interferon-β-1 therapy, too. However, three separate head-to-head studies comparing glatiramer acetate to two different interferon-β-1 preparations failed to show significant differences between the treatments in primary and most secondary endpoints.

Altogether, these studies suggest that all four of the injectable therapies have relatively similar efficacies, and any of them are reasonable first-line treatment for relapsing MS. The choice of therapy should be driven by individual patient preferences, such as frequent (every 1–3 days) subcutaneous versus less frequent (weekly) intramuscular injections, tolerance for skin reactions, and potential aggravation of preexisting conditions. Ongoing symptoms such as weakness, spasticity, depression, and pain syndromes suggest use of glatiramer acetate over interferon-β-1.

ADVANCED THERAPIES

Mitoxantrone

A synthetic anthracenedione, mitoxantrone intercalates into the DNA, causing cross-linking and strand breaks. It also interferes with RNA and topoisomerase II, an enzyme involved in DNA repair. The cytocidal effects of mitoxantrone lead to bone marrow suppression and immunosuppression. It is given by infusion once every 3 months. Controlled clinical trials found that mitoxantrone reduces clinical relapses and progressive disability. Mitoxantrone is approved for use in worsening RRMS or SPMS, although clinical experience has found its efficacy in SPMS is limited to very early SPMS, when active inflammation persists. Mitoxantrone is blue, which leads to a transient bluish discoloration of sclera, urine, and occasionally nail beds. Alopecia, nausea, leukopenia, and menstrual irregularities are also seen.

The main safety concerns with mitoxantrone are cardiotoxicity and leukemia. Decreased cardiac ejection fraction is observed in a cumulative dose-dependent fashion, requiring an echocardiogram or multiple uptake gated acquisition (MUGA) scan before every dose and limiting total exposure to 120 mg/m^2. Reduction of ejection fraction by 10% from baseline or below 50% suggests ongoing cardiotoxicity. Secondary acute myeloid leukemia is also a complication of mitoxantrone therapy, with several prospective studies finding an incidence of 1% to 2.5%. This toxicity has led some clinicians to use a short course as an induction agent. One clinical trial found that three monthly infusions followed by standard injectable MS therapy quickly controlled disease while minimizing total exposure to mitoxantrone. Nonetheless, the significant risks of mitoxantrone have rendered its use uncommon in the treatment of MS.

Natalizumab

α4-Integrin is an adhesion molecule on circulating leukocytes that mediates an important step in leukocytes, leaving the circulation and entering into the brain in response to inflammation. Natalizumab is a monoclonal antibody blocking α4-integrin. Natalizumab is administered by 1-hour intravenous infusion every 4 weeks. Controlled trials found natalizumab reduces clinical relapses by 68% compared with placebo, slows the progression of disability by 42%, and reduces the development of new brain lesions by 92%, all of which is significantly greater than that seen with any of the injectable therapies.

Natalizumab is generally well tolerated, with few side effects. One significant safety concern with natalizumab is infusion hypersensitivity reactions. Infusion hypersensitivity reactions occur within 2 hours of the start of infusion and include urticaria, pruritus, and rigors. Therefore, a 1-hour clinical observation is required after completion of every 1-hour infusion.

The other significant safety concern with natalizumab is progressive multifocal leukoencephalopathy (PML), a rare, destructive brain infection caused by the ubiquitous JC virus, which is carried by most adults. The estimated incidence of PML in natalizumab-treated patients is 1 per 1000 over 18 months of therapy. Immune reconstitution is the only treatment with demonstrated efficacy in PML, so it is hoped that the accelerated clearance of natalizumab by plasma exchange[1] can help MS patients who develop PML secondary to natalizumab treatment. Recognition of PML led to the development of a control system for natalizumab distribution in the United States. Patients, prescribing physicians, dispensing pharmacies, and infusion centers are required to register in the Tysabri Outreach Unified Commitment to Health (TOUCH) Program, which will help ensure appropriate use of the medication and monitor for PML and other possible opportunistic infections.

---

[1]Not FDA approved for this indication.

OTHER IMMUNOMODULATORY THERAPIES

Given the limited number of disease-modifying treatment options available for this lifelong disease, many other immunomodulating therapies have been used to treat MS. Oral weekly methotrexate (Trexall)[1] and bimonthly pulse corticosteroids are sometimes used for long-term therapy when standard injectable therapies do not sufficiently control disease, although a recent controlled trial showed them to be only marginally effective. Short-term (6–12 months) courses of monthly cyclophosphamide (Cytoxan)[1] have been used for several decades, but a controlled clinical trial showed only modest efficacy, which disappeared after treatment was stopped. Azathioprine (Imuran)[1] and mycophenolate mofetil (Cellcept)[1] are occasionally used, although their efficacy is supported only by small, mostly uncontrolled studies.

Rituximab (Rituxan)[1] is a monoclonal antibody that destroys B cells for 6 months or more following each course of treatment. Despite theories that MS is a T cell–mediated disease, a 6-month phase II trial of rituximab found that this anti–B cell therapy reduced MRI lesion activity by 91% and relapse rate by 56%.

In addition, several dozen new and old immunomodulating therapies are in various stages of development for the treatment of MS. These therapies include both oral and infusion treatments and target all forms of the disease, from clinically isolated syndrome to primary and secondary progressive MS. Many of these treatments should become available over the next several years.

DISEASE MONITORING

MS clinicians generally agree that MS therapies should be started immediately on the diagnosis of active RRMS. However, optimal monitoring and management of MS patients while they are receiving therapy, particularly regarding when to change therapies, are more controversial. Just as MRI has taken on an important role in the diagnosis of MS, MRI has also taken an on important role in the assessment of response to therapy. The familiar mantra "treat the patient, not the scan" is being replaced by recognition that MRI scans provide significant insight into disease activity. For example, recent studies found that new brain lesions on MRI are a stronger predictor of future disability than clinical relapses. There remains a significant disconnect between the total amount of injury on brain MRI and clinical disability, but measures of disease activity (gadolinium-enhancing lesions and new T2 lesions) have a stronger association with progressive clinical disability. In addition, a recent meta-analysis found that a therapy's effect on new MRI lesions accounted for 81% of the therapy's effect on clinical relapses. This observation provides clear evidence supporting the importance of routine MRI monitoring of patients during treatment.

Several factors should be weighed when assessing the efficacy of long-term disease-modifying therapy: frequency of clinical relapses, recovery from clinical relapses, progressive disability over time, and MRI activity. Over the course of 1 year, a single, mild relapse with good recovery would generally not merit a change in therapy. However, multiple mild relapses or a moderate to severe relapse with poor recovery would suggest that current therapy is inadequate.

Brain MRI can be used to confirm the clinical impression of disease activity. Although MRI does not always show new or enhancing lesions at the time of a clinical relapse, multiple relapses in the context of a stable MRI should raise the suspicion for an alternative diagnosis. Recurrent infections and emotional distress are two common causes of symptoms that mimic an MS clinical relapse.

The proper performance of MRI is crucial to accurate assessment of the MS disease state. Standard guidelines include sagittal FLAIR, axial FLAIR, T2-, and T1-weighted images, as well as T1-weighted images 5 or more minutes after gadolinium contrast injection. Because an important goal of monitoring MRI studies is to compare with previous images, MRIs should be performed using contiguous, nongapped slices. Ideally, imaging should be performed at the same imaging center over time so that comparable images are obtained and historical comparison can be performed by the radiologist. Multiple new or enhancing lesions over time suggest that current therapy is suboptimal in controlling disease activity. New brain lesions outnumber spine lesions by about 10 to 1, and new spine lesions typically cause clinical symptoms. Therefore, surveillance imaging is typically limited to brain MRI with and without gadolinium.

SYMPTOM MANAGEMENT

MS can cause a wide range of symptoms, affecting motor, sensory, coordination, gait, sphincter, sexual function, and psychiatric spheres. These symptoms can cause significant morbidity through impairment in quality of life and daily function. There are effective treatments for almost all of these symptoms, and symptomatic management should be part of routine management of MS patients (Box 1). Effective symptom management extends beyond medication alone, often involving physical or occupational therapy, psychotherapy, exercise and stretching programs, and the collaboration of other specialists such as urology and physical medicine and rehabilitation.

Special Clinical Circumstances

PROGRESSIVE MULTIPLE SCLEROSIS

Underlying both primary and secondary progressive forms of MS is thought to be a neurodegenerative process, for which no current therapies have demonstrated clinical efficacy. When active inflammation is present, as demonstrated by a clinical relapse or gadolinium-enhancing lesion, immunomodulating therapies can be partially effective. In the absence of active inflammation, numerous clinical trials have shown that immunomodulating therapies are ineffective, often causing only troublesome side effects. Intermittent pulses of corticosteroids can sometimes slow the progressive course of MS, which is often measured by patients through self-report of ambulatory function. Treatment of progressive MS should focus on symptomatic management, targeting spasticity, gait stability and mobility, pain, and sphincter dysfunction. Vigilance should be maintained for other contributing conditions, such as mechanical compressive myelopathy (disc herniation), vitamin B_{12} deficiency, and thyroid disorder.

NEUROMYELITIS OPTICA

Acute treatment of neuromyelitis optica is no different from that of a standard MS relapse. A rebound return of symptoms is common after the course of corticosteroids is complete, so prolonged prednisone taper over weeks or months can be helpful. Neuromyelitis optica typically does not respond to the standard long-term MS injectable therapies interferon-β-1 and glatiramer acetate. Azathioprine (Imuran)[1] 2–3 mg/kg/day is often effective in controlling disease, and case series have found rituximab (Rituxan)[1] is also effective. Discovery of a common pathogenic antibody against aquaporin-4 ion channels has led many clinicians to use plasma exchange as treatment for acute relapses and as long-term maintenance therapy.

PREGNANCY

MS typically starts in the third or fourth decade, making it commonly coincident with pregnancy. Observational studies found that MS often becomes quiescent during pregnancy, but then rebounds shortly following pregnancy. None of the long-term disease-modifying therapies is recommended for use during pregnancy, although glatiramer acetate is probably the best choice for patients who need treatment to continue during pregnancy. Clinical relapses with significant functional impairment can be treated with a course of methylprednisolone, and intermittent immune globulin[1] can be used as a maintenance therapy.

Long-term disease-modifying therapies are also not recommended while breast-feeding. Immune globulin[1] is again a treatment

---

[1]Not FDA approved for this indication.

[1]Not FDA approved for this indication.

BOX 1 Symptomatic Management of Multiple Sclerosis

Weakness

4-Aminopyridine,[1] 10–20 mg bid (available through compounding pharmacies)
Exercise program
Assistive devices: Ankle foot orthotic, cane, rolling walker

Spasticity

Stretching program twice daily
Baclofen (Lioresal) 5–20 mg bid-qid
Tizanidine (Zanaflex) 2–8 mg bid-qid
Gabapentin (Neurontin)[1] 100–600 mg bid-qid
Clonazepam (Klonopin)[1] 0.5–4 mg qhs
Diazepam (Valium) 2–10 mg qhs
Intrathecal baclofen pump
Botulinum toxin type A (Botox) injection (for focal spasticity)

Neuropathic Pain and Paresthesias

Pregabalin (Lyrica)[1] 50–100 mg tid
Gabapentin (Neurontin)[1] 100–600 mg bid-qid
Amitriptyline (Elavil)[1] 25–150 mg qhs
Nortriptyline (Pamelor)[1] 25–150 mg qhs
Phenytoin (Dilantin)[1] 150–300 mg daily-bid
Carbamazepine (Tegretol)[1] 200–400 mg tid
Duloxetine (Cymbalta)[1] 20–60 mg daily or divided bid

Fatigue

Routine exercise program
Good sleep hygiene
Amantadine (Symmetrel)[1] 100 mg bid
Modafinil (Provigil)[1] 100–200 mg qd-bid
Methylphenidate (Ritalin)[1] 10–20 mg bid-tid

Depression

Psychotherapy
SSRIs, such as citalopram (Celexa) 20–60 mg daily, fluoxetine (Prozac) 20–80 mg daily, or paroxetine (Paxil) 20–50 mg daily
SNRIs, such as venlafaxine (Effexor) 37.5–225 mg/d divided bid-tid, duloxetine (Cymbalta) 20–60 mg daily or divided bid
Bupropion (Wellbutrin SR) 100–400 mg/day divided bid

Urinary Frequency, Urgency, and Incontinence

Tolterodine (Detrol) 1–2 mg po bid (watch for acute retention)
Oxybutynin (Ditropan) 2.5–5 mg bid-qid (watch for acute retention)
Intermittent straight catheterization
Diverting suprapubic catheter

Recurrent Urinary Tract Infections

Nitrofurantoin (Macrodantin) 100 mg qhs
Diverting suprapubic catheter

Constipation

Bulk-forming agents
Stool softeners
Laxatives

Sexual Dysfunction

Phosphodiesterase 5 inhibitors: sildenafil (Viagra) 50–100 mg, tadalafil (Cialis) 10–20 mg, vardenafil (Levitra) 10–20 mg
Estrogen replacement: oral, topical, vaginal ring
Psychotherapy to improve communication
Avoidance of exacerbating medications (e.g., if using SSRIs, use bupropion [Wellbutrin] instead)
Devices: Mechanical vibrators and vacuum devices

Tremor

Very difficult to treat
Sometimes responds to levetiracetam (Keppra)[1] 500–1000 mg bid

Tonic Spasms

Spasms 10–60 seconds in duration, usually affecting the unilateral face, arm, and leg, without altered consciousness
Carbamazepine extended release (Tegretol XR)[1] 100–300 mg bid
Phenytoin extended release (Dilantin)[1] 100–300 mg daily

[1]Not FDA approved for this indication.
SNRI = serotonin-norepinephrine reuptake inhibitor; SSRI = selective serotonin reuptake inhibitor.

---

option. Low doses of corticosteroids diffuse freely in and out of breast milk within a few hours of administration, leaving little being passed on to the infant 4 hours after administration. However, no studies have been done with the very high doses of methylprednisolone typically used in MS. Therefore, breast milk should be pumped and discarded out to 24 hours after completion of a course of intravenous methylprednisolone.

MULTIPLE SCLEROSIS IN THE OLD AND YOUNG

MS can be seen in both children and the elderly, although both are uncommon. The formal diagnostic criteria were intended to be applied to persons ages 10 to 59 years, but they can be used in younger and older patients. Treatment options for children and adolescents are similar to those for adults, except that current FDA regulations prohibit use of natalizumab in patients younger than 18 years. Relapse recovery is generally very good in children and adolescents, but gradually progressive disability is common by the third or fourth decade. Therefore, aggressive treatment and monitoring are recommended.

The diagnosis of MS in the older adult is complicated by the increased frequency of other neurologic disorders, as well as nonspecific T2 lesions commonly seen on brain MRI. MS in persons beyond the seventh decade is typically a gradually progressive myelopathy, but some patients present with active inflammation requiring immunomodulating therapy.

REFERENCES

Francis GS, Rice GP, Alsop JC. Interferon beta-1a in MS: Results following development of neutralizing antibodies in PRISMS. Neurology 2005;65 (1):48–55.

Hauser SL, Waubant E, Arnold DL, et al. B-cell depletion with rituximab in relapsing-remitting multiple sclerosis. N Engl J Med. 2008;358 (7):676–88.

Kappos L, Weinshenker B, Pozzilli C, et al. Interferon beta-1b in secondary progressive MS: A combined analysis of the two trials. Neurology 2004;63(10):1779–87.

Lennon VA, Wingerchuk DM, Kryzer TJ, et al. A serum autoantibody marker of neuromyelitis optica: Distinction from multiple sclerosis. Lancet 2004;364(9451):2106–12.

Polman CH, O'Connor PW, Havrdova E, et al. A randomized, placebo-controlled trial of natalizumab for relapsing multiple sclerosis. N Engl J Med 2006;354(9):899–910.

Polman CH, Reingold SC, Edan G, et al. Diagnostic criteria for multiple sclerosis: 2005 revisions to the "McDonald Criteria" Ann Neurol 2005;58:840–6.

Rudick RA, Lee JC, Simon J, et al. Defining interferon beta response status in multiple sclerosis patients. Ann Neurol 2004;56(4):548–55.

Trapp BD, Peterson J, Ransohoff RM, et al. Axonal transection in the lesions of multiple sclerosis. New Engl J Med 1998;338:278–85.

Yousry TA, Major EO, Ryschkewitsch C, et al. Evaluation of patients treated with natalizumab for progressive multifocal leukoencephalopathy. N Engl J Med 2006;354(9):924–33.

Myasthenia Gravis and Related Disorders

Method of
Jenice Robinson, MD, and Milind J. Kothari, DO

Myasthenia gravis (MG) is a relatively uncommon disease of the postsynaptic neuromuscular junction (NMJ). Most patients with myasthenia have an acquired immunologic abnormality, but other uncommon inherited forms of myasthenia may result from structural abnormalities of the NMJ. The following discussion focuses on acquired (autoimmune) MG.

The physiologic abnormality in autoimmune MG results from the reduction in concentration of the nicotinic acetylcholine receptor (AChR) on the endplates of somatic muscles at the NMJ. Although the cause of the disorder is unknown, the pathogenesis of autoimmune MG is now well understood. Two antigens have been described: AChR and muscle-specific receptor tyrosine kinase (MuSK). Antibodies against AChR are found in 80% to 90% of patients with MG. Antibodies against MuSK are found in 40% of the remaining patients. Strong evidence supports the role of antibodies in the pathogenesis of MG. Anti-AChR antibodies cause disruption of myotubes in culture and cause myasthenic symptoms when transferred to experimental animals. Removal of anti-AChR antibodies results in clinical improvement. The thymus plays an important but incompletely understood role in MG.

Clinical Features

The hallmark of MG is fluctuating or fatigable weakness. MG presents with ocular symptoms of ptosis or diplopia in 60% of patients. Diplopia may not fluctuate, and an ocular misalignment may appear fixed. This presentation may mimic a neuropathy of the third, fourth, or sixth cranial nerves, or an internuclear ophthalmoplegia. Abnormalities of pupillary function should not be present in MG. Patients may present initially to an optometrist or ophthalmologist for these problems. Ocular symptoms eventually develop in almost all patients with MG. Presenting symptoms are bulbar (dysarthria, dysphagia, or facial weakness) in 10%, leg weakness in 10% to 20%, and generalized weakness in 10%. Symptoms often worsen with exercise and improve with rest. Symptoms are often most prominent late in the day. Weakness in MG arises from fluctuating strength of the voluntary muscles and always causes a functional deficit, such as an inability to hold the arms above the head when washing the hair or leg weakness resulting in sudden falls. If a patient has only generalized fatigue or tiredness, MG is unlikely. Chronic pain and sensory complaints are not features of MG. Respiratory dysfunction is the initial presenting symptom in only 1% of patients but, if present, requires admission to the hospital for monitoring and treatment because respiratory failure may occur rapidly. Weakness in MG can be worsened by infection, physical stress such as surgery, emotional stress, and medications. Medications that reportedly worsen strength in MG are listed in Table 1.

TABLE 1 Medications Reported to Exacerbate Myasthenia Gravis

Antibiotics
Aminoglycosides, ampicillin sodium, ciprofloxacin hydrochloride (Cipro), erythromycin, imipenem (Primaxin), kanamycin sulfate (Kantrex), pyrantel (Antiminth), chloroquine (Aralen)

Cardiovascular Agents
β-Blocking agents (propranolol hydrochloride [Inderal], oxprenolol hydrochloride[2] [Trasicor], timolol maleate [Blocadren]), procainamide (Procanbid), verapamil hydrochloride (Calan), propafenone hydrochloride (Rythmol), quinidine
Penicillamine (Cuprimine)
Corticosteroids (transiently when initiating therapy)
Magnesium salts and lithium carbonate (Eskalith)
Phenothiazine antipsychotics
Phenytoin sodium (Dilantin)

Neuromuscular Blocking Agents
Vecuronium bromide (Norcuron), succinylcholine chloride (Anectine)

Ocular Drugs
Timolol maleate (Timoptic), proparacaine hydrochloride (Alcaine), tropicamide (Mydriacyl)

Anticholinergic Agents
Trihexyphenidyl hydrochloride (Artane)
Acetazolamide (Diamox)

[2]Not available in the United States.

The prevalence of MG is estimated to be 14 per 100,000 people. MG may present at any age, but the most common ages of onset are in the second and third decades in women and in the seventh and eighth decades in men. In the past MG was more common in women than men, but with aging of the population, MG now is more common in men. Associated autoimmune diseases, such as thyroid disease, rheumatoid arthritis, lupus, and pernicious anemia, are present in 5% to 10% of patients. Approximately 10% of MG patients have an associated thymoma, and 50% to 70% of patients have thymic hyperplasia. Familial occurrence of autoimmune MG is rare, although the incidence of autoimmune diseases in first-degree relatives of patients with MG may be increased.

Diagnosis

An accurate diagnosis prior to initiating treatment for MG is crucial. A critical assessment of the patient's symptoms is the most important initial step in evaluation. The differential diagnosis of MG is quite limited in most patients. Disorders that may mimic MG are listed in Table 2.

All patients suspected of having MG should undergo testing consisting of a complete blood count (CBC), erythrocyte sedimentation rate, thyroid-stimulating hormone and thyroxine levels, rheumatoid factor concentration, and liver and renal profiles. Autoimmune thyroid disease may mimic or accompany MG. In addition to excluding other diagnoses, these tests are important because treatments of MG may have adverse effects on the bone marrow, liver, and kidneys.

The role of specific testing for MG is to confirm the clinical diagnosis. For a patient with ptosis, the ice test is easy and convenient. A small amount of ice is placed over the ptotic lid for a few minutes. Improvement of the ptosis with cooling is suggestive of a defect of neuromuscular transmission. Further testing should then be pursued.

EDROPHONIUM CHLORIDE (TENSILON) TEST

The edrophonium (Tensilon) test is readily available, but the result may be invalid if the test is not properly performed. A defined clinical endpoint is needed, and vague patient reports of improvement in strength are not acceptable. Cranial nerve deficits, such as ptosis, dysconjugate gaze, and limitation of extraocular movements, provide the most reliable endpoints. The test should be performed in a location where syncope, hypotension, or respiratory failure can be managed, as these

CURRENT DIAGNOSIS

- Hallmark of MG is fluctuating or fatigable weakness.
- Initial symptom is ptosis or diplopia in 60% of patients.
- Generalized fatigue or tiredness alone is not a symptom of MG.
- Diagnostic evaluation includes:
  - Laboratory evaluation: Thyroid-stimulating hormone level, complete blood count, erythrocyte sedimentation rate, rheumatoid factor, liver and renal function studies
  - Edrophonium chloride (Tensilon) test: >90% sensitivity, but be certain to choose a defined clinical endpoint (e.g., improvement in ptosis)
  - Antibody testing: Send AChR binding antibodies first. Binding antibodies are found in ~90% of patients with generalized MG, and 50% with ocular MG. If negative, send AChR modulating antibodies. If both are negative, send muscle-specific receptor tyrosine kinase antibody.
  - All patients with suspected MG should undergo chest computed tomography with contrast for thymoma
  - If antibodies are negative or if searching for evidence of generalized MG in a patient with pure ocular symptoms, obtain electromyography with repetitive nerve stimulation. This test result is abnormal in >70% of patients with generalized MG but is less sensitive in patients with pure ocular symptoms
  - If diagnosis remains unclear, refer to neuromuscular specialist.

Abbreviations: AChR = acetylcholine receptor; MG = myasthenia gravis.

TABLE 2 Clinical Presentations and Diagnostic Considerations in Myasthenia Gravis

Site of Predominant Weakness	Alternative Diagnoses
Ocular	Brainstem and cranial nerve disorders due to processes such as neoplasm, stroke, and multiple sclerosis Horner syndrome Oculopharyngeal muscular dystrophy Kearns-Sayre syndrome Graves' disease Congenital myasthenia Botulism (if symptom onset is acute) Miller-Fischer variant of GBS
Bulbar	Brainstem and multiple cranial nerve dysfunction due to processes such as neoplasm, stroke, and multiple sclerosis Bulbar-onset ALS Obstructive lesion of the oropharynx or laryngeal lesion Botulism (if symptom onset is acute)
Proximal extremity weakness	Inflammatory myopathies (e.g., polymyositis, dermatomyositis) LEMS GBS Periodic paralysis
Isolated respiratory weakness	Acid maltase deficiency ALS Polymyositis LEMS Myotonic dystrophy
Isolated neck weakness	ALS Inflammatory myopathies Paraspinous myopathy

Abbreviations: ALS = amyotrophic lateral sclerosis; GBS = Guillain-Barré syndrome; LEMS = Lambert-Eaton myasthenic syndrome.

complications can rarely occur in supersensitive individuals. Atropine sulfate 0.4 mg should be available in case of symptomatic bradycardia. An intravenous line is often started for the test, although some practitioners use a butterfly needle for administration. Edrophonium 10 mg (1 mL) is drawn up in a syringe. The strength or maximum excursion of the target muscles is assessed immediately prior to administration of the edrophonium. A 2-mg (0.2-mL) test dose is given to ensure that the patient is not supersensitive to the drug. If no respiratory or cardiac side effects occur, 3 mg (0.3 mL) of edrophonium is given. Re-examination of the target muscle is performed. If no definite improvement is observed at 60 seconds, the remaining 5 mg (0.5 mL) of edrophonium is given. If unequivocal improvement in the strength of the target muscle occurs within 60 seconds of administration of a dose of edrophonium, the test is considered positive. Edrophonium 10 mg will not weaken normal muscles, but the full dose may induce weakness in a patient with a defect in neuromuscular transmission. For this reason, the medication should be given in the manner described so that any improvement in muscle strength is not missed.

The edrophonium (Tensilon) test is positive in more than 90% of patients with MG, but a positive result is not specific for MG. Positive edrophonium tests have been reported in patients with the Lambert-Eaton myasthenic syndrome, motor neuron disease, lesions of the oculomotor nerves, and conditions affecting the extraocular muscles.

ANTIBODY TESTING

Acetylcholine receptor antibodies (AChR-Ab) are present in 90% of patients with generalized MG and in approximately 50% to 60% of patients with ocular myasthenia. They are the most specific test for MG. False-positive results can occur but are rare. Antibody levels are not predictive of the severity of MG in an individual patient.

Three different tests for AChR-Ab are available commercially: binding, modulating, and blocking antibodies. The binding antibody is the antibody most commonly found in MG and should be tested first. If the test result is negative, a modulating antibody test should be performed because this may be positive in a small number of patients who do not have binding antibodies. The blocking antibody titer adds little additional diagnostic value and is not generally indicated.

Recently, antibodies against muscle-specific receptor tyrosine kinase (MuSK-Ab) have been described in approximately 40% of patients with "seronegative" MG. Evidence indicates that MuSK is involved in the proper distribution of AChR at the muscle endplate, and some evidence indicates that MuSK-Abs are pathogenic in these patients. The MuSK-Ab test is commercially available. Patients with MuSK-Ab are almost always seronegative for AChR-Ab. For this reason, the MuSK-Ab test should be sent only if the patient has already been tested for AChR-Ab and is seronegative. MG in patients with MuSK-Ab may have a different natural history and response to treatment, and this is an area of active investigation. Patients with MuSK-Ab are more likely to be young women and present with bulbar, neck, or respiratory symptoms. Edrophonium (Tensilon) testing is less likely to yield a positive result. Whether thymectomy should be performed in patients with MuSK-Ab is unclear.

Striational antibodies are a marker for thymoma, although false-positive and false-negative results are common. Chest computed tomography (CT) with contrast to evaluate for possible thymoma is indicated for all patients diagnosed with MG. The added value of performing striational antibodies has not been definitely demonstrated.

ELECTROPHYSIOLOGIC TESTING

Electrophysiologic testing is indicated for evaluation of possible MG if the AChR-Ab test is negative. In antibody-positive patients, electrophysiologic testing is often not necessary unless the test is being performed to evaluate for evidence of generalized disease in those with purely ocular symptoms. Typically, routine nerve conduction studies and needle electromyography (EMG) are normal. These tests are performed to ensure that other disorders of the peripheral nerves or muscles are not present. Repetitive nerve stimulation (RNS) is then performed if the study was ordered to evaluate for an NMJ disorder. RNS has a sensitivity of approximately 50% to 60% in all patients with MG, with a higher yield in patients with generalized MG and a lower yield in patients with pure ocular MG. RNS of the spinal accessory and facial nerves may increase the yield of testing. It should be emphasized that abnormal RNS is not specific for MG, and routine nerve conduction studies and needle EMG must be performed to exclude other conditions. Single-fiber EMG (SFEMG) is a highly specialized and demanding technique with a sensitivity of approximately 90% to 95% in patients with MG. SFEMG is abnormal in many neuromuscular diseases and therefore should be performed only in the correct clinical context and after a routine EMG with RNS has been performed. Because of the demanding nature of the study, SFEMG is usually performed by a neuromuscular specialist.

OTHER INVESTIGATIONS

Currently all patients diagnosed with MG should undergo a CT scan of the chest with contrast to evaluate for an associated thymoma. Routine chest radiography or determination of antistriational antibodies is not an adequate substitute.

Prognosis

The natural history of MG is highly variable. Ocular symptoms are the presenting symptoms in approximately 50% to 60% of MG patients. Weakness subsequently develops in other muscles in most patients. Weakness remains restricted to the extraocular muscles for the entire course of MG in 15% to 20% of patients (pure ocular myasthenia). Patients with initial ocular involvement typically develop weakness in other muscles within the first year of having the disease. If no generalized symptoms develop after 2 years, subsequent generalization is unlikely. The maximal weakness from MG occurs within the initial 3 years of symptoms in 70% of patients. Mortality from MG is now low because of advances in critical care; however, quality of life is often affected by MG. Long-lasting remission occurs spontaneously in approximately 10% to 15% of patients if no immunosuppressive agents are used. Spontaneous remissions may be more frequent in patients with pure ocular myasthenia.

Treatment

CHOLINESTERASE INHIBITORS AS FIRST-LINE THERAPY

Cholinesterase inhibitors (ChEIs) are first-line therapy in all patients with MG. The commonly available ChEIs are listed in Table 3. Acetylcholinesterase (AChE) is anchored in the synaptic cleft on the postsynaptic membrane. AChE normally cleaves acetylcholine (ACh) released from the presynaptic nerve terminal, which normally prevents repeat binding of ACh to the AChR. ChEIs reduce the hydrolysis of ACh and increase the amount of ACh available at the postsynaptic membrane. ChEIs used for treatment of MG are reversible inhibitors of AChE and cause few central nervous system side effects because they do not cross the blood–brain barrier efficiently. Absorption from the gastrointestinal tract is inefficient, and oral bio-availability is low.

 CURRENT THERAPY

Be certain of the diagnosis
- Ocular symptoms only or mild weakness: Cholinesterase inhibitors
- Moderate to severe weakness:
  - Cholinesterase inhibitors, and
  - Thymectomy for patients younger than 60 years (with complete removal of the gland)
- If symptoms are uncontrolled with cholinesterase inhibitors, use immunosuppression:
  - Prednisone if urgent of severe
  - Azathioprine[1] (Imuran) or mycophenolate mofetil[1] (CellCept)
    - As a steroid-sparing agent to facilitate prednisone taper
    - Prednisone fails to elicit patient response
    - Prednisone contraindicated
    - Excessive prednisone side effects
- Plasma exchange or intravenous immune globulin[1]
  - Myasthenic crisis
  - Preoperative (i.e., before thymectomy)
- If the above measures fail:
  - Refer to neuromuscular specialist

[1]Not FDA approved for this indication.

TABLE 3 Commonly Available Cholinesterase Inhibitors

Medication	Route of Administration	Unit Dose	Average Dose (Adult)	Children's Dose
Pyridostigmine bromide tablet (Mestinon)	Oral	60-mg tablets, double-scored for splitting	30–60 mg every 4–6 hours, maximum 120 mg every 3 hours	1 mg/kg every 4–6 hours
Pyridostigmine bromide syrup	Oral	12 mg/mL	30–60 mg every 4–6 hours	1 mg/kg every 4–6 hours
Pyridostigmine bromide sustained-release (Mestinon Timespan)	Oral	180-mg tablet (not crushable)	1 table at bedtime	—
Pyridostigmine bromide	Intravenous	5-mg/mL ampules	1/30 of usual oral dose, i.e., 1–2 mg every 3–4 hours	—
Neostigmine bromide (Prostigmin)	Oral	15-mg tablets	7.5–15 mg every 3–4 hours	
Edrophonium (Tensilon)	Intravenous		Used for diagnosis	Used for diagnosis

Pyridostigmine bromide (Mestinon) is the most widely used ChEI. Onset of action is within 15 to 30 minutes of an oral dose, with peak action at 1 to 2 hours and gradual wearing off at 3 to 4 hours. All ChEI medications have muscarinic side effects, including cramping, diarrhea, salivation, lacrimation, and bradycardia. For this reason, the medication should always be introduced in low dose, preferably on the weekend. Pyridostigmine tablets are double scored and can be easily split. Start the patient with a half tablet (30 mg) of pyridostigmine once daily in the morning. The dose is then increased by a half tablet each day to a dose of a half tablet (30 mg) four times daily. Subsequently, the dose can be increased further to a full tablet (60 mg) four times daily. If necessary for symptom relief, pyridostigmine can be increased to a maximum dose of 120 mg every 3 to 4 hours, but 60 mg every 4 hours usually provides optimum benefit. If a patient has weakness while eating, pyridostigmine doses can be timed to be taken 1 hour before meals. If a patient has significant weakness upon awakening, the extended-release formulation of pyridostigmine (Mestinon Timespan) can be given at bedtime; however, absorption is too unpredictable for daytime use. If a patient requires parenteral dosing of medications, intravenous pyridostigmine is given at 1/30 the oral dose (usually 1–2 mg intravenously) every 3 to 4 hours.

When symptoms are not controlled with 60 to 120 mg of pyridostigmine every 4 hours, possible initiation of an immunosuppressive agent must be discussed fully with the patient. Most patients with generalized MG will require immunosuppressive treatment in order to induce a remission of symptoms. Pyridostigmine is often initially very effective, but therapeutic efficacy usually gradually diminishes. The immunosuppressive agents used in MG are corticosteroids, azathioprine[1] (Imuran), mycophenolate mofetil[1] (CellCept), cyclosporin A[1] (Neoral), and cyclophosphamide[1] (Cytoxan). Each of these agents is discussed separately in Table 4. Important considerations are the clinical severity of the MG, the patient's perception of his or her disability, any coexisting medical conditions, as well as the patient's age, gender, and overall lifestyle. For example, a physically active patient will be less tolerant of weakness than a patient with a sedentary lifestyle.

TREATMENT OF PURE OCULAR MYASTHENIA GRAVIS

From 15% to 20% of patients with MG have only visual symptoms for the entire course of their disease. Visual symptoms in patients with MG result from ptosis or ocular misalignment. Approximately 50% of patients will experience significant relief of visual symptoms with ChEIs alone and will be satisfied with their treatment. The effect on symptoms should be clear within 1 month of beginning pyridostigmine (Mestinon) therapy. In general, pyridostigmine provides significant relief of ptosis and is less helpful for ocular misalignment.

Among the 50% of patients who achieve significant control of ocular symptoms using pyridostigmine, this may be the only treatment necessary. If symptoms are not controlled, the patient's perception of his or her disability and lifestyle are very important to treatment. A patient who is unable to work because of visual misalignment will require further treatment. Nonpharmacologic options for symptom management include eyelid taping or eyelid crutches for ptosis and eye patching for ocular misalignment.

If the patient requests further treatment, prednisone[1] can be started at 10 mg/day, with an increase of 5 mg every other day until a dose of 40 to 60 mg/day is reached. This dose should be continued for approximately 1 month. The vast majority of patients will improve. At 1 month, a taper at 5 mg/wk can be started; at 20 mg the taper should be slowed to improve the chances of maintaining remission.

The role of corticosteroids in the treatment of pure ocular MG is controversial. Some data suggest that corticosteroids decrease the chance of developing generalized MG. However, corticosteroids have many undesired effects. In general, corticosteroids are used for ocular myasthenia only when the symptoms are significant to the patient and are uncontrolled by ChEIs.

CORTICOSTEROIDS

Corticosteroids are usually the first-line immunosuppressive agent. After 6 weeks of treatment with a corticosteroid, approximately 90% of patients have improvement in symptoms. Approximately 30% of patients treated with prednisone obtain remission, and 50% experience marked improvement. Paradoxically, 50% of patients have an initial increase in weakness during the first weeks of treatment with corticosteroids. The reasons for this effect are not well understood. Some practitioners begin treatment at the full therapeutic dose of prednisone 60 to 80 mg/day, with careful monitoring for increased weakness. If weakness worsens, the patient may require hospitalization and treatment with plasma exchange or intravenous immune globulin[1] (IVIG; Gamimune N). Others begin treatment at a lower dose with a gradual increase to the target dose over 1 month with the goal of avoiding the initial worsening of strength. An example of this method begins with a dose of prednisone 20 mg once daily. The dose is increased by 5 mg every third day until the target dose of 60 to 80 mg/day is reached. Alternate-day dosing with a target dose of 100 to 120 mg every other day can also be used. When beginning prednisone, calcium, vitamin D, and a bisphosphonate medication should be started at the same time unless a contraindication is present. This is appropriate because most patients will require long-term therapy with prednisone.

A clinical effect is typically seen within 6 weeks. If a remission is achieved, the full dose should be maintained for 6 weeks, followed by a slow taper. Initially the daily prednisone dose can be decreased by 5 mg/month. When the daily dose reaches 30 mg/day, the taper should be slowed, with further decreases in dose of 2.5 mg/month. Clinical exacerbations are frequent when the daily dose of prednisone reaches 20 to 30 mg/day, and a slower taper may prevent this problem. If an exacerbation occurs, the daily prednisone dose should be increased by 5 to 10 mg. The new dose can be maintained for 6 weeks, followed by a slower taper. Some practitioners use alternate-day dosing, with tapering from an initial dose of 100 to 120 mg every other day.

Long-term use of corticosteroids is associated with serious complications, including osteoporosis, fractures, medication-induced diabetes mellitus, obesity, glaucoma, cataracts, gastric and duodenal ulcers, anxiety or depression, myopathy, opportunistic infections, and avascular necrosis of the large joints. Most patients are not able to completely discontinue prednisone and require a minimum dose to maintain improvement of their MG. The decision to start a steroid-sparing agent is often not clear-cut. In general, if a patient has more than one relapse when tapering off steroids, therapy with a steroid-sparing agent should be considered. If a patient does not have a remission with steroids, combined therapy with a steroid-sparing agent should be considered. In the older patient population, treatment with a steroid-sparing agent should be considered early in the course. In a young patient, particularly a woman in her child-bearing years, steroid-sparing drugs should be avoided when possible because of teratogenicity and the increased risk of lymphoma with long-term use of these agents.

OTHER IMMUNOSUPPRESSIVE AGENTS

Azathioprine[1] (Imuran) has been extensively used in MG, usually as a steroid-sparing medication. Azathioprine is an inhibitor of purine synthesis and therefore affects rapidly dividing cell populations, such as lymphocytes. A large double-blind, randomized study demonstrated improvement in steroid tapering with the use of azathioprine. The major drawback of azathioprine is that a clinical effect may not be seen until 12 months. Side effects are less common than with steroids. Approximately 10% of patients have an idiosyncratic reaction in the first weeks of therapy, with fever, nausea, vomiting, and abdominal pain. Symptoms resolve with cessation of the drug but usually recur if azathioprine is restarted. Azathioprine may cause leukopenia or thrombocytopenia, vomiting, or hepatic

---

[1]Not FDA approved for this indication.

[1]Not FDA approved for this indication.

TABLE 4 Oral Immunosuppressive Agents Used on Myasthenia Gravis

Medication	Starting Dose	Therapeutic Dose	Time to Clinical Effect	Laboratory Monitoring	Side Effects	Advantages
Prednisone[1]	60–80 mg daily (see text)	60–80 mg daily (or 120 mg every other day)	Days to weeks	May need to follow blood glucose level; follow bone density every 6 mo	Many serious long-term side effects (see text); always start with calcium 1500 mg/day and vitamin D 400 IU/day; may also require bisphosphonate	Short time to clinical effect; long clinical experience in MG; not teratogenic, relatively safe in pregnancy; no increase in malignancy
Azathioprine[1] (Imuran)	50 mg daily	2–3 mg/kg/day in divided doses	4–12 mo	CBC, LFT weekly as dose increased; may then check once per month; if WBC <2500, stop azathioprine	~10% fever, nausea, abdominal pain during first weeks of treatment; increased risk of malignancy with long-term use; teratogenic	Long clinical experience; predictable; fewer long-term side effects than prednisone
Mycophenolate mofetil[1] (CellCept)	500 mg twice daily	1000–1500 mg twice daily	2–6 mo	CBC monthly, but significant myelosuppression is uncommon	Diarrhea; risk of malignancy with long-term use is currently unclear; should not be used in pregnancy because safety is unknown; clinical experience in MG is limited—randomized study is ongoing	Usually well tolerated; few serious side effects; faster onset of clinical effect than azathioprine
Cyclosporine[1] (Sandimmune, Neoral)	3–5 mg/kg/day in divided doses	3–5 mg/kg/day in divided doses	2–6 mo	Renal function, trough cyclosporine levels, electrolytes monthly; follow blood pressure	Significant renal toxicity is common and is a frequent reason to stop the drug; hypertension; should not be used in pregnancy; many drug interactions; use only under guidance of neuromuscular specialist	Faster onset of clinical effect than azathioprine
Cyclophosphamide[1] (Cytoxan)	25 mg/day orally; parenteral administration may be used in severe, refractory MG	2–5 mg daily		CBC monthly	Significant myelosuppression, hemorrhagic cystitis, risk of opportunistic infections; increased risk of malignancy; absolutely contraindicated during pregnancy; use only under guidance of neuromuscular specialist	May be effective in patients refractory to other treatments

[1]Not FDA approved for this indication.
Abbreviations: CBC = complete blood count; LFT = liver function test; MG = myasthenia gravis; WBC = white blood cell count.

dysfunction. Mild leukopenia occurs in 25% of patients but is usually not significant. Elevation of hepatic enzyme levels occurs in 5% of patients but is usually reversible with cessation of the drug. The risk of lymphoma increases slightly after 10 years of use. Azathioprine is potentially teratogenic and should be avoided in women of childbearing age. The initial dose is 50 mg/day (or 1 mg/kg/day). The dose is increased over a few months until the therapeutic dose of 2 mg/kg/day in divided doses is reached. CBC with differential and liver function tests initially should be tested weekly and monthly after the target dose has been reached. Leukopenia may develop even after several years of treatment. If the white blood cell count drops below 2500 cells/mm^3 or the absolute neutrophil count below 1000 cells/mm^3, the drug should be stopped. Overall, approximately 50% of patients improve with azathioprine therapy. Relapse after discontinuation of azathioprine occurs in more than 50% of patients.

Mycophenolate mofetil[1] (CellCept) is a newer immunosuppressant that inhibits proliferation of T and B lymphocytes by blocking de novo purine synthesis. Lymphocytes are selectively affected because they are unable to use the purine salvage pathway. The major advantages of mycophenolate are its relatively fast onset of clinical effect and its favorable side-effect profile. Side effects are usually mild and include diarrhea, abdominal pain, nausea, peripheral edema, and mild leukopenia. The long-term risk of malignancy with use of mycophenolate is unclear; however, an elderly MG patient who developed primary central nervous system lymphoma in association with mycophenolate use has been recently reported. Treatment trials of patients with MG are ongoing. Some practitioners use mycophenolate to induce remission without the concomitant use of steroids. Others use mycophenolate only as a steroid-sparing agent in steroid-dependent patients. The standard starting dose is 500 mg twice daily. The therapeutic dose for treatment of MG is 1000 to 1500 mg twice daily. Significant myelosuppression is uncommon; however, a monthly check of CBC with differential is standard practice.

Cyclosporine[1] (Sandimmune, Neoral) is an inhibitor of T-helper cell function through blockade of calcineurin-mediated cytokine signaling. Cyclosporine is of limited use for treatment of MG because of renal toxicity. Cyclosporine is used for cases of severe MG when steroids and azathioprine are not tolerated or are ineffective. The standard dosage for treatment of MG is 3 to 5 mg/kg/day in divided doses. Anecdotally, a lower target dose of 2 mg/kg/day may decrease the incidence of renal insufficiency while still achieving clinical improvement. A clinical effect is usually seen within the first 6 months of treatment. Renal function and trough cyclosporine levels should be followed monthly. Creatinine levels greater than 50% of the pretreatment levels are an indication to stop the drug. A rise in creatinine level typically occurs after several years of use. Hypertension is a frequent side effect, and blood pressure must be monitored regularly. In general, this medication should be used for treatment of MG under the guidance of a neuromuscular specialist.

Cyclophosphamide[1] (Cytoxan) is an alkylating agent that acts on DNA, inhibiting cell proliferation. Cyclophosphamide has limited use in MG because of multiple serious toxicities. Cyclophosphamide is used in patients with severe MG when steroids and azathioprine are ineffective or not tolerated. It appears effective at inducing remission when used in this manner. Cyclophosphamide has been used in combination with steroids for patients with severe disease who have not responded to steroids alone. The risk of side effects from cyclophosphamide is high. Cyclophosphamide may cause severe bone marrow suppression, severe opportunistic infections, bladder toxicity, and increased risk of neoplasm. Cyclophosphamide is a chemotherapeutic agent at higher doses, and parenteral high-dose administration has occasionally been used for patients with refractory, severe MG. In general, this medication should be used for treatment of MG only under the guidance of a neuromuscular specialist.

SHORT-TERM IMMUNOTHERAPY: PLASMA EXCHANGE AND INTRAVENOUS IMMUNE GLOBULIN

Plasma exchange (i.e., plasmapheresis) is a well-established intervention that produces short-term clinical improvement in patients with MG. Plasmapheresis is typically used in a MG patient with rapid worsening of weakness or myasthenic crisis. Plasma exchange treatments may be performed prior to an elective surgical procedure, such as thymectomy, to decrease the likelihood of a myasthenic exacerbation. Rarely a patient is refractory or intolerant of all long-term therapies and requires periodic plasma exchange on an ongoing basis. Typical treatment of a myasthenic exacerbation consists of five exchanges of 3 to 4 L each over a period of approximately 2 weeks. The effect is rapid and improvement is seen within days of starting therapy, but the effect is short lived. Typically the beneficial effects of plasma exchange last only a few weeks. Central venous access, typically with a large-bore catheter, is required. Complications of plasma exchange are usually related to the vascular access. Patients are at risk for significant iatrogenic infections, particularly because many of these patients are undergoing long-term therapy with immunosuppressive agents. Hematoma at the site of line placement, pulmonary embolism from venous thrombosis, electrolyte imbalance, pneumothorax, and hypotension during plasma exchange treatments can occur.

IVIG[1] is used for identical indications as plasma exchange. The standard dose is 400 mg/kg/day for 5 days. The only large, randomized study of IVIG in MG found IVIG equivalent to plasmapheresis for treatment of myasthenic crisis. Some practitioners anecdotally believe plasma exchange produces more rapid improvement in strength. The advantages of IVIG are that it is generally more widely available than is plasmapheresis, and it does not require central venous access. The most common side effects are headache and transient flulike symptoms. However, IVIG may cause volume overload, vascular events such as ischemic stroke, and venous thrombosis. IVIG should be used with caution in patients with risk factors for these conditions. IVIG cannot be used in patients with IgA deficiency, a relatively frequent condition. An IgA level must be determined prior to the first IVIG treatment to avoid a potentially serious allergic reaction. Anecdotally, some patients refractory to IVIG will have a good response to plasma exchange.

THYMECTOMY

Thymectomy has been standard therapy for treatment of MG for more than 50 years, but it has never been evaluated in a large, prospective, randomized controlled trial. Thymectomy appears to be effective in improving the course of MG in patients without thymoma. If a thymoma is present, thymectomy is mandatory. The procedure is not a cure for MG, but it appears to increase the likelihood of clinical remission, particularly if performed within the first year of symptom onset. Approximately 75% of patients appear to receive some benefit from the procedure, but the effect may be apparent only after several years. Thymectomy appears to be more effective in younger patients, which may reflect the involution of the thymus with aging. Patients younger than 60 years with moderate to severe MG are candidates for thymectomy. Patients with pure ocular myasthenia do not usually undergo thymectomy unless a thymoma is suspected. Thymic tissue may be present throughout the neck and the mediastinum. The majority of surgical centers perform a combined transsternal–transcervical exposure with en bloc removal of the thymus to ensure complete removal of the gland. Incomplete resections have been followed by persistent symptoms that were later relieved by removal of residual thymus at reoperation. Referrals for thymectomy should be made to an experienced surgeon willing to perform a maximal resection. In the days preceding thymectomy, patients often undergo plasma exchange to decrease the likelihood of an exacerbation due to the surgery. The surgery involves sternotomy and a

---

[1]Not FDA approved for this indication.

[1]Not FDA approved for this indication.

4- to 6-week convalescence. Serious complications are uncommon when the surgery is performed at an experienced center by anesthesiologists and neurologists familiar with the perioperative management of MG.

TREATMENT OF MYASTHENIC CRISIS

A myasthenic crisis is an exacerbation of MG producing respiratory weakness or profound muscle weakness. Myasthenic crisis is a neurologic emergency. Patients with worsening weakness should undergo tests including chest radiograph, blood and urine cultures, CBC with differential, and serum chemistries to screen for concurrent infections. The patient's medication list should be scrutinized and any recent additions or changes noted. Patients occasionally increase their ChEI dose to toxic levels without consulting their physician, resulting in increased muscle weakness and a "cholinergic crisis." This event is relatively uncommon, but recent consumption of ChEI must be determined in all myasthenic patients with increasing weakness. Signs of cholinergic crisis include abdominal cramps, diarrhea, nausea and vomiting, excessive secretions, and miotic pupils; these are not characteristics of myasthenic crisis. If cholinergic crisis is a consideration, the ChEI must be stopped. A patient in myasthenic crisis should be admitted to an intensive care unit if any signs of respiratory failure are present because respiratory deterioration may occur quickly. The vital capacity and peak negative inspiratory force should be followed as measures of respiratory strength. As a rule, elective intubation should be performed when the vital capacity falls below 15 mL/kg and peak negative inspiratory force below -20 cm H_2O. Arterial blood gas measurements do not accurately reflect the degree of respiratory muscle weakness in MG. Pco_2 and po_2 measurements may be normal until just prior to respiratory collapse. While a patient is ventilated, it is reasonable to discontinue pyridostigmine (Mestinon) because this medication may increase respiratory secretions. Any immunosuppressive agents should be continued. If the patient is a new-onset myasthenic, it is appropriate to begin prednisone therapy 60 to 80 mg/day while the patient is ventilated. Options for improving strength during crisis are plasma exchange treatments and IVIG (discussed earlier). Readiness for weaning from the ventilator can be assessed using the vital capacity and peak negative inspiratory force measurements. Weaning from the ventilator may otherwise be performed according to standard protocols. Once the patient is successfully extubated, treatment with ChEIs can be resumed. A treatment plan to prevent future myasthenic crises should be developed.

Other Issues

TRANSIENT NEONATAL MYASTHENIA

Transient neonatal myasthenia occurs in 10% of infants of mothers with autoimmune MG. Following delivery, the infant has a weak cry or suck, appears floppy, and may require mechanical ventilation. The symptoms result from maternal antibodies transferred across the placenta to the infant in utero and resolve within a few weeks. Infants with severe weakness can be treated with oral pyridostigmine 1 to 2 mg/kg every 2 hours.

LAMBERT-EATON MYASTHENIC SYNDROME

Lambert-Eaton myasthenic syndrome (LEMS) is an uncommon autoimmune disorder of the presynaptic NMJ. LEMS is characterized by fluctuating proximal extremity weakness. Symptoms typically include difficulty walking, standing up from a chair, and climbing stairs. Patients may complain of autonomic symptoms, such as dry mouth, blurry vision, anhidrosis, or constipation. Unlike MG, in LEMS ptosis, diplopia, dysphagia, and dysarthria are usually not prominent. Respiratory failure may occur but is uncommon. Patients may report improvement in muscle strength after sustained activity. Other frequent symptoms include myalgias, muscle stiffness, paresthesias, and a metallic taste in the mouth.

On examination, patients typically have proximal muscle weakness, more prominent in the lower extremities. The objective weakness may be less than expected given the patient's symptoms. Characteristically, muscle stretch reflexes are absent. Sustained muscle grip strength often increases over the first several seconds (Lambert's sign).

LEMS is a paraneoplastic syndrome in 60% of patients, most often due to a small cell carcinoma of the lung. In patients without malignancy, LEMS is often associated with other autoimmune conditions. Male patients older than 40 years are more likely to have an associated malignancy, whereas patients without malignancy are more often young women. All patients with suspected LEMS should undergo a thorough evaluation for malignancy, however. If no malignancy is found, the evaluation should be repeated at regular intervals. Presentation of LEMS may antedate the discovery of a malignancy by up to 2 years.

LEMS is believed to result from autoantibodies against the presynaptic voltage-gated calcium channels of cholinergic nerve terminals. At the NMJ, decreased release of acetylcholine from the presynaptic nerve terminal results in muscle weakness. The cholinergic nerve terminals of the autonomic nervous system are also affected. Seventy-five percent of patients with LEMS have detectable serum IgG antibodies against voltage-gated P/Q calcium channels. The diagnosis of LEMS should always be confirmed by electrophysiologic studies. Nerve conduction studies reveal diffusely low compound motor action potential (CMAP) amplitudes with normal sensory responses. RNS shows a CMAP decrement with slow rates of stimulation but marked increment of the CMAP response after brief exercise. A similar increment is seen with fast rates of RNS.

In LEMS with an associated malignancy, treatment of the malignancy may lead to improvement of LEMS symptoms. For symptomatic treatment, some patients achieve improvement with use of ChEIs such as pyridostigmine (Mestinon). 3,4-Diaminopyridine (DAP) increases release of ACh from the presynaptic nerve terminal by decreasing potassium conductance. 3,4-DAP is not approved by the Food and Drug Administration (FDA) for use in the United States. In countries where 3,4-DAP is approved, it represents the first-line symptomatic therapy for LEMS. The typical starting dose is 10 mg every 4 to 6 hours. In patients with disabling symptoms, immunosuppressive therapies such as long-term corticosteroids, plasma exchange treatments, and IVIG[1] can be used.

REFERENCES

Chaudry V, Cornblath DR, Griffin JW, et al. Mycophenolate mofetil: a safe and promising immunosuppressant in neuromuscular diseases. Neurology 2001;56:94–6.

Drachman DB. Myasthenia gravis. N Engl J Med 1994;330:1797–810.

Gajdos PH, Chevret S, Clair B, et al. Clinical trial of plasma exchange and high-dose intravenous immunoglobulin in myasthenia gravis. Ann Neurol 1997;41:789–96.

Jaretzki A, Steinglass KM, Sonett JR. Thymectomy in the management of myasthenia gravis. Semin Neurol 2004;24:49–62.

Kaminski HJ, editor. Current clinical neurology: myasthenia gravis and related disorders. Totowa, NJ: Humana Press; 2002.

Katirji B, Kaminski HJ. Electrodiagnostic approach to the patient with suspected neuromuscular junction disorder. Neurol Clin 2002;20:557–86.

Palace J, Newsom-Davis J, Lecky B. A randomized double-blind trial of prednisolone alone or with azathioprine in myasthenia gravis. Neurology 1998;50:1778–83.

Pascuzzi RM, Coslett HB, Johns TR. Long-term corticosteroid treatment of myasthenia gravis: Report of 116 patients. Ann Neurol 1984;15:291–8.

Richman DP, Agius MA. Treatment of autoimmune myasthenia gravis. Neurology 2003;61:1652–61.

Saperstein DS, Barohn RJ. Management of myasthenia gravis. Semin Neurol 2004;24:41–8.

Seybold ME, Drachman DB. Gradually increasing doses of prednisone in MG. N Engl J Med 1974;290:81–4.

Vincent A, Leite MI. Neuromuscular junction autoimmune disease: Muscle specific kinase antibodies and treatments for myasthenia gravis. Curr Opinion Neurol 2005;18:519–25.

[1]Not FDA approved for this indication.

Trigeminal Neuralgia

Method of
Ronald F. Young, MD

Trigeminal neuralgia (TN) is one of the most devastating pain conditions that people endure. The pain is frequently misdiagnosed as being of dental or paranasal sinus origin. Unnecessary dental procedures, such as root canals and extractions or sinus surgery, are often performed in misguided attempts to treat the pain. The condition is also referred to as *tic douloureux* because of the sudden facial grimacing that may be seen as a reaction to the pain. The illness is estimated to affect about 1 in 20,000 people and becomes more frequent with advancing age. TN may be of primary (idiopathic) origin or secondary origin due to a variety of structural conditions, such as tumors (meningiomas and vestibular schwannomas in particular), multiple sclerosis (MS), vascular malformations, and cysts of the posterior cranial fossa. The exact etiology of TN is still debated, but it is generally accepted that most cases of idiopathic TN are due to compression of the trigeminal nerve root near its entry into the brainstem at the pons by adjacent blood vessels, most commonly arteries. Such compression is thought to result in segmental demyelination due to the constant pulsatile forces directed against the nerve root. The underlying pathology is thought to be related to the aging process wherein arteries (particularly the superior cerebellar artery) that normally course superior to, but not in contact with, the nerve root gradually come into contact and then compress and distort the nerve root as a result of constant pulsatile pressure. Such pressure causes localized demyelination and loss of the normal insulating function of the myelin. Ephaptic or nonsynaptic transmission and abnormal local depolarization are then postulated to result in ectopic impulse generation. Such impulses are thought to activate nerve fibers in the trigeminal nerve root that generate the pain of TN. Ephaptic transmission is also thought to account for the "triggering" of pain by usually innocuous stimuli, such as lightly touching the face or brushing the teeth.

Diagnosis

In spite of modern technology, TN is a diagnosis based almost exclusively on the medical history. Neither laboratory nor imaging studies establish the diagnosis conclusively, although properly formatted magnetic resonance imaging (MRI) scans recently have been thought to contribute to the correct diagnosis if they demonstrate arterial compression of the trigeminal nerve root. Three aspects of the history are critical to the diagnosis: (1) the type of pain, (2) the location of the pain, and (3) the factors that trigger or activate the pain. The pain of TN is sharp, sudden, severe, and brief in character, usually lasting only a few seconds but often occurring in repeated bursts. The pain is often described as feeling like an electric shock or ice pick jabbing into the face. Pains that are of longer duration and described as burning, aching, boring, or like pressure are not typical of TN; when such symptoms are described, an alternative diagnosis should be considered. The pain of TN is confined within one or more of the major three peripheral divisions of the trigeminal nerve: the first division encompassing the anterior two thirds of the scalp, the forehead, the eye, and the upper portion of the nose; the second division encompassing the edges of the nares, the upper lip and cheek, the upper teeth, gums, and mucosal lining of the mouth; and the third division encompassing the skin over the mandible, including the lower lip as well as the lower teeth, gums, and anterior two thirds of the tongue. Pain that is located in the mastoid or occipital region, deep within the ear canal, extending below the edge of the mandible onto the neck or traversing the midline is not trigeminal in origin. TN is almost exclusively a unilateral condition. Bilateral pain is estimated to occur in less than 1% of cases; when bilateral the pain on

the two sides is often different with regard to the age of the patient at onset and the location of the pain. Most cases of bilateral TN occur in patients with MS wherein the pain is due to demyelination in the trigeminal nerve root secondary to an MS plaque. One of the most characteristic historical features of TN is the triggering of jabs or jolts of pain by stimuli that usually are innocuous. Such triggers include a variety of light mechanical stimuli, such as touching the face lightly, brushing the teeth, talking, attempting to eat and drink, and even a light breeze blowing against the face. Light, gentle stimuli are often more effective in eliciting the pain than are more forceful ones. Facial pain, even severe pain, probably is not TN if trigger phenomena are not described. The time course of TN is marked by unexplained, erratic exacerbations and remissions that may last days, weeks, months, or even years. The exacerbations tend to be less severe and shorter in duration at the onset of the illness and tend to become more severe and longer in duration and marked by shorter interval remissions as the illness persists over time. Patients who complain of persistent, unremitting facial pain, often with durations of weeks, months, or even years, probably do not suffer from TN. TN is often misdiagnosed as being of dental or paranasal sinus origin, but conversely other forms of facial pain are often misdiagnosed as TN. Most commonly misdiagnosed is so-called atypical facial pain. Such pain, often seen in young or middle-aged women but seen in men as well, usually is described as a strong, unremitting pressure or burning sensation that encompasses an area of the head and/or neck outside of the distribution of the trigeminal nerve, unassociated with trigger phenomena, often of prolonged durations (years), and usually unresponsive to a variety of medical interventions. Patients with atypical facial pain often express feelings of depression and hopelessness. Such pain is unresponsive to surgical intervention, and ill-advised surgical procedures often aggravate the pain and may leave the patient with new medical problems due to complications of the surgical procedures.

Physical Examination

In classic, or idiopathic, TN due to vascular compression of the trigeminal nerve root, the physical examination is usually completely unremarkable. Specifically, at least by the usual clinical examination techniques, facial sensation including the corneal reflex is normal. When loss of facial sensation to innocuous or painful stimuli is detected, a structural cause of TN should be sought. Tumors, vascular malformations, and MS are usually accompanied by other abnormal neurologic examination findings, including double vision, unilateral hearing loss, and facial weakness. MRI scanning is recommended in all patients with a suspected diagnosis of TN because even in some cases of TN caused by structural lesions, the examination may be normal, and the diagnosis of TN may be strengthened if an MRI scan demonstrates arterial compression of the trigeminal nerve root. Occasionally, an MRI scan discloses a completely unexpected cause of TN, such as a tortuous vertebrobasilar artery complex compressing the nerve root or even a large contralateral tumor or cyst displacing the brainstem. Such findings may radically alter any surgical recommendations made for treatment of TN. Patients who are unable to undergo MRI scanning because they have a cardiac pacemaker, for instance, should undergo thin-section computed tomography scanning, which cannot detect arterial vascular compression and small tumors but can detect larger tumors, vascular malformations, and vertebrobasilar artery compression.

Treatment

MEDICAL TREATMENT

The anticonvulsant family of drugs is the mainstay of medical treatment of TN. Carbamazepine (Tegretol) and oxcarbazepine (Trileptal)[1] are the best drugs for initial medical treatment of TN. Both should be started in relatively low doses, for example, 100 to 200 mg once or twice daily and then increased gradually and slowly until either satisfactory control of the pain or intolerable side effects occur. Such side effects include drowsiness, weakness, difficulty with recent memory, and unsteadiness of gait. Older patients are particularly sensitive to such side effects, and the initial dose and maximum tolerable dose are usually lower in older patients, particularly those in their 70s and older. From 5 to 7 days should elapse between dosing increments in order to allow development of a stable blood level of medication. Additional increments of 100 to 200 mg/day are recommended. Laboratory tests of serum levels of the medications are of little or no help in the treatment of TN. In order to establish a consistent blood level of these medications and to provide the best chance for achieving lasting pain relief with minimum side effects, counseling of the patient by the physician regarding the correct dosing regimen is essential. Patients often regard these medications as analgesics and vary the dosage on an as-needed basis, some days taking little or no medication and other days taking large amounts. Because of their pharmacokinetics, these medications must be taken in a consistent dosage on a daily basis in order to maximize the chance of success. It is surprising how hard it may be for patients to understand and adhere to such a regimen, but maintaining the regimen is essential for successful pain relief. Gabapentin (Neurontin)[1] has become popular for the treatment of TN, but experience indicates it is a secondary medication only. It may be useful when pain control cannot be achieved with carbamazepine (Tegretol) or oxcarbazepine (Trileptal) or when those medications cannot be tolerated because of side effects. Other potential second-line medications include a variety of other anticonvulsants (e.g., lamotrigine [Lamictal],[1] phenytoin [Dilantin][1]) as well as baclofen (Lioresal) A variety of toxicities, including liver dysfunction, bone marrow suppression, and allergic reactions, may accompany use of these medications, so appropriate laboratory surveillance should be performed per manufacturers' recommendations.

SURGICAL TREATMENT

In the past, surgery was reserved for patients who did not respond to medical management of TN because the medication was ineffective or the side effects or toxicities were intolerable. However, some studies suggest that the longer the illness persists, the smaller the chance

---

[1]Not FDA approved for this indication.

CURRENT THERAPY

- Usually responds to oral anticonvulsant medications, such as carbamazepine (Tegretol) or oxcarbazepine (Trileptal).[1]
- Early radiosurgical treatment offers a good chance of curing the illness with minimal side effects.
- Microvascular decompression is the most effective surgical treatment of TN, but it is associated with the greatest risk of serious complications.

---

[1]Not FDA approved for this indication.

for lasting successful surgical relief of the pain. Many patients considered the potential side effects and complications of the surgical procedures unacceptable, and neurologists often referred patients for surgical procedures only as a last resort. With the advent of radiosurgery as a viable, successful, and safe surgical treatment of TN, consideration of surgical intervention earlier rather than later in the disease course may be better. Microvascular decompression (MVD) is the most effective, yet most dangerous, of the surgical procedures for TN. About 90% of patients will achieve immediate relief of TN after MVD, but this success rate drops to about 75% in long-term follow-up. MVD is the only surgical procedure that treats the putative cause of TN, namely, vascular compression of the trigeminal nerve root. In the MVD procedure, a small posterior fossa craniotomy is performed. The trigeminal nerve root is visualized using the operating microscope, any compressing vessels are dissected free of the nerve, and future contact is prevented by placing a shock-absorbing material, usually shredded Teflon felt, between the vessel and the nerve. Fatal complications may occur in up to 1% of patients undergoing the MVD procedures. From 15% to 20% of patients who undergo MVD experience some complication of the procedure, such as cerebellar edema, brainstem infarction, subdural and epidural hematomas, facial paralysis, unilateral hearing loss, cerebrospinal fluid leakage, meningitis, and infection. Percutaneous procedures (e.g., radiofrequency electrocoagulation, glycerol rhizolysis, balloon compression) are considerably safer than MVD, but loss of facial sensation usually accompanies such procedures. Loss of facial sensation should be avoided in order to prevent secondary complications such as anesthesia dolorosa and loss of the corneal reflex with subsequent corneal ulceration or loss of vision. The initial success rate is about 90% with the percutaneous procedures, but recurrences are frequent. Serious side effects, such as meningitis, brain abscess or hematoma, and carotid artery to cavernous sinus fistulas, occasionally occur. One of the attractive features of percutaneous procedures is that they can be repeated fairly easily if pain recurs. Radiosurgery is gaining increased acceptance as a surgical method for treating TN. Although considered a form of surgery, the procedure is accomplished without an incision, instead using either gamma rays (Gamma Knife, Elekta, Inc.) or high-energy x-rays (linear accelerator [LINAC]) that are focused on the trigeminal nerve root adjacent to the brainstem. The treatment is planned using MRI or computed tomography scanning, and the radiation is guided to the target at the trigeminal nerve root in such a way as to avoid injury to adjacent structures. The procedure provides pain relief in about 60% of patients with TN without the need for medication; another 15% to 20% of patients experience pain relief with small tolerable doses of medication. Radiosurgery is attractive to patients and referring physicians because of the ease of performing the procedure and the minimum risk of side effects. Radiosurgery is a destructive form of treatment of TN, but the degree of damage to the nerve root is usually minimal enough that normal facial sensation is maintained. Permanent losses of facial sensation may occur in as few as 5% of patients treated with radiosurgery, depending on the dose of radiation used for the treatment. Drawbacks of radiosurgery include delayed onset of pain relief after treatment (usually a few months) and recurrences. Radiosurgery can be repeated in the event of initial failure of the treatment or in case of recurrence after an initially successful treatment. The reasonable success rate, the ease of performance of the procedure, and the minimal risk of side effects make radiosurgery a treatment that can be recommended early in the treatment of TN, once the diagnosis has been well established, because it may provide permanent cure of the disease with minimal risk.

REFERENCES

Bagheri SC, Fairhdvash F, Perciaccante VJ. Diagnosis and treatment of patients with trigeminal neuralgia. Am-Dent Assoc 2004;135:1713–17.

Kres B, Schindler M, Rasche D, et al. MRI volumetry for the preoperative diagnosis of trigeminal neuralgia. Eur Radiol 2005;15:1344–8.

Liu JK, Apfelbaum RI. Treatment of trigeminal neuralgia. Neurosurg Clin North Am 2004;15:319–34.

Shetter AG, Aabramisk JM, Speiser BL. Microvascular decompression after gamma knife surgery for trigeminal neuralgia: Intraoperative findings and treatment outcomes. J Neurosurg 2000;102(Suppl.):259–61.

Young RF. Stereotactic procedures for facial pain. In: Apuzzo M, editor. Brain Surgery: Complication Avoidance and Management. New York: Churchill Livingstone; 1993. p. 2097–114.

Young RF. Radiosurgery versus microsurgery for trigeminal neuralgia: Current techniques in neurosurgery. In: Salcman M, editor. Current medicine. New York: Springer; 1998. p. 35–43.

Young RF, Vermeulen SS, Grimm P, et al. Gamma knife radiosurgery for treatment of trigeminal neuralgia: Idiopathic and tumor related. Neurology 1997;48:608–14.

Young RF, Vermeulen SS, Posewitz A. Gamma knife radiosurgery for treatment of trigeminal neuralgia. Stereotact Funct Neurosurg 1998;70:192–9.

Acute Peripheral Facial Paralysis (Bell's Palsy)

Method of
Bryan K. Ward, MD, and Barry M. Schaitkin, MD

Acute facial nerve paralysis (i.e., Bell's palsy) manifests as an acute onset of facial muscle weakness. The condition is named for the Scottish surgeon Sir Charles Bell. In 1821, he described paralysis of the muscles of facial expression after facial trauma. The name *Bell's palsy* was later given to this common atraumatic cause of facial paralysis. Although there are numerous causes of facial paralysis, approximately two thirds of cases are idiopathic acute facial nerve paralysis, or Bell's palsy (Fig. 1).

DIFFERENTIAL DIAGNOSIS OF ACUTE FACIAL NERVE PARALYSIS

Idiopathic (65%)
- Bell's palsy

Infection (associated with Bell's palsy)
- Herpes zoster, herpes simplex, borreliosis (commonly associated)
- Epstein-Barr, HIV, cytomegalovirus virus, mycoplasma pneumonia, tuberculosis, Kawasaki syndrome (uncommonly associated)
- Acute and chronic suppurative otitis media (rare since introduction of antibiotics)

Trauma (25%)
- Temporal bone fracture, penetrating wound

Neoplasms (5%)
- Parotid gland, metastases (skin, breast, lung, kidney, colon), cholesteatoma, schwannoma

Metabolic and toxic
- Diabetes, thyroid disease, alcoholism, carbon monoxide

Other rare causes
- Sarcoidosis, multiple sclerosis, amyloidosis, Wegener's granulomatosis, Sjögren's disease, Guillain-Barré syndrome, Melkersson-Rosenthal syndrome

---

FIGURE 1. Causes of facial nerve palsy. *Abbreviation:* HIV = human immunodeficiency virus.

The incidence of Bell's palsy is 1 case per 3000 people per year. It occurs most commonly in persons between the ages of 15 and 40 years and less commonly in children younger than 15 years. Diabetics and pregnant women are at increased risk, with pregnant women three times as likely to develop Bell's palsy compared with nonpregnant women, particularly in the third-trimester and postpartum periods.

The mechanism of Bell's palsy is still unconfirmed, but there are hypotheses. One theory is that inflammation of the facial nerve causes entrapment along its course through the fallopian canal, leading to secondary ischemia and nerve damage. Another theory involves viral infection causing direct interference with neural function without nerve compression.

Numerous viruses have been associated with acute facial nerve paralysis. Evidence points to an association with herpesvirus, but no direct causality in humans has been shown. Using a mouse model, Sugita and colleagues were able to demonstrate transient facial weakness in mice inoculated with a strain of herpes simplex virus type 1 (HSV-1). The greatest evidence for a viral association with Bell's palsy in humans is the work by Murakami and associates, in which endoneural fluid from 10 of 13 patients tested positive by polymerase chain reaction (PCR) assay for HSV-1 DNA after surgical decompression of the facial nerve. PCR testing of endoneural fluid from 7 patients with Ramsay-Hunt syndrome showed the samples to be positive varicella-zoster virus (i.e., human herpesvirus 3).

A temporal relationship between viral reactivation and the onset of Bell's palsy has not been confirmed. PCR studies have demonstrated a link but cannot differentiate latent from active infections. Perhaps the strongest evidence for a viral cause of Bell's palsy comes from a clustering of cases in Switzerland after the administration of an inactivated nasal influenza vaccination. A matched case-control study showed that 27.7% of 68 patients with Bell's palsy during the study had received the vaccine, compared with 1.1% of controls. The risk for those who received the vaccination was highest at 30 to 60 days, and this increased risk did not exist for those who received the parenteral form.

Clinical Presentation

Bell's palsy has been described as "peas in a pod" because of its typical clinical presentation. Patients may initially experience pain behind the ear or in the ear canal that precedes facial muscle weakness. The patient may have a history of recent upper respiratory infection. Weakness progresses within 48 hours to complete or near-complete paralysis of all the muscles of facial expression, almost always unilaterally. Other possible symptoms include hyperacusis on the affected side due to paresis of the stapedius muscle, ipsilateral impaired taste in the anterior tongue due to dysfunction of the chorda tympani nerve, and decreased tearing from interrupted parasympathetic input to the lacrimal gland. Palsies of other cranial nerves have been associated with Bell's palsy, although this relationship is controversial.

Not all facial paralysis is Bell's palsy. Because the cause of Bell's palsy is probably viral, which has no available diagnostic test, other forms of acute facial paralysis must first be considered. Any patient with acute facial paralysis but without the typical clinical presentation of Bell's palsy should be further evaluated. Atypical presentations have been described by Mark May as lima beans in a pea pod, and they require further investigation. The time of onset of the facial weakness is important. Slowly progressive weakness and recurrent or persistent paralysis should raise suspicion of a neoplasm involving the facial nerve. Other findings suggesting a tumor include a parotid mass on physical examination, the isolated weakness of a single peripheral branch of the nerve, muscle twitching preceding paralysis, and a history of any previous malignancy. The patient should be asked about past trauma, a draining ear, vertigo, hearing loss, tinnitus, tick exposure, and other neurologic complaints.

Patients with more severe pain likely have herpes zoster oticus (i.e., Ramsay Hunt syndrome), which is diagnosed by the presence of vesicles that usually occur in the external auditory canal or on the auricle. Ramsay Hunt patients may also have vestibulocochlear nerve symptoms, such as hearing loss, vertigo, or tinnitus. These symptoms are not found in patients with Bell's palsy.

Lyme disease and sarcoidosis are two commonly discussed but uncommon causes of facial paralysis. Borreliosis can cause facial paralysis in up to 11% of all cases of Lyme disease, a third of which manifest bilaterally. If the patient does not demonstrate other symptoms of Lyme disease, it is unlikely to be the cause of facial paralysis. Lyme titers are not recommended unless a patient also has other symptoms, such as rash, arthritis, or heart block.

Sarcoidosis is another rare cause of bilateral facial paralysis; facial paralysis occurs in less than 5% of patients with sarcoidosis. Patients can present with a rare syndrome of sarcoidosis called Heerfordt's syndrome or uveoparotid fever, which includes uveitis, parotitis, and facial nerve paralysis.

Evaluation

When evaluating a patient for Bell's palsy, it is helpful to think about the course of the facial nerve. The commands for facial expression are initiated in the cerebral cortex at the lateral precentral gyrus and cross as corticobulbar fibers. The fibers supplying the lower face cross only once, whereas the fibers ultimately supplying the forehead cross twice and provide bilateral cortical innervation. A central cause of acute facial paralysis usually affects only the lower face on the contralateral side. Patients with cortical lesions may have some emotional or involuntary response in the affected side because these fibers are thought to arise more caudally in the thalamus.

From descending corticobulbar fibers, the facial nerve arises in the pons near the abducens nerve. Simultaneous facial muscle and lateral rectus muscle weakness suggests a pontine lesion. At the cerebellopontine angle, the facial nerve joins the vestibulocochlear nerve before entering the temporal bone. As a result of this proximity to other cranial nerves, performing a detailed cranial nerve examination is important for localizing mass lesions that may cause facial paresis.

The facial nerve then enters the temporal bone and travels 3 to 4 mm through the narrowest portion of the temporal bone, called the fallopian canal. The meatal segment is the narrowest portion of the canal and is a common site of injury during temporal bone fractures. This segment is thought to be the site of nerve compression by edema in Bell's palsy. Otoscopic examination of the auditory canal and tympanic membrane can help diagnose other causes of facial nerve damage in this area, such as acute or chronic otitis media, trauma, or masses such as cholesteatomas or glomus jugulare tumors.

The nerve exits the temporal bone through the stylomastoid foramen and enters the parotid gland, where it branches into terminal segments. Palpation of the parotid gland is important to evaluate for signs of neoplasms that can invade the facial nerve and cause paresis. Evaluation of the integrity of each of the five terminal branches is accomplished by asking the patient to elevate the brow, tightly close the eyes, show the teeth, pucker the lips, and tense the neck. Before emerging from the temporal bone, the facial nerve is not organized into distinct branches; therefore, any lesion with a distinct branch weakness can be caused only by parotid pathology.

Most patients with typical Bell's palsy do not require any additional work-up. In atypical cases, computed tomography (CT) or magnetic resonance imaging (MRI) may be beneficial for evaluating masses or other potential surgical causes of facial nerve paralysis. Electrodiagnostic testing can be performed on patients with acute facial nerve paralysis for diagnostic and prognostic purposes, but it is typically reserved for patients with complete paralysis. Electroneurography involves stimulating the facial nerve at the stylomastoid foramen and recording combined action potentials from electrodes placed over the affected muscles. This test is usually performed in the first 10 days after the onset of symptoms to evaluate nerve degeneration. More than 90% nerve degeneration combined with the absence of voluntary motor unit action potentials indicates a poor prognosis and a point at which surgical decompression may be beneficial, but surgery remains controversial.

CURRENT DIAGNOSIS

- Acute facial paralysis (Bell's Palsy) is a symptomatically defined diagnosis of exclusion.
- Full head and neck examination, including cranial nerves and House-Brackmann assessment, should be performed on all patients with acute facial paralysis.
- Patients with atypical features, such as prolonged paralysis, recurrent paralysis, or isolated branch weakness, should be evaluated with CT or MRI and evaluated by a specialist.

Clinical Course

Bell's palsy typically progresses to maximal weakness within 48 hours, but this progression may take up to 2 weeks. Approximately 85% of patients begin recovery within 3 weeks. No recovery within 3 weeks portends a poorer prognosis. Without treatment, 71% of patients with Bell's palsy will recover fully. An often-cited 1982 study by Pieterson and colleagues followed 1011 patients with Bell's palsy and revealed that the prognosis for full recovery depends on the severity of the initial paralysis. Clinically, the House-Brackmann (HB) scale is an accepted objective measure of this subjective clinical assessment of severity (Fig. 2).

In addition to severity of paralysis, other factors may affect the prognosis for recovery from facial paralysis. Ramsay Hunt syndrome causes more severe paralysis and has a poorer outcome. Gillman and coworkers showed that pregnant women who develop Bell's palsy might also have a poorer prognosis if complete paralysis develops (52% recovering to HB I or II, compared with 80% in a nonpregnant population). Diabetics may also have a poorer prognosis. Although the reason for this poorer prognosis is unknown, a possible explanation may involve patient compliance during steroid administration and resultant uncontrolled hyperglycemia.

Treatment

PHARMACOLOGIC THERAPY

The rationale for treatment with steroids originates with observations during surgery of facial nerve swelling in patients with Bell's palsy and the presumption that this edema contributes to facial paralysis.

HOUSE-BRACKMANN FACIAL NERVE GRADING SYSTEM

Grade I: Normal function

- Normal facial function in all areas

Grade II: Mild dysfunction

- Slight weakness noticeable on close inspection; may have very slight synkinesis

Grade III: Moderate dysfunction

- Obvious weakness or disfiguring asymmetry; normal symmetry and tone at rest; incomplete eye closure

Grade IV: Moderately severe dysfunction

- Obvious weakness or disfiguring asymmetry; normal symmetry and tone at rest; incomplete eye closure

Grade V: Severe dysfunction

- Only barely perceptible motion; asymmetry at rest

Grade VI: Total paralysis

- No movement

FIGURE 2. House-Brackmann facial nerve grading system.

Many studies have indicated a benefit for glucocorticoids over placebo in patients with Bell's palsy, although the data initially were conflicting. Because most patients with Bell's palsy do well without any intervention, demonstrating improvement requires much larger studies than were originally performed.

A double-blind, randomized, controlled trial by Sullivan and colleagues assessed the benefit of prednisolone (Millipred)[1] and acyclovir (Zovirax)[1] in the early treatment of Bell's palsy in a large population. The study had four arms consisting of acyclovir alone, prednisolone alone, acyclovir plus prednisolone, and placebo, with all treatments given within 72 hours of the development of symptoms. At 3 months and 9 months of follow-up, patients who received prednisolone were more likely to have a complete recovery than those who received placebo. The number of patients with facial paralysis needed to treat to obtain one additional full recovery was six at 3 months and eight at 9 months. As a result, early treatment with glucocorticoids for patients with Bell's palsy is recommended.

Results of trials of antiviral therapies have had conflicting results. Because Bell's palsy was strongly associated with viral infections, antiviral medications became a preferred treatment, regardless of the lack of evidence demonstrating their effectiveness. Numerous studies have indicated a role for early steroid treatment in improving long-term recovery of patients with Bell's palsy, but the role of antivirals remains controversial. The Sullivan study indicated no advantage for acyclovir over placebo, alone or combined with glucocorticoids. The results of this study, however, conflict with another large, randomized, controlled trial by Hato and associates, in which patients were given valacyclovir (Valtrex)[1] 500 mg twice daily for 5 days) or placebo and prednisolone. In this study, an overall benefit was seen for valacyclovir with prednisolone over prednisolone alone, including a marked improvement in percent of patients with complete facial paralysis who had full recovery among those (90.1% versus 75.0%). Although these outcomes are compelling, no study findings have been adopted as the gold standard. The use of valacyclovir should receive further investigation. Prednisone is used universally, and antivirals continue to be commonly employed.

Although the Sullivan study indicated no role for acyclovir in the treatment of Bell's palsy, valacyclovir may provide benefit because of its lack of first-pass metabolism and its better pharmacokinetic profile. Cost remains a factor because antivirals are considerably more expensive than corticosteroids. Valacyclovir may provide benefit, but it should be reserved for those with complete facial paralysis in the first 72 hours.

SURGICAL THERAPY

The surgical treatment of Bell's palsy is usually performed by a neuro-otologist who decompresses the facial nerve at its narrowest point in the fallopian canal using a middle fossa approach. Beginning with surgeons Balance and Duel in the 1930s, some of the earliest treatments for Bell's palsy were surgical decompression. These approaches began to wane as steroids became popular. Surgical decompression of the facial nerve is still performed, but it remains controversial. Electrical testing is used to determine potential surgical benefit, which is performed only in cases of complete facial paralysis. A retrospective study by Gantz and colleagues of 54 patients who elected to undergo decompression surgery demonstrated surgical benefit for those with complete facial paralysis and more than 90% degeneration as determined by electroneurography at 10 days and with no voluntary motor unit action potentials on electromyography. Of those who chose surgical decompression by a middle fossa approach, 91% achieved HB grade I or II results, compared with 42% who chose medical therapy with corticosteroids. The risks associated with this procedure include hearing loss, further facial nerve injury, cerebrospinal fluid leak, and seizures.

OTHER THERAPY

Eye care is needed. Patients for whom the eyelids cannot appose are at increased risk for drying and corneal ulceration. These patients need to be monitored for exposure keratitis, which may require referral to an ophthalmologist. Symptoms include blurred vision, photophobia, irritation, and epiphora (i.e., tearing). Use of artificial tears

CURRENT THERAPY

- Corticosteroid therapy initiated within 72 hours of the onset of paralysis increases the likelihood of recovery of patients with Bell's palsy (prednisolone[1] 20 mg twice daily for 7 days or prednisone 60–80 mg daily for 7 days).
- Although the use of acyclovir (Zovirax)[1] remains controversial, valacyclovir (Valtrex)[1] may provide benefit for patients with more severe facial paralysis (500 mg twice daily for 7 days).
- Eye care with artificial tears, barrier protection, and ophthalmic ointments at night can prevent exposure keratitis.

[1]Not FDA approved for this indication.

while awake and ophthalmic ointments at night can prevent drying. Protective glasses should be worn during the day. If necessary, a gold weight may aid in closing the affected eye.

Nerve stimulation has been used to aid recovery of facial nerve function; however, there have been no studies to show its effectiveness. Because cases of hemifacial spasm have been reported after electrical stimulation, it is not recommended for treatment of Bell's palsy. Management of Bell's palsy can usually be handled by the primary care physician in an outpatient setting. These patients should be followed for at least 6 months to monitor for improvement or progression of paralysis. Patients who fail to improve or who have atypical symptoms should be referred to an otolaryngologist with expertise in facial paralysis.

Although most patients with Bell's palsy recover without impairment, 30% suffer some permanent change, and 15% are left with substantial deficits. Facial paralysis greatly affects the individual's ability to interact socially. In addition to psychiatric concerns such as depressed mood and anxiety, patients may experience difficulty with maintaining employment and relationships. Regional centers offer facial physical therapy by therapists specializing in these problems. Facial reanimation procedures may aid cosmetically, but they are performed only in a small percentage of patients. Botulinum toxin (Botox)[1] injections and physical therapy are the primary therapies offered for late sequelae; nevertheless, patients with persistent paresis after Bell's palsy may require long-term psychosocial care.

REFERENCES

Gantz BJ, Rubinstein JT, Gidley P, Woodworth G. Surgical management of Bell's palsy. Laryngoscope 1999;109:1177–88.

Gillman GS, Schaitkin BM, May M, Klein SR. Bell's palsy in pregnancy: A study of recovery outcomes. Otolaryngol Head Neck Surg 2002;126:26–30.

Hato N, Yamada H, Kohno H, et al. Valacyclovir and prednisolone treatment for Bell's palsy: A multicenter, randomized, placebo-controlled study. Otol Neurotol 2007;28:408–13.

House JW, Brackmann DE. Facial nerve grading system. Otolaryngol Head Neck Surg 1985;93:146–7.

May M, Schaitkin BM. The Facial Nerve. 2nd ed. New York: Thieme Medical Publishers; 2000.

Murakami S, Mizobuchi M, Narashiro Y, et al. Bell's palsy and herpes simplex virus: Identification of viral DNA in endoneurial fluid and muscle. Ann Intern Med 1996;124:27–30.

Mutsch M, Zhou W, Rhodes P, et al. Use of the inactivated intranasal influenza vaccine and the risk of Bell's palsy in Switzerland. N Engl J Med 2004;350:896–903.

Peitersen E. The natural history of Bell's palsy. Am J Otol 1982;4:107–11.

Sugita T, Murakami S, Yanagihara N, et al. Facial nerve paralysis induced by herpes simplex virus in mice; an animal model of acute and transient facial paralysis. Ann Otol Rhinol Laryngol 1995;104:574–81.

Sullivan FM, Swan IRC, Donnan PT, et al. Early treatment with prednisolone or acyclovir in Bell's palsy. N Engl J Med 2007;357:1598–607.

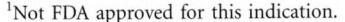

[1]Not FDA approved for this indication.

[1]Not FDA approved for this indication.

Parkinsonism

Method of
Rajesh Pahwa, MD, and Kelly E. Lyons, PhD

Clinical Features

Parkinsonism is a clinical syndrome with the cardinal motor signs of bradykinesia, rigidity, tremor and postural instability. A diagnosis of parkinsonism requires the presence of at least two of the four cardinal features. Other motor features can include hypomimia, decreased blink rate, speech difficulties including hypophonia and dysarthria, micrographia, no or reduced arm swing, shuffling and short steps, freezing, festination, difficulty turning in bed, and stooped posture or kyphosis. Common autonomic features include orthostatic hypotension, dysphagia, constipation, urinary frequency and urgency, incontinence, nocturia, sexual dysfunction, and thermoregulatory dysfunction. Sensory symptoms such as anosmia, visual difficulties, pain, and paresthesias can also occur with parkinsonism. Sleep disturbances including insomnia, fragmented sleep, excessive daytime sleepiness, vivid dreaming, and an increased incidence of sleep disorders are common. Finally, neuropsychiatric disturbances such as anxiety, depression, dementia, and psychosis are often seen with parkinsonism.

Differential Diagnosis

There are many possible causes of parkinsonism (Box 1). Diagnosis is based primarily on clinical examination, medical history, family history and past and current medication use. The most common cause of parkinsonism is Parkinson's disease (PD). PD is a slowly progressive neurodegenerative disease generally with unilateral onset. It is estimated that 0.03% of the general population, 3% older than 65 years and 10% older than 80 years develop PD, with an estimated 50,000 new cases diagnosed each year.

BOX 1   Causes of Parkinsonism

Degenerative Disorders
Parkinson's disease (sporadic and familial)
Parkinson-plus syndromes
• Progressive supranuclear palsy (PSP)
• Multiple system atrophy (MSA)
• Corticobasal degeneration (CBD)
• Dementia with Lewy bodies (DLB)

Other Degenerative Disorders
Hallervorden–Spatz disease
Huntington's disease
Lubag (X-linked dystonia–parkinsonism)
Neuroacanthocytosis
Parkinsonism–ALS–dementia complex of Guam
Spinocerebellar ataxias
Wilson's disease

Secondary Parkinsonism
Drug-induced
Infectious (e.g., Creutzfeld–Jakob disease)
Metabolic (e.g., parathyroidism)
Structural (e.g., hydrocephalus, trauma, tumor)
Toxin-induced
Vascular

ALS = amyotrophic lateral sclerosis.

 CURRENT DIAGNOSIS

Cardinal Motor Signs
- Bradykinesia
- Postural instability
- Rigidity
- Tremor

Autonomic Dysfunction
- Cardiovascular (e.g., orthostatic hypotension)
- Gastrointestinal (e.g., dysphagia, drooling, constipation, delayed gastric emptying)
- Sexual (e.g., erectile dysfunction, decreased desire and arousal)
- Thermoregulatory (e.g., hyperhydrosis)
- Urologic (e.g., increased frequency and urgency, incontinence, nocturia)

Neuropsychiatric Dysfunction
- Anxiety
- Depression
- Dementia
- Psychosis

Sensory Dysfunction
- Olfactory disturbance (e.g., anosmia)
- Pain
- Paresthesia
- Visual disturbances (e.g., abnormal eye movements, blurred or double vision)

Sleep Dysfunction
- Excessive daytime sleepiness
- Insomnia or fractionated sleep
- Sleep disorders (e.g., REM behavior disorder, sleep apnea, restless legs syndrome)

REM = rapid eye movement.

PD is a clinical diagnosis based on the presence of two of three cardinal symptoms of bradykinesia, rigidity, and tremor with a positive response to carbidopa/levodopa (Sinemet). Several features suggest a diagnosis of a form of parkinsonism other than PD (Table 1). The most common features include a poor response to levodopa, falling as an early symptom, symmetrical onset of symptoms, rapid progression, lack of tremor, and early autonomic symptoms such as urinary incontinence and symptomatic orthostatic hypotension.

PARKINSON-PLUS SYNDROMES

The Parkinson-plus syndromes, progressive supranuclear palsy (PSP), multiple system atrophy (MSA), corticobasal degeneration (CBD), and dementia with Lewy bodies (DLB), can be difficult to differentiate from PD and are often, especially early in the disease course, misdiagnosed as PD.

PSP is a slowly progressive neurodegenerative disease occurring after the age of 40 years; however, the disease course is generally more rapid than that of PD. It can manifest with bradykinesia, rigidity, hypomimia, hypophonia and postural instability with falling, often in the first year. The onset of PSP is often symmetrical, minimal to no rest tremor is observed, and the response to levodopa is poor. As the disease progresses, vertical gaze limitations and other eye movement abnormalities along with dysarthria and dysphagia generally occur. Neck rigidity is usually greater than limb rigidity, and the neck can be held in an extended posture. Frontal dementia and apathy are also commonly seen with PSP.

TABLE 1 Features Indicating a Form of Parkinsonism Other Than Parkinson's Disease

Feature	Possible Diagnosis
Acute onset	Vascular, drug or toxin-induced, psychogenic
Alien limb	Corticobasal degeneration
Apraxia	Corticobasal degeneration
Ataxia	Multiple system atrophy
Autonomic disturbances (early in disease course)	Multiple system atrophy
Dementia (within 1 y of parkinsonian signs)	Dementia with Lewy bodies
Gaze palsies	Progressive supranuclear palsy, corticobasal degeneration, multiple system atrophy, dementia with Lewy bodies
Hallucinations (unrelated to drug use)	Dementia with Lewy bodies
Pyramidal signs	Multiple system atrophy, vascular
Postural instability (early in disease course)	Progressive supranuclear palsy, multiple system atrophy
Symmetrical onset	Progressive supranuclear palsy, multiple system atrophy
Stepwise worsening	Vascular
Tremor minimal or absent	Progressive supranuclear palsy, vascular
Young onset (<40 y of age)	Drug induced, Wilson's disease

BOX 2 Medications That Can Cause Parkinsonism

Antipsychotics
Acetophenazine (Tindal)[2]
Chlorpromazine (Thorazine)
Chlorprothixene (Taractan)
Fluphenazine (Permitil, Prolixin)
Haloperidol (Haldol)
Loxapine (Loxitane)
Mesoridazine (Serentil)
Molindone (Moban)

Antiemetics
Metoclopramide (Reglan)
Ondansetron (Zofran)

Miscellaneous
Amiodarone (Cordarone)
Amoxapine (Asendin)
Divalproex (Depakote)
Lithium (Eskalith)
Olanzapine (Zyprexa)
Perphenazine (Trilafon)
Perphenazine + amitriptyline (Etafron, Triavil)
Procaine (Novocain)
Prochlorperazine (Compazine)
Promethazine (Phenergan)
Risperidone (Risperdal)
Thioridazine (Mellaril)
Thiothixene (Navane)
Trifluoperazine (Stelazine)
Trifluopromazine (Vesprin)
Ziprasidone (Geodon)

[2]Not available in the United States.

MSA is a neurodegenerative disorder with various combinations of parkinsonian, autonomic, cerebellar, and pyramidal signs. The disease course is generally more rapid than that of PD, and it generally affects people in their 50s and 60s. It is estimated that 80% of MSA patients have predominantly parkinsonian (MSA-P) features and 20% have predominantly cerebellar features (MSA-C). Autonomic symptoms most commonly include orthostatic hypotension, urinary incontinence or partial bladder emptying, and erectile dysfunction. Parkinsonian features can include bradykinesia, rigidity, postural instability, and tremor. In addition, orofacial dystonia, antecollis, and a jerky postural tremor can occur. MSA generally responds poorly to levodopa; an initial response may be observed, but it is rarely sustained. Cerebellar features include gait and limb ataxia, ataxic dysarthria, and sustained gaze-evoked nystagmus.

CBD is a progressive, asymmetric disorder affecting persons in their 60s and 70s. The cortical signs include cortical sensory loss, alien limb phenomenon, apraxia, frontal release reflexes, visual or sensory hemineglect, cognitive dysfunction, and dysphasia. The basal ganglia signs include akinesia, rigidity, action or postural tremor, limb dystonia, athetosis, postural instability, falling, and orolingual dyskinesia. Additional signs include hyperreflexia, impaired ocular motility, dysarthria, focal reflex myoclonus, blepharospasm, and dysphagia. CBD does not respond to levodopa.

DLB can be difficult to differentiate from PD dementia (PDD). In general, if the dementia and motor features occur within a year of each other, a diagnosis of DLB rather than PDD is made. DLB results in a progressive decline in cognition that is severe enough to interfere with activities of daily living. It is not uncommon to see fluctuations in cognition with significant variability in attention and alertness and recurrent visual hallucinations. Motor symptoms consistent with parkinsonism are also present. Additional supportive features include frequent falling, syncope, transient loss of consciousness, delusions, REM sleep behavior disorder, and depression. In DLB, the response to levodopa is variable, but few patients have the strong positive response seen in PD.

DRUG-INDUCED PARKINSONISM

Drug-induced parkinsonism occurs in 20% to 40% of patients taking dopamine-blocking agents. The most common offenders are antipsychotics and antiemetics, although other miscellaneous drugs have been reported to cause drug-induced parkinsonism (Box 2). Drug-induced parkinsonism generally has a subacute, asymmetrical onset and can resolve without discontinuation of the offending agent; however, it is best if the offending agent can be stopped. It also tends to be more common and more severe in older persons. Anticholinergics can be helpful with drug-induced symptoms in some patients, as can dopaminergic drugs; however, these drugs can worsen nausea and hallucinations.

Treatment

Although there are multiple treatment options that can improve PD symptoms, there is no known treatment for the other forms of parkinsonism. Often the same medications that are used for PD are tried for other forms of parkinsonism without significant improvement in symptoms. Occasionally, MSA initially responds to PD medications; however, the response is not sustained. In fact, a dramatic and sustained response to antiparkinsonian therapy usually confirms the diagnosis of PD. Symptomatic medical or surgical therapy is the basis of the management of PD. There is increasing attention being focused on the management of nonmotor symptoms of PD such as dementia, depression, psychosis, dysautonomia, and sleep disturbances.

MEDICATIONS

Currently available PD medications include carbidopa/levodopa, monoamine oxidase type B (MAO-B) inhibitors, dopamine agonists, catechol-O-methyl transferase (COMT) inhibitors, anticholinergics, and the antiviral drug amantadine (Symmetrel).

Levodopa

Dopamine is one of the main neurotransmitters that is reduced in PD, and treatment to date has focused on restoring or manipulating this neurotransmitter. Oral dopamine is metabolized and cannot be used as

CURRENT THERAPY

- Dopamine precursor (levodopa)
- MAO-B inhibitors
- Dopamine agonists
- COMT inhibitors
- Amantadine
- Anticholinergics

COMT = catechol-O-methyl transferase; MAO = monoamine oxidase.

treatment in PD. Levodopa, which is the precursor of dopamine, is considered the gold standard for the symptomatic treatment of PD. Orally administered levodopa is mainly absorbed in the upper gastrointestinal tract. Levodopa is metabolized in the periphery mainly to dopamine by aromatic amino acid decarboxylase (AAAD) and to 3-O-methyldopa (3-OMD) by the COMT enzyme. Once levodopa crosses the blood-brain barrier, it is converted to dopamine intraneuronally.

Orally administered levodopa is almost completely absorbed from the gut. Due to metabolism by AAAD and COMT, less than 5% of an oral dose of levodopa crosses the blood–brain barrier. Hence, levodopa is combined with carbidopa, an AAAD inhibitor. Because carbidopa does not cross the blood–brain barrier, it does not inhibit the conversion of levodopa to dopamine in the brain. The half-life of levodopa is approximately 50 minutes, but when administered with carbidopa it increases to 90 minutes. Approximately 70 to 100 mg of carbidopa is required to saturate peripheral decarboxylase to reduce the peripheral side effects of dopamine, such as nausea and vomiting.

Levodopa improves all the cardinal motor features of PD including tremor, bradykinesia, and rigidity. It is the most efficacious medication for PD. Levodopa does not generally improve nonmotor symptoms such as depression or dementia, nor does it improve axial motor symptoms such as speech or swallowing difficulties, freezing of gait and postural instability.

Carbidopa/levodopa is available in dosages of 10/100 mg, 25/100 mg, and 25/250 mg tablets. The initial dose of carbidopa/levodopa is generally one 25/100 mg tablet three times per day. It is advisable to initiate carbidopa/levodopa slowly, starting with one half of a 25/100 mg tablet twice a day for 1 week and then increasing by one-half tablet daily until symptoms are well controlled. Carbidopa/levodopa is also available in an orally dissolvable formulation (Parcopa). This formulation is available in the same strengths as immediate-release carbidopa/levodopa and has similar safety and efficacy. It is particularly useful in patients with swallowing difficulties.

There is also a controlled-release formulation of carbidopa/levodopa (Sinemet-CR) in doses of 25/100 mg and 50/200 mg. This formulation is generally started with 25/100 mg/day and increased to a typical dose of 25/100 mg three times per day or 50/200 mg twice a day. Controlled-release preparations are not as well absorbed, and the bioavailability is 20% to 30% lower than standard preparations. These formulations do not provide any major advantage over the standard formulations.

One of the biggest limitations to the long-term use of levodopa is the development of motor fluctuations and dyskinesia. Approximately 50% of PD patients develop these motor complications after 5 years of levodopa use. Motor fluctuations include end-of-dose wearing-off and random on/off phenomena. When levodopa is initiated, patients generally have a stable control of PD symptoms during the day. However, over a period of months to years, they experience improvement in the PD symptoms for only a few hours after levodopa ingestion and the effects of the drug wear off before the next dose, which is required before the symptoms improve again. This is known as *end-of-dose wearing off*. As the disease progresses, the number of hours of benefit with each dose of levodopa decreases and the patient often requires multiple doses throughout the day. Random on/off fluctuations are rapid transitions (over seconds) between the on state (when the PD symptoms are under good

control) and off state (when PD symptoms are present), and these are usually unpredictable and unrelated to the timing of levodopa.

Dyskinesia is another long-term motor complication of levodopa therapy. Dyskinesia involves involuntary movements such as chorea, dystonia, and ballismus. The most common types of dyskinesia are peak-dose dyskinesia, wearing-off dystonia, and diphasic dystonia/dyskinesia. Peak-dose dyskinesia is the most common form of dyskinesia and occurs when dopamine levels are at their peak. These movements consist of involuntary choreiform movements of the arms, legs, trunk, and head. Wearing-off dystonia is the painful dystonic movements that occur when dopamine levels are low, usually between levodopa dosing, in the middle of the night, or early in the morning before levodopa is taken. Diphasic dystonia/dyskinesia is uncommon and occurs when dopamine levels are rising or falling.

Common acute adverse effects with carbidopa/levodopa include nausea, vomiting, somnolence, and orthostatic hypotension. Other side effects include skin rash, diaphoresis, cardiac arrhythmias, and pedal edema. Psychiatric side effects include confusion, vivid dreams, nightmares, hallucinations, and delusions.

Dopamine Agonists

Dopamine agonists are drugs that directly stimulate the postsynaptic dopamine receptors. After levodopa, dopamine agonists are the most efficacious symptomatic therapy for PD. Dopamine agonists were initially used as an adjunctive therapy to levodopa; however, currently they are increasingly used as both initial monotherapy and as adjunctive therapy. Studies have demonstrated that initial use of dopamine agonists as monotherapy for PD delays the onset of motor fluctuations and dyskinesia. Dopamine agonists also reduce off time in PD patients on levodopa therapy with motor fluctuations.

Commonly used dopamine agonists include pramipexole (Mirapex) and ropinirole (Requip and Requip XL). Other dopamine agonists include bromocriptine (Parlodel), pergolide (Permax),[2] apomorphine (Apokyn), and the rotigotine transdermal system (Neupro).

Bromocriptine

Bromocriptine is an ergoline dopamine agonist and was the first dopamine agonist approved for use in the United States in 1978. Bromocriptine is mainly a D_2 agonist with weak D_1 antagonist properties. It is rapidly absorbed: Its half-life is between 3 and 8 hours and the peak drug plasma levels are reached in 1 to 2 hours. Due to the risk of ergot-related side effects, bromocriptine is rarely used in clinical practice. It is generally started at 1.25 mg once per day and titrated over several weeks to a maximum dose of 10 to 40 mg/day divided into three or four doses.

Pergolide

Pergolide is an ergot-derived dopamine agonist that was recently withdrawn from the United States market due to concerns of cardiac valvular fibrosis. Patients previously exposed to pergolide might be at risk and should undergo echocardiogram screening.

Pramipexole

Pramipexole is a nonergot dopamine agonist approved for use as monotherapy and adjunctive therapy in PD. Pramipexole mainly acts on the D_2, D_3, and D_4 dopamine receptors. It has a half-life of 8 to 12 hours and reaches peak drug plasma concentration in approximately 2 hours. Pramipexole is excreted in the urine mostly unchanged. It is initiated at 0.125 mg three times per day and slowly increased over several weeks to a maximum dose of 1.5 mg three times per day (Table 2).

Ropinirole

Ropinirole is also a nonergot dopamine agonist approved for both monotherapy and adjunctive therapy in PD. It has affinity for the D_2 family of dopamine receptors and no effect on the D_1 or D_5

---

[2]Not available in the United States.

TABLE 2 Dopamine Agonist Titration Schedules

Week	Pramipexole (Mirapex)	Ropinirole (Requip)	Ropinirole Extended Release (Requip XL)
1	0.125 mg tid	0.25 mg tid	2 mg qd
2	0.25 mg tid	0.5 mg tid	4 mg qd
3	0.5 mg tid	0.75 mg tid	6 mg qd
4	0.75 mg tid	1.0 mg tid	8 mg qd
5	1.0 mg tid	1.5 mg tid	12 mg qd
6	1.25 mg tid	2.0 mg tid	16 mg qd
7	1.5 mg tid	2.5 mg tid	20 mg qd
8		3.0 mg tid	24 mg qd
Maximum	1.5 mg tid	8.0 mg tid	24 mg qd

dopaminergic receptors. The plasma half-life of ropinirole is approximately 6 hours, and peak drug plasma concentrations occur in 1 to 2 hours. Ropinirole is initiated at 0.25 mg three times per day and gradually increased over several weeks to a maximum dose. An of 8 mg three times per day. An extended release formulation, ropinirole prolonged release (Requip XL) is also available, allowing once daily dosing (see Table 2).

Rotigotine

Rotigotine was the first transdermal PD medication approved for use in the United States; however, it was withdrawn from the market in 2008 due to manufacturing issues. It is a nonergot dopamine agonist currently approved for early PD. It mainly acts on the D_3, D_2, and D_1 receptors but also has action on the D_4 and D_5 receptors. It is continuously absorbed over 24 hours with stable plasma levels and a half-life of 5 to 7 hours. Rotigotine is initiated at 2 mg per 24 hours and over a period of 3 weeks can be increased to a maximum of 6 mg per 24 hours. The patch is changed daily. The transdermal patch is applied to different body locations, which should change daily, avoiding application to a previous location for at least 14 days to reduce the incidence of skin reactions.

Apomorphine

Apomorphine is approved for advanced PD as a rescue therapy for severe off periods. It is the only subcutaneous injection for PD available in the United States. It is a nonergot, fast-acting dopamine agonist with a high affinity for D_4 receptors, moderate affinity for D_2, D_3, D_5 receptors, and low affinity for D_1 receptors. Apomorphine is rapidly absorbed in 10 to 60 minutes, has a half-life of approximately 40 minutes, and provides an effect for up to 90 minutes. It can be given every 2 hours; however, there are limited data for use exceeding five times per day. A test dose of 2 mg (0.2 mL) is given under medical supervision during an off state, and the dose is titrated by 0.1 mL increments up to a maximum single dose of 0.6 mL.

Apomorphine is an emetic and can cause severe nausea and vomiting; therefore, an antiemetic such as trimethobenzamide (Tigan)[1] should be used for 3 days before administration and for at least 6 weeks after administration of apomorphine. Due to severe hypotension and possible loss of consciousness, apomorphine should not be used with 5-HT$_3$ antagonists like ondansetron (Zofran), granisetron (Kytril), dolasetron (Anzemet), palonosetron (Aloxi), and alosetron (Lotronex).[11]

Adverse Effects

All dopamine agonists have similar side effects except for the long-term risks of pulmonary fibrosis, retroperitoneal fibrosis, and cardiac valvular fibrosis associated only with the ergot dopamine agonists. Adverse effects may be dose and time dependent, and they often

---

[1]Not FDA approved for this indication.
[11]Required to enroll in the manufacturer's prescribing program.

---

occur when therapy is initiated. Common adverse effects include nausea, vomiting, dizziness, somnolence, insomnia, peripheral edema, and orthostatic hypotension. Central adverse effects are mainly psychiatric such as hallucinations, confusion, mood changes, depression, irritability, euphoria, vivid dreams, sleep disturbances, inappropriate sexual behavior, delusions, agitation, and paranoid psychosis. There have been reports of patients falling asleep during activities of daily living, including while operating motor vehicles, and of impulsive disorders like gambling, eating, shopping, and sexual behavior with dopamine agonists.

Catechol-O-Methyl Transferase Inhibitors

COMT inhibitors are drugs that increase the half-life of levodopa by reducing its metabolism. Using COMT inhibitors with levodopa prolongs the action of individual doses of levodopa. Tolcapone (Tasmar) and entacapone (Comtan) are both specific and reversible inhibitors of COMT, and they increase the area under the levodopa plasma concentration/time curve. At therapeutic doses, entacapone only acts peripherally and does not affect central COMT activity. Tolcapone can pass the blood-brain barrier and block central COMT in addition to its peripheral actions.

Tolcapone

Tolcapone (Tasmar) has a half-life of approximately 2 to 3 hours, and the time to maximum plasma concentration is approximately 2 hours. It is initiated at 100 mg three times a day and increased to 200 mg three times a day if needed. Tolcapone should always be used with levodopa.

The majority of the adverse effects related to tolcapone are dopaminergic in nature. Dyskinesia, nausea, hallucinations, insomnia, anorexia, and orthostatic hypotension are common. These adverse effects are usually improved by reduction in the levodopa dose. Diarrhea as an adverse effect usually begins at 6 to 12 weeks but can appear as early as 2 weeks after tolcapone is started. If the diarrhea is bothersome, therapy must be discontinued. Urine discoloration is a harmless side effect that occurs in less than 10% of patients.

Significant increases in liver enzymes have been reported, and after FDA approval, there were three cases of fatal liver injury reported with the use of tolcapone. This led to strict guidelines regarding the use of tolcapone: it may only be used in PD patients who have tried all other antiparkinsonian medications, and serum ALT and AST should be tested at baseline, every 2 to 4 weeks for the first 6 months, and then as clinically indicated. Tolcapone should be discontinued if the patient does not have a response or if there is a two times increase in the upper limit of ALT and AST.

Entacapone

Entacapone (Comtan) is approved for the management of motor fluctuations in PD. Its half-life is approximately one half hour (0.4–0.7 hours). It reduces the peripheral metabolism of levodopa and prolongs the levodopa half-life from 1.3 to 2.4 hours. It is initiated at 200 mg with each dose of levodopa for a maximum of eight doses per day.

The side effects of entacapone are similar to those of tolcapone and mostly related to increased dopaminergic stimulation. Dyskinesia, nausea, vomiting, and hallucinations are the most commonly seen dopaminergic adverse effects. These side effects can usually be reduced or eliminated by decreasing the levodopa dose. There is no known hepatotoxicity associated with entacapone and no requirement for liver enzyme monitoring.

Carbidopa/Levodopa/Entacapone

The triple combination carbidopa/levodopa/entacaopone (Stalevo) is available in six different combinations: Stalevo 50 (carbidopa 12.5 mg/levodopa 50 mg/entacapone 200 mg), Stalevo 75 (carbidopa 18.75 mg/levodopa 75 mg/entacapone 200 mg), Stalevo 100 (carbidopa 25 mg/levodopa 100 mg/entacapone 200 mg), Stalevo 125 (carbidopa 31.25 mg/levodopa 125 mg/entacapone 200 mg), Stalevo 150 (carbidopa 37.5 mg/levodopa 150 mg/entacapone 200 mg), and

Stalevo 200 (carbidopa 50 mg/levodopa 200 mg/entacapone 200 mg). This triple combination is indicated in PD patients as a substitute for immediate-release carbidopa/levodopa and entacapone previously administered separately. It can also replace immediate-release carbidopa/levodopa (without entacapone) in patients experiencing end-of-dose wearing-off who are taking 600 mg or less of levodopa and are not having dyskinesia. The adverse effects are similar to those seen with carbidopa/levodopa and entacapone used separately.

Monoamine Oxidase B (MAO-B) Inhibitors

Selegiline (Eldepryl), orally disintegrating selegiline (Zelapar), and rasagiline (Azilect) are the MAO-B inhibitors available in United States. They are selective irreversible MAO-B inhibitors. MAO-B inhibitors increase the half-life of levodopa by blocking the metabolism of dopamine by MAO-B.

Selegiline

Selegiline is an irreversible MAO-B inhibitor and has an elimination half-life of approximately 2 hours. However, because the drug irreversibly inhibits MAO-B, the therapeutic benefits are lost after the enzyme is regenerated. The major plasma metabolites of selegiline are N-desmethylselegiline (the only metabolite with MAO-B inhibiting properties), L-amphetamine, and L-methamphetamine. Selegiline is approved as an adjunct treatment to levodopa; however, it is also used as monotherapy in early disease. The typical dose is 5 mg with breakfast and lunch.

Selegiline is generally well tolerated. The most common adverse effects include nausea, dizziness, insomnia, constipation, excessive sweating, confusion, hallucinations, dry mouth, and orthostatic hypotension. When used as an adjunct to levodopa therapy, an increase in dyskinesia can occur, as well as increases in other levodopa-related side effects. As the dose of selegiline is increased, its selectivity to inhibit MAO-B is decreased, and inhibition of MAO-A can also occur.

Orally Disintegrating Selegiline

The orally disintegrating selegiline tablet is available for oral administration (not to be swallowed) in the strength of 1.25 mg. It is approved for use in advanced PD with motor fluctuations. The initial dose is 1.25 mg a day, which can be increased to 2.5 mg per day if clinically indicated. Selegiline disintegrates within seconds after placement on the tongue and is rapidly absorbed. The pregastric absorption of orally disintegrating selegiline and the avoidance of first-pass metabolism results in higher concentrations of selegiline and lower concentrations of its metabolites compared with the 5-mg swallowed selegiline tablet. Side effects are similar to those reported with selegiline tablets. There are no data on the use of orally disintegrating selegiline as monotherapy in PD.

Rasagiline

Rasagiline is an irreversible MAO-B inhibitor. It is rapidly absorbed and reaches peak plasma concentrations in approximately 1 hour. Its half-life is approximately 3 hours, but because it irreversibly inhibits MAO-B, the therapeutic benefit is not dependent on its half-life. It is approved as monotherapy in early disease (1 mg/day) and in PD patients with advanced disease experiencing motor fluctuations (0.5 mg/day, which can be increased to 1 mg/day as needed).

The most commonly observed adverse events with rasagiline monotherapy were flu syndrome, arthralgia, depression, dyspepsia, and falls. As an adjunct to levodopa, the common adverse effects included dyskinesia, accidental injury, weight loss, postural hypotension, vomiting, anorexia, arthralgia, abdominal pain, nausea, constipation, dry mouth, rash, ecchymosis, somnolence, and paresthesia.

Contraindications

Although MAO inhibitors used in the treatment of PD are specific MAO-B inhibitors, at higher than recommended doses or as an idiosyncratic reaction, MAO-A can also be inhibited. Hence, certain medications should not be used with these medications: analgesics such as meperidine (Demerol), tramadol (Ultram), methadone (Dolophine, Methadose), and propoxyphene (Darvon); the antitussive agent dextromethorphan (found in many over-the-counter cough medicines); St. John's wort, mirtazapine (Remeron), and cyclobenzaprine (Flexeril); sympathomimetic amines, including amphetamines as well as cold products and weight-reducing preparations that contain vasoconstrictors (e.g., pseudoephedrine, phenylephrine, phenylpropanolamine,[2] and ephedrine[2]); and other MAO inhibitors.

Anticholinergics

Anticholinergics were the first class of drugs used for the treatment of PD. They work mainly on the muscarinic acetylcholine receptors. The exact mechanism of action of anticholinergics is unclear. It is believed that there is antagonism between the effects of dopamine and acetylcholine in the basal ganglia and that anticholinergics work by correcting the disequilibrium between striatal dopamine and acetylcholine activity.

A number of anticholinergics are available. They are generally well absorbed after oral administration and usually require dosing two or three times a day. The commonly used anticholinergics for PD include biperiden (Akineton), trihexyphenidyl (Artane), benztropine (Cogentin), and procyclidine (Kemadrin). Anticholinergics should be started at low doses and increased very slowly. Anticholinergics are mildly beneficial in the management of PD and mainly help tremor without significantly affecting bradykinesia or rigidity. Anticholinergics are mainly used in young patients due to safety concerns.

Anticholinergics are contraindicated in patients with narrow-angle glaucoma, tachycardia, prostate hypertrophy, gastrointestinal obstruction, and megacolon. Common side effects include blurring of vision, nausea, constipation, urinary retention, and dry mucous membranes in the mouth and eyes. Acute confusion, hallucinations, psychosis, and sedation can occur. All central adverse effects are more likely to occur in patients with advanced age and in patients with impaired cognitive function.

Amantadine

Amantadine (Symmetrel) was initially marketed as an antiviral agent but was reported to be helpful for tremor, rigidity, and bradykinesia in PD. Since then, the efficacy of amantadine both as monotherapy and in combination with levodopa in the treatment of PD has been demonstrated. There are several modes of action of amantadine, but the exact mechanism in PD is unknown. Presynaptically, amantadine enhances the release of stored catecholamines from dopaminergic terminals and inhibits the reuptake process. Postsynaptically, amantadine exerts a direct effect on dopamine receptors. In addition, it is believed that amantadine has anticholinergic effects and N-methyl-D-aspartate (NMDA) glutamate receptor blockade.

Amantadine is quickly absorbed, with peak blood levels 2 to 4 hours after an oral dose. It should be used with caution in patients with impaired renal function and should not be used in patients with renal failure. The usual dose is 200 to 300 mg/day in divided doses. In early PD, amantadine has mild antiparkinsonian benefits on tremor, bradykinesia, and rigidity. In advanced PD, amantadine has been reported to be efficacious in improving dyskinesia. Common side effects include dizziness, anxiety, impaired coordination, insomnia, and nervousness. Nausea and vomiting occur in 5% to 10% of patients. In some patients, pedal edema and livedo reticularis can be bothersome and can lead to discontinuation of therapy.

DEEP BRAIN STIMULATION

When motor fluctuations and dyskinesia cannot be adequately controlled with medications, surgery may be an option for appropriate patients. Deep brain stimulation (DBS) involves implanting a stimulating electrode into the brain. There are three possible DBS targets for treating PD. DBS of the thalamus results in marked improvement in tremor but does not improve bradykinesia, rigidity, or drug-induced

---

[2]Not available in the United States.

dyskinesia and only minimally improves activities of daily living. DBS of the globus pallidus interna improves all of the cardinal symptoms of PD (tremor, rigidity, bradykinesia) and markedly reduces dyskinesia. DBS of the subthalamic nucleus is the most commonly performed DBS procedure for PD and results in improvements in all the cardinal motor symptoms of PD, motor fluctuations, and dyskinesia, while allowing a substantial decrease in antiparkinsonian medications.

Candidates for Deep Brain Stimulation

Thalamic stimulation is rarely used for PD and may be recommended for patients who have disabling, medication-resistant tremor with minimal signs of bradykinesia and rigidity. Patients who have levodopa-responsive PD and medication-resistant motor fluctuations and dyskinesia are appropriate candidates for pallidal or subthalamic stimulation. For DBS procedures, patients should not have significant cognitive, psychiatric, or behavioral problems, such as dementia or severe depression.

Adverse Events

In general, all DBS procedures have similar adverse effects. These adverse effects can be categorized as surgical, device-related, and stimulation-related complications. The experience of the neurosurgeon and proper patient selection generally reduce the occurrence of adverse events. Serious surgical complications can occur in 1% to 2% of patients and include intracranial bleeds, strokes, and seizures. Infections have been reported in 5% to 8% of patients. Device-related events can occur in up to 25% of patients. These include lead reposition due to incorrect placement, lead displacement, erosion of the skin over the lead or the extension, breakage of the lead or the extension, or malfunction of the implanted pulse generator. Adverse effects related to stimulation depend on the location of the electrode and the stimulus intensity, and they usually improve with stimulation adjustments.

MANAGEMENT

Early Disease

Multiple options are available in initiating therapy in a patient with newly diagnosed PD. Anticholinergics are rarely used due to concerns of adverse effects. Patients with mild symptoms are generally initiated with an MAO-B inhibitor and occasionally may be initiated on amantadine. However, if a patient has functional impairment, an MAO-B inhibitor, dopamine agonist, or levodopa is initiated. If the symptoms are causing significant functional disability, in young patients, a dopamine agonist such as ropinirole, ropinirole extended release, or pramipexole is initiated. In older patients, especially those with cognitive impairment, levodopa is initiated. As the disease progresses, patients often end up on combination therapy.

Advanced Disease

There are multiple treatment options for patients on levodopa who develop motor fluctuations. These include increasing the dose or dosing frequency of levodopa and providing adjunctive therapy with dopamine agonists, COMT inhibitors, or MAO-B inhibitors. Often, patients end up taking medications from each of these classes. Amantadine is the only drug reported to improve dyskinesia. If motor fluctuations and dyskinesia cannot be managed with medications, DBS may be considered in some patients.

REFERENCES

Litvan I. Atypical Parkinsonian Disorders: Clinical and Research Aspects. Totowa, NJ: Humana Press; 2005.
Miyasaki JM, Martin W, Suchowersky O, et al. Practice parameter: Initiation of treatment for Parkinson's disease: An evidence-based review. Neurology 2002;58:11–7.
Olanow CW, Watts RL, Koller WC. An algorithm (decision tree) for the management of Parkinson's disease (2001): Treatment guidelines. Neurology 2001;56(Suppl. 5):S1–8.
Pahwa R, Factor SA, Lyons KE, et al. Practice parameter: Treatment of Parkinson disease with motor fluctuations and dyskinesia (an evidence-based review). Neurology 2006;66:983–95.
Pahwa R, Lyons KE. Handbook of Parkinson's Disease. 4th ed. New York: Informa Healthcare; 2007.
Suchowersky O, Reich S, Perlmutter J, et al. Practice parameter: Diagnosis and prognosis of new onset Parkinson disease (an evidence-based review). Neurology 2006;66:968–75.

Peripheral Neuropathies

Method of
Kerrie Schoffer, MD, FRCPC

Disorders of the peripheral nerve system (PNS) include pathology affecting the spinal cord roots (radiculopathies), the dorsal root ganglia (neuronopathies), the brachial, lumbar, and sacral plexuses (plexopathies), and the terminal nerve (mononeuropathies) or nerves (polyneuropathies). They are among the most common and challenging problems in medical practice, with literally hundreds of conceivable causes. An organized diagnostic approach consists of first categorizing the neuropathy based on clinical and electrophysiologic assessments and then performing a tailored diagnostic evaluation. However astute the diagnostician, the cause of a neuropathy might not found in up to 20% of patients.

Anatomy

Four types of fibers are found in the PNS: motor, large fiber sensory, small fiber sensory, and autonomic. Motor fibers extend peripherally to the neuromuscular junction of their respective muscles and have their cell bodies in motor neurons located in the spinal cord. Conversely, sensory fibers receive information from peripheral sensory receptors and transfer this to cell bodies in the dorsal root ganglia, located near, but outside, the spinal cord. Large, myelinated sensory fibers supply information regarding position and vibration. Small myelinated axons, composed of autonomic and sensory fibers, are responsible for light touch, pain, temperature, and parasympathetic and sympathetic information.

Damage can occur to the cell bodies (neuronopathy), nerve fibers (axonopathy), or to the surrounding myelin sheath (myelinopathy). Myelinopathies principally affect only the coating around the nerve, and an axonopathy results in degeneration of both the axon and myelin. The most distal segments usually degenerate first, in a process termed *Wallerian degeneration*, resulting in a dying-back neuropathy and a stocking and glove clinical pattern. Neuronopathies affect either the motor neuron or dorsal root ganglion and result in degeneration of both peripheral and central processes.

Five-Step Approach to Neuropathies

When evaluating neuropathy, the differential diagnosis can be limited by asking five key questions:

- What is the *fiber type* involved (motor, large sensory, small sensory, autonomic, combination)?
- What is the *pattern of distribution* (distal or proximal, symmetric or asymmetric)?
- What is the *temporal course* (acute, chronic, progressive, stepwise, relapsing remitting)?
- Are there any *key features* pointing to a specific etiology?
- What is the *pathology* (axonal, demyelinating)?

FIBER TYPE

The PNS produces symptomatology in only two ways: negative symptoms (weakness, numbness), which reflects loss of nerve signaling; or positive symptoms (tingling, burning) due to inappropriate spontaneous nerve activity. Box 1 lists symptoms and signs that suggest localization to the peripheral nerves and point specifically to motor, sensory, or autonomic involvement. When inquiring about symptoms, it is important to ask the patient to be as specific as possible. Many patients simply describe an area as numb when, in fact, they are experiencing tingling or even weakness.

A detailed motor examination should include inspection for atrophy, particularly in the distal extensor digitorum brevis and first dorsal interosseous muscles, and for fasciculations (visible twitches of muscle), which are best seen using tangential light. Strength should be tested against resistance, as well as with active maneuvers such as walking on the heels and toes to assess distal strength, and rising from a squatting position to examine proximal muscles. Facial muscles should also be tested. When assessing deep tendon reflexes, ensure the reflex is truly absent by asking the patient to concurrently perform a Jendrassic maneuver (pulling against interlocking fingers) or clench the jaw. Note that the reflex arc consists of large-diameter afferent sensory input as well as motor nerve output, so that dysfunction of either can impair reflexes. Tone is sometimes reduced in peripheral nerve diseases.

On sensory examination, sensation should be tested with a pin and a 128-Hz vibratory tuning fork, beginning at the big toe level and moving progressively more proximal. Likewise, position testing should begin distally, with fingers placed on the lateral sides of the big toe and progressively smaller movements tested. Severe loss of position sense can result in athetoid movements of the fingers when the eyes are closed (pseudoathetosis) or a positive Romberg's sign. Temperature can be tested informally by placing

a cold tuning fork on the skin. Foot injuries may be apparent with severe sensory loss.

Other important signs include high arches and hammertoe deformities, which suggest a long-standing neuropathy causing differences in muscular force. Demyelinating neuropathies, amyloidosis, and leprosy can cause nerve thickening, which is felt best in the dorsal cutaneous nerve of the foot or the great auricular nerve. Superficial nerves, such as the ulnar nerve at the elbow, can be palpated when appropriate. Postural blood pressure should be assessed for a blood pressure drop more than 20 mm Hg systolic or more than 10 mm Hg diastolic, following 5 minutes of supine rest at a minimum, to test autonomic functioning.

Several other levels of the nervous system can mimic symptoms of PNS disease. Myelopathy and motor neuron disease can manifest with weakness similar to motor neuropathies, although upper motor neuron features such as spasticity and increased reflexes are clues. Myopathies can also cause weakness, but usually more proximal than distal and without any sensory impairment. Isolated sensory involvement should be a red flag that the dorsal root ganglia may be the site of involvement rather than the peripheral nerve, particularly important because neuronopathies have a limited differential.

PATTERN OF DISTRIBUTION

The pattern of distribution should be classified in two ways: symmetric or asymmetric and distal or proximal. Putting this together with the fiber type, six patterns of PNS disorders can be appreciated, with specific differentials (Table 1).

The symmetric distal sensorimotor neuropathy (pattern 1) manifests in a stocking-and-glove distribution and is the most common type of polyneuropathy. Once the level of the upper calves is reached, fibers of the same length in the fingertips begin to be affected. Sensorimotor polyneuropathies that affect both the distal and proximal nerves (pattern 2) should alert the physician to think of inflammatory neuropathies, such as Guillain-Barré syndrome (GBS) and chronic inflammatory demyelinating polyneuropathy (CIDP).

Asymmetric patterns (pattern 3) are often a result of trauma or compression, such as that seen in mononeuropathies, radiculopathies, and plexopathies. A pattern that affects multiple anatomically separated nerves is termed *mononeuritis multiplex* and is usually the result of a more diffuse process, such as diabetes or vasculitis.

Predominant motor neuropathies (pattern 4) are often proximal, such as diabetic amyotrophy. An exception is lead neuropathy, which affects motor fibers in a distal radial and peroneal distribution. Pure sensory neuropathies (pattern 5) are more likely to be distal, with the exception of a rare few such as Tangier disease, which manifests with a bathing-suit pattern. Neuropathies with autonomic impairment have a limited differential (pattern 6).

Additionally, involvement of the cranial nerves is only seen in a few causes of neuropathy. GBS, CIDP, Lyme disease, sarcoidosis, HIV-associated neuropathy, and Tangier disease are examples.

TEMPORAL COURSE

Acute neuropathies are relatively rare and suggest an etiology such as GBS, acute intermittent porphyria, ischemia, toxins (thallium toxicity), drugs, or infections (diphtheric neuropathy). Subacute onset (>8 weeks) is seen in nutritional deficiencies, metabolic neuropathies, paraneoplastic syndromes, and CIDP. A chronic course is typical of hereditary neuropathies, a stepwise pattern can be seen in mononeuropathy multiplex, and a relapsing-remitting course occurs with intermittent exposure to a toxin or drug and in CIDP.

KEY SIGNS

Sometimes, there is a key classic feature on history or examination that significantly narrows the differential immediately. Box 2 includes a checklist of items for inquiry and observation during assessment of neuropathy.

BOX 1   Signs and Symptoms of Peripheral Nervous System Disease by Fiber Type

Motor
- Cramps
- Fasciculations
- Hyporeflexia
- Hypotonia
- Muscle atrophy
- Myokymia
- Pes cavus
- Weakness

Large Fiber Sensory
- Decreased vibration and position
- Hyporeflexia
- Pins and needles
- Tingling
- Unsteady gait, especially at night or with eyes closed

Small Fiber Sensory
- Burning
- Decreased pain sensation
- Decreased temperature sensation
- Jabbing

Autonomic
- Decreased or increased sweating
- Heat intolerance
- Impotence
- Postural hypotension
- Urinary retention

TABLE 1 Causes of Neuropathy by Pattern Type

Causes	Potentially Useful Tests
Sensorimotor	
Symmetric and Distal	
Metabolic disorders	OGTT, LFT, creatinine, TSH, vitamin B$_{12}$
Hereditary disorders (CMT)	EMG/NCS
Infections (HIV, leprosy)	HIV test, review of medical and social history
Toxins (drugs, alcohol, arsenic, thallium)	
Symmetric and Proximal and Distal	
Inflammatory neuropathies (GBS, CIDP)	EMG/NCS, CSF
Asymmetric	
Mononeuropathy, radiculopathy, plexopathy	EMG/NCS
Mononeuritis multiplex	ANA, RF, ESR, ANCA, nerve bx
Vasculitis	
Diabetes	OGTT
HIV	HIV test
Multifocal CIDP	CSF
Rare: porphyria, leprosy, HNPP	
Pure Motor	
Proximal	
Diabetic amyotrophy	OGTT
MMNCB	EMG/NCS
Motor variants of GBS, CIDP, MGUS	CSF, SPE, IF
Lymphoma	CBC
Distal	
Rare: Lead toxicity, porphyria	
Pure Sensory	
Neuropathies	
Nonsystemic vasculitis neuropathy	Nerve bx
Chronic gluten enteropathy	Antigliadin antibodies
Vitamin E deficiency	Vitamin E level
Distal, demyelinating, symmetric neuropathy	SPE, IF
Rare: primary biliary cirrhosis, Crohn's disease	
Neuronopathies	
Paraneoplastic neuronopathy	Anti-Hu/CV2, Imaging
Sjögren's syndrome	Lip biopsy
HIV-related sensory neuronopathy	HIV test
Miller Fisher variant	EMG/NCS
Drugs (see Box 4)	Medication review
Autonomic	
Diabetes	OGTT
GBS	EMG/NCS
Paraneoplastic sensory neuropathy	Anti-Hu, CV2, imaging
HIV-related neuropathy	HIV test
Vincristine (Oncovin)	Medication review
Thiamine deficiency	Alcohol history
Rare: porphyria, hereditary autonomic neuropathy, amyloidosis	

Abbreviations: ANA = antinuclear antibodies; ANCA = antineutrophilic cytoplasmic antibodies; bx = biopsy; CBC = complete blood count; CIDP = chronic inflammatory demyelinating polyneuropathy; CMT = Charcot-Marie-Tooth disease; CSF = cerebrospinal fluid; EMG/NCS = electromyography/nerve conduction studies; ESR = erythrocyte sedimentation rate; GBS = Guillain-Barré syndrome; HIV = human immunodeficiency virus; HNPP = hereditary neuropathy with liability to pressure palsies; IF = immunofixation; LFT = liver function tests; MGUS = monoclonal gammopathy of unknown significance; MMNCB = multifocal motor neuropathy with conduction blocks; OGTT = oral glucose tolerance test; RF = rheumatoid factor; SPE = serum protein electrophoresis; TSH = thyroid-stimulating hormone.

BOX 2 Key Diagnostic Features

Medical History
- Connective tissue disease
- Diabetes
- Renal disease
- Thyroid disease

Surgical History, Trauma
- Compression neuropathies

Medication History
- Drug-induced neuropathy

Family History, High Arches
- Inherited neuropathy

Nutrition, Alcohol Use
- Alcoholic neuropathy
- Vitamin deficiency

Occupational Exposures
- Toxic neuropathy

History of Weight Loss
- Amyloidosis
- HIV
- Malignancy

Recent Infection, Travel
- Diphtheria
- Guillain-Barré syndrome
- HIV
- Leprosy
- Lyme disease

Dry Eyes and Mouth
- Sarcoidosis

Severe Pain
- Amyloidosis
- Diabetes
- Guillain-Barré syndrome
- HIV
- Vasculitis

Skin Lesions
- Anesthetic patches (leprosy)
- Bullous lesions (porphyria)
- Hyperpigmentation (osteosclerotic myeloma)
- Mee's lines (arsenic or thallium poisoning)
- Orange tonsils (Tangier disease)
- Angiokeratomas (Fabry's disease)

PATHOLOGY AND THE ROLE OF NEUROPHYSIOLOGY

Nerve conduction studies (NCSs) and electromyography (EMG) are highly specialized tests that are performed principally by neurologists. NCSs electrically activate peripheral nerves at particular sites and then assess for abnormal transmission from the stimulation point to the final muscle response. EMG involves placing a small needle into the muscle to observe both the sound and appearance of the muscle at rest and with motor units firing. Because NCSs can only be performed at points where the nerve is superficial (most often distal), EMG is needed to assess for more proximal damage such as radiculopathy. EMG can also rule out other mimics of PNS disease, such as myopathy.

BOX 3 Demyelinating Neuropathies

- Charcot-Marie-Tooth disease
- Hereditary neuropathy with liability to pressure palsies
- Inflammatory neuropathies
- Monoclonal gammopathies and paraproteinemias
- Multifocal motor neuropathy with conduction block
- Neuropathies caused by drugs such as amiodarone (Cordarone) and suramin[2]
- Neuropathies caused by infections (diphtheria) or toxins (arsenic)

[2]Not available in the United States.

For the general physician, the most important thing is being able to interpret the results of these tests. Often, a report will be received back such as: "There is evidence of a symmetric distal axonal sensorimotor neuropathy." An NCS/EMG study should be able to specify the distribution and if motor or sensory fibers are involved. Autonomic and small sensory fibers are not tested well by EMG, so the diagnosis of these types of neuropathies is often clinical or requires more specialized testing. Thus, a normal NCS/EMG does not rule out neuropathy.

A further feature that electrophysiology can add is whether the pathology is demyelinating or axonal. Demyelination is characterized by slowed conduction velocity, temporal dispersion of the muscle action potential, and conduction block. Hereditary demyelinating neuropathies, such as Charcot-Marie-Tooth disease, do not show the latter two features, which are only seen in acquired neuropathies. Axonal disease is characterized by modest slowing of velocities, and more marked reduction in the amplitudes of the muscle and sensory action potentials. On EMG, there are fibrillations within 3 weeks of the neuropathic injury, indicating spontaneous firing of denervated muscle. Enlarged and prolonged motor unit potentials indicate subsequent regeneration, which occurs after several weeks to months.

Demyelination has a limited differential (Box 3), and often a better prognosis, because myelin can start to regenerate within a few days. Axonal regeneration proceeds at a far slower rate of 1 to 3 μm/day, and nerves with proximal lesions must go a long distance to reinnervate their muscle and might never reach their goal.

Investigations

Once the neuropathy has been subclassified, investigations for the specific causes in that pattern class should be undertaken (see Table 1). Several recent papers suggest that 2-hour oral glucose tolerance testing (OGTT) is the best test for glucose intolerance due to the relatively low sensitivity of serum glucose levels and glycosylated hemoglobin (HbA1c). Likewise, vitamin B_{12} levels have a low sensitivity, and serum metabolites methylmalonic acid (MMA) and homocysteine (Hcy) should be measured in patients with a result less than 300 pg/mL to improve diagnostic accuracy. These metabolites can be falsely increased with hypovolemia, renal insufficiency, hypothyroidism, and increased age, but a return to normal levels 1 to 2 weeks after beginning replacement therapy indicates this is the cause. The combination of elevated gastrin and anti–parietal cell antibodies may be used to diagnose pernicious anemia. The yield of general testing for other vitamin deficiencies in polyneuropathy is relatively low.

Antinuclear antibodies (ANA) probably are usually only significant in the context of suggestive features (abrupt onset, mononeuropathy multiplex pattern, arthralgia or arthritis, fevers, rash, or renal abnormalities) because they are positive in about 3% of normal patients. However, referral to a rheumatologist should be considered with a very high titer (>1:1280).

The erythrocyte sedimentation rate (ESR) is often elevated, especially in older patients. Rates greater than 70 mm/hour tend to be more meaningful, particularly with a mononeuritis multiplex pattern.

CURRENT DIAGNOSIS

- The five-step approach to classify neuropathies based on fiber type, pattern of distribution, temporal course, pathology, and key features allows a tailored diagnostic evaluation.
- Electrodiagnostic testing provides a useful adjunct to the clinical evaluation.
- The cause of neuropathy might not be found in 20% of patients, but there are treatments for several known etiologies, as well as specific medications to treat neuropathic pain.

Serum protein electrophoresis lacks sensitivity, and immunofixation should be ordered if there is high suspicion of a paraproteinemia. If an elevated monoclonal antibody is found, a 24-hour urine test for Bence Jones proteinuria, skeletal survey, CBC, renal function tests, and serum calcium should be ordered. If the M protein is greater than 2.5 g/dL or if abnormalities are detected on these tests, referral to a hematologist for bone marrow aspiration is required. Polyclonal antibodies are not associated with neuropathy.

If there is suspicion of amyloidosis, a rectal, abdominal fat, or sensory nerve biopsy can be undertaken. Sural nerve biopsy is reserved for difficult diagnostic situations because it causes a permanent area of numbness with possible dysesthesias over the biopsied area. Suspicion of vasculitis is the most common indication, but pathology can also be seen in leprosy and with tumor infiltrate.

In approximately 20% of patients, an underlying cause of neuropathy is not found. These patients are said to have a cryptogenic sensory or sensorimotor neuropathy. A distinct clinical picture has emerged, most commonly of a patient in the sixth or seventh decade, manifesting with distal dysesthesias and possibly with mild weakness and sensory ataxia. These patients tend not to develop significant disability, and treatment is mainly for neuropathic pain.

Treatment

MONONEUROPATHIES

The most common cause of mononeuropathy is nerve compression, and surgical treatment is often a consideration for these patients. The four most common locations are median neuropathy at the wrist (carpal tunnel syndrome), ulnar neuropathy at the elbow, peroneal neuropathy at the fibular head, and facial nerve palsy (Bell's palsy).

Carpal tunnel syndrome manifests with pain and numbness principally in the first three digits, although it is often poorly localized. Classic features include pain at night and shaking out the hand to relieve pain. For milder symptoms, a nighttime splint, which prevents wrist flexion and high pressure in the carpal tunnel, is often helpful. Local corticosteroid injections can provide relief, and surgical decompression has a very high success rate.

Ulnar neuropathy manifests with numbness of the fourth and fifth digits and wasting of the interosseous muscles, often with pain localized to the elbow. Peroneal neuropathies manifest with foot drop and numbness on the dorsum of the foot. In both cases, avoidance of pressure over the nerve often leads to improvement. Surgery might improve symptoms, but less reliably so than carpal tunnel surgery.

Bell's palsy is an inflammatory rather than compressive process, presumably due to a viral etiology. Treatment is controversial, but early (within 14 days) use of prednisone[1] 60 mg daily, decreasing by 10 mg steps every 2 days, along with acyclovir (Zovirax)[1] 800 mg five times daily for 7 days has been advocated. About 15% of patients have residual facial weakness.

[1]Not FDA approved for this indication.

GUILLAIN-BARRÉ SYNDROME

GBS often begins following gastroenteritis with *Campylobacter jejuni*, or an upper respiratory tract infection, due to a presumed autoimmune response directed against myelin. The incidence is 1 or 2 per 100,000 persons per year. Characteristic features are ascending weakness, areflexia, and sensory and autonomic symptoms progressing over a few days up to 4 weeks. Facial diplegia and pain can occur. Electrophysiology shows acute demyelination with conduction blocks, and cerebrospinal fluid (CSF) reveals an increase in protein with a cell count of less than 5 white blood cells (cytoalbuminologic dissociation) in more than 80% of patients after 2 weeks. A CSF pleocytosis of more than 10 lymphocytes/mm^3 should alert the physician to another cause such as sarcoidosis, Lyme disease, or early HIV.

The Miller-Fisher variant is characterized by specific clinical features of sensory ataxia, areflexia, and ophthalmolplegia. *C. jejuni* infection has been correlated with more severe variants, such as acute motor axonal neuropathy (AMAN) and acute motor and sensory axonal neuropathy (AMSAM), which damage axons in addition to myelin. *C. jejuni*–related GBS correlates with anti-GM1 antibodies, although they are not prognostic or specific. Recovery can take months to years. Only 20% of patients are left without residual deficit. About 5% to 10% have significant persistent disability, and the mortality rate is 5%.

During early treatment, patients might require admission to intensive care, with close monitoring of pulmonary function tests for respiratory compromise. Diaphragmatic weakness correlates with neck flexion and extension and shoulder abduction. The patient should be intubated when the forced vital capacity (FVC) declines to less than 15 mL/kg or when negative inspiratory flow (NIF) is less than −20 to −30. Monitoring of the cardiac rhythm is important due to dysautonomia.

The preferred treatment is intravenous immunoglobulin (IVIg)[1] at a dose of 0.4 g/kg/day for 5 days. This is generally well tolerated, and adverse side effects such as myalgia, headache, or flu-like symptoms often resolve with a reduced infusion rate. If IVIg is contraindicated (renal failure, IgA deficiency), plasmapheresis can be initiated with four alternate-day exchanges over 7 to 10 days for a total of 200 to 250 mL/kg. Both plasmapheresis and IVIg continue to work for several weeks after the treatment period, but if patients experience a secondary worsening after successful treatment, a second dose may be initiated. Steroids were reviewed recently by a Cochrane systematic review and were not found to be of benefit in GBS.

CHRONIC INFLAMMATORY DEMYELINATING POLYNEUROPATHY

This neuropathy is pathologically similar to GBS, but progression is longer than 8 weeks, often with a relapsing-remitting course. Symmetric distal and proximal weakness and sensory impairment, hyporeflexia, and cytoalbuminergic dissociation in the CSF is the classic presentation, although there are variants.

Treatment is either IVIg[1] or prednisone. IVIg is given initially at 0.4 g/kg/day for 5 days, then the dose and frequency are reduced over time. Prednisone is given 1 mg/kg/day until improvement, followed by a slow tapering of 5 mg every 2 to 3 weeks over a period of months. Response is usually seen within 4 weeks. Refractory patients have been treated with repeated plasmapheresis treatments or immunosuppressive therapy with cyclosporine (Sandimmune).[1]

MULTIFOCAL MOTOR NEUROPATHY

Multifocal motor neuropathy (MMN) is not a common disorder but is important not to mistake for motor neuron disease because it has a very different prognosis and treatment. Patients present with progressive asymmetric distal weakness, often of the arm, without sensory loss and with less atrophy than would be expected for the degree of weakness. Unlike motor neuron disease, there are no upper motor neuron signs. It is different from multifocal acquired demyelinating sensory and motor neuropathy (MADSAM), an asymmetric variant of CIDP, in that loss of reflexes and weakness involves only the affected limb, there is a relatively normal CSF protein concentration, and sensory nerve conduction studies are normal. Diagnosis is supported by finding conduction blocks in sites not usually associated with compression. The GM1 antibody is elevated in 60% of cases. Repeated treatments with IVIg[1] or cyclophosphamide (Cytoxan)[1] are common choices. Rituximab (Rituxan),[1] a monoclonal antibody, has also been used. Prednisone classically worsens the condition.

DIABETIC NEUROPATHY

Diabetes is one of the most common causes of neuropathy. Patients can present with a symmetric distal neuropathy, autonomic proximal diabetic neuropathy, mononeuritis multiplex, compressive and cranial neuropathies, and trunk polyradiculopathies.

The distal symmetric sensory polyneuropathy (DSPN) correlates with the duration of the diabetes, control of hyperglycemia, and presence of retinopathy and nephropathy. The exact etiology is unknown, but theories include a metabolic process involving aldose reductase, ischemic damage, or an immunologic disorder. Typical symptoms include lancinating pains or burning, worse at night, and possible dysautonomia. Atrophy may be noted in the foot muscles, but severe weakness is atypical. NCS may be normal because small fibers are primarily affected. Treatment includes blood sugar control to limit progression and symptom control for neuropathic pain. Gabapentin (Neurontin)[1] and tricyclic antidepressants are common choices (see later). Drugs such as QR-333, a topical compound that contains quercetin, a flavonoid with aldose reductase–inhibitor effects, are being investigated specifically for diabetic neuropathy.

Autonomic neuropathy is treated symptomatically, with fludrocortisone (Florinef)[1] 0.1 mg/day for orthostatic hypotension metoclopramide (Reglan) 10 mg before meals for gastroparesis, and sildenafil (Viagra) 25 mg 1 hour before sexual intercourse for impotence.

Proximal diabetic neuropathy (diabetic amyotrophy) manifests typically with unilateral pain in the anterior thigh followed by stepwise progression over weeks to months of quadriceps weakness, atrophy of the proximal leg muscles, and a reduced knee reflex, with occasional contralateral leg involvement. The erythrocyte sedimentation rate (ESR) may be elevated and CSF protein mildly increased (120 mg/dL on average). NCS and EMG reflect multifocal active axonal damage (fibrillations) to the lumbar plexus and roots. Small retrospective studies have reported that IVIg[1] and other forms of immunosuppressive therapy are effective in treating patients with proximal diabetic neuropathy. A short course of corticosteroids (prednisone[1] 50 mg/day for 1 week, then tapering by 10 mg/week) can be used to ease pain in severe cases, with close monitoring of the glucose level, but overall prognosis is quite good, ranging from 1 to 18 months of recovery phase (mean of 6 months) and partial or complete restoration of strength in approximately 70% of patients.

PARAPROTEINEMIC NEUROPATHIES

Multiple myeloma, Waldenström's macroglobulinemia, cryoglobulinemia, osteosclerotic myeloma (POEMS syndrome), and monoclonal gammopathy of unknown significance (MGUS) are associated with monoclonal antibodies directed at PNS components, such as myelin-associated glycoprotein (MAG). Neuropathies associated with an immunoglobulin (Ig)M monoclonal protein (approximately 60%) are typically distal, demyelinating, and symmetric, whereas IgG (30%) and IgA (10%) gammopathies can be axonal or demyelinating. In terms of treatment, the distal demyelinating neuropathy of IgM paraproteinemias tends to be treatment refractory. IgG and IgA gammopathies can mimic the demyelination pattern seen in CIDP, and patients with any antibody and this pattern should receive immunotherapy as recommended for CIDP (see earlier). Axonal neuropathies and IgM, IgG, or IgA gammopathies have a less clear relationship and are typically not responsive to treatment.

---

[1]Not FDA approved for this indication.

[1]Not FDA approved for this indication.

HEREDITARY NEUROPATHIES

Charcot-Marie-Tooth (CMT) disease is among the most common of genetic neuromuscular disorders, and more than 30 genes have been identified. Clues are a history of difficulty running in childhood, high arches, hammertoes, ankle weakness, and nerve hypertrophy developing in teenage years. Depending on the subtype, the neuropathy may be axonal or demyelinating, but the most common type (CMT-1) is caused by an autosomal dominant gene encoding peripheral myelin protein 22 and is easily diagnosed by the relatively uniform slowing on nerve conduction velocities (<25% of lower limits of normal). Patients have a mild course and remain ambulatory throughout life in most cases.

Hereditary neuropathy with liability to pressure palsies (HNPP) is another dominantly inherited neuropathy in which patients have recurrent episodes of isolated mononeuropathies, typically affecting, in order of decreasing frequency, the common peroneal, ulnar, radial, and median nerves. Most attacks are sudden onset, painless, and followed by complete recovery. There is no treatment other than preventive measures.

TOXIC AND NUTRITIONAL NEUROPATHIES

Treatment of toxic and nutritional neuropathies involves detection and removal of the underlying cause. A thorough review of medications, occupational exposures, and nutritional risk factors is essential (Box 4). Drug toxicity is much more common than environmental toxicity. Incidence of neuropathy does not always correlate with the dosage and duration of exposure. For instance, amiodarone neuropathy has been reported with dosages as low as 200 mg/day and durations as short as 1 month. Symptoms might not improve, or might even worsen, for several weeks after the drug is stopped before improvement starts, a phenomenon known as *coasting*.

Cisplatin can cause a neuropathy that overlaps in symptomatology with paraneoplastic sensory neuronopathy, and dapsone is associated with a motor axonopathy. Gold neuropathy can have prominent myokymia and can mimic GBS.

Specific treatments for drug-induced neuropathies include cyanocobalamin (vitamin B_{12})[1] for nitrous oxide neuropathy and pyridoxine (vitamin B_6)[1] for hydralazine and isoniazid neuropathies. Excessive vitamin B_6 can also *cause* a neuropathy. Glutamine[7] and vitamin E[1] 300 mg twice a day has shown promise for paclitaxel neuropathy, and neuroprotective agents such as nerve growth factor are being investigated for cisplatin-induced neuropathy. Tacrolimus can cause a CIDP-like neuropathy that responds to IVIg[1] or plasmapheresis.

One of the most common nutritional neuropathies is caused by thiamine deficiency and is associated with alcohol consumption of at least 100 g per day. Patients present with burning feet, and early alcohol abstinence and treatment with thiamine denotes better chance of recovery. Vitamin B_{12} deficiency is vital not to miss and can manifest with a subacute combined degeneration, whereby patients have a superimposed myelopathy and neuropathy (spasticity but reduced reflexes). Sudden-onset symptoms, particularly in the feet and hands simultaneously, are also suggestive.

METABOLIC AND INFECTIOUS NEUROPATHIES

Peripheral neuropathy can complicate renal failure, hypothyroidism, biliary cirrhosis, porphyria, Tangier disease, Fabry's disease, and mitochondrial diseases.

Early in the course, HIV can manifest as a GBS-like syndrome, although with CSF pleocytosis. This typically responds to IVIg[1] and plasmapheresis. In later stages, patients might develop a distal symmetric polyneuropathy, although it is important to determine if this might be due to nucleoside reverse transcriptase inhibitors, nutritional deficiency, or infection. Cranial neuropathies, sensory neuronopathy, lumbosacral polyradiculopathies, and mononeuritis multiplex also occur.

Leprosy is the most common treatable neuropathy worldwide. Tuberculoid leprosy leads to hypopigmented patches with loss of

---

BOX 4 Causes of Toxic and Nutritional Neuropathies

Drug Toxins
Axonal
- Colchicine
- Dapsone
- Disulfiram
- Ethambutol
- Hyralazine
- Isoniazid
- Metronidazole
- Nitrofurantoin
- Nitrous oxide
- Nucleosides
- Paclitaxel
- Phenytoin
- Tacrolimus
- Vincristine

Demyelinating
- Amiodarone (Cordarone)
- Chloroquine (Aralen)
- Gold
- Suramin[2]

Neuronopathy
- Cisplatin (Platinol-AQ)
- Pyridoxine (vitamin B_6)
- Thalidomide (Thalomid)

Environmental Toxins
- Acrylamide (plastics)
- Allyl chloride (insecticides)
- Arsenic
- Carbon disulfide (cellophanes)
- Ethylene glycol (antifreeze)
- Ethylene oxide (sterilizer)
- Hexacarbons (glue)
- Lead
- Mercury
- Methyl bromide (fumigant)
- Organophosphates (insecticides)
- Thallium (pesticides)
- Trichloroethylene (drycleaning)
- Vacor (rodenticide)

Vitamin Deficiencies
- B_1 (alcoholism)
- B_3 (alcoholism)
- B_6 (isoniazid use)
- B_{12} (vegans, pernicious anemia)
- E (cholestasis and abetalipoproteinemia)

[2]Not available in the United States.

---

pain and temperature sensation. Lepromatous leprosy, a more severe form seen in immunosuppressed persons, can cause ulnar, common peroneal, and facial neuropathies. Treatment involves a long-term multidrug regimen of dapsone and rifampin (Rifadin).[1]

Herpes zoster can cause a postherpetic neuralgia, defined as pain persisting for more than 6 weeks after the rash appears. Early treatment with acyclovir (Zovirax) (800 mg five times daily for 7 days) can reduce the duration of the acute phase. Chronic discomfort is treated with medications for neuropathic pain (see later).

Lyme disease, caused by *Borrelia burgdorferi*, begins with erythema migrans, followed by multifocal peripheral and cranial neuropathies, particularly facial diplegia. CSF lymphocytic pleocytosis plus serologic demonstration of *B. burgdorferi* infection on serum or CSF are the diagnostic features. Early stages are treated with a 3-week course of doxycycline[1] 100 mg twice daily, and intravenous penicillin G[1] should be given in the late stages.

CARCINOMATOUS NEUROPATHY

Tumors can cause neuropathy by compression, metastatic spread, paraneoplastic antibodies, hemorrhage, and treatment with chemotherapy or radiation therapy. A distal sensorimotor neuropathy is associated with many different tumors and seldom precedes tumor diagnosis. Pathogenesis can include toxic, nutritional, and immunologic causes. A sensory neuronopathy is less common, but often precedes tumor diagnosis, thus warranting a careful work-up. Lung, breast, ovary, and gastrointestinal tract cancers are the most likely associated types. Imaging and paraneoplastic antibodies (particularly anti-Hu and anti-CV2, most commonly associated with lung cancer) may help in making the diagnosis. Treatment focuses on the underlying neoplasm.

VASCULITIC NEUROPATHY

Vasculitis can be primary (polyarteritis nodosa, Wegener's granulomatosis, Churg-Strauss syndrome, microscopic polyangitis) or secondary (connective tissue diseases, systemic infections, drug reactions). It classically manifests with a painful mononeuritis multiplex with asymmetric patchy features, reflecting multifocal ischemic damage. If the patient's vasculitis is restricted to the PNS, serologic testing for these disorders is often negative. In this case, a sural nerve biopsy might reveal fibrinoid necrosis and perivascular inflammation.

Treatment needs to be carefully undertaken with intravenous methylprednisolone (Solu-Medrol)[1] for 3 days followed by oral prednisone. In many cases, other immunosuppressive drugs are eventually used.

Neuropathic Pain

Often pain is the most predominant and distressing feature of neuropathy. Several classes of medications can be tried (Table 2), although it is important to counsel the patient that complete abolition of pain is unlikely. A trial period should be for at least 6 to 8 weeks before concluding that the patient does not respond. A combination of agents with different mechanisms can have an advantage over monotherapy for the nonresponsive patient.

First-line treatment is generally with tricyclic antidepressants. Serotonin and noradrenaline reuptake inhibitors such as amitriptyline[1] (Elavil), imipramine[1] (Tofranil), and clomipramine[1] (Anafranil) may be marginally more effective than those with relatively selective noradrenergic effects such as desipramine and nortriptyline. However, nortriptyline and desipramine are less sedating. Selective serotonin reuptake inhibitors appear to be less effective. Second-line antidepressants include venlafaxine[1] (Effexor), bupropion[1] (Wellbutrin), and the recently approved duloxetine (Cymbalta), which have the advantage of better tolerability due to less muscarinic, histaminergic, and α-adrenergic affinity.

The typical next class of medications to try is the antiepileptics. Gabapentin[1] is a common choice and is generally well tolerated. Pregabalin (Lyrica) is a newer related agent that, unlike gabapentin, exhibits linear pharmacokinetics and can be initiated at a therapeutic dose without a long titration. Second-line choices include lamotrigine[1] (Lamictal), carbamazepine[1] (Tegretol), and topiramate[1] (Topamax). Valproate[1] (Depacon) and zonisamide[1] (Zonegran) have limited evidence, and phenytoin[1] (Dilantin) can cause neuropathy. Oxcarbazepine[1] (Trileptal), like carbamazepine, slows the recovery rate of voltage-activated sodium channels, but it also inhibits high-threshold N-type and P/Q-type calcium channels and reduces glutamatergic transmission. As a result, it can modulate both peripheral and central neuropathic pain pathways, and several studies into its efficacy are under way.

Topical creams, such as capsaicin (Zostrix), an extract of chili, can be tried. Capsaicin works by depleting substance P and can temporarily worsen pain by causing a burning sensation. Lidocaine[1] (Xylocaine) can be also used topically.

Other agents for severe neuropathies include opioid agents, such as tramadol (Ultram), which has low-affinity binding for μ-opioid receptors coupled with mild inhibition of norepinephrine and serotonin reuptake. Slow-release opioids, such as oxycodone (OxyContin) 30 to 60 mg/day, can help, and risk of addiction is low in this population. Glutamate antagonists, such as dextromethorphan[1] (Delsym), have shown benefit in some studies, as has mexiletine[1] (Mexitil), a class IB antiarrhythmic agent and oral analogue of lidocaine. Nonpharmacologic therapies, such as transcutaneous electrical nerve stimulation (TENS) and acupuncture, might also provide adjunctive relief.

[1]Not FDA approved for this indication.

[1]Not FDA approved for this indication.

TABLE 2 Select Neuropathic Pain Medications

Drug	Dosage	Side Effects
Amitriptyline (Elavil)[1]	10 mg/d, increasing weekly by 10 mg, up to 150 mg/d	Dry mouth, sedation, urinary retention, cardiac arrhythmias, orthostatic hypotension, constipation, weight gain Contraindications: cardiac arrhythmias, CHF, recent MI, narrow angle glaucoma, urinary retention
Capsaicin (Zostrix)	0.075% cream applied tid to qid	Sneezing, coughing, rash, skin irritation
Carbamazepine (Tegretol)[1]	100 mg bid, increasing by 100 mg weekly Max: 1200 mg/d	Somnolence, dizziness, nausea, gait changes, urticaria, hyponatremia, pancytopenia, hepatic dysfunction Obtain baseline and 6-wk CBC and LFT
Gabapentin (Neurontin)[1]	300 mg on d 1, 600 mg on d 2, 900 mg on day 3 Max: 3600 mg/d	Sedation, fatigue, dizziness, confusion, tremor, weight gain, peripheral edema, headache Reduce dose in renal insufficiency
Lamotrigine (Lamictal)[1]	25 mg at night for 2 wk, increasing weekly by 25–50 mg Max: 400 mg/d	Severe rash (especially if increased too quickly), dizziness, unsteadiness, drowsiness, diplopia
Tramadol (Ultram)	50 mg bid Titrate 50 mg every 3–7 d, using a tid or qid schedule Max: 100 mg qid	Constipation, headache, nausea Risk of seizures with neuroleptics and antidepressants Reduce dose with hepatic or renal dysfunction

[1]Not FDA approved for this indication.
Abbreviations: CBC = complete blood count; CHF = congestive heart failure; LFT = liver function test; max = maximum; MI = myocardial infarction.

REFERENCES

Donofrio PD, Albers JW. AAEM minimonograph 34. Polyneuropathy: Classification by nerve conduction studies and electromyography. Muscle Nerve 1990;13:889–903.

Dworkin RH, Backonja M, Rowbotham MC, et al. Advances in neuropathic pain: Diagnosis, mechanisms, and treatment recommendations. Arch Neurol 2003;60:1524–34.

Grant I, Benstead TJ. Differential diagnosis of peripheral neuropathy. In: Dyck PK, Thomas PK, editors. Peripheral Neuropathy. Philadelphia: Saunders; 2005.

Poncelet AN. An algorithm for the evaluation of peripheral neuropathy. Am Fam Physician 1997;57(4):755–64.

Stewart JD. Focal peripheral neuropathies. New York: Raven; 1993.

Management of Head Injuries

Method of
Todd W. Vitaz, MD

Traumatic brain injury (TBI) most commonly results from motor vehicle crashes (MVC) and typically affects males in the 2nd through 4th decades of life. These sudden random acts can have long-lasting effects on the patient and family, but these events also impact society as a whole when a young, viable working-age individual becomes suddenly disabled and dependent on the care of others. TBI has no regard for age or gender, however, and can be seen in infants as a result of nonaccidental trauma as well as in geriatric patients following falls. The management of these patients can become extremely complicated and often requires the close interaction of numerous different health care providers ranging from trauma, orthopedic, and neurologic surgeons to nurses, social workers, speech, occupational, and physical therapists. Unfortunately, current interventions are still limited to the avoidance or minimization of secondary injury and rehabilitative intervention. However, when these patients are managed with aggressive, comprehensive, multidisciplinary approaches, the outcomes at times can be rewarding.

TBI can be categorized based on numerous factors. Most commonly it is differentiated based on mechanism and injury type (closed versus penetrating), whether it has occurred with or without systemic injuries (isolated versus multisystem), and the severity (mild, moderate, severe). The Glasgow Coma Scale (GCS) (Table 1), which was initially developed as a prognostic indicator following closed head injury, has become the principal triage tool for evaluating these patients. Patients are scored based on their best response in each of the three categories (eye opening, verbal responses, and motor score) and then subdivided into mild (13 to 15), moderate (9 to 12), and severe (3 to 8). One caveat to this assessment tool is that it can be affected by numerous alterations: hypoxia, hypotension, hypothermia, intoxication, infection, and other metabolic derangements, which are commonly seen in the trauma population.

Pathology

Another common classification system following TBI is based on pathophysiologic findings. Concussion commonly occurs following mild or moderate TBI as the result of transient (typically seconds to minutes) neurologic dysfunction in the setting of a normal computed tomography (CT) scan. Brief loss of consciousness, commonly with amnesia regarding the event, is not uncommon and is often associated with nausea, vomiting, headache, dizziness, and transient visual obscuration. These symptoms may persist for several hours to weeks as part of the *postconcussive syndrome* and, in rare instances, especially following repetitive injury, these alterations may become long-lasting. As a result of these persistent problems, in addition to a better understanding of the neurocognitive effects following this type of injury, there has been an enormous emphasis placed on their prevention (see text following).

Skull fractures may occur in isolation or be associated with other types of brain injuries. They are commonly classified based on whether they are open (overlying laceration) or closed, linear or comminuted, nondepressed or depressed. Skull fractures occur either as the result of a large force directed to a small area (i.e., depressed skull fracture following a blow to the head with a golf club) or when larger forces are dissipated throughout the skull resulting in fracture through the weakest area (linear fractures through frontal skull base, petrous, or squamous temporal bone). Linear fractures are commonly associated with raccoon eyes (frontal skull base fractures), Battle's sign (posterior skull base fracture), cerebrospinal fluid leak (otorrhea or rhinorrhea) or olfactory, facial or acoustic nerve injury (amnesia, facial palsy, sensorineuronal deafness).

In addition, temporal bone fractures may also be associated with epidural hematomas (EDHs). These extra-axial blood clots are most commonly caused by laceration of the middle meningeal artery and result in accumulation of *high-pressure arterial bleeding* in the potential space between the dura and skull. EDHs are more commonly seen in younger individuals probably because of the decreased skull thickness and lack of adhesions between the skull and dura mater in this population. Commonly, these lesions appear on CT scan as lens-shaped, extra-axial hematomas most often in the temporal region and can be rapidly expansive secondary to the high-pressure arterial bleeding. The clinical course in these patients is classically described by a brief loss of consciousness from the initial concussion, followed by a "lucid interval" in which the patient may be awake and alert, which then gives way to another episode of decreased mental status that may be rapidly progressive and associated with signs of brain stem compression (flexor or extensor posturing, dilated nonreactive pupil). EDHs are usually treated surgically unless they are extremely small and constitute one of the few true neurosurgical emergencies where mere minutes may make an enormous difference in the patient's outcome.

Unlike EDHs, subdural hematomas (SDHs) are often associated with other types of brain injury and thus typically involve an altered level of consciousness (LOC) from the onset. SDHs are typically caused by bleeding from bridging veins that get torn when the brain moves within its cerebrospinal fluid (CSF) buffer while the veins remain tethered at their dural insertions; however, other causes such as venous or arterial hemorrhage from a brain laceration also exist. CT scanning reveals that these lesions commonly appear more crescent-shaped but never cross the dural boundaries (falx or tentorium). Unlike the high-pressure EDHs, SDHs typically expand at a slower rate but still cause devastating neurologic dysfunction from compression of the underlying brain. In addition mortality rates tend to be higher with worse outcome for SDH as a result of the common underlying brain injury. Once again these extra-axial clots frequently

TABLE 1 Glasgow Coma Scale

Best Motor Score	Best Verbal Response	Best Eye Opening
6 Obeys commands	5 Normal speech	4 Spontaneous
5 Localizes to pain	4 Confused	3 To voice
4 Withdraws to pain	3 Inappropriate words	2 To pain
3 Flexor posturing	2 Incomprehensible sounds	1 No eye opening
2 Extensor posturing	1 No verbal response	
1 No motor response	Intubated patients receive a 1 with the suffix T added to score	

require surgical evacuation unless they are small and fail to have substantial compression on the underlying brain, where they are managed with serial imaging and close neurologic observation. In patients for whom a small SDH is not treated surgically, the physician must remain cognizant of the fact that a small proportion of these will increase in size between 1 and 4 weeks following the trauma and can be a cause of delayed deterioration or increased headache and new neurologic findings.

Intraparenchymal hematomas occur quite commonly following TBI and can be either hemorrhagic or nonhemorrhagic. These lesions range in size from 1 to 2 mm, up to several centimeters, and can cause a full range of symptoms and neurologic findings based on their location, size, and degree of compression on surrounding structures. Just like extra-axial hematomas, these lesions may increase in size and commonly coalesce or mature and *blossom* during the first 12 to 24 hours following the trauma. In addition, larger hematomas incite an inflammatory reaction in the surrounding brain resulting in increased edema around the lesion, which may result in increases in the intracranial pressure (ICP) (commonly seen on postinjury days [PIDs] 3 to 7). Management of these lesions depends on their size, location, and associated findings and ranges from serial observation and repeat imaging, surgical evacuation of the hematoma, or decompressive craniectomy with or without lobectomy.

The final category of pathologic abnormalities following TBI occurs as the result of shear injury to the axons themselves, called diffuse axonal injury (DAI). This is caused by either acceleration and deceleration or rotational forces to the axons resulting in micro- or macroscopic areas of injury and axonal transection. Most commonly this is encountered in the setting where a patient clinically has signs of a severe TBI, often with a GCS score less than 6; however, the CT scan is either unimpressive or shows only small areas of petechial hemorrhage. In addition ICP recording typically shows normal or only slightly elevated values. Magnetic resonance imaging (MRI) is commonly used in this subset of patients and can be used as a predictive indicator for determining the severity of injury, especially if CT is negative. MRI commonly shows areas of increased intensity on fluid attenuation inversion recovery (FLAIR) and T2-weighted sequences in the brainstem, diencephalon, deep white matter tracts, or corpus callosum. Recovery following this type of injury is variable and depends more on the injury location (reticular activating system of brainstem versus supratentorial white matter tracts) rather than the injury volume.

In addition to these abnormalities, patients with TBI are also at risk for damage to the spinal cord and vertebral and carotid arteries. Thus, patients with altered LOC should be assumed to have spinal instability and possible spinal cord injury (SCI); they should remain immobilized until the absence of these can be confirmed. The incidence of carotid and vertebral artery injury associated with severe TBI is unknown, but patients with facial or cervical fractures and those with soft tissue neck or chest injury (seat belt sign) have been found to be at higher risk. The appropriate screening for and treatment of these injuries have become a topic of intense debate in recent years but should be suspected in a patient with focal neurologic findings without identifiable cause on other imaging.

INTRACRANIAL PRESSURE AND THE MONROE-KELLIE DOCTRINE

Regardless of the pathophysiologic type of injury, the end result commonly is the generation of increases in the ICP, which can then lead to secondary brain injury. ICP dynamics are easily understood if one considers the principles of the volume pressure relationships outlined by the Monroe-Kellie doctrine. The basis of this principle resides on the fact that the skull is a fixed and rigid volume; because of this any changes to the volume of its contents will directly affect the pressure within this rigid space. In simplest terms the intracranial cavity contains blood, water, and tissue. Blood may be intravascular (IV) or extravascular (EV) in the case of extra-axial blood clots; water includes not only cerebrospinal fluid, which may build up in cases of hydrocephalus, but also edema following traumatic injuries; brain parenchyma typically compromises the tissue component but in select instances tumors or cysts may also fall into this category.

CURRENT DIAGNOSIS

Classification of Head Injuries

- Closed versus penetrating
- Isolated versus multisystem injuries
- Severity
  - Mild (GCS 13–15)
  - Moderate (GCS 9–12)
  - Severe (GCS 3–8)

Pathologic Findings with Closed Head Injuries

- Skull fractures
- Epidural hematomas
- Subdural hematomas
- Parenchymal contusions
- Intraparenchymal hematomas
- Diffuse axonal injury

As increases in any or all three of these categories occur, the pressure inside the cranial cavity increases proportionally. At first compensatory changes occur, which accommodate for these increases, resulting in only mild pressure changes; however, eventually a critical volume is reached where the compensatory mechanisms are saturated, resulting in rapid and dramatic pressure changes. The following scenario illustrates these principles. A patient is involved in a motor vehicle crash and suffers a head injury with a small epidural hematoma. Initially he is awake and alert without any focal neurologic findings. The epidural hematoma creates an increase in the EV blood component of the Monroe-Kellie doctrine; however, compensatory changes in intracranial CSF volume result in decreases in the water component, thus preventing significant changes in ICP. However, the hematoma continues to enlarge, causing increases in ICP exhibited clinically by slow deterioration in the patient's level of consciousness. The patient is now intubated and mildly hyperventilated causing vasoconstriction, therefore decreasing the intravascular blood component and reducing ICP with an improvement in the patient's neurologic condition. Unfortunately, as the operating room (OR) is being prepared, the patient suffers a rapid decrease in his level of conscious, becoming unresponsive with flexor posturing and a nonreactive pupil. Although the hematoma has expanded at a constant rate over time, the rapid change in the patient's condition is the result of him reaching the critical point where all compensatory mechanisms have been exhausted, thus causing profound rapid changes in the patient's ICP.

Treatment of Elevated Intracranial Pressure

Acute changes in ICP result in altered LOC, and at times other localizing neurologic findings such as *blown* (dilated, nonreactive) pupils and flexor or extensor posturing, and such findings may be the sign of impending herniation and death without immediate intervention. In a patient without a ventricular drain already in place, hyperventilation is the most rapid mechanism for acutely lowering elevated ICP. Currently, aggressive hyperventilation ($Pco_2 < 30$) is recommended only for short durations in cases of impending cerebral herniation while patients are being stabilized. As stated previously, hyperventilation causes vasoconstriction, which reduces intravascular blood within the cranial vault and almost instantaneously lowering ICP. However, several studies have now shown that the routine use of aggressive hyperventilation in the management of patients with severe closed head injury (CHI) results in decreased outcomes because of hypoxic injury and possible stroke caused by the sustained hyperventilation. Our current practice is to maintain Pco_2 values between 35 and 38 with controlled ventilation in all patients with severe CHI; because of this we leave all these patients intubated and mechanically ventilated until their ICPs normalize and all other therapies are withdrawn.

Adequate sedation and pain control are also important elements of ICP control. Patients who are restless and agitated will have higher ICPs than similar patients who are resting quietly in bed. Another important point is the prevention of venous congestion. This occasionally is evident in cervical collars, which are fastened too tight or with the use of trach ties that are wrapped too tightly around the neck to hold the endotracheal tube in place.

Several medications are available for the treatment of elevated ICP with the most common one being mannitol. Although this agent acts as an osmotic diuretic and helps pull excess interstitial fluid into the vascular space and thus lower ICP, there are several other hypothetical mechanisms that probably also increase its efficacy such as increasing RBC flexibility, decreasing RBC and platelet clumping in small arterioles and capillaries, and increasing intravascular volume, thus improving cardiac function. Other diuretics such as furosemide (Lasix)[1] or urea (Ureaphil) may also be used but have less dramatic effects on ICP. Hypertonic saline (NaCl 3% to 5%)[1] has also been used more recently by some physicians and has been shown to have many of the same effects as mannitol.

CSF diversion is one of the simplest, quickest acting methods for decreasing ICP especially if a ventricular drain is already in place. The emergent surgical evacuation of mass lesions such as large epidural, subdural, or intraparenchymal hematomas is also extremely effective for controlling ICP, and in many instances it is also life-saving. However, in some instances, underlying brain injury or stroke from prolonged brain compression may be exhibited as massive intraoperative brain swelling and in these instances may necessitate that the bone flap be left off (craniectomy).

Management of Severe Closed Head Injury

The current recommendations of the Brain Trauma Foundation Guidelines for the management of closed head injuries call for the placement of ICP monitors in all patients who fall into the severe category (GCS score <9). At our institution we routinely place combination intraventricular monitors and drains in all patients with a postresuscitation GCS score of less than 7. Monitors are inserted into patients with a GCS score of 7 to 9 on an individual basis depending on whether there are distracting reasons, such as intoxication, to cause the altered LOC. If patients are intubated and not following commands but are purposeful in their movements, we will sometimes elect not to place a ventriculostomy and follow the patient's clinical course over several hours. Other factors include CT findings and the need to go to the operating room during the acute period for the treatment of other life-threatening injuries, age, or for heavy sedation secondary to other injuries or pulmonary problems. At times patients in this GCS range will be given 6 to 12 hours and treated medically to see whether or not they improve prior to placement of an ICP monitor.

---

[1]Not FDA approved for this indication.

CURRENT THERAPY

Management of Elevated Intracranial Pressure

- Prevention of venous engorgement
- CO_2 control (mild hyperventilation)
- Sedation and pain control
- Cerebrospinal fluid drainage
- Mannitol
- Lasix
- Hypertonic saline
- Decompressive craniectomy
- Pentobarbital coma

Once an ICP monitor and drain have been placed elevations in ICP are treated in a systematic order. Target values include attempts to keep ICP less than 15 to 20 and cerebral perfusion pressure (CPP) greater than 60. Low CPP (CPP = mean arterial blood pressure [MAP] − ICP) is caused by either elevated ICP or low MAP. For patients with low MAP or uncontrolled ICP, vasopressors may be used to increase blood pressure (BP) and central venous pressure. At the University of Louisville, dopamine (Intropin) is used as a first line agent, followed by phenylephrine (Neo-Synephrine) and norepinephrine (Levophed) in refractory cases. ICP elevations are initially treated with adequate sedation and pain control, such as midazolam (Versed),[1] propofol (Diprivan), and/or morphine (Lioresal),[1] to prevent agitation and elevated airway pressures, which can further increase ICP and intermittent CSF diversion. In cases where this fails to control ICP, mannitol is then added to the treatment protocol along with more continuous CSF diversion and finally chemical paralysis. Mannitol is administered as a bolus infusion in doses ranging from 0.25 to 1.0 mg/kg body weight every 4 to 8 hours with the endpoints being either ICP control or measured serum osmolarity greater than 315 mOsmL.

Patients who continue to have sustained increases in their ICP despite these interventions are considered to have refractory ICP and at our facility are considered for one of two potential salvage treatments. Pentobarbital (Nembutal)[1] coma has been used successfully on occasion in young patients without mass lesions to decrease the metabolic demands of the brain during these periods of sustained ICP. Patients need to be chosen wisely for this therapy because it carries enormous risks in addition to the possibility of preserving the patient in a long-term, nonfunctional, persistent vegetative state. Initiation of pentobarbital (Nembutal)[1] coma causes severe hypotension, and patients almost always require the use of pressors in addition to volume expansion. At our facility we also place all of these patients on a Rotorest bed in an attempt to minimize the pulmonary complications that frequently occur with the use of this technique.

The second salvage therapy is decompressive craniectomy. This procedure involves the removal of a significant area of skull, typically almost an entire hemisphere or both frontal regions with opening of the dura. This permits the injured swollen brain to herniate through the opening and is the only intervention that increases the volume of the intracranial compartment, thereby reducing pressure. In addition this technique allows for the evacuation of large hemorrhagic contusions, or in cases of extreme ICP elevations it can be coupled with either frontal or temporal lobectomy. Once again, patients must be selected carefully for this intervention. Decompressive craniectomy is used much more frequently than pentobarbital (Nembutal)[1] coma at our institution. We use this strategy for patients with elevated ICP—more than 30 to 40 for more than 30 minutes—or a significant change in neurologic condition that is nonresponsive to all other interventions. In order for either of these two salvage approaches to be effective, they must be used at the first signs of refractory ICP prior to the occurrence of complications such as ischemic infarcts or brainstem compression or hemorrhage.

Patients treated with decompressive craniectomies are at risk for significant alterations in CSF dynamics that may result in delayed deterioration. Signs of hydrocephalus either in the form of ventriculomegaly or extra-axial or interhemispheric CSF fluid collections will be evident in 50% to 80% of these patients. When necessary these patients will be treated with external ventricular or subdural drains followed by early cranioplasty (replacement of the bone plate). In many instances these changes will resolve following cranioplasty and therefore avoid the need for ventriculoperitoneal shunting, with its associated risks and complications.

All patients with abnormal head CT scans (regardless of GCS score) are treated with close neurologic observation most commonly in an intensive care unit (ICU) setting, serial CT scans (4 to 6 hours later and on PID 1), and placed on 7 days of phenytoin (Dilantin). Temkin and colleagues showed that patients with post-traumatic

---

[1]Not FDA approved for this indication.

intracranial hemorrhage were at increased risk of suffering seizures in the acute period; treatment with antiepileptics beyond 7 days did not decrease the risk of these patients from developing epilepsy or delayed seizures but there were increased risks associated with side effects from medication administration. Patients who experience a seizure following CHI (with the exception of acute post-traumatic seizures) should be maintained on antiepileptics for at least 3 to 6 months and possible indefinitely depending on their clinical condition and EEG results. Patients with acute post-traumatic seizures (within the first several minutes following the event) are not felt to be at increased risk for developing further seizures and receive the routine 7-day treatment. At the University of Louisville we have found that changing phenytoin dosing to a weight-based schedule (15 mg/kg load, 2 mg/kg every 8 hours unless elderly [$\geq$70 years old], then 2 mg/kg every 12 hours) increases the chance of achieving a therapeutic dose earlier in the treatment course and lowers the costs of monitoring these agents.

Finally, the treatment of these patients requires a tight-knit group of specialists and ancillary service providers with open communication channels. We have found that the use of a time-independent phased outcome clinical pathway helps maximize the level of patient care and maintain cost-effectiveness. By using such an approach all routine interactions are initiated at the time of admission and each care provider has a clear role and responsibility; one of the most important aspects of this system is the creation of a clinical coordinator whose responsibility includes ensuring that all aspects of patient care and family education are completed at the appropriate intervals. We believe another key component of this is our philosophy toward early feeding (prior to PID 3) and early tracheotomy and percutaneous endoscopic gastrostomy (PEG) feeding tube placement in a majority of these individuals (PID 4). We have shown that such an aggressive approach to these issues helps reduce infectious complications and minimizes length of ICU stay.

Treatment of Mild and Moderate Traumatic Brain Injury

In many circumstances patients with moderate TBI are treated almost as though they had severe TBI, with the exception of invasive ICP monitoring. Many patients will be intubated at the time of admission and require sedation and adequate pain management. This can be difficult because it is of utmost importance to maintain the ability to perform serial neurologic examinations. Therefore, we commonly use a combination of propofol (Diprivan) infusions and intermittent morphine (Lioresal)[1] injections in these patients, thereby allowing hourly assessment of neurologic function. We have found that a subset of patients (older than age 45 years, multisystem trauma, presence of early pneumonia) with moderate TBI requires more aggressive treatment with early tracheotomy and PEG tube placement and at times ICP monitors.

The subset of patients with moderate TBI who are not intubated at the time of admission are also watched closely in the ICU. Once again, close monitoring of neurologic function and vigorous pulmonary toilet is of key importance because some patients may be lethargic and are at risk of pulmonary decompensation. We have found ipratropium (Atrovent)[1] and albuterol (Proventil)[1] nebulizers and early mobilization minimize pulmonary problems. Patients with progressive lethargy, worsening neurologic function, hypoxia, hypercapnia, or the inability to protect their airways are intubated and placed on mechanical ventilation. Once again, patients unable to tolerate a diet by PID 3 have a nasogastric feeding tube placed to allow for early enteral nutritional support; however, PEG tubes are not placed until later in the hospital course in the predischarge phase because many patients in this category will improve throughout their hospitalization and be able to tolerate an oral diet by the time of discharge.

Patients with mild TBI are treated over a much wider continuum, ranging from discharge from the emergency room (ER) with

appropriate adult supervision to observation in the ICU to immediate surgical treatment of surgical mass lesions. The two most important factors in determining treatment algorithms for these patients are presence or absence of abnormal CT findings and neurologic function, with associated symptoms such as nausea, vomiting, dizziness, or visual problems. Headache is a common complaint in all of these patients and must be taken in context with other complaints and imaging results. Patients with severe headaches, dizziness, and vomiting (postconcussive syndrome) may commonly require a brief hospital stay to allow for delayed imaging and at least partial resolution of some of the complaints.

Early and Delayed Neurologic Changes

Any patient suffering a significant neurologic injury requires close neurologic monitoring. Although most patients remain unchanged or show gradual improvement in the early phases, a small percentage will show signs of neurologic deterioration. At first these signs may be subtle (agitation, mild increase in lethargy, protracted vomiting); but eventually they may become more profound and can be precursors to impending neurologic demise and death. When these changes are the result of either expanding mass lesions or increases in ICP, treatment instituted in the early phases is more likely to be more successful compared to instances when interventions are performed under conditions associated with cerebral herniation syndromes. Thus any patient showing persistent signs of neurologic decline should be promptly evaluated by a physician and many may also require repeat CT scanning.

However, not all neurologic changes are the result of changes in ICP or expansion of mass lesions, and such irregularities may be caused by a long list of other metabolic or neurologic conditions. Some of the more common causes are seizures, strokes (especially from carotid or vertebral dissections), electrolyte imbalances, hypoxia, hypercarbia, fever, excess sedation, or drug and/or alcohol withdrawal.

Concussions and Sports-Related Injuries: Return to Play Guidelines

Over the past 2 decades, the knowledge regarding the detrimental effects of repetitive mild head injuries has led to intense public debate concerning whether athletes should be allowed to return to play following such injuries. Concussions are not uncommon among participants of competitive sports including football, hockey, baseball, and soccer. Concerns regarding the full negative impact of repetitive, almost innocuous injury have led many youth soccer leagues to ban or modify rules regarding *heading* of the ball. In addition, other concerns exist following more severe concussions such as development of other life-threatening neurologic injuries such as subdural or epidural hematomas, development of the double-impact syndrome (rapid uncontrolled increases in ICP following sequential minor traumas), and the long-term neuropsychological impact of these injuries. As a result of these concerns, the guidelines concerning when and if an athlete should be allowed to return to play have undergone modification since development of the earlier criteria. Because of these frequent changes, readers are encouraged to check with their local medical agencies or recent publications and Internet sources if faced with these issues. In short, if a player loses consciousness or has persistent symptoms (>15 to 20 minutes), he or she should not be allowed to return to play on that day or even not for 1 to 2 weeks following the complete resolution of all symptoms. It should also be stressed that an individual may have a concussion without loss of consciousness and that concussion is defined as any transient change in mental status. To this end many organizations including the National Football League have developed a sideline neuropsychological screening test that can often help illustrate these deficits even when the athlete appears normal.

---

[1]Not FDA approved for this indication.

Restorative Therapies

Patients suffering any type of TBI can have long-lasting cognitive, psychological, and emotional dysfunction in addition to their functional and neurologic deficits. Although most people assume that the resolution of decreased alertness and consciousness symbolizes resolution of the overall neurologic injury, this is not the case in most patients. In our series of patients with moderate TBI, we found that almost 50% of patients at median follow-up of 27 months complained of persistent emotional or cognitive problems that interfered with their lifestyle despite the fact that they all were discharged from the hospital with a GCS score of 14 to 15. Long-term speech and cognitive therapies as well as individual, group, and family counseling will be helpful for many of these patients.

In the late hospital and early rehabilitative stages, numerous pharmacologic agents may be helpful to overcome some of the neurologic side effects following TBI. Patients with autonomic storms (intermittent episodes of diaphoresis, tachycardia, fever, agitation) may respond to adrenergic antagonists such as clonidine (Catapres)[1] or propanolol (Inderal),[1] in addition to volume resuscitation, morphine (Lioresal),[1] baclofen,[1] and bromocriptine (Parlodel).[1] Patients with hypoarousal are treated with amantadine[1] (Symmetrel), 100 mg at 8 am and 12 pm, and bromocriptine,[1] 5 to 15 mg every day. Trazodone (Desyrel), 50 to 100 mg at bedtime, may be helpful in restoring sleep-wake cycles, whereas risperidone (Risperdal),[1] olanzapine (Zyprexa),[1] and quetiapine (Seroquel)[1] may be helpful to control agitation and combativeness during the subacute recovery phases.

Future Considerations

The previously mentioned treatment strategies include what is considered common practice at the University of Louisville; however, newer, more aggressive treatments and monitoring capabilities are always being developed. Some of the newer monitoring systems under development include cerebral oximetry measurements (frequently through invasive indwelling catheters) or cerebral microdialysis systems, in which continuous assessments are performed to determine the concentrations of critical markers such as lactate in the brain or CSF. Both of these methods provide physiologic feedback for the metabolic environment of the brain, are sensitive enough to predict changes in regional oxygenation, and have been found to be correlated with outcomes in small nonrandomized studies.

REFERENCES

Brain Trauma Foundation. Management and Prognosis of Severe Traumatic Brain Injury. New York: Brain Trauma Foundation; 2000.

Mcilvoy L, Spain DA, Raque G, et al. Successful incorporation of the Severe Head Injury Guidelines into a phased-outcome clinical pathway. J Neurosci Nurs 2001;33(2):72–8 82.

Miller PR, Fabian TC, Bee TK, et al. Blunt cerebrovascular injuries: Diagnosis and treatment. J Trauma 2001;51(2):279–86.

Temkin NR, Dikmen SS, Wilensky AJ, et al. A randomized, double-blind study of phenytoin for the prevention of post-traumatic seizures. N Engl J Med 1990;323:497–502.

Vitaz TW, McIlvoy L, Raque GH, et al. Development and implementation of a clinical pathway for severe traumatic brain injury. J Trauma 2001;51(2):369–75.

Vitaz TW, McIlvoy L, Raque GH, et al. Development and implementation of a clinical pathway for spinal cord injuries. J Spinal Disord 2001;14(3):271–6.

Vitaz TW, Jenks J, Raque GH, Shields CB. Outcome following moderate traumatic brain injury. Surg Neurol 2003;60(4):285–91.

---

[1]Not FDA approved for this indication.

Traumatic Brain Injury in Children

Method of
Stephen R. Deputy, MD

Traumatic brain injury (TBI) is one of the leading causes of death and disability among children, adolescents, and young adults. An estimated 185 per 100,000 children (ages 0 to 14 years) and 550 per 100,000 adolescents (ages 15 to 19 years) are hospitalized each year for TBI. The etiology of TBI varies depending on the age of the patient, with younger children more likely to be injured from falls and pedestrian injuries, and adolescents more often injured in motor vehicle accidents and assaults. Inflicted TBI (shaking-impact syndrome of infancy) is the leading cause of injury-related deaths in children younger than 4 years of age and accounts for 80% of deaths from head trauma in children younger than 2 years of age.

Types and Severity of Head Injury

Closed head injury is the most common type of TBI seen in children. Forces from rapid deceleration are applied diffusely throughout the brain and consciousness is frequently impaired. *Open head injuries*, in which the dura is breached, are caused by focal penetrating forces, and the risk of post-traumatic epilepsy is relatively high.

Primary brain injury is caused by the mechanical forces of the trauma itself. Diffuse axonal injury is an example of primary brain injury. During rapid deceleration, angular forces applied to the head cause the brain to rotate about its center of gravity. Shifting regions of differing densities within the brain itself result in shearing along planes such as the gray-white junction, corpus callosum, and brainstem. The shearing of axons effectively serves to "disconnect" the cortex from the brainstem and consciousness becomes impaired. Translational (straight-line) forces applied to the head produce impact-loading contact phenomena, resulting in focal injuries to the scalp, skull, and brain, such as lacerations, skull fractures, cerebral contusions, and epidural hematomas. *Subdural hematomas* may occur because of tearing of fragile dural bridging veins during rapid decelerations.

Secondary brain injury follows and is the consequence of primary injury. Examples include hypoxic-ischemic injury (secondary to low cerebral perfusion pressure or anoxia), disrupted cerebral autoregulation, seizures or status epilepticus, diffuse cerebral edema, hydrocephalus, and raised intracranial pressure. The goal of treatment for TBI is to reduce or prevent secondary brain injury from occurring because the primary brain injury has already happened at the time of trauma and cannot be altered.

The severity of TBI can be broken down into mild, moderate, and severe. *Mild* TBI is defined as head trauma with an initial Glasgow Coma Scale (GCS) score of 13 to 15. *Moderate* TBI occurs with an initial GCS score of 9 to 12. *Severe* TBI occurs with an initial GCS score of 8 or less. The GCS is modified for use in infants under the age of 36 months (Table 1).

Special attention should be given to those infants with TBI who do not show evidence of external facial or head trauma and who may not be presented by their caregivers as having a history of head injury. The *shaking-impact syndrome* is usually found in infants younger than 3 years of age with a peak incidence in infants younger than 1 year of age. Presenting symptoms include irritability, lethargy, or coma, apnea or breathing irregularities, and seizures. Retinal hemorrhages may be found in from 65% to 95% of these patients and should be actively looked for with a dilated funduscopic examination in any case where head trauma is suspected. Computed tomography (CT) imaging most commonly shows evidence of acute or remote subdural hematomas with or without evidence of cerebral infarction. Workup should include a skeletal survey to look for evidence of skull, posterior rib,

TABLE 1 Glasgow Coma Scale for Children

Score	Eyes Open	Best Verbal Response	Best Verbal Response	Best Motor Response (<36 mo)	Best Motor Response (<36 mo)
6	—	—	—	Follows commands	Normal spontaneous movements
5	—	Oriented and converses	Coos and babbles	Localizes pain	Withdraws to touch
4	Spontaneously	Confused	Irritable to pain	Withdraws to pain	Withdraws to pain
3	To verbal commands	Inappropriate words	Cries to pain	Flexor posturing	Flexor posturing
2	To painful stimuli	Nonspecific sounds	Moans to pain	Extensor posturing	Extensor posturing
1	None	None	None	No response	No response

or long bone fractures of different healing stages. Infants may be more susceptible to shaking-impact syndrome given their relatively large head size compared to their underdeveloped neck musculature. Infants also have thinner skulls, and translational forces may cause more severe contusions. Relatively longer subdural veins that bridge the infant's enlarged subarachnoid spaces can be easily lacerated from angular forces, resulting in subdural hematomas.

Management of Traumatic Brain Injury in Children

MILD TRAUMATIC BRAIN INJURY

Mild TBI accounts for more than 90% of all pediatric admissions for TBI. Children in this category should have a GCS score of 15 upon arrival to the emergency room, no focal neurologic deficits, and no signs of increased intracranial pressure (ICP). These children may have had a brief loss of consciousness (less than 1 minute), amnesia for the event, an immediate impact seizure, vomiting, or lethargy (as long as the GCS score is 15 during the evaluation). Children without loss of consciousness or amnesia may be observed or sent home with competent caregivers without performing neuroimaging studies. Vigilance for any change in the child's neurologic status should be maintained for up to 72 hours after the injury. If there has been a brief loss of consciousness or amnesia for the event, the risk of intracranial hemorrhage is still relatively low, and it is up to the discretion of the treating physician whether CT imaging is warranted.

Clinical predictors of intracranial hemorrhage are less reliable for children under the age of 2 years, and nonaccidental trauma also comes into consideration in this age group. Therefore, most children under the age of 2 years with TBI should undergo CT imaging followed by careful observation.

MODERATE TRAUMATIC BRAIN INJURY

Patients who fall within the moderate category generally need more intensive monitoring and medical management to avoid secondary brain injuries. As with all critical illness, attention should first be paid to following the ABCs (airway, breathing, circulation).

Airway

Patients with a GCS score of 9 or greater usually do not require endotracheal intubation for airway protection, although they should be kept NPO (nothing by mouth) in case of clinical deterioration.

Breathing

Hypoxemia and hypoventilation may increase ICP, so supplemental oxygen by nasal cannula may be helpful.

Circulation

It is important to avoid hypotension to maintain adequate cerebral perfusion pressure (CPP). Isotonic intravenous fluids should be provided with care to avoid fluid overload, hypoglycemia, or hyperglycemia.

Careful attention should be paid to fluid and sodium balance because these patients may be at risk for developing diabetes insipidus. Likewise, the head of the bed should be raised to 30 degrees and the patient's head kept midline to optimize venous return from the cranium to the right side of the heart. Sedation with short-acting sedatives (propofol [Diprivan] or midazolam [Versed]) or opioids may be necessary to avoid agitation, which can also reduce venous return to the heart.

Early post-traumatic seizures are fairly rare in children with moderate TBI. The need for empirical anticonvulsant therapy in this group remains controversial and should be reserved for those patients in whom raised intracranial pressure is of concern. Likewise, empirical use of mannitol has little clinical support for this group.

SEVERE TRAUMATIC BRAIN INJURY

Patients in the severe group are at the highest risk for secondary brain injuries. The following additional interventions are recommended.

Airway

By definition, these patients have a GCS score of 8 or lower and require endotracheal intubation for airway protection.

Breathing

Hyperventilation with a goal P_{CO_2} of 26 to 30 mm Hg should be performed only if there is impending brainstem herniation or to bridge the gap until more definitive neurosurgical intervention can be performed to lower intracranial pressure. The benefit of hyperventilation is generally short lived (1 to 24 hours) and may worsen local ischemia following trauma or acute stroke.

Circulation

In the setting of suspected raised intracranial pressure, the goal of fluid and blood pressure management should be to maintain the cerebral perfusion pressure greater than 50 to 70 mm Hg. Recall that CPP equals MAP (mean arterial blood pressure) minus ICP. Because children generally have a lower MAP than adults, it is not always necessary to provide vasopressor therapy to keep the CPP above 70 mm Hg unless there is evidence of raised ICP. Invasive intracranial pressure monitoring should be considered if the GCS score is lower than 8 or in the setting of elevated ICP to optimize CPP.

Other Techniques to Lower Intracranial Pressure

NEUROSURGICAL

Obvious mass lesions, such as hydrocephalus, subdural and epidural hematomas, and contused cortical tissue should be surgically evacuated whenever feasible. CT scanning is able to identify most of these surgical lesions. Decompressive craniectomy is now used more frequently to relieve pressure when multifocal contusions or diffuse cerebral edema is present. As mentioned earlier, ICP monitoring is usually warranted for all severe TBI patients.

CURRENT DIAGNOSIS

- Children under the age of 2 years with traumatic brain injury (TBI) may require neuroimaging because clinical predictors of intracranial hemorrhage are less reliable in this age group.
- Children under the age of 1 year presenting with lethargy, irritability, apnea, or seizures should be evaluated with computed tomography (CT) imaging and a dilated funduscopic examination to rule out shaking-impact syndrome.

OSMOTHERAPY

Mannitol (20% solution) may be given as an initial bolus of 0.5 to 1 g/kg. Repeat doses of 0.25 to 0.5 g/kg are given every 6 to 8 hours as needed to maintain the serum osmolality and sodium levels to less than or equal to 320 mOsmL and 150 mEq, respectively. Osmotic diuretics should be used with caution in patients with renal insufficiency. The beneficial effects occur within minutes, peak at 1 hour, and last 4 to 24 hours. Potential disadvantages include worsening of focal cerebral edema in areas where the blood-brain barrier is disrupted.

BARBITURATES

Sedating agents may lower ICP by reducing pain as well as by making the brain metabolically less active. Pentobarbital is given as a loading dose of 5 to 20 mg/kg, followed by a continuous infusion of 1 to 4 mg/kg per hour. Continuous EEG monitoring to maintain a burst suppression pattern is warranted with this therapy. Potential disadvantages include systemic hypotension and a long half-life that may interfere with the declaration of brain death.

ANTICONVULSANT THERAPY

Children with severe TBI are at a high risk for early post-traumatic seizures, which can further elevate the ICP. It is generally recommended empirically to load these children with 20 mg/kg of intravenous phenytoin (Cerebyx). Maintenance therapy can be achieved with 5 mg/kg per day divided every 8 hours with target blood levels of 10 to 20 mg/dL.

HYPOTHERMIA

More centers are including hypothermia as an option for patients with elevated ICP not responsive to medical or surgical management. The best method of cooling (i.e., whole body versus head only) and the optimal core temperature are not established for children.

CURRENT THERAPY

- Children with mild TBI and a GCS score of 15 at presentation can usually be observed clinically without the need for neuroimaging.
- The goal of treatment for TBI is to minimize *secondary* brain injury.
- In the setting of raised ICP, it is important to maintain CPP above 50 to 70 mm Hg.
- Early post-traumatic seizures are relatively frequent in open head injury and in severe TBI. They should be empirically treated in any patient in whom raised ICP is a concern.
- Direct intracranial pressure monitoring should be considered in any TBI patient with a GCS score of 8 or less.

Abbreviations: CPP = cerebral perfusion pressure; ICP = intracranial pressure; GCS = Glasgow Coma Scale; TBI = traumatic brain injury.

Of note, apart from neurosurgical interventions, none of the techniques just described are shown definitively to reduce morbidity or mortality in children with severe TBI.

REFERENCES

Annegers JF, Grabow JD, Grover RV, et al. Seizures after head trauma: A population study. Neurology 1980;30:683–9.

Bruce DA, Zimmerman RA. Shaken impact syndrome. Pediatr Ann 1989;18:482–94.

Committee on Quality Improvement. American Academy of Pediatrics: The management of minor closed head injury in children. Pediatrics 1999;104(6):1407–15.

Deputy SR. Shaking-impact syndrome of infancy. Semin Pediatr Neurol 2003;10(2):112–19.

Kraus JF, Nourjah P. The epidemiology of uncomplicated brain injury. J Trauma 1988;28:1637–43.

Schutzman SA, Barnes P, et al. Evaluation and management of children younger than two years old with apparently minor head trauma: Proposed guidelines. Pediatrics 2001;107:983–93.

Brain Tumors

Method of
Douglas E. Ney, MD, and Andrew B. Lassman, MD

More than 64,000 primary brain tumors were diagnosed between 1998 and 2002, yielding an incidence of 14.8 brain tumors per 100,000 people. For children and men between 20 and 39 years old, these tumors represent the second leading cause of death. Metastatic disease is much more common, with more than 100,000 symptomatic intracranial metastases diagnosed every year. Data suggest that the incidence of primary and metastatic tumors is increasing, although this may partially reflect advances in diagnosis.

Patients with brain tumors typically develop signs over a period of weeks to months, although occasionally onset is abrupt (e.g., seizure). Initial symptoms typically are nonspecific and are related to the anatomic location of the tumor. Frontal tumors may be particularly difficult to diagnosis because they may involve symptoms of personality or mood changes, which may be misdiagnosed as depression. Other common signs include headache, nausea, vomiting, seizures, weakness, double vision, tinnitus, personality change, confusion, and difficulty walking.

Magnetic resonance imaging (MRI) remains the gold standard for imaging brain tumors. It gives the best anatomic detail of the brain and enables superior localization. Ultimately, definitive diagnosis is based on histopathologic characteristics (Table 1). Noninvasive techniques being developed to assist in treatment planning include magnetic resonance spectroscopy, which allows biochemical measurement of a region of interest, and the findings may correlate with tumor histology. Perfusion MRI helps to determine tumor vascularity, which may be a marker for tumor grade. However, it is unclear how best to incorporate magnetic resonance spectroscopy or perfusion into routine clinical care. Computed tomography (CT) is helpful in characterizing calcification, which is more common in oligodendrogliomas than in astrocytomas, and identifying hemorrhage. It is also superior for determining bony involvement of the skull. Positron emission tomography (PET) provides metabolic imaging of tumors, and uptake of radiolabeled isotopes may increase in proportion to tumor grade.

Gliomas

Gliomas are tumors that resemble glia such as astrocytes, ependymal cells, and oligodendrocytes. Together, gliomas account for 40% of all primary brain tumors and 78% of all malignant brain tumors.

TABLE 1 WHO Classification of Common Primary Brain Tumors

Histologic Class	Subtype	WHO Grade
Astrocytic tumors	Subependymal giant cell astrocytoma	I
	Pilocytic astrocytoma	I
	Pleomorphic xanthoastrocytoma	I
	Astrocytoma	II
	Anaplastic astrocytoma	III
	Glioblastoma	IV
Oligodendroglial tumors	Oligodendroglioma	II
	Anaplastic oligodendroglioma	III
	Oligoastrocytoma	II
	Anaplastic oligoastrocytoma	III
Ependymal tumors	Subependymoma	I
	Myxopapillary ependymoma	I
	Ependymoma	II
	Anaplastic ependymoma	III
Meningeal tumors	Meningioma	I
	Atypical meningioma	II
	Anaplastic or malignant meningioma	III
	Hemangiopericytoma	II
	Anaplastic hemangiopericytoma	III
	Hemangioblastoma	I

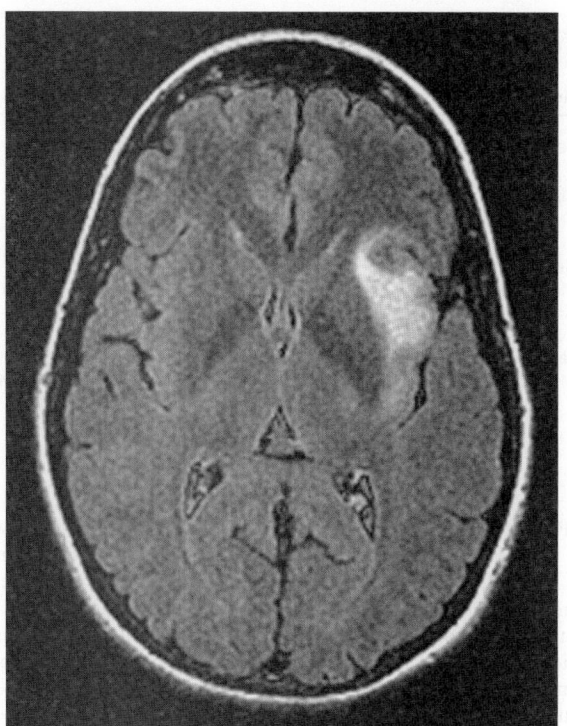

FIGURE 1. FLAIR MRI sequence of a brain shows a low-grade (WHO grade II) astrocytoma.

Gliomas are classified by histologic type and by levels of aggressiveness. Histologically, astrocytomas comprise most gliomas, and oligodendrogliomas represent only 10%.

LOW-GRADE GLIOMAS

World Health Organization (WHO) grade I astrocytomas, most commonly juvenile pilocytic astrocytomas, typically arise in the cerebellum of children and may be amenable to surgical cure. Their biology is different from the other gliomas (WHO grades II through IV), which are all diffusely infiltrating tumors without clean margins between tumor tissue and normal brain, making surgical cure impossible.

In adults, most low-grade gliomas are supratentorial, and they appear as nonenhancing masses on brain MRI (Fig. 1). After maximal surgical resection, low-grade (WHO grade II) astrocytomas and oligodendrogliomas usually are treated with radiation therapy (RT). A dose of approximately 50 Gy is standard because higher doses increase toxicity without improving survival. The timing of RT remains controversial because it may prolong progression-free survival but not overall survival. Observation may be a reasonable approach in young and otherwise healthy patients with small tumors that have predominantly oligodendroglial histology, who have undergone gross total resection, and who are asymptomatic. Older patients with poor performance status, neurologic symptoms, and large, bi-hemispheric tumors not amenable to extensive resection should undergo RT. Chemotherapy is not routinely used at diagnosis except in a research setting, although the use of temozolomide (Temodar), an oral alkylating agent that is generally well tolerated, is an emerging treatment (Table 2).

In almost all cases, WHO grade II gliomas are incurable diseases. With time, tumors accumulate molecular oncogenic abnormalities, leading to more aggressive behavior. In this manner, they transform into high-grade gliomas.

HIGH-GRADE GLIOMAS

Anaplastic (WHO grade III) astrocytomas are treated with RT, although some clinicians treat them analogously to glioblastoma (GBM) with irradiation and temozolomide. Treatment of anaplastic oligodendrogliomas or oligoastrocytomas is controversial, but commonly used approaches include RT, chemotherapy, and chemoradiation therapy. Two trials demonstrated that the addition of chemotherapy with the combination of procarbazine (Matulane),[1] lomustine (CCNU, CeeNU), and vincristine (Oncovin)[1] (PCV regimen) to RT likely prolongs progression-free but not overall survival (see Table 2). It remains controversial whether the improvement in progression-free survival outweighs the potential toxicity of the PCV regimen. Temozolomide has become the most commonly used form of chemotherapy for oligodendrogliomas, but a direct comparison with PCV has not been conducted.

GBM (WHO grade IV) is the most common glioma subtype (>50% of all gliomas), and it is also the most aggressive, with an average survival of about 1 year. GBMs can arise from lower-grade gliomas (i.e., secondary GBMs). Alternatively, tumors can manifest as GBM first without a history of a lower-grade glioma (i.e., *de novo* or primary GBMs). Primary and secondary GBMs are histologically identical and are treated in the same manner.

The current standard of care for patients with GBM who are younger than 70 years and have good baseline performance status is maximal surgical resection followed by RT to a dose of approximately 60 Gy, with concurrent and adjuvant temozolomide (see Table 2). The typical MRI appearance involves a contrast-enhancing abnormality with a necrotic center (Fig. 2). Fluid attenuation inversion recovery (FLAIR) imaging shows an abnormality encompassing a nonenhancing tumor and surrounding edema (Fig. 3). Compared with treatment with surgery and RT, the addition of temozolomide administered concurrently with RT and for 6 months after RT improves median survival from 12.1 to 14.6 months. Although modest, this benefit is sustained, with 2-year survival rates of 10% and 27% for those treated with RT alone and RT with temozolomide, respectively. Some advocate placement of carmustine (BCNU)-containing wafers (Gliadel) into the operative bed, and this approach is associated with a prolongation of survival, although it can also contribute to wound-healing difficulties.

Older patients or those with poor performance status may benefit from postoperative RT and temozolomide. However, they are sometimes treated with an abbreviated course of RT (fewer fractions and higher dose per fraction) or occasionally with temozolomide alone.

---

[1]Not FDA approved for this indication.

TABLE 2 Common Chemotherapy Regimens for Brain Tumors

Regimen	Generic Name	Trade Name	Dose
Temozolomide	Temozolomide	Temodar	75 mg/m^2 daily during radiotherapy for approximately 6 weeks 150–200 mg/m^2, days 1–5 of 28 not during radiotherapy
PCV	Procarbazine	Matulane[1]	60 mg/m^2/day (oral), days 8–21 of 56
	Lomustine	CCNU, CeeNU	110 mg/m^2 (oral), day 1 of 56
	Vincristine	Oncovin[1]	1.4 mg/m^2 (2-mg cap) IV, days 8 and 29 of 56
Bevacizumab +/–	Bevacizumab	Avastin	10 mg/kg, days 1 and 8 of 14
Irinotecan	Irinotecan	CPT-11, Camptosar[1]	125 mg/m^2* or 340 mg/m^2,[†] days 1 and 8 of 14

[1]Not FDA approved for this indication.
Patients not taking* or taking[†] concurrent hepatic P-450 enzyme-inducing antiseizure drugs such as phenytoin (Dilantin), fosphenytoin (Cerebyx), phenobarbital, primidone (Mysoline), carbamazepine (Tegretol, Carbatrol), or oxcarbazepine (Trileptal).

For recurrent or progressive disease, repeat resection with or without intracavitary carmustine wafer placement, intravenous carmustine (BiCNU), and temozolomide for naive patients are accepted standard options. However, their relatively poor efficacy rates lead many patients to participate in clinical trials. Results with antiangiogenic therapy, such as bevacizumab (Avastin) have generated enthusiasm, but serious toxicity (especially thromboembolic events) occurs in a substantial minority of patients. Bevacizumab recently received accelerated FDA approval for progressive GBM.

Brainstem gliomas are a heterogeneous group of tumors that account for less than 5% of all gliomas. Most occur in childhood, although the prognosis is usually better in adults. Imaging is usually sufficient for diagnosis. Surgery is restricted to biopsy alone, usually only when diagnosis is in question. Treatment for large or symptomatic lesions consists of RT. No chemotherapeutic regimens have been beneficial in treating brainstem gliomas.

Several factors are important in determining prognosis for patients with gliomas, including age, performance status, tumor histology and grade, extent of surgery, and presence of neurologic deficits. In adults, median survival for low-grade (WHO grade II) and anaplastic (WHO grade III) astrocytomas is about 5 and 2 years, respectively. Oligodendrogliomas are associated with longer survival times than astrocytomas of the same grade. For example, low-grade and anaplastic oligodendrogliomas have median survival times of about 10 and 4 years, respectively. However, there is a wide range of survival times for oligodendrogliomas, and the prognosis in part depends on molecular analysis of tumor tissue. Loss of heterozygosity of chromosomes 1p and 19q in oligodendrogliomas has been associated with better overall survival and better response to treatment. ^{O}6-Methylguanine DNA methyltransferase (MGMT) promoter methylation appears to correlate with increased sensitivity to temozolomide and improved prognosis, especially for GBM.

Meningiomas

Meningiomas account for approximately 30% of all brain tumors, with an incidence of 4.5 tumors per 100,000 people, and they represent the most common primary brain tumor. They occur most often in the elderly population and affect women two to three times more often than men. One identifiable risk factor is previous cranial irradiation.

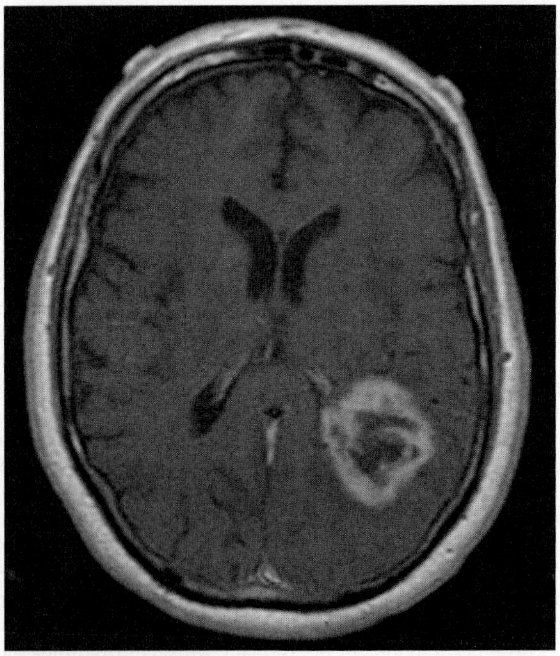

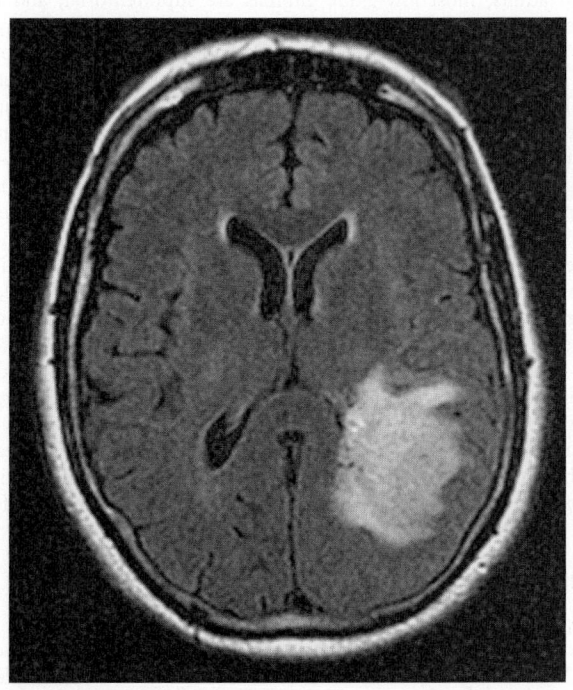

FIGURE 2. Contrast-enhanced MRI shows the typical appearance of a glioblastoma.

FIGURE 3. FLAIR MRI sequence (same patient as in Figure 2) shows a nonenhancing tumor and surrounding edema.

Meningiomas arise from arachnoid cap cells of the meninges. Loss of genetic material from chromosome 22 has been reported in the development of meningiomas. Accumulation of other chromosomal mutations may lead to the development of atypical or anaplastic meningiomas. Radiation-induced meningiomas usually are atypical or anaplastic.

Many histologic subtypes of meningioma exist, but grading has been the source of much debate. The WHO classifies meningiomas as benign (grade I), atypical (grade II), or anaplastic (grade III). Grading largely depends on the amount of mitotic activity in the tumor. Together, atypical and anaplastic meningiomas account for less than 10% of meningiomas.

Meningiomas are slow-growing tumors, and many are asymptomatic and discovered incidentally. In these cases, the decision to treat may be controversial, and observation is frequently recommended. However, treatment is usually indicated for patients presenting with neurologic symptoms or unusual radiographic features. Surgery remains the primary treatment modality. Surgery with curative intent requires complete excision. Because meningiomas are highly vascular tumors, they are sometimes embolized preoperatively.

After surgery, benign meningiomas undergoing complete excision usually do not warrant RT. However, RT may be useful for subtotal resections. If the tumor recurs, RT may be undertaken after a second resection. Atypical or malignant meningiomas always require RT. Chemotherapy has little established role in treatment of meningiomas. Hydroxyurea (Hydrea)[1] offers modest benefit for otherwise refractory disease. Other agents are under investigation.

Primary Central Nervous System Lymphoma

Primary central nervous system lymphoma (PCNSL) is a non-Hodgkin's lymphoma involving any part of the craniospinal axis and the eyes, usually without evidence of systemic disease. It accounts for 3% of all intracranial tumors and has an incidence of approximately 0.5 per 100,000 people. Two populations are affected by PCNSL: the immunocompetent and the immunocompromised. Whether congenital or acquired, immune suppression is the major established risk factor for this disease. Most PCNSLs in the immunosuppressed population are related to latent Epstein-Barr virus infection.

The treatment of PCNSL involves multiple modalities. Surgery is used only to make the diagnosis, usually by stereotactic biopsy. Debulking of tumor is not undertaken except when there is diagnostic confusion or impending herniation from large tumors causing increased intracranial pressure. In contrast to treatment of other brain tumors, corticosteroids can have a direct effect on lymphoma cells, leading to significant improvement and sometimes to resolution of the tumor burden. Corticosteroids should be withheld until after biopsy, if medically safe. The use of corticosteroids alone, however, rarely produces sustainable remission. Although it is a radiosensitive tumor, it is unclear whether whole-brain radiotherapy (WBRT) along with chemotherapy is superior to chemotherapy alone. Given the risk of delayed neurotoxicity, particularly in those older than 60 years, WBRT is often deferred and later used for relapsing disease. For ocular lymphoma, however, irradiation of the globes usually is typically considered mandatory.

The mainstay of chemotherapy is high-dose methotrexate, although ideal regimens continue to be under investigation. Doses from 3 to 8 g/m^2 are routinely used[3] to attain high tissue concentrations across the blood-brain barrier. Most regimens still use this as the basis of therapy, adding additional agents such as vincristine (Oncovin),[1] procarbazine (Matulane),[1] and cytarabine (Tarabine).[1] Other agents that cross the blood-brain barrier, such as temozolomide (Temodax)[1], are being investigated, as is the B-cell antibody rituximab (Rituxan).[1]

Outcome is worse for patients older than 60 years, those who are immunocompromised, and those with poor pretreatment performance status. WBRT produces a median survival of 12 to 18 months, whereas methotrexate-based regimens produce a median survival of 40 to 60 months. The risk of relapse approaches 50%, usually occurring within the first 2 years of diagnosis. There is no consensus strategy to manage relapsed PCNSL, but treatment may consist of any of the modalities used to treat a first occurrence, including prior chemotherapy.

Metastatic Disease

Metastatic disease remains the most common intracranial neoplasm, with approximately 200,000 people diagnosed every year. Approximately one half of patients have one metastasis, and the remaining patients have multiple lesions. Cancers of the lung, breast, and skin (melanoma) most commonly metastasize to the brain. Renal cell carcinoma and colon cancers also are common primary tumors. Diagnosis of a brain metastasis in a patient without a known primary cancer should always prompt a systemic evaluation.

Supportive treatment is based on the type and severity of symptoms. Symptomatic brain edema is frequently encountered in this population and usually is managed with corticosteroids such as dexamethasone (Decadron) in dosages between 16 and 100 mg/day.[3] Patients who are on corticosteroids for an extensive period (>6 weeks) should receive prophylaxis against *Pneumocystis jiroveci* pneumonia. Prophylactic anti-convulsants are not given unless the patient develops seizures.

Anti-convulsant use of surgery for patients with one brain metastasis is well established. Patients who undergo resection followed by WBRT (typically 30 to 35 Gy in 10 to 15 fractions) have improved survival, reduced local recurrence rates, and longer functional independence than patients undergoing WBRT alone. Whether patients who undergo complete resection should receive postoperative WBRT remains controversial because of concerns about long-term neurotoxicity from RT. However, postoperative WBRT clearly reduces local and whole-brain recurrence rates.

For patients with multiple metastases, WBRT is a standard approach, although surgical resection of up to three discrete lesions has been advocated by some, especially if there is a dominant lesion amenable to resection. Stereotactic radiosurgery (SRS) is increasingly used in the treatment of brain metastases. It involves high-dose radiation delivered to small areas of disease, and it may be most effective against tumors that are relatively resistant to standard RT. SRS is limited in that only lesions that are less than 3 cm (at most 4 cm) are amenable to treatment without substantially increasing the risk of toxicity. Chemotherapy may be beneficial, particularly among chemotherapy-naive patients and those with chemosensitive primary tumors (e.g., breast, lung). Standard regimens are those that are useful in the treatment of the underlying disease as long as they penetrate the blood-brain barrier. Agents such as temozolomide[1] and tyrosine kinase inhibitors are under investigation.

For untreated patients, median survival is 1 to 2 months. RT alone yields a meager median survival of 4 to 6 months, although most will experience neurologic improvement. Patients with a single brain metastasis that is excised, and who have systemic disease under good control, have a 10% to 15% 5-year survival rate.

Leptomeningeal Disease

Leptomeningeal disease results from infiltration of the covering of the brain with malignant cells, which usually are metastatic from an extrameningeal primary tumor. It can involve any area of the brain or spinal cord. Like solid brain metastases, the incidence of leptomeningeal metastases is increasing despite increased survival from systemic cancers. The increase is likely related to the poor penetrance

---

[1]Not FDA approved for this indication.
[3]Exceeds dosage recommended by the manufacturer.

[1]Not FDA approved for this indication.
[3]Exceeds dosage recommended by the manufacturer.

of systemic chemotherapies through the blood-brain barrier, allowing malignant cells to grow within the CNS as a sanctuary site.

Treatment of leptomeningeal disease is largely palliative. Corticosteroids and RT may alleviate neurologic symptoms. Despite the diffuse nature of the disease, focal RT to affected areas, such as WBRT for patients with headache or cranial neuropathies, may be helpful. In cases of cerebrospinal fluid blockade, hydrocephalus may develop, which sometimes requires ventriculoperitoneal shunting, although WBRT or focal RT to painful or bulky areas of spinal leptomeningeal disease may be helpful. Intrathecal treatment with methotrexate (Methotrexate LPF),[1] cytarabine (in free and depot formulations [Tarabine PFS, DepoCyt]),[1] and systemic chemotherapy have been used in patients able to tolerate such therapy. Ideally, intrathecal chemotherapy should be administered through an Ommaya reservoir. Systemic therapy with high-dose (3.5 g/m^2 body surface area)[3] intravenous methotrexate[1] may be helpful, especially for patients with breast cancer.

Prognosis depends performance status, bulk of CNS disease, extent of systemic cancer, and tumor type. Patients with breast cancer and lymphoma may survive longer than most, for whom the average is at best a few months.

REFERENCES

Abrey LE, Ben-Porat LL, Panageas KS, et al. Primary central nervous system lymphoma: The Memorial Sloan-Kettering Cancer Center prognostic model. J Clin Oncol 2006;24:5711–5.

Central Brain Tumor Registry of the United States. Statistical report: Primary brain tumors in the United States, 1998–2002, Available at http://www.cbtrus.org [accessed July 2009].

Gavrilovic IT, Posner J. Brain metastases: Epidemiology and pathophysiology. J Neurooncol 2005;75:5–14.

Gilbert MR, Lang FF. Anaplastic oligodendroglial tumors: A tale of two trials. J Clin Oncol 2006;24:2689–90.

Karim AB, Maat B, Hatlevoll R, et al. A randomized trial on dose-response in radiation therapy of low-grade cerebral glioma: European Organization for Research and Treatment of Cancer (EORTC) study 22844. Int J Radiat Oncol Biol Phys 1996;36:549–56.

Louis DN, Ohgaki H, Wiestler OD, et al. WHO Classification of Tumours of the Central Nervous System. 4th ed. Lyon: International Agency for Research on Cancer; 2007.

Patchell RA, Tibbs PA, Regine WF, et al. Postoperative radiotherapy in the treatment of single metastases to the brain: A randomized trial. JAMA 1998;280:1485–9.

Patchell RA, Tibbs PA, Walsh JW, et al. A randomized trial of surgery in the treatment of single metastases to the brain. N Engl J Med 1990;322:494–500.

Stupp R, Mason WP, van den Bent MJ, et al. Radiotherapy plus concomitant and adjuvant temozolomide for glioblastoma. N Engl J Med 2005;352:987–96.

van den Bent MJ, Afra D, de Witte O, et al. Long-term efficacy of early versus delayed radiotherapy for low-grade astrocytoma and oligodendroglioma in adults: The EORTC 22845 randomised trial. Lancet 2005;366:985–90.

Vredenburgh JJ, Desjardins A, Herndon JE, et al. Bevacizumab plus irinotecan in recurrent glioblastoma multiforme. J Clin Oncol 2007;25:4722–9.

Westphal M, Ram Z, Riddle V, et al. Gliadel wafer in initial surgery for malignant glioma: Long-term follow-up of a multicenter controlled trial. Acta Neurochir (Wien) 2006;148:269–75.

[1]Not FDA approved for this indication.
[3]Exceeds dosage recommended by the manufacturer.

The Locomotor System

Rheumatoid Arthritis

Method of
Arthur Kavanaugh, MD, and
Venkata Sri Cherukumilli, BS

Rheumatoid arthritis (RA) is a progressive, systemic inflammatory disease that affects about 0.5% to 1% of the population worldwide. RA is associated with substantial morbidity and accelerated mortality, and it exerts a tremendous economic toll on affected patients, their families, and society. Women are three to four times more likely to be affected than men. The peak age of onset is between 40 and 60 years, but it is possible to get RA at any age, and it affects the elderly and young children.

Even though there has been progress in deciphering the cellular and molecular mechanism of RA, the cause is still not fully defined. RA is characterized by synovial and vascular proliferation with the formation of pannus tissue, which results in damage to articular cartilage and adjacent subchondral bone. Activation of specific CD4$^+$ T cells, potentially in response to unidentified antigens, in an immunogenetically susceptible individual is hypothesized to be an early event in this process. Activated T cells orchestrate a cell-mediated immune response, stimulating and interacting with monocytes or macrophages, synovial fibroblasts, osteoclasts, B cells, and many other cell types. The cascade of inflammatory mediators that is released contributes to the sustenance of the ongoing immune activation and directly causes signs, symptoms, and sequelae of the disease, such as destruction of joints. Joint destruction, which

CURRENT DIAGNOSIS

- Morning stiffness in and around the joint that lasts for 1 hour before maximal improvement
- Arthritis (i.e., soft tissue swelling or fluid) in three or more joint areas simultaneously observed by a physician
- Arthritis involving the wrist, metacarpophalangeal, or proximal interphalangeal joints
- Symmetrical arthritis that involves same joint areas on both sides of the body
- Rheumatoid nodules (i.e., subcutaneous nodules over bony prominences, extensor surfaces, or in juxtaarticular regions) observed by a physician
- Positive serum rheumatoid factor test result
- Radiographic changes typical of RA on the posteroanterior hand and wrist

may be considered the sequela of untreated inflammation over time, correlates directly with functional disability. Impaired function correlates with many key outcomes, such as increased mortality and greater costs.

Diagnosis

RA diagnosis is mainly clinical based on physical findings, patient history, and ongoing observation of symptoms, signs, and response to therapy. The American College of Rheumatology (ACR) classification for the diagnosis of RA requires at least four of seven features to be present, and the first four criteria must be present for at least 6 weeks (see Current Diagnosis box).

Treatment

The main goals of treatment for RA are to alleviate pain, prevent or limit joint damage, optimize quality of life, avoid complications of therapy, and improve or preserve function. Novel therapies with specific targets are being designed based on the improved understanding of the pathophysiology of RA. Adoption of an aggressive approach early in the course of the disease is thought to be the best way to prevent irreversible joint damage and to spare patients years of pain and discomfort. Remission, once a purely hypothetical consideration, is now considered to be an appropriate and attainable goal, largely due to the introduction of new therapies, particularly biologic agents, and new treatment paradigms, particularly the frequent assessment of disease activity with resultant changes in treatment to achieve low disease activity.

Treatment response in clinical trials is typically measured using the ACR criteria for measuring improvement of arthritis. The ACR20 refers to 20% improvement in tender and swollen joint counts and 20% improvement in three of the five additional measures: patient and physician global assessments of arthritis, pain, disability, and an acute-phase reactant, such as the erythrocyte sedimentation rate (ESR) or C-reactive protein (CRP). Variations that define higher levels of response—the ACR50 and ACR70, which require improvements in individual measures exceeding 50% and 70%, respectively—are more stringent outcomes. The Health Assessment Questionnaire (HAQ) and Short Form 36 (SF-36) are used to calculate functional disability and health-related quality of life, respectively. Joint damage in patients with RA is assessed by quantifying radiographic changes characteristic of RA, including joint space narrowing and periarticular bony erosions.

Treatment of RA begins after the diagnosis is established, baseline activity is assessed, and prognosis is estimated. Therapy is initiated with patient education about the disease and the treatments available. Symptoms can be controlled to some extent with nonsteroidal anti-inflammatory drugs (NSAIDs) and low-dose oral glucocorticoids or glucocorticoid joint injections. Ideally, disease-modifying antirheumatic drugs (DMARDs) should be started soon after diagnosis is established (e.g., within 3 months). Further care is determined by assessing disease activity and response to treatment. The Current Therapy box lists commonly used treatments for RA and includes trade names and usual maintenance doses for these drugs.

ANALGESICS AND NONSTEROIDAL ANTIINFLAMMATORY DRUGS

Analgesics (e.g., acetaminophen, tramadol [Ultram], opioids) are used to relieve pain, but they do not reduce inflammation or prevent joint destruction. NSAIDs (e.g., aspirin, ibuprofen [Motrin], naproxen [Naprosyn], ketoprofen [Orudis], piroxicam [Feldene], diclofenac [Voltaren], celecoxib [Celebrex]) reduce pain and inflammation (at higher doses) but do not slow joint damage. These drugs are used as adjuncts but are not usually the sole treatment for RA because they do not prevent disease progression.

Although many analgesics and NSAIDs are available over the counter and are perceived by patients to be benign, they are not risk free. Narcotic analgesics should be used with caution because of their potential for habituation and toxicity with chronic use. NSAIDs work by inhibiting cyclooxygenase enzyme isoforms COX-1 and COX-2. COX-1 is constitutively expressed by many cells, whereas COX-2 production is usually increased at sites of inflammation. Side effects with chronic use of NSAIDs include gastrointestinal irritation, rash, fluid retention, and the potential for renal toxicity. Acetaminophen (Tylenol), a non-NSAID COX inhibitor, does not cause gastrointestinal irritation, but it may cause severe hepatotoxicity, and it potentially interacts with warfarin (Coumadin). The frequency of NSAID-induced ulcers can be reduced with concomitant use of proton pump inhibitors or misoprostol (Cytotec). COX-2 inhibitors were developed because their more specific activity was expected to control signs and symptoms of arthritis with less risk of gastrointestinal complications. However, two of the three COX-2 inhibitors approved in the United States were withdrawn due to concerns about thrombotic and atherosclerotic toxicities; the remaining available COX-2 inhibitor, celecoxib, seems to have a safety profile comparable to other NSAIDs in that regard.

GLUCOCORTICOIDS

Oral glucocorticoids at lower doses (e.g., <10 mg prednisone equivalent per day) are often used to control pain, inflammation, and stiffness, and they potentially can slow progression of joint damage. However, because of the possibility of significant side effects, especially with long-term use at a high dose, glucocorticoids are most commonly used for short-term treatment of very active or aggressive RA, usually in combination with NSAIDs and DMARDs. They are often tapered when the disease is under control.

Side effects of glucocorticoids include changes to appetite and weight, glucose intolerance or hyperglycemia, infection, osteoporosis, mood and sleep disturbances, hypertension, suppression of the hypothalamic-pituitary axis, and interference with wound healing, among others. Administering calcium and vitamin D supplementation, bisphosphonates, calcitonin (Miacalcin),[1] parathyroid hormone (teriparatide [Forteo]),[1] and estrogen[1] or testosterone[1] replacement can reduce the risk of bone loss in patients taking corticosteroids.

Intraarticular glucocorticoid injections can provide dramatic but usually temporary clinical improvement in patients who have a disease flare in a single or a few joints. Most clinicians think that no more than one injection in any 3-month period should be made in a given joint. The need for more repeated injections suggests that the overall treatment plan requires reevaluation.

DISEASE-MODIFYING ANTIRHEUMATIC DRUGS

DMARDs are the mainstay of treatment for RA because they can modify various aspects of the immune and inflammatory responses, potentially controlling signs and symptoms of disease and slowing its progression. Extensive clinical studies of DMARDs have

demonstrated reductions in joint damage, preservation of joint function, and higher rates of productivity. DMARDs are considered first-line therapy for all patients with newly diagnosed RA. The standard of care is to initiate DMARD therapy early, such as within the first 3 months of disease for patients with established RA who, despite adequate treatment with NSAIDs, have ongoing joint pain, significant morning stiffness or fatigue, active synovitis, evidence of active inflammation (e.g., persistent elevation of the ESR or CRP level, actively inflamed joints) or radiographic joint damage. Because DMARDs may take 2 to 6 months to reach full effect, NSAIDs and sometimes glucocorticoids can be used in the interim to reduce pain and swelling. The duration of DMARD use may be limited by loss of efficacy or development of toxicity.

Methotrexate (Rheumatrex) is the most commonly used DMARD because of its oral, once-weekly administration; well-defined safety profile; demonstrated efficacy; and low cost. Sulfasalazine (Azulfidine EN-tabs) or hydroxychloroquine (Plaquenil) tends to be used in persons whose disease is considered milder or more slowly progressive. They are also used in combination with methotrexate for aggressive disease. Leflunomide (Arava) was shown in several phase III trials to offer comparable efficacy to methotrexate and sulfasalazine against active RA. Older drugs in this class (e.g., parenteral or oral gold [aurothiomalate or auranofin], azathioprine [Imuran], D-penicillamine [Cuprimine]) were shown to be effective in older clinical trials, but they are less commonly used now largely due to tolerability issues.

In RA, methotrexate's mechanism of action may be related to its inhibition of inflammation, presumably by increasing the local release of adenosine. Clinical response may take 6 to 8 weeks to be seen. The mean dose used among RA patients worldwide is approximately 17.5 mg/week, although many clinicians initiate therapy at lower doses to help ensure tolerability. Most clinicians consider 25 mg/week to be a maximum dose. Higher doses are not clearly associated with better disease control but may be associated with more toxicity. Parenteral administration may be used at doses higher than 15 mg/week because of more predictable absorption. Many RA patients have taken methotrexate successfully for years, attesting to its efficacy and safety.

Leflunomide is a prodrug that is actively metabolized after oral administration. This active metabolite inhibits dihydroorotate dehydrogenase, which interferes with pyrimidine synthesis and ultimately leads to inhibition of activated T cells and other cells. To minimize toxicity, the maintenance dose of 20 mg/day can be reduced to 10 mg/day to improve tolerability.

Although DMARDs represent a major advance in the management of RA, they are not without risks or limitations. Methotrexate is associated with rare but serious side effects, including bone marrow suppression, hypersensitivity pneumonitis, and hepatotoxicity. It may also slightly increase the risk of infection. It must be used with caution in patients with preexisting liver disease, renal impairment, significant pulmonary disease, or alcohol abuse. Less serious but common side effects of methotrexate include stomatitis, gastrointestinal effects, headache, fatigue, and liver transaminase elevations. Folic acid supplementation can prevent many of the minor side effects. Leflunomide can lead to elevated liver enzyme levels, weight loss, hypertension, diarrhea, reversible alopecia, and myelosuppression. Leflunomide inhibits cytochrome P-450 (CYP) 2C9, so there is a theoretical potential for interactions with other drugs that are also CYP2C9 substrates. Methotrexate and leflunomide necessitate regular monitoring of liver enzymes and complete blood cell counts at regular intervals. Treatment should be stopped for any persistent or severe abnormalities.

Other side effects seen with various DMARDs include gastrointestinal intolerance and rash. Although antimalarial drugs (e.g., hydroxychloroquine) have been reported to cause ocular toxicity, with current dosages and preparations, this reaction is rare. Sulfasalazine may cause cutaneous adverse events (e.g., urticaria, maculopapular rash, photosensitivity) and hematologic side effects. Cyclosporine's use has been limited by its toxicity, which includes headache, tremors, hypertension, and renal insufficiency. Patients taking cyclosporine (Neoral) require regular monitoring of blood pressure and serum creatinine levels. Some DMARDs (e.g., cyclophosphamide

---

[1]Not FDA approved for this indication.

[Cytoxan],[1] chlorambucil [Leukeran],[1] azathioprine) may promote the development of secondary malignancies. Some DMARDs are teratogenic and abortifacient and therefore should not be used during pregnancy or breast-feeding and must be discontinued for an appropriate amount of time, typically 3 months or more, before any attempts to conceive.

BIOLOGIC RESPONSE MODIFIERS

The introduction of biologic agents was driven largely by three factors: recognition of the unmet clinical need for more effective treatments based on an appreciation of the significantly poor outcomes of uncontrolled RA; improved understanding of the immunopathogenesis of RA; and advances in biopharmaceutical science allowing the development of specific inhibitors of relevant targets within the dysregulated immune system.

Traditional therapies such as NSAIDs, corticosteroids, and DMARDs may help ameliorate the symptoms of RA, but they rarely induce sustained remission, and they can have toxicities that prevent their long-term use. Newer therapies, many of which are large protein molecules such as monoclonal antibodies or soluble receptor constructs, are referred to as biologic agents. Biologic agents, particularly inhibitors of tumor necrosis factor (TNF), have changed the treatment paradigm for RA. They can inhibit various components of the immune system and inflammatory response that are central to the pathogenesis of RA. The goal is to adopt an early, proactive approach to treatment to prevent the damage from chronic synovial inflammation. Studies have shown that biologic agents can slow disease progression, control signs and symptoms of disease, improve function, and improve quality of life. They are typically used in combination with DMARDs, most commonly methotrexate, to potentiate treatment responses. This newer class of antirheumatic drugs can be further subclassified according to their specific target or mechanism.

Tumor Necrosis Factor-α Inhibitors

Use of TNF-α inhibitors in combination with methotrexate is considered by many to be the gold standard for treatment of RA. TNF-α is a soluble 17-kDa protein homotrimer that binds to two receptors: type 1 TNF receptor and type 2 TNF receptor. A versatile, multipotent cytokine, it induces production of other inflammatory cytokines such as interleukin-1 (IL-1), IL-6, and granulocyte-monocyte colony-stimulating factor (GM-CSF) and chemokines such as IL-8. TNF-α causes tissue destruction by promoting release of matrix metalloproteinases, upregulates cell trafficking through adhesion molecules and chemokines, increases the breakdown of proteoglycans in the cartilage, and potentiates osteoclast differentiation and activation. There is abundant evidence that TNF inhibition dramatically improves patient outcomes for RA and other autoimmune systemic inflammatory conditions, including psoriasis, psoriatic arthritis, ankylosing spondylitis, and inflammatory bowel disease.

Most RA patients respond to TNF-α inhibitors with a reduction in signs and symptoms, improved quality of life, and preservation of functional status; some even achieve clinical remission of disease. Radiographic evidence shows that TNF-α inhibitors inhibit radiographic disease progression to an extent not seen with any previous agents. From an immunologic standpoint, TNF-α inhibitors do not represent a cure, and maintenance of clinical efficacy almost always requires continued therapy, certainly for patients with long-standing RA. Three of the available biologic agents are inhibitors of TNF-α: infliximab (Remicade), etanercept (Enbrel), and adalimumab (Humira).

Infliximab, a chimeric human/mouse monoclonal anti-TNF-α monoclonal antibody, was shown to be effective initially in open trials, followed soon by double-blind, placebo-controlled, randomized clinical trials. Inhibition in the progression of joint damage and improvement in health-related quality of life and functional status were observed in patients treated with infliximab. It is used mostly in combination with methotrexate, which decreases immunogenicity and produces synergy in clinical outcomes.

---

[1]Not FDA approved for this indication.

Etanercept is a recombinant form of the human receptor that is fused to the Fc fragment of the human immunoglobulin G1. Clinical trials have shown etanercept to be effective in improving the signs and symptoms of RA when used as monotherapy and in combination with methotrexate; it also inhibits disease progression and optimizes functional status and quality of life.

Adalimumab is a human anti-TNF-α monoclonal antibody. The efficacy of adalimumab on the signs and symptoms of RA has been proved in various studies, and it has demonstrated benefit in terms of improving quality of life and functional status and in attenuating the progression of joint damage.

TNF antagonists exhibit a rapid onset of action, provide significant clinical response, improve quality of life, and most importantly, substantially inhibit radiographic progression of disease. Most patients on TNF antagonists are still treated with methotrexate because studies have shown that TNF antagonists work better in this combination. There are some safety concerns because reports of opportunistic infections, tuberculosis, lymphoma, administration reactions, immune or autoimmune responses, and demyelinating syndromes have emerged with TNF antagonist treatment. Some patients do fail to respond or eventually lose the ability to respond. Other biologic agents can be effective for patients who fail anti-TNF therapy.

Interleukin-1 Receptor Antagonist

IL-1 appears to have a prominent role in synovial inflammation and displays many overlapping effects with TNF-α. RA patients have increased levels of IL-1 in the plasma and synovial fluid, and its concentration has been correlated with disease activity. Similar to TNF-α, IL-1 can activate a variety of inflammatory cells and mediators using some overlapping signal transduction pathways.

Anakinra is a subcutaneously administered IL-1 receptor antagonist. Anakinra has been shown in several studies to reduce the signs and symptoms of RA; however, the extent of improvement is less than that seen with TNF antagonists. Combination therapy with anti-IL-1 and anti-TNF is contraindicated because of an observed increase in the risk of adverse events in a study in which patients were treated with anakinra and etanercept. Anakinra usually is well tolerated, and the most common side effect is injection site reactions. The need for daily injectable administration and the modest efficacy compared with TNF inhibitors have limited the use of anakinra.

B-Cell Directed Therapy

Mounting evidence suggests that B cells play an active role in RA. B cells can accumulate in the synovium, form aggregates, produce autoantibodies such as rheumatoid factor (RF), and function as antigen-presenting cells that aid in the activation of CD4+ T cells. These findings provide the rationale for targeting B cells in RA patients. Rituximab (Rituxan) is a monoclonal antibody directed against the CD20 antigen found on the surface of B cells. When bound to CD20, rituximab depletes B cells through various mechanisms, including complement-mediated lysis, antibody-dependent cytotoxicity, and apoptosis.

Rituximab treatment induced depletion of peripheral-blood B cells for 6 months or longer, but the levels of immunoglobulins in the serum (IgG, IgA, IgM) did not change substantially. RF levels decreased substantially. Despite the prolonged depletion of peripheral-blood B cells, the overall incidence of infection was similar in the control group and the rituximab groups. However, an increased rate of infusion-related reactions was identified for the rituximab group compared with the placebo group. In patients with active RA who failed one or more anti-TNF-α therapies, rituximab significantly reduced signs, symptoms, fatigue, and disability and improved health-related quality of life.

T-Cell Directed Therapy

T-cell activation plays a central role in the pathogenesis of RA. For example, the rheumatoid synovium contains a preponderance of CD4+ T cells. It is thought that these cells are stimulated by

Nonpharmacologic Treatment

- Patient and family education and longitudinal supportive care by physicians and their staff
- Physical therapy and occupational therapy for patients with compromised activities of daily living
- Dynamic and aerobic conditioning exercises to improve mobility, strength, and psychological well-being

Pharmacologic Treatment

NSAIDs and Selective Cyclooxygenase 2 (COX-2) Inhibitors

- Improve joint function by reducing joint pain and swelling

Glucocorticoids

- Can relieve signs and symptoms of disease, and may slow progression
- Use low-dose glucocorticoids, such as <10 mg of prednisone daily or the equivalent
- Local injections of depot formulations of corticosteroids
- Bridge therapies for flares or when starting treatment

Disease-Modifying Antirheumatic Drugs (DMARDs)

- Can preserve joint integrity and function by reducing joint damage
- Commonly used DMARDs:
  - Methotrexate (Rheumatrex) PO 7.5 to 25 mg/week; injectable 7.5 to 25 mg/week
  - Hydroxychloroquine (Plaquenil) 200 mg twice daily
  - Sulfasalazine (Azulfidine-EN Tabs)[3] 1000 mg twice or three times daily
  - Leflunomide (Arava) 20 mg/day in a single dose, if tolerated; otherwise, 10 mg/day
  - Cyclosporine A (Neoral)[3] ≈2.5 to 4.5 mg/kg/day in divided doses (twice daily)
  - Combinations of DMARDs that have been effective in RA include methotrexate plus cyclosporine, methotrexate plus leflunomide, and methotrexate plus sulfasalazine plus hydroxychloroquine.

[3]Exceeds dosage recommended by the manufacturer.

Biologic Response Modifiers (Biologics)

- Commonly used in combination with methotrexate or less commonly with other DMARDs
- Slow or prevent disease progression (particularly TNF inhibitors) and can induce remission
- TNF-α inhibitors:
  - Infliximab (Remicade) intravenous infusion of doses between 3 and 10 mg/kg (mean dose, ≈5 mg/kg) with additional similar doses at 2 and 6 weeks after the first infusion and then every 8 weeks thereafter
  - Etanercept (Enbrel) = SQ injection 50 mg/week (given as a single dose of 50 mg once per week or 25 mg biweekly)
  - Adalimumab (Humira) SQ injection 40 mg every other week (also approved for use weekly)
- Interleukin-1 receptor antagonist: anakinra (Kineret) SQ injection 100 mg/day
- Anti-CD20 antibody: rituximab (Rituxan) two 1000-mg IV infusions separated by 2 weeks; further treatments are typically given after 6 months when disease activity recurs
- CTLA-4-immunoglobulin: abatacept (Orencia) IV infusion for initial dose, followed by doses 2 and 4 weeks later, with further doses every 4 weeks thereafter; dosage between 500 and 1000 mg based on weight (dose approximates 10 mg/kg)

Surgical Treatment

- Surgery is used for patients with intolerable pain, loss of range of motion, or structural joint damage that leads to limitation of function.
- Procedures include joint fusion, synovectomy, total joint arthroplasty, and partial joint replacement or remodeling.

---

arthritogenic antigens to initiate synovial inflammation. Cytotoxic T lymphocyte–associated antigen 4 (CTLA4) is expressed on the surface of T cells within days after they have become activated. CTLA4 binds to and prevents CD80 and CD86 from binding to CD28, thereby effectively blocking the costimulatory signal required for activation of T cells. Blocking CD28 costimulation has been shown to induce T-cell anergy.

Abatacept (Orencia), an inhibitor of T-cell costimulation, is a fusion protein construct consisting of the extracellular component of CTLA4 fused to the Fc region of human IgG, which increases its half-life. The high affinity of CTLA4-Ig for CD28 prevents B7-mediated costimulation. Abatacept has improved signs and symptoms of disease, helped to maintain physical function, and reduced progression of joint damage in patients with active disease despite concomitant methotrexate. Similarly, it improved signs and symptoms, physical function, and health-related quality of life in RA patients refractory to TNF-α inhibition.

Biologic agents have different mechanisms, methods of delivery, and side effects. A patient who does not respond to or cannot tolerate one may still have a good outcome with another. Although they are commonly used in combination with methotrexate, biologic agents usually are not given in combination with each other, because this approach may increase risk without much increase in benefit. Because biologic agents modulate part of the immune response, there is concern about potential side effects related to impaired immune function, such as increased risk of minor and serious infections and secondary malignancies.

Biologic agents require parenteral administration: subcutaneous injections (e.g., etanercept, adalimumab, anakinra) or intravenous infusions (e.g., infliximab, abatacept, rituximab). These routes are less convenient than orally administered drugs and can be associated with administration reactions, such as injection-site or infusion reactions. Biologic agents are also more expensive than traditional DMARDs, which has affected their use. However, the increased clinical benefit seen with these agents needs to be considered in any comprehensive cost-efficacy analysis.

Conclusions

RA is a prevalent disease and a leading cause of physical disability. There is no cure for RA. However, with available agents applied appropriately, clinical remission is the goal of therapy and is a realistic expectation for some patients. When remission is not achieved, the rheumatologist must look for the most effective combination of therapies to alleviate pain, maintain function, and maximize quality of life. Methotrexate is still the mainstay of long-term care, but newer biologic DMARDs provide additional benefits. The role of biologic agents is still evolving. Their use is often reserved for patients who fail to respond to methotrexate, but the trend is toward earlier use of these agents. NSAIDs and glucocorticoids are useful for bridge therapy in patients with acute symptoms, especially while waiting for DMARDs to reach their maximal effect. Patients should be evaluated periodically for evidence of disease activity and progression and for drug toxicity. The management strategy should be changed if there is progressive joint damage, evidence of ongoing activity after 3 months of maximal treatment, or if treatment is poorly tolerated.

REFERENCES

American College of Rheumatology Subcommittee on Rheumatoid Arthritis Guidelines. Guidelines for the management of rheumatoid arthritis: 2002 update. Arthritis Rheum 2002;46:328–46.

Arnett FC, Edworthy SM, Bloch DA, et al. The American Rheumatism Association 1987 revised criteria for the classification of rheumatoid arthritis. Arthritis Rheum 1988;31:315–24.

Chang J, Kavanaugh A. Novel therapies for rheumatoid arthritis. Pathophysiology 2005;12:217–25.

Doan QV, Chiou CF, Dubois RW. Review of eight pharmacoeconomic studies of the value of biologic DMARDs (adalimumab, etanercept, and infliximab) in the management of rheumatoid arthritis. J Manag Care Pharm 2006;12:555–69.

Felson DT, Anderson JJ, Boers M, et al. for the American College of Rheumatology: Preliminary definition of improvement in rheumatoid arthritis. Arthritis Rheum 1995;38:727–35.

Olsen NJ, Stein M. New drugs for rheumatoid arthritis. N Engl J Med. 2004;350:2167–79.

Scott D, Kingsley G. Biologics in Rheumatoid Arthritis. Inflammatory Arthritis in Clinical Practice. London: Springer; 2007.

Juvenile Idiopathic Arthritis

Method of
Terry L. Moore, MD

Juvenile rheumatoid arthritis (JRA), now mainly known by the International League of Associations of Rheumatologists (ILAR) classification as juvenile idiopathic arthritis (JIA), is a protean disorder whose variable modes of onset and patterns of disease course are accompanied by a myriad of diverse signs, symptoms, and manifestations. JIA affects approximately 250,000 children in the United States. No distinct race predilection is noted at this time. It is the most common disease cause of children missing school in the United States. It is also the second leading cause of eye pathology in children. JIA presents a difficult diagnostic problem because of its lack of specific serologic abnormalities. This represents a dual problem to a clinician in that it makes it difficult to establish an early diagnosis of JIA when the clinical picture is not clear, and even after the diagnosis is established, it is difficult to know when the disease has remitted or an exacerbation is beginning. The

CURRENT DIAGNOSIS

- Diagnose early and treat aggressively.
- Reduce inflammation and symptoms.
- Suppress joint activity and reduce erosions to prevent disability.
- Establish a team approach with pediatric rheumatologist, ophthalmologist, physical therapist, and occupational therapist.

diagnosis of JIA is usually made clinically. Serologic studies can be informative, but in the past no routine laboratory tests have been diagnostic.

Diagnostic criteria for JIA include children younger than 16 years with persistent arthritis of one or more joints for at least 6 weeks. Arthritis is defined as swelling of a joint or limitation of motion with heat, pain, and tenderness.

JIA Subtypes

These are the seven basic subgroups or categories of JIA:

1. *Polyarthritis (RF positive)*: 19S IgM rheumatoid factors (RF) are present in the peripheral blood on testing and usually anticyclic citrullinated peptide antibodies (αCCP Ab). This group is manifested by arthritis in five or more joints in the first 6 months of disease. The joints most commonly affected are peripheral joints, including the knees, ankles, wrists, and fingers, but all synovial joints can become involved. There may also be an associated tendonitis. The classical joints involved are predominantly the metacarpophalangeal (MCP) and proximal phalangeal (PIP) joints producing fusiform-shaped swelling of the fingers. The knees are usually the first joints to limit function. They may exhibit deformity and flexion contractures. Polyarthritis (RF positive) is seen in approximately 5% to 10% of the children with JIA. The incidence of this type increases with age with the highest incidence found in adolescent females. The disease course in these children is generally believed to be one of a lifelong constantly active, or recurrent, relapsing pattern. It is associated with subcutaneous nodules and a higher incidence of vasculitis than the other forms of JIA. Radiograph films may show erosions with greater frequency than other forms of arthritis in children and may be helpful in diagnosis. Antinuclear antibodies (ANA) are present in approximately 80%.

2. *Polyarthritis (RF negative)*: This group by definition also has arthritis in five or more joints involved during the first 6 months; however, RF testing is negative, but αCCP Ab may be present. The disease pattern is similar to that of the RF-positive polyarthritis group. The course of these patients may be long term; however, most improve over a period of time. This type of onset occurs in approximately 20% to 30% of children with JIA. This type also shows female predominance.

3. a. *Oligoarthritis (pauciarthritis) with iridocyclitis* (inflammation of the iris and ciliary body in the posterior uveal tract of the eye): Oligoarthritis is manifested by arthritis of one or more joints involved in the first 6 months, but less than five joints. This type of onset is seen in approximately 50% of children with JIA and again shows female predominance. The most common children presenting are younger than 4 years at onset and have ANA present on testing. The ANA positivity is found in approximately 90% of the children developing chronic iridocyclitis. This group has a very good prognosis with little residual joint damage. There may be occasional asymmetric growth and leg length differences that develop; however, the process usually produces no long-term abnormalities. Approximately 50% of these children develop some type of iridocyclitis. Most children with iridocyclitis are easily controlled with anti-inflammatories such as naproxen, local steroid drops, or mydriatics (dilators). Therefore, any child being considered for a diagnosis of JIA requires frequent slit-lamp examinations by an ophthalmologist. b. *Extended oligoarthritis*: This type has an oligoarticular onset and then becomes more widespread, developing polyarthritis with five or more joints involved after the first 6 months of disease.

4. *Enthesitis related*: This category is predominantly seen in males who may later develop sacroiliitis and ankylosing spondylitis. This type of onset is associated with an enthesitis such as Achilles tendonitis or arthritis of the lower extremities again involving fewer than five joints in the first 6 months. The large joints, such as knees, ankles, hips, and sacroiliac joints, are usually involved. Anterior uveitis may be associated. The onset type is predominantly male, usually from 8 to 14 years of age, and may progress on to true ankylosing spondylitis. It is seen in approximately 10% to 15% of children with JIA. There is a high incidence of

familial predisposition in these patients with an 80% to 95% occurrence of the HLA-B27 antigen found. Sacroiliitis is often present on radiographs before symptoms develop and precedes the development of real limitation of motion of the spine.

5. *Systemic arthritis*: Initially seen with daily temperatures rises usually late afternoon from normal to exceeding 39°C (103°F) in an intermittent, spiking pattern. This usually occurs for more than 2 weeks. The onset of this type may include a salmon-colored, transient skin rash, lymphadenopathy, splenomegaly, hepatomegaly, pleuritis, pericarditis, or abdominal pain. It is seen in approximately 20% of children with JIA. RF, αCCP Ab, and ANA are usually negative, but white blood cell counts may exceed 30 to 40,000/mm[3]. Erythrocyte sedimentation rate (ESR) and C-reactive protein (CRP) are elevated and anemia may rapidly develop. This group also shows a male predominance. Approximately 50% of children develop an oligoarticular pattern and remit quickly, but many of the children go on to develop a long-term symmetric polyarthritis. This type of onset causes the most consternation in the diagnosis because it may mimic severe localized infections, sepsis, or neoplasms, such as lymphomas or leukemias.

6. *Psoriatic arthritis*: Arthritis and psoriasis or dactylitis with nail pitting and onycholysis. Usually there is a first-degree relative with a psoriasis. RF is negative.

7. *Other arthritis*: Children with arthritis of unknown cause that persists for at least 6 weeks and does not fulfill criteria for any of the other categories or fulfills criteria for more than one of the other categories.

JIA Evaluation

The workup on a JIA patient includes a complete blood count (CBC) that may show an anemia, leukocytosis, and thrombocytosis in systemic onset. ESR and CRP are quite high in systemic and polyarticular disease but may be minimally elevated or normal in oligoarticular disease. RF is only positive in the late-onset polyarticular patients and αCCP Ab also mainly appears in this group but may be seen in a small number of RF-negative polyarticular and oligoarticular patients. ANA are found in the polyarticular group and also in the oligoarticular group, associated with the presence of iridocyclitis. Other immunologic testing and liver, muscle, and kidney function tests should be in the normal range. Radiographs should be performed of involved joints looking for periarticular demineralization, joint space narrowing, and/or erosions.

JIA Prognosis

The course and outcome of JIA is generally good, however, the disease needs to be treated early and aggressively to prevent asymmetrical skeletal development, osteopenia, chronic eye disease, or systemic manifestations. Approximately 75% of the children do well long term, with the oligoarticular group rarely having any residual damage. Approximately 25%, usually found in the polyarthritis and systemic groups, develop continuous arthritis with some long-term disability.

JIA Therapy

The therapy of JIA begins with the use of physical and occupational therapy (PT/OT). The object of PT is to strengthen muscles, improve range of motion, and decrease the impact loading on the joints. The object of OT is to improve body mechanics, posture, and other modalities to decrease any kind of impact loading on the joints. Medical therapy begins with the judicious use of nonsteroidal anti-inflammatory drugs (NSAIDs). Oligoarthritis patients are usually placed on a NSAID, usually naproxen (Naprosyn), at a dosage of

[3]Exceeds dosage recommended by the manufacturer.

10 to 20 mg/kg in two divided doses. Naproxen has an advantage over other NSAIDs in that it comes in both a tablet and a liquid form at 125 mg/5 mL and has a long half-life so it can be given in two doses, which is more amenable to taking before and after school for compliance. The other nonsteroidal in tablet form generally used is tolmetin sodium (Tolectin) at a dosage of 20 to 30 mg/kg in three to four divided doses. One other medication, meloxicam (Mobic), comes in a tablet and a liquid form. It has an advantage of a long half-life and can be given once daily at dosages of 0.125 to 0.25 mg/kg. The liquid form is 7.5 mg/5 mL. Two other medications are approved for the use of children with JIA including aspirin (dosages of 80 to 120 mg/kg in four divided doses) and ibuprofen at 30 to 40 mg in three or four divided doses. A liquid preparation comes at 100 mg/5 mL. Other NSAIDs recently used in trials in JIA include nabumetone (Relafen),[1] at 30 mg/kg. This medication has an advantage in that it is only once a day and also can be used in a liquid form by crushing the tablet and dissolving in warm water. Other agents are occasionally used such as oxaprozin (Daypro), at 10 to 20 mg/kg in one to two doses; fenoprofen (Nalfon), at 40 to 50 mg/kg three to four times per day; diclofenac sodium (Voltaren), 20 to 40 mg/kg twice to three times per day; sulindac (Clinoril), 4 to 6 mg/kg in a twice daily dosage; or celecoxib (Celebrex), a cyclooxygenase-2 (COX-2) inhibitor, at 4 to 6 mg/kg in two doses. Laboratory studies including CBC, urinalysis, and comprehensive metabolic panel should be drawn every 4 months to monitor medication toxicity.

Children who have erosions on radiograph or show more aggressive disease at time of onset, usually those with polyarthritis, with systemic disease with polyarthritis, or with very aggressive oligoarticular disease, benefit greatly by combination therapy to reduce long-term disability. This means being aggressive with therapy in the first 2 years of disease. The first 2 years of disease are the period in which the most erosions and joint damage occurs. Combination therapy has become the standard of care of patients with JIA. The most common combination is the use of two or more of the disease-modifying antirheumatic agents (DMARDs), which include methotrexate (MTX), hydroxychloroquine (Plaquenil) [HCQ], or some of the new biologic preparations. MTX, a purine inhibitor, in dosages of 10 to 20 mg/m[2] once weekly along with folic acid at 400 µg to 1 mg daily is a very efficacious DMARD with little toxicity. MTX can be given orally or by intramuscular (IM) or subcutaneous (SC) injection. Orally, the liquid preparation at 25 mg/mL can be given in 0.1 mL/2.5 mg increments from 5 mg (0.2 mL) to 20 mg (0.8 mL) or in pill form of 2.5 mg tablets from 5 mg (2 tablets) to 20 mg (8 tablets) once per week. Dosages more than 20 mg should always be administered IM or SC. These children, however, do need to be monitored monthly to every 6 weeks with CBC, urinalysis, and liver and kidney function tests to monitor the medication toxicity. The combination of MTX and HCQ is the most common with the addition of HCQ in dosages of 6 mg/kg as an excellent adjunct

[1]Not FDA approved for this indication.

CURRENT THERAPY

- Anti-inflammatory agents (NSAIDs: naproxen [Naprosyn], ibuprofen [Advil], tolmetin [Tolectin], meloxicam [Mobic]) and intra-articular steroids for oligoarticular disease
- Disease-modifying agents (methotrexate [Rheumatrex], hydroxychloroquine [Plaquenil], sulfasalazine [Azulfidine], etc.) and/or biologics (etanercept, adalimumab, abatacept) for polyarticular and systemic disease

Abbreviation: NSAIDs = nonsteroidal anti-inflammatory drugs.

along with the NSAID. Eye exams every 6 months to monitor HCQ toxicity are indicated. MTX is also monitored once a year with a chest radiograph and also if any cough is present. The toxicities of these medications are relatively minimal in patients with JIA. Other DMARDs, although not approved by the FDA in children, are cyclosporine (Neoral)[1] at 2.5 to 3 mg/kg, intramuscular gold[1] at a dosage of 1 mg/kg weekly for 20 weeks, and sulfasalazine (Azulfidine) (SSZ) at doses of 50 mg/kg beginning at 500 mg per day and up to 2 g twice a day.[3] These are used with efficacy in JIA patients. Also, leflunomide (Arava),[1] a pyrimidine synthetase inhibitor, is effective in children. It also has liver toxicity, so it should be monitored like MTX. Abdominal complaints such as diarrhea are the most common side effects. The drug has a long half-life and potential teratogenicity, so it should be used with caution in females of childbearing age. Recently, the use of biologics or anticytokines in JIA has brought about a great deal of improvement in some of the patients. One medication is etanercept (Enbrel) at 0.4 mg/kg SC two times per week or 0.8 mg/kg SQ once per week. It has brought about marked improvement in many patients with long-standing polyarthritis. Efficacy has been sustained for up to 10 years now. This medication has caused marked decrease in joint swelling, tenderness, decreased sedimentation rate, and marked improvement in fatigue. The mechanism of action is that of blocking tumor necrosis factor (TNF), a cytokine that increases the inflammatory response in joints. Etanercept is produced to function like the p75 receptor for TNF. It binds to TNF and keeps it from binding to its own receptor and increasing the inflammatory response. It is well tolerated with the main side effect injection site reactions. TNF blockers can exacerbate an underlying tuberculosis infection, so before starting the medication a chest radiograph and purified protein derivative (PPD) skin test should be performed and then yearly while on the medication. Its counterpart, infliximab (Remicade), a chimeric monoclonal antibody to TNF, though not FDA approved, also is very efficacious in JIA. It is used as an intravenous (IV) preparation at 3 mg/kg given at baseline, 2 weeks, 6 weeks, and 8 eight weeks thereafter in an IV infusion over a 2-hour period. The dosage may be increased to 5 to 8 mg/kg and the interval shortened to every 4 to 6 weeks if needed. This agent markedly decreases the inflammatory response. It has mainly been used in older children with polyarticular disease. Recently, also now FDA approved, a fully humanized monoclonal antibody to TNF, adalimumab (Humira) is given at 20 mg SC every 2 weeks for children 15 to 20 kg and at 40 mg SC every 2 weeks for children greater than 30 kg. Also, studies are being run on the interleukin (IL)-1 receptor antagonist, anakinra (Kineret), in children. It is given daily at 1 to 2 mg/kg SC up to 100 mg SC per day. This medication shows a more favorable response in children with systemic-onset than with polyarticular or oligoarticular disease. A high number of children experience injection site reactions. Also, recently FDA approved for children is abatacept (Orencia), which blocks T-cells from proliferating and producing inflammatory cytokines. It is given as an IV infusion at 10 mg/kg on days 1, 15, and 30 and then monthly. Other biologic medications are in trials, including an IL-6 receptor antagonist (tocilizumab)[2] in systemic onset JIA, anti-B cell therapy (rituximab) (Rituxan), and an IL-1 trap medication (rilonacept).

Prednisone still may be used in severe systemic disease to control fever, rash, and/or other systemic manifestations in dosages of 1 to 2 mg/kg. The possibility of long-term side effects such as growth retardation, avascular necrosis, osteoporosis, weight gain, and acneiform lesions from steroids make their long-term use tentative in children. If disease is controlled, steroids should be tapered. Steroid eye drops may be used at times for severe iridocyclitis or orally in those patients with severe eye disease. Intra-articular (IA) steroids may be used in all onset-types if one or more joints are severely involved at one point in time. Local injections of 10 to 40 mg of triamcinolone hexacetonide may provide symptomatic relief in one specific joint.

In the long course of the disease, other immunosuppressives such as cyclophosphamide (Cytoxan), azathioprine (Imuran), and chlorambucil (Leukeran)[1] are used in certain cases of severe systemic or polyarthritis, but the use of these has waned with the new biologic medication.

The use of PT and OT is indicated at the first onset of disease. The child, after being evaluated, is sent to PT for instructions in the use of moist heat to the joints such as hot packs, the judicial use of rest, and two to three periods each day of passive or active assisted exercises performed by the patient or aided by the parent. Splints that protect joints may be prescribed to decrease the development of deformities. Splints can be made out of lightweight plastic that is molded while warm to fit the child in the desired position. The wrists and knees are the most amenable to splinting, but finger splints may hold the entire hand in slight dorsiflexion to decrease ulnar drift. If flexion contractures occur, splints can be used to hold the joint in maximum extension. The use of OT begins with the instructions for the patient in posture, body mechanics, improvement in activities of daily living, and instructions in joint protection. These instructions help the patient learn to protect and not increase the impact loading on the joints. Exercises are important in all stages of the care of the child with arthritis. During appearance of disease activity, excessive exercises exacerbate the inflammation. In these stages, passive range of motion exercise should maintain range of motion along with active assistive exercise. As joints improve and the inflammation is reduced, the exercise should be increased to a more active form. Resistive and strengthening exercises should be introduced along with isometric exercises to help provide muscle tone. Swimming or hydrotherapy or water aerobics for exercise may greatly aid in improving muscle strength. The use of regular cycling exercises may also be helpful. If the child has a lot of morning stiffness in the hands, the use of paraffin baths may be of great help, and the use of Theraputty to squeeze and improve muscle strength in the hands is indicated.

In conclusion, children with JIA should be diagnosed as soon as possible and treated aggressively. It is not a benign condition if left partially treated or untreated. Early treatment prevents further disease progression, maintains range of motion of the joints, and promotes normal growth and development. Combination therapy of NSAIDs, DMARDs, and/or biologics should be used early in those patients identified with aggressive disease. The team approach of the pediatric rheumatologist, ophthalmologist, and physical and occupational therapists will best benefit the JIA patient for a good long-term outcome.

REFERENCES

Cassidy JT, Petty RE. Chronic arthritis. In: Cassidy JT, Petty RE, editors. Textbook of Pediatric Rheumatology. WB Saunders: Philadelphia; 2005. p. 206–341.

Kietz DA, Pepmueller PH, Moore TL. Therapeutic use of etanercept in polyarticular course juvenile rheumatoid arthritis over a two-year period. Ann Rheum Dis 2002;61:171–3.

Lovell D, Giannini EH, Reiff A, et al. Etanercept in children with polyarticular juvenile rheumatoid arthritis. N Engl J Med 2000;342:763–9.

Low JM, Chauhan AK, Kietz DA, et al. Determination of anti-cyclic citrullinated peptide antibodies in sera of patients with juvenile idiopathic arthritis. J Rheumatol 2004;31:1829–833.

Moore TL. Immunopathogenesis of juvenile rheumatoid arthritis. Curr Opin Rheumatol 1999;11:377–83.

Petty JE, Southwood TR, Manners P, et al. International League of Associations for Rheumatology classification of juvenile idiopathic arthritis; Second revision, Edmonton, 2001. J Rheumatol 2004;31:390–2.

Syed RH, Gilliam BE, Moore TL. Rheumatoid factors and anticyclic citrullinated peptide antibodies in pediatric rheumatology. Curr Rheumatol Rep 2008;10:156–63.

Wallace CA, Huang B, Bandeira M, et al. Patterns of clinical remission in select categories of juvenile idiopathic arthritis. Arthritis Rheum 2005; 52:3554–62.

---

[1]Not FDA approved for this indication.
[2]Not available in the United States.
[3]Exceeds dosage recommended by the manufacturer.

---

[1]Not FDA approved for this indication.

Ankylosing Spondylitis

Method of
*Finbar D. O'Shea, MB, MRCPI, and
Robert D. Inman, MD*

Ankylosing spondylitis (AS) is a chronic inflammatory rheumatic disease characterized by inflammatory back pain due to sacroiliitis and spondylitis, restricted spinal mobility due to the formation of syndesmophytes, and often peripheral arthritis, enthesitis, and acute anterior uveitis (iritis). Symptoms commonly begin in late adolescence and early adulthood. With an estimated prevalence of 0.9% in northern European white populations, AS is a significant health burden to the community.

AS has long been a therapeutic challenge for the clinician. Exercise and nonsteroidal antiinflammatory drugs (NSAIDs) have been the mainstays of symptom control for decades, but there has until recently been a dearth of effective disease-modifying treatments. The advent of biological treatments (specifically anti–tumor necrosis factor [TNF] agents) is currently revolutionizing the management of AS.

AS belongs to a group of related diseases termed *spondyloarthropathies* (SpA), which also comprises conditions such as arthritis/spondylitis associated with psoriasis, arthritis/spondylitis associated with inflammatory bowel disease, reactive arthritis, and undifferentiated spondyloarthritis (uSpA). They share many clinical manifestations and an association with human leukocyte antigen (HLA)-B27. The SpA group as a whole is one of the most common rheumatic diseases, with a prevalence of up to 1.9%, and this makes them at least as common as rheumatoid arthritis. The most common subgroups of SpA are AS and uSpA. It appears that all SpA subsets can progress to full-blown AS.

Diagnosis

DIFFICULTIES AND DELAYS IN DIAGNOSIS

Among the inflammatory rheumatic diseases there is a long delay between the onset of symptoms and the time of diagnosis for AS; in several studies an average duration of about 7 years has been reported. The mean age at onset of symptoms is in the mid-20s, thus at the normally most productive time of life. If AS is undiagnosed and untreated, or not treated effectively, continuous pain, stiffness, and fatigue are the consequences. Furthermore, a potentially progressive loss of spinal mobility and function cause a reduction in the quality of life and an increase in direct and indirect medical costs.

There are two major reasons for the long delay in the diagnosis of AS. First, the established classification criteria for AS, which date back more than 20 years, rely on the combination of clinical symptoms plus unequivocal radiographic sacroiliitis of at least grade 2 bilaterally or grade 3 unilaterally (see Box 1 for the modified New York criteria for the diagnosis of AS). The radiographs are often normal when symptoms arise, and it usually takes several years for definite radiographic sacroiliitis to evolve. Second, there is no unique clinical symptom or laboratory test to make the diagnosis of AS; thus it is a huge challenge to attempt to identify the estimated 5% of patients with SpA (including AS) among the great number of patients with chronic low back pain seen by the primary care physician.

Efforts have been made to try to address these issues. MRI has been used successfully to detect the presence of spinal and sacroiliac inflammation in early disease. However, until MRI detection of sacroiliitis is shown to be sensitive and specific for early AS, and until the availability of MRI greatly improves, most clinicians are left with plain radiography as the diagnostic test.

CLINICAL FEATURES

Choosing clinical parameters for screening patients for underlying AS is attractive because their determination is not expensive. The clinical symptom of inflammatory back pain has been suggested as a cardinal symptom for AS for years, and assessment requires neither laboratory testing nor x-ray. It has been estimated that when symptoms of inflammatory back pain are present in a patient with chronic low back pain, the post-test probability for this patient of having axial SpA is 14%.

Recent refinement of these clinical features has identified a new set of criteria for inflammatory back pain. The new criteria consist of morning stiffness for longer than 30 minutes, improvement in back pain with exercise but not with rest, awakening because of back pain during the second one half of the night only, and alternating buttock pain. These features were defined by a study that sought to identify the most sensitive and specific combination of parameters for inflammatory back pain using a cohort of patients with an established diagnosis of AS. Fulfillment of at least two of these four parameters yielded a sensitivity of 70% and a specificity of 81%, with a

CURRENT DIAGNOSIS

- Screen all patients younger than 40 years who have back pain longer than 3 months for features of IBP. IBP features include:
  - Early morning stiffness longer than 30 min
  - Improved back pain with exercise, not rest
  - Nocturnal pain, especially the second half of the night
  - Alternating buttock pain
- Screen for history of psoriasis, inflammatory bowel disease, iritis and any family history of these conditions
- Search for restriction in spinal mobility
  - Forward flexion (Schober's test)
  - Lateral spinal flexion
  - Chest expansion
- AP pelvic x-ray if IBP suspected for presence or absence of sacroiliitis
- If conventional radiography is not diagnostic and clinical suspicion remains, consider MRI (STIR sequence required). MRI allows direct visualization of inflammation in the spine and sacroiliac joints before conventional radiography shows any abnormality.

Abbreviations: AP = anteroposterior; IBP = inflammatory back pain; MRI = magnetic resonance imaging; STIR = short T1 inversion recovery.

positive likelihood ratio of 3.7. If at least three of the four parameters were fulfilled, the positive likelihood ratio increased to 12.4. However, how these discriminating features perform in a large non-specific back pain population has yet to be examined.

Treatment

Until recently, the treatment options for AS were limited. Regular physiotherapy and treatment with NSAIDs were the only available options. Approximately one half of AS patients are adequately managed with this regimen. However, conventional disease-modifying antirheumatic drugs, which are effective in other chronic inflammatory diseases such as rheumatoid arthritis, have only a very limited effect on spinal inflammation. Local injections of corticosteroids can be used effectively if inflammation is confined to a small number of joints. Thus, although an early and accurate diagnosis has been recognized as important in these patients, this seemed less urgent for many physicians because of the lack of therapeutic options.

This treatment approach has now changed. NSAIDs should probably be taken more regularly once a diagnosis has been made. Tumor necrosis factor (TNF) blockers offer an exciting new possibility for effective treatment and possibly for arresting disease progression. It has been shown that the anti-TNF agents infliximab (Remicade), etanercept (Enbrel), adalimumab (Humira), and golimumab (Simponi) have a prompt and robust effect on almost all aspects of active disease—most notably pain and fatigue, but also function, spinal mobility, peripheral arthritis, enthesitis, bone density, and acute inflammation as reflected by acute-phase reactants and MRI. In studies using these compounds, a 50% improvement of the disease activity could be demonstrated in about one half of the treated patients whose disease had proved refractory to NSAIDs and physiotherapy. In 72% of patients with a disease duration of less than 10 years there was at least 50% improvement of the Bath AS Disease Activity Index (BASDAI), clearly higher than patients with a longer disease duration. This finding supports the essential need for early diagnosis.

Recent studies have shown a sustained response among AS patients with the anti-TNF agents superior even to that seen in rheumatoid arthritis. Short- to medium-term data show them to be well tolerated. On the basis of the MRI changes, it is believed that the anti-TNF agents will have a positive effect on long-term radiographic progression, however, this has yet to be proved.

Infliximab, adalimumab, and golimumab are monoclonal antibodies directed against the proinflammatory cytokine TNF-α. Etanercept is a fusion protein of the p75 TNF receptor linked to the Fc portion of an immunoglobulin (Ig) G1 molecule that binds and inactivates TNF-α. Inflixiamb is administered intravenously in three loading doses and then every 8 weeks at a dose of 3 to 5 mg/kg.

Etanercept is administered subcutaneously once weekly (50-mg injection). Adalimumab is administered subcutaneously every other week (40-mg injection). Golimumab is administered subcutaneously every 4 weeks (50-mg injection). All four agents appear to have similar efficacy and tolerability. The most serious potential side effect with any of these agents is infection, specifically tuberculosis (TB). This has been greatly minimized by screening for any evidence of latent TB infection with a chest x-ray and a TB skin (PPD) test before commencing these agents. The issue of altered rates of malignancies with these agents in AS has not been resolved and is being addressed with monitoring of biologics registries in several countries.

Prognosis and Long-Term Outcomes

AS is a chronic condition with no predictable pattern of progression, and the disease does not follow a single defined course. Although many outcomes are possible, findings from previous prospective studies suggest that a pattern of AS emerges within the first 10 years of disease. About 74% of patients who had mild spinal restriction after 10 years did not progress to severe spinal involvement. In contrast, 81% of patients who had severe spinal restriction had been severely restricted within the first 10 years. What differentiates the rapid progression group has not been completely resolved. Hip involvement has repeatedly been shown to be an indicator of more severe disease. Other predictors of a poor outcome include a raised erythrocyte sedimentation rate (ESR), poor response to NSAIDs and peripheral oligoarthritis. Cigarette smoking is associated with worse clinical, functional, and radiologic outcomes. Early age at onset has been recently shown to be associated with a worse prognosis.

Men are afflicted with AS approximately 2 to 3 times more often than women. The disease pattern also varies by sex. The spine and pelvis are more commonly affected in men. In contrast, women have less severe involvement of the spine and more symptoms in the knees, ankles, and hips. It has been shown that women have a later age at onset. It was previously believed that women also had milder disease than men, but this view has been questioned recently.

With the advent of new effective therapies for AS, it has become important to identify predictors of response to these agents. This is important because the anti-TNF agents are expensive for the health care system and have potential side effects for the patient. It has been shown that younger patients with shorter disease duration, raised acute phase markers, and a higher disease activity at initiation do better. However, it has also been shown that patients with long-standing disease and established radiographic changes can also respond to these agents, and these patients should be also afforded a trial if conventional treatments have proved inadequate.

REFERENCES

Davis JC, van der Jeijde DM, Braun J, et al. Sustained durability and tolerability of etanercept in ankylosing spondylitis for 96 weeks. Ann Rheum Dis 2005;64(11):1557–62.

Inman RD, Davis JC Jr, Heijde D, et al. Efficacy and safety of golimumab in patients with ankylosing spondylitis: Results of a randomized, double-blind, placebo-controlled, phase III trial. Arthritis Rheum 2008;58(11):3402–12.

Maksymowych WP, Landewe R. Imaging in ankylosing spondylitis. Best Pract Res Clin Rheumatol 2006;20(3):507–19.

Rudwaleit M, van der Heijde D, Khan MA, et al. How to diagnose axial spondyloarthritis early. Ann Rheum Dis 2004;63:535–43.

Rudwaleit M, Metter A, Listing J, et al. Inflammatory back pain in ankylosing spondylitis: A reassessment of the clinical history for application as classification and diagnostic criteria. Arthritis Rheum 2006;54(2):569–78.

Sieper J, Braun J, Rudwaleit M, et al. Ankylosing spondylitis: An overview. Ann Rheum Dis 2002;61(Suppl. 3):iii8–18.

Sieper J, Rudwaleit M. Early referral recommendations for ankylosing spondylitis (including pre-radiographic and radiographic forms) in primary care. Ann Rheum Dis 2005;64:659–63.

Sieper J, Rudwaleit M, Khan MA, Braun J. Concepts and epidemiology of spondyloarthritis. Best Pract Res Clin Rheumatol 2006;20(3):401–17.

CURRENT THERAPY

- Physical therapy and a regular stretching program are important in all AS patients.
- NSAIDs are first-line therapy.
- Use a second NSAID even if the first has not achieved control of symptoms.
- Consider local corticosteroid injection if few joints involved.
- Ongoing disease activity is best reflected by the Bath Ankylosing Spondylitis Disease Activity Index (BASDAI). If the patient scores at least 4 out of 10 despite a full trial of two NSAIDs, an anti-TNF agent should be considered.

Abbreviations: NSAID = nonsteroidal anti-inflammatory drug; TNF = tumor necrosis factor.

Stone M, Warren RW, Bruckel J, et al. Juvenile-onset ankylosing spondylitis is associated with worse functional outcomes than adult-onset ankylosing spondylitis. Arthritis Rheum 2005;53(3):445–51.

van der Heijde D, Dijkmans B, Geusens P, et al. Efficacy and safety of infliximab in patients with ankylosing spondylitis: Results of a randomized, placebo-controlled trial (ASSERT). Arthritis Rheum 2005;52(2):582–91.

van der Heijde D, Kivitz A, Schiff MH, et al. Efficacy and safety of adalimumab in patients with ankylosing spondylitis: Results of a multicenter, randomized, double-blind, placebo-controlled trial. Arthritis Rheum 2006;54 (7):2136–46.

van der Linden S, Valkenburg HA, Cats A. Evaluation of diagnostic criteria for ankylosing spondylitis: A proposal for modification of the New York criteria. Arthritis Rheum 1984;27(4):361–8.

Zochling J, van der Heijde D, Burgos-Vargas R, et al. ASAS/EULAR recommendations for the management of ankylosing spondylitis. Ann Rheum Dis 2006;65:442–52.

Temporomandibular Disorders and Orofacial Pain

Method of

Richard Ohrbach, DDS, PhD, and Jeffrey Burgess, DDS, MSD

Temporomandibular disorder (TMD) and orofacial pain include pain in the oral, facial, or head regions. TMD is a collection of conditions that affect the muscles of mastication, the temporomandibular joint (TMJ), or both. The primary symptom is pain localized most often in the muscles of mastication or the preauricular area. Associated pain symptoms can involve the ear or cervical area and often include headache. The other major symptoms include limitation in jaw functioning (e.g., restriction in range of motion, difficulty with mastication) or noises or altered functioning in the TMJ.

In contrast, orofacial pain disorders are *not* typically associated with alterations in mandibular function but extend diagnostically across the disciplines of neurology, otolaryngology, psychiatry, and dentistry. The pain complaint is primarily located within the orofacial area, but the distribution (as well as underlying pathology) can extend beyond the orofacial area in either a caudal or cephalad direction. Contrasting TMDs and orofacial pain disorders, diagnostic distinctions are generally clear given a careful history. Many of the orofacial pain disorders represent diagnostic red flags for the TMDs.

Epidemiology

TMDs are relatively common; estimated U.S. prevalences are about 12% for TMD-related pain (6 months' duration) and about 8% for a diagnosed TMD requiring treatment. Any of the three major characteristics of a TMD (pain, limitation in motion, joint noise) occur in 5% to 50% of the population, and treatment-seeking appears to be primarily related to pain severity and limited jaw functioning. The modal patient is 18 to 45 years old, and the prevalence is much lower for late adolescents, the middle-aged, and elderly; women present for treatment 4 to 7 times more often than men, whereas the population gender prevalence is only 2:1. Emerging evidence suggests that genetic sensitivity for pain is a primary risk factor for TMD, and hormonal factors might account for the gender disparity, although an explanatory mechanism remains absent.

The orofacial pain conditions, excluding toothache and sinusitis, are much less common. Orofacial pain manifesting as facial migraine variants is probably less common than migraine headache but are also probably underdiagnosed.

Clinical Features and Diagnosis

Psychosocial factors are central in the diagnosis and treatment for the TMDs and are presumed to also play a role in the treatment of orofacial pain disorders when they have become chronic (i.e., at least 3–6 months in duration) or refractory to initial treatment. Thus, a dual-axis approach including biomedical and biobehavioral aspects is standard.

BIOMEDICAL EVALUATION

History

The pain history includes assessment of pain location, referral patterns, quality (e.g., ache, throb, burning, electrical), duration (e.g., brief, hours, days, months), temporal (e.g., intermittent, paroxysmal, recurrent, constant), patterning (e.g., morning, evening, during sleep), modifying factors (e.g., cold, chewing, head or body movement), and associated symptoms (e.g., dysesthesia, photophobia, phonophobia). A pain description that appears atypical should not be discounted but approached carefully because it can reflect multiple diagnoses or etiologies: central (e.g., intracranial), nonfacial (e.g., cardiac, oncologic, neck), or biobehavioral etiology.

A past or present history of TMJ noises such as clicking, popping, or crepitus may be important. A distinct click or pop occurring in the TMJ might suggest internal derangement of the disk, but nonpainful TMJ noise is considered to be benign, self-limited, and not needing intervention. In contrast, significant TMJ dysfunction involves intermittent or persistent locking for longer than 24 hours. Crepitus suggests degenerative disease. A history of intermittent joint noise (click or pop) followed by sudden opening limitation, pain, absence of noise, and severe opening deviation suggest nonreducing disk displacement and can be treated acutely. Chronic nonreducing disk displacement, ruled out by magnetic resonance imaging (MRI), might or might not be symptomatic and is significant only if opening continues to be limited.

Orofacial trauma involving jaw fracture is typically associated with acute malocclusion and severe pain at the fracture site; it might also be associated with limited jaw opening and lateral movement, and the patient may be able to partially occlude the teeth. TMJ intracapsular injury is more complex, if not controversial, and assessment of function takes priority. Complaint of progressive change in the bite, such as an opening between the posterior or anterior teeth, can indicate the presence of significant joint (e.g., rheumatoid or degenerative) or endocrine (e.g., acromegaly) disease. A perceived malocclusion (in the absence of objective evidence of such) coupled with facial or head pain suggests the presence of a myofascial or dysesthesia condition.

Physical Examination

Physical examination includes vital signs, general inspection of the head, and otologic and cranial nerve examination. Palpation of the neck, including the musculature, is also recommended because pain can be referred from this region to the cranium. Lack of published

---

   CURRENT DIAGNOSIS

- Primary symptoms of TMD are pain localized to the face and temple area coupled with some limitation in mandibular function; the clinical examination confirms limitation of mobility, interference in function, and regional pain from movement or palpation.
- Pain history supports the diagnosis of orofacial pain disorders, and examination is used to rule out other possible diagnoses.
- For these primarily pain disorders, biobehavioral factors are also assessed.

criteria for performing neck muscle palpation can limit its reliability and validity, and results should be interpreted cautiously, particularly in the absence of accompanying history. It is generally accepted that if pain in the head is being caused by the neck musculature, repeated palpation of identified trigger points should reproduce the phenomena. Neurophysiologic linkage between masticatory and cervical muscles during function can support a causal relationship between regional pain disorders; referred pain can also produce overlap.

A standardized examination (e.g., Research Diagnostic Criteria, RDC/TMD) has become the norm for TMD assessment, in part to prevent overdiagnosis. Although initially intended as a more reliable research instrument, the RDC is also time efficient in the clinical setting. Jaw opening is reliably measured with a millimeter ruler, and less than 35 mm is generally considered limited for both male and female patients. Jaw opening is evaluated for deviation and for disk movement by the application of light pressure over the TMJs. A stethoscope is probably more reliable for detection of crepitus. For palpation, 2 pounds of pressure to the primary extraoral masticatory muscles and 1 pound to the TMJs and the intraoral muscles appear to have appropriate sensitivity and specificity. The teeth, mucosa, and posterior pharynx should always be evaluated. Excessive tooth wear indicates past or present parafunctional behavior. Although TMD is not generally associated with malocclusion, malocclusion may be significant in certain circumstances.

Panography is sufficient for initial screening of maxillomandibular pathology and may be the only imaging necessary for most patients. CT is useful for confirming the diagnosis and extent of disease with suspected developmental abnormalities, neoplasm, trauma or fracture, sinus pathology, degenerative disease, chronic infection (e.g., osteomyelitis), and TMJ ankylosis. MRI of the TMJs should be ordered when jaw locking does not respond to initial treatments. SPECT, although not specific, can be helpful with suspected inflammatory disorders. Orofacial pain problems, depending on history and examination findings, often warrant greater use of regional imaging and laboratory and serologic assessment.

BIOBEHAVIORAL EVALUATION

Chronic TMD is similar to other chronic pain conditions such as headache and back pain with respect to psychophysiologic mechanisms, coping, behavioral manifestations, and impact. In contrast, these aspects can require less consideration in diagnosis and management of acute TMDs. Orofacial pain problems appear to be independent of these processes with respect to diagnosis, but they can become relevant in treatment when the orofacial pain disorder has become more persistent or refractory.

TMD characteristics shared with other chronic musculoskeletal pain disorders include poor correspondence between subjective complaints of pain and suffering versus the identifiable pathophysiology; impact of psychosocial stress in effecting nonfunctional increases in muscle activity; more frequent distress and greater difficulty in coping, which may be either a premorbid style or emerging from the chronic pain; greater prevalence of clinically diagnosable depression, anxiety, or somatization, the latter referring to the reporting of multiple somatic problems simultaneous with significant life disarray; disruption in usual performance at home, work, or school; and frequent health care visits, previous treatment successes now no longer effective, medication abuse, pursuing treatments that are exclusively somatic, and avoiding biobehavioral treatments. These similarities suggest that the following four domains be evaluated as potential yellow flags (summarized in Box 1).

Subjective Aspects of the Condition

The *pain complaint* should be evaluated for its relationship to relevant anatomy and physiology, which factors (physical, psychosocial) alter it, and what activities have been altered due to it. *Treatment history* should be evaluated with respect to which types of treatments were successful or unsuccessful, whether there was a preponderance or avoidance of any particular type (e.g., medications, behavioral treatment), whether there was premature abandonment of a treatment, and what factors were involved with resuming treatment when

---

BOX 1 Diagnostic Yellow Flags for Temporomandibular Disorder and Chronic Orofacial Pain

Subjective

Pain complaint: Anatomic correlates, whether altered by physical or psychosocial factors, and behavioral consequences.

Treatment history: Types of treatment previously effective or not, adherence, triggers for treatment cycles

Illness explanatory model: Symptom origin and meaning, expected outcome of physical or psychological treatments

Receptiveness to psychological referral

Behavior

Oral parafunctional behavior
Covariance of symptoms with other behavior

Psychological Status

Depression and anxiety
Somatization and somatoform disorders
Spectrum of nonspecific physical symptoms

Psychosocial Status

Activities of daily living
Mastication and speech
Social interaction
Intimate behavior

---

prior treatment-seeking was intermittent. The patient's *explanatory model* should be explored regarding the origin of the problem, the meaning of the symptoms, and the role of physical versus psychological treatments, with respect to etiology, maintenance, and exacerbation of the problem.

Referral for biobehavioral treatment should be considered at the outset rather than waiting until all physical diagnostic or therapeutic approaches have been tried and *then* referring the patient to a psychologist or psychiatrist. That latter approach to intervention gives the implicit message that the pain was initially real but, with the failure of treatment, has become imaginary. A patient with a rigid explanation that the problem is completely of physical origin is often highly reluctant, perhaps even resistant, to consider a biobehavioral perspective, and such patients have been reinforced to hold such views by repeated evaluations that are somatically focused and that exclude the biobehavioral domain.

Behavior

Oral parafunctional behavior during the waking state often indicates response to psychosocial stress. Psychosocial stress can also affect the related cervical muscles and contribute to the pain. Other potentially important behaviors, such as whether changes in pain are associated with specific home or work situations, are often best assessed via a self-report diary containing columns for the desired information coupled with specific instructions and follow-up by the physician. For example, a patient who reports no linkage of symptomatology to daily events (especially when the pain is daily and purportedly unchanging) might, after maintaining a diary for a week, report a very different symptom picture.

Psychological Status

Psychological status includes depression, anxiety, and somatization. These can be assessed through a standard clinical interview or standardized questionnaires such as the Symptom Checklist (SCL)-90R. Other measures can be used for depression and anxiety, but the SCL-90R is perhaps the best current tool for assessing the continuum underlying nonspecific physical symptoms. All TMD patients should receive the same screening evaluation in order to more consistently identify changes in psychological status that often escape detection by clinical interview.

The question is the extent and manner in which changes in psychological status manifest in this particular patient and contribute to the pain-related suffering, and whether to refer the patient for more specialized evaluations through referral to either a clinical psychologist or psychiatrist who specializes in chronic pain. Depression is common in the TMD population, is often comorbid with elevated anxiety, and responds to treatment (either pharmacologic or behavioral), which often alters the reported pain as well.

Somatization as a formal disorder is rare, but as a continuum it is present surprisingly often, and when present it can significantly influence treatment outcome and increase doctor shopping and treatment-seeking behaviors.

Psychosocial Status

Interference in psychosocial function (activities of daily living, mastication and speech, social interaction, oral intimate behavior) and increased health care use lead to a worse prognosis.

DIAGNOSTIC INTEGRATION

For the TMDs, a dual-axis system—the physical diagnosis and the biobehavioral implications for treatment—has been used for 20 years. The dual-axis system is probably applicable to orofacial pain disorders. One common practice is to escalate diagnostic testing for the physical disorder without equal consideration of the biobehavioral domain; both areas should be investigated equally from the outset.

TEMPOROMANDIBULAR DISORDERS

The most common TMDs are described in Box 2. Not included in this box are some potential disorders not yet well described in the literature and without clear inclusion criteria: muscle contracture, spasm, splinting, inflammatory disease (synovitis), and ligamentous injury (perforation, tearing).

OROFACIAL PAIN DISORDERS

Orofacial pain differential diagnosis is confounded by the anatomic complexity and potential for noncranial referral. In patients with chronic orofacial pain, the diagnosis may be further complicated by multiple overlapping diagnoses and emergence of biobehavioral factors.

Facial pain conditions are presented in Table 1. Of the many intracranial problems causing facial pain, cerebellar pontine angle meningioma (versus neuralgia or pulpal pathology) should be considered when there is paroxysmal pain plus patient description of dysesthesia (i.e., tingling or numbness) confirmed by cranial nerve examination. Other conditions associated with neuralgia-like pain include cranial tumor (e.g., epidermoid, metastatic, brainstem glioma), acoustic neuroma, nasopharyngeal carcinoma, vascular lesions (e.g., arteriovenous malformation), scleroderma, and Paget's disease. Neuralgia-like pain can also follow orthognathic and third molar surgery in a small number of cases.

Neurovascular problems presenting diagnostic difficulty include the atypical migraine variants, paroxysmal hemicrania, cluster-tic syndromes, temporal arteritis, carotodynia, and chronic cluster where pain may be perceived in the mid-face, cheek, or temple. The epidemiology, precipitating factors, and associated symptoms assist in differentiating between these conditions. For example, patients with nonchronic cluster are typically men ages 18 to 40 years, and ipsilateral nasal discharge, lacrimation, conjunctival injection, and facial flushing occurs with pain. Patients with temporal arteritis, in contrast, are typically older men or women who report pain and feeling ill, and the pain location and scalp hyperpathia in conjunction with muscle palpation tenderness could be misdiagnosed as a TMD.

Atypical neurogenic conditions including neuralgias and deafferentation syndromes can be confused with pain of odontogenic or intracranial etiology. Orofacial pain associated with TMD must be

---

BOX 2   Temporomandibular Disorders: Diagnostic Criteria

Group I: Muscle Disorders

Myofascial pain (pain in the muscles of mastication)
Pain or ache at rest or during function in the jaw, temples, face, preauricular area, inside the ear, *plus*
Palpation pain in at least three of 20 muscle sites
- Posterior, middle, anterior temporalis
- Origin, body, insertion of masseter
- Stylohyoid, digastric, lateral pterygoid, temporalis tendon)
Palpation pain must be at least present on the side of pain complaint

Group II: Disk Displacements

Disk displacement with reduction
- Reciprocal clicking in the TMJ
  - Click on both opening and closing or a click on either opening or closing
  - Click during lateral or protrusive excursions
Disk displacement without reduction, with limited opening
- Report of significant limitation of mandibular opening *plus*
- Maximum unassisted opening ≤35 mm *plus*
- Passive stretch increases opening 4 mm or less beyond unassisted opening *plus*
- Contralateral excursion <7 mm and/or uncorrected deviation to the ipsilateral side on opening *plus*
- Absence of joint sounds, or presence of joint sounds not meeting criteria for disk displacement with reduction
Disk displacement without reduction, without limited opening
- Report of significant limitation of mandibular opening *plus*
- Maximal unassisted opening >35 mm *plus*
- Passive stretch increases opening at least 5 mm *plus*
- Contralateral excursion ≥7 mm *plus*
- Presence of joint sounds not meeting criteria for disk displacement with reduction *plus*
- If joint imaging is requested, it should image the disk in closed and open mouth positions with arthrography or MRI

Group III: Arthralgia, Arthritis, Arthrosis

Arthralgia (pain in the joint)
- Pain in one or both joint sites during palpation *plus*
- One or more self-reports of pain in the region of the joint, pain in the joint during maximum unassisted or assisted opening, or lateral excursions *plus*
- Absence of coarse crepitus
Osteoarthritis of the TMJ (inflammatory changes in the joint)
- Arthralgia (see-above) *plus*
- Coarse crepitus in the joint or joint imaging showing erosions, sclerosis of condylar head or articular eminence, or flattening of the joint surfaces
Osteoarthrosis of the TMJ (remodeling of the articulating surfaces)
- Absence of arthralgia *plus*
- Coarse crepitus or joint imaging showing joint changes

Data from Dworkin SF, LeResche L. Research diagnostic criteria for temporomandibular disorders: Review, criteria, examinations and specifications, critique. J Craniomandib Disord 1992;6:301–355.

TABLE 1 Orofacial Pain Disorders: Characteristics and Differential Diagnosis

Condition	Pathognomonic Pain Characteristics	Pathognomonic Nonpain Characteristics	Differential Diagnosis
Intracranial			
Aneurysm	Throbbing with rapid increase in severity worsened with exertion	Neurologic signs, gastrointestinal upset	Odontogenic pathology, TMD, sinus disease, Tolosa–Hunt syndrome, migraine
Cerebellar pontine angle tumor	Constant ache exacerbated by head movement or coughing, neuralgia-like pain	Dysesthesia, paresthesia	Trigeminal neuralgia, odontogenic pathology
Neurovascular (Throbbing, Midface or Temporal)			
Migraine variant*	Pain intensity exacerbated by physical activity or triggered by stress or alcohol	Autonomic dysfunction, somatosensory hyperesthesia	Common migraine, Chiari malformation, Tolosa–Hunt syndrome, Raeder's syndrome
Chronic paroxysmal hemicrania	3- to 5-min paroxysms, 5–20 episodes/day, pain-free intervals between paroxysms; no known trigger. Unremitting form: daily at least for 1 y. Remitting form: daily for days to months, with remissions and recrudescence	Responsive to indomethacin (Indocin)	Cluster headache, neuralgia, sinusitis, odontogenic pain
Cluster headache†	Burning or sharp, unilateral, eye region	Nocturnal episodes, Horner's facial flushing, tearing, conjunctival injection	Atypical cluster, cluster-tic syndrome,† sinusitis, odontogenic pain, atypical migraine, chronic paroxysmal hemicrania (remitted form)†
Atypical cluster headache†	Throbbing, bilateral, not eye region	Not nocturnal, infrequent ocular or nasal signs	Same as cluster; chronic paroxysmal hemicrania (unremitted form)†
Temporal arteritis	Burning, associated claudication	Scalp allodynia, hyperesthesia, pain in maxillary teeth, positive sedimentation rate	Migraine, sinusitis, odontogenic pain, TMD
Neurogenic			
Neuralgia (trigeminal, glossopharyngeal)	Stabbing or electrical quality, paroxysms triggered by trivial sensation in associated distribution, duration of seconds with complete remission between episodes	Absence of sensory or reflex deficit by neurologic testing	Tumor (epidermoid, metastatic), brainstem glioma, acoustic neuroma, nasopharyngeal carcinoma, vascular lesion, CT disease, Paget's disease, syphilis, toxins, MS
Postherpetic	Distribution of V3, burning/ache with allodynia (cold), dysesthesia	Preceded by vesicular disease	Odontogenic pain, post trauma, jaw surgery
Other			
Odontogenic pathology (pain in jaw, teeth, midface)	Pain with chewing, intraoral hot or cold	Caries, exposed cementum or dentin, mucosal swelling, acute malocclusion	Neurogenic, neurovascular pain, TMD, sinusitis
Stylohyoid process syndrome†	Deep throbbing pain (mandible or throat region) evoked by swallowing or head turning or by palpation of stylohyoid ligament or carotid trunk	Dizziness	TMD, glossopharyngeal neuralgia, carotid arteritis, tonsillitis, parotitis, osteomyelitis
Salivary disease (pain in cheek, inferior mandible)	Pain with introduction of food or drink, sour taste	Associated swelling in region of gland with resolution and recrudescence	TMD, odontogenic pathology
Sinus pathology (pain in midface)	Constant or intermittent ache aggravated by postural change involving head movement; maxillary tooth pain	Facial flushing, positive imaging	Migraine variants, odontogenic pathology

TMD |

*Classic and common migraine should also be considered in the differential when TMD or craniofacial pain is located in or refers to the temporal region.
†Per taxonomy from the International Association for the Study of Pain, 2nd edition.
MS = multiple sclerosis; TMD = temporomandibular disorder.

differentiated from tension headache; the migraine variants; odontogenic pain caused by pulpal or periapical pathology (abscess); neurovascular or inflammatory headache with facial involvement; lesions of the parotid, ear, nose, and pharynx; and pain referred from the cervical musculature. A TMD diagnosis does not rule out non-TMD pain conditions. With traumatic injury, the differential diagnosis must contend with overlapping of multiple conditions causing pain.

Treatment

BIOMEDICAL TREATMENT

The management of TMD varies depending on the pain history and presence of biobehavioral factors but generally consists of treatments used in managing other musculoskeletal conditions as listed in Box 3. Normally, TMD is self-limited and symptoms can be effectively

---

BOX 3   Initial Symptomatic Treatment for Temporomandibular Disorder

Jaw rest and pain-free chewing for 14 days
Nonsteroidal antiinflammatory drugs at clinical dosage for 7–14 days
Cyclobenzaprine (Flexeril), 5–10 mg hs, or diazepam (Valium) 5 mg hs, for 7–14 days
Monitor red flags (see Table 1)
Monitor yellow flags (see Box 1)
Monitor symptom response at 2–4 weeks and determine whether other diagnostic tests or biobehavioral factors warrant further investigation
Refer to appropriate specialist if symptoms are not responding appropriately

---

reduced with assurance, accurate information regarding the disease and prognosis, instructions regarding behavior modification, and short-term use of medications. If parafunctional behavior such as nail biting, daytime tooth clenching, gum chewing, or habitual jaw popping are identified, they should be managed. Because habitual behavior is often stress related, the environmental factors that initiate or perpetuate the activity should be explored.

Pharmacologic management includes use of analgesics, nonsteroidal antiinflammatory drugs (NSAIDs), anxiolytics, muscle relaxants, and occasionally corticosteroids. Antidepressants, specifically the tertiary tricyclics (e.g., amitriptyline (Elavil)[1], nortriptyline (Pamelor)[1]), are especially useful for TMD because in addition to analgesic activity, they improve sleep and can suppress sleep bruxism; dosages are typically in the range of 10 to 25 mg at bedtime. In contrast, the SSRI antidepressants have been linked to increased sleep bruxism and could aggravate TMD unless combined with sleep medication.

Narcotic analgesics are discouraged in cases other than trauma because other approaches are generally available, but aggressive analgesics are important. NSAIDs are particularly effective for managing acute joint and muscle pain; dosages at the maximum recommended level should be considered. If one drug is ineffective, additional trials with others is appropriate. To prevent abuse, muscle-relaxant medication such as cyclobenzaprine (Flexeril) or anxiolytics such as diazepam (Valium) should be prescribed using a time-dependent administration. Therapeutic benefit may be increased by coupling these drugs with physical medicine intervention or a treatment contract.

In the patient with severe joint inflammation, pain relief is facilitated with corticosteroid (dexamethasone (Decadron) delivered via iontophoresis, injection (4–8 mg), or by mouth (40–60 mg tapered over 7–10 days).

If trigger points are identified in the masticatory muscles, 0.5% procaine in isotonic saline or isotonic saline alone can be delivered via local injection. Dry needling of trigger points can also be efficacious.

Physical therapy can reduce symptoms in TMD but should be prescribed carefully in order to avoid dependence. The main modality with proved efficacy is repetitive active or passive jaw exercises;

---

[1]Not FDA approved for this indication.

 CURRENT THERAPY

- Temporomandibular disorder is managed using symptomatic treatments according to a rehabilitation model for orthopedic type problems, and pharmacotherapy provides the primary management route for orofacial pain disorders.
- Behavioral management for pain disorders is included as indicated.

---

physical therapy modalities are commonly used, but efficacy data are poor. A home program in which the patient opens slowly in the midline 10 times, three times a day, coupled with thermal agents may be as useful in reducing pain as physical therapy. Active jaw stretching is contraindicated with acute nonreducing disk displacement. Continuous passive jaw movement may be helpful following TMJ surgery and in cases of chronic nonreducing disk displacement and osteoarthritis.

Intraoral appliances (splints, orthotics, nightguards), used historically to treat TMD, are constructed of soft or hard acrylic, fit over maxillary or mandibular teeth, and can protect the joint(s) in cases of trauma or TMJ injury or assist in controlling sleep bruxism. No additional benefit is gained with the appliance for sleep bruxism by repositioning the jaw. Intraoral appliances are an active treatment that can alter the occlusion; hence, this treatment should only be used by a knowledgeable clinician. Orthodontics, dental reconstruction, and bite adjustment are unlikely to cause greater symptom reduction than reversible treatment, are expensive, and create additional risks that might outweigh any long-term benefits. They are appropriate therapies only when symptoms are confounded by dental pathology or significant tooth loss.

At present, the use of botulinum toxin to treat orofacial pain associated with TMD is not well supported by randomized, controlled trials.

Arthrocentesis for acute locking TMJs involves joint lavage coupled with corticosteroids and appears to be useful. Arthroscopic surgery, in addition to irrigating the joint, allows visualization of the superior synovial space, débridement of minor adhesions, and biopsy. Arthroscopic surgery is not useful for changing disk position in cases of locking, but it can increase associated hypomobility. Arthrotomy or open joint surgery may be helpful for fibrous ankylosis, suspected neoplasm, and severe osteoarthritis.

TMJ surgery for internal derangements (displacement without reduction) should be approached rarely and generally only if jaw disability is high and after failure of standard office treatments coupled with sufficient treatment adherence. In sum, surgery should be considered if identifiable disease has failed medical management and disability is increasing. Independent of surgical indications, refractory pain warrants additional medical (e.g., neurosurgical, neurologic) and biobehavioral assessment.

The treatment of orofacial pain is predicated on the identified pathology, clinical diagnosis and, if chronic, biobehavioral components. For most orofacial pain conditions not involving frank pathology, initial therapy is pharmacologic. Specific therapies, including drug protocols, are outlined in the specific disease chapters (e.g., migraine and variants, neuralgias, odontogenic disease, mucosal diseases). Adjunctive therapy can include biobehavioral, nutritional, and preventive treatments and, in limited cases, surgery such as for trigeminal neuralgia.

BIOBEHAVIORAL TREATMENT

Although acute orofacial pain disorders may be appropriately treated with medical management, chronic orofacial pain disorders as well as both acute and chronic TMDs are best managed, like all chronic pain conditions, using a rehabilitation approach. More reliance is placed on the patient acquiring self-management skills, including pain-coping behavior, cognitive skills, adaptive responses to emotional states, and managed medications.

Biobehavioral treatments are effective and based on two fundamental aims: change the perception of the pain, and modify the action pattern. Similar to its impact in back pain and headache, a single psychoeducational session for TMD pain reduces pain-related interference at 1-year follow-up. Relaxation and biofeedback have clear beneficial effects in reducing both the psychophysiologic activation generally present with TMD pain and in promoting general self-regulation.

Premorbid psychosocial characteristics often influence the patient's adherence in using these two methods, and these characteristics often become the focus of the biobehavioral therapy. In that case, biobehavioral therapy focuses on the interactions among emotional reactivity, pain, suffering, and coping. Rapid improvement in general functioning as well as in pain can be observed in as few as six sessions when the patient is motivated. Motivation, in turn, is often influenced by the character of the referral and the patient's relationship with his or her primary physician. These approaches appear to have significant and enduring benefits compared with the usual clinical treatment for TMD.

Very little is known about which aspect of treatment—medical or biobehavioral—is responsible for changes in clinical symptoms. Thus, multimodal approaches are recommended, because we do not currently understand which patient will respond to which treatment. Before escalating either diagnostic intervention or treatment within the biomedical domain, the biobehavioral domain should be equally included at the outset and its diagnostic or treatment escalation should proceed in parallel with that in the biomedical domain. Outcome assessment has almost exclusively been focused on physical parameters and not psychosocial ones. We suspect that failure to incorporate the biobehavioral domain into treatment results in greater likelihood of relapse if not increased invasiveness of treatment in certain patients.

For orofacial pain disorders, biobehavioral treatments have been poorly studied and used. Although their role is likely small for the acute orofacial pain disorder, it is also likely that biobehavioral approaches for TMD are just as useful for chronic or refractory orofacial pain disorders.

REFERENCES

Cheung LK, Lo J. The long-term effect of transport distraction in the management of temporomandibular joint ankylosis. Plast Reconstr Surg 2007; 119:1003–9.

Clark GT, Stiles A, Lockerman LZ, Gross SG. A critical review of the use of botulinum toxin in orofacial pain disorders. Dent Clin North Am 2007;51:245–61.

DiFabio RP. Physical therapy for patients with TMD: A descriptive study of treatment, disability, and health status. J Orofac Pain 1998;12:124–35.

Dworkin SF, LeResche L. Research diagnostic criteria for temporomandibular disorders: Review, criteria, examinations and specifications, critique. J Craniomandib Disord 1992;6:301–55.

Herman CR, Schiffman EL, Look JO, Rindal DB. The effectiveness of adding pharmacologic treatment with clonazepam or cyclobenzaprine to patient education and self-care for the treatment of jaw pain upon awakening: A randomized clinical trial. J Orofac Pain 2002;16:64–70.

Johansson CB, Samuelsson N, Dahlstrom L. Utilization of pharmaceuticals among patients with temporomandibular disorders: A controlled study. Acta Odontol Scand 2006;64:187–92.

Ohrbach R. Biobehavioral therapy. In: Laskin DM, Greene CS, Hylander WL, editors. TMDs: An Evidence-Based Approach to Diagnosis and Treatment. Hanover Park, IL: Quintessence Publishing; 2006. p. 391–403.

Schiffman EL, Look JO, Hodges JS, et al. Randomized effectiveness study of four therapeutic strategies for TMJ closed lock. J Dent Res 2007;86:58–63.

Truelove E, Huggins KH, Mancl L, Dworkin SF. The efficacy of traditional, low-cost and nonsplint therapies for temporomandibular disorders: A randomized controlled trial. J Am Dent Assoc 2006;137:1099–107.

Bursitis, Tendinitis, Myofascial Pain, and Fibromyalgia

Method of
*Russell D. White, MD, and
Miguel Angel Solis, Jr., MD*

Musculoskeletal pain has many causes. The term *soft tissue rheumatism* is often used to describe musculoskeletal pain not caused by arthritis. The pain may be localized or diffuse, and it may affect muscle, fascia, tendon, or bursae. *Bursitis, tendinitis, myofascial pain syndrome*, and *fibromyalgia* are terms used to describe these soft tissue disorders.

The causes of these disorders vary. Most are caused by overuse from sports, occupational stress, trauma, or mechanical abnormalities. These disorders constitute a common chief complaint of patients who visit their primary care physicians. It is important to recognize them and their physical findings because imaging studies and laboratory work have a limited role in diagnosis. The diagnosis is made through key physical findings, and the mainstay of therapy is rest, ice, nonsteroidal antiinflammatory drugs (NSAIDs), and corticosteroid injections. The following sections review some of the more common soft tissue disorders affecting these patients.

Bursitis and Tendinitis: Tendinopathy

The body contains many bursae located between bony surfaces and overlying tendons. The name is Latin for purse. These sacs are filled with viscous synovial fluid, and their role is to "lubricate" the movement of tendons over bony surfaces. Bursitis is commonly caused by repetitive movement or excessive pressure. It is associated with local tenderness, swelling, or pain with specific movements and occasional accumulation of fluid. Tendons are tough bands of connective tissue made up of tight parallel-aligned collagen fibers. These are primarily type I collagen, proteoglycans, and glycoproteins. Tendons connect muscle to bone and transmit pulling forces.

The junction of bone and tendon is the most common site of overuse injuries. Historically, these injuries are referred to as tendinitis, suggesting inflammation. Histologic studies have shown that most overuse tendon injuries are degenerative, not inflammatory. The injury is characterized by collagen degradation, neovascularization, and absent inflammatory cells. The abnormal vascularity has been associated with tendon pain. Most patients report new or increased activity regimens before symptoms start. *Tendinopathy* is the preferred descriptor of overuse injury, with *tendinitis* reserved for histopathologic diagnosis.

SHOULDER

Subacromial Bursitis and Rotator Cuff Tendinitis

The subacromial bursa is located under the acromial arch and deltoid and above the superior surface of the rotator cuff tendons. It protects the rotator cuff tendons from friction during overhead shoulder movement. Disorders of the shoulder are common, and they increase with age. Repetitive activities can lead to inflammation and subsequent pain. Bursitis is often associated with rotator cuff tendinopathy due to its proximity. Patients complain of lateral shoulder pain with abduction.

Shoulder strength and range of motion should be evaluated on physical examination. The empty can or Jobe test is used to test supraspinatus strength. Both shoulders are abducted to 90 degrees with 30 degrees of forward flexion and thumbs turned down; the patient then resists the downward force applied by the examiner. Normal strength compared with the contralateral shoulder indicates an intact rotator cuff. Pain may be reproduced with the Hawkins test (i.e., passive internal rotation with the shoulder in 90 degrees of forward flexion). Imaging studies are usually not indicated unless underlying rotator cuff pathology is suspected.

Management begins with conservative treatment that includes avoidance of exacerbating factors, NSAIDs, ice, and physical therapy. If symptoms do not resolve after a trial period, an injection of corticosteroids and lidocaine is helpful.

Biceps Tendinitis

Biceps tendinitis is inflammation of the long head of the biceps tendons. Patients complain of pain with overhead activity or heavy lifting. Pain along the bicipital groove is exacerbated by resisted supination of the forearm (i.e., Yergason's test). The Speeds test (i.e., forward flexion of the shoulder against resistance while maintaining the elbow in extension and the forearm in supination) may produce pain in the bicipital groove.

Management is similar to that for subacromial bursitis: limitation of lifting by the affected arm, ice, and NSAIDs. Corticosteroid injection into the biceps tendon sheath may be attempted if no relief is achieved.

ELBOW

Olecranon Bursitis

The olecranon bursa is superficial to the olecranon process and is extra-articular to the elbow. Bursitis can result from acute or repetitive trauma to the elbow and inflammatory conditions such as gout, pseudogout, and rheumatoid arthritis. On physical examination, the posterior aspect of the elbow is swollen with fluctuance and may or may not have pain. Because of the superficial nature of this bursa, infection is possible, with erythema, increased swelling, and pain.

Aspiration of the bursa can be performed for acute relief of the swelling and pain. The patient may be placed in a supine position with the elbow in flexion to allow easier aspiration. An 18- to 20-gauge needle may be used with a 30- to 60-mL syringe. The needle is inserted directly into the bursa from the posterior aspect. The aspirate fluid should be sent for Gram stain, culture, cell count, and crystal analysis when appropriate. An elastic wrap should be applied to exert compression and prevent re-accumulation. Avoidance of exacerbating factors and use of NSAIDs and ice may be beneficial. For cases with re-accumulation, corticosteroids may be injected after repeat aspiration. This may be accomplished with a hemostat to change syringes while leaving the needle in place.

Medial and Lateral Epicondylitis

The lateral epicondyle is the origin of the extensor and supinator muscles of the forearm. Pain is caused by overuse of extension and/or supination. The condition is frequently associated with tennis players (i.e., tennis elbow). Patients have tenderness 1 cm distal to the lateral epicondyle. Pain is reproduced with resisted extension and supination. The chair test result may be positive. To perform the test, the patient is asked to stand behind a chair and grasp the top of the chair back and lift; pain is reproduced in the lateral epicondyle.

Management of lateral epicondylitis includes the use of a tennis brace, NSAIDs, and ice and avoidance of aggravating factors. A corticosteroid injection may be performed if symptoms persist. When conservative treatment has failed, surgery may be indicated to débride inflammatory tissue.

The medial epicondyle is the origin of the flexor and pronator muscles of the forearm. Pain is caused by overuse of flexion and pronation. The condition is frequently associated with golfers (i.e., golfer's elbow), but it may be present in manual laborers from repetitive use of screwdrivers or hammers. Patients have tenderness 1 cm distal to the medial epicondyle. Pain is reproduced with resisted flexion and pronation. Occasionally, patients may complain of numbness or tingling in the fourth and fifth digits, suggesting ulnar involvement with a positive Tinel sign (i.e., reproduces symptoms with light tapping over the nerve). If ulnar neuropathy is suspected, nerve conduction studies may be useful.

Management of medial epicondylitis includes the use of NSAIDs, ice, and physical therapy and avoidance of aggravating factors. A corticosteroid injection may be performed if symptoms persist. Special care must be taken to avoid the ulnar nerve. When conservative treatment has failed, surgery may be indicated to débride inflammatory tissue or release the ulnar entrapment.

HAND AND WRIST

De Quervain's Tenosynovitis

De Quervain's tenosynovitis occurs with repetitive use of the thumb (i.e., pinching or grasping). The term was coined by Swiss surgeon Fritz de Quervain. The tenosynovitis is common in factory workers, nursing mothers, people who text message on hand-held devices or cellular phones, people who knit, and video game players. The two tendon sheaths involved with the inflammation are the abductor pollicis longus and extensor pollicis brevis. Pain is present along the radial styloid. The Finkelstein test result is positive; the patient makes a fist on top of the thumb in ulnar deviation, reproducing pain. Management includes thumb spica splints, NSAIDs, ice, physical therapy, and avoidance of aggravating factors. A corticosteroid injection may be performed if symptoms do not resolve.

Trigger Finger: Digital Flexor Tenosynovitis

Trigger finger usually occurs in the third and fourth digits and is a result of overuse activities, but patients with diabetes mellitus, rheumatoid arthritis, and gout are at higher risk. Inflammation and stenosis of the flexor digitorum superficialis and profundus tendon sheaths cause this condition. The inflammatory response is thought to cause stenosis of the sheath below the A1 pulley. The tendon can form a nodule distal to the pulley, and as the finger flexes, the nodule becomes trapped proximally to the narrowing. A tender nodule can be palpated distal or at the metacarpal-phalangeal (MCP) joint.

Management includes splinting the digit in extension, NSAIDs, and avoidance of aggravating factors. A corticosteroid injection may be performed into the sheath if symptoms do not resolve.

Carpal Tunnel Syndrome

Carpal tunnel syndrome is a condition of median nerve compression at the wrist. It leads to numbness, weakness, and atrophy of the hand. The carpal tunnel is formed by the carpal bones dorsally and the transverse carpal ligament (i.e., flexor retinaculum) on the volar aspect. The contents of the carpal tunnel are the flexor tendons (i.e., flexor digitorum profundus and superficialis and the flexor pollicis longus) of the hand and the median nerve. Tenosynovitis of the flexors causes compression of the median nerve and symptoms. The causes include repetitive activities, pregnancy, hypothyroidism, diabetes, and inflammatory arthritis. Patients complain of pain at night and with repetitive activities. Numbness or tingling can be felt along the median nerve distribution (i.e., thumb, index, middle and fourth finger). Atrophy of the thenar muscles and decreased grip may be chronic.

Physical examination reveals a positive Tinel's sign (i.e., reproduces symptoms with light tapping over the nerve), Phalen sign (i.e., wrist flexion at 90 degrees for 1 minute produces numbness), and carpal compression test or Durkan test (i.e., compression of the carpal tunnel for 30 seconds reproduces symptoms). Nerve conduction studies may be helpful in grading the severity.

Management includes splinting in a neutral position (especially at night to avoid inadvertent flexion), use of NSAIDs, and avoidance of aggravating factors. If symptoms persist, a corticosteroid injection may be performed, or a surgical release of the carpal ligament may be necessary.

HIP

Trochanteric Bursitis

Trochanteric bursitis is a painful inflammation of the bursa over the greater trochanter of the femur. Patients complain of lateral hip pain, although the hip is not actually affected, and the inability to sleep on affected side. This condition is caused by direct trauma or repetitive trauma. On physical examination, patients have point tenderness over the greater trochanter and on resisted abduction of the hip. Radiographs of the hip may be helpful to rule out osteoarthritis or possible fracture. Management includes NSAIDs, physical therapy, iliotibial band stretching, and corticosteroid injection.

Ischial Bursitis

The ischial bursa is located between the ischial tuberosity and the gluteus muscle. Inflammation is usually caused by prolonged sitting in the same or hard position. Pain can be exacerbated by walking and may radiate down the leg. On physical examination, pain is reproduced by palpation of the ischial tuberosity ("pain in the butt").

Management includes sitting on a cushion, NSAIDs, physical therapy, and corticosteroid injection. When injecting, it is important to avoid injury to the sciatic nerve.

KNEE

Prepatellar and Infrapatellar Bursitis

The prepatellar bursa is located between the skin and patella, and it does not communicate with the joint space. The function of this bursa is to reduce friction with motion of the knee. Prepatellar bursitis occurs with repetitive kneeling. Some occupations that require frequent kneeling are carpet layers, tile workers, and maids (i.e., housemaid's knee). On physical examination, there is an obvious swelling shaped like an egg on the anterior patella.

The infrapatellar bursa can be divided into two components: deep and superficial. The deep component is between the patellar tendon and the proximal anterior tibia. The superficial component is between the skin and the patellar tendon, and it is the one affected in most cases. The cause of superficial infrapatellar bursitis is from kneeling in an upright position (i.e., clergyman's knee). On physical examination, a dumbbell-like swelling is palpable on each side of the tendon below the patella. The differential diagnosis includes Osgood-Schlatter apophysitis.

Because of the superficial location of these bursae, infection is possible. Management includes avoidance of exacerbating factors, ice, NSAIDs, and aspiration of the fluid. The aspirate fluid should be sent for Gram stain, culture, cell count, and crystal analysis when appropriate. An elastic wrap should be applied to exert compression and prevent re-accumulation. A corticosteroid injection may be performed if symptoms do not resolve.

Quadriceps and Patellar Tendinitis (Jumper's Knee)

Jumper's knee is an overuse injury caused by repetitive stress on the patellar and quadriceps tendons during jumping. Patients complain of anterior knee pain that has persisted for months and that worsens with running or climbing down stairs. In the past, jumper's knee was used to describe injury of the patellar tendon attached to the inferior pole, but the designation now includes the superior attachment by the quadriceps tendon. Injury is usually seen in sports that require frequent running and jumping, such as volleyball, basketball, and soccer. On physical examination, the inferior or superior pole of the patella is tender.

Management includes rest, ice, NSAIDs, quadriceps strengthening, and physical therapy. Rehabilitation and recovery may take up to 6 months. If no improvement is achieved with conservative measures, surgery may be necessary. Corticosteroid injection is contraindicated because of the risk of tendon rupture.

Pes Anserine Bursitis

The pes anserine bursa is formed by the tendinous insertion of the sartorius, gracilis, and semitendinosus muscles at the anteromedial aspect of the proximal tibia. The bursa lies under the tendons and is 4 to 5 cm below the joint line and superficial to the medial collateral ligament. Inflammation of the bursa can be caused by overuse or direct trauma. This condition is commonly seen in overweight, middle-aged women. Patients complain of medial knee pain, which may worsen with climbing stairs and when participating in sports that require side-to-side movement. On physical

examination, there is tenderness over the bursa and occasionally crepitance.

Management includes rest, ice, NSAIDs, quadriceps strengthening, hamstring stretching, and physical therapy. A corticosteroid injection with lidocaine is often performed early in the course of this condition and offers prompt relief.

Biceps Femoris and Semimembranosus (Hamstring) Tendinitis

The biceps femoris and semimembranosus make up the hamstring (along with the semitendinosus) in the posterior thigh. These muscles serve as knee flexors and hip extensors. This form of tendinitis is caused by overuse injury from running, jumping, kicking, and bursts of speed. Patients complain of pain in the posterior thigh, especially with sitting and climbing stairs. With biceps femoris tendinitis, pain is felt in the posterolateral aspect of the knee, and with semimembranosus tendinitis, pain is felt in the posteromedial aspect of the knee. On physical examination, pain is reproduced with resisted knee flexion. Management includes rest, ice, NSAIDs, strengthening exercises, and physical therapy.

Iliotibial Band Syndrome

The iliotibial band (ITB) is a fascial band that originates at the lateral iliac crest and inserts on the lateral aspect of the proximal tibia (i.e., Gerdy's tubercle). ITB syndrome is a common cause of lateral knee pain, and it results from excessive friction of the band over the lateral femoral condyle. Activities that involve repetitive flexion and extension, such as running and cycling, can cause inflammation. On physical examination, the patient has point tenderness at the lateral femoral condyle or over Gerdy's tubercle. The result of Ober's test is positive. To perform the test, the patient lies on the unaffected side while the affected hip is abducted against gravity and the knee is flexed at 90 degrees. The leg is then allowed to adduct beyond the midline. If pain or the inability to cross the midline is present, it implies inflammation of the ITB.

Management includes physical therapy to stretch the ITB and the use of ice and NSAIDs. A corticosteroid injection may be performed if symptoms do not resolve.

ANKLE

Retrocalcaneal Bursitis

As the Achilles tendon courses distally over the posterior calcaneus, it is sandwiched between two bursae, one deep (subtendinous) to the tendon and one superficial (subcutaneous). The tendon then inserts onto the posteroinferior calcaneus. Superficial bursitis is common with direct irritation over this area from improper footwear. In contrast, deep bursitis is often associated with inflammatory or crystalline-induced arthritis.

Symptoms include exquisite pain over the posterior heel with walking and dorsiflexion of the foot. Swelling and rubor may develop, and proximal radiation of pain in the Achilles tendon frequently occurs. The differential diagnosis includes Achilles tendonitis, Achilles tendon partial tear, and Haglund's abnormality (i.e., abnormal prominence of the posterior calcaneal tuberosity).

Initial treatment includes rest, ice, and NSAIDs, along with properly fitting shoes. In recalcitrant cases, corticosteroids may be administered into the bursa under imaging (e.g., fluoroscopy, ultrasound) or by means of iontophoresis.

Achilles Tendinitis

Tendonitis of the calcaneal (Achilles) tendon is caused by overuse, direct trauma, excessive incline walking or running, and inflammatory arthritis (e.g., rheumatoid arthritis). Although the Achilles tendon is the thickest and strongest tendon in the body, it can rupture from chronic inflammation or from the use of fluoroquinolone anti-biotics, especially if combined with systemic steroid administration in the elderly population.

Although patients complain of calf pain and heel pain, localized tenderness occurs at the insertion of the Achilles tendon on the pos-teroinferior region of the calcaneus. Thompsons's test (i.e., squeezing of the gastrocnemius with the patient lying prone produces plantar flexion of the foot) confirms an *intact* Achilles tendon. The differential diagnosis includes Achilles tendon partial tear, hematoma, or deep venous thrombosis. Ultrasonography or magnetic resonance imaging (MRI) can clarify the pathology.

Management includes relative rest, ice, NSAIDs, stretching exercises, and a heel lift to decrease tension on the tendon. Steroid administration may be attempted in recalcitrant cases, but many physicians avoid this modality unless surgery is being considered.

Posterior Tibial Tendinitis

The tibialis posterior tendon travels behind the medial malleolus, crosses the deltoid ligament, and inserts into the navicular tuberosity. This tendon stabilizes the arch and decreases flatfoot by distributing weight among the metatarsal heads, and it plantar flexes and inverts the foot by shifting weight to the lateral aspect of the foot. Posterior tibial tendonitis is an overuse syndrome caused by overpronation of the foot.

Symptoms include pain posterior to the medial malleolus and proximal radiation. On examination, there is localized tenderness posterior to the medial malleolus, and pain is reproducible with resisted inversion of the foot. If the flexor retinaculum that overlies this tendon is torn, subluxation of this tendon occurs.

Management includes rest, ice, NSAIDs, and orthotics to correct the overpronation. Moleskin applied over the flexor retinaculum and the tendon as it passes behind the medial malleolus can limit subluxation of the tendon. Steroid injection into the tibialis posterior tendon sheath may be considered in intractable cases.

FOOT

Plantar Fasciitis

The plantar fascia originates from the medial tubercle of the calcaneus and inserts distally onto the proximal phalanges. This thick fibrous tissue supports the arch of the foot. Plantar fasciitis occurs with prolonged standing or walking, running, obesity, and in those with pes planus. Often, an increase or change in activity, such as exercising on a different surface, can initiate symptoms. It can be associated with seronegative spondyloarthropathy.

Symptoms include exquisite plantar surface pain with initial walking after resting for hours or walking barefoot on firm, hard surfaces. Pain can be localized to the origin of the fascia. The cycle includes contraction of the fascia area during periods of prolonged inactivity (sleep), followed by tearing and bleeding of the fibrotic area with initial stretching (on arising). Stretching before and after sleep or sleeping with the ankle at 90 degrees can help break this vicious cycle.

Management includes ice massage, passive stretching of the fascia, firm heel cups and cushioned arch supports, physical therapy (cross-friction massage), and avoidance of aggravating activities. Late evening and early morning stretching using a Thera-Band or bath towel (before arising) limits the cycle. Stretching of the posterior leg complex (i.e., hamstrings, calf muscles, and plantar structures) promotes relief. Although no evidence-based medicine has demonstrated benefit from NSAIDs, it is a reasonable treatment choice. In one study, this syndrome had a 12-month self-limited course from onset to resolution, although treatment may ameliorate the symptoms. Careful corticosteroid injection into the origin of the plantar fascia may hasten symptom improvement (Box 1). The plantar fascia may rupture spontaneously without specific intervention and relieve symptoms. Ironically, surgical intervention is partial plantar fasciotomy.

CURRENT DIAGNOSIS

Tendinitis and Bursitis

- Caused by overuse from sports, occupation, trauma, mechanical abnormalities, and repetitive movement
- Bursitis is commonly caused by repetitive movement or excessive pressure.
- Tendinopathy is the preferred descriptor of overuse injury, with tendinitis reserved for histopathologic diagnosis.
- Localized pain at tendinous insertion, especially with active range of motion
- Localized swelling over superficial bursa

Myofascial Pain

- Trigger point is palpated in a muscle with focal induration or nodule.
- Palpation of the trigger point reproduces the referred pain in a distant or remote area.

Fibromyalgia

- History of chronic (>3 months), idiopathic, nonarticular pain involving both sides of the body and areas above and below the waist
- Pain with digital palpation in 11 or 18 defined tender points
- Associated symptoms of sleep disturbance, fatigue, depression, anxiety, headaches
- Irritable bladder
- Absence of articular pain, fever, chills, or skin changes
- Normal results for laboratory evaluation (complete blood cell count, urinalysis, chemistry panel, liver function tests, thyroid-stimulating hormone, erythrocyte sedimentation rate, creatine phosphokinase)
- Avoid ordering specialized tests (rheumatoid factor, antinuclear antibody, Lyme disease titer) unless indicated by specific history or physical examination findings.

Myofascial Pain Syndrome

Myofascial pain syndrome is defined as sensory, motor, and autonomic symptoms that are produced by myofascial trigger points. A myofascial trigger point is a tender, irritable focus in skeletal muscle that is associated with a palpable hypersensitive nodule (knot) identified on examination. When the trigger point is palpated, pain is produced in a referral area or zone often remote from the point of origin. The common sensory symptoms commonly are hyperalgesia and referred pain. Although the reproducible pain follows a consistent pattern, it is rarely consistent with dermatomal or neuronal distribution patterns. This pattern of referred pain differentiates myofascial pain syndrome from fibromyalgia.

The diagnosis is made through careful examination, and the patient frequently has localized the palpable, tender nodule. Examination is often done by one of three methods: flat palpation, deep palpation, and pincer palpation. Flat palpation involves sliding a fingertip across the muscle area, pushing the skin aside, and then feeling a tight muscle band with a localized trigger point. Deep palpation involves deep palpation with the fingertip over the attachment of the suspected muscle area and localizing a trigger point. A trigger point is located when the patient's symptoms (e.g., pain) are

---

BOX 1   Techniques for Injection of Common Bursitis and Tendinitis Conditions

Injection Principles
- Perform all injections with sterile technique.
- Other doses of injectable steroids may be substituted for triamcinolone (Kenalog-40) 40 mg/mL.
- Ethyl chloride topical spray may be used for surface anesthesia before injection.
- The injection should flow freely without resistance (which may indicate intratendinous insertion).
- Avoid pressure on the plunger of the syringe when withdrawing and steroid tracking into the skin to prevent atrophy and pigment changes.

Injection Technique
Subacromial Bursitis
- Inject 20 to 40 mg triamcinolone with 1 to 2 mL 1% lidocaine (Xylocaine) using a 1.5-inch, 25-gauge needle.
- Insert 1 to 2 cm below the point of the posterior acromion, and angle and direct it medially, anteriorly, and slightly superior into the subacromial bursa (i.e., posterior approach).

Supraspinatus Tendinitis
- Same procedures as for subacromial bursitis

Biceps Tendinitis
- Inject 20 to 40 mg triamcinolone with 1 to 2 mL 1% lidocaine using a 1.5-inch, 25-gauge needle.
- The tendon is palpated in the bicipital groove with the shoulder in external rotation. The needle is then inserted into the anterior shoulder toward the tendon at a 30- to 45-degree angle.

Lateral Epicondylitis
- Inject 1 to 2 mg dexamethasone (Decadron) with 1 to 2 mL 1% lidocaine using a 1.5-inch, 25-gauge needle.
- Locate the point of maximal tenderness over the epicondyle, and insert the needle until it touches the epicondyle; withdraw 1 mm, and inject.

De Quervain's Tenosynovitis
- Inject 1 to 2 mg dexamethasone with 0.5 to 1 mL 1% lidocaine using a 1.5-inch, 25-gauge needle.
- Insert at the lateral wrist distal to the radial styloid, and inject following the extensor tendon course.

Trigger Finger
- Inject 1 to 2 mg dexamethasone with 0.5 to 1 mL 1% lidocaine using a tuberculosis syringe.
- Insert distal to the proximal flexor crease toward the nodule at a 45-degree angle.

Carpal Tunnel Syndrome
- Inject 10 to 20 mg triamcinolone with 0.5 to 1 mL 1% lidocaine using a 1.5-inch, 25-gauge needle.
- Insert the needle distal to the proximal wrist crease and ulnar to the palmaris longus tendon; aim toward the middle finger.

Pes Anserine Bursitis
- Inject 10 to 20 mg triamcinolone with 1 to 2 mL 1% lidocaine using a 1.5-inch, 25-gauge needle.
- Insert into the area of maximal tenderness until the needle touches the tibia; withdraw 1 mm, and inject.

Trochanteric Bursitis
- Inject 20 to 40 mg triamcinolone with 1 to 2 mL 1% lidocaine using a 1.5-inch, 25-gauge needle; use a 3- to 4-inch spinal needle in obese patients.
- With the patient lying on the unaffected side, insert into the lateral hip until the trochanter is reached; withdraw 1 mm, and inject.

Plantar Fasciitis
- Inject 10 to 20 mg triamcinolone with 1 to 2 mL 1% lidocaine (Xylocaine) using a 1.5-inch, 25-gauge needle.
- Insert parallel to the floor of the foot at the medial side of the foot, aiming toward the medial tubercle of the calcaneus.
- Inject into the space superior to the proximal origin of the plantar fascia.

---

reproduced by pressing in one direction. Pincer palpation involves squeezing a suspected muscle between the thumb and index finger and rolling the tissue fibers while searching for a tense band. Specialized instruments and electromyography can assist in the diagnosis and in quantifying abnormalities.

Treatment involves injection of the inciting trigger points, avoiding aggravating activities and noninvasive maneuvers. Injections include lidocaine, corticosteroids, botulinum toxin (Botox),[1] normal saline, and dry needling. Noninvasive measures include spray (i.e., topical freeze) and stretch, physical therapy, ultrasound, transcutaneous electrical stimulation, and massage therapy combined with ischemic compression therapy (i.e., topical pressure application over the trigger point).

---

[1]Not FDA approved for this indication.

CURRENT THERAPY

Bursitis and Tendinitis

- Avoidance of exacerbating factors
- Ice for 15 to 20 minutes three times daily
- NSAIDs: Naproxen (Naprosyn) 500 mg PO twice daily, meloxicam (Mobic) 7.5 to 15 mg once daily; may consider proton pump inhibitors (e.g., lansoprazole [Prevacid], omeprazole [Prilosec], esomeprazole [Nexium]) for gastrointestinal protection
- Rest and immobilization with splints or bracing
- Physical therapy to strengthen muscle groups
- If symptoms do not resolve after a trial period of 1 to 2 weeks, an injection of corticosteroids and lidocaine may be performed (see Box 1). Injection of the patellar, quadriceps, and Achilles tendon is contraindicated because of risk of tendon rupture.

Myofascial Pain

- Avoidance of aggravating activities
- Consider referral to physical therapy for noninvasive modalities.
- Injection: 1 to 2 mL of 1% lidocaine (Xylocaine) directly into the trigger point

Fibromyalgia

- Demonstrate concern, compassion, and support while focusing on the most troublesome symptoms, such as restoring restful sleep and reducing painful symptoms.
- Adopt a multidisciplinary approach to management, and emphasize patient and family education in dealing with the disease process and treatment.
- Prescribe an exercise program. Outline aerobic activity for a minimum period (10 minutes) three times weekly and then gradually increase. Involve physical therapist in monitoring activities such as walking, swimming, stationary cycling, or aerobics. Support regular activity as the symptoms improve.
- Medications:
  - Pregabalin (Lyrica) 50 mg at bedtime and titrate up to 300 to 450 mg/day, used for treatment of pain, first FDA-approved agent for the treatment of fibromyalgia (not all patients respond to this agent)

- Tricyclic antidepressants (TCAs), start low and increase every 2 to 4 weeks. Examples include amitriptyline (Elavil)[1] 10 mg 1 to 2 hours before bedtime and increase slowly to 50 to 75 mg; doxepin (Sinequan)[1] 25 mg 1 hour before bedtime and titrate slowly; used for treatment of insomnia, pain, and depression
- Structurally related to TCAs, cyclobenzaprine (Flexeril)[1] 5 mg at bedtime and increase every 2 weeks to 10 to 15 mg; for treatment of insomnia, pain, and depression
- An alternative to TCAs, trazodone (Desyrel)[1] 25 mg 1 hour before bedtime and titrate slowly to 50 to 75 mg; for treatment of insomnia, pain, and depression
- Selective serotonin reuptake inhibitors (SSRIs): Sertraline (Zoloft)[1] 25 mg/day in the morning and increase to 50 to 150 mg/day. Alternatively, fluoxetine (Prozac)[1] 10 mg daily in the morning and increase to maximum dose of 20 to 60 mg daily. Often, a combination of a TCA and SSRI provides additional benefit over monotherapy with either group. Use for treatment of insomnia, pain, and depression.
- Consider serotonin-norepinephrine reuptake inhibitors (SNRIs) instead of TCAs: venlafaxine (Effexor)[1] 75 to 150 mg PO daily or duloxetine (Cymbalta) 40 to 60 mg PO daily
- Gabapentin (Neurontin)[1] 300 mg at bedtime; titrate up by 300 mg every 2 weeks. The usual effective dose is 300 mg three times daily to 600 mg three times daily. Alternatively, consider tramadol (Ultram) 50 mg PO every 6 hours, acetaminophen (Tylenol), or NSAIDs for treatment of pain.
- Minimize use of narcotic agents.
- Avoid use of corticosteroids. There are no evidence-based studies to support the use of these agents.
- For psychological support, consider referral for cognitive-behavioral therapy.

---

[1]Not FDA approved for this indication.

For education, refer to the Arthritis Foundation website (www.arthritis.org) and local self-help programs for fibromyalgia.

Fibromyalgia

Fibromyalgia is a chronic, idiopathic nonarticular pain syndrome with specifically defined tender points. It affects 2% of Americans, and women are 10 times more often affected than men. Patients frequently complain of sleep disorders, anxiety, depression, headaches (including migraine syndrome), inflammatory bowel disease, irritable bladder, restless leg syndrome, and noncardiac chest pain.

Diagnostic criteria from the American College of Rheumatology include a minimum duration of 3 months of diffuse pain involving the upper and lower body bilaterally, with axial involvement and with at least 11 of 18 specific tender points on examination (Fig. 1). The specific cause is not clear, but it seems to involve central nervous system alterations in processing pain and a heightened response to stress. Because of associated anxiety and depression, altered sleep patterns, functional bowel syndrome, and migraine headaches, abnormalities of the serotonin and adrenergic pathways are implicated. Specific triggers often include acute trauma, viral infections, severe medical illnesses, and chronic stress.

The differential diagnosis for fibromyalgia includes chronic fatigue syndrome, hypothyroidism, and myofascial pain syndrome. Because of the vague initial symptoms and an association with autoimmune diseases (e.g., rheumatoid arthritis, systemic lupus erythematosus), specific historical data, examination, and laboratory testing must be undertaken to rule out these possible diseases.

The only specific diagnostic examination criterion is the presence of multiple tender points in specific areas (see Fig. 1). Examination consists of sufficient digital pressure (4 kg/cm^2) to blanch the thumbnail. Laboratory testing includes a complete blood cell count, urinalysis, chemistry panel with liver tests, and determinations of thyroid-stimulating hormone, erythrocyte sedimentation rate, creatine phosphokinase, and serum aldolase. Most physicians usually obtain rheumatoid agglutinin titers, antinuclear antibodies, and serologic tests for Lyme disease, but these studies are rarely helpful. Fibromyalgia does not cause articular pain, fever, chills, or skin changes. The diagnosis of fibromyalgia should be based on the defined criteria and not on the exclusion of other diseases.

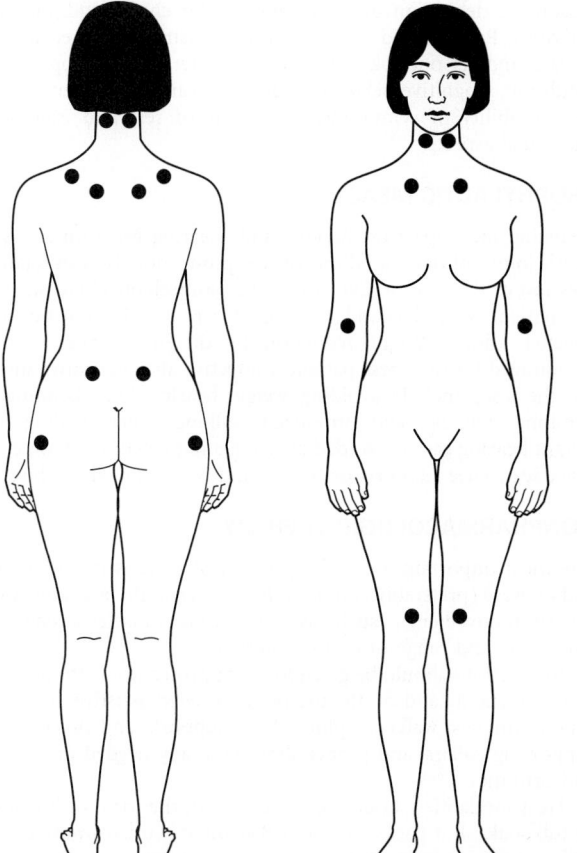

FIGURE 1. The location of the nine paired tender points that comprise the 1990 American College of Rheumatology criteria for fibromyalgia. (From the National Institute of Arthritis and Musculoskeletal and Skin Diseases: Questions and Answers about Fibromyalgia. Bethesda, MD, National Institute of Arthritis and Musculoskeletal and Skin Diseases, 2004. Available at http://www .niams.nih.gov/hi/topics/fibromyalgia/fibrofs.htm [accessed July 2009]).

After the diagnosis of fibromyalgia is made, management involves a multidisciplinary approach, including cognitive-behavioral therapies, patient education, physical therapy, and medical treatment. Educating and supporting the patient who has feared an alternate diagnosis (e.g., cancer) often bring reassurance. The primary goal should focus on the sleep disorder, followed by treating depression or anxiety along with the specific pain syndromes. Referring the patient to websites, the American College of Rheumatology, or a community fibromyalgia program is very useful. Often, treatment is initiated with low-dose amitriptyline (Elavil)[1] (or a structurally related compound, cyclobenzaprine [Flexeril][1]) at bedtime to restore a normal sleep pattern; a selective serotonin reuptake inhibitor (fluoxetine [Prozac] or venlafaxine [Effexor]) in the morning for anxiety and depression; and an appropriate exercise program. Specific analgesics for the pain syndromes include tramadol (Ultram), acetaminophen (Tylenol), NSAIDs, or limited use of narcotic analgesics. Although injection of tender points benefits some patients, systemic corticosteroids have not been found to be helpful. Additional agents for managing discomfort include gabapentin (Neurontin)[1] and duloxetine HCl (Cymbalta). Pregabalin (Lyrica) is an FDA-approved agent for fibromyalgia, but not all patients respond to it; Cymbalta has recently been approved for fibromyalgia. Nonpharmacologic management includes structured aerobic exercise, flexibility, balance and strength conditioning, cognitive-behavioral therapy, patient education, massage therapy, yoga, and acupuncture.

---

[1]Not FDA approved for this indication.

REFERENCES

Burbank KM, Stevenson JH, Czarnecki GR, et al. Chronic shoulder pain. Part I. Evaluation and diagnosis. Am Fam Physician 2007;77:453.

Calmbach WI, Hutchens M. Evaluation of patients presenting with knee pain. Part II. Differential diagnosis. Am Fam Physician 2003;68:917.

Cardone DA, Tallia AF. Diagnostic and therapeutic injection of the elbow region. Am Fam Physician 2002;66:2097.

Cardone DA, Tallia AF. Diagnostic and therapeutic injection of the hip and knee. Am Fam Physician 2003;67:2147.

Chakrabarty S, Zoorob R. Fibromyalgia. Am Fam Physician 2002;76:247.

Cosca DD, Navazio F. Common problems in endurance athletes. Am Fam Physician 2007;76:237.

Hyman GS, Malanga GA, Alladin I. Jumper's knee, eMedicine 2008. Available at http://www.emedicine.com/sports/topic56.htm [accessed July 2009].

Lavelle ED, Lavelle W, Smith HS. Myofascial trigger points. Anesthesiol Clin 2007;25:841.

League AC. Current concepts review: Plantar fasciitis. Foot Ankle Int 2008;29:358.

Riley G. Tendinopathy—From basic science to treatment. Nat Clin Pract Rheumatol 2008;4:82.

Ruiz HB, Zaffer SM. Hamstring injury, eMedicine 2008. Available at http://www.emedicine.com/sports/topic45.htm [accessed July 2009].

Tallia AF, Cardone DA. Diagnostic and therapeutic injection of the wrist and hand region. Am Fam Physician 2003;67:745.

Osteoarthritis

Method of
David H. Neustadt, MD

Osteoarthritis (OA) (degenerative joint disease) is the most commonly encountered rheumatic disorder and the major cause of disability and reduced activity after 50 years of age. Radiographic evidence of OA is found in up to 85% of people older than 65 years. Autopsies indicate evidence of OA in weight-bearing joints of almost all persons by the age of 45 years.

In spite of the evidence of pathologic changes of OA found in Java and Neanderthal human skeletons and dinosaur skeletons, OA was confused with rheumatoid arthritis (RA) until the turn of the 20th century. It is characterized pathologically by involvement of cartilage, varying from fissures and microfibrillations in early disease to erosive destruction in advanced disease. Weight-bearing or shearing forces are transmitted to the subchondral bone, leading to sclerosis, cyst formation, and bone remodeling. Osteophytes (spurs) develop at the margins of joints, and new cartilage proliferates over these bony spurs.

An inflammatory component is present in most patients with symptomatic OA. The traditional belief that OA is simply a wear-and-tear condition associated with the stress of advancing years is not tenable. This mistaken belief is considered the major reason for the relatively slow progress of cartilage and bone research and investigation into the etiology and pathogenesis of OA. During the past decade, much new knowledge on cartilage, including metabolic changes, genetic mutations, metalloproteinases, and possible diagnostic biomarkers and inflammatory mediators, has fostered considerable excitement and interest in new approaches for the prevention, monitoring, and treatment of OA.

Although the cause of OA is unknown, contributing factors include heredity, trauma, overweight, overuse of joints, and aging. OA may be classified into primary (idiopathic) and secondary forms. Secondary OA results from trauma or repetitive overuse of a specific joint; in an inflammatory form of arthritis such as RA, repeated attacks of gout, or septic arthritis; developmental problems such as congenital dysplasia of a hip or slipped capital femoral epiphysis; or metabolic and miscellaneous causes including hemophiliac arthropathy, ochronosis (alkaptonuria), and osteonecrosis. Thus, OA may be considered a (final) common pathway resulting from a host of many different problems.

CURRENT DIAGNOSIS

- Enhanced understanding and knowledge of the pathogenesis of osteoarthritis have led to increasing optimism for the 20 to 30 million osteoarthritis sufferers in the United States.
- Osteoarthritis is now known to involve inflammatory mechanisms, not mechanical wear and tear, as believed in the past.

Joints commonly affected in OA include the large weight-bearing and frequently used joints, such as the hips and knees, spine, distal interphalangeal (DIP) joints (Heberden's nodes), and trapeziometacarpal (carpometacarpal thumb base) and first metatarsophalangeal joint (bunion). Joints often spared in OA include the metacarpals, the wrists, the shoulders, and the ankles (except in ballet dancers).

Clinical Features

The onset of OA is insidious, and the course is slowly progressive. Clinical features include variable pain and mild stiffness, with associated limited motion; bony enlargement with or without tenderness; synovitis of the knees; and functional impairment with malalignment (varus or valgus deformities) when advanced involvement of the knees or hips develops. There are no specific laboratory abnormalities or specific (disease) markers of the disease, except in ochronosis.

Radiographs and other imaging procedures demonstrate evidence of OA, manifested chiefly by a narrowed joint space (loss of cartilage), osteophyte formation, and secondary subchondral sclerosis. There may be a poor correlation between symptoms and underlying abnormal structural findings on x-ray images. Special subsets of OA and significant associated conditions include inflammatory (cystic erosive) OA, calcium pyrophosphate dihydrate disease (chondrocalcinosis), and diffuse idiopathic skeletal hyperostosis (DISH).

Treatment

The optimal management program for OA should be individualized to the specific problems and clinical syndromes presented by each patient (Box 1).

GENERAL CONSIDERATIONS

Realistic reassurance that the patient does not have a serious, potentially crippling disease such as RA and adequate understanding of what to expect are of paramount importance for successful management. Education of the patient is the basic foundation of the treatment program. The updated OA booklet provided by the National Arthritis Foundation is an available useful supplement to education. Involving spouses and other family members in coping skills training may be helpful. Understanding the patient's problem permits reasonable delegation of responsibilities for chores and engaging in activities. Patients and spouses who are better informed about the disease and its outlook are generally better able to cope with the condition. Cognitive behavior techniques can help patients confront the variability of symptoms, the effects of rest and exercise, and emotional aspects.

PROPHYLACTIC MEASURES

Reducing the impact of the load and shearing force on an osteoarthritis joint not only can diminish symptoms but also can retard progression of the disease. Explaining the biomechanical factors enables the patient to understand the need for rest and protection of the affected joints. Weight reduction by dietetic means is strongly encouraged for the obese patient. Protective and preventive measures for the knee include avoiding weight-bearing knee bending, stair climbing, jogging, and prolonged walking. Knee loading during weight bearing can be avoided by using a high chair or stool, elevated toilet seat, knee supports or braces, and walking devices (Box 2).

NONPHARMACOLOGIC THERAPY

The most important aspect is specific instructions for balanced rest and exercise (preferably at home). Exercises should be mainly isometric (nonmovement), such as quadriceps muscle strengthening, stretching, and range-of-motion exercises.

Instructions should be given for joint protection with measures to conserve energy and on the use of any needed assistive aids, such as canes, crutches, walkers, splints, back supports and braces, cervical supporting collars, and proper shoes with any needed modifications and orthotics.

Heat modalities should be prescribed in the form of hot showers or tub soaks, hot packs such as a Bed Buddy (microwavable cervical collar or back wrap), and a warm pool for water aerobic exercises. These measures ameliorate discomfort and facilitate the exercise program. Diathermy, short wave, and ultrasound methods are relatively expensive and of questionable benefit. The use of a hot tub or whirlpool bath, especially after exercise or work, may be of palliative benefit.

Job and recreational activities must be assessed and modified if necessary to avoid overuse of affected joints. Sexual counseling may be needed, especially in some patients with severe knee, hip, or back involvement.

PHARMACOTHERAPY

The basic program of education and reassurance of the patient, joint rest and protection, and physical measures can control symptoms in some patients with early mild OA. Many patients, however, require drug therapy. Although no available drugs predictably reverse or halt the inexorable progression of the disease, the drugs do reduce pain and inflammation, enhancing the patient's quality of life.

Analgesics

Some patients with OA have minimal inflammation and can be managed with analgesics alone. Analgesic agents (non-narcotic) currently available include acetaminophen (Tylenol), propoxyphene (Darvon), and tramadol (Ultram). Effective dosages of acetaminophen are 1.0 to 1.3 g administered every 8 hours or three or four times daily (do not exceed 4 g/day). Adverse effects are rare, but caution must

---

BOX 1 **Comprehensive Management Program for Osteoarthritis**

Education of the patient and family
Coping measures: Rest and modification of activities of daily living
Measures to reduce joint loading
Physical therapy, occupational therapy, assistive devices
Pharmacotherapy
Intraarticular therapy (steroids, hyaluronan)
Surgery

BOX 2 **Measures to Protect Knees**

Avoid knee bending when weight bearing
Avoid steps when possible
Use high chair or high stool
Use elevated toilet seat
Use cane, crutches, or walker for prolonged walking
Do isometric quadriceps muscle-strengthening exercises

CURRENT THERAPY

- Although there is no cure for osteoarthritis, coping strategies including simple measures such as weight reduction and modification of activities to reduce stress and load on the joints should be emphasized.
- Pharmacotherapy includes acetaminophen (Tylenol), other simple analgesics, and judicious use of nonsteroidal antiinflammatory drugs. Opioids should be avoided.
- When usual medical measures fail to control the pain of osteoarthritis, intraarticular injections of a corticosteroid is the next step.
- A painful effusion is the major indication for arthrocentesis, aspiration, and if fluid is not infectious, instillation of a corticosteroid preparation.
- After a corticosteroid injection for knee osteoarthritis, increased therapeutic response results if a postinjection rest regimen is imposed. The patient remains in bed or at rest for 3 days and then uses walking devices (cane or crutches) for 2 to 3 weeks.
- The main factors that influence the therapeutic response from a series of hyaluronan injections are the extent of loss of cartilage and severity of the osteoarthritis disease in the affected knee.
- Total knee and hip replacement procedures are considered when nonoperative management fails to adequately control symptoms and pain.

be exercised in patients who have preexisting renal or liver conditions. Propoxyphene is effective, especially in combination with acetaminophen (Darvocet-N 100), and may be given in a dosage of 1 tablet every 4 to 6 hours for supplementary analgesia. Side effects are usually minimal, with the patient occasionally intolerant because of nausea or lightheadedness. Tramadol can be given in 50-, 100-, 200-, or 300-mg tablets up to two to three times daily for pain relief (do not exceed 400 mg of immediate-release tablets per day or 300 mg of extended-release tablets per day). These drugs are generally well tolerated, and nausea, vomiting, and dizziness are the most common adverse effects. A combination preparation, Ultram 37.5 plus acetaminophen (Ultracet), is available. I advise avoiding regular use of opioids. Opioids may be needed occasionally for intense pain, but the benefits are limited owing to the common gastrointestinal adverse events and the potential for addiction.

Antiinflammatory Agents

A much-discussed report compared acetaminophen 4 g/day with ibuprofen (Advil, Motrin) 1200 to 2400 mg/day, in OA of the knee. The clinical results demonstrated no significant difference in efficacy among the three treatment groups. Critical analysis of this comparative study, however, discloses a short duration of the treatment trial (4 weeks) and a relatively low antiinflammatory dosage (up to 2400 mg) of ibuprofen. In my experience and that of many others, pain in OA patients is often not adequately controlled with pure analgesics, whereas nonsteroidal antiinflammatory drugs (NSAIDs) in adequate dosage can provide significant clinical improvement.

Nonacetylated salicylates are widely used in OA. Compounds currently available include salsalate, choline magnesium trisalicylate, and magnesium salicylate. These agents are weak prostaglandin (cyclooxygenase) inhibitors, thus avoiding the anticlotting effect and potential adverse effect on the gastrointestinal tract and kidneys. Side effects are relatively uncommon and minor with nonacetylated salicylates when administered in a dosage of 1 to 1.5 g twice daily. Gastrointestinal and cardiovascular problems have not been reported. Salicylism with ototoxicity is a rare side effect.

If simple analgesics and salsalate fail to provide adequate relief, one of the many currently available NSAIDs may be selected for a therapeutic trial. Clinical trials with naproxen, diclofenac, and sulindac showed significantly greater improvement of the NSAID when compared with high-dose acetaminophen. The chief limiting factor in the use of NSAIDs is the possible induced gastric pathologic changes, disturbed renal function, and potential increased cardiac events.

Cost and compliance also must be given consideration. Many of the NSAIDs are now available in dosage forms that can be given once or twice daily, which helps overcome the compliance problem.

Currently available NSAIDs are all similar in their proposed mechanism of action but vary considerably in their pharmocokinetics, dosage, clinical response, and side effects. The variability of the effects of different NSAIDs in patients is significant and unpredictable. All NSAIDs are metabolized in the liver, except two available compounds, sulindac (Clinoril) and nabumetone (Relafen), which are prodrugs that are not converted to active drugs until after absorption and hepatic biotransformation. The prodrug effect might partially spare the gastrointestinal tract and also produces less suppression of renal prostaglandins. Etodolac (Lodine) reportedly has fewer gastric complications, and endoscopy does not demonstrate the typical gastric erosions found in the gastric mucosa of the majority of patients taking older NSAIDs.

Concomitant prophylactic use of misoprostol (Cytotec) has been recommended to protect gastric mucosa in patients with a previous history of peptic ulcer or gastrointestinal bleeding. Unfortunately, misoprostol causes cramps and diarrhea in a relatively high percentage of patients. A gastroprotective agent, such as a proton pump inhibitor, will reduce the risk of gastrointestinal adverse effects.

The question of potential deleterious effect on cartilage versus chondroprotective properties by various NSAIDs remains controversial.

Cyclooxygenase 2 Inhibitors

Prostaglandin synthesis in humans is catalyzed by two enzyme forms of cyclooxygenase: cyclooxygenase 1 (COX-1) and cyclooxygenase 2 (COX-2).

COX-1 is constitutively expressed and is considered responsible for suppression of physiologic functions including gastric mucosal protection. In contrast, COX-2 is induced by inflammatory mediators and is responsible for inflammation without any significant effect on the gastric mucosa. The development of agents that selectively inhibit the COX-2 pathway without significant gastrointestinal adverse effects was considered an extremely important advance.

Currently only one COX-2–specific inhibiting NSAID is FDA approved and available. Celecoxib (Celebrex) is equivalent to the older nonselective NSAIDs with regard to therapeutic effectiveness, but the risk of gastrointestinal toxicity and adverse effects on platelet aggregation is lessened. The risk of renal side effects is probably comparable with that of the conventional NSAIDs. A trial assessing the effect of celecoxib on cardiovascular events found a slightly higher risk of cardiovascular events but chiefly only at higher doses (400 mg/day or greater). Celecoxib can be used with low-dose aspirin (81 mg) daily and anticoagulants including warfarin (Coumadin).

INTRAARTICULAR INJECTIONS

Corticosteroids

After many years of controversy concerning intraarticular corticosteroid therapy in OA, there is now consensus that this form of therapy is of considerable value when it is indicated and skillfully administered. Although early on it is still preferable to attempt to control symptoms by simple measures with oral therapy, rather than by local injection, when faced with relatively acute painful conditions such as synovitis of the knee or inflamed Heberden's nodes, quick and sometimes lasting relief can be obtained with intrasynovial steroid injection. This form of treatment is considered an adjunct to a conventional management program.

A painful knee effusion is the most common indication for arthrocentesis followed by a local corticosteroid injection. The remote potential deleterious effect of instability developing in the knee can be avoided by giving injections at infrequent intervals and prescribing a strict postinjection rest regimen. Specific instructions are given to the patient to refrain from weight-bearing activity for 3 days, except getting up for meals and going to the bathroom. The patient is advised to reduce loading of the injected knee by using a cane or crutches with a three-point gait during weight bearing for 2 to 3 weeks after the procedure. This rest regimen delays escape of the steroid suspension from the joint cavity and promotes a longer duration of response to the injection. I have observed numerous patients with OA of the knee associated with large recurrent synovitis who had been given three to five or more local injections with only transient benefit. When a strict postinjection rest program was imposed, these patients obtained substantial improvement in the duration of the effect, and some achieved indefinite "cures." The remote risk of introducing infection from the procedure is minimized by adhering to a meticulous aseptic technique.

Another important indication for arthrocentesis and intraarticular steroid therapy is OA associated with crystal synovitis due to calcium pyrophosphate dihydrate disease (CPPD) or pseudogout. Diagnosis is confirmed by radiographic findings of chondrocalcinosis and polarized microscopic identification of the specific crystals in the fluid. Treatment, including aspiration and administration of intraarticular steroids, is usually successful in controlling the acute synovitis.

Hyaluronans (Hyaluronic Acid, Hyaluronate)

Intraarticular hyaluronan, approved by the FDA in 1997 as a new procedure for clinical use in OA of the knee, represents a valuable addition to the therapeutic armamentarium for the treatment of OA. The clinical use of intraarticular hyaluronan in painful OA of the knee was introduced in Europe in the 1990s. The mechanism of action of hyaluronate is termed *viscosupplementation* in an effort to restore normal viscoelastic properties to the pathologically altered synovial fluid. Other possible beneficial effects include protection of the chondrocytes, antiinflammatory effects, and improvement of the mechanics of joint motion.

Numerous preparations of FDA approved hyaluronan preparations are in wide use in the United States. Initially, all hyaluronans were extracted from rooster combs. Table 1 lists the more common hyaluronans that are available for injecting knee osteoarthritis. The hyaluronan products are injected in a series of three, four, or five at weekly intervals in accordance with the patient's response. All the hyaluronans are highly purified natural preparations except Hylan G-F20, which is cross-linked with added formaldehyde and vinyl sulfone in an effort to increase retention in the joint cavity. Effectiveness and duration of improvement are similar with all the products. Undesirable complications and adverse effects are limited to rare local mild pain, with the exception of the cross-linked Hylan G-F20, which can cause a severe acute inflammatory reaction (SAIR, or pseudoseptic reaction) in approximately 2% to 8% of patients injected with the product.

Newer hyaluronan products are non–animal-derived preparations that are developed from biological fermentation of streptococcal origin. Until recently, these hyaluronans have been available only in Europe. One of these products (Euflexxa) has been approved by the

FDA for use in the United States. This preparation would be especially useful in the rare patient who is allergic to avian products. Hyaluronan therapy has been studied in other specific joints including the hip, shoulder, ankle, and first carpometacarpal joints. Approval from the FDA is expected. Drawbacks of intraarticular hyaluronan include difficulty injecting and limited response in patients with extreme obesity and severe advanced osteoarthritis of the knee (grade 4 Kellgren classification). Re-treatment with intraarticular hyaluronic acid 1 year after the first series is safe and effective in patients whose initial course of therapy was successful. A new hyaluronan preparation (Monovisc) has been developed, containing 4 or 5 times the amount of hyaluronan used in the usual knee injection, which is given in a series of 3 or 4 weekly injections. The approach, if effective, would simplify the procedure, especially for "needle shy" patients. The treatment is available in Europe but is not FDA approved as yet for use in the United States.

JOINT LAVAGE AND ARTHROSCOPY

Lavage of the arthritic knee may be performed with arthroscopic visualization. The authors of a recent double-blind sham-controlled evaluation concluded that "most, if not all" of the effects of tidal irrigation seem to be attributable to a placebo effect. Arthroscopy permits inspection of the joint cavity. Associated abnormalities such as ligamentous and meniscal tears can be observed in conjunction with osteoarthritis. Calcified loose bodies can be removed, and débridement can be carried out.

TREATMENT OF CYSTIC EROSIVE (INFLAMMATORY) OSTEOARTHRITIS

Cystic erosive OA is the genetically determined clinical syndrome manifested by the lumpy-bumpy fingers with involvement of the DIP joints (Heberden's nodes) and proximal interphalangeal joints (Bouchard's nodules). It rarely causes significant pain except during the early developing stage. It is important to strongly reassure the patient that this is not a serious crippling disease, emphasizing the distinction of the knobby nodes from the swelling of the synovitis of RA. However, if the thumb base joint (trapeziometacarpal, first carpometacarpal) is involved, abduction splinting or local injection may be necessary for relief of pain.

Occasionally, when OA of the fingers is symptomatic, warm soaks; application of an analgesic balm, such as triethanolamine, after the warm soaks; and the wearing of spandex gloves during sleep at night are sometimes useful. When a digital node is inflamed, local instillation of a few drops of a corticosteroid suspension often provides prompt relief.

If symptoms persist, a cautious trial with one of the topical analgesic pepper plant creams (capsaicin) such as Zostrix may be worthwhile. Capsaicin is an inhibitor of substance P, the neuropeptide pain mediator. The topical cream is safe, and a local burning or transient stinging sensation during application is the only troublesome adverse effect. The stinging diminishes with use after a few days.

NEW APPROACHES

Disease-Modifying Drugs

The purpose of the investigational disease-modifying drugs is to play a role in either enhancing the biosynthesis of cartilage matrix or preventing enzymatic degradation and inhibiting catabolic cytokine activity in an attempt to induce cartilage repair and restore joint homeostasis.

Tetracycline (Sumycin)[1] and its congeners (doxycycline (Vibramycin),[1] minocycline (Dynacin)[1]) have shown evidence of inhibiting enzymatic degradation of cartilage, including that by stromelysin, collagenase, and gelatinase, in dog, guinea pig, and rabbit models of OA. A proposed long-term clinical trial in human subjects is in progress.

Hydroxychloroquine (Plaquenil)[1] and chloroquine (Aralen)[1] have been administered successfully for many years in RA and systemic

TABLE 1 Some Common FDA-Approved Hyaluronans and Their Molecular Weights

Product	MW (kDa)	Dose (Weekly)
Hylan G-F20 (Synvisc)	5000–6000	3 × 16 mg
High-molecular-weight hyaluronan (Orthovisc)	1000–2900	3–4 × 30 mg
Sodium hyaluronate (Hyalgan)	500–720	3–5 × 20 mg
Sodium hyaluronate (Supartz)	620–1200	5 × 25 mg
1% Sodium hyaluronate (Euflexxa)*	2400–3600	3 × 20 mg

*Derived from biological fermentations.

[1]Not FDA approved for this indication.

lupus erythematosus. Recently, anecdotal and retrospective uncontrolled studies have reported the efficacy of hydroxychloroquine in retarding the progression of inflammatory (cystic) erosive OA. It has been suggested that the beneficial action of hydroxychloroquine is due to its inhibitory effects on lysosomal enzymes and the secretion of interleukin-1. Experience thus far suggests that this agent may be promising in inflammatory OA.

Other novel therapeutic approaches that are under study but lack conclusive significant data at this time include insulin-like growth factors, transforming growth factor-β, and glucosamine, a proteoglycan component and a growth factor for cartilage. In ongoing studies, an antinerve growth factor antibody, fully humanized, effectively reduces pain and improves function in subjects with knee osteoarthritis. Undesirable effects so far are minor, including a rare transient mild peripheral neuritis.

Chondrocyte Transplantation

Chondrocyte transplantation was initially developed and carried out in Sweden for localized cartilage damage resulting from trauma in young subjects. A subsequent report described relatively successful treatment of 23 patients who had chondral defects of the knee and were given autologous chondrocyte transplantation combined with periosteal grafting. The expectation that the procedure will "cure" OA lesions remains an unmet possibility for the future. Regeneration of articular cartilage is a complex process and will require long-term evaluation of the function of the new cartilage and prospective controlled clinical studies to confirm the value of the procedure.

Gene Therapy

Gene therapy is an exciting new technology that holds promise for the future but requires considerable further investigation and refinement. Techniques to introduce gene transfer in conjunction with autologous cultured chondrocytes are being explored.

Glucosamine and Chondroitin Sulfate

Glucosamine[7] and chondroitin[7] sulfate are over-the-counter nutraceuticals (dietary supplements) that have considerable anecdotal data touting their symptom-modifying effects. Some reports have suggested that glucosamine can retard or modify structural changes of OA, but convincing evidence for this effect is lacking. The drugs are well tolerated and have no significant adverse effects. Recently published studies have no evidence or significant data demonstrating that either of these preparations used alone or in combination prevents or reduces pain in osteoarthritis of the knee. Further observations with long-term randomized, double-blind studies are needed to confirm any value of these popular but unproved medications.

SURGERY

When appropriate medical (nonoperative) management fails to adequately control pain, and functional disability significantly interferes with lifestyle, surgical options should be considered.

Available procedures include osteotomy for joint malalignment (varus knee deformities); arthroscopy, especially for specific lesions such as calcified loose bodies or meniscal tears; and arthrodesis (fusion) for unstable joints, when joint replacement is not indicated or declined. Arthrodesis may be the optimal procedure in young, overweight, active patients with severe OA involving a single knee.

Partial or total arthroplasty, especially total knee and hip replacement, may be carried out in patients in whom medical management fails to adequately control symptoms. An estimated 125,000 total hip replacements, most of which are for OA, are performed each year in the United States. Total knee replacement (total knee arthroplasty) is an increasingly gratifying operation for advanced knee OA. Innovative approaches and new techniques, including the development of minimal invasive procedures (MIS), bodes well for the future.

---

[7]Available as a dietary supplement.

REFERENCES

Mandell BF, Lipani J. Refractory osteoarthritis. Differential diagnosis and therapy. Rheum Dis Clin North Am 1995;21:163–78.

Neustadt DH. Intra-articular injections for osteoarthritis of the knee. Cleve Clin J Med 2006;73:897–910.

Neustadt DH. Current approach to therapy for osteoarthritis of the knee. Louisville Med 2004;51:341–3.

Neustadt DH, Altman RD. Intra-articular therapy. In: Moskowitz RW, Howell DS, Goldberg VM, et al., editors. Osteoarthritis, Diagnosis and Medical/Surgical Management. 4th ed. Philadelphia: Lippincott Williams & Wilkins; 2007. p. 287–301.

Poole AR, Howell DS. Etiopathogenesis of osteoarthritis. In: Moskowitz RW, Howell DS, Goldberg VM, et al., editors. Osteoarthritis, Diagnosis and Medical/Surgical Management. 4th ed. Philadelphia: Lippincott Williams & Wilkins; 2007. p. 27–49.

Sharma L, Kapoor D, Issa S. Epidemiology of osteoarthritis. In: Moskowitz RW, Howell DS, Goldberg VM, et al., editors. Osteoarthritis, Diagnosis and Medical/Surgical Management. 4th ed. Philadelphia: Lippincott Williams & Wilkins; 2007. p. 1–26.

Steinbrocker O, Neustadt DH. Aspiration and Injection Therapy. Arthritis and Musculoskeletal Disorders: A Handbook on Technique and Management. Hagerstown MD: Harper & Row; 1972.

Polymyalgia Rheumatica and Giant Cell Arteritis

Method of

Maria C. Cid, MD, Georgina Espígol-Frigolé, MD, Ana García-Martínez, MD, and José Hernández-Rodríguez, MD

Giant cell arteritis (GCA), the most common form of systemic vasculitis in Western countries, is a chronic granulomatous inflammatory disease that preferentially involves large and medium-sized arteries in individuals older than 50 years. It affects mostly white populations and is two or three times more common in women than in men.

The classic clinical manifestations of GCA derive from symptomatic involvement of the cranial arteries and include headache, jaw claudication, scalp tenderness, and a variety of craniofacial aches, including otalgia, odynophagia, carotodynia, toothaches, and tongue pain. Vascular occlusion leads to ischemic complications in 15% to 20% of patients. Complete or partial visual loss due to anterior ischemic optic neuritis (AION) and, less frequently, to occlusion of the central retinal artery or its branches is the most common ischemic complication of GCA. Stroke due to occlusion of vertebral or carotid artery branches may occur in 2% to 3% of patients. Inflammation of large arteries is usually silent, but up to 22.5% of patients develop significant aortic dilatation over the years, and 5% may die of dissection or rupture. Stenosis of supra-aortic branches or arteries supplying the extremities leading to limb claudication may occur in 5% to 15% of patients.

About 50% of GCA patients have polymyalgia rheumatica (PMR), a syndrome characterized by pain and stiffness in the upper and lower girdles and mainly derived from inflammation of the periarticular structures in proximal joints. PMR may appear concurrently with vascular symptoms, may precede clinically apparent vascular involvement by months or even years, or may appear during relapses in patients who presented with cranial symptoms only at the time of diagnosis. PMR may occur as an isolated entity, with no evidence of vascular inflammation. Isolated PMR is about three times more common than GCA.

GCA and PMR are characterized by a prominent acute-phase reaction, including systemic symptoms (i.e., low-grade fever and weight loss), anemia of the chronic disease type, accelerated erythrocyte sedimentation rate, and increased concentration of acute-phase proteins such as C-reactive protein. Thrombocytosis and increased alkaline phosphatase levels may be observed. The intensity of the acute-phase response varies among patients, and a small percentage of individuals with GCA or PMR may have near-normal or normal acute-phase reactants.

Diagnosis

Histopathologic examination of a biopsy of the superficial temporal artery provides the definitive diagnosis of GCA. Typical changes consist of mononuclear cell inflammation of the artery wall, internal elastic lamina disruption, intimal hyperplasia, and presence of the characteristic multinucleated giant cells in about 50% of cases. The extent of the inflammatory infiltrates varies, and sometimes, there are incomplete features that need to be recognized, such as mild adventitial inflammation or inflammation limited to the vasa vasorum. Although the specificity of the temporal artery biopsy approaches 100%, the sensitivity is lower because of the segmental nature of the lesions, which may sometimes spare the segment excised. Occasionally, the temporal artery or its branches may be involved by other systemic vasculitis.

The diagnostic usefulness of vascular imaging techniques has been evaluated. Although sensitivity is lower, color duplex ultrasonography of the temporal artery may disclose a hypoechoic halo surrounding the lumen, and high-resolution magnetic resonance imaging (MRI) may reveal thickening and contrast enhancement of the temporal artery wall. Both findings have a remarkable specificity for GCA.

CURRENT THERAPY

Starting Therapy

- GCA: Prednisone or prednisolone[1] 40 to 60 mg/day for 4 weeks. Low-dose aspirin 80 to 100 mg/day is recommended if transient or permanent ischemic events are present.
- Isolated PMR: Prednisone or prednisolone 10 to 20 mg/day for 4 weeks

Remission Maintenance and Glucocorticosteroid Tapering

- GCA: Reduction of 5 to 10 mg/week until dose is 15 mg/day. Subsequent reduction must be slower and aimed to achieve a maintenance dose of 5 to 10 mg/day at 12 months. Attempt to slowly discontinue prednisone or prednisolone after 2 years.
- PMR: Reduction of 2.5/day per month until a maintenance dose of 5 to 7.5 mg/day is achieved. Attempt to slowly discontinue prednisone after 2 years.

Disease Flares

- GCA: Increase 10 mg/day above the previously effective dose.
- PMR: Increase 2.5 to 5 mg above the previously effective dose.
- Adjuvant therapy: Methotrexate (Trexall)[1] at 10 to 15 mg/week; azathioprine (Imuran)[1] at 100 mg/day if there are contraindications for methotrexate. Adjuvant therapy must be considered in patients requiring maintenance glucocorticosteroid doses higher than those recommended previously or patients with difficult-to-manage glucocorticosteroid-related side effects.

Supportive Therapy

- Bone protection
- Control and treatment of conditions increasing vascular risk

---

[1]Not FDA approved for this indication.

The diagnosis of PMR is based on clinical criteria, which are being revised and validated by an international group of experts. Bilateral shoulder and pelvic aches and stiffness, systemic complaints, elevation of acute-phase reactants, and exclusion of other diseases are important clues for diagnosis. Ultrasonography and MRI may disclose subacromial or subdeltoid bursitis in the upper girdle and trochanteric bursitis as a substrate for symptoms in the lower girdle. Interspinous bursitis can be seen and may account for neck pain and stiffness, which are common in PMR.

Treatment

Glucocorticoids efficiently abrogate the clinical manifestations of GCA and prevent progression of visual loss in patients with transient blindness (i.e., amaurosis fugax) or partial defects. Treatment with glucocorticoids should be promptly started as soon as the diagnosis of GCA is established or when the diagnosis of GCA is strongly suspected and visual symptoms are present. Prednisone[1] and prednisolone (Millipred)[1] are widely used preparations, and the initial dose usually is 40 to 60 mg/day. This dose is maintained for 4 weeks, until remission of all symptoms and laboratory abnormalities is achieved. Glucocorticoids must be subsequently tapered, but the optimal tapering schedule has not been defined. Prednisone or prednisolone is commonly reduced at a rate of 5 to 10 mg/week until a daily dose of 15 mg is attained. Subsequent reductions must be slower and individualized, and they are aimed at achieving a maintenance dose of 5 to 7.5 mg/day 8 to 12 months after starting treatment. Isolated PMR also responds quickly to glucocorticoids at doses between 10 and 20 mg/day, which are usually maintained for 4 weeks, with subsequent slow tapering. Alternate-day administration is not advised because it is less effective than daily administration to control disease activity.

Disease flares during glucocorticoids reduction are common in GCA and PMR, occurring in 40% to 60% of patients. Flares usually appear when glucocorticoids are reduced below 15–20 mg/day and are exceptional while patients are receiving higher doses. Relapses are typically accompanied by a rebound in acute-phase reactants. Some patients maintain slightly elevated levels of acute-phase reactants with no clinical symptoms. Subclinical activity does not require an increase in glucocorticoids unless anemia or malaise not attributable to other causes occurs. About 40% to 60% of patients with GCA or PMR are able to discontinue glucocorticoids after 2 to 3 years of treatment. The remaining patients need more prolonged therapy.

Glucocorticoid-related adverse events are common in patients with GCA and PMR. Bone fractures, hypertension, diabetes, hypercholesterolemia, infections, myopathy, gastrointestinal bleeding, and cataracts are the more frequent effects. Weight increase, easy bruising, and sleep disturbances are also common.

TREATMENT OF VISUAL IMPAIRMENT

Visual loss is the most common and dreaded ischemic complication in GCA. It is frequently an early event in the course of the disease and is often preceded by transient symptoms (amaurosis fugax). When partial deficits occur, the probability of progression and involvement of the second eye is very high. Sight impairment is a medical emergency requiring immediate treatment. When visual loss is established, chances of recovery with any treatment are low. Objective improvement is observed in only 4% of patients. The main goal of intensive therapy is preserving the remaining vision rather than recovery. Pulsed intravenous treatment with 1 g of methylprednisolone (Solu-Medrol)[1] for 3 days is frequently advised, but there is no objective proof that this treatment achieves better results than the standard therapy. Low-dose aspirin[1] is also recommended. About 10% of patients presenting with visual symptoms have continuing deterioration of vision despite treatment during the first 1 to 2 weeks. When remission is attained, the probability of subsequent vision loss due to GCA is about 1% during a median follow-up of 5 years.

---

[1]Not FDA approved for this indication.

GLUCOCORTICOID-SPARING AGENTS

The high incidence of glucocorticoid-related side effects has motivated a search for glucocorticoid-sparing agents. A meta-analysis of three randomized, controlled trials demonstrated a modest effect of methotrexate[1] in reducing the likelihood of relapses and cumulated glucocorticoid doses. Azathioprine (Imuran)[1] may have some effect, as indicated by a randomized, controlled trial that included a small number of patients. Evidence supporting the usefulness of other immunosuppressive agents is weak. A randomized, controlled trial enrolling newly diagnosed patients failed to demonstrate the benefit of infliximab (Remicade)[1] over placebo in maintaining glucocorticoid-induced disease remission. Similar findings were obtained for patients with isolated PMR. A randomized, controlled trial of etanercept (Enbrel)[1] showed a trend toward benefit in GCA patients with relapsing disease or with glucocorticoid-related side effects, but the number of patients enrolled was insufficient to draw solid conclusions.

VASCULAR INTERVENTION: ANGIOPLASTY AND SURGERY

About 22.5% of patients with GCA develop significant aortic dilatation or aneurysms, mostly in the thoracic aorta. About one fourth of them are candidates for surgical repair due to the diameter of the aneurysm and the consequent risk of rupture or due to aortic valve insufficiency. Patients with GCA should be routinely screened for aortic dilatation. The frequency and method of screening have not been defined. Physical examination in search for aortic murmur, chest radiograph, and abdominal ultrasonography may be useful for routine screening of significant aortic dilatation. There is no evidence supporting any change in glucocorticoid doses when an aneurysm is discovered.

A less defined proportion of patients, about 5% to 15%, suffer from large-vessel stenosis leading to limb claudication or ischemia. When claudication occurs in the lower limbs, its relationship with GCA is difficult to define due to the age of the population targeted by GCA and the frequent coexistence of vascular risk factors. Large-vessel stenosis may partially respond to glucocorticoid therapy, but it may eventually require angioplasty, stenting, or bypass surgery.

PREVENTION OF CARDIOVASCULAR RISK FACTORS

The existence of vascular risk factors at diagnosis is associated with a higher frequency of GCA-related ischemic events. Although some studies indicate that patients with GCA may have an increased incidence of cardiovascular events, this has not been confirmed in other studies. However, appropriate control of diabetes, hypertension, hypercholesterolemia, and overweight is advisable, particularly in patients subjected to long-term use of glucocorticoids, which by themselves may cause or worsen these conditions. Low-dose aspirin is not indiscriminately advised, but it seems reasonable in patients with vascular risk factors and patients who have presented with transient or permanent disease-related ischemic complications. Proton pump inhibitors are recommended when using aspirin and glucocorticoids in this population.

BONE PROTECTION

GCA is a disease preferentially targeting elderly white women who are particularly prone to have low bone mass and to develop glucocorticoid-induced osteoporosis. Appropriate calcium and vitamin D supplements and bisphosphonates are advised during glucocorticoid treatment.

REFERENCES

Blockmans D, Bley T, Schmidt W. Imaging for large vessel vasculitis. Curr Opin Rheumatol 2009;21:19–28.

Cid MC, García-Martínez A, Lozano E, et al. Five clinical conundrums in the management of giant-cell arteritis. Rheum Clin Dis North Am 2007;33:819–34.

García-Martínez A, Hernández-Rodríguez J, Arguis P, et al. Development of aortic aneurysm/dilatation during the followup of patients with giant cell arteritis: A cross-sectional screening of fifty-four prospectively followed patients. Arthritis Rheum 2008;59:422–30.

Hoffman GS, Cid MC, Hellmann DB, et al. A multicenter, randomized, double-blind, placebo-controlled trial of adjuvant methotrexate treatment for giant-cell arteritis. Arthritis Rheum 2002;46:1309–18.

Hoffman GS, Cid MC, Rendt-Zagar K, et al. Infliximab for maintenance of glucocorticoid-induced remission of giant-cell arteritis. Ann Intern Med 2007;146:621–30.

Mahr AD, Jover JA, Spiera RF, et al. Adjunctive methotrexate for treatment of giant cell arteritis: An individual patient data meta-analysis. Arthritis Rheum 2007;56:2789–97.

Michet CJ, Matteson EL. Polymyalgia rheumatica. Br Med J 2008;336:765–9.

Mukhtyar C, Guillevin L, Cid MC, et al. EULAR recommendations for the management of large vessel vasculitis. Ann Rheum Dis 2009;68:318–23.

Proven A, Gabriel SE, Orces C, et al. Glucocorticoid therapy in giant-cell arteritis. Duration and adverse outcomes. Arthritis Rheum 2003;49:703–8.

Salvarani C, Cantini F, Hunder GG. Polymyalgia rheumatica and giant-cell arteritis. Lancet 2008;372:234–45.

Osteomyelitis

Method of
*Brian K. Albertson, MD, and
George D. Harris, MD, MS*

Osteomyelitis is a disease of the bone that has changed over the years from a primarily hematogenous disease with high mortality to one of high morbidity. Since the introduction of antibiotics, the incidence of hematogenous osteomyelitis has declined, whereas infection from direct inoculation has increased, especially in those with diabetes. Several methods are used to classify osteomyelitis; most separate the illness into acute or chronic types and hematogenous or contiguous types. Local extension may occur from spread from adjacent structures, or direct implantation of organisms may occur, as seen in cases of trauma or surgical procedures.

The Cierny-Mader system assigns the patient to one of several groups based on the anatomy of the infection and health of the host, including the increased risk for patients who have peripheral arterial obstructive disease or diabetes mellitus. Patients are further separated according to systemic and local factors that may influence disease progression or healing, such as diabetes, extremes of age, and tobacco use. In diabetic patients, osteomyelitis is most commonly caused by overlying lower limb cellulitis. In the nondiabetic adult patient, vertebral osteomyelitis is most common.

The Cierny-Mader classification allows the clinician to use tested treatment protocols, including chemotherapy, surgery, and adjunctive therapies, that are most effective for a specific class of disease and for the host status. The Cierny-Mader system divides the patients into four anatomic groups. Stage 1, or medullary osteomyelitis, is confined to the endosteum of the bone and is often hematogenous. State 2, or superficial osteomyelitis, is localized to the surface of the bone. This is a true contiguous lesion. Stage 3, or localized osteomyelitis, involves cortical sequestration or cavitation, or both, and is a full-thickness lesion that extends into the medullary region. Stage 4, or diffuse osteomyelitis, involves the hard and soft tissues ("through and through"), and it requires surgical débridement of the affected bone to remove all the infected tissue.

For treatment to be successful, the patient must be physiologically able to heal any wounds, defend against contamination or infection,

---

TABLE 1   Cierny-Mader Classification System

Feature	Examples
Anatomic type	Stage 1: medullary osteomyelitis
	Stage 2: superficial osteomyelitis
	Stage 3: localized osteomyelitis
	Stage 4: diffuse osteomyelitis
Physiologic class	A: normal (healthy) host
	B: compromised host
	B_S: systemically compromised
	B_L: locally compromised
	C: treatment worse than disease
Factors affecting host status	
Systemic	Malnutrition
	Renal and hepatic failure
	Diabetes mellitus
	Chronic hypoxia
	Immune disease
	Malignancy
	Extremes of age
	Immunosuppression
Local	Chronic lymphedema
	Venous stasis
	Major vessel compromise
	Arteritis
	Extensive scarring
	Radiation fibrosis
	Small-vessel disease
	Neuropathy
	Tobacco use

and tolerate the stress of treatment. The hosts are classified as A, B, or C, depending on the ability to resist infections. Those with good immunity are classified as an A host, whereas a B host is compromised locally (B_L) or systemically (B_S); Table 1 shows the physiologic classifications. The final class assigns a C rating to patients whose treatment is more detrimental than the disability from the disease. These patients may require suppressive or no treatment. The clinical stages are adjusted during the course of therapy as conditions change, allowing adjustment of the treatment protocol to optimize therapy.

A much simpler system described by Waldvogel classifies the patient by duration (i.e., acute or chronic) and the mechanism of inoculation (i.e., hematogenous or contiguous). Contiguous infections are further classified as those with or without vascular insufficiency. However, this classification does not provide guidance for specific surgical or antibiotic therapy.

Epidemiology

Acute hematogenous osteomyelitis is usually seen in male children of lower socioeconomic class before the age of 2 years or between 8 and 12 years. There may be some genetic influences. Aboriginal children in Western Australia are known to suffer from acute hematogenous osteomyelitis at a rate nearly four times that of Western European children living in the same neighborhood. An acute infection will progress to chronic osteomyelitis if it is not treated.

Chronic osteomyelitis is usually the result of direct inoculation (e.g., trauma, surgery). Its epidemiology is less clearly described, except in diabetic foot infections. It is estimated that 11 million people in the United States suffer from diabetes. Annually, more than 300,000 of them develop a foot ulcer, and nearly one third of those require amputations. In 2002, osteomyelitis was estimated to cost the citizens of the United States more than $2.3 billion dollars. This major public health problem is expected to increase as the incidence of adults with diabetes increases. Because chronic infection can persist for life, it is important to have early identification and treatment to ensure the best possible outcome.

Pathogenesis

The presence of bacteria in an open wound is not sufficient to cause infection. It is the compromised blood supply of traumatized tissue leading to necrosis and subsequent bacterial adherence that promotes the infection. Trauma can delay the inflammatory response to bacteria, depress cell-mediated immunity, and impair chemotaxis, superoxide production, and the microbial killing capacity of polymorphonuclear neutrophils (PMNs). Osteomyelitis usually involves the metaphysic, which is well vascularized and has significant bone growth.

In acute osteomyelitis, signs or symptoms are usually abrupt. Local infection is characterized by edema, vascular congestion, and small-vessel thrombosis. This leads to increased pressure within the intramedullary canal, allowing extravasation through the Havers and Volkmann canals to the periosteum. In children, the periosteum is usually more flexible and easier to detect radiographically; in adults, the bone matrix is more firmly attached to the periosteum. Untreated, the suppurative infection can reach adjacent soft tissue, leading to a cellulitis. The presence of a Brodie or intraosseous abscess without extravasation into surrounding tissue is classified as subacute pyogenic osteomyelitis. The resulting infection can lead to sequestration involving large areas of bone destruction and dead bone, with reactive bone formation leading ultimately to chronic osteomyelitis.

Chronic osteomyelitis is usually polymicrobial and is characterized by the presence of necrotic bone, new bone growth, and exudation of polymorphonuclear leukocytes, plasma cells, and other infection-fighting cells. The involucrum (i.e., layer of reactive competent bone that covers dead bone) is often dotted with tracts that allow pus to pass into surrounding tissue or to form a sinus tract to the skin surface. These sinus tracts are often contaminated with numerous organisms that do not reflect those found with direct sampling. This repetitive process of bone loss and growth and the involucrum explains why chronic osteomyelitis is difficult to eradicate with antibiotics alone. The antibiotics cannot penetrate avascular areas.

Etiology

CHILDREN

In children of all ages, the most common bacterial pathogen is *Staphylococcus aureus,* followed by *Streptococcus pneumoniae* and *Kingella kingae.* However, age and chronic illness allow other organisms to flourish; *Salmonella* and pneumococcal disease (*S. pneumoniae*) are common in patients with sickle cell disease. *Pasteurella multocida, Streptococcus* species, and anaerobes often are identified after animal or human bites. In children, most cases arise hematogenously and are characteristically seen in the metaphysis of long bones (i.e., femur, tibia, and humerus), accounting for 68% of childhood infections.

The exact mechanism is unclear, but it is thought that the extensive branching of the nutrient-rich arteries at the metaphyses of the long bones leads to sluggish blood flow and ultimate bacterial seeding. Possible routes include the formation of small hematomas in the metaphysis, allowing microbial seeding after transient bacteremia; penetrating injuries or surgical manipulation, causing direct inoculation of bacteria into bone; and local invasion from a contiguous focus of infection.

ADULTS

Most infections in adults arise by direct inoculation from sources such as trauma, prosthetic joints, open fractures, and diabetic foot infections. The most common organism remains *S. aureus.* Other organisms to consider include *Staphylococcus epidermis, Pseudomonas aeruginosa, Escherichia coli,* and *Serratia marcescens.* Most contiguous, related infections are polymicrobial.

Clinical Manifestations

The severity of the signs and symptoms depends on the location of the infection, the patient's age, and any comorbidities. Patients may experience many, few, or no symptoms. Classically, there are marked pain, tenderness, and swelling. Fever and leukocytosis are also common.

Vertebral osteomyelitis often causes severe pain, fever, and disability, whereas osteomyelitis of the foot rarely causes pain. An epidural abscess causes pain and neurologic deficits, whereas vertebral osteomyelitis without abscess formation has no neurologic deficits.

Children often present with systemic symptoms (e.g., fever, weight loss, pain). Pseudoparalysis may be the only sign in a newborn, but toddlers often exhibit pain, fever, erythema, edema, or warmth, or they may suddenly stop walking. In contrast, patients with chronic osteomyelitis may exhibit localized signs and symptoms, including nonhealing ulcers, purulence from sinus tracts, soft tissue edema and pain, abscesses, erythema, pain, and fatigue. Generalized signs and symptoms may be seen early in the disease, but they are unlikely in the later or chronic stages.

Diagnosis

LABORATORY TESTS

A bone biopsy remains the gold standard when diagnosing osteomyelitis. However, there is a high false-negative rate, and the negative predictive value is close to 65%, mainly due to the organism's patchy distribution. No specific laboratory test can be recommended. However, testing acute-phase reactants (e.g., erythrocyte sedimentation rate [ESR], C-reactive protein [CRP], leukocyte count with a differential count) can strongly suggest (positive predictive value of 100%) osteomyelitis if the ESR value is greater than 70 mm/hour in the absence of an inflamed ulcer. However, these tests lack specificity, and it may take several days to demonstrate significantly elevated levels. All patients should have blood cultures performed. A positive blood culture with a suspicious physical finding can suggest a bone infection, but only one half of the cases have a positive test result. Blood cultures, like bone biopsies, can be affected by recent antibiotic exposure.

RADIOLOGY

There is no one imaging modality routinely recommended to diagnose osteomyelitis, often requiring more than one technique. Plain film radiography should always be the initial study, and the result can be diagnostic if positive. However, changes (usually along the metaphysic) typically require at least 1 to 2 weeks to be seen radiographically.

Positive emission topography (PET) is the most specific and sensitive of imaging techniques, but its high cost and lack of availability makes it impractical for most clinicians. The best choice for imaging depends on the age of the patient, duration of symptoms, suspected location of infection (if known), and concurrent or previous medical conditions.

Plain radiographs are the most available, least expensive, and easiest to obtain, but they lack sensitivity (43%–75%), and a negative result does not exclude the diagnosis. However, they have reasonable specificity (75%–83%), and a positive finding can confirm the diagnosis or provide clues to alternative pathology, such as a tumor. Bony changes can take between 10 and 21 days to become visible on plain films; however, soft tissue changes can be seen in as little as 3 days. The soft tissue changes are especially important in neonates and children because focal soft tissue swelling around the bony metaphysis may be the first sign of bone involvement.

Radionuclide imaging (i.e., triple-phase bone scan, leukocyte scintigraphy, and PET) is a preferred method of advanced imaging, and it has several advantages compared with other techniques. Young children often complete the examination without sedation, and

prosthetic joints do not produce the artifact commonly seen on magnetic resonance imaging (MRI) and computed tomography (CT) scans. Positive results can be seen 24 to 48 hours after onset of symptoms, and a negative examination result effectively rules out osteomyelitis.

The triple-phase bone scan (technetium 99m diphosphonate) is often the examination of choice (sensitivity of 73%–100%), and it can distinguish between cellulitis and osteomyelitis when complications are absent. However, the sensitivity decreases dramatically when other conditions are present (i.e., trauma, diabetes, or recent surgery), and it has been reported to be as low as 38%. Bone scans usually lack the specificity (25%–90%) of other modalities, fail to provide detailed pictures of complex anatomy, and can be influenced by poor circulation. The examination takes up to 48 hours to complete and often requires the patient to make many trips to the facility. In the early phase, uptake is greatest in areas of acute inflammation. In the next phase, uptake occurs in areas of soft tissue inflammation, and in the late (delayed) phase, uptake remains in the presence of osteomyelitis.

Leukocyte scintigraphy using gallium 67 has a higher specificity (80%–90%) than triple-phase scanning (67%) in the peripheral skeleton, but it decreases to 25% when looking at the axial skeleton. Leukocyte scintigraphy is the preferred method when evaluating patients with previous joint replacements, diabetes, or trauma.

MRI can detect acute osteomyelitis as early as 3 days. It is nearly as sensitive (82%–100%) and specific (75%–96%) as radionuclide studies. MRI allows tracking of disease progress and response to treatment. MRI can be used to date osteomyelitis. Some patients with osteomyelitis are treated and later develop another episode. The MRI can distinguish whether the second episode is a new infection or a recurrence of the previous infection. It also provides detailed visualization of complex anatomy and critical structures, allowing surgeons to map any planned surgical intervention.

CT is rarely used for osteomyelitis, except when sequestered bone is suspected or for interventional procedures. Sinography can be used to map sinus tracts with fluoroscopy or combined with CT. Ultrasound is sometimes used in children and can be helpful in differentiating acute from chronic infections. It provides guidance during drainage, aspirations, or biopsies of the affected bone, and it is a noninvasive method to monitor soft tissue involvement in chronic illness.

CURRENT DIAGNOSIS

- A bone biopsy remains the gold standard when diagnosing osteomyelitis.
- All patients should have blood cultures performed.
- No one imaging modality is routinely recommended to diagnose osteomyelitis.
- Plain film radiography should always be the initial study and can be diagnostic if positive.
- Magnetic resonance imaging (MRI) can detect acute osteomyelitis as early as 3 days.

CURRENT THERAPY

- The Cierny-Mader classification system provides an easy-to-use algorithm for treatment (Box 1).
- The most important factor in any treatment is identification of the organism.
- The optimal duration of antibiotic therapy remains undefined, with most authorities recommending treatment for about 6 weeks.
- Hematogenous osteomyelitis is usually monomicrobial, whereas contiguous infections are usually polymicrobial.

BOX 1 Management of Suspected Osteomyelitis

History and physical findings suggesting osteomyelitis
Nonhealing ulcer present
Yes
Is bone visible or accessible by sterile probe?
Yes
Osteomyelitis
No
No
Plain radiography
Positive
Osteomyelitis
Treat empirically
Bone biopsy
Adjust treatment if appropriate
No
Highly suspicious
Further evaluation
Less suspicious
Repeat radiologic examination in 2 weeks
Further evaluation
ESR >70 mm/h
Yes
Osteomyelitis
No
Blood cultures
Positive
Treat accordingly
Source suspected
MRI of suspected part
Source site unknown
Bone scan
Negative
Bone scan
Bone scan
Source located
Yes
Bone biopsy
Treat accordingly
Treat empirically until biopsy or culture provides sensitivities
Consider MRI or CT scan if surgery considered
No source
Consider alternative pathology

Treatment

Older methods, such as closed suction drains, are no longer commonly used because of long hospital stays and the risk of contamination, and newer modalities, such as hyperbaric oxygen therapy, have failed to live up to expectations. The Cierny-Mader classification system provides a straightforward algorithm for treatment. However, the most important factor in any treatment is the identification of the causative organism.

ANTIBIOTIC THERAPY

Unlike chronic infections, acute infections require hospitalization for initiation of therapy and supportive care. Serial examinations should be undertaken to assess the success of treatment and monitor for systemic signs or symptoms. Cultures of blood and bone should be obtained to guide therapy. Laboratory studies can be followed, but other than CRP levels, they fail to provide significant data. The CRP value can be expected to decrease 24 to 48 hours after initiation of appropriate antibiotic therapy. A lack of response may indicate inappropriate therapy or an occult abscess, and the physician should reconsider surgery if previously delayed.

The medical literature remains inconclusive about the antibiotic treatment of osteomyelitis, especially when trying to determine the best agents, route, or duration of antibiotic therapy. Although the optimal duration of antibiotic therapy remains undefined, most authorities recommend treatment for about 6 weeks (Table 2). After the infection is under control, the physician may switch the patient to an oral antibiotic for 3 to 12 months (i.e., a fluoroquinolone with or without rifampin [Rifadin][1]). However, treatment can be as short as 3 weeks for uncomplicated acute, hematogenous osteomyelitis. Management can include oral preparations after a short parenteral course, provided the drug has high bioavailability and the organism is susceptible. A microbiologic diagnosis (preferably by bone biopsy) is essential so the choice of antibiotic accounts for the specific organism, the host status, and least toxic medication for the individual. Hematogenous osteomyelitis is usually monomicrobial, whereas contiguous infections are usually polymicrobial and may include *Pseudomonas* in certain populations.

For methicillin-sensitive *S. aureus*, nafcillin (Unipen) or a first- or second-generation cephalosporin can be implemented. For methicillin-resistant *S. aureus*, vancomycin (Vancocin) is recommended. For an anaerobic infection, clindamycin (Cleocin) is a good choice.

---

[1]Not FDA approved for this indication.

TABLE 2 Antibiotics for Osteomyelitis

Organism	Preferred Drug	Alternative Drugs
Staphylococcus aureus	Nafcillin (Unipen) 1–2 g IV or IM q4h	Cefazolin, vancomycin, clindamycin
Methicillin-resistant *S. aureus*	Vancomycin (Vancocin) 1 g q8h	Trimethoprim-sulfamethoxazole (Bactrim)[1] plus rifampin (Rifadin)[1]
Streptococcus pneumoniae, group A β-hemolytic streptococci	Penicillin G (Pfizerpen)[1] 2 million units IV q4h	Cefazolin, vancomycin, clindamycin
Enterococci, *Haemophilus influenzae* β-lactamase negative	Cefotaxime (Claforan) 2 g q6h	Trimethoprim-sulfamethoxazole, ceftriaxone
H. influenzae β-lactamase positive, *Klebsiella pneumoniae*	Ceftriaxone (Rocephin) 2 g q24h	Trimethoprim-sulfamethoxazole, ciprofloxacin, piperacillin (Pipracil), imipenem (Primaxin)
Escherichia coli	Cefazolin (Ancef) 2 g q8h	Ciprofloxacin, ceftriaxone, imipenem
Pseudomonas aeruginosa	Ciprofloxacin (Cipro) 400 mg q12h	Piperacillin plus aminoglycoside, aztreonam (Azactam)[1]
Salmonella	Choose ampicillin, ceftriaxone, imipenem (Primaxin), or ciprofloxacin, depending on sensitivities	
Bacteroides spp.	Clindamycin (Cleocin) 600 mg q6h	Imipenem, metronidazole (Flagyl)
Serratia marcescens	Ceftriaxone (Rocephin) 2 g q24h	Imipenem, trimethoprim-sulfamethoxazole, ciprofloxacin

Modified from Cohen J, Powderly WG (eds): Infectious Diseases, 2nd ed. St Louis, Mosby, 2003.
[1]Not FDA approved for this indication.

SURGERY

Bones can heal in the presence of active infection. However, in the presence of obvious signs of infection, such as an abscess or Cierny-Mader stage 3 or 4 disease, acute surgical débridement and irrigation are warranted. The goals of surgery include drainage, débridement, and stabilization. After successful débridement and stabilization, antibiotic therapy is initiated and continued until adequate healing has occurred, usually 6 weeks. If débridement is unsuccessful, inert substances must be completely removed and tissue débrided. Antibiotics should be placed in contact with the bone using a polymethylmethacrylate antibiotic (PMMA) bead chain or other biodegradable delivery systems to achieve higher local antibiotic concentrations. The site needs to be stabilized with an external fixator, and staged reconstruction should be initiated.

REFERENCES

Berendt A, Norden C. Acute and chronic osteomyelitis. In: Cohen J, Powderly WG, editors. Infectious Diseases, 2nd ed. St Louis: Mosby; 2003.

Cierny GIII, Mader JT, Pennick JJ. A clinical staging system for adult osteomyelitis. Contemp Orthop 1985;10:17–37.

Kaplan SL. Osteomyelitis in children. Infect Dis Clin North Am 2005;19:787–97.

Krogstad P. Osteomyelitis and septic arthritis. In: Feigin RD, Cherry JD, Demmler GJ, et al., editors. Textbook of Pediatric Infectious Diseases, 5th ed. Philadelphia: WB Saunders; 2004. p. 713–36.

Lampe RM. Osteomyelitis. In: Behrman RE, Kliegman RM, Jenson HB, Stanton BF, editors. Nelson Textbook of Pediatrics, 18th ed. Philadelphia: WB Saunders; 2007.

Lazzarini L, Lipsky BA, Mader JT. Antibiotic treatment of osteomyelitis: What have we learned from 30 years of clinical trials? Int J Infect Dis 2005;9:127–38.

Lipsky B, Weigelt J, Gupta V, et al. Skin, soft tissue, bone, and joint infections in hospitalized patients: Epidemiology and microbiological, clinical, and economic outcomes. Infect Control Hosp Epidemiol 2007;28:1290–8.

Pineda C, Vargas A, Rodriguez A. Imaging of osteomyelitis: Current concepts. Infect Dis Clin North Am 2006;20:789–825.

Waldvogel FA, Medoff G, Swartz MN. Osteomyelitis: A review of clinical features, therapeutic considerations and unusual aspects. N Engl J Med 1970;282:198–206.

White LM, Schweitzer ME, Deely DM, Gannon F. Study of osteomyelitis: Utility of combined histologic and microbiologic evaluation of percutaneous biopsy samples. Radiology 1995;197:840–2.

Ziran BH. Osteomyelitis. J Trauma 2007;62(Suppl.):S59–60.

Common Sports Injuries

Method of
Douglas DiOrio, MD, and Julie Shott, MD

Ankle Injuries

The ankle is the most frequently injured joint among athletes. In the primary care setting, the ankle sprain is the most commonly presenting musculoskeletal injury and accounts for 30% of all musculoskeletal visits.

Understanding the anatomy of the ankle is important for evaluating ankle injuries. The ankle is a hinge joint where three bones come together: the fibula, the tibia, and the talus. The lateral stability of the ankle is provided by the anterior talofibular ligament (ATFL), the calcaneofibular ligament (CFL), and the posterior talofibular ligament (PTFL). The ATFL is the most commonly injured ligament in the ankle. The medial stability of the ankle comes from the deltoid ligament.

When a patient presents with ankle pain, a complete history is necessary. This includes determining the mechanism of injury, such as whether the injury resulted from an inversion, eversion, plantar, or dorsiflexion mechanism. It is also important to know if the patient

could bear weight on the affected ankle immediately after the injury, where the patient felt the pain, when the swelling began, and a description of the type of pain.

A thorough examination of the injured ankle should be undertaken. The normal ankle also should always be examined and compared with the injured one. The ankle examination begins with a visual inspection for swelling, deformity, or ecchymosis. Passive and active range of motion and strength should be ascertained, although it is likely to be abnormal in most acute ankle sprains. Palpation of the ankle ligaments usually can pinpoint the source of injury in ankle sprains. Palpation of the medial and lateral malleoli and their physes and palpation of the proximal fifth metatarsal and the navicular should be done to rule out injury to the bones. Not all ankle injuries necessitate a radiograph. The Ottawa Ankle Rules can aid decision making about whether a foot or ankle radiograph is needed. These rules state that films are recommended if any of the following are positive: inability to walk four steps immediately after injury or in the office, tenderness of the distal 6 cm of the tibia or fibula, midfoot or navicular tenderness, tenderness over the proximal fifth metatarsal, age older than 55 years, or skeletal immaturity. A positive history of weight bearing immediately after the injury followed by a later increase in pain and swelling suggests an ankle sprain over a fracture.

LATERAL INVERSION SPRAIN

The lateral inversion sprain accounts for 80% to 85% of all ankle sprains. The mechanism of injury with a lateral inversion sprain is plantar flexion, inversion, and internal rotation of the ankle, which results in stretching and tearing of the three lateral ligaments. In a lateral inversion sprain, the ligaments are usually torn in the same order: ATFL, CFL, and PTFL. The patient often has acute pain after "twisting" the ankle. The area is tender over the ATFL and possibly over the CFL and the PTFL if those ligaments are involved.

MEDIAL EVERSION SPRAIN

Although the medial eversion sprain accounts for less than 10% of all ankle sprains, it accounts for more than 75% of all ankle fractures. The mechanism of injury with the medial eversion sprain is external rotation of the leg and dorsiflexion of the ankle and pronation, leading to injury of the deltoid ligament. The patient has pain over the deltoid ligament. It is important to rule out a fracture with any medial compartment injury, including a medial eversion sprain.

Treatment of medial and lateral ankle sprains includes protecting the joint and controlling the pain and swelling with RICE maneuvers: rest, ice, compression, and elevation. Patients may need crutches, an air cast, or a lace-up ankle brace to assist with ambulation.

For an adult, pain control can be initiated with acetaminophen (Tylenol) 1000 mg PO every 6 to 8 hours or ibuprofen (Motrin) 600 mg PO every 8 hours. For stable ankle sprains, adequate pain control is important to ensure that the patient begins early mobilization and rehabilitation. Rehabilitation of the ankle injury progresses to include regaining full motion, strength, and proprioception. This can be achieved through formal physical therapy or a home exercise program. The exercises focus on range of motion, resisted strength, and proprioception. They include a specific progression of exercises from standing on one foot with eyes open and then with eyes closed, to standing on uneven surfaces, and to standing on one foot and squatting. After the injured ankle has regained full range of motion and strength, the patient can gradually return to sport-specific activities. Appropriate and complete rehabilitation limits the chances the patient will repeatedly sprain his or her ankles.

Knee Injuries

ANTERIOR CRUCIATE LIGAMENT TEAR

The anterior cruciate ligament (ACL) is the key stabilizing ligament in the knee. Tears of the ACL are common among patients engaging in sports. Although ACL tears are seen in all agility sports, they occur most commonly in football, basketball, soccer, and gymnastics. Female athletes have a higher incidence of ACL tears (2.4–9.7 times) than their male counterparts. The ACL tear can be an isolated injury to the knee, or it can also involve meniscal or medial collateral ligament (MCL) injury. Fifty percent of ACL tears are associated with a meniscal tear, with the lateral meniscus tearing four times more commonly than the medial meniscus. Most commonly, the mechanism of an ACL tear involves a noncontact situation in which the athlete pivots on a planted foot, lands from a jump, or decelerates suddenly. It also can occur after a sudden valgus impact to the knee.

The classic history for a patient with an ACL tear is that the patient hears an audible "pop" or feels the knee "give out," and the patient has immediate pain and is unable to continue the activity. A thorough examination of the injured knee is important. The normal knee should always be examined and compared with the injured one. With an ACL tear, the patient often develops a hemarthrosis that is seen as a large, tense effusion. Athletes with an ACL tear have a positive Lachman's test result, although the effusion and muscle spasm may limit the examination. The Lachman's test is performed by flexing the knee to 15 degrees, holding the femur stable, and then drawing the tibia forward, assessing for laxity and the quality of the end point of the ACL. A positive test result has laxity and no discrete end point compared with the uninjured side. The athlete also has restricted movement, especially a loss of extension of the knee. There may be diffuse, mild tenderness of the knee. Medial or lateral joint line tenderness may be seen if there is an associated medial or lateral meniscal tear. Lateral joint line tenderness may also be seen because the subluxing knee stretches the lateral joint capsule.

If an ACL rupture is suspected, anteroposterior and lateral radiographs of the knee should be obtained to rule out the possibility of a tibial spine avulsion. Magnetic resonance imaging (MRI) may be needed if the diagnosis of ACL rupture is not clear or if associated injury to the cartilage is suspected. Eighty percent of ACL tears have a bone bruise visible on MRI, and most of these involve the lateral femoral condyle.

Treatment of patients with ACL tears includes referral to an orthopedic surgeon to discuss the possibility for reconstructive surgery. Athletes who wish to return to competitive sports participation are candidates for surgery. Not all patients with ACL tears need surgery. Depending on the patient's age and activity level, the patient may be treated conservatively without surgery. Until the patient is seen by the orthopedic surgeon, he or she can be placed on crutches and in a knee brace, as needed for comfort. The patient should be instructed to ice the injured knee several times each day for 20 minutes per session. Range-of-motion exercises are essential in the first week after the injury to ensure that the patient regains full extension of the knee. The patient can also do exercises to contract the hamstring and quadriceps muscles to help preserve muscle mass.

MEDIAL COLLATERAL LIGAMENT SPRAIN

An MCL sprain is another common injury to the knee. It results from a valgus stress to a partially flexed knee. It is common in football, wrestling, and basketball. If the force to the knee is severe, the ACL also may be injured. Patients with an MCL sprain present with pain over the medial aspect of the knee. MCL tears are graded I through III, depending on their severity. Stretching of the MCL fibers without an increase in joint laxity is classified as a grade I sprain. A grade II MCL sprain has partial tearing of the MCL fibers with increased laxity on valgus stress testing. A grade III sprain is a complete rupture of the MCL ligament fibers.

On examination, a patient with a grade I sprain has point tenderness along any point on the MCL but does not have swelling or increased laxity of the joint with valgus testing. A patient with a grade II MCL sprain presents with pain and swelling over the medial aspect of the knee, with point tenderness over the MCL and with pain and increased laxity with valgus stress testing at 30 degrees of knee flexion. On examination, an end point of the MCL is felt. A grade III MCL sprain is complete rupture of the MCL ligament fibers, and no end point of the MCL is felt with valgus stress testing. Any increased laxity at 0 degrees of flexion with valgus stress testing

points to a coexisting ACL injury. Radiographs are indicated if the patient has significant swelling to rule out an avulsion fracture.

Treatment of isolated MCL tears is conservative. The more severe the MCL injury, the longer the period of rehabilitation will be. The patient should be instructed to ice his or her knee three times each day for 20 minutes per session during the initial injury period. The patient should use crutches until he or she is able to walk with a normal gait. A hinged knee brace can provide support and protection to the knee during the healing process. During the first week after the injury, it is important to control swelling, work on range-of-motion exercises, and develop quadriceps strength. By 2 weeks after the injury, all swelling should be gone, and the patient should have full flexion range of motion. The patient should work on quadriceps strength after the injury, and a stationary bike is an excellent rehabilitation tool. The patient can return to sports when he or she has full range of motion, has full strength (compared with the uninjured side), and is able to do sport-specific drills with proper form. Rehabilitation times vary and may take 6 to 8 weeks for grade II sprains and up to 12 weeks for grade III sprains.

Hand Injuries

SCAPHOID FRACTURES

The most common carpal bone fractured is the scaphoid, accounting for 70% of all carpal fractures. Patients present with wrist pain after a fall on an outstretched hand. Many patients have a delay in presentation because they think they "sprained" their wrist and it will get better. It is important to diagnose this problem because a fractured scaphoid is vulnerable to nonunion and avascular necrosis. The blood supply to the scaphoid is from a recurrent interosseous blood supply that enters the bone distally and runs proximally. A more proximal fracture has a higher chance of delayed healing and a higher risk of avascular necrosis.

On physical examination, the hallmark sign of a scaphoid fracture is tenderness in the anatomic snuffbox, an area on the hand bordered ulnarly by the tendons of the extensor pollicis longus and the abductor pollicis longus and radially by the tendons of the extensor pollicis brevis. Other physical signs include possible pain with palpation of the scaphoid tubercle, swelling, and a loss of grip strength. If the patient has tenderness in the snuffbox, radiographs are mandated. Posteroanterior, lateral, and scaphoid views are recommended. A negative radiographic result *cannot* rule out a clinically suspected scaphoid fracture. If this occurs, initial treatment for a possible scaphoid fracture is indicated with a thumb spica splint or thumb spica cast. The patient is reassessed at 2 weeks, and radiographs are again obtained.

Treatment of a scaphoid fracture is based on the fracture location and whether there is any degree of displacement. If a suspected fracture does not have a radiographic abnormality, initial treatment for a scaphoid facture is begun; early immobilization with a short-arm thumb spica cast is maintained for 2 weeks. After 2 weeks, repeat radiographs are obtained. If a fracture is seen, definitive treatment for the scaphoid fracture is followed. If the radiographs are still negative but the physical examination still shows signs of a possible scaphoid fracture (i.e., snuffbox tenderness), a computed tomography (CT) scan or MRI should be obtained. If radiographs are negative and the physical examination is improved (i.e., no pain in the anatomic snuffbox), concern about a possible scaphoid fracture drops.

A patient with a stable, nondisplaced fracture (<1 mm of displacement) of the distal third of the scaphoid should be placed in a short-arm thumb spica cast for 6 weeks. A patient with a nondisplaced fracture of the middle or proximal third of the scaphoid should be placed in a long-arm thumb spica cast for 6 weeks, followed by a short-arm thumb spica cast until healing is visible on radiographs. Typically, these patients have a total of approximately 10 to 12 weeks of immobilization.

An unstable, displaced scaphoid fracture is a fracture that has a step-off or angulation of 1 mm or more. Patients with these fractures should be referred for an orthopedic consultation, as should patients with nonunion fractures and patients showing signs of early avascular necrosis.

After successful treatment of a scaphoid fracture, mobilization and strengthening of the wrist are necessary. Rehabilitation should begin immediately after cast removal.

Finger Injuries

MALLET FINGER

A mallet finger has an extension lag at the distal interphalangeal (DIP) joint caused by a loss of continuity of the terminal extensor digitorum tendon (EDT) at its insertion. This can be the result of stretching, rupture, or avulsion of the EDT, or it can be caused by a fracture of the distal phalange where the EDT inserts. The most common mechanism of injury is a blunt force to a slightly flexed fingertip, such as when a ball hits a distal finger. Often, the patient thinks he or she "jammed" the finger. The most common finger to be involved is the middle finger, although any finger can be affected. Although this is not a common sports injury, it is important because prompt diagnosis of the condition is necessary to ensure a full recovery for the patient.

When the patient presents for evaluation of this injury, each joint of the finger should be isolated and examined separately. The physical examination of a mallet finger shows that the affected joint sits in an abnormally flexed position, and the patient is unable to actively extend the DIP joint from this flexed position. Passive extension of the joint should be normal. Radiographs (i.e., anteroposterior, lateral, and oblique) are necessary to check for a possible avulsion fracture.

Treatment of a mallet finger is done by splinting the digit in hyperextension at the DIP joint. This can be accomplished by using a stack splint. If there is a bony avulsion, the patient should wear the stack splint continuously for 6 weeks. If there is no bony avulsion, the splint should be worn continuously for 8 weeks, followed by an additional 6 to 8 weeks with splinting at night and during athletic activities. Surgery is indicated if there is volar subluxation of the distal phalanx and a bony avulsion. The joint must be maintained in hyperextension at all times, even when taking the splint off to clean the finger. Any bending of the affected joint will restart the time of treatment to time zero and affect the chances for full healing.

JERSEY FINGER

Jersey finger is the term used to describe the disruption of the flexor digitorum profundus (FDP) tendon from the distal phalangeal base on the volar aspect of the hand. Typically, the mechanism of injury is an actively flexed DIP joint that is forcibly extended, as can occur when an athlete grabs onto another player's jersey. The usual history is that the patient hears a snap at the time of the injury. Although this type of injury can occur on any finger, in 75% of cases, the injury involves the fourth finger.

The patient presents with pain and swelling and an inability to actively flex the DIP joint of the affected finger. There may be fullness or pain proximal to the insertion of the DIP if the tendon retracted proximally. There may also be a palpable nodule, which represents the tendon at any point from the palm up to the DIP joint. Radiographs should be obtained to rule out the possibility of an avulsion fracture of the proximal DIP where the FDP inserts.

Treatment of a Jersey finger injury is surgery. The patient should be referred to an orthopedic surgeon so that repair of the finger can occur within 7 to 10 days of the injury. Operative intervention is less successful when the injury was initially missed and it became chronic in nature.

Overuse Syndromes

PATELLOFEMORAL PAIN SYNDROME

Patellofemoral pain syndrome (PFPS) is the most common diagnosis for patients with anterior knee pain who present to a primary care office. PFPS accounts for 25% to 40% of all knee problems of persons presenting to sports medicine centers. The terms *chondromalacia patella* and *runner's knee* are common synonyms for PFPS.

The patella is controlled by the quadriceps muscles as it moves through the femoral groove during flexion and extension of the knee. There can be a lack of control with quadriceps weakness or inhibition due to pain around the knee. This can cause PFPS and propagate it. Further pain leads to further inhibition of the quadriceps, which leads to further abnormal patellar tracking. Risk factors for PFPS include muscle dysfunction; patellar hypermobility; poor quadriceps, hamstring, or iliotibial band flexibility; training errors or overuse; trauma; malalignment; and altered biomechanics of the lower extremity.

The patient with PFPS presents to the physician complaining of unilateral or bilateral anterior knee pain. The pain is described as "all around," "behind," or "underneath" the patella. Rarely, an intraarticular effusion may be present. The pain is typically worse with walking, running, ascending or descending stairs, squatting, and sitting for prolonged periods (i.e., theatre sign). Patients may also complain of stiffness. Knee locking is not characteristic of PFPS and points to another diagnosis. The physical examination may reveal tenderness at the medial or lateral patellar facets. If the patient has pain only after activity, the examination findings may be benign, and the diagnosis needs to be based on the patient's history alone. Radiographs are not routinely indicated for PFPS but may be used for patients with a history of trauma or surgery, those with an effusion, or those who are not getting better after initial treatment.

Treatment of patellofemoral pain syndrome is done primarily through strengthening the quadriceps muscles and hip rotators. This can be accomplished through physical therapy. While the exercises are being done to strengthen the muscles, other activities are undertaken to reduce the pain of PFPS: resting from aggravating activities, using ice and nonsteroidal antiinflammatory medications as needed, and participating in other modalities such as ultrasound for pain relief. Runners may benefit from being properly fitted for running shoes.

ILIOTIBIAL BAND SYNDROME

The most common cause of lateral knee pain in an athlete is iliotibial band syndrome. Although any athlete who that participates in repetitive knee flexion activities can develop iliotibial band syndrome, it is most commonly seen in long distance runners and cyclists. The iliotibial band is made up of fascia from the hip abductors, extensors, and flexors. It originates at the anterior iliac crest outer lip and runs distally to insert at Gerdy's tubercle over the lateral aspect of the proximal tibia. The functions of the iliotibial band include helping with hip abduction, hip internal rotation, and knee flexion and extension, depending on the angle of the knee.

The patient with iliotibial band syndrome presents with pain or an ache over the lateral aspect of the knee that is worse with running, especially during long runs or downhill running. Risk factors for the development of iliotibial band syndrome include having iliotibial band tightness, putting in high weekly mileage (with running or biking), and having muscle weakness of the knee flexors, knee extensors, and hip abductors.

On physical examination, the patient may have tenderness over the lateral epicondyle of the femur about 1 inch above the joint line and at Gerdy's tubercle on the proximal tibia. Repeatedly flexing and extending the knee may reproduce the patient's symptoms. Ober's test may demonstrate iliotibial band tightness. The strength of the major muscle groups in the lower extremity must be tested, because hip abduction weakness may be identified. Radiographic imaging is usually not necessary for iliotibial band syndrome.

Iliotibial band syndrome is treated by physical therapy to strengthen the hip abductors, internal rotators, and knee flexors and extensors. Symptomatic relief of pain can be obtained through routine icing, antiinflammatory medications (e.g., ibuprofen [Motrin] 600 mg PO every 8 hours as needed), and physical therapy modalities such as ultrasound or electrical stimulation. The patient with iliotibial band syndrome may also use a foam roller on the lateral thigh along the length of the iliotibial band to stretch it. Runners should wear properly fitting running shoes.

LATERAL EPICONDYLITIS: TENNIS ELBOW

The patient who presents with lateral elbow pain may have lateral epicondylitis, also called *tennis elbow*. Tennis elbow is a tendinopathy of the extensor tendons that occurs from repeated wrist extension against resistance. This is a common injury for racket sport participants and for individuals who participate in occupational activities such as computer use and recreational activities such as sewing and knitting. Many processes can lead to the development of this tendinopathy, including overuse, poor technique, heavy racquets, grips that are too small, and a poor blood supply to the extensor tendons. When the tendinopathy becomes a chronic problem, it becomes a tendinosis. Although tendinosis may affect patients of any age, its peak incidence occurs between the ages of 40 and 50 years.

The patient with lateral epicondylitis usually describes a gradual onset of pain after the start of a new activity that involved repeated wrist extension or the sudden onset of pain after the patient overexerted his or her wrist extensors by lifting a heavy object. On physical examination, the patient has maximal point tenderness approximately 1 to 2 cm distal to the lateral epicondyle. The extensor muscles may also be tight and hypersensitive. The patient may have pain with resisted wrist extension, especially with the wrist pronated and radially deviated (i.e., Mill's test), and with resisted third digit extension. Occasionally, grip strength testing can cause pain.

No single treatment has been found to be 100% effective in treating lateral epicondylitis. A combination of several treatments results in resolution of symptoms in most cases. As with most soft tissue injuries, the treatment goals are pain control, restoration of range of motion and strength, correction of the predisposing factors (e.g., poor racquet technique), and a gradual return to full activity. Regular icing decreases inflammation. Physical therapy can help a patient with stretching and strengthening, and pain management can be achieved through physical therapy modalities such as ultrasound and electrical stimulation. Strengthening treatment initially focuses on isometric contraction of the wrist extensors and progresses to concentric and then to eccentric exercises. Soft tissue therapy such as myofascial release has been helpful. Acupuncture has provided short-term relief of lateral elbow pain. Corticosteroid injections are controversial and should be reserved for the patient who does not improve after 3 months of rehabilitation. Surgery should be reserved for patients with pain that lasts through at least 12 months of conservative treatment. Surgery involves the release of the tendon from the lateral epicondyle.

MEDIAL EPICONDYLITIS: GOLFER'S ELBOW

Although medial epicondylitis is not as common as lateral epicondylitis, it is still a fairly common injury seen in participants of certain sports such as golf, tennis, and racquetball. It is an injury that occurs in individuals who have had excessive activity of the wrist flexors and pronator teres.

The patient presents with a history of medial elbow pain. On physical examination, the patient has localized tenderness at or below the medial epicondyle. The patient has pain with resisted wrist flexion and pain with resisted forearm pronation. The flexor muscle group may have tight banding.

Treatment is the same as that for lateral epicondylitis. Athletes in golf and tennis also need to ensure that they are using appropriate technique (e.g., golf swing technique, the tennis forehand shot). Entrapment of the ulnar nerve in the scar tissue of an individual with medial epicondylitis is a concern, and it can be treated with neural stretching exercises.

REFERENCES

Brucker P, Khan K. Clinical Sports Medicine. 3rd ed. Sydney, Australia: McGraw-Hill; 2006.

Dixit S, DiFiori JP, Burton M, Mines B. Management of patellofemoral pain syndrome. Am Fam Physician 2007;75:194–202.

Eiff MP, Hatch RL, Calmbach WL. Fracture Management for Primary Care. 2nd ed. Philadelphia: WB Saunders; 2003.

McKeag DB, Moeller JL, editors. ACSM's Primary Care Sports Medicine. New York: Lippincott Williams & Wilkins; 2007.

Peterson JJ. Injuries of the fingers and thumb in the athlete. Clin Sports Med 2006;25:527–42.

Pommering TL, Kluchurosky L, Hall SL. Ankle and foot injuries in the pediatric and adult athlete. Prim Care 2005;32:133–61.

Obstetrics and Gynecology

Antepartum Care

Method of
Kirk D. Ramin, MD, and Jessica P. Swartout, MD

Antepartum Care

Ideally, antepartum care commences 3 months before actual conception with the recommendation that women who are sexually active and not using contraception should begin taking daily multivitamin or folic acid supplements. The most convincing trials of this were performed in Europe and China when it was concluded that women of reproductive age should take multivitamin supplements containing 0.4 mg of folate daily. Women with histories of children with neural tube defects or other anomalies should increase this dose to 4 mg of folate in the periconceptional period to reduce risks of recurrence.

Preconception counseling should also include an accurate assessment of preexisting maternal medical conditions. This is the ideal time to stress changes in factors that respond to early intervention: quitting smoking, refraining from alcohol or drug abuse, treating gum disease, and avoiding teratogens. Alcohol is a known teratogen. Immunization status should be reviewed and vaccines should be administered as appropriate. Special consideration is given to patients with thyroid disease. Concern focuses on associations with low intelligence quotients (IQs) in children conceived by hypothyroid mothers. Patients with diabetes should be counseled that the increased risk of birth defects is directly related to the level of glucose control at conception.

High-risk obstetric referrals may be offered to women with potential for obstetric complications suggested by conditions listed in Box 1. Identification of the high-risk patient is critical to avoiding adverse outcomes.

In most cases, a woman's pregnancy is a normal event that is complicated by potentially dangerous disease in a minority of cases. The physician who manages pregnant patients must follow the normal changes that occur during antepartum care, so that abnormalities can be recognized and treated appropriately. Additionally, routine prenatal care offers multiple opportunities for patient education, primary intervention, and appropriate monitoring of the low-risk pregnancy in the setting of the family and community. For some women, antepartum care is part of their own continuum in a long-term primary care relationship with caregivers.

Timeline of Routine Antepartum Care

FIRST VISIT AND EARLY CARE
History

After pregnancy is confirmed, it is extraordinarily important to determine the duration of pregnancy and the estimated date of confinement (EDC). Further care is heavily predicated on this estimate. The history begins with ascertaining the first day of the last menstrual period and calculating the EDC by assuming duration of pregnancy averages 280 days (40 weeks).

The documentation of prior obstetric history includes prior complications, route of delivery, and estimated birth weights. Maternal medical disorders are often exacerbated by pregnancy; cardiovascular, renal, and endocrine disorders require evaluation and counseling concerning possible treatments required. A history of previous gynecologic surgery, including cesarean delivery, is important to consider. A family history of twinning, diabetes mellitus, familial disorders, or hereditary disease is relevant.

Current medications (prescription and nonprescription) are reviewed. Certain prescription medications are known teratogens and should be discontinued. Examples include isotretinoin (Accutane), tetracycline (Sumycin), quinolone antibiotics (ciprofloxacin [Cipro], levofloxacin [Levaquin]), and warfarin (Coumadin). Angiotensin-converting enzyme (ACE) inhibitors should not be used during the second and third trimesters, and the FDA has recently raised doubt

---

BOX 1 Potential Indications for High-Risk Referral

- Current disease involving renal, cardiac, or endocrine systems
- Fetal anomalies
- History of preterm delivery
- Incompetent cervix
- Isoimmunization
- Known carrier of genetic disorder
- Multiple gestation
- Placenta previa after 28 weeks
- Prior intrauterine fetal demise or stillbirth
- Systemic diseases such as hypertension, diabetes, or asthma
- Third-trimester bleeding

about their use in the first trimester. According to the approved label, ACE inhibitors are labeled pregnancy category C for the first trimester and pregnancy category D during the second and third trimesters. On June 8, 2006, the FDA issued an alert that infants whose mothers had taken an ACE inhibitor during the first trimester had an increased risk of major congenital malformations.

Honest discussion of substance abuse (alcohol, tobacco, and illicit drugs) is an integral part of the patient interview. Counseling patients about smoking cessation is vital in early pregnancy. Smoking increases the risk of fetal death or damage in utero. It is also associated with increased risk of placental abruption and placenta previa, each of which put both mother and child at risk.

Examination

Physical examination begins with a thorough general examination to assess maternal well-being including body mass index (BMI) and blood pressure (BP). The BMI is calculated by dividing weight in kilograms by height in meters squared. The BMI of a patient is categorized as underweight (under 19.8), normal weight (19.8 to 25), overweight (25 to 30), or obese (over 30). A brief fundoscopic examination might reveal signs of hypertension-induced changes.

Breast examination may be significant for changes in pregnancy that result from hormonal responses by the mammary ducts. These changes include engorgement and vascular prominence, occasionally resulting in mastodynia. Enlargement of areolar sebaceous glands (Montgomery's tubercles) occurs between 6 and 8 weeks' gestation.

A pelvic examination is performed with attention to the adequacy of pelvis and evaluation for adnexal masses. Numerous changes in the pelvic organs occur in pregnancy. For example, congestion of the pelvic vasculature (Chadwick's sign) causes bluish discoloration of the vagina and cervix. Softening of the cervix due to increased vascularity of the cervical tissue (Goodell's sign) can occur as early as 4 weeks. The uterus is palpable at the pubic symphysis at 8 weeks.

Portable devices using Doppler effect will reliably detect fetal heart tones at a rate of 120 to 160 beats per minute as early as 8 weeks.

Laboratory Studies

Routine laboratory studies ordered at the first visit include complete blood count (CBC) with differential, ABO and Rh typing, red cell antibody screen, rubella immunoglobulin (Ig)G, hepatitis B surface antigen (HBsAg), syphilis serology, and HIV 1 and HIV 2 antibody screens. Patients may refuse HIV testing, but all patients are counseled and offered the option for screening. A Papanicolaou (Pap) smear is performed in conjunction with cultures for chlamydia and gonorrhea.

A midstream urinalysis checks for the presence of protein or glucose. A microscopic examination of the urine is performed to rule out infection or asymptomatic bacteriuria. A baseline 24-hour urine protein collection and serum creatinine should be collected from all patients with hypertension, diabetes, or other preexisting renal disease.

Other Studies

Special-purpose studies are also considered in early gestation. First-trimester screening with nuchal translucency should be offered to all women older than 35 years between 11 and 14 weeks. The first-trimester screen uses the nuchal translucency and maternal serum-free β—human chorionic gonadotropin (hCG) and pregnancy-associated plasma protein A (PAPP-A) and detects up to 85% of Down syndrome and trisomy 18 cases.

Chorionic villus sampling (CVS) may be offered at 10 to 13 weeks to women older than 35 years, to those with abnormal first-trimester screens, and to those with abnormal pedigrees. From this, placental tissue may be subjected to chromosomal, metabolic, or DNA study. CVS cannot be used for diagnosis of neural tube defects, because this requires measuring alpha fetoprotein (AFP) levels in maternal serum at a later date.

Patients with tuberculosis exposure may be assessed for active tuberculosis with skin testing (if not vaccinated with bacille Calmette-Guérin [BCG]) and chest x-ray. Serologic assessment for toxoplasmosis, cytomegalovirus, and varicella immunity is not routinely indicated.

Screening for genetic disorders may be undertaken if concern exists based on racial or ethnic background (hemoglobinopathies, β-thalassemia, α-thalassemia, Tay-Sachs disease) or familial background (cystic fibrosis, fragile X, Duchenne's muscular dystrophy).

Follow-up

Follow-up visits are scheduled once monthly until 28 weeks' gestation, and then patients are followed twice monthly until 36 weeks. Visits are then scheduled at weekly intervals until delivery. At each visit, weight gain, edema, BP, fundal height, Leopold's maneuvers, and fetal heart tones are recorded. Because BP tends to decrease during the second trimester, increases of 30 mm Hg systolic or 15 mm Hg diastolic over first trimester pressures are abnormal. Interval history includes questions about diet, sleeping patterns, and fetal movement. Warning signs such as bleeding, contractions, leaking of fluid, headache, or visual disturbances are reviewed.

15 TO 18 WEEKS' GESTATION

Alpha Fetoprotein Testing

Maternal serum AFP testing is offered for all pregnancies at 16 to 18 weeks as a means of screening for open neural tube defects or chromosomal trisomy. In pregnancy, AFP is produced in sequence by the fetal yolk sac, the fetal gastrointestinal tract, and the fetal liver. AFP in the maternal serum occurs via placental exchange and transamniotic diffusion.

High levels of AFP are associated with various fetal anomalies including neural tube defects, multiple gestations, and ventral wall defects. Unexplained elevation of AFP has been associated with poor fetal growth, fetal loss, and preeclampsia. In cases with unexplained elevation of AFP, maternal and fetal surveillance should be increased. Low levels of AFP are associated with increased risk of Down syndrome.

The interpretation of this test depends on the gestational age; even if timed correctly, it is known to have a moderate level of false-positive results. Expanded serum markers of AFP, unconjugated estriol, inhibin A, and β-hCG are available to more accurately screen for Down syndrome, but detection is only about 60%, and false-negative results remain at 5%.

Amniocentesis

A more certain diagnosis is available via ultrasound-guided transabdominal amniocentesis at 16 to 18 weeks. Chromosomes from fetal cells are subjected to fluorescent in-situ hybridization (FISH) analysis, which detects trisomies 13, 18, 21, and abnormal numbers of sex chromosomes.

Physical Findings

Interval changes in the physical examination now include the start of colostrum secretion, which can begin as early as 16 weeks' gestation.

Chloasma is darkening of the skin over the forehead, bridge of the nose, or cheekbones and is more obvious in those with dark complexions. It can begin to manifest at this time, and is intensified by exposure to sunlight. Darkening of the skin in the areolae and nipples becomes more accentuated. A darkened line appears in the lower midline of the abdomen from the umbilicus to the pubis (linea nigra). The basis of these changes is stimulation of melanophores by increased melanocyte-stimulating hormone.

At 15 to 20 weeks, abdominal enlargement can appear more rapid as the uterus rises out of the pelvis and into the abdomen.

18 TO 20 WEEKS' GESTATION

Physical Findings

The mother might detect fetal movements (quickening) at around 20 weeks. The uterus is palpable at 20 weeks at the umbilicus, and ballottement reveals a fetus floating in amniotic fluid. Measurements that are 2 cm smaller than expected for week of gestation are suspicious for oligohydramnios, intrauterine growth restriction, fetal anomaly, or abnormal fetal lie. Conversely, measurements 2 cm larger than expected can indicate multiple gestation, polyhydramnios, or fetal macrosomia. These rules apply for the gestational ages of 18 to 32 weeks. Either condition can be fully evaluated with ultrasound examination.

Laboratory Studies

Increased surveillance for preeclampsia includes testing for urine protein in patients with BP greater than 140/90 mm Hg or in those with weight gains greater than 3 pounds/week. Evaluation is also necessary for clinical signs of upper extremity edema, right upper quadrant tenderness, headaches, or vision changes. Proteinuria of more than 300 mg in 24 hours can indicate renal dysfunction or the onset of preeclampsia.

Ultrasonography

Sonography has long established itself as the single most useful technology in monitoring pregnancy and diagnosing complications. It is for this reason that basic level ultrasound is offered at 18 to 20 weeks to evaluate growth, placentation, amniotic fluid volume, and fetal anatomy. If earlier dating of the pregnancy is uncertain, this is an opportunity to confirm or refute prior estimates. If anomalous conditions are discovered, more comprehensive ultrasonography becomes necessary.

28 WEEKS' GESTATION

Physical Findings

New physical examination findings at this time include the onset of stretch marks (striae) of the breasts and abdomen. These are caused by separation of underlying collagen tissue, a response to increased adrenocorticosteroid. The ligamentous structures of the pelvis also undergo slight but definite relaxation of the joints, a progesterone effect. As the uterus enlarges, it often rotates to the right. Fundal size roughly correlates with the estimated gestational age at 26 to 34 weeks. Braxton Hicks contractions, characterized as painless uterine tightening, increase in regularity. The fetal outline can be easily palpated through the maternal abdominal wall.

Laboratory Studies

A CBC for anemia and a 1-hour glucose tolerance test (after ingestion of 50 g of glucose) is scheduled to detect patients at risk for developing gestational diabetes. If the screening test is abnormal, a 3-hour test is performed to confirm the diagnosis. Two or more abnormal values on this test are considered diagnostic of gestational diabetes mellitus.

A repeat Rh antibody is checked at this time in Rh-negative mothers. Those who remain unsensitized in the third trimester receive a first dose of Rho(D) immune globulin (RhoGAM) to prevent maternal isoimmunization to fetal red blood cells. A 300 µg dose is sufficient for 15 mL of red cells (equivalent to 30 mL of whole blood).

Follow-up

Return visits at 2-week intervals are now initiated, and the patient is oriented to the labor and delivery ward. Precautions are given regarding the onset of conditions listed in Box 2. The onset of any of these should prompt immediate medical attention.

36 WEEKS' GESTATION

Physical Findings

Patients might complain of increased vaginal discharge at this time in their pregnancy, a physiologic consequence of hormone stimulation. The discharge consists mainly of epithelial cells and cervical mucus and is treated with reassurance. Discharge accompanied by itching, burning, or malodor should be evaluated and treated accordingly, however.

BOX 2 Warning Signs and Symptoms Prompting Medical Attention

- Burning with urination
- Chills or fever
- Prolonged vomiting or inability to keep liquids down
- Pronounced decrease in fetal movements
- Rhythmic cramping pains (>6/h)
- Rupture of membranes
- Severe abdominal, pelvic, or back pain
- Signs of preeclampsia (headache, edema, right upper quadrant pain)
- Vaginal bleeding

Laboratory Studies

Vaginal and rectal cultures are collected to evaluate for the presence of group B streptococcus (GBS) at 35 to 37 weeks. GBS organisms are implicated in preterm labor, amnionitis, endometritis, and wound infection. If cultures are positive, the patient will be given antibiotic prophylaxis during active labor in efforts to protect the newborn against vertical transmission, resulting in newborn sepsis.

Follow-up

Follow-up visits are planned on a weekly basis with emphasis on weight gain, BP, and signs of preeclampsia. Review of precautions regarding infection, pregnancy loss, and symptoms of preeclampsia completes the visit.

POST-TERM GESTATION

About 3% to 12% of pregnancies continue beyond 43 weeks of gestation and are considered post-term. Although some of these may be due to inaccurate dating, some patients clearly progress to excessively long gestations that are a significant risk to the fetus. Increased antepartum surveillance by cervical examination, fetal heart rate testing (see the discussion of contraction stress testing), and biophysical profile should be initiated between 41 and 42 weeks. Even if fetal testing is reassuring, patients with reliable dating greater than 41 weeks are candidates for induction of labor.

Common Concerns of the Antenatal Period

BLEEDING

About one half of pregnant women experience some form of bleeding during the pregnancy; often this is benign. Patients also have a heightened awareness of symptoms that previously may have gone unnoticed in the nonpregnant state. Efficient and competent evaluation, followed by compassion and reassurance when prudent, allays many fears and provides clear direction. Spotting due to bleeding at the implantation site occurs from the time of implantation (about 6 days after fertilization) until 29 to 35 days after the last menstrual period in many women. Some women have unexplained cyclic bleeding throughout pregnancy. Usually, cardiac activity on ultrasound and appropriate β-hCG levels confirm a viable early pregnancy. First-trimester bleeding in lieu of these findings may be a sign of spontaneous miscarriage or ectopic pregnancy. Vaginal bleeding in late pregnancy is covered in other articles.

NAUSEA

Nausea is a common symptom that occurs in most pregnancies. It is heightened before 14 weeks' gestation and is largely benign. The etiology is not well understood but likely is related to elevating levels of β-hCG. Its moniker "morning sickness" is misleading, because nausea of pregnancy can occur at any time during the day. Aggravating factors vary with the individual patient; success varies with interventions designed to reduce symptoms.

Uncomplicated nausea may be responsive to small nonfatty portions at mealtime. Pyridoxine (vitamin B$_6$)[1] tablets 12.5 mg twice a day or doxylamine (Unisom)[1] 12.5 mg twice a day are safe in pregnancy and may be helpful. Antiemetic drugs in the outpatient setting are a measure of last resort.

Inability to control protracted vomiting in conjunction with clinical dehydration can require hospitalization for intravenous fluids and treatment of hyperemesis gravidarium. Extreme nausea and vomiting or nausea and vomiting that persists beyond 18 to 20 weeks' gestation may be signs of multiple gestation, thyroid disease, or molar pregnancy.

NUTRITION AND WEIGHT GAIN

The mother's nutrition is a vital factor in the development of the fetus from preconception through the postpartum period. Therefore, the pregnant woman should be advised to eat a balanced diet and should be informed of the additional 300 kcal/day needed during pregnancy. The American College of Obstetricians and Gynecologists (ACOG) recommends a target weight gain of 10 to 12 kg (22–27 lb) during pregnancy. They also advise that underweight women might need to gain more and obese women should gain less. Nutritional requirements for protein are 80 g/day, for calcium are 1500 mg/day, for iron are 30 mg/day, and for folate are 0.4 mg/day (4 mg/day in some cases). Patients with seizure disorders managed with valproic acid (Depakene) or carbamazepine (Tegretol) are also at risk and might benefit from the higher dose of folate.

HEARTBURN

Heartburn in the form of reflux esophagitis is caused by the enlarging uterus displacing the stomach and by progesterone's relaxation of the lower esophageal sphincter. Treatment consists of taking antacids, decreasing exacerbating factors such as spicy foods, eating more frequently but in smaller quantities, limiting eating before bedtime, and taking H$_2$-receptor inhibitors.

URINARY SYMPTOMS

Urinary frequency, nocturia, and bladder irritability are common complaints due to progesterone-mediated relaxation of smooth muscle and subsequent altered bladder function. Later in pregnancy, urinary frequency becomes even more prominent from pressure on the bladder by the enlarging uterus and the fetal presenting parts, such as when the fetal head descends into the pelvis.

Dysuria, however, is often a sign of infection that requires antibiotic treatment. Bacteriuria combined with urinary stasis from altered bladder function predisposes the patient to pyelonephritis. Although simple urinary tract infections are treated on an outpatient basis, pyelonephritis remains the most common nonobstetric cause for hospitalization during antenatal care.

Patients with a diagnosis of pyelonephritis require hospitalization, aggressive fluid replacement, and IV antibiotics until they remain afebrile for longer than 24 hours. Close monitoring of maternal respiratory status is important because these women are at risk for acute respiratory distress syndrome (ARDS). All patients should complete a 10-day course of antibiotic treatment. After treatment has been completed, suppressive therapy should be continued until delivery.

INFECTION

Two infections of special note are HIV and bacterial vaginosis (BV). HIV transmission to the newborn can be reduced significantly with appropriate infectious disease and maternal-fetal medicine specialty management. Appropriate treatment of BV in women at high risk for preterm delivery or recurrent loss can significantly reduce either of these untoward outcomes. Debate exists as to whether or not low-risk women should be screened.

---

[1]Not FDA approved for this indication.

Chlamydia trachomatis is an obligate intracellular bacterium and is the most common sexually transmitted bacterial infection in women of reproductive age. It may be associated with urethritis, mucopurulent cervicitis, and acute salpingitis, or it may be clinically silent. Perinatal transmission is clearly associated with neonatal conjunctivitis (leading to blindness) and pneumonia and is likely associated with preterm delivery, premature rupture of membranes, and perinatal mortality. Diagnosis is confirmed by polymerase chain reaction (PCR) during routine screening. Doxycycline should be avoided in pregnancy, and erythromycin is associated with gastrointestinal upset, so treatment with azithromycin is often appropriate.

Gonococcal infection is associated with concomitant chlamydia infection in about 40% of infected pregnant women. It is usually limited to the lower genital tract, including the cervix, urethra, and periurethral or vestibular glands. Because of an association between gonococcal cervicitis and septic spontaneous abortion, and because preterm delivery, premature rupture of membranes, and postpartum infection are more common with gonococcal infection, routine cultures are appropriate at the first antenatal visit. Because some strains have rendered some β-lactam drugs ineffective for therapy, the recommendation for uncomplicated gonococcal infection is intramuscular ceftriaxone 125 mg.

Vaginosis due to *Candida albicans* can become symptomatic with caseous white discharge and vaginal itching or burning, and it may be associated with red satellite lesions on the vulva. Marked inflammation of the vagina and introitus may be noted. Topical application of over-the-counter antifungal creams such as miconazole nitrate (Monistat) or nystatin (Mycostatin) is generally helpful in controlling the imbalance of vaginal flora.

Cytomegalovirus is a ubiquitous DNA herpes virus that is transmitted horizontally between humans by droplet infection. It is transmitted vertically from mother to fetus and is the most common cause of perinatal infection. The virus becomes latent after primary infection, with periodic reactivation and viral shedding. Infection is usually clinically silent. Many of the affected infants have died from infection, and most of the survivors have severe handicaps, including mental retardation, blindness, and deafness. Serious sequelae are more common among primary infections. The syndrome of congenital cytomegalovirus infection includes low birth weight, microcephaly, intracranial calcifications, chorioretinitis, mental and motor retardation, sensorineural deficits, hepatosplenomegaly, jaundice, hemolytic anemia, and thrombocytopenic purpura. Confirmation of primary infection is suggested by a fourfold increase of IgG titers in paired acute and convalescent sera or by detecting IgM cytomegalovirus antibodies. There is no effective therapy for maternal infection.

Human parvovirus B19 causes erythema infectiosum, or fifth disease. This is a single-stranded DNA virus that is heralded by the appearance of clinical findings of bright red macular rash and accompanying arthralgias. Acute infection is confirmed by IgM-specific antibody and can prompt adverse pregnancy outcomes, including spontaneous miscarriage and fetal death.

Rubella, also known as German measles, is directly responsible for spontaneous miscarriage and severe congenital malformations. Although large epidemics of rubella are nonexistent in the United States because of immunization, the disease can still affect the up to 25% of susceptible women. Absence of rubella antibody indicates susceptibility. Vaccination involves an attenuated live virus (MMR) and therefore is avoided in pregnancy. Vaccination of nonpregnant susceptible women (including those during the postpartum period) and hospital personnel continues to be the mainstay of therapy. Detection by IgM-specific antibody confirms recent infection. Congenital rubella syndrome (CRS) is a severe example of antenatal infection and includes one or more of the conditions listed in Box 3.

Varicella-zoster virus, the etiologic agent of childhood chickenpox, is a DNA herpes virus that remains latent in the dorsal root ganglia and may be reactivated years later to cause herpes zoster or shingles. Infection early in pregnancy can lead to severe congenital malformations including chorioretinitis, cerebral cortical atrophy, hydronephrosis, and cutaneous and bony leg defects. Varicella-zoster immunoglobulin (VZIg) 125 U/10 kg can attenuate varicella infection if given within 96 hours.

BOX 3 Conditions Associated with Congenital Rubella Syndrome

- Central nervous system defects (meningoencephalitis)
- Chromosomal abnormalities
- Chronic diffuse interstitial pneumonitis
- Eye lesions
  - Cataracts
  - Glaucoma
  - Microphthalmia
- Heart disease
  - Patent ductus arteriosus
  - Septal defects
  - Pulmonary artery stenosis
- Hepatic dysfunction
  - Hepatitis
  - Hepatosplenomegaly
  - Jaundice
- Osseous changes
- Retarded growth
- Sensorineural deafness
- Thrombocytopenia and anemia

Genital herpes simplex virus (HSV) may be confirmed by tissue culture if active lesions are present; in this event, cesarean delivery is indicated because the fetus is at risk for acquiring the virus during passage through the birth canal. Oral or topical acyclovir can improve symptoms. If no lesions and no prodromal symptoms are present, vaginal delivery is recommended.

Trichomonas vaginalis can be found in 20% to 30% of pregnant patients, but only a small number complain of discharge or irritation. This flagellated, oval, motile organism can be seen on normal saline wet prep and is evident clinically by presence of a foamy or greenish discharge accompanied by multiple cervical petechiae. Treatment is oral metronidazole.

Prenatally acquired infection caused by the protozoan parasite *Toxoplasma gondii* can result in the presence of abnormalities such as microcephalus or hydrocephalus at birth, development of jaundice with hepatosplenomegaly or meningoencephalitis in early childhood, or delayed appearance of ocular lesions such as chorioretinitis in later childhood. Exposure to the parasite is through eating undercooked meat, gardening in soil that is potentially contaminated by mammalian feces, or cleaning a cat's litter box.

VARICOSE VEINS

Pressure by the enlarged uterus on venous return from the legs and progesterone-mediated vasodilation can lead to prominent varicosities and edema of the legs or vulva. Any concern for deep vein thrombosis should be ruled out by examination for erythema, edema, cords, or tenderness. Doppler ultrasound may be indicated in equivocal findings of the lower extremities. Benign varicosities almost invariably return to normal after delivery, thus limiting the need for intervention in the antepartum period. Edema of the lower extremities is common, responds to elevation, and must be differentiated from facial or hand edema accompanying preeclampsia. Hemorrhoids are manifestations of the varicosities of the rectal veins. Treatment focuses on stool softeners, sitz baths, and over-the-counter topical preparations.

CONSTIPATION

Bowel transit time and relaxation of intestinal smooth muscle are both increased due to progesterone effects, resulting in overall slowing of bowel function. If pronounced, this can lead to constipation. Dietary management of this condition is centered around recommendations for increased fluids and high-fiber foods. Enemas and laxatives are avoided.

UPPER EXTREMITY DISCOMFORT

Periodic numbness and tingling of the fingers is due to exacerbations of carpal tunnel compression exacerbated by tissue edema. Splinting of the affected hand at night is indicated, with anticipation of resolution during postpartum diuresis.

 ## CURRENT DIAGNOSIS

- Pregnancy evaluation should begin 3 months before conception with optimization of underlying medical conditions and commencement of prenatal vitamins with 400 μg of folic acid.
- Preconception counseling with a specialist in high-risk pregnancies should be considered in all patients with underlying medical conditions, if possible.
- The first prenatal visit should include a review of the medical and obstetric histories, current medications, herbal remedies, and tobacco, alcohol, and drug use.
- Prenatal laboratory studies should be done at the first visit after a pregnancy is confirmed with a urine pregnancy test. These studies include hemoglobin, platelet count, type and screen, rubella status, and hepatitis B testing. All women should be offered screening for HIV. High-risk patients should be screened for hepatitis C, gonorrhea, and chlamydia.
- Genetic screening should be offered based on ethnic background and family history.
- Both first-trimester screening (nuchal translucency combined with maternal serum PAPP-A/free β-hCG) and second-trimester quadruple screen should be offered to all patients. These tests aid in diagnosis of chromosome abnormalities. If a patient opts for a first-trimester screen, it is important to perform an AFP screen in the second trimester to screen for neural tube defects.
- Appropriate weight gain in pregnancy depends on maternal BMI before pregnancy. In patients with a normal BMI, a 25- to 35-pound weight gain is recommended. Underweight patients are encouraged to gain 30 to 40 pounds, and overweight patients are encouraged to gain no more than 25 pounds.
- Prenatal visits should begin at 8 to 12 weeks' gestation and continue monthly until 24 weeks. Visits should then be every 2 weeks until 36 weeks and then weekly. Each visit should include assessment of maternal weight, BP, urinalysis for protein and glucose, fundal height measurement, documentation of fetal heart tones, and review of symptoms of preterm labor and preeclampsia.
- All patients should undergo a glucose challenge test at 24 to 28 weeks. This is done by administering a 50-g load of glucose and obtaining a serum sample 1 hour after administration. A level greater than 140 mg/dL is considered abnormal, and a 3-hour glucose tolerance test is indicated. If a woman demonstrates abnormalities in two of the four values, gestational diabetes is diagnosed.

Abbreviations: AFP = alpha fetoprotein; BMI = body mass index; BP = blood pressure; hCG = human chorionic gonadotropin; PAPP-A = pregnancy-associated plasma protein A.

CURRENT THERAPY

- Administration of the inactivated influenza vaccine (Fluzone, Fluvirin, Fluvarix) is recommended in all pregnant patients, regardless of trimester, who will be pregnant during the flu season.
- Folic acid supplementation should begin before conception. The recommended dose is 400 µg daily. In patients with a previous pregnancy complicated by a neural tube defect, 4 mg daily is recommended to prevent recurrence of a neural tube defect.
- Pyelonephritis requires hospitalization and IV antibiotics in all pregnant patients. IV antibiotics should be continued until the patient is afebrile for longer than 24 hours. Oral antibiotics should then be commenced to complete a 10-day course. All patients should continue on suppressive antibiotic therapy until delivery.
- All patients with HIV should be treated with antiretroviral therapy regardless of gestation. Intrapartum zidovudine is recommended for all patients with HIV.

BACKACHE AND PELVIC DISCOMFORT

Endocrine relaxation of ligamentous structures coupled with an offset center of gravity create exaggerated spinal curve, joint instability, and compensatory back pain. Most women experience some form of this discomfort as pregnancy progresses. Advice given for improvements in posture, local heat, acetaminophen, and massage may be helpful. Minimizing the time spent standing can have a positive effect. Round ligament pain usually occurs during the second trimester and is described as sharp bilateral or unilateral groin pain. It may be exacerbated by change in position or rapid movement and might respond to similar measures. These routine aches and pains of pregnancy must be differentiated from rhythmic cramping pains originating in the back. The latter may be a sign of preterm labor requiring appropriate evaluation.

LEG CRAMPS

Leg cramps in the form of recurrent muscle spasms in pregnancy are believed to be due to lower levels of serum calcium or higher levels of serum phosphorus. The calves are most commonly involved and attacks are more frequent at night and in the third trimester. There are no data from controlled trials to show benefit over placebo for treatment targeted toward reduced phosphate and increased calcium or magnesium intake. Local heat, putting the affected muscle on stretch, acetaminophen, and massage can be helpful in acute events.

INTERCOURSE

In general, intercourse is considered safe in pregnancy. The exception to this rule is found in patients who are experiencing uterine bleeding, or postcoital cramps, and spotting. It may be wise to avoid intercourse in couples who are at risk for special circumstances. Firmer recommendations can be made in instances of placenta previa or known rupture of membranes; in these instances intercourse should not occur.

DENTAL CARE

Ideally, women should have dental care completed before conception. However, dental procedures under local anesthesia may be carried out at any time during the pregnancy. Use of nitrous oxide inhalants is to be avoided, however. Long procedures should be postponed until the second trimester. Antibiotics are given for dental abscesses and in cases of rheumatic heart disease or mitral valve prolapse.

X-RAYS, IONIZING RADIATION, AND IMAGING

The adverse effects of ionizing radiation are dose dependent, but there is no single diagnostic procedure that results in a dose of radiation high enough to threaten the fetus or embryo. Diagnostic radiation of less than 5000 mrad is considered by ACOG to have minimal teratogenic risk, and if medically indicated, x-ray imaging may be performed safely. For example, patients may undergo chest x-rays as indicated; a dose of 0.05 mrad is typical exposure. Patients receiving dental x-rays are additionally protected by a lead apron. Still, the need for x-ray films should be evaluated for risks and potential benefits in the individual pregnant patient to conservatively protect the mother and fetus from theoretical genetic or oncogenic risk. MRI is considered safe due to its mechanism of action, which is a nonionizing form of radiation. Radioactive iodine (^{131}I) is contraindicated in pregnancy.

IMMUNIZATION

Live virus vaccines must be avoided during pregnancy because of possible effects on the fetus. These include measles, mumps, rubella (MMR) and yellow fever (VF-Vax). The risks to the fetus from the administration of rabies vaccine (RabAvert, IMOVAX) are unknown. The varicella vaccine (Varivax) is not recommended in pregnancy.

Diphtheria and tetanus toxoid (Td) may be administered in pregnancy if exposure to pathogens is likely. The hepatitis B vaccine (Engerix B, Recombivax HB) series is safe and may be given in pregnancy to women at risk. The inactivated influenza vaccine (Fluzone, Fluvirin, Fluvarix) is also recommended in all women during any trimester they will be pregnant during the flu season.

Tests of Fetal Well-Being

A primary goal in antepartum care is the competent management of patient care extended to both mother and baby in order to reduce the risk of fetal demise after 24 weeks, ensure optimal conditions for term delivery after 37 weeks, and intervene for evolving conditions threatening the well-being of either patient. Any pregnancy that may be at increased risk for antepartum fetal compromise is a candidate for tests of fetal well-being performed weekly, beginning at 28 to 32 weeks. Some conditions requiring antepartum testing are listed in Box 4.

NONSTRESS TEST

The nonstress test consists of fetal heart rate monitoring in the absence of uterine contractions. A reactive tracing is one in which heart rate accelerations of 15 bpm above the baseline of 120 to 160 bpm are of at least 15 seconds' duration. Two of these accelerations must be observed in a 20-minute period. False-positive nonreactive tracings are more common before 28 weeks' gestation.

CONTRACTION STRESS TEST

The requirements for a reactive tracing are combined with tocodynamometer recordings of three contractions of 40 seconds or more duration in a 10-minute period. If no contractions are present, they may be induced via nipple stimulation or intravenously administered oxytocin. Relative contraindications to this test are preterm premature rupture of membranes, classic uterine incision scar, placenta

---

BOX 4   Conditions That Prompt Further Testing

- Decreased fetal movements
- Fetal growth restriction
- Hypertensive disorders
- Insulin-dependent diabetes mellitus
- Multiple gestation with discordant fetal growth
- Oligohydramnios or polyhydramnios
- Post-term pregnancy
- Prior loss or stillbirth

TABLE 1 Possible Results of the Contraction Stress Test

Result	Description
Negative	No late decelerations
Positive	Late decelerations follow 50% of contractions
Equivocal	Intermittent or variable decelerations
Unsatisfactory	<3 contractions in 10 minutes

previa, and unexplained vaginal bleeding. The results of the contraction stress test are categorized in Table 1.

BIOPHYSICAL PROFILE

The biophysical profile consists of a nonstress test with ultrasound observations. A total of ten points is given for the following elements (two points each):

- Reactive nonstress test
- Presence of fetal breathing movements of 30 seconds or more in 30 minutes
- Fetal movement defined as three or more discrete body or limb movements within 30 minutes
- Fetal tone defined as one or more episodes of fetal extremity extension and return to flexion
- Quantification of amniotic fluid volume, defined as a pocket of fluid that measures at least 2 cm by 2 cm

Antepartum Hospitalization

Pregnant patients with complications requiring hospitalization are admitted to a high-risk antepartum floor in close proximity to the labor and delivery area. Specialists in maternal-fetal medicine are intimately involved in the care plans of these patients.

REFERENCES

American College of Obstetricians and Gynecologists. Compendium of Selected Publications. Atlanta: American College of Obstetricians and Gynecologists; 2007.

Carpenter MW, Coustan DR. Criteria for screening tests for gestational diabetes. Am J Obstet Gynecol 1982;144(7):763–73.

Centers for Disease Control and Prevention. Influenza: Information for Health Professionals, Available at http://www.cdc.gov/flu/ [accessed July 13, 2007].

Cunningham FG, Leveno KL, Bloom SL, et al. Williams Obstetrics. 22nd ed. New York: McGraw-Hill; 2005.

Lopez A, Dietz VJ, Wilson M, et al. Preventing congenital toxoplasmosis. MMWR Recomm Rep 2000;49(RR-2):59–68.

Wald NJ, Rodeck C, et al. First and second trimester antenatal screening for Down's syndrome. The results of the Serum, Urine and Ultrasound Screening Study. J Med Screen 2003;10(2):56–104.

Ectopic Pregnancy

Method of
Gary H. Lipscomb, MD

In the United States, the incidence of ectopic pregnancies has increased dramatically during the last several decades. Commonly cited risks include prior pelvic inflammatory disease (PID), previous tubal surgery, intrauterine device (IUD) use, previous ectopic pregnancy, ovulation induction and in vitro fertilization, progestin-containing contraceptives, smoking, previous abdominal surgery, in utero diethylstilbestrol (DES) exposure, and previous induced abortion.

A high degree of suspicion is necessary for the early diagnosis of an ectopic pregnancy. Almost all ectopic pregnancies have episodes of vaginal bleeding or lower abdominal pain prior to rupture. Such patients are appropriate candidates to evaluate for ectopic pregnancy. Figure 1 illustrates a diagnostic algorithm that is useful in efficiently coordinating and interpreting the tests used in the diagnosis of ectopic pregnancy.

Diagnosis

Serum progesterone levels are helpful as an initial screening test for ectopic pregnancy. Levels higher than 25 ng/mL are associated with ectopic pregnancy in only 1% to 2% of cases; levels less than 5 ng/mL are associated with a nonviable pregnancy (either intrauterine or ectopic) more than 99% of the time. If progesterone levels are not readily available in a timely manner, however, human chorionic gonadotropin (hCG) levels alone may be used.

Levels of hCG rise in an essentially linear fashion until after 41 days of gestation. By this gestational age, an intrauterine pregnancy (IUP) should be seen on ultrasound. In 85% of normal pregnancies, hCG doubles approximately every 2 days, rising at least 66% in 48 hours. However, 15% of normal IUPs rise less than this in 48 hours. Conversely, 15% of ectopic pregnancies rise more than 66%. But a rise of less than 50% is associated with an abnormal pregnancy 99.9% of the time.

Because the interassay variability of hCG is 15%, a change of less than this amount is considered a plateau. Plateaued levels are the most predictive of ectopic pregnancy. The use of a urine pregnancy test to rule out the possibility of phantom hCG is strongly recommended prior to surgical or medical treatment. This phenomenon, caused by heterophilic serum antibodies, produces false-positive hCG levels usually less than 1000 IU/L.

The sonographic identification of an intrauterine gestational sac essentially excludes an ectopic pregnancy. A viable IUP should always be visualized at an hCG titer of 2000 IU/L by transvaginal scan and by 6500 IU/L with transabdominal ultrasound. An adnexal mass, in a patient with a presumed ectopic pregnancy and hCG levels less than 2000 IU/L, should not automatically be assumed to be an ectopic without the presence of a yolk sac, fetal pole, or cardiac activity. Such masses are frequently corpus luteum cysts associated with an early IUP.

Except in the rare case of heterotopic pregnancy, the identification of chorionic villi in uterine contents essentially eliminates the diagnosis of ectopic pregnancy. The use of dilation and curettage (D&C) also eliminates giving methotrexate unnecessarily to a patient with a failed IUP.

A D&C is particularly important in patients with hCG titers below the discriminatory zone of ultrasound. In these patients, the appropriate use of hCG doubling times and serum progesterone levels is necessary to avoid interrupting a viable IUP. Patients with

CURRENT DIAGNOSIS

- Screening for symptomatic patients or those with risk factors
- Diagnostic algorithm to coordinate testing
- hCG titers every 48 hours
- Ultrasound at hCG level of 2000 mIU/mL
- D&C for inappropriate hCG rise (<50% in 48 hours) below 2000 mIU/mL

Abbreviations: D&C = dilation and curettage; hCG = human chorionic gonadotropin.

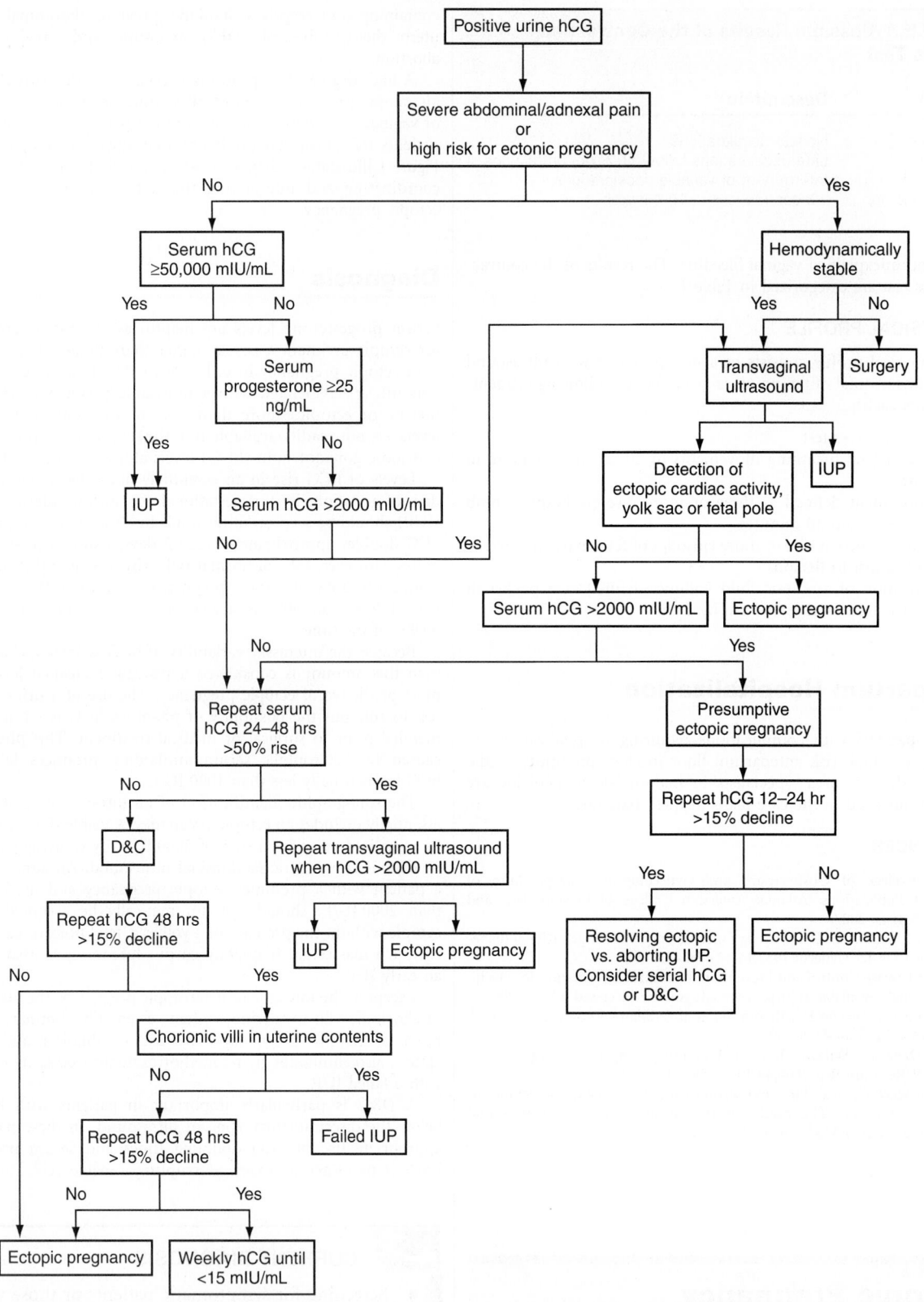

FIGURE 1. University of Tennessee Diagnostic Algorithm. D&C = dilation and curettage; hCG = human chorionic gonadotropin.

hCG titers that plateau (less than 15% change) or an hCG rise of less than 50% in 48 hours should undergo D&C to differentiate between a failed IUP and an ectopic pregnancy. Villi is absent on final histology in up to 50% of these cases. Because only the presence of villi is diagnostic, those without villi require serial hCG titers. While awaiting final histologic pathology, hCG titers are also followed. As noted in the ectopic algorithm, a serum hCG drawn after D&C is followed by a repeat level in 12 to 24 hours. Rising or inappropriately falling levels after D&C are considered diagnostic of an ectopic pregnancy.

Laparoscopy remains the gold standard for the diagnosis of ectopic pregnancy. It should be employed in any patient with suspected ectopic rupture, unreliable patients, or any others suspected of ectopic pregnancy for which the diagnostic algorithms are inappropriate.

CURRENT THERAPY

- Surgery: treatment of choice for unstable patients
- Methotrexate success: correlation with hCG levels
- Multidose methotrexate: 1 mg/kg body weight IM alternate days with leucovorin 0.1 mg/kg IM until hCG declines 15%
- Multidose treatment follow-up: daily hCG until decline, then weekly
- Single-dose methotrexate: 50 mg/m^2 based on actual body weight
- Single-dose treatment follow-up: hCG on days 1, 4, 7, then weekly if 15% decline between days 4 and 7

Abbreviations: hCG = human chorionic gonadotropin; IM = intramuscularly.

Treatment

Surgery is the classic treatment for ectopic pregnancy and remains the treatment of choice in hemodynamic unstable patients, those desiring no further pregnancies, or those who are unsuitable or unwilling to risk medical therapy.

Medical therapy with methotrexate[1] is an acceptable option to surgical therapy. Reported success rates range from 75% to 96%, with an average of approximately 90%. Whether a multidose or single-dose methotrexate protocol is most effective remains debatable, but single-dose methotrexate is the most popular because of its ease of use and low incidence of side effects.

Contraindications to medical therapy remain ill defined, but Boxes 1 and 2 note frequently used contraindications. The hCG level is the single factor most predictive of failure. With hCG levels of 5000 to 9999, success rates fall to approximately 87%, further dropping to 82% for levels 10,000 to 14,999 and 68% if more than 15,000. These levels can be used to counsel patients about the risk of failure.

MULTIDOSE METHOTREXATE

Intramuscular methotrexate, 1 mg/kg of actual body weight, alternating with citrovorum rescue factor (Leucovorin), 0.1 mg/kg, is given daily and continued until a 15% decline in two consecutive daily hCG titers. Human chorionic gonadotropin levels are then followed weekly. A repeat course of methotrexate/citrovorum is given if levels fall to less than 15% or rise between two consecutive hCG titers.

SINGLE-DOSE METHOTREXATE PROTOCOL

Methotrexate, 50 mg/m^2 based on actual body weight, is given intramuscularly. The day methotrexate is given is considered day 1. A repeat hCG is performed on days 4 and 7. If there is an appropriate decline, hCG levels are followed weekly. If the hCG level declines less

[1]Not FDA approved for this indication.

BOX 1   Generally Accepted Contraindications to Medical Therapy

White blood count <1500 cells/mL
Alanine aminotransferase (ALT) >twice upper limit normal
Creatinine >twice upper limit normal
Ectopic size >4 cm
Ectopic size >3.5 cm if cardiac activity present the upper limit of normal, hemodynamically unstable
Immunocompromised status

BOX 2   Relative Contraindications to Medical Therapy

Ectopic cardiac activity*
Serum hCG level >15,000†

─────────────

*Controversial; however, when corrected for hCG level, no longer a risk factor.
†Acceptable if patients are counseled on failure rate.
Abbreviation: hCG = human chorionic gonadotropin.

than 15% between days 4 and 7, a second dose of methotrexate is given and the protocol restarted at a new day 1. Although this protocol is referred to as "single-dose methotrexate," approximately 20% of patients require more than one treatment cycle.

In conclusion, the incidence of ectopic pregnancy has reached epidemic proportions in the United States. Nevertheless, the mortality associated with this disease is steadily declining. This decline is primarily because of earlier diagnosis that allows treatment prior to rupture. This earlier diagnosis is the result of improved assays for progesterone, hCG, transvaginal ultrasound, and the use of diagnostic algorithms that do not require the use of laparoscopy. Once diagnosed, numerous treatment options are now available, including the option of medical therapy. Future developments ideally will provide for an even earlier diagnosis as well as data on the optimum candidates for each form of treatment.

REFERENCES

Brenaschek G, Rudelstorfer R, Csaicsich P. Vaginal sonography versus serum human chorionic gonadotropin in early detection of pregnancy. Am J Obstet Gynecol 1988;158:608–12.

Kadar N, Freedman M, Zacher M. Further observation on the doubling time of human chorionic gonadotropin in early asymptomatic pregnancy. Fertil Steril 1980;54:783–7.

Lipscomb GH, McCord ML, Huff G, et al. Predictors of success of methotrexate treatment in women with tubal ectopic pregnancies. N Engl J Med 1999;341:1874–8.

Lipscomb GH, Stovall TS, Ling FW. Nonsurgical treatment of ectopic pregnancy. N Engl J Med 2000;343:1325–9.

Stovall TS, Ling FW, Buster JE. Nonsurgical diagnosis and treatment of tubal pregnancy. Fertil Steril 1990;54:537–8.

Stovall TG, Ling FW, Gray LA, et al. Methotrexate treatment of unruptured ectopic pregnancy: A report of 100 cases. Obstet Gynecol 1991;77:749–53.

Vaginal Bleeding in Late Pregnancy

Method of
Jami Star Zeltzer, MD

Vaginal bleeding in late pregnancy complicates approximately 6% of pregnancies and is associated with increased maternal and fetal morbidity and mortality. Excluding labor, the most likely causes are placenta previa and placental abruption, followed by uterine rupture and vasa previa; less common etiologies include trauma, cervical lesions, and coagulopathy. The primary focus in obstetric hemorrhage, regardless of cause, is maternal hemodynamic assessment and stabilization. Given the extraordinary blood flow to the uterus at term (600 to 800 mL/min), exsanguination can occur rapidly. Additionally, redistribution of maternal blood flow may lead to fetal hypoxia.

Early maternal signs of hemodynamic compromise include tachycardia and tachypnea; later, hypotension, weakened pulses, and oliguria ensue, along with evidence of fetal compromise. Further decompensation can ultimately result in the death of both mother and fetus. Guidelines for restoration of maternal circulating volume are approximately 3 mL of intravenous crystalloid, (i.e., normal saline or Ringer's solution) per 1 mL of blood lost (often underestimated). Laboratory evaluation includes a complete blood count, blood type, and crossmatch; in the setting of thrombocytopenia (less than 100,000 platelets), coagulation studies (prothrombin time [PT], partial thromboplastin time [PTT], fibrinogen, fibrin degradation products [FDPs]) are recommended. Packed red blood cells, fresh-frozen plasma, platelets, and/or cryoprecipitate are given to maintain maternal hemoglobin near 10 g/dL and correct coagulopathy (unlikely if whole blood is observed to clot in less than 8 minutes). Additional measures include administration of oxygen, lateral displacement of the uterus and, rarely, vasopressors. Fetal evaluation and treatment, including consideration of delivery, follow stabilization of the mother.

Placenta Previa

Placenta previa, or the implantation of the placenta adjacent to or covering the internal os, complicates approximately 0.5% of all deliveries. The degree of placenta previa may be:

- Complete (internal os covered entirely)
- Partial (portion of internal os covered)
- Marginal (placental edge at cervix or less than 2 cm away)
- Low lying (not a true previa, where the placental edge implants in the lower uterine segment but doesn't reach the cervix)

Box 1 lists the risk factors. The pathophysiology appears to involve endometrial damage, with resulting limitation of healthy uterine tissue for implantation.

The hallmark symptom is painless vaginal bleeding, presumably initiated by development of the lower uterine segment. Usually, this occurs by 29 to 30 weeks of gestation, although in approximately 33% of cases, there is no bleeding until labor. The first bleed may be self-limited, but rebleeding complicates approximately 60% of cases. The diagnosis is often made in the absence of symptoms on routine ultrasound. The incidence of placenta previa is 5% to 10% in mid-gestation; this resolves in most cases with development of the lower uterine segment (*placental migration*). When asymptomatic, expectant management is appropriate, although vaginal precautions after 28 weeks' gestation may be advised.

When a patient presents with third-trimester bleeding, speculum exams are contraindicated until placenta previa is ruled out. The most accurate method of diagnosis is transvaginal ultrasound, which is safe in experienced hands; transperineal or transabdominal ultrasound carry greater risks of false-positive and false-negative results.

Observation in the hospital is recommended following a bleed, during which time approximately 50% of patients will deliver. Steroids are indicated for enhancement of fetal lung maturation. Tocolysis can

be administered if the mother and fetus are stable, but betasympathomimetics should be avoided in order to minimize cardiovascular effects. Outpatient management is acceptable if bleeding ceases, as long as the patient is compliant and has ready access to a hospital. Serial ultrasound assessment is recommended because there is an increased risk of intrauterine growth restriction. Transfusion should be offered to maintain hemoglobin greater than 10 mg/dL.

Urgent delivery by cesarean section is indicated when there is ongoing maternal hemorrhage or evidence of fetal compromise. In the stable patient, a planned cesarean section can be performed at 35 to 36 weeks, generally after an amniocentesis is performed to confirm fetal lung maturity. Vaginal delivery may be attempted if delivery is imminent, or with marginal previa, although a double setup for emergent cesarean section is advised. In the setting of fetal demise, vaginal delivery is preferable.

Placenta previa predisposes to postpartum hemorrhage, either from atony of the lower uterine segment or inability to remove the placenta because of absence of the decidua basalis. The most common form of this latter condition is placenta accreta, where the trophoblast adheres to the myometrium. Less common forms include placenta increta (the trophoblast invades the myometrium) and placenta percreta (trophoblast invades uterine serosa and/or adjacent organs). The primary risk factor for placenta accreta is the number of previous cesarean sections, with an incidence approaching 40% in patients with two prior cesarean sections and a placenta previa. Other risk factors include age, parity, and history of curettage. Color Doppler ultrasound and magnetic resonance imaging (MRI) are helpful but not always definitive for diagnosis. If placenta accreta is suspected, preparations can be made for scheduled delivery with trained personnel and blood products available. At delivery, the placenta should be left in place if a cleavage plane cannot be developed easily. Cesarean–hysterectomy is often required for hemostasis, although conservative management, including preoperative and intraoperative selective embolization and/or use of methotrexate, has been reported. With placenta percreta, bladder invasion may require cystoscopy and urologic repair.

Placental Abruption

Abruption of the placenta, or separation of the normally implanted placenta before birth, complicates 1% to 2% of pregnancies. Bleeding into the decidua basalis, with subsequent separation of varying amounts of placental tissue from the endometrium, may result in fetal compromise and/or demise. The exact pathophysiology is unclear. Box 2 lists the risk factors.

Vaginal bleeding in the second half of pregnancy is assumed to be caused by placental abruption, once placenta previa and other rare

---

BOX 1   Risk Factors for Placenta Previa

- Advancing maternal age
- Ethnic background (increased in Asians)
- Multiparity
- Multiple gestation
- Previous curettage
- Prior cesarean section (increases with number of sections)
- Prior placenta previa
- Smoking

BOX 2   Risk Factors for Placental Abruption

- Chorioamnionitis
- Cocaine use
- Ethnic background (highest in blacks)
- Hypertension
- Male fetal gender
- Multiple gestation
- Parity
- Polyhydramnios (rapid decompression at membrane rupture and/or therapeutic amniocentesis)
- Preterm premature rupture of membranes
- Previous cesarean section
- Smoking
- Trauma, including domestic violence
- Unexplained elevated second trimester alpha-fetoprotein
- Uterine anomalies/short umbilical cord

causes are ruled out. Concealed hemorrhage, present in 10% to 20% of cases, can complicate the diagnosis. Abdominal pain, back pain, uterine contractions (often described as low amplitude, high frequency), hypertonus, uterine tenderness, and/or idiopathic premature labor may be present. While ultrasound can identify placenta previa, it cannot be relied upon to definitively diagnose abruption, as clot is sonographically visible in less than 50% of cases. The differential diagnoses include uterine rupture, appendicitis, and chorioamnionitis, as well as other causes of abdominal pain.

Most commonly, bleeding is not profuse and, if the episode is self-limited, expectant management of a preterm gestation includes observation, serial fetal growth assessment, fetal well-being testing, and steroid therapy to accelerate fetal lung maturation. With ongoing significant blood loss, stabilization of the mother, fetal assessment, and laboratory evaluation are indicated. Coagulopathy is rare in the absence of fetal demise. If tocolysis is required, betasympathomimetics should be avoided, as they may mask maternal cardiovascular decompensation.

Vaginal delivery is appropriate if mother and fetus are stable. Amniotomy may decrease extravasation of blood into the myometrium by head compression. Not uncommonly, effacement will precede dilatation; oxytocin (Pitocin) is acceptable for labor dysfunction. In the event of an intrauterine demise, vaginal delivery is preferred. Acute hemorrhage requires immediate cesarean delivery, with blood and coagulation factor replacement as needed.

Potential complications of abruption include hemorrhagic shock, disseminated intravascular coagulation (unlikely unless there is greater than 2000 mL blood loss and/or fetal demise), ischemic necrosis of maternal organs (especially kidney), and Couvelaire uterus (extravasation of blood into uterine muscle). Recurrence is approximately 5% to 15%, increasing with each subsequent event. There are no known preventive measures other than correcting modifiable risk factors. Research into the association between thrombophilia and abruption is ongoing, but in absence of other risk factors, a work-up for hypercoagulability may be considered.

Vasa Previa

Vasa previa is a rare condition (estimated 1 in 2500 deliveries) in which fetal blood vessels cross over the membranes in advance of the presenting part. This is most often associated with velamentous insertion of the umbilical cord (vessels reach the placenta after coursing through the membranes rather than by direct insertion); Box 3 lists the risk factors. Vasa previa carries a profound risk of fetal mortality from exsanguination, particularly at the time of membrane rupture (fetal blood volume at term is approximately 250 mL). Even in the absence of bleeding, vessel compression may result in compromise of the fetal circulation.

Signs include hemorrhage, as well as fetal heart rate abnormalities. A high index of suspicion is required, and advances in imaging techniques (color Doppler, transvaginal ultrasound) make prenatal diagnosis possible. If there is unexplained bleeding, an Apt test or Kleihauer-Betke test can identify fetal red blood cells. If the diagnosis of vasa previa is strongly suspected at term, or if hemorrhage is significant, prompt cesarean delivery is recommended, followed by neonatal resuscitation.

BOX 3　Risk Factors for Vasa Previa

- Bilobed placenta
- In vitro fertilization
- Low-lying placenta
- Multiple pregnancy
- Succenturiate lobe
- Velamentous insertion of umbilical cord

BOX 4　Uterine Rupture

Risk Factors	Differential Diagnoses
Previous cesarean section (especially classical)	Appendicitis
Use of oxytocin, prostaglandins, or misoprostol	Biliary colic
Multiparity	Pancreatitis
Midforceps application	Peptic ulcer disease
Breech version/extraction	Intestinal obstruction
Placental abruption	Ovarian torsion
Shoulder dystocia	Placental abruption
Placenta percreta	Urinary tract disorders
Müllerian duct anomalies	
History of pelvic radiation	

Uterine Rupture

Most often reported following prior cesarean section, uterine rupture can also occur in an unscarred uterus (1 in 8000 to 1 in 15,000 deliveries). This phenomenon implies complete separation of the uterine wall (as compared to uterine dehiscence), with or without expulsion of the fetus. Box 4 lists risk factors and differential diagnoses.

Common signs and symptoms include abdominal pain/tenderness and vaginal bleeding; additional complaints include epigastric or shoulder pain, abdominal distention, and constipation. The fetal tracing may show sudden variable decelerations or abrupt and prolonged bradycardia, often accompanied by recession of the presenting part. Maternal and fetal morbidity and mortality are high, particularly with delayed diagnosis. Treatment is urgent cesarean delivery, with repair of the uterus and/or hysterectomy as needed. Repeat cesarean section is advised in the future because of the risk for recurrence.

Hypertensive Disorders of Pregnancy

Method of
Brenda Stokes, MD

Hypertensive disorders of pregnancy are the most common medical disorder in pregnancy. Hypertension is estimated to occur in 5% to 12% percent of all pregnancies. It is a major cause of maternal and fetal morbidity and mortality. The hypertensive disorders of pregnancy are classified as shown in Box 1.

Pregnancy-induced or gestational hypertension is the most common cause of hypertension in pregnancy. It is defined as a systolic blood pressure of more than 140 mm Hg and diastolic blood pressure

---

BOX 1　Hypertensive Disorders of Pregnancy

- Gestational (pregnancy-induced) hypertension
- Preeclampsia and eclampsia
- Chronic hypertension
- Preeclampsia superimposed on chronic hypertension

of more than 90 mm Hg on two different measurements at least 6 hours apart. The measurements should be done no more than 1 week apart. This is further classified as mild or severe disease. Mild disease usually develops later in pregnancy. The pregnancy outcomes with mild disease usually are good. Severe disease is associated with a higher morbidity in pregnancy than women with mild preeclampsia. Women with severe disease have rates of preterm delivery, small for gestational age infants, and abruption similar to those for women with severe preeclampsia.

Clinical Characteristics and Diagnosis

Preeclampsia is defined as hypertension developing after 20 weeks' gestation and with proteinuria. Hypertension is defined the same for preeclampsia as for gestational hypertension. Proteinuria is defined as excretion of 300 mg or more of protein in a 24-hour urine collection. Preeclampsia is further divided into mild or severe disease. Multiple risk factors have been associated with the development of preeclampsia. Box 2 lists some of the common risk factors.

There are many theories about the cause of preeclampsia. For example, ongoing investigations suggest that preeclampsia may be an autoimmune disorder caused by pregnancy-induced autoantibodies that activate the angiotensin II receptor type 1a (AT1 receptor). Women with preeclampsia have been found to have autoantibodies that bind and stimulate AT1 receptors. In one study, injection of these AT1 autoantibodies into pregnant mice caused all of the main features of preeclampsia, including hypertension, glomerular endotheliosis, proteinuria, placental abnormalities, and reduced fetal size. There is definitely a relationship between abnormal placentation and preeclampsia, but it is unclear if this is a cause or an effect. For example, a genetic deficiency of an estradiol metabolite, 2-methoxyestradiol (2-ME), may underlie the placental effects in preeclampsia, suggesting that therapeutic supplementation may prevent or treat the disorder. Serum levels of 2-ME were greatly reduced in a model of preeclampsia, resulting from a lack of placental catechol-O-methyltransferase (COMT) expression. In normal pregnant women, levels of 2-ME are elevated during the third trimester, but in women with preeclampsia, 2-ME levels are lower, and placental expression of COMT protein expression is reduced. This suggests that the actions of COMT and 2-ME are central to proper vascular function in the placenta.

Preeclampsia affects multiple maternal organ systems. It causes proteinuria and can rarely lead to renal failure. Hyperreflexia, grand mal seizures, hemorrhagic stroke (rare), and visual disturbances, including transient blindness, can occur. The vascular system becomes contracted, which increases the hematocrit. Thrombocytopenia, coagulation abnormalities, and hemolysis can occur. Heart failure and pulmonary edema are late complications. Abnormal liver transaminase levels with hepatic congestion and hepatic rupture can also occur.

CURRENT DIAGNOSIS

- Hypertensive disorders of pregnancy are the most common medical disorder in pregnancy.
- Hypertensive disorders of pregnancy are a major cause of maternal and fetal morbidity and mortality.
- Clinicians providing care for pregnant patients should be aware of the signs and symptoms of preeclampsia and screen for them at every visit.

Preeclampsia also affects the developing fetus. Decreased placental perfusion leads to an increased incidence of intrauterine growth restriction and placental abruption. Oligohydramnios can develop as a result of the poor placental perfusion.

The initial signs and symptoms of preeclampsia vary. Patients typically present with increased blood pressure and proteinuria. Peripheral nondependent edema is common, as is weight gain. Symptoms may include epigastric or right upper quadrant abdominal pain, headaches, and visual disturbances. Most patients present with mild preeclampsia. However, some present with severe disease, which requires prompt diagnosis and treatment. Preeclampsia can manifest antepartum, intrapartum, or postpartum.

An increased rate of maternal and fetal morbidity and mortality is associated with preeclampsia. The rate depends on the severity of maternal disease and the gestational age of the fetus at diagnosis. Mild preeclampsia has been associated with fetal outcomes similar to those for normotensive patients. Patients with mild preeclampsia have a higher rate of cesarean delivery. Severe disease is associated with an increased risk of maternal morbidity and mortality and a higher rate of premature delivery, abruption, and small for gestational age infants. Because of the potential morbidity and mortality associated with preeclampsia, there is interest in early diagnosis and primary prevention in patients at high risk for the disease.

Prevention and Treatment

Many different therapies have been studied for primary prevention of preeclampsia in patients who are at high risk for the disease. Calcium[1] supplementation of 2 g/day or less has been studied, and the incidence of preeclampsia and gestational hypertension has been reduced. The benefit is seen more in patients at high risk for gestational hypertension and in women with a low dietary intake of calcium. Antioxidant supplementation, mostly with vitamins C[1] and E,[1] during pregnancy has been evaluated for preventing preeclampsia. A Cochrane systematic review of many studies failed to show any benefits for using antioxidants in pregnancy to prevent preeclampsia or its complications. A prospective cohort study showed a reduction in preeclampsia with supplementation of a multivitamin with folic acid[1] in the second trimester. Antiplatelet therapy, mainly low-dose aspirin,[1] has been moderately effective in reducing the incidence of preeclampsia and its complications in women at high risk for the disease. Physical activity has been studied for the prevention of preeclampsia, but the results have been inconclusive.

Preeclampsia can occur as mild or severe disease. Table 1 shows the clinical manifestations for each type. Disease is considered mild unless any of the criteria is met for severe disease.

The management of preeclampsia, especially severe disease, is controversial. Suggested management plans for mild and severe disease are presented in Figure 1. The recommendations are based on the best available data of maternal and fetal outcomes. The management of preeclampsia depends on the gestational age of the fetus at diagnosis and the severity of illness in the mother. Although some cases can occur in the postpartum period, delivery of the fetus is the definitive treatment for preeclampsia in other situations. Conservative management is

---

[1]Not FDA approved for this indication.

BOX 2   Risk Factors for the Development of Preeclampsia

- Nulliparity
- New partner
- Obesity
- Multiple gestation
- Family history of preeclampsia
- Chronic hypertension
- Renal disease
- Diabetes mellitus
- Presence of thrombophilias
- Previous history of preeclampsia
- Abnormal uterine Doppler studies at 18 and 24 weeks' gestation
- Maternal age ≥40 years

TABLE 1 Classification of Preeclampsia

Feature	Mild Disease	Severe Disease
CNS symptoms	Headache, hyperreflexia	Seizures, blurred vision, scotomas, headache, clonus, irritability
Proteinuria	≥300 mg/24 hours	>5 g/24 hours
Liver function	Normal transaminase levels	Elevated transaminase levels, epigastric pain, liver rupture
Platelet level	>100,000/hpf	<100,000/hpf
Hemoglobin level	Normal	Elevated level, hemolysis, DIC
Blood pressure	<160/110 mm Hg	>160/110 mm Hg
Fetal status	Normal AFI, fetal testing, and growth	IUGR, oligohydramnios, signs of fetal distress, abruption, fetal demise

Abbreviations: AFI = amniotic fluid index; CNS = central nervous system; DIC = disseminated intravascular coagulation; hpf = high-power field; IUGR = intrauterine growth restriction.

recommended in pregnancies less than 38 weeks' gestation and mothers with mild disease. Although bed rest is recommended, there is no evidence to support this. Care includes daily blood pressure checks and urine dipstick determinations for protein. Patients with mild disease can be managed on an inpatient or outpatient basis. Laboratory evaluation, which includes a 24-hour urine collection for total protein and blood testing, should be obtained for all patients at least twice weekly. Daily fetal kick counts are advised with antenatal fetal testing twice weekly. Serial obstetric ultrasound evaluations are recommended to monitor fetal growth at baseline and then every 3 weeks.

Severe preeclampsia is managed aggressively because of the increased risk of maternal and fetal morbidity. The primary goal in management is the health and well-being of the mother and then the delivery of a mature fetus. All patients with severe preeclampsia require immediate hospitalization. Intravenous magnesium sulfate infusion is recommended for seizure prophylaxis. Antihypertensive medications are recommended to treat systolic blood pressure higher than 160 mm Hg and diastolic blood pressure higher than 110 mm Hg. Corticosteroids are recommended for patients at gestational ages between 22 and 34 weeks. Daily maternal and fetal evaluations with laboratory testing and antepartum fetal testing are recommended. Obstetric ultrasound scans are used to evaluate intrauterine fetal growth restriction (IUGR), oligohydramnios, and abruption.

Choice of the mode of delivery of the fetus is based on the gestational age and the maternal and fetal status. Vaginal delivery is the preferred route of delivery in a patient with preeclampsia. Cesarean delivery should be considered for premature infants, for severe IUGR, and for severe disease with an unfavorable cervix. Continuous fetal monitoring should be instituted intrapartum. Epidural or spinal anesthesia is preferred for cesarean delivery. If necessary, maternal transfer should be considered to an institution that has the ability to care for the newborn infant, who may be premature, and the mother, who may need intensive care monitoring after delivery.

Intravenous magnesium sulfate infusion is typically initiated for seizure prophylaxis intrapartum and continued postpartum. Its use in mild preeclampsia is controversial because the data are not clear about whether the benefits outweigh the risks. The total intravenous fluid rate needs to be monitored closely and usually does not exceed 150 mL/hour. Magnesium sulfate is started as a bolus infusion of 4 to 6 g over 15–20 minutes and then continued at a rate of 1–2 g/hour. Magnesium toxicity needs to be monitored. Box 3 lists clinical signs of magnesium toxicity. Therapeutic levels are 4 to 8 mg/dL. Urine output should be monitored closely. Calcium gluconate should be available to reverse toxicity if needed. It is administered intravenously as 1 g over 2 minutes. The magnesium sulfate infusion is usually continued for 24 hours postpartum but should be continued longer if clinically indicated.

Blood pressure is monitored closely in the patient with preeclampsia. Treatment is indicated for systolic blood pressure higher than 160 mm Hg and diastolic blood pressure higher than 110 mm Hg. Traditionally, intravenous hydralazine (Apresoline) or labetalol (Trandate) have been used. Oral nifedipine (Procardia) also has been effective.

Eclampsia occurs in the setting of preeclampsia when seizures or coma develop without other identified causes. It can be associated with mild or severe disease, and it can occur antepartum, intrapartum,

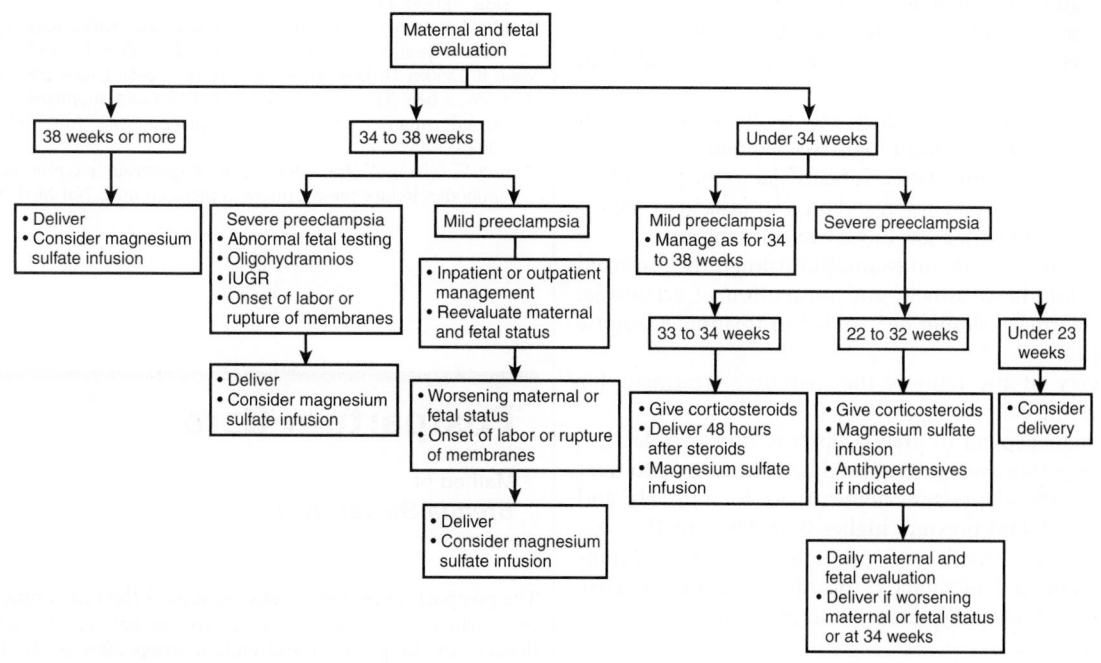

FIGURE 1. Management of preeclampsia. *Abbreviation:* IUGR = intrauterine growth restriction.

BOX 3 Signs of Magnesium Toxicity, Listed Progressively with Increasing Magnesium Levels

- Loss of deep tendon reflexes
- Somnolence and slurred speech
- Decreased respiratory rate <12 breaths/min
- Decreased urine output
- Pulmonary edema

or postpartum. The pathophysiology is unknown but is thought to include cerebral edema, ischemia, hemorrhage, or transient cerebral arterial vasospasm.

Eclampsia is managed by controlling blood pressure and preventing recurrent seizures. Intravenous magnesium sulfate infusion is the agent of choice for treatment of eclampsia and prevention of recurrent seizures. The maternal airway should be protected and supplemental oxygen given. Fetal heart rate abnormalities, usually fetal bradycardia, may occur but heart rate typically returns to baseline after the seizure. Immediate delivery is not always necessary if the infant and mother are stabilized. Polypharmacy to treat the seizures should be avoided because it only increases maternal side effects.

HELLP syndrome, a form of severe preeclampsia, is defined as hemolysis, elevated liver enzymes, and low platelets. It can sometimes be misdiagnosed when it occurs early in pregnancy and the blood pressure is not elevated. It should be managed the same as severe preeclampsia.

Chronic hypertension occurs in approximately 1% to 5% of pregnancies. Patients with chronic hypertension are at increased risk for complications in pregnancy, including preeclampsia. It is defined as hypertension diagnosed before pregnancy or before 20 weeks' gestation. It can also be diagnosed retrospectively postpartum when elevated blood pressure persists. It is associated with an increased risk of abruption, poor perinatal outcomes, and superimposed preeclampsia. Early prenatal care and close maternal and fetal monitoring are required.

CURRENT THERAPY

- Mild to moderate hypertension in pregnancy does not require treatment.
- Antihypertensive drug selection should be based on the clinician's familiarity with the medication.
- Angiotensin-converting enzyme (ACE) inhibitors and angiotensin receptor blockers are contraindicated in pregnancy.
- Low-dose aspirin[1] is beneficial in the prevention of preeclampsia in selected high-risk women.
- Calcium[1] supplementation is beneficial in the prevention of gestational hypertension and preeclampsia in women at high risk and with a low dietary calcium intake.
- Magnesium sulfate intravenous infusion is the preferred agent for the treatment and prevention of eclampsia. Polypharmacy should be avoided in treating eclamptic seizures.
- Delivery of the fetus is the definitive treatment for preeclampsia.
- The management of preeclampsia is controversial.
- Antihypertensive agents should be used acutely to treat systolic blood pressure higher than 160 mm Hg and diastolic blood pressure higher than 110 mm Hg.
- Intravenous hydralazine (Apresoline), labetalol (Trandate), and oral nifedipine (Procardia) have been effective in treating severe hypertension in pregnancy.

[1]Not FDA approved for this indication.

It is unclear whether treatment of chronic hypertension affects pregnancy outcomes, especially for women with mild hypertension. Maternal and fetal outcomes are generally good despite mild hypertension. Antihypertensive medications can reduce the risk of severe hypertension but do not reduce other complications. Medications usually can be discontinued in early pregnancy. Antihypertensive medication is chosen based on the clinician's preference and experience if indicated. Angiotensin-converting enzyme (ACE) inhibitors and angiotensin receptor blockers are contraindicated in pregnancy.

Summary

Hypertensive disorders of pregnancy are the most common medical problems encountered during pregnancy. Hypertension is associated with increased maternal and fetal morbidity and mortality. Close monitoring and appropriate timing of delivery are required to ensure the best possible maternal and fetal outcomes.

REFERENCES

Abalos E, Duley L, Steyn DW, Henderson-Smart DJ. Antihypertensive drug therapy for mild to moderate hypertension during pregnancy. Cochrane Database Syst Rev 2006;(1):CD002252.

Askie LM, Duley L, Henderson-Smart DJ, Stewart L, for the PARIS Collaborative Group. Antiplatelet agents for prevention of preeclampsia: A meta-analysis of individual patient data. Lancet 2007;369:1791–8.

Duley L, Henderson-Smart DJ, Meher S. Drugs for treatment of very high blood pressure during pregnancy. Cochrane Database Syst Rev 2006;(3): CD001449.

Duley L, Meher S, Abalos E. Management of preeclampsia. BMJ 2006;332: 463–538.

Hofmeyr GJ, Atallah AN, Duley L. Calcium supplementation during pregnancy for preventing hypertensive disorders and related problems. Cochrane Database Syst Rev 2006;(3):CD001059.

Leeman L, Fontaine P. Hypertensive disorders of pregnancy. Am Fam Physician 2008;78:93–100.

Kanasaki K, Palmsten K, Sugimoto H. Deficiency in catechol-O-methyltransferase and 2-methoxyoestradiol is associated with pre-eclampsia. Nature 2008;453: 1117–21.

Meher S, Duley L. Exercise or other physical activity for preventing preeclampsia and its complications. Cochrane Database Syst Rev 2006;(2): CD005942.

Roberts JM, Pearson G, Cutler J, Lindheimer M. Summary of the NHLBI working group on research on hypertension during pregnancy. Hypertension 2003;41:437–45.

Rumbold A, Duley L, Crowther CA, Haslam RR. Antioxidants for preventing preeclampsia. Cochrane Database Syst Rev 2008;(1):CD004227.

Sabai B, Dekker G, Kupferminc M. Pre-eclampsia. Lancet 2005;365:785–99.

Wen SW, Chen XK, Rodger M, et al. Folic acid supplementation in early second trimester and the risk of preeclampsia. Am J Obstet Gynecol 2008;198:45.

Zhou CC, Zhang Y, Irani RA, et al. Angiotensin receptor agonistic auto-antibodies induce pre-eclampsia in pregnant mice. Nat Med 2008;14:810–2.

Postpartum Care

Method of
Brenda Stokes, MD

The postpartum period, or puerperium, is the time immediately after birth when the uterus returns to its normal size. It starts with the delivery of the placenta and ends 6 weeks after birth. This chapter reviews specific concerns and problems that arise in the postpartum period.

BOX 1   Etiology of Postpartum Hemorrhage

Uterine atony
Lacerations
Retained products of conception
Coagulation disorders

Postpartum Hemorrhage

The World Health Organization defines postpartum hemorrhage as 500 mL or more of blood loss in the first 24 hours after delivery. Postpartum hemorrhage occurs in approximately 30% to 40% of all deliveries. It continues to be a major cause of maternal morbidity and mortality in both developed and developing countries.

Early recognition and treatment are essential in preventing complications from postpartum hemorrhage. The amount of blood loss following a delivery is difficult to measure accurately. It is typically estimated by visual inspection. Brisk vaginal bleeding following birth should trigger an investigation for its etiology.

The etiology of postpartum hemorrhage is shown in Box 1. Uterine atony is the most common cause of immediate postpartum hemorrhage. Once brisk bleeding is identified, a careful examination for the cause is performed. Palpation of the uterine fundus is done to assess the tone of the uterus. Bimanual uterine massage both confirms and treats uterine atony. The medications listed in Table 1 are oxytocics used to control vaginal bleeding due to uterine atony. Emptying the bladder with catheterization is useful to keep the uterus contracted. Surgical methods are considered if medications and uterine massage fail to control the bleeding. A careful inspection of the vagina and cervix for lacerations needs to be done. Manual curettage of the uterus can be performed immediately postpartum under appropriate anesthesia.

Breast-Feeding

Breast-feeding has many benefits for both the infant and mother. Breast milk provides the proper nutrition for the infant and protection against certain infectious diseases. Breast-feeding enhances maternal infant bonding and can delay ovulation.

Mothers need support for initiation and continuation of breast-feeding. Both social and professional support systems are invaluable resources for lactating mothers.

Common breast-feeding problems include sore nipples, breast engorgement, blocked milk ducts, and infections. Sore nipples are usually due to improper latch-on of the infant during feeding. This will improve after correction of the latch-on. Breast engorgement usually responds to emptying the breasts by feeding or pumping.

Blocked milk ducts can be confused with infections. A blocked milk duct appears as a localized area of tenderness and erythema in one breast. It responds to warm compresses and gentle massage to express the breast milk and unclog the duct. Mastitis manifests as an erythematous, tender, hard area on one breast. Most women have systemic symptoms, such as fever and chills. Narrow-spectrum

CURRENT DIAGNOSIS

- Recognize and treat postpartum hemorrhage early.
- Uterine atony is the most common cause of immediate postpartum hemorrhage.
- Return to normal diet and physical activity can occur just after birth.
- Endometritis is the most common cause of puerperal fever.
- Screen for postpartum depression several times throughout the postpartum period.
- Address postpartum contraception early after delivery.

antibiotics can be used in most cases. Breast-feeding should be continued on both breasts. If the mother is unable to breast-feed, both breasts should be emptied by a breast pump. A breast abscess can develop as a complication of mastitis and must be surgically drained.

Nutrition and Activity

There are no dietary restrictions in healthy women in the postpartum period. Lactating women need to increase the protein, calories, and calcium in their diet. Physical activity is recommended in pregnancy and should be continued in the postpartum period. Less active women tend to retain more weight at 1 year postpartum than active women.

Puerperal Infections

Uterine infection, which is referred to as *endometritis*, is a common cause of puerperal fever. It is more common following a cesarean delivery. Diagnosis is made from history and physical examination. Fever is the typical manifesting symptom. Uterine tenderness is usually present. Endometritis is a polymicrobial infection. Broad-spectrum intravenous antibiotics are required for treatment. Intravenous antibiotics should be continued for 24 hours after defervescence. Oral antibiotics are not needed following the initial intravenous antibiotics. Complications of endometritis include pelvic infections, pelvic abscess, and septic pelvic thrombophlebitis.

Contraception

Postpartum contraception needs to be addressed with every patient because most will become sexually active before the traditional 6-week postpartum visit. The choice of contraception depends on patient preference, desire for future fertility, and clinical considerations. Table 2 lists methods of postpartum contraception and precautions specific to the postpartum period.

TABLE 1   Medications Used in the Treatment of Postpartum Hemorrhage

Medication	Dosage	Route	Dosing Interval	Cautions and Contraindications
Oxytocin (Pitocin)	10 units IM, 10–40 units/ 1000 mL IV fluids	IV, IM	One dose IM, IV rate as needed to control bleeding	Hypersensitivity to drug or class
Carboprost tromethamine (Hemabate)	250 μg	IM	Every 15–90 min up to 2 mg total	Active cardiac, pulmonary, liver, or renal disease
Methylergonovine (methergine)	0.2 mg	IM, oral	Every 2–4 h up to 5 doses IM, oral tid-qid for 3–7 d	Hypertension

TABLE 2 Methods of Postpartum Contraception

Method of Contraception	When to Start	Precautions in Postpartum Period
Barrier methods: Condoms, diaphragm, cervical cap	At the resumption of sexual activity	Diaphragm or cervical cap will need to be refitted about 6 wk postpartum
Progesterone-only pills (Micronor), injectable (Depo-Provera), or implant (Implanon)	Any time after 24 h postpartum	Pills need to be taken the same time every d Can cause irregular prolonged bleeding postpartum Does not interfere with lactation
Combined oral contraceptive pills, patch (Ortho-Evra), or vaginal ring (NuvaRing)	4 wk postpartum	Decreases breast milk production Not advised if high risk of thromboembolic disease
Intrauterine device or system, progesterone containing (Mirena) or copper T (ParaGard)	Immediately postpartum or 6 wk postpartum	Increased risk of expulsion if inserted immediately postpartum Not advised if high risk of infection or previous ectopic pregnancy
Sterilization: Male or female (transabdominal or transcervical (Essure))	Male anytime, but ideally during the antepartum period. Female after delivery but before hospital discharge or 6 wk postpartum	Future fertility not desired Requires surgery Transcervical sterilization is an outpatient procedure but requires follow-up testing
Lactational amenorrhea method	Can be effective if exclusively breastfeeding up to 6 mo	Not reliable Ovulation can resume at any time
Natural family planning	After onset of first menses	None

Medical Complications

Hypertension and preeclampsia can occur in the postpartum period with persistently elevated blood pressures. Blood pressure is highest 3 to 6 days postpartum. According to a 2005 Cochrane review of trials for treatment and prevention of postpartum hypertension, there are no reliable data to guide its treatment. Significantly elevated blood pressures should be treated as indicated. Evaluation for preeclampsia should be performed postpartum when suspected based on typical symptoms.

Peripartum cardiomyopathy can occur any time from the last month of pregnancy to 5 months postpartum. Diagnosis is made when heart failure develops during this time with no other identifiable cause or preexisting heart failure. Echocardiography is used to document left ventricular systolic dysfunction.

Gestational diabetes complicates approximately 2% to 14% of all pregnancies. Postpartum glucose tolerance testing in gestational diabetics is recommended by the American College of Obstetricians and Gynecologists and the American Diabetes Association. This can be completed at the 6-week postpartum visit.

Other medical problems that can occur in the postpartum period include venous thromboembolic disease, urinary retention, and other infections. These should be identified and treated as appropriate based on the patient's symptoms.

CURRENT THERAPY

- Postpartum hemorrhage usually responds to uterine massage and oxytocics.
- Social and professional support systems are key factors in successful continuation of breast-feeding.
- Oral antibiotics are not necessary after intravenous treatment of endometritis.
- All methods of contraception are acceptable choices postpartum with a few special considerations.

Mood Disorders

Postpartum depression is a common problem that can negatively affect both the mother and infant. Early diagnosis and treatment are important to prevent any negative effects on the child or mother. It is important to screen for depression several times during the postpartum period. The baby blues is very common in the first week after birth and resolves without treatment. Symptoms in patients at high risk for postpartum depression or those that persist after the first week should be treated.

Treatment of postpartum depression should be individualized. Treatment consists of social support and counseling with or without medications. Psychosocial and psychological interventions are associated with a decreased likelihood of depressive symptoms at 1 year postpartum. Antidepressants may be used in the postpartum period but might need to be adjusted during lactation.

Postpartum psychosis is uncommon but potentially dangerous for the mother and infant. The risk of suicide and homicide is high. Inpatient treatment is recommended for postpartum psychosis.

REFERENCES

Britton C, McCormick FM, Renfrew MJ, et al. Support for breastfeeding mothers. Cochrane Database Syst Rev 2007;(1):CD001141.

Committee on Health Care for Underserved Women; Committee on Obstetric Practice. Breastfeeding: Maternal and infant aspects. Int J Gynaecol Obstet 2001;74:217–32.

Dennis CL, Hodnett E. Psychosocial and psychological interventions for treating postpartum depression. Cochrane Database Syst Rev 2007;(4):CD006116.

French LM, Smaill FM. Antibiotic regimens for endometritis after delivery. Cochrane Database Syst Rev 2004;(4):CD001067.

Grimes DA, Schulz KF, Van Vliet H, et al. Immediate post-partum insertion of intrauterine devices. Cochrane Database Syst Rev 2001;(2):CD003036.

Magee L, Sadeghi S. Prevention and treatment of postpartum hypertension. Cochrane Database Syst Rev 2005;(1):CD004351.

Olson CM, Strawderman MS, Hinton PS, Pearson TA. Gestational weight gain and postpartum behaviors associated with weight change from early pregnancy to 1 year postpartum. Int J Obes Relat Metab Disord 2003;27:117–27.

Oyelese Y, Scorza WE, Mastrolia R, Smulian JC. Postpartum hemorrhage. Obstet Gynecol Clin North Am 2007;34:421–41.

Ro A, Frishman WH. Peripartum cardiomyopathy. Cardiol Rev 2006;14:35–42.

Russell MA, Phipps MG, Olson CL, et al. Rates of postpartum glucose testing after gestational diabetes mellitus. Obstet Gynecol 2006;108:1456–62.

Resuscitation of the Newborn

Method of
Stacey Hinderliter, MD, and David Gregory, MD

The changes that occur in the transition from fetus to newborn are unmatched in any other time of life. Most newborns manage to make this transition on their own, but about 10% require some assistance. Approximately 1% of newborns require extensive resuscitative measures to survive. The approach to resuscitation in infants is similar to that in adults, consisting of evaluation and intervention when needed for the infant's airway, breathing, and circulation. Every birth should be attended by personnel trained in neonatal resuscitation. Specific training and certification are offered by the American Heart Association's Neonatal Resuscitation Provider (NRP) course.

Transition from Fetal to Extrauterine Life

The environment of the fetus differs greatly from that of the infant after birth. The fetus depends on receiving oxygen and nutrients from the mother through the placental circulation. The fetus experiences relative hypoxia and almost constant body temperature in the amniotic fluid. The fetal lungs are filled with fluid and do not participate in the exchange of oxygen and carbon dioxide. Several adaptations in the fetus permit survival in this environment.

Oxygenated blood from the mother enters the fetus by means of the placenta through the umbilical vein. Most of this oxygenated blood bypasses the liver through the ductus venosus and enters the inferior vena cava. On entering the right atrium, this oxygenated blood is directed toward the patent foramen ovale into the left atrium, bypassing the fetal lungs. Fetal blood also passes through the right atrium into the right ventricle and then into the pulmonary artery. The vascular resistance and blood pressure of the pulmonary vessels in the fetal lung are higher than in the aorta and systemic circulation; most of the blood is therefore shunted away from the lungs through the ductus arteriosus into the ascending aorta. Only a small amount of fetal blood passes through the lungs to the left atrium and then to the left ventricle. The umbilical arteries branch off from the internal iliac arteries and return fetal blood to the placenta. The functional organ for gas exchange of oxygen and carbon dioxide in the fetus is the placenta.

At birth, the newborn is no longer connected to the placenta, and the lungs become the only source of oxygen. The first breaths of the infant cause the fluid in the lung alveoli to be replaced with air. The umbilical arteries and veins constrict at birth and are eventually clamped. This increases the vascular resistance and blood pressure of the systemic circulation. As the oxygen level in the alveoli increases, the blood vessels in the lung start to relax, decreasing pulmonary vascular resistance. Blood in the pulmonary artery travels toward the lung and away from the ductus arteriosus because the blood pressure in the systemic circulation is higher than that in the pulmonary circulation. Increased blood flow to the lungs allows the oxygen from the alveoli to enter the infant's blood, increasing the Po_2. Oxygenated blood enters the left heart through the pulmonary vein and is delivered to the rest of the infant's tissues through the aorta.

Although the initial steps in this transition occur within a few minutes of birth, the entire process may not be completed for several hours to days. The ductus venosus, foramen ovale, and ductus arteriosus remain potentially patent and do not completely involute for days or weeks. Changes in the infant's systemic and pulmonary pressures can result in blood flow through these channels in the infant.

Transition can be prevented or delayed in several circumstances. The infant may not breathe adequately, in which case the lung fluid is not forced out of the alveoli. Material such as meconium may block air from entering the alveoli. If the lungs do not fill with air, hypoxia will quickly develop. Systemic hypotension due to excessive blood loss, poor cardiac function, or bradycardia prevents the change in the direction of blood flow that is necessary to promote blood flow into the lungs. Failure of the lungs to expand or hypoxia can prevent relaxation of the pulmonary blood vessels, resulting in a high pulmonary vascular resistance. This leads to decreased blood flow to the lungs and worsening of hypoxia.

Risk Factors for Newborn Resuscitation

A number of prenatal and intrapartum factors are associated with a higher chance that the infant will have a delay in transition and require resuscitation. These characteristics are summarized in Table 1. Some, such as severe maternal hypertension or toxemia, can directly affect the placenta blood vessels, resulting in decreased oxygen delivery to the fetus. Complications during labor, including placental abruption, chorioamnionitis, and premature labor, can affect the condition of the infant at the time of birth. Symptoms of fetal compromise, such as fetal bradycardia and meconium staining of the amniotic fluid, are warning signs for a possible need for resuscitation. Maternal age, lack of prenatal care, substance use, and other maternal issues can also affect the newborn infant in a multifactorial fashion. However, some infants *with no risk factors* need resuscitation; therefore, preparations for neonatal resuscitation should be made during all deliveries.

TABLE 1 Risk Factors for Newborn Resuscitation

Prenatal Factors	Intrapartum Factors
Maternal	Placental
Diabetes, preexisting	Placenta previa
Chronic hypertension	Abruption of the placenta
Infection	Premature or prolonged
Cardiac, renal, pulmonary,	rupture of membranes
thyroid, or neurologic	Chorioamnionitis
disease	Fetal
Drug therapy	Macrosomia
Substance use	Low birth weight
Lack of prenatal care	Breech or other abnormal
Age <16 or >35 years	presentation
Previous fetal or neonatal	Persistent fetal bradycardia
death	Non-reassuring fetal heart
Pregnancy	rate patterns
Bleeding in second or third	Labor
trimester	Premature labor
Pregnancy-induced	Precipitous labor
hypertension	Prolonged labor (>24 h)
Toxemia	Prolonged second stage of
Gestational diabetes	labor (>2 h)
Fetal anemia or	Prolapsed cord
isoimmunization	Emergency cesarean section
Polyhydramnios	Forceps or vacuum-assisted
Oligohydramnios	delivery
Fetal hydrops	Other
Postterm gestation	Meconium-stained amniotic
Multiple gestation	fluid
Size-date discrepancy	General anesthesia
Diminished fetal activity	Narcotics given within 4 h of
Fetal malformation or	delivery
abnormality	Uterine hyperstimulation
	Severe intrapartum bleeding

Reaction to Hypoxia and Asphyxia

Normally at birth, the newborn makes vigorous efforts to breathe. The process of leaving the warm, dark, and liquid environment in utero is replaced by cold air, dryness, and bright lights. Drying the infant with towels and suctioning the mouth and nose are all the assistance that most newborns require. The end result of any mechanism that delays transition is a period of hypoxia for the fetus or newborn infant. Laboratory studies have shown that the first sign of oxygen deprivation in the newborn is a change in the breathing pattern. After an initial period of rapid breathing attempts, cessation of breathing occurs. This is called *primary apnea*. Stimulation by drying the infant or slapping the feet can cause breathing to resume. If hypoxia continues after primary apnea has occurred, the infant will make attempts at gasping and then stop breathing. This is called *secondary apnea*. Stimulation does not affect secondary apnea. Assisted ventilation is necessary to provide breaths to the newborn to reverse the hypoxia. The infant's heart rate starts to decrease when primary apnea occurs. The heart rate increases with stimulation if the infant has primary apnea, and blood pressure is maintained. With continued hypoxia, the heart rate continues to drop, and hypotension develops. If assisted ventilation is not adequate to increase the infant's heart rate, chest compressions will be required.

When a newborn becomes apneic, it is not readily apparent whether the infant has primary or secondary apnea. The approach to resuscitation therefore requires that any apneic event in a newborn be treated using the same sequence of interventions. If the apneic infant responds to simple stimulation, the diagnosis is primary apnea, and no further intervention is required. If the infant does not improve with stimulation, secondary apnea has occurred, and more intensive intervention is needed.

CURRENT DIAGNOSIS

- The transition from intrauterine to extrauterine life at birth requires effective breathing by the infant to expand the lungs and oxygenate the blood. All newborn infants are at risk for delays in this process, prompting a need for resuscitation.
- The fetal and newborn response to hypoxia is to develop apnea. If primary apnea is diagnosed, it can be corrected by gentle stimulation and oxygen delivery. If hypoxia persists, secondary apnea will occur. It is not readily apparent whether a newborn has primary or secondary apnea, and the approach to resuscitation therefore requires that any apneic event be treated using the same sequence of interventions.
- Basic newborn resuscitation includes drying the infant, providing warmth, suctioning the airway, and providing gentle stimulation. Infants who do not respond to these interventions need more assistance. Establishment of effective ventilation spontaneously by the newborn or with assistance by positive-pressure ventilation is the most important step in newborn resuscitation.
- Reassessment of the infant's heart rate, respiratory effort, color, and tone every 30 seconds during resuscitation is crucial to determine the next appropriate intervention. Apgar scoring should *not* be used to guide newborn resuscitation.
- If application of positive-pressure ventilation does not improve the infant's heart rate, chest compressions or drug therapy, or both, may be required. A team approach is needed to coordinate these interventions, and ongoing reassessment is necessary to determine cardiorespiratory and hemodynamic status. Subsequent assessment and treatment should be performed in an intensive care setting.

Sequence of Newborn Resuscitation

INITIAL STEPS AND BASIC RESUSCITATION

Resuscitation of the newborn starts with knowledge of two essential risk factors: Is the infant at *term gestation*, and is the amniotic fluid stained with *meconium*? The answers to these questions will affect the approach to care. Resuscitation when fluid is meconium stained is discussed later in this chapter. The information presented here refers to term infants with clear amniotic fluid. More information regarding the care of premature infants is discussed in a later section.

The next step is to determine whether the infant is crying vigorously and whether there is good muscle tone. This quick assessment should be performed simultaneously with the initial steps of resuscitation: providing warmth, positioning and clearing (if needed) the airway, drying and stimulating the infant.

The newborn should be placed under a radiant warmer to prevent heat loss and to allow easy observation. Although warm blankets or towels can be used to dry the infant, they should not be left in place to cover the infant. The newborn should be placed on the back with the neck slightly extended in the "sniffing" position (Fig. 1). This facilitates air entry into the lungs by lining up the posterior pharynx, larynx, and trachea. Hyperextension or hyperflexion of the neck can obstruct air entry into the lungs.

If the newborn is crying vigorously, secretions can be removed by wiping the nose and the mouth with a towel or gentle suctioning of the mouth and nose with a bulb syringe or suction catheter. Deep or vigorous suctioning can be detrimental to the infant because of stimulation of the vagus nerve, causing bradycardia or apnea.

Drying the infant, slapping the feet, and rubbing the back are appropriate forms of stimulation. More forceful methods of stimulation can harm the infant. Primary apnea, if present, will respond to stimulation in less than 30 seconds. Prolonged apnea will require positive-pressure ventilation (PPV).

Evaluating the infant's response to resuscitation is essential. The Apgar score is a traditional method for evaluating newborn status at 1 and 5 minutes after delivery. However, effective resuscitation demands that evaluation of the newborn's status not be delayed until 1 minute of age, and Apgar scores therefore should *not* be used to guide resuscitative efforts. Within 30 seconds of delivery, the infant's need for PPV must be assessed. Establishment of effective ventilation spontaneously by the newborn or with assistance by PPV is the most important step in newborn resuscitation. The respiratory status, heart rate, and color should be determined. The chest wall should move with each breath, and the newborn should be breathing spontaneously. Heart rate can be assessed by feeling for a pulse at the base

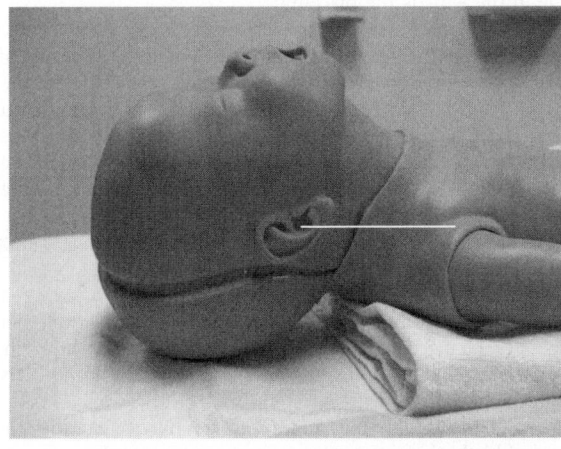

FIGURE 1. The sniffing position. Positioning the infant on the back with the neck slightly extended brings the posterior pharynx, larynx, and trachea in line (*white line*) to facilitate air entry into the lungs.

of the umbilical cord. If this pulse cannot be felt, a stethoscope can be used to listen for the heartbeat. The heart rate should be greater than 100 beats/min. Peripheral cyanosis (i.e., blueness of the hands and feet) is acceptable in the initial period after delivery. Central cyanosis in which the lips and trunk are blue indicates hypoxemia and the need for more resuscitation efforts.

RESPIRATORY SUPPORT AND POSITIVE-PRESSURE VENTILATION

If the infant is breathing with a heart rate higher than 100 beats/min but has central cyanosis, free-flowing oxygen delivery is indicated. This can be administered with a facemask or by holding oxygen tubing or a flow-inflating bag and mask close to the infant's face. *A self-inflating bag and mask cannot be used to give free-flowing oxygen.* If the newborn is apneic, not breathing effectively, or has a heart rate less than 100 beats/min, PPV using a self-inflating bag, flow-inflating (or anesthesia) bag, or a T-piece resuscitator is required. Use of a flow-inflating bag requires a compressed gas source and considerable practice to be used effectively. A T-piece resuscitator needs special equipment and a compressed gas source. Most delivery rooms are equipped with self-inflating bags (Fig. 2) because they are easy to use and can be fitted with a pressure-release valve to decrease overinflation. A reservoir must be used with a self-inflating bag to provide 100% oxygen.

The facemask should cover the infant's nose, mouth, and tip of chin, but not the eyes (Fig. 3). Multiple sizes should be available. A tight seal between the infant's skin and the facemask is needed, but excessive pressure can bruise the face. The mask can be held in place using the thumb and index finger in a C-shaped position on top of the mask, with the remaining fingers in an E-shaped position below the infant's chin (Fig. 4). Inspiratory pressures of 20 to 30 cm H_2O are usually needed when squeezing the bag to make the infant's chest rise. A pressure gauge can be connected to the self-inflating bag for monitoring inspiratory pressure. The heart rate and color of the infant should rapidly improve if enough pressure is being given. An assistant can also use a stethoscope to listen to breath sounds for air movement. Breaths should be given at a rate of 40 to 60 breaths/min.

Traditionally, 100% oxygen has been used in newborn resuscitation. However, several randomized, controlled studies enrolling term and near-term infants have shown that room air can be used initially with oxygen as a backup if room air fails. A meta-analysis of these trials showed a benefit for the use of room air. Providing oxygen at concentrations between room air and 100% requires the use of compressed air, oxygen, and blenders by experienced personnel. Not all facilities have these items available. The current recommendation is that initially using room air or 100% oxygen is acceptable and that ensuring adequate ventilation is the priority.

After 30 seconds of PPV, the infant should be reevaluated. Ventilation with a bag and mask can be stopped when the newborn has a

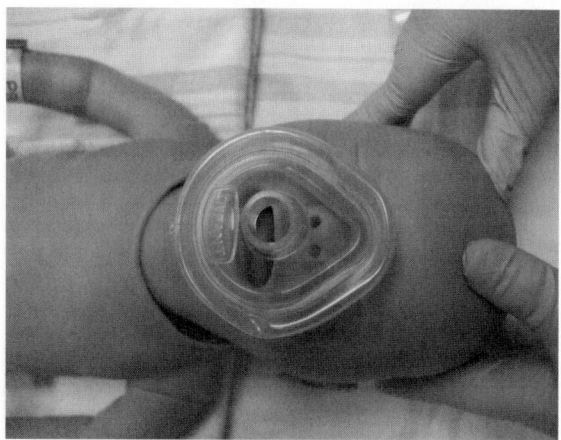

FIGURE 3. Facemask. Choose a size that covers the infant's mouth and nose.

heart rate higher than 100 beats/min, spontaneous breathing, improved color, and good muscle tone. Supplemental oxygen should still be given to the infant. If the newborn is not improving, reassess the seal between the face mask and the infant's skin, look for airway blockage by repositioning and suctioning, or increase the pressure being used to inflate the bag. If these steps do not improve the infant's heart rate and color, endotracheal (ET) intubation may be required.

ET intubation is a technical skill that must be learned and practiced to maintain competency. Effective ventilation can be given with a bag and mask approach to most newborns. This skill is easily mastered and maintained. If an infant is responding well to bag and mask ventilation, it can be continued for longer periods; however, some air may escape into the esophagus and into the stomach. This may cause gastric distention, which can prevent full expansion of the lungs and cause vomiting and aspiration. An orogastric tube can be placed in the stomach and left open to air to vent any air introduced into the infant's stomach during bag and mask ventilation.

CHEST COMPRESSIONS

After 30 seconds of effective PPV, the heart rate should be assessed. If the heart rate dips below 60 beats/min, chest compressions are needed to support the circulation. The thumb technique (Fig. 5) is preferred, but the two-finger technique (Fig. 6) can be used, especially when placement of an umbilical venous catheter is required. Two people are required to give PPV and chest compressions effectively. To coordinate the breaths and chest compressions, three compressions are given followed by one breath, and this sequence is repeated to give the infant

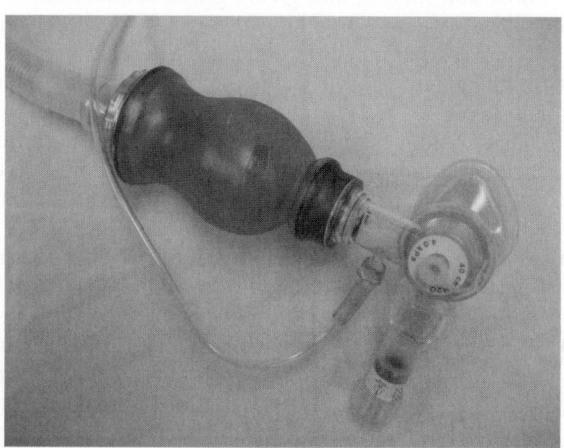

FIGURE 2. Self-inflating bag with infant mask and reservoir. This type of device is available in most delivery rooms.

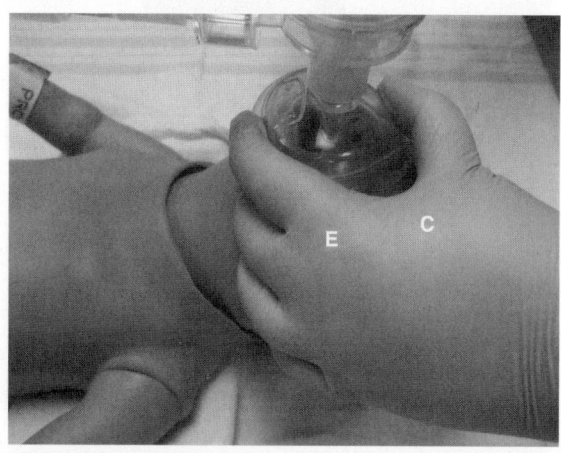

FIGURE 4. Facemask placement. The thumb and index finger are held in a C-shaped position on top of the mask, and the remaining fingers are held in an E-type position under the chin.

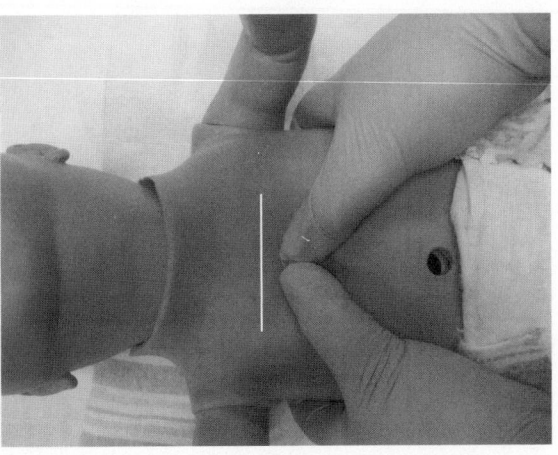

FIGURE 5. Thumb technique. The hands encircle the torso, and the thumbs are placed on top of the lower sternum above the xyphoid process and below a line drawn between the nipples (*white line*).

90 compressions and 30 breaths/min. The thumb or fingers are placed on the lower third of the infant's sternum but above the xyphoid process. The sternum is depressed to a depth of one third of the infant's anteroposterior chest diameter. The purpose of chest compressions is to squeeze the heart between the sternum and the spine, forcing blood in and out of the heart and to the body. The direction of the compressions should be perpendicular to the chest surface, and the fingers should not be lifted off of the chest after the correct placement is obtained. Incorrect methods during chest compressions can cause rib fracture and liver laceration.

After 30 seconds of chest compressions, the infant's heart rate, color, breathing, and tone are reassessed. If the heart rate is higher than 60 beats/min, chest compressions can be stopped, although PPV may still be needed. If the heart rate is not improving, the following problems must considered: ventilation is not adequate, 100% oxygen concentration is not being given, or the compressions may not be deep enough or well coordinated with the breaths.

MEDICATIONS FOR NEWBORN RESUSCITATION

If the newborn heart rate remains below 60 beats/min despite PPV and chest compressions, epinephrine (Adrenalin) can be used to stimulate the newborn heart. Fewer than 2 of 1000 infants will require this step in resuscitation. Epinephrine can be administered by ET tube, but *intravenous administration is preferred*.

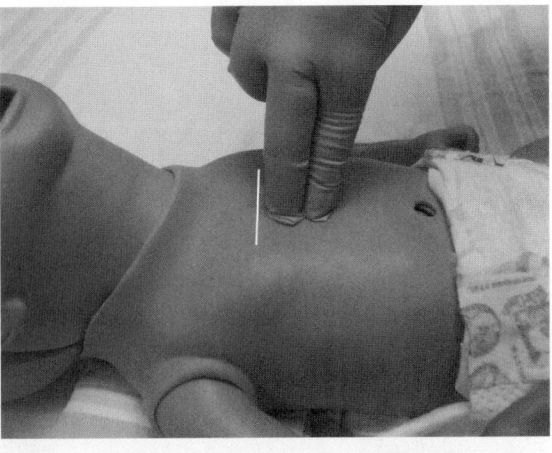

FIGURE 6. Two-finger technique. The index and middle finger are used to apply pressure on the lower third of the sternum above the xyphoid process and below a line drawn between the nipples (*white line*).

A catheter can be quickly inserted into the umbilical vein for intravenous access. A 3.5 or 5 F catheter prefilled with saline and connected to a 3-way stopcock is inserted about 2 to 4 cm into the umbilical vein using sterile technique. After blood is aspirated, insertion of the catheter is stopped, and the epinephrine is given, followed by a saline flush. The concentration of epinephrine used in neonatal resuscitation is 1:10,000. The intravenous dose is 0.01 to 0.03 mg/kg (0.1 to 0.3 mL/kg) (Table 2). A dose of epinephrine can be given through the ET tube during the umbilical vein catheterization. The ET dose of epinephrine is 0.03 to 0.1 mg/kg (0.3 to 1 mL/kg). *These higher doses are for ET use only.* Because lung absorption of epinephrine varies, the intravenous route using the umbilical vein is preferred.

During umbilical vein cannulation, PPV and chest compressions are continued. More personnel will be needed to place the catheter and draw up the medications and saline flushes. After an intravenous dose of epinephrine, the infant's heart rate, respirations, color, and tone are reevaluated. The heart rate should increase to more than 60 beats/min. If the heart rate does not respond, the dose of epinephrine can be repeated every 3 to 5 minutes. The effectiveness of ventilation and compressions should be reassessed. If the infant appears pale, has delayed capillary refill, or decreased pulses, shock may be present. Infant blood loss might have occurred during delivery from placental problems or other sources. Administration of a volume expander such as normal saline or Ringer's lactate at 10 mL/kg over 5 to 10 minutes can improve circulation. If anemia is suspected, O negative blood can be given. Volume expansion should be used cautiously because there is evidence from animal studies for poorer outcomes when volume expansion is used in the absence of hypovolemia.

Newborns, especially premature infants, are at risk for hypoglycemia. Blood from the infant's heel or the umbilical vein can be tested at the bedside and intravenous 10% dextrose (2 to 5 mL/kg) given for glucose levels below 40 g/dL. In cases of severe metabolic acidosis, administration of sodium bicarbonate may be considered, but only if ventilation is adequate because sodium bicarbonate produces carbon dioxide. It is also caustic and should *never* be given in the ET tube. There is no evidence that use of sodium bicarbonate benefits the neonate, and its use during resuscitation in the delivery room is not recommended.

After resuscitation, newborns should be monitored in an intensive care setting. These infants are at risk for several complications, such as infection, metabolic abnormalities, and seizures.

 CURRENT THERAPY

- Initial resuscitation therapy for all newborns includes drying the infant, providing warmth, suctioning the nose and mouth, and giving gentle stimulation.
- If the infant is breathing vigorously but has central cyanosis, oxygen should be administered.
- If the infant is apneic, breathing slowly, or gasping, positive-pressure ventilation (PPV) with a mask and bag should be administered. Infants with meconium-stained amniotic fluid who are apneic should receive suctioning of the trachea by endotracheal intubation before PPV.
- If the infant's heart rate drops below 60 beats/min, chest compressions should be initiated using the thumb or two-finger technique.
- If the heart rate remains less than 60 beats/min despite PPV and chest compressions, IV epinephrine (Adrenalin) and other medications should be given using an umbilical venous catheter.
- Reassessment of the newborn every 30 seconds during resuscitation is required to adjust therapy as indicated.

TABLE 2 Drugs for Newborn Resuscitation

Drug	Concentration	Dose	Indications	Comments
Epinephrine	1:10,000	0.01–0.03 mg/kg IV = 0.1–0.3 mL/kg IV route preferred 0.03–0.1 mg/kg ETT	Asystole Bradycardia that does not improve with PPV and chest compressions Shock	May repeat every 3–5 min
Volume expanders	Normal saline Ringer's lactate O negative blood	10 mL/kg IV	Hypovolemia	Crossmatch blood to mother if possible Repeat if needed
Glucose	10% Dextrose	2–5 mL/kg IV	Hypoglycemia	Monitor glucometer or venous glucose levels
Naloxone (Narcan)		0.1 mg/kg IV	Maternal administration of narcotics <4 h before delivery and newborn respiratory depression	Use PPV first, then give naloxone; repeated doses may be needed May cause opioid withdrawal in newborns born to addicted mothers
Sodium bicarbonate	0.5 mEq/mL	1–2 mEq/kg IV	Severe metabolic acidosis with adequate ventilation	Infuse slowly No evidence of benefit

Abbreviations: ETT = endotracheal tube; IV = intravenous; PPV = positive-pressure ventilation.

Special Considerations

Some newborns do not respond to resuscitation because of specific problems. Infants with upper airway obstruction from micrognathia can be helped by a nasopharyngeal airway and placement of the infant in the prone position. Choanal atresia can be treated by placing an oral airway. Absence of breath sounds on one side of the chest can indicate a pneumothorax, requiring needle aspiration of the chest. An infant with a scaphoid abdomen and decreased breath sounds may have a diaphragmatic hernia. These infants should be intubated, and PPV by mask and bag should not be used. If the mother has received narcotics shortly before the delivery, the narcotic may be the cause of respiratory depression in the infant. These infants need *PPV and respiratory support first.* After resuscitation, intravenous naloxone (Narcan) at 0.1 mg/kg can be given. Prolonged ventilation and multiple doses of naloxone may be needed.

ENDOTRACHEAL INTUBATION

Intubation of the newborn requires preparation that can be performed while the infant is being ventilated by bag and mask. The ET tube should not be placed unless the glottis is visualized by direct laryngoscopy. To ensure that the tube is in the trachea, a carbon dioxide (CO_2) detector should be used. Listening for equal breath sounds and looking for vapor condensation in the ET tube during exhalation can help, but an increase in the infant's heart rate or a positive detection of CO_2 is most reliable.

Intubation should be performed as quickly as possible, with a goal of 20 seconds from insertion of the laryngoscope to the connection of the ET tube to the resuscitation bag. Complications of intubation include worsening of hypoxia and bradycardia, pneumothorax, contusions, perforation of the trachea or esophagus, and infection. After the infant has been intubated, deterioration in the infant's status should prompt an organized sequence to assess the adequacy of ventilation using the mnemonic DOPE:

Dislodged (D): Is the tube in the right bronchus or out of the trachea?
Obstructed (O): Is the tube obstructed by secretions or blood?
Pneumothorax (P) and *esophagus* (E): Is the tube in the esophagus?

An alternative to intubation is placement of a laryngeal mask airway. This type of airway does not require laryngoscopy. A soft inflatable mask that is attached to a flexible airway tube is placed in the hypopharynx such that the air in the tube is directed into the larynx and away from the esophagus. However, this type of airway cannot be used to suction meconium from the trachea.

PREMATURE INFANTS

Infants born before 37 weeks' gestation are at increased risk for complications and the need for resuscitation. Premature lungs may lack surfactant, making ventilation difficult. Immature brain development may decrease the drive to breathe. Weak muscles make respiratory efforts less effective. Thin skin and decreased subcutaneous fat make temperature regulation a challenge. Premature infants often have infections such as pneumonia or sepsis. The blood vessels in their brains are fragile and can easily bleed during periods of blood pressure variation. The lower birth weights of premature newborns also require smaller sizes of equipment for resuscitation such as facemasks, suction catheters, endotracheal tubes, and umbilical catheters. Oxygen concentrations less than 100% are often used to protect the premature infant from oxygen toxicity. Many personnel trained in newborn resuscitation should be present at the delivery of a high-risk premature infant.

MECONIUM STAINING OF THE AMNIOTIC FLUID

Meconium is formed in the newborn gastrointestinal system during gestation. Intrauterine stress can cause release of meconium into the amniotic fluid. Aspiration of meconium-stained amniotic fluid into the lungs can result in severe pneumonitis and lung injury. The approach to resuscitation for an infant with meconium-stained fluid depends on the *condition of the infant immediately after birth.* There is no evidence that the consistency of meconium-stained fluid (i.e., thick or thin) should change these approaches.

Crying and Vigorous Infant

If the newborn with meconium-stained amniotic fluid has normal respiratory effort and muscle tone with a heart rate higher than 100 beats/min, *gentle* mouth and nose suctioning can be performed using a bulb syringe or suction catheter, similar to the initial resuscitation steps for all infants. Deep and prolonged suctioning should be avoided. ET intubation is not required for vigorous infants with meconium-stained amniotic fluid.

Depressed Infant

Newborns who are gasping or apneic, have poor muscle tone, and have a heart rate less than 100 beats/min require direct suctioning of the trachea to prevent aspiration of the meconium-stained fluid. A laryngoscope is inserted, and a 12- or 14-F catheter is used to suction the mouth and posterior pharynx. After visualizing the glottis, an ET tube is inserted and attached to a suction source. Suction is applied as the ET tube is withdrawn (Fig. 7). This maneuver may

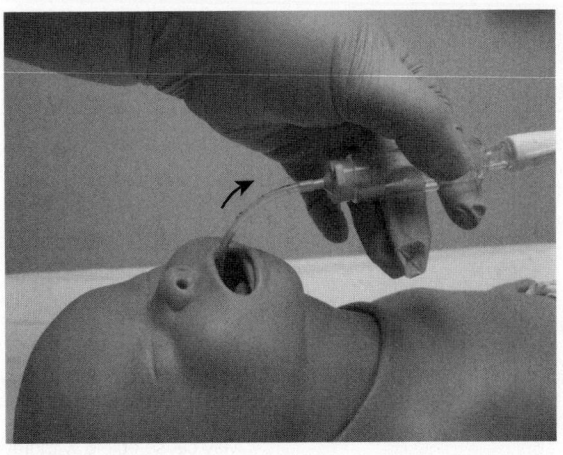

FIGURE 7. The meconium aspirator is attached to a suction source and connected to the endotracheal (ET) tube inserted into the infant's trachea. The thumb is used to occlude the suction-control port to apply suction to the ET tube while gradually withdrawing the ET tube from the trachea (*arrow*).

be repeated until the suctioned fluid is clear unless the infant requires resuscitation (e.g., apneic, heart rate <100 beats/min, decreased muscle tone, cyanotic). After ET suctioning, a bag and mask can be used to provide PPV for the infant if needed. The usual sequence of newborn resuscitation is then followed.

NEWBORN RESUSCITATION OUTSIDE OF THE DELIVERY ROOM

Resuscitation of infants born at home, in an emergency room, in an ambulance, or otherwise outside of a delivery room setting should proceed according to the same principles as in the delivery room. Providing warmth, suctioning the airway, and providing stimulation

TABLE 3 Equipment for Newborn Resuscitation

Type of Use	Equipment
General	Sterile towels
	Radiant warmer or heat lamps
	Pulse oximeter
	Cardiorespiratory monitor
	Sterile gowns, gloves
Airway	Bulb syringe
	Suction catheters (5, 8, 10, 12, 14 F)
	Suction source with manometer
	Oral and nasopharyngeal airways (newborn sizes)
	Laryngoscope and straight blades sizes 0 and 1
	Endotracheal tubes (sizes 2.5, 3.0, 3.5, 4.0)
	Meconium suction device
Ventilation	Face masks (premature, newborn, and infant sizes)
	Self-inflating bag (450–750 mL) with oxygen reservoir and manometer
	Oxygen source
	Orogastric tubes (8, 10 F)
	Carbon dioxide (CO_2) indicator
	Chest tubes (8 and 10 F)
Circulation	Umbilical catheters (3.5 and 5 F)
	Umbilical catheter tray (sterile scissors, scalpel, forceps, umbilical tape)
	Three-way stopcock
	Syringes (1, 3, 5, 10 mL)
	Normal saline
	Epinephrine 1:10,000
	10% Dextrose
	Naloxone (Narcan)
	Sodium bicarbonate (0.5 mEq/mL)
	Ringer's lactate

are usually adequate measures. Establishing effective ventilation using a bag and mask is the most important step if the infant fails to breathe on its own. Emergency providers should be familiar with resuscitation of the newborn, and basic equipment (Table 3) should be available.

WITHHOLDING AND WITHDRAWING NEWBORN RESUSCITATION

Newborns should be offered resuscitation at delivery except in extreme circumstances. Newborn resuscitation should not be used if the infant has a condition that is incompatible with survival, such as a confirmed gestational age of less than 23 completed weeks, birth weight less than 400 g, or congenital anomalies associated with certain death or extreme morbidity.

In most situations, initial resuscitation can provide time to observe the infant's response to interventions and to discuss the infant's condition with the parents. Techniques for obstetric dating of pregnancies are accurate only to ±1 to 2 weeks, and estimates of fetal weight are accurate only to ±100 to 200 g. Care must be taken before deciding to withhold resuscitation from a newborn. Ongoing conversation between parents and medical caregivers allows mutual decision making. Withdrawal of care is indicated if continued support is futile. After 10 minutes of asystole (heart rate of 0), newborns are very unlikely to survive.

REFERENCES

American Academy of Pediatrics Committee on Fetus and Newborn. Bell EF. Noninitiation or withdrawal of intensive care for high-risk newborns. Pediatrics 2007;119:401.

American Heart Association. 2005 American Heart Association (AHA) guidelines for cardiopulmonary resuscitation (CPR) and emergency cardiovascular care (ECC) of pediatric and neonatal patients: Neonatal resuscitation guidelines. Pediatrics 2006;117:e1029.

Aschner JL, Poland RL. Sodium bicarbonate: Basically useless therapy. Pediatrics 2008;122:831.

Bassam H, Mercer BM, Livingston JC, et al. Outcome after successful resuscitation of babies born with Apgar scores of 0 at both 1 and 5 minutes. Am J Obstet Gynecol 2000;182:1210.

Escobedo M. Moving from experience to evidence: Changes in US Neonatal Resuscitation Program based on International Liaison Committee on Resuscitation Review. J Perinatol 2008;28:835.

Field DJ, Dorling JS, Manktelow BN, et al. Survival of extremely premature babies in a geographically defined population: Prospective cohort study of 1994–99 compared with 2000–05. BMJ 2008;336:1221.

Halliday HL. Endotracheal intubation at birth for preventing morbidity and mortality in vigorous, meconium-stained infants born at term. Cochrane Database Syst Rev 2001;(1):CD000500.

Jain L, Ferre C, Vidyasagar D, et al. Cardiopulmonary resuscitation of apparently stillborn infants: Survival and long-term outcome. J Pediatr 1991;118:778.

Wiswell TE, Gannon CM, Jacob J, et al. Delivery room management of the apparently vigorous meconium-stained neonate: Results of the multicenter, international collaborative trial. Pediatrics 2000;105:1.

Care of the High-Risk Neonate

Method of
Dilcia McLenan, MD

Despite advances in prenatal care and diagnosis, the overall prematurity rate has not changed in the past two decades. The rate remains at 10% to 12% of all births in the United States. Although the overall mortality rate and the short-term morbidity rate have improved with the advances in neonatal care, premature births are still responsible for 75% to 85% of neonatal deaths. Congenital anomalies are associated with 20% to 30% of perinatal deaths. The early identification of the high-risk neonate is essential to improve outcome. The goal is to prevent the development or progression of more serious illnesses and to minimize the risk of both morbidity and mortality.

The definition of the high-risk neonate can be applied in the prenatal, perinatal or postnatal period. Approximately 75% of risk factors affecting the fetus are identified in the prenatal period. Maternal high-risk factors include age, race, socioeconomic status, nutrition and past obstetric history, current pregnancy problems, and maternal drug use. Maternal acute and chronic illness can also adversely affect the fetus. The placenta is considered fetal tissue; all conditions that affect the placenta will also affect the fetus, and vice versa. Fetal factors are limited to genetic conditions (chromosomal and nonchromosomal), and metabolic.

The prenatal diagnosis of the high-risk neonate uses many tools, such as chorionic villus sampling (CVS), amniocentesis, maternal serum screening, and cordocentesis. With the use of cytogenetics, molecular biology, and the fluorescence in situ hybridization, many genetic disorders and infectious conditions can be diagnosed. Fetal ultrasonography is another valuable tool in diagnosing high-risk conditions, including fetal growth abnormalities, which are associated with increased perinatal morbidity and mortality. The Doppler can assess blood velocity in the umbilical and fetal vessels. There is increased morbidity and mortality in fetuses with absent umbilical artery flow or with reverse end diastolic flow. The measurement of the nuchal translucency, done between 10 and 14 weeks of gestation by fetal ultrasound (US) in conjunction with the maternal serum markers, increases the detection rate of Down syndrome and other chromosomal and genetic syndromes, fetal structural malformations, and adverse pregnancy outcome.

Prenatal care facilitates the diagnosis and care of the high-risk neonate through a multidisciplinary approach. This multidisciplinary approach sets the stage for counseling, referrals, and the plan of care pre- and postnatally. When counseling the family, consider the gestational age at diagnosis, effect on maternal outcome and neonatal prognosis with or without therapy, plans for delivery, intrapartum management, and surgical intervention when applicable. General discussion with the parents during the intrapartum period regarding the preterm or high-risk neonate will include such things as anticipated birth weight and gestational age, the need for respiratory support, procedures to be expected, the need for transfusion of blood products, short- and long-term complications of each problem or condition, the need for other specialists, and morbidity and mortality. Involving the neonatologist in the counseling can aid families in making difficult decisions. One should also explain the need for transport, if delivered at a nontertiary care center, and the role the parents will have while their infant is in the neonatal intensive care unit (NICU).

The delivery management of the high-risk neonate is influenced by the factors identified in the antepartum and intrapartum period. In the intrapartum period, neonatal resuscitation facilitates the transition from the intrauterine to the extrauterine life. Approximately 5% to 10% of all newborns need help making this transition; 1% of all newborns need a more extensive intervention. The fetus is dependent on its mother and the placenta for the delivery of oxygen and nutrients as well as removal of carbon dioxide. After the umbilical cord is clamped and cut, the newborn needs to expand its lungs, establishing respirations and convert from a fetal (parallel) to an adult (in series) circulation for a successful transition, and avoid the development of asphyxia.

Resuscitation aims at facilitating the transition and reversing the process of asphyxia by clearing the airway, providing adequate oxygenation and ventilation, ensuring adequate cardiac output, and keeping oxygen consumption to the minimum. These objectives can be achieved by adhering to the initial steps and the four principles of neonatal resuscitation.

Principles of Neonatal Resuscitation

The American Heart Association (AHA) and the American Academy of Pediatrics (AAP) Neonatal Resuscitation Program (NRP) have defined the following principles of neonatal resuscitation:

- **Anticipation.** Risk factors in the antepartum and intrapartum history help identify instances that may potentially require intervention (Box 1).
- **Preparation.** In preparing the area, equipment should be assembled and checked, and drugs should be readied.
- **Availability of qualified personnel.** At every delivery there should be at least one person skilled in neonatal resuscitation whose only responsibility is the newborn; skills include the proper use of the bag and mask. In cases of emergency or if further intervention is needed, additional competent personnel should be immediately available.
- **Organized response to the emergencies—evaluation, decision, and action.** The ABCs (airway, breathing, and circulation) of resuscitation is the order in which assessment and needed intervention will be evaluated. The evaluation assesses the breathing, heart rate, and color, then the decision or diagnosis is made followed by the action or treatment.

BOX 1   Antepartum/Intrapartum Factors Associated with Potential Asphyxia

Antepartum Factors

Age >35 years
Maternal diabetes
Pregnancy-induced hypertension
Chronic hypertension
Anemia or isoimmunization
Previous fetal or neonatal death
Bleeding in 2nd or 3rd trimester
Maternal infection
Hydramnios
Oligohydramnios
Premature rupture of membranes
Post-term gestation
Multiple gestation
Size-date discrepancy
Drug therapy, e.g.:
    Lithium carbonate
    Magnesium
    Adrenergic blocking drugs
Maternal substance abuse
Fetal malformation
Diminished fetal activity
No prenatal care

Intrapartum Factors

Emergency cesarean section
Breech or other abnormal presentation
Premature labor
Prolonged rupture of membranes >24 h before delivery
Precipitous labor
Prolonged labor (>24 h)
Prolonged second stage of labor (>2 h)
Nonreassuring fetal heart rate pattern
Use of general anesthesia
Uterine tetany
Narcotics administered to mother within 4 h of delivery
Meconium-stained amniotic fluid
Prolapsed cord
Abruptio placentae
Placenta previa

Note: Keep these factors in mind because they will alert you that depression and possibly asphyxia are potential problems.
From Bloom RS, Cropley C: The AHNAAP Neonatal Resuscitation Program Steering Committee. Textbook of Neonatal Resuscitation. Dallas, TX, 1994, Copyright American Heart Association.

TABLE 1 At Birth

Initial Step	Objective
Provide warmth	Prevent heat loss, maintain oxygen consumption at a minimum, and prevent hypoglycemia
Position, clear the airway (as necessary)	Establish an airway
Dry stimulate and reposition	Initiate breathing and open the airway

The initial steps of resuscitation provide the support needed to make the transition from the intrauterine to the extrauterine life (Table 1).

Shortcutting these steps prolongs the resuscitation process, increases the risk for asphyxia, and increases the likelihood of morbidity and mortality. In cases where further intervention is needed beyond the initial steps of resuscitation, a thorough evaluation should be done to diagnose conditions that might have contributed to the need for further resuscitation, such as congenital abnormalities of the airway, heart, gastrointestinal (GI) tract, genitourinary (GU) system, or secondary cardiopulmonary disorders. Infants with Apgar scores below 7 at 10 minutes should be admitted to the NICU for further observation and management.

Asphyxia

Asphyxia is the result of prolonged decrease of oxygen delivery to the tissues. During the event, there is redistribution of blood flow to the heart, brain, and adrenals. The continuation of the insult results in bradycardia, impaired gas exchange, and reduced tissue perfusion. These series of events can occur prenatally, intrapartum, or postnatally. In severe cases of asphyxia almost every organ of the body is affected:

- Central nervous system (CNS): hypoxic ischemic encephalopathy
- Cardiovascular: myocardial dysfunction
- Renal: renal dysfunction and or acute renal failure
- GI: liver dysfunction and increased risk of necrotizing enterocolitis
- Hematologic: coagulopathy
- Pulmonary: activation of the mechanisms that cause persistent pulmonary hypertension of the newborn, surfactant (Survanta) deficiency, and meconium aspiration syndrome (MAS)
- Metabolic: acidosis, hypoglycemia, and hypocalcemia

After birth the normal newborn goes through a period of transition that lasts for several hours. During this period the cardiovascular, pulmonary, and sympathetic systems regulate themselves to adjust to extrauterine life. During the transition, abnormalities in color, respirations, heart rate, sleep state, motor activity, GI function, and temperature stability can be identified and will require care in the NICU. Clinical manifestations of abnormal transition include persistent tachypnea, nasal flaring, grunting, retractions, persistent cyanosis, apnea and bradycardia, pallor, temperature instability, blood pressure (BP) instability, lethargy, and other neurologic symptoms.

Postnatal Care

The postnatal care of the high-risk neonate is extremely important. There are interventions and supportive care that are common to the high-risk neonates to ensure the best possible outcome. These include thermoregulation, nutrition, developmental care, and parental involvement. Notwithstanding, individualized care that will address specific needs of each infant should always be kept in mind.

THERMOREGULATION

Thermoregulation is the balance between heat production and heat loss. It is closely linked to morbidity and mortality. In the neonate, heat loss can exceed heat production because of larger surface area to body mass ratio, decreased subcutaneous (SC) tissue or fat, increased permeability to water and small radius of curvature of exchange surfaces.

The newborn generates heat by nonshivering mechanisms—brown fat, increased muscular activity, flexion, and increased metabolic rate with increased oxygen consumption. The newborn loses heat through conduction, convection, evaporation, and radiation (Table 2).

In the neonate there is always a combination of types and mechanism of heat loss. The prevention of cold stress and hypothermia is critical for intact survival of the neonate (Figure 1).

Heat production is a result of metabolic processes that generate energy by oxidative metabolism of glucose (most efficient in the premature infant), fat, and protein. In the newborn, heat or energy production is low relative to heat or energy losses. Brown adipose tissue generates more energy than any other tissue in the body. The brown adipose tissue cells begin to differentiate by 26 to 30 weeks of gestation and continue to develop until 3 to 5 weeks after birth; they constitute 10% of the adipose tissue in term infants.

Thermoregulation is achieved by providing the appropriate thermal environment to prevent heat loss, hypothermia, and cold stress. The neutral thermal environment (NTE) is an idealized range of ambient temperature at which the body temperature is normal, metabolic rate or oxygen consumption is minimal, and thermoregulation is achieved by basal nonevaporative physical processes. It promotes growth and stability and minimizes heat (energy) and water loss.

TABLE 2 Thermoregulation: Types, Mechanisms, and Management

Type/Definition	Mechanism	Prevention
Conduction, transfer of heat from the body core to surface, and object in contact with body	Cold surfaces, cold objects in contact with the body	Use rubber mattresses, warm blankets, and warm mattresses.
Convection, heat transfer from the body surface to the surrounding air	Cool rapid air flow, cold oxygen flow	Swaddle using a cap, warm oxygen, and placing infant away from draft. Servo control air or skin incubators, warm room temperature.
Evaporation, moisture on the body surface or respiratory tract evaporates. Major source of heat loss after delivery or during bath. Inversely related to gestational age	Wet skin, increase of activity, tachypnea, under radiant warmer and phototherapy	Dry infant immediately after birth and bath; increase humidity, use warm soaks and solutions; use polyethylene wraps, warm and humidified oxygen.
Radiation, transfer of heat from the body to surrounding cooler surfaces not in contact with the infant	Dependent on ambient temperature, air speed and other heat loss mechanisms	Double-wall incubators, radiant warmer, and heat shield.

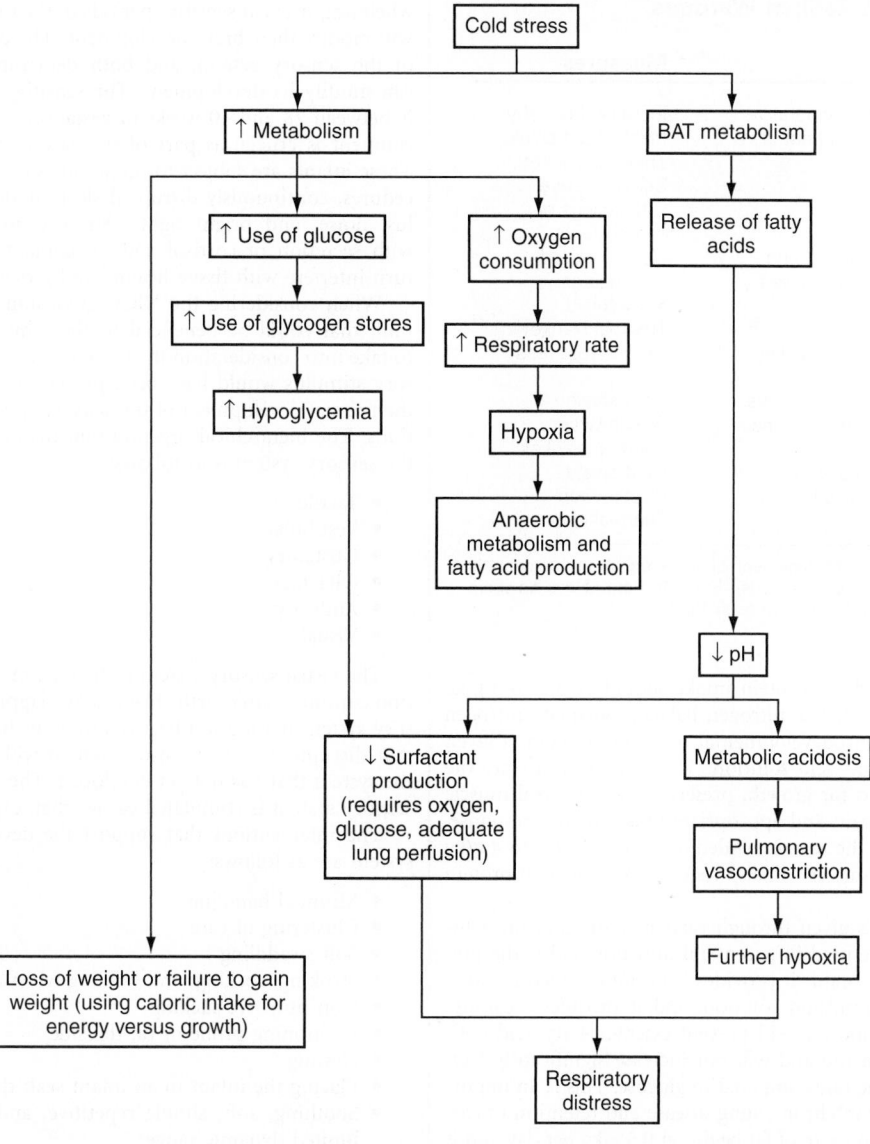

FIGURE 1. Physiologic consequences of cold stress. BAT = Brown adipose tissue.

Newborns have a narrow control range that make them vulnerable to alterations in the thermal environment. The NTE is achieved for the:

- Term infant at 32°C (89.6°F) to 33.5°C (92.3°F)
- Preterm infant greater than 1500 g at 34°C (93.2°F) to 35°C (95°F)
- Preterm infant less than 1500 g at 36.7°C (98.1°F) to 37.3°C (99.1°F)

The two common methods of supporting thermoregulation are the radiant warmer and the incubator (Table 3).

NUTRITION

Proper nutrition is essential for adequate growth, development, and healing. Protein and lipid stores are decreased in the neonate, who has a higher baseline energy requirement compared to children and adults. The low-birth-weight (LBW) infant and the premature infant have even higher baseline requirements. The premature infant has minimal stores of fat and carbohydrates and rapidly develops nutritional deficiencies in calcium, phosphorus, iron trace elements, and vitamins. Nutritional requirements of calories and protein increase even further in the critically ill neonate with overwhelming infections, severe lung disease, and major surgical conditions. These conditions obviate the enteral route of delivering adequate nutrition as well as the immature digestive pathways of the GI tract. In these cases parenteral nutrition is the only option. In premature infants nutritional support is aimed at achieving an intrauterine growth pattern of 15 to 30 g per day. To achieve comparable weight at term-corrected age, compared to a term infant, the daily growth rate would have to be higher to achieve catch-up growth, which usually happens after the time of discharge. When there is early positive nitrogen balance, weight loss is less, there is a better rate of growth, and healing and recovery are faster.

With parenteral nutrition the fluid requirement starts at 80 mL/kg per day and increases daily up to 100 to 180 mL/kg per day. Infants with increased fluid losses, in addition to their maintenance fluid requirement, will require replacement fluid with specific electrolytes to offset their losses. The caloric requirement varies from 90 kcal to 120 kcal/kg per day. Higher caloric needs of 20% to 30% more are required in the extremely premature infants and in the critically ill neonate. To achieve the expected postnatal growth pattern, the total nonprotein calorie requirement should be at least 70 to

TABLE 3 Measures to Promote Thermoregulation in Incubators and Radiant Warmers

Bed	Basis	Measures
Incubator	Decrease evaporative water and heat loss	Increase humidity
		Plastic heat shield
		Thermal blanket
		Semiocclusive dressings or emollients
	Reduce radiant and convective losses	Double-walled incubator
		Heat shield
		Thermal blanket
	Promote conductive heat gain	Heated mattress
Radiant warmer	Decrease evaporative water and heat loss	Heat shield
		Plastic wrap
		Thermal blanket
	Reduce radiant or convective losses	Heat shield
		Plastic wrap
		Thermal blanket

Modified from Sinclair, J. Management of the thermal environment. In J.C. Sinclair and M.B. Brocker (eds). Effective Care of the Newborn Infant. Oxford: Oxford University Press; 1992.

105 kcal/kg per day, and the protein intake should be 3.2 to 4 g/kg per day of protein for positive nitrogen balance, adequate nitrogen accretion, and good neurodevelopmental outcome. Protein is given in the form of an amino acid solution. These amino acids are the building blocks required for growth, preservation of skeletal muscle protein mass, tissue repair, and appropriate inflammatory response. Protein intake starts at the recommended daily intake of 3 to 4 g/kg per day. Critically ill neonates will also require an increase in protein intake by 10% to 20%.

Calories or energy is given through carbohydrates and fat. Glucose is the carbohydrate used in parenteral nutrition and is the preferred substrate for the brain. It provides 3.4 cal/g of glucose. Fat is given as a 20% lipid emulsion solution, and it provides 2 cal/mL. The use of the lipid emulsion will prevent essential fatty acid deficiency, improve protein use and will not increase significantly CO_2 production or metabolic rate compared to glucose. This is an important factor in infants with chronic lung disease and retention of carbon dioxide. The infusion rate of fat begins at 0.5 g/kg per day and is advanced by 0.5 g daily up to 2 to 3 g/kg per day. Close monitoring of triglycerides is required. A level above 250 mg/dL is considered high, so the rate of infusion should then be cut back. Adequate energy intake will promote or facilitate positive nitrogen balance and nitrogen accretion. Other components of parenteral nutrition are calcium, phosphorus, vitamins, and trace minerals. Sodium and potassium are added based on the serum electrolyte results. Carnitine is added when premature infants are on prolonged parenteral nutrition (>14 days) with no enteral feedings.

The task of providing adequate nutrition is multidisciplinary; the neonatologist, pharmacist, and nutritionist form part of the team. Close metabolic monitoring for glucose, electrolytes, urea, lipids, and acid–base balance is an integral part of the nutritional management of the high-risk neonates. This will help assess and meet nutritional needs as well as monitor for complications such as metabolic acidosis, electrolyte imbalance, cholestatic jaundice, increased triglyceride levels, and infection. When enteral feeding is possible, human milk should be considered. Although it may not provide adequate caloric and protein intake, it has many other assets that are important in promoting growth, healing, neurodevelopment, and protection against infection.

DEVELOPMENTAL CARE

The NICU environment plays a major role in the growth and development of the high-risk neonate and may contribute to the morbidity of these fragile infants. The amount of abnormal sensory stimulus that these fragile beings are exposed to is the source of overwhelming stress at sensitive periods of their development, and in turn will modify their brain development. The cortex of the brain is part of the sensory system, and both deprivation and overstimulation can modify its development. The sensitive period when this occurs is between 28 and 40 weeks of gestation. Therefore the NICU environment is crucial as part of the care of the sick newborn infant. These infants are subject to numerous stress factors, unpleasant procedures, continuously disrupted sleep, frequent noxious oral stimulus, noise, and bright lights. Stress causes autonomic instability, with secretion of cortisol and catecholamines. These hormones in turn interfere with tissue healing and growth.

When considering the NICU environment and the input or stimuli that could be beneficial to these high-risk neonates, one has to take into consideration the in utero environment and how the sensory stimulus would have been perceived in that environment, and the normal development of the sensory system for planned interventions. The hierarchical organization, maturation, and integration of the sensory system is as follows:

- Tactile
- Vestibular
- Gustatory
- Olfactory
- Auditory
- Visual

The visual sensory system is the least mature at term and maturation continues after birth. There is overlapping regarding when a sensory system maturation begins and ends, but there is clear evidence that disruption of one sensory system will affect the maturation of the system that has not yet developed. The same is true when a later sensory system is stimulated earlier than expected.

The interventions that support the development of the sensory system are as follows:

- Minimal handling
- Clustering of care
- Soft swaddling
- Stroking, rocking, and holding when appropriate
- Non-nutritive sucking
- Positioning prone or on the side
- Nesting
- Placing the infant in an infant seat; then swaddle and nest
- Soothing, soft, simple repetitive, and harmonic sounds with limited dynamic range
- Limit ambient light
- Shield eyes and chest from bright lights
- Limit the initial visual stimulus to the human face
- Massage therapy

These suggested interventions should take into consideration the gestational age and the clinical acuity of the high-risk patient. The goal is to improve growth and neurodevelopmental outcome of the high-risk neonate.

PARENTAL INVOLVEMENT

When looking at specific high-risk situations, one can appreciate the scope of support needed by these high-risk neonates from various subspecialists and ancillary health care professionals. One of the things often forgotten is the major role the parents play in the healing and development of their sick infant. Parents have a sense of loss from the time their sick newborn has to be resuscitated and/or is admitted to the NICU. They have a sense of loss for delivering prematurely, for not having a healthy full-term infant, loss of self-esteem, and social status as parents. Involving the parents in the care of their infant will provide some emotional, psychosocial, and spiritual support to the parents. The literature continues to support the need for and the benefits of parental involvement in the NICU as part of the care of the high-risk neonate.

Kangaroo care, or skin-to-skin contact between the parent and the infant, provides sustained multimodal stimulation of tactile, vestibular, proprioceptive, olfactory, and auditory sensory systems. Physiologic benefits such as stable temperature; stable oxygen consumption; higher saturation levels; increased quiet sleep, which lowers cortisol levels resulting in fewer infections; and better growth have been described. It promotes non-nutritive sucking, and there is a better letdown in breast-feeding mothers. Kangaroo care acts as a behavioral organizer or facilitator, decreases motor activity, increases the quiet state in stable preterm infants, and reduces the effect of painful stimuli. These infants are also discharged sooner.

Parents can also participate in massage therapy. It has a calming effect on infants; they express fewer stress behaviors, are more alert, actively respond to face and voice, and show more organized limb movements on the Brazelton behavioral scale. Better weight gain and early discharge have been reported. At 8 months these infants continue to show better weight gain and higher scores on the Bayley Scales of Infant Development.

Conditions Associated with Abnormal Transition

A few conditions associated with abnormal transition are described in the following text.

HYALINE MEMBRANE DISEASE

Hyaline membrane disease (HMD) is the result of surfactant deficiency. Surfactant reduces the surface tension of the alveoli and prevents them from collapsing. This disorder is common to preterm infants. The clinical presentation of HMD is that of respiratory distress characterized by grunting, retractions, and flaring. Grunting is used to maintain the intra-alveoli pressure and prevent it from collapsing. The blood gas typically has hypoxemia and to a lesser degree respiratory acidosis. Radiographically the lungs have a ground glass appearance (this represents microatelectasis) and air bronchograms (the contrast of the air-filled bronchi against the collapse parenchyma). These infants are managed with ventilator support and/or continuous positive airway pressure (CPAP), and surfactant (Survanta) replacement therapy. The use of antenatal steroids has decreased the incidence of HMD and the need for exogenous surfactant in the premature newborn, especially in infants who are 28 weeks' gestation or more.

TRANSIENT TACHYPNEA OF THE NEWBORN

Transient tachypnea of the newborn (TTN) is described as the retention of lung fluid or transient pulmonary edema. In some cases, there may be mild surfactant deficiency. During labor the increased level of prostaglandins causes dilation of the lymphatic vessels in the lungs promoting the absorption of the pulmonary interstitial fluid. After birth, this process is further accelerated by the expansion of the lungs with air-filled alveoli and increased pulmonary circulation. Any delay in this process will result in tachypnea and occasional grunting and flaring. This is common after elective cesarean section. The arterial blood gas shows various degrees of respiratory acidosis and some hypoxemia. The typical chest radiographic findings reveal increased interstitial marking with fluid in the fissure and on occasion pleural effusion. This condition is self-limited, resolving in 1 to 2 days. These infants are managed with oxygen support by hood and rarely require ventilator support.

MECONIUM ASPIRATION SYNDROME

Meconium staining of the amniotic fluid occurs in 10% to 25% of all deliveries. It is seen in fetuses beyond 35 weeks of gestation. Passage of meconium in utero is often the result of a hypoxemic event. Meconium can be aspirated before, during, or after delivery. Meconium aspiration syndrome occurs in 0.5% of live births. Once

aspirated it can cause obstruction of the airway and pulmonary air leak, chemical pneumonitis and secondary bacterial infection, secondary surfactant deficiency, and pulmonary hypertension of the newborn (PPHN) if hypoxemia persists. After birth, a depressed neonate with poor or no respiratory effort should be intubated and suctioned immediately after being placed under the radiant warmer. This action will clear the airway and prevent aspiration or any further aspiration. When the infant's head is delivered, routine care by the obstetrician is all that is required. The severity of the disease varies. The arterial blood gas pictures vary from mild respiratory acidosis with mild hypoxemia to severe respiratory failure with marked hypoxemia. The classic radiographic finding of the lungs is that of patchy infiltrates throughout the lung fields with areas of hyperlucency; air leak is seen in 10% to 20% of these cases. Postnatal management consists of support to minimize all factors that will perpetuate asphyxia and trigger pulmonary hypertension. Decrease energy loss and oxygen consumption by providing warmth, oxygen, and glucose. Aggressive respiratory support is needed, providing a high concentration of oxygen in a hood or through the ventilator, and surfactant replacement therapy. In cases associated with severe PPHN, inhaled nitric oxide (iNO [INO$_{max}$]), and ultimately extracorporeal membrane oxygenation (ECMO) may become part of the management.

PERSISTENT PULMONARY HYPERTENSION OF THE NEWBORN

Persistent pulmonary hypertension of the newborn is the result of severe hypoxemia because of right-to-left shunting through the foramen ovale and ductus arteriosus, without associated structural heart abnormality. The pulmonary hypertension results from increased pulmonary vasoreactivity and increased muscle mass of the pulmonary arterial vessels. The increase in pulmonary smooth arterial muscle mass seen in term infants is triggered by intrauterine stress or hypoxemia. The vasoreactive response seen after birth is caused by alteration of the balance between the circulating pulmonary vasodilator (endothelium-derived relaxing factor or endogenous nitric oxide) and pulmonary vasoconstrictors (endothelin). This vasoreactive response is seen also in preterm and term infants with primary lung disease, such as surfactant deficiency, pneumonia, or MAS. Tachypnea and cyanosis are the clinical presentations. The blood gas has severe hypoxemia and combine metabolic and respiratory acidosis. In primary PPHN, the chest radiograph is normal; in secondary PPHN, it will be characteristic of the disease in question. The diagnosis of PPHN is made with the aid of the echocardiogram, which will exclude structural heart disease, measure the pulmonary artery pressure and resistance, and visualize the right-to-left shunts and tricuspid regurgitation that are commonly present.

The management of neonates with PPHN can be challenging. The goal is to correct the hypoxemia and acidosis, both of which cause pulmonary vasoconstriction. The acidosis can be managed with hyperventilation using conventional or high-frequency ventilator (to achieve a Paco$_2$ close to 30 mm Hg) and/or infusion of sodium bicarbonate to maintain the arterial pH around 7.40. The hypoxemia is more difficult to manage because these infants do not always respond to high concentrations of oxygen with high ventilator support. The Pao$_2$ should be maintained above 80 mm Hg. Concurrent metabolic derangement, such as hypoglycemia and hypocalcemia, and polycythemia should be corrected. The systemic arterial BP should be maintained in the high range of normal. The use of vasopressor agents (dopamine [Intropin] or dobutamine [Dobutrex]) is recommended in achieving this goal, as opposed to volume expansion. The increase in the systemic BP may decrease the right-to-left shunt through the ductus arteriosus and improve pulmonary blood flow and in turn improve the hypoxemia.

When the previously described management fails, the use of iNO at a dose of 20 ppm or less will cause selective pulmonary vasodilatation. Because many infants respond to iNO, the need for ECMO has decreased. Extracorporeal membrane oxygenation is available only in a few medical centers for those cases that fail to respond to maximum ventilator support and iNO.

The Infant with Surgical Conditions

Infants before, during, or after surgery require special consideration regarding management and support of the cardiopulmonary system, thermoregulation, fluid and electrolyte management, nutritional support, and infection control.

GASTROSCHISIS

The combined incidence of omphalocele and gastroschisis is 1:4000 live births. Of these two abdominal wall defects, gastroschisis is the more common. It is a cleft in the abdominal wall to the right of the umbilical cord with herniation of the bowel. The association of other congenital and chromosomal anomalies is rare compared with omphalocele. Common associated problems seen in gastroschisis are malrotation of the bowel, undescended testes, stenosis, and atresia of the bowel, all of which are the result of vascular injury. In 20% of the patients, necrotizing enterocolitis has been reported postoperatively.

Gastroschisis can be diagnosed in the prenatal period. This will allow for proper counseling of the family as well as the plans for intrapartum and postnatal management. The intrapartum and postnatal management consist of preventing further injury to the bowel, temperature stabilization, fluid and electrolyte management, antibiotic therapy, nutritional support, and surgical correction. The exposed bowel is at risk for further circulatory compromise. This may be avoided by having the infant lie on his or her side. Because there is a large surface area exposed to the environment, heat and fluid losses are increased. The bowel should be wrapped in cephalexin (Keflex) soaked in warm normal saline, and then covered with a plastic barrier. The prolonged exposure of the bowel to the amniotic fluid causes a severe inflammatory response that results in ileus. In addition to the increased fluid losses through the exposed bowel, there is intraluminal loss of fluid and electrolyte because of the severe ileus. In these patients 1.5 to 2 times their fluid maintenance is needed for fluid resuscitation. The bowel should be decompressed using a nasogastric or orogastric tube connected to intermittent low suction. Close monitoring of vital signs, intake and output, and serum electrolytes will give indications of the fluid and electrolyte status of these infants.

Nutritional support in infants with gastroschisis is crucial for healing and to decrease morbidity and mortality. Prior to parenteral nutrition, the mortality in these infants was very high, malnutrition and complications associated with infection being major causes. These infants may go for several weeks before enteral feedings can be attempted or tolerated. Early placement of central venous access will facilitate the long-term nutritional support and the overall management. Long-term parenteral nutrition is the key for full recovery of these infants.

The surgical approach considers two options: primary or secondary closure. Secondary closure creates an enclosed hernia, a silo with the bowel content. The bowel is then slowly returned to the abdominal cavity over several days. Antibiotics are continued until the abdominal wall is closed. Primary closure returns the bowel into the abdominal cavity in one step. It is not uncommon, especially with large defects, to have respiratory compromise requiring ventilator support. Be conscious of the need for pain management in these infants, more so in those with respiratory compromise. Other complications seen with primary closure are further bowel compromise with bloody drainage, acidosis, infection, and increased intra-abdominal pressure that causes decrease renal and or central venous perfusion.

CONGENITAL DIAPHRAGMATIC HERNIA

The incidence of congenital diaphragmatic hernia (CDH) is 1:2000 to 5000 live births. This condition can be diagnosed in the prenatal period. When diagnosed in the prenatal period the plan of management begins. The infant should be delivered at a tertiary care center experienced in counseling and treatment of CDH. In these patients, further workup should be done to exclude other malformations of the heart, GI tract, GU system, and CNS and chromosomal anomalies. Associated malformations should be taken into account when counseling the family and when developing the postnatal plan of management. Plans to deliver at term, and at a center where there is a pediatric surgeon, capability for iNO (INO$_{max}$) and ECMO is desired. Once delivered, the infant should be intubated immediately, venous access obtained in case of needed circulatory support, and a nasogastric or orogastric tube placed to decompress the bowel. Bowel distention can further compromise respiration and cardiac function.

The infant should be transferred to the NICU, an arterial line should be placed and blood obtained for blood gas and crossmatch. Obtain a chest and abdominal radiograph to confirm the diagnosis and line placement. An echocardiogram should be done to assess for structural abnormalities of the heart and to estimate the degree of pulmonary hypertension. A head US should be obtained if the infant will be placed on ECMO, because of the risk of intracranial hemorrhage in patients on ECMO.

Skilled ventilator management is important because of the coexisting pulmonary hypertension. Barotrauma and volutrauma should be avoided in these patients. Permissive hypercapnia is permitted once there is adequate preductal oxygenation (preductal oxygenation is measured or obtained from the right upper extremity; the preductal blood perfuses the heart and brain). The highest rates of survival result in patients in whom barotrauma and volutrauma are avoided and permissive hypercapnia is allowed.

A patient is considered unstable or to have failed ventilator support when the pH is <7.25, a peak inspiratory pressure of >30 cm H$_2$O is needed, and preductal saturation is <90% on 60% oxygen. The use of iNO (INO$_{max}$) may be considered in these cases, but the direct effect on pulmonary vascular resistance and right heart function need to be monitored closely. Therapy should be discontinued if no response is demonstrated. Extracorporeal membrane oxygenation is a reasonable choice for patients that have received maximum medical intervention. A venous-venous shunt is preferred unless there is significant cardiac instability.

Surgical correction is done if the infant is stable after the honeymoon period (the first 24 hours). Achievement of 90% survival is possible in a nonselect group of patients with the combination of careful ventilator management, attention to the pulmonary hypertension, delayed surgery, and aggressive early nutrition support. Survival rates are also dependent on the presence or absence of associated abnormalities and their severity. Long-term follow-up beyond the neonatal period is necessary for accurate estimation of morbidity and mortality in patients who are placed on ECMO.

The Extremely Low Birth Weight Infant

A premature infant is a neonate who is delivered before 37 completed weeks of gestation. These infants can be further classified according to their birth weight:

- Low birth weight (LBW) if less than 2500 g
- Very low birth weight (VLBW) if less than 1500 g
- Extremely low birth weight (ELBW) if less than 1000 g

Special consideration needs to be given to late preterm infants, those delivered between 34 and 36 weeks of gestation. These infants have higher morbidity, mortality, and rate of re-hospitalization after the initial discharge throughout the first year of life. They are at high risk for cardiopulmonary (HMD, apnea, SIDS, severe infection with RSV [respiratory syncytial virus]); immune (infections); endocrine (hypoglycemia); temperature regulation (hypothermia); hepatic (prolonged jaundice); and feeding (failure to thrive, feeding difficulties, electrolyte disturbances, dehydration) problems.

Within the ELBW infants is a subgroup called the micropremie, if birth weight is less than 750 g. The need for intrapartum and postnatal intervention and support is inversely proportional to gestational age as well as the morbidity and mortality associated with these infants. The increased risks for asphyxia, heat and water loss, intraventricular hemorrhage, and respiratory distress increase with decreasing gestational age. In the delivery room, the initial steps of

TABLE 4 Common Problems and Management of the Extremely Low Birth Weight Infant

Problems	Management
Delivery Room. It is anticipated that a complete team will be needed for resuscitation: neonatal nurse, respiratory therapist, and neonatologist.	Prevent heat loss, provide respiratory support, prevent asphyxia, and avoid trauma. Place under radiant warmer and dry well, warm all objects that come in contact with the baby, use thermal mattress or warm blankets and cap. Use bag and mask properly and prompt intubation when needed. Properly position the ETT; avoid high inspiratory pressure with overdistention of the lungs. Follow the ABCs of resuscitation.
NICU. The management in the delivery room and the first hours of life sets the stage for the rest of the NICU care.	In the NICU, the infant is placed under a radiant warmer for easy access and thermoregulation. Connect to all monitors, insert umbilical venous and arterial catheters for fluid management, BP monitoring, and to facilitate blood draw. Obtain chest and abdominal radiograph to assess the severity of lung disease and position of the ETT, venous, and arterial catheters. Cover infant with plastic wrap to decrease evaporative heat and fluid loss. Frequent weighing with a bed scale will estimate hydration status. There should be minimal handling and clustered care in the first week of life.
Fluid and Electrolytes. The high insensible water loss in the ELBW infant increases the risk for dehydration, hypernatremia, and hyperkalemia.	Fluid requirements range from 100–150 mL/kg/d, given as D5W with no added electrolytes in the first 24–48 h. Monitoring of the electrolytes and strict I&O will estimate the hydration status. Monitor blood draw and replace with PRBC from a single donor, CMV negative, when 10% of blood volume is removed. Hypernatremia is caused by increased water loss and corrected with increased intake of free water. Risk of hyperkalemia is caused by water loss and increases if there is extravascular blood collection; this is corrected using insulin infusion with glucose, correcting acidosis with sodium bicarbonate, calcium gluconate to stabilize the myocardium, and a cation exchange resin per rectum–sodium polystyrene sulfonate (Kayexalate).
Nutrition. Long-term parenteral nutrition is required in these infants. Good nutritional support is necessary for growth and neurodevelopment.	Beginning early parenteral nutrition within the first 24 h will provide a source of energy (glucose) protein to decrease the risk of negative nitrogen balance, calcium, vitamins, and trace minerals. Placement of percutaneous CVC should be done early in the course. Please refer to the section on nutrition in this article for further nutrition management.
CNS. There is an increased risk of developing IVH in unstable infants in the first few days of life.	To prevent IVH, stressful conditions like cold stress, hypoxemia, acidosis swing in BP, and increased intrathoracic pressure should be avoided. Initial US in the first 3 d if unstable and at the end of the first week if stable. Follow-up will depend on findings. Infants with no IVH should have a repeat at 36 weeks postmenstrual age. The use of sedation in the first week of life has not shown significant changes in the incidence of IVH.
Respiratory. HMD is the most common condition. Avoid complications associated with the disease (air leaks and pulmonary emphysema, pulmonary hemorrhage, ICH, and CLD).	Use of exogenous surfactant when indicated and rapid weaning of PIP and O_2 and close monitoring to avoid complications. Blood gas is obtained 10–15 min after each change. Use high ventilator rate and the lowest PIP to maintain saturation 88%–93%, permissive hypercapnia ($Paco_2$ 50–60), mild acidosis (pH 7.25–7.35), and Po_2 50–70 are the goal. When stable, extubate to NCPAP. Apnea is common in these infants; they are treated with caffeine citrate (Cafcit). An initial bolus of 20 mg/kg is given followed by maintenance of 5–10 mg/kg every 24 h.
Cardiovascular. PDA occurs in >50% of ELBW infants. Appearing when the lung disease is improving, clinically there is increased need for respiratory support associated with desaturation, active precordium, bounding pulses, and wide pulse pressure. The diagnosis is confirmed by echocardiogram. The ductus arteriosus of the preterm responds less to the vasoconstrictive effect of oxygen.	Medical treatment consists of fluid restriction, maintenance of hematocrit around 40%, and the use of indomethacin (Indocin IV). Complications of indomethacin (Indocin IV) are decreased GFR causing fluid retention, and platelet dysfunction (contraindicated in renal failure, bleeding disorders, and low platelets). The dose is 0.2 mg/kg daily for three doses and a diuretic such as furosemide (Lasix) at 1 mg/kg/dose to try to prevent oliguria. If there is no response, additional dosing or courses can be given. The definitive treatment would be ligation of the ductus. Some centers use prophylactic indomethacin (Indocin IV).
Skin. Underdevelopment of the stratum corneum causes increased transepidermal water loss → dehydration → electrolyte imbalance and evaporative heat loss. Traumatized skin is the port of entry for many infectious organisms. Acceleration of skin maturation occurs after birth over the next 10–14 d.	Use of plastic shields, increased humidity, and topical skin emollient will decrease heat and water loss and may be protective to the skin.
Glucose. Hyperglycemia is secondary to high glucose-infusion rates. When an infant becomes hyperglycemic on a stable glucose-infusion rate, consider infection and or IVH. Early hypoglycemia is common in this group of infants due to poor glycogen stores and immature hormonal adaptation of the endocrine system.	Glucose level should be >45 mg/dL in the first 48–72 h and >50 mg/dL after 72 h. When hypoglycemic, a bolus of D10W at 200 mg/kg (2 mL/kg) is given. Glucose level is obtained in 30 min, frequent monitoring is continued every 1–3 h, and further boluses are given as needed. Maintenance fluid provides 4–6 mg/kg/min of glucose infusion. This rate of infusion should be increased by 2 mg/kg/min with every need for D10W bolus. Refer to specific text for detailed management.
Calcium. The stores of calcium are limited and the reserves are rapidly depleted after birth.	Higher intake of calcium with adequate phosphorus intake is required for bone formation and growth.
Jaundice. These infants are at increased risk for brain toxicity from high bilirubin levels. High bilirubin level develops due to hepatic immaturity, shorter RBC life span, extravasation of blood, and increased enterohepatic circulation, coupled with lower serum albumin level.	The level that causes toxicity is lower in these infants. A crude method to determine the need for phototherapy at 50% the weight in kg: A 0.9 Kg infant is placed under phototherapy for a bilirubin level of 4.5 mg/dL. Exchange level is determined by the weight, in this case 9 mg/dL. The risk for toxicity increases in the unstable infant, the reason why lower levels should be used when managing.

Abbreviations: ABC = airway, breathing, and circulation; BP = blood pressure; CLD = chronic lung disease; CMV = cytomegalovirus; CVC = central venous catheter; ELBW = extremely low birth weight infant; ETT = endotracheal tube; GFR = glomerular filtration rate; HMD = hyaline membrane disease; I&O = intake and output; ICH = intracranial hemorrhage; IV = intravenous; IVH = intraventricular hemorrhage; NCPAP = nasal continuous positive airway pressure; NICU = neonatal intensive care unit; PDA = patent ductus arteriosus; PIP = peak inspiratory pressure; PRBC = packed red blood cells; RBC = red blood cell; US = ultrasound.

CURRENT DIAGNOSIS

- Review of risk factors: antenatal, perinatal, and postnatal
- Assessment of infants in the delivery room: airway, breathing and circulation—respiration, heart rate, and color
- Continued assessment in the nursery: respirations, heart rate, color, temperature, and CNS
- Common problems: pulmonary, circulatory, gastrointestinal, metabolic, surgical, and temperature instability

Abbreviation: CNS = central nervous system.

resuscitation will support transition by preventing heat and water loss and asphyxia. The use of surfactant (Survanta) should be considered in ELBW infants. In infants more than 1000 g, surfactant replacement therapy should be done as soon as the neonate presents a clinical picture of surfactant deficiency (HMD). Surfactant should be given with the proper ventilator support and, it is not uncommon to require multiple doses. With delay in therapy the morbidity and mortality associated with HMD increases.

The ELBW infants are a special group within the premature infants because the advances in health care and technology seem to have had less of an impact on this group of infants. The overall morbidity and mortality continue to be comparatively high in these infants and more so in the micropremie or infants less than 27 weeks of gestation. Table 4 lists the common problems faced by the ELBW infants and their management.

Special Therapy

Although there are continued attempts to provide care for the ELBW infant, there are infants outside the scope of *viability*—infants with complex congenital malformations, including those labeled as *incompatible with life*, and those whose condition is irreversible and ultimately will lead to death. For such infants, we see the need for

CURRENT THERAPY

- Use functioning equipment and qualified personnel in the delivery room: initial steps and ABCs of neonatal resuscitation.
- Provide neutral thermal environment.
- Respiratory and cardiovascular support: oxygen, mechanical ventilation, vasopressor agent (dopamine).
- Infuse bolus of D10W and glucose at 6–8 mg/kg per minute or higher if needed.
- Use phototherapy for early jaundice and the bruised ELBW infant.
- Transfer to appropriate level of care when indicated.
- Monitor closely fluid and electrolytes and decreased IWL. Provide good nutritional support beginning in the first 24 hours and closely monitor for complications and tolerance.
- Provide family-centered care and appropriate environment to promote growth and development.
- Benefit special cases, especially those deemed futile, with a multidisciplinary approach.

Abbreviations: ABC = airway, breathing, and circulation; ELBW = extremely low birth weight; IWL = insensible water loss.

comfort care or palliative care. In these situations both the health care professional and parents find themselves in an awkward position. The family remains hopeful based on the perceived information that the health care professional gives, or the family goes through turmoil when interventions seem endless in a situation that they perceive as hopeless.

The decision for palliative care is made through collaboration between the health care team and the parents. The two factual considerations in making the decision for palliative care are pertinent medical facts (diagnosis, response to treatment given potential response to other treatments, and prognosis) and the human value (what the parents anticipate, expect, and desire for their infant) and what motivates these values in the parents. The values of the health care team involved in the care of the infant are also considered.

Palliative care, as defined by the World Health Organization (WHO), is care for patients for whom cure is no longer a reasonable expectation or possibility. It is an active and comprehensive management of the entire patient, and not abandonment of care.

Practical considerations that need to be taken into account, and specific components of the palliative care that are appropriate for each individual high-risk neonate, are considered before a specific plan can be put in place. The application of palliative care in the NICU is not only possible, but necessary.

REFERENCES

Aly H. Respiratory disorders in the newborn: Identification and diagnosis. Pediatr Rev 2004;25:201–8.

Avery GB, Fletcher MA, Macdonald MG, editors. Neonatology: Pathophysiology and Management of the Newborn. 5th ed. Philadelphia: Lippincott Williams & Wilkins; 1999, pp. 143–73.

Blackburn ST, Maternal F, et al. Neonatal Physiology: A Clinical Perspective. 2nd ed. Philadelphia: WB Saunders; 2003, pp. 707–30.

Carter BS. Comfort care principles for the high-risk newborn. NeoReviews 2004;e484–90.

Chescheir NC, Harsen WF. What's new in perinatology. Pediatr Rev 1999;20:57–63.

Downard CD, Wilson JM. Current therapy of infants with congenital diaphragmatic hernia. Semin Neonatol 2003;8:215–21.

Field TM. Stimulation of preterm infants. Pediatr Rev 2003;24:4–10.

Heird WC. Determination of nutritional requirements in preterm infants, with special reference to "catch-up" growth. Semin Neonatol 2001;6:365–75.

Klaus MH, Fanaroff MB. Care of the High-Risk Neonate. 5th ed. Philadelphia: WB Saunders; 2001, pp. 195–215.

Kattwinkel J, editor. Neonatal Resuscitation Textbook. 5th ed. Elk Grove Village, Ill.: American Heart Association.

Kleinman RE, editor. Pediatric Nutrition Handbook. 6th ed. Philadelphia: WB Saunders; 2009, pp. 79–112.

Welch KK, Malone FD. Advances in prenatal screening: Nuchal translucency ultrasonography in the first trimester. NeoReviews 2002;3:e202–8.

Welch KK, Malone FD. Advances in prenatal screening: Maternal serum screening for Down syndrome. Neoreviews 2002;3:e209–13.

Normal Infant Feeding

Method of
Meg Begany, RD, CSP, LDN, and
Maria Mascarenhas, MBBS

Adequate and appropriate nutrition is especially critical during infancy. Infancy, defined as birth to 1 year of age, is characterized by the period of most rapid growth and development during the life cycle. In addition, recent research shows that nutrition during infancy can influence risk factors for disease at other stages of the life cycle.

Infant Feeding

For the healthy term infant, the suck-swallow and rooting reflexes are present at birth, and thus liquid feedings can be initiated almost immediately following delivery.

BREAST-FEEDING

The American Academy of Pediatrics (AAP) recommends human milk as the feeding of choice for nearly all infants whenever possible and mutually desirable for the mother and infant. Successful lactation and breast-feeding requires a supportive environment for the mother provided by the medical practitioner, including instruction and counseling. The World Health Organization (WHO) Expert Consultation on the Optimal Duration of Exclusive Breastfeeding, which considered the results of a systematic review of the evidence, concluded that human milk is recommended as the exclusive source of nutrition for the first 6 months and continuing human milk in combination with complementary foods until at least 12 months of age. The nutrient needs of the full-term normal birth weight infant can be met by human milk alone, with few exceptions, for the first 6 months if the mother is well nourished. The benefits of breast-feeding over formula feeding are well established and include enhanced maturity and motility of the gastrointestinal tract; maternal–infant bonding; monetary savings; facilitated fat, protein, and carbohydrate digestion and absorption; passive immunity; improved cognitive development; and decreased incidence of otitis media and respiratory and gastrointestinal disease. Further potential benefits, such as lower risk of overweight in children and adults, as well as decreased risk of cardiovascular disease in adulthood, were demonstrated in recent research.

Breast-feeding should be offered as early as possible after birth and then every 2 to 3 hours until satiety for approximately 10 to 15 minutes per breast during the first few weeks. Less frequent feedings may occur once breast-feeding is established. Intervals of more than 5 hours in between breast-feeding should be avoided during the first few weeks, including at night. Adequacy of breast-feeding is demonstrated when the infant has feedings 8 to 12 times per day, at least 6 to 8 wet diapers per day, regular stooling pattern, and is growing along established growth curves.

The composition of breast milk varies from individual to individual, as well as within the same individual, with composition changes occurring with stage of lactation, time of day, maternal diet, and time elapsed since feeding began. Milk production tends to be higher during the daytime, and fat content is increased toward the end of a feeding. On average, breast milk provides approximately 20 calories per ounce.

Contraindications to breast-feeding include maternal infections by organisms known to be transmitted to the infant via breast milk (e.g., HIV); maternal exposure to drugs, foods, or environmental agents that are excreted in human milk and harmful to the infant; and inborn errors of metabolism that are exacerbated by components present in human milk (e.g., galactosemia).

INFANT FORMULA

When a mother chooses not to breast-feed or human milk is not an option, infant formula is an appropriate substitute. Although the composition of infant formula does not exactly duplicate that of breast milk, the composition of infant formulas continues to evolve in an effort to do so. The addition of docosahexaenoic acid (DHA) and arachidonic acid (ARA) is a recent modification to infant formula. Unlike breast milk, infant formulas prior to 2002 contained only the precursor essential fatty acids, linoleic and α-linolenic acids, from which DHA and ARA had to be synthesized. Multiple studies in both preterm and term infants have demonstrated significantly lower levels of DHA and ARA in the erythrocytes of formula-fed infants compared to their breast-fed counterparts. This suggested that infant formula containing only the precursors, α-linolenic acid and linoleic acid, could be ineffective in allowing adequate synthesis of DHA and ARA. Thus multiple studies have been published comparing visual acuity, developmental outcomes, and growth of infants fed DHA and ARA supplemented feeding and unsupplemented formula or breast milk. Some of these studies, but not all, found short-term improvements in visual and cognitive functions in both preterm and term infants. However, no long-term benefits were demonstrated. Although the single supplementation of DHA alone resulted in ARA deficiency status and poor growth in premature infants, the balanced supplementation of both DHA and ARA consistently do not show any adverse effect on growth.

Both iron-fortified and low-iron formulas are commercially available. The AAP has stated that there is no role for the use of low-iron formulas in infant feeding and recommends that all formulas fed to infants be fortified with iron. Well-controlled studies failed to show a benefit, in terms of feeding tolerance, related to the use of low-iron formula. The amount of iron present in iron-fortified formulas meets the iron requirements through the entire first year.

Infant formula should be prepared and stored with careful attention to the manufacturer's guidelines to prevent the risk of bacterial growth.

VITAMIN AND MINERAL SUPPLEMENTATION

The majority of vitamin and mineral requirements for infants are met in full by breast milk or infant formula. Guidelines for supplementation of vitamin K, vitamin D, iron, and fluoride are established. A single dose of vitamin K is typically given to all infants intramuscularly at birth to prevent hemorrhagic disease of the newborn.

In a 2008 report, the AAP advised that all infants and children have a minimum daily intake of 400 IU of vitamin D beginning in the first few days of life. This new recommendation replaces the prior report that recommended 200 IU of vitamin D per day. Adequate vitamin D is essential for the prevention and treatment of rickets, and evidence has shown that supplementation may have lifelong health benefits. A multivitamin or tri-vitamin preparation can be used. Alternatively, solitary vitamin D drops are now available in a cost-effective, easy-to-dose form (Carson Laboratories).

The iron requirements for formula-fed infants are met through iron-fortified formula. Although the iron content of human milk is minimal, its bioavailability is high. However, the iron body stores of the breast-fed infant diminish by 4 to 6 months of age, and thus an additional iron source is recommended at this age. Iron needs of the breast-fed infant can be met with the introduction of complementary foods when foods with good sources of iron are included (e.g., meat, fish, iron-fortified cereal, whole grains, and dark leafy green vegetables).

Fluoride supplementation is recommended at 6 months of age for both breast-fed infants and formula-fed infants who receive exclusively ready-to-feed formulas or whose water supply contains less than 0.3 ppm of fluoride.

INTRODUCTION OF COMPLEMENTARY FOODS

At approximately 6 months of age, human milk or infant formula can no longer supply all of an infant's nutrition requirements, and complementary foods are needed to ensure adequate nutrition and growth. It is the micronutrients, rather than energy and protein, which are likely to become lacking. The ability to digest and absorb carbohydrates, proteins, and fats is mature by 6 months of age. Trypsin and chymotrypsin activities increase during the first 4 months of life. Age should not be the only factor in determining the timing of introduction of complementary feeding, but rather the timing should be determined by individual physical and psychological readiness of the infant, as well as rate of maturation of the nervous system, intestinal tract, and kidneys. Before spoon feedings are introduced, the infant should exhibit trunk stability, head control, and disappearance of the extrusion reflex. At approximately 5 to 6 months, an infant is able to indicate a desire for food by leaning forward and opening his or her mouth to indicate hunger and leaning back and turning away to show disinterest or satiety. Muraro et al. state that introduction of complementary feedings prior to 4 months of age is associated with an increased risk of atopic eczema and cow's milk protein allergy. There are presently no controlled studies showing an allergy preventative effect of restrictive diets after 6 months of age. Studies suggest that introducing complementary foods prior to 6 months does not result in increased caloric intake and has no growth advantage because the infant will displace breast milk to maintain the same level of caloric intake. Although it is possible to meet the nutrition needs of the infant solely from infant formula through the entire first year, delay of introduction of solids can lead to feeding aversions and food refusal. All infants need exposure to a variety of tastes, textures, and foods to develop appropriate feeding practices and a wider acceptance of new foods. In addition to adequate nutrition, the feeding relationship between the infant and caregiver is vital for normal growth and development.

 CURRENT THERAPY

Infant Formula Composition and Indications

FORMULA	EXAMPLES	INDICATIONS	CHARACTERISTICS
Milk based	Enfamil LIPIL, Similac Advance Early Shield, Nestle Good Start Gentle PLUS, Nestle Good Start Protect PLUS, Nestle Good Start Nourish PLUS, Enfamil Gentlease, Similac Organic, Enfamil LactoFree, Similac Sensitive, Enfamil PREMIUM, Enfamil A.R., Similac Sensitive RS (thickens with gastric pH)	Breast milk substitute for term infants	Ready to feed, powder, or liquid concentrate Variable whey-to-casein ratio 20 kcal/oz May contain DHA/ARA
Soy based	Enfamil ProSobee, Similac Isomil Advance Nestle Good Start Soy PLUS Similac Isomil DF	Breast milk substitute for infants with lactose intolerance or milk protein allergy*	Lactose free; some sucrose free Ready to feed, powder, or liquid concentrate 20 kcal/oz May contain DHA/ARA May contain fiber
Premature (hospital grade)	Enfamil Premature, Similac Special Care, Good Start Premature 24	Breast milk substitute for low-birth-weight hospitalized preterm infants	Low lactose High calcium and phosphorus Contain MCT 20, 24, or 30 kcal/oz Contain DHA/ARA
Human milk fortifiers	Similac Human Milk Fortifier, Enfamil Human Milk Fortifier, Similac Special Care 30	Fortification of human milk for low-birth-weight preterm infants	Increase calorie, protein, and vitamin/mineral content of breast milk Contain MCT
Premature transitional	Similac NeoSure, Enfamil EnfaCare	Breast milk substitute for preterm infants >2.5 kg or discharge formula for preterm infants (used until 6–12 mo corrected age or until catch-up growth is completed)	22 kcal/oz Ready to feed or powder Contain DHA/ARA Vitamin and mineral content between that of term and premature formulas
Hypoallergenic	Nutramigen, Nutramigen AA, Nutramigen with Enflora LGG	Milk or soy protein allergy	Hydrolyzed protein or free amino acids Ready to feed, powder, or liquid concentrate Sucrose free, lactose free No MCT May contain DHA/ARA
Protein hydrolysate with MCT	Similac Alimentum, Enfamil Pregestimil	Malabsorption Short bowel syndrome Allergy	Lactose free Hydrolyzed protein Contain MCT May contain DHA/ARA Ready to feed or powder
Amino-acid based	Neocate, EleCare	Malabsorption Short bowel syndrome Allergy	Lactose free Free amino acids May contain MCT May contain DHA/ARA Powder only
Fat modified	Monogen, Portagen (no longer recommended for infants), Enfaport, Similac Alimentum, Enfamil Pregestimil	Defects in digestion, absorption, or transport of fat	Contain increased % of kcals as MCT

FORMULA	EXAMPLES	INDICATIONS	CHARACTERISTICS
Carbohydrate modified	RCF, 3232 A, Keto Cal	Simple sugar intolerance Ketogenic diet	Requires addition of complex carbohydrate to be complete
Amino acid modified	Multiple products (e.g., Cyclinex, MSUD Analog, Phenyl-Free)	Inborn errors of metabolism	Low or devoid of specific amino acids that cannot be metabolized
Electrolyte modified	Similac PM 60/40	Renal or other disease, state requiring low renal solute load	Decreased potassium content
			Decreased calcium and phosphorus content
			May be low iron content

*Children allergic to milk protein may also be allergic to soy protein.
Abbreviations: ARA = arachidonic acid; DHA = docosahexaenoic acid; MCT = medium chain triglycerides; MSUD = maple syrup urine disease.

To observe for symptoms of intolerance, only one new food should be introduced every 3 days. Because of its hypoallergenicity, infant rice cereal is often introduced as the first feeding. However, if spoon feeding is initiated at 6 months of age, gastrointestinal and renal development is mature enough to allow feedings from multiple food groups. Despite enhanced bioavailability, breast milk is relatively low in iron and zinc. Because low liver reserves of zinc at birth may predispose some infants to zinc deficiency, similar to the situation for iron, meat may be the ideal first food to provide these nutrients at the levels needed. Dr. Samuel Fomon states that unless there is a strong family history of allergy, introduction of soft-cooked red meats is desirable by 5 to 6 months of age. Furthermore, the proportion of Dietary Reference Intakes that needs to be supplied by complementary foods is highest for iron, zinc, phosphorus, and magnesium. Regardless of the food choice for the first feeding, the consistency should be thin and liquid/pureed. Thinning foods with breast milk or infant formula can enhance acceptability of the food by the infant. Repeated exposure to a new food may be necessary before it is accepted.

By 9 months of age, finely chopped foods and finger foods can be added to the infant's diet. At 12 months of age, rotary chewing is well controlled, and many infants can progress to table foods. Choking hazards that are round and hard, such as grapes, nuts, popcorn, hot dogs, and hard candy, should be avoided.

For the average healthy infant, meals of complementary foods should be provided two to three times per day from 6 to 8 months of age and three to four times per day from 9 to 12 months of age, with addition of nutritious snacks once or twice per day as desired. Vegetarian diets cannot meet nutrient needs at this age unless fortified products or nutrient supplements are provided. Estimates of the energy gap that must be filled by complementary food in industrialized countries is approximately 130 kcal/day at 6 to 8 months, 310 kcal/day at 9 to 11 months and 580 kcal/day at 12 to 23 months of age.

Juice is not a necessary component of the diet and may displace the intake of nutrient-dense breast milk or formula. In addition, offering juice by bottle can contribute to dental caries. If juice is provided, it should be limited to 4 to 8 ounces per day and should not be given prior to 6 months of age.

Whole cow's milk should not be introduced before 12 months of age because of its low iron content, high renal solute load, potential for causing gastrointestinal bleeding, and increased risk of cow's milk protein allergy. Furthermore, cow's milk is a poor source of vitamin C, vitamin E, and essential fatty acids. Breast-fed infants weaned before 12 months of age should receive an iron-fortified infant formula rather than cow's milk.

Nutritional Requirements

Because of the rapid rate of growth and development during infancy, nutrient needs per unit of body weight are very high in comparison to that of the older child or adult. An infant's energy or caloric requirement depends on many factors, including resting energy expenditure, body size and composition, physical activity, age, sex, and genetics. In general, an infant's hunger and satiety cues should guide decisions on when and how much to feed because infants are capable of regulating their intake to meet their caloric needs. The dietary reference intakes (DRIs) for healthy term infants provide the following equations to calculate estimated energy requirements (EERs):

$$0-3 \text{ months } (89 \times \text{weight [kg]} - 100) + 175 \text{ kcal}$$
$$4-6 \text{ months } (89 \times \text{weight [kg]} - 100) + 56 \text{ kcal}$$
$$7-12 \text{ months } (89 \times \text{weight [kg]} - 100) + 22 \text{ kcal}$$

Based on the above equations and reference weights ranging from 4.2 to 10.3 kg, estimated energy requirements for the healthy term infant range from 438 to 572 kcal/day (95 to 107 kcal/kg) at birth to 3 months, from 508 to 645 kcal/day (~82 kcal/kg) at 4 to 6 months, and from 608 to 844 kcal/day (~80–82 kcal/kg) at 7 to 12 months of age. Individual needs and growth patterns may necessitate modification of these requirements. The DRIs for protein were based on protein intake of the exclusively breast-fed infant from 0 to 6 months of age. Infant formula provides higher levels of protein than breast milk, which accounts for the decreased efficiency of absorption compared with that of breast milk. The contribution of complementary foods to total protein intake in the latter 6 months of infancy was considered in establishing the DRIs for this age. The DRI for protein is 9.1 g/day (~1.52 g/kg) from birth to 6 months and 11 g/day (~1.22 g/kg) from 7 to 12 months. Caloric distribution during infancy is recommended to be 40% to 50% fat, 7% to 11% protein, and 40% to 55% carbohydrate. The water-to-energy ratio should be 1.5 mL/kcal. Both human milk and infant formulas are models of this distribution. Hydration requirements are met by breast milk or infant formula without further addition of water to the diet, except potentially during periods of illness with fever, diarrhea, or emesis.

Growth

Growth velocity of weight, length, and head circumference is a general indicator of adequacy of kilocalorie, protein, and micronutrient intakes during infancy. Weight, length, and head circumference should be monitored serially during infancy and plotted on the gender-specific 2000 CDC (Centers for Disease Control and Prevention) Growth Charts. Breast-fed infants tend to gain less weight and usually are leaner than formula-fed infants in the second half of infancy. This difference does not seem to be the result of nutritional deficits but rather infant self-regulation of energy intake.

Obesity is increasing among children in the United States. High rates of weight gain during the first few months of life are associated with obesity in childhood and early adulthood. Optimal nutrition

Expected Growth Velocity during Infancy

Age	Weight Gain (g/d)	Length (cm/mo)	Head Circumference (cm/wk)
0–3 mo	25–35	2.5–3.5	0.3–0.6
3–6 mo	15–21	1.6–2.5	0.2–0.5
6–12 mo	10–13	1.2–1.7	0.1–0.4

and growth during infancy should be promoted by encouraging healthy eating patterns in the infant to prepare for a healthy lifestyle later in life. Early identification and intervention may be a key component for establishing appropriate weight gain patterns.

Although no consensus exists on universal criteria to define failure to thrive, careful evaluation should occur when weight is less than the 5th percentile or falls more than two major percentiles from a previously established growth channel. In addition, relationship of weight to height must be considered. Prompt intervention with nutritional rehabilitation is essential to prevent illness, growth stunting, cognitive delay, and social and behavioral problems.

For the treatment of either over- or undernutrition, a multidisciplinary team approach involving the physician, dietitian, psychologist, and social worker, along with community services, can often be beneficial and necessary.

In conclusion, infant feeding during the first year of life is a complex process, and guidelines are based on developmental, nutritional, and social factors. Human milk is superior to infant formula and should be the feeding of choice for all infants. Although infant formulas do not exactly duplicate breast milk, the composition of infant formulas continues to evolve in an effort to do so. Complementary foods should be introduced at 6 months of age. Cow's milk should not be introduced until 1 year of age. Careful attention should be paid to growth and nutritional status throughout infancy, with prompt attention to any deviation from expected growth patterns.

REFERENCES

American Academy of Pediatrics, Committee on Nutrition. Iron fortification of infant formulas. Pediatrics 1999;104:119–23.

American Academy of Pediatrics, Section on Breastfeeding. Breastfeeding and the use of human milk. Pediatrics 2005;115:496–506.

Dewey KG. Nutrition, growth and complementary feeding of the breastfed infant. Pediatr Clin North Am 2001;48:87–104.

Foman SJ. Feeding normal infants: Rationale for recommendations. J Am Diet Assoc 2001;101:1002–5.

Institute of Medicine, Food and Nutrition Board. Dietary Reference Intakes for Energy, Carbohydrate, Fiber, Fat, Fatty Acids, Cholesterol, Protein, and Amino Acids. Washington, DC: National Academies Press; 2005.

Kleinman RE, editor. Pediatric Nutrition Handbook. 5th ed. Elk Grove Village, Ill: American Academy of Pediatrics, Committee on Nutrition; 2003.

Michaelsen KF. Cows' milk in complementary feeding. Pediatrics 2000;106: 1302–3.

Muraro A, Dreborg S, Halken S, et al. Dietary prevention of allergic diseases in infants and small children. Part III: Critical review of published peer-reviewed observational and interventional studies and final recommendations. Pediatr Allergy Immunol 2004;15:291–307.

National Center for Health Statistics in collaboration with the National Center for Chronic Disease Prevention and Health Promotion. (2000). Clinical Growth Charts. Retrieved from http://www.cdc.gov/GrowthCharts.

PAHO and WHO. Guiding Principles for Complementary Feeding of the Breastfed Child. Washington, DC: Pan American Health Organization and World Health Organization; 2003.

Samour PQ, King K, editors. Handbook of Pediatric Nutrition. 3rd ed. Sudbury, Mass.: Jones and Bartlett; 2005.

Slaughter CW, Bryant AH. Hungry for love: The feeding relationship in the psychological development of young children. Permanente J 2004;8:23–9.

Wagner CL, Greer FR, et al. Prevention of rickets and vitamin D deficiency in infants, children, and adolescents. Pediatrics 2008;122:1142–52.

WHO Working Group on the Growth Reference Protocol and the WHO Task Force on Methods for the Natural Regulation of Fertility. Growth of healthy infants and the timing, type, and frequency of complementary foods. Am J Clin Nutr 2002;76:620–7.

Diseases of the Breast

Method of
Paniti Sukumvanich, MD, and
Patrick Borgen, MD

Benign Diseases of the Breast

Benign diseases of the breast historically are subdivided into proliferative and nonproliferative lesions (Table 1). In a study by Dupont and Page, patients with breast biopsies yielding nonproliferative lesions had no increased risk of subsequent breast cancer. In contrast, proliferative lesions were associated with a minimal to a fivefold increased risk of breast cancer. In clinical practice, of the proliferative lesions, only atypical epithelial lesions increase breast cancer risk significantly. Appropriate treatment and counseling of patients depend on the risk of breast cancer associated with these benign breast diseases.

Nonproliferative Lesions

Nonproliferative lesions comprise mild hyperplasia without atypia, squamous or apocrine metaplasia, duct ectasia, mastitis, and cysts. In the study of 3303 patients by Dupont and Page, only 2.2% of patients with nonproliferative lesions had breast cancer following a benign breast biopsy with a mean follow-up time of 17 years (Figure 1).

BREAST CYSTS AND FIBROCYSTIC BREAST DISEASE

Fibrocystic breast disease is a benign process in which generalized microcystic formation with stromal proliferation leads to increased breast nodularity. Cysts within the breast are most common in perimenopausal women 50 to 59 years of age as well as premenopausal women. Postmenopausal women not on hormone replacement therapy are unlikely to develop cysts in their breasts. Benign cysts are often tender and fluctuate in size with the menstrual cycle. Cysts may be detected either on physical examination as a palpable, smooth, mobile nodule or by breast ultrasound. They may appear as a solitary nodule or in a cluster. Ultrasonographic appearance of simple benign cysts is that of an anechoic, round or oval, well-circumscribed mass with posterior enhancement. If the mass has all

TABLE 1 Benign Diseases of the Breast

	Increase in Breast Cancer Risk
Nonproliferative Lesions	
Mild hyperplasia without atypia	None
Squamous or apocrine metaplasia	None
Duct ectasia	None
Mastitis	None
Cysts	None
Proliferative Lesions	
Fibroadenoma	None
Moderate or florid hyperplasia	Minimal
Microglandular adenosis	Minimal
Sclerosing adenosis	Minimal
Papilloma	Minimal
Atypical ductal hyperplasia	4- to 5-fold
Atypical lobular hyperplasia	5.8-fold

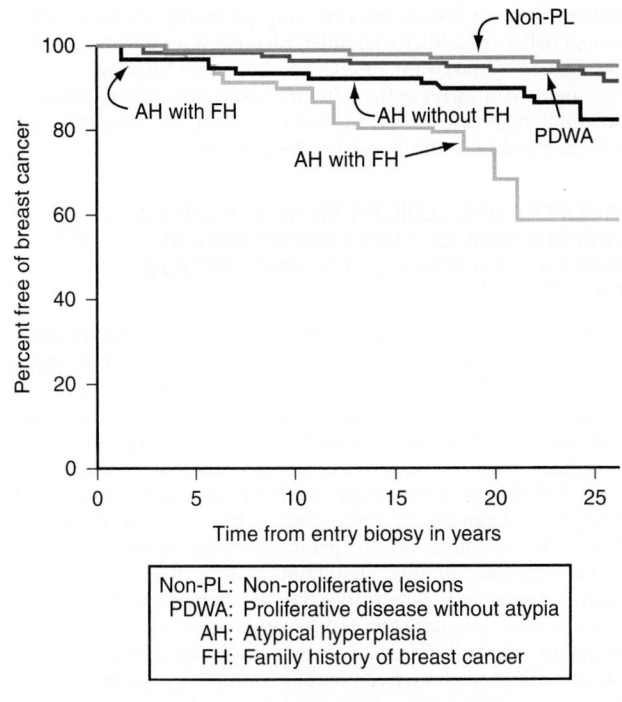

Non-PL: Non-proliferative lesions
PDWA: Proliferative disease without atypia
AH: Atypical hyperplasia
FH: Family history of breast cancer

FIGURE 1. Nonproliferative lesions in breast cancer.

four criteria, the accuracy of ultrasound is close to 100% for the diagnosis of a simple benign cyst. Cysts that appear complex, with internal echoes, thick septations, and irregular walls, are suspicious for breast carcinoma and should be examined surgically or with an ultrasound-guided biopsy. Confirmation of the diagnosis can be made by fine-needle aspiration (FNA) of the cystic fluid. Bloody fluid may be an indication for a biopsy. In a study of 6782 cyst aspirates, Ciatto and colleagues found that cytologic examination identified atypical cells in 1677 specimens. Of these specimens, only 0.3% of these cases had clinically and radiologically negative intracystic papillomas. Cytologic examination was positive in only 0.1% of these cases. Thus fluid from cyst aspirations are not sent routinely for cytologic examination. Figure 2 describes the management of suspected cysts.

MASTITIS AND DUCT ECTASIA

Mastitis is divided into lactational or nonlactational. Lactational mastitis can occur from the reflux of bacteria into the breast during breast-feeding. The causative bacteria are usually gram-positive cocci. Patients should be treated with antibiotics with the appropriate coverage and can continue to nurse or pump the breast to prevent engorgement. Nursing mothers can continue to breast-feed because the infant is not at risk for infection. Nonlactational (periductal) mastitis can be caused by duct ectasia, which occurs when the milk ducts become congested with secretions and debris, resulting in a periductal inflammation. These patients may present with greenish nipple discharge, nipple retraction, and subareolar noncyclical pain. The treatment of nonlactational mastitis includes broad-spectrum antibiotics to cover for gram-positive cocci and skin anaerobes. Total duct excision and eversion of the nipple may be necessary to treat recurrent periductal mastitis.

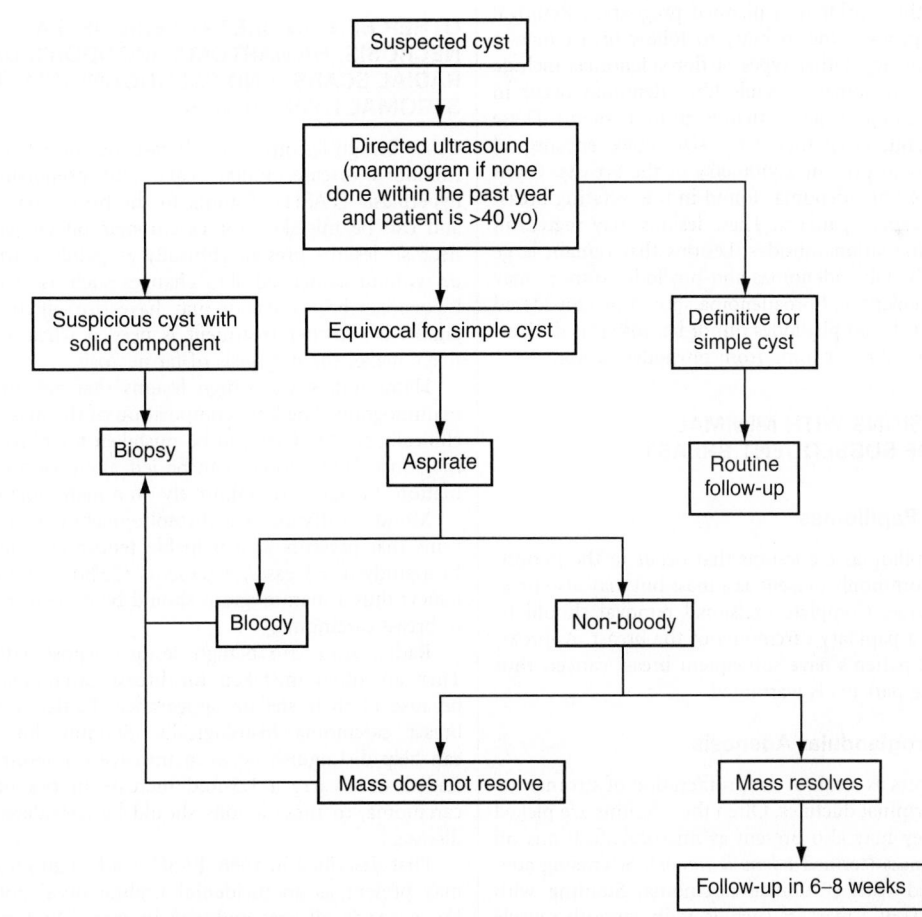

FIGURE 2. Algorithm for the management of suspected cysts.

Proliferative Benign Breast Diseases

Proliferative breast diseases include moderate or florid hyperplasia, microglandular and sclerosing adenosis, papilloma, fibroadenoma, and atypical ductal and lobular hyperplasia. All proliferative lesions have an increased risk of subsequent breast cancer after biopsy except for fibroadenoma. Overall, with a median follow-up of 17 years, 5.3% of patients with proliferative lesions develop breast cancer. This percentage increases to 12.9% in the presence of atypia (see Figure 1). Patients with moderate or florid hyperplasia, sclerosing adenosis, and solitary papilloma without atypia carry a minimal increase in risk of developing breast cancer over the general population. These patients are not classified as high risk. But the risk of subsequent breast cancer is increased by four- to fivefold in the presence of atypia. Atypical lobular hyperplasia carries a higher risk than atypical ductal hyperplasia, with a relative risk as high as 5.8. This increased risk applies to the contralateral breast because subsequent breast carcinomas are evenly divided between both breasts.

PROLIFERATIVE LESIONS WITH NO INCREASED RISK OF SUBSEQUENT CANCER: FIBROADENOMA

Fibroadenomas are benign tumors commonly found in young women (less than 30 years of age with a peak incidence at 21 to 25 years of age). They are characteristically detected on physical examination as well-circumscribed, rubbery, highly mobile, palpable masses. On mammograms, these lesions may appear as a well-circumscribed mass. Involution of fibroadenomas in the elderly can lead to hyalinization and dense popcorn-like calcification on mammograms. Fibroadenomas pose no increased risk of breast cancer and do not mandate surgical removal unless desired by the patient. Pregnancy can increase the size of these lesions; thus it may be reasonable to remove them prior to a planned pregnancy. Removal may facilitate follow-up, given the inability to follow breast masses adequately during pregnancy. Other types of fibroadenomas include juvenile and giant fibroadenomas. Juvenile fibroadenomas occur in adolescent women and can grow larger than 5 cm in diameter. These lesions are not malignant; given their large size, however, surgical excision may be needed to prevent asymmetry of the breasts. Giant fibroadenomas are large fibroadenomas found in the lactating breast or in the breasts of pregnant patients. These lesions may regress in size once hormonal stimulation subsides. Lesions that remain large can be excised surgically. Fibroadenomas and phyllodes tumors may be linked. Any rapidly enlarging fibroadenoma should be considered for surgical excision to rule out phyllodes tumor because it is difficult clinically to differentiate fibroadenoma from phyllodes tumor.

PROLIFERATIVE LESIONS WITH MINIMAL INCREASED RISK OF SUBSEQUENT BREAST CANCER

Multiple Peripheral Papillomas

Multiple peripheral papillomas are lesions that occur in the peripheral ducts. They most commonly present as a mass but may also present with nipple discharge. Complete excisional removal should be considered to rule out a papillary carcinoma of the breast. Approximately 10% to 33% of patients have subsequent breast cancer; thus close follow-up of these patients is warranted.

Sclerosing and Microglandular Adenosis

Sclerosing adenosis occurs as result of the proliferation of stromal tissue along with small terminal ductules. Often these lesions are picked up incidentally, but they may also present as microcalcifications on mammogram or as a mass (termed *adenosis tumor*). Sclerosing adenosis may be confused with a tubular carcinoma. Staining with immunohistochemical (IHC) markers such as actin, smooth muscle myosin heavy chain p63, or calponin may be helpful in distinguishing

between the two lesions because only sclerosing adenosis contains myoepithelial cells. Microglandular adenosis is an uncommon lesion that may be mistaken for tubular carcinoma on histologic examination, and it can increase the patient's subsequent breast cancer risk. Concomitant breast cancer has been reported, so complete surgical excision should be considered for these lesions.

PROLIFERATIVE LESIONS WITH A FOUR- TO FIVEFOLD RISK OF SUBSEQUENT BREAST CANCER: ATYPICAL DUCTAL AND LOBULAR HYPERPLASIA

Atypical ductal and lobular hyperplasia are very similar to their in situ counterparts. These lesions are termed *atypical hyperplasia* because they lack some of the microscopic features of in situ disease. The distinction between atypical hyperplasia and carcinoma in situ is sometimes hard to make. In a study by Rosai, five expert breast cancer pathologists reviewed 17 cases of ductal or lobular lesions. In no case did all five agree on a diagnosis. Four out of the five were able to agree on a diagnosis in three cases (18%). In one third of the patients, the diagnosis ran the gamut from hyperplasia without atypia to carcinoma in situ. Despite such difficulty, the diagnosis of atypical hyperplasia is on the rise as mammographic screening becomes more popular. Atypical hyperplasia, which is detected secondary to microcalcifications or by serendipity, carries the highest risk of subsequent breast carcinoma among all proliferative lesions of the breast, with a four- to fivefold increased risk over the general population. Atypical lobular hyperplasia carries a higher risk than atypical ductal hyperplasia, with a relative risk as high as 5.8. This risk applies to the contralateral breast as well as the ipsilateral breast. Surgical excision of atypical hyperplasia on a core biopsy is recommended because 20% of patients are found to have breast cancer at time of surgical excision for atypical hyperplasia. It is not necessary to achieve negative margins for these lesions.

OTHER BENIGN BREAST LESIONS: FAT NECROSIS, HAMARTOMA, MONDOR'S DISEASE, RADIAL SCARS, AND PSEUDOANGIOMATOUS STROMAL HYPERPLASIA

Other benign lesions of the breast include fat necrosis, hamartoma, Mondor's disease, radial scars, and pseudoangiomatous stromal hyperplasia (PASH). Trauma to the breast may lead to fat necrosis and can be mistaken for carcinomas on clinical examination. Fat necrosis lesions present clinically as painless, irregular masses with or without associated skin changes such as skin thickening. These lesions can be normal or may have rim calcifications on mammograms. No further treatment is needed when a core biopsy definitively makes the diagnosis of fat necrosis.

Hamartomas are benign lesions that are often picked up on a mammogram. The fatty composition of the mass makes these lesions clinically occult. They can be mistaken for fibroadenomas on mammograms. Hamartomas can be left alone without histologic confirmation if diagnosed definitively on a mammogram.

Mondor's disease is a thrombophlebitis of the superficial breast veins that presents as a palpable tender cord leading to the axilla. In a study of 63 cases, 8 patients (25%) had an underlying malignancy; thus a mammogram should be done to rule out the presence of breast carcinoma.

Radial scars are benign lesions whose etiology is unknown. They are often mistaken for breast carcinoma on mammograms because of their stellate appearance. Radial scars may also mimic breast carcinoma histologically. Staining for myoepithelial cells can help distinguish between invasive carcinoma and a radial scar. Radial scars carry a 1.5-fold increase in risk of subsequent breast carcinoma, so these lesions should be considered markers of future disease.

First described in 1986, PASH is a benign proliferative lesion that may present as an incidental finding or a mobile breast mass. It can occur in all ages and also in men. On a mammogram, PASH appears as a round noncalcified mass. Histologically, PASH may be mistaken for low-grade angiosarcoma. Unlike angiosarcoma, however, there should be no evidence of mitosis or cytologic atypia in PASH specimens. The role of hormones in the pathogenesis of PASH is controversial. Although these lesions tend to occur in young patients or in elderly patients on hormone therapy, most cases tend to be negative for estrogen receptors. The treatment for PASH is complete surgical excision. Approximately 7% of cases recur despite adequate treatment.

Risk Factors for Breast Cancer

An estimated 80% of women in whom breast cancer develops have no documented risk factors or determinants. Risk factors cannot be changed, whereas risk determinants can be altered to decrease a person's risk of subsequent breast cancer. Common risk factors include a familial history of breast cancer, personal breast biopsy history, menarche before 12 years of age, menopause after 55 years of age, increasing age, geographical location, and mutations of the BRCA1 or BRCA2 genes. Women known to have the BRCA1 or BRCA2 genetic mutation have an 85% lifetime risk of breast cancer as well as an increased risk of ovarian cancer. BRCA1 carriers are at a higher risk for developing ovarian cancer than BRCA2 (60% versus 20%, respectively). The risk determinants for breast cancer include reproductive factors such as nulliparity and first pregnancy after the age of 30 years and previous radiation exposure. Previous therapy for lymphoma, especially during adolescence, elevates a woman's risk of subsequent breast cancer.

Screening Techniques

Screening for breast cancer includes mammography, ultrasound, breast self-examination (BSE), and physical examination by a physician. Multiple studies such as the Göthenborg and Malmö trials show a reduction in breast cancer mortality from 30% to 40% in patients 40 to 49 years of age who undergo screening mammograms. A meta-analysis of six randomized trials indicates a 30% reduction in breast cancer mortality in patients 50 to 69 years of age. The sensitivity of mammograms depends on the patient's age and ranges from 53% to 81% in women 40 to 49 years of age to 73% to 81% in patients 50 years of age or older. An estimated 10% to 15% of breast cancer cases are not detectable on screening mammography, thus emphasizing the importance of physical breast examination by a physician and BSE that include both visual inspection and manual examination of the breast. On inspection, signs of breast malignancy include skin or nipple retraction or discoloration, nipple discharge/crusting, or peau d'orange edema of the breast. On palpation, any asymmetric mass of the breast or axilla may be regarded as a potential malignancy that deserves further evaluation.

Current recommendations are for a woman to start performing BSE at 18 years of age, have a yearly physical exam, and initiate annual mammography at 40 years of age. Little data exist on what should be the upper age limit of mammogram screening. Given that breast density decreases with age and breast cancer increases with age, mammograms should be even more sensitive and specific in the older age group. For these reasons, mammograms may be continued in very elderly patients as long as the patient is not suffering from any major co-morbidities. In patients who have a very high risk of breast cancer, such as BRCA carriers, screening should start 10 years earlier than the age of onset of an affected relative or at the age of 35. Kriege screened 1909 patients (including 358 BRCA mutation carriers) who had more than a 15% lifetime risk of developing breast cancer. These patients had a biannual breast exam as well as annual mammogram and breast magnetic resonance imaging (MRI). In this population, mammograms had a sensitivity of 33% with a specificity of 95%. Breast MRI had significantly higher rates of sensitivity and specificity at 80% and 90%, respectively. Given these findings, breast MRI should be a part of the screening exam for these high-risk patients. MRI is recommended as a standard screening test in BRCA

heterozygotes. Routine surveillance in high-risk patients includes a 6-month interval alternating between breast MRI and mammograms. Patients with a history of mantle radiation for lymphoma should start annual screening at 25 years of age and biannual screening 10 years after receiving radiation therapy.

Workup of a Breast Mass

DOMINANT PALPABLE MASS

The workup of a dominant palpable breast mass depends on the patient's menopausal status and the degree of suspicion. It is not unreasonable to follow a premenopausal patient with a nonsuspicious mass over one menstrual cycle and then reexamine her. Suspicious lesions present as a hard, nontender, irregular mass or as a mass in a high-risk patient. Palpable masses in postmenopausal patients may also warrant a workup. FNA should not be performed prior to diagnostic imaging because it may result in a hematoma that could obscure the image of the mass. Certain benign lesions on core biopsy should be excised, including lobular carcinoma in situ (LCIS), atypical ductal hyperplasia (ADH), radial scars, sclerosing papillary lesions, columnar cell hyperplasia with atypia, and PASH (Figure 3). Twenty percent of surgeries performed for atypical ductal hyperplasia have concurrent carcinoma in the specimen. Patients with a high-risk proliferative lesion should have close follow-up after surgery including physical examinations. Negative findings on a mammogram do not preclude the diagnosis of cancer because 10% of cancers are occult mammographically. This number drops to 3% when a lesion is occult both mammographically and ultrasonographically. An alternative to core biopsies in younger women is the use of the triple test: a physical exam in conjunction with breast imaging (mammogram or ultrasound) and FNA. When all three components indicate the mass is benign, the negative predictive value is 100%. In a study by Morris, a triple test score assigns points to each component of the test. One point is given for benign findings, 2 points for suspicious findings, and 3 points for malignant findings. When added together, masses with scores of 4 or less are found to be benign. The triple test should only be used in women 40 years of age or younger because the incidence of breast cancer increases dramatically after that cutoff.

MASSES REVEALED ON SCREENING MAMMOGRAMS

The American College of Radiology's classification lexicon, the Breast Imaging Reporting and Data System (BI-RADS), is used in breast imaging (Table 2). BI-RADS 0 means the assessment is incomplete and more workup is needed. BI-RADS 1 indicates a normal mammogram. Mammograms with BI-RADS 2 signify benign findings. Patients with BI-RADS 3 have a 1% to 2% risk of malignancy and should have short-term follow-up with another mammogram in 6 months. BI-RADS 4 indicates the presence of suspicious lesions with a 20% to 40% probability of a malignant lesion. BI-RADS 5 is highly suggestive of cancer with a greater than 95% chance of harboring an underlying malignant lesion. BI-RADS 6, recently added as a category, indicates known malignant disease. BI-RADS 4 and 5 both indicate a biopsy.

A core biopsy via ultrasound guidance may be attempted first. A stereotactic core biopsy should be considered if this is not possible. Stereotactic biopsies may be impossible in patients with lesions that are very superficial or close to the chest wall or in patients with very small breasts that compress to less than 3 cm or who are unable to lie still for the procedure. In such situations, surgical excision with needle localization is warranted. In studies comparing surgical excision to core biopsies, the concordance rate is close to 100%. The surgeon can obviate the need for multiple surgeries in the same patient by performing a core biopsy for diagnosis. High-risk proliferative lesions, such as LCIS, atypical ductal hyperplasia, radial scars, sclerosing papillary lesions, columnar cell hyperplasia with atypia, and PASH, should be considered for an excisional biopsy if the diagnosis is made by a core biopsy.

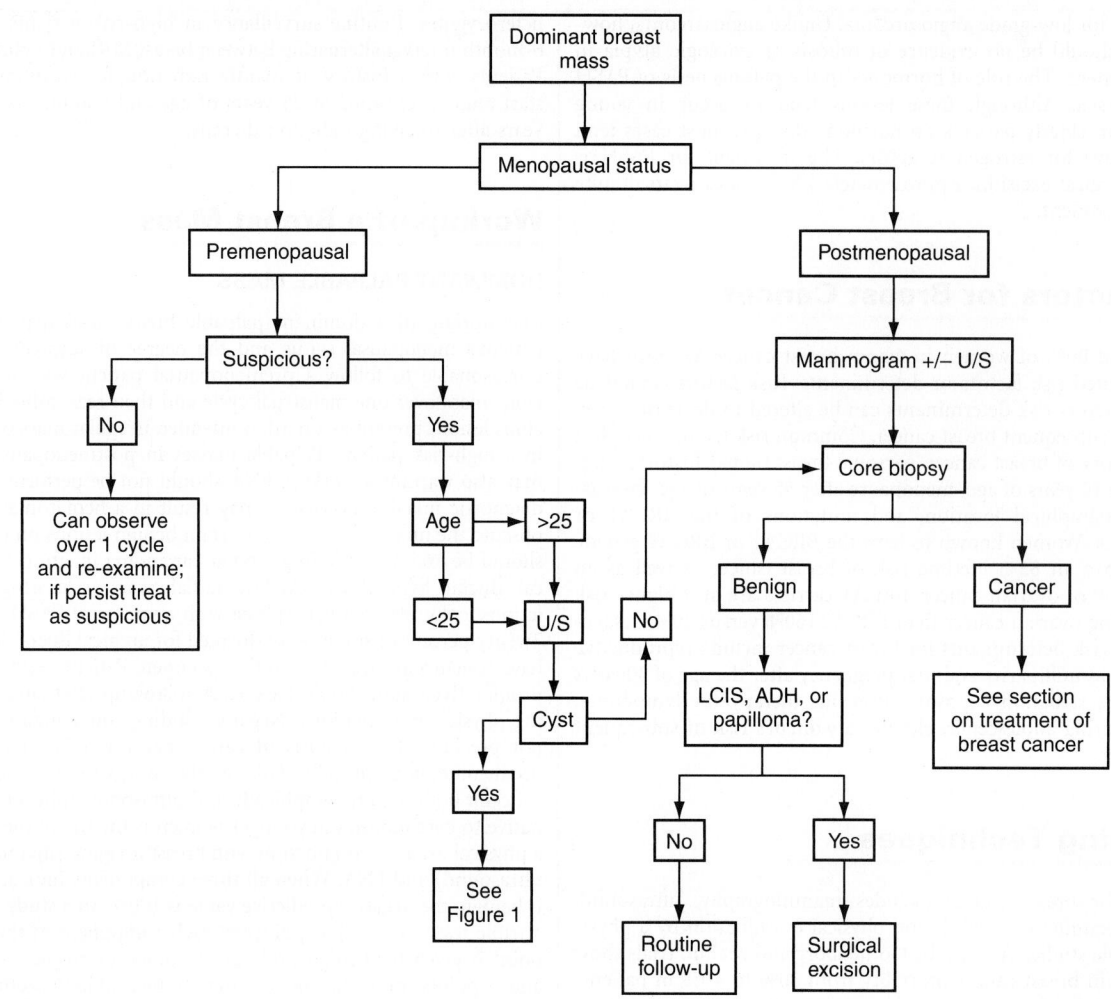

FIGURE 3. Algorithm for workup of a breast mass. ADH = atypical ductal hyperplasia; LCIS = lobular cancer in situ; U/S = ultrasound.

In Situ Diseases

LOBULAR CARCINOMA IN SITU

Lobular carcinoma in situ (LCIS) should be considered a marker for future breast cancer risk and not an early noninvasive lobular cancer. This disease is most commonly seen in premenopausal women, with a peak incidence in women 40 to 50 years of age. Only 10% of LCIS occurs in postmenopausal women. Unlike ductal carcinoma in situ, LCIS is often found incidentally because typically no clinical or radiologic abnormalities are seen at time of diagnosis. In 50% of patients, LCIS is a multifocal finding. In 30% of patients, it can be found in the contralateral breast. Patients with LCIS are at 8 to 10 times the risk of the general population for subsequent breast cancer. Their

overall lifetime risk is as high as 30% to 40% for the development of invasive breast cancer. In a meta-analysis, 15% of patients developed breast cancer in the ipsilateral breast, and 9.3% of patients developed cancer in the contralateral breast. The type of breast cancer can be either ductal or lobular, although the majority is ductal.

DUCTAL CARCINOMA IN SITU

Ductal carcinoma in situ (DCIS), or intraductal carcinoma, is a noninvasive breast cancer and designated stage 0. Historically, DCIS represented only approximately 5% of breast cancer cases, whereas today it constitutes 20% to 30% of all cases. This rise is predominantly attributed to the increasing use of screening mammography because DCIS is most often detected as mammographic microcalcifications. It tends to

TABLE 2 BI-RADS Mammography Classification

BI-RADS Category	Definition	Risk of Malignancy	Recommended Follow-Up
0	Incomplete assessment	N/A	Further workup
1	Negative study	N/A	Repeat mammogram in 1 y
2	Benign	N/A	Repeat mammogram in 1 y
3	Probably benign	<2%	Repeat mammogram in 6 mo
4	Suspicious	20%	Biopsy should be considered
5	Highly suggestive of malignancy	90%	Appropriate action should be taken
6	Known biopsy-proven malignancy	N/A	Appropriate action should be taken

Abbreviation: BI-RADS = Breast Imaging Reporting and Data System.

occur at a later age than LCIS and is not considered a multifocal or bilateral disease. Unlike LCIS, DCIS should be considered a true precursor lesion because if left untreated, approximately 60% to 100% of DCIS cases progress to invasive carcinoma.

TREATMENT FOR IN SITU DISEASE

Lobular Carcinoma in Situ

LCIS should be treated as a marker for increased breast cancer risk. Surgery in an attempt to achieve negative margins is not warranted for LCIS. The NSABP P-1 (the National Surgical Adjuvant Breast and Bowel Project) randomized trial examined the role of tamoxifen (Nolvadex) as a chemopreventive agent in high-risk patients, including those with LCIS. Women taking tamoxifen had a 50% reduction in the subsequent risk of breast cancer without any improvement in overall survival. The main risks of tamoxifen include increased risk of thromboembolic disease and endometrial cancer. The rate of pulmonary embolism was 3 in 1000 patients in the tamoxifen group versus 1 in 1000 in the placebo group. The rate of deep-vein thromboembolism was 5 in 1000 patients in the tamoxifen group versus 3 in 1000 in the placebo group. Endometrial cancer was seen in 9 in 1000 patients in the tamoxifen group versus 3.5 in 1000 in the placebo group. The decision to use tamoxifen as a chemopreventive agent should be made on an individual basis given these side effects. The highest reduction in breast cancer occurred in the LCIS group with a 70% reduction in risk. Despite this, no difference in survival was seen between the tamoxifen and placebo group.

Ductal Carcinoma in Situ

Treatment of DCIS has evolved from simple mastectomy to lumpectomy with radiation therapy. A simple mastectomy is associated with a 1% local recurrence rate. Thus it is still considered a viable option in patients who do not desire or are ineligible for breast conservation therapy (BCT). No difference in survival is seen in patients treated with mastectomy versus BCT. The NSABP B-17 randomized trial examined the role of lumpectomy with and without radiotherapy for the treatment of DCIS. The addition of radiotherapy decreased the recurrence rate from 16.4% to 7% with 8 years of follow-up. More importantly, it decreased the rate of invasive carcinoma from 8% to 2%. The 5-year event-free survival with lumpectomy and radiation is 84%. Limited data support excision alone in small well-differentiated DCIS with surgical margins of at least 1 cm. Silverstein showed in retrospective studies that the recurrence rate in such patients is approximately 4%. Routine axillary lymph node dissection (ALND) is not recommended for DCIS because only 1% of patients have positive axillary nodes. Recent studies, however, show that sentinel lymph node biopsy may have a role in the management of selected patients with DCIS. This is especially true in patients receiving a mastectomy as definitive treatment or if there is a question of microinvasion on the core biopsy. Patients with DCIS and microinvasion can have anywhere from a 3% to 20% incidence of nodal involvement. Indications for a sentinel node biopsy include extensive calcifications, a palpable lesion, patients undergoing mastectomy as treatment for DCIS, and lesions for which the pathology reads "can not rule out microinvasion." Tamoxifen (Nolvadex) can also be considered in cases of DCIS that are estrogen receptor positive. The NSABP B-24 randomized trial examined the utility of tamoxifen in patients treated with lumpectomy and radiotherapy. Ipsilateral tumor recurrences decreased from 13.4% without tamoxifen to 8.2% with tamoxifen. The incidence of invasive cancer was reduced by 47%. No difference in survival was observed between the placebo and the tamoxifen group. Side effects are similar to that of the NSABP P-1 trial.

Invasive Breast Cancer

INCIDENCE

An estimated 1 in 9 women living in the United States if they survive to 90 years of age will develop breast cancer. The average age at diagnosis is 64 years of age and increases along with age.

TABLE 3 Overall Survival in Breast Cancer Patients

Stage	10-Year Overall Survival	15-Year Overall Survival
I	74%–95%	64%
II	76%	62%
IIA	81%	72%
IIB	70%	52%
III	50%	40%
IIIA	59%	49%
IIIB	36%	18%
IIIC	36%	18%
IV	18%	18%

Adapted from Rosen PP, et al. J Clin Oncol 1989;355–366; Woodward WA, Strom EA, Tucker SL, et al. Changes in the 2003 American Joint Committee on Cancer staging for breast cancer, dramatically affect stage-specific survival. J Clin Oncol 2003;21:3244–3248.

The American Joint Committee on Cancer TMN (tumor, metastasis, node) system designates breast cancer as stage 0, I, II, III, or IV. This system categorizes breast cancer by its invasive or noninvasive character, tumor size, axillary lymph node status, and the presence of metastatic disease (see Table 2). Overall survival with breast cancer is related to stage (Table 3).

HISTOLOGY

The most common type of infiltrating carcinoma is ductal carcinoma-not otherwise specified (IFDC-NOS), which represents 85% of all invasive breast cancer. Infiltrating lobular carcinoma originates from the lobular structures of the breast and accounts for 15% of all invasive breast cancer. Other less common subtypes represent less than 10% and include tubular, medullary, mucinous, and papillary carcinoma. Additional rare subtypes of breast cancer include inflammatory carcinoma, malignant phyllodes tumor, sarcoma, lymphoma, and Paget disease.

BREAST CANCER STAGING

In 2003 the American Joint Committee on Cancer (AJCC) revised their staging system on breast cancer. This latest revision stresses the importance of nodal status as a prognostic factor by making several changes in how it is classified within the staging system. Major changes to the staging system include the following:

- Designation is made for isolated tumor cells (ITCs), which are differentiated from micrometastasis and defined as "single tumor cells or small cell clusters not greater than 0.2 mm, usually detected only by IHC (immunohistochemistry) or molecular methods, but which may be verified on H&E (hematoxylin-eosin) stains. ITCs do not usually show evidence of malignant activity, e.g., proliferation or stromal reaction." ITCs are designated as pN0 with modifiers for positive or negative IHC (i−, i+) and molecular findings (mol−, mol+).
- Internal mammary nodes (IMNs) are reclassified based on how they are detected and whether or not there is concomitant axillary lymph node metastasis. Detection of IMNs by sentinel node biopsy alone is classified as pN1b in the absence of positive axillary nodes or pN1c in the presence of positive axillary nodes. Internal mammary nodes detected by imaging studies (excluding lymphoscintigraphy) or by clinical exam are classified as pN2b in the absence of positive axillary nodes or pN3b in the presence of positive axillary nodes.
- Supraclavicular nodal involvement is now reclassified as N3 disease; thus a patient with supraclavicular nodal involvement does not automatically have stage IV disease.
- Infraclavicular nodal involvement is added as N3 disease.
- Axillary lymph node involvement is now classified by the number of nodes involved. Involvement of 1 to 3 axillary nodes is considered pN1 disease. Involvement of 4 to 9 axillary nodes is considered pN2 disease. Involvement of greater than 10 axillary nodes is considered pN3 disease.

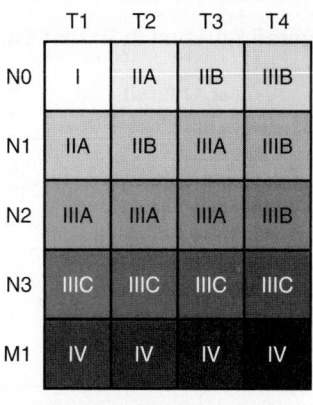

	T1	T2	T3	T4
N0	I	IIA	IIB	IIIB
N1	IIA	IIB	IIIA	IIIB
N2	IIIA	IIIA	IIIA	IIIB
N3	IIIC	IIIC	IIIC	IIIC
M1	IV	IV	IV	IV

FIGURE 4. Pathologic staging of breast cancer.

Staging of breast cancer can be divided into clinical staging versus pathologic staging. Factors used for clinical staging include the size of the tumor within the breast, presence or absence of pathologically confirmed lymph nodes, and presence or absence of distant metastasis. There are five stages for breast cancer. Stage 0 is defined as the presence of in situ disease only, without evidence of nodal or distant metastasis. Stage I is considered breast cancer confined to the breast, regardless of tumor size. Exception to this general characterization includes tumors with extension to the chest wall or skin or inflammatory breast cancers. These tumors are at least stage IIIB. Stage II is considered a breast cancer of any size with pathologically positive ipsilateral mobile axillary nodes. Stage IIIA is considered a breast cancer of any size with pathologically positive ipsilateral fixed axillary nodes or clinically apparent internal mammary nodes in the absence of positive axillary nodes. Also any large tumors (bigger than 5 cm) with any type of positive axillary or internal mammary nodes are considered stage IIIA. Stage IIIB tumors are breast tumors with extension to the skin or chest wall or inflammatory breast cancer. Involvement of the pectoralis major or minor muscle does not constitute chest wall involvement. Stage IIIC tumors are breast cancers of any size with either positive infraclavicular or supraclavicular nodes or positive internal mammary nodes in the presence of positive axillary nodes. Stage IV connotes any breast cancers with distant metastasis (see Figure 3).

Pathologic staging of breast cancer is more complicated and differs from clinical staging in that the number of nodes involved as well as how nodal metastasis is detected are used in stage designation of nodal status (Figures 4 and 5).

SURGICAL TREATMENT OF THE BREAST

A significant paradigm shift in the treatment of breast cancer has occurred over the past several decades. The Halsted paradigm, popularized at the beginning of the 20th century, hypothesized that breast cancer spreads in a contiguous fashion from the breast to the axillary lymph nodes and then to distant sites elsewhere in the body. The Fisher paradigm, which views breast cancer as systemic from very early in the course of the disease, modified this theory; the axillary lymph nodes act not as a barrier but as indicators of disease aggressiveness. Both paradigms are correct and incorrect. At a certain point in the evolution of a breast cancer, the disease changes from a local disease to a systemic disease. The Halsted paradigm promotes more intensive local treatment to eradicate the cancer, whereas the Fisher paradigm promotes less aggressive local treatment with the addition of systemic treatment in most women, even with relatively early disease. Because of this philosophy change and the detection of earlier disease through diligent screening techniques, surgical treatment of breast cancer is progressing toward less radical surgery and more adjuvant therapy, with equal or better outcomes. Recent mammograms of both breasts should be reviewed for any other suspicious lesions. There may be a slight increase in synchronous breast cancer in patients with invasive lobular cancer, although the rate of contralateral breast cancer is equal to that of invasive ductal carcinoma over the lifetime of the patient. The risk of distant metastasis is 25% to 50% in patients with inflammatory breast cancer.

Breast Conservation Therapy

Most small noninvasive and invasive breast cancers are treated by BCT, which consists of wide local excision with negative surgical margins and irradiation of the breast. The NSABP B-06, Milan I

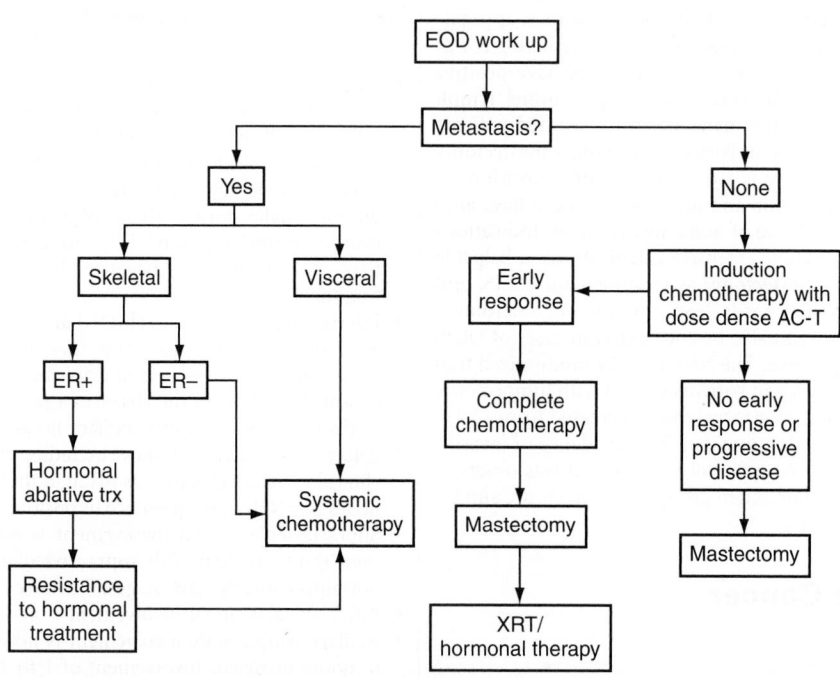

FIGURE 5. Algorithm for treatment of locally advanced breast cancer (LABC). AC-T = Adriamycin and cyclophosphamide plus Taxol; EOD = extent-of-disease; trx = treatment; XRT = x-radiation therapy.

and Milan II, as well as other clinical trials, show no statistically significant difference in patient survival with mastectomy or BCT.

The addition of radiation treatment to wide local excision in patients with noninvasive and invasive carcinoma is currently the standard of treatment. The NSABP B-06 randomized trial evaluated local recurrence of small invasive tumors with and without irradiation after lumpectomy. It found that patients who did not undergo radiation therapy had significantly higher rates of local recurrence. With BCT, incidence of recurrence in the treated breast is 7% at 5 years, 14% at 10 years, and 20% at 20 years. Local recurrence rate is much lower in patients treated with mastectomy, with an overall incidence of 5% to 10%. The majority of recurrences occur in the first 3 years after surgery. Contraindications to BCT include tumor of any size that can not be adequately excised with significant deformity to the breast, multicentric disease, noncompliant patient, first- or second-trimester pregnant patient, history of significant collagen vascular disease, and history of previous radiation therapy to the chest wall. If both BCT and mastectomy are viable options, the patient's preference should also play a role in the decision to proceed with BCT versus a mastectomy.

MASTECTOMY

A patient with contraindications to breast conservation should have a mastectomy with or without immediate reconstruction. Total mastectomy surgically removes the breast parenchyma, pectoral fascia, nipple, and the areola complex. A modified radical mastectomy includes axillary dissection. A radical mastectomy, rarely done today, includes removal of the pectoralis major and minor muscles and axillary dissection.

BREAST RECONSTRUCTION

Any patient recommended to have a mastectomy should be offered the option of immediate or delayed reconstruction and referred to a plastic and reconstructive surgeon to discuss which techniques are appropriate. One commonly used method of breast reconstruction is a tissue expander breast implant. A tissue expander is placed beneath the pectoralis muscles, and expansions are performed over a period of several weeks to months to stretch the subpectoral pocket to accommodate the permanent implant. The permanent saline or silicone implant is then inserted as a secondary procedure.

Another method of breast reconstruction is the transverse rectus abdominis myocutaneous (TRAM) flap, which involves the transfer of skin, fat, and muscle from the lower part of the abdomen to create a reconstructed breast. This procedure can be performed as a free flap with the arterial and venous supply anastomosed to vessels in the axilla or as a pedicle flap with the arterial and venous supply from the superior epigastric vessels. Other types of flap reconstructions include latissimus dorsi or gluteal flaps. Reconstruction of the nipple and areola is often performed as a later procedure.

SURGICAL TREATMENT OF THE AXILLA

The status of the axilla should be assessed for metastases in any patient with invasive breast cancer for several reasons. The status of the axillary lymph nodes is important in determining the patient's stage of disease. The presence or absence of axillary lymph node metastases is predictive of the prognosis and facilitates decisions by the medical oncology team regarding adjuvant therapy. Relapse-free survival is closely related to the number of lymph nodes that are positive. In a study of 2873 patients, Hilsenbeck found that the relapse-free survival at 5 years was 80% in patients with node-negative disease. This number decreased to 70%, 60%, and 40% with 1 to 3 positive nodes, 4 to 9 positive nodes, and more than 10 positive nodes, respectively. Nodal status is now incorporated into the sixth revision of the AJCC staging system. Surgical removal of metastatic nodes in the axilla significantly decreases the possibility of axillary recurrence. ALND may improve overall survival, but this issue is debated in the medical literature.

Sentinel Lymph Node Biopsy

Axillary dissection traditionally was performed on all patients with invasive breast cancer. Today, sentinel lymphadenectomy, or sentinel lymph node (SLN) biopsy, identifies the first, or sentinel, lymph node or nodes in the axillary chain to receive drainage from the breast cancer and thus the most likely to contain metastases. The SLN biopsy is performed by injecting isosulfan blue dye and/or radioactive isotope to localize the sentinel lymph node.

The sentinel node can be identified in 95% of all cases. Multiple studies show that SLN biopsy can predict accurately the presence of axillary metastases in T1-2 breast cancer with a false-negative rate of 5% and an accuracy rate of 95%. The false-negative rate of SLN biopsy can be decreased to 1% to 3% if any palpable node is removed along with any hot or blue nodes. The SLN biopsy, a less invasive way to assess the status of the axilla, is associated with fewer complications than an axillary node dissection. Areas of controversy in SLN biopsy include T3, palpable suspicious axillary lymph nodes, and previous neoadjuvant therapy. In a study by Specht, 25% of palpable suspicious axillary lymph nodes proved benign on final pathology. Previous axillary dissection is not a strict contraindication per se because 75% of these patients can still have an identifiable sentinel node. The success rate depends on the number of nodes previously removed, with a success rate of 87% when fewer than 10 nodes are removed versus a success rate of 47% when more than 10 nodes are removed. Contraindications to SLN biopsy include T4 breast cancer and pregnancy. SLN biopsy is contraindicated in pregnancy because of the lack of data regarding fetal safety, although computer models suggest the amount of radiation exposure to the fetus is negligible.

Axillary Dissection

Patients who have metastatic cells on SLN biopsy typically undergo complete ALND. Alternatively, if a patient is not a candidate for SLN biopsy, ALND should be considered. Axillary dissection involves the removal of 10 to 30 lymph nodes from the axilla. The potential risk of axillary dissection includes the accumulation of a seroma, ipsilateral arm lymphedema, and numbness around the area of the intercostal brachial innervation if the nerve is sacrificed at the time of surgery. Because of the lifetime increased chance of arm lymphedema and possible infection, patients should avoid any trauma or procedures such as venipuncture or blood pressure measurements on the ipsilateral arm.

Adjuvant Therapy

Adjuvant therapy is used to treat patients with a demonstrable likelihood for the development of metastatic disease. Most medical oncologists consider this risk sufficient in node-negative patients with a tumor diameter of 1 cm or larger and in those with nodal metastases to justify adjuvant chemotherapy or hormonal therapy. Most commonly used cytotoxic regimens include CMF (cyclophosphamide [Cytoxan], methotrexate, and 5-FU [fluorouracil]) for 6 cycles or AC-T for 8 cycles (4 cycles of doxorubicin [Adriamycin] and cyclophosphamide followed by 4 cycles of paclitaxel [Taxol]). There appears to be a slight improvement of 3% in overall survival favoring the anthracycline-containing regimen over the CMF regimens. In the elderly population, the CMF regimen may be easier to tolerate than the AC-T regimens. In a recent study, a dose dense regimen of AC-T results in a slight improvement of disease-free and overall survival. Dose-dense regimen involves giving the chemotherapy in cycles every 2 weeks, with bone marrow support such as G-CSF (Neupogen), as opposed to the traditional cycles every 3 weeks. The improvement in survival is approximately 3%. In the Early Breast Cancer Trialists' Collaborative Group (EBCTCG) meta-analysis, adjuvant chemotherapy appears the most beneficial for women younger than 50 years of age. Combination chemotherapy resulted in the improvement of 10-year-overall survival from 71% in node-negative patients not receiving chemotherapy to 78% in those that did receive chemotherapy. This increase was even more dramatic in node-positive patients, with an improvement of overall survival from 42% to 53%. A much smaller effect was seen in patients older than 50 years of age. In this group of patients, survival was increased from 67% to 69% when node-negative patients not receiving chemotherapy were compared to those receiving chemotherapy. In node-positive elderly patients, improvement in overall survival was also minimal, with an increase of survival from 47% to 49% with chemotherapy.

Hormonal therapy, such as tamoxifen, is a commonly used adjuvant treatment in early breast cancer patients with estrogen receptor–positive tumors. The EBCTCG meta-analysis looking at the role of tamoxifen in the premenopausal patients found that tamoxifen results in an absolute improvement of 10-year overall survival of 5.6% in node-negative patients and 10.9% in node-positive patients. This effect is even greater in the postmenopausal population, with a 26% proportional reduction in 10-year mortality rates. The recommended length of treatment for node-negative patients is 5 years. Additionally, tamoxifen can be used as a chemopreventive agent to decrease the chance of an additional ipsilateral tumor developing in patients undergoing breast conservation or to decrease the possibility of contralateral breast cancer.

More recently, three large randomized trials of aromatase inhibitors, such as anastrozole (Arimidex), exemestane (Aromasin), and letrozole (Femara), was published. In the ATAC (Arimidex, Tamoxifen, Alone or in Combination) trial, patients on anastrozole had a statistically significant longer disease-free interval when compared with patients on tamoxifen alone (hazard ratio of 0.83). No difference in survival was seen between the two groups. In another large study, patients on tamoxifen for 2 to 3 years were randomized to continuing tamoxifen versus switching to exemestane for a total of 5 years of therapy. There appeared to be an improvement in disease-free survival in the aromatase inhibitor arm (hazard ratio of 0.68). No difference in survival was seen, and given the early stoppage and cross-over of patients, no survival data will be obtainable from this study. Yet another large double-blinded randomized trial involved patients who had finished a 5-year course of tamoxifen and were then randomized to receiving letrozole versus placebo. The trial was stopped at a mean follow-up of 2.4 years secondary to a significant improvement in disease-free survival in the letrozole arm (hazard ratio of 0.57). Again, no difference in survival was seen. Aromatase inhibitors are useful only in postmenopausal patients. Premenopausal patients may benefit from an aromatase inhibitor only after ovarian ablation.

Recommendations regarding tamoxifen, aromatase inhibitors, and chemotherapy depend on the clinical judgment of the treating medical oncologist. In general, if adjuvant chemotherapy is given, it should take place prior to the initiation of radiotherapy. Consideration should be given to the likelihood of systemic recurrence based on nodal status, tumor size, and tumor grade. Estrogen receptor positivity of the tumor is predictive of a response to hormonal therapy, and HER2-neu may determine the type of appropriate chemotherapy. Another factor is the patient's age and any co-morbid diseases that would decrease the patient's tolerance to a course of chemotherapy.

Surveillance After a Diagnosis of Breast Cancer

Surveillance should continue alter diagnosis and treatment of breast cancer to detect local recurrence or a new primary breast cancer in either the ipsilateral or contralateral breast. The National Comprehensive Cancer Network guidelines recommend that patients continue diligent monthly self-examinations and that a physician perform a physical examination at 6-month intervals to assess for evidence of local recurrence and symptoms of metastatic disease. The ipsilateral arm should be evaluated to detect early signs of lymphedema and initiate appropriate management. Bilateral mammograms should be obtained every year. Bone and computed tomographic scans and other tumor markers should be performed only on patients with symptomatic systemic disease because of the lack of evidence of improved survival with early detection of distant metastases.

Special Topics in Breast Disease

PHYLLODES TUMOR

Phyllodes tumor (cystosarcoma phyllodes) is a fibroepithelial lesion that can be either benign or malignant. It is a rare tumor of the breast accounting for 1% of all cases. The mean age of patients is 54 years of age. These tumors often present as a breast mass on clinical and mammographic examination, and they are considered benign or malignant depending on stromal cellularity, mitotic activity, presence of necrosis, and type of borders. Treatment is complete excision without axillary node dissection. Metastases secondary to malignant phyllodes are hematogenous and primarily travel to the lungs. It is important to obtain negative margins. A mastectomy occasionally may be warranted for large lesions. Patients with malignant phyllodes have an 80% chance of 5-year survival as opposed to more than 95% for benign phyllodes.

NIPPLE DISCHARGE

Nipple discharge can occur at any age and presents as a bloody, serous, or milky discharge. Only 6% to 12% of patients with a nipple discharge are found to have an underlying malignancy. This risk is slightly elevated if the discharge is bloody. The most common cause of serous or serosanguineous nipple discharge is a benign intraductal papilloma. Numerous drugs can also cause nipple discharge, such as phenothiazine, tricyclic antidepressants, reserpine, butyrophenones, cimetidine (Tagamet), verapamil (Calan), metoclopramide (Reglan), thiazides, and hormone replacement therapy. The most common underlying malignancy is DCIS. Ductograms may be useful in locating the papilloma. When the nipple discharge is unilaterally persistent, spontaneous, or postmenopausal, further workup may be considered. Other suspicious nipple discharges are those confined to one duct or that are bloody or serous. In general, the evaluation of nipple discharge should begin with a clinical examination and a mammogram. Cytologic examination of the discharge has a low sensitivity for detection of underlying malignancy and should be not be used in the workup. Treatment consists of a major duct excision.

GYNECOMASTIA

Gynecomastia is the unilateral or bilateral benign enlargement of male breast tissue. The etiology is often related to various substances, including exogenous hormones, cimetidine (Tagamet), thiazides, digoxin, theophylline, phenothiazines, alcohol, and marijuana use; it may also be idiopathic. The main concern is to rule out the diagnosis of male breast cancer. Once breast cancer is excluded, no treatment is indicated. If medication and lifestyle etiologies are eliminated without remission of the gynecomastia, the excess breast tissue may be surgically removed for cosmetic considerations or for breast pain.

MALE BREAST CANCER

Carcinoma of the male breast represents 1% of all breast cancers. Because men are not routinely screened for breast cancer, the diagnosis is often delayed. The most common manifestation of male breast cancer is a painless, firm, subareolar breast mass. The differential diagnosis includes gynecomastia. Breast imaging with mammography and/or ultrasound may be helpful in rendering a diagnosis inasmuch as the appearance of male breast cancer is a stellate, irregular solid mass. Any suspicious breast mass in a male patient should undergo diagnostic biopsy. If a malignancy is diagnosed, standard treatment is mastectomy with assessment of the axillary nodes by SLN biopsy or ALND. Most cases of male breast cancer are estrogen receptor positive, and recommendations for adjuvant chemotherapy or hormonal therapy should be based on criteria similar to those for breast cancer in female patients.

BREAST CANCER IN PREGNANCY

Pregnancy-associated breast cancer represents less than 2% of all breast cancer diagnoses. The breast cancer frequently is diagnosed at a late stage because of the difficulty of examining the breast in pregnant women and the avoidance of mammography during pregnancy. Any suspicious lesion noted during pregnancy should be subjected to biopsy in the same fashion as in a nongravid woman. Radiation therapy should not be administered during pregnancy, so breast conservation is generally contraindicated unless the diagnosis is made within a few weeks of delivery. Surgical treatment with mastectomy and ALND is the standard treatment of breast cancer during pregnancy. Adjuvant chemotherapy can be delivered with selective agents during the second and third trimesters. The prognosis is similar to that of nongravid women in whom breast cancer is diagnosed at a comparable stage.

INFLAMMATORY BREAST CANCER

The classic manifestation of inflammatory breast cancer is erythema, edema, peau d'orange, and color of the breast resembling an infectious process. Malignant cells within the dermal lymphatic vessels of the breast confirm the diagnosis. The usual pathology of the associated carcinoma is IFDC-NOS. Inflammatory carcinoma is a very aggressive type of breast cancer, with over 90% of patients having positive axillary lymph nodes at diagnosis. The recommended treatment is multimodality therapy, with chemotherapy preceding surgery. Surgical treatment is mastectomy followed by radiation therapy and often additional chemotherapy.

LOCALLY ADVANCED BREAST CANCER

Patients with N2 or N3 nodal status or those with four or more positive axillary nodes, T3 or T4 tumors, or involvement of the pectoralis fascia have locally advanced breast cancer (LABC). The recommended treatment for patients is neoadjuvant chemotherapy, which is administered before surgical treatment, although it has no impact on overall survival. An extent-of-disease (EOD) workup should be done in patients with LABC and includes a computed tomography (CT) of the chest, abdomen, and pelvis along with a bone scan. Figure 5 provides an algorithm for the treatment of LABC.

Endometriosis

Method of
David L. Olive, MD

Endometriosis is one of the most common diseases encountered by the practicing gynecologist, yet it is also one of the most vexing. Researchers have been searching for answers to even the most fundamental questions regarding this disease for well over a century; even today huge gaps remain in the understanding of this disorder.

Definition

Endometriosis is defined as the presence of endometrial glands and stroma outside the endometrial cavity and uterine musculature. The requirement for both glands and stroma is an arbitrary standard, and it is unclear whether either component of endometrium alone, if placed ectopically, can result in the symptoms and signs of endometriosis.

Two related diseases are also frequently observed. Adenomyosis is the presence of endometrial glands and stroma within the myometrium. This disorder is epidemiologically and pathogenically distinct from endometriosis, but the resulting symptoms (and medical treatments) are similar. Endosalpingiosis is identical to endometriosis in location and appearance but histologically resembles tubal glands and stroma. This latter abnormality has been poorly studied, and to date, little is known regarding the distinction between endometriosis and endosalpingiosis.

Genetics

Evidence continues to accumulate that endometriosis has a genetic basis. Evidence for this includes familial clustering, concordance in monozygotic twins, and increased prevalence among first-degree relatives. A search was recently undertaken to identify the gene or genes responsible for susceptibility to endometriosis. Although suggestive linkages were discovered, no genes have been firmly identified as instrumental in this disorder. It is hoped, however, that genetic research will eventually uncover information critical to understanding the molecular and cellular basis of this disease.

Pathogenesis

The pathogenesis of endometriosis is a controversial subject inspiring many researchers to investigate it. Over the last 25 years considerable advancement has been made, providing solid clues to the understanding of the disease process. Today, a clear picture is beginning to emerge regarding how women develop endometriosis.

HISTOGENESIS

Leading researchers in the field have proposed numerous theories of histogenesis. The primary theory of histogenesis is transplantation of shed uterine endometrium to ectopic locations. A number of routes of dissemination of the tissue are proposed, including lymphatic dissemination, vascular spread, iatrogenic transplantation, and retrograde menstruation.

A critical aspect of this theory is that cast-off endometrium cells remain viable and capable of implanting. Furthermore, it proposes that the tissue distribution has the capacity to sustain implantation. Considerable research has established that shed endometrial cells are viable in vitro. In vitro studies of endometrial attachment to peritoneum also support the concept of transplantation, attachment, and invasion.

Additional theories of histogenesis include coelomic metaplasia and induction of endometriosis. However, little scientific evidence indicates that either route is a viable etiology of the disease, much less a common method for development.

ETIOLOGY AND MAINTENANCE

Retrograde menstruation is a well-established phenomenon. Data available from women undergoing peritoneal dialysis and laparoscopy at the time of menses suggest that 76% to 90% of women have retrograde flow. This mechanism is considered a critical first step in the initiation of much if not most endometriosis by a wide variety of epidemiologic and anatomic data. However, the majority of women do not have endometriosis. The question that arises is "Why not?"

Because the placement of menstrual debris into the peritoneal cavity happens with each menses, a mechanism must exist to eliminate this tissue. The prime candidate for removal of endometrial cells is cell-mediated cytotoxicity. Deficient cytotoxic response to ectopic endometrium is suggested as a mechanism for allowing implantation and growth. It is also postulated that factors positively affecting growth and maintenance may be altered to enhance the risk of endometriosis. Current evidence suggests that a variety of cytokines, including monocyte chemotactic protein-1, interleukin-8, and regulated on activation, T-cell expressed and secreted (RANTES) are overexpressed in women with endometriosis, resulting in the attraction and activation of macrophages. The source of this cytokine increase could be one or more of several tissues: Endometrium, peritoneal mesothelium, and macrophages themselves could be the primary aberrancy by which this cascade is begun.

Other abnormalities are speculated to promote endometriosis. These include abnormal expression of matrix metalloproteinases and the enzyme aromatase, which could locally produce a hyperestrogenic proimplantation environment. The mechanisms by which these abnormalities may cause disease as well as the source of such alterations are under investigation.

Prevalence and Epidemiology

Endometriosis is a disease found almost exclusively in reproductive-age women. The mean age at diagnosis is reported to be from 25 to 29 years, although this figure depends on the diagnostic method. Because traditional diagnosis requires laparoscopy, it is likely that the disease is frequently present in even younger patients for whom many gynecologists do not readily schedule surgery.

Although rare in the premenarcheal female, adolescent endometriosis is a relatively common entity. Endometriosis is found in 47% to 65% of women younger than 20 years with chronic pelvic pain or dyspareunia.

Endometriosis is associated with increased exposure to menstruation typified by earlier menarche, more frequent menses, longer menses, fewer pregnancies, later initial pregnancy, and less breastfeeding. In addition, factors known to decrease the amount of menses or lower estrogen levels also reduce the risk: oral contraceptive use, irregular menses/oligomenorrhea, stress, exercise, and cigarette smoking (Box 1).

Postmenopausal endometriosis seldom occurs; this age group represents only 2% to 4% of all women requiring laparoscopy for endometriosis. The majority of such cases are a sequela to reactivation of disease by hormone replacement therapy; this is not true in all cases.

Clinical Presentation

Endometriosis is associated with a wide array of presenting signs and symptoms, although many women with physical manifestations of the disease remain completely asymptomatic. Commonly, the severity of symptoms does not correlate with the stage of endometriosis; extensive disease sometimes causes only minimal symptoms, and in others, minimal disease can be associated with severe symptoms. Some symptoms may strongly suggest the presence of endometriosis, but none are pathognomonic of this disorder. Because endometriosis most commonly involves the pelvis, infertility, dysmenorrhea, pelvic pain, dyspareunia, and menstrual dysfunction are common clinical presentations. When the ovary is severely involved, an ovarian cyst or pelvic mass may be the initial sign of endometriosis.

Pelvic pain is the most frequent complaint for endometriosis patients. This generally presents as secondary dysmenorrhea, worsening primary dysmenorrhea, dyspareunia, or even noncyclic lower abdominal pain, chronic pelvic pain, and backaches. In addition, pain may be site specific when endometriosis is found in unusual locations outside of the pelvis.

Only rarely are physical findings specific for endometriosis. Localized cul-de-sac and uterosacral ligament tenderness may frequently be detected. Thickened, nodular uterosacral ligaments or rectovaginal masses may be palpable. Adnexal enlargement or tenderness may reflect ovarian involvement. Retroverted fixation of the uterus may be noted with posterior cul-de-sac obliteration by the disease.

Cutaneous manifestations may be present, with apparent lesions on the perineum or vagina, or, less commonly, in the inguinal region, the umbilical area, or at the site of surgical scars. They should be suspected whenever a scar or lesion is associated with cyclical pain, tenderness, swelling, or bleeding.

Diagnosis

The current gold standard for the definitive diagnosis of endometriosis is laparoscopy. However, because of the heterogeneity in appearance of endometriosis lesions, the accuracy of laparoscopic diagnosis is variable and depends on the ability of the surgeon to recognize the disease. Although histologic confirmation would be ideal to ensure the presence of disease, this is infrequently accomplished because of the reticence of surgeons to excise endometriosis lesions.

Ultrasound is most useful for the detection of ovarian endometriomas, although the appearance of a cystic structure with heightened echogenicity is certainly not limited to this form of endometriosis. Structures often confused with endometriomas include corpora lutea, hemorrhagic cysts, unilocular dermoid cysts, and other benign cystic neoplasias. Ultrasound is not currently useful for identifying focal implants.

Magnetic resonance imaging (MRI) demonstrates significant potential in the diagnosis of endometriosis. MRI is clearly of value in diagnosing the ovarian endometrioma, and as technology improves, the potential for detecting peritoneal lesions will increase.

Treatment

MEDICAL THERAPY

The first drug to be approved for the treatment of endometriosis in the United States was danazol (Danocrine), a derivative of testosterone. It was originally thought to produce a pseudomenopause, but subsequent studies have revealed that the drug acts primarily by diminishing the midcycle luteinizing hormone (LH) surge, creating a chronic anovulatory state. The recommended dosage of danazol for the treatment of endometriosis is 600 to 800 mg/day; however, these doses have substantial androgenic side effects such as increased hair growth, mood changes, adverse serum lipid profiles, deepening of the voice (possibly irreversible), and, rarely, liver damage (possibly irreversible and life threatening) and arterial thrombosis. Studies of lower doses as primary treatment for endometriosis-associated pain have been uncontrolled or with small numbers and thus contain information of limited value.

Progestogens are a class of compounds that produce progesterone-like effects on endometrial tissue. A large number of progestogens exist, ranging from those chemically derived from progesterone (progestins), such as medroxyprogesterone acetate (MPA), to 19-nortestosterone derivatives such as norethindrone and norgestrel. The proposed mechanism of action of these compounds causes initial

---

> **BOX 1   Epidemiology of Endometriosis**
>
> Increased risk with:
> - Menses >6 d
> - More menses
>
> Decreased risk with:
> - Increased parity
> - Irregular menses
> - Oral contraceptives
> - Late menarche
> - Exercise
> - Smoking

CURRENT DIAGNOSIS

- Symptoms associated with endometriosis are primarily those of pain and infertility, although site-specific symptoms and signs may exist when the disease is in unusual locations.
- The standard for diagnosis is laparoscopic visualization; however, this method has a high false-positive and false-negative rate. The only method to confirm the disease absolutely is excisional biopsy.

CURRENT THERAPY

- Both medical and surgical therapies are efficacious in the treatment of endometriosis-associated pain. It is unclear which offers the better approach.
- Combined medical/surgical therapy may offer an advantage over surgery alone, if the medication is used at least 6 months postoperatively.
- Medical therapy has no role in the treatment of endometriosis-associated infertility.
- Surgical therapy for endometriosis-associated infertility appears to be of value for all stages of disease, but its relative value compared to assisted reproduction is not yet determined.

shedding of endometrial tissue followed by eventual atrophy. The most extensively studied progestational agent for the treatment of endometriosis is medroxyprogesterone (dep-subQ Provera 104), which is currently approved by the Food and Drug Administration (FDA) for use in treating endometriosis in a depot subcutaneous form. A common side effect is transient breakthrough bleeding, which occurs in 38% to 47% of patients. This is generally well tolerated and, when necessary, can be adequately treated with supplemental estrogen or an increase in the progestogen dose. Other side effects include nausea (0% to 80%), breast tenderness (5%), fluid retention (50%), and depression (6%). A recent approach to treating endometriosis with progestogen is the use of a progestogen-containing intrauterine contraceptive device[1] (Mirena).

The combination of estrogen and progestogen for therapy of endometriosis, the so-called pseudopregnancy regimen, has been used for 40 years. The most commonly used pseudopregnancy regimen today is the oral contraceptive pill[1] (OCP); in fact, it is the most commonly prescribed treatment for endometriosis symptoms. Like progestational therapy, pseudopregnancy is believed to produce initial decidualization and growth of endometrial tissue, followed in several months by atrophy.

Gonadotropin-releasing hormone (GnRH) agonists are analogues of the hormone GnRH. This hypothalamic hormone is responsible for stimulating the pituitary gland to secrete follicle-stimulating hormone (FSH) and LH, two hormones necessary for normal ovarian function. GnRH is secreted in a pulsatile manner; the correct pulse results in stimulation of FSH and LH release, whereas too high or too low a pulse rate results in a decrease in pituitary hormone secretion. GnRH agonists are modified forms of GnRH that bind to the pituitary receptors and remain for a lengthy period. Thus, they are identified by the pituitary as rapidly pulsatile GnRH, and after initial stimulation of FSH and LH secretion, result in a shutdown (downregulation) of the pituitary and no stimulation of the ovary. The result is a hypoestrogenic state similar to that of menopause, producing endometrial atrophy and amenorrhea. The agonist can be given intranasally (naferelin [Synarel]), subcutaneously (goserelin [Zoladex]), or intramuscularly (IM) (leuprolide acetate [Lupro Depot]), depending on the specific product, with frequency of administration ranging from twice daily to every 3 months. The side effects are those of hypoestrogenism such as transient vaginal bleeding, hot flashes, vaginal dryness, decreased libido, breast tenderness, insomnia, depression, irritability and fatigue, headache, osteoporosis, and decreased skin elasticity; these are dose dependent.

A recent modification of GnRH agonist treatment is to add back small amounts of steroid hormone in a manner similar to that used in the treatment of postmenopausal women. The theory is that the requirement for estrogen is greater for endometriosis than is needed by the brain (to prevent hot flashes), the bone (to prevent osteoporosis), and other tissues deprived of this hormone. With this approach

---

[1]Not FDA approved for this indication.

there is an equivalent rate of pain relief with far fewer side effects than GnRH agonist alone. Estrogen as a solitary add-back, however, is less effective and thus not indicated.

SURGICAL THERAPY

Most surgeons performing surgery for endometriosis must choose one of two possibilities: conservative surgery, where the patient's future fertility remains an option, or definitive surgery. The latter procedure generally involves removal of the female gonads, a hysterectomy, or a combination of the two. The general perception is that definitive surgery is more effective over time than conservative treatment, but it must be reserved for patients in whom fertility or continued endocrine function is deemed less important than relief of pain symptoms.

When conservative surgery is desired, the first technical issue confronted is method of access. Traditionally, laparotomy was used for endometriosis surgery. However, recently, most surgeons performing extensive surgery for endometriosis have favored a laparoscopic approach because of improved magnification of disease with a resulting increase in surgical precision.

Surgical destruction of endometriosis lesions can be accomplished in a variety of ways: Excision, vaporization, and fulguration/desiccation have all been used. Excision is generally thought to be the most complete of these techniques, but no comparative trials have assessed the relative efficacy of each approach.

Endometriomas, or ovarian cysts formed from endometriosis, are commonly present in the patient with endometriosis. The ovaries should first be freed of all adhesions when operating on endometriomas. The endometrioma may open spontaneously during this process; if not, incision and drainage is indicated. At this point, the cyst wall may be stripped, excised, or drained.

TREATMENT RESULTS

Medical therapy is effective against endometriosis-associated pain. Placebo-controlled randomized clinical trials (RCTs) have proven that danazol and medroxyprogesterone reduce pain significantly better than no treatment for up to 6 months following discontinuation of the drug. No good data exist for longer follow-up periods. Numerous randomized trials have compared medical therapies to one another. In 15 RCTs comparing danazol to GnRH agonists, no difference was demonstrated between the two as first-line drugs. Similarly, little difference was seen when GnRH agonists were compared to oral contraceptives, progestogens, or gestrinone.

Several trials have addressed the efficacy of combined add-back therapy and GnRH agonist treatment during 6-month treatment periods. In general, pain was relieved as effectively with the combination as with GnRH agonist alone, and it significantly reduced the side effects of the GnRH agonist. The results were similar in three longer trials of approximately 1-year duration (Figure 1). The amelioration of side effects with maintenance of efficacy seems to be even when the add-back therapy is begun during the first month of treatment, suggesting that an add-back-free interval at the beginning of a treatment cycle is unnecessary.

Although the studies just described randomize patients for initial therapy of endometriosis-associated pain, one study examined the value of GnRH agonist in patients failing primary therapy. Ling and colleagues treated women having failed to obtain relief with OCPs with either GnRH agonist or placebo. Those treated with active drug responded significantly better than those given placebo, with more than 80% experiencing pain relief in 3 months (Figure 2). Of interest is the fact that the therapy seemed to be beneficial whether or not endometriosis was seen at laparoscopy.

Most of the established medical therapies used to treat endometriosis have been applied to the problem of subfertility in women with this disease. These medications inhibit ovulation, and thus they are used to treat the disease for a period of time prior to allowing an attempt at conception. Five randomized trials with six treatment arms have compared one of these medical treatments for endometriosis to placebo or no treatment with fertility as the outcome measure. Another eight RCTs compared danazol to a second medication. These

Endometriosis

1061

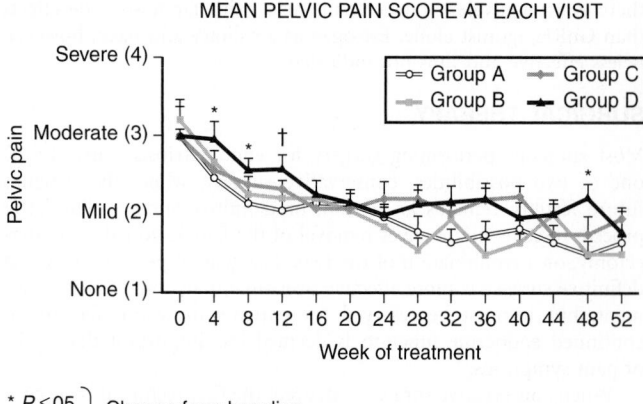

MEAN PELVIC PAIN SCORE AT EACH VISIT

* $P \le 05$ — Change from baseline
† $P \le 01$ — compared with Group A

FIGURE 1. Pain relief from gonadotropin-releasing hormone (GnRH) agonist (Group A) and three different add-back therapies. (High dose progestin, low dose estrogen/progestin, higher dose estrogen/progestin). No difference is seen among the groups in the amount of pain relief. (From Hornstein MD, Surrey ES, Weisberg GW, Casino LA: et al: Leuprolide acetate depot and hormonal add-back in endometriosis: A 12-month study. Lupron Add-Back Study Group. Obstet Gynecol 1998;91(1):16–24.)

latter trials were summarized by a meta-analysis by Hughes et al. and modified by Olive and Pritts to include loss of fertility while on the medications (Figure 3). The data clearly show that medical therapy for endometriosis has not proven to be of value, and in fact may be counterproductive, to the subfertile patient.

Only two studies have investigated surgery for endometriosis-associated pain versus sham surgery. Sutton and colleagues assessed the efficacy of laser laparoscopic surgery in the treatment of pain associated with minimal, mild, or moderate endometriosis. They found that there was no difference in pain at 3 months follow-up, but by 6 months a clear-cut advantage was seen for surgery. Abbott and colleagues evaluated excision of endometriosis versus diagnostic laparoscopy and had nearly identical results at 6 months. Thus, both techniques were proven better than no therapy.

Conservative surgery was used extensively in an attempt to enhance fertility. Most studies, however, are uncontrolled and of poor quality. Two randomized trials were performed to examine the value

Study	Medical	No treatment	Relative risk (95% CL)	
Bayer	11/37	17/36		0.63 (0.32–1.22)
Fedele	10/35	13/36		0.79 (0.36–1.68)
Telimaa	4/35	5/14		0.32 (0.08–1.24)
Thomas	4/20	4/17		0.85 (0.20–3.69)
Total	29/127	39/103		0.60 (0.39–0.93)

FIGURE 3. Meta-analysis of all randomized trials comparing medical therapy versus no treatment or placebo for endometriosis-associated infertility. Note that the untreated group has a significantly better pregnancy rate.

of ablation of early-stage endometriosis versus sham surgery, with contradictory results. When combined into a meta-analysis, surgical treatment of early-stage endometriosis still appears to provide a significant improvement in pregnancy rates. No such trials exist for more extensive disease; expert opinion would suggest that surgery will enhance fertility but may be inferior to advanced reproductive technologies.

The use of medical therapies for endometriosis is not restricted to their use as stand-alone agents. Clinicians frequently have used drugs in combination with surgical treatment of the disease. Numerous trials have examined the issue of postoperative medical therapy as an effective adjunct for pain. Those that have treated patients for at least 6 months after surgery showed efficacy, but in those studies where only 3 months of postoperative treatment was performed, no benefit was seen. Results are similar for all medications (Table 1).

In summary, endometriosis is an enigmatic disease that has long frustrated clinicians and patients. However, great strides in the understanding of this disorder are being made. The coming years are likely to produce a plethora of new treatment approaches targeting the biologic basis of this disease. In this regard, better understanding will undoubtedly result in renewed hope for the patient suffering from the ravages of endometriosis.

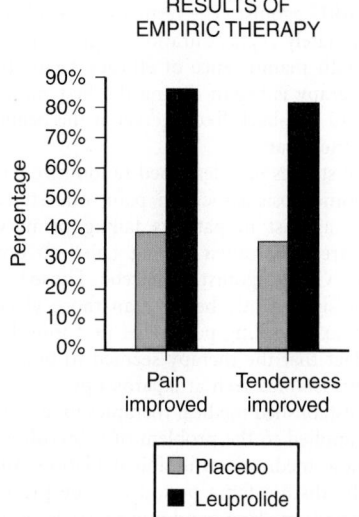

RESULTS OF EMPIRIC THERAPY

FIGURE 2. Patients with pain relief from empirical gonadotropin-releasing hormone (GnRH) agonist or placebo.

TABLE 1 Postoperative Medical Therapy

Drug	Duration of Treatment	Studies	Findings
OCPs	6 mo	1	NS at 24, 36 mo
Medroxy-progesterone, 100 mg/d	6 mo	1	$p < 0.05$ at 6 mo
Danazol, 600 mg/d	3 mo	1	NS at 6 mo
Danazol, 600 mg/d	6 mo	1	$p < 0.05$ at 6 mo
Danazol, 100 mg/d	6 mo	1	$p < 0.05$ at 24 mo
GnRH-a	3 mo	1	NS at 6 mo
GnRH-a	6 mo	2	$p = 0.008$ at 12 mo

Abbreviations: GnRH = gonadotropin-releasing hormone; NS = no sample; OCP = oral contraceptive pill.

REFERENCES

Abbott JA, Hawe J, Hunter D, et al. Laparoscopic excision of endometriosis: A randomized, placebo controlled trial. Fertil Steril 2004;82:878–84.

Hornstein MD, Surrey ES, Weisberg GW, Casino LA. Lupron Add-Back Study Group. Leuprolide acetate depot and hormonal add-back in endometriosis: a 12-month study. Obstet Gynecol 1998;91:16–24.

Hughes E, Ferorkow D, Collins J, Vandekerckhone P. Ovulation suppression for endometriosis (Cochrane review). In: The Cochrane Library (issue 1). Oxford, England: Update Software; 2000.

Jacobson TZ, Barlow DH, Koninclex PR, et al. Laparoscopic surgery for subfertility associated with endometriosis. Cochrane Database Syst Rev 2002; (4):CD001398.

Jansen RPS, Russel P. Nonpigmented endometriosis: Clinical, laparoscopic and pathologic definition. Am J Obstet Gynecol 1986;155:1154.

Ling FW. Randomized controlled trial of depot leuprolide in patients with chronic pelvic pain and clinically suspected endometriosis. Obstet Gynecol 1999;93:51–8.

Moghissi KS, Schlaff WD, Olive DL, et al. Goserelin acetate (Zoladex) with or without hormone replacement therapy for the treatment of endometriosis. Fertil Steril 1998;69:1056–62.

Olive DL, Pritts EA. The treatment of endometriosis: a review of the evidence. Ann NY Acad Sci 2002;955:360–72.

Olive DL, Pritts EA. Treatment of endometriosis. N Engl J Med 2001;345:266–75.

Sampson JA. Perforating hemorrhagic (chocolate) cysts of the ovary. Arch Surg 1921;3:245.

Sutton CJG, Ewen SP, Whitelaw N, Haines P. Prospective, randomized, double-blind, controlled trial of laser laparoscopy in the treatment of pelvic pain associated with minimal, mild, or moderate endometriosis. Fertil Steril 1994;62:696.

Abnormal Uterine Bleeding

Method of
Beth W. Rackow, MD, and Aydin Arici, MD

Abnormal uterine bleeding is a common disorder among reproductive-age women. Although abnormal bleeding often occurs due to a congenital or anatomic disorder, approximately 33–50% of women with abnormal bleeding are found to have a systemic disorder that affects the hypothalamic-pituitary-ovarian axis and hence makes them anovulatory. Normal menstrual bleeding predictably occurs at the end of an ovulatory cycle because of estrogen and progesterone withdrawal; the bleeding lasts up to 7 days, with a cycle interval of 24 to 35 days. Abnormal bleeding may present with altered intervals between menstrual cycles or changes in volume or duration of menstrual blood flow.

Evaluation of the woman with abnormal uterine bleeding must consider a broad differential diagnosis that includes a complication of pregnancy, cervical and uterine pathology (polyps, fibroids, adenomyosis, malignancies, chronic endometritis, congenital anomalies), infectious etiologies (sexually transmitted infections, vaginitis), endocrinopathies (thyroid or androgen disorders, hyperprolactinemia), medications (exogenous hormonal therapy, anticoagulants, antibiotics, glucocorticoids, tamoxifen [Nolvadex], herbal supplements), bleeding diathesis, systemic illness (liver or renal disease), and genital trauma or foreign bodies. A thorough menstrual history is essential and should include details about past and present length of intermenstrual intervals, regularity of menses, volume and duration of bleeding, onset of abnormal bleeding, factors associated with change in bleeding (postcoital, contraceptive method, postpartum, new medical diagnosis, change in weight), and associated symptoms (premenstrual symptoms, dysmenorrhea, dyspareunia, pelvic pain, hirsutism, galactorrhea). A complete medical history, list of medications, and review of systems help identify any systemic illness or medication effect contributing to the abnormal bleeding. The physical exam should include careful inspection of the external genitalia, vagina, and cervix and a bimanual exam to palpate the uterus and adnexa to assess size, contour, and tenderness.

Laboratory evaluation provides further information. A negative pregnancy test (preferably quantitative) rules out bleeding because of a pregnancy complication. A complete blood count evaluates for anemia and thrombocytopenia, and is important with prolonged or heavy bleeding. Endocrine testing may include serum thyroid stimulating hormone, prolactin, testosterone levels, and further evaluation as indicated. Coagulation studies (prothrombin, partial thromboplastin, bleeding time, and von Willebrand disease testing) should be performed in adolescents, women with unexplained menorrhagia, and those with a personal or family history concerning for a bleeding disorder. In the setting of a systemic disorder such as chronic liver or renal disease, appropriate testing should be performed.

An endometrial biopsy should be performed in women at high risk for hyperplasia and cancer based on age (35 years and older) and duration of unopposed estrogen exposure. Young women (less than 35 years old) with chronic anovulation, thus prolonged estrogen exposure, should also undergo endometrial biopsy because they can develop endometrial hyperplasia and cancer. If the biopsy reveals secretory endometrium, and not proliferative endometrium, this suggests that ovulation has occurred. A Pap smear, cervical cultures, and wet mount should also be performed as indicated.

A history of regular menstrual cycles with an increasing volume or duration of bleeding, or intermenstrual bleeding, is suggestive of an anatomic cause of abnormal bleeding. Transvaginal ultrasonography provides detailed assessment of the uterus and endometrium. Pathology such as leiomyomas and polyps can be identified, and size and location determined. Although an endometrial biopsy may not be necessary if the endometrium is thin (less than 5 mm), clinical suspicion of endometrial pathology takes precedence. Sonohysterography (or saline-infusion sonography) involves ultrasonographic assessment of the uterus and endometrium while sterile saline distends the uterine cavity. This procedure has high sensitivity and specificity for identifying uterine and endometrial pathology and is comparable to hysteroscopy. Hysteroscopy can simultaneously diagnose and treat intrauterine pathology, but involves an invasive procedure. During assessment of uterine anatomy, it is important to recognize when anatomic abnormalities, such as leiomyomas, are present but not contributing to the bleeding.

Anovulatory Uterine Bleeding

A menstrual history that reveals irregular, infrequent, unpredictable bleeding, a varying amount and duration of bleeding, and no reliable premenstrual symptoms is often sufficient to diagnose anovulatory bleeding. Considered a systemic disorder, anovulatory bleeding occurs because of a variety of endocrinologic, neurochemical, and pharmacologic processes. Estrogen breakthrough is the most common scenario: persistently high estrogen levels stimulate overgrowth of an endometrium that is fragile without the stabilizing, growth-limiting effects of progesterone, and focal areas of the endometrium breakdown, bleed, and subsequently heal because of estrogen effect. This abnormal bleeding is common in women with polycystic ovary syndrome, in postmenarchal adolescents, and in perimenopausal women. Other conditions associated with anovulation include thyroid disorders, hyperprolactinemia, androgen disorders, psychological or physical stress, eating disorders, dramatic weight changes, and insulin resistance.

Management of anovulatory bleeding involves treating both the cause of anovulation and the abnormal bleeding. Progestins are the foundation of this medical therapy. Cyclic courses of progestin stabilize the estrogen-stimulated endometrium and result in withdrawal bleeding after the progestin course. Medications used for a 10–14 day course each month include medroxyprogesterone acetate (Provera), 10 mg, and norethindrone acetate (Aygestin), 5 mg. If bleeding does not occur after progestin withdrawal, the woman may also be hypoestrogenic, and further evaluation is indicated. Estrogen-progestin contraceptives effectively cause regular withdrawal bleeding and may decrease the volume of bleeding and also provide contraception. Combined contraceptives are available in pill, patch, and vaginal ring preparations. Medroxyprogesterone acetate (Depo-Provera),[1] 150 mg intramuscularly every 3 months, can also be used to manage anovulatory bleeding, especially if women cannot take combined contraceptives. This therapy may cause irregular bleeding in the first few months, but 50% of women report amenorrhea by 12 months of use. Treatment of prolonged heavy anovulatory bleeding can be achieved with either low-dose monophasic combined contraceptives,[1] one pill twice daily for 5 to 7 days until the bleeding slows or stops, followed by routine daily use if desired, or with a higher-dose course of progestin therapy. Once the heavy bleeding is controlled, further evaluation is warranted.

Estrogen therapy is indicated for the treatment of abnormal bleeding with a thinned endometrium due to low estrogen levels or prolonged bleeding. This can be accomplished with conjugated estrogens (Premarin),[1] 1.25 mg, or micronized estradiol (Estrace),[1] 2 mg daily for 7 to 10 days. Similarly, estrogen (a 7- to 10-day course) can be used to treat progestin breakthrough bleeding in the setting of long-acting progestin therapy (medroxyprogesterone acetate [Depo-Provera]).

Ovulatory Uterine Bleeding

Heavy or prolonged bleeding may occur during ovulatory cycles, and often no specific etiology is identified; local defects in endometrial hemostasis are implicated. A number of medical and surgical therapies are effective in this situation. Nonsteroidal anti-inflammatory drugs (NSAIDs), such as ibuprofen (Motrin),[1] naproxen (Aleve),[1] or mefenamic acid (Ponstel),[1] decrease menstrual blood loss by inhibiting prostaglandin synthesis, and thus altering the balance of factors required for endometrial hemostasis. NSAIDs may decrease blood loss by 20% to 40%, and should be initiated just prior to the onset of menses and continued for 3 to 5 days. Similarly, combined contraceptives can reduce menstrual flow by 40% to 60%. Another option is the levonorgestrel-releasing intrauterine system (Mirena)[1]; the local progestin effect on the endometrium is profound and can reduce menstrual blood loss by 75% to 90% in women with heavy bleeding. Gonadotropin-releasing hormone agonists produce a hypoestrogenic state and thus cause amenorrhea as well as shrinkage of myomas, if present. This therapy is best reserved for short-term management of heavy bleeding and severe anemia prior to a surgical procedure because of its cost and significant side effects such as menopausal symptoms and bone demineralization. Less commonly employed therapies include tranexamic acid (Cyklokapron),[1] an antifibrinolytic agent used in Europe to treat menorrhagia (1 g every 6 hours for the first few days of bleeding), and danazol (Danocrine),[1] a therapy that inhibits ovulation and decreases menstrual blood loss but involves androgenic side effects (200 mg daily).

Intermenstrual bleeding can also occur during ovulatory cycles. This abnormal bleeding can be caused by anatomic abnormalities, infection, or the preovulatory decline in estrogen. Conjugated estrogens (Premarin),[1] 1.25 mg, or micronized estradiol (Estrace), 2 mg for 2 to 3 days midcycle or 7 to 10 days for persistent break-through bleeding, may be effective.

For women who fail medical therapy or for those who do not desire future fertility, surgical management is appropriate. The definitive procedure is hysterectomy, but this surgery carries a significant risk of complications and involves longer recovery time. Endometrial ablation by hysteroscopic, thermal, or cryosurgical techniques is a less invasive procedure for the management of abnormal bleeding in women who do not desire future fertility. These techniques can result in significantly reduced bleeding and dysmenorrhea, and even amenorrhea, but approximately 20% of women require additional procedures. Women with menorrhagia attributed to uterine myomas can be managed with myomectomy (hysteroscopic, laparoscopic, or abdominal procedures as indicated) or

[1]Not FDA approved for this indication.

CURRENT DIAGNOSIS

- Detailed medical and menstrual history
- Thorough physical and gynecologic examination
- Pregnancy test for all reproductive-age women
- Determination of ovulatory status based on menstrual history
- Laboratory evaluation: complete blood count, endocrine studies, coagulation profile
- Endometrial sampling if high risk for hyperplasia or cancer
- Imaging studies to evaluate anatomy

uterine artery embolization. Pregnancy is not recommended after the latter option because few data are available on postprocedure pregnancy outcomes.

Uterine Hemorrhage

Acute heavy bleeding requires high-dose estrogen therapy. Women who need inpatient management should receive conjugated estrogens (Premarin), 25 mg intravenously every 4 hours for 24 hours or until the bleeding decreases. A Foley catheter balloon (30 cc) can be placed in the uterine cavity to tamponade the bleeding. Additionally, dilation and curettage can be performed to help stop acute uterine hemorrhage. If stable for outpatient management, women can receive conjugated estrogens (Premarin),[1] 1.25 mg, or micronized estradiol (Estrace),[1] 2 mg every 4 to 6 hours for 24 hours, and when the bleeding is controlled, the dose is tapered to once daily for 7 to 10 days. Another effective regimen uses high-dose combination contraceptives[1] (3 to 4 pills daily) until the bleeding is decreased, followed by a taper to 1 pill daily for several weeks. Estrogen therapy should be followed by progestins or combined contraceptives to stabilize the estrogen-stimulated endometrium.

[1]Not FDA approved for this indication.

CURRENT THERAPY

- Progestins
  Cyclic or intermittent use
  Prolonged therapy
  Progestin-releasing intrauterine device (IUD) (Mirena)[1]
- Estrogens[1]
  Intermittent use
  High-dose course for acute heavy bleeding
- Estrogen-progestin contraceptives[1]
  Cyclic use
  High-dose course with taper for heavy bleeding
- Other therapies
  Nonsteroidal anti-inflammatory drugs[1]
  Tranexamic acid (Cyklokapron)[1]
  Danazol (Danocrine)[1]
  Gonadotropin-releasing hormone agonists
- Surgical options
  Endometrial ablation
  Myomectomy
  Uterine artery embolization
  Hysterectomy

[1]Not FDA approved for this indication.

When evaluating a woman with abnormal uterine bleeding, a thorough history and evaluation are essential to help narrow the differential diagnosis. A number of medical and surgical treatments are available for the management of abnormal uterine bleeding, but the range of options may be limited by a woman's fertility plans.

REFERENCES

American College of Obstetricians and Gynecologists. Management of anovulatory bleeding. ACOG Practice Bulletin, no. 14, March 2000.

Bayer SR, DeCherney AH. Clinical manifestations and treatment of dysfunctional uterine bleeding. JAMA 1993;269:1823–8.

Berek JS, editor. Benign diseases of the female reproductive tract. In: Berek JS, editor. Novak's Gynecology. Philadelphia: Lippincott Williams & Wilkins; 2002. p. 351–73.

Farquhar CM, Lethaby A, Sowter M, et al. An evaluation of risk factors for endometrial hyperplasia in premenopausal women with abnormal menstrual bleeding. Am J Obstet Gynecol 1999;181:525–9.

Kouides PA, Conard J, Peyvandi F, et al. Hemostasis and menstruation: Appropriate investigation for underlying disorders of hemostasis in women with excessive menstrual bleeding. Fertil Steril 2005;84:1345–51.

Munro MG. Dysfunctional uterine bleeding: Advances in diagnosis and treatment. Curr Opin Obstet Gynecol 2001;13:475–89.

Munro MG. Medical management of abnormal uterine bleeding. Obstet Gynecol Clin North Am 2000;27:287–304.

Shwayder JM. Pathophysiology of abnormal uterine bleeding. Obstet Gynecol Clin North Am 2000;27:219–34.

Speroff L, Fritz M. Dysfunctional uterine bleeding. In: Clinical Gynecologic Endocrinology and Infertility. Philadelphia: Lippincott Williams & Wilkins; 2005. p. 548–71.

Infertility

Method of
Steven R. Williams, MD

Absence of desired conception despite 12 months of unprotected intercourse generally defines infertility. Historical and physical factors allow the physician to adjust this definition to the individual patient. For example, women with longstanding amenorrhea or known distal hydrosalpinges should consider intervention before 12 months, time has elapsed. However, the couple, 22 years of age, with a negative history can be encouraged to try a bit longer than 12 months before evaluation begins. After 6 months of trying, approximately 45% of couples achieve pregnancy, and after 12 months of trying, approximately 85% will conceive. Pregnancy can occur with sex 6 days before ovulation, although one study found no pregnancies were conceived from sex the day after ovulation. Thus we recommend couples trying for a baby should plan to be active together every other day starting about 6 days before ovulation is expected (cycle day 8) until 2 to 3 days after ovulation has happened (cycle day 18). If the mood were to strike more often, that's fine with us; if the mood strikes less often, we can still be comfortable given the 6-day interval previously described. As in all of medicine, important historical points can guide the direction of the evaluation and treatment of the infertile couple.

Male-factor historical points include fathering past pregnancies or miscarriages, sexual function, urologic or hernia surgery, infections, medications, and tobacco use. Semen analysis remains the most important test for male factor evaluation. The World Health Organization (WHO) reports normal males to have more than 20 million sperm per cc with greater than 50% motility. It is probably best to advise 48 hours of abstinence before collection of the sample. A urologic exam and evaluation is indicated with abnormal counts. Modern in vitro fertilization (IVF) treatments can achieve pregnancies as long as any sperm at all can be isolated, even if that means

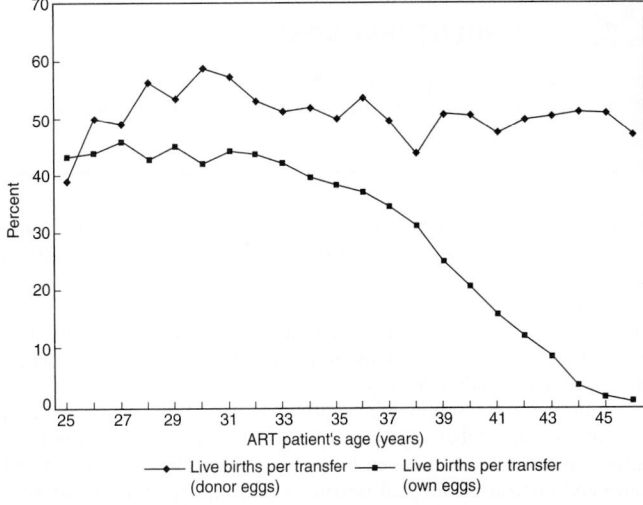

FIGURE 1. Live births per transfer for ART cycles using fresh embryos from own and donor eggs, by ART patient's age, 2002. ART = assisted reproductive technology.

surgical aspiration. Before pursuing assisted reproduction for severely low counts, genetic testing will be recommended because severely low counts can predict higher rates of cystic fibrosis carrier status, balanced translocation, and perhaps microdeletions of the Y chromosome.

A women's age has a strong correlation with fertility success. Figure 1 compares the live birth rate when IVF patients used their own eggs fertilized with their partner's sperm compared to the rate when young oocyte donor's eggs are fertilized with the IVF patient's partner's sperm and the resultant embryos transferred into the IVF patient's uterus. One must conclude from these data that the majority of the decline in success is related to oocyte quality, as anyone can expect the success of a woman 25 years of age who uses the oocytes from a woman 25 years of age! Follicle-stimulating hormone (FSH) measured on day 3 of the menstrual cycle correlates well with ovarian reserve and is commonly ordered for women more than 30 years of age with infertility. In our office, day-3 FSH values lower than 9 mU/mL are reassuring with respect to ovarian reserve, whereas values greater than 20 mU/mL are rarely associated with future fertility success using that patient's eggs.

Previous full-term deliveries are reassuring, whereas recurrent abortions or preterm deliveries can predict a uterine issue. Pelvic infections, intrauterine device (IUD) use, previous abdominal surgery, dysmenorrhea, or dyspareunia can predict tubal obstruction. This is explored with hysterosalpingography (HSG). After sterile preparation of the cervix, a sterile cannula is inserted, and under fluoroscopic guidance radiograph contrast is injected. The dye reveals the contour of the uterine cavity and displays uterine septa and intracavitary lesions such as fibroids or polyps. It then fills into the fallopian tubes and spills into the abdominal cavity. Most women describe the discomfort of the test as a severe menstrual cramp that lasts for several minutes. Pain is reduced by slow injection of the dye, gentle tissue handling, and pretreatment with nonsteroidal anti-inflammatory drugs (NSAIDs). Many authors suggest that the procedure itself has a fertility-enhancing effect. The American College of Obstetricians and Gynecologists (ACOG) suggests prophylaxis with doxycycline (Vibramycin)[1] 100 mg twice daily orally for 5 days after HSG if dilated tubes are demonstrated; no prophylaxis is indicated in a normal study. Abnormal uterine cavities can be further evaluated with saline infusion hysterograms or magnetic resonance imaging (MRI). Many uterine abnormalities can be treated completely with hysteroscopic surgery. Unilateral tubal disease noted on the HSG predicts subtle decreases in future fertility in these

---

[1]Not FDA approved for this indication.

CURRENT DIAGNOSIS

- Medical history can guide fertility testing.
- Simple laboratory and radiograph tests can determine infertility causes.

women compared with women with normal tubes. Bilateral tubal disease discovered on HSG predicts dramatic declines in fertility. Tubal patency established by HSG does not rule out peritubal adhesions that can affect fertility. Laparoscopy is an outpatient surgical procedure that can be used to further evaluate tubal abnormalities seen on HSG or to look for undetected peritubal adhesions. Laparoscopy also will detect endometriosis.

Endometriosis is noted in approximately 1 in 30 laparoscopies performed for tubal ligation (presumably for fertile women), although one third of women undergoing infertility evaluations will have endometriosis. Surgical treatment of minimal or mild endometriosis does appear to help with subsequent fertility somewhat. A prospective study of infertile women found to have mild or minimal endometriosis noted at laparoscopy showed a 31% pregnancy rate in the next 9 months for patients randomized to treatment versus a 17% pregnancy rate in the next 9 months for women randomized to no treatment.

Irregular menstruation generally indicates irregular ovulation and diminished fertility. Even with regular menstruations, serum progesterone measurements in the luteal phase (6 to 8 days after ovulation) should be greater than 10 ng/mL for the "most fertile" of ovulations. If it is not, thyroid and prolactin studies should be ordered and induction of ovulation with clomiphene citrate (Clomid) considered. Clomiphene citrate in a 50-mg dose is taken orally for 5 days starting on menstrual day 3, Serum luteal phase progesterone is drawn 7 days after ovulation and is expected to be greater than 10 ng/dL. If it is, refills for 2 more months of treatment are written. If it is not, we recommend increasing the dose of clomiphene citrate to 100 mg daily for 5 days and repeating the luteal phase progesterone assay. If still not greater than 10 ng/dL, clomiphene citrate at 150 mg daily can be tried. If the patient is still anovulatory, referral to a gynecologist or reproductive endocrinologist is considered. For resistant patients, adjunctive treatments with the clomiphene citrate can include ultrasound monitoring with HCG injections when mature follicles are noted or adding insulin-sensitizing agents or glucocorticoids. Clomiphene ovulation induction yields approximately a 70% ovulation rate and, in young couples, approximately an 8% pregnancy rate per month. One in ten clomiphene citrate pregnancies are twins, although triplets and quadruplets are very rare on this therapy. Side effects of clomiphene citrate include hot flushes, emotional lability, mittelschmerz, headache, and sleep disturbance. Discontinue the drug if the patient experiences severe visual disturbance. Because the majority of clomiphene citrate pregnancies happen early in treatment, referral to reproductive specialists should be considered if the patients is not pregnant after 3 months of treatment.

Gonadotropin ovulation induction is available for women who failed to ovulate using clomiphene citrate or did not conceive on that therapy. This medication is the natural hormone used to initiate ovulation; therefore, response and pregnancy rates are better than with clomiphene citrate. Unfortunately, dramatic increases in multiple pregnancy are associated with these medications, and often they are quite expensive. One large study reviewed success and multiple pregnancy rates in patients treated with gonadotropin ovulation induction.

CURRENT THERAPY

- Clomiphene citrate is a low risk treatment option when indicated.
- Assisted reproduction is delivering more and more babies with fewer multiples.

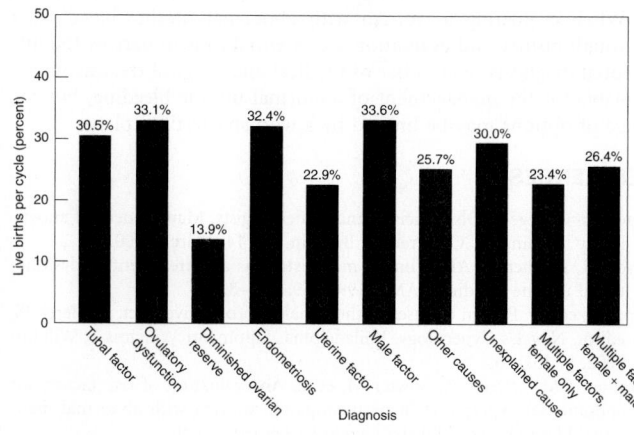

FIGURE 2. Live birth rates among women who had ART cycles using fresh nondonor eggs or embryos, by diagnosis, 2002. ART = assisted reproductive technology.

The authors concluded the protocols employed with gonadotropin ovulation induction lead to an unacceptably high incidence of higher-order multiple pregnancies and raised the question whether that treatment could be replaced by IVF.

IVF involves induction of ovulation with gonadotropin in hopes of retrieving multiple oocytes. Ovarian response is monitored with pelvic ultrasounds and serum estradiol measurements. When the oocytes are mature, HCG is given to trigger the completion of oocyte development. Then transvaginal ultrasound is used to guide an aspirating needle through the posterior cul-de-sac and into the ovaries for aspiration of the oocytes. The procedure takes approximately 15 minutes under local anesthesia and is often performed in an office setting. Oocytes are then inseminated in the lab with the husband's sperm and cultured. In certain circumstances (vey low sperm count, surgically aspirated sperm, previous failed fertilization) the oocytes can be directly injected with the sperm via intracytoplasmic sperm injection (ICSI). The resultant embryos are then cultured for 2 to 5 days and then transferred into the uterus via a simple transcervical approach. IVF thus allows embryo development without tubal ovarian interaction, making it a great choice for patients with tubal disease or endometriosis. In fact, nothing we can find at laparoscopy that was not discovered by pelvic ultrasound and HSG will affect IVF success (Figure 2). We are developing protocols that reduce the numbers of embryos transferred for couples at high risk for multiple pregnancy to one. I believe that in the future IVF will replace both gonadotropin ovulation induction and the need for laparoscopy for treatment of infertility. The 2001 Centers for Disease Control (CDC) report on assisted reproductive technology (ART) success reported national average live birth rates in the high 30% per cycle start for women younger than 35 years of age. Some individual centers are reporting live birth rates in the 50% range. IVF is a very effective and increasingly safer alternative to older treatments for refractory infertility.

REFERENCES

American College of Obstetrics and Gynecology. Antibiotic prophylaxis for gynecologic procedures. ACOG Practice Bulletin 2003;23.

Centers of Disease Control. 2002 Assisted reproductive technology success rates, National summary and fertility clinic reports. Atlanta: Center for Disease Control; 2002.

Gleicher N, Oleske DM, Tur-Kaspa I, et al. Reducing the risk of higher order multiple pregnancy after ovarian stimulation with gonadotropins. N Engl J Med 2000;343:2–7.

Jain T, Soules MR, Collins JA. Comparison of basal follicle-stimulating hormone versus the clomiphene citrate challenge test for ovarian reserve testing. Fertil Steril 2004;82:180–225.

Jordan J, Craig K, Clifton DK, et al. Luteal phase defect: The sensitivity and specificity of diagnostic methods in common clinical use. Fertil Steril 1995;63:427–8.

Marcoux S, Maheux R, Berube S. Laparoscopic surgery in infertile women with minimal or mild endometriosis. Canadian collaborative group on endometriosis. N Engl J Med 1997;337:217–22.

Mol BW, Swart P, Bossuyt BM, et al. Is hysterosalpingography an important tool in predicting fertility outcome? Fertil Steril 1997;67:663–9.

Schwabe MG, Shapiro SS, Haning RV Jr. Hysterosalpingography with oil contrast medium enhances fertility in patients with infertility of unknown etiology. Fertil Steril 1983;40:604–6.

Trimbos JB, Trimbos-Kemper GC, Peters AA, et al. Findings in 200 consecutive asymptomatic women, having a laparoscopic sterilization. Arch Gynecol Obstet 1990;247:121–4.

Wilcox AJ, Weinberg CR, Baird DD. Timing of sexual intercourse in relation to ovulation. Effects on the probability of conception, survival of the pregnancy, and sex of the baby. N Engl J Med 1995;333:1517–21.

Amenorrhea

Method of
Vickie Martin, MD, and Robert L. Reid, MD

Amenorrhea, simply put, is the absence of menses. It can be classified as either primary (when a woman of reproductive age has never had menstruation) or secondary (when amenorrhea occurs after menstruation has been established). There are normal situations in which amenorrhea is expected (physiologic amenorrhea): during pregnancy, during lactation, and at the onset of menopause. Approximately 5% of reproductive-age women experience amenorrhea at times other than these, which warrants investigation. Women with amenorrhea often present with significant apprehension and anxiety. Thus, an appropriate but timely work-up and diagnosis are required. The clinician must have a systematic approach for evaluating such women to ensure that important causes of amenorrhea are identified. As always, a detailed history, a targeted physical examination, and selective use of simple diagnostic tests are required.

Definition

Amenorrhea may be defined as the absence of menstruation for 3 or more months in women with past menses (secondary amenorrhea) or the absence of menarche by the age of 16 years in girls who have never menstruated (primary amenorrhea). Infrequent menstruation, termed *oligomenorrhea*, may have similar causes and also warrants investigation.

Menstrual Cycle

A clear working knowledge of the menstrual cycle and its physiology is mandatory for the clinician in these circumstances. Menstruation normally results when a cascade of hormonal signals from the hypothalamus (gonadotropin-releasing hormone [GnRH]) to cause pituitary release of luteinizing hormone (LH) and follicle-stimulating hormone (FSH). These in turn stimulate the development of an egg-containing ovarian follicle. Estrogen from this follicle results in steady growth of the endometrial lining over a 2-week period (follicular phase). When ovulation occurs, the follicle (now called the corpus luteum) develops the ability to produce a second hormone, progesterone.

The secretion of estrogen and progesterone for the next 2-week period causes the endometrial lining to become lush (decidualized) in preparation for implantation of a pregnancy. If pregnancy fails to occur, the corpus luteum undergoes a spontaneous demise, the endometrium no longer has adequate hormonal support to survive,

and the tissue is sloughed synchronously over the next 5 to 7 days as menstrual flow. The final steps of this process require a means of egress for blood, implying a normal uterus with a patent cervix and vagina (the outflow tract).

Etiology

Different classification systems have been employed. One system defines the type of amenorrhea based on the level of FSH in circulation. For example, high FSH levels indicate that the hypothalamus and pituitary are fully functioning but that the ovary is not responding (similar to menopause). The gonadotropin (FSH) levels are high and the ovary (gonad) is not functioning, which is termed *hypergonadotropic hypogonadism*. *Hypogonadotropic hypogonadism* refers to the situation where FSH levels are very low due to some central disturbance of hypothalamic or pituitary function. The problem with this classification is that normal FSH levels are often low and the distinction between hypogonadotropic and eugonadotropic causes of amenorrhea can be difficult.

A simple way to consider causes of amenorrhea is to divide the processes that regulate menstruation (the hypothalamic-pituitary-ovarian axis [HPO axis]) into compartments (Figure 1) and then consider possible contributory factors for disruption of normal processes at each of these levels. Always consider the possibility that amenorrhea may be due to unexpected pregnancy before moving on to a full investigation.

HYPOTHALAMIC COMPARTMENT

The hypothalamus integrates a wide variety of signals from the brain and is ultimately responsible for turning on or off the hormonal cascade necessary for triggering ovulatory and menstrual function. In adolescents, the development of breasts (thelarche) between ages 8 and 10 years is usually the first sign that the HPO axis has turned on and first menstruation (menarche) typically follows within 3 to 5 years. All girls with primary amenorrhea by age 14 years, particularly if 5 or more years have passed since the first evidence of pubertal development, warrant careful investigation, because girls with primary amenorrhea on the basis of constitutional delay cannot readily be differentiated on clinical history from the two thirds of patients

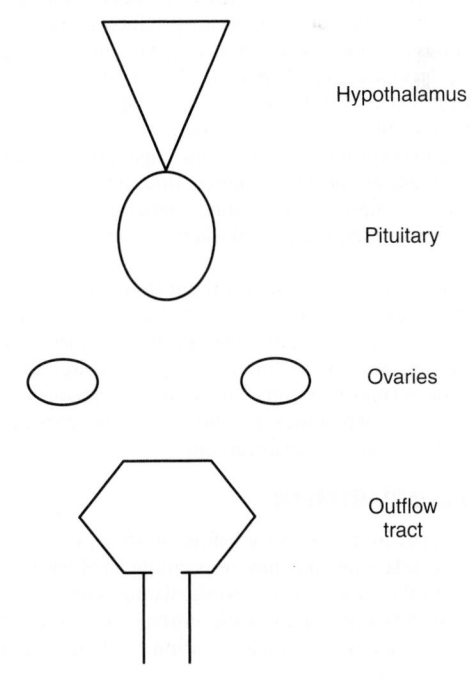

FIGURE 1. The four compartments to consider when evaluating amenorrhea.

with primary amenorrhea who have irreversible causes of reproductive failure.

Constitutional Delay

One third of young women presenting with primary amenorrhea have constitutional delay of puberty, meaning that they are undergoing a normal sequence of pubertal development at a rate that falls 2.5 standard deviations behind the mean. Girls with constitutional delay often present between ages 13 and 16 with primary amenorrhea and only early signs of breast development. Investigation reveals low to low-normal levels of gonadotropins and an otherwise negative work-up.

Congenital Causes

A variety of unusual congenital conditions result in hypogonadotropic hypogonadism and primary amenorrhea. These conditions may be caused by deficiency of GnRH production or by abnormalities of the GnRH receptor. A Kallman's-like syndrome has been identified in some affected women who present with anosmia and a complete lack of pubertal development.

Acquired Causes

Acquired diseases can lead the hypothalamus to shut down the reproductive hormonal cascade, resulting in amenorrhea, which may be primary or secondary, depending on when they develop. Nutritional deprivation (including eating disorders), excessive caloric demand due to participation in demanding sports, and extreme psychological stress are common reasons for delayed activation of reproductive processes by the hypothalamus. Less commonly, systemic illnesses, including malabsorption states, active autoimmune diseases, and rare hypoxemic states related to congenital heart malformations or severe anemias (sickle cell disease), can lead to amenorrhea.

PITUITARY COMPARTMENT

Lesions of the pituitary stalk that interrupt normal delivery of GnRH to the pituitary include those resulting from head trauma, rare stalk tumors such as craniopharyngiomas, or from the surgery to remove these.

Pituitary causes of amenorrhea are almost always due to oversecretion of prolactin. Hyperprolactinemia resulting in amenorrhea, if associated with central retro-orbital headache and bitemporal hemianopia, can result from a prolactin-producing tumor.

Other causes of hyperprolactinemia originate outside the pituitary. For example, primary hypothyroidism, breast or chest wall lesions (or piercings) in the T4-6 dermatome, renal failure, and a variety of medications have all been linked to hyperprolactinemia. Medications that can cause hyperprolactinemia include dopamine receptor antagonists (phenothiazines, butyrophenones, thioxanthenes, risperidone, metoclopramide, sulpiride,[2] pimozide), dopamine-depleting agents (e.g., methyldopa, reserpine), H$_2$-blockers (cimetidine), opiates, and cocaine.

Rarely, other pituitary conditions result in amenorrhea. In empty sella syndrome, radiologic examination reveals an apparently empty sella due to pituitary regression from some vascular or other insult. Other conditions include Sheehan syndrome (postpartum pituitary necrosis), pituitary apoplexy (massive pituitary infarction), and radiation-induced hypopituitarism. In each of these situations, amenorrhea is usually part of a larger picture of endocrine disruption.

OVARIAN COMPARTMENT

Depletion of eggs from the ovary before or after puberty results in primary or secondary amenorrhea, respectively. FSH levels are markedly elevated in these cases, as the hypothalamus and pituitary try to elicit follicular development from the unresponsive ovary. Destruction of oocytes by any of several environmental insults, including

ionizing radiation, various chemotherapeutic (especially alkylating) agents, and certain viral infections can accelerate follicular atresia.

Primary amenorrhea in a woman with evidence of gonadal failure should elicit a search for a chromosomal abnormality. It is known that two intact X chromosomes are needed for maintenance of ovarian function. A variety of X chromosome structural abnormalities have been identified in women with premature ovarian failure, including complete absence of one X chromosome (Turner's syndrome).

Elevated FSH occurs in association with a normal karyotype. These women have normal 46,XY or 46,XX karyotypes without the phenotypic abnormalities of Turner's syndrome. Those with a Y chromosome should have their gonads removed because of the potential for malignant transformation.

Several rare inherited enzymatic defects also may be associated with premature ovarian failure. These include partial deficiencies in four enzymes in the steroidogenic pathway—17α-hydroxylase, 17,20-desmolase, 20,22-desmolase, and aromatase—and galactosemia.

Premature ovarian failure may be associated with a number of autoimmune disorders. Most commonly associated with thyroiditis, ovarian failure also occurs in women with polyglandular failure, including hypoparathyroidism, hypoadrenalism, and mucocutaneous candidiasis.

Though it is not exclusively an ovarian disorder, it is useful to consider polycystic ovary syndrome (PCOS) in the ovarian compartment for the purpose of completeness in considering possible diagnoses. PCOS is one of the most common causes of secondary amenorrhea. Typically, women suffering from this condition are overweight (although one third have normal body weight) and have clinical features of hyperandrogenism (acne and hirsutism), hyperinsulinism (acanthosis nigricans), and hyperestrogenism (watery cervical mucus). Months of amenorrhea may be punctuated by episodes of heavy and prolonged menstrual bleeding as an estrogen-thickened endometrium sheds irregularly over several weeks.

OUTFLOW TRACT COMPARTMENT

Congenital abnormalities of development of the reproductive outflow tract can cause amenorrhea. Complete absence of a uterus can be due to isolated müllerian agenesis or it can manifest in phenotypic females with a 46,XY karyotype who have complete androgen insensitivity. Developmental abnormalities can include cervical atresia, tranverse vaginal septum, and imperforate hymen. These latter abnormalities may be associated with cyclic menstrual pain in the absence of bleeding (cryptomenorrhea). Similarly, monthly cramps can occur with cervical stenosis following trachelectomy or conization. Uterine synechiae due to a vigorous curettage in the face of a postpartum or postabortion endometritis can result in obliteration of the uterine cavity and secondary amenorrhea with or without monthly menstrual-like cramps.

OTHER CAUSES

Pregnancy must always be considered in a sexually active female patient presenting with secondary amenorrhea. Hormonal suppression of the endometrium can be accomplished with a variety of medications. The progestin component of the cyclic oral contraceptive gradually results in a thinner and thinner endometrium, which can ultimately result in pill-withdrawal amenorrhea. Other medications, including danazol, medroxyprogesterone, and long-acting GnRH agonists can result in amenorrhea.

Diagnosis

HISTORY

A search for clues as to the etiology should start with a personal developmental history in the amenorrheic teen and with a menstrual and reproductive history in the older amenorrheic woman. Events in the 3 to 6 months preceding the onset of amenorrhea are often critical. Rapid weight gain or loss or a marked change in energy

---

[2]Not available in the United States.

BOX 1 A Compartmental Approach to Systems Review

Hypothalamic Compartment
- Changes in temperature regulation, sleep, appetite, thirst
- Headache or visual field defects

Pituitary Compartment
- Central retro-orbital headache, bitemporal hemianopia
- Galactorrhea
- Features of hypothyroidism
- Medications affecting prolactin

Ovary Compartment
- Hot flushes
- Insomnia
- Night sweats
- Vaginal dryness

Outflow Compartment
- Cyclic cramps
- Possibility of pregnancy
- Recent gynecologic procedures (dilation and curettage, cervical laser or conization)

CURRENT DIAGNOSIS

- Always consider the possibility of pregnancy in any woman presenting with secondary amenorrhea.
- Secondary amenorrhea is most commonly the result of some significant lifestyle change (weight gain or loss, stress, excessive exercise) or illness (with marked weight loss) in the preceding 6 months.
- Obesity and features of androgen excess are most often related to polycystic ovary syndrome (PCOS).
- Because constitutional delay of puberty is found in only one third of girls presenting with delayed menarche, an investigation should be initiated at the time of presentation rather than waiting until the girl is 16 years old (meeting the definitional criteria).
- Primary amenorrhea, particularly with the absence of other features of pubertal development (breasts and pubic and axillary hair) suggests ovarian failure.
- When amenorrhea due to ovarian failure (high FSH) occurs before age 35 years, a karyotype is indicated. If Y chromosome material is identified on karyotype, gonadectomy is required to reduce the risk of malignancy in the gonadal tissues.

expenditure through exercise may be important. Systems review should examine possible disruption to any of the compartments (Box 1). Inquiry about general health, risk of pregnancy, and use of medication (including illicit drugs) is important.

PHYSICAL EXAMINATION

Height, weight, and body mass index (BMI) should be determined. Body habitus often provides an important clue to which patients are amenorrheic due to excessive physical or nutritional stress (eating disorder or malnutrition). In primary amenorrhea, examination for the stage of breast and pubic hair development (Tanner staging) can indicate whether there has been delay or disruption to the entire process of pubertal development. Restriction of later visual fields to examination by confrontation, the presence of galactorrhea, or evidence of recent scars or lesions in the region of the breast (such as zoster) can implicate hyperprolactinemia. The thyroid gland should be palpated and features of hypothyroidism sought. A lower abdominal mass may be due to pregnancy, hematocolpos or hematometra.

The gynecologic examination should be tailored to the patient. The external genitalia should be evaluated for pubic hair, acanthosis nigricans, and clitoral size. The hymen should be visualized; an imperforate hymen usually shows a bluish central bulge. Estrogenization of the tissues (presence of leukorrhea, thickened mucosa, or watery cervical mucus) can be assessed with speculum examination (choosing a speculum size appropriate to the sexual maturity of the patient). Visualization of the cervix in most circumstances is sufficient to rule out an outflow compartment problem.

INVESTIGATIONS

Initial Investigations

Initial investigation for any patient with amenorrhea or oligomenorrhea includes follicle-stimulating hormone (FSH), prolactin (PRL), thyroid stimulating hormone (TSH), and a sensitive pregnancy test if pregnancy is a possibility.

Ultrasonography can be helpful when an internal examination cannot be performed. When a congenital anomaly is considered, magnetic resonance imaging (MRI) can provide more definitive information.

Follow-up Investigations

A low normal FSH in the presence of a normal outflow tract should elicit a more detailed search for hypothalamic disruptors (such as nutritional, physical, or psychological stress). In a patient who has low FSH in conjunction with an elevated PRL and who is not taking medications known to increase PRL and whose TSH is normal, lesions of the hypothalamus or pituitary should be excluded with CT or MRI.

An elevated FSH indicates ovarian failure and should elicit a search for possible explanations such as past surgery, exposure to radiation or chemotherapy, or genetic causes. With an elevated FSH, a karyotype is usually indicated unless there is some obvious cause for loss of ovarian function. If the karyotype reveals any Y chromosome material, then, at the appropriate age, referral to a gynecologist is necessary for counseling and gonadectomy to reduce the risk of gonadoblastoma and dysgerminoma.

Evidence of outflow tract obstruction on pelvic examination or the possibility of cervical stenosis (cyclic dysmenorrhea without bleeding after a cervical surgical procedure such as a loop excision, cone biopsy, or trachelectomy) or Asherman's syndrome (obliteration of the endometrial cavity following a postpregnancy or postabortion dilation and curettage) merits referral to a gynecologist for further assessment and management.

Secondary amenorrhea related to weight gain or obesity, particularly when associated with features of acne and hirsutism, suggests the polycystic ovary syndrome. Management depends on whether the patient is seeking menstrual cycle regulation and relief from hirsutism (cyclic progestational therapy or an oral contraceptive plus an anti-androgen) or pregnancy (weight loss and fertility medication such as clomiphene citrate [Clomid]).

REFERENCES

Rebar RW. Evaluation of amenorrhea, anovulation and abnormal bleeding. March 26, 2006. Available at http://endotext.org/female/female4/female-frame4.htm [accessed June 15, 2007].

Reid RL. Amenorrhea. In: Copeland L, Jarrell J, McGregor J, editors. Textbook of Gynecology. 2nd ed. Philadelphia: WB Saunders; 1997. p. 365–90.

Reindollar R, Lalwani S. Abnormalities of female pubertal development. November 21, 2002. Available at http://endotext.org/female/female2/femaleframe2.htm [accessed June 15, 2007].

Dysmenorrhea

Method of
David R. Harnisch, Sr., MD

Dysmenorrhea, which is difficult and painful menstruation, is the most common gynecologic problem in menstruating women. It is divided into primary and secondary forms. *Primary dysmenorrhea* is dysmenorrhea due to a functional disturbance and not to inflammation, new growths, or anatomic factors. It may be referred to as intrinsic, functional, or essential. *Secondary dysmenorrhea* results from inflammation, infection, tumor, or anatomic factors. Primary dysmenorrhea is so common as to be normative, and in some published studies, it has been prevalent in 90% of the studied population. It becomes significant when it leads to loss of pleasure or diminishment in functional capacity. At worst, it can lead to significant absenteeism from school, work, or other social obligations or activities.

Primary Dysmenorrhea

Primary dysmenorrhea, or a painful cramping sensation in the lower abdomen, may be accompanied by a variety of other symptoms, including nausea, vomiting, headaches, malaise, dizziness, sweating, fatigue, bowel changes, and anxiety associated with the anticipation and experience of the pain. These symptoms occur just before the onset of menses and usually resolve within 48 to 72 hours.

Primary dysmenorrhea usually begins within 6 to 12 months of menarche and is associated with the establishment of ovulatory cycles. It has a greater prevalence in adolescence, with some easing of symptoms in adulthood and often a significant decrease in prevalence after childbirth.

The primary mechanism of the pain of primary dysmenorrhea is thought to be a prostaglandin-mediated event. Prostaglandins are produced during the secretory phase of the cycle, leading to uterine contractions and vasoconstriction with an associated degree of uterine ischemia. Vasopressin and leukotrienes may also play a role in generating the symptoms of primary dysmenorrhea and may ultimately lead to some novel therapies.

Significant risk factors for developing dysmenorrhea include tobacco use, heavy menses, depression or anxiety, attempts at weight loss, age younger than 20 years, and disruption of a patient's social supports. If the standard treatment measures instituted for the management of primary dysmenorrhea are successful in relieving the symptoms, the diagnostic evaluation may end there. If the symptoms do not resolve simply, secondary causes should be investigated.

DIAGNOSIS

The initial approach to the diagnosis and ultimately to treatment is a thorough history. Patients with a classic history of onset of pain with regard to menarche and timing of pain with regard to the menstrual flow and an otherwise noncontributory review or systems and past

CURRENT DIAGNOSIS

- Painful cramping sensation in the lower abdomen
- Occurs just before or during the menses and lasts 1 to 3 days
- Usually unaccompanied by other pathologic pelvic conditions

medical history may not need an extensive physical examination or laboratory testing. This is especially significant for the young, virginal patient because a complete gynecologic examination may be extremely disconcerting to her. Because pain is often a symptom found in young girls, parental assistance in obtaining the history may be necessary. One of the risk factors is a positive family history of primary dysmenorrhea. If the history deviates from the classic script of primary dysmenorrhea, a more detailed evaluation of the patient may be necessary before starting a trial of therapy.

TREATMENT

Treatment for primary dysmenorrhea involves patient education and reassurance and the use of antiprostaglandins in the form of non-steroidal antiinflammatory drugs (NSAIDs). Many young women have already begun self-treatment with NSAIDs before visiting the physician, but it is the provider's responsibility to ensure that adequate appropriate treatment regimens are instituted and followed.

Although research has been done implicating many different NSAIDs as possible treatment agents, starting with mefenamic acid (Ponstel), experience shows that any of the NSAIDs may be effective in the treatment of primary dysmenorrhea. However, some patients may find that they respond better to a nonsteroidal drug of a different class. The key to successful institution of therapy is to get therapy started before the typical symptoms of dysmenorrhea begin. Therapy is less successful after dysmenorrhea has begun. Table 1 lists some of the NSAIDs for the treatment of dysmenorrhea and their effective dosage ranges. This is not an inclusive listing, but representatives of each of the six classes of NSAIDs are listed. Notice that aspirin typically is not used because it is not potent enough in the standard dosage.

Effectiveness varies for drugs within each class. Therapy should be tailored to the individual. If a patient does not respond to one of the classes of NSAIDs, an agent from another class should be substituted and trialed. As a group, NSAIDs are 65% to 100% effective in treating the symptoms of dysmenorrhea.

Although NSAIDs are the mainstay of treatment, have a relatively low cost, and can be used on an intermittent basis with ease, some patients may be candidates for or desire to use other therapies, especially if the NSAID trials are ineffective. Alternate therapies may include oral contraceptive pills or injectable contraceptives if the patient has no contraindication to them. Decreased ovulation and thinning of the endometrial lining of the uterus may result in a decrease in endometrial volume, along with a decrease in prostaglandin levels. These hormonal options may be more effective when used in combination with NSAIDs. Alternate therapies are listed in Table 2.

TABLE 1 Nonsteroidal Antiinflammatory Drugs for the Treatment of Dysmenorrhea

Drug Class	Medication Name	Typical Dosages	Maximum Dosages
Propionate	Ibuprofen (Motrin, Advil)	400–800 q4–6h	2400 mg/d
Propionate	Naproxen (Naprosyn)	500 mg first dose, then 250 mg q6–8h prn	1250 mg/d
Acetic acid	Indomethacin (Indocin)[1]	25–50 mg PO tid	150 mg
Fenamate	Mefenamic acid (Ponstel)	500 mg first dose, then 250 mg q6h	For 3 days
Oxicam	Piroxicam (Feldene)[1]	20 mg qd	20 mg/d
Cyclooxygenase type 2 (COX-2) inhibitor	Celecoxib (Celebrex)	400 mg load, then 200 mg bid; may take additional 200 mg on day 1	Varies
Salicylate	Aspirin[1]	325–650 mg q4–6h	4 g/d

TABLE 2 Potential Therapeutic Options for Dysmenorrhea

Type of Interaction	Therapy
Surgical	Presacral neurectomy, laparoscopic uterosacral nerve ablation, oophorectomy, hysterectomy
Electrical	Transcutaneous electrical nerve stimulation (TENS)
Manual	Acupuncture, acupressure, heat-producing patches
Complementary and alternative	Omega-3 fatty acids,[1,7] exercise, Toki-shakuyaku-san[1,7]
Traditional medications	Transdermal nitroglycerin (NitroDur),[1] thiamine,[1] magnesium supplements,[1] vitamin E,[1] terbutaline (Brethine),[1] nifedipine (Procardia),[1] danazol (Danocrine),[1] leuprolide (Lupron),[1] levonorgestrel-releasing intrauterine device (Mirena),[1] glyceryl trinitrate (nitroglycerin),[1] selective serotonin reuptake inhibitors[1]

[1]Not FDA approved for this indication.
[7]Available as a dietary supplement.

CURRENT THERAPY

- Nonsteroidal antiinflammatory drugs
- Hormonal modalities
- Complementary and alternative medicines

Secondary Dysmenorrhea

Dysmenorrhea that does not resolve with NSAIDs or hormonal agents or that a comprehensive evaluation links to inflammation, infection, tumor, or anatomic factors is referred to as secondary dysmenorrhea. Causes include endometriosis, cervical stenosis, pelvic inflammatory disease, ovarian cysts, imperforate hymen, congenital obstruction of the vaginal outflow tract, adenomyosis, endometrial polyps, pelvic congestion, intrauterine devices, fibroids, and pelvic adhesions.

Characteristics that may point to a diagnosis of secondary dysmenorrhea include dysmenorrhea beginning during the first one or two cycles after menarche, pain that begins after age 25, later onset after a history of painless menstruation, any pelvic abnormality identified on the physical examination, infertility, heavy menstrual flow or irregular cycles, nulliparity, depression, and dyspareunia.

Some nongynecologic entities can manifest with or mimic dysmenorrhea. A partial list includes irritable bowel syndrome, psychogenic disorders, interstitial cystitis, inflammatory bowel syndrome, conditioned behavior, stress, and tension.

If primary treatments fail to relieve symptoms, a more extensive work-up is indicated. It can encompass a complete physical examination, including a complete gynecologic rectovaginal examination and cytologic and microbiologic testing. Pelvic ultrasound or computed tomography may be used for the evaluation, and the patient may be referred for laparoscopy or sonohysterography. Magnetic resonance imaging can be done, but it is less sensitive than other modalities, especially in the diagnosis of endometriosis. In the evaluation for secondary dysmenorrhea, it is important to rule out causes such as tumors or cysts. If the history or physical examination findings suggest further evaluation, cystoscopy or colonoscopy may be in order.

REFERENCES

American College of Obstetricians and Gynecologists (ACOG). Practice Bulletin Number 51: Chronic Pelvic Pain. Washington, DC: ACOG; 2004.
Coco AS. Primary dysmenorrhea. Am Fam Physician 1999;60:489–96.
Edmundson LD. Dysmenorrhea. Available at http://www.emedicine.com/emerg/topic156.htm [accessed July 2009].
French L. Dysmenorrhea. Am Fam Physician 2005;71:285–91, 292.
Smith RP, Kaunitz AM. Pathogenesis, clinical manifestations, and diagnosis of primary dysmenorrhea in adult women. Available at http://www.uptodate.com/online/index.do [accessed September 2008].
Smith RP, Kaunitz AM, et al. Treatment of primary dysmenorrhea in adult women. Available at http://www.uptodate.com/online/index.do [accessed September 2008].
Stenchever A. Primary and secondary dysmenorrhea and premenstrual syndrome. In: Stenchever A, Droegemueller W, Herbst AL, Mishell DR, editors. Comprehensive Gynecology. 4th ed. St Louis: Mosby; 2001. p. 1065–70.
Wellberry C. Diagnosis and treatment of endometriosis. Am Fam Physician 1999;60:1753–68.

Premenstrual Syndrome

Method of
Ellen W. Freeman, PhD

The premenstrual syndromes (PMS) are characterized by mood, behavioral, and physical symptoms that occur from several days to 2 weeks before menses and remit with the menstrual flow. The term *PMS* as used by clinicians and the general public is generic, imprecise, and commonly applied to numerous symptoms. Included symptoms range from the mild and normal physiologic changes of the menstrual cycle to clinically significant symptoms that limit or impair normal functioning. In recent years, randomized controlled trials and other well-designed studies have defined diagnostic criteria for PMS and identified effective treatments for this disorder.

Based on scientific evidence at this time, serotonergic antidepressants are considered the primary treatment for clinically significant PMS, and particularly its severe form termed premenstrual dysphoric disorder (PMDD). This review focuses on PMS and its treatment with serotonergic antidepressants. It is not a comprehensive review of all treatments or associated literature. Other recent reviews may guide the reader to further information and other treatments for PMS and PMDD.

Symptoms

Numerous symptoms were traditionally attributed to PMS. This plethora is related in part to the absence of a clear diagnosis that distinguishes PMS from other co-morbid conditions. Many disorders, both physical and psychiatric, are exacerbated premenstrually or occur as a co-morbid disorder with PMS. When a careful diagnosis is made to distinguish PMS from other conditions, a much smaller group of symptoms appear to be typical of the disorder (Box 1).

Mood symptoms are usually the main complaint (irritability, anxiety, tension, mood swings, feeling out of control, depression), but behavioral symptoms (e.g., decreased interest, fatigue, poor concentration, poor sleep) and physical symptoms, most commonly breast tenderness and abdominal swelling, are also present. Several recent

BOX 1   Symptoms of Premenstrual Syndrome

Affective
• Irritability
• Anxiety
• Angry outbursts
• Confusion
• Social withdrawal
• Depression
Somatic
• Bloating
• Swelling
• Breast tenderness
• Headache

From American College of Obstetricians and Gynecologists (ACOG) Practice Bulletin 15, 2001.

BOX 2   Diagnosis of Premenstrual Syndrome

Presenting symptoms:
• Consistent with premenstrual syndrome
• Restricted to the luteal phase
• Cause impairment or distress
• Not an exacerbation of another disorder
• Confirmed by 2 cycles of daily symptom rating

From American College of Obstetricians and Gynecologists (ACOG) Practice Bulletin 15, 2001.

studies suggest that irritability is the cardinal symptom of PMS. Although depressive symptoms such as low mood, fatigue, sleep difficulties, and poor concentration are frequent complaints of women with PMS, the growing evidence indicates that PMS is not a simple variant of depression but has distinct mechanisms that differ from those of depressive disorders.

Prevalence

Surveys indicate that PMS is among the most common health problems reported by reproductive-age women. Current estimates from epidemiologic data indicate that approximately 25% of women experience severe and clinically significant premenstrual symptoms, although only 6% to 8% of menstruating women meet the stringent and predominantly dysphoric criteria for PMDD.

Morbidity

The morbidity of PMS is related to its severity, chronicity, and resulting distress that affect work, personal relationships, or daily activities. The level of impairment is significantly above community norms and similar to that of other health problems such as major depressive disorder. Studies consistently demonstrate that the greatest impairment or distress resulting from PMS is in relationships with the partner or children and in the effectiveness of work.

Etiology

The etiology of PMS remains undefined, although the monthly cycling of the reproductive hormones appears to have an essential role in the disorder. While circulating levels of the hormones are in normal range, the dominant theory is that some women have an underlying vulnerability to the normal fluctuations of one or more of these hormones. It is further believed that PMS involves central nervous system–mediated interactions of the reproductive steroids with neurotransmitters. The principal research evidence at this time supports the involvement of reproductive hormones, serotonergic dysregulation, and possibly dysregulation of GABAergic receptor functioning.

Diagnosis

A diagnosis of PMS is determined primarily by the *timing* and the *severity* of the symptoms. These factors, together with an assessment of whether other physical or psychiatric disorders may account for the symptoms, are more important for the diagnosis than the particular symptoms, which are typically nonspecific and must be assessed for their relationship to the menstrual cycle.

Box 2 lists the diagnostic criteria for PMS presented by the American College of Obstetricians and Gynecologists in 2000. These criteria indicate that PMS symptoms must be experienced during the 5 days before menses and abate during the menstrual flow. The symptoms should cause identifiable impairment or distress, be confirmed by prospective reports recorded daily by the woman for at least two menstrual cycles, and not be accounted for by other disorders.

The diagnostic criteria for premenstrual dysphoric disorder (PMDD) are listed in the *Diagnostic and Statistical Manual of Mental Disorders,* Fourth Edition (*DSM-IV*). Importantly, the Food and Drug Administration (FDA) has approved medications only for the indication of PMDD and not for the indication of PMS at the present time. The PMDD criteria are intended to diagnose a severe, dysphoric form of PMS and require 5 of 11 listed symptoms including at least one of the mood symptoms. Physical symptoms, regardless of the number, are considered a single symptom in meeting the diagnostic criteria. The 11 PMDD symptoms are depressed mood, anxiety or tension, mood swings, anger or irritability, decreased interest, concentration difficulties, fatigue, appetite change or food cravings, sleep disturbance, feeling overwhelmed, and physical symptoms. At least five of these symptoms must each be severe premenstrually and abate with the menstrual flow. The symptoms must markedly interfere with functioning, be confirmed by daily symptom reports for at least two menstrual cycles, and not be an exacerbation of another physical or mental disorder.

CURRENT DIAGNOSIS

■ Confirm that symptoms occur premenstrually and abate following menses.
■ Confirm that symptoms are clinically significant and impair daily activities and/or cause problems for the woman.
■ Obtain a medical history and conduct a physical examination to determine that other disorders are not causing the symptoms.
■ Query depression, stress, substance abuse, and other diagnoses that could cause the symptoms.
■ Ask the woman to maintain a daily symptom report for two or more menstrual cycles to confirm the reported symptoms and their relation to the menstrual cycle.
■ Perform laboratory tests only as needed to confirm general good health or rule out other suspected conditions.

To diagnose PMS, a medical history should be obtained and a complete physical with gynecologic examination performed. PMS is understood to occur in ovulatory menstrual cycles; cycles that are irregular or outside the normal range are an indication for further gynecologic investigation. Co-morbid conditions such as dysmenorrhea, endometriosis, uterine fibroids, pelvic inflammatory disease, thyroid disorders, migraine, diabetes, mood disorders, substance abuse, and numerous other possibilities should be identified. It may be difficult to determine whether the symptoms under investigation are an exacerbation of a co-morbid condition or superimposed on another condition. In either case, the usual recommendation is to treat the ongoing condition first, then reassess and possibly add treatment for the symptoms that arise premenstrually.

No laboratory test identifies PMS and none should be routinely performed for diagnosis. Laboratory tests that indicate or confirm other possible disorders are useful if suggested by the individual woman's symptom presentation or medical findings.

The key diagnostic tool for evaluating premenstrual symptoms is the daily symptom report. The diagnostic criteria for both PMS and PMDD include a daily symptom report that is kept by the woman for at least two menstrual cycles to confirm that the woman's reported symptoms are linked to the menstrual cycle in the requisite pattern. Numerous symptom reports appropriate for this diagnosis are identified in the medical literature on PMS and PMDD. It is important that the ratings indicate the severity of each symptom (and not simply check the presence or absence of symptoms).

It is informative to use two visits for the diagnostic evaluation. Although counterintuitive, seeing the patient following menses when PMS symptoms have abated is instructive. If symptoms are absent, it provides strong evidence for the diagnosis. If symptoms are present in the follicular phase, the type and severity of the symptoms are important diagnostic information for identifying other physical or mental disorders that may be the primary focus of treatment.

Treatment

SELECTIVE SEROTONIN REUPTAKE INHIBITORS

Serotonergic antidepressants are the primary treatment for severe PMS and PMDD at this time. Modulating serotonergic function is consistent with a leading theoretical view that the normal gonadal steroid fluctuations of the menstrual cycle are associated with an abnormal serotonergic response in vulnerable women. A meta-analysis of randomized controlled trials of selective serotonin reuptake inhibitors (SSRIs) in treatment of PMS and PMDD determined that these drugs were an effective first-line therapy, with both a statistically significant and clinically meaningful difference from placebo. The FDA has approved fluoxetine (Sarafem), sertraline (Zoloft), and paroxetine (Paxil) for the indication of PMDD. Other randomized, placebo-controlled, double-blind trials showed efficacy for citalopram (Celexa[1]), venlafaxine (Effexor[1]) (a selective serotonin-norepinephrine reuptake inhibitor [SNRI]), and clomipramine (Anafranil[1]) (a tricyclic antidepressant) for treatment of PMS and PMDD.

Effective doses of SSRIs are consistently at the low end of the dose range for depressive disorders in all reports of PMS and PMDD treatments. Significant response is often seen in the first menstrual cycle of treatment, with smaller increments with or without dose adjustments in the second and third treatment cycles. If there is not sufficient response in the first treated menstrual cycle, the dose should be increased in the next cycle unless precluded by side effects.

Side effects are common with the initiation of an SSRI but are usually transient and abate within 1 to 2 weeks of continued treatment. The most common side effects include headache, nausea, insomnia, fatigue or lethargy, diarrhea, decreased concentration, dizziness, and decreased libido or delayed orgasm. The sexual side effects of SSRIs have received considerable attention, although it is often difficult to determine the extent to which sexual effects are related to the

SSRI	Range Studied (mg)	Mean Dose (mg/d)
Citalopram (Celexa[1])	10–30	20
Escitalopram (Lexapro[1])	10–20	15
Fluoxetine (Prozac,[1] Sarafem*)	10–60	20
Paroxetine (Paxil[1])	10–30	20
Paroxetine-CR* (Paxil-CR)	12.5, 25	NA[†]
Sertraline (Zoloft*)	50–150	75
SNRI		
Venlafaxine (Effexor[1])	37.5–200	112.5

[1]Not FDA approved for this indication.
*FDA approved for the indication of premenstrual dysphoric disorder (PMDD).
[†]Not applicable because of fixed-dose study.

medication or to preexisting conditions. The incidence of decreased sexual interest or delayed orgasm in the few published reports of PMS patients is approximately 9% to 16%, which is notably lower than the rates reported with the use of SSRIs by depressed patients. Another important issue is the lack of any well-controlled clinical trials of SSRI treatment for PMS and PMDD in adolescents. Whether SSRIs are safe and effective for this indication in women younger than 18 years is not demonstrated.

Luteal Phase Dosing

The use of medication only in the symptomatic luteal phase of the menstrual cycle is particularly important in PMS because of the cyclic pattern of the symptoms, which occur only in the premenstrual phase and abate following menses. Efficacy of luteal phase administration of the SSRIs is demonstrated in multiple trials: three large multicenter, randomized, placebo-controlled trials that examined fluoxetine (Sarafem), paroxetine (Paxil), and sertraline (Zoloft); a trial that directly compared continuous and luteal phase administration of sertraline; and multiple preliminary studies.

Luteal phase administration of an SSRI is typically initiated 14 days prior to the expected onset of menstrual bleeding and concluded within several days of bleeding, using a taper for increased doses. As with continuous dosing, the SSRI doses are usually at the low end of the dose range.

One preliminary study compared symptom-onset dosing (mean of 6 days before menses) to luteal phase dosing and found no difference between the two dosing regimens in improvement overall, although there was suggestion that women with more severe symptoms may respond better to full luteal phase dosing.

Side effects may be less frequent with an intermittent dosing regimen because they may not occur when not taking the medication. However, some women experience recurring side effects when dosing is resumed, and discontinuation symptoms might also occur with the stop-start dosing pattern. At this time, no systematic data confirm discontinuation symptoms with the intermittent dosing regimen.

Insufficient Response to Selective Serotonin Reuptake Inhibitors

Approximately 60% of PMS and PMDD patients in controlled studies respond well to an SSRI. There are no clear predictors of response. An adequate trial of an SSRI for PMS and PMDD is at least two menstrual cycles at a dose level of demonstrated efficacy, with a third cycle when there is partial response. If a woman has an insufficient response or unacceptable side effects, it is reasonable to try another SSRI. Although the SSRIs are similar in their structure and have similar response rates and side-effect profiles, an individual patient may respond better to one SSRI versus another.

[1]Not FDA approved for this indication.

Other approaches to a poor treatment response include augmenting the SSRI with another medication to address the nonresponding symptoms, but there is no systematic information on this in PMS or PMDD treatment. Switching to another class of medication, such as anxiolytics, is suggested, but no data indicate whether nonresponders to SSRIs will respond to another class of medication. Nonresponse may also be related to other co-morbid disorders. A thorough review of the diagnosis and adjustments of the premenstrual doses of medication for both the primary disorder and PMS should be considered before pursuing other treatments.

OTHER TREATMENTS

Hormonal

In spite of the evidence for hormonal involvement in PMS and PMDD, traditional oral contraceptives (OCs) do not show efficacy for the disorder. However, recent data indicate that shortening or omitting the placebo week in the traditional OC pill pack may effectively treat PMS and PMDD. The FDA has approved the oral contraceptive YAZ, a 24/4-day combination pill, to treat PMDD.

Gonadotropin-releasing hormone (GnRH) agonists such as depot leuprolide[1] (Lupron) and buserelin[2] (Suprefact) are effective for PMS and PMDD but are of limited usefulness because of the risks associated with low estrogen levels that result from these treatments. Although add-back therapy using low-lose estrogen and progesterone together with the GnRH agonist did not appear to reduce efficacy in a meta-analysis, there are no definitive data on the safety and efficacy of this approach in long-term treatment. The historic use of progesterone has failed to show efficacy for the mood and behavioral symptoms of PMS in numerous controlled trials.

Anxiolytics

Alprazolam[1] (Xanax) and buspirone[1] (Buspar) showed modest efficacy for PMS in some studies but not others. Although these medications offer an alternative to antidepressants, the response rates appear much lower, and it is not known whether a PMS patient who does not respond to antidepressants will respond to an anxiolytic. The risk of dependency with alprazolam should be considered. Dosing should be strictly limited to the luteal phase, and the patient should have no history of substance abuse.

Nonpharmacologic

Calcium supplementation[1] (600 mg twice daily) reduced PMS symptoms significantly more than placebo. Calcium offers a dietary supplement approach that may be beneficial for some women with PMS, although there are no predictors of which women will respond well to this therapy. Other complementary and alternative therapies may be helpful for some women, but there is no convincing evidence of their efficacy for PMS.

Behavioral treatments that facilitate coping or reduce stress may reduce PMS symptoms. Cognitive-behavioral therapy is effective for PMS, and in one study it was as effective as the SSRI fluoxetine after 6 months of treatment.

TREATMENT DURATION

All published studies of treatment efficacy for PMS and PMDD are based on acute treatment of 2 to 3 months' duration. Several small pilot investigations suggest that PMS symptoms are likely to return within several months after medication is stopped. It also appears that PMS symptoms do not resolve spontaneously but continue for many years. These observations of PMS as a chronic condition and the swift return of symptoms following the cessation of medication suggest that treatment can be expected to be long term; notably, there are no data from long-term maintenance studies at this time.

The SSRIs are currently the first-line treatment for severe PMS and PMDD. Continuous dosing and luteal phase dosing regimens

[1]Not FDA approved for this indication.
[2]Not available in the United States.

are similarly effective for these disorders when the symptoms are clearly limited to the luteal phase of the menstrual cycle. Hormonal treatments have lacked consistent scientific evidence of their efficacy or safety or both for PMS treatment. Several new oral contraceptives that decrease or omit the placebo interval may provide an effective alternative to antidepressant medications. Preliminary evidence indicates that long-term maintenance of the medication may be required for PMS and PMDD, but currently, there are no studies of the effectiveness, costs, and benefits of long-term treatment.

REFERENCES

ACOG Practice Bulletin. Premenstrual syndrome. Int J Gynecol Obstet 2001;73(2):183–90.

Dell DL. Premenstrual syndrome, premenstrual dysphoric disorder, and premenstrual exacerbation of another disorder. Clin Obstet Gynecol 2004;47 (3):568–75.

Dimmock PW, Wyatt KM, Jones PW, O'Brien PM. Efficacy of selective serotonin-reuptake inhibitors in premenstrual syndrome: A systematic review. Lancet 2000;356(9236):1131–6.

Freeman EW. Luteal phase administration of agents for the treatment of premenstrual dysphoric disorder. CNS Drugs 2004;18(7):453–68.

Girman A, Lee R, Kligler B. An integrative medicine approach to premenstrual syndrome. Am J Obstet Gynecol 2003;188(5 Suppl.):S56–65.

Grady-Weliky TA. Premenstrual dysphoric disorder. N Engl J Med 2003;348 (5):433–8.

Halbreich U. The etiology, biology, and evolving pathology of premenstrual syndromes. Psychoneuroendocrinology 2003;28(Suppl. 3):55–99.

Johnson SR. Premenstrual syndrome, premenstrual dysphoric disorder, and beyond: A clinical primer for practitioners. Obstet Gynecol 2004;104 (4):845–59.

Stevinson C, Ernst E. Complementary/alternative therapies for premenstrual syndrome: A systematic review of randomized controlled trials. Am J Obstet Gynecol 2001;185(1):227–35.

Menopause

Method of
Irina Burd, MD, PhD, Stacey A. Scheib, MD, and Krystene I. Boyle, MD

Menopause is the physiologic process characterized by a marked decrease in the number of oocytes, subsequent follicular depletion, decreased ovarian estrogen secretion, and finally cessation of menses. For 95% of women, menopause occurs between the ages of 45 and 55, with a mean age of 51. Time of menopause is influenced by genetic as well as environmental factors (Box 1). Menopause before age 40 years is considered premature ovarian failure.

Diagnosis

Menopause is defined clinically as 12 months of amenorrhea following the last menstrual period in the absence of other causes. The Staging of Reproductive Aging Workshop (STRAW) has provided a beneficial staging system to help categorize patients (Box 2).

The differential diagnosis for menopause includes thyroid disease, pregnancy, hyperprolactinemia, medications, carcinoid, pheochromocytoma, or underlying malignancy, which are important in considering the diagnosis algorithm (Box 3). Follicle-stimulating hormone (FSH) and estradiol are commonly measured to diagnose menopause and are often misleading because they can fluctuate vastly in the perimenopausal period.

BOX 1 Factors That Influence the Timing of Menopause

- Alcohol abuse
- Chemotherapy
- Cigarette smoking
- Contraception
- Family history of early menopause
- Galactose consumption
- Obesity
- Parity
- History of pelvic irradiation
- Physiologic and psychological stresses (e.g., living at high altitudes, depression)
- Race
- Shorter cycle length during adolescence
- Type 1 diabetes mellitus

BOX 2 STRAW Staging System

- Perimenopause
  - Stage −2 (early): Variable cycle length (>7 days from normal cycle)
  - Stage −1 (late): ≥2 skipped cycles and amenorrhea interval ≥60 days
- Menopause
  - Stage +1 (early): First 5 years after final menstrual period
  - Stage +2 (late): 5 years after final menstrual period until death

Abbreviation: STRAW = Stages of Reproductive Aging Workshop.

BOX 3 Algorithm for the Diagnosis of Menopause

Older than 45 years
- No symptoms suggestive of hyperthyroidism: No further diagnostic evaluation
- With symptoms suggestive of hyperthyroidism: Check serum TSH, T3, free T4

Younger than 45 years
- Oligomenorrhea or amenorrhea work-up: Check serum hCG, prolactin, TSH, FSH

Younger than 40 years
- Complete evaluation for premature ovarian failure

Abbreviations: FSH = follicle-stimulating hormone; hCG = human chorionic gonadotropin; T3 = triiodothyronine; T4 = thyroxine; TSH = thyroid-stimulating hormone.

Systemic Manifestations of Menopause

VASOMOTOR SYMPTOMS

Hot flushes are the most common symptom associated with menopause. They are self-limited sensations of generalized heat that last 2 to 4 minutes and vary widely among people and across cultures. Without treatment, they resolve within 1 to 5 years.

CURRENT DIAGNOSIS

- For women older than 45 years who have menopausal symptoms, no further work-up is necessary unless there are symptoms of hyperthyroidism.
- For women younger than 45 years, proceed with an oligomenorrhea or amenorrhea work-up: Check serum hCG, prolactin, TSH, and FSH.
- Women younger than 40 years should have a complete evaluation for premature ovarian failure.
- Common symptoms of menopause include abnormal bleeding, hot flushes, genitourinary complaints, sleep disturbances, mood disturbances, joint pain, and difficulty concentrating.
- FSH and estradiol levels can be misleading and so should not be used to make the diagnosis.

Abbreviations: FSH = follicle-stimulating hormone; hCG = human chorionic gonadotropin; TSH = thyroid-stimulating hormone.

SLEEP DISTURBANCES

Sleep disturbances often occur in menopause as a result of hot flushes arousing the woman from sleep. When the hot flushes are treated, sleep usually improves. Persistent sleep disturbances can lead to more serious symptoms such as difficulty concentrating, fatigue, mood disturbances, depression, and other psychological symptoms.

GENITOURINARY SYMPTOMS

Estrogen deficiency leads to atrophy of the urethral and vaginal epithelium. Vaginal atrophy can result in vaginal dryness, itching, irritation, and dyspareunia. The pH in the vagina also increases and, with vaginal atrophy, can lead to recurrent vaginal infections. Decreasing elasticity of the vaginal wall elasticity can result in a shorter and narrower vagina, especially without continued sexual activity. The lack of estrogen affects blood flow to the vagina and vulva, which in turn causes decreased lubrication and neuropathy. These are both reversible with estrogen replacement therapy, especially vaginal therapy.

Incontinence incidence increases with age but has not been clearly associated with menopause. The theory is that atrophy of the urethral epithelium results in diminished urethral mucosal seal, loss of compliance, and irritation. These are believed to contribute to stress and urge incontinence. These patients also report recurrent urinary tract infections; this is probably related to the increase in vaginal pH.

ABNORMAL BLEEDING

Even though most postmenopausal bleeding is due to atrophy, during the perimenopausal period the endometrium may be exposed to unopposed estrogen that can result in anovulatory bleeding or endometrial hyperplasia. If this occurs, endometrial biopsy is needed to rule out endometrial hyperplasia or cancer. A transvaginal ultrasound can also be used as a screening tool first and then be followed by an endometrial biopsy if the endometrial thickness is greater than 4 mm.

MOOD DISTURBANCES

In the Study of Women's Health Across the Nation (SWAN), higher risks of mood symptoms were found in perimenopausal women. The strongest risks of depression associated with menopause are a prior history of depression and premenstrual syndrome. Depression might not be entirely related to the physiology of menopause but may be a result of stressors concomitantly occurring around the time of menopause, such as children leaving home, dealing with aged parents, and midlife adjustment.

BOX 4 Risk Factors for Osteoporosis

Modifiable Risk Factors
- Chronic corticosteroid use
- Cigarette smoking
- Early menopause (before age 45 years)
- High alcohol intake
- High caffeine intake
- Low body weight (<127 pounds)
- Low dietary calcium intake
- Low vitamin D intake
- Premenopausal amenorrhea (>1 y)
- Sedentary lifestyle

Nonmodifiable Risk Factors
- Dementia
- Family history of osteoporosis
- Poor general health
- White or Asian ethnicity

MENSTRUAL MIGRAINES

Menstrual migraines are believed to be related to decreased estrogen levels around the time of menses. Because menopause is related to a decrease in estrogen, menstrual migraines can increase in intensity and frequency.

BALANCE AND OSTEOPOROSIS

Estrogen deficiency can have an effect on the central nervous system by impairing balance. Along with osteoporosis, loss of balance remains one of the big causes of fractures in menopausal women. There are multiple risk factors for osteoporosis, modifiable and non-modifiable (Box 4).

OTHER EFFECTS

Other long-term issues that are believed to be related to menopause include cardiovascular disease and dementia.

Treatment

HORMONE REPLACEMENT THERAPY

Until relatively recently, long-term estrogen and combined estrogen and progestin therapy was routinely given to postmenopausal women. Hormone replacement therapy (HRT) was believed to prevent cardiovascular disease and osteoporosis. The Women's Health Initiative (WHI) was a set of clinical trials, whose results were first published in 2002, that resulted in a dramatic change in clinical practice. The study was designed to see if there was a decrease in cardiovascular risk with conjugated equine estrogen (CEE [Premarin]) in patients without a uterus or in combination with medroxyprogesterone acetate (MPA [Provera]). The CEE-MPA (Prempro) arm of the trial was stopped early after 5 years because of the increased risks for breast cancer, coronary heart disease (CHD) (29%), stroke (41%) and venous thromboembolism (VTE) (33%), even though there was a reduction in risk of hip and vertebral fractures and colon cancer. There was also an increased risk of stroke (39%) and VTE (33%) in the CEE-alone arm after 7-year follow-up, but there was no difference in heart disease.

The Heart and Estrogen/progestin Replacement Studies (HERS I and II trials) looked at secondary prevention in postmenopausal women with known CHD, which showed that there was not a reduction of CHD events with CEE-MPA. Both the WHI and HERS studies revealed an increase in the number of VTEs.

 CURRENT THERAPY

- CEE or 17-β estradiol plus MPA, as either continuous or cyclic short-term therapy lasting no more than 5 years is a first-line treatment for vasomotor symptoms in a patient with no contraindications.
- Locally active estrogen-containing compounds are available for treating urogenital symptoms.
- SERMs provide an alternative for treating menopausal symptoms, specifically osteoporosis. Raloxifene has less antiresorptive action than the bisphosphonates (e.g., alendronate) and should be given to patients who do not tolerate bisphosphonates.
- Alendronate increases BMD in the vertebral spine and femoral neck more than raloxifene, but patients taking both alendronate and raloxifene increased their BMD the most.
- More research is needed in the use of androgen replacement in menopause, although some evidence suggests that it might improve libido.

Abbreviations: BMD = bone mineral density; CEE = conjugated equine estrogen; MPA = medroxyprogesterone acetate; SERM = selective estrogen-receptor modulator.

In the WHI Memory Study (WHIMS), with CEE and CEE-MPA there was an increased risk of dementia compared with placebo, but this was in an older postmenopausal population. Epidemiologic studies indicate that estrogen may be neuroprotective if initiated earlier. Therefore, therapy should not initiated after age 65 years.

As a result of these studies and the recommendations of the North American Menopause Society, the only use for estrogen therapy, either alone or combined with progestin, is for control of menopausal symptoms, particularly hot flushes, vaginal dryness, urinary symptoms, joint pain, skin changes, and emotional lability. Studies are inconclusive whether CEE alone or CEE-MPA is beneficial for incontinence. Contraindications to estrogen therapy are a history of endometrial cancer, liver disease, breast cancer, CHD, history of VTE or stroke, or high risk of any of the above. In the Nurses' Health Study, an increased incidence of new onset of asthma that may be dose related and development of systemic lupus erythematosus might result from estrogen therapy.

The absolute risk of an adverse event is extremely low. For a 50-year-old woman on combined estrogen-progestin, estimated risk is 1:1000 at 1 year and 1:200 at 5 years. This absolute risk doubles for a 60 year-old woman. The goal of treatment is a short-term therapy, lasting no more than 5 years. Therapy should be tapered, decreasing by one pill every 1 or 2 weeks, so that there is no rebound in menopausal symptoms.

Progestin should be added to HRT for any woman with a uterus in order to prevent endometrial hyperplasia and cancer. The Postmenopausal Estrogen/Progestin Interventions (PEPI) trial showed a statistically significant reduction in the incidence of simple, complex, and atypical endometrial hyperplasia with CEE-MPA therapy compared with CEE alone. The only recommended progestin at this time is MPA 2.5 mg/day. Alternative progestin doses, less frequent administration, and alternative routes of administration have not been studied and thus might not be able to prevent endometrial hyperplasia or cancer; if these are used, closer endometrial surveillance is necessary.

Women with premature ovarian failure should be given hormonal therapy, and risks and benefits should be reassessed at age 50 years.

More research is needed the in use of androgen replacement in menopause, although some evidence suggests that it might improve libido.

Alternative therapy has been proposed for menopausal symptoms (Table 1 and Box 5).

TABLE 1 Treatment of Vasomotor Symptoms

Treatment	Suggested Dose	Possible Side Effects
Hormones		
CEE (Premarin) or 17-β estradiol, plus MPA (Provera), either continuous or cyclic	CEE 0.3 mg/d *or* Estradiol 0.5 mg PO qd *or* Estradiol 0.05 mg patch qd *plus* MPA 2.5 mg/d or for 12–14 d/mo	See text
MPA	20 mg/d[3] oral or 150 mg IM (Depo-Provera)[1] q3 mo	Mood disturbances, breast tenderness, alopecia
Megestrol acetate (Megace)[1]	20 mg bid	Vomiting, diarrhea, flatulence
Selective Serotonin Reuptake Inhibitors		
Paroxetine (Paxil, Paxil CR)[1]	10–20 mg/d or 12.5–25 mg CR/d	Fatigue, dry mouth, nausea, decreased libido
Fluoxetine (Prozac)[1]	20 mg/d	
Venlafaxine (Effexor, Effexor XR)[1]	37.5–75 mg XR/d	
Other Medications		
Gabapentin (Neurontin)[1]	300–900 mg/d	Dizziness, somnolence, peripheral edema
Clonidine (Catapres TTS)[1]	0.1 mg/24 h wk patch	Orthostatic hypotension, drowsiness
Dietary Supplements		
Vitamin E[1]	800 IU/d	Fatigue, weakness, diarrhea
Black cohosh[7]		Gastrointestinal complaints, dizziness
Evening primrose oil[7]		
Other Interventions		
Acupuncture or acupressure		
Exercise		
Lifestyle interventions (e.g., layered clothing, fans, air conditioners)		

[1]Not FDA approved for this indication.
[3]Exceeds dosage recommended by the manufacturer.
[7]Available as a dietary supplement.
Abbreviations: CEE = conjugated equine estrogen; MPA = medroxyprogesterone acetate.

BISPHOSPHONATES

Bisphosphonates impair osteoclastic bone resorption and are used to treat osteoporosis (Box 6). The most common side effects are bone pain and upper gastrointestinal disorders such as dysphagia, esophagitis, and esophageal or gastric ulcer. They are contraindicated in patients with renal impairment, uncorrected hypocalcemia, or sensitivity to the drug components. There have been no randomized, controlled studies comparing one type of bisphosphonate with another.

SELECTIVE ESTROGEN RECEPTOR MODULATORS

Selective estrogen receptor modulators (SERMs) provide an alternative for treating menopausal symptoms, specifically osteoporosis (Box 6). SERMs bind to the estrogen receptor, but they have tissue-specific properties. The two SERMs that have been studied the most are raloxifene (Evista) and tamoxifen (Nolvadex). Raloxifene's mechanism for tissue-specific activity is not fully clear. Tamoxifen probably works by variable gene expression in different cell types.

Raloxifene

Two major double-blinded, placebo-controlled trials, one in the United States and one in Europe, have looked at raloxifene versus placebo, measuring bone mineral density (BMD), markers of bone turnover, and serum lipid levels. In all treatment arms in both studies, BMD was significantly increased and serum concentrations of both total and low-density lipoprotein (LDL) cholesterol were significantly decreased compared with placebo. In both trials there was no difference in complaints of breast pain or vaginal bleeding and no difference in endometrial thickness.

In the longer-term Multiple Outcomes of Raloxifene Evaluation (MORE) study, there was a relative risk reduction in vertebral fractures but not for nonvertebral fractures. The risk of invasive, but not noninvasive, breast cancer appeared to decrease, most likely due to the antagonistic effect of raloxifene. There was no increase in endometrial cancer. The relative risk of thromboembolic disease was 3.1 compared with placebo, but it appears that the risk is less than that with tamoxifen. There was no difference in cardiovascular events, except there was a decrease in the subset of women at greatest risk.

BOX 5   Treatment of Urogenital Atrophy Symptoms

- Systemic estrogen therapy alone or combined with progestin
- Estrogen cream (Estrace Vaginal, Premarin Vaginal): 0.5–1 g biw-tiw
- Estradiol vaginal tablet (Vagifem): 1 tablet tiw
- Estrogen-containing vaginal ring (Estring): 1 ring inserted every 3 mo
- Lubricants with intercourse as needed

BOX 6   Treatments for Osteoporosis

Bisphosphonates
- Alendronate (Fosamax) 70 mg/wk or 70-mg oral solution weekly or 10 mg/d
- Risedronate (Actonel) 35 mg/wk
- Ibandronate (Boniva) 150 mg/mo or 3-mg injection once every 3 mo

Selective Estrogen-Receptor Modulators
- Raloxifene 60 mg/d

- Perform annual gynecologic examinations.
- Monitor for signs or symptoms of endometrial hyperplasia or cancer.
- Investigate any abnormal vaginal symptoms.
- Reassess use if atypical hyperplasia develops and proceed with appropriate gynecologic management.
- Discontinue tamoxifen after 5 years because benefit has not been demonstrated beyond 5 years of use.

Abbreviation: ACOG = American College of Obstetricians and Gynecologists.

In a study looking at osteoporosis in postmenopausal women, patients on alendronate (Fosamax) increased their BMD in the vertebral spine and femoral neck more than patients on raloxifene, but patients taking both medications increased their BMD the most. CEE had a better effect on BMD compared with raloxifene in hysterectomized postmenopausal women. Raloxifene has less antiresorptive action than the bisphosphonates (e.g., alendronate) and should be given to patients who do not tolerate bisphosphonates.

Raloxifene significantly increased the occurrence of hot flushes compared with placebo in all the studies. Other side effects of raloxifene noted were influenza-like symptoms, peripheral edema, and leg cramps. It does not appear to affect vaginal symptoms, urinary symptoms, gallbladder disease, cognitive decline, or cataracts.

The recommended starting dose is 60 mg/day.

Tamoxifen

Tamoxifen[1] has demonstrated some benefit for osteoporosis, but estrogen and bisphosphonates have shown a greater increase in lumbar spine BMD. In the National Surgical Adjuvant Breast and Bowel Project (NSABP) P-1 Trial, women on tamoxifen had fewer hip, wrist, and vertebral fractures at 7-year follow-up. In this study there was not a significant difference in the occurrence of cardiovascular events. Total and LDL cholesterol were significantly decreased on tamoxifen.

In combination with adjuvant therapy for estrogen receptor–positive breast cancer, tamoxifen can decrease the risk of recurrence and death and aid those with metastatic disease.

As with raloxifene, patients taking tamoxifen have a greater risk for VTE. This association is found particularly in patients who are concomitantly receiving chemotherapy.

The main difference between raloxifene and tamoxifen is that tamoxifen use is associated with a greater risk of endometrial cancers, especially uterine sarcoma. This risk depended on length of treatment. As a result, the American College of Obstetrics and Gynecologists (ACOG) has recommendations regarding monitoring women taking tamoxifen (Box 7), but these are not evidence based. For prevention, an intrauterine levonorgestrel could be placed. Even though there is evidence to suggest that tamoxifen is effictive in preventing and treating osteoporosis, it is not approved by the FDA except for the prevention and treatment of breast cancer.

REFERENCES

American College of Obstetricians and Gynecologists. Tamoxifen and endometrial cancer. ACOG Committee Opinion 232. Washington, DC: American College of Obstetricians and Gynecologists; 2000.

American College of Obstetricians and Gynecologists Task Force. Hormone Therapy. Obstet Gynecol 2004;104(Suppl. 4):S1–129.

Barnabei VM, Cochrane BB, Aragaki AK, et al. Menopausal symptoms and treatment-related effects of estrogen and progestin in the Women's Health Initiative. Obstet Gynecol 2005;105:1063–73.

Barrett-Connor E, Cauley JA, Kulkarni PM, et al. Risk-benefit profile for raloxifene: 4-Year data from the Multiple Outcomes of Raloxifene Evaluation (MORE) randomized trial. J Bone Miner Res 2004;19:1270–15.

Grady D, Herrington D, Bittner V, et al. Cardiovascular disease outcomes during 6.8 years of hormone therapy: Heart and Estrogen/Progestin Replacement Study follow-up (HERS-II). JAMA 2002;288:49–57.

Hulley S, Grady D, Bush T, et al. for the Heart and Estrogen/Progestin Replacement Study (HERS) Research Group. Randomized trial of estrogen plus progestin for secondary prevention of coronary heart disease in postmenopausal women. JAMA 1998;280:605–13.

North American Menopause Society. Treatment of menopause-associated vasomotor symptoms: Position statement of The North American Menopause Society. Menopause 2004;11:11–33.

Soules MR, Sherman S, Parrott E, Rebar R. Executive summary: Stages of Reproductive Aging Workshop (STRAW). Fertil Steril 2001;76:874–8.

Women's Health Initiative Steering Committee. Effects of conjugated equine estrogen in postmenopausal women with hysterectomy. JAMA 2004;291:1707–12.

Writing Group for the PEPI Trial. Effects of estrogen or estrogen/progestin regimens on heart disease risk factors in postmenopausal women. The Postmenopausal Estrogen/Progestin Interventions (PEPI) Trial. JAMA 1995;273:199–208.

Writing Group for the Women's Health Initiative Investigators. Risks and benefits of estrogen plus progestin in healthy postmenopausal women: Principal results from the Women's Health Initiative randomized controlled trial. JAMA 2002;288:321–33.

Vulvovaginitis

Method of
Christine Hudak, MD

From a medical perspective, it is tempting to consider vulvovaginitis a minor problem. However, to the woman affected, getting relief is quite important. In addition to the immediate physical discomfort and potential risks in pregnancy, those with untreated vaginitis can experience body image issues and sexual problems. Evaluation of vaginitis accounts for more than 10 million office visits a year in the United States, so proper diagnosis and management are essential. This article addresses the most common causes of vaginitis: bacterial vaginosis (40%–50% of cases), candidiasis (20%–25%), and trichomoniasis (15%–20%.) Of these three, only trichomoniasis is sexually transmitted, although all have been associated with other sexually transmitted infections.

Symptoms of vaginitis most commonly include vaginal redness, itching, and discharge that may be malodorous. Trichomoniasis can also cause dysuria, dyspareunia, and postcoital bleeding. Candidal infections can also produce vulvar redness, itching, dysuria, and dyspareunia.

Identifying the etiology of vaginitis is primarily based on patient history, pelvic examination, vaginal pH measurement, and microscopic evaluation of the discharge. Even in expert hands, the sensitivity of a 0.9% normal saline and 10% KOH slide preparations is 50% to 60%. Culture and newer office-based testing options are also available.

Bacterial Vaginosis

Bacterial vaginosis is not an infection but rather a shift in the normal bacterial vaginal flora. There is a decrease of lactobacilli and an overgrowth of *Gardnerella vaginalis*, *Mycoplasma hominus*, and anaerobes. Factors that are associated with bacterial vaginosis include multiple sex partner, a new sex partner, and douching.

Clinical indicators of bacterial vaginosis include Amsel's criteria: abnormal gray discharge, vaginal pH greater than 4.5, a positive

[1]Not FDA approved for this indication.

amine test, and more than 20% clue cells on normal saline microscopy. If two or three of the criteria are present, the clinical diagnosis of bacterial vaginosis can be made with a 90% sensitivity and 77% specificity. (The amine test is commonly referred to as the *whiff test* and is positive if the addition of KOH to a sample of the discharge produces a strong fishy odor.) Additional microscopic findings can include a large amount of coccobacillary bacteria and a lack of lactobacilli.

A recent meta-analysis evaluating the accuracy of signs and symptoms of vaginitis to determine etiology found that in patients with the symptom of vaginal odor, the likelihood ratio for having bacterial vaginosis was 1.6 with a sensitivity of 97% and a specificity of 40%. The use of culture for the diagnosis of bacterial vaginosis is not recommended because the organisms in question are all normal vaginal flora. There is also a rapid office test available (QuickVue Advance *G. vaginalis* test) for CLIA (Clinical Laboratory Improvement Admendment) moderately complex labs. Changes suggesting bacterial vaginosis reported on a Papanicolaou (Pap) smear do not require treatment unless the patient is symptomatic.

In addition to causing vaginitis, bacterial vaginosis has also been associated with pelvic inflammatory disease, infections after gynecologic surgery, and acquisition of sexually transmitted infections such as herpes and HIV. Treatment for bacterial vaginosis prior to hysterectomy and abortion decreases the postoperative infection rate.

In pregnant patients, bacterial vaginosis has been associated with premature rupture of membranes (PROM), prematurity, chorioamnionitis, and low birth weight. In symptomatic patients, the treatment of bacterial vaginosis decreases those risks, though the current data do not support screening asymptomatic patients during pregnancy. The exception may be for women at high risk for preterm delivery. Several studies demonstrated that screening and treating asymptomatic pregnant women for bacterial vaginosis decreased the risk of prematurity and PROM, although one study did not show a benefit.

Box 1 summarizes the 2006 Centers for Disease Control and Prevention (CDC) recommendations for treating bacterial vaginosis. Because this is not a sexually transmitted infection, treatment of the partner is not recommended.

Vulvovaginal Candidiasis

Vulvovaginal candidiasis is the second most common etiology of clinical vaginitis. Symptoms of candidiasis are vaginal itching, irritation, a thick white discharge, dysuria, and dyspareunia. With the availability of over-the-counter antifungal treatments, many women self-diagnose and treat their symptoms. Unfortunately, the accuracy of self-diagnosis is not very good. If women have had a prior episode of candidiasis, they correctly identify recurrence 36% of the time. With no prior episode, self-diagnosis accuracy drops to 9%. Women treating themselves empirically for candidiasis can delay treatment of other more serious disorders. Although self-treatment may be a good option for some, it is important for patients to be evaluated by a physician if the initial treatment fails.

Similarly, physicians are not very accurate at making the diagnosis from symptoms and physical examination findings alone. The most predictive signs and symptoms are thick white curdlike discharge and vulvar inflammation. Microscopy with 10% KOH demonstrates blastospores or pseudohyphae and few (if any) leukocytes. Vaginal pH is typically normal in the presence of candidiasis, 4 to 4.5. The sensitivity of microscopy has been estimated at 65% and varies with the experience of the physician.

Most candidiasis is caused by *Candida albicans*, although non-albicans types can also cause symptoms. *Candida* is normal flora in the vagina and so is not a sexually transmitted infection but rather an overgrowth phenomenon like bacterial vaginosis. Culture is typically reserved for women who do not respond to treatment and is especially helpful when identifying non-albicans infections. *Candida glabrata* does not form the typical pseudohyphae seen on microscopy of *C. albicans*.

The CDC divides candidiasis into two categories: complicated and uncomplicated. Patient risk factors for complicated candidiasis include pregnancy, diabetes (or other serious medical conditions) and immunocompromised status. Other characteristics of complicated candidiasis are the suspicion of a non-albicans infection, a severe infection, or infection that recurs four or more times a year. Treatment recommendations are different for complicated and uncomplicated candidiasis. Partners of women with candidiasis do not need to be treated because this is not a sexually transmitted infection. Candidiasis has not been associated with any pregnancy risks.

Boxes 2 and 3 summarize the 2006 CDC recommendations for treatment of candidiasis.

Non-albicans infections such as those caused by *C. glabrata* are only about 50% responsive to the azoles. For azole treatment failure, 600 mg vaginal boric acid capsules[6] can be used daily for 14 days. Topical flucytosine cream[1,6] has also been used successfully in resistant infections. For recurrent candidiasis, maintenance regimens are suggested by the CDC, although there is a high rate of relapse once the medications are discontinued.

Trichomonas Vaginitis

Trichomoniasis is sexually transmitted and caused by the flagellated protozoan, *Trichomonas vaginalis*. Women may be asymptomatic (as their partners often are) or report symptoms of malodorous yellow-green discharge, itching, dysuria, dyspareunia, and postcoital bleeding.

Diagnosis in women is most commonly made by viewing motile trichomonads microscopically, which has a sensitivity of 60% to

---

[1]Not FDA approved for this indication.
[6]May be compounded by pharmacists.

CURRENT DIAGNOSIS

- Bacterial vaginosis: pH, >4.5; 20% clue cells, malodorous discharge
- Vulvovaginal candidiasis: pH, 4–4.5; pseudohyphae, blastospores, thick curdlike discharge, vulvar inflammation
- *Trichomonas* vaginitis: pH, >4.5; motile, flagellated trichomonads, many WBCs, yellow discharge, vulvovaginal inflammation

---

BOX 1   Treatment of Bacterial Vaginosis

Nonpregnant Patients
Recommended Regimens
Metronidazole (Flagyl): 500 mg PO bid × 7 days
Metronidazole gel 0.75% (MetroGel-Vaginal): 1 applicator (5 g) intravaginally qhs × 5 days
Clindamycin cream 2% (Cleocin): 1 applicator (5 g) intravaginally qhs × 7 days

Alternative Regimens
Clindamycin (Cleocin): 300 mg PO bid × 7 days
Clindamycin ovules (Cleocin): 100 g intravaginally qhs × 3 days

Pregnant Patients
Metronidazole (Flagyl): 500 mg PO bid × 7 days
Metronidazole: 250 mg PO tid × 7 days
Clindamycin (Cleocin): 300 mg PO bid × 7 days

BOX 2 Treatment of Uncomplicated Vulvovaginal Candidiasis

1-Day Therapy

Fluconazole (Diflucan): 1 150-mg tablet PO
Butoconazole 2% SR cream (Gynazole-1): 1 applicator (5 g) intravaginally × 1
Tioconazole 6.5% cream (Monistat-1, Vagistat-1): 1 applicator (4.6 g) intravaginally × 1
Miconazole 1200 mg suppository (Monistat-1 Combination Pack): 1 suppository intravaginally × 1

3-Day Therapy

Butoconazole 2% cream (Femstat-3, Mycelex 3) 1 applicator (5 g) intravaginally qhs × 3 days
Terconazole 0.8% cream (Terazol-3), 1 applicator (5 g) intravaginally qhs × 3 days
Clotrimazole 200 mg vaginal tablet (Gyne-Lotrimin-3) 1 tablet intravaginally qhs × 3 days
Miconazole 200 mg suppository (M-zole 3 combo pack) 1 suppository intravaginally qhs × 3 days
Terconazole 80 mg suppository (Terazol-3) 1 suppository intravaginally qhs × 3 days

7-Day+ Therapy

Clotrimazole 1% cream (Gyne-Lotrimin 7, Mycelex-7): 1 applicator (5 g) intravaginally qhs × 7–14 days
Miconazole 2% cream Femizol-M, Monistat-7): 1 applicator (5 g) intravaginally qhs × 7 days
Terconazole 0.4% cream (Terazol-7) 1 applicator (5 g): intravaginally × 7 days
Clotrimazole 100 mg tab (Mycelex-7 Combo pack): 1 tab intravaginally qhs × 7 days
Miconazole 100 mg suppository (Monistat 7): 1 suppository intravaginally qhs × 7 days
Nystatin 100,000 U tab: 1 tab intravaginally qhs × 14 days

70%. A large number of white blood cells can also be seen on the wet preparation. Vaginal pH is typically higher than normal. Office point-of-care testing kits are available, including the OSOM Trichomonas Rapid Test and the Affirm VP III (the last tests for *T. vaginalis*, *G. vaginalis*, and *C. albicans*). Samples may also be sent for culture of trichomonas, although they are not commonly used clinically.

In men, urethral swab, urine, or semen can be cultured if necessary because the wet preparation and microscopy are not sensitive. Physicians might consider empirically treating the partner to decrease the rate of reinfection.

BOX 3 Treatment of Complicated Vulvovaginal Candidiasis

Treatment Regimens

Fluconazole (Diflucan) 100-, 150-, or 200-mg tablet: 1 tablet PO q 3 days × 3 doses
Topical azole cream, tablet or suppository: 1 dose intravaginally qhs × 7–14 days

Maintenance Regimens

Fluconazole 100-, 150-, or 200-mg tablet: 1 tablet PO every week × 6 months
Clotrimazole 200-mg suppository (Gyne-Lotrimin 3): 1 suppository intravaginally qhs 2×/week
Butoconazole 2% cream (Femstat-3, Mycelex-3): 1 applicator (5 g) intravaginally qhs × 3 days

BOX 4 Treatment of Trichomoniasis

Recommended Regimens

Metronidazole (Flagyl) 2 g PO × 1 dose *or*
Tinidazole (Tindamax) 2 g PO × 1 dose

Alternative Regimen

Metronidazole 500 mg PO bid × 7 days

In pregnant patients, *Trichomonas* infection is associated with harmful outcomes such as PROM, preterm delivery, and low-birth-weight babies. Curiously, studies that have been done to date do not show a decrease in these outcomes when women have been treated. Those studies had some limitations, and there is no current recommendation about the necessity of treatment in pregnancy. However, the most common medication for treatment, metronidazole (Flagyl), is Category B and considered safe for use in all trimesters.

Box 4 summarizes the 2006 CDC recommendations for treatment of *Trichomonas* vaginitis.

Tinidazole (Tindamax) is newly approved in the United States for the treatment of trichomoniasis and is as efficacious as metronidazole. Resistance to metronidazole is estimated to be less than 5%, and this can often be overcome with a higher dose of metronidazole or by treating with tinidazole due to its longer half-life. Topical preparations of metronidazole (MetroGel-Vaginal, Vandazole) are not very successful in treating *Trichomonas* and are not recommended. Follow-up testing is not required for patients who are asymptomatic after treatment.

REFERENCES

ACOG Committee on Practice Bulletins—Gynecology. ACOG Practice Bulletin. Clinical management guidelines for obstetrician-gynecologists, Number 72, May 2006: Vaginitis. Obstet Gynecol 2006;107:1195–206.

Anderson MR, Klink K, Cohrssen A. Evaluation of vaginal complaints. JAMA 2004;291(11):1368–79.

Centers for Disease Control and Prevention. Workowski KA, Berman SM. Sexually transmitted diseases treatment guidelines, 2006. MMWR Recomm Rep 2006;55(RR-11):1–94.

Owen MK, Clenney TL. Management of vaginitis. Am Fam Physician 2004;70:2125–32, 2139–40.

Chlamydia trachomatis

Method of
*Catherine Stevens-Simon, MD**

The Scope of the Problem

Responsible for more than 3 million infections each year in the United States, *Chlamydia trachomatis* poses a public health problem of epidemic proportions. Because of the large reservoir of undiagnosed, asymptomatic infections, the number of reported cases significantly underestimates the true prevalence of this infection. Nonetheless, *C. trachomatis* is not only the most commonly reported bacterial sexually transmitted disease (STD) in the United States but also the nation's most commonly reported bacterial infection. It is difficult to give meaningful prevalence figures because the proportion

---

*Deceased.

of infected individuals depends on the characteristics of the population studied and how they are studied. In addition, whereas passive surveillance systems indicate that the prevalence of this infection has risen precipitously over the last decade, studies conducted at sentinel surveillance sites demonstrate a decline, which suggests that expanded screening, increased reporting, and improved test sensitivity mask a true decrease in prevalence in some sectors of American society. The epidemiologic characteristics and clinical manifestations of chlamydial infections in the United States reflect the fact that most infections are sexually transmitted and that prevalent stereotypes have an affinity for columnar epithelium. Teenage girls are most susceptible to these infections because of the following factors:

- At their age, the columnar epithelium is prominent on the ectocervix.
- Some experience a high level of unprotected, serially monogamous sexual activity with older men whose sexual risk profiles they rarely investigate.

With these two factors combined, teenage girls are at maximal biologic and social risk. Although the national prevalence of chlamydial infections in this population is unknown, school- and clinic-based studies suggest a range of 8% to 26% (compared to 3% to 5% in sociodemographically similar young adult women), with the highest age-specific prevalence reported among adolescents ages 14 to 15 years. Although readily eradicable, the economic and human costs of these infections are staggering. Annual expenditures are estimated to exceed $1.5 billion, with 75% of the cost devoted to treating sequelae of cervical infections that were initially uncomplicated. Because the majority of severe consequences of untreated infections occur in women, and as much as 66.6% of tubal factor infertility and 33.3% of ectopic pregnancies in the United States are attributed to chlamydial infections, it is estimated that every dollar spent on screening and treating asymptomatic young women and their sex partners saves approximately $12. Although this uniquely positions primary health care providers to prevent the costly sequelae of chlamydial infections, given their prevalence among teenagers, expansion of screening and treatment programs to nontraditional settings such as schools, juvenile detention centers, and drug treatment facilities is likely to be a critical component of any national strategy to ontrol this infection.

Clinical Presentation

Chlamydial infections are an excellent example of the dependence of the clinical manifestations of disease on the intrinsic properties of the pathogen and host. In Western industrialized countries, virtually all chlamydial infections are either sexually transmitted or vertically transmitted at birth. They are caused by nonlymphogranuloma venereum stereotypes that have an affinity for columnar epithelium and can only survive by a cytotoxic, replicative cycle that evokes a variable immune response in the host. Hence, in the United States, the endocervix, urethra, rectum, and conjunctiva are preferentially affected, and clinical manifestations range from asymptomatic to florid inflammatory conditions with severe reproductive consequences. *Chlamydia* should be suspected in these populations:

- Women and men with dysuria and pyuria
- Women with dyspareunia; abnormal vaginal discharge; postcoital, irregular menstrual, or breakthrough contraceptive bleeding; and lower abdominal or pelvic pain
- Infants with conjunctivitis or a staccato cough

These signs and symptoms are neither a sensitive nor a specific indication of infection, however. Indeed, because nearly 90% of chlamydial infections are asymptomatic and *C. trachomatis* is isolated from less than 33.3% of women with mucopurulent cervicitis and less than 50% of men with nongonococcal urethritis, such complaints are unreliable predictors of infection. In women, the most common sign is mucopurulent cervicitis, a nonspecific clinical syndrome characterized by erythema, edema, and friability of the ectocervix and purulent endocervical exudate. Mucopurulent cervicitis, however, is also caused by other STDs and noninfectious factors (i.e., cyclical fluctuations in gonadal hormones), which increase the size of the cervical ectropion or the resident population of cervical leukocytes. Other clinical manifestations of lower genital tract chlamydial infections in women include urethritis and bartholinitis. Although pelvic inflammatory disease (PID) is a polymicrobial infection, *C. trachomatis* is also often involved, and, conversely, PID is the most common complication of chlamydial cervicitis. The estimated incidence ranges from 10% to 40% in untreated women. Young age and prolonged or recurrent infection significantly increase, whereas treatment of asymptomatic infections significantly decreases both disease severity and sequelae, such as salpingo-oophoritis, perihepatitis (Fitz-Hugh-Curtis syndrome), infertility, ectopic pregnancy, and chronic pelvic pain. Adverse outcomes associated with chlamydial infections during pregnancy include preterm labor, premature rupture of the placental membranes, low-birth-weight delivery, neonatal death, postpartum or postabortal endometritis, and vertical transmission to infants. In the infected infants, 30% to 50% develop conjunctivitis, 15% to 20% develop nasopharyngitis, and 5% to 10% develop pneumonia.

In men, the most common clinical manifestation is urethritis, the symptoms of which typically commence 1 to 3 weeks after exposure and range from mild dysuria to frank penile discharge. Other clinical syndromes in men include epididymitis, prostatitis, acute proctocolitis, and Reiter syndrome (urethritis, conjunctivitis, arthritis, and mucocutaneous lesions). These suppurative complications rarely require inpatient therapy and are far less common than those encountered in women. Nonetheless, sequelae ranging from urethral strictures to infertility do occur. Nongenital clinical manifestations, such as conjunctivitis, tenosynovitis, and arthritis, are uncommon among adults in the United States.

Diagnosis and Screening

In the United States, testing for both symptomatic and asymptomatic chlamydial infections is done with ligase chain reaction (LCR), polymerase chain reaction (PCR), and other nucleic acid amplification techniques (NAATs) because they do not require the presence of intact organisms. Urine, cervical, vaginal, or urethral fluids can be used as the analyte for these tests; specimens are stable and easy to transport; and results can be obtained within a day. This is a major advantage over the stringent collection, transport, and 3-day growth period culturing requirements associated with this fastidious organism. Although nonculture assays, non-NAATs, and rapid diagnostic tests capable of making a diagnosis within 30 minutes are available, these assays are too insensitive to be recommended for routine testing.

The signs and symptoms of chlamydial infection are nonspecific and often persist for weeks after documented eradication of the pathogen. Because of this, leukocyte, esterase-positive urine dipsticks, leukocyte-laden vaginal wet mounts, and endocervical Gram stains should be regarded as no more than a trigger for testing. Although concerns about the consequences of underdiagnosis and undertreatment typically overshadow concerns about the consequences of overdiagnosis and overtreatment, therapeutic decisions should not be based on these poorly standardized tests. Indeed, given their low positive predictive value for chlamydial infections, the adverse psychological effects of being diagnosed with an STD, and the serious public health problems that the indiscriminate use of antibiotics creates—even in settings where the prevalence of chlamydial infections is high and patient follow-up is uncertain and in resource-poor clinics where NAATs are unavailable—enthusiasm for the practice of diagnosing chlamydial infections empirically. This must be tempered by the knowledge that to prevent one individual from suffering the sequelae of an untreated infection, hundreds will needlessly suffer the adverse psychosocial consequences of an STD diagnosis. This is true even when the diagnosis is made based on characteristic symptom complexes, suggestive leukocyte esterase urine dipsticks, and/or

CURRENT DIAGNOSIS

- Signs and symptoms are neither a sensitive nor a specific indication of chlamydial infection and often persist for weeks after documented eradication of the pathogen.
    Most chlamydial infections are asymptomatic.
    Chlamydia trachomatis is isolated from less than half of women and men with the most common signs and symptoms (mucopurulent cervicitis and urethritis).
- *Chlamydia* should be suspected in:
    Women and men with dysuria and pyuria.
    Women with dyspareunia, abnormal vaginal discharge, abnormal bleeding, and lower abdominal or pelvic pain; infants with conjunctivitis or a staccato cough
- Routine periodic screening with nucleic acid amplification techniques (NAATs) is the only reliable way to diagnose this infection.

vaginal wet mounts. Thus, with sensitivities and specificities fluctuating approximately 98% on male urethral and urine specimens as well as on female cervical specimens, NAATs are currently the best chlamydial tests available. However, because the sensitivity of these assays for detecting infections in women is significantly lower when urine (80% to 95%) or patient- or provider-collected vaginal fluid (70% to 85%) is the analyte, endocervical specimens should be used, except in screening situations where it is impractical to perform pelvic examinations. Thus every case diagnosed on a urine or vaginal specimen is a bonus.

Despite consensus about how to screen, uncertainty continues about whom to screen and how frequently to screen them. Pregnant women and sexually active women younger than 25 years of age are the only groups for whom there is good evidence that the benefits of screening outweigh the harms. Specifically, when prevalence rates exceed 2%, testing and treating these individuals for asymptomatic chlamydial infections is a cost-effective preventive measure that:

- Averts PID and associated medical complications.
- Reduces transmission to sex partners.
- Reduces the risk of acquiring HIV.
- Lowers the prevalence of *Chlamydia* in the community.

It is unlikely that these benefits reflect factors other than screening (i.e., increased condom use) because knowledge of sexual risk behavior adds nothing to predictive algorithms that include age and prior STD history. However, because of the highly infectious nature of this bacterium, the lack of a vaccine, and the failure of the human immune system to build up resistance to the bacteria, reinfection of effectively treated individuals tends to diminish short-term efficacy, making long-term periodic screening a prerequisite of cost efficacy.

The only other caveat is that most cost-effectiveness analyses are based on culture-proven disease and therefore may reflect a larger inoculum than infections diagnosed by NAAT assays, which can detect extremely low levels of viable and nonviable organisms. Thus further research is needed to determine if and how inoculum size affects disease presentation and to define the clinical and public health significance of NAAT-detectable infections. Specifically, studies comparing transmission rates and the clinical consequences of infections that are detected only by NAAT assay versus those that are detected by traditional assays are still needed to prove that routine, periodic, urine-based screening of asymptomatic individuals is a cost-effective way to control chlamydial infections at the population level. Moreover, because identifying infected individuals is only the first step in effective disease control, it is also important to demonstrate that once identified, the majority of these asymptomatically infected individuals and their sex partners can be contacted and treated. The randomized trial data that determine how frequently community members should be screened to lower chlamydial infections

at the population level are lacking; however, observational studies consistently indicate that among sexually active teens the median time between first and repeat infections is approximately 6 months. Based on these data, biannual screening seems reasonable for women at this age (older than 25 years). Because the risk of reinfection is inversely related to age, it is unclear if this recommendation should be extended to young adults. Nevertheless, a history of prior infection predicts reinfection regardless of sexual risk behavior, and in women repeat infections are implicated in the pathogenesis of upper genital tract damage. It may be wise, therefore, to rescreen all women who were treated for chlamydial infections at 6-month intervals.

Developing selective screening criteria is a vigorously pursued public health goal. With the exception of age, however, no single demographic or behavioral risk factor or combination of risk factors consistently identifies a group of young, sexually active women who should not be screened. The utility of more selective screening is limited by the high proportion of missed infections.

Parallel evidence to support screening asymptomatic men may be lacking because before the introduction of urine screening men were not routinely tested for chlamydial infection. But because the cost of treating men is lower than the cost of treating women, a greater proportion of infected men are symptomatic than women, and the harm associated with misdiagnoses is not inconsequent, it will undoubtedly be more difficult to justify routine periodic male screening. However, false-negative test results create a reservoir of untreated disease that is likely to contribute disproportionately to the spread of *C. trachomatis*; but the psychosocial consequences of false-positive test results can range from dysphoric feelings and decreased self-esteem to the disruption of romantic relationships and domestic violence. Moreover, if treatment is initiated inappropriately, the adverse effects of drug reactions and bacterial resistance caused by antibiotic overuse must be taken into account. Thus, until more data become available, the United States Preventive Services Task Force recommends symptom-based screening for all men and for women older than 25 years of age who do not exhibit other characteristics associated with a high prevalence of chlamydial infections (i.e., unmarried status, African American race, a history of STDs, a history of new or multiple sex partners, cervical ectopy, and inconsistent condom use).

Treatment

Recommendations for antibiotic treatment of chlamydial infections depend on the clinical syndrome. Box 1 summarizes the options for outpatient therapy of uncomplicated genital tract infections in men and women. However, because humans do not develop a natural immunity to chlamydia, treated patients remain at risk for reinfection. For this reason therapy should not be considered complete until all recent sexual contacts are treated and the patient is counseled about future disease prevention. An estimated 70% of the male partners of women with chlamydial cervicitis are infected, and, conversely, approximately 30% of the female partners of *Chlamydia*-infected men are infected. Treatment is recommended for the most recent sex partner and all other individuals who had sexual contact with the infected person during the 60 days preceding the onset of symptoms or diagnosis. Also, partners should abstain from sexual intercourse for a week after they complete treatment.

Although patient-delivered partner treatment is as effective as partner notification, partners are more likely to be treated if informed by physicians rather than by the patients. This is because only 65% (approximately) of women with known chlamydial infections refer their sex partners for therapy, and even fewer (approximately 45%) infected men do so. Because the cure rate for single-dose azithromycin (Zithromax) therapy is close to 100% and the medication can easily be administered under medical supervision, a test of cure 3 weeks after treatment—NAATs remain positive for this long despite successful eradication of infection—is only recommended for pregnant women (among whom antibiotic efficacy may be reduced) and when compliance is in doubt.

BOX 1 *Chlamydia trachomatis:* Recommended Treatment Regimens by Clinical Syndrome

Asymptomatic, Cervicitis, Urethritis*
- First-choice regimen
- Azithromycin (Zithromax), 1 g orally in a single dose
  or
- Doxycycline (Vibramycin), 100 mg orally twice a day for 7 days

Alternative Regimens (One of the Following)
- Erythromycin base (E-Mycin), 500 mg orally four times a day for 7 days
- Erythromycin ethylsuccinate (EES), 800 mg orally four times a day for 7 days
- Ofloxacin (Floxin), 300 mg orally twice a day for 7 days
- Levofloxacin (Levaquin),[1] 500 mg orally for 7 days

Epididymitis
- Ceftriaxone (Rocephin),[1] 250 mg intramuscularly (single dose)
  or
- Doxycycline,[1] 100 mg orally twice a day for 7 days

Outpatient Pelvic Inflammatory Disease
- Ceftriaxone, 250 mg intramuscularly (single dose)
  plus
- Doxycycline, 100 mg orally twice a day for 14 days *with or without*
- Metronidazole (Flagyl), 500 mg orally twice a day for 14 days

Alternative Regimens
- Ceftriaxone, 250 mg intramuscularly (single dose)
  or
- Cefoxitin (Mefoxin), 2 g intramuscularly (single dose)
  plus
- Probenecid, 1 g orally
  plus
- Doxycycline, 100 mg orally twice a day for 14 days *with or without*
- Metronidazole, 500 mg orally twice a day for 14 days

Inpatient Pelvic Inflammatory Disease[†]
- Cefotetan (Cefotan), 2 g intravenously every 12 hours
  or
- Cefoxitin, 2 g intravenously every 6 hours
  plus
- Doxycycline,[1] 100 mg orally or intravenously every 12 hours

Alternative Regimens
- Clindamycin, 900 mg intravenously every 8 hours
  plus
- Gentamicin,[1] 2 g/kg of body weight loading dose, then 1.5 mg/kg of body weight every 8 hours. Treatment should be continued for 24 to 48 hours after significant clinical improvement occurs and then should consist of oral therapy with doxycycline, 100 mg orally twice a day for 14 days, or clindamycin, 450 mg orally four times a day, for a total of 14 days.

Providers should consult the Centers for Disease Control and Prevention's website at: http://www.cdc.gov/std/treatment/for up-to-treatment recommendations.
[1]Not FDA approved for this indication.
*Pregnancy: Doxycycline, erythromycin estolate (Ilosone), and ofloxacin are contraindicated, and repeat testing 3 weeks after completion of therapy is recommended because antibiotics may be less efficacious. HIV infection: Patients who have chlamydial infection and who also are infected with HIV should receive the same treatment regimen as those who are HIV-negative.
[†]Studies indicate that the efficacy of inpatient and outpatient treatment is comparable in terms of fertility and other long-term health outcomes. Criteria for inpatient treatment include surgical emergencies, pregnancy, unresponsive to oral antimicrobial therapy, unable to follow or tolerate an outpatient oral regimen, severe illness, nausea and vomiting, high fever, or tubo-ovarian abscess.

 CURRENT THERAPY

- Antibiotic treatment is easy to summarize in tabular form but is ineffective if given in isolation of sexual network.
  - Large reservoir of asymptomatically infected partners and potential partners undermines the effectiveness of individual treatments.
  - Half of all chlamydial infections occur in previously treated persons.
- Therapy is not complete until all recent sexual contacts are treated and the patient is counseled about disease prevention.
- Prevalence of *Chlamydia trachomatis* in the sexual network is the best predictor of infection.
- Whom an individual has sexual intercourse with puts him or her at higher risk for acquisition of this infection than how they do so.
- For disease prevention, condoms are plan B. Plan A is choosing low-risk sexual partners.

Approximately 50% of all chlamydial infections occur in previously treated persons. Demographic characteristics, such as age and a past history of chlamydial infection, are better predictors of infection than behavioral risk factors, such as multiple sexual partners and the failure to use condoms consistently. Being involved with a sexual network in which *Chlamydia* is hyperendemic appears to put individuals at greater risk for infection than unsafe sexual behavior in the general population. Hence, to control the spread of *C. trachomatis*, it may be necessary to:

- Extend screening and treatment beyond recent partners to include the group of core transmitters in the infected individual's sexual network.
- Help STD patients learn to choose less risky sex partners by promoting sexual health communication within partnerships.

Although the debate about the content and duration of counseling necessary to achieve this goal is ongoing, there is a growing consensus that brief (5 minutes), personalized (provider-delivered and client-centered) counseling sessions—aimed at personal risk reduction and increasing awareness of partner risk behavior—are more effective than the conventional didactic approach to STD prevention education. They are certainly as effective as more prolonged sessions, which are difficult to conduct in busy public health clinics.

REFERENCES

Aral SO, Hughes JP, Stoner B, et al. Sexual mixing patterns in spread of gon-ococcal and chlamydial infections. Am J Pub Health 1999;89:825–33.

Biro F, Workowski K, Blythe MJ, Lara-Torre E. NASPAG/JPAG roundtable discussion annual clinical meeting 2003. Philadelphia, PA: Sexually transmitted diseases (STD) treatment guidelines 2002. J Pediatr Adolesc Gynecol 2004;17:143–6.

Cates Jr W. Contraception, unintended pregnancies, and sexually transmitted diseases: Why isn't a simple solution possible? Am J Epidemiol 1996;143:311–8.

Critchlow CW, Wolner-Hanssen P, Eschenbach DA, et al. Determinants of cervical ectopia and cervicitis: Age, oral contraception, specific cervical infection, smoking, and douching. Am J Obstet Gynecol 1995;173:534–43.

Duncan B, Hart G, Scoular A, Bigrigg A. Qualitative analysis of psychosocial impact of diagnosis of Chlamydia trachomatis. Implications for screening. BMJ 2001;322:195–229.

Ford CA, Viadro CI, Miller WC. Testing for chlamydial and gonorrheal infections outside of clinic settings. A summary of the literature. Sex Transm Dis 2004;31:38–51.

Kamb ML, Fishbein M, Douglas Jr JM, et al. Efficacy of risk-reduction counseling to prevent human immunodeficiency virus and sexually transmitted diseases: A randomized controlled trial for the Project RESPECT Study Group. JAMA 1998;280:1161–7.

Peipert JF. Clinical practice. Genital chlamydial infections. N Engl J Med 2003;349:2424–30.

Rietmeijer CA, Van Bemmelen R, Judson FN, Douglas JM. Incidence and repeat infection rates of Chlamydia trachomatis among male and female patients in an STD clinic. Sex Transm Dis 2002;29:65–72.

U.S. Preventive Services Task Force. Screening for chlamydial infection: Recommendations and rationale. Am J Prev Med 2001;20(3S):90–4.

Pelvic Inflammatory Disease

Method of
Adrianne Williams Bagley, MD, and
Maria Trent, MD, MPH

Pelvic inflammatory disease (PID) is a spectrum of disorders characterized by an infection of the female upper genital tract. Organs that may be affected include the uterus (endometritis, parametritis), fallopian tubes (salpingitis), and ovaries (oophoritis, tubo-ovarian abscesses [TOAs]), or the infection may involve the pelvic peritoneum.

Epidemiology

Approximately 800,000 women per year are diagnosed with PID. Up to 20% of cases occur in teenagers. Risk factors associated with development of PID mirror the risk factors that increase the likelihood of acquiring a sexually transmitted infection. These risk factors include having multiple sex partners and inconsistent or incorrect use of condoms. Douching and use of intrauterine devices are also associated with PID. Women with a prior diagnosis of PID are at higher risk of developing future episodes.

Pathophysiology

The infection of the female upper genital tract that characterizes PID is caused by the ascent of infectious organisms from the vagina and cervix. It is postulated that the ascent of organisms may occur more readily during menses because of reflux of blood in the fallopian tubes, and studies show a temporal relationship between menses and the subsequent diagnosis of PID.

The infectious agents most often implicated in PID are the sexually transmitted organisms *Neisseria gonorrhoeae* and *Chlamydia trachomatis*. However, PID may be a polymicrobial infection. Other contributing infectious etiologies include anaerobic bacteria such as *Bacteroides* and *Peptostreptococcus* species, *Gardnerella vaginalis*, *Haemophilus influenzae*, *Streptococcus* species, *Mycoplasma hominis*, *Ureaplasma urealyticum*, enteric gram-negative bacilli, and cytomegalovirus.

Diagnosis

The diagnosis of PID is made based on clinical assessment; therefore, a detailed history, careful examination, and the use of additional supportive diagnostic tests are warranted. Patients may present with varied nonspecific complaints including lower abdominal pain, vaginal discharge, and irregular menses or bleeding with sexual intercourse. Patients may or may not be febrile, experience vomiting or diarrhea, or have urinary symptoms. The differential diagnosis includes processes that affect not only the reproductive tract but also the gastrointestinal and urinary tracts. The differential diagnosis includes but is not limited to ovarian cyst, endometriosis, dysmenorrhea, ectopic pregnancy, septic or threatened abortion, gastroenteritis, appendicitis, diverticulitis, constipation, inflammatory bowel disease, irritable bowel syndrome, urethritis, cystitis, pyelonephritis, and nephrolithiasis.

The 2006 Centers for Disease Control and Prevention (CDC) guidelines recommend empirical treatment for PID in sexually active women with minimum diagnostic criteria of uterine tenderness, adnexal tenderness, or cervical motion tenderness, in whom no other cause can be identified. Additional supportive criteria may be used to increase the specificity of diagnosis; these criteria include oral temperature greater than 38°C (101°F), abnormal cervical or vaginal mucopurulent discharge, presence of white blood cells on saline wet mount of vaginal secretions, elevated erythrocyte sedimentation rate (ESR) or Creactive protein (CRP), and documented cervical infection with *N. gonorrhoeae* or *C. trachomatis*. However, if cervical infection with *N. gonorrhoeae* or *C. trachomatis* is not found, these organisms can still be responsible for upper genital tract infection. Additional diagnostic tests may include complete blood cell count (CBC) with differential, urine dipstick or urinalysis, urine culture, and urine pregnancy test. Pelvic ultrasonography should be obtained if there is evidence of a pelvic mass on examination or if there is adnexal tenderness in the setting of high fever, elevated white blood cell count, or elevated CRP or ESR; this constellation of findings may suggest a TOA.

Treatment

Treatment should be initiated promptly for the patient with suspected PID to prevent complications, which include chronic pelvic pain, ectopic pregnancy, and infertility. Antibiotic treatment is broad spectrum to ensure coverage of typical pathogens, namely *N. gonorrhoeae*, *C. trachomatis*, and anaerobes. With prompt appropriate medical treatment, the future reproductive ability of the patient may be protected.

 CURRENT DIAGNOSIS

- Pelvic inflammatory disease is a clinical diagnosis.
- The minimum diagnostic criterion is one or more of the following clinical findings: uterine tenderness, adnexal tenderness, *or* cervical motion tenderness in the patient in whom no other cause can be identified.
- The use of additional supportive criteria can increase the accuracy of the diagnosis.

The Current Therapy box outlines the 2006 CDC treatment guidelines for inpatient treatment. Hospitalization for parenteral treatment is reserved for patients for whom surgical causes of abdominal pain cannot be excluded, patients who are pregnant, patients who fail outpatient regimens (unable to follow or tolerate an outpatient regimen, no clinical response to oral antibiotics after 72 hours), patients with severe illness, nausea, vomiting, or high fever, and patients with a TOA. Patients younger than 16 years and those with extenuating social circumstances may also be candidates for inpatient treatment.

 CURRENT THERAPY

Inpatient Treatment for Pelvic Inflammatory Disease

Regimen A:
- Cefotetan (Cefotan), 2 g IV q12h, *or* cefoxitin (Mefoxin), 2 g IV q6h, *plus* doxycycline (Vibramycin), 100 mg PO or IV q12h

Regimen B:
- Clindamycin (Cleocin), 900 mg IV q8h, *plus* gentamicin (Garamycin) loading dose: 2 mg/kg IV/IM, followed by maintenance dose: 1.5 mg/kg IV q8h. Single daily dosing may be substituted.

Alternative Regimen:
- Ampicillin/Sulbactam (Unasyn) 3 g IV q6h *plus* doxycycline (Vibramycin) 100 mg PO or IV q12h.

Note: Parenteral therapy for PID should be considered for 24 h following clinical improvement, and patients should be discharged home on an oral course of doxycycline (Vibramycin) 100 mg PO bid, or clindamycin (Cleocin) 450 PO qid to complete 14 d.

Outpatient Treatment for Pelvic Inflammatory Disease

Recommended Oral Regimens:
- Ceftriaxone (Rocephin), 250 mg IM in a single dose, *or*
- Cefoxitin (Mefoxin), 2 g IM in a single dose, with probenecid, 1 g PO in a single dose, *or*
- Other parenteral third-generation cephalosporins (ceftizoxime [Cefizox] or cefotaxime [Claforan]) *plus* doxycycline (Vibramycin), 100 mg PO bid for 14 d, *with or without* metronidazole (Flagyl), 500 mg PO bid for 14 d.

Alternative Oral Regimens:
- Levofloxacin (Levaquin) 500 mg PO once daily for 14 d or ofloxacin (Floxin) 400 mg PO bid for 14 d with or without metronidazole (Flagyl) 500 mg PO bid for 14 d, if the community prevalence and individual risk of gonorrhea are low (see CDC Sexually Transmitted Disease Treatment Guidelines, 2006). Testing for N. gonorrhoeae must be performed prior to treatment. If NAAT test is positive, parental cephalosporin is recommended. If culture is positive for *N. gonorrhoeae*, treatment should be based on antimicrobial susceptibility. If antimicrobial susceptibility cannot be obtained or culture is quinolone resistant *N. gonorrhoeae* (QRNG), parenteral cephalosporin is recommended.

Note: Recommendations from the Centers for Disease Control and Prevention 2006 Sexually Transmitted Diseases Treatment Guidelines are available at http://www.cdc.giv/std/treatment.
Abbreviations: IM = intramuscular; IV = intravenous; PO = orally.

Outpatient treatment for PID is appropriate in most cases for patients who do not meet the criteria for hospitalization. Metronidazole (Flagyl) is often included as part of the treatment regimen to provide anaerobic coverage, and it is an appropriate adjunct medication in patients who also have evidence of bacterial vaginosis on saline wet mount.

FOLLOW-UP

Patients treated with outpatient therapy should be reevaluated in 48 to 72 hours to assess response to treatment. At this visit, the medical provider can review medication adherence, readdress partner notification, review the importance of safe sexual practices, discuss related family planning issues, answer questions that the patient may have about the diagnosis, and reexamine the patient to ensure that she is improving on the current therapeutic regimen. Patients who are not improving on oral antibiotics or who have been unable to adhere with the outpatient regimen may need additional diagnostic testing for complications and hospitalization for parental treatment.

Patients being treated for PID should be advised to abstain from sexual intercourse throughout the course of treatment. All sexual partners within the past 60 days should be tested and empirically treated for both *N. gonorrhoeae* and *C. trachomatis*.

Potential Complications

Short-term complications of PID include TOA and Fitz-Hugh–Curtis syndrome. Patients with TOA require hospitalization for parenteral treatment. Fitz-Hugh–Curtis syndrome is a perihepatitis that may result from spread of *N. gonorrhoeae* or *C. trachomatis* and is characterized by right upper quadrant pain.

Long-term complications of PID include chronic pelvic pain, tubal infertility secondary to scarring, and ectopic pregnancy. Patients with a history of PID have a 6- to 10-fold increased risk of ectopic pregnancy.

Prevention

Primary prevention of PID can be best accomplished by prevention of sexually transmitted infections. Sexually active women should undergo routine screening for gonorrhea and *Chlamydia* and be instructed about the importance of proper condom usage. Secondary prevention can be accomplished with partner notification and empirical treatment using antibiotics with adequate coverage for infections caused by *N. gonorrhoeae* and *C. trachomatis*.

REFERENCES

American Academy of Pediatrics. Pelvic inflammatory disease. In: Pickering LK, editor. Red Book: 2003 Report of the Committee on Infectious Diseases. 26th ed. Elk Grove Village, Ill: American Academy of Pediatrics; 2003. p. 468–72.

Centers for Disease Control and Prevention. Sexually transmitted disease treatment guidelines 2006. MMWR 2006;55(No. RR-11):56–61.

Ness RB, Soper DE, Holley RL, et al. Effectiveness of inpatient and outpatient treatment strategies for women with pelvic inflammatory disease: Results from the pelvic inflammatory disease evaluation and clinical health (PEACH) randomized trial. Am J Obstet Gynecol 2002;186(5):929–37.

Rein DB, Kassler WJ, Irwin KL, et al. Direct medical costs of pelvic inflammatory disease and its sequelae: Decreasing, but still substantial. Obstet Gynecol 2000;95(3):397–402.

Shrier LA. Bacterial sexually transmitted infections: Gonorrhea, chlamydia, pelvic inflammatory disease, and syphilis. In: Emans SJ, Laufer MR, Goldstein DP, editors. Pediatric and Adolescent Gynecology. 5th ed. Lippincott-Raven; 2004. p. 583–98.

Trent M, Chung S, Forrest L, Ellen JE. Subsequent pelvic inflammatory disease (PID) and sexually transmitted infections after outpatient treatment for PID in pediatric ambulatory settings. Arch Pediatr Adolesc Med 2008;162(11):1022–5.

Trent MA, Ellen JM, Walker A. Pelvic Inflammatory disease in adolescents—care delivery in pediatric ambulatory settings. Pediatr Emerg Care 2005;21(7):431–6.

Trent M, Judy SL, Ellen JM, Walker A. Use of an institutional intervention to improve quality of care for adolescents treated in pediatric ambulatory settings for pelvic inflammatory disease. J Adolesc Health 2006;39(1):50–6.

Update to CDC's sexually transmitted diseases treatment guidelines, 2006. Fluoroquinolones no longer recommended for treatment of gonococcal infections. MMWR Weekly April 13, 2007;56(14):332–6.

Uterine Leiomyomas

Method of
Tod C. Aeby, MD, and Stella Dantas, MD

Epidemiology

Uterine leiomyomas are the most common pelvic tumor in women. They affect approximately 20% of women older than 35 years of age and 40% of women older than 50 years of age, although they are found any time from puberty through menopause. Survey studies involving histologic examination of the uterus suggest they are present in more than 80% of women. Nulliparity, early menarche, and African American ethnicity increase the risk of developing leiomyomas. The incidence among women of African descent is not as high in countries other than the United States, which suggests possible dietary, environmental, and genetic influences on development. Risk is also increased in women with a higher body mass index, presumably because of the increased estrogen production in adipocytes. Pregnancy reduces the risk of developing leiomyomas.

Pathophysiology

The etiology of uterine leiomyomas is not completely understood, but development is thought to be a multistep process. They are benign monoclonal tumors of the smooth muscle of the myometrium that presumably derive from a normal myocyte. Estrogen and progesterone, in concert with local growth factors, lead to a somatic mutation of normal myometrium to a leiomyoma. Some growth factors that cause leiomyoma proliferation are epidermal growth factors, insulin-like growth factors, heparin-binding growth factors, and transforming growth factor-β. Leiomyomas develop during the reproductive years and increase in size during pregnancy. Growth usually ceases in menopause, and leiomyomas then decrease in volume. This supports the theory that estrogen and progesterone promote growth.

Symptoms and Signs

Most uterine leiomyomas are asymptomatic. They are categorized into subgroups based on their anatomic relationship and position in the uterus, and symptoms usually depend on those relationships. They can be subserosal, intramural, submucosal, or pedunculated. The most common symptom is abnormal uterine bleeding, usually menorrhagia, occurring in 30% of women with leiomyomas. The cause of the abnormal bleeding is not totally clear but may be the result of abnormal growth and function of the endometrium near the leiomyoma and local interference with normal physiologic mechanisms for hemostasis.

Pelvic pain and increasing pelvic pressure occur in 30% of women with leiomyomas. Other symptoms include dysmenorrhea, postcoital bleeding, and dyspareunia. Pain can be caused by leiomyomas outgrowing their blood supply and becoming necrotic. This red degeneration is common in pregnancy. Patients may have an increasing

CURRENT DIAGNOSIS

- Abnormal uterine bleeding, postcoital spotting
- Pelvic pain, pressure, dysmenorrhea and dyspareunia
- Urinary frequency and urgency, constipation
- Lethargy
- Infertility
- Physical findings: Enlarged, irregular, and firm uterus
- Ultrasound: Diagnostic imaging modality of choice
- Saline infusion sonohysterography and/or hysteroscopy: Used to evaluate the uterine cavity

abdominal girth and pressure symptoms as a result of large fibroids. Pressure on adjacent organs such as the bladder or bowel can cause urinary frequency and urgency or constipation. Rarely, an enlarged uterus causes a palpable kidney secondary to hydronephrosis from ureteral obstruction. Patients also may be lethargic from anemia secondary to menorrhagia. Leiomyomas may also be associated with infertility, although the relationship is controversial.

A rapidly enlarging uterus should raise concern for malignant transformation. But leiomyosarcomas are extremely rare, occurring in less than 0.1% of women operated on for presumed leiomyomas.

Diagnosis

Uterine leiomyomas are typically diagnosed at pelvic exam when an enlarged and irregularly shaped uterus is noted. Abdominal and transvaginal ultrasound is often helpful in making the diagnosis and in differentiating leiomyomas from adnexal masses or other pelvic pathology. Serial ultrasounds also can be used to monitor their growth. During a pelvic exam, it may not be possible to palpate ovaries next to an enlarged uterus, but an adnexal tumor can be suspected if the mass moves independently of the uterus. Submucosal leiomyomas are diagnosed using saline infusion sonohysterography and hysteroscopy. Definitive diagnosis requires histologic examination.

Management

For the most part, asymptomatic leiomyoma should be managed expectantly. The approaches to the patient experiencing problems fall into the three general categories of medical management, conservative procedures, and hysterectomy. The choice should be individualized to the patient, based on the severity of her symptoms, her plans for future childbearing, and her personal interest in retaining her uterus. Other causes of abnormal bleeding should be considered.

Current medical therapy is limited to the use of gonadotropin-releasing hormone (GnRH) analogues and antagonists (i.e., leuprolide acetate [Lupron Depot], 3.75 mg monthly; nafarelin acetate [Synarel],[1] 200 µg intranasally twice a day; and goserelin acetate implant [Zoladex],[1] 3.6-mg implant monthly, cetrorelix [Cetrotide]).[1] These expensive medications are shown to decrease the uterine size by up to 65%, allowing for easier or more conservative surgical treatments. The progesterone antagonist mifepristone (Mifeprex)[1] is also effective but not currently available for this purpose in the United States. GnRH therapy has significant side effects, mostly related to the induced hypoestrogenic state. To preserve bone density the duration of therapy must be limited. Additionally, the uterus rapidly returns to its enlarged size when the therapy is discontinued. These medications are a very effective means of inducing amenorrhea to allow for correction of an anemia prior to surgery.

---

[1]Not FDA approved for this indication.

TABLE 1 Comparison of Various Procedures for the Treatment of Symptomatic Uterine Leiomyoma

Therapy	Success Rate	Complication Rate	Possibility of Future Childbearing	Comments
Hysterectomy	100%	40%	No	Recovery time varies depending on the route of removal.
Myomectomy and myolysis	75%	39%	Yes	Can be associated with significant blood loss and can result in an unplanned hysterectomy. Recurrent leiomyomas are common.
Myolysis	62%–97%*	3%*	Not currently recommended	Several methods for myolysis are available, including bipolar electrocautery, laser energy, and cryotherapy.
Uterine artery embolization	77%–91%	5%	Not currently recommended	Complication rates are low but can be severe, including infection, sepsis, and nontarget tissue necrosis. A few deaths have been reported.
Hydrothermal endometrial ablation	80%–91%*	1%–2%	No	Hysteroscopic resection of submucosal leiomyomas, prior to endometrial ablation, improves success rates. Several methods are available, including hydrothermal, balloon, bipolar electrocautery, cryotherapy, and microwave endometrial ablation. Pregnancies have occurred after these procedures, so contraception is still required.

*Best estimate based on limited studies.

CURRENT THERAPY

- Only symptomatic leiomyomas require treatment.
- Medical therapy is for temporizing and making invasive procedures easier or more effective.
- Conservative procedures include myomectomy, myolysis, hydrothermal endometrial ablation, and uterine artery embolization.
- Hysterectomy is the only definitive therapy for leiomyomata.
- Choice of treatment should be made considering the severity of symptoms and respecting the patient's preferences.

Conservative procedures include myomectomy or myolysis (surgical removal or destruction of the individual fibroids while preserving the uterus), uterine artery embolization, and endometrial ablation. Each of these approaches has different risks, benefits, and complications (Table 1).

Hysterectomy remains the most common treatment for women with symptomatic leiomyoma and offers the advantage of a complete and definitive cure. The uterus can be removed through the vagina (with or without the aid of laparoscopic techniques) or through an abdominal incision. The route of removal largely depends on the size of the uterus, the patient's medical and surgical history, and the experience and preference of her surgeon.

REFERENCES

Buttram Jr VC, Reiter RC. Uterine leiomyomata: Etiology, symptomatology, and management. Fertil Steril 1981;36:433–45.

Felberbaum RE, Germer U, Ludwig M, et al. Treatment of uterine fibroids with a slow-release formulation of the gonadotrophin-releasing hormone antagonist Cetrorelix. Hum Reprod 1998;13(6):1660–8.

Goldfarb HA. Bipolar laparoscopic needles for myoma coagulation. J Am Assoc Gynecol Laparosc 1995;2(2):175–9.

Lethaby A, Vollenhoven B, Sowter M. Pre-operative GnRH analogue therapy before hysterectomy or myomectomy for uterine fibroids. The Cochrane Database Syst Rev 2001;(2):CD000547. DOI: 10.1002/14651858. CD000547.

Parker WH, Fu YS, Berek JS. Uterine sarcoma in patients operated on for presumed leiomyoma and rapidly growing leiomyoma. Obstet Gynecol 1994;83:414.

Pron G, Bennett J, Common A, et al. Ontario Uterine Fibroid Embolization Collaboration Group. The Ontario Uterine Fibroid Embolization Trial: II. Uterine fibroid reduction and symptom relief after uterine artery embolization for fibroids. Fertil Steril 2003;79(1):120–7.

The Hydro Therm Ablator system for management of menorrhagia in women with submucous myomas: 12- to 20-month follow-up. J Am Assoc Gynecol Laparosc 2003;10(4):521–7.

Cancer of the Endometrium

Method of
*D. Scott McMeekin, MD, and
Tashanna K. N. Myers, MD*

Epidemiology

Endometrial cancer is the most common gynecologic cancer facing women in the United States. The lifetime risk of endometrial cancer is currently 1 in 38. In 2007, approximately 39,000 women were found to have endometrial cancer, and 7400 (3%) women died from the disease. Endometrial cancer is the eighth leading cause of cancer death for women in the United States. African American women appear to have a poorer prognosis: Nearly twice than many (1.8:1) African American women die from endometrial cancer than white women.

Endometrial cancer primarily occurs in postmenopausal women, and the average age at onset is 60 years. Only 25% of patients are premenopausal, and of these, only 5% are younger than 40 years.

Etiology

Endometrial cancer is classically divided into two types (Table 1). Type I, the more common form, is associated with estrogen excess and often arises in the background of a precursor lesion, atypical hyperplasia. Type II tumors are rarer and more aggressive, and they arise in a background of atrophic endometrium or polyps.

TABLE 1 Comparison Between Type I and Type II Endometrial Cancers

Factor	Type I	Type II
Clinical Features		
Risk factors	Unopposed estrogen	Age
Race	White > African American	White = African American
Differentiation	Well differentiated	Poorly differentiated
Histology	Endometrioid	PS, CC, Grade 3
Stage	Early	Advanced
Prognosis	Favorable	Poorer
Molecular Features		
Ploidy	Diploid	Aneuploid
K-ras over expression	Yes	Yes
her-2/neu over expression	No	Yes
p53 mutation	No	Yes
PTEN mutation	Yes	No
Microsatellite instability	Yes	No

Abbreviations: CC = clear cell; PS = papillary serous.

The etiology is unclear. Despite the broad generalizations of the two categories, molecular and genetic changes differentiate these two groups as well. For example, mutations of *p53* are common in papillary serous tumors and are rare in type I tumors. *PTEN* mutations are common in type I tumors but are rare in papillary serous tumors. Global gene expression profiles also differ between type I and type II tumors.

Increased exposure to endogenous or exogenous estrogen increases the risk of developing type I cancers. Since the 1970s, unopposed estrogen use has been a known risk factor, prompting the routine addition of a progestin in combination with hormone replacement therapy regimens. Endogenous exposure to estrogens associated with obesity or chronic anovulation (polycystic ovary syndrome) are believed to be more common etiologies.

Other factors associated with an increased risk of developing endometrial cancer include late menopause (older than 52 years), nulliparity, diabetes, hypertension, or a diagnosis of complex atypical hyperplasia. In contrast, normal weight, oral contraceptives, progestin use, cigarette smoking, and multiparity have been associated with a decreased incidence of endometrial cancer. Type II tumors account for a small percentage of endometrial cancers, occur in an older population, and account for nearly one half of all relapses. Papillary serous, clear cell, and perhaps, grade 3 tumors fit into the type II category. Tamoxifen (Nolvadex) used in the prophylaxis of, or treatment for, breast cancer is an established risk factor for developing either type I or type II tumors.

Presentation and Diagnosis

Patients with endometrial cancer most commonly present with abnormal bleeding. Papanicolaou (Pap) smears detect only 30% to 50% of endometrial cancers and are not useful for diagnosing endometrial cancer. The diagnosis of endometrial cancer is most commonly made by biopsy. An endometrial biopsy can usually be performed in the office and has greater than 90% diagnostic accuracy. The histologic classification of endometrial cancers is listed in Box 1. Ultrasound has also been used to evaluate abnormal bleeding. Studies show that endometrial cancers are exceedingly uncommon if the endometrial thickness is less than 5 mm on ultrasound in postmenopausal women. Symptomatic patients with a thickened endometrium or patients with persistent bleeding despite a thin lining should have a histologic evaluation.

Currently there is no good screening test for endometrial cancer, and thus there are no screening recommendations. A high degree of suspicion should be maintained for women who have received unopposed estrogens or for patients with vaginal bleeding who are

---

BOX 1 Histologic Classification of Endometrial Cancers

- Endometrioid adenocarcinoma (includes adenosquamous carcinoma)
- Mucinous carcinoma
- Serous carcinoma
- Clear cell carcinoma
- Squamous carcinoma
- Undifferentiated carcinoma
- Mixed carcinoma

---

postmenopausal, obese, or taking tamoxifen. Hereditary syndromes (Lynch's) account for 3% to 5% of endometrial cancers and are seen in patients with strong familial histories of hereditary nonpolyposis colorectal, ovarian, and pancreatic cancers.

Staging

Endometrial cancer is surgically staged according to the 1988 criteria established by the International Federation of Gynecology and Obstetrics (FIGO) (Table 2). Staging includes collection of pelvic washings for cytology, a hysterectomy with removal of bilateral fallopian tubes and ovaries, and pelvic and para-aortic lymph node dissection. Controversies currently exist as to who should undergo lymph node dissection (all, some, or few patients), the type of nodal dissection (sampling or complete lymphadenectomy), and when to use adjuvant therapies.

The most important pathologic prognostic indicators include histologic grade, depth of invasion and lymph node status. The Gynecologic Oncology Group (GOG) performed a surgical pathologic study evaluating 621 patients with endometrial cancer and demonstrated important associations between grade, depth of myometrial invasion, and nodal involvement. For example, patients with deeply invasive (extending into the outer two thirds of the myometrium) tumors had pelvic nodal metastases between 11% and 34%, depending on tumor grade.

Fortunately, most women with endometrial cancer have stage I disease and have a favorable prognosis (Table 3). The 5-year survival for stage I disease approaches 90%, but the 5-year survival for women with stage IV (abdominal or distant spread) disease is only about 10%.

TABLE 2 FIGO (1988) Surgical Staging System for Endometrial Cancer

Stage	Description
IA	Tumor is confined to the endometrium
IB	Tumor is confined to less than one half of the myometrium
IC	Tumor is confined to more than one half of the myometrium
IIA	Cervical involvement is limited to the endocervical glands
IIB	Cervical involvement includes cervical stroma
IIIA	Tumor involves uterine serosa or adnexa or positive peritoneal cytology
IIIB	Vaginal metastases
IIIC	Tumor involves pelvic or para-aortic lymph nodes
IVA	Tumor involves bladder or bowel mucosa
IVB	Distant metastases including intra-abdominal and inguinal lymph node involvement

Abbreviation: FIGO = International Federation of Gynecology and Obstetrics.

Treatment

SURGICAL MANAGEMENT

Surgical management continues to evolve. The GOG has recently completed a large prospective trial evaluating the role of laparoscopic hysterectomy and nodal dissection compared with an abdominal approach. The study, evaluating more than 2500 patients, found that laparoscopic management was feasible, and 76% of the time patients randomized to laparoscopy could have the procedure performed without conversion to laparotomy. The numbers of nodes removed and the frequency of finding positive lymph nodes were similar in the two treatment arms. Despite an increased operative time, results showed that laparoscopic surgery resulted in a shorter hospital stay.

The benefits of routine nodal dissection include better stratification of patients into high-, intermediate-, or low risk-categories, reduced use of postoperative therapies for most node-negative patients, and improved identification of a subset of patients with nodal metastases who might benefit from adjuvant therapies. Information from a lymph node dissection is prognostic, but a lymphadenectomy is potentially therapeutic. Today, the more frequent use of nodal dissection has resulted in the less-frequent use of postoperative pelvic irradiation therapy.

Without information on nodal status, physicians and patients must decide whether or not to use postoperative therapies based on perceived risk determined from the hysterectomy findings. Because of this, many have recommended that a second surgery to complete the surgical staging be performed when only a hysterectomy was performed. Laparoscopic restaging is often a feasible approach. The risk

TABLE 3 Estimates of Distribution and Survival of Endometrial Cancer by Stage

Stage	Distribution of Cases (%)	5-Year Survival (%)
Stage IA	22	92
Stage IB	37	88
Stage IC	13	78
Stage II	9	72
Stage III	15	53
Stage IV	4	10

CURRENT DIAGNOSIS

- Patients with postmenopausal bleeding warrant endometrial biopsy.
- Patients at risk include those with abnormal bleeding and obesity, chronic anovulation, and unopposed estrogen or tamoxifen (Nolvadex) exposure.
- Office biopsy should be performed when possible, and D&C should be performed if office biopsy is not available or biopsy results are equivocal.
- Malignancy is unlikely if the endometrial stripe/thickness is less than 5 mm on ultrasound.

Abbreviation: D&C = dilation and curettage.

of nodal dissection must be balanced by the information provided. Serious complications related to nodal dissection include bleeding and visceral injury, and complications have been reported to occur in less than 2% of surgeries. Lower extremity lymphedema appears to be more common but is rarely severe.

ADJUVANT THERAPY

Early Stage Disease

Two large trials have evaluated the role of post-operative pelvic radiation in patients with early stage (stage I to occult stage II) endometrial cancer. In the PORTEC trial, 715 patients were randomized to pelvic radiation or surveillance. Lymph node dissection was not performed. Most patients had low-grade tumors (90% grade 1–2), and about 50% had superficial myometrial invasion (<50% invasion). Results showed that although radiation could reduce local and

CURRENT THERAPY

- Surgical therapy is the mainstay of endometrial cancer treatment. Laparoscopic surgery is increasingly being used.
- Surgical staging, including pelvic and para-aortic lymph node dissection, is recommended.
- The best way to define risk is to identify patients with nodal disease.
- Staging typically requires referral to a gynecologic oncologist.
- Unstaged patients may be considered for a restaging operation.
- Most patients have stage I (uterine-confined) disease.
- Low-risk patients—stages IA and IB, grades 1 or 2—require no additional therapy.
- Intermediate-risk patients—stage IB grade 3 and stage IC grades 1 or 2—require no additional therapy or vaginal cuff brachytherapy.
- High-intermediate-risk patients are those 50 years old with two risk factors or older than 70 years with one risk factor. Risk factors are:
  - Grade 2 or 3 tumor
  - Lymphovascular space involvement
  - Outer one third myometrial invasion
  - Stage I plus papillary serous or clear cell histology
- Treatment of these patients is controversial. There is no clear consensus regarding performing no additional therapy, performing vaginal cuff brachytherapy with or without chemotherapy, or performing pelvic radiation therapy.

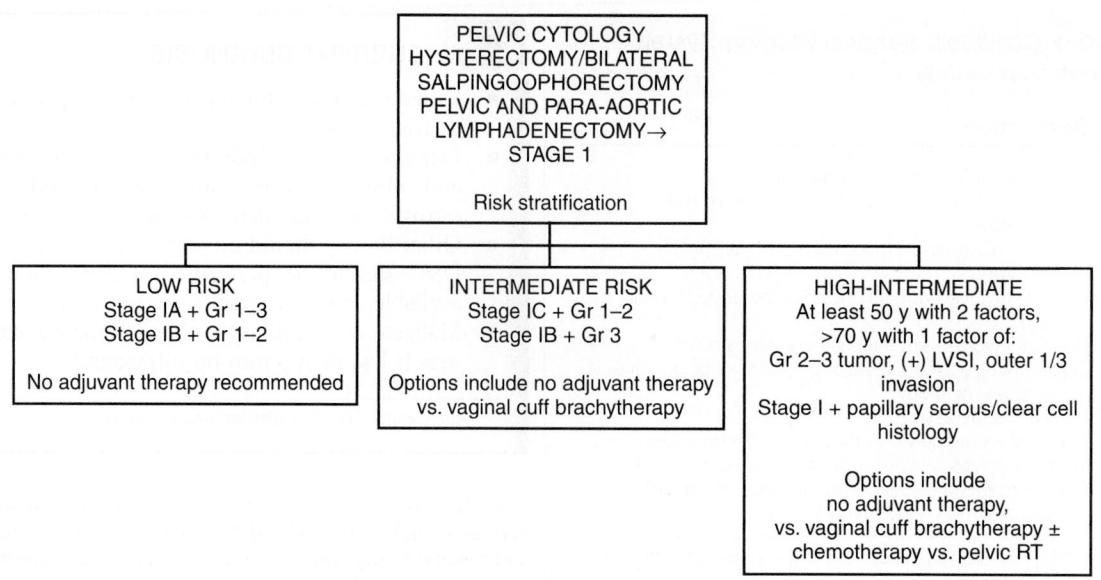

FIGURE 1. Postoperative treatment algorithm used at the University of Oklahoma for surgical staged endometrial carcinoma. Surgical staging allows risk stratification based on pathologic factors. *Abbreviations:* Gr = grade; LVSI = lymphovascular space involvement, RT = radiation therapy.

regional recurrences (14% vs. 4% with radiation), 5-year survival was 81% with and 85% without radiation. Similarly, the GOG performed a study with 392 patients with grades 1 to 3 tumors and any amount of myometrial invasion. All patients had a specified lymph node dissection and received either pelvic radiation or no additional therapy. Results showed that radiation reduced local recurrences but did not appreciably affect survival (4-year survival was 92% with radiation, 86% without radiation).

The lack of benefit from pelvic radiation in these studies may be due to the excellent outcomes seen in the low-risk populations enrolled in these studies. For example, in the GOG trial, only 18% of patients had grade 3 tumors, and 31% had deep myometrial invasion. The GOG trial did suggest that a subgroup of patients at higher risk for recurrence could be defined based on age, tumor grade, depth of invasion, and the presence of lymph-vascular space invasion. These high-intermediate risk patients represented one third of the total population but accounted for two thirds of recurrences, suggesting that it might be possible to identify some patients for whom radiation might offer a benefit.

The PORTEC and GOG studies also showed that vaginal cuff recurrences were the most common site of failure without radiation, and authors for both studies suggested that vaginal cuff brachytherapy might be a reasonable alternative to for pelvic radiation. Several studies have demonstrated excellent vaginal cuff control with the use of less toxic and more tolerable vaginal cuff brachytherapy. A proposed treatment algorithm is shown in Figure 1.

Patients with papillary serous and clear cell tumors are believed by many to be at particularly increased risk for recurrence. Extrauterine disease spread is common at initial presentation, making complete surgical staging especially important in these patients. Even patients with stage I disease have a risk of failure near 30% to 50%. Chemotherapy has been increasingly advocated for this group of patients.

Advanced and Recurrent Disease

Radiation therapy (pelvic, pelvic with an extended field to treat para-aortic nodes, and whole abdominal) has been the treatment of choice for patients with disease spread outside of the uterus. Recently, the GOG presented data showing improved progression-free and overall survival when chemotherapy (doxorubicin and cisplatin) was used compared with whole abdominal radiation in patients with stage III or IV disease. As a result, chemotherapy has been increasingly used in first-line management. Combining radiation with chemotherapy is being actively explored in clinical trials.

For patients with bulky advanced or recurrent disease, hormone therapy with progestins has been a long-standing treatment. Patients with grade 1 tumors, or those with estrogen- and progesterone-receptor positive tumors have shown the greatest likelihood of benefit. Chemotherapy has been increasingly integrated in a first-line setting for many patients due to the identification of several active agents. The most active agents include paclitaxel,[1] doxorubicin,[1] and platinum analogues.[1] Combinations of these agents have resulted in improved response rates, and the three-drug paclitaxel plus doxorubicin plus cisplatin regimen has been shown to have improved survival over the two-drug doxorubicin plus cisplatin regimen. Given the advanced age and concurrent medical comorbidities that are seen in patients with endometrial cancer, a careful balance between treatment objectives and toxicity must be made.

Future Directions

Increasing the understanding of endometrial cancer at a genetic and molecular level is a primary goal of current research. This information might provide insights into the prognosis and predict benefits of particular therapies. Targeted biological agents are currently being explored in patients with endometrial cancer, and their use in combination with cytotoxic chemotherapy agents might result in improved outcomes, as seen in other solid tumors such as breast and colon cancers.

REFERENCES

American College of Obstetricians and Gynecologists. ACOG practice bulletin, management guidelines for obstetrician-gynecologists, number 65, August 2005: Management of endometrial cancer. Obstet Gynecol 2005;106:413–25.

Cragun J, Havrilesky L, Calingaert B, et al. Retrospective analysis of selective lymphadenectomy in apparent early-stage endometrial cancer. J Clin Oncol 2005;23:3668–75.

Creasman W, Kohler M, Odicino F, et al. Prognosis of papillary serous, clear cell, and grade 3 stage I carcinoma of the endometrium. Gynecol Oncol 2004;95:593–6.

Creasman WT, Morrow CP, Bundy BN, et al. Surgical pathologic spread patterns of endometrial cancer. Cancer 1987;60:2035–41.

Creutzberg C, van Putten W, Koper P, et al. Surgery and post-operative radiotherapy versus surgery alone for patients with stage 1 endometrial carcinoma: Multi-center randomized trial. Lancet 2000;355:1404–11.

---

[1]Not FDA approved for this indication.

Fleming G, Brunetto V, Cella D, et al. Phase III trial of doxorubicin plus cisplatin with or without paclitaxel plus filgrastim in advanced endometrial cancer: A Gynecologic Oncology Group study. J Clin Oncol 2004;22:2159–66.

Keys H, Roberts J, Brunetto V, et al. A phase III trial of surgery with or without adjuvant external pelvic radiation therapy in intermediate risk endometrial adenocarcinoma: A Gynecologic Oncology Group study. Gynecol Oncol 2004;92:744–51.

Kilgore LC, Partridge EE, Alvarez RD, et al. Adenocarcinoma of the endometrium: Survival comparisons of patients with and without pelvic node sampling. Gynecol Oncol 1995;56:29–33.

Randall M, Filiaci G, Muss H, et al. Whole abdominal radiotherapy versus combination doxorubicin-cisplatin chemotherapy in advanced endometrial carcinoma: A randomized phase III trial of the Gynecologic Oncology Group. J Clin Oncol 2006;24:36–44.

Straughn JM, Huh WK, Kelly FJ, et al. Conservative management of stage I endometrial carcinoma after surgical staging. Gynecol Oncol 2002;84:191–3.

Cancer of the Uterine Cervix

Method of
Nader Husseinzadeh, MD

Invasive cervical cancer accounts for 2% to 3% of all cancers in women in the United States. Incidence and mortality from cervical cancer have declined dramatically with early detection and treatment of preinvasive disease. It is estimated that approximately 11,070 new cases will be diagnosed and 3870 patients died from cervical cancer in 2008 worldwide. Both incidence of and mortality from cervical cancer are second to breast cancer. Cervical cancer is a largely preventable disease with a known causative agent, the human papillomavirus (HPV), especially types 16 and 18.

Epidemiology

Age-specific incidences for white women are lower than those for African American women. Major risk factors for cervical cancer are listed in Box 1.

Some epidemiologic studies have shown that women using oral contraceptives tend to have more sexual contacts. Cigarette smoking has been linked to an increased risk of squamous cell carcinoma, and presence of nicotine byproduct as a carcinogen in cervical mucous or the partner's semen are possible explanations. Reduced risk of cervical cancer is noted in virgins and in women whose sexual partners were circumcised.

Etiology and Pathogenesis

The etiology of cervical cancer is unknown. Numerous studies have indicated a close association between HPV and cervical cancer.

BOX 1   Major Risk Factors for Cervical Cancer

- Immunosuppression (e.g., transplant, infection with HIV)
- Multiple pregnancies
- Multiple sexual partners
- Promiscuous sexual activity
- Sexually transmitted disease (herpes simplex virus, chlamydia, and human papillomavirus)
- Smoking
- Sexual activity at a young age

Although HPV appears to be the causative agent, many other changes at the molecular level have been identified that might not directly involve HPV. The molecular oncogenesis in cervical carcinoma can be explained to a degree by the regulation and function of two viral proteins, E6 and E7. The *E6* gene binds to the *p53* tumor suppressor gene and induces degradation. The *E7* gene binds another tumor suppressor, the retinoblastoma gene *(Rb)*. By binding to it, it functionally inactivates the protein, which like p53, works in cell cycle. There are more than 100 types of HPV, stratified into low-, intermediate-, and high-risk categories based on the strength of their association with invasive lesions. High-risk HPV types exhibit greater inactivation of *p53* and *Rb* genes.

The link between human leukocyte antigens (HLAs) and HPV might help to explain why the same HPV type leads to invasive cancer in one patient but not in another. It has been established that cervical dysplasia in HIV-infected women is associated with higher incidence, more rapid progression, and higher recurrence rates when compared with HIV-negative women.

Staging

Cervical cancer is staged clinically. Surgical-pathologic staging is superior to clinical staging. It provides useful information regarding the extent of disease and status of pelvic and para-aortic lymph nodes (Box 2).

BOX 2   FIGO Staging for Carcinoma of the Cervix

- Stage 0: Carcinoma in situ, intraepithelial carcinoma
- Stage I: The carcinoma is strictly confined to the cervix; extension to the corpus should be disregarded.
  - Stage IA: Invasive carcinoma diagnosed only by microscopy; all visible lesions, even with superficial invasion, are stage IB.
  - Stage IA1: Invasion of stroma is less than 3.0 mm^2, and the horizontal spread must not exceed 7.0 mm^2.
  - Stage IA2: Invasion of stroma is greater than 3.0 mm^2 and not more than 5.0 mm, and the horizontal spread is 7.0 mm or less. Larger lesions should be classified as stage IB.
  - Stage IB: Clinically visible lesions confined to the cervix or lesions of greater dimensions than stage IA2
  - Stage IB1: Clinically visible lesions no greater than 4.0 cm or less in greatest dimension
  - Stage IB2: Clinically visible lesions greater than 4.0 cm
- Stage II: The carcinoma extends beyond the cervix but not to the pelvic wall or to the lower one third of the vagina.
  - Stage IIA: Without parametrial invasion, involving upper one half of the vagina
  - Stage IIB: Tumor with parametrial invasion
- Stage III: The tumor extends to the pelvic wall or involves the lower one third of the vagina or causes hydronephrosis or nonfunctioning kidney.
  - Stage IIIA: Tumor involves lower one third of the vagina, no extension to the pelvic wall
  - Stage IIIB: Tumor extends to pelvic wall and/or causes hydronephrosis or nonfunctioning kidney
- Stage IV: The tumor has extended beyond the true pelvis or has involved the mucosa of the bladder or rectum. A bullous edema does not qualify as a criterion for stage IV disease.
  - Stage IVA: Tumor spread to adjacent organs (bladder, rectum, or both)
  - Stage IVB: Distant metastasis

Abbreviation: FIGO = International Federation of Gynecology and Obstetrics.

SYMPTOMATOLOGY

The symptoms related to cervical cancer vary according to the extent of the disease. Symptomatic patients with early-stage disease usually present with watery, blood-tinged, purulent (malodorous) discharge or commonly postcoital bleeding. Advanced-stage patients usually have leg and flank pain, leg edema, constipation, rectal bleeding, or hematuria.

PHYSICAL FINDINGS

The gross appearance of cervical cancer varies depending on whether the lesion is exophytic, endophytic, or ulcerative. Exophytic growths that characteristically bleed on contact are the most common type of cervical cancer. Sometimes the cancer develops entirely within the endocervical canal, manifesting as a hard, indurated, and often barrel-shaped lesion. The cancer can also appear as a small, shallow ulcer.

HISTOPATHOLOGY

Squamous cell carcinoma is the most common type of cervical cancer. Adenocarcinoma and other carcinomas are less common (Box 3).

PATHOPHYSIOLOGY

Cervical cancer in the early stage invades lymphatics in the parametrium and pelvic lymph nodes through tumor emboli. As the primary lesion progresses, the tumor extends to the pelvic side wall laterally, to the bladder base anteriorly, and, less frequently, to the rectum posteriorly.

SPREAD PATTERN

Cervical cancer exhibits three spread patterns. Direct extension is to parametrial tissue and the pelvic wall (ureter), to the bladder and rectum, or to the uterine corpus and vagina. Lymphatic spread is of two kinds. The primary group involves the paracervical, obturator, hypogastric, and external iliac lymph nodes, and the secondary group involves the common iliac, inguinal, and aortic lymph nodes. Hematogenous spread is to the lung, liver, bone, and brain.

EXAMINATION AND TESTING

The initial work-up includes history and physical examination; chest x-ray, intravenous pyelogram (IVP), or computed tomography (CT); and HIV testing (Box 4). Some centers do not routinely use IVP and CT or cystoscopy and protosigmoidoscopy for early-stage disease because of relatively low yield. In patients who are not candidates for surgery, a CT scan can be helpful in assessing nodal disease. Enlarged lymph nodes should be studied histocytologically by either surgical excision or fine-needle aspiration because of the 5% to 10% false-positive rate of a CT scan. More recently, magnetic resonance imaging (MRI) has been studied for early parametrial and nodal

---

BOX 3 Histopathology of Cervical Cancer

- Squamous cell carcinoma (80%)
- Nonsquamous carcinoma (15%)
  - Adenocarcinoma
  - Adenosquamous carcinoma
  - Clear cell adenocarcinoma
  - Glassy cell carcinoma
  - Small cell (neuroendocrine) carcinoma
- Other carcinomas (5%)
  - Choriocarcinoma
  - Melanoma
  - Metastatic: uterus (most common), then breast, stomach, and bladder; leukemia and lymphoma are rare
  - Sarcoma: stromal sarcoma, leiomyosarcoma, mixed mesodermal sarcoma, rhabdomyosarcoma

---

BOX 4 Cervical Cancer Work-up

- History and physical
- Chest x-ray
- Intravenous pyelogram
- Computed tomography of the abdomen and pelvis
- Cystoscopy or proctosigmoidoscopy
- Magnetic resonance imaging (possibly)
- Positron emission tomography (possibly)

---

disease. Positron emission tomography (PET) has been reported as useful to predict para-aortic disease. Because of infrequent colon involvement, sigmoidoscopy or barium enema should be restricted to symptomatic patients or those with a positive guaiac test.

Treatment

SURGERY AND RADIATION

In general, early-stage cervical cancer can be treated with radical hysterectomy or radiation. However, surgery is preferred for premenopausal women to preserve ovarian function and a functioning vagina following surgery. In patients with high-risk criteria—positive surgical margin, parametrial involvement, and positive pelvic nodes—cisplatin-based chemoradiation is usually recommended. Those with intermediate risk factors such as tumor size greater than 4 cm, deep cervical stromal invasion greater than 50%, or lymphovascular invasion might also benefit from chemoradiation.

Radical trachelectomy is a reasonable alternative treatment for select young patients who desire to maintain their childbearing capacity. The criteria include early-stage cervical cancer with a lesion less than 2 cm, no lymphovascular invasion, and no lymph node metastasis.

Laparoscopic-assisted radical vaginal hysterectomy (LARVH), like other surgical procedures, may be considered in select patients with early-stage cervical cancer. Reported advantages are less blood loss, better cosmetic results, shorter hospitalization, and earlier recovery.

CHEMORADIATION THERAPY

Squamous cell carcinoma of the cervix is a chemosensitive malignancy, particularly when cisplatinum-based chemotherapy is being used. In February 1999, the National Cancer Institute published a consensus statement demonstrating superiority of platinum-based chemoradiation compared with radiation alone for locally advanced cervical cancer (stage IIB-IVA), high-risk early-stage cervical cancer (IA2-IIA2), or bulky stage IB cervical cancer (Table 1).

Since then, chemoradiation has become the standard of care, and cisplatinum has shown the best activity as a single agent in cervical cancer, with a 20% to 30% objective response. Tumor cytotoxicity is intensified when cisplatinum is combined with radiation at the same time. Clinical studies have chiefly included neoadjuvant chemotherapy or a combination of chemotherapy and radiation when given together.

Although chemoradiation is associated with higher toxicity and increased cost, there is some economic benefit from less disease recurrence and subsequent medical costs.

THERAPY BY STAGE

Stage IA1

Patients with no lymphovascular invasion and tumor invasion to less than 3 mm (stage IA1) have less than 1% risk of nodal metastasis. The decision to proceed with conization versus abdominal or vaginal hysterectomy is based on the patient's desire for childbearing. Women with stage IA1 cancer may be treated by conization alone, provided that all cone margins are free of disease and endocervical curettage is negative. When lymphovascular invasion is present and tumor invasion is less than 3 mm, most physicians prefer modified radical hysterectomy over radiation.

TABLE 1 Concurrent Chemoradiation for Cervical Cancer

Reference	Study	FIGO Stages	Patients	Treatment Regimen	Overall Survival
Whitney et al	GOG 85	IIB-IVA	368	Cisplatin[1]/5-FU[1] + RT	67%
				Hydroxyurea[1] + RT	57%
Rose et al	GOG 120	IIB-IVA	526	Weekly cisplatin + RT	65%
				Cisplatin/5-FU/hydroxyurea + RT	65%
				Hydroxyurea + RT	47%
Morris et al	RTOG 9001	IB2-IVA*	388	Cisplatin/5-FU + RT	75%
				RT alone	63%
Keys et al	GOG 123	IB2[†]	369	Weekly cisplatin + R	83%
				RT	74%
Peters et al	GOG 109, SWOG 8797	IA2-IIA	243	Cisplatin/5-FU + RT	81%
				RT	71%

Data from National Cancer Institute: Concurrent chemoradiation for cervical cancer. Clinical announcement, Washington, DC, February 22, 1999.
[1]Not FDA approved for this indication.
*Stages IB and IIA required positive pelvic nodes or tumor size >5 cm.
[†]Extrafascial hysterectomy followed by chemoradiation or radiation.
References cited in the table:
Keys HM, Bundy BN, Stehman FB, et al. Cisplatin, radiation and adjuvant hysterectomy compared with radiation and adjuvant hysterectomy for bulky stage IB cervical carcinoma. N Engl J Med 1999;340(15):1154–1161.
Morris M, Eifel PJ, Lu J, et al: Pelvic radiation with concurrent chemotherapy compared with pelvic and para-aortic radiation for high-risk cervical cancer. N Engl J Med 1999;340(15):1137–1143.
Peters WA 3rd, Liu PY, Barrett RJ 2nd, et al. Concurrent chemotherapy and pelvic radiation therapy compared with pelvic radiation therapy alone as adjuvant therapy after radical surgery in high-risk early-stage cancer of the cervix. J Clin Oncol 2000;18(8):1606–1613.
Rose PG, Bundy BN, Watkins EB, et al. Concurrent cisplatin-based radiotherapy and chemotherapy for locally advanced cervical cancer. N Engl J Med 1999;340 (15):1144–1153.
Whitney CW, Sause W, Bundy BN, et al. Randomized comparison of fluorouracil plus cisplatin versus hydroxyurea as an adjunct to radiation therapy in stage IIB-IVA carcinoma of the cervix with negative para-aortic lymph nodes: A Gynecologic Oncology Group and Southwest Oncology Group study, J Clin Oncol 1999;17(5):1339–1348.
Abbreviations: FIGO = International Federation of Gynecology and Obstetrics; 5-FU = 5-fluorouracil; GOG = Gynecologic Oncology Group; RT = radiation therapy; RTOG = Radiation Therapy Oncology Group; SWOG = SouthWest Oncology Group.

Stage IA2

For patients with stroma invasion more than 3 mm or those with lymphovascular space involvement, the preferred treatment is modified or radical hysterectomy with pelvic lymphadenectomy. Radical trachelectomy with pelvic lymphadenectomy has been performed in women who desire further childbearing, with some women successfully becoming pregnant.

Stage IB

Patients with stage IB1 (tumor size <4 cm) can effectively be treated by radical hysterectomy with or without pelvic or para-aortic lymphadenectomy. Radiation therapy can be used in patients with stage 1A2 or 1B, particularly in those who are not medically suitable for radical surgery.

Treatment for patients with Stage 1B2 (bulky or barrel-shaped lesions) is the same as for stage 1B1. However, many of these tumors extend anatomically beyond the curative isodose curve of the radiation field and have significant central recurrences. Therefore, preoperative radiation therapy followed by extrafascial hysterectomy has been recommended.

Because nodal metastases are present in 20% to 25% of patients with stage 1B2 cervical cancers, para-aortic lymph node dissection should be considered at the time of hysterectomy if the para-aortic nodes were not included in the preoperative radiation fields.

Stage IIA

The optimal treatment for most patients with stage IIA cervical cancer is similar to that for stage 1B: Patients may be treated effectively by radical hysterectomy with pelvic and para-aortic lymphadenectomy and upper vaginectomy, provided that all surgical margins are free of disease. Many authors recommend postoperative whole pelvic radiation for patients with microscopic parametrial invasion, nodal metastasis, and involvement of resection margins. Morbidity from radiation therapy limited to 4500 to 5000 cGy appears acceptable; however, local recurrence is decreased, and the survival advantage, if any, is not known.

Stages IIB to IVA

For patients with locally advanced cervical cancer, primary radiation therapy (external beam and brachytherapy) and concomitant chemotherapy is recommended. Para-aortic nodal involvement is the most important prognostic factor in patients' survival. In the absence of para-aortic nodal metastasis, transposition of both ovaries in young women should be considered.

Elective para-aortic radiation is an alternative to surgical para-aortic lymphadenectomy. The two main methods of radiation for cervical cancer are external beam radiation and brachytherapy. Brachytherapy can be performed by either the intracavity technique or by the interstitial technique, using needles or after-loading catheters. Interstitial brachytherapy is used when cervical cancer cannot be optimally encompassed by intracavity applications.

Potential complications of radiation therapy can be acute occurring during treatment or they can be delayed, usually occurring 1.5 to 2 years after treatment is completed (Boxes 5 and 6).

Recurrence

It is estimated that approximately 35% of patients with invasive cervical cancer will have recurrent or persistent disease following therapy. Recurrence can be expected in 10% to 20% of patients treated with radical hysterectomy and lymphadenectomy. Most recurrences are distant metastasis involving the lung, bone, abdominal cavity, and supraclavicular lymph nodes.

Prognosis for patients with recurrent disease is more favorable in those with a small (<3 cm) central recurrence, no sidewall involvement, and longer disease-free interval.

SURGERY

Patients with central pelvic recurrences after primary treatment with radiation therapy may be salvaged with surgery. Those with small recurrences limited to the cervix or upper vagina can occasionally be treated with modified radical hysterectomy and upper vaginectomy

---

BOX 5 Complications of Radiation Therapy in Cervical Cancer

Intestinal
- Abdominal cramps, diarrhea
- Malabsorption
- Nausea and vomiting
- Stricture causing bowel obstruction
- Ulceration, bleeding, and perforation causing rectovaginal fistula

Urinary
- Dysuria and urinary frequency
- Hematuria that can progress to perforation, causing vesicovaginal fistula or scarring, resulting in smaller bladder capacity and incontinence
- Ureteral stricture, hydroureter, and hydronephrosis

Vaginal
- Decreased vaginal lubrication
- Dyspareunia
- Shortening and stenosis

Vascular
- Fibrosis and thrombosis of pelvic vessels, causing leg edema

---

with excellent results. Patients with larger central recurrences or those who have received previous high-dose radiation require pelvic exenteration for salvage therapy.

Recently, more attention has been directed to reconstructive procedures performed at the time of pelvic exenterations to improve quality of life. These include performing continent urinary diversion, primary colon reanastomosis, and vaginal reconstructions with myocutaneous flap.

RADIATION THERAPY

Radiation therapy may be useful in patients with localized central pelvic recurrence after radical hysterectomy or as palliation to control symptoms such as bleeding and pelvic pain.

BOX 6 Complications of Radical Hysterectomy in Cervical Cancer

Intestinal
- Ileus, bowel obstruction
- Rectal atony, rectal injury
- Rectovaginal fistula

Urinary
- Bladder atony, bladder injury resulting in vesicovaginal fistula
- Ureteral injury causing stricture or hydroureter and ureterovaginal fistula

Vaginal
- Dyspareunia
- Shortening vagina

Vascular
- Vascular injury, deep vein thrombosis, causing leg edema and pulmonary embolism
- Lymphocyst formation and lymphedema exist but are uncommon

CHEMOTHERAPY

Cervical cancer is a slow-growing neoplasm with poor response to chemotherapy. Cisplatinum (cisplatin)[1] remains the drug of choice for treating recurrences, although phase II trials are currently examining the efficacies of a broad range of compounds such as topotecan, paclitaxel,[1] and gemcitabine.[1] Combination therapy with agents such as paclitaxel and cisplatinum has been studied in phase II trials of recurrent or advanced squamous cell cancer of the cervix with 12% complete responses and 34% partial responses, although 61% of patients experienced severe neutropenia. Given the palliative nature of chemotherapy in recurrent disease, the quality of life and drug toxicity must be factored into the choice of agents.

The encouraging activity of topotecan plus cisplatin in phase II trials led to the comparison of this combination against single-agent cisplatin in GOG 179. The main goals of this trial were overall response rate, progression-free survival, and quality of life.

GOG 204 is a randomized phase III trial with four treatment arms designed to evaluate the efficacy and tolerability of cisplatin-based doublets in the treatment of primary stage IVB, recurrent, or persistent cervical cancer (Figure 1).

In addition to the exploration of new doublets, the incorporation of biological agents such as erlotinab[1] and bevacizumab[1] into the treatment of cervical cancer are ongoing as GOG phase II multicenter trials.

FOLLOW-UP

Most recurrence occurs in the first 2 years following primary therapy. Therefore, physical examination with nodal assessment, abdominal examination, pelvic examination including rectovaginal examination, and Pap smear should be done at 3-month intervals for the first year, at 4-month intervals for the second year, and at 6-month intervals thereafter. After 5 years, an annual examination appears to be appropriate. Interval chest x-ray and abdominal CT scanning should be considered. Symptoms of pain, bleeding, and gastrointestinal or genitourinary dysfunction should be investigated for possible recurrence.

Preliminary results did indicate that the paclitaxel and cisplatin arm was superior to other combinations.

---

[1]Not FDA approved for this indication.

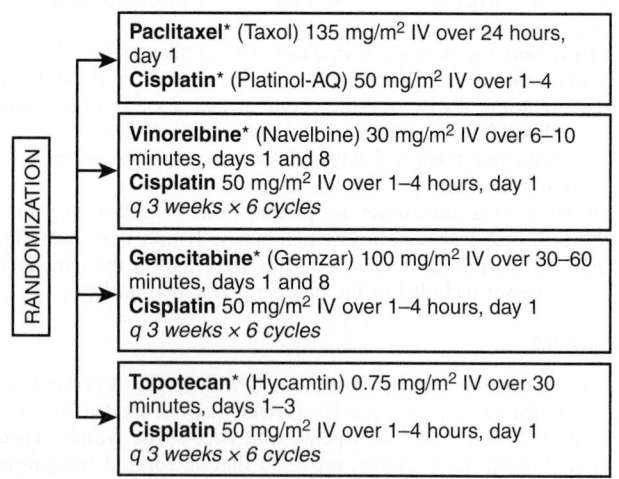

FIGURE 1. Treatment schema of the Randomized Phase III Study of Paclitaxel Plus Cisplatin vs. Vinorelbine Plus Cisplatin vs. Gemcitabine Plus Cisplatin vs. Topotecan Plus Cisplatin in Stage IVB, Recurrent, or Persistent Carcinoma of the Cervix (GOG 204). *Abbreviation:* GOG = Gynecologic Oncology Group.

Special Categories

CARCINOMA OF THE CERVICAL STUMP

Although supracervical hysterectomy is now rarely performed, carcinoma of the cervical stump is still encountered. Stage for stage, it is treated the same as cervical carcinoma of the intact uterus; for early stages, radical cervicectomy and parametrectomy with pelvic and possible para-aortic lymphadenopathy is performed. When radiation therapy is required, the short cervix often limits the amount of intracavitary radiation, therefore requiring higher-dose external irradiation.

INVASIVE CERVICAL CANCER AFTER HYSTERECTOMY

Occasionally, diagnosis of unsuspected invasive cervical cancer is made after a hysterectomy for a benign disease. Those with microinvasive disease do not require additional therapy. Those with invasive cancer confined to the cervix can be treated with radical parametrectomy, upper vaginectomy, and pelvic and para-aortic lymphadenopathy. The alternative is radiation therapy with or without chemotherapy.

INVASIVE CERVICAL CANCER DURING PREGNANCY

Pregnancy does not appear to affect the prognoses of patients with cervical cancer, and the fetus is not affected by maternal cervical cancer. However, the fetus might suffer consequences from treatment.

Patients with microinvasion diagnosed with conization can continue pregnancy until term and deliver vaginally. Before fetal maturity, patients should be treated individually, and the concerns for fetal survival must be weighed against the risk of delayed therapy.

Patients with stages IA2 to IIA can be treated by radical hysterectomy and pelvic lymphadenectomy with the fetus in situ. If the patient does not want to terminate the pregnancy or if she is close to term, then the fetus can be delivered with classic cesarean section followed by radical hysterectomy and pelvic lymphadenectomy.

Patients with larger tumors or locally advanced disease can be treated with chemoradiation. Those close to term or with fetal lung maturity can be delivered by cesarean section and surgical staging followed by chemoradiation. In a patient who declines pregnancy termination, consideration may be given to neoadjuvant chemotherapy to prevent progression of disease and time for fetal lung maturity.

ADENOCARCINOMA OF THE CERVIX

The management of adenocarcinoma of the cervix is similar to that for squamous cell carcinoma. The worse prognosis reported in some cases is attributed to a higher rate of distant metastasis.

Adenocarcinoma In Situ

Adenocarcinoma in situ (ACIS) may be identified from investigation of an abnormal Pap smear. When diagnosed on biopsy, conization is required because ACIS can be diffuse or multifocal and may be associated with underlying adenocarcinoma. The differential diagnosis includes well-differentiated adenocarcinoma (adenoma malignum or minimal deviation adenocarcinoma) and microglandular hyperplasia, which is associated with oral contraceptives and Arias-Stella changes of pregnancy. Simple hysterectomy is the treatment of choice for women who have no desire for further childbearing. Otherwise, cone biopsy may be adequate if the margins are clear and endocervical curettage is negative.

Microinvasive Adenocarcinoma

Patients with stage IA1 can be managed with simple hysterectomy. However, conization can be done for young women who desire to preserve fertility. Therefore, treatment should be individualized according to depth of invasion, margin of resection, and lymphovascular invasion.

Invasive Adenocarcinoma

Invasive adenocarcinoma accounts for approximately 5% to 10% of all cervical carcinomas. Adenocarcinoma has been classified into five subtypes: endocervical, endometrioid, clear cell, adenocystic, and adenosquamous.

Cervical adenocarcinoma usually originates from the endocervical canal. Vaginal bleeding and discharge are the most common symptoms. Endocervical and endometrial curettage are essential in the evaluation of patients if the results of gross examination of the cervix, colposcopy, and cervical biopsy are negative.

The recommended treatment for stage IA2 microinvasion is modified radical hysterectomy and pelvic lymphadenectomy. For stages IB and IIA, radical hysterectomy and pelvic lymphadenopathy are recommended. Adjuvant pelvic radiation should be considered for patients with nodal metastasis, lymphovascular invasion, poorly differentiated tumor, or larger lesions. When radiation is the primary treatment, an adjuvant simple hysterectomy is recommended. Follow-up CEA (carcinoembryonic antigen) and CA-125 (cancer antigen 125) are of value in cervical adenocarcinoma.

Adenosquamous Carcinoma

Adenosquamous carcinoma represents 20% to 30% of cervical adenocarcinomas. Overall 5-year survival and disease-free survival rates are not significantly different from those of other adenocarcinomas.

Clear Cell Adenocarcinoma

In clear cell adenocarcinoma, the tumor occurs in two distinct groups of patients—those younger than 24 years and those older than 45 years. Cancer in the older group is unrelated to diethylstilbestrol (DES) exposure in utero. Unlike uterine clear cell adenocarcinoma, the prognosis is the same as for other adenocarcinomas.

Glassy Cell Carcinoma

Glassy cell carcinoma is a poorly differentiated adenosquamous (or large cell undifferentiated) carcinoma with a moderate amount of cytoplasm and a typical ground glass appearance. The prognosis is poor. Reported survival for stage IB cancer treated with radical hysterectomy was 55%.

Small Cell Carcinoma

Small cell (neuroendocrine) carcinoma is very rare, only 0.6% of cervical cancers. Small cell carcinoma histologically stains for neuroendocrine markers. These cells can synthesize amines and hence are also called amine precursor uptake and decarboxylation (APUD) cells. Small cell carcinoma has a tendency to a higher lymphovascular invasion, resulting in higher recurrence and lower survival because of their propensity for early systemic spread. Chemotherapy is usually recommended in addition to surgery and radiation.

A larger study involving 23 women compared adjuvant chemotherapy with cisplatin,[1] vinblastine,[1] and bleomycin[1] (PVB) against vincristine,[1] doxorubicin,[1] and cyclophosphamide[1] (VAC) alternating with cisplatin[1] and etoposide[1] (PE) after radical hysterectomy. The reported survival was higher in the VAC/PE group (10 of 14) compared with the PVB group (3 of 9), with median follow-up of 41 months.

Chemoprevention and Vaccination

Due to the relatively long premalignant phase of cervical carcinogenesis (5–10 years), some investigators are studying the effect of chemoprevention or vaccination on disease progression. Investigators have

---

[1]Not FDA approved for this indication.

focused on the retinoids as chemoprevention agents for cervical dysplasia based on their cell-differentiating properties.

Topical *trans*-retinoic acid[1] (tretinoin) in a randomized phase III clinical trial has been shown to induce regression of mild and moderate dysplasias, but not of severe dysplasias. Other suitable agents for chemoprevention include difluoromethylornithine,[5] beta-carotene,[7] and cyclooxygenase-2 inhibitors.[1]

HPV vaccines are focused on targeting the oncogenic E6/E7 proteins as therapeutic vaccines. These peptide vaccines are designed to stimulate cytotoxic T lymphocytes against specific E6/E7 epitopes. HPV16 and HPV18 together cause about 70% of cervical cancers. It is estimated that 20 million people are infected worldwide and 6.2 million people in the United States get a new infection of HPV each year. Two new vaccines, Gardasil (Merck) and Cervarix[5] (GlaxoSmithKline) reported 100% protection against HPV 16 and HPV 18 infection. To improve that effort, researchers are already working on second-generation vaccines and exploring the possibility of a therapeutic vaccine that could help prevent HPV-related cancers in those who are already being infected by the virus.

REFERENCES

Boss EA, van Golde RI, Beerendonk CC, Massuger LE. Pregnancy after radical trachelectomy: A real option? Gynecol Oncol 2005;99(3 Suppl. 1): S152–6.

Dargent D, Martin X, Sacchetoni A, Mathevet P. Laparascopic vaginal radical trachelectomy: A treatment to preserve the fertility of cervical cancer carcinoma patients. Cancer 2000;88:1877–82.

Delgado G, Bundy B, Zaino R, et al. Prospective surgical-pathological study of disease-free interval in patients with stage IB squamous cell carcinoma of the cervix: A Gynecologic Oncology Group study. Gynecol Oncol 1990;38:352–7.

Giacalone PL, Laffargue E. Neoadjuvant chemotherapy in the treatment of locally advanced cervical carcinoma in pregnancy: A report of two cases and review of issues specific to the management of cervical carcinoma in pregnancy including planned delay of therapy. Cancer 1999;85:1203–4.

Hopkins MP, Lavin JP. Cervical cancer in pregnancy. Gynecol Oncol 1996;63:293.

Jemal A, Siegel R, Ward E, et al. Cancer statistics, 2008. CA Cancer J Clin 2008;58:71–96.

Jensen PT, Groenvold M, Klee MC, et al. Early-stage cervical carcinoma, radical hysterectomy, and sexual function: A longitudinal study. Cancer 2004;100:97–106.

Lertsanguansinchai P, Lertbutsayanukul C, Shotelersuk K, et al. Phase III randomized trial comparing LDR and HDR brachytherapy in treatment of cervical carcinoma. Int J Radiat Oncol Biol Phys 2004;59: 1424–31.

Monk BJ, Sill M, McMeekin DS, et al. A randomized phase III trial of four cisplatin (CIS) containing doublet combinations in stage IVB, recurrent or persistent cervical carcinoma: A gynecologic oncology group (GOG) study. J Clin Oncol 2008;26(May 20 Suppl.); abstr LBA5504.

Plante M, Renaud MC, FranAois H, Roy M. Vaginal radical trachelectomy: An oncologically safe fertility-preserving surgery: An updated series of 72 cases and review of the literature. Gynecol Oncol 2004;94:614–23.

Roman LD, Felix JC, Muderspach LL, et al. Risk of residual invasive disease in women with microinvasive squamous cancer in a conization specimen. Obstet Gynecol 1997;90:759–64.

Sedlis A, Bundy BN, Rotman MZ, et al. A randomized trial of pelvic radiation therapy versus no further therapy in selected patients with stage IB carcinoma of the cervix after radical hysterectomy and pelvic lymphadenectomy: A Gynecologic Oncology Group Study. Gynecol Oncol 1999;73:177–83.

Steed H, Rosen B, Murphy J, et al. A comparison of laparoscopic-assisted radical vaginal hysterectomy and radical abdominal hysterectomy in the treatment of cervical cancer. Gynecol Oncol 2004;93:588–93.

---

[1]Not FDA approved for this indication.
[5]Investigational drug in the United States.
[7]Available as dietary supplement.

Neoplasms of the Vulva

Method of
Susan A. Davidson, MD

The female external genitalia includes the mons pubis, labia majora, labia minora, clitoris, perineal body, and the structures of the vaginal introitus or vestibule. Whether benign or malignant, vulvar neoplasms are uncommon, occur at all ages, and have varying characteristics. Therefore liberal use of biopsies is usually required for diagnosis and to guide treatment.

Benign Cystic Neoplasms

Benign cystic lesions of the vulva include Bartholin's duct cyst, sebaceous and epidermal inclusion cysts, mucinous cysts, Skene duct cysts, and cysts of the canal of Nuck. Bartholin's duct cyst, located in the posterior labia near the vaginal introitus, is most common. Treatment is usually not required in asymptomatic young women (<40 years). If the cyst is symptomatic or infected, however, drainage by marsupialization or use of a Word catheter, is indicated. Bartholin's gland carcinomas are rare, especially in women younger than 40 years of age. But if the mass feels firm or nodular, it should be biopsied.

Sebaceous and epidermal inclusion cysts are also common. They are prone to infection but rarely malignant. If an infection develops, they should be incised and drained. Mucinous cysts are rare and possibly arise from the minor vestibular glands. They are located anteriorly on the vulva, typically on the inner labia minora. Skene duct cysts are located next to the urethra. Excision of these cysts is necessary only if symptomatic.

Cysts of the canal of Nuck are located in the anterior portion of the labia majora at the termination of the insertion of the round ligament. These cysts represent herniation of the peritoneum through the inguinal canal and contain peritoneal fluid. If symptomatic, excision must be accompanied by closure of the fascial defect to prevent recurrence.

Benign Solid Neoplasms

The benign solid tumors of the vulva include fibromas, myomas, lipomas, hidradenomas, syringomas, myoblastomas, vestibular adenomas, and angiomas, among others. Benign pigmented lesions, such as nevi and seborrheic keratoses, may occasionally be found. Malignancy is rare, but most should be excised for diagnostic and therapeutic purposes.

CONDYLOMA ACUMINATUM

Vulvar condyloma acuminatum is a sexually transmitted verrucous lesion of the vulva caused by human papilloma virus (HPV), most frequently types 6 and 11. These lesions are warty growths that frequently cover large areas of the vulva. Smoking and immunosuppression are risk factors. Representative biopsies should be obtained to document disease and rule out malignancy. Wide local excision can be used for small lesions, although these growths are usually best treated by ablation.

Chemical ablative techniques include topical application of trichloroacetic acid (Tri-Chlor), podofilox (0.5%, Condylox), 5-fluorouracil[1] (1%, Fluoroplex or 5%, Efudex),[1] or imiquimod (5%, Aldara). Podophyllin can be applied twice daily for 3 days, repeated weekly for 4 weeks. Imiquimod can be applied three times per week

---

[1]Not FDA approved for this indication.

for up to 16 weeks. Podophyllin and 5-fluorouracil should not be used in women who could become pregnant. Surgical ablative therapies include CO_2 laser vaporization and use of the Cavitron ultrasonic aspirator (CUSA), especially for extensive disease.

Intraepithelial Neoplasms of the Vulva

VULVAR INTRAEPITHELIAL NEOPLASIA

Vulvar intraepithelial neoplasia (VIN) is a dysplastic condition of the squamous epithelium whose incidence is increasing, especially in younger women. Risk factors are HPV types 16 and 18, smoking, and immunosuppression. Symptoms include pruritus (most common), pain, a noticeable lesion, and discoloration. Most patients with HPV-related disease have multifocal lesions including vaginal and cervical dysplasia. The most common location is in the area of the posterior fourchette and perineal body. Typical findings are raised white, gray, red, or mottled lesions; application of 4% acetic acid for several minutes can help identify faint lesions and outline abnormal vascular patterns. Diagnosis of VIN is made by punch biopsies through full thickness of the epithelium to rule out invasion, present in 20% of patients with VIN III (full-thickness dysplasia or carcinoma in situ). Of those patients with invasion, half (10% of VIN III) have invasion more than 1 mm.

Treatment of VIN can be categorized into excisional and ablative therapies. Patients at risk for microinvasion (unifocal disease, raised lesions, older age, and prior radiation) should have the lesion excised completely if possible. Skinning vulvectomy is rarely used because of psychological and sexual consequences related to scarring and disfigurement.

The ablative therapies can be divided into mechanical and chemical. The mechanical method most commonly used is the CO_2 laser, although use of the CUSA is also described. Both can ablate large or multifocal lesions successfully with an excellent cosmetic and functional outcome. The chemical method most commonly used is topical 5-fluorouracil (5%, Efudex).[1] Because of its teratogenic potential, it should not be used in women who could become pregnant. It can be applied on two consecutive nights weekly for 10 weeks. An alternative ablative therapy is use of imiquimod[1] (Aldara), as described earlier. Because of the irritation caused by these topical therapies, many patients have problems with treatment compliance. Residual disease should be excised to rule out invasion.

Patients with VIN frequently have recurrent disease, regardless of the treatment method used (Table 1). Continued smoking increases this risk, so patients should be counseled in smoking cessation. In those patients whose cancers recur and are retreated, subsequent 5-fluorouracil prophylaxis, with a single application biweekly, is used successfully to minimize further recurrences.

PAGET'S DISEASE

Paget's disease of the vulva is an uncommon condition characterized by a patchy, eczematoid lesion that frequently covers much of the vulva. Most patients are postmenopausal and present with

[1]Not FDA approved for this indication.

TABLE 1 Recurrence of Vulvar Intraepithelial Neoplasia III

Treatment Method	% Recurrence
Chemical ablation	20–40
Mechanical ablation	20–40
Wide local excision	
Negative margin	15–25
Positive margin	30–45

TABLE 2 Incidence of Regional Node Metastases by Tumor Diameter

Tumor Diameter (cm)	% Positive Inguinal Nodes
<1	0–15
5–20	
25–35	
35–50	
≥50	≥50

complaints of pruritus. Although Paget's disease is an in situ disease process, 15% to 25% of patients have an underlying malignancy, usually an adenocarcinoma of the apocrine glands but occasionally an invasive Paget's. In addition, up to 30% of patients have a synchronous adenocarcinoma of the breast, colon, rectum, or upper genital tract. Screening for these cancers is therefore recommended. To assess for invasion, the lesion should be excised via wide local excision or simple vulvectomy with at least 5 mm of the adjacent subcutaneous tissue. Achieving negative margin status is frequently difficult. However, the risk of recurrence is approximately 30% whether margins are negative or positive. Thus expectant management, reserving treatment for symptomatic recurrences, is usually recommended.

Invasive Vulvar Lesions

Less than 5% of gynecologic cancers arise on the vulva. Approximately 85% are squamous cell carcinomas. The etiology of this type appears mixed. Up to 50% evolve from VIN III and are usually associated with HPV-16. These women are slightly younger (age 45–52 years). Most arise in older women (mean age 60–69 years), and suggested risk factors include immunosuppression, hypertension, diabetes mellitus, obesity, and chronic vulvar inflammation. Other histologic types are melanomas (5% to 10%), basal cell carcinomas (2% to 3%), adenocarcinomas (1%), and sarcomas (1% to 2%). Most patients present with a combination of symptoms, including pruritus, discomfort, and complaints of a mass. Examination frequently reveals a suspicious lesion, which should be biopsied for diagnosis. Vulvar cancers typically spread by local extension and lymphatic dissemination. Factors that influence dissemination include tumor size (Table 2), depth of invasion (Table 3), lymphovascular space invasion, and tumor grade. Staging is surgical and classified using the tumor, nodes, and metastasis (TNM) system (Box 1) as well as the International Federation of Gynecology and Obstetrics (FIGO) system (Box 2).

SQUAMOUS CELL CARCINOMAS AND ADENOCARCINOMAS

Surgical management of squamous cell carcinomas and adenocarcinomas depends on the size, depth of invasion, and location of the lesion. The vulvar lesion is managed with a radical excision. Management of the groins is based on depth of invasion. Lesions with invasion of <1 mm have minimal risk of lymphatic spread and do not require lymphadenectomy. All others require surgical assessment of the lymph nodes. Lesions located in the midline structures require bilateral groin dissection, whereas lateral lesions are managed with

TABLE 3 Incidence of Regional Node Metastases by Depth of Tumor Invasion

Depth of Invasion (mm)	% Positive Inguinal Nodes
<1	1–5
1–3	10–15
3–5	15–30
5–10	30–45
>10	>40

BOX 1   TNM Classification of Vulvar Carcinoma

T	Primary tumor
Tis	Carcinoma in situ
T1	Confined to vulva, diameter ≤2 cm
T2	Confined to vulva, diameter >2 cm
T3	Adjacent spread to urethra, vagina, perineum, or anus (any size)
T4	Infiltration of upper urethral mucosa, bladder, rectum, or bone
N	Regional lymph nodes
N0	No lymph node metastases
N1	Unilateral regional lymph node metastasis
N2	Bilateral regional lymph node metastasis
M	Distant metastases
M0	No clinical metastases
M1	Distant metastasis (including pelvic lymph node metastasis)

Abbreviation: TNM = tumor, node, metastasis.

ipsilateral groin dissection. This surgical approach is associated with significant morbidity including disfigurement, wound breakdown, and problems with lymphocysts and chronic lymphedema. For patients with very large lesions or lesions in sensitive areas such as the clitoris, preoperative radiation, followed by less radical excision of residual disease, may minimize problems with the vulvar wound. Current investigations are ongoing in the use of sentinel lymph node dissections as a method of minimizing the groin morbidity without sacrificing survival. Positive vulvar margins or metastases to lymph nodes are managed with postoperative radiation. Survival depends on stage at diagnosis (Table 4).

BOX 2   FIGO Classification (With Corresponding TNM Classification) for Vulvar Carcinoma

Stage I (T1N0M0)	Tumor confined to vulva and/or perineum, 2 cm in greatest dimension; nodes are negative
Stage IA	Stromal invasion no greater than 1 mm
Stage IB	Stromal invasion >1 mm
Stage II (T2N0M0)	Tumor confined to the vulva and/or perineum, >2 cm in greatest dimension; nodes are negative
Stage III	
T3N0M0	Tumor of any size with adjacent spread to the lower urethra and/or the vagina or the anus
T3N1M0	Unilateral regional lymph node metastasis
T2N1M0	
Stage IVA	
T1N2M0	Tumor invades any of the following: upper urethra, bladder mucosa, rectal mucosa, pelvic bone, and/or bilateral regional node metastasis
T2N2M0	
T3N2M0	
T4 any N M0	
Stage IVB	
Any T any N M1	Any distant metastasis including pelvic lymph nodes

Abbreviations: FIGO = International Federation of Gynecology and Obstetrics; TNM = tumor, node, metastasis.

TABLE 4   Survival Rate by FIGO Stage for Patients With Invasive Squamous Cell Vulvar Cancer

FIGO Stage	% Surviving 5 Years
I	70–90
II	50–80
III	30–50
IV	10–15

Abbreviation: FIGO = International Federation of Gynecology and Obstetrics.

MALIGNANT MELANOMA

Malignant melanoma is the second most common vulvar malignancy. Most patients have disease on the mucosal surfaces of the vulvar introitus, clitoris, and labia minora. The vulvar lesion is treated by radical excision, but management of the groins is controversial. The risk of spread is significant with a tumor thickness greater than 0.75 mm, but survival at 5 years is only approximately 10% with groin node metastases. Some argue against node dissection for this reason. However, given some long-term survivors with modern melanoma therapy, either lymphadenectomy or sentinel lymph node dissection, as is done for other cutaneous melanomas, appears indicated.

VERRUCOUS CARCINOMA

Verrucous carcinoma is a large exophytic tumor that resembles giant condyloma acuminatum. It is a variant of squamous carcinomas but has an excellent prognosis because of the lack of metastases. Verrucous carcinomas have a high tendency to recur and should be managed with radical local excision.

 CURRENT DIAGNOSIS

- Most cystic lesions are benign. Excision is reserved for symptomatic cysts and suspicious Bartholin's gland cysts, especially in women older than 40 years of age.
- All solid lesions should be biopsied for diagnostic purposes.
- Multifocal disease requires multiple biopsies to rule out invasive disease.
- Most premalignant and malignant lesions cause pruritus, discomfort, or a noticeable lesion.
- The vagina and cervix in women with dysplastic or malignant vulvar lesions should be evaluated.

 CURRENT THERAPY

- Benign solid lesions should be excised.
- After ablative treatment of vulvar intraepithelial neoplasia (VIN), excise any residual lesions to rule out occult invasive disease.
- Avoid podophyllin and 5-fluorouracil in women of reproductive potential.
- Rule out synchronous neoplasms in women with Paget's disease.
- Invasion more than 1 mm requires radical excision and lymph node evaluation.

BASAL CELL CARCINOMA

Basal cell carcinomas typically occur in elderly white women, are commonly located on the labia majora, and have characteristics similar to basal cell carcinomas at other sites. Treatment is wide local excision only because metastases are rare. Basal cell carcinomas are prone to local recurrence, however. A malignant squamous component must be ruled out because it should be managed as a squamous cell carcinoma.

SARCOMAS

Leiomyosarcoma is the most common vulvar sarcoma and usually arises in the labia majora. Malignant fibrous histiocytoma is the second most common. Management of these lesions is radical vulvar excision.

REFERENCES

Garland SM. Imiquimod. Curr Opin Infect Dis 2003;16:85–9.
Homesley HD, Bundy BN, Sedlis A, et al. Prognostic factors for groin node metastasis in squamous cell carcinoma of the vulva (a Gynecologic Oncology Group study). Gynecol Oncol 1993;49:279–83.
Krebs HB. The use of topical 5-fluorouracil in the treatment of genital condylomas. Obstet Gynecol Clin North Am 1987;14(2):559–68.
Modesitt SC, Waters AB, Walton L, et al. Vulvar intraepithelial neoplasia III: Occult cancer and the impact of margin status on recurrence. Obstet Gynecol 1998;92(6):962–6.
Phillips GL, Bundy BN, Okagaki T, et al. Malignant melanoma of the vulva treated by radical hemivulvectomy, a prospective study of the Gynecologic Oncology Group. Cancer 1994;73:2626–32.
Tebes S, Cardosi R, Hoffman M. Paget's disease of the vulva. Am J Obstet Gynecol 2002;187:281–4.
Trimble CL, Trimble EL, Woodruff JD. Diseases of the vulva. In: Hernandez E, Atkinson BE, editors. Clinical Gynecologic Pathology. Philadelphia: WB Saunders; 1995. p. 1–90.
Wright VC, Chapman WB. Colposcopy of intraepithelial neoplasia of the vulva and adjacent sites. Obstet Gynecol Clin North Am 1993;20:(1):231–55.

Ovarian Cancer

Method of
Peter G. Rose, MD

Ovarian cancer is the seventh most common cancer and the fourth most common cause of cancer death for women. It is the second most common gynecologic cancer and the deadliest.

Epidemiology

Ovarian cancers are heterogeneous tumors. Germ cell tumors occur most frequently in the second and third decades of life, stromal tumors occur in a bimodal distribution, and epithelial tumors increase in frequency with increasing age, with the median occurrence in frequency with increasing age, with the median occurrence in the sixth and seventh decades of life. Approximately 10% of epithelial ovarian cancers are related to the *BRCA* gene mutation, and a small percentage of the tumors are associated with the hereditary nonpolyposis colon cancer (HNPCC) syndrome.

Screening

No effective screening programs have been established for ovarian cancer because of its rarity and nonspecific symptoms. Most ovarian cancer patients present with symptoms of dyspepsia, vague abdominal discomfort, gas, distention, early satiety, anorexia, increasing abdominal girth, change in bowel pattern, urinary frequency, and pain. However, in a primary care setting, 72% of women had recurring symptoms, with a median number of two symptoms. Goff and colleagues found that the most common were back pain (45%), fatigue (34%), bloating (27%), constipation (24%), abdominal pain (22%), and urinary symptoms (16%). A prospective study of screening by symptoms is planned.

Because patients with early-stage disease have a significantly better prognosis, identifying the disease as early as possible would be ideal. Most of the cancers diagnosed in screening studies were advanced-stage disease. Screening based on high-risk family history or *BRCA* gene mutation status also resulted in most detected cancers being advanced stage. Because of this pattern of late detection, prophylactic surgery to remove the fallopian tubes and ovaries remains the most effective way to reduce the risk of gynecologic cancer among high-risk patients. Patients with the HNPCC syndrome are at increased risk for uterine and ovarian cancer, and therefore removal of the uterus, fallopian tubes, and ovaries is advised.

Germ Cell Tumors

Germ cell tumors comprise 2% of ovarian cancers and are usually seen in adolescents and young adults. Treatment involves oophorectomy and staging surgery (Table 1), including omentectomy, peritoneal biopsies, and pelvic and paraaortic lymphadenectomy. These tumors are usually unilateral, and conservation of the uterus and contralateral ovary is the standard of care. Because these tumors are most often found unexpectedly, staging surgery is rarely performed.

Tumor histologies include dysgerminoma (40%), endodermal sinus tumor (22%), immature teratoma (20%), mixed tumors (14%), polyembryoma (<1%), and choriocarcinoma (<1%). Dysgerminomas have the best prognosis. They can be observed during the early stage and can be effectively treated with chemotherapy without bleomycin in the advanced stage. For patients with nondysgerminomatous tumors without gross residual disease, prospective trials have demonstrated that bleomycin (Blenoxane),[1] etoposide (Toposar),[1] and cisplatin (Platinol AQ) chemotherapy is associated

---

[1]Not FDA approved for this indication.

TABLE 1 FIGO Staging for Carcinoma of the Ovary

Stage	Description
I	Growth limited to the ovaries
Ia	Growth limited to one ovary
Ib	Growth limited to both ovaries
Ic	Stage Ia or Ib with tumor on surface of ovaries, or with capsule ruptured, or with ascites present containing malignant cells
II	With pelvic extension
IIa	Extension to reproductive organs
IIb	Extension to other pelvic tissues
IIc	Stage IIa or IIb with tumor on surface of ovaries, or with capsule(s) ruptured, or with ascites present containing malignant cells
III	Tumor outside the pelvis or positive retroperitoneal or inguinal nodes
IIIa	Microscopic seeding of abdominal peritoneal surfaces
IIIb	Macroscopic disease measuring less than 2 cm in diameter
IIIc	Macroscopic disease measuring greater than 2 cm in diameter or positive retroperitoneal or inguinal nodes
IV*	Extraabdominal extension

*If a pleural effusion is present, there must be positive cytology or parenchymal liver metastasis.
Abbreviation: FIGO = International Federation of Gynecology and Obstetrics.

with a survival rate of 98%. Low-grade and low-stage immature teratomas can be observed.

Stromal Tumors

Stromal tumors comprise 2% of ovarian cancers and are seen in young and older patients. Their treatment depends on the extent of disease and the reproductive potential of the patient. Conservation of the uterus and contralateral ovary is usually appropriate for young patients. Staging surgery, including omentectomy, peritoneal biopsies, and pelvic and paraaortic lymphadenectomy, is usually recommended. However, based on the patterns of recurrence, the role of lymphadenectomy has been questioned. Advanced-stage and recurrent stromal tumors are often treated like germ cell tumors, using a chemotherapy regimen of bleomycin,[1] etoposide,[1] and cisplatin. Paclitaxel (Taxol) is also active against stromal tumors, and some investigators have used carboplatin (Paraplatin) and paclitaxel for therapy.

Epithelial Ovarian Cancer

Epithelial ovarian cancer, also known as ovarian carcinoma, arises from the surface epithelium of the ovary. This epithelium is derived from pelvic peritoneum that envelops the ovarian tissue as it migrates during embryologic development from the supragonadal ridge to the pelvis. The ovarian epithelium is identical to other peritoneum, and peritoneal carcinomas are biologically equivalent to ovarian carcinoma. Approximately 15% of all ovarian carcinomas are borderline tumors, which are noninvasive and indolent in their behavior.

Borderline and invasive epithelial tumors of the ovary can be classified by their stage, histologic type, and histologic grade. Molecular studies have demonstrated that borderline and low-grade tumors are similar and distinct from high-grade carcinomas. Low-grade tumors are characterized by *KRAS* and *BRAF* mutations, whereas high-grade tumors have *TP53* mutations. Ovaries and tubes removed prophylactically in genetically predisposed individuals demonstrate frequent *TP53* mutations in the fallopian epithelium but not the ovarian surface epithelium, and the tubal epithelium has been proposed as the source of high-grade serous carcinomas.

The distinction of ovarian, peritoneal, and tubal carcinomas is more anatomic than functional, because these tumors are treated and behave similarly. Tumor histologies include serous (60%), endometrioid (20%), mucinous (3%), clear cell (2%), transitional (1%), and Brenner (1%). Advanced-stage or recurrent mucinous and clear cell tumors respond poorly to chemotherapy and have a poorer prognosis compared with other histologies.

CURRENT DIAGNOSIS

- Evaluate patients by family history of breast and ovarian cancer; seek genetic consultation.
- Evaluate for symptoms of ovarian cancer, including back pain, fatigue, bloating, constipation, abdominal pain, and urinary symptoms.
- Perform a follow-up assessment for any abnormal imaging results.
- Routine screening is not recommended.

Treatment

SURGERY

Ovarian cancer is typically treated with primary surgery to establish the diagnosis, determine the extent of disease, and remove as much cancer as possible before initiation of chemotherapy for advanced-stage disease. The surgical procedure indicated depends on the disease extent at presentation. For patients with apparent early-stage disease, staging surgery, including omentectomy, peritoneal biopsies, and pelvic and paraaortic lymphadenectomy, should be performed. For patients with limited metastatic disease, omentectomy and pelvic and paraaortic lymphadenectomy may affect staging and prognosis. For patients with advanced-stage disease, the goal of surgery is maximal tumor resection (i.e., cytoreduction or debulking). Retrospective data demonstrate improved survival for patients with no or minimal residual disease. The extent of surgery necessary to accomplish maximal tumor reduction varies from patient to patient. Intestinal surgery is often required, and sigmoid resection is the most common intestinal procedure.

After surgery, patients are evaluated for adjuvant chemotherapy based on disease stage and histologic findings. Borderline tumors are observed unless they have invasive metastatic implants. Patients with invasive tumors at low risk for recurrence (i.e., stage IA or IB with low-grade histology) are also observed. In view of the similar molecular profile of grade 2 and 3 histologies, treatment of grade 2 tumors should be considered.

CHEMOTHERAPY

Based on the results of randomized trials, primary chemotherapy consists of a platinum compound (i.e., carboplatin or cisplatin) and a taxane (i.e., paclitaxel or docetaxel [Taxotere][1]). In cases of advanced-stage disease, a minimum of six courses of a platinum/taxane doublet is given. For patients with suboptimal stage III and IV disease (i.e., residual tumor or tumors >1 cm in the greatest dimension), the median progression-free and overall survival times are 18 and 38 months, respectively. For patients with optimal residual disease (i.e., residual tumor or tumors <1 cm in greatest diameter), the median progression-free and overall survival times are 20.7 and 57.4 months, respectively.

In the late 1990s, several active second-line chemotherapy agents were approved for ovarian cancer. A very large, five-arm, randomized trial evaluating these agents in triplet or doublet combinations with carboplatin and paclitaxel failed to demonstrate an improvement. The number of courses of treatment is individualized based on radiologic and tumor marker response. After a complete clinical response, patients are observed. Clinical factors affecting survival after treatment for advanced-stage disease included no or minimal residual disease, germline *BRCA* mutation, nonmucinous or non–clear cell tumor histology, better performance status, and younger age.

Neoadjuvant chemotherapy with a platinum/taxane doublet for patients with apparent advanced-stage disease is used for those who are elderly and compromised or those with serious medical comorbidities. Neoadjuvant chemotherapy is also used by some investigators for patients with extensive disease. Patients who respond favorably can then be considered for interval debulking surgery. A randomized trial comparing primary surgery with neoadjuvant chemotherapy demonstrated similar progression-free and overall survival times of 12 and 30 months, respectively.

Intraperitoneal chemotherapy has demonstrated efficacy in three large randomized trials and has been advocated by a National Cancer Institute Clinical Alert. The latest study, which used intraperitoneal cisplatin[1] and intravenous paclitaxel on day 1 and intraperitoneal paclitaxel[1] on day 6, reported progression-free and overall survival times of 23.8 and 65.6 months, respectively, compared with 18.3 and 49.7 months for the control group. However, trial design

---
[1]Not FDA approved for this indication.

---
[1]Not FDA approved for this indication.

and increased toxicity with the most recent intraperitoneal regimen has limited its acceptance in clinical practice.

Second-look laparotomy or laparoscopy used in the past to determine pathologic response has not been shown to affect disease outcome.

CONSOLIDATION OR MAINTENANCE THERAPY

Despite the high response rate to primary chemotherapy, advanced-stage ovarian cancer patients are at significant risk for recurrent disease. Maintenance therapy with paclitaxel for 12 months produced a superior progression-free survival compared with treatment for 3 months. However, seven other maintenance trials with paclitaxel, topotecan (Hycamtin),[1] or biologic agents have had negative results. An ongoing trial powered to evaluate progression-free and overall survival is evaluating maintenance therapy with one of two taxane compounds compared with observation.

BIOLOGIC THERAPY

Among the numerous biologic agents that have been studied in ovarian cancer, bevacizumab (Avastin),[1] an antibody against the vascular endothelial growth factor (VEGF), has demonstrated the most activity. After demonstration of activity against recurrent disease, ongoing trials in the United States and Europe are evaluating its role in combination with carboplatin and paclitaxel and as single-agent maintenance.

TREATMENT OF RECURRENT DISEASE

Although recurrent disease is incurable, patients may benefit from interventions. The potential for successful treatment of recurrent ovarian carcinoma is determined by response to prior therapy and the duration of the treatment-free interval. Secondary cytoreductive surgery has been used and is most effective for patients with a long treatment-free interval (>12 months), isolated site of recurrence, prior complete response to chemotherapy, and good performance status. Very late recurrences may represent second primaries.

CURRENT THERAPY

Primary Disease

- Primary surgery with comprehensive staging or maximal cytoreduction
- Intravenous platinum or taxane, or both (patients with optimal and suboptimal residual disease)
- Intraperitoneal platinum with intravenous or intraperitoneal taxane (patients with optimal residual stage III disease)
- Neoadjuvant chemotherapy with interval debulking

Recurrent Disease

- Platinum combination for recurrence after more than 6 months off therapy
- Nonplatinum single-agent therapy for recurrence after less than 6 months off therapy
- Radiation therapy as needed for disease palliation

---

[1]Not FDA approved for this indication.

Second-line chemotherapy that includes retreatment with a platinum compound is most effective in patients with a treatment-free interval of 6 months or more, and better response rates have been seen with longer treatment-free intervals. In this patient population, platinum in combination with paclitaxel or gemcitabine (Gemzar) is appropriate based on randomized trial data.

Patients can be repeatedly treated with a platinum compound until they develop resistant disease or intolerance to the adverse effects. Numerous other agents may be effective in controlling disease progression. Radiation therapy is used as needed for disease palliation.

End-of-Life Care

Progressive disease can manifest as intestinal obstruction, unrelenting ascites, or pleural effusions. Percutaneous gastrostomy for drainage of effusions or ascites may provide symptomatic relief. Shifting from active treatment to a goal of palliation with attention to quality of life is appropriate at this point.

REFERENCES

Armstrong DK, Bundy B, Wenzel L, et al. for the Gynecologic Oncology Group. Intraperitoneal cisplatin and paclitaxel in ovarian cancer. N Engl J Med 2006;354:34–43.

Bookman MA, Brady MF, McGuire WP, et al. Evaluation of new platinum-based treatment regimens in advanced-stage ovarian cancer: A phase III trial of the Gynecologic Cancer Intergroup. J Clin Oncol 2009;27:1419–25.

Brown J, Sood AK, Deavers MT, et al. Patterns of metastasis in sex cord-stromal tumors of the ovary: Can routine staging lymphadenectomy be omitted? Gynecol Oncol 2009;113:86–90.

Fishman DA, Cohen L, Blank SV, et al. The role of ultrasound evaluation in the detection of early-stage epithelial ovarian cancer. Am J Obstet Gynecol 2005;192:1214–22.

Goff BA, Mandel LS, Melancon CH, Muntz HG. Frequency of symptoms of ovarian cancer in women presenting to primary care clinics. JAMA 2004;291:2705–12.

Markman M, Liu PY, Wilczynski S, et al. Phase III randomized trial of 12 versus 3 months of maintenance paclitaxel in patients with advanced ovarian cancer after complete response to platinum and paclitaxel-based chemotherapy: A Southwest Oncology Group and Gynecologic Oncology Group trial. J Clin Oncol 2003;21:2460–5.

McGuire WP, Hoskins WJ, Brady MF, et al. Cyclophosphamide and cisplatin versus paclitaxel and cisplatin: A phase III randomized trial in patients with suboptimal stage III/IV ovarian cancer. N Engl J Med 1996;334:1–6.

Ozols RF, Bundy BN, Greer BE, et al. Phase III trial of carboplatin and paclitaxel compared with cisplatin and paclitaxel in patients with optimally resected stage III ovarian cancer: A Gynecologic Oncology Group study. J Clin Oncol 2003;21:3194–200.

Parmar MK, Ledermann JA, Colombo N, et al. ICON and AGO Collaborators. Paclitaxel plus platinum-based chemotherapy versus conventional platinum-based chemotherapy in women with relapsed ovarian cancer: The ICON4/AGO-OVAR-2.2 trial. Lancet 2003;361:2099–106.

Partridge E, Kreimer AR, Greenlee RT, et al. Results from four rounds of ovarian cancer screening in a randomized trial. Obstet Gynecol 2009;113:775–82.

Pfisterer J, Plante M, Vergote I, et al., for AGO-OVAR; NCIC CTG; EORTC GCG. Gemcitabine plus carboplatin compared with carboplatin in patients with platinum-sensitive recurrent ovarian cancer: An intergroup trial of the AGO-OVAR, the NCIC CTG, and the EORTC GCG. J Clin Oncol 2006;24:4699–707.

Vergote I, Trope CG, Amant F, et al. EORTC-GCG/NCIC-CTG randomized trial comparing primary debulking surgery with neoadjuvant chemotherapy in stage IIIC-IV ovarian, fallopian tube and peritoneal cancer. Presented at the International Gynecologic Cancer Society (IGCS) Meeting, October 25, 2008, Bangkok, Thailand.

Winter WE, Maxwell GL, Tian C, et al. Prognostic factors for stage III epithelial ovarian cancer: Gynecologic Oncology Group Study. J Clin Oncol 2007;25:3621–7.

Psychiatric Disorders

Alcoholism

Method of
Richard N. Rosenthal, MD

Epidemiology

Alcohol-use disorders are among the most prevalent mental disorders in the population, occurring at frequencies that rival those of mood and anxiety disorders. In any year, almost 8½% of the U.S. population older than 18 years meets criteria for a formal alcohol use disorder (alcohol abuse or dependence), and almost 4% meets criteria for alcohol dependence.

Economic and Medical Sequelae

Alcohol use disorders are important to identify and treat for several reasons. The first is the direct negative impact of chronic heavy alcohol exposure on cognitive, physical, social, and vocational functioning. The second is the well-described long-term medical sequelae of alcohol dependence such as hepatic cirrhosis, pancreatitis, and dementia. Chronic heavy drinking, even in the absence of a formal diagnosis of alcohol dependence, is associated with an increased risk of diabetes mellitus, hypertension, gastrointestinal bleeding, hemorrhagic stroke, and several forms of carcinoma. The third reason for identification and treatment is the public impact of alcohol use disorders, which covers associated traumatic injuries from motor vehicle and job-related accidents, alcohol-related crime, and their associated economic costs. More than $180 billion is lost to the U.S. economy each year due to alcohol-related crime, injury, health care costs, and lost productivity in the workplace.

Screening

SCREENING RATIONALE

Screening for alcohol problems arrays patients on a continuum from abstinence to dependence and is a highly efficient way to identify patients who are at acute risk for the effects of alcohol abuse and dependence as well as those who do not currently meet formal alcohol-related diagnoses but who are at risk for long-term medical and social consequences of heavy alcohol exposure (Box 1). The U.S. Preventative Services Task Force (USPSTF) found that screening could accurately identify patients whose levels or patterns of alcohol consumption do not meet criteria for alcohol dependence but that place them at risk for increased morbidity and mortality. The USPSTF also found good evidence that brief interventions that consist of behavioral counseling and follow-up can reduce alcohol consumption for 6 to 12 months or longer and that the benefits outweigh any potential harms. Thus, it is recommended that alcohol screening and brief interventions be performed in primary care settings to reduce alcohol problems for adults, including pregnant women.

BRIEF SCREENING

Every patient should be asked about alcohol use. Because drinking is normative in the United States, if drinking is denied, it is useful to determine if the patient used to drink but has stopped because of a past problem. After determining if a patient currently uses any alcohol, the simplest strategy is to ask about the number of heavy drinking days in the past year, where heavy drinking is defined as more than four drinks for men and more than three drinks for women in one day. If that threshold is reached, which corresponds to at-risk or hazardous drinking, then further evaluation of alcohol-related problems is indicated through the use of screening instruments. A standard drink is the same amount of alcohol contained in different volumes of alcoholic beverages (Box 2).

BOX 1   Current Risk Terms

Abstinence
- No alcohol use

Moderate Drinking
- Men: No more than 2 standard drinks per drinking d
- Women: No more than 1 standard drink per drinking d
- Elderly persons (>65 y): No more than 1 standard drink per drinking d

Risky or Hazardous Drinking
- Men
  - More than 4 standard drinks per drinking d
  - More than 14 standard drinks per wk
- Women
  - More than 3 standard drinks per drinking d
  - More than 7 standard drinks per wk
- Elderly persons (>65 y):
  - More than 3 standard drinks per drinking d
  - More than 7 standard drinks per wk

BOX 2 Standard Drinks

Each equivalent drink contains about 14 g of pure alcohol:
- 12 oz of beer or wine cooler
- 8–9 oz of malt liquor
- 5 oz of wine
- 3 to 4 oz of fortified wine (e.g., port)
- 1½ oz of 80-proof distilled spirits (or 1 jigger of liquor before mixing)

The Alcohol Use Disorders Identification test (AUDIT) (Table 1) is a 10-item screen developed by the World Health Organization. Given its length, the AUDIT can be used as a self-report screener that patients can fill out in the waiting area before seeing the clinician. The minimum score is 0 and the maximum score is 40. A score of 8 or more for men or 4 or more for women, adolescents, and persons older than 65 years, like a positive endorsement of any heavy drinking days, indicates the need for further evaluation of alcohol use and an increased risk of an alcohol use disorder. For brevity, the AUDIT-C, a truncated version of the AUDIT consisting of the first three AUDIT questions focused on alcohol consumption, can be used as a part of a waiting-room health history form. A score of 6 or more for men or 4 or more for women on the AUDIT-C indicates a need for further evaluation.

Asking about alcohol consumption during a routine clinical interview is best bundled with other questions about lifestyle and health, such as diet, smoking, and exercise. In addition to giving the patient a pre-examination questionnaire to fill out such as the AUDIT, another screening strategy is to ask the CAGE questions (Box 3) during the clinical examination. A positive answer to any of these questions also indicates the need for further evaluation of alcohol use. Two or more CAGE questions answered affirmatively identifies a patient at high risk for alcohol dependence. Because the CAGE screens for consequences, it is not as sensitive for risky drinking.

There are other question sets that are more sensitive than the CAGE in specific demographic subsets, and these can also be easily asked during a routine history. The five-item TWEAK questionnaire (Table 2) may be a more optimal screening questionnaire for identifying women (including pregnant women) with risky drinking or alcohol-use disorders in racially mixed populations. The CRAFFT (Box 4) is a 6-item question set that has high sensitivity in screening adolescents for alcohol and other substance-abuse problems. For patients older than 65 years, the Short Michigan Alcoholism Screening Test—Geriatric (S-MAST-G) (Box 5) is useful in identifying those at risk for alcohol problems, because these patients might not need the same volumes of alcohol intake as others to develop alcohol-related problems. To complete the initial screening, one should compute the average number of drinks per week by multiplying the days per week on average that the patient drinks by the number of drinks consumed on a typical drinking day.

Laboratory testing for elevations of alanine aminotransferase (ALT), aspartate aminotransferase (AST), γ-glutamyltransferase (GGT), or carbohydrate-deficient transferrin (CDT) have no incremental sensitivity over those of validated screening instruments, and they may be better suited to monitoring patients already in treatment for alcohol-use disorders. The patient must still be asked about quantity and frequency of alcohol use. However, laboratory testing can provide indicators of covert heavy drinking (e.g., elevated GGT

TABLE 1 Alcohol Use Disorders Identification Test (AUDIT)

Questions	Scoring				
	0	1	2	3	4
Consumption (AUDIT-C)					
How often do you have a drink containing alcohol?	Never	Monthly or less	2 to 4 times a mo	2 to 3 times a wk	4 or more times a wk
How many drinks containing alcohol do you have on a typical day when you are drinking?	1 or 2	3 or 4	5 or 6	7 to 9	10 or more
How often do you have five or more drinks on one occasion?	Never	Less than monthly	Monthly	Weekly	Daily or almost daily
Personal Consequences					
How often during the last year have you found that you were not able to stop drinking once you had started?	Never	Less than monthly	Monthly	Weekly	Daily or almost daily
How often during the last year have you failed to do what was normally expected of you because of drinking?	Never	Less than monthly	Monthly	Weekly	Daily or almost daily
How often during the last year have you needed a first drink in the morning to get yourself going after a heavy drinking session?	Never	Less than monthly	Monthly	Weekly	Daily or almost daily
How often during the last year have you had a feeling of guilt or remorse after drinking?	Never	Less than monthly	Monthly	Weekly	Daily or almost daily
How often during the last year have you been unable to remember what happened the night before because of your drinking?	Never	Less than monthly	Monthly	Weekly	Daily or almost daily
Social Consequences					
Have you or someone else been injured because of your drinking?	No		Yes, but not in the last y		Yes, during the last y
Has a relative, friend, doctor, or other health care worker been concerned about your drinking or suggested you cut down?	No		Yes, but not in the last y		Yes, during the last y

Scoring and Interpretation
Add all scores to obtain a total: >8 points for men or >4 points for women indicates a high risk of alcohol use disorder.
AUDIT-C (first three AUDIT questions): >6 points for men or >4 points for women indicates a need for further evaluation.

and CDT) when the patient does not reveal the extent of alcohol intake. CDT, which is perturbed less than other indices by nonalcoholic liver disease, may be a more specific and sensitive indicator of heavy drinking.

Diagnosis

Screening can identify those who are at risk for the sequelae of risky or hazardous drinking and who might benefit from a brief intervention conducted in the primary care office, but only a diagnostic evaluation can confirm the clinician's suspicion that the patient's use of alcohol meets syndromal criteria and warrants specific medical and psychosocial treatment beyond the brief intervention. If, during the last 12 months, alcohol has contributed to repeated episodes of failure to fulfill obligations at home, school or work, episodes of increased risk of physical harm, arrests or other legal problems, or recurrent problems with significant others, then the patient has a diagnosis of alcohol abuse, according to *Diagnostic and Statistical Manual of Mental Disorders*, fourth edition (text revision) (DSM-IV TR) criteria (Table 3). The patient has a diagnosis of alcohol dependence if he or she has three or more of the following criteria over a 12-month period: physical tolerance, symptoms of withdrawal, repeatedly drinking more than intended, unsuccessful reduction or quit attempts, increased time drinking or recovering from drinking, reduced time in other pleasurable or important activities, and continued drinking despite physical or psychological problems.

Rates of co-occurring mood and anxiety disorders are especially high among those with alcohol-use disorders. Untreated mood and anxiety disorders tend to have a negative impact on alcoholism recovery. Among treatment-seeking patients in the National Epidemiologic Survey on Alcohol and Related Conditions (NESARC) sample with a current alcohol use disorder, 40% had at least one current independent mood disorder, and more than one third had at least one current independent anxiety disorder. Heavy alcohol intake can also induce symptoms of mood and other mental disorders. To differentiate alcohol-induced symptoms from independent disorders, it is optimal to reassess symptoms of a mental disorder several weeks after cessation or significant reduction of alcohol intake.

CURRENT DIAGNOSIS

Risky or Hazardous Drinking (Need Further Evaluation)

- Men who drink more than four standard drinks per day or 14 standard drinks per week
- Women and those older than 65 years who drink more than three standard drinks per day or more than seven standard drinks per week
- Drinking concurrent with any medical condition where alcohol is contraindicated

Alcohol Abuse

- Repeated failure to fulfill obligations at home, school, or work
- Increased risk of physical harm
- Legal problems or interpersonal problems in any year

Alcohol Dependence (Three or More in Any Year)

- Cannot cut down or stop
- Decreased time spent in other usual activities
- Drinking despite physical or psychological consequences
- Drinking more than intended
- Physical tolerance
- Preoccupied with drinking
- Withdrawal episodes

Brief Intervention

INTENTION

Although risky or hazardous drinking is not a formal diagnosis, it describes a group with a higher likelihood to develop alcohol problems with risk for accidents, injuries, and social and health problems compared with the general population (see Box 1). Thus, even without a formal diagnosis, it is beneficial to help the patient with risky drinking to change his or her drinking behavior. Several well-described short interchanges between the clinician and the patient, organized under the rubric of *brief interventions*, have been validated in randomized trials as decreasing alcohol intake in those who drink too much but do not have a diagnosis of alcohol dependence. Brief intervention has been demonstrated to reduce weekly alcohol use, frequency of binging, liver enzymes associated with heavy drinking, blood pressure, emergency department visits, hospital days, and psychosocial problems, typically for 6 to 12 months, and to reduce drinking and hospital days at up to 4 years in one study. Because most at-risk patients seen in primary care settings are subsyndromal for alcohol-use disorders, the typical clinical interaction related to alcohol will be that of screening and then a brief intervention for positive cases. The two are typically referred to together under the acronym SBI (screening and brief intervention).

The basic intention of a brief intervention is to educate the patient about the risks of heavy alcohol use in such a way as to motivate him or her to reduce weekly alcohol consumption. The standard

TABLE 2 TWEAK Questionnaire

Feature	Question	Answer	Score
Tolerance	How many drinks does it take before you begin to feel the first effects of alcohol?	≥3	2
Worry	Have your friends or relatives worried or complained about your drinking in the past year?	Yes	2
Eye-opener	Do you sometimes take a drink in the morning when you first get up?	Yes	1
Amnesia	Are there times when you drink and afterward you can't remember what you said or did?	Yes	1
Kut	Do you sometimes feel the need to cut down on your drinking?	Yes	1

Scoring and interpretation: Two or more points indicate a possible alcohol problem.

BOX 4   CRAFFT Questionnaire

- Have you ever ridden in a **C**ar driven by someone (including yourself) who was high or had been using alcohol or drugs?
- Do you ever use alcohol or drugs to **R**elax, feel better about yourself, or fit in?
- Do you ever use alcohol or drugs while you are **A**lone?
- Do you ever **F**orget things you did while using alcohol or drugs?
- Do your **F**amily or **F**riends ever tell you that you should cut down on your drinking or drug use?
- Have you ever gotten into **T**rouble while you were using alcohol or drugs?

One yes response indicates need for further assessment. Two yes responses indicate risk of alcohol-use disorder.

---

initial brief intervention takes about 15 minutes and consists of feedback, advice, and goal setting. It can be performed wholly in the primary care setting by the physician or other members of the health delivery team. Including alcohol screening, the USPSTF suggests five as to conducting SBI: *assess* the patient's alcohol consumption with a screening tool and clinical evaluation as indicated; *advise* reduction of alcohol consumption to appropriate levels, including abstinence if indicated; *agree* on individual goals for reducing alcohol use, including abstinence if indicated; *assist* patients in obtaining the motivation, skills, or supports needed to institute changes in drinking; and *arrange* for follow-up support, including specialty treatment referral for dependent patients. The most effective interventions are multicontact ones that provide ongoing assistance and follow-up.

PROCEDURE

Assess

Screen patients with the AUDIT or with the CAGE, TWEAK, CRAFFT, or S-MAST-G questionnaires as appropriate, and compute average drinks per week.

BOX 5   S-MAST-G Questionnaire

- When talking with others, do you ever underestimate how much you actually drink?
- After a few drinks, have you sometimes not eaten or been able to skip meals because you didn't feel hungry?
- Does having a few drinks help decrease your shakiness or tremors?
- Does alcohol sometimes make it hard for you to remember parts of the day or night?
- Do you usually take a drink to relax or calm your nerves?
- Do you drink to take your mind off your problems?
- Have you ever increased your drinking after experiencing a loss in your life?
- Has a doctor or nurse ever said that he or she was worried or concerned about your drinking?
- Have you ever made rules to manage your drinking?
- When you feel lonely, does having a drink help?

Two or more yes responses indicate a probable alcohol problem.

Abbreviation: S-MAST-G = Short Michigan Alcoholism Screening Test—Geriatric.

Advise

Give feedback in the form of expression of concern, direct conclusions, and recommendations. Present medical findings, such as elevated liver enzymes, to back up conclusive statements such as "I'm concerned that your alcohol intake exceeds safe limits." Show the patient information comparing use with population norms and the associated health risks. Educate the patient about how alcohol can lead to medical, psychosocial, and legal consequences. Where possible, link the patient's current symptoms to alcohol use. Recommend appropriate and specific changes in behavior, such as "I strongly recommend you cut down your drinking," or in the case where any drinking places the patient at high risk, "I strongly suggest you quit drinking."

Agree

Determine the patient's readiness to change drinking behavior, such as asking, "Do you think that cutting down on your drinking is something you are willing to talk about?" If the patient is ambivalent, avoid labeling the patient's behavior with a diagnosis at this stage, which can increase resistance to change, but encourage the patient to reflect on the positive reasons for drinking and the negative consequences of drinking. Offer concerns that continued drinking at the same level will impede the patient's achievement of goals such as decreased gastric distress or improved sleep patterns.

Empathic listening is generally more effective than a confrontational approach, and it is useful to express optimism about the patient's capacity to change. Elicit what the patient's concerns are about cutting down or quitting. Avoid arguing or challenging when the patient is unready to change, but schedule a follow-up visit to continue the dialogue and reassess drinking behavior. Restate your commitment to help when the patient is ready and that you remain open to questions.

When the patient concurs that a change in drinking would be beneficial, agree on a specific goal to cut down to particular daily and weekly limits for low-risk drinking or to stop drinking, if indicated, for a specific period of time. The agreement should be recorded and a copy given to the patient both as a reminder and motivator for behavioral change.

Assist

Work with the patient to formulate concrete steps to implement the drinking reduction plan. These steps include how to avoid high-risk drinking situations, how to keep a record of alcohol intake, and who can support the patient in meeting his or her goals. Provide resources in the form of patient educational materials, examples of which can be downloaded from the National Institute of Alcohol Abuse and Alcoholism (NIAAA) website (www.niaaa.nih.gov).

Arrange

Set up follow-up support and counseling visits or refer patients meeting dependence criteria for specialty treatment. Advise the patient to seek immediate medical treatment if withdrawal symptoms occur.

Treatment

DETOXIFICATION

Put simply, detoxification is medical stabilization that offers an opportunity to engage patients in alcoholism treatment, but it is not in itself treatment for alcohol dependence. Patients who drink more than 250 grams of alcohol daily are likely to experience physiologic withdrawal symptoms on cessation of drinking, but volume is not the only predictor of withdrawal severity. Although often mild, untreated alcohol withdrawal can result in seizures or delirium tremens (DTs), with increased risk of mortality.

TABLE 3 Diagnosis of Alcohol-Use Problems

Criteria	Typical Symptoms and History
Alcohol Abuse (≥1 in the last 12 mo)	
Alcohol has caused or contributed to repeated:	
Failure to fulfill obligations at home, school, or work	Hangovers at work, truancy at school, missing appointments
Episodes of increased risk of physical harm	Drinking and driving, swimming, or operating machinery
Arrests or other legal problems	Public intoxication, DUI or DWI
Problems with significant others	Spousal strife, physical fights
Alcohol Dependence (≥3 in the last 12 mo)	
Development of physical tolerance	Drinks more for the same effect
Episodes of withdrawal syndrome (see below)	Morning shakes, nausea, anxiety
Drinking more than intended repeatedly	Binging episodes
Unsuccessful efforts to cut down or stop drinking	Failed New Year's resolution
Increased time planning for drinking, drinking, or recovering from drinking	Instead of being with kids, spends weekend mornings sleeping in
Reduced time in other pleasurable or important activities	Stopped socializing with friends, withdrew from hobby group
Drinking persists despite physical or psychological problems	Developed depressed mood, but kept on drinking
Alcohol Withdrawal (≥2 within h to d after lowered blood alcohol levels)	
Autonomic hyperactivity	Heart rate ≥100 bpm, diaphoresis
Hand tremor	Hands shake when extended
Insomnia	Difficulty falling asleep
Nausea or vomiting	Feels queasy
Anxiety	Spontaneous report of fear
Psychomotor agitation	Inability to keep still, pacing
Hallucinations or illusions	Reports visual disturbances
Seizures	Tonic-clonic movements

Assessment

The Clinical Institute Withdrawal Assessment—Alcohol Revised (CIWA-Ar) is a public domain scale that scores 10 signs and symptoms of withdrawal by severity ranging from not present to severe (Box 6). A score of less than 8 indicates mild withdrawal, characterized by increased autonomic activity with low-grade anxiety, diaphoresis, agitation, nausea, and elevated blood pressure, temperature, and heart rate. Scores of 8 to 15 indicate moderate withdrawal, and scores of 15 or more indicate more severe withdrawal states. In severe withdrawal, in the context of autonomic hyperarousal, the patient can become disoriented and have a clouded sensorium, the hallmarks of delirium.

Prior history of severe withdrawal, such as DTs, is a reasonable predictor of similar future responses to alcohol withdrawal. Risk for withdrawal delirium is increased if the patient has a heart rate of greater than 120 bpm before treatment, a current infectious disease, withdrawal symptoms in the context of a blood alcohol concentration greater than 100 mg/dL, a prior history of either delirium or seizures, or a high CIWA-Ar score, indicating severe autonomic hyperactivity. Patients who have severe withdrawal symptoms, who are at high risk for seizures, or who have a medical condition likely to be exacerbated by withdrawal, such as type 1 diabetes or coronary artery disease, should have medically supervised inpatient detoxification.

 CURRENT THERAPY

All At-Risk Patients

- Assess: Screen patients with standard instruments and compute average standard drinks per week.
- Advise: Give feedback, express concern, present findings and conclusions, and recommend specific behavioral changes.
- Agree: Determine the patient's readiness to change, encourage reflection, listen empathically, elicit patient concerns, avoid arguing, express optimism, set a specific reduction or abstinence goal.
- Assist: Formulate concrete implementation plan, including avoiding high-risk situations, recording alcohol intake, and eliciting family and community support for patient goals.
- Arrange: Set up follow-up visits and refer patients meeting dependence criteria for specialty treatment.

Additionally for Alcohol-Dependent Patients

- Offer or arrange for detoxification if indicated.
- Offer or arrange for specialty alcoholism treatment and/or mutual help groups.
- Offer pharmacotherapy to support maintenance of abstinence: naltrexone, acamprosate, or disulfiram.
- Offer medication management support during follow-up visits.

Pharmacologic Therapy

Alcohol withdrawal is best treated with sedative hypnotic medications that are cross-tolerant with alcohol, such as benzodiazepines. Longer-acting benzodiazepines such as diazepam (Valium) and chlordiazepoxide (Librium) are easier to titrate against withdrawal symptoms and give a gradual offset in plasma concentration, but shorter-acting benzodiazepines such as lorazepam (Ativan)[1] are less likely to oversedate the patient. Rapid-onset benzodiazepines have a higher abuse liability and are generally best avoided. However, patients with severe hepatic impairment (elevated total bilirubin) are best treated with benzodiazepines that are not oxidized by the liver, such as oxazepam (Serax) or lorazepam.

Typical dosing is chlordiazepoxide 50 to 100 mg, diazepam 10 to 20 mg, oxazepam 20 to 40[3] mg, or lorazepam[1] 2 to 4 mg. The typical front-loading style of dosing is to administer medication at the higher end of the dose range every 1 to 2 hours so that the CIWA-Ar score is less than 8 for 24 hours.

With long-acting medications, once symptoms subside, there is often no need to taper doses. The short-acting benzodiazepines and long-acting benzodiazepines given to patients at high-risk for seizures

---

[1]Not FDA approved for this indication.
[3]Exceeds dosage recommended by the manufacturer.

BOX 6 Clinical Institute Withdrawal Assessment of Alcohol Scale, Revised (CIWA-Ar)

Patient:_____ Date:_____ Time:_____ (24 hour clock, midnight = 00:00)

Pulse or heart rate, taken for one minute:_____ Blood pressure:_____ mm Hg

Nausea and Vomiting – Ask "Do you feel sick to your stomach? Have you vomited?" Observation:
0 no nausea and no vomiting
1 mild nausea with no vomiting
2
3
4 intermittent nausea with dry heaves
5
6
7 constant nausea, frequent dry heaves, and vomiting

Tremor – Arms extended and fingers spread apart. Observation:
0 no tremor
1 not visible, but can be felt fingertip to fingertip
2
3
4 moderate, with patient's arms extended
5
6
7 severe, even with arms not extended

Paroxysmal Sweats – Observation:
0 no sweat visible
1 barely perceptible sweating, palms moist
2
3
4 beads of sweat obvious on forehead
5
6
7 drenching sweats

Anxiety – Ask "Do you feel nervous?" Observation:
0 no anxiety, at ease
1 mild anxious
2
3
4 moderately anxious, or guarded, so anxiety is inferred
5
6
7 equivalent to acute panic states as seen in severe
   delirium or acute schizophrenic reactions

Agitation – Observation:
0 normal activity
1 somewhat more than normal activity
2
3
4 moderately fidgety and restless
5
6
7 paces back and forth during most of the interview or
   constantly thrashes about

Tactile Disturbances – Ask "Have you any itching, pins and needles sensations, any burning, any numbness, or do you feel bugs crawling on or under your skin?" Observation:
0 none
1 very mild itching, pins and needles, burning, or numbness
2 mild itching, pins and needles, burning, or numbness
3 moderate itching, pins and needles, burning, or numbness
4 moderately severe hallucinations
5 severe hallucinations
6 extremely severe hallucinations
7 continuous hallucinations

Auditory Disturbances – Ask "Are you more aware of sounds around you? Are they harsh? Do they frighten you? Are you hearing anything that is disturbing to you? Are you hearing things you know are not there?" Observation:
0 not present
1 very mild harshness or ability to frighten
2 mild harshness or ability to frighten
3 moderate harshness or ability to frighten
4 moderately severe hallucinations
5 severe hallucinations
6 extremely severe hallucinations
7 continuous hallucinations

Visual Disturbances – Ask "Does the light appear to be too bright? Is its color different? Does it hurt your eyes? Are you seeing anything that is disturbing to you? Are you seeing things you know are not there?" Observation:
0 not present
1 very mild sensitivity
2 mild sensitivity
3 moderate sensitivity
4 moderately severe hallucinations
5 severe hallucinations
6 extremely severe hallucinations
7 continuous hallucinations

Headache, Fullness in Head – Ask "Does your head feel different? Does it feel like there is a band around your head?" Do not rate for dizziness or lightheadedness. Otherwise, rate severity:
0 not present
1 very mild
2 mild
3 moderate
4 moderately severe
5 severe
6 very severe
7 extremely severe

Orientation and Clouding of Sensorium – Ask "What day is this? Where are you? Who am I?"
0 oriented and can do serial additions
1 cannot do serial additions or is uncertain about date
2 disoriented for date by no more than 2 calendar d
3 disoriented for date by more than 2 calendar d
4 disoriented for place or person

Total CIWA-Ar Score_____
Rater's Initials_____
Maximum Possible Score: 67

The CIWA-Ar *is not* copyright and may be reproduced freely. This assessment for monitoring withdrawal symptoms requires approximately 5 minutes to administer.

From Sullivan JT, Sykora K, Schneiderman J, Naranjo CA, Sellers EM: Assessment of alcohol withdrawal: The revised Clinical Institute Withdrawal Assessment for Alcohol scale (CIWA-Ar). Br J Addiction 1989;84:1353–1357.

or DTs are best given on a fixed-dose regimen of four times daily for the first 24 hours, with the patient reassessed 1 to 2 hours after each dose, and additional medication given as needed. On days 2 and 3, 50% of the dose can be given four times daily.

Long-acting barbiturates, such as phenobarbital,[1] can be also used on a fixed-dose regimen of 60 mg every 4 to 6 hours, with a loading dose of 120 mg orally or intramuscularly every hour for acute withdrawal symptoms (e.g., pulse >110 bpm) or a CIWA-Ar score of 10 or more.

Anticonvulsants such as carbamazepine (Tegretol),[1] valproate (Depakote),[1] or gabapentin (Neurontin)[1] have also been used effectively in uncomplicated withdrawal, but they are unproved in preventing withdrawal-related seizures and in treating DTs.

Although phenothiazines and haloperidol are somewhat effective compared with benzodiazepines in reducing withdrawal symptoms such as agitation, they are not as protective against seizures or delirium and thus are not recommended.

Thiamine (vitamin B$_1$) supplementation of 100 mg/day for 3 days can counteract the thiamine deficiencies that are common in alcoholic patients.

PSYCHOSOCIAL INTERVENTIONS FOR ALCOHOL DEPENDENCE

In addition to brief interventions for risky alcohol use, the most opportune and practical psychosocial intervention that the primary care office can provide is clinical behavioral support for pharmacotherapy for alcohol dependence. Simply put, medication management support consists initially of feedback to the patient of screening and medical evaluation results and the negative health effects of continued heavy drinking, as in a brief intervention. The patient is then given the basis for the diagnosis of alcohol dependence, the rationale for abstinence, and recommendation for pharmacotherapy. The patient is given information about medication and the appropriate prescriptions and is encouraged to seek community support for sobriety in mutual help groups such as Alcoholics Anonymous or to follow a plan such as Rational Recovery. Follow-up visits consist of assessment of medication side effects, patient adherence to the medication regimen, assessment of abstinence or quantity and pattern of alcohol intake, and assessment of overall functioning. Problems with medication adherence are identified and addressed.

There are evidence-based psychosocial interventions that are typically performed in the context of specialty programs for alcohol dependence, but they can be offered by clinical personnel in the context of the physician's office. Cognitive behavior therapy, network therapy, behavioral family therapy, and motivational interviewing are effective approaches for the treatment of alcohol dependence. Motivational interviewing is especially adaptable for use in primary care settings in that it is an approach to interacting with the alcohol-dependent patient that can be learned quickly and executed by any staff with clinical contact. A motivational enhancement manual can be accessed at the NIAAA website (http://www.niaaa.nih.gov/).

MEDICATION MANAGEMENT OF ALCOHOL DEPENDENCE

There are currently four FDA-approved medications for the treatment of alcohol dependence. Any of these medications can and should be given concurrently with other interventions such as psychosocial treatment or mutual help groups.

Disulfiram (Antabuse) works by inhibiting the metabolism of ethyl alcohol, causing a buildup of acetaldehyde, a noxious substance, which causes a strong stereotypic aversive response (flushing, diaphoresis, nausea, tachycardia) in the patient. Standard dosing is 250 mg/day (range, 125–500 mg). The major clinical concern with disulfiram is patient noncompliance with the medication regimen. Thus, it is most likely to be effective when there is a concrete method for supporting compliance in place, such as directly observed therapy by a spouse or in a clinic.

More recently, the opioid antagonist naltrexone (ReVia, Depade) was approved for the treatment of alcohol dependence. It is dosed at 50 mg once daily. Naltrexone reduces days of heavy drinking and can reduce alcohol craving. Naltrexone in a long-acting intramuscular formulation (Vivitrol) allows once-monthly dosing (380 mg) and reduces the risk of noncompliance. It reduces heavy drinking overall and helps maintain abstinence in those who are abstinent at initial drug administration. Both oral and IM naltrexone formulations carry FDA black-box warnings related to findings of reversible elevations of liver enzymes at three to six times the standard dosage; however, naltrexone is safe at the recommended dose.

Acamprosate (Campral) is a taurine analogue that has been demonstrated to reduce relapse to any drinking as well as reducing heavy drinking in nonabstinent patients. It is dosed as two 333-mg tablets three times a day to patients who have ceased alcohol intake. It is excreted unchanged through the kidneys and has no interactions with other medications. Side effects are benign, and the most frequent is loose stools, which are mild to moderate and self-limited.

Topiramate[1] (Topamax) titrated over 5 weeks between 50 mg and 300 mg daily appears to reduce heavy drinking and days of any drinking over the short term (12 weeks) in alcohol-dependent patients who have not established abstinence prior to treatment. Common side effects include paresthesias, taste perversion, decreased appetite, and difficulty concentrating.

REFERENCES

American Psychiatric Association. Diagnostic and statistical manual of mental disorders. 4th ed. text revision. Washington, DC: American Psychiatric Association; 2000.

Bertholet N, Daeppen J-B, Wietlisbach V, et al. Reduction of alcohol consumption by brief alcohol intervention in primary care systematic review and meta-analysis. Arch Intern Med 2005;165:986–95.

Bradley KA, Boyd-Wickizer J, Powell SH, Burman ML. Alcohol screening questionnaires in women: A critical review. JAMA 1998;280:166–71.

Chang G, Kosten TR. Detoxification. In: Lowinson JH, Ruiz P, Millman RB, Langrod JG, editors. Substance Abuse: A Comprehensive Textbook. Philadelphia: Lippincott Williams & Wilkins; 2004. p. 579–87.

Fleming MF, Mundt MP, French MT, et al. Brief physician advice for problem drinkers: Long-term efficacy and cost-benefit analysis. Alcohol Clin Exp Res 2002;26:36–43.

Grant BF, Stinson FS, Dawson DA, et al. Prevalence and co-occurrence of substance use disorders and independent mood and anxiety disorders: Results from the National Epidemiologic Survey on Alcohol and Related Conditions. Arch Gen Psychiatry 2004;61:807–16.

Johnson BA, Rosenthal N, Capece JA, et al. Topiramate for treating alcohol dependence: A randomized controlled trial. JAMA 2007;298:1641–51.

Knight JR, Sherritt L, Shrier LA, et al. Validity of the CRAFFT substance abuse screening test among adolescent clinic patients. Arch Pediatr Adolesc Med 2002;156(6):607–14.

Maisto SA, Saitz R. Alcohol use disorders: Screening and diagnosis. Am J Addict 2003;12(Suppl. 1):S12–25.

McCaul ME, Petry NM. The role of psychosocial treatments in pharmacotherapy for alcoholism. Am J Addict 2003;12(Suppl. 1):S41–52.

National Institute on Alcohol Abuse and Alcoholism. Helping patients who drink too much: a clinician's guide, Rockville, MD: National Institute on Alcohol Abuse and Alcoholism; 2005. Available at http://pubs.niaaa.nih .gov/publications/Practitioner/CliniciansGuide2005/guide.pdf (accessed June 15, 2007).

Saitz R. Unhealthy alcohol use. N Engl J Med 2005;352:596–607.

Saunders JB, Aasland OG, Babor TF, et al. Development of the Alcohol Use Disorders Screening Test (AUDIT) WHO collaborative project on early detection of persons with harmful alcohol consumption. Addiction 1993;88:791–804.

Sullivan JT, Sykora K, Schneiderman J, et al. Assessment of alcohol withdrawal: The revised Clinical Institute Withdrawal Assessment for Alcohol scale (CIWA-Ar). Br J Addict 1989;84:1353–7.

U.S. Preventive Services Task Force. Screening and behavioral counseling interventions in primary care to reduce alcohol misuse: Recommendation statement. Ann Intern Med 2004;140:554–6.

---

[1]Not FDA approved for this indication.

---

[1]Not FDA approved for this indication.

Treatment for Addiction

Method of
Ari Kalechstein, PhD, Richard De La Garza, PhD, and Thomas Newton, MD

Addiction is a major public health concern in the United States. This assertion is supported by the data from various epidemiologic studies. For example, the 2007 National Survey on Drug Use and Health revealed that 18,900,000 individuals 12 years old or older were using illegal drugs or misusing licit medications at the time of the study (http://www.oas.samhsa.gov/nsduh/2k7nsduh/2k7Results.pdf). In 2006, the Drug Abuse Warning Network reported that approximately 1,700,000 emergency room visits were the result of misuse of alcohol, abuse of licit medications, or the use of illicit drugs (http://dawninfo.samhsa.gov/files/ED2006/DAWN2k6ED.pdf). In 2007, 1,817,577 treatment-seeking addicts were admitted to treatment facilities that receive state alcohol or drug agency funds (including federal block grant funds) for the provision of alcohol and drug treatment services (http://wwwdasis.samhsa.gov/teds07/tedshigh2k7.pdf).

Given the prevalence of drug use in 2007, the number of emergent situations in 2006, and the number of treatment admissions to publicly funded treatment agencies, it is imperative that efficacious treatment regimens be available for remediation of addiction. For the purpose of this chapter, *efficacious* is defined as demonstrated validity and reliability through the process of peer review. Double-blind, placebo-controlled studies are considered to be the gold standard of treatment efficacy, whereas case-control studies and anecdotal evidence, although informative, are not.

Because the focus of the chapter is treatment outcome, several issues are not addressed. For instance, the diagnostic criteria for particular disorders, the consequences of short- and long-term use, and the prevalence of misuse or abuse of particular substances are not discussed. Coverage of treatments for the most prevalent drugs of abuse, including alcohol, cocaine, heroin, marijuana, methamphetamine, and nicotine, is limited.

Alcohol

Alcohol, along with nicotine, has been the focus of the greatest number of treatment-outcome studies. A PubMed search using the search terms *alcoholism, treatment outcome,* and *pharmacotherapy* yielded 996 studies; one using the search terms *alcoholism, treatment outcome,* and *behavioral therapy* yielded 1496 studies; and another using the search terms *alcoholism, treatment outcome,* and *alcoholics anonymous* yielded 226 studies.

With respect to pharmacologic interventions, peer-reviewed research consistently identified disulfiram (Antabuse), acamprosate (Campral), topiramate (Topamax),[1] and naltrexone (ReVia) as effective adjuvant therapies approved by the FDA for the treatment of alcoholism. A subset of more refined analyses showed that acamprosate was effective in maintaining abstinence, whereas naltrexone was effective in ensuring that a single incident of alcohol use did not result in full-blown relapse to dependence. Several studies reported favorable findings regarding the use of injectable (Vivitrol) or oral (ReVia) naltrexone. Antidepressants and anxiolytics have received only limited attention in the research literature, and the studies did not yield positive findings.

Psychosocial interventions represent an effective form of treatment for alcoholism. The methodologies for these studies vary considerably, although the primary objective for these studies was that behavioral interventions reduce alcohol consumption or relapse to dependence. Despite variability in study findings, participants receiving cognitive-behavioral therapy (CBT) tended to use less alcohol. Investigators have not identified the specific factors that underlie the effectiveness of these treatments. Motivational interviewing techniques, contingency management, and relapse prevention also have demonstrated efficacy, even with the use of relatively brief interventions. With the exception of data obtained from Project MATCH, the efficacy of Alcoholics Anonymous as an intervention remains unclear and unproven; this outcome is not surprising given the lack of experimental controls.

Psychiatric comorbidity, such as the presence of thought disorder, mood disorders, or anxiety disorders, negatively affected treatment success. A subset of studies also reported that neurocognitive impairment was an obstacle to positive treatment outcomes. Identification and treatment of these co-occurring disorders, particularly mood and anxiety disorders, tend to enhance treatment outcome.

Other work has targeted the issue of pharmacogenetics. For example, associations between genetic profiles and metabolism of alcohol have been identified. It is likely that this work holds great promise with regard to explaining, at least in part, the variability in alcoholics' response to treatment.

Cocaine

There are no FDA-approved treatments for cocaine dependence, although there are preliminary indications for off-label use of candidate medications. As evidenced by the volume of peer-review studies, there exists a keen level of interest on this topic. A PubMed search using the search terms *cocaine, treatment outcome,* and *pharmacotherapy* yielded 626 studies; one using the search terms *cocaine, treatment outcome,* and *behavioral therapy* yielded 511 studies; and another using the search terms *cocaine, treatment outcome,* and *cocaine anonymous* yielded 21 studies, although there was considerable overlap between these studies and those culled using the other searches.

Despite the initial promise of the results of phase I and II safety trials used to identify candidate medications for the treatment of cocaine dependence, outpatient clinical trials have not yielded any consistent findings to suggest that a particular candidate medication or combination thereof can provide effective treatment. The lack of positive findings is not a reflection of the lack of effort by the National Institute on Drug Abuse (NIDA) or associated investigators. Numerous medications, including amantadine (Symmetrel),[1] cabergoline (Dostinex),[1] co-enzyme Q10,[1] disulfiram (Antabuse),[1] donepezil (Aricept),[1] gabapentin (Neurontin),[1] ergoloid mesylates (Hydergine),[1] lamotrigine (Lamictal),[1] levodopa/carbidopa (Sinemet),[1] modafinil (Provigil),[1] olanzapine (Zyprexa),[1] paroxetine (Paxil),[1] pentoxifylline (Trental),[1] propranolol (Inderal),[1] reserpine,[1] risperidone (Risperdal),[1] sertraline (Zoloft),[1] tiagabine (Gabitril),[1] valproate (Depacon),[1] and venlafaxine (Effexor),[1] were tested without success. Preliminary results suggest that modafinil is effective when used in a cocaine-dependent person who was not abusing alcohol. There was an initial indication that disulfiram and modafinil effectively treated cocaine dependence, but this finding was not replicated.

Whereas limited efficacy has been obtained using medications, behavioral treatments for cocaine dependence have consistently demonstrated positive results. For example, CBT implementation is associated with effective treatment outcomes at 1 year after treatment. The use of various forms of contingency management, including those using treatment vouchers, has resulted in positive treatment outcomes. Contingency management has been applied effectively in dually diagnosed, treatment-refractory individuals. Limited data preliminarily suggest that motivational interviewing is also useful, although the findings need to be replicated.

A subset of studies sought to identify factors that moderated treatment outcome. In relapse prevention studies, dispensation of higher-value vouchers was associated with increased treatment efficacy. Moreover, posttreatment care in the form of follow-up counseling

---

[1]Not FDA approved for this indication.

[1]Not FDA approved for this indication.

sessions was related to increased rates of abstinence. Treatment of co-occurring illnesses, such as depression, enhanced the effectiveness of treatment. In contrast, individuals with a positive urine toxicology screen at the beginning of treatment, those who exhibited increased impulsivity, and those with impaired neurocognition were individually associated with poorer treatment outcomes.

Over the past 8 to 10 years, there has been considerable interest in pinpointing the genetic underpinnings of cocaine dependence. For instance, catechol-O-methyltransferase (COMT) and other enzymes have been preliminarily implicated as risk factors for the onset of cocaine addiction. There is interest in the development of a vaccine using cocaine antibodies that would inoculate addicts against relapse, although there have not been tests in human study participants.

Heroin

Much emphasis has been placed on the development of treatments for heroin addiction. A PubMed search using the search terms *heroin, treatment outcome*, and *pharmacotherapy* yielded 501 studies, and one using the search terms *heroin, treatment outcome*, and *behavioral therapy* yielded 288 studies.

There are four FDA-approved pharmacologic treatments for heroin dependence: methadone (Dolophine), buprenorphine (Subutex), buprenorphine/naloxone (Suboxone), and levo-α-acetylmethadol (LAAM [Orlaam]).[2] Methadone has been the treatment of choice since the early 1970s, but Subutex and Suboxone have become increasingly popular choices for addiction specialists. The buprenorphine-based treatments have a relatively more benign side effect profile than methadone. Although LAAM is considered to be an effective treatment, it has been characterized as a second-line treatment, which means that the medication should be prescribed only when buprenorphine and methadone have been shown to be ineffective.

The available research shows that CBT and contingency management are efficacious treatment modalities. They seem to be most effective when used as adjuncts to pharmacotherapy, although the results of other studies suggest that contingency management is as effective as pharmacotherapy with respect to the promotion of abstinence. In contrast, motivational interviewing techniques have not been validated as an intervention for heroin addiction.

With regard to variables that moderate treatment effectiveness, the extant research yielded mixed findings about the influence of demographic indices, co-occurring illness, and co-occurring substance use on treatment outcome. For example, co-occurring depression, novelty seeking, and decreased life satisfaction were associated with poorer treatment outcomes. The number of years of heroin use and previous entry into treatment were negatively associated with treatment outcome. Although there is interest in the identification of specific genetic profiles and treatment outcomes in humans, none has been detected.

Marijuana

The spelling of *marihuana* as *marijuana* became popular in the 1930s, when drug control advocates decided that the major influx of the illicit drug was from south of the border: "marijuana from Tijuana." Despite long-standing concerns regarding the public health consequences of marijuana (more accurately referred to as *cannabis*) abuse and dependence, which date back to the production of *Reefer Madness*, marijuana abuse has received relatively little attention in the treatment-outcome literature. This is particularly surprising given that published epidemiologic data showed that the number of treatment admissions for marijuana dependence at publicly funded treatment facilities doubled from 1993 to 2005. A PubMed search using the search terms *marijuana, treatment outcome*, and *pharmacotherapy*

yielded 55 studies, and another using the search terms *marijuana, treatment outcome*, and *behavioral therapy* yielded 58 studies.

There are no FDA-approved pharmacologic treatments for marijuana dependence. Few candidate medications have been tested, although there is preliminary interest in several. The findings of these studies showed that bupropion (Wellbutrin),[1] divalproex (Depakote),[1] naltrexone (ReVia),[1] and nefazodone (Serzone)[1] did not influence treatment outcomes. One study, which used lithium carbonate (Eskalith),[1] provided preliminary results that were positive. Another series of studies showed that orally administered Δ^9-tetrahydrocannabinol (dronabinol [Marinol])[1] effectively eliminated withdrawal symptoms, but the data did not address the maintenance of abstinence. A case study suggested dronabinol as a candidate medication for these patients.

The available research shows greater emphasis has been placed on the use of behavioral therapies to promote abstinence from marijuana use. The available literature showed that use of CBT, contingency management, and motivational interviewing resulted in superior outcomes compared with placebo or basic drug counseling. More refined studies showed that combination-treatment approaches, such as motivational interviewing plus contingency management or CBT plus contingency management, produced enhanced treatment outcomes relative to motivational interviewing alone or CBT alone.

One of the few studies that addressed variables that moderate treatment effectiveness reported that other drug use does not influence marijuana use. The presence of co-occurring mental health conditions, such as major depression and attention-deficit/hyperactivity disorder, were associated with poorer treatment outcomes. Demographic indices such as younger age, lower income, and financial difficulties portended earlier treatment attrition. The cannabinoid receptor 1 (CNR1) and fatty acid amide hydrolase (FAAH) were identified as potential mediators of the onset of marijuana dependence, although this has not been verified in longitudinal studies.

Methamphetamine

There are no FDA-approved treatments for methamphetamine dependence. Compared with the studies on cocaine and treatment outcome, fewer studies have been published on methamphetamine and treatment outcome. A PubMed search using the search terms *methamphetamine, treatment outcome*, and *pharmacotherapy* yielded 54 studies, and another using the search terms *methamphetamine, treatment outcome*, and *behavioral therapy* yielded 37 studies.

Despite the relative paucity of studies on methamphetamine, pharmacotherapy, and treatment outcome, identification of a medication-based treatment for methamphetamine is considered to be a priority. The FDA and NIDA have placed a fast-track designation on candidate medications for the treatment methamphetamine (and cocaine) dependence, because methamphetamine addiction is considered to be a major public health problem. Similar to cocaine, despite the initial promise of the results of phase I and II safety trials used to identify candidate medications for the treatment of methamphetamine dependence, field trials have yielded nonsignificant results. Field trials have been attempted with baclofen (Lioresal),[1] imipramine (Tofranil),[1] mirtazapine (Remeron),[1] ondansetron (Zofran),[1] paroxetine (Paxil),[1] quetiapine (Seroquel),[1] sertraline (Zoloft),[1] and topiramate (Topomax),[1] but none has provided convincing evidence of efficacy. One study suggested that modafinil (Provigil)[1] is effective, and confirmatory studies are in progress to determine if the finding can be replicated. Two separate field studies suggested that bupropion (Wellbutrin)[1] may serve as an effective off-label treatment for methamphetamine dependence.

Although none of the candidate medications modulated methamphetamine use, behavioral treatments for methamphetamine dependence have consistently demonstrated positive results. For example, CBT implementation and contingency management were associated with increased levels of abstinence. In the one study that compared the two approaches, contingency management was superior to

---

CBT across various measures of treatment outcome. One study has evaluated the efficacy of motivational interviewing, and the findings preliminarily suggest that this approach is effective.

A subset of studies sought to identify factors that moderated treatment outcome. More time spent in treatment and participation in contingency management was related to increased levels of abstinence. One study reported that female gender, lifetime use for more than 2 years, and use of methamphetamine by smoking or injection was associated with an inability to maintain abstinence during treatment. Individuals with greater levels of education and those who demonstrated the capacity to maintain abstinence during treatment were more likely to complete treatment. Posttreatment use was associated with injection use, pretreatment use longer than 2 years, prior history of drug use treatment, and psychiatric comorbidity (e.g., depression).

Nicotine

Other than alcohol, nicotine has been the focus of the greatest number of treatment-outcome studies. A PubMed search using the search terms *nicotine, treatment outcome,* and *pharmacotherapy* yielded 624 studies, and another using the search terms *nicotine, treatment outcome,* and *behavioral therapy* yielded 925 studies.

There are seven FDA-approved pharmacologic treatments for nicotine dependence. Five are characterized as nicotine replacement therapy: transdermal patch (Nicoderm CQ), nasal spray (Nicotrol NS), lozenge (Commit), inhaler (Nicotrol Inhaler), and gum (Nicorette). Two other treatments, bupropion (Zyban, a dopamine and norepinephrine transport inhibitor) and varenicline (Chantix, an agonist at the α4-β2 nicotine receptor), have been quite efficacious. Meta-analyses revealed that each of these treatments was superior to the benefits conferred by placebo, and available data suggest that varenicline demonstrated superior efficacy relative to bupropion and placebo, making it the best current treatment for nicotine dependence.

The available research shows that behavioral therapy and self-help materials are effective treatment modalities. These approaches demonstrate greater efficacy than placebo, but they are less effective than the pharmacologic interventions detailed earlier. Not surprisingly, therapeutic approaches that combine medication and behavioral interventions are most effective.

With respect to variables that moderate treatment effectiveness, the extant research yielded mixed findings regarding the influence of demographic indices, co-occurring illness, and co-occurring substance use on treatment outcome. For example, increased alcohol use is a risk factor for continued nicotine use. Increased levels of depression and anxiety are associated with poorer treatment outcome. Remarkably, a diagnosis of cancer is not associated with a clear trend in reduction of use. Neither increased age nor increased education was associated with improved outcomes; however, lack of financial coverage and inadequate training of medical providers was identified as a barrier to successful outcome.

Considerable progress has been made in the identification of the genetic underpinnings of nicotine dependence. Publications in 2009 reported that studies of genes associated with smoking cessation success in clinical trial participants might also apply to smokers who are more or less able to initiate and sustain abstinence outside of clinical trial settings.

Summary

Taken together, the available research reveals progress with respect to the treatment of addictive disorders, with variable efficacy across disorders and treatment modalities. Implementation of behavioral treatments was associated with improved treatment outcomes, particularly when contingency management was the treatment of choice. In contrast, despite the popularity of the approach, the efficacy of Alcoholics Anonymous and Narcotics Anonymous is questionable.

Pharmacotherapeutic approaches have demonstrated the greatest efficacy for individuals dependent on alcohol, heroin, and nicotine. Not surprisingly, these substances have received the greatest level of attention from researchers and clinicians over the past 60 years. Over time, it is likely that similar gains will be obtained in the identification of effective pharmacotherapies for the treatment of cocaine and methamphetamine dependence.

Technologic advances have facilitated the study of genetic risk factors for the onset of addiction to alcohol and drugs. Detection of the genetic underpinnings of addiction should be useful for identifying individuals who are at risk for alcohol and drug addictions. The capacity to identify the specific physiologic mechanisms by which addiction emerges may allow us to circumvent or remedy them.

Anxiety Disorders

Method of
Ellen J. Teng, PhD, and Thomas R. Kosten, MD

Anxiety disorders are the most prevalent psychiatric disorder, affecting approximately 40 million American adults each year. It is a common disorder found in medical settings because the nature of panic and anxiety symptoms cause most people to present to the emergency room or primary care doctor. Causes of anxiety include medication side effects, underlying organic disorders, and substance use and withdrawal. Anxiety stemming from concerns about a medical illness or procedure is a normal reaction and typically transient; however, anxiety can also take the form of a more pathologic state of disabling fear that warrants careful assessment and diagnosis. Underrecognition and misdiagnoses of these problems lead to high rates of health care use, medical expenditures, and poor patient outcomes.

Primary anxiety disorders include panic disorder with or without agoraphobia, social phobia, generalized anxiety disorder, obsessive-compulsive disorder, specific phobia, and posttraumatic stress disorder. These disorders share in common increased physiologic activity and dysregulation of emotional, cognitive, and behavioral processes.

Panic Disorder With or Without Agoraphobia

Panic disorder involves recurring, unexpected panic attacks followed by at least 1 month of worry about additional attacks, implications of the attacks, or a significant change in behavior because of the attacks. Agoraphobic avoidance can accompany panic attacks, in which situations or places are avoided in fear that a panic attack may occur where escape or obtaining help would be difficult. Panic attacks are characterized by sudden and intense fear that usually peaks within minutes and is accompanied by a number of symptoms that may last 30 minutes to several hours. Panic attacks consist mostly of physical symptoms, which make this disorder common in the general medical setting. Cardiac, respiratory, neurologic, and gastrointestinal symptoms are common during a panic attack, whereas cognitive symptoms center on concerns about losing control, going crazy, and dying. Panic attacks also occur in other anxiety disorders on exposure to a feared stimulus. Onset typically occurs in late adolescence and

TABLE 1 Treatment of Anxiety Disorders

Anxiety Disorder	Drug Type	Medication	Initial Dose (mg)	Dose Range (mg/day)
Panic disorder	SSRI	Citalopram (Celexa)[1]	20	20–60
		Escitalopram (Lexapro)[1]	10	5–20
		Paroxetine (Paxil)	10	10–60
		Clomipramine (Anafranil)[1]	25	25–75
	TCA	Imipramine (Tofranil)[1]	10–25	150–300
	MAOI	Phenelzine (Nardil)[1]	15–30	45–90
	BZ	Alprazolam (Xanax)	0.25 tid	2–10
Social phobia	SSRI	Paroxetine (Paxil)	10	10–60
	SNRI	Venlafaxine (Effexor XR)[1]	75	75–300
	MAOI	Phenelzine (Nardil)[1]	15–30	45–90
	β-Blocker	Propranolol (Inderal)[1]	10	10–40
Generalized anxiety disorder	SSRI	Paroxetine (Paxil)	10	10–60
		Escitalopram (Lexapro)	10	5–20
	SNRI	Venlafaxine XR (Effexor XR)[1]	75	75–225
	TCA	Imipramine (Tofranil)[1]	10–25	150–300
	Other	Buspirone (Buspar)	5 tid	10–60
		Hydroxyzine (Vistaril)	25 tid	75–600
Obsessive-compulsive disorder	SSRI	Sertraline (Zoloft)	50	50–200
		Fluvoxamine (Luvox)	50	50–300
		Fluoxetine (Prozac)	5–10	10–80
	TCA	Clomipramine (Anafranil)	25	25–75
	ANTIPSY	Risperidone (Risperdal)[1]	1 bid	2–6
Specific phobia	BZ	Lorazepam (Ativan)[1]	0.5 tid	3–12
	SSRI	Paroxetine (Paxil)[1]	10	10–60
Posttraumatic stress disorder	SSRI	Paroxetine (Paxil)	10	10–60
	SNRI	Venlafaxine (Effexor)[1]	37.5 bid	75–300
	MAOI	Phenelzine (Nardil)[1]	15–30	45–90
	TCA	Amitriptyline (Elavil)[1]	75	150–200
	Other	Mirtazapine (Remeron)[1]	15	30–45

[1]Not FDA approved for this indication.
Abbreviations: ANTIPSY = antipsychotic; β-Blocker = beta-blocker; BZ = benzodiazepine; MAOI = monoamine oxidase inhibitor; SNRI = serotonin-norepinephrine reuptake inhibitor; SSRI = selective serotonin reuptake inhibitor; TCA = tricyclic antidepressant.

the mid-30s, and panic disorder is more prevalent among women than men.

Cognitive-behavioral therapy (CBT) is effective in treating panic disorder (Table 1). Treatment is typically delivered once per week over a period of 10 to 12 sessions. Sessions are structured to provide education about the nature of anxiety and panic, correct mistaken and maladaptive thoughts about anxiety, teach techniques to decrease sympathetic arousal, and engage in exposure exercises to bodily sensations resembling the symptoms experienced during an actual panic attack. Pharmacotherapy includes the use of high-potency benzodiazepines and antidepressants, particularly tricyclic antidepressants (TCAs) and monoamine oxidase inhibitors (MAOIs).

CBT for panic disorder offers distinct advantages over pharmacotherapy because patients acquire skills that can continue to be applied after completing treatment. Although combining psychosocial treatments with pharmacotherapy for panic disorder has shown modest advantages over the short term compared with either treatment alone, these gains diminish over the long term. In most instances, combining CBT with pharmacotherapy is not warranted except for short-term symptom management during CBT.

Social Phobia

Social phobia is characterized by overwhelming anxiety and extreme self-consciousness in situations in which an individual may be evaluated by others. Patients with social phobia experience intense and persistent fear that they will behave in a way that will embarrass or humiliate them. This fear may be limited to one type of situation, such as eating in front of others, or it may manifest across multiple domains of social functioning, including meeting new people and speaking in public. Because intense anxiety is typically experienced on exposure to these situations despite the person's awareness that the fear is unreasonable, such instances are avoided entirely or endured with great distress. Although some anxiety related to performance situations is common, the fear and anxiety associated with social phobia cause severe distress or problems in functioning. Children may be diagnosed with this disorder, because the onset of social phobia typically occurs during adolescence.

Treatment is based on a combination of exposure and cognitive techniques. Sessions begin with a treatment rationale, followed by teaching cognitive restructuring techniques to examine and challenge negative thoughts in social situations. These techniques are combined with systematic exposure to the feared social situations. Improved outcomes are associated with producing cognitive change and reducing the fear of negative evaluation. Evidence also suggests that behavioral therapy combined with pharmacotherapy can facilitate willingness to engage in exposure exercises and improve overall response to treatment. Pharmacotherapy for social phobia includes MAOIs, selective serotonin reuptake inhibitors (SSRIs), high-potency benzodiazepines, and β-adrenergic blockers. Choice of medication depends on the degree and subtype of social phobia. Fear limited to performance situations (e.g., public speaking) can be treated as needed with β-blockers or a benzodiazepine. The more generalized type of social phobia responds well to MAOIs, although SSRIs have become the first line of treatment because of their overall efficacy and fewer side effects.

CURRENT DIAGNOSIS

- Anxiety can mimic medical conditions.
- Adaptive anxiety should be differentiated from maladaptive anxiety.
- Anxiety disorders result from excessive and unreasonable fear and significantly impair normal functioning.
- Patients with anxiety disorders frequently present to medical settings for help.
- Psychiatric comorbidity is common in anxiety disorders.

Generalized Anxiety Disorder

Generalized anxiety disorder (GAD) involves excessive anxiety and pathologic worry about a variety of everyday problems that are present most of the day for at least 6 months. The worry is difficult to control and is accompanied by irritability, concentration problems, somatic symptoms of restlessness or fatigue, muscle tension, or disrupted sleep. Onset typically occurs during childhood or adolescence but can also occur in adulthood, and GAD is the most common anxiety disorder among the elderly. GAD is a chronic disorder that is more commonly diagnosed in women and that fluctuates and worsens during stressful times. It is also highly comorbid with other anxiety and mood disorders.

GAD can be effectively treated with 12 to 15 sessions of CBT, which incorporates psychoeducation, self-monitoring to increase awareness of when worry occurs, cognitive restructuring, relaxation methods, worry exposure, and worry behavior control. Cognitive restructuring is focused on identifying distorted thinking patterns concerning the patient's ability to cope effectively in difficult situations and on reducing overestimations of perceived negative outcomes. Worry exposure entails patients exposing themselves to their worry and imagining the worst possible outcome for some period to process the worry and achieve habituation. Pharmacotherapy includes buspirone (Buspar), benzodiazepines, hydroxyzine (Vistaril), and antidepressants such as SSRIs and dual serotonin-norepinephrine reuptake inhibitors (SNRIs). Given the problems associated with long-term use of benzodiazepines and the high rate of comorbidity, antidepressants should be considered first-line agents in treating GAD.

Obsessive-Compulsive Disorder

Obsessive-compulsive disorder (OCD) is a chronic disorder characterized by persistent and recurrent intrusive thoughts or images (i.e., obsessions) that cause significant anxiety or driven repetitive behaviors (i.e., compulsions) that occur overtly (e.g., checking) or covertly (e.g., counting). Compulsions are aimed at decreasing or preventing anxiety associated with an obsession or rigid set of rules. Obsessive content commonly centers on themes of contamination; somatic, sexual, or aggressive obsessions; and pathologic doubt. To be diagnosed with OCD, the obsessions or compulsions must cause significant distress or impairment in functioning or consume more than 1 hour per day. During the course of the disorder, adults recognize that the obsessions or compulsions are unreasonable and excessive, although children may not. OCD is equally common in adult men and women but is more prevalent among male children and adolescents. Evidence suggests that OCD is associated with chronic tic disorders and Tourette's syndrome.

Behavioral therapy has the most empiric support for treating OCD. Most forms of behavioral therapy incorporate exposure and response prevention techniques used in conjunction with a fear hierarchy. Patients purposely induce anxiety by systematically exposing themselves to triggers of obsessions or compulsions using imaginal or in vivo exercises, and they are not permitted to engage in rituals or compulsions to decrease their distress. After habituation occurs and the discomfort diminishes significantly, they can move to the

CURRENT THERAPY

- Cognitive-behavioral therapy effectively treats anxiety disorders.
- Exposure and cognitive restructuring techniques are key components.
- Pharmacotherapy includes selective serotonin reuptake inhibitors, tricyclic antidepressants, monoamine oxidase inhibitors, and benzodiazepines.
- Combination drug and behavioral therapies have limited utility in treating anxiety.
- D-Cycloserine (Seromycin)[1] may be a useful adjunct for exposure therapy.

next item on the hierarchy. Duration of treatment sessions depends on the process of habituation. Sessions usually last 90 minutes to 2 hours, and a full course of treatment requires at least 15 sessions.

Pharmacotherapy includes SSRIs and clomipramine (Anafranil). Patients with OCD and a comorbid tic disorder may benefit from an SSRI plus a low-dose antipsychotic such as risperidone (Risperdal)[1] or quetiapine (Seroquel).[1] In OCD treatment, medication can be a useful adjunct to improve compliance with behavioral therapy. However, treatment gains after behavioral therapy last longer than the effects of pharmacotherapy when discontinued.

Specific Phobia

Specific phobia is a relatively common anxiety disorder that involves excessive and unreasonable fear in response to a specific object or situation. Common phobic stimuli include airplanes, tight spaces, heights, and blood or injections. The fear is present for at least 6 months, and the phobic object or situation is avoided or endured with significant distress that interferes with normal functioning. Onset of specific phobias occurs in early adolescence, although the timing varies and depends on the type of phobia. For instance, animal and blood or injection phobias tend to develop in childhood, whereas claustrophobia typically develops in early adulthood. Traumatic experiences may be a predisposing factor in the development of a specific phobia.

Exposure-based treatments are highly effective, and successful results can often be achieved in one intensive session. The basis of treatment is to prevent the patient from avoiding the feared stimulus to learn that there is no basis for the feared outcome. Exposure can take many forms, including flooding, in vivo exposure, and systematic desensitization. In vivo exposure involves real-life exposure to the feared stimulus in gradated steps to reach habituation. Systematic desensitization uses imaginal exposure techniques paired with progressive muscle relaxation to manage anxiety stemming from exercises generated in a fear hierarchy. Pharmacotherapy may involve the use of benzodiazepines to help the patient tolerate exposure to the feared stimuli; however, successful outcomes for specific phobias are derived from behavioral therapy.

Posttraumatic Stress Disorder

Posttraumatic stress disorder (PTSD) can develop after an event involving serious injury or death or threat to physical integrity that results in feelings of intense fear, helplessness, or horror. This is accompanied by persistently re-experiencing symptoms through intrusive thoughts, nightmares, flashbacks, psychological distress, or physiologic reactivity in response to reminders of the traumatic

---

[1]Not FDA approved for this indication.

event. The individual also experiences at least three symptoms associated with avoidance and numbing, including avoidance of feelings and situations associated with the trauma, amnesia regarding the trauma, emotional blunting and social detachment, having a sense of a foreshortened future, and an inability to enjoy activities that were once pleasurable. At least two symptoms of hyperarousal involving insomnia, poor concentration, irritability or anger dyscontrol, hypervigilance, and exaggerated startle reaction must be present. This combination of symptoms must be present for more than 1 month and cause significant impairment or distress in daily functioning to warrant a PTSD diagnosis.

Onset of symptoms usually occurs within 3 months of the stressor but can be delayed by several months or years. PTSD can occur in childhood and adulthood, and it is more prevalent among combat veterans and victims of sexual assault and natural disasters. Mood disorders, panic disorder, and substance abuse are highly comorbid conditions in PTSD, and they can complicate the course of treatment and outcome.

Psychosocial treatments for PTSD based on an information-processing model typically include components of exposure and cognitive therapy. Cognitive processing therapy is one such approach that elicits memories of the trauma by having patients write about the traumatic event, and it directly challenges specific cognitions that are disrupted as a result of the event. In this 12-session treatment, patients are taught how to challenge maladaptive thinking patterns and learn ways to cope with distressing emotions. The themes of safety, trust, power or control, esteem, and intimacy are addressed during the course of treatment. Prolonged exposure is another highly effective treatment that uses imaginal and in vivo exposure to elicit emotional processing so that disrupted memories of the trauma can consolidate and habituate.

Pharmacologic treatment for PTSD includes the use of SSRIs, MAOIs, TCAs, and mood stabilizers such as valproate (Depakote)[1] and carbamazepine (Tegretol).[1] Evidence suggests that TCAs and MAOIs (e.g., phenelzine [Nardil][1]) are effective in treating combat veterans with PTSD, whereas SSRIs appear to be of more benefit to civilians and to women more than men.

Conclusions

Anxiety disorders affect a disproportionate number of individuals each year and are costly to the individual and society. Primary care physicians are likely to be the ones who first encounter patients with these types of problems. Patients must be carefully evaluated and recommended for appropriate treatment in a timely manner. Table 1 lists the psychopharmacologic agents recommended to treat specific anxiety disorders.

Among the available psychosocial treatments, cognitive and behavioral therapy approaches produce some of the best outcomes for anxiety disorders and offer a number of advantages over pharmacotherapy, including the absence of adverse physical side effects, increased self-efficacy, and maintenance of treatment gains. However, CBT requires more time and effort from patients and providers, and exposure exercises can be extremely uncomfortable. Attempts to use adjunctive pharmacotherapy to enhance the effects of psychotherapy by reducing the discomfort associated with cognitive processing and exposure exercises have been discouraging. However, emerging data suggest that D-cycloserine (DCS [Seromycin][1]), a partial N-methyl-D-aspartate (NMDA) receptor agonist, can facilitate fear extinction and exposure therapy across several anxiety disorders. Due to tolerance and its short duration of action, the use of DCS appears to be most effective with acute administrations immediately before or after exposure sessions to facilitate memory consolidation. Future research needs to examine the efficacy of DCS as an adjunctive treatment across a broader range of disorders along the anxiety spectrum.

---

[1]Not FDA approved for this indication.

REFERENCES

American Psychiatric Association. Diagnostic and statistical manual of mental disorders. 4th ed. text revision (DSM-IV-TR). Washington, DC: American Psychiatric Association; 2000.

Barlow DH, Gorman JM, Shear MK, et al. Cognitive-behavioral therapy, imipramine, or their combination for panic disorder: A randomized controlled trial. JAMA 2000;283:2529–36.

Barlow DH. Anxiety and its disorders. 2nd ed. New York: Guilford Press; 2002.

Foa E, Liebowitz M, Kozak MJ, et al. Randomized, placebo-controlled trial of exposure and ritual prevention, clomipramine and their combination in the treatment of OCD. Am J Psychiatry 2005;162:151–61.

Otto MW, Basden SL, Leyro TM, et al. Clinical perspectives on the combination of D-cycloserine and cognitive-behavioral therapy for the treatment of anxiety disorders. CNS Spectr 2007;12:51–66.

Resick P, Galovski T, O'Brien Uhlmansiek M, et al. A randomized clinical trial to dismantle components of cognitive processing therapy or posttraumatic stress disorder in female victims of interpersonal violence. J Consult Clin Psychol 2008;76:243–58.

Roy-Byrne PP, Craske MG, Stein MB, et al. A randomized effectiveness trial of cognitive-behavioural therapy and medication for primary care panic disorder. Arch Gen Psychiatry 2005;62:290–338.

Simon NM, Connor KM, Lang AJ, et al. Paroxetine CR augmentation for posttraumatic stress disorder refractory to prolonged exposure therapy. J Clin Psychiatry 2008;69:400–5.

Bulimia Nervosa

Method of
James Lock, MD

Bulimia nervosa is characterized by binge eating episodes, followed by inappropriate compensatory behaviors, such as self-induced vomiting, laxative or diuretic misuse, fasting, and excessive exercise. A sense of loss of control about overeating accompanies these episodes of binge eating. These behaviors are associated with overvaluation of shape and weight. The episodes must occur at a frequency of two times per week for 3 months to meet diagnostic thresholds.

Bulimic behaviors usually have their onset during middle adolescence (14–16 years old). Full-syndrome bulimia nervosa is most common during late adolescence and young adulthood (17–24 years old). Onset of bulimia nervosa is rare in younger children, although not unknown. The point prevalence of bulimia nervosa is 1% to 2% among females. Male patients account for about 10% of bulimia nervosa cases.

It is common for other psychiatric disorders to coexist with bulimia nervosa, particularly depression, anxiety disorders, and substance use. Common physical health problems associated with bulimia nervosa include electrolyte disturbances, loss of dental enamel, and esophageal tears. The use of ipecac to induce vomiting can lead to serious cardiac and skeletal myopathies. Frequent laxative use can cause metabolic acidosis and elevated serum amylase levels, and it can lead to dependence on laxatives for bowel emptying. Amenorrhea, infertility, osteoporosis, and dehydration are other possible outcomes.

Common characteristics associated with bulimia nervosa include impulsivity, interpersonal problems, substance use, and personality disorders. These related problems usually occur about the same time or after the onset of bulimia nervosa and many remit after treatment. In patients who abuse substances, most begin substance use as a means to control appetite and weight.

Etiology

Bulimia nervosa is best understood as a multiply determined phenomenon that includes biologic, psychological, familial, and sociocultural factors. Evidence for a biologic basis can be found in genetic, neurotransmitter, and neuroimaging studies. Bulimia nervosa clusters in families, supporting a genetic basis for the disorder. Twin studies document that one half of the variance in heritability is accounted for by genetic factors. There is also evidence of reduced serotonin levels in individuals with bulimia nervosa. Imaging studies have found disturbances in the orbital-frontal serotonergic circuits in these patients. These areas of the brain are associated with behavioral dyscontrol.

Psychological factors likely contribute to the cause of bulimia nervosa. Low self-esteem and increased sensitivity to peer rejection are highly associated with the disorder, as are personality characteristics of impulsivity, perfectionism, and interpersonal relationship instability. Family dynamics are also implicated. Parental obesity and familial criticism about weight, shape, and eating, as well as familial emphasis on appearance and achievement, appear to increase risk for the disorder. Families of patients are often characterized as unorganized, conflict ridden, and lacking in warmth.

Sociocultural factors appear to contribute to the increased risk for bulimia nervosa. Intensified pressures for women to be thin, as portrayed in magazine and television advertisements, contribute to increased rates of the disorder. These pressures may be increasing for men as the print and video media present male models with increased muscularity and less body fat.

Diagnosis

Clinicians must review the history and current status of the patient's eating disorder pathology, such as restriction, binge eating, purging, and other compensatory behaviors; height and weight trends; weight and shape concerns; history of weight control measures; and motivation for seeking current treatment. Examination of possible triggers for dieting and weight concerns should be explored, including past experiences with teasing about weight; family culture around food, weight, and eating; interpersonal relationship stressors; and occupational risks (e.g., food service worker, model, athlete). It is important to review any contributing medical symptoms, such as fatigue, headaches, bloating, constipation, and irregular menstrual status. Common comorbid mental health problems, particularly depression, anxiety, substance abuse, and personality disorders, must also be assessed.

Several self-report standardized interviews may be useful in making the diagnosis. Two of the most widely used measures are the Eating Attitudes Test and the Eating Disorders Inventory-2. A third commonly used self-report measure is the Bulimia Test-Revised. These self-report measures are best used to augment the clinical interview to refine information specific to eating-related symptoms and psychopathology.

Treatment

THERAPY FOR ADOLESCENT BULIMIA NERVOSA

Because bulimia nervosa has the potential for serious physical, emotional, and social consequences, treatment entails attention to this range of possible difficulties. Research has focused almost exclusively on adults with the disorder. More than 70 controlled treatment trials

CURRENT DIAGNOSIS

- Binge eating episodes (i.e., eating more than an average person would in the same setting) accompanied by a sense of being unable to cease eating occur at least twice each week for 3 months.
- Purging episodes (i.e., vomiting, laxative use, diuretics, enemas, overexercise) occur at least twice each week for 3 months.
- Overvaluation of shape and weight is a source of self-worth and self-esteem.
- Weight is in the normal range (i.e., patient is not experiencing an episode of anorexia nervosa).

have enrolled adults with bulimia nervosa, whereas only two randomized trials have enrolled adolescents. Treatment studies have focused on psychotherapy, mostly cognitive-behavioral therapy (CBT), and medications. Both approaches appear to be efficacious.

The main premise of CBT is that dysfunctional attitudes toward body shape and weight are the maintaining factors for the bulimia nervosa. As a result of these distorted ideas, there is an overvaluing of appearance, particularly thinness. This overvaluation leads to dissatisfaction with current body weight and shape, which is followed by attempts to control shape and weight by excessive dieting. Excessive dieting triggers a sense of psychological deprivation and real physiologic deprivation. Excessive dieting also increases feelings of hunger. Feelings of hunger increase the need to eat, which increases the probability of binge eating. After a binge has been completed, fears of weight gain are followed by purging (e.g., vomiting, laxatives, diuretic, enemas, extreme exercise) as an attempt to allay these anxieties. The combination of psychological and physical stresses often increases moodiness and depression.

CBT has been subjected to a large number of randomized, controlled trials and is considered the most effective psychotherapeutic approach for bulimia nervosa. Studies have found that CBT is more effective than no therapy, nondirective therapy, pill placebo, manualized psychodynamic therapy (i.e., supportive-expressive), stress management, and antidepressant treatment. Treatment response to CBT is generally good, with 50% of patients recovered and an additional 20% much improved by the end of treatment. Longer-term follow-up studies suggest that these improvements are sustained over time. At 5 years after treatment, about 60% of patients no longer had bulimia nervosa. In a meta-analysis of nine double-blind, placebo-controlled medication trials (870 subjects) and 26 randomized psychosocial studies (460 subjects), CBT was found to produce significantly greater improvements in binge eating, purging frequency, depression, and eating attitudes than comparison treatments.

The use of CBT for adolescents with bulimia nervosa treated with CBT has limited systematic support. Only two studies are available, but both provide preliminary evidence that CBT is acceptable and feasible as a treatment for these patients. Case series data on 40 adolescents treated with CBT found that 56% were recovered (i.e., absence of binge eating or purging) at the end of treatment. One randomized, controlled trial compared a self-help version of CBT (CBT-GSC) with family therapy. This study concluded that CBT-GSC was as effective (with rates of recovery of 36%) as family therapy for adolescent bulimia nervosa and was a more cost-effective treatment.

Interpersonal psychotherapy (IPT) modified for bulimia nervosa has been shown to be an effective therapy for the disorder. IPT focuses on the interpersonal context within which the eating disorder developed and is maintained with the aim of helping the patient make specific changes in identified interpersonal problem areas. Little attention is paid to eating habits or attitudes toward weight and shape, nor does the treatment contain any of the specific behavioral or cognitive procedures that characterize CBT. Because interpersonal success is closely linked to societal mandates about physical attractiveness, body shape and weight become critical determinants of self-esteem for adolescents, especially for girls. The relevance of IPT is supported by the findings of laboratory research showing that individuals with eating disorder symptoms seem particularly vulnerable to interpersonal stressors.

CBT was compared with IPT in a large, multisite trial enrolling 220 patients with bulimia nervosa. In this trial, CBT was superior to IPT at the end of treatment, but on follow-up, no differences were found between the two treatments. These studies suggested that bulimia nervosa was responsive to IPT and CBT, but that the improvements associated with IPT were slower to develop. IPT for adolescents with the disorder remains unexamined.

An approach specifically designed for adolescents is family-based treatment for bulimia nervosa (FBT-BN). The use of families to directly change dysfunctional eating behaviors in adolescents was used first with adolescents with anorexia nervosa. FBT-BN used parents to help their adolescent children stop binge eating and purging by directly monitoring these behaviors to prevent and disrupt them. This form of family therapy does not focus on the cause of bulimia

CURRENT THERAPY

- Cognitive-behavioral therapy (CBT) is the best-evidenced approach for bulimia nervosa.
- Interpersonal psychotherapy may be an alternative treatment if CBT is not effective or acceptable.
- Family-based treatment for bulimia nervosa is useful for adolescents.
- Antidepressants are useful but are not as effective as CBT and are a second-line treatment. However these medications may be used to augment psychological treatments or as an alternative when psychological treatments are not effective, are refused, or are not available.
- Serotonin reuptake inhibitors (SSRIs) are the recommended antidepressants. Relatively high doses are used, similar to the dosages used in the treatment of obsessive-compulsive disorder.

nervosa, but it assumes that most of the challenges of adolescence (e.g., peer relationships, increased autonomy, increased risk taking) are adversely affected by the disorder. Limited data are available to support the use of this approach with adolescents with bulimia nervosa in the form of pilot studies and two randomized clinical trials of moderate size. One study found that FBT-BN was superior to individual therapy for patients achieving abstinence at the end of treatment (40% versus 18%) and at follow-up (30% versus 10%).

PHARMACOTHERAPY

The use of antidepressant medications has also been examined. Studies include double-blind, placebo-controlled trials of antidepressants for adults. Most types of antidepressants are superior to placebo in reducing binge frequency. Mood disturbance, which is commonly associated with bulimia nervosa, improved with medication. However, controlled studies that examined the relative contributions to symptomatic change in combined treatment with CBT and antidepressants suggest that the additional benefit of medications over CBT alone is quite small. Unfortunately, only one small case series examined the use of antidepressants in adolescents. This pilot study found that fluoxetine (Prozac) was well tolerated, appeared to decrease binge eating and purging, and was acceptable to the patients and their parents.

REFERENCES

Agras WS, Walsh BT, Fairburn CG, et al. A multicenter comparison of cognitive-behavioral therapy and interpersonal psychotherapy for bulimia nervosa. Arch Gen Psychiatry 2000;57:459–66.

Bulik CM. Genetic and biological risk factors. In: Thompson J, editor. Handbook of Eating Disorders and Obesity. Hoboken, NJ: John Wiley & Sons; 2004. p. 3–16.

Fairburn CG, Brownell K. Eating Disorders and Obesity: A Comprehensive Handbook. New York: Guilford Press; 2002.

Fairburn CG, Marcus MD, Wilson GT. Cognitive-behavioral therapy for binge eating and bulimia nervosa: A comprehensive treatment manual. In: Fairburn GT, Wilson GT, editors. Binge Eating: Nature, Assessment, & Treatment. New York: Guildford Press; 1993. p. 361–404.

Hoek H, Hoeken DV. Review of prevalence and incidence of eating disorders. Int J Eat Disord 2003;34:383–96.

Le Grange D, Crosby R, Rathouz P, Leventhal B. A randomized controlled comparison of family-based treatment and supportive psychotherapy for adolescent bulimia nervosa. Arch Gen Psychiatry 2007;64:1049–56.

Le Grange D, Lock J. Treating Bulimia in Adolescence. New York: Guilford Press; 2007.

Lilenfeld L, Kaye WH, Greeno C, et al. A controlled family study of anorexia nervosa and bulimia nervosa: Psychiatric disorders in first-degree relatives and effects of proband comorbidity. Arch Gen Psychiatry 1998;55:603–10.

Lock J. Adjusting cognitive behavioral therapy for adolescent bulimia nervosa: Results of a case series. Am J Psychother 2005;59:267–81.

Stein D, Kaye WH, Matsunaga H, et al. Eating-related concerns, moods, personality traits in recovered bulimia nervosa subjects: A replication study. Int J Eat Disord 2002;32:225–9.

Delirium

Method of
Arna Banerjee, MD, and
Pratik Pandharipande, MD, MSCI

Delirium is defined by the *Diagnostic and Statistical Manual of Mental Disorders*, fourth edition (DSM-IV), as a disturbance of consciousness with inattention, accompanied by a change in cognition or perceptual disturbances that develop over a short period (hours to days) and that fluctuate over time (Box 1). Although dysfunction of other organ systems continues to receive more clinical attention, delirium is recognized to be a significant contributor to morbidity, including longer hospitalizations, higher costs, and prolonged cognitive impairment. More alarmingly, delirium is an independent predictor of higher mortality for hospitalized and critically ill patients. Data show that patients who manifest some but not all the diagnostic features of delirium (i.e., subsyndromal delirium) have higher morbidity and mortality rates than those who are normal, although they fare better than those meeting the full criteria for delirium.

Prevalence and Subtypes

The prevalence of delirium at hospital admission ranges from 14% to 24%, with incident rates up to 60% among general hospital populations, especially in older patients and those in nursing homes or postacute care settings. Although the overall prevalence of delirium in the community is only 1% to 2%, the prevalence increases with age, rising to 14% among those older than 85 years. The prevalence of delirium in medical and surgical intensive care unit (ICU) cohort studies is 20% to 80%, depending on the severity of illness and the need for mechanical ventilation. Despite high prevalence rates in the ICU, delirium often goes unrecognized by clinicians, or its symptoms are incorrectly attributed to dementia or depression, or they are considered an expected, inconsequential complication of critical illness.

Delirium can be categorized according to psychomotor behavior (Table 1). In non-ICU settings, the prevalences are 30% for the hyperactive subtype, 24% for the hypoactive subtype, and 46% for the mixed subtype. In the ICU, the rates are 1.6% for the hyperactive subtype, 43.5% for the hypoactive subtype, and 54.1% for the mixed subtype.

Pathogenesis and Risk Factors

The pathophysiology of delirium is poorly understood, although there are several hypotheses. Imbalance or derangement of multiple neurotransmitter systems has been implicated in the pathophysiology of

---

BOX 1   DSM-IV Criteria for Delirium

- Disturbance of consciousness (i.e., reduced clarity of awareness of the environment) with reduced ability to focus, sustain, or shift attention)
- A change in cognition (e.g., memory deficit, disorientation, language disturbance) or development of a perceptual disturbance that is not better accounted for by a preexisting, established, or evolving dementia
- The disturbance develops over a short period (usually hours to days) and tends to fluctuate during the course of the day.

Abbreviation: DSM-IV = *Diagnostic and Statistical Manual of Mental Disorders*, fourth edition.

TABLE 1 Subtypes of Delirium

Subtype	Characteristics
Hyperactive	Agitation Restlessness Attempts to remove catheters and tubes Hitting Biting Emotional lability
Hypoactive	Withdrawal Flat affect Apathy Lethargy Decreased responsiveness
Mixed	Concurrent or sequential appearance of hyperactive and hypoactive delirium

CURRENT DIAGNOSIS

- Delirium is a disturbance of consciousness with inattention, accompanied by a change in cognition or perceptual disturbances that develop over a short period and fluctuate over days.
- Three delirium subtypes depend on the psychomotor behavior: hyperactive, hypoactive, and mixed.
- The pathophysiology of delirium is poorly understood, although inflammation, cholinergic imbalances, and neurotransmitter disturbances are leading hypotheses.
- Delirium affects more than one third of hospitalized patients, but it remains underdiagnosed and often is inappropriately evaluated and managed.
- Diagnosis of delirium is a two-step process. Level of arousal is measured, and if the patient is arousable, delirium evaluation is performed using instruments such as the Confusion Assessment Method or the Delirium Rating Scale-Revised 98 (DRS-R 98).

delirium, with the greatest focus on dopamine, γ-aminobutyric acid (GABA), and acetylcholine. Dopamine is thought to increase the excitability of neurons, and acetylcholine and GABA decrease neuronal excitability. An excess of dopamine or depletion of acetylcholine has been associated with delirium. Other postulated mechanisms of delirium include serotonin imbalance, endorphin hyperfunction, and increased central noradrenergic activity.

Another hypothesis enlists inflammatory mediators. The inflammatory mediators produced during critical illness (e.g., tumor necrosis factor-α, interleukin-1, other cytokines and chemokines) potentially initiate a cascade of endothelial damage, thrombin formation, and microvascular compromise that may play a role in delirium.

Impaired oxidative metabolism may play a role in the pathophysiology of delirium. Early hypotheses attempted to explain delirium as a behavioral manifestation of a "widespread reduction of cerebral oxidative metabolism resulting in an imbalance of neurotransmission." Investigators hypothesized that delirium was the result of "cerebral insufficiency" (i.e., global failure of cerebral oxidative metabolism), a factor that is known to be important in the pathogenesis of multiple organ dysfunction in critical illness.

Other investigators looked at cholinergic deficiency. Impaired oxidative metabolism in the brain results in a cholinergic deficiency. The finding that hypoxia impairs acetylcholine synthesis supports this hypothesis. The reduction in cholinergic function results in an increase in the levels of glutamate, dopamine, and norepinephrine in the brain. Serotonin and GABA are reduced, contributing to delirium.

Neurotransmitter levels and function can be affected by changes in the plasma concentrations of various amino acid precursors. Amino acid entry into the brain is regulated by a sodium-independent large neutral amino acid transporter type 1 (LAT1). Increased cerebral uptake of tryptophan and phenylalanine, compared with that of other large neutral amino acids, can lead to elevated levels of dopamine and norepinephrine, two neurotransmitters that have been implicated in the pathogenesis of delirium.

The causes of delirium are multifactorial. The risk factors can be divided into predisposing factors (i.e., host factors) and precipitating factors (Table 2).

Diagnosis

Delirium affects more than one third of hospitalized patients, but it remains underdiagnosed and is often inappropriately evaluated and managed. The diagnosis of delirium is primarily clinical and is based on careful bedside observation of key features (Table 3).

Diagnosis of delirium is a two-step process. Level of arousal is first measured, and if the patient is arousable, delirium evaluation can be performed by instruments such as the Confusion Assessment Method (Table 4) or the Delirium Rating Scale-Revised 98 (DRS-R 98). The DRS-R 98 provides a measure of severity of delirium in addition to being used to diagnose delirium. It is a 16-item, clinician-rated scale with 13 severity items and 3 diagnostic items. In the ICU, delirium can be diagnosed by using a sedation scale to assess arousal, followed by the Confusion Assessment Method for the ICU (CAM-ICU) or the Intensive Care Delirium Screening Checklist (ICDSC); both instruments are reliable and have been validated in critically ill patients.

Prevention

Nonpharmacologic and pharmacologic approaches have been studied to prevent delirium in hospitalized patients (Table 5). A study in 1999 demonstrated that a unit-based proactive multicomponent

TABLE 2 Risk Factors for Delirium

Host Factors	Factors of Critical Illness	Iatrogenic Factors
Age 65 years or older Male sex Alcoholism ApoE4 polymorphism Cognitive impairment Dementia History of delirium Depression Hypertension Smoking Vision or hearing impairment	Acidosis Anemia Fever, infection, sepsis Hypotension Metabolic disturbances (e.g., sodium, calcium, blood urea nitrogen, bilirubin) Respiratory disease Great severity of illness	Immobilization Medications (e.g., opioids, benzodiazepines) Anticholinergic drugs Alcohol or drug withdrawal Sleep disturbances

TABLE 3 Clinical Features of Delirium

Feature	Description
Acute onset	Occurs abruptly, usually over a period of hours to days
Fluctuating course	Symptoms seem to come and go or increase and decrease in severity over a 24-hour period
	Characteristic lucid intervals
Inattention	Difficulty focusing, sustaining, and shifting attention
	Difficulty maintaining conversation or following commands
Disorganized thinking	Disorganized or incoherent speech
	Rambling, irrelevant conversation
	Unclear or illogical flow of ideas
Altered level of consciousness	Reduced clarity of awareness of the environment
Cognitive deficits	Disorientation, memory deficits, and language impairment
Perceptual disturbances	Illusions and hallucinations in 30% of patients
Psychomotor disturbances	Hypoactive, hyperactive, and mixed
Altered sleep-wake cycle	Daytime drowsiness, nighttime insomnia, fragmented sleep
Emotional disturbances	Symptoms of fear, paranoia, anxiety, depression, irritability, apathy, anger, or euphoria

TABLE 4 Confusion Assessment Method Diagnostic Algorithm

Feature*	Description	Diagnostic Relevance
1	Acute onset or fluctuating course	This feature is usually obtained from a family member or nurse and is shown by positive responses to the following questions: Is there evidence of an acute change in mental status from the patient's baseline? Did the (abnormal) behavior fluctuate during the day; that is, did it tend to come and go or increase and decrease in severity?
2	Inattention	This feature is demonstrated by a positive response to the following question: Did the patient have difficulty focusing attention, such as being easily distractible or having difficulty keeping track of what was being said?
3	Disorganized thinking	This feature is shown by a positive response to the following question: Was the patient's thinking disorganized or incoherent, such as rambling or irrelevant conversation, unclear or illogical flow of ideas or unpredictable switching from subject to subject?
4	Altered level of consciousness	This feature is demonstrated by any answer other than "alert" to the following question: Overall, how would you rate this patient's level of consciousness? Possible answers: alert (normal), vigilant (hyperalert), lethargic (drowsy, easily aroused), stupor (difficult to arouse), or coma (unarousable)

*Diagnosis of delirium by the Confusion Assessment Method requires the presence of features 1 and 2 plus feature 3 or 4.

TABLE 5 Models of Care for Delirium: Summary of Evidence

Model	Approach	Outcome	Comments
Hospital Elder Life Program (HELP)	Proactive	40% Reduction in incident delirium	No benefit in shortening the duration or severity of delirium
Geriatric consultation for hip fracture patients	Proactive	36% Reduction in incident delirium	No benefit in shortening the duration or severity of delirium
Re-organization of care: nurse-led programs, patient-centered care	Proactive	No reduction in incidence / Reduced severity and duration of delirium	Overall hospital length of stay shortened; some mortality benefit
Low-dose prophylactic haloperidol (Haldol)[1] in high-risk hip surgery patients	Proactive	No reduction in delirium incidence / Reduced severity and duration of delirium	Haloperidol (1.5 mg/d) well tolerated, with minimal side effects
Specialized delirium management team	Treatment	No significant benefit in any outcomes measured	Intervention may have been of insufficient duration or intensity; no difference observed

[1]Not FDA approved for this indication.

intervention, the Hospital Elder Life Program (HELP), reduced the incidence of delirium by 40% among hospitalized patients 70 years old or older. The protocol focused on optimization of risk factors with the following methods: repeated reorientation of the patient by trained volunteers and nurses, provision of cognitively stimulating activities for the patient three times per day, a nonpharmacologic sleep protocol to enhance normalization of sleep-wake cycles, early mobilization activities and range-of-motion exercises, timely removal of catheters and physical restraints, early correction of dehydration, earwax disimpaction, and institution of the use of eyeglasses, magnifying lenses, and hearing aids. Other studies have had similar or limited benefits in reducing the incidence of delirium or the severity and duration (see Table 5).

Treatment

A multidisciplinary, multifactorial approach to treatment is the most successful, because many factors contribute to delirium. Several interventions, even if individually small, may yield marked clinical improvement. Medications should be used only after giving adequate attention to correction of modifiable contributing factors (e.g., sleep disturbance, deliriogenic medications, restraints).

Delirium may be a manifestation of an acute, life-threatening problem that requires immediate attention (e.g., hypoxia, hypercarbia, hypoglycemia, metabolic derangements, shock). After addressing these concerns, delirious patients should be considered for nonpharmacologic interventions and their acute symptoms managed by pharmacologic protocols if necessary (Table 6 and Fig. 1). Although the agents used to treat delirium are intended to improve cognition, they

TABLE 6 Pharmacologic Treatment of Delirium in Hospitalized patients

Class and Drug	Dose
Antipsychotics	
Haloperidol (Haldol)[1]	0.5–1.0 mg PO twice daily, with additional doses every 4 hours as needed up to a maximum to 20 mg 0.5–1.0 mg IM; observe after 30–60 min and repeat if needed.
Atypical Antipsychotics	
Risperidone (Risperdal)[1]	0.25–1 mg PO daily or twice daily
Olanzapine (Zyprexa)[1]	2.5–10 mg PO daily or twice daily
Quetiapine (Seroquel)[1]	25–50 mg PO daily or twice daily
Ziprasidone (Geodon)[1]	20–40 mg PO once daily to twice daily
Benzodiazepines	
Lorazepam (Ativan)[1]	0.5–1 mg PO, with additional doses every 4 hours as needed. Reserve for use in alcohol withdrawal, Parkinson's disease, and neuroleptic malignant syndrome.
Antidepressants	
Trazodone (Desyrel)[1]	25–150 mg PO at bedtime

[1]Not FDA approved for this indication.

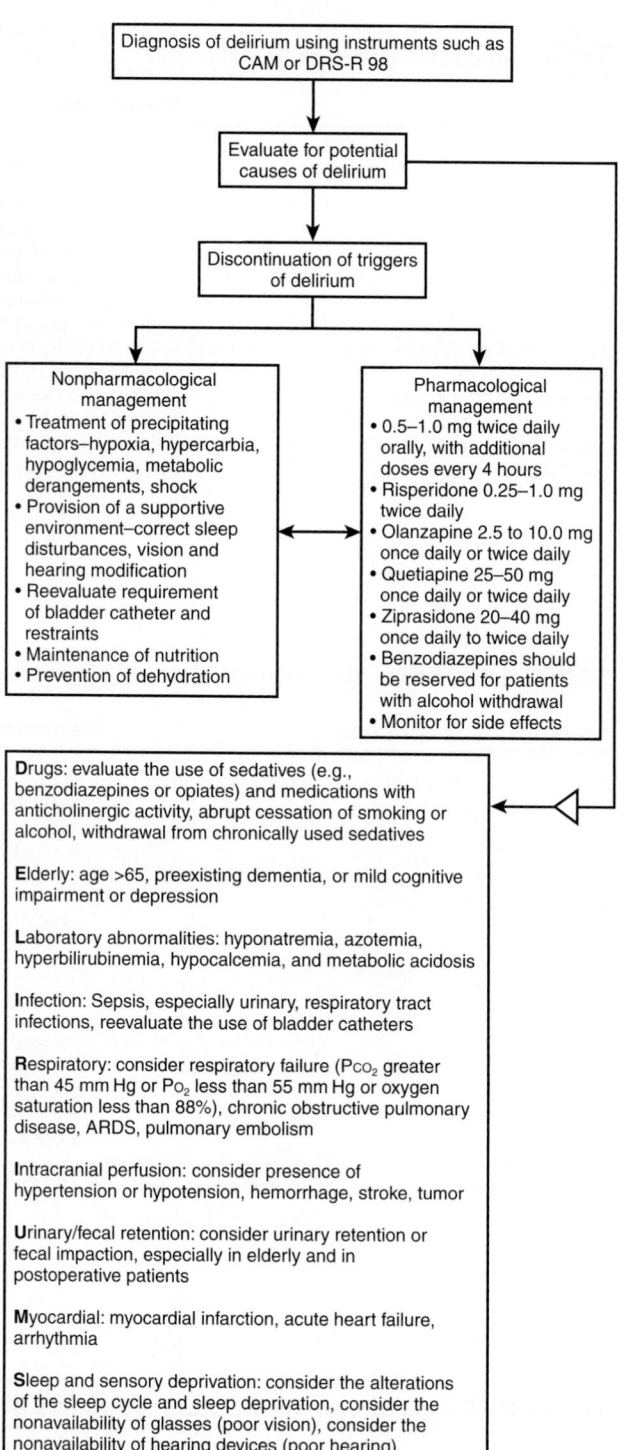

FIGURE 1. Treatment algorithm for hospitalized patients with delirium. *Abbreviations:* ARDS = acute respiratory distress syndrome; CAM = Confusion Assessment Method; DRS-R 98 = Delirium Rating Scale-Revised 98,

have psychoactive effects that may further cloud the sensorium and promote a longer overall duration of cognitive impairment. All typical and atypical antipsychotics can cause extrapyramidal symptoms and prolonged QT on electrocardiogram.

CURRENT THERAPY

- A multidisciplinary, multifactorial approach is the most successful, because many factors contribute to delirium.
- Medications should be used only after giving adequate attention to correction of modifiable contributing factors.
- The nonpharmacologic components of treatment include
  - Treatment of precipitating factors such as hypoxia, hypercarbia, hypoglycemia, metabolic derangements, and shock
  - Provision of a supportive environment (correction of sleep disturbance, restraints, maintaining familiar surroundings)
  - Maintenance of nutrition
  - Prevention of dehydration
  - Discontinuation of pharmacologic agents known to cause delirium
- Pharmacologic treatments include the following:
  - Haloperidol (Haldol)[1] is considered to be the first-line drug and should be started at a low dose.
  - Atypical antipsychotics have been used when the risk for adverse events such as QTc prolongation or extrapyramidal side effects are estimated to be high. These drugs include olanzapine (Zyprexa),[1] risperidone (Risperdal),[1] quetiapine (Seroquel),[1] and ziprasidone (Geodon).[1]
  - Benzodiazepines should be used only in cases of delirium associated with alcohol withdrawal.

---

[1]Not FDA approved for this indication.

Conclusions

Delirium is a common brain dysfunction in hospitalized and critically ill patients contributing to increased morbidity and mortality. The pathophysiology of delirium remains unclear and is the focus of ongoing research. Protocols and evidence-based strategies for prevention and treatment of delirium will emerge from ongoing randomized clinical trials of nonpharmacologic and pharmacologic strategies.

REFERENCES

American Psychiatric Association. Diagnostic and statistical manual of mental disorders. 4th ed. text revision (DSM-IV-TR). Washington, DC: American Psychiatric Association; 2000.

Ely EW, Shintani A, Truman B, et al. Delirium as a predictor of mortality in mechanically ventilated patients in the intensive care unit. JAMA 2004;291(14):1753–62.

Engel GL, Romano J. Delirium, a syndrome of cerebral insufficiency. J Chronic Dis 1959;9(3):260–77.

Girard T, Pandharipande P, Ely EW. Delirium in the intensive care unit. Crit Care 2008;12(Suppl. 3):S3.

Inouye SK. Delirium in older persons. N Engl J Med 2006;354(11):1157–65.

Maldonado JR. Delirium in the acute care setting: Characteristics, diagnosis and treatment. Crit Care Clin 2008;24(4):657–722.

Marcantonio ER. Clinical management and prevention of delirium. Psychiatry 2005;4(1):68–72.

Meagher DJ, Hanlon DO, Mahony EO, et al. Relationship between symptoms and motoric subtype of delirium. J Neuropsychiatry Clin Neurosci 2000;12:51–6.

Morandi A, Gunther ML, Ely EW, Pandharipande P. The pharmacological management of delirium in critical illness. Current Drug Ther 2008;3: 148–57.

Nayeem K, O'Keeffe ST. Delirium. Clin Med 2003;3(5):412–5.

Peterson JF, Pun BT, Dittus RS, et al. Delirium and its motoric subtypes: A study of 614 critically ill patients. J Am Geriatr Soc 2006;54(3):479–84.

Tropea J, Slee J-A, Brand CA, et al. Clinical practice guidelines for the management of delirium in older people in Australia. Australas J Ageing 2008;27:150–6.

Truman B, Ely EW. Monitoring delirium in critically ill patients: Using the Confusion Assessment Method for the ICU. Crit Care Nurse 2003;23: 25–36.

Trzepacz PT. General instructions for use of the DRS-R-981998.

Trzepacz PT. Update on the neuropathogenesis of delirium. Dement Geriatr Cogn Disord 1999;10:330–4.

Mood Disorders

Method of
Bret R. Rutherford, MD, and
Steven P. Roose, MD

Major Depression

Depressive disorders are highly prevalent and impose significant social and economic burdens on patients and society. Major depression alone affects approximately 15% of people at some point in their lives, resulting in 340 million cases worldwide. Depression is twice as common in women and is prevalent from childhood through late life.

DIAGNOSIS

Diagnosis of major depression is based on a clinical interview. As shown in Box 1, the diagnosis of a major depressive episode requires that the patient have a depressed mood or loss of pleasure or interest in usual activities for a period of at least 2 weeks. Patients may report their depressed mood in different ways, from feeling sad, blue, or anxious to numb or not having any feelings. Loss of interest typically manifests in a change in patients' daily activities: They might withdraw socially, cease participating in previously pleasurable pastimes, or socially isolate themselves.

Patients with depression often report changes in appetite, with accompanying weight gain or loss. They might have difficulty falling

---

BOX 1 DSM Criteria for Major Depressive Episode

Depressed mood most of the day, nearly every day, as indicated by either subjective report or observation made by others

Markedly diminished interest or pleasure in all, or almost all, activities most of the day, nearly every day

Significant weight loss when not dieting or significant weight gain, or decrease or increase in appetite nearly every day

Insomnia or hypersomnia nearly every day

Psychomotor agitation or retardation nearly every day

Fatigue or loss of energy nearly every day

Feelings of worthlessness or excessive or inappropriate guilt nearly every day

Diminished ability to think or concentrate, or indecisiveness, nearly every day

Recurrent thoughts of death, recurrent suicidal ideation without a specific plan, or suicide attempt or a specific plan for committing suicide

---

DSM = *Diagnostic and Statistical Manual of Mental Disorders,* fourth edition (text revision).

asleep or staying asleep or wake too early in the morning, or else they might find themselves oversleeping. Depressed persons can experience psychomotor slowing (manifested in slow, mumbled speech with long pauses, slowed thinking, and slow body movements) or agitation (motor restlessness manifested in pacing, wringing hands, or other repetitive movements). Many patients also report having low energy and being more easily fatigued than is usual for them.

Cognitive changes are often observed in patients with depression. Patients can feel worthless or inferior and tend to evaluate external events in unrealistically pessimistic or hopeless ways. Memory and concentration are often affected, and patients might find themselves unable to function at work, making careless mistakes at home, and being more forgetful than usual. Patients might report feeling helpless and that they must push themselves to do activities that previously did not require effort (e.g., bathing, dressing).

In every patient with depression, it is critical to assess for the presence of suicidal thoughts. Clinicians must ask whether patients have had thoughts of death, whether they ever think of harming themselves, and if so, in what ways they have thought of harming themselves. Intent to commit suicide should be evaluated by asking patients whether they intend to carry out a suicidal plan, or if not, what stops them and how close they have come to implementing such a plan in the past. Patients should be asked about their access to lethal means, such as firearms, lethal supplies of medications, and other weapons. If a patient has a history of suicide attempts, careful consideration should be given to discovering the circumstances and stressors precipitating the event, what the patient was thinking as the attempt was made, and the patient's reactions to surviving.

Additionally, clinical and demographic factors placing patients at increased risk for suicide should be carefully assessed and combined with these data to generate a suicide risk assessment. Clinical factors associated with increased suicide risk are the presence of mood or psychotic disorders (psychotic depression having particularly high risk), ongoing substance abuse (especially alcohol), medical illness, global insomnia, anhedonia, anxiety, impulsivity and aggressiveness, hopelessness, recent loss, history of trauma or abuse, a personal history of prior suicide attempts, and a family history of suicide. Demographic risk factors include age older than 65 years, male gender, white race, and divorced or widowed marital status. In summary, clinicians may use the helpful mnemonic SIGECAPS to remember the DSM criteria for depression: *s*leep, *i*nterest, *g*uilt, *e*nergy, *c*oncentration, *a*ppetite, *p*sychomotor agitation or retardation, and *s*uicidality.

In the differential diagnosis of patients with depression, it is critical to rule out medical illness manifesting with depressed mood. Some neurodegenerative conditions (e.g., Alzheimer's disease, Parkinson's disease, Huntington's disease), endocrine disorders (e.g., thyroid, parathyroid, adrenocortical system abnormalities), infectious diseases (e.g., HIV, AIDS), malignancies, and vascular disease (e.g., stroke) can manifest with depressed mood. Patients seeking help at unusual ages or with atypical presentations should be carefully screened for medical problems. For this reason, medical histories and physical examinations must be performed in patients with depression, and a laboratory work-up must be performed including complete blood count, basic metabolic panel, liver function tests, and thyroid function panel.

Although most patients with mood disorder have unipolar depression, the accurate diagnosis of bipolar disorder is essential. Bipolar depression does not respond well to treatment with antidepressants alone, and this can lead to increased frequency of cycling and switches to mania. Bipolar disorder should be specifically ruled out in patients presenting with highly recurrent major depression and in those with family histories of bipolar disorder or postpartum depression.

Ongoing substance abuse or dependence is also important to discover and quantify when treating depression. Although in the past it was widely thought that treatments for depression would be less effective in patients with current drug or alcohol abuse, more recent data have suggested depression may be successfully treated even in the context of heavy substance use. However, treatment can require specific modifications to ensure compliance and safe treatment.

TREATMENT

Phases of Treatment

One major development in the past 20 years regarding the pharmacologic treatment of depression is the shift in treatment goals from response to remission. Response refers to significant improvement in depressive symptoms without complete relief, and it is typically defined in terms of a 50% or more decrease from baseline scores on standardized measurements such as the Beck Depression Inventory (BDI) or the Hamilton Rating Scale for Depression (HRSD). Remission denotes a clinical situation of minimal or no symptoms and return to functional normality, and it is often measured by scores below a certain threshold on standardized measures. The term *recovery* is used to describe a patient in full remission for a period of time.

The goal of treatment has shifted from achieving response to remission in light of greater recognition of the consequences of persistent symptoms: increased risks of relapse and treatment resistance, continued psychosocial limitations and decreased work productivity, cardiovascular morbidity and mortality, and sustained risk of suicide and substance abuse.

With respect to the phases of depression treatment, as shown in Figure 1, the acute phase begins when the patient presents with an episode of major depression. The goal of treatment in this phase is to achieve remission. In the continuation phase, medication treatment is continued at the same dose required to achieve remission for 6 to 9 months to prevent relapse. Maintenance treatment continues indefinitely in patients with recurrent illness to prevent new episodes.

Antidepressant Drugs

Few data are available to guide clinicians in the selection of one particular agent over another, although a patient's personal history of response to a medication, family history of good response, or history

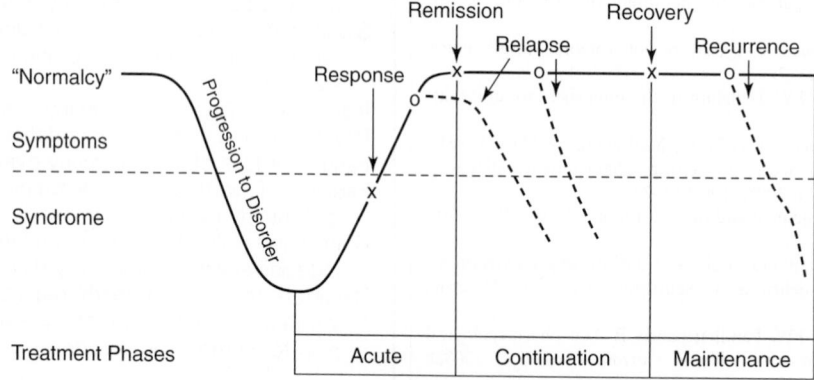

FIGURE 1. Phases of depression treatment. Modified from Kupfer DJ: Long-term treatment of depression. J Clin Psychiatry 1991;52(suppl 5):28–34.

of side effects might incline clinicians toward or away from certain agents. Additionally, the presence of significant anxiety comorbid with depression can influence clinicians to choose an agent with a serotoninergic mechanism of action, such as a selective serotonin reuptake inhibitor (SSRI) or serotonin–norepinephrine reuptake inhibitor (SNRI). Furthermore, certain medications may be relatively contraindicated in the presence of some medical comorbidities (e.g., tricyclic antidepressants [TCAs] and intraventricular conduction delay).

Selective Serotonin Reuptake Inhibitors

Introduced in the late 1980s, the SSRIs rapidly became the most prescribed antidepressant class owing to their relative tolerability and safety profiles. There is no consistent evidence that the SSRIs differ in efficacy or side effects. However, some, but not all, SSRIs significantly inhibit the action of hepatic cytochrome P-450 isoenzymes in addition to acting as a substrate for them and therefore have the potential for drug–drug interactions (see Box 2).

The most common side effects of SSRI treatment in the acute phase are gastrointestinal (nausea, vomiting, diarrhea), central nervous system (jitteriness, anxiety, akathisia), and sexual side effects (anorgasmia, erectile difficulty, decreased desire). Long-term treatment can be associated with significant weight gain. A rare but serious complication (and usually happening only when SSRIs are given in combination with another medication that enhances serotonin) is serotonin syndrome. Clinical signs and symptoms of serotonin syndrome include mental status changes (delirium, agitation), autonomic instability (diaphoresis, tachycardia, hyperpyrexia), and neuromuscular symptoms (rigidity, tremor). The combination of SSRIs and MAOIs is contraindicated due to the risk of serotonin syndrome. A major benefit to the SSRIs is that they are relatively safe in overdose.

SSRIs are started at the lowest effective dose and then titrated upward as required for clinical response. There may be a significant delay between starting an SSRI and achieving clinical effect, although some evidence suggests that patients who show benefit in the first 1 or 2 weeks of treatment might have a more positive long-term prognosis. Typical starting dosages are fluoxetine (Prozac) 10 to 20 mg, sertraline (Zoloft) 50 mg, paroxetine (Paxil) 20 mg, citalopram (Celexa) 20 mg, escitalopram (Lexapro) 10 mg, and fluvoxamine 100 mg. Children and adolescents, the elderly, and patients with panic or significant anxiety might require lower starting dosages. Initial doses are maintained for 1 to 2 weeks and then increased weekly as required for clinical benefit to maximum dosages of fluoxetine 80 mg, sertraline 200 mg, paroxetine 60 mg,[3] citalopram 60 mg, escitalopram 20 mg, and fluvoxamine 300 mg.

Serotonin–Norepinephrine Reuptake Inhibitors

SNRIs share the serotonin reuptake inhibition that is a hallmark of the SSRIs while also having strong affinity for the norepinephrine transporter. Venlafaxine appears to have a dual effect, whereby it primarily inhibits the serotonin transporter at lower doses and affects both the norepinephrine and serotonin transporters at doses greater than 150 mg/day. Venlafaxine is typically started at a dose of 37.5 mg daily and increased by 37.5 to 75 mg per week to a maximum of 300 mg daily.

Duloxetine is usually started at a dose of 30 mg daily and raised to 60 mg. If there is no clinical response at 60 mg, the dose could be raised to 120 mg,[3] which has been safely used in clinical and research populations. However, as with all the SSRIs and SNRIs, the benefits of increasing the dose above the minimally effective dose are unproved.

SNRIs share many aspects of their side-effect profile with SSRIs owing to their similar mechanisms of action. However, possibly due to their effects on norepinephrine reuptake, at higher doses these medications can result in mild elevations in blood pressure. For this reason, baseline blood pressures should be documented, followed by ongoing monitoring of blood pressure as long as the patient is taking an SNRI.

Buproprion

The aminoketone buproprion (Wellbutrin) is an interesting antidepressant whose mechanism of action is poorly understood, although it appears to reduce dopamine and norepinephrine reuptake. Buproprion is typically started at 150 mg/day and increased by 150 mg/week to a maximum of 450 mg daily. Some studies have reported that buproprion is less likely to cause manic switching in patients with bipolar disorder. It is also approved as a treatment for smoking cessation and may be a good choice in patients with depression and comorbid nicotine dependence. Typical adverse effects with buproprion include anxiety, insomnia, palpitations, dry mouth, and nausea.

Tricyclics

TCAs include imipramine, amitriptyline (Elavil), desipramine (Norpramin), maprotiline, protriptyline (Vivactil), and doxepin (Sinequan). Despite robust efficacy and the ability to regulate dose by monitoring plasma levels, the TCAs are generally less used due to their higher frequency of troublesome side effects and high mortality rate in overdose. All TCAs bring about norepinephrine transporter reuptake inhibition, and some have strong affinity for the serotonin transporter as well. TCAs are well absorbed in the small intestine and reach peak plasma levels 2 to 6 hours after oral administration. Metabolism is by hepatic microsomal enzymes, often to active metabolites. For example, imipramine's primary metabolite is desipramine, and amitriptyline's major metabolite is nortriptyline.

Anticholinergic side effects due to blockade of muscarinic receptors can be significant problems with TCAs. These can include decreased salivation, constipation, urinary retention, blurry vision and mydriasis, tachycardia, and impaired memory and cognition. Sympathomimetic side effects caused by inhibition of norepinephrine reuptake can cause anxiety, tremors, tachycardia, and diaphoresis. α-Receptor blockade can result in postural hypotension and falls in the elderly.

Starting doses for TCAs are generally 50 to 75 mg/day, with the exception of nortriptyline (25–50 mg/day) and protriptyline (10–15 mg/day). Dosages are titrated to achieve a therapeutic plasma level. Nortriptyline is the only TCA known to have a therapeutic window of blood plasma levels, making regular laboratory monitoring helpful. Plasma levels of 50 to 150 ng/mL appear optimal for nortriptyline, and imipramine and desipramine have a curvilinear dose-response curve with optimum blood levels from 150 to 300 ng/mL.

Monoamine Oxidase Inhibitors

Monoamine oxidase inhibitors (MAOIs), the first antidepressants discovered, inhibit the action of monoamine oxidase, which is the enzyme carrying out catabolism of the monoamines. MAO-A is the enzyme subtype located primarily in the brain, and MAO-B is localized to the gut. Enzymatic inhibition is irreversible for most MAOIs, meaning that new MAO enzyme must be synthesized to restore functioning, a process that can take approximately 2 weeks.

The use of MAOIs requires dietary restriction to avoid hypertensive crises. Inhibition of MAO prevents the metabolism of tyramine, which stimulates the release of norepinephrine from sympathetic terminals. Increased norepinephrine levels precipitate hypertension and hypertensive crises, which generally manifest clinically in pounding headaches. Obviously, extensive education about dietary requirements is necessary before patients begin an MAOI (see http://patienteducation.upmc.com/Pdf/MaoiDiet.pdf), and many clinicians supply their patients with 10 mg nifedipine (Adalat) tablets that may be taken in the case of a severe headache.

Phenelzine (Nardil) is started at a dose of 30 mg/daily and increased by 15 mg weekly to a target dose of 45 to 90 mg daily. Tranylcypromine (Parnate) may be started at 10 mg daily and increased by 10 mg weekly to 30 to 60 mg/day. The recent introduction of transdermal selegiline offers the potential for a better tolerated MAOI with fewer dietary restrictions. This patch is available in 6-, 9-, and 12-mg/day dosages, with only the latter two appearing to require dietary restrictions on tyramine-containing foods.

---

[3]Exceeds dosage recommended by the manufacturer.

BOX 2   Table of Substrates, Inhibitors, and Inducers of Cytochrome P-450 Isoenzymes

SUBSTRATES

1A2
clozapine
cyclobenzaprine
omipramine
mexiletine
naproxen
riluzole
tacrine
theophylline

2B6
bupropion
cyclophosphamide
efavirenz
ifosfamide
methadone

2C8

2C19
Proton Pump Inhibitors
omeprazole
lansoprazole
pantoprazole
rabeprazole

Anti-epileptics
diazepam
phenytoin
phenobarbitone
amitriptyline
clomipramine
clopidogrel
cyclophosphamide
progesterone

2C9
NSAIDs
diclofenac
ibuprofen
piroxicam

Oral Hypoglycemic Agents
tolbutamide
glipizide

Angiotensin II Blockers
NOT candesartan
irbesartan
losartan
NOT valsartan
celecoxib
fluvastatin
naproxen
phenytoin
sulfamethoxazole
tamoxifen
tolbutamide
torsemide
warfarin

2D6
Beta Blockers
S-metoprolol
propafenone
timolol

Antidepressants
amitriptyline
clomipramine
desipramine
imipramine
paroxetine

Antipsychotics
haloperidol
risperidone
thioridazine
aripiprazole
codeine
dextromethorphan
duloxetine
flecainide
mexiletine
ondansetron
tamoxifen
tramadol
venlafaxine

2E1
acetaminophen
chlorzoxazone
ethanol

3A4,5,7
Macrolide Antibiotics
clarithromycin
erythromycin
NOT azithromycin
telithromycin

Anti-arrhythmics
quinidine

Benzodiazepines
alprazolam
diazepam
midazolam
triazolam

Immune Modulators
cyclosporine
tacrolimus (FK506)

HIV Protease Inhibitors
indinavir
ritonavir
saquinavir

Prokinetic
cisapride

Antihistamines
astemizole
chlorpheniramine

Calcium Channel Blockers
amlodipine
diltiazem
felodipine
nifedipine
nisoldipine
nitrendipine
verapamil

HMG CoA Reductase Inhibitors
atorvastatin
cerivastatin
lovastatin
NOT pravastatin
simvastatin
aripiprazole
buspirone
gleevec
haloperidol (in part)
methadone
pimozide
quinine
NOT rosuvastatin
sildenafil
tamoxifen
trazodone
vincristine

INHIBITORS

1A2
cimetidine
fluoroquinolones
fluvoxamine
ticlopidine

2B6
thiotepa
ticlopidine

2C8
gemfibrozil
montelukast

2C19
fluoxetine
fluvoxamine
ketoconazole
lansoprazole
omeprazole
ticlopidine

2C9
amiodarone
fluconazole
isoniazid

2D6
amiodarone
buproprion
chlorpheniramine
cimetidine
clomipramine
duloxetine
fluoxetine
haloperidol
methadone
mibefradil
paroxetine
quinidine
ritonavir

2E1
disulfiram

3A4,5,7
HIV Protease Inhibitors
indinavir
nelfinavir
ritonavir
amiodarone
NOT azithromycin
cimetidine
clarithromycin
diltiazem
erythromycin
fluvoxamine
grapefruit juice
itraconazole
ketoconazole
mibefradil
nefazodone
troleandomycin
verapamil

INDUCERS
1A2
tobacco

2B6
phenobarbital
phenytoin
rifampin

2C8

2C19
N/A

2C9
rifampin
secobarbital

2D6
N/A

2E1
ethanol
isoniazid

3A4,5,7
carbamazepine
phenobarbital
phenytoin
ethanol
rifampin
St. John's wort
troglitazone

Adapted from Flockhart DA. Drug Interactions: Cytochrome P450 Drug Interaction Table. Indiana University School of Medicine (2007). Available at http://www.medicine.iupui.edu/flockhart/clinlist.htm (accessed June 13, 2008).

Other Antidepressants

Other antidepressant medications have numerous mechanisms of action. Nefazodone exhibits norepinephrine and serotonin reuptake inhibition, while also antagonizing 5-HT$_{2A}$ and α1-receptors. Nefazodone has a black box warning for the risk of liver failure due to the 1 in 250,000 to 300,000 patient-years risk of this outcome. This medication is usually given twice daily starting at 100 mg twice a day. Titration is done at a rate of 100 to 200 mg weekly to reach a maximum of 600 mg total daily. Mirtazapine (Remeron) appears to work through the blockade of α2-autoreceptors on presynaptic noradrenergic neurons and 5-HT$_2$ and 5-HT$_3$ receptors. It can be started at doses of 15 mg daily and increased by 15 mg weekly to a maximum of 45 mg/day. Paradoxically, doses lower than 15 mg daily may be more sedating than doses greater than 15 mg. Trazodone has been associated with penile priapism at a rate of 1 in 6000 to 8000 men. It is started at dosages of 50 to 75 mg/day and increased to a maximum of 400 to 600 mg/day. Currently, it is primarily used at lower doses for its hypnotic effect.

Psychotherapy

A number of specific psychotherapies are effective for treating depression. However, no single psychotherapy has been demonstrated to be superior to another, and many studies have shown nonspecific supportive psychotherapy to be as effective as the specific psychotherapies.

Cognitive Behavior Therapy

Developed by Aaron Beck and his colleagues in the 1960s, cognitive behavior therapy (CBT) is based on the cognitive model of mood disorders, which posits that the way people interpret their experiences influences how they feel and behave. For example, patients with depression typically have negative views of themselves, how others view them, and their future prospects. CBT focuses on identifying and changing these negative cognitions, which cause people to feel depressed or anxious. Patients learn to monitor these automatic thoughts and examine the evidence for and against them, alternative ways of thinking about the situation, and how different ways of thinking might influence the way they feel and behave.

This cognitive work is complemented by behavioral homework assignments, which require patients to keep a log of their daily activities, undertake graded exposure exercises to challenge maladaptive automatic thoughts, and role play new ways of thinking with their therapists. These behavioral experiments help patients develop a better sense of self-efficacy and mastery in addition to providing corrective experiences to counter maladaptive automatic thoughts. CBT is often undertaken one or more times weekly for 12 to 16 weeks, after which continuing meetings or booster sessions may be helpful.

Interpersonal Psychotherapy

Interpersonal psychotherapy (IPT) was developed by Klerman and colleagues in the 1970s to treat depression. IPT begins with a thorough evaluation, diagnosis, and assigning the patient the sick role. Patients' difficulties are then classified into one of four domains: grief, interpersonal role disputes, role transitions, and interpersonal deficits. Specific strategies to address the main problem areas (e.g., facilitate mourning in the case of grief) are then pursued with attention to improving the patient's interpersonal relationships. Termination is addressed explicitly, and the progress made by the patient is reviewed. IPT is usually conducted in 12 to 20 sessions over a 4- to 5-month period and may be individual or in a group.

Psychodynamic Psychotherapy

The overall goal of this psychotherapy is to increase patient's self-awareness, improve personal satisfaction, and resolve difficulties in interpersonal and romantic relationships. This treatment shares a theoretical framework with psychoanalysis, including the concepts of transference, countertransference, resistance, and unconscious conflict. Psychodynamic psychotherapy makes use of the techniques of clarification, confrontation, and interpretation and is usually undertaken at a frequency of one or more times weekly for a period of months or years.

Treatment-Resistant Depression

Many patients with major depression do not experience remission with the first antidepressant medication or course of psychotherapy. Patients are typically considered to have treatment-resistant depression when a minimum of two treatments at adequate dosage and duration have failed. One influential nomenclature for treatment-resistant depression developed by Thase and Rush relies on nonresponse to sequential trials of antidepressants with varying mechanisms of action. Stage I resistance is defined as lack of response to an adequate trial of one antidepressant; stage II resistance is defined as stage I resistance plus failure to respond to a second antidepressant having a different mechanism of action; stage III resistance is stage II resistance plus nonresponse to a tricyclic medication; stage IV resistance is stage III plus nonresponse to an MAOI; and stage V resistance is stage IV followed by nonresponse to electroconvulsive therapy (ECT).

Patients with treatment-resistant depression are among the most disabled persons with major depressive disorder, which itself ranks fourth among diseases worldwide in accounting for disability-adjusted life-years. Persistence of depressive symptoms can lead to continued psychosocial limitations and decreased work productivity, cardiovascular morbidity and mortality, and sustained risks of suicide and substance abuse. Due to the immense burden associated with treatment-resistant depression, there is consensus that the goal of treatment for patients is to achieve remission, defined as a final score of 10 on the HRSD or some comparable scale.

A unique perspective on the use of medications and psychotherapy to treat depression has been provided by the National Institute of Mental Health–sponsored Sequenced Treatment Alternatives to Relieve Depression (STAR*D) study, which is the largest prospective trial for depression ever conducted. Patients presented to one of 41 sites seeking treatment, and inclusion or exclusion criteria were structured so as to promote maximum generalizability. As shown in Figure 2, all 3271 patients received monotherapy with citalopram in level 1, and those whose depressions did not remit were encouraged to proceed with additional trials until remission was achieved. At level 2, patients were allowed to express preference for medication or psychotherapy and for switching treatments or augmenting treatment. Switch options were randomization to bupropion, sertraline, venlafaxine, and CBT; augmentation options were randomization to bupropion, buspirone, or CBT in addition to citalopram. Patients whose depressions still did not remit could be randomized at level 3 to either of two switch options (nortriptyline or mirtazapine) or two augmentation options (adding lithium or triiodothyronine (T$_3$) to whatever antidepressant they were taking). The final step, level 4, involved randomizing patients to tranylcypromine or the combination of venlafaxine and mirtazapine.

After initial treatment with citalopram, 37% of patients achieved remission. In level 2, patients who switched medications received either sustained-release bupropion up to 400 mg/day, sertraline up to 200 mg/day, or extended-release venlafaxine up to 375 mg/day. Remission rates, as measured by HRSD scores less than 7 on these medications, were 21% for bupropion, 18% for sertraline, and 25% for venlafaxine, which were not significantly different from one another. Augmentation of citalopram was with sustained-release bupropion up to 400 mg/day or buspirone up to 60 mg/day, and remission rates were identical (30% in each). In the level 3 augmentation trial, 16% of patients achieved remission with lithium compared to 25% of patients receiving T$_3$, which was not a significant difference. However, there was a suggestion that T$_3$ was better tolerated than lithium. In the level 4 trial, 7% of patients receiving tranylcypromine and 14% of patients receiving combined venlafaxine and mirtazapine remitted, which were not significantly different results.

Brain Stimulation

When patients fail multiple pharmacologic and psychotherapeutic trials, or when rapid control of depressive, manic, or psychotic symptoms is necessary, ECT should be strongly considered. ECT remains a

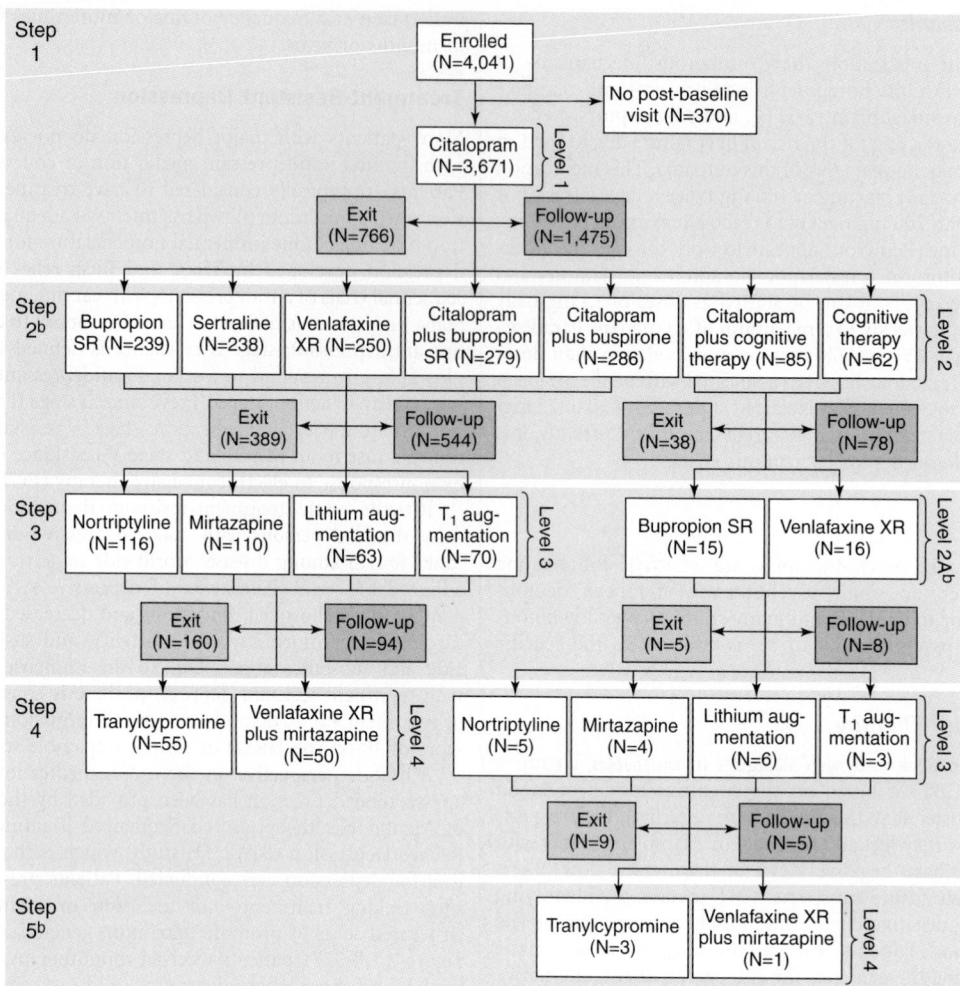

FIGURE 2. Sequenced Treatment Alternatives to Relieve Depression (STAR*D) study design. Adapted from Rush AJ, Trivedi MH, Wisniewski SR, et al: Acute and longer-term outcomes in depressed outpatients requiring one or several treatment steps: A STAR*D Report. Am J Psychiatry 2006;163:1905–17.

safe and effective treatment for mood disorders, and new protocols for treatment delivery aim to minimize cognitive side effects. Other brain stimulation treatments being studied as possible therapeutic tools include vagal nerve stimulation, deep brain stimulation, transcranial magnetic stimulation, and magnetic seizure therapy.

Bipolar Disorder

Epidemiologic studies show that 0.5% to 1.5% of people suffer from bipolar disorder, although up to 5% of the population might have bipolar spectrum illnesses. Patients usually present with a mood episode in their teens or 20s, and the risk of developing bipolar disorder dramatically decreases after the age of 50 years. Men and women are affected equally, and most persons go on to suffer a chronic course of repeated mood episodes.

DIAGNOSIS

Patients with bipolar spectrum disorders must meet diagnostic criteria for a hypomanic, manic, or mixed episode, and they often have had one or more major depressive episodes in the past. A manic episode is characterized by a period lasting at least 1 week of persistently elevated, expansive, or irritable mood (Box 3). Elevated moods are clearly recognized as excessive by persons close to the patient, and

---

BOX 3   DSM Criteria for Manic Episode

Distinct period of abnormally and persistently elevated, expansive or irritable mood, lasting at least 1 week (or any duration if hospitalization is necessary) and accompanied by:

Inflated self-esteem or grandiosity

Decreased need for sleep (e.g., feels rested after only 3 hours of sleep)

More talkative than usual or pressure to keep talking

Flight of ideas or subjective experience that thoughts are racing

Distractibility (i.e., attention too easily drawn to unimportant or irrelevant external stimuli)

Increase in goal-directed activity (at work, at school, or sexually) or psychomotor agitation

Excessive involvement in pleasurable activities that have a high potential for painful consequences (e.g., engaging in unrestrained buying sprees, sexual indiscretions, or foolish business investments)

DSM = *Diagnostic and Statistical Manual of Mental Disorders*, fourth edition (text revision).

the expansiveness of manic episodes is manifested in much increased enthusiasm for new projects or interpersonal interactions. Patients often have increased self-esteem, which may become psychotic as in grandiose delusions. Most persons experiencing a manic episode demonstrate a decreased need for sleep and increased energy.

Mental status examination of patients who are manic often reveals loud, rapid, poorly interruptible speech of dramatically increased productivity. Patients might report racing thoughts, which are experienced as moving faster than they can articulate or fully understand. Increased goal-directed activity refers to the excessive planning of and participation in activities such as new business ventures, housecleaning, hypergraphia, and calling people on the telephone. This activity is often coupled with impulsivity and poor judgment, as when patients engage in risky or dangerous activities such as spending sprees, violence, dangerous driving, and substance misuse.

To meet criteria for a manic episode, the impairment due to the mood disturbance must be severe enough to bring about marked difficulty functioning or require hospitalization. Hypomanic episodes are less severe than manic episodes, involving at least 4 days of elevated or irritable mood, fewer accompanying manic symptoms, and less severe functional impairment. Mixed episodes are 1-week periods during which the diagnostic criteria for both a major depressive episode and a manic episode are met. Clinicians may use the mnemonic DIGFAST to easily remember the list of DSM manic symptoms: *d*istractibility, *i*llegal (risky) activities, *g*randiosity, *f*light of ideas, increased goal-directed *a*ctivities, decreased *s*leep, and *t*alkativity.

As in the case of depressive disorders, suicide must be carefully evaluated in patients with bipolar disorder, because their risk of suicide is among the highest of all psychiatric patients. Medical conditions causing the manic, hypomanic, or mixed episode must be carefully ruled out, and other possible diagnoses such as substance-induced mood disorders and attention-deficit/hyperactivity disorder must be considered.

TREATMENT

Overview

Bipolar disorder is a chronic illness requiring lifelong management. Therefore, conducting an extensive process of patient education, facilitating treatment compliance, and developing a good therapeutic alliance are of great importance. Clinicians and patients have more information on which to base treatment decisions if continuous monitoring of the patient's mood (whether depressed or euphoric) is conducted using mood journals. Triggers for mood disturbance in each patient (e.g., long plane flight, fight with spouse, use of alcohol) should be carefully attended to and taken seriously when evident.

Given the highly recurrent nature of bipolar disorder and the severity of the disruption it typically causes, most experts agree that maintenance treatment is indicated after an acute manic, mixed, or depressive state resolves. A common practice in preventing future episodes of bipolar disorder is to continue the medication that resolved an acute episode. Many patients with bipolar disorder continue to experience significant symptoms even after they are considered to have remitted from an acute episode of depression or mania. These must be carefully assessed and treated to promote functional recovery and a good quality of life.

Mood Stabilizers

Phases of treatment for bipolar disorder include treatment of acute mania, prevention of mania, treatment of acute depression, and prevention of depression. Available mood-stabilizing agents are generally better in one phase than another, and no treatment is available that treats all phases of bipolar disorder.

Lithium

Lithium has been studied as a treatment for mania since the late 1940s. Several good-quality randomized, controlled trials demonstrate its efficacy in treating acute mania in bipolar patients; there is more limited evidence supporting the efficacy of lithium in patients with acute depression. Lithium appears effective in preventing both manic and depressive episodes, although some studies suggest more limited usefulness for lithium in preventing depression.

Lithium has good oral absorption, reaching peak plasma levels 1 to 3 hours after ingestion. It is excreted renally, which necessitates dosing modifications in older patients and in the setting of medications affecting tubular reabsorption. Lithium's exact mechanism of action is unknown, but it may be related to effects on noradrenergic and dopaminergic transmission or on complex transduction pathways.

Before a patient starts taking lithium, it is necessary to perform a medical work-up including medical history, physical examination with weight, blood urea nitrogen and creatinine, thyroid-function studies, complete blood count, and pregnancy testing for women of childbearing age. Lithium is usually started between 600 and 1200 mg daily for acute mania, with blood level determination (sampled 12 hours after last dose) after 4 days of treatment. A blood concentration between 0.8 and 1.2 mmol/L is desirable for acute mania, with toxic effects generally starting at blood levels of 1.5 and above. Patients with hypomania or in need of mania prophylaxis are started on lower doses of lithium, 300 to 600 mg daily, and titrated up more slowly to achieve blood levels of 0.6 to 0.8 mmol/L.

Common lithium side effects include nausea, vomiting, fine tremor, diarrhea, polydipsia, and polyuria. These are often transient and can be mitigated by dosage changes and slower titration strategies. Side effects of chronic treatment can include acne, psoriasis, hypothyroidism, and nephrogenic diabetes insipidus. Lithium toxicity is always a serious and potentially fatal condition. Signs and symptoms of toxic blood levels include mental status changes, ataxia, coarse tremor, and bradycardia. Treatment can require renal dialysis.

Anticonvulsants

Anticonvulsants have been used in patients with bipolar disorder since the 1960s, when "kindling" as a shared pathologic process with seizure disorders was purported to be the cause of disordered mood states. Not all anticonvulsants have proved effective for bipolar disorder, and those that have exhibit a wide range of mechanisms of action.

Divalproex sodium (Depakote) was the first anticonvulsant approved to treat acute mania and remains a first-line treatment for preventing and treating mania. However, this medication does not appear as effective for treating and preventing depression. Treatment of acutely manic patients with divalproex is typically begun with an oral loading dose of 15 to 20 mg/kg body weight divided into two or three daily doses, which is then continued for 4 days before checking a drug plasma level. Less urgently ill patients might have fewer side effects with more gradual titrations, starting at 250 to 500 mg daily and titrated up as needed. Blood levels of 50 to 125 mg/L represent the therapeutic range for this medication. Gastrointestinal side effects such as nausea and diarrhea are often observed with divalproex, as are sedation, weight gain, and tremor. Rare but potentially life-threatening adverse effects are hepatic failure, hemorrhagic pancreatitis, and encephalopathy caused by high ammonia levels.

Carbamazepine (Tegretol) has proved efficacy for mania in a number of randomized, controlled trials, but it too is of unclear benefit in treating and preventing depressive episodes. This medication is generally started at 200 to 600 mg daily in divided doses, then increased by 200 mg weekly to therapeutic effect or a maximum of 1600 mg/day. An extended-release form of carbamazepine is available that allows once-daily dosing. Therapeutic blood levels for epilepsy are 4 to 12 mg/L. The most commonly observed adverse effects with carbamazepine are nausea, sedation, blurred vision, and ataxia. Rare but serious side effects include hyponatremia due to secretion of inappropriate antidiuretic hormone (SIADH), liver transaminase elevations, aplastic anemia, and rash.

After being used off-label for several years for the prevention and treatment of bipolar depression, lamotrigine (Lamictal) received FDA approval in 2003 as a maintenance treatment for bipolar disorder. It has been shown in multiple randomized, controlled trials to be significantly superior to placebo in bipolar patients with recently resolved depression or mania in delaying the recurrence of a mood episode. Lamotrigine appears to be more effective in preventing episodes of depression than mania. Its value in the treatment of acute depressive episodes is much less clear. An initial randomized, controlled trial of lamotrigine versus placebo in patients with bipolar I depression revealed significant improvement in patients receiving 200 mg of lamotrigine compared with placebo. However, several more recent randomized, controlled trials have failed to replicate this finding, and the usefulness of this medication for patients with acute bipolar depression remains unclear.

Lamotrigine is generally started at doses of 25 mg daily for 2 weeks, followed by 50 mg for 2 weeks, and then 100 mg daily, with future titration of approximately 50 mg every 2 to 4 weeks. This slower titration schedule is thought to be helpful in reducing the risk of treatment-emergent rash, which can occur in up to 10% of patients on lamotrigine, and the rarer but more serious Stevens–Johnson syndrome. In patients who develop a rash and systemic signs such as fever or lymphadenopathy while taking lamotrigine, the medication should be immediately discontinued and the patient should be evaluated in an emergency room. The most common side effects observed with lamotrigine are dizziness, headache, blurred vision, and gastrointestinal distress.

Atypical Antipsychotics

All currently available atypical antipsychotics have now been approved by the FDA for managing acute bipolar mania, and quetiapine (Seroquel) is now appoved for bipolar depression. Many atypicals have proved efficacy as monotherapies for mania but also show improvement versus placebo when added on to other mood stabilizers. Most atypicals have high affinity for dopamine, serotonin, and α-adrenergic receptors, and some have additional high affinity for histamine. The exact mechanism of action of atypical antipsychotics in treating mania is unclear, although those that exert D_2-blocking effects might work by this route. Atypicals shown to be effective in treating depression might work by means of D2 and 5-HT_{2A} blockade.

Olanzapine (Zyprexa) is started at 10 to 15 mg daily and increased to 20 to 30 mg[3] daily as needed to control acute mania. An intramuscular form of olanzapine is also available for use in hospitalized patients with severe agitation. It is administered in a 10-mg dose that can be repeated 2 and 4 hours later for a total daily dose of 30 mg. Concomitant treatment with lorazepam is contraindicated due to reported cases of profound respiratory depression.

Quetiapine is started at 25 to 50 mg twice daily and titrated up as tolerated over the course of 1 to 2 weeks to approximately 600 mg daily. Evidence exists for the use of quetiapine in acute mania, and more recently two randomized, controlled trials have demonstrated significant antidepressant benefits for quetiapine monotherapy of patients with bipolar I or II depression. Apart from olanzapine and quetiapine, very limited evidence exists for the efficacy of other atypical antipsychotics in bipolar depression.

There is good evidence of efficacy for risperidone (Risperdal) as monotherapy for acute mania and as add-on treatment to lithium or an anticonvulsant. Risperidone is generally started at 1 to 2 mg/day in divided doses and titrated up by 1 to 2 mg daily to a range of 4 to 6 mg/day. Risperidone is currently the only atypical antipsychotic available in a long-acting preparation, which is injected intramuscularly[1] to provide slow release of risperidone over 3 weeks. Clinicians may start with 12.5 to 25 mg IM every 2 weeks, with increases of 12.5 mg every 4 weeks as needed up to 50 mg IM every 2 weeks.

Ziprasidone (Geodon) should be started at 40 mg twice daily, given with meals to increase the absorption of medication. Ziprasidone should be titrated up to a total of 160 mg/day within the first week of treatment, because some reports of activation in the lower dosing range have been reported. It is available in an intramuscular[1] form to assist in the management of acute agitation, with 10 to 20 mg given every 2 to 4 hours as needed up to a maximum of 40 mg daily.

Aripiprazole (Abilify) is the newest atypical antipsychotic approved for use in acute mania. As opposed to other atypicals, aripiprazole is a partial agonist at the D2 receptor. It can be started at 10 to 15 mg daily and titrated up over the course of a week to approximately 30 mg daily. An intramuscular form of aripiprazole is now available to treat acute agitation, and this injected form is given at a dose of 9.75 mg every 2 hours to a maximum of 30 mg daily.

The most significant category of side effects noted with the use of atypical antipsychotics is weight gain, dyslipidemia, and onset of type 2 diabetes mellitus. Management of patients taking these medications must include monitoring of waist circumference, fasting glucose, weight, and lipid profile.

Conclusions

Unipolar and bipolar mood disorders are often observed in clinical practice and have serious negative psychosocial and health consequences. Treatment must follow a structured approach beginning with comprehensive evaluation and diagnosis, proceeding through informed consent and patient education, and culminating in the initiation of treatment. In addition to several evidence-based psychotherapeutic modalities, numerous antidepressant and mood-stabilizing medications are available in a number of classes for treating depression and mania. The careful use of these treatments may be of considerable benefit for most patients with these disorders.

REFERENCES

Bowden CL, Calabrese JR, Sachs G, et al. A placebo-controlled 18-month trial of lamotrigine and lithium maintenance treatment in recently manic or hypomanic patients with bipolar I disorder. Arch Gen Psychiatry 2003;60:392–400.

Calabrese JR, Bowden CL, Sachs G, et al. A placebo-controlled 18-month trial of lamotrigine and lithium maintenance treatment in recently depressed patients with bipolar I disorder. J Clin Psychiatry 2003;64:1013–24.

Calabrese JR, Bowden CL, Sachs GS, et al. A double-blind placebo-controlled study of lamotrigine monotherapy in outpatients with bipolar I depression. Lamictal 602 Study Group. J Clin Psychiatry 1999;60:79–88.

Calabrese JR, Keck Jr PE, Macfadden W, et al. A randomized, double-blind, placebo-controlled trial of quetiapine in the treatment of bipolar I or II depression. Am J Psychiatry 2005;162:1351–60.

Frank E. Treatment outcomes for depression in primary care. Arch Gen Psychiatry 1991;48:851–95.

Greden JF. The burden of disease for treatment-resistant depression. J Clin Psychiatry 2001;62(Suppl. 16):26–31.

Judd LL, Paulus MJ, Schettler PJ, et al. Does incomplete recovery from first lifetime major depressive episode herald a chronic course of illness? Am J Psych 2000;157:1501–4.

Kessler RC, Berglund P, Demier O, et al. The epidemiology of major depressive disorder: Results from the National Comorbidity Survey Replication (NCS-R). JAMA 2003;289:3095–31105.

Kupfer DJ. Long-term treatment of depression. J Clin Psychiatry 1991;52 (Suppl. 5):28–34.

McGrath PJ, Stewart JW, Fava M, et al. Tranylcypromine versus venlafaxine plus mirtazipine following three failed antidepressant medication trials for depression: A STAR*D report. Am J Psychiatry 2006;163:1531–41.

Murray CJL, Lopez AD. The global burden of disease: A comprehensive assessment of mortality and disability from disease, injuries, and risk factors in 1990 and projected to 2020, vol 1. World Health Organization. Cambridge, Mass.: Harvard University Press; 1996.

Nierenberg AA, Fava M, Trivedi MH, et al. A comparison of lithium and T3 augmentation following two failed medication treatments for depression: A STAR*D report. Am J Psychiatry 2006;163:1519–30.

Nierenberg AA, Wright EC. Evolution of remission as the new standard in the treatment of depression. J Clin Psychiatry 1999;60(Suppl. 22):7–11.

Paykel ES, Ramana R, Cooper Z, et al. Residual symptoms after partial remission: an important outcome in depression. Psychol Med 1995;25:1171–80.

Thase ME, MacFadden W, Weisler RH, et al. Efficacy of quetiapine monotherapy in bipolar I and II depression: A double-blind, placebo-controlled study (the BOLDER II study). J Clin Psychopharmacol 2006;26:600–9.

Thase ME, Ninan PT. New goals in the treatment of depression: Moving toward recovery. Psychopharmacol Bull 2002;36(Suppl. 2):24–35.

---

[1]Not FDA approved for this indication.
[3]Exceeds dosage recommended by the manufacturer.

Thase ME, Rush HA. Treatment-resistant depression. In: Bloom FE, Kupfer DJ, editors. Psychopharmacology. New York: Raven, The 4th Generation of Progress; 1995. p. 1081–98.

Trivedi MH, Rush AJ, Wisniewski SR, et al. Evaluation of outcomes with citalopram for depression using measurement-based care in STAR*D: implications for clinical practice. Am J Psychiatry 2006;163:28–40.

Schizophrenia

Method of
Brian Miller, MD, MPH, and Peter Buckley, MD

Schizophrenia is a complex, chronic, and often severe psychiatric disorder that is a leading cause of disability worldwide. Although the literal translation of the word *schizophrenia* is "split mind," patients with this disorder do not have a "split personality" or a multiple personality disorder. Schizophrenia is a psychotic disorder that interferes with a person's thinking, mood, behavior, and interpersonal relations. Schizophrenia often has devastating, lifelong consequences for affected individuals and their families, and it is associated with an increased risk of premature mortality, including deaths from suicide and cardiovascular disease. In this chapter, the epidemiology and diagnosis of schizophrenia are reviewed. We then discuss pharmacologic and psychosocial treatments for schizophrenia in the context of a chronic disease model. The risks of medical and substance-use comorbidity and suicidality are also highlighted.

Epidemiology and Risk Factors

The cause of schizophrenia is not known, but it is thought to involve interactions between genetic (or epigenetic) and environmental factors, including developmental problems that occur during gestation. The lifetime prevalence of schizophrenia is approximately 1% and is equal for men and women. The usual age of onset is in the late teens or early 20s to late 30s, although schizophrenia can have onset before age 10 (early onset) or after age 45 (late onset). The age of onset is usually younger for men than women.

Several lines of evidence support a genetic contribution to the risk of schizophrenia. There is a 40% lifetime risk of schizophrenia in a child of two parents with schizophrenia. Twin-twin concordance is 50% for monozygotic twins and 12% for dizygotic twins. A meta-analysis found "strong epidemiologic credibility" for four candidate genes: *DRD1*, *DTNBP1*, *MTHFR*, and *TPH1*, although numerous other genes have been implicated. There are likely multiple candidate genes that increase the risk of schizophrenia, each with a small effect size.

Replicated environmental risk factors for schizophrenia include season of birth (i.e., winter), advanced paternal age, prenatal stress throughout gestation (e.g., famine and acute maternal stress in the first trimester, second-trimester influenza exposure, loss of the father in the second or third trimester), obstetric complications (e.g., gestational diabetes, low birth weight, asphyxia), severe childhood abuse, and cannabis use. It remains unclear whether some of these risk factors are causal or represent early manifestations of schizophrenia.

Diagnosis

There are three primary symptom domains in schizophrenia: positive, negative, and cognitive. Positive symptoms are abnormalities of thought content, including hallucinations (i.e., abnormal sensory perceptions in the absence of external stimuli) and delusions

CURRENT DIAGNOSIS

- Three primary symptom domains:
  - Positive (i.e., hallucinations, delusions, and disorganized thought and behavior)
  - Negative (i.e., blunted affect, anhedonia, alogia, and avolition)
  - Cognitive (i.e., attention, language, memory, and processing speed)
- Symptoms lasting for 1 month and continuous signs of illness for 6 months
- Significant impairment of one or more major areas of functioning (work, interpersonal relations, or self-care)
- Ensure that psychosis is not caused by a primary mood disorder, schizoaffective disorder, substance intoxication or withdrawal, or a general medical condition

(i.e., fixed, false beliefs) and disorganized thinking and behavior. Hallucinations are most commonly auditory, but they can occur in any sensory modality. Negative symptoms include impairments in motivation (i.e., avolition), emotional expression (i.e., blunted affect), speech (i.e., alogia), and the ability to experience pleasure (i.e., anhedonia). Cognitive symptoms include impairments in attention, language, memory, processing speed, and executive function.

The most commonly used diagnostic criteria for schizophrenia are derived from the *Diagnostic and Statistical Manual of Mental Disorders*, fourth edition, text revision (DSM-IV-TR). These criteria include the presence of two or more characteristic symptoms (i.e., delusions, hallucinations, disorganized speech, disorganized behavior, or negative symptoms) for a significant portion of time during a 1-month period, with continuous signs of the disturbance persisting for at least 6 months. During this period, there is significant impairment in one or more major areas of functioning, including work, interpersonal relations, and self-care. It must also be established that the disorder is not better accounted for by a primary mood disorder, schizoaffective disorder, substance intoxication or withdrawal, or another general medical condition. Delusions and hallucinations, although common, are not required for the diagnosis. Although cognitive symptoms are not required for the diagnosis, they are a significant cause of illness-related disability. A diagnosis of schizophrenia is most definitively made by interviewing the patient, obtaining collateral history from family and friends, and completing a medical work-up (i.e., physical examination with routine blood and urine tests).

Treatment

There is no cure for schizophrenia. Although there is significant clinical heterogeneity within the disorder, schizophrenia is usually a chronic condition that requires long-term treatment. Comprehensive treatment involves outpatient medication management and therapy, psychosocial interventions, involvement of the family and other support system, inpatient care for acute crisis intervention or illness exacerbation, and collaboration with primary care physicians.

Antipsychotic medications play an important role in the pharmacologic management of schizophrenia. First-generation antipsychotics have been in clinical use since the introduction of chlorpromazine (Thorazine) in the 1950s. These agents block the dopamine D_2 receptor, and common side effects include extrapyramidal side effects (e.g., parkinsonism, dystonia). The second-generation antipsychotics (SGAs), in addition to D_2 receptor blockade, are also serotonin 5-HT_2 receptor antagonists. Although the risk of extrapyramidal side effects is lower with the use of SGAs than with first-generation antipsychotics, the SGAs are associated with a heightened risk of weight gain and the metabolic syndrome. Table 1 provides a more detailed description of antipsychotic medications. The Texas Medication Algorithm Project (TMAP) recommends a trial of a single (non-clozapine)

TABLE 1 Antipsychotic Medications

Agent	Mechanism of Action*	Typical Dosing	Side Effects†	Side Effects†	Comments
First Generation					
Haloperidol (Haldol)	D_2-antagonist	1.5–15 mg/d	EPS/TD Akathisia	NMS Hyperprolactinemia	PO, IM, IV, and long-acting injection formulations
Second Generation					
Aripiprazole (Abilify)	Partial D_2-agonist and antagonist	10–30 mg/d	Weight gain (+) Dyslipidemia (+) Glucose dysregulation (+)	Sedation EPS/TD Akathisia	PO, rapid-dissolving PO, and IM formulations
Clozapine (Clozaril)	D_2-antagonist/5-HT_2 antagonist	300–900 mg/d	Weight gain (+++) Dyslipidemia (+++) Glucose dysregulation (++) Agranulocytosis Sedation	Orthostatic hypotension Seizures Myocarditis EPS/TD	PO and rapid-dissolving PO formulations
Olanzapine (Zyprexa)	D_2-antagonist/5-HT_2 antagonist	5–20 mg/d	Weight gain (+++) Dyslipidemia (+++) Glucose dysregulation (++)	Sedation EPS/TD	PO, rapid-dissolving PO, and IM formulations
Paliperidone (Invega)	D_2-antagonist/5-HT_2 antagonist	6–12 mg/d	Weight gain (+) Dyslipidemia (+) Glucose dysregulation (+)	EPS/TD	PO formulation Active metabolite of risperidone (Risperdal)
Quetiapine (Seroquel)	D_2-antagonist/5-HT_2 antagonist	400–800 mg/d	Weight gain (++) Dyslipidemia (+) Glucose dysregulation (+)	Sedation EPS/TD Orthostatic hypotension	PO, ER formulations
Risperidone (Risperdal)	D_2-antagonist/5-HT_2 antagonist	2–6 mg/d	Weight gain (++) Dyslipidemia (+) Glucose dysregulation (+)	EPS/TD Hyperprolactinemia	PO, PO liquid, rapid-dissolving PO, and long-acting injection formulations
Ziprasidone (Geodon)	D_2-antagonist/5-HT_2 antagonist	80–160 mg/d with food	Weight gain (+) Dyslipidemia (+) Glucose dysregulation (+)	QTc prolongation EPS/TD	PO and IM formulations

Abbreviations: D_2 = dopamine D_2 receptor; EPS = extrapyramidal side effects; ER, extended release; 5-HT_2 = serotonin 5-HT_2 receptor; NMS = neuroleptic malignant syndrome; TD = tardive dyskinesia; + = mild or low risk; ++ = moderate risk; +++ = severe risk.
*All first-generation and second-generation antipsychotics have an FDA black box warning for an "association with an increased risk of mortality in elderly patients treated for dementia-related psychosis."
†EPS and TD are possible side effects with all antipsychotics, but they occur less frequently with second-generation than first-generation drugs.

SGA for newly diagnosed patients with schizophrenia or for patients never before treated with an SGA. However, neither the TMAP nor the American Psychiatric Association (APA) guidelines for the treatment of schizophrenia preferentially endorse a particular antipsychotic. Clozapine (Clozaril) is primarily used for treatment-refractory schizophrenia, usually defined as a lack of or partial response to an adequate trial of two or three antipsychotics.

Adjunctive medications may play an important role in the pharmacologic treatment of some patients with schizophrenia. The drugs include antidepressants for depression and anxiety, mood stabilizers for depression or mood elevation, benzodiazepines for anxiety or agitation, β-blockers for akathisia, and anticholinergics for extrapyramidal side effects.

Medication nonadherence is a major treatment issue for patients with schizophrenia at all phases of the illness. Reasons for nonadherence are complex and multifaceted but may include medication side effects, impaired insight into illness, psychopathology in all three symptom domains, lack of efficacy, and comorbid substance use. More than 70% of patients in the Clinical Antipsychotic Trials of Intervention Effectiveness (CATIE) schizophrenia trial discontinued medication within the first 18 months of treatment. Medication nonadherence leads to dramatically increased risk of illness relapse, hospitalization, and suicidal behavior, and it should be routinely assessed in clinical visits. The use of rapid-dissolving oral or long-acting injectable medications may improve adherence for some patients.

Psychosocial interventions are a cornerstone of the comprehensive treatment of patients with schizophrenia, and when used in combination with medication, they are more effective than antipsychotics alone. Psychotherapy, including cognitive-behavioral therapy, supportive therapy, and group therapy, promotes improved illness management and medication adherence. Involvement of the patient's family or support system in care, including family-based therapies and psychoeducation, has increased medication adherence and decreased illness relapse rates. Psychosocial rehabilitation, which may include assertive community treatment, social skills training, vocational rehabilitation, and cognitive remediation, can help maximize patients' psychosocial function.

Although there is no typical patient with schizophrenia, the clinical course is often characterized by acute relapses of illness with interepisode absence or attenuation of symptoms. Many factors increase a patient's risk of illness relapse, including medication nonadherence, psychosocial stressors, substance use, medical illnesses such as infections, and the natural history of the disorder itself. Hospitalization may be required for acute exacerbations of psychotic symptoms, including hallucinations, delusions, and impaired self-care. Hospitalization may also be required if patients represent an acute danger to themselves or others.

CURRENT THERAPY

- Antipsychotic medication, with monitoring for medication adherence and side effects
- Adjunctive medications as needed, including antidepressants, mood stabilizers, benzodiazepines, β-blockers, and anticholinergics
- Aggressive monitoring for and management of medical comorbidities, substance use disorders, and suicidality, including collaboration with a primary care physician
- Psychosocial interventions
- Involvement of family and support system in care
- Long-term treatment, including outpatient medication management and therapy, with inpatient care for acute crisis intervention or illness exacerbation

The concept of the recovery model and recovery-oriented care is a movement that is transforming the delivery of mental health services. Integral to the recovery model are certified peer specialists (CPSs). CPSs are licensed professionals who have progressed in their own recovery from mental illness and work to assist patients with schizophrenia and other mental illness in regaining control over their own lives and over their own recovery process. CPSs provide peer support services, serve as consumer advocates, are a resource for psychoeducation, and offer the unique perspective of their individual experiences.

Comorbidity

Schizophrenia is associated with an increased risk of premature mortality, and cardiovascular disease is a leading cause of death in this patient population. Many factors contribute to this risk, including a high prevalence of smoking, poor health habits, poor health care, medication side effects, and perhaps the pathophysiology of the disorder itself. SGAs as a class are associated with weight gain and an increased risk of the metabolic syndrome. More than 40% of the 1460 patients in the CATIE schizophrenia trial met the criteria for the metabolic syndrome at baseline. Recommendations for monitoring of patients on SGAs, based on a consensus statement from the American Diabetes Association and the American Psychiatric Association, are described in Table 2. Primary care physicians play an important collaborative role with psychiatrists in the detection and management of metabolic disturbances in patients with schizophrenia to minimize the cardiovascular risks associated with these comorbidities.

Patients with schizophrenia are at an increased risk for suicide, which is a leading cause of premature mortality. The prevalence of completed suicide attempts among patients with schizophrenia is about 10%, and suicide attempts occur with even greater frequency. Clinicians should routinely assess patients for suicidal ideation, and if present, explore risk factors for completed suicide, which include a suicidal plan and intent, previous suicide attempts, a family history of suicide, access to lethal means, social isolation, and comorbid substance use. Medications, psychotherapy, and hospitalization may be required.

Comorbid substance-use disorders predominate among patients with schizophrenia; the estimated prevalence is 40% to 50%. Common substances of abuse include alcohol, marijuana, and cocaine. Patients with schizophrenia and comorbid substance use are at increased risk for medication nonadherence, illness relapse, hospitalization, suicidal and violent behavior, and an overall poor response to treatment. Up to 90% of patients with schizophrenia are tobacco users, which contributes to the increased risk of medical comorbidity. Clinicians are encouraged to routinely screen for and address substance use in their treatment plans.

Conclusions

Schizophrenia is a complex, heterogeneous, and chronic psychiatric disorder. Comprehensive treatment usually involves long-term medication management and therapy, education for patients and their families, and psychosocial interventions. Primary care physicians play an important collaborative role in the detection and management of medical comorbidities, substance-use disorders, and suicidality.

1131

TABLE 2 Monitoring Second-Generation Antipsychotics (Excluding Clozapine)

Feature	Baseline	4 Weeks	8 Weeks	12 Weeks	Quarterly	Annually	If Symptoms Arise	Every 5 Years	Other
Personal and family history*	X					X			
Pregnancy test†	X						X		
Weight and body mass index	X	X	X	X	X				
Waist circumference	X					X			
Blood pressure	X			X		X			
Fasting glucose and HgbA$_{1C}$	X			X		X			
Fasting lipid panel	X			X				X	
Electrocardiogram‡	X						X		
Prolactin	X						X		
Complete blood cell count with differential§	X								X

*Including obesity, diabetes, hypertension, and dyslipidemia.
†In all women of childbearing age.
‡For patients taking ziprasidone (Geodon), which may prolong the QTc interval, and clozapine (Clozaril).
§For patients taking clozapine (Clozaril). Complete blood cell count with a differential cell count is required at baseline, then weekly for 6 months, then every other week for 6 months, and then monthly thereafter. White blood cell count must be ≥3500/mm³, and absolute neutrophil count must be ≥2000/mm³ due to risk of agranulocytosis. More frequent assessments may be warranted based on clinical status.

Physicians, patients, and families are encouraged to become involved in the National Alliance on Mental Illness (NAMI; www.nami.org), which is a tremendous resource for help, support, education, and advocacy for patients with schizophrenia and other mental illness.

REFERENCES

Allen NC, Bagade S, McQueen MB, et al. Systematic meta-analyses and field synopsis of genetic association studies in schizophrenia: The SzGene database. Nat Genet 2008;40:827.

American Diabetes Association, American Psychiatric Association, American Association of Clinical Endocrinologists, North American Association for Studies on Obesity. Consensus development conference on antipsychotic drugs and obesity and diabetes. J Clin Psychiatry 2004;65:267.

American Psychiatric Association. Practice guideline for the treatment of patients with schizophrenia, 2nd edition. Am J Psychiatry 2004;161 (Suppl):1717.

Brown S. Excess mortality of schizophrenia. A meta-analysis. Br J Psychiatry 1997;171:502.

Buchanan RW, Carpenter WT. Schizophrenia and other psychotic disorders. In: Sadock BJ, Sadock VA, editors. Kaplan and Sadock's Comprehensive Textbook of Psychiatry. 8th ed. Philadelphia: Lippincott Williams & Wilkins; 2005. p. 1329–45.

Green A. Schizophrenia and comorbid substance use disorder: Effects of antipsychotics. J Clin Psychiatry 2005;66:21.

Leucht S, Corves C, Arbter D, et al. Second-generation versus first-generation antipsychotic drugs for schizophrenia: A meta-analysis. Lancet 2009; 373:31.

Lieberman JA, Stroup TS, McEvoy JP, et al. Effectiveness of antipsychotic drugs in patients with chronic schizophrenia. N Engl J Med 2005; 353:1209.

McEvoy JP, Meyer JM, Goff DC, et al. Prevalence of the metabolic syndrome in patients with schizophrenia: Baseline results from the clinical antipsychotic trials of intervention effectiveness (CATIE). Schizophr Res 2005;80:19.

Messias EL, Chen CY, Eaton WW. Epidemiology of schizophrenia: Review of findings and myths. Psychiatr Clin North Am 2007;30:323.

Panic Disorder

Method of
Lakshmi Ravindran, MD, and Murray B. Stein, MD

Lifetime prevalence estimates of panic disorder (PD), with or without agoraphobia, vary worldwide from 1.6% to 2.2%, but epidemiologic studies suggest that approximately 5% of U.S. adults will meet the criteria for panic disorder in their lifetimes. Although reasons for this discrepancy are not clear, differences in study methodology, diagnostic criteria, and cultural manifestations of panic may play a role.

Diagnosis

Panic attacks, the core feature of PD, are abrupt surges in anxiety characterized by physical and cognitive symptoms (Box 1). These symptoms build to a climax, usually within 10 to 15 minutes, before eventually dissipating over the next several minutes or hours. Although isolated panic attacks are not uncommon, with a lifetime prevalence of up to 23% reported for the general population, the attacks seen in PD are recurrent, may not have a precipitant, and are accompanied by persistent concerns and changes in behavior. Characteristic concerns seen in PD include fear of having more attacks or fears about what the attacks mean for the person's medical or mental health, whereas behavioral changes usually involve avoidance of activities or places that become associated with the attack itself or with its perceived triggers.

When avoidance becomes excessive, agoraphobia ("fear of the marketplace") may be diagnosed; it can be found in up to 50% of people with PD. Individuals with agoraphobia often restrict their excursions into novel or public places for fear of experiencing and displaying panic symptoms in front of strangers without possibility of escape. In extreme cases, individuals may become housebound. If left untreated, PD may cause considerable losses in quality of life and overall function, not to mention the societal costs that result.

Lifetime prevalence rates of PD are consistently greater in females, with reports of a twofold greater risk compared with males. Although the onset of PD may occur across a wide age span, the age of onset commonly reported is late adolescence and the early 20s. The National Comorbidity Survey-Replication (NCS-R) reports a median age of onset for PD of 24 years. Rarely, PD may begin in childhood and early adolescence, although this has been associated with the subsequent development of comorbid psychiatric illness. The new onset of panic attacks in older adults (>60 years) is also atypical and more likely to be related to another psychiatric or medical illness rather than primary PD.

The risk for development of PD has a genetic component. Evidence from twin and family studies suggests the heritability of PD is approximately 40%, with first-degree relatives of probands with PD at a sevenfold greater risk of also developing PD compared with the general population. This risk is substantially higher in families in which the proband had early-onset PD.

Because genetic patterns do not fully explain the incidence of PD, a stress-diathesis model has been proposed in which environmental stressors are presumed to play a role in precipitating and maintaining the illness in at-risk individuals. Some studies have reported that up to 80% of individuals described the occurrence of a stressful life event in the year preceding the onset of PD, with most subjects believing a direct connection existed between the two events.

Several other risk factors for PD have been identified. Anxiety sensitivity is a traitlike construct referencing an individual's tendency to specifically fear the physiologic symptoms of anxiety (e.g., palpitations, shortness of breath, sweating) because of the concern that they represent indications of a harmful or negative consequence (e.g., "I am having a heart attack."). Elevated anxiety sensitivity

---

BOX 1   Typical Symptoms of a Panic Attack

Physical Symptoms
- Palpitations, pounding heart, or rapid heartbeat
- Difficulty breathing (e.g., feeling smothered)
- Choking
- Chest pain
- Sweating
- Chills or hot flushes
- Nausea or abdominal discomfort
- Difficulty swallowing
- Dizziness, lightheadedness, or feeling faint
- Paresthesias (i.e., numbness, prickling, or tingling) in the extremities or the face
- Trembling or shaking

Cognitive Symptoms
- Fear of going crazy
- Fear of dying
- Fear of losing control
- Perceptual abnormalities
- Feeling detached from one's body (i.e., depersonalization)
- Feelings of unreality regarding objects outside one's body (i.e., derealization)
- Sense of impending doom
- Feelings of paralyzing terror

CURRENT DIAGNOSIS

- Presence of recurrent unexpected panic attacks
- Anticipatory anxiety about future attacks
- Fears about medical or psychological implications of an attack
- May engage in avoidance behavior
- Frequently presents with concern about somatic symptoms rather than panic
- New-onset panic attacks common in people in their late teens or early 20s but rare in older adults
- Commonly comorbid with other psychiatric disorders
- Always should assess suicide risk
- Panic attacks occurring in psychiatric disorders other than panic disorder

is a risk factor for different anxiety disorders, including PD, as is the personality trait of neuroticism (i.e., tendency to readily experience negative emotions such as anger or anxiety). Other risk factors for PD include a history of heavy smoking in adolescence or a history of childhood abuse.

Psychiatric comorbidity with PD is extremely common, with more than 83% reporting one or more lifetime comorbid conditions (NCS-R), although rates are even higher with a diagnosis of PD with agoraphobia. Other anxiety disorders were identified as the most frequent lifetime comorbidity, followed by mood disorders. Much attention has been focused on comorbidity with major depressive disorder (MDD) because 34.1% of individuals with PD report a lifetime history of MDD, and there is a higher risk for PD with agoraphobia (38.5%). In one third of cases, PD precedes MDD; the reverse occurs in another third; and in the final third, the two conditions may occur together. Comorbid depression is also associated with poorer outcomes in both conditions, including worse levels of disability, greater time to response, lower rates of remission, increased risk of substance abuse or additional comorbidity, and greater suicide risk. PD itself is associated with elevated risk of suicide attempts within the past year, independent of the presence of depression. A suspected diagnosis of PD should include a thorough suicide risk assessment.

Differential Diagnosis

A variety of medical and psychiatric illnesses may manifest with panic attacks or panic-like symptoms. Differentiating between these isolated panic attacks and PD poses a diagnostic challenge. Isolated panic attacks are discrete attacks that are not followed by persistent concerns about more attacks or avoidant behavior, nor are there any resultant changes in the patient's overall level of functioning. Distinguishing PD from other disorders may be more difficult (Table 1). The frightening presence of chest pain, palpitations, or respiratory difficulties during a panic attack may be why individuals with PD present with somatic symptoms as their primary complaint.

A complete history and thorough physical examination are key in ruling out the possibility of underlying medical illness, substance intoxication, or drug withdrawal. Simple laboratory investigations may be helpful in initially ruling out serious illness. For instance, a preliminary work-up that includes a complete blood cell count, basic chemistry panel, thyroid-stimulating hormone (TSH) determination, chest radiograph, electrocardiogram or Holter monitor, and urine toxicology screen can rule out a large number of the differential diagnoses. More complex investigations, such as electroencephalography, computed tomography, or assay of urinary catecholamines, may be performed based on specific indications from the clinical examination. Atypical symptoms, new-onset symptoms in older individuals, and accompanying physical signs may suggest an underlying medical cause.

Although medical illness can mimic, precipitate, or exacerbate preexisting panic symptoms, PD may also aggravate perception of

TABLE 1 Differential Diagnosis of Panic Attacks

Diagnostic Feature	Possible Diagnoses
Psychiatric	Mood disorder (e.g., major depression, bipolar disorder)
	Other anxiety disorder (e.g., social anxiety disorder, specific phobia, posttraumatic stress disorder, generalized anxiety disorder, obsessive-compulsive disorder)
	Agoraphobia without panic disorder
	Psychotic disorder
	Somatoform disorder
	Factitious disorder
Cardiac	Angina or myocardial infarction
	Arrhythmia
	Mitral valve prolapse
	Labile hypertension
	Congestive heart failure
Endocrine	Adrenal dysfunction
	Thyroid disorder (i.e., hypothyroid or hyperthyroid)
	Hypoglycemia
	Hyperparathyroidism
Respiratory	Chronic obstructive pulmonary disease
	Asthma
	Pulmonary embolus
Neurologic	Seizure disorder (e.g., temporal lobe epilepsy)
	Pheochromocytoma
	Vestibular dysfunction
Substance intoxication	Excess caffeine use
	Psychostimulants (e.g., L-dopa, cocaine, amphetamines)
	Cannabis use
Substance withdrawal	Caffeine withdrawal
	Nicotine withdrawal
	Alcohol or sedative withdrawal
	Opioid withdrawal

and vigilance about medical symptoms and may influence the outcome of physical illness. For instance, PD in patients with comorbid asthma has been associated with worse quality of life, increased use of respiratory medication, and increased hospitalization rates. The presence of comorbid PD is more frequently found in certain medical illnesses, such as respiratory disease, vestibular dysfunction, thyroid disorders (i.e., hypothyroidism and hyperthyroidism), cardiac disease, chronic pain, migraines, and irritable bowel syndrome.

Panic attacks often form part of the presentation of psychiatric illnesses, particularly of other anxiety disorders and major depression. A careful history documenting the onset, course, possible triggers, and accompanying symptoms is vital in establishing the diagnosis. For instance, the presence of situationally specific panic attacks can suggest a specific phobia or may occur as part of posttraumatic stress disorder when individuals are exposed to reminders of traumatic events, whereas new-onset panic attacks and excessive worry in a 50-year-old patient with accompanying symptoms of disturbances in sleep and appetite and with psychomotor changes may suggest MDD. Although uncommon (U.S. lifetime prevalence estimated at 0.17%–0.8%), some individuals may be diagnosed with agoraphobia without ever meeting the criteria for PD; this diagnosis remains controversial in the psychiatric community.

Treatment

Effective pharmacologic and psychotherapeutic strategies exist for the treatment of PD. Regardless of the modality chosen, aims of treatment include decreased frequency and eventual elimination of panic attacks, eradication of anticipatory anxiety and associated phobic avoidance, correction of faulty cognitions about panic, and return to optimal psychosocial function. Initial choice of treatment

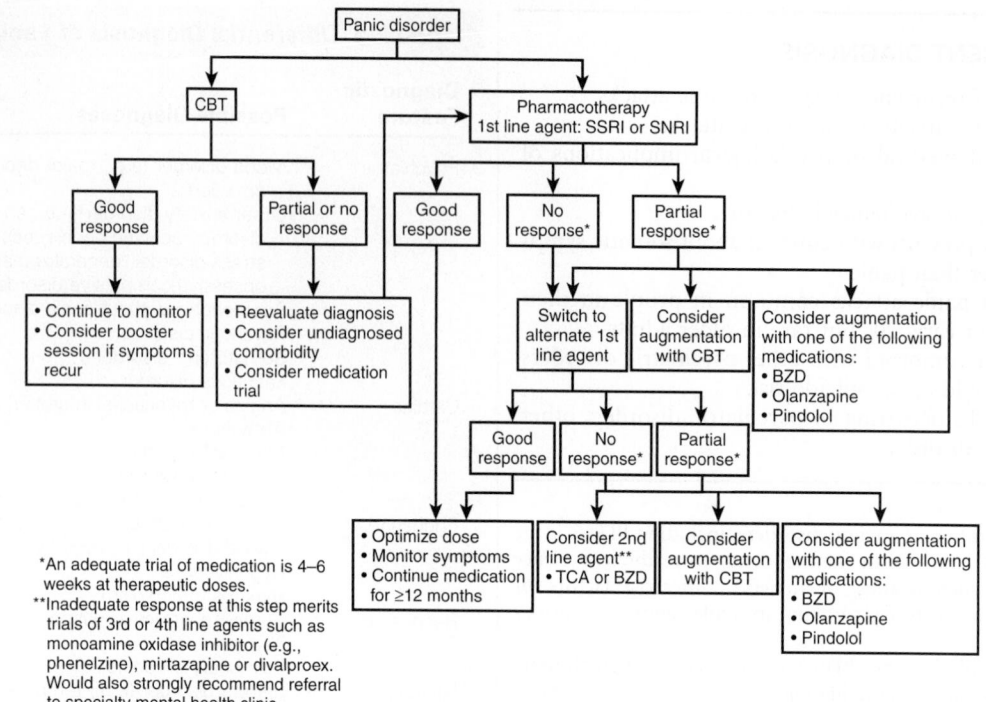

FIGURE 1. Suggested algorithm for the acute treatment of panic disorder. *Abbreviations:* BZD = benzodiazepine; CBT = cognitive-behavioral therapy; SNRI = serotonin-norepinephrine reuptake inhibitor; SSRI = selective serotonin reuptake inhibitor; TCA = tricyclic antidepressant.

modality may depend on a number of factors, including patient and physician preference, severity of symptoms, presence of comorbidity, availability of a therapist, and cost. There is insufficient evidence to recommend one modality (psychotherapy versus medication) over another as a first-line intervention during the acute phase. Figure 1 provides a suggested algorithm for the acute treatment of PD.

PHARMACOTHERAPY

Table 2 summarizes common medications used in the treatment of PD. A meta-analysis showed that selective serotonin reuptake inhibitors (SSRIs), tricyclic antidepressants (TCAs), and benzodiazepines had similar tolerability and efficacy in the treatment of PD. However, there may be clinical rationale for the choice of one medication class over another. Because benzodiazepines have limited benefit for mood symptoms, have the potential to be abused, and may cause psychomotor side effects, antidepressants may be the preferred treatment for patients with psychiatric comorbidity (particularly depressive or anxious disorders), a history of past or present substance abuse, older patients, or those with a history for a specific antidepressant agent. In contrast, benzodiazepines may be preferred in patients with severe physical symptoms of anxiety or with comorbid bipolar disorder or where there is an urgent need for onset of action. A temporary course of benzodiazepines may be prescribed at the time of SSRI initiation to provide some symptomatic relief while the SSRI takes effect and to alleviate potential SSRI side effects that mimic anxiety (e.g., nausea, dizziness, agitation). In some cases as-needed use of benzodiazepines may be helpful, such as in patients with rare panic symptoms that are otherwise not troublesome or for periodic breakthrough symptoms. However, using benzodiazepines on a regular schedule usually is preferred. Monotherapy with β-blockers or the partial 5-HT$_{1A}$ agonist, buspirone (BuSpar),[1] has not shown efficacy for PD.

If symptom remission and return to optimal psychosocial function are achieved, clinicians should maintain patients on the optimized dose of medication for a minimum of 12 months. At that time, the clinician may attempt a very slow taper off medication

(to minimize discontinuation or withdrawal symptoms) with close monitoring for symptom recurrence. A reasonable taper schedule may be 25% decreases in dose every 4 to 8 weeks, with an even slower taper for benzodiazepines (e.g., 10% decreases every 1 to 2 weeks).

TABLE 2 Common Medications Used to Treat Panic Disorder

Medication (Trade Name)	Recommended Initial Dose (mg/day)	Recommended Dose Range (mg/day)
Citalopram (Celexa)[1]	5–10	20–60
Escitalopram (Lexapro)[1]	5	10–20
Fluoxetine (Prozac)	5–10	20–60
Fluvoxamine (Luvox)[1]	50	100–300
Paroxetine (Paxil)	5–10	20–60
Paroxetine (Paxil CR)	6.25	25–75
Sertraline (Zoloft)	25	50–200
Venlafaxine XR (Effexor XR)	37.5	75–225
Tricyclic Antidepressants		
Clomipramine (Anafranil)[1]	25	75–250
Imipramine (Tofranil)[1]	25	75–250
Monoamine Oxidase Inhibitors		
Phenelzine* (Nardil)[1]	15	45–90†
Benzodiazepines		
Alprazolam (Xanax)	0.25 tid	2–4‡
Lorazepam (Ativan)[1]	0.25 tid	2–8‡
Clonazepam (Klonopin)	0.25 bid	1–2‡

[1]Not FDA approved for this indication.
*Dietary restrictions required (low-tyramine diet); 2-week washout required before initiation and after termination of monoamine oxidase inhibitor trial.
†Usually administered three times daily.
‡Total daily dosage is divided across 2 to 4 doses/day.

---

[1]Not FDA approved for this indication.

PSYCHOTHERAPY

Among the psychotherapies available, cognitive-behavioral therapy (CBT) has the greatest evidence to support its use. Two schools of CBT for PD predominate (i.e., panic control treatment [PCT] and cognitive therapy for panic [CTP]), although many therapists use elements of both. PCT, developed by Barlow and Craske, consists of three key components. First, psychoeducation provides patients with an understanding of the pathophysiology underlying panic attacks. This allows patients to link physiologic system changes with the production of somatic symptoms (e.g., palpitations, dizziness) and accompanying anxious thoughts (e.g., "I am going to lose consciousness.") and to understand how these factors may interact to reinforce each other. Second, cognitive restructuring teaches patients to identify erroneous beliefs about panic and to use logic and reasoning to correct distorted cognitions that overestimate the threat and consequences of panic attacks. Third, patients undergo interoceptive exposure—systematic, repeated exposure to feared internal cues (i.e., physical symptoms of panic)—which facilitates progressive desensitization and normalization of these sensations. Additional relaxation strategies, such as progressive muscle relaxation or deep breathing, which are useful for lowering general anxiety, may be used. When agoraphobia is also present, graded in vivo exposure of avoided situations may be incorporated into the treatment.

CTP, developed by Clark, is based on the premise that recurrent panic attacks are common in individuals with a habitual tendency to misinterpret normal bodily sensations (e.g., dizziness) as signs of imminent, potentially harmful events (e.g., a stroke). A positive-feedback loop is created when these misperceptions result in intense anxiety, which reinforces the intensity of the physical symptoms and arousal until a panic attack results. Although more reliant on cognitive techniques to correct misappraisals of physical symptoms, CTP also emphasizes psychoeducation to explain the creation of the vicious cycle. Patients become more aware of the sequence of events leading to the panic attack through the explanation of the vicious cycle. As with PCT, patients are encouraged to logically examine the basis of their fears and realistically evaluate their likelihood. Patients are taught to develop alternative rational explanations for the symptoms. Over time, the strength of beliefs that perpetuate the cycle is weakened and may be eliminated. CTP may also involve the use of exposure-based behavioral experiments to reinforce corrective learning.

PCT and CTP are time-limited interventions accomplished over 12 to 16 1-hour sessions. Periodic "booster" sessions, usually yearly, may be of benefit in cases of symptom recurrence.

Course and Prognosis

PD tends to follow a chronic course with a waxing and waning pattern. During periods of stress, the chance of recurrence or exacerbation is high. Follow-up studies of patients treated for PD suggest that at 4-year follow-up, about 30% of patients maintain remission, 40% to 50% continue to experience mild to moderate symptoms, and approximately 20% report persistent and more severe symptoms. Although CBT and pharmacotherapy appear to be relatively equivalent during the acute phase of treatment, some evidence suggests that CBT may prolong periods of remission in patients with PD but may not necessarily prevent recurrence. Among patients who were treated with CBT, 39% experienced a recurrence at 10 years, whereas among those treated with medications, the same proportion relapsed within 6 months. A meta-analysis did find an advantage for combined treatment (i.e., psychotherapy and pharmacotherapy) delivered in the acute phase over either psychotherapy or pharmacotherapy alone; however, after treatments were discontinued, no differences were observed between those who received combined treatment and those who received psychotherapy alone, although both groups did better than those on pharmacotherapy alone.

It has been suggested that rather than the duration of treatment, the level of symptom severity at the time of treatment discontinuation is the key factor in reducing recurrence, highlighting the importance of aiming for symptomatic remission. A course of CBT provided before medication discontinuation may enhance the odds of longer-term remission.

Among adults with PD, several negative prognostic factors have been identified: presence of comorbid depression, generalized anxiety, or personality disorder; longer duration of illness; greater levels of avoidance; low levels of social support; and more intense fears about social catastrophes after a panic attack (e.g., "People will laugh at me."). The presence of agoraphobia with PD has been associated with more severe symptoms, chronicity, and limited response to treatment.

CURRENT THERAPY

- Pharmacotherapy and cognitive-behavioral therapy (CBT) are effective for panic disorder.
- Recommended first-line antidepressant agents include selective serotonin reuptake inhibitors or venlafaxine XR (Effexor XR).
- To maximize tolerability, initiate antidepressants at 25% to 50% of the usual starting dose, but aim to reach antidepressant dose ranges similar to those used in major depression.
- To minimize side effects of agitation when antidepressants are initiated, consider temporary use of a benzodiazepine.
- Goal is symptom remission to minimize risk of relapse.
- If patients improve, treat for a minimum of 12 months.
- If discontinuing medications, use a very slow taper while monitoring closely for recurrence.
- In cases of treatment resistance, consider treatment noncompliance and undiagnosed comorbid disorders (e.g., substance use, medical illness), and consider reevaluation of the diagnosis.

REFERENCES

Barlow DH, Craske MG. Mastery of Your Anxiety and Panic. Albany, NY: Graywind Publications; 1989.

Clark DM. A cognitive approach to panic. Behav Res Ther 1986;24:461–70.

Furukawa TA, Watanabe N, Churchill R. Psychotherapy plus antidepressant for panic disorder with or without agoraphobia: Systematic review. Br J Psychiatry 2006;188:305–12.

Grant BF, Hasin DS, Stinson FS, et al. The epidemiology of DSM-IV panic disorder and agoraphobia in the United States: Results from the National Epidemiologic Survey on Alcohol and Related Conditions. J Clin Psychiatry 2006;67:363–74.

Kessler RC, Berglund P, Demler O, et al. Lifetime prevalence and age-of-onset distributions of DSM-IV disorders in the National Comorbidity Survey Replication. Arch Gen Psychiatry 2005;62:593–602.

Kessler RC, Chiu WT, Jin R, et al. The epidemiology of panic attacks, panic disorder, and agoraphobia in the National Comorbidity Survey Replication. Arch Gen Psychiatry 2006;63:415–24.

Manfro GG, Otto MW, McArdle ET, et al. Relationship of antecedent stressful life events to childhood and family history of anxiety and the course of panic disorder. J Affect Disord 1996;41:135–9.

Mitte K. A meta-analysis of the efficacy of psycho- and pharmacotherapy in panic disorder with and without agoraphobia. J Affect Disord 2005;88:27–45.

Smoller JW, Gardner-Schuster E, Covino J. The genetic basis of panic and phobic anxiety disorders. Am J Med Genet C Semin Med Genet 2008;148:118–26.

Stein MB, Goin MK, Pollack MH, et al. Practice guidelines for the treatment of patients with panic disorder, Washington, DC: American Psychiatric Publishing; 2009. Available at http://www.psychiatryonline.com/pracGuide/pracGuideTopic_9.aspx (accessed July 2009).

Physical and Chemical Injuries

Burn Treatment Guidelines

Method of
Barbara A. Latenser, MD

The initial management of the severely burned patient follows guidelines established by the American College of Surgeons (ACS). It is crucial that the patient be managed properly in the early hours after injury because the initial management of a seriously burned patient can significantly affect the long-term outcome. Optimal burn-care criteria have been established and refined by the American Burn Association (ABA) over the past 20 years.

Because of regionalization, it is common for the initial care of the seriously burned patient to occur outside the burn center. Burns are a specialized form of trauma. Therefore, the ABCs (airway, breathing, circulation) are the same as for the trauma patient: airway with cervical spine immobilization if appropriate, breathing, circulation, disability, and exposure. Also, the burn patient could be a victim of associated trauma. It is easy to be sidetracked by the obvious thermal injury. Only after the primary and secondary surveys have been performed should you evaluate the severity of the burn injury. Obtain as much information as possible regarding the incident and about the patient. An easy way to remember the information is the mnemonic AMPLE:

- Allergies
- Medications
- Past medical history
- Last meal
- Events

Universal precautions appropriate for each burn patient must be implemented by every member of the health care team.

The most commonly used guide for making an initial estimate of the second- and third-degree burns is the Rule of Nines (Figure 1). Various anatomic regions are roughly 9% of the total body surface area (TBSA) or multiples thereof. To calculate scattered burn areas, the patient's palm, including fingers, represents approximately 1% of the TBSA. A much more precise estimate of TBSA burn is provided by the Lund-Browder Classification (Figure 2). By drawing in the areas that are burned, the TBSA burn necessary for calculating resuscitation requirements can be determined. The consensus formula for the first 24 hours postburn is:

4 mL lactated Ringer's × body weight in kg × percent BSA burn

Half the calculated amount is given in the first 8 hours and the rest over the remaining 16 hours. Patients with burns on more than 20% TBSA are prone to gastric dilatation and should have a nasogastric (NG) tube. To determine hourly urine output, a urinary catheter is necessary. Intravenous (IV) morphine sulfate is indicated for control of pain associated with burns. Intramuscular (IM) or subcutaneous (SC) routes of drug administration should not be used as absorption is erratic. To calculate fluid needs, weigh the patient or estimate the pre-injury weight. Reliable peripheral veins should be used to establish an IV line. Use vessels underlying burned skin if necessary. If it is impossible to establish peripheral IV access, an intraosseous line may be necessary, and may be used in any age patient. If unable to insert an intraosseous line, central venous access may be necessary using a short, fluid infusion line made specifically for large volume resuscitations.

The burn wound should be covered with a clean, dry sheet to prevent air currents from causing pain in partial-thickness burns and to decrease fluid losses and hypothermia. Although there are many common topical antimicrobials in use, the optimal dressing prior to burn center transfer is plastic wrap such as Saran Wrap. Topical antimicrobials will just have to be washed off on arrival to the burn center, causing patient discomfort and mechanical trauma to the wound. Cold applications are appropriate only in small burns because they rapidly lead to hypothermia. Ice should never be applied because it will deepen the zone of ischemia in a thermal injury.

Escharotomies and/or fasciotomies are rarely required prior to burn center transfer, unless transfer is delayed beyond 24 hours. Patients most at risk are those with large TBSA burns, circumferential full-thickness burns, and those with electrical injury. Circumferential chest/abdominal burns may restrict ventilatory excursion. A child has a more pliable rib cage and may need an escharotomy earlier than an adult burn. If you are considering performing an escharotomy, confer with the accepting burn physician before proceeding.

So how do you know which patients should be referred to a burn center? To guide your decision making there are currently 10 burn unit referral criteria. You should have a written transfer agreement in place with a referral burn unit. The agreement should specify which patients will be referred, what stabilization is expected, who arranges transportation, and what the patient will need during transport.

Partial-Thickness Burns on More Than 10% Total Body Surface Area

Second-degree or partial-thickness burns involve a variable portion of dermis. The skin may be red, blistered, and edematous. Because sensory nerves are damaged and/or exposed, these wounds are typically extremely painful. Healing time is proportional to the depth of dermal injury. Scarring is minimal if healing occurs in 14 days or less. With closure time beyond 3 weeks, scarring will occur, the degree being greater in darker skinned individuals.

Proper fluid management is critical to the survival of patients with extensive burns. Fluid resuscitation is aimed at maintaining tissue perfusion and organ function while avoiding the complications of inadequate or excessive fluid therapy. Shock and organ failure, most commonly acute renal failure, may occur as a consequence of hypovolemia in a patient with an extensive burn who is inadequately

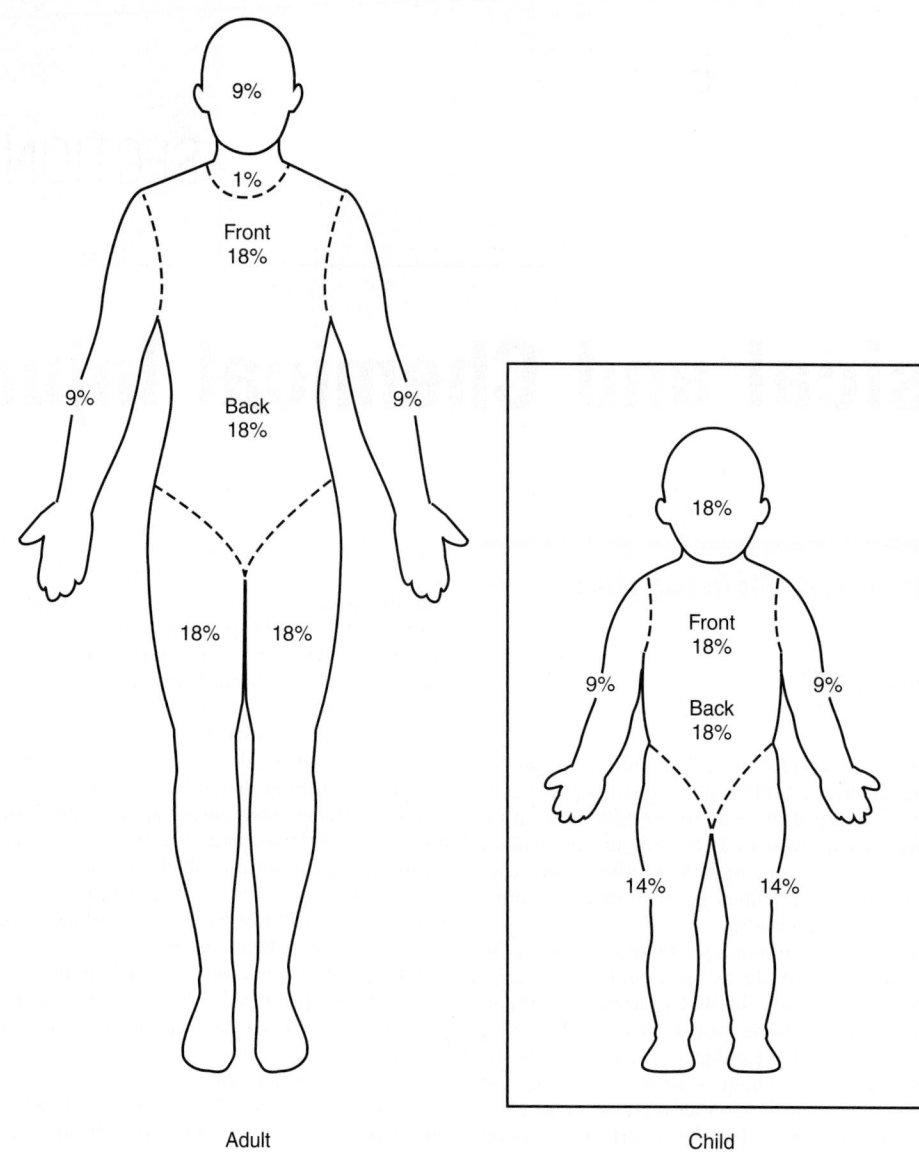

FIGURE 1. Rule of Nines.

resuscitated. The increase in capillary permeability caused by the burn is greatest in the immediate postburn period and diminution in effective blood volume is most rapid at that time. A marked increase in peripheral vascular resistance accompanied by a decrease in cardiac output occurs in the first 18 to 24 hours postinjury.

In the presence of increased capillary permeability, colloid content of the resuscitation fluid exerts little influence on intravascular retention during the initial hours postburn. Crystalloid fluid is the initial resuscitation of burn patients. *Always* remember, estimates are inexact. Each patient reacts differently to burn injury and resuscitation. The actual volume of fluid infused should be varied from the calculated volume as indicated by physiologic monitoring. The patient's general condition reflects the adequacy of fluid resuscitation and should be assessed and reassessed. Mental status, anxiety, and restlessness may be signs of hypoxemia, hypovolemia, or pain.

Although urine output does not guarantee tissue perfusion, it remains the most readily available and generally reliable guide to resuscitation. Adults should produce 0.5 mL/kg per hour of urine. Children should produce 1.0 mL/kg per hour of urine, and infants 12 months or younger should produce 2.0 mL/kg per hour of urine. Oliguria is most frequently the result of inadequate fluid administration. Diuretics are contraindicated; the rate of resuscitation should be increased. During the first 24 hours, neither the hemoglobin nor the hematocrit is a reliable guide to resuscitation, and using either leads

to over-resuscitation. For resuscitation failures or patients with large burns (>30% TBSA burn), colloid should be added. One method is hetastarch at 20 mL/kg/day for adults and 15 mL/kg/day for children. Hetastarch should be given only for 24 hours due to the increased bleeding risks.

Measuring blood pressure (BP) by a sphygmomanometer may be misleading in a burned limb with progressive edema formation. As the swelling increases, the signal becomes diminished. If fluid infusion is increased based on this finding, edema formation may be exaggerated. Even intra-arterial monitoring may be unreliable in patients with massive burns because of peripheral vasoconstriction secondary to marked elevation of catecholamines. Heart rate is also of limited usefulness in monitoring fluid therapy. The level of tachycardia depends on the normal heart rate in each child.

Burns That Involve the Face, Hands, Feet, Genitalia, Perineum, or Major Joints

Facial burns are considered a serious injury. The possibility of respiratory tract damage must be considered. Because of the rich blood supply and loose areolar tissue of the face, facial burns are associated

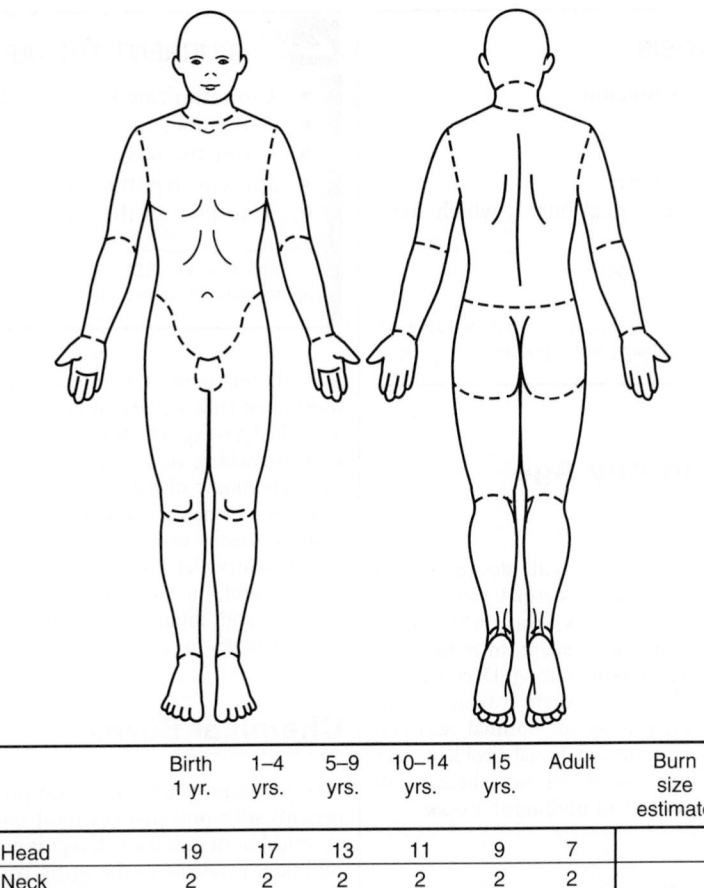

	Birth 1 yr.	1–4 yrs.	5–9 yrs.	10–14 yrs.	15 yrs.	Adult	Burn size estimate
Head	19	17	13	11	9	7	
Neck	2	2	2	2	2	2	
Anterior trunk	13	13	13	13	13	13	
Posterior trunk	13	13	13	13	13	13	
Right buttock	2.5	2.5	2.5	2.5	2.5	2.5	
Left buttock	2.5	2.5	2.5	2.5	2.5	2.5	
Genitalia	1	1	1	1	1	1	
Right upper arm	4	4	4	4	4	4	
Left upper arm	4	4	4	4	4	4	
Right lower arm	3	3	3	3	3	3	
Left lower arm	3	3	3	3	3	3	
Right hand	2.5	2.5	2.5	2.5	2.5	2.5	
Left hand	2.5	2.5	2.5	2.5	2.5	2.5	
Right thigh	5.5	6.5	8	8.5	9	9.5	
Left thigh	5.5	6.5	8	8.5	9	9.5	
Right leg	5	5	5.5	6	6.5	7	
Left leg	5	5	5.5	6	6.5	7	
Right foot	3.5	3.5	3.5	3.5	3.5	3.5	
Left foot	3.5	3.5	3.5	3.5	3.5	3.5	

Total BSAB ——————————

FIGURE 2. Lund-Browder Classification Burn Size and Diagram.

with extensive edema formation. To minimize this edema, keep the head of the bed elevated at 30°. Cool saline compresses on the face may also help. Careful examination of the eyes should be completed as soon as possible because the rapid onset of eyelid swelling will make this difficult. Fluorescein should be used to identify corneal injury. Chemical burns to the eyes should be rinsed with copious amounts of saline. Burns of the ears require examination of the external auditory canal and ear drum before swelling occurs.

Minor burns of the hands may result in only temporary disability and inconvenience. More extensive thermal injury may cause permanent loss of function. Monitoring the digital and palmar pulses with an ultrasonic flowmeter is the most accurate means of assessing perfusion of the tissues in the hand. The burned extremity should be elevated above the heart to minimize edema formation. Digital escharotomies are not indicated prior to transfer to a burn center. Contact the accepting burn center physician if you are concerned about the extent of the digital injury. As with burns of the upper extremity, it is important to assess the circulation and neurologic function of the feet on an hourly basis.

CURRENT DIAGNOSIS

- Maintain a high index of suspicion
- Remember the ABCs
- Rule out concomitant trauma
- Establish size and depth of burn
- Be wary of chemical and electrical burns, which may be misleading
- Establish resuscitation requirements

Abbreviations: ABC = airway with cervical spine immobilization if appropriate, breathing, circulation, disability, and exposure.

CURRENT THERAPY

- Communicate with your burn center early and often
- Remember the ABCs
- Cover the wound with Saran Wrap
- Prevent hypothermia
- Transport to the burn center

Abbreviations: ABC = airway with cervical spine immobilization if appropriate, breathing, circulation, disability, and exposure.

Third-Degree Burns in Any Age Group

A full-thickness or third-degree burn occurs with destruction of the entire epidermis and dermis, leaving no dermal elements to repopulate. A characteristic initial appearance is a waxy white color. Full-thickness injuries require emergent management. In most cases, treatment of the wound requires surgical skin grafting. Deep partial-thickness and full-thickness burns heal with severe scarring if not treated by surgical excision and skin grafting for optimal recovery. Disfigurement is common, and long-term functional problems can persist for years. There is also a high risk of infection, because an unexcised full-thickness burn behaves like an undrained abscess.

Electric Burns, Including Lightning Injury

Electrical burns can be divided into flash (typical thermal injury) and high-tension injury. The latter, caused by more than 1000 volts, produces clinically characteristic entry and exit wounds. They are usually ischemic, painless, and dry; wounds of entry may appear charred and the exit explosive. Deep-muscle injury may be present even when skin appears normal. Findings that suggest electrical injury include loss of consciousness, paralysis or mummification of an extremity, loss of peripheral pulses, flexor surface burns, myoglobinuria, serum creatine kinase (CK) more than 1000, and cardiopulmonary arrest at the scene. Electrical injuries can produce vascular thrombosis, muscle tetany causing fractures, and internal organ damage. In addition to other interventions, obtain a 12-lead electrocardiogram (ECG), cardiac enzymes, and evaluate the urine for myoglobin. If there is evidence of myoglobin from muscle damage, the urine output should be maintained at 2 mL/kg per hour until the urine grossly clears to prevent acid hematin deposition in the kidney and irreversible renal damage. Compartment pressures must be monitored. If a compartment syndrome develops, contact your burn center physician because fasciotomy may be required. The most serious immediate problem associated with electrical injuries is ventricular fibrillation, asystole, or other dysrhythmias. Life-threatening arrhythmias are treated according to advanced cardiac life support (ACLS) protocols. Survival of contact with voltage greater than 70,000 volts is uncommon.

The approximate electrical potential of a lightning bolt is 20 million volts. Lightning injury can produce an enormous spectrum of clinical symptoms and signs ranging from common (cardiac asystole, respiratory arrest, arborescent markings) to the rare (disseminated intravascular coagulation [DIC], intracerebral hemorrhage). Immediate neurologic manifestations include agitation, amnesia, loss of consciousness, or motor disturbances. The eyes are particularly vulnerable to injury from electrical current, and symptoms closely correlate with the extent of the central nervous system (CNS) injury. Vitreous hemorrhage, iridocyclitis, retinal tear, macular puncture, and retinal detachment have been reported.

Lightning injuries are not usually associated with deep burns but most often with superficial injury to the skin and underlying soft tissue called *ferning*. The feathering type of burn appears as an arborescent, branching skin marking that disappears within a few hours. Pathognomonic of lightning injury, they may be of great diagnostic value in a comatose patient. Often the respiratory arrest lasts longer than the cardiac arrest. Severely injured victims often present in asystole or ventricular fibrillation. Cardiac resuscitation may occasionally be successful; but direct brain trauma as well as blunt trauma, skull fracture, and intracranial injuries, are common in these patients. The prognosis for recovery in this group is usually poor.

Chemical Burns

Health care providers must wear protective clothing when caring for patients with potential chemical injury. The initial appearance of a chemical burn is usually deceptively benign. The severity of a chemical injury is related to the agent, concentration, volume, duration of contact, and mechanisms of action of the agent. Immediate irrigation decreases the concentration and duration of contact, reducing the severity of injury. If the agent is a powder, brush it off and irrigate with water. Irrigation should continue through emergency evaluation in the hospital and in general until evaluation in a burn center, especially for an alkali or if an unknown agent. Neutralizing agents are contraindicated because of the potential for heat generation, thereby giving the patient both a chemical and a thermal injury!

Acid burns are less severe than alkali burns. They are found in many household products including bathroom cleansers, drain cleaners, and swimming pool acidifiers. Tissue is damaged by coagulation necrosis and protein precipitation. Once a layer of eschar is formed, the burning process is self-limiting. The exception to this rule is hydrofluoric acid (HA), which is used to etch glass, make Teflon, and to remove rust. The pathogenesis of tissue damage in HA burns is distinct from other acids. HA readily crosses lipid membranes and has a potent diffusing capacity into the tissues. The molecule releases the freely dissociable fluoride ion, which produces extensive liquefactive necrosis of the soft tissues. Fluoride rapidly binds free calcium in the blood, and death from hypocalcemia may occur. Treatment is intra-arterial calcium gluconate[1] (or calcium chloride)[1] administered until the characteristic *pain out of proportion to the burn* has resolved. Even small areas of contact may result in profound hypocalcemia and death. Cardiac monitoring and frequent serum calcium determinations are indicated.

Alkalis damage tissue by liquefaction necrosis and protein denaturation. Tissue pH abnormalities may persist for 12 hours postburn, allowing deeper spread of the chemical and more severe burns. Examples would include the hydroxides, caustic sodas, and ammonium compounds found in oven cleaners, fertilizer, and cement. Wet cement damages skin in three ways: allergic dermatitis as a reaction to chromate ions, abrasions caused by the gritty nature of the cement, and as an alkali with a pH of 12.5. The ability of cement to cause such injury is not well recognized, even by professional users. With the

---

[1]Not FDA approved for this indication.

increased media interest in do-it-yourself projects, it is likely this problem will increase.

Organic compounds such as creosote and petroleum products produce contact chemical burns as well as systemic toxicity. Gasoline and diesel fuel are petroleum products that may produce a full-thickness burn that initially appears as only partial thickness. Organic compounds cause cutaneous damage by delipidation because of their fat solvent action on cell membranes. After a motor vehicle crash involving petroleum products, always look for petroleum exposure in the lower extremities, back, and buttocks. Systemic effects include elevated liver enzymes and decreased urinary output.

Inhalation Injury

Smoke inhalation injuries are the leading cause of fatalities from burn injuries, accounting for some 80% of all fire-related deaths. The major forms of inhalation injuries are carbon monoxide (CO) toxicity, injury to the upper airway, and pulmonary parenchymal damage. Each has different symptoms and signs, treatment, and prognosis. The compromised airway is protected by tracheal intubation, and respiratory failure is treated with assisted ventilation. Inhalation injury is manifested by the pathology and dysfunction that rapidly become evident in the airways, lungs, and respiratory system after inhaling the products of incomplete combustion. Patients receiving massive fluid resuscitation can develop upper airway edema with subsequent asphyxiation.

Immediate medical attention and diagnosis depend on a high index of suspicion, an appropriate history, careful examination of the upper airway, the presence of clinical symptoms, and suggestive arterial blood gases. An inhalation injury is suspected in any patient with full-thickness facial burns or with any burns combined with a history of being confined within an enclosed space. Other classic signs are soot or carbonaceous sputum, stridor or hoarseness, or blistering of the pharynx or vocal cords. Late signs include grunting, nasal flaring, retractions, wheezes, and rales. Use of prophylactic antibiotics and steroids is discouraged.

The effect of CO poisoning may be exhibited by respiratory symptoms and CNS findings such as altered level of consciousness, seizures, or coma. Cardiovascular effects include diminished cardiac output evidenced by decreased perfusion and hypotension. There is much controversy regarding hyperbaric oxygen therapy, but there are no objective data proving the efficacy of hyperbaric oxygen in CO poisoning. At this time, hyperbaric oxygen treatment for acute CO toxicity should be restricted to randomized prospective studies. The correct treatment is administering 100% oxygen, thereby decreasing the CO half-life from 4 hours to 45 minutes.

Burn Injury in Patients with Preexisting Medical Disorders That Could Complicate Management, Prolong Recovery, or Affect Mortality

Peripheral vascular disease can lead to a decrease in wound blood flow. Diabetes, through high glucose, will impede capillary flow. Optimum control of the blood glucose is needed to optimize blood flow. A local decrease in wound-tissue oxygen tension is recognized to be a major wound-healing impediment because all phases of healing are oxygen dependent, including local infection control. Most common causes are a decrease in systemic blood volume and oxygen delivery, decrease in hemoglobin saturation, eschar on the wound surface, or infection. Treatment modalities need to focus first on correction of systemic abnormalities: correct cardiovascular and lung function, correct large vessel obstructive disease impeding wound

flow, aggressive wound débridement, and eliminate tissue exudates. Patients with preexisting cardiac disease are particularly sensitive to fluids and may tolerate the necessary fluid resuscitation poorly.

Any Patient With Burns and Concomitant Trauma (Such as Fractures) in Which the Burn Injury Poses the Greatest Risk of Morbidity and Mortality

In such cases, if the trauma poses the greater immediate risk, the patient may be initially stabilized in a trauma center before being transferred to a burn unit. Physician judgment will be necessary in such situations and should be in concert with the regional medical control plan and triage protocols.

Most burn-trauma publications cite a 5% frequency of burn-trauma patient. Because burn trauma is rare outside of a major conflict or disaster, most centers see only a few patients annually. By definition, child abuse falls into the burn-trauma category. It may be the burn injury that prompts relatives or neighbors to bring the child to the hospital or report the family to authority. The visibility of the injury may instigate corrective action. In a 44-month review we saw 120 cases of burns and trauma. Although motor vehicle crashes (MVCs) can result in fracture, soft tissue, and thermal injury, unique to this burn-trauma population was that the MVC injury was frequently a result of assault. With the graying of America, elder abuse may become a larger societal problem.

Burned Children in Hospitals Without Qualified Personnel or Equipment for the Care of Children

Each year more than 2500 children die and 10,000 more sustain permanent disability from thermal injury. Children are not just little adults! They respond differently than adults to severe trauma, maintaining normal vital signs longer but decompensating rapidly. Because of the smaller cross-sectional diameter of the pediatric airway, it takes much less edema to compromise a pediatric airway. If intubation is required, the most experienced pediatric airway manager should intubate the child because repeated attempts may create sufficient airway edema as to cause obstruction. Anatomical airway differences make intubation by the inexperienced even more difficult.

The greater surface area per unit of body mass of children necessitates the administration of relatively greater amounts of resuscitation fluid. The surface area/body mass relationship of the child also defines a lesser intravascular volume per unit surface area burned. This makes the burned child more susceptible to fluid overload and hemodilution. Hypoglycemia may occur if the limited glycogen stores of the child are rapidly exhausted by the early postburn elevation of circulating levels of steroids and catecholamines. Infants should receive maintenance fluids with 5% dextrose in addition to the resuscitation fluids outlined in the consensus formula. Children younger than 2 years of age have disproportionally thin skin so that exposures that would produce only partial-thickness burns in older patients produce full-thickness injuries. Children have a relatively small muscle mass, hampering intrinsic heat generation. Children younger than 6 months of age are unable to shiver and thus are even more prone to develop hypothermia.

Stress for the burned child not only includes the body surface area (BSA) burn and the pain that is involved but also the separation from parents and loved ones. This escalates especially if the parents were also burned in the fire. Emergency management of each pediatric burn patient requires an individual care plan. Early consultation with the burn center physician is advised.

Burn Injury in Patients Who Will Require Special Social, Emotional, and/or Long-Term Rehabilitative Intervention

Failure to recognize the thermal manifestations of child abuse not only negates protection of the child but predicates potential lethal injury. Awareness of the patterns of abuse, the behavior patterns of the parents, and the physical manifestations will protect the child by early recognition and reporting. Physical child abuse victims frequently present with thermal injuries of varying degrees. The history of injury should correlate with the physical findings. The history also becomes important in identifying repetitious hospital visits for accidental injury. Not infrequently, the hospital visits will be made at different hospitals to avoid disclosure and identification.

The events leading to an injury are extremely important in the initial evaluation of an infant or child. *Always* consider the potential for child abuse. The incidence of child abuse is approximately 10% of all children presenting to an emergency department (ED), with a mortality rate less than 1%. Abused children present with a higher median Injury Severity Score, more severe injuries of the head and integument, longer hospital lengths of stay, and a high mortality rate.

A burn of any magnitude can be a serious injury. Health care providers must be able to assess the injuries rapidly and develop a priority-based plan of care. The plan of care is determined by the type, extent, and degree of burn as well as by available resources.

Burn care is complex. It involves a multisystem assessment and appropriate intervention. The first 24 hours of management are perhaps the most critical for patient survival. Burn centers provide optimal care in a cost-effective, multidisciplinary manner. Every health care provider must know how and when to contact the closest burn center. If the attending physician determines that the patient should be treated at the burn center, the extent of treatment provided at the referring hospital—and the method of transport to the burn center—should be decided in consultation with the burn center physician. A complete list of verified burn centers is available at http://ameriburn.org.

REFERENCES

Advanced Burn Life Support Course. American Burn Association, 625 N. Michigan Ave., Suite 1530, Chicago, IL. 60611. 2001.

American College of Surgeons Committee on Trauma. Resources for optimal care of the injured patient: 1999. Chicago: American College of Surgeons; 1999.

Andrews CJ, Cooper MA, Darveniza M, Mackerras D, editors. Lightning injuries: Electrical, medical, and legal aspects. Boca Raton, Fla: CRC Press; 1992.

Burd A. Hydrofluoric acid—revisited. Burns 2004;30(7):720–2.

Chang DC, Knight V, Ziegfeld S, et al. The tip of the iceberg for child abuse: The critical roles of the pediatric trauma service and its registry. J Trauma 2004;57(6):1189–98.

Heimbach DM. Regionalization of burn care: A concept whose time has come. J Burn Care Rehabil 2003;24(3):173–4.

Latenser BA, Iteld L. Smoke inhalation injury. Seminars in Respiratory and Critical Care Medicine 2001;22(1):13–22.

Luce EA, editor. Clinics in plastic surgery. An international quarterly. Burn care and management. Philadelphia: WB Saunders; 2000.

Varghese TK, Kim AW, Kowal-Vern A, Latenser BA. Frequency of burn-trauma patients in an urban setting. Arch Surg 2003;138:1292–6.

High-Altitude Illness

Method of
James A. Litch, MD, DTMH

Decreased partial pressure of oxygen at high altitude results in pronounced physiologic responses that range from beneficial to pathologic. Slow ascent normally leads to acclimatization. High-altitude illness is a collective term for a cluster of acute clinical syndromes that are a direct consequence of rapid ascent to high altitude above 2500 m. The acute syndromes affecting the brain include acute mountain sickness (AMS) and high-altitude cerebral edema (HACE). The acute syndrome affecting the lung is high-altitude pulmonary edema (HAPE). All unacclimatized sojourners to high altitude are potentially at risk. The characteristic cerebral and pulmonary abnormalities are not subtle, but when unrecognized or ignored, they may progress to death. Each year millions travel to high-altitude locations on every continent, resulting in morbidity and mortality with associated economic consequences.

Normal Acclimatization

It is not uncommon for normal acclimatization of novice healthy visitors to high altitude to cause concern that they are experiencing a health problem. Normal acclimatization includes immediate hyperventilation, shortness of breath with moderate excursion, and a decreased work capacity. These are followed by diuresis, disturbed sleep (including periodic breathing), and peripheral/facial edema. It is important to recognize the signs of normal acclimatization so reassurance and education may be appropriately provided.

Incidence and Risk Factors

Determinants of whether high-altitude illness will occur are individual susceptibility, rate of ascent, altitude reached, and sleep altitude. Incidence rates of AMS reported in literature are difficult to compare because of variability in methodology and rates of ascent. Reported incident figures for AMS following ascent by hiking, vehicle, or flying range from 10% to 40% at 2700 to 3000 m, and from 40% to 95% at 3800 to 4000 m. HACE and HAPE are both far less common than mild AMS, but actual incident rates are unavailable. HAPE can occur as low as 2500 m. HACE is rare below 3600 m. Most cases of HACE and HAPE are preceded by AMS.

Risk factors for altitude illness include a history of previous high-altitude illness, residence at altitude below 1000 m, physical exertion, and preexisting cardiopulmonary conditions. Traveling in a large group presents a risk because a tight itinerary often does not allow time for acclimatization, and members are reluctant to declare symptoms for fear of being left behind. Children appear to carry the same risk for altitude illness as adults, but persons over 50 years of age seem less susceptible, possibly because of a more cautious ascent profile. There appears to be little or no gender difference for AMS, but women may be less susceptible to HAPE. Heavy physical exertion at exceedingly high altitude appears to be an important risk factor for HAPE. Rapid ascent, especially by flying or driving to altitude, places sojourners at risk for altitude illnesses.

Prevention of Altitude Illnesses

Gradual ascent to altitude over several days to allow for acclimatization reduces the likelihood of acute mountain sickness. Ascent rates of less than 300 m per day at altitudes of more than 2500 m is a common recommendation; but individuals will still experience altitude illness when abiding to this recommendation. However, the critical understanding to prevent serious life-threatening altitude illness (HAPE and HACE) is to halt further ascent until symptoms resolve.

Medications are available to help prevent the symptoms of AMS when rapid ascent (<24 hours) to altitudes more than 3000 m is anticipated, or for those with a past history of AMS with a similar ascent profile. These agents are started the evening before ascent and continued for 2 to 3 days. The most commonly used medications are acetazolamide (Diamox) (125 to 250 mg twice a day), acetaminophen[1] (325 mg four times a day), or aspirin[1] (325 mg three

---

[1]Not FDA approved for this indication.

times a day). Acetazolamide (Diamox) is particularly useful because it actually improves oxygenation, has a positive impact on the quality of sleep at high altitude, and is effective for periodic breathing that occurs during sleep. However, these medications do not protect against the development of life threatening altitude illness: HAPE and HACE. Other medications have been suggested for use in preventing altitude illness. Randomized double blinded placebo-controlled trails of ginkgo biloba[1] and acetazolamide (Diamox) have shown no benefit from ginkgo biloba over placebo, and reduced incidence and severity of AMS symptoms from acetazolamide (Diamox). Dexamethasone (Decadron),[1] a potent steroid, is generally best avoided as a prevention measure against AMS during ascent so it may be used, if needed, for treatment of HACE along with descent.

Nifedipine (Adalat, Procardia)[1] has been studied for use in prevention of HAPE and found to be of benefit for persons with a history of recurrent HAPE. Studies are under way to evaluate sildenafil citrate (Viagra),[1] an agent that selectively lowers pulmonary artery pressure, in the prevention of HAPE. In addition, inhaled salmeterol (Serevent)[1] has been found effective for the prevention of HAPE in a small group of climbers who had previously shown susceptibility to HAPE. However, these high-risk individuals would do far better with cautious gradual ascent, rather than relying on a medication with limited effect for a life-threatening condition.

Several nonmedication measures that can prevent or ameliorate symptoms of high-altitude illness include the following:

- Begin a high-carbohydrate diet one or two days before the climb and maintain during the ascent
- Adapt plans to realistically reflect the decreased work capacity at high altitude
- Reschedule or slow the ascent should an upper respiratory or other active infection present
- Avoid overexertion during ascent by maintaining a reasonable pace and not overloading with nonessential gear
- Maintain adequate hydration on the climb to offset increased fluid loss at altitude
- Avoid nonessential medications and remedies
- Provide good ventilation for camp stoves used in confined places
- Allow for several days of altitude exposure the week prior to ascent to high altitude

Acute Mountain Sickness and High-Altitude Cerebral Edema

AMS is defined as a headache in the setting of recent altitude gain and typical symptoms which include anorexia, nausea, vomiting, insomnia, dizziness, or fatigue (Current Diagnosis box). Symptoms are nonspecific, and there is an absence of physical findings. The differential diagnosis is extensive and other conditions should be considered (Box 1). Pulse oximetry values may be high, normal, or low for the altitude and do not correlate to severity of symptoms. A careful and detailed history is essential to steer diagnostic decision making. Often in outdoor settings multiple conditions can be present such as AMS and dehydration. Rapid resolution of symptoms during treatment with oxygen is very specific to AMS. Early recognition of AMS is a key principle in remote areas with limited support.

AMS is not life threatening, but ignoring it can be. Progressive neurologic deterioration may occur over hours or days as dangerous collections of fluid develop in the brain leading to HACE. HACE presents with truncal ataxia, confusion, and hallucination in the setting of recent altitude gain. The period of time from initial ataxia and confusion to onset of coma may be as little as 8 to 12 hours. If descent or oxygen supplementation is not accomplished within hours, coma and death can ensue from brain herniation. A presumptive and/or rigid diagnosis of HACE in the setting of progressive neurologic

---

BOX 1 Differential Diagnosis of High-Altitude Illnesses

Acute Mountain Sickness and High-Altitude Cerebral Edema
- Alcohol intoxication
- Brain tumor
- CO inhalation
- CNS infection
- Cerebral vascular accident
- Dehydration
- Diabetic ketoacidosis
- Exhaustion
- Hypoglycemia and insulin shock
- Hyponatremia
- Hypothermia
- Migraine
- Narcotics
- Poisoning
- Psychosis
- Sedatives overdose
- Seizures
- Subarachnoid hemorrhage
- Transient ischemic attack

High-Altitude Pulmonary Edema
- Adult respiratory distress syndrome
- Asthma
- Bronchitis
- Congestive heart failure
- Myocardial infarction
- Pneumonia (infection or aspiration)
- Poisoning
- Pulmonary embolus
- Respiratory failure

Abbreviations: CNS = central nervous system; CO = carbon monoxide.

deterioration has led to tragic situations when other life-threatening conditions were actually present (see Box 1). Details of the initial presentation, response to immediate descent/supplemental oxygen, and recognition of additional signs can guide clinical decision making while maintaining a high index of suspicion for other neurologic conditions. Patients with persistent symptoms after descent require prompt evacuation and thorough evaluation. In addition, HAPE may develop concurrently with HACE resulting in shortness of breath while at rest and a further reduction of oxygen delivery to the body.

Definitive diagnosis is available using imaging studies such as CT and MRI. However, these have limited application, because the condition should have greatly improved from oxygen/descent before the opportunity presents to obtain the study. Neuroimaging demonstrates vasogenic edema in individuals with moderate to severe AMS or HACE.

Management of AMS is directed at limiting further hypoxia by halting ascent, and providing additional oxygen should symptoms persist or progress to HACE. Acetazolamide (Diamox) is helpful for the treatment of AMS. For the management of HACE improved oxygenation is the definitive treatment. There are several methods of oxygen delivery: (1) descent, (2) supplemental oxygen via cylinder or concentrator, and/or (3) portable hyperbaric bag. These may be combined or applied in series depending on resources, location, and logistic support. Concomitant pharmacologic treatment with dexamethasone (Decadron)[1] and acetazolamide (Diamox) aid recovery. Persons with suspected HACE who do not rapidly recover during

---

[1]Not FDA approved for this indication.

[1]Not FDA approved for this indication.

CURRENT DIAGNOSIS

- Acute Mountain Sickness—In the setting of a recent gain in altitude, the presence of headache and at least one of the following: GI symptoms (anorexia, nausea, or vomiting), fatigue or weakness, dizziness or lightheadedness, or difficulty sleeping
- High-Altitude Cerebral Edema—In the setting of a recent gain in altitude, the presence of a change in mental status and/or ataxia in a person with AMS, or the presence of both mental status change and ataxia in a person without AMS
- High-Altitude Pulmonary Edema—In the setting of a recent gain in altitude, the presence of at least two of the following symptoms: dyspnea at rest, cough, weakness or decreased exercise performance, chest tightness, or congestion; and two of the following signs: rales or wheezing in at least one lung field, central cyanosis, tachypnea, or tachycardia

*The Lake Louise Consensus on the Definition and Quantification of Altitude Illness.
Abbreviations: AMS = acute mountain sickness; GI = gastrointestinal.

treatment or those with focal neurologic deficits should be hospitalized and undergo comprehensive neurologic evaluation including magnetic resonance imaging (MRI). The Current Therapy box summarizes management of HACE.

High-Altitude Pulmonary Edema

HAPE is defined as noncardiogenic edema resulting from hypoxia-induced changes in the pulmonary circulation. HAPE is commonly preceded by AMS, and 20% of individuals with HAPE develop HACE. Early symptoms of HAPE include decreased exercise performance beyond that expected for the altitude, often accompanied with a dry cough (see Current Diagnosis Box). Progression is rapid with even minimal continued physical activity without descent. The hallmark of progression requiring prompt action is dyspnea at rest. Rales are present at this stage. Resting pulse oximetry reveals below-normal oxygen saturation for the altitude. Tachypnea and tachycardia beyond that expected for the altitude also are present. Pink, frothy sputum develops late in the illness. Early diagnosis is important because progression of the illness further limits oxygenation and worsens the degree of hypoxemia causing the condition.

HAPE is a life-threatening emergency; immediate improvement in oxygenation is critical to arrest the progression and is the definitive treatment. In medical facilities high-flow supplemental oxygen while at rest and sitting in an upright position should be initiated immediately during the initial assessment of the patient. Response may be assessed by pulse oximetry and resting respiratory rate. Despite prompt improvement during the first few hours of treatment, maintenance of oxygenation (oxygen saturation greater than 90%) with low-flow supplemental oxygen and rest is often required for 2 to 3 days unless descent is achieved. For vacationers to high-altitude resort areas, this oxygen requirement can be maintained outside the hospital using a cylinder or concentrator as an alternative to descent for informed individuals that wish to remain in the locale of family and friends. A continued requirement of high-flow oxygen of 4 to 5 L per minute or more to maintain oxygen saturation greater than 90%, or concurrent HACE, requires hospitalization. Antibiotics are indicated if infection is suspected. Endotracheal intubation and mechanical ventilation are rarely indicated. The differential diagnosis is extensive, and a high index of suspicion for other conditions should be maintained throughout the treatment course (see Box 1).

CURRENT THERAPY

Acute Mountain Sickness

- Halt ascent, do not exceed light activity level, oral hydration.
- Administer acetazolamide (Diamox) 250 mg PO bid.
- Administer analgesics and antiemetics.
- If readily available, administer oxygen 1 to 2 L per minute as needed to resolve symptoms.
- If no improvement after 24 hours, descend to altitude where person last slept without symptoms until fully recovered.

High-Altitude Cerebral Edema

- Administer oxygen 2 to 4 L per minute.
- In remote mountain areas, prepare for immediate descent of at least 600 m by ground or aircraft, and if oxygen unavailable, use portable hyperbaric chamber.
- Monitor at all times, and replenish/maintain hydration as needed.
- Administer dexamethasone (Decadron) 8 mg IM, IV, or PO × 1 dose, then 4 mg q6h.
- Administer acetazolamide (Diamox) 250 mg PO bid.

High-Altitude Pulmonary Edema

- Administer oxygen initially 4 to 6 L per minute, then titrate to keep arterial oxygen saturation more than 90%.
- In remote mountain areas, prepare for immediate descent of at least 600 m by ground or aircraft; and if oxygen unavailable, use portable hyperbaric chamber on incline with head end elevated.
- Sit upright at 45 degree angle, strict rest, and monitor at all times.
- Administer nifedipine (Adalat, Procardia) 10 mg PO initially, then 30 mg extended release q12h IF oxygen unavailable AND IV fluid resuscitation immediately available.
- Administer salmeterol (Serevent) inhaler, 1 puff bid OR albuterol (Proventil) inhaler, 4 to 6 puffs q4h.
- Administer dexamethasone (Decadron) 8 mg IM, IV or PO × 1 dose, then 4 mg q6h IF suspect or unsure if HACE is also present.

Abbreviations: bid = twice daily; IM = intramuscular; IV = intravenous; PO = orally; q = every.

In remote areas oxygen may be administered by:

- Descent with minimal exertion
- Supplemental oxygen via cylinder or concentrator
- Portable hyperbaric bag placed on an incline to keep the head elevated

Because of a lack of equipment, immediate descent may be the only option available. In late stages more than one oxygen modality may need to be employed concurrently. These efforts place great strain on the limited resources of groups traveling in remote areas. It is common for the shared concern and cooperation among group members (tourists/staff/porters) to disintegrate or for groups to discover that they are woefully unequipped to handle HAPE. As a result fatal outcomes are common when HAPE presents in remote settings.

Pharmacologic treatment is directed at agents that reduce pulmonary artery pressure and thereby may improve oxygenation in HAPE. Medications including nifedipine (Adalat, Procardia),[1] nitric oxide

[1]Not FDA approved for this indication.

(INO$_{max}$),[1] epoprostenol (Flolan),[1] and sildenafil (Viagra)[1] have been studied for use in treatment of HAPE. Current clinical experience warrants consideration of nifedipine (Adalat, Procardia) as an adjunct treatment for HAPE when immediate supplemental oxygen is unavailable or descent is delayed. Vascular access and intravenous (IV) fluid should be immediately available if nifedipine (Adalat, Procardia) is administered because patients are often intravascularly depleted and risk a severe hypotensive event that could be devastating in the setting of concomitant HACE. Sildenafil citrate (Viagra)[1] can also selectively lower pulmonary artery pressure with less effect on systemic blood pressure, and is under study for the treatment of HAPE. Inhaled β-agonists, salmeterol (Serevent),[1] and albuterol (Proventil)[1] are currently under study for treatment of HAPE because β-agonists increase the clearance of fluid from the alveolar space and might lower pulmonary artery pressure. The Current Therapy Box summarizes the management of HAPE.

Reascent After Altitude Illness

Mild AMS is common and indicative of an ascent rate that is too rapid for a given person. Further ascent should not resume until full resolution of all symptoms. Future trips with similar ascent profiles warrant consideration of prophylaxis with acetazolamide (Diamox).

After episodes of HACE and HAPE resolve fully, reascent has been successful for many patients, some reaching exceptionally high summits. Caution is warranted, however. Persons should be advised to ascend more slowly and to recognize and act appropriately for early signs of altitude illness. Persons with multiple episodes of HAPE may benefit during subsequent ascent from prophylaxis with nifedipine (Adalat, Procardia)[1] and potentially with salmeterol (Serevent)[1] while stressing the value of cautious gradual ascent over medication. Recurrent HAPE or HAPE occurring at altitudes below 3000 m should prompt evaluation to rule out cardiac or pulmonary shunts, valvular disease, or pulmonary hypertension.

REFERENCES

Bartsch P, Merki B, Hofstetter D, et al. Treatment of acute mountain sickness by simulated descent: A randomized controlled trial. BMJ 1993;306: 1098–101.
Chow T, Browne V, Heileson HL, et al. Ginkgo biloba and acetazolamide prophylaxis for acute mountain sickness: A randomized placebo-controlled trial. Arch Intern Med 2005;165:296–301.
Consensus Group. The Lake Louise consensus on the definition and quantification of altitude illness. In: Sutton JR, Coates G, Houston CS, editors. Hypoxia and mountain medicine. Burlington, VT: Queen City Printers; 1992. p. 327–30.
Litch JA. Endotracheal intubation and mechanical ventilation following respiratory arrest from high altitude pulmonary edema. West J Med 1999;170 (3):174–6.
Litch JA, Basnyat B, Zimmerman M. Subarachnoid hemorrhage at high altitude. West J Med 1997;167(3):180–1.
Litch JA, Bishop RA. Re-ascent following resolution of high altitude pulmonary edema (HAPE). High Alt Med Biol 2001;2(1):53–5.
Litch JA, Bishop RA. Oxygen concentrators for the delivery of supplemental oxygen in remote high altitude areas. Wilderness Environ Med 2000;11 (3):189–91.
Larson EB, Roach RC, Schoene RB, Hornbein TF. Acute mountain sickness and acetazolamide—Clinical efficacy and effect on ventilation. JAMA 1982;248:328–32.
Oelz O, Maggiorini M, Ritter M, et al. Prevention and treatment of high altitude pulmonary edema by a calcium channel blocker. Int J Sports Med 1992;13(Suppl. 1):S65–8.
Pollard AJ, Niermeyer S, Barry P, et al. Children at high altitude: An international consensus statement by an ad hoc committee of the International Society of Mountain Medicine. High Alt Med Biol 2001;2(3):389–403.
Rabold MB. Dexamethasone for prophylaxis and treatment of acute mountain sickness. West J Med 1992;3:54–60.
Sartori C, Allemann Y, Duplain H, et al. Salmeterol for the prevention of high-altitude pulmonary edema. N Engl J Med 2002;346(21):1631–6.

[1]Not FDA approved for this indication.

Disturbances Due to Cold

Method of
Frederick K. Korley, MD, and
Jerrold B. Leikin, MD

Accidental Hypothermia

Hypothermia is classically defined as a reduction in the body's core temperature below 95.0°F (35.0°C). Most reported cases of hypothermia are due to exposure to low ambient temperatures (accidental hypothermia). Other causes of hypothermia include sepsis, severe hypothyroidism, diabetic ketoacidosis, multisystem trauma, and prolonged cardiac arrest.

EPIDEMIOLOGY

Risk factors for developing hypothermia include extremes of age (the elderly might not be able to remove themselves from cold environments, and young children lose heat more rapidly due to their increased total body surface area), major trauma, homelessness, psychiatric illness, and drug and alcohol abuse (Box 1). Cold-related deaths also are reported in military combatants and outdoor winter sports participants. Several drugs and chemicals can predispose to hypothermia (Box 2). Alcohol is the most common intoxicant associated with hypothermia due to its ability to cause cutaneous vasodilation, impairment of shivering, and impairment of adaptive behavior.

Between 1979 and 2002, a total of 16,555 deaths in the United States, an average of 689 per year, were attributed to exposure to low environmental temperatures. In 2002, of the 646 hypothermia-related deaths reported, 66% occurred in male patients, 52% of all decedents were aged 65 years or younger, 45% of the deaths occurred among white male patients, and 14% occurred among black male patients. The states of Alaska, New Mexico, North Dakota, and Montana had the largest overall death rates due to hypothermia in 2002. The lowest recorded core temperature in a pediatric survivor of accidental hypothermia is 57.9°F (14.4°C) and the lowest is 56.7°F (13.7°C) in an adult survivor.

PATHOPHYSIOLOGY

The normal range of human core temperature is 97.5°F (36.4°C) to 99.5°F (37.5°C). Humans are thus warm-blooded and are normally able to maintain their body temperature by heat-generating mechanisms and heat-conserving behavior. These compensatory responses, however, can be overwhelmed under extreme environmental conditions, leading to hypothermia. Each organ system is affected uniquely by hypothermia.

The anterior hypothalamus coordinates the nonshivering heat conservation and dissipation mechanisms, and the posterior hypothalamus coordinates shivering thermogenesis. Heat loss usually occurs by four mechanisms: About 55% to 65% of heat is lost by radiation, 25% to 30% by evaporation from the skin and respiratory tract, and 10% to 15% by conduction and convection. The amount of heat lost via conduction is markedly increased in cold-water immersion (by about 32 times). Each organ system is affected uniquely by hypothermia.

The Cardiovascular System

One of the initial heat-conserving mechanisms is peripheral vasoconstriction to decrease blood flow to the skin. There are also initial increases, in heart rate and blood pressure due to a catecholamine surge. At core temperatures below 82.4°F (28.0°C), bradycardia can occur. The myocardium also becomes irritable, predisposing it to arrhythmias. Atrial arrhythmias can occur with a slow ventricular response and they can precede ventricular arrhythmias and asystole at core temperatures below 77.0°F (25.0°C). The characteristic Osborn

BOX 1 Factors Predisposing to Hypothermia or Frostbite

Physiologic

Decreased Heat Production

Age extremes (infants, elderly)
Dehydration or nalnutrition
Diaphoresis or hyperhidrosis
Endocrinologic insufficiency
Hypoxia
Insufficient fuel
Overexertion
Physical conditioning
Prior cold injury
Trauma (multisystem or extremity)

Increased Heat Loss

Burns
- Dermatologic malfunction
- Cold infusions
- Emergency resuscitation
- Poor acclimatization or conditioning
- Shock
- Vascular diseases

Impaired Thermoregulation

- Central nervous system trauma or disease
- Metabolic disorders
- Pharmacologic or toxicologic agents
- Sepsis
- Spinal cord injury

Psychological

- Fatigue
- Fear or panic
- Hunger
- Intense concentration on tasks
- Intoxicants
- Mental status or attitude
- Peer pressure

Environmental

- Altitude with or without associated conditions
- Ambient temperature or humidity
- Duration of exposure
- Heat loss (conductive, evaporative, radiative, convective)
- Quantity of exposed surface area
- Wind chill factor

Mechanical

- Constricting or wet clothing or boots
- Inadequate insulation
- Immobility or cramped positioning

or J waves (a hump seen at the QRS-ST junction) may be seen on the electrocardiogram (ECG) at core temperatures below 89.6°F (32.0°C).

The Renal System

Renal blood flow is increased by peripheral vasoconstriction, leading to cold-induced diuresis. Antidiuretic hormone activity is usually inhibited. This results in intravascular volume depletion, subsequent vasodilation, to increase renal blood flow, and ultimately acute renal failure.

The Respiratory System

At core temperatures below 82.4°F (28°C), minute ventilation is reduced; bronchorrhea can occur, with a loss of cough and gag reflexes leading to an increased risk for aspiration. Apnea can then result.

The Central Nervous System

Cerebral metabolism is depressed 6% to 7% per 1°C decrease in core temperature. Cerebrovascular autoregulation remains intact until below 77.0°F (25.0°C), which helps maintain cortical blood flow. Electroencephalographic activity is clearly not prognostic, and it silences around 66.2°F to 68.0°F (19.0°C–20.0°C).

CLINICAL PRESENTATION

Accidental hypothermia is classified as mild at body temperatures of 90°F (32.2°C) to 95°F (35°C), moderate at body temperatures of 82.4°F (28.0°C) to 90°F (<32.2°C), or severe at body temperatures less than 28°C (82.4°F).

In general, a patient's symptoms depend on the severity of the temperature drop. Patients with mild hypothermia can develop vigorous shivering and cold diuresis. Those with moderate hypothermia can have a paradoxical decrease in shivering, slurred speech, hyporeflexia, and confusion. They may have Osborn J waves on the ECG. They are also at risk for intravascular thrombosis. Splanchnic vasoconstriction, gastric erosions, hepatic necrosis, and pancreatitis can occur.

During severe hypothermia, shivering gives way to rigor, minute ventilation decreases, and heart rate and cardiac output decrease. Cardiac instability can be seen at this stage and can manifest in the form of arrhythmias, heart blocks, and eventually asystole. Neurologically, the patient's mental status declines. He or she might attempt to undress (paradoxical undressing) and might respond only to painful stimuli, have decreased gag reflexes, and eventually become apenic. Generally, at about 68.0°F (20.0°C), patients become totally neurologically unresponsive, lose corneal and ocular reflexes, and can have a flat electroencephalograph (EEG).

EMERGENCY DEPARTMENT EVALUATION

Typically, the source of hypothermia is revealed from the patient's history; however, it is very important to rule out secondary causes of hypothermia such as sepsis, hypothyroidism, central nervous system (CNS) lesions, and hypoglycemia among others. All patients arriving in the emergency department with hypothermia need a complete evaluation to rule out traumatic injuries and drug or toxin ingestion or overdose.

As in all resuscitation, attention should be paid to the ABCs (airway, breathing and circulation). Respiratory failure should be treated with endotracheal intubation and mechanical ventilation. Hypotension can be treated initially with warmed fluids. Placing the patient in a warm environment, removing all cold and wet clothes, and remembering to cover up the patient after he or she has been exposed should help avoid further heat loss.

The temperature should be confirmed by checking a core temperature (e.g., rectal, bladder, or esophageal), using a thermometer capable of recording very low temperatures. Patients should be placed on a cardiac monitor and an ECG should be obtained. Laboratory testing is especially useful in the postresuscitative period when complications begin. Laboratory tests should include a complete blood count (CBC), a chemistry panel, creatine phosphokinase (CPK) to evaluate for rhabdomyolysis, a coagulation profile, blood type and screen, an arterial blood gas (ABG), and a drug screen. A Foley catheter should be placed to access urinary output.

REWARMING STRATEGIES

There are several methods of rewarming. The method of choice usually depends on the severity of hypothermia. During rewarming, the patient should be placed on a cardiac monitor with frequent measurements of blood pressure and temperature (via a rectal probe) for easy detection of complications of rewarming such as rewarming-related hypotension, arrhythmias, and core temperature after-drop.

BOX 2   Drugs and Chemicals That Can Cause Hypothermia

Medicinals

Acetaminophen (Tylenol)
Amphotericin B (Fungizone)
Azithromycin (Zithromax)
Baclofen (Lioresal)
Barbiturates
Benzodiazepines
β-Adrenergic blocking agents
Bethanechol (Urecholine)
Biperiden (Akineton)
Bromocriptine (Parlodel)
Carbamazepine (Tegretol)
Chloral hydrate (Noctec)
Chlorpromazine (Thorazine)
Clonidine (Catapres)
Colchicine
Diltiazem (Cardizem)
Ethchlorvynol (Placidyl)
Ethyl alcohol
Fenoprofen (Nalfon)
Fluphenazine (Prolixin)
Fosphenytoin (Cerebyx)
Gallium nitrate (Ganite)
Glutethimide (Doriden)[2]
Guanabenz (Wytensin)
Guanfacine (Tenex)
Haloperidol (Haldol)
Heroin
Ibuprofen (Advil, Motrin)
Insulin preparations
Interferon-β-1 b (Betaseron)
Lithium (Eskalith, Lithobid)
Loxapine (Loxapac, Loxitane)
Magnesium sulfate
Maprotiline (Ludiomil)
Mefenamic acid (Ponstel)
Methyldopa (Aldomet)
Methyprylon (Noludar)[2]
Moricizine (Ethmozine)

Morphine sulfate
Naphazoline (Naphcon)
Omeprazole (Prilosec)
Oxymetazoline (Afrin)
Phencyclidine
Phenol
Phenytoin (Dilantin)
Pilocarpine (Salagen)
Prazosin (Minipress)
Propoxyphene (Darvon)
Rauwolfia serpentine
Reserpine
Salicylate
Terazosin (Hytrin)
Tetracycline (Sumycin)
Tetrahydrozoline (Visine, Opti-Clear)
Thioridazine (Mellaril)
Tretinoin (Topical) (Retin A)
Tricyclic antidepressants
Valproic acid and derivatives
   (Depakene)
Zinc sulfate

Nonmedicinals

Acrylamide
Aldicarb
Amitraz
Barium
Bromophos
Carbon disulfide
Carbon monoxide
Chloralose
Chlorfenvinphos
Chloryrifos
Coumaphos
Cyanide
Diazinon
Dichlorvos

Dicrotophos
Dioxathion
Disulfoton
Ether
Ethion
Fensulfothion
Fenthion
Hexachlorobenzene
Hydrogen sulfide
Isopropyl alcohol
Lewisite
Malathion
Methidathion
Methiocarb
Methomyl
Methylparathion
Nickel
Parathion
Profenofos
Pyrimidifen
Sodium azide
Terbufos
Tetraethyl-pyrophosphate

Biologicals

Ackee fruit poisoning
Ciguatera food poisoning
Delphinium
Lobelia
Marijuana (*Cannabis*)
Monkshood
Nutmeg
Star of Bethlehem (*Hippobroman longiflora*)
Tetrodotoxin food poisoning
White chameleon

[2]Not available in the United States.

Passive External Warming

Passive external warming is ideal for patients with mild hypothermia who are otherwise healthy. It uses the patient's endogenous heat production for rewarming and it involves simple, logical passive maneuvers that minimize heat dissipation. When using this method, all wet clothing should be removed, the ambient core temperature should exceed 70.0°F (21.0°C), and the patient should be covered with insulating materials. Patients warmed easily using this method can be safely discharged.

Active External Rewarming

Active external rewarming is controversial. It involves exposing the skin of the patient to exogenous heat sources. Radiant heat, thermal mattresses, electric heating blankets, and forced-air heating blankets are some of the available techniques.

This method has a number of disadvantages. First, burn injuries can occur to the vasoconstricted skin. Second, any sort of immersion can hinder monitoring and other resuscitative activities. Finally and most important, active external rewarming produces a phenomenon called *core temperature after-drop*. This refers to a drop in core temperature as a result of sudden peripheral vasodilation. This causes cold, acidic blood to return to the core. Hypotension and potentially fatal dysrhythmias can result. Focusing on rewarming the trunk only (rather than the trunk and extremities) can prevent these temperature gradients. In general, active external rewarming is used in conjunction with active core rewarming.

Active Core Rewarming

Active core rewarming involves techniques to deliver direct heat internally. It should be used in patients with moderate to severe hypothermia. The simplest method entails the administration of

 ## CURRENT DIAGNOSIS

- Accidental hypothermia may be classified as mild, moderate, or severe.
- The measured temperature should be the core body temperature.
- The method of rewarming depends on the severity of the temperature drop.
- The complications of rewarming include arrhythmias, rewarming-related hypotension, core temperature after drop, and rhabdomyolysis.
- Patients can only be declared dead after they are warm and dead.

heated, humidified oxygen at 107.6°F to 114.8°F (42.0°C–46.0°C) and intravenous saline solution warmed to 109.4°F (43.0°C). Saline should be administered via a central line at 150 to 200 mL/hour. Gastric, bladder, and colonic irrigations have been used but their relatively small surface areas usually limit their effect.

Another method of active core rewarming is pleural irrigation using two large-bore (36°F or greater) thoracostomy tubes. One tube is placed at the midclavicular line and is connected to saline to 107.6°F (42.0°C). The other tube is placed at the posterior axillary line and connected to a chest tube drainage kit.

A more aggressive method of active core rewarming is via peritoneal lavage and dialysis. This can be accomplished using a standard diagnostic peritoneal lavage (DPL) kit and introducing an 8-F catheter into the peritoneum using Seldinger's technique. The crystalloid dialysate should be warmed to 104.0°F to 113.0°F (40.0°C–45.0°C). This method affords the added advantage of allowing the serum potassium level to be adjusted.

The most efficient and physiologic active core rewarming method is via extracorporeal warming or heated cardiopulmonary bypass. This is the method of choice for the most severe cases, patients with severe rhabdomyolysis, and for patients who require cardiopulmonary resuscitation.

Most arrhythmias are corrected by rewarming. Atropine is typically ineffective for associated bradydysrhythmias. Ventricular tachycardia and fibrillation require electrocardioversion and the use of bretylium,[2] if it is available. The safety of amiodarone (Cordarone) in these situations is questionable. Dopamine (Intropin) may be an effective vasopressor. Empiric antibiotics may be given. However, the empiric use of levothyroxine (Synthroid)[1] and corticosteroids may be hazardous. Phenytoin (Dilantin)[1] might have cardiac-depressant qualities in the moderately hypothermic patient. Box 3 demonstrates drugs with possible decreased metabolism or clearance with increase in toxicity in hypothermia.

Indicators of grave prognosis include development of profound hyperkalemia (serum potassium >10 mEq/L), underlying medical conditions, intravascular thrombosis (fibrinogen <59 mg/dL), pH less than 6.5, and a core temperature less than 50.0°F to 53.6°F (10.0°C–12.0°C).

Peripheral Cold Injuries

Peripheral cold injuries span a spectrum ranging from minimal to severe tissue damage. Freezing and nonfreezing syndromes can cause these injuries. Frostnip and frostbite are caused by exposure to freezing temperatures. *Frostnip* refers to the numbness and blue-white discoloration of the face and extremities that occur during exposure to freezing temperatures. It is a precursor to frostbite. It is characterized by reversible skin changes including blanching and numbness with no permanent tissue damage, unlike frostbite. Nonfreezing injuries depend on whether the ambient environment during exposure was wet (trench or immersion foot) or dry (pernio or chilblain).

---

[1]Not FDA approved for this indication.
[2]Not available in the United States.

BOX 3	Drugs Displaying Reduced Metabolism or Clearance in Hypothermia

- Atropine
- Digoxin
- D-Tubocurarine
- Fentanyl (Sublimaze, Duragesic)
- Gentamicin (Garamycin)
- Lidocaine (Xylocaine)
- Phenobarbital
- Procaine
- Propranolol (Inderal)
- Sulfanilamide (AVC Cream)
- Suxamethonium (Succinylcholine, Anectine)

PATHOPHYSIOLOGY

During exposure to cold temperatures, the core body temperature is preserved to the detriment of the extremities. Frostbite occurs in four stages: prefreeze, freeze-thaw, vascular stasis, and late ischemic stages. The prefreeze phase occurs when the temperature of the extremities falls below 50.0°F (10.0°C) and cutaneous sensation is lost. Vasoconstriction also occurs along with leakage of intracellular fluid into the interstitium. The freeze-thaw phase begins at the freezing point of water (32.0°F or 0°C) with the formation of ice crystals extracellularly. This further enhances the exit of water from the intracellular space under osmotic forces, resulting in cell shrinkage and ultimately damage. During the vascular stasis phase, plasma leakage and formation of ice crystals continue. Arachidonic acid break down products are then released from underlying damaged tissue. Both prostaglandin $F_{2\alpha}$ and thromboxane A_2 produce platelet aggregation, leukocyte immobilization, and vasoconstriction. Endothelial cells are sensitive to cold injury, and the microvasculature becomes distorted and clogged, leading to tissue ischemia. The late ischemic phase is characterized by ischemia, thrombosis, continued shunting, gangrene, autonomic dysfunction, and denaturation of tissue proteins. The tissue can eventually mummify and demarcate more than 60 to 90 days later.

CLINICAL PRESENTATION

The face and ears are the most common sites prone to cold injury, followed by the hands and feet.

Frostnip and Frostbite

Patients with frostnip usually have blanching and numbness of their fingertips. Frostbite has been classified as superficial, affecting the skin and subcutaneous tissue, or deep, affecting the bones, joints, and tendons. When a superficial frostbite is rewarmed, the skin can form a clear blister; however, when a deep frostbite is rewarmed, it can form a hemorrhagic blister. This classification, however, has no therapeutic or prognostic value given that frostbites can initially appear benign. Many weeks can pass before the demarcation between viable and nonviable tissues becomes apparent.

Although no prognostic factors can be entirely predictive, favorable factors include retained sensation, normal skin color, and clear rather than cloudy fluid in the blisters, if present. Poor prognostic features include nonblanching cyanosis, firm skin, and dark, fluid-filled blisters. Patients can present with pain, numbness, and a clumsy "chunk of wood" sensation in the affected extremity. The pain is initially described as a dull ache and evolves to become a throbbing sensation in about 48 to 72 hours.

Chilblain

Chilblain results from repetitive exposure to cold dry air. It manifests as erythematous or cyanotic lesions often referred to as *cold sores*. These lesions usually develop on exposed surfaces after a delay of 12 to 14 hours and are characterized by pruritus and burning paresthesias. Young women, especially those with Raynaud's phenomenon, are at risk.

Trench Foot and Immersion Foot

Trench foot occurs as a result of prolonged exposure to a damp, cold, nonfreezing environment. It has been classically described among soldiers in World War I, many of whom were confined to cold and damp trenches for prolonged periods. Symptoms include numbness and painful paresthesias that can progress to a throbbing and burning sensation. Initial evaluation reveals a cold, pale extremity, with or without vesicles or bullae.

Immersion foot may be considered the sailor's counterpart to trench foot. It occurs after prolonged immersion in cold water at temperatures above freezing.

TREATMENT

Treatment of frostbite should begin with removing all wet or frozen clothing. For patients with moderate and severe hypothermia as described above, initial resuscitative efforts should be geared toward

CURRENT THERAPY

Mild Hypothermia: 32.2°C (90°F) to 35°C (95°F)

- Passive external rewarming
  - Remove wet clothing.
  - Ambient temperature should exceed 21.0°C (70.0°F).
  - Cover patient with insulating material.

Moderate Hypothermia: 28°C (82.4°F) to 32.2°C (90°F)

- Active external rewarming
  - Radiant heat
  - Thermal mattresses
  - Electric heating blankets
  - Forced-air heating blankets
- Active core rewarming
  - Warmed humidified oxygen
  - Warmed intravenous saline
  - Bladder, colonic, and gastric irrigation
  - Pleural cavity lavage

Severe Hypothermia: Less than 28°C (82.4°F)

- Aggressive active core rewarming
  - Warmed, humidified oxygen
  - Warmed intravenous saline
  - Bladder, colonic, and gastric irrigation
  - Pleural cavity lavage
  - Peritoneal lavage or dialysis
  - Extracorporeal warming or heated cardiopulmonary bypass

Frostnip

- Gentle rewarming
- Usually self-resolving

Frostbite

- Warm-water immersion
- Débride broken vesicles
- Apply topical aloe vera or antibiotic ointment
- Use NSAIDs for pain
- Update tetanus status

Chilblain

- Gentle rewarming
- Nifidipine (procardia)

Trench Foot

- Dry the foot
- Gentle rewarming

Abbreviation: NSAID = nonsteroidal antiinflammatory drug.

raising their core temperature. The patient should be moved to a warm environment and all wet clothing should be removed. The frozen extremity should be rewarmed by immersion in circulation water at 104.0°F to 108.0°F (40.0°C–42.0°C) for about 15 to 30 minutes. Given the risks of thermal injury, the frozen parts should not be exposed to direct or dry heat (such as hair dryers, heating pads, or heat lamps). Do not rub or massage the affected area. The process should be continued until the extremity appears warm and well perfused. Due to the pain associated with reperfusion, there may be the temptation to abruptly abort the rewarming process. This can, however, promote further tissue damage. Parenteral analgesic medications (nonsteroidal antiinflammatory drugs [NSAIDs] and opioids) may be administered as needed to make this process more tolerable.

Almost all authors agree that hemorrhagic blisters should not be débrided because of the risk of secondary desiccation of deep dermal layers, extending the injury. Débriding broken vesicles or bullae is also widely accepted; however, clear, intact vesicles may be broken and débrided or left intact. Topical aloe vera ointment (Dermaide Aloe) (a thromboxane inhibitor) or topical antibiotic ointments may be applied. The injured tissue should be loosely covered with sterile, dry, nonadherent dressing. Hands and feet may be splinted and elevated to reduce edema. Because the damaged tissue is tetanus prone, patients whose tetanus status has not been updated need a tetanus shot (Td).

Adjunctive agents that have been used for their antithrombotic and vasodilative properties with varying success include heparin,[1] steroids,[1] NSAIDs,[1] dimethylsulfoxide (DMSO),[1] nonionic detergents,[1] dipyridamole (Persantine),[1] calcium channel blockers,[1] pentoxifylline (Trental),[1] and phenoxybenzamine (Dibenzyline).

Surgical consultation is appropriate for guiding long-term management, because some patients might need débridement of infections or skin grafts for nonhealing wounds. A sympathetic nerve block can relieve painful and refractory vasospasms.

Chilblain (pernio) may be treated with nifidipine (Procardia)[1] at an oral dose of 20 to 60 mg daily.

SEQUELAE

Late sequelae of frostbite include cold hypersensitivity, numbness, pain, and decreased sensation. This is a result of early neuronal damage and abnormal sympathetic tone. Patients with chronic symptoms should be advised to avoid nicotine and cold exposure while using NSAIDs. Tissue demarcation can occur 60 to 90 days after initial injury. Amputation decisions should be deferred unless there is supervening sepsis or gangrene. The ultimate tissue salvage after a spontaneous slough usually far exceeds the most optimistic initial estimates.

Therapeutic Hypothermia

Therapeutic hypothermia for reducing anoxic brain injury has been increasingly used in clinical practice in post–cardiac arrest states. The usual scenarios for such a practice are in patients with suspected postanoxic injuries following cardiopulmonary resuscitation, traumatic brain injuries associated with elevation of intracranial pressure, stroke, and various perioperative situations (such as vascular surgery). Hypothermia can reduce the metabolic oxygen utilization rate in the brain by 6% for every 1°C reduction in brain temperature (over 82.4°F or 28°C) due to reduced normal cerebral electrical activity and suppression of chemical reactions (such as free radical and glutamate production along with calcium shifts) associated with reperfusion injury. Cooling is usually initiated within 6 hours following return of spontaneous circulation, with moderate hypothermia (82.4°F to 90°F or 28°C to 32.2°C) for induction. Intravenous cooling techniques (infusion of 30 mL/kg of crystalloid solution at 4°C over 30 minutes) or extracorporeal cooling methods have been used. An intravascular heat-exchange device has also been developed. Shivering is prevented via neuromuscular blockade and sedation. Temperature can be monitored by a bladder temperature probe or through a central pulmonary catheter.

REFERENCES

Aslam AF, Aslam AK, Vasavada BC, Khan IA. Hypothermia: Evaluation, electrocardiographic manifestations, and management. Am J Med 2006;119(4): 297–301.

Bhagat H, Bithal PK, Chouhan RS, Arora R. Is phenytoin administration safe in a hypothermic child? J Clin Neurosci 2006;13(9):953–5.

Centers for Disease Control and Prevention (CDC). Hypothermia-related deaths—United States, 2003–2004. MMWR Morb Mortal Wkly Rep 2005;54(7):173–5.

[1]Not FDA approved for this indication.

Danzl DF. Hypothermia. Semin Respir Crit Care Med 2002;23(1):57–68.

Danzl DF, Pozos RS. Accidental hypothermia. N Engl J Med 1994;331(26): 1756–60.

Ervasti O, Juopperi K, Ketlumen P, et al. The occurance of frostbite and its risk factors in young men. Int J Circumpolar Health 2004;63(1):71–80.

Gilbert M, Busund R, Skagseth A, et al. Resuscitation from accidental hypothermia of 13.7 degrees C with circulatory arrest. Lancet 2000;355 (9201):375–6.

Lloyd EL. Accidental hypothermia. Resuscitation 1996;32:111–24.

McCauley RD, Smith DJ, Robson MC, et al. Frostbite and other cold-induced injuries. In: Auerbach PS, editor. Wilderness medicine: Management of wilderness and environmental emergencies. 3rd ed. St Louis: Mosby; 1995. p. 129–45.

McDonagh DL, Allen IN, Keifer JC, Warner DS. Induction of hypothermia after intraoperative hypoxic brain insult. Anesth Analg 2006;103(1):180–1.

Nolan JP, Morley PT, Vanden Hoek TL, Hickey RW, et al. International Liaison Committee on Resuscitation: Therapeutic hypothermia after cardiac arrest: An advisory statement by the advanced life support task force of the International Liaison Committee on Resuscitation. Circulation 2003;108:118–21.

Ulrich AS, Rathlev NK. Hypothermia and localized cold injuries. Emerg Med Clin North Am 2004;22(2):281–98.

Disturbances Caused by Heat

Method of
John F. Coyle II, MD

Exertional Heat Stroke

Heat stroke is an illness caused by failure of thermoregulation with elevation of core temperature to 40.6°C (105°F) or more, associated with central nervous system dysfunction. Heat stroke is traditionally subdivided into *exertional* and *classic* (or nonexertional) forms.

Exertional heat stroke is a sporadic illness triggered by exercise in warm environmental conditions that add to the thermal load produced by muscular contraction. It mainly strikes manual laborers, soldiers in training, and athletic competitors; indeed, it is the third leading cause of death among high school and college athletes in the United States. Exertional heat stroke may occur at moderate temperatures, especially if humidity is high, but both exertional and classic heat strokes most likely develop in conditions of high heat. The incidence of heat stroke increases exponentially when heat stress exceeds a boundary value. Appearance of the first case should sound an alarm that conditions have become dangerous, and more cases should be anticipated. The typical heat stroke victim is highly motivated, poorly conditioned, obese, and not acclimatized. Fatigue and sleep deprivation are commonly encountered, and recent or ongoing febrile or dehydrating illness increases risk. Dehydration may play a role, especially if severe. The use of certain medicines also increases risk, most notably those that decrease cardiac output (β-blockers), promote dehydration (diuretics), affect hypothalamic control (major tranquilizers, neuroleptics, alcohol), inhibit sweating (anticholinergics, tricyclic antidepressants, antihistamines), or increase thermogenicity (amphetamines, cocaine).

Prevention is the ideal treatment. Because behavior is the most powerful thermoregulatory mechanism, education and empowerment have the greatest preventive potential. To avoid exertional heat stroke, organizers should schedule vigorous exercise in the coolest hours of the day (shortly after dawn or after nightfall, in difficult seasons). Exercise level should be governed by athlete fitness, acclimatization, hydration status, and freedom from intercurrent illness. Clothing should be appropriate for exercise conditions. Medication use that might interfere with effective thermoregulation should be recognized, and medical personnel must be charged with the responsibility for stopping any participant who appears to be decompensating.

Triage of those with exertional heat stroke is highly variable. Runners who are plunged unconscious into an ice water bath at the end of a race often respond promptly to treatment, reawaken, and are sometimes sent home without hospitalization. A less-favorable response necessitates hospital admission.

Classic (Nonexertional) Heat Stroke

Classic (nonexertional) heat stroke usually occurs during heat waves that cause passive warming by exposure to unrelenting hot and humid conditions, afflicting urban dwellers who are elderly, infirm, solitary, and poor. Heat waves tend to be "silent and invisible killers of silent and invisible people." Their housing lacks air-conditioning or they do not use it because of expense or confusion. Alcoholism and chronic illness, especially mental illness, predispose people to heat stroke. Young children are susceptible, reflecting their high surface-to-volume ratio, relatively inefficient sweat glands, and dependent status. Classic heat stroke requires preventive measures at the community level. Those with chronic illness and substance abuse history are at highest risk, and they may be the most difficult to contact. Although ventilation fans are of little help in hot and humid conditions, a few hours spent in air-conditioned rooms each day can significantly reduce the likelihood of heat stroke. Whether this is primarily a physiologic or a sociologic effect is unclear. Patients with classic heat stroke usually respond slowly to treatment and require hospital admission.

Pathophysiology

The pathophysiology of heat stroke is incompletely understood. Although a vast number of runners in a marathon may develop dehydration and a high core temperature, very few proceed to heat stroke. Excessive heat is a noxious agent that causes direct cell injury. The severity of heat stroke is related to the degree and duration of temperature elevation above 41.6°C (106.9°F). Exercise lowers the thermal threshold for heat stroke because of hormonal effects and

---

 CURRENT DIAGNOSIS

- Heat stroke often occurs in the first 2 hours of exercise and may occur in so-called moderate heat stress conditions.
- Heat stroke may occur in sedentary urban dwellers during heat waves, especially in the presence of drug or alcohol use, senility, or in young children.
- Abnormal mental status (coma, delirium, agitation, confusion, combativeness) is a constant feature of heat stroke.
- Rectal temperature should be checked immediately. Axillary and aural temperatures may be misleadingly low. A rectal temperature of 40.6°C (105°F) or more is required for diagnosis of heat stroke, but delayed measurement may produce a misleadingly low temperature.
- The trap of proceeding with complex diagnostic procedures (such as computed tomographic scans) before core temperature is assessed and lowered to less than 39°C (102.2°F) should be avoided.
- After cooling measures are instituted, blood samples should be obtained to assess coagulation status, hepatic function, renal function, likelihood of infection, acid-base status, and muscle injury.

competing demands of organ systems as blood flow is directed away from the viscera to the active muscles and the skin. Gut ischemia may result in release of bacterial polysaccharides into the blood. What happens next is a complex interplay of factors including cytokines, bacterial polysaccharides, and heat shock proteins. As endothelial abnormalities accumulate, there is precipitation of a cascade of events including activation of the coagulation system and vascular dilation, resulting in hypotension and coagulation disorders. These events in many respects mimic sepsis.

Because the brain is extremely sensitive to heat stress, the first signs of heat stroke are neurologic. Judgment is impaired, and the chance for self-diagnosis is greatly reduced. After loss of consciousness, muscular activity is markedly diminished, but temperature may remain elevated for hours. Multisystem injury may follow, with the possibility of neurologic, pulmonary, cardiac, hepatic, renal, vascular, hematologic, and immunologic damage. A high percentage of classic heat stroke patients suffer infection within 36 hours of hospital admission.

Treatment

Treatment of heat stroke can be summarized easily:

- Lower rectal temperature immediately to 39°C (102.2°F).
- Support organ systems injured by heat, hypotension, inflammation, and coagulopathy.

There is a *golden hour* after the onset of heat stroke in which therapy can be extremely effective. When treating a patient outside of the hospital, the patient should be moved to a shaded area, clothes removed, and the person covered with water and fanned. When resources become available, the simplest treatment appears to be cold-water immersion in a shallow tub, with patient head, arms, and lower legs outside the tub. The high efficiency of this method comes from two properties of water: It has 25 times the thermal conductivity of air, and it makes perfect contact with all skin surfaces. In addition, the hydrostatic properties of water tend to reduce the risk of hypotension. Other methods of cooling include skin wetting with fanning, application of total-body ice packs (24 ice packs, with special emphasis on the neck, armpits, and groin), or use of a body-cooling unit (evaporation and convection).

Assessment of the patient with presumed heat stroke should be delayed pending initiation of cooling. Determination of rectal temperature, heart rate, and blood pressure can be carried out while the patient is being cooled. Oral and tympanic membrane temperatures cannot be used because they may be misleadingly low. Rectal temperature should be measured every 5 to 10 minutes, and the patient should be removed from cooling when 39°C (102.2°F) is reached, to avoid overshoot hypothermia. Hydration with normal saline or lactated Ringer's solution should be started after initiation of cooling, and most patients require 1 L in the first hour of treatment. Further rehydration needs to be guided by estimated water losses, and in difficult cases placement of a central venous monitoring catheter may be needed. Overhydration may promote cerebral edema, pulmonary edema, and hyponatremia.

Seizures, which occur commonly, should be managed with diazepam (Valium), 5 mg intravenously (IV). Shivering may also be treated with diazepam. The patient must be monitored closely with use of this medication, which occasionally promotes hypotension. Hypotension should be treated with cooling and volume expansion. If blood pressure remains depressed, pressors may be needed. For patients with prolonged exertional heat stroke, mannitol, 0.25 g/kg, or furosemide (Lasix), 0.5 to 1 mg/kg, should be given after volume expansion is carried out to minimize the adverse effects of rhabdomyolysis on renal function.

In patients with severe multiorgan damage, disseminated intravascular coagulation (DIC) is a common finding. Bleeding in DIC should be treated with transfusion of fresh-frozen plasma, cryoprecipitate, and platelet concentrates as needed. There is no role for heparin or thrombolytics in DIC in this setting. Adult respiratory distress

CURRENT THERAPY

- Injury because of heat stroke is related to both the magnitude and duration of core temperature elevation.
- After elevated rectal temperature is documented, treatment should not be delayed. In particular, it should not be delayed to start an intravenous line or to carry out advanced testing such as computed tomography or other radiograph study.
- Ideal treatment for heat stroke is cold-water immersion in a low tub, such as a child's wading pool, with the patient's arms, legs, and head hanging out of the tub.
- If low tub immersion is not available, constant flowing of cold water from a tap over the patient with drainage through a slotted Gurney cart in the presence of constant high-velocity electric fanning can be effective.
- Applying ice packs to the axillae, groins, trunk, and as many other skin surfaces as possible can be useful, but this method of cooling is not as efficient as cold-water immersion or constant cold-water flow because of reduced contact surface and limited thermal gradient.
- Rectal temperature should be checked every 5 minutes during cooling. Cooling measures are discontinued when rectal temperature reaches 39°C (102.2°F) to avoid excessive cooling. Clinicians should watch for rebound temperature elevation after cooling is discontinued.
- Clinicians should be prepared to support the patient through multisystem organ failure. Hemorrhage should be treated with transfusion of red blood cells, platelets, fresh-frozen plasma, and clotting factors. Heparin has no role in treatment of this consumptive coagulopathy. Volume expansion may be needed. Prolonged ventilator support and hemodialysis may be required.
- Medications that may be needed are diazepam (Valium), 5 mg intravenously (IV), for seizures; pressors; and mannitol, 0.25 g/kg IV, and furosemide (Lasix), 0.5 to 1.0 mg/kg IV, for renal protection from rhabdomyolysis, but only after adequate volume expansion is achieved.

syndrome tends to occur in conjunction with DIC, and prolonged ventilator support may be required. Hepatic failure in heat stroke is usually transient. Renal failure may necessitate emergency hemodialysis. No evidence supports use of anti-inflammatory agents or antipyretic agents in heat stroke. Use of strategies that are helpful in sepsis may ultimately find a role in treatment of heat stroke, but such treatments should be considered experimental at this time.

Prognosis can be estimated by time to recovery of consciousness (shorter is better) and elevation of liver enzymes (lactate dehydrogenase [LDH] at 24 hours less than three times normal is a good prognostic sign).

Heat stroke should usually be regarded as an accident, like drowning. The population at highest risk is readily defined, but because of the rarity of this ailment it is difficult to maintain a high level of preparedness for its prevention and treatment. Once encountered, heat stroke must be treated with much the same urgency as cardiac arrest because prompt cooling can sometimes make the crisis little more than an inconvenience. After the process of systemic injury becomes established, heat stroke's cascade of microvascular dysfunction can take on a life of its own, eventuating in a desperate struggle against multisystem failure and a high mortality rate.

REFERENCES

Bouchama A, Knochel JP. Heat stroke. N Engl J Med 2002;346(25):1978–88.

Crandall CG, Vongpatanasin W, Victor RG. Mechanism of cocaine-induced hyperthermia in humans. Ann Intern Med 2002;136(11):785–91.

Dematte JE, O'Mara K, Buescher J, et al. Near-fatal heat stroke during the 1995 heat wave in Chicago. Ann Intern Med 1998;129(3):173–81.

Eichner ER. Treatment of suspected heat illness. Int J Sports Med 1998;19 (Suppl. 2):S150–3.

Epstein Y, Moran DS, Shapiro Y. Exertional heatstroke in the Israeli Defence Forces. In: Pandolf KB, Burr RE, editors. Medical aspects of harsh environments. U.S. Defense Dept., Army, Office of the Surgeon General; 2001. p. 281–92. Available free online: http://www.bordeninstitute.army.mil/medaspofharshenvrnmnts/

Gaffin SL, Hubbard RW. Pathophysiology of heatstroke, In: Pandolf KB, Burr RE, editors. Medical aspects of harsh environments. U.S. Defense Dept., Army, Office of the Surgeon General; 2001. p. 161–208. Available free online: http://www.bordeninstitute.army.mil/medaspofharshenvrnmnts/.

Gardner JW, Kark JA. Clinical diagnosis, management and surveillance of exertional heat illness, In: Pandolf KB, Burr RE, editors. Medical aspects of harsh environments. U.S. Defense Dept., Army, Office of the Surgeon General; 2001. p. 221–79. Available free online: http://www.bordeninstitute.army.mil/medaspofharshenvrnmnts/

Klinenberg E. Review of heat wave: Social autopsy of disaster in Chicago. N Engl J Med 2003;348(7):666–7.

Shephard RJ, Shek PN. Immune dysfunction as a factor in heat illness. Crit Rev Immunol 1999;19(4):285–302.

Spider Bites and Scorpion Stings

Method of

Rachel Haroz, MD, and James R. Roberts, MD

Spider Bites

Most of the approximately 34,000 species of spiders are considered to be venomous, but their short and delicate jaws generally prevent significant human envenomation. Approximately 200 species, however, do possess the ability to envenomate humans, resulting in symptoms ranging from minor to occasionally serious skin lesions to neurotoxicity, systemic illness, multiorgan dysfunction, and death. Spider identification after a bite is desirable but usually impossible. Here we discuss features, symptoms of envenomation, and treatment for bites from the *Loxosceles, Latrodectus,* and tarantula spiders.

LOXOSCELES ENVENOMATION

Relatively small (approximately 1.5 cm in leg span), *Loxosceles* spiders are light brown in color with darker brown markings on their dorsal surface. The most distinctive identifying characteristic appears on the female brown recluse (*L. reclusa*), which is described as violin shaped. Eleven native species of *Loxosceles* exist in the United States in the southern, southwestern, and central states. Most confirmed necrotic arachnidism in the United States is caused by *L. reclusa*. *Loxosceles* spiders have six eyes, which differs from the typical eight eyes found in most other spiders. Females are usually larger than males, which are rarely considered venomous. Considered nonaggressive and nocturnal, most *Loxosceles* bites occur when the spider is inadvertently caught between clothing or bedding and the victim's skin. Perineal and genital bites can occur in outhouses. The bite may be minimally painful or go totally unnoticed.

The initial skin manifestation is a small, erythematous, flat lesion surrounded by a light-colored ring. Within hours to days this lesion becomes bluish with a deepening of the color of the ring and

CURRENT DIAGNOSIS

- *Loxosceles* spider bites generally result in local symptoms, whereas *Latrodectus* and scorpion stings have predominantly systemic manifestations, which may be severe.
- The spider or scorpion should be identified if at all possible.
- Not all necrotic wounds are spider bites; therefore a differential diagnosis should be entertained.

progressing to a blister/bleb. A necrotic eschar with an ulcerative base may develop, which rarely becomes quite extensive. The lesion is minimally painful but often takes several weeks to heal, occasionally requiring extensive débridement or skin grafting. Some ulcerated wounds (approximately 10%) produce permanent scarring. *Loxosceles* venom contains various toxic enzymes, most notably sphingomyelinase D, that contribute to cellular destruction and tissue damage.

Systemic symptoms are rare (1% to 3% of all bites) but may include hemolysis, platelet aggregation, hemoglobinuria, myoglobinuria, maculopapular rash, nausea, vomiting, renal failure, disseminated intravascular coagulation, fever, seizures, coma, and death. These symptoms are more common in children and following South American *Loxosceles* bites.

There is little the clinician can do to affect favorably the course of a *Loxosceles* bite, with the ultimate outcome dependent on the amount and potency of the venom and host factors. Local wound care includes antisepsis, immobilization, and elevation of the affected extremity, cool compresses, appropriate analgesics, antihistamines for itching, and tetanus prophylaxis. Envenomation is difficult to differentiate from infection, but antibiotics may be necessary for secondarily infected wounds. Débridement of necrotic tissue is performed as needed. Delayed excision and wound grafting may be indicated. Once recommended, early wound excision and intrawound steroid injections should be avoided. Several other treatments to ameliorate tissue necrosis are advocated, including dapsone,[1] colchicine,[1] topical nitroglycerin,[1] high-dose vitamin C,[1] electric shock therapy, cyproheptadine (Periactin),[1] and hyperbaric oxygenation, but none has proven effective. Patients exhibiting systemic symptoms should be hospitalized and receive supportive care.

Absent a witnessed attack, a spider bite is usually a clinical diagnosis made by exclusion. *Loxosceles* and other spider bites are overreported and occur far less frequently than suspected by the lay public or diagnosed by clinicians. Outside of the endemic areas, *Loxosceles* bites are highly unlikely. Importantly, if the spider was not positively identified, a differential diagnosis should be entertained. Entities confused with a spider bite include clandestine drug injection (especially cocaine and amphetamines), methicillin-resistant *Staphylococcus aureus* (MRSA) skin infections, early shingles lesions, other bug bites, self-induced trauma, and infectious embolic lesions (such as endocarditis and gonococcemia).

NON-*LOXOSCELES* NECROTIC ARACHNIDISM

Several other species of spiders in the United States (*Cheiracanthium* species and *Tegenaria agrestis* [hobo] spiders) are associated with necrotic lesions. *Cheiracanthium* spiders are widespread and usually found indoors (e.g., in the folds of curtains or on warm windowsills). They are aggressive night foragers and produce painful, pruritic bites, usually resolving within several days. Their bites rarely result in ulceration and necrosis. Hobo spiders inhabit the Pacific Northwest to where they recently emigrated from Western Europe. They are large, aggressive, and inhabit woodpiles, subfloors, and baseboards. Their bites are usually painless but may lead to multiple ruptured blisters within 1 to 2 days and a necrotic wound. Hobo spider bites

---

[1]Not FDA approved for this indication.

CURRENT THERAPY

- Conservative wound care is essential in all envenomations, particularly for a *Loxosceles* spider bite.
- Particular care should be given to the very young, elderly, and patients with comorbidity. In the setting of significant systemic symptoms, the administration of antivenom, if available, should be considered.
- Patients with ocular symptoms after exposure to a tarantula spider must be promptly referred to an ophthalmologist.
- Supportive care is often more valuable than antivenom administration, particularly considering the relatively high rate of both immediate and delayed hypersensitivity reactions.

are probably responsible for necrotic arachnidism in the colder areas of the United States where the brown recluse spider is not found. Treatment of hobo spider bites is similar to that of *Loxosceles* bites.

LATRODECTUS ENVENOMATION

Latrodectus species (widow spiders) are found worldwide. In the United States, five widow spiders are endemic. These spiders are generally dark with various ventral patterns; the most well known is the red hourglass figure found on the female black widow spider. Females are larger (16- to 20-mm leg span) and more venomous than males. *Latrodectus* spiders generally inhabit outdoor dark spaces and are nonaggressive, but they do bite if provoked. The initial bite may be mildly painful, resulting in a small raised wheal. The neurotoxicity associated with these bites results from α-latrotoxin in the venom that causes a large calcium-dependent presynaptic terminal release of neurotransmitters including norepinephrine, glutamate, acetylcholine, and dopamine. The reuptake of choline is simultaneously inhibited. Symptoms begin approximately 30 minutes to an hour after the bite, and patients can appear quite ill. Muscle cramps and pain spread from the bite site and can be severe. Facial contortion and periorbital swelling, *facies latrodectismica*, may occur. Abdominal rigidity mimicking an acute abdomen, thoracic muscle spasm leading to hypoventilation and respiratory failure, diaphoresis, hypertension, nausea, vomiting, diffuse skin erythema, tremor, priapism, headache, tachycardia, paresthesias, and coma have been described. Lower extremity pain and diaphoresis, even in upper extremity bites, seem to be characteristic features. Symptoms resolve over 3 to 7 days, and death is rare.

Local wound care includes thorough cleansing, appropriate analgesics, ice application, and tetanus prophylaxis. Severe pain and muscle spasms are treated with intravenous opioids and benzodiazepines. Intravenous calcium, although recommended in the past, is ineffective. *Latrodectus* antivenom (antivenin *Lactrodectus mactans*) is horse based and may cause anaphylaxis and serum sickness in allergic persons. It should be reserved for patients with severe systemic symptoms or those with potential for complications, such as the elderly, young children, pregnant patients, and patients with severe cardiovascular disease. Patients who manifest refractory pain, autonomic instability, respiratory distress, or significant neurologic changes should be treated with antivenom. The clinical response to antivenom can be dramatic even when administered 24 hours or more after envenomation.

TARANTULAS

Approximately 1500 species of tarantulas are found worldwide, with 40 species endemic to the southwestern United States. Tarantulas are also now popular household pets because many are considered harmless and nonvenomous. Relatively large spiders (18- to 24-cm leg span), tarantulas live in underground burrows and are night foragers.

Tarantula envenomations in humans often cause mild pain with some surrounding inflammation, but necrotic wounds and systemic symptoms are rare. Bites in dogs, however, are usually rapidly fatal.

Several tarantula species possess urticating hairs, which they launch to incapacitate their enemy. These hairs may penetrate the human skin and cause intense inflammation or lodge in the cornea leading to keratitis, uveitis, and ophthalmia nodosa, a condition characterized by granulomatous lesions in the cornea. Case reports generally describe patients who developed eye symptoms after cleaning tarantula cages or handling the tarantulas. Treatment involves wound care including cleansing, elevation, and immobilization of the affected extremity, tetanus prophylaxis, and appropriate analgesics. Hairs embedded in the cornea that are readily identified should be removed and the patient promptly referred to an ophthalmologist. Antihistamines and corticosteroids may be necessary for pruritus and inflammation. Patients with ophthalmia nodosa may require prolonged topical corticosteroids. Tarantula owners should be cautioned to wear gloves and eye protection when handling their pets and to wash their hands and avoid any eye rubbing after such interactions.

Scorpion Stings

Scorpions range in size from several millimeters to 15 cm. They have a lobster-like appearance with a small head, two front claws, eight paired legs, and a segmented abdomen ending in a venom-containing tail consisting of a storage vesicle and a stinger. Scorpions are typically night stalkers and often found hidden under rocks, in shallow burrows, and in shoes, clothing, and cooking pots. Most of the severe envenomations in the United States are caused by stings by *Centruroides exilicauda* (*sculpturata*), a small (4 to 7 cm long) yellowish brown scorpion.

Scorpion stings are usually very painful, quickly causing local paresthesias and edema. In adults, this usually resolves in several hours. Systemic effects are usually seen in the elderly and in infants and children. Scorpion venom blocks sodium and potassium channels and causes marked acetylcholine and catecholamine release. This leads to an initial cholinergic toxidrome characterized by the SLUDGE syndrome: salivation, lacrimation, urination, defecation, gastroenteritis, and emesis. Subsequently, catecholamine release leads to anxiety, tachycardia, hypertension, pulmonary edema, confusion, dystonic and myoclonic movements, seizures, ataxia, hyperglycemia, hyperpyrexia, and pancreatitis. Neuromotor hyperactivity is common, as are oculomotor abnormalities (nystagmus and rotary movements). Respiratory compromise may occur, especially in children. Myocardial depression, myocardial infarctions without thrombosis, and ischemic strokes are rarely described.

Wound care should encompass thorough cleansing, elevation and immobilization of the affected extremity, cool compresses, tetanus prophylaxis, and appropriate analgesics. Patients should be observed for a period of 6 hours after the sting for the development of systemic symptoms.

Supportive care is the mainstay of treatment. Sympathetic symptoms should be blunted aggressively in an intensive care environment. Benzodiazepines, especially intravenous midazolam, are the mainstay to ameliorate systemic symptoms. β-blockers, diuretics, digoxin (Lanoxin),[1] and nitroprusside (Nitropress) may be useful. Dopamine (Intropin) and dobutamine (Dobutrex) may be necessary for the hypotensive patient, and mechanical ventilation may be required for respiratory failure. Angiotensin-converting enzyme inhibitors, opioids, and nifedipine may be detrimental and should be avoided.

There are currently no FDA-approved therapies, and previously used goat-derived antivenom is controversial and no longer produced. The incidence of immediate and delayed hypersensitivity with this product is relatively high (3% and 60%, respectively). Although helpful with pain, antivenom may not reverse cardiovascular and respiratory compromise because these are secondary to massive catecholamine release. In one small prospective study in critically ill

---

[1]Not FDA approved for this indication.

children, systemic neurotoxicity produced by envenomation from the North American scorpion *Centruroides sculpturatus* was rapidly and markedly reduced by the administration of a scorpion-specific F(ab′)2 antivenom. The need for concomitant benzodiazepine sedation was reduced, as were levels of circulating unbound venom. This product is not currently FDA approved in the United States, nor commercially available except in Mexico (Anascorp, Centruroides immune F(ab)2 intravenous [equine], Instituto Bioclon), but the use of this novel treatment appears safe, and its efficacy is quite promising.

REFERENCES

Blaikie AJ, Ellis J, Sanders R, et al. Eye disease associated with handling pet tarantulas: Three case reports. BMJ 1997;314:1524–5.

Boyer LV, Theodorus AA, Berg RA, et al. Antivenom for critically ill children with neurotoxicity from scorpion stings. N Engl J Med 2009;360:2090.

Clark RF, Wethern-Kestner S, Vance MV, et al. Clinical presentation and treatment of black widow spider envenomations: A review of 163 cases. Ann Emerg Med 1992;21:782–7.

Diaz HJ. The global epidemiology, syndromic classification, management, and prevention of spider bites. Am J Trop Med Hyg 2004;71:239–50.

Hered RW, Spaulding AG, Sanitato JJ, et al. Ophthalmia nodosa caused by tarantula hairs. Ophthalmology 1988;95:166–9.

LoVecchio F, Welch S, Klemens J, et al. Incidence of immediate and delayed hypersensitivity to Centruroides antivenom. Ann Emerg Med 1999;5:615–9.

Mazzei de Davila CA, Davila DF, Donis JH. Sympathetic nervous system activation, antivenin administration and cardiovascular manifestations of scorpion envenomation. Toxicon 2002;40:1339–46.

Merchant ML, Hinton JF, Geren CR. Effect of hyperbaric oxygen on sphingomyelinase D activity of brown recluse spider (*Loxosceles reclusa*) venom as studied by ^{31}P nuclear magnetic resonance spectroscopy. Am J Trop Med Hyg 1997;56:335–8.

Mold JW, Thompson DM. Management of brown recluse spider bites in primary care. J Am Board Fam Pract 2004;17:347–52.

Saucier JR. Arachnid envenomation. Emerg Med Clin North Am 2004;22:405–22.

Suntorntham S, Roberts JR, Nilsen GJ. Dramatic clinical response to the delayed administration of black widow spider antivenom. Ann Emerg Med 1994;24:1198–9.

Swanson DL, Vetter RS. Bites of brown recluse spiders and suspected necrotic arachnidism. N Engl J Med 2005;352:700–7.

Venomous Snakebite

Method of
Steven A. Seifert, MD, FAACT, FACMT

Two families of venomous snakes are native to the United States. The Viperidae family (viperids) is composed of three genera and more than 30 species of rattlesnakes, copperheads, and cottonmouths. The Elapidae family (elapids) is composed of two genera and several species of coral snakes.

Each year, there are approximately 4750 venomous bites by native species reported to U.S. poison centers, with fewer than 10 deaths. Ninety-eight percent of these bites are from viperids, and a single Crotalidae polyvalent immune FAB (ovine) antivenom (CroFab, Protherics, Brentwood, TN) is effective against all native species in this family. There is also a single antivenom (Antivenin [*Micrurus fulvius*] equine origin, Wyeth Laboratories, Marietta, PA) against coral snakes, which are usually easily recognized by their distinctive markings. After a bite, it is not necessary to capture or further identify the snake, because this will only increase the likelihood of additional envenomations and victims.

There are approximately 50 additional bites per year by a wide variety of nonnative venomous species of snakes housed in zoos, academic institutions, and private collections. Identification of the biting species in these cases is usually not an issue.

Diagnostic and Management Overview

TAKING ACTION

Only a few actions can be undertaken in the field to reduce morbidity or mortality from a venomous snakebite. Most "treatments" that have been advocated—cutting, sucking, or applying tourniquets, heat, cold, or electricity—have no proven efficacy and are much more likely to result in additional tissue injury and delay of definitive therapy. Appropriate local injury management—primarily removal of jewelry, splinting of the extremity, and measures to retard venom entry into central circulation until definitive therapy can be undertaken *in carefully selected cases*—and expeditious transport to a health care facility can produce optimal outcomes.

Definitive management for native venomous snakes in the United States is achieved with appropriate local wound care and antivenom, which is composed of antibodies raised in a host animal (i.e., horses or sheep) against snake venom components. Because native viperids inhabit every state except Maine, every hospital should stock or have ready access to this antivenom.

No FDA-approved elapid antivenom is currently being manufactured in the United States. Older stocks of a previously produced antivenom (Antivenin) are still available at many hospitals in endemic areas (e.g., Florida, Georgia, Alabama, Louisiana, Texas), but they are rapidly being depleted, and existing stocks eventually will be consumed or pass their expiration dates. Foreign-produced antivenoms against related coral snake species may have efficacy against U.S. snakes.

An even more difficult situation results from exotic envenomations, for which the appropriate antivenom (if one exists) is certain to be a non–FDA-approved product and may be located at a zoo or other non–health care source quite distant from the location of the envenomation.

Antivenom, local wound care, and symptomatic and supportive care are the mainstays of envenomation management. A regional poison center should be contacted for information and assistance in managing any venomous snake exposure, including locating an appropriate antivenom. Poison centers have personnel who are experienced at assessing and managing envenomations and have access to a database, the Antivenom Index, which lists sources of non–FDA-approved antivenoms. Poison centers can be contacted from anywhere in the United States by calling 800-222-1222.

SNAKE IDENTIFICATION

Beyond determining whether the victim has been bitten by a coral snake or a viperid, it is relatively immaterial to know the species of the offending snake. A photo taken with a cell phone may be of some value to the treating physician, but it should be obtained only if it can be done safely and without causing a delay in transporting the patient. Viperid snakes are easily differentiated from coral snakes by virtue of the latter's distinctive color pattern of red, yellow, and black bands. It can be difficult to differentiate a coral snake from nonvenomous snakes that have similar markings. The ditty "red on yellow, kill a fellow; red on black, venom lack," which describes the red band being surrounded on either side by yellow or black, is accurate only for North American coral snakes. South American coral snakes have the opposite pattern.

Because all viperid envenomations are treated with a single product and the physical findings or laboratory evaluation is all that is required to determine that the snake is venomous, attempting to kill or capture the snake is unlikely to add additional information to treatment decisions but is likely to result in the individual being bitten a second time or other individuals becoming bite victims. Differences in the appearance of the bite wound (e.g., fang punctures, swelling, ecchymosis) and the observation of signs and symptoms are usually sufficient to determine whether the biting snake was venomous and to guide therapy.

For future reference, remember this advice: "Red on yellow, leave it alone. Red on black, leave it alone. Slithers on the ground, LEAVE IT ALONE."

FACTORS AFFECTING TOXICITY AND THE SEVERITY OF ENVENOMATION

Many factors govern whether an envenomation occurs after a bite, the signs and symptoms that develop, and the overall severity of effects. Up to 25% of viperid bites and up to 50% of elapid bites do not result in an envenomation. Barriers to fang penetration and other factors may result in no venom being injected. Patients must be watched for a sufficient length of time (i.e., 8 hours in a viperid bite and 24 hours in a coral snakebite) to ensure that this has been the case.

If an envenomation has occurred, the family and species of snake generally determines the spectrum of symptoms and signs. The amount of venom, specific venom components, and the underlying health status of the victim determine severity.

Viperid Envenomations

EPIDEMIOLOGY AND RECOGNITION

Viperid snakes are distributed throughout North America, with the apparent exception of Maine. Bites are more common in southern states and during summer months, but they occur year-round and may occur at any time and in any location with captive collections. The various genera and species of viperids in the United States have relatively stable geographic ranges, with much overlap. Many different species of venomous snakes may inhabit any given area. Nonvenomous or mildly venomous colubrid snakes are also native to the United States. Viperids, also called pit vipers (i.e., rattlesnakes, copperheads, and cottonmouths), may be recognized by a generally triangular-shaped head, the so-called pit (an infrared heat-detection organ) located approximately midway between the nostril and the eye, and pupils shaped like those of a cat (not round).

Pit vipers have large, movable fangs through which venom is injected into the victim. Because fangs are curved, venom is usually injected subcutaneously, rather than into deeper muscle compartments. Because of anatomic and other physical factors, bite wounds may appear as scratches or as one or more punctures. Envenomation may occur with a break in the skin.

Viperid venom is complex, consisting of dozens of proteolytic enzymes, small peptides, phospholipases, and other elements responsible for the spectrum of clinical effects seen. There is a great variability in this complex poison between species, within species, and even within a single specimen over the course of a season and lifespan.

CLINICAL EFFECTS

The spectrum of clinical effects is based on the specific genus or species of viperid and is unpredictable, ranging in any given event from a nonenvenomation (up to 25% of bites) to life-threatening reactions. Viperid snake envenomation invariably results in tissue injury, manifested by pain and progressive swelling, and it may include ecchymosis, elevated tissue and compartment pressures, tissue necrosis, and tissue loss. The complete absence of local effects can be used as a reliable marker of nonenvenomation in a viperid bite as long as a sufficient period (8–10 hours) of observation has occurred.

Systemic effects may occur, including hematologic, neurologic, cardiovascular, and nonspecific findings. Rattlesnake envenomations are more likely to result in hematologic effects, such as thrombocytopenia, hypofibrinogenemia, or prolongation of the prothrombin time (PT) or activated partial thromboplastin time (aPTT), and are more likely to produce neurologic effects, such as muscle fasciculation or weakness, compared with copperhead or cottonmouth envenomations, but these effects can be seen with any viperid snake. Hypotension from direct myocardial depression or from type 1 hypersensitivity (i.e., anaphylactic or anaphylactoid) reactions may occur with any viperid exposure. Nausea, vomiting, diaphoresis, anxiety, and other nonspecific effects may be seen.

DURATION OF CLINICAL EFFECTS

Local effects may develop rapidly or may not be apparent for many hours. Progression may occur for 24 to 36 hours, with resolution of tissue injury occurring over 3 to 6 weeks. Complications of tissue necrosis or infection have their own time frame of resolution. Hematologic effects usually begin within 1 to 2 hours of envenomation. If antivenom is given within this time frame, the detection of those effects may be masked and become apparent only after unbound antivenom has been eliminated from the body, usually 2 to 4 days after treatment. Hematologic effects may persist for 1 to 3 weeks after an envenomation. Neurologic and other systemic effects tend to occur within a few hours of envenomation and resolve over 24 to 36 hours.

SEVERITY OF ENVENOMATION

Untreated, local injury worsens over time, with proximal progression of tissue injury. Hematologic effects can be profound, resulting in spontaneous hemorrhage. Hypotension may be profound and can result in death. Neurologic and other systemic effects are rarely life-threatening events. Because of changes in basic medical care and health care systems, it is not directly applicable to compare case-fatality rates before the introduction of antivenom (1950) with what can be expected today. However, at that time, there were several hundred deaths per year in the United States from viperid envenomations.

MANAGEMENT

Determining Whether Envenomation Has Occurred and Its Severity

Because of the unpredictability of envenomation and the variability of possible clinical effects, each viperid bite must be assessed and responded to individually (Box 1). It is important to determine whether an envenomation has occurred. If there are no signs or symptoms of envenomation, there is no indication for antivenom or other specific treatment. The severity of the envenomation helps to determine the amount of antivenom required to counter and neutralize venom effects, but this may not be immediately apparent, because envenomations tend to progress over time, and what may at first appear to be mild venom effects may progress to a severe envenomation.

Initial Hospital Management

On arrival at the hospital, jewelry should be removed and the bitten extremity loosely splinted. The wound should be cleaned, and a radiograph should be obtained to rule out a foreign body (Box 2). Tetanus status should be updated if needed. In the absence of other factors, the extremity should be maintained slightly below heart level until antivenom is started and then should be elevated. If there are immediate life-threatening effects (e.g., anaphylaxis, hypotension), the extremity should be placed in an inferior position and consideration given to impeding venom entry into central circulation by means of a lymphatic constriction band or pressure immobilization bandage, weighing the potential benefit against the possible risk of

---

> **BOX 1 Prehospital Management of Viperid Envenomation**
>
> - Remove jewelry.
> - Splint the extremity and maintain just below heart level.
> - Expeditiously transport to a health care facility.
> - Consider use of lymphatic constriction band (blood pressure cuff at 15–25 mm Hg) *for life-threatening effects only.*
> - Obtain intravenous access if possible.
> - Do not use cutting, sucking, heat, cold, or other local "therapies."

increased local tissue injury from increasing venom concentration and duration in the tissues. Patients often require opioid-level pain relief.

At least one large intravenous line should be initiated and crystalloid infused as needed. Initial hospital therapy, including a first dose of antivenom, should be provided in an area capable of close monitoring of vital signs and capable of managing life-threatening reactions; this usually is an emergency department. Whether an intensive care unit (ICU) or similar patient care area is used for subsequent management depends on the clinical situation.

Indications for Antivenom

Because of the safety of the current FDA-approved antivenom and its ability to stop proximal progression of local tissue injury, all patients with signs of progressive local envenomation effects and those with significant systemic effects are candidates for treatment with antivenom.

Depending on the original indication for treatment, initial control of envenomation effects is the goal of the loading dose of antivenom. The only FDA-approved viperid antivenom for North American pit viper envenomation is Crotalidae Polyvalent Immune Fab (ovine) Antivenin (CroFab), which is an ovine-based Fab antivenom. The incidence of type 1 hypersensitivity reactions is approximately 6%. There are rare reports of IgE-mediated type 1 hypersensitivity reactions on repeat exposure in individuals who were previously treated with CroFab, but most people who have been previously treated do not develop an adverse reaction to subsequent administrations. The incidence of type 3 hypersensitivity reactions ("serum sickness") is also approximately 6%. Pretreatment sensitivity testing is not required or recommended. The half-life of this antivenom is approximately 18 to 24 hours, which is considerably shorter than IgG or F(ab')2 antivenoms, and it is responsible for the recurrence of hematologic effects in approximately 70% of patients with an initial coagulopathy.

For moderate to severe envenomations, antivenom is administered as an intravenous solution, with 4 to 6 vials diluted into 250 to 500 mL of D₅W or normal saline. Treatment of life-threatening envenomations may be started with 10 to 12 vials. The infusion should be run slowly for the first 5 to 10 minutes, and the patient should be observed closely for a type 1 hypersensitivity reaction. If such a reaction occurs, the infusion should be slowed or stopped, depending on the severity, and appropriate symptomatic treatment should be started with H₁- and H₂-blockers, epinephrine, corticosteroids, and other supportive measures, as needed. It should be determined whether antivenom is still required, and if so, it should be restarted at a slower rate or higher dilution, or both. If a reaction does not occur, the infusion is concluded over 1 hour.

Treatment of Local Tissue Injury

If the antivenom is given exclusively for local findings, the syndromic response to envenomation is deemed to be controlled if there is cessation of proximal progression of edema at the end of the infusion. There is often some redistribution of existing tissue edema, and continued proximal progression is usually distinguishable by a raised, tender, and perhaps erythematous leading edge of edema. If antivenom is being given for hematologic effects, cessation of worsening or reversal should be seen. Often, thrombocytopenia rebounds dramatically. Hypofibrinogenemia may not rebound as quickly or merely stabilize, because the liver must manufacture new fibrinogen. Although an elevated D-dimer value indicates fibrinogenolytic activity, it is not an independent indicator for antivenom treatment.

Other systemic effects may serve as indicators for antivenom use, and they should show control by the end of the initial infusion. If initial control is not deemed to have occurred, additional doses of antivenom should be administered until initial control is determined to have occurred. Most patients achieve initial control with 4 to 12 vials of antivenom, although more may be required.

Maintenance Doses

Because of the rapid decline of antivenom levels resulting from the larger volume of distribution of Fab antivenoms, after initial control is achieved, maintenance dosing of 2 vials every 6 hours for three doses is commenced. This usually maintains adequate antivenom serum levels to prevent recurrence of local tissue injury progression. If progression does recur, an additional 2 vials of antivenom usually are sufficient to control local worsening. Tissue pressures may be increased, and elevated muscle compartment pressures may be identified when measured directly. My colleagues and I do not routinely measure tissue or compartment pressures. When pressures are measured and demonstrated to be elevated, it should be remembered that the mechanisms of these phenomena are different from other muscle compartment syndromes. For example, extensive edema in the subcutaneous space circumferentially in an extremity may elevate compartment pressures by extrinsic compression. Case reports and series suggest that additional antivenom and extremity elevation result in reduced tissue and compartment pressures. Intracompartmental injection of venom can result in a true compartment syndrome. However, there is no evidence that fasciotomy is beneficial in this setting, and there are animal data to suggest that it may result in worse clinical outcomes.

Bleb formation at the site of a bite is not an important sign in and of itself, although it may suggest significantly elevated tissue pressures resulting in dermal-epidermal separation or the presence of tissue necrosis. Bleb fluid may contain unneutralized venom. It is reasonable to unroof blebs at or near the bite site and to débride obviously necrotic tissue that usually becomes apparent several days after the bite.

Antibiotics

The incidence of culture-proven infection in U.S. viperid bites is low, probably less than 5%. There are no data to support the use of prophylactic antibiotics, and it is best to limit the opportunities for adverse drug effects. It is often difficult to distinguish inflammatory venom effects from infection starting on the second day after an envenomation. If antibiotics are prescribed, a first-generation, broad-spectrum agent should be used.

Long-Term Local Tissue Effects

The edema and tissue injury produced by most North American viperid envenomations usually resolves within 1 to 2 months, and a return to normal function can be anticipated. However, tissue necrosis or deep tissue injury may result in longer-term or even permanent structural and functional disability. Loss of tissue may occur, including digits and other parts of extremities, although this is rare and may be associated with prehospital application of tourniquets or other imprudent surgical interventions, delayed care, or complications such as infections. Some victims engage in behaviors that result in multiple envenomations, and this may increase the risks of long-term tissue injury.

Hematologic Abnormalities and Bleeding

One or more hematologic abnormalities may occur with native viperid envenomation (Box 3). Significant decreases in platelet count or fibrinogen concentrations are independent indications for antivenom treatment. Isolated, mild prolongations of PT or aPTT may not require antivenom treatment. However, these effects may be progressive or indicate an impending hypofibrinogenemia, and early antivenom treatment may prevent severe abnormalities. Even if

platelets, fibrinogen, and intrinsic and extrinsic clotting systems are involved, the end result is not a true disseminated intravascular coagulopathy, because there is no true intravascular coagulation. Sufficient platelets, fibrinogen, and thrombin are usually available for hemostasis, and clinically significant bleeding is rarely seen. However, severe depletion of individual clotting elements or a combination of hematologic abnormalities can result in bleeding.

The management of initial or persistent laboratory abnormalities is achieved with additional antivenom. Administration of blood products (e.g., fresh-frozen plasma [FFP], platelet concentrates, other blood products) should be reserved for clinically significant bleeding and be given in conjunction with additional antivenom, because transfused elements are similarly likely to be consumed by venom activity. Ecchymoses in damaged tissues, expansion of the vascular volume from crystalloid administration, and red blood cell hemolysis from hemolytic venom factors may produce an anemia that may rarely require a red blood cell transfusion.

Recurrence of Hematologic Effects

Approximately 70% of patients who develop an initial hematologic effect will have a recurrence of those effects 2 to 4 days after initial treatment. The severity of the recurrence is usually similar to the initial effects. A person who presented with a severe thrombocytopenia is likely to return with recurrent severe thrombocytopenia. The mechanism is recurrent unneutralized venomemia after elimination of unbound Fab antivenom. The recurrent effects may be milder, because there is less venom in the body and severity is a function of venom effect and the body's ability to produce factors such as platelets or fibrinogen in excess of their rate of consumption. Recurrent effects may be more severe, however, or even appear to be occurring de novo if the patient was treated soon after envenomation, blunting the acute effects of the venom and masking the true severity of the envenomation.

Patients who present with severe early hematologic effects or who are treated with antivenom within 1 to 2 hours of envenomation are at risk for severe recurrent effects and should be followed closely after discharge. Although the incidence of significant bleeding is low, even with profound laboratory abnormalities, it seems prudent to administer additional antivenom if the platelet count is less than 25,000, the fibrinogen level is less than 50 mg/dL, the PT or PTT values indicate nonclotting, there is a combination of significant defects in coagulation, or there are underlying medical conditions that make hemorrhage more likely, such as advanced age, hypertension, or a bleeding diathesis. Additional antivenom can be given on an outpatient basis, although patients with any significant bleeding or at high risk for bleeding should be readmitted. Two vials of antivenom should be given, with daily follow-up until hematologic laboratory values are improving, which may take 2 to 3 weeks in some cases.

DISPOSITION

Patients whose local effects are regressing and do not have complications, such as infection or necrosis, and whose hematologic and other systemic effects are controlled may be discharged. Typically, this occurs between 36 and 48 hours after envenomation. Ongoing pain relief may be required, with an effort to transition to nonopioid agents during the first week, and the patient should be warned to watch for signs of serum sickness. Occupational or physical therapy should be arranged to maximize return of function, and follow-up for local and systemic effects should be arranged.

Elapid Envenomations

EPIDEMIOLOGY AND RECOGNITION

U.S. coral snakes can be recognized by their distinctive band pattern, with a red band seeming to be placed on top of a larger yellow band. This color pattern applies only to North American coral snakes. Each year, there are approximately 75 to 100 bites by coral snakes in the United States. Two genera and several species inhabit the United States, with the *Micrurus* genus responsible for most bites in Florida,

---

BOX 3   Management of Hematologic Effects and Recurrence in Viperid Envenomation

- Administer 4 to 6 vials of antivenom (Crotalidae polyvalent immune Fab [Ovine]) for significant abnormalities of platelet count, PT or INR, aPTT, or fibrinogen. An elevated D-dimer value indicates accelerated fibrinogen breakdown and should prompt close monitoring of the fibrinogen concentrations, but it is not an independent indication to treat with antivenom.
- Administer additional antivenom in 4- to 6-vial increments until there is reversal of hematologic abnormalities. Replacement of platelets, clotting factors, or fibrinogen may be gradual, and a positive trend indicates neutralization of venom or replacement in excess of venom effect.
- Patients with initial hematologic effects or who were treated within 1 to 2 hours of envenomation are at risk for recurrent effects 2 to 4 days after treatment and should be followed closely: every other day until no recurrence at 4 days or daily for declining parameters.
- Consider treating recurrent hematologic abnormalities with additional antivenom. Indications include platelets <25,000/mm^3; fibrinogen <50 mg/dL; INR >5; aPTT >150 seconds; and lesser abnormalities involving more than one parameter.
- Consider readmission for severe abnormalities, other risk factors (e.g., uncontrolled hypertension, advanced age, other bleeding diatheses), or clinically significant bleeding.
- Administer blood products *plus* additional antivenom for significant bleeding.

Abbreviations: aPTT = activated partial thromboplastin time; INR = International Normalized Ratio; PT = prothrombin time.

Texas, Georgia, Louisiana, Alabama, and some neighboring states. A smaller genus, *Micruroides*, is found in Arizona and New Mexico, but it is responsible for very few bites, and there have been no reports of serious envenomations in recent years. Bites are more common during the warmer months.

Elapids have relatively short, fixed fangs, which may decrease the rate of envenomation. More than one puncture, deep punctures, and a history of the snake hanging on increases the risk of envenomation.

CLINICAL EFFECTS

Envenomation by the coral snake produces primarily neurologic toxicity from presynaptic toxins initially producing bulbar muscle weakness, ptosis, diplopia, and dysphagia. These effects can begin within 15 to 30 minutes or may be delayed up to 24 hours after an envenomation. Muscle weakness and paralysis progress to include respiratory muscles, and they can result in respiratory arrest and death. Typical of presynaptic toxins, effect progression can be arrested with the use of antivenom, but the effects are not rapidly reversed. Typically, there is no or little local tissue injury, and the absence of local injury cannot be used to exclude envenomation. Likewise, there is usually no effect on hematologic function, and other systemic effects are rare. Patients cannot be assumed to have eluded envenomation by a coral snake because they lack these symptoms, and patients should be observed for at least 24 hours before concluding that an envenomation has not occurred.

Because of changes in basic medical care and health care systems, it is not directly applicable to compare case-fatality rates before the introduction of antivenom (1967) with what can be expected today. However, at that time, the case-fatality rate was approximately 10%.

MANAGEMENT

Because of the potential for rapid progression of motor paralysis and respiratory compromise, the difficulty of reversing paralysis after it is established, and the lack of local effects, it is reasonable to attempt to retard venom progression into the circulation until a decision regarding antivenom can be made. A pressure immobilization band (i.e., elastic bandage wrapped from an extremity's tip to trunk with the degree of tension used for sprains) is used for this purpose for elapid envenomations elsewhere in the world (Boxes 4 and 5). However, the proper technique requires training, and the infrequency of these bites makes teaching and retention of such skills problematic. A blood pressure cuff inflated to 15 to 25 mm Hg may also retard venom entry into circulation, and it can be a more reliable and easily taught technique, although it has not been validated in clinical studies.

Standard wound care should be performed, including cleansing the wound, obtaining a radiograph, and updating the tetanus status, if needed. Wound infection is uncommon, and prophylactic antibiotics are not recommended.

Because the first signs of envenomation can be rapidly progressive neurotoxicity and because of the difficulty of reversing paralysis, some authorities have proposed administering antivenom in cases in which an envenomation is possible, before the appearance of any

---

BOX 4   Prehospital Management of Elapid Envenomation

- Remove jewelry.
- Splint the extremity and maintain just below heart level.
- Expeditiously transport to a health care facility.
- Apply a pressure immobilization bandage (i.e., 3- to 4-inch crepe bandage at lymphatic pressure from the tip of the extremity to the trunk) or a lymphatic constriction band (i.e., wide rubber band or blood pressure cuff at 15–25 mm Hg) proximal to the bite site.
- Obtain intravenous access if possible.
- Do not use cutting, sucking, heat, cold, or other local "therapies."

BOX 5   Hospital Diagnosis and Initial Management of Elapid Envenomation

- Remove jewelry.
- If an arterial or venous tourniquet has been placed, convert to a lymphatic constriction band.
- Obtain intravenous access, and use crystalloid as indicated.
- Determine whether an envenomation has occurred.
- Determine severity based on the family or species of snake, the age and health status of the victim, and the rate of progression of signs or symptoms (i.e., paralysis and other neurologic effects).
- Determine the tetanus vaccination status and update if necessary.
- Seek consultation from a poison center: 800-222-1222.
- If a pressure immobilization band or lymphatic constriction band has been placed before arrival at the hospital, determine whether antivenom is needed, and begin antivenom infusion before removing the band.
- Determine whether antivenom is indicated, and administer per protocol.
- Provide basic wound care (i.e., cleaning and radiograph), and determine whether local injury requires specific management.
- Determine whether other systemic effects require specific management.

---

clinical symptoms. Others have pointed to the infrequency of respiratory muscle paralysis resulting in the need for intubation and respiratory support and to possible geographic differences in snake toxicity, and they have counseled observation and antivenom treatment only after envenomation has been confirmed by progressive symptoms. Recent analysis of the national database has not demonstrated a significant difference in clinical severity between Florida and Texas coral snake envenomations, which supports early treatment. However, the impending loss of an FDA-approved coral snake antivenom (Antivenin)[2] is likely to result in delays of many hours before antivenom can be administered, if it is available at all. Aggressive and meticulous respiratory support, including intubation and ventilation that may be needed for days to weeks, should ultimately result in survival of even severe neurotoxic envenomations.

Exotic Snakebite

EPIDEMIOLOGY AND CLINICAL EFFECTS

In the United States, most exotic snake envenomations occur in private collections. These are not usually known to authorities or health care providers until an envenomation occurs, and they may involve the collection owner or family members, including children. They may occur in any locale, and victims may present to any health care facility.

Viperid and elapid snakes, which account for the bulk of venomous bites worldwide, have patterns of venom activity similar to those of their North American counterparts, with some variation and with generally greater toxicity for some non-U.S. species. Some nonnative elapids, such as cobras, mambas, black snakes, or taipans, produce much higher rates of respiratory paralysis and may produce much greater local tissue injury than U.S. coral snakes. Similarly, envenomation from some nonnative viperids, such as *Bothrops*, *Echis*, or *Bitis* species, or from an African colubrid, such as the boomslang, results in a greater risk of bleeding. Some of these species may directly activate prothrombin (e.g., *Echis* species, *Bothrops* species) and factor X (e.g., *Vipera* species, *Dispholidus* species), leading to a true disseminated intravascular coagulopathy with intravascular thrombosis, marked organ dysfunction, and potentially, death.

---

[2]Not available in the United States.

MANAGEMENT

The specific management of exotic envenomations is beyond the scope of this chapter. Not all venomous exotic snakes have antivenoms, and even for snakes with antivenoms, none may be available in the United States, but zoos stock antivenoms for snakes in their collections. An updateable online database, the Antivenom Index, lists these antivenoms and is accessible by regional poison centers. For information on exotic antivenoms and assistance in managing an exotic snake envenomation, the regional poison center should be contacted (1-800-222-1222).

REFERENCES

Boyer LV, Seifert SA, Cain JS. Recurrence phenomena after immunoglobulin therapy for snake envenomations. Part 2. Guidelines for clinical management with Crotaline Fab antivenom. Ann Emerg Med 2001;37:196–201.

Boyer LV, Seifert SA, Clark RF, et al. Recurrent and persistent coagulopathy following pit viper envenomation. Arch Intern Med 1999;159(7):706–10.

Gold BS, Barish RA, Dart RC. North American snake envenomation: Diagnosis, treatment, and management. Emerg Med Clin North Am 2004;22(2):423–43 ix.

Kitchens CS, Van Mierop LH. Envenomation by the Eastern coral snake (*Micrurus fulvius fulvius*). A study of 39 victims. JAMA 1987;258(12):1615–8.

Seifert SA, Boyer LV. Recurrence phenomena after immunoglobulin therapy for snake envenomations. Part 1. Pharmacokinetics and pharmacodynamics of immunoglobulin antivenoms and related antibodies. Ann Emerg Med 2001;37(2):189–95.

Seifert SA, Boyer LV, Dart RC, et al. Relationship of venom effects to venom antigen and antivenom serum concentrations in a patient with *Crotalus atrox* envenomation treated with a Fab antivenom. Ann Emerg Med 1997;30(1):49–53.

Seifert SA, Oakes JA, Boyer LV. Toxic Exposure Surveillance System (TESS)-based characterization of U.S. non-native venomous snake exposures, 1995–2004. Clin Toxicol (Phila) 2007;45(5):571–8.

Marine Poisonings, Envenomations, and Trauma

Method of
Allen Perkins, MD, MPH

The United States has more than 80,000 miles of coastline, and more people are enjoying water-dependent recreation activities such as scuba diving, snorkeling, and surfing. As a consequence, people are more likely to suffer trauma, envenomation, or poisoning related to an encounter with a marine creature, which will come to the attention of a physician. The science of marine medicine is limited; hence, treatment of these conditions is largely based on case reports and expert opinion; very few randomized, controlled studies are available. Misdiagnosis is common, especially when the patient has returned from vacationing or when the patient has been poisoned by improperly handled seafood. This article describes common ailments and injuries occurring as a consequence of direct contact with sea creatures and discusses management and prevention.

Ingestions

CIGUATERA

Epidemiology

Ciguatera poisoning is the most commonly reported marine toxin disease in the world. It is caused by human ingestion of reef fish that have bioaccumulated sufficient amounts of the dinoflagellate *Gambierdiscus toxicus*, either through direct ingestion or through ingestion of smaller reef fish. Although limited to tropical regions, it is heat and cold tolerant, is lipid soluble, and can survive transport to other areas. The toxin becomes more concentrated as it passes up the food chain; fish such as amberjack, grouper, and snapper pose less of a risk than predatory fish such as barracuda and moray eel. Ciguatera poisoning affects at least 50,000 people worldwide annually, and there are several thousand cases of poisoning in Puerto Rico, the U.S. Virgin Islands, Hawaii, and Florida each year.

Clinical Features

Patients can exhibit a primarily gastrointestinal (diarrhea, abdominal cramps, and vomiting), neurologic (parasthesias, diffuse pain, blurred vision), cardiac (bradycardia), or mixed pattern of symptoms. Additionally, a cold sensation reversal, in which a patient perceives the cold temperatures as a hot sensation and vice versa, occurs in 80% of patients and is considered pathognomonic for ciguatera poison (Box 1).

The attack rate is high. As many as 80% to 100% of people who ingest affected fish develop symptoms depending on the size of the fish and the toxin load. Ingestion of internal organs where the toxin accumulates (e.g., liver, roe) is associated with more severe symptoms, but avoiding these organs is not protective. The symptoms are also related to the number of exposures over time, and patients typically have more severe symptoms with subsequent exposures. There is no age-related susceptibility, and no immunity is acquired through exposure.

Symptoms typically begin 1 to 6 hours after ingestion, although a delay of 12 to 24 hours can occur. Duration is 7 to 14 days, and neurologic symptoms occasionally persist for months to years. Chronic ciguatera syndrome can also occur as a constellation of symptoms such as general malaise, depression, headaches, muscle aches, and dysesthesias in the extremities. Patients with chronic disease report recurrences with ingestion of fish, ethanol, caffeine, and nuts up to 6 months after the acute illness resolves.

Diagnosis

The diagnosis should be entertained in any patient who has neurologic, gastrointestinal, or cardiac symptoms and a history of ingesting predatory fish within the past 24 hours. The symptom constellation can be

---

BOX 1	Symptom Patterns Associated With Ciguatera Poisoning

Gastrointestinal Pattern

Onset 15 minutes to 24 hours, typically worsens, lasts 1–2 days and resolves
- Nausea and/or vomiting
- Profuse, watery diarrhea
- Abdominal pain

Neurologic Pattern

Onset up to 24 hours after ingestion, commonly nonphysiologic pattern, can last several months
- Numbness and paresthesias
- Vertigo
- Ataxia
- Severe weakness or lethargy
- Severe myalgia
- Decreased vibration and pain sensations
- Diffuse pain pattern
- Cold sensation reversal
- Coma

Cardiovascular Pattern

Onset up to 24 hours after ingestion is uncommon but occurs rapidly
- Bradycardia
- Hypotension
- Cardiovascular collapse

CURRENT DIAGNOSIS

- History of exposure is necessary for diagnosis.
- Ingested toxins can cause unusual symptoms, predominately gastrointestinal.
- Jellyfish envenomation is very painful but almost always self-limited.
- Trauma management follows principles of dirty wounds.
- Specific marine pathogens should be covered if contamination is suspected.

similar to other ingestions, such as certain shellfish toxins, and differentiation requires knowledge of the patient's diet for the previous day. Additionally, scombroid and type E botulinum poisoning should be considered, but these are unlikely if the patient did not ingest ill-appearing game. Other poisonings, such as organophosphates, can produce a similar symptom complex. There are no currently available clinical assays to assist in making the diagnosis, which is based on clinical suspicion and knowledge of the patient's diet history.

Treatment

If ciguatera poisoning is suspected soon after ingestion, I would consider gut decontamination with activated charcoal (Actidose-Aqua) because it can reduce the toxin load and subsequent symptoms. Initial symptomatic treatment typically consists of fluid replacement to replace gastrointestinal losses.

Atropine (AtroPen) is used in patients who have bradycardia. Temporary electrical pacing may be used for refractory symptoms, and pressors may be needed in cases of severe hypotension. Neurologic symptoms are problematic because of their extended course as well as their severity. Mannitol (Osmitrol)[1] is often cited as effective in reducing the duration of neurologic symptoms, but I would use it with caution because the only double-blind trial failed to show any benefit. Nifedipine (Procardia)[1] (adult dose 10–20 mg three times daily) shows some theoretical promise in this regard, but there have been no studies in humans at this time. There are many local remedies used throughout the world that are said to be successful, which

---

[1]Not FDA approved for this indication.

likely attests to the self-limited course of the ingestion in most cases. Table 1 offers more details regarding treatments currently used for ciguatera poisoning.

Prevention

Prevention is difficult except by avoiding ingestion of affected reef fish. The toxin is not deactivated by cooking, freezing, smoking, or salting. There are no outward signs of ciguatera: The fish look, taste, and smell normal. Although several commercial assays are available, they are neither sensitive nor specific enough to be relied on to prevent ciguatera poisoning.

To decrease the risk of ciguatera poisoning, I recommend the following steps: Avoid warm-water reef fish, especially those caught where ciguatera poisoning is known to occur; avoid moray eel injection; avoid ingesting large game fish; avoid consuming the internal organs; and limit the amount of initial ingestion if you are in an area where ciguatera is known to occur. Additionally, patients travelling to distant locales should be made aware that, although the vast majority of cases result from direct ingestion, there have been cases of ciguatera passed through sexual contact and through breast milk, so they should be wary of body fluid contact if ciguatoxin is endemic to the area, if for no other reasons.

SCOMBROID

Epidemiology

Scombroid poisoning (also known as histamine fish poisoning) results from improper handling of certain fish between the time the fish is caught and the time it is cooked. In the United States it is most common in Hawaii and California. Improper preservation and refrigeration lead to histamine and histamine-like substances being produced in the dark meat of certain fish through a conversion of histadine to histamine by bacterial decarboxylases. Members of the family Scombridae, such as tuna and mackerel, contain the highest amounts of this substance, but both scombroid and nonscombroid fish have been associated with the disease. The production of toxins requires the introduction of bacteria during the handling process, primarily during storage at high temperatures. It is the total amount of histamine, the presence of other biogenic amines, and individual susceptibility that determine the severity of the symptoms.

Clinical Features

The patient develops a histamine reaction 20 to 30 minutes after ingestion. Symptoms can be cutaneous, gastrointestinal, neurologic,

---

TABLE 1 Treatment for Ciguatera Poisoning

Drug	Dose	Indication
Activated charcoal (Actidose-Aqua)	Children <1 y: 1 g/kg Children 1–12 y: 25–50 g Adults: 25–100 g	Gut emptying and decontamination More effective in first h
Antiemetics (no preference)	Administer per dosing recommendations	Intractable nausea and/or vomiting
Intravenous fluid bolus and infusion (normal saline or lactated Ringer's as initial)	Per volume replacement protocols	Hypovolemia
Atropine (AtroPen)	0.5–1.0 mg IV every 3–5 min to a maximum dose of 0.04 mg/kg per episode Maximum total dose: 3 mg for adults, 2 mg for adolescents, 1 mg for young children	Bradycardia
Pressors: Dopamine (Intropin), dobutamine (Dobutrex), epinephrine	Varies with clinical response	Hypotension, shock
Antihistamines (no preference)	Administer per dosing recommendations	Pruritis
Mannitol (Osmitrol)[1]	1 g/kg of a 20% solution given IV over several h Adult dose 25–100 g, titrate to urinary output of 100 mL/h	Neurologic symptoms, double-blind study did not show benefit
Amitriptyline (Elavil)[1]	25–75 mg PO bid for patients >25 kg	Pruritis, dysesthesias

[1]Not FDA approved for this indication.

or hemodynamic or any combination of these. Cutaneous (flushing, urticaria and conjunctival injection, and localized edema; gastrointestinal symptoms include dry mouth, nausea, vomiting, diarrhea, and abdominal cramping; neurologic symptoms include severe headache and dizziness; and hemodynamic symptoms include palpitations and hypotension. In severe cases there can be bronchospasm and respiratory distress. These symptoms typically come on rapidly (within several minutes) and last less than 6 to 8 hours. Flushing is the most consistent clinical sign, occurring on exposed areas so it typically resembles sunburn. Diarrhea is also very common, occurring in 75% of symptomatic patients.

Diagnosis

As with ciguatera, the diagnosis is one of history. If the time between ingestion and illness is short and the patient has ingested a type of fish previously implicated in scombroid, then a tentative diagnosis can be made. The diagnosis is often confused with an allergic reaction. It can be distinguished from allergy by the lack of a previous allergic reaction as well as by testing the remaining fish for histamine, although testing is rarely warranted.

Treatment

Treatment is the same as for any histamine reaction, the cornerstone of which is antihistamine. Diphenhydramine (Benadryl) 50 mg for adults and 0.5–1 mg/kg/dose for children, repeated every 4 hours until symptoms abate, is delivered either intravenously or intramuscularly in severe cases and orally for milder cases. For severe cases, cimetidine (Tagamet)[1] 300 mg for adults, 20 mg/kg for children, either orally or intravenously, might be added for more complete histamine-receptor blockade. In cases where ingestion was recent, consider induced emesis using syrup of ipecac: 15 mL for children younger than 12 years or 30 mL otherwise. Most patients require only reassurance, and pharmacologic treatment will be unnecessary. It should be stressed to the patient that this is not an *allergic* reaction to fish, because the histamine is exogenous. Prevention is possible in regions where food storage and preparation are monitored through identification and removal of suspect fish.

OTHER INGESTED TOXINS

In addition to the toxins just discussed, ingestion of certain other marine creatures can lead to problems.

Ingestion of bivalves harvested from contaminated waters has been associated with hepatitis A, Norwalk virus, *Vibrio parahaemolyticus* and *Vibrio vulnificans* infections, the latter two particularly problematic and occasionally fatal in immunocompromised patients. I counsel patients likely to be immunocompromised, including diabetics and those with known liver disease, to avoid uncooked bivalves.

Shellfish are occasionally known to contain one or more of several toxins acquired through bioaccumulation of certain algae. These dinoflagellates tend to bloom in summer months. The symptoms occur immediately after ingestion and last several hours and are typically neurologic or gastrointestinal, or both. The shellfish poisoning syndromes are known as paralytic, neurologic, diarrheal, or amnestic depending on the predominant symptom. The care is typically supportive. Public health officials typically monitor local mollusk populations fairly carefully and alert the public to possible hazards.

Ingestion of the flesh of certain puffer fish has been associated with tetrodotoxin poisoning. The flesh of the fish (fugu) is considered a delicacy. The toxin builds up in internal organs such as the liver and the roe. If the toxin is ingested, it is likely to be fatal but there are certified chefs who are trained in avoiding the toxin when preparing the dish. Despite this precaution, as many as 50 deaths occur in Japan annually from exposure to this toxin. Avoiding this puffer fish and avoiding the ingestion of certain other exotic animals (such as the blue-ringed octopus) eliminate the risk of acquiring this toxin.

Envenomations

Many marine creatures are venomous, and beachgoers experience clinically significant envenomations with some regularity. Jellyfish and related creatures (Cnidarians), sea urchins (Echinodermata), and stingrays (Chondrichthyes) are some of the more commonly identified marine animals involved with envenomations.

JELLYFISH

These invertebrates have stinging cells called *nematocytes*, which carry nematocysts that continue to function when separated from the larger organism. For example, jellyfish nematocysts can sting if the tentacle is separated and after the jellyfish is dead. The venom is antigenic and causes a reaction of a dermatonecrotic, hemolytic, cardiopathic, or neurotoxic nature. The severity of the reaction depends on several variables, including the number of nematocysts that discharge, the toxicity of the coelenterate involved, and each patient's unique antigenic response.

Clinical Features

Although occasionally fatal as a consequence of an anaphylactic response in the United States and Caribbean, the primary concern in these areas with contact is pain, which is almost always self-limiting. Other less common symptoms include parasthesias, nausea, headaches, and chills. The symptoms may last up to 2 to 3 days. Certain Pacific jellyfish primarily found in the waters around Australia have a more potent toxin and are much more likely to cause death (which is still very uncommon). Additionally, the Irukandji syndrome, which occurs in the Pacific, is a suite of symptoms including muscle spasms, vomiting, hypertension, incessant coughing, and occasionally heart failure and brain hemorrhage. Almost all exposed people, regardless of the geographic location, do not have a severe reaction, and the principles of first aid are primarily the same throughout the world.

Treatment

In my experience, treatment is mostly concerned with limiting pain and neurologic symptoms, because anaphylaxis and other severe reactions are rare, and the following general guidelines can be applied. In the field, either the victim or a companion should remove any visible tentacles. To do so requires using care, with gloves or forceps being optimal to prevent further stings. If a towel is used, any nematocysts remaining on the towel can still discharge. Household vinegar will prevent discharge of the remaining nematocysts on the skin and should be applied liberally when available. If vinegar is not available in the field, salt water can be used to wash off the nematocysts. Urine, fresh water, and rubbing with sand should be avoided.

Should the victim present to the physician's office or emergency department, household vinegar (5% acetic acid)[1] should be liberally applied for 30 minutes or until the pain subsides followed by removal of the nematocysts, usually through use of the gloved hand or with forceps. Another method for removing the nematocysts is to apply shaving cream or baking soda slurry to the area and scrape off the nematocysts with a razor. Applications of cold, in the form of an ice pack, and immesion in hot water have variously been shown to improve pain, but because of the self-limited nature of the discomfort it is hard to gauge an optimum therapy. Either is probably acceptable until the patient is comfortable. Meat tenderizer has been found to be ineffective. Local anesthetics, antihistamines, and steroids are all used to control prolonged symptoms based on anecdotal experience. Antibiotics are not generally necessary. In the rare cases of cardiovascular collapse, supportive care and principles of treatment of anaphylaxis should be followed. A delayed hypersensitivity reaction can occur 1 to 3 days out, which will almost certainly be self-limited and can be treated with oral antihistamines and topical steroids if symptoms are severe.

---

[1]Not FDA approved for this indication.

[1]Not FDA approved for this indication.

CURRENT THERAPY

Ingestions

- Avoidance is the best strategy.
- Early decontamination with activated charcoal (Actidose-Aqua) can reduce duration of symptoms.
- Symptomatic care is generally sufficient.

Jellyfish

- Remove visible stingers.
- Acetic acid 5%[1] can be used to denature stingers on skin.
- Control pain with topical analgesia.

Trauma

- Avoiding water at feeding time can help to avoid injury.
- If envenomation is suspected, consider hot water immersion.
- Tetanus status should be checked.
- Antibiotic coverage should take marine pathogens into account.

[1]Not FDA approved for this indication.

Sea bather's itch is a form of jellyfish sting caused by the larvae of the thimble jellyfish. It is characterized by a painful, itchy rash under the edges of the bathing suit or wet suit. It can occasionally progress to a popular rash. Topical steroids can be used to relieve symptoms.

Prevention

Prevention is mostly a matter of common sense. Staying away from the organism (the tentacles can extend several meters from the body of the organism) and staying out of the water when jellyfish are known to be present are the most effective. There is a commercially available product, Safe Sea, which has been shown to reduce the number of nematocyst discharges and thus the severity of the sting should a swimmer need to be in the water when jellyfish are present. Wetsuits and other protective gear are ineffective.

ECHINODERMS

The Echinoderm family includes sea urchins. Urchins have toxin-coated spines that break off, leaving calcareous material in the wound, which can potentially cause infection. Symptoms include local pain, burning, and local discoloration. The discoloration is thought to be a temporary tattooing of the skin resulting from dye in the spines; absence of a spine is indicated if the discoloration spontaneously resolves within 48 hours. Theoretically, hot water disables the toxin, although there is no evidence in humans that it is effective. If a spine is present and easily accessible, it should be removed with fingers or forceps. If it is close to a joint or neurovascular structure it should be surgically removed. If the spines do not cause symptoms, retained pieces will likely reabsorb into the skin.

STINGRAYS

Although many fish are venomous, stingrays are the most clinically important, accounting for an estimated 1500 mostly minor injuries in the United States annually. These creatures partially bury themselves in the shallow, sandy bottom of the ocean, leading water enthusiasts to accidentally step on them or grab at what they think is a seashell.

Clinical Features

Stingrays have a spine at the base of their tail, which contains a venom gland. The spine, including the venom gland, is broken off and may be left in the resulting wound. The venom has vasoconstrictive properties that can lead to cyanosis and necrosis with poor wound healing and infection. Symptoms can include immediate and intense pain, salivation, nausea, vomiting, diarrhea, muscle cramps, dyspnea, seizures, headaches, and cardiac arrhythmias. Fatalities are rare and mostly a consequence of exsanguination at the scene or penetration of a vital organ.

Treatment

Home care should include rinsing the area thoroughly with fresh water if available (salt water if not) and removing any foreign body. If the damage is minimal the victim may soak the wound in warm water at home. The victim should watch for signs of infection and seek care for excessive bleeding, retained foreign body, or infection.

For severe wounds that lead the victim to seek medical attention, treatment should include achieving hemostasis followed by submersion of the affected region in hot but not scalding water (42–45°C, 108–113°F) for 30 to 90 minutes or until the pain resolves. Spines and stingers are typically radiopaque, so radiographs or an ultrasound should be obtained if a retained spine is suspected. The wound should be thoroughly cleansed, and delayed closure should be allowed. Tetanus immunization status should be reviewed and updated as appropriate. Surgical exploration may be necessary to remove residual foreign bodies. Prophylactic antibiotics are typically not necessary unless there is a residual foreign body or if the patient is immunosuppressed. If the wound becomes infected, *Staphylococcus* and *Streptococcus* species are the most common pathologic organisms. Unique to the marine environment are *Vibrio vulnificus* and *Mycobacterium marinum*, and antibiotic coverage should include coverage for all of these (Table 2).

OTHER VENOMOUS SEA CREATURES

Seasnakes are venomous creatures found most commonly in the Indo-Pacific area. Bites are uncommon (and envenomation is even less common), but should they occur, the toxin is very potent. The care is supportive. There is antivenom, which may be available in areas where the snakes are endemic.

Certain other fish and octopi have been associated with envenomation and occasional death. Most are tropical such as the stonefish, scorpionfish, and rabbitfish and the blue-ringed octopus. Certain varieties of catfish have venom as well. Envenomations, are rare and if they occur, treatment is based on good first-aid principles and antivenom where available (mostly in tropical areas).

Certain cone shells contain a toxin that can be fatal. This toxin is injected by the mollusk into the victim from a proboscis which it extends from the small end of the cone. Treatment is primarily supportive.

Trauma

Abrasions, bites, and lacerations are usually the result of a marine animal's instinct to protect itself against a perceived danger. The most commonly involved marine animals are octopi, sharks, moray eels, and barracuda. The trauma alone creates problems for patients but the trauma can be further complicated by envenomation. It is often difficult to identify the marine animal involved in the attack. Treatment is for the most part symptomatic, with local cleansing and topical dressing usually sufficing. If the wound becomes infected, antibiotics should cover common organisms (see Table 2).

ENVIRONMENTAL HAZARDS

Abrasions from the ambient environment are also common. These wounds should be thoroughly cleansed with soap and water and a topical antibiotic applied, because the wounds can contain toxins

TABLE 2 Antibiotic Choices in Marine Injuries

Drug	Dosage	
	Pediatric	Adult
Outpatient Management		
Ciprofloxacin (Cipro)	20–30 mg/kg/day PO × 14 d[1]	500 mg PO bid × 14 d
Levofloxin (Levaquin)		750 mg PO qd × 14 d
Doxycycline (Vibramycin, Doryx)	>8 y: 2.2 mg/kg PO qd × 14 d	100 mg bid × 14 d
Inpatient Management		
Preferred		
Ceftazidime (Fortaz, Tazicef)	150 mg/kg/d q8h	1 g IV q8h
plus		
PO or IV quinolone or doxycycline	150 mg/kg/d q8h	1 g IV q8h
Alternative		
Gentamicin *plus*	Typically based on institutional protocol and adjusted based on serum levels	Typically based on institutional protocol and adjusted based on serum levels
TMP-SMX (Bactrim, Cotrim, Septra)	8–10 mg/kg/d TMP	8–10 mg/kg (lean body mass)/d TMP

[1]Not FDA approved for this indication.
TMP-SMX = trimethoprim-sulfamethoxazole.

and are commonly contaminated with bacteria. Coral contains nematocysts and also has very sharp edges. Scuba divers in particular suffer from coral cuts in the course of their recreational diving. If these wounds become infected, coverage for *Vibrio* species should be included as well.

SHARKS

Although sharks attacks receive a lot of publicity, there are only around 50 such attacks worldwide annually and they result in fewer than 10 deaths. The majority of the deaths are in South Africa. Typically these attacks involve the tiger, great white, gray reef, and bull sharks. Attacks occur in shallow water within 100 feet of shore during the evening hours when sharks tend to feed. Common sense dictates avoiding areas where aggressive shark feeding has been noted.

Sequelae of a shark attack range from abrasions to death from hemorrhage. Abrasions and lacerations can occur when sharks brush or aggressively investigate humans. Soft tissue damage, fractures, and neurovascular damage result from such attacks. The majority of

attacks result in minor injuries that require simple suturing. Morbidity increases in wounds that are greater than 20 cm or where more than one myofascial compartment is lost. General principles of first aid in marine animal injuries are found in Box 2. Although it would seem self-evident, practices such as urinating on the injury, applying oil or gasoline to injuries, and application of any strong oxidizing agents, such as strong bases or acids should be counseled against when doing patient education regarding self-care.

REFERENCES

Centers for Disease Control and Prevention. Management of *Vibrio vulnificus* wound infection. Available at http://www.bt.cdc.gov/disasters/hurricanes/katrina/vibriofaq.asp (accessed June 13, 2008).

Edmonds C. Marine animal injuries. In: Bove AA, editor. Bove and Davis' Diving Medicine. 4th ed. Philadelphia: Saunders; 2004. p. 287–318.

Fleming LE. Ciguatera fish poisoning. Miami, FL: National Institute of Environmental Health Sciences, Marine and Freshwater Biomedical Sciences Center; 2006 available at http://www.rsmas.miami.edu/groups/niehs/science/ciguatera.htm (accessed June 14, 2008).

Isbister GK. Venomous fish stings in tropical northern Australia. Am J Emerg Med 2001;19:561–5.

Lahey T. Invasive *Mycobacterium marinum* infections, Emerg Infect Dis [serial online] 2003 November; Available at http://www.cdc.gov/ncidod/EID/vol9no11/03-0192.htm (accessed June 14, 2008).

Lehane L, Olley J. Histamine (scombroid) fish poisoning: A review in a risk-assessment framework. Canberra, Australia: National Office of Animal and Plant Health; 1999.

Lynch PR, Bove AA. Marine poisonings and intoxications. In: Bove AA, editor. Bove and Davis' Diving Medicine. 4th ed. Philadelphia: Saunders; 2004. p. 287–318.

Nomura JT. A randomized paired comparison trial of cutaneous treatments for acute jellyfish (*Carybdea alata*) stings. Am J Emerg Med 2002;20:624–6.

Perkins A, Morgan S. Poisonings, envenomations, and trauma from marine creatures. Am Fam Physician 2004;69:885–90.

Thomas C, Scott SA. All Stings Considered: First Aid and Medical Treatment of Hawaii's Marine Injuries. Honolulu: University of Hawaii Press; 1997.

Thomas CS, Scott SA, Galanis DJ, Goto RS. Box jellyfish *Carybdea alata* in Waikiki. The analgesic effect of Sting-Aid, Adolph's meat tenderizer and fresh water on their stings: A double-blinded, randomized, placebo-controlled clinical trial. Hawaii Med J 2001;60:205–10.

Thomas CS, Scott SA, Galanis DJ, Goto RS. Box jellyfish *Carybdea alata* in Waikiki. Their influx cycle plus the analgesic effect of hot and cold packs on their stings to swimmers at the beach: A randomized, placebo-controlled, clinical trial. Hawaii Med J 2001;60:100–7.

BOX 2   Management of Marine Trauma

Remove the victim from the water.
Ensure airway control.
Control bleeding.
Do not remove the wet suit if the victim is wearing one.
Attempt to identify the animal involved in the injury.
If the injury is severe, transport the victim to a hospital.
If envenomation is suspected, consider hot water immersion.
Irrigate the wound with normal saline.
Perform surgical débridement of the wound as appropriate.
If sutures must be placed, place them loosely and allow drainage. Primary suturing should be avoided in puncture wounds, crush injuries, and wounds in the distal extremities.
Start appropriate antibiotics if indicated.

Medical Toxicology: Ingestions, Inhalations, and Dermal and Ocular Absorptions

Method of

Howard C. Mofenson, MD, Thomas R. Caraccio, PharmD, Michael McGuigan, MD, and Joseph Greensher, MD

Introduction and Epidemiology

According to the national Toxic Exposure Surveillance System (TESS), over 2.4 million potentially toxic exposures were reported last year to Poison Control Centers throughout the United States. Poisonings were responsible for 1183 deaths and more than 500,000 hospitalizations. Poisoning accounts for 2% to 5% of pediatric hospital admissions, 10% of adult admissions, 5% of hospital admissions in the elderly (>65 years of age), and 5% of ambulance calls. In one urban hospital, drug-related emergencies accounted for 38% of the emergency department visits. An evaluation of a medical intensive care unit and step-down unit over a 3-month period indicated that poisonings accounted for 19.7% of admissions.

The largest number of fatalities resulting from poisoning reported to the TESS are caused by analgesics. The other principal toxicologic causes of fatalities are antidepressants, sedative hypnotics/antipsychotics, stimulants/street drugs, cardiovascular agents, and alcohols. Less than 1% of overdose cases reaching the hospitals result in fatality. However, patients presenting in deep coma to medical care facilities have a fatality rate of 13% to 35%. The largest single cause of coma of inapparent etiology is drug poisoning.

Pharmaceutical preparations are involved in 50% of poisonings. The number one pharmaceutical agent involved in exposures is acetaminophen. The severity of the manifestations of acute poisoning exposures varies greatly depending on whether the poisoning was intentional or unintentional. Unintentional exposures make up 85% to 90% of all poisoning exposures. The majority of cases are acute, occurring in children younger than 5 years of age, in the home, and resulting in no or minor toxicity. Many are actually ingestions of relatively nontoxic substances that require minimal medical care. Intentional poisonings, such as suicides, constitute 10% to 15% of exposures and may require the highest standards of medical and nursing care and the use of sophisticated equipment for recovery. Intentional ingestions are often of multiple substances and frequently include ethanol, acetaminophen, and aspirin. Suicides make up 54% of the reported fatalities. About 25% of suicides are attempted with drugs. Sixty percent of patients who take a drug overdose use their own medication and 15% use drugs prescribed for close relatives. The majority of the drug-related suicide attempts involve a central nervous system (CNS) depressant, and coma management is vital to the treatment.

Assessment and Maintenance of the Vital Functions

The initial assessment of all patients in medical emergencies follows the principles of basic and advanced cardiac life support. The adequacy of the patient's airway, degree of ventilation, and circulatory status should be determined. The vital functions should be established and maintained. Vital signs should be measured frequently and should include body core temperature. The assessment of vital functions should include the rate numbers (e.g., respiratory rate) and indications of effectiveness (e.g., depth of respirations and degree of gas exchange). Table 1 gives important measurements and vital signs.

Level of consciousness should be assessed by immediate AVPU (Alert, responds to Verbal stimuli, responds to Painful stimuli, and Unconscious). If the patient is unconscious, one must assess the severity of the unconsciousness by the Glasgow Coma Scale (Table 2).

If the patient is comatose, management requires administering 100% oxygen, establishing vascular access, and obtaining blood for pertinent laboratory studies. The administration of glucose, thiamine, and naloxone, as well as intubation to protect the airway, should be considered. Pertinent laboratory studies include arterial blood gases (ABG), electrocardiography (ECG), determination of blood glucose level, electrolytes, renal and liver tests, and acetaminophen plasma concentration in all cases of intentional ingestions. Radiography of the chest and abdomen may be useful. The severity of a stimulant's effects can also be assessed and should be documented to follow the trend.

The examiner should completely expose the patient by removing clothes and other items that interfere with a full evaluation. One should look for clues to etiology in the clothes and include the hat and shoes.

TABLE 1 Important Measurements and Vital Signs

Age	Body Surface Area (m²)	Weight (kg)	Height (cm)	Pulse (bpm) Resting	Blood Pressure Hypotension	Hypertension Significant	Hypertension Severe	Respiratory Rate (rpm)
Newborn	0.19	3.5	50	70–190	<60/40	>96	>106	30–60
1 mo–6 mo	0.30	4–7	50–65	80–160	<70/45	>104	>110	30–50
6 mo–1 y	0.38	7–10	65–75	80–160	<70/45	>104	>110	20–40
1–2 y	0.50–0.55	10–12	75–85	80–140	<74/47	>112/74	>118/82	20–40
3–5 y	0.54–0.68	15–20	90–108	80–120	<80/52	>116/76	>124/84	20–40
6–9 y	0.68–0.85	20–28	122–133	75–115	<90/60	>122/82	>130/86	16–25
10–12 y	1.00–1.07	30–40	138–147	70–110	<90/60	>126/82	>134/90	16–25
13–15 y	1.07–1.22	42–50	152–160	60–100	<90/60	>136/86	>144/92	16–20
16–18 y	1.30–1.60	53–60	160–170	60–100	<90/60	>142/92	>150/98	12–16
Adult	1.40–1.70	60–70	160–170	60–100	<90/60	>140/90	>210/120	10–16

Data from Nadas A: Pediatric Cardiology, 3rd ed. Philadelphia, WB Saunders, 1976; Blumer JL (ed): A Practice Guide to Pediatric Intensive Care. St Louis, Mosby, 1990; AAP and ACEP: Respiratory Distress in APLS Pediatric Emergency Medicine Course, 1993; Second Task Force: Blood pressure control in children– 1987, Pediatr 79:1, 1987; Linakis JG: Hypertension. In Fliesher GR, Ludwig S (eds); Textbook of Pediatric Emergency Medicine, 3rd ed. Baltimore, Williams & Wilkins, 1993.

TABLE 2 Glasgow Coma Scale

Scale	Adult Response	Score	Pediatric, 0–1 Years
Eye opening	Spontaneous	4	Spontaneous
	To verbal command	3	To shout
	To pain	2	To pain
	None	1	No response
Motor response			
To verbal command	Obeys	6	
To painful stimuli	Localized pain	5	Localized pain
	Flexion withdrawal	4	Flexion withdrawal
	Decorticate flexion	3	Decorticate flexion
	Decerebrate extension	2	Decerebrate flexion
	None	1	None
Verbal response: adult	Oriented and converses	5	Cries, smiles, coos
	Disoriented but converses	4	Cries or screams
	Inappropriate words	3	Inappropriate sounds
	Incomprehensible sounds	2	Grunts
	None	1	Gives no response
Verbal response: child	Oriented	5	
	Words or babbles	4	
	Vocal sounds	3	
	Cries or moans to stimuli	2	
	None	1	

Data from Teasdale G, Jennett B: Assessment of coma impaired consciousness. Lancet 2:83, 1974; Simpson D, Reilly P: Pediatric coma scale. Lancet 2:450, 1982; Seidel J: Preparing for pediatric emergencies. Pediatr Rev 16:470, 1995.

Prevention of Absorption and Reduction of Local Damage

EXPOSURE

Poisoning exposure routes include ingestion (76.8%), dermal (8%), ophthalmologic (5%), inhalation (6%), insect bites and stings (4%), and parenteral injections (0.5%). The effect of the toxin may be local, systemic, or both.

Local effects (skin, eyes, mucosa of respiratory or gastrointestinal tract) occur where contact is made with the poisonous substance. Local effects are nonspecific chemical reactions that depend on the chemical properties (e.g., pH), concentration, contact time, and type of exposed surface.

Systemic effects occur when the poison is absorbed into the body and depend on the dose, the distribution, and the functional reserve of the organ systems. Shock and hypoxia are part of systemic toxicity.

DELAYED TOXIC ACTION

Therapeutic doses of most pharmaceuticals are absorbed within 90 minutes. However, the patient with exposure to a potential toxin may be asymptomatic at this time because a sufficient amount has not yet been absorbed or metabolized to produce toxicity at the time the patient presents for care.

Absorption can be significantly delayed under the following circumstances:

1. Drugs with anticholinergic properties (e.g., antihistamines, belladonna alkaloids, diphenoxylate with atropine [Lomotil], phenothiazines, and tricyclic antidepressants).
2. Modified release preparations such as sustained-release, enteric-coated, and controlled-release formulations have delayed and prolonged absorption.
3. Concretions may form (e.g., salicylates, iron, glutethimide, and meprobamate [Equanil]) that can delay absorption and prolong the toxic effects. Large quantities of drugs tend to be absorbed more slowly than small quantities.

Some substances must be metabolized into a toxic metabolite (acetaminophen, acetonitrile, ethylene glycol, methanol, methylene chloride, parathion, and paraquat). In some cases, time is required to produce a toxic effect on organ systems (*Amanita phalloides* mushrooms, carbon tetrachloride, colchicine, digoxin [Lanoxin], heavy metals, monoamine oxidase inhibitors, and oral hypoglycemic agents).

Initial Management

1. Stabilization of airway, breathing, and circulation and protection of same.
2. Identification of specific toxin or toxic syndrome.
3. Initial treatment: D50W; consider thiamine, naloxone (Narcan), oxygen, and antidotes if needed.
4. Physical assessment.
5. Decontamination: Gastrointestinal tract, skin, eyes.

DECONTAMINATION

In the asymptomatic patient who has been exposed to a toxic substance, decontamination procedures should be considered if the patient has been exposed to potentially toxic substances in toxic amounts.

Ocular exposure should be immediately treated with water irrigation for 15 to 20 minutes with the eyelids fully retracted. One should not use neutralizing chemicals. All caustic and corrosive injuries should be evaluated with fluorescein dye and by an ophthalmologist.

Dermal exposure is treated immediately with copious water irrigation for 30 minutes, not a forceful flushing. Shampooing the hair, cleansing the fingernails, navel, and perineum, and irrigating the eyes are necessary in the case of an extensive exposure. The clothes should be specially bagged and may have to be discarded. Leather goods can become irreversibly contaminated and must be abandoned. Caustic (alkali) exposures can require hours of irrigation. Dermal absorption can occur with pesticides, hydrocarbons, and cyanide.

Injection exposures (e.g., snake envenomation) can be treated with venom extracts. Venom extractors can be used within minutes of envenomation, and proximal lymphatic constricting bands or elastic wraps can be used to delay lymphatic flow and immobilize the extremity. Cold packs and tourniquets should not be used and incision is generally not recommended. Substances of abuse may be injected intravenously or subcutaneously. In these cases, little decontamination can be done.

Inhalation exposure to toxic substances is managed by immediate removal of the victim from the contaminated environment by protected rescuers.

Gastrointestinal exposure is the most common route of poisoning. Gastrointestinal decontamination historically has been done by gastric emptying: induction of emesis, gastric lavage, administration of activated charcoal, and the use of cathartics or whole bowel irrigation. No procedure is routine; it should be individualized for each case. If no attempt is made to decontaminate the patient, the reason should be clearly documented on the medical record (e.g., time elapsed, past peak of action, ineffectiveness, or risk of procedure).

Gastric Emptying Procedures

The gastric emptying procedure used is influenced by the age of the patient, the effectiveness of the procedure, the time of ingestion (gastric emptying is usually ineffective after 1 hour postingestion), the patient's clinical status (time of peak effect has passed or the patient's condition is too unstable), formulation of the substance ingested (regular release versus modified release), the amount ingested, and the rapidity of onset of CNS depression or stimulation (convulsions). Most studies show that only 30% (range, 19% to 62%) of the ingested toxin is removed by gastric emptying under optimal conditions. It has not been demonstrated that the choice of procedure improved the outcome.

A mnemonic for gathering information is STATS:

S—substance
T—type of formulation
A—amount and age
T—time of ingestion
S—signs and symptoms

The examiner should attempt to obtain AMPLE information about the patient:

A—age and allergies
M—available medications
P—past medical history including pregnancy, psychiatric illnesses, substance abuse, or intentional ingestions
L—time of last meal, which may influence absorption and the onset and peak action
E—events leading to present condition

The intent of the patient should also be determined.

The Regional Poison Center should be consulted for the exact ingredients of the ingested substance and the latest management. The treatment information on the labels of products and in the Physician's Desk Reference are notoriously inaccurate.

Ipecac Syrup

Syrup of ipecac–induced emesis has virtually no use in the emergency department. Although at one time it was considered most useful in young children with a recent witnessed ingestion, it is no longer advised in most cases. Current guidelines from the American Association of Poison Control Centers have significantly limited the indications for inducing emesis because the risk most often exceeds the benefit derived from this procedure. The Poison Control Center should be called if inducting emesis is being considered.

Contraindications or situations in which induction of emesis is inappropriate include the following:

- Ingestion of caustic substance
- Loss of airway protective reflexes because of ingestion of substances that can produce rapid onset of CNS depression (e.g., short-acting benzodiazepines, barbiturates, nonbarbiturate sedative-hypnotics, opioids, tricyclic antidepressants) or convulsions (e.g., camphor [Ponstel], chloroquine [Aralen], codeine, isoniazid [Nydrazid], mefenamic acid, nicotine, propoxyphene [Darvon], organophosphate insecticides, strychnine, and tricyclic antidepressants)
- Ingestion of low-viscosity petroleum distillates (e.g., gasoline, lighter fluid, kerosene)

- Significant vomiting prior to presentation or hematemesis
- Age under 6 months (no established dose, safety, or efficacy data)
- Ingestion of foreign bodies (emesis is ineffective and may lead to aspiration)
- Clinical conditions including neurologic impairment, hemodynamic instability, increased intracranial pressure, and hypertension
- Delay in presentation (more than 1 hour postingestion)

The dose of syrup of ipecac in the 6- to 9-month-old infant is 5 mL; in the 9- to 12-month-old, 10 mL; and in the 1- to 12-year-old, 15 mL. In children older than 12 years and in adults, the dose is 30 mL. The dose can be repeated once if the child does not vomit in 15 to 20 minutes. The vomitus should be inspected for remnants of pills or toxic substances, and the appearance and odor should be documented. When ipecac is not available, 30 mL of mild dishwashing soap (not dishwasher detergent) can be used, although it is less effective.

Complications are very rare but include aspiration, protracted vomiting, rarely cardiac toxicity with long-term abuse, pneumothorax, gastric rupture, diaphragmatic hernia, intracranial hemorrhage, and Mallory-Weiss tears.

Gastric Lavage

Gastric lavage should be considered only when life-threatening amounts of substances were involved, when the benefits outweigh the risks, when it can be performed within 1 hour of the ingestion, and when no contraindications exist.

The contraindications are similar to those for ipecac-induced emesis. However, gastric lavage can be accomplished after the insertion of an endotracheal tube in cases of CNS depression or controlled convulsions. The patient should be placed with the head lower than the hips in a left-lateral decubitus position. The location of the tube should be confirmed by radiography, if necessary, and suctioning equipment should be available.

Contraindications to gastric lavage include the following:

- Ingestion of caustic substances (risk of esophageal perforation)
- Uncontrolled convulsions, because of the danger of aspiration and injury during the procedure
- Ingestion of low-viscosity petroleum distillate products
- CNS depression or absent protective airway reflexes, without endotracheal protection
- Significant cardiac dysrhythmias
- Significant emesis or hematemesis prior to presentation
- Delay in presentation (more than 1 hour postingestion)

Size of Tube

The best results with gastric lavage are obtained with the largest possible orogastric tube that can be reasonably passed (nasogastric tubes are not large enough to remove solid material). In adults, a large-bore orogastric Lavacuator hose or a No. 42 French Ewald tube should be used; in young children, orogastric tubes are generally too small to remove solid material and gastric lavage is not recommended.

The amount of fluid used varies with the patient's age and size. In general, aliquots of 50 to 100 mL per lavage are used in adults. Larger amounts of fluid may force the toxin past the pylorus. Lavage fluid is 0.9% saline.

Complications are rare and may include respiratory depression, aspiration pneumonitis, cardiac dysrhythmias as a result of increased vagal tone, esophageal-gastric tears and perforation, laryngospasm, and mediastinitis.

Activated Charcoal

Oral activated charcoal adsorbs the toxin onto its surface before absorption. According to recent guidelines set forth by the American Academy of Clinical Toxicology, activated charcoal should not be used routinely. Its use is indicated only if a toxic amount of substance has been ingested and is optimally effective within 1 hour of the

TABLE 3 Substances Poorly Adsorbed by Activated Charcoal

C   Caustics and corrosives
H   Heavy metals (arsenic, iron, lead, mercury)
A   Alcohols (ethanol, methanol, isopropanol) and glycols (ethylene glycols)
R   Rapid onset of absorption (cyanide and strychnine)
C   Chlorine and iodine
O   Others insoluble in water (substances in tablet form)
A   Aliphatic hydrocarbons (petroleum distillates)
L   Laxatives (sodium, magnesium, potassium, and lithium)

ingestion. Because of the slow absorption of large quantities of toxin, activated charcoal may be beneficial after 1 hour postingestion.

Activated charcoal does not effectively adsorb small molecules or molecules lacking carbon (Table 3). Activated charcoal adsorption may be diminished by milk, cocoa powder, and ice cream.

There are a few relative contraindications to the use of activated charcoal:

1. Ingestion of caustics and corrosives, which may produce vomiting or cling to the mucosa and falsely appear as a burn on endoscopy.
2. Comatose patient, in whom the airway must be secured prior to activated charcoal administration.
3. Patient without presence of bowel sounds.

Note: Activated charcoal was shown not to interfere with effectiveness of *N*-acetylcysteine in cases of acetaminophen overdose, so it is no longer contraindicated as was thought in the past.

The usual initial adult dose is 60 to 100 g and the dose for children is 15 to 30 g. It is administered orally as a slurry mixed with water or by nasogastric or orogastric tube. *Caution:* Be sure the tube is in the stomach. Cathartics are not necessary.

Although repeated dosing with activated charcoal may decrease the half-life and increases the clearance of phenobarbital, dapsone, quinidine, theophylline, and carbamazepine (Tegretol), recent guidelines indicate there is insufficient evidence to support the use of multiple-dose activated charcoal unless a life-threatening amount of one of the substances mentioned is involved. At present there are no controlled studies that demonstrate that multiple-dose activated charcoal or cathartics alter the clinical course of an intoxication. The dose varies from 0.25 to 0.50 g/kg every 1 to 4 hours, and continuous nasogastric tube infusion of 0.25 to 0.5 g/kg/h has been used to decrease vomiting.

Gastrointestinal dialysis is the diffusion of the toxin from the higher concentration in the serum of the mesenteric vessels to the lower levels in the gastrointestinal tract mucosal cell and subsequently into the gastrointestinal lumen, where the concentration has been lowered by intraluminal adsorption of activated charcoal.

Complications of treatment with activated charcoal include vomiting in 50% of cases, desorption (especially with weak acids in intestine), and aspiration (at least a dozen cases of aspiration have been reported). There are many cases of unreported pulmonary aspirations and "charcoal lungs," intestinal obstruction or pseudoobstruction (three case reports with multiple dosing, none with a single dose), empyema following esophageal perforation, and hypermagnesemia and hypernatremia, which have been associated with repeated concurrent doses of activated charcoal and saline cathartics. Catharsis was used to hasten the elimination of any remaining toxin in the gastrointestinal tract. There are no studies to demonstrate the effectiveness of cathartics, and they are no longer recommended as a form of gastrointestinal decontamination.

Whole-Bowel Irrigation

With whole bowel irrigation, solutions of polyethylene glycol (PEG) with balanced electrolytes are used to cleanse the bowel without causing shifts in fluids and electrolytes. The procedure is not approved by the U.S. Food and Drug Administration for this purpose.

Indications

The procedure has been studied and used successfully in cases of iron overdose when abdominal radiographs reveal incomplete emptying of excess iron. There are additional indications for other types of ingestions, such as with body-packing of illicit drugs (e.g., cocaine, heroin).

The procedure is to administer the solution (GoLYTELY or Colyte), orally or by nasogastric tube, in a dose of 0.5 L per hour in children younger than 5 years of age and 2 L per hour in adolescents and adults for 5 hours. The end point is reached when the rectal effluent is clear or radiopaque materials can no longer be seen in the gastrointestinal tract on abdominal radiographs.

Contraindications

These measures should not be used if there is extensive hematemesis, ileus, or signs of bowel obstruction, perforation, or peritonitis. Animal experiments in which PEG was added to activated charcoal indicated that activated charcoal-salicylates and activated charcoal-theophylline combinations resulted in decreased adsorption and desorption of salicylate and theophylline and no therapeutic benefit over activated charcoal alone. Polyethylene solutions are bound by activated charcoal in vitro, decreasing the efficacy of activated charcoal.

Dilutional treatment is indicated for the immediate management of caustic and corrosive poisonings but is otherwise not useful. The administration of diluting fluid above 30 mL in children and 250 mL in adults may produce vomiting, reexposing the vital tissues to the effects of local damage and possible aspiration.

Neutralization is not proven to be either safe or effective.

Endoscopy and surgery have been required in the case of body-packer obstruction, intestinal ischemia produced by cocaine ingestion, and iron local caustic action.

Differential Diagnosis of Poisons on the Basis of Central Nervous System Manifestations

Neurologic parameters help to classify and assess the need for supportive treatment as well as provide diagnostic clues to the etiology. Table 4 lists the effects of CNS depressants, CNS stimulants, hallucinogens, and autonomic nervous system anticholinergics and cholinergics.

Central nervous system depressants are cholinergics, opioids, sedative-hypnotics, and sympatholytic agents. The hallmarks are lethargy, sedation, stupor, and coma. In exception to the manifestations listed in Table 4, (a) barbiturates may produce an initial tachycardia; (b) convulsions are produced by codeine, propoxyphene (Darvon), meperidine (Demerol), glutethimide, phenothiazines, methaqualone, and tricyclic and cyclic antidepressants; (c) benzodiazepines rarely produce coma that will interfere with cardiorespiratory functions; and (d) pulmonary edema is common with opioids and sedative-hypnotics.

The CNS stimulants are anticholinergic, hallucinogenic, sympathomimetic, and withdrawal agents. The hallmarks of CNS stimulants are convulsions and hyperactivity.

There is considerable overlapping of effects among the various hallucinogens, but the major hallmark manifestation is hallucinations.

Guidelines for In-Hospital Disposition

Classification of patients as high risk depends on clinical judgment. Any patient who needs cardiorespiratory support or has a persistently altered mental status for 3 hours or more should be considered for intensive care.

TABLE 4   Agents with Central Nervous System (CNS) Effects

Agents	General Manifestations	Agents	General Manifestations
CNS Depressants	Bradycardia	**Hallucinogens**‡	Tachycardia and dysrhythmias
Alcohols and glycols (S-H)	Bradypnea	Amphetamines‡	Tachypnea
Anticonvulsants (S-H)	Shallow respirations	Anticholinergics	Hypertension
Antidysrhythmics (S-H)	Hypotension	Cardiac glycosides	Hallucinations, usually visual
Antihypertensives (S-H)	Hypothermia	Cocaine	Disorientation
Barbiturates (S-H)	Flaccid coma	Ethanol withdrawal	Panic reaction
Benzodiazepines (S-H)	Miosis	Hydrocarbon inhalation (abuse)	Toxic psychosis
Butyrophenones (Syly)	Hypoactive bowel sounds	Mescaline (peyote)	Moist skin
β-Adrenergic blockers (Syly)		Mushrooms (psilocybin)	Mydriasis (reactive)
Calcium channel blockers (Syly)		Phencyclidine	Hyperthermia
Digitalis (Syl)			Flashbacks
Opioids			
Lithium (mixed)			
Muscle relaxants			
Phenothiazines (Syly)		**Anticholinergics**	Tachycardia, dysrhythmias (rare)
Nonbarbiturate/benzodiazepine		Antihistamines	Tachypnea
glutethimide, methaqualone,		Antispasmodic gastrointestinal preparations	Hypertension (mild)
methyprylon, sedative-hypnotics		Antiparkinsonian preparations	Hyperthermia
(chloral hydrate, ethchlorvynol, bromide)		Atropine	Hallucinations ("mad as a hatter")
Tricyclic antidepressants (late Syly)		Cyclobenzaprine (Flexeril)	Mydriasis (unreactive)
		Mydriatic ophthalmologic agents	("blind as a bat")
		Over-the-counter sleep agents	Flushed skin ("red as a beet")
CNS Stimulants	Tachycardia	Plants (Datura spp)/mushrooms	Dry skin and mouth ("dry as a bone")
Amphetamines (Sy)	Tachypnea and dysrhythmias		Hypoactive bowel sounds
Anticholinergics*	Hypertension	Phenothiazines (early)	Urinary retention
Cocaine (Sy)	Convulsions	Scopolamine	Lilliputian hallucinations ("little people")
Camphor (mixed)	Toxic psychosis	Tricyclic/cyclic antidepressants (early)	
Ergot alkaloids (Sy)	Mydriasis (reactive)		
Isoniazid (mixed)	Agitation and restlessness		
Lithium (mixed)	Moist skin	**Cholinergics**	Bradycardia (muscarinic)
Lysergic acid diethylamide (H)	Tremors	Bethanechol (Urecholine)	Tachycardia (nicotinic effect)
Hallucinogens (H)		Carbamate insecticides (Carbaryl)	Miosis (muscarinic)
Mescaline and synthetic analogs		Edrophonium	Diarrhea (muscarinic)
Metals (arsenic, lead, mercury)		Organophosphate insecticides (Malathion, parathion)	Hypertension (variable)
Methylphenidate (Ritalin) (Sy)		Parasympathetic agents (physostigmine, pyridostigmine)	Hyperactive bowel sounds
Monoamine oxidase inhibitors (Sy)		Toxic mushrooms (Clitocybe spp.)	Excess urination (muscarinic)
Pemoline (Cylert) (Sy)			Excess salivation (muscarinic)
Phencyclidine (H)†			Lacrimation (muscarinic)
Salicylates (mixed)			Bronchospasm (muscarinic)
Strychnine (mixed)			Muscle fasciculations (nicotinic)
Sympathomimetics (Sy) (phenylpropanolamine,			Paralysis (nicotinic)
theophylline, caffeine, thyroid)			
Withdrawal from ethanol, β-adrenergic blockers,			
clonidine, opioids, sedative-hypnotics (W)			

*Anticholinergics produce dry skin and mucosa and decreased bowel sounds.
†Phencyclidine may produce miosis.
‡The amphetamine hybrids are methylene dioxymethamphetamine (MDMA, ecstasy, "ADAM") and methylene dioxyamphetamine (MDA, "Eve"), which are associated with deaths.
Abbreviations: H = hallucinogen; S-H = sedative-hypnotic; Sy = sympathomimetic; Syly = sympatholytic; W = withdrawal.

Guidelines for admitting patients older than 14 years of age to an intensive care unit, after 2 to 3 hours in the emergency department, include the following:

1. Need for intubation
2. Seizures
3. Unresponsiveness to verbal stimuli
4. Arterial carbon dioxide pressure greater than 45 mm Hg
5. Cardiac conduction or rhythm disturbances (any rhythm except sinus arrhythmia)
6. Close monitoring of vital signs during antidotal therapy or elimination procedures
7. The need for continuous monitoring
8. QRS interval greater than 0.10 second, in cases of tricyclic antidepressant poisoning
9. Systolic blood pressure less than 80 mm Hg
10. Hypoxia, hypercarbia, acid-base imbalance, or metabolic abnormalities
11. Extremes of temperature
12. Progressive deterioration or significant underlying medical disorders

Use of Antidotes

Antidotes are available for only a relatively small number of poisons. An antidote is not a substitute for good supportive care. Table 5 summarizes the commonly used antidotes, their indications, and their methods of administration. The Regional Poison Control Center can give further information on these antidotes.

Enhancement of Elimination

The acceptable methods for elimination of absorbed toxic substances are dialysis, hemoperfusion, exchange transfusion, plasmapheresis, enzyme induction, and inhibition. Methods of increasing urinary excretion of toxic chemicals and drugs have been studied extensively, but the other modalities have not been well evaluated.

In general, these methods are needed in only a minority of cases and should be reserved for life-threatening circumstances when a definite benefit is anticipated.

DIALYSIS

Dialysis is the extrarenal means of removing certain substances from the body, and it can substitute for the kidney when renal failure occurs. Dialysis is not the first measure instituted; however, it may be lifesaving later in the course of a severe intoxication. It is needed in only a minority of intoxicated patients.

Peritoneal dialysis uses the peritoneum as the membrane for dialysis. It is only 1/20 as effective as hemodialysis. It is easier to use and less hazardous to the patient but also less effective in removing the toxin; thus it is rarely used except in small infants.

Hemodialysis is the most effective dialysis method but requires experience with sophisticated equipment. Blood is circulated past a semipermeable extracorporeal membrane. Substances are removed by diffusion down a concentration gradient. Anticoagulation with heparin is necessary. Flow rates of 300 to 500 mL/min can be achieved, and clearance rates may reach 200 or 300 mL/min.

Dialyzable substances easily diffuse across the dialysis membrane and have the following characteristics: (a) a molecular weight less than 500 daltons and preferably less than 350; (b) a volume of distribution less than 1 L/kg; (c) protein binding less than 50%; (d) high water solubility (low lipid solubility); and (e) high plasma concentration and a toxicity that correlates reasonably with the plasma concentration. Considerations for hemodialysis and hemoperfusion are cases of serious ingestions (the nephrologist should be notified immediately), and cases involving a compound that is ingested in a potentially lethal dose and the rapid removal of which may improve the prognosis. Examples of the latter are ethylene glycol 1.4 mL/kg

100% solution or equivalent and methanol 6 mL/kg 100% solution or equivalent. Common dialyzable substances include alcohol, bromides, lithium, and salicylates.

The patient-related criteria for dialysis are (a) anticipated prolonged coma and the likelihood of complications; (b) renal compromise (toxin excreted or metabolized by kidneys and dialyzable chelating agents in heavy metal poisoning); (c) laboratory confirmation of lethal blood concentration; (d) lethal dose poisoning with an agent with delayed toxicity or known to be metabolized into a more toxic metabolite (e.g., ethylene glycol, methanol); and (e) hepatic impairment when the agent is metabolized by the liver, and clinical deterioration despite optimal supportive medical management. Table 6 gives plasma concentrations above which removal by extracorporeal measures should be considered.

The contraindications to hemodialysis include the following: (a) substances are not dialyzable; (b) effective antidotes are available; (c) patient is hemodynamically unstable (e.g., shock); and (d) presence of coagulopathy because heparinization is required.

Hemodialysis also has a role in correcting disturbances that are not amenable to appropriate medical management. These are easily remembered by the "vowel" mnemonic:

A—refractory acid-base disturbances
E—refractory electrolyte disturbances
I—intoxication with dialyzable substances (e.g., ethanol, ethylene glycol, isopropyl alcohol, methanol, lithium, and salicylates)
O—overhydration
U—uremia

Complications of dialysis include hemorrhage, thrombosis, air embolism, hypotension, infections, electrolyte imbalance, thrombocytopenia, and removal of therapeutic medications.

HEMOPERFUSION

Hemoperfusion is the parenteral form of oral activated charcoal. Heparinization is necessary. The patient's blood is routed extracorporeally through an outflow arterial catheter through a filter-adsorbing cartridge (charcoal or resin) and returned through a venous catheter. Cartridges must be changed every 4 hours. The blood glucose, electrolytes, calcium, and albumin levels; complete blood cell count; platelets; and serum and urine osmolarity must be carefully monitored. This procedure has extended extracorporeal removal to a large range of substances that were formerly either poorly dialyzable or nondialyzable. It is not limited by molecular weight, water solubility, or protein binding, but it is limited by a volume distribution greater than 400 L, plasma concentration, and rate of flow through the filter. Activated charcoal cartridges are the primary type of hemoperfusion that is currently available in the United States.

The patient-related criteria for hemoperfusion are (a) anticipated prolonged coma and the likelihood of complications; (b) laboratory confirmation of lethal blood concentrations; (c) hepatic impairment when an agent is metabolized by the liver; and (d) clinical deterioration despite optimally supportive medical management.

The contraindications are similar to those for hemodialysis.

Limited data are available as to which toxins are best treated with hemoperfusion. Hemoperfusion has proved useful in treating glutethimide intoxication, phenobarbital overdose, and carbamazepine, phenytoin, and theophylline intoxication.

Complications include hemorrhage, thrombocytopenia, hypotension, infection, leukopenia, depressed phagocytic activity of granulocytes, decreased immunoglobulin levels, hypoglycemia, hypothermia, hypocalcemia, pulmonary edema, and air and charcoal embolism.

HEMOFILTRATION

Continuous arteriovenous or venovenous hemodiafiltration (CAVHD or CVVHD, respectively) has been suggested as an alternative to conventional hemodialysis when the need for rapid removal of the drug is less urgent. These procedures, like peritoneal dialysis, are minimally invasive, have no significant impact on hemodynamics, and can be carried out continuously for many hours. Their role in the management of acute poisoning remains uncertain, however.

TABLE 5 Initial Doses of Antidotes for Common Poisonings

Antidote	Use	Dose	Route	Adverse Reactions/Comments
N-Acetyl Cysteine (NAC, Mucomyst): Stock level to treat 70 kg adult for 24 h: 25 vials, 20%, 30 mL	Acetaminophen, carbon tetrachloride (experimental)	140 mg/kg loading, followed by 70 mg/kg every 4 h for 17 doses. 150 mg/kg in 200 mL of D₅W over 1 hr, then 50 mg/kg in 1 liter D₅W over 16 hrs	PO IV	Nausea, vomiting. Dilute to 5% with sweet juice or flat cola. Useful for those who cannot tolerate oral route.
Atropine: Stock level to treat 70 kg adult for 24 h: 1 g (1 mg/mL in 1, 10 mL)	Organophosphate and carbamate pesticides: bradydysrhythmics, β-adrenergics, calcium channel blockers/nerve agents	*Child*: 0.02–0.05 mg/kg repeated q5–10 min to max of 2 mg as necessary until cessation of secretions *Adult*: 1–2 mg q5–10 min as necessary. Dilute in 1–2 mL of 0.9% saline for ET instillation. *IV infusion dose*: Place 8 mg of atropine in 100 mL D₅W or saline. Conc. = 0.08 mg/mL; dose range = 0.02–0.08 mg/kg/h or 0.25–1 mL/kg/h. Severe poisoning may require supplemental doses of IV atropine intermittently in doses of 1–5 mg until drying of secretions occurs.	IV/ET	Tachycardia, dry mouth, blurred vision, and urinary retention. Ensure adequate ventilation before administration.
Calcium Chloride (10%): Stock level to treat 70 kg adult for 24 h: 10 vials 1 g (1.35 mEq/mL)	Hypocalcemia, fluoride, calcium channel blockers, β-blockers, oxalates, ethylene glycol, hypermagnesemia	0.1–0.2 mL/kg (10–20 mg/kg) slow push every 10 min up to max 10 mL (1 g). Since calcium response lasts 15 min, some may require continuous infusion 0.2 mL/kg/h up to maximum of 10 mL/h while monitoring for dysrhythmias and hypotension.	IV	Administer slowly with BP and ECG monitoring and have magnesium available to reverse calcium effects. Tissue irritation, hypotension, dysrhythmias from rapid injection. Contraindications: digitalis glycoside intoxication.
Calcium Gluconate (10%): Stock level to treat 70 kg adult for 24 h: 20 vials 1 g (0.45 mEq/mL)	Hypocalcemia, fluoride, calcium channel blockers, hydrofluoric acid; black widow envenomation	0.3–0.4 mL/kg (30–40 mg/kg) slow push; repeat as needed up to max dose 10–20 mL (1–2 g).	IV	Same comments as calcium chloride.
Infiltration of Calcium Gluconate	Hydrofluoric acid skin exposure	Dose: Infiltrate each square cm of affected dermis/ subcutaneous tissue with about 0.5 mL of 10% calcium gluconate using a 30-gauge needle. Repeat as needed to control pain.	Infiltrate	
Intra-arterial Calcium Gluconate	Hydrofluoric acid skin exposure	Infuse 20 mL of 10% calcium gluconate (not chloride) diluted in 250 mL D₅W via the radial or brachial artery proximal to the injury over 3–4 hours.		Alternatively, dilute 10 mL of 10% calcium gluconate with 40–50 mL of D₅W.
Calcium Gluconate Gel: Stock level: 3.5 g	Hydrofluoric acid skin exposure	2.5 g USP powder added to 100 mL water-soluble lubricating jelly, e.g., K-Y Jelly or Lubifax (or 3.5 mg into 150 mL). Some use 6 g of calcium carbonate in 100 g of lubricant. Place injured hand in surgical glove filled with gel. Apply q4h. If pain persists, calcium gluconate injection may be needed (above).	Dermal	Powder is available from Spectrum Pharmaceutical Co. in California: 800-772-8786. Commercial preparation of Ca gluconate gel is available from Pharmascience in Montreal, Quebec: 514-340-1114.

Antidote	Indication	Route	Dose	Comments
Cyanide Antidote Kit: Stock level to treat 70 kg adult for 24 h: 2 Lilly Cyanide Antidote kits	Cyanide Hydrogen sulfide (nitrites are given only) Do not use sodium thiosulfate for hydrogen sulfide Individual portions of the kit can be used in certain circumstances (consult PCC)	Inhalation	Amyl nitrite: 1 crushable ampule for 30 sec of every min. Use new amp q3 min. May omit step if venous access is established.	If methemoglobinemia occurs, do not use methylene blue to correct this because it releases cyanide.
	Cyanide Hydrogen sulfide (nitrites are given only) Do not use sodium thiosulfate for hydrogen sulfide Individual portions of the kit can be used in certain circumstances (consult PCC)	IV	Sodium nitrite: *Child:* 0.33 mL/kg of 3% solution if hemoglobin level is not known, otherwise based on tables with product. *Adult:* up to 300 mg (10 mL). Dilute nitrite in 100 mL 0.9% saline, administer slowly at 5 mL/min. Slow infusion if fall in BP.	If methemoglobinemia occurs, do not use methylene blue to correct this because it releases cyanide.
	Cyanide Hydrogen sulfide Do not use sodium thiosulfate for hydrogen sulfide Individual portions of the kit can be used in certain circumstances (consult PCC)	IV	Sodium thiosulfate: *Child:* 1.6 mL/kg of 25% solution, may be repeated every 30–60 min to a maximum of 12.5 or 50 mL in adult. Administer over 20 min.	Nausea, dizziness, headache.
Dantrolene Sodium (Dantrium): Stock level to treat 70 kg adult for 24 h: 700 mg, 35 vials (20 mg/vial)	Malignant hyperthermia	IV/PO	2–3 mg/kg IV rapidly. Repeat loading dose every 10 min. If necessary up to a maximum total dose of 10 mg/kg. When temperature and heart rate decrease, slow the infusion 1–2 mg/kg every 6 hours for 24–28 h until all evidence of malignant hyperthermia syndrome has subsided. Follow with oral doses 1–2 mg/kg four times a day for 24 h as necessary.	Tachycardia, muscle rigidity, and bronchospasm (rapid administration). Hepatotoxicity occurs with cumulative dose of 10 mg/kg. Thrombophlebitis (best given in central line). Available as 20 mg lyophilized dantrolene powder for reconstitution, which contains 3 g mannitol and sodium hydroxide in 70-mL vial. Mix with 60 mL sterile distilled water without a bacteriostatic agent and protect from light. Use within 6 hours after reconstituting.
Deferoxamine (Desferal): Stock level to treat 70 kg adult for 24 h: 17 vials (500 mg/amp)	Iron	Preferred IV: avoid therapy >24 h	IV infusion of 15 mg/kg/h (3 mL/kg/h: 500 mg in 100 mL D₅W) max 6 g/d Rates of >45 μg/kg/h if cone >1000 μg/dL.	Hypotension (minimized by avoiding rapid infusion rates) DFO challenge test 50 mg/kg is unreliable if negative.
Diazepam (Valium): Stock level to treat 70 kg adult for 24 h: 200 mg, 5 mg/mL; 2, 10 mL	Any intoxication that provokes seizures when specific therapy is not available, e.g., amphetamines, PCP, barbiturate and alcohol withdrawal.	IV	Adult, 5–10 mg IV (max 20 mg) at a rate of 5 mg/min until seizure is controlled. May be repeated 2 or 3 times. Child, 0.1–0.3 mg/kg up to 10 mg IV slowly over 2 min.	Confusion, somnolence, coma, hypotension. Intramuscular absorption is erratic. Establish airway and administer 100% oxygen and glucose.
Digoxin-Specific Fab Antibodies (Digibind): Stock level to treat 70 kg adult for 24 h: 20 vials	Chloroquine poisoning. Digoxin, digitoxin, oleander tea with the following: (1) Imminent cardiac arrest or shock, (2) hyperkalemia >5.0 mEq/L. (3) serum digoxin >5 ng/mL (child) at 8–12 h post ingestion in adults, (4) digitalis delirium, (5) ingestion over 10 mg in adults or 4 mg in child, (6) bradycardia or second- or third-degree heart block unresponsive to atropine.	IV	(1) If amount ingested is known total dose × bioavailability (0.8) = body burden. The body burden + 0.6 (0.5 mg of digoxin is bound by 1 vial of 38 mg of Fab) = # vials needed. (2) If amount is unknown but the steady state serum concentration is known in ng/mL: Digoxin: ng/mL: (5.6 L/kg Vd) × (wt kg) = μg body burden. Body burden + 100 = mg body burden/0.5 = # vials needed. Digitoxin body burden = ng/mL × (0.56 L/kg Vd) × (wt kg)	Allergic reactions (rare), return of condition being treated with digitalis glycoside. Administer by infusion over 30 min through a 0.22-μ filter. If cardiac arrest imminent, may administer by bolus. Consult PCC for more details.

Continued

TABLE 5 Initial Doses of Antidotes for Common Poisonings—Cont'd

Antidote	Use	Dose	Route	Adverse Reactions/Comments
	(7) life-threatening digitoxin or oleander poisoning	Body burden ÷ 1000 = mg body burden/0.5 = # vials needed. (3) If the amount is not known, it is administered in life-threatening situations as 10 vials (400 mg) IV in saline over 30 min in adults. If cardiac arrest is imminent, administer 20 vials (adult) as a bolus.		
Dimercaprol (BAL in Peanut Oil): Stock level to treat 70 kg adult for 24 h: 1200 mg (4 amps—100 mg/mL 10% in oil in 3 mL amp)	Chelating agent for arsenic, mercury, and lead	3–5 mg/kg q4h usually for 5–10 d	Deep IM	Local infection site pain and sterile abscess, nausea, vomiting, fever, salivation, hypertension, and nephrotoxicity (alkalinize urine).
2,3 Dimercaptosuccinic Acid (DMSA Succimer): 100 mg/capsule: 20 capsules	Used as a chelating agent for lead, especially blood lead levels >45 μg/dL. May also be used for symptomatic mercury exposure	10 mg/kg 3 × daily for 5 days followed by 10 mg/kg 2 × daily for 14 days.	PO	Precautions: monitor AST/ALT; use with caution in G6PD-deficient patients. Avoid concurrent iron therapy. Relatively safe antidote, rarely severe, uncommon minor skin rashes may occur.
Diphenhydramine (Benadryl): Antiparkinsonian action. Stock level to treat a 70 kg adult for 24 h: 5 vials (10 mg/mL, 10 mL each)	Used to treat extrapyramidal symptoms and dystonia induced by phenothiazines, phencyclidine, and related drugs	*Children:* 1–2 mg/kg IV slowly over 5 min up to maximum 50 mg followed by 5 mg/kg/24 h orally divided every 6 h up to 300 mg/24 h *Adults:* 50 mg IV followed by 50 mg orally four times daily for 5–7 d. *Note:* Symptoms abate within 2–5 min after IV.	IV	Fatal dose: 20–40 mg/kg. Dry mouth, drowsiness.
Ethanol (Ethyl Alcohol): Stock level to treat 70 kg adult for 24 h: 3 bottles 10% (1 L each)	Methanol, ethylene glycol	10 mL/kg loading dose concurrently with 1.4 mL/kg (average) infusion of 10% ethanol (consult PCC for more details)	IV	Nausea, vomiting, sedation. Use 0.22 μm filter if preparing from bulk 100% ethanol.
Flumazenil (Romazicon): Stock level to treat 70 kg adult for 24 h: 4 vials (0.1 mg/mL, 10 mL)	Benzodiazepines (may also be beneficial in the treatment of hepatic encephalopathy)	Administer 0.2 mg (2 mL) IV over 30 sec (pediatric dose not established, 0.01 mg/kg). then wait 3 min for a response, then if desired consciousness is not achieved, administer 0.3 mg (3 mL) over 30 sec, then wait 3 min for response, then if desired consciousness is not achieved, administer 0.5 mg (5 mL) over 30 sec at 60-sec intervals up to a maximum cumulative dose of 3 mg (30 mL) (1 mg in children). Because effects last only 1–5 h, if patient responds monitor carefully over next 6 h for resedation. If multiple repeated doses, consider a continuous infusion of 0.2–1 mg/h.	IV	Nausea, vomiting, facial flushing, agitation, headache, dizziness, seizures, and death. It is not recommended to improve ventilation. Its role in CNS depression needs to be clarified. It should not be used routinely in comatose patients. It is **contraindicated** in cyclic antidepressant intoxications, stimulant overdose, long-term benzodiazepine use (may precipitate life-threatening withdrawal, if benzodiazepines are used to control seizures, in head trauma.
Folic Acid (Folvite): Stock level to treat 70 kg adult for 24 h: 4 100-mg vials	Methanol/ethylene glycol (investigational)	1 mg/kg up to 50 mg q4h for 6 doses.	IV	Uncommon

Antidote	Indication	Route	Dose	Notes
Fomepizole (4-MP, Antizol): Stock level to treat 70 kg adult: 4 1.5-mL vials (1 g/mL)	Ethylene glycol	IV	Loading dose: 15 mg/kg (0.015 mL/kg) IV followed by maintenance dose of 10 mg/kg (0.01 mL/kg) every 12 h for 4 doses, then 15 mg/kg every 12 h until ethylene glycol levels are <20 mg/dL. Fomepizole can be given to patients undergoing hemodialysis (dose q4h).	Suggested: co-administer folate 50 mg IV (child 1 mg/kg), thiamine 100 mg/d (child 50 mg), and pyridoxine 50 mg IV/IM q6h until intoxication is resolved. Monitor for urinary oxalate crystals. Adverse reactions include headache, nausea, and dizziness. Antizole should be diluted in 100 mL 0.9% saline or D_5W and mixed well. Antizole should not be given undiluted.
	Methanol			
Glucagon: Stock level to treat 70 kg adult for 24 h: 10 vials, 10 units	β-Blocker, calcium channel blocker	IV	3–10 mg in adult, then infuse 2–5 mg/h (0.05–0.1 mg/kg in child, then infuse 0.07 mg/kg/h) Large doses up to 100 mg/24 h used	Use D_5W, not 0.9% saline, to reconstitute the glucagon (rather than diluent of Eli Lilly, which contains phenol). Vomiting precautions.
Magnesium Sulfate: Stock level to treat 70 kg adult for 24 h: approx 25 g (50 mL of 50% or 200 mL of 12.5%)	Torsades de pointes	IV	*Adult:* 2 g (20 mL or 20%) over 20 min. If no response in 10 min, repeat and follow by continuous infusion 1 g/h. *Children:* 25–50 mg/kg/24 h) (0.25–0.5 mEq/kg/24 h) up to 1000 mg/24 h. (Dose not studied in controlled fashion.)	Use with caution if renal impairment is present.
Methylene Blue: Stock level to treat 70 kg adult for 24 h: 5 amps (10 mg/10 mL)	Methemoglobinemia	IV	0.1–0.2 mL/kg of 1% solution, slow infusion, may be repeated every 30–60 min	Nausea, vomiting, headache, dizziness.
Naloxone (Narcan): Stock level to treat 70 kg adult for 24 h: 3 vials (1 mg/mL, 10 mL)	Comatose patient; decreased respirations <12; opioids	IV, ET	In postoperative opioid depression reversal, IV 0.1–0.5 μg/kg every 2 min as needed and may repeat up to a total dose of 1 μg/kg. In **suspected overdose,** administer IV 0.1 mg/kg in a child younger than 5 years of age up to 2 mg, in older children and adults administer 2 mg every 2 min up to a total of 10–20 mg. Can also be administered into the endotracheal tube. If no response by 10 mg, a pure opioid intoxication is unlikely. If **opioid abuse** is suspected, **restraints** should be in place before administration; **initial dose** 0.1 mg to avoid withdrawal and violent behavior. The initial dose is then doubled every minute progressively to a total of 10 mg. A **continuous infusion** has been advocated because many opioids outlast the short half-life of naloxone (30–60 min). The **naloxone infusion hourly rate** to produce a response is equal to the effective dose required (improvement in ventilation and arousal). An additional dose may be required in 15–30 min as a bolus.	**Larger doses** of naloxone may be required for more poorly antagonized synthetic opioid drugs: buprenorphine (Buprenex), codeine, dextromethorphan, fentanyl, pentazocine (Talwin), propoxyphene (Darvon), diphenoxylate, nalbuphine (Nubain), new potent "designer" drugs, or long-acting opioids such as methadone (Dolophine). **Complications.** Although naloxone is safe and effective, there are rare reports of complications (<1%) of pulmonary edema, seizures, hypertension, cardiac arrest, and sudden death. The infusions are titrated to avoid respiratory depression and opioid withdrawal manifestations. Tapering of infusions can be attempted after 12 h and when the patient is stable.

Continued

TABLE 5 Initial Doses of Antidotes for Common Poisonings—Cont'd

Antidote	Use	Dose	Route	Adverse Reactions/Comments
Physostigmine (Antilirium): Stock level to treat 70 kg adult for 24 h: 2–4 mg (2 mL each)	Anticholinergic agents (not routinely used, only indicated if life-threatening complications)	*Child:* 0.02 mg/kg slow push to max 2 mg q30–60 min *Adult:* 1–2 mg q5 min to max 6 mg.	IV	Bradycardia, asystole, seizures, bronchospasm, vomiting, headaches. Do not use for cyclic antidepressants.
Pralidoxime (2PAM, Protopan): Stock level to treat 70 kg adult for 24 h: 12 vials (1 g per 20 mL)	Organophosphates/nerve agents	Child ≤12 y, 25–50 mg/kg max (4 mg/min); >12 y, 1–2 g/dose in 250 mL of 0.9% saline over 5–10 min. Max 200 mg/min. Repeat q6–12h for 24–48h. Max adult 6 g/d. Alternative: Maintenance infusion 1 g in 100 mL, of 0.9% saline at 5–20 mg/kg/h (0.5–12 mL/kg/h) up to max 500 mg/h or 50 mL/h. Titrate to desired response. End point is absence of fasciculations and return of muscle strength.	IV	Nausea, dizziness, headache; tachycardia, muscle rigidity, bronchospasm (rapid administration).
Pyridoxine (Vitamin B₆): Stock level to treat 70 kg adult for 24 h: 100 mg/mL 10% solution. For a 70 kg patient, 10 g = 10 vials	Seizures from isoniazid or *Gyromitra* mushrooms, ethylene glycol	*Isoniazid: Unknown amt ingested:* 5 g (70 mg/kg) in 50 mL D₅W over 5 min + diazepam 0.3 mg/kg IV at rate of 1 mg/min in child or 10 mg dose at rate up to 5 mg/min in adults. Use different site (synergism). May repeat q5–20 min until seizure controlled. Up to 375 mg/kg have been given (52 g). *Known amount:* 1 g for each gram isoniazid ingested over 5 min with diazepam (dose above) *Gyromitra mushroom:* Child 25 mg/kg or 2–5 g, adults IV over 15–30 min to max 20 g.	IV	After seizure is controlled, administer remainder of pyridoxine 1 g/1 g isoniazid total 5 g as infusion over 60 min. Adverse reactions uncommon; do not administer in same bottle as sodium bicarbonate. For *Gyromitra* mushrooms, some use PO 25 mg/kg/d early when mushroom ingestion is suspected.
Sodium Bicarbonate (NaHCO₃): Stock level to treat 70 kg adult for 24 h: 10 ampules or syringes (500 mEq)	Tricyclic antidepressant cardiotoxicity (QRS >0.12 sec; ventricular tachycardia, severe conduction disturbances); metabolic acidosis; phenothiazine toxicity *Salicylate:* to keep blood pH 7.5–7.55 (not >7.55) and urine pH 7.5–8.0. Alkalinization recommended if salicylate conc. >40 mg/dL in acute poisoning and at lower levels if symptomatic in chronic intoxication, 2 mEq/kg will raise blood pH 0.1 unit	*Ethylene glycol:* 100 mg IV daily. 1–2 mEq/kg undiluted as a bolus. If no effect on cardiotoxicity, repeat twice a few minutes apart *Adult* with clear physical signs and laboratory findings of acute moderate or severe salicylism: Bolus 1–2 mEq/kg followed by infusion of 100–150 mEq NaHCO₃ added to 1 L of 5% dextrose at rate of 200–300 mL/h *Child:* Bolus same as adult followed by 1–2 mEq/kg in infusion of 20 mL/kg/h 5% dextrose in 0.45% saline.	IV	Monitor sodium, potassium, and blood pH because fatal alkalemia and hyponatremia have been reported. Monitor both urine and blood pH. Do not use the urine pH alone to assess the need for alkalinization because of the paradoxical aciduria that may occur. Adjust the urine pH to 7.5–8 by NaHCO₃ infusion. After urine output established, add potassium 40 mEq/L.

		Add potassium when patient voids. Rate and amount of the initial infusion, if patient is volume depleted: 1 h to achieve urine output of 2 mL/kg/h and urine pH 7–8. In mild cases without acidosis and urine pH >6 administer 5% dextrose in 0.9% saline with 50 mEq/L or 1 mEq/kg NaHCO$_3$ as maintenance to replace ongoing renal losses. If acidemia is present and pH <7.2, add 2 mEq/kg as loading dose followed by 2 mEq/kg q3–4h to keep pH at 7.5–7.55. If acidemia is present, recommend isotonic NaHCO$_3$, 3 ampules to 1 L of D$_5$W @ 10–15 mL/kg/h or sufficient to produce normal urine flow and a urine pH of 7.5 or higher.
Long-acting barbiturates: Phenobarbital and primidone (Mysoline). *Note*: Alkalinization is ineffective for the short- or intermediate-acting barbiturates	IV	NaHCO$_3$: 2 mEq/kg during the first hour or 100 mEq in 1 L of D$_5$W with 40 mEq/L potassium at a rate of 100 mL/h in adults. Adequate potassium is necessary to accomplish alkalinization Additional sodium bicarbonate and potassium chloride may be needed. Adjust the urine pH to 7.5–8 by NaHCO$_3$ infusion.
Thiamine: 100 mg/mL, 2 vials	Thiamine deficiency, ethylene glycol poisoning, alcoholism	IV/IM	100 mg IV followed with 100 mg V/IM for 5–7 days in an alcoholic and followed by 100 mg/d orally.
Vitamin K$_1$ (Aqua Mephyton): 10 mg/1–5 mL; 5-mg tablets	Warfarin anticoagulant or rodenticide toxicity	PO/SC, IV	Oral 0.4 mg/kg/dose child, 10–25 mg adults. If evidence of bleeding administer vitamin K$_1$ SC, IV 0.6 mg/kg/dose child and up to 25–50 mg adults for 6 hours depending on severity. Give vitamin K daily until PT/INR are normal. Examine stools and urine for evidence of bleeding.

Abbreviations: ALT = alanine aminotransferase; amp = ampule; AST = aspartate aminotransferase; BAL = British anti-Lewisite; BP = blood pressure; Conc. = concentration; ECG = electrocardiogram; ET = endotracheal; G6PD = glucose-6-phosphate dehydrogenase; IM = intramuscular; IV = intravenous; PCC = poison control center; PO = oral; PT = prothrombin time; SC = subcutaneous.

TABLE 6 Plasma Concentrations Above Which Removal by Extracorporeal Measures Should Be Considered

Drug	Plasma Concentration	Protein Binding (%)	Volume Distribution (L/kg)	Method of Choice
Amanitin	NA	25	1.0	HP
Ethanol	500–700 mg/dL	0	0.3	HD
Ethchlorvynol	150 µg/mL	35–50	3–4	HP
Ethylene glycol	25–50 µg/mL	0	0.6	HD
Glutethimide	100 µg/mL	50	2.7	HP
Isopropyl alcohol	400 mg/dL	0	0.7	HD
Lithium	4 mEq/L	0	0.7	HD
Meprobamate (Equanil)	100 µg/mL	0	NA	HP
Methanol	50 mg/dL	0	0.7	HD
Methaqualone	40 µg/dL	20–60	6.0	HP
Other barbiturates	50 µg/dL	50	0–1	HP
Paraquat	0.1 mg/dL	poor	2.8	HP > HD
Phenobarbital	100 µg/mL	50	0.9	HP > HD
Salicylates	80–100 mg/dL	90	0.2	HD > HP
Theophylline		0	0.5	
Chronic	40–60 µg/mL			HP
Acute	80–100 µg/mL			HP
Trichlorethanol	250 µg/mL	70	0.6	HP

Data from Winchester JF: Active methods for detoxification. In Haddad LM, Winchester JF (eds). Clinical Management of Poisoning and Drug Overdose, 2nd ed. Philadelphia, WB Saunders, 1990; Balsam L, Cortitsidis GN, Fienfeld DA: Role of hemodialysis and hemoperfusion in the treatment of intoxications. Contemp Manage Crit Care 1:61, 1991.

Note: Cartridges for charcoal hemoperfusion are not readily available anymore in most locations. So hemodialysis may be substituted in these situations. In mixed or chronic drug overdoses, extracorporeal measures may be considered at lower drug concentrations.

Abbreviations: HD = hemodialysis; HP = hemoperfusion; HP > HD hemoperfusion preferred over hemodialysis.

PLASMAPHERESIS

Plasmapheresis consists of removal of a volume of blood. All the extracted components are returned to the blood except the plasma, which is replaced with a colloid protein solution. There are limited clinical data on guidelines and efficacy in toxicology. Centrifugal and membrane separators of cellular elements are used. It can be as effective as hemodialysis or hemoperfusion for removing toxins that have high protein binding, and it may be useful for toxins not filtered by hemodialysis and hemoperfusion.

Plasmapheresis has been anecdotally used in treating intoxications with the following agents: paraquat (removed 10%), propranolol (removed 30%), quinine (removed 10%), L-thyroxine (removed 30%), and salicylate (removed 10%). It has been shown to remove less than 10% of digoxin, phenobarbital, prednisolone, and tobramycin. Complications include infection; allergic reactions including anaphylaxis; hemorrhagic disorders; thrombocytopenia; embolus and thrombus; hypervolemia and hypovolemia; dysrhythmias; syncope; tetany; paresthesia; pneumothorax; acute respiratory distress syndrome; and seizures.

Supportive Care, Observation, and Therapy for Complications

ALTERED MENTAL STATUS

If airway protective reflexes are absent, endotracheal intubation is indicated for a comatose patient or a patient with altered mental status. If respirations are ineffective, ventilation should be instituted, and if hypoxemia persists, supplemental oxygen is indicated. If a cyanotic patient fails to respond to oxygen, the practitioner should consider methemoglobinemia.

HYPOGLYCEMIA

Hypoglycemia accompanies many poisonings, including with ethanol (especially in children), clonidine (Catapres), insulin, organophosphates, salicylates, sulfonylureas, and the unripe fruit or seed of a Jamaican plant called ackee. If hypoglycemia is present or suspected, glucose should be administered immediately as an intravenous bolus. Doses are as follows: in a neonate, 10% glucose (5 mL/kg); in a child, 25% glucose 0.25 g/kg (2 mL/kg); and in an adult, 50% glucose 0.5 g/kg (1 mL/kg).

A bedside capillary test for blood glucose is performed to detect hypoglycemia, and the sample is sent to the laboratory for confirmation. If the glucose reagent strip visually reads less than 150 mg/dL, one administers glucose. Venous blood should be used rather than capillary blood for the bedside test if the patient is in shock or is hypotensive. Large amounts of glucose given rapidly to nondiabetic patients may cause a transient reactive hypoglycemia and hyperkalemia and may accentuate damage in ischemic cerebrovascular and cardiac tissue. If focal neurologic signs are present, it may be prudent to withhold glucose, because hypoglycemia causes focal signs in less than 10% of cases.

THIAMINE DEFICIENCY ENCEPHALOPATHY

Thiamine is administered to avoid precipitating thiamine deficiency encephalopathy (Wernicke-Korsakoff syndrome) in alcohol abusers and in malnourished patients. The overall incidence of thiamine deficiency in ethanol abusers is 12%. Thiamine 100 mg intravenously should be administered around the time of the glucose administration but not necessarily before the glucose. The clinician should be prepared to manage the anaphylaxis that sometimes is caused by thiamine, although it is extremely rare.

OPIOID REACTIONS

Naloxone (Narcan) reverses CNS and respiratory depression, miosis, bradycardia, and decreased gastrointestinal peristalsis caused by opioids acting through µ, κ, and δ receptors. It also affects endogenous opioid peptides (endorphins and enkephalins), which accounts for the variable responses reported in patients with intoxications from ethanol, benzodiazepines, clonidine (Catapres), captopril (Capoten), and valproic acid (Depakote) and in patients with spinal cord injuries. There is a high sensitivity for predicting a response if pinpoint pupils and circumstantial evidence of opioid abuse (e.g., track marks) are present.

In cases of suspected overdose, naloxone 0.1 mg/kg is administered intravenously initially in a child younger than 5 years of age. The dose can be repeated in 2 minutes, if necessary up to a total dose of 2 mg. In older children and adults, the dose is 2 mg every 2 minutes for five doses up to a total of 10 mg. Naloxone can also be administered into an endotracheal tube if intravenous access is unavailable. If there is no response after 10 mg, a pure opioid intoxication is unlikely. If opioid abuse is suspected, restraints should be in place before the administration of naloxone, and it is recommended that the initial dose be 0.1 to 0.2 mg to avoid withdrawal and violent behavior. The initial dose is then doubled every minute progressively to a total of 10 mg. Naloxone may unmask concomitant sympathomimetic intoxication as well as withdrawal.

Larger doses of naloxone may be required for more poorly antagonized synthetic opioid drugs: buprenorphine (Buprenex), codeine, dextromethorphan, fentanyl and its derivatives, pentazocine (Talwin), propoxyphene (Darvon), diphenoxylate, nalbuphine (Nubain), and long-acting opioids such as methadone (Dolophine).

Indications for a continuous infusion include a second dose for recurrent respiratory depression, exposure to poorly antagonized opioids, a large overdose, and decreased opioid metabolism, as with impaired liver function. A continuous infusion has been advocated because many opioids outlast the short half-life of naloxone (30 to 60 minutes). The hourly rate of naloxone infusion is equal to the effective dose required to produce a response (improvement in ventilation and arousal). An additional dose may be required in 15 to 30 minutes as a bolus. The infusions are titrated to avoid respiratory depression and opioid withdrawal manifestations. Tapering of infusions can be attempted after 12 hours and when the patient's condition has been stabilized.

Although naloxone is safe and effective, there are rare reports of complications (less than 1%) of pulmonary edema, seizures, hypertension, cardiac arrest, and sudden death.

AGENTS WHOSE ROLES ARE NOT CLARIFIED

Nalmefene (Revex), a long-acting parenteral opioid antagonist that the Food and Drug Administration has approved, is undergoing investigation, but its role in the treatment of comatose patients and patients with opioid overdose is not clear. It is 16 times more potent than naloxone, and its duration of action is up to 8 hours (half-life 10.8 hours, versus naloxone 1 hour).

Flumazenil (Romazicon) is a pure competitive benzodiazepine antagonist. It has been demonstrated to be safe and effective for reversing benzodiazepine-induced sedation. It is not recommended to improve ventilation. Its role in cases of CNS depression needs to be clarified. It should not be used routinely in comatose patients and is not an essential ingredient of the coma therapeutic regimen. It is contraindicated in cases of co-ingestion of cyclic antidepressant intoxication, stimulant overdose, and long-term benzodiazepine use (may precipitate life-threatening withdrawal) if benzodiazepines are used to control seizures. There is a concern about the potential for seizures and cardiac dysrhythmias that may occur in these settings.

Laboratory and Radiographic Studies

An electrocardiogram (ECG) should be obtained to identify dysrhythmias or conduction delays from cardiotoxic medications. If aspiration pneumonia (history of loss of consciousness, unarousable state, vomiting) or noncardiac pulmonary edema is suspected, a chest radiograph is needed. Electrolyte and glucose concentrations in the blood, the anion gap, acid-base balance, the arterial blood gas (ABG) profile (if patient has respiratory distress or altered mental status), and serum osmolality should be measured if a toxic alcohol ingestion is suspected. Table 7 lists appropriate testing on the basis of clinical toxicologic presentation. All laboratory specimens should be carefully labeled, including time and date. For potential legal cases, a "chain of custody" must be established. Assessment of the laboratory studies may provide a clue to the etiologic agent.

TABLE 7 Patient Condition/Systemic Toxin and Appropriate Tests

Condition	Tests
Comatose	Toxicologic tests (acetaminophen, sedative-hypnotic, ethanol, opioids, benzodiazepine), glucose.
Respiratory toxicity	Spirometry, FEV_1, arterial blood gases, chest radiograph, monitor O_2 saturation
Cardiac toxicity	ECG 12-lead and monitoring, echocardiogram, serial cardiac enzymes (if evidence or suspicion of a myocardial infarction), hemodynamic monitoring
Hepatic toxicity	Enzymes (AST, ALT, GGT), ammonia, albumin, bilirubin, glucose, PT, PTT, amylase
Nephrotoxicity	BUN, creatinine, electrolytes (Na, F, Mg, Ca, PO_4), serum and urine osmolarity, 24-hour urine for heavy metals if suspected, creatine kinase, serum and urine myoglobin, urinalysis and urinary sodium
Bleeding	Platelets, PT, PTT, bleeding time, fibrin split products, fibrinogen, type and match

Abbreviations: ALT = alanine aminotransaminase; AST = aspartate aminotransaminase; BUN = blood urea nitrogen; ECG = electrocardiogram; FEV_1 = forced expiratory volume at 1 second; GGT = γ-glutamyltransferase; PT = prothrombin time; PTT = partial thromboplastin time.

ELECTROLYTE, ACID-BASE, AND OSMOLALITY DISTURBANCES

Electrolyte and acid-base disturbances should be evaluated and corrected. Metabolic acidosis (usually low or normal pH with a low or normal/high $Paco_2$ and low HCO_3) with an increased anion gap is seen with many agents in cases of overdose.

The anion gap is an estimate of those anions other than chloride and HCO_3 necessary to counterbalance the positive charge of sodium. It serves as a clue to causes, compensations, and complications. The anion gap (AG) is calculated from the standard serum electrolytes by subtracting the total CO_2 (which reflects the actual measured bicarbonate) and chloride from the sodium: $(Na - [Cl + HCO_3]) = AG$. The potassium is usually not used in the calculation because it may be hemolyzed and is an intracellular cation. The lack of anion gap does not exclude a toxic etiology.

The normal gap is usually 7 to 11 mEq/L by flame photometer. However, there has been a "lowering" of the normal anion gap to 7 ± 4 mEq/L by the newer techniques (e.g., ion selective electrodes or colorimetric titration). Some studies have found anion gaps to be relatively insensitive for determining the presence of toxins.

It is important to recognize anion gap toxins, such as salicylates, methanol, and ethylene glycol, because they have specific antidotes, and hemodialysis is effective in management of cases of overdose with these agents.

Table 8 lists the reasons for increased anion gap, decreased anion gap, or no gap. The most common cause of a decreased anion gap is laboratory error. Lactic acidosis produces the largest anion gap and can result from any poisoning that results in hypoxia, hypoglycemia, or convulsions.

Table 9 lists other blood chemistry derangements that suggest certain intoxications.

Serum osmolality is a measure of the number of molecules of solute per kilogram of solvent, or mOsm/kg water. The osmolarity is molecules of solute per liter of solution, or mOsm/L water at a specified temperature. Osmolarity is usually the calculated value and osmolality is usually a measured value. They are considered interchangeable where 1 L equals 1 kg. The normal serum osmolality is 280 to 290 mOsm/kg. The freezing point serum osmolarity measurement specimen and the serum electrolyte specimens for calculation should be drawn simultaneously.

TABLE 8 Etiologies of Metabolic Acidosis

Normal Anion Gap Hyperchloremic	Increased Anion Gap Normochloremic	Decreased Anion Gap
Acidifying agents	Methanol	Laboratory error†
Adrenal insufficiency	Uremia*	Intoxication—bromine, lithium
Anhydrase inhibitors	Diabetic ketoacidosis*	Protein abnormal
Fistula	Paraldehyde,* phenformin	Sodium low
Osteotomies	Isoniazid	
Obstructive uropathies	Iron	
Renal tubular acidosis	Lactic acidosis†	
Diarrhea, uncomplicated*	Ethanol,* ethylene glycol*	
Dilutional	Salicylates, starvation solvents	
Sulfamylon		

*Indicates hyperosmolar situation. Studies have found that the anion gap may be relatively insensitive for determining the presence of toxins.
†Lactic acidosis can be produced by intoxications of the following: carbon monoxide, cyanide, hydrogen sulfide, hypoxia, ibuprofen, iron, isoniazid, phenformin, salicylates, seizures, theophylline.

TABLE 9 Blood Chemistry Derangements in Toxicology

Derangement	Toxin
Acetonemia without acidosis	Acetone or isopropyl alcohol
Hypomagnesemia	Ethanol, digitalis
Hypocalcemia	Ethylene glycol, oxalate, fluoride
Hyperkalemia	β-Blockers, acute digitalis, renal failure
Hypokalemia	Diuretics, salicylism, sympathomimetics, theophylline, corticosteroids, chronic digitalis
Hyperglycemia	Diazoxide, glucagon, iron, isoniazid, organophosphate insecticides, phenylurea insecticides, phenytoin (Dilantin), salicylates, sympathomimetic agents, thyroid vasopressors
Hypoglycemia	β-Blockers, ethanol, insulin, isoniazid, oral hypoglycemic agents, salicylates
Rhabdomyolysis	Amphetamines, ethanol, cocaine, or phencyclidine, elevated creatine phosphokinase

The serum osmolal gap is defined as the difference between the measured osmolality determined by the freezing point method and the calculated osmolarity. It is determined by the following formula:

$$(\text{Sodium} \times 2) + (\text{BUN}/3) + (\text{Glucose}/20)$$

(where BUN is blood urea nitrogen).

This gap estimate is normally within 10 mOsm of the simultaneously measured serum osmolality. Ethanol, if present, may be included in the equation to eliminate its influence on the osmolal gap (the ethanol concentration divided by 4.6; Table 10).

The osmolal gap is not valid in cases of shock and postmortem state. Metabolic disorders such as hyperglycemia, uremia, and dehydration increase the osmolarity but usually do not cause gaps greater than 10 mOsm/kg. A gap greater than 10 mOsm/mL suggests that unidentified osmolal-acting substances are present: acetone, ethanol, ethylene glycol, glycerin, isopropyl alcohol, isoniazid, ethanol, mannitol, methanol, and trichloroethane. Alcohols and glycols should be sought when the degree of obtundation exceeds that expected from the blood ethanol concentration or when other clinical conditions exist: visual loss (methanol), metabolic acidosis (methanol and ethylene glycol), or renal failure (ethylene glycol).

A falsely elevated osmolar gap can be produced by other low molecular weight un-ionized substances (dextran, diuretics, sorbitol,

ketones), hyperlipidemia, and unmeasured electrolytes (e.g., magnesium).

Note: A normal osmolal gap may be reported in the presence of toxic alcohol or glycol poisoning, if the parent compound is already metabolized. This situation can occur when the osmolar gap is measured after a significant time has elapsed since the ingestion. In cases of alcohol and glycol intoxication, an early osmolar gap is a result of the relatively nontoxic parent drug and delayed metabolic acidosis, and an anion gap is a result of the more toxic metabolites. The serum concentration is calculated as

$$\text{mg/dL} = \text{mOsm gap} \times \text{MW of substance divided by 10.}$$

RADIOGRAPHIC STUDIES

Chest and neck radiographs are useful for suspected pathologic conditions such as aspiration pneumonia, pulmonary edema, and foreign bodies and to determine the location of the endotracheal tube. Abdominal radiographs can be used to detect radiopaque substances.

The mnemonic for radiopaque substances seen on abdominal radiographs is CHIPES:

C—chlorides and chloral hydrate
H—heavy metals (arsenic, barium, iron, lead, mercury, zinc)

TABLE 10 Conversion Factors for Alcohols and Glycols

Alcohols/Glycols	1 mg/dL in Blood Raises Osmolality mOsm/L	Molecular Weight	Conversion Factor
Ethanol	0.228	40	4.6
Methanol	0.327	32	3.2
Ethylene glycol	0.190	62	6.2
Isopropanol	0.176	60	6.0
Acetone	0.182	58	5.8
Propylene glycol	not available	72	7.2

Example: Methanol osmolality. Subtract the calculated osmolality from the measured serum osmolarity (freezing point method) = osmolar gap × 3.2 (one-tenth molecular weight) = estimated serum methanol concentration.
Note: This equation is often not considered very reliable in predicting the actual measured blood concentration of these alcohols or glycols.

I—iodides

P—PlayDoh, Pepto-Bismol, phenothiazine (inconsistent)

E—enteric-coated tablets

S—sodium, potassium, and other elements in tablet form (bismuth, calcium, potassium) and solvents containing chlorides (e.g., carbon tetrachloride)

TOXICOLOGIC STUDIES

Routine blood and urine screening is of little practical value in the initial care of the poisoned patient. Specific toxicologic analyses and quantitative levels of certain drugs may be extremely helpful. One should always ask oneself the following questions: (a) How will the result of the test alter the management? and (b) Can the result of the test be returned in time to have a positive effect on therapy?

Owing to long turnaround time, lack of availability, factors contributing to unreliability, and the risk of serious morbidity without supportive clinical management, toxicology screening is estimated to affect management in less than 15% of cases of drug overdoses or poisonings. Toxicology screening may look specifically for only 40 to 50 drugs out of more than 10,000 possible drugs or toxins and more than several million chemicals. To detect many different drugs, toxic screens usually include methods with broad specificity, and sensitivity may be poor for some drugs, resulting in false-negative or false-positive findings. On the other hand, some drugs present in therapeutic amounts may be detected on the screen, even though they are causing no clinical symptoms. Because many agents are not sought or detected during a toxicologic screening, a negative result does not always rule out poisonings. The specificity of toxicologic tests is dependent on the method and the laboratory. The presence of other drugs, drug metabolites, disease states, or incorrect sampling may cause erroneous results.

For the average toxicologic laboratory, false-negative results occur at a rate of 10% to 30% and false-positives at a rate of 0% to 10%. The positive screen predictive value is approximately 90%. A negative toxicology screen does not exclude a poisoning. The negative predictive value of toxicologic screening is approximately 70%. For example, the following benzodiazepines may not be detected by some routine immunoassay benzodiazepine screening tests: alprazolam (Xanax), clonazepam (Klonopin), temazepam (Restoril), and triazolam (Halcion).

The "toxic urine screen" is generally a qualitative urine test for several common drugs, usually substances of abuse (cocaine and metabolites, opioids, amphetamines, benzodiazepines, barbiturates, and phencyclidine). Results of these tests are usually available within 2 to 6 hours. Because these tests may vary with each hospital and community, the physician should determine exactly which substances are included in the toxic urine screen of his or her laboratory. Tests for ethylene glycol, red blood cell cholinesterase, and serum cyanide are not readily available.

For cases of ingestion of certain substances, quantitative blood levels should be obtained at specific times after the ingestion to avoid spurious low values in the distribution phase, which result from incomplete absorption. The detection time for drugs is influenced by many variables, such as type of substance, formulation, amount, time since ingestion, duration of exposure, and half-life. For many drugs, the detection time is measured in days after the exposure.

Common Poisons

ACETAMINOPHEN (PARACETAMOL, N-ACETYL-PARAAMINOPHENOL)

Toxic Mechanism

At therapeutic doses of acetaminophen, less than 5% is metabolized by P450-2E1 to a toxic reactive oxidizing metabolite, N-acetyl-p-benzoquinoneimine (NAPQI). In a case of overdose, there is insufficient glutathione available to reduce the excess NAPQI into nontoxic conjugate, so it forms covalent bonds with hepatic intracellular proteins to produce centrilobular necrosis. Renal damage is caused by a similar mechanism.

Toxic Dose

The therapeutic dose of acetaminophen is 10 to 15 mg/kg, with a maximum of five doses in 24 hours for a maximum total daily dose of 4 g. An acute single toxic dose is greater than 140 mg/kg, possibly greater than 200 mg/kg in a child younger than age 5 years. Factors affecting the P450 enzymes include enzyme inducers such as barbiturates and phenytoin (Dilantin), ingestion of isoniazid, and alcoholism. Factors that decrease glutathione stores (alcoholism, malnutrition, and HIV infection) contribute to the toxicity of acetaminophen. Alcoholics ingesting 3 to 4 g/d of acetaminophen for a few days can have depleted glutathione stores and require N-acetylcysteine therapy at 50% below hepatotoxic blood acetaminophen levels on the nomogram.

Kinetics

Peak plasma concentration is usually reached 2 to 4 hours after an overdose. Volume distribution is 0.9 L/kg, and protein binding is less than 50% (albumin).

Route of elimination is by hepatic metabolism to an inactive nontoxic glucuronide conjugate and inactive nontoxic sulfate metabolite by two saturable pathways; less than 5% is metabolized into reactive metabolite NAPQI. In patients younger than 6 years of age, metabolic elimination occurs to a greater degree by conjugation via the sulfate pathway.

The half-life of acetaminophen is 1 to 3 hours.

Manifestations

The four phases of the intoxication's clinical course may overlap, and the absence of a phase does not exclude toxicity.

- Phase I occurs within 0.5 to 24 hours after ingestion and may consist of a few hours of malaise, diaphoresis, nausea, and vomiting or produce no symptoms. CNS depression or coma is not a feature.
- Phase II occurs 24 to 48 hours after ingestion and is a period of diminished symptoms. The liver enzymes, serum aspartate aminotransferase (AST) (earliest), and serum alanine aminotransferase (ALT) may increase as early as 4 hours or as late as 36 hours after ingestion.
- Phase III occurs at 48 to 96 hours, with peak liver function abnormalities at 72 to 96 hours. The degree of elevation of the hepatic enzymes generally correlates with outcome, but not always. Recovery starts at about 4 days unless hepatic failure develops. Less than 1% of patients with a history of overdose develop fulminant hepatotoxicity.
- Phase IV occurs at 4 to 14 days, with hepatic enzyme abnormalities resolving. If extensive liver damage has occurred, sepsis and disseminated intravascular coagulation may ensue.

Transient renal failure may develop at 5 to 7 days with or without evidence of hepatic damage. Rare cases of myocarditis and pancreatitis have been reported. Death can occur at 7 to 14 days.

Laboratory Investigations

The therapeutic reference range is 10 to 20 µg/mL. For toxic levels, see the nomogram presented in Figure 1.

Appropriate and reliable methods for analysis are radioimmunoassay, high-pressure liquid chromatography, and gas chromatography. Spectroscopic assays often give falsely elevated values: bilirubin, salicylate, salicylamide, diflunisal (Dolobid), phenols, and methyldopa (Aldomet) increase the acetaminophen level. Each 1 mg/dL increase in creatinine increases the acetaminophen plasma level 30 µg/mL.

If a toxic acetaminophen level is reached, liver profile (including AST, ALT, bilirubin, and prothrombin time), serum amylase, and blood glucose must be monitored. A complete blood cell count (CBC); platelet count; phosphate, electrolytes, and bicarbonate level measurements; ECG; and urinalysis are indicated.

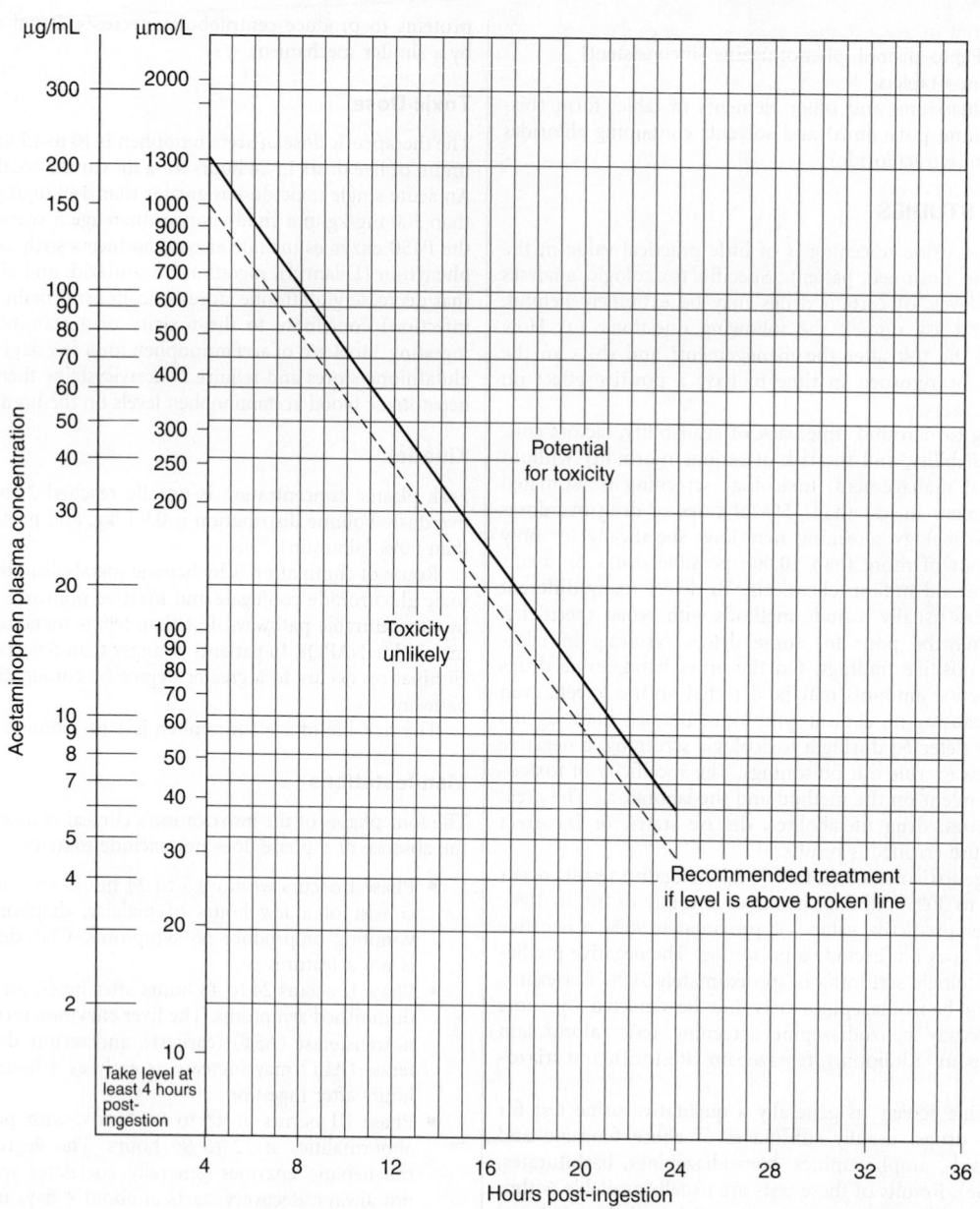

FIGURE 1. Nomogram for acetaminophen intoxication. *N*-acetylcysteine therapy is started if levels and time coordinates are above the lower line on the nomogram. Continue and complete therapy even if subsequent values fall below the toxic zone. The nomogram is useful only in cases of acute single ingestion. Levels in serum drawn before 4 hours may not represent peak levels. (From Rumack BH, Matthew H: Acetaminophen poisoning and toxicity. Pediatrics 55:871, 1975.)

Management

Gastrointestinal Decontamination

Although ipecac-induced emesis may be useful within 30 minutes of ingestion of the toxic substance, we do not advise it because it could result in vomiting of the activated charcoal. Gastric lavage is not necessary. Studies have indicated that activated charcoal is useful within 1 hour after ingestion. Activated charcoal does adsorb *N*-acetylcysteine (NAC) if given together, but this is not clinically important.

However, if activated charcoal needs to be given along with NAC, separate the administration of activated charcoal from the administration of NAC by 1 to 2 hours to avoid vomiting.

N-Acetylcysteine (Mucomyst)

NAC (Table 11), a derivative of the amino acid cysteine, acts as a sulfhydryl donor for glutathione synthesis, as surrogate glutathione, and may increase the nontoxic sulfation pathway resulting in conjugation of NAPQI. Oral NAC should be administered within the first 8 hours

TABLE 11 Protocol for *N*-Acetylcysteine Administration

Route	Loading Dose	Maintenance Dose	Course	FDA Approval
Oral	140 mg/kg	70 mg/kg every 4 h	72 h	Yes
Intravenous	150 mg/kg over 15 min	50 mg/kg over 4 h followed by 100 mg/kg over 16 h	20 h	Yes

after a toxic amount of acetaminophen has been ingested. NAC can be started while one awaits the results of the blood test for acetaminophen plasma concentration, but there is no advantage to giving it before 8 hours. If the acetaminophen concentration result after 4 hours following ingestion is above the upper line on the modified Rumack-Matthew nomogram (see Figure 1), one should continue with a maintenance course. Repeat blood specimens should be obtained 4 hours after the initial level is measured if it is greater than 20 mg/mL, which is below the therapy line, because of unexpected delays in the peak by food and co-ingestants. Intravenous NAC (see Table 11) is approved in the United States.

There have been a few cases of anaphylactoid reaction and death by the intravenous route.

Variations in Therapy

In patients with chronic alcoholism, it is recommended that NAC treatment be administered at 50% below the upper toxic line on the nomogram.

If emesis occurs within 1 hour after NAC administration, the dose should be repeated. To avoid emesis, the proper dilution from 20% to 5% NAC must be used, and it should be served in a palatable vehicle, in a covered container through a straw. If this administration is unsuccessful, a slow drip over 30 to 60 minutes through a nasogastric tube or a fluoroscopically placed nasoduodenal tube can be used. Antiemetics can be used if necessary: metoclopramide (Reglan) 10 mg per dose intravenously 30 minutes before administration of NAC (in children, 0.1 mg/kg; maximum, 0.5 mg/kg/d) or ondansetron (Zofran) 32 mg (0.15 mg/kg) by infusion over 15 minutes and repeated for three doses if necessary. The side effects of these antiemetics include anaphylaxis and increases in liver enzymes.

Some investigators recommend variable durations of NAC therapy, stopping the therapy if serial acetaminophen blood concentrations become nondetectable and the liver enzyme levels (ALT and AST) remain normal after 24 to 36 hours.

There is a loss of efficacy if NAC is initiated 8 or 10 hours postingestion, but the loss is not complete, and NAC may be initiated 36 hours or more after ingestion. Late treatment (after 24 hours) decreases the rates of morbidity and mortality in patients with fulminant liver failure caused by acetaminophen and other agents.

Extended relief formulations (*ER* embossed on caplet) contain 325 mg of acetaminophen for immediate release and 325 mg for delayed release. A single 4-hour postingestion serum acetaminophen concentration can underestimate the level because ER formulations can have secondary delayed peaks. In cases of overdose of the ER formulation, it is recommended that additional acetaminophen levels be obtained at 4-hour intervals after the initial level is measured. If any level is in the toxic zone, therapy should be initiated.

It is recommended that pregnant patients with toxic plasma concentrations of acetaminophen be treated with NAC to prevent hepatotoxicity in both fetus and mother. The available data suggest no teratogenicity to NAC or acetaminophen.

Indications for NAC therapy in cases of chronic intoxication are a history of ingestion of 3 to 4 g for several days with elevated liver enzyme levels (AST and ALT). The acetaminophen blood concentration is often low in these cases because of the extended time lapse since ingestion and should not be plotted on the Rumack-Matthew nomogram. Patients with a history of chronic alcoholism or those on chronic enzyme inducers may also present with elevated liver enzyme levels and should be considered for NAC therapy if they have a history of taking acetaminophen on a chronic basis, because they are considered to be at a greater risk for hepatotoxicity despite a low acetaminophen blood concentration.

Specific support care may be needed to treat liver failure, pancreatitis, transient renal failure, and myocarditis.

Liver transplantation has a definite but limited role in patients with acute acetaminophen overdose. A retrospective analysis determined that a continuing rise in the prothrombin time (4-day peak, 180 seconds), a pH of less than 7.3 2 days after the overdose, a serum creatinine level of greater than 3.3 mg/dL, severe hepatic encephalopathy, and disturbed coagulation factor VII/V ratio greater than 30 suggest a poor prognosis and may be indicators for hepatology consultation for consideration of liver transplantation.

Extracorporeal measures are not expected to be of benefit.

Disposition

Adults who have ingested more than 140 mg/kg and children younger than 6 years of age who have ingested more than 200 mg/kg should receive therapy within 8 hours postingestion or until the results of the 4-hour postingestion acetaminophen plasma concentration are known.

AMPHETAMINES

The amphetamines include illicit methamphetamine ("Ice"), diet pills, and formulations under various trade names. Analogues include MDMA (3,4 methylenedioxymethamphetamine, known as "ecstasy," "XTC," "Adam") and MDA (3,4-methylenedioxyamphetamine, known as "Eve"). MDA is a common hallucinogen and euphoriant "club drug" used at "raves," which are all-night dances. Use of methamphetamine and designer analogues is on the rise, especially among young people between the ages of 12 and 25 years. Other similar stimulants are phenylpropanolamine and cocaine.

Toxic Mechanism

Amphetamines have a direct CNS stimulant effect and a sympathetic nervous system effect by releasing catecholamines from α- and β-adrenergic nerve terminals but inhibiting their reuptake.

Hallucinogenic MDMA has an additional hazard of serotonin effect (refer to serotonin syndrome in the SSRI section). MDMA also affect the dopamine system in the brain. Because of its effects on 5-hydroxytryptamine, dopamine, and norepinephrine, MDMA can lead to serotonin syndrome associated with malignant hyperthermia and rhabdomyolysis, which contributes to the potentially life-threatening hyperthermia observed in several patients who have used MDMA.

Phenylpropanolamine stimulates only the β-adrenergic receptors.

Toxic Dose

In children, the toxic dose of dextroamphetamine is 1 mg/kg; in adults, the toxic dose is 5 mg/kg. The potentially fatal dose of dextroamphetamine is 12 mg/kg.

Kinetics

Amphetamine is a weak base with pKa of 8 to 10. Onset of action is 30 to 60 minutes, and peak effects are 2 to 4 hours. The volume distribution is 2 to 3 L/kg.

Through hepatic metabolism, 60% of the substance is metabolized into a hydroxylated metabolite that may be responsible for psychotic effects.

The half-life of amphetamines is pH dependent—8 to 10 hours in acid urine (pH <6.0) and 16 to 31 hours in alkaline urine (pH >7.5). Excretion is by the kidney—30% to 40% at alkaline urine pH and 50% to 70% at acid urine pH.

Manifestations

Effects are seen within 30 to 60 minutes following ingestion.

Neurologic manifestations include restlessness, irritation and agitation, tremors and hyperreflexia, and auditory and visual hallucinations. Hyperpyrexia may precede seizures, convulsions, paranoia, violence, intracranial hemorrhage, psychosis, and self-destructive behavior. Paranoid psychosis and cerebral vasculitis occur with chronic abuse.

MDMA is often adulterated with cocaine, heroin, or ketamine, or a combination of these, to create a variety of mood alterations. This possibility must be taken into consideration when one manages patients with MDMA ingestions, as the symptom complex may reflect both CNS stimulation and CNS depression.

Other manifestations include dilated but reactive pupils, cardiac dysrhythmias (supraventricular and ventricular), tachycardia, hypertension, rhabdomyolysis, and myoglobinuria.

Laboratory Investigations

The clinician should monitor ECG and cardiac readings, ABG and oxygen saturation, electrolytes, blood glucose, BUN, creatinine, creatine kinase, cardiac fraction if there is chest pain, and liver profile. Also, one should evaluate for rhabdomyolysis and check urine for myoglobin, cocaine and metabolites, and other substances of abuse. The peak plasma concentration of amphetamines is 10 to 50 ng/mL 1 to 2 hours after ingestion of 10 to 25 mg. The toxic plasma concentration is 200 ng/mL. When the rapid immunoassays are used, cross-reactions can occur with amphetamine derivatives (e.g., MDA, "ecstasy"), brompheniramine (Dimetane), chlorpromazine (Thorazine), ephedrine, phenylpropanolamine, phentermine (Adipex-P), phenmetrazine, ranitidine (Zantac), and Vicks Inhaler (L-desoxyephedrine). False-positive results may occur.

Management

Management is similar to management for cocaine intoxication. Supportive care includes blood pressure and temperature control, cardiac monitoring, and seizure precautions. Diazepam (Valium) can be administered. Gastrointestinal decontamination can be undertaken with activated charcoal administered up to 1 hour after ingestion.

Anxiety, agitation, and convulsions are treated with diazepam. If diazepam fails to control seizures, neuromuscular blockers can be used and the electroencephalogram (EEG) monitored for nonmotor seizures. One should avoid neuroleptic phenothiazines and butyrophenone, which can lower the seizure threshold.

Hypertension and tachycardia are usually transient and can be managed by titration of diazepam. Nitroprusside can be used for hypertensive crisis at a maximum infusion rate of 10 µg/kg/minute for 10 minutes followed with a lower infusion rate of 0.3 to 2 mg/kg/minute. Myocardial ischemia is managed by oxygen, vascular access, benzodiazepines, and nitroglycerin. Aspirin and thrombolytics are not routinely recommended because of the danger of intracranial hemorrhage. It is important to distinguish between angina and true ischemia. Delayed hypotension can be treated with fluids and vasopressors if needed. Life-threatening tachydysrhythmias may respond to an α-blocker such as phentolamine (Regitine) 5 mg IV for adults or 0.1 mg/kg IV for children and a short-acting β-blocker such as esmolol (Brevibloc) 500 µg/kg IV over 1 minute for adults, or 300 to 500 µg/kg over 1 minute for children. Ventricular dysrhythmias may respond to lidocaine or, in a severely hemodynamically compromised patient, immediate synchronized electrical cardioversion.

Rhabdomyolysis and myoglobinuria are treated with fluids, alkaline diuresis, and diuretics. Hyperthermia is treated with external cooling and cool 100% humidified oxygen. More extensive therapy may be needed in severe cases. If focal neurologic symptoms are present, the possibility of a cerebrovascular accident should be considered and a CT scan of the head should be obtained.

Paranoid ideation and threatening behavior should be treated with rapid tranquilization using a benzodiazepine. One should observe for suicidal depression that may follow intoxication and may require suicide precautions.

Extracorporeal measures are of no benefit.

Disposition

Symptomatic patients should be observed on a monitored unit until the symptoms resolve and then observed for a short time after resolution for relapse.

ANTICHOLINERGIC AGENTS

Drugs with anticholinergic properties include antihistamines (H_1 blockers), neuroleptics (phenothiazines), tricyclic antidepressants, antiparkinsonism drugs (trihexyphenidyl [Artane], benztropine [Cogentin]), ophthalmic products (atropine), and a number of common plants.

The antihistamines are divided into the sedating anticholinergic types, and the nonsedating single daily dose types. The sedating types include ethanolamines (e.g., diphenhydramine [Benadryl], dimenhydrinate [Dramamine], and clemastine [Tavist]), ethylenediamines (e.g., tripelennamine [Pyribenzamine]), alkyl amines (e.g., chlorpheniramine [Chlor-Trimeton], brompheniramine [Dimetane]), piperazines (e.g., cyclizine [Marezine], hydroxyzine [Atarax], and meclizine [Antivert]), and phenothiazine (e.g., Phenergan). The nonsedating types include astemizole (Hismanal), terfenadine (Seldane), loratadine (Claritin), fexofenadine (Allegra), and cetirizine (Zyrtec).

The anticholinergic plants include jimsonweed (*Datura stramonium*), deadly nightshade (*Atropa belladonna*), henbane (*Hyoscyamus niger*), and antispasmodic agents for the bowel (atropine derivatives).

Toxic Mechanism

By competitive inhibition, anticholinergics block the action of acetylcholine on postsynaptic cholinergic receptor sites. The toxic mechanism primarily involves the peripheral and CNS muscarinic receptors. H_1 sedating-type agents also depress or stimulate the CNS, and in large overdoses some have cardiac membrane–depressant effects (e.g., diphenhydramine [Benadryl]) and α-adrenergic receptor blockade effects (e.g., promethazine [Phenergan]). Nonsedating agents produce peripheral H_1 blockade but do not possess anticholinergic or sedating actions. The original agents terfenadine (Seldane) and astemizole (Hismanal) were recently removed from the market because of the severe cardiac dysrhythmias associated with their use, especially when used in combination with macrolide antibiotics and certain antifungal agents such as ketoconazole (Nizoral), which inhibit hepatic metabolism or excretion. The newer nonsedating agents, including loratadine (Claritin), fexofenadine (Allegra), and cetirizine (Zyrtec), have not been reported to cause the severe drug interactions associated with terfenadine and astemizole.

Toxic Dose

The estimated toxic oral dose of atropine is 0.05 mg/kg in children and more than 2 mg in adults. The minimal estimated lethal dose of atropine is more than 10 mg in adults and more than 2 mg in children. Other synthetic anticholinergic agents are less toxic, and the fatal dose varies from 10 to 100 mg.

The estimated toxic oral dose of diphenhydramine (Benadryl) in a child is 15 mg/kg, and the potential lethal amount is 25 mg/kg. In an adult, the potential lethal amount is 2.8 g. Ingestion of five times the single dose of an antihistamine is toxic.

For the nonsedating agents, an overdose of 3360 mg of terfenadine was reported in an adult who developed ventricular tachycardia and fibrillation that responded to lidocaine and defibrillation. A 1500-mg overdose produced hypotension. Cases of delayed serious dysrhythmias (torsades de pointes) have been reported with doses of more than 200 mg of astemizole. The toxic doses of fexofenadine (Allegra), cetirizine, and loratadine (Claritin) need to be established.

Kinetics

The onset of absorption of intravenous atropine is in 2 to 4 minutes. Peak effects on salivation after intravenous or intramuscular administration are at 30 to 60 minutes.

Onset of absorption after oral ingestion is 30 to 60 minutes, peak action is 1 to 3 hours, and duration of action is 4 to 6 hours, but symptoms are prolonged in cases of overdose or with sustained-release preparations.

The onset of absorption of diphenhydramine is in 15 minutes to 1 hour, with a peak of action in 1 to 4 hours. Volume distribution is 3.3 to 6.8 L/kg, and protein binding is 75% to 80%. Ninety-eight percent of diphenhydramine is metabolized via the liver by N-demethylation. Interactions with erythromycin, ketoconazole (Nizoral), and derivatives produce excessive blood levels of the antihistamine and ventricular dysrhythmias.

The half-life of diphenhydramine is 3 to 10 hours.

The chemical structure of nonsedating agents prevents their entry into the CNS. Absorption begins in 1 hour, with peak effects in 4 in 6 hours. The duration of action is greater than 24 hours.

These agents are metabolized in the gastrointestinal tract and liver. Protein binding is greater than 90%. The plasma half-life is

3.5 hours. Only 1% is excreted unchanged; 60% of that is excreted in the feces and 40% in the urine.

Manifestations

Anticholinergic signs are hyperpyrexia ("hot as a hare"), mydriasis ("blind as a bat"), flushing of skin ("red as a beet"), dry mucosa and skin ("dry as a bone"), "Lilliputian type" hallucinations and delirium ("mad as a hatter"), coma, dysphagia, tachycardia, moderate hypertension, and rarely convulsions and urinary retention. Other effects include jaundice (cyproheptadine [Periactin]), dystonia (diphenhydramine [Benadryl]), rhabdomyolysis (doxylamine), and, in large doses, cardiotoxic effects (diphenhydramine).

Overdose with nonsedating agents produces headache and confusion, nausea, and dysrhythmias (e.g., torsades de pointes).

Laboratory Investigations

Monitoring of ABG (in cases of respiratory depression), electrolytes, glucose, and the ECG should be undertaken. Anticholinergic drugs and plants are not routinely included on screens for substances of abuse.

Management

For patients in respiratory failure, intubation and assisted ventilation should be instituted. Gastrointestinal decontamination can be instituted. Caution must be taken with emesis in cases of diphenhydramine (Benadryl) overdose because of the drug's rapid onset of action and risk of seizures. If bowel sounds are present for up to 1 hour after ingestion, activated charcoal can be given. Seizures can be controlled with benzodiazepines (diazepam [Valium] or lorazepam [Ativan]).

The administration of physostigmine (Antilirium) is not routine and is reserved for life-threatening anticholinergic effects that are refractory to conventional treatments. It should be administered with adequate monitoring and resuscitative equipment available. The use of physostigmine should be avoided if a tricyclic antidepressant is present because of increased toxicity. Urinary retention should be relieved by catheterization to avoid reabsorption of the drug and additional toxicity.

Supraventricular tachycardia should be treated only if the patient is hemodynamically unstable. Ventricular dysrhythmias can be controlled with lidocaine or cardioversion. Sodium bicarbonate 1 to 2 mEq/kg IV may be useful for myocardial depression and QRS prolongation. Torsades de pointes, especially when associated with terfenadine and astemizole ingestion, has been treated with magnesium sulfate 4 g or 40 mL 10% solution intravenously over 10 to 20 minutes and countershock if the patient fails to respond.

Hyperpyrexia is controlled by external cooling. Hemodialysis and hemoperfusion are not effective.

Disposition

Antihistamine H₁ Antagonists

Symptomatic patients should be observed on a monitored unit until the symptoms resolve, then observed for a short time (3 to 4 hours) after resolution for relapse.

Nonsedating Agents

All asymptomatic children who acutely ingest more than the maximum adult dose and all symptomatic children should be referred to a health care facility for a minimum of 6 hours' observation as well as cardiac monitoring. Asymptomatic adults who acutely ingest more than twice the maximum adult daily dose should be monitored for a minimum of 6 hours. All symptomatic patients should be monitored for as long as there are symptoms present.

BARBITURATES

Barbiturates have been used as sedatives, anesthetic agents, and anticonvulsants, but their use is declining as safer, more effective drugs become available.

Toxic Mechanism

Barbiturates are γ-aminobutyric acid (GABA) agonists (increasing the chloride flow and inhibiting depolarization). They enhance the CNS depressant effect of GABA and depress the cardiovascular system.

Toxic Dose

The shorter-acting barbiturates (including the intermediate-acting agents) and their hypnotic doses are as follows: amobarbital (Amytal), 100 to 200 mg; aprobarbital (Alurate), 50 to 100 mg; butabarbital (Butisol), 50 to 100 mg; butalbital, 100 to 200 mg; pentobarbital (Nembutal), 100 to 200 mg; secobarbital (Seconal), 100 to 200 mg. They cause toxicity at lower doses than long-acting barbiturates and have a minimum toxic dose of 6 mg/kg; the fatal adult dose is 3 to 6 g.

The long-acting barbiturates and their doses include mephobarbital (Mebaral), 50 to 100 mg, and phenobarbital, 100 to 200 mg. Their minimum toxic dose is greater than 10 mg/kg, and the fatal adult dose is 6 to 10 g. A general rule is that an amount five times the hypnotic dose is toxic and an amount 10 times the hypnotic dose is potentially fatal. Methohexital and thiopental are ultrashort-acting parenteral preparations and are not discussed.

Kinetics

The barbiturates are enzyme inducers. Short-acting barbiturates are highly lipid-soluble, penetrate the brain readily, and have shorter elimination times. Onset of action is in 10 to 30 minutes, with a peak at 1 to 2 hours. Duration of action is 3 to 8 hours. The volume distribution of short-acting barbiturate is 0.8 to 1.5 L/kg; pKa is about 8. Mean half-life varies from 8 to 48 hours.

Long-acting agents have longer elimination times and can be used as anticonvulsants. Onset of action is in 20 to 60 minutes, with a peak at 1 to 6 hours. In cases of overdose, the peak can be at 10 hours. Usual duration of action is 8 to 12 hours. Volume distribution is 0.8 L/kg, and half-life is 11 to 120 hours. The pKa of phenobarbital is 7.2. Alkalinization of urine promotes its excretion.

Manifestations

Mild intoxication resembles alcohol intoxication and includes ataxia, slurred speech, and depressed cognition. Severe intoxication causes slow respirations, coma, and loss of reflexes (except pupillary light reflex).

Other manifestations include hypotension (vasodilation), hypothermia, hypoglycemia, and death by respiratory arrest.

Laboratory Investigations

Most barbiturates are detected on routine drug screens and can be measured in most hospital laboratories. Investigation should include barbiturate level; ABG; toxicology screen, including acetaminophen; glucose, electrolyte, BUN, creatinine, and creatine kinase levels; and urine pH. The minimum toxic plasma levels are greater than 10 μg/mL for short-acting barbiturates and greater than 40 μg/dL for long-acting agents. Fatal levels are 30 μg/mL for short-acting barbiturates and 80 to 150 μg/mL for long-acting agents. Both short-acting and long-acting agents can be detected in urine 24 to 72 hours after ingestion, and long-acting agents can be detected up to 7 days.

Management

Vital functions must be established and maintained. Intensive supportive care including intubation and assisted ventilation should dominate the management. All stuporous and comatose patients should have glucose (for hypoglycemia), thiamine (if chronically alcoholic), and naloxone (Narcan) (in case of an opioid ingestion) intravenously and should be admitted to the intensive care unit. Emesis should be avoided especially in cases of ingestion of the shorter-acting barbiturates. Activated charcoal followed by MDAC (0.5 g/kg) every 2 to 4 hours has been shown to reduce the serum half-life of phenobarbital by 50%, but its effect on clinical course is undetermined.

Fluids should be administered to correct dehydration and hypotension. Vasopressors may be necessary to correct severe hypotension, and hemodynamic monitoring may be needed. The patient must be observed carefully for fluid overload. Alkalinization (ion trapping) is used only for phenobarbital (pKa 7.2) but not for short-acting barbiturates. Sodium bicarbonate, 1 to 2 mEq/kg IV in 500 mL of 5% dextrose in adults or 10 to 15 mL/kg in children during the first hour, followed by sufficient bicarbonate to keep the urinary pH at 7.5 to 8.0, enhances excretion of phenobarbital and shortens the half-life by 50%. Diuresis is not advocated because of the danger of cerebral or pulmonary edema.

Hemodialysis shortens the half-life to 8 to 14 hours, and charcoal hemoperfusion shortens the half-life to 6 to 8 hours for long-acting barbiturates such as phenobarbital. Both procedures may be effective in patients with both long-acting and short-acting barbiturate ingestion. If the patient does not respond to supportive measures or if the phenobarbital plasma concentration is greater than 150 μg/mL, both procedures may be tried to shorten the half-life.

Bullae are treated as a local second-degree skin burn. Hypothermia should be treated.

Disposition

All comatose patients should be admitted to the intensive care unit. Awake and oriented patients with an overdose of short-acting agents should be observed for at least 6 asymptomatic hours; overdose of long-acting agents warrants observation for at least 12 asymptomatic hours because of the potential for delayed absorption. In the case of an intentional overdose, psychiatric clearance is needed before the patient can be discharged. Chronic use can lead to tolerance, physical dependency, and withdrawal and necessitates follow-up.

BENZODIAZEPINES

Benzodiazepines are used as anxiolytics, sedatives, and relaxants.

Toxic Mechanism

The GABA agonists produce CNS depression and increase chloride flow, inhibiting depolarization.

Flunitrazepam (Rohypnol; street name "roofies") is a long-acting benzodiazepine agonist sold by prescription in more than 60 countries worldwide, but it is not legally available in the United States.

Toxic Dose

The long-acting benzodiazepines (half-life >24 hours) and their maximum therapeutic doses are as follows: chlordiazepoxide (Librium), 50 mg; clorazepate (Tranxene), 30 mg; clonazepam (Klonopin), 20 mg; diazepam (Valium), 10 mg in adults or 0.2 mg/kg in children; flurazepam (Dalmane), 30 mg; and prazepam, 20 mg.

The short-acting benzodiazepines (half-life 10 to 24 hours) and their doses include the following: alprazolam (Xanax), 0.5 mg, and lorazepam (Ativan), 4 mg in adults or 0.05 mg/kg in children, which act similar to the long-acting benzodiazepines.

The ultrashort-acting benzodiazepines (half-life <10 hours) are more toxic and include temazepam (Restoril), 30 mg; triazolam (Halcion), 0.5 mg; midazolam (Versed), 0.2 mg/kg; and oxazepam (Serax), 30 mg.

In cases of overdose of short- and long-acting agents, 10 to 20 times the therapeutic dose (>1500 mg diazepam or 2000 mg chlordiazepoxide) have been ingested with resulting mild coma but without respiratory depression. Fatalities are rare, and most patients recover within 24 to 36 hours after overdose. Asymptomatic unintentional overdoses of less than five times the therapeutic dose can be seen. Ultrashort-acting agents have produced respiratory arrest and coma within 1 hour after ingestion of 5 mg of triazolam (Halcion) and death with ingestion of as little as 10 mg. Midazolam (Versed) and diazepam (Valium) by rapid intravenous injection have produced respiratory arrest.

Kinetics

Onset of CNS depression is usually in 30 to 120 minutes; peak action usually occurs within 1 to 3 hours when ingestion is by the oral route. The volume distribution varies from 0.26 to 6 L/kg (LA, 1.1 L/kg); protein binding is 70% to 99%. For flunitrazepam, the onset of action is in 0.5 to 2 hours, oral peak is in 2 hours, and duration 8 hours or more. The half-life of flunitrazepam is 20 to 30 hours, volume distribution is 3.3 to 5.5 L/kg, and 80% is protein bound. Flunitrazepam can be identified in urine 4 to 30 days after ingestion.

Manifestations

Neurologic manifestations include ataxia, slurred speech, and CNS depression. Deep coma leading to respiratory depression suggests the presence of short-acting benzodiazepines or other CNS depressants. In elderly persons, the therapeutic doses can produce toxicity and can have an additive effect with other CNS depressants. Chronic use can lead to tolerance, physical dependency, and withdrawal.

Laboratory Investigations

Most benzodiazepines can be detected in urine drug screens. Quantitative blood levels are not useful. Some of the immunoassay urinary screens cannot detect all of the new benzodiazepines currently available. A consultation with the laboratory analyst is warranted if a specific case occurs in which the test result is negative but benzodiazepine use is suspected by the patient's history. Situations in which benzodiazepines may not be detected include ingestion of a low dose (e.g., <10 mg), rapid elimination, and a different or no metabolite. Some immunoassay methods can produce a false-positive finding for the benzodiazepines when nonsteroidal anti-inflammatory drugs (tolmetin [Tolectin], naproxen [Aleve], etodolac [Lodine], and fenoprofen [Nalfon]) are used. If this is a concern, the laboratory analyst should be consulted.

In cases in which "date rape" drugs such as flunitrazepam are suspected, a police crime or reference laboratory should be consulted for testing.

Management

Emesis and gastric lavage should be avoided. Activated charcoal can be useful only if given early before the peak time of absorption occurs. Supportive treatment should be instituted but rarely requires intubation or assisted ventilation.

Flumazenil (Romazicon) is a specific benzodiazepine receptor antagonist that blocks the chloride flow and inhibitor of GABA neurotransmitters. It reverses the sedative effects of benzodiazepines, zolpidem (Ambien), and endogenous benzodiazepines associated with hepatic encephalopathy. It is not recommended to reverse benzodiazepine-induced hypoventilation. The manufacturer advises that flumazenil be used with caution in cases of overdose with possible benzodiazepine dependency (because it can precipitate life-threatening withdrawal), if cyclic antidepressant use is suspected, or if a patient has a known seizure disorder.

Disposition

If the patient is comatose, he or she must be admitted to the intensive care unit. If the overdose was intentional, psychiatric clearance is needed before the patient can be discharged.

β-ADRENERGIC BLOCKERS (β-BLOCKERS)

β-Blockers are used in the treatment of hypertension and of a number of systemic and ophthalmologic disorders. Properties of β-blockers include the factors listed in Table 12.

Lipid-soluble drugs have CNS effects, active metabolites, longer duration of action, and interactions (e.g., propranolol). Cardioselectivity is lost in overdose. Intrinsic partial agonist agents (e.g., pindolol) may initially produce tachycardia and hypertension. Cardiac membrane depressive effect (quinidine-like) occurs in cases of overdose but not at therapeutic doses (e.g., with metoprolol or sotalol). α-Blocking effect is weak (e.g., with labetalol or acebutolol).

TABLE 12 Pharmacologic and Toxic Properties of β-Blockers

Blocker	Maximum Solubility	Therapeutic Plasma Level	Lipid Solubility	Intrinsic Sympathomimetic Activity (Partial Agonist)	Membrane Stabilizing Effect	β-Selective β1	β2	Cardiac Selectivity α-Selective
Acebutolol (Sectral)	800 mg	200–2000 ng/mL	Moderate	+	+	–	+	+
Alprenolol²	800 mg	50–200 ng/mL	Moderate	2+	+	–	–	–
Atenolol (Tenormin)	100 mg	200–500 ng/mL	Low	–	–	–	2+	–
Betaxolol (Kerlone)	20 mg	NA	Low	+	–	–	+	–
Carteolol (Cartrol)	10 mg	NA	No	+	–	–	+	–
Esmolol (Brevibloc) (Class II antidysrhythmic, IV only)			Low	–	–	–	+	–
Labetalol (Trandate)	800 mg	50–500 ng/mL	Low	+	+/–	–	–	+
Levobunolol (AKBeta eyedrop) (Eye drops 0.25% and 0.5%)	20 mg	NA	No	–	–	–	–	–
Metoprolol (Lopressor)			Moderate	–	–	–	2+	–
Nadolol (Corgard)	320 mg	20–40 ng/mL	Low	–	–	–	–	–
Oxyprenolol²	480 mg	80–100 ng/mL	Moderate	2+	+	–	–	–
Pindolol (Visken)	60 mg	50–150 ng/mL	Moderate	3+	+/–	–	–	–
Propranolol (Inderal) (Class II antidysrhythmic)	360 mg	50–100 ng/mL	High	–	2+	–	–	–
Sotalol (Betapace) (Class II antidysrhythmic)	480 mg	500–4000 ng/mL	Low	–	–	–	–	–
Timolol (Blocadren)	60 mg	5–10 ng/mL	Low	–	+/–	–	–	–

²Not available in the United States.

Toxic Mechanism

β-Blockers compete with the catecholamines for receptor sites and block receptor action in the bronchi, the vascular smooth muscle, and the myocardium.

Toxic Dose

Ingestions of greater than twice the maximum recommended daily therapeutic dose are considered toxic (see Table 12). Ingestion of 1 mg/kg propranolol in a child may produce hypoglycemia. Fatalities have been reported in adults with 7.5 g of metoprolol. The most toxic agent is sotalol, and the least toxic is atenolol.

Kinetics

Regular-release formulations usually cause symptoms within 2 hours. Propranolol's onset of action is 20 to 30 minutes and peak is at 1 to 4 hours, but it may be delayed by co-ingestants. The onset of action with sustained-release preparations may be delayed to 6 hours and the peak to 12 to 16 hours. Volume distribution is 1 to 5.6 L/kg. Protein binding is variable, from 5% to 93%.

Metabolism

Atenolol (Tenormin), nadolol (Corgard), and santalol (Betapace) have enterohepatic recirculation. The duration of action for regular-acting agents is 4 to 6 hours, but in cases of overdose it may be 24 to 48 hours. The duration of action for sustained-release agents is 24 to 48 hours.

The regular preparation with the longest half-life is nadolol, at 12 to 24 hours, and the one with the shortest half-life is esmolol, at 5 to 10 minutes.

Manifestations

See "Toxic Properties" and Table 12.

Highly lipid soluble agents produce coma and seizures. Bradycardia and hypotension are the major cardiac symptoms and may lead to cardiogenic shock. Intrinsic partial agonists initially may cause tachycardia and hypertension. ECG changes include atrioventricular conduction delay or asystole. Membrane-depressant effects produce prolonged QRS and QT interval, which may result in torsades de pointes. Sotalol produces a very prolonged QT interval. Bronchospasm may occur in patients with reactive airway disease with any β-blocker because the selectivity is lost in overdose. Other manifestations include hypoglycemia (because β-blockers block catecholamine counter-regulatory mechanisms) and hyperkalemia.

Laboratory Investigations

Measurements of blood levels are not readily available or useful. ECG and cardiac monitoring should be maintained, and blood glucose and electrolytes, BUN, and creatinine levels should be monitored, as well as ABG if there are respiratory symptoms.

Management

Vital functions must be established and maintained. Vascular access, baseline ECG, and continuous cardiac and blood pressure monitoring should be established. A pacemaker must be available. Gastrointestinal decontamination can be undertaken initially with activated charcoal up to 1 hour after ingestion. MDAC is no longer recommended, based on the latest guidelines. Whole-bowel irrigation can be considered in cases of large overdoses with sustained-release preparations, but there are no studies evaluating the efficacy of intervention.

If there are cardiovascular disturbances, a cardiac consultation should be obtained. Class IA antidysrhythmic agents (procainamide, quinidine) and III (bretylium) are not recommended. Hypotension is treated with fluids initially, although it usually does not respond. Frequently, glucagon and cardiac pacing are needed. Bradycardia in asymptomatic, hemodynamically stable patients requires no therapy. It is not predictive of the future course of the disease. If the patient is unstable (has hypotension or a high-degree atrioventricular block), atropine 0.02 mg/kg (up to 2 mg) in adults, glucagon, and a pacemaker can be used. In case of ventricular tachycardia, overdrive pacing can be used. A wide QRS interval may respond to sodium bicarbonate. Torsades de pointes (associated with sotalol) may respond to magnesium sulfate and overdrive pacing. Prophylactic magnesium for prolonged QT interval has been suggested, but there are no data. Epinephrine must not be used because an unopposed α effect may occur.

Hypotension and myocardial depression are managed by correction of dysrhythmias, Trendelenburg position, fluids, glucagon, or amrinone (Inocor), or a combination of these. Hemodynamic monitoring with a Swan-Ganz catheter or arterial line may be necessary to manage fluid therapy.

Glucagon is the initial drug of choice. It works through adenyl cyclase and bypasses catecholamine receptors; therefore, it is not affected by β-blockers. Glucagon increases cardiac contractility and heart rate. It is given as an intravenous bolus of 5 to 10 mg[3] over 1 minute and followed by a continuous infusion of 1 to 5 mg/h (in children, 0.15 mg/kg followed by 0.05 to 0.1 mg/kg/h). In large doses and in infusion therapy D_5W, sterile water, or saline should be used as a dilutant to reconstitute glucagon in place of the 0.2% phenol diluent provided with some drugs. Effects are seen within minutes. It can be used with other agents such as amrinone.

Amrinone (Inocor) inhibits phosphodiesterase enzyme, which metabolizes cyclic AMP. It is administered as a bolus of 0.15 to 2 mg/kg (0.15 to 0.4 mL/kg) intravenously, followed by infusion of 5 to 10 µg/kg/min.

Hypoglycemia should be treated with intravenous glucose. Life-threatening hyperkalemia is treated with calcium (avoid if digoxin is present), bicarbonate, and glucose or insulin. Convulsions can be controlled with diazepam or phenobarbital. If bronchospasm is present, β_2 nebulized bronchodilators are given.

Extraordinary measures such as intra-aortic balloon pump support can be instituted. Extracorporeal measures can be undertaken. Hemodialysis for cases of atenolol, acebutolol, nadolol, and sotalol (low volume distribution, low protein binding) ingestion may be helpful, particularly when there is evidence of renal failure. Hemodialysis is not effective for propranolol, metoprolol, and timolol.

Prenalterol[2] has successfully reversed both bradycardia and hypotension but is not currently available in the United States.

Disposition

Asymptomatic patients with history of overdose require baseline ECG and continuous cardiac monitoring for at least 6 hours with regular-release preparations and for 24 hours with sustained-release preparations. Symptomatic patients should be observed with cardiac monitoring for 24 hours. If seizures or abnormal rhythm or vital signs are present, the patient should be admitted to the intensive care unit.

CALCIUM CHANNEL BLOCKERS

Calcium channel blockers are used in the treatment of effort angina, supraventricular tachycardia, and hypertension.

Toxic Mechanism

Calcium channel blockers reduce influx of calcium through the slow channels in membranes of the myocardium, the atrioventricular nodes, and the vascular smooth muscles and result in peripheral, systemic, and coronary vasodilation, impaired cardiac conduction, and depression of cardiac contractility. All calcium channel blockers have vasodilatory action, but only bepridil, diltiazem, and verapamil depress myocardial contractility and cause atrioventricular block.

Toxic Dose

Any ingested amount greater than the maximum daily dose has the potential of severe toxicity. The maximum oral daily doses in adults and toxic doses in children of each are as follows: amlodipine (Norvasc), 10 mg for adults and more than 0.25 mg/kg for children; bepridil (Vascor), 400 mg for adults and more than 5.7 mg/kg for children; diltiazem (Cardizem), 360 mg for adults (toxic dose >2 g) and more

than 6 mg/kg for children; felodipine (Plendil), 40 mg for adults and more than 0.56 mg/kg for children; isradipine (DynaCirc), 40 mg for adults and more than 0.4 mg/kg for children; nicardipine (Cardene), 120 mg for adults and more than 0.85 mg/kg for children; nifedipine (Procardia), 120 mg for adults and more than 2 mg/kg for children; nimodipine (Nimotop), 360 mg for adults and more than 0.85 mg/kg for children; nitrendipine (Baypress),[1] 80 mg for adults and more than 1.14 mg/kg for children; and verapamil (Calan), 480 mg for adults and 15 mg/kg for children.

Kinetics

Onset of action of regular-release preparations varies: for verapamil it is 60 to 120 minutes, for nifedipine 20 minutes, and for diltiazem 15 minutes after ingestion. Peak effect for verapamil is 2 to 4 hours, for nifedipine 60 to 90 minutes, and for diltiazem 30 to 60 minutes, but the peak action may be delayed for 6 to 8 hours. Duration of action is up to 36 hours. The onset of action for sustained-release preparations is usually 4 hours but may be delayed, and peak effect is at 12 to 24 hours. In cases of massive overdose, concretions and prolonged toxicity can develop.

Volume distribution varies from 3 to 7 L/kg. Hepatic elimination half-life varies from 3 to 7 hours. Patients receiving digitalis and calcium channel blockers run the risk of digitalis toxicity, because calcium channel blockers increase digitalis levels.

Manifestations

Cardiac manifestations include hypotension, bradycardia, and conduction disturbances occurring 30 minutes to 5 hours after ingestion. A prolonged PR interval is an early finding and may occur at therapeutic doses. Torsades de pointes has been reported. All degrees of blocks may occur and may be delayed up to 16 hours. Lactic acidosis may be present. Calcium channel blockers do not affect intraventricular conduction, so the QRS interval is usually not affected.

Hypocalcemia is rarely present. Hyperglycemia may be present because of interference in calcium-dependent insulin release. Mental status changes, headaches, seizures, hemiparesis, and CNS depression may occur.

Laboratory Investigations

Specific drug levels are not readily available and are not useful. Monitor blood sugar, electrolytes, calcium, ABG, pulse oximetry, creatinine, and BUN, and also use hemodynamic monitoring, ECG, and cardiac monitoring.

Management

Vital functions must be established and maintained. Baseline ECG readings should be obtained and continuous cardiac and blood pressure monitoring maintained. A pacemaker should be available. Cardiology consultation should be sought.

Gastrointestinal decontamination with activated charcoal is recommended. If a large dose of a sustained-release preparation was ingested, whole-bowel irrigation can be considered, but its effectiveness has not been investigated.

If the patient is symptomatic, immediate cardiology consult must be obtained, because a pacemaker and hemodynamic monitoring may be needed. In the case of heart block, atropine is rarely effective and isoproterenol (Isuprel) may produce vasodilation. The use of a pacemaker should be considered early.

Hypotension and bradycardia can be treated with positioning, fluids, and calcium gluconate or chloride, glucagon, amrinone (Inocor), and ventricular pacing. Calcium salts must be avoided if digoxin is present. Calcium usually reverses depressed myocardial contractility but may not reverse nodal depression or peripheral vasodilation. Calcium chloride can be given in a 10% solution, 0.1 to 0.2 mL/kg up to 10 mL in an adult, or calcium gluconate in a 10% solution 0.3 to 0.4 mL/kg up to 20 mL in an adult. Administration is intravenous, over 5 to 10 minutes. One should monitor for dysrhythmias, hypotension, and the serum ionized calcium. The aim is to increase

---

[2]Not available in the United States.
[3]Exceeds dosage recommended by the manufacturer.

[1]Not available in the United States.

calcium 4 mg/dL to a maximum of 13 mg/dL. The calcium response lasts 15 minutes and may require repeated doses or a continuous calcium gluconate infusion 0.2 mL/kg/h up to maximum of 10 mL/h.

If calcium fails, glucagon can be tried for its positive inotropic and chronotropic effect, or both. Amrinone (Inocor), an inotropic agent, may reverse the effects of calcium channel blockers. An effective dose is 0.15 mg to 2 mg/kg (0.15 to 0.4 mL/kg) by intravenous bolus followed by infusion of 5 to 10 µg/kg/min.

In case of hypotension, fluids, norepinephrine (Levophed), and epinephrine may be required. Amrinone and glucagon have been tried alone and in combination. Dobutamine and dopamine are often ineffective.

Extracorporeal measures (e.g., hemodialysis and charcoal hemoperfusion) are not useful, but extraordinary measures such as intra-aortic balloon pump and cardiopulmonary bypass have been used successfully.

For cases of calcium channel blocker toxicity that fail to respond to aggressive management, recent studies demonstrate that insulin and glucose have therapeutic value. The suggested dose range for insulin is to infuse regular insulin at 0.5 IU/kg/h with a simultaneous infusion of glucose 1 g/kg/h, with glucose monitoring every 30 minutes for at least the first 4 hours of administration and subsequent glucose adjustment to maintain euglycemia (70 to 100 mg/dL). Potassium levels should be monitored regularly, as they may shift in response to the insulin.

Disposition

Patients who have ingested regular-release preparations should be monitored for at least 6 hours and those who have ingested sustained-release preparations should be monitored for 24 hours after the ingestion. Intentional overdose necessitates psychiatric clearance. Symptomatic patients should be admitted to the intensive care unit.

CARBON MONOXIDE

Carbon monoxide is an odorless, colorless gas produced from incomplete combustion; it is also an in vivo metabolic breakdown product of methylene chloride used in paint removers.

Toxic Mechanism

Carbon monoxide's affinity for hemoglobin is 240 times greater than that of oxygen. It shifts the oxygen dissociation curve to the left, which impairs hemoglobin release of oxygen to tissues and inhibits the cytochrome oxidase enzymes.

Toxic Dose and Manifestations

Table 13 describes the manifestations of carbon monoxide toxicity. Exposure to 0.5% for a few minutes is lethal. Sequelae correlate with the patient's level of consciousness at presentation. ECG abnormalities may be noted. Creatine kinase is often elevated, and rhabdomyolysis and myoglobinuria may occur.

The carboxyhemoglobin (CoHB) expresses in percentage the extent to which carbon monoxide has bound with the total hemoglobin. This may be misleadingly low in the anemic patient with less hemoglobin than normal. The patient's presentation is a more reliable indicator of severity than the CoHB level. The manifestations listed in Table 13 for each level are in addition to those listed at the level above. The CoHB may not correlate reliably with the severity of the intoxication, and linking symptoms to specific levels of CoHB frequently leads to inaccurate conclusions. A level of carbon monoxide greater than 40% is usually associated with obvious intoxication.

Kinetics

The natural metabolism of the body produces small amounts of CoHB, less than 2% for nonsmokers and 5% to 9% for smokers.

Carbon monoxide is rapidly absorbed through the lungs. The rate of absorption is directly related to alveolar ventilation. Elimination also occurs through the lungs. The half-life of CoHB in room air (21% oxygen) is 5 to 6 hours; in 100% oxygen, it is 90 minutes; in hyperbaric pressure at 3 atmospheres oxygen, it is 20 to 30 minutes.

TABLE 13 Carbon Monoxide Exposure and Possible Manifestations

CoHB Saturation (%)	Manifestations
3.5	None
5	Slight headache, decreased exercise tolerance
10	Slight headache, dyspnea on vigorous exertion, may impair driving skills
10–20	Moderate dyspnea on exertion, throbbing, temporal headache
20–30	Severe headache, syncope, dizziness, visual changes, weakness, nausea, vomiting, altered judgment
30–40	Vertigo, ataxia, blurred vision, confusion, loss of consciousness
40–50	Confusion, tachycardia, tachypnea, coma, convulsions
50–60	Cheyne-Stokes, coma, convulsions, shock, apnea
60–70	Coma, convulsions, respiratory and heart failure, death

Laboratory Investigations

An ABG reading may show metabolic acidosis and normal oxygen tension. In cases of significant poisoning, the ABG, electrolytes, blood glucose, serum creatine kinase and cardiac enzymes, renal function tests, and liver function tests should be monitored. A urinalysis and test for myoglobinuria should be obtained. Chest radiograph can be useful in cases of smoke inhalation or if the patient is being considered for hyperbaric chamber. ECG monitoring should be maintained, especially if the patient is older than 40 years, has a history of cardiac disease, or has moderate to severe symptoms. Which toxicology studies are used is based on symptoms and circumstances. CoHB should be monitored during and at the end of therapy. The pulse oximeter has two wavelengths and overestimates oxyhemoglobin saturation in carbon monoxide poisoning. The true oxygen saturation is determined by blood gas analysis, which measures the oxygen bound to hemoglobin. The co-oximeter measures four wavelengths and separates out CoHB and the other hemoglobin binding agents from oxyhemoglobin. Fetal hemoglobin has a greater affinity for carbon monoxide than adult hemoglobin and may falsely elevate the CoHB as much as 4% in young infants.

Management

The first step is to adequately protect the rescuer. The patient must be removed from the contaminated area, and his or her vital functions must be established.

The mainstay of treatment is 100% oxygen via a non-rebreathing mask with an oxygen reservoir or endotracheal tube. All patients receive 100% oxygen until the CoHB level is 5% or less. Assisted ventilation may be necessary. ABG and CoHB should be monitored and the present CoHB level determined. *Note:* A near-normal CoHB level does not exclude significant carbon monoxide poisoning, especially if the measurement is taken several hours after termination of exposure or if oxygen has been administered prior to obtaining the sample.

The exposed pregnant woman should be kept on 100% oxygen for several hours after the CoHB level is almost 0, because carbon monoxide concentrates in the fetus and oxygen is needed longer to ensure elimination of the carbon monoxide from fetal circulation. The fetus must be monitored, because carbon monoxide and hypoxia are potentially teratogenic.

Metabolic acidosis should be treated with sodium bicarbonate only if the pH is below 7.2 after correction of hypoxia and adequate ventilation. Acidosis shifts the oxygen dissociation curve to the right and facilitates oxygen delivery to the tissues.

The decision to use the hyperbaric oxygen chamber must be made on the basis of the ability to handle other acute emergencies that may coexist in the patient and of the severity of the poisoning. The standard of care for persons exposed to carbon monoxide has yet to be determined, but most authorities recommend using the hyperbaric oxygen chamber under any of the following conditions:

- If the patient is in a coma or has a history of loss of consciousness or seizures
- If there is cardiovascular dysfunction (clinical ischemic chest pain or ECG evidence of ischemia)
- If the patient has metabolic acidosis
- If symptoms persist despite 100% oxygen therapy
- In a child, if the initial CoHB is greater than 15%
- In symptomatic patients with preexisting ischemia
- If there are signs of maternal or fetal distress regardless of CoHB level (infants and fetus are a special problem because fetal hemoglobin has greater affinity for carbon monoxide)

Although controversial, a neurologic-cognitive examination has been used to help determine which patients with low carbon monoxide levels should receive more aggressive therapy. Testing should include the following: general orientation memory testing involving address, phone number, date of birth, and present date; and cognitive testing, involving counting by 7s, digit span, and forward and backward spelling of three-letter and four-letter words. Patients with delayed neurologic sequelae or recurrent symptoms up to 3 weeks may benefit from hyperbaric oxygen chamber treatment.

Seizures and cerebral edema must be treated.

Disposition

Patients with no or mild symptoms who become asymptomatic after a few hours of oxygen therapy and have a carbon monoxide level less than 10%, and normal physical and neurologic-cognitive examination findings can be discharged, but they should be instructed to return if any signs of neurologic dysfunction appear. Patients with carbon monoxide poisoning requiring treatment need follow-up neuropsychiatric examinations.

CAUSTICS AND CORROSIVES

The terms *caustic* and *corrosive* are used interchangeably and can be divided into acids and alkalis. The U.S. Consumer Product Safety Commission Labeling Recommendations on containers for acids and alkalis indicate the potential for producing serious damage, as follows:

- Caution—weak irritant
- Warning—strong irritant
- Danger—corrosive

Some common acids with corrosive potential include acetic acid, formic acid, glycolic acid, hydrochloric acid, mercuric chloride, nitric acid, oxalic acid, phosphoric acid, sulfuric acid (battery acid), zinc chloride, and zinc sulfate. Some common alkalis with corrosive potential include ammonia, calcium carbide, calcium hydroxide (dry), calcium oxide, potassium hydroxide (lye), and sodium hydroxide (lye).

Toxic Mechanism

Acids produce mucosal coagulation necrosis and may be absorbed systemically; they do not penetrate deeply. Injury to the gastric mucosa is more likely, although specific sites of injury for acids and alkalis are not clearly defined.

Alkalis produce liquefaction necrosis and saponification and penetrate deeply. The esophageal mucosa is likely to be damaged. Oropharyngeal and esophageal damage is more frequently caused by solids than by liquids. Liquids produce superficial circumferential burns and gastric damage.

Toxic Dose

The toxicity is determined by concentration, contact time, and pH. Significant injury is more likely with a substance that has a pH of less than 2 or greater than 12, with a prolonged contact time, and with large volumes.

Manifestations

The absence of oral burns does not exclude the possibility of esophageal or gastric damage. General clinical findings are stridor; dysphagia; drooling; oropharyngeal, retrosternal, and epigastric pain; and ocular and oral burns. Alkali burns are yellow, soapy, frothy lesions. Acid burns are gray-white and later form an eschar. Abdominal tenderness and guarding may be present if perforation has happened.

Laboratory Investigations

If acid ingestion has taken place, the patient's acid-base balance and electrolyte status should be determined. If pulmonary symptoms are present, a chest radiograph, ABG measurement, and pulse oximetry are called for.

Management

It is recommended that the container be brought to the examination, as the substance must be identified and the pH of the substance, vomitus, tears, or saliva tested.

If the acid or alkali has been ingested, all gastrointestinal decontamination procedures are contraindicated except for immediate rinse, removal of substance from the mouth, and dilution with small amounts (sips) of milk or water. The examiner should check for ocular and dermal involvement. Contraindications to oral dilution are dysphagias, respiratory distress, obtundation, or shock. If there is ocular involvement one should immediately irrigate the eye with tepid water for at least 30 minutes, perform fluorescein stain of eye, and consult an ophthalmologist. If there is dermal involvement, one should immediately remove contaminated clothes and irrigate the skin with tepid water for at least 15 minutes. Consultation with a burn specialist is called for.

In cases of acid ingestion, some authorities advocate a small flexible nasogastric tube and aspiration within 30 minutes after ingestion.

Patients should receive only intravenous fluids following dilution until endoscopic consultation is obtained. Endoscopy is valuable to predict damage and risk of stricture. The indications are controversial, with some authorities recommending it in all cases of caustic ingestions regardless of symptoms, and others selectively using clinical features such as vomiting, stridor, drooling, and oral or facial lesions as criteria. We recommend endoscopy for all symptomatic patients or patients with intentional ingestions. Endoscopy may be performed immediately if the patient is symptomatic, but it is usually done 12 to 48 hours postingestion.

The use of corticosteroids is considered controversial. Some feel they may be useful for patients with second-degree circumferential burns. They recommend starting with hydrocortisone sodium succinate (Solu-Cortef) intravenously 10 to 20 mg/kg/d within 48 hours and changing to oral prednisolone 2 mg/kg/d for 3 weeks before tapering the dose. We do not usually recommend using corticosteroids because they have not been shown to be effective.

Tetanus prophylaxis should be provided if the patient requires it for wound care. Antibiotics are not useful prophylactically. Contrast studies are not useful in the first few days and may interfere with endoscopic evaluation; later, they can be used to assess the severity of damage.

Emergency medical therapy includes agents to inhibit collagen formation and intraluminal stents. Esophageal and gastric outlet dilation may be needed if there is evidence of stricture. Bougienage of the esophagus, however, has been associated with brain abscess. Interposition of the colon may be necessary if dilation fails to provide an adequate-sized passage.

Management of inhalation cases requires immediate removal from the environment, administration of humid supplemental oxygen, and observation for airway obstruction and noncardiac pulmonary edema. Radiographic and ABG evaluation should be obtained when appropriate. Intubation and respiratory support may be required.

Certain caustics produce systemic disturbances. Formaldehyde causes metabolic acidosis, hydrofluoric acid causes hypocalcemia and renal damage, oxalic acid causes hypocalcemia, phenol causes hepatic and renal damage, and picric acid causes renal injury.

Disposition

Infants and small children should be medically evaluated and observed. All symptomatic patients should be admitted. If they have severe symptoms or danger of airway compromise, they should be admitted to the intensive care unit. After endoscopy, if no damage is detected, the patient may be discharged when he or she can tolerate oral feedings. Intentional exposures require psychiatric evaluation before the patient can be discharged.

COCAINE (BENZOYLMETHYLECGONINE)

Cocaine is derived from the leaves of *Erythroxylum coca* and *Truxillo coca*. "Body packing" refers to the placement of many small packages of contraband cocaine for concealment in the gastrointestinal tract or other areas for illicit transport. "Body stuffing" refers to spontaneous ingestion of substances for the purpose of hiding evidence.

Toxic Mechanism

Cocaine directly stimulates the CNS presynaptic sympathetic neurons to release catecholamines and acetylcholine, while it blocks the presynaptic reuptake of the catecholamines; it blocks the sodium channels along neuronal membranes; and it increases platelet aggregation. Long-term use depletes the CNS of dopamine.

Toxic Dose

The maximum mucosal local anesthetic therapeutic dose of cocaine is 200 mg or 2 mL of a 10% solution. Although CNS effects can occur at relatively low local anesthetic doses (50 to 95 mg), they are more common with doses greater than 1 mg/kg; cardiac effects can occur with doses greater than 1 mg/kg. The potential fatal dose is 1200 mg intranasally, but death has occurred with 20 mg parenterally.

Kinetics

Cocaine is well absorbed by all routes, including nasal insufflation, and oral, dermal, and inhalation routes (Table 14). Protein binding is 8.7%, and volume distribution is 1.5 L/kg.

Cocaine is metabolized by plasma and liver cholinesterase to the inactive metabolites ecgonine methyl ester and benzoylecgonine. Plasma pseudocholinesterase is congenitally deficient in 3% of the population and decreased in fetuses, young infants, the elderly, pregnant people, and people with liver disease. These enzyme-deficient individuals are at increased risk for life-threatening cocaine toxicity.

Ten percent of cocaine is excreted unchanged. Cocaine and ethanol undergo liver synthesis to form cocaethylene, a metabolite with a half-life three times longer than that of cocaine. It may account for some of cocaine's cardiotoxicity and appears to be more lethal than cocaine or ethanol alone.

Manifestations

The CNS manifestations of cocaine ingestion are euphoria, hyperactivity, agitation, convulsions, and intracranial hemorrhage. Mydriasis and septal perforation can occur, as well as cardiac dysrhythmias, hypertension, and hypotension (with severe overdose). Chest pain is frequent, but only 5.8% of patients have true myocardial ischemia and infarction. Other manifestations include vasoconstriction, hyperthermia (because of increased metabolic rate), ischemic bowel perforation if the substance is ingested, rhabdomyolysis, myoglobinuria, and renal failure. In pregnant users, premature labor and abruptio placentae can occur.

Body cavity packing should be suspected in cases of prolonged toxicity.

Mortality can result from cerebrovascular accidents, coronary artery spasm, myocardial injury, or lethal dysrhythmias.

Laboratory Investigations

Monitoring of the ECG and cardiac rhythms, ABG, oxygen saturation, electrolytes, blood glucose, BUN, creatinine, and creatine kinase levels should be maintained. One should monitor cardiac fraction if the patient has chest pain, as well as the liver profile, and the urine for myoglobin. Intravenous drug users should have HIV and hepatitis virus testing.

Urine should be tested for cocaine and metabolites and other substances of abuse, and abdominal radiographs or ultrasonogram should be ordered for body packers. If the urine sample was collected more than 12 hours after cocaine intake, it will contain little or no cocaine. If cocaine is present, cocaine has been used within the past 12 hours. Cocaine's metabolite benzoylecgonine may be detected within 4 hours after a single nasal insufflation and for up to 114 hours. Cross-reactions with some herbal teas, lidocaine, and droperidol (Inapsine) may give false-positive results by some immunoassay methods.

Management

Supportive care includes blood pressure, cardiac, and thermal monitoring and seizure precautions. Diazepam (Valium) is the drug of choice for treatment of cocaine toxicity agitation, seizures, and dysrhythmias; doses are 10 to 30 mg intravenously at 2.5 mg per minute for adults and 0.2 to 0.5 mg/kg at 1 mg per minute up to 10 mg for a child.

Gastrointestinal decontamination should be instituted, if the cocaine was ingested, by administration of activated charcoal. MDAC may adsorb cocaine leakage in body stuffers or body packers. Whole-bowel irrigation with polyethylene glycol solution (PEG) has been used in body packers and stuffers if the contraband is in a firm container. If the packages are not visible on plain radiographs of the abdomen, a contrast study or CT scan can help to confirm successful passage. Cocaine in the nasal passage can be removed with an applicator dipped in a non–water-soluble product (lubricating jelly) if this is done within a few minutes after application.

In body packers and stuffers, venous access must be secured, and drugs must be readily available for treating life-threatening manifestations until the contraband is passed in the stool. Surgical removal may be indicated if the packet does not pass the pylorus, in an asymptomatic body packer, or in the case of intestinal obstruction.

Hypertension and tachycardia are usually transient and can be managed by careful titration of diazepam. Nitroprusside may be used for severe hypertension. Myocardial ischemia is managed by oxygen, vascular access, benzodiazepines, and nitroglycerin. Aspirin and thrombolysis are not routinely recommended because of the danger of intracranial hemorrhage.

Dysrhythmias are usually supraventricular (SVT) and do not require specific management. Adenosine is ineffective. Life-threatening tachydysrhythmias may respond to phentolamine (Regitine) 5 mg IV

TABLE 14 The Different Routes and Kinetics of Cocaine

Type	Route	Onset	Peak (min)	Half-Life (min)	Duration (min)
Cocaine leaf	Oral, chewing	20–30 min	45–90	NA	240–360
Hydrochloride	Insufflation	1–3 min	5–10	78	60–90
	Ingestion	20–30 min	50–90	54	Sustained
	Intravenous	30–120 sec	5–11	36	60–90
Freebase/crack	Smoking	5–10 sec	5–11	–	Up to 20
Coca paste	Smoking	Unknown	–	–	–

bolus in adults or 0.1 mg/kg in children at 5- to 10-minute intervals. Phentolamine also relieves coronary artery spasm and myocardial ischemia. Electrical synchronized cardioversion should be considered for patients with hemodynamically unstable dysrhythmias. Lidocaine is not recommended initially but may be used after 3 hours for ventricular tachycardia. Wide complex QRS ventricular tachycardia may be treated with sodium bicarbonate 2 mEq/kg as a bolus. β-Adrenergic blockers are not recommended.

Anxiety, agitation, and convulsions can be treated with diazepam. If diazepam fails to control seizures, neuromuscular blockers can be used. The EEG should be monitored for nonmotor seizure activity. For hyperthermia, external cooling and cool humidified 100% oxygen should be administered. Neuromuscular paralysis to control seizures will reduce temperature. Dantrolene and antipyretics are not recommended. Rhabdomyolysis and myoglobinuria are treated with fluids, alkaline diuresis, and diuretics.

If the patient is pregnant, the fetus must be monitored and the patient observed for spontaneous abortion.

Paranoid ideation and threatening behavior should be treated with rapid tranquilization. The patient should be observed for suicidal depression that may follow intoxication and may require suicide precautions. If focal neurologic manifestations are present, one should consider the possibility of a cerebrovascular accident and obtain a CT scan.

Extracorporeal clearance techniques are of no benefit.

Disposition

Patients with mild intoxication or a brief seizure that does not require treatment who become asymptomatic may be discharged after 6 hours with appropriate psychosocial follow-up. If cardiac or cerebral ischemic manifestations are present, the patient should be monitored in the intensive care unit. Body packers and stuffers require care in the intensive care unit until passage of the contraband.

CYANIDE

Hydrogen cyanide is a byproduct of burning plastic and wools in residential fires. Hydrocyanic acid is the liquefied form of hydrogen cyanide. Cyanide salts can be found in ore extraction. Nitriles, such as acetonitrile (artificial nail removers) are metabolized in the body to produce cyanide. Cyanogenic glycosides are present in some fruit seeds (such as amygdalin in apricots, peaches, and apples). Sodium nitroprusside, the antihypertensive vasodilator, contains five cyanide groups.

Toxic Mechanism

Cyanide blocks the cellular electron transport mechanism and cellular respiration by inhibiting the mitochondrial ferricytochrome oxidase system and other enzymes. This results in cellular hypoxia and lactic acidosis. *Note:* Citrus fruit seeds form cyanide in the presence of intestinal β-glucosidase (the seeds are harmful only if the capsule is broken).

Toxic Dose

The ingestion of 1 mg/kg or 50 mg of hydrogen cyanide can produce death within 15 minutes. The lethal dose of potassium cyanide is 200 mg. Five to 10 mL of 84% acetonitrile is lethal. Infusions of sodium nitroprusside in rates above 2 μg/kg per minute may cause cyanide to accumulate to toxic concentrations in critically ill patients.

Kinetics

Cyanide is rapidly absorbed by all routes. In the stomach, it forms hydrocyanic acid. Volume distribution is 1.5 L/kg. Protein binding is 60%. Cyanide is detoxified by metabolism in the liver via the mitochondrial thiosulfate-rhodanase pathway, which catalyzes the transfer of sulfur donor to cyanide, forming the less toxic irreversible thiocyanate that is excreted in the urine. Cyanide is also detoxified by reacting with hydroxocobalamin (vitamin B_{12a}) to form cyanocobalamin (vitamin B_{12}).

The cyanide elimination half-life from the blood is 1.2 hours. The elimination route is through the lungs.

Manifestations

Hydrogen cyanide has the distinctive odor of bitter almonds or silver polish. Manifestations of cyanide intoxication include hypertension, cardiac dysrhythmias, various ECG abnormalities, headache, hyperpnea, seizures, stupor, pulmonary edema, and flushing. Cyanosis is absent or appears late.

Laboratory Investigations

The examiner should obtain and monitor ABGs, oxygen saturation, blood lactate, hemoglobin, blood glucose, and electrolytes. Lactic acidemia, a decrease in the arterial-venous oxygen difference, and bright red venous blood occurs. If smoke inhalation is the possible source of cyanide exposure, CoHB and methemoglobin (MetHb) concentrations should be measured.

Cyanide levels in whole blood, red blood cells, or serum are not useful in the acute management because the determinations are not readily available. Specific cyanide blood levels are as follows: smokers have less than 0.5 μg/mL; a patient with flushing and tachycardia has 0.5 to 1.0 μg/mL, one with obtundation has 1.0 to 2.5 μg/mL, and one in coma or who has died has more than 2.5 μg/mL.

Management

If the cyanide was inhaled, the patient must be removed from the contaminated atmosphere. Attendants should not administer mouth-to-mouth resuscitation. Rescuers and attendants must be protected. Immediate administration of 100% oxygen is called for and oxygen should be continued during and after the administration of the antidote. The clinician must decide whether to use any or all components of the cyanide antidote kit.

The mechanism of action of the antidote kit is twofold: to produce methemoglobinemia and to provide a sulfur substrate for the detoxification of cyanide. The nitrites make methemoglobin, which has a greater affinity for cyanide than does the cytochrome oxidase enzymes. The combination of methemoglobin and cyanide forms cyanomethemoglobin. Sodium thiosulfate provides a sulfur substrate for the rhodanese enzyme, which converts cyanide into the relatively nontoxic sodium thiocyanate, which is excreted by the kidney.

The procedure for using the antidote kit is as follows:

Step 1: Amyl nitrite inhalant perles is only a temporizing measure (forms only 2% to 5% methemoglobin) and it can be omitted if venous access is established. Alternate 100% oxygen and the inhalant for 30 seconds each minute. Use a new perle every 3 minutes.

Step 2: Sodium nitrite ampule is indicated for cyanide exposures, except for cases of residential fires, smoke inhalation, and nitroprusside or acetonitrile poisonings. It is administered intravenously to produce methemoglobin of 20% to 30% at 35 to 70 minutes after administration. A dose of 10 mL of 3% solution of sodium nitrite for adults and 0.33 mL/kg of 3% solution for children is diluted to 100 mL 0.9% saline and administered slowly intravenously at 5 mL/min. If hypotension develops, the infusion should be slowed.

Step 3: Sodium thiosulfate is useful alone in cases of smoke inhalation, nitroprusside toxicity, and acetonitrile toxicity and should not be used at all in cases of hydrogen sulfide poisoning. The administration dose is 12.5 g of sodium thiosulfate or 50 mL of 25% solution for adults and 1.65 mL/kg of 25% solution for children intravenously over 10 to 20 minutes.

If cyanide symptoms recur, further treatment with nitrites or the perles is controversial. Some authorities suggest repeating the antidotes in 30 minutes at half of the initial dose, but others do not advise this for lack of efficacy. The child dosage regimen on the package insert must be carefully followed.

One hour after antidotes are administered, the methemoglobin level should be obtained and should not exceed 20%. Methylene blue should not be used to reverse excessive methemoglobin.

Gastrointestinal decontamination of oral ingestion by activated charcoal is recommended but is not very effective because of the rapidity of absorption. Seizures are treated with intravenous diazepam. Acidosis should be treated with sodium bicarbonate if it does not rapidly resolve with therapy. There is no role for hyperbaric oxygen or hemodialysis or hemoperfusion.

Other antidotes include hydroxocobalamin (vitamin B_{12a}) (Cyanokit), which has proven effective when given immediately after exposure in large doses of 4 g (50 mg/kg) or 50 times the amount of cyanide exposure with 8 g of sodium thiosulfate. Hydroxocobalamin has FDA orphan drug approval.

Disposition

Asymptomatic patients should be observed for a minimum of 3 hours. Patients who ingest nitrile compounds must be observed for 24 hours. Patients requiring antidote administration should be admitted to the intensive care unit.

DIGITALIS

Cardiac glycosides are found in cardiac medications, common plants, and the skin of the Bufo toad.

Toxic Mechanism

Cardiac glycosides inhibit the enzyme sodium/potassium-adenosine triphosphatase (NA^+, K^+, ATPase), leading to intracellular potassium loss and increased intracellular sodium, and producing phase 4 depolarization, increased automaticity, and ectopy. There is increased intracellular calcium and potentiation of contractility. Pacemaker cells are inhibited, and the refractory period is prolonged, leading to atrioventricular blocks. There is increased vagal tone.

Toxic Dose

Digoxin total digitalizing dose, the dose required to achieve therapeutic blood levels of 0.6 to 2.0 ng/mL, is 0.75 to 1.25 mg or 10 to 15 µg/kg for patients older than 10 years of age; 40 to 50 µg/kg for patients younger than 2 years of age; and 30 to 40 µg/kg for patients 2 to 10 years of age.

The acute single toxic dose is greater than 0.07 mg/kg or greater than 2 or 3 mg in an adult, but 2 mg in a child or 4 mg in an adult usually produces only mild toxicity. One to 3 mg or more may be found in a few leaves of oleander or foxglove. Serious and fatal overdoses are more than 4 mg in a child and more than 10 mg in an adult.

Acute digitoxin ingestion of 10 to 35 mg has produced severe toxicity and death. Digitoxin therapeutic steady state is 15 to 25 ng/mL. In cases of chronic or acute-on-chronic ingestions in patients with cardiac disease, more than 2 mg may produce toxicity; however, toxicity can develop within therapeutic range on chronic therapy.

Patients at greatest risk of overdose include those with cardiac disease, those with electrolyte abnormalities (low potassium, low magnesium, low T_4, high calcium), those with renal impairment, and those on amiodarone (Cordarone), quinidine, erythromycin, tetracycline, calcium channel blockers, and β-blockers.

Kinetics

Digoxin is a metabolite of digitoxin. In cases of oral overdose, the typical onset is 30 minutes, with peak effects in 3 to 12 hours. Duration is 3 to 4 days. Intravenous onset is in 5 to 30 minutes; peak level is immediate, and peak effect is at 1.5 to 3 hours.

Volume distribution is 5 to 6 L/kg. The cardiac-to-plasma ratio is 30:1. After an acute ingestion overdose, the serum concentration is not reflective of tissue concentration for at least 6 hours or more, and steady state is 12 to 16 hours after last dose.

Sixty percent to 80% of the parent compound is excreted unchanged in the urine. The elimination half-life is 30 to 50 hours.

Manifestations

Onset of manifestations is usually within 2 hours but may be delayed up to 12 hours.

Gastrointestinal effects of nausea and vomiting are frequently present in cases of acute ingestion but may also occur in cases of chronic ingestion. The "digitalis effect" on ECG is scooped ST segments and PR prolongation; in cases of overdose, any dysrhythmia or block is possible but none are characteristic. Bradycardia occurs in patients with acute overdose with healthy hearts; supraventricular tachycardia occurs in patients with existing heart disease or chronic overdose. Ventricular tachycardia is seen only in cases of severe poisoning.

The CNS effects include headaches, visual disturbances, and colored halo vision. Hyperkalemia occurs following acute overdose and correlates with digoxin level and outcome. Among patients with serum potassium levels of less than 5.0 mEq/L, all survive. If the level is 5 to 5.5, 50% survive, and if the level is greater than 5.5, all die. Hypokalemia is commonly seen with chronic intoxication. Patients with normal digitalis levels may have toxicity in the presence of hypokalemia.

Chronic intoxications are more likely to produce scotoma, color perception disturbances, yellow vision, halos, delirium, hallucinations or psychosis, tachycardia, and hypokalemia.

Laboratory Investigations

Continuous monitoring of ECG, pulse, and blood pressure is called for. Blood glucose, electrolytes, calcium, magnesium, BUN, and creatinine levels should also be monitored. An initial digoxin level should be measured on patient presentation and repeated thereafter. Levels should be measured more than 6 hours postingestion because earlier values do not reflect tissue distribution. Digoxin clinical toxicity is usually associated with serum digoxin levels of greater than 3.5 ng/mL in adults.

An endogenous digoxin-like substance cross-reacts in most common immunoassays (not with high-pressure liquid chromatography) and values as high as 4.1 ng/mL have been reported in newborns, patients with chronic renal failure, patients with abnormal immunoglobulins, and women in the third trimester of pregnancy.

Management

A cardiology consult should be obtained and a pacemaker should be readily available.

In undertaking gastrointestinal decontamination, excessive vagal stimulation should be avoided (e.g., emesis and gastric lavage). Activated charcoal should be administered, and if a nasogastric tube is required for the activated charcoal, pretreatment with atropine (0.02 mg/kg in children and 0.5 mg in adults) should be considered.

Digoxin-specific antibody fragments (Fab, Digibind) 38 mg binds 0.5 mg digoxin and then is excreted through the kidneys. The onset of action is within 30 minutes. Problems associated with Fab therapy are mainly from withdrawal of digoxin and worsening heart failure, hypokalemia, decrease in glucose (if the patient has low glycogen stores), and allergic reactions (very rare). Digitalis administered after Fab therapy is bound and may be inactivated for 5 to 7 days.

Absolute indications for Fab therapy include the following:

- Life-threatening malignant (hemodynamically unstable) dysrhythmias
- Ventricular dysrhythmias, unstable severe bradycardia, or second- or third-degree blocks unresponsive to atropine or rapid deterioration in clinical status
- Life-threatening digitoxin and oleander poisonings
- Relative indications for Fab therapy include the following:
- Ingestions greater than 4 mg in a child and 10 mg in an adult
- Serum potassium level greater than 5.0 mEq/L
- Serum digoxin level greater than 10 ng/mL in adults or greater than 5 ng/mL in children 6 hours after an acute ingestion
- Digitalis delirium and thrombocytopenia response

Digoxin-specific Fab fragments therapy can be administered as a bolus through a 22-µm filter if the case is a critical emergency. If the case is less urgent, then it can be administered over 30 minutes. An empiric dose is 10 vials in adults and 5 vials in a child for an unknown amount ingested in a symptomatic patient with history of a digoxin overdose.

To calculate the dose in the case of a known ingestion, the following equation is used:

$$\text{Amount (total mg)} \times (0.8)\ \text{body burden}$$

If liquid capsules were taken or the substance was given intravenously the 80% bioavailability figure is not used. Instead, the body burden divided by 0.5 (0.5 mg digoxin is bound by 1 vial of 38 mg of Fab) equals the number of vials needed.

If the amount is unknown but the steady state serum concentration is known, the following equations are used:

For digoxin:

$$\text{Digitoxin ng/mL} \times (5.6\ \text{L/kg Vd}) \times (\text{wt kg}) = \text{mg body burden}$$
$$\text{Body burden} \div 1000 = \text{mg body burden}$$
$$\text{Body burden}/0.5 = \text{number of vials needed}$$

For digitoxin:

$$\text{Digitoxin ng/mL} \times (0.56\ \text{L/kg Vd}) \times (\text{wt kg}) = \text{mg body burden}$$
$$\text{Body burden} \div 1000 = \text{mg body burden}$$
$$\text{Body burden}/0.5 = \text{number of vials needed}$$

Antidysrhythmic agents or a pacemaker should be used only if Fab therapy fails. For ventricular tachydysrhythmias, electrolyte disturbances should be corrected by the administration of lidocaine or phenytoin. For torsades de pointes, magnesium sulfate 20 mL 20% IV can be given slowly over 20 minutes (or 25 to 50 mg/kg in a child), titrated to control the dysrhythmia. Magnesium should be discontinued if hypotension, heart block, or decreased deep tendon reflexes are present. Magnesium is used with caution if the patient has renal impairment.

Unstable bradycardia and second-degree and third-degree atrioventricular block should be treated by Fab first. A pacemaker should be available if necessary. Isoproterenol should be avoided because it causes dysrhythmias. Cardioversion is used with caution, starting at a setting of 5 to 10 joules. The patient should be pretreated with lidocaine, if possible, because cardioversion may precipitate ventricular fibrillation or asystole.

Potassium disturbances are caused by a shift, not a change, in total body potassium. Hyperkalemia (>5.0 mEq/L) is treated with Fab only. Calcium must never be used, and insulin/glucose and sodium bicarbonate should not be used concomitantly with Fab because they may produce severe life-threatening hypokalemia. Sodium polystyrene sulfonate (Kayexalate) should not be used. Hypokalemia must be treated with caution because it may be cardioprotective. Treatment can be administered if the patient has ventricular dysrhythmias or a serum potassium level less than 3.0 mEq/L and atrioventricular block.

Extracorporeal procedures are ineffective. Hemodialysis is used for severe or refractory hyperkalemia.

One must never use antidysrhythmic types Ia (procainamide, quinidine, disopyramide [Norpace], amiodarone [Cordarone]), Ic (propafenone [Rythmol], flecainide [Tambocor]), II (β-blockers), or IV (calcium channel blockers). Class Ib drugs (lidocaine, phenytoin [Dilantin], mexiletine [Mexitil], and tocainide [Tonocard]) can be used.

Disposition

Consultation with a poison control center and a cardiologist experienced with digoxin-specific Fab fragments is warranted. All patients with significant dysrhythmias, symptoms, elevated serum digoxin concentration, or elevated serum potassium level should be admitted to the intensive care unit.

ETHANOL

Table 15 lists the features of alcohols and glycols.

Toxic Mechanism

Ethanol has CNS depressant and anesthetic effects. Ethanol stimulates the γ-aminobutyric acid (GABA) system. It promotes cutaneous vasodilation (contributes to hypothermia), stimulates secretion of gastric juice (gastritis), inhibits the secretion of the antidiuretic hormone, inhibits gluconeogenesis (hypoglycemia), and influences fat metabolism (lipidemia).

Toxic Dose

A dose of 1 mL/kg of absolute ethanol (100% ethanol, or 200 proof) gives a blood ethanol concentration of 100 mg/dL. A potentially fatal dose is 3 g/kg for children or 6 g/kg for adults. Children are more prone to developing hypoglycemia than adults.

Kinetics

Onset of action is 30 to 60 minutes after ingestion; peak action is 90 minutes on empty stomach. Volume distribution is 0.6 L/kg. The major route of elimination (>90%) is by hepatic oxidative metabolism. The first step is by the enzyme alcohol dehydrogenase, which converts ethanol to acetaldehyde. Alcohol dehydrogenase metabolizes ethanol at a constant rate of 12 to 20 mg/dL/h (12 to 15 mg/dL/h in nondrinkers, 15 to 30 mg/dL/h in social drinkers, 30 to 50 mg/dL/h in heavy drinkers, and 25 to 30 mg/dL/h in children). At very low blood ethanol concentration (>30 mg/dL), the metabolism is by first-order kinetics. In the second step, acetaldehyde is metabolized by acetaldehyde dehydrogenase to acetic acid, which is metabolized by the Krebs cycle to carbon dioxide and water. The enzyme steps are nicotinamide adenine dinucleotide-dependent, which interferes with gluconeogenesis. Less than 10% of ethanol is excreted unchanged by the kidneys. The relationship between blood ethanol concentration (BEC) and dose (amount ingested) can be calculated as follows:

TABLE 15 Summary of Alcohol and Glycol Features

	Methanol	Isopropanol	Ethanol	Ethylene Glycol
Principal uses	Gas line antifreeze, Sterno, windshield de-icer	Solvent jewelry cleaner, rubbing alcohol	Beverage, solvent	Radiator antifreeze, windshield de-icer
Specific gravity	0.719	0.785	0.789	1.12
Fatal dose	1 mL/Kg 100%	3 mL/kg 100%	5 mL/kg 100%	1.4 mL/kg
Inebriation	±	2+	2+	1+
Metabolic change		Hyperglycemia		
Metabolic acidosis	4+	0	Hypoglycemia	Hypocalcemia
Anion gap	4+	±	1+	2+
Ketosis	Ketobutyric	Acetone	2+	4+
Gastrointestinal tract	Pancreatitis	Hemorrhagic gastritis	Hydroxybutyric	None
Osmolality*	0.337	0.176	Gastritis	
			0.228	0.190

*1 mL/dL of substances raises freezing point osmolarity of serum. The validity of the correlation of osmolality with blood concentrations has been questioned.

TABLE 16 Clinical Signs in the Nontolerant Ethanol Drinker

Ethanol Blood Concentration (mg/dL)*	Manifestations
>25	Euphoria
>47	**Mild incoordination,** sensory and motor impairment
>50	Increased risk of motor vehicle accidents
>100	Ataxia (legal toxic level in many localities)
>150	*Moderate incoordination,* slow reaction time
>200	Drowsiness and confusion
>300	Severe incoordination, stupor, blurred vision
>500	*Flaccid coma,* respiratory failure, hypotension; may be fatal

*Ethanol concentrations sometimes reported in %.
Note: mg% is not equivalent to mg/dL because ethanol weighs less than water (specific gravity 0.79). A 1% ethanol concentration is 790 mg/dL and 0.1% is 79 mg/dL. There is great variation in individual behavior at different blood ethanol levels. Behavior is dependent on tolerance and other factors.

$$BEC \, (mg/dL) = amount \, ingested \, (mL) \times$$
$$\% \, ethanol \, product \times SG \, (0.79)/Vd \, (0.6 \, L/kg) \times body \, wt \, (kg)$$
$$Dose \, (amount \, ingested) = BEC \, (mg/dL) \times$$
$$Vd \, (0.6) \times body \, wt \, (kg)/\% \, ethanol \times$$
$$specific \, gravity \, (0.79)$$

Manifestations

Table 16 lists the clinical signs of acute ethanol intoxication.

Chronic alcoholic patients tolerate higher blood ethanol concentration, and correlation with manifestations is not valid. Rapid interview for alcoholism is the CAGE questions:

- C—Have you felt the need to Cut down?
- A—Have others Annoyed you by criticism of your drinking?
- G—Have you felt Guilty about your drinking?
- E—Have you ever had a morning Eye-opening drink to steady your nerves or get rid of a hangover?

Two affirmative answers indicate probable alcoholism.

Laboratory Investigations

The blood ethanol concentration should be specifically requested and followed. Gas chromatography or a breathalyzer test gives rapid reliable results if no belching or vomiting is present. Enzymatic methods do not differentiate between the alcohols. ABG, electrolytes, and glucose should be measured, the anion and osmolar gaps determined (measure by freezing point depression, not vapor pressure), and a check for ketosis made.

Management

The examiner should inquire about trauma and disulfiram use. The patient must be protected from aspiration and hypoxia. Vital functions must be established and maintained. The patient may require intubation and assisted ventilation.

Gastrointestinal decontamination plays no role in the management of ethanol intoxication.

If the patient is comatose, glucose should be administered intravenously, 1 mL/kg 50% glucose in adults and 2 mL/kg 25% glucose in children. Thiamine, 100 mg intravenously, is administered if the patient has a history of chronic alcoholism, malnutrition, or suspected eating disorders to prevent Wernicke-Korsakoff syndrome. Naloxone (Narcan) has produced a partial inconsistent response but is not recommended for known alcoholics.

General supportive care includes administration of fluids to correct hydration and hypotension and correction of electrolyte abnormalities and acid-base imbalance. Vasopressors and plasma expanders may be necessary to correct severe hypotension. Hypomagnesemia is frequent in chronic alcoholics. In case of hypomagnesemia, a loading dose of 2 g magnesium sulfate 10% is administered by intravenous solution over 5 minutes in the intensive care unit with blood pressure and cardiac monitoring and calcium chloride 10% on hand in case of overdose. This is followed with constant infusion of 6 g of 10% solution over 3 to 4 hours. Caution must be taken with the use of magnesium if renal failure is present.

Hypothermic patients should be warmed. See the section on disturbances caused by cold.

Hemodialysis can be used in severe cases when conventional therapy is ineffective (rarely needed).

Repeated or prolonged seizures should be treated with diazepam (Valium). The brief "rum fits" do not need long-term anticonvulsant therapy. Repeated seizures or focal neurologic findings may warrant skull radiographs, lumbar puncture, and CT scan of the head, depending on the clinical findings. Withdrawal is treated with hydration and large doses of chlordiazepoxide (Librium) 50 to 100 mg or diazepam (Valium) 2 to 10 mg intravenously; these doses may be repeated in 2 to 4 hours. Very large doses of benzodiazepines may be required for delirium tremens. Withdrawal can occur in presence of elevated blood ethanol concentration and can be fatal if left untreated.

Chest radiograph is warranted to determine whether aspiration pneumonia is present. Renal and liver function tests and bilirubin level measurement should be made.

Disposition

Clinical severity (e.g., intubation, assisted ventilation, aspiration pneumonia) should determine the level of hospital care needed. Young children with significant unintentional exposure to ethanol (calculated to reach a blood ethanol concentration of 50 mg/dL) should have blood ethanol concentration obtained and blood glucose levels monitored for hypoglycemia frequently for 4 hours after ingestion. Patients with acute ethanol intoxication seldom require admission unless a complication is present. However, intoxicated patients should not be discharged until they are fully functional (can walk, talk, and think independently), have suicide potential evaluated, have proper disposition environment, and have a sober escort.

ETHYLENE GLYCOL

Ethylene glycol is found in solvents, de-icers, radiator antifreeze (95%), and air-conditioning units. Ethylene glycol is a sweet-tasting, colorless, water-soluble liquid with a sweet aromatic fragrance.

Toxic Mechanism

Ethylene glycol is oxidized by alcohol dehydrogenase to glycolaldehyde, which is metabolized to glycolic acid and glyoxylic acid. Glyoxylic acid is metabolized to oxalic acid via a pyridoxine-dependent pathway to glycine and by thiamine and magnesium-dependent pathways to α-hydroxy-ketoadipic acid. The metabolites of ethylene glycol produce a profound metabolic acidosis, increased anion gap, hypocalcemia, and oxalate crystals, which deposit in tissues (particularly the kidney).

Toxic Dose

The ingestion of 0.1 mL/kg 100% ethylene glycol can result in a toxic serum ethylene glycol concentration of 20 mg/dL. Ingestion of 3.0 mL (less than 1 teaspoonful or swallow) of a 100% solution in a 10-kg child or 30 mL of 100% ethylene glycol in an adult produces a serum ethylene glycol concentration of 50 mg/dL, a concentration that requires hemodialysis. The fatal amount is 1.4 mL/kg of 100% solution.

Kinetics

Absorption is via dermal, inhalation, and ingestion routes. Ethylene glycol is rapidly absorbed from the gastrointestinal tract. Onset is usually in 30 minutes but may be delayed by co-ingestion of food and ethanol. The usual peak level is at 2 hours. Volume distribution is 0.65 to 0.8 L/kg.

For metabolism, see *Toxic Mechanism*.

The half-life of ethylene glycol without ethanol is 3 to 8 hours; with ethanol, it is 17 hours, and with hemodialysis it is 2.5 hours. Renal clearance is 3.2 mL/kg/minute. About 20% to 50% is excreted unchanged in the urine. The relationship between serum ethylene glycol concentration (SEGC) and dose (amount ingested) can be calculated as follows:

$$0.12 \text{ mL/kg of } 100\% = \text{SEGC } 10 \text{ mg/dL}$$

Manifestations

Phase I

The onset of manifestations is 30 minutes to several hours longer after ingestion with concomitant ethanol ingestion. The patient may be inebriated. Hypocalcemia, tetany, and calcium oxalate and hippuric acid crystals in urine can be seen within 4 to 8 hours but are not always present. Early, before metabolism of ethylene glycol, an osmolal gap may be present (see *Laboratory Investigations*). Later, the metabolites of ethylene glycol produce changes starting 4 to 12 hours following ingestion, including an anion gap, metabolic acidosis, coma, convulsions, cardiac disturbances, and pulmonary and cerebral edema. Because fluorescein is added to some antifreeze, the presence of fluorescence may be a clue to ethylene glycol exposure. However, it has been shown that fluorescent urine is not a reliable indicator of ethylene glycol ingestion and should not be used as a screen.

Phase II

After 12 to 36 hours, cardiopulmonary deterioration occurs, with pulmonary edema and congestive heart failure.

Phase III

Phase III occurs 36 to 72 hours after ingestion, with pulmonary edema and oliguric renal failure from oxalate crystal deposition and tubular necrosis predominating.

Phase IV

Neurologic sequelae may occur rarely, especially in patients who fail to receive early antidotal therapy. The onset ranges from 6 to 10 days after ingestion. Findings include facial diplegia, hearing loss, bilateral visual disturbances, elevated cerebrospinal fluid pressure with or without elevated protein levels and pleocytosis, vomiting, hyperreflexia, dysphagia, and ataxia.

Laboratory Investigations

Blood glucose and electrolytes should be monitored. Urinalysis should look for oxalate ("envelope") and monohydrate ("hemp seed") crystals. Urine fluorescence is not reliable as a screen. ABG, ethylene glycol, and ethanol levels, plasma osmolarity (using freezing point depression method), calcium, BUN, and creatinine should be measured. A serum ethylene glycol concentration of 20 mg/dL is toxic (ethylene glycol levels are very difficult to obtain). If possible, a glycolate level should be obtained. Cross-reactions with propylene glycol, a vehicle in many liquids and intravenous medications (phenytoin [Dilantin], diazepam [Valium]), other glycols, and triglycerides may produce spurious ethylene glycol levels. False-positive ethylene glycol values may occur with colorimetric or gas chromatography using an OV-17 column in the presence of propylene glycol.

The following equations can be used to calculate the osmolality, osmolal gap, and ethylene glycol level:

$$2(Na + mEq/L) + (\text{Blood glucose mg/dL})/20 + (\text{BUN mg/dL})/3 =$$
Total calculated osmolality (mOsm/L)

Osmolar Gap = measured osmolality (by freezing point depression method) − calculate osmolality

A gap greater than 10 is abnormal. *Note:* if ethanol is involved, add ethanol level/4.6 to the calculated equation.

An increased osmolal gap is produced by the following common substances: acetone, dextran, dimethyl sulfoxide, diuretics, ethanol, ethyl ether, ethylene glycol, isopropanol, paraldehyde, mannitol, methanol, sorbitol, and trichloroethane. Table 10 gives the conversion factors for these substances.

Although a specific blood level of ethylene glycol in milligrams per deciliter can be estimated using the equation below, this is not considered to be a reliable method and should not take the place of obtaining a measured ethylene glycol blood concentration.

$$\text{osmolar gap} \times \text{conversion factor} = \text{serum concentration}$$

Caution: The accuracy of the ethylene glycol estimated decreases as the ethylene glycol levels decrease. The toxic metabolites are not osmotically active, and patients presenting late may show signs of severe toxicity without an elevated osmolar gap.

The anion gap can be calculated using the following equation:

$$Na - (Cl + HCO_3) = \text{anion gap}$$

The normal gap is 8 to 12. Potassium is not used because it is a small amount and may be hemolyzed. Table 8 lists factors that may account for an increased or a decreased anion gap.

Management

Vital functions should be established and maintained. The airway must be protected, and assisted ventilation can be used, if necessary. Gastrointestinal decontamination has a limited role. Only gastric aspiration can be used within 60 minutes after ingestion. Activated charcoal is not effective.

Baseline measurements of serum electrolytes and calcium, glucose, ABGs, ethanol, serum ethylene glycol concentration (may be difficult to obtain readily in some institutions), and methanol concentrations should be obtained. In the first few hours, the measured serum osmolality should be determined and compared to calculated osmolality (see osmolality equation, earlier). If seizures occur, one should measure serum calcium (preferably ionized calcium) and treat with intravenous diazepam. If the patient has hypocalcemic seizures, he or she should also be treated with 10 to 20 mL 10% calcium gluconate (0.2 to 0.3 mL/kg in children) slowly intravenously, with the dose repeated as needed. Metabolic acidosis should be corrected with intravenous sodium bicarbonate.

Ethanol therapy should be initiated immediately if fomepizole (Antizol) is unavailable (see next paragraph). Alcohol dehydrogenase has a greater affinity for ethanol than ethylene glycol. Therefore, ethanol blocks the metabolism of ethylene glycol. Ethanol therapy is called for if there is a history of ingestion of 0.1 mL/kg of 100% ethylene glycol, serum ethylene glycol concentration is greater than 20 mg/dL, there is an osmolar gap not accounted for by other alcohols or factors (e.g., hyperlipidemia), metabolic acidosis is present with an increased anion gap, or there are oxalate crystals in the urine. Ethanol should be administered intravenously (the oral route is less reliable) to produce a blood ethanol concentration of 100 to 150 mg/dL. The loading dose is 10 mL/kg of 10% ethanol intravenously, administered concomitantly with a maintenance dose of 10% ethanol of 1.0 mL/kg/h. This dose may need to be increased to 2 mL/kg/h in patients who are heavy drinkers. The blood ethanol concentration should be measured hourly and the infusion rate should be adjusted to maintain a blood ethanol concentration of 100 to 150 mg/dL.

Fomepizole (Antizol, 4-methylpyrazole) inhibits alcohol dehydrogenase more reliability than ethanol and it does not require constant monitoring of ethanol levels and adjustment of infusion rates. Fomepizole is available in 1 g/mL vials of 1.5 mL. The loading dose is 15 mg/kg (0.015 mL/kg) IV; maintenance dose is 10 mg/kg (0.01 mL/kg) every 12 hours for four doses, then 15 mg/kg every 12 hours until the ethylene glycol levels are less than 20 mg/dL. The solution is prepared by being mixed with 100 mL of 0.9% saline or D$_5$W (5% dextrose in water). Fomepizole can be given to patients requiring hemodialysis but should be dosed as follows:

Dose at the beginning of hemodialysis:

- If <6 hours since last Antizol dose, do not administer dose
- If >6 hours since last dose, administer next scheduled dose

Dosing during hemodialysis:

- Dose every 4 hours

Dosing at the time hemodialysis is completed:

- If <1 hour between last dose and end of dialysis, do not administer dose at end of dialysis
- If 1 to 3 hours between last dose and end of dialysis, administer one half of next scheduled dose
- If >3 hours between last dose and end of dialysis, administer next scheduled dose

Maintenance dosing off hemodialysis:

- Give the next scheduled dose 12 hours from the last dose administered

Hemodialysis is indicated if the ingestion was potentially fatal; if the serum ethylene glycol concentration is greater than 50 mg/dL (some recommend at levels of >25 mg/dL); if severe acidosis or electrolyte abnormalities occur despite conventional therapy; or if congestive heart failure or renal failure is present. Hemodialysis reduces the ethylene glycol half-life from 17 hours on ethanol therapy to 3 hours. Therapy (fomepizole and hemodialysis) should be continued until the serum ethylene glycol concentration is less than 10 mg/dL, the glycolate level is nondetectable (not readily available), the acidosis has cleared, there are no mental disturbances, the creatinine level is normal, and the urinary output is adequate. This may require 2 to 5 days.

Adjunct therapy involving thiamine, 100 mg/d (in children, 50 mg), slowly over 5 minutes intravenously or intramuscularly and repeated every 6 hours and pyridoxine, 50 mg IV or IM every 6 hours, has been recommended until intoxication is resolved, but these agents have not been extensively studied. Folate, 50 mg IV (child 1 mg/kg), can be given every 4 hours for 6 doses.

Disposition

All patients who have ingested significant amounts of ethylene glycol (calculated level above 20 mg/dL), have a history of a toxic dose, or are symptomatic should be referred to the emergency department and admitted. If the serum ethylene glycol concentration cannot be obtained, the patient should be followed for 12 hours, with monitoring of the osmolal gap, acid-base parameters, and electrolytes to exclude development of metabolic acidosis with an anion gap. Transfer should be considered for fomepizole therapy or hemodialysis.

HYDROCARBONS

The lower the viscosity and surface tension of hydrocarbons or the greater the volatility, the greater the risk of aspiration. Volatile substance abuse has produced the "Sudden Sniffing's Death Syndrome," most likely caused by dysrhythmias.

Toxicologic Classification and Toxic Mechanism

All systemically absorbed hydrocarbons can lower the threshold of the myocardium to dysrhythmias produced by endogenous and exogenous catecholamines.

Aliphatic hydrocarbons are branched straight chain hydrocarbons. A few aspirated drops are poorly absorbed from the gastrointestinal tract and produce no systemic toxicity by this route. However, aspiration of very small amounts can produce chemical pneumonitis. Examples of aliphatic hydrocarbons are gasoline, kerosene, charcoal lighter fluid, mineral spirits (Stoddard's solvent), and petroleum naphtha. Mineral seal oil (signal oil), found in furniture polishes, is a low-viscosity and low-volatility oil with minimum absorption that never warrants gastric decontamination. It can produce severe pneumonia if aspirated.

Aromatic hydrocarbons are six carbon ring structures that are absorbed through the gastrointestinal tract. Systemic toxicity includes CNS depression and, in cases of chronic abuse, multiple organ effects such as leukemia (benzene) and renal toxicity (toluene). Examples are benzene, toluene, styrene, and xylene. The seriously toxic ingested dose is 20 to 50 mL in adults.

Halogenated hydrocarbons are aliphatic or aromatic hydrocarbons with one or more halogen substitutions (Cl, Br, Fl, or I). They are highly volatile and are abused as inhalants. They are well absorbed from the gastrointestinal tract, produce CNS depression, and have metabolites that can damage the liver and kidneys. Examples include methylene chloride (may be converted into carbon monoxide in the body), dichloroethylene (also causes a disulfiram [Antabuse] reaction known as "degreaser's flush" when associated with consumption of ethanol), and 1,1,1-trichloroethane (Glamorene Spot Remover, Scotchgard, typewriter correction fluid). An acute lethal oral dose is 0.5 to 5 mL/kg.

Dangerous additives to the hydrocarbons can be summed up with the mnemonic CHAMP: C, camphor (demothing agent); H, halogenated hydrocarbons; A, aromatic hydrocarbons; M, metals (heavy); and P, pesticides. Ingestion of these substances may warrant gastric emptying with a small-bore nasogastric tube.

Heavy hydrocarbons have high viscosity, low volatility, and minimal gastrointestinal absorption, so gastric decontamination is not necessary. Examples are asphalt (tar), machine oil, motor oil (lubricating oil, engine oil), home heating oil, and petroleum jelly (mineral oil).

Laboratory Investigations

The ECG, ABG, pulmonary function, serum electrolytes, and serial chest radiographs should be continuously monitored. Liver and renal function should be monitored in cases of inhalation of aromatic hydrocarbons.

Management

Asymptomatic patients who ingested small amounts of aliphatic petroleum distillates can be followed at home by telephone for development of signs of aspiration (cough, wheezing, tachypnea, and dyspnea) for 4 to 6 hours. Inhalation of any hydrocarbon vapors in a closed space can produce intoxication. The victim must be removed from the environment, have oxygen administered, and receive respiratory support.

Gastrointestinal decontamination is not advised in cases of hydrocarbon ingestion that usually do not cause systemic toxicity (aliphatic petroleum distillates, heavy hydrocarbons). In cases of ingestion of hydrocarbons that cause systemic toxicity in small amounts (aromatic hydrocarbons, halogenated hydrocarbons), the clinician should pass a small-bore nasogastric tube and aspirate if the ingestion was within 2 hours and if spontaneous vomiting has not occurred. Some toxicologists advocate ipecac-induced emesis under medical supervision instead of small-bore nasogastric gastric lavage; we do not.

Patients with altered mental status should have their airway protected because of concern about aspiration. The use of activated charcoal has been suggested, but there are no scientific data as to effectiveness and it may produce vomiting. Activated charcoal may, however, be useful in adsorbing toxic additives such as pesticides or co-ingestants.

The symptomatic patient who is coughing, gagging, choking, or wheezing on arrival has probably aspirated. The clinician should provide supportive respiratory care and supplemental oxygen, while monitoring pulse oximetry, ABG, chest radiograph, and ECG. The patient should be admitted to the intensive care unit. A chest radiograph for aspiration may be positive as early as 30 minutes after ingestion, and almost all are positive within 6 hours. Negative chest radiographs within 4 hours do not rule out aspiration.

Bronchospasm is treated with a nebulized β-adrenergic agonist and intravenous aminophylline if necessary. Epinephrine should be avoided because of susceptibility to dysrhythmias. Cyanosis in the presence of a normal arterial Pao_2 may be a result of methemoglobinemia that requires therapy with methylene blue. Corticosteroids and prophylactic antimicrobial agents have not been shown to be beneficial. (Fever or leukocytosis may be produced by the chemical pneumonitis itself.)

Most infiltrations resolve spontaneously in 1 week; lipoid pneumonia may last up to 6 weeks. It is not necessary to surgically treat pneumatoceles that develop because they usually resolve. Dysrhythmias may require α- and β-adrenergic antagonists or cardioversion.

There is no role for enhanced elimination procedures.

Methylene chloride is metabolized over several hours to carbon monoxide. See treatment of carbon monoxide poisoning. Halogenated hydrocarbons are hepatorenal toxins; therefore, hepatorenal function should be monitored. N-acetylcysteine therapy may be useful if there is evidence of hepatic damage.

Extracorporeal membrane oxygenation (ECMO) has been used successfully for a few patients with life threatening respiratory failure. Surfactant used for hydrocarbon aspiration was found to be detrimental.

Disposition

Asymptomatic patients with small ingestions of petroleum distillates can be managed at home. Symptomatic patients with abnormal chest radiographic, oxygen saturation, or ABG findings should be admitted. Patients who become asymptomatic and have normal oxygenation and a normal repeat radiograph can be discharged.

IRON

There are more than 100 iron over-the-counter preparations for supplementation and treatment of iron deficiency anemia.

Toxic Mechanism

Toxicity depends on the amount of elemental iron available in various salts (gluconate 12%, sulfate 20%, fumarate 33%, lactate 19%, chloride 21% of elemental iron), not the amount of the salt. Locally, iron is corrosive and may cause fluid loss, hypovolemic shock, and perforation. Excessive free unbound iron in the blood is directly toxic to the vasculature and leads to the release of vasoactive substances, which produces vasodilation. In cases of overdose, iron deposits injure mitochondria in the liver, the kidneys, and the myocardium. The exact mechanism of cellular damage is not clear but is thought to be related to free radical formation.

Toxic Dose

The therapeutic dose is 6 mg/kg/d of elemental iron. An elemental iron dose of 20 to 40 mg/kg may produce mild self-limited gastrointestinal symptoms, 40 to 60 mg/kg produces moderate toxicity, more than 60 mg/kg produces severe toxicity and is potentially lethal, and more than 180 mg/kg is usually fatal without treatment. Children's chewable vitamins with iron have between 12 and 18 mg of elemental iron per tablet or 0.6 mL of liquid drops. These preparations rarely produce toxicity unless very large quantities are ingested and have never caused death.

Kinetics

Absorption occurs chiefly in the upper small intestine. Ferrous (+2) iron is absorbed into the mucosal cells, where it is oxidized to the ferric (+3) state and bound to ferritin. Iron is slowly released from ferritin into the plasma, where it binds to transferrin and is transported to specific tissues for production of hemoglobin (70%), myoglobin (5%), and cytochrome. About 25% of iron is stored in the liver and spleen. In cases of overdose, larger amounts of iron are absorbed because of direct mucosal corrosion. There is no mechanism for the elimination of iron (elimination is 1 to 2 mg/d) except through bile, sweat, and blood loss.

Manifestations

Serious toxicity is unlikely if the patient remains asymptomatic for 6 hours and has a negative abdominal radiograph. Iron intoxication can produce five phases of toxicity. The phases may not be distinct from one another.

Phase I

Gastrointestinal mucosal injury occurs 30 minutes to 12 hours postingestion. Vomiting starts within 30 minutes to 1 hour of ingestion and is persistent; hematemesis and bloody diarrhea may occur; abdominal cramps, fever, hyperglycemia, and leukocytosis may occur. Enteric-coated tablets may pass through the stomach without causing symptoms. Acidosis and shock can occur within 6 to 12 hours.

Phase II

A latent period of apparent improvement occurs over 8 to 12 hours postingestion.

Phase III

Systemic toxicity phase occurs 12 to 48 hours postingestion with cardiovascular collapse and severe metabolic acidosis.

Phase IV

Two to 4 days postingestion, hepatic injury associated with jaundice, elevated liver enzymes, and prolonged prothrombin time occur. Kidney injury with proteinuria and hematuria occur. Pulmonary edema, disseminated intravascular coagulation, and Yersinia enterocolitica sepsis can occur.

Phase V

Four to 8 weeks postingestion, pyloric outlet or intestinal stricture may cause obstruction or anemia secondary to blood loss.

Laboratory Investigations

Iron poisoning produces anion gap metabolic acidosis. Monitoring should include complete blood cell counts, blood glucose level, serum iron, stools and vomitus for occult blood, electrolytes, acid-base balance, urinalysis and urinary output, liver function tests, and BUN and creatinine levels. Blood type and match should be obtained.

Serum iron measurements taken at the proper time correlate with the clinical findings. The lavender top Vacutainer tube contains EDTA, which falsely lowers serum iron. One must obtain the serum iron measurement before administering deferoxamine. Serum iron levels of less than 350 µg/dL at 2 to 6 hours predict an asymptomatic course; levels of 350 to 500 µg/dL are usually associated with mild gastrointestinal symptoms; those greater than 500 µg/dL have a 20% risk of shock and serious iron toxicity. A follow-up serum iron measurement after 6 hours may not be elevated even in cases of severe poisoning, but a serum iron measurement taken at 8 to 12 hours is useful to exclude delayed absorption from a bezoar or sustained-release preparation. The total iron-binding capacity is not necessary.

Adult iron tablet preparations are radiopaque before they dissolve by 4 hours postingestion. A "negative" abdominal radiograph more than 4 hours postingestion does not exclude iron poisoning.

Patients who develop high fevers and signs of sepsis following iron overdose should have blood and stool cultures checked for Yersinia enterocolitica.

Management

Gastrointestinal decontamination should involve immediate induction of emesis in cases of ingestions of elemental iron of greater than 40 mg/kg if vomiting has not already occurred. Activated charcoal is ineffective. An abdominal radiograph should be obtained after emesis to determine the success of gastric emptying. Children's chewable vitamins and liquid iron preparations are not radiopaque. If radiopaque iron is still present, whole-bowel irrigation with polyethylene glycol solution should be considered. In extreme cases, removal by endoscopy or surgery may be necessary because coalesced iron tablets produce hemorrhagic infarction in the bowel and perforation peritonitis.

Deferoxamine (Desferal) in a dose of about 100 mg binds 8.5 to 9.35 mg of free iron in the serum. The deferoxamine infusion should not exceed 15 mg/kg/h or 6 g daily, but faster rates (up to 45 mg/kg) and larger daily amounts have been administered and tolerated in extreme cases of iron poisoning (>1000 mg/dL). The deferoxamine-iron complex is hemodialyzable if renal failure develops.

Indications for chelation therapy are any of the following:

- Very large, symptomatic ingestions
- Serious clinical intoxication (severe vomiting and diarrhea [often bloody], severe abdominal pain, metabolic acidosis, hypotension, or shock)
- Symptoms that persist or progress to more serious toxicity
- Serum iron level greater than 500 mg/dL

Chelation should be performed as early as possible within 12 to 18 hours to be effective. One should start the infusion slowly and gradually increase to avoid hypotension.

Adult respiratory distress syndrome has developed in patients with high doses of deferoxamine for several days; infusions longer than 24 hours should be avoided.

The endpoint of treatment is when the patient is asymptomatic and the urine clears if it was originally a positive "vin rosö" color.

For supportive therapy, intravenous bicarbonate may be needed to correct the metabolic acidosis. Hypotension and shock treatment may require volume expansion, vasopressors, and blood transfusions. The physician should attempt to keep the urinary output at greater than 2 mL/kg/h. Coagulation abnormalities and overt bleeding require blood products or vitamin K. Pregnant patients are treated in a fashion similar to any other patient with iron poisoning.

Hemodialysis and hemoperfusion are ineffective. Exchange transfusion has been used in single cases of massive poisonings in children.

Disposition

The asymptomatic or minimally symptomatic patient should be observed for persistence and progression of symptoms or development of toxicity signs (gastrointestinal bleeding, acidosis, shock, altered mental state). Patients with mild self-limited gastrointestinal symptoms who become asymptomatic or have no signs of toxicity for 6 hours are unlikely to have a serious intoxication and can be discharged after psychiatric clearance, if needed. Patients with moderate or severe toxicity should be admitted to the intensive care unit.

ISONIAZID

Isoniazid is a hydrazide derivative of vitamin B_3 (nicotinamide) and is used as an antituberculosis drug.

Toxic Mechanism

Isoniazid produces pyridoxine deficiency by increasing the excretion of pyridoxine (vitamin B_6) and by inhibiting pyridoxal 5-phosphate (the active form of pyridoxine) from acting with L-glutamic acid decarboxylase to form γ-aminobutyric acid (GABA), the major CNS neurotransmitter inhibitor, resulting in seizures. Isoniazid also blocks the conversion of lactate to pyruvate, resulting in profound and prolonged lactic acidosis.

Toxic Dose

The therapeutic dose is 5 to 10 mg/kg (maximum 300 mg) daily. A single acute dose of 15 mg/kg lowers the seizure threshold; 35 to 40 mg/kg produces spontaneous convulsions; more than 80 mg/kg produces severe toxicity. A fatal dose in adults is 4.5 to 15 g. The malnourished patients, those with a previous seizure disorder, alcoholic patients, and slow acetylators are more susceptible to isoniazid toxicity. In cases of chronic intoxication, 10 mg/kg/d produces hepatitis in 10% to 20% of patients but less than 2% at doses of 3 to 5 mg/kg/d.

Kinetics

Absorption from intestine occurs in 30 to 60 minutes, and onset is in 30 to 120 minutes, with peak levels of 5 to 8 µg/mL within 1 to 2 hours. Volume distribution is 0.6 L/kg, with minimal protein binding.

Elimination is by liver acetylation to a hepatotoxic metabolite, acetyl-isoniazid, which is then hydrolyzed to isonicotinic acid. In slow acetylators, isoniazid has a half-life of 140 to 460 minutes (mean 5 hours), and 10% to 15% is eliminated unchanged in the urine. Most (45% to 75%) whites and 50% of African blacks are slow acetylators, and, with chronic use (without pyridoxine supplements), they may develop peripheral neuropathy. In fast acetylators, isoniazid has a half-life of 35 to 110 minutes (mean 80 minutes), and 25% to 30% is excreted unchanged in the urine. About 90% of Asians and patients with diabetes mellitus are fast acetylators and may develop hepatitis on chronic use.

In patients with overdose and hepatic disease, the serum half-life may increase. Isoniazid inhibits the metabolism of phenytoin (Dilantin), diazepam, phenobarbital, carbamazepine (Tegretol), and prednisone. These drugs also interfere with the metabolism of isoniazid. Ethanol may decrease the half-life of isoniazid but increase its toxicity.

Manifestations

Within 30 to 60 minutes, nausea, vomiting, slurred speech, dizziness, visual disturbances, and ataxia are present. Within 30 to 120 minutes, the major clinical triad of severe overdose includes refractory convulsions (90% of overdose patients have one or more seizures), coma, and resistant severe lactic acidosis (secondary to convulsions), often with a plasma pH of 6.8.

Laboratory Investigations

Isoniazid produces anion gap metabolic acidosis. Therapeutic levels are 5 to 8 µg/mL and acute toxic levels are greater than 20 µg/mL. These levels are not readily available to assist in making decisions in acute overdose situations. One should monitor the blood glucose (often hyperglycemia), electrolytes (often hyperkalemia), bicarbonate, ABGs, liver function tests (elevations occur with chronic exposure), BUN, and creatinine.

Management

Seizures must be controlled. Pyridoxine and diazepam should be administered concomitantly through different IV sites. Pyridoxine (vitamin B_6) is given in a dose of 1 g for each gram of isoniazid ingested. If the dose ingested is unknown, at least 5 g of pyridoxine should be given intravenously. Pyridoxine is administered in 50 mL D_5W or 0.9% saline over 5 minutes intravenously. It must not be administered in the same bottle as sodium bicarbonate. Intravenous pyridoxine is repeated every 5 to 20 minutes until the seizures are controlled. Total doses of pyridoxine up to 52 g have been safely administered; however, patients given 132 and 183 g of pyridoxine have developed a persistent crippling sensory neuropathy.

Diazepam is administered concomitantly with pyridoxine but at a different site. They work synergistically. Diazepam should be administered intravenously slowly, 0.3 mg/kg at a rate of 1 mg/min in children or 10 mg at a rate of 5 mg/min in adults. After the seizures are controlled, the remainder of the pyridoxine is administered (1 g/1 g isoniazid) or a total dose of 5 g.

Phenobarbital or phenytoin is ineffective and should not be used.

In asymptomatic patients or patients without seizures, pyridoxine has been advised by some toxicologists prophylactically in gram-for-gram doses in cases of large overdoses (<80 mg/kg per dose) of isoniazid, although there are no studies to support this recommendation. In comatose patients, pyridoxine administration may result in the patient's rapid regaining of consciousness. Correction of acidosis may occur spontaneously with pyridoxine administration and correction of the seizures. Sodium bicarbonate should be administered if acidosis persists.

Hemodialysis is rarely needed because of antidotal therapy and the short half-life of isoniazid, but it may be used as an adjunct for cases of uncontrollable acidosis and seizures. Hemoperfusion has not been adequately evaluated. Diuresis is ineffective.

Disposition

Asymptomatic or mildly symptomatic patients who become asymptomatic can be observed in the emergency department for 4 to 6 hours. Larger amounts of isoniazid may warrant pyridoxine administration and longer periods of observation. Intentional ingestions necessitate psychiatric evaluation before the patient is discharged. Patients with convulsions or coma should be admitted to the intensive care unit.

ISOPROPANOL (ISOPROPYL ALCOHOL)

Isopropanol can be found in rubbing alcohol, solvents, and lacquer thinner. Coma has occurred in children sponged for fever with isopropanol. See Table 10 for ethanol features of alcohols and glycols.

Toxic Mechanism

Isopropanol is a gastric irritant. It is metabolized to acetone, a CNS and myocardial depressant. It inhibits gluconeogenesis. Normal propyl alcohol is related to isopropyl alcohol but is more toxic.

Toxic Dose

A toxic dose of 0.5 to 1 mg/kg of 70% isopropanol (1 mL/kg of 70%) produces a blood isopropanol plasma concentration of 70 mg/dL. The CNS depressant potency is twice that of ethanol.

Kinetics

Onset of action is within 30 to 60 minutes, and peak is 1 hour postingestion. Volume distribution is 0.6 kg/L. Isopropyl alcohol metabolizes to acetone. Its excretion is renal.

Note: The serum isopropyl concentration and amount ingested can be estimated using the same equation as is used in ethanol kinetics and substituting the specific gravity of 0.785 for isopropyl alcohol.

Manifestations

Ethanol-like inebriation occurs, with an acetone odor to the breath, gastritis, occasionally with hematemesis, acetonuria, and acetonemia without systemic acidosis.

Depression of the CNS occurs: lethargy at blood isopropyl alcohol levels of 50 to 100 mg/dL, coma at levels of 150 to 200 mg/dL, potentially death in adults at levels greater than 240 mg/dL.

Hypoglycemia and seizures may occur.

Laboratory Investigation

Monitoring of blood isopropyl alcohol levels (not readily available in all institutions), acetone, glucose, and ABG should be maintained. The osmolal gap increases 1 mOsm per 5.9 mg/dL of isopropyl alcohol and 1 mOsm per 5.5 mg/dL of acetone. The absence of excess acetone in the blood (normal is 0.3 to 2 mg/dL) within 30 to 60 minutes or excess acetone in the urine within 3 hours excludes the possibility of significant isopropanol exposure.

Management

The airway must be protected with intubation, and assisted ventilation administered if necessary. If the patient is hypoglycemic, glucose should be administered. Supportive treatment is similar to that for ethanol ingestions.

Gastrointestinal decontamination has no role in the treatment of isopropanol ingestion. Hemodialysis is warranted in cases of life-threatening overdose but is rarely needed. A nephrologist should be consulted if the bloodisopropanol plasma concentration is greater than 250 mg/dL.

Disposition

Symptomatic patients with concentrations greater than 100 mg/dL require at least 24 hours of close observation for resolution and should be admitted. If the patient is hypoglycemic, hypotensive, or comatose, he or she should be admitted to the intensive care unit.

LEAD

Acute lead intoxication is rare and usually occurs by inhalation of lead, resulting in severe intoxication and often death. Lead fumes can be produced by burning of lead batteries or use of a heat gun to remove lead paint. Acute lead intoxication also occurs from exposure to high concentrations of organic lead (e.g., tetraethyl lead).

Chronic lead poisoning occurs most often in children 6 months to 6 years of age who are exposed in their environment and in adults in certain occupations (Table 17). In the United States, the prevalence in children aged 1 to 5 years with a venous blood lead greater than 10 µg/dL decreased from 88.2% in a 1976–1980 survey to 8.9% in a 1988–1991 survey as a consequence of measures to reduce lead in the environment, particularly leaded gasoline. However, an estimated 1.7 million children between 1 and 5 years of age and more than 1 million workers in over 100 different occupations still have blood lead levels greater than 10 µg/dL.

Toxic Dose

In cases of chronic lead poisoning, a daily intake of more than 5 µg/kg/d in children or more than 150 µg/d in adults can give a positive lead balance. In 1991, the Centers for Disease Control and Prevention (CDC) recommended routine screening for all children younger than 6 years of age. In children a venous blood level greater than 10 µg/dL was determined to be a threshold of concern. The average venous blood level in the United States is 4 µg/dL. In cases of occupational exposure (see Table 17), a venous blood level greater than 40 µg/dL is indicative of increased lead absorption in adults.

Toxic Mechanism

Lead affects the sulfhydryl enzyme systems, the immature CNS, the enzymes of heme synthesis, vitamin D conversion, the kidneys, the bones, and growth. Lead alters the tertiary structure of cell proteins by denaturing them and causing cell death. Risk factors are mouthing behavior of infants and children and excessive oral behavior (pica), living in the inner city, a poorly maintained home, and poor nutrition (e.g., low calcium and iron). The CDC questionnaire given in Table 18 is recommended at every pediatric visit. If any answers to the CDC questionnaire are "positive," a blood screening test for lead should be administered. To be more accurate, however, identifying lead exposure studies have suggested that the questionnaire will have to be modified for each individual community because it has had poor sensitivity (40%) and specificity (60%) as it stands.

Table 19 lists sources of lead. The number one source is deteriorating lead-based paint, which forms leaded dust. Lead concentrations in indoor paint were not reduced to safer (0.06%) levels until 1978. Lead can also be produced by improper interior or exterior home renovation (scraping or demolition). It is found in pre-1960 built homes. The use of leaded gasoline (limited in 1973) resulted in residue from leaded motor vehicle emissions. Lead persists in the soil near major highways and in deteriorating homes and buildings. Vegetables grown in contaminated soil may contain lead.

TABLE 17 Occupations Associated With Lead Exposure

Lead production or smelting	Demolition of ships and
Production of illicit whiskey	bridges
Brass, copper, and lead	Battery manufacturing
foundries	Machining/grinding lead
Radiator repair	alloys
Scrap handling	Welding of old painted
Sanding of old paint	metals
Lead soldering	Thermal paint stripping
Cable stripping	of old buildings
Worker or janitor at a firing	Ceramic glaze/pottery
range	mixing

Modified from Rempel D: The lead-exposed worker. JAMA 262:533, 1989.

TABLE 18 CDC Questionnaire: Priority Groups for Lead Screening

1. Children age 6–72 months (was 12–36 months) who live in or are frequent visitors to older, deteriorated housing built before 1960.
2. Children age 6–72 months who live in housing built prior to 1960 with recent, ongoing, or planned renovation or remodeling.
3. Children age 6–72 months who are siblings, housemates, or playmates of children with known lead poisoning.
4. Children age 6–72 months whose parents or other household members participate in a lead-related industry or hobby.
5. Children age 6–72 months who live near active lead smelters, battery recycling plants, or other industries likely to result in atmospheric lead release.

BOX 1 Hobbies Associated With Lead Exposure

Casting of ammunition
Collecting antique pewter
Collecting/painting lead toys (e.g., soldiers and figures)
Ceramics or glazed pottery
Refinishing furniture
Making fishing weights
Home renovation
Jewelry making, lead solder
Glass blowing, lead glass
Bronze casting
Print making and other fine arts (when lead white, flake white, chrome yellow pigments are involved)
Liquor distillation
Hunting and target shooting
Painting
Car and boat repair
Burning/engraving lead-painted wood
Making stained leaded glass
Copper enameling

Oil refineries and lead-processing smelters produce lead residue. Food cans produced in Mexico contain lead solder (95% do not in United States). Lead water pipes (until 1950) and lead solder (until 1986) deliver lead-containing drinking water (calcium deposits, however, may offer some protection). Water at a consumer's tap should contain less than 15 parts per billion (ppb) of lead (Table 20).

For occupational exposure, see Table 17. The Occupational Safety and Health Administration (OSHA) standards require employers to provide showering and clothes changing facilities for personnel working with lead; however, businesses with fewer than 25 employees are exempt from the regulation. The OSHA lead standard of 1978 set a limit of 60 μg/dL for occupational exposure to lead. At a blood lead level of 60 μg/dL, a worker should be removed from lead exposure and not allowed back until his or her lead level is below 40 μg/dL. Many authorities believe that this level should be lower. The lead residue on the clothes of the workers may represent a hazard to the family. Other occupations that are potential sources of lead exposure include plumbers, pipe fitters, lead miners, auto repairers, shipbuilders, printers, steel welders and cutters, construction workers, and rubber product manufacturers.

Leaded pots to make molds for "kusmusha" tea represent lead exposure. Imported pottery lined with ceramic glaze can leach large amounts of lead into acids (e.g., citrus fruit juices).

Hobbies associated with lead exposure are listed in Box 1. Some "traditional" folk remedies or cosmetics that contain lead include the following:

- "Azarcon por empacho" ("Maria Louisa" 90% to 95% lead trioxide): a bright orange powder used in Hispanic culture, especially Mexican, for digestive problems and diarrhea.
- "Greta" (4% to 90% lead): a yellow powder "por empacho" ("empacho" refers to a variety of gastrointestinal symptoms), used in Hispanic cultures, especially Mexican.

TABLE 19 Sources of Lead

Product	Lead Content (%) by Dry Weight
Paint	0.06
Solder	0.6
Plastic additives	2.0
Priming inks	2.0
Plumbing fixtures	2.0
Pesticides	0.1
Stained glass cames	0.1
Wine bottle foils	0.1
Construction material	0.1
Fertilizers	0.1
Glazes, enamels	0.06
Toys/recreational games	0.1
Curtain weights	0.1
Fishing weights	0.1

TABLE 20 Agency Regulations and Recommendations Concerning Lead Content

Agency	Specimen	Level	Comments
CDC	Blood (child)	10 μg/dL	Investigate community
OSHA	Blood (adult)	60 μg/dL	Medical removal from work
OSHA	Air	50 μg/m³	PEL*
	Air	0.75 μg/m³	Tetraethyl or tetramethyl
ACGIH	Air	150 μg/m³	TWA†
EPA	Air	1.5 μg/m³	Three-month average
EPA	Water	15 μg/L (ppb)	5 ppb circulating
EPA	Food	100 μg/d	Advisory
FDA	Wine	300 ppm	Plan to reduce to 200 ppm
EPA	Soil/dust	50 ppm	
CPSC	Paint	600 ppm (0.06%) by dry weight	

*PEL = permissible exposure limit (highest level over an 8-hour workday).
†TWA = time-weighted average (air concentration for 8-hour workday and 40 hour workweek).
Abbreviations: ACGIH = American Conference of Governmental Industrial Hygienists; CDC = Centers for Disease Control and Prevention; CPSC = Consumer Product Safety Commission; EPA = Environmental Protection Agency; FDA = Food and Drug Administration; OSHA = Occupational Safety and Health Administration.

- "Pay-loo-ah": an orange-red powder used for rash and fever in Southeast Asian cultures, especially among Northern Laos Hmong immigrants.
- "Alkohl" (Al-kohl, kohl, suma 5% to 92% lead): a black powder used in Middle Eastern, African, and Asian cultures as a cosmetic and an umbilical stump astringent.
- "Farouk": an orange granular powder with lead used in Saudi Arabian culture.
- "Bint Al Zahab": used to treat colic in Saudi Arabian culture.
- "Surma" (23% to 26% lead): a black powder used in India as a cosmetic and to improve eyesight.
- "Bali goli": a round black bean that is dissolved in "grippe water," used by Asian and Indian cultures to aid digestion.

Cases of substance abuse involving lead poisoning have been reported, in which the patient sniffs leaded gasoline or uses improperly synthesized amphetamines.

Kinetics

Absorption of lead is 10% to 15% of the ingested dose in adults; in children, up to 40% is absorbed, especially in cases of iron deficiency anemia. With inhalation of fumes, absorption is rapid and complete. Volume distribution in blood (0.9% of total body burden) is 95% in red blood cells. Lead passes through the placenta to the fetus and is present in breast milk.

Organic lead is metabolized in the liver to inorganic lead. Its half-life is 35 to 40 days in blood; in soft tissue, the half-life is 45 days and in bone (99% of the lead), the half-life is 28 years. The major elimination route is the stool, 80% to 90%, and then renal 10% (80 g/d) and hair, nails, sweat, and saliva. Nine percent of organic lead is excreted in the urine per day.

Manifestations

Adverse health effects are given in Table 21 and include the following.

Hematologic

Lead inhibits γ-aminolevulinic acid dehydratase (early in the synthesis of heme) and ferrochelatase (transfers iron to ferritin for incorporation of iron into protoporphyrin to produce heme). Anemia is a late finding. Decreased heme synthesis starts at >40 µg/dL. Basophilic stippling occurs in 20% of severe lead poisoning.

Neurologic

Segmental demyelination and peripheral neuropathy, usually of the motor type (wrist and ankle drop), occurs in workers. A venous blood level of lead greater than 70 µg/dL (usually >100 µg/dL), produces encephalopathy in children (symptom mnemonic "PAINT": P, persistent forceful vomiting and papilledema; A, ataxia; I, intermittent stupor and lucidity; N, neurologic coma and refractory convulsions; T, tired and lethargic). Decreased cognitive abilities have been reported with a venous blood level of lead greater than 10 µg/dL, including behavioral problems, decreased attention span, and learning disabilities. IQ scores may begin to decrease at 15 µg/dL. Encephalopathy is rare in adults.

Renal

Nephropathy as a result of damaged capillaries and glomerulus can occur at a venous blood level of lead greater than 80 µg/dL, but recent studies show renal damage and hypertension with low venous blood levels. A direct correlation between hypertension and venous blood level over 30 µg/dL has been reported. Lead reduces excretion of uric acid, and high-level exposure may be associated with hyperuricemia and "saturnine gout," Fanconi's syndrome (aminoaciduria and renal tubular acidosis), and tubular fibrosis.

Reproductive

Spontaneous abortion, transient delay in the child's development (catch up at age 5 to 6 years), decreased sperm count, and abnormal

TABLE 21 Summary of Lead-Induced Health Effects in Adults and Children

Blood Lead Level (µg/dL)	Age Group	Health Effect
>100	Adult	Encephalopathic signs and symptoms
>80	Adult	Anemia
	Child	Encephalopathy
		Chronic nephropathy (e.g., aminoaciduria)
>70	Adult	Clinically evident peripheral neuropathy
	Child	Colic and other gastrointestinal symptoms
>60	Adult	Female reproductive effects
		CNS disturbance symptoms (i.e., sleep disturbances, mood changes, memory and concentration problems, headaches)
>50	Adult	Decreased hemoglobin production
		Decreased performance on neurobehavioral tests
	Adult	Altered testicular function
		Gastrointestinal symptoms (i.e., abdominal pain, constipation, diarrhea, nausea, anorexia)
	Child	Peripheral neuropathy*
>40	Adult	Decreased peripheral nerve conduction
		Hypertension, age 40–59 years
		Chronic neuropathy*
>25	Adult	Elevated erythrocyte protoporphyrin in males
15–25	Adult	Elevated erythrocyte protoporphyrin in females
>10	Child	Decreased intelligence and growth
		Impaired learning
		Reduced birth weight*
		Impaired mental ability
	Fetus	Preterm delivery

From Anonymous: Implementation of the Lead Contamination Control Act of 1988. MMWR Morb Mortal Wkly Rep 41:288, 1992.
*Controversial.

sperm morphology can occur with lead exposure. Lead crosses the placenta and fetal blood levels reach 75% to 100% of maternal blood levels. Lead is teratogenic.

Metabolic

Decreased cytochrome P450 activity alters the metabolism of medication and endogenously produced substances. Decreased activation of cortisol and decreased growth is caused by interference in vitamin conversion (25-hydroxyvitamin D to 1,25 hydroxyvitamin D) at venous blood levels of 20 to 30 µg/dL.

Other Manifestations

Abnormalities of thyroid, cardiac, and hepatic function occur in adults. Abdominal colic is seen in children at doses greater than 50 µg/dL. "Lead gum lines" at the dental border of the gingiva can occur in cases of chronic lead poisoning.

Laboratory Investigations

Serial venous blood lead measurements are taken on days 3 and 5 during treatment and 7 days after chelation therapy, then every 1 to 2 weeks for 8 weeks, and then every month for 6 months. Intravenous infusion should be stopped at least 1 hour before blood lead levels are measured. Table 22 gives a classification of blood lead concentrations in children.

TABLE 22 Classification of Blood Lead Concentrations in Children

Blood Lead (μg/dL)	Recommended Interventions
<9	None
10–14	Community intervention
	Repeat blood lead in 3 months
15–19	Individual case management
	Environmental counseling
	Nutritional counseling
	Repeat blood lead in 3 months
20–44	Medical referral
	Environmental inspection/abatement
	Nutritional counseling
	Repeat blood lead in 3 months
45–69	Environmental inspection/abatement
	Nutritional counseling
	Pharmacologic therapy
	DMSA succimer oral or CaNa$_2$EDTA parenteral
	Repeat every 2 weeks for 6–8 weeks, then monthly for 4–6 months
>70	Hospitalization in intensive care unit
	Environmental inspection/abatement
	Pharmacologic therapy
	Dimercaprol (BAL in oil) IM initial alone
	Dimercaprol IM and CaNa$_2$EDTA together
	Repeat every week

Abbreviations: BAL = British anti-Lewisite; CaNa$_2$EDTA = edetate calcium disodium; DMS = dimercaptosuccinic acid; IM = intramuscular.

One should evaluate CBC, serum ferritin, erythrocyte protoporphyrin (>35 μg/dL indicates lead poisoning as well as iron deficiency and other causes), electrolytes, serum calcium and phosphorus, urinalysis, BUN, and creatinine. Abdominal and long bone radiographs may be useful in certain circumstances to identify radiopaque material in bowel and "lead lines" in proximal tibia (which occur after prolonged exposure in association with venous blood lead levels greater than 50 μg/dL).

Neuropsychological tests are difficult to perform in young children but should be considered at the end of treatment, especially to determine auditory dysfunction.

Management

The basis of treatment is removal of the source of lead. Cases of poisoning in children should be reported to local health department and cases of occupational poisoning should be reported to OSHA. The source must be identified and abated, and dust controlled by wet mopping. Cold water should be let to run for 2 minutes before being used for drinking. Planting shrubbery (not vegetables) in contaminated soil will keep children away.

Supportive care should be instituted, including measures to deal with refractory seizures (continued antidotal therapy, diazepam, and possibly neuromuscular blockers), with the hepatic and renal failure, and intravascular hemolysis in severe cases. Seizures are treated with diazepam followed by neuromuscular blockers if needed.

Lead does not bind to activated charcoal. One must not delay chelation therapy for complete gastrointestinal decontamination in severe cases. Whole-bowel irrigation has been used prior to treatment. Some authorities recommend abdominal radiographs followed by gastrointestinal decontamination if necessary before switching to oral therapy. Chelation therapy can be used for patients in whom venous blood level of lead is greater than 45 μg/dL in children and greater than 80 μg/dL in adults or in adults with lower levels who are symptomatic or who have a "positive" lead mobilization test result (not routinely performed at most centers) (Table 23).

Succimer (dimercaptosuccinic acid, DMSA, Chemet), a derivative of British anti-Lewisite (BAL), is an oral agent for chelation in children with a venous blood level of greater than 45 μg/dL. The recommended dose is 10 mg/kg every 8 hours for 5 days, then every 12 hours for 14 days. DMSA is under investigation to determine its role in children with a venous blood level less than 45 μg/dL. Although not approved for adults, it has been used in the same dosage. Monitoring should be maintained by CBC, liver transaminases, and urinalysis for adverse effects.

D-Penicillamine (Cuprimine) is another oral chelator that is given in doses of 20 to 40 mg/kg/d not to exceed 1 g/d. However, it is not FDA approved and has a 10% adverse reaction rate. Nevertheless, D-penicillamine has been used infrequently in adults and children with elevated venous blood lead levels.

Edetate calcium disodium (ethylene diaminetetra-acetic acid or CaNa$_2$EDTA Versenate) is a water-soluble chelator given intramuscularly (with 0.5% procaine) or intravenously. The calcium in the compound is displaced by divalent and trivalent heavy metals, forming a soluble complex, which is stable at physiologic pH (but not at acid pH) and enhances lead clearance in the urine. EDTA usually is administered intravenously, especially in severe cases. It must not be administered until adequate urine flow is established. It may redistribute lead to the brain; therefore, BAL may be given first at a venous blood lead level of greater than 55 μg/dL in children and greater than 100 μg/dL in adults. Phlebitis occurs at a concentration greater than 0.5 mg/mL. Alkalinization of the urine may be helpful. CaNa$_2$EDTA should not be confused with sodium EDTA (disodium edetate), which is used to treat hypercalcemia; inadvertent use may produce severe hypocalcemia.

TABLE 23 Pharmacologic Chelation Therapy of Lead Poisoning

Drug	Route	Dose	Duration	Precautions	Monitor
Dimercaprol (BAL in oil)	IM	3–5 mg/kg q4–6h	3–5 days	G6PD deficiency Concurrent iron therapy	AST/ALT enzymes
CaNa$_2$ EDTA (calcium disodium versenate)	IM/IV	50 mg/kg per day	5 days	Inadequate fluid intake Renal impairment Penicillin allergy	Urinalysis, BUN Creatinine Urinalysis, BUN
D-Penicillamine (Cuprimine)	PO	10 mg/kg per day increase 30 mg/kg over 2 weeks	6–20 weeks	Concurrent iron therapy; lead exposure Renal impairment	Creatinine, CBC
2,3-Dimercaptosuccinic acid (DMSA; succimer)	PO	10 mg/kg per dose 3 times daily 10 mg/kg per dose twice daily for 14 days	19 days	AST/ALT Concurrent iron therapy G6PD deficiency lead exposure	AST/ALT

Abbreviations: ALT = alanine aminotransferase; AST = aspartate transaminase; BAL = British anti-Lewisite; bid = twice daily; BUN = blood urea nitrogen; CBC = complete blood count; G6PD = glucose-6-phosphate dehydrogenase; IM = intramuscular; IV = intravenous; PO = oral; tid = three times daily.

Dimercaprol (BAL) is a peanut oil–based dithiol (two sulfhydryl molecules) that combines with one atom of lead to form a heterocyclic stable ring complex. It is usually reserved for patients in whom venous blood lead is greater than 70 μg/dL, and it chelates red blood cell lead, enhancing its elimination through the urine and bile. It crosses the blood-brain barrier. Approximately 50% of patients have adverse reactions, including bad metallic taste in the mouth, pain at the injection site, sterile abscesses, and fever.

A venous blood lead level greater than 70 μg/dL or the presence of clinical symptoms suggesting encephalopathy in children is a potentially life-threatening emergency. Management should be accomplished in a medical center with a pediatric intensive care unit by a multidisciplinary team including a critical care specialist, a toxicologist, a neurologist, and a neurosurgeon. Careful monitoring of neurologic status, fluid status, and intracranial pressure should be undertaken if necessary. These patients need close monitoring for hemodynamic instability. Hydration should be maintained to ensure renal excretion of lead. Fluids, renal and hepatic function, and electrolyte levels should be monitored.

While waiting for adequate urine flow, therapy should be initiated with intramuscular dimercaprol (BAL) only (25 mg/kg/d divided into 6 doses). Four hours later, the second dose of BAL should be given intramuscularly, concurrently with CaNa$_2$EDTA 50 mg/kg/d as a single dose infused over several hours or as a continuous infusion. The double therapy is continued until the venous blood level is less than 40 μg/dL.

As long as the venous blood level is greater than 40 μg/dL, therapy is continued for 72 hours and followed by two alternatives: either parenteral therapy with two drugs (CaNa$_2$EDTA and BAL) for 5 days or continuation of therapy with CaNa$_2$EDTA alone if a good response is achieved and the venous blood level of lead is less than 40 μg/dL. If one cannot get the venous blood lead report back, one should continue therapy with both BAL and EDTA for 5 days. In patients with lead encephalopathy, parenteral chelation should be continued with both drugs until the patient is clinically stable before changing therapy. Mannitol and dexa-methasone can reduce the cerebral edema, but their role in lead encephalopathy is not clear. Surgical decompression is not recommended to reduce cerebral edema in these cases.

If BAL and CaNa$_2$EDTA are used together, a minimum of 2 days with no treatment should elapse before another 5-day course of therapy is considered. The 5-day course is repeated with CaNa$_2$EDTA alone if the blood lead level rebounds to greater than 40 μg/dL or in combination with BAL if the venous blood level is greater than 70 μg/dL. If a third course is required, unless there are compelling reasons, one should wait at least 5 to 7 days before administering the course.

Following chelation therapy, a period of equilibration of 10 to 14 days should be allowed and a repeat venous blood lead concentration should be obtained. If the patient is stable enough for oral intake, oral succimer 30 mg/kg/d in three divided doses for 5 days followed by 20 mg/kg/d in two divided doses for 14 days has been suggested, but there are limited data to support this recommendation. Therapy should be continued until venous blood lead level is less than 20 μg/dL in children or less than 40 μg/dL in adults.

Chelators combined with lead are hemodialyzable in the event of renal failure.

Disposition

All patients with a venous blood lead level of greater than 70 μg/dL or who are symptomatic should be admitted. If a child is hospitalized, all lead hazards must be removed from the home environment before allowing the child to return. The source must be eliminated by environmental and occupational investigations. The local health department should be involved in dealing with children who are lead poisoned, and OSHA should be involved with cases of occupational lead poisoning. Consultation with a poison control center or experienced toxicologist is necessary when chelating patients. Follow-up venous blood lead concentrations should be obtained within 1 to 2 weeks and followed every 2 weeks for 6 to 8 weeks, then monthly for 4 to 6 months if the patient required chelation therapy. All patients with venous blood level greater than 10 μg/dL should be followed at least every 3 months until two venous blood lead concentrations are 10 μg/dL or three are less than 15 μg/dL.

LITHIUM (ESKALITH, LITHANE)

Lithium is an alkali metal used primarily in the treatment of bipolar psychiatric disorders. Most intoxications are cases of chronic overdose. One gram of lithium carbonate contains 189 mg (5.1 mEq) of lithium; a regular tablet contains 300 mg (8.12 mEq) and a sustained-release preparation contains 450 mg or 12.18 mEq.

Toxic Mechanism

The brain is the primary target organ of toxicity, but the mechanism is unclear. Lithium may interfere with physiologic functions by acting as a substitute for cellular cations (sodium and potassium), depressing neural excitation and synaptic transmission.

Toxic Dose

A dose of 1 mEq/kg (40 mg/kg) of lithium will give a peak serum lithium concentration about 1.2 mEq/L. The therapeutic serum lithium concentration in cases of acute mania is 0.6 to 1.2 mEq/L, and for maintenance it is 0.5 to 0.8 mEq/L. Serum lithium concentration levels are usually obtained 12 hours after the last dose. The toxic dose is determined by clinical manifestations and serum levels after the distribution phase.

Acute ingestion of twenty 300-mg tablets (300 mg increases the serum lithium concentration by 0.2 to 0.4 mEq/L) in adults may produce serious intoxication. Chronic intoxication can be produced by conditions listed below that can decrease the elimination of lithium or increase lithium reabsorption in the kidney.

The risk factors that predispose to chronic lithium toxicity are febrile illness, impaired renal function, hyponatremia, advanced age, lithium-induced diabetes insipidus, dehydration, vomiting and diarrhea, and concomitant use of other drugs, such as thiazide and spironolactone diuretics, nonsteroidal antiinflammatory drugs, salicylates, angiotensin-converting enzyme inhibitors (e.g., captopril), serotonin reuptake inhibitors (e.g., fluoxetine [Prozac]), and phenothiazines.

Kinetics

Gastrointestinal absorption of regular-release preparations is rapid; serum lithium concentration peaks in 2 to 4 hours and is complete by 6 to 8 hours. The onset of toxicity may occur at 1 to 4 hours after acute overdose but usually is delayed because lithium enters the brain slowly. Absorption of sustained-release preparations and the development of toxicity may be delayed 6 to 12 hours.

Volume distribution is 0.5 to 0.9 L/kg. Lithium is not protein bound. The half-life after a single dose is 9 to 13 hours; at steady state, it may be 30 to 58 hours. The renal handling of lithium is similar to that of sodium: glomerular filtration and reabsorption (80%) by the proximal renal tubule. Adequate sodium must be present to prevent lithium reabsorption. More than 90% of lithium is excreted by the kidney, 30% to 60% within 6 to 12 hours.

Manifestations

The examiner must distinguish between side effects, acute intoxication, acute or chronic toxicity, and chronic intoxications. Chronic is the most common and dangerous type of intoxication.

Side effects include fine tremor, gastrointestinal upset, hypothyroidism, polyuria and frank diabetes insipidus, dermatologic manifestations, and cardiac conduction deficits. Lithium is teratogenic.

Patients with acute poisoning may be asymptomatic, with an early high serum lithium concentration of 9 mEq/L, and deteriorate as the serum lithium concentration falls by 50% and the lithium distributes to the brain and the other tissues. Nausea and vomiting may occur within 1 to 4 hours, but the systemic manifestations are usually delayed several more hours. It may take as long as 3 to 5 days for serious symptoms to develop. Acute toxicity and acute on chronic toxicity are manifested by neurologic findings, including weakness, fasciculations, altered mental state, myoclonus, hyperreflexia, rigidity, coma, and convulsions with limbs in hypertension. Cardiovascular effects are nonspecific and occur at therapeutic doses, flat T or inverted T waves, atrioventricular block, and prolonged QT interval. Lithium is not a primary cardiotoxin. Cardiogenic shock occurs secondary to CNS toxicity. Chronic intoxication is associated with manifestations at lower serum lithium concentrations. There is some correlation with manifestations, especially at higher serum lithium concentrations. Although the levels do not always correlate with the manifestations, they are more predictive in cases of severe intoxication. A serum lithium concentration greater than 3.0 mEq/L with chronic intoxication and altered mental state indicates severe toxicity. Permanent neurologic sequelae can result from lithium intoxication.

Laboratory Investigations

Monitoring should include CBC (lithium causes significant leukocytosis), renal function, thyroid function (chronic intoxication), ECG, and electrolytes. Serum lithium concentrations should be determined every 2 to 4 hours until levels are close to therapeutic range. Cross-reactions with green-top Vacutainer specimen tubes containing heparin will spuriously elevate serum lithium concentration 6 to 8 mEq/L.

Management

Vital function must be established and maintained. Seizure precautions should be instituted and seizures, hypotension, and dysrhythmias treated. Evaluation should include examination for rigidity and hyperreflexia signs, hydration, renal function (BUN, creatinine), and electrolytes, especially sodium. The examiner should inquire about diuretic and other drug use that increase serum lithium concentration, and the patient must discontinue the drugs. If the patient is on chronic therapy, the lithium should be discontinued. Serial serum lithium concentrations should be obtained every 4 hours until serum lithium concentration peaks and there is a downward trend toward almost therapeutic range, especially in sustained-release preparations. Vital signs should be monitored, including temperature, and ECG and serial neurologic examinations should be undertaken, including mental status and urinary output. Nephrology consultation is warranted in case of a chronic and elevated serum lithium concentration (>2.5 mEq/L), a large ingestion, or altered mental state.

An intravenous line should be established and hydration and electrolyte balance restored. Serum sodium level should be determined before 0.9% saline fluid is administered in patients with chronic overdose because hypernatremia may be present from diabetes insipidus. Although current evidence supports an initial 0.9% saline infusion (200 mL/h) to enhance excretion of lithium, once hydration, urine output, and normonatremia are established, one should administer 0.45% saline and slow the infusion (100 mL/h) for all patients.

Gastric lavage is often not recommended in cases of acute ingestion because of the large size of the tablets, and it is not necessary after chronic intoxication. Activated charcoal is ineffective. For sustained-release preparations, whole-bowel irrigation may be useful but is not proven. Sodium polystyrene sulfonate (Kayexalate), an ion exchange resin, is difficult to administer and has been used only in uncontrolled studies. Its use is not recommended.

Hemodialysis is the most efficient method for removing lithium from the vascular compartment. It is the treatment of choice for patients with severe intoxication with an altered mental state, those with seizures, and anuric patients. Long runs are used until the serum lithium concentration is less than 1 mEq/L because of extensive re-equilibration. Serum lithium concentration should be monitored every 4 hours after dialysis for rebound. Repeated and prolonged hemodialysis may be necessary. A lag in neurologic recovery can be expected.

Disposition

An acute asymptomatic lithium overdose cannot be medically cleared on the basis of single lithium level. Patients should be admitted if they have any neurologic manifestations (altered mental status, hyperreflexia, stiffness, or tremor). Patients should be admitted to the intensive care unit if they are dehydrated, have renal impairment, or have a high or rising lithium level.

METHANOL (WOOD ALCOHOL, METHYL ALCOHOL)

The concentration of methanol in Sterno fuel is 4% and it contains ethanol, in windshield washer fluid it is 30% to 60%, and in gas-line antifreeze it is 100%.

Toxic Mechanism

Methanol is metabolized by alcohol dehydrogenase to formaldehyde, which is metabolized to formate. Formate inhibits cytochrome oxidase, producing tissue hypoxia, lactic acidosis, and optic nerve edema. Formate is converted by folate-dependent enzymes to carbon dioxide.

Toxic Dose

The minimal toxic amount is approximately 100 mg/kg. Serious toxicity in a young child can be produced by the ingestion of 2.5 to 5.0 mL of 100% methanol. Ingestion of 5-mL 100% methanol by a 10-kg child produces estimated peak blood methanol of 80 mg/dL. Ingestion of 15 mL 40% methanol was lethal for a 2-year-old child in one report. A fatal adult oral dose is 30 to 240 mL 100% (20 to 150 g). Ingestion of 6 to 10 mL 100% causes blindness in adults. The toxic blood concentration is greater than 20 mg/dL; very serious toxicity and potential fatality occur at levels greater than 50 mg/dL.

Kinetics

Onset of action can start within 1 hour but may be delayed up to 12 to 18 hours by metabolism to toxic metabolites. It may be delayed longer if ethanol is ingested concomitantly or in infants. Peak blood methanol concentration is 1 hour. Volume distribution is 0.6 L/kg (total body water).

For metabolism, see *Toxic Mechanism*.

Elimination is through metabolism. The half-life of methanol is 8 hours, with ethanol blocking it is 30 to 35 hours, and with hemodialysis 2.5 hours.

Manifestations

Metabolism creates a delay in onset for 12 to 18 hours or longer if ethanol is ingested concomitantly. Initial findings are as follows:

- 0 to 6 hours: Confusion, ataxia, inebriation, formaldehyde odor on breath, and abdominal pain can be present, but the patient may be asymptomatic. Note: Methanol produces an osmolal gap (early), and its metabolite formate produces the anion gap metabolic acidosis (see later). Absence of osmolar or anion gap does not always exclude methanol intoxication.
- 6 to 12 hours: Malaise, headache, abdominal pain, vomiting, visual symptoms, including hyperemia of optic disc, "snow vision," and blindness can be seen.
- More than 12 hours: Worsening acidosis, hyperglycemia, shock, and multiorgan failure develop, with death from complications of intractable acidosis and cerebral edema.

Laboratory Investigation

Methanol can be detected on some chromatography drug screens if specified. Methanol and ethanol levels, electrolytes, glucose, BUN, creatinine, amylase, and ABG should be monitored every 4 hours. Formate levels correlate more closely than blood methanol concentration with severity of intoxication and should be obtained if possible.

Management

One should protect the airway by intubation to prevent aspiration and administer assisted ventilation as needed. If needed, 100%

oxygen can be administered. A nephrologist should be consulted early regarding the need for hemodialysis.

Gastrointestinal decontamination procedures have no role.

Metabolic acidosis should be treated vigorously with sodium bicarbonate 2 to 3 mEq/kg intravenously. Large amounts may be needed.

Antidote therapy is initiated to inhibit metabolism if the patient has a history of ingesting more than 0.4 mL/kg of 100% with the following conditions:

- Blood methanol level is greater than 20 mg/dL
- The patient has osmolar gap not accounted for by other factors
- The patient is symptomatic or acidotic with increased anion gap and/or hyperemia of the optic disc.

The ethanol or fomepizole therapy outlined below can be used.

Ethanol Therapy

Ethanol should be initiated immediately if fomepizole is unavailable (see *Fomepizole Therapy*). Alcohol dehydrogenase has a greater affinity for ethanol than ethylene glycol. Therefore, ethanol blocks the metabolism of ethylene glycol.

Ethanol should be administered intravenously (oral administration is less reliable) to produce a blood ethanol concentration of 100 to 150 mg/dL. The loading dose is 10 mL/kg of 10% ethanol administered intravenously concomitantly with a maintenance dose of 10% ethanol at 1.0 mL/kg/h. This dose may need to be increased to 2 mL/kg/h in patients who are heavy drinkers. The blood ethanol concentration should be measured hourly and the infusion rate should be adjusted to maintain a concentration of 100 to 150 mg/dL.

Fomepizole Therapy

Fomepizole (Antizol, 4-methylpyrazole) inhibits alcohol dehydrogenase more reliably than ethanol and it does not require constant monitoring of ethanol levels and adjustment of infusion rates. Fomepizole is available in 1 g/mL vials of 1.5 mL. The loading dose is 15 mg/kg (0.015 mL/kg) IV, maintenance dose is 10 mg/kg (0.01 mL/kg) every 12 hours for 4 doses, then 15 mg/kg every 12 hours until the ethylene glycol levels are less than 20 mg/dL. The solution is prepared by being mixed with 100 mL of 0.9% saline or D$_5$W. Fomepizole can be given to patients requiring hemodialysis but should be dosed as follows:

Dose at the beginning of hemodialysis:

- If less than 6 hours since last Antizol dose, do not administer dose
- If more than 6 hours since last dose, administer next scheduled dose

Dosing during hemodialysis:

- Dose every 4 hours

Dosing at the time hemodialysis is completed:

- If less than 1 hour between last dose and end dialysis, do not administer dose at end of dialysis
- If 1 to 3 hours between last dose and end dialysis, administer one half of next scheduled dose
- If more than 3 hours between last dose and end dialysis, administer next scheduled dose

Maintenance dosing off hemodialysis:

- Give the next scheduled dose 12 hours from the last dose administered

Hemodialysis increases the clearance of both methanol and formate 10-fold over renal clearance. A blood methanol concentration greater than 50 mg/dL has been used as an indication for hemodialysis, but recently some toxicologists from the New York City Poison Center recommended early hemodialysis in patients with blood methanol concentration greater than 25 mg/dL because it may be able to shorten the course of intoxication if started early. One should continue to monitor methanol levels and/or formate levels every 4 hours after the procedure for rebound. Other indications for early

hemodialysis are significant metabolic acidosis and electrolyte abnormalities despite conventional therapy and if visual or neurologic signs or symptoms are present.

A serum formate level greater than 20 mg/dL has also been used as a criterion for hemodialysis, although this is often not readily available through many laboratories. If hemodialysis is used, the infusion rate of 10% ethanol should be increased 2.0 to 3.5 mL/kg/h. The blood ethanol concentration and glucose level should be obtained every 2 hours.

Therapy is continued with both ethanol and hemodialysis until the blood methanol level is undetectable, there is no acidosis, and the patient has no neurologic or visual disturbances. This may require several days.

Hypoglycemia is treated with intravenous glucose. Doses of folinic acid (Leucovorin) and folic acid have been used successfully in animal investigations to enhance formate metabolism to carbon dioxide and water. Leucovorin 1 mg/kg up to 50 mg IV is administered every 4 hours for several days.

An initial ophthalmologic consultation and follow-up are warranted.

Disposition

All patients who have ingested significant amounts of methanol should be referred to the emergency department for evaluation and blood methanol concentration measurement. Ophthalmologic follow-up of all patients with methanol intoxications should be arranged.

MONOAMINE OXIDASE INHIBITORS

Nonselective monoamine oxidase inhibitors (MAOIs) include the hydrazines phenelzine (Nardil) and isocarboxazid (Marplan), and the nonhydrazine tranylcypromine (Parnate). Furazolidone (Furoxone) and pargyline (Eutonyl)[2] are also considered nonselective MAOIs. Moclobemide,[2] which is available in many countries but not the United States, is a selective MAO-A inhibitor. MAO-B inhibitors include selegiline (Eldepryl), an antiparkinsonism agent, which does not have similar toxicity to MAO-A and is not discussed. Selectivity is lost in an overdose. MAOIs are used to treat severe depression.

Toxic Mechanism

Monoamine oxidase enzymes are responsible for the oxidative deamination of both endogenous and exogenous catecholamines such as norepinephrine. MAO-A in the intestinal wall also metabolizes tyramine in food. MAOIs permanently inhibit MAO enzymes until a new enzyme is synthesized after 14 days or longer. The toxicity results from the accumulation, potentiation, and prolongation of the catecholamine action followed by profound hypotension and cardiovascular collapse.

Toxic Dose

Toxicity begins at 2 to 3 mg/kg and fatalities occur at 4 to 6 mg/kg. Death has occurred after a single dose of 170 mg of tranylcypromine in an adult.

Kinetics

Structurally, MAOIs are related to amphetamines and catecholamines. The hydrazine peak levels are at 1 to 2 hours; metabolism is hepatic acetylation; and inactive metabolites are excreted in the urine. For the nonhydrazines, peak levels occur at 1 to 4 hours, and metabolism is via the liver to active amphetamine-like metabolites.

The onset of symptoms in a case of overdose is delayed 6 to 24 hours after ingestion, peak activity is 8 to 12 hours, and duration is 72 hours or longer. The peak of MAO inhibition is in 5 to 10 days and lasts as long as 5 weeks.

---

[2]Not available in the United States.

Manifestations

Manifestations of an acute ingestion overdose of MAO-A inhibitors are as follows:

Phase I

An adrenergic crisis occurs, with delayed onset for 6 to 24 hours, and may not reach peak until 24 hours. The crisis starts as hyperthermia, tachycardia, tachypnea, dysarthria, transient hypertension, hyperreflexia, and CNS stimulation.

Phase II

Neuromuscular excitation and sympathetic hyperactivity occur with increased temperature greater than 40°C (104°F), agitation, hyperactivity, confusion, fasciculations, twitching, tremor, masseter spasm, muscle rigidity, acidosis, and electrolyte abnormalities. Seizures and dystonic reactions may occur. The pupils are mydriatic, sometimes nonreactive with "ping-pong gaze."

Phase III

CNS depression and cardiovascular collapse occur in cases of severe overdose as the catecholamines are depleted. Symptoms usually resolve within 5 days but may last 2 weeks.

Phase IV

Secondary complications occur, including rhabdomyolysis, cardiac dysrhythmias, multiorgan failure, and coagulopathies.

Biogenic interactions usually occur while the patient is on therapeutic doses of MAOI or shortly after they are discontinued (30 to 60 minutes), before the new MAO enzyme is synthesized. The following substances have been implicated: indirect acting sympathomimetics such as amphetamines, serotonergic drugs, opioids (e.g., meperidine, dextromethorphan), tricyclic antidepressants, specific serotonin reuptake inhibitors (SSRI; e.g., fluoxetine [Prozac], sertraline [Zoloft], paroxetine [Paxil]), tyramine-containing foods (e.g., wine, beer, avocados, cheese, caviar, chocolate, chicken liver), and L-tryptophan. SSRIs should not be started for at least 5 weeks after MAOIs have been discontinued.

In mild cases, usually caused by foods, headache and hypertension develop and last for several hours. In severe cases, malignant hypertension and severe hyperthermia syndromes consisting of hypertension or hyperthermia, altered mental state, skeletal muscle rigidity, shivering (often beginning in the masseter muscle), and seizures may occur.

The serotonin syndrome, which may be a result of inhibition of serotonin metabolism, has similar clinical findings to those of malignant hyperthermia and may occur with or without hyperthermia or hypertension.

Chronic toxicity clinical findings include tremors, hyperhidrosis, agitation, hallucinations, confusion, and seizures and may be confused with withdrawal syndromes.

Laboratory Investigations

Monitoring of the ECG, cardiac monitoring, CPK, ABG, pulse oximeter, electrolytes, blood glucose, and acid-base balance should be maintained.

Management

In the case of MAOI overdose, ipecac-induced emesis should not be used. Only activated charcoal alone should be used.

If the patient is admitted to the hospital and is well enough to eat, a nontyramine diet should be ordered.

Extreme agitation and seizures can be controlled with benzodiazepines and barbiturates. Phenytoin is ineffective. Nondepolarizing neuromuscular blockers (not depolarizing succinylcholine) may be needed in severe cases of hyperthermia and rigidity. If the patient has severe hypertension (catecholamine mediated), phentolamine (Regitine), a parenteral β-blocking agent, 3 to 5 mg intravenously, or labetalol (Normodyne), a combination of an α-blocking agent

and a β-blocker, 20-mg intravenous bolus, should be given. If malignant hypertension with rigidity is present, a short-acting nitroprusside and benzodiazepine can be used. Hypertension is often followed by severe hypotension, which should be managed by fluid and vasopressors. *Caution:* Vasopressor therapy should be administered at lower doses than usual because of exaggerated pharmacologic response. Norepinephrine is preferred to dopamine, which requires release of intracellular amines.

Cardiac dysrhythmias are treated with standard therapy but are often refractory, and cardioversion and pacemakers may be needed.

For malignant hyperthermia, dantrolene (Dantrium), a nonspecific peripheral skeletal relaxing agent, is administered, which inhibits the release of calcium from the sarcoplasm. Dantrolene is reconstituted with 60 mL sterile water without bacteriostatic agents. Glass equipment must not be used, and the drug must be protected from light and used within 6 hours. Loading dose is 2 to 3 mg/kg intravenously as a bolus, and the loading dose is repeated until the signs of malignant hyperthermia (tachycardia, rigidity, increased end-tidal CO_2, and temperature) are controlled. Maximum total dose is 10 mg/kg to avoid hepatotoxicity.

When malignant hyperthermia has subsided, 1 mg/kg IV is given every 6 hours for 24 to 48 hours, then orally 1 mg/kg every 6 hours for 24 hours to prevent recurrence. There is a danger of thrombophlebitis following peripheral dantrolene, and it should be administered through a central line if possible. In addition one should administer external cooling and correct metabolic acidosis and electrolyte disturbances. Benzodiazepine can be used for sedation. Dantrolene does not reverse central dopamine blockade; therefore, bromocriptine mesylate (Parlodel) 2.5 to 10 mg should be given orally or through a nasogastric tube three times a day.

Rhabdomyolysis and myoglobinuria are treated with fluids. Urine alkalinization should also be treated.

Hemodialysis and hemoperfusion are of no proven value.

Biogenic amine interactions are managed symptomatically, similar to cases of overdose. For the serotonin syndrome cyproheptadine (Periactin), a serotonin blocker, 4 mg orally every hour for three doses, or methysergide (Sansert), 2 mg orally every 6 hours for three doses, should be considered. The effectiveness of these drugs has not been proven.

Disposition

All patients who have ingested more than 2 mg/kg of an MAOI should be admitted to the hospital for 24 hours of observation and monitoring in the intensive care unit because the life-threatening manifestations may be delayed. Patients with drug or dietary interactions that are mild may not require admission if symptoms subside within 4 to 6 hours and the patients remain asymptomatic. Patients with symptoms that persist or require active intervention should be admitted to the intensive care unit.

OPIOIDS (NARCOTIC OPIATES)

Opioids are used for analgesia, as antitussives, and as antidiarrheal agents and are illicit agents (heroin, opium) used in substance abuse. Tolerance, physical dependency, and withdrawal may develop.

Toxic Mechanism

At least four main opioid receptors have been identified. The μ receptor is considered the most important for central analgesia and CNS depression. The κ and δ receptors predominate in spinal analgesia. The σ receptors may mediate dysphoria. Death is a consequence of dose-dependent CNS respiratory depression or secondary to pulmonary aspiration or noncardiac pulmonary edema. The mechanism of noncardiac pulmonary edema is unknown.

Dextromethorphan can interact with MAOIs, causing severe hyperthermia, and may cause the serotonin syndrome (see *Selective Serotonin Reuptake Inhibitors*). Dextromethorphan inhibits the metabolism of norepinephrine and serotonin and blocks the reuptake of serotonin. It is found as a component of a large number of nonprescription cough and cold remedies.

TABLE 24 Doses and Onset and Duration of Action of Common Opioids

Drug	Adult Oral Dose	Child Oral Dose	Onset of Action	Duration of Action	Adult Fatal Dose
Camphored tincture of opium	25 mL	0.25–0.50 mL/kg (0.4 mg/mL)	15–30 min	4–5 h	NA
Codeine	30–180 mg	0.5–1 mg/kg	15–30 min	4–6 h	800 mg
		>1 mg/kg is toxic in a child, above 200 mg in adult >5 mg/kg fatal in a child			
Dextromethorphan	15 mg 10 mg/kg is toxic	0.25 mg/kg	15–30 min	3–6 h	NA
Diacetylmorphine; street heroin is less than 10% pure	60 mg	NA	15–30 min	3–4 h	100 mg
Diphenoxylate atropine (Lomotil)	5–10 mg	NA	120–240 min	14 h	300 mg
	7.5 mg is toxic in a child, 300 mg is toxic in adult				
Fentanyl (Duragesic)	0.1–0.2 mg	0.001–0.002 mg/kg	7–8 min	Intramuscular: 1/2–2 h	1.0 mg
Hydrocodone with APAP (Lortab)	5–30 mg	0.15 mg/kg	30 min	3–4 h	100 mg
Hydromorphone (Dilaudid)	4 mg	0.1 mg/kg	15–30 min	3–4 h	100 mg
Meperidine (Demerol)	100 mg	1–1.5 mg/kg	10–45 min	3–4 h	350 mg
Methadone (Dolophine)	10 mg	0.1 mg/kg	30–60 min	4–12 h	120 mg
Morphine	10–60 mg	0.1–0.2 mg/kg	<20 min	4–6 h	200 mg
	Oral dose is 6 times parenteral dose, MS Contin sustained-release prep				
Oxycodone APAP (Percocet)	5 mg	NA	15–30 min	4–5 h	NA
Pentazocine (Talwin)	50–100 mg	NA	15–30 min	3–4 h	NA
Propoxyphene (Darvon)	65–100 mg	NA	30–60 min	2–4 h	700 mg

Toxic Dose

The toxic dose depends on the specific drug, route of administration, and degree of tolerance. For therapeutic and toxic doses, see Table 24. In children, respiratory depression has been produced by 10 mg of morphine or methadone, 75 mg of meperidine, and 12.5 mg of diphenoxylate. Infants younger than 3 months of age are more susceptible to respiratory depression. The dose should be reduced by 50%.

Kinetics

Oral onset of analgesic effect of morphine is 10 to 15 minutes; the action peaks in 1 hour and lasts 4 to 6 hours. With sustained-release preparations, the duration is 8 to 12 hours. Opioids are 90% metabolized in the liver by hepatic conjugation and 90% excreted in the urine as inactive compounds. Volume distribution is 1 to 4 L/kg. Protein binding is 35% to 75%. The typical plasma half-life of opiates is 2 to 5 hours, but that of methadone is 24 to 36 hours. Morphine metabolites include morphine-3-glucuronide (inactive) and morphine-6-glucuronide (active) and normorphine (active). Meperidine (Demerol) is rapidly hydrolyzed by tissue esterases into the active metabolite normeperidine, which has twice the convulsant activity of meperidine. Heroin (diacetylmorphine) is deacetylated within minutes to 6-monacetylmorphine and morphine. Propoxyphene (Darvon) has a rapid onset of action, and death has occurred within 15 to 30 minutes after a massive overdose. Propoxyphene is metabolized to norpropoxyphene, an active metabolite with convulsive, cardiac dysrhythmic, and heart block properties. Symptoms of diphenoxylate overdose appear within 1 to 4 hours. It is metabolized into the active metabolite difenoxin, which is five times more active as a regular respiratory depressant agent. Death has been reported in children after ingestion of a single tablet.

Manifestations

Initially, mild intoxication produces miosis, dull face, drowsiness, partial ptosis, and "nodding" (head drops to chest then bobs up). Larger amounts produce the classic triad of miotic pupils (exceptions below), respiratory depression, and depressed level of consciousness (flaccid coma). The blood pressure, pulse, and bowel activity are decreased.

Dilated pupils do not exclude opioid intoxication. Some exceptions to the miosis effect include dextromethorphan (paralyzes iris), fentanyl, meperidine, and diphenoxylate (rarely). Physiologic disturbances including acidosis, hypoglycemia, hypoxia, and postictal state, or a co-ingestant may also produce mydriasis.

Usually, the muscles are flaccid, but increased muscle tone can be produced by meperidine and fentanyl (chest rigidity). Seizures are rare but can occur with ingestion of codeine, meperidine, propoxyphene, and dextromethorphan. Hallucinations and agitation have been reported.

Pruritus and urticaria are caused by histamine release by some opioids or by sulfite additives.

Noncardiac pulmonary edema may occur after an overdose, especially with intravenous heroin abuse. Cardiac effects include vasodilation and hypotension. A heart murmur in an intravenous addict suggests endocarditis. Propoxyphene can produce delayed cardiac dysrhythmias.

Fentanyl is 100 times more potent than morphine and can cause chest wall muscle rigidity. Some of its derivatives are 2000 times more potent than morphine.

Laboratory Investigations

For patients with overdose, one should obtain and monitor ABG, blood glucose, and electrolyte levels; chest radiographs; and ECG. For drug abusers, one should consider testing for hepatitis B, syphilis, and HIV antibody (HIV testing usually requires consent). Blood opioid concentrations are not useful. They confirm diagnosis (morphine therapeutic dose, 65 to 80 ng/mL; toxic, <200 ng/mL), but are not useful for making a therapeutic decision. Cross-reactions can occur with Vick's Formula 44, poppy seeds, and other opioids (codeine and heroin are metabolized to morphine). Naloxone 4 mg IV was not associated with a positive enzyme multiplied immunoassay technique urine screen at 60 minutes, 6 hours, or 48 hours.

Management

Supportive care should be instituted, particularly an endotracheal tube and assisted ventilation. Temporary ventilation can be provided by a bag-valve mask with 100% oxygen. The patient should be placed on a cardiac monitor, have intravenous access established, and have specimens for ABG, glucose, electrolytes, BUN, and creatinine levels, CBC, coagulation profile, liver function, toxicology screen, and urinalysis taken.

For gastrointestinal decontamination, emesis should not be induced, but activated charcoal can be administered if bowel sounds are present.

If it is suspected that the patient is an addict, he or she should be restrained first and then 0.1 mg of naloxone (Narcan) should be administered. The dose should be doubled every 2 minutes until the patient responds or 10 to 20 mg has been given. If the patient is not suspected to be an addict, then 2 mg every 2 to 3 minutes to total of 10 to 20 mg is administered.

It is essential to determine whether there is a complete response to naloxone (mydriasis, improvement in ventilation), because it is a diagnostic therapeutic test. A continuous naloxone infusion may be appropriate, using the "response dose" every hour. Repeat doses of naloxone may be necessary because the effects of many opioids can last much longer than naloxone does (30 to 60 minutes). Methadone ingestions may require a naloxone infusion for 24 to 48 hours. Half of the response dose may need to be repeated in 15 to 20 minutes, after the infusion has been started.

Acute iatrogenic withdrawal precipitated by the administration of naloxone to a dependent patient should not be treated with morphine or other opioids. Naloxone's effects are limited to 30 to 60 minutes (shorter than most opioids) and withdrawal will subside in a short time.

Nalmefene (Revex), an FDA-approved long-acting (4 to 8 hours) pure opioid antagonist, is being investigated, but its role in cases of acute intoxication is unclear and it could produce prolonged withdrawal. It may have a role in place of naloxone infusion.

Noncardiac pulmonary edema does not respond to naloxone, and the patient needs intubation, assisted ventilation, positive end-expiratory pressure, and hemodynamic monitoring. Fluids should be given cautiously in patients with opioid overdose because opioids stimulate the antidiuretic hormone.

If the patient is comatose, 50% glucose (3% to 4% of comatose opioid overdose patients have hypoglycemia) and thiamine should be given prior to naloxone. If the patient has seizures that are unresponsive to naloxone, one administers diazepam and examines for metabolic (hypoglycemia, electrolyte disturbances) causes and structural disturbances.

Hypotension is rare and should direct a search for another etiology. If the patient is agitated, hypoxia and hypoglycemia must be excluded before opioid withdrawal is considered as a cause. Complications to consider include urinary retention, constipation, rhabdomyolysis, myoglobinuria, hypoglycemia, and withdrawal.

Disposition

If a patient responds to intravenous naloxone, careful observation for relapse and the development of pulmonary edema is required, with cardiac and respiratory monitoring for 6 to 12 hours. Patients requiring repeated doses of naloxone or an infusion, or those who develop pulmonary edema, require intensive care unit admission and cannot be discharged from the intensive care unit until they are symptom free for 12 hours. Intravenous overdose complications are expected to be present within 20 minutes after injection, and discharge after 4 symptom-free hours has been recommended. Adults with oral overdose have delayed onset of toxicity and require 6 hours of observation. Children with oral opioid overdose should be admitted to the hospital for observation because of delayed toxicity. Some toxicologists advise restraining a patient who attempts to sign out against medical advice after treatment with naloxone, at least until the patient receives psychiatric evaluation.

ORGANOPHOSPHATES AND CARBAMATES

Cholinergic intoxication sources are insecticides (organophosphates or carbamates), some medications, and some mushrooms. Examples of organophosphate insecticides are malathion (low toxicity, median lethal dose [LD$_{50}$] 2800 mg/kg), chlorpyrifos, which has been removed from market (moderate toxicity), and parathion (high toxicity, LD$_{50}$ 2 mg/kg). Carbamate insecticides include carbaryl (low toxicity, LD$_{50}$ 500 mg/kg), propoxur (moderate toxicity, LD$_{50}$ 95 mg/kg), and aldicarb (high toxicity, LD$_{50}$ 0.9 mg/kg). Pharmaceuticals with carbamate properties include neostigmine (Prostigmin) and physostigmine (Antilirium). Cholinergic compounds also include the "G" nerve war weapons tabun (GA), sarin (GB), soman (GB), and venom X (VX).

Toxic Mechanism

Organophosphates phosphorylate the active site on red cell acetylcholinesterase and pseudocholinesterase in the serum, neuromuscular and parasympathetic neuroeffector junctions, and in the major synapses of the autonomic ganglia, causing irreversible inhibition. There are two types of organophosphate intoxication: (a) direct action by the parent compound (e.g., tetraethylpyrophosphate), or (b) indirect action by the toxic metabolite (e.g., parathoxon or malathoxon).

Carbamates (esters of carbonic acid) cause reversible carbamylation of the active site of the enzymes. When a critical amount, greater than 50%, of cholinesterase is inhibited, acetylcholine accumulates and causes transient stimulation at cholinergic synapses and sympathetic terminals (muscarinic effect), the somatic nerves, the autonomic ganglia (nicotinic effect), and CNS synapses. Stimulation of conduction is followed by inhibition of conduction.

The major differences between the carbamates and the organophosphates are as follows: (a) carbamate toxicity is less and the duration is shorter; (b) carbamates rarely produce overt CNS effects (poor CNS penetration); (c) carbamate inhibition of the acetylcholinesterase enzyme is reversible and activity returns to normal rapidly; (d) pralidoxime, the enzyme regenerator, may not be necessary in the management of mild carbamate intoxication (e.g., carbaryl).

Toxic Dose

Parathion's minimum lethal dose is 2 mg in children and 10 to 20 mg in adults. The lethal dose of malathion is greater than 1375 mg/kg and that of chlorpyrifos is 25 g; the latter compound is unlikely to cause death.

Kinetics

Absorption is by all routes. The onset of acute ingestion toxicity occurs as early as 3 hours, usually before 12 hours and always before 24 hours. Lipid-soluble agents absorbed by the dermal route (e.g., fenthion) may have a delayed onset of more than 24 hours. Inhalation toxicity occurs immediately after exposure. Massive ingestion can produce intoxication within minutes.

Metabolism is via the liver. With some pesticides (e.g., parathion, malathion), the effects are delayed because they undergo hepatic microsomal oxidative metabolism to their toxic metabolites, the -oxons (e.g., paroxon, malaoxon).

The half-life of malathion is 2.89 hours and that of parathion is 2.1 days. The metabolites are eliminated in the urine and the presence of p-nitrophenol in the urine is a clue up to 48 hours after exposure.

Manifestations

Many organophosphates produce a garlic odor on the breath, in the gastric contents, or in the container. Diaphoresis, excessive salivation, miosis, and muscle twitching are helpful clues to diagnosis.

Early, a cholinergic (muscarinic) crisis develops that consists of parasympathetic nervous system activity. DUMBELS is the mnemonic for defecation, cramps, and increased bowel motility; urinary incontinence; miosis (mydriasis may occur in 20%); bronchospasm and bronchorrhea; excess secretion; lacrimation; and seizures. Bradycardia, pulmonary edema, and hypotension may be present.

Later, sympathetic and nicotinic effects occur, consisting of MATCH: muscle weakness and fasciculation (eyelid twitching is often present), adrenal stimulation and hyperglycemia, tachycardia, cramps in muscles, and hypertension. Finally, paralysis of the skeletal muscles ensues.

The CNS effects are headache, blurred vision, anxiety, ataxia, delirium and toxic psychosis, convulsions, coma, and respiratory depression. Cranial nerve palsies have been noted. Delayed hallucinations may occur.

Delayed respiratory paralysis and neurologic and neurobehavioral disorders have been described following certain organophosphate ingestions or dermal exposure. The "intermediate syndrome" is paralysis of proximal and respiratory muscles developing 24 to

96 hours after the successful treatment of organophosphate poisoning. A delayed distal polyneuropathy has been described with ingestion of certain organophosphates, such as triorthocresyl phosphate, bromoleptophos, and methomidophos.

Complications include aspiration, pulmonary edema, and acute respiratory distress syndrome.

Laboratory Investigations

Monitoring should include chest radiograph, blood glucose (nonketotic hyperglycemia is frequent), ABG, pulse oximetry, ECG, blood coagulation status, liver function, hyperamylasemia (pancreatitis reported), and urinalysis for the metabolite alkyl phosphate paranitrophenol. Blood should be drawn for red blood cell cholinesterase determination before pralidoxime is given. The red blood cell cholinesterase activity roughly correlates with clinical severity. Mild poisoning is 20% to 50% of normal, moderate poisoning is 10% to 20% of normal, and severe poisoning is 10% of normal (>90% depressed). A post-exposure rise of 10% to 15% in the cholinesterase level determined at least 10 to 14 days after the exposure confirms the diagnosis.

Management

Protection of health care personnel with clothing (masks, gloves, gowns, goggles) and respiratory equipment or hazardous material suits, as necessary, is called for. General decontamination consists of isolation, bagging, and disposal of contaminated clothing and other articles. Vital functions should be established and maintained. Cardiac and oxygen saturation monitoring are needed. Intubation and assisted ventilation may be needed. Secretions should be suctioned until atropinization drying is achieved.

Dermal decontamination involves prompt removal of clothing and cleansing of all affected areas of skin, hair, and eyes. Ocular decontamination involves irrigation with copious amounts of tepid water or 0.9% saline for at least 15 minutes. Gastrointestinal decontamination, if the ingestion was recent, involves the administration of activated charcoal.

Atropine sulfate can be given as an antidote. It is both a diagnostic and a therapeutic agent. Atropine counteracts the muscarinic effects but is only partially effective for the CNS effects (seizures and coma). Preservative-free atropine (no benzyl alcohol) should be used. If the patient is symptomatic (bradycardia or bronchorrhea), a test dose should be administered, 0.02 mg/kg in children or 1 mg in adults, intravenously. If no signs of atropinization are present (tachycardia, drying of secretions, and mydriasis), atropine should be administered immediately, 0.05 mg/kg in children or 2 mg in adults, every 5 to 10 minutes as needed to dry the secretions and clear the lungs. Beneficial effects are seen within 1 to 4 minutes and maximum effect in 8 minutes. The average dose in the first 24 hours is 40 mg, but 1000 mg or more has been required in severe cases. Glycopyrrolate (Robinul) can be used if atropine is not available. The maximum dose should be maintained for 12 to 24 hours, then tapered and the patient observed for relapse. Poisoning, especially with lipophilic agents (e.g., fenthion, chlorfenthion), may require weeks of atropine therapy. An alternative is a continuous infusion of atropine 8 mg in 100 mL 0.9% saline at rate of 0.02 to 0.08 mg/kg/h (0.25 to 1.0 mL/kg/h) with additional 1 to 5 mg boluses as needed to dry the secretions.

Pralidoxime chloride (Protopam) has both antinicotinic and antimuscarinic effects and possibly also CNS effects. Successful treatment with pralidoxime chloride may allow a reduction in the dose of atropine. Pralidoxime acts to reactivate the phosphorylated cholinesterases by binding the phosphate moiety on the esteritic site and displacing it. It should be given early before "aging" of phosphate bond produces tighter binding. However, recent reports indicate that pralidoxime chloride is beneficial even several days after the poisoning. Improvement is seen within 10 to 40 minutes. The initial dose of pralidoxime chloride is 1 to 2 g in 250 mL 0.89% saline over 5 to 10 minutes, maximum 200 mg/minute, in adults or 25 to 50 mg/kg, maximum 4 mg/kg/minute, in children younger than 12 years of age. The dose can be repeated every 6 to 12 hours for several days.

An alternative is a continuous infusion of 1 g in 100 mL 0.89% saline at 5 to 20 mg/kg/h (0.5 to 12 mL/g/h) up to 500 mg/h and titrated to desired response. Maximum adult daily dose is 12 g. Cardiac and blood pressure monitoring are advised during and for several hours after the infusion. The end point is absence of fasciculations and return of muscle strength.

Contraindicated drugs include morphine, aminophylline, barbiturates, opioids, phenothiazine, reserpine-like drugs, parasympathomimetics, and succinylcholine.

Noncardiac pulmonary edema may require respiratory support. Seizures may respond to atropine and pralidoxime chloride but often require anticonvulsants. Cardiac dysrhythmias may require electrical cardioversion or antidysrhythmic therapy if the patient is hemodynamically unstable. Extracorporeal procedures are of no proven value.

Disposition

Asymptomatic patients with normal examination findings after 6 to 8 hours of observation may be discharged. In cases of intentional poisoning, the patients require psychiatric clearance for discharge. Symptomatic patients should be admitted to the intensive care unit. Observation of milder cases of carbamate poisoning, even those requiring atropine, for 6 to 8 hours symptom-free may be sufficient to exclude significant toxicity. In cases of workplace exposure, OSHA should be notified.

PHENCYCLIDINE (ANGEL DUST)

Phencyclidine is an arylcyclohexylamine related to ketamine and chemically related to the phenothiazines. Originally a "dissociative" anesthetic banned in United States since 1979, it is now an illicit substance, with at least 38 analogs. It is inexpensively manufactured by "kitchen chemists" and is mislabeled as other hallucinogens. Improper phencyclidine synthesis may release cyanide when heated or smoked and can cause explosions.

Toxic Mechanism

The mechanism of phencyclidine is complex and not completely understood. It inhibits some neurotransmitters and causes a loss of pain sensation without depressing the CNS respiratory status. It stimulates α-adrenergic receptors and may act as a "false neurotransmitter." The effects are sympathomimetic, cholinergic, and cerebellar.

Toxic Dose

The usual dose of phencyclidine mixed with marijuana joints is 100 to 400 mg of phencyclidine. Joints or leaf mixtures contain 0.24% to 7.9% of PCP, 1 mg of PCP/150 leaves. Tablets contain 5 mg (the usual street dose). CNS effects at doses of 1 to 6 mg include hallucinations and euphoria, 6 to 10 mg produces toxic psychosis and sympathetic stimulation, 10 to 25 mg produces severe toxicity, and more than 100 mg has resulted in fatalities.

Kinetics

Phencyclidine is a lipophilic weak base, with a pKa of 8.5 to 9.5. It is rapidly absorbed when smoked and snorted, poorly absorbed from the acid stomach, and rapidly absorbed from the alkaline middle small intestine. It has an enterogastric secretion and is reabsorbed in the small intestine. The onset of action when smoked is 2 to 5 minutes, with a peak in 15 to 30 minutes. With oral ingestion, the onset is in 30 to 60 minutes and when taken intravenously it is immediate. Most adverse reactions in cases of overdose begin within 1 to 2 hours. Its duration of action at low doses is 4 to 6 hours and normality returns in 24 hours; in large overdoses, fluctuating coma may last 6 to 10 days.

Volume distribution is 6.2 L/kg. Phencyclidine concentrates in brain and adipose tissue. Protein binding is 70%. The route of elimination is by gastric secretion, liver metabolism, and 10% urinary excretion of conjugates and free phencyclidine. Renal excretion may be increased 50% with urinary acidification. The half-life is 1 hour (in cases of overdose, it is 11 to 89 hours).

Manifestations

The classic picture is bursts of horizontal, vertical, and rotary nystagmus, which is a clue to diagnosis (occurs in 50% of cases), miosis, hypertension, and fluctuating altered mental state. There is a wide spectrum of clinical presentations.

Mild intoxication with 1 to 6 mg produces drunken and bizarre behavior, agitation, rotary nystagmus, and blank stare. Violent behavior and sensory anesthesia make these patients insensitive to pain, self-destructive, and dangerous. Most are communicative within 1 to 2 hours, are alert and oriented in 6 to 8 hours, and recover completely in 24 to 48 hours.

Moderate intoxication with 6 to 10 mg produces excess salivation, hypertension, hyperthermia, muscle rigidity, myoclonus, and catatonia. Recovery of consciousness occurs in 24 to 48 hours and complete recovery in 1 week.

Severe intoxication with 10 to 25 mg results in opisthotonus, decerebrate rigidity, convulsions, prolonged fluctuating coma, and respiratory failure. Patients in this category have a high rate of medical complications. Recovery of consciousness occurs in 24 to 48 hours, with complete normality in a month. Medical complications include apnea, aspiration pneumonia, cardiac arrest, hypertensive encephalopathy, hyperthermia, intracerebral hemorrhage, psychosis, rhabdomyolysis and myoglobinuria, and seizures. Loss of memory and "flashbacks" last for months. Phencyclidine-induced depression and suicide have been reported.

Fatalities occur with ingestions of greater than 100 mg and with serum levels greater than 100 to 250 ng/mL.

Laboratory Investigations

Marked elevation of creatine kinase level may occur. Values greater than 20,000 units have been reported. Urinalysis should be monitored and urine tested for myoglobin. One should monitor the blood for creatine kinase, uric acid (an early clue to rhabdomyolysis), BUN, creatinine, electrolytes (hyperkalemia), blood glucose (20% of patients have hypoglycemia), urinary output, liver function tests, ECG, and ABG if the patient has any respiratory manifestations. Measurement of phencyclidine in the gastric juice is called for because concentrations are 10 to 50 times higher than in blood or urine. Phencyclidine blood concentrations are not helpful. Phencyclidine may be detected in the urine of the average user for 10 days to 3 weeks after the last dose. In chronic users, it can be detected for over 1 month. The analogs of phencyclidine may not produce positive test results for phencyclidine in the urine. Cross-reactions with bleach and dextromethorphan may cause false-positive urine test results on immunoassay, and cross-reaction with doxylamine may produce a false-positive finding on gas chromatography.

Management

The patient should be observed for violent, self-destructive, bizarre behavior and paranoid schizophrenia. Patients should be placed in a low sensory environment and dangerous objects should be removed from the area.

Gastrointestinal decontamination is not effective because phencyclidine is rapidly absorbed from intestines. Overtreating the mild intoxication should be avoided. There is insufficient evidence to support the use of MDAC. In cases of severe toxicity (stupor or coma), continuous gastric suction can be tried (with protection of the airway) because the drug is secreted into the gastric juice. The value of this procedure is controversial because of limited data.

The patient must be protected from harming himself or herself or others. Physical restraints may be necessary, but they should be used sparingly and for the shortest time possible because they increase risk of rhabdomyolysis. Metal restraints such as handcuffs should be avoided. For behavioral disorders and toxic psychosis, diazepam is the agent of choice. Pharmacologic intervention includes diazepam (Valium) 10 to 30 mg orally or 2 to 5 mg intravenously initially and titrated upward to 10 mg; however, up to 30 mg may be required. "Talk down" technique is usually ineffective and dangerous. Phenothiazines and butyrophenones should be avoided in the acute phase because they lower the convulsive threshold; however, they may be needed later for psychosis. Haloperidol (Haldol) administration has been reported to produce catatonia.

Seizures and muscle spasm are managed with diazepam, from 2.5 mg up to 10 mg. Hyperthermia (>38.5°C [101.3°F]) is treated with external cooling measures. Hypertension is usually transient and does not require treatment. In the case of emergent hypertensive crisis (blood pressure >200/115 mm Hg) nitroprusside can be used in a dose of 0.3 to 2 µg/kg/min. Maximum infusion rate is 10 µg/kg/min for only 10 minutes.

Acid ion trapping diuresis is not recommended because of the danger of myoglobin precipitation in the renal tubules. Rhabdomyolysis and myoglobinuria are treated by correcting volume depletion and insuring a urinary output of greater than 2 mL/kg/h. Alkalinization is controversial because of reabsorption of phencyclidine.

Hemodialysis is beneficial if renal failure occurs; otherwise, the extracorporeal procedures are not beneficial.

Disposition

All patients with coma, delirium, catatonia, violent behavior, aspiration pneumonia, sustained hypertension greater than 200/115, and significant rhabdomyolysis should be admitted to the intensive care unit until asymptomatic for at least 24 hours. If patients with mild intoxication are mentally and neurologically stable and become asymptomatic (except for nystagmus) for 4 hours, they may be discharged in the company of a responsible adult. All patients must be assessed for suicide risk before discharge. Drug counseling and psychiatric follow-up should be arranged. Patients should be warned that episodes of disorientation and depression may continue intermittently for 4 weeks or more.

PHENOTHIAZINES AND NONPHENOTHIAZINES (NEUROLEPTICS)

Toxic Mechanism

Neuroleptics have complex mechanisms of toxicity, including (a) block of the postsynaptic dopamine receptors; (b) block of peripheral and central α-adrenergic receptors; (c) block of cholinergic muscarinic receptors; (d) quinidine-like antidysrhythmic and myocardial depressant effect in cases of large overdose; (e) lowering of the convulsive threshold; (f) effect on hypothalamic temperature regulation (Table 25).

Toxic Dose

Extrapyramidal reactions, anticholinergic effects, and orthostatic hypotension may occur at therapeutic doses. The toxic amount is not established, but the maximum daily therapeutic dose may result in significant side effects, and twice this amount may be potentially fatal. Chlorpromazine (Thorazine), the prototype, may produce serious hypotension and CNS depression at doses greater than 200 mg (17 mg/kg) in children and 3 to 5 g in an adult. Fatalities have been reported after 2.5 g of loxapine (Loxitane) and mesoridazine (Serentil) and 1.5 g of thioridazine (Mellaril).

Kinetics

These agents are lipophilic and have unpredictable gastrointestinal absorption. Peak levels occur 2 to 6 hours postingestion and have enterohepatic recirculation.

The mean serum half-life in phase 1 is 1 to 2 hours and the biphasic half-life is 20 to 40 hours. Volume distribution is 10 to 40 L/kg; protein binding is 92% to 98%. Chlorpromazine taken orally has an onset of action in 30 to 60 minutes, peak in 2 to 4 hours, and duration of 4 to 6 hours. With sustained-release preparations, the onset is in 30 to 60 minutes and duration 6 to 12 hours.

Elimination is by hepatic metabolism, which results in multiple metabolites (some are active). Metabolites can be detected in urine months after chronic therapy. Only 1% to 3% is excreted unchanged in the urine.

TABLE 25 Neuroleptics and Properties

Compound	Antipsychotic	Anticholinergic	Extrapyramidal	Hypotensive and Cardiotoxic	Sedative
Phenothiazine					
Aliphatic	1+	3+	2+	2+	3+
Chlorpromazine (Thorazine)					
Promethazine (Phenergan)					
Piperazine	3+	1+	3+	1+	1+
Fluphenazine (Prolixin)					
Perphenazine (Trilafon)					
Prochlorperazine (Compazine)					
Trifluoperazine (Stelazine)					
Piperidine	1+	2+	1+	3+	3+
Mesoridazine (Serentil)					
Thioridazine (Mellaril)					
Nonphenothiazine					
Butyrophenone	3+	1+	3+	1+	1+
Haloperidol (Haldol)					
Dibenzoxazepine	3+	1+	3+	1+	2+
Loxapine (Loxitane)					
Dihydroindolone	3+	1+	3+	1+	1+
Molindone (Moban)					
Thioxanthenes	3+	1+	3+	3+	1+
Thiothixene (Navane)					
Chlorprothixene (Taractan)					

1+ = very low activity; 2+ = moderate activity; 3+ = very high activity.

Manifestations

In cases of phenothiazine overdose, anticholinergic symptoms may be present early but are not life-threatening. Miosis is usually present (80%) if the phenothiazine has strong α-adrenergic blocking effect (e.g., chlorpromazine), but anticholinergic activity mydriasis may occur. Agitation and delirium rapidly progress into coma. Major problems are cardiac toxicity and hypotension. The cardiotoxic effects are seen more commonly with thioridazine and its metabolite mesoridazine. These agents have produced the largest number of fatalities in patients with phenothiazine overdose. Cardiac conduction disturbances include prolonged PR, QRS, and QTc intervals, U- and T-wave abnormalities, and ventricular dysrhythmias, including torsades de pointes. Seizures occur mainly in patients with convulsive disorders or with administration of loxapine. Sudden death in children and adults has been reported.

Idiosyncratic dystonic reactions are most common with the piperidine group. Reactions are not dose-dependent and consist of opisthotonos, torticollis, orolingual dyskinesia, or oculogyric crisis (painful upward gaze). These reactions are more frequent in children and women. Neuroleptic malignant syndrome occurs in patients on chronic therapy and is characterized by hyperthermia, muscle rigidity, autonomic dysfunction, and altered mental state. There is one case reported with acute overdose. The loxapine syndrome consists of seizures, rhabdomyolysis, and renal failure.

Laboratory Investigations

Monitoring should include arterial blood gases, renal and hepatic function, electrolytes, blood glucose, and creatine kinase and myoglobinemia in neuroleptic malignant syndrome. Most of these agents are detected on routine screening. Quantitative serum levels are not useful in management. Cross-reactions with enzyme multiplied immunoassay technique tests occur with cyclic antidepressants. Phenothiazines give false-negative results on pregnancy urine tests using human chorionic gonadotropin as an indicator, and give false-positive results for urine porphyrins, indirect Coombs test, urobilinogen, and amylase.

Management

Vital functions must be established and maintained. All overdose patients require venous access, 12-lead ECG (to measure intervals), cardiac and respiratory monitoring, and seizure precautions. One should monitor core temperature to detect poikilothermic effect. If the patient is comatose, intubation and assisted ventilation may be required, as well as 100% oxygen, intravenous glucose, naloxone (Narcan), and thiamine.

Emesis is not recommended. Activated charcoal can be administered if ingestion was within 1 hour. MDAC has not been proven beneficial. A radiograph of the abdomen may be useful, if the phenothiazine is radiopaque. Haloperidol (Haldol) and trifluoperazine (Stelazine) are most likely to be radiopaque. Whole-bowel irrigation may be useful when a large number of pills are visualized on radiograph or if sustained-release preparations were taken, but whole-bowel irrigation has not been evaluated in patients with phenothiazine overdose.

Convulsions are treated with diazepam or lorazepam (Ativan). Loxapine (Loxitane) overdose may result in status epilepticus. If nondepolarizing neuromuscular blockade is required, pancuronium (Pavulon) or vecuronium (Norcuron) should be used (not succinylcholine [Anectine], which may cause malignant hyperthermia), and EEG should be monitored during paralysis.

Patients with dysrhythmias should be monitored with serial ECGs. Unstable rhythms can be treated with electrical cardioversion. Class 1a antidysrhythmics (procainamide, quinidine, and disopyramide [Norpace]) must be avoided.

Hypokalemia predisposes to dysrhythmias and should be corrected aggressively. Supraventricular tachycardia with hemodynamic instability is treated with electrical cardioversion. The role of adenosine has not been defined. Calcium channel and β-blockers should be avoided.

Prolongation of the QRS interval is treated with sodium bicarbonate 1 to 2 mEq/kg by intravenous bolus over a few minutes. Torsades de pointes is treated with magnesium sulfate IV 20% solution 2 g over 2 to 3 minutes. If there is no response in 10 minutes, the dose is repeated and followed by a continuous infusion of 5 to 10 mg/min or given as an infusion of 50 mg/minute for 2 hours followed by 30 mg/minute for 90 minutes twice a day for several days, as needed. The dose in children is 25 to 50 mg/kg initially and maintenance dose is 30 to 60 mg/kg per 24 hours (0.25 to 0.50 mEq/kg per 24 hours) up to 1000 mg per 24 hours. Serum magnesium levels should be monitored.

To treat ventricular tachydysrhythmias in a stable patient, lidocaine is used. If the patient is unstable, electrical cardioversion is used. Patients with heart block with hemodynamic instability should be managed with temporary cardiac pacing.

Hypotension is treated with the Trendelenburg position and 0.9% saline. If the condition is refractory to treatment or there is a danger of fluid overload, vasopressors are administered. The vasopressor of choice is α-adrenergic agonist norepinephrine (Levophed), titrated to response. Epinephrine and dopamine should not be used because β-receptor stimulation in the presence of α-receptor blockade may provoke dysrhythmias and phenothiazines are antidopaminergic.

Hypothermia and hyperthermia are treated with external warming and cooling measures, respectively. Antipyretic drugs must not be used.

Management of the neuroleptic malignant syndrome includes the following actions:

- Immediately discontinuing the offending agent
- Hyperventilating the patient, using 100% humidified, cooled oxygen at high gas flows (at least 10 L/min) because of rapid breathing
- Administering a benzodiazepine to control convulsions and facilitate cooling measures
- Initiating appropriate mechanical cooling measures, which may include intravenous cold saline (not lactated Ringer's), ice baths, cold lavage of the stomach, bladder, and rectum, and a hypothermic blanket
- Correcting acid-base and electrolyte disturbances and treating significant hyperkalemia with hyperventilation, calcium, sodium bicarbonate, intravenous glucose, and insulin; hemodialysis may be necessary

In addition, dysrhythmias usually respond to correction of the underlying acid-base disturbances and hyperkalemia. If antidysrhythmic agents are required, calcium channel blockers must be avoided because they may precipitate hyperkalemia and cardiovascular collapse. Dantrolene sodium (Dantrium), which is a phenytoin derivative, inhibits calcium release from the sarcoplasmic reticulum and results in decreased muscle contraction. Dantrolene acts peripherally and does not reverse the rigidity or psychomotor disturbances resulting from the central dopamine blockade; it therefore is often used in combination with bromocriptine. Bromocriptine mesylate (Parlodel) acts centrally as a dopamine agonist, as does amantadine hydrochloride (Symmetrel). Bromocriptine and dantrolene have been reported to be successful in combination with cooling and good supportive measures in malignant hyperthermia.

Dosing for these agents is as follows: dantrolene sodium at 2 to 3 mg/kg IV as a bolus, then 1 mg/kg/minute to a maximum of 10 mg/kg or until the tachycardia, rigidity, increased end-tidal CO_2, and temperature elevation are controlled. *Note:* Hepatotoxicity occurs with doses greater than 10 mg/kg. To prevent symptom recurrence, 1 mg/kg should be administered every 6 hours for 24 to 48 hours after the episode. After that time, oral dantrolene can be used at a dose of 1 mg/kg every 6 hours for 24 hours as necessary. The patient should be observed for thrombophlebitis following intravenous dantrolene. It is best administered via a central line. Bromocriptine mesylate at 2.5 to 10 mg orally or via a nasogastric tube, three times a day, should be used in combination with dantrolene.

Idiosyncratic dystonic reaction can be treated with diphenhydramine (Benadryl) 1 to 2 mg/kg/dose intravenously over 5 minutes up to maximum of 50 mg intravenously; a response is noted within 2 to 5 minutes. This can be followed with oral doses for 4 to 6 days to prevent recurrence.

Extracorporeal measures (hemodialysis, hemoperfusion) are not effective in removing these agents.

Disposition

Asymptomatic patients should be observed for at least 6 hours after gastric decontamination. Symptomatic patients with cardiotoxicity, hypotension, and convulsions should be admitted to the intensive care unit and monitored for 48 hours.

SALICYLATES (ACETYLSALICYLIC ACID, SALICYLIC ACID)

Toxic Mechanism

The primary toxic mechanisms include (a) direct stimulation of the medullary chemoreceptor trigger zone and respiratory center; (b) uncoupling oxidative phosphorylation; (c) inhibition of the Krebs cycle enzymes; (d) inhibition of vitamin K dependent and independent clotting factors; (e) alteration of platelet function; and (f) inhibition of prostaglandin synthesis.

Toxic Dose

Acute mild intoxication occurs at a dose of 150 to 200 mg/kg, moderate intoxication at 200 to 300 mg/kg, and severe intoxication at 300 to 500 mg/kg. Acute salicylate plasma concentration greater than 30 mg/dL (usually >40 mg/dL) may be associated with clinical toxicity. Chronic intoxication occurs at ingestions greater than 100 mg/kg/d for more than 2 days because of accumulation kinetics. Methyl salicylate (oil of wintergreen) is the most toxic form of salicylate. A dose of 1 mL of 98% contains 1.4 g of salicylate. Fatalities have occurred with ingestion of 1 teaspoonful in children and 1 ounce in adults. It is found in topical ointments and liniments (18% to 30%).

Kinetics

Acetylsalicylic acid and salicylic acid are weak acids with a pKa of 3.5 and 3.0, respectively. Acetylsalicylic acid is absorbed from the stomach, from the small bowel, and dermally. Onset of action is within 30 minutes. Methyl salicylate and effervescent tablets are absorbed more rapidly. Salicylate plasma concentration is detectable within 15 minutes after ingestion and peaks in 30 to 120 minutes. The peak may be delayed 6 to 12 hours in cases of large overdose, overdose with enteric-coated or sustained-release preparations, and development of concretions. The therapeutic duration of action is 3 to 4 hours but is markedly prolonged in cases of overdose.

Volume distribution is 0.13 L/kg for salicylic acid but increases as the salicylate plasma concentration increases. Protein binding is greater than 90% for salicylic acid at pH 7.4 and a salicylate plasma concentration of 20 to 30 mg/dL, 75% at a salicylate plasma concentration greater than 40 mg/dL, 50% at a salicylate plasma concentration of 70 mg/dL, and 30% at a salicylate plasma concentration of 120 mg/dL.

The half-life for salicylic acid is 3 hours after a 300 mg dose, 6 hours after a 1 g overdose, and greater than 10 hours after a 10-g overdose. Elimination includes Michaelis-Menten hepatic metabolism by three saturable pathways: (a) glycine conjugation to salicyluric acid (75%); (b) glucuronyl transferase to salicyl phenol glucuronide (10%); and (c) salicyl aryl glucuronide (4%). Nonsaturable pathways are hydrolysis to gentisic acid (<1%). Ten percent is excreted unchanged.

Acidosis increases the severity of the intoxication by increasing the non-ionized salicylate that can cross membranes and enter the brain cells. In kidneys, the unionized salicylic acid undergoes glomerular filtration, and the ionized portion undergoes tubular secretion in proximal tubules and passive reabsorption in the distal tubules. Renal excretion of salicylate is enhanced by alkaline urine.

Manifestations

The ingestion of concentrated topical salicylic acid preparations (e.g., wart remover) can cause mucosal caustic injury to the gastrointestinal tract. Occult salicylate overdose should be considered in any patient with unexplained acid-base disturbance.

The manifestations of acute overdose of salicylates are as follows:

Minimal Symptoms

Tinnitus, dizziness, and deafness may occur at high therapeutic salicylate plasma concentrations of 20 to 30 mg/dL. Nausea and vomiting may occur immediately because of local gastric irritation.

Phase I. Mild manifestations occur at 1 to 12 hours after ingestion with a 6-hour salicylate plasma concentration of 45 to 70 mg/dL. Nausea and vomiting followed by hyperventilation are usually present within 3 to 8 hours after acute overdose. Hyperventilation, an increase in both rate (tachypnea) and depth (hyperpnea), is present but it may be subtle. It results in a mild respiratory alkalosis with a serum pH greater than 7.4 and urine pH greater than 6.0. Some patients may have lethargy, vertigo, headache, and confusion. Diaphoresis may be noted.

Phase II. Moderate manifestations occur at 12 to 24 hours after ingestion with a 6-hour salicylate plasma concentration of 70 to 90 mg/dL. Serious metabolic disturbances, including a marked respiratory alkalosis with anion gap metabolic acidosis, dehydration, and urine pH less than 6.0, may occur. Other metabolic disturbances include hypoglycemia or hyperglycemia, hypokalemia, decreased ionized calcium, and increased BUN, creatinine, and lactate. Mental disturbances (confusion, disorientation, hallucinations) may occur. Hypotension and convulsions have been reported.

Phase III. Severe intoxication occurs more than 24 hours after ingestion with a 6-hour salicylate plasma concentration of 90 to 130 mg/dL. In addition to the above clinical findings, coma and seizures develop and indicate severe intoxication. Pulmonary edema may occur. Metabolic disturbances include metabolic acidemia (pH <7.4) and aciduria (pH <6.0). In adults, alkalosis may persist until terminal respiratory failure.

In children younger than 4 years of age, a mixed metabolic acidosis and respiratory alkalosis develop earlier (within 4 to 6 hours) than in adults because children have less respiratory reserve and accumulate lactate and other organic acids. Hypoglycemia is more common in children.

Fatalities occur at 6-hour salicylate plasma concentrations greater than 130 to 150 mg/dL and result from CNS depression, cardiovascular collapse, electrolyte imbalance, and cerebral edema.

Chronic salicylism is more serious than acute intoxication and the 6-hour salicylate plasma concentration does not correlate well with the manifestations in both acute and chronic cases of intoxication. Chronic intoxication usually occurs with therapeutic errors in young children or the elderly with underlying illness, and the diagnosis is delayed because it is not recognized. Noncardiac pulmonary edema is a frequent complication in the elderly. The mortality rate is about 25%. Chronic salicylate poisoning in children may mimic Reye syndrome. It is associated with exaggerated CNS findings (hallucinations, delirium, dementia, memory loss, papilledema, bizarre behavior, agitation, encephalopathy, seizures, and coma). Hemorrhagic manifestations, renal failure, and pulmonary and cerebral edema may occur. The metabolic picture is hypoglycemia and mixed acid-base derangements. A chronic salicylate plasma concentration greater than 60 mg/dL with metabolic acidosis and an altered mental state is very serious.

Laboratory Investigations

All patients with intentional salicylate overdoses should have acetaminophen plasma level measured after 4 hours.

One should continuously monitor ECG, urine output, urine pH, and specific gravity. Every 2 to 4 hours in cases of severe intoxication, salicylate plasma concentration, glucose (in a case of salicylism, CNS hypoglycemia may be present despite normal serum glucose), electrolytes, ionized calcium, magnesium and phosphorous, anion gap, ABGs, and pulse oximeter should be monitored. Daily monitoring of BUN, creatinine, liver function tests, and prothrombin time should take place.

The therapeutic salicylate plasma concentration is less than 10 mg/dL for analgesia and 15 to 30 mg/dL for anti-inflammatory effect. Cross-reaction with diflunisal (Dolobid) will give a falsely high salicylate plasma concentration. The Done nomogram is not considered accurate in evaluating acute or chronic salicylate intoxications.

Management

Treatment is based on clinical and metabolic findings, not on salicylate levels. Continuous monitoring of the urine pH is essential for successful alkalinization treatment. One should always obtain an acetaminophen plasma level.

Vital functions must be established and maintained. If the patient is in an altered mental state, glucose, naloxone, and thiamine are administered in standard doses. Depending on the severity, the initial studies include an immediate and a 6-hour postingestion salicylate plasma concentration, ECG and cardiac monitoring, pulse oximeter, urine (analysis, pH, and specific gravity), chest radiograph, ABGs, blood glucose, electrolytes and anion gap calculation, calcium (ionized), magnesium, renal and liver profiles, and prothrombin time. Gastric contents and stool should be tested for occult blood. Bismuth and magnesium salicylate preparations may be radiopaque on radiographs. Consultation with a nephrologist is warranted in cases of moderate, severe, or chronic intoxication.

For gastrointestinal decontamination, activated charcoal is useful (each gram of activated charcoal binds 550 mg of salicylic acid) if a toxic dose was ingested up to 4 hours postingestion. MDAC is not recommended for salicylate intoxication.

Concretions may occur with massive (usually >300 mg/kg) ingestions. If blood levels fail to decline, prompt contrast radiography of the stomach may reveal concretions that have to be removed by repeated lavage, whole-bowel irrigation, endoscopy, or gastrostomy.

Fluids and electrolyte treatment of salicylate poisonings is given in Table 26. For shock, perfusion and vascular volume should be established with 5% dextrose in 0.9% saline, then the treatment can proceed with correction of dehydration and alkalinization.

TABLE 26 Fluid and Electrolyte Treatment of Salicylate Poisoning

Type of Salicylism	Metabolic Disturbance	Blood pH	Urine pH	Hydrating Solution	Amount of NaHCO₃ (mEq/L)	Amount of Potassium (mEq/L)
Mild	Respiratory alkalosis	>7.4	>6.0	5% Dextrose, 0.45% saline	50 (adult) 1 mEq/kg (child)	20
Moderate Chronic Child <4 years	Respiratory alkalosis Metabolic acidosis	>7.4 or <7.4	<6.0	5% Dextrose in water	100 (adult) 1–2 mEq/kg (child)	40
Severe Chronic Child <4 years	Metabolic acidosis Respiratory alkalosis	<7.4	<6.0	5% Dextrose in water	150 (adult) 2 mEq/kg (child)	60
CNS Depressant Co-ingestant	Respiratory acidosis	<7.4	<6.0	5% Dextrose in water	100–150*	60

Modified from Linden CH, Rumack BH: The legitimate analgesics, aspirin and acetaminophen. In Hansen W Jr (ed): Toxic Emergencies. New York, Churchill Livingstone, 1984.
*Correct hypoventilation.

For cases of acute moderate or severe salicylism (see Table 26), adults should receive a bolus of 1 to 2 mEq/kg of sodium bicarbonate ($NaHCO_3$) followed by an infusion of 100 to 150 mEq $NaHCO_3$ added to 500 to 1000 mL of 5% dextrose and administered over 60 minutes. Children should receive a bolus of 1 to 2 mEq/kg of $NaHCO_3$ followed by an infusion of 1 to 2 mEq/kg added to 20 mL/kg of 5% dextrose administered over 60 minutes. Potassium is added after the patient voids. The goal is to achieve a urine output of greater than 2 mL/kg/hr and a urine pH of greater than 8. The initial infusion is followed by subsequent infusions (two to three times normal maintenance) of 200 to 300 mL/h in adults or 10 mL/kg/h in children. If the patient is acidotic and has a serum pH of less than 7.15, an additional 1 to 2 mEq/kg of $NaHCO_3$ is given over 1 to 2 hours; persistent acidosis may require 1 to 2 mEq/kg of bicarbonate every 2 hours. The infusion rate, the amount of bicarbonate, and the electrolytes should be adjusted to correct serum abnormalities and to maintain the targeted urine output and urinary pH. Diuresis is not as important as the alkalinization. Careful monitoring for fluid overload should take place for patients at risk of pulmonary and cerebral edema (e.g., the elderly) and because of inappropriate secretion of the antidiuretic hormone.

In patients with mild intoxication who are not acidotic and have a urine pH greater than 6, 5% dextrose in 0.45% saline should be administered as maintenance to replace ongoing fluid loss. Some toxicologists may consider adding sodium bicarbonate 50 mEq/L or 1 mEq/kg in some cases.

To achieve alkalinization, sodium bicarbonate is administered to produce a serum pH 7.4 to 7.5 and a urine pH greater than 8. Carbonic anhydrase inhibitors (acetazolamide [Diamox]) should not be used. If the patient is acidotic, additional bicarbonate may be required. About 2 mEq/kg raises the blood pH 0.1. In children, alkalinization may be a difficult problem because of the organic acid production and hypokalemia. Hypokalemic and fluid-depleted patients cannot be adequately alkalinized. Alkalinization is usually discontinued in asymptomatic patients with a salicylate plasma concentration less than 30 to 40 mg/dL but is continued in symptomatic patients regardless of the salicylate plasma concentration. A decreased serum bicarbonate but normal or high blood pH indicates respiratory alkalosis predominating over metabolic acidosis, and the bicarbonate should be administered cautiously. An alkalemic pH of 7.40 to 7.50 is not a contraindication to bicarbonate therapy because these patients have a significant base deficit in spite of elevated blood pH.

Potassium is added, 20 to 40 mEq/L, to the infusion after the patient voids. In cases of severe, late, and chronic salicylism, 60 mEq/L of potassium may be needed. When the serum potassium is below 4.0 mEq/L, 10 mEq/L should be added over the first hour. If the patient has hypokalemia less than 3 mEq/L and flat T waves and U waves, 0.25 to 0.5 mEq/kg up to 10 mEq/h is administered. Potassium should be administered under ECG monitoring. Serum potassium is rechecked after each rapidly administered dose. A paradoxical urine acidosis (alkaline serum pH and acid urine pH) indicates that potassium is probably needed.

Convulsions are treated with diazepam or lorazepam, but hypoglycemia, low ionized calcium, cerebral edema, and hemorrhage should first be excluded with a CT scan. If tetany develops, the $NaHCO_3$ therapy is discontinued and calcium gluconate 0.1 to 0.2 mL/kg 10% administered.

Pulmonary edema management consists of fluid restriction, high FIO_2, mechanical ventilation, and positive end-expiratory pressure.

Cerebral edema management consists of fluid restriction, elevation of the head, hyperventilation, osmotic diuresis, and administration of dexamethasone. Vitamin K_1 is administered parenterally to correct an increased prothrombin time (>20 seconds) and coagulation abnormalities. If the patient has active bleeding, fresh plasma and platelets are administered as needed. Hyperpyrexia is managed by external cooling measures, not antipyretics.

Hemodialysis is the choice for removal of salicylates because it corrects the acid-base, electrolyte, and fluid disturbances as well. The indications for hemodialysis include the following:

- Acute poisoning with salicylate plasma concentration greater than 100 mg/dL without improvement after 6 hours of appropriate therapy
- Chronic poisoning with cardiopulmonary disease and a salicylate plasma concentration as low as 40 mg/dL with refractory acidosis, severe CNS manifestations (coma and seizures), and progressive deterioration, especially in elderly patients
- Impairment of vital organs of elimination
- Clinical deterioration in spite of good supportive care and alkalinization
- Severe refractory acid-base or electrolyte disturbances despite appropriate corrective measures

Disposition

There are limitations of salicylate plasma levels and patients are treated on the basis of clinical and laboratory findings. Patients who are asymptomatic should be monitored for a minimum of 6 hours, and longer if enteric-coated tablets or massive overdose was taken or if there is suspicion of concretions. Those who remain asymptomatic with a salicylate plasma concentration less than 35 mg/dL may be discharged following psychiatric evaluation, if indicated. Chronic salicylate-intoxicated patients with acidosis and an altered mental state should be admitted to the intensive care unit. Patients with acute ingestion and a salicylate plasma concentration less than 60 mg/dL and mild symptoms may be able to be treated in the emergency department. Patients with moderate and severe intoxications should be admitted to the intensive care unit.

SELECTIVE SEROTONIN REUPTAKE INHIBITORS

Selective serotonin reuptake inhibitors (SSRIs) are primarily prescribed as antidepressants. SSRIs include fluoxetine (Prozac), paroxetine (Paxil), and sertraline (Zoloft).

Toxic Mechanism

The SSRIs interfere with the neuron reuptake of serotonin (5-hydroxytryptamine) at the presynaptic ganglia sites in the brain, increasing the activity of serotonin. SSRIs should not be used within 5 weeks of when a MAOI is given, nor should MAOI therapy be initiated or discontinued within 5 weeks of SSRI therapy.

Toxic Dose

The therapeutic oral dose of fluoxetine is 20 to 80 mg/d. No toxicity is seen in children with up to 3.5 mg/kg/dose orally. A fatal dose for adults is 6 g. The therapeutic dose for paroxetine is 20 to 50 mg/d. In 35 adult patients, none developed serious side effects after the ingestion of 10 to 1000 mg, and a study involving 35 children failed to demonstrate serious adverse effects at doses less than 180 mg. The therapeutic dose for sertraline is 50 mg to 200 mg/d. Patients have ingested up to 2.6 g without serious side effects. Overdose involving children who ingested less than 100 mg failed to cause adverse events.

Kinetics

Fluoxetine is well absorbed from the gastrointestinal tract, and has a peak plasma concentration at 6 to 8 hours. Volume distribution is 20 to 42 L/kg; 95% is protein bound. The half-life is 4 days (for the demethylated active metabolite norfluoxetine, the half-life is 7 to 15 days). Elimination is 80% renal. Fluoxetine and other serotonin inhibitors are inhibitors of the cytochrome P450, CYP 2D6 enzyme. Therefore interactions may occur with many other medications, such as antidysrhythmic class IC drugs (quinidine), phenytoin (Dilantin), haloperidol, lithium, tricyclic antidepressants (TCAs), β-blockers, codeine, and carbamazepine (Tegretol).

Paroxetine is almost completely absorbed from the gastrointestinal tract, with a peak in 2 to 8 hours. Protein binding is greater than 90%; volume distribution is 13 L/kg. Paroxetine undergoes extensive first-pass liver metabolism by oxidation and methylation to inactive metabolites. It inhibits the P450 system (see fluoxetine metabolism). The average half-life is 21 hours.

Sertraline peaks in 8 to 12 hours. Its volume distribution is 20 L/kg and protein binding is 98%. The average half-life of sertraline is 26 hours. It is metabolized to form a less-active metabolite, *N*-desmethylsertraline (half-life of 62 to 104 hours).

Manifestations

All SSRIs may cause serotonin syndrome, a potentially life-threatening reaction, if they are administered concurrently with an MAOI. Serotonin syndrome is caused by cerebral serotonergic stimulation and can cause severe hyperthermia, myoclonus, rhabdomyolysis, confusion, tremors, and a variety of psychological disturbances. In addition, cardiovascular complications and extrapyramidal side effects, including akathisia, dyskinesia, and Parkinson-like syndromes may occur. Also, increased suicidal ideation, seizures, sexual disorders, and hematologic disorders (platelet serotonin activity blockade leading to prolonged bleeding times) may develop. Inappropriate secretion of antidiuretic hormone resulting in hyponatremia may occur when SSRIs are administered to the elderly. This effect is usually seen within the first week of therapy.

Overdose effects are similar to the serotonin syndrome.

Laboratory Investigations

One should obtain a complete blood count (CBC), electrolytes, glucose levels, a coagulation profile, liver function tests, creatine kinase level, and an ECG.

Management

There is no specific antidote to SSRI intoxication.

Initial management consists of stabilizing vital functions, including thermoregulation. Supportive therapy and anticipation of potential life-threatening manifestations (hypotension, hyperthermia, seizures, coma, disseminated intravascular coagulation, ventricular tachycardia, and metabolic acidosis), are essential. Vital signs, EEG, creatine kinase, and blood chemistry should be monitored.

Benzodiazepines are administered to prevent and control muscle hyperactivity (diazepam [Valium] for seizures, clonazepam [Klonopin] for myoclonus). If benzodiazepine therapy fails to control muscle activity or seizures, anesthesia or nondepolarizing neuromuscular blockade may be necessary.

Electrolyte abnormalities and acid-base balance should be corrected. Fluids are used to maintain a urine output of greater than 2 mL/kg/h if there is a risk of myoglobinuria.

There are no data to support the use of gastrointestinal decontamination, although activated charcoal may be used if an ingestion has occurred within 1 hour. Hemodialysis and charcoal hemoperfusion are unlikely to be beneficial. Haloperidol (Haldol), phenothiazines, and other highly protein-bound drugs are to be avoided.

Benzodiazepine and cooling therapy can be used for hyperthermia. Serotonin antagonists, such as cyproheptadine (Periactin), may be useful in treating serotonin syndrome, although there are no controlled data. Dantrolene (Dantrium) and bromocriptine (Parlodel) are not recommended and may actually precipitate serotonin syndrome.

Disposition

Cases of ingestions in children up to 5 years of age of less than 180 mg of paroxetine (Paxil), less than 3.5 mg/kg of fluoxetine (Prozac), or less than 100 mg of sertraline (Zoloft) can be observed at home. Symptomatic patients should be admitted to the intensive care unit until asymptomatic for 24 hours. Asymptomatic patients should be observed for 6 hours. All patients should be assessed for risk of suicide before discharge. When taken chronically, SSRIs may increase cholesterol and triglycerides and decrease uric acid, so these test results should be followed.

THEOPHYLLINE

Theophylline (Slo-Phyllin) is a methylxanthine alkaloid similar to caffeine and theobromine. Aminophylline is 80% theophylline.

Theophylline is used in the acute treatment of asthma, pulmonary edema, chronic obstructive pulmonary disease, and neonatal apnea.

Toxic Mechanism

The proposed mechanisms of action include phosphodiesterase inhibition, adenosine receptor antagonism, inhibition of prostaglandins, and increase in serum catecholamines. Theophylline stimulates the central nervous, respiratory, and emetic centers and reduces the seizure threshold. It has positive cardiac inotropic and chronotropic effects, acts as a diuretic, relaxes smooth muscle, and causes peripheral vasodilation but cerebral vasoconstriction. Gastric secretions, gastrointestinal motility, lipolysis, glycogenolysis, and gluconeogenesis are all increased.

Toxic Dose

A single dose of 1 mg/kg produces a theophylline plasma concentration of approximately 2 μg/mL. The therapeutic range usually is 10 to 20 μg/mL. An acute, single dose greater than 10 mg/kg causes mild toxicity, a dose greater than 20 mg/kg causes moderate toxicity, and a dose greater than 50 mg/kg causes serious, possibly fatal toxicity. Fatalities occur at lower doses in patients with chronic toxicity, especially those with risk factors (see *Kinetics*).

Kinetics

The pKa is 9.5. Absorption from the stomach and upper small intestine is complete and rapid, with onset in 30 to 60 minutes. Peak theophylline plasma concentration occurs within 1 to 2 hours after ingestion of liquid preparations, 2 to 4 hours after ingestion of regular tablets, and 7 to 24 hours after ingestion of slow-release formulations. Volume distribution is 0.3 to 0.7 L/kg. Protein binding is 40% to 60% in adults, mainly to albumin (low albumin increases free active theophylline).

Elimination is 90% by hepatic metabolism to an active metabolite, 2-methyl xanthine. The half-life is 3.5 hours in a child and 4 to 6 hours in an adult. The half-life is shorter in smokers and patients taking enzyme-inducing drugs. Only 8% to 10% of the drug is excreted unchanged in the urine.

Risk factors that produce a longer half-life include age younger than 6 months or older than 60 years, use of enzyme-inhibitor drugs (calcium channel blockers, oral contraceptives, cimetidine [Tagamet], ciprofloxacin [Cipro], erythromycin, macrolide antibiotics, isoniazid), illness (persistent fever >38.9°C [>102°F]), viral illness, liver impairment, heart failure, chronic obstructive pulmonary disease, and influenza vaccination.

Manifestations

Acute toxicity generally correlates with blood levels; chronic toxicity does not (Table 27).

In the case of an acute, single, regular-release overdose, vomiting and occasionally hematemesis occur at low theophylline plasma concentrations. CNS stimulation includes restlessness, muscle tremors, and protracted tonic–clonic seizures, but coma is rare. Convulsions are a sign of severe toxicity and usually are preceded by gastrointestinal symptoms (except with sustained-release and chronic intoxications). Cardiovascular disturbances include cardiac dysrhythmias (supraventricular tachycardia) and transient hypertension with mild overdoses, but hypotension and ventricular dysrhythmias with severe intoxications. Rhabdomyolysis and renal failure are occasionally seen. Children tolerate higher serum levels, and cardiac dysrhythmias and seizures occur at theophylline plasma concentrations greater than 100 μg/mL. Possible metabolic disturbances include hyperglycemia, pronounced hypokalemia, hypocalcemia, hypomagnesemia, hypophosphatemia, increased serum amylase, and elevation of uric acid.

Chronic intoxication, defined as multiple doses of theophylline over 24 hours, or cases in which interacting drugs or illness interfere with theophylline metabolism are more serious and difficult to treat. Cardiac dysrhythmias and convulsions may occur at theophylline plasma concentrations of 40 to 60 μg/mL and there is no correlation with TPC. The seizures occur without warning and are protracted

TABLE 27 Theophylline Blood Concentrations and Acute Toxicity

Plasma Concentration (µg/mL)	Toxicity Degree	Manifestations
8–10	None	Bronchodilation
10–20	Mild	Therapeutic range: nausea, vomiting, nervousness, respiratory alkalosis, tachycardia
15–25		35% have mild manifestations of toxicity
20–40	Moderate	Gastrointestinal complaints and central nervous system stimulation
		Transient hypertension, tachypnea, tachycardia; 80% will have some manifestations of toxicity
60	Severe	Convulsions, dysrhythmias
100		Hypokalemia, hyperglycemia Ventricular dysrhythmias, protracted convulsions, hypotension, acid-base abnormalities

Reprinted and modified from Linden CH, Rumack BH. In Toxic Emergencies (Honser W Jr [ed]): The legitimate analgesics, aspirin and acetaminophen, copyright 1984, with permission from Elsevier.

and repetitive and may produce status epilepticus. Vomiting and typical metabolic disturbances do not occur.

Differences with slow-release preparations are that few or no gastrointestinal symptoms occur, peak concentrations and convulsions may be delayed 12 to 24 hours postingestion, and convulsions occur without warning.

Laboratory Investigations

Monitoring includes vital signs, pulse oximeter, ABG, hemoglobin, hematocrit (for gastrointestinal hemorrhage), ECG and cardiac monitor, renal and hepatic function, electrolytes, blood glucose, acid-base balance, and serum albumin. Gastric contents and stools should be tested for occult blood. Samples for theophylline plasma concentration measurement should be drawn within 1 to 2 hours after ingestion of liquid preparations, 2 to 4 hours after ingestion of regular-release formulations, and 4 hours after ingestion of slow-release formulations. One should check the serum albumin level because a decrease in albumin levels may cause manifestations of toxicity despite normal theophylline plasma concentration. A single theophylline plasma concentration reading may be misleading; therefore, theophylline plasma concentration measurement should be repeated every 2 to 4 hours to determine the trend until a declining trend is reached and then monitored every 4 to 6 hours until it is below 20 µg/mL.

Management

Vital functions must be established and maintained. If the patient is in a coma or has convulsions or vomiting, he or she should be intubated immediately. The theophylline plasma concentration is obtained and repeated every 2 to 4 hours to determine peak absorption, and a theophylline bezoar should be considered if the theophylline plasma concentration fails to decline. Consultation with a nephrologist about charcoal hemoperfusion is recommended.

Gastrointestinal decontamination is warranted in the case of an acute overdose, but emesis must not be induced. Activated charcoal is the choice decontamination procedure in a dose of 1 g/kg to all patients, followed with MDAC 0.5 g/kg every 2 to 4 hours until the theophylline plasma concentration is less than 20 µg/mL. MDAC is

effective in treating acute, chronic, and intravenous overdoses. Activated charcoal shortens the half-life of theophylline by about 50% and may be indicated up to 24 hours following ingestion.

Whole-bowel irrigation with polyethylene-electrolyte solution has been recommended for cases of massive overdose, possible concretions, and ingestion of sustained-release preparations. If intractable vomiting occurs, the antiemetic metoclopramide (Reglan) (0.1 mg/kg adult dose), droperidol (Inapsine) (2.5 to 10 mg IV), or ondansetron (Zofran) (8 to 32 mg IV) is administered. Ondansetron, however, inhibits metabolism of theophylline after a few doses.

Convulsions are controlled with lorazepam (Ativan) or diazepam (Valium) and phenobarbital. Phenytoin (Dilantin) is ineffective. The convulsions in patients with chronic intoxication are often refractory and may require, in addition to anticonvulsants, neuromuscular paralyzing agents, sedation, assisted ventilation, and EEG monitoring.

Hypotension is treated with fluids and vasopressors, if necessary. Norepinephrine (Levophed) 0.05 µg/kg/min is preferred as the vasopressor over dopamine.

Supraventricular tachycardia with hemodynamic instability requires cardioversion. Low-dose β-blockers may be used but should not be used in patients with reactive airway disease or hypotension. Adenosine (Adenocard) is ineffective. For ventricular dysrhythmias, electrolyte disturbances should be corrected. Lidocaine is the treatment of choice but has the potential to cause seizures at toxic concentrations. Cardioversion may be needed.

Hematemesis is managed with sucralfate (Carafate) 1 g four times daily and/or Maalox TC 30 mL every 2 hours and blood replacement, if necessary. H_2 antihistamine blockers that are enzyme inhibitors are not used.

Fluid and metabolic disturbances should be corrected. Hyperglycemia does not require insulin therapy. Hypokalemia should be corrected cautiously, as it may be largely an intracellular shift and not total body loss. Usually adding 40 mEq potassium to a liter of fluid will suffice. The serum potassium level must be monitored closely.

Charcoal hemoperfusion is the management of choice for patients with serious intoxications. Hemoperfusion can increase the clearance twofold to threefold over hemodialysis, but hemodialysis can be used if hemoperfusion is not available. Criteria for charcoal hemoperfusion are as follows:

- Life-threatening events such as convulsions or dysrhythmias
- Intractable vomiting refractory to antiemetics
- Acute intoxications with a theophylline plasma concentration greater than 80 µg/mL or greater than 70 µg/mL 4 hours after overdose with a sustained-release formulation and greater than 40 µg/mL in the case of chronic intoxication
- Acute or chronic overdoses with a theophylline plasma concentration greater than 40 µg/mL, especially if the patient has risk factors that lengthen the half-life of the drug (see Kinetics).

Disposition

Patients with mild symptoms and a theophylline plasma concentration less than 20 µg/mL can be treated in emergency department and discharged when asymptomatic for a few hours. Any patient with acute ingestion and a theophylline plasma concentration greater than 35 µg/mL should be admitted to a monitored bed with seizure precautions and suicide precautions, if needed. If neurologic or cardiotoxic effects or a theophylline plasma concentration greater than 50 µg/mL is present, the patient should be admitted to the intensive care unit. A patient with an overdose of a sustained-release preparation, regardless of symptoms or initial theophylline plasma concentration, requires admission, monitoring, activated charcoal, and MDAC. In patients on chronic therapy, toxicity may occur at a lower theophylline plasma concentration, and these patients should not be discharged until they are asymptomatic for several hours.

TRICYCLIC AND CYCLIC ANTIDEPRESSANTS

Historically, tricyclic antidepressants are an important cause of pharmaceutical overdose fatalities. The mortality rate was reduced from 15% in the 1970s to less than 1% in the 1990s because of a better

TABLE 28 Cyclic Antidepressants, Daily Dose and Their Major Properties

Generic Name	Adult Daily Dose (mg)	Therapeutic Range (ng/mL)	Half-Life (hours)	Toxicity* Antichol	Toxicity* CNS	Toxicity* Cardiac
Tertiary Amines						
Amitriptyline (Elavil)	75–300	120–250	31–46	3+	3+	3+
Imipramine (Tofranil)	75–300	125–250	9–24	3+	3+	3+
Doxepin (Sinequan)	75–300	30–150	8–24	3+	3+	2+
Trimipramine (Surmantil)	75–200	10–240	16–18	3+	3+	2+
Secondary Amines						
Nortriptyline (Pamelor)	75–150	50–150	18–93	2+	3+	3+
Desipramine (Norpramin)	75–200	75–160	14–62	1+	3+	3+
Protriptyline (Vivactil)	20–60	70–250	54–198	2+	3+	3+
Newer Cyclic Antidepressants						
Teracyclic			30–60	1+	2+	3+
Maprotiline (Ludiomil)	75–300	—	30–60	1+	2+	3+
Trizolopyridine, a noncyclic, produces less serious cardiac and CNS toxicity						
Trazodone (Desyrel)	50–600	700	4–7	1+	1+	1+
Monocyclic Aminoketones						
Bupropion (Wellbutrin)	200–400	—	8–24	1+	3+	1+
Dibenzazepine						
Clomipramine (Anafranil)	100–250	200–500	21–32	2+	2+	2+
Dibenoxazepine						
Amoxapine (Ascendin)	150–300	200–500	6–10	1+	3+	2+

*Antichol = anticholinergic effect; CNS = central nervous system effect primarily seizures; Cardiac = cardiac effect.
Other drugs with similar structures are cyclobenzaprine, a muscle relaxant (similar to amitriptyline), and carbamazepine, an anticonvulsant (similar to imipramine); however, they cause less cardiac toxicity.

understanding of the pathophysiology of these agents and improvements in management (Table 28).

Toxic Mechanism

The major mechanisms of toxicity of the tricyclic antidepressants are (a) central and peripheral anticholinergic effects; (b) peripheral α-adrenergic blockade; (c) quinidine-like cardiac membrane stabilizing action blockade of the fast inward sodium channels; and (d) inhibition of synaptic neurotransmitter reuptake in the CNS presynaptic neurons. The tetracyclics, monocyclic aminoketones, and dibenzoxazepines possess convulsive activity and less cardiac toxicity in overdose than the older tricyclic antidepressants. Triazolopyridine has less serious cardiac and CNS toxicity.

Toxic Dose

The therapeutic dose of imipramine (Tofranil) is 1.5 to 5 mg/kg; a dose greater than 5 mg/kg may be mildly toxic; 10 to 20 mg/kg may be life threatening, although less than 20 mg/kg has produced few fatalities; greater than 30 mg/kg carries a 30% mortality rate; and at a dose greater than 70 mg/kg, patients rarely survive. In children 375 mg and in adults as little as 500 mg have been fatal. In adults, five times the maximum daily dose is toxic and 10 times is potentially fatal. Although major overdose symptoms are associated with plasma concentrations greater than 1 μg/mL (>1000 ng/mL), plasma tricyclic levels do not correlate well with toxicity; clinical signs and symptoms should guide therapy.

The relative dosage or potency equivalents are as follows: amitriptyline (Elavil) 100 mg = amoxapine (Asendin) 125 mg = desipramine (Norpramin) 75 mg = doxepin (Sinequan) 100 mg = imipramine (Tofranil) 75 mg = maprotiline (Ludiomil) 75 mg = nortriptyline (Pamelor) 50 mg = trazodone (Desyrel) 200 mg. This allows one to determine an equivalent dosage of an agent compared with another (see Table 28).

Kinetics

The tricyclic and cyclic antidepressants are lipophilic. They are rapidly absorbed from the alkaline small intestine, but absorption may be prolonged and delayed in cases of massive overdose owing to anticholinergic action. Onset varies from less than 1 hour (30 to 40 minutes) to, rarely, 12 hours. The peak serum levels are reached in 2 to 8 hours and the peak effect is in 6 hours but may be delayed 12 hours because of erratic absorption. The clinical effects correlate poorly with plasma levels.

Cyclic antidepressants are highly protein-bound to plasma glycoproteins, 98% at a pH 7.5 and 90% at 7.0. Volume distribution is 10 to 50 L/kg. The elimination route is by hepatic metabolism. The tertiary amines are metabolized into active demethylated secondary amine metabolites. The active secondary amine metabolites undergo a 15% enterohepatic recirculation and are metabolized over a period of days into nonactive metabolites. The intestinal bacterial flora may reconstitute the metabolites, which are active.

The half-life varies from 10 hours for imipramine to 81 hours for amitriptyline and 100 hours for nortriptyline. The active metabolites have longer half-lives.

Only 3% of the ingested dose is excreted in the urine unchanged.

Manifestations

There are reports of asymptomatic patients who, upon arrival to an emergency department, suddenly have a seizure, develop hemodynamically unstable dysrhythmias, and die shortly thereafter from ingestion of a tricyclic antidepressant. Most patients with severe toxicity develop symptoms within 1 to 2 hours, but symptoms may be delayed 6 hours after overdose.

Small overdoses produce early anticholinergic effects, agitation, and transient hypertension, which are not life-threatening. Large overdoses produce depression of the CNS and myocardium, convulsions, and hypotension. Death can occur within the first 2 to 6 hours following ingestion.

Some ECG screening tools for predicting cardiac or neurologic toxicity from ingestion of a tricyclic antidepressant have been developed: (a) A QRS greater than 0.10 second may produce seizures, and if greater than 0.16 second, 50% of patients may develop ventricular dysrhythmias (20% of these may be life-threatening) and seizures; (b) a terminal 40 msec of the QRS axis greater than 120 degrees in the right frontal plane may be associated with toxicity; or (c) a large

R wave greater than 3 mm in ECG lead aVR may predispose the patient to toxicity. The quinidine cardiac membrane stabilizing effect produces depression of myocardium, conduction, and ECG changes. The peripheral α-adrenergic blockade produces hypotension.

The secondary amines are metabolized to inactive metabolites. The tetracyclics produce a high incidence of cardiovascular disturbances and seizures. Monocyclic aminoketones produce seizures in doses greater than 600 mg. Dibenzoxazepines produce a syndrome of convulsions, rhabdomyolysis, and renal failure.

Laboratory Investigations

If the patient has altered mental status or ECG abnormalities, ABG, ECG, chest radiograph, blood glucose, serum electrolytes, calcium, magnesium, blood urea nitrogen, and creatinine levels, liver profile, creatine kinase level, urine output, and, in severe cases, hemodynamic monitoring are indicated. Levels of the tricyclic and cyclic antidepressants less than 300 ng/mL are therapeutic; levels greater than 500 ng/mL indicate toxicity, and levels greater than 1000 ng/mL indicate serious poisoning and are associated with QRS widening.

Management

Vital functions must be established and maintained. Even if the patient is asymptomatic, intravenous access should be established, vital signs and neurologic status monitored, and baseline 12-lead ECG and continuous cardiac monitoring obtained for at least 6 hours from admission or 8 to 12 hours postingestion. QRS interval should be measured on a limb lead ECG every 15 minutes for 6 hours postingestion.

For gastrointestinal decontamination, emesis should not be induced and gastric lavage should not be used. Activated charcoal is preferable. If the patient is in an altered mental state, the airway must be protected. Activated charcoal 1 g/kg is recommended up to 1 hour postingestion. Benefit from MDAC has not been demonstrated.

Alkalinization does not control seizures; diazepam or lorazepam should be used. Status epilepticus may require high-dose barbiturates or neuromuscular blockers with intravenous diazepam. If not successful, the patient can be paralyzed with short-term nondepolarizing neuromuscular blockers such as vecuronium (Norcuron), intubation, and assisted ventilation. A bolus of sodium bicarbonate is recommended as an adjunct to correct the acidosis produced by the seizures.

Sodium bicarbonate is administered in a dose of 1 to 2 mEq/kg undiluted as a bolus and repeated twice a few minutes apart, if needed, for "sodium loading" and alkalinization, which may increase protein binding from 90% to 98%. The sodium loading overcomes the sodium channel blockage and is more important than the alkalinization. Indications include (a) a QRS complex greater than 0.12 second, (b) ventricular tachycardia, (c) severe conduction disturbances, (d) metabolic acidosis, (e) coma, and (f) seizures. A continuous infusion of sodium bicarbonate is of limited usefulness for controlling dysrhythmias. Bolus therapy should be used as needed.

Hyperventilation alone has been recommended, but the pH elevation is not as instantaneous and there is compensatory renal excretion of bicarbonate; therefore, we do not recommend it. The combination of hyperventilation and sodium bicarbonate has produced fatal alkalemia and is not recommended. One should monitor serum potassium level (the sudden increase in blood pH can aggravate or precipitate hypokalemia), serum sodium, and ionized calcium levels (hypocalcemia may occur with alkalinization) and blood pH.

Specific cardiovascular complications should be treated as follows: Hypotension is treated with norepinephrine, a predominantly α-adrenergic drug, which is preferred over dopamine. Hypertension that occurs early rarely requires treatment. Sinus tachycardia usually does not require treatment. Supraventricular tachycardia in a patient who is hemodynamically unstable requires synchronized electrical cardioversion, starting at 0.25 to 1.0 watt-second per kg, after sedation. Ventricular tachycardia that persists after alkalinization requires intravenous lidocaine or countershock if the patient is hemodynamically unstable. Ventricular fibrillation should be treated with defibrillation. Torsades de pointes is treated with magnesium sulfate IV 20% solution, 2 g over 2 to 3 minutes, followed by a continuous infusion of 1.5 mL 10% solution or 5 to 10 mg per minute. For the treatment of bradydysrhythmias, atropine is contraindicated because of the anticholinergic activity. Isoproterenol 0.1 µg/kg/minute, used with caution, may produce hypotension. If the patient is hemodynamically unstable, a pacemaker is used.

Extraordinary measures, such as aortic balloon pump and cardiopulmonary bypass, have been successful.

Investigational treatments include FAB fragments specific for tricyclic antidepressant, which have been successful in animals. Prophylactic NaHCO3 to prevent dysrhythmias is also being investigated.

Physostigmine has produced asystole, and flumazenil has produced seizures. Both are contraindicated.

Disposition

A patient with an antidepressant overdose who meets any of the following criteria should be admitted to the intensive care unit for 12 to 24 hours: (a) ECG abnormalities except sinus tachycardia, (b) altered mental state, (c) seizures, (d) respiratory depression, and (e) hypotension. Low-risk patients include those in whom the above symptoms are absent at 6 hours postingestion, those who present with minor transient manifestations such as sinus tachycardia who subsequently become and remain asymptomatic for a 6-hour period, and asymptomatic patients who remain asymptomatic for 6 hours. These patients may be discharged if the ECG remains normal, they have normal bowel sounds, and they undergo psychiatric disposition.

Even if the patient is asymptomatic upon presentation to the health care facility, intravenous access should be established, vital signs and neurologic status monitored, a baseline 12-lead ECG obtained, and cardiac monitoring continued for at least 6 hours. Caution: in 25% of fatal cases, the patients were initially alert and awake at presentation. However, in most cases of fatality initially deemed as sudden cardiac death, the patient, upon reexamination, actually had symptoms that were missed.

Children younger than 6 years of age with non-intentional (accidental) exposures to amitriptyline (Elavil), desipramine (Norpramin), doxepin (Sinequan), imipramine (Tofranil), or nortriptyline (Aventyl) in a dose less than 5 mg/kg, who are asymptomatic and have what are deemed reliable caregivers, can be observed at home, with close poison control follow-up for 6 hours. Parents or caregivers should be given instructions regarding signs and symptoms to be alert for. Children who are symptomatic, or who ingested greater than 5 mg/kg, should be referred to the emergency department for monitoring, observation, and activated charcoal treatment.

Appendices and Index

Reference Intervals for the Interpretation of Laboratory Tests

Method of
Laura J. McCloskey, PhD

Most of the tests performed in a clinical laboratory are quantitative; that is, the amount of a substance present in blood or serum is measured and reported in terms of concentration, activity (e.g., enzyme activity), or counts (e.g., blood cell counts). The laboratory must provide reference intervals to assist the clinician in the interpretation of laboratory results. These reference intervals represent the physiologic quantities of a substance (concentrations, activities, or counts) to be expected in healthy persons. Deviation above or below the reference range may be associated with a disease process, and the severity of the disease process may be associated with the magnitude of the deviation. Unfortunately, a sharp demarcation rarely exists to distinguish between physiologic and pathologic values, and the time of transition between the two is often gradual as the disease process progresses.

Defining Normal Values

The terms "normal" and "abnormal" have been used to describe laboratory values that fall inside and outside the reference range, respectively. Use of these terms is inappropriate because no good definition of normality exists in the clinical sense, and the term "normal" may be confused with the statistical term "gaussian." Reference ranges are established from statistical studies in groups of healthy volunteers. These study subjects must be free of disease, but they may have lifestyles or habits that result in variations in certain laboratory values. Examples of these variables include diet, body mass, exercise, and geographic location. Age and gender can also affect reference values.

When the data from a large cohort of healthy subjects fit a gaussian distribution, the usual statistical approach is to define the reference limits as 2 standard deviations (SD) above and below the mean. By definition, the reference range excludes the 2.5% of the population with the lowest values and the 2.5% with the highest values. Nongaussian distributions are handled by different statistical methods, but the result is similar, in that the reference range is defined by the central 95% of the population. In other words, the probability that a healthy person has a laboratory result falling outside the reference range is 1 in 20. If 12 laboratory tests are performed, the probability that at least one of the results is outside the reference range increases to about 50%, which means that all healthy persons are likely to have a few laboratory results that are unexpected. The clinician must then integrate these data with other clinical information, such as the history and physical examination, to arrive at an appropriate clinical decision.

The reference intervals for many tests (especially enzyme and immunochemical measurements) vary with the method used. Accordingly, each laboratory must establish its own reference intervals that are appropriate for the methods used.

International System of Units

During the 1980s, a concerted effort was made to introduce the International System of Units (Systéme International d'Unités; SI units). The rationale for conversion to SI units is sound. Laboratory data are scientifically more informative when the units are based on molar concentration rather than on mass concentration. For example, the conversion of glucose to lactate and pyruvate or the binding of a drug to albumin is more easily understood in units of molar concentration. Another example is illustrated as follows:

Conventional Units	SI Units
1.0 g of hemoglobin:	4.0 mmol of hemoglobin:
Combines with 1.37 mL of oxygen	Combines with 4.0 mmol of oxygen
Contains 3.4 mg of iron	Contains 4.0 mmol of iron
Forms 34.9 mg of bilirubin	Forms 4.0 mmol of bilirubin

The use of SI units would also enhance the standardization of nomenclature to facilitate global communication of medical and scientific information. The units, symbols, and prefixes used in the international system are shown in Tables 1, 2, and 3.

TABLE 1 Base SI Units

Property	Unit	Symbol
Length	Meter	m
Mass	Kilogram	kg
Amount of substance	Mole	mol
Time	Second	s
Thermodynamic temperature	Kelvin	K
Electrical current	Ampere	A
Luminous intensity	Candela	cd
Catalytic amount	Katal	kat

Abbreviation: SI = International System of Units.

TABLE 2 Derived SI Units and Non-SI Units Retained for Use with SI Units

Property	Unit	Symbol
Area	Square meter	m^2
Volume	Cubic meter	m^3
	Liter	L
Mass	Kilograms per cubic meter	kg/m^3 concentration
	Grams per liter	g/L
Substance concentration	Moles per cubic meter	mol/m^3
		mol/L
Temperature	Degree Celsius	C = K-273.15
Dynamic viscosity	Pascal-second	$Pa\text{-}s = 1\ kg \cdot m^{-1} \cdot s^{-1}$

Abbreviation: SI = International System of Units.

Unfortunately, problems have arisen with the implementation of SI units in the United States. The introduction of this system in 1987 prompted many medical journals to report laboratory values in both SI and conventional units in anticipation of complete conversion to SI units in the early 1990s. The lack of a coordinated effort toward this goal forced a retrenchment on the issue. Physicians continue to think and practice with laboratory results expressed in conventional units, and few, if any, hospitals or clinical laboratories in the United States use SI units exclusively. Complete conversion to SI units is not likely to occur in the foreseeable future, but most medical journals will probably continue to publish both sets of units.

TABLE 3 Standard Prefixes

Prefix	Multiplication Factor	Symbol
yocto	10^{-24}	y
zepto	10^{-21}	z
atto	10^{-18}	a
femto	10^{-15}	f
pico	10^{-12}	p
nano	10^{-9}	n
micro	10^{-6}	μ
milli	10^{-3}	m
centi	10^{-2}	c
deci	10^{-1}	d
deca	10^{1}	da
hecto	10^{2}	h
kilo	10^{3}	k
mega	10^{6}	M
giga	10^{9}	G
tera	10^{12}	T

For this reason, the values in the tables of reference ranges in this appendix are given in both conventional units and SI units.

Tables of Reference Intervals

Some of the values included in the tables that follow have been established by the Clinical Laboratories at the Thomas Jefferson University Hospital in Philadelphia and have not been published elsewhere. Other values have been compiled from the sources cited in the suggested readings. These tables are provided for information and educational purposes only. Laboratory values must always be interpreted in the context of clinical data derived from other sources, including the medical history and physical examination. One must exercise individual judgment when using the information provided in this appendix.

REFERENCES

American Medical Association. Drug evaluations annual. Chicago: American Medical Association; 1994.

Bick RL, editor. Hematology: Clinical and laboratory practice. St Louis: Mosby—Year Book; 1993.

Borer WZ. Selection and use of laboratory tests. In: Tietz NW, Conn RB, Pruden E, editors. Applied laboratory medicine. Philadelphia: WB Saunders; 1992. p. 1–5.

Campion EW. A retreat from SI units. N Engl J Med 1992;327:49.

Friedman RB, Young DS. Effects of disease on clinical laboratory tests. 3rd ed. Washington, DC: American Association for Clinical Chemistry Press; 1997.

Henry JB. Clinical diagnosis and management by laboratory methods. 19th ed. Philadelphia: WB Saunders; 1996.

Hicks JM, Young DS. DORA 97–99: Directory of rare analyses. Washington, DC: American Association for Clinical Chemistry Press; 1997.

Jacob DS, Demott WR, Grady HJ, et al., editors. Laboratory test handbook. 4th ed. Baltimore: Williams & Wilkins; 1996.

Kaplan LA, Pesce AJ. Clinical chemistry: Theory, analysis, and correlation. 3rd ed. St Louis: Mosby—Year Book; 1996.

Kjeldsberg CR, Knight JA. Body fluids: Laboratory examination of amniotic, cerebrospinal, seminal, serous and synovial fluids. 3rd ed. Chicago: ASCP Press; 1993.

Laposata M. SI Unit Conversion Guide. Boston: NEJM Books; 1992.

Scully RE, McNeely WF, Mark EJ, McNeely BU. Normal reference laboratory values. N Engl J Med 1992;327:718–24.

Speicher CE. The right test: A physician's guide to laboratory medicine. 3rd ed. Philadelphia: WB Saunders; 1998.

Tietz NW, editor. Clinical guide to laboratory tests. 3rd ed. Philadelphia: WB Saunders; 1995.

Wallach J. Interpretation of diagnostic tests: A synopsis of laboratory medicine. 6th ed. Boston: Little, Brown; 1996.

Young DS. Effects of Preanalytical variables on clinical laboratory tests. 2nd ed. Washington, DC: American Association for Clinical Chemistry Press; 1997.

Young DS. Effects of drugs on clinical laboratory tests. 4th ed. Washington, DC: American Association for Clinical Chemistry Press; 1995.

Young DS. Determination and validation of reference intervals. Arch Pathol Lab Med 1992;116:704–9.

Young DS. Implementation of SI units for clinical laboratory data. Ann Intern Med 1987;106:114–29.

Reference Intervals* for Hematology

Test	Conventional Units	SI Units
Acid hemolysis (Ham test)	No hemolysis	No hemolysis
Alkaline phosphatase, leukocyte	Total score, 14–100	Total score, 14–100
Cell counts		
Erythrocytes		
Males	4.6–6.2 million/mm^3	4.6–6.2 × 10^{12}/L
Females	4.2–5.4 million/mm^3	4.2–5.4 × 10^{12}/L
Children (varies with age)	4.5–5.1 million/mm^3	4.5–5.1 × 10^{12}/L
Leukocytes, total	4500–11,000/mm^3	4.5–11.0 × 10^9/L
Leukocytes, differential counts*		
Myelocytes	0%	0/L
Band neutrophils	3–5%	150–400 × 10^6/L
Segmented neutrophils	54–62%	3000–5800 × 10^6/L
Lymphocytes	25–33%	1500–3000 × 10^6/L
Monocytes	3–7%	300–500 × 10^6/L
Eosinophils	1–3%	50–250 × 10^6/L
Basophils	0–1%	15–50 × 10^6/L
Platelets	150,000–400,000/mm^3	150–400 × 10^9/L
Reticulocytes	25,000–75,000/mm^3 (0.5%–1.5% of erythrocytes)	25–75 × 10^9/L
Coagulation tests		
Bleeding time (template)	2.75–8.0 min	2.75–8.0 min
Coagulation time (glass tube)	5–15 min	5–15 min
D dimer	<0.5 µg/mL	<0.5 mg/L
Factor VIII and other coagulation factors	50–150% of normal	0.5–1.5 of normal
Fibrin split products (Thrombo-Welco test)	<10 µg/mL	<10 mg/L
Fibrinogen	200–400 mg/dL	2.0–4.0 g/L
Partial thromboplastin time, activated (aPTT)	20–25 s	20–35 s
Prothrombin time (PT)	12.0–14.0 s	12.0–14.0 s
Coombs' test		
Direct	Negative	Negative
Indirect	Negative	Negative
Corpuscular values of erythrocytes		
Mean corpuscular hemoglobin (MCH)	26–34 pg/cell	26–34 pg/cell
Mean corpuscular volume (MCV)	80–96 µm^3	80–96 fL
Mean corpuscular hemoglobin concentration (MCHC)	32–36 g/dL	320–360 g/L
Haptoglobin	20–165 mg/dL	0.20–1.65 g/L
Hematocrit		
Males	40–54 mL/dL	0.40–0.54 g/L
Females	37–47 mL/dL	0.37–0.47 g/L
Newborns	49–54 mL/dL	0.49–0.54 g/L
Children (varies with age)	35–49 mL/dL	0.35–0.49 g/L
Hemoglobin		
Males	13.0–18.0 g/dL	8.1–11.2 mmol/L
Females	12.0–16.0 g/dL	7.4–9.9 mmol/L
Newborns	16.5–19.5 g/dL	10.2–12.1 mmol/L
Children (varies with age)	11.2–16.5 g/dL	7.0–10.2 mmol/L
Hemoglobin, fetal	<1.0 of total	<0.01 of total
Hemoglobin A1c	3–5% of total	0.03–0.05 of total
Hemoglobin A2	1.5–3.0% of total	0.015–0.03 of total
Hemoglobin, plasma	0.0%–5.0 mg/dL	0.0–3.2 µmol/L
Methemoglobin	30%–130 mg/dL	19–80 µmol/L
Erythrocyte sedimentation rate (ESR)		
Westergren		
Males	0–15 mm/h	0–15 mm/h
Females	0–20 mm/h	0–20 mm/h
Wintrobe		
Males	0–5 mm/h	0–5 mm/h
Females	0–15 mm/h	0–15 mm/h

*Conventional units are percentages; SI units are absolute cell counts.
Abbreviation: SI = International System of Units.

Reference Intervals* for Clinical Chemistry (Blood, Serum, and Plasma)

Analyte	Conventional Units	SI Units
Acetoacetate plus acetone		
Qualitative	Negative	Negative
Quantitative	0.3–2.0 mg/dL	30–200 mol/L
Acid phosphatase, serum (thymolphthalein monophosphate substrate)	0.1–0.6 U/L	0.1–0.6 U/L
ACTH (see Corticotropin)		
Alanine aminotransferase (ALT), serum (SGPT)	1–45 U/L	1–45 U/L
Albumin, serum	3.3–5.2 g/dL	33–52 g/L
Aldolase, serum	0.0–7.0 U/L	0.0–7.0 U/L
Aldosterone, plasma		
Standing	5–30 ng/dL	140–830 pmol/L
Recumbent	3–10 ng/dL	80–275 pmol/L
Alkaline, phosphatase (ALP), serum		
Adult	35–150 U/L	35–150 U/L
Adolescent	100–500 U/L	100–500 U/L
Child	100–350 U/L	100–350 U/L
Ammonia nitrogen, plasma	10–50 µmol/L	10–50 µmol/L
Amylase, serum	25–125 U/L	25–125 U/L
Anion gap, serum calculated	8–16 mEq/L	8–16 mmol/L
Ascorbic acid, blood	0.4–1.5 mg/dL	23–85 µmol/L
Aspartate aminotransferase (AST), serum (SGOT)	1–36 U/L	1–36 U/L
Base excess, arterial blood, calculated	0±2 mEq/L	0±2 mmol/L
Bicarbonate		
Venous plasma	23–29 mEq/L	23–29 mmol/L
Arterial blood	21–27 mEq/L	21–27 mmol/L
Bile acids, serum	0.3–3.0 mg/dL	0.8–7.6 mmol/L
Bilirubin, serum		
Conjugated	0.1–0.4 mg/dL	1.7–6.8 µmol/L
Total	0.3–1.1 mg/dL	5.1–19.0 µmol/L
Calcium, serum	8.4–10.6 mg/dL	2.10–2.65 mmol/L
Calcium, ionized, serum	4.25–5.25 mg/dL	1.05–1.30 mmol/L
Carbon dioxide, total, serum or plasma	24–31 mEq/L	24–31 mmol/L
Carbon dioxide tension (Pco_2), blood	35–45 mm Hg	35–45 mm Hg
β-Carotene, serum	60–260 µg/dL	1.1–8.6 µmol/L
Ceruloplasmin, serum	23–44 mg/dL	230–440 mg/L
Chloride, serum or plasma	96–106 mEq/L	96–106 mmol/L
Cholesterol, serum or EDTA plasma		
Desirable range	<200 mg/dL	<5.20 mmol/L
Low-density lipoprotein (LDL) cholesterol	60–180 mg/dL	1.55–4.65 mmol/L
High-density lipoprotein (HDL) cholesterol	30–80 mg/dL	0.80–2.05 mmol/L
Copper	70–140 µg/dL	11–22 µmol/L
Corticotropin (ACTH), plasma, 8 AM	10–80 pg/mL	2–18 pmol/L
Cortisol, plasma		
8:00 AM	6–23 µg/dL	170–630 µmol/L
4:00 PM	3–15 µg/dL	80–410 µmol/L
10:00 PM	<50% of 8:00 AM value	<50% of 8:00 AM value
Creatine, serum		
Males	0.2–0.5 mg/dL	15–40 µmol/L
Females	0.3–0.9 mg/dL	25–70 µmol/L
Creatine kinase (CK), serum		
Males	55–170 U/L	55–170 U/L
Females	30–135 U/L	30–135 U/L
Creatine kinase MB isoenzyme, serum	<5% of total CK activity	<5% of total CK activity
	<5% of ng/mL by immunoassay	<5% of ng/mL by immunoassay
Creatinine, serum	0.6–1.2 mg/dL	50–110 µmol/L
Erythrocytes	145–540 ng/mL	330–120 nmol/L
Estradiol-17β, adult		
Males	10–65 pg/mL	35–240 pmol/L
Females		
Follicular	30–100 pg/mL	110–370 pmol/L
Ovulatory	200–400 pg/mL	730–1470 pmol/L
Luteal	50–140 pg/mL	180–510 pmol/L
Ferritin, serum	20–200 ng/mL	20–200 µg/L
Fibrinogen, plasma	200–400 mg/dL	2.0–4.0 g/L
Folate, serum	3–18 ng/mL	6.8–4.1 nmol/L
Follicle-stimulating hormone (FSH), plasma		
Males	4–25 mU/mL	4–25 U/L
Females, premenopausal	4–30 mU/mL	4–30 U/L
Females, postmenopausal	40–250 mU/mL	40–250 U/L
Gastrin, fasting, serum	0–100 pg/mL	0–100 mg/L
Glucose, fasting, plasma or serum	70–115 mg/dL	3.9–6.4 nmol/L
γ-Glutamyltransferase (GGT), serum	5–40 U/L	5–40 U/L
Growth hormone (hGH), plasma, adult, fasting	0–6 ng/mL	0–6 µg/L
Haptoglobin, serum	20–165 mg/dL	0.20–1.65 g/L

Reference Intervals* for Clinical Chemistry (Blood, Serum, and Plasma)—Cont'd

Analyte	Conventional Units	SI Units
Immunoglobulins, serum (see table, Reference Intervals for Tests of Immunologic Function)		
Iron, serum	75–175 µg/dL	13–31 µmol/L
Iron-binding capacity, serum		
Total	250–410 µg/dL	45–73 µmol/L
Saturation	20–55%	0.20–0.55
Lactate		
Venous whole blood	5.0–20.0 mg/dL	0.6–2.2 mmol/L
Arterial whole blood	5.0–15.0 mg/dL	0.6–1.7 mmol/L
Lactate dehydrogenase (LD), serum	110–220 U/L	110–220 U/L
Lipase, serum	10–140 U/L	10–140 U/L
Lutropin (LH), serum		
Males	1–9 U/L	-9 U/L
Females		
Follicular phase	2–10 U/L	2–10 U/L
Midcycle peak	15–65 U/L	15–65 U/L
Luteal phase	1–12 U/L	1–12 U/L
Postmenopausal	12–65 U/L	12–65 U/L
Magnesium, serum	1.3–2.1 mg/dL	0.65–1.05 mmol/L
Osmolality	275–295 mOsm/kg water	275–295 mOsm/kg water
Oxygen, blood, arterial, room air		
Partial pressure (PaO_2)	80–100 mm Hg	80–100 mm Hg
Saturation (SaO_2)	95–98%	95–98%
pH, arterial blood	7.35–7.45	7.35–7.45
Phosphate, inorganic, serum		
Adult	3.0–4.5 mg/dL	1.0–1.5 mmol/L
Child	4.0–7.0 mg/dL	1.3–2.3 mmol/L
Potassium		
Serum	3.5–5.0 mEq/L	3.5–5.0 mmol/L
Plasma	3.5–4.5 mEq/L	3.5–4.5 mmol/L
Progesterone, serum, adult		
Males	0.0–0.4 ng/mL	0.0–1.3 mmol/L
Females		
Follicular phase	0.1–1.5 ng/mL	0.3–4.8 mmol/L
Luteal phase	2.5–28.0 ng/mL	8.0–89.0 mmol/L
Prolactin, serum		
Males	1.0–15.0 ng/mL	1.0–15.0 µg/L
Females	1.0–20.0 ng/mL	1.0–20.0 µg/L
Protein, serum, electrophoresis		
Total	6.0–8.0 g/dL	60–80 µg/L
Albumin	3.5–5.5 g/dL	35–55 µg/L
Globulins		
α_1	0.2–0.4 g/dL	2.0–4.0 g/L
α_2	0.5–0.9 g/dL	5.0–9.0 g/L
β	0.6–1.1 g/dL	6.0–11.0 g/L
γ	0.7–1.7 g/dL	7.0–17.0 g/L
Pyruvate, blood	0.3–0.9 mg/dL	0.03–0.10 mmol/L
Rheumatoid factor	0.0–30.0 IU/mL	0.0–30.0 kIU/L
Sodium, serum or plasma	135–145 mEq/L	135–145 mmol/L
Testosterone, plasma		
Men	300–1200 ng/dL	10.4–41.6 nmol/L
Women	20–75 ng/dL	0.7–2.6 nmol/L
Pregnant	40–200 ng/dL	1.4–6.9 nmol/L
Thyroglobulin	3–42 ng/mL	3–42 µg/L
Thyrotropin (hTSH), serum	0.4–4.8 µIU/mL	0.4–4.8 mIU/L
Thyrotropin-releasing hormone (TRH)	5–60 pg/mL	5–60 ng/L
Thyroxine, free (FT_4), serum	0.9–2.1 ng/dL	12–27 pmol/L
Thyroxine (T_4), serum	4.5–12.0 µg/dL	58–154 nmol/L
Thyroxine-binding globulin (TBG)	15.0–34.0 µg/mL	15.0–34.0 mg/L
Transferrin	250–430 mg/dL	2.5–4.3 g/L
Triglycerides, serum, after 12-h fast	40–150 mg/dL	0.4–1.5 g/L
Triiodothyronine (T_3), serum	70–190 ng/dL	1.1–2.9 nmol/L
Triiodothyronine uptake, resin (T_3RU)	25–38%	0.25–0.38
Troponin I	0.05–0.50 ng/mL	0.05–0.50 ng/mL
Urate		
(FT_4) Males	2.5–8.0 mg/dL	150–480 µmol/L
(FT_4) Females	2.2–7.0 mg/dL	130–420 µmol/L
Urea, serum or plasma	24–49 mg/dL	4.0–8.2 nmol/L
Urea nitrogen, serum or plasma	11–23 mg/dL	8.0–16.4 nmol/L
Viscosity, serum	1.1–1.8 cP	1.1–1.8 mPas-s
Vitamin A, serum	20–80 µg/dL	0.70–2.80 µmol/L
Vitamin B_{12}, serum	180–900 pg/mL	133–664 pmol/L

*Reference values can vary depending on the method and sample source used.
Abbreviations: EDTA = ethylenediaminetetraacetic acid; SI = International System of Units.

Reference Intervals for Therapeutic Drug Monitoring (Serum or Plasma)*

Analyte	Therapeutic Range	Toxic Concentrations	Proprietary Analyte Name(s)
Analgesics			
Acetaminophen	10–40 µg/mL	>150 µg/mL	Tylenol, Datril
Salicylate	100–250 µg/mL	>300 µg/mL	Aspirin, Bufferin
Antibiotics			
Amikacin	20–30 µg/mL	Peak >35 µg/mL	Amkin
		Trough >10 µg/mL	
Gentamicin	5–10 µg/mL	Peak >10 µg/mL	Garamycin
		Trough >2 µg/mL	
Tobramycin	5–10 µg/mL	Peak >10 µg/mL	Nebcin
		Trough >2 µg/mL	
Vancomycin	5–35 µg/mL	Peak >40 µg/mL	Vancocin
		Trough >10 µg/mL	
Anticonvulsants			
Carbamazepine	5–12 µg/mL	>15 µg/mL	Tegretol
Ethosuximide	40–100 µg/mL	>250 µg/mL	Zarontin
Phenobarbital	15–40 µg/mL	40–100 ng/mL (varies widely)	Luminal
Phenytoin	10–20 µg/mL	>20 µg/mL	Dilantin
Primidone	5–12 µg/mL	>15 µg/mL	Mysoline
Valproic acid	50–100 µg/mL	>100 µg/mL	Depakene
Antineoplastics and Immunosuppressives			
Cyclosporine A	150–350 ng/mL	>400 ng/mL	Sandimmune
Methotrexate, high-dose, 48 h	Variable	>1 µmol/L, 48 h after dose	
Sirolimus (within 1 h of 2-mg dose)	4.5–14 ng/mL	Variable	Rapamune
Sirolimus (within 1 h of 5-mg dose)	10–28 ng/mL	Variable	Rapamune
Tacrolimus (FK-506), whole blood	3–20 µg/L	>15 µg/L	Prograf
Bronchodilators and Respiratory Stimulants			
Caffeine	3–15 ng/mL	>30 ng/mL	Elixophyllin
Theophylline (aminophylline)	10–20 µg/mL	>30 µg/mL	Quibron
Cardiovascular Drugs			
Amiodarone (obtain specimen more than 8 h after last dose)	1.0–2.0 µg/mL	>2.0 µg/mL	Cordarone
Digoxin (obtain specimen more than 6 h after last dose)	0.8–2.0 ng/mL	>2.4 ng/mL	Lanoxin
Disopyramide	2–5 µg/mL	>7 µg/mL	Norpace
Flecainide	0.2–1.0 µg/mL	>1 µg/mL	Tambocor
Lidocaine	1.5–5.0 µg/mL	>6 µg/mL	Xylocaine
Mexiletine	0.7–2.0 µg/mL	>2 µg/mL	Mexitil
Procainamide	4–10 µg/mL	>12 µg/mL	Pronestyl
Procainamide plus NAPA (N-acetyl procainamide)	8–30 µg/mL	>30 µg/mL	
Propranolol	50–100 ng/mL	Variable	Inderal
Quinidine	2–5 µg/mL	>6 µg/mL	Cardioquin, Quinaglute
Tocainide	4–10 ng/mL	>10 ng/mL	Tonocard
Psychopharmacologic Drugs			
Amitriptyline	120–150 ng/mL	>500 ng/mL	Elavil, Triavil
Bupropion	25–100 ng/mL	Not applicable	Wellbutrin
Desipramine	150–300 ng/mL	>500 ng/mL	Norpramin
Imipramine	125–250 ng/mL	>400 ng/mL	Tofranil
Lithium (obtain specimen 12 h after last dose)	0.6–1.5 mEq/L	>1.5 mEq/L	Lithobid
Nortriptyline	50–150 ng/mL	>500 ng/mL	Aventyl, Pamelor

*Values can vary depending on the method and sample collection device used. Always consult the reference values provided by the laboratory performing the analysis.

Reference Intervals* for Clinical Chemistry (Urine)

Analyte	Conventional Units	SI Units
Acetone and acetoacetate, qualitative	Negative	Negative
Albumin		
Qualitative	Negative	Negative
Quantitative	10–100 mg/24 h	0.15–1.5 μmol/d
Aldosterone	3–20 μg/24 h	8.3–55 nmol/d
δ-Aminolevulinic acid (δ-ALA)	1.3–7.0 mg/24 h	10–53 μmol/d
Amylase	<17 U/h	<17 U/h
Amylase-to-creatinine clearance ratio	0.01–0.04	0.01–0.04
Bilirubin, qualitative	Negative	Negative
Calcium (regular diet)	<250 mg/24 h	<6.3 nmol/d
Catecholamines		
Epinephrine	<10 μg/24 h	<55 nmol/d
Norepinephrine	<100 μg/24 h	<590 nmol/d
Total free catecholamines	4–126 μg/24 h	24–745 nmol/d
Total metanephrines	0.1–1.6 mg/24 h	0.5–8.1 μmol/d
Chloride (varies with intake)	110–250 mEq/24 h	110–250 mmol/d
Copper	0–50 μg/24 h	0.0–0.80 μmol/d
Cortisol, free	10–100 μg/24 h	27.6–276 nmol/d
Creatine		
Males	0–40 mg/24 h	0.0–0.30 mmol/d
Females	0–80 mg/24 h	0.0–0.60 mmol/d
Creatinine	15–25 mg/kg/24 h	0.13–0.22 mmol/kg/d
Creatinine clearance (endogenous)		
Males	110–150 mL/min/1.73 m^2	110–150 mL/min/1.73 m^2
Females	105–132 mL/min/1.73 m^2	105–132 mL/min/1.73 m^2
Cystine or cysteine	Negative	Negative
Dehydroepiandrosterone		
Males	0.2–2.0 mg/24 h	0.7–6.9 μmol/d
Females	0.2–1.8 mg/24 h	0.7–6.2 μmol/d
Estrogens, total		
Males	4–25 μg/24 h	14–90 nmol/d
Females	5–100 μg/24 h	18–360 nmol/d
Glucose (as reducing substance)	<250 mg/24 h	<250 mg/d
Hemoglobin and myoglobin, qualitative	Negative	Negative
Hemogentisic acid, qualitative	Negative	Negative
17-Hydroxycorticosteroids		
Males	3–9 mg/24 h	8.3–25 μmol/d
Females	2–8 mg/24 h	5.5–22 μmol/d
5-Hydroxyindoleacetic acid		
Qualitative	Negative	Negative
Quantitative	2–6 mg/24 h	10–31 μmol/d
17-Ketogenic steroids		
Males	5–23 mg/24 h	17–80 μmol/d
Females	3–15 mg/24 h	10–52 μmol/d
17-Ketosteroids		
Males	8–22 mg/24 h	28–76 μmol/d
Females	6–15 mg/24 h	21–52 μmol/d
Magnesium	6–10 mEq/24 h	3–5 mmol/d
Metanephrines	0.05–1.2 ng/mg creatinine	0.03–0.70 mmol/mmol creatinine
Osmolality	38–1400 mOsm/kg water	38–1400 mOsm/kg water
pH	4.6–8.0	4.6–8.0
Phenylpyruvic acid, qualitative	Negative	Negative
Phosphate	0.4–1.3 g/24 h	13–42 mmol/d
Porphobilinogen		
Qualitative	Negative	Negative
Quantitative	<2 mg/24 h	<9 μmol/d
Porphyrins		
Coproporphyrin	50–250 μg/24 h	77–380 nmol/d
Uroporphyrin	10–30 μg/24 h	12–36 nmol/d
Potassium	25–125 mEq/24 h	25–125 mmol/d
Pregnanediol		
Males	0.0–1.9 mg/24 h	0.0–6.0 μmol/d
Females		
Proliferative phase	0.0–2.6 mg/24 h	0.0–8.0 μmol/d
Luteal phase	2.6–10.6 mg/24 h	8–33 μmol/d
Postmenopausal	0.2–1.0 mg/24 h	0.6–3.1 μmol/d
Pregnanetriol	0.0–2.5 mg/24 h	0.0–7.4 μmol/d
Protein, total		
Qualitative	Negative	Negative
Quantitative	10–150 mg/24 h	10–150 mg/d
Protein-to-creatinine ratio	<0.2	<0.2

Continued

Reference Intervals* for Clinical Chemistry (Urine)—Cont'd

Analyte	Conventional Units	SI Units
Sodium (regular diet)	60–260 mEq/24 h	60–260 mmol/d
Specific gravity		
Random specimen	1.003–1.030	1.003–1.030
24-h collection	1.015–1.025	1.015–1.025
Urate (regular diet)	250–750 mg/24 h	1.5–4.4 mmol/d
Urobilinogen	0.5–4.0 mg/24 h	0.6–6.8 μmol/d
Vanillylmandelic acid (VMA)	1.0–8.0 mg/24 h	5–40 μmol/d

*Values can vary depending on the method used.
Abbreviation: SI = International System of Units.

Reference Intervals for Toxic Substances

Analyte	Conventional Units	SI Units
Arsenic, urine	<130 μg/24 h	<1.7 μmol/d
Bromides, serum, inorganic	<100 mg/dL	<10 mmol/L
Toxic symptoms	140–1000 mg/dL	14–100 mmol/L
Carboxyhemoglobin, blood	Saturation, percent	
Urban environment	<5%	<0.05
Smokers	<12%	<0.12
Symptoms		
Headache	>15%	>0.15
Nausea and vomiting	>25%	>0.25
Potentially lethal	>50%	>0.50
Ethanol, blood	<0.05 mg/dL, <0.005%	<1.0 mmol/L
Intoxication	>100 mg/dL, >0.1%	>22 mmol/L
Marked intoxication	300–400 mg/dL, 0.3%–0.4%	65–87 mmol/L
Alcoholic stupor	400–500 mg/dL, 0.4%–0.5%,	87–109 mmol/L
Coma	>500 mg/dL, >0.5%	>109 mmol/L
Lead, blood		
Adults	<20 μg/dL	<1.0 μmol/L
Children	<10 μg/dL	<0.5 μmol/L
Lead, urine	<80 μg/24 h	<0.4 μmol/d
Mercury, urine	<10 μg/24 h	<150 nmol/d

Abbreviation: SI = International System of Units.

Reference Intervals for Tests Performed on Cerebrospinal Fluid

Test	Conventional Units	SI Units
Cells	<5 mm³; all mononuclear	<5 × 10⁶/L, all mononuclear
Protein electrophoresis	Albumin predominant	Albumin predominant
Glucose	50–75 mg/dL (20 mg/dL less than in serum)	2.8–4.2 mmol/L (1.1 mmol/L less than in serum)
IgG		
Children <14 y	<8% of total protein	<0.08 of total protein
Adults	<14% of total protein	<0.14 of total protein
IgG index	0.3–0.6	0.3–0.6
Oligoclonal banding on electrophoresis	Absent	Absent
Pressure, opening	70–180 mm H₂O	70–180 mm H₂O
Protein, total	15–45 mg/dL	150–450 mg/L

Abbreviations: Ig = immunoglobulin; SI = International System of Units.

Reference Intervals for Tests of Gastrointestinal Function

Test	Conventional Units
Bentiromide	6-h urinary arylamine excretion >57% excludes pancreatic insufficiency
β-Carotene, serum	60–250 ng/dL
Fecal fat estimation	
Qualitative	No fat globules seen by high-power microscope
Quantitative	<6 g/24 h (>95% coefficient of fat absorption)
Gastric acid output	
Basal	
Males	0.0–10.5 mmol/h
Females	0.0–5.6 mmol/h
Maximum (after histamine or pentagastrin)	
Males	9.0–48.0 mmol/h
Females	6.0–31.0 mmol/h
Ratio: basal/maximum	
Males	0.0–0.31
Females	0.0–0.29
Secretin test, pancreatic fluid	
Volume	>1.8 mL/kg/h
Bicarbonate	>80 mEq/L
D-Xylose absorption test, urine	>20% of ingested dose excreted in 5 h

Reference Intervals for Tests of Immunologic Function

Test	Conventional Units	SI Units
Autoantibodies, Serum, Adult		
Anti-CCP antibody	0–19 U	
Anti-dsDNA antibody	0–40 IU	0–40 IU
Antinuclear antibody	<1:40	
Rheumatoid factor (total IgG, IgA, IgM)	0–30 mg/dL	
Complement, Serum		
C3	85–175 mg/dL	0.85–1.75 g/L
C4	15–45 mg/dL	150–450 mg/L
Total hemolytic (CH_{50})	150–250 U/mL	150–250 U/mL
Immunoglobulins, Serum, Adult		
IgA	70–310 mg/dL	0.70–3.1 g/L
IgD	0.0–6.0 mg/dL	0.0–60 mg/L
IgE	0.0–430 ng/dL	0.0–430 mg/L
IgG	640–1350 mg/dL	6.4–13.5 g/L
IgM	90–350 mg/dL	0.90–3.5 g/L

Helper-to-suppressor ratio: 0.8–1.8.
Abbreviations: anti-CCP = anticyclic citrullinated peptide; dsDNA = double-stranded DNA; Ig = immunoglobulin; SI = International System of Units.

Reference Intervals for Lymphocyte Subsets, Whole Blood, Heparinized

Antigen(s) Expressed	Cell Type	Percentage	Absolute Cell Count
CD2	E rosette T cells	73–87%	1040–2160
CD3	Total T cells	56–77%	860–1880
CD3 and CD4	Helper-inducer cells	32–54%	550–1190
CD3 and CD8	Suppressor-cytotoxic cells	24–37%	430–1060
CD3 and DR	Activated T cells	5–14%	70–310
CD16 and CD56	Natural killer (NK) cells	8–22%	130–500
CD19	Total B cells	7–17%	140–370

Reference Values for Semen Analysis

Test	Conventional Units	SI Units
Volume	2–5 mL	2–5 mL
Liquefaction	Complete in 15 min	Complete in 15 min
pH	7.2–8.0	7.2–8.0
Leukocytes	Occasional or absent	Occasional or absent
Spermatozoa		
Count	$60–150 \times 10^6$ mL	$60–150 \times 10^6$ mL
Fructose	>150 mg/dL	>8.33 mmol/L
Morphology	80–90% normal forms	>0.80–0.90 normal
Motility	>80% motile	>0.80 motile

Abbreviation: SI = International System of Units.

Toxic Chemical Agents Reference Chart: Symptoms and Treatment

Method of
James J. James, MD, DrPH, MHA, and
James M. Lyznicki, MS, MPH

Toxic chemical agents are poisonous vapors, aerosols, gasses, liquids, or solids that have toxic effects on people, animals, or plants. Most of these agents are liquid at room temperature and are disseminated as vapors and aerosols. They may be released as bombs, sprayed from aircraft and boats, or disseminated by other means to intentionally create a hazard to people and the environment. Some of these agents are highly toxic and persistent, features that can render a site uninhabitable and require costly and potentially hazardous decontamination and remediation. Health effects range from irritation and burning of skin and mucous membranes to rapid cardiopulmonary collapse and death.

Efficient deployment of hazardous materials (HazMat) teams is critical to control a chemical agent attack. Although all major cities and emergency medical systems have plans and equipment in place to address this situation, physicians and other health professionals must be aware of principles involved in managing a patient or multiple patients exposed to these agents. Chemical weapon agents have a high potential for secondary contamination from victims to responders. This requires that medical treatment facilities have clearly defined procedures for handling contaminated casualties, many of whom will transport themselves to the facility. Precautions must be used until thorough decontamination has been performed or the specific chemical agent is identified. Health care professionals must first protect themselves (e.g., by using protective suits, respiratory protection, and chemical-resistant gloves) because secondary contamination with even small amounts of these substances (particularly nerve agents such as VX) may be lethal.

Primary detection of exposure to chemical agents will be based on the signs and symptoms of the potential victim (Table 1). Confirmation of a chemical agent, using detection equipment or laboratory analyses, will take considerable time and will not likely contribute to the early management of mass casualty victims. Several patients presenting with the same symptoms should alert physicians and hospital staff to the possibility of a chemical attack. If a chemical attack occurs, most victims will likely arrive within a short time. This situation differentiates a chemical attack from a biological attack involving infectious microorganisms. Additional diagnostic clues include:

- Unusual temporal or geographic clustering of illness
- Any sudden increase in illness in previously healthy persons
- Sudden increase in non-specific syndromes (e.g., sudden unexplained weakness in previously healthy persons; dimmed or blurred vision; hypersecretion, inhalation, or burn-like syndrome)

A coordinated communication network is critical for transmitting reliable information from the incident scene to treatment facilities. Any suspicious or confirmed exposure to a chemical weapons agent should be reported to the local health department, local Federal Bureau of Investigations office, and the Centers for Disease Control and Prevention (1-770-488-7100).

TABLE 1 Quick Reference Chart on Chemical Weapon Agents

Chemical Agent	Diagnostic Considerations	Treatment Considerations*
Cyanides Cyanogen chloride (CK) Hydrogen cyanide (AC)	• Symptom onset: rapid, seconds to minutes • Odor: bitter almond, musty, or chlorine-like • Nonspecific hypoxic and hypoxemic symptoms • Binds cellular cytochrome oxidase causing chemical asphyxia • Respiratory: shortness of breath, chest tightness, hyperventilation, respiratory arrest • GI: nausea, vomiting • Cardiovascular: ventricular arrhythmias, hypotension, cardiac arrest, shock • CNS: anxiety, headache, drowsiness, weakness, apnea, convulsions, seizure, coma • CNS effects may be confused with carbon monoxide and hydrogen sulfide poisoning • Metabolic acidosis and increased concentration of venous oxygen (patient also may present with cyanosis) • Laboratory testing: cyanide, thiocyanate, serum lactate levels; venous and arterial partial oxygen pressure	• Immediate treatment of symptomatic patients is critical • Antidote: sodium nitrite and sodium thiosulfate; repeat one-half initial doses of both agents in 30 minutes if there is inadequate clinical response • Amyl nitrate capsules are available for first aid until intravenous access is achieved • Cyanide antidone kits are commercially available • Investigational in the United States, available in Europe: hydroxycobalamin (vitamin B_{12a}) administered with thiosulfate • Activated charcoal[A] for oral exposure • Mechanical ventilation as needed • Circulatory support with crystalloids and vasopressors • Metabolic acidosis corrected with IV sodium bicarbonate • Seizures controlled with benzodiazepines
Incapacitating Agents Agent 15 3-quinuclidinyl benzilate (BZ)	• Symptom onset: hours 0–4 h: parasympathetic blockade and mild CNS effects 4–20 h: stupor with ataxia and hyperthermia 20–96 h: full-blown delirium Resolution phase: paranoia, deep sleep, reawakening, crawling, climbing automatisms, eventual reorientation • Odorless • Competitive inhibitor of acetylcholine muscarinic receptor • Mydriasis, blurred vision, dry mouth, dry skin, possible atropine-like flush, initial rise in heart rate, decreased level of consciousness, confusion, disorientation, visual hallucinations, impaired memory	• Antidote: physostigmine salicylate (Antilirium)[A] • Support, intravenous fluids

TABLE 1 Quick Reference Chart on Chemical Weapon Agents—Cont'd

Chemical Agent	Diagnostic Considerations	Treatment Considerations*
Nerve Agents Cyclohexyl sarin (GF) Sarin (GB) Soman (GD) Tabun (GA) VX	• Symptom onset: vapor (seconds), liquid (minutes or hours); symptom onset may be delayed up to 18 hours particularly for localized exposures • Odor: none (GB, VX), fruity (GA), camphor-like (GD) • Most toxic of known chemical agents • Irreversible acetylcholinesterase inhibitors • Eyes: excessive lacrimation, miosis may be present • Respiratory: rhinorrhea, bronchospasm, respiratory failure • GI: hypersalivation, nausea, vomiting, diarrhea • Skin: localized sweating • Cardiac: sinus bradycardia • Skeletal muscles: fasciculations followed by weakness, flaccid paralysis • CNS: loss of consciousness, convulsions, apnea, seizures • May be confused with organophosphate and carbamate pesticide poisoning • Laboratory testing: erythrocyte or serum cholinesterase activity to confirm exposure	• Rapid establishment of patent airway • Antidote: Atropine[A] and pralidoxime[A] chloride (Protopam chloride, 2-PAM); additional doses until bronchial secretions are cleared and ventilation improved • Early administration of 2-PAM is critical to minimize permanent agent inactivation of acetylcholinesterase (i.e., "aging") • Benzodiazepines to control nerve agent-induced seizures • Airway and ventilatory support as needed • Atropine,[A] pralidoxime,[A] and diazepam[A] are available in autoinjector kits through the U.S. military
Pulmonary or Choking Agents Acrolein Ammonia (NH3) Chlorine (CL) Choloropicrin (PS) Diphosgene (DP) Nitrogen oxides (NO_x) Perfluoroisobutylene (PFIB) Phosgene (CG) Sulfur dioxide (SO_2)	• Symptom onset: rapid or delayed; 1–24 h (rarely up to 72 h) • Odor (CG): freshly mown hay or grass • Easily absorbed via mucous membranes of eyes, nose, oropharynx. Degree of water solubility of the agent influences onset and severity of respiratory injury. • Eye and airway irritation, dyspnea, chest tightness, rhinorrhea, hypersalivation, cough, wheezing • High-dose inhalation may produce laryngospasm, pneumonitis, and acute lung injury with delayed onset ($\leq$48 h) of acute respiratory distress syndrome • Chest radiograph: hyperinflation, noncardiogenic pulmonary edema • May be confused with inhalation exposure to industrial chemicals (e.g., HCl, Cl_2, NH_3)	• No specific antidote • Supportive measures; specific treatment depends on the agent • IV fluids for hypotension; no diuretics • Ventilation with or without positive airway pressure • Bronchodilators for bronchospasm • Methylprednisolone[A] may be effective in preventing noncardiogenic pulmonary edema
Riot Control Agents Mace (CN) Tear gas (CS)	• Symptom onset: immediate • Odor: apple blossom (CN); pepper (CS) • Metallic taste • SN_2 alkylating agents • Burning and pain on mucosal membranes and skin • Eyes: irritation, pain, tearing, blepharospasm • Airways: burning in nose and mouth, respiratory discomfort, bronchospasm (may be delayed 36 h) • Skin: tingling, erythema • Nausea and vomiting common • CN can cause corneal opacification • No specific laboratory tests	• Supportive care • Irrigation as necessary • Persons with asthma, emphysema may need oxygen, inhaled bronchodilators, steroids, assisted ventilation • Lotions, such as calamine,[A] for persistent erythema
Vesicant or Blister Agents	• Symptoms onset: immediate (L, CX); delayed 2–48 h (H, HD) • Primary liquid hazard • May be confused with skin exposure to caustic irritants (e.g., sodium hydroxide, ammonia) • Intracellular enzyme and DNA alkylating agents • Clinical effects dependent on extent and route of exposure; effects may be delayed, appearing hours after exposure	• Immediate decontamination • Supportive care • Thermal burn-type treatment • Symptomatic management of lesions
Sulfur mustard (H) Distilled mustard (HD)	• Odor: garlic, horseradish, or mustard • Skin: erythema and blisters (may be delayed $\leq$8 h), pruritus • Eye: irritation, conjunctivitis, corneal damage, lacrimation, pain, blepharospasm • Respiratory: mild to marked acute airway damage, pneumonitis within 1–3 d, respiratory failure • GI effects (nausea, vomiting diarrhea) may be present	• No specific antidote • Skin: silver sulfadiazine[A] • Eye: homatropine[A] ophthalmic ointment • Pulmonary: antibiotics, bronchodilators, steroids • Colony stimulating factor may be helpful for leukopenia • Systemic analgesic and antipruritics • Early use of positive-end expiratory pressure or continuous positive airway pressure

Continued

TABLE 1 Quick Reference Chart on Chemical Weapon Agents—Cont'd

Chemical Agent	Diagnostic Considerations	Treatment Considerations*
	• Bone marrow stem cell suppression leading to pancytopenia and increased susceptibility to infection • Fever, sputum production • Combination with Lewisite (called mustard-Lewisite or HL) results in rapid effects of Lewisite and delayed effects of mustard agents	• Maintain fluid and electrolyte balance (do not excessively fluid resuscitate as in thermal burns)
Lewisite (L)	• Odor: fruity or geranium • More volatile than mustard • Damages eyes, skin, and airways by direct contact • Skin: gray area of dead skin within 5 min, erythema within 30 min, blistering 2–3 h, immediate irritation or burning pain on contact, severe tissue necrosis • Eye: pain, blepharospasm, conjunctival and lid edema • Airway: pseudomembrane formation, nasal irritation • Intravascular fluid loss, hypovolemia, shock, organ congestion, leukocytosis	• Antidote: British anti-Lewisite (BAL or Dimercaprol)
Phosgene oxime (CX)	• Odor: freshly mown hay • Urticant, nonvesicant agent • Vapor extremely irritating; vapor and liquid cause tissue damage upon contact • Immediate burning, irritation, wheal-like skin lesions, eye and airway damage, conjunctivitis, lacrimation, lid edema, blepharospasm • No distinctive laboratory findings	• No antidote • Parenteral methylprednisolone[A] may be effective in preventing noncardiogenic pulmonary edema • Experimental: aerosolized dexamethasone[A] and theophylline[A] for pulmonary involvement
Vomiting (Arsine-Based) Agents Adamsite (DM) Diphenylchlorarsine (DA) Diphenylcyanoarsine (DC)	• Symptom onset: All rapidly acting within minutes • Odor: none (DA), garlic (DC), burning fireworks (DM) • Primary route of absorption is through respiratory system • Arsine gas depletes erythrocyte glutathione and causes hemolysis • Eyes: conjunctival irritation, tearing, and blepharospasm • Airways: sneezing, mucosal lung irritation, edema, progressive cough, wheezing • Cardiac: tachypnea, tachycardia • GI: intestinal cramps, emesis, diarrhea • Skin: erythema, edema at the site of dermal contact • CNS: depression, syncope • Chest radiograph to rule out chemical pneumonitis	• Supportive care • Monitor for hemolysis • Wheezing or dyspnea; may need albuterol inhalation • Eye irrigation (water, normal saline, lactated Ringer's solution) in patients sustaining ocular exposure • Treat repetitive emesis with IV hydration and antiemetics • Blood transfusion may be required • Exchange transfusion may be required • Hemodialysis may be useful in decreasing arsenic level and treating renal failure

[A]Not FDA approved for this indication.
*Different situations may require different treatment and dosage regimens. Please consult other references as well as a regional poison control conter (1-800-222-1222), medical toxicologist, clinical pharmacologist, or other drug information specialist for definitive dosage information, especially dosages for pregnant women and children.
Abbreviations: CNS = central nervous system; GI = gastrointestinal.

Biologic Agents Reference Chart—Symptoms, Tests, and Treatment

Method of
James J. James, MD, DrPH, MHA, and
James M. Lyznicki, MS, MPH

Biologic weapons are devices used intentionally to cause disease or death through dissemination of microorganisms or toxins in food and water, by insect vectors, or by aerosols. Potential targets include human beings, food crops, livestock, and other resources essential for national security, economy, and defense. Unlike nuclear, chemical, and conventional weapons, the onset of a biological attack will probably be insidious. For some infectious agents, secondary and tertiary transmission may continue for weeks or months after the initial attack.

Initial detection of an unannounced biological attack will likely occur when an astute health professional notices an unusual case or disease cluster and reports his or her concerns to local public health authorities. Physicians and other health professionals should be alert to the following:

- Unusual temporal or geographic clustering of illnesses
- Sudden increase of illness in previously healthy persons
- Sudden increase in non-specific illnesses (e.g., pneumonia, flulike illness; bleeding disorders; unexplained rashes, particularly in adults; neuromuscular illness; diarrhea)

To enhance detection and treatment capabilities, physicians and other health professionals in acute care settings should be familiar with the clinical manifestations, diagnostic techniques, isolation precautions, treatment, and prophylaxis for likely causative agents (e.g., smallpox, pneumonic plague, anthrax, viral hemorrhagic fevers). Table 1 provides a quick summary of diagnostic and treatment considerations for various infectious and toxic biological agents. For some of these agents, delay in medical response could result in a potentially devastating number of casualties. To mitigate such consequences, early identification and intervention are imperative. Front-line physicians must have an increased level of suspicion regarding the possible intentional use of biological agents as well as an increased sensitivity to reporting those suspicious to public health authorities, who, in turn, must be willing to evaluate a predictable increase in false positive reports.

Medical response efforts require coordination and planning with emergency management agencies, law enforcement, health care facilities, and social services agencies. Health care agencies should ensure that physicians know whom to call with reports of suspicious cases and clusters of infectious diseases, and should work to build a good relationship with the local medical community. Resource integration is absolutely necessary to:

- Establish adequate capacity to initiate rapid investigation of an outbreak
- Educate the public
- Begin mass distribution of antibiotics and vaccines
- Ensure mass medical care
- Control public anger and fear

In an epidemic, overwhelming numbers of critically ill patients will require acute and follow-up medical care. Both infected persons and the *worried well* will seek medical attention, with a corresponding need for medical supplies, diagnostic tests, and hospital beds. The impact—or even the threat—of an attack can elicit widespread panic and civil disorder, overwhelm hospital resources, and disrupt social services.

Any suspicious or confirmed exposure to a biological weapons agent should be reported immediately to the local health department, local Federal Bureau of Investigation office, and the Centers of Disease Control and Prevention (1-770-488-7100).

1231

TABLE 1 Quick Reference Chart on Biological Weapon Agents

Disease/Agent	Diagnostic Considerations	Treatment Considerations[1]	Prophylaxis
Bacteria Anthrax *Bacillus anthracis*	Incubation period: 1–5 d (perhaps ≤60 d)[2] *Cutaneous* • Evolving skin lesion (face, neck, arms), progresses to vesicle, dispressed ulcer, and black necrotic lesions • Lethality: 20% if untreated, otherwise rarely fatal *Gastrointestinal* • Nausea, vomiting, abdominal pain, bloody diarrhea, sepsis • Lethality: approaches 100% if untreated but data are limited; rapid, aggressive treatment may reduce mortality *Inhalational* • Abrupt onset of flu-like symptoms, fever with or without chills, sweats, fatigue or malaise, non- or minimally productive cough, nausea, vomiting, dyspnea, headache, chest pain, followed in 2–5 d by severe respiratory distress, mediastinitis, hemorrhagic meningitis, sepsis, shock.[3] • Widened mediastinum on chest radiograph is characteristic for inhalational and occasionally GI anthrax.[4]	Combination therapy of ciprofloxacin (Cipro) or doxycycline (Vibramycin) plus one or two other antimicrobials should be considered with inhalational anthrax[6] Penicillin[A] should be considered if strain is susceptible and does not possess inducible β-lactamases If meningitis suspected, doxycycline (Vibramycin) may be less optimal because of poor CNS penetration Steroids may be considered for severe edema and for meningitis	Ciprofloxacin (Cipro) or doxycycline (Vibramycin) with or without vaccination If strain is susceptible, penicillin[A] or amoxicillin[A] (Amoxil) should be considered Inactivated vaccine (licensed but not readily available); six injections and annual booster

Continued

TABLE 1 Quick Reference Chart on Biological Weapon Agents—Cont'd

Disease/Agent	Diagnostic Considerations	Treatment Considerations[1]	Prophylaxis
	• Lethality: Once respiratory distress develops, mortality rates may approach 90%; begin treatment when inhalational anthrax is suspected; do not wait for confirmatory testing.[5] Gram stain and culture of blood, pleural fluid, cerebrospinal fluid, ascitic fluid, vesicular fluid or lesion exudate; sputum rarely positive; confirmatory serological and PCR tests available through public health laboratory network		
Brucellosis *B. abortus* *B. canis* *B. mellitensis* *B. suis*	Incubation period: 5–60 d (usually 1–2 mo) • Non-specific flu-like symptoms, fever, headache, profound weakness and fatigue, GI symptoms such as anorexia, nausea, vomiting, diarrhea, or constipation • Osteoarticular complications common • Lethality: less than 5% even if untreated; tends to incapacitate rather than kill. Blood and bone marrow culture (may require 6 wk to grow *Brucella*), confirmatory culture and serological testing available through public health laboratory network	Doxycycline (Vibramycin) plus streptomycin or rifampin[A] (Rifadin) *Alternative therapies:* Ofloxacin (Floxin)[A] plus rifampin[A] (Rifadin) Doxycycline (Vibramycin) plus gentamicin (Garamycin) TMP/SMX (Bactrim,[A] Septra) plus gentamicin (Garamycin)	Doxycycline (Vibramycin) plus streptomycin or rifampin (Rifadin) No approved human vaccine
Inhalational (Pneumonic) Tularemia *Francisella tularensis*	Incubation period: 3–5 d (range of 1–21 d) • Sudden onset of acute febrile illness, weakness, chills, headache, generalized body aches, elevated WBCs • Pulmonary symptoms such as dry cough, chest pain or tightness with or without objective signs of pneumonia • Progressive weakness, malaise, anorexia, and weight loss occurs, potentially leading to sepsis and organ failure • Largely clinical diagnosis • Lethality: ≈30–60% fatal if untreated Culture of blood, sputum, biopsies, pleural fluid, bronchial washings (culture is difficult and potentially dangerous); confirmatory testing available through public health laboratory network	Streptomycin or gentamicin (Garamycin) *Alternative therapies:* Ciprofloxacin (Cipro)[A] Doxycycline (Vibramycin) Chloramphenicol[A] (Chloromycetin)	Tetracycline Doxycycline (Vibramycin) Ciprofloxacin (Cipro)[A] Live attenuated vaccine (USAMRIID, IND) given by scarification; currently under FDA review, limited availability
Pneumonic Plague *Yersinia pestis*	Incubation period: 1–10 d (typically 2–3 d) • Acute onset of flu-like prodrome: fever, myalgia, weakness, headache; within 24 h of prodrome, chest discomfort, cough with bloody sputum, and dyspnea. By day 2 to 4 of illness, symptoms progressing to cyanosis, respiratory distress, and hemodynamic instability • Lethality: almost 100% if untreated; 20–60% if appropriately treated within 18–24 h of symptoms; begin treatment when diagnosis of plague is suspected; do not wait for confirmatory testing Gram stain and culture of blood, CSF, sputum, lymph node aspirates, bronchial washings; confirmatory serological and bacteriological tests available through public health laboratory network	Streptomycin; gentamicin (Garamycin) *Alternative therapies:* Doxycycline (Vibramycin) Tetracycline Ciprofloxacin[A] (Cipro) Chloramphenicol[A] (Chloromycetin) is first choice for meningitis except for pregnant women	Tetracycline Doxycycline (Vibramycin) Ciprofloxacin[A] (Cipro) Inactivated whole cell vaccine licensed but not readily available; injection with boosters Vaccine not effective against aerosol exposure

TABLE 1 Quick Reference Chart on Biological Weapon Agents—Cont'd

Disease/Agent	Diagnostic Considerations	Treatment Considerations[1]	Prophylaxis
Rickettsia Q-Fever *Coxiella burnetii*	Incubation period: 2–14 d (may be ≤40 days) • Nonspecific febrile disease, chills, cough, weakness and fatigue, pleuritic chest pain, pneumonia possible • Lethality: 1–3%, fatalities are uncommon even if untreated but relapsing symptoms may occur Isolation of organism may be difficult; confirmatory testing via serology or PCR available through public health laboratory network	Tetracycline Doxycycline (Vibramycin)	Tetracycline Doxycycline (Vibramycin) Inactivated whole cell[B] vaccine (IND) Skin test to determine prior exposure to *C. burnetii* recommended before vaccination
Viruses Smallpox Variola major virus	Incubation period: 7–17 d • Prodrome of high fever, malaise, prostration, headache, vomiting, delirium followed in 2–3 d maculopapular rash uniformly progressing to pustules and scabs, mostly on extremities and face • Requires astute clinical evaluation; may be confused with chickenpox, erythema multiforme with bullae, or allergic contact dermatitis • Lethality: 30% in unvaccinated persons Pharyngeal swab, vesicular fluid, biopsies, scab material for electron microscopy and PCR testing through public health laboratory network Notify CDC Poxvirus Section at 1-404-639-2184	Supportive care Cidofovir (Vistide) shown to be effective in vitro and in experimental animals infected with surrogate orthopox virus	Live attenuated vaccinia vaccine derived from calf lymph; given by scarification (licensed, restricted supply) New vaccine being developed from tissue culture Vaccination given within 3–4 d following exposure can prevent or decrease the severity of disease
Viral Encephalitis Eastern (EEE) Western (WEE) Venezuelan (VEE)	Incubation period: 2–6 d (VEE); 7–14 d (EEE, WEE) • Systemic febrile illness, with encephalitis developing in some populations • Generalized malaise, spiking fevers, headache, myalgia • Incidence of seizures and/or focal neurologic deficits may be higher after biological attack • White blood cell count may show striking leukopenia and lymphopenia • Clinical and epidemiologic diagnosis • Lethality: <10% (VEE); 10% (VVEE); 50–75% (EEE) Confirmatory test and viral isolation available through public health laboratory network	Supportive care Analgesics, anticonvulsants as needed	Several IND vaccines, poorly immunogenic, highly reactogenic
Viral Hemorrhagic Fevers (VHFs) Arenaviruses (Lassa, Junin, and related viruses) Bunyaviruses (Hanta, Congo-Crimean, Rift Valley) Filoviruses (Ebola, Marburg) Flaviviruses (yellow fever, dengue, various tick-borne disease viruses)	Incubation period: 4–21 d • Fever with mucous membrane bleeding, petechiae, thrombocytopenia, and hypotension in patients without underlying malignancies • Malaise, myalgias, headache, vomiting, diarrhea possible • Lethality: Variable depending on viral strain; 15–25% with Lassa fever to ≤90% with Ebola Confirmatory testing and viral isolation available through public health laboratory network Call CDC Special Pathogens Office at 1-404-639-1115	Supportive therapy Ribavirin (Virazole) A may be effective for Lassa fever, Rift Valley fever, Argentine hemorrhagic fever, and Congo-Crimean hemorrhagic fever	Ribavarin (Virazole)[A] is suggested for Congo-Crimean hemorrhagic fever and Lassa fever Yellow fever vaccine is the only licensed vaccine available Vaccines for some of the other VHFs exist but are for investigational use only
Biological Toxins Botulism *Clostridium botulinum* toxin	Symptom onset: 1–5 d (typically 12–36 h) • Blurred vision, diploplia, dry mouth, ptosis, fatigue • As disease progresses, acute bilateral descending flaccid paralysis, respiratory paralysis resulting in death • Clinical diagnosis	Intensive and prolonged supportive care; ventilation may be necessary Trivalent equine antitoxin (serotypes A, B, E, – licensed, available from the CDC) should be administered immediately after clinical diagnosis	Pentavalent toxoid (A–E), yearly booster (IND, CDC) Not available to the public Antitoxin may be sufficient to prevent illness following exposure but is not recommended until patient is showing symptoms

TABLE 1 Quick Reference Chart on Biological Weapon Agents—Cont'd

Disease/Agent	Diagnostic Considerations	Treatment Considerations[1]	Prophylaxis
	• Lethality: 60% without ventilatory support Serum and stool should be assayed for toxin by mouse neutralization bioassay, which may require several days	Anaphylaxis and serum sickness are potential complications of antitoxin Aminoglycosides and clindamycin (Cleocin) A must not be used	
Enterotoxin B *Staphylococcus aureus*	Symptom onset: 3–12 h • Acute onset of fever, chills headache, nonproductive cough • Normal chest radiograph • Clinical diagnosis • Lethality: probably low (few data available for respiratory exposure) Serology on acute and convalescent serum can confirm diagnosis	Supportive care	No vaccine available
Ricin Toxin *Ricinus communis*	Symptom onset: ≤6–24 h • Weakness, nausea, chest tightness, fever, cough, pulmonary edema, respiratory failure, circulatory collapse, hypoxemia resulting in death (usually within 36–72 h) • Clinical and epidemiological diagnosis • Lethality: mortality data not available but is likely to be high with extensive exposure Confirmatory serological testing available through public health laboratory network	Supportive care Treatment for pulmonary edema Gastric decontamination if toxin ingested	No vaccine available
T-2 Mycotoxins *Fusarium* *Myrothecium* *Trichoderma* *Stachybotrys* Other filamentous fungi	Symptom onset: minutes to hours • Abrupt onset of mucocutaneous and airway irritation and pain • May include skin, eyes, and GI tract; systemic toxicity may follow • Lethality: severe exposure can cause death in hours to days Consult with local health department regarding specimen collection and diagnostic testing procedures; confirmation requires testing blood, tissue, and environmental samples	Clinical support Soap and water washing within 4–6 h reduces dermal toxicity; washing within 1 h may eliminate toxicity entirely	No vaccine available

Adopted for *Biological Weapons: Quick Reference Guide*. American Medical Association; 2002. Available at http://www.amaassn.org/ama1/pub/upload/mm/415/quickreference0902.pdf.

[A]Not FDA approved for this indication.

[B]Not available in the United States.

[1]Different situations may require different dosage and treatment regimens. Please consult other references and an infectious disease specialist for definitive dosage information, especially dosages for pregnant women and children.

[2]Data from 22 patients infected with anthrax in October and November 2001 indicate a median incubation period of 4 d (range 4–7 d) for inhalational anthrax and a mean incubation of 5 d (range 1–10 d) for cutaneous anthrax.

[3]Limited data from the October/November 2001 anthrax infections indicate hemorrhagic pleural effusions to be strongly associated with inhalational anthrax; rhinorrhea was present in only 1/10 patients.

[4]Chest radiograph abnormalities include paratracheal and hilar fullness and may be subtle. Consider chest computed tomography if diagnosis is uncertain.

[5]Limited data from the 2001 terrorist-related anthrax infections indicate that early treatment significantly decreased the mortality rate.

[6]Other agents with in vitro activity suggested for use in conjunction with ciprofloxacin (Cipro) or doxycycline (Vibramycin) for treatment of inhalational anthrax include rifampin (Rifadin), vancomycin (Vancocin), imipenem (Primaxin), chloramphenicol (Chloromycetin), penicillin and ampicillin, clindamycin (Cleocin), and clarithromycin (Biaxin).

Abbreviations: CDC = Centers for Disease Control and Prevention; CNS = central nervous system; CSF = cerebrospinal fluid; GI = gastrointestinal; IND = investigational new drug; PCR = polymerase chain reaction; TMP-SMX = trimethoprim-sulfamethoxazole; USAMRIID, U.S. Army Medical Research Institute of Infectious Diseases; WBC = white blood cell.

Popular Herbs and Nutritional Supplements

Method of
Miriam M. Chan, BSc, PharmD

Common Herbs and Nutritional Supplements

Herb or Nutritional Supplement	Common Uses	Reasonable Adult Oral Dosage*	Precautions and Drug Interactions
Bilberry fruit	Often used orally to improve visual acuity and to treat degenerative retinal conditions Used orally to treat chronic venous insufficiency, varicose veins, and hemorrhoids Approved in Germany to use orally for acute diarrhea and topically for mild inflammation of the mucous membranes of mouth and throat	For eye conditions and circulation, 80–160 mg tid of the extract standardized to at least 25% anthocyanosides For diarrhea, 20–60 g/d of the dried, ripe berries or as a tea preparation (5–10 g of crushed dried berries in 150 mL water, brought to a boil for 10 min and then strained) For external use, 10% decoction	No known side effects reported with bilberry fruit and extract However, bilberry leaf taken in large quantities or used long term has caused wasting, anemia, jaundice, acute excitation, disturbances of tonus, and death in animals. The anthocyanidin extracts from bilberry may increase the risk of bleeding in those taking warfarin or other blood thinners.
Black cohosh root	Commonly used to relieve hot flashes and other menopausal symptoms Used to treat premenstrual discomfort and dysmenorrhea	20 mg bid of the rhizome extract standardized to triterpene glycosides German guidelines do not recommend its use for >6 mo.	Black cohosh may have an estrogen-like effect and should be avoided in women with breast cancer. Large doses may induce miscarriage, and it is contraindicated during pregnancy. It may cause GI disturbances, headache, and hypotension. International case reports of liver dysfunction suspected to be associated with its use
Black haw	To relieve uterine cramps and painful periods To prevent miscarriage and ease pain that followed childbirth	For menstrual pain, 5 mL of tincture in water, taken 3–5 times daily For prevention of miscarriage, 1–2 cups of tea per day (1 tsp of dried herb in 1 cup of boiling water, steeped for 10 min)	Black haw should not be used in pregnancy because of its uterine relaxant effects. The salicylate constituent in black haw can trigger allergic reactions in individuals with aspirin allergies or asthma. Black haw may aggravate tinnitus. Large doses may prolong bleeding time. The oxalic acid component of black haw may increase kidney stone formation in susceptible individuals. Black haw may interact with warfarin and increase risk of bleeding.
Chamomile flower	Used orally to calm nerves and treat GI spasms and inflammatory diseases of the GI tract Used topically to treat wounds, skin infections, and skin or mucous membrane inflammation	1 cup of freshly made tea 3–4 times daily (1 Tbsp or 3 g of dried flower in 150 mL boiling water for 5–10 min)	Chamomile may cause an allergic reaction, especially in people with severe allergies to ragweed or other members of the daisy family (e.g., echinacea, feverfew, milk thistle). It should not be taken concurrently with other sedatives, such as alcohol or benzodiazepines.
Chaste tree berry (chasteberry, *Vitex agnus-castus*)	For normalizing irregular menstrual periods and relieving premenstrual complaints For relieving menopausal symptoms For restoring fertility in women For treating acne associated with menstrual cycles For increasing breast milk production in lactating women	For menstrual irregularities and premenstrual complaints, 30–40 mg/d of the dried berries or an equivalent amount of aqueous-alcoholic extracts (50%–70% v/v) Dried fruit extract, standardized to 0.6% agnusides, is used in doses of 175–225 mg/d. For other conditions, no established dosage is documented.	Chaste tree berry can have uterine stimulant properties and should be avoided in pregnancy. Women with hormone-dependent conditions (i.e., breast, uterine, and ovarian cancers and endometriosis and uterine fibroids) and men with prostate cancer should avoid chaste tree berry because it contains progestins.

Continued

Herb or Nutritional Supplement	Common Uses	Reasonable Adult Oral Dosage*	Precautions and Drug Interactions
			Side effects include intramenstrual bleeding, dry mouth, headache, nausea, rash, alopecia, and tachycardia.
			High doses (≥480 mg/d extract) can paradoxically decrease lactation.
			Chaste tree berry is thought to have dopaminergic effects and may interact with dopamine antagonists, such as antipsychotics and metoclopramide.
			Chaste tree berry may decrease the effects of oral contraceptives and hormone replacement therapy.
Chondroitin	Orally, used frequently in combination with glucosamine for osteoarthritis Topically, in combination with sodium hyaluronate, as a viscoelastic agent in cataract surgery	Oral: 200–400 mg tid	Occasional mild side effects include nausea, indigestion, and allergic reactions. Chondroitin derived from bovine cartilage may carry a potential risk of contamination with diseased animals.
Chromium	For diabetes For hypercholesterolemia Commonly found in weight-loss products Also promoted for body building	For diabetes, 100 μg bid for ≤4 mo or 500 μg bid for 2 mo For hypercholesterolemia, 200 μg tid or 500 μg bid for 2–4 mo For body building, 200–400 μg/d Chromium picolinate has been used in most studies, even though the chloride form is also available.	Adverse effects are rare, but they may include headaches, insomnia, sleep disturbances, irritability and mood changes. Some patients may also experience cognitive, perceptual, and motor dysfunction. Long-term use of high doses (600–2400 μg/d) can cause anemia, thrombocytopenia, hemolysis, hepatic dysfunction, and renal failure. Interstitial nephritis has been reported A few studies suggest that chromium may cause DNA damage Chromium competes with iron for binding to transferrin and can cause iron deficiency. Antacids, H_2-blockers, and proton pump inhibitors can decrease the absorption of chromium.
Coenzyme Q10	As adjunctive treatment for congestive heart failure, angina, hypertension, and diabetes Used for reducing cardiotoxicity associated with doxorubicin Used to treat statin-induced myopathy	For heart failure, 100 mg/d in two or three divided doses For angina, 50 mg tid For hypertension, 60 mg bid For diabetes, 100–200 mg/d	Mild adverse events include gastric distress, nausea, vomiting, and hypotension. Doses >300 mg/d may cause elevated liver enzyme levels. Coenzyme Q10 may reduce the anticoagulation effects of warfarin. Oral hypoglycemic agents and HMG-CoA reductase inhibitors may reduce serum coenzyme Q10 levels.
Cranberry	To prevent and treat UTIs or *Helicobacter pylori* infections that can lead to stomach ulcers To prevent dental plaque As an antioxidant to prevent cardiovascular disease and cancer	For UTIs, 150–600 mL of cranberry juice daily or 300–400 mg of standardized extract bid For other conditions, no dosage determined	Drinking excessive amounts of juice can cause GI upset or diarrhea. Prolonged use of cranberry juice in large doses may increase the risk of kidney stone formation due to its high oxalate content. Cranberry may interact with warfarin and cause an increase in INR. The effectiveness of proton pump inhibitors may be reduced by cranberry due to its acidity.

Herb or Nutritional Supplement	Common Uses	Reasonable Adult Oral Dosage*	Precautions and Drug Interactions
Creatine	To enhance muscle performance, especially during short-duration, high-intensity exercise	Loading dose of 20 g/d for 5–7 d, followed by a maintenance dose of ≥2 g/d Alternative dosing of 3 g/d for 28 d has been suggested.	Creatine can cause gastroenteritis, diarrhea, heat intolerance, muscle cramps, and elevated serum creatinine levels. Creatine is contraindicated in patients taking diuretics. Concurrent use with cimetidine, probenecid, or NSAIDs increases the risk of adverse renal effects. Caffeine may decrease creatine's ergogenic effects.
Dehydroepiandrosterone (DHEA)	Replace low serum DHEA levels in adrenal insufficiency Treat SLE Reverse aging Used in many other conditions, including Alzheimer's disease, depression, diabetes, menopause, osteoporosis, impotence, and AIDS Used to promote weight loss Used by bodybuilders to increase muscle mass	For replacement therapy, 25–50 mg/d For SLE, 200 mg/d For antiaging and osteoporosis, 50 mg/d For other conditions, no established dosage documented	Most common side effects are androgenic in nature and include acne, hair loss, hirsutism, and deepening of the voice. Cases of hepatitis have been reported. When used in high doses, DHEA can cause insomnia, manic symptoms, and palpitations. DHEA at physiologic doses increases circulating androgens in women but not in men; it increases circulating estrogens in men and women. Avoid use of DHEA in individuals with a history of sex hormone–dependent malignancy. Safety of DHEA in individuals <30 y is unknown. DHEA inhibits the cytochrome P-450 3A4 isoenzyme and can increase serum concentrations of drugs metabolized by this isoenzyme (e.g., lovastatin, ketoconazole, itraconazole, and triazolam).
Dong quai root	Commonly used for the relief of premenstrual and menopausal symptoms Used as a "blood tonic" and a strengthening treatment for the heart, spleen, liver, and kidneys	For premenstrual and menopausal symptoms, 3–4 g/d in three divided doses For other conditions, no established dosage documented	Dong quai should not be used in pregnant women due to its uterine stimulant and relaxant effects. Women with hormone sensitive conditions (i.e., breast, uterine, and ovarian cancers and endometriosis and uterine fibroids) should avoid dong quai because of its estrogenic effects. Drinking the essential oil of dong quai is not recommended because it contains a small amount of carcinogenic constituents. Dong quai contains psoralens that can cause photosensitivity and photodermatitis. Dong quai contains natural coumarin derivatives that can increase the risk of bleeding in those who are taking anticoagulant or antiplatelet drugs.
Echinacea	As an immune stimulant, particularly for the prevention and treatment of the common cold and influenza Supportive therapy for lower urinary tract infections Used topically to treat skin disorders and promote wound healing	300 mg tid of *Echinacea pallida* root or 2–3 mL tid of expressed juice of *Echinacea purpurea* herb Do not use for >8 wk because echinacea may suppress immunity if used long term.	Echinacea should not be used in transplant patients and those with autoimmune disease or liver dysfunction. Allergic reactions have been reported. Adverse events are rare and may include mild GI effects. It should be discontinued as far in advance of surgery as possible. Echinacea may decrease the effectiveness of immunosuppressants.

Continued

Herb or Nutritional Supplement	Common Uses	Reasonable Adult Oral Dosage*	Precautions and Drug Interactions
Ephedra (ma huang)	For diseases of the respiratory tract with mild bronchospasm Promoted for weight loss and performance enhancement	1 tsp or 2 g of dried herb (15–30 mg of ephedrine) in 240 mL boiling water for 10 min In Canada, the maximum allowable dosage of ephedrine is 8 mg per dose or 32 mg/d.	Ephedra contains ephedrine, which has sympathomimetic activities; consequently, it should not be used in patients who have cardiovascular disease, diabetes, glaucoma, hypertension, hyperthyroidism, prostate enlargement, psychiatric disorders, or seizures. Serious adverse effects, including seizures, arrhythmias, heart attack, stroke, and death, have been associated with the use of ephedra; as a result, the FDA has banned the sale of ephedra products in the United States. Because of the cardiovascular effects of ephedrine, patients taking ephedra should discontinue use at least 24 h before surgery. Concurrent use of ephedra and digitalis, guanethidine, monoamine oxidase inhibitors, or other stimulants, including caffeine, is not recommended.
Evening primrose oil	For PMS, especially if mastalgia is present For treatment of atopic eczema Used for other medical conditions, including rheumatoid arthritis, menopausal symptoms, Raynaud's phenomenon, Sjögren's syndrome, and diabetic neuropathy	For PMS, 2–4 g/d For atopic eczema, 6–8 g/d For rheumatoid arthritis, 2.8 g/d These doses are based on products standardized to 9% γ-linolenic acid. Daily dose can be given in divided doses.	Evening primrose oil may increase the risk of pregnancy complications. Side effects may include indigestion, nausea, soft stools, and headache. Seizures have been reported in patients with schizophrenia who were taking phenothiazines and evening primrose oil concomitantly. Evening primrose oil may interact with anesthesia and cause seizures. Concomitant use of evening primrose oil with anticoagulant and antiplatelet drugs can increase the risk of bleeding.
Fenugreek seed	For diabetes and hypercholesterolemia Used for constipation, dyspepsia, gastritis, and kidney ailments Approved in Germany for use orally for loss of appetite and topically as a poultice for local inflammation	For loss of appetite, 1–2 g of the seed tid or 1 cup of tea (500 mg seed in 150 mL cold water for 3 h) several times per day Maximum 6 g/d For other conditions, no established dosage documented For topical use, 50 g powdered seed in 0.25 L of hot water to form a paste	Fenugreek may cause uterine contractions and should be avoided in pregnancy. Individuals who have allergies to peanuts or soybeans may also be allergic to fenugreek. Fenugreek can cause diarrhea and flatulence; it may also make the urine smell like maple syrup. Hypoglycemia may occur if fenugreek is taken in large amounts. Repeated external applications can result in undesirable skin reactions. Fenugreek contains small amounts of coumarins and may interact with anticoagulants and antiplatelet drugs. High mucilage content of fenugreek can affect the absorption of oral drugs; therefore, fenugreek should not be taken within 2 h of other drugs.
Feverfew	For migraine headache prophylaxis For treatment of fever, menstrual problems, and arthritis	25–75 mg bid of the encapsulated dried leaf extract standardized to 0.2% parthenolide	Feverfew may induce menstrual bleeding and is contraindicated in pregnancy. Fresh leaves may cause oral ulcers and GI irritation. Sudden discontinuation of feverfew can precipitate rebound headache. Feverfew may interact with anticoagulants and potentiate the antiplatelet effect of aspirin.

Herb or Nutritional Supplement	Common Uses	Reasonable Adult Oral Dosage*	Precautions and Drug Interactions
Fish oils (omega-3 fatty acids)	Commonly used in the treatment of hypertriglyceridemia Used to prevent CHD and stroke Used in many noncardiac conditions, including depression, diabetes, dysmenorrhea, rheumatoid arthritis, and IgA nephropathy Used to reduce the risk of developing age-related maculopathy, Alzheimer's disease, and cancer Promotes visual and mental development in children	For hypertriglyceridemia, 3–5 g/d For cardioprotection, 1 g/d for patients with CHD; oily fish at least twice per week, or about 0.5 g/d for people with no known heart disease For other conditions, no established dosage documented Fish oils are composed of EPA and DHA. Fish oil capsules vary widely in amounts and ratios of EPA and DHA. The most common fish oil capsules in the United States provide 180 mg of EPA and 120 mg DHA per capsule, and three capsules provide about 1 g/d of omega-3 fatty acids.	Common side effects include fishy aftertaste, GI disturbances, belching, halitosis, and heartburn. High doses can cause nausea and loose stools. Doses >3 g/d can inhibit platelet aggregation, suppress immune function, worsen glycemic control, and raise LDL cholesterol levels. Long-term use may be associated with weight gain. Less well-controlled preparations can contain appreciable amount of organochloride contaminants. Fish oil may increase the risk of bleeding in patients taking warfarin, an antiplatelet agent, or herbs that have antiplatelet constituents (e.g., garlic, ginkgo, red clover). Fish oils can lower blood pressure and may have additive effects with antihypertensive agents. Oral contraceptives may interfere with the triglyceride lowering effects of fish oils
Flaxseed	Orally, approved in Germany for chronic constipation, irritable bowel, and other colon disorders Often used orally for hypercholesterolemia and atherosclerosis Topically, approved in Germany for painful skin inflammation	For constipation, 1 Tbsp (5 g) of whole or "bruised" seeds (not ground) in 150 mL of liquid 2–3 times daily For bowel inflammation, soak 2–3 Tbsp of milled flaxseed soaked in 200–300 mL water and strain after 30 min For hypercholesterolemia, 1–2 Tbsp flaxseed oil daily Topical: 30–50 g flaxseed flour as poultice or compress for a moist heat application directly to the skin	Flaxseed should be taken with plenty of water to prevent possible intestinal blockage. Patients with ileus should not take flaxseed. High mucilage content of flaxseed may delay absorption of other drugs taken at the same time.
Garlic	To lower blood pressure and serum cholesterol To prevent atherosclerosis	Fresh clove: one 4-g clove per day Tablet: 300 mg bid to tid standardized to 0.6%–1.3% allicin	Intake of large quantities can lead to stomach complaints. Garlic has antiplatelet effects, so patients should discontinue use of garlic at least 7 d before surgery. Concomitant use of garlic and anticoagulants may increase the risk of bleeding.
Ginger root	As an antiemetic For prevention of motion sickness	Fresh rhizome: 2–4 g/d Powdered ginger: 250 mg 3 to 4 times daily Tea: 1 cup of tea tid (0.5–1 g dried root in 150 mL boiling water for 5–10 min)	Ginger should not be used by patients with gallstones because of its cholagogic effect. Can inhibit platelet aggregation; cases of postoperative bleeding have been reported. Large doses of ginger may increase bleeding time in patients taking antiplatelet agents.
Ginkgo biloba leaf	To slow cognitive deterioration in dementia To increase peripheral blood flow in claudication To treat sexual dysfunction associated with the use of SSRIs	60–120 mg bid of extract Egb761 standardized to 24% flavonoids and 6% terpenoids	Adverse effects are rare and may include mild stomach or intestinal upset, headache, or allergic skin reaction. Ginkgo can inhibit platelet aggregation; reports of spontaneous bleeding have been published. Patients should discontinue ginkgo at least 36 h before surgery. Concurrent use of ginkgo and anticoagulants, antiplatelet agents, vitamin E, or garlic may increase the risk of bleeding.

Continued

Herb or Nutritional Supplement	Common Uses	Reasonable Adult Oral Dosage*	Precautions and Drug Interactions
Ginseng root	As a tonic during times of stress, fatigue, disability, and convalescence To improve physical performance and stamina	Root: 1–2 g/d Tablet: 100 mg bid of extract standardized to 4%–7% ginsenosides A 2- to 3-week period of using ginseng followed by a 1- to 2-week "rest" period is generally recommended Ginseng is commonly adulterated, especially Siberian ginseng (eleuthero) products.	Ginseng has a mild stimulant effect and should be avoided in patients with cardiovascular disease. Tachycardia and hypertension can occur. Overdosages can lead to ginseng abuse syndrome, characterized by insomnia, hypotonia, and edema. Ginseng has estrogenic effects and may cause vaginal bleeding and breast tenderness. Ginseng has been shown to inhibit platelets, so patients should discontinue ginseng use at least 7 d before surgery. Ginseng should not be used with other stimulants. Patients taking antidiabetic agents and ginseng should be monitored to avoid the hypoglycemic effects of ginseng. Ginseng may interact with warfarin and cause a decreased INR. Siberian ginseng may increase digoxin levels. Ginseng can interact with phenelzine (an MAOI), resulting in insomnia, headache, tremulousness, and manic-like symptoms.
Glucosamine	For osteoarthritis	500 mg tid with meals Glucosamine is available in the form of sulfate, hydrochloride, or N-acetyl salt. Glucosamine sulfate is the form that has been used in most clinical studies.	Side effects are generally limited to mild GI symptoms, including stomach upset, heartburn, diarrhea, nausea, and indigestion. Glucosamine derived from marine exoskeletons may cause reactions in people allergic to shellfish. Glucosamine may raise blood glucose level in patients with diabetes.
Goldenseal	Often combined with echinacea to treat colds and other upper respiratory infections Used for diarrhea, dyspepsia, and gastritis Used topically as an eyewash, mouthwash, feminine cleansing product, and skin remedy	Oral: 0.5–1 g of the dried rhizome/root or 2–4 mL tincture (1:10, 60% ethanol) or 0.3–1 mL fluid extract (1:1, 60% ethanol) tid Eyewash: For trachoma infections, 2 drops of a 0.2% aqueous berberine solution tid × 3 wk	Avoid using goldenseal during pregnancy and breast-feeding. Berberine, the principal constituent in goldenseal, can cause uterine contractions and neonatal jaundice. Avoid using goldenseal in kidney failure due to inadequate urinary excretion of its alkaloids. High dosages or long-term usage can lead to nausea, vomiting, headache, hypotension, bradycardia, leukopenia, and mucosal irritation. Berberine may increase the risk of bleeding in patients taking warfarin or an antiplatelet agent. Be aware that other herbs containing berberine, including Chinese goldthread and Oregon grape, are sometimes substituted for goldenseal.
Grape seed	For conditions related to the heart and blood vessels, such as atherosclerosis, high blood pressure, high cholesterol, and poor circulation For vision problems, diabetic neuropathy or retinopathy, and swelling after an injury or surgery For cancer prevention and wound healing	For general health purposes, 100–300 mg daily of a standardized extract (95% oligomeric proanthocyanidin complexes)	Side effects include headache, dizziness, nausea, and dry, itchy scalp. Concomitant use with warfarin or antiplatelet agents may increase risk of bleeding due to the tocopherol content of grape seed oil.

Common Herbs and Nutritional Supplements—Cont'd

Herb or Nutritional Supplement	Common Uses	Reasonable Adult Oral Dosage*	Precautions and Drug Interactions
Hawthorn leaf with flower	Commonly used in Germany to increase cardiac output in patients with New York Heart Association stage I and II heart failure	160–900 mg water-ethanol extract (30–169 mg procyanidins or 3.5–19.8 mg flavonoids) divided into 2–3 doses	Side effects include GI upset, palpitations, hypotension, headache, dizziness, and insomnia. Concomitant use with CNS depressants may have additive CNS effects. Hawthorn may potentiate effects of digoxin and vasodilators.
Hops	For mood disturbances such as restlessness and anxiety For sleep disturbances Commonly found in combination products with other herbal sedatives	0.5 g of cut or powdered strobile in a single dose; can be taken as tea (0.5 g in 150 mL water), fluid extract 1:1 (0.5 mL), tincture 1:5 (2.5 mL), or dry extract 6–8:1 (60–80 mg) The preparation contains at least 0.35% (v/w) essential oil.	Side effects are rare but may include drowsiness and allergic reactions. Hops is not recommended for use during pregnancy and lactation. It may potentiate the sedative effect of CNS depressants (e.g., benzodiazepines, alcohol) and other herbal tranquilizers.
Horse chestnut seed	To relieve symptoms of chronic venous insufficiency	250 mg bid of extract standardized to 50 mg aescin (escin). in delayed-release form Unsafe to ingest the raw seed, which contains significant amounts of the most toxic constituent, esculin	Mild GI symptoms, headache, dizziness, and pruritus have been reported. Ingestion of high doses may cause renal, hepatic, and hematologic toxicity. Concomitant use with anticoagulants may increase the risk of bleeding. Horse chestnut may potentiate the effects of hypoglycemic drugs.
Kava kava	As an anxiolytic for nervous anxiety, stress, and restlessness As a sedative to induce sleep	Herb and preparations equivalent to 60–120 mg/d of kava pyrones Most clinical trials have used 100 mg tid of extract standardized to 70% kava pyrones for anxiety disorders.	Kava should not be used by patients with depression. Kava should be avoided in pregnant or nursing women. Kava may affect motor reflexes and judgment, so it should not be taken while driving or operating heavy machinery. Accommodative disturbances have been reported; kava may exacerbate Parkinson's disease. Extended use can cause a temporary yellow discoloration of skin, hair, and nails. Reports have linked kava use to at least 25 cases of severe liver toxicity; sale of products containing kava has been banned in Canada and several European countries. Kava has additive CNS depressant effects with benzodiazepines, alcohol, and herbal tranquilizers. Kava may potentiate the sedative effects of anesthetics, so kava should be discontinued at least 24 h before surgery.
Lutein	Commonly used to prevent AMD and cataracts Used to prevent skin cancer, breast cancer, and colon cancer Used to protect against cardiovascular disease	For AMD and cataracts, 6–20 mg/d of lutein from diet For other uses, no established dosage documented Foods containing high concentrations of lutein include kale, spinach, broccoli, and romaine lettuce. Not known if supplemental lutein is as effective as natural lutein Supplemental lutein in the form of esters may require a higher fat intake for effective absorption than purified lutein.	No major adverse effects and drug interactions have been reported.

Continued

Common Herbs and Nutritional Supplements—Cont'd

Herb or Nutritional Supplement	Common Uses	Reasonable Adult Oral Dosage*	Precautions and Drug Interactions
Lycopene	Commonly used to prevent and treat prostate cancer Used for cancer prevention, arthrosclerosis prevention, and reduction of asthma symptoms	For decreasing the growth of prostate cancer, 15 mg supplement bid For prostate cancer prevention, at least 6 mg/d from tomato products (or ≥10 servings/wk) For other uses, no established dosage documented Heat processing converts lycopene in fresh tomatoes from the *trans* to the *cis* configuration. The *cis* isomer has better bioavailability. Lycopene supplements usually do not specify the type and amount of isomers in their product labeling	Lycopene, when consumed in amounts found in foods, is generally considered to be safe. Concomitant ingestion of beta-carotene may increase lycopene absorption. Lycopene may reduce cholesterol levels and potentiate the effects of statins.
Melatonin	For jet lag, insomnia, shift-work disorder, and circadian rhythm disorders For other medical conditions, including depression, multiple sclerosis, tinnitus, headache, and cancer	For jet lag, 5 mg at bedtime for 2–5 d beginning the day of return For sleep disorders, 0.3–5 mg taken 2 hrs before bedtime Avoid melatonin from animal pineal gland due to possibility of contamination.	Avoid use in pregnancy because melatonin decreases serum luteinizing hormone concentrations and increases serum prolactin levels. The common adverse reactions include headache, transient depressive symptoms, daytime fatigue and drowsiness, dizziness, abdominal cramps, irritability, and reduced alertness. Concomitant use of melatonin with alcohol, benzodiazepines, or other CNS depressants may cause additive sedation. Melatonin can affect immune function and may interfere with immunosuppressive therapy. Concomitant use with other herbs that have sedative properties (e.g., chamomile, goldenseal, hop, kava, valerian) may produce additive CNS-impairing effects.
Milk thistle fruit	As a hepatoprotectant and antioxidant, particularly for treatment of hepatitis, cirrhosis, and toxic liver damage Used in Europe for the treatment of hepatotoxic mushroom poisoning from *Amanita phalloides*	Average daily dose is 12–15 g of crude drug or formulations equivalent to 200–400 mg of silymarin	Adverse effects are rare but may include diarrhea and allergic reactions. Milk thistle may potentiate the hypoglycemic effect of antidiabetic agents.
Probiotics	Prevent and treat antibiotic-associated diarrhea and acute infectious diarrhea Relieve symptoms of irritable bowel syndrome Treat atopic dermatitis for at-risk infants	Dosage varies based on preparations *Lactobacillus* sp., *Bifidobacterium* sp., and *Saccharomyces boulardii* are the most widely used organisms. For *Lactobacillus* sp., 10 billion CFUs/d For *Lactobacillus* sp./ *Bifidobacterium* sp., 100 million to 35 billion CFUs/d For *S. boulardii*, 250–500 mg/d Quality of products varies among brands Refrigeration is required to maintain potency.	Avoid use in short-gut syndrome and severe immunocompromised condition. Common adverse effects include flatulence, mild abdominal discomfort, and rarely septicemia.

Common Herbs and Nutritional Supplements—Cont'd

Herb or Nutritional Supplement	Common Uses	Reasonable Adult Oral Dosage*	Precautions and Drug Interactions
Red clover flower	Commonly used for conditions associated with menopause, such as hot flashes, cardiovascular health, and osteoporosis Also used for PMS, benign prostate hyperplasia, and cancer prevention Used topically to treat psoriasis, eczema, and other rashes	For hot flashes, 40 mg/d of the isoflavone extract (Promensil) For other conditions, no established dosage documented	Red clover has estrogenic activity and should be avoided during pregnancy and lactation. Women with hormone-dependent conditions (i.e., breast, uterine, and ovarian cancer and endometriosis and uterine fibroids) and men with prostate cancer should avoid taking red clover. Side effects include headache, myalgia, nausea, and rash. Red clover contains coumarin derivatives and may increase the risk of bleeding in those who are taking anticoagulants or antiplatelet drugs. Preliminary report suggests that red clover may antagonize the effects of tamoxifen. Some evidence suggests that red clover can increase the levels of drugs that metabolized by the cytochrome P-450 3A4 isoenzyme (e.g., lovastatin, ketoconazole, itraconazole, fexofenadine, triazolam).
SAMe (S-adenosyl-L-methionine)	For treatment of osteoarthritis, depression, fibromyalgia, and liver disease	For osteoarthritis, 200 mg tid For depression and fibromyalgia, 800 mg bid For liver disease, 600–800 mg bid	Common side effects include flatulence, nausea, vomiting, and diarrhea. SAMe can cause anxiety in people with depression and hypomania in people with bipolar disorder. Concurrent use of SAMe and other antidepressants may cause serotonin syndrome.
Saw palmetto berry	To treat symptomatic benign prostatic hyperplasia and irritable bladder	160 mg bid of extract standardized to 85%–95% fatty acids and sterols	Adverse effects are rare but may include headache, nausea, and upset stomach. High doses can cause diarrhea.
Soy	Commonly used for cholesterol reduction in combination with a low-fat diet Used for menopausal symptoms and for prevention of osteoporosis and cardiovascular disease in postmenopausal women	For lowering cholesterol, 25–50 g/d of soy protein For hot flashes, 20–60 g/d of soy protein For osteoporosis, 40 g/d of soy protein containing 90 mg isoflavones	Soy, when consumed as whole foods (e.g., tofu, soy milk), has minimal adverse effects. Consumption of large amounts soy may cause gastric complaints such as constipation, bloating, and nausea. Long-term use of soy tablets containing isoflavones (150 mg/d for 5 y) can cause endometrial hyperplasia.
St. John's wort	Effective for treatment of mild to moderate depression May have antiinflammatory and antiinfective activities	300 mg tid of Hypericum extract standardized to 0.3% hypericin	St. John's wort should not be used in pregnancy. Side effects include dry mouth, GI upset, dizziness, fatigue, and constipation. St. John's wort may induce photosensitivity, especially in fair-skinned individuals. It may cause serotonin syndrome if used with other antidepressants, including SSRIs, or other serotonergic drugs. It has been shown to induce CYP3A4 and decrease blood levels of many drugs such as indinavir, nevirapine, cyclosporine, digoxin, theophylline, simvastatin, oral contraceptive pills, and warfarin.

Continued

Common Herbs and Nutritional Supplements—Cont'd

Herb or Nutritional Supplement	Common Uses	Reasonable Adult Oral Dosage*	Precautions and Drug Interactions
			St. John's wort should be discontinued at least 5 d before surgery to avoid any potential drug interactions.
Stinging nettle root	Approved in Germany for difficulty in urination in BPH stage 1 and 2	4–6 g per day of cut root; can be taken as tea (1.5 g in 150 mL boiling water for 10–20 min, tid), fluid extract 1:1 (1.5 mL tid), tincture 1:5 (5–7.5 mL tid), or dry extract 5.4–6.6:1 (0.22–0.33 g tid)	Occasionally, mild GI upsets may occur. No known interactions with drugs.
Valerian root	Used as a mild sedative for insomnia and anxiety	2–3 g of dried root or 1–3 mL of tincture, qd to several times per day Two clinical trials found 400–450 mg of the root extract effective for insomnia.	Valerian has a bad odor and can cause morning drowsiness. Long-term administration may lead to paradoxical stimulation, including restlessness and palpitations. Because of the risk of benzodiazepine-like withdrawal, valerian should be tapered over a period of several weeks before surgery. It may potentiate the sedative effect of CNS depressants (e.g., benzodiazepines, alcohol) and other herbal tranquilizers.

*Doses presented in the table are adapted from the German Commission E Monographs and data from clinical trials. Products from different manufacturers vary considerably. A reliable product should have a label clearly stating the botanical name of the herb and milligram amount contained in the product. Standardized extracts should be used whenever possible, and information is often disclosed on the label of quality products.

Abbreviations: AIDS = acquired immunodeficiency syndrome; AMD = age-related macular degeneration; BPH = benign prostatic hyperplasia; CFU = colony-forming unit; CHD = coronary heart disease; CNS, central nervous system; DHA = docosahexaenoic acid; EPA = eicosapentaenoic acid; FDA = Food and Drug Administration; GI = gastrointestinal; HMG-CoA = 3-hydroxy-3-methylglutaryl coenzyme A; INR = International Normalized Ratio; LDL = low-density lipoprotein; MAOI = monoamine oxidase inhibitor; NSAIDs = nonsteroidal antiinflammatory drugs; PMS = premenstrual syndrome; SLE = systemic lupus erythematosus; SSRIs = selective serotonin reuptake inhibitors; UTIs = urinary tract infections.

REFERENCES

Ang-Lee MK, Moss J, Yuan C. Herbal medicines and perioperative care. JAMA 2001;286:208–16.

Blumenthal M, editor. Herbal Medicines: Expanded Commission E Monographs. Austin, TX: American Botanical Council; 2000.

Blumenthal M, editor. The ABC Clinical Guide to Herbs. Austin, TX: American Botanical Council; 2003.

Cupp MJ. Herbal remedies: Adverse effects and drug interactions. Am Fam Physician 1999;59:1239–44.

Ernst E. The risk-benefit profile of commonly used herbal therapies: Ginkgo, St. John's Wort, Ginseng, Echinacea, Saw Palmetto, and Kava. Ann Intern Med 2002;136:42–53.

Fleming T, editor. PDR for Herbal Medicines. 3rd ed. Montvale, NJ: Medical Economics; 2004.

Jellin JM, Gregory P, Batz F, et al. Pharmacist's letter/prescriber's letter natural medicines comprehensive database. 7th ed. Stockton, CA: Therapeutic Research Faculty; 2005.

Klepser TB, Klepser ME. Unsafe and potentially safe herbal therapies. Am J Health Syst Pharm 1999;56:125–38.

Kligler B, Cohrssen A. Probiotics. Am Fam Physician 2008;78:1073–8.

Kronenberg F, Fugh-Berman A. Complementary and alternative medicine for menopausal symptoms: A review of randomized controlled trials. Ann Intern Med 2002;137:805–13.

Mar C, Bent S. An evidence-based review of the 10 most commonly used herbs. West J Med 1999;171:168–71.

O'Hara MA, Kiefer D, Farrell K, Kemper K. A review of 12 commonly used medicinal herbs. Arch Fam Med 1998;7:523–36.

Rotblatt MD. Cranberry, feverfew, horse chestnut, and kava. West J Med 1999;171:195–228.

Smet P. Herbal remedies. N Engl J Med 2002;2046–56.

New Drugs in 2008 and Agents Pending FDA Approval

Method of
Miriam Chan, BSc, PharmD

New Drugs Approved in 2008

Generic Name	Trade Name (Manufacturer)	Strength	Dosage Form	Normal Dosage Range	Pregnancy Rating*	FDA Approval Date	Indication	Classification
New Molecular Entity								
Alvimopan	Entereg (GlaxoSmithKline, Adolor)	12 mg	Capsule	12 mg given 30 min to 5 h before surgery; followed by 12 mg bid beginning the day after surgery, for up to 7 d for a max of 15 doses	B	5/20/08	For short-term hospital use only to accelerate the time to upper and lower gastrointestinal recovery following partial large or small bowel resection surgery with primary anastomosis	Opioid antagonist, peripherally acting μ-opioid receptor antagonist
Bendamustine hydrochloride	Treanda (Cephalon)	100 mg vial	Injection	100 mg/m² IV infusion over 30 min on days 1 and 2 of a 28-day cycle, up to 6 cycles; adjust dose based on patient response and drug toxicity	D	3/20/08	Treatment of patients with chronic lymphocytic leukemia (CLL)	Antineoplastic, alkylating agent
C1 inhibitor (human)	Cinryze (Lev Pharm)	500 U in an 8-mL vial	Injection	Infuse 1000 U IV over 10 min at 1 mL/min q3–4d	C	10/10/08	Routine prophylaxis against angioedema attacks in adolescent and adult patients with hereditary angioedema	Blood product, C1 inhibitor
Certolizumab pegol	Cimzia (UCB)	200-mg vial	Injection	400 mg SC initially and at wk 2 and 4; if response occurs, follow with 400 mg SC q4wk	B	4/22/08	Reducing signs and symptoms of Crohn's disease and maintaining clinical response in adult patients with moderately to severely active disease who have had an inadequate response to conventional therapy	Immunomodulator, tumor necrosis factor (TNF) blocker
Clevidipine butyrate	Cleviprex (Medicines)	0.5 mg/mL in 50-, 100-mL vial	Injection	Initiate IV infusion at 1–2 mg/h and titrate by doubling the dose q90sec When blood pressure approaches goal, titrate q 5–10 min at less than double the dose Max dose is 16 mg/h Max duration of therapy is 72 h	C	8/1/08	For the reduction of blood pressure when oral therapy is not feasible or not desirable	Antihypertensive, dihydropyridine calcium channel blocker

New Drugs in 2008 and Agents Pending FDA Approval

Continued

New Drugs Approved in 2008—Cont'd

Generic Name	Trade Name (Manufacturer)	Strength	Dosage Form	Normal Dosage Range	Pregnancy Rating*	FDA Approval Date	Indication	Classification
Degarelix acetate	Trade name pending	80-, 120-mg vial	Injection	Starting dose: 240 mg given as 2 SC injections of 120 mg each Maintenance doses: 80 mg SC q28d	X	12/24/08	Treatment of patients with advanced prostate cancer	Hormone, gonadotropin-releasing hormone (GnRH) receptor antagonist
Desvenlafaxine	Pristiq (Wyeth)	50, 100 mg	Extended-release tablet	50 mg once daily	C	2/29/08	Treatment of major depressive disorder	Antidepressant, serotonin-norepinephrine reuptake inhibitor (SNRI)
Difluprednate	Durezol (Sirion Therapeutics)	0.05%, 2.5, 5 mL in 5-mL bottle	Ophthalmic emulsion	1 drop into the conjunctival sac of the affected eye qid beginning 24 h after surgery and continuing throughout the first 2 wk of the postoperative period, followed by bid × 1 wk and then a taper based on the response	C	6/23/08	Treatment of inflammation and pain associated with ocular surgery	Ocular antiinflammatory, corticosteroid
Eltrombopag	Promacta (GlaxoSmithKline)	25, 50 mg	Tablet	50 mg once daily on an empty stomach	C	11/20/08	Treatment of thrombocytopenia in patients with chronic immune (idiopathic) thrombocytopenic purpura who have had an insufficient response to corticosteroids, immunoglobulins, or splenectomy.	Platelet production stimulator, thrombopoietin receptor agonist
Etravirine	Intelence (Tibotec)	100 mg	Tablet	200 mg bid after a meal	B	1/18/08	In combination with other antiretroviral agents for the treatment of human immunodeficiency virus type 1 (HIV-1) infection in treatment-experienced adult patients, who have evidence of viral replication and HIV-1 strains resistant to an non-nucleoside reverse transcriptase inhibitor (NNRTI) and other antiretroviral agents	Antiretroviral, NNRTI

Generic	Brand (Manufacturer)	Strength	Dosage form	Dose	Preg	Date	Indication	Drug class
Fesoterodine	Toviaz (Pfizer)	4 mg	Extended-release tablet	4 mg once daily; may increase dose to 8 mg once daily	C	10/31/08	Treatment of overactive bladder with symptoms of urge urinary incontinence, urgency, and frequency	Urinary antispasmodics, competitive muscarinic receptor antagonist
Fospropofol	Lusedra (Eisai)	35-mg/mL single-use vial	Injection	6.5 mg/kg followed by supplemental doses of 1.6 mg/kg as needed. No initial dose should exceed 16.5 mL; no supplemental dose should exceed 4 mL.	B	12/12/08	For monitored anesthesia care (MAC) sedation in adult patients undergoing diagnostic or therapeutic procedures	Sedative-hypnotic, phenol derivative
Gadofosveset	Vasovist (Epix)	244 mg/mL (0.25 mmol/mL) in 10-, 15-mL vial	Injection	0.12 mL/kg (0.03 mmol/kg)	C	12/22/08	A contrast imaging agent for use with magnetic resonance angiography for the visualization of abdominal or limb vessels in patients with suspected or known vascular disease	Diagnostic agent, contrast agent
Gadoxetate disodium	Eovist (Bayer)	181.43 mg/mL (0.25 mol/L), 10-mL vial	Injection	0.1 mL/kg (0.025 mmol/kg) given IV push at 2 mL/sec, following with a saline flush	C	7/3/08	A gadolinium-based contrast agent for T1-weighted magnetic resonance imaging of the liver to detect and characterize lesions in adults with known or suspected focal liver disease	Diagnostic agent, contrast agent
Iobenguane sulfate I 123	AdreView (GE Healthcare)	5-mL single-use vial (2 mCi/mL at calibration time)	Injection	For patients ≥16 y or <16 y and ≥70 kg: 10 mCi dose. For patients <16 y and <70 kg: amount scaled to the adult reference activity based on weight	C	9/19/08	For the detection of primary or metastatic pheochromocytoma or neuroblastoma as an adjunct to other diagnostic tests	Diagnostic agent, radiopharmaceutical agent for gamma-scintigraphy
Lacosamide	Vimpat (Schwarz)	50-, 100-, 150-, 200-mg tablets for oral use; 200-mg/20-mL vial for IV use	Tablet, injection	Start at 50 mg PO bid; increase at weekly intervals to a max daily dose of 100–200 mg PO bid. May administer IV over 30–60 min at an equivalent daily dose and frequency when PO administration is temporarily not feasible	C	10/28/08	Adjunctive therapy for partial-onset seizures in patients ≥17 y	Anticonvulsant, functionalized amino acid
Methylnaltrexone bromide	Relistor (Wyeth)	12-mg/0.6-mL vial	Injection	Dose is weight based, given SC every other day as needed. Adults <38 kg: 0.15 mg/kg	B	4/24/08	Treatment of opioid-induced constipation in patients with advanced illness who are receiving	Laxative, opioid receptor antagonist

Continued

New Drugs Approved in 2008—Cont'd

Generic Name	Trade Name (Manufacturer)	Strength	Dosage Form	Normal Dosage Range	Pregnancy Rating*	FDA Approval Date	Indication	Classification
							palliative care, when response to laxative therapy has not been sufficient	
Plerixafor	Mozobil (Genzyme)	20-mg/mL single-use vial	Injection	Adults 38–61 kg: 8 mg Adults 62–114 kg: 12 mg Adults >114 kg: 0.15 mg/kg	D	12/15/08	With granulocyte colony-stimulating factor (G-CSF) to mobilize stem cells for autologous transplantation in patients with non-Hodgkin's lymphoma and multiple myeloma	Hematologic drug, hematopoietic stem cell mobilizer
Regadenoson	Lexiscan (Astellas)	0.4-mg/5-mL vial 0.4-mg/5-mL prefilled syringe	Injection	0.4 mg/5 mL rapid IV injection; following immediately by saline flush and radiopharmaceutical	C	4/10/08	A pharmacologic stress agent for radionuclide myocardial perfusion imaging in patients unable to undergo adequate exercise stress	Diagnostic agent, adenosine A_{2a} receptor agonist
Rilonacept	Arcalyst (Regeneron)	220-mg in single-use 20-mL vial	Injection	Adults ≥18 y: loading dose of 320 mg, delivered as two 160 mg/2 mL SC injections given at two different sites; then 160 mg/2 mL SC injection once weekly Children 12–17 y: loading dose of 4.4 mg/kg up to a max of 320 mg, delivered as 1–2 SC injections with a max volume of 2 mL/injection; then 2.2 mg/kg, up to a max dose of 160 mg/2 mL SC injection once weekly	C	2/27/08	Treatment of cryopyrin-associated periodic syndromes (CAPS), including familial cold autoinflammatory syndrome (FCAS) and Muckle-Wells syndrome (MWS) in adults and children ≥12 y	Immunosuppressant, an interleukin-1 blocker
Romiplostim	Nplate (Amgen)	250-, 500-µg vial	Injection	Initially, 1 µg/kg SC once weekly. Adjust dose as needed in increments of 1 µg/kg to maintain platelet count of ≥50 × 10^9/L to reduce the risk of bleeding	C	8/22/08	Treatment of thrombocytopenia in patients with chronic immune (idiopathic) thrombocytopenic purpura (ITP) who have had an insufficient response	Antithrombocytopenic, thrombopoietin receptor agonist

Generic	Brand (Manufacturer)	Strength	Form	Dosing	Pregnancy Category	FDA Approval	Indication	Class
				Max dose: 10 µg/kg. Withhold drug if platelet count >400 × 10^9/L. Stop drug if platelet count does not increase after 4 wk at the max dose				to corticosteroids, immunoglobulins, or splenectomy
Rotavirus vaccine, live, oral	Rotarix (GlaxoSmithKline)	1-mL single-use vial	Oral	Children ages 6–24 wk: give first 1-mL dose beginning at age 6 wk. Allow at least 4 wk before giving the second 1-mL dose. The two-dose series must be completed before age 24 wk	C	4/3/08	To prevent rotavirus gastroenteritis caused by GI and non-GI types	Vaccine, live virus antigen
Rufinamide	Banzel (Eisai)	200, 400 mg	Tablet	≥4 y: start at 10 mg/kg/d given in 2 equally divided doses, then increase dose by 10-mg/kg increments qod to a target dose of 45 mg/kg/d or 3200 mg/d, whichever is less. Adults: start at 400–800 mg/d given in 2 equally divided doses, then increase dose by 400–800 mg/d q2d until a max daily dose of 3200 mg/d	C	11/14/08	Adjunctive treatment of seizures associated with Lennox-Gastaut syndrome in children ≥4 y and adults	Antiepileptic agent, triazole derivative
Silodosin	Rapaflo (Watson)	4, 8 mg	Capsule	8 mg once daily	B	10/8/08	Treatment of the signs and symptoms of benign prostatic hyperplasia	Antiadrenergics, α$_1$-receptor antagonist
Tapentadol	Nucynta (Johnson & Johnson)	50, 75, 100 mg	Tablet	Start at a dose of 50, 75, or 100 mg q4–6h, depending on pain intensity	C	11/20/08	For the relief of moderate to severe acute pain in patients ≥18 y	Centrally acting analgesic, µ-opioid receptor agonist and norepinephrine reuptake inhibitor
Tetrabenazine	Xenazine (Biovail Americas)	12.5, 25 mg	Tablet	Start at 12.5 mg qam; may increase dose to 12.5 mg bid after 1 wk. Titrate dose by 12.5 mg at weekly intervals, as needed. Max single dose is 25 mg.	C	8/15/08	For the treatment of chorea associated with Huntington disease	Anti-chorea, depletes monoamine

Continued

New Drugs Approved in 2008—Cont'd

Generic Name	Trade Name (Manufacturer)	Strength	Dosage Form	Normal Dosage Range	Pregnancy Rating*	FDA Approval Date	Indication	Classification
Thrombin, topical (Recombinant)	Recothrom (ZymoGenetics)	5000-, 20,000-IU vial	Topical solution	Apply Recothrom solution (1000 IU/mL) directly to bleeding site surface or in conjunction with absorbable gelatin sponge; amount needed varies with the area of tissue to be treated.	C	1/17/08	As an aid to hemostasis whenever oozing blood and minor bleeding from capillaries and small venules are accessible and control of bleeding by standard surgical techniques is ineffective or impractical	Hemostatic agent, thrombin
Significant New Ester, New Salt, or Other Derivative								
Bupropion hydrobromide	Aplenzin (Biovail Labs Intl)	174, 348, 522 mg	Extended-release tablet	Start: 174 mg/d Usual target: 348 mg/d	C	4/23/08	Treatment of major depressive disorder	Antidepressant, aminoketone
Fosaprepitant dimeglumine	Emend for Injection (Merck)	115-mg/10-mL vial	Injection	115-mg IV infusion over 15 min on day 1 only of the 3-day chemotherapy-induced nausea and vomiting regimen, 30 min before chemotherapy	B	1/25/08	In combination with other antiemetic agents for the prevention of acute and delayed nausea and vomiting associated initial and repeat courses of highly and moderately emetogenic cancer chemotherapy	Antiemetic, prodrug to aprepitant (a substance NK1 receptor antagonist)
Palonosetron	Aloxi (Helsin Healthcare)	0.5 mg	Capsule	1 cap taken 1 h before the start of chemotherapy	B	8/22/08	Prevention of acute nausea and vomiting associated with initial and repeat courses of moderately emetogenic cancer chemotherapy	Antiemetic, serotonin subtype 3 (5-HT3) receptor antagonist
Synthetic conjugated estrogens, A	SCE-A Vaginal Cream (Duramed)	0.625 mg/g, 30-g tube	Vaginal cream	1 g intravaginally daily for 1 wk followed by 1 g intravaginally 2 ×/wk	Not recommended	11/28/08	Treatment of moderate to severe vaginal dryness, a symptom of vulvar and vaginal atrophy, due to menopause Treatment of moderate to severe dyspareunia, a symptom of vulvar and vaginal atrophy, due to menopause	Sex hormone, plant-derived conjugated estrogen

Significant New Combination

Generic	Brand (Manufacturer)	Form	Strength	Administration/Dosage	Preg. Cat.	Date	Indication	Class
Adapalene/benzoyl peroxide gel	Epiduo (Galderma Laboratories)	Topical gel	0.1%/2.5%	Apply a thin film to affected areas of the face and/or trunk once daily after washing. Use a pea-sized amount for each area of the face (e.g., forehead, chin, each cheek). Avoid the eyes, lips, and mucous membranes	C	12/8/08	Topical treatment of acne vulgaris in patients ≥12 y	Anti-acne, retinoid/anti-infective
Aliskiren/hydro-chlorothiazide	Tekturna HCT (Novartis)	Tablet	150-mg/12.5 mg, 150 mg/25 mg, 300 mg/12.5 mg, 300 mg/25 mg	1 tab once daily; adjust as needed to max dose of 300 mg/25 mg	D	1/18/08	Treatment of hypertension	Antihypertensive, renin inhibitor, diuretic
Diphtheria and tetanus toxoids and acellular pertussis absorbed and inactivated poliovirus vaccine (DTaP)	Kinrix (GlaxoSmithKline)	Injection	0.5-mL suspension in single-dose vial	0.5 mL IM × 1	C	6/24/08	Active immunization against diphtheria, tetanus, pertussis, and poliomyelitis as the fifth dose in the DTaP vaccine series and the fourth dose in the IPV series in children 4–6 y whose previous DTaP vaccine doses have been with Infanrix and/or Pediarix for the first 3 doses and Infanrix for the fourth dose	Vaccine, bacteria and virus antigen
Diphtheria and tetanus toxoids and acellular pertussis adsorbed, inactivated poliovirus and Haemophilus influenzae type b conjugate (tetanus toxoid conjugate) vaccine	Pentacel (Sanofi Pasteur)	Injection	Single-dose vial	Give IM, as a 4 dose series at 2, 4 and 6, and 15–18 months of age	C	6/20/08	Active immunization against diphtheria, tetanus, pertussis, poliomyelitis and invasive disease due to H. influenzae type b. Pentacel vaccine is approved for use in children 6 wk–4 y (before fifth birthday)	Vaccine, bacteria and virus antigen
Insulin aspart protamine suspension/insulin aspart (rDNA origin)	Novolog Mix 50/50 (Novo Nordisk)	Injection	100 U/mL in 3-mL PenFill cartridge 100 U/mL in 3-mL FlexPen	Give SC within 15 min before a meal up to 3 × daily Calculate dose according to the patient's metabolic needs, eating habits, and other lifestyle variables	C	8/26/08	As an adjunct to diet and exercise to improve glycemic control in patients with diabetes mellitus	Antidiabetic agent, insulin

Continued

New Drugs Approved in 2008—Cont'd

Generic Name	Trade Name (Manufacturer)	Strength	Dosage Form	Normal Dosage Range	Pregnancy Rating*	FDA Approval Date	Indication	Classification
Niacin/simvastatin	Simcor	500 mg/20 mg, 750 mg/20 mg, 1000 mg/20 mg	Film-coated tablet	500/20 mg to 2000/40 mg once daily	X	2/15/08	Reduce elevated total cholesterol, LDL-C, Apo B, non-HDL-C, triglycerides (TG) or to increase HDL-C in patients with primary hypercholesterolemia and mixed dyslipidemia when treatment with simvastatin monotherapy or niacin extended-release monotherapy is considered inadequate Reduce TG in patients with hypertriglyceridemia (Fredrickson type IV hyperlipidemia) when treatment with simvastatin monotherapy or niacin extended-release monotherapy is considered inadequate	Antilipemic, HMG coenzyme A inhibitor/ vitamin
Repaglinide/ metformin	PrandiMet (Novo Nordisk)	1 mg/500 mg, 2 mg/500 mg	Tablet	Start with 1 mg/500 mg bid, 15 min before meals Max 10 mg/2500 mg per day or 4 mg/1000 mg per meal	C	6/23/08	As an adjunct to diet and exercise to improve glycemic control in adults with type 2 diabetes mellitus who are already treated with a meglitinide and metformin or who have inadequate glycemic control on a meglitinide alone or metformin alone	Antidiabetic agent, meglitinide/biguanide
Sumatriptan succinate/ naproxen sodium	Treximet (GlaxoSmithKline)	85 mg sumatriptan/ 500 mg naproxen	Tablet	Recommended dose is 1 tab Do not take >2 tab/24 h Dosing of tab should be ≥2 h apart	C	4/15/08	Acute treatment of migraine attacks with or without aura in adults.	Migraine agent, serotonin 5-HT₁ receptor agonist, NSAID

Significant New Formulation

Generic Name	Trade Name (Manufacturer)	Strength	Dosage Form	Normal Dosage Range	Pregnancy Rating*	FDA Approval Date	Indication	Classification
Amoxicillin extended release	Moxatag (Middlebrook Pharms)	775 mg	Tablet	Tonsillitis and/or Pharyngitis: 775 mg once daily for 10 d with a meal Do not chew or crush tablet	B	1/23/08	Treatment of tonsillitis or pharyngitis from *Streptococcus pyogenes* in adults and pediatric patients ≥12 y	Antibacterial, penicillin

Continued

Drug	Brand (Manufacturer)	Strength	Form	Dosing	Preg. Cat.	Indication	Classification	Approval
Antihemophilic factor (Recombinant), plasma/albumin free	Xyntha (Wyeth)	250-, 500-, 1000-, 2000-IU vial	Injection	Body wt (kg) × desired factor VIII rise (IU/dL or % of normal) × 0.5 (IU/kg per IU/dL); repeat dose as necessary	C	Control and prevention of bleeding episodes in patients with hemophilia A; Surgical prophylaxis in patients with hemophilia A	Hemostasis, coagulation factor	2/21/08
Bimatoprost ophthalmic solution 0.03%	Latisse (Allergan)	0.3 mg/mL, 3-mL bottle	Ophthalmic solution	Apply nightly directly to the skin of the upper eyelid margin at the base of the eyelashes using the accompanying applicators	C	To treat hypotrichosis of the eyelashes by increasing their growth including length, thickness, and darkness	Ophthalmic, prostaglandin analogue	12/24/08
Ciclesonide inhalation aerosol	Alvesco (Nycomed)	80-, 160-μg/actuation	Oral inhalation	If previously received bronchodilators alone, give inhaled dose of 80 μg bid, to a max of 160 μg bid; If previously received inhaled corticosteroids, give inhaled dose of 80 μg bid, to a max of 320 μg bid; If previously received oral corticosteroids, give inhaled dose of 320 μg bid	C	Maintenance treatment of asthma as prophylactic therapy in adult and adolescent patients ≥12 y	Antiasthmatic, corticosteroid	1/10/08
Choline fenofibrate	Trilipix (Abbott)	45, 135 mg	Delayed-release capsule	Mixed dyslipidemia: 135 mg once daily; Hypertriglyceridemia: 45 to 135 mg once daily; Renally impaired patients: 45 mg once daily; Maximum dose: 135 mg once daily	C	In combination with a statin to reduce TG and increase HDL-C in patients with mixed dyslipidemia and coronary heart disease (CHD) or a CHD risk equivalent who are on optimal statin therapy to achieve their LDL-C goal; As monotherapy to reduce TG in patients with severe hypertriglyceridemia; As monotherapy to reduce elevated LDL-C, Total-C, TG, and Apo B and to increase HDL-C in patients with primary hyperlipidemia or mixed dyslipidemia	Antihyperlipidemic, fibric acid derivatives	12/15/08

New Drugs Approved in 2008—Cont'd

Generic Name	Trade Name (Manufacturer)	Strength	Dosage Form	Normal Dosage Range	Pregnancy Rating*	FDA Approval Date	Indication	Classification
Granisetron Transdermal System	Sancuso (Strakan)	34.3-mg patch delivering 3.1 mg/24 h	Transderm patch	Apply 1 patch to the upper outer arm a min of 24 h before chemotherapy Remove the patch a min of 24 h after completion of chemotherapy May wear patch for up to 7 d depending on the duration of the chemotherapy regimen	B	9/12/08	For the prevention of nausea and vomiting in patients receiving moderately and/or highly emetogenic chemotherapy for up to 5 consecutive days	Antiemetic, serotonin subtype 3 (5-HT$_3$) receptor antagonist

*FDA pregnancy categories:
A: Adequate studies in pregnant women have not demonstrated a risk to the fetus in the first trimester of pregnancy, and there is no evidence of risk in later trimesters.
B: Animal studies have shown an adverse effect, but adequate studies in pregnant women have not demonstrated a risk to the fetus during the first trimester of pregnancy, and there is no evidence of risk in later trimesters.
C: Animal studies have shown an adverse effect on the fetus, but there are no adequate studies in humans; the benefits from the use of the drug in pregnant women may be acceptable despite its potential risks.
D: There is evidence of human fetal risk, but the potential benefits from the use of the drug in pregnant women may be acceptable despite any possible benefit.
X: Adverse reaction reports indicate evidence of fetal risk; the risk of use in a pregnant woman clearly outweighs any possible benefit.
No drug should be administered during pregnancy unless it is clearly needed and the potential benefit outweighs the potential hazard to the fetus, regardless of the pregnancy category.

Agents Pending FDA Approval

Generic Name	Trade Name (Manufacturer)	Indication
ABT-335/Rosuvastatin	No brand name (Abbott & AstraZeneca)	Treatment of mixed dyslipidemia
Albiglutide	Syncria (GlaxoSmithKline)	Treatment of type 2 diabetes
Almorexant	No brand name (Actelion)	Treatment of primary insomnia
Alopliptin	No brand name (Takeda)	Treatment of type 2 diabetes
Apixaban	No brand name (Bristol-Myers Squibb/Pfizer)	Prevention of venous thromboembolism and prevention of stroke
Bazedoxifene	Viviant (Wyeth)	Prevention of postmenopausal osteoporosis
17α-Hydroxyprogesterone caproate	Gestiva (Adeza)	Prevention of preterm delivery (<35 weeks) in women with a history of prior preterm delivery
Ceftobiprole	Zeftera (Johnson & Johnson)	Treatment of complicated skin and soft tissue infections, including diabetes-related foot infections
Cilomilast	Ariflo (GlaxoSmithKline)	Treatment of patients with chronic obstructive pulmonary disease (COPD) who are poorly responsive to albuterol
Clodronate	Bonefos (Berlex Laboratories)	Adjuvant oral treatment for reducing the occurrence of bone metastases in stage II or III breast cancer patients
Denosumab	No brand name (Amgen)	Treatment and prevention of postmenopausal osteoporosis in women; treatment and prevention of bone loss in patients undergoing hormone ablation for prostate or breast cancer
Dextromethorphan/quinidine	Zenvia (Avanir)	Treatment of involuntary emotional expression disorder Treatment of diabetic peripheral neuropathic pain
Ecallantide	Kalbitor (Dyax)	Treatment of acute attacks of hereditary angioedema
Efaproxiral	Efaproxyn (Allos Therapeutics)	An adjunct agent to whole brain radiation therapy for the treatment of brain metastases in patients with breast cancer
Garenoxacin mesylate	Geninax (Schering)	Treatment of acute bacterial exacerbation of chronic bronchitis, acute bacterial sinusitis, community acquired pneumonia, complicated and uncomplicated skin and skin structure infections, and complicated intraabdominal infections
Icatibant	Firazyr (Jerini)	Treatment of hereditary angioedema
Lasofoxifene	Fablyn (Prizer)	Treatment of osteoporosis in postmenopausal women at increased risk of fracture
Liraglutide	Victoza (Novo Nordisk)	Treatment of type 2 diabetes
Mepolizumab	Bosatria (GlaxoSmithKline)	An anti-IL5 monoclonal antibody for treatment of hypereosinophilic syndrome
Odanacatib	No brand name (Merck)	Treatment of osteoporosis in postmenopausal women
Ofatumumab	Arzerra (GlaxoSmithKline)	An anti-CD20 human monoclonal antibody refractory for the treatment of chronic lymphocytic leukemia
Rivaroxaban	Xarelto (Johnson & Johnson, Bayer)	Venous blood clot prevention after elective total knee and hip replacement surgery
Sitaxsentan sodium	Thelin (Encysive Pharmaceuticals)	Treatment of pulmonary arterial hypertension
SnET2 (tin ethyl etiopurpurin)	No brand name (Miravent Medical Technologies)	Slow the progression of wet age-related macular degeneration
Tocilizumab	Actemra (Chugai/Roche)	Treatment of moderate to severe rheumatoid arthritis
Trabectedin	Yondelis (Ortho Biotech)	In combination with doxorubicin hydrochloride liposome injection for the treatment of women with relapsed ovarian cancer
Ustekinumab	No brand name (Johnson & Johnson)	Treatment for patients with chronic, moderate to severe plaque psoriasis
Vapreotide	Sanvar IR (H3 Pharma)	Treatment of acute esophageal variceal bleeding from portal hypertension
Venakalant	No brand name (Astellas Pharma)	For conversion of atrial fibrillation to normal sinus rhythm
Vildagliptin	Galvus (Novartis)	Treatment of type 2 diabetes

Note: Page numbers followed by *b*, *f*, and *t* indicate boxes, figures, and tables, respectively.

Index

1264

Index

1303